Pediatric Emergency Medicine

Pediatric Emergency Medicine

Jill M. Baren, MD, MBE, FACEP, FAAP

Associate Professor of Emergency Medicine and Pediatrics
University of Pennsylvania School of Medicine
Department of Emergency Medicine
Hospital of the University of Pennsylvania
Department of Pediatrics
Division of Emergency Medicine
The Children's Hospital of Philadelphia
Philadelphia, Pennsylvania

Steven G. Rothrock, MD, FACEP, FAAP

Professor of Emergency Medicine
University of Florida
Associate Professor of Clinical Sciences
Florida State University
Orlando Regional Healthcare System
Orlando, Florida

John A. Brennan, MD, FACEP, FAAP

Executive Director, Newark Beth Israel Medical Center
and the Children's Hospital of New Jersey
Newark, New Jersey
Senior Vice President for Clinical and Emergency Services
Director, Pediatric Emergency Medicine
Saint Barnabas Health Care System
West Orange, New Jersey

Lance Brown, MD, MPH, FACEP, FAAP

Chief, Division of Pediatric Emergency Medicine
Associate Professor of Emergency Medicine and Pediatrics
Loma Linda University Medical Center and Children's Hospital
Loma Linda, California

Pharmacology Editor

Ran D. Goldman, MD
Division Head and Medical Director, Division of Pediatric Emergency Medicine
British Columbia Children's Hospital
Associate Professor, Department of Pediatrics
University of British Columbia
Senior Associate Clinician Scientist
Child & Family Research Institute (CFRI)
Vancouver, British Columbia, Canada

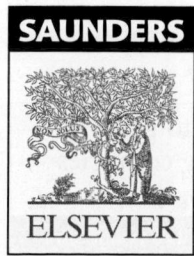

SAUNDERS

ELSEVIER

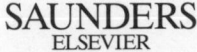

SAUNDERS
ELSEVIER

1600 John F. Kennedy Blvd.
Ste 1800
Philadelphia, PA 19103-2899

Notice

Knowledge and best practice in this field are constantly changing. As new research and experience broaden our knowledge, changes in practice, treatment and drug therapy may become necessary or appropriate. Readers are advised to check the most current information provided (i) on procedures featured or (ii) by the manufacturer of each product to be administered, to verify the recommended dose or formula, the method and duration of administration, and contraindications. It is the responsibility of the practitioner, relying on their own experience and knowledge of the patient, to make diagnoses, to determine dosages and the best treatment for each individual patient, and to take all appropriate safety precautions. To the fullest extent of the law, neither the Publisher nor the Editors assumes any liability for any injury and/or damage to persons or property arising out or related to any use of the material contained in this book.

The Publisher

Library of Congress Cataloging-in-Publication Data
Pediatric emergency medicine / [edited by] Jill M. Baren . . . [et al.].
     p. ; cm.
   Includes bibliographical references and index.
   ISBN-13: 978-1-4160-0087-7
   ISBN-10: 1-4160-0087-9
   1. Pediatric emergencies.   I. Baren, Jill M.
   [DNLM: 1. Emergencies.   2. Child.   3. Critical Care—methods.   4. Infant.   WS
205 P3712 2007]
RJ370.P45153 2007
618.92′0025—dc22

2007018571

Acquisitions Editor: Maria Lorusso
Developmental Editor: Joanie Milnes
Project Manager: David Saltzberg
Design Direction: Steven Stave

Printed in China

Last digit is the print number: 9   8   7   6   5   4   3   2   1

Working together to grow
libraries in developing countries

www.elsevier.com | www.bookaid.org | www.sabre.org

ELSEVIER   BOOK AID International   Sabre Foundation

To my husband Kenneth—I am truly grateful for your endless love, support of our family life, and pride in my career, for without those things, this book and all of my work would not exist.

To my sons Noah and Andrew—I am continually amazed by your gifts of love, patience, and wisdom beyond your years. You have made every minute of my life worthwhile.

To my parents—you gave me the right start and never stopped encouraging me to be what I wanted to be.

To an extraordinary mentor, James S. Seidel, MD, PhD, who opened many doors in the world of pediatric emergency medicine and encouraged me to go through them.

To my co-editors John, Lance, and Steve—thank you for your friendship, creativity, humor, persistence, high standards, and the countless hours you spent making this a reality.

Jill Baren

I dedicate this work to the two loves of my life—my wife Angela, and my daughter Ava. It is my hope that this text serves to help protect, repair and sustain the health and lives of children and parents everywhere.

Steve Rothrock

To my wife, Mary Beth, and our children, Kelly, Matthew and Colleen for all their help, love and patience. To my friends and colleagues for all the support and mentoring they have given me over the past 25 years. Especially to all the children and parents who, in a time of crisis, put their faith and confidence in our care.

John A. Brennan

To acutely ill and injured children and the professionals who care for them.

Lance Brown

Contributors

Fredrick M. Abrahamian, DO, FACEP
Assistant Professor of Medicine, UCLA School of Medicine, Los Angeles; Director of Education, Department of Emergency Medicine, Olive View-UCLA Medical Center, Sylmar, California
Tetanus Prophylaxis; Rabies Postexposure Prophylaxis

Thomas J. Abramo, MD, FAAP, FACEP
Professor of Emergency Medicine and Pediatrics, Director, Pediatric Emergency Department, Medical Director of Pediatric Transport, and Pediatric Emergency Phyisician-in-Chief, Department of Emergency Medicine, Vanderbilt University Medical Center, Monroe Carell Jr. Children's Hospital at Vanderbilt, Nashville, Tennessee
Monitoring in Critically Ill Children

Robert Acosta, MD
Assistant Professor, Department of Pediatrics, Albert Einstein College of Medicine; Attending Physician, Department of Pediatric Emergency Medicine, Jacobi Medical Center, Bronx, New York
Rhinosinusitis

Paula Agosto, RN, MHA
Director of Nursing, Emergency, Critical Care, and Transport, The Children's Hospital of Philadelphia, Philadelphia, Pennsylvania
Burns

Coburn Allen, MD
Assistant Professor of Pediatrics, Baylor College of Medicine; Attending Physician, Texas Children's Hospital, Houston, Texas
Bone, Joint, and Spine Infections

Elizabeth R. Alpern, MD, MSCE
Assistant Professor, Department of Pediatrics, University of Pennsylvania School of Medicine; Attending Physician, Division of Emergency Medicine, Department of Pediatrics, The Children's Hospital of Philadelphia, Philadelphia, Pennsylvania
Bacteremia

Jesus M. Arroyo, MD
Assistant Professor of Emergency Medicine, Department of Emergency Medicine, University of Texas Medical School at Houston, Houston, Texas
Sepsis

Miriam Aschkenasy, MD, MPH
Assistant Professor, Boston University School of Medicine; Attending Physician, Boston Medical Center, Boston, Massachusetts
Ear Diseases

Peter S. Auerbach, MD, FAAEM, FAAP
Attending Physician, Department of Emergency Medicine, Inova Fairfax Hospital and Inova Fairfax Hospital for Children, Falls Church, Virginia
Pelvic and Genitourinary Trauma

Franz E. Babl, MD, MPH
Clinical Associate Professor, University of Melbourne; Pediatric Emergency Physician, Royal Children's Hospital, Melbourne, Victoria, Australia
Central Nervous System Vascular Disorders; Vaccination-Related Complaints and Side Effects

Michael C. Bachman, MD, MBA
Assistant Medical Director, Department of Pediatric Emergency Medicine, and Pediatric Emergency Medicine Fellowship Director, Newark Beth Israel Medical Center, Newark, New Jersey
Eye Disorders

Megan H. Bair-Merritt, MD, MSCE
Assistant Professor, Division of General Pediatrics and Adolescent Medicine, Johns Hopkins School of Medicine, Baltimore, Maryland
Interpersonal and Intimate Partner Violence

Roger A. Band, MD
Department of Emergency Medicine, Hospital of the University of Pennsylvania, Philadelphia, Pennsylvania
Penile and Testicular Disorders

Isabel Barata, MD
Assistant Professor of Pediatrics, New York University Medical School, New York; Director of Pediatric Emergency Medicine, North Shore University Hospital, Manhasset, New York
Neurovascular Injuries

Besh Barcega, MD, MBA
Assistant Professor, Emergency Medicine and Pediatrics, Loma Linda University School of Medicine; Medical Director, Pediatric Emergency Department, Loma Linda University Children's Hospital and Medical Center, Loma Linda, California
Lower Extremity Trauma

Jill M. Baren, MD, MBE, FACEP, FAAP
Associate Professor of Emergency Medicine and Pediatrics, University of Pennsylvania School of Medicine; Department of Emergency Medicine, Hospital of the University of Pennsylvania; Division of Emergency Medicine, Department of Pediatrics, The Children's Hospital of Philadelphia, Philadelphia, Pennsylvania
End-of-Life Issues

Beverly H. Bauman, MD
Department of Emergency Medicine, Oregon Health and Sciences University, Portland, Oregon
Ovarian Disorders; Vaginal and Urethral Disorders

Lee S. Benjamin, MD
Assistant Professor, Division of Emergency Medicine, Department of Surgery, and Division of Pediatric Emergency Medicine, Department of Pediatrics, Duke University School of Medicine; Interim Associate Medical Director of Pediatric Emergency Medicine, Duke University Medical Center, Durham, North Carolina
Serum Sickness

Suzanne M. Beno, MD
Assistant Professor, Faculty of Medicine and Dentistry, University of Alberta; Faculty, Division of Pediatric Emergency Medicine, The Stollery Children's Hospital, Edmonton, Alberta, Canada; Formerly Clinical Instructor, University of Pennsylvania School of Medicine; Fellow, Pediatric Emergency Medicine, The Children's Hospital of Philadelphia, Philadelphia, Pennsylvania
Anaphylaxis; Renal Disorders

Deena Berkowitz, MD, MPH
Adjunct Professor, Department of Pediatrics, George Washington University of Medicine; Attending, Emergency Department, Children's National Medical Center, Washington, DC
Lumbar Puncture

Jason E. Bernad, MD
Attending Physician—Emergency Medicine, Saratoga Hospital, Saratoga Springs, New York
Wound Management

Daan Biesbroeck, MD
Attending Emergency Department Staff, OLVG Hospital, Amsterdam, The Netherlands
Urinary Tract Infections in Children and Adolescents

Jeffrey S. Blake, MD
Pediatric Emergency Medicine Fellow, Division of Emergency Medicine, Children's National Medical Center, Washington, DC
Gastrointestinal Bleeding

Frederick C. Blum, MD, FACEP
Associate Professor of Emergency Medicine and Pediatrics, West Virginia University School of Medicine, Department of Emergency Medicine, Ruby Memorial Hospital, Morgantown, West Virginia
Abdominal Trauma

Boura'a Bou Aram, MD
Department of Pediatrics, State University of New York Upstate Medical University, Syracuse, New York
Hemolytic-Uremic Syndrome; Utilizing Blood Bank Resources/Transfusion Reactions and Complications

John C. Brancato, MD
Assistant Professor of Pediatrics and Emergency Medicine, University of Connecticut School of Medicine, Farmington; Attending Physician, Division of Emergency Medicine, Connecticut Children's Medical Center, Hartford, Connecticut
Abdominal Hernias; Metabolic Acidosis; Metabolic Alkalosis

Daniel F. Brennan, MD
Clinical Associate Professor, Department of Emergency Medicine, University of Florida College of Medicine, Gainesville; Clinical Associate Professor, Department of Clinical Sciences, Florida State University College of Medicine, Orlando Campus, Tallahassee; Attending Physician, Department of Emergency Medicine, Emergency Medicine Residency Program, Orlando Regional Medical Center, Orlando, Florida
Ectopic Pregnancy

John A. Brennan, MD, FACEP, FAAP
Executive Director, Newark Beth Israel Medical Center and the Children's Hospital of New Jersey, Newark, New Jersey; Senior Vice President for Clinical and Emergency Services, and Director, Pediatric Emergency Medicine, Saint Barnabas Health Care System, West Orange, New Jersey
The Sick or Injured Child in a Community Hospital Emergency Department; Patient Safety, Medical Errors, and Quality of Care; Hernia Reduction

Allison V. Brewer, MD
Attending Physician, Mercy Hospital, Portland, Maine
Musculoskeletal Disorders in Systemic Disease

Kenneth B. Briskin, MD, FACS
Associate Clinical Professor, Temple University, Philadelphia; Assistant Clinical Professor, University of Pennsylvania, Philadelphia, Pennsylvania; Chief, Division of Otolaryngology, Crozer-Chester Medical Center, Upland, Pennsylvania
Epistaxis; Epistaxis Control

Kathleen Brown, MD
Assistant Professor of Pediatrics and Emergency Medicine, George Washington University School of Medicine; Medical Unit Director, Pediatric Emergency Medicine, Children's National Medical Center, Washington, DC
Lumbar Puncture

Lance Brown, MD, MPH, FACEP, FAAP
Chief, Division of Pediatric Emergency Medicine, and Associate Professor of Emergency Medicine and Pediatrics, Loma Linda University Medical Center and Children's Hospital, Loma Linda, California
Approach to Multisystem Trauma; Excessive Crying

Linda L. Brown, MD, MSCE
Assistant Professor of Pediatrics, Yale University School of
Medicine; Attending, Pediatric Emergency Medicine,
Yale-New Haven Children's Hospital, New Haven,
Connecticut
Dental Disorders

Michael D. Burg, MD, FACEP
Assistant Clinical Professor of Emergency Medicine,
Department of Emergency Medicine, University of
California, San Francisco-Fresno, University Medical
Center, Fresno, California
Upper Extremity Trauma

Sean P. Bush, MD, FACEP
Professor of Emergency Medicine, Department of
Emergency Medicine, Loma Linda University School of
Medicine; Director, Fellowship of Envenomation
Medicine, Department of Emergency Medicine, Loma
Linda University Medical Center, Loma Linda,
California
Snake and Spider Envenomations

James M. Callahan, MD
Associate Professor of Clinical Pediatrics, Department of
Pediatrics, Division of Emergency Medicine, University
of Pennsylvania School of Medicine; Director, Medical
Education, Emergency Department, The Children's
Hospital of Philadelphia, Philadelphia, Pennsylvania
Wound Management

Richard M. Cantor, MD
Associate Professor of Emergency Medicine and Pediatrics,
Upstate Medical University; Director, Pediatric
Emergency Services, University Hospital, Syracuse, New
York
Neonatal Resuscitation; Common Pediatric Overdoses

Nicole P. Carbonell, MD
Resident, School of Medicine, University of Alabama at
Birmingham; Resident, Department of Emergency
Medicine, University Hospital, University of Alabama at
Birmingham, Birmingham, Alabama
Thoracostomy

Eric T. Carter, MD
Assistant Medical Director, Emergency Department, South
Lake Hospital, Clermont, Florida
Hypokalemia; Hyperkalemia; Hypocalcemia

David D. Cassidy, MD
Clinical Assistant Professor, Department of Emergency
Medicine, University of Florida College of Medicine,
Gainesville; Clinical Assistant Professor, Department of
Clinical Sciences, Florida State University College of
Medicine, Tallahassee; Assistant Director, Department
of Emergency Medicine, and Attending and Ultrasound
Director, Emergency Medicine Residency Program,
Orlando Regional Medical Center, Orlando, Florida
Pyloric Stenosis; Constipation

Marina Catallozzi, MD
Assistant Professor of Clinical Pediatrics and Population
and Family Health, Columbia University—College of
Physicians and Surgeons, Mailman School of Public
Health, New York, New York
*Human Immunodeficiency Virus Infection and Other
Immunosuppressive Conditions*

Esther H. Chen, MD
Assistant Professor, University of Pennsylvania; Attending
Physician, Hospital of the University of Pennsylvania,
Philadelphia, Pennsylvania
Postexposure Prophylaxis

Richard E. Chinnock, MD
Professor and Chair of Pediatrics, Loma Linda University
School of Medicine; Physician-in-Chief, and Director,
Pediatric Heart Transplant Program, Loma Linda
University Children's Hospital, Loma Linda, California
Postsurgical Cardiac Conditions and Transplantation

Christine S. Cho, MD, MPH
Assistant Clinical Professor, Department of Pediatrics,
University of California San Francisco, San Francisco;
Attending Physician, Children's Hospital and Research
Center, Oakland, California
Circulatory Emergencies: Shock

Thomas H. Chun, MD
Assistant Professor, Departments of Emergency Medicine
and Pediatrics, Brown University; Attending Physician,
Emergency Department, Hasbro Children's Hospital,
Providence, Rhode Island
Psychobehavioral Disorders

Mark C. Clark, MD, FACEP, FAAP
Clinical Associate Professor, Department of Emergency
Medicine, University of Florida College of Medicine,
Gainesville; Medical Director, Department of
Emergency Medicine, Arnold Palmer Hospital for
Children, Orlando; Clinical Associate Professor,
Department of Clinical Sciences, Florida State University
College of Medicine, Tallahassee, Florida
Hernia Reduction

Robert L. Cloutier, MD
Assistant Professor, Department of Emergency Medicine &
Pediatrics, Oregon Health & Science University,
Portland, Oregon
Ovarian Disorders; Vaginal and Urethral Disorders

Teresa J. Coco, MD
Assistant Professor of Pediatric Emergency Medicine,
University of Alabama at Birmingham School of
Medicine; Administrator, After Hours Clinic Children's
South, Children's Hospital of Alabama, Birmingham,
Alabama
General Approach to Poisoning

Arthur Cooper, MD, MS
Professor of Surgery, Columbia University College of
Physicians & Surgeons; Director of Trauma & Pediatric
Surgical Services, Harlem Hospital Center, New York,
New York
Thoracic Trauma; Abdominal Trauma

James D'Agostino, MD
Assistant Professor of Emergency Medicine and Pediatrics, Department of Emergency Medicine, Upstate Medical University, Syracuse, New York
Malrotation and Midgut Volvulus

Elizabeth M. Datner, MD
Associate Professor, University of Pennsylvania School of Medicine; Medical Director, Department of Emergency Medicine, Hospital of the University of Pennsylvania, Philadelphia, Pennsylvania
Pregnancy-Related Complications

Sergio V. Delgado, MD
Associate Professor, Child and Adolescent Psychiatry, Department of Psychiatry, University of Cincinnati School of Medicine; Medical Director, Outpatient Services, Department of Psychiatry, Cincinnati Children's Hospital Medical Center, Cincinnati, Ohio
Major Depression and Suicidality

T. Kent Denmark, MD
Associate Professor of Emergency Medicine and Pediatrics, and Medical Director, Medical Simulation Center, Loma Linda University School of Medicine; Program Director, Pediatric Emergency Medicine, Attending Physician, Pediatric Emergency Department, Loma Linda University Medical Center and Children's Hospital, Loma Linda, California
Inborn Errors of Metabolism; Near Drowning and Submersion Injuries

Andrew DePiero, MD
Assistant Professor of Pediatrics, Jefferson Medical College, Philadelphia, Pennsylvania; Attending Physician, Division of Emergency Medicine, A.I. duPont Hospital for Children, Wilmington, Delaware
Apparent Life-Threatening Events

Stephanie J. Doniger, MD, FAAP
Pediatric Emergency Medicine Fellow, Children's Hospital and Health Center/University of California, San Diego, San Diego, California
Dysrhythmias

Aaron J. Donoghue, MD, MSCE
Assistant Professor of Pediatrics and Anesthesia, University of Pennsylvania School of Medicine; Attending Physician, Division of Emergency Medicine and Critical Care Medicine, The Children's Hospital of Philadelphia, Philadelphia, Pennsylvania
Intubation, Rescue Devices, and Airway Adjuncts

Gregory M. Enns, MB, ChB
Associate Professor of Pediatrics, and Director, Biomedical Genetics Program, Division of Medical Genetics, Stanford University, Stanford, California
Hypoglycemia

Mirna M. Farah, MD
Assistant Professor, Division of Emergency Medicine, Department of Pediatrics, University of Pennsylvania School of Medicine; Attending Physician, The Children's Hospital of Philadelphia, Philadelphia, Pennsylvania
Family Presence

Joel A. Fein, MD, MPH
Associate Professor of Pediatrics and Emergency Medicine, University of Pennsylvania School of Medicine; Attending Physician, Emergency Department, The Children's Hospital of Philadelphia, Philadelphia, Pennsylvania
Interpersonal and Intimate Partner Violence

George L. Foltin, MD
Associate Professor of Pediatrics and Emergency Medicine, New York University School of Medicine; Director, Center for Pediatric Emergency Medicine, Bellevue Hospital Center, New York, New York
Thoracic Trauma; Abdominal Trauma; Emergency Medical Services and Transport

Eron Y. Friedlaender, MD, MPH
Assistant Professor of Clinical Pediatrics, University of Pennsylvania School of Medicine; Attending Physician, Division of Emergency Medicine, Department of Pediatrics, The Children's Hospital of Philadelphia, Philadelphia, Pennsylvania
Cystic Fibrosis

Susan Fuchs, MD
Professor of Pediatrics, Feinberg School of Medicine, Northwestern University; Associate Director, Division of Pediatric Emergency Medicine, Children's Memorial Hospital, Chicago, Illinois
The Child-Friendly Emergency Department: Practices, Policies, and Procedures

Gregory Garra, DO
Assistant Clinical Professor of Emergency Medicine, Stony Brook University School of Medicine; Emergency Medicine Residency Program Director, Stony Brook University Hospital, Stony Brook, New York
Removal of Ocular Foreign Bodies; Fracture Reduction and Splinting Techniques

Marianne Gausche-Hill, MD
Professor of Clinical Medicine, David Geffen School of Medicine at UCLA, Los Angeles; Director, EMS and Pediatric Emergency Medicine Fellowships, Harbor-UCLA Medical Center, Torrance, California
Respiratory Distress and Respiratory Failure

Barry G. Gilmore, MD, MSW
Associate Professor of Pediatrics, Department of Pediatrics, University of Tennessee Health Sciences Center College of Medicine; Attending Physician, and Director of Emergency Services, Division of Emergency Services, LeBonheur Children's Medical Center, Memphis, Tennessee
Disorders of Movement; Ultrasonography

Timothy G. Givens, MD
Associate Professor, Emergency Medicine and Pediatrics, Vanderbilt University Medical Center; Associate Medical Director, and Fellowship Director, Pediatric Emergency Medicine, Monroe Carell Jr. Children's Hospital at Vanderbilt, Nashville, Tennessee
Sickle Cell Disease

Nicole Glaser, MD
Associate Professor of Pediatrics, University of California, Davis, School of Medicine; Department of Pediatrics, University of California, Davis, Medical Center, Sacramento, California
Diabetic Ketoacidosis; Hypoglycemia

Theodore E. Glynn, MD
Department of Emergency Medicine, Ingham Regional Medical Center, Lansing; Assistant Clinical Professor, Michigan State University, East Lansing, Michigan
Syncope

Ran D. Goldman, MD
Division Head and Medical Director, Division of Pediatric Emergency Medicine, BC Children's Hospital; Associate Professor, Department of Pediatrics, University of British Columbia; Senior Associate Clinician Scientist, Child & Family Research Institute (CFRI), Vancouver, British Columbia, Canada
Oral, Ocular, and Maxillofacial Trauma

Marc H. Gorelick, MD, MSCE
Professor of Pediatrics and Population Health, Medical College of Wisconsin; Jon E. Vice Chair in Emergency Medicine, Children's Hospital of Wisconsin, Milwaukee, Wisconsin
Urinary Tract Infection in Infants

Vincent J. Grant, MD, FRCP(C), FAAP
Assistant Professor, Division of Pediatric Emergency Medicine, Department of Pediatrics, University of Ottawa; Medical Director, Trauma Program, Children's Hospital of Eastern Ontario, Ottawa, Ontario, Canada
Head Trauma

Steven M. Green, MD
Professor of Emergency Medicine and Pediatrics, Loma Linda University, Loma Linda, California
Procedural Sedation and Analgesia

Victoria S. Gregg, MD
Assistant Professor of Pediatrics, Baylor College of Medicine; Attending Physician, Emergency Department, Texas Children's Hospital, Houston, Texas
Overuse Syndromes and Inflammatory Conditions

Jacqueline Grupp-Phelan, MD, MPH
Associate Professor of Clinical Pediatrics, University of Cincinnati College of Medicine; Assistant Professor of Clinical Pediatrics, Division of Emergency Medicine, Cincinnati Children's Hospital Medical Center, Cincinnati, Ohio
Major Depression and Suicidality

Martin I. Herman, MD
Professor of Pediatrics, University of Tennessee Health Sciences Center College of Medicine; Attending Physician, Director of Urgent Care Services, and Assistant Director, Emergency Services, LeBonheur Children's Medical Center, Memphis, Tennessee
Disorders of Movement; Testicular Torsion

Marilyn P. Hicks, MD*
Director of Pediatric Emergency Medicine Education, Department of Emergency Medicine, WakeMed Health Systems, Raleigh; Adjunct Assistant Professor of Emergency Medicine, University of North Carolina at Chapel Hill, Chapel Hill, North Carolina
Excessive Crying

Nancy E. Holecek, RN
Senior Vice President for Patient Care Services, Saint Barnabas Health Care System, West Orange New Jersey
Patient Safety, Medical Errors, and Quality of Care

Mark A. Hostetler, MD, MPH, FACEP, FAAP
Associate Professor, Department of Pediatrics, and Chief, Section of Pediatric Emergency Medicine, The University of Chicago, Pritzker School of Medicine; Medical Director, Pediatric Emergency Department, The University of Chicago Comer Children's Hospital, Chicago, Illinois
Inhalation Exposures

Vivian Hwang, MD
Assistant Clinical Professor of Emergency Medicine, The George Washington University School of Medicine and Health Sciences, Washington, DC; Attending Physician, Inova Fairfax Hospital, Falls Church, Virginia
Muscle and Connective Tissue Disorders

Alson S. Inaba, MD, PALS-NF
Associate Professor of Pediatrics, University of Hawaii John A. Burns School of Medicine; Pediatric Emergency Medicine Attending Physician and Course Director, Kapiolani Medical Center for Women and Children; Course Director, Pediatric Advanced Life Support, The Queen's Medical Center; Pediatric Advanced Life Support National Faculty and PROAD Subcommittee, American Heart Association National ECC Committee, Honolulu, Hawaii
Congenital Heart Disease

Sean F. Isaak, MD
Clinical Assistant Professor, Department of Clinical Sciences, Florida State University College of Medicine, Tallahassee; Attending Emergency Medicine, Department of Emergency Medicine, Orlando Regional Healthcare, Orlando, Florida
Incision and Drainage

Paul Ishimine, MD
Assistant Clinical Professor, Departments of Medicine and Pediatrics, University of California, San Diego, School of Medicine; Director, Pediatric Emergency Medicine, Department of Emergency Medicine, University of California, San Diego, Medical Center; Associate Fellowship Director, Division of Pediatric Emergency Medicine, Rady Children's Hospital—San Diego, San Diego, California
Hyperthermia; Hypothermia

---

*Deceased

Cynthia R. Jacobstein, MD, MSCE
Clinical Assistant Professor of Pediatrics, University of
Pennsylvania School of Medicine; Attending Physician,
Emergency Department, The Children's Hospital of
Philadelphia, Philadelphia, Pennsylvania
Issues of Consent, Confidentiality and Minor Status

Gloria Cecelia C. Jacome, MD
Emergency Medical Associates, Long Branch, New Jersey
Digital Injuries and Infections

David M. Jaffe, MD
Dana Brown Professor of Pediatrics, and Director, Division
of Emergency Medicine, Washington University, and St.
Louis Children's Hospital, St. Louis, Missouri
Fever in the Well-Appearing Young Infant

David P. John, MD
Director of Quality and Risk Management, Department of
Emergency Medicine, Middlesex Healthcare System,
Middletown, Connecticut
Patient Safety, Medical Errors, and Quality of Care

Madeline Matar Joseph, MD
Associate Professor of Emergency Medicine and Pediatrics,
Chief, Pediatric Emergency Medicine Department, and
Medical Director, Pediatric Emergency Department,
University of Florida Health Science Center, Jacksonville,
Florida
Gastrointestinal Foreign Bodies; Hepatitis; Pancreatitis

Kelly A. Keogh, MD
Assistant Professor of Paediatrics, University of Toronto;
Division of Pediatric Emergency Medicine, Hospital for
Sick Children Toronto, Ontario, Canada
Enterostomy Tubes

Nazeema Khan, MD
Pediatric Emergency Medicine Attending, Joe DiMaggio
Children's Hospital, Hollywood, Florida
Hypertensive Emergencies; Valvular Heart Disease

Grace J. Kim, MD
Assistant Professor of Emergency Medicine, Loma Linda
University School of Medicine; Assistant Program
Director, Pediatric Emergency Medicine Fellowship, Loma
Linda University Medical Center, Loma Linda, California
Postsurgical Cardiac Conditions and Transplantation

Tommy Y. Kim, MD
Assistant Professor, Department of Pediatric Emergency
Medicine, Loma Linda University Medical Center, Loma
Linda, California
*Headaches; Conditions Causing Increased Intracranial
Pressure*

Brent R. King, MD
Professor of Emergency Medicine and Pediatrics, and
Chairman, Department of Emergency Medicine, The
University of Texas Medical School at Houston; Chief of
Emergency Services, Memorial Hermann Hospital;
Attending Physician, Department of Emergency
Medicine, Lyndon B. Johnson General Hospital,
Houston, Texas
Sepsis

Christopher R. King, MD, FACEP
Associate Professor of Emergency Medicine and Pediatrics,
University of Pittsburgh School of Medicine, UPMC
Presbyterian Hospital, Children's Hospital of Pittsburgh,
Pittsburgh, Pennsylvania
Local and Regional Anesthesia

Niranjan Kissoon, MD, FRCP(C), FAAP, FCCM, FACPE
Professor and Associate Head, Department of Pediatrics,
Faculty of Medicine, University of British Columbia;
Senior Medical Director, Acute and Critical Care
Program, BC Children's Hospital, Vancouver, British
Columbia, Canada
Jaundice

Craig A. Kizewic, DO
Pediatric Emergency Medicine Fellow, Department of
Emergency Medicine, University of Florida Health
Science Center—Shands Jacksonville, Jacksonville, Florida
Gastrointestinal Foreign Bodies

Ann Klasner, MD, MPH
Associate Professor of Pediatrics, University of Alabama at
Birmingham; Co-Director, Pediatric Emergency
Fellowship Program, and Attending Physician,
Emergency Department, The Children's Hospital of
Alabama, Birmingham, Alabama
Brain Tumor

Terry P. Klassen, MD, MSc, FRCPC
Professor and Chair, Department of Pediatrics, University
of Alberta; Regional Program Clinical Director,
Department of Child Health, Stollery Children's
Hospital, Capital Health, Edmonton, Alberta, Canada
Upper Airway Disorders

Stephen R. Knazik, DO, MBA
Clinical Associate Professor of Pediatrics and Emergency
Medicine, Wayne State University School of Medicine;
E.D. Medical Director and Chief of Pediatric Emergency
Medicine, Children's Hospital of Michigan, Detroit,
Michigan
Chest Pain

Paul Kolecki, MD, FACEP
Associate Professor, Department of Emergency Medicine,
Thomas Jefferson University; Consultant, Philadelphia
Poison Control Center, Philadelphia, Pennsylvania
Adverse Effects of Anticonvulsants and Psychotropic Agents

Baruch Krauss, MD, EdM
Assistant Professor of Pediatrics, Harvard Medical School
and Children's Hospital, Boston, Massachusetts
Procedural Sedation and Analgesia

Kelly L. Kriwanek, MD
Attending Physician, Children's Hospital Central
California, Madera, California
Peripheral Neuromuscular Disorders

Nathan Kuppermann, MD, MPH
Professor of Emergency Medicine and Pediatrics, University
of California, Davis, School of Medicine, Sacramento,
California
Diabetic Ketoacidosis

Kenneth T. Kwon, MD, FACEP, FAAP
Associate Clinical Professor, Department of Emergency
    Medicine, University of California, Irvine, School of
    Medicine, Irvine; Director of Pediatric Emergency
    Medicine, Department of Emergency Medicine,
    University of California, Irvine, Medical Center, Orange,
    California
Electrical Injury

Steve Levi, MD
Assistant Clinical Professor of Medicine, Robert Wood
    Johnson School of Medicine; Chief, Electrophysiology,
    Our Lady of Lourdes Medical Center, Camden, New
    Jersey
Pacemakers and Internal Defibrillators

Deborah A. Levine, MD
Clinical Assistant Professor of Pediatrics and Emergency
    Medicine, New York University School of Medicine;
    Attending Physician, Bellevue Hospital Center, New
    York, New York
Bronchiolitis

Stuart Lewena, MBBS, BMedSci, FRACP
Honorary Fellow, Department of Pediatrics, Melbourne
    University, Melbourne; Pediatric Emergency Physician,
    Royal Children's Hospital, Victoria, Australia
*Central Nervous System Vascular Disorders; Vaccination-
    Related Complaints and Side Effects*

Erica L. Liebelt, MD
Associate Professor of Pediatrics and Emergency Medicine,
    University of Alabama at Birmingham School of
    Medicine; Director, Medical Toxicology Services,
    Children's Hospital and University of Alabama at
    Birmingham Hospital, Birmingham, Alabama
General Approach to Poisoning

Marc Y. R. Linares, MD
Director, Pediatric Emergency Fellowship Program, and
    Attending Physician, Emergency Department, Miami
    Children's Hospital, Miami, Florida
Gallbladder Disorders

Robert Luten, MD
Professor of Pediatrics and Emergency Medicine,
    Department of Emergency Medicine, University of
    Florida School of Medicine, Shands Hospital,
    Jacksonville, Florida
*Approach to Resuscitation and Advanced Life Support for
    Infants and Children*

Sharon E. Mace, MD
Associate Professor, Department of Emergency Medicine,
    The Ohio State University School of Medicine,
    Columbus; Faculty, and Emergency Medicine Residency,
    MetroHealth Medical Center, Cleveland; Director,
    Pediatric Education/Quality Improvement, and Director,
    Observation Unit, Cleveland Clinic, Cleveland, Ohio
Triage

Charles G. Macias, MD, MPH
Associate Professor of Pediatrics, Baylor College of
    Medicine; Attending Physician, Emergency Department,
    Texas Children's Hospital, Houston, Texas
*Bone, Joint, and Spine Infections; Overuse Syndromes and
    Inflammatory Conditions*

Ian Maconochie, MBBS, FRCPCH, FCEM
Honorary Senior Lecturer, Imperial College; Lead
    Clinician, Paediatric Emergency Department, St. Mary's
    Hospital, St. Mary's Trust, London, United Kingdom
Dehydration and Disorders of Sodium Balance

William K. Mallon, MD, FACEP, FAASM
Associate Professor of Clinical Emergency Medicine, Keck
    School of Medicine of University of Southern California;
    Director, Division of International Emergency Medicine,
    Department of Emergency Medicine, Los Angeles
    County + University of Southern California Medical
    Center, Los Angeles, California
Neck Trauma

Courtney H. Mann, MD
Adjunct Instructor, University of North Carolina at Chapel
    Hill, Chapel Hill; Medical Director, Pediatric Emergency
    Department, WakeMed Health and Hospitals, Raleigh,
    North Carolina
Vomiting and Diarrhea

Deborah J. Mann, MD
Assistant Professor, Emergency Medicine, State University
    of New York Upstate Medical University, Syracuse,
    New York
Common Pediatric Overdoses

Jonathan Marr, MD
Pediatric Emergency Medicine Fellow, University of Texas
    Southwestern Medical School, and Children's Medical
    Center Dallas, Dallas, Texas
Monitoring in Critically Ill Children; Seizures

Nestor Martinez, MD
Fellow, Pediatric Emergency Medicine, Miami Children's
    Hospital, Miami, Florida
Gallbladder Disorders

Andrew D. Mason, MD
Division of Pediatric Emergency Medicine, Hospital for
    Sick Children, Toronto, Ontario, Canada
Enterostomy Tubes

Todd A. Mastrovitch, MD
Instructor of Emergency Medicine in Clinical Pediatrics,
    Weill Medical College of Cornell University, New York;
    Academic Pediatric Emergency Medicine Attending, and
    Director, Pediatric Education, Department of Emergency
    Medicine, New York Hospital Queens, Flushing, New
    York
Failure to Thrive

Thom A. Mayer, MD
Chairman of Emergency Medicine, Fairfax Medical Center,
    Fairfax, Virginia
Triage

James J. McCarthy, MD, FACEP
Assistant Professor, Department of Emergency Medicine,
  University of Texas at Houston Medical School; Medical
  Director, Emergency Center, Memorial Hermann
  Hospital, Houston, Texas
Sepsis

Maureen McCollough, MD, FACEP
Associate Professor of Emergency Medicine and Pediatrics,
  Keck School of Medicine of University of Southern
  California; Medical Director, Department of Emergency
  Medicine, and Director, Pediatric Emergency
  Department, Los Angeles County + University of
  Southern California Medical Center, Los Angeles,
  California
The Critically Ill Neonate

Ryan S. McCormick, BS, EMT-P
Director, Office of Emergency Management, and Director,
  Center for Healthcare Preparedness, Saint Barnabas
  Health Care System, West Orange, New Jersey
Disaster Preparedness for Children

Barbara E. McDevitt, MD
Director of Pediatric Emergency Services, Saint Barnabas
  Medical Center, Livingston, New Jersey
*Thoracic Trauma; Vomiting, Spitting Up, and Feeding
  Disorders*

William M. McDonnell, MD, JD
Assistant Professor of Pediatrics, Division of Pediatric
  Emergency Medicine, University of Utah School of
  Medicine; Primary Children's Medical Center, Salt Lake
  City, Utah
High Altitude–Associated Illnesses

Mark S. McIntosh, MD, MPH, FAAP, FACEP
Clinical Assistant Professor, Department of Emergency
  Medicine, University of Florida, Jacksonville, Florida
Valvular Heart Disease

Francis Mencl, MD, MS, FACEP
Associate Professor of Emergency Medicine, Northeastern
  Ohio Universities College of Medicine, Rootstown;
  Director of EMS, and Attending Emergency Department
  Staff, Summa Health Systems, Akron, Ohio
Urinary Tract Infections in Children and Adolescents

Russell Migita, MD
Clinical Assistant Professor, Division of Emergency
  Medicine, Department of Pediatrics, University of
  Washington School of Medicine; Clinical Director,
  Emergency Services, Children's Hospital and Regional
  Medical Center, Seattle, Washington
Ventriculoperitoneal and Other Intracranial Shunts

Angela M. Mills, MD, FACEP
Assistant Professor, University of Pennsylvania School of
  Medicine; Attending Physician, Department of
  Emergency Medicine, Hospital of the University of
  Pennsylvania, Philadelphia, Pennsylvania
Pregnancy-Related Complications

Lilit Minasyan, MD
Fellow, Pediatric Emergency Medicine, Loma Linda
  University Children's Hospital and Medical Center,
  Loma Linda, California
Lower Extremity Trauma

Rakesh D. Mistry, MD, MS
Assistant Professor of Pediatrics, University of Pennsylvania
  School of Medicine; Attending Physician, Division of
  Emergency Medicine, The Children's Hospital of
  Philadelphia, Philadelphia, Pennsylvania
Urinary Tract Infection in Infants

Ameer P. Mody, MD, MPH
Assistant Professor of Emergency Medicine and Pediatrics,
  Loma Linda University School of Medicine, Loma Linda;
  Clinical Director, Pediatric Emergency Medicine,
  Emergency Medicine Specialists of Orange County,
  Children's Hospital of Orange County, Orange,
  California
*Trauma in Infants; The Steroid-Dependent Child; Addisonian
  Crisis; Thyrotoxicosis*

Cynthia J. Mollen, MD, MSCE
Assistant Professor, Pediatrics, University of Pennsylvania;
  Attending Physician, Emergency Medicine, The
  Children's Hospital of Philadelphia, Philadelphia,
  Pennsylvania
Sexually Transmitted Infections

James A. Moynihan, MS, DO, FAAP
Assistant Residency Director for Pediatric Emergency
  Medicine Fellowship, and Assistant Professor of
  Emergency Medicine, Division of Pediatric Emergency
  Medicine, Department of Emergency Medicine, Loma
  Linda University School of Medicine; Assistant Medical
  Director, Department of Emergency Medicine, Loma
  Linda University Medical Center and Children's
  Hospital, Loma Linda, California
Snake and Spider Envenomations

Antonio E. Muñiz, MD, FACEP, FAAP, FAAEM
Associate Professor of Emergency Medicine and Pediatrics,
  The University of Texas Medical School at Houston;
  Medical Director of Pediatric Emergency Medicine,
  Children's Memorial Hermann Hospital, Houston, Texas
*Stridor in Infancy; Neonatal Skin Disorders; Erythema
  Multiforme Major and Minor; Henoch-Schönlein Purpura;
  Classic Viral Exanthems; Dermatitis; Infestations; Other
  Important Rashes*

Stacey Murray-Taylor, MD
Associate Director, Adult Emergency Department, Newark
  Beth Israel Medical Center, Newark, New Jersey
*Access of Ports and Catheters and Management of
  Obstruction*

Michael J. Muszynski, MD
Professor of Clinical Sciences, and Orlando Regional
  Campus Dean, Florida State University College of
  Medicine, Tallahassee, Florida
Skin and Soft Tissue Infections

Frances M. Nadel, MD, MSCE
Assistant Professor of Clinical Pediatrics, University of
Pennsylvania School of Medicine; Attending Physician,
Division of Emergency Medicine, The Children's
Hospital of Philadelphia, Philadelphia, Pennsylvania
Vascular Access

Alan L. Nager, MD
Assistant Professor of Pediatrics, Department of Pediatrics,
Keck School of Medicine of University of Southern
California; Director, Department of Emergency and
Transport Medicine, Children's Hospital Los Angeles,
Los Angeles, California
Dehydration and Disorders of Sodium Balance

John F. O'Brien, MD, FACEP
Associate Clinical Professor, Department of Emergency
Medicine, University of Florida Gainesville, Gainesville;
Orlando Regional Medical Center, Associate Residency
Director, Department of Emergency Medicine, Orlando
Regional Medical Center, Orlando, Florida
Incision and Drainage

Pamela J. Okada, MD
Associate Professor of Pediatrics, University of Texas
Southwestern Medical Center at Dallas; Attending
Physician, Emergency Department, Children's Medical
Center Dallas, Dallas, Texas
Seizures

Robert P. Olympia, MD
Assistant Professor of Emergency Medicine and Pediatrics,
Penn State College of Medicine; Attending Physician,
Department of Emergency Medicine, Penn State Milton
S. Hershey Medical Center, Hershey, Pennsylvania
Selected Infectious Diseases

Kevin C. Osterhoudt, MD, MSCE
Associate Professor of Pediatrics, University of
Pennsylvania School of Medicine; Medical Director, The
Poison Control Center, The Children's Hospital of
Philadelphia, Philadelphia, Pennsylvania
Toxic Alcohols

Patricia S. Padlipsky, MD
Fellow in Pediatric Emergency Medicine, Harbor-UCLA
Medical Center, Torrance, California
Respiratory Distress and Respiratory Failure

Joe Pagane, MD
Department of Emergency Medicine, Orlando Regional
Medical Center, Orlando, Florida
Foreign Body Removal

Ruth Ann Pannell, MD
Resident, Emergency Medicine, Orlando Regional Medical
Center, Orlando, Florida
Foreign Body Removal

Norman A. Paradis, MD
Senior Medical Director, Emergency Medicine, and
Professor of Surgery and Medicine, University of
Colorado Health Sciences Center, Denver, Colorado
Cerebral Resuscitation

Ronald I. Paul, MD
Professor of Pediatrics, and Chief, Division of Pediatric
Emergency Medicine, University of Louisville; Chief,
Pediatric Emergency Medicine, Kosair Children's
Hospital, Louisville, Kentucky
Diseases of the Hip

Barbara M. Garcia Peña, MD, MPH
Research Director, Assistant Fellowship Director,
Emergency Department, Miami Children's Hospital,
Miami, Florida
Inflammatory Bowel Disease

Jay Pershad, MD, FAAP
Associate Professor of Pediatrics, and Co-Director,
Pediatric Emergency Fellowship Program, University of
Tennessee Health Sciences Center; Attending Physician,
Emergency Department, and Associate Medical Director,
EMSC Education, and Sedationist, Radiology
Department, LeBonheur Children's Medical Center,
Memphis, Tennessee
Peripheral Neuromuscular Disorders; Ultrasonography

Shari L. Platt, MD, FAAP
Associate Professor of Clinical Pediatrics, Weill Cornell
College of Medicine; Director, Pediatric Emergency
Service, New York Presbyterian Hospital, New York,
New York
Pneumonia

Jill C. Posner, MD, MSCE
Assistant Professor of Pediatrics, University of Pennsylvania
School of Medicine, University of Pennsylvania;
Attending Physician, Pediatric Emergency Medicine, The
Children's Hospital of Philadelphia, Philadelphia,
Pennsylvania
Menstrual Disorders; Replacing a Tracheostomy Tube

Amy L. Puchalski, MD
Assistant Professor of Pediatrics and Emergency Medicine,
Medical College of Georgia; Attending Physician,
Children's Medical Center, Augusta, Georgia
Neck Infections; Neck Masses

Earl J. Reisdorff, MD
Director of Medical Education, Department of Emergency
Medicine, Ingham Regional Medical Center, Lansing;
Associate Professor, Michigan State University, East
Lansing, Michigan
Syncope; Chest Pain

Mark G. Roback, MD
Professor of Pediatrics, and Associate Director, Division of
Emergency Medicine, University of Minnesota Medical
School, Minneapolis, Minnesota
High Altitude–Associated Illnesses

Steven C. Rogers, MD
Fellow, Pediatric Emergency Medicine, University of Utah
Health Sciences Center, Salt Lake City, Utah
Near Drowning and Submersion Injuries

Genie E. Roosevelt, MD, MPH
Assistant Professor, Section of Emergency Medicine,
Department of Pediatrics, University of Colorado at
Denver and Health Sciences Center; Attending
Physician, Emergency Department, The Children's
Hospital, Denver, Colorado
Cerebral Resuscitation

Lazaro G. Rosales, MD
Department of Pathology, State University of New York
Upstate Medical University, Syracuse, New York
*Utilizing Blood Bank Resources/Transfusion Reactions and
Complications*

Kimberly R. Roth, MD
Assistant Professor, Division of Pediatric Emergency
Medicine, University of Pittsburgh School of Medicine,
Children's Hospital of Pittsburgh, Pittsburgh,
Pennsylvania
Local and Regional Anesthesia

Steven G. Rothrock, MD, FACEP, FAAP
Professor of Emergency Medicine, University of Florida;
Associate Professor of Clinical Sciences, Florida State
University, Orlando Regional Healthcare System,
Orlando, Florida
*Approach to Resuscitation and Advanced Life Support for
Infants and Children; Rapid Sequence Intubation;
Neonatal Resuscitation; The Critically Ill Neonate;
Circulatory Emergencies: Shock; Oral, Ocular, and
Maxillofacial Trauma; Appendicitis*

Alfred Sacchetti, MD
Assistant Clinical Professor, Emergency Medicine, Thomas
Jefferson University, Philadelphia, Pennsylvania; Chief,
Emergency Services, Our Lady of Lourdes Medical
Center, Camden, New Jersey
*The Sick or Injured Child in a Community Hospital
Emergency Department; Pacemakers and Internal
Defibrillators*

Peter D. Sadowitz, MD
Associate Professor of Pediatric Emergency Medicine and
Associate Professor of Medicine, State University of New
York, Syracuse, New York
*Cancer and Cancer-Related Complications in Children; Acute
Childhood Immune Thrombocytopenic Purpura and
Related Platelet Disorders*

Esther Maria Sampayo, MD
Assistant Professor of Pediatrics and Pediatric Emergency
Medicine, University of Pennsylvania; Children's
Hospital of Philadelphia, Philadelphia, Pennsylvania
Oral Lesions

John P. Santamaria, MD
Affiliate Professor, Department of Pediatrics, University of
South Florida School of Medicine, Tampa, Florida
Dysbarism

Neil Schamban, MD
Associate Clinical Professor, Emergency Medicine, Mount
Sinai School of Medicine, New York, New York; Vice
Chairman, Department of Emergency Medicine, Newark
Beth Israel Medical Center, Newark, New Jersey
*Eye Disorders; The Sick or Injured Child in a Community
Hospital Emergency Department; Access of Ports and
Catheters and Management of Obstruction*

Carl H. Schultz, MD, FACEP
Professor of Clinical Emergency Medicine, and Co-
Director, EMS and Disaster Medical Sciences Fellowship,
Department of Emergency Medicine, University of
California, Irvine, School of Medicine, Irvine; Director,
Disaster Medical Services, Department of Emergency
Medicine, University of California, Irvine, Medical
Center, Orange, California
Electrical Injury

Sandra H. Schwab, MD
Assistant Professor, Department of General Pediatrics,
University of Pennsylvania; Attending Physician,
Department of General Pediatrics, Division of
Emergency Medicine, The Childrens Hospital of
Philadelphia, Philadelphia, Pennsylvania
Menstrual Disorders

Fred Schwartz, MD
Attending Physician, Pediatric Emergency Medicine, Saint
Barnabas Medical Center, Livingston, New Jersey
Paraphimosis Reduction

Deborah Scott, RN, ARNP
Nurse Examiner, Arnold Palmer Hospital Child Advocacy
Center, Orlando, Florida
Sexual Abuse

Matthew A. Seibel, MD
Clinical Professor, Florida State University; Pediatric
Hospitalist, Arnold Palmer Hospital for Children,
Orlando, Florida
Sexual Abuse

Samir S. Shah, MD
Assistant Professor of Pediatrics and Epidemiology,
University of Pennsylvania School of Medicine;
Attending Physician, Divisions of Infectious Diseases
and General Pediatrics, The Children's Hospital of
Philadelphia, Philadelphia, Pennsylvania
Post-Liver Transplantation Complications

Ghazala Q. Sharieff, MD, FACEP, FAAEM, FAAP
Associate Clinical Professor, Children's Hospital and
Health Center, University of California, San Diego;
Director of Pediatric Emergency Medicine, Palomar-
Pomerado Hospitals, California Emergency Physicians,
San Diego, California
Dysrhythmias; Pericarditis, Myocarditis, and Endocarditis

Richard D. Shih, MD, FAAEM, FACEP
Associate Professor of Surgery, New Jersey Medical School,
UMDNJ, Newark; Residency Director, Emergency
Medicine, Morristown Memorial Hospital, Morristown,
New Jersey
Adverse Effects of Anticonvulsants and Psychotropic Agents

Jan M. Shoenberger, MD, FACEP, FAAEM
Assistant Professor of Clinical Emergency Medicine, Keck School of Medicine of University of Southern California; Associate Residency Director, Department of Emergency Medicine, Los Angeles County + University of Southern California Medical Center, Los Angeles, California
Neck Trauma

Ian Shrier, MD, PhD, Dip Sport Med (FACSM)
Associate Professor, Department of Family Medicine, SMBD-Jewish General Hospital, McGill University; Investigator, Centre for Clinical Epidemiology and Community Studies, Montréal, Québec, Canada
Compartment Syndrome

Jonathan I. Singer, MD, FAAP, FACEP
Professor of Emergency Medicine and Pediatrics, Vice Chair, and Associate Program Director, Department of Emergency Medicine, Boonshoft School of Medicine, Wright State University; Staff Physician, Children's Medical Center, Dayton, Ohio
Intussusception

Sharon R. Smith, MD
Associate Professor of Pediatrics, Department of Pediatrics, University of Connecticut Health Center, Farmington; Associate Professor of Pediatrics, Department of Emergency Medicine, Connecticut Children's Medical Center, Hartford, Connecticut
Management of Acute Asthma

Abdul-Kader Souid, MD, PhD
Professor of Pediatrics and Biochemistry, State University of New York Upstate Medical University, Syracuse, New York
Cancer and Cancer-Related Complications in Children; Acute Childhood Immune Thrombocytopenic Purpura and Related Platelet Disorders; Disorders of Coagulation; Hemolytic-Uremic Syndrome; Utilizing Blood Bank Resources/Transfusion Reactions and Complications

Blake Spirko, MD, FACEP, FAAP
Pediatric Emergency Medicine Fellowship Director, and Assistant Professor, Department of Emergency Medicine, Tufts University School of Medicine, Boston; Pediatric Emergency Medicine Fellowship Director, and Assistant Professor, Department of Emergency Medicine, Baystate Medical Center, Springfield, Massachusetts
Musculoskeletal Disorders in Systemic Disease

Nicole S. Sroufe, MD, MPH
Pediatric Emergency Medicine Fellow, Department of Emergency Medicine, University of Michigan, Ann Arbor, Michigan
Rhabdomyolysis

Rachel M. Stanley, MD, MHSA
Assistant Professor, University of Michigan; Department of Emergency Medicine, University of Michigan Health Center, Ann Arbor, Michigan
Rhabdomyolysis

Robert Steele, MD, FACEP
Associate Professor, Loma Linda University Medical School; Interim Medical Director, Department of Emergency Medicine, Loma Linda University Medical Center, Loma Linda, California
Pericardiocentesis

Mardi Steere, MBBS, FAAP
Staff Specialist, Pediatric Emergency, Women's and Children's Hospital, North Adelaide, South Australia, Australia
Pancreatitis

Gail M. Stewart, DO, FAAP
Associate Professor of Emergency Medicine and Pediatrics, Loma Linda University School of Medicine; Attending Physician, Pediatric Emergency Department, Loma Linda University Medical Center and Children's Hospital, Loma Linda, California
Trauma in Infants; Conditions Causing Increased Intracranial Pressure

Patricia Sweeney-McMahon, RN, MS
Assistant Vice President, Clinical and Emergency Services, Saint Barnabas Health Care System, West Orange, New Jersey
Patient Safety, Medical Errors, and Quality of Care; Digital Injuries and Infections

David A. Talan, MD, FACEP, FIDSA
Professor of Medicine, UCLA School of Medicine, Los Angeles; Chairman, Department of Emergency Medicine, and Faculty, Division of Infectious Diseases, Olive View-UCLA Medical Center, Sylmar, California
Tetanus Prophylaxis; Rabies Postexposure Prophylaxis

Todd B. Taylor, MD
Adjunct Associate Professor, Department of Emergency Medicine, Vanderbilt University School of Medicine, Vanderbilt University, Nashville, Tennessee
Emergency Medical Treatment and Labor Act (EMTALA)

Stephen J. Teach, MD, MPH
Professor of Pediatrics and Emergency Medicine, Department of Pediatrics, George Washington University School of Medicine and Health Sciences; Associate Chief, Division of Emergency Medicine, Children's National Medical Center; Associate Director, Center for Clinical and Community Research, Children's National Medical Center, Washington, DC
Gastrointestinal Bleeding

Sieuwert-Jan C. ten Napel, MD
Resident, Emergency Medicine, Emergency Department, Onze lieve Vrouwe Gasthuis-Hospital, Amsterdam, The Netherlands
Upper Extremity Trauma

Thomas E. Terndrup, MD, FACEP, FAAEM
Professor and Chair, Emergency Medicine, and Associate Dean for Clinical Research, Penn State Milton S. Hershey Medical Center, Penn State College of Medicine, Hershey, Pennsylvania
Thoracostomy

Tonya M. Thompson, MD, MA
Assistant Professor, Departments of Pediatrics and
  Emergency Medicine, University of Arkansas for
  Medical Sciences; Associate Pediatric Emergency
  Medicine Fellowship Director, Department of Pediatrics,
  Arkansas Children's Hospital, Little Rock, Arkansas
Headaches

Andrea Thorp, MD
Fellow in Pediatric Emergency Medicine, Loma Linda
  University Medical Center and Children's Hospital,
  Loma Linda, California
Pericardiocentesis

Irene Tien, MD, MSc
Assistant Professor, Boston University School of Medicine,
  Boston; Staff Physician, Newton-Wellesley Hospital,
  Newton, Massachusetts
Ear Diseases; Physical Abuse and Child Neglect

John A. Tilelli, MD
Clinical Assistant Professor, Florida State University,
  Tallahassee; Intensivist, Division of Pediatric Critical
  Care Medicine, Arnold Palmer Children's Hospital,
  Orlando Regional Healthcare System, Orlando, Florida
*Drugs of Abuse; Cardiovascular Agents; Ventilator
Considerations*

Nicholas Tsarouhas, MD
Associate Professor of Clinical Pediatrics, Department of
  Pediatrics, University of Pennsylvania School of
  Medicine; Medical Director, Emergency Transport
  Services, and Attending Physician, Emergency
  Department, The Children's Hospital of Philadelphia,
  Philadelphia, Pennsylvania
Burns

Michael G. Tunik, MD
Associate Professor of Pediatrics and Emergency Medicine,
  New York University School of Medicine; Research
  Director, and Associate Director, Pediatric Emergency
  Medicine, Bellevue Hospital Center, New York, New York
Emergency Medical Services and Transport

Christian Vaillancourt, MD, MSc, FRCPC
Assistant Professor, Department of Emergency Medicine,
  The Ottawa Hospital, University of Ottawa; Associate
  Scientist, Ottawa Health Research Institute, Ottawa,
  Ontario, Canada
Compartment Syndrome

Jonathan H. Valente, MD, FACEP
Assistant Professor, Departments of Emergency Medicine
  and Pediatrics, Brown Medical School, Brown
  University; Attending Physician, Rhode Island Hospital
  and Hasbro Children's Hospital, Providence, Rhode
  Island
Minor Infant Problems

Peter Viccellio, MD
Clinical Professor of Emergency Medicine, Stony Brook
  University Medical Center, Stony Brook, New York
Spinal Trauma

Andrew Wackett, MD
Assistant Clinical Professor of Emergency Medicine, Stony
  Brook University Medical Center, Stony Brook, New
  York
Spinal Trauma

Ron M. Walls, MD
Professor of Medicine, Department of Emergency
  Medicine, Harvard Medical School; Chairman,
  Department of Emergency Medicine, Brigham and
  Women's Hospital, Boston, Massachusetts
Intubation, Rescue Devices, and Airway Adjuncts

Jennifer L. Waxler, DO
Emergency Medical Associates, Long Branch, New Jersey
Digital Injuries and Infections

Evan J. Weiner, MD, FAAP
Fellow, Pediatric Emergency Medicine, University of
  Florida Health Science Center; Physician, Pediatric
  Emergency Medicine, Wolfson Children's Hospital,
  Jacksonville, Florida
Hepatitis

Stuart B. Weiss, MD
Partner, MedPrep Consulting Group, LLC, New York, New
  York
Disaster Preparedness for Children

James A. Wilde, MD, FAAP
Associate Professor of Emergency Medicine and Pediatrics,
  and Director, Pediatric Emergency Medicine, Medical
  College of Georgia, Augusta, Georgia
Central Nervous System Infections

Kristine G. Williams, MD, MPH
Instructor, Pediatrics, Washington University School of
  Medicine; Instructor, Pediatrics, Division of Emergency
  Medicine, St. Louis Children's Hospital, St. Louis,
  Missouri
Fever in the Well-Appearing Young Infant

Michael Witt, MD, MPH
Instructor in Pediatrics, Harvard Medical School;
  Attending Physician, Children's Hospital, Boston,
  Massachusetts
Abdominal Hernias

Aaron Wohl, MD
Clinical Assistant Professor, Department of Emergency
  Medicine, University of Florida College of Medicine,
  Gainesville; Attending Physician, Department of
  Emergency Medicine, Lee Memorial Hospital, Fort
  Myers, Florida
Constipation

Tony Woodward, MD, MBA
Professor, Division of Emergency Medicine, Department of
Pediatrics, University of Washington School of
Medicine; Director, Emergency Services, Children's
Hospital and Regional Medical Center, Seattle,
Washington
Ventriculoperitoneal and Other Intracranial Shunts

Robert Bruce Wright, MD, FAAP, FRCPC
Assistant Professor, Division of Pediatric Emergency
Medicine, Department of Pediatrics, University of
Alberta; Assistant Director, Division of Pediatric
Emergency Medicine, Stollery Children's Hospital,
Edmonton, Alberta, Canada
Upper Airway Disorders

Todd Wylie, MD, MPH
Assistant Professor, Program Director Pediatric Emergency
Medicine Fellowship, Department of Emergency
Medicine, University of Florida, Jacksonville, Florida
*Pericarditis, Myocarditis, and Endocarditis; Hypertensive
Emergencies*

Kelly D. Young, MD, MS
Associate Clinical Professor of Pediatrics, David Geffen
School of Medicine at UCLA, Los Angeles; Director,
Pediatric Emergency and Pain Management Education,
Department of Emergency Medicine, Harbor-UCLA
Medical Center, Torrance, California
Approach to Pain Management

Joseph J. Zorc, MD
Associate Professor of Pediatrics and Emergency Medicine,
University of Pennsylvania School of Medicine;
Attending Physician, The Children's Hospital of
Philadelphia, Philadelphia, Pennsylvania
Altered Mental Status/Coma

Alexander Zouros, MD, FRCS(C)
Assistant Professor, Department of Neurosurgery, Loma
Linda University Medical Center, Loma Linda,
California
Conditions Causing Increased Intracranial Pressure

Preface

Societies are often judged by the care they provide for the young and the weak. The quality of care for injured and ill children has grown tremendously since the formation and growth of pediatric emergency medicine as a subspecialty within the pediatric and emergency medicine communities. The body of knowledge that defines pediatric emergency medicine is deep in breadth and wide in scope. Those who practice it are energetic, intelligent, and caring. They come from diverse backgrounds and share the common goal of providing safe, comprehensive, high quality, cost-effective care. Because children are treated in many venues ranging from the prehospital setting, to urgent care clinics, community hospital emergency departments, academic medical centers and pediatric specialty care hospitals, the provision of excellent pediatric emergency care is of great interest to many.

This text is designed to meet the needs of anyone who cares for childhood emergencies. It is a highly practical and clinically useful reference organized in a logical fashion – according to the way one would think and problem solve when confronted with any emergency in a child. The emphasis is on information that has an impact in real-time care at the bedside and therefore helps the emergency practitioner at the moment help is most required. The book includes 200 chapters replete with clinical algorithms, tables, photos, figures, and expert commentary. The information is presented in a format which highlights key points, important clinical features, potential pitfalls, and delineates the diagnostic approach and specific management for a myriad of pediatric emergency problems.

The sections of the book are divided according to the typical way that one experiences patients in an emergency department – by level of acuity, type of disease, and patient characteristics. Section I: *Immediate Approach to the Critical Patient* addresses life-threatening presentations of medical and surgical disease and contains crucial information on providing immediate and life-saving therapies. Section II: *Approach to the Trauma Patient*, provides similar information when dealing with acute injury as well as definitive management recommendations for a wide range of traumatic conditions. Section III: *Approach to Unique Problems of Infancy* highlights important clinical features and critical management information for conditions which specifically affect this high-risk population of emergency patients. Sections IV and V: *Approach to the Acutely Ill Patient and Approach to Envi-*

ronmental Illness and Injury cover the wide spectrum of conditions encountered on a regular basis in the emergency care of children. Section VII: *Procedures, Sedation, Pain Management and Devices*, provides step by step techniques, important clinical considerations, and helpful illustrations for performing procedures and managing devices in children in the emergency department.

Several unique features of this text will prove invaluable to busy clinicians. Section VI: *The Practice Environment*, explicitly discusses difficult issues such as triage, the care of minors, end of life care, and family presence during resuscitation and offers practical and workable solutions. Section VIII: *Quick Looks*, offers an immediate differential diagnosis to common pediatric emergency department symptom-oriented complaints ranging from abdominal pain and cyanosis to jaundice and lymphadenopathy. The text is extensively cross referenced to provide the most rapid and useful assistance to the reader.

The creation of the first edition of *Pediatric Emergency Medicine* was borne out of the desire to synthesize and disseminate the evidence based practice of emergency care for children, where such evidence exists. There has been an explosive amount of research in the last several years on many aspects of pediatric emergency medicine, with findings that challenge current practices on a regular basis. Much is still to be learned, however, each year therapies based on anecdotal evidence or opinion are replaced with evidence based guidelines and validated decision rules. When evidence to support a particular diagnostic strategy or treatment could not be found, this text makes the best possible recommendation based on current literature and expert opinion or consensus, referencing statements in text for our readers' convenience. It also highlights controversies, cutting edge developments and areas that are in need of further study.

Our goal is to assure that a scientifically sound rationale is used as the basis for the management of ill and injured children. We hope to further such care on a regular basis in emergency departments everywhere to individuals of all backgrounds who provide pediatric emergency care. It is our intention that this first edition of *Pediatric Emergency Medicine* will become an invaluable resource in this capacity. With the knowledge and insight gained from the experts who have written on these pages, we sincerely hope that this text will promote and advance excellent emergency care to the young and vulnerable.

We gratefully acknowledge the work of Joanie Milnes, our developmental editor. Joanie was the ultimate professional, gently guiding us through every stage of publication. She was tough and persistent when we needed her to be but always kind, and remarkably hard working. We also appreciate the guidance and assistance of other Elsevier staff, particularly Todd Hummel who gave us a great start, and Maria Lorusso who gave us a great finish.

Ran D. Goldman, our pharmacology editor, did us a tremendous service and we are indebted to him for providing an efficient and thorough review of our chapters and for checking every medication dose and reference contained within. Ran, we thank you for that extra reassurance and for your tremendous hard work.

We pay tribute to all our contributors who authored chapters and put up with many requests and deadlines. Their level of excitement about the project as well as their knowledge and commitment to creating a high quality, thoroughly referenced work was unsurpassed. Several colleagues volunteered above and beyond the call of duty to author multiple chapters and we are indebted to them for the volume of work they embraced in a short period of time.

We especially thank our colleagues at The Children's Hospital of Philadelphia, the Hospital of the University of Pennsylvania, Saint Barnabas Health Care System, Loma Linda University Medical Center and Children's Hospital, and Orlando Regional Healthcare for their willingness to become authors and for the daily privilege of working with them in our respective emergency departments.

And finally, the motivation to create this book comes in large part, from our patients. They are a constant source of learning and inspiration and we thank them for the opportunity to care for them. It is our intention and hope that this text will improve the health and well being of those we are privileged to serve.

Jill M. Baren, MD, MBE, FACEP, FAAP
Steven G. Rothrock, MD, FACEP, FAAP
John A. Brennan, MD, FACEP, FAAP
Lance Brown, MD, MPH, FACEP, FAAP

Contents

SECTION III
Approach to Unique Problems of Infancy

SECTION IV
Approach to the Acutely Ill Patient

Central Nervous System

HEENT/Neck

SECTION VIII
Quick Looks

Immediate Approach to the Critical Patient

Chapter 1

Approach to Resuscitation and Advanced Life Support for Infants and Children

Robert Luten, MD and Steven G. Rothrock, MD

Key Points

Both shock and respiratory failure can be diagnosed and treated in a timely fashion utilizing simple bedside clinical parameters.

With the exception of infants with cardiac failure, clinicians are most likely to under-resuscitate infants and children with shock (i.e., they do not administer enough fluids in a timely manner).

A clear understanding of technique and equipment for BVM ventilation *before,* and maintenance of endotracheal tube position *after,* intubation is crucial.

Eliminate unnecessary mental activity so that time can be used for assessing the priorities of resuscitation. Use printed material or cards to facilitate dosing and equipment selection and age-specific algorithms to improve management of resuscitation and evaluation of critically ill infants and children.

The practice of fundamental mock scenarios and treatment modalities can provide confidence when addressing the rare critically ill child.

Introduction and Background

Survival following cardiac arrest in children is poor. As opposed to adults, in whom cardiac arrest is frequently a primary event brought on by ischemic heart disease, in children cardiac arrest is a secondary phenomenon, usually the result of profound metabolic disturbances from untreated shock or respiratory failure. In the early 1980s, the American Heart Association, through the creation of the Pediatric Advanced Life Support (PALS) course, aimed its educational emphasis at the recognition and treatment of respiratory

failure and shock as its principal resuscitative thrust. The treatment of pediatric cardiac arrest, although included, needs to be seen in perspective relative to the larger picture, the priority for recognition of and resuscitation from shock and respiratory failure. Although the science of resuscitation therapy is continually evolving and requires periodic review, management of a pediatric resuscitation is a skill that changes little over time. Certain practical issues that are inherent in the treatment of respiratory failure, shock, and cardiac arrest in children are discussed in this chapter.

Survival with normal neurologic function following inhospital cardiac arrest is 14% to 15% and less than 3% after out-of-hospital pediatric cardiac arrest.[1-5] Studies have delineated markers for poor outcome and no survival. It is helpful to know these probability markers to guide appropriateness of ongoing resuscitation and to quickly prepare and console parents in dealing with the death of their child. Also, in an effort to prevent cardiac survival in the presence of probable devastating neurologic outcome, it is helpful to have guidelines for termination of resuscitative efforts. Most authors agree that, in the absence of extenuating circumstances such as profound hypothermia, resuscitative efforts beyond two to three doses of epinephrine are unlikely to be successful.[3,6,7] Other markers for poor probability of survival include drowning requiring chest compressions and advanced life support medications at the scene, lack of cardiac activity on arrival to the emergency department (ED), and prolonged (>30 minutes) resuscitation.[3,6,7]

Approach

A recent review of the pediatric resuscitation process attempted to define elements of the mental (cognitive) burden of providers when dealing with critically ill children.[8] An increase in logistical time is inherent in pediatric resuscitation compared to adult resuscitation. One of the reasons for this increased logistical time is the age- and size-related variations unique to children, which introduce the need for more complex, "nonautomatic" mental activities, such as calculating drug doses and selecting equipment. These activities may subtract from other important mental activities such as assessment, evaluation, prioritization, and synthesis of information, which can be referred to in the resuscitative process as "critical thinking activity." Summation of these logistical difficulties leads to inevitable time delays, and a corresponding increase in the potential for decision-making errors in the pediatric resuscitative process. This is in sharp contrast to adult resuscitation. One way of understanding this differences is to examine the adult resuscitation process. Medications used frequently (e.g., epinephrine, atropine, glucose, bicarbonate, and lidocaine) are packaged in prefilled syringes containing the exact adult dose, making their ordering and administration "automatic" (i.e., not requiring mental effort beyond the decision to order one ampule or one unit dose of the drug). The same concept is seen in equipment selection, where the usual necessary equipment is laid out for immediate access and use. It is also common to have preprinted algorithms readily available to guide drug selection, drug dosing, equipment selection, and administration decisions, even though the provider frequently has a good working knowledge of these issues. The end result is that the adult provider's time is freed up for critical thinking, and is not occupied with these other decisions.

The use of resuscitation aids in pediatric resuscitation can significantly reduce the cognitive load caused by obligatory calculations of dosage and equipment selection. These aids relegate these activities to a lower order of mental function. In other words, the use of resuscitation aids in pediatric resuscitation transforms nonautomatic activities into automatic activities, decreasing logistical time, thereby increasing critical thinking time. An example is the Broselow-Luten system that codifies children to a color by a single length measurement. The color then serves as a code for preselected equipment, precalculated medications, and other age/size-related variables such as fluids and ventilator settings (Fig. 1–1).

Evaluation and Management

The ABCs

Standard preliminary treatment is usually initiated prior to arrival of critically ill or arrested children in the ED. Laypeople and emergency medical services (EMS) providers have been shown inaccurate at detecting breathlessness and the presence of a pulse in patients with cardiac arrest.[9] For this reason, a complete cardiopulmonary re-evaluation is essential upon patient arrival in the ED. Head tilt and chin lift (jaw thrust without head tilt if cervical spine injury is possible) are initiated to open an obstructed airway while rescue breaths are given for apneic patients. Upon ED arrival, more advanced airway techniques, subsequently described, are applied. As respiratory failure is the most common precipitating event in childhood cardiac arrest, attention to properly opening the airway, adequate ventilation, and oxygenation are key resuscitation techniques.

Clinicians should be aware that the infant's heart is below the lower third of the sternum in 88% of cases.[10] For this reason, chest compressions over the lower third of the sternum generate a higher mean arterial pressure compared to the midsternum[11] (Fig. 1–2). Additionally, using both hand to encircle the chest while applying chest compressions to

infants (<1 year old) results in a higher arterial pressure than two-finger compressions during CPR.[12] For rescuers who are on their own, compression of the sternum with two fingers may be an appropriate alternative to allow for rapid transition between ventilation and compressions.[13] While estimates of appropriate compression depths for different ages are suggested (Table 1–1), an increase in end-tidal CO_2 ($ETCO_2$) is seen with more effective chest compressions and may guide the efficacy of these efforts.[14]

Expert recommendations and advanced life support courses require a considerable amount of memorization of specific time intervals, depth of compression, and frequency of ventilation and chest compression, contributing to an excess cognitive burden during resuscitation efforts (Table 1–1). In reality, no specific ventilation rate or ratio has been shown to result in superior outcome during cardiopulmonary resuscitation (CPR). In fact, during bystander CPR, chest compressions may be all that are required to ensure adequate ventilation.[15,16] Moreover, recommended compression rates of 100 beats/min in infants and children may be too low as rates of compression of 120 beats/min result in higher aortic and coronary perfusion pressures, and these rates barely approach normal heart rates at their recommended ages.[17,18] Realistically, attention to properly opening the airway and to appropriately located and rapid compressions augmented by monitoring $ETCO_2$ will provide the best chance for intact survival in cardiac arrest while limiting the cognitive burden of adhering to a set of rigid, inflexible ratios and numbers that have limited scientific validity.

Two additional tools that may aid in the diagnosis and management of patients in cardiac arrest include $ETCO_2$ monitoring and ultrasonography (US). During CPR, a sudden rise in $ETCO_2$ to greater than 15 mm Hg predicts a return of spontaneous circulation (ROSC), while persistence of $ETCO_2$ less than 10 mm Hg for 20 or more minutes predicts a near-zero probability of ROSC.[18,19] $ETCO_2$ also may discriminate between true pulseless electrical activity (PEA) and patients with true cardiac activity and a low blood pressure with nonpalpable pulses.[20] Bedside US in the ED can be used to identify cardiac activity during cardiac arrest. Adults with any cardiac activity on US during resuscitation have a 26% rate of survival to hospital admission compared to 3% for those with no cardiac activity.[21] While this study has not been replicated in children, it is likely that US has some ability to predict survivors in this population. Ultrasonography has been used to detect ventricular fibrillation in patients initially thought to have asystole and, thus, guide appropriate management.[22] Like capnography, US can be used to discriminate between patients with true PEA and those with a low blood pressure.[21]

After ED arrival, the first few seconds of evaluation determine the priorities and management over the next few minutes. Referred to as the "ABCs," the initial clinical evaluation of the airway (A), breathing (B), and circulation (C) determines whether the child is suffering from respiratory failure (abnormal A and B), shock (abnormal C), or cardiopulmonary failure or arrest (abnormal or absent ABC). The presence of normal ABCs in the unresponsive patient eliminates respiratory failure (CO_2 retention and narcosis) and shock (decreased cerebral perfusion) as causes of the altered mental status and also eliminates the majority of critical pediatric diseases since children tend follow the pathways of

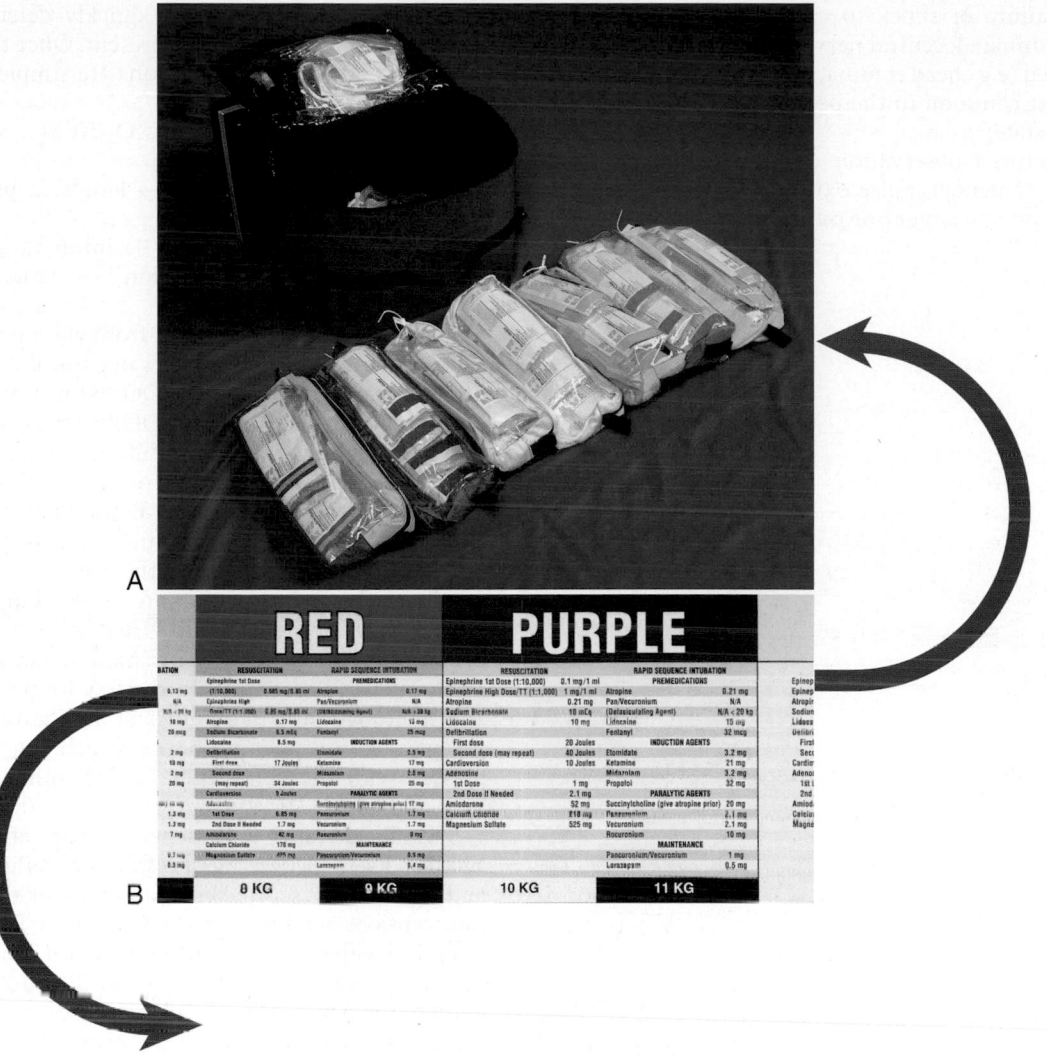

FIGURE 1–1. For situations in which a patient cannot be weighed, an accurate prediction of a patient's color zone can be determined using the Broselow tape. Once a color has been obtained, it references precalculated drug doses and drug volumes as well as appropriately preselected equipment. **A,** Equipment storage system. **B,** Broselow tape. **C,** Medication label, the Broselow-Luten system.

respiratory failure or shock to cardiac arrest. Once these causes are eliminated, central nervous system disorders need to be addressed (e.g., head trauma, medication overdose, and, probably most common in the pediatric emergency setting, the postictal state).

Brief, structured observation of breathing difficulty to assess airway (patency), pulse oximetry to assess breathing (adequacy), and assessment of pulses and capillary refill to assess circulation (perfusion) quickly determines whether respiratory failure or shock is present. Once recognized, subsequent therapeutic interventions are simple but effective if appropriately applied:

Respiratory Failure → O₂/BVM ventilation → Intubation

Shock → Vascular access → Fluids, ± pressors or antibiotics or blood

Arrest → BVM ventilation → intubation → chest compressions → defibrillation → vascular access → fluids/medications

Anywhere in the treatment, from the initial diagnosis to subsequent unexpected changes in clinical course, regardless of the disease, the mnemonic DOPE must be considered following patient deterioration. DOPE refers to **D**islodgement of the endotracheal tube (ET) into the esophagus or a mainstem bronchus, **O**bstruction of the ETT from debris or kinking, **P**neumothorax, or **E**quipment malfunction. A sequential approach to evaluation and treatment using the mnemonic (1–disconnecting the patient from mechanical ventilation and 2–auscultation of the lungs, followed by 3–suctioning of the ETT and visual inspection of the glottic opening) may be warranted in a more structured setting such as an intensive care unit. In the ED, immediate extubation and reintubation is more efficient and eliminates all causes except a tension pneumothorax, which can then be decompressed with the confidence that all other etiologies have been addressed.

Specific therapy will depend upon etiology (e.g., β-agonists for the wheezing of respiratory failure or antibiotics and steroids for septic shock). Details of these therapeutic interventions are found in other chapters. The following sections deal with some of the major practical issues and pitfalls in the initial treatment of the critically ill child based on evaluation of the ABCs. Many etiologies traditionally are listed in the differential diagnosis of the critically ill child, some of which are extremely rare. The approach described herein

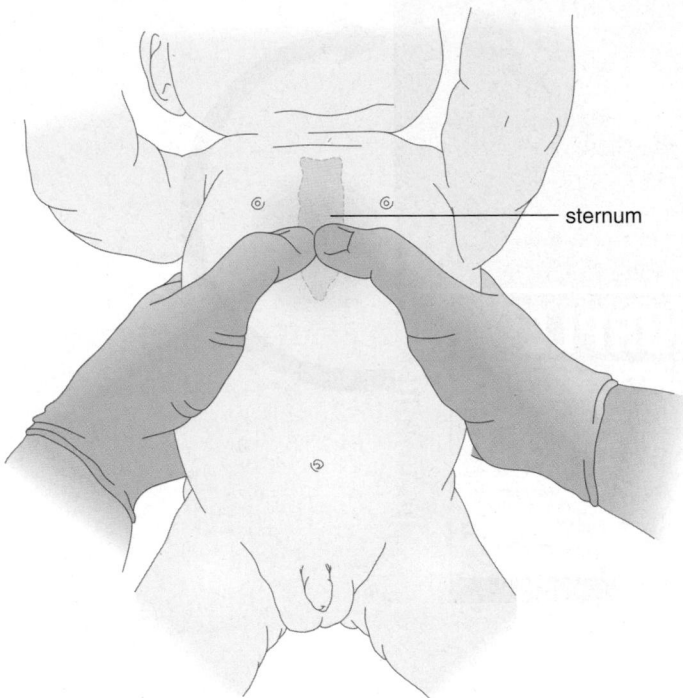

sternum

FIGURE 1–2. Optimum cardiac compressions (with two-person CPR) in infants (<1 year old) with thumbs compressing lower third of sternum and hands encircling chest.

Table 1–1	CPR Maneuvers and Techniques in Newborns, Infants, and Children		
Maneuver	**Newborn/Neonate**	**Infant (<1 yr)**	**Child (1–8 yr)**
Open Airway **Breathing**	Head tilt–chin lift (jaw lift without head tilt if trauma)—all ages		
Initial	May require 30–40 cm H₂O pressure	Two breaths to make chest rise	Two breaths to make chest rise
Subsequent			
if no CPR	30–60 breaths/min	12–20 breaths/min	12–20 breaths/min
during CPR	30–60 breaths/min	8–10 breaths/min	8–10 breaths/min
Circulation*			
Check pulse	Umbilical/brachial	Brachial or femoral	Carotid
Compress at	Lower ½ sternum	Lower ½ sternum	Lower ½ sternum
Compress with	Two thumbs, encircling chest with hands	Two thumbs, encircling chest with hands	Heel of one hand
Depth	One third to one half of depth of chest for all listed ages		
Rate†	120/min @ 3 : 1	100/min 15 : 2	100/min @ 15 : 2
Ratio†	3 : 1 (interposed breath)	15 : 2 (interposed breaths)	15 : 2 (interposed breaths)
Foreign Body **Airway** **Obstruction**§	Back blows Chest thrusts	Back blows Chest thrusts	Abdominal thrust (Heimlich maneuver). Chest thrust or back blow is acceptable alternative.

*Also check for normal breathing, movement, or coughing. Laypeople do not check pulse.
†Total number of events: compressions plus breaths.
‡Ratios are for two-person CPR.
§Only if the obstruction is severe, such that the victim is unable to make a sound.
From Rothrock SG (ed): Pediatric Emergency Pocketbook, 5th ed. Lompac, CA: Tarascon Publishing Inc, 2007.

addresses the physiologic derangements common to multiple causes. Some etiologies, although uncommon, become apparent within the context of the evaluative process or "secondary survey" (e.g., hypothermia, hyperthermia, hyperkalemia).

Respiratory Failure—The Basics

The major advance in the emergency management of respiratory failure in children is the implementation by emergency physicians of rapid sequence intubation (RSI), the use of potent sedatives and muscle relaxants in a defined procedure that facilitates intubation while reducing complications of intubation such as aspiration. Children requiring resuscitation from cardiac arrest are not intubated with RSI, however, as this procedure is usually reserved for patients not in cardiac arrest (see Chapters 2, Respiratory Distress and Respiratory Failure; and Chapter 3, Rapid Sequence Intubation). Appropriate bag-valve-mask (BVM) ventilation, ETT placement, and maintenance of ETT position are important components of successful advanced resuscitation.

Why Is BVM Ventilation So Important in Children and Why Is It Recommended in Arrest from "Total Airway Obstruction"?

BVM ventilation is a proven technique. In emergencies, for providers who rarely encounter critically ill children, it may be as effective as endotracheal intubation as a short-term rescue/temporizing measure. In fact, some subsets of infants and children undergoing prehospital endotracheal intubation (e.g., those with head trauma) have a worse outcome compared to those receiving only BVM ventilation. Importantly, BVM ventilation also can be effective in children with airway obstruction. Efforts by the patient to alleviate airway obstruction can cause worsening of the obstruction (i.e., forced inspiration worsens obstruction as *negative* extrathoracic pressure is generated, collapsing the airway). A respiratory arrest occurs secondary to fatigue from increased work of breathing (note, *not* from total obstruction as the obstruction has both a fixed and a dynamic and reversible component in children). Application of *positive* pressure via BVM causes the opposite effect by stenting or relieving the dynamic component of obstruction. Hence, experts recommend BVM ventilation as a temporizing measure even if the patient arrests from obstruction. Case reports of successful resuscitation after respiratory arrest from epiglottitis have born this out.

BVM Size and Safety Features

For emergency airway management, a self-inflating BVM is preferred over an anesthesia ventilation bag. The BVM apparatus should have an oxygen reservoir so that a fraction of inspired oxygen of 90% to 95% is obtained when 10 to 15 L of oxygen is administered. The smallest bag that should be used is the 450-mL BVM device. Neonatal bags that are smaller (250 mL) do not provide effective tidal volume for small infants. Many BVM devices have a pop-off valve. The pop-off valve is usually set around 35 to 45 cm of water and is used to prevent barotrauma by providing a release of excessive pressure generated during BVM ventilation. Since a higher respiratory pressure is needed to ventilate a patient in some emergent airway situations, the bag should either have no pop-off valve or a valve that is easily adjusted or occluded. A new "old problem" occurs because of lack of familiarity by

staff with this safety feature. If the bag is stored with the valve unoccluded (i.e., as packaged from the manufacturer), it is common for staff to begin ventilating with the valve set in that position. As a result of the higher pressures required for initial ventilation, either because of increased lung compliance or poor positioning of the airway, oxygen escapes from the valve and is not delivered to the patient.[23] Critical time is lost until staff realize what is happening since the sensation of a leak from a poor seal of the mask over the face is lost as oxygen escapes from the valve. Another, even more dangerous possibility is the escape of oxygen from an unoccluded manometer port, as the resistance is much lower than 35 to 45 cm H_2O. Both possibilities can be prevented if providers perform a "leak test," similar to checking laryngoscope blade lights before intubation. This test is performed by compressing the bag with one hand while simultaneously occluding the patient connection port with other. If the pop-off valve, and other valves are in the occluded position, no air can be expressed and the bag remains full or tight, avoiding the pitfall of failure to deliver oxygen to the patient. A flow of at least 10 to 15 L/min of oxygen must be maintained into a reservoir attached to a pediatric bag, and at least 15 L/min must be supplied for an adult bag.

Many infants and children requiring mask ventilation will ultimately require endotracheal intubation, in many cases using RSI. Advanced airway techniques and maintenance of a controlled airway are described in Chapter 2 (Respiratory Distress and Respiratory Failure) and Chapter 3 (Rapid Sequence Intubation).

Achievement and Maintenance of Endotracheal Tube Position

Ideal placement of the ETT in the trachea is approximately midway between the vocal cords and the carina. A common occurrence when intubating a child is right mainstem intubation. Once correctly positioned, maintenance of the desired postintubation position is challenging in children. One method used to prevent mainstem intubation is to place one of the ETT insertion lines (near the distal tip of the tube) at the level of the cords during intubation. If the tube is maintained at that level, it will be positioned correctly. This placement, however, does not always occur in emergency intubations. Even if the tube is placed at one of the ETT distal insertion lines and it becomes dislodged during treatment, there is no simple method to detect this displacement or realign the tube at the insertion line without repeat laryngoscopy. Cole's formula for ETT size and depth, a more reliable method, is to insert the tube until the lip-to-tip distance is reached (a defined centimeter mark for each tube size), and secure the tube at that level. The lip-to-tip distance is approximately three times the internal diameter of the tube size in centimeters for a given patient. For example, the lip-to-tip distance for a 3.5-mm tube is approximately 10.5 cm. The actual distance is a range that can be obtained from reference materials. When a smaller size tube is used for a given patient—for example, in a patient with subglottic stenosis— the lip-to-tip distance for that tube would be the distance of the tube that would fit in a patient without the stenosis. That is, if a 3.0-mm tube is used instead of a 3.5-mm tube, which is the normally recommended tube for the patient, then the lip-to-tip distance would be still be 10.5, even though the patient is intubated with the smaller tube. A word of caution:

This formula may overestimate ETT depth in infants and children under age 2 by 0.5 to 1.0 cm.

Following intubation, two factors lead to ETT dislodgement. The first is the ease with which the tube slides in and out, since it is not anchored by an inflated cuff as in the adult, and the second is the movement of the tube within the trachea as a consequence of the large range of movement of the head and neck. Anesthesiologists have evaluated the average movement of the ETT with head movement in young infants. In 16- to 19-month-old infants, flexion of the neck by 30° to 45° causes insertion of the ETT 0.9 to 1.7 cm deeper into the trachea, while extension by 30° causes the tube to move out of the trachea by a mean 1 cm.[24] Others have found that head flexion in children weighing more than 10 kg produces a mean downward displacement of the ETT by 1 cm, and head extension produces a mean upward displacement of 1.4 cm.[25] As the trachea is short at this age, this amount of head or neck movement can lead to extubation or mainstem intubation (Fig. 1–3). To ensure the tube does not slide in and out, adequate securing of the tube at the mouth is required.

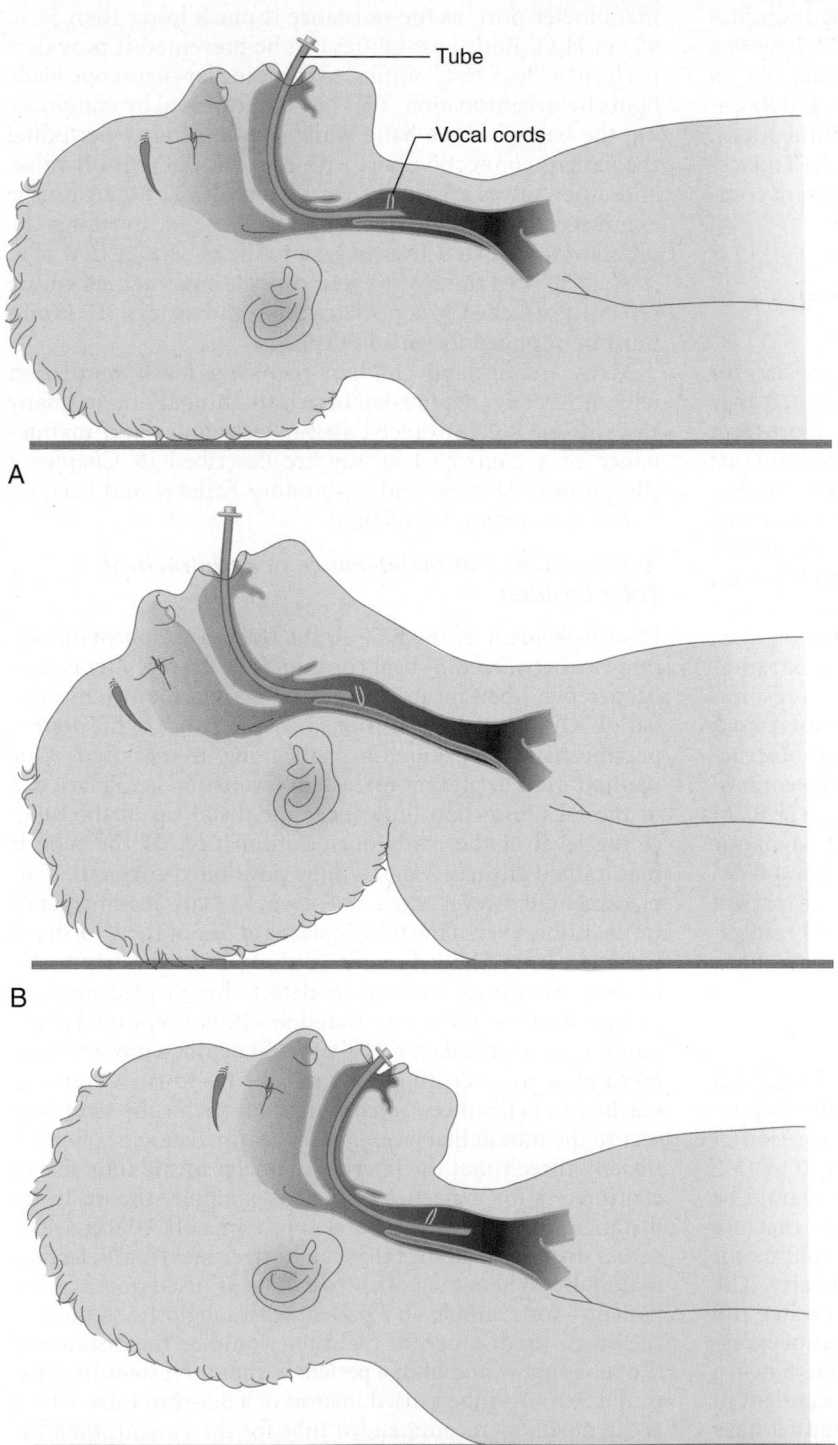

FIGURE 1–3. Position of endotracheal tube in normal position (A), with head and neck extended (B), and with head and neck flexed (C).

Inexperienced providers can apply commercial tube holders, which hold the tube adequately. Movement of the tube secondary to head and neck movement can be prevented by application of a cervical collar. Once the head and neck are immobilized, the most common complications of pediatric intubation (extubation and mainstem intubation) can be minimized.

Shock—The Basics

The recognition and treatment of shock has been identified as a pediatric resuscitation priority since the initial PALS effort.[26] Early studies identified adequate fluid resuscitation as a key to enhanced survival.[27] This concept, as well as aggressive intensive care management, has dramatically reduced mortality from septic shock.[28] The emergency physician's role is that of early recognition, initial aggressive management, and transfer to a higher level of care. Initial fluid and pressor therapy is guided by clinical determination of the type of shock and appropriate therapy. One of the misconceptions of pediatric care in general is that clinicians must be very cautious with fluids in children. In the setting of noncardiogenic shock, fluid needs are often great, especially in small children. A barrier to effective treatment is the tendency to "err on the side of less, rather than more" during fluid resuscitation. The patient in shock, hypovolemic and septic, may require repeated boluses totaling 100 to 200 mL/kg in the stabilization process (the total blood volume of a child is approximately 80 mL/kg).

The first steps in the resuscitative process for shock are simultaneous vascular access for the administration of an initial isotonic fluid bolus of 20 mL/kg and clinical evaluation to determine the cause of shock. Because fluid administration may be detrimental in cardiogenic shock, this condition must be excluded prior to initiation of large volumes. Cardiogenic shock can usually be ruled out most easily by the presence of a large liver on palpation, and to a lesser extent by the presence of rales in the lungs, and probably least often by the presence a murmur. A chest radiograph with normal lung fields and a normal-sized heart also makes cardiogenic shock unlikely. The second decision point comes when shock persists despite three to four boluses of isotonic fluid (Fig. 1–4). This state is sometimes referred to as "fluid-refractory" shock. This step is the clinical differentiation of septic versus hypovolemic shock, which determines which patients would benefit from pressor support in addition to aggressive fluid resuscitation (septic) and which patients require fluid (or blood) management alone (hypovolemic) (see Fig. 1–4). This differentiation becomes especially important when massive volumes of fluid are required to reverse a poorly perfused state. Importantly, the distinction between septic and hypovolemic is arbitrary in the sense that both can be considered hypovolemic, requiring large fluid volumes as part of the therapy. The term *hypovolemic* generally refers to the state of intravascular and interstitial fluid depletion usually resulting from fluid loss (e.g., diarrhea). The clinical signs associated with hypovolemic shock correlate with the severity of the interstitial fluid deficit, and permit a reliable clinical diagnosis. The term *septic* refers to the state of hypovolemia resulting from vascular permeability and fluid leakage, leading in many cases to interstitial hypervolemia manifested early on by warm skin and strong central pulses associated with intravascular depletion and late hypotension

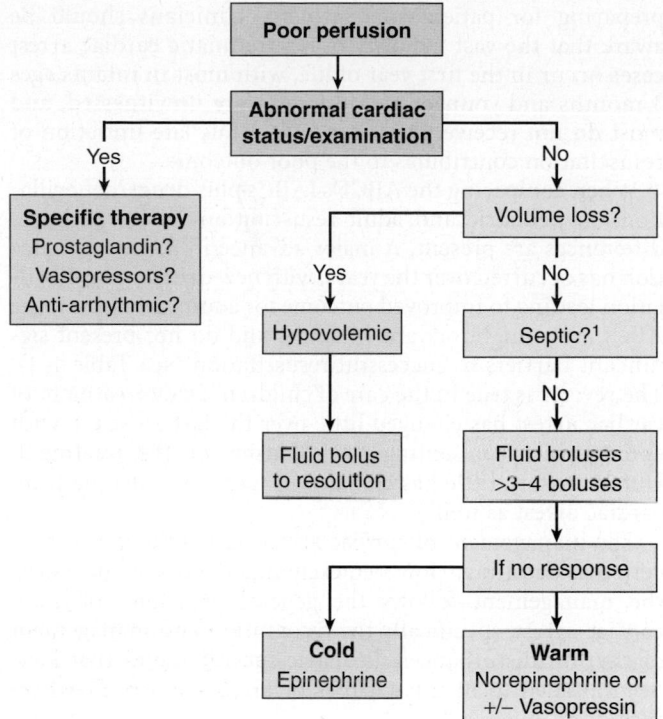

¹Administer empiric antibiotics and consider steroids.

FIGURE 1–4. Clinical differentiation of shock types and initial management.

and more obvious signs of shock. Anaphylactic shock and spinal cord injury also manifest features of early hyperdynamic shock as seen in early sepsis. (See Chapter 8, Circulatory Emergencies: Shock, for a more detailed review of shock.)

Vascular Access

Although central venous access is ideal during critical resuscitations, it is rarely feasible. Most resuscitations occur in the prehospital or ED environment where rapid peripheral access may be problematic, limiting the ultimate success of resuscitation. The intraosseus (IO) route provides a rapid, reliable, alternate method of gaining vascular access when peripheral access cannot be achieved rapidly. IO access can usually be rapidly achieved even in relatively inexperienced hands.[29] A new intraosseus innovation has the potential to make mastery of this technique even more certain.[30] The Bone Injection gun (BIG) IO device is a spring-loaded cylinder that, when activated, "injects" the IO needle into the bone at a predetermined adjustable level (see Chapter 161, Vascular Access). If time permits, central venous (e.g., femoral vein) access may be an appropriate alternative. Ultrasound guidance can improve speed of this technique and decrease complications related to central venous access.

ABCDs of Resuscitation from Cardiac Arrest in Children

The most common causes of pediatric cardiac arrest include sudden infant death syndrome (SIDS), trauma, submersion, cardiac disorders, and sepsis.[7] While knowledge of the specific precipitant resulting in cardiac arrest is important, attention to airway management and early CPR are vital to increasing the probability of ROSC regardless of cause. In preparing for patient management, clinicians should be aware that the vast majority of nontraumatic cardiac arrest cases occur in the first year of life, with most in infants ages 3 months and younger.[7,31] Most cases are unwitnessed, and most do not receive bystander CPR. Thus late initiation of resuscitation contributes to the poor outcome.[7]

When comparing the ABCDs (ABCs plus drugs/defibrillation) in pediatric and adult resuscitation, major practical differences are present. A major advance in adult resuscitation has occurred over the years, with new drugs and defibrillation leading to improved outcome for adults. Moreover, the ABCs are straightforward in adults and do not present significant barriers to successful resuscitation (see Table 1–1). The reverse is true in the care of children. Drug treatment of cardiac arrest has changed little over the last 25 years, with epinephrine representing the mainstay of the treatment. Unfortunately, little has changed in terms of outcome from cardiac arrest as well.

The management of cardiac arrest in a child can be perceived as daunting. However, excluding child-specific issues, the management follows the general principles of adult cardiac arrest, specifically the recognition and management of rhythm disturbances. Pediatric-specific issues that have been alluded to in this chapter or are discussed elsewhere include

- Eliminating age- and size-related issues, which can cause error, time delay, and confusion
- The rapid recognition and aggressive treatment of respiratory failure and shock (preventing cardiac arrest)
- The psychological overlay of dealing with a critically ill child

Once the ABCs have been addressed in critically ill or arrested patients, subsequent therapy (Ds) relates to the management of the cardiac rhythm. The goal of rhythm therapy is the achievement of adequate cardiac output (CO). Utilizing the formula CO = heart rate (HR) × stroke volume (SV) as a guide, one can see that rhythm disturbances that alter either HR or SV and thus affect CO must be changed, and this usually done with drugs. Rhythm disturbances can be classified as fast, slow, or absent (collapse) rhythms (Table 1–2). In an unstable patient, slow rhythms must be "sped up," and they are generally all treated the same way, regardless of specific rhythm. Fast rhythms need to be "slowed down," and in general, treatment in unstable patients consists of electrical cardioversion. Collapse rhythms must be converted to viable rhythms, and the treatment of these is specific, though not complicated. If perfusion remains poor in spite of rate normalization, a vasopressor may then be initiated.

For the purposes of resuscitation, rhythms in childhood cardiac arrest can be divided into shockable (ventricular fibrillation [VF] and ventricular tachycardia [VT]) and nonshockable (asystole and PEA) arrhythmias (Fig. 1–5). Asystole is by far the most common cardiac arrest rhythm noted in children, accounting for nearly two thirds of all cases.[3] In general, asystole outcome is dismal as this rhythm occurs late and rarely responds to interventions. PEA is the second most common pediatric arrest rhythm and is the initial rhythm found in nearly one quarter of out-of-hospital pediatric cardiac arrest cases.[3] PEA is defined as organized electrical activity on a cardiac monitor without pulses or any detectable cardiac output. Reversible causes of PEA include the 4 Hs (hypovolemia, hypoxia, hypothermia, hyperkalemia and other metabolic disoders), and the 4 Ts (tension pneumothorax, pericardial tamponade, thromboembolism and toxins).[32] Importantly, $ETCO_2$ and cardiac US can be used to identify a subset of patients with cardiac activity that is not evident on physical examination who may respond to fluids, acute intervention (pericardiocentesis, needle thoracotomy), or pressure support. Management consists of airway support, ventilation, chest compressions, and reversing any identifiable cause (see Fig. 1–5). Epinephrine is also recommended to increase cardiac activity, coronary perfusion, and diastolic blood pressure, which are associated with improved ROSC. The recommended dose of epinephrine is 0.01 mg/kg intravenously (IV) or IO or 0.1 mg/kg intratracheally repeated every 3 to 5 minutes. Earlier studies that evaluated escalating doses of epinephrine have not been supported by evidence of improved outcome and cannot be recommended. Importantly, above 8 years, adult PEA and asystole algorithms are recommended. The primary difference is the use of vasopressin (40 units IV), which may improve survival to hospital discharge compared to epinephrine for the subset of adult cardiac arrest patients with asystolic cardiac arrest.

Shockable rhythms (VF or pulseless VT) are present in nearly 10% of out of hospital pediatric cardiac arrest cases.[3] If cases of SIDS are excluded, this number may be as high as 19% to 24%.[33] These rhythms have the highest rate of neurologically intact survival of all arrest rhythms in children.[33] Ideally, patients with these rhythms are identified as early as possible and treated with immediate defibrillation at 2 joules/kg. If unsuccessful, they are defibrillated with another 2 to 4 joules/kg, then with 4 joules/kg. Either a monophasic or biphasic shock may be administered.[13] To achieve appropriate variable dose, a manual defibrillator or an automated external defibrillator (AED) that can recognize pediatric VT and VF and that is equipped with dose attenuation can be used

Table 1–2	Classification of Arrest/Prearrest Rhythms by Heart Rate				
Heart Rate	**Cardiac Output**	**HR × SV**	**Example**	**Rationale**	
Fast	↓	↓	SVT, VT	HR is too fast for diastolic filling of heart	
Slow	↓	Normal	Blocks and bradycardia	Self-explanatory	
Absent	↓	↓	PEA* and VFib	Self-explanatory	

*This classification is based on pulse rate, the absence of which gives the clinical diagnosis of pulseless electrical activity (PEA). PEA due to an ischemic, hypoxic myocardium or electromechanical disassociation (EMD) has no pulse and an almost universally poor prognosis. In a poorly perfused infant or child, pulses are difficult to palpate and the child's rhythm may not be truly pulseless. Cardiac activity with a low blood pressure may be present, with an improved prognosis mandating aggressive therapy compared to a patient who is truly in PEA.
Abbreviations: HR, heart rate; PEA, pulseless electrical activity; SV, stroke volume; SVT, supraventricular tachycardia; VFib, ventricular fibrillation; VT, ventricular tachycardia.

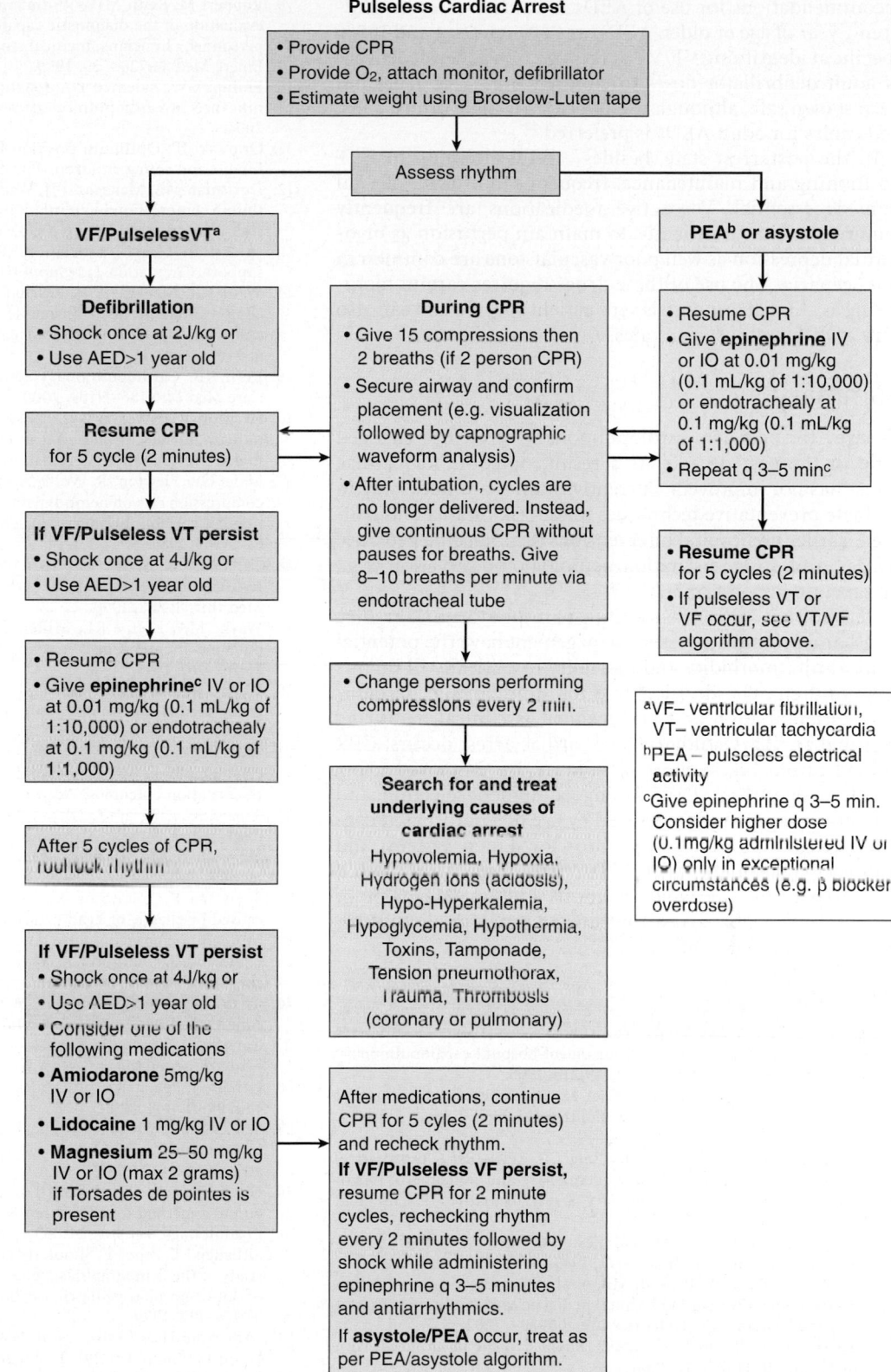

FIGURE 1–5. Pulseless cardiac arrest management.

in children 1 to 8 years old. Subsequently, ventilation and cardiac compressions are initiated and medications, including epinephrine and antiarrhythmics, are given. As for asystole and PEA, adult arrest protocols are recommended for children over 8 years old with VF/pulseless VT, the primary

difference being the use of vasopressin for these arrest rhythms instead of or in addition to epinephrine. Following drug administration, repeat defibrillation at 4 joules/kg is followed by CPR and further drug administration (see Fig. 1–5). Clinicians need to be aware of prehospital provider recommendations for use of AEDs in cardiac arrest in children 1 year of age or older. AEDs are 96% sensitive and 100% specific at identifying VF/VT at this age.[34] In general, delivery of adult defibrillator doses to children over 1 year old has been shown safe, although use of pediatric algorithms, pads, and cables for adult AEDs is preferred.[33]

In the postarrest state, besides careful attention to ETT positioning and maintenance, frequent monitoring of vital signs is essential. Vasoactive medications are frequently required, at least transiently, to maintain perfusion as myocardial depression as well poor vascular tone are common in this scenario. The use of these drugs requires careful monitoring as clinical response is very patient specific and can also vary at different infusion rates.

Summary

Therapy for pediatric cardiopulmonary arrest has changed little in the past decade. As a result, outcome for cardiac arrest has not improved. Currently, studies are underway to evaluate preventative techniques for at-risk infants and children, earlier prehospital interventions (e.g., specific pediatric AEDs), and postresuscitation neurologic preservation (e.g., therapeutic hypothermia).

Recognition of disorders leading to respiratory and cardiac arrest and prompt aggressive management have the potential to minimize morbidity and mortality in critically ill infants and children. The decision tree for simultaneous recognition, differentiation and management is clinical, requiring minimal ancillary studies. Once cardiac arrest occurs, CPR and advanced life support techniques are employed using standard algorithms. Drug dosing, equipment selection, and patient management is enhanced by use of length-based cognitive resuscitation aids (e.g., Broselow-Luten system) and printed management guides. Newer techniques of US and ETCO$_2$ may aid in rapid diagnosis and management of patients with viable arrest rhythms and may predict return of spontaneous circulation.

REFERENCES

1. Ronco R, King W, Donley DK, et al: Outcome and cost at a children's hospital following resuscitation for out-of-hospital cardiopulmonary arrest. Arch Pediatr Adolesc Med 149:210, 1995.
2. Schindler MB, Bohn D, Cox PN, et al: Outcome of out-of-hospital cardiac or respiratory arrest in children. N Engl J Med 335:1473, 1996.
3. Young KD, Gasuche-Hill M, McClung CD, Lewis RJ: A prospective, population based study of the epidemiology and outcome of out of hospital pediatric cardiopulmonary arrest. Pediatrics 114:157–164, 2004.
4. Gills J, Dickson D, Rieder M, et al: Results of inpatient pediatric resuscitation. Crit Care Med 14:469–471, 1986.
5. Reis AG, Nadkarni V, Perondi MB, et al: A prospective investigation into the epidemiology of in hospital pediatric cardiopulmonary arrest using the Utstein style. Pediatrics 109:200–209, 2002.
6. Zarirsky A, Nadkarni V, Getson P, Kuehl K: CPR in children. Ann Emerg Med 16:1107–1111, 1998.
*7. Young KD, Seidel JS: Pediatric cardiopulmonary resuscitation: a collective review. Ann Emerg Med 33:195, 1999.
*8. Luten R, Wears R, Broselow J, et al: Managing the unique size related issues of pediatric resuscitation: reducing cognitive load with resuscitation aids. Acad Emerg Med 9:840–847, 2002.
9. Ruppert M, Reith MW, Widmann JH, et al: Checking for breathing: evaluation of the diagnostic capability of emergency medical services personnel, physicians, medical students, and medical laypersons. Ann Emerg Med 34:720–729, 1999.
10. Phillips GW, Zideman DA: Relationship of infant to sternum: its significance in cardiopulmonary resuscitation. Pediatrics 114:157–164, 2004.
11. Orlowski JP: Optimum position for external cardiac compression in infants and young children. Ann Emerg Med 15:667–673, 1986.
12. Dorfsman ML, Menegazzi JJ, Wadas RJ, Auble TE: Two finger vs. two thumb compression in an infant model of prolonged cardiopulmonary resuscitation. Acad Emerg Med 7:1077–1082, 2000.
*13. American Heart Association: Pediatric basic and advanced life support. Circulation 112(Suppl III):III-73–III-90, 2005.
14. Ward KR, Menegazzi JJ, Zelenak RR, et al: A comparison of chest compressions between mechanical and manual CPR by monitoring end-tidal CO$_2$ during human cardiac arrest. Ann Emerg Med 22:669–674, 1993.
15. Kern KB: Cardiopulmonary resuscitation without ventilation. Crit Care Med 28:N186–N189, 2000.
16. Swenson RD, Weaver WD, Niskanen RA, et al: Hemodynamics in humans during conventional and experimental methods of cardiopulmonary resuscitation. Circulation 78:630–639, 1988.
17. Maier GW, Newton JR, Wolfe JA, et al: The influence of manual cardiac compression rate on hemodynamic support during cardiac arrest: high impulse cardiopulmonary resuscitation. Circulation 74(Suppl IV):IV-51–IV-59, 1986.
18. Callaham M, Barton C: Prediction of outcome of cardiopulmonary resuscitation from end-tidal carbon dioxide concentration. Crit Care Med 18:358–362, 1990.
19. Wayne MA, Levine RL, Miller CC: Use of end tidal CO$_2$ to predict outcome in prehospital cardiopulmonary arrest. Ann Emerg Med 25:762–767, 1995.
20. Ward KR, Yealy DM: End tidal carbon dioxide monitoring in emergency medicine: clinical applications. Acad Emerg Med 5:637–646, 1998.
21. Salen PO, O'Connor R, Sierzenski P, et al: Can cardiac sonography and capnography be used independently and in combination to predict resuscitation outcomes? Acad Emerg Med 8:610–615, 2001.
22. Amaya SC, Langsam A: Ultrasound detection of ventricular fibrillation disguised as asystole. Ann Emerg Med 33:344–346, 1999.
23. Hirschman AM, Krauath RE: Venting vs. ventilating: a danger of manual resuscitation. Chest 82:369–370, 1982.
24. Sugiyama K, Yokoyama K: Displacement of the endotracheal tube caused by change of head position in pediatric anesthesia: evaluation by fiberoptic bronchoscopy. Anesth Analg 82:251–253, 1996.
25. Olufolabi AJ, Charlton GA, Spargo PM: Effect of head posture on tracheal tube position in children. Anaesthesia 59:1069–1072, 2004.
26. Chameides L (ed): Textbook of Pediatric Life Support. Dallas, TX: American Heart Association, 1987.
27. Carcillo JA, Davis AL, Zaritsky A: Role of early fluid resuscitation in pediatric septic shock. JAMA 266:1242–1245, 1991.
28. Carcillo J: Pediatric septic shock and multiple organ failure. Crit Care Clin 19:413–440, 2003.
29. Seigler RS, Tecklenburg F, Shealy R: Prehospital intraosseus infusions by emergency medical services personnnel: a prospective study. Pediatrics 84:173–177, 1989.
30. Olsen D, Packer BE, Perrett J, et al: Evaluation of the bone injection gun as a method for intraosseous cannula placement for fluid therapy in adult dogs. Vet Surg 31:533–540, 2002.
31. Sirbaugh PE, Pepe PE, Shook JE, et al: A prospective, population-based study of the demographics, epidemiology, management, and outcome of out-of-hospital pediatric cardiopulmonary arrest. Ann Emerg Med 33:174–184, 1999.
*32. American Heart Association: Pediatric advanced life support. Circulation 102(Suppl I):I-291–I-342, 2000.
33. Samson RA, Berg RA, Bingham R, et al: Use of automated external defibrillators for children: an update. An advisory statement from the Pediatric Advanced Life Support Task Force, International Liaison Committee on Resuscitation. Circulation 107:3250–3255, 2003.
34. Ceechin F, Jorgenson JB, Berul CI, et al: Is arrhythmia detection by automatic external defibrillator accurate for children? Sensitivity and specificity of an automatic external defibrillator algorithm in 696 pediatric arrhythmias. Circulation 103:2483–2488, 2001.

*Selected readings.

Chapter 2

Respiratory Distress and Respiratory Failure

Patricia S. Padlipsky, MD and Marianne Gausche-Hill, MD

Key Points

Pediatric airway differences are most pronounced in infants. By 8 years of age the pediatric airway is anatomically like the adult airway.

Respiratory distress is a state of increased work of breathing, whereas respiratory failure is a state of inadequate oxygenation or ventilation. Respiratory failure may or may not be preceded by respiratory distress.

Assessment of the respiratory status of an infant or child begins with the Pediatric Assessment Triangle. A rapid general impression directs immediate airway management.

Infants and children have unique clinical scenarios and conditions that may lead to a difficult airway.

Introduction and Background

Respiratory problems or complaints are one of the most common reasons for infants and children seeking medical care in an emergency department (ED). Children represent about 10% of all prehospital care transports, and of these about 10% are due to respiratory complaints.[1-3] In the ED, respiratory complaints account for approximately 10% to 20% of the pediatric visits.[4] Respiratory compromise is the leading cause of death in children less than 1 year of age. Children often go through a period of respiratory distress prior to respiratory failure, but respiratory failure may exist without signs of respiratory distress. The survival of children from cardiopulmonary arrest (9%) is dismal compared to those in respiratory failure alone (80%); therefore, it is imperative that the emergency physician anticipate and recognize early signs and symptoms of respiratory failure and intervene quickly to prevent further deterioration to cardiopulmonary failure/arrest.[5,6]

Recognition and Approach

There are anatomic, physiologic, and behavioral differences between the adult and pediatric airway that affect the risk of airway obstruction, the risk of the development of respiratory compromise, and the approach to management. The transition from neonatal to adult airway anatomy is completed by 8 to 10 years of age. By this time the airway is similar to that of the adult, only smaller. Anatomic, physiologic, and behavioral differences with their impact on patient care are summarized in Table 2-1.

Anatomic Differences

Neonates (defined as < 1 month of age) have large heads in relation to their body size. The relatively large occiput can result in natural flexion of the neck when lying supine, which can lead to airway obstruction. A towel roll placed under the infant's shoulders will elevate the patient's torso and result in a neutral position (Fig. 2–1). The neonate's chest muscles are not well developed, and the diaphragm and abdominal muscles are the main muscles of respiration. Abdominal breathing is normal in infants, but it often becomes exaggerated and faster as the infant has increasing respiratory difficulty. With increasing respiratory distress, the abdominal muscles may become fatigued, leading to seesawing respirations that may precede respiratory failure. Also, factors that impede diaphragmatic excursion, such as a distended gastric air bubble, severe pneumoperitoneum, or ascites, can also result in respiratory failure.

The differences in anatomy of the upper airway in infants and children versus adults result in increased susceptibility to respiratory distress and failure. For example, children have a relatively *larger volume of tongue* intraorally, which can lead to airway obstruction especially if there is loss of muscle tone and the tongue relaxes in a posterior position, obstructing the upper airway. This obstruction can be overcome by making sure that the head is repositioned to the midline and in the sniffing position. If necessary, an airway adjunct (oropharyngeal or nasopharyngeal) can be inserted. The *narrow upper airway* passage can also be obstructed by a foreign body or an infection that may cause inflammation and excess secretions. The *large mass of tonsilar and adenoidal tissue* can result in trauma to these tissues during nasotracheal

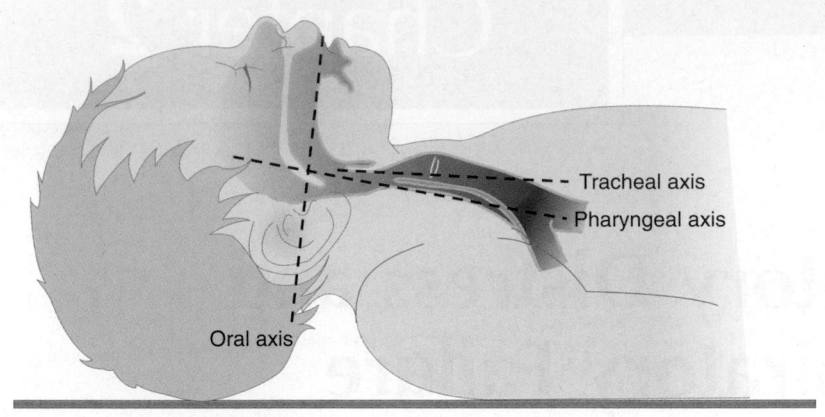

A

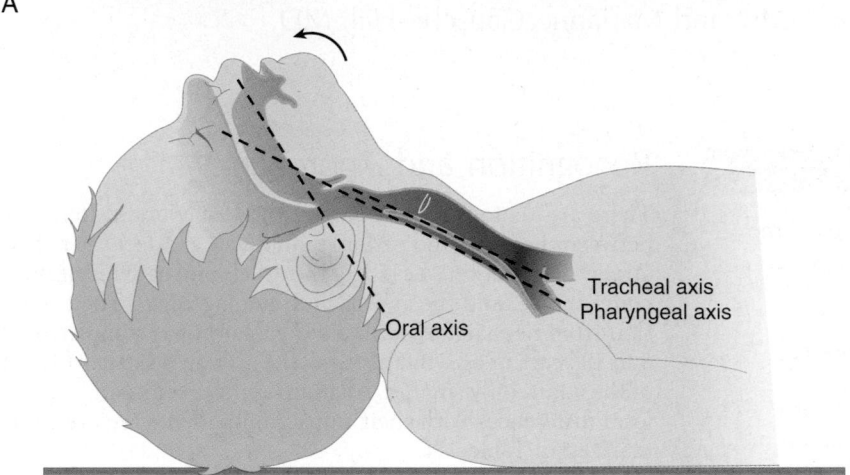

B

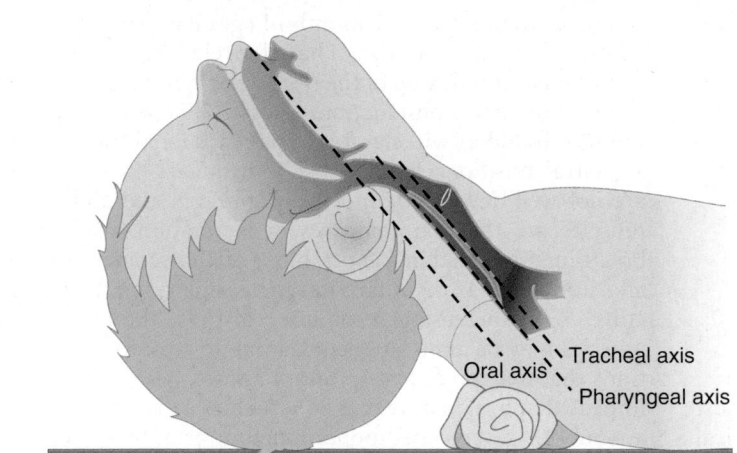

C

FIGURE 2–1. Alignment of the tracheal, pharyngeal, and oral axes. **A,** Alignment of airway axes with neck flexion. **B,** Alignment of airway axes with head extension and neck flexion—the "sniffing position." **C,** Alignment of airway axes in supine position. (From Hazinski MF [ed]: PALS Provider Manual. Dallas: American Heart Association, 2002, p 95.)

intubation or nasopharyngeal airway placement. Therefore, emergency nasotracheal intubation is rarely performed in infants and children, and caution must be exercised in placing a nasopharyngeal airway in an infant.

Other airway differences that can result in additional challenges to successful endotracheal intubation include the following: 1) the pediatric *epiglottis is floppy, soft, and omega or U-shaped* as compared to the adult epiglottis, and 2) the *larynx is higher and more cephalad* (the glottis is located at C3-4 in the newborn, at C4-5 by 2 years of age, and at C5-6

for an adult) (Fig. 2–2). Use of a Miller or Wis-Hipple laryngoscope blade is often helpful in these situations. A straight laryngoscope blade is used in young children during laryngoscopy because of the acute epiglottic angle and shallow vallecula (Fig. 2–3). The straight blade is recommended for use until approximately 3 to 5 years of age but may be used in any age child or adolescent. Also, placing a towel under the patient's shoulders until age 2 years and under the head in older children (with head in the sniffing position) will help align the tracheal, pharyngeal, and oral axes, facilitating

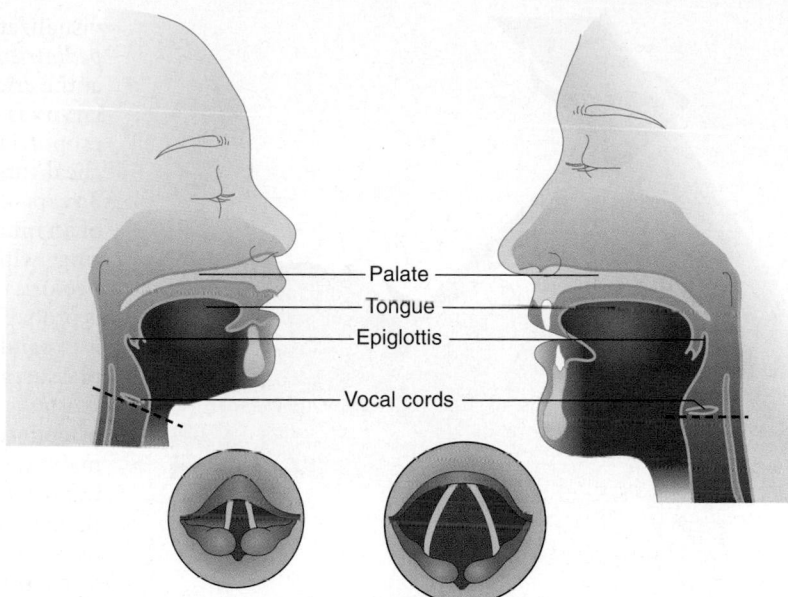

Palate
Tongue
Epiglottis
Vocal cords

FIGURE 2–2. Comparison of adult and pediatric airway structures. (Modified from Riazzi J: The difficult pediatric airway. *In* Benumof JL [ed]: Airway Management: Principles and Practice. St. Louis: Mosby Year Book, 1996, p 587.)

Table 2–1	Anatomic and Physiologic Airway Differences between Children and Adults That Impact Emergency Airway Management	
	Impact	**Action**
Anatomic Differences		
Large occiput	Flexion of the neck with possible airway obstruction	Reposition head, towel under shoulders
Large tongue	Airway obstruction, especially with loss of muscle tone	Reposition head, sniffing position, towel under shoulders, airway adjuncts
Larger adenoids and tonsils	May obstruct airway, hemorrhage into the airway if injured	Caution with use of nasopharyngeal airway; reposition head
Floppy and long epiglottis	Visualization of vocal cords difficult	Use straight blade to intubate
Larynx cephalad and anterior	Vocal cords more difficult to visualize	Positioning and use of straight blade
Narrowest portion of larynx at the cricoid ring	Use of cuffed tubes may cause pressure damage to cartilage	Use uncuffed tubes until about 8 years of age or, if cuffed tube used, do not overinflate cuff
Narrower tracheal diameter, shorter distance between rings	Needle cricothyrotomy preferred surgical airway in infants and small children	Consider needle cricothyrotomy if cannot bag-mask ventilate, intubate, or use LMA
Shorter tracheal length	Intubation of the right mainstem; dislodgement	Use length-based resuscitation tape for ETT size and depth of ETT placement, or estimate by 3 times the ETT size; reassess frequently
Narrower airway	Greater airway resistance	Suction liberally; remove foreign material; use bronchodilators for lower airway obstruction
Fewer alveoli	Increase respiratory rate to increase minute ventilation	Provide supplemental oxygen; assist ventilation when respiratory rates too slow
Underdeveloped chest and abdominal muscles	Easy fatigability, increased abdominal breathing, increased respiratory rate	Early oxygen with signs/symptoms of respiratory distress, bag-mask ventilation with poor tidal volume or respiratory failure
Physiologic Differences		
Preferential nose breathers	Mucus or blood may obstruct nares, causing respiratory distress	Suction nares liberally
Increased metabolism and reduced FRC*	Shortened period of protection from hypoxia	Oxygenate; bag-mask ventilation and cricoid pressure may be necessary prior to intubation
Immature immune system	At greater risk for respiratory infections	Assess for infections with fever or signs of respiratory illness
Behavioral Differences		
Inability to verbalize distress or pain	Practitioner must rely on signs based on developmental milestones	Recognize signs of respiratory distress and failure

*Functional residual capacity is the lung volume at the end of a normal expiration, when the muscles of respiration are completely relaxed; at FRC, *and at FRC only,* the tendency of the lungs to collapse is exactly balanced by the tendency of the chest wall to expand (see Johns Hopkins School of Medicine Interactive Respiratory Physiology website at *http://oac.med.jhmi.edu/res_phys/Dictionary.html*).
Abbreviations: ETT, endotracheal tube; LMA, laryngeal mask airway.

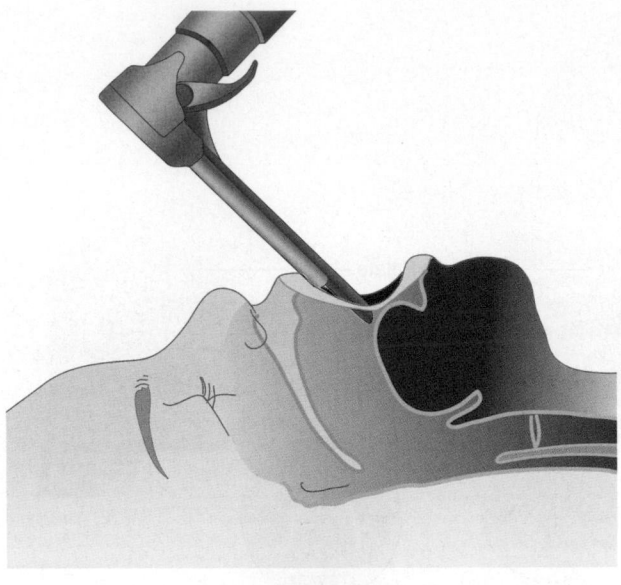

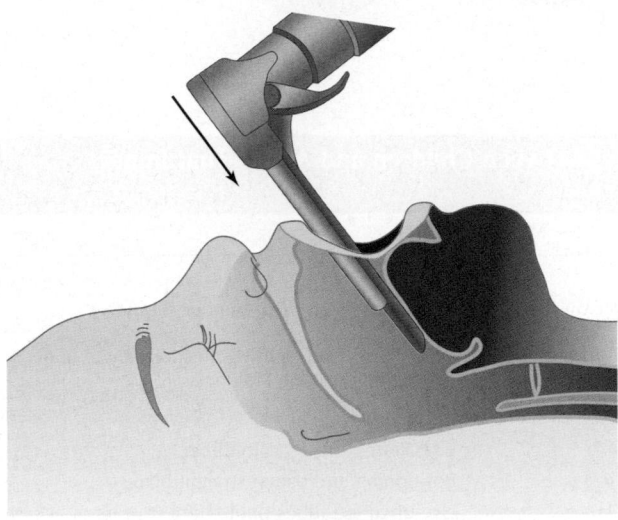

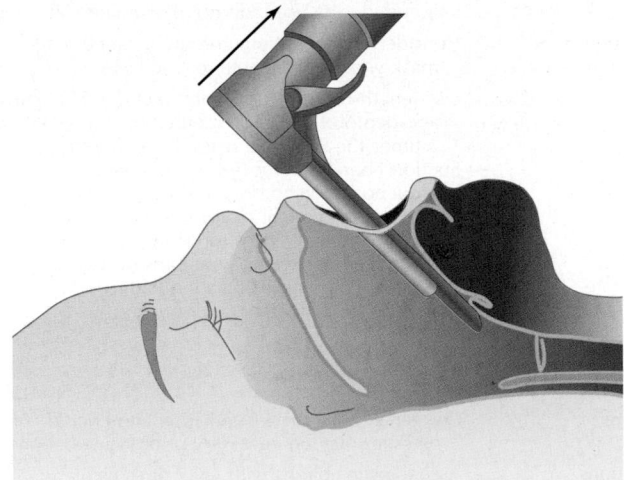

FIGURE 2–3. Proper use of and blade position for laryngoscope. (Modified from Gausche-Hill M, Henderson DP, Goodrich SM, et al [eds]: Pediatric Airway Management for the Prehospital Professional. Sudbury, MA: Jones & Bartlett, 2004, p 84.)

visualization of the glottis with intubation (Fig. 2–1). *The pediatric larynx is funnel shaped,* with the narrowest portion at the cricoid ring (below the vocal cords), whereas the adult larynx is cylinder shaped, with the glottis being the narrowest portion. Therefore, uncuffed rather than cuffed endotracheal tubes (ETTs) are often used in children younger than 8 years of age or until a size 6.0-mm ETT is needed. The use of an inflated cuff on the ETT can put pressure on the cricoid ring, which may limit blood supply and lead to pressure necrosis of the cartilage. This complication of cuffed tube use is probably less important than once believed, and now there is expanded use of cuffed ETTs in children who require high pressures to ventilate (e.g., asthma, submersion injury). The *shorter tracheal length* predisposes the child to complications of endotracheal intubation such as intubation of the right maintain bronchus or ETT dislodgement. Therefore, it is important to know how to estimate depth of placement of the ETT (three times the interior diameter of the ETT or by use of the Broselow tape), to check placement by auscultation or capnography, and to reassess the patient's clinical status frequently. The *narrower trachea and shorter distance between tracheal rings,* as well as the short neck and increased subcutaneous tissue in infants and young children, result in greater difficulty in locating anatomic landmarks to perform surgical cricothyrotomy and in increased likelihood of severe complications such creation of a false tract, pneumomediastinum, infection, or bleeding. Needle cricothyrotomy is recommended in these infants and children if an immediate surgical airway is needed.

Differences between the adult and pediatric airway are also seen in the lower airways and in the lung. The *large airways of the pediatric patient are narrower* than those of an adult. This leads to greater susceptibility to obstruction by mucus, edema or foreign bodies, which then leads to greater airway resistance. This is explained by looking at Poiseuille's law, which states that resistance to flow (R) is inversely proportional to the fourth power of the radius (r) of the lumen ($R = 1/r^4$). Therefore, if the radius is halved, the resistance increases by 16-fold. This is especially true for children with a tracheostomy because insertion of the tracheostomy tube narrows the airway opening further. Therefore, the tracheostomy lumen can easily become blocked by secretions.[7] It is important to suction all patients liberally, particularly if they are producing large amounts of secretions. In the lung, *infants and children have less alveoli* than adults. Several studies have shown that neonates have only one third to one half of the number of alveoli in the adult human lung. The number of alveoli reaches adult values by age 8.[8,9] The fewer number of alveoli results in decreased area for gas exchange. Because they do not have extra alveoli for recruitment, young children increase their respiratory rate to increase minute ventilation and oxygenation, and to eliminate carbon dioxide, making tachypnea a hallmark sign of respiratory distress. This is more pronounced in children with lung disease (e.g., reactive airway disease, bronchopulmonary dysplasia). Early intervention with supplemental oxygen and bronchodilators and support of ventilation with a bag-mask device may prevent progression of the clinical status to respiratory failure.

Physiologic Differences

It has been demonstrated that neonates and infants (1 month to 1 year) may be *preferential nose breathers,*[10] thus making them susceptible to nasal obstruction (choanal atresia, mucus, blood). Miller and colleagues[11] noted that 8% of infants at 30 to 32 weeks' postconceptual age and 78% of term infants were capable of oral breathing in response to nasal occlusion. The ability to tolerate complete nasal occlusion occurs in most infants by 5 months of age. Therefore, if a neonate or infant is having any respiratory difficulty, it is important to suction out both nares to relieve any obstruction.

Children have a *basal oxygen consumption rate two to three times that of adults*.[12,13] Adults consume 2 to 3 mL of oxygen per kilogram per minute under normal basal conditions. Infants and young children metabolize 4 to 9 mL of oxygen per kilogram per minute.[12,13] Infants and young children also have a diminished functional residual capacity as compared to adults. This is quite significant because it means that, during apnea, children will maintain "normal" oxygenation for less than half the time of an adult; in other words, children will experience desaturation with shorter times of apnea. Therefore, it is important to supply oxygen to all children showing any signs of respiratory distress. It is also probable that bag-mask ventilation may be required to maintain "normal" oxygenation during periods of apnea prior to intubation.[14]

Behavioral/Developmental Issues

Infants and young children are not able to communicate like an older child or an adult. They cannot tell you how they feel or verbalize that they are short of breath or in pain. Therefore, attainment of knowledge of normal behavioral milestones is imperative so that an alteration of these behaviors may be recognized and signs of respiratory failure managed promptly.

Evaluation

Evaluation of a child in respiratory distress must begin with understanding of physiologic states of respiratory compromise and characterization of the anatomic site of that compromise.

Respiratory distress: A condition characterized by increased work of breathing. It is often associated with increase in respiratory rate, but in later stages rates may fall and be less than normal. Signs of airway obstruction such as change in body positioning, nasal flaring, grunting, retractions, stridor, or wheezing may be present. Nonspecific signs of anxiety, restlessness, and irritability with any of the previous signs may be seen and can indicate the need for immediate intervention to avoid the progression to respiratory failure.

Respiratory failure: A condition in which the compensatory mechanisms are no longer able to maintain adequate oxygenation or ventilation. Respiratory failure is characterized by poor appearance, including decrease in muscle tone, poor interactiveness, "glassy-eyed" stare and inability to focus, and weak or absent speech or cry. Changes in skin color may occur and vary from pale to cyanotic.

Respiratory arrest: A condition characterized by absence of respiratory effort (prolonged apnea).

Upper airway obstruction: Obstruction of the flow of air/oxygen from the oropharynx to the carina of the trachea.

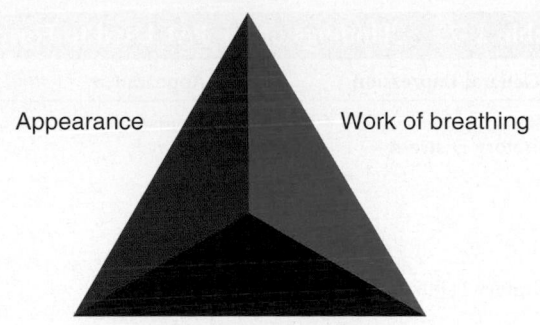

FIGURE 2–4. Pediatric Assessment Triangle. (From Gausche-Hill M, Henderson DP, Goodrich SM, et al [eds]: Pediatric Airway Management for the Prehospital Professional. Sudbury, MA: Jones & Bartlett, 2004, p 15.)

Lower airway obstruction: Obstruction of flow of air/oxygen within the bronchi and/or bronchioles from distal to the mainstem bronchi to the aveoli.

Diseases of the lung: Inflammation, infection, or scarring of the aveoli or interstitium of the lung.

Assessment

Any child with respiratory complaints, or any child about whom the parent expresses concerns regarding respiratory status, however mild, requires a rapid and thorough evaluation. The initial overall evaluation should contain two parts: the Pediatric Assessment Triangle (PAT), which is used to obtain an immediate general impression of the seriousness of the illness or injury, and the initial physical assessment. Based on these assessment steps, the examiners, within seconds, will have a general impression of how ill the child is and whether they need to intervene with treatment immediately or if they can continue further evaluation with the focused history and physical examination.[14,15]

The PAT offers an orderly approach that can be used to assess children of all ages. It allows one to gather visual and auditory clues without touching the child. This "hands-off" assessment can allow the examiner to gather critical information from a distance without upsetting the child with an invasive physical examination.[14] The PAT focuses on general appearance, work of breathing, and the circulatory status of the patient (Fig. 2–4).

General Appearance

How a child appears to an examiner demonstrates in part the adequacy of ventilation, oxygenation, brain perfusion, body homeostasis, and central nervous system function. The components of the assessment of the general appearance are summarized in the TICLS (pronounced "tickles") mnemonic: **t**one, **i**nteractiveness, **c**onsolability, **l**ook/gaze, and **s**peech/cry.[14]

These five characteristics (TICLS) offer a quick way to assess a patient's general appearance. If the patient's appearance seems normal, then it is likely that oxygenation, ventilation, and brain perfusion are at least adequate. However, if a child's general appearance is grossly abnormal, immediate efforts must be made to assess and treat abnormalities in oxygenation, ventilation, and perfusion while completing the initial assessment. There is still the potential for serious illness, so frequent reassessment is mandatory (Table 2–2).

Table 2–2	Findings of the PAT Used to Form a General Impression of the Physiologic State		
PAT General Impression	**Appearance**	**Work of Breathing**	**Circulation to the Skin**
Stable	Normal	Normal	Normal
Respiratory Distress	Normal	Abnormal Nasal flaring Grunting Stridor Wheezing Retractions	Normal
Respiratory Failure	Abnormal Poor tone Combative Listless Lethargic	Abnormal Grunting Stridor Retractions Tachypnea Bradypnea Apnea	Normal/abnormal* Pale Cyanotic
Shock	Normal/abnormal* Poor tone Listless Lethargic	Normal	Abnormal Pale Mottled
CNS/Metabolic Disorder	Abnormal Poor tone, interactiveness Inconsolability Abnormal speech or cry	Normal	Normal
Cardiopulmonary Failure	Abnormal Unresponsive	Abnormal Apneic	Abnormal Cyanotic

*In early stages will be normal and later progresses to abnormal.

Work of Breathing

Work of breathing reflects the child's attempt to compensate for abnormalities in oxygenation and ventilation. Assessing work of breathing requires looking for signs of increased work of breathing and listening for abnormal airway sounds.

VISUAL SIGNS

Abnormal positioning, respiratory rate, retractions, head bobbing and nasal flaring, are all visual signs that indicate increased work of breathing in an effort to improve oxygenation and ventilation. A few postures indicate compensatory efforts to increase airflow. A child who is in the "sniffing" position (child sits leaning forward) is trying to open up his or her airway and increase airflow. It is usually a result of severe upper airway obstruction (retropharyngeal abscess, foreign body, epiglottitis). A child who refuses to lie down or who leans forward on outstretched arms (tripod position) is attempting to use accessory muscles to improve breathing (severe bronchoconstriction; asthma, bronchiolitis).

Respiratory rate changes with sleep and wake states, and normal rates vary with age. The goal of the PAT assessment of respiratory rate is to determine if the rate is slow, fast, or absent.

Retractions are a common physical sign of increased work of breathing. They represent the use of accessory muscles to help breathing. **Retractions can be easily missed unless they are looked for with the child undressed.** They can occur in the supraclavicular area, intercostal area, and substernal area. When a child is approaching respiratory failure, retractions can decrease. This is an ominous sign and occurs when a child has exhausted compensatory mechanisms.

Head bobbing is the use of accessory neck muscles in infants to increase inspiratory pressure and improve breathing. The child extends the neck while inhaling, then the head falls forward during exhalation. This visual sign suggests moderate to severe hypoxia.

Nasal flaring is the exaggerated opening of the nostrils during labored breathing and indicates another form of accessory muscle use that reflects significant increase in the work of breathing.

AUDIBLE AIRWAY SOUNDS

Abnormal airway sounds provide information about breathing effort and anatomic location of airway obstruction. Normally, the movement of air in and out of the airway cannot be heard without a stethoscope. Airway sounds that can be heard without the use of a stethoscope are abnormal and indicate obstruction to the passage of air through the airway structures. The type of abnormal airway sound is related to the location of the disease process. Table 2–3 lists abnormal airway sounds and their location, causes, and possible interventions.[15]

Circulatory Status

The third part of the PAT is a rapid evaluation of the circulatory system to determine the adequacy of cardiac output and perfusion of vital organs. The most important part of this assessment is to observe the skin. When there is inadequate blood volume or when the heart is unable to maintain output to the body, blood supply to vital organs is conserved by shunting blood away from less essential areas of the body such as the skin and mucous membranes, resulting in mottling, pallor, and/or cyanosis. Patients in respiratory failure may also show changes in skin color. Pallor is seen in early stages and cyanosis in late stages.

Using the PAT gives the clinician a rapid overall impression of whether the child's illness or injury is severe and life threatening before a more thorough hands-on evaluation is done.

Table 2–3	Abnormal Airway Sounds: Possible Causes and Immediate Management			
Airway Sound	**Description**	**Location**	**Causes**	**Immediate Management**
Gurgling	Heard without a stethoscope; gurgling or bubbling	Posterior pharynx Upper airway	Inability to clear secretions or excessive fluid in upper airway	Provide oxygen; suctioning
Snoring	Heard without a stethoscope; low-pitched nasal sound	Upper airway	Oropharynx partically obstructed by tongue or soft tissues (adenoids, tonsils)	Head positioning; airway adjuncts
Muffled Speech	Heard without a stethoscope; "hot potato" voice	Upper airway	Peritonsilar abscess; epiglottitis	Head positioning; support ventilation as needed
Hoarse Speech	Heard without a stethoscope; raspy voice with changes in volume and pitch	Upper airway	Glottic inflammation from URI; croup, nodules, GE reflux	No immediate treatment needed. Specific treatment dependent on cause
Stridor	High-pitched sound usually heard during inspiration; may also be heard on expiration	Upper airway	Air passing through narrowed laryngeal or subglottic areas; foreign body, obstruction, croup, epiglottitis, allergic reaction	Allow patient to stay in position of comfort; provide oxygen. Support ventilation if in respiratory failure or severe distress. Specific treatment dependent on cause.
Rhonchi	Low-pitched musical, rough, rattling sounds	Upper airway; mainstem bronchus	Secretions, fluids, or narrowing in the large airways	Provide oxygen; suctioning. Observe for adequate oxygenation and ventilation. Bronchodilator
Grunting	Brief, vocalization on expiration against a partially closed glottis. Low-pitched sound.	Upper or lower airway	Produces positive end-expiratory pressure (PEEP) to keep alveoli open; pneumonia, pulmonary contusion, pulmonary edema	Usually indicative of moderate to severe hypoxia. Provide oxygen. Support ventilation as needed.
Wheezing	Whistling, musical sound usually present on expiration but may also be present on inspiration	Lower airway; bronchioles; alveoli	Partially obstructed lower airway; edema, secretions, spasm. Asthma most common cause, infection, reactive airway disease, pneumonia, allergic reaction	Provide oxygen. Bronchodilator with MDI or by nebulization. Steroids. Support of ventilation as needed.
Rales (Crackles)	Fine, high-pitched crackling sounds heard mid to late inspiration	Alveoli	Fluid or mucus in air sacs. Pneumonia most common cause; also pneumonitis.	Provide oxygen. Observe for adequate oxygenation and ventilation
Absence of Breath Sounds	No sound on auscultation	Severe partial or complete airway obstruction; severe lung disease	Obstructed airway due to foreign body or airway disease	Provide oxygen. Foreign body removal maneuvers. Trial of bronchodilator. Support of ventilation as needed.

Abbreviations: GE, gastroesophageal; MDI, metered-dose inhaler; URI, upper respiratory infection.

A child, who is alert and anxious, is breathing rapidly, and has retractions and normal skin color is a child in respiratory distress. If this child's appearance becomes abnormal (i.e., listless, lethargic), then the child's condition has deteriorated to respiratory failure. The PAT helps to determine how rapidly intervention is needed and what treatments may be needed immediately. For example, a child with respiratory failure or cardiopulmonary failure will need immediate support of ventilation and oxygenation, whereas a child who has respiratory distress initially may require only supplemental oxygen.

The ABCDEs

The second part of the initial assessment includes a physical evaluation of the ABCDEs: airway, breathing, circulation, disability, and exposure.[14,15] After the PAT and the physical examination, it should be evident whether the patient is stable or unstable. As one proceeds through the ABCDE evaluation, it is often necessary to start interventions prior to completing the evaluation. This can be done by delegating the task while the examination is being completed.

A—Airway

The PAT may identify the presence and possibly the location of airway obstruction but not necessarily the degree of obstruction. It is during this "hands-on" part of the initial evaluation that one assesses the severity of the illness. If the airway is not open, one must immediately perform maneuvers to attempt to open the airway.

B—Breathing

During the PAT, the child's rate of breathing is assessed as either slow, fast, or absent. During the breathing examination, the number of breaths per minute is determined and the child's chest is auscultated with a stethoscope. When determining an infant's respiratory rate, it is important to actually count the number of respirations for at least 30 to 60 seconds because infants often have periodic breathing. *Increased respiratory rate* can indicate a number of conditions, including respiratory illness, and is a sign of respiratory distress. However, in and of itself respiratory rate can be misleading. Pain, cold, exercise, anxiety, and fever can lead to an increase in respiratory rate in the absence of hypoxia. For example, for every degree in temperature elevation, respiratory rate can increase up to 5 respirations per minute. Respiratory rate can also be increased in metabolic acidosis as a buffering mechanism and might not represent a primary respiratory abnormality at all. It is also important to realize that a child who has been showing evidence of increased work of breathing and who now has a normal respiratory rate may be becoming fatigued. Because respiratory rates may vary with external or internal stimuli, recording several rates may be more useful. The trend of the results is often more accurate than the initial documented rate. A normal respiratory rate must be placed in context with other clinical signs to determine if breathing is adequate. Finally, the normal respiratory rate slows as the patient ages (Table 2–4). Increases in vital capacity allow for increased tidal volume with growth and therefore slower rates to maintain minute ventilation. Unfortunately, most references have defined normal respiratory rates for well children without anxiety, pain, respiratory complaints (without pneumonia), or fever. Moreover, the cutoffs for defining tachypnea are much higher than most published standards.[16] In fact, the cutoffs for defining an abnormal respiratory rate indicative of pneumonia are much higher. The World Health Organization defines tachypnea as ≥ 60 breaths per minute (bpm) for neonates (birth to 30 days), ≥ 50 bpm for infants 1 month to 1 year old, and ≥ 40 bpm for children 1 to 5 years old.[17] Others have evaluated febrile children and found that a respiratory rate ≥ 59 at birth to 6 months old, ≥ 52 at 6 to 12 months old, and ≥ 49 at 1 to 2 years old was the optimum cutoff for predicting pneumonia in febrile infants and children.[18]

Minute ventilation is equal to tidal volume times respiratory rate ($MV = TV \times RR$). Generally, young infants respond by increasing respiratory rate but have a limited ability to increase tidal volume. As respiratory rates increase in response to hypoxia, there is not enough time during a respiratory cycle to achieve adequate tidal volume or to allow oxygen to move from the alveoli into capillaries, and respiratory failure ensues.

During *auscultation,* it is important to note the absence of breath sounds or any abnormal lungs sounds during inhalation or exhalation. It is also important to evaluate air movement and effectiveness of the work of breathing (see Table 2–3). Absence of breath sounds may indicate severe airway obstruction (upper or lower), consolidation, effusion, or pneumo- or hemothorax.

C—Circulation

A general impression of the circulatory status of the patient is made from looking at the skin during the PAT. A more in-depth "hands-on" assessment is then made by measuring the rate and quality of the child's pulse, skin temperature, capillary refill time, and blood pressure. The environmental temperature must be considered when evaluating skin temperature, capillary refill time, and skin color in children. Young children and infants are very susceptible to changes in temperature. It has been documented that capillary refill time is prolonged in cool temperatures, even in children with normal circulatory status.[19]

D—Disability

Assessment of disability is the evaluation of the child's neurologic status. This evaluation includes level of consciousness, motor movements, and typically pupillary status. Hypoxia, hypercarbia, and poor perfusion along with acute central nervous system injury can result in altered levels of consciousness. Assessments of level of consciousness in children are age dependent and may include the use of the AVPU (**A**lert, responsive to **V**oice, responsive to **P**ain, **U**nresponsive) scale or the modified Glasgow Coma Scale (GCS).[14,15,20] Children who are only responsive to pain or who are unresponsive on the AVPU scale, and certainly children with a GCS score less than 9, if as a result of trauma, should undergo rapid sequence intubation (RSI) to control their airway, and provide neurologic resuscitation as needed to avert herniation. Children with a medical condition resulting in severe alteration of consciousness should be considered for RSI if their condition is not quickly reversible (see Chapter 3, Rapid Sequence Intubation).

E—Exposure

The PAT requires that the child's clothing be removed enough to evaluate their face, chest, and skin. When completing the initial assessment, during the ABCDE evaluation, the clothing needs to be removed enough so the child can be fully evaluated for other physiologic and anatomic abnormalities.

Ancillary Studies

Assessment is ongoing and, depending on patient stability, includes a secondary assessment, focused history, and complete physical examination. For children who require stabilization or resuscitation, initial assessment and critical interventions take place simultaneously. Tools such as the Broselow-Luten tape have been developed to provide a rapid and accurate method of estimating weight, necessary drug dosages, and sizes of airway equipment.[21,22]

Table 2–4	Normal Respiratory Rates in Children*	
Age	**Respiratory Rate (per minute)**
0–6 month	30–55
6–12 months	24–50
1–3 years	16–46
4–6 years	14–36
7–9 years	12–40
10–14 years	15–32
14–18 years	14–32

Adapted from Hooker EA, Danzl DF, Brueggmeyere M, Harper E: Respiratory rates in pediatric emergency patients. J Emerg Med 10:407–410, 1992.
*Cutoffs for febrile infants and children may be slightly higher.

Pulse Oximetry

Pulse oximetry can be used to determine the child's oxygen saturation level (SaO_2) and estimates the adequacy of the child's oxygenation. It does not reflect ventilation. Its use is indicated in any patient with cardiopulmonary arrest; in unstable or critically ill patients; in patients with cardiopulmonary disease; and in patients with or with the potential for hypoxia, apnea, respiratory distress/failure, or shock. Continuous pulse oximetry is recommended in the care of critically ill or injured patients, as well as those patients for whom the potential for respiratory failure exists, as it has been shown that health care providers cannot detect hypoxemia by clinical examination alone.[23] A pulse oximetry reading above 94% indicates oxygenation is probably adequate; however, a child in respiratory distress or early respiratory failure might be able to maintain oxygenation by increasing work of breathing and respiratory rate. Interpretation of pulse oximetry readings should be combined with the assessment of respiratory rate, work of breathing, and chest auscultation to obtain an accurate idea of respiratory status. Chapter 5 (Monitoring in Critically Ill Children) discusses the utility of and pitfalls associated with pulse oximetry in more detail.

Carbon Dioxide (CO_2) Detection/Monitoring

End-tidal CO_2 detectors are often used to confirm placement of an ETT in the trachea. If the ETT is placed correctly, as the patient is ventilated the CO_2 detector should turn from its baseline purple color to yellow with expiration, and return to purple when 100% oxygen passes across the filter paper. These detectors have been shown to be reliable in non–cardiac arrest states and can be used in infants weighing as little as 2 kg.[24] A pediatric-size detector should be used for infants and children who weigh 2 to 15 kg. For children who weigh more than 15 kg, an adult-size detector should be used. If an adult-size detector is used in an infant, it can be used to confirm tracheal placement of the ETT but must not be left in-line as the device has a large amount of dead space (38 mL), which could lead to hypoventilation in the small infant[25] (see Chapter 5, Monitoring in Critically Ill Children).

Capnography

Capnography or continuous end-tidal CO_2 monitoring is a noninvasive method for continuously assessing the level of CO_2. Carbon dioxide is produced during cellular metabolism, transported to the heart, and exhaled via the lung. Continuous monitoring of end-tidal CO_2 can provide information on adequacy of ventilation, metabolism, and circulation. Capnograpy has most commonly been used to verify ETT placement and monitor ventilation in the emergency department, operating room, and intensive care unit and during transport of critically ill patients.[26-29] During cardiopulmonary resuscitation (CPR), continuous end-tidal CO_2 concentrations vary directly with cardiac output produced by precordial compressions.[30] During effective CPR, end-tidal CO_2 correlates with the efficacy of cardiac compressions and identifies the return of spontaneous circulation and likelihood of survival.[31,32] Continuous CO_2 monitoring also may assist in detecting hypercapnic episodes and episodes of ETT dislodgement in mechanically ventilated patients.[33] Finally, end-tidal CO_2 measurement may provide an earlier indication of respiratory failure versus that provided by pulse oximetry or measure of respiratory rate alone during procedural sedation.[34]

Arterial Blood Gas Measurement

As the use of pulse oximetry monitoring has become standard in most emergency departments, there is much less need for arterial blood gas measurement. Arterial blood gases are rarely needed in the evaluation of children for respiratory failure but may assist in assessment of shock states or presence of acidosis (metabolic or respiratory).

Radiography

In the emergency department, chest radiographs are often obtained on children with asthma, acute lower respiratory infections, foreign bodies, and hypoxia and to check ETT placement. Chest radiographs are of overall limited value and should be ordered and interpreted in the context of a complete medical history and physical examination. For example, experts have found that there is no evidence that chest radiography improves the outcome of ambulatory children with acute lower respiratory infection.[35,36] In children with foreign bodies, the sensitivity and specificity of the chest radiograph in identifying the presence of an airway foreign body are 73% and 45%, respectively.[37] Therefore, one should not rely on chest radiography for making a diagnosis if the clinical suspicion is high.

Chest radiographs are often ordered in children with wheezing. Most children with wheezing have normal chest radiographs, and those with positive findings on chest radiograph have either increased respiratory rate, increased pulse, localized rales, or decreased breath sounds.[38] Dalton found that only 14% of asthmatics have abnormal radiography findings that may change management and concluded that chest radiographs should be taken in children with asthma only if the child does not respond to initial therapy.[39] Lastly, routine chest radiographs in infants with bronchiolitis are usually unnecessary; fever ($\geq 38°$ C) and oxygen saturation less than 94% were findings most often associated with infiltrates on radiographs in this population.[40]

Chest radiography has also been utilized to evaluate children with high fever. Bachur et al. demonstrated that pneumonia was diagnosed by chest radiography in 38 of 146 children (26%) with fever (>39° C) and an elevated peripheral white blood cell (WBC) count (>20,000/μL). Of note is that these children with occult pneumonia did not have hypoxia or tachypnea.[41]

Routine chest radiographs for asthma or acute respiratory infections without other signs (e.g., tachypnea, tachycardia, hypoxia, fever, elevated WBC) are unnecessary unless a patient is failing management, has chronic symptoms, has localized symptoms, or is at high risk (e.g., very young, immunocompromised).

Etiologies of Respiratory Distress or Failure

Many different diseases and conditions can lead to respiratory distress and/or failure. These processes often involve the respiratory system, but many systemic and neurologic processes can also lead to respiratory distress and/or failure. These etiologies are listed in Table 2–5. Many of these processes are discussed in detail in other chapters throughout this book.

Table 2–5	Etiologies of Respiratory Distress and Failure in Infants and Children	

Upper Airway	Lower Airway
Laryngotracheobronchitis (croup)	Asthma
Epiglottitis	Reactive airway disease
Foreign body aspiration	Bronchiolitis
Adenotonsilar hypertrophy	Tracheobronchomalacia
Peritonsilar, parapharyngeal, or retropharyngeal abscess	Foreign body aspiration
	α_1-Antitrypsin deficiency
Subglottic stenosis, web, hemangiomas	Hydrocarbon aspiration
Tracheomalacia	
Laryngoedema	
Congenital anomalies	
Anaphylaxis	
Disease of the Lung	**Systemic**
Bronchopulmonary dysplasia	Central Nervous System
Cystic fibrosis	Status epilepticus
Submersion injury	Encephalopathy
Congestive heart failure	Meningoencephalitis
Pneumonia	Brain abscess, hematoma, tumor
Pneumonitis	Brain stem injury
	Drug intoxication
	Arnold-Chiari malformation
	Medication induced
Chest Wall Conditions	Spinal/Anterior Horn Cell
Diaphragmatic hernia	Poliomyelitis
Pneumothorax/hemothorax/chylothorax	Guillain-Barré disease
	Wernig-Hoffmann disease
Severe kyphoscoliosis	
Severe pectus excavatum	
Other Diseases	Neuromuscular junction
Cardiac disease	Myasthenia gravis
Sepsis	Botulism
Obstructive sleep apnea (pickwickian syndrome)	Tetanus
	Myopathy/neuropathy
	General anesthesia
	Organophosphates

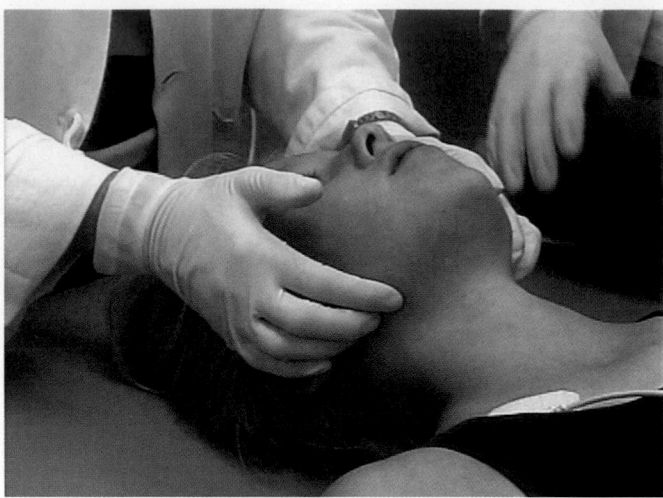

FIGURE 2–5. Jaw-thrust maneuver to open the airway.

The initial diagnostic evaluation is used to determine if the patient is stable or unstable and to identify the category of respiratory disorder. If the patient is stable, then the physician can continue with the secondary assessment, complete history, and physical examination. Interventions may proceed based on physiologic dysfunction and category of respiratory dysfunction. It is important to reassess the patient frequently so that, if the patient becomes unstable, immediate management occurs. If the patient is unstable (respiratory distress, respiratory failure, respiratory arrest, cardiopulmonary failure or cardiopulmonary arrest), then the physician should begin immediate interventions to support oxygenation and perfusion.

Management

Management proceeds based on assessment of need and in a logical fashion from the least to most invasive and complex interventions. These interventions may include all or some of the following:

1. Positioning of the head in the midline position with a towel under the shoulders or head.

2. Opening the airway by performing a head tilt–chin lift in the medical patient or a jaw-thrust maneuver in the trauma patient (Fig. 2–5).
3. Suctioning the airway if the patient has oral or nasal secretions or blood.
4. Providing oxygen supplementation, either by low-flow systems such as a nasal cannula, or by simple face masks, which provide a low fraction of inspired oxygen (FiO_2) (but greater than ambient FiO_2), or systems that provide inspired oxygen levels of 95% or greater. These systems include partial non-rebreather masks for infants or full non-rebreather masks for older children.
5. Placing airway adjuncts such as a nasopharyngeal airway (can be used in the semiconscious patient) or an oropharyngeal airway (only used in the unconscious patient without a gag reflex).
6. Performing bag-mask ventilation to support ventilation and oxygenation for patients requiring assisted ventilation or neurologic resuscitation.
7. Considering advanced airway techniques when the management techniques listed previously do not improve the patient's clinical status: RSI, and laryngoscopy and foreign body removal with Magill forceps.
8. Placing a laryngeal mask airway or performing cricothyrotomy (needle or surgical) for patients who cannot be ventilated with bag-mask ventilation or whose airway cannot be secured by endotracheal intubation (see Chapter 3, Rapid Sequence Intubation; and Chapter 4, Intubation, Rescue Devices, and Airway Adjuncts).

Initial intervention will include *positioning the head, opening the airway, and providing supplemental oxygen. Suctioning* may be added for signs of increased secretions or blood in the airway. If positioning and suctioning do not open the airway, one should consider upper airway obstruction from a foreign body and perform age-specific obstructed airway techniques (back blows and chest thrusts for infants or abdominal thrusts for children > 1 year of age). Consider *direct laryngoscopy with Magill forceps* for possible foreign body removal. If airway obstruction continues, a surgical airway can be attempted with *needle or surgical cricothyrotomy.*

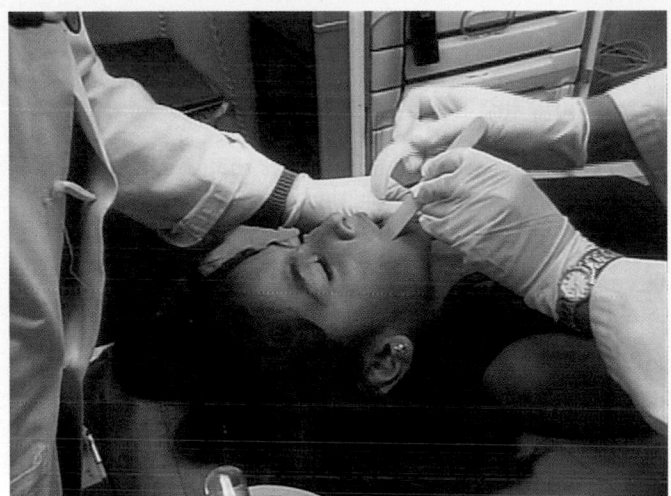

FIGURE 2–6. Placement of an oropharyngeal airway.

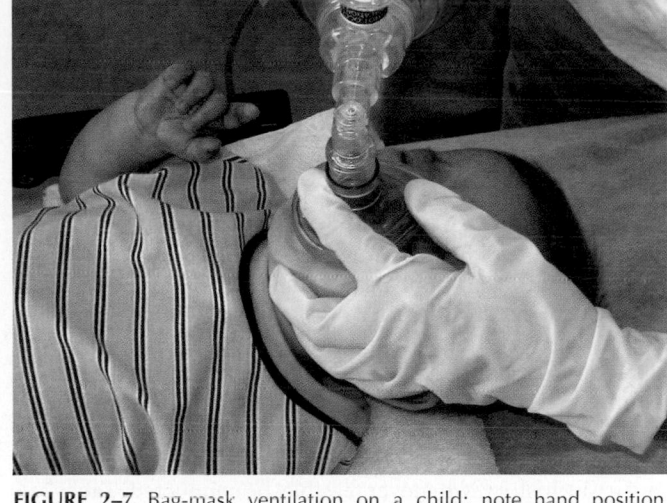

FIGURE 2–7. Bag-mask ventilation on a child; note hand position (EC clamp).

For patients *without* foreign body obstruction but who are unable to maintain a patent airway with positioning, the physician should place an airway adjunct such as a *nasopharyngeal airway* or an oropharyngeal airway. Nasopharyngeal airways are used in semiconscious patients and should be avoided in young infants, patients with bleeding disorders, or those with craniofacial injury. *Oropharyngeal airways* are used in unconscious patients without a gag reflex to keep the airway open, usually during bag-mask ventilation. Figure 2–6 demonstrates placement of the oropharyngeal airway in a pediatric patient.

Bag-mask ventilation is indicated for the initial support of ventilation and oxygenation when compensatory mechanisms fail and the patient is in respiratory failure. If positioning, suctioning, adding airway adjuncts, or providing supplemental oxygen are not successful in improving a patient's condition and assisted ventilation is needed, then bag-mask ventilation should begin without delay. The first step is to ensure the correct size of face mask is used. The correct size mask will measure from the bridge of the nose to the cleft of the chin. Once the mask is attached to the elbow adapter on the bag, a "C" is formed with the physician's thumb and index finger. The mask is placed on the patient's face, the physician's thumb is wrapped around the mask at the end of the mask that lies on the bridge of the nose, and the index finger is placed around the lower part of the mask at the chin. The third, fourth, and fifth digits are placed along the angle of the patient's jaw, forming an "E," and the chin is pulled into the mask to ensure a seal. The entire hand position is called the "EC clamp" (Fig. 2–7).[42] It is important *not* to place the "E" fingers in the soft tissue under the chin as pressure in this area can compress the airway or cause the tongue to fall back against the posterior pharynx, leading to airway obstruction. The Sellick maneuver (cricoid pressure) may be used if significant pressure is needed to ventilate, but it is possible to place too much pressure on the cricoid membrane and collapse the airway, leading to airway obstruction. To begin ventilation, the physician squeezes the bag for 1 to 2 seconds and with only enough force to cause chest rise, then releases the pressure on the bag. It is important to realize that the volume of air needed to provide adequate chest rise is

between 8 and 10 mL/kg. For a neonate only about 30 mL (2 tablespoons) of air is needed to cause adequate chest rise; a 1-year-old requires only about 105 mL (7 tablespoons). Excessive volume instilled with the bag-mask device can lead to gastric insufflation and vomiting.[43]

Gausche and colleagues showed that using the "squeeze, release, release" technique for bag-mask ventilation, versus using endotracheal intubation to ventilate infants and children in the prehospital setting, can lead to improved outcomes for children in respiratory failure.[44] The person providing bag-mask ventilation should allow for slightly longer inspiratory times and then the patient is allowed time to passively exhale. The respiratory rate should be between 30 and 40 breaths/min in a neonate, 20 and 30 breaths/min in an infant, and no more than 20 breaths/min in a child. Modifications of this technique can be considered in patients when it is difficult to maintain a seal with one hand. In these cases, a two-person technique, with one person holding the mask with the EC clamp using both hands and the other squeezing the bag-mask device, may be used. In a case of upper airway obstruction, it has been shown that bag-mask ventilation with the patient in the prone position may be useful.[45]

Endotracheal intubation and RSI are utilized in patients requiring long-term support of oxygenation and ventilation; in patients requiring neurologic resuscitation (GCS score < 9); in patients requiring airway protection, such as those with burns, anaphylaxis, or overdose; and in patients in whom bag-mask ventilation fails to support oxygenation and ventilation. (Endotracheal intubation and RSI are discussed in more detail in Chapter 3 Rapid Sequence Intubation; and Chapter 4, Intubation, Rescue Devices, and Airway Adjuncts.)

The Difficult Airway

When dealing with children in an emergency department setting, it is imperative that one be able to anticipate a potentially difficult airway and have a backup plan if bag-mask ventilation and endotracheal intubation are unsuccessful. It is also necessary to have backup management plans when one comes across an unanticipated difficult airway.

Unlike the adult difficult airway, evaluation and management strategies for the difficult airway in children are not well described. This section discusses the evaluation, history, and physical examination of a patient prior to airway management to look for features that may indicate a difficult airway.

History

The American Society of Anesthesiologists Task Force on Management of the Difficult Airway stated that, although there is insufficient published evidence to evaluate the effect of a bedside medical history on predicting the presence of a difficult airway, there is suggestive evidence that some features of a patient's medical history (congenital syndromes, acquired or traumatic disease states, or history of prior difficult intubation) may be related to the likelihood of encountering a difficult airway.[46] Therefore, it is recommended that an airway history, whenever feasible, be conducted. Table 2–6 lists features that may be evident from the history that can indicate the possibility of encountering a difficult airway. Importantly, there are multiple congenital disorders and syndromes associated with anatomic and physiologic disorders that make airway management difficult (e.g., micrognathia, macroglossia, cervical spine disorders, hypotonia, midface disorders).[47]

Physical Examination

According to the American Society of Anesthesiologists Task Force, an airway physical examination should be conducted, whenever feasible, prior to the initiation of airway management in all patients. The intent of this examination is to detect physical characteristics that may indicate the presence of a difficult airway.[46] Physical findings that may predict airway difficulty are listed in Table 2–7, and some are discussed below.[47-52]

The oropharyngeal examination is the first step to examining the airway. If possible, the patient's oral cavity should be examined with his or her mouth open and tongue maximally protruded. If the patient is uncooperative or too young to cooperate, this can be done with a tongue blade with the patient lying down. The degree of mouth opening and the size of the tongue in relation to the oral cavity are assessed. Mallampati et al.[53] classified airways on the basis of the degree of visualization of the faucial pillars, soft palate, and uvula. This classification has been used extensively in adults to predict the degree of difficulty with endotracheal intubation. Whether it can successfully predict difficulty in children is not known. Other findings in the oropharyngeal examination that may suggest difficult laryngoscopy and intubation are outlined in Table 2–7.

After the oropharyngeal examination, the ability to extend the patient's neck should be assessed. Neck extension is often necessary during laryngoscopy to be able to visualize the vocal cords. Obviously, neck extension should not be evaluated in a trauma patient when cervical spine trauma is suspected. However, the inability to extend the neck as a result of trauma or congenital syndromes, such as trisomy 21 or Goldenhar and Klippel-Feil syndromes, or acquired conditions, such as juvenile rheumatoid arthritis or prior cervical spine fixation, is a predictor of the possibility of difficult laryngoscopy and intubation.[49,51] A short mandible, micrognathia, or a small oral cavity make visualization of the airway challenging due to the anterior location of the airway

Table 2–6	Historical Features That May Indicate a Difficult Airway
Feature	**Anatomic Correlate**
Prior history of difficult intubation	Narrow epiglottic angle; anterior vocal cords
Snoring/noisy breathing/obstructive sleep apnea	Enlarged adenoidal/tonsillar tissue
Difficulty feeding secondary to cough or cyanosis	Possibly reduced oxygen reserve
Difficulty breathing with URI	Enlarged adenoidal/tonsillar tissue
Recurrent croup	Narrow glottic area, hemangioma
Juvenile rheumatoid arthritis	Limited mouth opening
TMJ syndrome	Limited mouth opening
Acquired conditions Croup Epiglottis Retropharyngeal abscess Ludwig's angina Thermal injury Caustic ingestion	Normal anatomy is altered, usually by swelling, leading to upper airway obstruction
Facial or neck trauma	Variety of reasons: obstruction, loss of landmarks, blood in airway, cervical spine stabilization
Foreign body	Upper airway obstruction

Abbreviations: TMJ, temporomandibular; URI, upper respiratory infection.

Table 2–7	Findings on Physical Examination That May Predict a Difficult Airway

Trauma

Facial and/or neck trauma
Blood in airway
Facial or oral burns

Oropharyngeal

Mallampati class III and class IV
Macroglossia
Small mouth
Prominent central incisors
Limited mouth opening (e.g., limited TMJ mobility, trismus from deep space infections, maxillofacial trauma)
Laryngeal edema (e.g., infection, inhalation injury, caustic ingestion)
Enlarged tonsils
High-arched palate
Foreign body
Secretions in upper airway
Swelling of intraoral structures (e.g., anaphylaxis, congenital syndromes)

Other

Short neck
Limited neck extension or flexion
Micrognathia (short mandible)
Obesity

Abbreviation: TMJ, temporomandibular.

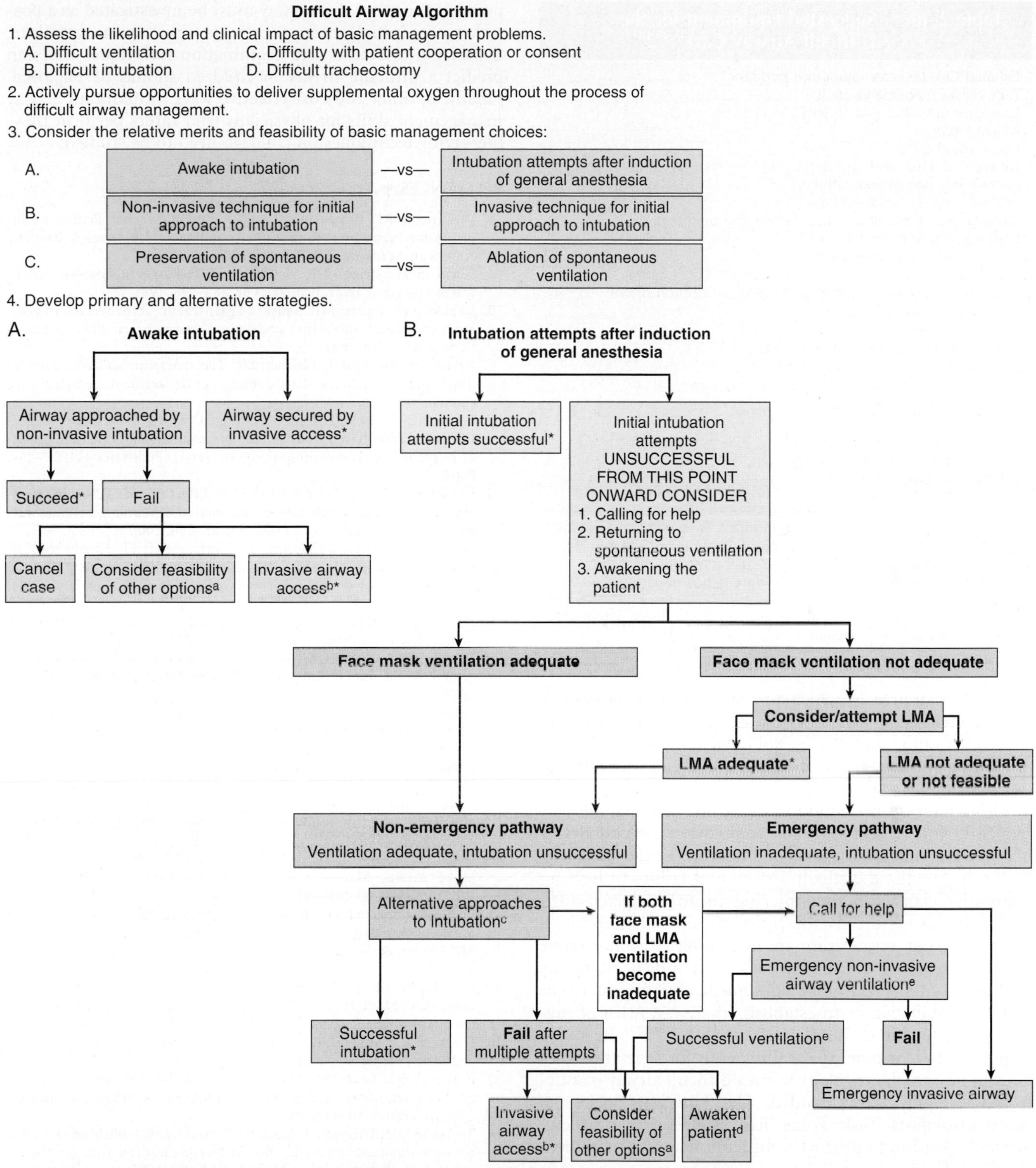

Difficult Airway Algorithm

1. Assess the likelihood and clinical impact of basic management problems.
   A. Difficult ventilation
   B. Difficult intubation
   C. Difficulty with patient cooperation or consent
   D. Difficult tracheostomy

2. Actively pursue opportunities to deliver supplemental oxygen throughout the process of difficult airway management.

3. Consider the relative merits and feasibility of basic management choices:

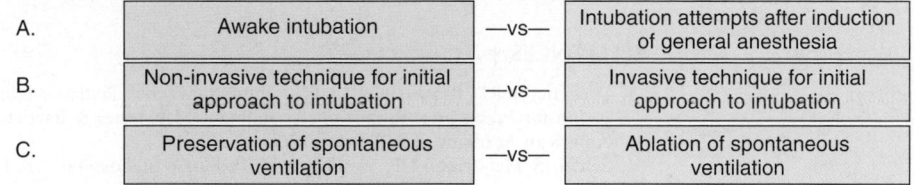

A. | Awake intubation | —vs— | Intubation attempts after induction of general anesthesia |

B. | Non-invasive technique for initial approach to intubation | —vs— | Invasive technique for initial approach to intubation |

C. | Preservation of spontaneous ventilation | —vs— | Ablation of spontaneous ventilation |

4. Develop primary and alternative strategies.

A. Awake intubation

- Airway approached by non-invasive intubation
  - Succeed*
  - Fail
    - Cancel case
    - Consider feasibility of other options[a]
    - Invasive airway access[b]*
- Airway secured by invasive access*

B. Intubation attempts after induction of general anesthesia

- Initial intubation attempts successful*
- Initial intubation attempts UNSUCCESSFUL FROM THIS POINT ONWARD CONSIDER
  1. Calling for help
  2. Returning to spontaneous ventilation
  3. Awakening the patient

Face mask ventilation adequate

Face mask ventilation not adequate
- Consider/attempt LMA
  - LMA adequate*
  - LMA not adequate or not feasible

Non-emergency pathway
Ventilation adequate, intubation unsuccessful

Emergency pathway
Ventilation inadequate, intubation unsuccessful

- Alternative approaches to Intubation[c]
  - Successful intubation*
  - Fail after multiple attempts

If both face mask and LMA ventilation become inadequate

- Call for help
  - Emergency non-invasive airway ventilation[e]
    - Successful ventilation[e]
    - Fail
      - Emergency invasive airway

- Invasive airway access[b]*
- Consider feasibility of other options[a]
- Awaken patient[d]

[a] Other options include (but are not limited to): surgery utilizing face mask or LMA anesthesia, local anesthesia infiltration or regional nerve blockade. Pursuit of these options usually implies that mask ventilation will not be problematic. Therefore, these options may be of limited value if this step in the algorithm has been reached via the Emergency Pathway.

[b] Invasive airway access includes surgical or percutaneous tracheostomy or cricothyrotomy.

[c] Alternative non-invasive approaches to difficult intubation include (but are not limited to): use of different laryngoscope blades, LMA as an intubation conduit (with or without fiberoptic guidance), fiberoptic intubation, intubating stylet or tube changer, light wand, retrograde intubation, and blind oral or nasal intubation.

[d] Consider re-preparation of the patient for awake intubation or canceling surgery.

[e] Options for emergency non-invasive airway ventilation include (but are not limited to): rigid bronchoscope, esophageal-tracheal combitube ventilation, or transtracheal jet ventilation.

FIGURE 2–8. Guideline for management of the difficult airway. (Adapted from American Society of Anesthesiologists Task Force on Management of the Difficult Airway: Practice guidelines for management of the difficult airway. an updated report. Anesthesiology 95:1269–1277, 2003.)

Table 2–8	Suggested Equipment for the Difficult Airway Cart[46,49,50]

Exhaled CO_2 detector (adult and pediatric)
Face masks (neonate to adult)
Laryngoscope blades of all sizes and styles
Magill forceps
Local anesthetics
All sizes of naso- and oropharyngeal airways
Suction equipment and catheters
Self-inflating resuscitation bags
Endotracheal tubes of all sizes, cuffed and uncuffed
Endotracheal tube guides:
   Semirigid intubation stylets
   Light wand
   Forceps designed to manipulate the distal portion of the
      tracheal tube
Gum elastic bougie
Laryngeal mask airways, assorted sizes
Flexible fiberoptic intubation equipment
Emergency nonsurgical ventilation (at least one):
   Transtracheal jet ventilation
   Hollow jet ventilation stylet
   Tracheoesophageal Combitube
Emergency surgical airway access:
   Cricothyrotomy equipment
   Commercially available cricothyrotomy kit for children

The items listed represent only suggestions as some of these items will be available in standard intubation/airway trays. The contents of the difficult airway cart should be customized to meet the needs, preferences, and skills of the emergency department physicians.[46]
From Behringer EC: Approaches to managing the upper pathway. Anesthesiol Clin North America 20:813–832, 2002.

and the small area in which to manipulate the structures with laryngoscopy. Micrognathia is a prominent feature in Treacher-Collins and Pierre Robin syndromes.[49,51] Micrognathia can also make it difficult to achieve an adequate seal during bag-mask ventilation.

Although it is uncommon to encounter a difficult airway in a child, it is critical to be able to predict a difficult airway before using induction agents and neuromuscular blockade. Failure to predict a difficult airway and failure to have an alternative plan when encountering an unanticipated difficult airway can result in a life-threatening situation in which ventilation and oxygenation are impossible. It is imperative that emergency physicians have access to a difficult airway cart that contains additional equipment used to perform or facilitate intubation or to establish an airway. A list of suggested equipment is found in Table 2–8.[46,48,49,51] It is also important to remember that calling early for assistance from anesthesia or otolaryngology when a difficult airway is anticipated is highly recommended. The American Society of Anesthesiologists Task Force has established a difficult airway algorithm to help with difficult airway management (Fig. 2–8).[46]

Summary

Early recognition of respiratory distress and failure in an infant or child with appropriate interventions will optimize outcomes. Additional research is needed to identify factors leading to respiratory failure and devices that may accurately predict the need for early intervention. The role of the laryngeal mask airway in emergency settings is ill-defined at this point in time, but this airway must be investigated as a possible tool to initially manage patients with respiratory failure. Evaluation of factors and examination techniques that can predict a difficult airway in children should be explored. Finally, optimal and cost-effective ways to maintain airway management skills for physicians who rarely perform these life-saving techniques on children need to be studied.

REFERENCES

1. Dieckmann RD, Brownstein DR, Gausche-Hill M (eds): Pediatric Education for Prehospital Professionals. Sudbury, MA: Jones & Bartlett/American Academy of Pediatrics, 2000.
2. Seidel JS, Henderson DP, Ward P, et al: Pediatric prehospital care in urban and rural areas. Pediatrics 88:681–690, 1991.
3. Isaacman DJ, Poirier MP, Gausche-Hill M, et al: Controversies in pediatric emergency medicine: prehospital emergencies. Pediatr Emerg Care 20:135–149, 2004.
4. Krauss BS, Harakal T, Fleisher GR: The spectrum and frequency of illness presenting to a pediatric emergency department. Pediatr Emerg Care 7:67–71, 1991.
5. Young KD, Gausche-Hill M, McClung CD, Lewis RJ: A large prospective population-based study of the epidemiology and outcome of out-of-hospital pediatric cardiopulmonary arrest. Pediatrics 114:157–164, 2004.
6. Gausche M, Lewis RJ, Stratton SJ, et al: Effect of out-of-hospital pediatric endotracheal intubation on survival and neurological outcome: a controlled clinical trial. JAMA 283:783–790, 2000.
7. Gausche-Hill M: Introduction. In Gausche-Hill M, Henderson DP, Goodrich SM, et al (eds): Pediatric Airway Management for the Prehospital Professional. Sudbury, MA: Jones & Bartlett, 2004, pp 1–11.
8. Hislop AA, Wigglesworth JS, Desai R: Alveolar development in the human fetus and infant. Early Human Dev 13:1–11, 1986.
9. Zeltner TB, Caduff JH, Gehr P, et al: The postnatal development and growth of the human lung. Morphometry Respir Physiol 67:247–267, 1987.
10. Berry FA, Yemen TA: Pediatric airway in health and disease. Pediatr Clin North Am 41:153–180, 1994.
11. Miller MJ, Carlo WA, Strohl KP, et al: Effect of maturation on oral breathing in sleeping premature infants. J Pediatr 109:515–519, 1986.
12. Hill JR, Rahimtulla KA: Heat balance and the metabolic rate of newborn babies in relation to environmental temperatures and the effect of age and of weight on basal metabolic rate. J Physiol (Lond) 180:239–265, 1965.
13. Luten RC: The pediatric patient. In Walls RM (ed): Manual of Emergency Airway Management. Philadelphia: Lippincott, Williams & Wilkins, 2000, pp 143–152.
14. Pediatric assessment. In Dieckmann RD, Brownstein DR, Gausche-Hill M (eds): Pediatric Education for Prehospital Professionals. Sudbury, MA: Jones & Bartlett/American Academy of Pediatrics, 2000, pp 33–55.
15. Henderson DP: Assessment. In Gausche-Hill M, Henderson DP, Goodrich SM, et al (eds): Pediatric Airway Management for the Prehospital Professional. Sudbury, MA: Jones & Bartlett, 2004, pp 14–27.
16. Hooker EA, Danzl DF, Brueggmeyer M, Harper E: Respiratory rates in pediatric emergency patients. J Emerg Med 10:407–410, 1992.
17. Rothrock SG, Green SM, Fanelli JM, et al: Do published guidelines predict pneumonia in children presenting to an urban ED? Pediatr Emerg Care 17:240–243, 2001.
18. Taylor JA, Del Beccaro M, Done S, Winters W: Establishing clinically relevant standards for tachypnea in febrile children younger than 2 years. Arch Pediatr Adolesc Med 149:283–287, 1995.
19. Gorelick MH, Shaw KN, Baker MD: Effect of ambient temperature on capillary refill in healthy children. Pediatrics 92:699–702, 1993.
20. Trauma resuscitation and spinal immobilization. In Hazinski MF, Zaritsky AL, Nadkarni VM, et al (eds): PALS Provider Manual. Dallas, TX: American Heart Association, 2002, pp 253–286.
21. Lubitz DS, Seidel JS, Chameides L, et al: A rapid method for estimating weight and resuscitation drug dosages from length in the pediatric age group. Ann Emerg Med 17:576–581, 1988.
22. Luten R: Error and time delay in pediatric trauma resuscitation: addressing the problem with color-coded resuscitation aids. Surg Clin North Am 82:303–314, 2002.

23. Brown LH, Manring EA, Komegay HB, et al.: Can prehospital personnel detect hypoxemia without the aid of pulse oximeters? Am J Emerg Med 14:43–44, 1996.
24. Bhende MS, Thompson AE, Orr RA: Utility of an end-tidal CO_2 detector in verifying endotracheal tube placement in infants and children. Ann Emerg Med 21:142–145, 1992.
25. Endotracheal intubation. In Gausche-Hill M, Henderson DP, Goodrich SM, et al (eds): Pediatric Airway Management for the Prehospital Professional. Sudbury, MA: Jones & Bartlett, 2004, pp 79–95.
26. Bhende MS: End-tidal carbon dioxide monitoring in pediatrics—clinical applications. J Postgrad Med 47:215–218, 2001.
27. Bhende MS, Thompson AE, Orr RA: Utility of an end-tidal CO_2 detector during stabilization and transport of critically ill children. Pediatrics 89:1042–1044, 1992.
28. Palmon SC, Liu M, Moore LE, Kirsch JR: Capnography facilitates tight control of ventilation during transport. Crit Care Med 24:608–611, 1996.
29. Tobias JD, Lynch A, Garrett J: Alterations of end-tidal carbon dioxide during the intrahospital transport of children. Pediatr Emerg Care 12:249–251, 1996.
30. Falk JL, Rackow EC, Weil MH: End-tidal carbon dioxide concentration during cardiopulmonary resuscitation. N Engl J Med 318:607–611, 1988.
31. Sanders AB, Ewy GA, Bragg S, et al: Expired PCO_2 as a prognostic indicator of successful resuscitation from cardiac arrest. Ann Emerg Med 14:948–952, 1985.
32. Garnett AR, Ornato JP, Gonzalez ER, Johnson EB: End-tidal carbon dioxide monitoring during cardiopulmonary resuscitation. JAMA 257:512–515, 1987.
33. Bhende MS: Capnography in the paediatric emergency department. Pediatr Emerg Care 15:64–69, 1999.
34. Hart LS, Berns SD, Houck CS, Boenning DAI: The value of end-tidal CO_2 monitoring when comparing three methods of procedural sedation for children undergoing painful procedures in the emergency department. Pediatr Emerg Care 13:189–193, 1997.
35. Swingler GH, Hussey GD, Zwarenstein M: Randomised controlled trial of clinical outcome after chest radiograph in ambulatory acute lower-respiratory infection in children. Lancet 351:404–408, 1998.
36. Swingler GH, Zwarenstein M: Chest radiograph in acute respiratory infections in children. Cochrane Database Syst Rev 2:CD001268, 2000.
37. Silva AB, Muntz HR, Clary R: Utility of conventional radiography in the diagnosis and management of pediatric airway foreign bodies. Ann Otol Rhinol Laryngol 107:834–838, 1998.
38. Gerohel JC, Goldman HS, Stein RE, et al: The usefulness of chest radiographs in first asthma attacks. N Engl J Med 309:336–339, 1983.
39. Dalton AM: A review of radiological abnormalities in 135 patients presenting with acute asthma. Arch Emerg Med 1:36–40, 1991.
40. Garcia Garcia ML, Calvo Rey C, Quevedo Teruel S, et al: Chest radiograph in bronchiolitis: is it always necessary? An Pediatr (Barc) 61:219–225, 2004.
41. Bachur R, Perry H, Harper MB: Occult pneumonias: empiric chest radiographs in febrile children with leukocytosis. Ann Emerg Med 33:166–173, 1999.
42. Cooper A, Tunik M, Foltin G, et al: Teaching paramedics to ventilate infants: preliminary results of a new method. In Chameides L (ed): Proceedings of the International Conference on Pediatric Resuscitation. Washington, DC: Washington National Center for Education in Maternal and Child Health, June, 1994, p 8.
43. Melker RJ, Banner MJ: Ventilation during CPR: two-rescuer standards reappraised. Ann Emerg Med 14:397–402, 1985.
44. Gausche M, Lewis RJ, Stratton SJ, et al: Effect of out-of-hospital pediatric endotracheal intubation on survival and neurological outcome: A controlled clinical trial. JAMA 283:783–790, 2000.
45. Ghirga G, Ghirga P, Palazzi C, et al: Bag-mask ventilation as a temporizing measure in acute infectious upper-airway obstruction: does it really work? Pediatr Emerg Care 17:444–446, 2001.
*46. American Society of Anesthesiologists Task Force on Management of the Difficult Airway: Practice guidelines for management of the difficult airway. an updated report. Anesthesiology 95:1269–1277, 2003.
47. Walker RW: Management of the difficult airway in children. J R Soc Med 94:341–344, 2001.
48. Jones KL (ed): Smith's Recognizable Patterns of Human Malformation. Philadelphia: WB Saunders, 1997.
*49. Sullivan KJ, Kissoon N: Securing the child's airway in the emergency department. Pediatr Emerg Care 18:108–120, 2002.
50. Behringer EC: Approaches to managing the upper airway. Anesthesiol Clin North America 20:813–832, 2002.
51. Tobias JD: Airway management for pediatric emergencies. Pediatr Ann 25:323–328, 1996.
52. Kaide CG, Hollingsworth JC: Current strategies for airway management in the trauma patient, part II: managing difficult and failed airways. Trauma Reps 4:1–12, 2003.
53. Mallampati Sr, Gatt SP, Gugino LD, et al: A clinical sign to predict difficult tracheal intubation: a prospective study. Can Anaesth Soc J 32:429–434, 1985.

*Selected readings.

Chapter 3

Rapid Sequence Intubation

Steven G. Rothrock, MD

Key Points

Immaturity of the autonomic nervous system in neonates and infants increases their propensity to develop bradycardia with airway manipulation, hypoxia, and succinylcholine use.

Unique anatomic and physiologic properties require a different approach, medication dosing, and techniques for rapid sequence intubation in neonates, young infants, children, and adolescents.

Preoxygenation for 2 minutes with 100% oxygen allows for only 2 minutes of apnea before desaturation occurs in healthy infants and even less time in ill infants.

To ensure success, clinicians must use a consistent stepwise methodology for intubation that includes personnel and patient preparation, medication and equipment selection, procedural performance, confirmation of correct tube placement, and advancement to rescue techniques when appropriate.

Introduction and Background

Airway manipulation during endotracheal intubation is associated with adverse cardiovascular effects (hypertension, bradycardia, tachycardia, arrhythmias) and increased intracranial, intraocular, and intragastric pressure in addition to airway trauma and hypoxia. Rapid sequence induction is the process of providing rapid sedation during general anesthesia in unprepared patients at risk for aspiration. Rapid sequence intubation (RSI) is used to describe rapid sequence induction using sedation and paralysis during endotracheal intubation while minimizing trauma, time to airway control, and complications of intubation and airway manipulation. Emergency medicine and pediatric emergency medicine physicians using RSI have ≥ 99% success rates for controlling an airway in children with traumatic and medical disorders without requiring surgical rescue techniques.[1-3]

Recognition and Approach

Several features make the technique of rapid sequence induction more difficult in infants and children compared to adults. Infants and young children have less rigid support to their major airway structures.[4] The soft palate and epiglottis obstruct the airway more commonly than the tongue in patients with an altered level of consciousness and in those undergoing anesthesia.[5-7] In infants and children, these structures have less cartilaginous support than found in adults, increasing the propensity to collapse and obstruct during sedation. The tongue also encompasses a proportionately larger amount of the oropharynx, increasing the difficulty of mask ventilation and passage of airway devices. Immature diaphragmatic and intercostal muscle composition and positioning lead to more rapid fatigue and respiratory decompensation, accelerating the need to make airway decisions in the very young.[4]

The physiologic response to hypoxia and laryngeal manipulation is exaggerated in young infants. The neonatal cardiac conduction system has predominant intrinsic sympathetic activity within the sinus and atrioventricular nodes, resulting in a high resting heart rate.[8] In contrast, little sympathetic innervation of the ventricles and bundle branches exists in neonates and young infants.[9] The absence of nerves that directly supply the ventricles makes them less electrically stable and exaggerates the cardiac response to stress.[8] This effect is offset by a predominant vagal nerve influence mediated by cholinergic fibers that directly supply the atrial and ventricular conduction systems.[8,10] This autonomic imbalance predisposes the heart to profound accelerations and decelerations with stress. Bradycardia is induced by airway manipulation, hypoxia, and succinylcholine administration in infants ≤ 1 year old. By 1 year, autonomic imbalances diminish, limiting these adverse effects and limiting the theoretical basis for using atropine as a premedication.[11,12]

Neonates and young infants differ from older children and adults in their responses to many anesthetic agents. In the neonate, relatively larger extracellular fluid volume and blood volume, smaller muscle mass and fat stores, and greater blood flow to the central organs influence the effect and metabolism of drugs.[8] Drug metabolism is less effective in neonates than in children due to incompletely developed hepatic enzyme systems and glomerular filtration. These factors contribute to increased toxicity and sensitivity to a variety of agents used during airway management (e.g., benzodiazepines and narcotics) and a requirement for different drug doses. A smaller muscle mass and a larger volume of distribution require use of higher relative doses of succinylcholine at younger ages.[13] Knowledge of these physiologic differences allows for selection of safer, rational choices during RSI.

Prior to performing RSI, patients are preoxygenated with 100% O_2 to create an oxygen reservoir. In healthy adults, the effect of this nitrogen washout is a maintenance of oxygen saturation greater than 90% for up to 8 minutes of apnea.[14] Infants and young children consume more oxygen and have a smaller functional residual capacity compared to older children, adolescents, and adults.[12,15] For this reason, infants and children will desaturate more quickly, resulting in a shortened window of opportunity for endotracheal intubation before hypoxia occurs.[14]

Selection of patients requiring RSI is one of the most important decisions made in the emergency department (ED). This technique should be considered in every patient requiring definitive airway control (e.g., respiratory failure, shock, altered mental status) in an emergency fashion in whom no contraindications exist.

Evaluation

If time permits, obtain a brief history including allergies, prior problems with anesthesia, medications, time of last meal, and associated medical conditions. Disorders placing patients at risk for complications from RSI require immediate identification. Subacute or chronic burns and neurologic or muscle disease (e.g., muscular dystrophy) increase the risk of fatal hyperkalemia following succinylcholine administration and require use of nondepolarizing agents.[16] Children with prior reactions to anesthetics or a family history of malignant hyperthermia or neuroleptic malignant syndrome should not receive succinylcholine.[16] The presence of an upper respiratory infection or airway irritation (e.g., trauma, blood) increases the risk of laryngospasm and decreases the time to desaturation.[17]

Prior to paralysis, clinicians must make a determination of their ability to manually intubate and ventilate the patient based upon history, clinical features, and anatomic variables. Authors have analyzed the ability of intraoral (incisor-to-incisor) distance, mandibular length, Mallampatti score, and thyromental distance to predict difficult intubations in adults undergoing general anesthesia. These parameters have poor utility in the ED. Only an intraoral distance less than 2.5 cm is statistically associated with difficult intubations in adult ED patients.[18] No studies have analyzed the ability of any of these criteria to predict difficult intubations in infants or children. Children at risk for difficult intubations include those with a history of micrognathia, macroglossia, prominent dentition, cleft palate, limited temporomandibular joint mobility or congenital cervical spine disorders. Acquired abnormalities associated with difficult intubations include any disorder that distorts the neck, oral, or facial anatomy (e.g., burns, edema, blood, vomitus, infection), temporomandibular joint immobility (e.g., lateral airway abscess or trauma), or potential cervical spine trauma requiring immobility. Intrinsic or acquired airway and lung disease may make bag-mask ventilation difficult in patients who are sedated and paralyzed. Depending upon the urgency for airway control,

immediate surgical or alternate airway techniques (e.g., awake intubation, bronchoscopy) may be required in patients at risk for difficult intubations. A significant number of children with difficult intubations have no identifiable risk factors; therefore, rescue devices and alternative techniques must be prepared for every patient undergoing RSI (see Chapter 4, Intubation, Rescue Devices, and Airway Adjuncts).

Management

Equipment Preparation

Equipment preparation prior to patient arrival is essential to satisfactory completion of RSI. Every ED should be equipped with appropriate ventilation and bag-mask devices, oxygen masks, laryngoscope blades, oral airways, suctioning devices, endotracheal tubes (ETTs), laryngeal mask airways, and other rescue devices for all ages and sizes. A color-coded system (e.g., drawers in a cart or wall shelving) based on weight and age helps to rapidly select appropriately sized equipment. Monitoring devices, including cardiac monitors, pulse oximetry, and ETT placement confirmation devices (e.g., end-tidal CO_2 monitors), should be available and checked systematically for proper functioning. Length-based estimates (e.g., Broselow-Luten tape) are a rapid and accurate means of equipment selection (Table 3–1).

Age-based equipment selection may be employed, although this technique may be slightly less accurate than length-based estimates (Table 3–1). Straight laryngoscope blades are used until age 2 years, with either curved (e.g., McIntosh) or straight blades used above this age. For the youngest infants (<1 year old), straight laryngoscope blades with the widest flange (e.g., Oxford, Wis-Hipple, Wisconsin, Flagg) are best for controlling the relatively large tongue.[19,20] Above 1 year, blades with a narrower flange (e.g., Miller) can control the tongue and decrease trauma to the gingiva and teeth.[20] Further modification with a curve at the tip allows for the options of either direct elevation of the epiglottis via the blade or blade insertion into the vallecula (e.g., modified Miller, Phillips) in older infants.[20]

Cole's age-based formula can be used to select an appropriate-sized ETT, although length-based estimates will select tubes less likely to produce an air leak.[21] Preterm neonates require ETTs with an internal diameter (ID) of 2.5 to 3.0 mm, birth to 3-month-olds require 3 to 3.5 mm ID, 3- to 9-month-olds require 3.5 to 4.0 mm ID, greater than 9-month-olds to 18-month-olds require 4 to 4.5 mm ID, and 18- to 24-month-olds require 4.5 to 5 mm ID. Above 24 months, an appropriate tube size can be estimated by using the formula: [age (in years) ÷ 4] + 4 mm (Table 3–1).[21] Modification of Cole's formula to [age (in years) ÷ 3] + 4 mm identifies cuffed ETTs that can be inserted (with or without blowing up the balloon) to decrease the amount of air leak compared to uncuffed tubes.[22] Alternate methods for estimating ETT sizes (e.g., fifth finger width, fifth finger diameter, fifth finger nail width, naris diameter) are all less accurate than length-based and age-based formula estimates and should not be used.[23] In general, uninflated or uncuffed ETTs are used for children ≤ 8 years old. At this age, the area below the vocal cords, the cricoid ring, is the narrowest part of the airway, precluding the need for a cuff and leading to pressure-induced complications if a cuff is used. New low-pressure, high-volume cuffs (using Cole's formula minus 0.5 to 1.0 mm ID for ETT size)

Table 3–1	Rapid Sequence Intubation Protocol*

Preparation of Equipment

Apply cardiac monitor, pulse oximeter, spine immobilization devices.
Ready suctioning devices, postintubation confirmation device.
Ready backup devices (laryngeal mask airway, bougie, surgical equipment).
Ready appropriate-size blades and endotracheal (ET) tubes (and tubes $1/2$ size above/below with stylets).

Age	Laryngoscope[†]	ET tube (mm)[‡]	ET depth (cm)[§]
Premature	0 straight	2.5–3.0	8
Newborn	0–1 straight	3.0–3.5	9–10
3 mo	0–1 straight	3.0–3.5	9–10
6 mo	1–1.5 straight	3.5–4.0	10
1 yr	1–1.5 straight	4.0–4.5	11–12
2 yr	1–2 straight or curved	4.0–4.5	11–13
5 yr	2 straight or curved	5.0–5.5	15–16.5
12 yr	3 straight or curved	6.5–7.0	19–21

Preparation of Personnel

Identify personnel for directing intubation, monitoring, applying cricoid pressure, medication, and ventilation.

Preparation of Patient and Medications

Immobilize cervical spine.
Preoxygenate—3 min of 100% O_2 or 4–8 deep breaths over 30–60 sec
Premedication/medications* (calculate and prepare doses in labeled syringes): atropine, lidocaine, sedatives, cardioprotective agents, defasciculating or priming agent, paralytic

Sedation and Paralysis and Timing of Events: (–) signifies time agent given prior to laryngoscopy*

(–) 7 min	Preoxygenation for 3 min if spontaneously breathing
(–) 4 min	Atropine (esp. ≤1 year old, ketamine use, second dose succinylcholine)
(–) 4 min	Defasciculating/priming agent (optional) (Observe for rare respiratory depression)
(–) 3 min	Lidocaine (esp. if weaker sedating agent)
(–) 2 min	Sedation or induction agent and application of cricoid pressure
(–) 1 min	Succinycholine or paralytic agent (administer 90 sec preintubation if defasciculating or priming agent used)
0 min	Laryngoscopy and intubation

Postintubation Evaluation

Confirm ET tube position—capnographic waveform analyis is most accurate. Alternately, use colorimetric end-tidal CO_2 device or, in adolescents, esophageal detection device.
Reexamine patient and obtain chest radiograph. Secure ET tube with taping that ensures tube will not move when head and neck move, and consider administration of sedative or sedative with paralytic.

*See Table 3–2 for medication dosage and timing.
[†]French size of laryngoscope blades.
[‡]ET tube internal diameter (ID) is estimated by: [age (in years) ÷ 4] + 4 if age >2.
[§]Distance from incisors or gum line to midtrachea in centimeters. If patient is ≥2 years, ET ID × 3 estimates correct ET tube depth in centimeters.

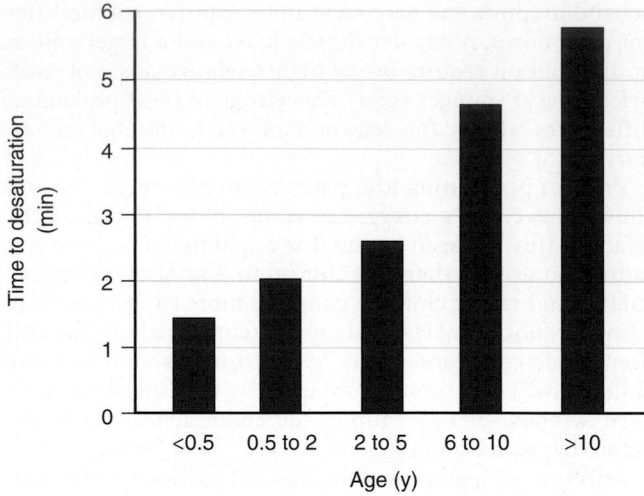

FIGURE 3–1. Time to arterial desaturation (<90% SaO_2) in apneic healthy infants and children preoxygenated at 100% O_2 for 2 to 3 minutes.[14,30,31]

handle equipment (e.g., ETT, suction devices, rescue devices), watch monitoring devices, confirm intubation, and prepare and administer medications (see Table 3–1).

Patient Preparation and Preoxygenation

Upon patient arrival and during initial resuscitation, the patient's spine is immobilized if trauma is suspected. A cardiac monitor and pulse oximeter are applied and one or more intravenous cannulas inserted. Apneic patients require bag-mask ventilation with 100% oxygen, whereas those in cardiac arrest require endotracheal intubation without the RSI technique.

If time permits, patients who are spontaneously breathing require administration of 100% oxygen with a tight-fitting non-rebreather mask. This will assist in displacing nitrogen and creating an oxygen reservoir for patients subjected to prolonged apnea due to sedation and paralysis during RSI. Under optimum conditions, the alveolar oxygen saturation rises to at least 87% to 90%.[26] With application of 100% oxygen via a tightly sealed mask and an anesthesiology closed system that actively removes expired gases, this target is reached within 2 minutes in almost all healthy infants and children breathing spontaneously.[27] In the ED, a tight-fitting non-rebreather mask with at least 10-L/min oxygen flow will lead to an adequate alveolar saturation within 3 minutes.[28,29] This will allow for maintenance of arterial saturation greater than 90% during apnea for 1.5 to 2 minutes in healthy infants ≤ 6 months old, 2 to 3.5 minutes in 7-month-old to 5-year-old children, 3.5 to 5 minutes in 6- to 10-year-old children, and over 6 minutes in children and adolescents older than 10 years (Fig. 3–1).[14,30,31] For obese or ill children (e.g., those with lung disease or higher oxygen consumption), the time to desaturation will be shorter. For apneic patients, ventilation with 100% oxygen (applying cricoid pressure) will build oxygen reserves in a similar fashion and allow for some degree of apnea during sedation, paralysis, and intubation but will increase the risk of vomiting and aspiration.

Premedication

Laryngoscopy and endotracheal intubation can lead to a variety of adverse physiologic effects, including increased

may reduce these complications and provide a safe alternate to using uncuffed ETTs.[24,25]

Personnel Preparation

Prior to patient arrival, personnel are to intubate, apply cricoid pressure, immobilize the neck, bag-mask ventilate,

intracranial pressure, increased intragastric pressure with vomiting, increased intraocular pressure, elevated blood pressure, tachycardia or bradycardia, laryngospasm, and bronchospasm. Many of these effects are exacerbated by administration of succinylcholine. To diminish these effects, a variety of medications can be given prior to sedation and paralysis (Table 3–2).

Atropine has been used for over 50 years to decrease salivation and prevent bradycardia associated with airway manipulation and succinylcholine use. Initial studies that evaluated the cardiovascular complications of endotracheal intubation and succinylcholine use demonstrated that most of these complications were due to volatile anesthetics (e.g., halothane) or hypoxia that occurred during intubation.[32-34] Children ≤1 year old have a more pronounced bradycardic response to intubation and to succinylcholine administration. At this age, atropine use prior to intubation (especially if succinylcholine is used) is often recommended.[35-37] Many experts also recommend use of atropine in older children (i.e., up to 5 to 10 years).[20,35-37] Reasons for this recommendation are less clear. The sympathetic-parasympathetic imbalance disappears in the first year of life.[38] When less cardioactive anesthetic agents (e.g., isoflurane) are administered to children receiving succinylcholine, the typical response is an

Table 3–2	Medications Used for Rapid Sequence Intubation					
	Intravenous Dose*	Onset† (min)	Duration (min)	Indications	Select Contraindications (Relative and Absolute)	Prominent Side Effects
Premedication						
Atropine	0.02 mg/kg	2–4	>120	Infants ≤1 yr old, all requiring >1 dose of succinylcholine	Extreme tachycardia or tachycardic arrhythmia	Agitation, tachycardia, arrhythmias, seizures, hyperthermia, urine retention
Lidocaine	1.5–2.0 mg/kg	3	Only useful 3 min before intubation	Head injury suspected and weak sedative given	High-degree atrioventricular block, amide anesthetic allergy	Bradycardia, heart block, seizures, altered mental status, respiratory depression
Defasciculating or priming agent	1/10th paralytic dose below	3–4	N/A	Consider if >5 yr & possible increased intracranial pressure	See succinylcholine and nondepolarizing agents below	Respiratory arrest; see paralytic side effects below
Induction						
Etomidate	0.3–0.4 mg/kg	0.25–0.5	5–15	Trauma, head injury, hypovolemia	Adrenal suppression, underlying seizures	Painful injection, myoclonus, vomiting, adrenal suppression
Thiopental	3–5 mg/kg	0.5–1.0	10–30	Head injury, normal blood pressure	Hypotension, barbiturate allergy, porphyria	Hypotension, bronchospasm (esp. if asthma), local necrosis
Ketamine (with atropine)	1–2 mg/kg	0.5–1.0	10	Asthma, noncardiac hypotension	Head injury, glaucoma, cardiogenic shock	Vomiting, hypersalivation, hypertension, tachycardia
Midazolam	0.1–0.3 mg/kg	1–5	20–30	Absence of shock (do not use in preterm infants)	Shock, hypersensitive to midazolam, narrow-angle glaucoma	Hypotension, bradycardia
Propofol	2.5 mg/kg	0.5–1.0	3–10	Useful if paralytics contraindicated, age ≥3 years, and blood pressure is OK	Hypotension; hypersensitive to sulfites, soybean oil, egg yolk, or egg lectithin	Hypotension, bradycardia, flushing, acidosis, muscular twitching, pain on injection
Paralytic						
Succinylcholine	0–1 year: 2–3 mg/kg 1–5 year: 1.5–2 mg/kg >5 years: 1–1.5 mg/kg	0.5–1	3–8	Rapid paralysis	Cannot ventilate, neurologic or muscle disease, subacute-chronic burn, hyperkalemia	Hyperkalemia; increased intracranial, gastric, and ocular pressure; fasciculations
Rocuronium	0.6 mg/kg (0.9 mg/kg)	1–1.5 (<1)	30–45 (>60)	Priming or defasciculating agent, cannot use succinylcholine	Unable to mask ventilate; use half dose if liver disease	Hypotension, tachycardia or bradycardia, arrhythmias, bronchospasm
Mivacurium	0.15–0.25 mg/kg	2–2.5	10–20	See above	Unable to mask ventilate	See above
Vecuronium	0.1–0.2 mg/kg	2–5	30–45	See above	Unable to mask ventilate	See above

*Dose for rapid sequence intubation.
†See Table 3–1 for exact timing of medication administration.

increased heart rate or tachycardia in 88% to 95%, with a decreased heart rate in 12% and bradycardia in 0 to 2%[39-41] In contrast, use of halothane with succinycholine in children leads to bradycardia in 14% to 30% of cases.[32,40,42] Addition of atropine to succinylcholine may increase the overall number of dysrhythmias compared to use of succinycholine alone.[17,43] Adding sedatives to the intubating regimen further diminishes the cardiovascular response and side effects from laryngoscopy and succinylcholine. Other important considerations include the ability of atropine to mask significant physiologic changes (e.g., assessing shock management, intracranial pressure changes, airway complications, pain, sedation level). Moreover, atropine increases temperature and the risk of malignant hyperthermia, increases ventricular arrhythmias, relaxes the lower esophageal sphincter with increased risk of aspiration, lowers the seizure threshold, induces confusion, and increases urinary retention. Atropine also has a narrow therapeutic index, increasing the potential for dosing errors.[39,43,44]

Despite prior recommendations, atropine use is no longer considered routine in infants and children undergoing intubation among many neonatologists and anesthesiologists in the United States, Canada, Europe, and Australia.[43-47] As no controlled studies have proven when atropine is beneficial, evidence-based recommendations cannot be given. Atropine should always be readily available with appropriate dosing calculated prior to all intubations as its use may become necessary. If no contraindications exist prior to intubation, atropine should be administered to all infants ≤ 1 year old, to all patients receiving a second dose of succinylcholine regardless of age, and to all patients receiving ketamine, an agent that causes prominent airway secretions. Moreover, children who are already bradycardic require atropine prior to intubation, especially when succinylcholine is used. For all other cases, ED personnel should be prepared to administer atropine if bradycardia develops during or after intubation with the realization that bradycardia may be a clue to a coexisting physiologic derangement (e.g., airway blockage, hypoxia, increased intracranial pressure, profound shock) or prolonged airway manipulation. The correct dose of atropine is 0.02 mg/kg intravenously (IV), with a minimum of 0.1 mg and maximum of 0.6 mg per single dose.

Lidocaine is a cardioactive agent that has been recommended by some experts to reduce intracranial pressure in patients with possible head trauma or space-occupying intracranial lesions who require endotracheal intubation.[36,48,49] This recommendation has been based, in part, on adult studies that evaluated the intracranial pressure response to endotracheal suctioning in patients with tumors or a recent neurosurgical procedure.[50-53] Lidocaine has been shown to suppress the cough reflex, and this mechanism may explain its benefit during endotracheal suctioning.[50-52] Others have examined the effect of IV lidocaine administration on hemodynamic parameters during intubation, assuming that blunting the hemodynamic response to intubation would correlate with a diminished intracranial pressure response. Conflicting studies have found that IV lidocaine either has no effect on blood pressure[54-63] or heart rate[55-57,60-64] or attenuates a rise in blood pressure[65-68] and heart rate[58,59,65-68] during laryngoscopy and intubation. Upon further analysis of these studies, it appears that the addition of lidocaine to a strong sedating agent (e.g., thiopental, propofol) has minimal

to no additional hemodynamic blunting effect.[57-59,61,63-65,69,70] A hemodynamic blunting effect is more likely when agents with less sedating or less cardiovascular effects are used (e.g., midazolam, etomidate).[61,71,72] The optimum lidocaine dose is 1.5 to 2 mg/kg IV.[66,68,73-75] To be effective, lidocaine must be given precisely 3 minutes prior to laryngoscopy.[67,76] If given at 1, 2, or 5 minutes preintubation, its effects are diminished or absent.[67,76] Lidocaine should be considered in patients who receive etomidate or midazolam as induction agents.

Other cardioactive agents (especially β-blockers, calcium channel blockers, and short-acting narcotics) have been used to blunt the heart rate and blood pressure response to endotracheal intubation and lower the intracranial pressure response to intubation. Of these, esmolol has been shown most useful at blunting hemodynamic parameters.[55,62] However, no pediatric studies have shown this to be a safe addition to RSI in the ED setting. Short-acting narcotics (e.g., fentanyl, alfentanil, sufentanil) also increase intracranial pressure and should be avoided during RSI if a head injury is possible.[77,78]

A "defasciculating" dose of a neuromuscular blocking agent is often administered prior to succinylcholine in adults to diminish side effects during RSI. Generally, this involves administration of a 1/10th intubating dose of a nondepolarizing agent or a 1/10th dose of succinylcholine IV 3 to 4 minutes prior to administration of a full dose of succinylcholine to decrease muscle fasciculations and intracranial, intragastric, and intraocular pressure. Children 5 years old and younger have less muscle mass and have minimal to no risk of fasciculations with succinylcholine administration. Thus, defasciculating agents are not recommended at this age. For children older than 5 years, use of a defasciculating agent is controversial. Importantly, experts have found that it is not the fasciculations that determine the cerebral response to succinylcholine. Instead, it is the effect of succinylcholine on muscle spindle afferent fibers that correlates with peak cerebral pressure and flow responses regardless of whether or not fasciculations occur.[79] It is unclear if this muscle afferent signal is blocked by administration of a defasciculating agent.[79,80] Moreover, administration of a defasciculating dose of a paralytic rarely can cause paralysis, adds to the multidrug cocktail given for RSI and thus increases the risk for dosing errors, and increases the time to intubation during RSI with succinycholine. This technique is best reserved for relatively stable patients older than 5 years when a 3- to 4-minute delay will not affect outcome.

Alternately, a similar priming dose (1/10th of paralytic dose) of a nondepolarizing agent can be administered 3 to 4 minutes prior to the intubating dose of a nondepolarizing paralytic agent. This priming dose will decrease the time required to wait for complete paralysis by nearly one half depending upon which agent is administered.

Medications (Sedatives and Paralytics)

Multiple drugs can be used to induce anesthesia or unconsciousness during RSI. Clinicians need to be fully aware of indications, contraindications, side effects, and dosing for each of these medications (see Table 3–2).

Sodium thiopental is a barbiturate that depresses the patient's reticular activating system. This agent has a rapid uptake within the brain, producing a rapid onset, usually within 30 seconds. It also causes cerebral vasoconstriction, decreasing blood flow and intracranial pressure. It is ideal for patients with isolated increased intracranial pressure without hypotension. It should be avoided in patients with hypotension, hypovolemia, or cardiovascular instability.[35]

Etomidate is a carboxylated imidazole with sedative-hypnotic properties that produces unconsciousness within 15 to 30 seconds of administration. It is not an analgesic, has little effect on blood pressure, and causes a slight decrease in systemic vascular resistance, cerebral blood flow, and intracranial pressure.[37,81] Due to its cardiovascular and central nervous system protective effects, it is an ideal induction agent in trauma patients with and without head injury.[82] Side effects include pain on injection, adrenocortical suppression (minimal with a single dose), hypertonicity, coughing, laryngospasm, hiccoughing, vomiting, occasional involuntary muscle movements, and muted ability to blunt blood pressure and heart rate responses to laryngeal manipulation.[37,81] Due to these effects, many experts recommend adding other cardioprotective agents (e.g., benzodiazepines, lidocaine) when etomidate is used as an induction agent.[37,81] The typical RSI dose is 0.3 to 0.4 mg/kg IV.[81,82]

Ketamine is a dissociative sedative that produces profound analgesia and amnesia. When used alone, it results in protective airway reflexes, spontaneous respirations, and cardiopulmonary stability. Its bronchodilating effects make it an ideal agent for intubation of asthmatics. Its hemodynamic protective effects allow for use in patients who are hypotensive due to volume depletion. Prominent salivation requires coadministration with atropine, although ketamine's catecholamine stimulatory effects limit bradycardia when coadministered with succinylcholine. Ketamine raises intracranial pressure and intraocular pressure and should be avoided if either of these effects is a concern. Ketamine may have adverse effects if cardiogenic shock is present and should be avoided in most patients with cardiac related hypotension. A typical IV dose is 1 to 2 mg/kg (administered with atropine), with an onset of less than 1 minute.[83]

Midazolam is a rapid-acting benzodiazepine that can be used as an induction agent in select cases. It has no analgesic properties and may worsen hypotension. It is most appropriately used in hemodynamically stable patients. Its dose should be reduced or an alternate agent selected in patients with severe cardiovascular instability. The typical induction dose is 0.1 to 0.3 mg/kg IV.[35]

Propofol is an IV anesthetic that can be used an induction agent. It has a rapid onset (<30 seconds) and brief duration of action. A major side effect limiting its use is hypotension. For this reason, it should be avoided in patients with multisystem trauma, hypovolemia, cardiac compromise, or hypotension from any cause. Due to prominent relaxation of pharynx and laryngeal reflexes, some authors recommend propofol in patients in whom neuromuscular blockade cannot be used.[37] Intubating conditions with propofol alone (i.e., no paralytics) are superior to those obtained while using thiopental alone for RSI.[84] Others have found that administration of a short-acting narcotic (e.g., alfentanil 20 or 40 mcg/kg IV) prior to propofol improves intubating conditions to near those of RSI with paralytic agents.[85] Since experience with propofol alone or coadministered with alfentanil is limited in the ED setting, this regimen cannot be recommended as routine at this time. The typical dose of propofol

used with RSI is 2.5 mg/kg IV given 30 to 60 seconds prior to succinylcholine.

Neuromuscular Blocking Agents

Succinylcholine is a neuromuscular blocking agent that acts by depolarizing the neuromuscular end plate and sympathetic and parasympathetic ganglia.[16] Initial muscular contractions may cause fasciculations followed by muscle relaxation until the muscle membrane repolarizes following hydrolysis of succinylcholine by plasma cholinesterase. Muscle contraction and muscle spindle afferent activity can cause increased intracranial, gastric, and ocular pressure. Hyperkalemia with cardiac arrest can occur in patients who are susceptible, including those with myopathies, neuromuscular disease, denervation injuries, shock, metabolic acidosis, crush injuries, renal failure, and subacute or chronic burns.[16,20] Patients who deteriorate immediately after succinycholine administration require confirmation of ETT position and function. If tube function and position are adequate, treatment should be directed at reversing hyperkalemia (IV calcium, sodium bicarbonate, glucose, and insulin). Bradycardia also is prominent in children ≤ 1 year old, and in children at all ages receiving more than one dose. In these instances, atropine is administered prior to succinylcholine. Disorders that affect plasma cholinesterase levels (e.g., liver disease, hereditary deficiency, anemia, renal failure, connective tissue disorders, or pregnancy) increase the duration of action of succinylcholine. The recommended dose of succinycholine is 2 to 3 mg/kg in neonates and young infants (<1 year), 1.5 to 2 mg/kg at 1 to 5 years, and 1 to 1.5 mg/kg above 5 years.[16,81] If a defasciculating agent is administered, the higher end of the dosing range should be administered. A final alternative for patients requiring rapid airway control without IV access (e.g., patients with laryngospasm) is 4 mg/kg administered intramuscularly (IM). Maximum paralysis with IM dosing occurs in 3 to 4 minutes with a duration of 19 to 23 minutes.[37]

Rocuronium is a nondepolarizing neuromuscular blocking agent. It has a rapid onset (70 to 90 seconds) and relatively short duration (≤45 minutes) following a 0.6 mg/kg dose.[16] The time to onset is comparable to succinycholine (<60 seconds) if a higher dose (0.9 mg/kg) is administered, although this regimen results in a longer duration of action (>60 minutes).[86,87] Alternately, the typical RSI dose may be split into a priming dose (1/10th original dose) and an intubating dose (9/10th original dose). The priming dose of 0.06 mg/kg can be given 3 minutes prior to the intubating dose (0.54 mg/kg) with an onset of paralysis in less than 1 minute after administration of the intubating dose.[37] Care must be used with this technique as the priming dose rarely can cause neuromuscular depression requiring mask ventilation, as well as anxiety and aspiration. In general, this drug has few hemodynamic effects making it relatively safe in critically ill patients. Since rocuronium is metabolized hepatically, duration of action is up to 50% longer if liver disease is present.[16]

Mivacurium is a short-acting nondepolarizing neuromuscular blocking agent. The recommended dose of mivacurium for RSI is 0.15 to 0.25 mg/kg IV.[16,37] Onset is 1 to 2 minutes with a typical duration of 15 to 20 minutes.[12,88] It is rapidly hydrolyzed by plasma cholinesterase, resulting in a shorter duration of action compared to other nondepolarizing neuromuscular blockers. Administration of a priming dose (0.025 mg/kg) followed 3 minutes later by an intubating dose (0.225 mg/kg) results in a more rapid onset of paralysis (~1 minute).[89] An important side effect that occasionally occurs with higher doses is cutaneous flushing and mild hypotension due to histamine release.

Vecuronium is a nondepolarizing neuromuscular blocking agent with few hemodynamic effects. A dose of 0.1 to 0.2 mg/kg IV produces adequate paralysis within 2 to 2.5 minutes, with a duration of greater than 60 minutes in infants and 25 to 55 minutes in children and adolescents.[90] A 0.01-mg/kg priming dose followed in 3 minutes by 0.15 mg/kg produces adequate paralysis in 90 seconds.

Techniques and Sequencing

All spontaneously breathing patients require preoxygenation with 100% oxygen via tight-fitting non-rebreather mask for at least 2 to 3 minutes. For patients requiring atropine, this agent should be administered 4 minutes prior to anticipated laryngoscopy (see Table 3–1). Priming or defasciculating doses of neuromuscular blocking agents, if used, are given 3 minutes prior to administration of the intubating dose of paralytic (~4 minutes prior to intubation). For optimum effect, if administered, lidocaine must be given 3 minutes prior to intubation. Sedating agents are administered 2 minutes prior to intubation, with succinylcholine or nondepolarizing paralytic administered approximately 1 minute prior to intubation (90 seconds prior to intubation if a defasciculating agent is used) (see Table 3–1). Once sedatives are injected, cricoid pressure is applied and maintained until intubation is confirmed. Spontaneously breathing patients who are able to maintain an oxygen saturation of 100% do not require assisted ventilation. Bag-mask ventilation, in this instance, may cause vomiting and aspiration. Patients who are hypoxic, in respiratory distress, or hypoventilating prior to medication administration require bag-mask ventilation while waiting for maximum sedation and paralysis.

Several techniques assist in visualization of the vocal cords and passage of the ETT. If cervical spine trauma is not a concern, the patient is placed in a sniffing position (depending upon occiput size and patient age) for a more direct view of the glottic structures. If a cervical collar is in place, removal of the collar with manual immobilization of the cervical spine allows for more movement of the mandible. Use of the BURP technique (**b**ackward, **u**pward, **r**ightward **p**ressure on the larynx) by an assistant will increase glottic visualization. Moreover, external laryngeal manipulation with the nonintubating hand by the intubator allows for a more direct view of the vocal cords. During intubation, the physician should limit intubation attempts to 30 seconds and prevent and treat hypoxia via bag-mask ventilation if attempts are unsuccessful. Tube insertion is stopped once the double lines at the end of the ETT pass the vocal cords. Correct tube depth (distance from incisors or gum line to midtrachea) can be estimated by multiplying the ETT internal diameter by 3, although this formula may cause ETTs to be placed 0.5 to 1.0 cm too deep in infants less than 2 years old (see Table 3–1).

Disposition (Postintubation)

Following intubation, placement of the ETT should immediately be confirmed. The most accurate method for confirma-

tion is capnographic waveform analysis. The presence of a waveform assures tube placement within the trachea.[91] Alternately, a colorimetric end-tidal CO_2 detection device can be attached to the endotracheal tube. A color change from purple to yellow with each breath after an initial six breaths confirms tracheal tube placement.[91] A false positive (permanent yellow) is seen if acid (vomitus) or epinephrine contaminates the colorimetric device. While ventilating, the physician should listen over the stomach for bowel sounds with bagging, and over the lateral aspects of the chest for bilateral breath sounds. Clinicians should be aware that auscultation can be inaccurate (especially in younger children) and will reveal bilateral breath sounds at the axilla in up to 15% and vapor condensation of the ET tube in 85% with esophageal intubations.[92] An alternate confirmation device that may be used in older children and adolescents is the esophageal detector device. With this device, clinicians attempt to aspirate 10 mL of air from the endotracheal tube. Ten milliliters is easily aspirated from the trachea, but will cause collapse of the esophagus and inhibit aspiration of air. After tube confirmation, the tube is immediately taped in place so that it will not move with head movement. Sedation is continued in all patients, and paralysis is considered if indicated.

Clinicians need to be prepared for deterioration before, during, and after intubation. If a patient cannot be intubated or ventilated following administration of sedating and paralytic agents, a stepwise approach must be taken.[93] The first step is to attempt insertion of a laryngeal mask airway (LMA) with ventilation via the mask. If successful, endotracheal intubation can be attempted via a conduit present in intubating LMA devices. If the patient still cannot be intubated or ventilated, trans-tracheal jet ventilation or an alternate surgical airway procedure will be required depending upon the patient's age and clinical circumstances (see Chapter 4, Intubation, Rescue Devices, and Airway Adjuncts).

Borland detailed the most common complications during pediatric intubations. These include hypoxia (4.3%), laryngospasm (2.3%), hypotension (0.6%), and cardiac arrest, aspiration, wrong drug administration, dislodged ETT, and dental injuries (0.1% to 0.2% each).[94] Prevention of these complications involves adequate preoxygenation, appropriate medication dosing, and intensive monitoring. Capnography can aid in diagnosis of many of these conditions. Tube dislodgement causes a loss of the waveform, whereas hypotension causes a gradual decrease in the height of the waveform. Malignant hyperthermia causes an increasing end-tidal CO_2 and increased height of the capnographic waveform in addition to the typical signs of dark urine, increased temperature, and muscle rigidity.

Summary

Successful rapid sequence intubation requires a stepwise algorithmic approach to preparation, patient monitoring, medication selection, dosing and administration, procedural performance, and confirmation of completion. A complete understanding of every step and every medication is essential to successful completion of this procedure. Clinicians must be prepared for deterioration at any time and the inability to intubate or ventilate after medication administration. A thorough knowledge of each of these factors will protect the patient and ensure the best possible outcome.

REFERENCES

1. Gnauck K, Lungo JB, Scalzo A, et al: Emergency intubation of the pediatric medical patient: use of anesthetic agents in the emergency department. Ann Emerg Med 23:1242–1247, 1994.

2. Marvez-Valls E, Houry D, Ernst AA, et al: Protocol for rapid sequence intubation in pediatric patients—a four year study. Med Sci Monit 8:229–234, 2002.

3. Sagarin MJ, Chiang V, Sakles JC, et al: Rapid sequence intubation for pediatric emergency airway management. Pediatr Emerg Care 18:417–423, 2002.

4. McDowall RH: Anesthesia for the pediatric patient. Chest Surg Clin N Am 7:831–848, 1997.

5. Abernathy LJ, Allan PL, Drummond GB: Ultrasound assessment of the position of the tongue during induction of anaesthesia. Br J Anaesth 65:744–748, 1990.

6. Boidin MP: Airway patency in the unconscious patient. Br J Anesth 57:306–310, 1985.

7. Nandi PR, Charlesworth CH, Taylor SJ, et al: Effect of general anaesthesia on the pharynx. Br J Anaesth 66:157–162, 1991.

8. Chow LTC, Chow SSM, Anderson RH, Gosling JA. Autonomic innervation of the human cardiac conduction system: changes from infancy to senility—an immunohistochemical and histochemical analysis. Anat Record 264:169–182, 2001.

9. Friedman WF, Pool PE, Jacobowitz D, et al: Sympathetic innervation of the developing rabbit heart: biochemical and histochemical comparisons of fetal, neonatal, and adult myocardium. Circ Res 23:25–32, 1968.

10. Kent DM, Epstein SE, Cooper T, Jacobowitz DM: Cholinergic innervation of the canine and human ventricular conducting system: anatomic and electrophysiologic correlation. Circulation 50:948–955, 1974.

11. Goudsouzian NG: Mivacurium in infants and children. Paediatr Anaesth 7:183–190, 1997.

12. Goudsouzian NG: Anatomy and physiology in relation to pediatric anesthesia. In Katz J (ed): Anesthesia and Uncommon Pediatric Diseases, 2nd ed. Philadelphia: WB Saunders, 1993, pp 1–18.

13. Cook DR. Paediatric anaesthesia: pharmacological considerations. Drugs 12:212-221, 1976.

*14. Benumof JL, Dagg R, Benumof R: Critical hemoglobin desaturation will occur before return to an unparalyzed state following 1 mg/kg intravenous succinylcholine. Anesthesiology 87:979–982, 1997.

*15. Thorsteinsson A, Jonmarker C, Larsson A, et al: Functional residual capacity in anesthetized children: normal values and values in children with cardiac anomalies. Anesthesiology 73:876–881, 1990.

16. Gronert BJ, Brandom BW: Neuromuscular blocking drugs in infants and children. Pediatr Clin North Am 41:73–91, 1994.

17. Kinouchi K, Tanigami H, Tashiro C, et al: Duration of apnea in anesthetized infants and children required for desaturation of hemoglobin to 95%: the influence of upper respiratory infection. Anesthesiology 77:1105–1107, 1992.

18. Macchiarroli R, Rothrock SG, McCoy K, Green SM: An assessment of the Mallampati criteria, incisor distance, mandibular distance and modified thyromental distance for predicting difficult intubations in the emergency department [abstract]. Acad Emerg Med 7:527, 2000.

19. Levitan R, Ochroch EA: Airway management and direct laryngoscopy: a review and update. Crit Care Clin 16:373–388, 2000.

20. Gronert BJ, Motoyama EK: Induction of anesthesia and endotracheal intubation. In Motoyama EK, Davis PJ (eds): Smith's Anesthesia for Infants and Children, 6th ed. St. Louis: Mosby, 1996, pp 281–312.

21. Luten RC, Wears RL, Broselow J, et al: Length based endotracheal tube and emergency equipment in pediatrics. Ann Emerg Med 21:900–904, 1992.

22. Khinc IIII, Corddy DH, Kettrick RG, et al: Comparison of cuffed and uncuffed endotracheal tubes in young children during general anesthesia. Anesthesiology 86:627–631, 1997.

23. King BR, Baker MD, Braitman LE, et al: Endotracheal tube selection in children: a comparison of four methods. Ann Emerg Med 22:530–534, 1993.

24. Fine GF, Borland LM: The future of the cuffed endotracheal tube. Paediatr Anaesth 14:38–42, 2004.

25. Newth CJ, Rachman B, Patel N, Hammer J: The use of cuffed vs. uncuffed endotracheal tubes in pediatric intensive care. J Pediatr 144:333–337, 2004.

26. Benumof JL: Preoxygenation: best method for both efficacy and efficiency. Anesthesiology 9:603–605, 1999.

*27. Morrison JE Jr, Collier E, Friesen RH, Logan L: Preoxygenation before laryngoscopy in children: how long is enough? Paediatr Anaesth 8:293–298, 1998.

28. Drummond GB, Park GR: Arterial oxygen saturation before intubation of the trachea: an assessment of oxygenation techniques. Br J Anaesth 56:987–993, 1984.

29. Videira RL, Neto PP, do Amaral RV, Freeman JA: Preoxygenation in children: for how long? Acta Anaesthesiol Scand 36:109–111, 1992.

30. Xue FS, Luo LK, Tong SY, et al: Study of the safe threshold of apneic period in children during anesthesia induction. J Clin Anesth 8:568–574, 1996.

31. Patel R, Lenczyk M, Hannallah RS, McGill WA: Age and the onset of desaturation in apnoeic children. Can J Anaesth 41:771–774, 1994.

32. Friesen RH, Lichtor JL: Cardiovascular depression during halothane anesthesia in infants: study of three induction techniques. Anesth Analg 61:42–45, 1982.

33. Leigh MD, McCoy DD, Belton MK, Lewis GB: Bradycardia following intravenous administration of succinylcholine chloride to infants and children. Anesthesiology 18:698–702, 1957.

34. Magee DA, Sweet PT, Holland AJ: Effect of atropine on bradydysrhythmias induced by succinylcholine following pretreatment with D-tubocurarine. Can Anaesth Soc J 29:573–576, 1982.

35. Bledsoe GH, Schexnayder SM: Pediatric rapid sequence intubation: a review. Pediatr Emerg Care 20:339–344, 2004.

36. Gerardi MJ, Sacchetti AD, Cantor RM, et al: Rapid sequence intubation of the pediatric patient. Ann Emerg Med 28:55–74, 1996.

37. Wadbrook PS: Advances in airway pharmacology: emerging trends and evolving controversy. Emerg Med Clin North Am 18:767–788, 2000.

38. Guyton DC, Scharf SM: Should atropine be routine in children? Can J Anaesth 43:754–755, 1996.

*39. Blanc VF: Atropine and succinylcholine: beliefs and controversies in paediatric anaesthesia. Can J Anaesth 42:1–7, 1995.

40. Lerman J, Robinson S, Willis MM, et al: Succinylcholine-induced heart rate changes in children during isoflurane and halothane. Anesthesiology 59:A443, 1983.

41. Thurlow AC: Cardiac dysrhythmias in outpatient dental anaesthesia in children: the effect of prophylactic intravenous atropine. Anaesthesia 27:429–435, 1972.

42. Annila P, Rorarius M, Reinikainen P, et al: Effect of pre-treatment with atropine or glycopyrrolate on arrhythmias during halothane anaesthesia for adenoidectomy in children. Br J Anaesth 80:756–760, 1998.

43. McAuliffe G, Bissonnette B, Boutin C: Should the routine use of atropine before succinylcholine in children be reconsidered? Can J Anaesth 42:724–729, 1995.

44. Johr M: Is it time to question the routine use of anticholinergic agents in paediatric anaesthesia? Paediatr Anaesth 9:99–101, 1999.

45. Mirakhur RK: Preanaesthetic medication: a survey of current usage. J R Soc Med 84:481–483, 1991.

46. Morris J, Cook TM: Rapid sequence induction: a national survey. Anaesthesia 56:1090–1097, 2001.

47. Parnis SJ, van der Walt JH: A national survey of atropine use by Australian anaesthetists. Anaesth Intensive Care 22:61–65, 1994.

48. Lev R, Rosen P: Prophylactic lidocaine use preintubation: a review. J Emerg Med 12:499–506, 1994.

49. O'Connor RE, Levine BJ: Airway management in the trauma setting. In Ferrera PC, Colucciello SA, Marx JA, et al (eds): Trauma Management: An Emergency Medicine Approach. St. Louis: Mosby, 2000, pp 52–74.

50. Donegon MF, Bedford RF: Intravenously administered lidocaine prevents intracranial hypertension during endotracheal suctioning. Anesthesiology 52:516–518, 1980.

51. White PF, Schlobohm RM, Pitts LH, Lindauer JM: A randomized study of drugs for preventing increases in intracranial pressure during endotracheal suctioning. Anesthesiology 57:242–244, 1982.

52. Yano M, Nishiyama H, Yokota H, et al: Effect of lidocaine on ICP response to endotracheal suctioning. Anesthesiology 64:651–653, 1986.

53. Hamill JF, Bedford RF, Weaver DC, Colohan AR: Lidocaine before endotracheal intubation: intravenous or laryngotracheal? Anesthesiology 55:578–581, 1981.

54. Chraemmer-Jorgensen B, Hoilund-Carlsen PF, Marving J, Christensen V: Lack of effect of intravenous lidocaine on hemodynamic responses

---

*Selected reading.

to rapid sequence induction of general anesthesia: a double-blind controlled clinical trial. Anesth Analg 65:1037–1041, 1986.

55. Feng CK, Chan KH, Liu KN, et al: A comparison of lidocaine, fentanyl, and esmolol for attenuation of cardiovascular response to laryngoscopy and tracheal intubation. Acta Anaesthesiol Sin 34:61–67, 1996.

56. Inada E, Cullen DJ, Nemeskal AR, Teplick R: Effect of labetalol or lidocaine on the hemodynamic response to intubation: a controlled randomized double-blind study. J Clin Anesth 1:207–213, 1989.

57. Kindler CH, Schumacher PG, Schneider MC, Urwyler A: Effects of intravenous lidocaine and/or esmolol on hemodynamic responses to laryngoscopy and intubation: a double-blind, controlled clinical trial. J Clin Anesth 8:491–496, 1996.

58. Liu J, Latson TW, Wu G, White PF: Effects of IV and or aerosolized lidocaine on the hemodynamic and EEG responses to laryngoscopy and tracheal intubation [abstract]. Anesthesiology 79:A157, 1993.

59. Miller CD, Warren SJ: IV lignocaine fails to attenuate the cardiovascular response to laryngoscopy and tracheal intubation. Br J Anaesth 65:216–219, 1990.

60. Pathak D, Slater RM, Ping SS, From RP: Effects of alfentanil and lidocaine on the hemodynamic responses to laryngoscopy and tracheal intubation. J Clin Anesth 2:81–85, 1990.

61. Roelofse JA, Shipton EA, Joubert JJ, Grotepass FW: A comparison of labetalol, acebutolol, and lidocaine for controlling the cardiovascular responses to endotracheal intubation for oral surgical procedures. J Oral Maxillofac Surg 45:835–841, 1987.

*62. Singh H, Vichitvejpaisal P, Gaines GY, White PF: Comparative effects of lidocaine, esmolol, and nitroglycerin in modifying the hemodynamic response to laryngoscopy and intubation. J Clin Anesth 7:5–8, 1995.

63. Splinter WM: Intravenous lidocaine does not attenuate the haemodynamic response of children to laryngoscopy and tracheal intubation. Can J Anaesth 37(4 Pt 1):440–443, 1990.

64. Lin PL, Wang YP, Chou YM, et al: Lack of intravenous lidocaine effects on HRV changes of tracheal intubation during induction of general anesthesia. Acta Anaesthesiol Sin 39:77–82, 2001.

65. Hamaya Y, Dohi S: Differences in cardiovascular response to airway stimulation at different sites and blockade of the responses by lidocaine. Anesthesiology 93:95–103, 2000.

66. Levitt MA, Dresden GM: The efficacy of esmolol versus lidocaine to attenuate the hemodynamic response to intubation in isolated head trauma patients. Acad Emerg Med 8:19–24, 2001.

67. Tam S, Chung F, Campbell M: Intravenous lidocaine: optimal time of injection before tracheal intubation. Anesth Analg 66:1036–1038, 1987.

68. Warner LO, Balch DR, Davidson PJ: Is intravenous lidocaine an effective adjuvant for endotracheal intubation in children undergoing induction of anesthesia with halothane-nitrous oxide? J Clin Anesth 9:270–274, 1997.

69. Helfman SM, Gold MI, DeLisser EA, Herrington CA: Which drug prevents tachycardia and hypertension associated with tracheal intubation: lidocaine, fentanyl, or esmolol? Anesth Analg 72:482–486, 1993.

70. Mulholland D, Carlisle RJ: Intubation with propofol augmented with intravenous lignocaine. Anaesthesia 46:312–313, 1991.

71. Nishiyama T, Misawa K, Yokoyama T, Hanaoka K: Effects of combining midazolam and barbiturate on the response to tracheal intubation: changes in autonomic nervous system. J Clin Anesth 14:344–348, 2002.

72. Papazian L, Albanese J, Thirion X, et al: Effect of bolus doses of midazolam on intracranial pressure and cerebral perfusion pressure in patients with severe head injury. Br J Anaesth 71:267–271, 1993.

73. Lev R, Rosen P: Prophylactic lidocaine use preintubation: a review. J Emerg Med 12:499–506, 1994.

74. Skinner HJ, Biswas A, Mahajan RP: Evaluation of intubating conditions with rocuronium and either propofol or etomidate for rapid sequence induction. Anaesthesia 53:702–710, 1998.

75. Weiss-Bloom LJ, Reich DL: Haemodynamic responses to tracheal intubation following etomidate and fentanyl for anaesthetic induction. Can J Anaesth 39:780–785, 1992.

76. Takita K, Morimoto Y, Kemmotsu O: Tracheal lidocaine attenuates the cardiovascular response to endotracheal intubation. Can J Anaesth 48:732–736, 2001.

77. Albanese J, Viviand X, Potie F, et al: Sufentanil, fentanyl, and alfentanil in head trauma patients: a study on cerebral hemodynamics. Crit Care Med 27:407–411, 1999.

78. DeLima LGR: Cerebrovascular autoregulation may be the probable mechanism responsible for fentanyl and sufentanil induced increases in ICP in patients with head trauma. Anesthesiology 79:186–187, 1993.

79. Lanier WL, Iaizzo PA, Milde JH: Cerebral function and muscle afferent activity following intravenous succinylcholine in dogs anesthetized with halothane: the effects of pretreatment with a defasciculating dose of pancuronium. Anesthesiology 71:87–95, 1989.

80. Stirt JA, Grosslight KR, Bedford RF, Vollmer D: "Defasciculation" with metocurine prevents succinylcholine-induced increases in intracranial pressure. Anesthesiology 67:50–53, 1987.

81. Rodricks MB, Deutschman CS: Emergency airway management: indications and methods in the face of confounding conditions. Crit Care Clin 16:389–409, 2000.

*82. Sokolove PE, Price DD, Okada P: The safety of etomidate for emergency rapid sequence intubation of pediatric patients. Pediatr Emerg Care 16:18–21, 2000.

83. Green SM, Krauss B: Procedural sedation terminology: moving beyond "conscious sedation." Ann Emerg Med 39:433–435, 2002.

84. McKeating K, Bali IM, Dundee JW: The effects of thiopentone and propofol on upper airway integrity. Anaesthesia 43:638–640, 1988.

85. Hiller A, Klemola UM, Saarnivaara L: Tracheal intubation after induction of anaesthesia with propofol, alfentanil, and lidocaine without neuromuscular blocking drugs in children. Acta Anaesthesiol Scand 37:725–729, 1993.

86. Cheng CA, Aun GS, Gin T: Comparison of rocuronium and suxemethonium for rapid tracheal intubation in children. Paediatr Anaesth 12:140–145, 2002.

87. Weiss JH, Gratz I, Goldberg ME, et al: Double blind comparison of two doses of rocuronium and succinylcholine for rapid sequence intubation. J Clin Anesth 9:379–382, 1997.

88. Ostergaard D, Gatke MR, Berg H, et al: The pharmacodynamics and pharmacokinetics of mivacurium in children. Acta Anaesthesiol Scand 46:512–518, 2002.

89. Chu YC, Lim SM, Huang YC, et al: Priming technique accelerates the onset time of mivacurium in children undergoing halothane anesthesia. Acta Anaesthesiol Sin 35:15–20, 1997.

90. Kalli I, Meretoja OA: Duration of action of vecuronium in infants and children anesthetized without potent inhalational agents. Acta Anaesthesiol Scand 33:29–33, 1989.

91. Bhende M: Capnography in the pediatric emergency department. Pediatr Emerg Care 15:64–69, 1999.

92. Andersen KH, Hald A: Assessing the position of the tracheal tube: the reliability of different methods. Anaesthesia 44:984–985, 1989.

93. Combes X, Le Roux B, Suen P, et al: Unanticipated difficult airway in anesthetized patients: prospective validation of a management algorithm. Anesthesiology 100:1146–1150, 2004.

94. Borland LM: Complications of 9615 anesthetics given over one year. Anesthesiology 71:A920, 1989.

Intubation, Rescue Devices, and Airway Adjuncts

Aaron J. Donoghue, MD, MSCE and Ron M. Walls, MD

Key Points

Preservation of oxygenation of the brain and vital organs is the most important step in pediatric resuscitation.

The most prominent anatomic differences of a pediatric airway are the relatively large tongue, the superior larynx, and the narrowest point of the airway being at the cricoid cartilage. Respiratory physiologic differences in young children result in a greater tendency for hypoxemia.

Failure of oral intubation is uncommon, but several rescue devices and alternative approaches exist and are well validated.

Indications

The emergency physician is responsible for airway management for patients in the emergency department (ED), and therefore has a responsibility for the decision making, drugs, and techniques that constitute the armamentarium of modern airway management. The challenge in caring for the acutely ill or injured child lies in determining which interventions are needed, and in balancing the risks and benefits of these interventions. The need for intubation can be obvious, as when the child presents in cardiopulmonary arrest, but it is in the more subtle cases that the judgment of the provider is most important. In general, intubation is safe and highly effective, with a low rate of adverse events, and patient outcome is more often threatened by a delay in intubation than by an intubation that might have been unnecessary or undertaken too early. The key management decision is whether, and when, to intubate the patient with serious illness, but whose airway or respirations have not yet failed. There is no easy way to determine which patients should be intubated, or when; however, the decision to undertake intubation or another form of active airway management is based

on an assessment of the patient with respect to three central issues:

I. Failure of airway maintenance or protection
   A. Coma
   B. Loss of intrinsic tone of airway musculature (e.g., from critical illness, intoxication)
   C. Loss of airway protective reflexes
      1. Inability to swallow/expectorate secretions adequately (more reliable measure than the gag reflex)
      2. Inability to cough
      3. Inability to keep airway patent (upper airway obstruction from tongue, foreign body, inflammatory or infectious process)
II. Failure of oxygenation or ventilation
   A. Ventilatory failure that is not reversible by other means (e.g., opioid respiratory depression is reversible by administration of naloxone)
   B. Hypoxemia that is not responsive to supplemental oxygen (e.g., pneumonia with persistent hypoxemia despite high flow oxygen)
III. Anticipatory management: What is the patient's anticipated clinical course? Is it likely that deterioration will occur, and threaten either the airway or the patient?
   A. Injury/illness with foreseeable need to control airway (e.g., septic shock with concern for metabolic debt and work of breathing, anterior neck injury with potential for worsening airway obstruction, multiply injured trauma patient with shock or need for multiple invasive procedures)
   B. Need for diagnostic or interventional procedure requiring patient cooperation (e.g., computed tomography, magnetic resonance imaging, painful procedures) when procedural sedation is not possible or is contraindicated (e.g., patient too ill or unstable for sedation without airway control)
   C. Securing of airway for interfacility transport or transport to an area of the hospital where resuscitation will be difficult if the patient deteriorates (e.g., computed tomography, magnetic resonance imaging)

A recent summary of pediatric data from the National Emergency Airway Registry (NEAR) project reported on the indications for intubation in 156 pediatric patients in 11 hospitals. A total of 77 (49%) were intubated as a result of trauma (38 of 77 sustained traumatic brain injury), 25 (16%) were intubated during management of status epilepticus, and 9 (6%) were intubated during management of a toxic ingestion. Other diagnoses included asthma, congestive heart failure, sepsis, pneumonia, and coma (Table 4–1).[1]

Contraindications

- There are no contraindications for airway management in general, but patient condition might dictate which approach is best.
- Cricothyrotomy is contraindicated in children under 10 years old, in whom it is technically difficult. In this age group, needle cricothyrotomy is preferable when access from above the glottis is not possible.
- Identification of attributes that predict difficult intubation (Box 4–1), especially when accompanied by attributes of difficult bag-mask ventilation, is a relative

contraindication for rapid sequence intubation (RSI; see Chapter 3 Rapid Sequence Intubation), unless as part of a double setup in which the backup, or rescue, maneuver is planned for and readily available.

Preparation/Consent

Pertinent Past Medical History

It is often impossible to obtain detailed historical information before intubating a critically ill child. If time permits, however, a past medical history should focus on whether the patient has been intubated before and if any problems were experienced. The patient's birth history may be contributory: former premature infants have a higher incidence of subglottic stenosis and of chronic respiratory insufficiency. Patients with certain genetic syndromes (e.g., Down syndrome, mucopolysaccharidoses) may be predisposed to distorted airway anatomy. It is essential to seek any history compatible with muscular dystrophy, the presence of which contraindicates the use of succinylcholine. If the current indication for endotracheal intubation (ETI) is trauma, maintaining cervical spine immobility is paramount, and an additional operator will be required for ETI. Likewise, certain preexisting diagnoses (e.g., Down syndrome) may predispose the patient to atlantoaxial instability, in which case cervical spine precautions should be employed. A list of preexisting medical diagnoses that should alert the emergency physician to the possibility of a difficult airway is provided in Table 4–2.[2]

All patients should be assumed to have a full stomach, and planning should account for this. In the absence of an identified difficult airway, RSI is the procedure of choice.

Box 4–1 *The Intubation Difficulty Scale**

- **Number of intubation attempts > 1**
- **Number of intubators > 1**
- **Number of alternative techniques used**
- **Cormack glottic visualization score (0 = complete, 3 = nonvisualization)**
- **Lifting force for laryngoscopy (0 or 1)**
- **External laryngeal pressure to visualize cords (0 or 1)**
- **Vocal cords abducted? (0 or 1)**

*An ideal intubation would receive a score of zero.

Table 4–1   Indications for Intubation: NEAR I

Trauma	
Head injury	38
General management	24
Airway problem	9
Face/neck trauma	2
Burn/inhalational injury	2
Traumatic arrest	2
Total (trauma)	**77**
Medical	
Status epilepticus	25
Toxin	9
Cardiac arrest	7
Asthma	6
Pneumonia	3
Sepsis	3
Coma	2
Congestive heart failure	2
Other	20
Total (medical)	**77**
Unknown	2
Total Overall	**156**

From Sagarin MJ, Chiang V, Sakles JC, et al: Rapid sequence intubation for pediatric emergency airway management. Pediatr Emerg Care 18:417–423, 2002.

Table 4–2   Preexisting Conditions That May Predispose to Difficult Airway Management in Children

Newborn Period	Trauma
Tracheal agenesis	Cervical spine injury
Laryngeal atresia	Face/neck trauma
Congenital fusion of jaws	Burn/inhalational injury
Congenital laryngeal stenosis	**Mass Lesions**
Laryngeal web	Head/neck tumors
Congenital ankylosis of	Hematoma/hemangiomas
temporomandibular joint	Lingual thyroid, epiglottic cyst
Cystic hygroma	
Craniofacial Dysmorphology	**Metabolic/Musculoskeletal**
Cleft lip/palate	**Disorders**
Micrognathic disorders (Pierre-	Mucopolysaccharidoses
Robin, Treacher-Collins, etc.)	Mucolipidoses
Goldenhar syndrome	Beckwith-Wiedemann syndrome
	Arthrogryposis
	Achondroplasia
Acute/Chronic Inflammatory	**Other**
Diseases	Trisomy 21
Epiglottitis	Cri-du-chat syndrome
Tonsillitis	Russell-Silver syndrome
Head/neck abcess	Klippel-Feil syndrome
(retropharyngeal,	Cockayne syndrome
peritonsillar,	
submandibular)	
Gangrenous stomatitis	
Ludwig's angina	

From Frei FJ, Ummenhofer W: Difficult airway in pediatrics. Paediatr Anaesth 6:251–263, 1996.

Anatomy

Pediatric intubation is, in general, easily accomplished, and the incidence of difficult intubation is less than in adults, who have many more acquired conditions that make intubation difficult. Important anatomic differences, however, distinguish the pediatric intubation from the adult, and, to a lesser degree, intubation of the infant from that of the older child. Age-related variations in size also mandate careful equipment selection and drug dosing. Specific considerations related to pediatric intubation are as follows:

- **Size**—airway structures are smaller and the field of vision with laryngoscopy is more narrow
- **Adenoidal hypertrophy** is common in young children, leading to:
  - Greater difficulty with nasotracheal intubation
  - Greater risk for injury to adenoidal tissue with resultant bleeding in the hypopharynx when laryngoscopy is performed
- The **tongue is large** relative to the size of the oropharynx.
- **Superior larynx** (Fig. 4–1)—often imprecisely referred to as "anterior," the laryngeal opening in infants and young children is actually located in a *superior* position (in infants, the larynx is opposite C3-4 as opposed to C4-5 in adults). This makes the angle of the laryngeal opening with respect to the base of the tongue more acute and visualization by direct laryngoscopy more difficult.
- The **hyoepiglottic ligament** (connects base of tongue to epiglottis) is more elastic in young children; thus, a laryngoscope blade in the vallecula may not elevate the epiglottis as efficiently as in an adult.
- The **epiglottis** of children is narrow and angled acutely with respect to the tracheal axis; thus the epiglottis covers the tracheal opening to a greater extent and can be more difficult to mobilize.
- The **narrowest point** of the young child's airway occurs at the level of the *cricoid cartilage* instead of at the level of the glottic opening itself.

Physiology

Respiratory Physiology

LUNG

Infants have fewer and smaller alveoli than young children, and their overall gas exchange surface area is disproportionately small. Surface area reaches proportions similar to adulthood by 8 years of age. Channels for collateral ventilation (pores of Kuhn and Lambert's channels) are absent in infancy. The overall effect of these phenomena is a greater tendency for alveolar hypoventilation and for the development of atelectasis during a respiratory illness.[3]

RESPIRATORY MECHANICS

The pediatric thoracic skeleton is largely cartilaginous and much more compliant than the adult skeleton. Elastic recoil of the chest wall in the young child is essentially absent. A given change in thoracic pressure will result in a larger change in lung volume, similar to the physiology seen in an adult with emphysema. A given change in volume is associated with little or no change in pressure, so that a greater amount of work is required to generate a tidal breath.

The high compliance of the pediatric chest wall results in a closing volume (CV) (volume at which terminal bronchioles collapse because they are no longer supported by elastic recoil) that can be elevated with respect to functional residual capacity (FRC). If the already diminished elastic recoil is impaired (e.g., by supine positioning), CV can exceed FRC to an even greater extent, resulting in the absence of ventilation of some lung segments during normal tidal breathing. Young patients therefore have a greater tendency for intrapulmonary shunting and hypoxemia with the positioning required for airway management.

Accessory respiratory muscles in young children are composed of a lower percentage of slow-twitch muscle fibers and are more susceptible to fatigue compared to the diaphragm. Also, the architecture of the pediatric thorax (horizontal rib orientation with extensive cartilage composition) is such that

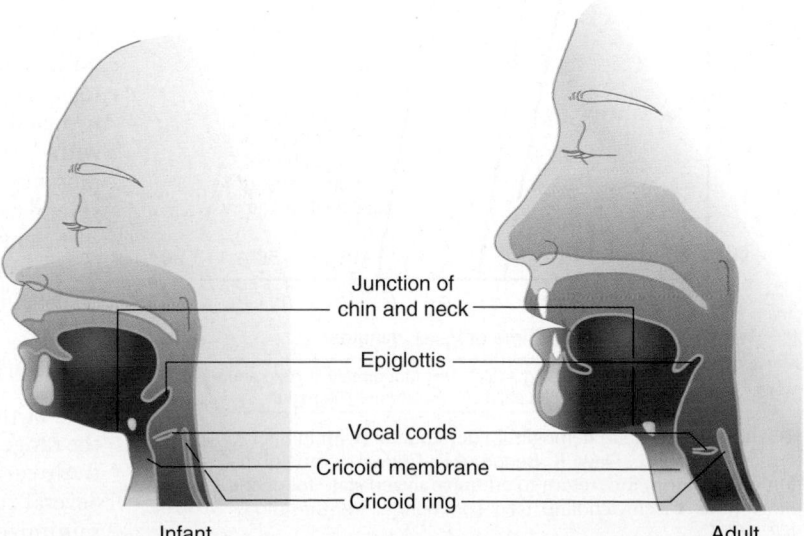

FIGURE 4–1. Relative position of the pediatric larynx in the neck compared to that in the adult. (Adapted from Walls RA [ed]: Manual of Emergency Airway Management. Philadelphia: Lippincott Williams & Wilkins, 2000.)

Junction of chin and neck

Epiglottis

Vocal cords

Cricoid membrane

Cricoid ring

Infant

Adult

intercostal and suprasternal muscles are poorly recruited to assist in respiratory effort.

AIRWAY

Airway diameter and length increase with age. The distal airway (bronchioles) lags in growth behind the proximal airway during the first few years of life. Poiseuille's law states that airway resistance is inversely proportional to the fourth power of the radius of the airway. Thus young children have higher resistance to airflow at baseline in their lower airways, and a change in airway diameter of a given dimension will have a much more profound effect on airway resistance in a small child than in an older child or adult. Such a change can occur as a result of edema, obstruction, or excess secretions. Illnesses that affect the caliber of small airways (such as asthma and viral bronchiolitis) produce a disproportionate increase in work of breathing in infants and children.[3]

CELLULAR OXYGENATION

Resting oxygen consumption in the newborn is twice that of an adult (6 mL/kg/min vs. 3 mL/kg/min), and increased adipose tissue provides a greater mass per volume of FRC than in the adult. Oxygen consumption in infants is extremely sensitive to physiologic derangements such as fever and hypothermia. The oxyhemoglobin dissociation curve for young infants is shifted to the left (greater affinity of hemoglobin for oxygen and poorer tissue oxygen delivery) by the presence of elevated amounts of fetal hemoglobin.[3]

Combined Effects of Respiratory Physiologic Factors

The summary effects of the various respiratory physiologic phenomena described previously are a greater tendency for hypoxemia and arterial desaturation. Figure 4–2 shows a

model of oxyhemoglobin desaturation[4] to demonstrate the time to critical desaturation of several classes of patients, including children. According to this model, a healthy 10-kg child will desaturate to 90% after approximately 3 minutes of apnea, much more quickly than healthy or even moderately ill adults.[5] This rapid desaturation is a product of two attributes: the greater oxygen consumption in children (described earlier) and the greater body mass index of young children, placing a greater relative demand on their pulmonary oxygen capacity. Desaturation rates vary with age. Infants preoxygenated with 100% oxygen for 2 minutes can maintain their oxyhemoglobin saturation above 90% for approximately 2 minutes, compared with almost 2.5 minutes for toddlers and over 4 minutes for children greater than 3 years of age. The time required for the saturation to fall from 95% to 90% is significantly shorter in infants than older children as well (8 seconds compared with 16 seconds).[6] The rate of oxyhemoglobin desaturation has not been determined for children with varying degrees of systemic or pulmonary illness or injury, but it is logical to assume that it is even more rapid than described here, reinforcing the requirement for continuous monitoring of oxyhemoglobin saturation during intubation, as during all phases of the management of a seriously ill or injured child. When oxyhemoglobin saturation falls to 90%, intubation attempts are paused to permit bag-mask ventilation to restore adequate (>95%) oxygen saturation.

Cardiovascular Physiology

Children have higher vagal tone than older patients, so laryngoscopy has a much greater tendency to produce vagally mediated bradycardia in young children. Succinylcholine, which is formed by joining two acetylcholine molecules, can have significant cardiac muscarinic effect in children, aggravating the vagal effects of the laryngoscopy. Atropine, 0.02 mg/kg, should be administered to children under 10 years of age who are to receive succinylcholine for intubation. Children have a limited ability to vary stroke volume in order to maintain cardiac output, and, as a result, tachycardia is often the sole compensatory mechanism in low cardiac output states. Vagally mediated bradycardia can have a significantly deleterious effect on cardiac output.

Neonatal Physiology

Neonates in particular have significantly fragile cardiopulmonary adaptive mechanisms. Hypoxia is very poorly tolerated and causes paradoxical bradycardia. Additionally, neonatal respiratory control is immature and uncoordinated, with newborns typically exhibiting periodic breathing (absence of respiratory effort for up to 15 seconds) for up to several weeks of life. Minute ventilation does not increase sufficiently in response to hypercarbia, so hypoxemia results in transient hyperventilation and actually progresses to respiratory depression as oxygen tension falls.

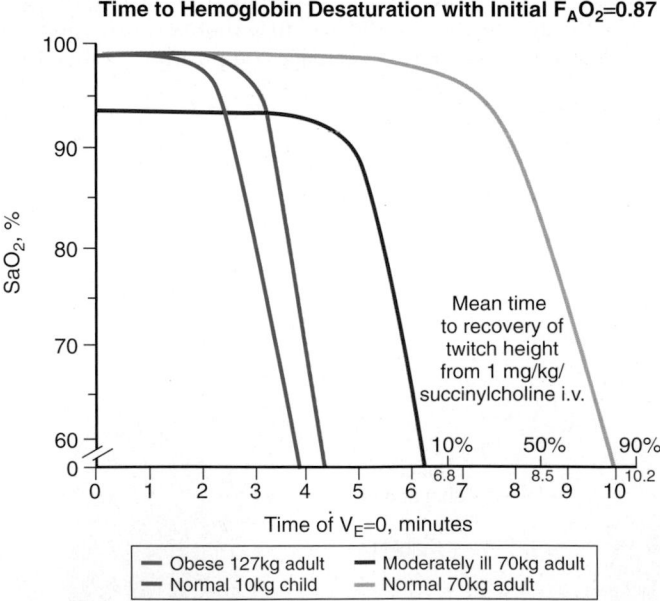

Time to Hemoglobin Desaturation with Initial F_AO_2=0.87

Mean time to recovery of twitch height from 1 mg/kg/ succinylcholine i.v.

— Obese 127kg adult   — Moderately ill 70kg adult
— Normal 10kg child   — Normal 70kg adult

FIGURE 4–2. Time to hemoglobin desaturation with initial F_AO_2 = 0.87. (From Benumof JL, Dagg R, Benumof R: Critical hemoglobin desaturation will occur before return to an unparalyzed state following 1 mg/kg intravenous succinylcholine [see comment]. Anesthesiology 87:979–982, 1997.)

Equipment

One of the challenges in airway management of children is the range of sizes of equipment necessary for safely and effectively caring for patients throughout the pediatric age range. Several rules of thumb have been designed and validated to minimize confusion pertaining to this issue; among the most prevalently used is the length-based equipment selection, commonly accomplished through use of the Broselow-Luten tape and color-coding system. This and other sizing schema are discussed in more detail in this section as well as in Chapter 2 (Respiratory Distress and Respiratory Failure).

Ventilation Equipment

Bag-Valve-Mask Devices (Anesthesia vs. Self-inflating)

Bag-valve-mask (BVM) devices fall into two broad classes. Self-inflating bags, or Ambu bags, are semirigid plastic elliptical bags that return to their original shape spontaneously after being compressed. A properly configured self-inflating bag has a one-way exhalation valve, requiring the bag to replenish itself from a high-flow oxygen supply, often combined with a reservoir system, to deliver high concentrations of oxygen (>90%). These bags can also deliver high concentrations of oxygen during active breathing by the patient.

Anesthesia circuits consist of collapsible bags connected to an expiratory limb and a venting mechanism, most often a one-way valve allowing the egress of exhaled gases. Advantages to the use of anesthesia bags include the ability to provide 100% oxygen without a reservoir and a greater sensitivity to detect changes in airway pressure, with both spontaneous and assisted breaths. Most anesthesia circuits have an adjustable valve incorporated into the venting mechanism, allowing the operator to adjust the maximum amount of inspiratory pressure delivered to the patient; this may enable the operator to minimize barotrauma from elevated inflating pressures. Disadvantages of anesthesia circuits include the fact that they are more difficult to use by inexperienced personnel and the fact that they cannot be used in the absence of an air or oxygen source.

Suctioning

Ideally two separate suction devices should be available and opened to maximal suction. One should have a rigid tonsillar suction (Yankauer) tip attached for suctioning the mouth and oropharynx, and the second should have a smaller caliber flexible catheter for suctioning thin secretions in the hypopharynx or via the endotracheal tube, after intubation. If only one suction source is available, both suction tip devices should be at hand so that they can be interchanged if necessary.

Endotracheal Intubation

Laryngoscope

The two predominant types of laryngoscope blades used in pediatric airway management are the straight (Miller, Wisconsin) and curved (MacIntosh). Both types can be used in children and adults successfully depending on operator experience. Most pediatric practitioners favor the use of straight blades when intubating young children because of the laxity of the supporting structures of the epiglottis discussed previously. For infants less than 1 year, straight laryngoscope blades with the widest flange (e.g., Wis-Hipple, Wisconsin, Flagg) are best for controlling the relatively large tongue.[7,8] For older children, blades with a narrower flange (e.g., Miller) can control the tongue and decrease trauma to the gingiva and teeth. Further modification with a curve at the tip allows for the options of either direct elevation of the

Table 4–3	Laryngoscope Blades and Sizes	
Laryngoscope Blade	Patient Age	Patient Length (Broselow-Luten Tape Color)
Miller 0	Newborns up to 2.5 kg	NA
Miller 1	0–3 mo	60.75–85 cm (pink, red, purple)
Wis-Hipple 1.5 Miller 2	3 mo–3 yr >3 yr	85–132.5 cm (yellow, white, blue, orange)
Miller 3	Large adolescents	137.5–155 cm (green)

epiglottis via the blade or blade insertion into the vallecula (e.g., modified Miller, Phillips) in older infants.[8] Appropriate sizes of blades for children of different ages, according to both age and Broselow-Luten sizing, are shown in Table 4–3.

When properly inserted, the tip of a straight laryngoscope blade rests underneath the tip of the epiglottis, and, when upward force is applied, the blade physically lifts the epiglottis out of the way to expose the glottic opening, as depicted in Figure 4–3A. The curved blade can be used in exactly the same manner, but usually the blade is positioned such that the tip lies in the vallecula, anterior to the epiglottis, and upward traction pulls the epiglottis up and exposes the glottic opening, as shown in Figure 4–3B.

Endotracheal Tubes

The two most commonly applied rules of thumb for sizing of endotracheal tubes (ETTs) are the age-based rule and selection based on body length (the Broselow-Luten tape). The age-based rule is

$$[\text{Age in years}/4] + 4 = \text{ETT size}$$

The Broselow-Luten tape selects the size of ETT based on the length of the patient. Both age- and length-based rules have been shown to be accurate in the majority of patients, and both can be used depending on operator preference. Some data have shown that the age-based rule tends to overestimate ETT size, whereas the Broselow tape tends to underestimate it.[9-12] Application of age-based sizing criteria to children younger than 2 years of age is less accurate; recommendations for ETT sizing in this age range are detailed in Chapter 2 (Respiratory Distress and Respiratory Failure).

Another unvalidated "rule" that is often applied to children is that the diameter of a child's airway is approximately the same diameter as the child's fifth digit, and that an ETT with an outer diameter of that same size is an accurate choice of size. This simple guideline has unfortunately not stood up to validation testing, and cannot be recommended. It may be that the width of the *nail* of the fifth digit is a more accurate predictor of ETT size than the diameter of the finger itself.[11,13]

As mentioned earlier, the narrowest point in the airway of the young child occurs at the level of the cricoid cartilage, below the insertion of the vocal cords. In these patients, uncuffed endotracheal tubes are often the most appropriate

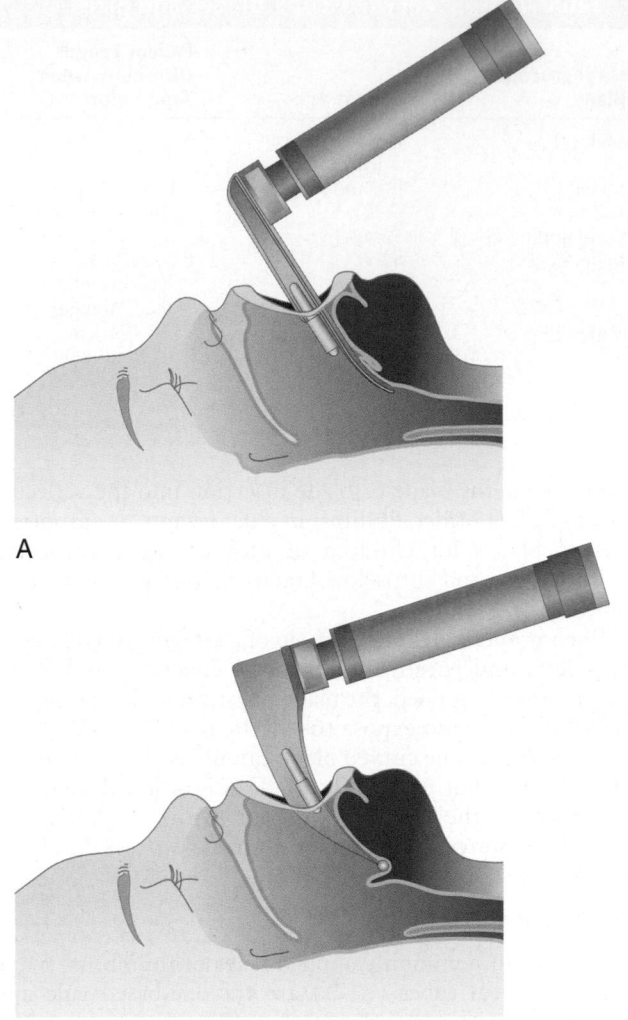

A

B

FIGURE 4–3. A, Correct position and exposure of glottic opening with a straight laryngoscope blade. **B,** Correct position and exposure of glottic opening with a curved laryngoscope blade.

tubes to achieve easy passage through the upper airway and the ability to ventilate effectively without excessive air leak. The conformation of the airway approximates that of an adult by about age 8 years; children beyond that age most often require cuffed endotracheal tubes to achieve a good fit in the trachea. Multiple studies have shown that cuffed ETTs can be safely used in small children, and that the likelihood of postextubation stridor is not significantly increased by their use; additionally, anesthesia studies have shown decreased need for gas flow with cuffed ETT use, suggesting a better fit to the tracheal lumen with cuffed than uncuffed ETTs.[14,15] Current recommendations state that "cuffed endotracheal tubes . . . may be appropriate under circumstances in which high inspiratory pressure is expected."[16]

Airway Adjuncts (Oral Airways, Nasopharyngeal Airways)

Oropharyngeal (OP) and nasopharyngeal (NP) airways can be used to maintain airway patency, particularly during BVM ventilation, but provide no airway protection. In general, a patient who requires a device to maintain airway patency may also require intubation for airway protection. Both devices exist in a range of sizes suitable for all pediatric ages. The correct size of an OP airway for a patient can be estimated by the distance from the patient's central incisors to the angle of the mandible; for NP airways, the correct size is estimated by the distance from the naris to the earlobe. OP airways, when properly positioned, tend to rest against the base of the tongue and, in conscious patients, can induce gagging and vomiting so they should be used only in the unconscious patient. An OP airway should always be used when an unconscious patient is undergoing bag-mask ventilation.

Alternative Airway Techniques[17]

A number of devices and techniques have been used successfully in the operating room for ventilation during general anesthesia, and have also been used for both primary and rescue airway management in emergency patients. Some are specific devices that are placed into the airway, and these can be thought of as supraglottic (e.g., laryngeal mask airway [LMA]), infraglottic (e.g., Combitube), or surgical (e.g., percutaneous transtracheal jet ventilation, cricothyrotomy), to distinguish them from the glottic placement of an endotracheal tube. Other devices assist in the placement of an ETT by improving visualization of the glottic aperature, and include fiberoptic (both flexible and rigid) and video devices. LMAs (see discussion of use later) are available in multiple sizes and from multiple manufacturers to accommodate patients from newborn through adulthood. The Combitube (see discussion of use later) is available in sizes appropriate for patients of at least 48 inches in height. Newer supraglottic devices such as the cuffed oropharyngeal airway (COPA), the laryngeal tube (King LT), and the pharyngeal-tracheal lumen (PTL), exist in sizes appropriate for use in larger patients.

Monitoring

A patient undergoing emergency ETI is potentially critically ill, and should have single-lead electrocardiography, oximetry, and blood pressure monitoring. Many operators find it helpful to have the tone of the oximeter made audible so that a change in heart rate (cadence) or saturation (pitch of tone) can be appreciated without viewing the readout. Bradycardia during laryngoscopy is usually caused by vagal influence, but hypoxemia must always be excluded by oximetry. Monitoring should continue from the preparatory phases through the intubation and throughout the period of postintubation care.

Detection of exhaled carbon dioxide is the standard of care for confirmation of tracheal placement of an ETT, and should be performed in every case. This can be done using a colorimetric device, or by continuous capnography. Capnography can be useful in circumstances in which noninvasive continuous monitoring of alveolar ventilation is desirable (e.g., status asthmaticus, traumatic brain injury).

In cases of prolonged cardiac arrest, when CO_2 exchange has ceased, end-tidal CO_2 ($ETCO_2$) detection can be falsely negative, indicating esophageal placement when the tube is in the trachea. In cardiac arrest resuscitation, if $ETCO_2$ is detected and the tube is inserted to the proper depth, tracheal placement is assured. When $ETCO_2$ detection is negative during circulatory arrest, alternate means of tube placement confirmation are required.

Techniques

Orotracheal Intubation

Airway Positioning

ANATOMIC ASPECTS

Numerous anatomic features unique to children must be recognized with regard to airway positioning. Elevation of the occiput with respect to the shoulders, commonly employed in adults and adolescents, may worsen the view of the glottic opening in infants and toddlers. The infant or toddler should be supine on a flat surface with the head in a neutral position or with a small degree of extension at the neck. Excessive flexion or extension can result in airway obstruction in small children.

CERVICAL SPINE PRECAUTIONS

When necessary, cervical spine immobilization requires the presence of an assistant maintaining the head in a neutral position. This can be performed by kneeling or standing at the intubator's side and holding the child's head from above the patient, or by standing at one side of the patient and reaching from below to hold the sides of the head. The purpose of the immobilization is to both prevent and detect any movement that might be occurring during that intubation that is changing the relationship between the head, neck, and torso. During intubation, the front of the cervical collar is opened to prevent restriction of jaw opening produced by the collar.

JAW THRUST AND CHIN LIFT

Maintaining a patent airway in the supine patient involves displacing the mandibular block of tissue (jaw, floor of mouth, and tongue) anteriorly away from the posterior oropharynx. This can be accomplished by one or a combination of numerous techniques. Most commonly applied are the jaw thrust, in which the operator applies upward pressure behind the angle of the mandible on one or both sides of the patient, and the chin lift, in which the apex of the mandible is grasped and lifted upward. These techniques can be applied with one or two hands and with or without a mask in place. Difficulty maintaining airway patency with these techniques may be indicative of the need for an airway adjunct, or (worst case) a surgical approach to the airway.

Preoxygenation

As discussed previously, the time to desaturation of healthy, fully preoxygenated children is on the order of 2 to 3 minutes. Critically ill children have a shorter desaturation time. Preoxygenation is essential for children undergoing ETI, unless it is not possible. Despite adequate preoxygenation, a critically ill child can desaturate very quickly after apnea is induced, and continuous oximetry is essential. Critically ill children may require assisted ventilation during their apneic period to maintain arterial saturation, which makes good BVM technique as well as properly applied cricoid pressure (see next) of paramount importance.[5,6,18,19]

Cricoid Pressure/Laryngeal Manipulation

The technique of cricoid pressure was initially described by Sellick in 1961 as a technique to prevent aspiration of regurgitated gastric contents during anesthesia induction and intubation.[20] Sellick's maneuver also prevents insufflation of air into the stomach with positive pressure ventilation. The technique is performed by applying firm pressure on the cricoid ring, displacing it backward to occlude the posterior esophagus. Sellick's maneuver is applied as soon as the patient loses consciousness and is continued vigilantly until the endotracheal tube is placed, with the cuff inflated (if applicable) and position confirmed by $ETCO_2$ detection. The generally accepted standard in adults is to apply 10 pounds (4.5 kg, 44 N) of pressure continuously. Published reports have shown that cricoid pressure is often applied incorrectly or ineffectively, and cases of vocal cord and glottis distortion and even airway obstruction due to improperly performed cricoid pressure maneuvers have been reported.[21-23] Those performing the maneuver should be trained to do so.

Current literature has not specifically examined the use of cricoid pressure for RSI in the ill child. While it is logical to extrapolate that decreased pressure is required for children, no data exist as to the optimal pressure required to occlude the pediatric esophagus. The pressure typically applied by anesthesiologists has been shown to be less than for adults (5 to 5.5 pounds), but whether this pressure is clinically appropriate is unknown.[24] The theoretical rationale for the use of cricoid pressure in pediatric intubation is very strong. In addition to reducing the likelihood of gastric regurgitation with aspiration during intubation, Sellick's maneuver also minimizes entry of air into the stomach during bag-mask ventilation. It is very often necessary to support ill children with positive pressure ventilation during RSI, and the prevention of gastric insufflation with cricoid pressure can be of great importance to minimize gastric distention and risk of regurgitation of gastric contents.

Application of backward-upward-rightward pressure on the larynx—commonly referred to as "BURP"—optimizes the view of the glottic opening in cases of difficult laryngoscopy.[20] An assistant applies direct pressure on the thyroid cartilage, displacing it dorsally, rostrally, and to the patient's right. The BURP maneuver is superior to simple cricoid pressure in improving glottic visualization in difficult laryngoscopy cases.[25] External laryngeal manipulation is a technique wherein the intubator uses his/her right hand to maneuver the laryngeal structures while maintaining his/her own line of sight with the airway opening.[26] Once an optimal position is found, the intubator ensures that an assistant maintains that position of the larynx while the patient is intubated. This technique has been validated using videographic imaging in adults intubated by emergency medicine interns.[27]

Neither of these techniques has been studied in children, but both could be logically extrapolated to the pediatric patient as long as gentle external forces are used, as the amount of pressure needed to occlude or distort the pediatric airway is likely much less than that needed for an adult.

Laryngoscopy (see Table 4-2, Fig. 4-1)

The laryngoscope is held in the intubator's left hand and the right hand is used to open the mouth. The blade is advanced into the oropharynx in such a way as to sweep the tongue to the left side of the mouth and hold it there. Passing the blade to a midline position and gently down the esophagus will allow the intubator to visualize the glottis during gentle withdrawal of the blade. As the blade is withdrawn, the first structure that comes into view is the glottis, with the epiglottis held in an anterior position by the blade. Figure 4–3A and Figure 4-3B show the proper positioning of straight and curved laryngoscope blades. In the former case, the tip goes under the epiglottis, lifting it out of the way; in the latter, the tip rests in the vallecula and upward traction pulls the epiglottis up out of the line of sight. The curved blade can also be used to actively lift the epiglottis if necessary.[16]

Tube Insertion

The ETT is held by the right hand and inserted while line of sight to the glottic opening is maintained with the laryngoscope. It is important not to allow the tube to obstruct the intubator's view of the vocal cords. A common error that leads to obstruction of the line of sight during direct laryngoscopy is sliding the tube along the channel of the blade instead of at the right side of the mouth away from the blade. If a video laryngoscope is used (e.g., DCI Video MacIntosh, Karl Storz North America), the tube is placed by passing it along the channel of the blade and through the glottis under video visualization. In children with small mouths, an assistant can stretch the right corner of the mouth laterally to provide more space for the ETT. Midtracheal placement of the ETT tip is usually assured when the "double black line" (marked on the outside of an uncuffed ETT) is aligned with the vocal cords. Additionally, multiplying the inner diameter of the ETT by a factor of 3 gives the depth of insertion in centimeters (measured at the lip) that usually gives proper midtracheal positioning (this rule of thumb may incorrectly overestimate depth of placement in children younger than 2 years old).

Confirmation of Placement

$ETCO_2$ detection is the standard of care to confirm proper ETT placement. Several types of $ETCO_2$ detectors are commercially available. Most EDs use disposable colorimetric devices, which register exhaled CO_2 by a change in color of an indicator, but some use capnometry, which digitally displays the exact partial pressure of exhaled CO_2, or capnography, which provides a waveform.

Several studies have supported the specificity and sensitivity of confirmation of placement of ETTs using $ETCO_2$ in infants and children.[28,29] In the patient in cardiopulmonary arrest, the absence of pulmonary blood flow may limit the amount of carbon dioxide in the alveoli, making $ETCO_2$ prone to false-negative results (the tube is in the trachea, but the test indicates the tube is in the esophagus), but this occurs in only a subset of patients. Persistent detection of CO_2, however, reliably indicates that the tube is in the airway.[30] Concomitant physical examination will address the possibility that the tube, while in the airway, has been inadvertently placed in the supraglottic larynx, or in a mainstem bronchus.

The imperfect specificity of $ETCO_2$ in the arrested patient occasionally will require use of alternative devices to confirm ETT placement. Air aspirators, or esophageal detection devices (EDD), are one common class of such devices. The principle behind the use of the EDD relies on the collapsibility of the esophagus compared to the cartilage-reinforced trachea. EDDs attempt to aspirate air from the endotracheal tube by negative pressure (examples include a syringe-like device and a semirigid plastic bulb that reinflates when squeezed). If negative pressure is applied to a tube in the trachea, the reinforced trachea will resist collapse and the EDD will fill with air, confirming that the tube is in the trachea. Negative pressure applied to a tube in the esophagus, on the other hand, will collapse the esophagus around the end of the tube and result in slow or incomplete filling of the EDD with air.

EDDs have been shown to be accurate in older children.[31] Some studies have shown their accuracy to be poor in children under 1 year of age and when used with uncuffed ETTs.[32-34] At present, no recommendations exist for the routine use of EDDs in children, and these devices should be used only when there is uncertainty about tube position after use of $ETCO_2$ detection.

There is no method of confirming proper placement of an ETT that is 100% reliable. A combination of the techniques described here and clinical examination will provide the correct information in the vast majority of cases. Physical examination should not be used to overrule a "negative" $ETCO_2$ detection (tube in esophagus) unless the patient is in cardiac arrest and clinical evidence strongly supports tracheal placement.

Securing the ETT

Securing an ETT is most often accomplished by one of two methods. Strips of adhesive tape can be torn longitudinally to allow half of each piece to attach to the patient's face and the other to the shaft of the ETT. Alternatively, a number of prefabricated tube devices are commercially available. In the conscious or responsive patient, it may be necessary to place an adjunctive device between the incisors (a "bite block") to prevent the patient from biting against the tube and occluding it. Oropharyngeal airways may be used for this purpose, along with rolls of gauze or other prefabricated devices.

Alternative Intubation Techniques

Blind Nasotracheal Intubation

Blind nasotracheal intubation (BNTI) has little role in the modern ED, particularly in children, in whom it is more difficult than in adults because of the wider discrepancy between the pharyngeal and laryngeal axes, as well as the presence of large adenoidal tissue. BNTI is reserved for those cases in which oral intubation is deemed to be unlikely to succeed and alternative techniques, including fiberoptic intubation, are not available. The patient must be cooperative and spontaneously breathing to allow appreciation of breath sounds through the ETT as the tip is blindly inserted through one naris and advanced to just above the glottic opening. Pediatric experience with this technique is extremely limited. The anterosuperior location of the glottic opening with respect to the nasopharynx in infants and young children make the blind placement of a tube through a naris and into the trachea extremely difficult. Therefore, this technique is not recommended in children less than 10 years old.

Lighted Stylet

The lighted stylet relies on the characteristic appearance of light transilluminating the larynx through the anterior neck.

The ETT is threaded over the light wand, which is bent almost to a right angle to direct the lighted tip anteriorly toward the glottic opening. The wand-tube combination is then advanced blindly over the tongue and directed anteriorly toward the vocal cords. When the visible illumination goes from a diffuse circle of light to a more focused and clearly delineated outline of the glottic opening (sometimes called "coning"), the tube is advanced off the device into the trachea. Both reuseable and disposable light wand devices exist that can accommodate ETTs down to infant and pediatric sizes. Literature on the emergent use of this technique is limited.

Fiberoptic Intubation

Equipment for fiberoptic laryngoscopy exists in sizes small enough that fiberoptic techniques can be employed in any age of patient. Fiberoptic intubation requires training and experience, and can be acquired as a skill through training courses or in a simulation laboratory. It is uncommonly used in children, but offers the added advantage of a detailed airway examination that may avert intubation altogether (e.g., in smoke inhalation).

Digital Intubation

This technique, which also has little role in modern airway management, is performed by advancing the index finger of one hand into the patient's mouth and palpating the tip of the epiglottis. The intubator then pushes the epiglottis anteriorly with that fingertip while sliding an ETT along the side of the finger with the opposite hand. There is very little human, and even less pediatric, experience with this method.

Retrograde Intubation

This technique is rarely used in the ED in pediatric or adult patients, and involves percutaneously inserting a needle through the cricothyroid membrane and inserting a guidewire cephalad through the needle lumen until it can be pulled through the patient's open mouth. An ETT is then threaded over the wire and advanced into the trachea. There is virtually no experience or study related to the use of this approach in the pediatric age group.

Rescue Devices

Rescue devices are those that are used when intubation has failed or the operator judges that further attempts at orotracheal intubation are likely to be futile.

Laryngeal Mask Airway

The LMA consists of a teardrop shaped inflatable cuff surrounding a fenestrated latex window that faces the glottic opening when properly positioned (Fig. 4–4A). The device is inserted into the open mouth of the patient and advanced until resistance is felt, at which point the cuff is inflated. Studies of the use of the LMA by various classes of personnel have shown that it is easy to place and rarely associated with significant complications.[35,36] LMAs are made in a range of sizes that are appropriate for all ages from neonate to adult. A summary of appropriate sizes and cuff volumes for LMAs is given in Table 4–4.

The LMA does not result in the placement of a cuffed ETT in the trachea, so it is generally believed that the device does not protect against aspiration. It appears that aspiration

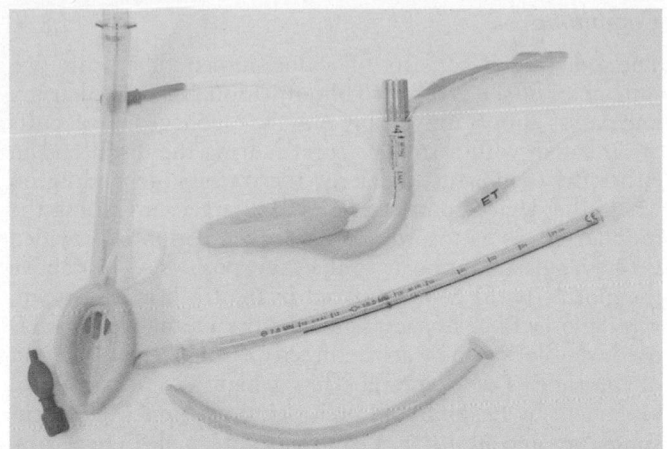

A

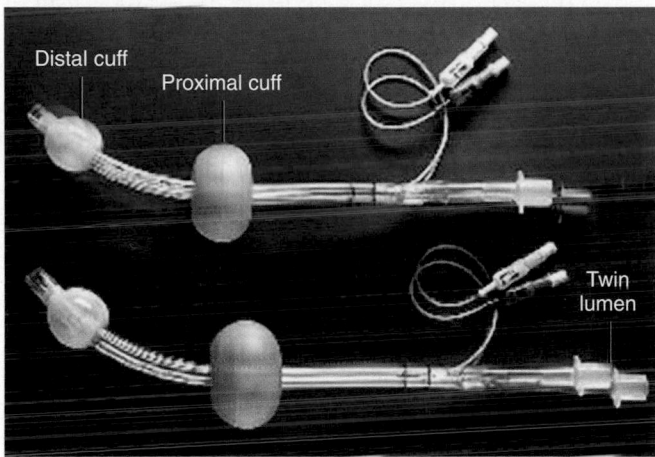

B

FIGURE 4–4. Rescue devices. **A,** LMA classic (left) and the Fastrach intubating LMA. The former is available in sizes from neonate to large adult. The intubating LMA should only be used in patients over 30 kg. **B,** The Combitube is available in two sizes, SA (small adult) on left, and standard on right. Patients must be over 48 inches tall if a Combitube is to be used.

Table 4–4	Laryngeal Mask Airway Sizes	
Size	Patient Weight	Amount of Air in Cuff (mL)
1	<5 kg	4
1½	5–10 kg	7
2	10–20 kg	10
2½	20–30 kg	14
3	Children >30 kg; small adult	20
4	Normal adult	30
5	Large adult	40

risk may approximate that when bag-mask ventilation is employed.[37] Data comparing LMA use to ETI and BVM ventilation are children is limited[16]; nonetheless, LMAs are widely used in operating room settings, EDs, and by some prehospital care communities.[17] The patent for the original LMA has run out, and numerous products are now available, some claiming improvements over the original design.

Combitube

The Combitube consists of a dual-lumen tube with two inflatable cuffs. It is inserted blindly through the oropharynx and passes almost universally into the esophagus. Both cuffs are inflated, with a smaller cuff securing the distal end in either the esophagus or, rarely, the trachea (depending on where the device comes to lie) and a larger cuff filling the oropharynx so as to provide a seal. Ventilation is provided through sidestream ports in the tube, positioned just above the glottis. If the tube is placed in the trachea, sidestream ventilation will be unsuccessful, and the alternative lumen is used, ventilating the trachea directly through the distal end of the tube. The Combitube has a high rate of successful placement by hospital and prehospital personnel in patient simulators and adults.[38,39] Combitubes are made in two sizes, and only the "SA" (small adult) size is suitable for pediatric use (Fig. 4–4B). The Combitube is restricted to patients greater than 48 inches in height, (typical size and weight of a 10 year old). No sizes of Combitube currently exist for pediatric patients of younger age.[40] The PTL tube is a device similar to the Combitube, inserted via a blind technique and shown to be relatively easy to use.[39] The PTL is also unavailable in pediatric sizes. Both the PTL and Combitube are safe to use in adolescent patients.

Surgical and Transtracheal Airway Procedures

Emergency surgical airway management is rare, and particularly so in pediatrics. In the first phase of the multihospital NEAR study, only 1 of 156 emergency pediatric airways was managed by cricothyrotomy.[1] The small size of the cricothyroid membrane, incomplete development of the normal external laryngeal landmarks, excessive mobility of the airway, and lack of rigidity of the structures make surgical airways particularly challenging in small children. Although tracheostomy is possible in even very small neonates under highly controlled conditions, emergency airway management accesses the airway through the cricothyroid membrane. Cricothyrotomy can be performed using an open surgical technique, percutaneously using a Seldinger technique, or by using a cricothyrotome (an instrument designed to access the membrane and provide an airway, usually in one or two steps.) There is no evidence in support of using any of the cricothyrotomes, including those represented as being specially designed for the pediatric airway. In general, such devices should be avoided. For children greater than 10 years old, surgical cricothyrotomy can be performed, particularly in older children, whose airway dimensions approach those of adults. Under age 10 years, needle cricothyrotomy is preferable; this can be accomplished using an angiocatheter of reasonable size. Jet ventilation requires the use of a special apparatus that incorporates a regulator to control pressure to limit barotrauma, and can be provided through this catheter. In infants less than 1 year old, bag ventilation is performed through the catheter by incorporating the ETT adaptor from a 3-mm ETT. Use of the bag in the small child minimizes the risks of barotrauma.

There are no studies to clearly delineate the role of emergency transtracheal ventilation in pediatric patients, and the technique is rarely if ever used. It is relatively simple, however, and may be valuable in those small patients for whom a surgical airway is not feasible.

The Difficult Pediatric Airway

Difficulty in intubation in children can be due to chronic or acute conditions as discussed briefly earlier (see Table 4–2). A recent clinical review provides a detailed list of conditions that may predispose a child to a difficult intubation.[2] Anticipating that a child will be difficult to intubate is hard to do with any degree of specificity or sensitivity. Predictors shown to be useful in adults, such as Mallampati and Cormack and Lehane scoring, have not been shown to be specific in children for predicting difficulty in ETI. Some empiric observations such as inability to move the neck (rheumatic disease, Klippel-Feil syndrome, arthrogryposis) or potential for morbidity from neck motion (trauma, Down syndrome), a small or distorted mandibular space (Pierre-Robin syndrome, Treacher-Collins syndrome), and tongue size are of predictive value for children in need of airway management.

The difficult pediatric airway is a very rare clinical phenomenon. This very fact also means that not even experienced emergency medicine practitioners frequently manage the difficult pediatric airway. The need for fiberoptic or surgical management of a pediatric airway is most commonly encountered in the operating room, and therefore it is those subspecialists that frequently manage children via these techniques (anesthesiologists, otorhinolaryngologists) that are most likely to have enough experience to intervene in a facile manner.

Two mnemonics often used for identifying difficult intubation in adults are presented here. The abnormalities identified by these rules of thumb are uncommon in children, but the general principles of signs of potential difficulty can be applied in a manner nonspecific to age. Thinking through these mnemonics may help the emergency medicine practitioner to identify children for whom paralysis (RSI) should be avoided or subspecialist assistance might be warranted.[41,42] It must be noted that these mnemonics are derived from adult studies and have not been shown to be specific or sensitive in children. In general, when developing a system for identification of a potentially difficult intubation, sensitivity is much more important than specificity; that is, it is more valuable to identify every difficult airway at the expense of considering some to be difficult when they are not. The mnemonics are presented here as a representative framework for anticipating difficulty with a pediatric airway.

Lemon

- Look externally for signs of procedural difficulty (facial/oral characteristics, habitus, etc.) and potential difficulty with bag-mask ventilation (obesity, poor mask seal, airway obstruction, high ventilatory resistance [e.g., asthma])
- Evaluate the "3-3-2" rule (the interincisor gap of an open mouth should approximate three of the patient's finger breadths; the distance from the mentum to the hyoid bone should also be three of the patient's finger breadths; the distance from the thyroid notch to the floor of the mouth should be two of the patient's finger breadths). While these measurements are not specifically validated in small children, they can serve as a guide to judge the accessibility of the upper airway for direct laryngoscopy.
- Mallampati score (Fig. 4–5)

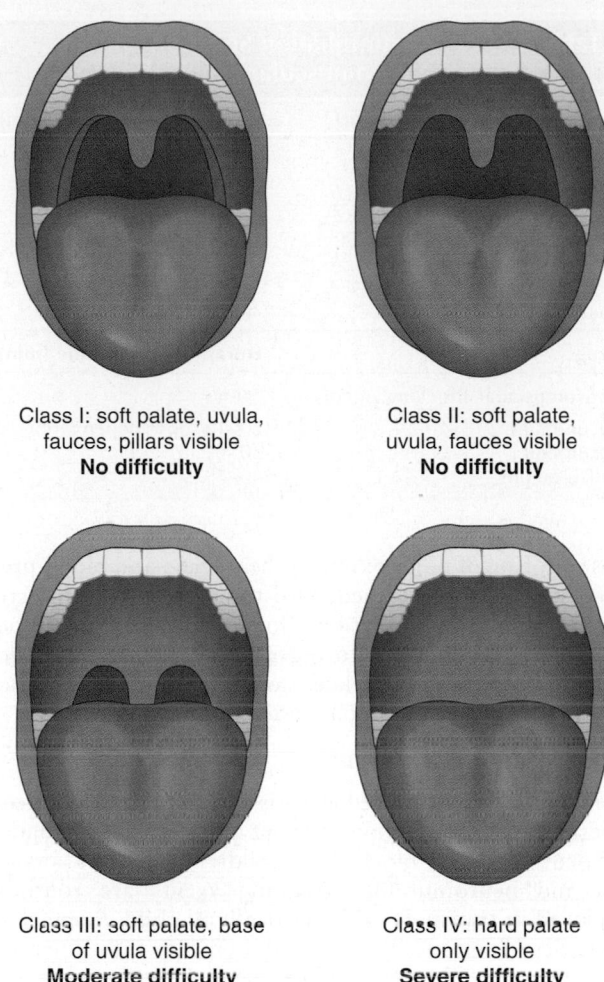

Class I: soft palate, uvula, fauces, pillars visible
No difficulty

Class II: soft palate, uvula, fauces visible
No difficulty

Class III: soft palate, base of uvula visible
Moderate difficulty

Class IV: hard palate only visible
Severe difficulty

FIGURE 4–5. Mallampati scoring system for visualization of pharyngeal structures. Easy intubation is anticipated by a score of 1 or 2, some difficulty is expected with a score of 3, and great difficulty or impossible intubation is associated with a score of 4. (From Whitten CE: Anyone can Intubate, 4th ed. San Diego: Mooncat Publications, 2004.)

- **O**bstruction (any evidence/suspicion for airway obstruction)
- **N**eck mobility (i.e., reduction of neck mobility that limits the ability to put the neck in extended position for direct laryngoscopy)

The Four Ds
- **D**istortion of facial/neck/oral anatomy by disease process
- **D**isproportion of neck, mandible, submandibular space
- **D**ysmobility of jaw, neck
- **D**entition—edentulous adults are difficult to maintain a sealed bag-valve mask on; this seldom is true for edentulous infants

Success Rates and Complications

Incidence of Complications

Estimates of the incidence of complications of ETI vary.[43-45] The definition of "complication" related to ETI is inconsistent across studies, encompassing such phenomena as predictable changes in physiology, imperfect fit of selected equipment, and adverse events attributable directly to the process of laryngoscopy and ETT placement. The NEAR registry has employed a strict definitional scheme to differentiate between "true" complications (resulting from the procedure itself) and "technical problems" (cuff leak, detected ETI, equipment failure, etc.) or "physiologic alteration" (changes in physiology during or after ETI that may or may not be attributable to the intubation).[1] This new nomenclature, while sensible, was not available at the time of publication of most other studies. Such phenomena as mainstem intubations, gastric distention, and failure to place a gastric tube for stomach decompression are cited as complications in other studies, resulting in misleading reports of complication rates that are higher than would have occurred had only true complications been included.

Failure of Procedure

Failure of laryngoscopy and ETI in children varies with the setting, patient age, and training and experience of the intubator. Prehospital studies of ETI in children have found success rates varying from 18% to 30% in infants and young children and 71% to 90% in older children and adolescents.[46,47] ED-based studies of pediatric ETI show that success rates vary with age as well. Data from the NEAR study found that the first intubation attempt was successful in 60% of patients less than 5 years old, while success rates for older children ranged from 71% to 85%. In the same study, the first intubator was successful in 74% to 79% of children less than 5 years old and in 86% to 94% of children 6 to 18 years old.[1]

A landmark study comparing BVM ventilation to ETI in the prehospital management of children in need of respiratory support demonstrated no benefit of ETI over BVM, although the paramedics studied rarely undertook pediatric intubation in the large, urban center studied. In that study, unrecognized esophageal intubation occurred in 15 children, and 14 of these children died.[48] Uniform use of $ETCO_2$ detection is meant to reduce the occurrence of this event.

Trauma (Oral, Pharyngeal, Laryngeal)

Trauma to the oropharynx, teeth, lip, tongue, and larynx have been reported with ETI, but is uncommon and generally mild. The NEAR study identified direct trauma in only 1 of 156 intubation attempts; other studies of prehospital and ED pediatric intubations found a range of similarly infrequent incidences (0.5% to 4%).[45,48,49] Young children have primary teeth, which are easily injured and avulsed and can pose an aspiration risk. Primary teeth overlie secondary tooth buds that can be damaged by forces exerted on primary teeth. Other pertinent anatomic features in children include the small mouth, large tongue, and prominent adenoidal tissue.

Respiratory Complications (Aspiration, Air Leak Syndrome/Pneumothorax)

The conversion from native negative pressure breathing to positive pressure ventilation via an ETT is associated with a significant increase in intrathoracic pressure, particularly in clinical situations in which lung or chest wall compliance is decreased. Complications from barotrauma, such as pneumothorax, interstitial emphysema, and subcutaneous air, can result from positive pressure ventilation. It is difficult to determine whether such phenomena, when observed, result from the intubation or from the condition for which intubation was required.

Emesis and aspiration of gastric contents are uncommon but significant events that can occur before, during, or after ETI. The common use of BVM ventilation for preoxygenation and for maintenance of arterial oxygen saturation during RSI may put small children at a greater risk of these complications. The use of cricoid pressure to prevent both gastric insufflation and regurgitation is designed for the prevention of these complications.

Physiologic Complications

Vagally mediated bradycardia related to laryngoscopy in children is discussed earlier in this chapter and in Chapter 2 (Respiratory Distress and Respiratory Failure).

Cardiopulmonary interactions following the conversion from spontaneous negative pressure ventilation to positive pressure ventilation involve an increase in intrathoracic pressure resulting in a decrease in preload and possibly left ventricular afterload. The compliance of the chest wall in small children results in the need for greater changes in pressure to yield a given tidal volume, and so it can be extrapolated that the resultant preload changes may be more dramatic in young children. Left ventricular function in young children is affected more drastically by metabolic disturbances (hypoglycemia, acidosis, hypocalcemia), states that commonly accompany clinical situations in which ETI is necessary. Additionally, lower respiratory illnesses such as bronchiolitis and pneumonia, common indications for pediatric ETI, result in increased pulmonary vascular resistance, increased right ventricular diameter, and consequently (via ventricular interdependence) decreased left ventricular preload.[50] Anyone performing ETI on a critically ill child should be wary of the concurrent presence of any disease state resulting in decreased preload (hypovolemia, capillary leak, blood loss), as well as whether the metabolic milieu can be optimized prior to ETI.

Equipment-Related Complications

Children who undergo intubation with ETTs of the wrong size or type can experience difficulty with maintaining appropriate oxygenation and ventilation. The rules of thumb commonly used for selection of types and sizes of equipment related to ETI are imperfect and yield estimates that are incorrect in certain circumstances. Additionally, and probably more commonly, availability of or practitioner familiarity with appropriate equipment is suboptimal. ETTs of incorrect size have been shown to be frequently used by both ED physicians and prehospital care providers, although such equipment variances have not been correlated with adverse patient outcomes.[45,49]

Postprocedural Care and Disposition

A chest radiograph should be obtained following all intubations to confirm that endobronchial intubation is not present, and that the tube is well positioned below the glottis. Placement of the tip of an ETT either too deep (right mainstem bronchus) or too shallow (high in the trachea near the glottis) can predispose the patient to complications such as tube dislodgement, obstruction, and barotrauma.

Table 4–5	Postintubation Sedation and Neuromuscular Blockade	
Drug	**$t_{1/2}$ (hr)**	**Clearance (mL/kg/min)**
Sedatives and Analgesics		
Midazolam	1.7–2.6	6.4–11
Lorazepam	11–22	0.8–1.8
Diazepam	20–50	0.2–0.5
Fentanyl	1.7–2.6	6.4–11
Morphine	2–4	10–40
Meperidine	2–5	10–20
Drug		**Duration of Blockade (min)**
Neuromuscular Blocking Agents		
Rocuronium		20–30 (dose dependent)
Vecuronium		30–60
Pancuronium		40–75

Monitoring of pulse oximetry, heart rate, and blood pressure should be maintained until the patient is transferred from the ED or resuscitation efforts are terminated. When possible, continuous monitoring of ETCO₂ is a useful adjunct, both for complications related to the ETT and ventilation system and for underlying disease processes.

Issues Related to Transport

Transport of the intubated child is a difficult task requiring expertise with airway management and the use of sedation and neuromuscular blockade in children. Sedatives, analgesics, and neuromuscular blocking agents are routinely employed in transport of the critically ill child. Some characteristics of commonly employed agents for these purposes are shown in Table 4–5; which agent is appropriate will depend on the individual child's situation.

Monitoring in transport can be more difficult due to the inability to auscultate heart and breath sounds, as well as the presence of movement artifacts in electrocardiography leads. Continuous monitoring of pulse oximetry, heart rate, blood pressure, and neurologic status are essential to safely transporting such patients. Bhende and colleagues examined the use of colorimetric ETCO₂ detection for evaluating placement of ETTs in 58 intubated children while in transport; in all cases in which tube position was checked while en route, the location of the tube was correctly identified.[28] Transport teams caring for intubated children must be able to at least intermittently (if not continuously) monitor the presence of ETCO₂ as evidence of correct placement of the ETT.

REFERENCES

1. Sagarin MJ, Chiang V, Sakles JC, et al: Rapid sequence intubation for pediatric emergency airway management. Pediatr Emerg Care 18:417–423, 2002.
2. Frei FJ, Ummenhofer W: Difficult intubation in paediatrics. Paediatr Anaesth 6:251-63, 1996.
3. Helfaer MA, Nichols DG, Rogers MC: Developmental physiology of the respiratory system. In Rogers MC (ed): Textbook of Pediatric Intensive Care. Baltimore: Williams & Wilkins, 1996, pp 97–126.
4. Farmery AD, Roe PG: A model to describe the rate of oxyhaemoglobin desaturation during apnoea. Br J Anaesth 76:284–291, 1996. [Published erratum appears in Br J Anaesth 76:890, 1996.]
5. Benumof JL, Dagg R, Benumof R: Critical hemoglobin desaturation will occur before return to an unparalyzed state following 1 mg/kg intravenous succinylcholine [see comment]. Anesthesiology 87:979–982, 1997.

6. Xue FS, Luo LK, Tong SY, et al: Study of the safe threshold of apneic period in children during anesthesia induction. J Clin Anesth 8:568–574, 1996.

7. Levitan RM, Ochroch EA: Airway management and direct laryngoscopy: a review and update. Crit Care Clin 16:373–388, 2000.

8. Gronert BJ, Motoyama EK: Induction of anesthesia and endotracheal intubation. In Motoyama EK, Davis PJ (eds): Smith's Anesthesia for Infants and Children. St. Louis: Mosby, 1996 pp 281–312.

9. Davis D, Barbee L, Ririe D: Pediatric endotracheal tube selection: a comparison of age-based and height-based criteria. AANA J 66:299–303, 1998.

10. Hofer CK, Ganter M, Tucci M, et al: How reliable is length-based determination of body weight and tracheal tube size in the paediatric age group? The Broselow tape reconsidered. Br J Anaesth 88:283–285, 2002.

11. King BR, Baker MB, Braitman LE, et al: Endotracheal tube selection in children: a comparison of four methods. Ann Emerg Med 22:530–534, 1993.

12. Luten RC, Wears RL, Broselow J, et al: Length-based endotracheal tube and emergency equipment in pediatrics. Ann Emerg Med 21:900–904, 1992. [Published erratum appears in Ann Emerg Med 22:155, 1993.]

13. van den Berg AA, Mphanza T: Choice of tracheal tube size for children: finger size or age-related formula? Anaesthesia 52:701–703, 1997.

14. Khine HH, Corddry DH, Kettrick RG, et al: Comparison of cuffed and uncuffed endotracheal tubes in young children during general anesthesia. Anesthesiology 86:627–631; discussion 27A, 1997.

15. Deakers TW, Reynolds G, Stretton M, Newth CJ: Cuffed endotracheal tubes in pediatric intensive care. J Pediatr 125:57–62, 1994.

*16. Part 10: Pediatric Advanced Life Support. Circulation 102:291I–342I, 2000.

17. Airway, ventilation, and mangement of respiratory distress and failure. In Hazinski MF, Zaritsky AL, Nadkarni VM, et al (eds): PALS Provider Manual. Dallas, TX: American Heart Association, 2002, pp 81–126.

18. Xue FS, Tong SY, Wang XL, et al: Study of the optimal duration of preoxygenation in children. J Clin Anesth 7:93–96, 1995.

19. Patel R, Lenczyk M, Hannallah RS, McGill WA: Age and the onset of desaturation in apnoeic children. Can J Anaesth 41:771–774, 1994.

20. Sellick B: Cricoid pressure to control regurgitation of stomach contents during induction of anesthesia. Lancet 2:404–406, 1961.

21. Brock-Utne JG: Is cricoid pressure necessary? [see comment]. Paediatr Anaesth 12:1–4, 2002.

22. Hartsilver EL, Vanner RG: Airway obstruction with cricoid pressure. Anaesthesia 55:208–211, 2000.

23. Palmer JHM, Ball DR: The effect of cricoid pressure on the cricoid cartilage and vocal cords: an endoscopic study in anesthetised patients. Anaesthesia 55:263–268, 2000.

24. Francis S, Enani S, Shah J, et al: Simulated cricoid force in paediatric anesthesia. Br J Anaesth 85:164P, 2000.

25. Takahata O, Kubota M, Mamiya K, et al: The efficacy of the "BURP" maneuver during a difficult laryngoscopy. Anesth Analg 84:419–421, 1997.

26. Benumof JL, Cooper SD: Quantitative improvement in laryngoscopic view by optimal external laryngeal manipulation. J Clin Anesth 8:136–140, 1996.

27. Levitan RM, Mickler T, Hollander JE: Bimanual laryngoscopy: a videographic study of external laryngeal manipulation by novice intubators.[see comment]. Ann Emerg Med 40:30–37, 2002.

28. Bhende MS, Thompson AE, Orr RA: Utility of an end-tidal carbon dioxide detector during stabilization and transport of critically ill children. Pediatrics 89(6 Pt 1):1042–1044, 1992.

29. Bhende MS, Thompson AE, Cook DR, Saville AL: Validity of a disposable end-tidal CO_2 detector in verifying endotracheal tube placement in infants and children [see comment]. Ann Emerg Med 21:142–145, 1992.

30. Bhende MS: End-tidal carbon dioxide monitoring in pediatrics—clinical applications. J Postgrad Med 47:215–218, 2001.

31. Morton NS, Stuart JC, Thomson MF, Wee MY: The oesophageal detector device: successful use in children. Anaesthesia 44:523–524, 1989.

32. Haynes SR, Morton NS: Use of the oesophageal detector device in children under one year of age. Anaesthesia 45:1067–1069, 1990.

33. Wee MY, Walker AK: The oesophageal detector device: an assessment with uncuffed tubes in children. Anaesthesia 46:869–871, 1991.

34. Sharieff GQ, Rodarte A, Wilton N, Bleyle D: The self-inflating bulb as an airway adjunct: is it reliable in children weighing less than 20 kilograms? Acad Emerg Med 10:303–308, 2003.

35. Lopez-Gil M, Brimacombe J, Alvarez M: Safety and efficacy of the laryngeal mask airway: a prospective survey of 1400 children. Anaesthesia 51:969–972, 1996.

36. Lopez-Gil M, Brimacombe J, Cebrian J, Arranz J: Laryngeal mask airway in pediatric practice: a prospective study of skill acquisition by anesthesia residents. Anesthesiology 84:807–811, 1996.

37. Brimacombe JR, Berry A: The incidence of aspiration associated with the laryngeal mask airway: a meta-analysis of published literature. J Clin Anesth 7:297–305, 1995.

38. Dorges V, Ocker H, Wenzel V, et al: Emergency airway management by non-anaesthesia house officers—a comparison of three strategies. Emerg Med J 18:90–94, 2001.

39. Rumball CJ, MacDonald D: The PTL, Combitube, laryngeal mask, and oral airway: a randomized prehospital comparative study of ventilatory device effectiveness and cost-effectiveness in 470 cases of cardiorespiratory arrest [see comment]. Prehospital Emerg Care 1:1–10, 1997.

40. Murphy MF: Special devices and techniques for managing the difficult or failed airway. In Walls RM (ed): Manual of Emergency Airway Management. Philadelphia: Lippincott, Williams & Wilkins, 2000, pp 68–81.

41. Murphy MF, Walls RM: The difficult and failed airway. In Walls RA (ed): Manual of Emergency Airway Management. Philadelphia: Lippincott Williams & Wilkins, 2000, pp 31–39.

42. Levitan RM: Practical Emergency Airway Management. Wayne, PA: Airway Cam Technologies, Inc., 2003.

43. Gnauck K, Lungo JB, Scalzo A, et al: Emergency intubation of the pediatric medical patient: use of anesthetic agents in the emergency department. Ann Emerg Med 23:1242–1247, 1994.

44. Nakayama DK, Gardner MJ, Rowe MI: Emergency endotracheal intubation in pediatric trauma. Ann Surg 211:218–223, 1990.

45. Easley RB, Segeleon JE, Haun SE, Tobias JD: Prospective study of airway management of children requiring endotracheal intubation before admission to a pediatric intensive care unit. Crit Care Med 28:2058–2063, 2000.

46. Aijian P, Tsai A, Knopp R, Kallsen GW: Endotracheal intubation of pediatric patients by paramedics [see comment]. Ann Emerg Med 18:489–494, 1989.

47. Kumar VR, Bachman DT, Kiskaddon RT: Children and adults in cardiopulmonary arrest: are advanced life support guidelines followed in the prehospital setting? [see comment]. Ann Emerg Med 29:743–747, 1997.

48. Gausche M, Lewis RJ, Stratton SJ, et al: Effect of out-of-hospital pediatric endotracheal intubation on survival and neurological outcome: a controlled clinical trial [see comment]. JAMA 283:783–790, 2000. [Published erratum appears in JAMA 283:3204, 2000.]

49. Brownstein D, Shugerman R, Cummings P, et al: Prehospital endotracheal intubation of children by paramedics [see comment]. Ann Emerg Med 28:34–39, 1996.

50. Robotham JL, Peters J, Takata M, Wetzel RC: Cardiorespiratory interactions. In Rogers MC (ed): Textbook of Pediatric Intensive Care. Baltimore: Williams & Wilkins, 1996, pp 369–396.

---

*Selected reading.

Chapter 5

Monitoring in Critically Ill Children

Jonathan Marr, MD and Thomas J. Abramo, MD

Key Points

Cyanosis is not an early or reliable indicator of hypoxemia in anemic children.

Pulse oximetry is accurate when saturations are greater than 70%.

Capnographic end-tidal CO_2 is the most reliable method for confirming endotracheal tube placement.

Oscillometric blood pressure measurements are accurate in pediatric patients.

Introduction

Improved EMS systems and the development of transport medicine have increased the need for real-time information. Caring for the ill or injured child can be difficult since invasive blood draws (e.g., arterial blood gas) are not always easy to obtain and may not be tolerated if performed multiple times. Thus a noninvasive means of patient monitoring is a promising area of emergency pediatrics. Physicians must be aware of how new devices impact their clinical decision making and of the limitations of the information these devices provide.

Noninvasive monitoring of critically ill children in the emergency department (ED) includes pulse oximetry, capnography, cardiac telemetry, and oscillometric blood pressure measurement. In the ED, invasive monitoring is usually limited to blood gases and occasionally continuous indwelling arterial pressure monitoring. Central venous pressure and mixed venous oxygen monitoring may become more common in the future.

Recognition and Approach

Identification of the seriously ill and injured child in the ED requires rapid cardiopulmonary assessment and has become the foundation of pediatric advanced life support. Goals are to assess for respiratory failure, shock, and the impact on end-organ function. An orderly approach that assesses the triad of respiratory effort, perfusion, and mental status will allow for early identification of critically ill children (see Chapter 2, Respiratory Distress and Respiratory Failure; Chapter 8, Circulatory Emergencies: Shock; and Chapter 9, Cerebral Resuscitation). Addition of noninvasive and invasive monitoring techniques will allow for early recognition of patient deterioration and rapid determination of response to therapy.

Evaluation and Management

Noninvasive Monitoring

Pulse Oximetry

Pulse oximetry has become an essential tool in the ED and is often referred to as the fifth vital sign. Furthermore, continuous evaluation of arterial oxygen saturation remains an important monitoring technique during stabilization and transport since providers cannot reliably detect hypoxemia by clinical examination alone.[1] Historically, the pulse oximeter has been utilized in research since 1935. The principle of pulse oximetry is based on the Beer-Lambert law, which states that the concentration of an absorbing substance in solution can be determined from the intensity of light transmitted through that solution.[2] Simply stated, arterial oxygen saturation is based on the differential absorption of red and infrared photons by oxyhemoglobin and deoxyhemoglobin measured by the pulse oximeter.

Two light-emitting diodes (LEDs) in the pulse oximeter probe each emit light of specific wavelength from one side of the oximeter that passes through locations such as the digits or earlobe, with cutaneous *pulsatile* blood flow. Other possible monitoring sites include the nares, the cheek at the corner of the mouth, and the tongue.[3] A photodiode detector at the far side of the oximeter measures the intensity of transmitted light at each wavelength. Oxygen saturation is derived from calibration curves that associate the absorbance ratios to arterial oxygen saturation.

Initial calibration curves were derived from Beer-Lambert calculations, but more accurate calibration curves have come

Table 5–1	Sources of Errors in Pulse Oximetry

Light interference	Venous pulsations
• Ambient light	• Obstructed venous return
• Penumbra effect	• Severe right heart failure
Optical shunting	• Tricuspid regurgitation
• Probe malposition	• Dependent limb
• Oversized probe	• Tourniquet constriction
Motion artifact	• High positive pressure ventilation
Low signal-to-noise ratio	
• Shock	
• Cardiac arrest	
Dyshemoglobinemias	
• Carboxyhemoglobin	
• Methemoglobin	
• Sickle cell anemia (crisis)	
Dyes	
Other	
• Anemia	
• Blue or black nail polish	

from experimentally derived data. These curves are based on measurements in healthy young volunteers after induction of hypoxemia with coincident determination of oxygen saturation by both pulse oximeter and in vitro laboratory co-oximeter.[2] Due to limitations in the degree of hypoxemia induced in volunteers, levels below 75% to 80% are extrapolated and thus subject to significant bias as oxygen saturation decreases. In general, pulse oximeters are accurate to within ± 3% at arterial saturations greater than 70%.[4,5]

Pulse oximetry error can come from a variety of sources (Table 5–1). The most common cause of an erroneous reading is related to false signals caused by the detection of nontransmitted light. Ambient light is a major source of interference, and sources include fluorescent lighting, surgical lamps, infrared heating lamps, fiberoptic instruments, and sunlight.[6,7] Optical shunting occurs when light reaches the photodetector without passing through an arterial bed, and takes place when probes are malpositioned or oversized. This is also called the *penumbra effect,*[8] and yields a calculated saturation in the low 80s despite normal saturations. In hypoxic patients, however, the penumbra effect from ambient light and optical shunt will lead to *overestimation* of their oxygen saturation.[9]

Movement creates high-amplitude signals that are mistaken for arterial pulsations and cause erroneous calculations in saturation values. The net effect of motion artifact is to factitiously lower pulse the oximeter saturation. Internal algorithms in newer generation oximeters have attempted to attenuate errors due to motion artifact. Similarly, states of venous pulsation causing congestion also cause false signals that artificially lower oxygen saturation readings.[10] These states include obstructed venous return, severe right heart failure, tricuspid regurgitation, measurements in a dependent limb, constrictive tourniquets, and high positive pressure ventilation.

States of absent or low-amplitude pulses create a low signal-to-noise ratio, causing the pulse oximeter to "search" for a saturation reading. This will occur in the seriously ill patient, in whom such information is essential. Fortunately, in most instances the failure to detect signal is more often due to local vasoconstriction rather than systemic hypotension. Earlobe probes have been suggested to produce better

signals compared to digit probes.[11] Their use is supported by evidence that the earlobe is less vasoactive than the nail bed and thus less susceptible to vasoconstrictive effects.[12]

Carboxyhemoglobin and methemoglobin are *dyshemoglobinemias* not capable of carrying oxygen and thus affect oxygen-carrying capacity. Hemoglobin exists in varying states: bound to oxygen (oxyhemoglobin or O_2Hb), unbound to oxygen (reduced hemoglobin or Hb), bound to carbon monoxide (carboxyhemoglobin or COHb), and altered to a ferric state (methemoglobin or MetHb). Dyshemoglobinemias absorb light used by the pulse oximeter and will produce false absorptions attributed to O_2Hb and Hb. High levels of COHb will cause pulse oximeter saturations to be overestimated.[13-15] Methemoglobin, formed as iron is oxidized to the ferric state, occurs congenitally or from exposure to anesthetics, sulfa drugs, or nitrites.[2] Increasing levels of MetHb lead to concomitant decreases in pulse oximetry saturations to a plateau of 82% to 85%.[16,17]

Intravenous dyes are known to cause falsely low measured oxygen saturations by pulse oximeter. Methylene blue has been documented to cause profound decrease in measured oxygen saturations with pulse oximetry.[18] Indocyanine green is used in angiography of the retina, and indigo carmine to evaluate for dysplasia in ulcerative colitis. These dyes can cause falsely low pulse oximeter readings that occur 35 to 40 seconds after dye administration.[18]

Pulse oximetry readings have reportedly underestimated the degree of hypoxemia in severe anemia,[19] but one study found pulse oximetry to be accurate down to a Hb level of 2.3 g/dl in nonhypoxic adult patients.[20] Skin pigmentation has had variable effects on pulse oximetry and likely has negligible effects on accuracy. Nail polish, specifically black or blue colors, demonstrated the most interference with pulse oximeter readings, lowering oximetry values by 6% in one study.[2,16] Solutions to this problem include removing the nail polish or placing the probe sideways to remove the nail from the transmission path.

In the ED, pulse oximetry serves to detect arterial hypoxemia from respiratory, cardiac, infectious, and metabolic etiologies while facilitating timely intervention before a patient deteriorates. Furthermore, pulse oximetry is used to monitor patients who are sedated for imaging or who undergo procedural sedation and analgesia for painful procedures. The Joint Commission on Accreditation of Healthcare Organizations has recognized the need for noninvasive monitors to improve patient safety.

Current-generation pulse oximeters have improved algorithms that improve accuracy with patient movement while continuing to use *transmitted* light to determine saturations. Other advances include recent Food and Drug Administration approval of a new method for continuous, noninvasive measurement of carbon monoxide in blood (*http://masimo.com/Rainbow/rb-overview.htm*). *Reflectance* oximeters provide innovative technology that detects "backscatter" of light from LEDs and estimates arterial oxygen saturations. Testing of reflection oximetry of retinal blood to measure cerebral oxygenation and perfusion has been in development for the last decade.[21] Unfortunately, reflectance oximeters lack accuracy and have increased susceptibility to noise, and have remained inappropriate for current clinical practice. Near-infrared technology is a noninvasive and relatively low-cost optical technique that is used to measure tissue O_2 saturation,

Table 5–2	Colorimetric Device Color	
Color	**Percent CO$_2$**	**Memory Aid**
Purple	<0.5%	Purple = Problem
Tan	0.5–2%	Tan = Think
Yellow	>2%	Yellow = YES!

*Normal expired end-tidal CO$_2$ is 5%.

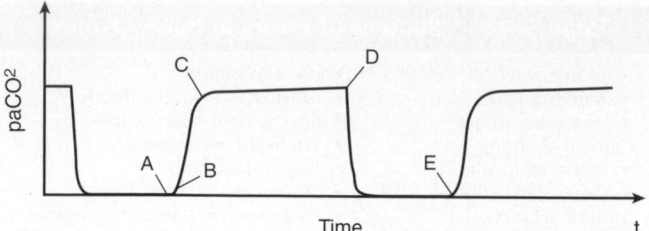

FIGURE 5–1. Capnogram showing the typical curves and loops seen in mechanical ventilation.[87] Point A, end of inhalation; point B, beginning of expiration; segment B–C, appearance of CO$_2$; segment C–D, flow in uniformly ventilated alveoli with near-constant CO$_2$; point D, end-tidal CO$_2$; segment D–E, inspiratory phase. Abnormal shapes can provide clues to clinical findings. A rising segment C–D with no plateau is suggestive of prolonged expiration and differential emptying of alveoli, as noted with asthma or partially obstructed endotracheal tubes (ETTs). Sudden decrease in CO$_2$ with no waveform suggests dislodged ETT, esophageal intubation, obstructed ETT, or ventilator disconnection.

changes in hemoglobin volume, and, indirectly, brain/muscle blood flow and muscle O$_2$ consumption.[22] Currently, this technology remains in development with ongoing research.[23,24]

Capnography/End-Tidal CO$_2$

While pulse oximeters measure oxygenation, the other functional component of the respiratory system that can be non-invasively measured is ventilation, or elimination of CO$_2$. Diseases that cause respiratory distress or failure interfere with exchange of oxygen and carbon dioxide via ventilation/ perfusion mismatch, loss of lung compliance, increased airway resistance, or impairment of respiratory drive.

End-tidal CO$_2$ (ETCO$_2$) monitoring is a noninvasive means for following levels of CO$_2$ in the exhaled breath.[25] Carbon dioxide can be measured qualitatively by colorimetric CO$_2$ detectors or quantitatively by infrared capnometers.[26,27] Since CO$_2$ is the by-product of cellular metabolism and is transported by the circulatory system to be eliminated via exhalation, measurement by capnometry provides an indirect measure of systemic metabolism, cardiac output, and ventilation.[28,29]

Either colorimetric detector or infrared spectroscopy achieves confirmation of CO$_2$ in the ED. Colorimetric devices have a pH-sensitive paper that produces a reversible color scale based on the concentration of CO$_2$ (Table 5–2).[30] Accuracy is affected by humidity, secretions, or contamination with gastric contents or acidic drugs, but is safe in brief use in infants and children greater than 1 kg.[26] Colorimetric detectors are semiquantitative and cannot detect hypo- or hypercarbia, right mainstem bronchus intubation, or oropharyngeal intubation in a spontaneously breathing patient.[26] False-negative results occur during cardiac arrest, severe airway obstruction, pulmonary edema, and severely hypocarbic infants. Despite these limitations, colorimetric detectors have shown prognostic value in pediatric cardiopulmonary resuscitation (CPR), while a capnometric or capnographic rise in ETCO$_2$ to greater than 15 mm Hg precedes return of spontaneous circulation in adults.[31]

Carbon dioxide molecules absorb infrared radiation at a specific wavelength; thus, when filtered infrared light passes through a CO$_2$-containing sample and is compared with a known standard, the concentration of ETCO$_2$ is obtained.[26,27] A capnogram is a graphic display of the CO$_2$ waveform over time (Fig. 5–1).

ETCO$_2$ measurement has been found to be the most reliable method of confirming endotracheal tube position and can distinguish between endotracheal and esophageal intubation.[26,29,32,33] Furthermore, continuous ETCO$_2$ monitoring can detect airway obstruction and inadvertent extubation more rapidly than pulse oximetry.[34] Thus, the American Heart Association guidelines require secondary confirmation of proper tube placement in all patients with a perfusing rhythm by capnography or exhaled CO$_2$ detection immediately following intubation and during transport.[35]

Although an exponential decrease in ETCO$_2$ occurs in cardiac arrest or severe sudden hypotension, it remains a valuable clinical tool during CPR. During effective CPR, ETCO$_2$ has been shown to correlate with cardiac output,[36] efficacy of cardiac compression, return of spontaneous circulation (ROSC), and survival.[37] ETCO$_2$ greater than 10 mm Hg during the first 20 minutes was shown to be associated with ROSC,[38] whereas a value less than 10 mm Hg at 20 minutes predicted death.[39] Following ROSC, ETCO$_2$ values return to normal.[40,41]

Recently, continuous ETCO$_2$ monitoring in *nonintubated* pediatric patients has been shown to be useful for monitoring respirations during seizures[42,43] and sedation and monitoring acid-base status in diabetic ketoacidosis.[44] Other studies have shown that ETCO$_2$ correlates with arterial partial pressure of CO$_2$ (Pco$_2$) measurements.[45-47]

Blood Pressure Oscillometry

Oscillometry is based on the principle that the artery wall oscillates when blood flows through an artery during cuff deflation.[48] The rapid increase in oscillation amplitude estimates *systolic* pressure, while the sudden decrease in oscillation approximates *diastolic* pressure; the period of maximal oscillation is used to estimate *mean* intra-arterial blood pressure.[49] The estimation of systolic and diastolic values is determined indirectly from an empirically derived manufacturer-specific algorithm.[50] Noninvasive oscillometric (automated) blood pressure measurements are as accurate as auscultatory measurements, with less interobserver variability in children.[51]

Oscillometry-derived blood pressures have limitations. Large differences in estimated pressure readings between various manufacturers' devices are thought to be secondary to proprietary algorithms that provide blood pressure estimates. However, systolic blood pressure can average as much as 10 mm Hg above that obtained by auscultation, while diastolic blood pressure measurements are 5 mm Hg higher in children.[12] For this reason, standard blood pressure tables that define normal values for children may not apply to blood pressure measurements obtained by oscillometric methods.[52] Others note poor correlation with diastolic blood pressures. In addition, the devices do not perform well in the presence of limb movement or dysrhythmias.[53] Finally, mean arterial pressures may be significantly underestimated in patients with widened pulse pressures.[54]

Ultrasonic Doppler devices for blood pressure measurement have recently been developed, but have not become established in clinical practice. The probe is placed over an extremity artery while a proximal cuff is slowly deflated; systolic pressure is estimated with appearance of the first Doppler signal, and diastolic pressure is read when the strength and quality of the signal decrease.[55] This technique may be helpful for intermittent blood pressure measurements when the oscillometric device is not able to provide pressure readings and an arterial line is not available.

Another method to *estimate* systolic blood pressure includes the *needle-bounce technique,* which is used by anesthesiologists and flight nurses/physicians and obviates the need to auscultate Korotkoff sounds.[55] Using a sphygmomanometer, the inflated cuff is slowly deflated and the first visible bounce of the needle correlates with systolic blood pressure. Pulse oximetry can estimate systolic blood pressure by the reappearance of waveforms during deflation[56] or by the disappearance of waveform during inflation.[57] Inflation and deflation, however, must be performed slowly (2 to 3 mm Hg/sec) in order for this technique to be accurate.[2]

A continuous partial radial artery compression device has been developed utilizing an oscillometric technique to indirectly measure blood pressure. Continual variable pressure is placed over the radial artery, and pulse pressure waveforms are measured and recorded in real time. This information is processed through a proprietary algorithm generating systolic, diastolic, and mean pressures. A recent study demonstrated that this device performed as well as oscillometric assessment and arterial line pressures.[58] Pediatric studies are currently ongoing.

Continuous ECG Monitoring

Continuous electrocardiographic (ECG) monitoring is required in all patients at risk for cardiac, pulmonary, or neurologic deterioration in the ED. All systems use electrodes that transmit potentials from the heart through the tissues. The ECG signal is then amplified, filtered, and displayed on an oscilloscope. Three- and five-lead systems are available. Lead II can be used to detect most arrhythmias, while the CM5 configuration (right arm electrode at the manubrium, left arm at the V_5 position, and final lead at the left shoulder) detects most left ventricular ischemic events.

Electrical interference and artifacts can occur from several sources (any electrical device powered by alternating current, shivering, movement). Placement of electrodes over bony prominences reduces some of the artifacts. High skin impedance is another common cause of poor signals. Removing skin oils with alcohol diminishes this interference.

Tissue Perfusion Monitoring

The assessment of perfusion status in critically ill patients traditionally has been obtained by global indices such as blood pressure, heart rate, urine output, and mental status. These indices, however, are delayed in exhibiting *early* signs of severe perfusion defects.[59] Early detection of tissue hypo-

perfusion by regional monitoring is based on the concept that blood flow is the primary determinant of tissue carbon dioxide.[60] Gastric tonometry indirectly assesses the splanchnic circulation, which receives up to 25% of cardiac output and contains 20% to 25% of the systemic blood volume.[61] During low-flow states (i.e., shock), large areas become hypoperfused, increasing anaerobic metabolism, lactate, and CO_2 production.[62] Tonometry measures the partial pressure of CO_2 that freely diffuses across gastric mucosa, providing early and accurate information about tissue perfusion.[63] Pediatric studies, however, are limited and gastric tonometry has not been widely implemented in younger age groups due to technical and artifact problems.

Sublingual capnometry has emerged as an alternative to monitoring tissue perfusion. The carbon dioxide–sensing optode (optical sensor) forms carbonic acid upon exposure to carbon dioxide. The pH change causes a shift in the fluorescence of the indicator and is converted to a carbon dioxide concentration. Multiple studies have suggested that sublingual capnometry is predictive of severity of shock[64] and outcome.[65] These studies are small and primarily reflect adult findings. Nonetheless, sublingual capnometry has emerged as a promising technique of noninvasive monitoring of perfusion and hemodynamic disturbances.

Invasive Testing/Monitoring

Critical Lab Monitoring

Arterial blood gas (ABG) analysis is the most commonly used tool for monitoring the effectiveness of oxygenation, ventilation, quantification of acid-base status, and response to therapy. Measured variables are partial pressures of oxygen (Po_2) and carbon dioxide (Pco_2) and hydrogen ion concentration (pH), while other values, such as concentration of total hemoglobin (tHb), O_2Hb saturation, saturations of the dyshemoglobins (COHb and MetHb), plasma bicarbonate, and base excess/deficit, are calculated.[66] In clinical practice, Pco_2 is the best measure of ventilation and adequacy of breathing. The Po_2 represents oxygen dissolved in the blood and can be low secondary to low atmospheric pressure (e.g., high altitude), hypoventilation, lung disease causing ventilation/perfusion (V/Q) mismatch (e.g., asthma, pneumonia), loss of pulmonary architecture (e.g., emphysema), and shunt (e.g., cyanotic heart disease). Distinguishing between hypoventilation and V/Q mismatch can be accomplished by calculating the alveolar-arterial (A-a) gradient using the fraction of inspired oxygen (FiO_2), Po_2, and Pco_2:

$$FiO_2 \times \text{air pressure } (713 \times 0.21 \text{ or } 150 \text{ at sea level, room air}) - (Po_2 + Pco_2/0.8)$$

Contemporary research has shown comparable accuracy of venous blood gases with ABGs for measuring pH and bicarbonate (HCO_3) in adult diabetic ketoacidosis.[67] Studies also have shown a correlation between arterial and capillary pH and Pco_2 in acutely ill children.[68,69] Others have shown a correlation between pH, Pco_2, base excess (BE), and HCO_3 in ABG, capillary blood gas, and venous blood gas values.[70]

The accuracy of arterial blood gases is influenced by air bubbles within the sample; the resultant gas equilibrium between air and arterial blood lowers arterial carbon dioxide pressure and increases arterial oxygen pressure.[71] Time and

Table 5–3	Unmeasured Anions

Organic acids
- Lactate
- Ketoacids
- Albumin

Inorganic acids
- Phosphates
- Sulfates

Exogenous
- Salicylate
- Formate
- Nitrate
- Penicillin

Miscellaneous
- Acetate
- Paraldehyde
- Ethylene glycol
- Methanol
- Ethanol
- Urea
- Glucose

Data from Rhodes and Cusack[76] and Balasubramanyan et al.[72]

temperature are other variables that affect accuracy. If the sample cannot be analyzed quickly, it should be placed on ice and cooled to 5°C, at which it can be stored for up to an hour. Complications associated with arterial punctures include pain, arterial injury, thrombosis, hemorrhage, and aneurysm formation.

The BE has traditionally been used to assess acid-base status and estimate unmeasured anion concentrations (Table 5–3). First, *standard bicarbonate* is calculated from measured blood gas pH using the Henderson-Hasselbalch equation; the P_{CO_2} is kept constant at 40 torr to isolate the metabolic contribution and remove the respiratory component.[72] Next the difference between standard bicarbonate and 22.9, multiplied by a factor of 1.2, calculates the BE.[73] A BE values ≤–5 is considered a clinically significant metabolic acidosis. Moreover, BE values ≤–8 predict a higher mortality (23% vs. 6% if BE >–8) in pediatric trauma victims.[74] One limitation is that the calculations of BE assume normal water content, electrolytes, and albumin; these values are more than likely altered in critically ill children and are more apt to introduce error.

The presence in critically ill patients of metabolic acidosis based on BE values was thought to reflect elevated lactic acid levels, poor perfusion, and concomitant organ dysfunction. This principle has since been challenged[75-77] because hyperchloremia skews the BE to suggest false acidosis,[78] and BE poorly correlates with lactic acidosis.[72,77]

In adults, a strong ion gap (SIG) greater than 2 mEq/L is more accurate than BE in detecting true tissue acidosis,[77] identifying patients with lactic acidosis and splanchnic hypoperfusion with multiorgan dysfunction, and predicting mortality.[72] The SIG represents a complex calculation that measures the difference between strong anions and strong cations and is the mathematical difference between the apparent strong ion difference (SIDa) and the effective strong ion difference (SIDe).[79] An elevated SIG greater than 2 mEq/L signifies that unmeasured strong anions are present in the bloodstream:

$$SIDa = [Na^+ + K^+ + Ca^{2+} + Mg^{2+} - Cl^- - lactate - urate]$$
$$SIDe = [albumin \times (0.123 \times pH - 0.631)] + [PO_4 \times (0.309 \times pH - 0.469)] + HCO_3$$
$$SIG = SIDa - SIDe \text{ (abnormal SIG is } > 2 \text{ mEq/L)}$$

In the absence of oxygen, lactate is a by-product of glycolysis to maintain energy production (ATP) when pyruvate cannot enter the Krebs cycle.[80] Lactate abruptly increases when oxygen delivery falls to a critical level and concomitant decrease in oxygen extraction occurs.[81] Clearance occurs via the liver and kidneys, and normal arterial lactate levels are between 0.5 and 1 mEq/L. Traditionally, elevated blood lactate levels in hemodynamically unstable patients are thought to reflect circulatory shock, arterial hypoxemia, or both. Elevated lactate levels are described in circulatory shock, acute lung injury, sepsis, and multiorgan failure, and are an indicator of severe inflammatory cascade. Increasing lactate levels are associated with organ dysfunction, adverse events, and mortality in adult patients with shock, trauma, and sepsis.[76] Nonetheless, lactate levels remain useful indicators for indirectly monitoring perfusion and oxygen delivery/consumption.

Continuous Indwelling Arterial Monitoring

Patients requiring close arterial blood pressure monitoring or frequent arterial blood gas analysis may require arterial cannulation for continuous monitoring. The transducer that translates the blood pressure into a waveform can be set to alarm if specific high or low values for mean arterial pressure, systolic blood pressure, or diastolic blood pressure are reached. The dicrotic notch signifying aortic valve closure should be greater than one third of the height of the systolic pressure unless cardiac output is depressed (Fig. 5–2A). The slope of the upstroke reflects myocardial contractility, with a diminished slope indicating shock (Fig. 5–2B). Formulas can be used to estimate stroke volume by measuring the area from the beginning of the upstroke to the dicrotic notch. Multiplying this value by the heart rate will estimate the cardiac output. Finally, the downward slope during diastole indirectly assesses resistance to cardiac outflow. Vasoconstriction causes a slow fall in this slope. Importantly, mean arterial pressure will be higher when measured at the periphery (e.g., distal lower extremity) compared to more centrally obtained pressures. Auscultatory measurements may give a slightly lower value than continuous indwelling catheter measurements. Falsely lowered values may be present if vasoconstriction occurs (e.g., severe shock, hypothermia, or vasopressor administration). Importantly, loss of a normal waveform or any distal extremity problems (pain, blanching, loss of pulse) may indicate thrombotic obstruction and the need to remove the cannula. A dampened waveform (increased diastolic and decreased systolic blood pressure) can be due to air bubbles, blood clots, soft tubing, or a soft diaphragm within the pressure transducer.

Central Venous Pressure Monitoring

Central venous pressure monitoring is used in critically ill patients who are in circulatory failure, require massive fluid or blood replacement, or have a compromised cardiovascular system. New interest in goal-directed therapy for septic shock

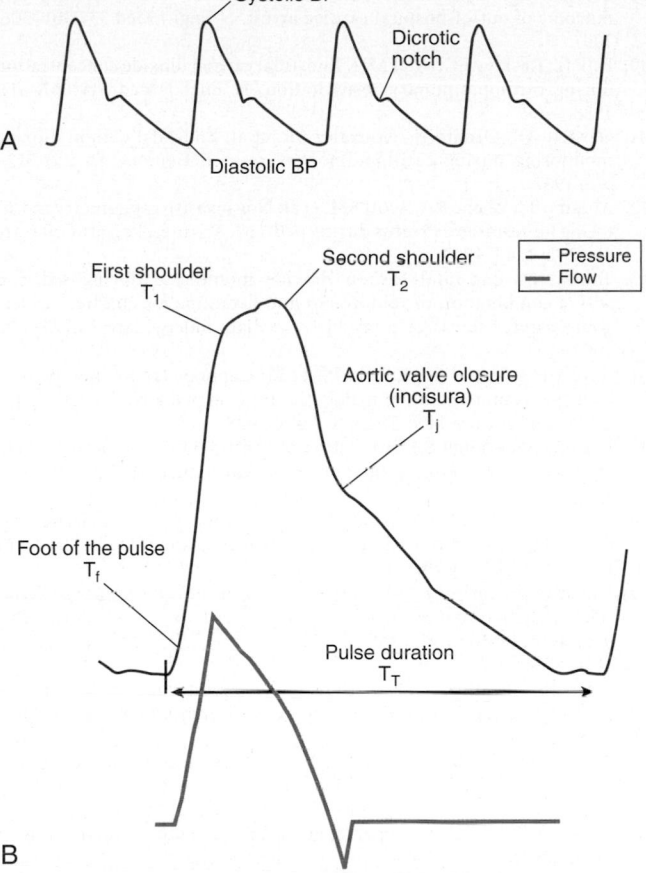

Figure 5–2. A, Blood pressure (BP) translated to waveform during continuous BP monitoring. **B,** Correlation of blood pressure and arterial blood flow.

has increased the potential use of this tool in critically ill infants and children presenting to the ED.[82]

Following placement of a central venous catheter (see Chapter 161, Vascular Access), measurement of central venous pressure (CVP) can be used to diagnose disorders and guide treatment. A normal CVP is 5 to 12 cm H_2O, with low values indicating a low right atrial pressure and hypovolemic or distributive shock. High values indicate cardiogenic shock, overhydration, pulmonary embolism, tension pneumothorax, valvular heart disease (e.g., pulmonary stenosis), pericardial tamponade, or restrictive pericarditis. Importantly, changes in CVP readings following infusion of a fluid bolus reflect intravascular volume and are more important predictors of volume abnormalities. Following a 10-ml/kg fluid bolus, the CVP is expected to rise 3 to 4 cm H_2O. If this number drops rapidly (in <5 to 10 minutes) to its baseline or only rises 1 to 2 cm with a fluid bolus, hypovolemia is probable and further fluid administration is usually indicated. A rise greater than 5 cm H_2O indicates overfilling and the potential for development of pulmonary edema.

During treatment of septic shock, one goal is to maintain a normal perfusion pressure (mean arterial pressure minus CVP) for an infant or child's age: 55 cm H_2O for infants up to 1 year old, 60 cm H_2O for those from 1 to 2 years old, and 65 cm H_2O for those who are greater than 2 to 15 years old[81] (see Chapter 8, Circulatory Emergencies: Shock).

Inaccurate CVP monitoring can result from a malpositioned catheter tip within the internal jugular vein, subclavian vein, or right ventricle or migration between discordant locations. Radiographic confirmation can limit this complication. Readings must be obtained using the same reference level at the midaxillary line with the patient supine. Measurements are taken at rest and during exhalation. Coughing, straining, positive pressure ventilation, air bubble within the catheter, and possibly vasopressors can falsely raise CVP values. Falsely low readings occur with catheter obstruction or contact with the vessel wall.

Mixed Venous Oxygen Saturation

Superior vena cava or mixed venous oxygen saturation (SvO_2) can serve as a guide to therapy in septic shock. When oxygen saturation, oxygen consumption, and hemoglobin are stable, this parameter indirectly measures cardiac output. Patients in septic shock often have a low SvO_2 due to decreased cardiac output and increased consumption. One goal in managing septic shock is to achieve an SvO_2 greater than 70% using a combination of volume, vasopressors, vasodilators, and type III phosphodiesterase inhibitors depending upon the clinical scenario (see Chapter 8, Circulatory Emergencies: Shock; and Chapter 13, Sepsis). While interpreting SvO_2 values, clinicians should be aware that many parameters decrease this value, including low cardiac output, decreased arterial saturation, anemia, and increased oxygen extraction (e.g., early sepsis, agitation).

Pulmonary capillary wedge pressure monitoring for infants is generally not undertaken in the ED. As more accurate, less invasive means of monitoring cardiac output/cardiac index become available, it is expected that these tools will assist in diagnosing and managing critically ill patients in the ED.

Summary

Hemodynamic monitoring in the ED is vital, since the condition of an ill child may change quickly. Emergency physicians are multitasking and caring for multiple patients simultaneously, thus real-time information must be readily available and accessible. Recognition and rapid assessment can be accomplished in a few minutes using noninvasive monitoring techniques. Knowledge of the utility and limitations of critical monitoring techniques will enhance patient care and potentially improve outcome for seriously injured and ill children.

REFERENCES

1. Brown LH, Manring EA, Kornegay HB, Prasad NH: Can prehospital personnel detect hypoxemia without the aid of pulse oximeters? Am J Emerg Med 14:61–65, 1996.
2. Sinex JE: Pulse oximetry: principles and limitations. Am J Emerg Med 17:59–67, 1999.
3. Epstein RA, Hyman AI: Ventilatory requirements of critically ill neonates. Anesthesiology 53:379–384, 1980.
4. Severinghaus JW, Kelleher JF: Recent developments in pulse oximetry. Anesthesiology 76:1018–1038, 1992.
5. Severinghaus JW: History and recent developments in pulse oximetry. Scand J Clin Lab Invest Suppl 53:105–111, 1993.
6. Grace RF: Pulse oximetry: gold standard or false sense of security? Med J Aust 160:638–644, 1994.
7. Costarino AT, Davis DA, Keon TO: Falsely normal saturation with the pulse oximeter. Anesthesiology 67:830–831, 1987.

8. Kelleher JF, Ruff RH: The penumbra effect: vasomotion-dependent pulse oximeter artifact due to probe malposition. Anesthesiology 71:787–791, 1989.

9. Barker SJ, Hyatt J, Shah NK, et al: The effect of sensor malpositioning on pulse oximeter accuracy during hypoxemia. Anesthesiology 79:248–252, 1993.

10. Schnapp LM, Cohen NH: Pulse oximetry—uses and abuses. Chest 98:1244–1250, 1990.

11. Kelleher JF: Pulse oximetry. J Clin Monit 5:37–62, 1989.

12. Evans ML, Geddes LA: An assessment of blood vessel vasoactivity using photoplethysmography. Med Instrument 22:29–32, 1988.

13. Barker SJ, Temper KK: The effect of carbon monoxide inhalation on pulse oximetry and transcutaneous PO$_2$. Anesthesiology 66:677–679, 1987.

14. Vegfors M, Lennmarken C: Carboxyhaemoglobinaemia and pulse oximetry. Br J Anaesth 66:625–626, 1991.

15. Buckley RG, Aks SE, Eshom JL, et al: The pulse oximetry gap in carbon monoxide intoxication. Ann Emerg Med 24:252–255, 1994.

16. Ralston AC, Webb RK, Runciman WB: Potential errors in pulse oximetry. III: effects of interferences, dyes, dyshaemoglobinemias, and other pigments. Anaesthesia 46:291–295, 1991.

17. Watcha MF, Connor MT, Hing AV: Pulse oximetry in methemoglobinemia. Am J Dis Child 143:845–847, 1989.

18. Scheller MS, Unger RJ, Kelner MJ: Effects of intravenously administered dyes on pulse oximetry readings. Anesthesiology 65:550–552, 1986.

19. Severinghaus JW, Koh SO: Effect of anemia on pulse oximeter accuracy at low saturation. J Clin Monit 6:85–88, 1990.

20. Jay GD, Hughes L, Renzi FP: Pulse oximetry is accurate in acute anemia from hemorrhage. Ann Emerg Med 24:32–35, 1994.

21. Nelson DA, Krupsky S, Pollack A, et al: Special report: noninvasive multiparameter functional optical imaging of the eye. Ophthalmic Surg Lasers Imaging 36:57–66, 2005.

22. Ferrari M, Mottola L, Quaresima V: Principles, techniques, and limitations of near infrared spectroscopy. Can J Appl Physiol 29:463–487, 2004.

23. Madsen PL, Secher NH: Near-infrared oximetry of the brain. Prog Neurobiol 58:541–560, 1999.

24. Frangioni JV: In vivo near-infrared fluorescence imaging. Curr Opin Chem Biol 7:626–634, 2003.

25. Bhende MS, LaCovey DC: End-tidal carbon dioxide monitoring in the prehospital setting. Prehospital Emerg Care 5:208–213, 2001.

26. Bhende MS: Capnography in the pediatric emergency department. Pediatr Emerg Care 15:1–6, 1999.

27. Ward KR, Yealy D: End-tidal CO$_2$ monitoring in emergency medicine. Part I: basic principles. Acad Emerg Med 5:628–636, 1998.

28. Szaflarski NL, Cohen NH: Use of capnography in critically ill adults. Heart Lung 20:363–372, 1991.

29. Sanders AB: Capnometry in emergency medicine. Ann Emerg Med 18:1287–1290, 1989.

30. Nellcor: EasyCap ET CO$_2$ detector product information. Hayward, CA: Nellcor, Inc, 1992.

31. Bhende MS, Thompson AE: Evaluation of an end-tidal CO$_2$ detector during pediatric cardiopulmonary resuscitation. Pediatrics 95:395–399, 1995.

32. Gravenstein JS, Paulus DA, Hayes TJ: Clinical indications. In Gravenstein JS, Paulus DA, Hayes TJ (eds): Capnography in Clinical Practice. Stoneham, MA: Butterworth, 1989, pp 43–49.

33. Birmingham PK, Cheney FW, Ward RJ: Esophageal intubation: a review of detection techniques. Anesth Analg 65:886–891, 1986.

34. Poirier MP, Gonzalez Del-Rey JP, Del-Rey JA, et al: Utility of monitoring capnography, pulse oximetry, and vital signs in the detection of airway mishaps: a hyperoxemic animal model. Am J Emerg Med 16:350–352, 1998.

35. Cummins RO, Hazinski MF: New guidelines on tracheal tube confirmation and prevention of dislodgement. Circulation 102(Suppl I):I380–I384, 2000.

36. Weil MH, Bisera J, Trevino RP, et al: Cardiac output and end-tidal carbon dioxide. Crit Care Med 13:907–909, 1985.

37. Sanders AB, Ewy GA, Bragg S, et al: Expired PCO$_2$ as a prognostic indicator of successful resuscitation from cardiac arrest. Ann Emerg Med 14:948–952, 1985.

38. Cantineau JP, Lambert Y, Merckx P, et al: End-tidal carbon dioxide during cardiopulmonary resuscitation in humans presenting mostly with asystole: a predictor of outcome. Crit Care Med 24:791–796, 1997.

39. Levine RL, Wayne MA, Miller CC: End-tidal carbon dioxide and outcome of out-of-hospital cardiac arrest. N Engl J Med 337:301–306, 1997.

40. Falk JL, Rackow EC, Weil MH: End-tidal carbon dioxide concentration during cardiopulmonary resuscitation. N Engl J Med 318:607–611, 1988.

41. Garnett AR, Ornato JP, Gonzalez ER, et al: End-tidal carbon dioxide monitoring during cardiopulmonary resuscitation. JAMA 257:512–515, 1987.

42. Abramo TJ, Wiebe RA, Scott SM, et al: Noninvasive capnometry monitoring for respiratory status during pediatric seizures. Pediatr Crit Care 25:1242–1246, 1997.

43. Tobias JD: End-tidal carbon dioxide monitoring during sedation with a combination of midazolam and ketamine for children undergoing painful, invasive procedures. Pediatr Emerg Care 15:173–175, 1999.

44. Garcia E, Abramo TJ, Okada PJ, et al: Capnometry for noninvasive continuous monitoring of metabolic status in pediatric diabetic ketoacidosis. Crit Care Med 31:2539–2543, 2003.

45. Barton CW, Wang ESJ: Correlation of end-tidal CO$_2$ measurements to arterial CO$_2$ in non-intubated patients. Ann Emerg Med 23:560–563, 1994.

46. Abramo TJ, Cowan MR, Scott SM, et al: Comparison of pediatric end-tidal CO$_2$ measured with nasal/oral cannula circuit and capillary PCO$_2$. Am J Emerg Med 13:30–33, 1995.

47. Flanagan JF, Garrett JS, McDuffee A: Non-invasive monitoring of end-tidal carbon dioxide tension via nasal cannulas in spontaneously breathing children with profound hypocarbia. Crit Care Med 23:1140–1142, 1995.

48. Mark JB, Slaughter TF: Cardiovascular monitoring. In Miller RD: Miller's Anesthesia, 6th ed. Philadelphia, Churchill Livingstone, 2005, pp 1265–1362.

49. Mauck GW, Smith CR, Geddes LA, et al: The meaning of the point of maximum oscillations in cuff pressure in the indirect measurement of blood pressure—part II. J Biomech Eng 102:28–33, 1980.

50. Pickering TG, Hall JE, Appel LJ, et al: AHA Scientific Statement: Recommendations for blood pressure measurements in humans and experimental animals. Hypertension 45:142–161, 2005.

51. Mattu GS, Heran BS, Wright JM: Comparison of the automated non-invasive oscillometric blood pressure monitor (BpTRU) with the auscultatory mercury sphygmomanometer in a paediatric population. Blood Press Monit 9:39–45, 2004.

52. Park MK, Menard SW, Yuan C: Comparison of auscultatory and oscillometric blood pressures. Arch Pediatr Adolesc Med 155:50–53, 2001.

53. Stanford TJ, Jones BR, Ty Smith N: Noninvasive blood pressure measurement. Anesthesiol Clin North Am 6:721, 1988.

54. van Montfrans GA: Oscillometric blood pressure measurement: progress and problems. Blood Press Monit 5:81–89, 2001.

55. Sweeney MF, Madsen MS, Belani KG, Swedlow DB: Noninvasive vital monitoring in children. In Fuhrman BP, Zimmerman JJ (eds): Pediatric Critical Care, 2nd ed. St. Louis: Mosby, 1998, pp 95–105.

56. Talke P, Nichols RJ, Traber DL: Monitoring patients during helicopter flight. J Clin Monit 6:139–140, 1990.

57. Chawla R, Kumarvel V, Girdhar KK, et al: Can pulse oximetry be used to measure systolic blood pressure? Anesth Analg 74:196–200, 1992.

58. Thomas SH, Winsor GR, Pang PS, et al: Use of radial artery compression device for noninvasive, near-continuous blood pressure monitoring in the ED. Am J Emerg Med 22:474–478, 2004.

59. Brown SD, Gutierrez G: Does gastric tonometry work? Yes. Crit Care Clin 12:569–585, 1996.

60. Maciel AT, Creteur J, Vincent JL: Tissue capnometry: does the answer lie under the tongue? Intensive Care Med 30:2157–2165, 2004.

61. Garrett SA, Pearl RG: Improved gastric tonometry for monitoring tissue perfusion: the canary sings louder. Anesth Analg 83:1–3, 1996.

62. Maynard N, Bihari D, Beale R, et al: Assessment of splanchnic oxygenation by gastric tonometry in patients with acute circulatory failure. JAMA 270:1203–1210, 1993.

63. Huang, CC, Tsai YH, Lin MC, et al: Gastric intramucosal PCO$_2$ and pH variability in ventilated critically ill patients. Crit Care Med 29:88–95, 2001.

64. Weil MH, Nakagawa Y, Tang W, et al: Sublingual capnometry: a new noninvasive measurement for diagnosis and quantitation of severity of circulatory shock. Crit Care Med 27:1225–1229, 1999.

65. Marik PE, Bankov A: Sublingual capnometry versus traditional markers of tissue oxygenation in critically ill patients. Crit Care Med 31:818–822, 2003.

66. Blood gas analysis and hemoximetry: 2001 revision and update. Respir Care 46:498–505, 2001.

67. Brandenburg MA, Dire DJ: Comparison of arterial and venous blood gas values in the initial emergency department evaluation of patients with diabetic ketoacidosis. Ann Emerg Med 31:459–465, 1998.

68. Harrison AM, Lynch JM, Dean JM, et al: Comparison of simultaneously obtained arterial and capillary blood gases in pediatric intensive care unit patients. Crit Care Med 25:1904–1908, 1997.

69. Kirubakaran C, Gnananayagam JE, Sundaravalli EK: Comparison of blood gas values in arterial and venous blood. Ind J Pediatr 70:781–785, 2003.

70. Yildizdas D, Yapicioglu H, Yilmaz HL, et al: Correlation of simultaneously obtained capillary, venous, and arterial blood gases of patients in a paediatric intensive care unit. Arch Dis Child 89:176–180, 2004.

71. Williams AJ: ABC of oxygen: assessing and interpreting arterial blood gases and acid-base balance. BMJ 317:1213–1216, 1998.

72. Balasubramanyan N, Havens PL, Hoffman G: Unmeasured anions identified by the Fencl-Stewart method predict mortality better than base excess, anion gap, and lactate in patients in the pediatric intensive care unit. Crit Care Med 27:1577–1581, 1999.

73. Siggaard-Anderson O: Acid-base terminology. Lancet 2:1010–1012, 1965.

74. Peterson DL, Schinco MA, Kerwin AJ, et al: Evaluation of initial base deficit as a prognosticator of outcome in the pediatric trauma population. Am Surg 70:326–328, 2004.

75. Fencl V, Jabor A, Kazda A, Figge J: Diagnosis of metabolic acid-base disturbances in critically ill patients. Am J Respir Crit Care Med 162:2246–2251, 2000.

76. Rhodes A, Cusack RJ: Arterial blood gas analysis and lactate. Curr Opin Crit Care 6:227–231, 2000.

77. Murray DM, Olhsson VZ, Fraser JI: Defining acidosis in postoperative cardiac patients using Stewart's method of strong ion difference. Pediatr Crit Care Med 5:240–245, 2004.

78. Skellett S, Mayer A, Durward A, et al: Chasing the base deficit: hyperchloremic acidosis following 0.9% saline resuscitation. Arch Dis Child 83:514–516, 2000.

79. Kaplan LJ, Kellum JA: Initial pH, base deficit, lacate, anion gap, strong ion difference and strong ion gap predict outcome from major vascular injury. Crit Care Med 32:1120–1124, 2004.

80. De Backer D: Lactic acidosis. Intensive Care Med 29:699–702, 2003.

81. Vincent JL, De Backer DD: Oxygen transport—the oxygen delivery controversy. Intensive Care Med 30:1990–1996, 2004.

82. Carcillo JA, Fields AI: Clinical practice parameters for hemodynamic support of pediatric and neonatal patients in septic shock. Crit Care Med 30:1365–1378, 2002.

83. Rittner F, Doring M: Curves and loops in mechanical ventilation. Draeger Medical, 2006. Available at *http://www.draeger.com/MT/internet/pdf/CareAreas/CriticalCare/cc_loops_book_en.pdf*

Chapter 6

Neonatal Resuscitation

Richard M. Cantor, MD and Steven G. Rothrock, MD

Key Points

Neonatal resuscitation rarely occurs within most emergency departments; therefore, appropriate personnel, equipment, and medications must be readily available.

More than 90% of newly born infants respond well to basic and standardized resuscitative efforts.

A decreasing heart rate is a sign of clinical deterioration; assisted ventilation is required if the heart rate is less than 100 beats per minute (bpm) and cardiac compression is required if it is less than 60 bpm.

Direct tracheal suction is required in newly born infants with absent or depressed respirations, poor muscle tone, or a heart rate less than 100 bpm.

Introduction and Background

When discussing neonatal resuscitation, it is important to define the age range that is being discussed. To avoid confusion with terminology, the International Liaison Committee on Resuscitation has defined "newly born" as an infant in the first minutes to hours after birth to focus attention on the needs of the infant who has just been born. A "neonate" is defined as being 0 to 28 days old, while the term *newborn* is no longer used.[1]

There are approximately 4.1 million infants born each year in the United States. Ninety percent of newly born infants (first hours after birth) are capable of transitioning from intrauterine to extrauterine life without any difficulty. They will require little or no assistance to initiate spontaneous and regular respirations. Nearly 10% of newly born infants require some degree of assistance to begin breathing at birth.[2] Approximately 1% will require extensive resuscitative measures to survive.[3,4]

The priorities of resuscitation in the newly born mimic those in adults. The airway must be open and clear. Breathing must be guaranteed, whether spontaneous or assisted. Oxygenated blood must adequately circulate centrally and to the periphery. An additional stressor for the newly born involves the maintenance of thermal regularity. The large surface area of these infants combined with exposure to wet surfaces facilitates the development of hypothermia.

When considering procedures to initiate while attending the delivery, the following measures are listed in order of required frequency[5,6]:

- Adequate assessment of the baby's response to birth
- Maintenance of thermal regularity
- Positioning, clearing the airway, stimulation to breath by drying, and the provision of oxygen if necessary
- Establishment of effective ventilation whether by bag, bag-mask, or endotracheal intubation
- Institution of chest compressions
- Administration of resuscitative medications

Recognition and Approach

Pathophysiologic Factors

Prenatally, only a small fraction of fetal blood passes through the fetal lungs. While in utero, the potential air sacs within the alveoli are filled with fluid rather than air. The pulmonary vasculature is constricted prenatally and diminished in importance. After delivery, the lungs expand with oxygen and there is global relaxation of the pulmonary vascular network.

Three major changes take place within seconds after birth:

- Fluid in the alveoli is absorbed into lung tissue and replaced by air.
- Clamping of the umbilical arteries and vein results in a dramatic increase in systemic blood pressure.
- As a result of utilization of the alveolar potential space, the blood vessels in the lung tissue relax. This facilitates a decrease in flow through the ductus arteriosis. The eventual closure of the ductus is directly related to the rapidly rising partial pressure of oxygen in neonatal blood.

At the completion of this normal transition, the infant's initial cries and deep breaths will assist the movement of fluid from the airways.[7] This facilitates the resolution of any cyanosis in the child into an oxygenated state. There is a gradual improvement in oxygenation and pH over the first 24 hours, while there is relatively high hematocrit (Table 6–1).

An infant may encounter difficulty before labor, during labor, or after birth. Processes that began in utero usually manifest themselves in compromised blood flow within the placenta or the umbilical cord. Fetal bradycardia will often be present in the distressed newly born. Problems that occur after birth are more likely to involve the infant's airway. Specifically, the infant may not manifest a sufficient breath to adequately force fluid from the alveoli.[8] In addition, foreign material, such as meconium, may block air from entering the alveoli. In any event, the lungs will not fill with air and the body will be deprived of oxygen. A relatively rare complication of a term delivery is the existence of persistent pulmonary hypertension. This entity represents an intrauterine lack of oxygen, which results in sustained constriction of the pulmonary arterials. This manifests itself with profound cyanosis.

Multiple risk factors are associated with the need for resuscitation in the newly born (Table 6–2). Infants who are compromised may exhibit one or more of the following symptoms and signs:
- Cyanosis
- Bradycardia
- Hypotension
- Depression of the respiratory drive
- Poor muscle tone

To identify hypotension, clinicians must be aware of age- and weight-based normal blood pressures for newly born infants (Table 6–3). The mean arterial pressure for premature newly born infants should be greater than their gestational age in weeks.

Personnel Required at Anticipated Delivery

At every delivery, there should be one identified person primarily responsible for initiating resuscitation. This person should have the skills necessary to perform a complete resuscitation, including endotracheal intubation and supervision of emergent medications. When resuscitation is necessary, it must be initiated immediately.

If a high-risk delivery is anticipated, at least two people must be present solely to manage the baby—one with the full compliment of resuscitation skills and the other to provide assistance. In high-risk cases, the primary resuscitator will serve as the leader of the team and will be responsible for opening the airway and intubation if necessary. Other personnel will be needed to assist with positioning, suctioning, drying, administering oxygen, ventilating, or applying chest compressions. One staff member should be available for drawing up and administering medications.[6] In all cases, personnel must observe appropriate precautions to protect against exposure to infectious agents.

All necessary equipment for a complete resuscitation must be readily available and operational at all times (Table 6–4).

Evaluation

In general, determining the need for resuscitative efforts begins immediately after birth. Most newly born infants respond to the extrauterine environment by demonstrating a vigorous cry, movement of all extremities, and a strong respiratory effort. With these responses in place, early cyanosis improves to duskiness and finally to a pink color. Infants who do not meet these criteria require intervention (Fig. 6–1).

Table 6–1	Normal Arterial Blood/Hct Values in Full-Term Newly Born				
Age	PaO$_2$	PaCO$_2$	pH	Base Excess	Hct (vol %)
1 hr	63 mm Hg	36 mm Hg	7.33	−6.0 mEq/L	53
24 hr	73 mm Hg	33 mm Hg	7.37	−5.0 mEq/L	55

Abbreviations: Hct, hematocrit; PaCO$_2$, arterial partial pressure of carbon dioxide; PaO$_2$, arterial partial pressure of oxygen.

Table 6–2	Risk Factors Associated with the Need for Neonatal Resuscitation

Antepartum Factors

Maternal diabetes (esp. if poor control)	Multiple gestation
Preeclampsia or eclampsia	Size-dates discrepancy
Chronic hypertension	Medication & drug use
Chronic anemia or isoimmunization (if Rh−)	Illicit drugs (e.g., cocaine, amphetamines)
Prior late fetal demise or neonatal death	Lithium carbonate
Late-trimester bleeding	Sedatives, narcotics
Maternal infection or fever	Magnesium
Maternal underlying disease (e.g., heart, lungs, kidney, thyroid, or neurologic)	Adrenergic blocking drugs
Polyhydramnios	Maternal cigarette or alcohol use
Oligohydramnios	Fetal malformation
Premature rupture of membranes	Diminished fetal activity
Postterm gestation	No prenatal care
	Age <16 or >35 yr

Intrapartum Factors

Emergency cesarean section or general anesthesia	Fetal bradycardia
Assisted delivery (forceps or vacuum extraction)	Abnormal fetal heart rate patterns
Breech or other abnormal lie/presentation	Uterine tetany or atony
Premature labor	Maternal narcotics administration within 4 hr of delivery
Precipitous delivery	Meconium-stained umbilical cord
Chorioamnionitis	Placental abruption—stained amniotic fluid
Prolonged rupture of membranes (>18 hr before delivery)	Prolapsed uterus
Prolonged labor (>24 hr)	Placenta previa
Prolonged second stage of labor (>2 hr)	

Table 6–3	Normal Blood Pressure (BP) for Different Birth Weights			
	Weight			
	<1 kg	1–2 kg	2–3 kg	>3 kg
Systolic BP (mm Hg)	40–60	50–60	50–70	50–80
Diastolic BP (mm Hg)	15–35	20–40	25–45	30–50

Table 6–4	Equipment and Supplies Used during Resuscitation

Self-inflating bag with reservoir *or* flow-inflating bag and mask with an oxygen source
Masks (term and preterm sizes)
Laryngoscope straight blades (0, 1)
Endotracheal tubes (2.5, 3, 3.5 internal diameter)
Oxygen source
Bulb suction, or DeLee suction trap and meconium aspirator
Wall suction device with attachments
1-, 3-, and 20-ml syringes
Three-way stopcock
3.5F or 5F umbilical catheters
5F feeding tube or catheter with connector to accommodate syringe (for endotracheal medicines)
Normal saline flush
Povidone-iodine applicator (or similar sterilizing fluid)
Sterile gloves
Umbilical tape and scissors
Scalpel handle and blade
Curved hemostat
Forceps
Normal saline for volume expansion
Dry, warm blankets
Radiant warmer
Medication labels
Code sheet for recording medication

In a fairly rapid manner, the healthy newly born infant should establish regular respirations sufficient to maintain a heart rate greater than 100 beats per minute (bpm). The need for assisted ventilation is indicated by the presence of gasping, apnea, or a heart rate less than 100 bpm.

The heart rate can be estimated by listening directly to the precordium or feeling pulsations at the base of the umbilical cord. Central and peripheral pulses in the neck and extremities are often difficult to feel in infants.[9,10] An additional benefit to palpating the umbilical base is the avoidance of interference with respiratory assistance. The heart rate should consistently remain above 100 bpm. Any changes in the heart rate may indicate improvement or deterioration of the clinical status.

A stable, fully perfused newly born infant should maintain a pink color in the mucous membranes without supplemental oxygen. The face, trunk, and mucous membranes are examined for central cyanosis. Acrocyanosis is considered a normal finding at birth and is not a reliable indicator of central hypoxemia. In most cases it is more a sign of cold stress. Decreased cardiac output, severe anemia, hypovolemia, and acidosis are associated with the development of pallor. Capillary refill should not be relied upon to diagnose hypovolemia or shock at this age. Normal newly born capillary refill time can be greater than 3 to 4 seconds.[11]

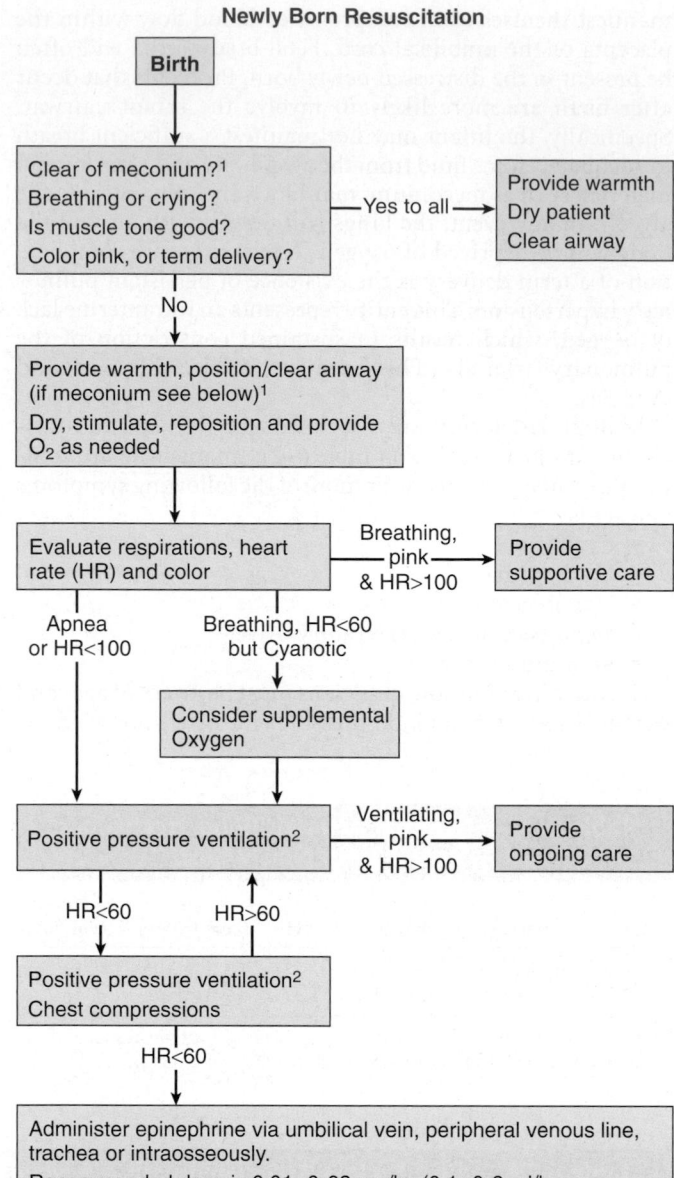

Newly Born Resuscitation

[1]Meconium management: *Intrapartum*—Suctioning the mouth, pharynx, and nose is no longer recommended after delivery of the head.

Following delivery—Perform immediate direct laryngoscopy with suctioning ONLY if (1) depressed respirations (2) absent of diminished muscle tone or (3) HR<100 beats/minute. Repeat until little meconium is recovered or HR<60–80 (indicating need for resuscitation). Perform tracheal suctioning before initiating positive pressure ventilation (PPV). If patient becomes severely distressed, positive pressure ventilation may be required even if all of meconium is not suctioned out.

[2]Consider endotracheal intubation if positive pressure ventilation is ineffective at this step.

FIGURE 6–1. Decision chart for newly born resuscitation.

Management

Thermal Regularity

Cold stress will increase oxygen consumption and impede effective resuscitation.[12] The goal is to avoid overshoot hyperthermia since it may favor the development of respiratory depression. It is important to provide a warm, draft-free environment for the infant. Normothermia is facilitated by placing the infant under a radiant warmer, drying the skin, removing wet linen, and wrapping the infant in prewarmed blankets. Plastic bags or plastic (food-grade, heat-resistant) wrapping applied to neonates placed under a radiant heat source will aid in maintaining temperature.[13] An additional mechanism for the prevention of heat loss involves placing the infant directly on the mother's chest or abdomen.

Positioning of the Airway

The newly born infant is placed supine or lying on one side with the head in a neutral position. It is important at this point to rule out airway obstruction as manifested by respiratory effort without air movement. In this case, the head position is readdressed by placing a blanket or towel under the shoulders to facilitate air entry.

Suctioning

In most deliveries, there is enough time to suction the infant's nose and mouth with a bulb syringe. Secretions are wiped from the nose with gauze or a towel. If suctioning is necessary, first the mouth and then the nose is suctioned with a bulb syringe or a suction catheter. Aggressive pharyngeal suction must be avoided since this may cause laryngeal spasm and bradycardia, delaying the onset of spontaneous breathing.[14,15]

Meconium Aspiration

Approximately 12% to 14% of deliveries are complicated by the presence of meconium in the amniotic fluid. There is evidence from a randomized trial that intrapartum (after delivery of the head) suctioning of meconium does not reduce the incidence of meconium aspiration syndrome. For this reason, routine intrapartum oropharyngeal and nasopharyngeal suction of neonates with meconium-stained fluid is no longer recommended.[13] Tracheal suctioning is recommended after delivery *if cardiorespiratory depression is present.* If meconium and depressed respirations are present, direct laryngoscopy is performed immediately after birth for suctioning of residual meconium from both the hypopharynx and the trachea. Suctioning is then applied directly to the tracheal tube as it is withdrawn from the airway. This combination of intubation and suctioning is repeated until little additional meconium is removed or bradycardia precludes any further interventions. In cases in which severe bradycardia or bradypnea is present, it may be necessary to begin positive pressure ventilation despite the presence of meconium in the airway. In contrast, clinical studies have suggested that tracheal suctioning of the vigorous infant does not improve outcome and may cause complications. Therefore, acute interventions are reserved for those infants who have signs of cardiopulmonary depression.

Physical Stimulation

In most cases, drying and suctioning produce enough stimulation to begin effective respirations. If these maneuvers fail, flicking the soles of the feet may initiate spontaneous respiration. If these efforts are unsuccessful, positive pressure ventilation is begun. It is important to avoid forms of stimulation that may be hazardous to the infant (Table 6–5).

Ventilation

A bag and mask will often be sufficient in ventilating infants who require positive pressure breaths.[16] Proper ventilation

Table 6–5	Forms of Stimulation That May Be Hazardous to the Newly Born	
Harmful Actions	**Potential Consequences**
Slapping the back	Bruising
Squeezing the rib cage	Fractures, pneumothorax, respiratory distress, death
Forcing thighs onto abdomen	Rupture of liver or spleen
Dilating anal sphincter	Tearing of anal sphincter
Using hot or cold compresses or baths	Hyperthermia, hypothermia, burns
Shaking	Brain damage

may be one of the most important skills required for resuscitating newly born infants. One study found that improper ventilation was the cause of or contributed to neonatal cardiorespiratory depression in more than 60% of newly born infants requiring chest compressions.[4] Indications for positive pressure ventilation include apnea or gasping respirations, a heart rate below 100 bpm, and persistent central cyanosis. Failure to improve or deterioration during ventilation should prompt immediate reassessment of airway positioning and ventilation techniques.

When delivering the first several breaths, it is important to consider utilizing higher inflation pressures (30 to 40 cm H_2O in full-term and 20 to 25 cm H_2O in preterm newly born infants). Lower pressures can be used with subsequent breaths. If pressure is not being monitored, the minimal inflation needed to increase the heart rate should be used.[13] A rate of 30 to 60 breaths/min should be attempted. Adequate ventilation is demonstrated by bilateral expansions of the lungs and improvement of heart rate and skin color. It is important to check the seal between the mask and face and clear any airway obstructions to assure the delivery of an adequate breath. Abdominal distention is an indication of air in the stomach, which can impede ventilatory sufficiency. It is important in this scenario to insert an 8-French orogastric tube and aspirate with a syringe. Subsequently the tube may be left open to air. If these maneuvers do not result in sufficient air entry, the patient must be endotracheally intubated.

Either a self-inflating bag, a flowinflating bag or a T-piece mechanical device designed to regulate pressure can be used to ventilate a newly born infant. Clinicians should be knowledgeable about the use of devices they choose to use during resuscitation.

A T-piece connection to a face mask can deliver a flow-regulated, pressure-limited, oxygen supply to the baby and enable application of prolonged initial inflation breaths. Use of a T-piece connector more consistently delivers target pressures and prolonged inflation independent of the operator's expertise. Some experts believe that this technique can reduce the need for endotracheal intubation, although this opinion has not been formally investigated in any subsequent studies.[17]

Resuscitation bags larger than 750 ml should be avoided. Self-inflating bags refill independently of gas flow based on surface tension of the bag. When using self-inflating bags, to assure the delivery of high concentrations of oxygen, an oxygen reservoir is attached. The pressure release valve is set at a pressure of approximately 30 to 35 cm of H_2O. An override feature should be in place to deliver higher pressures if necessary. As mentioned previously, self-inflating bags should not be used to deliver oxygen passively through the mask.

Flow-inflating (anesthesia) bags have a long history in neonatal resuscitation. They only inflate when compressed gas is flowing and the patient outlet is partially occluded. The appropriate use of this equipment requires a more complex skill set on the part of the care provider. Since high pressures can be delivered, a manometer is used at all times. High concentrations of oxygen may be moved passively through the mask of a flow-inflating bag.

With few exceptions, clinicians should avoid hypocarbia during newly born resuscitation after correcting hypoxia. Every 1 mm Hg drop in the partial pressure of carbon dioxide during ventilation decreases cerebral blood flow by 3%, potentially worsening cerebral ischemia associated with birth asphyxia.[18] While the use of hyperventilation (and hypocarbia) for treating persistent pulmonary hypertension of the newborn is unproven, many centers employ modest hyperventilation in this instance.[19] Hypocarbia also may benefit a subset of neonates with worsening cerebral edema and intracranial bleeding. However, benefits from this practice are small and transitory.[18]

Endotracheal Intubation

Fortunately, most newly born infants will respond to bag-valve-mask ventilation alone.[20] Relative indications for endotracheal intubation include ineffective bag-valve-mask ventilation, prolonged need for positive pressure ventilation, meconium clearance, and the administration of resuscitative medications. Guidelines for choosing airway equipment size exist (Table 6–6). An additional method for determining endotracheal tube (ETT) size is to divide the gestational age (in weeks) by 10. Most practitioners favor the orotracheal route for intubation. In more than 10% of newly born infants who deteriorate and require chest compression, an improperly placed ETT (esophageal or mainstem intubation) is the cause.[4] The "1,2,3, . . . 7,8,9" rule is used to estimate proper depth of the ETT in centimeters at the lip. For a 1-kg infant, the proper ETT depth is 7 cm, while a 2-kg infant requires an 8-cm depth and a 3-kg infant requires a 9-cm depth at the lips.[18] Proper positioning must be ascertained by direct auscultation, chest wall movements, end-tidal capnography, and radiography. Clinicians should be aware that there are two sizes of colorimetric end-tidal CO_2 devices: one is used in children greater than 15 kg (Easy Cap II, Nellcor) and one is used in young children and infants 1 to 15 kg (Pedi-Cap).[21] False-negative colorimetric end-tidal CO_2 confirmation can occur with very small neonates (<1 kg) and neonates who are

in shock (see Chapter 5, Monitoring in Critically Ill Children). Once the ETT position is confirmed, the tube must be securely taped in place.

If bag-mask ventilation and tracheal intubation are unsuccessful, a laryngeal mask airway (LMA) can be inserted during resuscitation. A size 1 LMA can be used in neonates up to 5 to 6.5 kg.

Oxygen Administration

Experts have found that air is as effective as 100% oxygen for most resuscitations following delivery. There is evidence that 100% oxygen has detrimental effects on breathing physiology and cerebral circulation, and causes damage from oxygen free radicals.[13] For this reason, adequate lung inflation, ventilation, and support of cardiac output should take priority. Supplemental oxygen should be considered for neonates with persistent central cyanosis. If administered, blow-by oxygen may be delivered through a face mask, an oxygen mask, or a hand cupped around oxygen tubing. Self-inflating bags cannot reliably deliver significant oxygen flow without compression. The goal is to deliver sufficient oxygen to achieve a resolution of cyanosis in the mucous membranes. Reliance on pulse oximetry to determine adequate oxygenation is problematic since it normally takes 20 to 60 minutes after birth to achieve an oxygen saturation above 95%.[22,23]

Chest Compressions

The provision of adequate ventilation and oxygenation will restore vital signs in most newly born infants. Decisions to initiate chest compressions involve consideration of the heart rate, responsiveness of the heart rate, and the time elapsed after measures have been initiated. Ventilatory sufficiency must be assured before chest compressions are instituted.

Chest compressions should begin if the heart rate remains below 60 bpm despite adequate ventilation for 30 seconds. Ventilation is of paramount importance and should not be compromised by compressive efforts.

Compressions are delivered on the lower third of the sternum.[24] An accepted technique involves two thumbs on the sternum superimposed on or adjacent to each other depending on the size of the infant. The fingers should encircle the chest and support the back at the same time. An additional method involves two fingers of one hand placed on the sternum at right angles to the chest with the other hand supporting the back. Investigators have determined that the two-hand encircling technique may deliver improved systolic and coronary perfusion pressures.[25]

The depth of compressions should approximate one third of the anterior-posterior diameter of the chest. Palpable

Table 6–6	Equipment Size by Weight					
Weight (g)	Gestational Age (wk)	ETT Size (mm)	ETT Depth (cm)*	Suction Catheter (Fr)	Oral Airway	Laryngoscope Straight Blade
<1000	<28	2.5	6.5–7	5	000	0
1000–1250	28–30	2.5, 3.0	7	5, 6	000	0
1250–2500	31–36	3.0	7–8	6	00	0, 1
2500–3000	36–38	3.0, 3.5	8–9	6, 8	0	1
>3000	>38	3.5, 4.0	>9	8	0	1

*Depth at the lips.

pulses should be generated, and compressions and ventilations coordinated to avoid simultaneous delivery. A 3 : 1 ratio of compressions to ventilation is maintained, with 90 compressions and 30 breaths achieving 120 events per minute. Personnel must remember to reassess the heart rate approximately every 30 seconds. Chest compressions may be discontinued when the heart rate is over 60 bpm.

Medication and Fluid Administration

In general, bradycardia in the newly born is the result of inadequate lung inflation or hypoxemia. Medications are administered only when adequate ventilation and compressions fail.[26] Several potential routes for medication delivery exist, including tracheal, peripheral venous, umbilical vein, and intraosseous (IO) (see Chapter 161, Vascular Access). The tracheal route can be used for intubated patients to administer epinephrine and naloxone (although the subcutaneous route is recommended for naloxone administration if no intravenous [IV] line is available). However, absorption is variable and umbilical and peripheral venous routes are preferred if available. Umbilical vein cannulation is ideal for administration of fluids and resuscitation medications. For clinicians who rarely perform this procedure, the time to insertion may be unacceptably long. Therefore, if umbilical and peripheral routes are not easily achieved, IO access is an appropriate alternative for fluid and medication delivery.[27] Use of this route may cause fractures (especially in preterm newly born infants and neonates) and tissue damage if extravasation occurs. Therefore, the IO access should be removed as soon as an acceptable alternate site is obtained.

Epinephrine

Administer epinephrine when the heart rate remains less than 60 bpm after a minimum of 30 seconds of adequate ventilation and compressions. Asystole and profound bradycardia are the primary indications for the administration of epinephrine.

The recommended IV dose is 0.01 to 0.03 mg/kg of a 1 : 10,000 solution (0.1 to 0.3 ml/kg) repeated every 3 to 5 minutes.[28] The use of high-dose intravenous epinephrine is not indicated at this age. However, a higher dose (0.1 mg/kg) is recommended if the tracheal route is used for epinephrine administration.

Volume Expanders

Hypovolemic newly born infants require the administration of volume expanders. Clinical situations that suggest volume loss include heavy perinatal bleeding, cyanosis, pallor, apnea, extreme tachycardia or bradycardia, loss of muscle tone, and absence of response to other resuscitative measures (e.g., ventilation, oxygenation, drying, stimulation). Normal saline or lactated Ringer's solution is the fluid of choice for volume expansion. Large-volume blood loss may be corrected by the administration of O-negative blood. The use of albumin-containing solutions should be avoided.[29] The initial dose of volume expanders is 10 ml/kg given over 5 to 10 minutes. Volumes greater than this may result in complications such as intracranial hemorrhaging or volume overload in asphyxiated or premature neonates. The response and clinical scenario will dictate the need for additional fluids, blood, or pressors.

Glucose

Hypoglycemia is an important cause of clinical deterioration in newly born infants who are premature or who have diabetic mothers. Stressed neonates can quickly deplete their glycogen stores and develop hyperinsulinemia.[30] Neonates who have perinatal asphyxia also may develop hyperinsulinemia and have a worsened prognosis if they are hypoglycemic.[31,32] Signs of hypoglycemia include irritability, hypotonia, seizures, depressed mentation, and shock. Normal values for glucose vary with the infant's gestational age. While debate exists as to the cutoff that defines hypoglycemia, most experts define any value less than 40 to 47 mg/dl as abnormal for a full-term infant.[33] As bedside glucose testing can be inaccurate, all values less than 50 mg/dl are considered abnormal. Management consists of 2 ml/kg of a 10% glucose solution administered intravenously. A continuous IV solution initially may be required, with conversion to oral solutions containing glucose once stabilized.

Bicarbonate

The routine of use of bicarbonate in resuscitation of the newly born is unsupported. It should only be given after full cardiopulmonary resuscitation is in progress and only after prolonged efforts. A dose of 1 to 2 mEq/kg (diluted to 0.5 mEq/ml in solution) may be given by slow IV push.

Naloxone

Naloxone hydrochloride is a pure narcotic antagonist. It will reverse respiratory depression in the newly born infant whose mother has received opioids within 4 to 6 hours of delivery. However, naloxone may exacerbate neurologic injury during asphyxia and cause seizures in infants born to mothers with opioid addiction. In adults and adolescents, arrhythmias, hypertension, and pulmonary edema have occurred following its use. For this reason, naloxone is not recommended during the initial resuscitation of newborns with respiratory depression. Before naloxone is administered, ventilation should be attempted first to restore heart rate and color. If used, the recommended dose of naloxone is 0.1 mg/kg given intravenously or intramuscularly. It is important to realize that repeated does of naloxone may be necessary since the half-life of the offending agent is often prolonged.

Postresuscitation Care

After resuscitation, personnel must continue monitoring heart rate, respiratory rate, administered oxygen concentration, and arterial oxygen saturation. Blood pressure should be documented and the blood glucose level checked during stabilization after resuscitation. Chest radiography will help rule out any correctible complications (Tables 6–7 and 6–8), such as the presence of a pneumothorax.

One randomized prospective trial evaluated the effect of whole-body hypothermia on neonates with hypoxic-ischemic encephalopathy and acidosis or perinatal complications who required resuscitation at birth. Hypothermia (33.5°C for 72 hours) decreased the risk of death and disability in this population.[34] Confirmation of this study and implementation of a practical, widely available method for delivery of hypothermia may make this treatment standard in the future.

Table 6–7	Complications of Resuscitation	
Complication	**Possible Causes**	**Prevention or Corrective Action to Be Considered**
Hypoxia	Taking too long to intubate	Preoxygenate with bag and mask.
		Provide free-flow oxygen during procedure.
		Halt intubation attempt after 20 sec.
Bradycardia/apnea	Incorrect placement of tube	Reposition tube.
	Hypoxia	Preoxygenate with bag and mask.
	Vagal response from laryngoscope or suction catheter	Provide free-flow oxygen during procedure.
		Oxygenate after intubation with bag and tube.
Pneumothorax	Overventilation of one lung due to tube in right main bronchus	Place tube correctly.
	Excessive ventilation pressures	Use appropriate ventilating pressures.
Contusions or lacerations of tongue, gums, or airway	Rough handling of laryngoscope or tube	Obtain additional practice/skill
	Inappropriate "rocking" rather than lifting of laryngoscope	
	Laryngoscope blade too long or too short	Select appropriate equipment.
Perforation of trachea or esophagus	Too vigorous insertion of tube	Handle gently.
	Stylet protrudes beyond end of tube	Place stylet properly.
Obstructed endotracheal tube	Kink in tube or tube obstructed with secretions	Try to suction tube with catheter.
		If unsuccessful, consider replacing tube.
Infection	Introduction of organisms via hands or equipment	Pay careful attention to clean/sterile technique.

Table 6–8	Postresuscitation Considerations	
Organ System	**Potential Complication**	**Postresuscitation Action**
Brain	Apnea	Monitor for apnea.
	Seizures	Support ventilation as needed.
		Monitor glucose and electrolytes.
		Avoid hyperthermia.
		Consider anticonvulsant therapy.
Lungs	Pulmonary hypertension	Maintain adequate oxygenation and ventilation.
	Pneumonia	Consider antibiotics.
	Pneumothorax	Obtain radiograph if respiratory distress is present.
	Transient tachypnea	Consider surfactant therapy.
	Meconium aspiration syndrome	Delay feedings if respiratory distress is present.
	Surfactant deficiency	
Cardiovascular	Hypotension	Monitor blood pressure and heart rate.
		Consider inotrope (e.g., dopamine) and/or volume replacement.
Kidneys	Acute tubular necrosis	Monitor urine output.
		Restrict fluids if oliguric volume and vascular volume are adequate.
		Monitor serum electrolytes.
Gastrointestinal	Ileus	Delay initiation of feedings.
	Necrotizing enterocolitis	Give intravenous fluids.
		Consider parenteral nutrition.
Metabolic/Hematologic	Hypoglycemia	Monitor blood sugar
	Hypocalcemia; hyponatremia	Monitor electrolytes
	Anemia	Monitor hematocrit
	Thrombocytopenia	Monitor platelets

Termination of Resuscitation

During resuscitation, clinicians must be aware of factors that are associated with high mortality and little chance of survival. Extreme prematurity (gestational age <23 weeks, or birth weight <400 g) and anomalies such as anencephaly and known trisomy 13 and 18 have been shown to have a uniformly poor prognosis, and experts do not recommend initiating resuscitation.[13] In conditions with an unknown prognosis associated with borderline survival and high morbidity with a high burden to the child, experts recommend supporting the parent's views regarding the initiation of resuscitation.[13]

For neonates who are born without signs of life, a uniformly poor prognosis is associated with a gestational age less than 26 weeks (even if there is return of spontaneous circulation), weight less than 750 g, or no signs of life after 10 minutes of resuscitation.[35,36]

Summary

Neonatal resuscitation is a skill set that all emergency physicians must maintain. Most newly born infants will respond well to simple therapeutic interventions. Chest compression and medications are required in only a small subset of infants. Proper personnel, training, equipment and preparation, and adherence to protocols, will prevent complications and optimize outcome for distressed newly born infants.

REFERENCES

1. American Heart Association: Neonatal resuscitation. Circulation 102(Suppl I):I343–I357, 2000.
2. Saugstad OD: Practical aspects of resuscitating asphyxiated newborn infants. Eur J Pediatr 157:S11–S15, 1998.
3. Palme-Kilander C: Methods of resuscitation in low Apgar score newborn infants. Acta Pediatr 81:739–744, 1992.
4. Perlman JM: Cardiopulmonary resuscitation in the delivery room: associated clinical events. Arch Pediatr Adolesc Med 149:20–25, 1995.
5. Kattwinkel J: ILCOR advisory statement: resuscitation of the newly born infant. An advisory statement from the pediatric working group of the International Committee on Resuscitation. Circulation 99:1927–1938, 1999.
6. Bloom RS, Cropley C, and the AHA/AAP Neonatal Resuscitation Program Steering Committee: Textbook of Neonatal Resuscitation, rev ed. Elk Grove Village, IL: AAP, 1994.
7. Vyas H: Determinants of the first inspiratory volume and functional residual capacity at birth. Pediatr Pulmonol 2:189–193, 1986.
8. Gregory GA: Meconium aspiration in infants: a prospective study. J Pediatr 85:848–52, 1974.
9. Whitelaw CC: Comparison of two techniques for determining the presence of a pulse in an infant. Acad Emerg Med 4:153–154, 1997.
10. Theophilopoulos DT: Accuracy for different methods for heart rate determination during simulated neonatal resuscitations. J Perinatol 18:65–67, 1998.
*11. Leflore JL, Engle WD: Capillary refill time is an unreliable indicator of cardiovascular status in term neonates. Adv Neonatal Care 5:147–154, 2005.
12. Dahm LS: Newborn temperature and calculated heat loss in the delivery room. Pediatrics 49:504–513, 1972.
13. American Heart Association: Neonatal resuscitation. Circulation 112(Suppl III):III91–III99, 2005.
14. Estol PC: Oro-naso-pharyngeal suction at birth: effects on respiratory adaptation of normal term vaginally born infants. J Perinatal Med 20:297–305, 1992.
15. Cordero L: Neonatal bradycardia following nasopharyngeal stimulation. J Pediatr 78:441–447, 1971.
16. Kanter RK: Evaluation of mask-bag ventilation in resuscitation of infants. Am J Dis Child 141:761–763, 1987.
17. Allwood AC, Madar RJ, Baumer JH, et al: Changes in resuscitation practice at birth. Arch Dis Child Fetal Neonatal Ed 88:F375–379, 2003.

*18. Hermansen MC, Hermansen MG: Pitfalls in neonatal resuscitation. Clin Perinatol 32:77–95, 2005.
19. Ambalavanan N: The mismatch between evidence and practice: common therapies in search of evidence. Clin Perinatol 30:305–331, 2003.
20. Rotschild A: Optimal positioning of endotracheal tubes for ventilation of preterm infants. Am J Dis Child 145:1007–1012, 1991.
21. Sullivan KJ, Kissoon N, Goodwin SR: End-tidal carbon dioxide monitoring in pediatric emergencies. Pediatr Emerg Care 21:327–332, 2005.
22. Reedy VK, Holzman IR, Wedgwood JF: Pulse oximetry saturations in the first 6 hours of life in normal term infants. Clin Pediatr 38:87–92, 1999.
23. Toth B, Becker A, Seelbach-Gobel B: Oxygen saturation in healthy newborn infants immediately after birth measured by pulse oximetry. Arch Gynecol Obstet 266:105–107, 2002.
24. Orlowski JP: Optimum position for external cardiac compression in infants and young children. Ann Emerg Med 15:667–673, 1986.
25. Houri PK: A randomized, controlled trial of two-thumbed vs. two-finger chest compression in a swine infant model of cardiac arrest. Prehosp Emerg Care 1:65–67, 1997.
26. Burchfield DJ: Medication use in neonatal resuscitation. Clin Perinatol 26:683–691, 1999.
27. Abe KK, Blum GT, Yamamoto LG: Intraosseous is faster and easier than umbilical venous catheterization in newborn emergency vascular access models. Am J Emerg Med 18:126–129, 2000.
28. Lucas VW: Epinephrine absorption following endotracheal administration: effects of hypoxia induced low pulmonary blood flow. Resuscitation 27:31–34, 1994.
29. Cochrane Injuries Group, Albumin Reviewers: Human albumin administration in critically ill patients: systematic review of randomized controlled trials. BMJ 317:235–240, 1998.
30. Clark W, O'Donovan D: Transient hyperinsulinism in an asphyxiated newborn infant with hypoglycemia. Am J Perinatol 18:175–178, 2001.
31. Davis DJ, Creery WD, Radziuk J: Inappropriately high plasma insulin levels in suspected perinatal asphyxia. Acta Paediatr 88:76–81, 1999.
32. Salhab WA, Wyckoff MH, Laptook AR, et al: Initial hypoglycemia and neonatal brain injury in term infants with severe fetal acidemia. Pediatrics 114:361–366, 2004.
33. Lteif AN: Hypoglycemia in infants and children. Endocrinol Metab Clin North Am 28:619–646, 1999.
34. Shankaran S, Laptook AR, Ehrenkranz RA, et al: Whole body hypothermia for neonates with hypoxic-ischemic encephalopathy. N Engl J Med 353:1619–1620, 2005.
35. Haddad B, Mercer BN, Livingston JC, et al: Outcome after successful resuscitation of babies born with Apgar scores of 0 at both 1 and 5 minutes. Am J Obstet Gynecol 182:1210–1214, 2000.
36. Jain L, Ferre C, Vidyasagar D, et al: Cardiopulmonary resuscitation of apparently stillborn infants: survival and long term outcome. J Pediatr 118:778–782, 1991.

---

*Selected readings.

Chapter 7

The Critically Ill Neonate

Maureen McCollough, MD and Steven G. Rothrock, MD

Key Points

All emergency departments should be prepared to care for a critically ill infant, including having the appropriate-sized equipment.

Knowledge of the normal findings on examination, vital signs, and serum parameters will allow for early identification of neonates at risk for serious illness.

Understanding the anatomic and physiologic changes that occur in the first month of life will aid physicians in understanding the unique disease processes that occur at this age.

Early treatment to maintain normothermia and normal blood glucose levels is an important goal that is easily overlooked in critically ill neonates.

Introduction and Background

Knowing the anatomic and physiologic changes that occur in the first month of life is critical to understanding the pathophysiology of many neonatal disorders. For example, the ductus arteriosus that shunted blood away from the lungs during fetal development closes during the first few days of life. Pulmonary vascular resistance also falls for several weeks as blood flow improves to the lungs. This increased flow can unmask disorders placing neonates at risk for congestive heart failure (e.g., large ventricular septal defect).

Most term infants will lose weight (10%) during the first few days of life, but this will level off by day 5 to 7. Most will regain their birth weight by day 10 to 14, and then will gain 20 to 30 g (~$1/2$ to 1 ounce) per day for the first few weeks of life. In general, the normal respiratory rate (RR) of a newborn is 30 to 40 breaths/min, although the World Health Organization defines an abnormal value as any RR ≥60 breaths/min. Neonates are obligate nose-breathers. Because of this nasal dependency, use of a nasal cannula can sometimes worsen a newborn's respiratory distress. A newborn infant's ribs are aligned horizontally, so in order to increase thoracic capacity, the infant must lower his diaphragm. If the stomach is distended with air, the diaphragm will not function properly, leading to poor ventilation. A nasogastric or orogastric tube can decompress the stomach in order to improve ventilation.

Periodic breathing, which occurs during the first few months of life, is the cessation of breathing for 5 to 10 seconds followed by a burst of more rapid breathing with more than 50 to 60 breaths/min for 10 to 15 seconds. This pattern repeats over and over for a period of time. With periodic breathing, the cessation of breathing is not associated with cyanosis, bradycardia, limpness, or altered mental status. Because of periodic breathing, newborns should have respiratory rates recorded for at least 30-second intervals to avoid falsely high or low counts. Normal heart rates range from 90 to 180 beats per minute (bpm); the average is 120 to 150 bpm.[1] The normal systolic blood pressure is 60 mm Hg. For premature neonates, the mean arterial pressure is usually greater than or equal to their gestational age in weeks. Acrocyanosis (cyanotic distal extremities) is common. At birth, newborns have a relatively thick right ventricular wall and elevated pulmonary vascular resistance, with a rapid decrease by 6 to 8 weeks and a more gradual decrease to adult levels by age 6 years.

Guidelines have been published for interpreting the neonatal electrocardiogram (ECG), with normal values defined as all values between the 2nd and 98th percentiles.[1] The ECG normally will show a right axis deviation, ranging from +60 to +180 degrees.[1] The normal heart rate for a neonate is 90 to 180 while values >220 to 230 are associated with supraventricular tachycardia. Due to the normal right axis, tall R waves are normally seen in leads V_1, V_2, and rV_4. QRS and T waves show small voltages. The normal QRS interval is 0.02 to 0.08 seconds.[1] Since the normal QRS value is narrow, ventricular tachycardia may appear narrower than typically expected, leading to misinterpretation as supraventricular tachycardia. The normal value for a corrected QT interval (QTc) is 440 msec.[1]

The normal point of maximal impulse where the left ventricle pushes against the chest is at the left lower sternal border. A normal early systolic murmur caused by the normal persistent patency of the ductus arteriosus may be heard in the first few days of life. An innocent pulmonary flow murmur can be heard radiating to sides of the chest and back, usually less than grade 2/6. Peripheral pulses, including a dorsalis pedis pulse, should be palpable in all normal neonates. On chest radiography, the normal cardiothoracic ratio is less than 0.57 to 0.65 as both inspiration and the size of the thymus will affect this.[2,3] The liver is palpable 1 to 2 cm below the right costal margin in newborns, and the spleen tip is often palpable.

Formula-fed newborns will consume 2 to 4 ounces every 3 to 4 hours by the end of the first week of life. Breast-fed infants will generally empty a breast within 7 to 8 minutes, so switching breasts is recommended. Young infants may stop middle-of-the-night feeds by 3 to 6 weeks of age, while others continue until 4 to 6 months of age. Clinicians should always ask about feeding parameters when assessing for adequate weight gain.

The first meconium stool should be passed within 24 hours of birth. If stool is not passed, Hirschsprung's disease, congenital colon disorders, or hypothyroidism may be present. After mild feedings begin, transitional stools will start on the third to fourth day that are greenish brown and may contain milk curds. Soon after, stools of breast-fed infants will become stringy, loose, yellow, and sweet smelling. Formula-fed babies will produce stool that is more pasty, homogeneous, yellow-brown, and more foul smelling. Stool frequency often corresponds to the number of feeds but is usually 3 to 5 per day. Breast-fed babies may stool after every feed. Infants born in the breech position, especially male infants, may have significant bruising to the genital area.

Normal hemoglobin values for a newborn range from 13 to 20 g/dl. This will generally decrease during the first month of life. Infants reach their "physiologic nadir" around 2 to 3 months old with hemoglobin values averaging 11.4 g/dl; then erythropoesis resumes. The amount of fetal hemoglobin varies from infant to infant, disappearing by 7 months. The white blood cell (WBC) count may also range at birth from 8000 to 35,000, with a gradual decline over the first month. Cerebrospinal fluid (CSF) in a neonate may show up to 22 WBCs/mm³ with a predominance of lymphocytes.[4-6]

Recognition and Approach

Managing a critically ill neonate in the emergency department (ED) is challenging. Because of anatomic and physiologic changes that are occurring in the neonate, unique diseases will occur in the neonatal period (Table 7–1). Young neonates (<7 to 10 days old) who present to the ED have a particularly high incidence of serious illness, with 10% to 33% requiring hospital admission.[7,8] The most common diagnoses in admitted patients include respiratory infections, sepsis, dehydration, congenital heart disease, bowel obstruction, hypoglycemia, and seizures.[7,8]

Evaluation of a critically ill neonate who presents to the ED begins with placement of a cardiac monitor and pulse oximeter; assessment of vital signs, including blood pressure, temperature, heart rate, and respiratory rate; and bedside testing for blood glucose. The temperature must be determined as neonates may be hypothermic or hyperthermic. The temperature of the undressed neonate should be rechecked periodically as young infants have difficulty with temperature regulation due to large body surface areas. For this reason, radiant warming for normothermic and hypothermic neonates should be considered.

Delivery of oxygen by high-flow mask may be sufficient to reverse hypoxia in ill neonates. If not, intubation and assisted ventilation are required. Scalp veins can be used to deliver

Table 7–1	Important Causes of Critical Illness in Neonates

Infectious

Sepsis due to bacteria (*E. coli*, group B streptococcus, *Listeria*) or viruses (herpes, enteroviruses)
Meningitis
Omphalitis

Neurologic

Seizures
Central nervous system hemorrhage
  Birth injury
  Spontaneous (e.g., arteriovenous malformation)
  Trauma—accidental and nonaccidental
Hydrocephalus

Respiratory Disease

Upper airway disorders (e.g., vocal cord paralysis, laryngomalacia, papillomas)
Lower airway disorders
  Pneumonia (viral and bacterial)
  Bronchiolitis
  Bronchopulmonary dysplasia
  Aspiration

Cardiac

Dysrhythmias
Congenital left ventricular outflow obstruction (e.g., hypoplastic left heart, critical aortic stenosis, interrupted aortic arch)
Congenital cyanotic heart defects
  with diminished pulmonary flow (e.g., tetralogy of Fallot)
  with increased pulmonary flow (e.g., transposition of the great arteries)
Congenital acyanotic heart defects (e.g., large ventricular septal defect)
Cardiomyopathies

Intestinal Disorders

Volvulus
Necrotizing enterocolitis
Hirschsprung's enterocolitis
Incarcerated hernias

Metabolic/Endocrine

Inborn errors of metabolism or other metabolic derangements— hyponatremia, hypocalcemia, hypomagnesemia
Hypoglycemia
Congenital adrenal hyperplasia
Hypothyroidism
Formula mix-ups with electrolyte abnormalities (e.g., hyponatremia)

Other Disorders

Vitamin K deficiency (hemorrhagic disease of the newborn)
Toxins and other home remedies

both fluid boluses and medications. If no intravenous (IV) lines can be established, either an intraosseous (IO) line or umbilical vein catheter must be placed (see Chapter 161, Venous Access). For most physicians who do not frequently care for very young infants, an IO line may be easier to establish. Because of the limited ability for neonates to maintain normal glucose, a rapid bedside measure of serum glucose is mandatory. Blood glucose concentrations below 40 mg/dl are considered abnormal in neonates, while a blood glucose concentration between 40 to 50 mg/dl can be normal or abnormal (see Chapter 106, Hypoglycemia). Due to the inaccuracy of bedside tests, levels below 50 mg/dl mandate intervention. Management consists of 5 ml/kg of IV 10% dextrose (D_{10}). The serum glucose should be remeasured within 5 to 10 minutes to check for effectiveness of the glucose, and periodically during the resuscitation and ED stay.

If saline boluses are required, the clinician should begin with 20 ml/kg, and then reassess vital signs and clinical signs of perfusion (e.g., capillary refill, mental status). For premature neonates and neonates with asphyxia or suspected cardiac disorders, fluid boluses should be limited to 10 ml/kg. Maintenance fluids for normally perfused neonates can be sustained with 5% dextrose in $\frac{1}{4}$ normal saline ($D_{5\ 1/4}NS$) at 4 ml/kg/hr while in the ED. If packed red blood cells, platelets, or fresh frozen plasma is needed, it should be administered in 10-ml/kg dosages. Early communication with a neonatal intensive care unit or pediatric intensive care unit will help expedite a potential transfer of the critically ill neonate, and a critical care team or personnel experienced with caring for young infants will be needed during transport.

Evaluation and Management

The presenting features of many serious neonatal disorders are nonspecific. Respiratory distress can signify both respiratory and nonrespiratory disease. Neurologic complaints, including altered mentation and seizures, can be due to serious intracranial disorders (e.g., bleeding, infection, hydrocephalus, encephalopathy) and non-neurologic disorders (e.g., metabolic disease, toxins, hypoxia, hypotension). The differential diagnosis of shock is extensive and includes sepsis, congenital obstructive left heart syndromes, arrhythmias, volume or blood loss, metabolic disease, and endocrine disorders. Vomiting may be due to multiple disorders, including gastrointestinal disorders, intracranial disease, infections, metabolic abnormalities, and toxins. Knowledge of typical and atypical presentations can improve the accuracy of diagnosis of critical illness in neonates.

Selected Disorders Causing Respiratory Distress in Neonates

Difficulty breathing and respiratory distress are among the most common reasons for ill neonates to be brought to the ED. Clinicians must be able to distinguish between upper airway disorders causing stridor, lower respiratory disorders (e.g., pneumonia, bronchiolitis, bronchopulmonary dysplasia), and nonrespiratory disorders (e.g., congenital heart disease).

Neonatal Stridor

Neonates with upper airway obstruction present with respiratory distress and stridor (see Chapter 34, Stridor in Infancy). Stridor is primarily inspiratory with supraglottic disorders (e.g., laryngomalacia), biphasic or inspiratory and expiratory with glottic and subglottic disorders (e.g., vocal cord disease, subglottic stenosis), and expiratory with tracheal disease (e.g., tracheomalacia).[9] Contrary to classic teaching,[9] the pitch is not a useful discriminator between diseases causing stridor and wheezing.[10]

Laryngomalacia is the most common cause of stridor in neonates.[11] Onset of stridor occurs within the first 2 to 4 weeks of life; stridor is worse with crying and agitation, and is relieved by lying in the prone position. Gastroesophageal reflux often accompanies laryngomalacia. The second most common cause of neonatal stridor is vocal cord paralysis,

with nearly one quarter of cases bilateral. Unilateral paralysis leads to a weak cry and aspiration since the affected vocal cord is abducted. If paralysis is bilateral, stridor is usually severe, the cry may be strong, and aphonia is present since the vocal cords are usually paralyzed in the midline. Bilateral vocal cord paralysis can cause apnea, severe stridor, and respiratory arrest. While most cases are idiopathic, vocal cord paralysis, especially if bilateral, may be due to intracranial disease (hemorrhage, hydrocephalus, Arnold-Chiari malformation, meningoencephalocele). Other less common causes of neonatal stridor include tracheomalacia, laryngeal webs, subglottic stenosis (postintubation), hemangiomas, papillomas, abscesses, and vascular slings.[9]

While management of stridor depends on the underlying cause, neonates with new-onset stridor require admission for diagnostic evaluation (e.g., laryngoscopy, bronchoscopy) and treatment. Although laryngomalacia is usually benign and self-limited, occasionally stridor is severe and requires emergent intervention. Pulling the tongue and mandible forward and placing the neonate in the prone position may improve symptoms. Bag-mask ventilation or endotracheal intubation also may be required.

Lower Respiratory Tract Infections

Respiratory infections are an important cause of severe illness in neonates (see Chapter 57, Bronchiolitis; and Chapter 58, Pneumonia/Pneumonitis). Early-onset pneumonia that occurs within 7 days of birth is most commonly due to group B streptococcus. Organisms causing early-onset pneumonia are contracted congenitally or via the intrauterine route (herpes simplex, cytomegalovirus, adenovirus, *Treponema pallidum*, *Listeria monocytogenes*, *Mycobacterium tuberculosis*) or after birth (group B streptococcus, *Escherichia coli*, *Klebsiella pneumoniae*, *Ureaplasma urealyticum*). Risk factors include maternal amnionitis, prolonged rupture of membranes, low Apgar scores, prematurity, and placental abruption. Late-onset pneumonia in the discharged neonate begins more than 7 days after birth. In addition to the organisms causing early-onset pneumonia, late-onset pneumonia may be due to respiratory syncytial virus, *Streptococcus pneumoniae*, *Staphylococcus aureus* (often acquired nosocomially), and both nontypable and type B *Haemophilus influenzae*.

Manifestations of neonatal pneumonia include respiratory difficulty (e.g., tachypnea, retractions, grunting, respiratory distress, rales, wheezing, cyanosis) and nonspecific symptoms (e.g., temperature instability, feeding difficulty, irritability). Group B streptococcus can produce a rapid onset of respiratory distress and hypotension, often with coexisting sepsis and meningitis. Chest radiography may show diffuse bilateral granular infiltrates or patchy infiltrates with occasional pleural effusions. Respiratory syncytial virus (RSV) often causes bronchiolitis with wheezing, tachypnea, and feeding difficulty. Radiography may be normal or reveal hyperinflation, interstitial infiltrates, or atelectasis. This virus has the potential to cause severe disease in premature neonates, or those with underlying cardiac or pulmonary disease. *Chlamydia trachomatis* is an important cause of pneumonia in neonates 3 weeks old and older. Onset is insidious, fever is uncommon, and conjunctivitis is present in half of all cases.[12] Radiography typically shows bilateral interstitial infiltrates with hyperinflation. *Bordatella pertussis* may be one of the most common causes of death from community-acquired infections in infants under 2 months old.[13] Most cases of pertussis are acquired from an infected mother.[14] The classic stages of pertussis (asymptomatic, catarrhal, and paroxysmal cough) often do not occur in neonates.[15] The catarrhal stage (nasal discharge, sneezing) is often brief or absent.[15] Most neonates do not develop a paroxysmal cough or inspiratory whooping. Symptoms include tachypnea, recurrent gagging, apnea, cyanosis, feeding difficulty, and post-tussive emesis.[15] Radiography may show perihilar infiltrates and atelectasis. Pneumothorax, pneumomediastinum, and bronchiectasis may be seen. Lymphocytosis, which is common in older children and adults, is usually absent in neonates. Complications of pertussis include ventricular fibrillation, cardiac arrest, seizures, subarachnoid hemorrhage, rectal prolapse, hernias, and dehydration.[15]

Laboratory testing is often not useful in diagnosing neonatal pneumonia. An elevated serum WBC count is nonspecific, and blood cultures are positive in a minority of neonates with bacterial pneumonia.[16] Urine latex agglutination testing for group B streptococcus is available but has limited sensitivity.[16] A nasopharyngeal swab can be obtained and tested via enzyme immunoassay or polymerase chain reaction for RSV or direct fluorescent antibody (DFA) for pertussis. Serologic confirmation of pertussis can be performed via enzyme-linked immunoassay (ELISA). Any conjunctival discharge in a neonate with pneumonia should be tested for *Chlamydia trachomatis* via DFA or ELISA. However, neither test is as sensitive as a culture.

Management of lower respiratory infection (pneumonia and bronchiolitis) in neonates includes administration of oxygen and IV fluids, continuous cardiac monitoring, and pulse oximetry. For neonates who are wheezing, a trial of inhaled β-agonists or epinephrine may be useful. Use of steroids for wheezing is controversial. Broad-spectrum IV antibiotics are indicated for pneumonia, including ampicillin plus gentamicin or cefotaxime. *Chlamydia trachomatis* is treated with a macrolide. Treatment of pertussis may only be effective during the catarrhal stage, with antibiotic options including macrolides and trimethoprim-sulfamethoxazole.

Bronchopulmonary Dysplasia

By definition, infants with bronchopulmonary dysplasia (BPD) have required oxygen for at least 28 days after birth at least up to 36 weeks of age (gestational age at birth plus postnatal age). BPD usually develops in premature neonates being treated with oxygen and positive pressure ventilation for respiratory insufficiency. Pulmonary damage causes increased airway resistance, decreased lung compliance, increased airway reactivity, and increased airway obstruction. Increased pulmonary vascular resistance, right and left ventricular hypertrophy, and systemic hypertension can also occur. Infants may present with respiratory distress, tachypnea, and wheezing. Congestive heart failure may also occur. Many infants have baseline hypoxemia and cannot maintain their oxygen saturation above 90% without supplementation. Arterial blood gas analysis may reveal hypoxia, elevated bicarbonate levels, or elevated partial pressure of carbon dioxide due to chronic respiratory insufficiency. Acute exacerbations of illness may be associated with viral infections (e.g., RSV) with an increased risk of respiratory failure, apnea, and pneumonia. Chest radiography may be difficult to interpret due to chronic changes. By the time patients are discharged home from their initial hospitalization, cystic lucencies, increased lung volumes, and fibrotic scarring are present on plain radiographs. It is important to compare current radiographs to prior films to assess for interval changes (e.g., new infiltrate). Treatment consists of bronchodilators (albuterol, ipratropium), and steroids for acute wheezing. If fluid overload is present, diuretics are administered. All infants with BPD and acute respiratory symptoms require hospital admission.

Cardiac Disease

Neonates with congenital heart disease (CHD) often present in the first month of life (see Chapter 30, Congenital Heart Disease). Congenital heart disease occurs in 8 of every 1000 live births. Most infants with cardiac emergencies who present in the neonatal period will have *cyanosis, cardiovascular collapse, congestive heart failure*, or an *arrhythmia*. Disorders causing these symptoms present at different times during the first month of life (Table 7–2).[17]

Structural abnormalities of the heart, if presenting during the neonatal period, will generally present in one of three ways: (1) cyanosis due to right-to-left shunting of blood within the heart; (2) a mottled or gray appearance due to outflow obstruction, with shock often mimicking sepsis; or (3) congestive heart failure due to left-to-right intracardiac shunting.

Chest radiography, arterial blood gases, and clinical evaluation can discriminate between disorders with these features. Left-to-right shunt lesions (e.g., ventricular septal defect) cause pulmonary congestion (Table 7–3) These patients will

---

Table 7–2   Most Common Congenital Cardiac Defects Diagnosed at Different Neonatal Ages

0–6 Days		7–13 Days		14–28 Days	
D-Transposition of great arteries	19%	Coarctation of aorta	16%	VSD	16%
Hypoplastic LH	14%	VSD	14%	Coarctation of aorta	12%
Tetralogy of Fallot	8%	Hypoplastic LH	8%	Tetralogy of Fallot	7%
Coarctation of aorta	7%	D-Transposition of great arteries	7%	D-Transposition of great arteries	7%
VSD	3%	Tetralogy of Fallot	7%	Patent ductus	5%
Other defects	49%	Other defects	48%	Other defects	53%

Abbreviations: LH, left heart; VSD, ventricular septal defect.
From Marino BS, Bird GL, Wernovsky G: Diagnosis and management of the newborn with suspected congenital heart disease. Clin Perinatol 28:91–136, 2001.

Table 7–3	Causes of Congestive Heart Failure in Neonates

Noncardiac disorders (the most common cause of CHF in the first 24 hr of life)
  Severe anemia
  Sepsis
  Metabolic disorders (acidosis, hypothermia, hypoglycemia, hypocalcemia)
Left-to-right intracardiac shunt
  Ventricular septal defect, large
  Arteriovenous malformations
  Complete atrioventricular canal
  Patent ductus arteriosus, large
Right-to-left intracardiac shunts
  Transposition of the great arteries
  Total anomalous pulmonary venous return
  Truncus arteriosus
Diminished left ventricular function or output (less common and often associated with shock)
  Hypoplastic left heart syndrome
  Critical aortic stenosis
  Interrupted aortic arch
Cardiomyopathies
Tachyarrhythmias (most commonly supraventricular tachycardia)
Anomalous coronary artery origin
Coronary artery fistulas

usually be able to increase their partial pressure of oxygen (Po_2) to greater than 60 to 70 mm Hg (saturation >90% to 95%) when 100% oxygen is administered for 10 minutes (hyperoxia test). In contrast, patients with cyanotic heart disease usually cannot increase their Po_2 above 60 mm Hg (85% to 90% saturation) during a hyperoxia test. Moreover, chest radiography in patients with cyanotic CHD may reveal oligemia (e.g., tetrology of Fallot) or congestive heart failure (e.g., transposition of the great arteries or total anomalous pulmonary venous return). Management of left-to-right heart lesions causing congestive heart failure consists of oxygen administration, diuretics, vasopressors for hypotension, and vasodilators for afterload reduction (e.g., hypertension, vasoconstriction). Infants with right-to-left cyanotic heart disease with ductus-dependent pulmonary flow (e.g., tetralogy of Fallot, Ebstein's anomaly, critical pulmonary stenosis) or shock due to outflow obstruction require prostaglandin E₁ (see Chapter 30, Congenital Heart Disease).

Selected Disorders Causing Shock in Neonates

Sepsis

Any ill-appearing young infant should be considered septic until proven otherwise (See Chapter 8, Circulatory Emergencies: Shock; and Chapter 13, Sepsis). "Late-onset" sepsis usually occurs after 1 week of age, develops more gradually, and is less associated with perinatal risk factors. Meningitis is a common presentation, and thus a lumbar puncture is indicated in all septic-appearing neonates. Group B streptococcus is the most common bacterial cause of sepsis in the United States. *Listeria monocytogenes, E. coli, Klebsiella,* enterococcus, non–group D α-hemolytic streptococcus, and *H. influenzae* are other bacterial causes. Viral causes include herpes simplex, enteroviruses (coxsackievirus, ECHO virus), and adenovirus (liver and central nervous system [CNS] are usually involved). The mother of a newborn infected with herpes may be asymptomatic.

In an ill-appearing neonate, the diagnosis of sepsis is often straightforward. However, the clinical signs of sepsis may be more subtle. Lethargy, irritability, and decreased oral intake are common. Other clinical features include vomiting, diarrhea, temperature instability (high or low), abdominal distention or ileus, apnea, tachypnea, cyanosis, respiratory distress, tachycardia, bradycardia, jaundice, pallor, petechiae, and poor perfusion.

The evaluation of a critically ill-appearing neonate requires a physical examination to look for sources of infection such as herpes lesions or omphalitis. Neonates with herpes may present with a disseminated infection involving multiple organ systems, or encephalitis with or without a rash, or less commonly with disease localized to the skin, eyes, or mouth. If lesions are to be found, they will usually appear on the birth "presenting" portion of the baby. If the child was delivered head first, the scalp must be thoroughly examined for lesions, especially where a fetal scalp electrode may have been inserted. If the CSF has many WBCs or a predominance of red blood cells but no organisms on Gram stain, herpesvirus infection should be considered. If herpesvirus is suspected, a polymerase chain reaction assay for herpes can be obtained on a sample of the CSF. This test is more than 95% sensitive for herpes meningitis and encephalitis.[18]

Several serum parameters are elevated in neonatal sepsis. An immature neutrophil–to–total neutrophil ratio greater than 0.2 is 60% to 90% sensitive and 70% to 80% specific for diagnosing neonatal sepsis, while an abnormal C-reactive protein is 75% sensitive and 86% specific for this disorder.[19-21] Limited studies have found that an elevated interleukin-6 level (100 or 135 pg/ml cutoff) is 81% to 93% sensitive and 86% to 96% specific, a procalcitonin level greater than 0.5 μg/L is 93% to 100% sensitive and 92% to 98% specific, and an elevated tumor necrosis factor-α level is 72% to 95% sensitive and 43% to 78% specific for diagnosing neonatal sepsis.[22]

Any ill-appearing infant who is considered septic needs all body fluids cultured, including CSF. Positioning the infant in a sitting position or lateral nonflexed position may be less likely to make the child hypoxic during lumbar puncture (LP). All young infants should be placed on a pulse oximeter during the LP. Be wary of performing an LP on a critically ill-appearing young infant as the risk of apnea is higher. It may be better to forego the LP, administer antibiotics, and examine the CSF when the infant is more hemodynamically stable. A urinalysis is insufficient to rule out a urinary tract infection in very young infants. A culture must be sent at the same time. A chest radiograph can be obtained but is unlikely to have significant findings if the child has no signs of respiratory or cardiac disease.

All critically ill-appearing neonates should be admitted to the hospital. Management includes correction of hypovolemia, hypoglycemia, electrolyte disorders, and hypothermia. If sepsis is a consideration, antibiotics should be administered in the ED. Ampicillin 200 mg/kg/day IV every 6 hours (to treat gram-positive organisms, *Listeria,* and enterococcus) plus gentamicin (synergism plus broad gram-negative coverage) are recommended in the treatment of neonatal sepsis. Gentamicin is nephrotoxic and ototoxic; therefore, the exact dosage depends on the neonate's gestational age and weight:

1. If the neonate is 0 to 4 weeks old and the birth weight was <1200 g, administer 2.5 mg/kg IV every 18 to 24 hours.
2. If the neonate is <1 week old and the birth weight was >1200 g, administer 2.5 mg/kg IV every 12 hours.
3. If the infants age is >1 week and the birth weight was 1200 to 2000 g, administer 2.5 mg/kg IV every 8 to 12 hours.
4. If the infant is >1 week old and the birth weight was >2000 g, administer 2.5 mg/kg every 8 hours.

If the CSF is positive or suspicious for infection, then the infant should receive ampicillin (200 mg/kg/day divided q 6 hours) plus cefotaxime (100 mg/kg/day divided q 12 hours). A recent study questioned the use of ampicillin as *Listeria* did not seem to be a consideration today in septic neonates; however, the sample size was too small to definitively exclude *Listeria* as a pathogen.[23] Acyclovir 20 mg/kg per dose every 8 hours (every 12 hours if gestational age plus age in weeks = 34 weeks) IV is administered to cover herpesvirus infections in the following situations[24,25]:

- WBCs or high protein but no organisms are found on CSF.
- CSF pleocytosis is present with vesicular rash on infant, focal neurologic signs, pneumonitis or hepatitis, or a maternal history of herpes.
- There is an elevated red blood cell count in the CSF.

Congenital Obstructive Left Heart Syndromes

Patients with congenital obstructive left heart syndromes (e.g., hypoplastic left heart, coarctation of the aortic, interrupted aortic arch) present dramatically with shock that is often mistaken for sepsis (see Chapter 30, Congenital Heart Disease). Importantly, 85% manifest cardiomegaly, 70% have diminished lower extremity pulses (and lower arterial saturation in the feet compared to the hands), and over half have a murmur noted on examination.[26] Clinicians must be aware that prostaglandin E$_1$ may be life saving in patients with ductus-dependent systemic flow (hypoplastic left heart, interrupted aortic arch, critical coarctation of the aorta, transposition of the great arteries with tricuspid atresia) and pulmonary flow (tetrology of Fallot, Ebstein's anomaly, critical pulmonic stenosis, tricuspid atresia, and pulmonary valve atresia).

Congenital Adrenal Hyperplasia

Congenital adrenal hyperplasia (CAH) occurs in approximately 1 of every 15,000 live births (see Chapter 108, Addisonian Crisis). CAH is adrenal insufficiency resulting from deficient activity of one of the five enzymes required to produce cortisol. The most commonly deficient enzyme is 21-hydroxylase. This results in decreased conversion of 17-hydroxyprogesterone to 11-desoxycortisol in the glucocorticoid pathway. This decreased conversion leads to a *deficiency in cortisol* synthesis, which results in cardiovascular collapse. Hyperplasia of the adrenal gland develops as a result of overstimulation by adrenocorticotropic hormone (ACTH) (which has no negative feedback from cortisol).

Most infants affected by this enzyme deficiency have decreased conversion of progesterone to 11-desoxycorticosterone in the mineralocorticoid pathway. This leads to a *deficiency of aldosterone* synthesis with urinary salt wasting.

Aldosterone deficiency results in classic electrolyte findings and also contributes to cardiovascular collapse.

As a result of elevated ACTH stimulation, adrenal *steroid precursors accumulate* and are metabolized to *androgens,* resulting in the virilization of the external genitalia in female infants. Female infants are more likely to be found to have this disorder in the neonatal nursery because of the external findings. Since male infants' genitalia usually are not affected, this disorder may go unrecognized, putting male infants at greater risk for presentation to the ED.

Clinical signs include total body salt depletion, vomiting, and dehydration that may lead to circulatory collapse and death during the initial 2 to 3 weeks of life (commonly at the end of the first week of life). Females may have enlarged clitoris and fusion of labial folds; in some, the female infant may be mistaken for a male. An affected male infant may have a small phallus.

Laboratory tests may reveal hyponatremia, hyperkalemia, azotemia, and metabolic acidosis. Potassium levels can be as high as 9. Hypoglycemia can also be present. When blood is drawn for testing, an additional 5 ml should be saved (in a red-topped tube) so that blood can be sent for 17-hydroxyprogesterone, dehydroepiandrosterone, androstenedione, and testosterone levels. If possible, this sample should be drawn before giving hydrocortisone. Volume is restored with 0.9% normal saline boluses, and then D$_5$ $_{1/4}$NS is administered at 1 to 1^1/$_2$ times the maintenance rate. Cortisol replacement is accomplished with hydrocortisone 1 to 2 mg/kg IV for term infants, then 25 to 100 mg/m^2/day divided into three to four doses every 6 to 8 hours. Extreme hyperkalemia is usually well tolerated, and saline is usually the only measure needed to lower potassium. Intravenous 10% calcium gluconate, β-agonists, insulin, and glucose may be used if arrhythmias occur (see Chapter 114, Hyperkalemia). As in any critically ill infant, the temperature and glucose must be monitored throughout the resuscitation and ED stay.[4,6]

Other important disorders causing shock in neonates include hypovolemia from gastroenteritis, gastrointestinal bleeding (see Chapter 75), arrhythmias (see Chapter 63), inborn errors of metabolism (see Chapter 29 and "Neurologic Presentation of Serious Illness in Neonates" later in this chapter), and abdominal catastrophes.

Serious Disorders Causing Gastrointestinal Complaints in Neonates

Vomiting (bilious and nonbilious), diarrhea, gastrointestinal bleeding, and jaundice are important clinical features that may indicate critical illness in neonates. It is important to differentiate between bilious and nonbilious vomiting. In a neonate, bilious vomiting is a surgical emergency until proven otherwise. Studies have shown that 20% to 50% of neonates presenting with bilious emesis within the first week of life have a surgical condition.[27-29] For example, bilious vomiting is common symptoms in infants who have malrotation with volvulus.

Volvulus

Volvulus begins with congenital malrotation of the midgut portion of the intestine (see Chapter 83, Malrotation and Midgut Volvulus). During the fifth to eighth week of embryonic life, the embryonic intestine rotates 270 degrees. If there is no rotation or incomplete rotation, the intestine will not be attached correctly at the mesentery. This puts the bowel at risk for volvulus or twisting of a loop of bowel about its mesenteric base attachment. This is a true surgical emergency because bowel necrosis can occur within hours of onset of the twisting.

Infants with malrotation can present with (1) a sudden onset of bilious vomiting and abdominal pain consistent with an acute volvulus; (2) duodenal obstruction due to obstructing Ladd bands; or (3) intermittent vomiting, constipation, and failure to thrive due to feeding intolerance from an internal hernia.[30-33] Bilious vomiting in neonates is always worrisome and should be considered a true emergency until proven otherwise. Most neonates with volvulus are described as well appearing; however, if the bowel is already ischemic or necrotic, they may develop shock. The abdomen is usually not distended. The pain is a constant pain, not usually intermittent, although this finding is difficult to discern in neonates. Jaundice and hematochezia are late and ominous signs.

Laboratory tests in cases of volvulus may show dehydration and acidosis. With a volvulus, plain abdominal radiography may be normal or show a small bowel obstruction. If a duodenal obstruction is present, abdominal radiography may show the classic "double bubble sign" (a paucity of gas [airless abdomen] with two air bubbles—one in the stomach and one in the duodenum).

An upper gastrointestinal contrast study is the procedure of choice for diagnosing a volvulus. The small intestine is rotated to the right side of the abdomen with a midgut volvulus. Contrast will be seen to narrow at the site of obstruction ("cork-screwing"). Ultrasound may show spiraling of the small bowel about the superior mesenteric artery. Ultrasound may also show a distended, fluid-filled duodenum; increased peritoneal fluid; and dilated loops of small bowel to the right of the spine.[34-36]

The diagnosis of volvulus needs to be made rapidly. Rehydration of the infant is important, using 20-ml/kg boluses of normal saline as needed. A nasogastric tube is placed. Antibiotics effective against enteric organisms (e.g., ampicillin, clindamycin, gentamicin) should be administered if shock or peritonitis is present. When the diagnosis is being considered, a surgeon should be contacted immediately, prior to contrast imaging or ultrasonography. Some pediatric surgeons may take an ill-appearing neonate with bilious vomiting to the operating room directly without additional diagnostic radiologic tests.

Necrotizing Enterocolitis

Necrotizing enterocolitis (NEC) is usually seen in premature infants but can be seen in term infants, usually in first 10 days of life. Often these infants have a history of an anoxic event or stress at birth. Infants with NEC can appear ill, with lethargy, irritability, anorexia, a distended abdomen, and bloody stools. Plain abdominal radiography usually shows pneumatosis cystoides intestinalis caused by gas in the intestinal wall. Antibiotics such as ampicillin, clindamycin, and gentamicin are administered to cover bowel flora. Admission to an intensive care unit and consultation with a pediatric surgeon are imperative. Surgery is generally indicated for perforation, abdominal wall cellulitis, portal vein gas, a fixed abdominal mass, or clinical deterioration indicating intestinal gangrene.

Intestinal Obstruction

Failure to pass meconium within 24 hours of birth, distention, refusal to feed, and bilious vomiting are signs of lower intestinal obstruction in neonates. While many of these infants are detected in the neonatal nursery, occasional cases are discharged home and present acutely to the ED in the first month of life. Disorders causing neonatal lower intestinal obstruction include Hirschsprung's disease (see Chapter 77, Constipation), anorectal malformations, meconium plug syndrome, small left colon syndrome, hypoganglionosis, neuronal intestinal dysplasia, and megacystis-microcolon–intestinal hypoperistalsis syndrome. Management is medical or surgical depending upon the cause of obstruction.[37]

Neonates with duodenal atresia can present in a manner similar to those with midgut volvulus. Vomiting is bilious in up to 85% of cases, since the duodenal web or the area of atresia is distal to the ampulla of Vater in most cases. The abdomen may be scaphoid due to a paucity of distal gas or may be distended due to a dilated duodenal loop. Plain abdominal radiography may reveal a double bubble with air in the stomach and in the proximal duodenal loop. Importantly, associated genetic (trisomy 21), congenital cardiac, and gastrointestinal disorders (e.g., imperforate anus) are present in a large number of cases. Preoperative management consists of nasogastric tube placement and fluid resuscitation.

Other disorders causing bowel obstruction in neonates include pyloric stenosis (see Chapter 76), jejunoileal atresia, and rarely appendicitis (see Chapter 73).

Incarcerated Hernia

Incarcerated hernias are more common in premature infants (see Chapter 84, Hernia). The parent may notice swelling in the groin area at the time of diaper change. Incarcerated hernias should be included in the differential diagnosis for an inconsolable crying infant. Gentle reduction (see Chapter 169, Hernia Reduction) can be attempted in the ED after administration of analgesia and sedation. If the hernia is not reducable or ischemic or necrotic bowel is suspected, consultation with a pediatric surgeon is required.

Jaundice

Hyperbilirubinemia with jaundice is an important clinical feature in certain neonates with serious illness. While elevated unconjugated bilirubin is usually physiologic, abnormally high levels can damage the brain, especially in neonates who are premature, or those with hypoxia, hypercarbia, and acidosis.[38] Exact levels of unconjugated bilirubin that are of concern at different gestational ages are discussed elsewhere (see Chapter 38, Jaundice). Moreover, pathologic causes of elevated unconjugated bilirubin exist, including ABO incompatibility, inherited red cell disorders, extravasated blood or hematomas, and bowel obstruction (e.g., pyloric stenosis, large or small bowel obstruction). Hemolytic disorders are often associated with anemia (hemoglobin <13 g/dl) and a reticulocyte count greater than 6%. If Rh or ABO blood type incompatibility is present, a Coombs test will be positive. Elevated conjugated bilirubin, defined as greater than 2 mg/dl or greater than 20% of the total bilirubin, is always abnormal. Serious underlying causes include biliary obstruction, infections (e.g., sepsis, urinary tract infections, TORCH syndrome diseases), toxins, hypothyroidism, hypoadrenalism, and inherited metabolic disorders.[39] In addition to high unconjugated bilirubin, jaundice occurring before 24 hours or at greater than 1 week of age, or increasing more than 5 mg/dl/day, or associated with persistent vomiting, ill appearance, or suspected gastrointestinal tract obstruction requires a comprehensive evaluation to exclude serious pathologic causes.

Neurologic Presentation of Serious Illness in Neonates

Seizures

Generalized tonic-clonic, jacksonian march, and absence seizures are rarely seen in neonates (see Chapter 40, Seizures). Electrical discharges are incompletely spread and tend to remain localized due to anatomic and physiologic CNS immaturity. Many neonatal seizures involve subtle motor automatisms. "Electroclinical dissociation" is common as neonates may have clinical seizures without electroencephalographic (EEG) correlation. There are few idiopathic seizures in neonates; a search for the etiology is mandatory. Focal seizures can be caused by metabolic disorders in neonates, and do not necessarily imply a focal CNS lesion. Seizures occur in 0.2% to 1.4% of all newborns; mortality ranges from 15% to 40%.[40]

Seizures may be subtle in the neonate and include multifocal movement, asynchronous bilateral clonic activity, motor automatisms, and the absence of generalized tonic-clonic seizures seen in older infants and children. Examples of motor automatisms include oral buccal-lingual movements (e.g., lip smacking, tongue thrusting), progressive limb movements (stepping, bicycling, pedaling), and ocular movements (e.g., staring spells, prolonged eye deviation, nystagmus). Nonmotor seizure activity can include vasomotor changes, apnea, pallor, pupillodilation, changes in respiration, changes in heart rate, excessive salivation, and elevation in blood pressure. Clonic seizures may be focal and migratory (first one leg, then the opposite arm), and consciousness is usually maintained. The clonic movement of neonatal seizures is slower and more rhythmic than an older child's clonic movements. Tonic seizure with hyperextension of the trunk, neck, or limbs is another variant. Neonatal jitteriness (nonseizure) will involve fast movements of all extremities; stimulation will induce movements, movements will stop with restraint or passive flexion, eye movement and gaze are normal, and rarely does jitteriness have autonomic signs or symptoms.

The list of disorders that can cause seizures is extensive (Table 7–4). Clues as to the etiology can be found based on the age of the infant at presentation. Seizures in the first 48 hours are usually due to birth trauma, pyridoxine dependency, hypoxic encephalopathy, or hypoglycemia. Benign familial neonatal seizures usually begin on the second or third day of life and resolve by 1 to 6 months. Infants who present at 4 to 7 days old may be hypocalcemic due to a high phosphate load from formula. Benign idiopathic "fifth day fits" start on the fifth day of life and cease by day 15. Seizures that present after 7 days of age are more likely due to infection.

The prenatal and intrapartum history are important in determining infection risks, prenatal STORCH (syphilis, toxoplasmosis, other infections, rubella, cytomegalovirus,

Table 7–4	Etiology of Neonatal Seizures

Central Nervous System

Hemorrhage—subdural, intracortical, intraventricular, subarachnoid (15%–20%)
   Consider abuse as an etiology of intracranial hemorrhage
Hypoxic encephalopathy/birth trauma (30%–65% of cases)
Hydrocephalus
Congenital anomalies or developmental brain disorder*
Cerebral necrosis/infarcts
Cortical vein thrombosis
Neurodegenerative disorders

Metabolic and Systemic

Hypertension
Hypoglycemia
Electrolyte imbalance (hypernatremia, hyponatremia, hypocalcemia, hypomagnesemia)
Inborn errors of metabolism*
Hyperthermia
Pyridoxine (vitamin B_6) deficiency/dependency
   Related to maternal use of isoniazid*

Infections (10%–15%)

Bacterial or viral meningitis*
Cerebral abscess
Viral encephalitis (herpesvirus, coxsackievirus)
Congenital (STORCH: syphilis, toxoplasmosis, other infections, rubella, cytomegalovirus, herpesvirus)

Drug Withdrawal*

Narcotics (e.g., methadone, propoxyphene, heroin)
Barbiturates

Toxins

Local anesthetic
Bilirubin*

Familial Seizures

Benign familial neonatal seizures*
Benign idiopathic neonatal ("fifth day fits") seizures*

*Unique to or of particular concern in the neonatal period.

and herpes simplex) studies, substance abuse, perinatal asphyxia, or family history of seizures. Opiate withdrawal seizures can present up to several weeks postbirth. If the infant is bottle fed, it is important to ask how the caregiver mixes the formula. If the caregiver has supplemented or replaced the infant's diet with free water or tea or other home remedies such as baking soda for colic, hyponatremic seizures can result.

The physical examination should include a blood pressure check for hypertension. An unusual odor of sweat or urine can indicate inborn errors of metabolism. A cranial bruit may be an indication of an intracranial arteriovenous malformation. The skin should be evaluated for jaundice, café-au-lait spots, or herpes vesicles (look at scalp electrode sites). The neurologic examination should include cranial nerves, motor nerves, and neonatal reflexes such as the Moro reflex. Laboratory tests should include glucose, sodium, calcium, and magnesium levels. Other tests to consider include hematocrit, electrolytes, blood urea nitrogen, phosphate, serum ammonia, arterial blood gases, and possibly blood cultures (bacterial and viral), and STORCH titers. Urine should be sent for urinalysis, culture, and toxicology screening. Suspicion of an inborn error of metabolism requires specialized testing (see Chapter 29, Inborn Errors of Metabolism). If another etiology is not found, then CSF will need to be sent for glucose, protein, cell count, differential, Gram stain, bacterial and viral cultures, polymerase chain reaction for viruses (especially herpesviruses), lactate and pyruvate, and glycine. Cranial computed tomography (CT) is required if an obvious cause is not found on initial evaluation. Head ultrasound can be performed at the bedside to identify hemorrhage (e.g., intraventricular hemorrhage) and hydrocephalus. Magnetic resonance imaging can also identify most acute intracranial disorders; however, this test takes time and requires patient stability. Therefore, it usually not performed on critically ill neonates.

For actively seizing and postictal patients, management consists of first supporting the airway, breathing, and circulation. A bedside glucose must immediately be checked and, if low, corrected with a glucose bolus of 0.5 g/kg (5 ml/kg D_{10}). Standard anticonvulsant therapy, such as benzodiazepines, should be initiated, followed by phenobarbital or dilantin if there is no response to benzodiazepines (see Chapter 40, Seizures). Traditionally, phenobarbital has been preferred over phenytoin for treating neonatal seizures. However, limited studies suggest that both drugs are equally effective in treating neonatal seizures.[41] Antiseizure drug treatment options for seizing neonates include the following:

1. Lorazepam (Ativan) 0.05 to 0.1 mg/kg IV or rectally over 2 to 5 minutes; may repeat 0.05 mg/kg IV once in 10 to 15 minutes
2. Phenobarbital 15 to 20 mg/kg IV (infuse no faster than 1 mg/kg/min); may repeat 5-mg/kg/dose every 15 to 30 minutes, up to total dose of 30 mg/kg
3. Diazepam (Valium) 0.1 mg/kg IV given over 3 to 5 minutes or every 15 to 30 min for two to three doses, or 0.5 mg/kg rectally
4. Phenytoin (or fosphenytoin PE) 15 to 20 mg/kg IV, infusing phenytoin no faster than 0.5 mg/kg/min and fosphenytoin no faster than 2 mg/kg/min

The clinician should use caution when administering benzodiazepines to neonates since they have greater respiratory depression compared to older infants and children. Calcium gluconate 10%, 50 to 200 mg/kg IV (0.5 to 2 ml/kg at 1 ml/min), should be administered if seizing persists after standard therapy and hypocalcemia is suspected or proven. If there is no response to calcium, a slow infusion of magnesium sulfate (25 to 50 mg/kg IV) should be considered since hypocalcemia may not be reversed until hypomagnesemia is corrected. Pyridoxine (vitamin B_6) 50 to 100 mg IV should be administered if the infant is still seizing after standard anticonvulsant therapy, glucose, and calcium infusion. Pyridoxine is a cofactor for the synthesis of the inhibitory neurotransmitter γ-aminobutyric acid. Infants whose mothers are on isoniazid are at risk for vitamin B_6 deficiency. Hypertension-induced seizures are treated with antihypertensive medications. EEG monitoring may be required during intensive anticonvulsant therapy to verify whether or not seizures are present. Antibiotics (i.e., cefotaxime and ampicillin) should be administered to septic neonates. Acyclovir 20 mg/kg per dose every 8 hours (every 12 hours if gestational age plus age in weeks = 34 weeks) IV should be considered if there are WBCs or high protein but no organisms on CSF assay, pleocytosis, vesicular rash on the infant, or focal neurologic signs; if pneumonitis or hepatitis is present; or if there is a maternal history of herpes. All neonates with seizures require admission to a monitored bed.[42,43]

Central Nervous System Disorders

Neonates with an intracranial bleed also can appear critically ill. Symptoms include vomiting, lethargy, seizures, and an altered mental status (see Chapter 42, Conditions Causing Increased Intracranial Pressure). Birth-related trauma can cause parenchymal and intraventricular hemorrhage, especially if the neonate was premature or underwent a precipitous delivery. Infarction occurs in up to 15% of neonates with intracranial bleeding.[44] Delayed development of hydrocephalus may occur in 5% of cases.[45] CT is required if bleeding or hydrocephalus is a concern, while magnetic resonance imaging may be required to make the diagnosis of infarction. Young infants also can be victims of nonaccidental trauma. CT findings suggestive of nonaccidental trauma include subarachnoid hemorrhage, interhemispheric subdural hematomas, and multiple skull fractures (especially in different stages of healing) (see Chapter 119, Physical Abuse and Child Neglect).

Hemorrhagic disease of the newborn can manifest as intracranial bleeding. At birth, neonates receive an intramuscular (IM) injection of vitamin K to combat the normal transient decrease in vitamin K–dependent coagulation factors (II, VII, IX, X) that occurs 48 to 72 hours after birth, with gradual return to normal by 7 to 10 days. This decrease is probably due to lack of free vitamin K in the mother and an absence in the newborn of bacterial intestinal flora normally responsible for synthesis of vitamin K. Infants born at home may not receive regular neonatal care, or the hospital nursery may fail to give vitamin K as an oversight. Breast milk has minimal vitamin K (15 mcg/ml); infant formulas are fortified with 50 to 100 mcg/ml. Breast-fed infants' intestines are colonized with lactobacilli, which are incapable of synthesizing vitamin K; formula-fed infants' intestines are colonized with E. coli, which produces vitamin K.

Neonates who do not receive IM vitamin K at birth are at risk for hemorrhagic disease of the newborn. Early presentation occurs at less than 24 hours of age and may be due to maternal drugs that interfere with vitamin K metabolism (phenobarbitol, dilantin, rifampin, isoniazid, coumadin). These patients may present with umbilicial or circumcision site bleeding.

Classic presentations occur on the second to fifth day of life and are found in breast-fed infants who did not receive vitamin K at birth. Infants present with spontaneous bruising and gastrointestinal, nasal, subgaleal, intracranial, or cirumcision site bleeding. Late presentation develops after 2 weeks in breast-fed infants who did not receive vitamin K at birth. Infants can present as late as 1 to 2 months old with pallor, intracranial hemorrhage, deep ecchymosis, or nodular purpura, which may be mistaken for child abuse. During evaluation of infants with spontaneous bleeding, the clinician should examine the midthigh area for evidence of a vitamin K needle stick. Laboratory results include a normal platelet count, prolonged partial thromboplastin time, and prolonged prothrombin time. Resuscitation is directed at correcting respiratory insufficiency and hypovolemia with administration of packed red blood cells (type O, Rh negative), 10 ml/kg over 20 to 30 minutes. For severe bleeding, the coagulopathy is corrected with fresh frozen plasma,

10 ml/kg. The infant should be given 1 mg vitamin K and admitted for observation.[4]

Inborn Errors of Metabolism

Inborn errors of metabolism refer to the hundreds of hereditary biochemical disorders resulting in the alteration of a protein structure or the amount of a protein being synthesized (see Chapter 29, Inborn Errors of Metabolism). Inborn errors are usually caused by deficiency of an enzyme needed to convert one metabolite to another. This results in the accumulation in body fluids of a metabolic intermediate that is normally present in low concentrations. Normally these metabolic intermediates are not toxic, but high levels can cause serious effects. The usual target organ affected is the CNS, followed by the gastrointestinal tract, with up to 93% of infants manifesting signs and symptoms related to one of these systems.[46] Most inborn errors manifest themselves in the newborn period or soon after.

The most common inherited metabolic disorders presenting with acute, life-threatening encephalopathy are organic acidemias, urea cycle defects, and specific amino acid defects.[47] Hypotonia, lethargy, coma, seizures, cerebral edema, intracranial bleeding, or other neurologic abnormalities occur in 85% of cases. In addition to neurologic features, neonates frequently manifest gastrointestinal symptoms, including vomiting, hepatic dysfunction, feeding difficulty, and diarrhea.[46] Hepatomegaly, jaundice, and a coagulopathy may be present. Many of these infants will have a peculiar odor associated with a particular inborn error. In general, patients have either a metabolic acidosis, elevated ammonia, hyperglycemia, hypoglycemia, or a combination of these serum abnormalities (Table 7–5). More intensive testing will reveal elevated levels of a particular metabolite in the serum or urine (specific amino acids, pyruvate, organic acids, carnitine, galactose). Tissue biopsy, fibroblast culture for enzyme assay, and DNA studies may be required to confirm the diagnosis. Viral or bacterial infection, introduction of a new food, or high protein ingestion can trigger the presentation of the inborn error. Because these disorders run in families, the clinician should ask about previous siblings, especially males, who died in infancy. A history of deterioration in a previously well neonate should be considered sepsis or an inborn error until proven otherwise. Specific management is directed at treating precipitants and reversing hypoglycemia, hypovolemia, and acidosis (administering vitamin B_{12} for methylmalonic academia, biotin for carboxylase deficiency). Ammonia may be reduced by arginine in a urea cycle defect. Dialysis to lower ammonia levels may be needed.

Neonatal Hypocalcemia

Neonatal hypocalcemia is more often seen in the first few days of life but can occur later as a result of high phosphate levels in cow's milk formula, maternal hypoparathyroidism, maternal diabetes, congenital hypoparathyroidism, immature renal function, hypomagnesemia, or maternal vitamin D deficiency (see Chapter 115, Hypocalcemia). Hypocalcemia is defined as plasma calcium less than 7 mg/dl; clinical signs include jitteriness and poor feeding. Tetany may occur with increased muscle activity, twitching, vomiting, carpal pedal spasm, clonus, laryngospasm, or stridor (most classically, the neonate presents only with a weak cry, like a baby lamb.) Young infants with hypocalcemia do not have the classic hypocalcemic tetany signs as in adults. Hypocalcemia can account for up to 34% of neonatal seizures. These seizures can be multifocal or migratory clonic seizures. An ECG showing a QTc interval greater than 0.44 to 0.46 seconds supports the diagnosis of hypocalcemia. Serum calcium, magnesium, and ionized calcium levels should be determined before treatment if possible. Calcium gluconate 10%, 50 to 200 mg/kg IV (0.5 to 2 ml/kg at 1 ml/min), can be administered for hypocalcemic seizures. It should be infused slowly to prevent bradycardia, and repeated as needed. Hypomagnesemia (<1 mEq/L) can be treated with 25 to 50 mg/kg IV or IM magnesium sulfate.

Other Disorders Causing Neurologic Manifestations

Occasionally and unknowingly, a parent may be to blame for a child's seizures. Young infants can be exposed to a variety

Table 7–5			Laboratory Parameters in Inborn Errors of Metabolism
MA*	NH₄†	Glu‡	Specific Inborn Errors of Metabolism§
↔	↔	↔	Nonketotic hyperglycinemia
↔	↑	↔	*Citrulline normal:* transient hyperammonemia of newborn or HHH (hyperornithinemia, hyperammonemia, & homocitrullinuria)
			Urea cycle disorders: *low citrulline* (↓ ornithine transcarbamylase or ↓ carbamyl phosphate synthetase), *mild ↑ citrulline* (↓argininosuccinate lyase), *↑ citrulline* (citrullinemia)
↑	↑	↓	**Fatty acid oxidation:** carnitine deficiency, medium/long/short-chain acyl coenzyme A dehydrogenase
			Organic acidemia: dicarboxylic aciduria, glutaric acidemia type II (K), methylmalonic acidemia (K,L), propionic acidemia (K,L), congenital lactic acidosis (K,L)
↑	↑	↔	Periodic hyperlysinemia
			Organic acidemia: ketothiolase deficiency
↑	↑	↑	**Organic acidemias:** isovaleric acidemia (K,L), methylmalonic acidemia (K,L), propionic acidemia (K,L)
↑	↔	↔	**Organic acidemia:** isovaleric acidemia
↑	↔	↓	**Carbohydrate metabolism:** fructose-1,6-diphosphatase deficiency (L)
			Glycogen storage diseases: type I, III (K)
			Aminoaciduria: maple syrup urine disease (early onset), glutaric aciduria type I

*Metabolic acidosis with anion gap (↑) vs. no metabolic acidosis (↔).
†Hyperammonemia (↑) vs. normal ammonia (↔).
‡Hyperglycemia (↑) vs. normoglycemia (↔) vs. hypoglycemia (↓).
§K, ketonuria; L, lactic acidosis.
From Rothrock SG: Inborn errors of metabolism. *In* Rothrock SG (ed): Pediatric Emergency Pocketbook, 5th ed. Lompac, CA: Tarascon Publishing (*www.tarascon.com*), 2007, p 116, with permission.

of substances that can alter their electrolytes, calcium, or magnesium. Parents may also inappropriate mix formula, using more water than is needed. Infant formula comes in three standard preparations: ready-to-eat liquid, which should not be mixed with water; liquid concentrate, which should be mixed 1 : 1 with water; and powdered formula, which should be mixed 1 scoop to 2 ounces of water.

Home remedies for a variety of ailments may also be given to young infants, causing severe consequences. The clinician must ask about additional liquids, powders, herbs, or other substances given to the neonate since parents will not always volunteer this information. Examples of inappropriate substances given by parents include baking soda for colic or herbal teas for constipation or colic.[48]

Unlike older children, infants can become colonized after ingesting spores of *Clostridium botulinum*. Botulism has been reported in neonates as young as 3 days old,[49] although the disease peaks in the 2- to 4-month age range. Risk factors include parents who work with soil and who live in a rural area. In the past, ingestion of honey was a common cause; however, educational efforts have diminished this risk factor in the United States. Symptoms are due to cholinergic blockade and include hypotonia, constipation, descending flaccid paralysis, autonomic instability, and absence of cranial nerve reflexes (with dilated pupils). While serum tests are available to aid in diagnosis, these tests are insensitive. Diagnosis is usually made by an assay performed on stool. This may need to be sent to a state health department. Management requires prolonged support of ventilation and nutritional support. Medications that prolong cholinergic blockade (e.g., gentamicin) should be avoided. Human botulinum immune globulin (Baby-BIG), pooled from adults immunized with pentavalent botulinum toxin, is available for infant botulism treatment and can decrease the length of hospitalization by over 50%. It is active against the type A and B toxin but not against types C through F. Trivalent equine immunoglobulin to toxins A, B, and E is available for adults, but is not recommended for use in infants due to a high hypersensitivity rate and short duration of action.[49]

Summary

Managing a critically ill newborn is difficult. Understanding the anatomic and physiologic changes that are occurring can improve the ability to diagnose and manage many disorders at this age. Considering the unique disease processes that present in the neonatal period is also imperative. Preestablished communication between the ED and the neonatal or pediatric intensive care unit is vital for streamlining the transfer for ongoing critical care.

REFERENCES

1. Schwartz PJ, Garson A, Paul T, et al: Guidelines for the interpretation of the neonatal electrocardiogram. Eur Heart J 23:1329–1344, 2002.
2. Jaffe RB, Condon VR, Reid BS, et al: Normal lung and clinical anatomy. *In* Kuhn JP, Slovis T, Haller J (eds): Caffey's Pediatric Diagnostic Imaging, 10th ed. Philadelphia: Elsevier, 2004, pp 1230–1236.
3. Crummy AB, McDermott JC, Baron MG: The cardiovascular system. *In* Juhl JH, Crummy AB, Kuhlman JE (eds): Essentials of Radiologic Imaging, 7th ed. Philadelphia: Lippincott, 1998, pp 1197–1265.
4. Donn S, Faix R: Neonatal Emergencies. New York: Futura, 1991.
5. Schreiner R, Bradburn N: Care of the Newborn, 2nd ed. New York: Raven Press, 1988.
6. Avery M, Taeusch H (eds): Schaffer's Disease of the Newborn, 5th ed. Philadelphia: WB Saunders, 1984.
*7. Millar KR, Gloor JE, Wellington N, Joubert G: Early neonatal presentations to the pediatric emergency department. Pediatr Emerg Care 16:145–152, 2000.
8. Sacchetti AD, Berardi M, Sawchuk P, Hibl I: Boomerang babies: emergency department utilization by early discharge neonates. Pediatr Emerg Care 13:365–368.
9. Mancuso RF: Stridor in neonates. Pediatr Clin North Am 43:1339–1356, 1996.
10. Baughman RP, Loudon RG: Stridor: differentiation from asthma or upper airway noise. Am Rev Respir Dis 139:1407–1409, 1989.
11. Holinger LD: Etiology of stridor in the neonate, infant, and child. Ann Otol Rhinol Laryngol 89:397–400, 1980.
12. Tipple MA, Beem MO, Saxon EM: Clinical characteristics of the afebrile pneumonia associated with *Chlamydia trachomatis* infection in infants less than 6 months of age. Pediatrics 63:192–197, 1979.
13. Floret D: Pediatric deaths due to community-acquired bacterial infection: survey of French pediatric intensive care units. Arch Pediatr 8:705s–711s, 2001.
14. Izurieta HS, Kenyon TA, Strebel PM, et al: Risk factors for pertussis in young infants during an outbreak in Chicago in 1993. Clin Infect Dis 22:503–507, 1966.
15. Hoppe JE: Neonatal pertussis. Pediatr Infect Dis J 19:244–247, 2000.
16. Gerdes JS: Diagnosis and management of bacterial infections in the neonate. Pediatr Clin North Am 51:939–959, 2004.
17. Marino BS, Bird GL, Wernovsky G: Diagnosis and management of the newborn with suspected congenital heart disease. Clin Perinatol 28:91–136, 2001.
18. Whitley RJ, Gnann JW: Viral encephalitis: familiar infections and emerging pathogens. Lancet 359:507–513, 2002.
19. Berger C, Uehlinger J, Ghelfi D, et al: Comparison of C-reactive protein and white blood cell count with differential in neonates at risk for septicaemia. Eur J Pediatr 154:138–144, 1995.
20. Griffin MP, Lake DE, Moorman JR: Heart rate characteristics and laboratory tests in neonatal sepsis. Pediatrics 115:937–941, 2005.
21. Manucha V, Rusia U, Sikka M, et al: Utility of haematological parameters and C-reactive protein in the detection of neonatal sepsis. J Paediatr Child Health 38:459–464, 2002.
22. Malk A, Hui CPS, Pennie RA, Kirpalani H: Beyond the complete blood cell count and C-reactive protein. Arch Pediatr Adolesc Med 57:511–516, 2003.
23. Sadow KB, Derr R, Teach SJ: Bacterial infections in infants 60 days and younger Arch Pediatr Adolesc Med 153:611–614, 1999.
24. Poland R., Watterberg K: Sepsis in the newborn. Pediatr Rev 14:262–263, 1993.
25. Baraff LJ: Editorial: clinical policy for children younger than three years presenting to the emergency department with fever. Ann Emerg Med 42:546–549, 2003.
26. Pickert CB, Moss MM, Fiser DH: Differentiation of systemic infection from congenital obstructive left heart disease in the very young infant. Pediatr Emerg Care 14:263–267, 1998.
27. Godbole P: Bilious vomiting in the newborn: how often is it pathologic? J Pediatr Surg 37:909–911, 2002.
28. Lilien LD, Srinivasan G, Pyati SP, et al: Green vomiting in the first 72 hours in normal infants. Am J Dis Child 140:662–664, 1986.
29. Kao H-A: Bilious vomiting during the first week of life. Acta Paediatr Sin 35:202–207, 1994.
30. Swischuk L: Acute onset vomiting in a 15 day old infant. Pediatr Emerg Care 8:359–360, 1992.
31. Swischuk L: Vomiting in a nine-day-old infant. Pediatr Emerg Care 11:131–132, 1995.
32. Lin JN, Lou CC, Wang KL: Intestinal malrotation and midgut volvulus: a 15-year review. J Formos Med Assoc 94:178–181, 1995.
33. Ilce Z, Celayir S, Akova F, et al: Intestinal rotation anomalies in childhood: review of 22 years' experience. Surg Today 33:893–895, 2003.
34. Shimianuki Y, Aihara T, Takano H, et al: Clockwise whirlpool sign at color Doppler US: an objective and definite sign of midgut volvulus. Radiology 199:261–264, 1999.
35. Pracros JP, Sann L, Genin G, et al: Ultrasound diagnosis of midgut volvulus: the whirlpool sign. Pediatr Radiol 22:18–20, 1992.

*Selected reading.

36. Patino M, Munden M: Utility of the sonographic whirlpool sign in diagnosing midgut volvulus in patients with atypical clinical presentations. J Ultrasound Med 23:397–401, 2004.

37. Loeing-Baucke V, Kimura K: Failure to pass meconium: diagnosing neonatal intestinal obstruction. Am Fam Physician 60:2042–2050, 1999.

38. Hansen TW: Mechanisms of bilirubin toxicity: clinical implications. Clin Perinatol 29:765–768, 2002.

39. McKiernan P: Neonatal cholestasis. Semin Neonatol 7:153–165, 2002.

40. Mizrahi EM: Neonatal seizures and neonatal nonepileptic syndromes. Neurol Clin 19:427–463, 2001.

*41. Painter MJ, Sher MS, Stein AD, et al: Phenobarbital compared with phenytoin for the treatment of neonatal seizures. N Engl J Med 341:485–489, 1999.

42. Bernes S., Kaplan A: Evolution of neonatal seizures. Pediatr Clin North Am 41:1069–1104, 1994.

43. Sfafstrom C: Neonatal seizures. Pediatr Rev 16:248–256, 1995.

44. Guzetta F, Shackelford GD, Volpe S, et al: Periventricular intraparenchymal echodensities in the premature newborn: critical determinant of neurological status. Pediatrics 78:995–1006, 1990.

45. Perlman JM, Lynch B, Volpe JJ: Late hydrocephalus after arrest and resolution of neonatal posthemorrhagic hydrocephalus. Dev Med Child Neurol 32:725–729, 1990.

46. Calvo M, Artuch R, Macia E, et al: Diagnostic approach to inborn errors of metabolism in an emergency unit. Pediatr Emerg Care 16:405–408, 2000.

*47. Burton BK: Inborn errors of metabolism in infancy: a guide to diagnosis. Pediatrics 102:e69, 1998.

48. Nichols M, Wason S, Gonzalez del Rey J, et al: Baking soda: a potentially fatal home remedy. Pediatr Emerg Care 11:109, 1995.

49. Fox CK, Keet CA, Stroker JB: Recent advances in infant botulism. Pediatr Neurol 32:149–154, 2005.

Chapter 8

Circulatory Emergencies: Shock

Christine S. Cho, MD, MPH and Steven G. Rothrock, MD

Introduction and Background

Shock is an abnormal physiologic state in which there is an inability to deliver adequate oxygen to meet the metabolic needs of the body. At the cellular level, impairment of oxygen delivery leads to ischemia, a transition from aerobic to anaerobic metabolism, lactic acidosis, and ultimately organ dysfunction and failure. If interventions are not made in a timely, aggressive manner, individual organ failure will progress to multisystem organ failure and eventual death.

Mortality from septic shock has decreased from 97% to 9% over the last 40 to 50 years due to improved hemodynamic monitoring, advanced life support, and the advent of critical care units.[1] However, infants (especially premature infants) continue to have the highest morbidity and mortality. Racial and regional disparities also exist in shock mortality.[2,3]

The early recognition of shock can be challenging. Reliance on the development of hypotension before making the diagnosis of shock will lead to underrecognition. This is especially true in children because of their increased physiologic reserve and their ability to maintain a normal blood pressure despite moderate to profound hypovolemia. In fact, children can lose up to 25% to 30% of their blood volume with only minimal changes in vital signs.[4,5] The term *compensated shock* is used for patients with shock physiology, but preservation of normal blood pressure. *Decompensated shock* is used when the patient has hypotension, and is usually a late sign of shock. If untreated, decompensated shock will become irreversible, leading to eventual death.

Physiologic subtypes of shock include hypovolemic, cardiogenic, distributive, and obstructive shock. Hypovolemic shock is due to a deficiency in intravascular volume either through insufficient intake or excessive loss of fluid. Cardiogenic shock is due to failure of the heart to provide sufficient cardiac output. Distributive shock is defined as a change in vascular capacitance resulting in peripheral vasodilation and abnormal redistribution of blood flow. Obstructive shock is due to an obstruction of outflow from the heart. The differential diagnosis for each type of shock is extensive (Table 8–1).

While it is useful to distinguish between the physiologic subtypes of shock, recognition and treatment of the specific disorders that lead to shock is equally important. In addition, some diseases have multisystem involvement with several different subtypes of shock. For example, children with septic shock may be hypovolemic from fluid loss and inadequate intake, and may have sepsis-induced myocardial depression that directly limits contractility and cardiac output.

Recognition and Approach

Knowledge of physiologic compensatory responses can help clinicians identify shock subtypes and initiate appropriate management. Cardiac output is regulated by both the heart rate and the stroke volume of each contraction. Preload, cardiac contractility, and afterload determine stroke volume. Preload reflects both the absolute intravascular volume and changes in venous capacitance. Afterload is related to systemic vascular resistance. The primary physiologic response to compensate for shock is via the sympathetic nervous system. Baroreceptors in the carotid sinus and chemoreceptors in the aorta and carotid bodies sense hypovolemia and hypoxemia, respectively, and activate the sympathetic adrenergic response. The release of catecholamines activates α_1 receptors in peripheral vascular smooth muscle, causing peripheral vasoconstriction.[6] Presynaptic α_2 receptors in the heart and vasculature are activated by norepinephrine released from sympathetic nerves and mediate negative feedback inhibition of further norepinephrine release.

Table 8–1	Differential Diagnosis of Shock by Physiologic Subtypes

Hypovolemic Shock

Decreased Intake
Increased Loss
Intravascular
  Blood
    External trauma (wounds, open fracture)
    Internal trauma (thorax, abdomen, pelvis, long bone fractures, nonaccidental trauma)
    Surgical blood loss
    Gastrointestinal bleed
  Nonblood
    Vomiting
    Diarrhea
    Diabetes mellitus
    Diabetes insipidus
    Heat exhaustion
Interstitial (third spacing)
  Burns
  Sepsis
  Nephrotic syndrome
  Protein-losing enteropathy
  Intestinal obstruction

Distributive Shock

Anaphylaxis
Neurogenic (spinal cord or head injury)
Medication
Sepsis*

Obstructive Shock

COLHS
HLHS
Interrupted aortic arch
Critical aortic stenosis
Pericardial Tamponade
Tension Pneumothorax
Hemothorax

Cardiogenic Shock

Congenital
Obstructive heart disease (see Obstructive Shock)
Congestive heart failure
  VSD
  Endocardial cushion defect
  TAPVR
  Arrythmia
    SVT from WPW syndrome
Ischemia
  Kawasaki disease
  Anomalous coronary artery
Heart block
  Neonatal lupus
Sick sinus syndrome
Acquired
High-output failure
  Severe anemia
  AVM
    Intracranial
    Intra-abdominal
    Kasabach-Merritt syndrome
Heart block
  Lyme carditis
Myocarditis
  Viral
  Acute rheumatic fever
Toxin-mediated
  Calcium channel blocker
  Beta-blocker

*Although sepsis is classically considered a form of distributive shock secondary to endotoxin-mediated vasodilation, septic shock also comprises elements of hypovolemia and cardiac dysfunction. In addition, septic shock can manifest with either low or high systemic vascular resistance.
Abbreviations: AVM, arteriovenous malformation; COLHS, congenital obstructive left heart syndromes; HLHS, hypoplastic left heart syndrome; SVT, supraventricular tachycardia; TAPVR, total anomalous pulmonary venous return; VSD, ventricular septal defect; WPW, Wolff-Parkinson-White.

Table 8–2	Adrenergic Receptor Actions as They Relate to Treatment of Shock

Receptor	Receptor Actions
α_1	Peripheral vascular, including pulmonary vascular, smooth muscle constriction
α_2	Presynaptic receptors in heart and vasculature are activated by norepinephrine released by sympathetic nerve and mediate negative feedback on further release of norepinephrine
	Postsynaptic receptors mediate vasoconstriction
β_1	Increased heart rate (chronotropy), AV node conduction (dromotropy), and cardiac contractility (inotropy)
	Increased renin secretion
β_2	Peripheral vascular and bronchiolar smooth muscle relaxation
β_3	Decreased cardiac contractility (inotropy)
D_1	Renal, coronary, and mesenteric vasodilation
	Stimulate natriuresis
D_2	Inhibit norepinephrine release from nerve endings

Abbreviations: α, alpha; β, beta; AV, atrioventricular; D, dopamine.

Postsynaptic α_1 and α_2 receptors in peripheral vessels mediate vasoconstriction. In the heart, β_1 receptors are activated to increase heart rate (chronotropy), conduction velocity (dromotropy), and contractility (inotropy). In the failing heart, β_3 receptors are upregulated and cause negative inotropic effects mediated by nitric oxide and cyclic GMP (Table 8–2). Peripheral dopamine$_1$ (D_1) receptors mediate dilation of coronary and mesenteric arteries and stimulate a natriuretic response. Dopamine$_2$ (D_2) receptors exist on nerve endings and inhibit norepinephrine release from synaptic nerve endings, inhibit release of prolactin, and induce vomiting. Stimulation of either D_1 or D_2 receptors suppresses gastrointestinal (GI) tract function and may precipitate an ileus. Phosphodiesterase (PDE) inhibitors increase contractility by increasing cyclic AMP and potentiating the delivery of calcium into myocardial cells. At the same time, PDE inhibitors dilate peripheral blood vessels. Knowledge of individual receptor functions and the mechanism of different vasoactive agents allows clinicians to tailor therapy to the specific disease (Tables 8–2 and 8–3).

Individual organs control delivery of oxygen by autoregulation of regional blood flow. Each organ has a critical perfusion pressure below which it cannot maintain adequate oxygen delivery through autoregulation. An important treatment goal in shock is to maintain an adequate perfusion pressure (mean arterial pressure–central venous pressure difference) (Table 8–4). Autoregulation also helps to preferentially perfuse organs that are more vital for survival (e.g., brain, heart, kidneys).

In addition to the sympathetic nervous system, endocrine-mediated mechanisms help maintain perfusion in shock. Atrial receptors in the heart sense decreased volume and stimulate the release of antidiuretic hormone, which acts as a peripheral vasoconstrictor and increases water reabsorption at the renal collecting ducts. The renin-angiotensin-aldosterone system is activated in shock when the kidneys release renin in response to decreased renal blood flow. Angiotensin II is a peripheral vasoconstrictor, and aldoste-

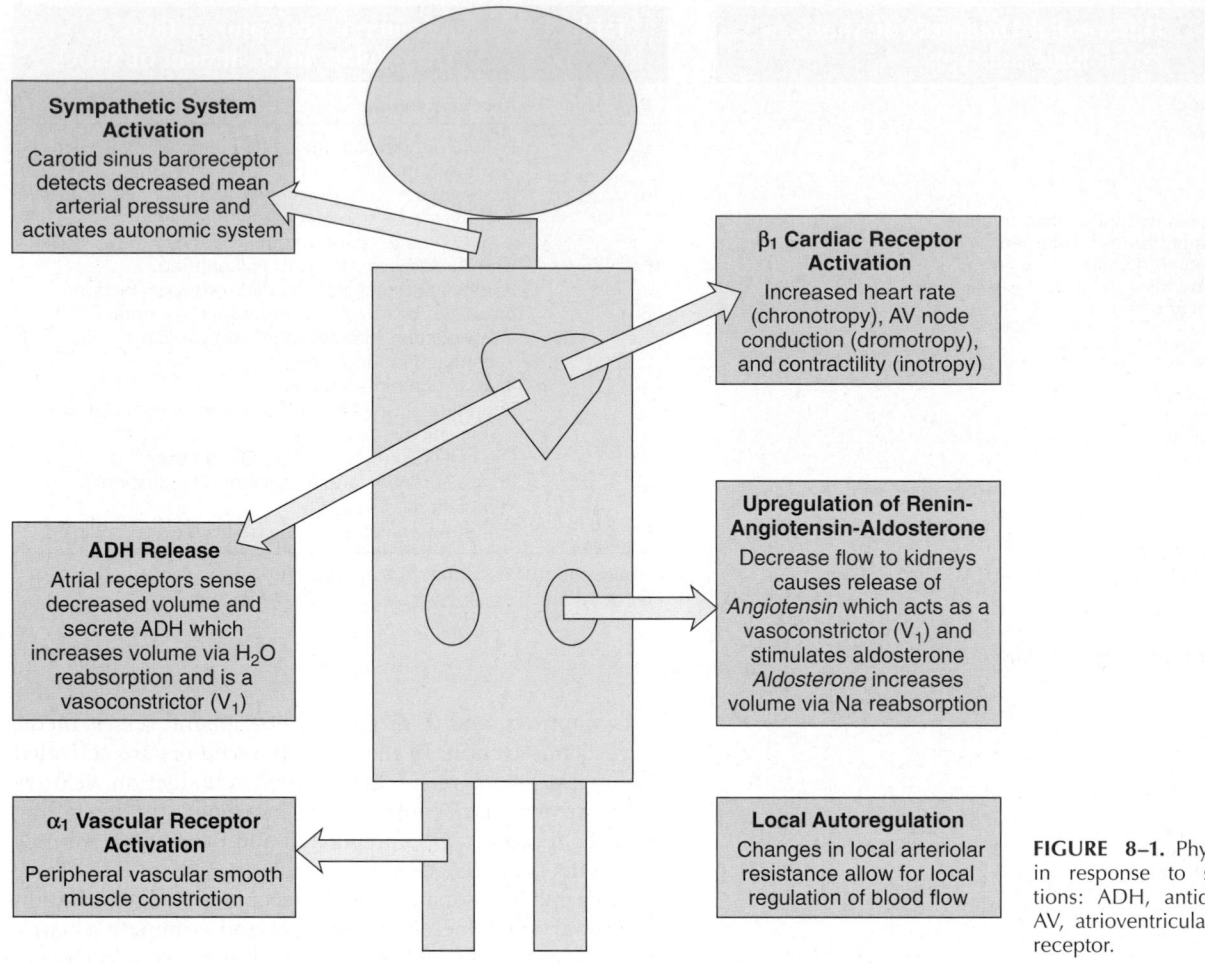

FIGURE 8–1. Physiologic changes in response to shock. Abbreviations: ADH, antidiuretic hormone; AV, atrioventricular; V_1, vasopressin receptor.

Table 8–3	Common Vasoactive Medications Used in Treatment of Shock		
Drug	**Receptor Activation***	**Dose (mcg/kg/min)**	**Physiologic Result†**
Dopamine	D_1, β_1, α_1 (α at high doses)	<5	Predominately increased renal, mesenteric, and coronary beds
		5–10	Cardiac stimulation (inotropy or contractility, heart rate)
		>10	Peripherally vasoconstricts to increase blood pressure
Dobutamine	β_1, β_2 > > α_1	2–20	Cardiac stimulation, vasodilator
Epinephrine	β_1, β_2, > $\alpha_{1/2}$ (α at high doses)	Low: 0.01–0.3	Cardiac stimulation
		High: >0.3	Cardiac stimulation and vasopressor
Norepinephrine	$\alpha_{1/2}$, β_1	0.05–2	Vasopressor, cardiac stimulation
Isoproterenol	β_1, β_2	0.1–2	Cardiac stimulation
Phenylephrine	α_1	0.1–0.5	Vasopressor
Milrinone	PDE inhibitor	Loading: 50 mcg/kg Then 0.5–1	Cardiac stimulation, vasodilator
Nitroprusside	Activation of NO	0.3–10	Vasodilator

*β_1, Beta$_1$-adrenergic receptor; β_2, beta$_2$-adrenergic receptor; α_1, alpha$_1$-adrenergic receptor; $\alpha_{1/2}$, alpha$_1$- and alpha$_2$-adrenergic receptors; D_1, dopaminergic receptor; PDE, phosphodiesterase; NO, nitric oxide.
†Cardiac stimulation: increases cardiac contractility, heart rate, and atrioventricular nodal conduction; Vasopressor: peripheral vasoconstriction (increasing systemic vascular resistance); Vasodilator: peripheral vasodilation (decreasing systemic vascular resistance).

rone will increase volume via sodium reabsorption at the kidneys (Fig. 8–1).

Various physiologic parameters can be directly or indirectly measured during shock resuscitation. If a central line is placed into the superior vena cava, central venous pressure and venous oxygen saturation can be monitored. If a pulmonary artery catheter is placed, cardiac index and systemic venous resistance can be calculated to help in the selection of vasoactive agents (Figs. 8–2 and 8–3) (see Chapter 5, Monitoring in Critically Ill Children).

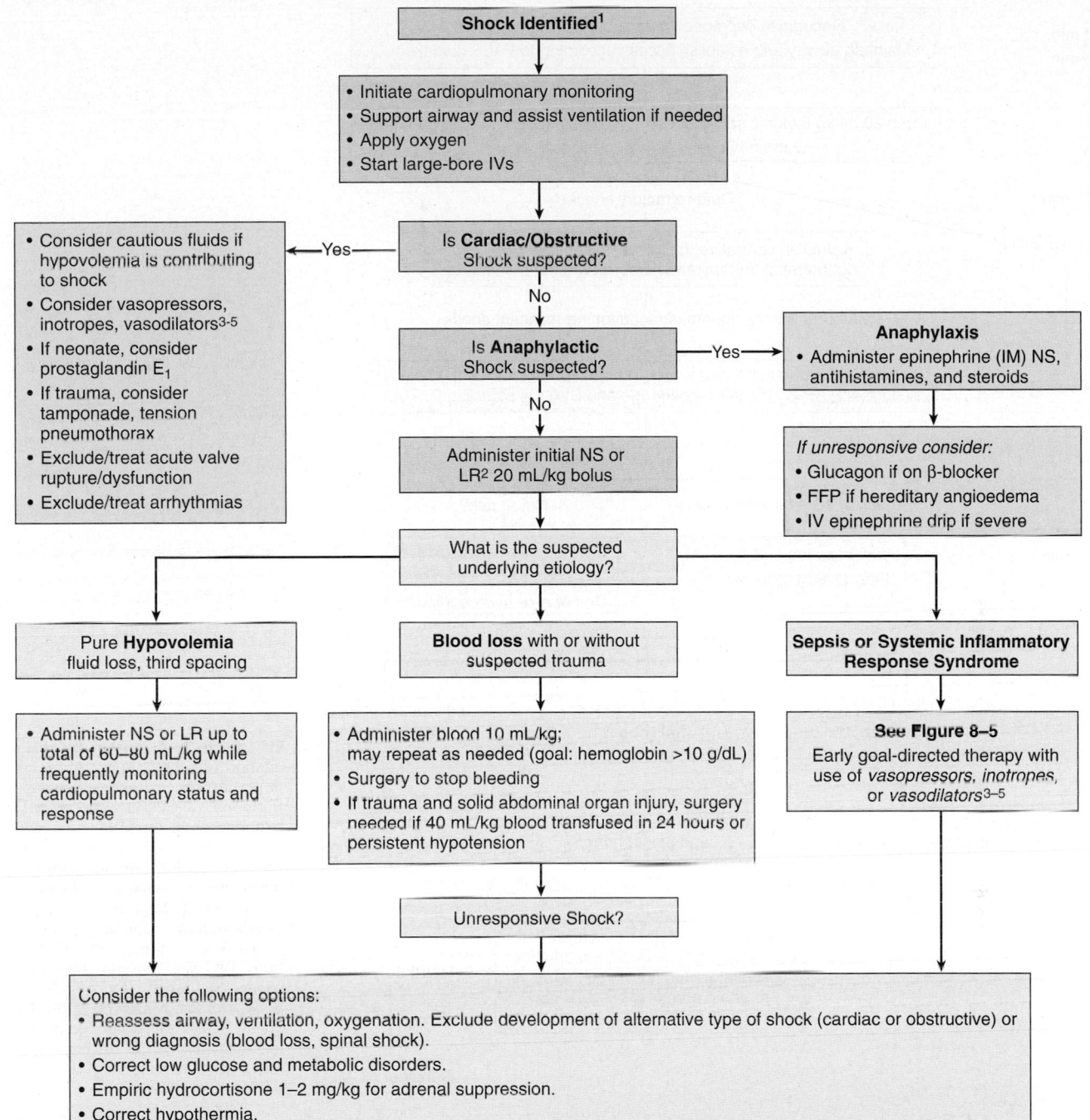

Shock Identified[1]

- Initiate cardiopulmonary monitoring
- Support airway and assist ventilation if needed
- Apply oxygen
- Start large-bore IVs

Is Cardiac/Obstructive Shock suspected? — Yes →

- Consider cautious fluids if hypovolemia is contributing to shock
- Consider vasopressors, inotropes, vasodilators[3-5]
- If neonate, consider prostaglandin E_1
- If trauma, consider tamponade, tension pneumothorax
- Exclude/treat acute valve rupture/dysfunction
- Exclude/treat arrhythmias

No ↓

Is Anaphylactic Shock suspected? — Yes →

Anaphylaxis
- Administer epinephrine (IM) NS, antihistamines, and steroids

If unresponsive consider:
- Glucagon if on β-blocker
- FFP if hereditary angioedema
- IV epinephrine drip if severe

No ↓

Administer initial NS or LR[2] 20 mL/kg bolus

What is the suspected underlying etiology?

Pure Hypovolemia fluid loss, third spacing

Blood loss with or without suspected trauma

Sepsis or Systemic Inflammatory Response Syndrome

- Administer NS or LR up to total of 60–80 mL/kg while frequently monitoring cardiopulmonary status and response

- Administer blood 10 mL/kg; may repeat as needed (goal: hemoglobin >10 g/dL)
- Surgery to stop bleeding
- If trauma and solid abdominal organ injury, surgery needed if 40 mL/kg blood transfused in 24 hours or persistent hypotension

See Figure 8–5
Early goal-directed therapy with use of *vasopressors, inotropes,* or *vasodilators*[3-5]

Unresponsive Shock?

Consider the following options:
- Reassess airway, ventilation, oxygenation. Exclude development of alternative type of shock (cardiac or obstructive) or wrong diagnosis (blood loss, spinal shock).
- Correct low glucose and metabolic disorders.
- Empiric hydrocortisone 1–2 mg/kg for adrenal suppression.
- Correct hypothermia.
- Institute invasive monitoring (central venous pressure, oxygenation, pulmonary capillary wedge pressure, arterial line).
- Assess for technical malfunctions (e.g., cuff, monitors, lines).
- Contact consultants for assistance (e.g., intensivist, cardiologist, pulmonologist, infectious disease specialist, surgeons).

[1] Algorithm is a suggested general approach that does not cover all diagnoses, scenarios, and management options. Clinicians should use their judgment and frequently reassess the response to therapy.

[2] LR, Lactated Ringer's solution; NS, normal saline.

[3] *Inotropes:* dopamine (5 and 10 mcg/kg/min), dobutamine, amrinone, milrinone, epinephrine (< 0.3 mcg/kg/min or > 0.3 mcg/kg/min with a vasodilator) to increase the cardiac index (CI) and reverse shock if CI < 3.3 L/min/m² after fluid resuscitation.

[4] *Vasopressors:* dopamine (≥10 mcg/kg/min), norepinephrine, phenylephrine, epinephrine (> 0.3 mcg/kg/min), or vasopressin to increase systemic vascular resistance (SVR) and reverse shock if SVR <800 dyne-sec/cm⁵/m² after fluid resuscitation.

[5] *Vasodilators:* nitroprusside, nitroglycerin, or phentolamine to decrease SVR if there is a CI < 3.3 L/min/m² and an SVR > 1600 dyne-sec/cm⁵/m² after fluid resuscitation.

FIGURE 8–2. General approach to management of shock based on etiology. Abbreviations: FFP, fresh frozen plasma; IM, intramuscular; IV, intravenous.

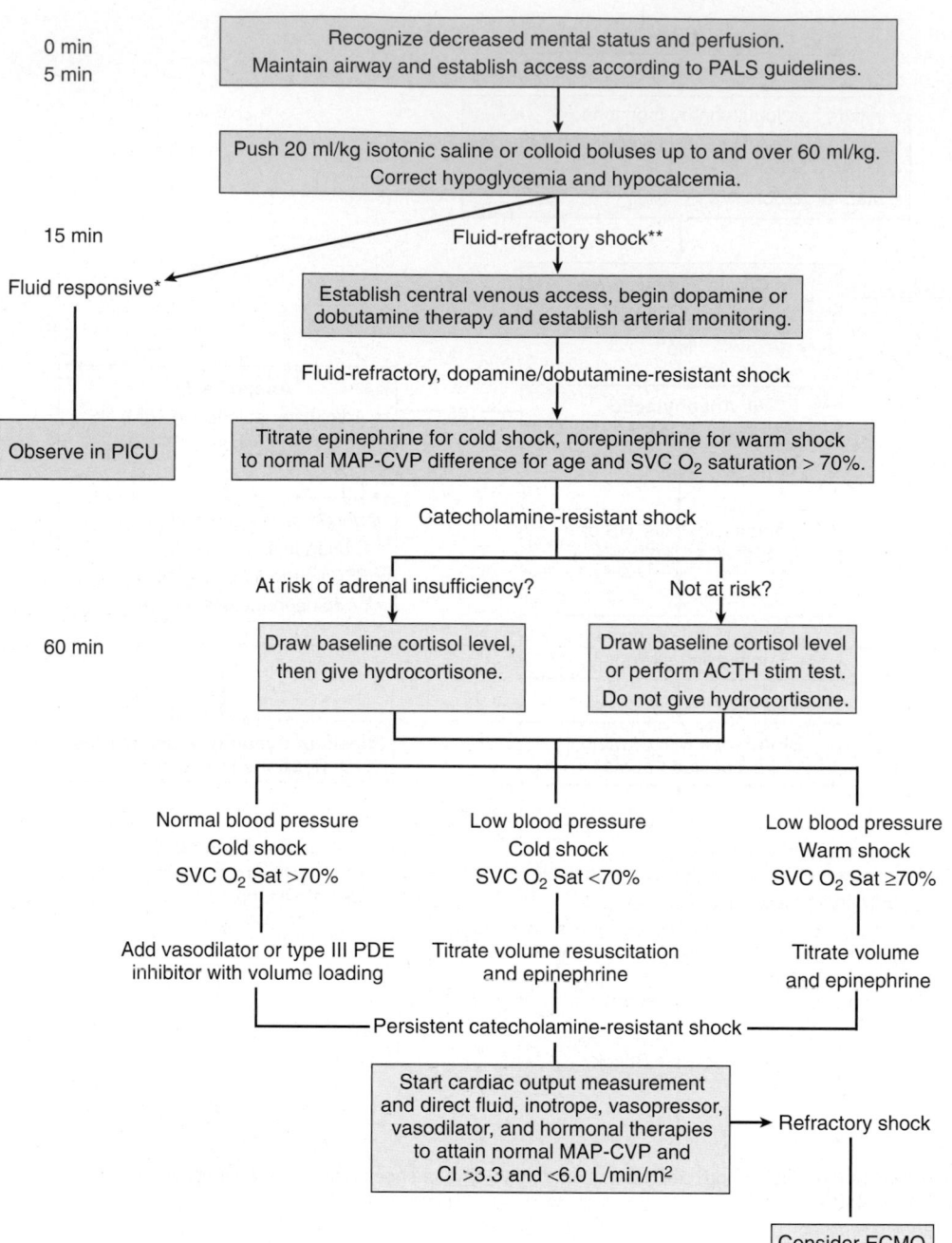

0 min
5 min

Recognize decreased mental status and perfusion.
Maintain airway and establish access according to PALS guidelines.

Push 20 ml/kg isotonic saline or colloid boluses up to and over 60 ml/kg.
Correct hypoglycemia and hypocalcemia.

15 min

Fluid-refractory shock**

Fluid responsive*

Establish central venous access, begin dopamine or
dobutamine therapy and establish arterial monitoring.

Fluid-refractory, dopamine/dobutamine-resistant shock

Observe in PICU

Titrate epinephrine for cold shock, norepinephrine for warm shock
to normal MAP-CVP difference for age and SVC O_2 saturation > 70%.

Catecholamine-resistant shock

At risk of adrenal insufficiency?

Not at risk?

60 min

Draw baseline cortisol level,
then give hydrocortisone.

Draw baseline cortisol level
or perform ACTH stim test.
Do not give hydrocortisone.

Normal blood pressure
Cold shock
SVC O_2 Sat >70%

Low blood pressure
Cold shock
SVC O_2 Sat <70%

Low blood pressure
Warm shock
SVC O_2 Sat ≥70%

Add vasodilator or type III PDE
inhibitor with volume loading

Titrate volume resuscitation
and epinephrine

Titrate volume
and epinephrine

Persistent catecholamine-resistant shock

Start cardiac output measurement
and direct fluid, inotrope, vasopressor,
vasodilator, and hormonal therapies
to attain normal MAP-CVP and
CI >3.3 and <6.0 L/min/m²

Refractory shock

Consider ECMO

FIGURE 8–3. Algorithm for resuscitation of septic shock. Abbreviations: ACTH, adrenocorticotropic hormone; CI, cardiac index; ECMO, extracorporeal membrane oxygenation; MAP-CVP, mean arterial pressure–central venous pressure difference; PALS, Pediatric Advanced Life Support; PDE, phosphodiesterase; PICU, pediatric intensive care unit; stim., stimulation; SVC O_2, superior vena cava oxygen saturation. (From Dellinger RP, Carlet JM, Masur H, et al: Surviving sepsis campaign guidelines for management of severe sepsis and septic shock. Crit Care Med 32:858–873, 2004.)

Table 8–4	Threshold Heart Rate and Perfusion Pressure for Age	
Current Age (yr)	**Heart Rate (beats/min)**	**MAP-CVP (cm H₂O)**
Term Neonate	120–180	55
≤1	120–180	60
≤2	120–160	65
≤7	100–140	65
≤15	90–140	65

Abbreviation: MAP-CVP, mean arterial pressure–central venous pressure difference.
From Carcillo JA, Fields AI, American College of Critical Care Medicine Task Force Committee Members: Clinical practice parameters for hemodynamic support of pediatric and neonatal patients in septic shock. Crit Care Med 30:1371, 2002.

Evaluation

Symptoms of disorders causing shock are disease specific (e.g., wheezing and rash in anaphylaxis, abdominal pain in traumatic hemorrhagic due to solid organ injury). Other important symptoms include change in mental status, dyspnea, and decreased urine output. The list of symptoms of organ system dysfunction is extensive and eventually involves most organ systems (Table 8–5).

Vital signs are extremely variable in shock. While isolated tachycardia may be an early and sensitive sign of impaired oxygen delivery, it has poor specificity. Bradycardia is a late finding in shock and indicates impending cardiac or pulmonary arrest. Tachypnea is an early manifestation of shock that is easily overlooked. While hypotension is a poor indicator of early shock, a widened pulse pressure in the setting of a

Table 8–5	Systemic Signs and Symptoms of Impaired Perfusion/Shock	
Organ	Early Impairment	Late Impairment
Brain	Change in mental status: irritability, anxiety, confusion, sleepiness, agitation	Lethargy, obtundation, coma
Kidney	Oliguria	Anuria
Liver	Transaminase elevation, hyperbilirubinemia	Liver failure, coagulopathy
Heart	Ischemia, tachycardia, widened pulse pressure	Dyspnea due to congestive failure, bradycardia, malignant arrhythmias
Gastrointestinal tract	Mucosal ischemia, emesis	Ileus, ascites, ischemia with bleeding
Lungs	Pulmonary edema, tachypnea, hypoxemia	Bradypnea, respiratory failure
Hematologic system	Mild bleeding due to coagulopathy, thrombocytopenia	Uncontrolled bleeding due to disseminated intravascular coagulopathy
Skin	Cool and pale, or warm (early sepsis)	Mottled, cold, pale, or purple discoloration

normal blood pressure may be a subtle early finding. Hyperthermia may be present in early septic shock, while hypothermia will eventually develop in all types of shock.

Physical examination findings consistent with shock vary depending on the primary etiology (see Table 8–5). Infants and children with early distributive shock (e.g., neurogenic, early sepsis, anaphylaxis) exhibit warm extremities, bounding peripheral pulses, and a brisk capillary refill time, while most other forms of shock lead to cool extremities, weak pulses, and a delayed capillary refill time. Capillary refill time should be interpreted within the context of the ambient room temperature. In one pediatric study, only 31% of healthy patients in a cold room had a normal capillary refill time.[7] Capillary refill time also has poor interobserver reliability when assessed in ill children.[8] In addition, a normal capillary refill time of ≤ 2 seconds is an inaccurate predictor of hemodynamic status in children in pediatric critical care units.[9] Recognition of physical examination patterns can aid in determining the etiology of shock (Figs. 8–4 and 8–5).

Prompt recognition of shock is important so that aggressive treatment can be initiated. One study found that delayed reversal of septic shock was associated with a greater than twofold increase in mortality for every hour that passed without reversal.[10] Knowledge of the limitations of the history and physical examination and of pattern recognition can assist in an early diagnosis of shock and can help identify the exact cause.

Hypovolemia

Hypovolemia is the most common cause of shock throughout the world. This is primarily due to the high incidence of and morbidity from dehydration due to gastroenteritis in developing countries. In addition to gastroenteritis, several other diseases result in excessive fluid loss and can lead to hypovolemic shock. Examples include hemorrhage from trauma or GI bleeding, as well as fluid loss from burns, diabetic ketoacidosis (DKA), and diabetes insipidus.

In gastroenteritis, a history of vomiting with diarrhea is typically present. Infants and children with shock will exhibit physical examination findings of severe dehydration: cool extremities, weak peripheral pulses, dry mucous membranes, a sunken fontanelle in infants, sunken eyes, diminished skin turgor, and a delayed capillary refill time (see Chapter 72, Vomiting and Diarrhea). The presence of three of four clinical features—ill appearance, dry mucous membranes, diminished capillary refill time, and absent tears—identifies most

children with ≥10% dehydration, signifying a population at high risk for hypovolemic shock.[11]

Patients with DKA are a unique population who often suffer from extreme dehydration. In young children, this can be particularly profound since symptoms of diabetes are difficult to recognize. In the past, there was concern that rapid correction of glucose, sodium, and serum osmolality might harm patients with DKA. However, development of cerebral edema is not associated with the rate of fluid administration or rate of change in serum glucose.[12] Children with DKA and hypotension require aggressive treatment with intravenous fluids in a manner similar to children with other types of hypovolemic shock (see Chapter 105, Diabetic Ketoacidosis).

In a patient who has suffered extensive full-thickness or deep partial-thickness burns, shock may result. The body has lost its protective shield and therefore has increased fluid losses. In addition, massive capillary leak of fluid leads to intravascular hypovolemia. Patients with burns may also have shock from infection and sepsis, although this is more likely in the subacute phase and not when the patient immediately presents to the emergency department (ED). All burns that total 15% of the total body surface area will require aggressive fluid management (see Chapter 26, Burns).

Another etiology of hypovolemic shock is massive GI bleeding. Causes include portal hypertension and esophageal varices from congenital or chronic liver disease, ulcer bleeding, platelet disorders, and coagulopathies. Bleeding from GI infection, inflammatory colitis, ischemic bowel, or surgical disorders (e.g., Meckel's diverticulum) may also lead to blood loss (see Chapter 75, Gastrointestinal Bleeding).

Septic Shock

Sepsis is an inflammatory state in the presence of infection. Five percent to 30% of children with sepsis will develop septic shock.[13] The systemic inflammatory response syndrome (SIRS) leads to shock through an interplay of mechanisms. Hypovolemia exists from decreased intake prior to presentation. Disruption of vascular integrity and increased vascular capacitance from cytokines also decreases preload and compromises stroke volume. Myocardial dysfunction from endotoxins contributes to decreased organ perfusion and compounds shock.

Severe sepsis and septic shock, as defined by a recent consensus conference, are overlapping syndromes[14,15] (Tables 8–6 and 8–7). Importantly, shock physiology can occur without hypotension.

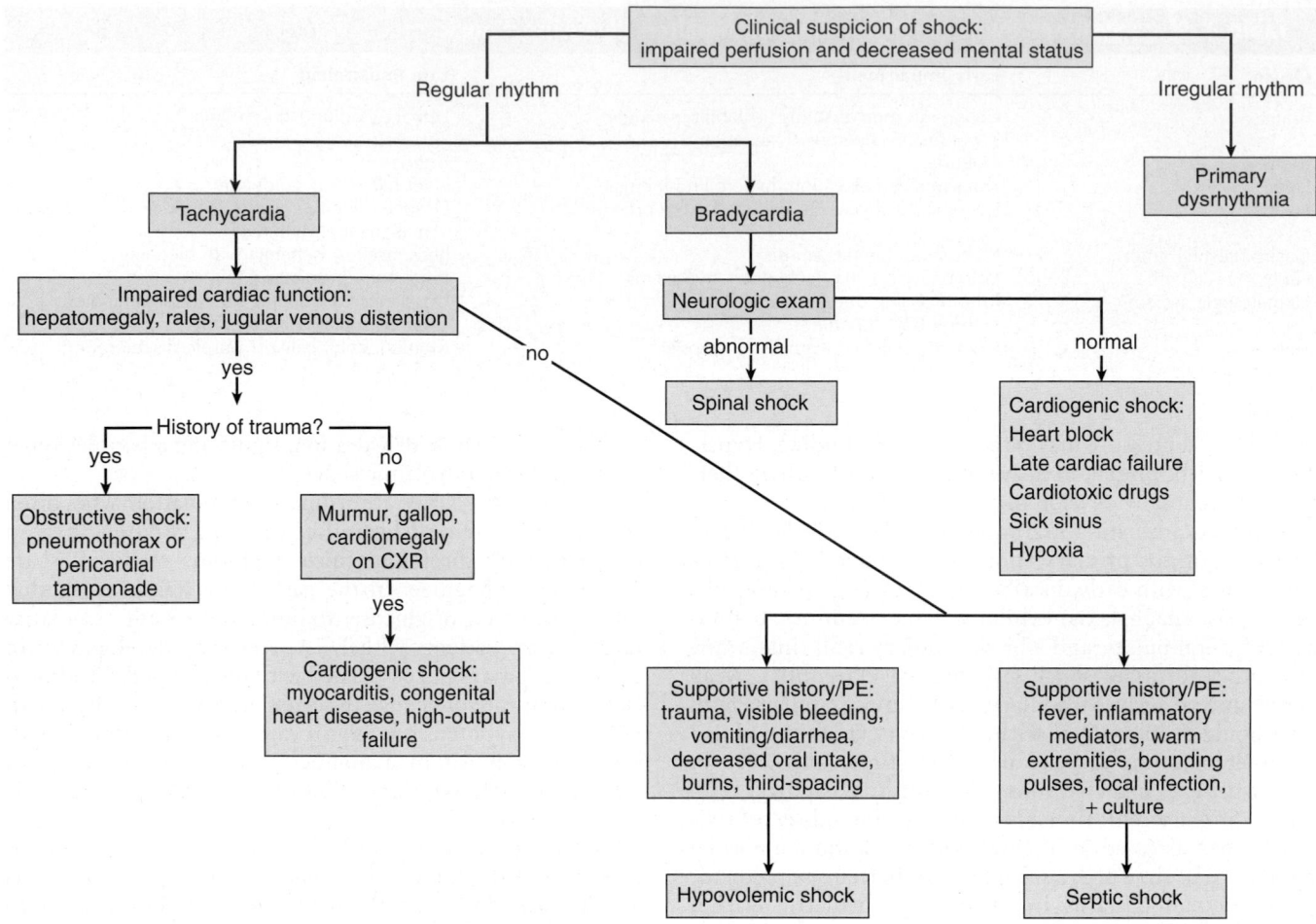

FIGURE 8–4. Algorithm for elucidating etiology of shock. Abbreviations: CXR, chest radiograph; PE, physical examination.

Table 8–6	Definitions of Sepsis-Related Terms
SIRS (systemic inflammatory response syndrome)*	Presence of 2 of the following: • Core (rectal, bladder, oral) temperature <36° C or >38.5° C • Heart rate > 2 standard deviations above percentile for age, or otherwise unexplained, persistent elevation for 0.5–4 hr; if <1 yr old, bradycardia < 10th percentile for age • Respiratory rate > 2 standards deviations above percentile for age, or need for mechanical ventilation • White blood cell count elevated or depressed for age or >10% bands
Sepsis*	SIRS + presence of infection (positive culture or clinical evidence with high probability of infection)
Severe Sepsis*	Sepsis + presence of 1 of the following: • Cardiovascular organ dysfunction • Acute respiratory distress syndrome • Dysfunction of 2 or more other organs (see Table 8–7)
Septic Shock*	Severe sepsis + cardiovascular organ dysfunction (see Table 8–7)
Cold Shock†	Septic shock with decreased capillary refill time and mottled, cool extremities (epinephrine)
Warm Shock†	Septic shock with warm extremities; strong, bounding pulses; and instant capillary refill (norepinephrine)
Fluid-Refractory/Dopamine-Resistant Shock†	Persistence of shock despite ≥ 60 ml/kg of fluid resuscitation in first hour and dopamine infusion to 10 mcg/kg/min
Catecholamine-Resistant Shock†	Persistence of shock despite use of epinephrine or norepinephrine for fluid-refractory, dopamine-resistant shock
Refractory Shock†	Persistence of shock despite goal-directed use of inotropic agents, vasopressors, vasodilators, and maintenance of metabolic (glucose and calcium) and hormonal (thyroid and hydrocortisone) homeostasis

*Data from Goldstein B, Grioir B, Randolph A, et al: International pediatric sepsis consensus conference: definitions for sepsis and organ dysfunction in pediatrics. Pediatr Crit Care Med 6:2–8, 2005.
†Modified from Carcillo JA, Fields AI, American College of Critical Care Medicine Task Force Committee Members: Clinical practice parameters or hemodynamic support of pediatric and neonatal patients in septic shock. Crit Care Med 30:1365–1378, 2002.

Recognize Shock: Poor Perfusion, Change in Mental Status, Decreased Urine Output

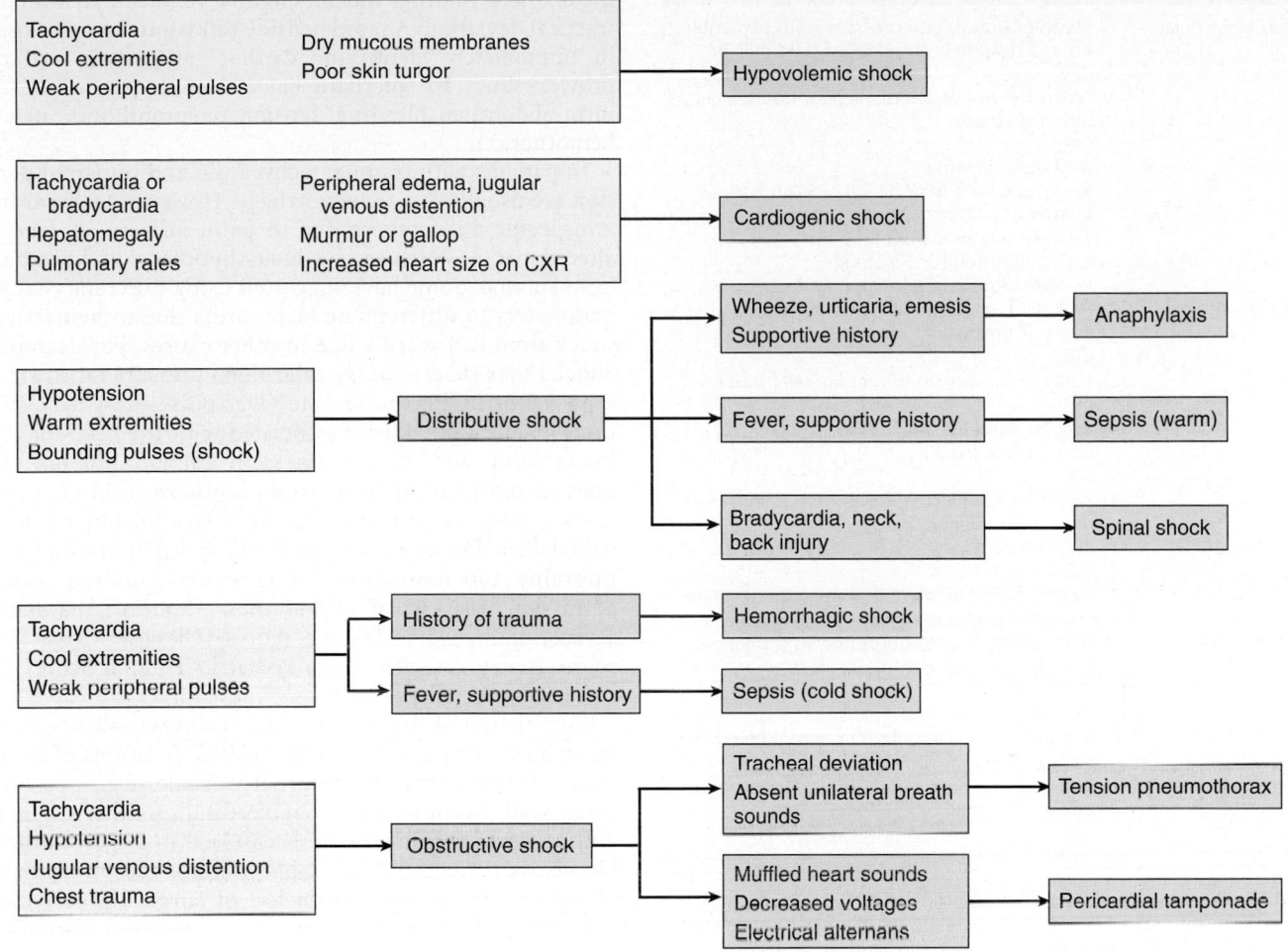

FIGURE 8–5. Pattern recognition for different types of shock. Abbreviation: CXR, chest radiograph.

Differentiating the clinical presentation into warm (early) or cold (late) shock can assist in management. Cold shock is accompanied by decreased capillary refill time, weak peripheral pulses, and mottled, cool extremities. Children with warm shock present with warm extremities, strong, bounding pulses, and normal capillary refill time. Abnormal endotoxin-mediated vasodilation causes warm shock and is the basis for the major categorization of septic shock as a distributive-type shock.

Elevated troponin[16,17] and B-type natriuretic peptide[18] levels can be used as a marker for cardiac compromise during septic shock, although it is unclear whether cardiac dysfunction is a result of poor perfusion during septic shock, or if cardiac compromise is due to the underlying cause of sepsis. Echocardiography can be used to diagnose or confirm diminished cardiac function.

Various studies have attempted to find prognostic factors for septic shock. In adults, elevated levels of tumor necrosis factor (TNF) and interleukin-1B have been found to be associated with a poor outcome.[19,20] High TNF levels are associated with higher probability of obtaining a positive blood culture in patients with shock.[20] Children with septic shock have higher levels of erythropoietin and interleukin-6[21,22] compared to those without septic shock. A C-reactive protein

level greater than 8 mg/dl is 94% sensitive and 87% specific for SIRS in adults, although cutoffs are less well defined for children.[23] However, procalcitonin is a more specific marker for children with septic shock and correlates with higher morbidity.[24-26] The median admission procalcitonin level for nonsurvivors with septic shock is significantly elevated (273 vs. 82 ng/ml) compared to survivors.[26] Children with shock have higher median levels of procalcitonin (39.1 vs. 15.0 ng/ml) compared to children without shock.[24]

The most studied marker for severity of septic shock is arterial lactate.[27,28] Normalization of lactate and base deficit has been associated with recovery from septic shock.[27] Noninvasive monitoring systems for impaired perfusion and shock include gastric tonometry and capnometry. In gastric tonometry, mucosal pH and partial pressure of carbon dioxide (Pco_2) are measured to identify splanchnic vasoconstriction, which occurs early in hypoperfused states. Importantly, adults and children with lower intramucosal pH have higher mortality,[27-29] although tonometry is not a feasible measurement tool for the ED. Elevated end-tidal CO_2 is also a marker for impaired tissue perfusion. In adults, elevated sublingual capnometry has been used as another noninvasive method of estimating lactate and severe shock.[30] One study found that sublingual CO_2 greater than

Table 8–7	Organ Dysfunction Criteria
Cardiovascular	1) Hypotension (blood pressure <5th percentile for age despite ≥ 40 ml/kg of fluid in 1 hr) OR 2) Need for vasoactive medication to maintain blood pressure OR 3) 2 of the following • Unexplained base deficit > 5.0 mEq/L • Arterial lactate > 2 times normal • Urine output < 0.5 ml/kg/hr • Capillary refill > 5 seconds • Core-to-peripheral temperature gap > 3° C
Respiratory	1) PaO_2/FIO_2 < 300 in absence of congenital heart or preexisting lung disease OR 2) $PaCO_2$ > 65 torr or 20 mm Hg over baseline OR 3) Proven need for 0.5 FIO_2 to maintain saturation ≥ 92% OR 4) Need for nonelective invasive or noninvasive mechanical ventilation
Neurologic	1) GCS score ≤ 11 OR 2) Acute change in mental status with decrease in GCS score to ≥ 3 points from baseline
Hematologic	1) Platelet count < 80,000/µl or 50% decline from highest value in past 3 days OR 2) INR > 2
Renal	Creatinine ≥ 2 times normal or twofold increase from baseline
Hepatic	1) Total bilirubin ≥ 4 mg/dl (excluding newborn infants) OR 2) ALT > 2 times normal

Abbreviations: ALT, alanine transaminase; FIO_2, fraction of inspired oxygen; GCS, Glasgow Coma Scale; INR, international normalized ratio; $PaCO_2$, arterial partial pressure of carbon dioxide; PaO_2, arterial partial pressure of oxygen.

70 mm Hg was associated with shock, a lactate level greater than 2.5 mmol/L, and an increased risk of death in adults presenting to an ED or admitted to an intensive care unit.[30] Useful cutoffs for clinical decision making in children are less well defined (see Chapter 5, Monitoring in Critically Ill Children).

Trauma

Trauma can affect an isolated organ system or may cause multisystem derangements. The trauma patient is best initially assessed using an algorithmic approach with sequential or simultaneous attention to airway, breathing, and then circulation (see Chapter 12, Approach to Multisystem Trauma). A trauma patient with signs of shock may have one or more of several causes to explain the shock. Patients with obstructive shock (manifesting as decreased perfusion and hypotension or, if severe, pulseless electrical activity) can have a tension pneumothorax, massive hemothorax, or pericardial tamponade. A tension pneumothorax is identified in a patient who is in extremis with hypotension and dyspnea (or difficulty bagging) by the absence of breath sounds and hyper-

resonance to percussion on the affected side. Late and inconsistent findings include jugular venous distention and tracheal deviation. A rapid bedside ultrasound may be useful in immediately identifying cardiac tamponade and may provide clues to alternate causes for hypotension (e.g., intra-abdominal bleeding, tension pneumothorax, massive hemothorax).

In patients with trauma, tachycardia and impaired perfusion are usually due to hemorrhage. However, tachycardia is nonspecific and may be due to pain, anxiety, or fear. An altered mental status can be due to hypotension, hypoxia, or head trauma. Some have suggested using different vital sign parameters to differentiate tachycardia due to hemorrhagic shock from tachycardia due to other causes. For example, a Shock Index (heart rate/systolic blood pressure ratio) greater than 0.9 or ROPE (pulse *Rate Over* pulse *Pressure Evaluation*) greater than 3.0 are associated with the need for acute intervention and critical illness in adults, although these markers have not yet been proven useful in children.[31] Prognosis of patients with trauma can be stratified by the initial base deficit. The more negative the base deficit, the higher the mortality and morbidity.[5,32] Infants and children with an admission base deficit of less than −5 mEq/L have more severe injury, worse trauma scores (Glasgow Coma Scale score, Injury Severity Score, Pediatric Trauma Score), and increased mortality.[5]

Completion of the primary and secondary survey during trauma evaluation will identify possible locations of hemorrhage. Actively bleeding external wounds (e.g., open fractures, scalp lacerations, arterial bleeding), solid organ injury, and pelvis and femur fractures can lead to large volumes of blood loss. Patients with unstable vital signs despite initiation of fluid therapy, and a suspicion of surgically correctable hemorrhage (e.g., splenic laceration, large vessel disruption), should go directly to the operating room. Abdominal bleeding is usually diagnosed by computed tomography (CT) or bedside ultrasonography (FAST examination), and the physical examination is often abnormal in these patients if they have a normal mental status. Abdominal tenderness, distention, and bruising of the abdominal wall are suggestive signs. In the past, diagnostic peritoneal lavage (DPL) was frequently used to diagnose intraperitoneal injury. Now that CT and bedside ultrasound are readily available, DPL is rarely used.

Several serum markers can guide therapy and predict outcome in patients with hemorrhagic shock due to trauma. While an initial elevated lactate level is associated with mortality from trauma, a response to therapy with a normalization of lactate by 24 hours signifies a diminished probability of death.[33] Initial ED pH of ≤7.25, lactate of ≥5 mmol/L, base excess of ≤−7.3 mEq/L, an elevated anion gap, and a strong ion gap of ≥5 mEq/L all signify a higher probability of death in adults with major trauma, while patients with none of these factors have a very low probability of trauma-associated death. The strongest predictor of mortality may be an elevated strong ion gap (SIG). The SIG represents a complex calculation that measures the difference between strong anions and strong cations and is the mathematical difference between the apparent strong ion difference (SIDa) and the effective strong ion difference (SIDe).[34] An elevated SIG (>2 mEq/L) signifies that unmeasured strong anions are present:

$$SIDa = [Na^+ + K^+ + Ca^{+2} + Mg^{+2} - Cl^- - lactate - urate]$$

$$SIDe = [albumin \times (0.123 \times pH - 0.631)] +$$
$$[PO_4 \times (0.309 \times pH - 0.469)] + HCO_3$$

$$SIG = SIDa - SIDe \text{ (abnormal SIG is >2 mEq/L)}$$

Cardiac Disorders

Neonates and young infants with congenital disorders that obstruct the left ventricular outflow tract or with congenital obstructive left heart syndromes (COLHS) usually present early in life with shock (see Chapter 30, Congenital Heart Disease). In older infants and children, a variety of disorders cause myocardial damage and diminished pump function. These include myocarditis (e.g., viral, autoimmune), primary cardiomyopathies, and secondary cardiomyopathies due to a variety of disorders, including hyperthyroidism, metabolic defects (e.g., carnitine deficiency), neuromuscular disease (e.g., Friedreich's ataxia, muscular dystrophy), glycogen storage disease, mucopolysaccharidoses, and medication toxicity (e.g., adriamycin). Chest radiography usually shows cardiomegaly and varying degrees of congestive heart failure. Electrocardiographic (ECG) abnormalities often reflect the underlying pathology, while echocardiography is often diagnostic. Cardiac troponins and brain natriuretic peptide may be elevated. When pump function is compromised and a stressor is added (e.g., respiratory infection), the heart often cannot increase contractility to meet the excess demands and cardiogenic shock may develop. While features of the underlying disorder are often present, these patients often present with profound shock with evidence of congestive heart failure. Importantly, the myocardium may be too diseased to respond to small fluid boluses or vasopressors.

Arrhythmias (including supraventricular and ventricular tachycardia and conduction blocks with bradycardia) can also lead to diminished cardiac output and cardiogenic shock. These disorders require prompt recognition and reversal to prevent cardiac arrest.

Anaphylaxis

Anaphylaxis is a systemic allergic response at the severe end of the allergic reaction spectrum. Signs and symptoms include generalized urticaria, wheezing, respiratory distress, hypotension due to distributive shock, emesis, and GI tract inflammation. Patients with anaphylactic shock classically have food or medication sensitization and immediate immunoglobulin E–mediated hypersensitivity reactions (see Chapter 14, Anaphylaxis/Allergic Reaction).

Neonatal Shock

Neonates (birth to 28 days old) comprise an important group of patients with unique disorders causing shock (see Chapter 7, The Critically Ill Neonate). Neonatal shock is less obvious and will manifest with subtle clinical features that differ from those in older infants and cause difficulty in discriminating between disorders causing shock. Typical features include temperature instability (hypothermia and hyperthermia), lethargy, apnea, hypotension, tachycardia, respiratory distress, and poor feeding. Blood pressure does not correlate well with systemic blood flow, and the goal for mean arterial pressure is to maintain it higher than the baby's gestational age at the time of birth.[35] Hypotension is defined as a blood pressure that is less than the 10th percentile for age. Normal capillary refill time for the neonate is greater than that of older infants (3 seconds), while normal capillary refill time for preterm babies can exceed 5 seconds.

Infections are an important and common cause of shock in neonates. Group B streptococcal (GBS) infections are unique, with early (48 hours postpartum) and late (2 to 90 days) presentations. Risk factors include prematurity, African American ethnicity, young maternal age (<20 years), and prior history of GBS. Meningitis manifests in one third of GBS cases, and a diffuse pneumonia with a ground-glass appearance on radiographs is common.

Several serum parameters are elevated in neonatal sepsis. An immature neutrophil–to–total neutrophil ratio greater than 0.2 is 60% to 90% sensitive and 70% to 80% specific for diagnosing neonatal sepsis, while an abnormal C-reactive protein is 75% sensitive and 86% specific for this disorder.[36-38] Limited studies have found that an elevated interleukin-6 level (100 or 135 pg/ml cutoff) is 81% to 93% sensitive and 86% to 96% specific, a procalcitonin level greater than 0.5 mcg/L is 93% to 100% sensitive and 92% to 98% specific, and an elevated TNF-α level is 72% to 95% sensitive and 43% to 78% specific for diagnosing neonatal sepsis.[39] Other elevated serum parameters in neonatal sepsis include neutrophil CD11b, interleukin-8, interleukin-1 receptor antagonist, fibronectin, neutrophil elastase inhibitors, and TNF receptors p55 and p75.[39]

Viral infections (especially perinatally acquired herpes simplex virus) may cause viremia and clinical sepsis. Neonates may have coexisting central nervous system (CNS) disease with seizures or disseminated disease with liver and pulmonary involvement. About 60% to 80% will have skin lesions when infected with herpes. Regardless of the responsible organism, hypovolemia, distributive mechanisms (third spacing of fluids), and cardiac dysfunction contribute to neonatal shock (see Chapter 13, Sepsis). Management is directed at each of these underlying pathologic entities in addition to the use of specific antimicrobials.

Neonates with COLHS (e.g., hypoplastic left heart, coarctation of the aorta, interrupted aortic arch, critical aortic stenosis) may present in the first 30 days of life with shock that initially appears indistinguishable from sepsis.[40] These neonates have an obstruction to cardiac outflow and present in profound shock once the ductus arteriosis closes (see Chapter 30, Congenital Heart Disease). Feeding difficulty, somnolence, cyanosis, tachycardia, delayed capillary refill time, significant upper and lower extremity blood pressures differences, and acidosis are common to both sepsis and COLHS. One study compared neonates with COLHS to those with sepsis and meningitis. Neonates with COLHS more frequently had respiratory distress (87% vs. 55%), cardiomegaly (85% vs. 5%), a murmur (53% vs. 5%), and diminished upper and lower extremity pulses (32% and 70% vs. 3% and 11%), while they less frequently had irritability (11% vs. 55%) and a fever history (0 vs. 63%).[40] Radiography shows cardiomegaly in up to 85% of cases, while ECG abnormalities are noted in 80% of cases.[40] Other cardiac disorders affecting cardiac output in neonates include arrhythmias and tamponade.

Gastrointestinal catastrophies, including necrotizing enterocolitis (in premature neonates), malrotation and midgut volvulus, and incarcerated hernias, must be considered in neonates with acute onset of vomiting (especially bilious), abdominal distention, or GI bleeding followed by shock (see Chapter 83, Malrotation and Midgut Volvulus; and Chapter 84, Hernia). Hypovolemia (including blood loss) and sepsis contribute to shock in these neonates and require correction, with concurrent administration of antibiotics directed against gram-negative enteric organisms.

Metabolic disturbances are an important and easily overlooked cause of shock in neonates. Hypoglycemia may accompany shock due to poor glycogen reserves, decreased muscle mass, inadequate intake, and increased glucose demand in stressed states. For this reason, a rapid bedside glucose check is mandatory in all neonates with shock. Immaturity of the endocrine axis (thyroid, parathyroid) and congenital abnormalities also require consideration of thyroid and calcium replacement.

Management

Shock therapy should proceed simultaneously with a directed clinical evaluation to determine the cause of a patient's clinical syndrome. Universal management for all types of shock includes support of airway and breathing (e.g., early intubation with assisted ventilation or supplemental oxygen); continuous monitoring of cardiopulmonary status (see Chapter 5, Monitoring in Critically Ill Children) with cardiac telemetry, oximetry, and/or capnography; frequent or continuous assessment of vitals signs; temperature support; and correction of underlying metabolic disorders (e.g., hypoglycemia, electrolyte disturbances). Blood pressure support and shock reversal measures are then directed at the underlying cause of shock (see Fig. 8–2).

Hypovolemia

In addition to airway management, aggressive fluid resuscitation is the most important therapy for treating hypovolemic shock. Optimally, two large-bore intravenous (IV) lines are placed, because repeated normal saline boluses of 20 ml/kg, up to a total of 60 to 80 ml/kg, may be needed to correct hypovolemia. Treatment goals include an improved mental status, capillary refill time less than 2 seconds, normal pulses, warm extremities, and a normal blood pressure. Glucose is checked as soon as IV access is obtained; ideally, blood glucose levels are maintained between 80 and 110 g/dl.[41] Electrolyte abnormalities also may require correction during management. With long-standing gastroenteritis, metabolic acidosis may develop. For patients with decompensated shock and severe acidosis, treatment with bicarbonate may help to improve cardiac function.[42] However, bicarbonate administration can worsen intracellular acidosis and cerebral acidosis and theoretically worsen shock, and cannot be routinely recommended.

For burn patients, 20-ml/kg crystalloid fluid boluses are administered in succession, with re-evaluation of hemodynamic, cardiac, and respiratory status. Lactated Ringer's solution is recommended for resuscitation in the first 24 hours after a significant burn. Lactated Ringer's solution contains physiologic concentrations of major electrolytes, and lactate serves as a buffer that lessens the risk of hyperchloremic acidosis. Large volumes of fluid are needed for burn patients since only 20% to 30% of administered isotonic fluids remain in the intravascular space. In general, potassium should not initially be added to fluids since cellular

breakdown will often lead to release of large amounts of this electrolyte. Also, albumin should not be administered in the first 24 hours after a burn since capillary leak of this colloid can markedly increased edema. Formulas used to calculate the amount of fluid required to replace losses over the first 24 hours include the Parkland formula (4 ml/kg per percent body surface area [%BSA] burned) and the Carvajal formula (5000 ml/m²/%BSA burn) (see Chapter 26, Burns). The Parkland formula may underestimate fluid losses in young children, while the Carvajal formula is ideal for use in children younger than 6 years old. Both formulas require addition of maintenance fluids, with administration of half of the total volume in the first 8 hours and the other half over the ensuing 16 hours. All fluid replacement regimens require monitoring for end points indicating adequate resuscitation, including adequate urine output (2 ml/kg/hr if <1 year old, 1.5 ml/kg if 1 to 3 years old, and 1 ml/kg if >3 years old), normal mental status, and improvement in vital signs. If these goals are not met, additional fluids above those dictated by burn formulas are indicated. Children with extensive burns may need massive quantities of fluid replacement, and the tendency to insufficiently fluid resuscitate patients with burns has been shown.[43]

Gastrointestinal bleeding with esophageal varices may be treated with octreotide, sclerotherapy, or surgical intervention. Coagulopathy is treated with appropriate blood products. A bleeding Meckel's diverticulum that is causing hemodynamic compromise needs to be surgically removed.

Septic Shock

The Golden Hour

Primary goals in treatment of septic shock include maintenance of ventilation, oxygenation, and perfusion through normalization and optimization of circulatory hemodynamics and blood pressure (see Table 8–4 and Fig. 8–3). Infants and young children are more likely to need early intubation due to their limited pulmonary reserve. Specifically, infants and young children have a relatively reduced functional residual capacity, increased oxygen consumption, immature intercostal and diaphragmatic muscles, inefficient intercostal muscle positioning, and diaphragmatic apposition to the chest wall.[44] Intubation and mechanical ventilation can decrease oxygen requirements since the excess metabolic demand for work of breathing is removed. Moreover, aggressive fluid therapy coupled with increased capillary permeability may lead to pulmonary edema, which may require mechanical ventilation with increased peak end-expiratory pressures.[45]

Inadequate early fluid resuscitation in the ED is associated with increased mortality in septic shock. One study found that children who died from septic shock only received 20 ml/kg of fluid in the first hour despite receiving more vasopressors than children who survived.[10] Administration of greater than 40 ml/kg of crystalloid fluid in the first hour is associated with improved survival and does not increase the incidence of acute respiratory distress syndrome.[46]

Ideally, crystalloid IV fluid should be administered in successive 20-ml/kg boluses over 5 to 10 minutes. Clinical end points of treatment include capillary refill time less than 2 seconds, normal pulses (without central-peripheral discordance), warm extremities, urine output greater than 1 ml/kg/hr, normal mental status, and normal blood pressure.[44,45] The patient should be monitored for the development of congestive heart failure (a gallop, rales, increased work of breathing, or hepatomegaly). Inotropic therapy should be initiated earlier in the presence of these clinical signs. If 60 ml/kg of fluid has been administered without reversal of shock, vasoactive agents should be administered. These medications can be started in a peripheral IV line, but establishment of central venous access is ideal (see Figs. 8–2 and 8–3).

Vasoactive medications are administered after fluid therapy has been maximized in septic shock. *Inotropes* are used to increase cardiac output and are particularly useful in patients with a diminished cardiac output (cardiac index <3.3 L/min/m^2). Inotropes include dopamine (5–10 mcg/kg/min), dobutamine, amrinone, milrinone, and epinephrine (<0.3 mcg/kg/min or > 0.3 mcg/kg/min when combined with a vasodilator). *Vasopressors* are added to increase systemic vascular resistance (SVR) in patients with peripheral vasodilation and a depressed SVR (<800 dyne-sec/cm^5/m^2). These agents include dopamine (≥ 10 mcg/kg/min), norepinephrine, phenylephrine, vasopressin, and epinephrine (>0.3 mcg/kg/min). *Vasodilators* (nitroprusside, nitroglycerin, or phentolamine) are used in patients with a high SVR (>1600 dyne-sec/cm^5/m^2) to decrease the pressure head against which the heart must pump blood to the body. Clinicians must remember that specific agents may have inotropic, vasodilator, and vasopressors effects at different doses (see Fig. 8–2 and Table 8–3).

Dopamine is the drug of choice for shock unresponsive to fluids. At low doses (<5 mcg/kg/min) it increases renal and mesenteric flow, at medium doses (5 to 10 mcg/kg/min) it has inotropic activity, and at higher doses (>10 mcg/kg/min) it acts as a vasopressor. Children with septic shock often have a diminished cardiac output due to direct endotoxic effects of bacteria as well as from acidosis- and electrolyte-induced cardiac dysfunction.[42]

Dobutamine can be used as a first-line vasoactive agent in septic shock. Its cardiac effect on contractility improves cardiac function. In patients with increased SVR, the β_2-agonist vasodilatory effects of dobutamine may be superior to dopamine. In a study of fluid-refractory septic shock, 58% of children responded to inotropic therapy, but half of those children needed an additional vasodilator. Twenty percent of children had a high cardiac index and low SVR and responded to vasopressor therapy, with half of those children requiring an additional inotrope.[50] Twenty percent of children had both low cardiac contractility and SVR and responded to inotropes and vasopressors (see Figs. 8–2 and 8–3).

Early goal-directed therapy decreases mortality in adult patients with septic shock.[47,48] This approach entails the use of central venous and arterial monitoring to titrate the use of fluids, vasoactive agents, airway support, and blood transfusion (if hemoglobin is <10 g/dl) to maintain normal central venous pressure (CVP), normal mean arterial pressure (MAP), and superior vena cava oxygen saturation (SVC O$_2$) greater than 70%.[47,48] Mixed venous oxygen saturation (SvO$_2$) can substitute for SVC O$_2$ saturation in the absence of a central catheter in the SVC. Additional goals include decreasing arterial lactate, normalizing base deficit, optimizing cardiac function by echocardiography, maximizing perfusion pressure (MAP-CVP difference), and maintaining

cardiac index between 3.3 and 6.0 L/min/m^2 if a pulmonary artery catheter is placed[1,44,45] (see Fig. 8–3).

After the initiation of dopamine, shock may persist (fluid-refractory/dopamine-resistant shock). It is necessary to differentiate between cold and warm shock at this point (see Table 8–6). For cold shock, epinephrine is added as a second agent. Norepinephrine is recommended for warm shock. Glucose and ionized calcium are measured and replaced as needed to maintain normal values (goal: glucose level of 80 to 100 g/dl and ionized calcium level of 1.14 to 1.29).[41] Stress-dose hydrocortisone (1 to 2 mg/kg) is administered to children who are known to have adrenal disorders or who are on chronic steroid medication (see Fig. 8–3).

In addition to supportive treatment, the suspected infection is empirically treated with broad-spectrum antimicrobials. If time permits, blood, urine, and tissue samples from potential sites of infection should be obtained prior to antibiotic administration. However, in an unstable child, initiation of antimicrobials takes precedence over culturing all sites (see Chapter 13, Sepsis). If meningitis is a possibility, higher doses of antibiotics may be required (see Chapter 43, Central Nervous System Infections). Atypical pathogens (e.g., *Pseudomonas*, gram-negatives, fungi) should be considered in immunocompromised patients, and skin flora (e.g., *Staphylococcus aureus*) should be considered if a chronic indwelling venous catheter is present.[49]

Beyond the Golden Hour

After the "golden hour" of septic shock management, goal-directed therapy is continued, aiming for an SVC or mixed venous saturation greater than 70%, and maintenance of normal perfusion using clinical examination, MAP, and perfusion pressures.

If shock persists despite fluids and catecholamine therapy, hydrocortisone should be considered. For children with catecholamine-resistant shock, baseline cortisol levels are obtained. If adrenal insufficiency is suspected (adrenal disorder, chronic steroid medication therapy, CNS disorders, or purpura that suggests meningococcemia and possible Waterhouse-Friderichsen syndrome), stress-dose hydrocortisone (at least 1 to 2 mg/kg) should be administered. Debate exists as to the proper dose of steroids in suspected adrenal insufficiency-associated shock, and recommendations vary from 1 to 2 mg/kg up to 50 mg/kg.[1,44]

After dopamine and catecholamines, several alternative vasoactive medications can be considered. For catecholamine-resistant shock with a non-hyperdynamic state (low cardiac output and high SVR), vasodilators (e.g., nitroprusside) can decrease afterload and optimize cardiac output. If blood pressure is normal and SVR is elevated, a PDE inhibitor (e.g., milrinone) may be of benefit.[1] Phosphodiesterase inhibitors in combination with catecholamines increase cardiac index and oxygen delivery[50]; however, clinicians must be aware of their prolonged half-life. Catecholamine-resistant shock with a hyperdynamic state (high cardiac output and low SVR) is more common in adults than children.[51] In adults, vasopressin improves hemodynamics,[42] but studies in children are limited to case reports and its routine use in the emergency department cannot be currently recommended.[52-54]

In refractory septic shock (see Table 8–6), extracorporeal membrane oxygenation (ECMO) should be considered.[1,44,45] ECMO has been used in neonates with persistent pulmonary hypertension and sepsis, and may be effective in cardiogenic shock. Further study is needed before its role in refractory septic shock is clear.[55,56]

Other treatments under investigation for pediatric shock include activated protein C, naloxone, plasmapheresis, and immunoglobulin therapy. In adults, activated protein C is recommended in patients at high risk for death from sepsis,[57] but in children, it is not yet well studied. Case reports and a limited Phase II trial have shown improved coagulopathy parameters and safety, but no studies have demonstrated improved outcome with this agent.[58,59]

Other treatments currently under investigation in children include plasmapheresis, IV immunoglobulins, naloxone, and recombinant bactericidal/permeability-increasing protein.[60-63]

Trauma

Patients with hemorrhagic shock require aggressive fluid resuscitation to treat hypovolemia and require blood products for hypotension that does not rapidly respond to fluids. Supplemental oxygen is an important adjunct in the setting of anemia. Dissolved oxygen will be a significant proportion of oxygen content in the anemic patient with a decreased hemoglobin. Traumatic injuries may require emergent surgery (e.g., thoracoabdominal vascular or viscus injury). These patients are identified by imaging that reveals a specific injury and hypotension that is unresponsive to blood and fluid administration, or the requirement for transfusion of more than 40 ml/kg of blood over 24 hours. Readily reversible causes of shock (e.g., cardiac tamponade, tension pneumothorax) require immediate recognition and reversal. Bedside ultrasonography may provide a rapid diagnosis.

Hypotension on ED arrival due to traumatic blood loss carries a mortality rate that may exceed 50%.[64] In hemorrhagic shock, the first-line therapy is IV crystalloid fluids. The clinician should administer 20 ml/kg of crystalloid fluid over 5 to 10 minutes using multiple large-bore IV sites, and consider administration of blood if vital signs do not improve rapidly. Colloids (e.g., albumin, blood, modified fluid gelatin, dextran, hydroxyethyl starch) are better retained in the intravascular space than crystalloids. Other than blood, colloids do not provide a mortality benefit compared to crystalloids in hemorrhagic shock.[65-68]

Although the generous administration of crystalloids and blood products seems logical, there is evidence to suggest that aggressive fluid management in uncontrolled hemorrhage may worsen a patient's condition by increasing blood pressure and disrupting a clot that has formed or by creating a dilutional coagulopathy that can worsen hemorrhage.[69] Several animal studies indicate that bleeding is increased with aggressive fluid resuscitation.[70] For this reason, patients with trauma-related hypotension require rapid evaluation to identify sites of bleeding and early surgical therapy to control those sites.

Although hemorrhage is the most common cause of shock in the trauma patient, hypotension in the setting of neck or back trauma, abnormal neurologic examination, or relative bradycardia may indicate distributive spinal shock. Diving, cervical flexion-extension, and back injuries should heighten the suspicion for spinal cord injury. In spinal shock, cord injury leads to abnormal neural regulation of the peripheral vasculature. This manifests as hypotension, peripheral vasodilation with warm skin, adequate peripheral pulses, and

inappropriate bradycardia or lack of expected tachycardia. Once hemorrhage has been excluded, agents with α_1-agonist properties (e.g., phenylephrine) will counteract the underlying peripheral vasodilation. Norepinephrine and high-dose dopamine have β_1-agonist action in addition to α_1 action and can be used if cardiac inotropy is also desired.

Cardiac Disorders

Caution is necessary when administering IV fluids to patients in shock with associated cardiac dysfunction. Depressed cardiac function may be the primary cause of shock or may coexist in patients with noncardiac shock. Patients with cardiac dysfunction require small fluid boluses if hypovolemia is a contributing factor, but aggressive fluid therapy is not used alone if cardiac dysfunction is suspected.

Myocarditis (usually from viral illness) is one of the most common causes of cardiogenic shock. Young infants and neonates may present with COLHS (e.g., hypoplastic left heart, coarctation of the aorta, an interrupted arch). In these patients, administration of prostaglandin E$_1$ to maintain a patent ductus arteriosus may be life saving (see Chapter 30, Congenital Heart Disease). Other important congenital heart diseases, such as left-to-right shunts (e.g., ventricular septal defect) and cyanotic heart defects (e.g., total anomalous pulmonary venous return), also may progress to congestive heart failure. Supraventricular and ventricular tachycardias and bradyarrythmias, especially in infants, can cause cardiogenic shock due to the overreliance on heart rate as a determinant of cardiac output at this age. Pharmacologic or electrical conversion may be required for tachyarrhythmias, while chronotropic agents or a pacemaker may be required to reverse hemodynamically significant bradyarrhythmias (see Chapter 63, Dysrhythmias). Ischemic heart disease from congenital or acquired abnormalities can cause cardiogenic shock. High-output cardiac failure can result from severe anemia or shunting of blood (e.g., arteriovenous malformation).

If cardiogenic shock is suspected or known, a 5- to 10-ml/kg saline bolus should be administered if hypovolemia coexists. Inotropic therapy must be initiated early in cardiogenic shock. Dobutamine is an ideal agent for its inotropic effect on β_1 receptors in the heart and afterload reduction via β_2 peripheral vasodilation. Dopamine is also effective, although at high doses vasoconstriction predominates. In the setting of cardiogenic shock, SVR is high to maintain adequate perfusion pressure. For this reason, decreasing afterload may improve hemodynamics, making dobutamine more ideal than dopamine. Phosphodiesterase inhibitors (e.g., milrinone) can also be useful in the treatment of cardiogenic shock if SVR is high.

A small case series including infants and children demonstrated a decreased mortality with use of ECMO rescue in refractory cardiogenic shock.[71] Further research is needed to study its benefit.

Anaphylaxis

Treatment for anaphylaxis includes supporting ventilation and oxygenation through treatment of bronchospasm with β_2-agonist respiratory therapy, IV fluids, and epinephrine. Cardiovascular collapse is treated with IV fluid boluses of 20 ml/kg and simultaneous administration of epinephrine. Depending upon the degree of hypotension, 0.1 mg/kg intramuscularly or 10 mcg/kg IV should be administered over 3 to 10 minutes, following by a continuous drip of 0.1 to 1 mcg/kg/min if needed. Adjunctive therapies include H_1-receptor histamine antagonists (e.g., diphenhydramine) and corticosteroids. H_2-receptor histamine antagonists (e.g., ranitidine) are often recommended for the treatment of allergic disorders. However, these agents have only been proven to ameliorate dermatologic symptoms and may worsen bronchospasm (see Chapter 14, Anaphylaxis/Allergic Reactions).

Shock in Neonates

While typical treatment for hypovolemic shock consists of aggressive fluid management, this approach is associated with higher pulmonary, cardiac, gastrointestinal, and CNS morbidity in premature infants.[72,73] High pulmonary vascular resistance and closure of shunts sets up a unique physiology during the transition from fetal to neonatal circulation. In the setting of shock, acidosis, and hypoxemia, increased pulmonary artery pressure may result in persistent pulmonary hypertension of the neonate (PPHN) and cardiac failure. Myocardial dysfunction frequently accompanies neonatal hypotension.[74] For this reason, neonates who receive IV fluid boluses require frequent cardiopulmonary assessment, while the use of 10-ml/kg boluses instead of 20 ml/kg is recommended in preterm neonates. Neonates with PPHN may also benefit from pulmonary vasodilation through inhaled nitric oxide therapy and metabolic alkalinization.

Vasopressors do not affect the neonatal cardiac system in a manner similar to older children and adults. Only one third of a neonate's heart is composed of contractile tissue, compared to two thirds of an adult heart. For this reason, neonates cannot alter their cardiac output by increasing contractility as well as adults and older children. Myocardial norepinephrine stores are also immature and become rapidly depleted, making dopamine less effective. Changes in adrenergic receptor expression during critical illness and production of local vasodilators during shock can make neonates appear unresponsive to dopamine. Dobutamine is less effective than dopamine in raising blood pressure[75] due to dopamine's α-adrenergic vasopressor activity.

Neonates with inborn metabolic errors can present with unexplained hypoglycemia, elevated ammonia levels, or an unexplained metabolic acidosis (see Chapter 29, Inborn Errors of Metabolism). These abnormalities may be associated with seizures, hypotension, hypotonia, or feeding difficulties. Therapy is directed at reversing the metabolic problem (e.g., administering glucose and bicarbonate, managing hyperkalemia). Ammonia is reduced by hemodialysis, administration of ammonia-scavenging agents, and repletion of arginine.

Infants with congenital adrenal hyperplasia (CAH) classically present with hypotension, acidosis, hyponatremia, and hyperkalemia in the second week of life (see Chapter 108, Addisonian Crisis). However, newborn screening has reduced morbidity from CAH. Once CAH is suspected, management consists of restoring fluid homeostasis with IV fluids, correcting hypoglycemia, and administering hydrocortisone while excluding other potential causes for symptoms (e.g., sepsis).

Summary

Shock is a dynamic physiologic state that is the final end point for various disease processes. Hypovolemic, cardio-genic, distributive, and obstructive shock are the major physiologic mechanisms by which we define shock. However, a combination of these mechanisms may play a role in individual patients with shock. If unrecognized or undertreated, shock will progress to death.

After securing an airway and maintaining adequate ventilation, the mainstay of shock treatment (excluding cardiogenic shock) is aggressive fluid resuscitation. Crystalloids should be administered in 20-ml/kg boluses up to 60 ml/kg as quickly as possible. The patient should be assessed for cardiac compromise in the form of murmurs or gallops, hepatomegaly, pulmonary rales, or jugular venous distention at the onset of treatment as well as during aggressive fluid therapy. Shock from cardiac dysfunction is treated with judicious use of fluids and the initiation of appropriate vasoactive medications.

In septic shock, after 60 ml/kg of fluid have been given, inotropes, vasopressors, or vasodilators are initiated using goal-directed parameters. Dopamine is a first-line agent that has cardiac stimulatory as well as peripheral vasoconstrictive properties. For fluid-refractory and dopamine-resistant patients, a second vasoactive agent is added. Epinephrine and norepinephrine are indicated for cold and warm shock, respectively. For catecholamine-resistant shock, relative adrenal suppression should be considered.

Mortality from shock has improved with the advent of goal-directed therapies and evidence-based guidelines. Prompt recognition with rapid and aggressive treatment will further improve outcome in children who present to the ED in shock.

REFERENCES

1. Carcillo JA, Fields AI, American College of Critical Care Medicine Task Force Committee Members: Clinical practice parameters for hemodynamic support of pediatric and neonatal patients in septic shock. Crit Care Med 30:1367–1378, 2002.
2. Stoll BJ, Holman RC, Shuchat A: Decline in sepsis associated neonatal and infant deaths: 1979 through 1994. Pediatrics 102:e18, 1998.
3. Watson RS, Carcillo JA, Linde-Zwirble WT, et al: The epidemiology of severe sepsis in children in the United States. Am J Respir Crit Care Med 167:695–701, 2003.
4. Partrick DA, Bensard DD, Janik JS, Karrer FM: Is hypotension a reliable indicator of blood loss from traumatic injury in children? Am J Surg 184:555–560, 2002.
5. Randolph LC, Takacs M, Davis KA: Resuscitation in the pediatric trauma population: admission base deficit remains an important prognostic indicator. J Trauma 53:838–842, 2002.
6. Miyagatani Y, Yukioka T, Ohta S, et al: Vascular tone in patients with hemorrhagic shock. Trauma 47:282–287, 1999.
7. Gorelick MH, Shaw KN, Baker MD: Effect of ambient temperature on capillary refill in healthy children. Pediatrics 92:699–702, 1993.
8. Otieno H, Were E, Ahmed I, et al: Are bedside features of shock reproducible between different observers? Arch Dis Child 89:977–979, 2004.
9. Tibby SM, Tatherill M, Murdoch IA: Capillary refill and core peripheral temperature gap as indicators of haemodynamic status in paediatric intensive care patients. Arch Dis Child 80:163–166, 1999.
10. Han YY, Carcillo JA, Dragotta MA, et al: Early reversal of pediatric-neonatal septic shock by community physicians is associated with improved outcome. Pediatrics 112:793–799, 2003.
11. Gorelick MH, Shaw KN, Murphy KO: Clinical reliability of clinical signs in the diagnosis of dehydration in children. Pediatrics 99:e6, 1997.
12. Glaser N, Barnet P, McCaslin I, et al: Risk factors for cerebral edema in children with diabetic ketoacidosis. N Engl J Med 344:264–269, 2001.
13. Kutko MC, Calarco MP, Flaherty MB, et al: Mortality rates in pediatric septic shock with and without multiple organ system failure. Pediatr Crit Care Med 4:333–337, 2003.

14. Brilli RJ, Goldstein B: Pediatric sepsis definitions: past, present, and future. Pediatr Crit Care Med 6:S6, 2005.
15. Goldstein B, Grioir B, Randolph A, et al: International pediatric sepsis consensus conference: definitions for sepsis and organ dysfunction in pediatrics. Pediatr Crit Care Med 6:2–8, 2005.
16. Gurkan F, Alkaya A, Ece A, et al: Cardiac troponin-I as a marker of myocardial dysfunction in children with septic shock. Swiss Med Weekly 134:593–596, 2004.
17. ver Elst KM, Spapen HD, Nguyen DN, et al: Cardiac troponins I and T are biological markers of left ventricular dysfunction in septic shock. Clin Chem 46:650–657, 2000.
18. Roch A, Allardet-Servent J, Michelet P, et al: NH₂ terminal pro-brain natriuretic peptide plasma level as an early marker for prognosis and cardiac dysfunction in septic shock patients. Crit Care Med 33:1001–1007, 2005.
19. Calandra T, Baumgartner JD, Grau GE, et al: Prognostic values of tumor necrosis factor/cachectin, interleukin-1, interferon-alpha, and interferon-gamma in the serum of patients with septic shock. J Infect Dis 161:982–987, 1990.
20. Cohen J, Abraham E: Microbiologic findings and correlations with serum tumor necrosis factor-alpha in patients with severe sepsis and septic shock. J Infect Dis 180:116–121, 1999.
21. Hazelzet JA, deGroot R, vanMierlo G, et al: Complement activation in relation to capillary leakage in children with septic shock and purpura. Infect Immun 66:5350–5356, 1998.
22. Krafte-Jacobs B, Bock GH: Circulating erythropoietin and interleukin-6 concentrations increase in critically ill children with sepsis and septic shock. Crit Care Med 24:1455–1459, 1996.
23. Sierra R, Rello J, Bailen MA, et al: C-reactive protein used as an early indicator of infection in patients with systemic inflammatory response syndrome. Intensive Care Med 30:2038–2045, 2004.
24. Casado-Flores J, Blanco-Quiros A, Asension J, et al: Serum procalcitonin in children with suspected sepsis: a comparison with C-reactive protein and neutrophil count. Pediatr Crit Care Med 4:190–195, 2003.
25. Han YY, Doughty LA, Kofos D, et al: Procalcitonin is persistently increased among children with poor outcome from bacterial sepsis. Pediatr Crit Care Med 4:21–25, 2003.
26. Hatherill M, Tibby SM, Turner C, et al: Procalcitonin and cytokine levels: relationship to organ failure and mortality in pediatric septic shock. Crit Care Med 28:2591–2594, 2000.
27. Dugas MA, Roulx F, deJager A, et al: Marker of tissue hypoperfusion in pediatric septic shock. Intesive Care Med 26:75–83, 1999.
28. Calvo C, Ruza F, Lopez-Herce J, et al: Usefulness of gastric intramucosal pH for monitoring hemodynamic complications in critically ill children. Intensive Care Med 23:1268–1274, 1997.
28. Hatherill M, Waggie Z, Purves L, et al: Mortality and the nature of metabolic acidosis in children with shock. Intensive Care Med 29:286–291, 2003.
29. Hatherill M, Tibby SM, Evans R, Murdoch IA: Gastric tonometry in septic shock. Arch Dis Child 78:155–158, 1998.
30. Weil MH, Nakagawa Y, Tang W, et al: Sublingual capnometry: a new noninvasive measurement for diagnosis and quantitation of severity of circulatory shock. Crit Care Med 27:1225–1229, 1999.
31. Ardagh MW, Hodgson T, Shaw L, Turner D: Pulse rate over pressure evaluation (ROPE) is useful in the assessment of compensated haemorrhagic shock. Emerg Med 13:43–46, 2001.
32. Peterson DL, Schinco MA, Kerwin AJ, et al: Evaluation of initial base deficit as a prognosticator of outcome in the pediatric trauma population. Am Surg 70:326–328, 2004.
33. Blow O, Magliore L, Claridge JA, et al: The golden hour and the silver day: detection and correction of occult hypoperfusion within 24 hours improves outcome from major trauma. J Trauma 47:964–969, 1999.
34. Kaplan LJ, Kellum JA: Initial pH, base deficit, lacate, anion gap, strong ion difference and strong ion gap predict outcome from major vascular injury. Crit Care Med 32:1120–1124, 2004.
35. Evans N, Seri I: Cardiovascular compromise in the newborn infant. *In* Taeusch HW, Brodsky D (eds): Avery's Disease of the Newborn, 8th ed. Philadelphia: Elsevier, 2005, pp 398–409.
36. Berger C, Uehlinger J, Ghelfi D, et al: Comparison of C-reactive protein and white blood cell count with differential in neonates at risk for septicaemia. Eur J Pediatr 154:138–144, 1995.
37. Griffin MP, Lake DE, Moorman JR: Heart rate characteristics and laboratory tests in neonatal sepsis. Pediatrics 115:937–941, 2005.
38. Manucha V, Rusia U, Sikka M, et al: Utility of haematological parameters and C-reactive protein in the detection of neonatal sepsis. J Paediatr Child Health 38:459–464, 2002.
39. Malk A, Hui CPS, Pennie RA, Kirpalani H: Beyond the complete blood cell count and C-reactive protein. Arch Pediatr Adolesc Med 57:511–516, 2003.
*40. Pickert CB, Moss MM, Fiser DH: Differentiation of systemic infection and congenital obstructive left heart disease in the very young infant. Pediatr Emerg Care 14:263–267, 1998.
41. Arnal LE, Stein F: Pediatric septic shock: why has mortality decreased? The utility of goal directed therapy. Semin Pediatr Infect Dis 14:165–173, 2003.
42. Tabbutt S: Heart failure in pediatric septic shock: utilizing inotropic support. Crit Care Med 29:S231–S236, 2001.
43. Holm C, Mayr M, Tegeler J, et al: A clinical randomized study on the effects of invasive monitoring on burn shock resuscitation. Burns 30:798–807, 2004.
*44. Parker MM, Hazelzet JA, Carcillo JA: Pediatric considerations. Crit Care Med 32:S591–S594, 2004.
45. Dellinger RP, Carlet JM, Masur H, et al: Surviving sepsis campaign guidelines for management of severe sepsis and septic shock. Crit Care Med 32:858–873, 2004.
46. Carcillo JA, Davis AL, Zaritsky A: Role of early fluid resuscitation in pediatric septic shock. JAMA 266:1242–1245, 1991.
47. Rhodes A, Bennett ED: Early goal-directed therapy: an evidence-based review. Crit Care Med 32:S448–S550, 2004.
*48. Rivers E, Nguyen B, Havstad S, et al: Early goal-directed therapy in the treatment of severe sepsis and septic shock. N Engl J Med 346:1368–1377, 2001.
49. Gea-Banacloche JC, Opal SM, Jorgensen J: Sepsis associated with immunosuppressive medications: an evidence-based review. Crit Care Med 32:S578–S590, 2004.
50. Barton P, Garcia J, Kouatli A, et al: Hemodynamic effects of IV milrinone lactate in pediatric patients with septic shock: a prospective, double-blinded, randomized, placebo-controlled, interventional study. Chest 109:1302–1312, 1996.
*51. Ceneviva G, Paschall JA, Maffei F, Carcillo JA: Hemodynamic support in fluid refractory pediatric septic shock. Pediatrics 102:e19, 1998.
52. Matok I, Leibovitch L, Vardi A, et al: Terlipressin as rescue therapy for intractable hypotension during neonatal septic shock. Pediatr Crit Care Med 5:116–118, 2004.
53. Peters MJ, Booth RA, Petros A: Terlipressin bolus induces systemic vasoconstriction in septic shock. Pediatr Crit Care Med 5:112–115, 2004.
54. Rodriguez-Nunez A, Fernandez-Sanmartin M, Martinon-Torres F, et al: Terlipressin for catecholamine-resistant septic shock in children. Intensive Care Med 30:477–480, 2004.
55. Dalton HJ, Siewers RD, Fuhrman BP, et al: Extracorporeal membrane oxygenation for cardiac rescue in children with severe myocardial dysfunction. Crit Care Med 21:1020–1028, 1997.
56. Meyer DM, Jessen ME: Results of extracorporeal membrane oxygenation in children with sepsis. Ann Thorac Surg 63:756–761, 1997.
57. de Kleijn ED, de Groot R, Hack E, et al: Activation of protein C following infusion of protein C concentrate in childen with severe meningococcal sepsis and purpura fulminans: a randomized, double-blinded, placebo-controlled, dose-finding study. Crit Care Med 31:1839–1847, 2003.
57. Fourrier F: Recombinant human activated protein C in the treatment of severe sepsis: an evidence based review. Crit Care Med 32:S534–S541, 2004.
59. Sajan I, Da-Silva SS, Dellinger RP: Drotrecogin alfa (activated) in an infant with gram-negative septic shock. J Intensive Care Med 19:56–57, 2004.
60. Busund R, Koukline V, Utrobin U, Nedashkovsky E: Plasmapheresis in severe sepsis and septic shock: a prospective, randomised, controlled trial. Intensive Care Med 28:1434–1439, 2002.
61. Alejandria MM, Lansang MA, Dans LF, Mantaring JBV: Intravenous immunoglobin for treating sepsis and septic shock. Cochrane Database Syst Rev (1):CD001090, 2002.
62. Boeuf B, Poirier V, Gauvin F, et al: Naloxone for shock. Cochrane Database Syst Rev (4):CD004443, 2003.

---

*Selected reading.

63. Levin M, Quint PA, Goldstein B, et al: Recombinant bactericidal/permeability-increasing protein (RBPI$_{21}$) as adjunctive treatment for children with severe meningococcal sepsis: a randomised trial. Lancet 356:961–967, 2000.

64. Heckbert SR, Vedder NB, Hoffman W, et al: Outcome after hemorrhagic shock in trauma patients. J Trauma 45:545–549, 1998.

65. Alderson P, Bunn F, Lefebvre C, et al: Human albumin solution for resuscitation and volume expansion in critically ill patients. Cochrane Database Syst Rev (4):CD001208, 2004.

66. Kwan I, Bunn F, Roberts I, et al: Timing and volume of fluid administration for patients with bleeding. Cochrane Database Syst Rev (3):CD002245, 2003.

67. Roberts I, Alderson P, Bunn F, et al: Colloids versus crystalloids for fluid resuscitation in critically ill patients. Cochrane Database Syst Rev (4):CD000567, 2004.

68. Wu JJ, Huang MS, Tang GJ, et al: Hemodynamic response of modified fluid gelatin compared with lactated Ringer's solution for volume expansion in emergency resuscitation of hypovolemic shock patients: preliminary report of a prospective, randomized trial. World J Surg 25:598–602, 2001.

69. Bickell WH, Wall MJ, Pepe PE, et al: Immediate versus delayed fluid resuscitation for hypotensive patients with penetrating torso injuries. N Engl J Med 331:1105–1109, 1994.

70. Burris D, Rhee P, Kaurmann C, et al: Controlled resuscitation for uncontrolled hemorrhagic shock. J Trauma 46:216–223, 1999.

71. Chen S, Wang MJ, Chou NK, et al: Rescue for acute myocarditis with shock by extracorporeal membrane oxgenation. Ann Thorac Surg 68:2220–2224, 1999.

72. Kavvadia V, Greenough A, Dimitrioe G, et al: Randomized trial of fluid restriction in ventilated very low birth weight infants. Arch Dis Child Fetal Neonatal Ed 83:F91–F96, 2000.

73. Lundstrom K, Pryds O, Greisen G: The hemodynamic effects of dopamine and volume expansion in sick preterm infants. Early Hum Dev 57:157–163, 2000.

74. Gill AB, Weindling AM: Echocardiographic assessment of cardiac function in shocked very low birthweight infants. Arch Dis Child 68:17–21, 1993.

75. Subhedar NV, Shaw: Dopamine versus dobutamine for hypotensive preterm infants. Cochrane Database Syst Rev (3):CD001242, 2005.

Chapter 9

Cerebral Resuscitation

Genie E. Roosevelt, MD, MPH and Norman A. Paradis, MD

Key Points

Adequate basic and advanced life support are important initial determinants of outcome during cerebral resuscitation.

Clinicians must promptly identify processes that place the cerebrum at risk (e.g., asphyxia, hypotension) in order to intervene early, prevent further deterioration, and limit the need for cerebral resuscitation.

Hyperventilation is not standard therapy for increased intracranial pressure and in some instances may be detrimental.

Background and Introduction

Cerebral resuscitation is required because the primary pathophysiologic process has placed neurologic tissue at risk secondary to ischemia. In children, this generally occurs because processes such as asphyxia or trauma, with secondary edema, threaten to interfere with delivery of oxygen to neurologic tissues that are intolerant of even brief periods of severe partial anoxia. Because cerebral oxygen delivery is wholly dependent on adequate cardiac output, advanced life support comes first. Failure to promptly restore systemic hemodynamics will render all secondary efforts at cerebral resuscitation ineffective. The apparent capacity of pediatric patients to recover from neurologic injury that initially appears devastating makes cerebral resuscitation particularly important in this population.

In infants and children, the two principal mechanisms resulting in cerebral edema requiring resuscitation are traumatic brain injury (TBI) and asphyxial cardiac arrest. Other less common mechanisms include ischemia, infection, and swelling due to mass effect. Prompt identification of pathophysiologic processes that place the cerebrum at risk and early intervention to counteract their effects are crucial to limit the need for cerebral resuscitation. Many mechanisms responsible for brain injury, including the molecular, cellular, and biochemical mechanisms that underlie neurologic injury, have been elucidated over the last 30 years. However, it has been very difficult to demonstrate the clinical efficacy of potential therapies. For this reason, pediatric cerebral resuscitation remains primarily empirical, supplemented with extrapolations from adult data. Improved understanding of the pathophysiology of cerebral ischemia, and in particular the importance of reperfusion injury, holds the promise of significantly more effective therapies in the future.

Most of the current data available focus on cerebral resuscitation after TBI, but some of these same therapies may also be applicable to cerebral resuscitation after cardiac arrest. Recent indications that hypothermia may be effective in the treatment of cerebral reperfusion injury after cardiac arrest hold particular promise, and pediatric trials are underway at the time of this writing. In 2003, guidelines for the management of pediatric severe TBI were published in both surgical and critical care journals.[1] These guidelines were an attempt to present current clinical data, combined with expert consensus, in a manner similar to adult guidelines originally developed originally in 1996 and revised in 2000.[2,3]

The achievement of optimal clinical outcomes will require coordination between prehospital providers, emergency department staff, intensivists, and rehabilitation health care providers. Protocols necessary to achieve this coordination should generally be in place beforehand, so that timely application of multiple interventions can be achieved. Prevention of neuronal cell death often requires that therapies be given at the injury scene or shortly after the initial insult. Prevention of insults that place neuronal tissue at risk is always preferable to cerebral resuscitation, and, in reality, such prevention is optimal resuscitation. Prevention of initial hypoxia-mediated pathways and later reperfusion-mediated pathways of neurologic injury is the foundation of cerebral resuscitation.

Recognition and Approach

There are over 150,000 pediatric head injuries per year, resulting in approximately 7000 deaths and 29,000 children with new, permanent disabilities.[4-6] Trauma is the leading cause of mortality and morbidity in children and is responsible for the majority of childhood deaths.[7] Even with minor traumatic head injuries, there can be significant long-term sequelae.[8,9] The most common cause of cardiac arrest in children is respiratory distress leading to respiratory failure, which accounts for the majority of admissions to pediatric intensive care units.[10] Other causes of prearrest states in children include, in descending order, cardiac failure, neurologic conditions such as seizures, and acute failure of the liver, kidney, or adrenals.[11]

While the exact mechanisms of cerebral edema are not fully delineated, they include cellular swelling, injury to the blood-brain barrier (BBB) or vasogenic edema, osmolar swelling, and increased cerebral blood volume (CBV).[12] Cellular swelling, which is probably more important in asphyxial cardiac arrest than in TBI, is mediated by acidosis, potassium, and arachidonic acid.[13] The swelling is predominantly in the astrocyte foot processes as the uptake of the excitatory amino acid (EAA) glutamate is coupled with sodium and water intake. The significance of BBB injury or vasogenic edema is now believed to have been overstated in the past and is probably more important in asphyxial cardiac arrest than in TBI.[14] More recently, osmolar swelling in an area of contusion necrosis, defined as a cerebral contusion in which the cellular elements undergo shrinkage, disintegration, and homogenization, seems to be a much more important mechanism in TBI.[15] The role of increased CBV in cerebral edema in adults has been challenged.[16] However, this mechanism may be more important in pediatric TBI and requires further study.

Although TBI and asphyxial cardiac arrest are different insults, two early important mechanisms of injury for both insults appear to be excitotoxicity and hypoperfusion. Both of these mechanisms may result in early cellular damage, and appear to set in motion the triggers that lead to programmed cell death (PCD). Excitotoxicity is the process by which EAAs cause neuronal damage after hypoxia or injury. Glutamate, in particular, appears to be the predominant excitatory neurotransmitter of the brain and acts through several receptors. In both animal models and clinical studies, pathologic levels of glutamate known to cause cell death in vitro are seen in the cerebrospinal fluid (CSF) after both TBI and asphyxial cardiac arrest.[17-19] EAA receptor antagonists have improved outcomes in experimental models.[20] The rise in glutamate occurs early, suggesting a potential role for early intervention in either field resuscitation or the emergency department. Current clinical therapies with anti-excitotoxic properties include hypothermia, barbiturates, inhaled anesthetics, calcium channel blockers, and anticonvulsants. Hypothermia reduces levels of glutamate in the cerebrospinal fluid.[21] Induction of a barbiturate coma can reduce the amount of glutamate and lactate in the extracellular space of the brain via microdialysis.[22]

Although both TBI and asphyxial cardiac arrest result in elevated EAAs, the mechanisms may differ. After TBI, excitotoxic damage is mediated by the N-methyl-D-aspartate (NMDA) receptor, one of the major glutamate receptors.[19] One study of a competitive NMDA antagonist (selfotel) was terminated due to safety concerns as this agent had important phencyclidine-like properties and side effects that limit its use in conscious patients.[23] The dramatic excitotoxic response to TBI, particularly in children less than 4 years of age,[24] would suggest that therapy preventing the insult from elevated glutamate levels may be important even if there are some concerns over side effects. Elevated EAAs appear to be important enough in acute neurologic injury that additional research directed at blocking EAA effects without undue toxicity is of particular importance.

Cerebral ischemia and hypoxia play a central role in the secondary neurologic damage after cardiac arrest or TBI. Immediately after cardiac arrest or TBI, there is a period of hypoperfusion in both adults and children,[25,26] which occurs at the same time as an increased metabolic rate termed *hyperglycolysis*.[27] In experimental models, cerebral hypoperfusion is seen for hours to days after global ischemia, while systemic oxygen utilization returns to normal, resulting in cerebral ischemia during reperfusion.[28] This suggests that increasing cerebral blood flow (CBF) after cardiac arrest may be beneficial. Experimental models suggest that L-arginine, endothelin-1 (vasoconstrictor) antagonist, and transient systemic hypertension increase CBF and may improve outcome in both TBI and cardiac arrest.[29-31]

An exciting future direction in cerebral resuscitation is to target both cerebral hypoperfusion and EAAs simultaneously. Although the systemic effects of adenosine limit its use, an adenosine agonist has been shown to be neuroprotective in experimental animal models when given locally through a ventriculostomy catheter.[32] The inhaled anesthetic isoflurane, which increases CBF while serving as a potent anti-excitotoxic agent, is associated with reduced neuronal damage after both TBI and cardiac arrest compared to fentanyl.[33,34] Ethanol has been shown to reduce hypoperfusion, excitotoxicity, and hyperglycolysis after TBI and cardiac arrest in rats.[35] However, no practical, single pharmacologic agent is effective in targeting both excitotoxicity and hypoperfusion.

While some neuronal death may occur immediately after TBI and cardiac arrest, additional neuronal death may occur after the insult secondary to PCD, or apoptosis.[36] PCD is regulated by genes and proteins, in contrast to immediate and delayed necrotic cell death, which is not regulated by proteins and is characterized by cellular and nuclear swelling with dissolution of membranes. Upstream regulators of PCD include the Bcl-2 family of proteins, some of which promote cell survival and some of which promote cell death.[37] In animal models, Bcl-2 protein is seen in neurons that survive compared to neurons that do not.[38] In addition, elevated levels of Bcl-2 in the CSF have been associated with improved survival in children and infants after TBI.[39] Administration of Bcl-2 analogues is protective in animal models, suggesting a potential clinical application.[40] Other upstream regulators of PCD are the tumor necrosis factor (TNF) superfamily cell surface receptors.[41] Binding of TNF or Fas ligand to their respective cell surface receptors activates the PCD cascade. Soluble Fas receptors are increased in the CSF after pediatric TBI,[41] suggesting a potential means to intervene in PCD by using soluble ligands or decoy Fas or TNF receptors. Alternative, potentially effective therapies might prevent PCD by stabilizing the mitochondrial membrane with cyclosporine[42] or antioxidants,[43] or might target the final pathways of the PCD cascade, particularly the caspase pathway. Several currently investigated clinical strategies, such as hypothermia and anti-excitotoxic therapies, may also work by reducing PCD.[44,45] Since PCD is also an essential part of human development and probably maintenance of biologic function, disrupting this cascade may have disruptive effects, and methods will need to be developed to target the effect on PCD specifically to the central nervous system during the vulnerable postinsult period.

Clinical Evaluation

Since cerebral edema is associated with a significant traumatic, asphyxial, or metabolic event or derangement, such as diabetic ketoacidosis, recognition relies on the practitioner anticipating the association of the primary condition with cerebral edema. This is vitally important since early identification of the inciting event makes prevention or early resuscitation possible. Signs and symptoms associated with cerebral edema include altered mental status, pupillary changes, and posturing. Any change in a child's level of alertness or a possible focal neurologic deficit, in the context of traumatic, hypoxic, or metabolic insult, should lead to immediate counter-insult interventions. An objective assessment of the child's level of consciousness may be accomplished with the AVPU system[46] (*A*lert, responds to *V*oice, responds to *P*ain, *U*nresponsive) or the Pediatric Glasgow Coma Scale.[47] Altered mental status is the first sign, with pupillary changes and posturing presenting as late signs of cerebral edema and impending herniation.

Early intracranial pressure (ICP) monitoring allows an objective measure of cerebral edema and an assessment of the effect of therapies. ICP monitoring in TBI is accepted as effective, although data are insufficient to support a treatment standard.[1] Generally, ICP monitoring is not recommended in cardiac arrest as animal models of cardiac arrest indicate that the insult necessary to produce vegetative outcome is below the threshold that results in intracranial hypertension, implying that ICP monitoring–directed therapy is unlikely to improve outcomes.[48,49] Recent guidelines suggest performing ICP monitoring in infants and children with severe TBI, defined as a Glasgow Coma Scale (GCS) score of 8. The presence of an open fontanelle and/or sutures does not preclude monitoring. ICP monitoring is not indicated in mild or moderate injury. Adult data support ICP monitoring in patients with severe TBI (GCS = 8 after cardiopulmonary resuscitation), and there is no evidence to suggest that this is not true in pediatrics. Monitoring is suggested in patients with severe TBI and an abnormal admission computed tomography (CT) scan demonstrating hematomas, contusions, cerebral edema, and/or compressed basal cisterns. In addition, monitoring is suggested even with a normal admission cranial CT scan if two or more of the following are present: motor posturing, systemic hypotension, or age greater than 40 years.[3]

Management

Cerebral resuscitation naturally falls into two broad areas: (1) therapies widely believed to be effective and that can be instituted in community emergency departments (Table 9–1, Fig. 9–1), and (2) advanced techniques that are applied only to subsets of patients and usually utilized only in tertiary centers by specialists.

Cerebral Resuscitation: Basic Techniques

As with any resuscitation, controlling and maintaining the airway, breathing, and circulation are the first priorities. In children with TBI, extreme care must be taken with respect to possible injury to the spine. There must be immediate attention to preventing additional primary insult, be it traumatic, hypoxic, or metabolic, contemporaneous with initiation of cerebral resuscitation. Early therapies such as the use of sedation and osmolar agents may be initiated prior to obtaining a CT scan in cases in which cerebral edema seems likely.

Sedation and Neuromuscular Blockade

Although data are insufficient to support a treatment standard for the use of sedation and neuromuscular blockade[1] once the airway has been established, these medications may be useful in maintaining the airway, during procedures, and in the reduction of pain and stress, and have some physiologic basis for their use. Painful or stressful stimuli are associated with increases in cerebral metabolic rate,[50] and it is reasonable to conjecture that ICP will increase during Valsalva-like events that occur during poorly controlled resuscitation. Although historical concerns related to the use of depolarizing agents and their effect on ICP may not be relevant during the initial resuscitation,[51] these agents are not generally used after the initial resuscitation. Suggested intravenous agents for neuromuscular blockade include rocuronium, vecuronium, and pancuronium.

There are no specific recommendations on the choice and dosing of sedation based on evidence; however, continuous propofol infusion should be avoided as it has been associated with increased mortality and morbidity (acidosis, rhabdomyolysis) when used for a prolonged period.[52,53] Suggested intravenous agents for sedation include morphine sulfate 0.1 to 0.2 mg/kg per dose every 2 to 4 hours, with continuous infusion to run at 0.1 mg/kg/hr; lorazepam 0.05 to 0.1 mg/kg per dose, with continuous infusion to run at 0.1 mg/kg/hr, which may be titrated to effect; and midazolam 0.05 to 0.1 mg/kg per dose, with continuous infusion to run at 2 mcg/kg/min, which may be titrated to desired effect (usually within the range 0.4 to 6 mcg/kg/min).[54] Fentanyl 1 to 2 mcg/kg per dose every 1 to 2 hours, with continuous infusion to run at 1 to 3 mcg/kg per dose, is another suggested agent; however, there is limited evidence that bolus dosing may transiently increase intracranial pressure.[55-57]

Hyperosmolar Therapy

Hyperosmolar therapies such as mannitol and hypertonic saline may be important adjuncts in cerebral resuscitation, especially in settings in which increased ICP is anticipated to be important. Data are insufficient to support a treatment standard directed at prevention of edema.[1] The absence of such data should not, however, prevent clinicians from initiating therapies intended to prevent potentially devastating increases in ICP. Consensus suggests that hyperosmolar therapy should be initiated if adequate sedation, analgesia, elevation of the head of the bed, and CSF drainage, if available, are ineffective in controlling ICP.[1]

Mannitol has long been accepted as clinically efficacious without significant scientific data to support its widespread use. Mannitol is believed to reduce ICP by two mechanisms: reduction of blood viscosity[58,59] and an osmotic effect.[60] The only scientific evidence for mannitol in pediatrics relies on two retrospective studies that involved adult patients as well.[61,62] Effective doses of mannitol range from 0.25 g/kg to 1 g/kg, with maintenance dosing 0.25 to 0.5 g/kg every 4 to 6 hours.[52] Serum osmolarity should be maintained below 320 mOsm/L.

In contrast, while there is limited clinical experience with hypertonic saline, recent studies suggest that it is effective

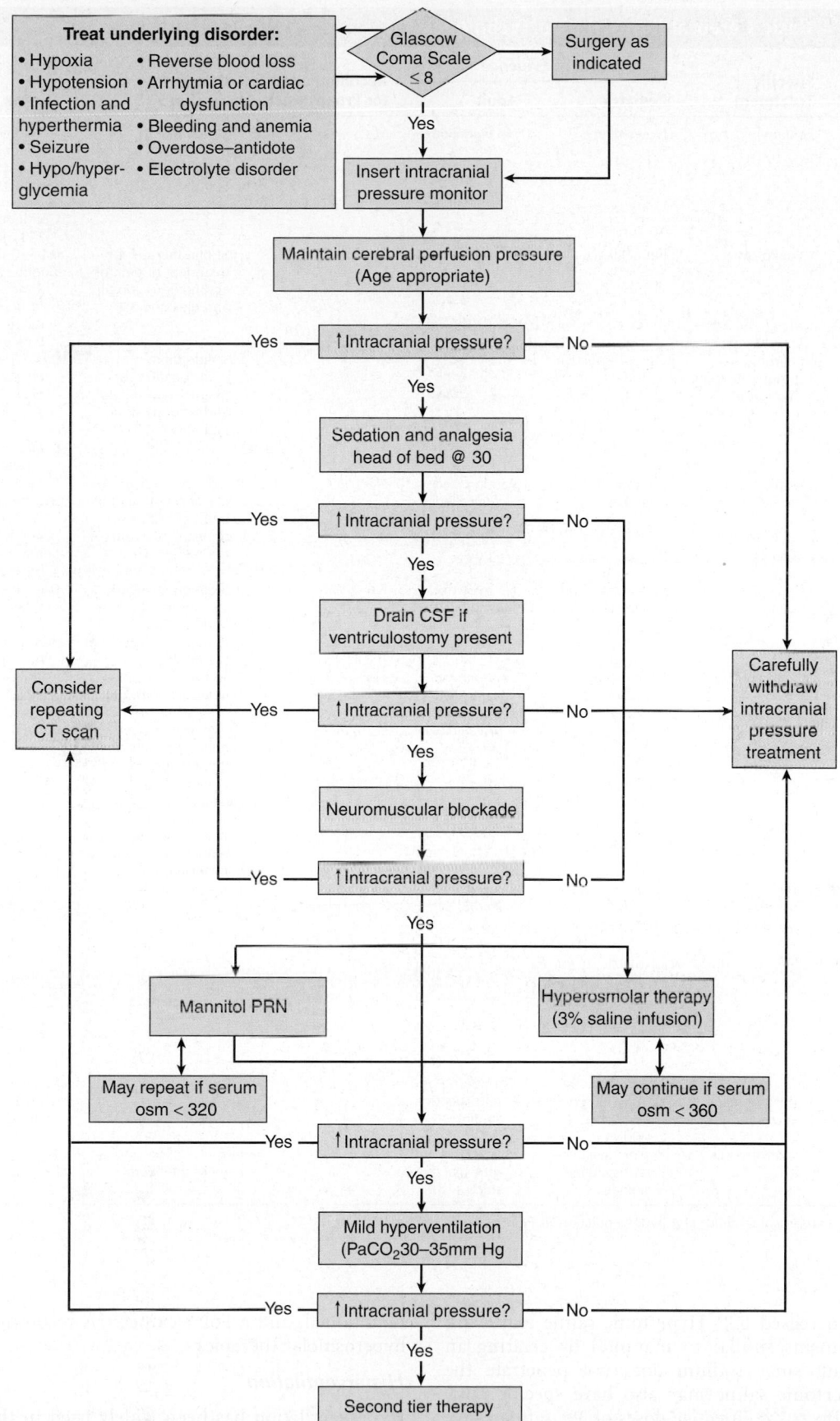

FIGURE 9–1. Algorithm for first-tier therapy. Abbreviations: CPP, cerebral perfusion pressure; CSF, cerebrospinal fluid; CT, computed tomography; GCS, Glasgow Coma Scale score; HOB, head of bed; ICP, intracranial pressure; PRN, as needed. (Adapted from Adelson PD, Bratton SL, Carney NA, et al: Guidelines for the acute medical management of severe traumatic brain injury in infants, children, and adolescents. Pediatr Crit Care Med 4[Suppl]:S1–S75, 2003.)

| Table 9–1 | Basic Cerebral Resuscitation Techniques |

Treatment Category	Specific Treatment	Level of Evidence		Recommended for Prophylaxis?	Treatment Indications	Dosing Regimens
		Pediatric	Adult			
Analgesia & Sedation	Fentanyl	No evidence	No evidence	Yes	First-line therapy for treatment of painful and noxious stimuli and elevated ICP	1–2 mcg/kg/dose (inconclusive data indicate bolus dosing may ↑ intracranial pressure). Continous infusion: 1–3 mcg/kg/hr.
	Midazolam	No evidence	No evidence	Yes	First-line therapy for treatment of painful and noxious stimuli and elevated ICP	0.05–0.1 mg/kg/dose. Continuous infusion: 2 mcg/kg/min, titrate to desired effect with range of 0.4–6 mcg/kg/min.
Paralysis (decreased muscular activity)	Rocuronium (neuromuscular blockade)	One prospective study	No evidence	Yes	First-line therapy with sedation for treatment of painful and noxious stimuli and elevated ICP	0.6–1.2 mg/kg/dose. repeat doses: 0.2 mg/kg every 20–30 min as needed. or Continuous infusion: 10–12 mcg/kg/min.
Hyperosmolar Therapy	Mannitol	Retrospective studies	Randomized, controlled trials and retrospective studies	No	If sedation, analgesia, elevation of head of bed, and CSF drainage (if available) are ineffective	0.25–1.0 g/kg bolus. Maintenance dosing: 0.25–0.5 g/kg every 4–6 hr. Serum osmolarity should be <320 mOsm/L.
	Hypertonic saline	Prospective and retrospective studies	No evidence	No	If sedation, analgesia, elevation of head of bed, and CSF drainage (if available) are ineffective	0.1–1.0 ml/kg/hr of 3% saline using minimal dose needed. Serum osmolarity should be <360 mOsm/L.
Cerebral Vasoconstriction	Hyperventilation	Prospective studies	Randomized, controlled trials and prospective studies	No	Mild HV if sedation, analgesia, elevation of head of bed, CSF, drainage (if available), and hyperosmolar therapy are ineffective. Aggressive HV may be considered as a second tier with refractory intracranial hypertension.	Mild HV: $PaCO_2$ 30–35 mm Hg Aggressive HV: $PaCO_2$ <30 mm Hg
Seizure Therapy & Prophylaxis	Early posttraumatic seizures	One prospective study	Prospective studies	May be considered	Seizures	First-line therapy: Fosphenytoin P.E. 15–20 mg/kg load with maintenance dosing of 4–6 mg/kg/24 hr divided 1–2 times a day. Second tier: Phenobarbital 15–20 mg/kg load with maintenance dosing of 3–5 mg/kg/24 hr divided 1–2 times a day.
	Late posttraumatic seizures	One prospective study, otherwise retrospectives studies	Prospective and retrospective studies	No	Seizures	Same as early posttraumatic seizure therapy
Anti-inflammatory	Corticosteroids	Prospective and retrospective studies	Prospective and retrospective studies	No	Not recommended	Not recommended

Abbreviations: CSF, cerebrospinal fluid; HV, hyperventilation; ICP, intracerebral pressure.

in controlling increased ICP. Hypertonic saline may work through mechanisms similar to mannitol by creating an osmolar gradient, since sodium does not penetrate the BBB well. Hypertonic saline may also have specific anti-inflammatory effects.[63,64] Effective doses of 3% saline range between 0.1 and 1.0 ml/kg/hr; clinicians should use the minimal dose needed. A higher level of serum osmolarity (360 mOsm/L) appears to be tolerated. Euvolemia must be maintained, and a Foley catheter is recommended with all hyperosmolar therapies.

Hyperventilation

Hyperventilation has been widely used in the past to treat ICP based on the assumption that cerebral hyperemia is a major component in secondary brain insults. The intact cerebral vasculature responds to decreasing CO_2 tension by vasoconstriction. Decreasing the volume of the intracerebral compartment can lower ICP. Hyperventilation was also thought to reduce cerebral acidosis, improve cerebral metabolism, and increase blood flow to ischemic areas of the brain. The mechanism of hyperventilation is the induction of hypocapnia, which leads to cerebral vasoconstriction and reduction in CBF. Although hypocapnia will reduce CBV, it also has the potential to induce ischemia.[65]

Recent studies show that hyperemia may not be that common[66] and that hyperventilation may cause cerebral ischemia.[67] Moreover, cerebral vasculature autoregulation is lost shortly after injury, and hyperventilation becomes ineffective in lowering ICP. There are no studies comparing hyperventilation with other therapies such as hyperosmolar agents, barbiturates, and hypothermia. Therefore, data are insufficient to support a treatment standard. Recent widespread use of noninvasive means of measuring carbon dioxide, such as end-tidal carbon dioxide monitors, enable health care workers to see the immediate effects of adjustments in ventilation.[68] Consensus of expert opinion suggests the following[1]:

- Prophylactic hyperventilation (arterial partial pressure of carbon dioxide [$Paco_2$] < 35 mm Hg) in children should be avoided.
- Mild hyperventilation ($Paco_2$ 30 to 35 mm Hg) may be considered for elevated ICP not responsive to sedation and analgesia, neuromuscular blockade, CSF drainage, and hyperosmolar therapy.
- Aggressive hyperventilation ($Paco_2$ < 30 mm Hg) may be considered as a second-tier option in the setting of refractory hypertension with monitoring to detect cerebral ischemia in place; also, aggressive hyperventilation may be necessary for brief periods of cerebral herniation or acute neurologic deterioration.

Because hyperventilation may be ineffective, and possibly deleterious, measurement of ICP should guide its application. After initial stabilization, the cervical spine should be kept in a neutral position to avoid venous outflow obstruction, which also can raise ICP.

After the initial insult, and especially during reperfusion, it is important to prevent secondary injury. In particular, it is vital that additional hypoxia and ischemia not happen. Clinicians often fail to realize that inadequate oxygen delivery can occur not only because of low delivery of oxygen, but also because of increased oxygen utilization. If oxygen delivery is limited because of shock, elevated ICP, or derangements in cerebral autoregulation, events that create any imbalance between delivery and utilization can cause a secondary injury. Examples of such events include processes that raise cerebral metabolism, such as fever or convulsion.

Seizure Therapy

Posttraumatic seizures (PTS) have been classified as early (occurring within 7 days) or late (occurring after 7 days) following injury.[3] Seizures may cause secondary injury through a number of pathways, including increased cerebral metabolism, increased ICP, systemic hypoxia, increased cerebral temperature, interference with venous return, and release of excitatory neurotransmitters. Early PTS are more common in pediatric patients (20% to 39%)[69,70] than adult patients after severe TBI. Both low GCS score and young age

(<2 years) are associated with an increased risk of early PTS.[70,71] Consensus suggests that prophylactic antiseizure therapy may be considered as a treatment option to prevent early PTS in young children and infants at high risk for PTS.[1] Adult evidence suggests that anticonvulsants (phenytoin and carbamazepine) reduce early PTS but do not improve long-term outcomes.[3] Suggested anticonvulsants include fosphenytoin and phenobarbital.[72]

Late PTS are slightly less common in children (7% to 12%)[73] than adults (9% to 13%),[74] and data are insufficient to recommend prophylactic use of antiseizure medicine for children after severe TBI for preventing late PTS.

Steroids

Corticosteroids have been used in TBI with the intent of reducing cerebral swelling due to inflammation.[75] While experimental data suggests that corticosteroids reduce cerebral edema and attenuate free radical production in the setting of TBI, clinical studies have not supported their use.[3] At least eight studies examined the effect of corticosteroids in pediatric patients after TBI, with some studies reporting a beneficial effect on outcome. These studies have, however, been difficult to synthesize into a standard recommendation because of heterogeneous mechanisms of injury, confounding bias, and variable complications.[76,77] Two studies showed a marked increase in bacterial infections, including pneumonia.[78,79] At this time, data are insufficient to support a treatment standard or guideline for the use of corticosteroids in the treatment of TBI in pediatric patients.[1]

Cerebral Resuscitation: Advanced Techniques
(Table 9–2, Fig. 9–2)

ICP Monitoring

In tertiary care centers, the ability to place ICP monitoring devices allows for more precise management of increased ICP. This may be most important in TBI, as ICP monitoring is not recommended in cardiac arrest. In animal models of cardiac arrest, the insult necessary to produce a poor outcome is below the threshold needed to result in intracranial hypertension, implying that ICP monitoring–directed therapy is unlikely to improve outcomes.[48,49] In addition to intracranial monitoring devices, adult studies suggest that monitoring cerebral extraction of oxygen via jugular bulb catheters in addition to cerebral perfusion pressure after TBI results in improved neurologic outcome.[80]

Unfortunately, the decision as to when to initiate treatment of ICP in the management of TBI is made more difficult by the lack of data to support a treatment standard or guideline.[1] The posttraumatic brain is most likely sensitive to the secondary ischemia that may develop due to loss of cerebral perfusion pressure (CPP). Therefore, CPP monitoring (mean arterial pressure minus intracranial pressure) may be helpful. As ICP increases secondary to cerebral edema, it can ablate adequate perfusion. CPP estimates the ability of CBF to deliver important metabolic substrates to the cerebral tissue. As with treatment of elevated increased ICP, data are insufficient to propose a specific guideline for an appropriate range to maintain for CPP.[1] Retrospective data suggest that prolonged increased ICP greater than 20 mm Hg, and in particular ICP greater than 40 mm Hg, are associated with poor long-term neurologic outcome and mortality.[81,82]

Table 9–2	Advanced Cerebral Resuscitation Techniques					
Treatment Category	**Specific Treatment**	**Level of Evidence**		**Recommended for Prophylaxis?**	**Treatment Indications**	**Dosing Regimens**
		Pediatric	**Adult**			
Invasive Monitoring	Treatment based on ICP ICP reading	Retrospective studies	One prospective study and retrospective studies	Not applicable	ICP ≥ 20 mm Hg	Not applicable
Diminished Metabolism	Barbiturates	Retrospective studies	One prospective study and retrospectives studies	No	Second-tier therapy if sedation, analgesia, elevation of head of bed, CSF drainage (if available), and mild hyperventilation are ineffective	Pentobarbital 10 mg/kg load, then 5 mg/kg every hour for 3 doses with a maintenance infusion of 1 mg/kg/hr. Thiopental 10–20 mg/kg with a maintenance infusion of 3–5 mg/kg/hr. Consider reducing dose with decreased blood pressure or ICP < 25 mm Hg.
	Hypothermia	Retrospectives studies	Prospective studies	No	Second-tier therapy if sedation, analgesia, elevation of head of bed, CSF drainage (if available), mild hyperventilation, and barbiturates are ineffective	Core body temperature < 35°C. Regimens must be established per institution.
Surgical Procedures	Ventricular drainage	Retrospective studies	2 prospective studies and retrospective studies	No	Second-tier therapy if sedation, analgesia, and elevation of head of bed are ineffective	Via ventriculostomy catheter
	Decompressive craniotomy	Retrospective studies	Retrospective studies	No	Second-tier therapy that may be considered if: diffuse cerebral swelling on CT, within 48 hr of injury, no episodes of ICP > 40 mm Hg before surgery, GCS score > 3 at some point after injury, secondary clinical deterioration, evolving cerebral herniation syndrome	Surgical technique left to the discretion of the surgeon

Abbreviations: CSF, cerebrospinal fluid; CT, computed tomography; GCS, Glascow Coma Scale; ICP, intracerebral pressure.

Additionally, an inverse relationship has been seen with CPP and increased ICP, such that patients with ICP readings above 20 mm Hg are likely to have depressed CPP.[83] Increased mortality is associated with a mean CPP less than 40 mm Hg.[84] Therefore, treatment of increased ICP should begin at an ICP of 20 mm Hg, and CPP should be maintained in the range of 40 to 65 mm Hg in children with TBI.[1] Treatment should be supported by close physiologic monitoring, frequent clinical examinations, and cranial imaging.

Barbiturates

High-dose barbiturates reduce ICP by reduction of resting cerebral metabolic rate and altering vascular tone.[85,86] The reduction in the metabolic rate is associated with a reduction in CBF and CBV. On a molecular level, induction of a barbiturate coma reduces the amount of glutamate and lactate (both excitotoxicity mediators that cause neuronal damage) in the extracellular space of the brain via microdialysis.[22] Improvement in clinical outcomes such as long-term neuro-

logic status, however, has not been documented, and barbiturate coma has been associated with hypotension,[87] decreased jugular venous saturations, and worse outcomes.[88] Barbiturate therapy may be divided into prophylactic use for prevention of intracranial hypertension, and therapeutic use for established and refractory intracranial hypertension. There are no pediatric studies investigating the prophylactic use of barbiturates, and adult studies suggest no benefit.[89] Therefore, induction of a barbiturate coma is not indicated to prevent the development of intracranial hypertension. Studies of the efficacy of high-dose barbiturates in refractory intracranial hypertension in children have been small case series showing a reduction of ICP but no improvement in long-term neurologic outcome.[90,91] Often therapy with barbiturates was complicated by significant hypotension requiring fluid resuscitation and the use of pressors.[90] Therefore, data are insufficient to support a treatment standard or guideline. However, expert opinion suggests that high-dose barbiturate therapy may be considered in hemodynamically stable patients with

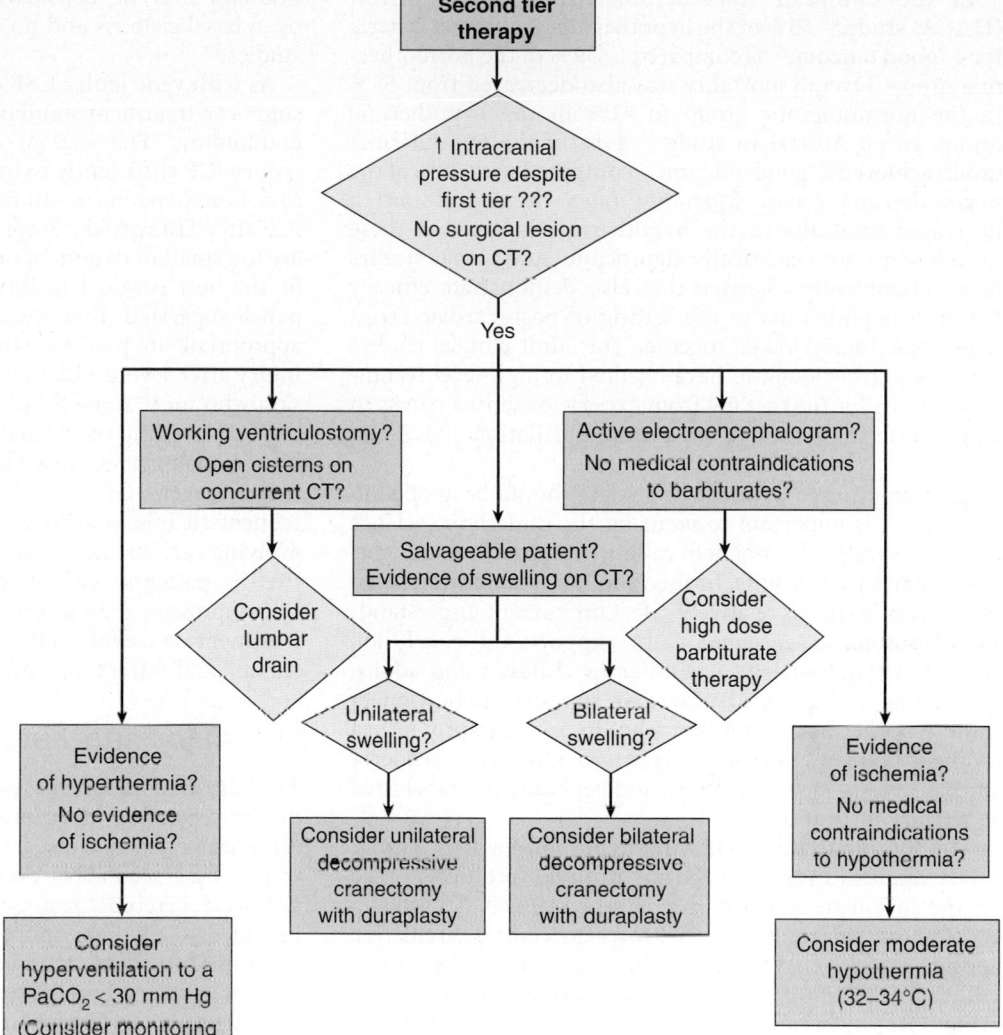

FIGURE 9–2. Algorithm for second-tier therapy. Abbreviations: AJDO2, arterial-jugular venous difference in oxygen content; CBF, cerebral blood flow; CT, computed tomography; EEG, electroencephalogram; ICP, intracranial pressure; SjO2, jugular venous oxygen saturation. (Adapted from Adelson PD, Bratton SL, Carney NA, et al: Guidelines for the acute medical management of severe traumatic brain injury in infants, children, and adolescents. Pediatr Crit Care Med 4[Suppl]:S1–S75, 2003.)

salvageable severe head injury and refractory intracranial hypertension with appropriate hemodynamic monitoring and cardiovascular support.[1] Therapeutic regimens that have been reported include pentobarbital with a loading dose of 10 mg/kg, then 5 mg/kg every hour for three doses with a maintenance drip of 1 mg/kg/hr,[92] or thiopental with a loading dose of 10 to 20 mg/kg followed by a maintenance drip of 3 to 5 mg/kg/hr.[93] Barbiturates are a second-tier therapy to consider when adequate sedation, analgesia, elevation of the head of the bed, CSF drainage if available, and mild hyperventilation are ineffective in controlling ICP.[1]

Therapeutic Hypothermia

Postinjury hypothermia, defined as a core body temperature less than 35° C, reduces apoptotic neuronal death in animal models.[44,94] Hypothermia also reducs levels of glutamate in the CSF.[21] Although two early studies showed promise in the use of hypothermia for the management of children after TBI, no additional work has been published between the 1970s and the 1990s. In the 1990s, several small adult studies showed improvements in CPP[95] and trends toward improved long-term neurologic outcome.[95-98] However, a multicenter

trial in adults after TBI was unable to show any benefit,[99] although a trend toward improved outcome existed in patients who presented hypothermic and were less than 40 years old. No child less than 16 years old was entered. Therefore, data are insufficient to support a treatment standard or guideline for the induction or maintenance of hypothermia after TBI. An expert consensus panel concluded that hypothermia may be considered in the setting of refractory intracranial hypertension.[1] Hyperthermia has been associated with poor outcome in experimental models and adult studies[100] and should be avoided.

Although no current studies support the application of hypothermia in children, the outcome of patients who remain in coma after resuscitation from cardiac arrest can be so poor that the therapy should be considered based on a reasonable extrapolation of laboratory and adult clinical data. The benefit of mild hypothermia after cardiac arrest in adults is supported by European and Australian randomized clinical trials published contemporaneously in 2002.[101,102] These studies indicated that mild hypothermia (32 to 34° C for 12 to 24 hours postarrest) is effective in preventing, or at least ameliorating, postanoxic encephalopathy in adults.

In the European Hypothermia After Cardiac Arrest (HACA) study,[102] 55% of the hypothermia group met criteria for a "good outcome" as compared to 39% of the normothermia group. Overall mortality was also decreased from 55% in the normothermic group to 41% in the hypothermic group. In an Australian study,[101] 49% of the hypothermia group achieved a "good outcome," compared with 29% of the normothermia group. Mortality rates trended toward a decreased mortality in the hypothermia group, but these results were not statistically significant. Additional studies have subsequently appeared that also demonstrate efficacy for mild hypothermia in the setting of post–cardiac arrest neurologic injury. Taken together, the adult clinical studies are persuasive enough to have resulted in high-level recommendations for the therapy from expert consensus panels in adults suffering witnessed ventricular fibrillation. (AHA and HACA).[102]

In attempting to decide if these data should be applied to children, it is important to focus on the underlying science and the overall risk-to-benefit ratio with respect to outcome. The experience in adults, limited though it is, indicates that mild hypothermia is relatively safe. Our current understanding of postanoxic encephalopathy supports the conclusion that its pathophysiology is similar in children and adults. Taken together, these assumptions support application of mild hypothermia in children who do not promptly return to their previous neurologic function after an episode of cardiac arrest. Such patients should generally be transferred to tertiary institutions.

The specific technique of mild hypothermia after cardiac arrest requires individualized institutional protocols based on the specific technology that will be utilized. Techniques range from surface cooling with ice to central circulation cooling catheters. Whatever technique is used, the patient will generally require sedation and paralysis to prevent shivering. Care must be taken to avoid temperature overshoot. This is best accomplished by measuring either central circulatory or bladder temperature and adjusting the cooling device carefully as the target temperature is approached. Some of the devices include a servo mechanism that controls temperature automatically. The most significant toxicities are infectious, so careful monitoring for early indicators of sepsis should be initiated.

Ventricular CSF Drainage and Decompression Craniotomy

Other advanced therapies applicable in tertiary centers that have been considered include ventricular CSF drainage and decompression craniotomy. Ventricular CSF drainage is used in conjunction with ICP monitoring and is thought to lower ICP by reducing intracranial volume and may remove clinically important detrimental mediators which cause neuronal death or damage. One retrospective study in children after TBI showed a reduction in ICP with CSF drainage.[103] Lumbar drainage in appropriate patients has been shown to reduce ICP in two small studies.[104,105] All of the pediatric studies are too small to show a difference in long-term neurologic outcome. Therefore, data are insufficient to support a treatment guideline for the role of CSF drainage in the management of TBI. The expert consensus panel recommended that CSF drainage may be considered as an option.[1] In addition to ventriculostomy catheter drainage, lumbar drainage may be considered in appropriate patients with open basal cisterns and no mass lesion or shift on radiology studies.[1]

As with ventricular CSF drainage, data are insufficient to support a treatment standard or guideline for decompressive craniotomy.[1] The goal of decompressive craniotomy is to reduce ICP sufficiently to maintain CPP and prevent herniation. Several pediatric studies have documented a decrease in ICP after TBI with decompressive craniotomy, but the studies are too small to comment on long-term neurologic outcomes or the best surgical technique.[106-108] The expert consensus panel suggested that decompressive craniotomy may be appropriate in patients with potentially recoverable brain injury after severe TBI and refractory intracranial hypertension who meet some or all of the following criteria: diffuse cerebral swelling on cranial CT imaging, within 48 hours of injury, no episodes of sustained ICP greater than 40 mm Hg before surgery, GCS score greater than 3 at some point subsequent to injury, secondary clinical deterioration, and/or evolving cerebral herniation syndrome. It appears less effective in patients with extensive secondary brain insults. Decompressive craniotomy should also be considered in the treatment of severe TBI in children with nonaccidental trauma and refractory intracranial hypertension.[1]

Summary and Future Directions

The improved understanding of the pathophysiology involved in the secondary deterioration that occurs after TBI and asphyxial cardiac arrest indicates that future therapies that target these secondary events may improve the efficacy of pediatric cerebral resuscitation. In particular, therapies intended to mediate apoptosis hold promise in preventing additional damage secondary to reperfusion injury. Future directions in cerebral resuscitation may also involve enhancing regeneration through administration of neurotrophic factors and cell transplantation.

Recovery from TBI has been shown to be enhanced by stimulation of the catecholamine systems.[109] Medications with catecholamine-like effects that have been studied include D-amphetamines, amantadine, and methylphenidate.[110-114] Increasing levels of the neurotransmitter acetylcholine attenuate memory deficits after experimental TBI.[115] Inhibiting cholinesterase with physostigmine also results in reduced memory and attention deficits after TBI.[116] Stimulation of the production of acetylcholine through cytidine diphosphoryl (CDP)-choline reduced postconcussion symptoms in adults after TBI when compared to placebo.[117] Unfortunately, no studies in children with neurotransmitter replacement therapy exist, and none of these agents can be recommended clinically at this time.

Neurotrophic factors (NTFs) are a family of proteins that are responsible for the growth and survival of neurons. They stimulate damaged neurons to regrow their axonal processes. Exogenous local infusion of NTFs improved memory retention[118] and attenuated neuronal loss in rats after TBI.[119] The clinical application of NTFs or NTF agonists has not yet occurred. Cell transplantation of genetically altered cells or cells transfected with viral vectors may allow the delivery of neuroactive substances to focal regions of the brain. Cells modified to produce nerve growth factor do support survival of cholinergic neurons after injury in models.[119]

Although TBI and cardiac arrest are two distinctly different insults, it is likely that many therapies targeted at preventing neuronal death will be applicable to both insults. The keys to treatment after brain injury will likely focus on prevention of secondary insults. Many therapies may need to be initiated early, perhaps in the field, to be effective. As in most areas of resuscitation, there continues to be a dearth of good scientific knowledge to guide the practitioner at this time. Children who have suffered a significant cerebral injury will not, however, wait for the clear delineation of effective therapies. Clinicians must decide which children's presentations demand intervention, and apply therapies intended to prevent, to the extent possible, additional loss of neurologic function.

REFERENCES

*1. Adelson PD, Bratton SL, Carney NA, et al: Guidelines for the acute medical management of severe traumatic brain injury in infants, children, and adolescents. Pediatr Crit Care Med 4(Suppl):S1–S75, 2003.
2. Bullock R, Chestnut R, Clifton GL, et al: Guidelines for the management of severe head injury. J Neurotrauma 13:641–734, 1996.
3. Bullock R, Chestnut R, Clifton GL, et al: Guidelines for the management of severe head injury. J Neurotrauma 17:449–627, 2000.
4. Luerssen TG, Klauber MR. Marshall LF: Outcome from head injury related to patient's age: a longitudinal prospective study of adult and pediatric head injury. J Neurosurg 68:409–416, 1988.
5. Wegman ME: Annual summary of vital statistics—1980. Pediatrics 68:755–762, 1981.
6. Kraus JF, Rock A, Hemyari P: Brain injuries among infants, children, adolescents, and young adults. Am J Dis Child 144:684–691, 1990.
7. Rivara FP: Childhood injuries. III. Epidemiology of non-motor vehicle head trauma. Dev Med Child Neurol 26:81–87, 1984.
8. Gronwell D, Wrightson P: Delayed recovery of intellectual function after minor head injury. Lancet 2:605–609, 1974.
9. Casey R, Ludwig S, McCormick MC: Morbidity following minor head trauma in children. Pediatrics 78:497–502, 1986.
10. Frankel LR: Respiratory distress and failure. In Behrman RE, Kliegman RM, Jenson JB (eds): Nelson Textbook of Pediatrics. Philadelphia: WB Saunders, 2003, pp 301–303.
11. Mathers LH, Frankel LR: Pediatric emergencies and resuscitation. In Behrman RE, Kliegman RM, Jenson JB (eds): Nelson Textbook of Pediatrics. Philadelphia: WB Saunders, 2003, pp 279–296.
12. Beaumont A, Marmarou A, Ward J: Intracranial hypertension mechanisms and management. In McClone DG (ed): Pediatric Neurosurgery. Philadelphia: WB Saunders, 2001, pp 619–633.
13. Baethmann A, Staub F: Cellular edema. In Welch KMA, Caplan LR, Reis EJ, et al (eds): Primer on Cerebrovascular Diseases. San Diego: Academic Press, 1997, pp 153–156.
14. Van Harreveld A, Fifkova E: Light and electron microscopic changes in central nervous tissue after electrophoretic injection of glutamate. Exp Mol Pathol 15:61, 1971.
15. Katayama Y, Mori T, Maeda T, et al: Pathogenesis of the mass effect of cerebral contusions: rapid increase in osmolality within the contusion necrosis. Acta Neurochir Suppl (Wien) 71:289–292, 1998.
16. Marmarou A, Fatouros PP, Brazos P, et al: Contribution of edema and cerebral blood volume to traumatic brain swelling in head-injured patients. J Neurosurg 93:183–193, 2000.
17. Benveniste HJ, Drejer A, Schousboe A, et al: Elevation of extracellular concentrations of glutamate and aspartate in rat hippocampus during transient cerebral ischemia monitored by intracerebral microdialysis. J Neurochem 43:1369–1374, 1984.
18. Choi DW: Ionic dependence of glutamate neurotoxicity in cortical cell culture. J Neurosci 7:369–379, 1987.
19. Palmer AM, Marion DW, Botscheller ML, et al: Traumatic brain injury-induced excitotoxicity assessed in a controlled cortical impact model. J Neurchem 61:2015–2024, 1993.
20. Faden AI, Demediuk P, Panter SS, et al: The role of excitatory amino acids and NMDA receptors in traumatic brain injury. Science 344:789–800, 1989.
21. Marion DW, Penrod LE, Kelsey SF, et al: Treatment of traumatic brain injury with moderate hypothermia. N Engl J Med 336:540–546, 1997.
22. Goodman JC, Valadka AB, Gopinath SP, et al: Lactate and excitatory amino acids measured by microdialysis are decreased by pentobarbital coma in head-injured patients. J Neurotrauma 13:549–556, 1996.
23. Morris GF, Bullock R, Marshall SB, et al: Failure of the competitive N-methyl-D-aspartate antagonist Selfotel (CGS 19755) in the treatment of severe head injury: Results of two Phase III clinical trials. J Neurosurg 91:737–743, 1999.
24. Ruppel RA, Kochanek PM, Adelson PD, et al: Excitotoxicity after severe traumatic brain injury in infants and children: the role of child abuse. J Pediatr 138:18–25, 2001.
25. Bouma GJ, Muizelaar JP, Stringer WA, et al: Ultra-early evaluation of regional cerebral blood flow in severely head-injured patients using xenon-enhanced computerized tomography. J Neurosurg 77:360–368, 1992.
26. Adelson PD, Clyde B, Kochanek PM, et al: Cerebrovascular response in infants and young children following severe traumatic brain injury: a preliminary report. Pediatr Neurosurg 26:200–207, 1997.
27. Hovda DA, Lee SM, Smith ML, et al: The neurochemical and metabolic cascade following brain injury: moving from animal models to man. J Neurotrauma 12:903–906, 1995.
28. Snyder JV, Nemoto E, Carroll RG, et al: Global ischemia in dogs: intracranial pressure, brain blood flow and metabolism. Stroke 6:21–27, 1975.
29. Armstead WM: Role of endothelin-1 in age-dependent cerebrovascular hypotensive responses after brain injury. Am J Physiol 277:H1884–H1894, 1999.
30. Cherian L, Chacko G, Goodman JC, et al: Cerebral hemodynamic effects of phenylephrine and l-arginine after cortical impact injury. Crit Care Med 27:2512–2517, 1999.
31. Safar P, Brown TC, Holtey WJ, et al: Ventilation and circulation with closed-chest cardiac massage in man. JAMA 176:92–94, 1961.
32. Headrick JP, Bendall MR, Faden AL, et al: Dissociation of adenosine levels from bioenergetic state in experimental brain trauma. J Cereb Blood Flow Metab 14:853–861, 1994.
33. Muira Y, Grocott HP, Bart RD, et al: Differential effects of anesthetic agents on outcome from near-complete but not complete global ischemia in the rat. Anesthesiology 89:391–400, 1998.
34. Statler KD, Kochanek PM, Dixon CE, et al: Fentanyl versus isoflurane anesthesia: effect on outcome after traumatic brain injury in rats. J Neurotrauma 17:1179–1189, 2000.
35. Kelly DF, Kozlowski DA, Haddad E, et al: Ethanol reduces metabolic uncoupling following experimental head injury. J Neurotrauma 17:261–272, 2000.
36. Kerr JF, Wyllie AH, Currie AR: Apoptosis: a basic biological phenomenon with wide-ranging implications in tissue kinetics. Br J Cancer 26:239–257, 1972.
37. Clark RSB, Chen J, Watkins SC, et al: Apoptosis-suppressor gene bcl-2 expression after traumatic brain injury in rats. J Neurosci 17:9172–9182, 1997.
38. Seidberg NA, Clark RSB, Kochanek PM, et al: Soluble Fas is increased in CSF from infants and children after head injury. Crit Care Med 27: A38, 2000.
39. Yin X-M, Oltvai ZN, Korsmeyer SJ: BH1 and BH2 domains of bcl-2 are required for inhibition of apoptosis and heterodimerization with bax. Nature 369:321–323, 1994.
40. Okonkwo DO, Povlishock JT: An intrathecal bolus of cyclosporin A before injury preserves mitochondrial integrity and attenuates axonal disruption in traumatic brain injury. J Cereb Blood Flow Metab 19:443–451, 1999.
41. Zamzami N, Marchetti P, Castedo M, et al: Sequential reduction mitochondrial transmembrane potential and generation of reactive oxygen species in early programmed cell death. J Exp Med 182:367–377, 1995.
42. Nicholson DW, Ali A, Thornberry NA, et al: Identification and inhibition of the ICE/CED-3 protease necessary for mammalian apoptosis. Nature 376:37–43, 1995.
43. Casciola-Rosen LA, Ahnalt GJ, Rosen A: DNA-dependent protein kinase is one of a subset of autoantigens specifically cleaved early during apoptosis. J Exp Med 182:1625–1634, 1995.
44. Choi DW: Ischemia-induced neuronal apoptosis. Curr Opin Neurobiol 6:667–672, 1996.

---

*Selected reading.

45. Deshmukh M, Johnson EM Jr: Evidence of a novel event during neuronal death: development of competence-to-die in response to cytoplasmic cytochrome c. Neuron 21:695–705, 1998.

46. Dieckmann R, Brownstein D, Gausche-Hill M (eds): Pediatric Education for Prehospital Professionals. Sudbury, MA: Jones and Bartlett Publishers/American Academy of Pediatrics, 2000, pp 30–57.

47. Dolan M: Head trauma. In Barkin RM (ed): Pediatric Emergency Medicine. St. Louis: Mosby, 1997, p 240.

48. Nemoto EM, Bleyaert AL, Stezoski SW, et al: Global brain ischemia: a reproducible monkey model. Stroke 8:558, 1977.

49. Safer P: Cerebral resuscitation after cardiac arrest: a review. Circulation 4:138, 1986.

50. Rehncrona A, Siesjo BK: Metabolic and physiologic changes in acute brain failure. In Grenvik A, Safar P (eds): Brain Failure and Resuscitation. New York: Churchill Linvingstone, 1981, pp 11–33.

51. DeGarmo BH, Dronen S: Pharmacologic and clinical use of neuromuscular blocking agents. Ann Emerg Med 12:48–55, 1983.

52. Hanna JP, Ramundo ML: Rhabdomyolysis and hypoxia associated with prolonged propofol infusion in children. Neurology 50:301–303, 1998.

53. Cray SH, Robinson BH, Cox PN: Lactate acidemia and bradyarrhythmia in a child sedated with propofol. Crit Care Med 26:2087–2092, 1998.

54. Milton J (ed): Formulary and Drug Dosing Handbook of The Children's Hospital of Denver. Hudson, OH: Lexi-Comp, 2000, pp 1-578.

55. Albanese J, Viviand X, Potie F, et al: Sufentanil, fentanyl, and alfentanil in head trauma patients: a study on cerebral hemodynamics. Crit Care Med 27:407–411, 1999.

56. de Nadal M, Ausina A, Sahuquillo J, et al: Effects on intracranial pressure of fentanyl in severe head injured patients. Acta Neurochir Suppl 71:10–12, 1998.

57. Sperry RJ, Bailey PL, Reichman MV, et al: Fentanyl and sufentanil increase intracranial pressure in head trauma patients. Anesthesiology 77:416–420, 1992.

58. Muizelaar JP, Wei EP, Kontos HA, et al: Cerebral blood flow is regulated by changes in blood pressure and in blood viscosity alike. Stroke 17:44–48, 1986.

59. Bouma GJ, Muizelaar JP: Cerebral blood flow, cerebral blood volume, and cerebrovascular reactivity after severe head injury. J Neurotrauma 9:S333–S348, 1992.

60. Kaieda R, Todd MM, Cook LN, et al: Acute effects of changing plasma osmolality and colloid oncotic pressure on the formation of brain edema after cryogenic injury. Neurosurgery 24:671–677, 1989.

61. James HE: Methodology for the control of intracranial pressure with hypertonic mannitol. Acta Neurochir 51:161–172, 1980.

62. Miller JD, Piper IR, Dearden NM: Management of intracranial hypertension in head injury: matching treatment with cause. Acta Neurochir 57:152–159, 1993.

63. Peterson B, Khanna S, Fisher B, et al: Prolonged hypernatremia controls elevated intracranial pressure in head-injured pediatric patients. Crit Care Med 28:1136–1143, 2000.

64. Khanna S, Davis D, Peterson B, et al: Use of hypertonic saline in the treatment of severe refractory posttraumatic intracranial hypertension in pediatric traumatic brain injury. Crit Care Med 28:1144–1151, 2000.

65. Muizelaar JP, Vanderpoel HG, Li Z, et al: Pial arteriolar diameter and CO_2 reactivity during prolonged hyperventilation in the rabbit. J Neurosurg 69:923–927, 1988.

66. Skippen P, Seear M, Poskitt K, et al: Effect of hyperventilation on regional cerebral blood flow in head-injured children. Crit Care Med 25:1402–1409, 1997.

67. Kiening KL, Hartl R, Unterberg AW, et al: Brain tissue pO_2 monitoring in comatose patients: implications for therapy. Neurol Res 19:233–240, 1997.

68. Yosefy C, Hay E, Nasri Y, et al: End tidal carbon dioxide as a predictor of the arterial PCO_2 in the emergency department setting. Emerg Med J 21:557–559, 2004.

69. Ratan SK, Kulshreshtha R, Pandey RM: Predictors of posttraumatic convulsions in head injured children. Pediatr Neurosurg 30:127–131, 1999.

70. Hahn YS, Fuchs S, Flannery AM, et al: Factors influencing posttraumatic seizures in children. Neurosurgery 22:864–867, 1988.

71. Lewis RJ, Yee L, Inkelis SH, et al: Clinical predictors of post-traumatic seizures in children with head trauma. Ann Emerg Med 22:1114–1118, 1993.

72. Fischer JH, Patel TV, Fischer PA: Fosphenytoin: clinical pharmacokinetics and comparative advantages in the acute treatment of seizures. Clin Pharmacokinet 42:33–58, 2003.

73. Young B, Rapp RP, Haack D, et al: Failure of prophylactically administered phenytoin to prevent post-traumatic seizures in children. Childs Brain 10:185–192, 1983.

74. Yablon SA: Posttraumatic seizures. Arch Phys Med Rehabil 74:983–1001, 1993.

75. Cooper PR, Moody S, Clark WK, et al: Dexamethasone and severe head injury. J Neurosurg 51:307–316, 1979.

76. Gobiet W: Advances in management of severe head injuries in childhood. Neurochirugica 39:201–210, 1977.

77. Kretschmer H: Prognosis of severe head injuries in childhood and adolescents. Neuropediatrics 14:176–181, 1983.

78. Kloti J, Fanconi S, Zachmann M, et al: Dexamethasone therapy and cortisol excretion in severe pediatric head injury. Childs Nerv Syst 3:103–105, 1987.

79. Fanconi S, Kloti J, Meuli M, et al: Dexamethasone therapy and endogenous cortisol production in severe pediatric head injury. Intensive Care Med 14:163–166, 1988.

80. Cruz J: The first decade of continuous monitoring of jugular bulb oxyhemoglobin saturation: management strategies and clinical outcome. Crit Care Med 26:344–351, 1998.

81. Pfenninger J, Kaiser G, Lutschg J, et al: Treatment and outcome of the severely head injured child. Intensive Care Med 9:13–16, 1983.

82. Esparza J, Portillo JM, Sarabia M, et al: Outcome in children with severe head injuries. Childs Nerv Syst 1:109–114, 1985.

83. Sharples PM, Stuart AG, Matthews DS, et al: Cerebral blood flow and metabolism in children with severe head injury. Part 1: Relation to age, Glasgow Coma Scale, outcome, intracranial pressure, and time after injury. J Neurosurg 58:145–152, 1995.

84. Downward C, Hulka F, Mullins RJ, et al: Relationship of cerebral perfusion pressure and survival in pediatric brain-injured patients. J Trauma 49:654–658, 2000.

85. Piatt JH, Schiff SJ: High dose barbiturate therapy in neurosurgery and intensive care. Neurosurgery 15:427–444, 1984.

86. Demopoulous HB, Flamm ES, Pietronigro DD, et al: The free radical pathology and the microcirculation in the major central nervous system. Acta Physiol Scand Suppl 492:91–119, 1980.

87. Ward JD, Becker DP, Miller JD, et al: Failure of prophylactic barbiturate coma in the treatment of severe head injury. J Neurosurg 62:383–388, 1985.

88. Cruz J: Adverse effects of a pentobarbital on cerebral oxygenation of comatose patients with acute traumatic brain swelling: relationship to outcome. J Neurosurg 85:758–761, 1996.

89. Schwartz ML, Tator CH, Rowed DW, et al: The University of Toronto head injury treatment study: a prospective randomized comparison of pentobarbital and mannitol. Can J Neurol Sci 11:434–440, 1984.

90. Kasoff SS, Lansen TA, Holder D, et al: Aggressive physiologic monitoring of pediatric trauma patients with elevated intracranial pressure. Pediatr Neurosci 14:241–249, 1988.

91. Pittman T, Bucholz R, Williams D: Efficacy of barbiturates in the treatment of resistant intracranial hypertension in severely head-injured children. Pediatr Neurosci 15:13–17, 1989.

92. Eisenberg HM, Frankowski RF, Contant CF, et al: High-dose barbiturate control of elevated intracranial pressure in patients with severe head injury. J Neurosurg 69:15–23, 1988.

93. Nordby HK, Nesbakken R: The effect of high dose barbiturate decompression after severe head injury: a controlled clinical trial. Acta Neurochir 72:157–166, 1984.

94. Rossiter JP, Riopelle RJ, Bisby MA: Axotomy-induced apoptotic cell death of neonatal rat facial motoneurons: time course analysis and relation to NADPH-diaphorase activity. Exp Neurol 138:33–44, 1996.

95. Marion DW, Obrist WD, Carlier PM, et al: The use of moderate therapeutic hypothermia for patients with severe head injuriers: a preliminary report. J Neurosurg 79:354–362, 1993.

96. Shiozaki T, Hisashi S, Taneda M, et al: Effect of mild hypothermia on uncontrollable intracranial hypertension after severe head injury. J Neurosurg 79:363–368, 1993.

97. Marion DW, Penrod LE, Kelsey SF, et al: Treatment of traumatic brain injury with moderate hypothermia. N Engl J Med 336:540–546, 1997.

98. Clifton GL, Allen S, Barrodale P, et al: A Phase II study of moderate hypothermia in severe brain injury. J Neurotrauma 10:263–271, 1993.

99. Clifton GL, Miller ER, Choi SC, et al: Lack of effect of induction of hypothermia after acute brain injury. N Engl J Med 344:556–563, 2001.

100. Jones PA, Andrews PJ, Midgley S, et al: Measuring the burden of secondary insults in head injured patients during intensive care. J Neurosurg Anesthesiol 6:4–14, 1994.

101. Bernard SA, Gray TW, Buist MD, et al: Treatment of comatose survivors of out-of-hospital cardiac arrest with induced hypothermia. N Engl J Med 346:557–563, 2002.

102. The Hypothermia after Cardiac Arrest Study Group: Mild therapeutic hypothermia to improve the neurologic outcome after cardiac arrest. N Engl J Med 346:549–556, 2002.

103. Shapiro K, Marmarou A: Clinical applications of the pressure-volume index in treatment of pediatric head injuries. J Neurosurg 56:819–825, 1982.

104. Baldwin HZ, Rekate HL: Preliminary experience with controlled external lumbar drainage in diffuse pediatric head injury. Pediatr Neurosurg 17:115–120, 1991–1992.

105. Levy DI, Rekate HL, Cherny WB, et al: Controlled lumbar drainage in pediatric head injury. J Neurosurg 83:452–460, 1995.

106. Taylor A, Warwick B, Rosenfeld J, et al: A randomized trial of very early decompressive craniectomy in children with traumatic brain injury and sustained intracranial hypertension. Childs Nerv Syst 17:154–162, 2001.

107. Hieu PD, Sizun J, Person H, et al: The place of decompressive surgery in the treatment of uncontrollable post-traumatic intracranial hypertension in children. Childs Nerv Syst 12:270–275, 1996.

108. Cho DY, Wang YC, Chi CS: Decompressive craniotomy for acute shaken/impact syndrome. Pediatr Neurosurg 23:192–198, 1995.

109. Feeney DM: Pharmacologic modulation of recovery after brain injury: a reconsideration of diaschisis. J Neuro Rehabil 5:113–128, 1991.

110. Feeney DM, Gonzalez A, Law WA: Amphetamine, haloperidol, and experience interact to affect rate of recovery after motor cortex injury. Science 217:855–857, 1982.

111. Gianutsos G, Chute S, Dunn JP: Pharmacological changes in dopaminergic systems induced by long-term administration of amantidine. Eur J Pharmacol 110:357–361, 0000.

112. Gualtieri T, Chandler M, Coons TB, et al: Amantidine: a new clinical profile for traumatic brain injury. Clin Neuropharmacol 12:258–270, 1989.

113. Kraus MF, Maki PM: Effect of amantadine hydrochloride on symptoms of frontal lobe dysfunction brain injury: case studies and review. J Neuropsychiatry Clin Neurosci 9:222–230, 1997.

114. Mooney GF, Haas LJ: Effect of methylphenidate on brain injury-related anger. Arch Phys Med Rehabil 74:153–160, 1993.

115. Dixon CE, Kochanek PM, Yan HQ, et al: One-year study of spatial memory performance, brain morphology, and cholinergic markers after moderate controlled cortical impact in rats. J Neurotrauma 16:109–122, 1999.

116. Levin HS, Peters BH, Kalisky A, et al: Effects of oral physostigmine and lecithin on memory and attention in closed head injury patients. Cent Nerv Syst Trauma 3:333–342, 1986.

117. Levin HS: Treatment of postconcussional symptoms with CDP-choline. J Neurol Sci 103:S39–S42, 1999.

118. Dixon CE, Flinn P, Bao J, et al: Nerve growth factor attenuates cholinergic deficits following traumatic brain injury in rats. Exp Neurol 146:479–490, 1997.

119. Zou L, Huang L, Hayes R, et al: Liposome-mediated NGF gene transfection following neuronal injury: potential therapeutic applications. Gene Ther 6:994–1005, 1999.

Chapter 10

General Approach to Poisoning

Teresa J. Coco, MD and Erica L. Liebelt, MD

Key Points

Although most unintentional ingestions in young children result in few sequelae, there are several medications and agents that are toxic or even fatal when ingested in small doses.

Identifying particular toxidromes is helpful in guiding management.

Preventing the absorption of a drug or substance with activated charcoal is the primary modality for gastrointestinal decontamination for most ingestions.

Qualitative drug screens provide minimal useful information that will change the acute management of most poisoned patients and do not always rule out a poisoning.

Most poisoned patients can be treated with supportive care alone; however, there are specific antidotes for certain drugs and toxicants that can greatly reduce the morbidity and mortality associated with the toxicity.

Introduction and Background

Childhood poisonings are among the most common presenting medical emergencies encountered in pediatrics. Fortunately, the majority of substances involved produce minimal or mild clinical toxic effects. However, certain toxic poisonings can lead to severe clinical deterioration and eventually death. Therefore, physicians and other health care providers should be knowledgeable and competent in the assessment and management of childhood ingestions.

According to the Toxic Exposure Surveillance System (TESS) of the American Association of Poison Control Centers (AAPCC), there were 2,438,644 human exposures reported to poison control centers in 2004, of which 51% occurred in children younger than 6 years of age.[1] Over 1.5 million exposure cases were reported in individuals less than 20 years of age. The most common route of exposure was by ingestion (77%), followed by dermal, inhalation, and ocular exposure. Of those cases treated in a health care facility, 10%

were less than 6 years of age, 13% were between 6 and 12 years of age, and 49% between 13 and 19 years of age. However, the majority of these cases were treated and released. There were 27 reported deaths in children younger than 6 years of age, 16 deaths in the age range 6 to 12 years, and 90 reported deaths in the age range 13 to 19 years.

Pediatric poisonings can be classified as intentional or unintentional. Unintentional ingestions occur more frequently in children less than 6 years of age. In 2004, the AAPCC reported that 61% of unintentional ingestions were in this age group.[1] Because of the inquisitive and exploratory nature of children at this developmental stage, unintentional ingestions are more common. Medication errors by caregivers have also been reported in several studies to be a frequent event in this population.[2-4] The possibility of malicious intent to harm or transplacental exposure must also be recognized.

Intentional ingestion becomes more likely in school-age children over the age of 6 years. Thirty percent of intentional exposures reported to the AAPCC occurred between the ages of 6 and 19 years.[1] Older children may have more experimentation behavior that leads to the intentional ingestion. Psychosocial issues such as peer pressure can contribute to this type of ingestion. Suicidal gestures and attempts are also a frequent basis for intentional ingestions in this age group.

Since the passage of the Poison Prevention Packaging Act of 1970, which mandated child-resistant closures on household products and prescription medications, morbidity and mortality of childhood poisoning has been significantly reduced.[5] The establishment of poison control centers in the 1950s with the assistance of the American Academy of Pediatrics has greatly improved the recognition, management, and prevention of pediatric poisonings. These poison control centers have developed into complex computerized systems with specially trained health professionals providing advice 24 hours a day. The TESS database has been instrumental in providing surveillance and identification of certain hazardous and toxic substances in pediatric poisonings, such as the 10 most common pediatric exposures (Table 10–1). Many common exposures, including personal care products, cosmetics, and cleaning substances, have a relatively low risk of causing serious systemic symptoms.[6]

Some of the most hazardous household products include hydrocarbons, pesticides, alcohols, drain and oven cleaners, and glue gun agents containing selenious acid.[7] Pharmaceutical agents associated with the greatest potential for severe

Table 10–1	The Top 10 Pediatric Exposures in Children Less Than 6 Years of Age as Reported by the AAPCC

Cosmetics and personal care products
Cleaning substances
Analgesics
Topicals
Foreign bodies
Cough and cold preparations
Plants
Pesticides
Vitamins
Antihistamines

Table 10–2	Drugs and Substances That Are Toxic in Small Amounts

Drug/Substance	Toxic Effects
Benzocaine	Methemoglobinemia
β-Blockers (propanolol)	Bradycardia, hypotension, seizures, hypoglycemia
Calcium channel antagonists (verapamil)	Bradycardia, hypotension, heart block
Camphor	Seizures, CNS depression
Chloroquine	Seizures, dysrhythmias
Clonidine	Bradycardia, hypotension, CNS depression
Cyclic antidepressants	Seizures, dysrhythmias, hypotension
Diphenoxylate and atropine (Lomotil)	CNS depression, respiratory depression
Lindane	Seizures, CNS depression
Methadone	CNS depression, respiratory depression
Methyl salicylate	Seizures, metabolic acidosis, cardiovascular collapse
Phenothiazines	Seizures, CNS depression, dysrhythmias
Quinidine/quinine	Seizures, dysrhythmias
Sulfonylureas (glyburide)	Hypoglycemia

Abbreviation: CNS, central nervous system.

Table 10–3	Substances and Drugs Toxic to the Respiratory System

Respiratory System Effect	Causative Substance/Drug
Airway obstruction	Caustics (acids and alkalis), ACE inhibitors
Increased secretions	Organophosphates, nerve gases
Loss of airway reflexes	
CNS depression	Sedative-hypnotics
Seizures	Isoniazid, bupropion, cyclic antidepressants
Respiratory failure	
Pneumonitis	Hydrocarbons, inhalants
Paralysis	Botulinum toxin, tetanus
Noncardiogenic pulmonary edema/acute lung injury	Opioids, salicylates

Abbreviations: ACE, angiotensin-converting enzyme; CNS, central nervous system.

ideation.[10] Clinicians must consider poisoning in any child presenting with a history or symptom complex that is atypical or confusing.[11]

The initial phase of management in a suspected poisoning involves simultaneous assessment and stabilization according to the traditional "ABCDEs" of emergency medicine:

Airway
Breathing
Circulation
Disability
    Mental Status—awake, lethargic or obtunded?
    Pupils—large or small?
Drug Therapy
    Oxygen—carbon monoxide poisoning
    Naloxone—opioid poisoning
    Glucose—insulin or sulfonylurea poisoning
Decontamination: ocular and skin
Exposure: undress the patient and minimize heat loss

Evaluation of the airway includes looking for signs of obstruction, loss of protective airway reflexes, risk of aspiration, increased secretions, or predicted rapid progression to respiratory failure. Multiple toxic substances can affect the respiratory system (Table 10–3). Elective endotracheal intubation is indicated for impending respiratory failure. Early establishment of intravenous access should be obtained for any symptomatic poisoned child.

The "D" in the mnemonic traditionally represents disability or the neurologic examination, but can also stand for life-saving drug therapy and initial decontamination. Empirical drug therapy in symptomatic patients may prove to be life saving. A potentially poisoned child who presents with altered mental status or respiratory depression should be given a trial of naloxone (0.01 mg/kg intravenously; give a subsequent dose of 0.1 mg/kg if inadequate response; use intramuscularly, subcutaneously, or endotracheal tube if intravenous is not available). Infants and young children are susceptible to drug-induced hypoglycemia due to their limited glycogen stores. Hypoglycemia is frequently reported in ingestions of ethanol, oral hypoglycemic agents, β-blockers, and salicylates (see Chapter 106, Hypoglycemia). A rapid bedside glucose test is useful in identifying hypoglycemia early. Anticonvulsants may be necessary to stabilize seizure activity. Children have a higher body surface area than adults

toxicity are iron supplements, antidepressants, cardiovascular medications, and salicylates.[6-8] There are several agents that have been identified as extremely toxic or even fatal in children less than 2 years of age or weighing less than 10 kg when ingested in one to two swallows or one to two tablets[9] (Table 10–2).

Recognition and Approach

Infants and children exposed to potentially toxic substances may present as an acute emergency with or without multisystem involvement. These patients may pose a diagnostic challenge for emergency physicians, depending on the substance involved and the complexity of its toxic effects. Young children with unintentional ingestions usually ingest a single known substance, making the history and evaluation more straightforward. The adolescent patient, on the other hand, usually presents with a polysubstance overdose. Caregivers may be unavailable or unwilling to provide pertinent historical information. Adolescents may withhold knowledge of ingestion in an effort to conceal substance abuse or suicidal

and are at a higher risk for toxicity in dermal exposures and for developing hypothermia. Therefore, evaluation of exposure is an important part of the initial assessment of any poisoned pediatric patient.

After the patient is stabilized, a more detailed history is needed to determine the nature of the potential poisoning. When the ingestion is not witnessed, it is difficult to predict what was ingested or available to the patient, when the ingestion occurred, and how much was ingested. However, identifying the potential severity of an ingestion will determine which therapeutic interventions will be necessary and which laboratory tests are indicated. Because children often present with an unclear history of ingestion, emergency physicians should be suspicious of ingestion when there is an acute onset of multisystem dysfunction, altered mental status, or a confusing clinical picture. If an ingestion has occurred, the clinician should assume that the child has consumed the maximum available amount of the substance that was taken. The potential milligram-per-kilogram quantity consumed is calculated based on the caregiver's description of the concentration of the type of pill or liquid. When two children have potentially co-ingested a substance, the milligram-per-kilogram quantity ingested is calculated for each child assuming that each child has ingested all the substance. The best estimation of the time of ingestion is important in determining the need for charcoal and the blood levels of specific drugs, and to estimate the length of observation needed in the emergency department. For example, a serum acetaminophen level is only predictive of hepatotoxicity if obtained at least 4 hours post-ingestion for plotting on the Rumack-Matthew nomogram or 2 hours post-ingestion for the elixir.[12] Exposures to toxins can be oral, ocular, dermal, or by inhalation. Knowing the route of exposure is important for the proper decontamination of the patient and for appropriate protection of the health care providers.

A physical examination should focus on vital signs, mental status, cardiovascular and respiratory function, pupils, skin changes, and bowel and bladder function. Specific physical findings may give the clinician clues as to the type of substance ingested. These characteristic features represent a *toxidrome*, which is a constellation of signs and symptoms that are suggestive of a certain class of toxicants/toxins. Recognition or exclusion of classic toxidromes is important when evaluating the poisoned pediatric patient (Table 10–4). Understanding the basic toxidromes can help the emergency physician determine if the patient was exposed to a drug/toxicant from one of the following classes: sympathomimetic, anticholinergic, cholinergic/anticholinesterase, sedative-hypnotic, opioid, or serotonin-like substances. However, it is important to note that exposures involving multiple substances may not develop as a classic toxidrome and that patients may not present with all of the findings associated with a single toxidrome. Therefore, in a suspected pediatric poisoning, it is essential to attempt to determine all the substances that may have been accessible at the time of ingestion. Even with an unknown ingestion, paying close attention to the presenting symptoms can direct the health care professional to the appropriate toxidrome. Patients may also present with a predominant symptom such as vomiting/diarrhea, seizures, or hyperthermia. It is helpful to go through a differential diagnosis of toxicants that can cause these predominant symptoms (Tables 10–5, 10–6, and 10–7).

Table 10–4	Toxidromes
Sympathomimetic	
Vital signs	Tachycardia, hypertension, tachypnea, hyperthermia
CNS	Agitation, hallucinations, psychosis, seizures
Pupils	Mydriasis
Skin	Diaphoresis

Examples: amphetamines, methamphetamine, methylphenidate, cocaine, MDMA (Ecstasy), pseudoephedrine, caffeine, albuterol, theophylline

Anticholinergic	
Vital signs	Hyperthermia, tachycardia, hypertension, tachypnea
CNS	Altered mental status, agitation, delirium, hallucinations, seizures, lethargy, coma
Pupils	Mydriasis
Skin/mucous membranes	Dry, flushed skin; dry mucous membranes
GI tract	Decreased bowel sounds
GU system	Urinary retention

Examples: atropine, antihistamines, antipsychotics, antispasmodics, cyclic antidepressants, jimsonweed

Cholinergic/Anticholinesterase	
Vital signs	Bradycardia or tachycardia, tachypnea
CNS	Confusion, coma, fasciculations, seizures
Pupils	Miosis
Skin	Sweating
GI tract	Vomiting, diarrhea
Lungs	Bronchorrhea, bronchospasm
Skin/mucous membranes	Diaphoresis, lacrimation, salivation

Examples: organophosphate pesticides and nerve agents/gases (sarin, soman); carbamate insecticides; nicotine

Opioid/Clonidine	
Vital signs	Bradycardia, hypotension, bradypnea/apnea, hypothermia
CNS	Euphoria, lethargy, coma
Pupils	Miosis

Examples: opiates, clonidine, other imidazolines (tetrahydrozoline eyedrops)

Serotonin Syndrome	
Vital signs	Tachycardia, blood pressure fluctuation, hyperthermia
CNS	Agitation, confusion, delirium, hallucinations, mania, mutism, coma
Pupils	Mydriasis
Neuromuscular abnormalities	Hyperreflexia, myoclonus, akathisia (restlessness), seizures, rigidity

Examples: SSRIs; combinations of serotonergic agents—MAOIs, dextromethorphan, meperidine, MDMA (Ecstasy)

Sedative-Hypnotic Syndrome	
Vital signs	Hypotension, bradypnea, hypothermia
CNS	Slurred speech, ataxia, depressed mental status, hyporeflexia, paradoxical excitement in very young children
Pupils	Normal to large, sluggishly reactive

Examples: barbiturates, benzodiazepines, buspirone, chloral hydrate, meprobamate, methaqualone

Abbreviations: CNS, central nervous system; GI, gastrointestinal; GU, genitourinary; MAOIs, monoamine oxidase inhibitors; SSRIs, selective serotonin reuptake inhibitors.

Table 10–5	Toxic Substances That Present with Vomiting and/or Diarrhea

Carbon monoxide
Caustic agents
Colchicine
Digoxin
Iron
Metals (arsenic, mercury, zinc)
Mushrooms
Nicotine
Organophosphate pesticides/insecticides
Salicylates
Theophylline

Table 10–6	Drugs and Substances That Induce Seizures

Amphetamines (MDMA)
Anticholinergic agents
Baclofen
β-Blockers
Bupropion
Camphor
Carbamazepine
Carbon monoxide
Cocaine
Cyanide
Ethanol withdrawal
GHB (γ-hydroxybutyrate)
Isoniazid
Lead
Lidocaine
Lindane
Lithium
Meperidine
Nerve agents (sarin, soman, tabun, VX gas, Substance 33)
Oral hypoglycemics
Organophosphates
Phencyclidine
Phenytoin
Propoxyphene
Salicylates
Sympathomimetic agents
Theophylline
Tricyclic antidepressants
Water hemolock plant

Table 10–7	Drugs That Cause Hyperthermia

Amphetamines
Anticholinergics
Antihistamines
Butyrophenones (haloperidol)
Cocaine
Cyclic antidepressants
Dinotrophenol
LSD
MAOIs
Methamphetamine/Ecstasy
Phencyclidine
Phenothiazines
Pseudoephedrine
Salicylates
SSRIs
Sympathomimetic agents
Theophylline
Thyroxine
Withdrawal of ethanol, dopamine agonists, sedative-hypnotic agents

Abbreviations: LSD, lysergic acid diethylamide; MAOIs, monoamine oxidase inhibitors; SSRIs, selective serotonin reuptake inhibitors.

Table 10–8	Laboratory Evaluation of the Poisoned Patient

Bedside blood glucose
Pulse oximetry
Electrocardiogram
Serum electrolytes and calculation of anion gap
Serum osmolality and calculation of osmolal gap
Urinalysis
Serum drug levels (e.g., acetaminophen, salicylate, digoxin)
Pregnancy test
Focused toxicology laboratory testing

Table 10–9	Toxic Substances That Cause a High-Anion-Gap Metabolic Acidosis

Cyanide
Ethanol
Ethylene glycol
Iron
Isoniazid
Metformin
Methanol
Paraldehyde
Phenformin
Salicylates

Evaluation

An understanding of laboratory assays, their indications, and their limitations is an important aspect of managing children with potential toxic exposures. Laboratory evaluation of potentially poisoned patients with systemic symptoms of an unknown ingestion should include a focused evaluation based on the clinical situation (Table 10–8). Any patient presenting with an altered mental status or the potential to develop hypoglycemia from a toxic substance or drug should have a bedside blood glucose determination. Serum electrolytes, calculation of an anion gap, and blood gas assessment can help determine if a high-anion-gap metabolic acidosis is present (Table 10–9). An elevated osmolal gap (difference between the measured and calculated serum osmolality) may be a helpful clue in determining whether a patient has ingested a toxic alcohol (isopropyl, ethylene glycol, or methanol). However, it is important to realize the limitations of this test.

Depending on the time of ingestion, little of the osmotically active parent alcohol may be present when a patient presents with signs of toxicity. The normal osmolal gap varies (−5 to 15 mOsm) depending on the equation used to determine the gap and the time the calculation was made.[13]

Acetaminophen is available in many single and multidrug over-the-counter and prescription medications. Consequently, many patients are unaware that they ingested acetaminophen. Because it is the most common co-ingestant in polydrug overdoses in the United States and there is an available antidote, all patients with intentional overdoses should be empirically tested for acetaminophen.[14] Quantitative serum concentrations of other specific drugs (digoxin, salicylate) can be important in determining the severity of the ingestion and to guide the management of interventions and specific antidotes.[15] Urinalysis may reveal important diagnostic clues. Calcium oxalate crystals are considered pathognomonic for ethylene glycol poisoning, but are usually discovered late in the clinical course. A pregnancy test is recommended in female patients of childbearing age, because of the possibility that the ingestion may be prompted by a wish to abort a fetus. Certain exposures warrant counseling regarding the potential for fetal loss or malformations, including retinoids, antineoplastic agents, selected anticonvulsants (phenytoin), and coumadin.

Routine qualitative drug screens provide minimal useful information that will change the acute management of most poisoned patients.[15] There is no standard definition of what constitutes a "toxicology drug screen." It is important for the emergency physician to understand the specific testing available at his or her facility. Most laboratory toxicology screens are immunoassays capable of screening for commonly abused drugs such as marijuana, opioids, amphetamines, benzodiazepines, and cocaine in the urine. In contrast, some laboratories can perform highly specific assays for hundreds of drugs on urine and blood specimens. These more complex toxicology screens can be important when an unknown substance has been ingested or child abuse is suspected.

It is important to understand the limitations of toxicology screens. They are only qualitative tests, detecting the presence of drugs. A drug that is present may not necessarily be causing the clinical symptomatology. Also, there are several dangerous drugs and substances not routinely detected by screens (Table 10–10). False-positive results are another limiting factor of broad toxicology screens. Finally, a negative toxicology screen does not rule out a poisoning for all of the reasons mentioned earlier. The majority of toxicologic diagnostic and therapeutic decisions can be made on a clinical or historical basis for most poisoned patients.

Additional tests that may be of benefit in an unknown ingestion include a 12-lead electrocardiogram to evaluate for a prolonged corrected QT interval, a widened QRS complex, or a dysrhythmia that may be caused by tricyclic antidepressants or other cardiotoxic agents.[16] Chest radiography may demonstrate pulmonary injury caused by respiratory irritants and other gases. Some agents are radiopaque and can be detected by the use of abdominal radiographs. Examples include chloral hydrate, iron, lead, enteric-coated preparations, drug-filled condoms, and foreign bodies. Computed tomography can help to document illicit drug–induced pathology (leakage or rupture of "body packers" and "body stuffers").[17]

Management

After the suspected toxin has been identified, decontamination can be directed to the particular area exposed. Ocular and dermal decontamination should be carried out immediately as the toxic substance needs to be removed promptly to prevent ongoing absorption. Ocular exposures accounted for 5.2% of exposures reported by the AAPCC in 2004.[1] Ocular toxins can produce permanent injury and blindness if not appropriately managed. Ocular injuries are considered ophthalmologic emergencies. Immediate decontamination with irrigation of the eyes with sterile water, lactated Ringer's solution, or sterile isotonic saline solution for 15 to 30 minutes is recommended. Suspected corrosive injuries require obtaining a pH of the ocular fluid. If the pH is greater than 7, irrigation should continue until that end point is reached. Ocular injuries with persistent pain should be referred for immediate consultation with an ophthalmologist.

Dermal exposures require immediate removal of all clothing and irrigation of the affected area with water. Significant absorption through the skin can occur with certain lipophilic compounds (e.g., organophosphates). A wide range of dermal toxins can produce corrosive injuries similar to burn injuries. These injuries may be treated with the same management strategy as burns. Of particular importance is the protection of health care professionals who come in contact with the toxic substance. Protective gear should be worn for suspected dermal toxins that may contaminate the air or be contacted through dermal exposure. For example, neoprene gloves should be worn if taking care of a patient with organophosphate exposure because organophosphates can penetrate through routine latex gloves.

Any patient with a suspected inhalation exposure should be removed from the source. Appropriate protective gear must be worn by any person that may come in contact with the same exposure. All clothing should be removed from the patient. Areas of the body possibly exposed to the inhalant should be decontaminated with abundant irrigation. Supplemental oxygen should be provided to any symptomatic patient.

The decision to perform gastrointestinal decontamination should be made only after initial stabilization has been initiated. Gastrointestinal decontamination is performed to prevent absorption after a substance has been ingested. The principal components of gastrointestinal decontamination include gastric emptying and administration of an absorbent compound. The benefit of gastric emptying decreases with time and is most effective if performed within an hour of ingestion. Induction of emesis in the hospital setting has not been shown to clinically improve the outcome of poisoned

Table 10–10	Drugs and Substances Not Routinely Detected on Comprehensive Toxicology Screen Testing

β-Agonists
β-Blockers
Calcium channel antagonists
Carbon monoxide
Clonidine
Cyanide
Digoxin
Dextromethorphan
Diphenhydramine
Ethylene glycol
GHB (γ-hydroxybutyrate)
Heavy metals
Hydrocarbons
Iron
Isoniazid
Ketamine
Methanol
Organophosphates
Sulfonylureas

pediatric patients and should not be performed as part of the routine management in the emergency department.[18-20] Ipecac may delay the administration or reduce the effectiveness of activated charcoal, oral antidotes, and whole-bowel irrigation.

Gastric lavage is no longer considered the standard of care for gastrointestinal decontamination and should not be routinely performed in the management of the poisoned patient. Lavage should be considered if a potentially life-threatening substance has been ingested (cyclic antidepressant, β-blocker, calcium channel antagonist) and if it can be undertaken within 1 hour of the ingestion. This change in clinical practice has evolved in the last 15 years.[18] There is little evidence that gastric lavage improves outcome even if performed within an hour of ingestion.[21,22] Gastric lavage is contraindicated in the unintubated patient with depressed consciousness, if there is potential for loss of airway protective reflexes, in cases of ingestion of a corrosive substance or hydrocarbon, and in patients at risk for hemorrhage or gastrointestinal perforation. Complications include aspiration, mechanical injury to the oropharynx, esophagus, and stomach, and electrolyte imbalances.[22] Substances for which gastric lavage may be useful for improving clinical outcome include sustained-release medications, agents that delay gastric emptying (opioids, anticholinergics), and substances not absorbed by activated charcoal (iron, lithium).

One limitation of gastric lavage in children is the diameter of the tube, which may not be large enough to accommodate pill fragments. A 16- to 28-French tube should be used in a child, and at least a 36-French tube in an adolescent. Gastric lavage is almost never warranted in young children.[18] In adolescents with intentional overdoses, each case should be assessed on an individual basis, but lavage should never be employed routinely.

Absorbents bind toxic substances within the gastrointestinal tract and reduce systemic absorption. Activated charcoal is extremely effective in binding a wide variety of substances ranging from pharmaceuticals to biologic agents. The absorptive capacity of activated charcoal is a function of its binding surface area, which ranges from 1000 to 2000 m²/g. The administration of activated charcoal is the most common method of gastrointestinal decontamination in poisoned children. The maximal benefit occurs when it is given within an hour of the ingestion. However, it may be given after an hour if the agent ingested delays gastric emptying. The recommended dose of charcoal is 1 g/kg in children up to the age of 1 year, 25 to 50 g in children 1 to 12 years, and 25 to 100 g in adolescents. Charcoal may be given orally or by a nasogastric tube. Activated charcoal must not be administered to patients with a depressed level of consciousness, to unintubated patients who may have loss of protective airway reflexes, in cases in which there is an increased risk of aspiration (i.e., household hydrocarbons), or in cases with suspected gastrointestinal hemorrhage or perforation. Charcoal is not indicated when the agent is nontoxic or when it is unable to bind to substances. The main adverse events associated with activated charcoal are vomiting and aspiration, which can lead to pulmonary injury and death.[8] Activated charcoal is not effective in binding ethanol, heavy metals, iron, caustics, lithium, hydrocarbons, and potassium. Any child suspected of ingesting a potentially life-threatening substance who has the ability to protect airway reflexes should receive a dose of activated charcoal unless there is a specific contraindication.

Cathartic agents are not recommended in the routine gastrointestinal decontamination of an infant or child. The major function of a cathartic is to rapidly move the toxin through the gastrointestinal tract, reducing the amount of time for absorption. There is no clinical evidence to support the use of cathartics as adjunctive decontamination therapy.[18] Adverse effects include vomiting, electrolyte imbalances, and hypovolemia.

Whole-bowel irrigation with balanced polyethylene glycol solutions (e.g., Golytely) given in large volumes aids in the rapid elimination of the toxicant through the gastrointestinal tract. These iso-osmotic solutions can be given safely in large volumes, without electrolyte imbalances or fluid shifts, even in small children. Typical rates of administration are 0.5 L/hr for children less than 6 years of age, 1 L/hr for children ages 6 to 12 years, and 1.5 L/hr for children older than 12 years of age, either orally or by nasogastric tube. This technique is most effective in eliminating sustained-release substances and substances poorly absorbed by activated charcoal, such as iron and lithium.[23] Knowing the potential toxicity of the toxicant, the ingestion time, the chemical nature of the toxicant, and the presence of contraindications will help direct the appropriate decontamination therapy. The risks and benefits must be weighed before institution of any therapy.

Supportive care is the mainstay of treatment for most patients with overdoses. Careful attention to the basic management of airway, ventilation, and hemodynamic support is adequate for most toxic exposures. However, there are toxicants for which a specific antidote can counteract the effects of the poison. A limited number of effective pharmaceutical antidotes are available, and it is important for clinicians to understand specific indications for their administration[24] (Table 10–11).

Although very few toxic exposures are effectively treated by extracorporeal techniques, these modalities are essential and life saving in the treatment of selected poisoned patients. Emergency physicians must be aware of when to initiate consultations for these interventions. The extracorporeal techniques most commonly employed for the removal of toxicants are hemodialysis and charcoal hemoperfusion, although exchange transfusion and continuous ultrafiltration techniques may also be used. Implementation of these invasive techniques requires the availability of nephrologists and pediatric critical care specialists on a 24-hour basis, as well as pediatric dialysis equipment and technicians who have expertise in the care of pediatric patients. In addition, it is essential that a reference laboratory also be able to monitor the efficacy of treatment on a 24-hour basis. Indications for extracorporeal removal of drugs and toxicants are ingestion of a substance whose removal can be enhanced 30% or more in a patient with a blood level or ingested quantity that is generally associated with severe toxicity, impaired natural removal mechanisms (i.e., renal failure), a deteriorating clinical condition despite supportive care (phenobarbitol), and clinical evidence of severe toxicity, such as metabolic acidosis (salicylates, methanol), dysrhythmias, or cardiac decompensation (theophylline).[25] A list of toxicants removed by hemodialysis is shown in Table 10–12. Continuous renal replacement therapies (e.g., continuous venovenous hemofiltration) may be more appropriate for removal of toxicants in patients who

Table 10–11	Selected Antidotes

Antidote	Indications
N-acetylcysteine	Acetaminophen
Atropine	Bradycardia due to cardiotoxic drugs, cholinergic poisoning (organophosphates, carbamates, nerve gas agents)
Bicarbonate, sodium and sodium chloride[26,27]	Cyclic antidepressants, salicylate, wide-complex dysrhythmias (cocaine, diphenhydramine, chloroquine)
Black widow spider antivenin[28]	Severe hypertension, muscle spasms not alleviated by analgesic and/or muscle relaxants
Calcium	Calcium channel antagonist poisoning, hydrofluoric acid burn
Crotaline antivenom[29,30]	Progressive and/or significant envenomation by rattlesnake, cottonmouth, copperhead snakes

Cyanide antidote kit
  Amyl nitrite
  Sodium nitrite
  Sodium thiosulfate
	Cyanide poisoning

Cyproheptadine[31,32]	Baclofen withdrawal, serotonin syndrome
Dantrolene	Muscle rigidity, hyperthermia, metabolic acidosis due to malignant hyperthermia, neuroleptic malignant syndrome
Deferoxamine	Iron toxicity
Digoxin-specific antibody fragments (Digibind, Digifab)[33]	Digoxin, cardiac glycoside toxicity
Ethanol	Methanol or ethylene glycol poisoning when fomepizole is not available
Flumazenil	Known, pure benzodiazepine overdose in a benzodiazepine-naive patient
Fomepizole (4-MP, Antizol)[34]	Methanol or ethylene glycol poisoning
Glucagon[24,35]	β-Blocker or calcium channel antagonist overdose with bradycardia/hypotension
Hyperinsulinemia/euglycemia[36,37]	Calcium channel antagonist overdose with severe hypotension/symptomatic bradycardia refractory to other therapies
Methylene blue	Methemoglobinemia with symptoms of hypoxia, other systemic toxicity, or level > 25%
Naloxone (Narcan)	Opioid, imidazoline (clonidine) poisoning
Octreotide[38,39]	Hypoglycemia due to oral hypoglycemic agent (sulfonylurea) toxicity
Oxygen, hyperbaric	Carbon monoxide toxicity
Physostigmine[40]	Pure anticholinergic poisoning
Pralidoxime (2-PAM, Protopam)	Organophosphate, nerve agent toxicity; use in conjunction with atropine
Pyridoxine (vitamin B₆)	Isoniazid-induced seizures, Gyromitra mushroom, monomethylhydrazine
Vitamin K₁	Clinical bleeding due to coumadin, brodifacoum toxicity

Table 10–12	Common Toxicants and Drugs Removed by Hemodialysis or Charcoal Hemoperfusion

Bromide
Carbamazepine
Chloral hydrate
Ethylene glycol
Isopropanol
Lithium
Metformin
Methanol
Phenobarbital
Salicylates
Theophylline
Valproic acid

Table 10–13	Suggested Guidelines on When to Consider Consulting a Medical Toxicologist

Calcium channel antagonist/β-blocker ingestion with hypotension and/or bradycardia
Cyclic antidepressant ingestion with coma, seizures, hypotension, and/or dysrhythmias
Toxic alcohol ingestion (ethylene glycol, methanol)
Organophosphates/carbamate exposure with symptoms
Acute heavy metal exposure (arsenic, mercury) with symptoms
Snake envenomation
Intractable seizures secondary to toxic substance
Critically ill patient requiring:
  Special antidote—digoxin Fab, methylene blue, glucagon, antivenom
  Hemodialysis
  Hyperbaric oxygen

are hemodynamically unstable and avoid the problem of rebound toxicity (i.e., lithium). Consultation with a medical toxicologist and nephrologist can help decide which modality is best for the clinical situation.

There are other mechanisms that can enhance the elimination of poisons. These include urinary alkalinization for salicylates and multiple doses of activated charcoal for theophylline, salicylates, and phenobarbital (see Chapter 133, Classic Pediatric Ingestions; and Chapter 136, Adverse Effects of Anticonvulsants and Psychotropic Agents).

Consider consulting a medical toxicologist for patients who are critically ill, who require specific antidotes, or who have ingested unusual or lethal toxins (Table 10–13).

Summary

Decision making regarding the disposition of a poisoned patient depends on numerous factors, including the type of exposure, the toxicant itself, the circumstances surrounding the exposure, and the child's social situation. Because most unintentional ingestions in young children result in either no or mild sequelae, these children can usually be discharged after an observation period of 4 to 6 hours. Utilization of the regional poison control center can help clinicians make these disposition decisions based on the particular exposure/ingestant. A common toll-free number is available nationally (1-800-222-1222) so that all health care providers as well as the public have 24-hour access to their regional poison control center for poison and drug information.

"Medical clearance" of a patient who has had a potentially toxic exposure sometimes can be more problematic in the pediatric population. Any child or adolescent who presents with an intentional ingestion/overdose and does not need to be admitted for a medical reason must have a psychiatric assessment to determine whether further inpatient hospitalization is warranted. Most intentional ingestions warrant inpatient psychiatric hospitalization. If the circumstances are carefully evaluated and it is believed that the patient can be safely discharged, urgent follow-up with mental health services must be assured.

Pediatric poisonings are a common cause of presentations to emergency departments. Very few unintentional ingestions in young children require hospitalization. Yet there is a selected list of drugs and substances that can cause serious toxicity even when ingested in small amounts. Fatalities in young children due to poisonings have decreased dramatically since the 1950s due to numerous factors—product reformulations, child-resistant packaging, heightened parental awareness of product toxic effects, intervention by poison information centers, and treatment by specially trained health care professionals. The profile of intentional overdoses in adolescents is similar to that of young adults in terms of intent, nature of polysubstance ingestion, and type of substances ingested. However, the prognosis of adolescents who seek health care because of available parental oversight is excellent.

Evaluation of the potentially poisoned patient relies primarily on the history and physical examination. Recognizing specific clinical toxidromes may help the clinician to recognize particular classes of drugs, which can then help guide further evaluation and therapy. The mainstay of therapy for most poisoned patients is supportive care. There are a limited number of antidotes that can limit the toxicity of specific drugs and toxicants. In addition, there are different modalities to enhance the elimination of a limited number of drugs and toxicants that may be initiated in the emergency department. Ocular, dermal, and/or gastrointestinal decontamination may be necessary depending on the route of exposure and time since the exposure took place. Research in the last 10 years has provided evidence to support the avoidance of routine gastric emptying for all ingestions in the emergency department. Whole-bowel irrigation is a new decontamination modality for selected ingestions that are not amenable to charcoal therapy.

It is important for the emergency physician to remember other resources available—particularly the regional poison control center and the medical toxicologist, who may be at the health care facility or available through the poison control center.

REFERENCES

1. Watson WA, Litovitz TL, Rodgers GC, et al: 2004 Annual Report of the American Association of Poison Control Centers Toxic Exposures Surveillance System. Am J Emerg Med 23:589–666, 2004.
2. Jonville AE, Autret E, Bavoux F, et al: Characteristics of medication errors in pediatrics. DICP Ann Pharmacother 25:1113–1118, 1991.
3. Santell JP, Cousins D: Medication errors—documenting and reducing medication errors. US Pharmacist 28(7), 2003. Available at *http://uspharmacist.com/index.asp?show=article&page=8-1120.htm*
4. Li SF, Lacher B, Crain EF: Acetaminophen and ibuprofen dosing by parents. Pediatr Emerg Care 16:394–397, 2002.
5. Rodgers GB: The safety effects of child-resistant packaging for oral prescription drugs: two decades of experience. JAMA 275:1661–1665, 1996.
6. Litovitz T, Manoguerra A: Comparison of pediatric poisoning hazards: an analysis of 3.8 million exposure incidents. A report from the American Association of Poison Control Centers. Pediatrics 89(6 Pt 1):999–1006, 1993.
7. Emery D, Singer JI: Highly toxic ingestions for toddlers: when a pill can kill. Pediatr Emerg Med Rep 3(12):111–119, 1998.
8. Shannon M: Ingestion of toxic substances by children. N Engl J Med 342:186–191, 2000.
*9. Bar-Oz B, Levichek Z, Koren G: Medications that can be fatal for a toddler with one tablet or teaspoonful: a 2004 update. Pediatr Drugs 6(2):123–126, 2004.
10. Gupta S, Taneja V: Poisoned child: emergency room management. Indian J Pediatr 70(Suppl 1):S2–S8, 2003.
11. Henretig FM: Special considerations in the poisoned pediatric patient. Emerg Med Clin North Am 12:549–567, 1994.
12. Anderson BJ, Holford NG, Armishaw JC, et al: Predicting concentrations in children presenting with acetaminophen overdose. J Pediatr 135:290–295, 1999.
13. Hoffman RS, Smilkstin MJ, Howland MA, et al: Osmol gaps revisited: normal values and limitations. Clin Toxicol 31:81–93, 1993.
14. Ashbourne JF, Olson KR, Khayam-Bashi H: Value of rapid screening for acetaminophen in all patients with intentional drug overdose. Ann Emerg Med 18:1035–1038, 1989.
*15. Belson MG, Simon HK, Sullivan K, Geller RJ: The utility of toxicologic analysis in children with suspected ingestions. Pediatr Emerg Care 15:383–387, 1999.
16. Liebelt EL, Francis PD, Woolf AD: ECG lead aVR versus QRS interval in predicting seizures and arrhythmias in acute tricyclic antidepressant overdose. Ann Emerg Med 18:348–351, 1989.
17. Traub SJ, Hoffman RS, Nelson LS: Body packing—the internal concealment of illicit drugs. N Engl J Med 349:2519–2526, 2003.
18. Liebelt EL, DeAngelis CD: Evolving trends and treatment advances in pediatric poisoning. JAMA 282:1113–1115, 1999.
19. Riordan M, Rylance G, Berry K: Poisoning in children: general management. Arch Dis Child 87:392–396, 2002.
20. American Academy of Clinical Toxicology, European Association of Poisons Centres and Clinical Toxicologist: Position statement: ipecac syrup. Clin Toxicol 35:699–709, 1997.
*21. Pond SM, Lewis-Driver DJ, William GM, et al: Gastric emptying in acute overdose: a prospective randomized controlled trial. Med J Aust 163:345–349, 1995.
22. American Academy of Clinical Toxicology, European Association of Poisons Centres and Clinical Toxicologist: Position statement: gastric lavage. Clin Toxicol 35:711–719, 1997.
23. Tenenbein M, Cohen S, Sitar DS: Whole bowel irrigation as a decontamination procedure after acute drug overdose. Arch Intern Med 147:905–907, 1987.
*24. Liebelt EL: Newer antidotal therapies for pediatric poisonings. Clin Pediatr Emerg Med 1:234–243, 2000.
25. Pond SM: Extracorporeal techniques in the treatment of poisoned patients. Med J Aust 154:617–622, 1991.
26. Blackman K, Brown SF, Wilkes GJ: Plasma alkalinization for tricyclic antidepressant toxicity: a systematic review. Emerg Med 13:204–210, 2001.
27. McKinney PE, Rasmussen R: Reversal of severe tricyclic antidepressant-induced cardiotoxicity with intravenous hypertonic saline solution. Ann Emerg Med 42:20–24, 2003.
28. Clark RF, Wethern-Kestner S, Vance MV, et al: Clinical presentation and treatment of black widow spider envenomation: a review of 163 cases. Ann Emerg Med 21:782–787, 1992.
29. Dart RC, Seifert SA, Boyer LV, et al: A randomized multicenter trial of Crotalidae Polyvalent Immune Fab (ovine) antivenom for the treatment for crotaline snakebite in the United States. Arch Intern Med 161:2030–2036, 2001.

*Selected readings.

30. Lavonas EJ, Gerardo CJ, O'Malley J, et al: Initial experience with Crotalidae Polyvalent Immune Fab (ovine) antivenom in the treatment of copperhead snakebite. Ann Emerg Med 43:200–206, 2004.

31. Graudins A, Stearman A, Chan B: Treatment of the serotonin syndrome with cyproheptadine. J Emerg Med 16:615–619, 1998.

32. Meythaler JM, Roper JF, Brunner RC: Cyproheptadine for intrathecal baclofen withdrawal. Arch Phys Med Rehabil 84:638–642, 2003.

33. Woolf AD, Wenger T, Smith TW, et al: The use of digoxin-specific Fab fragments for severe digitalis intoxication in children. N Engl J Med 326:1739–1744, 1992.

34. Brent J, McMartin K, Phillips S, et al: Fomepizole for the treatment of ethylene glycol poisoning. N Engl J Med 340:832–838, 1999.

35. White CM: A review of potential cardiovascular uses of intravenous glucagon administration. J Clin Pharmacol 39:442–447, 1999.

36. Yuan TH, Kerns WP, Tomaszewski CA, et al: Insulin-glucose as adjunctive therapy for severe calcium channel antagonist poisoning. J Toxicol Clin Toxicol 37:463–474, 1999.

*37. Boyer EW, Duic PA, Evans A: Hyperinsulinemia/euglycemia therapy for calcium channel blocker poisoning. Pediatr Emerg Care 18:36–37, 2002.

38. Boyle PJ, Justice K, Krentz AJ: Octreotide reverses hyperinsulinemia and prevents hypoglycemia induced by sulfonylurea overdoses. J Clin Endocrinol Metab 76:752–756, 1993.

39. Krentz AJ, Boyle PJ, Justice KM: Successful treatment of severe refractory sulfonylurea-induced hypoglycemia with octreotide. Diabetes Care 16:184–186, 1993.

*40. Burns MJ, Linden CH, Graudins A, et al: A comparison of physostigmine and benzodiazepines for the treatment of anticholinergic poisoning. Ann Emerg Med 35:374–381, 2000.

Chapter 11

Altered Mental Status/Coma

Joseph J. Zorc, MD

Key Points

The approach to a child with altered mental status requires an organized and prioritized process of stabilization, assessment, differential diagnosis, and definitive management.

In a patient with altered mental status, inability to provide a history or cooperate with assessment mandates a detailed physical examination with a particular focus on vital signs and neurologic examination.

Reversible causes of altered mental status such as hypoglycemia and opiate ingestion should be immediately identified and treated prior to further tests or interventions.

Multiple diagnostic tests may be indicated in the evaluation of a child with altered mental status. Consideration should be given to the appropriate sequence of tests based on suspicion of a focal central nervous system process versus a systemic process.

Introduction and Background

Altered mental status in a child is a particularly challenging clinical problem for an emergency physician. At initial presentation, the etiology is frequently unclear, and potential impairment of airway, breathing, and circulation requires a rapid and focused assessment. Reversible causes such as hypoglycemia and opioid ingestion need to be identified and treated prior to other procedures. History and physical examination are important and may provide key clues, but may be limited by the inability of the patient to cooperate with the evaluation. The differential diagnosis of a child with altered mental status is extensive and ranges in severity from self-limited processes requiring brief supportive care to life-threatening causes requiring aggressive intervention. Medications such as sedatives for radiographic tests or paralytics for intubation may interfere with later assessment and need to be considered carefully. For these reasons, an altered mental status requires a structured, ordered approach to evaluation and management.

Recognition and Approach

Altered mental status occurs when the ability of a child to arouse and interact with the external environment differs from normal. Abnormality in mental status must be interpreted in the context of normal stages of childhood development as well as the baseline functioning of the specific patient being evaluated. Careful assessment and documentation of the degree of alteration is important to identify changes in mental status over time. Terms for depressed mental status are often used loosely, although specific definitions over the spectrum of abnormality have been classically described.[1] *Confusion* is a state in which cognitive abilities are slowed and impaired. *Delirium* represents an increased level of disability with disordered thinking, delusion, and often agitated behavior. *Obtundation* is a state in which the patient is less alert and disinterested in the environment. *Stupor* is a further progression in which stimulation is required to obtain arousal. *Coma* is the end point on the spectrum in which the patient does not respond to stimulation. While these terms are often used to describe infants and children with an altered mental status, it is helpful for clinicians to describe the exact nature of the abnormal behavior and to attempt to apply objective descriptors or rating scales to their behavior.

Descriptive scales that numerically rate components of consciousness, such as eye opening, verbal, and motor activity, have been developed. One such example is the Glasgow Coma Scale (GCS).[2] Although originally developed for use after head injury, the GCS has been applied widely as a quantitative measure of altered mental status, and adaptations are available for preverbal children (Table 11–1).[3,4] Although useful in research and in the clinical setting to document trends in progression of symptoms over time, the reliability and validity of the GCS for use in the acute setting has been questioned.[5] Little information exists about the use of the GCS in young children. The GCS should be used as a supplement to a more detailed assessment and descriptive documentation of alteration in mental status.

The approach to a patient with altered mental status is typically dichotomized into two broad categories of etiology: disturbances localized within the central nervous system and systemic disorders (Table 11–2). Mass lesions within the central nervous system, such as tumor or hematoma, may be

Table 11–1	Glasgow Coma Scale (GCS) with Adaptations for Preverbal Children*		
Eye Opening	**Best Motor Response**	**Best Verbal Response**	
0–1 yr	**0–1 yr**	**0–2 yr**	
Spontaneous (4)	Spontaneous movement (6)	Normal cry, coos, smiles (5)	
To shout (3)	Localizes pain (5)	Cries (4)	
To pain (2)	Flexion withdrawal (4)	Inappropriate cry, screams (3)	
No response (1)	Flexor posturing (3)	Grunts (2)	
	Extensor posturing (2)	No response (1)	
	No response (1)		
>1 yr	**>1 yr**	**2–5 yr**	
Spontaneous (4)	Spontaneous movement (6)	Appropriate words (5)	
To verbal (3)	Localizes pain (5)	Inappropriate words (4)	
To pain (2)	Flexion withdrawal (4)	Cries or screams (3)	
No response (1)	Flexor posturing (3)	Grunts (2)	
	Extensor posturing (2)	No response (1)	
	No response (1)		
		>5 yr	
		Oriented (5)	
		Disoriented conversation (4)	
		Inappropriate words (3)	
		Incomprehensible, moans (2)	
		No response (1)	

*GCS scores ranges from 3 (worst) to 15 (best).

Table 11–2	Differential Diagnosis of Altered Mental Status

Central Nervous System Disturbances

Trauma
   Mass lesion (epidural, subdural, intracerebral hematoma)
   Diffuse or localized cerebral edema
   Cerebral contusion
Tumors (often with hemorrhage)
Hydrocephalus
Circulation disorders
   Cerebrovascular accident
   Cerebral venous thrombosis
Infection/inflammation
   Meningitis
   Encephalitis
   Cerebral abscess
   Subdural empyema
   Cerebritis
Seizure
   Subclinical status epilepticus
   Postictal state

Systemic Disorders

Hypoxemia
Hypo/hyperthermia
Hypoglycemia
Endocrine disorders
   Diabetic ketoacidosis
   Addisonian crisis
   Thyrotoxicosis, hypothyroidism
Electrolyte disorders: sodium, potassium, calcium, magnesium
Hepatic encephalopathy/Reye's syndrome
Uremic encephalopathy/hemolytic-uremic syndrome
Inborn errors of metabolism
Exogenous toxins
   Opiates
   Barbiturates/benzodiazepines
   Anticonvulsants: carbamazepine, phenytoin, valproic acid
   Organophosphate poisoning
   Anticholinergics: atropine, tricyclic antidepressants, phenothiazines
   Lead
   Metabolic acidosis ("MUDPILES")
     Methanol
     Uremia
     Paraldehyde
     Isoniazid, iron
     Lactic acidosis: carbon monoxide, cyanide
     Ethanol, ethylene glycol
     Salicylates
Systemic infection
   Sepsis
   Toxin-producing (e.g., *Shigella*)
Strangulated or herniated bowel
   Intussusception
   Volvulus

Adapted from Green M: Coma. *In* Pediatric Diagnosis, 6th ed. Philadelphia: WB Saunders, 1998, pp 338–345.

further subdivided into supra- and subtentorial based on the location of the lesion relative to the tentorium cerebelli, the dural fold that divides the anterior from the posterior fossa. This anatomy has clinical relevance because the midbrain at the level of the tentorium contains the reticular activating system, the network of neurons passing from spinal cord and brainstem to the cerebral cortex that plays a key role in maintaining consciousness. Mass lesions can compress this area and cause altered mental status, often accompanied by focal neurologic findings in nearby cranial nerves. In contrast, abnormalities causing altered mental status at the level of the cerebral cortex affect the brain diffusely through reduced delivery of a necessary substrate, effects of a toxin, or other widespread neuronal injury. The presence of focal findings may suggest a structural central nervous system lesion, although this is not entirely reliable as some systemic processes (e.g., hypoglycemia) may present with asymmetric findings.

Clinical Presentation

Evaluation of a child with altered mental status begins with a rapid assessment of airway, breathing, and circulation. Since unrecognized trauma is a concern, airway stabilization should be accomplished with manual stabilization of the cervical spine in the midline; a jaw thrust and other airway adjuncts such as a nasopharyngeal or oral airway may be useful depending upon the level of consciousness of the patient (see Chapter 2, Respiratory Distress and Respiratory Failure). Assessment of breathing, provision of 100% oxygen, and circulatory assessment of pulses, perfusion, and cardiac rhythm with continuous monitoring should follow.

A rapid determination of the level of consciousness should proceed while intravenous access is being obtained. A useful first assessment is guided by the acronym AVPU: *a*lert at baseline, requires *v*erbal stimuli to arouse, requires *p*ainful stimuli, or *u*nresponsive to painful stimuli. More formal assessment and documentation of the level of unconsciousness by description and numerical GCS can follow.

Diagnostic evaluation begins with measurement of serum glucose using a bedside glucometer. Conservative guidelines suggest that blood glucose concentrations below 40 mg/dl should be considered abnormal at any age; blood glucose concentration between 40 and 50 mg/dl require further evaluation at any age, but may possibly be normal in neonates; and blood glucose concentrations below 60 mg/dl beyond early infancy should be considered borderline, with further evaluation required. Inaccuracies of bedside glucose meters should be taken into account when determining whether to undertake further evaluation and treatment for hypoglycemia. Some texts actually recommend a trial of empirical treatment with glucose in patients with unknown coma for levels as high as 80 to 100 mg/dl, but individual circumstances must be accounted for.[6] Glucose can be given according to the "rule of 50," whereby the product of the volume (ml/kg) and the concentration of the glucose solution should be 50 (e.g., 2 ml/kg of 25% dextrose or 5 ml/kg of 10% dextrose). Common causes of hypoglycemia that may lead to altered mental status in a child are discussed more fully elsewhere (see Chapter 106, Hypoglycemia). Ketotic (starvation) hypoglycemia, sepsis, inborn errors of metabolism, and ingestions of ethanol or oral hypoglycemic agents are among the more common causes in children.[7]

Nalaxone should be administered to all patients with an altered mental status of unknown etiology or suspected opioid overdose. The clinician should not rely on the presence of pupillary constriction (miosis) to diagnose opioid overdose since meperidine, pentazocine, diphenoxylate/atropine (Lomotil), propoxyphene, and drug-induced hypoxia and co-ingestants may cause pupillary dilation (mydriasis). The empirical dose of naloxone is now recommended at 0.01 mg/kg intravenously. Give a subsequent dose of 0.1 mg/kg if there is an inadequate response. Use intramuscularly, subcutaneously or via endotracheal tube if the intravenous route is not available. Larger doses may be required for certain ingestions (e.g., diphenoxylate atropine [Lomotil], methadone, propoxyphene, pentazocine, fentanyl derivatives, and certain forms of heroin [black tar]). If a response is observed, the patient should be monitored closely with consideration for a naloxone infusion as the half-life of many ingested agents is longer than the 60- to 90-minute effect of naloxone.[8] Unlike adults, in whom withdrawal may be a concern, trial of an empirical dose of naloxone has little potential for adverse effects in children and may also produce a partial response in other situations such as clonidine overdose or intussusception (see discussion later). Other reversal agents, such as the benzodiazepine antagonist flumazenil, should not be given empirically in unknown cases due to the risk of seizure or interaction with other potential ingestions.[9] This agent should be reserved for situations in which an overdose of benzodiazepine alone is established, as in an iatrogenic overdose. Other agents typically administered empirically to adults, such as thiamine, are also generally not required in children.

The history should begin with a focused review of allergies, medications for the child or others in the household, and prior medical history. A thorough review of events leading up to the onset of symptoms should follow and may be best obtained by another clinician not involved in the acute stabilization. Frequently the caregiver most familiar with these events may not have accompanied the child, and reaching this person by telephone may provide key information. In particular, recent history of trauma and symptoms of infection or increased intracranial pressure should always be suspected. Many pediatric ingestions occur in new environments where the normal exploratory behavior of young children places them in contact with unsecured toxins; this may point toward a toxicologic cause.

Physical examination should begin with obtaining vital signs. Patterns of abnormalities in vital signs accompanying other clinical findings may indicate a "toxidrome" associated with classes of toxic ingestions (see Chapter 10, General Approach to Poisoning) that may be helpful in establishing a diagnosis. Cushing's triad is a classic pattern of bradycardia, bradypnea, and hypertension that has been described in association with elevated intracranial pressure. Patterns of abnormal respiration have also been described with various states of altered mental status. The Cheyne-Stokes variation is an alternation of deep and shallow breathing usually associated with metabolic encephalopathy. Central hyperventilation and "apneustic" inspiratory pauses have been described with various brainstem lesions.[1] The presence of fever may indicate an infection, exogenous heat exposure, and other potential diagnoses (e.g., thryotoxicosis; ingestion of salicylate or sympathomimetic or anticholinergic agents). Hypothermia may be associated with cold exposure or metabolic abnormalities such as hyponatremia. Hypertension may also cause altered mental status in the setting of hypertensive crisis (see Chapter 65, Hypertensive Emergencies). However, hypertension may also be a compensatory response to elevated intracranial pressure, in which case treatment of the primary process is indicated as a priority to maintain cerebral perfusion pressure.[10]

In summary, physical findings may provide important clues to a definitive diagnosis of altered mental status in children (Table 11-3).

Neurologic Examination

A thorough neurologic examination can aid in narrowing the differential diagnosis. In particular, the cranial nerves are of importance, as the nuclei of these nerves are located close to the reticular activating system in the brainstem and may indicate dysfunction due to a focal mass lesion compressing this area. Pupillary findings also aid in identifying the cause of altered mental status. Pupils can be small or mid-sized and symmetrically reactive in metabolic coma (e.g., hypoglycemia, encephalitis, ethanol poisoning). Constricted pupils may be seen with opioid ingestion, although some reactivity usually remains on close examination. Central lesions in the pons can also cause bilaterally constricted pupils. Asymmetrically reactive pupils should raise concern for a focal mass lesion unless there is a history of eye trauma or direct exposure to a mydriatic agent (e.g., ipratropium). Horner's syndrome occurs when there is injury to the hypothalamus or sympathetic chain nerves, resulting in a small but usually reactive pupil (miosis) associated with ptosis and anhidrosis.

Herniation syndromes are a constellation of findings that are the end result of significant elevation in intracranial pressure (see Chapter 42, Conditions Causing Increased Intracranial Pressure). The "uncal syndrome" occurs when the uncus, the medial part of the temporal lobe, herniates through the tentorium due to elevated pressure superiorly, causing compression of the oculomotor nerve and a unilateral dilated and fixed pupil, usually on the side of the mass lesion. Progression of elevated pressure on one side or symmetric elevation of intracranial pressure due to diffuse swelling or hydrocephalus can cause central herniation with bilateral pupillary and occulomotor impairment as well as decerebrate extensor

Table 11–3	Physical Clues to the Diagnosis of Infants and Children with Altered Mental Status*
Physical Finding	**Diagnosis**
Hypotension	• Any disease causing hypotension can directly cause an altered mental status (e.g., bleeding, sepsis, trauma) • Toxins: antihypertensive agents (e.g., β-blockers, calcium channel blockers), barbiturates, benzodiazepines, clonidine overdose (late), cyanide poisoning (late), narcotics
Hypertension	• Intracranial bleed • Intracranial mass • Hypertensive encephalopathy • Eclampsia • Postictal state • Hypoglycemia • Toxins: agents causing neuroleptic malignant syndrome and serotonin syndrome, clonidine overdose (early), cyanide poisoning (early), monoamine oxidase inhibitors, phencyclidine, sympathomimetics
Hyperthermia	• Meningitis • Encephalitis • Early sepsis • Malignant hyperthermia or neuroleptic malignant syndrome • Toxins: anticholinergics, nerve agents/gases (Sarin, Soman, Tabun, VX gas, Substance 33), organophosphates, sympathomimetics
Hypothermia	• Adrenal insufficiency, crisis • Prolonged hypoglycemia • Hypothyroidism • Sepsis (late) • Environmental exposure to cold • Toxins: barbiturates, benzodiazepines, hypoglycemic agents, or any toxin that causes patients to be immobilized and hypometabolic for prolonged periods
Tachycardia	Nonspecific and can occur with most diseases
Bradycardia	• Impending brainstem herniation • Respiratory failure of any etiology • Cardiac disorders • Toxins: β-blockers, calcium channel blockers, clonidine, cyanide, digoxin, γ-hydroxybutyrate (GHB), opioids, organophosphates
Tachypnea	• Metabolic acidosis from any cause • Toxins: isoniazid, nicotine, salicylates, theophylline, toxic alcohols
Bradypnea	• Respiratory failure of any etiology • Toxins: benzodiazepines, botulinum, GHB, narcotics, sedative-hypnotics
Diaphoresis	• Meningitis • Encephalitis • Sepsis • Toxins: nerve agents/gases (Sarin, Soman, Tabun, VX gas, Substance 33), organophophates, sympathomimetics
Mydriasis (bilateral)	• Toxins: anticholinergics, antihistamines, drug withdrawal, GHB, nerve agents/gases, organophosphates, and sympathomimetics rarely cause mydriasis when nicotinic effects exceed muscarinic effects
Miosis	• Pontine bleed or stroke • Coma from benzodiazepine, barbiturate or ethanol • Toxins: anticholinesterase, clonidone, narcotics, nicotine
Abdominal pain or rectal bleeding	• Intussuception • Volvulus • Strangulated or herniated bowel • Toxins: iron
Seizure	• Hypoxia • Hypoglycemia from any cause • Intracranial mass, bleed, or infection • Toxins: all drugs causing hypoxia, anticholinergics, antidepressants, amphetamines, baclofen, β-blockers, camphor, carbamazepine, carbon monoxide, cocaine, cyanide, ethanol withdrawal, GHB, hypoglycemic agents, isoniazid, lidocaine, lindane, lithium, meperidine, propoxyphene, phencyclidine, salicylates, sympathomimetics, theophylline, water hemlock plant

*List is not all inclusive.

posturing. Compression of the brainstem leads to altered respiratory and cardiovascular status and death. Other patterns of herniation occur elsewhere in the cranium, including across the midline falx cerebri or at the level of the brainstem into the foramen magnum. The presence of an open fontanelle in a young child may provide evidence of increased intracranial pressure but does not eliminate the risk of brain herniation from one compartment to another. Evidence of herniation calls for aggressive management of intracranial pressure with mannitol and emergent neurosurgical evalua-

tion (see Chapter 9, Cerebral Resuscitation). Recent evidence suggests that 3% saline may be useful in management of intracranial hypertension.[11] Since intracranial pressure rises dramatically once compensatory responses in the brain have been overcome, even small interventions to reduce intracranial volume may be effective. Controlled hyperventilation can reduce intracranial pressure in emergent situations by reducing cerebral blood flow, although this may have detrimental results if used for prolonged periods beyond the goal of a partial pressure of CO_2 of 35 mm Hg.[12]

Other important findings on neurologic examination include an assessment of tone, reflexes, and motor activity to detect seizure activity. Subclinical status epilepticus can be a cause of altered mental status. Decorticate posturing with flexion of the arms and extension of the legs may accompany lesions in the cerebral hemispheres.[1] Decerebrate extensor posturing of the arms and legs usually indicates dysfunction at the level of the midbrain or cerebellum or, alternatively, severe metabolic dysfunction. Funduscopic examination should be performed to detect retinal hemorrhages associated with shaken infant syndrome; papilledema may indicate long-standing increased intracranial pressure, although it is not a reliable early finding after an acute insult. Brainstem control of eye movements can be assessed with a "doll's-eye" maneuver of the head or cold caloric testing, although these interventions are not usually indicated during the initial assessment in the emergency department. The remainder of the physical examination involves a thorough head-to-toe secondary survey looking for subtle skin findings such as bruising or rash, abdominal mass associated with intussusception, or other abnormalities. Odors on the breath or in the urine may be indicative of diabetic ketoacidosis, ethanol ingestion, or various metabolic derangements. Psychogenic causes of coma due to conversion reaction or other causes are uncommon in children and typically can be identified on examination by the presence of voluntary responses such as resistance to movement or withdrawal from noxious stimuli.

Differential Diagnosis

The differential diagnosis of altered mental status is broad and may be organized in several ways. Categorization of physical findings into central nervous system versus systemic (see Table 11–2) is helpful from a pathophysiologic standpoint, although a mnemonic device may be most useful in the acute setting to ensure that all important diagnoses have been considered (Table 11–4). Vascular abnormalities causing altered mental status are uncommon in children and usually are associated with underlying chronic conditions such as sickle cell disease or prothrombotic states (see Chapter 44, Central Nervous System Vascular Disorders). Infection can alter mental status through direct involvement of the central nervous system from a variety of viral, bacterial, fungal, or parasitic causes (see Chapter 43, Central Nervous System Infections). Infections outside of the central nervous system can alter mental status via systemic effects or toxins produced by organisms such as the Shiga toxin from *Shigella*. Toxicologic causes of altered mental status are diverse and

are more fully discussed elsewhere (see Chapter 10, General Approach to Poisoning). Clues to presence of a toxic ingestion include the presence of clinical toxidromes such as bradycardia/bradypnea (opioid, sedative-hypnotic) or tachycardia/tachypnea (sympathomimetic, anticholinergic). Other findings such as the size of the pupils (usually small in opioid ingestions), the condition of the skin (dry in anticholinergic toxicity), or the presence of acidosis on laboratory evaluation can help to further specify the toxin involved.

Trauma can affect mental status by direct compression of the reticular activating system from an epidural or subdural hematoma with focal findings, or by intracerebral contusion, focal hemorrhage, or diffuse axonal injury (see Chapter 15, Trauma in Infants; and Chapter 17, Head Trauma). Epidural hematomas usually arise from injury to arterial vessels underlying a skull fracture; symptoms may progress rapidly to unconsciousness after an initial lucid period. Subdural hematomas are usually more indolent and may be a marker of diffuse axonal injury such as that seen in the shaken infant syndrome. These infants often appear to have a metabolic cause of altered mental status due to the nonfocal nature of the injury. If child abuse is suspected, a skeletal survey may identify occult injuries and assist with the diagnosis.

Metabolic causes of altered mental status are multiple and covered fully in Chapters 110 through 115. Young children are predisposed to hypoglycemia due to reduced glycogen stores that result in a risk for ketotic hypoglycemia with a prolonged fast. Absence of ketones in the urine in the setting of hypoglycemia should raise the concern of an inborn error of metabolism such as a fatty acid oxidation defect.[13] Inborn errors of metabolism typically present in newborns or in young infants at the time of an illness or when new foods are introduced, when catabolic processes fail and the body is unable to appropriately break down protein, fat, or carbohydrate. Inborn errors may require consultation with an endocrinology or metabolism specialist as well as detailed laboratory testing to make a complete diagnosis. Hepatomegaly or laboratory abnormalities such as hypoglycemia, hyperammonemia, and acidosis are clues to the presence of these disorders. Metabolic causes such as electrolyte abnormalities or hepatic, renal, or endocrine disorders will usually be detected on routine chemistry screening.

Infants with strangulated or incarcerated bowel (e.g., intussusception or volvulus) can present with lethargy. This unique presentation in infants and toddlers has been described in up to half of intussusception cases in one series.[14] These children are often initially considered to have systemic infections or toxic ingestions and often have significant delays in diagnosis and treatment.[15] The cause of altered mental status associated with intussusception is unclear. Case reports of reversal with naloxone indicate that this process may be mediated by the release of endogenous opioid substances in the gut[16] (see Chapter 74, Intussusception). Ruling out serious bowel disorders in a lethargic infant based on physical examination or plain radiographs may be difficult, and contrast or air enema, ultrasound, an upper gastrointestinal series, and/or surgical consultation may be required.[17]

Finally, other abnormalities in the central nervous system, such as intracranial mass lesions and hydrocephalus, should always be considered. Young infants with obstructive hydrocephalus may present with increased head circumference and

Table 11–4	VITAMINS Mnemonic for Altered Mental Status

Vascular: stroke, inflammatory cerebritis, migraine
Infection: meningitis, encephalitis, brain abscess, toxin-producing organism (e.g., *Shigella*)
Toxins
Accident/Abuse: traumatic epidural, subdural, or diffuse axonal injury
Metabolic: renal, hepatic, endocrine, electrolytes, inborn error
Intussusception
Neoplasm: tumor, hydrocephalus
Seizure: subclinical status epilepticus, postictal state

"sunsetting" of the eyes (paralysis of upward gaze) due to compression of the ocular nuclei. Various seizures may alter mental status during and following an ictal event. Generalized seizures often are accompanied by tonic-clonic activity, but subtle subclinical status epilepticus may require electroencephalography to make a definitive diagnosis. A seizure accompanied by a postictal state can be identified by the presence of an acidosis that clears rapidly. Empirical therapy with a benzodiazepine or other antiepileptic may be indicated if ongoing subclinical seizure is suspected. Absence seizures usually alter mental status for brief periods with return to baseline, as opposed to partial complex seizures, which usually are longer and may be followed by a postictal period. If a prolonged generalized tonic-clonic seizure has occurred, a postictal state may alter mental status for a period of several hours.

Management

Many potential etiologies can cause altered mental status, so an ordered process is required to organize diagnostic testing and management. If hypoglycemia and opioid ingestion have been ruled out, the next steps will be dictated by the depth of impairment and clues to the diagnosis on history and physical examination.[18] Multiple etiologies may occur simultaneously; for example, a postictal state may follow a seizure due to a toxic ingestion. For this reason, it is difficult to organize management into a simple algorithm. Investigation should be individualized, with multiple potential etiologies ruled out in parallel based on clinical judgment.

Initial laboratory tests are obtained after the secondary survey so that they can be processed while other examinations are being completed. Screening tests typically include serum electrolytes, renal and liver function tests, and a complete blood count. A venous blood gas determination of acid-base status/carboxyhemoglobin level may also be appropriate. Serum ammonia level may be considered if liver disease or an inborn error of metabolism is suspected. The laboratory evaluation should also include levels of any anticonvulsant medications prescribed or potentially ingested by the patient. Toxicology screens vary by institution, so it is important to be aware of what is being ordered. Utility in the acute setting varies greatly depending upon which test is ordered. Urine drugs of abuse screens are helpful in the initial evaluation to screen for opioids, barbiturates, cannabis, cocaine, amphetamines, phencyclidine, and benzodiazepines, although other important substances may be missed (e.g., some synthetic opiates, γ-hydroxybutyrate, lysergic acid diethylamide).[19] Serum toxicology screens include ethanol levels and may also include acetaminophen, salicylate, and other drugs that are appropriate for empirical testing. An electrocardiogram should be obtained if primary cardiac disease or a toxic ingestion is suspected.

Imaging of the brain is clearly indicated in altered mental status when there is a concern for an intracranial process (history of trauma, focal neurologic findings, signs of elevated intracranial pressure) or when the etiology is unknown. The usual initial study is computed tomography (CT) of the brain without contrast. Intravenous contrast can be added if tumor or an inflammatory process is suspected. CT may not identify posterior fossa masses, and further imaging may be required after the initial study.

Since imaging and other tests may require transport to another location, consideration should be given to the stability of the patient and the ability to protect the airway. The decision to control the airway should be individualized based on the patient's level of alertness, presence of airway reflexes, and expected course. If trauma is suspected, aggressive management should be considered, whereas self-limited processes such as seizure may require only monitoring and supportive care. Airway management should be performed under controlled circumstances with measures taken to avoid increases in intracranial pressure (see Chapter 3, Rapid Sequence Intubation). Short-acting sedatives and paralytics are preferred to allow for serial reassessment of mental status and neurologic examination.

For altered mental status due to suspected infection, the issue of when to obtain cerebrospinal fluid versus CT scan is controversial. Increased intracranial pressure from a mass lesion or obstruction of the ventricular system is a contraindication to lumbar puncture. Imaging is recommended prior to lumbar puncture for a patient with an undifferentiated cause of altered mental status, as clinical examination may not easily identify these contraindications.[20] In addition, some studies have described a temporal association between lumbar puncture and herniation in cases of severe meningitis, although the causal nature of this relationship is debated.[21] Imaging does not reliably predict marked elevation in intracranial pressure.[22] In general, when cerebrospinal fluid is obtained in a patient with altered mental status, caution is advised; close monitoring, measurement of cerebrospinal fluid pressure, and careful withdrawal of the minimal amount of fluid required with a small-bore needle are recommended. Empirical treatment with antibiotics should not be delayed for imaging or other procedures if intracranial infection is suspected.

If an etiology for altered mental status is still unclear after initial tests are completed, further tests for occult etiologies are appropriate. Since intussusception is difficult to rule out based on clinical findings, an ultrasound or barium enema may be indicated. Subclinical status epilepticus may require electroencephalographic monitoring for detection.[23] If this is not available, empirical treatment with anticonvulsant medications may be appropriate. It may not be possible to confirm encephalitis in the acute setting, and empirical treatment with intravenous acyclovir to treat herpes should be considered. In some cases no diagnosis can be made acutely, and supportive care can be provided with appropriate consultation with neurologists, toxicologists, or other consultants to further investigate other causes.

All of the above-mentioned measures can be incorporated into a general altered mental status management algorithm, although alternative management options should be tailored to the patient's presentation and the clinician's suspicion for specific disorders (Fig. 11–1).

Summary

Definitive management of a child with altered mental status will depend upon the etiology and the response to initial management. Patients with persistent symptoms or unclear etiology require hospitalization for close observation and specialty consultation. In many cases this will require admission to an intensive care unit. Prognosis of altered mental

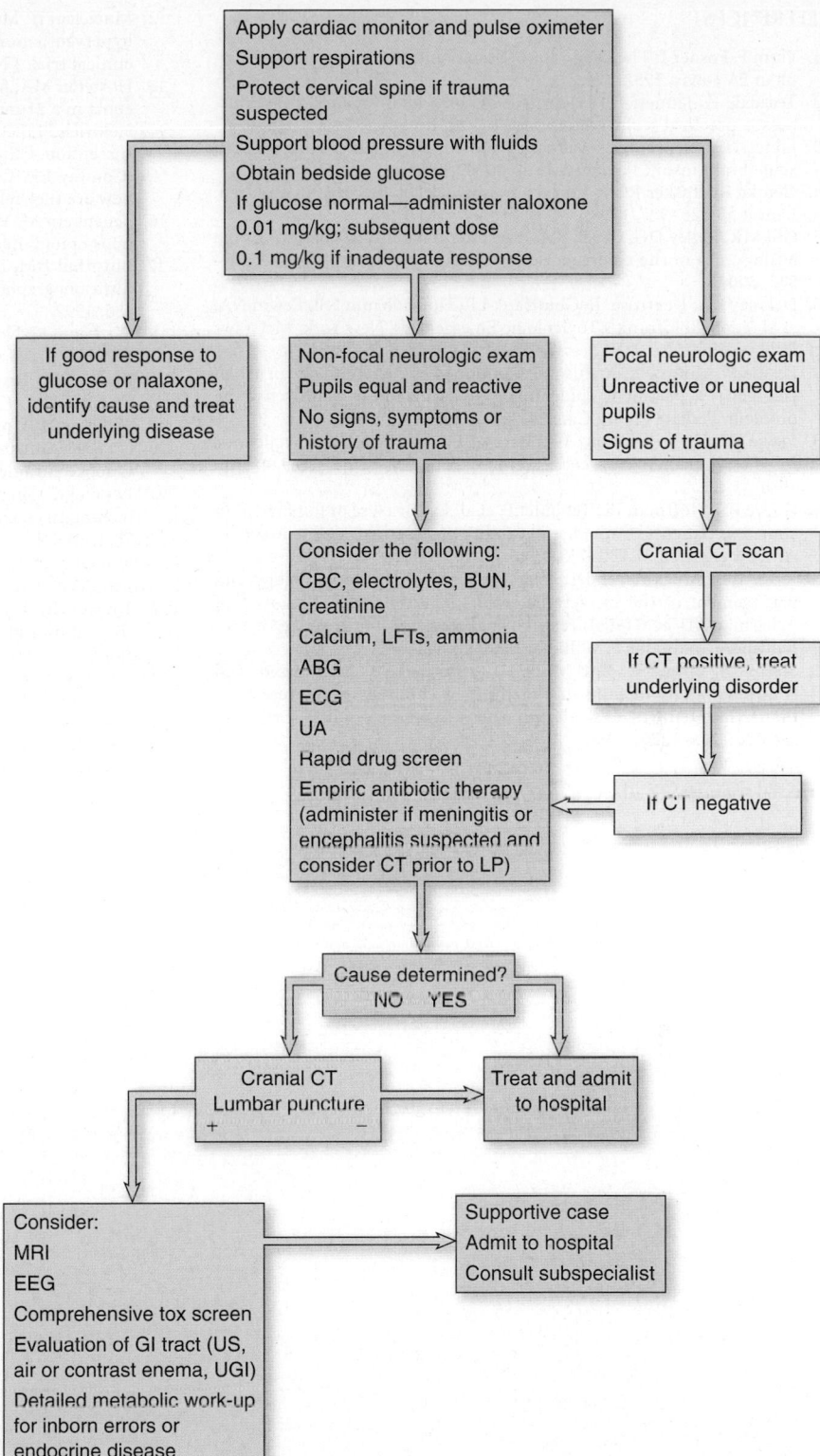

FIGURE 11–1. Approach to the infant or child with altered mental status of unknown cause. Abbreviations: ABG, arterial blood gases; BUN, blood urea nitrogen; CBC, complete blood count; CT, computed tomography; ECG, electrocardiogram; EEG, electroencephalogram; GI, gastrointestinal; LFT, liver function test; LP, lumbar puncture; MRI, magnetic resonance imaging; UA, urinalysis; US, ultrasound; UGI, upper gastrointestinal.

status varies widely based on the etiology; mortality ranges from 3% to 84% by diagnosis in children with nontraumatic coma.[24] The impression that young children recover more fully from coma than adults has been questioned as more detailed studies have explored cognitive outcomes in depth.[25]

Altered mental status in a child is a challenging clinical scenario for an emergency physician. With an organized process for evaluation and management, the physician should be able to detected and managed most causes effectively in the emergency department. Future research in this area will likely focus on improving descriptive scales for altered mental status in children and developing more accurate diagnostic testing and treatments for the multiple potential causes of altered mental status.

REFERENCES

*1. Plum F, Posner J: The Diagnosis of Stupor and Coma, 3rd ed. Philadelphia: FA Davis, 1982.

2. Teasdale G, Jennett B: Assessment of coma and impaired consciousness: a practical scale. Lancet 2:81–84, 1974.

3. James HE: Neurologic evaluation and support in the child with an acute brain insult. Pediatr Ann 15:16–22, 1986.

4. Gemke RJ, Tasker RC: Clinical assessment of acute coma in children. Lancet 35:926–927, 1998.

*5. Gill MR, Reiley DG, Green SM: Interrater reliability of Glasgow Coma Scale scores in the emergency department. Ann Emerg Med 43:215–223, 2004.

6. Delaney KA: Dextrose. *In* Goldfrank LR, Flomenbaum NE, Lewin NA, et al (eds): Goldfrank's Toxicologic Emergencies. New York: McGraw-Hill, pp 606–610.

7. Pershad J, Monroe K, Atchison J: Childhood hypoglycemia in an urban emergency department: epidemiology and a diagnostic approach to the problem. Pediatr Emerg Care 14:268–271, 1998.

8. Lewis JM, Klein-Schwartz W, Benson BE, et al: Continuous naloxone infusion in pediatric narcotic overdose. Am J Dis Child 138:944–946, 1984.

9. Gueye PN, Hoffman JR, Taboulet P, et al: Empiric use of flumazenil in comatose patients: limited applicability of criteria to define low risk. Ann Emerg Med 27:730–735, 1996.

*10. Poss WB, Brockmeyer DL, Clay B, Dean JM: Pathophysiology and management of the intracranial vault. *In* Rogers MC, Nichols DG, Ackerman AD, et al (eds): Textbook of Pediatric Intensive Care, 3rd ed. Baltimore: Williams & Wilkins, 1996, pp 645–665.

11. Simma B, Burger R, Falk M, et al: A prospective, randomized, and controlled study of fluid management in children with severe head injury: lactated Ringer's solution versus hypertonic saline. Crit Care Med 26:1265–1270, 1998.

_____

*Selected readings.

12. Muizelaar JP, Marmarou A, Ward JD, et al: Adverse effects of prolonged hyperventilation in patients with severe head injury: a randomized clinical trial. J Neurosurg 75:731–739, 1991.

13. Hostetler MA, Arnold GL, Mooney R, et al: Hypoketotic hypoglycemic coma in a 21-month-old child. Ann Emerg Med 34:394–398, 1999.

14. Heldrich FJ: Lethargy as a presenting symptom in patients with intussusception. Clin Pediatr 25:363–365, 1986.

*15. Conway EE: Central nervous system findings and intussusception: how are they related? Pediatr Emerg Care 9:15–18, 1993.

16. Tenenbein M, Wiseman NE: Early coma in intussusception: endogenous opioid induced? Pediatr Emerg Care 3:22–23, 1987.

17. Bhisitkul DM, Listernick R, Shkolnik A, et al: Clinical application of ultrasonography in the diagnosis of intussusception. J Pediatr 121:182–186, 1992.

*18. Kirkham FJ: Non-traumatic coma in children. Arch Dis Child 85:303–312, 2001.

19. Rainey PM: Toxicology screening. *In* Goldfrank LR, Flomenbaum NE, Lewin NA, et al (eds): Goldfrank's Toxicologic Emergencies. New York: McGraw-Hill, pp 82–89.

20. Quality Standards Committee of the American Academy of Neurology: Practice parameters: lumbar puncture. Neurology 43:625–627, 1993.

21. Rennick G, Shann F, de Campo J: Cerebral herniation during bacterial meningitis in children. BMJ 306:953–955, 1993.

22. Shetty AK, Desselle BC, Craver RW, et al: Fatal cerebral herniation after lumbar puncture in a patient with a normal computed tomography scan. Pediatrics 103:1284–1287, 1999.

23. Towne AR, Waterhouse EJ, Boggs JG, et al: Prevalence of nonconvulsive status epilepticus in comatose patients. Neurology 54:340–345, 2000.

*24. Wong CP, Forsyth RJ, Kelly TP: Incidence, aetiology, and outcome of non-traumatic coma: a population based study. Arch Dis Child 84:193–199, 2001.

25. Forsyth RJ, Wong CP, Kelly TP, et al: Cognitive and adaptive outcomes and age at insult effects after non-traumatic coma. Arch Dis Child 84:200–204.

Chapter 12

Approach to Multisystem Trauma

Lance Brown, MD, MPH

Key Points

Mechanism of injury is a relatively poor predictor of injury severity.

An age-appropriate primary survey facilitates the physical examination and limits unnecessary testing.

Laboratory studies have minimal utility in the management of most traumatized children.

Computed tomograpic scanning is indispensable in evaluating children at risk for multisystem trauma.

Nonoperative management of selected intra-abdominal and intracranial injuries is now common.

Introduction and Background

Using an evidence-based approach to pediatric multisystem trauma care is problematic. Due to the absence of agreed-upon definitions for "pediatric" and "multisystem," various age thresholds for considering a subject "pediatric" exist. Development progresses at a somewhat different rate for each child. Authors of "pediatric" studies have included individuals who present to a children's hospital without a specific age threshold identified[1-3] and individuals younger than 21 years of age,[4] 19 years of age,[5] 18 years of age,[6-9] 16 years of age,[10-12] 15 years of age,[13,14] or 11 years of age.[15] The inclusion of both preverbal infants and physiologic adults in many of these studies weakens the validity of proposed conclusions regarding "pediatric" trauma.[16]

The term *multisystem* and synonyms such as "polytrauma" lack agreed-upon definitions. "Multisystem" most appropriately refers to multiple, serious injuries sustained by a single child following blunt trauma, or to whole-body blunt forces that place a child *at risk* for multiple internal injuries.[17] This may partially explain why many studies from the pediatric trauma literature focus on injuries to a single body region.[2,3,5-9,18-39] Unfortunately, many injuries are unlikely to be found in isolation, making uniform management recommendations difficult.

The management of children who have sustained multisystem trauma involves coordinated care among multiple specialists. These children not only require the unique skills of the emergency physician, but may also require care by an orthopedic surgeon, neurosurgeon, pediatric or general surgeon, otolaryngologist, plastic surgeon, maxillofacial surgeon, or urologist. Given the difficulties in developing an evidence-based understanding of pediatric multisystem trauma, conflicts regarding management may arise among these specialties. Although still evolving, the science of pediatric trauma care offers reasonable evidence on which physicians can base their diagnostic and management plans.

Recognition and Approach

To some extent, the unique anatomic and physiologic features of children and the mechanism of injury predispose children to specific injuries. Pedestrian motor vehicle trauma victims often have multiple injuries, including injuries to the head, thorax, and pelvis. Unrestrained motor vehicle occupants are at significant risk for head, face, and cervical injuries, while restrained passengers are at risk for cervical spine, lumbar spine, and solid and hollow organ injury. Additionally, seat belts, when used without a booster seat for children 4 to 9 years of age, increase the risk of bowel/bladder rupture or hematoma.[40] Bicyclists who are injured are at risk for head injury (especially if unhelmeted), upper extremity trauma, and handlebar injuries to the pancreas and bowel.[40] Falls from the second story of a building or higher increase the risk of head injury, with long-bone fractures increasing with falls from the third story, and thoracoabdominal injuries dramatically rising at the fifth story.[41]

Anatomic and physiologic developmental differences help to identify distinct injuries and responses to injury within different age groups. Head injuries are common in younger infants and children. The relatively larger size of an infant's head dramatically increases the risk that the skull will be involved in most blunt force mechanisms. The skull is relatively soft in infants and toddlers. Forces are more easily transmitted through a weaker, immature skull to soft developing neural tissue. Unlike older children, infants with open fontanelles and sutures may actually develop hypotensive shock due to intracranial bleeding. Unlike adults, children frequently develop intracranial hyperemia following head injury, which increases cerebral blood flow, intracranial blood volume, and intracranial pressure.[42]

Thoracoabdominal injuries are an important cause of mortality in infants and children, accounting for 10% to 20% of all trauma-related deaths.[43] The greater pliability of the thoracic cage in young children permits the ribs to be easily compressed without fracturing and without obvious external evidence of trauma. As a result, pulmonary contusions occur without rib fractures.[44] As the bony rib cage ossifies, fractures and obvious chest wall trauma become more common. Since the chest is relatively small compared to the head and abdomen of infants and young children, isolated thoracic trauma is uncommon. Solid abdominal organs are larger in children compared to adolescents and adults, increasing their propensity to be traumatized during blunt force injuries. Infants and young children have poorly developed abdominal muscles, a more protuberant abdomen, and less fatty insulation compared to adults, thus increasing their risk for injury during blunt trauma. The pediatric kidney retains fetal lobulations, leading to a higher risk for fracture. The spleen's capsule is relatively thicker at younger ages, allowing for an increased ability to contain traumatic splenic bleeding and improving the possibility that injuries can be managed nonoperatively. Importantly, the bladder is an abdominal organ in young children, increasing the possibility for injury following abdominal trauma.[40]

A child's smaller body leads to traumatic forces that are often distributed over a smaller body mass, increasing the number of systems injured during trauma. A larger relative surface area and increased metabolic rate promote hypothermia, complicating the management of shock. Physiologic characteristics account for important cardiopulmonary responses to injury. A smaller functional residual capacity and increased oxygen consumption account for an increased risk of respiratory failure with blunt thoracic trauma and hypovolemic shock. Infants and children more readily maintain a normal blood pressure with significant bleeding, compared to adults and adolescents. As much as 25% to 30% of circulating blood volume might be lost before hypotension develops. As blood loss occurs, increases in systemic vascular resistance and peripheral vasoconstriction makes vascular access difficult. Tachycardia is a poor marker for blood loss due to the significant variability with age, pain, temperature, and stress. Capillary refill time is often cited as a useful marker for blood loss and shock in children. However, this test is an unreliable marker for hypovolemia due to high interobserver variation, large fluctuations with environmental temperatures, and variability in measurement techniques and individual responses to hypovolemia.[40]

Evaluation

Injury severity occurs along a continuum from minimal injury to full traumatic arrest. At either end of the spectrum, the evaluation is typically straightforward. When a child has obviously sustained minimal injury or is uninjured, a focused history and physical examination followed by reassurance or some basic first aid (e.g., abrasion care) is all that is typically required. When confronted with a critically injured child, a protocol-driven assessment with attention to definitive airway management, prompt vascular access, and the performance of any invasive, potentially life-saving procedures is warranted. Few would question the ordering of any radiographic or laboratory test deemed potentially useful in this extreme situation. Although emotionally and technically challenging, the decision-making processes in these cases can be formulaic. In contrast, cases with intermediate acuity or concern for subtle injuries offer a much greater challenge for the experienced emergency physician. In these cases, selective diagnostic testing is indicated and decision making is fairly complex. For emergency physicians more familiar with the resuscitation of traumatized adults, there are some important differences between children and adults that may have a substantial impact on the trauma evaluation (Table 12–1). Decision making in pediatric trauma requires knowledge of child development and proper resource utilization with regard to prehospital triage, trauma team activation, laboratory tests, and radiographic tests.

The primary survey has been considered a critical element to proper trauma care.[45,46] Although this sequential approach of progressing through airway, breathing, circulation, disability, and exposure (the ABCDEs) is simple and has been advocated for decades, it has not been evaluated in children. Nonetheless, it has been explicitly stated that children should simply be treated the same as adults with regard to the primary survey.[45] Clinical experience suggests that applying this approach to the awake, alert, traumatized child may complicate, rather than facilitate, the evaluation and management. The typical approach involves donning masks and gowns, using loud voices, promptly applying monitoring devices, cutting clothing off, and promptly attempting intravenous line placement while keeping a child tied to a board and telling them to hold still. This can be unkind and decreases the likelihood of a meaningful physical examination. Without a meaningful physical examination, assessment of the child's mental status, abdomen, and spine are less reliable. Prolonged immobilization in a cervical collar on a hard board may lead to iatrogenic neck pain, back pain, and impaired respiratory capacity.[47,48] This, in turn, may lead to unnecessary sedation and radiologic testing. The classically implemented primary survey is likely to be effective and appropriate for evaluating the traumatized child with grossly altered mental status, or who is critically ill or comatose. An alternative approach may be more successful in evaluating awake, alert, traumatized children (Table 12–2). Although this has not been prospectively evaluated for safety and efficacy, this approach can be considered in patients who appear to be stable and have normal mental status.

Predictors of Serious Injury

Identifying predictors of serious injury is needed for the development of decision rules for prehospital triage and trauma team activation. These two events have the greatest impact on overall trauma resource utilization. For example, a simple decision rule to determine which children are likely to require services available only at a specialty pediatric trauma center would likely reduce unnecessary transport to those centers. Similarly, for children brought to specialty trauma centers, identification of those at high risk for needing prompt surgical intervention would result in better use of surgical consultation and avoid disruption of other important patient care activities outside the emergency department.

Although there are no completely reliable predictors of the need for care at a trauma center, knowledge of trauma scores and their limitations may be useful. The Pediatric Trauma Score (PTS) was initially developed as a tool to quickly deter-

Table 12–1	Common Pediatric Characteristics That Impact Trauma Presentation, Management, and Outcome
Characteristics	**Potential Impact on Trauma Care**
Heart rate	• Tachycardia is common and is not specific for bleeding or hypotension. • Bradycardia is a prearrest event often signifying shock or respiratory failure.
Blood pressure	• Up to 25–30% of blood volume may be lost before significant hypotension develops.
Head	• Open fontanelle and sutures can lead to significant uncontrolled bleeding and cause hypotension in young infants. • Hyperermia/vasodilation is common in children with head injury, compared to vasoconstriction/ischemia in adults.
Cervical spine	• Immature and flexible ligaments lead to false appearance of subluxation C2-3, and disparity in growth rates at C1-2 leads to false appearance of C1 burst fracture (pseudo-Jefferson's fracture). • The relatively large head means that centrifugal and rotational forces more commonly lead to trauma at C1 and C2 in children under 8 years, while C5-7 injuries are more common at or above this age.
Myocardium and coronary arteries	• Myocardium and coronary arteries are normal, with less risk for myocardial contusion.
Lungs and ribs	• Less functional residual capacity and higher oxygen consumption (1) increase the risk for respiratory failure with chest trauma and with shock and (2) lead to quicker desaturation during rapid sequence intubation and sedation. • Pliant ribs are less able to protect the liver and spleen during blunt trauma.
Blood vessels	• Pliability means fewer aortic and major vascular injuries resulting from blunt trauma.
Bones	• Immaturity results in fewer rib fractures, less obvious chest wall trauma with significant pulmonary injury, and unique growth plate injuries.
Sold abdominal organs	• Relatively larger size, less fat insulation, and less well-developed abdominal muscles increase risk of blunt traumatic injury.
Kidneys	• Kidneys retain fetal lobulations and are less protected by location and musculature, increasing risk of fracture.
Spleen	• Relatively thicker capsule at younger ages may decrease risk for rupture and increase probability of successful nonoperative management.
Stomach	• More distended and less protected within the abdomen, increasing the propensity to perforation or respiratory compromise.
Bowel	• Small bowel is prone to injury, typically in 4- to 9-year-olds, with seat belt that encircles abdomen instead of pelvis.
Bladder	• Abdominal structure in the very young is more likely to rupture with blunt force.

Table 12–2	Suggested Principles for a Modified Evaluation of the Awake, Alert, Traumatized Child

- Number of individuals at the bedside can be minimized (one emergency physician and one nurse is ideal).
- Quiet voices should be used at all times.
- No commands should be directed at the child.
- Attachment of monitors to the child may be delayed if deemed appropriate by the emergency physician.
- Cutting off clothes may be deferred at the discretion of the emergency physician.
- All explanations provided to the child should be age appropriate.
- Analgesia should be provided as soon as possible.
- Techniques such as distraction should be used to calm the child as needed.
- Mental status should be continually assessed by having a conversation with the child.
- Removal of the cervical collar should take place safely but expeditiously.
- Removal from the spinal board should take place as soon as possible.
- Parents and guardians should be allowed to come to the bedside as soon as possible.

Table 12–3	Pediatric Trauma Score		
	Score		
Patient Feature	**+2**	**+1**	**−1**
Weight (kg)	>20	10–20	<10
Airway	Patent	Maintainable	Nonmaintainable
Systolic blood pressure (mm Hg)	>90	50–90	<50
Mental status	Awake	Obtunded	Comatose
Open wound	None	Minor	Major
Extremity fracture	None	Closed	Open or multiple

mine the need to transport children to a trauma center[49] (Table 12–3). Initial studies found that children with a PTS less than 0 had 100% mortality, those with a PTS of 1 to 4 had 40% mortality, those with a PTS of 5 to 8 had 7% mortality, and those with a PTS greater than 8 had virtually no mortality following trauma.[50,51] Based on these data, a PTS less than 8 is the recommended threshold for diverting children to a designated pediatric or adult trauma center.[49] The Revised Trauma Score (used in adults) is as accurate as the PTS for determining injury severity and is a better predictor of overall outcome in pediatric trauma[52 54] (Table 12–4). Supporters of the RTS believe it is easier to calculate and allows for a single score to be used by prehospital personnel for all ages.[52-54] An RTS less than 12 is the recommended threshold for diverting a child to a trauma center.[51] While the RTS and the PTS can stratify the risk of deterioration following trauma, it is important to note that children with isolated abdominal injuries may manifest initial vital sign stability and relatively normal trauma scores. Up to 86% of children with isolated spleen and liver trauma have a normal heart rate, 94% have a normal systolic blood pressure, and most have a PTS above 10,[55] signifying the limitations of trauma

Table 12–4	Revised Trauma Score		
Revised Trauma Score*	Glasgow Coma Scale Score	Systolic Blood Pressure (mm Hg)	Respiratory Rate (breaths/min)
4	13–15	>89	>29
3	9–12	76–89	10–29
2	6–8	50–75	6–9
1	4–5	1–49	1–5
0	3	0	0

*Add total points (0 to 4) for each category to obtain score.

scoring in identifying children who potentially require trauma center care.

There is a growing body of evidence that some of the traditionally accepted predictors of injury severity do not effectively risk-stratify traumatized children. Although frequently cited and historically relied upon, mechanism of injury tends to be a relatively poor predictor of injury severity. Still, published trauma team activation criteria include various mechanisms of injury.[13,56-59] These mechanisms typically include falls from a height greater than 3 to 6 m (10 to 20 feet), rollover motor vehicle accidents, pedestrian struck at greater than 16 to 32 km/hr (10 to 20 miles/hr), passenger ejection from the vehicle, death of a co-occupant of the same vehicle, and the need for a extrication from the vehicle lasting longer than 20 minutes.[13,54,55,60-62] These mechanisms have a certain degree of intuitive appeal; however, there is building evidence that they do not accurately predict serious injuries.[13,15,56,58,61-64] In addition, there is also a risk of false histories. It has been suggested that, if a short vertical fall is offered as the mechanism of injury and the child has sustained a serious injury, the history is most likely false[15,61] (see Chapter 119, Physical Abuse and Child Neglect). This concept that the mechanism of injury alone fails to predict serious injury is also supported by studies of adults.[58,65-69]

However, there is one mechanism of injury that is predictive of specific intra-abdominal injuries. A "handlebar injury" has been associated with pancreatic and bowel injuries in children in addition to liver and spleen injuries.[70-73] In these cases, a bicycle-riding child loses control and the end of the bicycle handlebar strikes the child directly in the epigastrium during the fall. Similar injuries occur when a child is struck in the abdomen with the end of a baseball bat or kicked in the epigastrium, for example. These types of injuries result in a substantial force being applied to a relatively small area of the abdomen. In addition to the more common solid organ injuries, particular attention should be given to diagnosing pancreatic and small bowel injuries in these children.

Another frequently cited predictor of serious injury is loss of consciousness. Brief loss of consciousness, as an isolated symptom, does not predict intracranial injury.[74-78] In one study, loss of consciousness had a positive predictive value of only 9%.[76] Although there is now compelling evidence to suggest that a history of brief loss of consciousness does not accurately predict intracranial injuries identifiable on computed tomography (CT) scan of the head, consensus groups persist in recommending CT scans of the head based solely on a history of loss of consciousness[79] (see Chapter 17, Head Trauma).

The use of seat belts and child safety seats, and placing children in the back seat of a vehicle, decrease the likelihood of morbidity and mortality for children who are passengers in motor vehicle crashes.[80,81] Properly restrained younger children are also less likely to require transport to the hospital.[82,83]

Laboratory Testing

A small body of literature has evaluated the utility of laboratory tests in evaluating cases of pediatric multisystem trauma. In general, the diagnostic utility of laboratory tests is minimal.[84-86] A substantial problem with evaluating laboratory tests is that the outcome of interest in cases of multisystem trauma is heterogeneous. The clinician desires to find all "serious injuries." In addition, because of differences in study design, authors of different studies may arrive at incompatible conclusions. While one author examines the utility of a test as a screening tool (thereby looking for high sensitivity), another author may examine that same test, but assess its utility as a diagnostic tool (thereby looking for high specificity). Their stated conclusions may be contradictory.

Ancillary laboratory tests rarely identify unsuspected injuries in awake, alert, cooperative children without severe trauma. One author evaluated 3939 laboratory screening tests obtained in 285 consecutive children with minimal to moderate injury admitted to a pediatric trauma center, and 91 patients with proven intra-abdominal injury.[86] The abdominal examination combined with a urinalysis detected 98% of all injuries and 100% of injuries requiring surgical intervention.[86] Laboratory values often provide only confirmatory evidence that an injury is present and are not diagnostic.[87]

Coagulation studies, including platelet count, prothrombin time, and partial thromboplastin time, are seldom useful in previously healthy children.[88] Children who receive multiple units of transfused blood are at risk for developing coagulopathies. Electrolyte abnormalities are uncommon in acute trauma. In children with shock due to acute blood loss, a metabolic acidosis can be expected.[89,90] Important electrolyte abnormalities that occur primarily following massive transfusions include hyperkalemia, metabolic alkalosis, hyperphosphatemia, and hypocalcemia.

Liver function tests are elevated in most cases of blunt hepatic trauma.[91] One study found that the presence of either a serum aspartate aminotransferase (AST) greater than 450 IU/L or a serum alanine aminotransferase (ALT) greater than 250 IU/L was 100% sensitive and 92% specific in detecting hepatic trauma in children with blunt abdominal trauma.[92] AST and ALT were highest in the first 12 hours, declining to normal within 5 days of injury.[92] A large review of adult and pediatric blunt abdominal trauma victims found that the presence of either an AST or ALT greater than 130 IU/L was 100% sensitive in detecting liver injuries.[93]

Since CT is recommended to identify and grade suspected liver injuries, liver function tests are generally not required in managing liver injuries. Their main use might be to identify unsuspected injuries in children who do not undergo CT or who are being evaluated for other disorders.

Amylase and lipase elevations are common in patients with blunt abdominal trauma. However, these tests have poor sensitivity, with elevations reported in only 13% to 77% of CT or laparoscopically proven cases of pancreatic trauma.[94-100] Repeat values over time may increase the sensitivity of these tests in detecting significant pancreatic injury.[98] Amylase and lipase levels cannot discriminate between pancreatic and nonpancreatic trauma. Pancreatic enzyme abnormalities are elevated in nearly half of all blunt trauma victims.[97] One study found than only 2% of patients with an elevated amylase or lipase level actually had a pancreatic injury.[97] Moreover, as few as 13% with pancreatic trauma have elevated pancreatic enzymes.[100] Because of the poor discriminatory ability of these tests, they should not be relied upon to diagnose or exclude pancreatic injury.

Hematuria is commonly seen in seriously injured children.[101] Hematuria can indicate trauma anywhere within the genitourinary system. Of note, hematuria is absent in up to 50% of patients with renal pedicle injuries (associated with massive trauma) and isolated ureteral injuries (e.g., gunshot and stab wounds).[102-104] In general, evaluation of these patients is straightforward, and all require radiologic evaluation. Importantly, most serious renal injuries occur in patients with other indications for CT of the abdomen/pelvis or gross hematuria. Debate has existed concerning the appropriate workup of patients with only minor blunt trauma, no lower genitourinary injury, minimal or no symptoms, and microscopic hematuria. In the past, radiologic evaluation was performed on all children with any degree of hematuria in the belief that minor degrees of hematuria might be the only indicator of serious renal injury or of hidden congenital renal disorders.[105] This approach is no longer universally accepted[106,107] (see Chapter 21, Pelvic and Genitourinary Trauma).

Most diagnostic laboratory studies provide no useful information in previously healthy children with blunt abdominal trauma. Laboratory studies might be helpful in children with an underlying disease, hypotension, or the need for multiple units of blood, or who are at risk for developing specific complications following admission (e.g., coagulopathy, electrolyte disorders).

Imaging Studies

The utility of the traditional "C-spine, chest, pelvis" set of plain radiographs has not been adequately studied in children. Understanding the role of these radiographs in the setting of alternative imaging modalities such as CT and magnetic resonance imaging (MRI) is becoming increasingly important.

Although large, well-designed studies have provided important information on when adults do not require cervical spine imaging, studies in children are limited.[108-110] A large prospective series of trauma patients found that adult trauma victims did not require imaging if they met the following NEXUS criteria: a normal mental status, no midline neck tenderness, no distracting injury, no intoxication with drugs or alcohol, and no motor or sensory deficits.[109] This study also included 2160 patients 8 to 17 years old and 817

patients 2 to 8 years old with a total of 30 cervical spine injuries.[111] Although the criteria were 100% sensitive in detecting all cervical spine injuries at these ages, there were too few injuries to adequately assess the NEXUS criteria for use with children. Importantly, this study only included 88 patients less than 2 years old, limiting the applicability of these criteria to this age group. The total number of cervical spine injuries was small, with only 30 document injuries (1% of cases). To verify that these criteria will be highly sensitive, they need to be done in larger studies that include more pediatric injuries.

Flexion-extension, oblique, and odontoid radiographs rarely reveal abnormalities in children.[112-114] However, the number of patients in each of these studies was small. Clinical experience supports the minimal utility of these studies for evaluating traumatized children.

In cases where the cervical spine cannot be cleared clinically or with plain radiographs, maintaining spinal precautions until an MRI can be obtained is prudent.[116] In essence, MRI is the criterion standard for evaluating the spine of the unconscious child.

Indications for obtaining a chest radiograph in pediatric trauma are not clear. In one case-control study, the presence of an abnormal respiratory rate for age, chest tenderness, or back abrasions was 100% sensitive for identifying children with abnormal chest radiographs.[117] Clinical experience suggests that grunting respirations, hypoxia, asymmetric breath sounds, and dyspnea are indications for chest radiography. Endotracheal intubation, thoracostomy tube insertion, and central vascular access in the internal jugular or subclavian veins are also indications for chest radiography. A single study examined whether CT of the chest should replace plain radiographs.[118] The authors concluded that plain radiographs should remain the primary imaging modality in the setting of blunt pediatric trauma.

Children are less likely to sustain pelvic fractures than adults.[36] This appears to be true regardless of the mechanism of injury. There is seldom the need for a rapid, bedside assessment of the pelvis using plain radiography.[36,119] It has been shown that pelvic fractures can be readily identified on CT scanning of the abdomen and pelvis.[120] The routine ordering of pelvic radiographs may be unnecessary, particularly in situations in which a child will be undergoing CT scanning of the abdomen and pelvis based on other indications.

CT scanning has been the greatest advance in pediatric trauma management in the last few decades. CT scanning offers a painless, noninvasive, detailed set of images of the interior of the head and torso. There is ongoing work to determine the exact indications for CT scanning of the head, abdomen, and pelvis in the setting of pediatric multisystem trauma. Although there are proposed indications for head CT scanning and for abdominal and pelvic CT scanning (see Chapter 17, Head Trauma; Chapter 24, Thoracic Trauma; and Chapter 25, Abdominal Trauma), abnormal mental status is an indication for all three scans since it is impossible to confidently rule out intracranial or intra-abdominal injuries based on the clinical examination. Other indications for CT scanning of the abdomen and pelvis include gross hematuria, lap belt injury, nonaccidental trauma, handlebar injury, and abdominal tenderness.[70-73,121] Although CT scanning of the abdomen and pelvis is very effective for evaluating injuries to solid organs such as the liver, spleen, and kidney, it is

Table 12–5	Selected General Concepts for the Emergency Department Management of Children at Risk for Multisystem Trauma

- **Whenever possible, prolonged chemical paralysis should be avoided.** Children who have sustained head injuries may develop seizures. If the child's muscle activity has been masked by medications, seizures may go unnoticed. This leaves a child as risk for unrecognized status epilepticus and severe brain injury. For the intubated child, adequate sedation should be provided rather than prolonged chemical paralysis whenever possible. (See Chapter 3, Rapid Sequence Intubation; and Chapter 40, Seizures.)
- **A negative CT scan does not rule out all intra-abdominal injuries.** Although CT scanning is excellent at identifying or ruling out most solid organ injuries, pancreatic and bowel injuries may not be apparent on initial scans.[9,34,35,37,122-124] If a child has persistent abdominal pain or tenderness, but a negative CT scan of the abdomen and pelvis, admission for observation and repeat evaluations is typically warranted. In this way, more subtle injuries such as those to the pancreas and bowel can be identified. (See Chapter 25, Abdominal Trauma.)
- **Hemodynamic instability warrants the prompt administration of packed red blood cells.** A child who has persistent tachycardia or hypotension after the administration of two or three 20-ml/kg boluses of crystalloid (usually normal saline, although lactated Ringer's solution is acceptable) should receive at least 10 ml/kg of packed red blood cells.[128,129] Since hemodynamic instability is often due to bleeding, the administration of packed red blood cells is also an appropriate initial treatment. (See Chapter 25, Abdominal Trauma; and Chapter 132, Utilizing Blood Bank Resources/Transfusion Reactions and Complications.)
- **Nonoperative management is becoming increasingly common.** The detailed and timely anatomic information available from CT scanning has allowed for nonoperative management of some intra-abdominal and intracranial injuries.[5,130-139] This trend has led to infrequent laparotomies at major pediatric trauma centers.[140] This trend will likely continue and will increase the role of emergency physicians in the management and study of pediatric multisystem trauma. (See Chapter 25, Abdominal Trauma; and Chapter 17, Head Trauma.)

Abbreviation: CT, computed tomography.

not sensitive in ruling out pancreatic, mesenteric, or bowel injuries.[9,34,35,37,122-124] Despite the valuable information gained, there are potential deleterious effects of radiation incurred to a child undergoing multiple CT scans in the setting of trauma. A risk:benefit analysis is indicated to minimize unnecessary CT scanning.

The utility of Focused Abdominal Sonography for Trauma (FAST), now widely used in the emergency department evaluation of adult trauma patients, is controversial in children who have sustained multisystem trauma. Ultrasound is an excellent test for identifying free fluid (i.e., blood) within the abdomen.[125] However, the presence or absence of free fluid does not necessarily impact management.[126,127] Since the presence of free fluid in a child's abdomen does not indicate the need for immediate laparotomy except in very rare instances, ultrasound rarely impacts the clinical management of children who are at risk for multisystem trauma. In addition, there are solid organ injuries identifiable on CT scanning that are clinically important to identify, but do not lead to free fluid in the abdomen. These injuries, therefore, will be missed on ultrasound. Those individuals for whom ultrasound might be useful are almost always the same children who meet the indications for CT scanning of the abdomen and pelvis (see Chapter 179, Ultrasonography).

Management

Management is guided by the results of the initial evaluation. The combination of individual injuries that can be identified during the evaluation of a child who is at risk for multisystem trauma is nearly infinite (see Section II, Approach to the Trauma Patient). However, a few general concepts are useful for managing a child who is at risk for multisystem trauma (Table 12–5).

Summary

Our understanding of pediatric multisystem trauma is evolving. This is reflected in the currently available literature. Traditionally accepted predictors of injury severity such as mechanism of injury and brief loss of consciousness have

been shown to have limited utility in risk-stratifying traumatized children. An age-appropriate evaluation offers the clinician the greatest opportunity for obtaining a meaningful physical examination and for minimizing unnecessary testing. The traditional "C-spine, chest, pelvis" set of radiographs is no longer universally accepted due to limited utility. MRI is the criterion standard for evaluating the spine of the unconscious child. When indicated, CT scanning is the most effective means of evaluating the head, abdomen, and pelvis. Nonoperative management of some intra-abdominal and intracranial injuries has become increasingly common. This necessitates that emergency physicians have a detailed, evidence-based knowledge of the evaluation and management of children who are at risk for multisystem trauma.

REFERENCES

1. Connors JM, Ruddy RM, McCall J, et al: Delayed diagnosis in pediatric blunt trauma. Pediatr Emerg Care 17:1–4, 2001.
2. Laham JL, Cotcamp DH, Gibbons PA, et al: Isolated head injuries versus multiple trauma in pediatric patients: do the same indications for cervical spine evaluation apply? Pediatr Neurosurg 21:21–226, 1994.
3. Brown RL, Brunn MA, Garcia VF: Cervical spine injuries in children: a review of 103 patients treated consecutively at a level 1 pediatric trauma center. J Pediatr Surg 36:1107–1114, 2001.
4. Danseco ER, Miller TR, Spicer RS: Incidence and costs of 1987–1994 childhood injuries: demographic breakdowns. Pediatrics 105:e27, 2000.
5. Davis DH, Localio AR, Stafford PW, et al: Trends in operative management of pediatric splenic injury in a regional trauma system. Pediatrics 115:89–94, 2005.
6. Baker C, Kadish H, Schunk JE: Evaluation of pediatric cervical spine injuries. Am J Emerg Med 17:230–234, 1999.
*7. Viccellio P, Simon H, Pressman BD, et al: A prospective multicenter study of cervical spine injury in children. Pediatrics 108:e20, 2001.
8. Palchak MJ, Holmes JF, Vance CW, et al: A decision rule for identifying children at low risk for brain injuries after blunt head trauma. Ann Emerg Med 42:492–506, 2003.
9. Jerby BL, Attorri RJ, Morton D Jr: Blunt intestinal injury in children: the role of the physical examination. J Pediatr Surg 32:580–584, 1997.
10. Holmes JF, Sokolove PE, Brant WE, et al: A clinical decision rule for identifying children with thoracic injuries after blunt torso trauma. Ann Emerg Med 39:492–499, 2002.

*Selected readings.

11. Holmes JF, Sokolove PE, Brant WE, et al: Identification of children with intra-abdominal injuries after blunt trauma. Ann Emerg Med 39:500–509, 2002.

12. Thompson EC, Perkowski P, Villarreal D, et al: Morbidity and mortality of children following motor vehicle crashes. Arch Surg 138:142–145, 2003.

*13. Qazi K, Wright MS, Kippes C: Stable pediatric blunt trauma patients: is trauma team activation always necessary? J Trauma 45:562–564, 1998.

14. Orzechowski KM, Edgerton EA, Bulas DI, et al: Patterns of injury to restrained children in side impact motor vehicle crashes: the side impact syndrome. J Trauma 54:1094–1101, 2003.

*15. Brown L, Moynihan JA, Denmark TK: Blunt pediatric head trauma requiring neurosurgical intervention: how subtle can it be? Am J Emerg Med 21:467–472, 2003.

16. Brown L: Heterogeneity, evidence, and salt. Can J Emerg Med 6:165–166, 2004.

17. Spady DW, Saunders DL, Schopflocher DP, et al: Patterns of injury in children: a population-based approach. Pediatrics 113:522–529, 2004.

18. Pang G, Wilberger JE: Spinal cord injury without radiographic abnormalities in children. J Neurosurg 57:114–129, 1982.

*19. Bosch PP, Vogt MT, Ward WT: Pediatric spinal cord injury without radiographic abnormality (SCIWORA): the absence of occult instability and lack of indication for bracing. Spine 27:2788–2800, 2002.

20. Bass DH, Semple PL, Cywes S: Investigation and management of blunt renal injuries in children: a review of 11 years' experience. J Pediatr Surg 26:196–200, 1991.

21. Fleisher G: Prospective evaluation of selective criteria for imaging among children with suspected blunt renal trauma. Pediatr Emerg Care 5:8–11, 1989.

22. Lieu TA, Fleisher GR, Mahboubi S, et al: Hematuria and clinical findings as indications for intravenous pyelography in pediatric blunt renal trauma. Pediatrics 82:216–222, 1988.

23. Morey AF, Bruce JE, McAninch JW: Efficacy of radiographic imaging in pediatric blunt renal trauma. J Urol 156:2014–2018, 1996.

24. Hashmi A, Klassen T: Correlation between urinalysis and intravenous pyelography in pediatric abdominal trauma. J Emerg Med 13:255–258, 1995.

25. Cass AS: Blunt renal trauma in children. J Trauma 23:123–127, 1983.

26. Stein JP, Kaji DM, Eastham J, et al: Blunt renal trauma in the pediatric population: indications for radiographic evaluation. Urology 44:406–410, 1994.

27. Taylor GA, Eichelberger MR, Potter BM: Hematuria: a marker of abdominal injury in children after blunt trauma. Ann Surg 208:688–693, 1988.

28. Stalker HP, Kaufman RA, Stedje K: The significance of hematuria in children after blunt abdominal trauma. AJR Am J Roentgenol 154:569–571, 1990.

29. Brown SL, Haas C, Dinchman KH, et al: Radiologic evaluation of pediatric blunt renal trauma in patients with microscopic hematuria. World J Surg 25:1557–1560, 2001.

30. Abou-Jaoude WA, Sugarman JM, Fallat ME, et al: Indicators of genitourinary tract injury or anomaly in cases of pediatric blunt trauma. J Pediatr Surg 31:86–90, 1996.

31. Smith EM, Elder JS, Spirnak JP: Major blunt renal trauma in the pediatric population: is a nonoperative approach indicated? J Urol 149:546–548, 1993.

32. Nance ML, Lutz N, Carr MC, et al: Blunt renal injuries in children can be managed nonoperatively: outcome in a consecutive series of patients. J Trauma 57:474–478, 2004.

33. Quinlan DM, Gearhart JP: Blunt renal trauma in childhood: features indicating severe injury. Br J Urol 66:526–531, 1990.

34. Nadler EP, Gardner M, Schall LC, et al: Management of blunt pancreatic injury in children. J Trauma 47:1098–1103, 1999.

35. Desai KM, Dorward IG, Minkes RK, et al: Blunt duodenal injuries in children. J Trauma 54:640–646, 2003.

36. Demetriades D, Karaiskakis M, Velmahos GC, et al: Pelvic fractures in pediatric and adult trauma patients: are they different injuries? J Trauma 54:1146–1151, 2003.

37. Jobst MA, Canty TG Sr, Lynch FP: Management of pancreatic injury in pediatric blunt abdominal trauma. J Pediatr Surg 34:818–824, 1999.

38. Lin PH, Barr V, Bush RL, et al: Isolated abdominal aortic rupture in a child due to all-terrain vehicle accident—a case report. Vasc Endovascular Surg 37:289–292, 2003.

39. Prasad VS, Schwartz A, Bhutani R, et al: Characteristics of injuries to the cervical spine and spinal cord in polytrauma patient population: experience from a regional trauma unit. Spinal Cord 37:560–568, 1999.

40. Rothrock SG, Green SM, Morgan R: Abdominal trauma in infants and children: prompt identification and early management of serious and life threatening injuries. Part I: Injury patterns and initial assessment. Pediatr Emerg Care 16:106–115, 2000.

41. Barlow B, Niemirska M, Gandhi R: Ten years of experience with falls from a height in children. J Pediatr Surg 18:509–511, 1983.

42. Vavilala MS, Lee LA, Boddu K, et al: Cerebral autoregulation in pediatric traumatic brain injury. Pediatr Crit Care Med 5:257–263, 2004.

43. Cooper A, Barlow B, DiScala C, String D: Mortality and truncal injury: the pediatric perspective. J Pediatr Surg 29:33–38, 1994.

44. Peclet MH, Newman KD, Eichelberger MR, et al: Thoracic trauma in children: an indicator of increased mortality. J Pediatr Surg 25:961–965, 1990.

45. American College of Surgeons, Committee on Trauma: Initial assessment and management. *In* Advanced Trauma Life Support Student Manual. Chicago: American College of Surgeons, 1997, p 26.

46. Tepas JJ III, Fallat ME, Moriarty TM: Trauma. *In* Gausche-Hill M, Fuchs S, Yamamoto L (eds): APLS: The Pediatric Emergency Medicine Resource. Sudbury, MA: Jones and Bartlett, 2004, pp 274–283.

*47. Schafermeyer RW, Ribbeck BM, Gaskins J, et al: Respiratory effects of spinal immobilization in children. Ann Emerg Med 20:115–117, 1991.

*48. Chan D, Goldberg R, Tascone A, et al: The effect of spinal immobilization on healthy volunteers. Ann Emerg Med 23:48–51, 1994.

49. Tepas JJ, Mollitt DL, Talbert JL, et al: The Pediatric Trauma Score as a predictor of injury severity in the injured child. J Pediatr Surg 22:14–18, 1987.

50. Tepas JJ, Ramenofsky ML, Mollitt DL, et al: The Pediatric Trauma Score as a predictor of injury severity: an objective assessment. J Trauma 28:425–427, 1988.

51. Ramnofsky M, Luterman A, Quindlen E, et al: Maximum survival in pediatric trauma: the ideal system. J Trauma 24:818–823, 1984.

52. Eichelberger MR, Gotschall CS, Sacco WJ, et al: A comparison of the Trauma Score, the Revised Trauma Score, and the Pediatric Trauma Score. Ann Emerg Med 18:1053–1058, 1989.

53. Kauffman CR, Maier RV, Rivara FP, et al: Evaluation of the Pediatric Trauma Score. JAMA 263:69–72, 1990.

54. Nayduch DA, Moilin J, Rugledge R, et al: Comparison of the ability of adult and pediatric trauma scores to predict pediatric outcome following major trauma. J Trauma 31:452–457, 1991.

55. Saladino R, Lund D, Fleisher G: The spectrum of liver and spleen injuries in children: failure of the Pediatric Trauma Score and clinical signs to predict isolated injuries. Ann Emerg Med 20:636–640, 1991.

56. Dowd MD, McAneney C, Lacher M, et al: Maximizing the sensitivity and specificity of pediatric trauma team activation criteria. Acad Emerg Med 7:1119–1125, 2000.

57. Sola JE, Scherer LR, Haller JA, et al: Criteria for safe cost-effective pediatric trauma triage: prehospital evaluation and distribution of injured children. J Pediatr Surg 29:738–741, 1994.

*58. Terregino CA, Reid JC, Marburger RK, et al: Secondary emergency department triage (supertriage) and trauma team activation: effects on resource utilization and patient care. J Trauma 43:61–64, 1997.

59. Chen LE, Snyder AK, Minkes RK, et al: Trauma stat and trauma minor: are we making the call appropriately? Pediatr Emerg Care 20:421–425, 2004.

60. Nuss KE, Dietrich AM, Smith GA: Effectiveness of a pediatric trauma team protocol. Pediatr Emerg Care 17:96–100, 2001.

61. Chadwick DL, Chin S, Salerno C, et al: Deaths from falls in children: how far is fatal? J Trauma 31:1353–1355, 1991.

62. Tarantino CA, Dowd D, Murdock TC: Short vertical falls in infants. Pediatr Emerg Care 15:5–8, 1999.

63. Newgard CD, Lewis RJ, Jolly BT: Use of out-of-hospital variables to predict severity of injury in pediatric patients involved in motor vehicle crashes. Ann Emerg Med 39:481–491, 2002.

64. Williams RA: Injuries in infants and small children resulting from witnessed and corroborated free falls. J Trauma 31:1350–1352, 1991.

65. Simon BJ, Legere P, Emhoff T, et al: Vehicular trauma triage by mechanism: avoidance of the unproductive evaluation. J Trauma 37:645–649, 1994.

66. Kohn MA, Hammel JM, Bretz SW, et al: Trauma team activation criteria as predictors of patient disposition from the emergency department. Acad Emerg Med 11:1–9, 2004.

67. Palanca S, Taylor DM, Bailey M, et al: Mechanisms of motor vehicle accidents that predict major injury. Emerg Med 15:423–428, 2003.

68. Shatney CH, Sensaki K: Trauma team activation for "mechanism of injury" blunt trauma victims: time for a change? J Trauma 37:275–281, 1994.

69. Goodacre S, Than M, Goyder EC, et al: Can the distance fallen predict serious injury after a fall from a height? J Trauma 46:1055–1058, 1999.

70. Erez I, Lazar L, Gutermacher M, et al: Abdominal injuries caused by bicycle handlebars. Eur J Surg 167:331–333, 2001.

71. Clarnette TD, Beasley SW: Handlebar injuries in children: patterns and prevention. Aust N Z J Surg 67:338–339, 1997.

72. Acton CH, Thomas S, Clark R, et al: Bicycle incidents in children—abdominal trauma and handlebars. Med J Aust 160:344–346, 1994.

73. Winston FK, Shaw KN, Kreshak AA, et al: Hidden spears: handlebars as injury hazards to children. Pediatrics 102:596–601, 1998.

74. Gruskin KD, Schutzman SA: Head trauma in children younger than 2 years: are there predictors for complications? Arch Pediatr Adolesc Med 153:15–20, 1999.

75. Dietrich AM, Bowman MJ, Ginn-Pease ME, et al: Pediatric head injuries: can clinical factors reliably predict an abnormality on computed tomography? Ann Emerg Med 22:1535–1540, 1993.

76. Quayle KS, Jaffe DM, Kuppermann N, et al: Diagnostic testing for acute head injury in children: when are head computed tomography and skull radiographs indicated? Pediatrics 99:e11, 1997.

77. Simon B, Letourneau P, Vitorino E, et al: Pediatric minor head trauma: indications for computed tomographic scanning revisited. J Trauma 51:231–238, 2001.

78. Palchak MJ, Holmes JF, Vance CW, et al: Does an isolated history of loss of consciousness or amnesia predict brain injuries in children after blunt head trauma? Pediatrics 113:e507–e513, 2004.

79. Schutzman SA, Barnes P, Duhaime AC, et al: Evaluation and management of children younger than two years old with apparently minor head trauma: proposed guidelines. Pediatrics 107:983–993, 2001.

80. Osberg JS, Di Scala C: Morbidity among pediatric motor vehicle crash victims: the effectiveness of seat belts. Am J Public Health 82:422–425, 1992.

81. Valent F, McGwin G, Hardin W, et al: Restraint use and injury patterns among children involved in motor vehicle collisions. J Trauma 52:745–751, 2002.

82. Caviness AC, Jones JL, Deguzman MA, et al: Pediatric restraint use is associated with reduced transports by emergency medical services providers after motor vehicle crashes. Prehosp Emerg Care 7:448–452, 2003.

83. Phelan KJ, Khoury J, Grossman DC, et al: Pediatric motor vehicle related injuries in the Navajo Nation: the impact of the 1988 child occupant restraint laws. Inj Prev 8:216–220, 2002.

84. Cotton BA, Beckert BW, Smith MK, et al: The utility of clinical and laboratory data for predicting intraabdominal injury among children. J Trauma 56:1068–1075, 2004.

85. Ford EG, Karamanoukian HL, McGrath N, et al: Emergency center laboratory evaluation of pediatric trauma victims. Am Surg 56:752–757, 1990.

86. Isaacman DJ, Scarfone RJ, Kost SI, et al: Utility of routine laboratory testing for detecting intra-abdominal injury in the pediatric trauma patient. Pediatrics 92:691–694, 1993.

87. Foltin GL, Cooper A: Abdominal trauma. *In* Barkin RM, Caputo GL, Jaffe DM, et al (eds): Pediatric Emergency Medicine: Concepts and Clinical Practice, 2nd ed. St. Louis: CV Mosby, 1997, pp 335–354.

88. Holmes JF, Goodwin H, Land C, et al: Coagulation studies in pediatric blunt trauma patients [Abstract]. Ann Emerg Med 32:S39, 1998.

89. Davis JW, Mackersie RC, Holbrook TL, et al: Base deficit as an indicator of significant abdominal injury. Ann Emerg Med 20:842–844, 1991.

90. Bannon MP, O'Neill CM, Martin M, et al: Central venous oxygen saturation, arterial base deficit, and lactate concentration in trauma patients. Am Surg 61:738–745, 1995.

91. Oldham KT, Guice KS, Kaufmann RA, et al: Blunt hepatic injury and elevated hepatic enzymes: a clinical correlation in children. J Pediatr Surg 19:457–461, 1984.

92. Hennes HM, Smith DS, Schneider K, et al: Elevated liver transaminase levels in children with blunt abdominal trauma: a predictor of liver injury. Pediatrics 86:87–90, 1990.

93. Sahdev P, Garramone RR, Schwartz RJ, et al: Evaluation of liver function tests in screening for intra-abdominal injuries. Ann Emerg Med 20:838–841, 1991.

94. Akhrass R, Kim K, Brandt C: Computed tomography: an unreliable indicator of pancreatic trauma. Am Surg 62:647–651, 1996.

95. Gorenstein A, O'Halpin D, Wesson DE, et al: Blunt injury to the pancreas in children: selective management based on ultrasound. J Pediatr Surg 22:1110–1118, 1987.

96. Smith SD, Nakayama DK, Gantt N, et al: Pancreatic injuries in children due to blunt trauma. J Pediatr Surg 23:610–614, 1988.

97. Buechter KJ, Arnold M, Steele B, et al: The use of serum amylase and lipase in evaluating and managing blunt abdominal trauma. Am Surg 56:204–208, 1990.

98. Shilyansky J, Sena LM, Kreller M, et al: Nonoperative management of pancreatic injuries in children. J Pediatr Surg 33:343–349, 1998.

99. Sivit CJ, Eichelberger MR, Taylor GA, et al: Blunt pancreatic trauma in children: CT diagnosis. AJR Am J Roentgenol 158:1097–1100, 1992.

100. Simon HK, Muehlberg A, Linakis JG: Serum amylase determinations in pediatric patients presenting to the ED with acute abdominal pain or trauma. Am J Emerg Med 12:292–295, 1994.

101. Taylor GA, Eichelberger MR, O'Donnell R, et al: Indications for computed tomography in children with blunt abdominal trauma. Ann Surg 213:212–218, 1991.

102. Boone TB, Gilling PJ, Husmann DA: Ureteropelvic junction disruption following blunt abdominal trauma. J Urol 150:33–36, 1993.

103. Cass AS: Blunt renal trauma in children. J Trauma 23:123–127, 1983.

104. Morey AF, Bruce JE, McAninch JW: Efficacy of radiologic imaging in pediatric blunt renal trauma. J Urol 156:2014–2018, 1996.

105. Emmanuel B, Weiss H, Gollm P: Renal trauma in children. J Trauma 17:275–278, 1977.

106. Holmes JF, Sokolove PE, Land C, et al: Identification of intra-abdominal injuries in children hospitalized following blunt torso trauma. Acad Emerg Med 6:799–806, 1999.

107. Perez-Brayfield MR, Gatti JM, Smith EA, et al: Blunt traumatic hematuria in children: is a simplified algorithm justified? J Urol 167:2543–2547, 2002.

108. Stiell IG, Wells GA, Vandemheen KL, et al: The Canadian c-spine rule for radiography in alert and stable trauma patients. JAMA 286:1841–1848, 2001.

109. Hoffman JR, Mower WR, Wolfson AB, et al: Validity of a set of clinical criteria to rule out injury to the cervical spine in patients with blunt trauma: National Emergency X-Radiography Utilization Study Group. N Engl J Med 343:94–99, 2000.

110. Slack SE, Clancy MJ: Clearing the cervical spine of paediatric trauma patients. Emerg Med J 21:189–193, 2004.

111. Viccellio P, Simon H, Pressman BD, et al: A prospective multicenter study of cervical spine injury in children. Pediatrics 108:e20, 2001.

112. Ralston ME, Chung K, Barnes PD, et al: Role of flexion-extension radiographs in blunt pediatric cervical spine injury. Acad Emerg Med 8:237–245, 2001.

113. Ralston ME, Ecklund K, Emans JB, et al: Role of oblique radiographs in blunt pediatric cervical injury. Pediatr Emerg Care 19:68–72, 2003.

114. Buhs C, Cullen M, Klein M, et al: The pediatric trauma c-spine: is the "odontoid" view necessary? J Pediatr Surg 35:994–997, 2000.

*115. Lee SL, Sena M, Greenholz SK, et al: A multidisciplinary approach to the development of a cervical spine clearance protocol: process, rationale, and initial results. J Pediatr Surg 38:358–362, 2003.

116. Launay F, Leet AL, Sponseller PD: Pediatric spinal cord injury without radiographic abnormality: a meta-analysis. Clin Orthop Relat Res 433:166–179, 2005.

117. Gittleman MA, Gonzalez-del-Rey J, Brody A, et al: Clinical predictors for the selective use of chest radiographs in pediatric blunt trauma evaluations. J Trauma 55:670–676, 2003.

118. Renton J, Kincaid S, Ehrlich PF: Should helical CT scanning of the thoracic cavity replace the conventional chest x-ray as a primary assessment tool in pediatric trauma? An efficacy and cost analysis. J Pediatr Surg 38:793–797, 2003.

*119. Guillamondegui OD, Mahboubi S, Stafford PW, et al: The utility of the pelvic radiograph in the assessment of pediatric pelvic fractures. J Trauma 55:236–239, 2003.

*120. Vo NJ, Gash J, Browning J, Hutson RK: Pelvic imaging in the stable trauma patient: is the AP pelvic radiograph necessary when abdominopelvic CT shows no acute injury? Emerg Radiol 10:246–249, 2004.

121. Taylor GA, Eichelberger MR, Potter BM: Hematuria: A marker of abdominal injury in children after blunt trauma. Ann Surg 208:688–693, 1988.

122. Kurkchubasche AG, Fendya DG, Tracy TF, et al: Blunt intestinal injury in children: diagnostic and therapeutic considerations. Arch Surg 132:652–658, 1997.

123. Frick EJ, Pasquale MD, Cipolle MD: Small-bowel and mesentery injuries in blunt trauma. J Trauma 46:920–926, 1999.

124. Graham JS, Wong AL: A review of computed tomography in the diagnosis of intestinal and mesenteric injury in pediatric blunt abdominal trauma. J Pediatr Surg 31:754–756, 1996.

125. Rathaus V, Zissin R, Werner M, et al: Minimal pelvic fluid in blunt abdominal trauma in children: the significance of this sonographic finding. J Pediatr Surg 36:1387–1389, 2001.

126. Coley BD, Mutabagani KH, Martin LC, et al: Focused abdominal sonography for trauma (FAST) in children with blunt abdominal trauma. J Trauma 48:902–906, 2000.

127. Benya EC, Lim-Dunham JE, Landrum O, et al: Abdominal sonography in examination of children with blunt abdominal trauma. AJR Am J Roentgenol 174:1613–1616, 2000.

128. Robinson WP 3rd, Ahn J, Stiffler A, et al: Blood transfusion is an independent predictor of increased mortality in nonoperatively managed blunt hepatic and splenic injuries. J Trauma 58:437–444, 2005.

129. Patrick DA, Bensard DD, Janik JS, et al: Is hypotension a reliable indicator of blood loss from traumatic injury in children? Am J Surg 184:555–560, 2002.

130. Rutledge R, Hunt JP, Lentz CW, et al: A statewide, population-based time-series analysis of the increasing frequency of nonoperative management of abdominal solid organ injury. Ann Surg 222:311–322, 1995.

131. Ceylan S, Kuzeyli K, Ilbay K, et al: Nonoperative management of acute extradural hematomas in children. J Neurosurg Sci 36:85–88, 1992.

132. Tuncer R, Kazan T, Uçar C, et al: Conservative management of epidural haematomas: prospective study of 15 cases. Acta Neurochir 121:48–52, 1993.

133. Paddock HN, Tepas JJ, Ramenofsky ML, et al: Management of blunt pediatric hepatic and splenic injury: similar process, different outcome. Am Surg 70:1068–1072, 2004.

134. Partrick DA, Moore EE, Bensard DD, et al: Operative management of injured children at an adult level I trauma center. J Trauma 48:894–901, 2000.

135. Rossi D, de Ville de Goyet J, de Cléty SC, et al: Management of intra-abdominal organ injury following blunt abdominal trauma in children. Intensive Care Med 19:415–419, 1993.

136. Fallat ME, Casale AJ: Practice patterns of pediatric surgeons caring for stable patients with traumatic solid organ injury. J Trauma 43:820–824, 1997.

137. Ozturk H, Dokucu AI, Onen A, et al: Non-operative management of isolated solid organ injuries due to blunt abdominal trauma in children: a fifteen-year experience. Eur J Pediatr Surg 14:29–34, 2004.

138. Leone RJ Jr, Hammond JS: Nonoperative management of pediatric blunt hepatic trauma. Am Surg 67:138–142, 2001.

139. Lahat E, Livne M, Barr J, et al: The management of epidural haematomas—surgical versus conservative treatment. Eur J Pediatr 153:198–201, 1994.

*140. Green SM, Rothrock SG: Is pediatric trauma really a surgical disease? Ann Emerg Med 39:537–540, 2002.

Chapter 13

Sepsis

Jesus M. Arroyo, MD, James J. McCarthy, MD, and Brent R. King, MD

Introduction and Background

Sepsis has long been recognized as a major cause of morbidity and mortality for both adults and children. In 1992, a consensus panel defined the clinical entity of "sepsis" for adults as a "systemic inflammatory response syndrome (SIRS) with infection"[1] This definition was reaffirmed in 2003.[2] In 2005 another consensus panel provided the medical community with the first pediatric-specific definitions of SIRS, infection, sepsis, severe sepsis, and septic shock[3] (Tables 13–1 and 13–2). These consensus definitions provide a clear and objective basis for the diagnosis of sepsis, which provides the framework for helping clinicians communicate particularly with regard to referrals between community hospitals and tertiary care settings.

The term *sepsis syndrome* describes a complex continuum of disease, the pathophysiology of which is still not fully understood. Although the word *sepsis* implies rampant infection, the actual clinical impact of the disease process goes far beyond the presence of bacteria in the bloodstream. There is still debate as to what actually causes the clinical syndrome, but there is general agreement that the presence of the bacteria and their products is only a part of the picture. Many of the clinical findings associated with sepsis are actually the result of the host's response to bacterial invasion. The body's initial and adaptive response to overwhelming infection goes awry and results in the simultaneous activation of the coagulation system and the proinflammatory network, which may progress to organ ischemia and multisystem organ failure and ultimately death.[4] The host's own defenses may pose a greater danger than the invading bacteria.[5]

More recently this theory has been challenged by the hypothesis that the sepsis syndrome is the result of the immune system becoming somehow compromised, leaving the patient unable to adequately respond to severe infection. Sepsis patients have features consistent with immunosuppression, such as loss of delayed hypersensitivity and a predisposition to nosocomial infection.[6,7] The syndrome of sepsis may, therefore, actually represent a continuum that begins with an inflammatory response and progresses to immunosuppression.

While our understanding of sepsis is growing, the precise etiology of organ failure and ultimately death is still poorly understood. Myocardial depression and refractory shock clearly play a major role, but the precise details have yet to be determined. Aside from antimicrobial therapy, the mainstays of sepsis management—circulatory support, respiratory support, and vasoactive drugs—are purely supportive. Though trials of novel therapies are underway, currently the emergency physician can rely only upon a few proven treatments along with careful attention to physiologic homeostasis.

Recognition and Approach

Epidemiology

The epidemiology of severe sepsis and septic shock differs across demographic regions worldwide and is influenced by many factors. In the United States, it is estimated that annually there are three cases of sepsis for every 1000 hospitalizations, or about 750,000 cases. Of these, nearly 200,000 are presumed to be cases of severe sepsis. The incidence of severe sepsis among children has been estimated to be as high as 42,000 cases per year with over 4000 deaths.[8]

Certain patient factors play a significant role. Sepsis is more common at the extremes of age. Almost half of the annual cases of severe sepsis in children occur in patients less than 1 year old and, of these, over two thirds are neonates. By comparison, the incidence of sepsis among older children is only 0.2 cases per 1000 patients per year. Gender is a factor in neonatal sepsis, with males being affected more often than females, but this difference diminishes with increasing age

Table 13–1	Classification of Severe Pediatric Sepsis by Vital Signs According to Age				
Age	Classification	Tachycardia (bpm)	Bradycardia (bpm)	Respiratory Rate (breaths/min)	SBP (mm Hg)
Birth–7 days	Newborn	>180	<100	>50	<65
1 wk–1 mo	Neonate	>180	<100	>40	<75
1 mo–1 yr	Infant	>180	<90	>34	<100
2–5 yr	Toddler	>140	NA	>22	<94
6–12 yr	School age	>130	NA	>18	<105
13–18 yr	Adolescent	>110	NA	>14	<117

*Lower values for heart rate and SPB are for the 5th percentile, and upper values for heart rate and respiratory rate and are for 95th percentile.
Abbreviations: bpm, beats per minute; NA, not applicable; SBP, systolic blood pressure.

Table 13–2	Pediatric-Specific Definitions of Sepsis and Related Terms
Term	Definition
Systemic inflammatory response syndrome (SIRS)	The presence of at least two of the following four criteria, one of which must be abnormal temperature or leukocyte count: • Core temperature of > 38.5° C or < 36° C. • Tachycardia, defined as a mean heart rate > 2 SD above normal for age in the absence of external stimulus, chronic drugs, or painful stimuli; or otherwise unexplained persistent elevation over a 0.5- to 4-hr time period OR for children < 1 yr old: bradycardia, defined as a mean heart rate < 10th percentile for age in the absence of external vagal stimulus, β-blocker drugs, or congenital heart disease; or otherwise unexplained persistent depression over a 0.5-hr time period. • Mean respiratory rate > 2 SD above normal for age or mechanical ventilation for an acute process not related to underlying neuromuscular disease or the receipt of general anesthesia. • Leukocyte count elevated or depressed for age (not secondary to chemotherapy-induced leukopenia) or > 10% immature neutrophils.
Infection	A suspected or proven (by positive culture, tissue stain, or polymerase chain reaction test) infection caused by any pathogen OR a clinical syndrome associated with a high probability of infection. Evidence of infection includes positive findings on clinical examination, imaging, or laboratory tests.
Sepsis	SIRS in the presence of or as a result of suspected or proven infection.
Severe sepsis	Sepsis plus one of the following: • Cardiovascular organ dysfunction • Acute respiratory distress syndrome • Two or more other organ dysfunctions
Septic shock	Sepsis and cardiovascular organ dysfunction

Modified from Goldstein B, Grior B, Randolph A, et al: International Pediatric Sepsis Consensus Conference: definitions for sepsis and organ dysfunction in pediatrics. Pediatr Crit Care Med 6:2–8, 2005.
Abbreviation: SD, standard deviation.

and becomes insignificant by adolescence. Among affected neonates, birth weight appears to be important. Studies of neonates who developed severe sepsis have found that 69.3% were low-birth-weight infants and, of these, fully one half were very-low-birth-weight infants.[8] In developing countries, sepsis has been shown to be more prevalent among those with poor nutrition. Patients with compromised immunity are at greater risk than their immunocompetent peers.

Among children with severe sepsis, it is estimated that 5% to 30% will develop septic shock. In a study of over 9600 patients with severe sepsis, the mortality rate was 10.3%.[8] This represents considerably fewer deaths than in previous studies, which reported mortality rates for septic shock exceeding 50% to 100%. Much of this difference can be attributed to the availability of newer therapies, including advanced anti-infective agents, and the use of more aggressive treatment protocols. With currently available care, mortality for severe sepsis and septic shock is thought to range from 10% to 40%, with overall mortality at 10% for pediatric patients and 40% in the elderly.[9] As might be expected, mortality and significant complications are higher in patients with underlying disease, in those who have undergone surgical procedures, and in immunosuppressed children (e.g., children infected with the human immunodeficiency virus [HIV] and bone marrow transplant recipients).

It has been estimated that the annual cost of treating severe sepsis is equivalent to roughly 1% of the annual gross national product. The average length of hospitalization for a child with severe sepsis is 31.2 days at a cost of approximately $47,000. When multiplied by the number of children who are treated each year, it is estimated that this disease process is responsible for 1.3 million hospital days and $1.97 billion in costs.

Pathophysiology

Severe sepsis is a process triggered by an infectious agent, a product produced by an infectious agent, and/or the host's response to infection. As bacterial antigens (exo- or endotoxins) enter the body and interact with cells of the immune system (macrophages, neutrophils, and dentritic cells), leukocytes release proinflammatory cytokines. These cytokines—tumor necrosis factor-α, interleukin-1 (IL-1), and interleukin-6 (IL-6)—have two principal effects: (1) they activate transcription genes that, in turn, produce more cytokines; and (2) they recruit more leukocytes to the site of infection.[10,11] Macrophages and dendritic cells also release interleukin-12, which activates CD4 T cells. These cells have two antagonistic functions. They can become either T helper type 1 (Th1) cells or T helper type 2 (Th2) cells. Investigations are underway to identify what determines the subtype of cell created by the CD4 T cells. Some have suggested that the subtype of cell is determined by the type of bacteria, the size of the inoculum, or the site of the infection.[12] Th1 cells release proinflammatory cytokines, which activate more macrophages and dentritic cells, creating a vicious cycle of inflammation. Previously activated neutrophils release more cytokines, which in turn activate more Th1 cells.

As the cascade progresses, inflammatory cytokines activate tissue factor in endothelial cells and monocytes. Tissue factor triggers the extrinsic coagulation pathway, activating thrombin, which has multiple physiologic effects.[4] Inflammatory cytokines also deplete activated protein C and antithrombin III (which inhibits thrombin and many of the clotting factors in both the intrinsic and extrinsic coagulation cascades), two of the body's natural anticoagulants. The result of this process is a state of diffuse inflammation and endothelial injury and thrombosis complicated by a disordered coagulation system that cannot maintain the homeostatic balance between its procoagulant and anticoagulant properties.[4,13,14] These processes create the final end point of sepsis pathophysiology: a state of microvascular thrombosis causing tissue ischemia and eventually cell necrosis, organ dysfunction, and, eventually, death.[15] A proposed second wave in the sepsis cascade has also been described such that the immune system changes from an inflammatory cascade to an anti-inflammatory system, with progression of disease.[13]

Direct effects of bacteria and exotoxins in combination with the inflammatory mediators create a clinical state of volume depletion, peripheral vasodilation, myocardial depression, and increased metabolism. The net result is an imbalance of oxygen delivery relative to oxygen demand, resulting in profound global tissue hypoxia.[16] The clinical manifestations of the processes described previously can be envisioned as follows. Bacteria enter the bloodstream, triggering an inflammatory immune response. If the process is not interrupted, the patient develops clinical evidence of diffuse systemic inflammation (SIRS) and the initial clinical manifestations of sepsis. As the process continues, the patient develops more severe symptoms that culminate in shock and multiple organ dysfunction syndrome (MODS).

Recognition of sepsis begins with a basic understanding of the physiology along with the understanding that sepsis is a disease process, rather than an isolated clinical syndrome. Patients may present for care at any point along a broad continuum of symptoms. At one end of the continuum are moribund patients with obvious systemic compromise. Many of these children even will die even with optimal management. On the other end of the continuum are those children who present so early in their course of illness that it may be impossible to distinguish them from patients with minor infections. Patients at this stage of illness will be identified by happenstance, if at all. The broad middle portion of the continuum contains those children who have some clinical symptoms of physiologic perturbation. If these children can be identified and treated promptly, they have a reasonable chance of survival.

Evaluation

Because sepsis has multiple physiologic effects, patients may present with myriad findings, but there are a few unifying themes. Recent literature has suggested that sepsis among children be defined as the presence of SIRS (see Table 13–2) with an identified infection. Clinical findings might include symptoms identified as a part of the SIRS syndrome, such as temperature elevation or depression, tachycardia or bradycardia, tachypnea, leukocytosis, and leukopenia or a "left shift"—an increase in immature white blood cells (i.e., "bands"). Physical and/or laboratory findings consistent with a specific infectious process such as pneumonia, urinary tract infection, or cellulitis are likely to be found as well. The definition of the syndrome includes some symptoms indicative of physiologic compromise. In its mildest expression this may take the form of subtle tachycardia or tachypnea, or a narrowed pulse pressure. The adolescent or older child may actually be able to describe a feeling that "something is wrong." As the disease process progresses, the patient will develop more extreme tachycardia and tachypnea, altered mental status, and hypotension.

It is probable that many cases of very early sepsis go unrecognized because the underlying infectious process is treated promptly and the cascade of sepsis physiology is aborted long before it becomes manifest as overt clinical symptoms. Likewise, many cases that have progressed beyond the very early stages are likely to be confused with other illnesses and nonetheless treated appropriately. An example of this latter scenario is the child with sepsis secondary to a urinary tract infection who presents to an emergency department with fever, tachycardia, and tachypnea along with a history of vomiting. The urinary tract infection is diagnosed and appropriately treated but the physiologic symptoms are attributed to dehydration rather than sepsis. However, antibiotics and intravenous fluids help to restore effective circulation and interrupt the physiologic processes that would have led to sepsis had intervention not occurred.

Subtle symptoms such as mild alteration in mental status (lethargy, irritability, unusual behavior) should prompt clinicians to consider the possibility of sepsis. Older children may demonstrate subtle cognitive deficits that can be recognized only by those who know the child well, thus parental concerns in this regard should be taken seriously. Parents of infants with early sepsis might report changes in the baby's feeding or sleeping patterns, excessive fussiness, or lethargy. Other early signs are body and joint aches, chills, rigors, and flushing. In some instances (e.g., meningococcemia), a characteristic rash will be present. As described earlier, laboratory findings are variable and might include elevated polymorphonuclear cell and/or total white blood cell counts, decreases in these counts, and a variety of electrolyte abnormalities, including hypoglycemia, hyperglycemia, and acidosis. As the disease progresses, signs of serious illness become more obvious. Respiratory compromise is manifest as tachypnea, tachycardia, grunting, or even apnea. Impaired circulation is manifest as prolonged capillary refill time, peripheral pallor, cool mottled skin, and decreased urine output. Further evolution leads to signs of end-organ dysfunction and failure.[17] The patient may develop seizures or experience a respiratory or cardiac arrest. In an otherwise healthy child with this presentation, sepsis should be the first major consideration.

Potential Pathogens

Because sepsis begins with infection, one must consider the most likely pathogens for each age group of patients as well as the ways in which such patients might present for medical care. The causative organism influences both symptoms and outcome. Patients with septic shock caused by gram-negative bacteria have a mortality of 20% to 50%, while those with gram-positive septic shock have mortality rate of only 10% to 20%.[18,19] While gram-negative bacteria are more likely to affect the gastrointestinal system, gram-positive organisms more often affect the lungs, adrenal glands, kidneys, and heart.

In neonates, the organisms most associated with sepsis are group B streptococcus, the Enterobacteriaceae, *Listeria monocytogenes,* and *Staphylococcus aureus,* but *Streptococcus pneumoniae* and *Neisseria meningitidis* should also be considered. Agents most likely to affect infants beyond the neonatal period include *S. pneumoniae, N. meningitidis,* and *S. aureus.* Signs and symptoms of sepsis in neonates and infants are nonspecific and may not offer the clinician any insight into the bacterial agent responsible for an individual case. The challenge lies in identifying the infant with early sepsis who may initially present with feeding difficulties, vomiting, irritability, lethargy, fever, hypothermia, or apnea. Depending upon the source of the infection, there may be few or no signs suggestive of infection. For example, infants with pneumonia may present with tachypnea, while those with urinary tract infection may have no specific symptoms attributable to the infectious process at all. Subtle signs might be present but not immediately appreciated. For example, omphalitis or an infected scalp probe site might initially be overlooked.

The bacteria most commonly responsible for sepsis in older infants and children are *S. pneumoniae, N. meningitidis,* and occasionally the Enterobacteriaceae. *Haemophilus influenzae* type B, once a common cause of severe infection, has been mostly eliminated by more than a decade of immunization. Severe infection in this age group is not likely to be missed but could be confused with another process. Such patients often have, in addition to fever, tachycardia, tachypnea, lethargy, confusion, vomiting, diarrhea, and abdominal distention. The source of their symptoms can generally be identified by physical examination or with a rudimentary laboratory evaluation. The occurrence of sepsis in healthy older children and adolescents is unusual. When it occurs, the source of infection is often apparent and, when such a source cannot be identified, the physician should consider an undiagnosed immunodeficiency syndrome or intravenous drug use.

There are some populations of patients in whom both the causative agents and the presentation of sepsis might be atypical. For example, sepsis should be a consideration in the child who has undergone an invasive procedure and experiences clinical deterioration hours or days later. Also, children with immunosuppression (e.g., HIV infection, leukemia, lymphoma, or sickle cell anemia) may have more subtle presentations and have infections caused by unusual bacteria. Children receiving lipids through central venous catheters

have been shown to be at greater risk from infections caused by coagulase-negative streptococci, enterococci, and *Enterobacter cloacae.*[17] Children with impaired immunity who present with fever but are otherwise well appearing can rapidly become gravely ill. For this reason, children with impaired immune systems require more careful attention and more conservative management when they present with evidence of infection. Similar consideration should be given to children with certain chronic illnesses, particularly when the patient has an indwelling central venous or urinary catheter or other medical appliance. Children with impaired mentation at baseline are also difficult to assess because of the lack of ability to communicate in an age-appropriate fashion. Additionally, they may be predisposed to problems such as decubitus ulcers that are not commonly encountered in children. Finally, there are some conditions that are actually less likely to cause sepsis but can serve to inappropriately narrow the physician's differential diagnosis. An example of this potential pitfall is the patient with a ventriculoperitoneal shunt. Except in the first few postoperative weeks, the shunt is unlikely to be the source of infection, but its presence can distract attention from the performance of an appropriate and thorough evaluation.

Clinical Assessment

Once sepsis is suspected, a multifaceted approach is warranted. This approach begins with stabilization of the patient but also includes a search for both the cause of the infection and evidence of physiologic compromise. Baseline laboratory studies should include blood cultures, with specimens drawn from at least two sites if possible, though this might be impractical in neonates and infants. If the child has an indwelling central venous catheter, culture samples should be drawn through the catheter and, if appropriate, the catheter should be removed. A complete blood count will identify neutropenia, thrombocytopenia, or anemia, any of which can contribute to a poor outcome. Because sepsis-associated microischemia can affect virtually any organ system, organ function should be assessed in a directed fashion (Table 13–3). Renal function, serum electrolytes, and calcium should be obtained along with measurements of serum glucose. Liver function studies should also be obtained to assess for sepsis-related liver injury. Serum prothrombin and partial thromboplastin times are excellent indicators of coagulation status and hepatic function. Markers of cardiac injury should be obtained in selected cases, and children at risk for thyroid dysfunction (e.g., trisomy 21, congenital heart disease) should undergo thyroid function studies, though the emergency physician can defer such testing to the inpatient setting. A urinalysis should be obtained in infants, young children, and those with impaired mental status or risk factors for urinary tract infection. Similarly, when meningitis cannot be reasonably excluded on clinical grounds, a lumbar puncture is mandatory. Children with open wounds should have wound cultures performed. In some cases, it might be possible to identify a specific causative agent early in the course of illness through the use of a rapid immune assay.

To offer the patient the best chance of survival, it is critical to identify sepsis and impending shock in its earliest stages. Prior to overt clinical findings of shock, microenvironments within the host are becoming ischemic, leading to acidosis. Therefore, any patient in whom the diagnosis of sepsis is

Table 13–3	Criteria for Defining Organ Dysfunction
Organ System	**Criteria**

Cardiovascular	• Hypotension—unresponsive to fluid challenge ≥ 60 ml/kg *or* requiring vasopressors
	• Cardiac arrest
	• Tachycardia/bradycardia
	  ○ Less than 12 mo: < 50 or > 220 beats/min
	  ○ Greater than 12 mo: < 40 or > 200 beats/min
	• Two of the following:
	  ○ Metabolic acidosis: base deficit > 5.0 mEq/L
	  ○ Elevated lactate > 2 × upper limit of normal
	  ○ Oliguria
	  ○ Capillary refill >5 sec
	  ○ Core-to-peripheral temperature gap > 3° C

Respiratory	PaO_2/FiO_2 < 300 $PaCO_2$ > 65 mm Hg PaO_2 < 40 mm Hg Requirement for mechanical ventilatory support
Neurologic	Intercranial hypertension requiring intervention Glasgow Coma Scale score <11 *or* acute change with decrease > 3 points
Hematologic	INR > 2 Platelets < 80,000/mm³ Hemoglobin < 5 g/dl White blood cell count < 3000
Renal	Creatine > 20 mg/dl
Hepatic	Total bilirubin ≥ 5 mg/dl ALS > 2 × normal

*Adapted from Goldstein B, Grior B, Randolph A, et al: International Pediatric Sepsis Consensus Conference: definitions for sepsis and organ dysfunction in pediatrics. Pediatr Crit Care Med 6:2–8, 2005; and from Tantaléan JA, Léon RJ, Santos AA, Sánchez E: Multiple organ dysfunction syndrome in children. Pediatr Crit Care Med 4:181–185, 2003.
Abbreviations: ALS, alanine aminotransferase; FiO₂, fraction of inspired oxygen; INR, international normalized ratio; PaCO₂, arterial partial pressure of carbon dioxide; PaO₂, arterial partial pressure of oxygen.

being seriously considered should undergo measurement of serum acid-base status and serum lactate determination. Some authors have suggested that mixed venous oxygen saturation be measured initially and later to gauge response to therapy. Since some children have risk factors for reduced cortisol levels and an impaired response to physiologic stress, many investigators have recommended that cortisol levels be drawn, and supplemental steroids be administered empirically to such children. Others have suggested that an adrenocorticotrophic hormone (ACTH) stimulation test be conducted before administration of steroids.[20] C-reactive protein plays a role in the sepsis cascade and is easily measured, but its utility as a marker of severity of illness or a guide to further therapy is unclear. Other more esoteric laboratory studies of mediators involved in the evolution of SIRS, sepsis, septic shock, and/or MODS (e.g., procalcitonin, IL-1, IL-6, nitric oxide metabolites) have been described in the literature, but currently these are utilized most often in research settings.

Imaging studies should be ordered as indicated by the clinical scenario, for example, obtaining a chest radiograph when pneumonia is suspected. Computed tomography may help to identify clinically occult abscesses and to delineate the extent to which a particular organ is involved. As described later, bedside ultrasonography can be used to evaluate cardiac function as myocardial depression is a well-recognized complication of sepsis.[21] More formal echocardiography might also be used to identify possible endocarditis.

Differential Diagnosis

Because the symptoms of sepsis are nonspecific, the differential diagnosis is necessarily broad. Many conditions that cause severe illness and shock can mimic sepsis, and some of these are, in fact, closely related conditions. Toxic shock syndrome must be considered in the infant or child presenting with a clinical picture consistent with septic shock. In certain infants, necrotizing enterocolitis might be confused with sepsis; meningitis or encephalitis might also resemble sepsis.

Because sepsis may ultimately cause shock, septic shock can be confused with other types of shock. While hemorrhagic and neurogenic shock are in the differential diagnosis, cardiogenic shock from congenital heart disease or viral myocarditis is most likely to be confused with sepsis. The child with cardiogenic shock is more likely to present with congestive heart failure. It has recently been demonstrated that emergency physicians using bedside ultrasonography can identify impaired cardiac wall motion and decreased ejection fraction with reasonable accuracy.[22] As this technology becomes more widely used, it may be possible to identify those patients whose symptoms are at least partially caused by cardiac dysfunction. Hemorrhagic and neurogenic shock generally follow significant trauma. Without such a history, with the exception of the adolescent female with a ruptured ectopic pregnancy, the clinician must consider inflicted injury.

Children who have impaired production of cortisol, and are less able to tolerate physiologic stress, may present with shock or a sepsis-like picture. Included are children with congenital adrenal hyperplasia and those with severe pituitary or adrenal dysfunction. It is important to note that a similar picture can be created by the chronic administration of steroid hormones. Any severe illness can mimic sepsis, but most such illnesses are rare in the pediatric age group and most present with clues that direct the clinician toward the specific etiology. Consider the possibility of rare conditions such as pulmonary embolus, acute renal failure, myocardial infarction, or aortic dissection when the clinical picture indicates such consideration or is confusing.

Management

The foundations of sepsis management are establishment and maintenance of a patent airway, effective ventilation and oxygenation, circulatory support, treatment of infection, and exclusion of alternative diagnoses. Adherence to rigorous treatment protocols, and awareness of the concept of early goal-directed therapy (EGDT) have resulted in a 92% decrease in sepsis-related mortality over the last 4 decades.[22a] It is critical to recognize that most of the recommendations noted in this section are derived from studies of adult patients. Few, if any, similar studies involving infants and children are available; therefore, these recommendations must be approached with caution. However, many have proven themselves in the clinical arena, and they represent the best therapy available for a potentially devastating disease process.

A 9-year retrospective review of infants transported a tertiary care center with sepsis and septic shock demonstrated that better survival was associated with aggressive resuscitation by the referring physicians.[23] Early aggressive treatment in the community was clearly beneficial, but many septic patients were frequently underresuscitated in community emergency departments.[23] When the diagnosis of sepsis is being considered, treatment must be instituted immediately. Circulatory and respiratory support are vitally important. Antimicrobial therapy plays an important role but is in and of itself insufficient. The progression of sepsis in children is different from that seen in adults. Whereas an adult patient might experience a gradual deterioration, children often appear stable for an extended period only to experience a precipitous decline in vital function.

Antimicrobial therapy is a key component of treatment and should be started as soon as possible. Treatment should include one or more antimicrobial agents with activity against the most likely pathogens, taking into account community- and facility-specific patterns of bacterial resistance, and mitigating host factors. Unless rapid testing has identified a specific agent, prudence dictates the selection of broad-spectrum agents until specific pathogens have been identified (Table 13–4). Patients who are immune deficient or who are at risk for particularly virulent bacteria (e.g., *Pseudomonas*) should be treated with several antibiotics appropriately, but broadly directed at the suspected pathogens. Additionally, in some cases, a potential source of infection can be eliminated. Abscesses can be drained, necrotic tissue can be incised, and indwelling catheters can be removed.

Circulatory support is critical and should be initiated before hypotension and other signs of shock have developed. Effectiveness of therapy should be monitored by evaluation of several parameters, including heart rate, urine output, mental status, respiratory rate, serum acid-base status, and serum lactate, in addition to blood pressure and pulse pressure. Some authors have advocated continuous measurement of central venous pressure and arterial pressure rather than blood pressure.

Aggressive early volume resuscitation is the cornerstone of initial therapy. While physicians often do an excellent job in the management of sepsis, they frequently do not administer enough volume when resuscitating septic patients and fail to follow the current advanced life support guidelines.[23] They should first administer 20 ml/kg of crystalloid and give subsequent boluses based upon patient response. Some authors advocate the administration of colloid after several boluses of crystalloid because it can provide similar clinical effects with a smaller volume of administration. However, no studies have demonstrated a definite benefit of one fluid type over another. The risk of overhydration is overstated. Aggressive fluid resuscitation in excess of 40 ml/kg in the first hour of treatment is associated with increased survival with no increased risk of acute respiratory distress syndrome (ARDS) or cardiogenic pulmonary edema.[24]

Evaluation of EGDT for severe sepsis and septic shock in a major adult sepsis clinical trial[16] suggested that initial therapy should be dictated by mixed venous oxygen saturation, hematocrit, and central venous pressure. The goal of volume expansion should be a central venous pressure of 8 to 12 mm Hg except in the case of mechanically ventilated patients, who require higher central venous pressure of 12 to 15 mm Hg due to elevated intrathoracic pressures. Volume expansion might help to restore systemic circulation and reverse the sepsis cascade, but alone may not be sufficient. Mixed venous oxygen saturation, measured by a Swan-Ganz catheter or other special measurement device, should be maintained above 70%. During the first 6 hours of treatment, if fluid therapy has achieved a central venous pressure of 8 to 12 mm Hg (12 to 15 mm Hg in mechanically ventilated patients) and the patient's mixed venous oxygen saturation remains below 70%, further therapy is guided by the hematocrit. For a hematocrit below 30%, blood is transfused. If the hematocrit is normal or if transfusion fails to achieve a mixed venous oxygen saturation of 70%, dobutamine is administered until this goal has been achieved or to a maximum dose of 20 mcg/kg/min (see Chapter 8, Circulatory Emergencies: Shock).

In the absence of mixed venous oxygen saturation, the treating physician should aim for a central venous pressure of 8 to 12 mm Hg (12 to 15 mm Hg if mechanically ventilated) and a hematocrit no less than 30%. Once these goals have been met, signs of poor perfusion should be treated with dobutamine as described. Dobutamine is recommended because it is assumed that, given adequate left ventricular filling pressures and red blood cell volume, the most likely source of impaired perfusion is depressed cardiac output. As described earlier, bedside ultrasound may allow the clinician to determine the effectiveness of cardiac activity and help guide therapy.

EGDT has been demonstrated to improve the mortality from sepsis in adults. These guidelines have not been tested in children, but several investigators have found that, in conjunction with goal-directed therapy, implementation of the American College of Critical Care Medicine Pediatric Advanced Life Support guidelines results in improved clinical outcomes.[25] Published guidelines for the treatment of pediatric and neonatal sepsis have incorporated these elements (Fig. 13–1).

Table 13–4	Age-Specific Recommendations for Initial Empiric Antibiotic Selection in Sepsis
Age	**Antibiotics**
Neonates < 1 wk old	Ampicillin 25 mg/kg q8h *and* Cefotaxime 50 mg/kg q8h
Neonates 1–4 wk	Ampicillin 25 mg/kg q8h *and* Cefotaxime 50 mg/kg q8h *or* ceftriaxone 75 mg/kg q24h
Children	Cefotaxime 50 mg/kg q8h *or* Ceftriaxone 100 mg/kg q24h
Adolescents/young adults	Cefepime 50 mg/kg q8h *or* Imipenem 25 mg/kg q6h *or* Meropenem 60 mg/kg q8h
Special considerations	Suspected MRSA—add vancomycin Suspected VRE—add linezolid Abdominal processes—add anaerobic coverage Urinary pathogen—add aminoglycoside Suspected pulmonary infection—add macrolide

*Selections should be tailored to suspected sources, local resistance patterns, and patient allergies.
Abbreviations: MRSA, methicillin-resistant *Staphylococcus aureus*; VRE, vancomycin-resistant enterococcus.

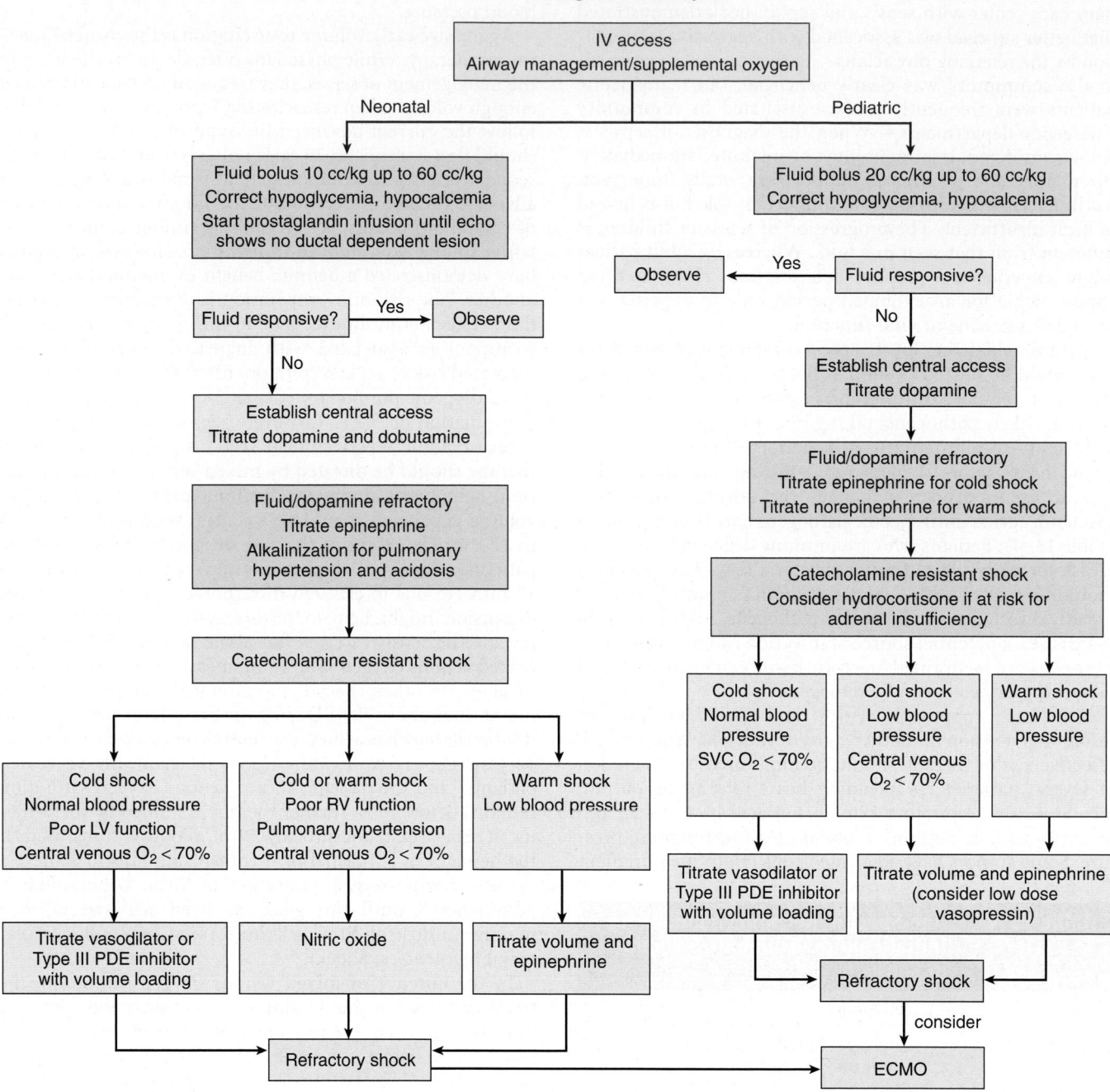

FIGURE 13–1. Algorithm for treatment of pediatric and neonatal sepsis. (Adapted from Carcillo JA, Fields AI; American College of Critical Care Medicine Task Force Committee Members: Clinical practice parameters for hemodynamic support of pediatric and neonatal patients in septic shock. Crit Care Med 30:1365–1378, 2002.)

Other vasopressors can be added to achieve specific desired effects. If cardiac output cannot be determined or is adequate after volume resuscitation, the physician should consider dopamine or norepinephrine. One of these drugs can be added to dobutamine for persistent hypotension despite correction of cardiac output. These agents are preferred over epinephrine because they cause less profound tachycardia and less vasoconstriction of the splanchnic bed. However, there is evidence of an age-dependent resistance to dopamine,[26] and failure to respond should prompt the clinician to employ another agent. Phenylephrine causes vasoconstric-

tion without tachycardia and could be chosen when vasodilatory shock is strongly suspected. Ideally, the administration of vasopressors should be guided by continuous arterial pressure monitoring. Such monitoring is not universally available in the emergency department. In its absence, the clinician should rely upon measurement of peripheral blood pressure, urine output, mental status, and systemic acid-base status until the patient can be transferred to an intensive care unit.

One should consider adding a short-acting, titratable vasodilator such as nitroprusside or nitroglycerine for patients with strong evidence of elevated peripheral vascular resistance and depressed cardiac output unresponsive to the previously discussed therapies. If these agents fail to improve cardiac output and peripheral perfusion, then milrinone or amrinone should be considered. Abnormally low cardiac output in pediatric patients is associated with increased mortality, so every effort should be made to ensure that it is normal.

Children with cortisol deficiency may be resistant to vasopressor therapy. At least one trial has demonstrated improved outcome when such children are identified and treated promptly.[25] Adrenal insufficiency can be the result of sepsis itself (e.g., Waterhouse-Friederichsen syndrome), but is more likely to be the result of a congenital or acquired endocrinopathy or chronic steroid use. Experts recommend administration of stress doses of corticosteroids (e.g., hydrocortisone 1 to 2 mg/m^2/hr) for children with potential adrenal insufficiency and higher doses (25 to 50 mg/m^2 loading dose followed by 1 to 2 mg/m^2/hr) for shock states associated with Waterhouse-Friderichsen syndrome. However, two adult studies have demonstrated worse outcomes in patients receiving high-dose corticosteroids (e.g., more than 300 mg/day), so excessively high doses are not recommended.[27-29]

When uncertainty exists regarding the state of the patient's pituitary-adrenal axis, a cortisol stimulation test can be obtained. Patients who have an adequate response to ACTH do not need exogenous steroids. This test is impractical in many emergency departments; dexamethasone (0.6 to 1 mg/kg) will not interfere with the stimulation test and can be safely given if this test is deemed necessary at a later point. Corticosteroids have not been demonstrated to be beneficial to patients who have normal cortisol production and should not be administered in this situation.

Priority should be given to the patient's electrolyte balance and glucose levels. Maintenance of serum glucose at levels between 80 and 150 mg/dl has been associated with improved survival.[29a] Hypoglycemia should be avoided and hyperglycemia should be treated with regular insulin, administered intravenously. Glucose levels should be monitored frequently. Calcium can be depleted during septic shock but should only be replaced if indicated by a low serum ionized calcium level.

Several immune-modulating agents that theoretically decrease the exogenous immune response and improve tissue ischemia have been investigated as potential therapies in pediatric sepsis. Thus far, only recombinant human activated protein C has shown minimal benefit, and only in adult patients.[30] Activated protein C decreases serum levels of activated factors V and VIII, thus decreasing thrombin formation and increasing fibrinolysis. Both tissue pathway factor inhibitor and interferon gamma have produced some promising early results in clinical trials. Studies of plasma filtration have demonstrated that this therapy can reduce amounts of circulating acute-phase reactants, but has thus far not been shown to improve outcomes.[30a]

Many children with sepsis will require mechanical ventilation. Recent literature suggests that ventilator-associated lung injury contributes to ARDS both by direct barotrauma and by increased pulmonary cytokine production. Experts now recommend ventilation with low tidal volumes (e.g., 6 ml/kg), low end-expiratory pressures, and, if necessary, permissive hypercapnia.[31-33] Because many of these patients will be intubated in the emergency department, emergency physicians must understand these issues and adhere to these principles during both manual and mechanical ventilation.

Neonates with advanced sepsis present some unique challenges. The acidosis associated with sepsis can lead to persistent patency of the ductus arteriosus and, in some cases, to persistent pulmonary hypertension. This disease state can create a vicious cycle of hypoxemia and worsening acidosis and can ultimately cause right ventricular failure. Inhaled nitric oxide is currently used in neonatal units and by many neonatal transport teams to avert this complication. In most emergency departments, treatment would primarily include supplemental oxygen and correction of acidosis.

Summary

Recognition and management of sepsis in the pediatric population requires early diagnosis and aggressive, goal-directed therapy. Emergency physicians must be very familiar with the specific criteria for SIRS, stay attuned to possible subtle presentations of infection in infancy and childhood, and be highly suspicious for the diagnosis of sepsis in infants and immunocompromised children. Effective initial stabilization can be performed in a variety of settings. However, with rare exceptions, all septic pediatric patients require prompt transfer to tertiary care centers, preferably those with pediatric-specific critical care units.

Isotonic intravenous fluids, blood product transfusions, ventilatory support, early appropriate antibiotics, and early surgical intervention for abscesses and acute abdominal processes are the mainstays of therapy. Initial therapeutic efforts should be focused on aggressive restoration of volume and, if necessary, ion-tropic support. Treatment decisions should be based on a balance between potential benefits and potential harms. Because septic children and adults have differing mortality rates, treatment-related morbidity may not always favor intervention.

Research in sepsis is particularly challenging, and is more so in children. The new consensus definition of sepsis helps to provide a framework to generate multicenter trials. As our knowledge and understanding of the pathophysiology of sepsis continue to grow, our ability to intervene will move beyond antibiotics and supportive therapy. Areas of promise and current trials include serum markers for sepsis, "designer antibiotics," and coagulation- and inflammatory–pathway specific therapies.

REFERENCES

1. Levy MM, Fink MP, Marshal JC, et al: 2001 SCCM/ESICM/ACCP/ATS/SIS International Sepsis Definitions Conference. Intensive Care Med 29:530–538, 2003.
2. Goldstein B, Grior B, Randolph A, et al: International Pediatric Sepsis Consensus Conference: definitions for sepsis and organ dysfunction in pediatrics. Pediatr Crit Care Med 6:2–8, 2005.
3. Bone RC, Sprung CL, Sibbald WJ: Definitions for sepsis and organ failure. Crit Care Med 20:724–726, 1992.
4. Burns JP: Septic shock in the pediatric patient: pathogenesis and novel treatments. Pediatr Emerg Care 19:112–115, 2003.
5. Thomas L: Germs. N Engl J Med 287:553–555, 1972.
6. Meakins JL, Pietsch JB, Bubenick O, et al: Delayed hypersensitivity: indicator of acquired failure of host defenses in sepsis and trauma. Ann Surg 186:241–250, 1977.

7. Oberholzer A, Olberholtzer C, Moldawer LL: Sepsis syndromes: understanding the role of innate immunity. Shock 16:83–96, 2001.

8. Watson RS, Carcillo JA, Linde-Zwirble WT, et al: The epidemiology of severe sepsis in children in the United States. Am J Respir Crit Care Med 167:695–701, 2003.

9. Angus DC, Linde Zwirble WT, Liddicker J, et al: Epidemiology of severe sepsis in the United States: analysis of incidence, outcome, and associated costs of care. Crit Care Med 29:1303–1310, 2001.

10. Parrillo JE: Pathogenetic mechanisms of septic shock. N Engl J Med 328:1471–1477, 1993.

11. Kurahashi K, Kajikawa O, Sawa T, et al: Pathogenesis of septic shock in *Pseudomonas aeruginosa* pneumonia. J Clin Invest 104:743–750, 1999.

12. Abbas AK, Murphy KM, Sher A: Functional diversity of helper T lymphocytes. Nature 383:787–793, 1996.

13. Hotchkiss RS, Karl IE: The pathophysiology and treatment of sepsis. N Engl J Med 384:138–150, 2003.

14. Levi M, Ten Cate H: Disseminated intravascular coagulation. N Engl J Med 341:586–592, 1999.

15. Despond O, Proulx F, Carcillo JA, Lacroix J: Pediatric sepsis and multiple organ dysfunction syndrome. Curr Opin Pediatr 13:247–253, 2001.

16. Rivers E, Nguyen B, Havstad S, et al: Early goal-directed therapy in the treatment of severe sepsis and septic shock. N Engl J Med 345:1368–1377, 2001.

17. Martinot A, Leclerc F, Cremer R, et al: Sepsis in neonates and children: definitions, epidemiology, and outcome. Pediatr Emerg Care 13:277–281, 1997.

18. Kreger BE, Craven DE, Carling P, et al: Gram-negative bacteremia. III. Reassessment of etiology, epidemiology and ecology in 612 patients. Am J Med 60:332–343, 1980.

19. Weinstein MP, Murphy JR, Reller LB, et al: The clinical significance of positive blood cultures: a comprehensive analysis of 500 episodes of bacteremia and fungemia in adults. II. Clinical observations, with special reference to factors influencing prognosis. Rev Infect Dis 5:54–70, 1983.

20. Dellinger RP, Carlet JM, Masur H, et al; Surviving Sepsis Campaign Management Guidelines Committee: Surviving Sepsis Campaign guidelines for management of severe sepsis and septic shock. Crit Care Med 32:858–873, 2004

21. Monsalve F, Rucabado L, Salvador A, et al: Myocardial depression in septic shock caused by meningococcal infection. Crit Care Med 12:1021–1023, 1984.

22. Moore CL, Rose GA, Tayal VS, et al: Determination of left ventricular function by emergency physician echocardiography of hypotensive patients. Acad Emerg Med 9:186–193, 2002.

22a. Arnal AE, Stein F: Pediatric septic shock: Why has mortality decreased?—The utility of goal directed therapy. Sem Pediatr Infect Dis 14:165–172, 2003.

23. Han YY, Carcillo JA, Dragotta MA, et al: Early reversal of pediatric-neonatal septic shock by community physicians is associated with improved outcome. Pediatrics 112:793–799, 2003.

24. Carcillo JA, Davis AL, Zaritsky A: Role of early fluid resuscitation in pediatric septic shock. JAMA 266:1242–1245, 1991.

25. Carcillo JA, Fields AI; American College of Critical Care Medicine Task Force Committee Members: Clinical practice parameters for hemodynamic support of pediatric and neonatal patients in septic shock. Crit Care Med 30:1365–1378, 2002.

26. Bhatt-Mehta V, Nahata MC, McClead RE, et al: Dopamine pharmacokinetics in critically ill newborn infants. Eur J Clin Pharmacol 40:593–597, 1991.

27. Cronin L, Cook DJ, Carlet J, et al: Corticosteroid treatment for sepsis: a critical appraisal and meta-analysis of the literature. Crit Care Med 23:1430–1439, 1995.

28. Veterans Administration Systemic Sepsis Cooperative Study Group: Effect on high-dose glucocorticoid therapy on mortality in patients with clinical signs of sepsis. N Engl J Med 317:659–665, 1987.

29. Bone RC, Fisher CJ, Clemmer TP: A controlled clinical trial of high-dose methyprednisolone in the treatment of severe sepsis and septic shock. N Engl J Med 317:653–658, 1987.

29a. Dellinger RP, Carlet JM, Masur H, et al: Surviving sepsis campaign management guidelines committee: Surviving sepsis campaign guidelines for management of severe sepsis and septic shock. Crit Care Med 32:858–873, 2004.

30. Bernard GR, Vincent JL, Laterre PF, et al: Efficacy and safety of recombinant human activated protein C for severe sepsis. N Engl J Med 344:699–709, 2001.

30a. Despond O, Proulx F, Carcillo JA, Lacroix J: Pediatric sepsis and multiple organ dysfunction syndrome. Curr Opin Pediatr 13:247–255, 2001.

31. Bidani A, Tzouanakis AE, Cardenas VJ, et al: Permissive hypercapnia in acute respiratory failure. JAMA 272:957–962, 1994.

32. Ventilation with lower tidal volumes as compared with the traditional tidal volume for acute lung injury and the acute respiratory distress syndrome. The Acute Respiratory Distress Syndrome Network. N Engl J Med 342:1301–1308, 2000.

33. Hickling KG, Walsh J, Henderson S, et al: Low mortality rate in adult respiratory distress syndrome using low-volume, pressure limited ventilation with permissive hypercapnia: a prospective study. Crit Care Med 22:1568–1578, 1994.

Chapter 14

Anaphylaxis

Suzanne M. Beno, MD

Key Points

Survival is dependent upon immediate recognition and intervention.

Rapid administration of intramuscular epinephrine is first-line therapy for anaphylaxis.

Children with asthma are at increased risk for delayed and more severe reactions.

Introduction and Background

Anaphylaxis has long been recognized as a severe, life-threatening reaction that involves multiple target organs, including skin, respiratory, gastrointestinal, cardiovascular, and neurologic systems.[1] Consensus regarding its exact definition currently does not exist and there is considerable disagreement about its prevalence, diagnosis, and management. A recent practice parameter addresses these issues and attempts to provide an evidence-based approach to the definition of this condition.[2] Anaphylaxis is considered to be highly likely when any one of the following three criteria is present:

1. Acute onset of an illness (minutes to hours) involving skin/mucosa and either respiratory compromise or hypotension (associated symptoms)
2. Two or more of the following that occur rapidly after exposure (minutes to hours) to a *likely* allergen for that patient: skin/mucosal involvement, respiratory compromise, hypotension and associated symptoms, and persistent gastrointestinal symptoms
3. Hypotension after exposure to *known* allergen for that patient (minutes to hours)

The term *anaphylaxis* encompasses both immunoglobulin E (IgE)–mediated reactions and non–IgE-mediated mechanisms (*anaphylactoid* reactions); the difference impacts allergen counseling but is of little consequence in the immediate management of the patient.[2]

Recognition and Approach

Epidemiology data in the general population are sparse and affected by variable definitions, coding, and misclassification errors. Population data from the 1980s estimated an annual occurrence rate of 30 per 100,000 person-years, while more recent literature suggests occurrence rates as high as 590 per 100,000 person-years.[3] The actual incidence, especially in children, remains uncertain as very few population-based studies exist. A prevalence study using rates of injectable epinephrine dispensing data in Manitoba supports various retrospective reviews suggesting a 1% prevalence in the community. This study specifically noted a peak in anaphylaxis from all triggers in early childhood with a gradual decline toward adolescence.[4]

Anaphylaxis is generally considered to be at the severe end of the generalized hypersensitivity spectrum, with respiratory and/or cardiovascular involvement denoting severity. Different grading systems have been explored, and are based upon the current proposed definition for anaphylaxis.[2] A systematic compilation of the frequency of signs and symptoms in anaphylaxis is shown in Table 14–1.

Evaluation

Anaphylaxis is an immediate uniphasic reaction invoking various end-organ responses in the skin, respiratory tract, and cardiovascular and gastrointestinal systems. Other patterns of anaphylaxis exist, and include delayed onset (>30 minutes postexposure), protracted or persistent reactions (can last up to 32 hours), and biphasic reactions in which recurrence of symptoms follows a symptom-free period (8 to 12 hours). The resultant reaction in a biphasic response is usually more severe and less amenable to treatment.[6,7]

The majority of anaphylaxis will present with some degree of cutaneous involvement, such as flushing, pruritus, urticaria, and angioedema, but these symptoms may be either overlooked or missed after epinephrine administration.[8] Other classic features include signs of upper and lower airway obstruction, gastrointestinal symptoms, syncope, hypotension, and dizziness. In its severe form, anaphylaxis can result in cardiovascular collapse and death.

The most common etiologies of anaphylactic reactions include reactions to food, medications, *Hymenoptera* stings, and latex.[2] Certain groups of children are more prone to anaphylaxis. Children with neural tube defects and/or genitourinary abnormalities requiring self-catheterization are at increased risk for latex allergy. Children with asthma, particularly if poorly controlled, have an increased incidence of fatal anaphylaxis.[6,9,10]

Table 14–1	Signs and Symptoms: Frequency of Occurrence in Anaphylaxis (%)		
	Lieberman et al.[5] (mostly adults)	Lee and Greenes[35] (children): N = 106	Dibs and Baker[36] (children): N = 55
Cutaneous	>90	92	93
Urticaria/angioedema	85–90		
Flushing	45–55		
Pruritis w/o rash	<5		
Respiratory	40–60		93
Upper airway	50–60	78	
Dyspnea, wheeze	45–50	58	
Rhinitis	15–20		
Gastrointestinal			
Nausea, vomiting, diarrhea	25–30	37	13
Dizziness, Syncope, Decreased Blood Pressure	30–35	30	26
Neurologic			
Seizure/HA	5–8	27	26
Seizure alone	1–2		
Miscellaneous			
Substernal chest pain	4–6		

Adapted from references 5, 35, 36.

Food-Induced Anaphylaxis

This is the single most common cause of anaphylaxis treated in emergency departments in the United States, particularly in children, and these reactions are mainly attributable to peanuts, tree nuts, fish, shellfish, milk, and eggs.[11] The prevalence of these reactions is rising and estimated to now affect 0.8% to 2.0% of the population.[12,13] Reactions tend to worsen in severity with age and the development of asthma. Food-associated exercise-induced anaphylaxis can occur when exercise takes place within 2 to 4 hours after ingestion of a specific food, but its pathogenesis and true incidence are unknown.[14]

Drug-Induced Anaphylaxis

A careful history is key to establishing the correct diagnosis, including when the exposure occurred, the interval to reaction, previous medications, and response to therapy. The development of drug-specific IgE antibodies during previous sensitization accounts for these reactions. Penicillin is the most common cause of drug-induced anaphylaxis, followed by aspirin and nonsteroidal anti-inflammatory medications. Validated tests for IgE-mediated reactions are available for penicillin and insulin, but largely unavailable for most drugs and biologic agents.[2] There is a 5% to 10% cross reactivity of penicillin with first-generation cephalosporins and less than 1% cross reactivity with third-generation cephalosporins. Some drugs cause anaphylactoid reactions, and do not require a preceding sensitization. Radiographic contrast material (RCM) is such an agent, and moderate reactions requiring treatment occur in about 1% of patients receiving RCM, while life-threatening reactions occur less than 0.1% of the time.[5] Pretreatment regimens in emergency situations include some combination of corticosteroids and H_1-receptor antagonists and possibly H_2-receptor antagonists (antihistamines).

Insect Sting–Induced Anaphylaxis

Self-administered epinephrine is critically important in this situation. Onset of anaphylaxis after an insect sting is rapid, with 96% of fatal reactions beginning within 30 minutes of the insect sting.[15] Unfortunately, most fatal reactions occur with the first sting reaction and thus are not preventable. Diagnostic skin testing for screening purposes lacks specificity as 25% of adults are positive, and its utility in children has not been established.[16] Immunotherapy is available for prevention of subsequent anaphylactic reactions, and individuals should be referred for this purpose.[17]

Latex-Induced Anaphylaxis

Latex-induced anaphylaxis is an IgE mast cell–mediated reaction. Its incidence has reached a plateau after a steady increase over the last 20 years; 6.5% in the general population are affected. Up to 17% of cases of intraoperative anaphylaxis are latex induced, and approximately 75% of the spina bifida population are sensitized.[5] The plateau and hopeful decline are likely secondary to the creation of latex-safe environments through increased awareness, decreased use of latex products, and Food and Drug Administration labeling warnings about the presence of latex in medical products.[18]

Idiopathic Anaphylaxis

This is a diagnosis of exclusion encompassing approximately 20% of cases of anaphylaxis, and is more common in adults than in children. It lacks distinguishing features, may be fatal, and is sometimes treated with prophylactic corticosteroid and antihistamine therapy.[19] Systemic mastocytosis should be ruled out in these patients.

Angioedema

Angioedema is a hypersensitivity disorder that manifests as an acute onset of noninflammatory edema in the subcutaneous tissues or mucosa, most often in the upper respiratory or gastrointestinal tracts. Children can present with life-threatening airway obstruction or with symptoms mimicking an acute abdomen. Urticaria is not typically seen. Both hereditary and acquired forms are clinically similar. Hereditary angioedema is an autosomal dominant disease characterized by an inherited defect in C_1 esterase inhibitor activity that disrupts regulation of the allergic cascade, and usually manifests in late childhood. Although standard anaphylaxis therapy is often not very helpful for this condition, antihistamines, corticosteroids, and epinephrine may be beneficial.[20] The treatment of choice is an intravenous concentrate of C_1 inhibitor.[21] Fresh frozen plasma contains C_1 inhibitor and can be helpful but occasionally paradoxically worsens angioedema.[22] Antifibrinolytic agents such as ε-aminocaproic acid are used in children in place of attenuated androgens, which increase complement levels and are standard treatment in adults.[20]

Anaphylaxis remains a clinical diagnosis, and laboratory tests are of little value. Two mediators that are currently available as serum levels are tryptase and histamine, both of which have unreliable diagnostic accuracy and poor predictive value. Additional biomarkers that are easily and rapidly measured may be of benefit in the future.[5]

The two major pitfalls in the management of an anaphylactic reaction are (1) failure to recognize anaphylaxis and (2) failure to administer epinephrine early in suspected anaphylaxis. Recognition failure can be the result of physician-related factors, such as failing to diagnose anaphylaxis in the absence of shock with subsequent failure to prescribe epinephrine for future reactions. Patient-related factors include not appreciating the significance of mild to moderate symptoms that often spontaneously resolve, and thus never seeking evaluation or treatment. Reported rates are thus believed to be an underestimate of the true prevalence of this condition mainly for these reasons.[4]

Table 14–2 illustrates many of the conditions that can be misinterpreted as anaphylaxis. One condition in particular, acute asphyxic asthma, may confound the diagnosis of anaphylaxis. Acute asphyxic asthma has recently been recognized as a subset of sudden and severe asthma exacerbations.[23] There exists concern that children presenting with typical symptoms of this disorder, particularly those with urticaria, hypotension, or a poor response to bronchodilators, may actually be experiencing anaphylaxis. This finding is supported by postmortem histologic examination. There may be a role for prescribing self-administered epinephrine devices, Medic Alert bracelets, and allergen counseling for survivors of this condition.[24]

Management

Immediate management in the emergency department includes ensuring a patent airway and adequate oxygenation, establishment of intravenous (IV) access for circulatory support, and early administration of epinephrine (Box 14–1). A multicenter emergency department–based study showed wide variability in treatment of allergic reactions and found that treatment was largely symptom based, with use of some combination of antihistamines, steroids, and epinephrine.[25]

Epinephrine is considered the drug of choice for anaphylaxis, and it should be given immediately. The recommended dose is 0.01 mg/kg (1:1000 solution) intramuscularly, with a minimum of 0.1 mg/dose and a maximum of 0.3 mg/dose. The dose can be repeated every 10 to 20 minutes if symptoms persist or worsen.[5] The lateral aspect of the thigh is considered the optimal location for administration in adults, and intramuscular injections are preferred to subcutaneous administration in both children and adults based on mean plasma concentrations in asymptomatic individuals.[26,27] Current outpatient formulations include (1) Epipen (0.3 mg) and EpiPen Jr (0.15 mg) for children weighing less than 25 kg, and (2) Twinject (0.3 mg and 0.15 mg) which recently came on the market and offers two doses of epinephrine in one device. Considerable discussion among experts regarding appropriate childhood dosing for injectable epinephrine has taken place and will hopefully result in availability of additional fixed-dose pens.[11,28] Alternative delivery methods of epinephrine include sublingual and inhaled administration. Inhaled epinephrine was recently studied prospectively in a small number of asymptomatic children who were unable to inhale sufficient quantities to significantly increase their plasma epinephrine concentration. Therefore, it may be beneficial for reversal of laryngeal edema or persistent

Table 14–2	Conditions Mimicking Acute Anaphylaxis

Vasodepressor (vasovagal) reactions
Flushing episodes (vancomycin-induced "red man" syndrome, alcohol intoxication or withdrawal, malignancy, autonomic epilepsy)
Postprandial syndromes (monosodium glutamate [MSG], sulfites, scombroid)
Asthma (acute asphyxic asthma)
Vocal cord dysfunction
Acute anxiety (panic attacks, hyperventilation)
Myocardial dysfunction
Pulmonary embolus
Shock (hemorrhagic, cardiogenic)
Systemic mast cell disorders
Foreign-body aspiration
Acute poisoning
Hypoglycemia
Erythema multiforme major

Box 14–1 *Therapeutics*

- Cardiac monitor, continuous pulse oximetry
- Supplemental oxygen
- Airway management
- IM epinephrine (0.01 mg/kg of 1:1000; max 0.3 mg per dose, min 0.1 mg per dose)
- IV epinephrine (0.01 mg/kg of 1:10,000 over 2–5 min) for patients in extremis or refractory shock
- IV fluid expansion (20 ml/kg NS or LR; repeat as needed)
- Consider Trendelenburg positioning
- Nebulized albuterol (0.5–1 ml 5% soln), ipratropium (125–500 mcg), or racemic epinephrine (0.25–0.5 ml 2.25% soln)
- H_1 antagonist (diphenhydramine 1 mg/kg up to 50 mg)
- H_2 antagonist (ranitidine 1–2 mg/kg); use with caution in children with bronchospasm
- Corticosteroids (1–2 mg/kg prednisone or methylprednisolone)
- Glucagon (20–30 mcg/kg up to 1 mg)

Abbreviations: IM, intramuscular; IV, intravenous; LR, lactated Ringer's solution; NS, normal saline; soln, solution.

bronchospasm but is not an equivalent substitute for injected epinephrine.[29] Intravenous epinephrine is reserved for patients in extremis, persistent hypotension, or shock. Although epinephrine injected early is more likely to reverse the reaction, as many as 10% of cases may not be reversible.[10] Epinephrine has no absolute contraindications in anaphylaxis; it is *relatively* contraindicated with concomitant cocaine use because of its sensitization of the myocardium. The dose *may* need to be halved for patients taking β-blocker agents, tricyclic antidepressants, and monoamine oxidase inhibitors because of the risk of unopposed α-adrenergic receptor activity and cardiac arrythmias.[1]

Patients with anaphylaxis should be placed in a supine position. A recent practice parameter also suggests elevation of the lower extremities to prevent orthostasis and to shunt effective circulation to the head, heart, and kidneys, but the Trendelenburg position has also been shown to worsen pulmonary hemodynamics.[5,30] A review of 214 cases of anaphylaxis noted a link in patients who, after assuming an upright posture, had immediate cardiovascular collapse.[31] Changes in vascular permeability in anaphylaxis can result in potential loss of 50% of an individual's intravascular fluid within 10 minutes.[32] Patients with persistent hypotension despite epinephrine need volume expansion, typically in the form of crystalloid solutions such as 0.9% saline or lactated Ringer's solution. Children require at least 20 ml/kg within the first hour of therapy.

Secondary therapeutic interventions include the use of histamine receptor antagonists, corticosteroids, β₂-agonists and glucagon therapy. Antihistamines are a useful adjunct in the management of anaphylaxis, specifically targeting urticaria-angioedema and pruritus. Diphenhydramine at 1 mg/kg (up to 50 mg) administered intravenously, intramuscularly, or orally has traditionally been used to block H₁ receptors. Second-generation agents such as loratidine and cetirizine are equally effective and have less sedating effects than first-generation antihistamines in urticaria, but their role in anaphylaxis has yet to be explored. The role of H₂ antagonists has yielded inconsistent results in the literature; however, recently an emergency department–based study of almost 100 adults demonstrated combining diphenhydramine with ranitidine resulted in superior resolution of cutaneous symptoms and tachycardia.[33]

Currently there is no evidence for use of H₂ antagonists in children experiencing anaphylaxis. If administered to children, ranitidine at 1 to 2 mg/kg per dose IV over 10 to 15 minutes is the agent of choice.[5] It can be repeated up to twice a day or to a maximum of 300 mg/day. H₁ and H₂ blockers have competing effects in the lungs, thus H₂ blockers can theoretically lead to bronchoconstriction. While H₂ blockers have been proven useful in cutaneous manifestations of anaphylaxis, they have not been proven to ameliorate other manifestations.

Corticosteroids, though commonly used in anaphylaxis, have never been evaluated in placebo-controlled trials. The effects of corticosteroids are believed to occur within 4 to 6 hours, potentially prevent protracted or biphasic anaphylaxis, and provide additional benefit for children with asthma. Methylprednisolone at 1 to 2 mg/kg/day administered intravenously every 6 hours or 1 to 2 mg/kg of oral prednisone for milder attacks are commonly used regimens.[5] Inhaled β₂-agonists, such as albuterol 0.5 to 1 ml of a 0.5% solution or racemic epinephrine 0.25 to 0.05 ml of 2.25% solution, should be administered for bronchospasm; ipratropium may also reverse bronchospasm. Children taking β-blockers are more likely to experience profound bradycardia, hypotension, and bronchospasm that is unresponsive, or only partially responsive, to epinephrine. These children and those whose hypotension is refractory require aggressive volume expansion and glucagon therapy (20 to 30 mcg/kg up to 1 mg in children) administered intramuscularly, intravenously, or subcutaneously followed by an infusion.

It is vital to immediately discontinue exposure to the suspected causal agent, such as avoiding all latex products in the treatment of latex-induced anaphylaxis. This problem is now easily obviated by the replacement of latex products in many emergency departments or the availability of latex-free treatment areas and emergency equipment carts. Bee sting–induced anaphylaxis can also benefit from local application of ice and removal of the stinger if feasible. Other therapeutic complications include improperly injected epinephrine resulting in ineffective drug delivery or tissue ischemia if inadvertently injected into a digit.

Summary

The prognosis of anaphylaxis is variable, ranging from immediate recovery to irreversible cardiovascular collapse. Children with asthma experience more severe and often delayed reactions, placing them at increased risk of death. Other predictors of severity include older age, insect venom, and iatrogenic causes; as well, some studies suggest the use of angiotensin-converting enzyme inhibitors and β-blockers as independent risk factors.[34]

Transportation to a facility with appropriate resources is mandatory for all prehospital-treated patients. Biphasic reactions with resultant death after premature discharge from the emergency department have been reported to occur between 1.3 and 28 hours after the first symptoms subside. Therefore, patients should be observed for at least 8 hours after the initial symptoms subside, or admitted for 24 hours based on severity, etiology, and underlying disease.[35] A history of a previous severe reaction or a patient's inability to return promptly if symptoms relapse mandates an admission to hospital for observation.[11] Treatment upon discharge should be continued for at least 48 hours. Standard treatment includes scheduled antihistamines and corticosteroids, although supportive evidence for the latter does not currently exist. Debate exists regarding prescription of injectable epinephrine or an anaphylaxis kit; however, any child having experienced an anaphylactic reaction secondary to food or insect venom *must* receive at least one on discharge with adequate instruction in its use. All children with anaphylaxis should be referred to an allergist for further counseling, diagnostic testing, or immunotherapy as applicable. Ideally children with a known allergen should wear a Medic Alert bracelet that will help identify their disease on presentation to the emergency department.

Currently there is no consensus regarding the definition and classification of anaphylaxis. Future research will explore the pathophysiology of why individuals have such variable responses and presentations, as well as identification of laboratory markers with high predictive values that identify both anaphylactic reactions and individuals at risk for them. Prospective evaluation of diagnostic and management algorithms, along with increased public and provider education, is greatly needed.

REFERENCES

1. McLean-Tooke APC, Bethune CA, Fay AC, Spickett GP: Adrenaline in the treatment of anaphylaxis: what is the evidence? BMJ 327:1332–1335, 2003.
*2. Sampson HA, Munoz-Furlong A, Campbell RL, et al: Second symposium on the definition and management of anaphylaxis: Summary report-Second National Institute of Allergy and Infectious Disease/Food Allergy and Anaphylaxis Network symposium. J Allergy Clin Immunol 117:391–397, 2006.
3. Sicherer SH, Simons FER: Quandaries in prescribing an emergency action plan and self-injectable epinephrine for first-aid management of anaphylaxis in the community. J Allergy Clin Immunol 115:575–583, 2005.
4. Simons FER, Peterson S, Black CD: Epinephrine dispensing patterns for an out-of-hospital population: a novel approach to studying the epidemiology of anaphylaxis. J Allergy Clin Immunol 110:647–651, 2002.
*5. Lieberman P, Kemp SF, Oppenheimer J, et al: The diagnosis and management of anaphylaxis: an updated practice parameter. J Allergy Clin Immunol 115:S483–S523, 2005.
6. Sampson HA, Mendelson LM, Rosen JP: Fatal and near-fatal anaphylactic reactions to food in children and adolescents. N Engl J Med 327:380–384, 1992.
7. Starks BJ, Sullivan TJ: Biphasic and protracted anaphylaxis. J Allergy Clin Immunol 78:76–83, 1986.
8. Simons FER: First-aid treatment of anaphylaxis to food: focus on epinephrine. J Allergy Clin Immunol 113:837–844, 2004.
9. Settipane G, Chafee R, Klein DE, et al: Anaphylactic reactions to *Hymenoptera* stings in asthmatic patients. Clin Allergy 10:659–665, 1980.
10. Bock SA, Munoz-Furlong A, Sampson HA: Fatalities due to anaphylactic reactions to foods. J Allergy Clin Immunol 107:191–193, 2001.
*11. Sampson HA: Anaphylaxis and emergency treatment. Pediatrics 111:1601–1608, 2003
12. Sicherer SH, Munoz-Furlong A, Sampson HA: Prevalence of peanut and tree nut allergy in the United States determined by means of a random digit dial telephone survey: a 5 year follow up study. J Allergy Clin Immunol 112:1203–1207, 2003.
13. Kagan RS, Joseph L, Dufresne C, et al: Prevalence of peanut allergy in primary-school children in Montreal, Canada. J Allergy Clin Immunol 112:1223–1228, 2003.
14. Romano A, Fonso M, Giuffreda F, et al: Diagnostic work-up for food-dependent, exercise-induced anaphylaxis. Allergy 50:817–824, 1995.
15. Barnard J: Studies of 400 *Hymenoptera* sting deaths in the United States. J Allergy Clin Immunol 52:259–264, 1973.
16. Golden DB, Marsh DG, Kagey-Sobotka A, et al: Epidemiology of insect venom sensitivity. JAMA 262:240–244, 1989.
17. Golden DB, Kagey-Sobotka A, Norman AP, et al: Outcomes of allergy to insect stings in children, with and without venom immunotherapy. N Engl J Med 351:668–674, 2004.
18. Hepner DL, Castells MC: Anaphylaxis during the perioperative period. Anesth Analg 97:1381–1395, 2003.
19. Lencher K, Grammar LC: A current review of idiopathic anaphylaxis. Curr Opin Allergy Clin Immunol 3:305–311, 2003
20. Cicardi M, Agostoni A: Hereditary angioedema. N Engl J Med 334:1666–1667, 1996.
21. Waytes AT, Rosen FS, Frank MM: Treatment of hereditary angioedema with a vapor-heated C1 inhibitor concentrate. N Engl J Med 334:1630–1634, 1996.
22. Karim MY, Masood A: Fresh-frozen plasma as a treatment of life-threatening ACE-inhibitor angioedema. J Allergy Clin Immunol 109:370–371, 2002.
23. Maffei FA, van der Jagt EW, Powers KS, et al: Duration of mechanical ventilation in life-threatening pediatric asthma: description of an acute asphyxial subgroup. Pediatrics 114:762–767, 2004.
24. Rainbow J, Browne GJ: Fatal asthma or anaphylaxis? Emerg Med J 19:415–417, 2002.
25. Clark S, Bock SA, Gaeta TJ, et al: Multicenter study of emergency department visits for food allergies. J Allergy Clin Immunol 113:347–352, 2004.
26. Simons FER, Gu X, Simons KJ: Epinephrine absorption in adults: intramuscular versus subcutaneous injection. J Allergy Clin Immunol 108:871–873, 2001.
27. Simons FER, Roberts JR, Gu X, et al: Epinephrine absorption in children with a history of anaphylaxis. J Allergy Clin Immunol 101:33–37, 1998.
28. Simons FER, Gu X, Silver NA, et al: Epipen Jr versus Epipen in young children weighing 15 to 30 kg at risk for anaphylaxis. J Allergy Clin Immunol 109:171–175, 2002.
29. Simons FER, Gu X, Johnston LM, et al: Can epinephrine inhalations be substituted for epinephrine injection in children at risk for systemic anaphylaxis? Pediatrics 106:1040–1044, 2000.
30. Sing RF, O'Hara D, Sawyer MA, et al: Trendelenburg position and oxygen transport in hypovolemic adults. Ann Emerg Med 23:564–567, 1994.
31. Pumphrey RSH: Fatal posture in anaphylactic shock. J Allergy Clin Immunol 112:451–452, 2003.
32. Fisher MM: Clinical observations on the pathophysiology and treatment of anaphylactic cardiovascular collapse. Anaesth Intensive Care 14:17–21, 1986.
*33. Lin RY, Curry A, Pesola GR, et al: Improved outcomes in patients with acute allergic syndromes who are treated with combined H_1 and H_2 antagonists. Ann Emerg Med 36:462–468, 2000.
34. Brown SGA: Clinical features and severity grading of anaphylaxis. J Allergy Clin Immunol 114:371–376, 2004.
35. Lee JM, Greenes DS: Biphasic anaphylactic reactions in pediatrics. Pediatrics 106:762–766, 2000.
36. Dibs DS, Baker MD: Anaphylaxis in children: a 5-year experience. Pediatrics 99:e7, 1997.

---

*Selected readings.

SECTION II

Approach to the Trauma Patient

Chapter 15

Trauma in Infants

Gail M. Stewart, DO and Ameer P. Mody, MD, MPH

Key Points

Although infant trauma is common, it is rarely associated with severe injury.

Infants are not "little children." Unique anatomic and physiologic variations result in distinct injury patterns.

Decision rules for management of infant trauma have not been developed.

Car seats have had a profound impact on decreasing the frequency and severity of infant injuries sustained during traffic collisions.

Introduction and Background

Evaluating and managing a screaming, wiggling 6-month-old who presents to the emergency department (ED) taped and strapped to her car seat following a traffic collision can be a challenge. Infants with traumatic injuries are in a special subset of pediatric patients. Their inability to cooperate or communicate makes it difficult to assess the severity of injury based on history or physical examination. Their preverbal and relatively immobile state makes them susceptible to nonaccidental trauma. Unique anatomic variations include a disproportionately large head, weak neck muscles, lack of complete skeletal ossification, relatively large body surface area, and immature central nervous system.

Generally, infants are defined as children younger than 12 months of age. There are some predictable patterns of injuries in this age group and a relatively low frequency of comorbid medical conditions. Regrettably, few papers have been published addressing how to manage traumatized infants. Most management principles are extrapolated from adult or pediatric literature that includes older children. This chapter focuses on accidental trauma in infants (see Chapter 119, Physical Abuse and Child Neglect). An overarching theme to this chapter is that "infants are not just little children."

Recognition and Approach

Infant trauma is a common occurrence. Ten percent of infant visits to EDs are for nonfatal injuries.[1] The most common mechanisms of injury are falls (50% to 60%), burns (5%), being struck by a falling object (5%), ingestions (5%), and traffic collisions (5%).[2-4] Hospitalization is uncommonly needed, occurring in approximately 5% of infants evaluated in an ED.[4,5] The infant mortality rate due to accidental injury is low, approximately 3%.[2] Epidemiologic studies of infant injuries suggest a bimodal distribution predominantly comprising minor injuries and severe, life-threatening injuries. Cases of intermediate acuity are less common than either of these two extremes.

The advent of the rear-facing infant car seat has significantly altered the mechanism and frequency of infant injury in traffic collisions.[6,7] The rear-facing position provides better support to the infant's head, neck, and back, and spreads the crash force more evenly over the entire body. Current guidelines recommend infants remain in the rear-facing position until reaching 1 year of age, or a minimum of 20 pounds (approximately 10 kg).[8] Car seat use has resulted in a 71% reduction in the number of serious injuries and deaths sustained by infants involved in motor vehicle accidents.[8]

Head trauma is the most frequently reported injury in infants. Up to 97% of falls result in injury to the head, which is disproportionately large compared to the body, and supported by weak neck muscles.[5,9] Distinctive features of the infant skull include a soft, thin, bone, unfused sutures and open fontanelles.[4] The infant skull fractures easily, even following relatively minor trauma.[10,11] Forces applied to the deformable skull are easily transmitted to the underlying brain, causing direct tissue damage.[12] Infants with a skull fracture are at an increased risk for having an associated intracranial bleed.[13] In the vast majority of infants, there will be soft tissue swelling overlying the site of the fracture.[10] It is important to document the presence of even seemingly clinically insignificant skull fractures because a leptomeningeal cyst (i.e., a "growing fracture") may develop later.[14] The infant scalp can develop significant extracranial hematomas following impact. Infantile extracranial hematomas may arise in one of two different anatomic locations resulting in either a subgaleal hematoma or a cephalohematoma. Subgaleal hematomas are composed of a collection of blood between the galea aponeurotica and the periosteum of the skull. These hematomas can become quite large, are not generally associated with skull fractures, and cross suture lines. Cephalohematomas form underneath the periosteum. These hematomas do not cross suture lines and have an association with underlying skull fractures.[15,16] Both subgaleal hematomas and cephalohematomas may cause clinically significant anemia.

The infant brain differs from that of older children in that myelination is incomplete, cerebral autoregulation is underdeveloped, and cerebrospinal fluid spaces are larger.[9] With impact, the brain has more motion within the calvarium, causing the dural veins to stretch and tear. Subdural hematomas in infants are common following high-velocity impact injury, and are typically associated with contusion, cerebral edema, or diffuse axonal injury.[9,15] Infants who sustain severe traumatic brain injury have a poor prognosis for recovery.[14]

Cervical spine injuries in infants are rare. In a study of 3065 pediatric patients who underwent imaging for a suspected neck injury, less than 1% had a cervical injury, and of these, none was less than 2 years of age.[17] Spinal cord injuries in infants most often result from abusive shaking, motor vehicle accidents, or falls from a height. Younger children tend to have upper cervical spine involvement compared to older children and adults.[18] Anatomic differences in the pediatric cervical spine include anterior wedging of the vertebral bodies, horizontal facet orientation, and absence of uncinate processes on the vertebral bodies. The net result is that infants have relatively more ligamentous injuries than bony injuries.[19] Infants are susceptible to hyperextension and flexion injuries, which can cause momentary dislocation followed by spontaneous reduction of the vertebrae.[19]

The bony and ligamentous spinal column of infants is quite elastic and can stretch up to a total of 50 mm vertically. However, the spinal cord can only tolerate about 5 mm of stretch without substantial disruption occurring.[18] Therefore, spinal cord injuries may occur without demonstrable bony injury. In 1982, Pang and Wilberger coined the term *spinal cord injury without radiographic abnormality* (SCIWORA) to describe this phenomenon.[20] With the advent of magnetic resonance imaging (MRI), which can allow for the visualization of ligamentous injuries and injuries to the spinal cord itself, the term *SCIWORA* is probably no longer clinically meaningful (see Chapter 23, Spinal Trauma).

Infant thoracic trauma usually results from a blunt force applied to the chest wall, resulting in pulmonary contusion, pneumothorax, or hemothorax. Injury to the heart, tracheobronchial tree, aorta, esophagus, or diaphragm is rare.[21] Pulmonary contusion is the most common, serious thoracic injury identified in infants, occurring when the anterior ribs are compressed against the posterior ribs.[22] Because infants' ribs are so pliable, internal thoracic injury often occurs without fracture.[23,24] Presence of rib fractures in infants indicates significant energy transfer, and should alert the physician to the possibility of child abuse and multisystem injuries[21,25] (see Chapter 12, Approach to Multisystem Trauma; Chapter 24, Thoracic Trauma; and Chapter 119, Physical Abuse and Child Neglect).

Management of an infant with a potential abdominal injury generally follows the same principles as those applicable to older children (see Chapter 25, Abdominal Trauma). In infants, the abdominal organs are proportionally larger and closer together. They are less protected due to weaker abdominal wall musculature and the higher position of the rib cage. The spleen and liver are the most frequently injured abdominal organs in infants. Up to 90% of abdominal organ injuries are managed nonoperatively.[26] Infants have a smaller total circulating blood volume, and therefore any particular volume loss is relatively larger for an infant than for older children.

Evaluation

In approaching the injured infant, an effort should be made to establish eye contact and calm the baby before assessing mental status. To the extent possible, the parent or caregiver should be allowed to be within eye and physical contact of the infant, and analgesia and sedation should not be withheld.

In recent years, some Emergency Medical Services providers have adopted a protocol that allows for an injured infant to be immobilized and transported in his or her car seat from the scene of an accident to the ED (Fig. 15–1). Once in the ED, if the infant appears stable, parts of the initial evaluation can be done with the infant remaining in the car seat. If significant injury is suspected, a two-person technique is used

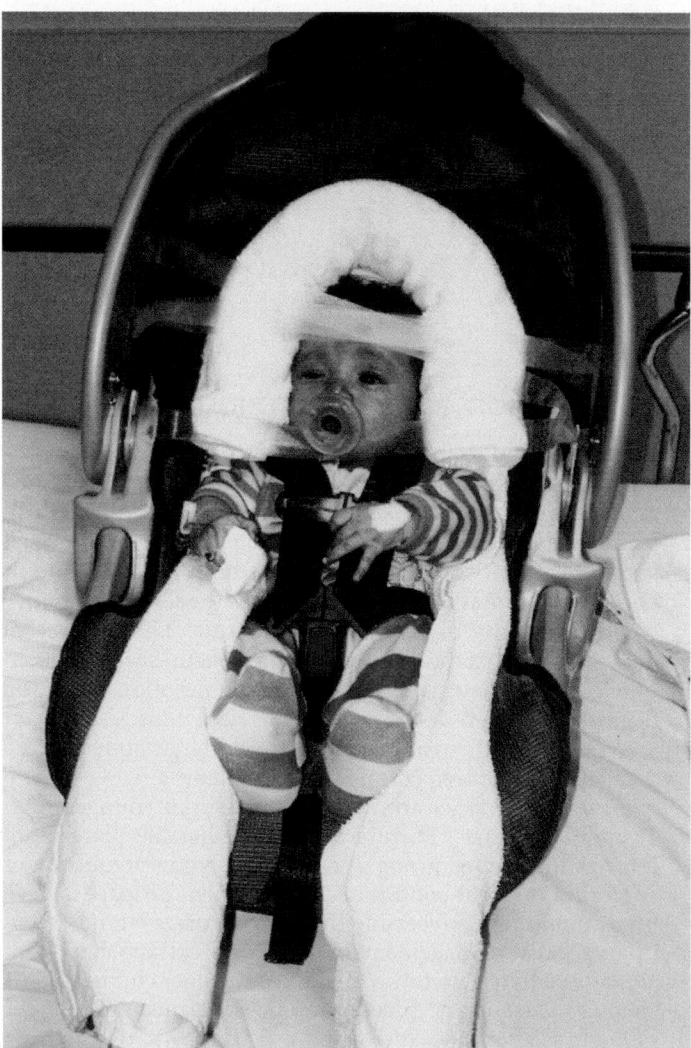

FIGURE 15–1. Typical car seat cervical spine immobilization of a young infant.

to carefully remove the baby from the car seat while maintaining spinal immobilization.

Just as in the evaluation of older children, the evaluation of an injured infant can be organized around primary and secondary surveys. The primary survey assesses and treats problems with the airway, breathing, and circulation. During the primary survey, a brief neurologic examination is performed and the infant is undressed. In the secondary survey, a complete head-to-toe assessment is undertaken. The physician should take advantage of the "windows of opportunity" that the infant offers. For example, the mouth can be examined when the baby is crying and the fontanelle can be assessed when the infant is quiet.

Physical Examination

The infant skull should be carefully palpated for swelling or bony step-offs. Hematomas should be identified because they can cause significant bleeding. Soft tissue swelling of the scalp may overlie a skull fracture. A bulging fontanelle in a quiet infant is associated with increased intracranial pressure and in the setting of trauma suggests intracranial hemorrhage. Small infants are sensitive to bright lights. It may be helpful to dim the lights before attempting to examine the pupillary response.

The cervical spine should be evaluated by palpation, assessing for tenderness, swelling, crepitus, or bony anomalies. A thorough neurologic examination should be done in conjunction with the neck examination. If the neck seems tender, or any focal neurologic anomalies are present, cervical immobilization should be maintained pending imaging studies. Unfortunately, the NEXUS criteria used to predict cervical spine injuries in adults cannot be applied to infants.[27]

The infant trachea is narrow, short, and compressible. Small changes in airway diameter can cause rapid respiratory embarrassment.[22] Frequent suctioning may be necessary. Because breath sounds are shallow and easily transmitted, the lung fields may sound equal on auscultation despite the presence of a pulmonary contusion or pneumothorax. Infants with respiratory distress from pulmonary contusions may demonstrate "abdominal" breathing, increased work of breathing, and grunting. The examination of the infant abdomen is not substantially different than the examination of older children. However, infants tend to cry more and can present with a distended abdomen secondary to aerophagia (i.e., excessive air in the stomach).[26] Extremities should be examined looking for bony deformities, swelling, or tenderness.

An initial neurologic examination of the infant should evaluate the infant's mental status, pupillary response, motor function, and deep tendon reflexes. A more detailed neurologic examination should be completed following stabilization.

Laboratory Testing

There is no routine "trauma panel" recommended for the injured infant. Laboratory tests should be tailored to individual circumstances (see Chapter 12, Approach to Multisystem Trauma).

Imaging Studies

Imaging studies may help elucidate anomalies detected on the primary or secondary survey. In the infant with major head trauma, an emergent computed tomography (CT) scan should be expediently obtained. The role for imaging studies in children with minor head trauma is controversial (see Chapter 17, Head Trauma). Some believe that skull radiographs are only indicated to confirm a depressed fracture, to evaluate a penetrating injury, or to help evaluate for nonaccidental trauma.[28] Guidelines published by the American Academy of Pediatrics for managing minor head injury in children only apply to those over 2 years of age.[29]

In a review by an expert panel, infants younger than 2 years with apparently minor head injury were designated as having a high, intermediate, or low risk for presence of intracranial injury based on history, mechanism of injury, and clinical parameters. Imaging recommendations were based on risk level (Table 15–1). Since the incidence of intracranial injury following minor head trauma is 3% to 6% in infants, a low threshold for head imaging is probably reasonable.

Table 15–1	Proposed Guidelines for Imaging Children <2 Years of Age with Apparently Minor Head Trauma			
		Intermediate Risk		
High Risk: CT Scan	**Subgroup 1*: Consider CT or Observation 4–6 hr**	**Subgroup 2†: Consider CT, Skull Radiograph, or Observation**	**Low Risk: Observation**
Depressed mental status	Vomiting 3–4 times	Higher force mechanism	Low-energy mechanism
Focal neurologic findings	Transient LOC	Falls onto hard surface	No signs or symptoms ≥2 hr after injury
Signs of depressed/basilar fracture	History of lethargy or irritability	Scalp hematomas	>3–6 mo of age
Skull fracture by radiograph	Behavior not at baseline	Unwitnessed trauma	
Irritability	Nonacute skull fracture (>24 hr old)	Vague or absent history of trauma	
Bulging fontanelle			
Seizure			
Progressive vomiting			
LOC >1 min			

*Children with clinical indicators of possible brain injury.
†Children with concerning or unknown mechanism.
Abbreviation: LOC, loss of consciousness.
Table adapted from Schutzman et al.[30]

Presence of a scalp hematoma is a predictor of a skull fracture and, if relatively large, predictive of intracranial hemorrhage.[30]

Cervical spine injuries in children are uncommon, occurring in about 1% of all pediatric trauma victims.[27,31] The incidence is undoubtedly lower in infants. Two proposed explanations for the low incidence are that (1) infants may not be exposed to the dangerous mechanisms that cause these injuries, or (2) infants with injuries to the upper cervical spine have lethal injuries that are never specifically identified, at least not in the ED.[27] There are few studies addressing infants with cervical spine injuries. Infants involved in a high-risk mechanism of injury should undergo a careful physical examination. Diagnostic imaging of the cervical spine should be obtained in the presence of cervical spine tenderness, crepitus or bony step-off, or altered mental status, or in patients with focal motor deficit or paralysis of an extremity. The assessment of tenderness is often impossible in infants. The choice of imaging study is controversial. Initially, a radiograph with anterior-posterior and lateral views is generally recommended. These radiographs will generally allow adequate visualization of the entire cervical spine.[18] The utility of the odontoid view radiograph in the presence of a normal lateral view is questionable and can be technically challenging in infants. A study of pediatric radiologists' practice in using the open-mouth odontoid view in young children found significant variability in its perceived utility.[32] If the plain radiographs are negative, an infant suspected of having a cervical spine injury should undergo MRI of the spine. MRI is sensitive for detecting ligament disruptions, and can define the extent of the any clinically significant spinal cord injury. MRI is also useful in the obtunded, intubated infant.[33] A CT scan of the cervical spine can be used to delineate and clarify anomalies detected on the plain film; however, CT scanning does not allow for imaging of the spinal cord. Clinical experience suggests that the traumatized infant who is awake, moving all extremities, easily consoled, and without neck pain or other major injury may be clinically cleared from cervical spine immobilization.

Indications for imaging the chest and extremities of the traumatized infant are similar to those for older children (see Chapter 12, Approach to Multisystem Trauma; Chapter 19, Upper Extremity Trauma; Chapter 20, Lower Extremity Trauma; and Chapter 24, Thoracic Trauma).

Infants who present to the emergency department with suspected abdominal trauma might have external bruising, abdominal distention, or tenderness on palpation. In the past, the hemodynamically unstable infant with abdominal trauma was taken directly to surgery, whereas the hemodynamically stable patient underwent laboratory evaluation and CT scan. The introduction of the "focused abdominal sonography for trauma" (FAST) scan to emergency medicine has altered how adults with blunt abdominal trauma are approached and managed. Using a portable ultrasound machine, the FAST scan quickly detects fluid in the abdomen, pelvis, or pericardium. It is gaining worldwide acceptance as an efficient screening tool. A positive scan in a hemodynamically unstable adult indicates the need for a laparotomy. The role of the FAST scan in pediatrics is currently being investigated.[34] The advantages to FAST scanning are the availability at the bedside, speed, low cost, and avoidance of exposure to ionizing radiation. CT scanning, in contrast, can be time consuming and expensive, may require sedation, and exposes the infant to ionizing radiation.[33] An advantage of the CT scan, however, is that it provides an accurate diagnosis of parenchymal and retroperitoneal injuries, whereas sonography is poor at identifying organ-specific injuries or injuries that do not produce free fluid (i.e., blood) in the abdominal cavity. Since most cases of pediatric abdominal organ injury are now managed nonoperatively, this may be a serious limitation to the use of FAST scanning in the evaluation of traumatized infants.[26]

Management

The management of traumatized infants should proceed efficiently. The bimodal distribution of injury severity should be kept in mind, necessitating early and aggressive treatment for clearly injured patients and a conservative approach to those who appear well. Because infants have a small blood volume and limited pulmonary reserve, they can progress rapidly to uncompensated shock and death (see Chapter 8, Circulatory Emergencies: Shock).

Securing the airway is the principal goal in the management of traumatized infants. Indications for intubation include unstable vital signs, respiratory distress, shock, and signs of significant head injury. In the obtunded infant with significant injury, head trauma should be presumed and rapid sequence intubation performed (see Chapter 3, Rapid Sequence Intubation). The use of lidocaine to decrease the risk of elevating the intracranial pressure during intubation[35,36] and atropine to avoid bradycardia[37] are both controversial. Due to the shortened length of the infant trachea, it is easy for the endotracheal tube to enter the right mainstem bronchus. If a postintubation chest radiograph shows a whiteout of the left hemithorax in the setting of a right mainstem intubation, the first consideration should be a right mainstem intubation and not massive hemothorax. A trial of pulling the endotracheal tube back into an appropriate position may resolve the radiographic whiteout and minimize iatrogenic trauma.

Fluid resuscitation requirements are based on the physical examination findings. The presence of poor perfusion and tachycardia indicates the need for fluid resuscitation. An intravenous or intraosseous bolus of 20 ml/kg crystalloid (e.g., normal saline) is the most readily available and appropriate initial management option. Re-evaluation after the initial fluid bolus can guide further management decisions. In the hemodynamically unstable patient, the need for colloid or blood products should be anticipated early to allow the blood bank adequate preparation time. Vascular access in the volume-depleted infant can be very challenging. Oftentimes an intraosseous needle is the most practical and efficient early option (see Chapter 161, Vascular Access).

Infants are prone to becoming hypothermic due to their relatively large body surface area. Replacing wet linens with warm blankets will assist in stabilization and assessment. Use of warming lights and warmed intravenous fluids may also be beneficial. Oftentimes a cold, crying, tachycardic infant with poor capillary refill will improve with these basic interventions. Infants also have relatively small glycogen stores and are prone to develop hypoglycemia when stressed and kept *nil per os* (NPO) (see Chapter 106, Hypoglycemia). Blood sugars should be frequently monitored and hypoglycemia should be treated promptly.

The pliable chest wall in infants makes rib fractures less common than pulmonary contusion, and also makes signs of external trauma unreliable in predicting deeper injury. On chest radiograph, pulmonary contusions can appear as scattered patchy infiltrates or a complete whiteout of the involved lung. Management requires early endotracheal intubation and application of sufficient positive end-expiratory pressure to open the alveoli. A pulmonary contusion that appears as a whiteout of one side of the chest must be differentiated from a hemothorax. However, pulmonary contusions are much more common than hemothoraces. Yet, when complete unilateral whiteout is seen, tube thoracostomy may be indicated (see Chapter 168, Thoracostomy Tube). A gentle approach, to avoid placing the thoracostomy tube directly into the injured lung parenchyma, is prudent.

Summary

Accidental injuries in infants most often result from falls, scald burns, falling objects, or motor vehicle accidents. Fortunately, these injuries are seldom severe. Primary preventative interventions have had a positive influence on the epidemiology of accidental infant trauma as evidenced by a decrease in the frequency and severity of injuries. Research into preventative measures has been successful in the past (e.g., car seats) and offers an excellent opportunity for the improvement in the health of infants.

The pronounced physiologic differences between adults and infants alter how injuries are managed in the ED. Trauma guidelines and protocols developed for management of adult trauma (i.e., the Advanced Trauma Life Support course) may not be applicable to the care of the injured infant. Research directed toward development of a tailored approach to the injured infant should include recognition of injuries, stabilization, appropriate diagnostic testing and treatment, and techniques for proper sedation and analgesia. Infants with major injuries will benefit from admission or transfer to a pediatric intensive care unit.

REFERENCES

1. Powell EC, Tanz RR: Adjusting our view of injury risk: the burden of nonfatal injuries in infants. Pediatrics 110:792–796, 2002.
2. Agran PF, Anderson C, Winn D, et al: Rates of pediatric injuries by 3-month intervals for children 0 to 3 years of age. Pediatrics 111:e683–e692, 2003.
*3. Stewart GM, Meert K, Rosenberg NM. Trauma in infants less than three months of age. Pediatr Emerg Care 9:199–201, 1993.
4. Pickett W, Streight S, Simpson K, et al: Injuries experienced by infant children: a population-based epidemiological analysis. Pediatrics 111: e365–e370, 2003.
*5. Warrington SA, Wright CM, ALSPAC Study Team: Accidents and resulting injuries in premobile infants: data from the ALSPAC study. Arch Dis Child 85:104–107, 2001.
*6. Berg MD, Corneli HM, Vernon DD, et al: Effect of seating position and restraint use on injuries to children in motor vehicle crashes. Pediatrics 105:831–835, 2000
7. Howard AW: Automobile restraints for children: a review for clinicians. CMAJ 167:769–773, 2002.
8. Arbogast KB, Cornejo RA, Morris SD, et al: Showing (motor vehicle) restraint: a primer for emergency physicians. Clin Pediatr Emerg Med 4:90–120, 2003.
9. Enrione MA: Current concepts in the acute management of severe pediatric head trauma. Clin Pediatr Emerg Med 2:28–40, 2001.
*10. Greenes DS, Schutzman SA: Infants with isolated skull fracture: what are their clinical characteristics, and do they require hospitalization? Ann Emerg Med 30:253–258, 1997.
11. Duhaime AC, Alario AJ, Lewander WF, et al: Head injury in very young children: mechanisms, injury types and ophthalmologic findings in 100 hospitalized patients younger than 2 years of age. Pediatrics 90:279–285, 1992.
12. Cantor RM, Leaming JM: Pediatric trauma. In Marx JA, Hockberger RS, Walls RM (eds): Rosen's Emergency Medicine: Concepts and Clinical Practice, 5th ed. St. Louis: Mosby, 2002, pp 267–281.
13. Gruskin KD, Schutzman SA: Head trauma in children younger than 2 years—are there predictors for complications? Arch Pediatr Adolesc Med 153:15–20, 1999.
14. Biros MH, Heegaard WG: Head trauma. In Marx JA, Hockberger RS, Walls RM (eds): Rosen's Emergency Medicine: Concepts and Clinical Practice, 5th ed. St. Louis: Mosby, 2002, pp 286–314.
15. Dias MS: Traumatic brain and spinal cord injury. Pediatr Clin North Am 51:271–303, 2004.
16. Hardwood-Nash DC, Hendrick EB, et al: The significance of skull fractures in children. Radiology 101:151–155, 1971.
*17. Hoffman JR, Mower WR, Wolfson AB, et al: Validity of a set of clinical criteria to rule out injury to the cervical spine in patients with blunt trauma. National Emergency X-Radiography Utilization Study Group. N Engl J Med 343:94–99, 2000.
18. Proctor MR: Spinal cord injury. Crit Care Med 30:S489–S499, 2002.
19. Kriss VM, Kriss TC: SCIWORA (spinal cord injury without radiographic abnormality) in infants and children. Clin Pediatr 35:119–124, 1996.
20. Pang D, Wilberger JE: Spinal cord injury without radiographic abnormalities in children. J Neurosurg 57:114–129, 1982.
21. Furnival RA: Controversies in pediatric thoracic and abdominal trauma. Clin Pediatr Emerg Med 2:48–62, 2001.
22. Bliss K, Silen M: Pediatric thoracic trauma. Crit Care Med 30:S409–S415, 2002.
23. Holmes JF, Sokolove PE, Brant WE, et al: A clinical decision rule for identifying children with thoracic injuries after blunt torso trauma. Ann Emerg Med 39:492–499, 2002.
24. Holmes JF, Sokolove PE, Brant WE, et al: Identification of children with intra-abdominal injuries after blunt trauma. Ann Emerg Med 39:500–509, 2002.
*25. Bulloch B, Schubert CJ, Brophy PD, et al: Cause and clinical characteristics of rib fractures in infants. Pediatrics 105:e48, 2001.
26. Gaines BA, Ford HR: Abdominal and pelvic trauma in children. Crit Care Med 30:S416–S423, 2002.
*27. Viccellio P, Simon H, Pressman BD, et al: A prospective multicenter study of cervical spine injury in children. Pediatrics 108:e20, 2001.
28. Lloyd DA, Carty H, Patterson M, et al: Predictive value of skull radiography for intracranial injury in children with blunt head injury. Lancet 349:821–824, 1997.
29. Committee on Quality Improvement, American Academy of Pediatrics, & Commission on Clinical Policies and Research, American Academy of Family Physicians: The management of minor closed head injury in children. Pediatrics 104:1407–1415, 1999.
*30. Schutzman SA, Barnes P, Duhaime AC, et al: Evaluation and management of children younger than two years old with apparently minor head trauma: proposed guidelines. Pediatrics 107:983–993, 2001.
31. Patel JC: Pediatric cervical spine injuries: defining the disease. J Pediatr Surg 36:373–376, 2001.
*32. Swischuk LE, John SD, Hendrick EP. Is the open mouth odontoid view necessary in children under 5 years? Pediatr Radiol 30:186–189, 2000.
33. Frank JB, Lim CK, Flynn JM, et al: The efficacy of magnetic resonance imaging in pediatric cervical spine clearance. Spine 27:1176–1179, 2002.
34. Soudack M, Epelman M, Maor R, et al: Experience with focused abdominal sonography for trauma (FAST) in 313 pediatric patients. J Clin Ultrasound 32:53–61, 2004.
35. Bozeman WP, Idris AM: Intracranial pressure changes during rapid sequence intubation: a swine model. J Trauma 58:278–283, 2005.
36. Robinson N, Clancy M: In patients with head injury undergoing rapid sequence intubation, does pretreatment with intravenous lignocaine/lidocaine lead to an improved neurologic outcome? A review of the literature. Emerg Med J 18:419, 2001.
37. Fastle RK, Roback MG: Pediatric rapid sequence intubation: incidence of reflex bradycardia and effects of pretreatment with atropine. Pediatr Emerg Care 20:651–655, 2004.

---

*Selected readings.

Chapter 16

Oral, Ocular, and Maxillofacial Trauma

Ran D. Goldman, MD and Steven G. Rothrock, MD

Key Points

Nasal bone and mandibular fractures are the most common facial fractures in children, while midface and Le Fort fractures are uncommon.

Head and face injuries occur in most infants and children who are abused.

Computed tomography scanning is the radiologic test of choice for most facial injuries in children.

Facial fractures that do not result in functional (e.g., limited eye movements, visual changes, malocclusion) or cosmetic problems are seldom serious.

Introduction and Background

The etiology of facial injury depends mostly on a child's age. In a large series from Austria, the main causes of facial trauma in children less than 15 years old were play (58%) and sports (32%). Half of all children had soft tissue injuries, and three quarters had dentoalveolar injuries.[1] Facial fractures only occur in a minority of children with facial injury and are most commonly due to motor vehicle accidents.[2-4] Other important fracture causes include falls, sports injuries, bicycle/motorcycle accidents, and assaults.[2-4] One easily overlooked mechanism is abuse, with facial bruising or abrasions occurring in the majority of abused infants and children.[5] Boys have a 1.5- to 3-fold greater risk of facial injury compared to girls.[1,3,4,6,7] In addition, the risk of facial fracture occurring with facial trauma rises with increasing age. While 5% to 15% of all facial fractures occur in children less than 16 years old, fewer than 1% occur in those less than 5 years old.[8-12]

While nasal bone fractures are the most common pediatric facial fracture, the most frequent fracture site in admitted patients is the mandible (Fig. 16–1), followed by the zygomatic arch and alveolar ridge.[3,4] Less common fracture sites include the orbital floor, the hard palate, and rarely the midface (Le Fort fractures). Importantly, Le Fort fractures almost never occur in children under 10 years old. Associated injuries occur in most children with facial trauma, including intracranial, spine, eye, dental, and nerve injuries. For those children with serious injury mechanisms, thoracoabdominal and orthopedic injuries must be excluded.

Recognition and Approach

While children under 7 years old are at risk for soft tissue injury, fractures are uncommon at this age.[13] Eighty percent of cranial growth occurs during the first years of life. After age 2, the face begins to grow faster than the skull. In a newborn infant, the ratio of cranial volume to facial volume is 8 : 1, while in adults this ratio is 2 : 1.[13] Therefore, trauma is more likely to impact the skull and forehead and less likely to injure midfacial structures in young children. This disproportionate growth results in more frequent orbital roof (cranial floor) fractures in infants and more frequent associated neurologic trauma. In contrast, lower orbital fractures generally occur after age 7, have less associated intracranial injury, and more often require surgical reconstruction.[13] Other protective features of a young child's face include underdeveloped paranasal sinuses, increased number of facial fat pads, unerupted dentition that strengthens the maxilla and mandible, and relatively flexible bone. In contrast to young children, adolescents have higher rates of facial trauma due to a mature facial skeleton and more adult activity profile.

Clinicians must be able to recognize the location of important structures when confronted with children with facial trauma (Fig. 16–2). The major portions of the facial nerve are posterior to a vertical line perpendicular to the lateral canthus.[14] Facial nerve injuries anterior to this line only require repair if they involve solitary terminal branches (i.e., marginal mandibular branch, frontal branch).[14] The parotid gland lies anterior to the sternomastoid and external auditory meatus and inferior to the posterior two thirds of the zygomatic arch. Stensen's duct exits the parotid and traverses along the middle third of a line drawn from the tragus to the midportion of the upper lip. This duct opens into the mouth opposite the secondary maxillary molar. The buccal branch

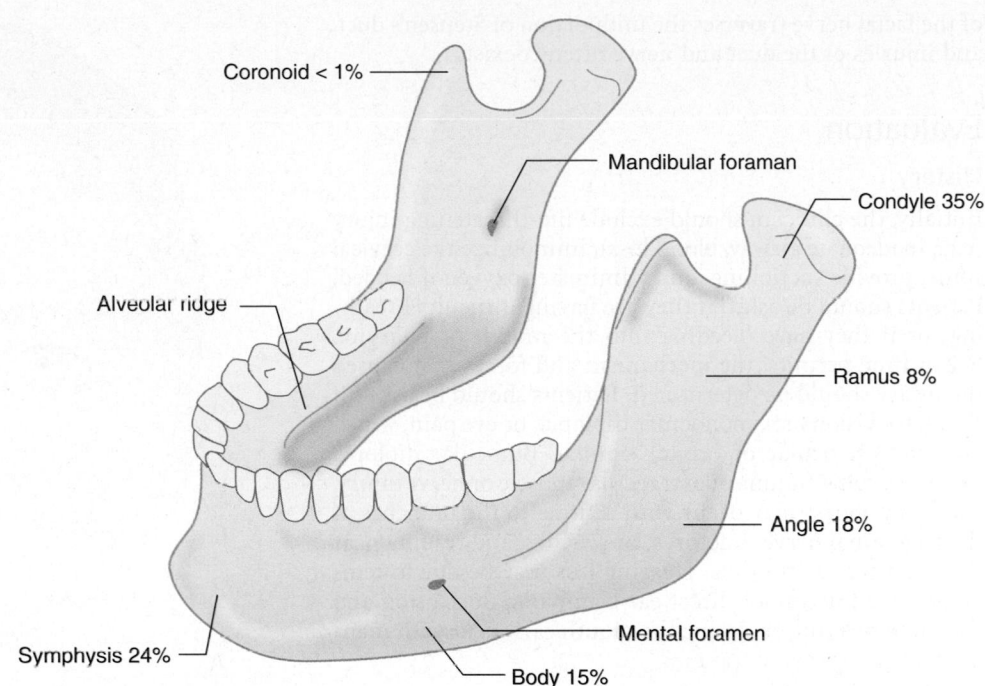

FIGURE 16–1. Most common location of mandibular fractures in children.

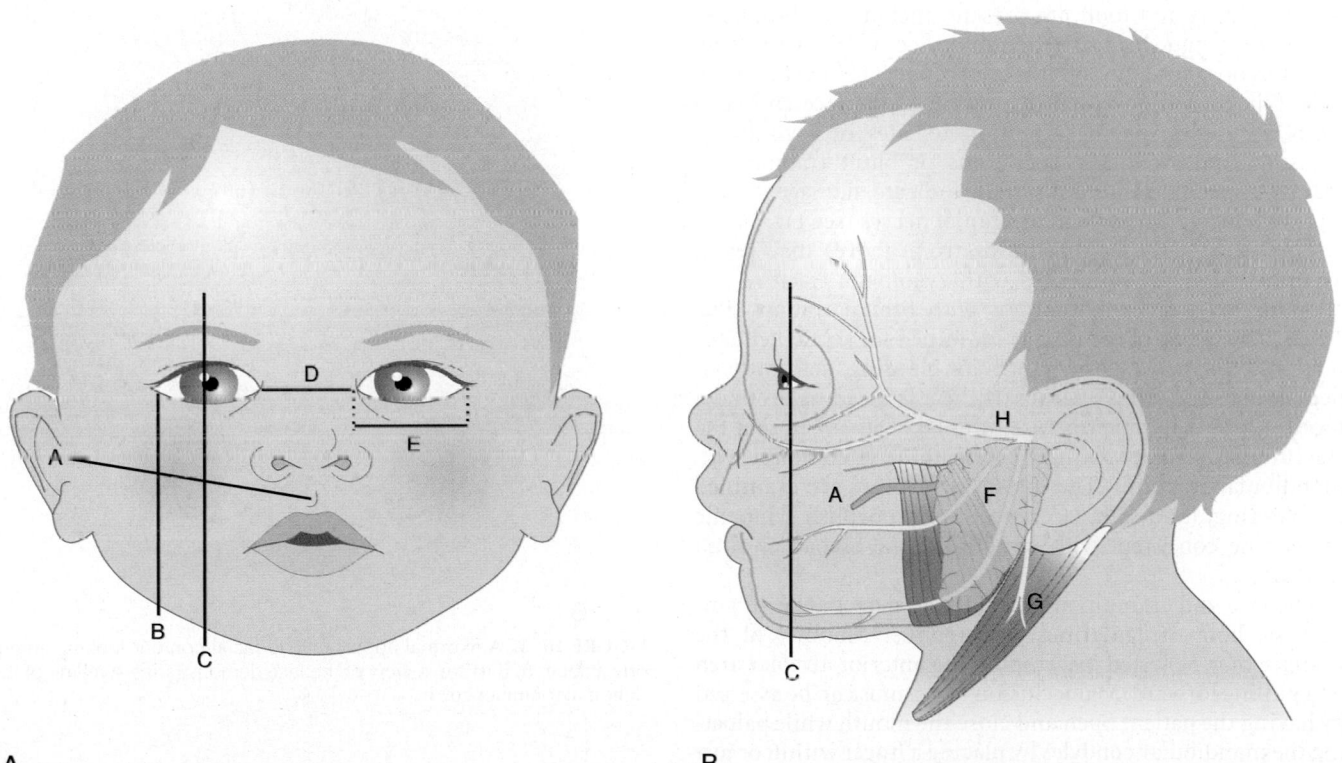

A

B

FIGURE 16–2. The parotid duct **(A)** traverses the middle third of a line connecting the tragus to the middle of the upper lip. Repair of facial nerve branches beyond a vertical line **(B)** originating at the lateral canthus is usually not required. Trigeminal nerve branches exit the face at foramina located along this line **(C)** (vertical line through pupil), including the supraorbital branch of the ophthalmic nerve (V1), the infraorbital branch of the maxillary nerve (V2), and the mental nerve (branches of the trigeminal nerve) (V3). The distance between the medial canthi of each eye **(D)** should be no greater than the size of the palpebral fissure (*red line*) **(E)**. The parotid gland **(F)** lies below the zygomatic arch and anterior to the sternomastoid muscle **(G)**. Major branches of the facial nerve **(H)** run through the parotid gland.

of the facial nerve traverses the midportion of Stensen's duct, and injuries of the duct and nerve often coexist.

Evaluation

History

Initially, the clinician should exclude life-threatening injury (e.g., inadequate airway, blood loss), immobilize the cervical spine, provide suctioning, and administer oxygen if needed. Patients should be asked if they are having difficulty breathing, or if they have bleeding into the mouth or pharynx. When time permits, the mechanism and forces that caused the injury should be determined. Patients should be asked if they have vision loss, monocular diplopia, or eye pain, which may suggest ocular or orbital trauma. Binocular diplopia suggests orbital trauma or extraocular muscle or nerve injury. Facial numbness may occur with trauma to the branches of the trigeminal nerve, fractures, or swelling and trauma near their respective foramina. Hearing loss may be due to temporal bone fracture or direct ear trauma. Malocclusion and difficulty opening or closing the mouth can occur with mandibular or zygomatic trauma.

Physical Examination

Prior to examination, the clinician should ensure that appropriate lighting and tools are present, including a headlamp or mirror, tongue blades, a suction device, a nasal speculum, an otoscope, and an ophthalmoscope. The examination should begin with a visual inspection of the face and skull from all angles, paying attention to sites of asymmetry, bruising, and swelling. Lacerations or blunt trauma that involves specific landmarks may indicate damage to the lacrimal duct, parotid duct, or cranial nerves (see Fig. 16–2). A bird's-eye view (looking down from above) may reveal asymmetric malar eminences with zygomatic fractures, or enophthalmos or exophthalmos with orbital trauma (Fig. 16–3). The inside of the nose is examined for septal hematomas, and the inside of the mouth for bleeding, deformity, or hematoma suggesting fracture. If there is bleeding around a tooth near a mandible fracture, it must be assumed that the fracture is open. A sublingual hematoma is common with mandibular fractures. The insides of the ears are examined for bleeding, fluid leak, lacerations, or a purplish tympanic membrane consistent with temporal bone or basilar skull fracture.

The face and cranium are palpated to detect areas of tenderness, bony irregularities, or crepitus. Mobility of the midface may be tested by grasping the anterior alveolar arch and pulling forward. Malocclusion or trismus can be assessed by having the patient open and close the mouth while palpating the mandibular condyles by placing a finger within or just below the external auditory canal. Cooperative patients can be asked to bite down on a tongue blade. In adolescents and adults, the inability to break the blade when it is twisted is 95% sensitive for mandibular fractures.[15] The patient should be asked to smile, frown, raise the eyebrows, and open and close the eyes tightly to assess facial nerve integrity. Sensation to terminal trigeminal nerve branches should be tested (see Fig. 16–2).

A thorough eye examination is required in all infants and children with facial trauma. The eyelids should be inspected

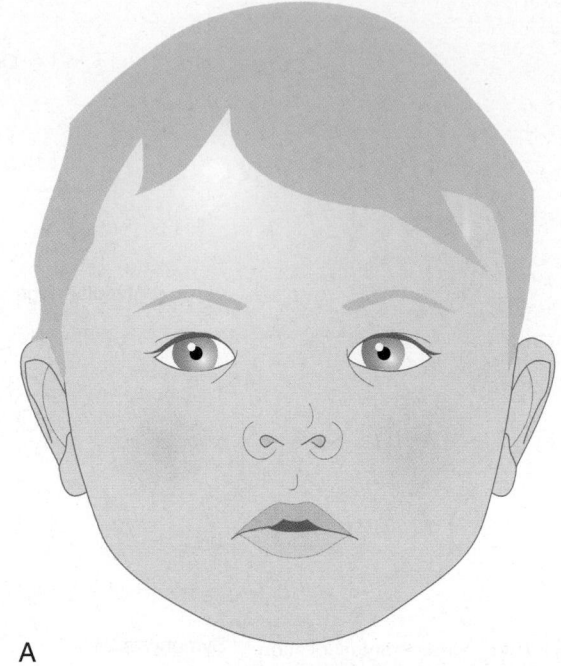

A

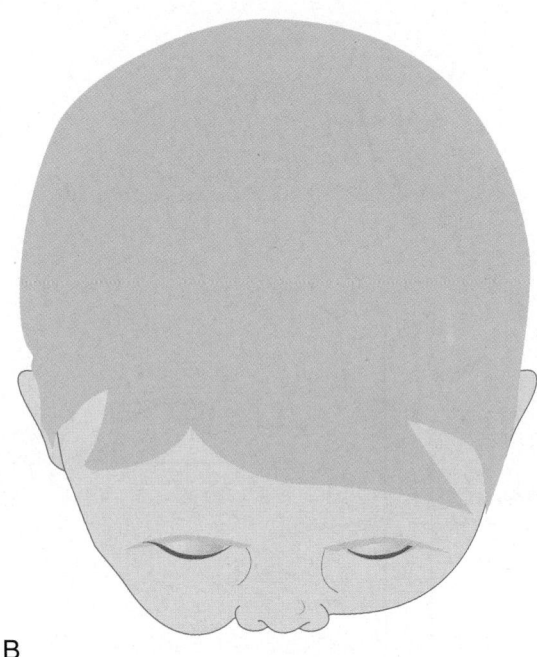

B

FIGURE 16–3. A, Normal appearance to facial contour looking anteriorly at face. **B,** Bird's-eye view of the face demonstrating swelling of the right malar eminence.

for lacerations that involve the tarsal plate, either the canthus or potentially the lacrimal duct. If the distance between the medial canthi is greater than the horizontal width of an orbit (or 35 to 40 mm in a child > 5 years old), *telecanthus* is present and a midfacial fracture is likely. Extraocular muscles are tested for entrapment (e.g., limited upward gaze with orbital blowout fracture). Visual acuities should be obtained in older, cooperative children. The clinician should assess pupil size, test direct and indirect pupillary reaction to light, and directly examine the cornea. Fluorescein administration and slit-lamp examination may be required.

Lack of cooperation, anxiety, pain, and limited communication skills can interfere with proper evaluation of infants and children with facial injuries. Appropriate analgesia and sedation should be administered depending upon the patient's airway, associated injuries, and medical condition (see Chapter 159, Procedural Sedation and Analgesia).

An integral part of evaluating infants and children with facial trauma includes a head-to-toe examination for nonfacial injuries.[16] Associated injuries are present in up to 87% of children facial fractures.[3] In addition, early photographs may be helpful in preoperative planning and patient counseling, as well as for prospective medicolegal matters.

Radiology

With the exception of a Panorex view, plain radiography usually provides limited diagnostic information to the clinical examination and limited information regarding facial fractures in children.[3] Nearly half of all significant facial fractures in children are missed by plain radiography.[3] For this reason, children with suspected facial bone injury usually require a computed tomography (CT) scan of the face. Typically, facial CT consists of 3-mm slices taken in the axial plane with both axial and coronal reconstruction.[10,17] Three-dimensional reconstruction can provide even more detail regarding fractures. One quick clue to the presence of a midface fracture is the presence of fluid within the paranasal sinuses. In adults, nearly 100% of all midface fractures (excluding nasal, and zyomatic fractures) have associated paranasal sinus fluid.[18] A panoramic view (*Panorex*) of the mandible can display upper and lower teeth and the mandibular condyles; however, full cooperation of the injured child is needed and an upright posture must be maintained. Supplemental oblique mandible views (*mandible series*) can be used to evaluate the mandibular condyles and rami. A *Towne's view* (anterior-posterior view 35 degrees caudad) can be helpful for zygoma and mandibular rami fractures. Other views, including the *Waters'* (occipitomental), *submentover-tex* (jug-handle), and *Caldwell's* (posterior-anterior) views, have largely been supplanted by facial CT due to its superior accuracy at identifying facial fractures.

Clinical features suggestive of the need for facial CT have been identified in adults and can be recognized by the mnemonic LIPS-N, which stand for *l*ip laceration, *i*ntra-oral laceration, *p*eriorbital contusion, *s*ubconjunctival bleeding, and *n*asal laceration.[19] Others have identified the following features in 96% of all orbital fractures and 98% of all orbital fractures requiring surgery: blepharohematoma, subcutaneous emphysema, a palpable deformity or gap, infraorbital anesthesia, enophthalmos, exophthalmos, abnormal ocular motility, diplopia, abnormal papillary reaction, or vision problems.[20] It is uncertain if the mnemonic LIPS-N or other identified features in adults are equally sensitive in identifying fractures in children. Children who require head CT are another population who are at high risk for facial fractures. Ten percent to 12% of patients requiring a head CT will have a facial fracture.[4,19,21] In the subset of patients with severe head injury (i.e., those who are intubated), up to 29% will have facial fractures; many of which are unsuspected.[22]

Management

Initial Management

Management of any child with facial injury initially begins with assessment of airway patency. Accompanying head injury may lead to apnea and decreased airway tone with obstruction. Contrary to popular belief, airway obstruction in patients with an altered mental status is more likely due to hypotonia with collapse of the hypopharynx, soft palate, and epiglottis and not obstruction by the tongue.[23-25] For this reason, airway maneuvers that move the tongue anteriorly (e.g., chin lift, jaw thrust) are not always successful at opening an obstructed airway. For the same reason, use of an oral airway in obstructed patients may be unsuccessful and oral intubation may be required at an early stage. Clinicians must realize that sedation and paralysis may be extremely difficult in patients with significant mandible or maxillary fractures. Blood and secretions should be gently suctioned from the mouth, and foreign bodies such as as teeth or bone fragments identified and removed. Intubation in cases of distorted anatomy might be necessary as a preventive measure and should not be delayed. Before intubation, a team experienced in difficult airway management and all the necessary equipment must be at the bedside (see Chapter 3, Rapid Sequence Intubation; and Chapter 4, Intubation, Rescue Devices, and Airway Adjuncts). Warning signs such as stridor, drooling, active bleeding, or hematoma on the face or neck indicate immediate or impending airway compromise and mandate intubation.

Cervical spine stabilization is crucial for children with facial injury, in order to prevent further damage to cervical structures affected by the trauma. A head-to-toe evaluation is required to exclude other life-threatening injuries (see Chapter 12, Approach to Multisystem Trauma).

Maxillofacial Fractures

Mandibular Fractures

Mandibular fractures are the most common facial fractures found in hospitalized children.[26] The mandible includes the condyle, ramus, body, angle, and arch (symphysis and parasymphysis) (see Fig. 16-1). Fractures of the mandible are relatively common compared to other bones in the face, mostly due to transferred force through the overlying fat tissue. Condylar fractures, in particular, are common since the condyles are heavily vascularized and thin in children.[26]

Most mandibular fractures with normal occlusion and movement are usually treated with a soft diet and movement exercise. Most condylar, body, and angle fractures fall within this category and are treated conservatively. If malocclusion or movement limitations are present or an open fracture is present, immobilization is required via surgery, or splinting.

Midface and Maxillary Fractures

Maxillary fractures are infrequent in young children and occur primarily in children ≥ 10 years old.[1,4] The Le Fort classification used to classify maxillary fractures in adolescents and adults is based on the horizontal level of the fracture. Le Fort I fractures result in separation of the maxilla from the palate. These fractures may result from a force on the maxillary alveolar rim in a descending direction. Le Fort

II fractures result in separation of the cranium from the midface. Le Fort III is the most severe fracture and results in complete separation of the facial bones from the cranium. Displaced midface fractures require open reduction and rigid internal fixation.[26]

Nasoethmoid Fractures

Nasoethmoid fractures occur when there is disruption at the nasofrontal suture, nasal bones, medial orbital rim, and infraorbital rim. If all four sides are involved, a central fragment may exist. Surgery will be required if telecanthus is present, or there is disruption of bony or soft tissue support for the eye.[13,26]

Nasal fractures are the most common facial bone injury in children. The younger the child, the lower the risk of nasal fracture since the cartilaginous part of the nose is larger and more elastic. Clinical interpretation of a nasal fracture is usually difficult in the emergency department (ED) due to swelling and hematoma in the area as a result of the injury. It may be necessary to wait a few days to determine if a fracture actually occurred.

Nasal radiographs are usually not necessary in the ED unless ordered for parental reassurance.[27] Radiographs are nonspecific, and even if a fracture is suspected, they do not alter subsequent management.

High vascularity of the nose cause significant bleeding even after minor soft tissue injury. Septal hematoma is one of the known complications after such bleeding, and is an indication for immediate evacuation. Unilateral nasal obstruction is common in septal hematoma, and rhinoscopy will show a bulging mass (usually purple) in one nostril. Evacuation of septal hematoma will relieve pain due to pressure in the area, and will also prevent septal deformity. Infection in the area is also possible. Once the hematoma is drained, oral antibiotics should be administered.

Zygomaticomaxillary Complex Fractures

Zygomaticomaxillary complex fractures are uncommon under the age of 5 years, before the maxillary sinus becomes aerated. Low-impact injuries often result in greenstick fractures, which are usually nondisplaced and often require no treatment. Open reduction and internal fixation is required for displaced, comminuted, or unstable fractures. Functional deficits (e.g., diplopia, or infraorbital sensory loss) also often require surgery.[26]

Frontal Bone/Sinus Fractures

The frontal sinus becomes developed by age 6 to 8 years. Before this age, frontal sinus fractures are uncommon. Anterior sinus table fractures that are not displaced can be observed, with most experts administering antibiotics since the fracture connects to a sinus. Because displaced anterior fractures are associated with mucocele formation, nasofrontal duct obstruction, and cosmetic deformity, surgical repair is generally required. Posterior wall fractures should be treated as an open skull fracture with the potential for associated cerebrospinal fluid leak. Neurosurgical consultation is required.

Orbital Trauma

Childhood is the most common period for serious eye injuries throughout life,[28,29] with the majority of injuries occur-

ring in boys. Ocular trauma is the leading cause of noncongenital unilateral blindness in children under 20 years old and the foremost cause for enucleation of the eye in children, especially in boys.[30] Most major eye trauma in children occurs during sports activities because proportionally more children and adolescents participate in high-risk activities. Basketball, baseball, racquet sports, martial arts, wrestling, and archery are the most frequent cause of injury. BB and pellet guns also present an extreme hazard to children.

Understanding the mechanism of injury is important for planning management better. Clinicians must determine if there is blunt or sharp object injury, if a foreign body is present in the eye, and if protected devices were used. As assessment of pain, photophobia, eye movements (diplopia), and visual acuity will aid in determining the nature of the injury. Visual acuity examination is the most important part of the physical examination and should be separately performed for each eye. Finger counting, the "E" chart, and a numeric chart can be used for examination of the injured child. If needed, a topical anesthetic (such as tetracaine or proparacaine) should be administered to ensure adequate examination.

During examination of the eyes and orbit, the emergency physician should examine the integrity of the orbital rims, orbital floor, vision, extraocular motion, position of the globe, and intercanthal distance. A complaint of diplopia or limited extraocular movements on examination is usually the result of entrapment and dysfunction of extraocular muscles with associated orbital floor blowout fractures. Cranial nerve palsy from associated head injury can also result in headache and diplopia. With globe or scleral rupture, severe external disruption of the eye is not always evident. With rupture, the iris or choroids will extent toward the wound, resulting in a dark (blue or black) spot on the sclera (Fig. 16–4). The pupil may take a dysmorphic or teardrop shape.

Pupils are usually examined as part of the neurologic evaluation in the primary survey. However, they should be examined carefully in any suspected injury. The clinician should assess size, shape, and direct plus indirect reaction to light.

While anisocoria could be a normal phenomenon in a small percentage of the population, this finding may indicate

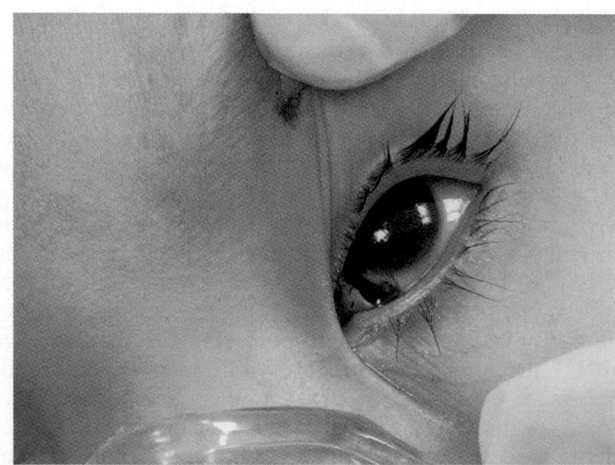

FIGURE 16–4. Scleral rupture with extruded uvea, which appears brown-black.

a possible injury to the third cranial nerve or increased intraocular pressure (IOP). A combination of ptosis, miosis, and anhydrosis, known as Horner's syndrome, suggests a lesion of the sympathetic pathway.

In the ED, direct ophthalmoscopy and slit-lamp examination may be required to evaluate the cornea, anterior and posterior chambers, and retina. Measurement of IOP is contraindicated in suspected globe rupture, but may help to identify retrobulbar hemorrhage causing increased IOP. Except for cases of large radiopaque foreign bodies, plain radiography of the ocular system is usually unhelpful. For sites with expertise, ultrasonography can be used to identifying ocular foreign bodies, retinal detachment, vitreous hemorrhage, and globe rupture.[31] For most other sites, CT with thin slices (1 to 1.5 mm) in the canthal-meatal plane, with sagittal and coronal reconstruction, is used for identification of potential intraocular injuries.[32] Orbital CT is 75% sensitive and 93% specific for identifying globe rupture.[33] CT is also accurate at identifying ocular foreign bodies.[32] Helical CT can detect all steel and copper foreign bodies larger than 1 mm^3 and most glass foreign bodies larger than 2 mm^3.[34] Wood and plastic can be difficult to visualize using typical bone and soft tissue CT windows since wood may be isodense with air and fat. To identify wooden foreign bodies, the CT window should be adjusted to allow visualization of soft tissue contrast and show an attenuation difference between the wood and surrounding tissue, or the alternating density pattern of the grain of the wood. Alternately, magnetic resonance imaging can be used to identify wood or plastic foreign bodies once metallic foreign bodies have been excluded.

Orbital Fractures

Following blunt compressive eye trauma, the eyeball may be pushed posteriorly and induce pressure that causes "blowout" of one or more bones of the orbital wall. Unlike adults, children are particularly susceptible to pure orbital fractures, usually of the "trapdoor" type.[35] Most of the orbital floor is immature in childhood, and this elasticity makes the orbital bones more susceptible to fractures when pushed against external force. The fracture is usually linear along the obliquely situated infraorbital canal, resulting in trapping of muscles. These fractures occur when a circular segment of the bony orbit fractures and becomes displaced, but remains attached on one side. Afterward, orbital contents can herniate through the fractured site, with entrapment of the herniated contents.[36]

Blowout fractures of the orbital wall are usually diagnosed clinically after observation of asymmetric and restricted eyeball movement. Trapping of the intraocular muscle prevents movement of the eye away from the fracture site. While orbital hemorrhage is a differential diagnosis in this clinical scenario, lack of normal range of motion should raise a high suspicion of orbital fracture in an injured child. Due to the disrupted wall, the eyeball might fall back into the fracture, and the eye will also look sunken.

Orbital roof fracture occurs mostly in children under 5 years, because of a proportionally larger cranium and the lack of frontal sinus pneumatization, while orbital floor fractures occur later in childhood, after facial growth and the pneumatization of the paranasal sinuses. *Orbital roof* fractures are particularly hazardous because of the possible communication between the orbit and the intracranial cavity.

Pulsating proptosis could serve as a clue to the presence of such a fracture. A history of a blow to the brow in conjunction with late periorbital ecchymosis may be an important clue to the injury. *Orbital floor* fractures are less common but could cause partial or complete injury to the infraorbital nerve, causing ipsilateral numbness of the malar region. This is usually a transient phenomenon. Periorbital ecchymosis, lid edema, subconjunctival hemorrhage, and diplopia are the most common presenting signs. Most patients have a severe limitation of ocular movement caused by direct entrapment of the inferior rectus muscle into the fracture site, and many patients, especially those with muscle entrapment, will suffer extreme pain with eye movements and will present with nausea and vomiting.[37]

Ophthalmologic consultation is important in cases of suspected orbital wall fracture since in some cases an intraorbital injury is accompanied by other skeletal fractures. CT scan is the radiologic test of choice for children with suspected orbital bony injury, and both axial and coronal views are necessary.[38]

The emergency physician should always consider the possibility of child abuse[30] in cases of orbital fracture in young children. The ED staff also has a role in teaching the young patient and the family how to effectively protect the eye from trauma, especially due to foreign bodies. The use of protective eyewear during activities associated with ocular trauma, such as sports, is of great importance.

Ruptured Globe

A rupture of the globe is rare and can occur after significant laceration of the cornea or sclera due to sharp objects or blunt trauma. The limbus (beneath the insertions of the rectus muscle) and the equator of the globe are the weakest areas of the sclera and most prone to rupture following blunt trauma. Visual loss, bloody chemosis (especially localized), a soft globe, and an abnormally deep anterior chamber are seen with rupture. The uvea may appear as a dark mass prolapsing through the ruptured site (see Fig. 16-4). Associated hyphema, lens dislocation, and vitreous hemorrhage also may occur.

When a rupture is suspected, a protective shield should be placed over the eye. Broad-spectrum intravenous antibiotics effective against skin flora (*Streptococcus* and *Staphylococcus aureus/epidermidis*) and tetanus prophylaxis should be administered, as well as analgesics and sedatives if needed. Antiemetics may be required to diminish increased IOP from vomiting. For children requiring intubation, debate exists as to the appropriate use of muscle relaxants. Succinylcholine can increase IOP by an average of 9 mm Hg following administration. However, these effects can be blunted by multiple medications (see Chapter 3, Rapid Sequence Intubation). Moreover, rare ocular injury following use of succinylcholine has primarily been reported in patients receiving light or inadequate sedation.[39] For this reason, some experts still recommend use of succinylcholine for patients at risk for a difficult airway due to its fast onset and short duration, as long as efforts are made to attenuate its IOP effects.[39] For all other patients, non-depolarizing muscle relaxants are recommended.[39] Following patient stabilization, immediate pediatric ophthalmologist consultation is required if scleral rupture is suspected since damage to the posterior segment of the eye can cause permanent visual loss.

Retrobulbar Hemorrhage

Retrobulbar hemorrhage can lead to rapid compression of the optic nerve and irreversible vision loss. Patients usually have severe blunt trauma, proptosis, vision loss with afferent pupillary defect, chemosis, and increased IOP. CT is often diagnostic. Treatment consists of a lateral canthotomy with lysis of the inferior lateral canthal tendon. Depending upon the availability of backup, severity of vision loss, and IOP, this procedure may need to be performed in the ED. This allows the orbital contents to move forward, releasing pressure on the optic nerve.

Optic Nerve Injury

The optic nerve is divided into a small intraocular portion and a long mobile intraorbital portion, and intracanalicular (within the bony canal) and intracranial segments. Fractures within the bony canal may occur with severe head or midface injury, with transection of the optic nerve. Alternately, shearing, compression, or tearing or arterioles along the course of the nerve from blunt trauma may disrupt the arterial supply. Depending upon the cause of trauma, the eye may have a normal appearance. Visual loss may be severe or complete, and an afferent pupillary defect may be present. Funduscopic examination may be normal, with eventual development of pallor. Orbital CT can identify the site of trauma. Surgical decompression may be necessary with disruption of the intracanalicular optic nerve, while the use of high-dose steroids is controversial for these injuries.

Posterior Eye Injuries (Vitreous and Retinal Trauma)

While the posterior segments of the eye are not involved in eye trauma as often as anterior structures, these injuries are more likely to result in permanent visual loss. The retina or vitreous is involved in half of all severe open and closed globe injuries.[40]

Retinal detachment can occur from blunt trauma deforming the eye with peripheral tears, while penetrating trauma can result in direct localized tears or rupture. While retinal detachments do not cause pain, associated ocular trauma may be painful. Symptoms of detachment include floaters due to bleeding, flashing lights, and variably decreased visual acuity depending upon the location of the detachment and amount of bleeding. Patients may complain of a curtain coming down, up, or across their visual field. The anterior segment is usually normal, while the red reflex may be absent with a hazy or gray appearance to the retina, on funduscopic examination. Importantly, direct ophthalmoscopy may not reveal the site of detachment. If an optic nerve injury or significant retinal detachment is present, an afferent pupillary defect may be present.[40]

Isolated vitreous hemorrhage or detachment can produce symptoms similar to retinal detachment. However, an afferent pupillary defect will not be present. Ophthalmologic consultation is required to exclude or treat associated retinal and optic nerve trauma.[40]

Iris and Ciliary Trauma

Traumatic iridocyclitis can occur from blunt trauma with contusion, causing inflammation of the iris and ciliary body with resulting ciliary spasm. Children complain of photophobia, redness, and pain with onset often delayed until 1 to 3 days after the injury. The pupil is usually constricted (*traumatic miosis*). However, if the sphincter is torn or injured, *traumatic mydriasis* or an irregular or scalloped pupil margin may be present. In iritis, slit-lamp examination will reveal flare and cells. Initially, the IOP may be low or normal. Treatment consists of a cycloplegic to relax the iris and ciliary body (e.g., homatropine) and pain medications.

If the iris root is separated from the ciliary body, *iridodialysis* is present. This results in the iris bowing toward the pupil. A coexisting hyphema is often present. Patients may complain of glare, photophobia, and monocular diplopia. A double-pupil appearance to the pupil may be present on examination. Initially, treatment is directed at managing the hyphema. Late surgical repair may be required for double vision, persistent glare, or cosmesis. While initial IOPs are often depressed, glaucoma often occurs in the ensuing 3 months.

Damage to the structures of the anterior chamber may impede drainage of aqueous humor from the eye and lead to *acute glaucoma*. Patients who present with eye pain following blunt trauma require measurement of IOP once rupture and cornea trauma have been excluded.

Lens Injury

Blunt lens trauma can lead to *cataract* formation. If the lens capsule is torn, swelling and opacification of the lens can occur.

Blunt injury to the lens also can disrupt the lens zonules that encircle the lens and anchor it to the ciliary body. The lens can fall partially (*subluxation*) or completely (*dislocation*) away. The edge of the lens may be at the pupillary border, or the entire lens may be dislocated into the anterior or posterior chamber. Patients may complain of visual blurring or monocular diplopia. *Iridodonesis* or trembling of the iris may be seen following rapid eye movements if the lens is dislocated. If the lens is trapped within the pupil or touching the cornea (anterior dislocation), acute glaucoma may occur and emergency surgery is required. Isolated posterior dislocations do not require emergency surgery.

Hyphema

A hyphema refers to accumulation of blood in the anterior chamber of the eye. The blood may be layered inferiorly or may be spread diffusely throughout the anterior chamber. Blood is normally caused by a tear in the iris root and bleeding from arterioles supplying the iris. Complications occur from obstruction of the outflow of the anterior chamber, with resulting inflammation and increased IOP. Patients with sickle cell disease or trait, those with thalassemia, or those taking anticoagulants are at risk for central retinal artery and optic nerve damage from less than severe elevations in IOP. Patients are at risk for rebleeding 3 to 5 days after the initial injury due to clot lysis and retraction.

Management should be coordinated with an ophthalmologist. Initial treatment consists of supportive care, with initial bed rest and elevation of the head of the bed 30 degrees and application of a protective barrier. Patients with large hyphemas (i.e., > 50% of the anterior chamber) may benefit from admission. Patients should avoid aspirin and nonsteroidal anti-inflammatory medications. Topical anticholinergics are administered to stabilize the blood-aqueous barrier and improve symptoms from associated iritis. Topical steroids are also administered. Patients at high risk for rebleeding are treated with oral steroids. Oral aminocaproic acid is administered to enhance clot lysis. Initially, IOP elevations may be treated with topical β-blockers, α-agonists, or carbonic anhydrase inhibitors. Surgery is indicated for persistent elevation of IOP, corneal blood staining, or select patients with sickle cell disease or trait.[41]

Corneal Injuries

Corneal injuries are one of the most common reasons for pediatric visits to the emergency department with ophthalmologic complaints. Self-inflicted injuries from fingers, chemicals, or contact lenses are common, as are injuries inflicted by foreign bodies in the eye. Pain is a prominent complaint in patients with corneal injury. Corneal injury should be part of the assessment of the crying infant since irritability is a common presenting symptom in this age group. Excessive tearing, photophobia, and complaints of a foreign body sensation are common.

While changes in visual acuity are hard to assess due to pain, tearing and frequent blinking are easily noticed on examination. Visual acuity is part of the eye physical examination in children with suspected injury. However, normal visual acuity does not rule out corneal trauma. Examination with fluorescein should follow. The first step should be administration of a topical anesthetic such as tetracaine or proparacaine, followed by a drop of fluorescein from a wet sterile paper strip in the inferior fornix. Foreign body or abrasion can easily be seen under cobalt blue light as corneal lesions will fluoresce brightly.

Corneal Abrasion

Corneal abrasions are the most common eye injury in all ages and are especially common among older children who wear contact lenses. Although found in about 10% of visits with a chief complaint related to eye problem in EDs, the actual estimated incidence of corneal abrasions in children is not known.

Current management of corneal abrasion in children is based on treatment established in adults. Recommended therapy consists of eye patching, cycloplegic drops, and antibiotics. Cycloplegic drops prevent discomfort from ciliary spasm, and antibiotics are administered to prevent infection.[42] In the past, patching was thought to facilitate healing and to relieve pain due to decreased shearing forces over the defect.[43] However, routine use of a patch has been questioned because it impairs binocular vision; obscures half of the visual field; may carry a risk for anaerobic infections, particularly in children using contact lenses; and does not improve the rate of healing.[44,45] Although no clear evidence exists, many ophthalmologists prescribe a topical antibiotic (e.g., fluroquinolone) for infection prophylaxis after corneal abrasion in children.

All children except those with a very mild corneal abrasion should have a slit-lamp examination. In all significant corneal injuries, examination by an ophthalmologist is desirable for management and further follow-up after discharge from the ED. Close follow-up care of children with corneal abrasions is necessary because of a possible progression of the abrasion to an ulcer.

Soft Tissue Injuries

Eyelid Lacerations

Eyelid lacerations are common in children with blunt and penetrating facial trauma. While relatively easy to detect externally, an underlying eye injury should always be suspected and skilled evaluation of the eye should take place before correction of the laceration. Ocular injury is assumed to be present in any full-thickness penetration of the eyelid. Importantly, visualization of fat from an eyelid injury indicates full-thickness injury with septal trauma and possible levator injury. The lids should be everted and the conjunctival surface examined in all eyelid injuries. If there is any suspicion that ocular penetration has occurred from penetrating trauma (e.g., pellets or BBs), an orbital CT should be obtained. Hyphema, orbital fractures, orbital penetration, and other ocular adnexal trauma often occurs with lid trauma. To test levator function, the position of the brow is fixed and the patient is asked to look up and down. If the canthal angles are rounded, medial or lateral canthus trauma is likely. With eyelid margin lacerations, there is often retraction of tissue due to orbicularis contraction, and the eyelid appears avulsed.[46] However, this tissue often stretches out to its normal size. Lacerations of the nasolacrimal duct puncta or medial to this site require probing of the canaliculus for possible injury. Sensation above the orbital rim should be tested to exclude supraorbital nerve injury.

Depending upon the child's age, anxiety level, and complexity of repair, eyelid lacerations may require moderate to deep sedation (see Chapter 159, Procedural Sedation and Analgesia). Simple partial-thickness lacerations may be repaired using 6-0 or 7-0 nylon sutures. However, plastic surgery or ophthalmology repair is required for full-thickness lacerations or those with a high potential for cosmetic deformity, canthal ligament involvement, lid margin involvement, lacrimal damage (e.g., medial lower eyelid), tissue avulsion, or levator involvement.

Ear Trauma

Blunt trauma to the external ear canal may result in hematoma, laceration to the auricle, cartilage trauma, and fractures of adjacent skull or facial bones. A subperichondrial hematoma may result from blunt trauma to the pinna. Failure to recognize and treat this condition early usually leads to a visual deformity. The pinna becomes a shapeless, reddish purple mass when blood collects between the perichondrium and the cartilage. Because the perichondrium carries the blood supply to the cartilage, avascular necrosis of the cartilage may occur. Organized, calcified hematoma may result in "cauliflower ear." Collection of blood or serous fluid between the perichondrium and cartilage may be successfully treated by needle aspiration under sterile conditions, followed by the application of a pressure dressing. If a hematoma recurs within 48 hours, formal incision and drainage are then required.

For lacerations of the pinna that penetrate the cartilage and skin on both sides, treatment is aimed at covering the exposed cartilage and minimizing deformity. Cartilage is avascular with a high risk of infection and minimal healing ability. Prior to any repair, devitalized tissue is removed. The cartilage is approximated with overlying perichondrium using 4-0 or 5-0 absorbable sutures. Next, the posterior skin surface is closed with 5-0 nonabsorbable sutures. Then the anterior surface is closed with 5-0 or 6-0 nonabsorbable sutures with attention to joining landmarks and everting wound edges along the rim of the ear so that notching does not occur. Following repair, a compression dressing is applied to ensure a hematoma does not develop. Antibiotics should be administered to patients with devitalized or contaminated wounds. If there is not enough skin to cover cartilage (i.e., indicating a need for a skin flap) or if there is a high potential for deformity, plastic surgical consultation should be obtained.[47]

Forceful blows to the mandible may be transmitted to the anterior wall of the ear canal (posterior wall of the glenoid fossa). Displaced fragments from a fractured anterior wall may cause stenosis of the canal and must be reduced or removed using a general anesthetic.

Abrasions and lacerations of the external auditory canal are common and may be caused either by the patient or iatrogenically while trying to remove wax. Eardrops containing antibiotics are usually effective in preventing an external otitis resulting from secondary infection. Aminoglycoside drops should be avoided in the presence of a tympanic membrane perforation.

Oral and Tongue Lacerations

Most inner lip and tongue lacerations do not require suturing. Importantly, lacerations that penetrate the oral mucosa require close inspection to exclude a tooth fragment or other foreign body. Patients with lacerations involving the gingiva also require evaluation to ensure that no associated fracture is present. Lacerations with large flaps and those with uncontrolled bleeding, that gape and are likely to collect food, or that involve an extensive amount of the tongue edge and may cause functional impairment require repair in the ED. The maxillary frenulum has no function and does not require repair unless trauma is extensive and extends into the surrounding mucosa. In contrast, the lingual frenulum is highly vascular and more likely to require repair to prevent continued bleeding. Lacerations that cause a degloving injury to the gum margin also require repair, usually by an oral surgeon.

For intraoral repair, absorbable sutures are used in all cases. For through-and-through tongue lacerations, the muscle layer is closed separately. Moderate sedation is often required for children who need tongue laceration repair (see Chapter 159, Procedural Sedation and Analgesia).

Other Structures

NASOLACRIMAL SYSTEM

Tears drain from the eye via puncta into the upper and lower canaliculi at the medial aspect of the eye. These puncta are directed posteriorly toward the globe and usually cannot be visualized unless the lids are everted. The upper and lower canaliculi merge to form a common canaliculus that drains into the lacrimal sac, which then drains into the nasolacrimal duct, which courses inferiorly and posteriorly through the maxilla, draining inferiorly to the inferior turbinate. Children with upper or lower eyelid trauma that is medial to the pupil require examination to exclude trauma to these structures. Moreover, if medial canthal disruption is present (e.g., rounded medial canthus), nasolacrimal trauma is also possible. In either instance, ophthalmology consultation is required.

NERVES

Five branches of the facial nerve supply motor innervation to facial muscles: the temporal, zygomatic, buccal, mandibular, and cervical branches. Paralysis of the facial nerve can affect the forehead, eyebrow, eye, nose, mouth, lips, or platysma, depending on the branches of the facial nerve affected. If hearing or taste is affected or decreased tear production is present in the ipsilateral eye, then facial nerve injury is localized to its intratemporal course (e.g., temporal bone fracture) where it give off branches involved in hearing and taste. The trigeminal nerve innervates the muscles of mastication (temporalis and masseter) and sensation to the face (see Fig. 16–2) In general, nerve injury due to penetrating trauma requires acute repair. Blunt traumatic injuries with associated fractures (e.g., temporal bone) may require decompression or may be managed conservatively depending upon the presence of associated facial injuries. In some instances, surgeons may base their decision to operate on the extent of injury noted during electrodiagnostic testing.

PAROTID DUCT

The parotid gland occupies a key location within the face, with important facial nerve branches and the parotid duct contained within its structure (see Fig. 16–2). It lies anterior to the sternomastoid muscle and inferior to the zygoma. Importantly, the buccal branch of the facial nerve, which supplies the buccinator, closely approximates the position of the parotid duct. Injury to the parotid duct or buccal branch of the facial nerve requires exploration for corresponding injury to the adjacent structure. In general, parotid duct injuries require exploration and repair by a plastic surgeon.

Summary

Oral, facial, and ocular injuries are common injuries that are easily overlooked. Clinical evaluation requires knowledge of important anatomic landmarks. While the clinical evaluation of infants and children with facial fractures can be difficult, CT is the ideal imaging study for evaluating children with potential fractures. Play, sports, and motor vehicle accidents are common causes of facial trauma in children. However, clinicians must consider and exclude the diagnosis of abuse in all cases. Importantly, patients with closed injuries and no functional deficit (e.g., visual loss, sensory/motor loss, malocclusion) usually require no acute intervention. Unless they are open, most facial fractures that are displaced or comminuted or that result in a functional deformity may wait until swelling subsides (2 to 4 days) before undergoing surgery.

REFERENCES

1. Gassner R, Tuli T, Hachl O, et al: Craniomaxillofacial trauma in children: a review of 3,385 cases with 6,060 injuries in 10 years. J Oral Maxillofac Surg 62:399–407, 2004.
2. Tanaka N, Uchide N, Suzuki K, et al: Maxillofacial fractures in children. J Craniomaxillofac Surg 21:289–293, 1993.
3. Holland AJ, Broome C, Steinberg A, Cass DT: Facial fractures in children. Pediatr Emerg Care 17:157–160, 2001.
4. Ferreira PC, Amarante JM, Silva PN, et al: Retrospective study of 1251 maxillofacial fractures in children and adolescents. Plast Reconstr Surg 115:1500–1508, 2005.

5. Cairns AM, Mok JY, Welbury RR: Injuries to the head, face, mouth, and neck in physically abused children in a community setting. Int J Paediatr Dent 15:310–318, 2005.

6. Zerfowski M, Bremerich A: Facial trauma in children and adolescents. Clin Oral Invest 2:120–124, 1998.

7. Lim LH, Kumar M, Myer CM 3rd: Head and neck trauma in hospitalized pediatric patients. Otolaryngol Head Neck Surg 130:255–261, 2004.

8. Gussack GS, Luterman A, Powell RW, et al: Pediatric maxillofacial trauma: unique features in diagnosis and treatment. Laryngoscope 97(8 Pt 1):925–930, 1987.

9. Kaban LB: Diagnosis and treatment of fractures of the facial bones in children 1943–1993. J Oral Maxillofac Surg 51:722–729, 1993.

10. Koltai PJ, Rabkin D, Hoehn J: Rigid fixation of facial fractures in children. J Craniomaxillofac Trauma 1:32–42, 1995.

11. McGraw BL, Cole RR: Pediatric maxillofacial trauma. Arch Otolaryngol Head Neck Surg 116:41–45, 1990.

12. Rowe NL: Fractures of the facial skeleton in children. J Oral Surg 26:505–515, 1967.

13. Koltai PJ, Amjad I, Meyer D, et al: Orbital fractures in children. Arch Otolaryngol Head Neck Surg 121:1375–1379, 1995.

14. Hogg NJV, Horswell BW: Soft tissue pediatric facial trauma: a review. J Can Dent Assoc 72:549–552, 2006.

15. Alonso LL, Purcell TB: Accuracy of the tongue blade test in patients with suspected mandibular fracture. J Emerg Med 13:297–304, 1995.

16. Sinclaire D, Schwartz M, Gruss J, McLellan B: A retrospective review of the relationships between facial fractures, head injuries and cervical spine injuries. J Emerg Med 6:109–112, 1988.

17. Koltai PJ, Wood GW: Three-dimensional CT reconstruction for the evaluation and surgical planning of facial fractures. Otolaryngol Head Neck Surg 95:10–15, 1986.

18. Lambert DM, Mirvis SE, Shanmuganathan K, Tilghman DL: Computed tomography exclusion of osseous paranasal sinus injury in blunt trauma patients: the clear sinus sign. J Oral Maxillofac Surg 55:1207–1211, 1997.

19. Holmgren EP, Dierks EJ, Assael LA, et al: Facial soft tissue injuries as an aid to ordering a combination head and facial computed tomography in trauma patients. J Oral Maxillofac Surg 63:651–654, 2005.

20. Exadatylos AK, Sclabas GM, Smolka K, et al: The value of computed tomographic scanning in the diagnosis and management of orbital fractures associated with head trauma: a prospective, consecutive study at a level I trauma center. J Trauma 58:336–341, 2005.

21. Holmgren EP, Dierks EJ, Homer LD, Potter BE: Facial computed tomography use in trauma patients who require a head computed tomogram. J Oral Maxillofac Surg 62:913–918, 2004.

22. Rehm CG, Ross SE: Diagnosis of unsuspected facial fractures on routine head computerized tomographic scans in the unconscious multiply injured patient. J Oral Maxillofac Surg 53:522–524, 1995.

23. Boidin MP: Airway patency in the unconscious patient. Br J Anaesth 57:306–310, 1985.

24. Nandi PR, Charlesworth CH, Taylor SJ, et al: Effect of general anaesthesia on the pharynx. Br J Anaesth 66:157–162, 1991.

25. Abernethy LJ, Allan PL, Drummond GB: Ultrasound assessment of the position of the tongue during induction of anaesthesia. Br J Anesth 65:744–748, 1990.

26. Zimmerman CE, Troulis MJ, Kaban LB: Pediatric facial fractures: recent advances in prevention, diagnosis and management. Int J Oral Maxillofac Surg 35:2–13, 2006.

27. Stucker FJ, Bryarly RC, Shockley WW: Management of nasal trauma in children. Arch Otolaryngol 110:190, 1984.

28. Apt L, Sarin LK: Causes for enucleation of the eye in infants and children. JAMA 181:948, 1962.

29. Macewen CJ: Eye injuries: a prospective survey of 5671 cases. Br J Ophthalmol 73:888, 1989.

30. Strahlman E, Elman M, Daub E, Baker S: Causes of pediatric eye injuries: a population-based study. Arch Ophthalmol 108:603–606, 1990.

31. Blaivas M, Theodoro D, Sierzenski PR: A study of bedside ocular ultrasonography in the emergency department. Acad Emerg Med 9:791–799, 2002.

32. Mafee MF, Mafee RF, Malik M, Pierce J: Medical imaging in pediatric ophthalmology. Pediatr Clin North Am 50:259–286, 2003.

33. Joseph DP, Pieramici DJ, Beauchamp NJ: Computed tomography in the diagnosis and prognosis of pen globe injuries. Ophthalmology 107:1899–1906, 2000.

34. Rhea JT: Helical CT and 3-dimensional CT of facial and orbital injury. Radiol Clin North Am 37:489–513, 1999.

35. Grant JH III, Patrinely JR, Weiss AH, et al: Trapdoor fracture of the orbit in a pediatric population. Plast Reconstr Surg 109:482–489, 2002.

36. Bansagi ZC, Meyer DR: Internal orbital fractures in the pediatric age group: characterization and management. Ophthalmology 107:829–836, 2000.

37. Egbert JE, May K, Kersten RC, Kulwin DR: Pediatric orbital floor fracture: direct extraocular muscle involvement. Ophthalmology 107:1875–1879, 2000.

38. Lee HJ, Jilani M, Frohman L, Baker S: CT of orbital trauma. Emerg Radiol 10:168–172, 2004.

39. Chidiac EJ, Raiskin AO: Succinylcholine and the open eye. Ophthalmol Clin North Am 19:279–285, 2006.

40. Pieramici DJ: Vitreoretinal trauma. Ophthalmol Clin North Am 15:225–234, 2002.

41. Kuhn F, Mester V: Anterior chamber abnormalities and cataract. Ophthalmol Clin North Am 15:195–203, 2002.

42. Dhillon B, Fleck B: Disease of the eye and orbit. In Barnard S, Edgar D (eds): Pediatric Eye Care. Cambridge: Blackwell Sciences, 1996, pp 243–267.

43. Levin AV: Eye emergencies: acute management in the pediatric ambulatory care setting. Pediatr Emerg Care 7:367–377, 1991.

44. Clemons CS, Cohen EJ, Arentsen JJ, et al: *Pseudomonas* ulcers following patching of corneal abrasions associated with contact lens wear. CLAO J 13:161–164, 1987.

45. Michael JG, Hug D, Dowd MD: Management of corneal abrasion in children: a randomized clinical trial. Ann Emerg Med 40:67–72, 2002.

46. Long J, Tann T: Adnexal trauma. Ophthalmol Clin North Am 15:179–184, 2002.

47. Park SS, Hood RJ: Management of facial cutaneous defects. Part II: auricular reconstruction. Otolaryngol Clin North Am 34:713–738, 2001.

Chapter 17

Head Trauma

Vincent J. Grant, MD

Key Points

Head trauma is common and a significant source of pediatric morbidity and mortality.

Injury prevention is the only intervention that can minimize primary traumatic brain injury.

The main goals of the emergency department management of head-injured children are to identify serious intracranial injuries and minimize secondary traumatic brain injury.

Signs and symptoms of head injury do not correlate well with the risk of intracranial injuries.

In the evaluation of most head-injured children, the greatest challenge is deciding when it is safe to evaluate these children without performing computed tomographic scanning of the head.

Introduction and Background

Emergency physicians treat children with head injuries every day.[1,2] These injuries range from trivial to fatal. Along this severity spectrum, many management issues and controversies arise. Familiarity with these issues and controversies allows emergency physicians to make rational and reasoned decisions in the face of conflicting or absent evidence.

One approach to categorizing head injuries is to group them according to the patient's Glasgow Coma Scale score[3] (Table 17–1). According to this scheme, children with mild injuries have Glasgow Coma Scale scores of 13, 14, and 15; those with moderate injuries have scores from 9 to 12; and those with severe injuries have a score of 8 or less.[4] Although relatively simple in concept, there are several problems with this approach. The Glasgow Coma Scale score seems to have only modest interrater reliability.[5] This calls into question the reproducibility of studies based on this categorization scheme. In addition, Glasgow Coma Scale scores do not adequately correlate with intracranial injuries identified on computed tomographic (CT) scanning of the head.[6] This suggests that this categorization scheme is not a valid surrogate for brain injuries. The Glasgow Coma Scale was intended for use in the era before the widespread availability of CT scanning. To consider a patient with a completely normal evaluation (Glasgow Coma Scale score 15) and a patient who is confused and localizes pain (Glasgow Coma Scale score 13) to both have the same category of head injury is counterintuitive. Nonetheless, this categorization scheme is commonly used. There have been modifications to the Glasgow Coma Scale to make it more applicable to children.[7,8] These modified scoring systems have the same problems as the original.

Recognition and Approach

Traumatic brain injury is the leading cause of death and disability in pediatric trauma.[9-11] In the United States, traumatic brain injury accounts for approximately 3000 deaths, 50,000 hospitalizations and 650,000 emergency department visits annually.[12,13] Most children have a greater propensity for head injuries than most adults. Children tend to have proportionately larger heads, relatively weaker neck musculature, and less refined coordination than adults. In addition, they participate in different daily activities, are less inclined to understand and use safety equipment, have underdeveloped judgment, and may lack the required supervision to keep them safe. Infants, in particular, are at risk for nonaccidental trauma and have relatively thin skulls (see Chapter 119, Physical Abuse and Child Neglect).

The mechanisms of injury for pediatric head injuries are age dependent. The majority of accidental head injuries in younger children are due to falls and motor vehicle accidents. Adolescents are more likely to have injuries related to sporting or recreational activities, although motor vehicle accidents are also a frequent cause of head injuries in this age group. Penetrating head injuries are relatively rare in children and uncommon in most populations of adolescents. Gang activities in some adolescents increases the risk of penetrating head injuries (see Chapter 157, Interpersonal and Intimate Partner Violence).

One conceptually simple approach to traumatic brain injuries categorizes them as either primary or secondary. Primary brain injury occurs at the time of the injury. At the time of impact, cellular and structural damage occurs. We currently have no effective treatments for primary brain injuries. The only effective intervention yet to be identified is injury prevention.[14] Effective interventions include laws mandating the use of seat belts, car seats, and bicycle helmets.[15,16] Although emergency physicians can play an important role in promoting injury prevention, this does not

Table 17–1	Glasgow Coma Score Scale	
		Score
Eye Opening		
Spontaneous		4
To verbal stimulation		3
To painful stimulation		2
No eye opening		1
Motor		
Obeys commands		6
Localizes pain		5
Withdraws to pain		4
Flexion posturing		3
Extension posturing		2
No motor response		1
Verbal		
Alert and oriented		5
Confused		4
Inappropriate language		3
Incoherent language		2
No verbal response		1

From Teasdale G, Jennett B: Assessment of coma and impaired consciousness: a practical scale. Lancet 2:81–84, 1974.

help the child who presents having already sustained a head injury. Secondary brain injury occurs after the time of the initial impact. The major causes of secondary brain injury include hypoxia, hypotension, and intracranial hypertension.[17] Examples of secondary brain injury include anoxic brain injury from hypoxia that occurs after an injury or brain herniation due to an expanding intracranial hemorrhage or brain swelling. Left untreated, secondary brain injury can lead to progressive neurologic deterioration and death. Prehospital and emergency department care is directed at minimizing secondary brain injury.

Evaluation

Several intuitively appealing signs and symptoms that potentially predict the presence of a clinically significant head injury have been studied. These include abnormal mental status, loss of consciousness, amnesia to the event, a Glasgow Coma Scale score less than 15, skull fracture, scalp hematoma, a focal neurologic examination, irritability, a bulging fontanelle, vomiting, seizure, and headache.[18-22] One meta-analysis found that loss of consciousness, skull fracture, focal neurologic signs, and a Glasgow Coma Scale score less than 15 are strong risk factors for intracranial injuries.[23] Another group found that loss of consciousness, amnesia to the event, or both did not correlate with traumatic brain injuries on CT scanning.[24] The NEXUS II investigators took another approach.[22,25] This group suggested that, if the following seven criteria were not present, the risk of clinically significant intracranial injury was very low: (1) evidence of significant skull fracture, (2) altered level of alertness, (3) neurologic deficit, (4) persistent vomiting, (5) presence of scalp hematoma, (6) abnormal behavior, and (7) coagulopathy.[22] The implication, of course, is that if these seven criteria are not present, CT scanning is not needed. Although the authors note that their decision criteria worked well in children younger than 3 years of age, the number of these young children in this study was small. After reviewing the available literature, one group proposing

a practice guideline for infants and young children determined that loss of consciousness and vomiting did not correlate with clinically significant findings on CT scanning.[26] Strangely, this group acknowledged this and yet still recommended CT scanning for children who lost consciousness for greater than 1 minute or who vomited five or more times.[26] One group suggested that infants could present in an "occult" manner without appreciable signs or symptoms of head injury.[27] Another group disputed the existence of "occult" head injuries.[21] The reasons for the variability in the findings of these studies are not entirely clear. It is conceivable that the heterogeneity of the injury types, the ages and development of the children in the study populations, and the outcomes of interest led to conflicting and confusing results.

The greatest advances in evaluating children with head injuries are in imaging. CT scanning has had the greatest impact. The decision about when to obtain a CT scan, however, is not always clear. The greatest controversy exists for those children at the less severe end of the injury spectrum. It is clear that a traumatized, comatose child requires CT scanning of the head. At the other end of the severity spectrum, the decision on when to perform CT scanning is controversial. It is probably reasonable to perform CT scanning on children who have abnormal mental status and infants with relatively large scalp hematomas.[23,24,28-31] Isolated, brief loss of consciousness is probably not an indication for CT scanning.[20] Beyond that, it is difficult to universally define when CT scanning is indicated. There is no role for skull radiographs in the identification of intracranial injuries as the intracranial contents are not seen on plain radiographs. Since intracranial injuries occur in the absence of skull fractures, skull radiographs poorly risk-stratify children for the presence of intracranial injuries. Magnetic resonance imaging is currently too time consuming for the evaluation of acutely injured children in the emergency department.[32]

Management

Management of head-injured children is directed at specific findings on physical examination and CT scanning results. The management of head-injured children needs to take into account the possibility of multisystem trauma and follow general principles of resuscitating children (see Chapter 1, Approach to Resuscitation and Advanced Life Support for Infants and Children; Chapter 3, Rapid Sequence Intubation; and Chapter 12, Approach to Multisystem Trauma). There has been some interest in using controlled hypothermia to treat severe brain injuries. Laboratory studies have shown that moderate hypothermia decreases neuronal loss, decreases excessive neurotransmitter release, and prevents disruption of the blood-brain barrier.[33] Hypothermia has not been adequately studied to recommend it at this time. More detailed basic and advanced cerebral resuscitation techniques are described in detail elsewhere (see Chapter 9, Cerebral Resuscitation).

Impending Herniation

In severely head injured children there is the possibility of impending brain herniation. This is usually evident on physical examination by the presence of a bulging fontanelle, unequal or fixed and dilated pupils, and posturing or coma. If the child is hemodynamically stable enough to undergo CT scanning, the scan may reveal intracranial bleeding or diffuse axonal injury. Diffuse axonal injury is the proposed mechanism for patients who suffer severe closed head injury without the presence of obvious macroscopic intracranial injuries, such as contusion, hematoma, or cerebral edema on CT scanning.[34] A few interventions have been recommended for decreasing intracranial hypertension. One is elevation of the head of the bed 30 degrees.[35] This has been recommended for children, but has not been studied in children. Although generally recommended several years ago, hyperventilation is to be avoided as it is now thought to lead to intracranial blood vessel constriction and brain ischemia.[36,37] Instead of the traditional mannitol used to treat adults, the use of 3% hypertonic saline (which can be given as a bolus of 3 ml/kg intravenously) is gaining acceptance as a means of treating and preventing intracranial hypertension[38,39] (see Chapter 9, Cerebral Resuscitation).

Scalp Injuries

Although it is a highly vascular structure that bleeds profusely when injured, the scalp is underestimated in its contribution to head injury morbidity. In young infants, scalp injuries, with or without an opening in the skin, can cause deterioration from hemorrhagic shock.[19,40] In particular, a subgaleal hematoma in an infant may be a significant source of hypovolemia from scalp hemorrhage without any signs of external bleeding.

Skull Fractures

There are four main types of skull fractures: linear, depressed, diastatic, and basilar. Linear skull fractures are the most common type of fracture seen in pediatrics, comprising approximately 75% to 90% of all fractures.[19] A depressed skull fracture includes any skull fracture in which the bone fragment is depressed below the inner table of the skull. A depressed skull fracture typically requires operative elevation if it is depressed to a depth greater than the thickness of the skull.[19] Diastatic fractures involve sutures. One common complication of both depressed and diastatic fractures is the leptomeningeal cyst or "growing" fracture. This complication arises when a tear in the dura allows the arachnoid membrane to penetrate the fracture, leading to demineralization of the bone fragments at the fracture site and penetration of cerebrospinal fluid into the subarachnoid space.[41] Healing is impaired, and therefore necessitates careful follow-up, with surgical repair being occasionally required if the fracture continues to "grow" 2 to 3 months following the injury. Basilar skull fractures account for up to 20% of all skull fractures, and classically have distinctive clinical features, including periorbital ecchymosis ("raccoon eyes"), postauricular mastoid ecchymosis (Battle's sign), hemotympanum, and cerebrospinal fluid rhinorrhea or otorrhea. In these cases, ecchymosis is not typically present on presentation to the emergency department. Complications of basal skull fractures include facial nerve palsy, cerebrospinal fluid fistulas, and meningitis. Antibiotic prophylaxis for basilar skull fractures is not recommended as this may lead to subsequent meningitis with resistant bacteria.[19]

Intracranial Hemorrhages

Intracranial hemorrhages represent the most common life-threatening complications of head injuries. As a group, these injuries occur in up to 12% of patients with mild head injuries alone.[41] Early diagnosis of intracranial hemorrhage is essential to allow identification of the subgroup that requires prompt neurosurgical management. Intracranial hemorrhages can be divided into four main types: parenchymal contusions, epidural hematomas, subdural hematomas, and subarachnoid hemorrhages.

Parenchymal contusions develop as a result of direct impact between the brain and the overlying skull, causing a focal area of bruising, hemorrhage, and edema. Contusions are either caused by abrupt acceleration of the head, causing a "coup" injury on the same side as impact, or by abrupt deceleration of the head, causing a "contrecoup" injury on the opposite side from impact. Immediate surgical intervention is not usually indicated for parenchymal contusions.

Epidural hematomas are collections of blood between the skull and the dura of the brain. Because the dura is tightly adhered to the skull in certain areas, the collection of hemorrhage grows in a characteristic lens-shaped pattern. The vessel injury in question can be either arterial or venous, but the most significant injuries are from arterial injury, typically the middle meningeal artery. There may be an associated skull fracture. The clinical presentation may lead to false reassurance, because the typical presentation usually includes a lucid interval of time between the initial injury and rapid neurologic deterioration associated with rapid expansion of the hematoma. Small epidural hematomas have been shown to occur after minor head trauma in alert children with no focal neurologic signs.[42] Larger epidural hematomas usually require urgent neurosurgical intervention.[31] Prognosis is excellent with early treatment.[31]

Subdural hematomas are collections of blood between the dura and the arachnoid membrane. This hemorrhage is most commonly a result of torn bridging veins in the subdural space, that present as crescent-shaped lesions on CT. Typically, these lesions are not associated with skull fractures, and occur most often as a result of rapid acceleration/deceleration.[43] Compared to epidural hematomas, subdural hematomas are less amenable to neurosurgical intervention, and outcomes may be poor, with up to 50% of patients developing profound disabilities regardless of the treatment provided.[43]

Subarachnoid hemorrhage occurs as a result of damage to superficial vessels running along the surface of the brain, underneath the arachnoid membranes. The blood is irritating to the meninges, sometimes causing nuchal rigidity and severe headache. These lesions can result in vasospasm and further ischemic injury, but rarely require acute intervention.

Posttraumatic Seizures

Posttraumatic seizures occur in as many as 5% to 10% of all head-injured children. The timing of the seizures is classified as immediate, early, and late. Immediate posttraumatic seizures occur at the time of injury, and are thought to be due to instant depolarization of the cortex in response to the injury. This type of seizure generally does not recur. These "impact seizures" are not predictive of clinically significant intracranial injuries, nor do they require any specific treatment or imaging. In contrast, early seizures occur after the impact, but within 24 hours of the injury. Early seizures are more likely to be a manifestation of an intracranial injury and therefore warrant imaging. Late seizures occur greater than 1 week after injury and are a result of scarring and mechanical irritation of the brain.[41] The routine use of prophylactic antiepileptic medications after minor head injuries is not necessary.[41,44] Children with repeated seizures or those in status epilepticus require prompt management of their seizures (see Chapter 40, Seizures).

Transient Cortical Blindness and Trauma-Triggered Migraine

Since the mid-1960s, with Bodian's original description of six children who had transient loss of vision for a few hours following trauma, transient cortical blindness has been recognized as a complication of head trauma.[45-49] Traumatic cortical blindness is typically seen in children and young adults who have sustained minor head injury, brief or no loss of consciousness, blindness occurring within hours of the head injury, normal pupils and fundi, and a normal CT scan of the head.[50] Particularly in the young child with limited language skills, assessing blindness may be exceedingly difficult and the patient may simply exhibit anxiety and agitation.[51] There appears to be some overlap with transient cortical blindness and what has been called "trauma-triggered migraine."[52,53] In these cases, a child sustains a blow to the head and then has a clinical presentation like that of a classic or complicated migraine (see Chapter 41, Headaches). Visual disturbances include scintillating scotoma, homonymous hemianopia, blurred vision, tunnel vision, or transient blindness. These symptoms usually resolve and are then replaced by headache, nausea, and vomiting. The patient may exhibit confusion or incoherence, paresthesias, dysphasia, and hemiparesis. Children may become agitated and combative.[52] The etiology of transient cortical blindness and trauma-triggered migraine is unknown. Theories to explain these events have centered on vasospasm and localized cerebral edema.[54] Although β-blocker therapy has been considered a treatment for posttraumatic migraines, there is currently no standard treatment.[53]

Summary

The disposition and prognosis for head-injured children is dependent on the type and degree of injury. Most children who have negative CT scans and have resolution of their symptoms in the emergency department can be safely discharged home. There is no need for awakening the child throughout the night as the likelihood of a missed clinically significant intracranial injury is very low. Exceptions to this include hemophiliacs and children on warfarin, in whom the risk of a delayed bleed is much greater. Children who are awake and have small intracranial bleeds may be admitted or transferred to a facility with a pediatric neurosurgeon and a monitored intensive care area. Severely injured children will require admission or transfer to a pediatric intensive care unit for pediatric neurosurgical evaluation.

An area of some controversy is the management of child diagnosed with a concussion who has a normal CT scan of the head. A concussion is a transient alteration in mental status following a blow to the head. The main controversy surrounds the decision as to when a child may return to sporting activities. There are no evidence-based guidelines; however, there are some consensus-based recommendations.[55] For children who experience transient confusion with resolution of symptoms within 15 minutes and without loss of consciousness, the recommendation is to have the child be immediately removed from play and return to play if his or her mental status is normal after 15 minutes on the sidelines. For children who experience transient confusion for longer than 15 minutes without loss of consciousness, the recommendation is to have the child sit out for the rest of the day and return to play in 1 week if the neurologic examination is normal at that point. For children who experience any loss of consciousness, the recommendation is for removal from play for 1 week if the loss of consciousness lasts for a few seconds or 2 weeks if the loss of consciousness lasts longer than that. For these children, the child needs to be asymptomatic at rest and with exertion to return to play after sitting out for a week or two.

Survivors of traumatic brain injury are at increased risk for long-term neuropsychological deficits in the areas of verbal reasoning, learning and recall, attention, executive functions, and constructional skills. If these functions recover, the recovery period may last years.[56] Children with traumatic brain injuries are also at risk of psychiatric disturbances, such as major depression and anxiety disorders, attention-deficit/hyperactivity disorder, and organic personality disorder.[57,58]

REFERENCES

1. Jager TE, Weiss HB, Coben JH, et al: Traumatic brain injuries evaluated in U.S. emergency departments, 1992–1994. Acad Emerg Med 7:134–140, 2000.
2. Thurman DJ, Alverson C, Dunn KA, et al: Traumatic brain injury in the United States: a public health perspective. J Head Trauma Rehabil 14:602–615, 1999.
3. Teasdale G, Jennett B: Assessment of coma and impaired consciousness: a practical scale. Lancet 2:81–84, 1974.
4. Kraus JF, Fife D, Conroy C: Pediatric brain injuries: the nature, clinical course, and early outcomes in a defined United States population. Pediatrics 79:501–507, 1987.
5. Gill MR, Reiley DG, Green SM: Interrater reliability of Glasgow Coma Scale scores in the emergency department. Ann Emerg Med 43:215–223, 2004.
6. Ratan SK, Pandey RM, Ratan J: Association among duration of unconsciousness, Glasgow Coma Scale, and cranial computed tomography abnormalities in head injured children. Clin Pediatr 40:375–378, 2001.
7. Durham SR, Clancy RR, Leuthardt E, et al: CHOP infant coma scale (Infant Face Scale): a novel coma scale for children less than two years of age. J Neurotrauma 17:729–737, 2000.
8. Hahn YS, Chyung C, Barthel MJ, et al: Head injuries in children under 36 months of age. Childs Nerv Syst 4:34–49, 1988.
9. National Vital Statistics System: Ten Leading Causes of Death, United States 1999. Atlanta, GA: National Center for Injury Prevention and Control, 1999.
10. Hoyert DL, Arias E, Smith B, et al: Final Data for 1999: National Vital Statistics Reports, Vol 49. Hyattsville, MD: National Center for Health Statistics, 2001.
11. National Center for Injury Prevention and Control: Traumatic Brain Injury in the United States: A Report to Congress. Atlanta: Centers for Disease Control and Prevention, 1999.
12. Centers for Disease Control and Prevention: 2000 National Hospital Ambulatory Medical Care Survey, Emergency Department File 2002 [on CD-ROM]. Vital Health Stat 13(33):1.
13. National Center for Injury Prevention and Control: Traumatic Brain Injury in the United States: Assessing Outcomes in Children. Atlanta, GA: Centers for Disease Control and Prevention, 2002.
14. McCaig LF, Burt CW: National Hospital Ambulatory Medical Care Survey: 2002 Emergency Department Summary. Adv Data 340:1.
15. National Center for Health Statistics: Healthy People 2010: Focus Area 15: Injury and Violence Prevention. Hyattsville, MD: Public Health Service, 2004.

16. National Center for Health Statistics: Healthy People 2000 Final Review. Hyattsville, MD: Public Health Service, 2001.

17. Kokoska ER, Smith GS, Pittman T, et al: Early hypotension worsens neurological outcome in pediatric patients with moderately severe head trauma. J Pediatr Surg 33:333–338, 1998.

18. Quayle KS, Jaffe DM, Kuppermann N, et al: Diagnostic testing for acute head injury in children: when are computed tomography and skull radiographs indicated? Pediatrics 99:e11, 1997.

19. Woestman R, Perkin R, Serna T, et al: Mild head injury in children: identification, clinical evaluation, neuroimaging, and disposition. J Pediatr Health Care 12:288–298, 1998.

*20. American Academy of Pediatrics; Commission on Clinical Policies and Research, American Academy of Family Physicians: The management of minor closed head injury in children. Pediatrics 104:1407–1415, 1999.

21. Brown L, Moynihan JA, Denmark TK: Blunt pediatric head trauma requiring neurosurgical intervention: how subtle can it be? Am J Emerg Med 21:467–472, 2003.

22. Oman JA, Cooper RJ, Holmes JF, et al: Performance of a decision rule to predict need for computed tomography among children with blunt head trauma. Pediatrics 117:238–246, 2006.

*23. Dunning J, Batchelor J, Stratford-Smith P, et al: A meta-analysis of variables that predict significant intracranial injury in minor head trauma. Arch Dis Child 89:653–659, 2004.

*24. Palchak MJ, Holmes JF, Vance CW, et al: A decision rule for identifying children at low risk for brain injuries after blunt head trauma. Ann Emerg Med 42:492–506, 2003.

25. Mower WR, Hoffman JR, Herbert M, et al, for the NEXUS II Investigators: Developing a decision instrument to guide computed tomographic imaging of blunt head injury patients. J Trauma 59:954–959, 2005.

*26. Schutzman SA, Barnes P, Duhaime AC, et al: Evaluation and management of children younger than two years old with apparently minor head trauma: proposed guidelines. Pediatrics 107:983–993, 2001.

27. Greenes DS, Schulzman SA: Occult intracranial injury in infants. Ann Emerg Med 32:680–686, 1998.

28. Greenes DS, Schutzman SA: Clinical indicators of intracranial injury in head-injured infants. Pediatrics 104:861–867, 1999.

29. Gruskin KD, Schulzman SA: Head trauma in children younger than 2 years: are there predictors for complications? Arch Pediatr Adolesc Med 153:15–20, 1999.

*30. Haydel MJ, Shembekar AD: Prediction of intracranial injury in children aged five years and older with loss of consciousness after minor head injury due to nontrivial mechanisms. Ann Emerg Med 42:507–514, 2003.

31. Beni-Adani L, Flores I, Spektor S, et al: Epidural hematoma in infants: a different entity? J Trauma 46:306–311, 1999.

32. American Academy of Pediatrics, Section on Radiology: Diagnostic imaging of child abuse. Pediatrics 105:1345–1348, 2000.

*33. Enrione MA: Current concepts in the acute management of severe pediatric head trauma. Clin Pediatr Emerg Med 2:28–40, 2001.

34. Mittl RL, Grossman RI, Hichle JF, et al: Prevalence of MR evidence of diffuse axonal injury in patients with mild traumatic brain injury and normal head CT findings. Am J Neuroradiol 15:1583–1589, 1994.

35. Feldman Z, Kanter MJ, Robertson CS, et al: Effect of head elevation on intracranial pressure, cerebral perfusion pressure, and cerebral blood flow in head-injured patients. J Neurosurg 76:207–211, 1992.

36. Skippen P, Seear M, Poskitt K, et al: Effect of hyperventilation on regional cerebral blood flow in head-injured children. Crit Care Med 25:1402–1409, 1997.

37. Sharples PM, Stuart AG, Matthews DS, et al: Cerebral blood flow and metabolism in children with severe head injury. Part 1: Relation to age, Glasgow coma score, outcome, intracranial pressure, and time after injury. J Neurol Neurosurg Psychiatry 58:145–158, 1995.

38. Khanna S, Davis D, Peterson B, et al: Use of hypertonic saline in the treatment of severe refractory posttraumatic intracranial hypertension in pediatric traumatic brain injury. Crit Care Med 28:1144–1151, 2000.

39. Peterson B, Khanna S, Fisher B, et al: Prolonged hypernatremia controls elevated intracranial pressure in head-injured pediatric patients. Crit Care Med 28:1136–1143, 2000.

40. Meyer P, Legros C, Orliaguet G: Critical care management of neurotrauma in children: new trends and perspectives. Childs Nerv Syst 15:732–739, 1999.

41. Savitsky EA, Votey SR: Current controversies in the management of minor pediatric head injuries. Am J Emerg Med 18:96–101, 2000.

42. Schutzman SA, Barnes PD, Mantello M, et al: Epidural hematoma in children. Ann Emerg Med 22:535–541, 1993.

43. Jayawant S, Rawlinson A, Gibbon F, et al: Subdural hemorrhage in infants: population based study. BMJ 317:1558–1561, 1998.

44. Dias MS, Carnevale F, Li V: Immediate posttruamtic seizures: is routine hospitalization necessary? Pediatr Neurosurg 30:232–238, 1999.

45. Bodian M: Transient loss of vision following head trauma. N Y State J Med 64:916–920, 1964.

46. Harrison DW, Walls RM: Blindness following minor head trauma in children: a report of two cases with a review of the literature. J Emerg Med 8:21–24, 1990.

47. Rodriguez A, Lozano JA, del Pozo D, et al: Post-traumatic transient cortical blindness. Int Ophthalmol 17:277–283, 1993.

48. Eldridge PR, Punt JA: Transient traumatic cortical blindness in children. Lancet 1:815–816, 1988.

49. Gleeson AP, Beatrie TF: Post-traumatic transient cortical blindness in children: a report of four cases and a review of the literature. J Accid Emerg Med 11:250–252, 1994.

50. Yamamoto LG, Bart RD: Transient blindness following mild head trauma: criteria for benign outcome. Clin Pediatr 27:479–483, 1988.

51. Woodward GA: Posttraumatic cortical blindness: are we missing the diagnosis in children? Pediatr Emerg Care 6:289–292, 1990.

52. Haas DC, Lourie H: Trauma-triggered migraine: an explanation for common neurological attacks after mild head injury. J Neurosurg 68:181–188, 1988.

53. Hochstetler K, Beals RD: Transient cortical blindness in a child. Ann Emerg Med 16:218–219, 1987.

54. Ferrera PC, Reicho PR: Acute confusional migraine and trauma-triggered migraine. Am J Emerg Med 14:276–278, 1996.

55. Practice parameter: The management of concussion in sports (summary statement)—report of the Quality Standards Subcommittee. Neurology 48:581–585, 1997.

56. Yeates KO, Taylor HG, Wade SI, et al: A prospective study of short and long-term neuropsychological outcomes after traumatic brain injury in children. Neuropsychology 16:514–523, 2002.

57. Swift EE, Taylor HG, Kaugars AS, et al: Sibling relationships and behavior after pediatric traumatic brain injury. J Dev Behav Pediatr 24:24–31, 2003.

58. Wase SL, Taylor HG, Drotar D, et al: Family burden and adaptation during the initial year after traumatic brain injury in children. Pediatrics 102:110–116, 1998.

*Selected readings.

Chapter 18

Neck Trauma

Jan M. Shoenberger, MD and William K. Mallon, MD

Key Points

Early definitive airway management with rapid sequence intubation can be lifesaving in blunt and penetrating neck trauma.

Identifying the zone of injury (I, II, and III) is important for determining the appropriate management plan.

Penetrating facial trauma below the horizon of the pupils may result in zone III neck injuries.

Neurologic deficits, even if transient, suggest a vascular or spinal cord injury.

Introduction and Background

The mechanisms of injury for cases of pediatric neck trauma are numerous and heterogeneous. The most common cause of both penetrating and blunt neck injuries is motor vehicle accidents. Penetrating injuries occur most frequently in adolescents, including accidental injuries and injuries received when they are victims of violent crime.[1,2] Penetrating neck wounds from impalement, dog and human bites, and fireworks are also reported.[3-5] Mechanisms of injury causing blunt neck trauma include bicycle injuries, sports injuries, falls, near-hangings, and scooter and in-line skating injuries.[6-14] Trampoline use is associated with both neck injuries and cervical spine injuries[15,16] (see Chapter 23, Spinal Trauma).

Recognition and Approach

Neck anatomy is complex, with many vital structures contained within a relatively small, flexible space. To describe neck injuries, a commonly accepted approach is to divide the neck into three anatomic zones designated I, II, and III (Fig. 18–1). The numbering is somewhat counterintuitive, with zone III being the most cephalad. Zone I extends inferiorly from the cricoid cartilage to the clavicles. Injuries in this region carry a higher mortality because they can involve major vessels, lung apices, and the esophagus, trachea, thyroid structures, and thoracic duct. Zone I is difficult to access

surgically. Zone II consists of the area between the cricoid cartilage and the angle of the mandible. Zone II is where the majority of neck wounds occur. The major structures in zone II include the trachea, esophagus, larynx, spinal cord, jugular veins, and carotid arteries. Injuries in zone II carry a lower mortality. The assessment and surgical management of zone II neck injuries is easier than that in the other two zones due to the absence of bony obstruction. Zone III comprises the area between the angle of the mandible and the base of the skull. The major structures in zone III include the pharynx, jugular veins, and vertebral and carotid arteries. Penetrating facial trauma as high as the horizon of the pupils may result in zone III neck injuries. Injuries to the spinal cord may occur in conjunction with injuries to any zone. Zone II injuries account for about 50% of neck injuries, with zones I and III accounting for about 25% each.[17,18]

The neck can also be divided into anterior and posterior triangles. Wounds in the anterior and lateral aspects of the neck pose the greatest threat to a patient's airway because of their proximity to the trachea, larynx, laryngeal nerves, and vessels of the neck.[19] Trauma involving the area posterior to the trapezius ridge is the least likely to involve vital structures. The neck is a three-dimensional structure, and the apparent depth of wounds contributes to the overall assessment and management plan. For example, for anterior penetrating wounds, if the platysma muscle has been violated, the management approach is much more aggressive than if it has not been violated.

The anatomic relationships in the pediatric neck differ from those seen in adults (Table 18–1). Because the pediatric neck is much shorter, the zones of the neck are less distinct; thus the surgeon will have less operative exposure. The vascular structures are proportionately larger and have less muscle and soft tissue protection than seen in most adults. Compared with adults, hematomas may expand and extend more rapidly in children due to greater tissue pliability. The larynx is in a more anterior position and the trachea is shorter.[20] A smaller mandible and chin result in children being less likely to "take it on the chin." The pediatric airway is more flexible and has bulkier adjacent soft tissues, increasing the potential for early obstruction.[21]

Evaluation

The prehospital care phase should include consideration of cervical immobilization. Clinical experience suggests that

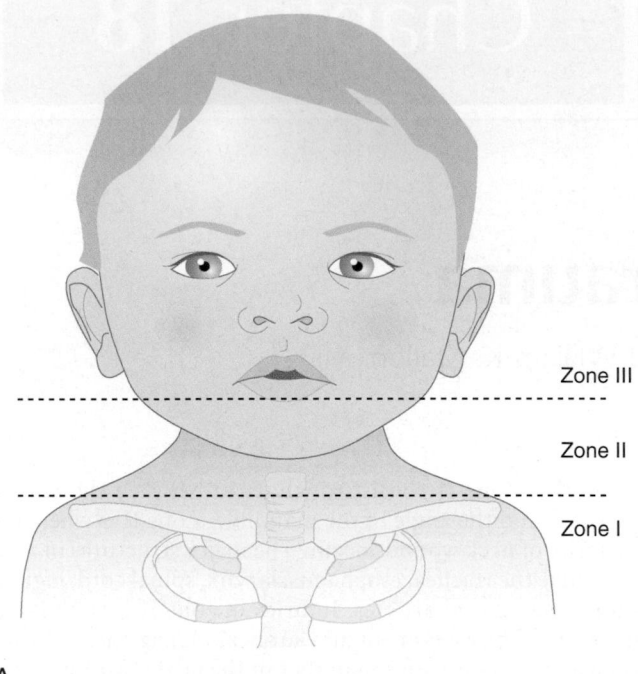

Zone III

Zone II

Zone I

A

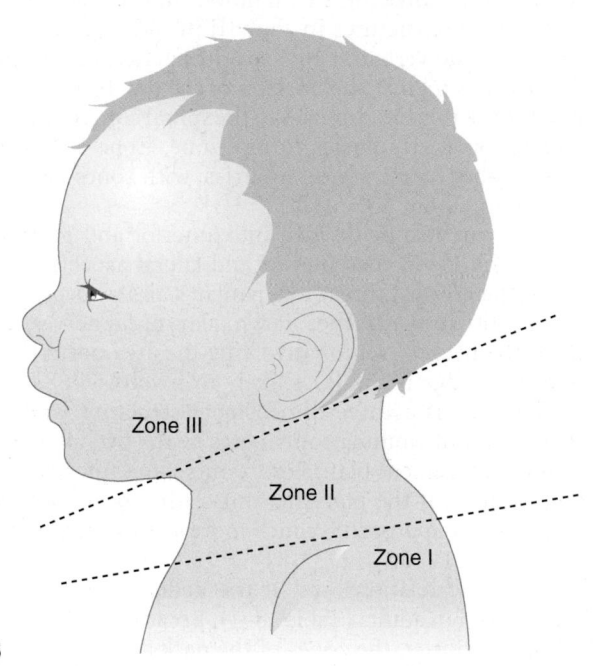

Zone III

Zone II

Zone I

B

FIGURE 18–1. Zones of the neck. **A,** Anterior view. **B,** Lateral view.

Table 18–1	Characteristics of the Pediatric Neck

Anterior airway
Indistinct transitions between the zones of the neck
Obscured laryngeal landmarks
Relatively small chin
Short neck
Small cricothyroid membrane
Small muscle mass

derangement of the airway structures developing in a dynamic fashion. False reassurance may develop because the skin overlying the neck may be relatively normal in appearance even in cases of substantial internal injury. An airway injury is suspected if the child exhibits stridor, hoarseness, subcutaneous emphysema, or air bubbling from any wound. Other signs of serious neck injuries include a vascular bruit, a pulse deficit, a neurologic deficit, hemoptysis, hematemesis, and crepitance.[23] In general, it is unwise to probe neck wounds. Probing blindly can disrupt hematomas, can cause new injuries, and is uncomfortable. Probing also can be misleading due to mobile tissue planes.

The major decision node for neck injuries relates to the airway and hemodynamic stability of the patient. Unstable patients generally require prompt surgical exploration. Previously, "all" zone II penetrating neck injuries underwent surgical exploration. This historical approach is increasingly uncommon.[24] For stable children, computed tomographic (CT) angiography is currently the imaging modality of choice for assessing vascular injuries.[25] Ultrasound with color flow Doppler technique is another valuable imaging tool, but has not been studied as extensively as CT angiography.[26,27] For serious, stable, penetrating injuries, CT angiography is often combined with esophagoscopy, laryngoscopy, and bronchoscopy to fully evaluate vital structures.[17]

Management

The primary tasks for emergency physicians in the setting of serious neck injuries are airway and hemorrhage control. Orotracheal intubation is the preferred route for definitive airway control. This can best be achieved with rapid sequence intubation[28] (see Chapter 3, Rapid Sequence Intubation). The decision on when to intubate is not always clear. In general, anticipating deterioration and airway occlusion is prudent. However, this must be balanced with the risk of performing an unnecessary intubation and causing airway trauma. If airway compromise is imminent and intubation is not successful, needle jet ventilation may be a reasonable temporizing measure pending definitive airway control. Similar to other body regions, active bleeding can usually be controlled with direct pressure. Obviously, applying excessive pressure to the structures of the neck can have deleterious effects. The balance between applying sufficient pressure to control hemorrhage and avoiding excessive pressure can be difficult. Acute anemia from hemorrhage may require the transfusion of packed red blood cells. Consultation with trauma surgeons and ear, nose, and throat surgeons is indicated in many cases of serious neck injuries. Consultation with a neurosurgeon for suspected spinal cord injuries is also indicated.

some prehospital care providers place all traumatized individuals in cervical spine precautions. This global approach has been challenged, particularly with regard to penetrating injuries.[22] The utility of cervical spine immobilization in most cases of neck injuries is probably very low. In addition, cervical collars make it difficult to visualize important life-threatening signs and hinder access to sites of bleeding.

In the emergency department, the assessment and management of the airway is the highest initial priority[21] (see Chapter 2, Respiratory Distress and Respiratory Failure). Patients with penetrating neck injuries may have an internal

Summary

Specific risk criteria that differentiate "minor" from "major" neck injuries have not been identified. Nonetheless, most blunt neck injuries in children require no imaging, require no testing, and have few complications. After a "brief" period of observation, these children can be discharged home with close follow-up. For moderate blunt injuries, there are no definitive pediatric studies. The utility of relatively prolonged observation or imaging is unclear. More severe blunt neck injuries and all but the obviously superficial penetrating injuries require multidisciplinary evaluation and management. Disposition depends on the results of imaging studies and visualization of structures with endoscopy. Given the heterogeneity of neck injuries, the prognosis of these children varies greatly.

REFERENCES

1. Freed HA, Milzman DP, Holt RW, et al: Age 14 starts a child's increased risk of major knife or gun injury in Washington, DC. J Natl Med Assoc 96:169–174, 2004.
2. Holland P, O'Brien DF, May PL: Should airguns be banned? Br J Neurosurg 18:124–129, 2004.
3. Feldman KA, Trent R, Jay MT: Epidemiology of hospitalizations resulting from dog bites in California. Am J Public Health 94:1940–1941, 2004.
4. Martinez-Lage JF, Mesones J, Gilabert A: Air-gun pellet injuries to the head and neck in children. Pediatr Surg Int 17:657–660, 2001.
5. Khan MS, Kirkland PM, Kumar R: Migrating foreign body in the tracheobronchial tree: an unusual case of firework penetrating neck injury. J Laryngol Otol 116:148–149, 2002.
6. Joffe M, Ludwig S: Stairway injuries in children. Pediatrics 82:457–461, 1988.
7. Digeronimo RJ, Mayes TC: Near-hanging injury in childhood: a literature review and report of three cases. Pediatr Emerg Care 10:150–156, 1994.
8. Nguyen D, Letts M: In-line skating injuries in children: a 10-year review. J Pediatr Orthop 21:613–618, 2001.
9. Parker JF, O'Shea JS, Simon HK: Unpowered scooter injuries reported to the Consumer Product Safety Commission: 1995–2001. Am J Emerg Med 22:273–275, 2004.
10. Claes I, Van Schil P, Corthouts B, et al: Posterior tracheal wall laceration after blunt neck trauma in children: a case report and review of the literature. Resuscitation 63:97–102, 2004.
11. Corsten G, Berkowitz RG: Membranous tracheal rupture in children following minor blunt cervical trauma. Ann Otol Rhinol Laryngol 111:197–199, 2002.
12. Starr BE, Shubert A, Baumann B: A child with isolated Horner's syndrome after blunt neck trauma. J Emerg Med 26:425–427, 2004.
13. Kadish H, Schunk J, Woodward GA: Blunt pediatric laryngotracheal trauma: case reports and review of the literature. Am J Emerg Med 12:207–211, 1994.
14. Ford HR, Gardner MJ, Lynch JM: Laryngotracheal disruption from blunt pediatric neck injuries: impact of early recognition and intervention on outcome. J Pediatr Surg 30:331–334, 1995.
15. Brown PG, Lee M: Trampoline injuries of the cervical spine. Pediatr Neurosurg 32:170–175, 2000.
16. Woodward GA, Furnival R, Schunk JE: Trampolines revisited: a review of 114 pediatric recreational trampoline injuries. Pediatrics 89:849–854, 1992.
17. Kim MK, Buckman R, Szermeta W: Penetrating neck trauma in children: an urban hospital's experience. Otolaryngol Head Neck Surg 123:439–443, 2000.
18. Mutabagani KH, Beaver BL, Cooney DR, et al: Penetrating neck trauma in children: a reappraisal. J Pediatr Surg 30:341–344, 1995.
19. Desjardins G, Varon AJ: Airway management for penetrating neck injuries: the Miami experience. Resuscitation 48:71–75, 2001.
20. Gerardi MJ, Sacchetti AD, Cantor RM, et al: Rapid-sequence intubation of the pediatric patient. Ann Emerg Med 28:55–74, 1996.
21. Lim LH, Kumar M, Myer CM 3rd: Head and neck trauma in hospitalized pediatric patients. Otolaryngol Head Neck Surg 130:255–261, 2004.
22. Barkana Y, Stein M, Scope A: Prehospital stabilization of the cervical spine for penetrating injuries of the neck—is it necessary? Int J Care Injured 31:305–309, 2000.
23. Goudy SL, Miller FB, Bumpous JM: Neck crepitance: evaluation and management of suspected aerodigestive tract injury. Laryngoscope 112:791–795, 2002.
24. Sriussadaporn S, Pak-Art R, Tharavej C, et al: Selective management of penetrating neck injuries based on clinical presentations is safe and practical. Int Surg 86:90–93, 2001.
25. Munera F, Soto JA, Palacio DM, et al: Penetrating neck injuries: helical CT angiography for initial evaluation. Radiology 224:366–372, 2002.
26. Corr P, Abdool Carrim AT, Robbs J: Colour-flow ultrasound in the detection of penetrating vascular injuries of the neck. S Afr Med J 89:644–646, 1999.
27. Demetriades D, Theodorou D, Cornwell E 3rd, et al: Penetrating injuries of the neck in patients in stable condition: physical examination, angiography, or color flow Doppler imaging. Arch Surg 130:971–975, 1995.
28. Mandavia DP, Qualls S, Rokos I: Emergency airway management in penetrating neck injury. Ann Emerg Med 35:221–225, 2000.

Chapter 19

Upper Extremity Trauma

Michael D. Burg, MD and Sieuwert-Jan C. ten Napel, MD

Key Points

Pediatric upper extremity trauma is extremely common and therefore a major source of morbidity.

Determining the need for radiographs in an acutely injured child is often difficult.

Radiographs comparing the injured arm to the uninjured arm are not routinely indicated.

Injuries may be produced by a single major trauma or accident, repeated minor trauma, nonaccidental trauma, or physiologic stress on a pathologic site.

Recognizing activity-injury patterns and the ages at which these injuries tend to occur may allow for the identification of subtle fractures and fracture-dislocations.

Selected Diagnoses

Shoulder Injuries
    Clavicular Fractures
    Acromioclavicular Separation
    Shoulder Dislocation
    Shoulder Injuries in the Child Athlete
    Upper Arm and Elbow Injuries
    Humeral Fractures
    Radial Head Subluxation
    Elbow Fractures
    Elbow Dislocation
    Elbow Injuries in the Child Athlete
Forearm Injuries
    Forearm Fractures
    Monteggia Fracture-Dislocation
    Galeazzi Fracture-Dislocation
    Greenstick Fractures
Wrist and Hand Injuries
    Wrist Fractures
    Hand Fractures
    Nail Bed Injuries

Discussion of Individual Diagnoses

Shoulder Injuries

Clavicular Fractures

In children, the clavicle is the most commonly broken bone in the shoulder region, accounting for 8% to 15% of all fractures in this population.[1,2] The clavicle may be injured during delivery (0.4% to 1.5% of all newborns), and accounts for nearly 90% of all obstetric fractures. Clavicle fractures in newborns are associated with shoulder dystocia, increased birth weight, and increased gestational age.[3,4] Clavicular fractures are classified by anatomic location: medial third, middle third, and distal third.[5] The middle third is the most frequently fractured, accounting for 80% of all clavicular fractures; most of them are nondisplaced.[2] Distal third fractures range from 15% in incidence.[2,6] Medial third fractures are relatively uncommon, accounting for 5% of all clavicle fractures in children and adolescents.[2] A fall on the shoulder is the most common injury mechanism. Others include a direct blow to the clavicle and a fall on an outstretched hand, the latter being a relatively uncommon cause.[7] Clavicle fractures also occur in multitrauma patients, in whom the injury is often a minor problem.[8]

A child with a broken clavicle will characteristically present supporting the elbow on the affected side with the contralateral hand. Often the head will be turned toward the fracture in order to relax the sternocleidomastoid muscle. Spasm of the sternocleidomastoid or trapezius muscle may lift the proximal fragment superiorly.[9,10] A visible and palpable deformity can be found along with variable degrees of tenderness. The skin overlying the fracture may be tented, and limited shoulder motion may be seen.[10] Assessment of distal neurovascular status is an important part of the evaluation. Plain radiographs are usually sufficient for diagnosis and management.[10] Ultrasound can be used to detect clavicle fractures in newborns.[11]

Most clavicular fractures are treated conservatively. A sling to support the elbow and forearm and pain medication are generally all that is required. A randomized controlled trial found that slings caused less discomfort and possibly fewer complications than treatment with a figure-of-eight bandage. The functional and cosmetic results were identical.[12] No statistically significant difference was found in the speed of recovery between these two conservative therapies.[13] The sling should be used during waking hours for at least 2 weeks, and longer in children older than 12 years. Parents should be advised about callus formation and resultant deformity, which can be visible for up to a year.[10] Clavicle fractures in children seldom require operative management. A study of 939 clavicular fractures reported a 1.6% operative rate. Operative indications included open fractures, soft tissue impingement, skin perforation potential, severe shortening of the shoulder girdle with or without displaced intermediate fragments, and displaced fractures with potential risk to the neurovascular bundle or mediastinal structures.[14] In another study, 2 of 26 children with distal clavicle fractures underwent operation; all others were treated conservatively with good results.[6] Excellent results were found in all of 25 children with conservative treatment of lateral clavicle fractures.[15]

Acromioclavicular Separation

True acromioclavicular separations in young children are rare. A fall on the point of the shoulder usually results in an acromioclavicular separation in the adult or older adolescent, but in children results in fractures through the physis or metaphysis.[10] Because distal clavicular epiphyseal ossification does not occur until the age of 18 or 19 years, fractures in this area appear as acromioclavicular dislocations or pseudodislocations.[16,17] Superior displacement of the lateral clavicle occurs due to a tear in the thick periosteal tube surrounding the distal clavicle. The lateral clavicular epiphysis, along with the acromioclavicular and coracoclavicular ligaments, usually remains intact.[10,17] Injury mechanisms include birth trauma, child abuse, falls, and motor vehicle crashes. Children will present with pain or tender-ness over the acromioclavicular region.[17] Nondisplaced to moderately displaced fractures require symptomatic treatment with a sling. Operative stabilization is required in injuries with marked displacement of the fracture fragments.[10,16-18]

Shoulder Dislocation

Limited recent literature exists concerning the incidence and presentation of shoulder dislocations in children. Optimal reduction techniques are also not well studied, so standard adult techniques are generally used. A 5-year survey study found a 4.2% incidence of primary anterior dislocation in children ages 12 to 17 years.[19] Anterior dislocations in children less than 10 years of age are uncommon.[20] Recent literature does address the incidence of re-dislocation after a primary dislocation in adolescents. The recurrence rates after primary dislocation range from 72% to 86% for teens.[19,21] Fewer re-dislocations were found in younger patients in two studies,[19,21] and it was hypothesized that this may be due to greater shoulder capsule elasticity in younger patients.[19] This finding contradicts that of a study reporting a 100% recurrence rate in 21 children with open physes.[22] Another study found that the type and duration of immobilization technique had no effect on re-dislocation rate.[23] The high incidence of re-dislocation or shoulder instability makes orthopedic follow-up after treatment in the emergency department prudent.

Shoulder Injuries in the Child Athlete

An ever-increasing number of children participate in organized sports and recreational programs. Over one third of young athletes will sustain injuries requiring medical attention.[24] Acute shoulder injuries are commonly seen in football, bicycling, snowboarding, skiing, wrestling, and baseball.[10] Injuries can also occur due to repetitive stress and are common in swimmers, gymnasts, cheerleaders, and baseball players (see Chapter 98, Overuse Syndromes and Inflammatory Conditions).[25]

One overuse injury in children is "little leaguer's shoulder." It represents a stress fracture of the proximal humerus growth plate.[25] The patient with this injury will complain of pain during throwing localized to the proximal humerus. On physical examination, tenderness to palpation over the proximal or lateral aspect of the humerus is found.[26] This condition is mostly seen between 11 and 13 years of age and can be treated with rest.[10] Ninety-one percent of those with little leaguer's shoulder were asymptomatic while playing baseball after a 3-month rest period.[26]

Upper Arm and Elbow Injuries

Humeral Fractures

PROXIMAL HUMERAL FRACTURES

Proximal humeral epiphyseal fractures are rare and occur more in adolescents than younger children.[27] If they occur, therapy is primarily conservative.[28,29] Patients present with shoulder swelling and pain, especially when moving the shoulder joint. A neurovascular examination is an important part of the evaluation, as are anteroposterior and lateral radiographs.[20,30,31] Nonoperative treatment is appropriate in almost all cases, even with severely displaced fractures, and consists of a hanging cast or simple sling.[27] The magnitude of displacement alone does not justify operative management.[32] Proximal humeral fractures have excellent remodeling capacity.[32,33] Open fractures, those causing neurovascular compromise, pathologic fractures in juvenile bone cysts, and displaced fractures of the articular surface are operative indications.[28,31,33]

HUMERAL SHAFT FRACTURES

Humeral shaft fractures comprise a small percentage of all fractures in children, with an increased incidence in adolescence.[34] Therapy is mainly conservative, and generally only angulations greater than 10 degrees need surgical stabilization, the preferred method being elastic-stable intramedullary nailing.[28] Humeral fractures can cause radial nerve palsy. Most have a good prognosis, and expectant management is advocated.[35,36] Impaired brachioradialis muscle functioning, wrist extension, and finger and thumb extension are seen with radial nerve injury.[35] Of 222 diaphyseal fractures in children, 8 patients had radial nerve palsy and 1 patient had ulnar nerve palsy; all were transitory.[36] The clinician must be alert to the possibility of child abuse in toddlers with humeral shaft fractures. Midshaft or metaphyseal humeral fractures were found to be a marker for abuse in those under 3 years of age.[37] A study in a similar population classified 18% of humeral shaft fractures as probably due to abuse but cautioned that neither fracture pattern nor age is diagnostic of abuse.[38]

SUPRACONDYLAR FRACTURES

The supracondylar humerus fracture is the most common elbow fracture in children, accounting for more than half of all pediatric elbow fractures[39,40] and 3% to 18% of all fractures seen in children.[1,34] Diagnosis of these fractures can be challenging, and, if missed or improperly treated, vascular, neurologic, and structural complications can occur. A fall on an outstretched hand with elbow extension is the main cause (70% to 90%) of these fractures.[41,42] The majority of supracondylar fractures occur in the first decade of life, with a peak incidence between ages 4 and 7 years.[34,39,42] The nondominant arm is more often injured than the dominant arm.[34,39,40,42] In children, ligamentous strength exceeds bone strength. When falling with the hand outstretched and the elbow extended, the collateral ligaments of the elbow prevent hyperextension at the joint space and the olecranon transmits the longitudinal force to the supracondylar region, which fractures.[41] These extension-type injuries account for almost all supracondylar fractures.[43] Extension-type supracondylar fractures are divided into three types based on displacement: type I, minimal or none; type II, partially intact posterior cortex with angulation but without complete displacement; and type III, completely displaced.[44] Flexion-type fractures are caused by a direct fall on the elbow with impact on the olecranon, resulting in a posterior cortical disruption and anterior displacement or angulation.[41,43]

Children with supracondylar fractures will complain of arm or elbow pain. They often hold the injured arm in an extended, pronated position. The elbow will be swollen and resistant to movement. The distal humerus will be focally tender.[41] Assessment and documentation of distal neurovascular status is critically important. The reported incidence of specific nerve injury varies widely.[41,45] The median nerve is most commonly injured (28% to 60%), with the anterior interosseous branch most commonly involved (80%). The radial nerve is involved in 26% to 61% of cases and the ulnar nerve in 11% to 15%.[45-47] Anterior interosseous nerve impairment results in mild weakness of forearm supination, of the flexor digitorum profundus to the index finger, and of the flexor pollicis longus. Nerve function is assessed by asking the patient to make an "OK" sign and testing this for strength.[41] Complete radial, median, and ulnar nerve functional testing are important, although this may be difficult in a child in pain. Type III fractures are those most often associated with neurovascular damage.[40,45-48] Vascular status is assessed by checking capillary refill, color, distal pulses, and skin temperature. The uninjured arm may serve as a control. A Doppler ultrasound device is used if the pulses are faint or nonpalpable. Vascular compromise is most often due to a brachial artery injury,[49] and immediate orthopedic consultation is warranted. If neurovascular compromise exists, the initial treatment is immediate reduction. If an orthopedist is not readily available, the emergency physician should perform the reduction.[41] If the radial pulse is not palpable while the hand stays well perfused, no consensus exists on optimal treatment. A strategy of closed reduction and internal fixation followed by close observation and neurovascular checks is advocated by some.[49,50] Others recommend a more aggressive approach: immediate surgical exploration.[51-53]

Radiographs of the elbow are obtained to confirm the diagnosis and estimate the degree of distraction and angulation. On a properly obtained, normal lateral radiograph, a line drawn down the anterior cortical margin of the humerus should intersect the middle third of the capitellum (Fig. 19–1). With extension-type fractures, the anterior humeral line will pass anterior to this area, and with flexion-type injuries

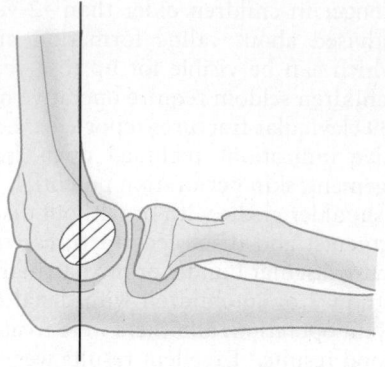

FIGURE 19–1. Radiographic line that is demonstrated on a lateral radiograph of the elbow. The anterior humeral line is drawn down the outer edge of the anterior cortex of the distal end of the humerus. As the line is drawn distally through the capitellum, it should pass through the middle of the capitellum. (From Green NE, Swiontkowski MF [eds]: Skeletal Trauma in Children, 3rd ed. Philadelphia: WB Saunders, 2003.)

the line will pass posteriorly. A line drawn along the midshaft of the proximal radius should intersect the capitellum in all radiographic views.[41] The significance of a positive posterior "fat pad sign" is uncertain. Only 9 of 54 children with joint effusions and no identifiable fracture immediately after elbow trauma ultimately had evidence of a healing fracture.[54] In a prospective study limited to children, the presence of a posterior fat pad was predictive of fracture in 76% of patients.[55] It seems prudent to continue to treat children with elbow trauma and posterior fat pad signs as though they have occult supracondylar fractures (Fig. 19–2). A comparison of radiography of traumatized elbows with magnetic resonance imaging (MRI) concluded that a less severe spectrum of injury occurred in children with normal findings on radiographs versus those with an effusion.[56] Studies show that comparison views of the uninjured elbow in children with a spectrum of injuries do not improve diagnostic accuracy and are unnecessary.[57,58]

Type I fractures are typically treated with a long arm posterior splint for 3 weeks with the elbow flexed to 90 degrees and the forearm in a neutral position. The most likely pitfall associated with type I fractures is missing the diagnosis.[41] Treatment of type II and III fractures depends on the degree of displacement and fracture stability. Definitive therapy includes closed reduction and internal fixation.[48] The distal neurovascular status of patients with supracondylar fractures must be reassessed in a timely fashion. For type I fractures this can be done on an outpatient basis, but for type II and III fractures, hospitalization is recommended.[41] Most nerve injuries due to supracondylar fractures are neurapraxias. Motor deficits typically resolve over 7 to 12 weeks; sensory recovery can take as long as 6 months.[46,59] A feared complication described after vascular injury is compartment syndrome (see Chapter 22, Compartment Syndrome). Untreated compartment syndrome may lead to Volkmann's ischemic contracture which is characterized by fixed elbow flexion, forearm pronation, wrist flexion, metacarpophalangeal joint extension, and interphalangeal joint flexion.[48] Immobilizing the elbow in a position more flexed than 90 degrees can lead to increased pressure in the antecubital region and increase the risk of compartment syndrome.[60] Inadequately reduced or stabilized fractures may heal with a varus deformity.[48,61]

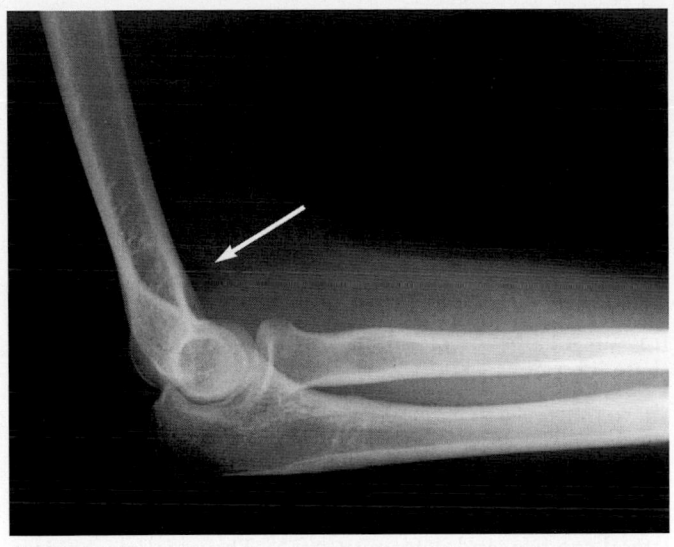

A

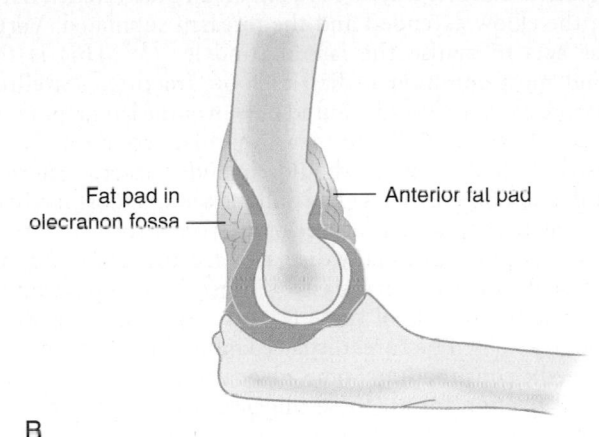

Fat pad in olecranon fossa — — Anterior fat pad

B

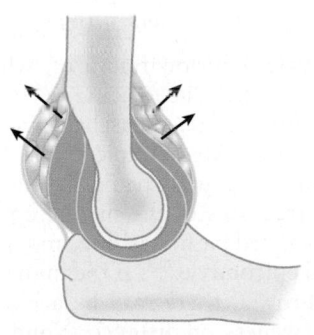

C

FIGURE 19–2. A, Anterior "fat pad sign" on lateral study *(white arrow).* **B,** The anterior fat pad is normally a thin radiolucent stripe, and the posterior fat pad is not seen. **C,** An effusion displaces both fat pads. This posterior fat pad is now visible. (From Marx JA, Hockberger RS, Walls RM, et al [eds]: Rosen's Emergency Medicine: Concepts and Clinical Practice, 5th ed. St. Louis: Mosby, 2002.)

Radial Head Subluxation

Radial head subluxation is also known as pulled elbow or nursemaid's elbow. Most radial head subluxations occur in children 1 to 3 years of age. The presumed pathophysiology of this injury is entrapment of the immature radial head

distal to the annular ligament that occurs during longitudinal traction on the arm.[62,63] This often happens when a child sinks toward the ground while being held at the wrist. However, in approximately 50% of cases, a "pull" mechanism of injury is not elucidated.[64] Parents or other caregivers are occasionally unable or unwilling to provide an accurate history either because they did not witness the injury or because they are afraid of being considered abusive. Simple observation will generally reveal a nondistressed child with the affected arm held immobile at the side, in minimal flexion at the elbow and pronation at the wrist. No deformity will be seen. The child will generally cry out if the elbow is moved or if pressure is placed on the radial head. Local swelling is uncommon. The remainder of the physical examination will be unremarkable. When the history and physical examination findings are consistent with radial head subluxation, radiographs are not required to confirm the diagnosis.[65] However, many physicians do order radiographs in children with arm injuries when the history is unclear or when the physical examination suggests an alternative diagnosis.[66]

Classically, reduction of a radial head subluxation is performed by supinating the patient's wrist and flexing the elbow while palpating the radial head.[67] A click over the radial head generally signifies successful reduction. Children less than 2 years of age may have a slower return to normal functioning.[68] Two relatively recent papers describe a hyperpronation method of reduction for radial head subluxations.[63,69] In this method, hyperpronation of the forearm is followed by elbow flexion. Both studies found hyperpronation to be superior to supination, with success rates of 80% versus 69% in one study[69] and 95% versus 77%[63] on first attempts. A trend toward less pain with the hyperpronation technique was reported in one study.[69] After a reduction attempt, the child is expected to begin using the injured arm, generally within 15 minutes. If this does not occur, there are three main possibilities: unsuccessful reduction, alternative diagnosis (fracture), or slow resolution. Second and even third attempts at reduction are completely acceptable. Fractures about the elbow and at more distant sites (especially the clavicle) should be considered as well. Children under the age of 2 years may take longer to begin using their injured arm even after successful reduction.[68] Immobilization with a collar and cuff or sling is a classic, non–evidence-based recommendation, but is impractical given the ages of children affected by this process and its benign course. No immobilization is needed. Parents should be cautioned not to pull on the child's arms. Analgesics are infrequently needed after reduction.

Elbow Fractures

The elbow consists of a complex series of three unions, the radiocapitellar and radioulnar articulations and the articulation of the distal humerus with the olecranon fossa of the ulna.[70,71] A large variety of elbow fractures have been described. Three of the more common periarticular elbow fractures are described in this section. Complicating the evaluation of the child with an elbow fracture is the fact that six ossification centers exist around the joint (Fig. 19–3). Knowing the location of the ossification centers and the age at which each appears is important when evaluating children with elbow trauma. The mnemonic CRMTOL (*C*ome *R*ead *M*y *T*ale *O*f *L*ove), standing for *c*apitellum, *r*adial head, *m*edial

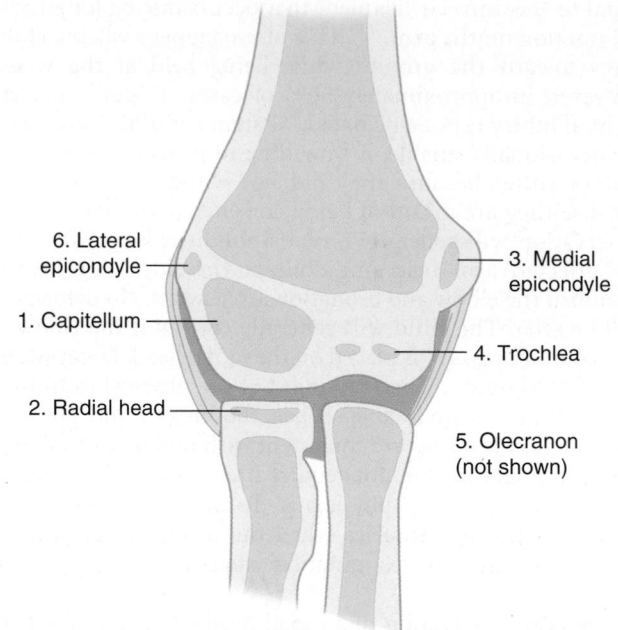

6. Lateral epicondyle

1. Capitellum

2. Radial head

3. Medial epicondyle

4. Trochlea

5. Olecranon (not shown)

FIGURE 19–3. The six ossification centers of the elbow: 1, capitellum; 2, radial head; 3, medial epicondyle; 4, trochlea; 5, olecranon (not shown); and 6, lateral epicondyle. (From Connolly JF [ed]: DePalma's The Management of Fractures and Dislocations: An Atlas. Philadelphia: WB Saunders, 1981.)

epicondyle, *t*rochlea, *o*lecranon, and *l*ateral epicondyle, can be used to recall the names of the ossification centers. The age in years at which each appears is variably quoted as: capitellum, 1 to 2; radial head, 4 to 5; medial epicondyle, 4 to 7; trochlea, 8 to 10; olecranon, 8 to 10; and lateral epicondyle, 10 to 11.[70-73] Ossification of these centers in boys tends to lag that in girls by about 1 year.[70]

The literature does not support the routine use of comparison radiographs of the contralateral, uninjured elbow to improve diagnostic accuracy.[57,58] However, in selected cases, comparison views may be helpful. In the case of a diagnostic dilemma, additional radiographs or alternate imaging techniques (computed tomography, MRI, bone scan, others) may be helpful. At least one study of children with elbow trauma demonstrated that MRI detected a wide spectrum of injuries not apparent on plain radiographs. However, this same study found that the additional sensitivity of MRI did little to alter treatment.[56] For the child with a worrisome mechanism of injury and physical examination, but with normal radiographs, a reasonable plan is to immobilize the elbow in a splint, prescribe analgesia, and arrange follow-up with an orthopedist.[74]

RADIAL HEAD AND NECK FRACTURES

These injuries constitute approximately 5% to 15% of all pediatric elbow fractures, and their optimal treatment is an area of active controversy.[75,76] Generally these fractures occur due to a fall on an outstretched hand.[75] Nine and one-half years is the mean age for radial neck fractures; 13 years is the mean age for radial head fractures.[75,76] Boys and girls are at equal risk.[75] The child with this injury usually holds the elbow slightly flexed. Flexion-extension, pronation-supination, and radial head palpation cause pain. There is no consensus among orthopedists regarding classification of these injuries. Even the terms *radial head* and *radial neck* are often used interchangeably in the literature. Additionally, identifying which injuries should be treated with closed reduction versus percutaneous versus open reduction is murky. Finally, definitive studies assessing functional outcomes, range of motion, and complications among the treatment options are lacking. Minimally displaced fractures can be treated with long arm immobilization with the elbow flexed to 90 degrees.[75] Orthopedic consultation is required for all other fractures involving the radial head and neck. Up to half of these patients will have other associated elbow fractures; elbow or radial head dislocation may accompany these injuries as well.[75]

FRACTURES OF THE LATERAL EPICONDYLE

This injury is difficult to diagnose and is fraught with a variety of complications including nonunion, malunion, late stiffness, late ulnar nerve palsy, avascular necrosis of the lateral condyle, and deformity.[71,72,77,78] The usual mechanism for a lateral condyle fracture is a fall on an outstretched hand with the elbow extended and the forearm supinated. Varus stress acts to avulse the lateral condyle.[71,72,77] This is the second most common pediatric elbow fracture.[72] Swelling and tenderness are usually found only over the lateral portion of the elbow, and acute neurovascular compromise is unusual.[72] Radiographs should include anteroposterior, lateral, and oblique views. The oblique view is most likely to show the injury and true degree of fracture displacement.[71,72] Nondisplaced or minimally displaced fractures (0 to 2 mm) are treated with a long arm cast.[71,72] Close follow-up is important since up to 10% of these fractures may displace while immobilized.[77,78] Fractures displaced more than 2 mm require orthopedic consultation. Some advocate open reduction and internal fixation for all these injuries, while some perform closed reduction and pinning for fractures displaced 2 to 4 mm and open procedures for more widely displaced fractures.[71,72,79]

FRACTURES OF THE MEDIAL EPICONDYLE

Medial epicondyle avulsion fractures, which occur at the growth plate, can occur due to acute or chronic valgus stress on the elbow. Throwers (e.g., baseball pitchers) are prone to this type of injury.[80] Medial epicondyle fractures are also commonly seen along with pediatric elbow dislocations.[81] Children with fractures of the medial epicondyle typically present with localized pain, swelling, and tenderness directly over the medial epicondyle.[70,80] If the injury is due to chronic overuse in a thrower, there may be a history of decreased throwing effectiveness or distance. Nondisplaced fractures are treated with a short period of immobilization and pain relief.[80] Those children with displaced fractures should be referred to an orthopedist for consideration of operative repair.[70,80,82] Controversy exists over operative indications in isolated, displaced medial humeral epicondyle fractures. One retrospective study found similar functional outcomes in nonsurgical versus surgical management of this injury.[83] Fracture fragments within the joint space require emergent extrication and fixation.[80,84]

Elbow Dislocation

This is an uncommon injury in children, with the peak incidence during the early teen years.[10,86] Contact sports and falls account for most of these injuries. Most dislocations are posterior and closed, but a wide spectrum of dislocation patterns has been described[10,81] (Fig. 19–4). A variety of associated fractures are seen with elbow dislocations.[81,85] Injuries to the median, ulnar, and radial nerves have been described, as well as vascular injuries. Nerve entrapment or a fracture fragment within the ulnohumeral joint mandates immediate surgery.[86] If elbow reduction attempts are unsuccessful, an entrapped fracture fragment or interposed soft tissue should be suspected.[10]

Elbow Injuries in the Child Athlete

Over 30 million children in the United States participate in organized sports. The incidence of upper extremity injury is second only to ankle and knee injuries in the child athlete.[87] Although a wide variety of acute elbow injuries can be sustained by the child athlete, one chronic overuse injury seen by emergency physicians is "little leaguer's elbow." The repetitive valgus stress induced by throwing or similar motions produces osseous damage of the elbow. While little leaguer's elbow was originally described in baseball pitchers, it is also seen in nonpitching baseball players, racquet sport players, football players, and others.[10] Most with this condition will complain of medial elbow pain. When questioned, the athlete with little leaguer's elbow will also report decreased throwing effectiveness or distance.[10,88] Radiographs may reveal hypertrophy or separation of the medial humeral condyle.[89] The optimal "treatment" is prevention, through a combination of rest, proper throwing mechanics, and avoidance of overexertion. Once little leaguer's elbow develops, rest—until there is complete resolution of pain—is important. When activity resumes, proper throwing mechanics are key to preventing recurrence.[90]

Forearm Injuries

Forearm Fractures

Distal forearm fractures occur most commonly at the time of the pubertal growth spurt in early adolescence. This is

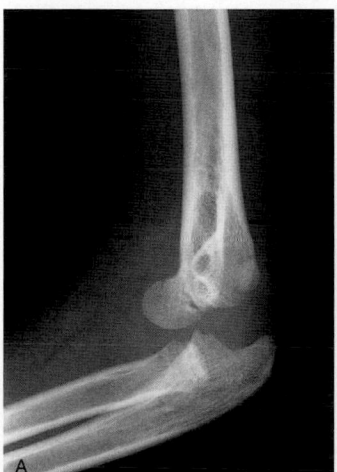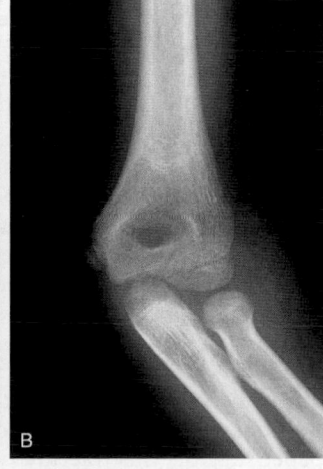

FIGURE 19–4. Posterior dislocation of the elbow. **A,** Lateral radiograph of the elbow. The ulna and radius are displaced posteriorly. **B,** Anteroposterior radiograph of the posterior dislocation of the elbow. (From Green NE, Swiontkowski MF [eds]: Skeletal Trauma in Children, 3rd ed. Philadelphia: WB Saunders, 2003.)

likely due to increased physical activity that occurs at this time of life and decreased bone strength due to enhanced bone turnover.[91] Most of these fractures occur due to a fall on an outstretched hand, although direct local trauma can produce them as well.[92] Acceptable pronation, supination, and cosmesis are the main treatment outcomes of interest.[92] Outcomes are largely dependent on fracture angulation at the time of fracture healing. Fracture angulation, in turn, depends on the quality and maintenance of the initial reduction.[93] Most pediatric forearm fractures can be successfully treated with a combination of reduction and immobilization. There is controversy regarding the treatment of completely displaced metaphyseal fractures of the distal radius. Since up to 21% of distal radius fractures displace after successful reduction,[94] some have suggested the use of percutaneous Kirschner wires to maintain reduction.[95]

For diaphyseal forearm fractures, failure of closed reduction is the most common surgical indication. Adolescents with these injuries are generally treated with internal fixation and early mobilization like adults with these injuries.[96] During the physical examination of these children, particular attention paid to the wrist and elbow will make missing a Monteggia or Galeazzi fracture-dislocation less likely.[97] Most nerve injuries resulting from forearm fractures are neuropraxias that typically resolve within several weeks without specific intervention.

Monteggia Fracture-Dislocation

Isolated ulna fractures in children are uncommon.[97] A Monteggia fracture-dislocation is an ulnar fracture in association with a radial head dislocation.[98] Four primary Monteggia-type injuries have been described, with the type dependent upon the fracture location and the direction of ulnar dislocation.[99] It is well established that Monteggia fracture-dislocations are misdiagnosed by both emergency physicians and radiologists.[99] The injury generally results from a fall on an outstretched hand. Boys more commonly sustain this injury, and the average age is approximately 7 years with a wide range.[100] The wrist and elbow must be carefully examined for fractures and dislocations. Patients with an isolated ulna fracture and radial head tenderness may have spontaneously reduced their dislocation. Neurologic deficits may be found in up to 17% of patients. They are generally neurapraxias and resolve over weeks to months.[100] If a Monteggia fracture-dislocation is suspected, radiographs of the wrist and elbow (in addition to the forearm) are indicated. To avoid missing this injury, it is essential to recognize that in normal radiographs, the midshaft of the proximal radius points at the capitellum in all views.[100] Closed reduction of both components of the fracture-dislocation and immobilization are used to treat most of these injuries. Open reduction may be required in the case of an otherwise irreducible radial head or an unstable ulna fracture.[99]

Galeazzi Fracture-Dislocation

The Galeazzi fracture-dislocation is an uncommon but important injury in children.[101] The Galeazzi fracture-dislocation is a radial shaft fracture in association with a distal radioulnar joint dislocation.[101] The injury is usually caused by a fall on an outstretched hand with the forearm in pronation. Careful examination of the wrist is helpful in avoiding missing this injury.[101] Children with a Galeazzi fracture dislocation will not be able to fully promote and supinate their forearms. Treatment involves closed reduction and immobilization.[101-103]

Greenstick Fractures

This fracture type involves a break in one bony cortex and compression of the bony cortex opposite the fracture site. In one large series of over 3300 pediatric patients with upper extremity fractures, greenstick fractures occurred in just over 5% of patients.[104] However, another large study found a nearly 52% incidence of greenstick fractures.[105] Subject selection for these studies likely explains this discrepancy. The decision to reduce these fractures generally depends on the amount of angulation present. If reduction is required, the angulation is overcorrected toward the cortical break, in essence completing the fracture so as to prevent persistent angulation and resultant deformity. A splint is then applied.

Wrist and Hand Injuries

Wrist Fractures

DISTAL RADIUS FRACTURES

These injuries are common in children and generally result from a fall onto an outstretched hand.[105] The most common type of distal radius fracture is the buckle fracture (also known as a torous fracture).[106-109] These minor fractures tend to do very well with a removable splint that can be worn for three to four weeks.[106-108] These fractures seldom have complications and can be managed by either primary care physicians or orthopedists. In more severe injuries, there may be a distal "both bones" fracture involving both the radius and ulna. Local tenderness and swelling are invariably present, but may be somewhat subtle. If angulated or displaced, these fractures typically require closed reduction that can be performed by the emergency physician or an orthopedist. There is no universally accepted degree of residual angulation after reduction and local standards tend to guide the acceptance of a reduction attempt. Younger children have greater degrees of acceptable residual angulation.[110] This is due to a greater capacity for remodeling in younger children. For very distal injuries that may involve the growth plate, orthopedic follow-up is prudent.[111] In general, children with distal radius fractures do well. Resultant traumatic arthritis is rare.[112]

CARPAL INJURIES

Pediatric carpal fractures are uncommon. This may be because the carpus is largely unossified throughout much of early childhood. Adolescents, whose carpal bones are nearly completely ossified, have adult-type injury patterns.[113] The scaphoid is the most commonly fractured carpal bone in children, as it is in adults, although the patterns of injury are different.[113] More are located distally, they more often involve a single cortex, and they are more often nondisplaced.[114] The peak incidence of scaphoid fractures occurs at age 12 years.[113] Radiographs done in the emergency department may easily miss scaphoid fractures. MRI is far more sensitive for fracture detection in this region.[115] However, no study has examined the benefit of early detection of scaphoid injuries, so long as they are suspected, immobilized in a thumb spica splint, and referred for follow-up. Scaphoid fractures have

been reported in association with distal radius fractures.[116] Tenderness in the anatomic snuffbox or scaphoid compression pain should cause the treating physician to consider a scaphoid fracture and treat for same. A wide variety of carpal fractures and dislocations have been described in children, all in small case series. Care is therefore individualized.

Hand Fractures

Hand injuries are common in children of all ages, and fractures make up 15% to 19% of all hand injuries.[117-119] Fracture incidence has a bimodal distribution, with distal phalanx injuries predominating at age 1 year and other phalangeal and metacarpal injuries peaking at age 12 years.[120,121] Most pediatric hand fractures heal uneventfully.[122] Open fractures, those involving articular surfaces, comminuted fractures, and markedly displaced and angulated fractures mandate the timely involvement of a hand surgeon or orthopedist experienced in caring for head injuries.

METACARPAL FRACTURES

The shaft is the most commonly fractured metacarpal region in children; however, articular and periarticular fractures do occur.[120,122] A volar angulated fracture involving the neck of the fourth or fifth metacarpal (i.e., a boxer's fracture) often occurs when a hard surface is punched. Evidence to guide the optimal treatment of these injuries is scant. Depending on community standards and degree of angulation, these fractures can be reduced[120] or left in place and the digit either buddy taped or placed in an ulnar gutter splint. Rotational deformity of the affected digit needs to be identified since healing and regrowth will not correct this abnormality. To check for rotational deformity, the patient should be asked to fully flex all the digits. In full flexion, all digit tips should point evenly at the thenar eminence. Overlap, indicating rotation, should prompt consultation with a hand surgeon. Similarly, fractures at the base of the thumb metacarpal require hand surgeon consultation.[120,123]

PROXIMAL PHALANX FRACTURES

Many of these fractures in children are articular or periarticular.[120,123] Radiographs including posteroanterior, lateral, and oblique views are helpful to avoid missing subtle injuries.[120] A common injury pattern is the Salter type II fracture at the phalangeal base[123] (see Fig. 20–2). If it involves the little finger, the digit is usually abducted and extended. Reduction is performed by using a pencil in the fourth web space to lever the fracture back into place. Reduction is maintained by buddy taping.[120,123] Fractures at the base of the thumb's proximal phalanx are often Salter type III fractures and can be considered the childhood equivalent of ulnar collateral ligament rupture (i.e., gamekeeper's or skier's thumb). Although experts are not in perfect agreement on treatment, in general, minimally displaced fractures can be immobilized without reduction. Displaced fractures require reduction and internal fixation.[120,123]

Distal periarticular or articular fractures can be easily overlooked. The mechanism of injury may be a tip-off. One paper suggests this fracture type occurs when a child's digit is closed in a car door and forcibly extracted. It further states that the fracture fragment may be purely cartilaginous, making radiographic visualization of it difficult.[120] Another suggests that oblique radiographs may be particularly helpful in diagnosing these injuries.[123] In any event, displaced distal fractures involving the articular surface must be reduced and internally fixed.[120,123]

MIDDLE PHALANX FRACTURES

Many of these fractures are similar to those seen in the proximal phalanges 2 through 5.[120] Nondisplaced articular fractures are treated with buddy taping. Fractures displaced more than 2 mm require reduction and internal fixation.[120,123]

DISTAL PHALANX FRACTURES

Many of these involve crush injury to the fingertip, nail, and nail bed and vary widely in severity.[120,123-125] As one would expect, outcome and degree of initial injury are correlated.[124] Traditionally, open crush injuries are treated with antibiotics to reduce the risk of osteomyelitis,[120] although this is not an evidence-based recommendation. A prescription for oral antibiotics is probably adequate. Mallet finger–type fractures are generally treated with closed reduction and immobilization in slight hyperextension.[123]

Nail Bed Injuries

For subungual hematomas larger than 25%, nail removal and nail bed repair is often advocated. However, a 1999 study has called this recommendation into question.[125] It found that, in children with an intact nail and nail margin and a subungual hematoma, trephination versus nail bed repair produced similarly excellent results (see Chapter 173, Management of Digit Injuries and Infections).

REFERENCES

*1. Landin LA: Epidemiology of children's fractures. J Pediatr Orthop B 6.79–83, 1997.
2. Nordqvist A, Petersson C: The incidence of fractures of the clavicle. Clin Orthop 300:127–132, 1994.
3. Many A, Brenner SH, Yaron Y, et al: Prospective study of incidence and predisposing factors for clavicular fracture in newborn. Acta Obstet Gynecol Scand 75:378–381, 1996.
4. Roberts SW, Hernandez C, Maberry MC, et al: Obstetric clavicular fracture: the enigma of normal birth. Obstet Gynecol 86:978–981, 1995.
5. Post M: Current concepts in the treatment of fractures of the clavicle. Clin Orthop 245:89–101, 1989.
6. Wilfinger C, Hollwarth M: Lateral clavicular fractures in children and adolescents. Unfallchirurgie 105:602–605, 2002.
7. Stanley D, Trowbridge EA, Norris SH: The mechanism of clavicular fractures: a clinical and biomechanical analysis. J Bone Joint Surg Br 70:461–464, 1988.
8. Rozycki GS, Tremblay L, Feliciano DV, et al: A prospective study for the detection of vascular injury in adult and pediatric patients with cervicothoracic seat belt signs. J Trauma 52:618–623, 2002.
9. Goddard NJ, Stabler J, Albert JS: Atlanto-axial rotatory fixation and fracture of the clavicle: an association and classification. J Bone Joint Surg Br 72:72–75, 1990.
*10. Kocher MS, Waters PM, Micheli LJ: Upper extremity injuries in the paediatric athlete. Sports Med 30:117–135, 2000.
11. Blab E, Geissler W, Rokitansky A: Sonographic management of infantile clavicular fractures. Pediatr Surg Int 15:251–254, 1999.
12. Andersen K, Jensen PO, Lauritzen J: Treatment of clavicular fractures: figure-of-eight bandage versus a simple sling. Acta Orthop Scand 58:71–74, 1987.
13. Stanley D, Norris SH: Recovery following fractures of the clavicle treated conservatively. Injury 19:162–164, 1988.
14. Kubiak R, Slongo T: Operative treatment of clavicle fractures in children: a review of 21 years. J Pediatr Orthop 22:736–739, 2002.
15. Nordqvist A, Petersson C, Redlund-Johnell I: The natural course of lateral clavicle fracture: 15 (11–21) year follow-up of 110 cases. Acta Orthop Scand 64:87–91, 1993.
16. Black GB, McPherson JA, Reed MH: Traumatic pseudodislocation of the acromioclavicular joint in children: a fifteen year review. Am J Sports Med 19:644–646, 1991.
17. Ogden JA: Distal clavicular physeal injury. Clin Orthop 188:68–73, 1984.
18. Havranek P: Injuries of distal clavicular physis in children. J Pediatr Orthop 9:213–215, 1989.
19. Postacchini F, Gumina S, Cinotti G: Anterior shoulder dislocation in adolescents. J Shoulder Elbow Surg 9:470–474, 2000.
20. Obremskey W, Routt ML: Fracture-dislocation of the shoulder in a child: case report. J Trauma 36:137–140, 1994.
21. Deitch J, Mehlman CT, Foad SL, et al: Traumatic anterior shoulder dislocation in adolescents. Am J Sports Med 31:758–763, 2003.
*22. Marans HJ, Angel KR, Schemitsch EH, et al: The fate of traumatic anterior dislocation of the shoulder in children. J Bone Joint Surg Am 74:1242–1244, 1992.
23. Hovelius L, Augustini BG, Fredin H, et al: Primary anterior dislocation of the shoulder in young patients: a ten year prospective study. J Bone Joint Surg Am 78:1677–1684, 1996.
24. Adirim TA, Cheng TL: Overview of injuries in the young athlete. Sports Med 33:75–81, 2003.
25. Paterson PD, Waters PM: Shoulder injuries in the childhood athlete. Clin Sports Med 19:681–692, 2000.
26. Carson WG, Gasser SI: Little Leaguer's shoulder: a report of 23 cases. Am J Sports Med 26:575–580, 1998.
27. Larsen CF, Kiaer T, Lindequist S: Fractures of the proximal humerus in children: nine-year follow up of 64 unoperated on cases. Acta Orthop Scand 61:255–257, 1990.
28. Schmittenbecher PP, Blum J, David S, et al: The treatment of humeral shaft and subcapital fractures in children: consensus report of the child trauma section of the DGU. Unfallchirurgie 107:8–14, 2004.
29. Kohler R, Trillaud JM: Fracture and fracture separation of the proximal humerus in children: report of 136 cases. J Pediatr Orthop 3:326–332, 1983.
30. te Slaa RL, Nollen AJ: A Salter type 3 fracture of the proximal epiphysis of the humerus. Injury 18:429–431, 1987.
31. Gregg-Smith SJ, White SH: Salter-Harris III fracture-dislocation of the proximal humeral epiphysis. Injury 23:199–200, 1992.
32. Beringer DC, Weiner DS, Noble JS, et al: Severely displaced proximal humeral epiphyseal fractures: a follow-up study. J Pediatr Orthop 18:31–37, 1998.
33. Baxter MP, Wiley JJ: Fractures of the proximal humeral epiphysis: their influence on humeral growth. J Bone Joint Surg Br 68:570–573, 1986.
34. Cheng JC, Ng BK, Ying SY, et al: A 10-year study of the changes in the pattern and treatment of 6,493 fractures. J Pediatr Orthop 19:344–350, 1999.
35. Larsen LB, Barfred T: Radial nerve palsy after simple fracture of the humerus. Scand J Plast Reconstr Hand Surg 34:363–366, 2000.
36. Machan FG, Vinz H: Humeral shaft fracture in childhood. Unfallchirurgie 19:166–174, 1993.
37. Leventhal JM, Thomas SA, Rosenfield NS, et al: Fractures in young children: distinguishing child abuse from unintentional injuries. Am J Dis Child 147:87–92, 1993.
38. Shaw BA, Murphy KM, Shaw A, et al: Humerus shaft fractures in young children: accident or abuse? J Pediatr Orthop 17:293–297, 1997.
39. Landin LA, Danielsson LG: Elbow fractures in children: an epidemiological analysis of 589 cases. Acta Orthop Scand 57:309–312, 1986.
40. Houshian S, Mehdi B, Larsen MS: The epidemiology of elbow fractures in children: analysis of 355 fractures, with special reference to supracondylar humerus fractures. J Orthop Sci 6:312–315, 2001.
41. Wu J, Perron AD, Miller MD, et al: Orthopedic pitfalls in the ED: pediatric supracondylar humerus fractures. Am J Emerg Med 20:544–550, 2002.
42. Farnsworth CL, Silva PD, Mubarak SJ: Etiology of supracondylar humerus fractures. J Pediatr Orthop 18:38–42, 1998.
43. De Boeck H: Flexion-type supracondylar elbow fractures in children. J Pediatr Orthop 21:460–463, 2001.
44. Gartland JJ: Management of supracondylar fractures of the humerus in children. Surg Gynecol Obstet 109:145–154, 1959.

45. Lyons ST, Quinn M, Stanitski CL: Neurovascular injuries in type III humeral supracondylar fractures in children. Clin Orthop 376:62–67, 2000.

46. Brown IC, Zinar DM: Traumatic and iatrogenic neurological complications after supracondylar humerus fractures in children. J Pediatr Orthop 15:440–443, 1995.

47. Campbell CC, Waters PM, Emans JB, et al: Neurovascular injury and displacement in type III supracondylar humerus fractures. J Pediatr Orthop 15:47–52, 1995.

48. Pirone AM, Graham HK, Krajbich JI: Management of displaced extension-type supracondylar fractures of the humerus in children. J Bone Joint Surg Am 70:641–650, 1988.

*49. Sabharwal S, Tredwell SJ, Beauchamp RD, et al: Management of pulseless pink hand in pediatric supracondylar fractures of humerus. J Pediatr Orthop 17:303–310, 1997.

50. Garbuz DS, Leitch K, Wright JG: The treatment of supracondylar fractures in children with an absent radial pulse. J Pediatr Orthop 16:594–596, 1996.

51. Wilkins KE: Supracondylar fractures: what's new? J Pediatr Orthop 6:110–116, 1997.

52. Shaw BA, Kasser JR, Emans JB, et al: Management of vascular injuries in displaced supracondylar humerus fractures without arteriography. J Orthop Trauma 4:25–29, 1990.

53. Clement DA: Assessment of a treatment plan for managing acute vascular complications associated with supracondylar fractures of the humerus in children. J Pediatr Orthop 10:97–100, 1990.

*54. Donnelly LF, Klostermeier TT, Klosterman LA: Traumatic elbow effusions in pediatric patients: are occult fractures the rule? AJR Am J Roentgenol 171:243–245, 1998.

55. Skaggs DL, Mirzayan R: The posterior fat pad sign in association with occult fracture of the elbow in children. J Bone Joint Surg Am 81:1429–1433, 1999.

56. Griffith JF, Roebuck DJ, Cheng JC, et al: Acute elbow trauma in children: spectrum of injury revealed by MR imaging not apparent on radiographs. AJR Am J Roentgenol 176:53–60, 2001.

57. Chacon D, Kissoon N, Brown T, et al: Use of comparison radiographs in the diagnosis of traumatic injuries of the elbow. Ann Emerg Med 21:895–899, 1992.

58. Kissoon N, Galpin R, Gayle M, et al: Evaluation of the role of comparison radiographs in the diagnosis of traumatic elbow injuries. J Pediatr Orthop 15:449–453, 1995.

59. The RM, Severijnen RS: Neurological complications in children with supracondylar fractures of the humerus. Eur J Surg 165:180–182, 1999.

60. Battaglia TC, Armstrong DG, Schwend RM: Factors affecting forearm compartment pressures in children with supracondylar fractures of the humerus. J Pediatr Orthop 22:431–439, 2002.

61. Ippolito E, Caterini R, Scola E: Supracondylar fractures of the humerus in children: analysis at maturity of fifty-three patients treated conservatively. J Bone Joint Surg Am 68:333–344, 1986.

62. Choung W, Heinrich SD: Acute annular ligament interposition into the radiocapitellar joint in children (nursemaid's elbow). J Pediatr Orthop 15:454–456, 1995.

63. Macias CG, Bothner J, Wiebe R: A comparison of supination/flexion to hyperpronation in the reduction of radial head subluxations. Pediatrics 102:e10, 1998.

64. Schutzman SA, Teach S: Upper-extremity impairment in young children. Ann Emerg Med 26:474–479, 1995.

65. Macias CG, Wiebe R, Bothner J: History and radiographic findings associated with clinically suspected radial head subluxations. Pediatr Emerg Care 16:22–25, 2000.

66. Snyder HS: Radiographic changes with radial head subluxation in children. J Emerg Med 8:265–269, 1990

67. Ufberg J, McNamara R: Management of common dislocations. In Roberts JR, Hedges JR (eds): Clinical Procedures in Emergency Medicine, 4th ed. Philadelphia: Elsevier Saunders, 2004, pp 946–988.

68. Schunk JE: Radial head subluxation: epidemiology and treatment of 87 episodes. Ann Emerg Med 19:1019–1023, 1990

69. McDonald J, Whitelaw C, Goldsmith LJ: Radial head subluxation: comparing two methods of reduction. Acad Emerg Med 6:715–718, 1999.

70. DaSilva MF, Williams JS, Fadale PD, et al: Pediatric throwing injuries about the elbow. Am J Orthop 27:90–96, 1998.

71. Do T, Herrera-Soto J: Elbow injuries in children. Curr Opin Pediatr 15:68–73, 2003.

72. Skaggs D, Pershad J: Pediatric elbow trauma. Pediatric Emerg Care 13:425–434, 1997.

73. Kelly Am, Pappas AM: Shoulder and elbow injuries and painful syndromes. Adolesc Med 9:569–587, 1998.

74. David T: Missed upper extremity fractures in athletes. Curr Sports Med Rep 1:327–332, 2002.

75. Radomisli TE, Rosen AL: Controversies regarding radial neck fractures in children. Clin Orthop 353:30–39, 1998.

76. Leung AG, Peterson HA: Fractures of the proximal radial head and neck in children with emphasis on those that involve the articular cartilage. J Pediatr Orthop 20:7–14, 2000.

77. Flynn JM, Sarwark JF, Waters PM, et al: The surgical management of pediatric fractures of the upper extremity. Instr Course Lect 52:635–645, 2003.

78. Beaty JH, Kasser JR: Fracture about the elbow. Instr Course Lect 44:199–215, 1995.

79. Mirsky EC, Karas EH, Weiner LS: Lateral condyle fractures in children: evaluation of classification and treatment. J Orthop Trauma 11:117–120, 1997.

80. Hutchinson MR, Ireland ML: Overuse and throwing injuries in the skeletally immature athlete. Instr Course Lect 52:25–36, 2003.

81. Rasool MN: Dislocations of the elbow in children. J Bone Joint Surg Br 86:1050–1058, 2004.

82. Case SL, Hennrikus WL: Surgical treatment of displaced medial epicondyle fractures in adolescent athletes. Am J Sports Med 25:682–686, 1997.

83. Farsetti P, Potenza V, Caterini R, et al: Long-term results of treatment of fractures of the medial humeral epicondyle in children. J Bone Joint Surg Am 83:1299–1305, 2001.

84. Papandrea R, Waters PM: Posttraumatic reconstruction of the elbow in the pediatric patient. Clin Orthop 370:115–126, 2000.

85. Fowles JV, Slimane N, Kassab MT: Elbow dislocation with avulsion of the medial humeral epicondyle. J Bone Joint Surg Br 72:102–104, 1990.

86. Carlioz H, Abols Y: Posterior dislocation of the elbow in children. J Pediatr Orthop 1:8–12, 1984.

87. Adirim TA, Cheng TL: Overview of injuries in the young athlete. Sports Med 33:75–81, 2003.

88. Kaeding CC, Whitehead R: Musculoskeletal injuries in adolescents. Prim Care 25:211–223, 1998.

89. Hang DW, Chao CM, Hang YS: A clinical and roentgenographic study of little league elbow. Am J Sports Med 32:79–84, 2004.

90. Klingele KE, Kocher MS: Little league elbow: valgus overload injury in the paediatric athlete. Sports Med 32:1005–1015, 2002.

*91. Khosla S, Melton LJ, Dekutoski MB, et al: Incidence of childhood distal forearm fractures over 30 years. JAMA 290:1479–1485, 2003.

92. Noonan KJ, Price CT: Forearm and distal radius fractures in children. J Am Acad Orthop Surg 6:146–156, 1998.

93. Younger AS, Tredwell SJ, Mackenzie WG: Factors affecting fracture position at cast removal after pediatric forearm fracture. J Pediatr Orthop 17:332–336, 1997.

94. Haddad FS, Williams RL: Forearm fractures in children: avoiding redisplacement. Injury 26:691–692, 1995.

95. McLauchlan GJ, Cowan B, Annan IH, et al: Management of completely displaced metaphyseal fractures of the distal radius in children. J Bone Joint Surg Br 84:413–417, 2002.

96. Flynn JM: Pediatric forearm fractures: decision making, surgical techniques, and complications. Instr Course Lect 51:355–360, 2002.

97. Goodwin RC, Kuivila TE: Pediatric elbow and forearm fractures requiring surgical treatment. Hand Clin 18:135–148, 2002.

98. Beaty JH: Elbow fractures in children and adolescents. Instr Course Lect 52:661–665, 2003.

99. Gleeson AP, Beattie TF: Monteggia fracture-dislocation in children. J Accid Emerg Med 11:192–194, 1994.

100. Kay RM, Skaggs DL: The pediatric Monteggia fracture. Am J Orthop 27:606–609, 1998.

101. Vorlat P, De Boeck H: Traumatic bowing and Galeazzi fracture-dislocation—a report of 2 children. Acta Orthop Scand 73:234–237, 2002.

102. Shonnard PY, DeCoster TA: Combined Monteggia and Galeazzi fractures in a child's forearm: a case report. Orthop Rev 23:755–759, 1994.

103. Walsh HP, McLaren CA, Owen R: Galeazzi fractures in children. J Bone Joint Surg Br 69:730–733, 1987.

104. Cheng JC, Shen WY: Limb fracture pattern in different pediatric age groups: a study of 3,350 children. J Orthop Trauma 7:15–22, 1993.

105. Worlock P, Stower M: Fracture patterns in Nottingham children. J Pediatr Orthop 6:656–660, 1986.

106. Symons S, Rowsell M, Bhowal B, et al: Hospital versus home management of children with buckle fractures of the distal radius. J Bone Joint Surg Br 83:556–560, 2001.

107. Plint AC, Perry JJ, Correll R, et al: A randomized, controlled trial of removable splinting versus casting for wrist buckle fractures in children. Pediatrics 117:691–697, 2006.

108. Davidson JS, Brown DJ, Barnes SN, et al: Simple treatment for torus fractures of the distal radius. J Bone Joint Surg Br 83:1173–1175, 2001.

109. Abraham A, Henman P: Interventions for treating wrist fractures in children (protocol). Cochrane Database Syst Rev (3):CD004576, 2004.

110. Overly F, Steele DW: Common pediatric fractures and dislocations. Clin Ped Emerg Med 3:106–117, 2002.

111. Huurman WW: Injuries to the wrist and hand. Adolesc Med 9:611–625, 1998.

112. Peljovich AE, Simmons BP: Traumatic arthritis of the hand and wrist in children. Hand Clin 16:673–684, 2000.

113. Light TR: Carpal injuries in children. Hand Clin 16:513–522, 2000.

114. Fabre O, De Boeck H, Haentjens P: Fractures and nonunions of the carpal scaphoid in children. Acta Orthop Belg 67:121–125, 2001.

115. Cook PA, Yu JS, Wiand W, et al: Suspected scaphoid fractures in skeletally immature patients: application of MRI. J Comput Assist Tomogr 21:511–515, 1997.

116. Albert MC, Barre PS: A scaphoid fracture associated with a displaced distal radial fracture in a child. Clin Orthop 240:232–235, 1989.

117. Bhende MS, Dandrea LA, Davis HW: Hand injuries in children presenting to a pediatric emergency department. Ann Emerg Med 22:1519–1523, 1993.

*118. Fetter-Zarzeka A, Joseph MM: Hand and fingertip injuries in children. Pediatr Emerg Care 18:341–345, 2002.

119. Ljungberg E, Rosberg HE, Dahlin LB: Hand injuries in young children. J Hand Surg Br 28:376–380, 2003.

120. Nofsinger CC, Wolfe SW: Common pediatric hand fractures. Curr Opin Pediatr 14:42–45, 2002.

121. Hastings H, Simmons BP: Hand fractures in children: a statistical analysis. Clin Orthop 188:120–130, 1984.

122. Mahabir RC, Kazemi AR, Cannon WG, et al: Pediatric hand fractures: a review. Pediatr Emerg Care 17:153–156, 2001.

123. Leclercq C, Korn W: Articular fractures of the fingers in children. Hand Clin 16:523–534, 2000.

124. O'Shaughnessy M, McCann J, O'Connor TP, et al: Nail re-growth in fingertip injuries. Ir Med J 83:136–137, 1990.

*125. Roser SE, Gellman H: Comparison of nail bed repair versus nail trephination for subungual hematomas in children. J Hand Surg Am 24:1166–1170, 1999.

Chapter 20

Lower Extremity Trauma

Besh Barcega, MD, MBA and Lilit Minasyan, MD

Key Points

A delayed diagnosis of slipped capital femoral epiphysis has a high likelihood of leading to avascular necrosis of the femoral head.

A saline arthrogram is useful for identifying knee lacerations that penetrate the joint space.

Tibia and fibula fractures place the child at risk for a compartment syndrome of the leg.

Selected Diagnoses

Traumatic hip dislocation
Slipped capital femoral epiphysis
Femur fractures
Knee injuries
Osgood-Schlatter disease
Tibia and fibula fractures
Ankle injuries
Foot injuries
Toe injuries
Approach to the special needs child

Discussion of Individual Diagnoses

Traumatic Hip Dislocation

Traumatic hip dislocations are relatively rare in children.[1] The mechanisms of injury involve high-energy events such as falls from substantial heights and motor vehicle accidents. Children generally present with groin and thigh pain, flexion and external rotation of the involved hip, and apparent shortening of the lower extremity. A small percentage of children with hip dislocations will also have associated acetabular fractures.[1] Posterior dislocations are the most common. Pain control and neurovascular assessment are important factors in the initial emergency department evaluation of these children. An anterior-posterior pelvis radiograph will usually confirm the diagnosis (Fig. 20–1). Closed reduction by the emergency physician is indicated. The use of procedure-related sedation for this procedure is prudent. Once success-

ful reduction has occurred, keeping the hips in abduction with a pillow or blankets between the thighs minimizes the risk of re-dislocation. Postreduction radiographs are indicated. Patients with traumatic hip dislocations are usually admitted to the hospital for spica casting or traction followed by early mobilization. Emergent orthopedic consultation is needed if initial reduction attempts are unsuccessful. A delay in diagnosis or successful reduction increases the risk of avascular necrosis of the femoral head. With prompt treatment, most children with traumatic hip dislocations do well and have minimal or no long-term sequelae.[1]

Slipped Capital Femoral Epiphysis

A slipped capital femoral epiphysis (SCFE, usually pronounced "skiffy") results from shearing forces through the proximal femoral physis. This is a type of Salter-Harris type I fracture (Fig. 20–2). SCFE is in the differential diagnosis of any child with a limp and no other constitutional symptoms.[2-4] The most commonly affected age group includes older school-age children and younger adolescents. Bone age is probably more important than chronological age.[5] There may be a history of relatively minor trauma. The onset may be sudden and rather obvious or indolent and subtle. The child may complain of groin, hip, or knee pain. In particular, an older school-age child who has seen multiple physicians for knee pain, has undergone multiple normal radiographs of the knee, and has a normal knee examination is a classic example of an indolent case of SCFE. More than 20% of children with SCFE will have bilateral disease at presentation or will develop SCFE on the contralateral side at some point in childhood.[6] Obese children are at higher risk for bilateral disease.[6]

When SCFE is suspected, anterior-posterior and frog-leg lateral hip radiographs and an anterior-posterior pelvis radiograph are indicated. The key finding on radiographs is an abnormal position of the proximal femoral epiphysis in relation to the metaphysis. This has been referred to as "the ice cream falling off the cone." When slippage is not obvious, evaluation of Klein's line is useful.[7] Klein's line is drawn along the superior aspect of the femoral neck and should intersect the femoral epiphysis. Failure of Klein's line to intersect the femoral epiphysis is supportive of the diagnosis of SCFE. Once SCFE is identified, orthopedic consultation is indicated. Operative stabilization is usually undertaken. The timing of this is controversial and is at the discretion of the orthopedist.[8] If radiographs are normal yet the diagnosis of

SCFE remains likely, one reasonable plan is to discharge the patient home with crutches and instructions for non–weight bearing on the involved extremity. Arrangements can then be made for an outpatient magnetic resonance imaging (MRI) study of the hip within 1 to 2 weeks.[9] Complications of SCFE include avascular necrosis of the femoral head and osteoarthritis of the hip. A delayed diagnosis increases the risk of complications. Even with appropriate management, avascular necrosis occurs in as many as 14% of children diagnosed with SCFE.[10]

Femur Fractures

Femur fractures are the most common traumatic orthopedic injuries requiring hospitalization.[11] Most femur fractures result from a high-impact mechanism, and the patients present with obvious swelling, deformity, pain, and tenderness in the affected thigh. Shortening of the involved extremity will be evident on physical examination. Infants and nonverbal children with femur fractures may present with a history of refusing to crawl, excessive crying, and swelling over the thigh or tenderness over the fracture site. Although femur fractures in nonambulatory infants and children are suggestive of nonaccidental trauma, they are not pathognomonic for child abuse[12] (see Chapter 119, Physical Abuse and Child Neglect).

Emergency department management of femur fractures generally involves splinting, analgesia, and monitoring the neurovascular status of the involved extremity. Radiographs of femur fractures are seldom subtle. Unlike adults, isolated, closed femur fractures have not been found to be a significant cause of hypotension in children.[13,14] If a child with a closed femur fracture is experiencing hemodynamic instability, alternative causes should be investigated. Orthopedic consultation in the emergency department is indicated for most

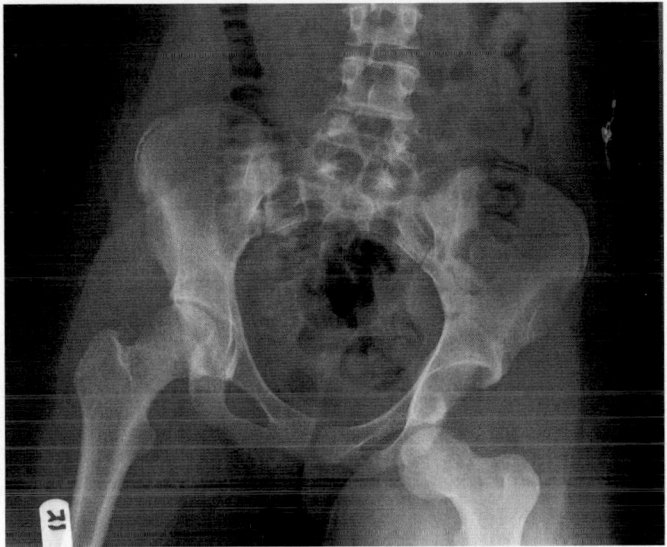

FIGURE 20–1. Radiograph of a traumatic hip dislocation.

Salter-Harris Classification of Growth Plate Fractures

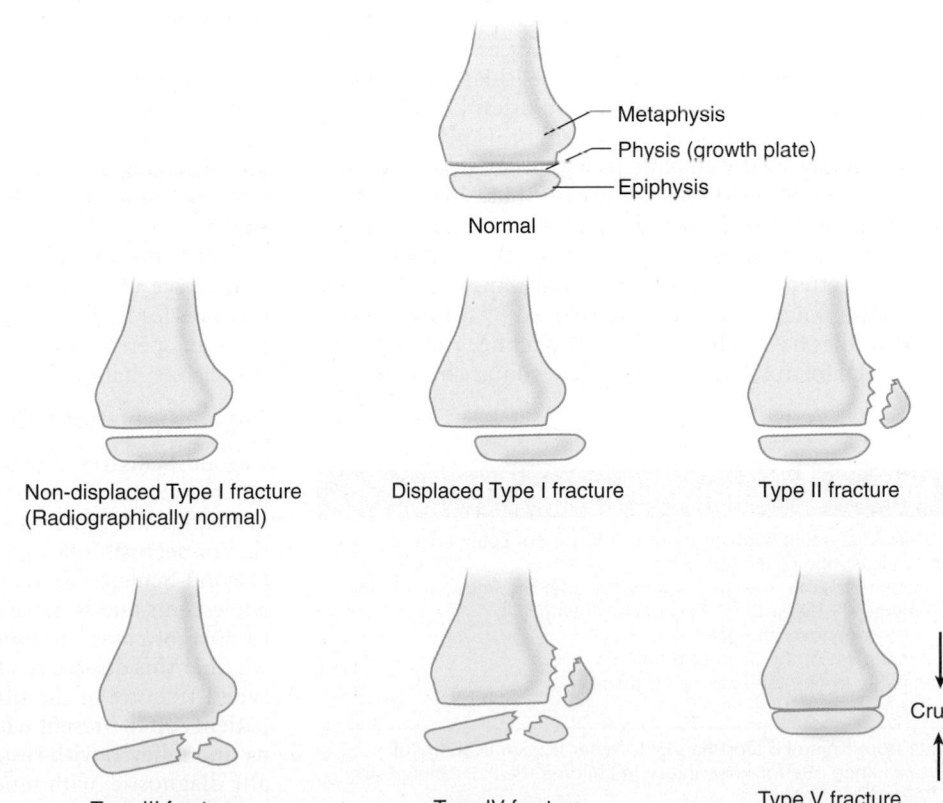

FIGURE 20–2. Salter-Harris classification of growth plate fractures. (Adapted from Salter RB, Harris WR: Injuries involving the epiphyseal plate. J Bone Joint Surg [Am] 45:587–622, 1963.)

femur fractures as most infants and children under age 6 are treated with spica casting and those over 6 years are typically treated with open reduction and internal fixation.[11] In certain circumstances, children with femur fractures can be discharged home from the emergency department without orthopedic consultation. Examples of these fractures include a child with a torus fracture of the femoral metaphysis without significant displacement or angulation and an adolescent with an avulsion fracture of the lesser trochanter.[15]

Knee Injuries

Urgent orthopedic consultation is seldom needed for knee injuries seen in the pediatric emergency department. Specific conditions managed by the emergency physician include patellar dislocations and injuries to the menisci and ligaments. In most patellar dislocations, the patella is displaced laterally. Reduction is straightforward and is accomplished by extending the knee. This reduction is somewhat painful, but mercifully brief and simple to perform. Procedural sedation is seldom needed. Prompt pain relief is expected. Discharge to home in a knee immobilizer is the usual disposition. Orthopedic or primary care follow-up for a gradual return to normal activities is appropriate.

Meniscal and ligamentous injuries are frequently due to a forced twisting motion of the knee. Frequently, the patient will have joint swelling due to hemarthrosis. Joint line tenderness is expected in most of these injuries. Injuries to the ligaments will result in a degree of joint laxity in the direction supported by the injured ligament. However, if the knee is excessively tender and swollen, testing for joint laxity will not be feasible. Radiographs typically will not reveal a fracture unless ligamentous disruption has resulted in a small avulsion fracture. Discharge to home in a knee immobilizer with or without crutches is the usual disposition. Orthopedic follow-up with the expectation of an outpatient MRI is a reasonable plan under most circumstances.[16,17] There has recently been some interest in using bedside ultrasound to evaluate ligamentous and meniscal injuries.[18] The role for ultrasound for this purpose is unclear at this point.

Traditionally, nearly all patients with injured knees underwent radiographs. Although obviously indicated in severe injuries, the utility of these radiographs on the less acute end of the continuum of injuries was frequently questionable at best. In an attempt to limit unnecessary knee radiographs, the Ottawa knee rules were developed[19-21] (Table 20–1). Recent studies have validated the Ottawa knee rules for children.[19-21] Unfortunately, relatively few young children were included in these studies, thus limiting the applicability of the rules to younger children. Applying the Ottawa knee rules to older school-age children and adolescents is probably reasonable.

Several conditions involving the knee require urgent orthopedic consultation. These include open fractures, displaced fractures involving the growth plate, penetrating injuries involving the joint space, significantly avulsed tibial spine fractures, and foreign bodies within the joint space.[22] Another injury pattern requiring prompt orthopedic consultation is the "floating knee," which results from ipsilateral femoral and tibial fractures. This fracture combination is relatively rare in children, arising in the setting of high-energy trauma such as occurs when pediatric pedestrians are struck by automobiles (i.e., "auto vs. pedestrian"). Children with floating knees present with pain, swelling, and obvious deformity over the fracture sites. There is substantial instability of the entire middle of the lower extremity. Bedside portable radiographs are usually sufficient to make the diagnosis. Emergent angiography, including assessment of the popliteal vessels, is indicated. The initial emergency department management of these injuries involves providing adequate analgesia, applying a posterior long-leg splint, and obtaining prompt orthopedic consultation. The definitive treatment is open reduction and internal fixation.[23,24]

The knee is the most common joint to sustain a penetrating injury. Treatment of children is similar to that of adults. Plain radiographs can be obtained to evaluate for associated fracture, air in the joint space indicating a violation of the joint, and the presence of a radiopaque foreign body. In addition, vascular trauma must be diagnosed in a timely manner to assure appropriate treatment. Bynoe et al. found duplex ultrasonography to accurately locate vascular injuries.[25] In appropriate hands, duplex ultrasonography may serve as a noninvasive alternative to arteriography. Deep lacerations in close proximity to the joint should raise suspicion for an open joint wound. This can be confirmed by performing an arthrogram of the joint. An arthrogram is performed by preparing a sterile field on a site distant from the laceration and inserting a relatively large-bore needle (e.g., 18 gauge) into the joint space. By infusing injectable, sterile normal saline (from a bag of normal saline used for intravenous infusion, not the saline used for wound irrigation) into the joint space until there is swelling, the emergency physician observes for fluid leakage from the wound. Fluid leakage suggests on open joint injury. This should prompt urgent orthopedic consultation for operative washout and repair.

Osgood-Schlatter Disease

Osgood-Schlatter disease refers to osteochondrosis of the anterior tuberosity of the tibia.[26] Osteochondrosis is a "disease of ossification centers in children that begins as a degeneration or necrosis followed by regeneration or recalcification."[26] Osgood-Schlatter disease is a relatively common condition in adolescents and is more common in boys.[27] As many as 25% to 50% of cases are bilateral.[27] There is some debate as to whether this disease is a form of tendonitis or a Salter-Harris type I fracture of the tibial tubercle[28] (see Fig. 20–1). These patients often present with knee pain that is worse with activity and relieved with rest. The physical examination is generally diagnostic, with tenderness and a bony bulge at the site of the tibial tuberosity. Radiographs are seldom needed for

Table 20–1	Ottawa Knee Rules

Obtain knee radiographs if there is a history of acute knee injury and at least one of the following:
- Inability to walk 4 steps immediately after the injury and in the emergency department (regardless of limp)
- Tenderness over the patella
- Tenderness of the head of the fibula
- Inability to flex the knee to 90 degrees
- Age greater than 55 yr

Data from Khine H, Dorfman DH, Avner JR: Applicability of Ottawa knee rule for knee injury in children. Pediatr Emerg Care 17:401–404, 2001.

the diagnosis or management of suspected Osgood-Schlatter disease. The usual treatment is conservative and consists of rest, anti-inflammatory/analgesic medications (e.g., ibuprofen), and follow-up with a primary care physician. For serious athletes, follow-up with a sports medicine physician is ideal to allow for maximum participation balanced with sufficient rest to minimize pain.

Tibia and Fibula Fractures

Most fractures of the fibula occur in association with tibia fractures. Isolated fibula fractures are rare in children. The location of the injury is usually clear from the physical examination, in which crepitus, a palpable step-off, bruising, and tenderness are expected at the fracture site. Radiographs of the entire tibia and fibula tend to offer adequate visualization of clinically important fractures. The identification of a fracture of both the tibia and fibula is straightforward. Emergency department management with a posterior molded splint is also straightforward. However, because of the relatively "tight" compartments of the leg, compartment syndrome may develop due to swelling at the fracture site (see Chapter 22, Compartment Syndrome). Prolonged periods of elevation are indicated during the first day or two after the injury. Admission to an observation unit or to the hospital overnight after reduction and splinting is suggested. Selected patients likely to be very compliant with the elevation requirement are the best candidates for discharge home from the emergency department.

A tibial fracture seen only in young children is the toddler's fracture. Toddler's fractures are oblique or spiral fractures in the middle or distal third of the tibia. These fractures are due to a twisting force. Classically, these fractures have no displacement and no angulation. The classic story is of a toddler limping or refusing to walk after getting the foot caught in something and falling while twisting about to release the foot. The child may present without a clear mechanism of injury, however. The physical examination findings may be subtle. If the child is able to tolerate the examination, pain may be elicited at the fracture site. There is typically little, if any, swelling. The overlying skin usually appears normal. Toddler's fractures are notoriously difficult to diagnose on plain radiographs: the fracture may appear to be a "nutrient vessel" with a dark, oblique line running through the tibial shaft without apparent violation of the cortex, or it may appear on only one view. The fracture may not be evident at all on initial radiographs, only appearing when repeat radiographs are obtained 7 to 10 days after the injury as callus formation becomes radiographically evident.[29] Treatment for toddler's fractures, both those clearly diagnosed and those merely suspected, is with a long-leg splint and close follow-up with a primary care physician or orthopedist in 7 to 10 days.[30-33]

Ankle Injuries

Ankle injuries are common. The ankle is a flexible, multidirectional, narrow joint that must support the body's entire weight while moving and changing direction over uneven surfaces. Ankle injuries can range from minor strains of the supporting ligaments to serious fractures requiring operative intervention.

At the more serious end of the injury spectrum are the Tillaux fracture and the Maisonneuve fracture. The Tillaux fracture is a Salter-Harris type III fracture of the lateral, distal tibia. This fracture appears to be unique to adolescents. The fracture pattern is thought to result from asymmetric closing of the growth plate with the medial aspect closing earlier than the lateral aspect. This fracture may be difficult to appreciate on plain radiographs. Computed tomographic (CT) scanning may be required to make the diagnosis.[34] Open reduction and internal fixation are usually required.[35] The Maisonneuve fracture is actually two fractures. The first is a medial malleolar fracture (of the distal tibia). The second is an oblique fracture of the proximal fibula. If the physical examination and plain radiographs focus exclusively on the ankle, this proximal fibula fracture might be missed. With most Maisonneuve fractures there is disruption of the interosseous membrane between the tibia and fibula. When this occurs, the ankle joint is unstable and subsequent diastasis of the joint is likely. Maisonneuve fractures typically require open reduction and internal fixation.[36]

Along the more minor end of the spectrum of ankle injuries are ankle sprains and "occult" distal fibula fractures. Classic teaching has suggested that the ligaments of pediatric ankles are stronger than the growth plate of the distal fibula. If true, nondisplaced Salter-Harris type I fractures of the distal fibula would be expected to be more common than ankle sprains in children. For children who have sustained inversion injuries to the ankle and have normal radiographs, the treatment recommendations have typically focused on immobilization with a posterior molded splint and avoidance of weight bearing. The recommended follow-up plan is then to have a primary care physician or orthopedist re-evaluate the child in about 10 days with the expectation of repeat radiographs to look for callus formation. Preliminary work with ultrasound suggests that it may be able to differentiate ankle sprains from occult distal fibula fractures.[37] Further study is required before ultrasound can be recommended for this purpose.

One area of controversy is the use of the Ottawa ankle rules for evaluating children with ankle injuries (Table 20-2). The Ottawa ankle rules were developed to minimize the use of unnecessary radiographs in the evaluation of relatively minor ankle injuries.[38] A few studies have supported the use of the Ottawa ankle rules in children,[39-41] and one study found the

Table 20–2	Ottawa Foot and Ankle Rules

Obtain ankle radiographs if there is acute ankle injury and at least one of the following:
- Inability to bear weight (4 steps) immediately after the injury and in the emergency department regardless of limp
- Tenderness to palpation over the posterior edge or tip of the lateral malleolus
- Tenderness to palpation over the posterior edge or tip of the medial malleolus

Obtain foot radiographs if there is a history of acute foot injury and at least one of the following:
- Inability to bear weight immediately after the injury and in the emergency department
- Tenderness to palpation over the base of the 5th metatarsal
- Tenderness to palpation over the navicular bone

Data from Stiell IG, McKnight RD, Greenberg GH, et al: Implementation of the Ottawa Ankle Rules. JAMA 271:827–832, 1994.

Ottawa ankle rules inappropriate for children.[42] Other decision rules have also been suggested for evaluating pediatric ankle injuries.[43,44] The clinical application of any of these decision rules is dependent on the emergency physician's tolerance for failing to identify a clinically insignificant ankle fracture. The use of radiograph-minimizing decision rules for children remains controversial. What is clear, however, is that skeletally mature adolescents with ankle injuries can be treated like adults with similar injuries.[38]

Foot Injuries

Pediatric midfoot and hindfoot fractures are relatively common. In younger children, these fractures often present with a chief complaint of limp and may be mistakenly diagnosed as a toddler's fracture or foot sprain as the initial radiographs may be normal at the time of the emergency department visit. In cases of subtle midfoot and hindfoot injuries, plain radiographs obtained 2 to 4 weeks after the initial visit will typically reveal sclerotic changes at the fracture sites.[45,46] The most commonly seen of these fractures involve the calcaneus or cuboid. Because of the difficulty in diagnosing subtle midfoot and hindfoot fractures, bone scans have been advocated for the early evaluation of these fractures.[45-47] However, the clinical outcomes of these injuries is generally excellent without any particular intervention suggesting that bone scans may only be indicated for serious athletes or other special groups. Displaced fractures of the calcaneus and the midfoot sustained under a high-impact mechanism require orthopedic consultation in the emergency department. Avascular necrosis is a serious complication of these fractures. Lisfranc-type injuries (tarsometatarsal joint injuries after a midfoot plantar-flexion injury) rarely occur in young children. Unlike adults and adolescents who require urgent orthopedic consultation in the emergency department, younger children with these injuries can be successfully managed with a short-leg walking cast for 3 to 7 weeks.[48] One complication of Lisfranc-type injuries is compartment syndrome. Therefore, elevation of the injured foot and monitoring for the development of compartment syndrome are indicated for these injuries.

Common foot injuries in all age groups are proximal fifth metatarsal fractures. These fractures arise from inversion injuries of the foot and may be missed if the physical examination and evaluation of the radiographs focuses exclusively on the ankle. This is reflected in the inclusion of these fractures in the Ottawa ankle rules (see Table 20–2). The location of the fracture determines the management and prognosis. The most proximal fractures are usually avulsion fractures and are often referred to as dancer's fractures. These fractures can usually be treated in a hard-soled shoe for a few weeks and seldom lead to complications. Follow-up with a primary care physician is reasonable for these common fractures. More distal fractures are usually referred to as Jones fractures. There is not a well-defined distinction between dancer's fractures and Jones fractures. In adults, dancer's fractures are thought to occur within 1.5 cm from the proximal tip of the fifth metatarsal, while Jones fractures occur more distally. Jones fractures do not heal as well as dancer's fractures and may require open reduction and internal fixation if closed treatment fails. A short-leg, posterior molded splint and the avoidance of weight bearing are usually indicated for Jones fractures. Alternatively, a walking boot may be used. Follow-up with an orthopedist is indicated for Jones fractures.

The approach to the patient with a puncture wound to the plantar surface of the foot depends on the mechanism of injury, the timing of the injury, and the possibility of a retained foreign body (see Chapter 160, Wound Management). Plain radiographs can aid in documenting the presence of radiopaque foreign bodies such as glass and metal. For wooden foreign bodies, ultrasound, CT scanning, and MRI may be reasonable imaging studies depending on the individual circumstances.[49-52] Lawnmower and bicycle spoke injuries can result in extensive bony and soft tissue damage and loss. Urgent orthopedic consultation is indicated.

Toe Injuries

Nondisplaced fractures of the toes are seldom serious and are generally treated with "buddy taping" the injured toe to the adjacent toe. For displaced fractures, closed reduction and buddy taping by the emergency physician is usually adequate. This is particularly important for fifth toe fractures. If reduction is not accomplished, the fifth toe will protrude laterally from the foot. This leads to the patient "catching" the toe on objects when walking barefoot at any point in the future. Orthopedic consultation in 1 to 2 weeks may be obtained on an outpatient basis for unstable fractures. Great toe injuries with bleeding around the nail bed are probably best treated as open fractures with irrigation and prophylactic antibiotics to minimize the risk of osteomyelitis.[53] Cephalexin (25 mg/kg per dose three times per day for 7 days) is a reasonable antibiotic choice.

Approach to the Special Needs Child

Technology-dependent children and those who are not ambulatory frequently have osteopenia that places them at high risk for fractures. Certain conditions are well known to predispose children to fractures. Examples include osteogenesis imperfecta and Ehlers-Danlos syndrome. Fracture of the lower extremity is included in the differential diagnosis for the fussy special needs child, especially if the examination reveals redness, swelling, or possible tenderness to palpation of the lower extremity. There may be a recent history of physical therapy or pain during patient transfer (such as in and out of a specialized wheelchair), but no history of any significant trauma, such as a fall. Plain radiographs of the involved extremity from the hip to the toes may be needed to locate the injury. Fractures in the nonambulating special needs child generally can be treated with splinting and pain control. Closed reduction of significantly displaced fractures is prudent. Procedural sedation may be required to accomplish these reductions (see Chapter 159, Procedural Sedation and Analgesia).

REFERENCES

1. Mehlman CT, Hubbard GW, Crawford AH, et al: Traumatic hip dislocation in children. Clin Orthopedics 376:68–79, 2000.
*2. Kocher MS, Bishop JA, Weed B, et al: Delay in the diagnosis of slipped capital femoral epiphysis. Pediatrics 113:322–325, 2004.
3. Ledwith CA, Fleisher GR: Slipped capital femoral epiphysis without hip pain leads to missed diagnosis. Pediatrics 89:660–662, 1992.

*Selected readings.

4. Matava MJ, Patton CM, Luhmann S, et al: Knee pain as the initial symptom of slipped capital femoral epiphysis: an analysis of initial presentation and treatment. J Pediatr Orthop 19:455–460, 1999.

5. Loder RT, Starnes T, Dikos G: The narrow window of bone age in children with slipped capital femoral epiphysis: a reassessment one decade later. J Pediatr Orthop 26:300–306, 2006.

*6. Bhatia NN, Pirpiris M, Otsuka NY: Body mass index in patients with slipped capital femoral epiphysis. J Pediatr Orthop 26:197–199, 2006.

7. Klein A, Joplin RJ, Reidy JA, et al: Roentgenographic features of slipped capital femoral epiphysis. Am J Roentgenol Radium Ther 66:361–374, 1951.

8. Kalogrianitis S, Tan CK, Kemp GJ, et al: Does slipped capital femoral epiphysis require urgent stabilization? J Pediatr Orthop B 16:6–9, 2007.

9. Umans H, Liebling MS, Moy L, et al: Slipped capital femoral epiphysis: a physeal lesion diagnosed by MRI with radiographic and CT correlation. Skeletal Radiol 27:139–144, 1998.

10. Krahn TH, Canale ST, Beaty JH, et al: Long-term follow-up of patients with avascular necrosis after treatment of slipped capital femoral epiphysis. J Pediatr Orthop 13:154–158, 1993.

11. Heyworth BE, Galano GJ, Vitale MA, et al: Management of closed femoral shaft fractures in children ages 6 to 10: national practice patterns and emerging trends. J Pediatr Orthop 24:455–459, 2004.

12. Scherl SA, Miller LM, Lively N, et al: Accidental and nonaccidental femur fractures in children. Clin Orthop 376:96–105, 2000.

13. Anderson WA: The significance of femoral fractures in children. Ann Emerg Med 11:174–177, 1982.

14. Ciarallo L, Fleisher G: Femoral fractures: are children at risk for significant blood loss? Pediatr Emerg Care 12:343–346, 1996.

15. Kim SS, Thomas M: A football player with thigh pain. Pediatr Emerg Care 17:267–268, 2001.

16. Stanitski CL: Correlation of arthroscopic and clinical examinations with magnetic resonance imaging findings of injured knees in children and adolescents. Am J Sports Med 26:2–6, 1998.

17. Wessel LM, Scholz S, Rusch, M, et al: Hemarthrosis after trauma to the pediatric knee joint: what is the value of magnetic resonance imaging in the diagnostic algorithm? J Pediatr Orthop 21:338–342, 2001.

18. O'Reilly MA, O'Reilly PM, Bell J: Sonographic appearances of medial retinacular complex injury in transient patellar dislocation. Clin Radiol 58:636–641, 2003.

*19. Bulloch B, Neto G, Plint A, et al: Validation of the Ottawa knee rule in children: a multicenter study. Ann Emerg Med 42:48–55, 2003.

20. Khine H, Dorfman DH, Avner JR: Applicability of Ottawa knee rule for knee injury in children. Pediatr Emerg Care 17:401–404, 2001.

*21. Stiell IG, Greenburg GH, McKnight RD, et al: Decision rules for the use of radiography in acute knee injuries: refinement and prospective validation. JAMA 269:1127–1132, 1994.

*22. Salter RB, Harris WR: Injuries involving the epiphyseal plate. J Bone Joint Surg [Am] 45:587–622, 1963.

23. Arslan H, Kapukaya H, Kesemenli C, et al: Floating knee in children. J Pediatr Orthop 23:458–463, 2003.

24. Yue JJ, Churchill RS, Copperman DR, et al: The floating knee in the pediatric patient. Clin Orthop 376:124–136, 2000.

25. Bynoe RP, Miles WS, Bell RM, et al: Noninvasive diagnosis of vascular trauma by duplex ultrasonography. J Vasc Surg 3:346–352, 1991.

26. Anderson DM, Novak PD, Keith J, et al (eds): Dorland's Illustrated Medical Dictionary, 30th ed. Philadelphia: WB Saunders, 2003, p 1333.

27. Osgood RB: Lesions of the tibial tubercle occurring during adolescence. Boston Med Surg J 148:114–117, 1903.

28. Rosenberg ZS, Kawelblum M, Cheung YY, et al: Osgood-Schlatter lesion: fracture or tendonitis? Scintigraphic, CT, and MR imaging features. Radiology 185:853–858, 1992.

*29. Oudjhane K, Newman B, Oh KS, et al: Occult fractures in preschool children. J Trauma 28:858–860, 1988.

30. Englaro EE, Gelfand MJ, Paltiel HJ: Bone scintigraphy in preschool children with lower extremity pain of unknown origin. J Nucl Med 33:351–354, 1992.

31. John SD, Moorthy CS, Swischuk LE: Expanding the concept of the toddler's fracture. Radiographics 17:367–376, 1997.

32. Mellick LB, Ressor K: Spiral tibial fractures of children: a common accidental spiral long bone fracture. Am J Emerg Med 8:234–237, 1990.

33. Tenenbein MH, Reed MH, Black GB: The toddler's fracture revisited. Am J Emerg Med 8:208–211, 1990.

34. Horn BD, Crisci K, Krug M, et al: Radiologic evaluation of juvenile Tillaux fractures of the distal tibia. J Pediatr Orthop 21:162–164, 2001.

35. Koury SI, Stone CK, Harrell G, et al: Recognition and management of Tillaux fractures in adolescents. Pediatr Emerg Care 15:37–39, 1999.

36. Duchesneau S, Fallat LM: The Maisonneuve fracture. J Foot Ankle Surg 34:422–428, 1995.

37. Farley PA, Kuhns L, Jacobson JA, et al: Ultrasound examination of ankle injuries in children. J Pediatr Orthop 21:604–607, 2001.

*38. Stiell IG, Greenburg GH, McKnight RD, et al: A study to develop clinical decision rules for the use of radiography in acute ankle injuries. Ann Emerg Med 21:384–390, 1992.

39. Chande VT: Decision rules of roentgenography of children with acute ankle injuries. Arch Pediatr Adolesc Med 149:255–258, 1995.

40. Libetta C, Burke D, Brennan P, et al: Validation of the Ottawa ankle rules in children. J Accid Emerg Med 16:342–344, 1999.

*41. Plint A, Bulloch B, Osmond M, et al: Validation of the Ottawa ankle rules in children with ankle injuries. Acad Emerg Med 6:1005–1009, 1999.

42. Clark KD, Tanner S: Evaluation of the Ottawa ankle rules in children. Pediatr Emerg Care 19:73–78, 2003.

43. Boutis K, Komar L, Jaramillo D, et al: Sensitivity of a clinical examination to predict the need for radiography in children with ankle injuries: a prospective study. Lancet 358:2118–2121, 2001.

44. Dayan PS, Vitale M, Langsam D, et al: Derivation of clinical prediction rules to identify children with fractures after twisting injuries of the ankle. Acad Emerg Med 11:736–743, 2004.

45. Blumberg K, Patterson RJ: The toddler's cuboid fracture. Radiology 179:93–94, 1991.

46. Schindler A, Mason DE, Allington NJ: Occult fracture of the calcaneus in toddlers. J Pediatr Orthop 16:201–205, 1996.

47. Lalotis N, Pennie BH, Carty H, et al: Toddler's fracture of the calcaneum. Injury 24:169–170, 1993.

48. Buoncristiani AM, Manos RE, Mills WJ: Plantar-flexion tarsometatarsal joint injuries in children. J Pediatr Orthop 21:324–327, 2001.

49. Mizel MS, Steinmetz ND, Trepman E: Detection of wooden foreign bodies in muscle tissue: experimental comparison of computed tomography, magnetic resonance imaging, and ultrasonography. Foot Ankle Int 15:437–443, 1994.

50. Yanay O, Vaughan, DJ Brownstein, D, et al: Retained wooden foreign body in a child's thigh complicated by severe necrotizing faciitis: a case report and a discussion of imaging modalities for early diagnosis. Pediatr Emerg Care 17:354–355, 2001.

51. Imoisili MA, Bonwit AM, Bulas DI: Toothpick puncture injuries of the foot in children. Pediatr Infect Dis J 23:80–82, 2004.

*52. Inaba AS, Zukin DD, Perro M: An update on the evaluation and management of plantar puncture wounds and Pseudomonas osteomyelitis. Pediatr Emerg Care 8:38–44, 1992.

53. Kensiger DR, Guille JT, Horn BD, et al: The stubbed great toe: importance of early recognition and treatment of open fractures of the distal phalanx. J Pediatr Orthop 21:31–41, 2001.

Chapter 21

Pelvic and Genitourinary Trauma

Peter S. Auerbach, MD

Key Points

In children, mortality directly related to pelvic fractures is very low.

"Routine" pelvic radiographs are no longer advocated.

Approximately 10% of children with pelvic fractures also have injuries to the genitourinary system.

The utility of a microscopic urinalysis is unclear.

Blood seen at the penile meatus is a contraindication to blindly placing a Foley catheter.

Introduction and Background

Pelvic fractures are relatively uncommon in children, occurring in 3% to 5% of children versus 6% to 10% of adult blunt trauma patients.[1,2] When fractures of the pelvis do occur in children, they are usually associated with a severe mechanism and multiple associated injuries. Mortality from pelvic fractures is lower in children than in adults due to differences in the types of fractures sustained and the inherent fracture resistance of the bony and ligamentous structures of the pediatric pelvis.

Although rarely life threatening, injuries to the genitourinary system often occur in children with pelvic trauma and are sometimes overlooked during the initial assessment due to the high incidence of higher priority, associated injuries. Lower genitourinary injuries (i.e., injuries to the bladder, urethra, and genitals) are seen in fewer than 5% of children with pelvic fractures.[3] Urethral injuries are difficult to diagnose. Serious renal injuries are seldom missed because of the high frequency with which abdominal and pelvic computed tomographic (CT) scanning are performed on traumatized children.

Recognition and Approach

The most common mechanism of injury resulting in pediatric pelvic fractures is a pedestrian struck by a motor vehicle.[4-7] In contrast, adults who sustain pelvic fractures are more likely to be the driver or passenger in a motor vehicle collision.[1,2] The most common significant injury associated with pelvic fractures in children is a head injury. Intra-abdominal solid organ injuries are also commonly associated with pelvic fractures.

The classification of pediatric pelvic fractures has not been standardized, which makes a direct comparison of published studies difficult. Of the classification systems used, the most widely accepted classifies pelvic fractures into three types based on structural integrity[8] (Fig. 21–1). Type A fractures spare the posterior pelvic arch and are therefore mechanically stable. Commonly seen type A fractures include those of the pubic rami. Type B fractures involve incomplete disruption of the posterior arch, making the pelvic ring horizontally unstable but vertically stable. Type B pelvic fractures are frequently the result of anterior-posterior compression. Type C fractures involve complete disruption of the posterior arch, often through the sacroiliac joint, rendering the pelvic ring both horizontally and vertically unstable. Type C pelvic fractures are frequently the result of vertical forces resulting from a fall. Type B and C fractures are relatively rare in children.[4,5]

The pediatric genitourinary system differs from that of adults in several important ways. The kidneys are more easily injured in children because they are relatively larger in size and less well protected by the ribs. Children tend to have less perirenal fat, weaker abdominal muscles, and a flexible rib cage. In addition, pediatric kidneys are more likely to contain persistent fetal lobulations, which may predispose to parenchymal disruption during blunt trauma.[9] The pediatric bladder is more susceptible to injury because it extends superiorly into the abdomen and is less well protected by the pelvic ring. The bladder wall musculature is weakest at the superior pole, where it lies in contact with the peritoneum, making intraperitoneal bladder rupture more likely. In boys, the urethra may also be more susceptible to injury because it is less elastic and less well protected by the prostate.[10]

Injuries may involve any portion of the genitourinary system. The kidney is the most commonly injured portion of the genitourinary system. The most widely accepted scoring system for kidney injuries is incorporated into the comprehensive Organ Injury Scoring and Scaling System[11] (Table 21–1). Most pediatric kidney injuries identified are grade I. The bladder is the second most frequently injured component of the genitourinary system. There is some utility in

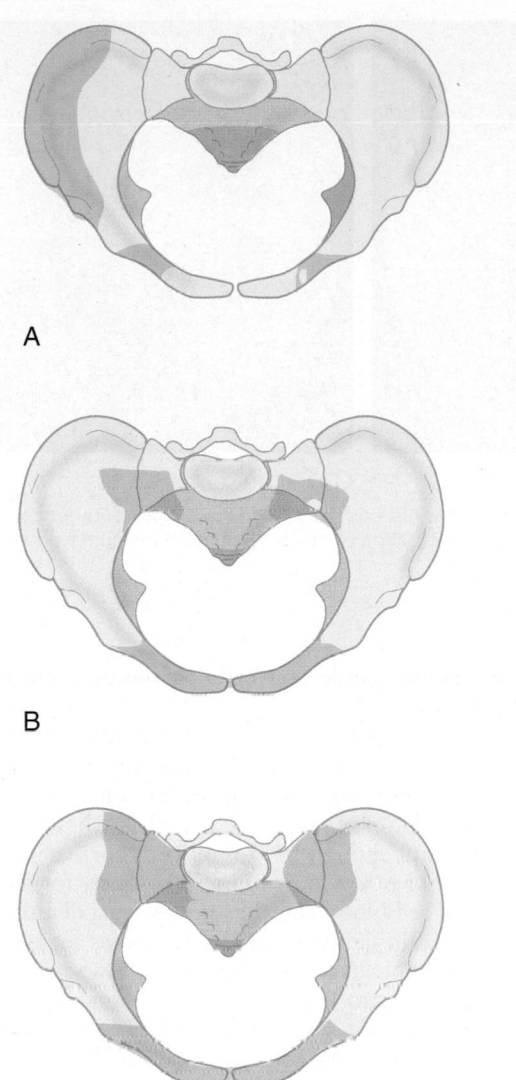

A

B

C

FIGURE 21–1. Classification of pelvic fractures. **Type A,** Lesions sparing (or with no displacement of) the posterior pelvic arch. **Type B,** Incomplete disruption of the posterior arch (partially stable). **Type C,** Complete disruption of the posterior arch (unstable). (Images courtesy of the Orthopedic Trauma Association.)

Table 21–1	Kidney Injury Scoring
Grade	**Description of Injury**
I	Contusion
	or
	Subcapsular hematoma
II	Nonexpanding perirenal hematoma confined to the retroperitoneum
	or
	<1.0-cm renal parenchymal laceration without urinary extravasation
III	>1.0-cm renal parenchymal laceration without urinary extravasation
	or
	Collecting system involvement
IV	Laceration extending into the collecting system
	or
	Renal artery or vein injury with contained hemorrhage
V	Shattered kidney
	or
	Avulsion of renal hilum, which devascularizes kidney

Adapted from the Organ Injury Scaling Committee of the American Association for the Surgery of Trauma.[11]

separating bladder injuries into three general categories: bladder contusions, extraperitoneal bladder rupture, and intraperitoneal bladder rupture. Contusions are partial tears of the bladder mucosa. Extraperitoneal bladder rupture usually occurs as a result of a displaced pelvic fracture lacerating the bladder. Intraperitoneal bladder rupture usually results from significant blunt trauma to a full bladder. Intraperitoneal bladder rupture is the most serious type of bladder injury and is the most likely type of bladder injury to require operative repair. Bladder injuries almost always present with gross hematuria, difficulty with urination, or significant abdominal pain.[3] The male urethra is susceptible to injury during pelvic and perineal trauma. The male urethra is anatomically divided into posterior and anterior segments by the urogenital diaphragm between the pubic rami. The posterior segment is proximal and the anterior segment is distal. The two segments of the male urethra have different patterns of

injury. Posterior urethral injuries result from high-energy blunt trauma and are often associated with pelvic fractures and bladder injuries (Fig. 21–2). In contrast, anterior urethral trauma usually results from straddle injuries. Anterior urethral injuries are associated with external genital injuries. Both types of urethral injuries almost always present with blood at the penile meatus. Accidental injuries to the female urethra are extremely rare and are almost always accompanied by pelvic fractures.[12]

Blunt trauma to the pelvis and perineum can also result in injury to the external genitalia. In males, the most common genital injuries occur to the testicles. Injuries to the testicle include testicular rupture, traumatic torsion, dislocation, hematomas, and hematoceles (see Chapter 87, Testicular Torsion). In females, the most common accidental injuries to the external genitalia involve minor vulvar lacerations from straddle injuries.

Evaluation

The initial approach to a child with possible pelvic or genitourinary trauma should begin with an accurate description of the mechanism of injury. A history of significant deceleration is associated with renal injuries even in the absence of abnormal physical findings or gross hematuria.[13-15] Physical examination findings associated with pelvic fractures include pelvic tenderness, instability on gentle compression, and ecchymoses or abrasions directly overlying the bony pelvis. In most children with serious pelvic injuries, CT scanning of the abdomen and pelvis is ostensibly performed for other indications (see Chapter 25, Abdominal Trauma). When CT scanning is performed, these images of the bony pelvis preclude the need for plain radiographs. If CT scanning is not planned, a single anterior-posterior pelvis radiograph may be obtained if indicated by the physical examination. Routine pelvis radiographs as part of a traditional "C-spine/chest/pelvis" set of radiographs are no longer advocated. Several recent pediatric studies of blunt trauma patients have

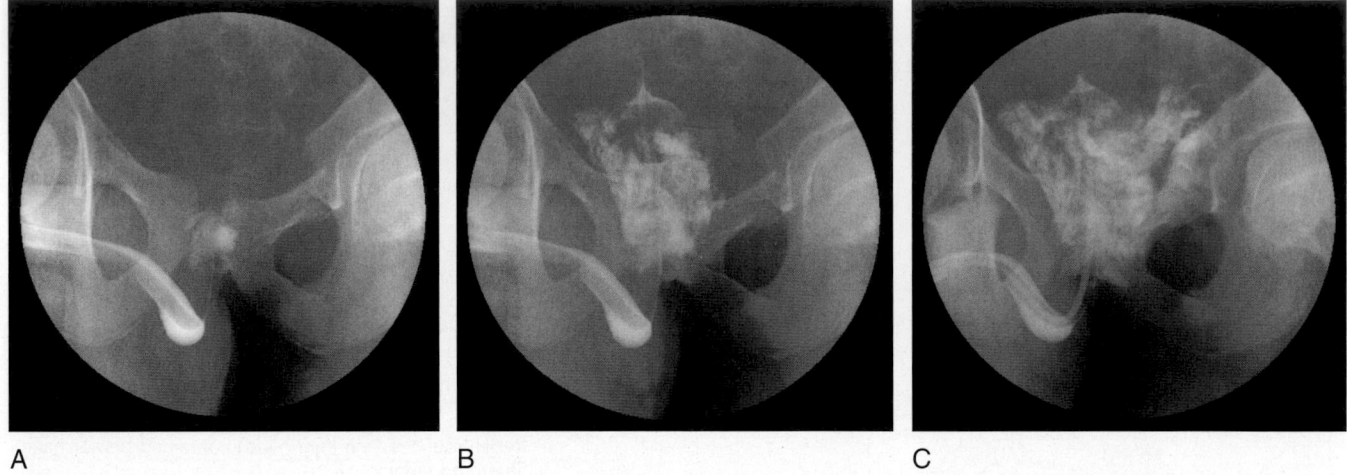

A   B   C

FIGURE 21–2. Retrograde urethrogram demonstrating posterior urethral tear in a 16-year-old boy. **A,** Immediate extravasation of contrast at the level of the prostatic urethra. **B** and **C,** Further retrograde dye injection demonstrates extravasation of nearly all contrast medium with no significant filling of the bladder.

demonstrated that the "routine" pelvis radiograph has extremely low yield and may be safely omitted in many patients. In particular, this is true for children with normal mental status, a normal physical examination of the pelvis, and no distracting injuries.[16-18]

Open pelvic fractures are rare in children but have a mortality rate of 20% or higher.[19] Open pelvic fractures must therefore be excluded through a detailed examination of the overlying skin. Any laceration near a fracture site, as well as on the buttocks, perineum, or genital area, is suspicious for an open fracture. Although rectal examinations are seldom indicated otherwise,[20,21] a careful rectal examination should be performed in patients with displaced pelvic fractures to exclude internal lacerations. Care must be taken by the examiner to avoid sustaining a finger laceration. These examinations may require procedural sedation or general anesthesia to be performed safely. Girls with displaced pelvic fractures should have a cautious manual vaginal examination. For prepubertal girls who are not comatose, it is prudent to perform these examinations with procedural sedation or under general anesthesia.

The physical examination may suggest particular genitourinary injuries. Physical findings suggestive of renal injury include flank or lateral abdominal tenderness, ecchymosis, hematomas, or a palpable mass. In the absence of such findings, gross hematuria alone is a highly sensitive sign of a serious renal injury and should prompt radiographic imaging. Patients with bladder or urethral injuries may complain of lower abdominal pain, urinary urgency, or the inability to void. Physical findings associated with lower genitourinary injuries include gross hematuria, blood at the penile meatus, suprapubic tenderness, and a palpable, tender bladder. Gross hematuria is seen in nearly all cases of lower genitourinary injuries, and its absence is enough to exclude significant bladder or urethral injury unless abnormal physical examination findings or multiple associated injuries are present.[3,22] The finding of blood at the penile meatus is highly sensitive for urethral injury and is a contraindication to blind urethral catheterization, even if a patient is able to spontaneously void. If catheterization is inappropriately attempted, the

urinary catheter could convert a partial urethral tear into a complete tear.

Historically, various degrees of microscopic hematuria have been used to screen for the presence of renal injury.[23-29] There continues to be debate in the literature over how many red blood cells on microscopic urinalysis should be considered significant enough to prompt genitourinary imaging in the absence of other indications. The quest for this "magic number" of red blood cells has not led to a definitive result. Data from multiple recent pediatric studies suggest that isolated microscopic hematuria has a very low yield when used as the sole indication for genitourinary imaging.[13-15,30-32] It is conceivable that the test characteristics of microscopic urinalysis for identifying genitourinary injuries are not good enough to advocate using microscopic hematuria for this kind of decision making.

Contemporary options for imaging children at risk for genitourinary injuries include CT scanning, ultrasound, cystograms, and urethrograms. The studies selected reflect the anatomic area of concern and, to some extent, the overall hemodynamic stability of the patients. Historically, the intravenous pyelogram was used to image the kidneys and ureters,[23,24] but CT scanning is now the imaging modality of choice. CT scanning leads to faster results, is more sensitive for identifying renal injuries, and can be used to identify injuries to other intra-abdominal and pelvic structures.[13,33] Ultrasound has a sensitivity for renal injury of only 70%, but can be performed rapidly at the bedside and does not require the use of intravenous contrast or radiation.[34] Ultrasound may have the greatest utility in pregnant girls and any child too hemodynamically unstable to tolerate CT scanning. Ultrasound is useful for follow-up imaging in patients with known injuries (Fig. 21–3). Ultrasound, particularly when Doppler flow is assessed, is also useful for evaluating testicular injuries. Bladder injuries can best be identified by performing a cystogram. Cystograms involve the retrograde injection of contrast material through the urethra into the bladder. Cystograms may be performed with plain radiographs or with CT scanning. Bladder rupture is diagnosed by observing extravasation of the contrast material. Urethral

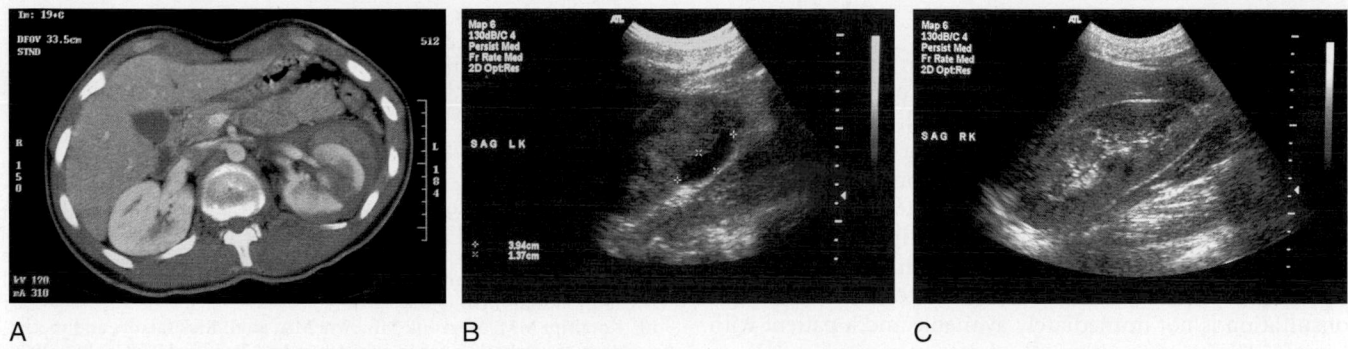

FIGURE 21–3. Renal laceration and perinephric hematoma in a 17-year-old boy. **A,** Computed tomography shows acute laceration of the left kidney with a large perinephric hematoma. **B,** Ultrasound image of same patient 3 weeks later shows resolving hematoma but does not reveal a laceration. **C,** Comparison view of right (normal) kidney ultrasound.

injuries are diagnosed in a similar manner by retrograde urethrogram. A urethrogram is performed by gently injecting a small amount of contrast material (usually 10 to 30 ml depending upon the size of the child) into the distal urethra under fluoroscopy or while obtaining a plain film radiograph. If a complete urethral tear is present, extravasation of contrast material will be seen without filling of the urethra or bladder proximal to the injury (see Fig. 21–2). If the bladder fills but extravasation is present, the likely diagnosis is a partial tear of the urethra. If no extravasation occurs and the bladder fills, then the examination is negative for urethral disruption.

Management

In general, the identification of pelvic fractures and genitourinary injuries takes place in the context of an evaluation for multisystem trauma (see Chapter 11, Approach to Multisystem Trauma). Treatments for specific pelvic and genitourinary injuries need to be incorporated into the overall management of the traumatized child.

Pelvic Fractures

If a pelvic fracture is closed and nondisplaced, and the pelvic ring is stable, then no immediate management of the fracture is indicated. In this circumstance, the priorities are analgesia and identification of associated injuries. Children rarely become hypotensive as a direct result of pelvic fractures, so children in shock should be presumed to have another source of bleeding. In the rare event that a severe pelvic fracture contributes to ongoing blood loss, immediate measures can be taken in the emergency department (ED) to stabilize the pelvis by reapproximating the fracture surfaces. This is most often necessary for "open book" pelvic fractures. The simplest means to reapproximate such fractures and control hemorrhage is to tighten a sheet around the pelvis. Commercial devices designed for this purpose may be inappropriately sized for most children. Urgent orthopedic consultation for internal or external fixation is then needed. Embolization performed by a interventional radiologist may also be indicated. This may require transfer of the patient to a pediatric trauma center.

Obvious or suspected open pelvic fractures require the prompt administration of intravenous antibiotics. Open pelvic fractures, particularly in children, are sufficiently rare

that no evidence-based recommendations on antibiotic selection can be made. In this context, the selection of antibiotics may be based on the degree of soft tissue injury and the likelihood of bowel perforation.[35,36] Relatively clean, open fractures of the iliac wing, for example, may do well with intravenous cefazolin. Open pelvic fractures with more extensive soft tissue damage may do well with intravenous cefazolin and gentamicin. Injuries likely to involve bowel perforation may do best with traditional "triple antibiotics" (i.e., cefazolin, gentimicin, and metronidazole).

Given that many pelvic fractures are associated with other internal injuries, most children with pelvic fractures will require hospitalization. Over 90% of pelvic fractures in children are treated nonoperatively.[4-6,37] Children with minor pelvic fractures and no other injuries may be candidates for discharge from the ED with close outpatient follow-up.

Renal and Ureteral Injuries

Almost 90% of blunt renal injuries, including severe ones, can be managed nonoperatively by hospitalization with close observation of hemodynamics, urine output, and hematocrit.[38,39] This may also be true for some penetrating renal injuries.[40] Immediate complications associated with renal injury include infection, urinary obstruction, persistent bleeding, and urinary extravasation. Ureteral injuries are generally managed surgically, either by reanastomosis or stent placement. When a delay in the diagnosis of a ureteral injury occurs, urinary diversion with delayed repair is usually necessary.

Bladder Injuries

The management of bladder injuries depends on the type and severity of the injury. Children with simple bladder contusions can be discharged with outpatient urologic follow-up if they can spontaneously void and have no other indications for admission. Extraperitoneal bladder rupture generally requires external urinary drainage. This can be accomplished by placement of a Foley or suprapubic catheter. If a displaced fragment of bone from the pelvis remains in the bladder wall, however, surgical removal and repair may be necessary. Intraperitoneal bladder rupture requires surgical repair. These injuries require suprapubic urinary diversion. Complications of bladder rupture include infection, vesicular fistula formation, and poor healing with the need for delayed surgical repair.

Urethral Injuries

Damage to the urethra may be managed in a number of ways depending upon the location and severity of injury. Posterior urethral injuries are typically treated with endoscopic catheterization using a guidewire. The urethra is then allowed to heal over the catheter. Severe posterior injuries require urinary diversion (e.g., suprapubic cystostomy) with delayed surgical reanastomosis. Anterior urethral injuries are treated by either long-term catheter placement, which allows healing of the urethra over the catheter, or reanastomosis. If urologic consultation is not immediately available and a patient with a urethral injury cannot void, then a suprapubic urinary catheter can be placed by the emergency physician to empty the bladder. This is most easily accomplished using a kit designed for this purpose, which usually includes a guidewire, dilator, and introducer sheath. Young children may require a smaller catheter size than is provided in standard kits. Procedural sedation may be needed to facilitate this procedure. Complications of urethral injury include stricture formation, infection, and impotence.

Testicular Injuries

Testicular rupture and traumatic torsion both require immediate operative intervention (see Chapter 87, Testicular Torsion). Testicular salvage rates decrease with time. If dislocation is suspected, the missing testis will likely be palpable superior to the scrotum. Manual reduction is typically indicated. Intravenous analgesia or procedural sedation is prudent for this procedure. Urologic consultation is required if attempts at reduction by the ED physician are unsuccessful. Large testicular hematomas and hematoceles may require surgical treatment. Children who have small scrotal hematomas, skin ecchymosis, or superficial lacerations without evidence of injury to the testicle can be discharged home with outpatient follow-up and oral analgesia as needed. More significant scrotal injuries, and any injury involving the testes, typically require urologic consultation.

Summary

Pelvic fractures are uncommon in children. Genitourinary injuries are more common, but seldom life threatening. Children with pelvic fractures and associated genitourinary injuries are usually also at risk for multisystem trauma. The prognosis of children with isolated pelvic fractures is generally excellent. Injuries to other anatomic systems usually dictate overall management and contribute strongly to the ultimate outcome.

REFERENCES

*1. Demetriades D, Karaiskakis M, Velmahos GC, et al: Pelvic fractures in pediatric and adult trauma patients: are they different injuries? J Trauma 54:1146–1151, 2003.
*2. Ismail BN, Bellemare JF, Mollitt DL, et al: Death from pelvic fracture: children are different. J Pediatr Surg 31:82–85, 1996.
3. Tarman GJ, Kaplan GW, Lerman SL, et al: Lower genitourinary injury and pelvic fractures in pediatric patients. Urology 59:123–126, 2002.
4. Chia JP, Holland AJ, Little, D, et al: Pelvic fractures and associated injuries in children. J Trauma 56:83–88, 2004.

*5. Silber JS, Flynn JM, Koffler KM, et al: Analysis of the cause, classification, and associated injuries of 166 consecutive pediatric pelvic fractures. J Pediatr Orthop 21:446–450, 2001.
6. Grisoni N, Connor S, Marsh E, et al: Pelvic fractures in a pediatric level I trauma center. J Orthop Trauma 16:458–463, 2002.
7. Rieger H, Brug E: Fractures of the pelvis in children. Clin Orthop 336:226–239, 1997.
8. Fracture and dislocation compendium. Orthopaedic Trauma Association Committee for Coding and Classification. J Orthop Trauma 10(Suppl 1):v–ix, 1–154, 1996.
9. Brown SL, Elder JS, Spirnak JP: Are pediatric patients more susceptible to major renal injury from blunt trauma? A comparative study. J Urol 160:138–140, 1998.
10. Koraitim MM, Marzouk ME, Atta MA, et al: Risk factors and mechanism of urethral injury in pelvic fractures. Br J Urol 77:876–880, 1996.
11. Moore EE, Shackford SR, Pachter HL, et al: Organ injury scaling: spleen, liver and kidney. J Trauma 29:1664, 1989.
12. Okur H, Kucukaydin M, Kazez A, et al: Genitourinary tract injuries in girls. Pediatr Urol 78:446–449, 1996.
13. Perez-Brayfield MR, Gatti JM, Smith EA, et al: Blunt traumatic hematuria in children: is a simplified algorithm justified? J Urol 167:2543–2547, 2002.
14. Santucci RA, Langenburg SE, Zachareas MJ: Traumatic hematuria in children can be evaluated as in adults. J Urol 171: 822–825, 2004.
15. Nguyen MM, Das S: Pediatric renal trauma. Urology 59:762–767, 2002.
16. Junkins EP, Furnival RA, Bolte RG: The clinical presentation of pediatric pelvic fractures. Pediatr Emerg Care 17:15–18, 2001.
17. Junkins EP, Nelson DS, Carroll KL, et al: A prospective evaluation of the clinical presentation of pediatric pelvic fractures. J Trauma 51:64–68, 2001.
18. Rees MJ, Aickin R, Kolbe A, et al: The screening pelvic radiograph in pediatric trauma. Pediatr Radiol 31:497–500, 2001.
19. Mosheiff R, Suchar A, Porat S, et al: The "crushed open pelvis" in children. Injury 30(Suppl 2):B14–B18, 1999.
*20. Esposito TJ, Ingraham A, Luchette FA, et al: Reasons to omit digital rectal exam in trauma patients: no fingers, no rectum, no useful information. J Trauma 59:1314–1319, 2005.
*21. Guldner G, Babbitt J, Boulton M, et al: Deferral of the rectal examination in blunt trauma patients: a clinical decision rule. Acad Emerg Med 11:635–641, 2004.
22. Iverson AJ, Morey AF: Radiographic evaluation of suspected bladder rupture following blunt trauma: critical review. World J Surg 25:1588–1591, 2001.
23. Fleisher G: Prospective evaluation of selective criteria for imaging among children with suspected blunt renal trauma. Pediatr Emerg Care 5:8–11, 1989.
24. Lieu TA, Fleisher GR, Mahboubi S, et al: Hematuria and clinical findings as indications for intravenous pyelography in pediatric blunt renal trauma. Pediatrics 82:216–222, 1988.
25. Bass DH, Semple PL, Cywes S: Investigation and management of blunt renal injuries in children: a review of 11 years' experience. J Pediatr Surg 26:196–200, 1991.
26. Hashmi A, Klassen T: Correlation between urinalysis and intravenous pyelography in pediatric abdominal trauma. J Emerg Med 13:255–258, 1995.
27. Miller KS, McAninch JW: Radiographic assessment of renal trauma: our 15-year experience. J Urol 154:352–355, 1995.
28. Eastham JA, Wilson TG, Ahlering TE: Radiographic evaluation of adult patients with blunt renal trauma. J Urol 148:266–267, 1992.
29. Stalker HP, Kaufman RA, Stedje K: The significance of hematuria in children after blunt abdominal trauma. AJR Am J Roentgenol 154:569–571, 1990.
30. Morey AF, Bruce JE, McAninch JW: Efficacy of radiographic imaging in pediatric blunt renal trauma. J Urol 156:2014–2018, 1996.
31. Abou-Jaoude WA, Sugarman JM, Fallat ME, et al: Indicators of genitourinary tract injury or anomaly in cases of pediatric blunt trauma. J Pediatr Surg 31:86–90, 1996.
32. Brown SL, Haas C, Dinchman KH, et al: Radiographic evaluation of pediatric blunt renal trauma in patients with microscopic hematuria. World J Surg 25:1557–1560, 2001.
33. Porter JM, Singh Y: Value of computed tomography in the evaluation of retroperitoneal organ injury in blunt abdominal trauma. Am J Emerg Med 16:225–227, 1998.
34. Yen K: Ultrasound applications for the pediatric emergency department: a review of the current literature. Pediatr Emerg Care 18:226–234, 2002.

*Selected readings.

35. Merritt K: Factors increasing the risk of infection in patients with open fractures. J Trauma 28:823–827, 1988.
36. Robinson D, On E, Hadas N, et al: Microbiologic flora contaminating open fractures: its significance in the choice of primary antibiotic agents and the likelihood of deep wound infection. J Orthop Trauma 3:283–286, 1989.
37. Blasier RD, McAtee J, White R, et al: Disruption of the pelvic ring in pediatric patients. Clin Orthop 376:87–95, 2000.
38. Margenthaler JA, Weber TR, Keller MS: Blunt renal trauma in children: experience with conservative management at a pediatric trauma center. J Trauma 52:928–932, 2002.
39. Wessel LM, Scholz S, Jester I, et al: Management of kidney injuries in children with blunt abdominal trauma. J Pediatr Surg 35:1326–1330, 2000.
40. Wessells H, McAninch JW, Meyer A, et al: Criteria for nonoperative treatment of significant penetrating renal lacerations. J Urol 157:24–27, 1997.

Chapter 22

Compartment Syndrome

Christian Vaillancourt, MD, MSc and Ian Shrier, MD, PhD

Key Points

Acute compartment syndrome is a limb-threatening condition.

This condition should be recognized early, before pulses are lost.

Significant necrosis can occur within 3 to 4 hours of the injury.

Compartment pressure should be measured when the diagnosis is clinically equivocal.

Definitive therapy is surgical fasciotomy.

Introduction and Background

Acute compartment syndrome is a limb-threatening condition in which increased pressure within closed tissue spaces compromises the nutrient blood flow to muscles and nerves such that necrosis will invariably occur if decompression is not performed.[1-4] This is in contrast to chronic (or recurrent) compartment syndrome, in which the mechanism of injury is usually exertional, symptoms most often subside at rest, and the condition is managed conservatively initially and by elective surgery when warranted.[5-8] Acute compartment syndrome was first described in 1881 by a German physician named Dr. Richard von Volkmann.[9] He reported on many cases of clawhand resulting from elbow injuries in children, which initially became known as "Volkmann's contracture."

A compartment is a functional unit usually containing muscles, nerves, veins, and arteries. Each compartment is surrounded by a thick fascia that lacks the ability to stretch. A limb can contain more than one compartment; the four leg compartments are depicted in Figure 22–1. Acute compartment syndrome is not limited to the extremities; for example, it has been reported in the orbit[10] as well as in the abdominal cavity.[11]

When pressure increases inside a closed compartment, it compresses both arterioles and venules. The increased venous resistance results in increased venular pressure, and presumably increased capillary pressure.[12] This may explain why one observes more serious injuries in acute compartment syndrome–induced ischemia compared to that produced by tourniquet-induced ischemia alone, a condition associated with decreased venular pressure.[13]

Recognition and Approach

As suggested by Matsen,[14] the numerous acute compartment syndrome etiologies can be classified within two categories: increased compartmental content and decreased compartmental volume (Table 22–1). Acute compartment syndrome is a well-recognized complication of revascularization surgery,[15,16] as well as pelvic surgery in the lithotomy position.[17,18] It has been described in a variety of other conditions, such as steroid use,[19] human immunodeficiency virus–induced myositis,[20] post–diagnostic electromyography,[21] and self-induced hand suction in children.[22] Because such a variety of circumstances can lead to acute compartment syndrome, it is important to maintain a high level of suspicion and inquire about the mechanism of injury. Most patients will be young males, will be involved in a traumatic incident, and will often have an associated fracture.[23,24]

The leg compartments are most often involved in the adult population[25] (Fig. 22–2). Perhaps because of their smaller stature or a different mechanism of injury, there seems to be a more equal distribution between upper and lower extremities in children.[23,24]

Evaluation

The presence of a tight compartment on palpation should alert emergency physicians to the possibility of acute compartment syndrome.[2] The hallmark presentation is that of pain out of proportion to the apparent injury (Table 22–2). Nerve structures are particularly sensitive to ischemia, leading to early paresthesia or paralysis. Particular attention should be given to agitated/uncooperative young patients,[23] those requiring increasing amounts of analgesia,[23,26] or those receiving continuous epidural analgesia.[27] The loss of peripheral pulses is a late and ominous sign; acute compartment syndrome should be diagnosed before pulses are lost.

It is often clinically easier to exclude the diagnosis of acute compartment syndrome than it is to confirm it.[28] While

Fascial Compartments of Leg

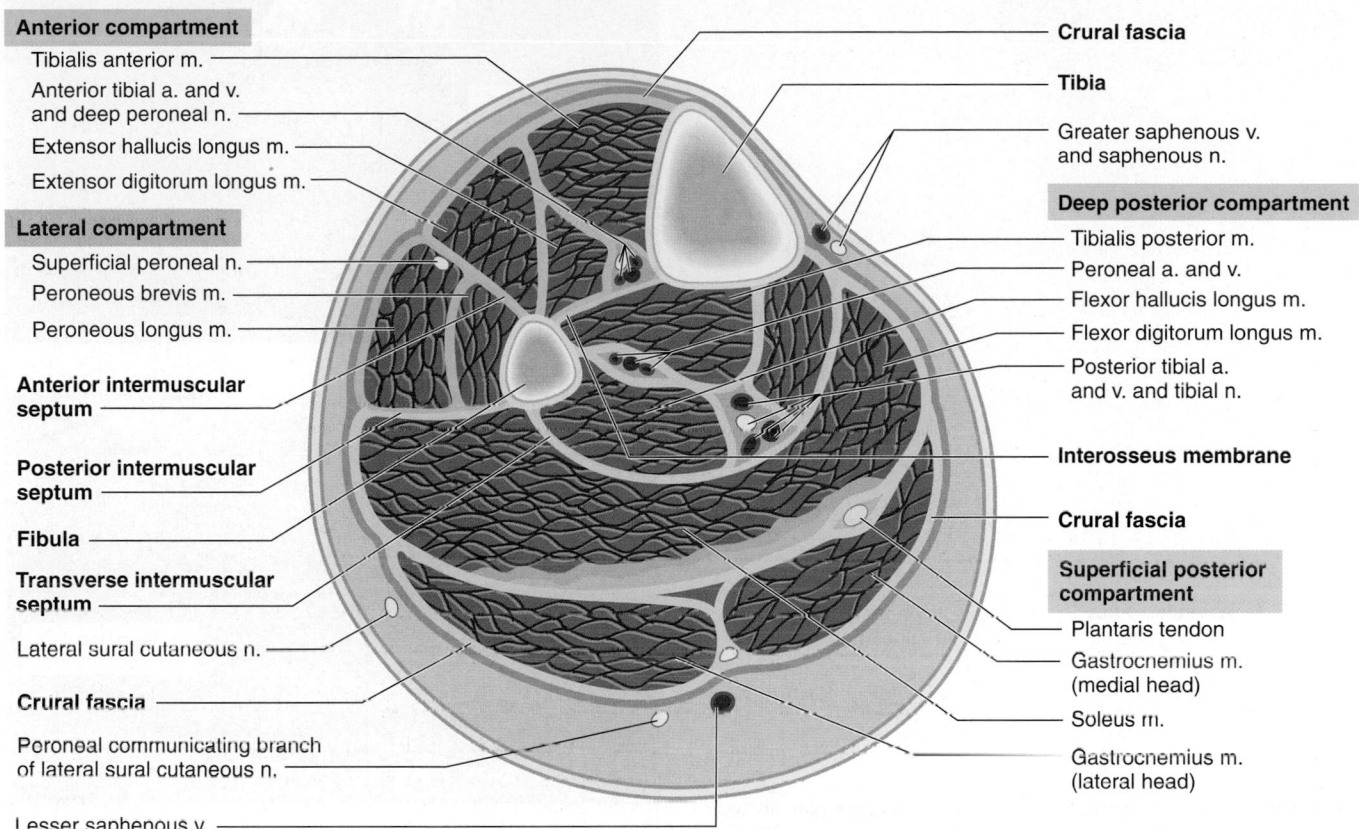

Anterior compartment
- Tibialis anterior m.
- Anterior tibial a. and v. and deep peroneal n.
- Extensor hallucis longus m.
- Extensor digitorum longus m.

Lateral compartment
- Superficial peroneal n.
- Peroneous brevis m.
- Peroneous longus m.

Anterior intermuscular septum

Posterior intermuscular septum

Fibula

Transverse intermuscular septum

- Lateral sural cutaneous n.

Crural fascia

- Peroneal communicating branch of lateral sural cutaneous n.

- Lesser saphenous v.

Crural fascia

Tibia

- Greater saphenous v. and saphenous n.

Deep posterior compartment
- Tibialis posterior m.
- Peroneal a. and v.
- Flexor hallucis longus m.
- Flexor digitorum longus m.
- Posterior tibial a. and v. and tibial n.

Interosseus membrane

Crural fascia

Superficial posterior compartment
- Plantaris tendon
- Gastrocnemius m. (medial head)
- Soleus m.
- Gastrocnemius m. (lateral head)

FIGURE 22–1. Cross-section of a leg illustrating its four compartments and their respective contents.

Table 22–1   Classification of Acute Compartment Syndrome Etiologies

Increased Content	Decreased Volume
Bleeding	Tight dressing or cast
Major vascular injuries	Military antishock trousers
Bleeding disorder or	(MAST)
anticoagulants	Burn eschars
Increased capillary permeability	Lying on a limb or localized
Postischemic swelling	external pressure
Muscle contraction (exercise,	Closure of fascial defects
seizure, tetany)	
Burns	
Intra-arterial drugs	
Envenomation	
Infiltrated infusion	
Nephrotic syndrome	

Table 22–2   Clinical Findings in Conscious Patients

Common Clinical Findings*	
Pain	95%
Neurologic abnormalities	53%
Pain on passive stretch	49%

*Pallor and pulselessness are late and ominous signs. Acute compartment syndrome should be diagnosed before they occur.

clinically obvious cases should be referred to an orthopedic surgeon without further delay,[29,30] up to 50% of cases will remain equivocal despite a thorough clinical evaluation.[25,31] Measurement of intracompartmental pressure can be achieved using one of three methods: the Stryker instrument, the manometric Intervenous Alarm Control (IVAC) pump, or the Whitesides method. The Stryker instrument is accurate and easy to use[32] (Fig. 22–3). If this instrument is not available, the pressure can just as accurately be measured using a method described by Uppal et al.[33]: (1) set up the

IVAC pump to manometric mode, (2) zero the IVAC pump with the pump placed at the same height as the limb compartment that is to be measured to ensure that there is no hydrostatic pressure gradient, (3) insert the 18-gauge needle into the compartment, (4) infuse 0.3 ml of normal saline, and (5) read the pressure measurement. The Whitesides method requires a complicated procedure that includes a mercury manometer and is not as reliable.[34] When measuring the pressure, the needle should be inserted within 5 cm of a suspected fracture, and measurements may have to be repeated if clinical suspicion is high.[35]

While it is accepted that normal compartment pressure should be less than 10 mm Hg, the pressure threshold for diagnosis of acute compartment syndrome is more controversial. Many surgeons make the diagnosis when an absolute pressure measurement of 30 to 40 mm Hg is reached.[31]

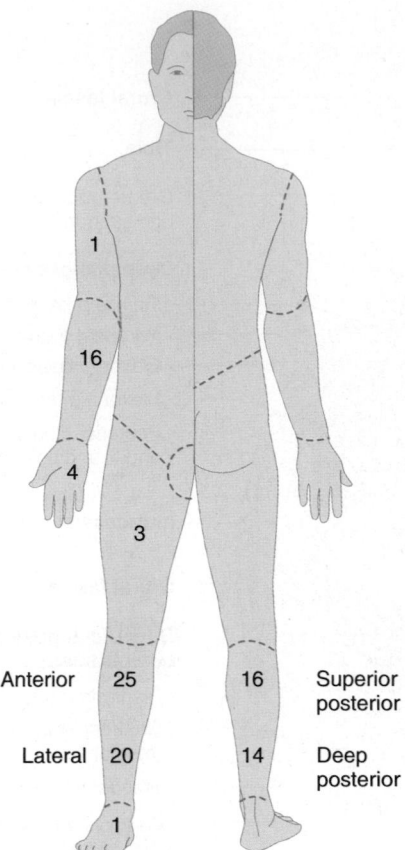

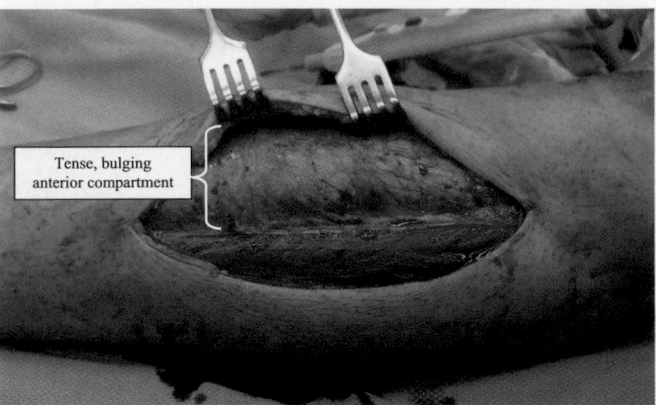

A

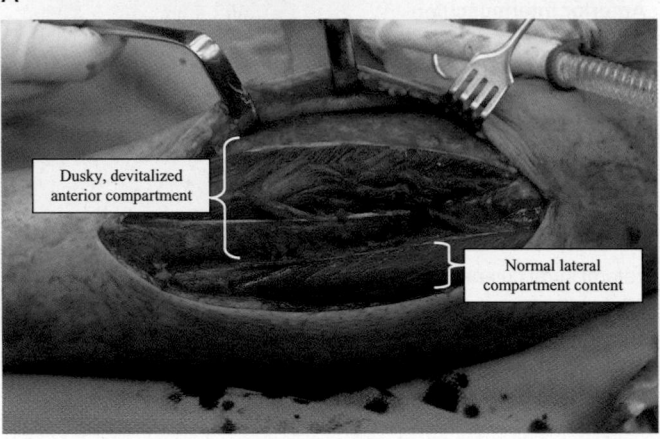

B

FIGURE 22–2. Distribution of involved compartments in patients with acute compartment syndrome confirmed at time of surgery (n = 76, age range 1 to 80 years). Some patients had more than one compartment involved. Numbers represent the percentage of of the total number of involved compartments (n = 140). Most injuries occurred in the lower extremities. (From Vaillancourt C, Shrier I, Vandal A, et al: Acute compartment syndrome: how long before muscle necrosis occurs? Can J Emerg Med 6:147–154, 2004.)

FIGURE 22–4. Acute compartment syndrome **(A)** immediately after anterolateral incision, anterior compartment is bulging and hard; and **(B)** after fasciotomy release of the anterior and lateral compartments, the lateral compartment content is normal and viable but the anterior compartment content is dusky and devitalized. (Images reproduced with permission from Dr. Steven Papp, Assistant Professor, Orthopedic Trauma, The Ottawa Hospital, University of Ottawa, Canada.)

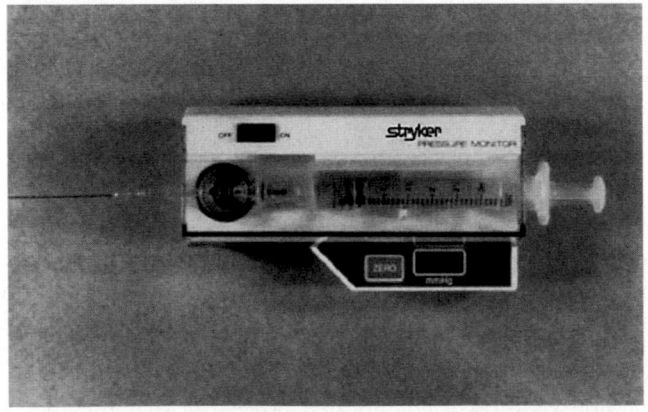

FIGURE 22–3. Using the Stryker instrument to measure the intracompartmental pressure: (1) assemble the needle, the diaphragm chamber, and the prefilled syringe on the pressure monitor as shown; (2) zero the Stryker instrument; (3) insert the needle in the compartment to be measured; (4) inject 0.3 ml of normal saline; and (5) read the pressure measurement. (Photo courtesy of the Stryker Corporation.)

Original work from McQueen and Court-Brown has shown that many unnecessary surgeries would result from using this absolute pressure measurement criterion, and that a differential pressure of 30 mm Hg (i.e., diastolic pressure—compartment pressure is < 30 mm Hg) is more appropriate and would have missed no case of acute compartment syndrome.[36]

Management

The only accepted therapy for acute compartment syndrome is urgent fasciotomy[2-4,29]; this should only be second to adequate narcotic pain control. Delays in diagnosis and compartment decompression can result in tissue necrosis, disability, or loss of limb[25,37-40] (Fig. 22–4). While basic science has determined that muscle can tolerate up to 3 hours of tourniquet-induced ischemia before necrosis occurs,[41] laboratory and clinical data on acute compartment syndrome have shown that muscle necrosis can occur well within that presumably safe 3-hour period.[13,25] In a recent review of 76 acute compartment syndrome cases, almost half suffered some level of muscle necrosis, 30% of those lost more than 25% of the muscle belly, and it is estimated that necrosis

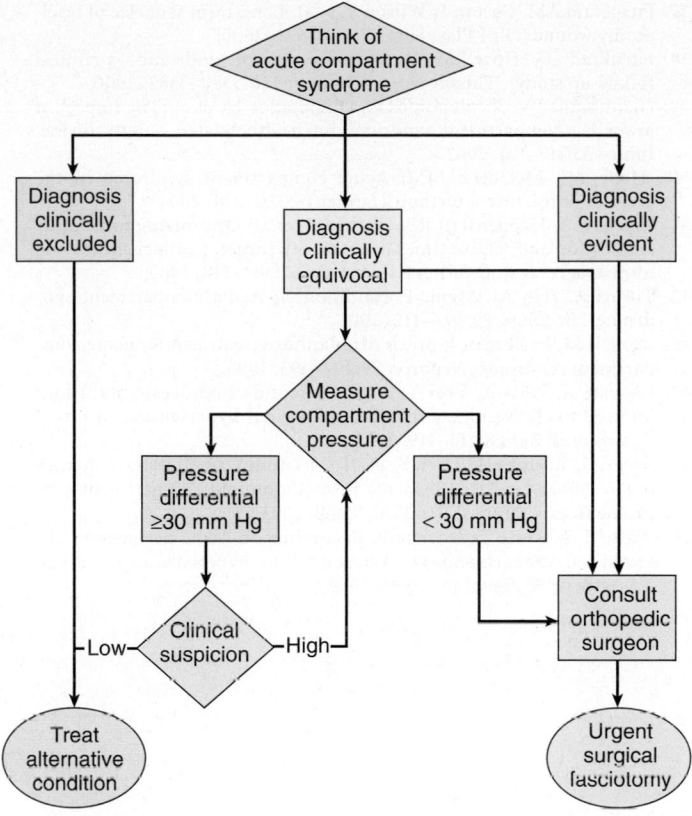

FIGURE 22–5. Diagnostic and therapeutic algorithm for acute compartment syndrome.

occurred within 3 hours of the initial injury in 37% of cases.[25]

Repeated or continuous monitoring of compartment pressure[36,42] should occur in suspected cases if the initial pressure measurement was normal, if the child's ability to communicate is limited due to age or other injuries, or if the child is receiving frequent or continuous narcotic analgesia. In the meantime, it is controversial whether the limb should be elevated or not; in acute compartment syndrome, limb elevation could lead to decreased perfusion pressure and more tissue damage.

A number of adjunct therapeutic modalities have been suggested. These include mannitol,[2,43] octreotide,[44] melatonin,[45] and hyperbaric oxygen.[46] Unfortunately, none of these measures can alleviate the need for a rapid surgical fasciotomy.

Summary

Acute compartment syndrome is a limb-threatening disease that can rapidly lead to permanent disability or lost of limb. A high level of suspicion for acute compartment syndrome should be maintained in appropriate cases. When in doubt, emergency physicians can easily confirm the diagnosis using needle pressure measurements (Fig. 22–5). Repeated or continuous pressure measurements should be performed in cases where suspicion for acute compartment syndrome remains high. Orthopedic surgeons should be consulted early, and urgent fasciotomy should take place when the diagnosis is confirmed.

REFERENCES

*1. McQueen M: Acute compartment syndrome. Acta Chir Belg 98:166–170, 1998.
 2. Mabee JR: Compartment syndrome: a complication of acute extremity trauma. J Emerg Med 12:651–656, 1994.
*3. Gulli B, Templeman D: Compartment syndrome of the lower extremity. Orthop Clin North Am 25:677–684, 1994.
*4. Matsen FA, Winquist RA, Krugmire R: Diagnosis and management of compartment syndromes. J Bone Joint Surg Am 62:286–291, 1980.
 5. Fehlandt A Jr, Micheli L: Acute exertional anterior compartment syndrome in an adolescent female. Med Sci Sports Exerc 27:3–327, 1995.
 6. Shrier I: Exercised-induced acute compartment syndrome: a case report. Clin J Sport Med 1:202–204, 1991.
 7. Hurschler C, Vanderby R Jr, Martinez DA: Mechanical and biochemical analysis of tibial compartment fascia in chronic compartment syndrome. Ann Biomed Eng 22:272–279, 1994.
 8. Turnipseed WD, Hurschler C, Vanderby R Jr: The effects of elevated compartment pressure on tibial arteriovenous flow and relationship of mechanical and biochemical characteristics of fascia to genesis of chronic anterior compartment syndrome. J Vasc Surg 21:810–816, 1995.
 9. Von Volkmann R: Die Ischämischen Muskellähmungen und Kontracturen. Centralbl Chir 51:801–803, 1881.
10. Prodhan P, Noviski NN, Butler WE, et al: Orbital compartment syndrome mimicking cerebral herniation in a 12-yr-old boy with severe traumatic asphyxia. Pediatr Crit Care Med 4:367–369, 2003.
11. Tao J, Wang C, Chen L, et al: Diagnosis and management of severe acute pancreatitis complicated with abdominal compartment syndrome. J Huazhong Univ Sci Technol 23:399–402, 2003.
12. Shrier I, Magder S: Pressure-flow relationships in in vitro model of compartment syndrome. J Appl Physiol 79:214–221, 1995.
13. Heppenstall RB, Scott R, Sapega A, et al: A comparative study of the tolerance of skeletal muscle to ischemia: tourniquet application compared with acute compartment syndrome. J Bone Joint Surg 68:820–828, 1986.
14. Matsen FA: Compartment syndromes. Hosp Pract 15:113–117, 1980.
15. Quinn RH, Ruby ST: Compartment syndrome after elective revascularization for chronic ischemia: a case report and review of the literature. Arch Surg 127:865–866, 1992.
16. Scott DJ, Allen MJ, Bell PR, et al: Does oedema following lower limb revascularisation cause compartment syndromes? Ann R Coll Surg Engl 70:372–376, 1988.
17. Meyer RS, White KK, Smith JM, et al: Intramuscular and blood pressures in legs positioned in the hemilithotomy position: clarification of risk factors for well-leg acute compartment syndrome. J Bone Joint Surg Am 84:1829–1835, 2002.
18. Peters P, Baker SR, Leopold PW, et al: Compartment syndrome following prolonged pelvic surgery. Br J Surg 81:1128–1131, 1994.
19. Bahia H, Platt A, Hart NB, Baguley P: Anabolic steroid accelerated multicompartment syndrome following trauma. Br J Sports Med 34:308–309, 2000.
20. Lam R, Lin PH, Alankar S, et al: Acute limb ischemia secondary to myositis-induced compartment syndrome in a patient with human immunodeficiency virus infection. J Vasc Surg 37:1103–1105, 2003.
21. Farrell CM, Rubin DI, Haidukewych GJ: Acute compartment syndrome of the leg following diagnostic electromyography. Muscle Nerve 27:374–377, 2003.
22. Shin AY, Chambers H, Wilkins KE, Bucknell A: Suction injuries in children leading to acute compartment syndrome of the interosseous muscles of the hand: case reports. J Hand Surg Am 21:675–678, 1996.
*23. Bae DS, Kadiyala RK, Waters PM: Acute compartment syndrome in children: contemporary diagnosis, treatment, and outcome. J Pediatr Orthop 21:680–688, 2001.
*24. McQueen MM, Gaston P, Court-Brown CM: Acute compartment syndrome: who is at risk? J Bone Joint Surg Br 82:200–203, 2000.
*25. Vaillancourt C, Shrier I, Vandal A, et al: Acute compartment syndrome: how long before muscle necrosis occurs? Can J Emerg Med 6:147–154, 2004.
26. Kadiyala RK, Waters PM: Upper extremity pediatric compartment syndromes. Hand Clin 14:467–475, 1998.

———————————————
*Selected readings.

27. Tang WM, Chiu KY: Silent compartment syndrome complicating total knee arthroplasty: continuous epidural anesthesia masked the pain. J Arthroplasty 15:241–243, 2000.

28. Ulmer T: The clinical diagnosis of compartment syndrome of the lower leg: are clinical findings predictive of the disorder? J Orthop Trauma 16:572–577, 2002.

29. Lagerstrom CF, Reed RL, Rowlands BJ, Fischer RP: Early fasciotomy for acute clinically evident posttraumatic compartment syndrome. Am J Surg 158:36–39, 1989.

30. Vaillancourt C, Shrier I, Falk M, et al: Quantifying delays in the recognition and management of acute compartment syndrome. Can J Emerg Med 3:26–30, 2001.

31. Sterk J, Schierlinger M, Gerngross H, Willy C: [Intracompartmental pressure measurement in in acute compartment syndrome: results of a survey of indications, measuring technique and critical pressure value]. Unfallchirurg 104:119–126, 2001.

32. Uliasz A, Ishida JT, Fleming JK, Yamamoto LG: Comparing the methods of measuring compartment pressures in acute compartment syndrome. Am J Emerg Med 21:143–145, 2003.

33. Uppal GS, Smith RC, Sherk HH, Mooar P: Accurate compartment pressure measurement using the Intervenous Alarm Control (IVAC) Pump: report of a technique. J Orthop Trauma 6:87–89, 1992.

34. Whitesides TE Jr, Haney TC, Harada H, et al: A simple method for tissue pressure determination. Arch Surg 110:1311–1313, 1975.

35. Menetrey J, Peter R: Syndrome de loge aigu de jambe post-traumatique. Rev Chir Orthop Reparatrice Appar Mot 84:272–280, 1998.

36. McQueen MM, Court-Brown CM: Compartment monitoring in tibial fractures: the pressure threshold for decompression. J Bone Joint Surg Br 78:99–104, 1996.

37. Fitzgerald AM, Gaston P, Wilson Y, et al: Long-term sequelae of fasciotomy wounds. Br J Plast Surg 53:690–693, 2000.

38. Furulund OK, Hove LM: [Acute compartment syndrome—a clinical follow-up study]. Tidsskr Nor Laegeforen 120:3380–3382, 2000.

39. Giannoudis PV, Nicolopoulos C, Dinopoulos H, et al: The impact of lower leg compartment syndrome on health related quality of life. Injury 33:117–121, 2002.

*40. Hope MJ, McQueen MM: Acute compartment syndrome in the absence of fracture. J Orthop Trauma 18:220–224, 2004.

41. Sapega AA, Heppenstall RB, Chance B, et al: Optimizing tourniquet application and release times in extremity surgery: a biochemical and ultrastructural study. J Bone Joint Surg 67:303–314, 1985.

42. Tiwari A, Haq AI, Myint F, Hamilton G: Acute compartment syndromes. Br J Surg 89:397–412, 2002.

43. Daniels M, Reichman J, Brezis M: Mannitol treatment for acute compartment syndrome. Nephron 79:492–493, 1998.

44. Kacmaz A, Polat A, User Y, et al: Octreotide improves reperfusion-induced oxidative injury in acute abdominal hypertension in rats. J Gastrointest Surg 8:113–119, 2004.

45. Sener G, Kacmaz A, User Y, et al: Melatonin ameliorates oxidative organ damage induced by acute intra-abdominal compartment syndrome in rats. J Pineal Res 35:163–168, 2003.

46. Wattel F, Mathieu D, Neviere R, Bocquillon N: Acute peripheral ischaemia and compartment syndromes: a role for hyperbaric oxygenation. Anaesthesia 53(Suppl 2):63–65, 1998.

Chapter 23

Spinal Trauma

Andrew Wackett, MD and Peter Viccellio, MD

Key Points

The management of a child with a potential spinal injury begins with the assessment of airway, breathing, and circulation while maintaining spinal immobilization.

Children are more susceptible to upper cervical spine injuries, which bring a greater risk for airway compromise.

Spinal cord injury without radiologic abnormality (SCIWORA) presentation ranges from subtle to obvious and may be delayed.

Neurogenic shock is characterized by hypotension and bradycardia, but it is a diagnosis that should be entertained only after hemorrhagic shock has been excluded.

Although controversial, steroid use in spinal cord injuries has become a standard of care in the United States.

Introduction and Background

The National Head and Spinal Cord Injury Survey indicates that there are approximately 11,200 new cases of acute spinal cord injury in the United States each year. Children account for 1065 (10%) of these cases. The mortality among spine-injured children is estimated at 25% to 32%. Costs of medical treatment for all spinal cord injury are estimated to be in excess of $380 million/year. Motor vehicle collisions are the most common etiology. They account for 36% to 54% of cases. Falls, diving injuries, sports-related injuries, birth injuries, penetrating injuries (knife and gunshot wounds), and child abuse account for the remaining precipitants.[1]

Recognition and Approach

There are several vertebral injury patterns that present in children. These patterns are best understood by three unifying concepts: the unique pediatric anatomy, Denis' three-column system, and Daffner's "fingerprints" of vertebral trauma.[1-3]

Pediatric Spinal Anatomy

Pediatric vertebral and spinal injuries have unique characteristics. Specifically, the type and distribution of vertebral injuries in young children, up to 8 to 12 years of age, are different from those of adolescents and adults. The fulcrum of cervical motion occurs at the C5-6 level in adolescents and adults, and it occurs at the C2-3 level in children, due to the relatively larger mass of the head. Thus the majority of spinal injuries in children involve the upper cervical spine and the cranio-vertebral junction, and the associated mortality is higher in children.[1]

Compared to adults, children have much more laxity in their spinal ligaments, weaker musculature, and more horizontally angled facet joints. Children can have significant spinal cord injuries without spinal fractures. This injury is referred to as a spinal cord injury without radiologic abnormality (SCIWORA). The reported incidence of SCIWORA is 16% to 19% in children compared to 0.2% in adults.[4]

During assessment of infants and children, including radiographic examination, clinicians must be aware of anatomic variation and age-related normal development (Tables 23–1 and 23–2).

Vertebral Functional Columns

The vertebrae can be divided into three distinct functional columns. The anterior column extends from the anterior longitudinal ligament to a line drawn vertically through the center of the vertebral body. The middle column begins at this line and extends to the posterior longitudinal ligament. The posterior column extends from the posterior longitudinal ligament to the supraspinous ligament (Fig. 23–1). All the major support structures for the vertebrae are contained within the middle and posterior columns. Thus any disruption extending through all three columns will produce an unstable injury.[3]

Mechanisms of Spine Injury

Spine injury mechanisms include flexion, extension, shearing, and rotational injuries.[2]

Flexion Injuries

Flexion injuries can be further divided into simple, burst, distraction, and dislocation patterns (Fig. 23–2). Simple flexion injuries demonstrate anterior compression of the superior aspect of the vertebral body. These injuries occur due to an anterior flexion force. There may or may not be narrowing of the disk space above the level of injury; however, the posterior vertebral body line and posterior ligamentous structures must remain intact. With up to 50% compression, the posterior and middle elements are not involved, thus leaving the injury both mechanically and neurologically stable. Greater than 50% compression should raise suspicion for posterior injury.

Burst injuries show a vertebra comminuted by compressive forces with retropulsion of fragments. The mechanism of injury involves an axial load. These fractures involve both the anterior and middle columns and are therefore usually unstable, especially when the middle column is retropulsed into the spinal canal.

Distraction injuries demonstrate widening of the interspinous and interfacet distance. Seat belt fractures, also known as Chance fractures, are examples of these injuries. These fractures involve failure of the middle and posterior columns and are thus unstable.

Finally, dislocation injuries display a complete loss of bone continuity at the articular surfaces. Since there is failure of all three columns, these fractures are always unstable.

Extension Injuries

The radiographic findings of extension injuries include compression, fragmentation, burst vertebral bodies, teardrop fragments, wide interspinous spaces, anterolisthesis, locked facets, and narrow disk spaces. Extension injuries result when the child hyperextends the vertebral column over a solid object. Like flexion injuries, they are also subdivided into simple, distraction, and dislocation injuries. The simple subtype leaves the posterior and middle columns intact and as such is a stable injury. Distraction and dislocation exten-

Table 23–1	Normal Cervical Spine Variants in Infants and Children
Age	**Feature**
<6 mo	C1 ring invisible and all synchondroses are open, vertebrae are normally wedged anteriorly, and there is often no lordosis to the uninjured spine
1 yr	Body of C1 becomes visible radiographically
3 yr	Posteriorly located spinous process synchondroses fuse
	Dens becomes ossified (visible radiographically)
3–6 yr	Neurocentral (body) and C2-odontoid synchondroses fuse
	Summit ossification center appears at the apex (top) of the odontoid
	Anterior wedging of the vertebral bodies resolves (wedging is not normal if seen now)
8 yr	Pseudosubluxation and predental widening resolve, lordosis is normal now
12–14 yr	Secondary ossification centers appear at spinous process tips (mistaken for fractures), summit ossification center of odontoid fuses (if it does not, os odontoideum is present), superior/inferior epiphyseal rings appear on body
25 yr	Secondary ossification centers at tips of spinous processes fuse
	Superior/inferior epiphyseal rings fuse to vertebral body

Table 23–2	Infant/Child Versus Adult Cervical Spine

- More horizontal facets allowing for increased mobility and spine injury
- Differential growth of C1 compared to C2 gives false appearance of burst fracture (pseudo-Jefferson's fracture)
- Increased predental space (up to 5 mm) compared to adults
- Normal lordosis to cervical spine is absent in 14% of children
- Normal posterior angulation of odontoid can be seen
- Majority of injuries occur at C1-2 in children ≤ 8 yr old and in lower cervical spine in those > 8 yr old
- Os odontoideum—congenital anomaly in which odontoid does not fuse with C2*
- Ossiculum terminale—a secondary center of ossification for odontoid tip; appears by age 3 yr (in 26% of children) and fuses with odontoid by age 12 yr (may never fuse)
- Prevertebral space at C3 is ≤ $\frac{1}{2}$–$\frac{1}{3}$ that of C3 vertebral body width or ≤ 5–7 mm†
- Prevertebral space at C5 is ≤ $\frac{5}{4}$ of (C5 or C6) vertebral body width or ≤ 14 mm†
- Predental space up to 5 mm in children ≤ 8 yr old (up to 3 mm in children > 8 yr old)
- Pseudo-Jefferson's fracture—C1 lateral masses grow faster than those of C2, so C1 overlaps C2 (usually < 6 mm); present in 90% of children age 1–2 yr, 18% of children age 7 yr
- Pseudosubluxation of C2/C3 or C3/C4 in 40% (normal variant in which anterior aspect of C2 spinolaminar line is ≤ 2 mm anterior or posterior to posterior cervical line)

*Injury can occur with minor trauma.
†These values can be unreliable in children.
Adapted from Rothrock SG: Pediatric Emergency Pocketbook, 5th ed. Tarascon Publishing, 2007, with permission.

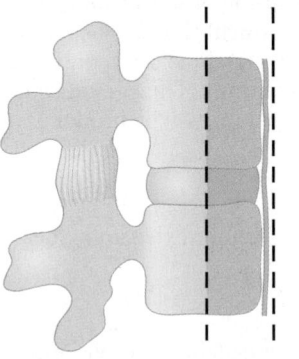
Anterior

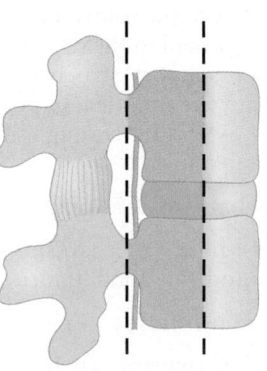
Middle

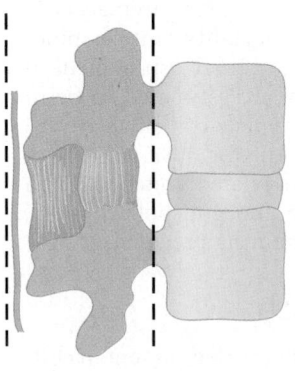
Posterior

FIGURE 23–1. The three-column model of Denis is shown with anterior, middle, and posterior columns. (From Garfin S, et al: Thoracic and upper lumbar spine injuries. *In* Browner BD, et al [eds]: Skeletal Trauma: Fractures, Dislocations, Ligamentous Injuries, 2nd ed. Philadelphia: WB Saunders, 1998.)

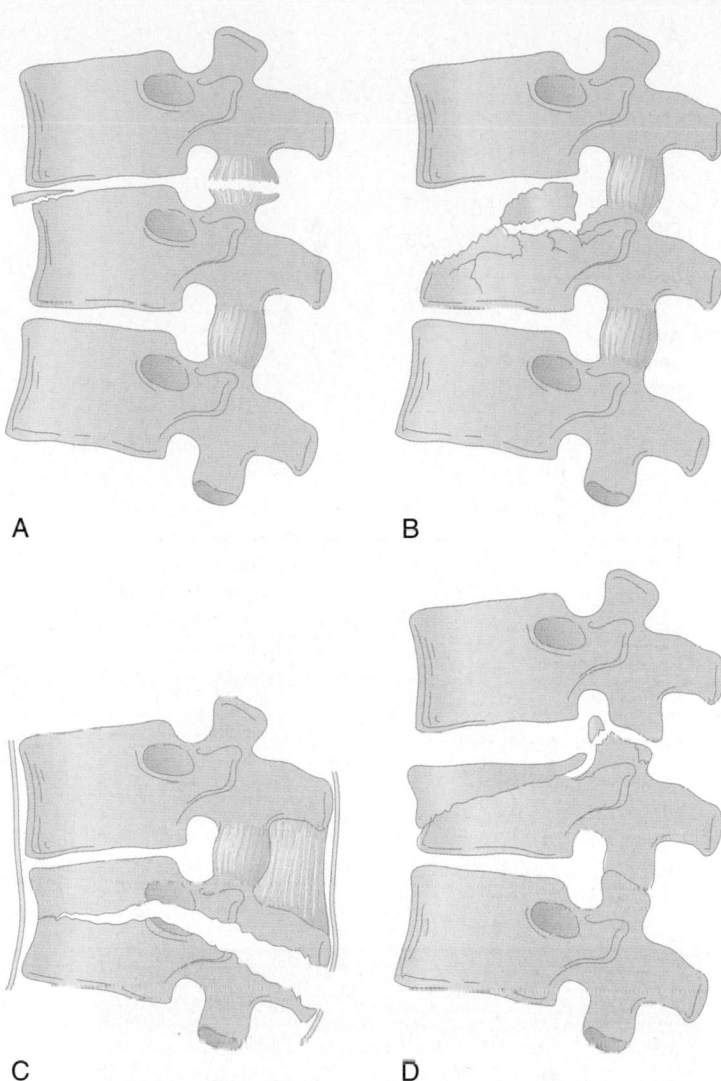

FIGURE 23–2. Daffner's flexion injuries can be further divided into simple (**A**), burst (**B**), distraction (**C**), and dislocation (**D**) patterns. (From Garfin S, et al: Thoracic and upper lumbar spine injuries. *In* Browner BD, et al [eds]: Skeletal Trauma: Fractures, Dislocations, Ligamentous Injuries, 2nd ed. Philadelphia: WB Saunders, 1998.)

sion injuries disrupt two or more columns and are unstable (Fig. 23–3). The radiographic findings of extension injuries include wide disk space, triangular avulsion fracture, retrolisthesis, neural arch fracture, and anterolithesis with normal interspinous space and spinolaminar line.

Shearing Injuries

Shearing injuries result from forces horizontally or obliquely directed upon the vertebral column with the lower body fixed. These injuries typically disrupt all three columns and are therefore unstable (Fig. 23–4). The radiographic findings demonstrate lateral distraction, lateral dislocation, and transverse process fractures.

Rotational Injuries

Rotational injuries result from a rotary or torsional force applied about the long axis of the vertebral column. An example is a heavy blow to the upper torso that compresses the vertebral column and flexes the torso laterally with the lower portion of the body in a fixed position. These injuries typically disrupt all three columns and are unstable (Fig. 23–5). The radiographic findings include rotation, dislocation, and facet/pillar fractures.

Spine Injuries Typically Seen in Children

Several specific injuries are seen in children. They include atlanto-occipital dislocation, atlas fractures, atlantoaxial subluxation, odontoid fractures, axis fractures, middle to lower cervical spine injuries, and thoracolumbar injuries.[5]

Atlanto-occipital dislocation is rarely seen as it is usually associated with brainstem injury and cardiorespiratory arrest. The atlanto-occipital articulation is less stable in children due to the relatively large head, small occipital condyles, and horizontal orientation of the joint. Therefore, the cranium moves with respect to the spine.

Fractures of the atlas are uncommon in young children, but are seen in teenagers after axial compression injuries such as those sustained while diving. Jefferson's or burst fracture involves fractures through the anterior and posterior arches.

Atlantoaxial subluxation occurs due to traumatic disruption of the transverse ligament. It is quite rare in children as an odontoid fracture is more likely to occur. The exception occurs in children with Down syndrome and connective tissue disorders.

Odontoid fractures occur uniquely in children. A cartilaginous synchondrosis between the odontoid and body

A

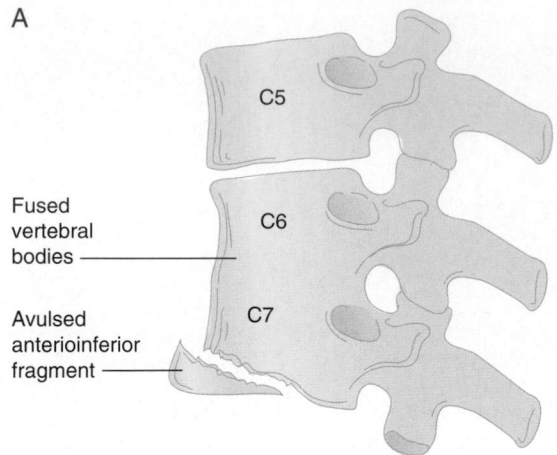

Fused vertebral bodies

Avulsed anterioinferior fragment

C5

C6

C7

B

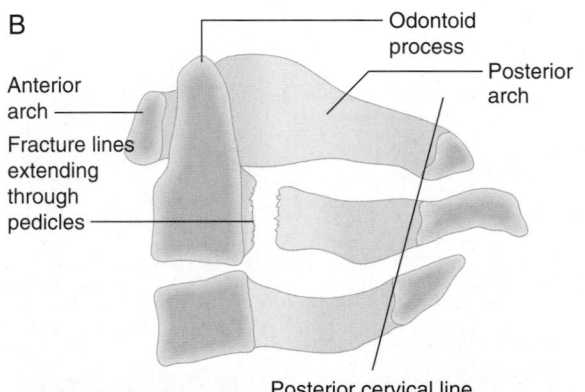

Anterior arch

Fracture lines extending through pedicles

Odontoid process

Posterior arch

Posterior cervical line

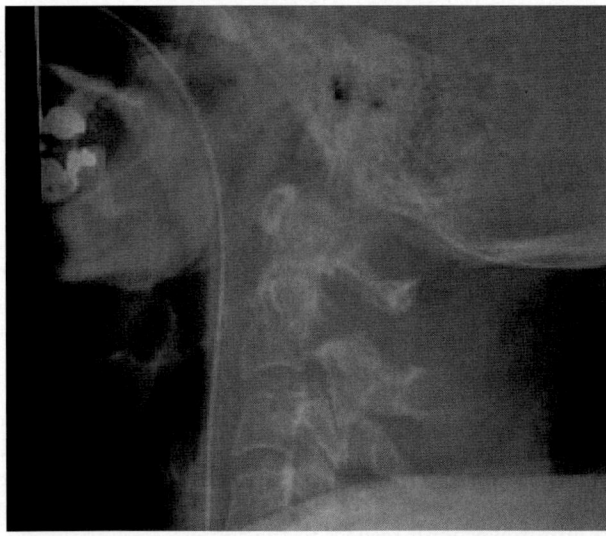

C

FIGURE 23–3. Extension injuries are stable if the posterior and middle columns remain intact. A small extension teardrop fracture is stable as it interrupts the anterior column only. This larger extension teardrop fracture (**A**) interrupts the anterior and middle column. The hangman's fracture (**B** and **C**) interrupts the middle column. Both are unstable. (**A** and **B** from Marx JA, Hockberger RS, Walls RM, et al [eds]: Rosen's Emergency Medicine: Concepts and Clinical Practice, 5th ed. St. Louis: Mosby, 2002; **C** courtesy of Stony Brook University Medical Center.)

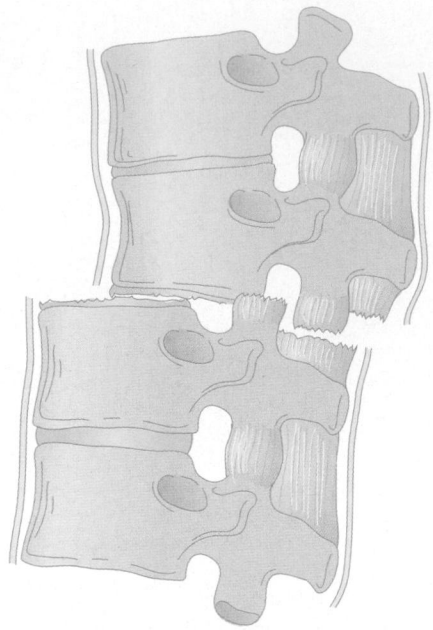

FIGURE 23–4. Shearing injuries disrupt all three columns and are unstable. (From Garfin S, et al: Thoracic and upper lumbar spine injuries. *In* Browner BD, et al [eds]: Skeletal Trauma: Fractures, Dislocations, Ligamentous Injuries, 2nd ed. Philadelphia: WB Saunders, 1998.)

exists until 5 to 7 years of age. Thus fractures occur through this growth plate until 7 years of age. They occur at the base of the odontoid in older children.[5]

The hangman's fracture is the typical axis fracture. It includes bilateral fracture of the pars interarticularis and anterior subluxation of C2 on C3.

Injuries to the middle and lower cervical spine are less common. They include facet disruption, compression fractures, and end plate injuries, of which injury of the inferior end plate is more common.

Vertebral injuries below the cervical spine are less common. Thoracic injuries predominately consist of compression fractures with anterior wedging. Lumbar injuries consist of anterior compression, burst fractures, isolated neural arch and transverse process fractures, Chance fractures, and Smith's fractures. Chance fractures were referred to earlier. They are horizontal fractures through the spinous process, pedicles, and posterior vertebral body. Smith's fractures are horizontal fractures through the spinous process, pedicles, and posterior spinal ligaments.

SCIWORA

Infants and children are prone to spinal cord injuries without radiologic abnormality (SCIWORA), meaning spinal cord injury without evidence of vertebral fracture or malalignment on plain radiographs or computed tomography (CT). The incidence is typically 16% to 19%, but has been reported as high as 65%.[4] It is predominately seen in children under 8 years.[4] SCIWORA likely occurs due to one of four mechanisms: longitudinal distraction, hyperflexion, hyperextension, or ischemic spinal cord injury.[4]

1. Longitudinal distraction causes SCIWORA by the following mechanism. The infantile bony spinal column is quite elastic and stretches approximately 5 cm prior

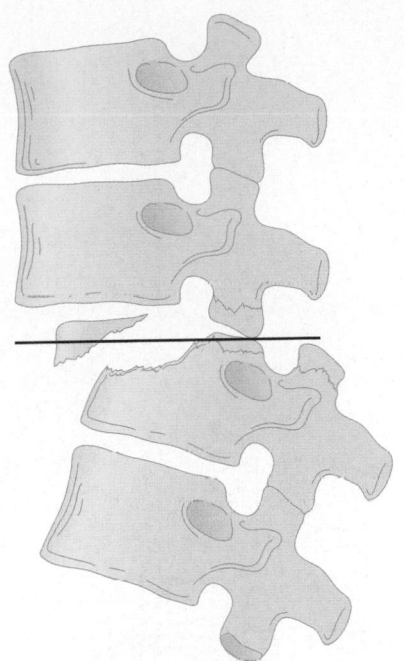 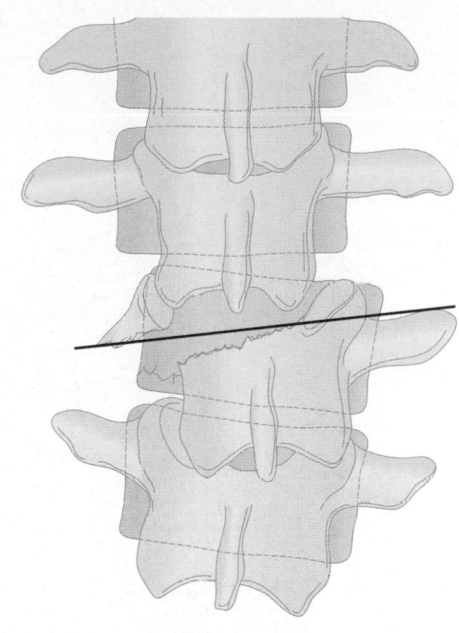

FIGURE 23–5. Rotational injuries injuries disrupt all three columns and are unstable. (From Garfin S, et al: Thoracic and upper lumbar spine injuries. *In* Browner BD, et al [eds]: Skeletal Trauma: Fractures, Dislocations, Ligamentous Injuries, 2nd ed. Philadelphia: WB Saunders, 1998.)

to disruption. The spinal cord is less pliable and is disrupted with as little as 5 mm of traction.

2. Hyperflexion can also contribute to SCIWORA. The combination of horizontally oriented facet joints and physiologic anterior wedging of the vertebral bodies allows for excessive forward flexion of the vertebrae, thus stretching the cord without disrupting the vertebral column.

3. Hyperextension of the cervical spine causes forward bulging of the interlaminar ligaments, which compress the cord without bony vertebral damage.

4. Direct vessel injury from compression, hypotension, and hypoperfusion can contribute to spinal cord infarction. Thus spinal cord injury can become apparent without bony trauma.

Injury to the spinal cord has the highest morbidity and mortality of vertebral trauma. The effect on the spinal cord includes both the direct trauma and the events that proceed the trauma. Spinal cord edema, decreased blood flow to the spinal cord, cell membrane disruption, ion and calcium fluxes, lipid peroxidation due to free radicals, and impaired prostaglandin synthesis produce secondary injury to the cord.[6,7] Appropriate evaluation and management are targeted toward reducing these secondary effects.

Evaluation

The evaluation of the patient with suspected vertebral or spinal cord injury begins during the initial stabilization. The child, guardian, and out-of-hospital providers should be questioned as to the mechanism of the injury, any neck or back pain, and any numbness or weakness, including transient symptoms. The complaint of transient pins and needles–like sensations to the extremities may represent SCIWORA.

The physical examination should include both a careful neck and neurologic evaluation. This examination should test for sensory and motor function (Fig. 23–6). By convention, a spinal cord injury is identified using the lowest functional level. Neurologic examination also includes a rectal examination, and evaluation for priapism and presence of the bulbocavernosus reflex. Absence of the bulbocavernosus reflex associated with hypotonia and areflexia indicates presence of spinal shock. Assessment of an injury level is unreliable until resolution of spinal shock, which may take up to 72 hours.[8]

Respiratory compromise is common after cervical spinal cord injuries and must be monitored. Normal breathing utilizes the diaphragm, intercostals, and abdominal muscles. When necessary, the accessory muscles can be recruited. With high cervical injuries, the accessory muscles operate alone, causing paradoxical abdominal breathing. The accessory muscles expand the thorax on inspiration, causing passive upward movement of the diaphragms and inversion of the abdomen. The reverse occurs with expiration. Paradoxical abdominal breathing is an ominous sign.[8]

Spinal cord injury may involve disruption in the descending sympathetic pathways. Hypotension can result from reduced vasomotor constrictor tone and bradycardia can result from unchecked vagal stimulation to the heart. Hypovolemic shock is another cause for hemodynamic instability.

Spinal Cord Injury Syndromes

There are five specific spinal cord injury syndromes: central cord syndrome, Brown-Séquard's syndrome, anterior spinal cord syndrome, complete spinal cord injury syndrome, and partial spinal cord injury syndrome.

In central cord syndrome, the damage involves the central part of the cervical spinal cord, thus interrupting the more medially placed fibers of the cervical roots. In this case the

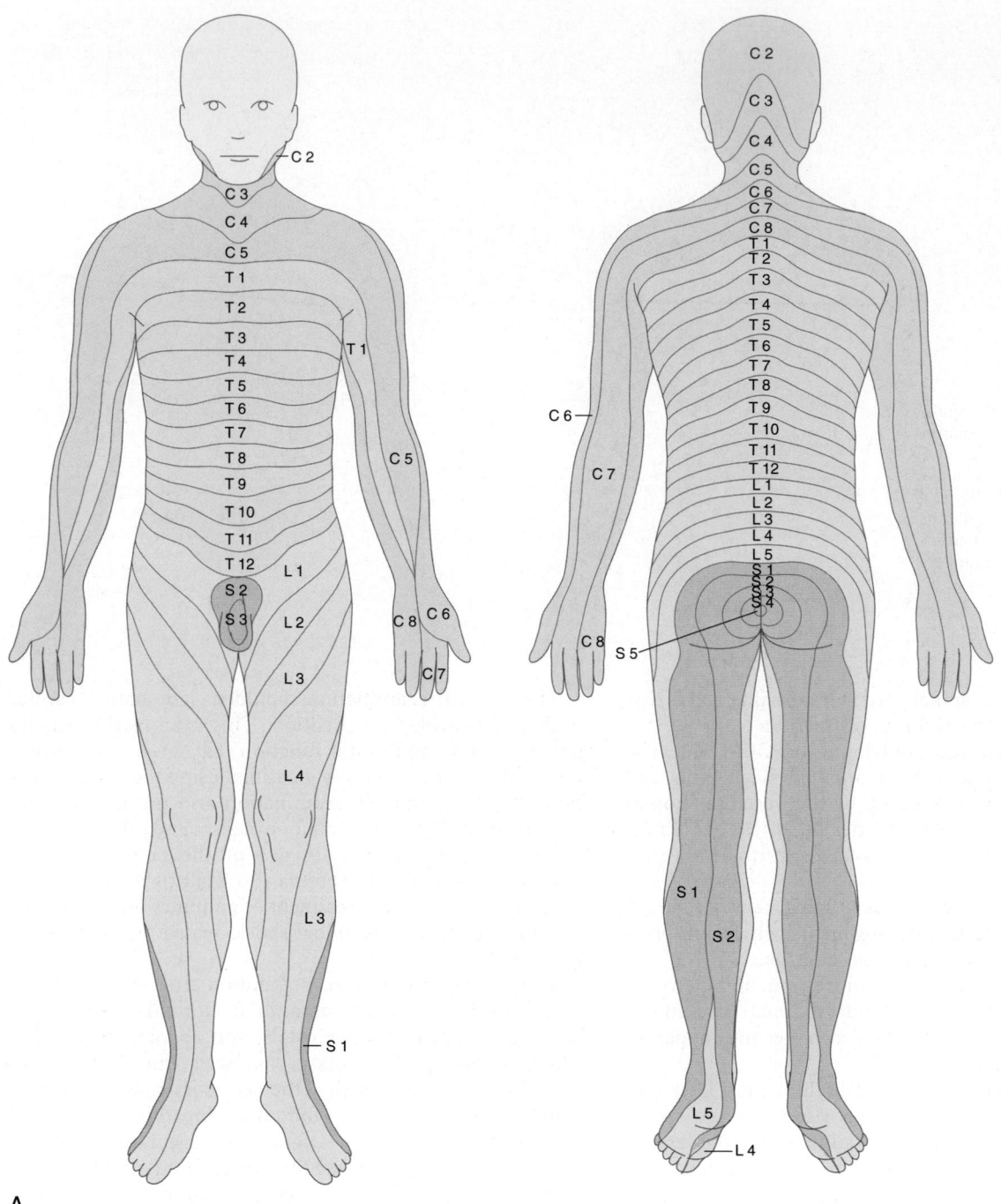

A

Cord Level	Muscles
C5	Elbow flexors (biceps, brachialis)
C6	Wrist extensors (extensor carpi radialis longus and brevis)
C7	Elbow extensors (triceps)
C8	Finger flexors to the middle finger (flexor digitorum profundus)
T1	Small finger abductors (abductor digiti minimi)
L2	Hip flexors (liliopsoas)
L3	Knee extensors (quadriceps)
L4	Ankle dorsiflextors (tibialis anterior)
L5	Long toe extensors (extensor hallucis longus)
S1	Ankle plantarflexors (gastrocnemius soleus)

B

FIGURE 23–6. The physical examination should test for sensory and motor function. **A,** Dermatomes of each spinal segment. **B,** Key muscles for testing motor function. (From Ferrera PC, et al [eds]: Trauma Management: An Emergency Medicine Approach. St. Louis: Mosby, 2001.)

upper limbs, especially the hands, are weaker than the lower limbs, which are often normal.

Brown-Séquard's syndrome is a situation in which damage produces a hemisection of the cord. There is motor loss on the ipsilateral side of the lesion and pain and temperature loss beginning one or two levels below the lesion on the opposite side.

If trauma produces disruption to the anterior spinal artery, there is an anterior spinal cord syndrome with only the dorsal columns being spared. These children may have complete paralysis and loss of pain and temperature sensation from that level down. Vibration, proprioception, and light touch are spared.

Complete spinal cord injury syndrome is the loss of function (motor, sensation, reflexes, rectal tone, and bowel/bladder function) below the injured level. Complete spinal cord injury is the most common spinal cord injury pattern in children. The reason for this is not completely clear, but it may be related to the immature spinal cord microvasculature in children.[1] Partial spinal cord injury syndrome includes a combination of symptoms that do not fit into any of the other syndromes.

Imaging Studies

The criteria for radiologic evaluation, as defined by the National Emergency X-Radiography Utilization Study (NEXUS) criteria,[9] include the presence of posterior midline tenderness, altered mental status due to either brain injury or intoxication, neurologic deficits, and distracting injuries.[10] This study, which evaluated presenting features of adults following trauma, also included 2160 patients 8 to 17 years old and 817 patients 2 to 8 years old with a total of 30 cervical spine injuries.[9] The criteria were 100% sensitive in detecting all cervical spine injuries at these ages. Importantly, only 88 patients less than 2 years old were included, limiting the applicability of these criteria to this age. For all infants and children, the total number of cervical spine injuries was small, with only 30 document injuries (1% of cases). To confirm that these criteria are highly sensitive, they need to be verified in large studies that include more injuries and a more diverse population.

To adequately evaluate the cervical spine, at least three views are required. The lateral view yields a sensitivity of 79% to 85% in children. The addition of the anteroposterior (AP) and open-mouth views increases sensitivity to 94%.[9] Thoracic and lumbar imaging includes AP and lateral views. If spinal injury is identified at one level, the entire spine should be imaged, as multilevel injury occurs in 16% of cases.[1]

CT should be employed in two situations: if additional detail of an injury is required for the management of the patient or to detect injuries that are highly suspect, but apparently absent on plain radiographs. The occiput through the second cervical level and the cervicothoracic junction are the anatomic areas where plain radiographs are not always reliable.[11]

Finally, children with neurologic deficits need the addition of magnetic resonance imaging. T1-weighting images emphasize the skeletal anatomy and demonstrate vertebral alignment and bony relationships to the spinal cord. T2-weighting images are useful for evaluating the interface of the cerebrospinal fluid and the extradural space, especially for patients with extradural compression from bone fragments.[12]

Evaluation of Spine Radiographs

Evaluation of spine radiographs should proceed in a systematic fashion. A useful system is the ABC'S[13,14]: adequacy and abnormalities of *a*lignment, abnormalities of *b*ony integrity, abnormalities of *c*artilage or joint space, and abnormalities of *s*oft tissues. First, the spine series must be adequate. On the lateral cervical view, all seven cervical vertebrae and the cervicothoracic junction should be visualized. If this is not the case, a swimmer's view or CT scan should be added.

Cervical spine radiographs are also inspected for alignment. On the lateral view, the anterior spinal line, the posterior spinal line, and the spinolaminar line should form smooth arcs. The spinolaminar line does not always intersect the base of the C2 spinous process, a normal variant called pseudosubluxation. Pseudosubluxation, an anterior displacement of C2 on C3 or of C3 on C4 of up to 4 mm, occurs in 40% of children up to age 7. The posterior cervical line (or line of Swischuk) helps differentiate pseudosubluxation from pathologic subluxation. A line drawn between the anterior cortices of the spinous processes of C1 and C3 should intersect or be less than 2 mm from the anterior cortex of the spinous process of C2; otherwise pathologic subluxation should be considered (Fig. 23–7).

Additionally, there should be no widening between spinous processes, the distance from the anterior arch of C1 to the odontoid should be no more than 5 mm, and the distance from the base of the clivus to the superior continuation of the line drawn from the posterior cortex of the body of C2 should be no more than 12 mm. On the AP projection, the spinous processes and facets should be in straight alignment and evenly spaced. Spinous process distance should vary by no more than 50% and should form a straight line. The open-mouth view is inspected for alignment of the lateral masses of C1 to the odontoid process and to the lateral margins of the articular surface of C2. The lateral masses may extend beyond these margins slightly, termed *pseudospread*, but should be less than 6 mm. Pseudospread is common up to 4 to 7 years of age.[8]

The lateral and AP views of the thoracic and lumbar spine are inspected for alignment. On the lateral view, the anterior, posterior, and spinolaminar lines should show parallel alignment. On the AP view, the lateral margins of the vertebral bodies, the position of the transverse processes, and the interspinous distance should be aligned.

Next, the bones are individually inspected. On the lateral projection of the cervical spine, the bones are inspected for superior or inferior end plate fractures. Also, the anterior vertebral body height should be no more than 3 mm less than the posterior height. Anterior wedging up to 3 mm may occur normally. In the lumbar and thoracic spines, abnormalities of bony integrity are usually obvious. The width of the interpediculate distance on the AP view and the posterior vertebral body line on the lateral view should be reviewed for any abnormalities. A difference of more than 3 mm between anterior and posterior vertebral body height is considered abnormal.

Cartilage and joint space abnormalities are considered next. The cervical, thoracic, and lumbar radiographs should be reviewed for widening or narrowing of the intervertebral disk space, widening of the facet joint, or widening of the interspinous distance on both AP and lateral views.

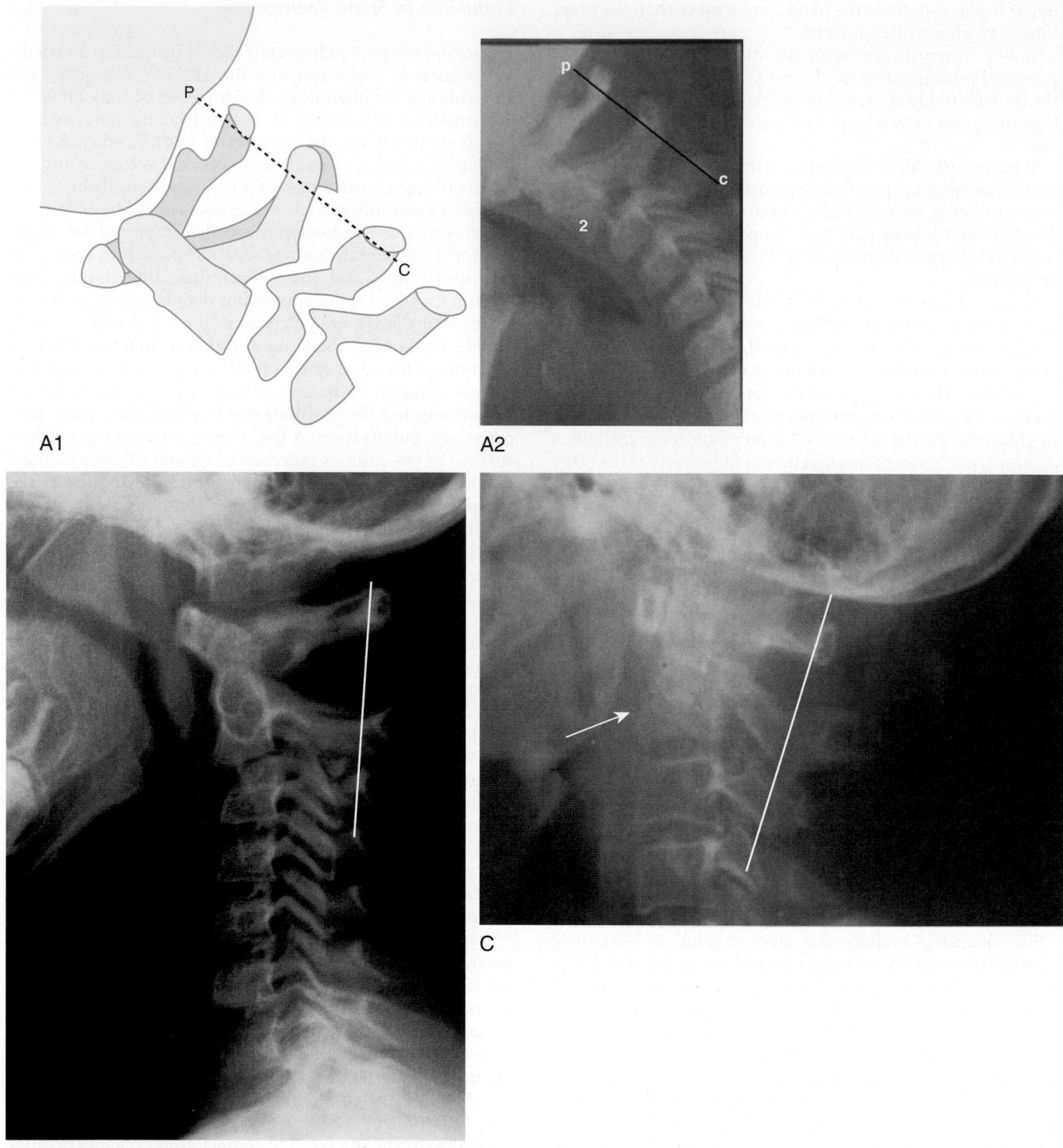

FIGURE 23–7. Spinolaminar line. **A,** Diagram of spinolaminar line. **B,** Radiograph demonstrating pseudosubluxation of C2 on C3. Note the the anterior cortex of the spinous process for C2 is less than 2 mm from the posterior cervical line (the line connecting the anterior cortex of the first and third cervical spinous processes). **C,** Odontoid fracture; note the abnormal spinolaminar line and the irregular suspicious line through the body of C2 *(arrow)*. (**A** and **C** courtesy of Stony Brook University Medical Center; **B** from Grainger RG, Allison DJ, Dixon AK [eds]: Grainger & Allison's Diagnostic Radiology: A Textbook of Medical Imaging, 4th ed. New York: Churchill Livingstone, 2001, p 2139. Copyright © 2001 Churchill Livingstone, Inc; from the MD Consult website.)

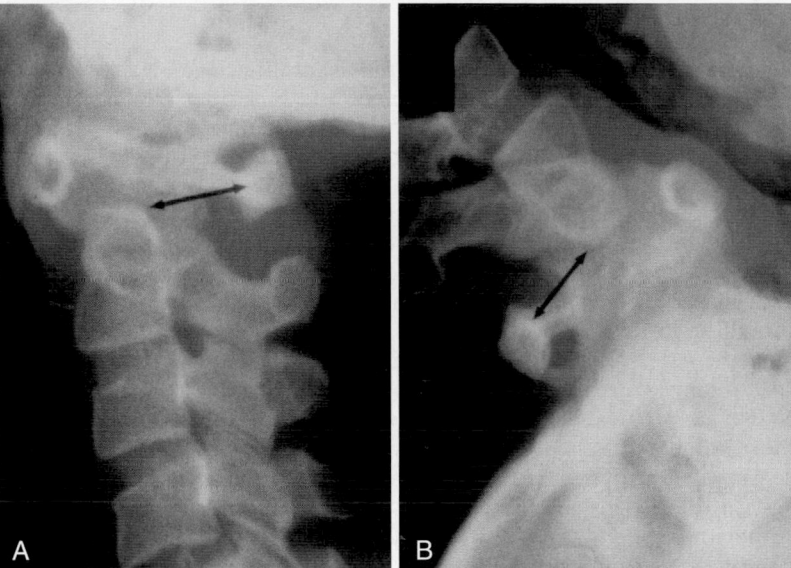

FIGURE 23–8. Extension **(A)** and flexion **(B)** lateral cervical radiographs of an adolescent boy with an os odontoideum and a progressive decrease in exercise tolerance. Note decrease in the space available for the spinal cord (*arrow*). Because the ossicle of the odontoid moves with the ring of C1, it is not possible to measure the atlantodential interval. (From Herman MJ, Pizzutillo PD: Cervical spine disorders in children. Orthop Clin North Am 30:460, 1999.)

Finally, the radiographs should be inspected for soft tissue abnormalities. The cervicocranial prevertebral soft tissue contour should follow the contour of the anterior cortex of the atlas and axis. The width of the soft tissues at C2 is no more than 7 mm, although this is influenced by neck posture or crying, and that at C6 should be no more than 14 mm. Thoracic and lumbar radiographs can demonstrate a paraspinal soft tissue mass or loss of the psoas stripe on the AP views.

Evidence of Spine Injuries Typically Seen in Children

Radiographic evidence of those injuries typically seen in children (atlanto-occipital dislocation, atlas fractures, atlantoaxial subluxation, odontoid fractures, axis fractures, middle to lower cervical spine injuries, and thoracolumbar injuries) is as follows.

Atlanto-occipital dislocation includes widening of the gap between the occipital condyles and the condylar surface of the atlas to more than 5 mm or a distance of greater than 12 mm between the tip of the clivus and a line drawn along the posterior cortex of the body of the axis.

Jefferson's or burst fractures show bilateral offset of the lateral masses with respect to the odontoid.

Atlantoaxial subluxation demonstrates greater than 5 mm of distance between the anterior arch of the atlas and the odontoid on the lateral view.

Odontoid fractures show prevertebral soft tissue swelling on the lateral radiograph and subtle lucency through the base of the odontoid on open-mouth view. The hangman's fracture is a fracture through the pedicle of C2 and is best seen on the lateral radiograph. Os odontoideum is a condition in which the dens is separated from the axis body. This disorder once was thought to be a congenital failure of fusion of the dens to the axis. Now, it is believed to be due to a prior fracture of the odontoid synchondrosis before its closure at age 5 to 6 years. Os odontoideum appears as an ossicle that is separated from the axis by a large gap (Fig. 23–8). The border of the ossicle does not directly match up with the axis body.

Impingement of the upper cervical cord or vertebral artery can occur due to hypermobility at C1-2. In contrast, ossiculum terminale is due to failure of the secondary ossification center of the dens to fuse with the base of the odontoid. Persistent ossiculum terminale is differentiated from os odontoideum by its ossicle, which is much smaller and is at the tip of the dens. Ossiculum terminale, unlike os odontoideum, is not associated with significant instability.

Compression fractures of the middle and lower cervical spine are seen on the lateral radiograph. Although underossification of growth plates can be misleading, greater than 50% of anterior wedging is pathologic. Vertebral end plate injuries are also obvious on lateral radiographs but should not be confused with secondary centers of ossification, which appear between 10 and 12 years of age.

Anterior wedge fractures are observed on the lateral thoracic spine radiograph when the difference in height between the anterior and posterior cortices is greater than 3 mm. Anterior wedge fractures are similarly observed on the lateral lumbar spine radiographs, and can be distinguished from burst fractures as the latter show disruption of the posterior cortex of the vertebral body, as well as widening of the interpedicular distance on the AP view.

Associated Injuries

Children with spinal injuries should also be evaluated for associated injuries. Children with spinal injuries have associated head injuries in 25% to 50% of cases, extremity fractures in 30% of cases, and chest and abdominal injuries in 21% of cases.[5] Abdominal injuries of the small bowel are associated with seat belt fractures of the thoracolumbar spine. Children who fall or jump from a height and land on their feet should be examined for calcaneal, ankle, and thoracolumbar spine injuries.[5] Finally, a high index of suspicion should be held for nonaccidental trauma in the setting of vertebral injuries. Both vertebral body fractures and subluxation have moderate specificity for child abuse. They are highly specific when the history of trauma is absent or inconsistent.[15]

Management

The management of vertebral trauma is multifaceted. It begins in the field. Airway management and breathing are the first clinical priorities. Adequate airway management also helps prevent secondary injury to the spinal cord from hypoxia.

During airway interventions, manipulation of the spine should be minimized. Basic airway techniques include chin lift, jaw thrust, and placement of oropharyngeal and nasopharyngeal airways. Placement of an oropharyngeal airway should be avoided in a patient with an intact gag reflex as movement during gagging and vomiting could worsen spinal cord injury. Initially, supplemental oxygen should be delivered by non-rebreather mask; if ventilations are not adequate, they should be assisted by a bag-valve mask. There is some degree of controversy as to which method of intubation is best in the patient with spinal cord injury. However, most authorities agree that the technique with which one is most familiar should be used.[16] This typically involves orotracheal intubation facilitated by rapid sequence induction. Manual in-line stabilization must be maintained by a second team member during any airway intervention.[16,17]

Circulation should also be attended to early in the management. Bleeding must be controlled, and volume replaced with crystalloid fluids initially and then blood, if indicated, to maintain hemodynamic stability.

Before transport, patients with suspected vertebral trauma should be properly immobilized. Immobilization includes a rigid cervical collar, short and long backboards, and cervical blocks. Ideally, if time allows and the child is without immediate life-threatening injuries, the cervical collar is placed and the short board immobilizer is used to maintain vertebral alignment during extrication. The child is then transferred to the long board, cervical blocks are placed, and straps are engaged. In children up to 6 years of age, the occiput is large relative to the torso and therefore a pad is placed behind the child's shoulders to prevent flexion of the spine.[18] Thus criteria for immobilizing the child's cervical spine should be evidence based, such as the criteria introduced by the NEXUS study.[10,18-20]

In the emergency department, airway, breathing, and circulation, with maintenance of spine stabilization, should again be evaluated. Hemodynamic instability can also occur after spinal cord trauma. Neurogenic shock is one possible etiology. Hypovolemic shock may be another cause for hemodynamic instability and should be ruled out systematically. The child should be placed on continuous cardiac monitoring, and either an indwelling arterial catheter or a noninvasive blood pressure cuff recording pressures every 5 minutes should be instituted. If neurogenic shock is considered and hemorrhagic shock has been excluded, bradycardia should be treated with atropine 0.02 mg/kg and hypotension managed initially with fluids and then α-agonists (e.g., phenylephrine).[21]

Neurologic deterioration occurs rostrally and may be due to spinal cord edema, hemorrhage, or mechanical and/or physiologic secondary insults. If deterioration is apparent, magnetic resonance imaging should be obtained to evaluate for disk herniation, epidural hematoma, or vascular injury to the vertebral arteries. Surgical intervention should be expedited in these circumstances.[12,22]

Next, the patient should be removed from the uncushioned backboard at the earliest convenience. Insensate skin of the child with spinal cord injury is rapidly susceptible to pressure sores.[8]

Finally, the pharmacologic therapy for spinal cord injury should be addressed. While pharmacology at this point can do little to reverse the primary injury to the spinal cord, it can be used to reduce secondary damage from spinal cord edema, cell membrane damage, lipid peroxidation, and prostaglandin synthesis. The second National Acute Spinal Cord Injury Study (NASCIS II) compared high-dose methylprednisolone with naloxone and placebo. The results demonstrated a statistically significant improvement in motor abilities after long-term follow-up. However, positive results were only found after post hoc subset analysis.[6] Recent studies have been less supportive of the benefits of steroids. They have shown no benefit from steroids and have shown an increased risk of pneumonia, sepsis, myopathy, myelopathy (nerve degeneration), decreased spinal blood flow, increased hospital length of stay, and increased cost. Moreover, no patients under 13 years old were included in these studies.

The treatment guidelines for spinal cord injuries should be multidisciplinary and institutionally supported.[23-25] Currently, several specialty societies state that steroid treatment is experimental and not the standard of care, including the American Academy of Emergency Medicine, the California Association of Emergency Physicians, the Canadian Association of Emergency Physicians, the Canadian Spine Society, and the Canadian Neurosurgical Society. Seventy-five percent of British and most European spine centers do not use steroids for acute spinal cord injury.[26] Due to the controversy surrounding the use of steroids, each institution should reach a consensus with its trauma and neurosurgical experts regarding their use. For those sites using steroids, ASCISS III further defined the duration of treatment based upon time of onset. Within 3 hours of injury, the child with spinal cord injury should receive 30 mg/kg of methylprednisolone over 15 minutes, followed in 45 minutes by a 23-hour infusion of 5.4 mg/kg/hr. If the patient is between 3 and 8 hours postinjury, a 48-hour course is given.[7]

The operative management of vertebral and spinal cord injuries is at the discretion of the spine surgeon or neurosurgeon. Nonoperative treatment is usually recommended for stable injuries such as compression fractures with less than 50% loss of body height or SCIWORA injuries with complete neurologic deficits. Unstable fractures and those with worsening neurologic deficits require surgical management.[27] The timing of the surgery depends on the overall condition of the patient and occurs after open fractures and head, thoracic, abdominal, tibia, femur, and pelvis injuries have been stabilized.[8]

Summary

Patterns of injury with vertebral and spinal cord injuries in children vary from those of adults. Knowledge of the anatomic differences in children helps in understanding these differences and predicting findings. Evaluation involves meticulous gathering of history and physical examination combined with radiologic imaging when indicated. Management should focus on airway, breathing, and circulation;

preventing and reducing secondary injuries; and identifying other threatening injuries.

The most effective strategy is prevention. As motor vehicle accidents are frequently responsible, attention has been paid to this mechanism. Proper child restraint mechanisms offer the greatest potential for reducing needless injuries. The appropriate restraint mechanism varies in infants, toddlers, school-age children, and adolescents as the center of gravity migrates from head to pelvis. Infants and toddlers (ages birth to 3 years) should be placed in a child safety seat. At this age, the proportionately larger head produces a high center of gravity. School-age children (ages 4 to 9 years) should be placed in a booster seat. The center of gravity moves toward the umbilicus at this age. Also, the iliac crests are not developed enough to hold the lap belt, and so it slides up over the abdomen if the child is placed in the standard seat. Adolescents (ages 10 years and up) can be restrained as would be an adult. Their center of gravity is lower and their iliac crests are adequately developed.[15]

REFERENCES

*1. Osenbach RK, Menezes AH: Pediatric spinal cord and vertebral column injury. Neurosurgery 30:385–390, 1992.
2. Daffner RH, Deeb ZL, Rothfus WE: "Fingerprints" of vertebral trauma—a unifying concept based on mechanism. Skeletal Radiol 15:518–525, 1986.
*3. Denis F: Spinal instability as defined by the three column spine concept in acute trauma. Clin Orthop 189:65, 1984.
4. Kriss VM, Kriss TC: SCIWORA (spinal cord injury without radiologic abnormality) in infants and children. Clin Pediatr 35:119–124, 1996.
5. Roche C, Carty H: Spinal trauma in children. Pediatr Radiol 31:677–700, 2001.
6. Bracken MB, Shepard MJ, Collins WF, et al: A randomized, controlled trial of methylprednisolone or naloxone in the treatment of acute spinal-cord injury. N Engl J Med 322:1405–1411, 1990.
*7. Bracken MB, Shepard MJ, Holford TR, et al: Administration of methylprednisolone for 24 to 48 hours or tirilazad mesylate for 48 hours in the treatment of acute spinal cord injury. JAMA 277:1597–1604, 1997.
*8. Patel RV, DeLong W, Vresilovic EJ: Evaluation and treatment of spinal injuries in the patient with polytrauma. Clin Orthop Rel Res 422:43–54, 2004.

*9. Viccellio P, Simon H, Pressman BD, et al: A prospective multicenter study of cervical spine injury in children. Pediatrics 108:e20, 2001.
*10. Hoffman JR, Wolfson AB, Todd K, Mower WR: Selective cervical spine radiography of blunt trauma victims: results of the National Emergency X-Radiography Utilization Study (NEXUS). Acad Emerg Med 6:451, 1999.
11. Cassar-Pullicino VN: Spinal injury: optimizing the imaging options. Eur J Radiol 42:85–91, 2002.
12. Keiper MD, Zimmerman RA, Bilaniuk LT: MRI in the assessment of the supportive soft tissues of the cervical spine in acute trauma in children. Neuroradiology 40:359–363, 1998.
*13. Driscoll PA, Ross R, Nicholson DA: ABC of emergency radiography: cervical spine I. BMJ 307:785–789, 1993.
*14. Driscoll PA, Ross R, Nicholson DA: ABC of emergency radiography: cervical spine II. BMJ 307:855–859, 1993.
15. Behrooz AA: Pediatric spine fractures. Orthop Clin North Am 30:521–536, 1999.
*16. Walls RM: Airway management in the blunt trauma patient: how important is the cervical spine? Can J Surg 35:27–34, 1992.
17. Rhee KJ, Green W, Holcroft JW, Mangili JA: Oral intubation in the multiply injured patient: the risk of exacerbating spinal cord damage. Ann Emerg Med 19:511–514, 1990.
18. Kish DL: Prehospital management of spinal trauma: an evolution. Crit Care Nurs Q 22:36–43, 1999.
19. Hauswald M, Ong G, Tandberg D, Omar Z: Out-of-hospital spinal immobilization: its effect on neurologic injury. Acad Emerg Med 5:214–218, 1998.
20. Orledge JD, Pepe PE: Out of hospital spinal immobilization: is it really necessary? Acad Emerg Med 5:203–204, 1998.
21. Vale FL, Burns J, Jackson AB, Hadley MN: Combined medical and surgical treatment after acute spinal cord injury: results of a prospective pilot study to assess the merits of aggressive medical resuscitation and blood pressure management. J Neurosurg 87:239–246, 1997.
22. Harrop JS, Sharan AD, Vaccaro AR, Przybylski GJ: The cause of neurologic deterioration after acute cervical spinal cord injury. Spine 26:340–346, 2001.
23. George ER, Scholten DJ, Buechler CM, et al: Failure of methylprednisolone to improve the outcome of spinal cord injuries. Am Surg 61:659–663, 1995.
24. Galandiuk S, Raque G, Appel S, Polk HC Jr: The two-edged sword of large dose steroids for spinal cord trauma. Ann Surg 218:419–425, 1993.
*25. Petitjean ME, Pointillart V, Dixmerias F, et al: Medical treatment of spinal cord injury in the acute stage. Ann Fr Anesth Reanim 17:114–122, 1998.
26. Nichols K, Brown A, Sett P: Special feature: spinal cord injury—the condition and its acute management. Hosp Pharmacist 12:91–94, 2005.
27. Vaccaro AR, Daugherty RJ, Sheehan TP, et al: Neurologic outcome of early versus late surgery for cervical spinal cord injury. Spine 22:2609–2613, 1997.

*Suggested readings.

Chapter 24

Thoracic Trauma

Barbara E. McDevitt, MD, George L. Foltin, MD,
and Arthur Cooper, MD, MS

Key Points

Thoracic trauma is the second leading cause of death in children after trauma to the central nervous system.

There are anatomic and physiologic differences between children and adults that impact on both diagnosis and management.

The chest roentgenogram remains the number one screening modality for the evaluation of thoracic injury, but it is crucial that evidence-based criteria be developed to select the most appropriate and sensitive of the rapidly developing armory of diagnostic modalities.

The physician assessing the pediatric patient must recognize the need for acute intervention in life-threatening thoracic injuries, particularly with regard to tracheal intubation, chest decompression and drainage, volume resuscitation, and, in rare instances, pericardial decompression and resuscitative thoracotomy.

The differential diagnosis of immediate life-threatening thoracic injuries is challenging, and is best accomplished through a systematic approach.

The majority of thoracic injuries can be managed conservatively, the most common intervention being a thoracostomy tube.

It is essential to be aware of the probability of coexisting injuries.

Pediatric patients with life-threatening thoracic injuries must be stabilized, then transported to trauma centers with pediatric capabilities, when such resources are not available on site.

Introduction and Background

Trauma remains the leading cause of death in the pediatric population between 1 and 14 years of age, resulting in more fatalities than all other diseases combined. Traumatic brain injury is the foremost killer in this age group, but thoracic trauma is the second most important source of lethal injury in children. Although it is important to recognize that, in contrast to adult trauma, pediatric trauma is primarily a disease of the airway and breathing, rather than of the circulation, it is also important to understand that the observed derangements of airway and breathing in injured children typically have a neuroventilatory cause, rather than a cardiorespiratory cause. In other words, observed derangements of airway and breathing in pediatric trauma patients stem far more often from the cardiorespiratory effects of traumatic brain injury than from thoracic injuries.

Historical data from the National Pediatric Trauma Registry, which was comprised mostly of pediatric trauma centers from children's specialty units, show that major thoracic trauma is relatively uncommon in children, occurring as the only body region injured in only 1%, but as the principal anatomic diagnosis in approximately 6%, of children admitted to pediatric trauma hospitals. Yet, the case fatality rates associated with these injuries have been shown to be as high as 15%, and may increase significantly when injury to other organ systems is present, although thoracic injury itself is rarely the proximate cause of death. Hence, physicians caring for injured children must be familiar with the recognition, evaluation, and management of thoracic injury in children, as well as the mechanisms of injury that result in thoracic trauma.[1-8] These will vary by age, geographic location, and trends in popular sports, as well as community compliance with injury prevention measures. Blunt trauma is the most frequent cause, though penetrating trauma regrettably afflicts the adolescent population. Because of anatomic, physiologic, and epidemiologic differences, children must be assessed and managed differently from adults. The development of a systematic diagnostic approach to the evaluation of thoracic injuries in children continues to evolve as better diagnostic modalities emerge.

Blunt thoracic injuries outnumber penetrating thoracic injuries by a ratio of 5 : 1. Together, motor vehicle occupant and pedestrian injuries account for about three fourths of all blunt thoracic injuries in children. Falls, bicycle and motorcycle accidents, and miscellaneous injuries account for the remainder. Gunshot and stab wounds are responsible for nearly all penetrating injuries, in a ratio of slightly less than 2 : 1. About one in six children with an intrathoracic injury will die, but those with blunt injuries die mostly from associated injuries, while those with penetrating injuries die nearly always from the injury itself.[1]

However, data from the National Trauma Data Bank™ (*http://www.ntdb.org*), which currently comprises the largest repository of pediatric trauma registry data available worldwide, reflect a somewhat older population than its forerunner, the National Pediatric Trauma Registry, consistent with the far greater number, and proportion, of general trauma centers that contribute to this database. As of 2006, this database contained 241,457 pediatric cases from 612 North American trauma centers, of whom 31,138 (13%) had thoracic injuries. Of these, 59% had injuries to the chest wall or diaphragm, 38% had injuries to the lungs, 3% had injuries to the heart, and <1% had injuries to the tracheobronchial tree or the esophagus. By contrast, among those who died with thoracic injuries, 51% had injuries to the chest wall or diaphragm, 39% had injuries to the lungs, 9% had injuries to the heart, and <1% had injuries to the tracheobronchial tree or the esophagus, findings which do not differ statistically versus survivors, but for the greater lethality of cardiac injuries.

Recognition and Approach

Specific attention to the diagnosis and treatment of the injured child has resulted in significant decreases in the morbidity and mortality of all traumatic injuries, including those to the pediatric cardiorespiratory system. This has been achieved by developing standards of care for injured children that build upon the American College of Surgeons Committee on Trauma's Advanced Trauma Life Support® (ATLS®) protocols for the injured adult, but address the special problems encountered in the pediatric population, best described in the American Heart Association and American Academy of Pediatrics Pediatric Advanced Life Support guidelines.[9,10] As a result, the primary survey in children, which remains directed toward priority assessment and stabilization of airway, breathing, and circulation, applies these principles based upon key pediatric differences in anatomy and physiology that require a modified approach. For this reason, a firm understanding of the pathophysiology unique to pediatric thoracic trauma is paramount.

As with other body regions in pediatric patients, the bony and cartilaginous structures of the chest wall in childhood are fairly flexible, and therefore less likely to fracture. However, the rarity of chest wall fractures in the pediatric population is a double-edged sword, for kinetic energy is absorbed when a bone breaks. Absent such fractures, forces of injury are not absorbed by the body's outer shell, but directed toward its inner assets. Since the child's thinner muscles also offer less protection to the thoracic and abdominal organs, underlying lung tissue is frequently bruised by the transmitted forces. As a result, pulmonary contusions,

which can cause ventilation-perfusion mismatch and arterial hypoxemia, are the most common life-threatening thoracic injuries found in the pediatric population, and threaten respiration in all children with major thoracic trauma.[11-13]

Another unique feature of the pediatric chest wall is the high elastin content of the mediastinum and its structures. This makes the mediastinum both more mobile and more susceptible to wide shifts, which can lead to a significant compromise of major organs and vessels in the presence of extrapulmonary collections of air or blood within the thorax, such as those associated with pneumothorax and hemothorax, especially if under tension. Tension pneumothorax, in particular, is especially poorly tolerated by children, and can predispose to rapid demise due to both ventilatory and circulatory compromise, as the contralateral lung is compressed and the venae cavae are torsed at the thoracic inlets, causing both profound respiratory distress, and obstructive shock due to impeded venous return.

Children sustaining blunt trauma also experience significant aerophagia, with subsequent gastric dilation. As children are diaphragmatic breathers, owing to the more horizontal alignment of their ribs and the relative weakness of their intercostal muscles, gastric dilation, by pushing upward on the diaphragm, decreases vital capacity and impairs both spontaneous and assisted ventilation. At the same time, since children have both a larger oxygen consumption and a smaller functional residual capacity than adults, they are more susceptible to hypoxemia. This is especially problematic in physiologically stressed infants, whose diaphragmatic muscles often tire quickly, causing sudden apnea.

Cardiac function in children initially may be able to compensate for hypoxemia. Cardiac output in children is maintained chiefly through increases in heart rate, since the smaller chamber size and thicker ventricular walls decrease myocardial compliance, thereby limiting the compensatory potential of Starling forces. When hypoxemia is present, the child's body first responds with a reflex tachycardia. Gastric dilation therefore further compromises resuscitation following major thoracic trauma through the vagally mediated decreases in heart rate commonly observed in small children with gastric distention.

Cardiac function in children may also be able to compensate for up to a 40% blood loss. This can lead to initial underestimation of the child's degree of hypovolemia due to major hemorrhage. Fortunately, most intrathoracic bleeding is self-limited. The lungs fill most of the thorax, hence are the most common source of hemorrhage. However, they contain an abundant supply of tissue thromboplastins in pulmonary parenchyma, with the result that most bleeding rapidly stops. Injuries to intrathoracic vessels, including both the heart and great vessels, well protected as they are by the sternum and the spine, and to the somewhat less well protected intercostal vessels, are the exception to the rule that most intrathoracic bleeding is self-limited, since vascular hemorrhage rarely stops spontaneously. Moreover, as children have a blood volume comprising some 8% of their total body mass, which slightly exceeds that of adults, a greater proportion of blood must be lost before hypovolemia becomes evident, which can also contribute to a missed diagnosis of shock. Thus, failure to account for the vigorous compensatory response to hypovolemia, and the proportionately larger blood loss needed to produce shock, may each forestall early intervention to prevent circulatory collapse.

Evaluation

Trauma to the chest may involve injury to the thoracic cage and its contents, including the lungs, heart, great vessels, tracheobronchial tree, and esophagus. Injuries to these organs may manifest acutely during the primary survey, or their presentation may be gradual and insidious and only diagnosed by a careful secondary survey. Continuous evaluations are mandatory once the child is admitted to the hospital for treatment.[14]

Injuries to the thorax can cause sudden and significant cardiorespiratory compromise almost immediately. If not recognized and promptly treated, the result may be lethal. It is therefore imperative for the treating physician to detect all underlying injuries, decide the priority of treatment, and begin to reverse the pathophysiologic changes induced by the injuries. The American College of Surgeons Committee on Trauma's ATLS® protocol includes a standardized assessment of the patient's airway, breathing, and circulation that should enable the treating physician to recognize, evaluate, and manage life-threatening thoracic injuries in priority sequence, as shown in Table 24–1.[9] Immediately life-threatening injuries to the airway (obstruction), breathing (tension pneumothorax, flail chest, open pneumothorax), and circulation (massive hemothorax, cardiac tamponade) can usually be detected during the primary survey. Potentially life-threatening injuries to the airway (tracheobronchial disruption), breathing (pulmonary contusion, traumatic diaphragmatic hernia, traumatic asphyxia), and circulation (blunt cardiac injury, aortic disruption) are more often detected during the secondary survey, as are injuries that affect multiple intrathoracic structures (such as mediastinal traversing injuries), and injuries that affect the integrity of the alimentary canal (esophageal disruption) and present with sepsis if initially overlooked.

Clinical Evaluation[9]

In performing the primary survey, the treating physician will look first for airway patency and maintainability, as judged by the absence of abnormal nasopharyngeal or oropharyngeal sounds (snoring, gurgling, stridor, or hoarseness) and the presence of spontaneous air movement at the nares. Next assessed is breathing, through evaluation of ventilation (chest rise, air entry, respiratory effort and rate) and oxygenation (central skin and mucous membrane color, sensorium). Last assessed is circulation, through examination for major hemorrhage (external and internal), as well as tissue perfusion (pulse rate and character, peripheral skin and mucous membrane color, temperature and moisture, capillary refill, urinary output). This is because hypotension (the cardinal sign of decompensated shock) does not occur until very late in the downward spiral of circulatory deterioration, when the opportunities for successful resuscitation are limited.

Ensuring an open airway and facilitating adequate gas exchange are the major goals of treatment during the primary survey. Failure to detect the most common immediate life-threatening thoracic injury, tension pneumothorax, which can cause sudden and severe respiratory and circulatory

Table 24–1 Principles of Advanced Trauma Life Support® (ATLS®)[9]

Primary Survey and Resuscitation

Airway/cervical spine
- Open: jaw thrust/spine stabilization
- Clear: suction/remove particulate matter
- Support: oropharyngeal/nasopharyngeal airway
- Establish: orotracheal/nasotracheal intubation*
- Maintain: primary/secondary confirmation†
- Bypass: needle/surgical cricothyroidotomy

Breathing/chest wall
- Ventilation: chest rise/air entry/effort/rate
- Oxygenation: central color/pulse oximetry
- Support: distress → NRB/failure → BVM
- Chest wall: ensure integrity/expand lungs
  - Tension pneumothorax: needle, chest tube§
  - Open pneumothorax: occlude, chest tube
  - Massive hemothorax: volume, chest tube

Circulation/external bleeding
- Stop bleeding: direct pressure, avoid clamps
- Shock evaluation: pulse, skin perfusion, CRT, LOC¶
- Blood pressure: avoid over/undercorrection
  - Infant/child: low normal ≥ 70 + (age × 2) mm Hg
  - Adolescent: low normal ≥ 90 mm Hg or significant change
- Volume resuscitation: Ringer's lactate (RL) → packed red blood cells (PRBC)
  - Infant/child: 20 ml/kg RL, repeat × 1–2 → 10 ml/PRBC
  - Adolescent: 1–2 L RL, repeat × 1–2 → 1–2 U PRBC

Disability/mental status
- Pupils: symmetry, reaction
- LOC: GCS
  - Track and trend as a vital sign
  - Significant change ≥ 2 points
  - Intubate for coma (GCS ≤ 8) or significant change
- Motor: strength, symmetry
- Abnormality/deterioration: call neurosurgeon
  - Mild TBI (GCS 14–15): observe, consider CT for history of LOC
  - Moderate TBI (GCS 9–13): admit, obtain CT, repeat CT 12–24 hr
  - Severe TBI (GCS 3–8): intubate, ventilate, obtain CT, repeat CT 12–24 hr

Exposure and environment
- Disrobe: cut off clothes
- Logroll: requires four people
- Screening examination: front and back
- Avoid hypothermia: keep patient warm!

Adjuncts (Primary Survey and Resuscitation)

Foley catheter unless contraindicated‡
Gastric tube unless contraindicated**

Secondary Survey and Re-evaluation

History and physical examination: SAMPLE history, complete examination

Adjuncts (Secondary Survey and Re-evaluation)

Imaging and laboratory studies: plain radiographs,†† special studies‡‡

---

*Rapid sequence induction technique: etomidate then succinylcholine.
†Primary: chest rise, air entry; secondary: exhaled CO_2 detector, esophageal detector device. Watch for DOPE: **D**islodgement, **O**bstruction, **P**neumothorax, **E**quipment failure.
§Do not wait for confirmatory chest x-ray!
¶Consider obstructive and neurogenic as well as hypovolemic shock; exclude tension pneumothorax, cardiac tamponade, spinal shock.
‡Contraindications: meatal blood, scrotal hematoma, high-riding prostate.
**Contraindications: cerebrospinal fluid oto/rhinorrhea, basilar skull fracture, midface instability.
††Chest, pelvis, lateral cervical spine; others as indicated
‡‡Focused Assessment by Sonography in Trauma (FAST), CT as indicated.
Abbreviations: BVM, bag-valve-mask; CRT, capillary refill time; CT, computed tomography; GCS, Glasgow Coma Scale; LOC, level of consciousness; NRB, non-rebreather mask; SAMPLE: **S**igns/symptoms, **A**llergies, **M**edications, **P**ertinent past history, **L**ast oral intake, **E**vents leading up to the injury; TBI, traumatic brain injury.

collapse, and to which infants and young children are especially prone, is catastrophic. Therefore, careful and frequent re-evaluations are required to ensure that tension pneumothorax is not overlooked.

Abnormalities in the primary survey are addressed as they arise, since accurate evaluation of each step in the delivery of oxygen to the tissues (airway/ventilation, breathing/oxygenation, circulation/perfusion) presumes the integrity of the previous step. Adjuncts to the primary survey that will assist in the evaluation of each of these steps include vital signs (appropriate for age), pulse oximetry (demonstrating adequate oxygen saturation [S_pO_2]), end-tidal capnography (confirming gas exchange [$ETCO_2$]), and, with respect to the thorax, a supine chest roentgenogram (identifying pathologic findings). Evidence of respiratory distress or compensated shock mandates urgent resuscitation. Evidence of respiratory failure or decompensated shock mandates emergent resuscitation.

In performing the secondary survey, the complete physical examination for thoracic injuries will assess for visible contusions, subcutaneous emphysema, chest wall stability, and other palpable abnormalities (by inspection and palpation), and for abnormal collections of air or blood within the thoracic cavity (by percussion and auscultation).

Injuries commonly requiring immediate intervention in the pediatric patient include immediate life-threatening thoracic injuries such as airway obstruction, tension pneumothorax with respiratory insufficiency, and massive hemothorax with shock. Less frequently encountered are open pneumothorax, flail chest, and cardiac tamponade. Clinical stabilization with appropriate interventions must be accomplished in an orderly and timely manner to prevent further respiratory or cardiac decompensation. Injuries requiring delayed intervention in the pediatric patient include potentially life-threatening thoracic injuries that in most cases will not be detected without radiographic or laboratory tests, or ongoing monitoring and continuous reassessment of the patient's clinical status.

Immediately Life-Threatening Thoracic Injuries[9]

AIRWAY

Airway obstruction most commonly results from passive closure of the upper airway due to unconsciousness, which leads to loss of tone in the muscles of the head and neck and subsequent collapse of hypopharyngeal soft tissues across the glottic inlet. It may also be caused by particulate matter that becomes lodged in the funnel-shaped upper airway above, at, or below the level of the vocal cords, but above the cricoid ring. Rare causes of airway obstruction include laryngeal hematoma and fracture. Most episodes of airway obstruction are relieved in the normal course of airway opening and positioning during the primary survey, but may not be recognized unless abnormal sounds, such as snoring (soft tissue obstruction), gurgling (excessive hypopharyngeal secretions), stridor (particulate matter obstruction), and hoarseness (direct laryngeal trauma) are present.

BREATHING

Tension pneumothorax develops when sufficient air accumulates in the pleural space to compress the ipsilateral lung and to shift the mediastinum toward the opposite side and compress the contralateral lung. It is often missed on initial examinations, and may only be diagnosed after assisted ventilation adds to the volume of the entrapped gas and leads to further deterioration. Confirmatory chest roentgenograms should not delay prompt intervention via needle decompression in patients who present with clinical symptoms and signs of tension pneumothorax. These include air hunger, decreased or absent breath sounds on the ipsilateral side, a hyperresonant percussion note on the ipsilateral side, shift of the trachea toward the contralateral side, and distention of neck veins (uncommonly observed in small children and those with short necks). Any patient with thoracic trauma who presents with severe respiratory and cardiovascular compromise should be considered for empirical needle decompression, which is both diagnostic and therapeutic.

Flail chest is uncommon in children, and results from two or more adjacent fractures in two or more adjacent ribs that cause instability in the chest wall and compromise in the ventilatory effort. Most flail segments in children are relatively small, and do not directly affect ventilation due to spasm of the adjacent muscles, but indirectly affect oxygenation owing to the sizeable pulmonary contusions that are invariably associated with flail chest. However, if flail segments are large and posterolateral, ventilation is adversely affected, as the damaged chest wall caves in during inspiration. Diagnosis is confirmed when bony crepitus is palpated in association with a free-floating segment of chest wall.

Open pneumothorax is recognized by the presence of a defect in the chest wall that allows air to move freely between the atmosphere and the pleural cavity. The result is paradoxical respiration, in which the lung collapses during inspiration, and expands during expiration, as air enters and exits the pleural cavity via the defect during inhalation and exhalation, rather than entering and exiting the lungs via the trachea and bronchi. It is uncommon in children, and results by definition from penetrating trauma. Open pneumothorax will exist whenever there is a defect in the chest wall that is larger than one half to two thirds the size of the corresponding intercostal space. Immediate treatment is needed to avoid rapid progression of respiratory failure to respiratory arrest.

CIRCULATION

Massive hemothorax develops as a result of either blunt or penetrating trauma that causes injury to lung parenchyma or intrathoracic vessels and leads to accumulation of blood in the pleural space. Bleeding is usually self-limited in parenchymal injury due both to the high concentration of pulmonary thromboplastins and the tamponading effect of entrapped blood, but may rapidly accumulate in vascular injury due to the ongoing hemorrhage that produces external manifestations of shock. Massive hemothorax is the leading thoracic cause of shock following thoracic injury. Massive hemothorax may also develop following inadvertent misplacement of a chest tube into the lung, liver, or spleen. Children with massive hemothorax may initially present with minimal symptoms but can rapidly progress to severe dyspnea, tachypnea, tachycardia, and cardiovascular collapse due to hypovolemic shock. Late presentations may include chronic atelectasis with ventilation-perfusion mismatch, pneumonia, empyema, sepsis, or fibrothorax. Initial evaluation includes chest roentgenograms with or without computed tomograms. Beyond these, minimally invasive techniques such as video-assisted thoracoscopic surgery (VATS) have been used to both diagnose and evacuate residual hematomas.[15-18]

Cardiac tamponade exists when a sufficient volume of blood accumulates in the nondistensible pericardial sac following penetrating trauma or blunt trauma (rarely in small children), thereby compressing the heart and compromising cardiac output. As blood further accumulates, the cardiac chambers become unable to fill, and cardiac output drops precipitously. Cardiac tamponade should be suspected whenever there is a penetrating injury to the imaginary square box bounded superiorly by the intermammary line, inferiorly by the costal margins, and bilaterally by lines running caudally from the nipples. It is heralded by the classic Beck's triad of muffled heart tones, jugular venous distention, and pulsus paradoxus, although pronounced tachycardia, followed by decompensated shock, are the most common and most consistent signs. The diagnosis is confirmed by the presence of fluid in the pericardial sac on Focused Assessment by Sonography in Trauma (FAST), or by pericardiocentesis, which is both diagnostic and therapeutic, should FAST not be available to the treating physician. When pericardiocentesis is performed, an alligator clip emanating from the V lead of an electrocardiograph should be attached to the metal part of the large-bore needle used for the procedure in an attempt to identify the current of injury, which appears as a spike in the tracing when the myocardium is touched by the needle tip. The classic teaching that pericardial blood does not clot is false, and cannot be relied upon in actual practice.

Potentially Life-Threatening Thoracic Injuries

AIRWAY

Tracheobronchial injury is rare in children. When found, it follows penetrating trauma or violent blunt force impact to the chest. Blunt tracheobronchial injuries are typically located adjacent to the carina, where shear forces will be the greatest, and large airways are their thinnest, and unprotected by lung. Injuries may be complete or incomplete, such that small tears may not be manifest for several days. Tracheobronchial injuries should be suspected whenever there exists a persistent massive air leak via a thoracostomy tube. If the tear is complete, the fatality rate is as high as 20%, in part due to the tear's association with concomitant injury to the head, neck, spine, and chest, and in part due to its relative inaccessibility. Evaluation of tracheobronchial injury may include bronchoscopy as well as computed tomography, although immediate thoracotomy may be needed for diagnosis and treatment if rapid deterioration occurs before diagnostic imaging can be obtained.

BREATHING

Pulmonary contusion remains the most common thoracic injury in childhood, although its incidence has decreased markedly over the past decade following the introduction of mandatory child restraint systems. Caused by a direct force to the lung that leads to parenchymal bleeding and interstitial edema, it first presents with mild symptoms, but as edema increases, ventilation-perfusion mismatch, hypoxemia, and hypoventilation may develop. Late complications may include atelectasis, pneumonia, and acute respiratory distress syndrome. Physical findings may include cyanosis, tachypnea, tachycardia, decreased breath sounds, and wheezing. Initial chest roentgenograms may not disclose the characteristic mixed alveolar and interstitial infiltrates for hours or days.

Traumatic diaphragmatic hernia is uncommon in children, but frequently occurs in association with penetrating trauma to the thoracoabdominal region, located between the intermammary line and the costal margins, and rarely occurs in blunt trauma, which often involves severe blunt force impact or improperly worn shoulder belts. In penetrating trauma, this injury is not readily revealed by diagnostic imaging, and may be found only upon surgical exploration. In blunt trauma, this injury is also commonly associated with multiple organ system trauma involving the liver, spleen, and gastrointestinal tract, and usually occurs on the left side, since a major etiology is pedestrian–motor vehicle crashes. Symptoms and signs of traumatic diaphragmatic hernia will not be immediately apparent unless associated with abdominal visceral herniation into the thorax. If present, they may include respiratory distress, decreased or atypical breath sounds, or a scaphoid abdomen. A chest roentgenogram will be diagnostic only with frank herniation, as manifested by the presence of the gastric bubble or gastric tube within the chest, but will be suspicious in the presence of an elevated or indistinct diaphragmatic silhouette. Definitive diagnosis may require evaluation by computed tomography or surgical exploration.

Traumatic asphyxia occurs more commonly in children than adults due to the increased compliance of their chest walls and the absence of fully developed valves in the superior and inferior venac cavae. It results from sudden massive compression of the chest. Direct compression on a closed glottis causes pressure to be transmitted to the heart, lungs, venae cavae, neck, and head. This increase in pressure may lead to bleeding in the brain and other organs. Physical examination typically reveals numerous petechiae of the head and neck, subconjunctival hemorrhages, and cyanosis above the clavicles. Diagnosis is directed toward underlying complications associated with massive blunt thoracic injury.

CIRCULATION

Blunt cardiac injury refers to a constellation of injuries to the heart, including myocardial contusion, valvular and ventricular injuries, and commotio cordis, all of which are unusual in children following blunt trauma.[19-24] Manifestations of myocardial contusion include dysrhythmias, hypotension, and elevated cardiac enzymes. Definitive diagnosis is controversial, in part because it has few clinical implications. Electrocardiography is most useful, since it will detect the rare cardiac arrhythmia. Echocardiography is also useful to evaluate ventricular function but is rarely abnormal, and even when abnormal, is not predictive of clinical deterioration. Cardiac enzymes are no longer used routinely as predictors of complications in blunt cardiac injury, and while troponin I may predict echocardiographic abnormalities, its clinical significance has yet to be defined. Valvular and ventricular injuries, including rupture of the chordae tendineae and the ventricular wall, are devastating events that can be diagnosed only by echocardiography. Commotio cordis is a unique pediatric traumatic cardiac event that usually results in sudden death. Associated with severe blunt force impact to the lower sternum, usually during a sports activity, it causes sudden ventricular fibrillation. Exact understanding of its mechanism remains to be delineated. Since the only effective interventions are immediate on-site cardiopulmonary resuscitation and automated external defibrillation, many jurisdictions are mandating that both be available at sports activities involving children.

Traumatic aortic disruption is rare in children, and when it occurs it is usually associated with significant injury to other intrathoracic organs following massive deceleration injury, although it is occasionally caused by penetrating injury, most often in adolescents. It carries a high mortality rate, as death often ensues prior to arrival at a treating facility. The chest roentgenogram remains the primary screening test, and typically demonstrates a widened mediastinum. However, it cannot be used for definitive diagnosis, since the portable anteroposterior supine film obtained per ATLS protocol is not accurate enough to supplant other tests. Actual aortic injury occurs in only 10% to 20% of patients with widened mediastinum on chest roentgenogram, while approximately 7% of aortic injuries are missed by chest roentgentogram. Thoracic aortography therefore remains the study of choice if traumatic aortic disruption is a likely possibility, as it establishes and defines the anatomy of the injury. However, it requires transport to the angiographic suite, and is therefore performed only if the screening film is abnormal, or it is clinically indicated. Computed tomography by rapid helical scanning with three-dimensional reconstruction may ultimately replace aortography. It is now used to exclude mediastinal hematoma in clinically stable patients with (1) equivocal chest roentgenograms, (2) negative chest roentgenograms but with signs of aortic disruption, and (3) suspected thoracic injuries who also require computed tomography of the abdomen. The roles of other imaging modalities are still being defined. Transthoracic echocardiography can rapidly detect pericardial tamponade and cardiac rupture in clinically unstable patients, but requires an experienced operator. Transesophageal echocardiography is a promising new technique, but it also requires an experienced operator. More invasive than computed tomography, it is both less invasive and less sensitive than thoracic aortography. The use of FAST is also rapidly evolving, but needs to be more specifically studied in its application to cardiac injuries in children.

Possibly Life-Threatening Thoracic Injuries

Simple pneumothorax may be caused by blunt or penetrating trauma, with or without fractured ribs. It occurs when air escapes into the pleural space due to a tear in the lung, tracheobronchial tree, esophagus, or chest wall, causing partial or complete lung collapse. As most pneumothoraces are due to lung injury, most seal quickly and do not progress to tension pneumothorax, causing increased intrathoracic pressure, mediastinal shift, both ipsilateral and contralateral lung collapse, and decreased cardiac output secondary to impaired venous return. As a result, the child with simple pneumothorax typically presents with mild to moderate symptoms, such as ipsilaterally decreased breath sounds, tachypnea, tachycardia, or pain, or may be completely asymptomatic. In such

circumstances, the injury may not be detected until a chest roentgenogram is obtained.

Simple hemothorax may also be caused by blunt or penetrating trauma, with or without fractured ribs. It occurs when blood leaks from injured lung parenchyma, but may also result from vascular or costal bleeding that stops spontaneously as increased intrathoracic pressure tamponades small bleeding veins or narrow venous plexuses. Bleeding arteries usually result in massive hemothorax rather than simple hemothorax, since intrathoracic pressure cannot exceed arterial pressure. Injuries to the great vessels are usually fatal at the scene, although patients with bleeding pulmonary veins occasionally survive.

Rib fractures are uncommon in young children, but incidence increases with age. The fourth through ninth ribs are most commonly fractured, and are associated with damage to abdominal organs. The first through the third ribs are less commonly fractured, but are associated with injuries to the trachea, bronchi, and great vessels. Manifestations may include bruising, localized pain, crepitus, or decreased respiratory effort and pain. Because the ribs are softer in children than adults, the presence of one or more rib fractures in children indicates that a substantial energy load was transferred to the chest. Rib fractures are therefore significant not only as a source of morbidity on their own, but also as a marker of severe injury, although recent evidence indicates that this association may not be consistent.[25-28] Multiple rib fractures in infancy may indicate child abuse, or an underlying organic disorder such as osteogenesis imperfecta.

Sternal fracture is rare in children. Older data indicated close correlation with cardiac injury. However, more current studies show a less conclusive association.[29] Diagnosis is made by lateral chest roentgenograms or computed thoracic tomography.

Esophageal injuries are also rare in children. Because the esophagus is a well-protected organ that is very flexible and capable of self-decompression, it rarely sustains blunt injury. However, penetrating injuries that transverse the mediastinum may lacerate the esophagus. Diagnostic modalities include contrast fluoroscopy and endoscopy, and should be considered whenever there is unexplained gas in the mediastinum, or if food or saliva are observed to be draining from a properly placed chest tube.

Mediastinal traversing injuries are increasingly recognized as a cause of significant morbidity and mortality, particularly in adolescent boys engaged in violent behavior involving firearms. Patients who are unstable on presentation require immediate surgical intervention. Patients who are stable on presentation require immediate surgical consultation, in case of unexpected sudden deterioration, and for treatment of associated injuries. Diagnostic tests typically employed to exclude injury in stable patients may include chest roentgenography, computed tomography, contrast fluoroscopy, rigid or flexible bronchoscopy or esophagoscopy, and echocardiography.

Diagnostic Modalities

Clinical Examination

Over the past several decades, multiple modalities have been developed to facilitate the prompt and accurate diagnosis of

Table 24–2	Differential Diagnosis of Immediately Life-Threatening Thoracic Injuries		
	Tension Pneumothorax	**Massive Hemothorax**	**Cardiac Tamponade**
Breath sounds	Ipsilaterally ↓	Ispilaterally ↓	Normal
Percussion note	Hyperresonant	Dull	Normal
Tracheal location	Contralaterally shifted	Midline	Midline
Neck veins	Distended	Flat	Distended
Heart tones	Contralaterally shifted	Normal	Muffled

thoracic injuries. Classic *clinical signs* remain reliable indicators of intrathoracic injuries, and are typically used to guide initial diagnosis and treatment, as shown in Table 24–2. Although many investigators have attempted to develop clinical prediction rules to identify children with these injuries, definitive evidence-based protocols are still undergoing investigation.[30] However, children undergoing evaluation for blunt trauma have been found to have an increased risk of thoracic injury if they present with certain clinical manifestations, including tachypnea, abnormal chest auscultation, low blood pressure, low Glasgow Coma Scale score, and femur fracture.

Use of FAST is rapidly evolving, but needs to be more specifically studied in its application to thoracic injuries. It consists of a bedside transabdominal sonographic examination for abnormal fluid collections in the pericardial cavity, the subhepatic pouch (of Morison), the splenic fossa, and the retrovesical space.

Imaging Studies

Beyond the physical examination, *chest roentgenography* remains the primary screening tool used for evaluation of thoracic injuries. It can rapidly identify most of the immediate, potential, and possible life-threatening thoracic injuries, it can localize tubes and catheters, and it has the advantage of being inexpensive, readily available, and associated with minimal morbidity.[31] Yet, while chest roentgenography remains an important screening tool, it can miss a significant number of injuries, and lacks specificity for mediastinal injuries. It can also underestimate the magnitude of pleural and parenchymal injuries, and incorrectly localize the placement of tubes.

For these reasons, *computed tomography* is increasingly used for definitive diagnosis of intrathoracic injuries in stable patients.[32-38] It is a better test for detection and quantification of abnormal collections of air or blood (which are often missed on supine chest roentgenography), for inclusion or exclusion of mediastinal hemorrhage due to aortic disruption (since mediastinal widening is typically exaggerated by supine chest roentgenography), and for documenting the position of tubes and catheters (which requires an additional lateral view on chest roentgenography that often proves difficult to obtain during initial evaluation and resuscitation). Yet, while it provides far greater sensitivity and specificity in the detection of thoracic trauma, its greater diagnostic accuracy must be weighed not only against its effect on the clinical management and outcome (recognizing that it is no more useful than other tests for most intrathoracic injuries), but also against its potential long-term radiologic side effects.[39] For example, computed tomography appears

to be more sensitive than chest roentgenography in the detection of small pneumothoraces, but the clinical import of this fact may be negligible, as most patients with small pneumothoraces are safely managed without tube thoracostomy.[40]

Transthoracic echocardiography is the radiographic study of choice for cardiac injuries, including cardiac tamponade. It is less useful for great vessel injuries, which are not optimally visualized via subxiphoid or intercostals windows. When immediately available, it is somewhat more accurate for diagnosis of pericardial fluid, and it is ideal for diagnosis of valvular disruption. Unfortunately, it is rarely available during evening and weekend hours when seriously injured children are most likely to present.

Transesophageal echocardiography is a relatively new technique for diagnosis of cardiac and great vessel injuries, but it requires an experienced operator. While it is more invasive than helical computed tomography with intravenous contrast, it may be more sensitive in skilled hands for the diagnosis of aortic disruption.[41,42] However, it is both less invasive and less sensitive than aortography for this purpose. Moreover, because it requires passage of a sonographic probe into the esophageal lumen, helical computed tomography with intravenous contrast may be preferred for most patients.

Thoracic aortography remains the "gold standard" for radiographic diagnosis of aortic disruption, since it establishes and defines the anatomy of the injury. It is not usually performed unless the chest roentgenogram shows a widened mediastinum or the computed tomogram shows a mediastinal hematoma and suggests aortic injury. Because it requires transfer to the angiographic suite for an invasive procedure that employs both an intra-arterial catheter and intravenous contrast, it is reserved for only high-risk patients, upon request of the thoracic surgeon who will perform the repair. The role of intra-arterial thoracic subtraction angiography needs further delineation.

Video-assisted thoracoscopic surgery is increasingly being used in diagnosis and treatment of intrapleural complications of intrathoracic trauma, such as trapped lung and empyema. Its role in diagnosis of major intrathoracic trauma is uncertain. Anecdotal reports of video-assisted thoracostomy and intracavitary missile retrieval have appeared. However, there currently appears to be no role for VATS in evaluation and management of thoracic injuries in the emergency department.

Laboratory Tests

Laboratory tests are of limited utility for the early diagnosis and treatment of thoracic injuries in childhood. *Hemoglobin concentration* and *hematocrit* are likely to be misleading during the initial phases of resuscitation, as dilutional anemia from endogenous fluid shifts and exogenous fluid administration will not as yet have occurred, although both tests will be useful as a baseline for further measurements. Similarly, *arterial blood gases* will serve as an initial indicator of ventilation, oxygenation, and perfusion, but are more useful in terms of their trend, since all three functions can be reliably assessed more quickly via bedside monitoring or clinical tests, such as end-tidal capnography ($ETCO_2$), pulse oximetry (SpO_2), and vital signs.[43] Blood type and crossmatch are routinely obtained in all children with significant injury.

Cardiac enzymes have played an important historical role in the diagnosis of blunt cardiac injury, particularly myocardial contusion. However, the clinical significance of this diagnosis in childhood is uncertain. As such, the role of cardiac enzymes has markedly decreased as a predictor of complications in patients with blunt myocardial contusion. Although abnormally high troponin I levels may predict echocardiographic abnormalities, the clinical importance of these findings has yet to be defined.[44]

Management

Thoracic injuries pose a major threat to the integrity of the airway, breathing, and circulation, hence to ventilation, oxygenation, and perfusion of core organs and body tissues, thence to vital functions. As such, resuscitation must proceed simultaneously with assessment. Abnormalities of the airway, breathing, and circulation must therefore be treated in sequence, as soon as they are recognized, both to restore flow of oxygen through the series circuit composed of the tracheobronchial tree, the lungs, and the bloodstream, and to ensure accurate assessment of downstream segments of this circuit. It is therefore important that the stepwise pathophysiologic assessment of airway, breathing, and circulation advocated by the ATLS® Course of the American College of Surgeons Committee on Trauma be followed in detail.

The six immediately life-threatening thoracic injuries described previously are recognized and treated during the primary survey, while potential and possible life-threatening thoracic injuries are recognized and treated during the secondary survey. Meticulous attention to the early detection and optimal management of these injuries is the ideal way to ensure effective restoration of ventilation, oxygenation, and perfusion, hence the best chance the seriously injured child has of a full and complete physical and neurologic recovery. Indications for both tube thoracostomy and urgent thoracotomy are delineated in Tables 24–3 and 24–4.

Major Chest Injuries

Immediately Life-Threatening Thoracic Injuries

AIRWAY

An injured child who cannot easily breathe, cough, cry, or speak has *upper airway obstruction* until proven otherwise. The airway must be opened and repositioned, with a modified jaw thrust maneuver and bimanual cervical spine stabilization. The quality of any abnormal sounds heard will dictate the correct initial treatment. Snoring suggests soft

Table 24–3	Indications for Tube Thoracostomy

Immediate Life-Threatening Thoracic Injuries (Addressed during Primary Survey)

Airway
- None

Breathing
- Tension pneumothorax (after immediate needle decompression)
- Open pneumothorax (after applying occlusive dressing)

Circulation
- Massive hemothorax (after initiating volume resuscitation)

Potential Life-Threatening Thoracic Injuries (Addressed during Secondary Survey)

Airway
- Tracheobronchial injury

Breathing
- None

Circulation
- None

Possible Life-Threatening Thoracic Injuries (Addressed during Secondary Survey)

Airway
- None

Breathing
- Simple pneumothorax

Circulation
- Simple hemothorax

Special Considerations (Addressed during Secondary Survey)
- Esophageal injuries
- Mediastinal traversing wounds
- Thoracoabdominal wounds

Table 24–4	Indications for Urgent Thoracotomy

Emergency Thoracotomy (in the Operating Room)

Airway
- Tracheobronchial injury with massive uncontrollable air leak

Breathing
- Open pneumothorax with large chest wall defect
- Traumatic diaphragmatic hernia

Circulation
- Massive hemothorax
  - Immediate drainage of 20–25 ml/kg blood from chest tube
  - Ongoing drainage of 2–2.5 ml/kg/hr blood from chest tube
- Cardiac tamponade (cardiopulmonary bypass advisable)
- Traumatic aortic disruption (cardiopulmonary bypass advisable)
- Blunt cardiac injuries needing surgical repair (cardiopulmonary bypass required)

Other
- Esophageal injury (if disruption evident)
- Mediastinal traversing injury (if hemodynamically unstable)
- Completion of thoracotomy following successful resuscitative thoracotomy

Resuscitative Thoracotomy (in the Emergency Department)

Airway
- None

Breathing
- None

Circulation
- Penetrating traumatic cardiac arrest with signs of life at the scene or thereafter

tissue obstruction for which airway opening and repositioning alone should be sufficient, followed in the absence of a gag reflex by insertion of an oropharyngeal airway that reaches from the mental foramen to the angle of the mandible. Gurgling suggests abundant pharyngeal secretions, which must be cleared through aggressive but gentle use of a large-bore oropharyngeal suction device. Stridor suggests a laryngeal foreign body, such as fractured dental fragments or small intraoral playtoys, that may require extraction under direct laryngoscopy using pediatric Magill or Rovenstine forceps, if a directly observable fingersweep is unsuccessful. Hoarseness suggests blunt laryngeal injury that may require medical or, rarely, surgical cricothyroidotomy if airway opening maneuvers fail, followed by definitive surgical repair if laryngeal fracture is present, a diagnosis that is made by computed tomography once definitive airway control has been obtained.

Endotracheal intubation using an uncuffed endotracheal tube will in due course be required for injured children under 8 years of age who present in respiratory failure, decompensated shock, or traumatic coma, or who cannot protect their own airway. An uncuffed tube is preferred for such children, not because of the "physiologic" mucosal "cuff" that is the serendipitous benefit of the funnel-shaped upper airway, the narrowest point of which is at the subglottic level of the cricoid ring, but because the larger outer diameter created by the plastic "balloon" cuff necessitates use of a tube with a smaller inner diameter than is ideal, thereby predisposing the tube to earlier obstruction from bloody or mucousy secretions than a tube of larger inner diameter. However, the tube need not be inserted the moment the need for it is recognized, so long as the airway can be temporarily maintained by other means. This gives time for the treating physician to rapidly assess the child for conditions such as tension pneumothorax that may worsen if the child is tracheally intubated before they are addressed.

Orotracheal intubation is the preferred approach in injured children requiring definitive airways. This is because the anterior, cephalad location of the larynx in children under 8 years of age precludes nasotracheal intubation in most emergent situations, while attempts at nasotracheal intubation may cause profuse adenoidal bleeding. In rare circumstances, tracheal intubation may not be possible due to laryngeal injury. Needle cricothyroidotomy followed by needle jet ventilation is preferred for such patients, since the hyoid bone is often more prominent than the thyroid cartilage in infants and young children, a fact that may predispose to misidentification of anatomic landmarks, which can lead to improper placement of the surgical cricothyroidotomy incision.

Rapid sequence intubation, using etomidate and succinylcholine after an adequate interval of suction and preoxygenation, is preferred for injured children requiring tracheal intubation, unless the Glasgow Coma Scale score indicates global unresponsiveness. Adjunctive use of lidocaine to blunt a potential rise in intracranial pressure remains controversial. Deterioration or desaturation of an intubated patient requires immediate re-evaluation of the airway. The mnemonic "Don't be a DOPE" may serve to remind the treating physician of common pitfalls of endotracheal intubation such as esophageal or right mainstem bronchial

*d*islodgement, particularly when a patient is moved from the ambulance to the hospital stretcher, or from gurney to gantry, or vice versa, when undergoing computed tomography; *o*bstruction by blood, secretions, kinking, or biting; tension *p*neumothorax, either from exacerbation of an existing or unrecognized tension pneumothorax, or creation of a new tension pneumothorax from overly zealous assisted bag-valve-mask or -tube ventilation, or ventilator-induced baro- or volutrauma; or *e*quipment failure, most commonly the result of failure of oxygen supply, either from an empty tank or, in rare instances, inadequate delivery of wall oxygen.

BREATHING

All children with potential thoracic injuries require immediate administration of high-concentration oxygen, preferably humidified oxygen. Supplemental oxygen should be administered by a non-rebreather mask for children in respiratory distress or by assisted bag-valve-mask or -tube ventilation for children in respiratory failure or arrest. Supplemental oxygen is required even if the arterial oxygen saturation, whether measured by pulse oximetry or arterial blood gas analysis, is normal. This is because coexistent volume deficits may lead to increased peripheral oxygen extraction, hence mixed venous oxygen desaturation, even when the arterial oxygen saturation is found to be normal.

Adequate oxygenation presupposes adequate ventilation. To determine if ventilation is adequate, the treating physician should observe for adequacy of chest rise; listen for the presence, quality, and equality of breath sounds; judge the adequacy of respiratory effort by observing for signs of increased, labored, decreased, or absent work of breathing, such as accessory muscle use, head bobbing, grunting, and fatigue; and count the respiratory rate to ensure that it lies within the normal range. To determine if oxygenation is adequate, the physician should look for central cyanosis or pallor, assess whether the sensorium is intact, and measure arterial oxygen saturation; in general, respiratory distress is present when the oxygen saturation falls below 95%, while respiratory failure is present when it falls below 90%.

Correct treatment of immediate life-threatening thoracic injuries requires immediate differentiation between tension pneumothorax, massive hemothorax, and cardiac tamponade. This can be difficult in the first few moments after presentation to the emergency department, and each requires a different approach to immediate treatment. Such distinction is further complicated when an endotracheal tube is in place, since right mainstem bronchial intubation can lead to decreased breath sounds on the left, which can mislead the inexperienced physician to suspect pneumo- or hemothorax. The differential diagnosis of these conditions, once again, is delineated in Table 24–2.

Tension pneumothorax is decompressed immediately using a large-bore over-the-needle catheter, without waiting for the chest radiograph that will confirm the diagnosis, but at the expense of inappropriate delay that may result in the rapid deterioration and death of the patient. This catheter should be inserted via the second interspace on the midclavicular line, just above the third rib, to avoid injury to the neurovascular bundles that run immediately below the second rib. If tension pneumothorax is present, a gush of entrapped air will be heard rushing from the catheter. The catheter should be left in place and attached to a Heimlich, or similar, one-way flap valve, until definitive tube thoracostomy can be performed (see Chapter 168, Thoracostomy). A chest roentgenogram can then be obtained to document lung re-expansion and correct tube placement.

Open pneumothorax is converted immediately to closed pneumothorax using an occlusive dressing. Classic teaching states that this presumably rectangular dressing should be taped only on three of its four sides, to allow escape of entrapped air that could lead to development of tension pneumothorax. This philosophy, however, is being replaced by the teaching that a tube thoracostomy should be immediately inserted to effectively drain any accumulated blood and/or intrapleural air. Definitive surgical repair will be required for open pneumothoraces caused by large defects in the chest wall.

The approach to management of *flail chest* is not infrequently misunderstood. Only rarely is it necessary to splint the chest wall since, barring the unusual circumstance when the floating segment is so large that it leads to paradoxical ventilation during inspiration, the muscles surrounding the "floating" segment become spastic, thereby splinting the chest wall without need for internal or external appliances. Moreover, the pathophysiology of open pneumothorax, excepting once again the presence of paradoxical ventilation, is related not to the "floating" chest wall segment, but to arterial hypoxemia due to the ventilation perfusion mismatch associated with the invariably coexistent pulmonary contusions. Thus the initial treatment of flail chest is supplemental oxygen and appropriate analgesia, unless the "floating" segment is of such a large size that paradoxical ventilation requires "internal" splinting via mechanical ventilation.

CIRCULATION

Immediate life-threatening thoracic injuries chiefly affecting the circulation require volume resuscitation in addition to temporizing management and definitive treatment. As with endotracheal intubation for definitive airway control, definitive treatment is often temporarily delayed until intravascular volume has been substantially restored. The pneumatic antishock garment or medical antishock trousers are no longer used for treatment of hypotension, except for selected patients with unstable pelvic fractures, and have always been contraindicated for patients with thoracic injuries. Although no data are available in pediatric patients, permissive hypotension has been employed with limited success in adult patients, provided blood pressure is adequate to maintain cerebral perfusion and definitive surgical management is readily available.

The importance of hemorrhage control cannot be sufficiently emphasized. Volume resuscitation may transiently restore core organ perfusion, but dilutional anemia is too often the result, particularly when bleeding patients are held in the emergency department in a futile attempt to achieve hemodynamic stability. If volume resuscitation must be employed in the absence of a surgeon, packed red blood cells, in boluses of 10 ml/kg, should be administered as soon as possible to patients who are hypotensive on arrival in the emergency department, or who do not respond immediately

to 40 to 60 ml/kg of normal saline or lactated Ringer's solution, rapidly infused in continuous aliquots of 20 ml/kg. Use of an autotransfuser should be considered for patients with intrathoracic hemorrhage.

Although *massive hemothorax* will often be detected during the breathing assessment on the basis of decreased breath sounds, it is on the circulation that it mostly impacts. Since children may sequester up to 40% of their blood volume in a hemithorax before the onset of cardiovascular collapse, due to the propensity of the mediastinum to shift when under tension from entrapped air or blood, volume resuscitation is essential. Once intravascular volume resuscitation is initiated and vital signs begin to normalize, tube thoracostomy should be expeditiously performed, followed by surgical intervention for cases in which the initial output from the chest tube exceeds some 25% to 30% of circulating blood volume, or 20 to 25 ml/kg, or the ongoing output from the chest tube exceeds approximately 2.5% to 3% of circulating blood volume per hour, or 2 to 2.5 ml/kg/hr. Due to the relatively high tissue thromboplastin content of pulmonary parenchyma, most bleeding from lung wounds will cease spontaneously. Hence, ongoing bleeding suggests vascular trauma, which in most cases results from injury to the intercostals vessels, typically the arteries.

Pericardial or *cardiac tamponade* must be treated expeditiously for a favorable outcome to be achieved. Since it can only result from a cardiac wound, immediate surgical repair is mandatory. Rarely seen following blunt thoracic trauma, penetrating trauma to the "box" that is bounded by the nipples superiorly and bilaterally and the costal margins inferiorly requires immediate FAST for diagnosis, followed by pericardiocentesis as soon as vital signs begin to destabilize, if a surgeon with experience in operative management of thoracic injuries is not immediately available. To perform pericardiocentesis safely, an alligator clip is attached to the needle of a large-bore through-the-needle catheter set, which in turn is attached to a V lead port of an electrocardiograph machine, and the needle is carefully inserted through the skin to the left of the xiphoid process under continuous electrocardiographic monitoring, and slowly advanced posterolaterally toward the tip of the scapula. Once blood is encountered, the physician can advance the catheter over the needle, withdraw the needle, remove whatever blood can be aspirated, and secure the catheter at skin level. While classic teaching states that pericardial blood does not clot, this is not true in the acute setting. Thus urgent surgical intervention is of the utmost importance.

Potentially Life-Threatening Thoracic Injuries

AIRWAY

Tracheobronchial injuries, although rare in children, must be urgently addressed. They are manifested chiefly by a continuous air leak through the waterseal chamber of the chest drainage collection device that persists once all external sources of air entrainment have been excluded, and are confirmed radiologically when a persistent pneumothorax is seen on chest roentgenography. Management consists first of increasing the suction on the chest drainage collection device from −10 cm H_2O pressure slowly to −25 cm H_2O pressure.

If this fails to resolve the pneumothorax, a second chest tube may be needed. Definitive treatment consists of bronchoscopic confirmation, followed by surgical repair if the air leak has not significantly decreased after 24 to 48 hours of conservative management, to which most tracheobronchial injuries will quickly respond.

BREATHING

Pulmonary contusions require adequate oxygenation and pulmonary toilet for effective treatment. The goal of therapy is to avoid progression to "adult" respiratory distress syndrome (ARDS), which now typically results from the development of ventilator associated pneumonia (VAP), although posttraumatic pulmonary insufficiency (PTPS), or "shock lung," due to massive isotonic crystalloid infusion, was a common cause in years past. Prevention of VAP is best accomplished through meticulous attention to aseptic suctioning of intubated, mechanically ventilated patients, and avoidance of prophylactic antibiotics. Prevention of PTPS and ARDS due to overly zealous fluid administration is best achieved through appropriate fluid management, and selective fluid restriction.

Traumatic diaphragmatic hernia requires immediate definitive surgical repair. Ipsilateral tube thoracostomy should be avoided, as this will suck abdominal contents into the involved hemithorax, markedly worsening respiratory status. Although blunt torso injuries are the cause of most traumatic diaphragmatic injuries, penetrating thoracoabdominal injuries occasionally cause traumatic diaphragmatic hernias if the diaphragmatic defect is large. All penetrating thoracoabdominal injuries require tube thoracostomy, followed by abdominal exploration and diaphragmatic repair, via laparotomy or laparoscopy.

Traumatic asphyxia requires no specific treatment. It serves chiefly as a marker of the severity of impacting forces. As such, its presence mandates a careful search for other thoracic injuries that may require treatment. Definitive treatment of the normally transient neurologic sequelae of severe traumatic asphyxia remains expectant.

CIRCULATION

Blunt cardiac injury encompasses a spectrum of injuries from myocardial contusion to valvular or ventricular rupture. Myocardial contusion is treated by observation and continuous electrocardiographic monitoring, reserving antidysrhythmic therapy for the rare patient who develops electrical instability. Commotio cordis requires immediate advanced cardiac life support, starting with automated external defibrillation rather than cardiopulmonary resuscitation for witnessed arrests. Valvular rupture, which presents with sudden cardiac failure, and ventricular rupture, which presents with sudden cardiac tamponade, require immediate surgical repair.

Traumatic aortic disruption, for the small number of cases not immediately fatal at the scene, requires immediate surgical repair. Most surgeons experienced with the treatment of this injury employ cardiopulmonary bypass, although a small minority continues to "clamp and sew." Preoperative management emphasizes controlled hypotension to avoid progressive dissection, or worse, intrathoracic rupture. A transfer agreement with a cardiac surgical center is obligatory where cardiopulmonary bypass is unavailable.

Possibly Life-Threatening Thoracic Injuries

Simple pneumothorax and *simple hemothorax* are both definitively treated by simple tube thoracostomy. Prophylactic antibiotic therapy should be avoided in both conditions. It is important that all air and blood collections be fully drained, but especially the latter, to prevent both empyema formation in the early postinjury stage or the late development of fibrothorax, or "trapped lung," both of which require VATS if not formal thoracotomy. In both conditions the tube should be left in place for an average of 5 days, and may be removed when a chest roentgenograph obtained on water seal drainage but off suction reveals no evidence of recollection of air or blood.

Rib fractures and *sternal fractures* require no specific treatment beyond appropriate analgesia. Intercostal nerve blocks are sometimes employed for the former, especially in older children and adolescents. Opioids should be avoided to the extent feasible, due to their propensity to depress ventilatory drive and predispose the patient to atelectasis and pneumonia, particularly since patients with rib and sternal fractures may be splinting during breathing due to pleuritic or costal pain, making them more susceptible to infection. Incentive spirometry and early ambulation should be used to encourage deep breathing.

Esophageal injuries require urgent surgical intervention. For such injuries, open thoracotomy, direct repair, and mediastinal drainage are required to prevent the inevitable subsequent development of mediastinitis, which remains a lethal illness if left untreated. Early treatment of esophageal injuries excludes oral intake but includes intravenous antibiotics. For iatrogenic injuries resulting from traumatic attempts at endotracheal intubation, gastric intubation, or rigid esophagoscopic procedures, a similar approach is followed, although minor mucosal repairs are increasingly managed nonoperatively.

Mediastinal traversing injuries require either immediate operative intervention if there is evidence of hemodynamic instability, or expectant management if all diagnostic tests are negative. A surgeon experienced in the management of these complex injuries should be involved from the earliest stages of management. If hemodynamic instability is present, time is of the essence, and operative intervention cannot be delayed, since the heart or great vessels have likely been injured. If not, management may proceed at a less urgent, but still timely, pace, since failure to expeditiously recognize and treat potential injuries to the airways, the lungs, the esophagus, or the chest wall can also be fatal.

Resuscitative Thoracotomy

"Resuscitative" or "emergency department" thoracotomy is utilized only in cases for which there is a chance of recovery. In general, patients who present in blunt traumatic cardiac arrest have such a dismal outcome that such a heroic measure cannot be justified, as costs are high and risk to treating physicians is potentially higher. By contrast, patients who present in traumatic arrest from penetrating injuries have a real chance for recovery, if signs of life were present in the field or are lost on arrival or during resuscitation in the emergency department. Even so, resuscitative thoracotomy remains an advanced technique that should be used only by trained physicians.[45,46]

The procedure is performed via left anterior thoracotomy through the fifth left intercostal space, extended as necessary across the midline, superiorly or inferiorly by sharply bisecting the costal cartilages, or further laterally. A rapid inspection is made for injury that may be amenable to temporary control. The pericardium is opened axially, parallel and anterior to the vagus nerve, and entrapped blood is rapidly evacuated with the hands and using suction. Open cardiac wounds may be controlled with a Foley catheter, or with skin staples, followed by aggressive resuscitation, and transfer to the operating room for definitive surgical management should the patient survive the resuscitation.

Resuscitative thoracotomy for massive intra-abdominal bleeding has largely been abandoned. While cross clamping of the distal thoracic aorta temporarily raises blood pressure in the upper body, it does so at tremendous expense. The lower half of the body receives no blood supply, except via collateral vessels, and the spinal cord may be grossly underperfused. The procedure also delays definitive control of intra-abdominal bleeding, which continues unabated until the abdomen is opened and packed, utilizing principles of damage control surgery that are far more likely to result in a favorable outcome.

An emergency department thoracotomy for penetrating injuries can be life saving. The pericardium is responsible for this, since without its presence, cardiac wounds would be uniformly fatal, from rapid exsanguination into the hemithorax. Neurologically intact survival is more difficult to achieve, but patients who present with a perfusing rhythm and acceptable, if marginal, vital signs can be expected to recover fully. Early involvement of a qualified surgeon is therefore essential to optimal results.

Minor Chest Injuries

Minor chest injuries are those confined to the soft tissues of the chest wall, and that in cases of penetrating trauma do not violate the parietal pleura. They are noteworthy chiefly because of their frequency. Blunt injury to the chest wall typically results in superficial contusions to the skin and subcutaneous tissues, most often overlying the bony prominences of the child's ribs, and does not require treatment beyond the symptomatic relief provided by warm compresses and oral analgesics. Penetrating injury to the chest wall is rarely associated with intrathoracic injury absent signs of respiratory distress, but great care is warranted during exploration of an apparently superficial penetrating wound.

Wounds that penetrate the deep fascia may require surgical exploration in the operating room. Likewise, contaminated wounds may also benefit from operative débridement by means of pulse jet irrigation prior to formal closure. Otherwise, superficial lacerations may be repaired in the emergency department, closing the wound in two layers whenever possible. Tetanus prophylaxis is given as appropriate.

Subcutaneous emphysema serves as an indicator of severe associated injury. Bone crepitus is associated with rib, sternal, or scapular fracture. Subcutaneous crepitus is associated with barotrauma. In either case, careful examination to rule out bone injury and pneumothorax is warranted.

Costochondral separation is a condition mainly affecting physically active children. It results when a shear force is applied to one or more adjacent costochondral junctions, causing separation of the bone and the cartilaginous rib elements adjacent to the sternum. The condition is fairly painful, and typically requires oral analgesic therapy. It is self-limiting, usually resolving within a month, if excessive physical activity is avoided.

Penetrating Injuries

When first encountered, all penetrating injuries to the thorax must be considered to have violated the parietal pleura. Great care must be taken during exploration of the wound to avoid such violation if it has not yet occurred. "Sucking" chest wounds must be covered immediately with an occlusive dressing, followed immediately by tube thoracostomy for drainage of entrapped air and blood. All penetrating thoracic injuries must be deemed contaminated, and must be thoroughly cleansed and débrided prior to suture repair, in addition to appropriate antibiotic and tetanus prophylaxis as indicated. As with abusive injuries, the history obtained following penetrating trauma is likely to be inaccurate. As such, hospital admission is warranted, both to ensure that the child receives a full course of antibiotics, and to allow full involvement of social work and pastoral care services, whose skills are critical in determining the circumstances surrounding the injury. Finally, all gunshot and stab wound injuries in children must be reported to the police, and to the local child protective services.

Thoracoabdominal Injuries

Thoracoabdominal injuries are penetrating injuries that traverse the diaphragm. They must be suspected whenever a penetrating injury is found anywhere between the nipples and the umbilicus. All potential thoracoabdominal injuries mandate immediate chest roentgenography, to identify possible intrathoracic air or blood, followed by insertion of a chest tube if present. All such injuries will also require exploratory laparotomy or laparoscopy, both to determine whether and where diaphragmatic penetration may have occurred, and to exclude other intra-abdominal injuries that also require operative repair.

Summary

Serious thoracic injuries occur in nearly 1 in 15 cases of major childhood trauma, but are second only to central neuraxis injuries in their lethality. Most pediatric thoracic injuries are initially managed conservatively or by tube thoracostomy, although major thoracic injuries typically coexist with immediate or potential life-threatening to other body regions. Still, a high level of vigilance for thoracic injuries is never misplaced, since derangements of ventilation, oxygenation, and perfusion resulting from injury to intrathoracic components of the airway, breathing, and circulation substantially worsen the prognosis of associated injuries, particularly central neuraxis injuries, due to inadequate delivery of oxygen to damaged brain tissue. A physiologic approach to the emergent management of thoracic trauma best serves the needs of the injured child, whose greater oxygen requirements, smaller oxygen reserves, and early fatigueability call for both rapid restoration and meticulous maintenance of oxygen saturation, such that cellular respiration can be supported and irreversible shock can be avoided.

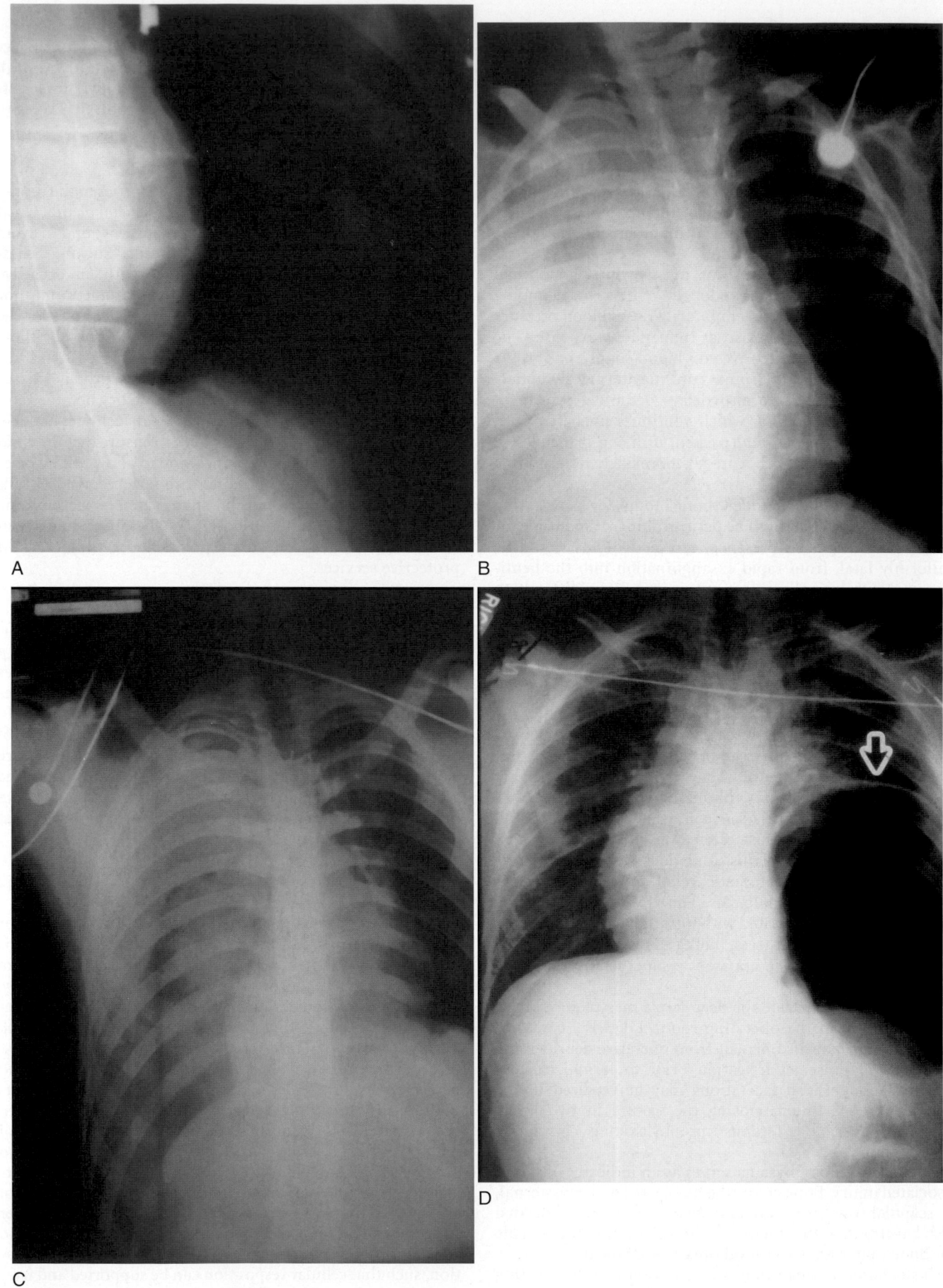

A

B

C

D

FIGURE 24–1. For legend see opposite page

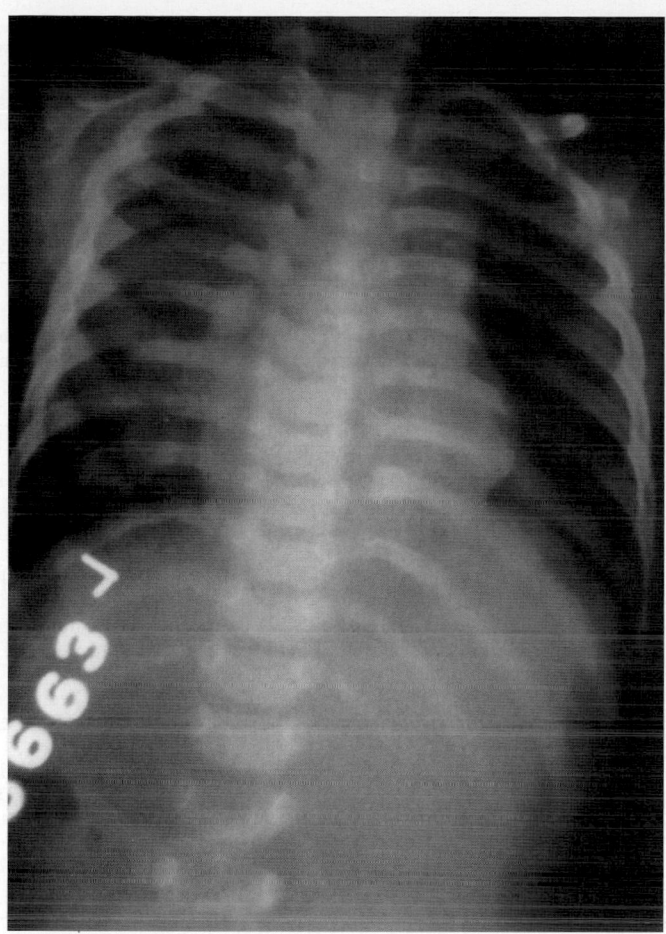

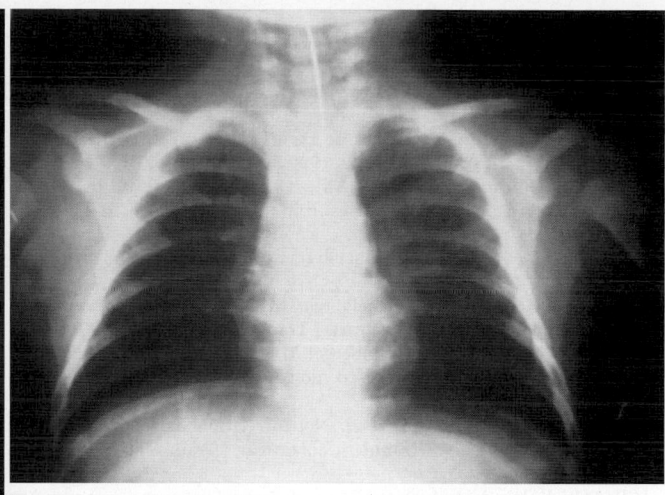

FIGURE 24–1. A, Classic radiographic appearance of tension pneumothorax. Treatment requires needle decompression followed by tube thoracostomy. **B,** Classic radiographic appearance of massive hemothorax. Treatment requires volume resuscitation followed by tube thoracostomy. **C,** Classic radiographic appearance of pulmonary contusion. Treatment requires adequate oxygenation and judicious fluid administration. **D,** Classic radiographic appearance of left traumatic diaphragmatic hernia. Treatment requires operative repair. **E,** Classic radiographic appearance of multiple fratures in various stages of healing due to child maltreatment. Treatment requires recognition and reporting. **F,** Classic radiographic appearance of hypovolemia with a small cardiac silhouette. Treatment requires volume resuscitation.

REFERENCES

*1. Cooper A, Barlow B, DiScala C, String D: Mortality and truncal injury: the pediatric perspective. J Pediatr Surg 29:33–38, 1994.
2. Smyth BT: Chest trauma in children. J Pediatr Surg 14:41–47, 1979.
3. Meller JL, Little AG, Shermeta DW: Thoracic trauma in children. Pediatrics 74:813–819, 1974.
4. Nakayama DK, Ramenofsky MI, Rowe MI: Chest injuries in children. Ann Surg 210:770–775, 1989.
5. Roux P, Fisher RM: Chest injuries in children: an analysis of 100 cases of blunt chest trauma from motor vehicle accidents. J Pediatr Surg 27:551–555, 1992.
6. Reilly JP, Brandt ML, Mattox KL, et al: Thoracic trauma in children. J Trauma 34:329–331, 1993.
*7. Peterson RJ, Tepas JJ, Edwards FH, et al: Pediatric and adult thoracic trauma: age-related impact on presentation and outcome. Ann Thorac Surg 58:14–18, 1994.
8. Reinhorn M, Kaufman HL, Hirsch EF, et al: Penetrating thoracic injury in a pediatric population. Ann Thorac Surg 61:1501–1505, 1996.
*9. Subcommittee on Advanced Trauma Life Support, American College of Surgeons Committee on Trauma: Advanced Trauma Life Support for Doctors Student Manual, 7th ed. Chicago: American College of Surgeons, 2004.

*10. Subcommittee on Pediatric Resuscitation, American Heart Association Committee on Emergency Cardiovascular Care: Textbook of Pediatric Advanced Life Support, 4th ed. Dallas: American Heart Association, 2006.
11. Bonadio WA, Hellmich T: Post-traumatic pulmonary contusion in children. Ann Emerg Med 18:1050–1052, 1989.
12. Allen GS, Cox CS, Moore FA, et al: Pulmonary contusions: are children different? J Am Coll Surg 85:229–233, 1997.
13. Allen GS, Cox CS: Pulmonary contusion in children: diagnosis and management. South Med J 91:1099–1106, 1998.
*14. Peery CL, Chendrasekhar A, Paradise NF, et al: Missed injuries in pediatric trauma. Am Surg 65:1067–1069, 1999.
15. Uribe RA, Pachon CE, Frame SB, et al: A prospective evaluation of thoracoscopy for the diagnosis of penetrating thoracoabdominal trauma. J Trauma 37:650–654, 1994.
16. Lang-Lazdunski L, Mouroux J, Pons F, et al: Role of videothoracoscopy in chest trauma. Ann Thorac Surg 63:327–333, 1997.
17. Meyer DM, Jessen ME, Wait MA, et al: Early evacuation of traumatic retained hemothoraces using thoracoscopy: a prospective, randomized trial. Ann Thorac Surg 64:1396–1401, 1997.
18. Mineo TC, Ambrogi V, Cristino B, et al: Changing indications for thoracotomy in blunt chest trauma after the advent of videothoracoscopy. J Trauma 47:1088–1091, 1999.
19. Tellez DW, Hardin WD, Takahashi M, et al: Blunt cardiac injury in children. J Pediatr Surg 22:1123–1128, 1987.
20. Dowd MD, Krug S: Pediatric blunt cardiac injury: epidemiology, clinical features, and diagnosis. J Trauma 40:61–67, 1996.

*Selected readings.

21. Bromberg BI, Mazziotti MV, Cante, CE, et al: Recognition and management of nonpenetrating cardiac trauma in children. J Pediatr 128:536–541, 1996.

22. Maron B: Cardiovascular risks to young persons on the athletic field. Ann Intern Med 129:379–386, 1998.

23. Fulterman L, Lenberg L: Commotio cordis: sudden cardiac death in athletes. Am J Crit Care 8:270–272, 1999.

*24. Maron BJ, Goldman TE, Estes NAM, et al: The clinical spectrum of commotio cordis: the first 100 cases from the US registry. Circulation 103:609, 2000.

25. Harris GJ, Soper RT: Pediatric first rib fractures. J Trauma 30:343–345, 1990.

26. Garcia VF, Gotschall CS, Eichelberger MR, et al: Rib fractures in children: a marker of severe trauma. J Trauma 30:695–700, 1990.

27. Peclet MH, Newman KD, Eichelberger MR, et al: Thoracic trauma in children: an indicator of increased mortality. J Pediatr Surg 25:961–965, 1990.

28. Lee J, Harris JH, Duke JH, et al: Noncorrelation between thoracic skeletal injuries and acute traumatic aortic tear. J Trauma 43:400–404, 1997.

29. Hills MW, Delprado AM, Deans SA, et al: Sternal fractures: associated injuries and management. J Trauma 35:55–60, 1993.

30. Holmes JF, Sokolove PE, Brant WE, et al: A clinical decision rule for identifying children with thoracic injuries after blunt torso trauma. Ann Emerg Med 39:492–499, 2002.

31. Renton J, Kincaid S, Ehrlich PF: Should helical CT scanning of the thoracic cavity replace the conventional chest x-ray as a primary assessment tool in pediatric trauma? An efficacy and cost analysis. J Pediatr Surg 38:793–797, 2003.

32. Sivit CJ, Taylor GA, Eichelberger MR: Chest injury in children with blunt abdominal trauma: evaluation with CT. Radiology 171:815–818, 1989.

33. Manson D, Babyn PS, Palder S, et al: CT of blunt chest trauma in children. Pediatr Radiol 23:1–5, 1993.

34. Spouge AR, Burrows PE, Armstrong D, et al: Traumatic aortic rupture in the pediatric population: role of plain films, CT and angiography in the diagnosis. Pediatr Radiol 21:324–328, 1991.

35. Smejkal R, O'Malley KF, David E, et al: Routine initial computed tomography of the chest in blunt torso trauma. Chest 100:667–669, 1991.

*36. Durham RM, Zuckerman D, Wolverson M, et al: Computed tomography as a screening exam in patients with suspected blunt aortic injury. Ann Surg 220:699–704, 1994.

37. Lowe LH, Bulas DI, Eichelberger MR, et al: Traumatic aortic injuries in children: radiologic evaluation. AJR Am J Roentgenol 170:39–42, 1998.

38. Fishman JE, Nunez D, Kane A, et al: Direct versus indirect signs of traumatic aortic injury revealed by helical CT: performance characteristics and interobserver agreement. AJR Am J Roentgenol 172:1027–1031, 1999.

*39. Jindal A, Velmahos GC, Rofougaran R, et al: Computed tomography for evaluation of mild to moderate pediatric trauma: are we overusing it? World J Surg 26:16, 2002.

40. Holmes JF, Brant WE, Bogren HG, et al: Prevalence and importance of pneumothoraces visualized on abdominal computed tomographic scan in children with blunt trauma. J Trauma 50:516–520, 2001.

41. Brook SW, Young YC, Cmolik B, et al: Use of transesophageal echocardiography in the evaluation of chest trauma. J Trauma 32:761–767, 1992.

42. Smith MD, Cassidy JM, Southern S, et al: Transesophageal echocardiography in the diagnosis of traumatic rupture of the aorta. N Engl J Med 332:356–362, 1995.

43. Parish RA, Watson M, Rivara FP: Why obtain arterial blood gases, chest x-rays, and clotting studies in injured children? Experience in a regional trauma center. Pediatr Emerg Care 2:218–222, 1986.

44. Hirsch R, Landt Y, Porter S, et al: Cardiac troponin I in pediatrics: normal values and potential use in the assessment of cardiac injury. J Pediatr 130:872–877, 1997.

45. Sheikh AA, Culbertson CB: Emergency department thoracotomy in children: rationale for selective application. J Trauma 34:323–328, 1993.

*46. Working Group, Ad Hoc Subcommittee on Outcomes, American College of Surgeons Committee on Trauma: Practice management guidelines for emergency department thoracotomy. J Am Coll Surg 193:303–307, 2001.

Chapter 25

Abdominal Trauma

Frederick C. Blum, MD, George L. Foltin, MD, and Arthur Cooper, MD, MS

Key Points

Abdominal trauma is the third leading cause of trauma death in children after trauma to the central nervous system and the thorax.

There are anatomic and physiologic differences between children and adults that impact on both diagnosis and management.

The computed tomogram remains the most specific test for the evaluation of abdominal injury, but it is crucial that evidence-based criteria be developed to determine the role of Focused Assessment by Sonography in Trauma (FAST) for diagnosis of abdominal trauma in children, which has largely supplanted the role of diagnostic peritoneal lavage in adults.

The physician assessing the pediatric patient must recognize the need for acute intervention in life-threatening abdominal injuries, particularly with regard to volume resuscitation, gastric decompression, pelvic stabilization, and, in rare instances, the pneumatic antishock garment.

The differential diagnosis of life-threatening abdominal injuries is challenging, but not of immediate importance in the emergency department, where the focus should be on resuscitation and stabilization.

The majority of blunt abdominal injuries can be managed conservatively, but life-threatening injuries require observation in a pediatric intensive care unit and availability of surgeons experienced in the management of abdominal injuries in childhood.

It is essential to be aware of the probability of coexisting injuries.

Pediatric patients with life-threatening abdominal injuries must be stabilized, then transported to trauma centers with pediatric capabilities, when such resources are not available on site.

Introduction and Background

Trauma remains the leading cause of death in the pediatric population between 1 and 14 years of age, resulting in more fatalities than all other diseases combined. Traumatic brain and thoracic injuries are the two foremost killers in this age group, but abdominal trauma is the third most important source of lethal injuries in children, and the main source of initially unrecognized injury leading to mortality in pediatric patients. Although it is important to recognize that, in contrast to adult trauma, pediatric trauma is primarily a disease of the airway and breathing, rather than of the circulation, it is also important to understand that, when a hemodynamic abnormality is added to the neuroventilatory abnormality from which most observed derangements of airway and breathing actually result, the observed mortality rate in pediatric trauma patients has been shown to double, and is worsened further still if a cardiorespiratory derangement is also found to coexist.[1,2]

Historical data from the National Pediatric Trauma Registry[3] and current statistics from the National Trauma Data Bank (http://www.ntdb.org) show that major abdominal trauma is relatively uncommon in children, occurring as the only body region injured in only 3%. Yet the case fatality rates associated with these injuries have been shown to be as high as 15%, and may increase significantly when injury to other organ systems is present. Hence, physicians caring for injured children must be familiar with the recognition, evaluation, and management of abdominal injury in children, as well as the mechanisms of injury that result in abdominal trauma. These will vary by age, geographic location, and trends in popular sports, as well as community compliance with injury prevention measures. Because of anatomic, physiologic, and epidemiologic differences, children must be assessed and managed differently than adults. The development of a systematic diagnostic approach to the evaluation of abdominal injuries in children continues to evolve as better diagnostic modalities emerge.

Blunt abdominal injuries outnumber penetrating abdominal injuries by a ratio of 6:1. Together, motor vehicle occupant and pedestrian injuries account for about three fifths of all blunt abdominal injuries in children. Fall, bicycle, and miscellaneous injuries account for the remainder. Gunshot and stab wounds are responsible for all but one fifth of penetrating injuries, in a ratio of slightly more than 2:1. About 1 in 12 children with an intra-abdominal injury will die, but

4 of every 5 children dying from blunt abdominal injuries die from associated injuries, most often to the head, while 2 of every 3 children dying from penetrating abdominal injuries die from the injury itself.[3]

Recognition and Approach

Specific attention to the diagnosis and treatment of the injured child has resulted in significant decreases in the morbidity and mortality of all traumatic injuries, including those to the pediatric alimentary tract and associated organs. This has been achieved by developing standards of care for injured children that build upon the American College of Surgeons Committee on Trauma Advanced Trauma Life Support (ATLS) protocols for the injured adult, but address the special problems encountered in the pediatric population best described in the American Heart Association and American Academy of Pediatrics Pediatric Advanced Life Support guidelines.[4,5] As a result, the primary survey in children, which remains directed toward priority assessment and stabilization of airway, breathing, and circulation, applies these principles based upon key pediatric differences in anatomy and physiology that require a modified approach. For this reason, a firm understanding of the pathophysiology unique to pediatric abdominal trauma is critical.

The pediatric abdomen is prone to injury for a number of reasons. The thinner layers of the abdominal wall provide less protection to underlying organs. Owing to the more horizontal orientation of the abdomen, the liver and spleen are not fully covered by the ribs, while the dome of the urinary bladder extends well above the pubic ramus. Most important, the abdomen cavity is more compact. Thus, impacting forces are concentrated in a smaller volume, such that intra-abdominal injuries are much more often multiple.

Perhaps the most important consideration in recognizing and approaching abdominal injuries is their propensity for delayed presentation. Injured children are frightened, and a tachycardic response to injury is to be expected. Therefore, tachycardia is not a reliable early indicator of intra-abdominal bleeding, although every child with intra-abdominal bleeding will certainly exhibit tachycardia. Moreover, the ability of the child's blood vessels, particularly the small arterioles, to vasocontrict in the presence of hypovolemia and hypothermia is well known, such that hypotension is a notoriously late sign of hemorrhagic shock, leading to what has been called the "deceptive" presentation of shock in infants and young children. Unfortunately, while the child's compensatory mechanisms are excellent, they are relatively short lived in terms of compensatory response. Thus a high index of suspicion for intra-abdominal injuries, and the understanding that hemodynamic changes may at first be subtle, are the treating physician's most vital tools in the recognition and approach to management of abdominal injuries in childhood.

Intra-abdominal organs are bluntly injured in one of three ways.[6] Solid organs can be compressed against the spine, followed by contusion, laceration, or disruption, with subsequent hemorrhage (Fig. 25–1A–C). Hollow organs can also be compressed against the spine, and can similarly rupture as intraluminal pressures increase (Fig. 25–1D, E, and M). Finally, the posterior attachments of both solid and hollow organs to the abdominal wall can be torn, leading to massive hemorrhage as hepatic and mesenteric vessels are torn from the larger vessels into which they drain by shearing forces that typically follow upon sudden deceleration injuries. By contrast, penetrating injuries damage tissue in one of two ways. Direct injury by the penetrating vector along the path of its trajectory is responsible for most damage in low-velocity injuries, such as those caused by knives or handguns. However, in high-velocity injuries, such as those cause by high-powered rifles or automatic weapons in which the muzzle velocity is much higher, energy transfer to injured tissues is greatly increased according to the familiar formula, $KE = \frac{1}{2} mv^2$, in which high missile velocity is far more deadly than high missile mass. The result is a conical shock wave that both devitalizes adjacent structures and causes much more tissue destruction at exit than at entrance sites.

The most common cause of major trauma in childhood is the motor vehicle. Injuries to pedestrians are slightly more common than injuries to occupants in most series.[7] The Waddell triad is perhaps the most widely known injury pattern of injury in childhood, and involves the head, abdomen, and thighs of the preschool or young school-age child who is struck by a moving vehicle. The bumper strikes the child in the thigh, causing a femur fracture, while the hood strikes the torso, causing a potential liver or spleen injury, depending upon whether the child is struck on the right or the left side. The triad is completed by the brain injury that results when the youngster's top-heavy body lands head first, after being thrown through the air following transfer of momentum from the moving vehicle to the injured child. Although the Waddell triad has been variously described to include the pelvis rather than the femurs or the abdomen, and while all components of the triad are present in no more than about 3% of cases, the illustrative value of the Waddell triad is self-evident.[8] The young child struck by a moving vehicle is at high risk for injuries to the head, torso, and femurs, because of the biomechanics of energy transfer. Thus the child struck by a moving vehicle who presents, for example, with an "isolated" femur fracture must also be suspected of having sustained significant, if subclinical, injuries to the brain and abdomen. A careful history will often disclose a probable loss of consciousness, confirming the former, while a biochemical profile may reveal a clinically or radiologically unsuspected hepatic contusion, confirming the latter.

The lap and shoulder belt complex of injuries has been recently recognized in children improperly restrained as motor vehicle occupants during a crash. The lap belt complex is heralded by the Chance fracture, a hyperflexion fracture of a lumbar vertebral body, coupled with hematoma or perforation of an upper intestinal loop. While either or both of these may occur, severe injuries are typically heralded by associated contusions of the abdominal wall.[9] The injury is the expected result of failure to use a booster seat for a toddler or preschooler, who is then improperly restrained solely by a lap belt that crosses the lower abdomen instead of the hips. The shoulder belt complex results from a similar failure to use proper restraints, and sometimes results in traumatic diaphragmatic hernia. Major blunt abdominal injuries in children due to airbag deployment are extremely rare.[10]

Another classic mechanism of injury commonly encountered in the injured child is the bicycle handlebar injury.[11]

The child's front bicycle wheel strikes a solid object or falls into a hole, causing the handlebar to suddenly rotate as the bicycle abruptly stops, while momentum thrusts the child's upper abdomen forward into the end of the handlebar.[12] The result may be a liver, spleen, gastric, duodenal, or pancreatic injury, which may not be initially detected unless the mechanism of injury is clearly understood by the treating physician. Similar injuries also occur as the result of sledding or tobogganing mishaps in which the child's abdomen is struck by tree stumps or branches hidden beneath the snow. In addition, straddle injuries often occur when the child's perineum strikes the transverse bar between the handlebar and the saddle, resulting in urethral injuries, chiefly in boys.

Sports-related injuries are an uncommon cause of major blunt abdominal trauma in childhood. Blows to the flank sustained during contact sports such as football can lead to significant renal injury. Unintentional blows to the lower ribs or upper abdomen, such as might occur when striking a fielder's foot while attempting to slide into a base, or being kicked by a horse or similarly large animal, have been reported to cause isolated hepatic and splenic injuries. In like manner, unintentional blows to the upper abdomen from a baseball bat or a hockey stick are known to have caused isolated intestinal perforations. Falls sustained during play are perhaps the most common recreational injuries that occur during childhood, but rarely result in abdominal injuries, unless from extreme heights.[13,14]

All-terrain vehicles are increasingly recognized as an important source of major blunt abdominal trauma in children.[15] The higher center of gravity of these vehicles, coupled with the immature motor skills of the young child, make them especially dangerous in the pediatric population. About 1 in 20 serious injuries sustained by children riding all-terrain vehicles involve the abdomen, the spectrum of which injuries closely parallels that observed in children with bicycle handlebar injuries, although injuries are usually more serious, given the higher velocities attained by all-terrain vehicles. For example, a recent case report described abdominal aortic rupture associated with all-terrain vehicle injury.[16]

Text continued on p. 233.

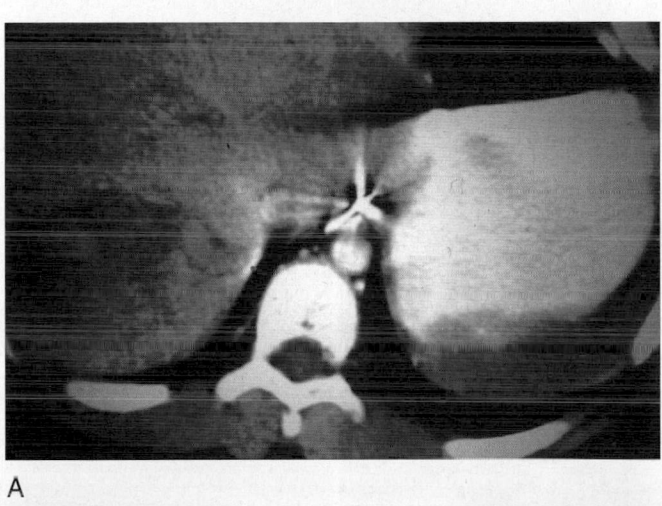

A

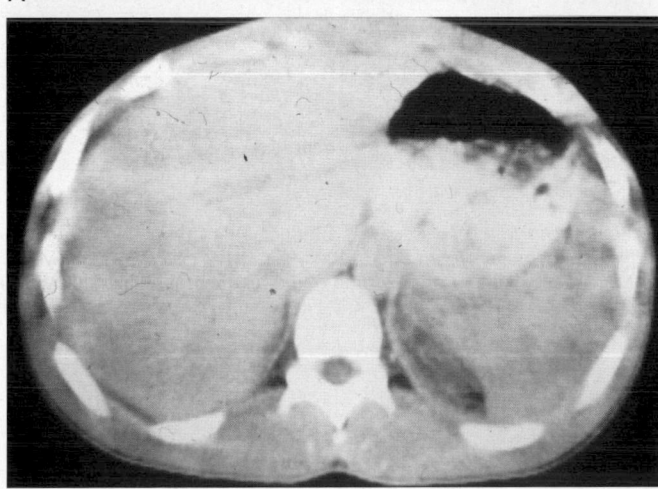

B

FIGURE 25–1. Typical radiographic and clinical appearance of commonly encountered diagnostic entities. **A,** Subcapsular hematoma of the liver following blunt trauma due to motor vehicle–pedestrian injury: tomographic and intraoperative findings. Treatment is mostly nonoperative. (From Barkin RM [ed]: Pediatric Emergency Medicine, 2nd ed. St. Louis: Mosby, 1997.) **B,** Stellate fracture of the kidney following blunt trauma due to motor vehicle–pedestrian injury: tomographic and intraoperative findings. Treatment is mostly nonoperative. (From Barkin RM [ed]: Pediatric Emergency Medicine, 2nd ed. St. Louis: Mosby, 1997.)   *Continued*

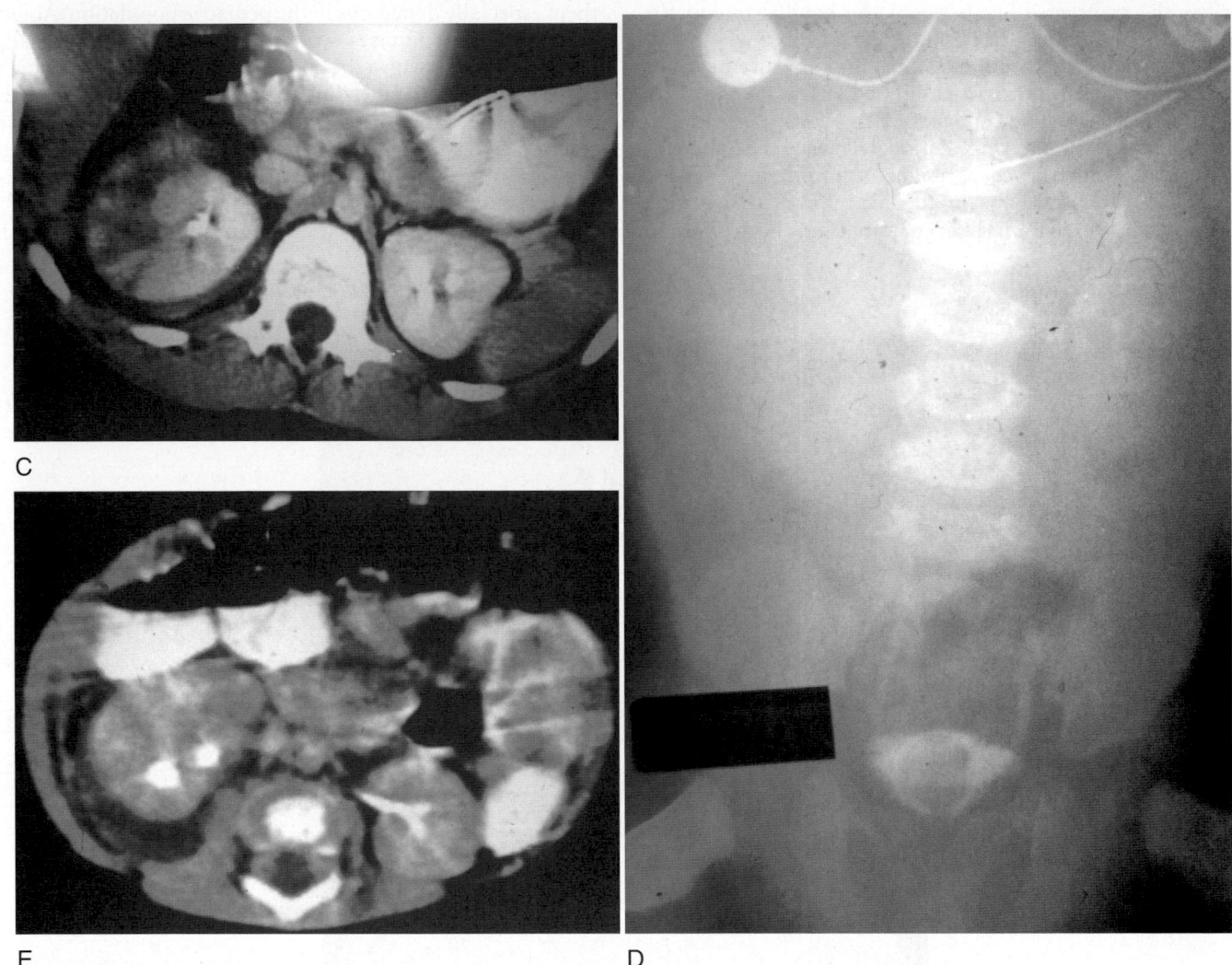

FIGURE 25–1 (cont.). C, Transverse laceration of the spleen following blunt trauma due to motor vehicle–pedestrian injury: tomographic and intraoperative findings. Treatment is mostly nonoperative. (From Barkin RM [ed]: Pediatric Emergency Medicine, 2nd ed. St. Louis: Mosby, 1997.)
D and **E,** Intraperitoneal extravasation of urine due to rupture of the dome of the bladder following blunt trauma: urographic and tomographic findings. Treatment requires operative repair. (From Barkin RM [ed]: Pediatric Emergency Medicine, 2nd ed. St. Louis: Mosby, 1997.)

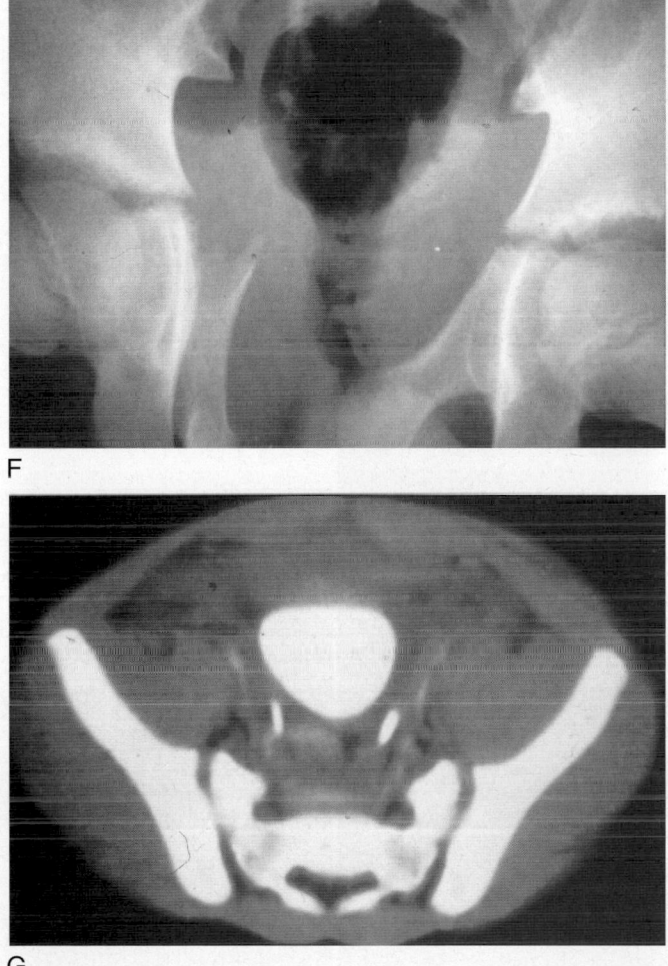

F

G

FIGURE 25–1 (cont.). **F** and **G,** Intraparenchymal hematoma of the liver following blunt trauma due to child abuse; roentgenographic and tomographic findings. Treatment is mostly nonoperative. (From Barkin RM [ed]: Pediatric Emergency Medicine, 2nd ed. St. Louis: Mosby, 1997.)

Continued

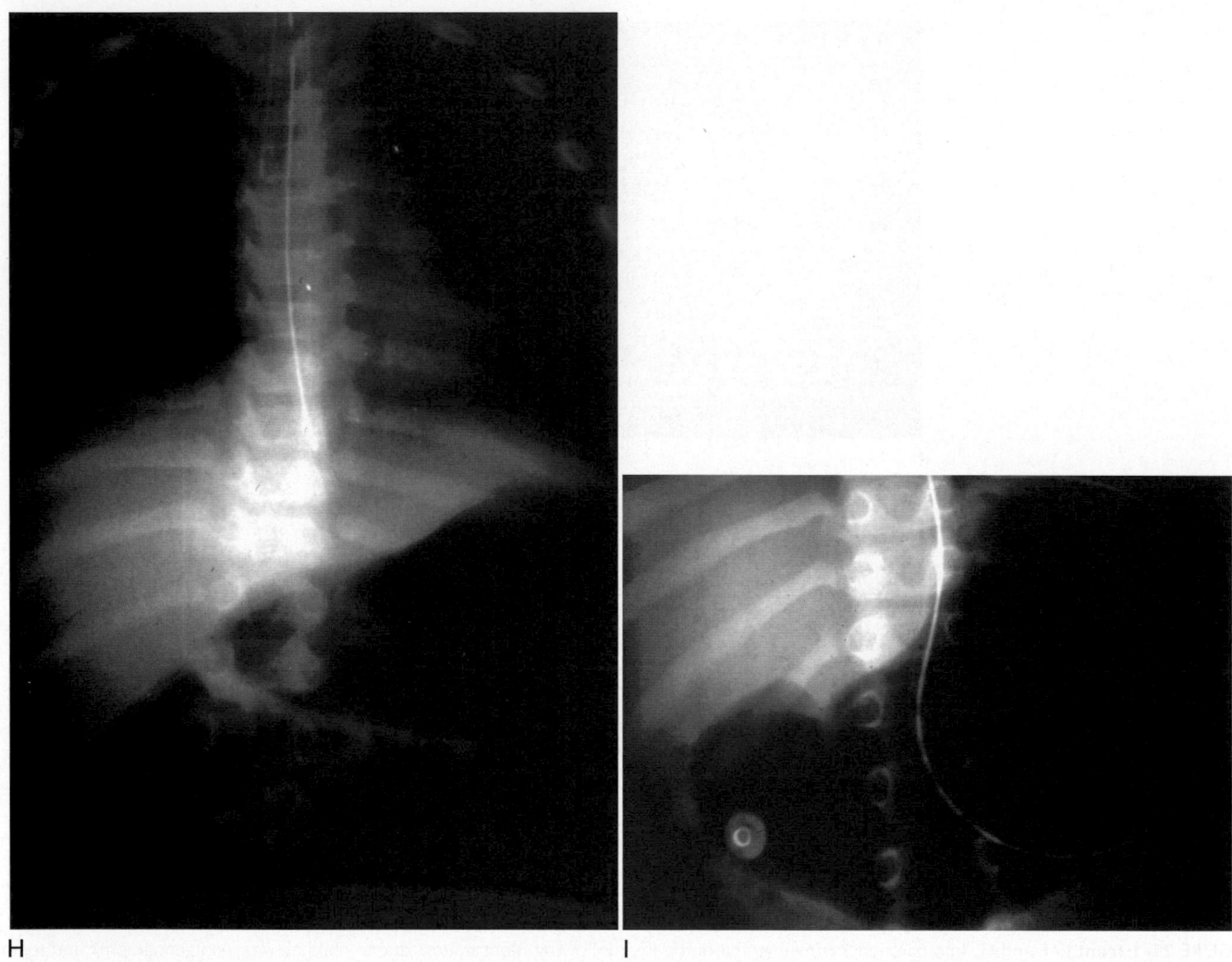

H   I

FIGURE 25–1 (cont.). H and **I,** Intramural hematoma of the duodenum following blunt trauma due to child abuse: fluoroscopic and intraoperative findings. Treatment is mostly nonoperative. (From Barkin RM [ed]: Pediatric Emergency Medicine, 2nd ed. St. Louis: Mosby, 1997.)

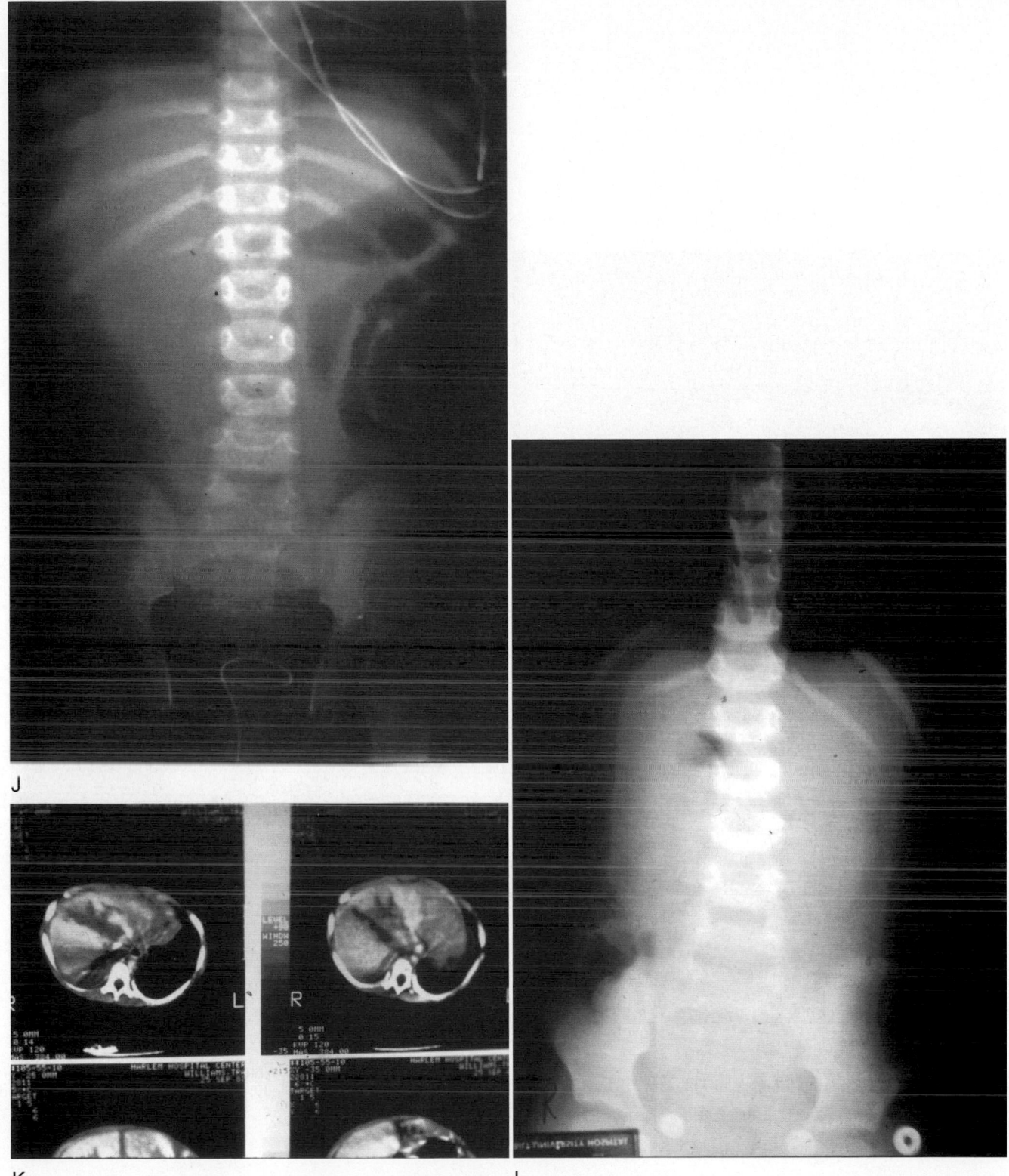

FIGURE 25–1 (cont.). J–L, Retroperitoneal hematoma and duodenal transection following blunt trauma due to child abuse: roentgenographic and intraoperative findings. Note the presence of both subdiaphragmatic and retroperitoneal gas on plain film. (From Barkin RM [ed]: Pediatric Emergency Medicine, 2nd ed. St. Louis: Mosby, 1997.)   *Continued*

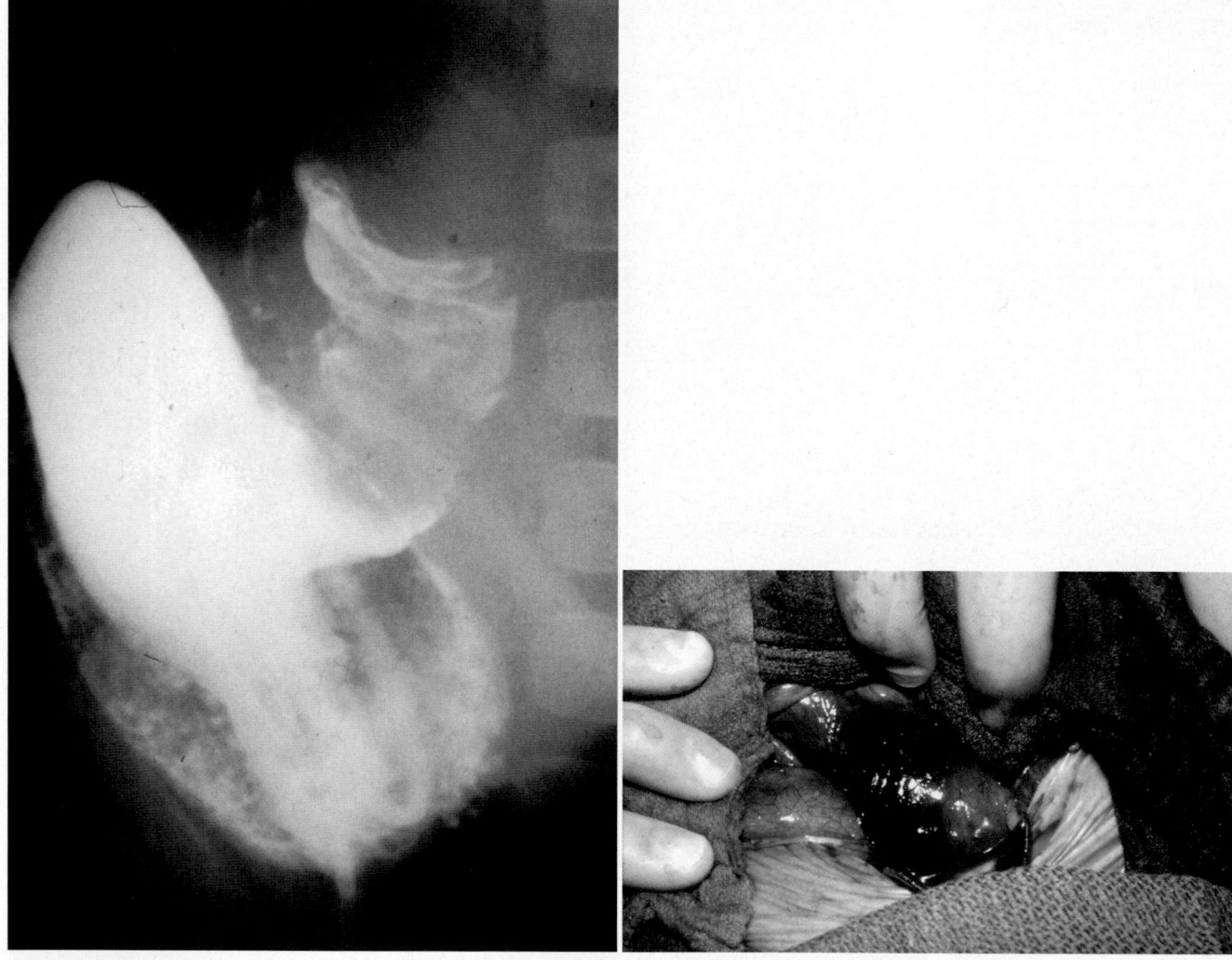

M

FIGURE 25–1 (cont.). M, Gastric dilation following blunt trauma due to motor vehicle–pedestrian injury. Note that gastric dilation remains unrelieved despite passage of nasogastric tube as tube was not advanced fully into stomach. (From Barkin RM [ed]: Pediatric Emergency Medicine, 2nd ed. St. Louis: Mosby, 1997.)

Abuse-related injuries merit special comment.[17] Major blunt abdominal trauma resulting from physical abuse is caused by a forceful blow to the upper abdomen (Fig. 25–1F–L), and occurs in four distinct patterns, readily identifiable by associated vital signs.[18] The first involves duodenal and jejunal hematomas. Such children typically present with bilious vomiting and stable vital signs in the absence of abdominal findings. The second is characterized by duodenal or jejunal perforations. These children also present with bilious vomiting, but are likely to be febrile and tachycardic, with the abdomen distended and tender on examination. The third involves significant disruption of solid organs, most often the liver, with associated intra-abdominal hemorrhage. These children usually present with acute anemia and compensated shock, which often, but not always, are self-limited owing to the thick, elastic capsules of the solid abdominal organs in children. The fourth is characterized by massive hepatic lacerations with or without cavohepatic or cavomesenteric disruptions. These children present in decompensated shock or in frank traumatic cardiopulmonary arrest, and are rarely salvageable. In none of these children will accurate histories be proffered, and most present 12 to 24 hours following injury. Unfortunately, no more than half of these children will have external marks to suggest the diagnosis of intra-abdominal injury. Thus a high index of suspicion is fundamental to making the correct diagnosis.

Evaluation

Trauma to the abdomen may involve injury to its muscular abdominal wall or the contents of any of its five distinct regions. The abdominal portion of the peritoneal cavity contains the liver, the gallbladder and biliary tree, the spleen, and most of the alimentary canal, including a short segment of distal esophagus, the entire stomach, the duodenal bulb, the entire jejunum and ileum, the transverse colon, and the anterior halves of the ascending and descending colons, as well as the dome of the urinary bladder in infants and younger children. The pelvic portion of the peritoneal cavity contains the sigmoid colon, the dome of the urinary bladder in older children and adolescents, and the supracervical uterus, fallopian tubes, and ovaries in girls. The central portion of the upper retroperitoneal space (designated as zone I) contains the great vessels of the abdomen, including the aorta and inferior vena cava and their major branches; the second, third, and fourth segments of the duodenum; the pancreas; and the retroperitoneal surface or "bare area" of the liver. The lateral portions of the upper retroperitoneal space (designated as zone II) contain the kidneys and adrenal glands, the upper two thirds of the ureters and gonadal vessels, and the posterior halves of the ascending and descending colons. The lower, or pelvic, retroperitoneal space, inferior and medial to the pelvic brim (designated as zone III), contains the iliac arteries and veins, the lower thirds of the ureters and gonadal vessels, the upper rectum, and the inferior surfaces of all sides of the urinary bladder (including the trigone). In addition, zone III contains the prostate gland, seminal vesicles, and vasa deferentia in boys; the cervix and upper vagina in girls; and, posterior to Waldeyer's fossa, an intricate plexus of lumbosacral vessels and nerves. Injuries to these organs may manifest acutely during the primary survey, or their presentation may be gradual and insidious in their

onset, hence found only by a careful secondary survey, or perhaps even a tertiary survey performed once the child is admitted to the hospital for treatment.[19]

Injuries to the abdomen can cause severe and substantial cardiovascular compromise that is rapidly progressive. At the same time they can cause equally serious and significant intra-abdominal infections and septic shock of often insidious onset. If these conditions are not recognized and promptly treated, the result may be lethal. It is therefore imperative for the treating physician to detect all underlying injuries, decide the priority of treatment, and begin to reverse the pathophysiologic changes induced by the injuries. The ATLS protocol includes a standardized assessment of the patient's airway, breathing, and circulation that should enable the treating physician to recognize, evaluate, and manage lifethreatening abdominal injuries in priority order, as shown in Table 25–1.[4] Immediately life-threatening abdominal injuries that derange the circulation (massive intra-abdominal bleeding, also called hemoperitoneum, or massive retroperitoneal bleeding, most often due to great vessel injury or unstable pelvic fracture) can usually be detected during the primary survey. Potentially life-threatening abdominal injuries to the circulation (solid organ injuries that do not cause decompensated shock) are more often detected during the secondary survey, as are injuries that affect the integrity of the alimentary canal (hollow organ disruption) and present with peritonitis, and finally sepsis if initially overlooked.

Clinical Evaluation

In performing the primary survey, the treating physician will look first for derangements of the airway and breathing, as delineated in Chapter 12 (Approach to Multisystem Trauma). Once these have been initially addressed, the treating physician looks next for derangements of the circulation. However, the abdomen discloses its secrets slowly and serially. Therefore, careful and frequent re-evaluations are required to ensure that such derangements are not overlooked.

Control of hemorrhage is the first goal of treatment during the primary survey, but intra-abdominal hemorrhage is internal rather than external, and is rarely detected by direct observation alone. Rather, it must first be suspected, then sequentially excluded, by means that involve indirect observations over time, such as those described later. Moreover, major intra-abdominal hemorrhage is detected chiefly through examination for circulatory instability, which requires ongoing evaluation of tissue perfusion (pulse rate and character, peripheral skin and mucous membrane color, temperature and moisture, capillary refill, urinary output). This is because frank hypotension (the cardinal sign of decompensated shock) does not occur until very late in the downward spiral of circulatory deterioration, when the opportunities for successful resuscitation are limited.

Abnormalities in the primary survey are addressed as they arise, since accurate evaluation of each step in the series circuit of substrate (oxygen/fuel) delivery to the tissues (airway/ventilation, breathing/oxygenation, circulation/perfusion) presumes the integrity of the previous step. Adjuncts to the primary survey that will assist in the evaluation of each of these include vital signs (appropriate for age), pulse oximetry (demonstrating adequate S_PO_2), end-tidal capnography (confirming gas exchange), and, with respect to the abdomen, a supine pelvic roentgenogram (identifying

Table 25–1	Principles of Advanced Trauma Life Support[4]

Primary Survey and Resuscitation

Airway/cervical spine
- Open: jaw thrust/spinal stabilization
- Clear: suction/remove particulate matter
- Support: oropharyngeal/nasopharyngeal airway
- Establish: orotracheal/nasotracheal intubation*
- Maintain: primary/secondary confirmation†
- Bypass: needle/surgical cricothyroidotomy

Breathing/chest wall
- Ventilation: chest rise/air entry/effort/rate
- Oxygenation: central color/pulse oximetry
- Support: distress—NRB/failure—BVM
- Chest wall: ensure integrity/expand lungs
  - Tension pneumothorax: needle, chest tube‡
  - Open pneumothorax: occlude, chest tube
  - Massive hemothorax: volume, chest tube

Circulation/external bleeding
- Stop bleeding: direct pressure, avoid clamps
- Shock evaluation: pulse, skin CRT, LOC§
- Blood pressure: avoid over/undercorrection
  - Infant/child: low normal = 70 + (age × 2) mm Hg
  - Adolescent: low normal = 90 mm Hg
- Volume resuscitation: RL → PRBC
  - Infant/child: 20 ml/kg RL, repeat × 1–2 → 10 ml PRBC
  - Adolescent: 1–2 L RL, repeat × 1–2 → 1–2 U PRBC

Disability/mental status
- Pupils: symmetry, reaction

- LOC: GCS score
  - Track and trend as a vital sign
  - Significant change = 2 points
  - Intubate for coma = GCS score ≤ 8
- Motor: strength, symmetry
- Abnormality/deterioration: call neurosurgeon
  - Mild TBI (GCS score 14–15): observe, consider CT for history of LOC
  - Moderate TBI (GCS score 9–13): admit, obtain CT, repeat CT 12–24 hr
  - Severe TBI (GCS score 3–8): intubate, ventilate, obtain CT, repeat CT 12–24 hr

Exposure and environment
- Disrobe: cut off clothes
- Logroll: requires four people
- Screening examination: front and back
- Avoid hypothermia: keep patient warm!

Adjuncts

Foley catheter unless contraindicated‖
Gastric tube unless contraindicated¶

Secondary Survey and Reevaluation

History and physical examination: SAMPLE history, complete examination

Adjuncts

Imaging and laboratory studies: plain radiographs,# special studies**

*Rapid sequence induction technique: etomidate, then succinylcholine.
†Primary: chest rise, air entry; secondary: exhaled CO_2 detector, esophageal detector device; watch for DOPE: dislodgement, obstruction, pneumothorax, equipment failure.
‡Do not wait for confirmatory chest x-ray!
§Consider obstructive and neurogenic as well as hypovolemic shock: exclude tension pneumothorax, cardiac tamponade, and spinal shock.
‖Contraindications include meatal blood, scrotal hematoma, and high-riding prostate.
¶Contraindications include cerebrospinal fluid oto/rhinorrhea, basilar skull fracture, and midface instability.
#Chest, pelvis, and lateral cervical spine; others as indicated.
**Focused Assessment by Sonography in Trauma, CT as indicated.
Abbreviations: BVM, bag-valve-mask; CRT, capillary refill time; CT, computed tomography; GCS, Glasgow Coma Scale; LOC, level of consciousness; NRB, non-rebreather mask; PRBC, packed red blood cells; RL, Ringer's lactate; TBI, traumatic brain injury.

unstable fractures). Evidence of simple hypovolemia (compensated shock) mandates urgent resuscitation. Evidence of frank hypotension (decompensated shock) mandates emergent resuscitation.

In performing the secondary survey, the complete physical examination for abdominal injuries will assess for visible contusions, peritoneal irritation, pelvic stability, and other palpable abnormalities (by inspection and palpation), and for abnormal collections or movement of gas within the gastrointestinal tract (by percussion and auscultation). Mechanisms of injury reliably predict patterns of injury and their clinical presentations, and should form the basis of informed diagnosis. Thus mechanisms known to produce intra-abdominal or pelvic bleeding, or peritonitis, should lead the treating physician to tailor the physical examination, the imaging studies, and the laboratory tests specifically to detect and confirm intra-abdominal injuries that predispose to these physical findings. For example, children who present immediately after high-speed motor vehicle–pedestrian injury with signs of compensated or decompensated shock, such as simple hypovolemia or frank hypotension with altered mental status, should be suspected of having sustained major solid organ disruption, for which volume resuscitation followed immediately by computed tomography

(CT) or emergent laparotomy are warranted. By contrast, children who present in delayed fashion several hours after seemingly trivial injury with signs of frank peritonitis, such as abdominal pain, distention, or tenderness, with or without fever, vomiting, or sepsis, should be suspected of gastrointestinal or pancreatic injury, or minor solid organ disruption associated with persistent oozing, for which volume resuscitation followed in a timely manner by urgent laparotomy or CT are needed. Physical signs of immediately life-threatening abdominal injuries are shown in Table 25–2.

Injuries commonly requiring immediate intervention in the pediatric patient include immediately life-threatening abdominal injuries such as massive, uncontrolled intra-abdominal hemorrhage, and peritonitis associated with septic shock. Far more often encountered but far less often lethal are potentially life-threatening abdominal injuries such as minor, self-limited solid organ hemorrhage. Clinical stabilization with appropriate interventions must be accomplished in an orderly and timely manner to prevent further deterioration. Injuries requiring delayed intervention in the pediatric patient include potentially life-threatening abdominal injuries that in most cases are manifested by abdominal tenderness, as well as those that will not be detected without radiographic or laboratory tests, or ongoing monitoring and

Table 25–2   Physical Diagnosis of Immediately Life-Threatening Abdominal Injuries

General Examination

- AMS
- Poor skin perfusion

Vital Signs

- Tachycardia: heart rate >150 − 5 × age in years
- Hypotension: blood pressure <70 + 2 × age in years

Abdominal Examination

- Abdominal distention unrelieved by gastric decompression
- "Doughy" abdomen, suggestive of intraperitoneal bleeding
- Pelvic instability or Cullen's sign, suggestive of retroperitoneal bleeding
- Abdominal rebound tenderness or involuntary guarding ("spasm")

continuous reassessment of the patient's clinical status, chiefly by means of abdominal examination. For the most part, mild to moderate intra-abdominal organ injuries are now managed nonoperatively, unless radiographic findings indicate that the injury is of such magnitude that operative intervention is indicated, so reliance upon sophisticated diagnostic tools, if available, is important. The American Association for the Surgery of Trauma (AAST) Organ Injury Scaling (OIS) system is now recognized as the standard for correlation of clinical and radiographic findings, although physiologic status remains the best guide for patient care decisions.[20-22] The grading system is applied both prospectively for description of injury severity based on radiographic findings, and retrospectively for performance improvement and research based on intraoperative findings when available, and is delineated in Table 25–3 for each of the major

Table 25–3   American Association for the Surgery of Trauma (AAST) Organ Injury Scaling (OIS)[13]

Liver

Grade I
- Nonexpanding subcapsular hematoma, <10% of surface area
- Capsular tear, nonbleeding, <1 cm in depth

Grade II
- Nonexpanding hematoma, subcapsular or intraparenchymal, 10–50% of surface area or <10 cm in diameter
- Bleeding capsular tear
- Laceration 1–3 cm in depth, <10 cm in length

Grade III
- Subcapsular hematoma >50% of surface area, expanding or ruptured with bleeding
- Intraparenchymal hematoma, >10 cm or expanding
- Laceration >3 cm deep

Grade IV
- Ruptured intraparenchymal hematoma with bleeding
- Parenchymal disruption involving 25–75% of lobe or 1–3 segments

Grade V
- Parenchymal disruption of >75% of lobe or more than 3 segments
- Juxtahepatic venous injury

Grade VI
- Hepatic avulsion

Spleen

Grade I
- Subcapsular hematoma, <10% of surface area
- Laceration/capsular tear, <1 cm in deep

Grade II
- Subcapsular hematoma, 10–50% of surface area
- Intraparenchymal hematoma, <5 cm
- Laceration 1–3 cm, without vessel involvement

Grade III
- Subcapsular hematoma, >50% of surface area or expanding
- Intraparenchymal hematoma, >5 cm
- Ruptured hematoma
- Laceration >3 cm or with trabecular vessel involvement

Grade IV
- Laceration of segmental or hilar vessels causing major devascularization >25% of spleen
- Parenchymal disruption involving 25–75% of lobe or 1–3 segments

Grade V
- Shattered spleen
- Injury of hilar vessels with completely devascularized spleen

Kidneys

Grade I
- Contusion: hematuria without radiographic abnormalities
- Subcapsular hematoma: no parenchymal laceration

Grade II
- Perinephric hematoma confined to the retroperitoneum
- Laceration of renal cortex <1 cm in depth

Grade III
- Laceration >3 cm in depth

Grade IV
- Laceration through collecting system
- Vascular injury with contained hemorrhage

Grade V
- Vascular avulsion
- Shattered kidney

Pancreas*

Grade I
- Hematoma: minor contusion without duct injury
- Laceration: superficial laceration without duct injury

Grade II
- Hematoma: major contusion without duct injury
- Laceration: major laceration without duct injury or tissue loss

Grade III
- Laceration: distal transection without duct injury or tissue loss

Grade IV
- Laceration: proximal transection or parenchymal injury involving ampulla

Grade V
- Laceration: massive disruption of the pancreatic head

Duodenum*

Grade I
- Hematoma: involving single portion of duodenum

Grade II
- Laceration: partial thickness, no perforation
- Hematoma: involving more than one portion

Grade III
- Laceration: disruption <50% of circumference
- Laceration: disruption 50–75% of circumference of D2

Grade IV
- Laceration: disruption 50–100% of circumference of D1, D3, D4
- Laceration: disruption >75% of circumference of D2
- Laceration: involving ampulla or distal common bile duct

Grade V
- Laceration: massive disruption of the duodenopancreatic complex
- Laceration: devascularization of duodenum

*Advance one grade for multiple injuries to same organ.

intrabdominal organs commonly found to be injured in pediatric patients.

Solid Organs

Together with the spleen, the *liver* is the most commonly injured solid abdominal organ, with each of these organs being damaged in 27% of children with abdominal injuries who historically have required admission to a pediatric trauma center. Its central position in the upper abdomen beneath the epigastrium is responsible for this fact, together with the lesser degree of protection afforded the liver by the ribs in pediatric patients. Most liver injuries in childhood are fairly minor, as 70% of these injuries are either contusions, hematomas, or minor lacerations (AAST grade I). Moderate and major lacerations (AAST grades II–III) account for almost all the rest. Only ruptured hematomas, parenchymal disruptions, juxtahepatic venous injuries, and hepatic avulsions (AAST grades IV–VI) are likely to fail nonoperative management, which is successful in about 90% of hepatic injuries.

Similar to the liver, the position of the *spleen* beneath the soft lower ribs of the left upper quadrant of the abdomen is responsible for its high incidence of injury. In addition, in North America motor vehicles occupy the right side of the road, giving their drivers less time to stop for children darting into the road from the right, thereby exposing the left sides of pedestrians struck by motor vehicles. Most spleen injuries in childhood are relatively minor, as 70% of these injuries are either limited subcapsular hematomas, capsular tears, or relatively superficial lacerations (AAST grades I–II). Extensive subcapsular hematomas, intraparenchymal hematomas, deep lacerations (AAST grade III), segmental or hilar vessel injuries with devascularization (AAST grade IV), and shattering injuries (AAST grade V) account for the remainder, but only the latter two are likely to fail nonoperative management, which is successful in 95% of splenic injuries.

The *kidneys* are the third most commonly injured solid abdominal organs in childhood, and are also damaged in 27% of children with abdominal trauma. This is somewhat surprising, given their relatively well-protected position beneath the paraspinous muscles and the fact that they are embedded in fat pads enclosed by the tough fibrous envelopes of Gerota's fascia. Fortunately, and perhaps as a result of their protected location, most renal injuries in childhood are minor, involving only hematomas and contusions (AAST grade I), lacerations not involving the collecting system (AAST grades II–III), and major lacerations involving the collecting system (AAST grade IV). Vascular injuries with contained hemorrhage, vascular avulsions, and renal disruptions or shattering (grade V) are rare. However, although serious renal injuries are uncommon, 80% of such injuries are associated with other serious intra-abdominal injuries. Therefore, serious renal injuries, heralded by hematuria, serve as a marker of serious intra-abdominal injuries.

The *pancreas* is the fourth most commonly injured solid abdominal organ in childhood, and is damaged in 5% of children with abdominal trauma. Given its well-protected location in the middle upper retroperitoneal space, it is not surprising that it is infrequently injured. However, its position overlying the spinal column makes it subject to frank transection when forceful blows are applied to the epigas-trium. Fortunately, most pancreatic injuries are minor and limited to mild traumatic pancreatitis. Pancreatic pseudocysts are the typical sequelae of pancreatic duct injuries, but rarely present before the third to the fifth postinjury day, and most ultimately resorb spontaneously. Pancreatic transections are rare, and many do not require operative management.

Hollow Organs

The *gastrointestinal tract* is the most commonly injured abdominal hollow organ in childhood, and is damaged in 21% of children with abdominal trauma. It is surprising that the gastrointestinal tract is not more frequently injured, given that it occupies both the greatest volume of the abdominal cavity and its most central location. Injuries to the stomach and duodenum represent about 25% of injuries to the gastrointestinal tract, with injuries to the small and large intestine representing the remainder, in roughly equal proportions. Most blunt injuries involve intramural contusions and hematomas, with disruptions being limited chiefly to fixed segments of intestine adjacent to bony prominences, such as the duodenum and proximal ileum. Most penetrating injuries involve transmural lacerations.

The *genitourinary tract*, exclusive of the kidneys, is the second most commonly injured hollow abdominal organ in childhood, and is damaged in 5% of children with abdominal trauma. The urinary bladder and urethra account for four fifths of these injuries and are usually associated with complex pelvic fractures. The ureters account most of the rest, as the genital organs in both boys and girls are small and primordial, and are rarely injured.

The *great vessels* of the abdomen and pelvis are the third most commonly injured hollow abdominal organs in childhood, and are collectively damaged in 5% of children with abdominal trauma, although no one blood vessel is individually damaged in more than 1% of children with abdominal trauma. However, mortality is high, approaching 50% overall, and approaching 90% for aortic injuries. Caval injuries are somewhat less lethal, with mortality in excess of 60%. Mortality in renal and iliac vessel injuries is 20% to 30%.

Bony Pelvis

The bony pelvis is the least commonly injured abdominal structure in childhood, accounting for less than 1% of abdominal injuries in children with abdominal trauma. The vast majority of pelvic fractures in childhood are simple and stable, and free of hemodynamic consequences.[23] However, as in adults, complex, unstable pelvic fractures are associated with life-threatening hemorrhage as well as damage to the genitourinary system. Most such injuries are associated with numerous other injuries, such as traumatic brain injury.

Diagnostic Modalities

Clinical Examination

The physical examination remains the cornerstone of timely diagnosis of intra-abdominal injuries in childhood. Classic *physical signs* remain reliable indicators of intra-abdominal injuries, and are typically used to guide initial diagnosis and treatment, as shown in Table 25–2. Although regarded as adjuncts to the primary survey, vital signs, especially heart rate and blood pressure, are critical components of the clinical examination of the abdomen. The limited role of blood pressure in early diagnosis of circulatory instability is well known, but less well known is the significance of heart rate. No doubt, heart rate is a poor indicator of instability in infants and children, in whom fear and anxiety alone can drive the heart rate to supranormal levels. By contrast, in adolescents and young adults, the heart rate is a highly reliable indicator of circulatory instability. Just as infants and children have the ability to maintain systolic blood pressure via intense vasoconstriction in the face of hypovolemia, adolescents and young adults do so as well. However, in infants and children, the marked associated tachycardia (the upper limit of normal heart rate being estimated at the bedside using the formula, $150 - 5 \times$ age in years) can result from causes other than hemorrhagic shock, while in the adolescent and young adult, a heart rate in excess of 100 beats/min indicates profound hypovolemia until proven otherwise, and should instigate an immediate search for an intra-abdominal source.

Much has been written about the technique of physical examination in childhood. Since the key information to be gleaned from the physical examination is a rapid determination of circulatory stability, vital signs and the status of tissue perfusion, as judged by pulse rate and character, skin color, temperature and moisture, and capillary refill time, are of paramount importance, recognizing that the latter is subject to environmental temperature in the examination room, which should be kept tolerably warm. Abdominal examination is secondary in importance to vital signs and tissue perfusion, and during the primary survey focuses only upon appreciation of findings that suggest blood loss, such as pelvic instability and abdominal distention. To detect the former, the pelvic wings should be compressed first bimedially to determine if the pelvis is grossly stable, then bilaterally to determine if the grossly stable pelvis is fully stable, since pelvic instability in the face of potential pelvic fracture connotes increased pelvic volume and extensive retroperitoneal bleeding. To detect the latter, the abdomen should be directly observed for signs of increased abdominal girth. If this is found, gentle percussion over the upper abdomen can be used to detect gastric dilation, a frequent concomitant of major trauma, particularly traumatic brain injury, in children due to associated aerophagia. If the percussion note is hyperresonant, the stomach should be intubated with a sump tube to decompress it. In most cases, the tube may be inserted via the nasogastric route, but if there is evidence of either basilar skull fracture or midface instability, the tube should be inserted via the orogastric route. If after careful gastric decompression, which in comatose patients should be undertaken only after an endotracheal tube has been placed to protect the airway, abdominal distention persists, the presence of intra-abdominal hemorrhage should be presumed until proven otherwise. However, neither the presence of intra-abdominal hemorrhage nor that of frank peritonitis can be excluded on the basis of a single abdominal examination, since such findings can develop over time. Therefore, serial abdominal examinations are mandatory, unless the findings on initial abdominal examination unequivocally indicate massive hemorrhage, frank peritonitis, or abdominal evisceration, all of which mandate emergent laparotomy.

Examination of the abdomen for signs of peritoneal irritation is performed as part of the secondary survey. Mild peritoneal irritation may indicate the presence of blood or chyme in the peritoneal cavity, but moderate to severe peritoneal irritation essentially always indicates hollow visceral disruption. Both altered mental status and painful distracting injuries, such as extremity fractures, can confound the abdominal examination, as can marked gastric dilation, which can mimic, as well as mask, the classic physical sign of peritonitis, parietal peritoneal irritation. This should be sought using gentle palpation that displaces the abdominal wall only minimally, and confirmed using gentle percussion. There is no need to confirm the presence of peritoneal irritation, also known as rebound tenderness, via marked displacement of the abdominal wall that is followed by rapid release. This will serve only to frighten the child, at best, or to cause the child extreme discomfort, at worst. Specific physical diagnosis of intra-abdominal injury is very difficult, if not impossible, in the emergency department. It is therefore sufficient in the emergency department to limit abdominal examination to simple maneuvers designed to detect findings that warrant emergent laparotomy, such as hemorrhage and peritonitis. This is true not only for the belly examination, but for the rectal examination as well, the purpose of which is to determine the presence or absence of blood or anterior tenderness.

Use of Focused Assessment by Sonography in Trauma (FAST) as an extension of the abdominal examination is rapidly evolving, but needs to be more specifically studied in its application to abdominal injuries. It consists of a bedside transabdominal sonographic examination for abnormal fluid collections in the pericardial cavity, the subhepatic pouch (of Morison), the splenic fossa, and the retrovesical space. Limited studies of abdominal FAST have been performed in children to date, but while initial studies suggested that its specificity and sensitivity were poor, recent studies suggest otherwise.[25-28] However, since the main purpose of FAST in abdominal trauma is to detect the presence of intra-abdominal fluid presumed to be blood, and since modern management of solid organ injury is dependent on the physiologic status of the patient rather than the presence or absence of blood, its role at present remains controversial. What can be said with certainty is that the role of FAST in the diagnosis of abdominal injury is increasing. The presence of small amounts of intraperitoneal fluid, presumably blood, is unlikely to be associated with significant injury, while the presence of large amounts of intraperitoneal fluid uniformly indicates severe injury.[29-31] Moreover, FAST has the additional advantage that assessments can be performed serially, at the patient's bedside, especially in equivocal cases, thereby improving diagnostic accuracy.[32]

In contrast to FAST, the role of diagnostic peritoneal lavage (DPL) is decreasing. DPL is highly sensitive for the presence of blood in the intraperitoneal cavity, but completely nonspecific with respect to its source. It may also fail to detect retroperitoneal bleeding, which further limits its utility. DPL is somewhat more useful in the diagnosis of hollow visceral injury, but most experts believe that serial physical examination is equally reliable. The procedure is ideally performed via an open technique, following decompression of the stomach and urinary bladder. It requires a small vertical cutdown on the abdominal midline just below the umbilicus.

Table 25–4	Criteria for Positive Diagnostic Peritoneal Lavage*

Intraperitoneal Blood
- Gross blood observed on paracentesis or in lavage effluent
- Inability to read standard newsprint through lavage effluent
- >100,000 RBCs/mm^3 in lavage effluent

Intraperitoneal Soilage
- Gross food particles in lavage effluent
- Gross bile staining of lavage effluent
- Gross chyme or fecal staining of lavage effluent
- >500 WBCs/mm^3 in lavage effluent
- >175 IU/dl amylase in lavage effluent
- >6 IU/dl alkaline phosphatase in lavage effluent
- Gram stain of lavage effluent positive for bacteria

*Blunt trauma.
Abbreviations: RBCs, red blood cells; WBCs, white blood cells.

The procedure is difficult for the inexperienced physician, and is best performed by the surgical consultant. The criteria for DPL to be deemed positive for bleeding or peritonitis are shown in Table 25–4.

Imaging Studies

Beyond the early identification of free intraperitoneal gas and subclinical pelvic fractures, the adjunctive supine chest and abdominal roentgenograms performed as part of the primary survey add little to the detection of abdominal injuries. However, they can occasionally reveal important clues to the differential diagnosis, particularly if there are physical signs of intra-abdominal injury, such as pelvic tenderness, ecchymosis or abrasions, hematuria or difficulty voiding, or abdominal distention.[33] They can also identify most rib, vertebral, and pelvic fractures, detect the presence of gastric dilation, and confirm the correct placement of gastric tubes. The abdominal roentgenogram can also suggest the presence of intraperitoneal or retroperitoneal blood or urine (ground-glass appearance of the abdominal cavity, blurring of psoas shadows), splenic laceration or hematoma (medial displacement of the lateral border of the stomach, as marked by the gastric tube, especially if the fundic mucosa has a sawtooth appearance, indicative of bleeding from the short gastric vessels), renal injury (scoliosis, obliteration of the nephric outlines and psoas shadows, in association with fractures of the lower ribs), and pancreatic contusion or hematoma (inferiorly displaced transverse colon). Unfortunately, the diagnosis of transmural duodenal injury (small retroperitoneal or perinephric gas bubbles or shadows on the right side of the abdomen, slightly below the liver) and duodenal or proximal jejunal hematoma (paucity of gas in the distal small intestine) are quite difficult, and the diagnosis of ileal, colonic, or vesical injury essentially impossible. Even so, the role of upper gastrointestinal contrast fluoroscopy, using air or sterile intravenous contrast administered perorally or via a gastric tube, is extremely limited, and reserved for stable patients suspected of duodenal or proximal jejunal injury, since extraluminal extravasation of contrast does not universally occur once it is given.

Intravenous urography, also known as intravenous pyelography, although largely supplanted by newer techniques, is still occasionally useful, and has two primary indications. The first is in penetrating abdominal injury, when a "one-shot" intravenous urogram is obtained immediately prior to operative intervention in conjunction with the abdominal or pelvic roentgenogram, to confirm the presence of two kidneys and detect extravasation of urine from the kidneys, ureters, and bladder. The second is in blunt abdominal injury in which the presentation is delayed, and manifested only by significant hematuria (>20 red blood cells per high-power field [RBCs/hpf] on microscopic urinalysis). In this situation, it is still acceptable to obtain an intravenous urogram rather than CT to decrease radiation exposure, provided that the patient is otherwise stable.

Retrograde cystourethrography is a vitally important test for male patients in whom pelvic instability, blood at the urinary meatus, perineal or scrotal hematoma, or, in adolescents, a high-riding prostate precludes safe insertion of a urinary (Foley) catheter when indicated. It is typically performed by mixing half-strength intravenous contrast with sterile lubricating jelly, which is then injected retrograde into the urethra as a plain roentgenogram is obtained. If the urethra is demonstrated to be intact, the treating physician may safely proceed with insertion of the urinary catheter. If not, suprapubic cystostomy may be needed, depending upon the physiologic status of the patient and the advice of a urology consultant experienced in the management of injured children.

Double (peroral and intravenous) and triple (per rectum as well, if clinically indicated by the possibility of rectosigmoid or desending colonic perforation) contrast-enhanced CT has become the "gold standard" for definitive diagnosis of intra-abdominal injuries in stable patients. It is a better test for detection and quantification of abnormal collections of air or blood in the lower chest or in the abdomen (which are often missed on supine chest and abdominal roentgenography).[34] It is also more accurate for inclusion or exclusion of contusion, laceration, disruption, or extravasation of intravenous contrast from solid organs, such as "splenic blush" (which indicates persistent bleeding from the spleen or its hilum, the clinical significance of which remains uncertain in the pediatric population), and intraperitoneal or retroperitoneal contrast seepage from the upper or lower tracts of the collecting system (which indicates urinary leak, and has the same clinical significance in children as it does in adults).[35] Finally, it is especially good for documenting the positions of tubes and catheters (which on abdominal roentgenography requires an additional lateral view that often proves difficult to obtain during initial evaluation and resuscitation). Unfortunately, it cannot predict the need for operation, as this judgment is made on clinical grounds.[36] Moreover, while it is more sensitive than plain roentgenography and contrast fluoroscopy for the diagnosis of duodenal and proximal jejunal injury, contrast-enhanced CT cannot definitively exclude such injuries, since leakage of contrast from the intestine may or may not occur.[37] Yet, while it provides far greater sensitivity and specificity in the detection of most abdominal trauma than most other tests, its greater diagnostic accuracy must be weighed not only against its effect on the clinical management and outcome in potentially labile patients (recognizing that the patient must be physiologically stable in terms of both cardiorespiratory and hemodynamic status to safely undergo CT, since it takes up to 1 hour for peroral contrast to suffuse through the entire intestine), but

Table 25–5	Doses of Peroral and Intravenous Contrast Agents for Computed Tomography

Peroral Contrast

Meglumine diatrizoate (Hypaque), 1.5%, by mouth or via gastric tube
- Birth–2 yr: 60 ml
- 3–5 yr: 120 ml
- 6–9 yr: 180 ml
- >9 yr: 300–400 ml

Intravenous Contrast

Meglumine diatrizoate (Hypaque), 60%, by vein
- Step 1: Small intravenous test dose
- Step 2: Intravenous bolus, 2 ml/kg, maximum 50 ml
- Step 3: Intravenous infusion, 50–100 ml, during scanning

also against its potential long-term radiologic side effects in terms of late development of malignant neoplasia (especially when the potential diagnostic benefits from CT are marginal).[38-40] Such risks are now being actively studied, and should lead to derivation and promulgation of a clinical decision rule that ascertains exactly which patients in whom the benefits exceed the risks. The preferred doses for peroral and intravenous contrast agents are shown in Table 25–5.

Abdominal ultrasonography also has a key role in the diagnosis of intra-abdominal injury in children. Not to be confused with FAST, abdominal ultrasonography, in the hands of a skilled ultrasonographer, is nearly as sensitive and specific as CT, and may be preferred for static imaging of the pancreas and kidneys. However, while it is both more time efficient than CT (when considering the added time for contrast suffusion), and obviates the need for administration of peroral or intravenous contrast (especially useful in patients with allergies to shellfish or iodinated contrast agents), it is more difficult for the novice physician to perform or read, and is less accurate than CT, although it is increasingly being used serially to follow healing of solid organ injuries.[41]

Laboratory Studies

Hematologic tests are of limited utility for the early diagnosis and treatment of abdominal injuries in childhood. Hemoglobin concentration and hematocrit are likely to be misleading during the initial phases of resuscitation, as dilutional anemia from endogenous fluid shifts and exogenous fluid administration will not as yet have occurred, although both tests will be useful as a baseline for further measurements. Similarly, arterial blood gases will serve as an initial indicator of core organ perfusion, but are more useful in terms of their trend, although they are more invasive than vital signs and urinary output.[42] However, blood type and crossmatch are routinely obtained in all children with significant injury, especially those with hepatic, splenic, or, rarely, renal injuries likely to require transfusion in lieu of, or in addition to, operative management.

After blood type and crossmatch, the most important biochemical test is urinalysis. The presence of blood in the urine (>20 RBCs/hpf on microscopic urinalysis, to ensure that failure to pursue microscopic hematuria does not result in failure to detect potential congenital anomalies or renal tumors) mandates CT if the child presents early (to exclude potential associated injuries as well as renal injuries), or intravenous urogram if the child presents late (for reasons noted earlier). However, some have argued that the standard used for adults (>50 RBCs/hpf) can also be applied to children.[43] Still others have suggested that CT may not be necessary at all if injuries appear minor.[44] The serum electrolytes (Na^+, K^+, Cl^-, HCO_3^-), blood urea nitrogen, and serum creatinine are valuable tests of renal function, and while they are virtually always normal in children with no previous history of kidney disease, they also serve as a baseline for management of fluids during and after resuscitation. Hepatic and pancreatic enzymes (serum aspartate aminotransferase, alanine aminotransferase, lactate dehydrogenase, total and direct bilirubin, and alkaline phosphatase, as well as amylase and lipase) also play an important role in the diagnosis of blunt abdominal injury in childhood. Hepatic enzymes can detect a subclinical hepatic contusion or biliary leak, while pancreatic enzymes can detect unsuspected pancreatic injury, and by inference, since the tail of the pancreas extends into the hilum of the spleen, possible splenic injury as well, although the latter do not appear cost effective.[45,46]

Management

Major Abdominal Injuries

Abdominal injuries pose an immediate threat to the integrity of the breathing (via associated gastric dilation) and circulation (via associated intra-abdominal hemorrhage), hence to ventilation, oxygenation, and perfusion of core organs and body tissues, thence to vital functions. As such, resuscitation must proceed simultaneously with assessment. Abnormalities of the airway, breathing, and circulation are therefore treated in sequence, as soon as they are recognized, both to restore flow of oxygen through the series circuit composed of the tracheobronchial tree, the lungs, and the bloodstream, and to ensure accurate assessment of downstream segments of this circuit. Of the three major functions—ventilation, oxygenation, and perfusion—evaluated during the primary survey, deficits of perfusion, although uncommon, are the most detrimental. Since most of these perfusion deficits are caused by intra-abdominal hemorrhage, the approach to resuscitation of the child with intra-abdominal injury must be timely, precise, and vigorous.

It is therefore vital that the stepwise pathophysiologic assessment of airway, breathing, and circulation advocated by the ATLS Course of the American College of Surgeons Committee on Trauma be followed in detail.[4] The key immediately life-threatening abdominal condition, intra-abdominal hemorrhage due to solid organ injury or unstable pelvic fracture, is recognized and treated during the primary survey. The key potentially life-threatening abdominal conditions, minor hemorrhage due to minor solid organ injuries, frank peritonitis due to gastrointestinal disruption, are recognized and treated during the secondary survey. Meticulous attention to the early detection and optimal management of these injuries is the ideal way to ensure effective restoration of core organ perfusion, thus the best chance the seriously injured child has of a full and complete physical and neurologic recovery.

With the sole exception of massive gastric dilation that significantly impairs the airway (by causing pulmonary aspiration of acidic gastric contents), the breathing (by limiting diaphragmatic excursion), and the circulation (by markedly increasing vagal tone, thereby causing reflex bradycardia in the infant and young child), immediately life-threatening intra-abdominal injuries result in intra-abdominal hemorrhage (hence deranged tissue perfusion), and require emergent volume resuscitation prior to definitive treatment.

However, major pediatric trauma is chiefly a disease of the airway and breathing (due to severe traumatic brain injury), rather than the circulation (due to ongoing major intra-abdominal hemorrhage), owing to the top-heavy body habitus of the infant and young child, which makes head injuries more common and torso injuries less common. Therefore, volume resuscitation must be guided by physical and laboratory signs of poor tissue perfusion: increased pulse rate; decreased pulse volume; pale, cool, skin that is mottled in infants and young children or clammy in older children and adolescents; increased capillary refill time; electrolytes that reveal high anion gap metabolic acidosis; arterial blood gases that reveal significant base deficit; and elevated serum lactate. In other words, the goal of volume resuscitation is not aggressive fluid administration, but appropriate fluid administration, since excessive water intake can significantly increase cerebral edema, and ultimately, intracranial pressure, complicating treatment of traumatic brain injury.

Volume resuscitation is administered via the intravenous or, in infants or young children in whom intravenous access is difficult, the anterior tibial intraosseous routes, unless the latter is contraindicated by ipsilateral lower extremity fracture. Intravenous access should always be attempted first (due to the serious, if rare, complications of intraosseous access such as osteomyelitis), using large-bore over-the-needle plastic catheters wide enough to rapidly deliver fluid or blood, but narrow enough to fit inside the preferred intravenous access site (either the median cubital veins in the antecubital fossae, or the greater saphenous veins just anterior to the medial malleoli). Insertion of two large-bore catheters above the diaphragm is preferred, although other sites may be used if these are unavailable. In general, peripheral intravenous access is favored over central venous access, although femoral venous access may be employed if there is no other option. Volume resuscitation is initiated using an isotonic balanced salt solution, such as lactated Ringer's solution, in continuously infused aliquots or "boluses" of 20 ml/kg (equivalent to 25% of the circulating blood volume of the infant or young child, the smallest volume reduction that typically results in systolic hypotension, defined by the formula, 70 + 2 × age in years). These boluses may repeated twice (administered thrice) before red blood cells must be transfused (in accordance with the 3 : 1 rule, which states that isotonic balanced salt solutions are only one third as effective as red blood cells as a plasma expander). Although no data are available in pediatric patients, permissive hypotension has been employed with limited success in adult patients, provided blood pressure is adequate to maintain cerebral perfusion, and definitive surgical management is readily available. The pneumatic antishock garment (PASG), or military antishock trousers (MAST), are no longer used for treatment of decompensated shock, except in selected hypotensive patients with unstable pelvic fractures, among whom the device is used not to correct abnormal hemodynamics, but to stabilize fracture fragments.[47,48]

However, as crucial as volume resuscitation may be in children with intra-abdominal hemorrhage, the importance of stopping the bleeding cannot be sufficiently emphasized. Volume resuscitation may transiently restore core organ perfusion, but dilutional anemia is too often the result, particularly when bleeding patients are held in the emergency department in a futile attempt to achieve hemodynamic stability. If volume resuscitation must be employed in the absence of a surgeon, packed red blood cells (type specific if available, or type O, ideally Rh negative, if not) in continuous aliquots of 10 ml/kg should be administered as soon as possible to patients who are hypotensive on arrival in the emergency department, or who do not respond immediately to 40 to 60 ml/kg of lactated Ringer's solution, rapidly infused, as stated, in continuous aliquots of 20 ml/kg. Use of an autotransfuser should be considered for patients with massive, ongoing intra-abdominal hemorrhage, but this is no substitute for emergent surgical consultation and intervention.

Detection of peritonitis is also vital to abdominal examination in the child. There is no test for peritonitis other than physical examination. Mild direct tenderness may indicate minor damage to an underlying organ, but does not indicate peritonitis. Marked direct tenderness, especially when associated with direct or referred rebound tenderness, are the key clinical signs of peritonitis, and together are called peritoneal irritation. The classic "boardlike" rigidity described in adult patients with peritonitis is rarely felt in pediatric patients. Instead, they present with involuntary guarding, termed *spasm*, which differs from boardlike rigidity in that the treating physician can displace the abdominal wall. Regardless, true peritoneal irritation always reflects an intra-abdominal catastrophe, and mandates emergent laparotomy, usually for repair of a ruptured hollow viscus.

Uncontrolled hemorrhage and frank peritonitis are the two main indications for emergent operative intervention in abdominal trauma, in children as well as adults. The former connotes solid visceral injury, and the latter hollow visceral injury. Other conditions mandate urgent laparotomy or laparoscopy as the situation warrants. The general indications for operative management in abdominal trauma are shown in Table 25–6.

Solid Organs

Modern management of nearly all solid organ injuries in childhood is nonoperative. Yet it is not nonsurgical, because operation is needed in a high proportion of pediatric trauma patients, and since, as with appendicitis, mature surgical judgment is required to decide whether, or when, operation may be indicated.[49,50] As a general rule, children with liver, spleen, and kidney injuries will not require operative intervention for hemorrhage control unless the transfusion requirement exceeds half the blood volume (40 ml/kg) within the first postinjury day. However, this statement is somewhat misleading, since most patients who require operation declare themselves in the first few hours after injury, while patients whose transfusion requirement slowly approaches this limit 24 hours after injury are unlikely to rebleed later. This has led in recent years to reconsideration of the traditional approach to nonoperative management of solid organ injuries in childhood, such that extended stays in the pediatric intensive care unit are no longer the norm across North

Table 25–6	General Indications for Operative Management of Abdominal Organ Injuries

Blunt Trauma

- Hemodynamic instability despite adequate volume resuscitation
- Decompensated shock on admission
- Transfusion requirement > 40 ml/kg
- Physical signs of peritonitis
- Positive findings on diagnostic peritoneal lavage (if so decided by the trauma surgeon)
- Radiologic evidence of pneumoperitoneum
- Radiologic evidence of intraperitoneal bladder rupture
- Radiologic evidence of renovascular pedicle injury

Penetrating Trauma

- All gunshot wounds
- All stab wounds associated with:
  - Physical signs of shock or peritonitis
  - Blood in the stomach, urine, or rectum
  - Evisceration
- Radiologic evidence of intraperitoneal or retroperitoneal gas
- Positive findings on diagnostic peritoneal lavage (if so decided by the trauma surgeon)
- All suspected thoracoabdominal injuries

America, provided that nonoperative management is conducted in a hospital with a pediatric intensive care unit and ready access to a pediatric surgeon, a pediatric anesthesiologist, and ample blood products to ensure their availability when needed.[51-53]

There is little doubt that general trauma surgeons with significant pediatric experience can successfully manage children with solid organ injuries using nonoperative treatment protocols.[54] However, neither a general trauma surgeon nor a pediatric trauma surgeon should attempt such management absent the availability of appropriate pediatric support, in terms of a pediatric intensive care unit and, most important, trained pediatric nursing. If these cannot be locally accomplished, and the injured child is stable enough for transfer to a pediatric-capable trauma center, transfer should be initiated as soon as possible after the primary survey has been completed, in accordance with preexisting transfer agreements well known to the treating physician. The time before transfer is effected is used to continue resuscitation, and to perform the secondary survey, without taking extra time to obtain imaging studies that will further delay transfer. However, if the child is unstable, operative management is appropriate. It is far better for such a child to safely remove a seriously damaged organ, even if likely salvageable under ideal circumstances, than to risk nonoperative management in an environment that is unprepared for it.

Liver injuries are suspected based upon clinical evaluation, and confirmed by abdominal CT. Upper abdominal tenderness, more right than left sided, may or may not be present. As stated, volume resuscitation is the foundation of early care, since nonoperative management will be successful in 90% of children with hepatic injuries. Operation is indicated in pediatric blunt trauma patients who are frankly hypotensive on arrival in the emergency department, or who respond only transiently to volume resuscitation, since patients with severe injuries, especially AAST OIS grade V injuries, have a poor outcome.[55] Urgent surgical consultation should be obtained on patient arrival in the emergency department, but in no case should it be delayed beyond definitive diagnosis by CT. It should also be obtained in patients who present after "successful" nonoperative management, since, as with splenic injuries, delayed bleeding is known to occur.[56] Operation is nearly always indicated in penetrating trauma.

Spleen injuries are likewise suspected based on clinical evaluation, and confirmed by abdominal CT. Left upper quadrant tenderness and left shoulder pain (Kehr's sign) may or may not be present. Once again, volume resuscitation is the foundation of early care, nonoperative management being successful in 95% of children with splenic injuries. The presence of a splenic blush on CT is not yet well studied in pediatric patients, but preliminary experience suggests that, as with FAST, it may add little to management of blunt trauma patients, since current treatment is physiologically based, and linked to transfusion requirement.[35] In the rare situation in which emergent operation is indicated, prior administration of multivalent pneumococcal vaccine could theoretically decrease the low incidence of overwhelming postsplenectomy infection, but there are no data proving this is so. Operation is nearly always indicated for penetrating trauma.

Kidney injuries are managed nonoperatively in virtually all instances. As with liver and spleen injuries, the diagnosis is suspected based on clinical evaluation, and confirmed by CT obtained on clinical grounds or for significant hematuria.[57] Renal injuries are typically minor, so volume resuscitation is needed only for severe injuries. This is also true of operative management, which is usually required for intraperitoneal leak from the collecting system, massive upper tract bleeding presenting as gross hematuria, severe disruption or shattering, and renal pedicle avulsion. Most blunt injuries with urinary leaks are managed nonoperatively, or by percutaneous nephrostomy, while most penetrating injuries with urinary leaks are managed by direct surgical repair. One-shot intravenous urography is mandatory whenever emergent surgical intervention is required and abdominal CT has not been, or should not, be obtained. Operation is needed in penetrating trauma only in severe cases (AAST OIS grade III–V).

Pancreatic injuries in children are also managed nonoperatively in virtually all instances. The diagnosis is suspected typically on clinical grounds, and confirmed by CT or ultrasonography and appropriate laboratory tests. Traumatic pancreatitis presents with epigastric pain, and is managed conservatively, giving nothing by mouth and administering intravenous fluids until pain disappears and biochemical abnormalities are resolved. Pancreatic pseudocysts present with soft but tender epigastric masses, and are also managed conservatively, substituting total parenteral nutrition for intravenous fluids if the pseudocyst is well established. Operative intervention is rarely required for blunt trauma, and is associated with complication rates that are significantly higher than nonoperative care, even in severe cases associated with transection of the pancreatic head, body, tail, or duct.[58-60] Operation is nearly always indicated for penetrating trauma.

Hollow Organs

Gastrointestinal tract injuries require operative intervention only if transmural disruption is present.[61] Unfortunately, it is prohibitively difficult to identify such injuries without an operation. Neither CT nor contrast fluoroscopy is sufficient valid and reliable to exclude the diagnosis, although risk is increased if more than one organ is found to be injured.[62] Thus the treating physician must wait for signs of peritoneal irritation to develop, or perform DPL, which can itself confound the abdominal examination if negative, and is no more accurate than CT or contrast fluoroscopy in ruling out intestinal perforation or laceration. Thus, in the absence of frank indications for laparotomy, serial abdominal examination, seeking signs of peritoneal information, is likely the most valid and reliable test available to the treating physician for diagnosis of gastrointestinal disruption. It is certainly the most cost effective. Gastrointestinal tract disruption is uncommon in blunt trauma but common in penetrating trauma. Signs of peritonitis always mandate urgent laparotomy.

Genitourinary injuries exclusive of the kidneys require organ-specific management. Ureteric injuries are detected by CT or intravenous urography, and require stented repair when involving the supravesical component or reimplantation when involving the intravescial component. Vesical injuries are detected by similar means, and confirmed by voiding cysturethrogram. Intraperitoneal injuries to the dome of the urinary bladder require direct operative repair. Extraperitoneal injuries to the base of the urinary bladder require catheter drainage. Injuries to the male and female genital tracts are rarely associated with blunt trauma, with the exception of urethral injury in boys, for which a transurethral stent, ideally a urinary catheter, is required. Injuries to the male and female genital tracts seldom occur in penetrating trauma, but require surgical repair.

Great vessel injuries always require operative repair, and are nearly universally detected at emergent laparotomy performed for massive, ongoing intra-abdominal hemorrhage that typically presents with decompensated shock.[63,64] No preoperative tests are necessary, practical, or desirable, save for the one-shot intravenous urogram obtained for penetrating trauma whenever feasible. Survival is dependent upon immediate repair.

Bony Pelvis

Unstable fractures of the bony pelvis are detected clinically as described previously, and confirmed by pelvic roentgenography. Clinically unstable pelvic fractures require a pelvic sling, or similar device, to decrease pelvic volume and stabilize fracture fragments in an attempt to limit bleeding in the emergent phase of treatment. As stated, unstable pelvic fractures associated with hypotension may benefit from application and inflation of a PASG or MAST device, but are used in this situation to stabilize fracture fragments, hence limit further bleeding. Most pelvic fractures in childhood are simple and stable, and rarely require volume resuscitation. However, complex pelvic fractures, though rare, are both biomechanically and hemodynamically unstable, and require massive volume resuscitation. Closed pelvic fractures, via tamponade, will limit the ultimate amount of blood lost, provided operative intervention, which opens tissue planes and counteracts this tamponade, is not required for other reasons. Open pelvic fractures present an extraordinary management challenge, for which interven-

tional radiology and external fixation are typically both required.

Abdominal Compartment Syndrome

A recent development in trauma surgery has been the recognition of abdominal compartment syndrome. Presumed to be due to reperfusion injury after prolonged operative treatment and resuscitation, and mediated by superoxide radicals, abdominal compartment syndrome results in massive edema of all intra-abdominal organs in the afflicted patient, impeding ventilation and oxygenation via upward pressure on the diaphragm, and impeding perfusion of intra-abdominal organs via compromised circulation. Rarely observed in the emergency department, the condition is recognized by intravesical pressures that exceed 25 cm H_2O, and treated by release of pressure, typically by reoperation for placement of a Bogota bag, much as a Silon pouch is used for neonates undergoing delayed primary closure of gastroschisis or omphalocele, until such time as edema resolves and delayed primary closure can be safely effected. It is mentioned here because some emergency departments may rarely receive patients with abdominal compartment syndrome in transfer from other hospitals.

Trauma Laparotomy

It is axiomatic that optimal stabilization of the trauma patient frequently requires surgical intervention. Contemporary surgical management of abdominal injuries therefore relies heavily on "damage control." A midline incision is swiftly made, and all four quadrants are packed. A rapid but careful inspection is then made for sources of bleeding and soilage. Sources of bleeding that can be readily controlled by repair or ligation are then addressed, leaving packing in place to apply direct pressure to other bleeding sites. Sources of soilage are then similarly readily controlled by stapling or ligation, after which the abdomen is speedily irrigated with warm saline solution, and temporarily closed with towel clips or Bogota bag. The patient is then fully resuscitated either in the operating room or the intensive care unit, until such time as normal body temperature is restored, metabolic derangements are corrected, and hematologic deficiencies are addressed, both in terms of oxygen-carrying capacity and with respect to blood clotting factors, which are adversely affected by hypothermia, hypocalcemia, dilution, and consumption. Once the patient is fully stabilized, definitive operation can proceed, and needed repairs can be performed.

Trauma Laparoscopy

The role of trauma laparoscopy is in evolution. To date, it has mostly been employed to determine whether abdominal penetration has occurred in questionable cases, and for diagnosis, and occasionally diaphragmatic repair, of potential or actual thoracoabdominal injuries. Theoretically, its application to trauma surgery is limited only by the speed and skill of the operating surgeon. However, at this point, its uses are limited to cases in which good visibility is assured, and active bleeding and soilage are not encountered.

Minor Abdominal Injuries

Minor abdominal injuries are those confined to the soft tissues of the abdominal wall, and which in cases of penetrating trauma do not violate the parietal peritonuem. They are noteworthy chiefly because of their frequency. Blunt injury to the abdominal wall typically results in superficial contusions to the skin and subcutaneous tissues, although occasionally the rectus muscles also, and does not require treatment beyond the symptomatic relief provided by warm compresses and oral analgesics. Penetrating injury to the abdominal wall is rarely associated with intra-abdominal injury absent signs of compensated or decompensated shock or parietal peritoneal irritation, but great care is warranted during exploration of an apparently superficial penetrating wound, since it is all too easy to explore a wound to such a depth that the abdomen is entered.

Wounds that penetrate the transversalis fascia may require surgical exploration in the operating room, either by laparotomy or by laparoscopy. Likewise, contaminated wounds may also benefit from operative débridement by means of pulse jet irrigation prior to formal closure. Otherwise, superficial lacerations may be repaired in the emergency department, closing the wound in a minimum of two layers whenever possible. Tetanus prophylaxis is indicated for all contaminated wounds.

Penetrating Injuries

When first encountered, all penetrating injuries to the abdomen must be considered to have violated the parietal peritoneum. Great care must be taken during exploration of the wound to avoid such violation if it has not yet occurred. All penetrating gunshot wounds to the abdomen require exploratory laparotomy, as do those stab wounds associated with shock, peritonitis, evisceration, or blood in the stomach, urine, or rectum on insertion of a gastric tube or urinary catheter or digital examination. The remainder may be observed via serial physical examination. All penetrating abdominal injuries must be deemed contaminated, and must be thoroughly cleansed and débrided prior to suture repair, in addition to appropriate antibiotic and tetanus prophylaxis as indicated. As with abusive injuries, the history obtained following penetrating trauma is likely to be inaccurate. As such, hospital admission is warranted, both to ensure that the child receives a full course of antibiotics, and to allow full involvement of social work and pastoral care services, whose skills are critical in determining the circumstances surrounding the injury and minimizing the likelihood of recidivism. Finally, all gunshot and stab wound injuries in children must be reported to the police, and to local child protective services as well, if there is any hint that the injuries may have resulted from parental abuse or neglect.

Thoracoabdominal Injuries

Thoracoabdominal injuries are penetrating injuries that traverse the diaphragm. They must be suspected whenever a penetrating injury is found anywhere between the nipples and the umbilicus. All potential thoracoabdominal injuries mandate immediate chest roentgenography, to identify possible intrathoracic air or blood, followed by insertion of a chest tube if present. All such injuries will also require exploratory laparotomy or laparoscopy, both to determine whether and where diaphragmatic penetration may have occurred, and to exclude other intra-abdominal injuries that also require operative repair.

Table 25–7	Triage Guidelines for Emergency Management of Abdominal Trauma

Blunt Trauma*

Hemodynamically stable patient
- Negative indications for CT → acute care area
- Positive indications for CT → CT negative → acute care area
- Positive indications for CT → CT positive → PICU vs. OR

Hemodynamically unstable patient
- Responds well to volume resuscitation → CT negative → PICU
- Responds well to volume resuscitation → CT positive → PICU vs. OR
- Responds poorly to volume resuscitation → OR

Penetrating Trauma*
- Gunshot wound → OR
- Stab wound → OR vs. PICU vs. acute care area
  - Hypotension or peritonitis → OR
  - Blood in the stomach, rectum, or urine → OR
  - Evisceration → OR
- Thoracoabdominal wounds → OR

*If signs of peritoneal irritation, a laparotomy or OR is indicated.
Abbreviations: CT, computed tomography; OR, operating room; PICU, pediatric intensive care unit.

Summary

Serious abdominal injuries occur in nearly 1 in 10 cases of major childhood trauma, and follow only central neuraxis injuries and intrathoracic injuries in their lethality. Most pediatric abdominal injuries are initially managed nonoperatively, although major abdominal injuries typically coexist with immediately or potentially life-threatening injuries to other body regions. A high index of suspicion for abdominal injuries is always warranted, since derangements of ventilation, oxygenation, and perfusion resulting from injury to intra-abdominal organs that affect the integrity of the airway, breathing, and circulation substantially worsen the prognosis of associated injuries, particularly central neuraxis injuries, due to inadequate delivery of blood to damaged brain tissue. A physiologic approach to the emergent management of abdominal trauma best serves the needs of the injured child, whose vigorous hemodynamic compensation but limited circulatory reserves call for both rapid restoration and meticulous maintenance of circulating volume, so cellular respiration is supported and irreversible shock is avoided (Table 25–7).

REFERENCES

1. Pigula FA, Wald SL, Shackford SR, et al: The effect of hypotension and hypoxia on children with severe head injuries. J Pediatr Surg 28:310–316, 1993.
2. Cooper A, Barlow B, DiScala C: Vital signs and trauma mortality: the pediatric perspective. Pediatr Emerg Care 16:66, 2000.
3. Cooper A, Barlow B, DiScala C, et al: Mortality and truncal injury: the pediatric perspective. J Pediatr Surg 29:33–38, 1994.
4. Subcommittee on Advanced Trauma Life Support, American College of Surgeons Committee on Trauma: Advanced Trauma Life Support for Doctors Student Manual, 7th ed. Chicago: American College of Surgeons, 2004.
5. Subcommittee on Pediatric Resuscitation, American Heart Association Committee on Emergency Cardiovascular Care: Textbook of Pediatric

Advanced Life Support, 4th ed. Dallas: American Heart Association, 2006.

6. Haller JA: Injuries of the gastro-intestinal tract in children: notes on recognition and management. Clin Pediatr 5:476–480, 1966.

7. Peng RY, Bongard FS: Pedestrian versus motor vehicle accidents: an analysis of 5,000 patients. J Am Coll Surg 189:343–348, 1999.

8. Orsborn R, Haley K, Hammond S, et al: Pediatric pedestrian versus motor vehicle patterns of injury: debunking the myth. Air Med J 18:107–110, 1999.

9. Campbell DJ, Sprouse LR, Smith LA, et al: Injuries in pediatric patients with seatbelt contusions. Am Surg 69:1095–1099, 2003.

10. Grisoni ER, Pillai SB, Volsko TA, et al: Pediatric airbag injuries: the Ohio experience. J Pediatr Surg 35:160–163, 2000.

11. Erez I, Lazar L, Gutermacher M, et al: Abdominal injuries caused by bicycle handlebars. Eur J Surg 167:331–333, 2001.

12. Winston FK, Shaw KN, Kreshak AA, et al: Hidden spears: handlebars as injury hazards to children. Pediatrics 102:596–601, 1998.

13. Lallier M, Bouchard S, St-Vil D, et al: Falls from heights among children: a retrospective review. J Pediatr Surg 34:1060–1063, 1999.

14. Wang MY, Kim KA, Griffith PM, et al: Injuries from falls in the pediatric population: an analysis of 729 cases. J Pediatr Surg 36:1528–1534, 2001.

15. Cvijanovich NZ, Cook LJ, Mann NC, et al: A population-based assessment of pediatric all-terrain vehicle injuries. Pediatrics 108:631–635, 2001.

16. Lin PH, Barr V, Bush RL, et al: Isolated abdominal aortic rupture in a child due to all-terrain vehicle accident: a case report. Vasc Endovasc Surg 37:289–292, 2003.

17. DiScala C, Sege R, Li G, et al: Child abuse and unintentional injuries: a 10-year retrospective. Arch Pediatr Adolesc Med 154:16–22, 2000.

18. Cooper A, Floyd T, Barlow B, et al: Fifteen years' experience with major blunt abdominal trauma due to child abuse. J Trauma 28:1483–1487, 1988.

19. Peery CL, Chendrasekhar A, Paradise NF, et al: Missed injuries in pediatric trauma. Am Surg 65:1067–1069, 1999.

20. Jacobs LM, Gross R, Luk S (eds): Advanced Trauma Operative Management. Woodbury, CT: Ciné-Med, Inc., 2004.

21. Hackam DJ, Potoka D, Meza M, et al: Utility of radiographic hepatic injury grade in predicting outcome for children after blunt abdominal trauma. J Pediatr Surg 37:386–389, 2002.

22. Potoka DA, Schall LC, Ford HR: Risk factors for splenectomy in children with blunt splenic trauma. J Pediatr Surg 37:294–299, 2002.

23. Ismail NH, Bellemare JF, Mollitt DL, et al: Death from pelvic fracture: children are different. J Pediatr Surg 31:82–85, 1996.

24. Holmes JF, Sokolove PE, Land C, et al: Identification of intra-abdominal injuries in children hospitalized following blunt torso trauma. Acad Emerg Med 6:799–806, 1999.

25. Patel JC, Tepas JJ: The efficacy of focused abdominal sonography for trauma (FAST) as a screening tool in the assessment of injured children. J Pediatr Surg 34:44–47, 52–54, 1999.

26. Mutabagani KH, Coley BD, Zumberge M, et al: Preliminary experience with Focused Abdominal Sonography in Trauma (FAST) in children: is it useful? J Pediatr Surg 34:48–54, 1999.

27. Corbett SW, Andrews HG, Baker EM, et al: ED evaluation of the pediatric trauma patient by ultrasonography. Am J Emerg Med 18:244–249, 2000.

28. Soudack M, Epelman M, Maor R, et al: Experience with focused abdominal sonography for trauma (FAST) in 313 pediatric patients. J Clin Ultrasound 32:53–61, 2004.

29. Holmes JF, London KL, Brant WE, et al: Isolated intraperitoneal fluid on abdominal computed tomography in children with blunt trauma. Acad Emerg Med 7:335–341, 2000.

30. Rathaus V, Zissin R, Werner M, et al: Minimal pelvic fluid in blunt abdominal trauma in children: the significance of this sonographic finding. J Pediatr Surg 36:1387–1389, 2001.

31. Holmes JF, Brant WE, Bond WF, et al: Emergency department ultrasonography in the evaluation of hypotensive and normotensive children with blunt abdominal trauma. J Pediatr Surg 36:968–973, 2001.

32. Pershad J, Gilmore B: Serial bedside emergency ultrasound in a case of pediatric blunt abdominal trauma with severe abdominal pain. Pediatr Emerg Care 16:375–376, 2000.

33. Kevill K, Wong AM, Goldman HS, et al: Is a complete trauma series indicated for all pediatric trauma victims? Pediatr Emerg Care 18:75–77, 2002.

34. Holmes JF, Brant WE, Bogren HG, et al: Prevalence and importance of pneumothoraces visualized on abdominal computed tomographic scan in children with blunt trauma. J Trauma 50:516–520, 2001.

35. Lutz N, Mahboubi S, Nance ML, et al: The significance of contrast blush on computed tomography in children with splenic injuries. J Pediatr Surg 39:491–494, 2004.

36. Sievers EM, Murray JA, Chen D, et al: Abdominal computed tomography scan in pediatric blunt abdominal trauma. Am Surg 65:968–971, 1999.

37. Strouse PJ, Close BJ, Marshall KW, et al: CT of bowel and mesenteric trauma in children. Radiographics 19:1237–1250, 1999.

38. Brenner D, Elliston C, Hall E, et al: Estimated risks of radiation-induced fatal cancer from pediatric CT. AJR Am J Roentgenol 176:289–296, 2001.

39. Brenner DJ: Estimating cancer risks from pediatric CT: going from the qualitative to the quantitative. Pediatr Radiol 32:228–231, 2002.

40. Jindal A, Velmahos GC, Rofougaran R: Computed tomography for evaluation of mild to moderate pediatric trauma: are we overusing it? World J Surg 26:13–16, 2002.

41. Minarik L, Slim M, Rachlin S, et al: Diagnostic imaging in the follow-up of nonoperative management of splenic trauma in children. Pediatr Surg Int 18:429–431, 2002.

42. Parish RA, Watson M, Rivara FP: Why obtain arterial blood gases, chest x-rays, and clotting studies in injured children? Experience in a regional trauma center. Pediatr Emerg Care 2:218–222, 1986.

43. Perez-Brayfield MR, Gatti JM, Smith EA, et al: Blunt traumatic hematuria in children: is a simplified algorithm justified? J Urol 167:2543–2547, 2002.

44. Brown SL, Haas C, Dinchman KH, et al: Radiologic evaluation of pediatric blunt renal trauma in patients with microscopic hematuria. World J Surg 25:1557–1560, 2001.

45. Puranik SR, Hayes JS, Long J, et al: Liver enzymes as predictors of liver damage due to blunt abdominal trauma in children. South Med J 95:203–206, 2002.

46. Adamson WT, Hebra A, Thomas PB, et al: Serum amylase and lipase alone are not cost-effective screening methods for pediatric pancreatic trauma. J Pediatr Surg 38:354–357, 2003.

47. Cooper A, Barlow B, DiScala C, et al: Efficacy of MAST use in children who present in hypotensive shock. J Trauma 33:151, 1992.

48. Garcia V, Eichelberger M, Ziegler M, et al: Use of military antishock trouser in a child. J Pediatr Surg 16:544–546, 1981.

49. Green SM, Rothrock SG: Is pediatric trauma really a surgical disease? Ann Emerg Med 39:537–540, 2002.

50. Tepas JJ, Frykberg ER, Schinco MA, et al: Pediatric trauma is very much a surgical disease. Ann Surg 237:775–781, 2003.

51. Mehall JR, Ennis JS, Saltzman DA, et al: Prospective results of a standardized algorithm based on hemodynamic status for managing pediatric solid organ injury. J Am Coll Surg 193:347–353, 2001.

52. Stylianos S: Evidence-based guidelines for resource utilization in children with isolated spleen or liver injury. J Pediatr Surg 35:164–169, 2000.

53. Stylianos S: Compliance with evidence-based guidelines in children with isolated spleen or liver injury: a prospective study. J Pediatr Surg 37:453–456, 2002.

54. Jacobs IA, Kelly K, Valenziano C, et al: Nonoperative management of blunt splenic and hepatic trauma in the pediatric population: significant differences between adult and pediatric surgeons? Am Surg 67:149–154, 2001.

55. Pryor JP, Stafford PW, Nance ML: Severe blunt hepatic trauma in children. J Pediatr Surg 36:974–979, 2001.

56. Fisher JC, Moulton SL: Nonoperative management and delayed hemorrhage after pediatric liver injury: new issues to consider. J Pediatr Surg 39:619–622, 2004.

57. Wessel LM, Scholz S, Jester I, et al: Management of kidney injuries in children with blunt abdominal trauma. J Pediatr Surg 35:1326–1330, 2000.

58. Shilyansky J, Sen LM, Kreller M, et al: Nonoperative management of pancreatic injuries in children. J Pediatr Surg 33:343–345, 1998.

59. Kouchi K, Tanabe M, Yoshida H, et al: Nonoperative management of blunt pancreatic injury in children. J Pediatr Surg 34:1736–1738, 1999.
60. Wales PW, Shuckett B, Kim PCW: Long-term outcome of nonoperative management of complete traumatic pancreatic transection in children. J Pediatr Surg 36:823–827, 2001.
61. Canty TG Sr, Canty TG Jr, Brown C: Injuries of the gastrointestinal tract from blunt trauma in children: a 12-year experience at a designated pediatric trauma center. J Trauma 46:234–240, 1999.
62. Nance ML, Keller MS, Stafford PW: Predicting hollow visceral injury in the pediatric blunt trauma patient with solid visceral injury. J Pediatr Surg 35:1300–1303, 2000.
63. Harris LM, Hordines J: Major vascular injuries in the pediatric population. Ann Vasc Surg 17:266–269, 2003.
64. Cox CS, Black CT, Duke JH, et al: Operative treatment of truncal vascular injuries in children and adolescents. J Pediatr Surg 33:462–467, 1998.

Chapter 26

Burns

Nicholas Tsarouhas, MD and Paula Agosto, RN, MHA

Key Points

Proper management of the burn patient requires the clinician to be comfortable with the classification of burns by both depth and body surface area.

It is crucial to anticipate and be able to manage the possibility of fulminant airway edema in the burn patient.

The profound fluid needs of the burn patient with circulatory impairment require familiarity with weight-based and body surface area–based calculations.

The goal of burn wound management is to reduce the risk of infection while minimizing the likelihood of an adverse cosmetic outcome.

The decision to admit and/or transfer a child to a burn center depends on many factors, including the risk of infection, cosmetic and functional outcomes, pain control, complexity of wound care, age, associated morbidities, underlying medical conditions, and social concerns.

Introduction and Background

Epidemiology

Burns continue to be a major source of morbidity and mortality in the pediatric population. In the United States in 2001, there were more than 181,000 fire- and burn-related injuries, and 672 deaths in children up to age 19 years.[1] In children 1 to 9 years old, burns rank third among injury-related deaths.[2] Most pediatric deaths occur as a result of house fires. Lower socioeconomic areas account for the highest death rates. While the incidence of burns continues to drop in the United States, it is important to remember that many burns are not reported; therefore, most data underestimate the true scope of this public health issue.[3]

Causes

The leading causes of burns in children are scalds, flame burns, and electrical injuries.[3] Children less than 5, especially boys, are the highest risk group. In toddlers, scald burns from hot liquids account for 80% of all thermal injuries.[3] Toddlers also are commonly burned from touching hot metals such as stoves, grills, and home space heaters. School-age children often sustain thermal burns from play with dangerous equipment such as matches and cigarette lighters. Teenagers are more commonly burned from risk-taking activities, fireworks, and careless use of flammable substances. Household fires caused by unattended cigarettes or candles are a major contributor to pediatric burn injuries and death in all age groups. Cigarettes alone are responsible for 35% of the fatal house fires in the United States.[4]

Anatomy and Physiology

The skin is the organ most visibly affected by burns. It consists of two main layers: the epidermis and the dermis. The epidermis (the outer layer of skin) is formed from several layers of stratified epithelium. The dermis is composed of connective tissue, which is tough and elastic. The nerve endings concerned with the sensation of touch and temperature are located in the dermis. Structures within the skin include sweat glands, hair follicles, and sebaceous glands. A layer of subcutaneous fat separates the skin from underlying structures. In addition to its cosmetic importance, the skin protects the body against infection, regulates body temperature, and serves as a barrier to prevent fluid loss.

Pathophysiology

Thermal Burns

The thinner skin of young children accounts for deeper burns as compared to adults. Thermal energy damages skin in proportion to intensity and duration. Once tissue is damaged, blood supply and cellular activity increase in the injured area, causing heat and redness. The damaged tissue and mast cells ooze various enzymes and histamine, which trigger vasodilation and increased capillary permeability. Swelling and edema then develop as the capillary walls leak inflammatory exudate (containing plasma, antibodies, and some red blood cells and white blood cells) into the surrounding tissue. Macrophage cells begin to arrive at the wound site to defend against bacteria and help clear blood clots, damaged tissue, and other debris.[5]

Inhalation Injury

While thermal burns account for major fire-related morbidity, mortality is intimately tied to inhalation injury and carbon monoxide (CO) poisoning. Inhalation of toxins associated with flame smoke accounts for 80% of burn-related deaths.[6] Direct thermal injury may lead to upper airway edema and obstruction. Some combustion of soot particles continues, and these small particles may be carried into the lung. Additional clinical consequences include systemic capillary leak, bronchospasm from aerosolized irritants, small airway occlusion from sloughed endobronchial debris, impaired ciliary clearance, loss of surfactant, increased dead space and intrapulmonary shunting from alveolar flooding, decreased lung compliance from interstitial and alveolar edema, decreased thoracic compliance from chest wall burns, and, later, infection of the denuded tracheobronchial tree (tracheobronchitis) or pulmonary parenchyma (pneumonia).[7] The evaluation and management of smoke inhalation is covered in detail in Chapter 143 (Inhalations and Exposures).

Carbon Monoxide Poisoning

Smoke inhalation is commonly associated with CO poisoning, as levels of CO may reach 10% in house fires.[8] CO impairs oxygen delivery and utilization. It binds tightly to hemoglobin with an affinity 250 times that of oxygen. CO also binds to cytochrome oxidase, thus interfering with cellular oxidative energy metabolism.[9] The net result of this impairment in the delivery, release, and use of oxygen is tissue and cellular hypoxia. The evaluation and management of CO poisoning is covered in detail in Chapter 143 (Inhalations and Exposures).

Electrical Injury

Electrical burns result in over 1500 deaths per year[10] and 2% to 3% of all admissions to hospital burn centers.[11] Electrical burns result from thermal energy that is produced as an electrical current passes through the body. The amount of thermal energy produced is directly proportional to the degree of the electric current. Nerves, muscles, and blood vessels have low electrical resistance, so electricity will preferentially flow through these structures. Alternating current, which is found in household electricity, produces muscle tetany caused by the continual contraction and relaxation of the muscle with each cycle. One of the most common pediatric electrical injuries occurs as a result of a child biting an electrical cord.

Direct current, found in lightning, poses its greatest risk when the current traverses the heart, resulting in ventricular fibrillation or asystole. While 70% to 80% of those struck by lightning survive,[12] 100 fatalities occur in the United States each year.[13] The major cause of arrest in these patients is the result of dysrhythmias, myocardial damage, or respiratory arrest with asphyxia. The evaluation and management of electrical injuries is covered in detail in Chapter 142 (Electrical Injury).

Chemical Burns

Nearly 100,000 chemical burns are reported in the United States each year.[11] Fortunately, the overwhelming majority of these prove to be relatively benign. In most cases, the burn is a result of a direct chemical injury. Acid burns result in coagulation necrosis, which usually limits the depth and penetration of the burn. Common household products that contain acids include drain cleaners (sulfuric acid or hydrochloric acid), toilet cleaners (hydrochloric acid or phosphoric acid), and car batteries (sulfuric acid).[14]

Alkalis produce liquefactive necrosis, thus causing deeper penetration and a more significant burn. Alkalis include lye (sodium hydroxide), fertilizers (anhydrous ammonia), oven and drain cleaners (sodium or potassium hydroxide), paint strippers (sodium hydroxide), and various detergents.[15] Consultation with a poison control center should be considered when evaluating children with chemical burns, to assess the possibility of associated systemic toxicities in addition to the cutaneous burn. The evaluation and management of chemical burns is covered in detail in Chapter 143 (Inhalations and Exposures).

Recognition and Approach

Classification of Thermal Burns

Depth

Traditionally, burns have been classified as first, second, third, and even fourth degree. Many experts now recommend that this nomenclature be replaced by the designations of superficial, superficial partial thickness, deep partial thickness, and full thickness (Table 26–1). It is often difficult to correctly identify the depth of the burn, however, and it is common to have several depths exhibited in one injury. The center usually has a higher degree of burn than the periphery.

First-degree or superficial burns are limited to the epidermis. They are characterized by painful, erythematous,

Table 26–1	Classification of Burns by Depth				
Burn Type	**Histology**	**Appearance**	**Pain?**	**Healing**	**Scarring?**
Superficial/first degree	Epidermis only	Painful, erythematous, nonblistered	Painful	3–5 days	None
Superficial partial thickness/second degree	Complete destruction of epidermis and <50% of dermis	Erythematous, blistering, moist	Painful	2 wk	Possible
Deep partial thickness/second degree	Complete destruction of epidermis and >50% of dermis	Paler, drier, blistering	May be less painful	Several weeks	Likely
Full thickness/third degree	Complete destruction of epidermis and dermis	Pale and white, or charred and leathery	May be painless	Months	Always

nonblistered areas of inflammation. An example is a severe sunburn. Importantly, when body surface area (BSA) calculations are performed to estimate the amount of burn, first-degree burns are not included. Generally, these burns heal within 3 to 5 days with no scarring.

Second-degree or partial-thickness burns extend into the dermis. Superficial partial-thickness burns result in the complete destruction of the epidermis and less than 50% of the dermis. These burns are erythematous, blistering, moist, and painful. There is pain because intact sensory nerve receptors are still exposed. These usually heal in 2 weeks, though scars are possible. Deep partial-thickness burns result in the complete destruction of the epidermis and greater than 50% of the dermis. They are often paler and drier, and may be less painful as there is some destruction of cutaneous nerves. These take many weeks to heal, and scars are likely.

Third-degree or full-thickness burns extend into the subcutaneous tissues. Full-thickness burns result in the complete destruction of the epidermis and the dermis. Their appearance may be pale and white, or charred and leathery. These are usually nontender as there is widespread destruction of cutaneous nerves. Healing is slow, and skin grafting is usually needed.

Some experts add an additional category of fourth-degree burns. These involve destruction of the underlying structures such as muscles, tendons, nerves, and bones. Severe electrical burns are an example of this type.

Body Surface Area

BSA estimates are important in the initial evaluation and management of burns. These calculations help guide volume resuscitation, decisions to admit, transfer to burn centers, and prognosis. Importantly, only second- and third-degree burns are included in the BSA calculation, because superficial burns have little impact on patient care and outcome.

The "rule of nines" (Table 26–2) is a convenient and rapid method of estimating the extent of BSA burned in adolescents. It divides the surface area of the body into areas of 9%. When all body areas of these 9% segments are summed, 1% remains, which is assigned to the genitalia and perineum. It is inaccurate for children, however, as they have relatively larger heads and smaller extremities.

The rule of nines is good for a quick estimate in children older than 9 years. For patients who are 9 years and younger, a more precise method of burn size estimation should ultimately be used. The Lund and Browder chart[16] (Fig. 26–1) subdivides body areas into segments and assigns a propor-

tionate percentage of body surface to each area, based on age. The lower extremity is divided into upper leg, lower leg, and foot, rather than being considered as a whole. The head of a baby is proportionately much larger than any other area of the body. As a child grows, the head becomes relatively smaller as compared with the rest of the body, and the lower extremities assume more BSA.

Another method of estimating burn injury extent uses the size of the child's hand. The BSA represented by the hand is set at 1%. Some experts advocate including the fingers, while others do not. A better estimate of the palm itself may be 0.5%[17]; one study estimated the palm at 0.4%, and the entire hand at 0.8%.[18] This method is both quick and useful for areas of irregular or nonconfluent burns.

Recognition of Child Abuse

Between 10% and 20% of burns in children are intentionally inflicted.[11] Most inflicted burns are scald or contact burns that have recognizable patterns (Table 26–3). Toddlers submerged in hot water, particularly as punishment for toilet training misfortunes, present with a characteristic scald burn to the buttocks, perineum, thighs, and feet (see Chapter 119, Physical Abuse and Neglect). The primary care provider needs to have a high index of suspicion when the history of the injury does not match the pattern of the burn, or is not consistent with the child's developmental age. While the burn needs to be promptly treated, the provider is mandated to report all suspicious injuries to the appropriate social services and child protective agencies.

Evaluation

Immediate Emergency Department Evaluation

Airway Assessment

Inhalation of hot gases can burn the airway, and lead to rapidly progressive airway edema and obstruction. The child's airway is exquisitely sensitive to swelling, as airway resistance increases as the fourth power of the radius. Thus even small degrees of edema may have catastrophic airway implications.

Every emergent evaluation, regardless of the injury, begins with an airway assessment. The evaluation commences with an "across the room" inspection of the child's airway patency. The crying child, at the very least, is able to maintain the airway at that point in time. The child who is quiet or exhibiting signs of distress is more ominous. The usual signs and symptoms of airway compromise should be sought: stridor, hoarseness, drooling, gagging, coughing, and increased work of breathing. Additional signs of concern include burns to the face, singed facial hairs, and carbonaceous sputum.

Table 26–2	Classification of Burns by Body Surface Area: "Rule of Nines"*
Body Area	**Relative Percent Burn**
Head and neck	9%
Anterior/posterior torso	18% each (36%)
Lower extremity	18% each (36%)
Upper extremity	9% each (18%)
Genitalia/perineum	1%
Total	100%

*Note: Less accurate for children 9 years and younger, who have relatively larger heads and smaller extremities.

Table 26–3	Recognizable Patterns of Intentionally Inflicted Burns

- Triangular shape from the tip of an iron
- Linear parallel lines from a radiator
- Hot water submersion burns to buttocks, thighs, feet
- Symmetric, well-demarcated stocking/glove burns to feet/hands
- Splash burns when a hot liquid is thrown
- Deep, small, circular cigarette burns

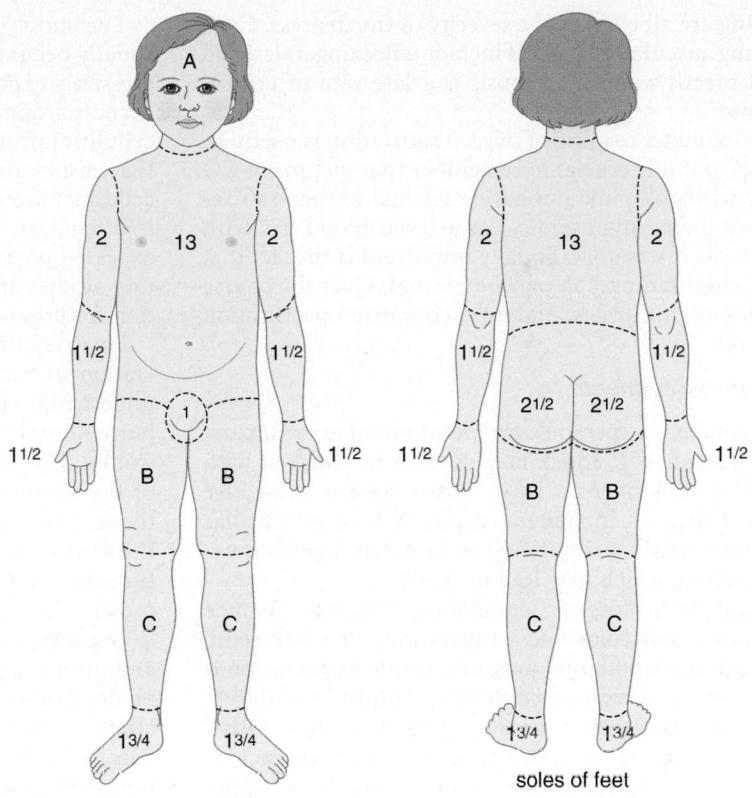

FIGURE 26–1. Classification of burns by body surface area: the Lund and Browder chart. (Adapted from Thermal injury. *In* Barkin RM [ed]: Pediatric Emergency Medicine, 2nd ed. St. Louis: Mosby, 1997, p 490.)

	< 1 yr	1 yr	5 yr	10 yr	15 yr	Adult
A half of head	9 1/2%	8 1/2%	6 1/2%	5 1/2%	4 1/2%	3 1/2%
B half of thigh	2 3/4%	3 1/4%	4%	4 1/4%	4 1/2%	4 3/4%
C half of leg	2 1/2%	2 1/2%	2 3/4%	3%	3 1/4%	3 1/2%
head	19%	17%	13%	11%	9%	
neck	2%	2%	2%	2%	2%	
half of trunk (ant or post)	13%	13%	13%	13%	13%	
one buttock	2.5%	2.5%	2.5%	2.5%	2.5%	
genitalia	1%	1%	1%	1%	1%	
upper (3) or lower (4) arm	3-4%	3-4%	3-4%	3-4%	3-4%	
one hand (2.5) or foot (3.5)	2.5-3.5%	2.5-3.5%	2.5-3.5%	2.5-3.5%	2.5-3.5%	
one thigh	5%	6.5%	8.5%	9%	9.5%	
one leg (below knee)	5%	5%	5.5%	6%	6.5%	

It is important to remember that cervical spine trauma may be present. Often, patients have jumped or have fallen from burning buildings. If the history is unclear or unknown, patients must be cervically immobilized until clinical or radiographic assessment and clearance is completed.

Breathing Assessment

Bronchospasm is very common from the extreme irritative properties of inhaled smoke and toxic gases. Once again, the patient in respiratory distress should be obvious at the onset. Tachypnea, retractions, grunting respirations, coughing, and nasal flaring are all clues to the severity of the distress. Concerning lung ausculatory sounds include wheezing, rales, and decreased breath sounds. Cyanosis is a late sign of critical compromise.

A pulse oximeter reading of oxygen saturation is useful in many cases, but it is crucial to remember that victims of CO poisoning will look pink and have a normal oxygen saturation, despite being hypoxemic. An arterial blood gas with co-oximetry is mandatory. Equally important is the fact that the initial chest radiograph may be normal. Over the course of a few hours, infiltrates, and even complete opacification may develop.

Circulation Assessment

Burn patients may experience profound circulatory impairment ("burn shock"). Shock may develop in children with 15% to 20% BSA burns.[11] Large burns release vasoactive mediators that result in systemic capillary leakage. Cardiac output is decreased by circulating factors that depress myocardial function, which may lead to shock.

Important indicators of circulatory integrity include mental status, skin color and temperature, capillary refill, pulses, heart rate, and blood pressure. While hypotension is a late and ominous sign of circulatory failure in children, hypertension is also seen in severely burned children. Other important parameters to guide fluid management include urine output and, in some cases, central venous pressures. Basic metabolic chemistries and blood gases for pH are also important to assist in the fluid management of these patients.

Mental Status Assessment

Alteration in mental status should prompt a thorough assessment for the underlying etiology. Possible life-threatening etiologies include anoxia from asphyxiation, hypercarbia from hypoventilation, CO intoxication, hypovolemia with resultant cerebral hypoperfusion, traumatic brain injury, and seizures. Other causes may include pain, anxiety, drugs, and alcohol.

Children with large burns, although alert in the first hours after injury, may become obtunded secondary to fluid shifts, pain medication, sleep deprivation, and exhaustion.[19] Nevertheless, computed tomography scans should be obtained when the etiology of the mental status aberration is unknown, to exclude occult head injury. Blood gases with co-oximetry, electrolytes, and toxicologic screens also add useful information.

Life-Threatening Complications

Infection

Infection remains the leading cause of morbidity and mortality in burn patients.[20] The overall reported incidence of infections in burned children is 13.6%.[21] Necrosis of burned tissue produces a protein-rich medium that encourages bacterial growth. Inevitably, all burns become colonized by skin flora and potentially pathogenic organisms that may invade this breached epithelial barrier and lead to infectious complications. Inhalation injury to the respiratory tract may lead to lethal pulmonary disease. Importantly, seriously burned children also have a global immunosuppression that compounds their infection susceptibility.[7]

The most common burn infection is a cellulitis. This usually occurs in the first few days after the burn. Any progressively expanding area of erythema, induration, and tenderness around a burn's margins should raise suspicion of a cellulitic infection. Unfortunately, the inflammatory response that ensues after a burn also may easily be confused with a cellulitis. Moreover, fever, which is common with cellulitis, is often seen in the setting of an uninfected burn, as an expected physiologic inflammatory response. While laboratory studies are occasionally helpful, close clinical observation for progression is crucial.

Invasive burn wound infections also occur. A rapid proliferation of bacteria in burn eschar may proceed to invade underlying viable tissues. Clinical signs of an invasive burn wound infection include (1) a change in color of the wound; (2) a dark brown, black, or violaceous discoloration of the wound; (3) hemorrhagic discoloration of subeschar tissue; (4) conversion of a burn from partial thickness to full thickness; (5) new drainage; and (6) a foul odor.[22] Additionally, fever and other systemic signs of toxicity may be present.

Gram-positive organisms, typically *Staphylococcus aureus* and group A β-hemolytic streptococcus (GABHS), are the predominate pathogens in *early* burn infections (Table 26–4). Gram-negative organisms, especially *Pseudomonas aeruginosa*, colonize the eschar and should be considered when infections develop after a week. *P. aeruginosa* infection classically presents with the green pigment pyocyanin. Ecthyma gangrenosum should also raise suspicion for *P. aeruginosa* infection. These deep cutaneous erosions, usually seen in immunocompromised patients, often begin as vesicles, which pustulate, and then progress rapidly to gangrenous ulcers. Sepsis is common.

Bacteroides and other anaerobic bacteria are occasional isolates from serious burn infections. In extensively burned patients who develop late infections, *Candida* and other fungi should be considered.[20] Viral infections of burns, most commonly herpes simplex virus (HSV) or cytomegalovirus, are usually heralded by a vesicular eruption.

Systemic Inflammatory Response Syndrome

Systemic inflammatory response syndrome may follow severe burns. The common presentation is fever, tachypnea, tachycardia, shock, and multisystem organ failure. The hyperactive immune response causes a generalized inflammation that damages healthy tissue as well as infected burn wounds. Microvascular permeability leads to decreased tissue oxygenation, and blood flow is reduced due to microthrombi. During

Table 26–4	Pathogens Responsible for Burn Infections

Early Infections

Staphylococcus aureus
Group A β-hemolytic streptococcus (GABHS)

Late Infections

Pseudomonas aeruginosa and other gram negatives
Bacteroides and other anaerobic bacteria
Candida and other fungi
Herpes simplex virus, cytomegalovirus, and other viruses

this reaction, the intestinal and, possibly, the respiratory barriers to infection are damaged, allowing the entry of additional bacteria into the circulation.[6] Aggressive supportive care remains the therapeutic mainstay.

Myoglobinuria

Myoglobinuria secondary to muscle breakdown and widespread cell death (rhabdomyolysis) is seen when BSA burns approach 30%. Myoglobin accumulates in the kidneys at alarming rates and may lead to fulminant renal failure. Strict attention to the urine output, urinalysis, and fluid therapy is crucial.

Special Considerations

Eye Burns

Serious corneal burns are generally obvious on physical examination, with the cornea having a clouded appearance. More subtle injuries can be detected after topical fluorescein application. In general, any burns of the eyes or eyelids require urgent ophthalmologic consultation.

Ear Burns

The most important aspect of managing deeply burned ears is to prevent auricular chondritis. This serious complication results from the poor blood supply of the cartilage of the external ear. The prevention of infection is paramount as infected cartilage liquefies, losing its structural integrity. Topical mafenide acetate has been shown to sharply reduce the incidence of auricular chondritis.[23]

Hand Burns

Preservation of the functional integrity of the hand mandates specialized attention. Hand surgery consultation is mandatory. During the first 24 to 48 hours, adequate blood flow must be ensured. The adequacy of perfusion can be judged by temperature and the presence of pulsatile flow detectable by Doppler in the digital pulp. If there is any question, escharotomy or fasciotomy should be done. Subsequently, the hands should be splinted in a position of function, with the metacarpophalangeal joints at 70 to 90 degrees, the interphalangeal joints in extension, the first web space open, and the wrist at 20 degrees of extension.[23]

Management

Emergency Stabilization

Airway

Humidified oxygen (100%) should be administered immediately to all burn patients. As burn patients may also have cervical spine trauma, the head should be maintained in neutral position, and any airway manipulation should presume the presence of a cervical spine injury. The jaw thrust should be the airway opening maneuver of choice, as opposed to the chin lift, which could extend the neck and damage the spinal cord. Endotracheal intubation should only occur with the assistance of someone maintaining in-line cervical stabilization.

Because the airway is so precarious, experts recommend early intubation, as edema and obstruction can develop rapidly.[24] In anticipation of a distorted and edematous airway,

endotracheal tubes (ETTs) with smaller diameter than usual for age should be readily available. Once the tube is in place, it should be very carefully secured, as reintubation may be impossible if it is dislodged. One safe method of securing the ETT in the burn patient is to tape both under and over the ears.[25]

Breathing

Once the airway is secure and oxygen is being delivered, attention turns to the adequacy of oxygenation and ventilation. The clinical assessment is augmented by electronic end-tidal CO_2 monitoring and pulse oximetry. It is vital to remember, however, that in the presence of elevated carboxyhemoglobin levels (common with smoke inhalation) pulse oximetry overestimates the true oxyhemoglobin saturation.[26] Thus, arterial blood gas determination (with co-oximetry) is mandatory.

If the patient's breathing is judged to be suboptimal, ventilatory support is necessary. Hand ventilation with a bag-valve-mask apparatus should be employed initially while preparations are made for endotracheal intubation. Ideally, an anesthesia (Mapleson) bag should be used to manually ventilate, as it allows one to assess lung compliance, which is often compromised in the setting of smoke inhalation. The bronchospasm that commonly accompanies smoke inhalation should be treated with aerosolized β_2-agonists (albuterol, levalbuterol), terbutaline, and/or epinephrine. Corticosteroids have not been shown to be of benefit in decreasing the tracheobronchial inflammation induced by smoke inhalation.[27]

If endotracheal intubation and mechanical ventilation are required, there are a few important medication selection considerations. The most common sedative choices are thiopental, midazolam, ketamine, and etomidate. Because thiopental is associated with hypotension, it should be avoided in the burn patient with circulatory insufficiency or shock. While etomidate and midazolam are fine choices, ketamine has the added benefit of being a bronchodilator, which may be useful in the setting of smoke-induced bronchospasm. The muscle relaxants of choices are usually the nondepolarizers (vecuronium, pancuronium, rocuronium). Nondepolarizing muscle relaxants are preferred over succinylcholine for burns that are more than 48 hours old.

Once mechanical ventilation is initiated, air trapping should be anticipated. Adequate expiratory times should be ensured, and one should be alert for dynamic hyperinflation.[28] Inflating pressures to greater than 40 cm H_2O should be avoided, unless there is severely impaired chest wall compliance.[7]

Circulation/Fluid Therapies

Adequate vascular access is required to support the resuscitation needs of the severely burned patient. Peripheral vascular access can be difficult to secure in hypovolemic burn patients, especially young children. When necessary, it is acceptable to place an intravenous (IV) line through the burn wound.[29] Central access is generally required in children with large burn injuries.[7] The intraosseous route should be used in the unstable child needing fluid therapy in whom rapid vascular access is not easily obtained.

Burns greater than 15% to 20% BSA will produce hypovolemic shock unless appropriately managed with crystalloid fluid replacement. Burns less than 15% are not associated with massive capillary leak; therefore, formal fluid resuscitation is not required.[30] Isotonic saline, most commonly lactated Ringer's solution, is recommended for resuscitation in the first 24 hours after a significant burn.[7] Lactated Ringer's solution contains physiologic concentrations of major electrolytes. The lactate serves as a buffer, which may lessen the propensity for hyperchloremic acidosis.[30] Normal saline, however, is an acceptable alternative. An initial fluid bolus of 20 ml/kg is recommended. Large volumes of fluid are needed, however, for proper resuscitation, because only 20% to 30% of the isotonic fluid remains in the intravascular space.[31]

The initial fluids should not contain potassium, as cell breakdown (common to massive burns) releases a large amount of intracellular potassium. This hyperkalemia could have devastating effects on both the heart and kidneys. Albumin also should be avoided initially, as edema may be increased by albumin use in the first 24 hours because of capillary leak. Once capillary integrity is restored and intravascular volume is replete, colloid may be helpful for volume expansion and preservation of serum oncotic pressure.

Some experts have recommended the use of 3% sodium chloride solution during resuscitation. The theory is that the hypertonic saline might preserve intravascular volume and decrease edema. However, other experts disagree. One particular study found that hypertonic sodium resuscitation was associated with renal failure and death.[32]

The Parkland formula[33] and its variations have become the standard method for calculating the initial fluid requirements of severely burned patients. During the initial 24 hours after injury, the patient receives 4 ml/kg/%BSA burn of lactated Ringer's solution in addition to maintenance fluids. Half of this total is given in the first 8 hours after injury, and the remainder is given in the subsequent 16 hours.

It is universally acknowledged that the Parkland formula, while quick and easy to use, underestimates the needs of young children, as it is strictly based on weight. Weight-based formulas are suboptimal because BSA correlates imprecisely with weight in growing children. Using weight-related formulas may lead to the administration of less than maintenance fluids to smaller children. Thus, maintenance fluids should be added to the Parkland calculation for children younger than 5 years.

An alternative is to use a surface area–related formula, such as the one devised by Carvajal.[34] The Carvajal formula recommends that, in the first 24 hours, in children less than 5 years old, the following formula be used: $5000\,ml/m^2/\%BSA$ burn, plus $2000\,ml/m^2$. As with the Parkland formula, half of this total is given in the first 8 hours after injury, and the remainder is given in the subsequent 16 hours.

Dextrose

Smaller children (<20 kg) are at risk for hypoglycemia. In cases of documented hypoglycemia, the child should receive a dextrose bolus of 0.5 g/kg. This is most easily accomplished by the administration of 5 ml/kg of a 10% dextrose solution. Euglycemic children less than 20 kg should receive lactated Ringer's solution with 5% dextrose at maintenance rates. The gluconeogenic capacity of older children and adolescents is such that no glucose-containing solutions are usually required during resuscitation.[7]

Environmental

Thermoregulation may be significantly affected due to the profound skin loss in extensive burns. It is important to maintain the body temperature within normal limits. This is especially crucial in infants and small children. In the hypothermic child, active warming should be initiated as soon as possible in an environmentally controlled room. Warming blankets, heat shields, and warm intravenous fluids may be necessary.[35]

Additional Interventions

Analgesics

Opiates continue to be the mainstay of analgesic therapy in burn patients. Burn patients are exquisitely sensitive to narcotics.[29] Basic science studies suggest that systemic opiates (in particular, morphine) have an added effect on burn pain, as inflammatory burn states may lead to an increased expression of peripheral opioid receptors. This enhanced potency of morphine is due to its action on these peripheral opioid receptors.[36] Morphine sulfate is most commonly used at 0.1 mg/kg. Multiple doses are often necessary. Side effects of morphine include hypotension and respiratory depression. The IV route is best, as systemic absorption is more variable by intramuscular and oral routes. Importantly, analgesics should be used not only at the initial burn presentation, but also with dressing changes.

Antibiotics

Prophylactic systemic antibiotics are contraindicated in burn care, as their use has been shown to increase the risk of more virulent and resistant organisms.[29,35,37,38] Antibiotic therapy should be initiated only if the clinical suspicion for an infected burn is high. A progressively expanding burn cellulitis should be treated with topical mafenide acetate and a systemic semisynthetic penicillin to cover for GABHS and *S. aureus,* or a broad-spectrum β-lactam antibiotic if culture results are unavailable.[22] Invasive burn wound infections can be life threatening, and generally require treatment with a combination of surgery and antibiotics.[23]

Topical antifungal agents (clotrimazole) are used for localized fungal infections, but any suspicion of disseminated fungal infection should be aggressively treated with IV amphotericin B, possibly with the addition of 5-flucytosine.[22] Topical acyclovir (5%) may be used in patients with documented localized HSV infections, but similarly, any suspicion of disseminated HSV infection should prompt treatment with IV acyclovir.[22] Routine use of topical antibacterials, such as silver sulfadiazine and mafenide acetate, is discussed later.

Nasogastric Tube

A nasogastric tube is usually recommended in children with large burns, as air swallowing and gastric dilation (especially in crying children) are common. Some guidelines recommend that children should be placed on "nothing by mouth" status for the first 24 to 48 hours to avoid complications associated with an intestinal ileus. However, there is evidence that the initiation of enteral feeding immediately after a burn has been shown to be safe and effective in patients with serious thermal injuries.[39,40]

Bladder Catheterization

Bladder catheterization (with a Foley catheter) is important in severely burned patients to monitor the adequacy of fluid resuscitation. The minimum acceptable urine output should be 1 ml/kg/min. Additionally, male patients with burns near the perineum should have a catheter placed as penile edema may ultimately complicate urination. Importantly, the foreskin should be over the bladder catheter after insertion to prevent the development of paraphimosis.[7]

Peptic Ulcer Prophylaxis

Reduced splanchnic blood flow is a common complication in patients with widespread burns.[7] Consequently, gastroduodenal ulcers ("Curling" ulcers) are common in these systemically stressed patients. Histamine$_2$ receptor antagonists (cimetidine, ranitidine, famotidine) are commonly recommended as prophylaxis against these peptic ulcers.

Tetanus Prophylaxis

As burns are tetanus-prone wounds, tetanus immunity must be addressed. In children who have completed their primary series of immunizations, active immunization with tetanus toxoid is indicated, unless one has been administered within the previous 5 years. If the primary series is incomplete, the patient should also receive passive immunization with tetanus immune globulin, especially in deep or heavily contaminated burns. If the immunization status is unknown or questionable, prophylaxis should be empirically administered.

Hyperbaric Oxygen Therapy

Hyperbaric oxygen therapy is frequently used in patients who are victims of smoke inhalation. Its primary purpose is to rapidly clear the blood of carboxyhemoglobin, thus minimizing the risk of permanent neurologic sequelae in patients who have been poisoned with CO. While carboxyhemoglobin levels are important, they cannot be used alone to dictate the need for hyperbaric therapy (see Chapter 143, Inhalations and Exposures).

Steroids

Most experts agree that there is no role for steroid use in the management of burn victims.[29,41,42] The use of prophylactic steroids increases both infectious complications and mortality. Table 26–5 summarizes the emergency management of the burn patient.

Burn Wound Management

Initial Care

The goal of burn wound management is to reduce the risk of infection while minimizing the likelihood of an adverse cosmetic outcome. Initially, any burnt clothing, debris, and jewelry must be gently removed. The wounds should be cleansed with warmed, sterile normal saline, and then covered loosely with clean sheets.

Escharotomy

Circumferential burns to the chest may interfere with the patient's ability to ventilate and may require an escharotomy. Circumferential burns of the extremities may warrant escharotomy to prevent distal tissue ischemia. Distal pulses should be monitored with Doppler ultrasound. Surgical consulta-

Table 26–5	Summary Emergency Management of the Burn Patient

Emergency Stabilization (ABCDEs)

Airway
Assess patency
Administer oxygen
Maintain cervical spine immobilization
Consider early endotracheal intubation with smaller than
  anticipated tube size based on age

Breathing
Assess adequacy
Assist mechanically if necessary
If smoke inhalation:
  Consider bronchodilators
  Monitor arterial blood gas with co-oximetry

Circulation
Assess integrity
Establish intravenous access (peripheral/central)
Give fluid bolus with lactated Ringer's solution
Calculate burn depth and body surface area:
  Lund and Browder chart
  Rule of nines
  Palm of hand
Calculate fluid requirements
  Parkland formula
  Carvajal formula

Dextrose
Check glucose level
Treat hypoglycemia

Disabilities (Neurologic)
Evaluate mental status
Check for smoke-related causes (carbon monoxide, etc.)
Perform head computed tomography scan if trauma a possibility

Environmental
Check body temperature
Maintain euthermia

Exposure
Evaluate for circumferential burns
Perform escharotomies when necessary
Institute initial burn wound management

Additional Interventions

Removal of rings and jewelry
Analgesics
Nasogastric tube
Bladder catheterization
Peptic ulcer prophylaxis
Tetanus prophylaxis
Hyperbaric oxygen therapy
Attention to psychosocial needs of patient/family

Disposition

Admission decision making
Arrangements for transfer to burn center
Social services (especially if child abuse concerns)

tion and intervention are mandatory when this is a concern.

Débridement

Loose necrotic tissue should be carefully débrided, using meticulous antiseptic technique, to reduce the risk of infection. One method involves using a saline-soaked gauze to gently wipe away the necrotic tissue of nonintact blisters. One should wipe in parallel to the periphery of the burn's margins, as opposed to wiping perpendicularly *toward* the margins, in order not to extend the wound further. Figure 26–2 depicts this wound débridement technique. The rest of the burn

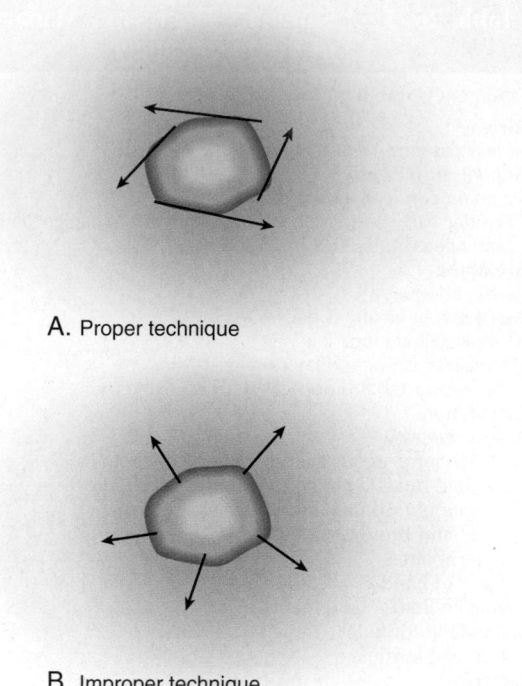

A. Proper technique

B. Improper technique

FIGURE 26–2. Wound débridement. **A,** Proper technique: one should débride in parallel to the periphery of the burn's margins. **B,** Improper technique: avoid débriding perpendicularly toward the margins, so as not to extend the wound further.

should also be gently débrided with gauze to remove additional wound debris and exudate. There appears to be no benefit to antimicrobial prophylaxis during débridement in children.[43]

Controversy still exists over the management of blisters. Many experts prefer to leave blisters intact, débriding only those blisters that have spontaneously broken. It is generally believed that the biologic dressing afforded by the intact blister outweighs other considerations. Others, however, believe that large blisters (>1 to 2 cm) should be broken and débrided.[35,42] These experts believe that leaving blisters intact may interfere with assessment and with joint mobility.[44] Still others advocate relieving uncomfortable pressure by aspirating the burn fluid from tense blisters, leaving the epithelium to act as a biologic dressing.[45,46]

Topical Antibiotics

After the burn has been cleaned and débrided, attention must be given to controlling bacterial density and decreasing the likelihood of a burn wound infection. A number of agents are effective as topical antimicrobials in burn wound care. They are generally divided into potent agents that are designed to prevent burn wound invasion (silver sulfadiazine, mafenide acetate, and silver nitrate), and milder agents (bacitracin, Neosporin, Polysporin, and mupirocin) that are used to treat small or superficial wounds. The more potent agents may delay epithelialization and should be reserved for use in managing more extensive and deeper burns. The milder agents, when used in combination with nonadherent gauze, provide a comfortable, protective environment that promotes epithelialization of the wound.[35]

Silver sulfadiazine (Silvadene) cream is the most commonly used topical agent. It is bacteriostatic, but poorly diffusible and limited in its penetration of the burn wound. It is painless upon application and has a soothing effect. It should not be used on the face secondary to the risk of skin discoloration. The bacterial spectrum of Silvadene includes *S. aureus,* GABHS, *Escherichia coli, Klebsiella* species, *P. aeruginosa, Proteus* species, and *Candida albicans.*[6] Side effects include transient leukopenia (5% to 15%),[6] rash (5%),[42] and hemolysis in patients with glucose-6-phosphate dehydrogenase deficiency.

Mafenide acetate 5% cream is bacteriostatic, freely soluble, and readily diffuses through burn eschar to the viable tissue interface. This antibiotic also has the broadest spectrum against *Pseudomonas* species and other gram-negative organisms. The principal limitations of this agent are (1) the pain produced when applied to partial-thickness wounds, and (2) the inhibition of carbonic anhydrase that predisposes to the development of metabolic acidosis. Use of this agent is generally limited to wounds with or at high risk for invasive infection.[35]

Silver nitrate solution (0.5%) is an effective agent, but has decreased in popularity over the past two decades. It is painless upon application, has a wide spectrum of antimicrobial activity, and has no known bacterial resistance. Its use is limited due to its staining, requirement for greater nursing care, and the leeching of electrolytes from the wound.[35]

Dressings

The use of light occlusive dressings is generally believed to prevent bacterial infection and enhance the rate at which wounds epithelialize. Additionally, optimal dressings should absorb exudates, prevent the wound from further damage, and cause minimal pain upon removal. Many centers use petroleum or mesh gauze as the first layer on the wound. This provides a moist environment that promotes healing, and doesn't stick to the wound upon removal. This gauze is then covered with multiple layers of absorbent padding to better protect the wound from additional trauma.

While not a standard for emergency department use, Biobrane, a bilaminar temporary skin substitute, is sometimes used. This biosynthetic wound dressing is constructed of a silicon film with a nylon fabric partially embedded in the film. The fabric presents to the wound bed a complex, three-dimensional structure of trifilament threads to which collagen has been chemically bound.[47] One prospective study found that the treatment of partial-thickness burns with Biobrane was superior to topical therapy with 1% silver sulfadiazine.[48] While different uses have been advocated for this dressing, its use in partial-thickness burns has remained controversial. One of the concerns that has been raised against the use of Biobrane in this setting is infection. Infection rates from 5% to 22.6% have been reported.[49-51]

Disposition

Indications for Admission

It is often difficult to decide the disposition of pediatric burn patients. While many guidelines exist that define specific BSA percentages, as well as wound severity, these alone cannot be the sole determinants. The risk of infection,

Table 26-6	Indications for Admission

Burn Depth/Body Surface Area (BSA)
Full thickness >2% BSA
Partial thickness >10% BSA
Burn Location
Face
Perineum and genitalia
Hands, feet, joints
Circumferential
Burn Mechanism
Inhalation
Electrical/high voltage
Chemical
Associated Issues
Serious trauma
Underlying medical problems
Social concerns
Very young age
Social/Environmental Issues
Neglect
Abuse
Unable to care for self

cosmetic and functional outcomes, pain control, complexity of wound care, age, associated morbidities, underlying medical conditions, and social concerns all must be factored into this complicated decision. Table 26-6 lists some useful parameters to assist with this decision making.

Indications for Transfer to a Burn Center

Most experts agree that burn centers have improved survival and reduced morbidity in burn patients. Many publications list factors to consider when deciding which children should be transferred to a burn center.[52] Many of these parallel the indications to admit noted previously. For example, burn patients with preexisting medical disorders often require transfer, as issues related to these disorders could complicate management, prolong recovery, and affect mortality. While trauma is often cited as a reason to transfer, the burned patient initially should be stabilized in a trauma center before being transferred to a burn center. Burned children in hospitals without qualified personnel or equipment should be transferred. Transfer should be considered in all children who will require special social, emotional, or long-term rehabilitative care. Importantly, these factors should be considered as guidelines, rather than rigid protocols.

Out-of-Hospital Care

Emergency Medical Services providers follow many of the management strategies outlined earlier. Most importantly, they must be cognizant of the risk of impending airway compromise; therefore, they must always be vigilant about the need for early endotracheal intubation. Oxygen (100%) should be administered and breathing should be supported, while maintaining cervical spine immobilization as necessary. At least one, but preferably two peripheral IV lines should be started in patients with significant burns. Lactated Ringer's solution should be infused, usually in boluses of 20 ml/kg. Great care must be taken to ensure that the patient's body temperature is maintained, as hypothermia is an important problem in young children with large burns.

Discharge Care
Medications

Acetaminophen or ibuprofen are commonly used analgesics at discharge. Narcotics, such as codeine or hydrocodone, however, may be necessary in cases of larger, painful burns. As burns are pruritic, medications such as hydroxyzine, diphenhydramine, and newer antihistamines may be helpful, especially when used in conjunction with moisturizing creams or lotions.[35]

Wound Infection

The parents should be advised to return with the patient if there are signs of infection: redness, swelling, tenderness, and purulent discharge. Of course, many of these signs are normal in the course of burn healing, so it is not always easy to distinguish a burn infection from a normally healing burn wound. It is common for Silvadene-treated burns to form a greenish serous drainage that is easily mistaken for purulence. Furthermore, while many associate the development of a fever with an infection, it is important to remember that burn patients may develop low-grade fevers a day or two after the burn—even in the absence of infection.

Wound Care

The parents should be instructed to keep the wound clean and dry. They can clean the wound with soap and lukewarm water. Some recommend saline solutions. The parents may debride loose nonviable tissue, and wash off accumulated exudates and topical antibiotic residues.

After the wound has been cleaned, topical antibiotic ointments or creams may be applied. These topical antibiotics, typically Silvadene or Polysporin, are usually applied twice daily until the wound has completely re-epithelialized. This process usually takes 5 to 10 days for superficial wounds and 10 to 14 days for medium-depth wounds.[35] It is important to use clean, but not necessarily sterile technique when performing burn wound care at home.[53]

The wound is dressed with a light, nonadherent dressing following the application of the topical antibiotic. Most experts recommend twice-daily dressing changes.[53] On smaller wounds, however, once daily should suffice.[37]

Follow-up Care

Follow-up care of all partial- and full-thickness burns is extremely important. The wound should be examined by a clinician every 2 to 3 days. The parents and patient should be instructed to return 4 to 6 weeks later to assess for hypertrophic scar and pigment changes. Patients should also be instructed to avoid ultraviolet light exposure (i.e., sunlight) during the time of wound maturation because the wound may become permanently hyperpigmented. The use of a sun block (>30 sun protection factor) is recommended for at least 1 year for any patient whose wounds are exposed to sunlight.[35]

Approach to the Child and Family

An important component to the management of the severely burned child centers around the psychosocial trauma that this injury has on the family. Parents may be experiencing feelings of guilt, anger, anxiety, and fear. These feelings are often sensed by the child. Gentle reassurance in a calm, quiet manner will assist in soothing those involved.

The age of the child will dictate the specific approach. For the child younger than 2 years, communication is most effective through the parents. Children of this age have little understanding of what is happening, but usually feel a sense of security when a parent is present. For the 2- to 7-year-old child, careful reassurance and explanation in words that the child can understand are vital, as these children often believe that injury, discomfort, and painful procedures are a punishment for bad behavior. For the 7- to 11-year-old, clear, simple explanations are required. Children who are ill or in pain often regress. They should be reassured that that it is acceptable to cry when they feel pain, otherwise they might feel ashamed and uncomfortable. Above 11 years, children are able to comprehend the outcome of their injuries, and will want precise information, particularly regarding potential scarring.[54]

The parents, also, will want clear information about what to expect. Parents often feel that they lose control of their child's well-being in the clinical environment. Including them in the care of their child, ensures partnership, and helps to give them control in the child's care.

Summary

Prognosis

A study looking at burn survival rates in children from 1974 to 1980, versus from 1991 to 1997, concluded that survival rates after burns have improved significantly for all children. Furthermore, even children with large burns should survive today.[55] Importantly, the large majority of those who survive serious burns have favorable long-term outcomes.[56-59] Even those who survive massive injuries can be expected to have a satisfying quality of life.[60-63] Advances in resuscitation, intensive care, mechanical ventilation, vascular access, antimicrobials, analgesia, nutrition, surgical intervention, and wound care have all contributed to improvements in survival and quality of life.[55]

Prevention

During the past two decades, fire-related deaths have declined. This is due to improved fire-fighting techniques, enhanced emergency medical services, and widespread educational programs aimed at both children and adults.[64] For example, the use of home smoke detectors has dramatically reduced the severity of burn injuries, resulting in an estimated 80% reduction in mortality and a 74% decrease in injuries from residential fires.[64,65] The use of flame-resistant childhood sleepwear has further contributed to these reductions.

Lowering the temperature of the water on the thermostats of water heating units has also made a significant impact. The contact time for a scald burn drops significantly as water temperature rises above 120° F. For this reason, it is recommended that hot water heaters be set at or below 120° F. A water temperature of greater than 140° F (common in hot water heaters) causes severe burns in less than 5 seconds in children.[66] The bath water temperature should always be checked first by an adult.

Parents and caregivers should be warned of the common summertime burn dangers from fireworks, barbecue grills, and campfires. Even excessive sun exposure can lead to sunburns with serious consequences. Winter burn threats include wood stoves and electric and kerosene space heaters.

Advances in our abilities to evaluate patients and manage their burn-related morbidities have led to dramatic improvements in the overall care of burned children. Nevertheless, prevention remains our first defense against these tragedies. Research should continue to focus on creative new strategies to ensure the safety of our children.

REFERENCES

1. Centers for Disease Control and Prevention, National Center for Injury Prevention and Control, WISQUARS: Overall fire/burn nonfatal injuries and rates per 100,000 and fire/burn deaths and rates per 100,000. Available at *http://webapp.cdc.gov/cgi-bin/broker.exe*
2. Centers for Disease Control and Prevention: Ten leading causes of injury death by age group—2001 highlighting unintentional injury deaths. Available at *ftp://ftp.cdc.gov/pub/ncipc/10LC-2001/PDF/10lc*
*3. Passaretti D, Billmire D: Management of pediatric burns. J Craniofac Surg 14:713–718, 2003.
4. McLoughlin E, McGuire A: The causes, cost and prevention of childhood burn injuries. Am J Dis Child 144:677–683, 1990.
*5. Taylor K: The management of minor burns and scalds in children. Nursing Standard 16(11):45–52, 54, 2001.
6. Klein G, Herndon D: Burns. Pediatr Rev 25:411–417, 2004.
*7. Sheridan RL: Burns. Crit Care Med 30:S500–S514, 2002.
8. Thom S, Keim L: Carbon monoxide poisoning: a review—epidemiology, pathophysiology, clinical findings and treatment options including hyperbaric oxygen therapy. Clin Toxicol 27:141, 1989.
9. Ryan C, Shankowsky H, Tredget E: Profile of the pediatric burn patient in a Canadian burn center. Burns 18:267–272, 1992.
10. Zubair M, Besner GE: Pediatric electrical burns: management strategies. Burns 23:413–420, 1997.
*11. Reed J, Pomerantz W: Emergency management of pediatric burns. Pediatr Emerg Care 21:118–129, 2005.
12. Otherson H: Burns and scalds. Pediatr Ann 12:753–760, 1983.
13. Thompson J, Ashwal K: Electrical burns in children. Am J Dis Child 137:231–235, 1983.
14. Bates N: Acid and alkali injury. Emerg Nurse 7(8):21–26, 2000.
15. Smith ML: Pediatric burns: management of thermal, electrical, and chemical burns and burn-like dermatologic conditions. Pediatr Ann 29:367–378, 2000.
16. Lund C, Browder N: The estimate of areas of burns. Surg Gynecol Obstet 79:352, 1944.
17. Sheridan RL, Petras L, Basha G, et al: Planimetry study of the percent of body surface represented by the hand and palm: sizing irregular burns is more accurately done with the palm. J Burn Care Rehabil 16:605–606, 1995.
18. Morgan E, Bledsoe S, Barker J: Practical therapeutics: ambulatory management of burns. Am Fam Physician 62:2015–2026, 2000.
19. Cohen BJ, Jordan MH, Chapin SD, et al: Pontine myelinolysis after correction of hyponatremia during burn resuscitation. J Burn Care Rehabil 12:153–156, 1991.
*20. Das A, Kim K: Infections in burn injury. Pediatr Infect Dis J 19:737–738, 2000.
21. Weber JM, Sheridan RL, Pasternack MS, Tompkins RG: Nosocomial infections in pediatric patients with burns. Am J Infect Control 25:195–201, 1997.
22. Pruitt BA Jr, McManus AT, Kim SH, Goodwin CW: Burn wound infections: current status. World J Surg 22:135–145, 1998.
23. Sheridan RL: Evaluating and managing burn wounds. Dermatol Nurs 12:17, 18, 21–28, 2000.
24. Grande C, Stene J, Bernhard W: Airway management: considerations in the trauma patient. Crit Care Clin 6:37–59, 1990.
25. Mlcak RP, Helvick B: Protocol for securing endotracheal tubes in a pediatric burn unit. J Burn Care 8:233–237, 1987.
26. Buckley RG, Aks SE, Eshorn JL, et al: The pulse oximetry gap in carbon monoxide intoxication. Ann Emerg Med 24:252, 1994.

*Selected readings.

27. Nieman GF, Clark WR, Hakim T: Methylprednisolone does not protect the lung from inhalation injury. Burns 17:384,1991.

28. Parker JC, Hernandez LA, Peevy KJ: Mechanisms of ventilator-induced lung injury. Crit Care Med 21:131–143, 1993.

29. Finkelstein J, Schwartz S, Madden M, et al: Pediatric emergency medicine. Pediatric burns: an overview. Pediatr Clin North Am 39:1145–1163, 1992.

30. Sheridan RL: The seriously burned child: resuscitation through reintegration—1. Curr Probl Pediatr 28:105–127, 1998.

31. Monafo WW: Initial management of burns. N Engl J Med 335:1581–1586, 1996.

32. Huang PP, Stucky FS, Dimick AR, et al: Hypertonic sodium resuscitation is associated with renal failure and death. Ann Surg 221:543, 1995.

33. Warden GD: Burn shock resuscitation. World J Surg 16:16–23, 1992.

34. Carvajal HF: Fluid resuscitation of pediatric burn victims: a critical appraisal. Pediatr Nephrol 8:357–366, 1994.

35. Kagan RJ, Smith SC: Evaluation and treatment of thermal injuries. Dermatol Nurs 12:334–350, 2000.

36. Hedderich R, Ness T: Analgesia for trauma and burns. Crit Care Clin 15:167–184, 1999.

37. Kao CC, Garner WL: Acute burns. Plast Reconstr Surg 101:2482–2493, 2000.

38. Palmieri T, Greenhalgh D: Topical treatment of pediatric patients with burns: a practical guide. Am J Clin Dermatol 3:529–534, 2002.

39. McDonald WS, Sharp CW, Deitch EA: Immediate enteral feeding in burn patients is safe and effective. Ann Surg 213:177–183, 1991.

40. Mainous MR, Block EF, Deitch EA: Nutritional support of the gut: how and why. New Horiz 2:193–201, 1994.

41. Deitch EA: The management of burns. N Engl J Med 323:1249–1253, 1990.

42. Schonfeld N: Outpatient management of burns in children. Pediatr Emerg Care 6:249–253, 1990.

43. Edwards-Jones V, Shawcross SG: Toxic shock syndrome in the burned patient. Br J Biomed Sci 54:110–117, 1997.

44. Bosworth C: Burns Trauma: Management and Nursing Care. London: Bailliere Tindall, 1997.

45. Flanagan M, Graham J: Should burn blisters be left intact or debrided? J Wound Care 10:41–45, 2001.

46. Gowar J, Lawrence J: The incidence, causes and treatment of minor burns. J Wound Care 4:71–74, 1995.

47. Kao CC, Garner W: Acute burns. Plast Reconstr Surg 105:2482–2493, 2000.

48. Barret JP, Dziewulski P, Ramzy P, et al: Biobrane versus 1% silver sulfadiazine in second-degree pediatric burns. Plast Reconstr Surg 105:62–65, 2000.

49. Demling RH: Use of Biobrane in management of scalds. J Burn Care Rehabil 16:329, 1995.

50. Phillips LG, Robson MC, Smith DJ: Uses and abuses of a biosynthetic dressing for partial-skin thickness burns. Burns 15:846, 1989.

51. Ou LF, Lee SY, Chen YC, et al: Use of Biobrane in pediatric scald burns: experience in 106 children. Burns 24:49, 1998.

52. Committee on Trauma, American College of Surgeons: Guidelines for the operations of burn units. In Resources for Optimal Care of the Injured Patient: 1999. Chicago: American College of Surgeons, 1999, pp 55–62.

53. Sheridan RL: The seriously burned child: resuscitation through reintegration—2. Curr Probl Pediatr 28:139–167, 1998.

54. Morgan M: Nursing management of the injured child in the A&E department. In Mead DM, Sibert JR (eds): The Injured Child: An Action Plan for Nurses. London: Scutari Press, 1991, pp 45–52.

55. Sheridan RL, Remensnyder JP, Schnitzer JJ, et al: Current expectations for survival in pediatric burns. Arch Pediatr Adolesc Med 154:245–249, 2000.

56. Andreasen NJ, Norris AS, Hartford CE: Incidence of long-term psychiatric complications in severely burned adults. Ann Surg 174:785–793, 1971.

57. Blades BC, Jones C, Munster AM: Quality of life after major burns. J Trauma 19:556–558, 1979.

58. Abdullah A, Blakeney P, Hunt R, et al: Visible scars and self-esteem in pediatric patients with burns. J Burn Care Rehabil 15:164–168, 1994.

59. Moore P, Blakeney P, Broemeling L, et al: Psychologic adjustment after childhood burn injuries as predicted by personality traits. J Burn Care Rehabil 14:80–82, 1993.

60. Herndon DN, LeMaster J, Beard S, et al: The quality of life after major thermal injury in children: an analysis of 12 survivors with greater than or equal to 80% total body, 70% third-degree burns. J Trauma 26:609–619, 1986.

61. Powers PS, Cruse CW, Daniels S, Stevens B: Posttraumatic stress disorder in patients with burns. J Burn Care Rehabil 15:147–153, 1994.

62. Tarnowski KJ, Rasnake LK, Linscheid TR, Mulick JA: Behavioral adjustment of pediatric burn victims. J Pediatr Psychol 14:607–615, 1989.

63. Sawyer MG, Minde K, Zuker R: The burned child: scarred for life? A study of the psychosocial impact of a burn injury at different developmental stages. Burns Incl Therm Inj 9:205–213, 1983.

64. Mallonee S, Istre GR, Rosenberg M, et al: Surveillance and prevention of residential-fire injuries. N Engl J Med 335:27, 1996.

65. Marshall SW, Runyan CK, Bangdiwala SI, et al: Fatal residential fires: who dies and who survives? JAMA 279:1633–1637, 1998.

66. American Burn Association: The Advanced Burn Life Support Course, Chicago: American Burn Association, 2000.

Neurovascular Injuries

Isabel Barata, MD

Introduction and Background

Traumatic injury disproportionately affects the young and is the leading cause of death and disability in the pediatric age group; however, vascular injuries in pediatric patients are rare. The majority of vascular injuries that occur in children are extremity injuries related to fractures[1] or broken glass.[2] Motor vehicle accidents, heavy machinery–related injuries, and falls cause a small proportion of blunt vascular injuries secondary to decelerating or crushing forces. Vascular injuries are usually caused by penetrating trauma from glass, bullets, and knives. Penetrating peripheral vascular injuries secondary to gunshots or stab wounds are more common in males than in females.

Recognition and Approach

Blunt trauma causes vascular injury due to either tensile or shear strain. Tensile strain leads to longitudinal forces causing vessel or intimal rupture, which exposes flowing blood to a large surface area rich in thrombogenic substances, resulting in a local thrombosis. Shear strain is secondary to lateral forces acting on the vessel wall and can result in partial or complete transection.

Penetrating injuries cause damage to vascular structures by direct injury secondary to stab or low-velocity missile wounds and/or high-velocity injury. Velocity and mass will influence the missile's destructive power. These types of injuries can cause severe damage, even in the absence of direct vascular trauma. Direct vascular injury can lead to partial or complete transection, contusion, laceration, and arteriovenous fistula formation. Indirect injuries can be more subtle in presentation and include vessel spasm, external compression, mural contusion, thrombosis, and aneurysm formation.

Peripheral vascular injuries to extremity tissues can be tolerated without ischemia when collateral vascular flow is present and adequate. This may not always be the situation, depending on the mechanism, location, and extent of injury and on the patient's baseline circulation to the involved extremity. In general, extremity tissues tolerate 4 to 6 hours of ischemia before irreversible injury occurs.

Evaluation

Vascular and Nerve Injury

Upper Extremity Injuries

FRACTURES

Approximately 75% of all fractures sustained by children occur in the upper extremities and frequently occur during a fall with an outstretched hand. Most of these injuries involve the wrist and forearm. The elbow accounts for approximately 3% to 7% of all fractures in children.[3] The majority of elbow fractures in children are supracondylar fractures of the humerus[4] (Fig. 27–1).

Elbow fractures are challenging due to the high potential for limb-threatening damage to neurovascular structures. The neurovascular examination is often difficult in a crying and frightened child; however, it must be done before the child is sent for radiographs. Pulses, capillary refill, and skin temperature of the extremity being evaluated should be checked. A brief overview of the sensorimotor evaluation of the hand is outlined in Table 27–1.[5,6] No one test has been accepted as the standard procedure for the evaluation of sensation. The various sensory tests available for patient assessment will yield different information regarding the integrity of the quickly and slowly adapting sensory receptors. Tests such as provocative maneuvers and sensory thresholds (cutaneous and vibration) will be more sensitive in the evaluation of patients with nerve compression, and will yield better functional information in patients with nerve injury. In adult patients, one of the preferred methods to assess sensation is two-point discrimination, which may be of limited value in children depending on the age and degree of cooperation. When diagnosis of vascular trauma is uncertain, the following signs and symptoms may indicate peripheral ischemia:

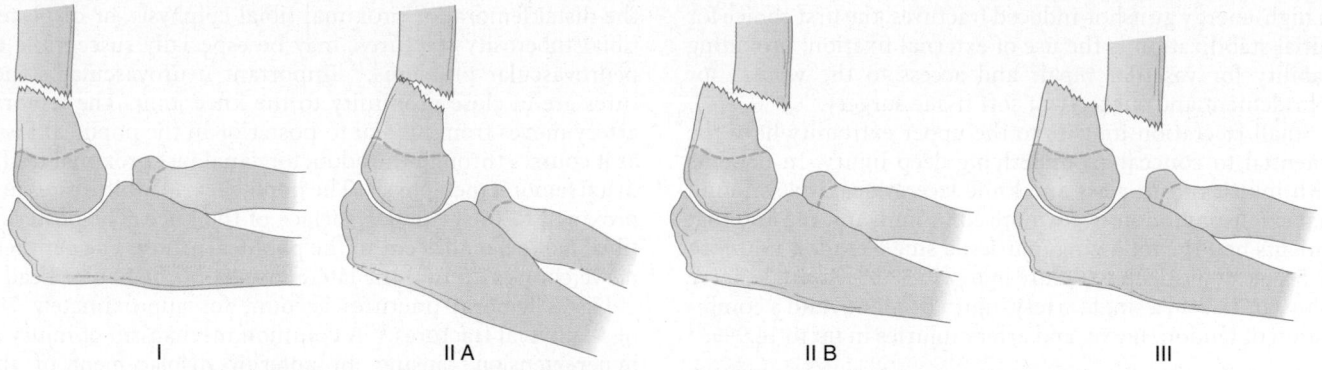

FIGURE 27–1. Modified Gartland grading of supracondylar fractures of the humerus in children.

Table 27–1	Neurovascular Examination of the Upper Extremity	
	Sensory	**Motor**
Radial nerve	Dorsal thumb web space	Raise the thumb (give "thumbs-up" sign) or raise the wrist
Median nerve	Volar tip of the index finger	Flex the thumb or index finger (make an "O" with the thumb and index finger)
Ulnar nerve	Volar tip of the lateral border of the small finger	Move the index finger medially and laterally, or flex the tip of the fifth finger

Table 27–2	Supracondylar Fracture Displacement Direction and Associated Nerve Injuries
Fracture Displacement	**Nerve Injury (Most Common)**
Posterolateral	Median nerve: Up to 80% Anterior interosseous nerve
Posteriomedial	Radial nerve
Anterolateral	Ulnar nerve

pain, pallor, paresthesias, pulselessness (palpable pulse does not exclude diagnosis), prolonged capillary refill, and paralysis (the 6 Ps). Increased pain and decreasing sensation are cardinal signs that a compartment syndrome is beginning.[7]

Vascular injury to the brachial artery and neural injury to the median, radial, and ulnar nerves can occur from stretching, entrapping, or disrupting the neurovascular structures. The incidence of neural and vascular injuries associated with humeral supracondylar fracture has been reported as nerve injury only in 6% to as high as 16% of patients,[8,9] vascular compromise only in 2.9% of patients, and combined nerve and vascular injury in 2.9%.[9] Median nerve injuries accounted for 58.9% of nerve injuries, followed by radial (26.4%) and ulnar (14.7%).[9] The supracondylar fracture of the humerus in children can be due to an extension-type fracture, in which the condylar complex shifts posterolaterally or posteromedially, or, in a smaller number of cases, a flexion-type fracture in which the condylar complex shifts anterolaterally.[10] Posterolateral fracture displacement correlates with median nerve and vascular compromise.[11] Up to 80% of median nerve injuries involve the anterior interosseous nerve.[9,12-14] Posteromedial fracture displacement correlates with radial nerve injury. Anterolateral fracture displacement in a flexion-type fracture is more frequently associated with ulnar nerve damage[15,16] (Table 27–2).

Secondary injuries can also occur in two primary ways: (1) during manipulation of the fracture, the nerves and/or vessels can be stretched or entrapped between the fracture ends; and (2) treatment in the hyperflexed position (used when only closed reduction is performed) can compromise the vascularity of the forearm, eventually resulting in Volkmann's contracture. The rate of iatrogenic nerve injury has been reported to be 2% to 3%.[17] The radial pulse is reported to be absent before reduction in 7% to 12% of all fractures and in up to 19% in displaced fractures. After reduction, the pulse is restored in 80% of cases. Injury to the nerves can also exist due to swelling of the tissues around the elbow irrespective of the treatment.

A wide variety of treatments has been recommended for displaced supracondylar fractures, ranging from nonoperative treatment through closed reduction and percutaneous Kirschner wire transfixation to open reduction with more or less stable internal fixation. The management is determined by the difficulty in obtaining and maintaining reduction and by the involvement of neurovascular structures.

BLUNT INJURIES

Blunt extremity vascular injury associated with blasts (e.g., fireworks) can be associated with fractures, amputations, dislocations, and digit neurovascular injury.[18]

PENETRATING INJURIES

A study of penetrating injuries of the upper extremity in which the mechanism of injury was stabbing in 39%, bullet in 51%, pellets in 4%, and dog bites in 6% found that the proximity of the injury to neurovascular bundles was a poor predictor of arterial injury, and long-term morbidity was mainly associated with nerve injuries.[19] Injuries to the upper extremity due to gunshot wounds are common.[20] The extent of soft tissue disruption and the type of fracture depends on the energy of the gunshot. Injuries resulting from low-energy gunshot wounds are more likely to have less soft tissue, bone, and neurovascular disruption. High-energy gunshot wounds cause more soft tissue disruption, bone loss, complex comminuted and unstable fractures, and neurovascular injuries.[21]

In high-energy gunshot-induced fractures, the first choice for initial stabilization is the use of external fixation, providing stability for vascular repair and access to the wound for débridement and subsequent soft tissue surgery.[21]

Small laceration injuries to the upper extremity have the potential to conceal an underlying deep injury. In patients with injuries from glass and knife lacerations, it was found that extensor tendons were more commonly injured and that patients had the following injuries: a single tendon injury in 92.5%, a single deep structure injury in 59.3%, a single nerve injury in 18.7%, a single artery injury in 14.9%, and a combination of tendon, nerve, and artery injuries in up to 14.9%.[22]

Lower Extremity Injuries

Fractures of the femoral supracondylar region are common in adolescents and middle-aged adults. Most often they are the result of high-energy blunt trauma such as motor vehicle collisions or industrial injuries. These fractures are usually associated with injuries to the neurovascular bundle. Blunt vascular injuries in the lower extremities occur most commonly in the anteroposterior tibial arteries.[23] The neurovascular injuries are even more complex when they are the result of penetrating trauma such as missile injuries.[24,25] Peripheral nerve injuries can result from either blunt or penetrating trauma with resulting injuries of the femoral, sciatic, peroneal, or tibial nerves. On physical examination, patients with femoral neuropathy demonstrate weakness on knee extension and sensory deficit in the area just superior and medial to the patella, with diminished or absent knee deep tendon reflexes. Findings in sciatic neuropathy are weakness of the hamstring muscle and all muscles below the knee, sensory loss in the posterior thigh and most of the leg below the knee, and absent or diminished ankle deep tendon reflexes. Peroneal nerve injuries are associated with weakness of the extensor hallucis longus muscle, with inability to dorsiflex the foot or move the toes, and sensory loss in the first toe and first web space (Table 27–3).

FRACTURES

Traumatic forces applied to the immature knee result in fracture patterns different from those in adults. Trauma that would result in a ligament injury in an adult is likely to cause in a child or adolescent an injury to the growth plate (physis) as well as the adjacent areas of the femur, tibia, or patella. The relative abundance of cartilage in the knee of the growing child may make the diagnosis of certain injuries more challenging. Certain fractures, such as hyperextension injuries to the distal femoral or proximal tibial epiphysis, or displaced tibial tuberosity fractures, may be especially susceptible to neurovascular problems.[26] Important neurovascular structures are in close proximity to the knee joint. The femoral artery moves from medial to posterior in the popliteal fossa as it courses through the adductor canal just proximal to the distal femoral metaphysis. The popliteal artery bifurcates just proximal to the articular surface of the knee. The posterior tibial nerve lies adjacent to the popliteal artery. The peroneal nerve courses around the lateral aspect of the fibular head.

Distal femoral fractures account for approximately 7% of all physeal fractures.[27] A common mechanism of injury is hyperextension causing an anterior displacement of the epiphysis. Displacement of the fracture in the sagittal plane may be associated with neurovascular injury in the popliteal fossa and instability on closed reduction. Physeal fracture displacement in the coronal plane is not associated with other injuries, and the joint may be stable after closed reduction.[28] Clinically, the thigh may appear angulated and shortened compared with the contralateral thigh. The pain, knee effusion, and soft tissue swelling usually are severe.

The Salter-Harris (SH) classification system (Fig. 27–2) provides general guidelines regarding the risk of growth disturbance, but there are no clinical methods for quantifying the true extent of physeal damage in an acute injury. Hemarthrosis may be more severe in SH III and SH IV fractures, and vascular examinations may reveal diminished or absent distal pulses. Neurologic symptoms also may be evident dis-

Table 27–3	Neurovascular Examination of the Lower Extremity	
	Sensory	**Motor**
Femoral nerve	Area superior and medial to the patella	Weakness on knee extension Diminished or absent knee deep tendon reflexes
Sciatic nerve	Posterior thigh and leg below the knee	Weakness of the hamstring muscle and all muscles below the knee Absent or diminished ankle deep tendon reflexes
Peroneal nerve	First toe and first web space	Inability to dorsiflex foot and move toes

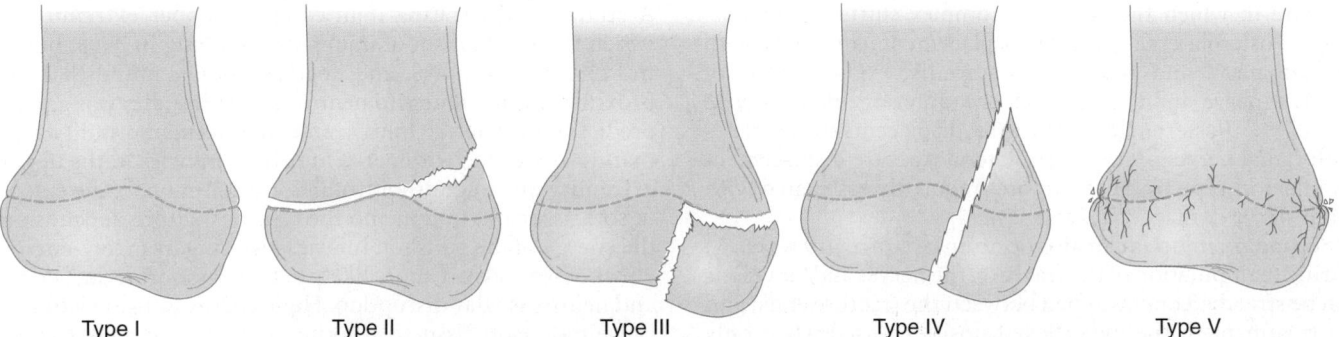

| Type I | Type II | Type III | Type IV | Type V |

FIGURE 27–2. Classification of epiphyseal fractures according to the Salter-Harris system.

tally due to disruption of the posterior tibial and common peroneal nerve distributions.

Treatment for distal femoral physeal fractures varies according to severity of injury. Displaced SH I or SH II fractures are treated with closed reduction and splinting with a hip spica cast. SH III and SH IV injuries usually require anatomic reduction, which cannot be obtained with closed reduction, and are very often unstable. Operative treatment is required since even slight residual displacement can result in formation of a bone bar that causes limb-length discrepancy and angular deformity. Whereas fractures involving the tibia and fibula are the most common lower extremity pediatric fractures, those involving the proximal tibial epiphysis are among the most uncommon, comprising less than 2% of all physeal injuries,[29] but have the highest rate of complications. The injury is usually due to anterior-posterior forces with increased risk of neurologic and/or vascular compromise, with the potential for the development of a compartment syndrome as well. When displacement occurs, the popliteal artery is vulnerable. At the tibial metaphysis, the artery is just posterior to the popliteus muscle. SH I injuries occur at an earlier age (average age 10 years). Half of SH I injuries are nondisplaced and diagnosed by stress radiographs only. SH II are the most common type, and one third are nondisplaced. SH III injuries are often associated with lateral condyle fractures or medial collateral ligament injuries. SH IV injuries are often associated with angular deformity. SH V injuries are usually diagnosed retrospectively. Anterior physis closure can cause significant genu recurvatum. Complications of these injuries include vascular insufficiency and peroneal nerve palsy.[28]

PENETRATING INJURIES

In a study of penetrating injuries, caused by gunshot wounds in 58.3% of patients and fragments of mines or other explosive devices in 41.7%, it was found that 18% of the injuries were supracondylar fractures, with associated neurovascular bundle injuries in 38% and vascular injuries in 34%. Patients required external fixation in 86% of cases and primary reconstruction of large blood vessels in 32% of limbs.[25] A similar study looking at injuries resulting from infantry weapon missiles in 70.7% of patients and explosive devices in 29.3% found that associated neurovascular bundle injuries were present in 26.8% of patients.[24]

Nerve and tendon lacerations of the foot and ankle region are relatively common. Acute nerve and tendon injuries should be repaired with appropriate techniques at the time of initial wound exploration. Primary nerve repair may help minimize the risk of painful neuroma formation; primary tendon repair can lead to better functional results than delayed repair.[30]

Compartment Syndrome

Acute compartment syndrome is a potentially devastating condition in which the pressure within an osseofascial compartment rises to a level that decreases the perfusion gradient across tissue capillary beds, leading to cellular anoxia, muscle ischemia, and death (see Chapter 22, Compartment Syndrome). A variety of injuries and medical conditions may initiate acute compartment syndrome, including fractures, contusions, bleeding disorders, burns, trauma, postischemic swelling, and gunshot wounds. Diagnosis is primarily clinical (pain out of proportion to the injury or

physical findings), supplemented by compartment pressure measurements. Nerve blocks and other forms of regional and epidural anesthesia may contribute to a delay in diagnosis. Basic science data suggest that the ischemic threshold of normal muscle is reached when pressure within the compartment is elevated to 20 mm Hg below the diastolic pressure or 30 mm Hg below the mean arterial blood pressure.[31] On diagnosis of impending or true compartment syndrome, immediate measures must be taken. Complete fasciotomy of all compartments involved is required to reliably normalize compartment pressures and restore perfusion to the affected tissues.

Recognizing compartment syndromes requires having and maintaining a high index of suspicion, performing serial examinations in patients at risk, and carefully documenting changes over time. In a retrospective study of upper extremity fasciotomy at a level I trauma center, it was found that the mechanism of injury was penetrating trauma (gunshot wounds in 37% and stab wounds in 11%), blunt or crush in 33%, and burns in 18% of cases. Fifty-six percent of patients had vascular injuries and 33% of patients had fractures. The decision to perform fasciotomy was clinical in 75% of patients, and only 22% of patients had compartment pressures measured (range, 40 to 87 mm Hg; mean, 52).[32]

Thoracic/Abdominal Injuries

Pediatric truncal vascular injuries are rare, but the reported mortality is high (35% to 55%) and similar to that in adults.[33] Thoracic injuries are primarily due to blunt rupture, which accounts for 85% of cases, 75% being motor vehicle collision related.[34] In contrast, penetrating thoracic injuries are rare in children less than 13 years old.[35] The most common thoracic vascular injury is to the aorta. Studies have shown that concomitant injuries such as traumatic brain injury, pulmonary contusion, rib fractures, hemothorax, cervicothoracic spine injury, femur fracture, and other orthopedic injuries occurred with 83% of thoracic aortic injuries and multiple vascular injuries occurred in 25% of cases.[32] Abdominal vascular injuries were primarily due to a penetrating mechanism, and the vessel most commonly involved was the inferior vena cava, followed by the aorta and less commonly the iliac artery/vein, superior mesenteric artery/vein, hepatic vein, portal vein, splenic artery/vein, and renal artery/vein.[33] Concomitant injuries associated with abdominal vascular injuries included small bowel, spleen, pancreas, large bowel, stomach, duodenum, liver, kidney, bile duct, bladder, diaphragm and orthopedic injuries. The survival and subsequent complications of patients with vascular injuries, regardless of which body cavity or vessel was injured, were related to the initial hemodynamic status. Patients presenting with blood pressure of less than 90 mm Hg had 100% mortality rate, and all patients with blood pressure greater than 90 mm Hg survived.[33,36] For further information on specific evaluation and management, see Chapter 24 (Thoracic Trauma) and Chapter 25 (Abdominal Trauma).

Neck

Vascular injuries of the neck are not as common in children as in adults; however, a delayed diagnosis of injury to a major cervicothoracic vessel from blunt trauma may cause significant adverse sequelae. The presence of cervicothoracic "seat belt sign" has been reported in the adult population to be

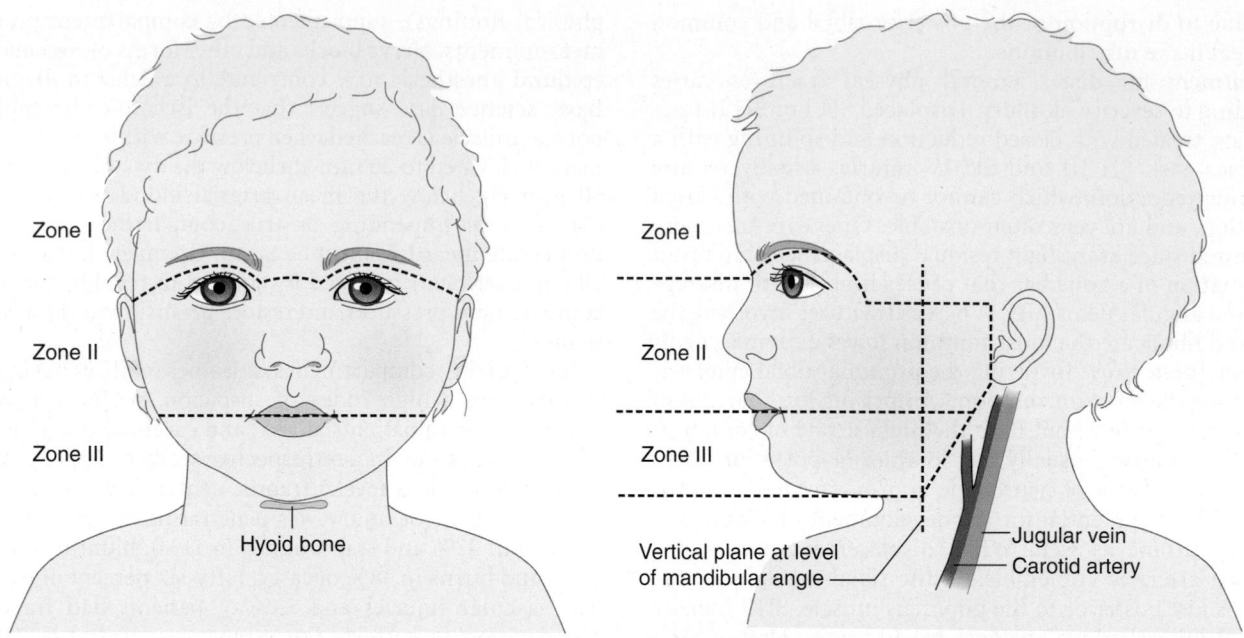

FIGURE 27–3. Anatomic divisions of the face into three areas for penetrating injuries: Zone I, above the angle of the mandible to the base of the skull; Zone II, from the angle of the mandible to the cricoid; and Zone III, below the cricoid to the suprasternal notch/clavicles.

associated with blunt vascular injury in anywhere from 0.24% to 3% of cases.[37,38] The presence of vascular injury was strongly associated with a Glasgow Coma Scale score less than 14, an Injury Severity Score greater than 16, and the presence of a clavicle and/or first rib fracture in adult patients. Pediatric patients have a higher incidence of seat belt sign as compared to adult patients; however, vascular injuries and cervical spine fractures are rare.[37]

Penetrating neck trauma in children may lead to potentially life-threatening injuries. Several studies of penetrating trauma to the head and neck in children have found that the risk for vascular and neurologic injuries is high.[33,39,40] The most commonly affected vessel is the carotid artery, followed by the vertebral artery, internal jugular vein, and facial artery. The immediate threats to life with neck injury are loss of airway due to expanding hematomas or laryngotracheal injuries, massive arterial bleed from neck or associated mediastinal/chest bleed, associated tension pneumothorax, and disruption of cerebral perfusion resulting in a cerebrovascular accident. The pediatric approach to patients with neck injuries emphasizes the selective approach to neck exploration.[39] Hemodynamically unstable patients, patients with expanding hematomas, air bubbling from a wound, or respiratory distress, and patients with suspected tracheal or esophageal injuries need emergency surgical exploration. Children who are hemodynamically stable should have an appropriate preoperative diagnostic evaluation followed by clinical observation. Nonoperative observation of penetrating zone II neck injuries (Fig. 27–3) is safe if active observation can be performed and the facilities for immediate operative intervention are available.[41,42]

Diagnostic Evaluation

Extremities

Careful neurologic (Table 27–4; see also Table 27–1) and vascular evaluation is important since many nerves and

Table 27–4	Orthopedic Injuries and Associated Nerve Injuries
Orthopedic Injury	**Nerve Injury**
Elbow supracondylar fracture	Median, radial, or ulnar
Acetabulum fracture	Sciatic
Hip dislocation	Femoral
Femoral shaft fracture	Peroneal
Femoral distal physeal fracture	Tibial or peroneal
Knee dislocation	Tibial or peroneal
Proximal tibial physeal fracture	Peroneal

arteries run within the same bundle. If a peripheral nerve injury is present, there is a good chance that the artery is also injured. Physical examination, as already mentioned, should look for the 6 Ps. However, the physical examination alone is often inadequate for predicting arterial trauma. Patients with a history of severe hemorrhage at the scene, diminished or unequal pulses, nonpulsatile hematoma, and decreased two-point discrimination in an anatomic nerve distribution should have a Doppler examination for pulses and arterial pressure index (API). The API can be used as a screening tool for clinically significant arterial compromise.[43-46] It is obtained by measuring systolic blood pressure in the injured and uninjured extremity and calculating brachial-brachial or ankle-ankle blood pressure ratios to detect penetrating vascular injury.[43-45] It can also be used in patients with blunt vascular injury.[43,46] If none of the hard signs of vascular injury, such as pulsatile hemorrhage, a palpable thrill or audible bruit, or a pulseless limb, is present, the cutoff for imaging is an API less than 0.9 between sides, which has a sensitivity of 95% to 97% and a negative predictive value of 99%.[43-45] This ratio is only useful for injuries proximal to the elbow or knee, as distal injuries do not require repair if hard signs are absent due to division of the blood supply into two main arteries with collateralization. Also, an API may be difficult to determine in certain injuries that preclude cuff placement at the wrist or ankle or in patients with hypovolemia. The API combined with physical examination was used in a study of penetrating extremity trauma to decide which patients needed angiography. In this study, 4% of patients with hard signs of vascular injury went to the operating room, 17% without vascular compromise underwent operative procedures or were admitted for other injuries, 23% with nonproximity wounds were discharged, and 55.7% with a negative physical examination and normal API were discharged from the emergency department. The authors concluded that angiography is only indicated for symptomatic patients or asymptomatic patients with abnormal APIs.[45] Also, the API can be used in patients with blunt trauma; an ankle-brachial index less than 0.9 suggests vascular injury.[46]

Plain radiographs help diagnose fractures, foreign bodies, or missiles that may be responsible for neurovascular compromise. If plain radiographs fail to reveal a fracture, a stress radiograph, computed tomography scan, or magnetic resonance imaging study may help to establish the diagnosis.

Duplex ultrasonography images the vessel and measures blood flow and velocity. Color flow duplex scanning has been shown to be useful postoperatively to manage children who have undergone various procedures to establish a radial pulse after type 3 supracondylar fractures of the humerus.[47] It is a noninvasive alternative to angiography in monitoring occult injuries. It may be particularly advantageous in small children since it can be performed serially at the bedside; however, it is an operator-dependent test.

Digital subtraction angiography is more sensitive than angiography in detecting extravasation of contrast material[48]; however, it is very sensitive to motion artifact. It involves manual contrast injection followed by immediate radiography.[49] It is rapid and accurate, and does not require transportation of an unstable patient to an angiography suite. Digital subtraction angiography is currently used in young children, as formal angiography is difficult to obtain in an uncooperative patient.

Multidetector-row helical computed tomographic arteriography (MDCTA) is emerging as a new way to study arterial anatomy. It is noninvasive and allows evaluation of different body areas simultaneously. In one study of adult patients, MDCTA adequately demonstrated the nature and location of all arterial injuries when compared with conventional arteriography or surgical exploration.[50] MDCTA is a reliable technique for the detection and characterization of traumatic extremity arterial injuries in adult patients; however, it has not been studied in children.

Angiography in pediatric patients under 5 years of age poses the risk of iatrogenic injury due to the small caliber of the vessels. In addition, arterial spasm is more common in the pediatric patient and can complicate the use of angiography. Therefore, angiography should be reserved for patients with suspected arterial injury with an equivocal vascular examination (decreased pulse, abnormal API, abnormal ankle-brachial index, and bruits).[51] Patients with obvious vascular injuries (bleeding or ischemia) should go to the operating room.

In summary, in the evaluation of blunt or penetrating vascular injury of the extremity, the following approach is indicated. If the patient has hard signs of vascular injury, such as pulsatile hemorrhage, an expanding hematoma, a palpable thrill or audible bruit, or a pulseless limb, the patient requires immediate surgical exploration and vascular repair. Patients with no hard signs but either soft signs (e.g., history of large blood loss, decreased two-point discrimination, decreased or unequal pulses, and nonpulsatile hematoma) or injuries that are known to be associated with a high incidence of arterial damage should be screened with an API. If the API is greater than 0.9, a serial clinical evaluation should be performed. If the API is less than 0.90, further evaluation is indicated with either duplex ultrasonography or MDCTA, if studies show the latter evaluation to be useful in children. If these diagnostic tests are abnormal, then angiography is indicated. In patients with low likelihood of vascular injury (proximity injury, penetrating wound in proximity to vascular structures without clinical findings to suggest vascular compromise), duplex ultrasonography follow-up may be used.

Compartment Syndrome

If the history and physical examination suggest compartment syndrome, an orthopedic consultation should be obtained, and compartment pressures measured with commercially available monitors. The patient should be carefully followed with serial examinations and pressure measurements (see Chapter 22, Compartment Syndrome).

Neck

Traumatic injury to the major vessels of the head and neck can result in potentially devastating neurologic sequelae. Carotid duplex ultrasound is a noninvasive, rapid screening test for arterial injury. Conventional angiography has been the primary imaging modality used to evaluate these often challenging patients with both blunt neck trauma and penetrating wounds in zone I or zone III (see Fig. 27–3), carotid bruit, large hematoma, and suspected arterial injury. The absence of hemorrhage, expanding hematoma, bruit, thrill, or neurologic (hard signs) deficit reliably excludes surgically significant vascular injuries in penetrating zone III neck trauma, suggesting that angiography is not necessary.[52] Hard signs in stable patients should mandate angiography because these vascular injuries may be amenable to endovascular therapy.[52] Advances in cross-sectional imaging have improved the ability to screen for these lesions, which have been found to be more common than previously thought.[53] MDCTA screening increases the detected incidence of blunt vascular neck injury eightfold, with rates similar to angiography-based screening protocols. MDCTA screening significantly decreases blunt vascular neck injury–related morbidity and mortality in an efficient manner, underscoring its utility in the early diagnosis of this injury.[54] Other studies of blunt and/or penetrating neck injuries showed that MDCTA is adequate for the initial evaluation and triage of patients to conventional angiography or surgery for appropriate treatment, and as a guide to conservative management when appropriate.[55,56]

In summary, if hard signs of vascular injury are present, the unstable patient requires operative management and the stable patient angiography. If the patient does not have hard signs of vascular injury, then MDCTA can be used as screening tool to guide further evaluation and intervention.

Management

After initial stabilization, a more detailed secondary evaluation is conducted to assess for vascular injury. Fractures are splinted and dislocations reduced since anatomic repositioning and splinting may help restore circulation in dislocations or fractures. If penetrating injuries, particularly high-velocity injuries, are near major vascular structures, the clinician should assume there is damage to those structures. It is important to control hemorrhage with direct pressure; however, blindly clamping a blood vessel should be avoided. Vascular status must be frequently reassessed and popliteal artery injuries carefully monitored because of minimal collateral circulation present in the lower extremity. Obvious vascular injury with evidence of ischemia is an indication for emergent surgical exploration. Prompt consultation with the trauma team is routine at most major urban trauma centers. If isolated peripheral vascular injury is present, the vascular surgeon should be consulted early in the management of the patient. Also, early intravenous antibiotics and tetanus immunization (if indicated) should be provided. If surgical consultation and appropriate diagnostic evaluation tools are not available at the primary institution, the patient must be transferred as quickly as possible after stabilization.

Summary

The goals in management of children with neurovascular injuries are stabilization of the patient and minimization of ischemic time. A thorough neurovascular examination is more difficult in young children. However, it should be performed and carefully documented. Children have a higher risk of developmental abnormalities secondary to ischemia. Prompt consultation, early intravenous antibiotics, and tetanus immunization if indicated are also important aspects of management. Prognosis depends upon ischemic time and number and extent of associated injuries. Associated nerve damage occurs in a large percentage of vascular injuries; 45% of those result in permanent deficits. After initial stabilization, if surgical consultation is not available, the clinician should arrange for transfer.

REFERENCES

1. Richardson JD, Fallat M, Nagaraj HS, et al: Arterial injuries in children. Arch Surg 116:685–690, 1981.
*2. Wolf YG, Reyna T, Schropp KP, Harmel RP: Arterial trauma of the upper extremity in children. J Trauma 30:903–905, 1990.
3. Landin LA: Fracture patterns in children: analysis of 8,682 fractures with special reference to incidence, etiology and secular changes in a Swedish urban population 1950–1979. Acta Orthop Scand Suppl 202:1–109, 1983.
4. Landin LA, Danielsson LG: Elbow fractures in children: an epidemiological analysis of 589 cases. Acta Orthop Scand 57:309, 1986.
5. Townsend DJ, Bassett GS: Common elbow fractures in children. Am Fam Physician 53:2031–2041, 1996.
6. Skaggs D, Pershad J: Pediatric elbow trauma. Pediatr Emerg Care 13:425–434, 1997.
7. Weinmann M: Compartment syndrome. Emerg Med Serv 32(9):36, 2003.
8. Culp RW, Osterman, AL, Davidson RS, et al: Neural injuries associated with supracondylar fractures of the humerus in children. J Bone Joint Surg Am 72:1211–1215, 1990.

*9. Lyons ST, Quinn M, Stanitski CL: Neurovascular injuries in type III humeral supracondylar fractures in children. Clin Orthop Relat Res (376):62–67, 2000.
10. Farnsworth CL, Silva PD, Mubarak SJ: Etiology of supracondylar humerus fractures. J Pediatr Orthop 18:38–42, 1998.
11. Rasool MN, Naidoo KS: Supracondylar fractures: posterolateral type with brachialis muscle penetration and neurovascular injury. J Pediatr Orthop 19:518–522, 1999.
12. Campbell CC, Waters PM, Emans JB, et al: Neurovascular injury and displacement in type III supracondylar humerus fractures. J Pediatr Orthop 15:47–52, 1995.
13. Cramer KE, Green NE, Devito DP: Incidence of anterior interosseous nerve palsy in supracondylar humerus fractures in children. J Pediatr Orthop 13:502–505, 1993.
14. Jones ET, Louis DS: Median nerve injuries associated with supracondylar fractures of the humerus in children. Clin Orthop Relat Res (150):181–186, 1980.
15. Wilkins KE: Residuals of elbow trauma in children. Orthop Clin North Am 21:291–314, 1990.
16. Wilkins KE: The operative management of supracondylar fractures. Orthop Clin North Am 21:269–289, 1990.
17. Rasool MN: Ulnar nerve injury after K-wire fixation of supracondylar humerus fractures in children. J Pediatr Orthop 18:686–690, 1998.
18. Moore RS, Tan V, Dormans JP, Bozentka DJ: Major pediatric hand trauma associated with fireworks. J Orthop Trauma 14:426–428, 2000.
19. Degiannis E, Levy RD, Sliwa K, et al: Penetrating injuries of the brachial artery. Injury 26:249–252, 1995.
*20. Hahn M, Strauss E, Yang EC: Gunshot wounds to the forearm. Orthop Clin North Am 26:85–93, 1995.
21. Johnson EC, Strauss E: Recent advances in the treatment of gunshot fractures of the humeral shaft. Clin Orthop Relat Res (408):126–132, 2003.
22. Tuncali D, Yavuz N, Terzioglu A, Aslan G: The rate of upper-extremity deep-structure injuries through small penetrating lacerations. Ann Plast Surg 55:146–148, 2005.
23. Rozycki GS, Tremblay LN, Feliciano DV, et al: Blunt vascular trauma in the extremity: diagnosis, management, and outcome. J Trauma 55:814–824, 2003.
24. Nikolic D, Jovanovic Z, Turkovic G, et al: Subtrochanteric missile fractures of the femur. Injury 29:743–749, 1998.
25. Nikolic DK, Jovanovic Z, Turkovic G, et al: Supracondylar missile fractures of the femur. Injury 33:161–166, 2002.
26. Zionts LE: Fractures around the knee in children. J Am Acad Orthop Surg 10:345–355, 2002.
27. Mann DC, Rajmaira S: Distribution of physeal and nonphyseal fractures in 2,650 long-bone fractures in children aged 0-16 years. J Pediatr Orthop 10:713–716, 1990.
28. Beaty JH, Kumar A: Fractures about the knee in children. J Bone Joint Surg Am 76:1870–1880, 1994.
29. Donahue JP, Brennan JF, Barron OA: Combined physeal/apophyseal fracture of the proximal tibia with anterior angulation from an indirect force: report of 2 cases. Am J Orthop 32:604–607, 2003.
30. Thordarson DB, Shean CJ: Nerve and tendon lacerations about the foot and ankle. J Am Acad Orthop Surg 13(3):186–196, 2005.
31. Gulli B, Templeman D: Compartment syndrome of the lower extremity. Orthop Clin North Am 25:677–684, 1994.
32. Dente CJ, Feliciano DV, Rozyck, GS, et al: A review of upper extremity fasciotomies in a level I trauma center. Am Surg 70:1088–1093, 2004.
*33. Cox CS, Black CT, Duke JH, et al: Operative treatment of truncal vascular injuries in children and adolescents. J Pediatr Surg 33:462–467, 1998.
34. Cooper A: Thoracic injuries. Semin Pediatr Surg 4:109–115, 1995.
35. Meller JL, Little AG, Shermeta DW: Thoracic trauma in children. Pediatrics 74:813–819, 1984.
36. Sirinek KR, Gaskill HV, Root HD, Levine BA: Truncal vascular injury—factors influencing survival. J Trauma 23:372–377, 1983.
37. Rozycki GS, Gaskill HV, Root HD, et al: A prospective study for the detection of vascular injury in adult and pediatric patients with cervicothoracic seat belt signs. J Trauma 52:618–623; discussion 623–624, 2002.
38. Fabian TC, Patton JH, Croce MA, et al: Blunt carotid injury: importance of early diagnosis and anticoagulant therapy. Ann Surg 223:513–522; discussion 522–555, 1996.
39. Cooper A, Barlow B, Niemirska M, et al: Fifteen years' experience with penetrating trauma to the head and neck in children. J Pediatr Surg 22:24–27, 1987.

---

*Selected readings.

40. Martin WS, Gussack GS: Pediatric penetrating head and neck trauma. Laryngoscope 100:1288–1291, 1990.

*41. Kim MK, Buckman R, Szeremeta W: Penetrating neck trauma in children: an urban hospital's experience. Otolaryngol Head Neck Surg 123:439–442, 2000.

42. Hall JR, Reyes HM, Meller JL: Penetrating zone-II neck injuries in children. J Trauma 31:1614–1617, 1991.

43. Levy BA, Zlowodzki MP, Graves M, Cole PA: Screening for extremity arterial injury with the arterial pressure index. Am J Emerg Med 23:689–695, 2005.

*44. Johansen K, Lynch K, Paun M, Copass M: Non-invasive vascular tests reliably exclude occult arterial trauma in injured extremities. J Trauma 31:515–519; discussion 519–522, 1991.

45. Conrad MF, Patton JH, Parikshak M, Kralovich KA: Evaluation of vascular injury in penetrating extremity trauma: angiographers stay home. Am Surg 68:269–274, 2002.

46. Mills WJ, Barei DP, McNair P: The value of the ankle-brachial index for diagnosing arterial injury after knee dislocation: a prospective study. J Trauma 56:1261–1265, 2004.

47. Sabharwa S, Tredwell SJ, Beauchamp RD, et al: Management of pulseless pink hand in pediatric supracondylar fractures of humerus. J Pediatr Orthop 17:303–310, 1997.

48. Sibbitt RR, Palmaz JC, Garcia F, Reuter SR: Trauma of the extremities: prospective comparison of digital and conventional angiography. Radiology 160:179–182, 1986.

*49. Itani KM, Rothenberg SS, Brandt ML, et al: Emergency center arteriography in the evaluation of suspected peripheral vascular injuries in children. J Pediatr Surg 28:677–680, 1993.

50. Busquets AR, Acosta JA, Colon E, et al: Helical computed tomographic angiography for the diagnosis of traumatic arterial injuries of the extremities. J Trauma 56:625–628, 2004.

51. de Virgilio C, Mercado PD, Arnell T, et al: Noniatrogenic pediatric vascular trauma: a ten-year experience at a level I trauma center. Am Surg 63:781–784, 1997.

52. Ferguson E, Dennis JW, Vu JH, Frykberg ER: Redefining the role of arterial imaging in the management of penetrating zone 3 neck injuries. Vascular 13:158–163, 2005.

53. Stallmeyer MJ, Morales RE, Flanders AE: Imaging of traumatic neurovascular injury. Radiol Clin North Am 44:13–39, 2006.

54. Schneidereit NP, Simons R, Nicolaou S, et al: Utility of screening for blunt vascular neck injuries with computed tomographic angiography. J Trauma 60:209–215; discussion 215–216, 2006.

*55. Stuhlfaut JW, Barest G, Sakai O, et al: Impact of MDCT angiography on the use of catheter angiography for the assessment of cervical arterial injury after blunt or penetrating trauma. AJR Am J Roentgenol 185:1063–1068, 2005.

56. Woo K, Magner DP, Wilson MT, et al: CT angiography in penetrating neck trauma reduces the need for operative neck exploration. Am Surg 71:754–758, 2005.

SECTION III

Approach to Unique Problems of Infancy

Approach to
Chronic Problems
of Urinary

Chapter 28

Apparent Life-Threatening Events

Andrew DePiero, MD

Key Points

The term *apparent life-threatening event* does not refer to a single diagnosis, but identifies a heterogeneous group of conditions with a common clinical presentation.

Potentially life-threatening conditions may present as apparent life-threatening events.

Infants who have experienced an apparent life-threatening event do not usually appear ill on presentation to the emergency department.

There is no standardized approach to the emergency department evaluation or management of infants who have experienced apparent life-threatening events.

Introduction and Background

Infants commonly present to the emergency department (ED) for evaluation of a possible apparent life-threatening event (ALTE). The term *apparent life-threatening event* does not refer to a single diagnosis, but identifies a heterogeneous group of conditions with a common clinical presentation. A formal definition from the National Institutes of Health in 1986 defined an ALTE as "an episode that is frightening to the observer and that is characterized by some combination of apnea (central or occasionally obstructive), color change (usually cyanotic or pallid but occasionally erythematous or plethoric), marked change in muscle tone (usually marked limpness), choking or gagging. In some cases the observer fears that the infant has died."[1] The term *apparent life-threatening event* replaces the previously used terms, "aborted crib death" and "near-miss SIDS," to avoid implying a close association with sudden infant death syndrome (SIDS).[1]

Despite this consensus definition of ALTE, controversy remains. Varying definitions lead to heterogeneity in clinical studies. Varying upper limits on age have been used. There are no generally accepted criteria for either the general appearance or the clinical stability of infants suspected of having experienced an ALTE. Some have proposed that the definition of ALTE be amended to include the lack of obvious physical examination findings.[2] An infant who is in moderate respiratory distress may fit some definitions of ALTE, whereas only well-appearing infants with an entirely normal physical examination fit other definitions. Practitioners and researchers continue to struggle with what constitutes an ALTE (Table 28–1). Substantial variability exists with respect to age and clinical presentation. The absence of a reproducible, widely accepted clinical definition complicates any interpretation of the existing literature on this topic. Therefore, basing clinical practice on available evidence is problematic. Nonetheless, the varied definitions of ALTE are sufficiently similar to offer information on which to base a reasonable approach to these infants when they present to the ED.[3-7]

Recognition and Approach

ALTEs are relatively uncommon. Limited epidemiologic data suggest the incidence is between 0.6 and 2.5 per 1000 live births.[7,8] Historically, ALTEs were thought to be episodes that would have resulted in SIDS if someone had not intervened. The link between SIDS and ALTEs is unclear. In particular, the "back to sleep" campaign aimed at increasing the number of infants placed supine to sleep appears to have decreased the incidence of SIDS, but not ALTEs.[9]

Clinical Presentation

An ALTE is most often identified from historical data provided by caregivers. Cyanosis, apnea, and difficulty breathing are the most frequently reported symptoms.[10,11] Other reported symptoms include abnormal movements, loss of consciousness, vomiting, choking, color change other than cyanosis (e.g., gray, red, or pale), gagging, and change in tone (i.e., limp or stiff). The episodes may occur while awake or asleep. Interventions by care providers range from vigorous stimulation to cardiopulmonary resuscitation. These events frighten most parents and care providers.

In the ED, personnel should obtain a history of the event, including a description of any associated symptoms and an account of any recent changes in the patient's health (e.g., fever, upper respiratory tract symptoms). The past medical history should focus on any prior unusual episodes or behaviors, a perinatal history, and a description of any respiratory symptoms or symptoms associated with gastroesophageal reflux (see Chapter 35, Vomiting, Spitting Up, and Feeding Difficulties). The clinician should inquire about a family

Table 28–1	Varying Definitions of Apparent Life-Threatening Events	
Working Definition		**Age Range of Study Subjects**
Apparent Life-Threatening Event (ALTE)—"An episode that is frightening to the observer and that is characterized by some combination of apnea (central or occasionally obstructive), color change (usually cyanotic or pallid but occasionally erythematous or plethoric), marked change in muscle tone (usually marked limpness), choking or gagging"[1]		Not defined
"sudden occurrence of one or more of the following: breathing irregularity (e.g., apnea, labored or shallow breathing, choking and gagging), color change indicative of decreased oxygenation (e.g., cyanosis, pallor), altered muscle tone or mental status (e.g., hypotonia, hypertonia, clonic movements, and unresponsiveness)"[11]		<12 mo
"apnea monitor alarm or an episode associated with two or more of the following factors: apnea, color change, change in muscle tone, choking/gagging or the performance of CPR at the time of the episode . . . . single episode within the previous 24 hours and presenting with stable vital signs"[13]		<6 mo
"one or more symptoms of apnea, color change, choking or abnormal limb movements and provided this has caused sufficient concern in the observer to seek medical attention"[10]		<12 mo
"unexpected change in behavior that alarmed the caregiver. The initial episodes can occur during sleep, awake or while feeding . . . some combination of apnea, color change, marked change in muscle tone, choking or gagging . . . . In most cases . . . prompt intervention was associated with normalization of the child's appearance."[24]		Not defined
"episodes of cyanosis or pallor for which vigorous stimulation had been given by the caregivers"[3]		<12 mo
"a cessation of breathing, cyanosis or change in the level of consciousness"[18]		1–604 days
"apneic episodes accompanied by one or more of the following manifestations: cyanosis, hypotonia, loss of consciousness necessitating vigorous stimulation or resuscitation"[4]		25 days–6 mo
"an event of prolonged apnea, hypotonia and cyanosis or pallor"[14]		2–36 wk
"attack of an infant who, during presumed sleep, is found not breathing, cyanotic or pale, often limp and who has to be vigorously stimulated or ventilated mouth-to-mouth to be resuscitated"[5]		Birth–24 wk

Abbreviation: CPR, cardiopulmonary resuscitation.

history of SIDS or other causes of infant deaths, ALTEs, seizures, metabolic disorders, and cardiac or respiratory abnormalities.

Infants who have experienced an ALTE typically appear well at the time of the ED evaluation. The physical examination of these infants is usually normal. Close monitoring may reveal further ALTEs in the ED. Some of the etiologies of ALTE can lead to rapid deterioration after a period of relatively well appearance. Being prepared for this eventuality is prudent and might be life saving (see Chapter 5, Monitoring in Critically Ill Children; and Chapter 7, The Critically Ill Neonate).

Important Clinical Features and Considerations

Serious etiologies of ALTEs may not be identified by a thorough history and careful physical examination. Because of this, the diagnosis of a truly life-threatening condition may be delayed as testing is undertaken. In particular, patients with infectious, traumatic, cardiac, and respiratory etiologies for their ALTEs are at risk for poor outcomes if the diagnosis is substantially delayed.

Many infectious diseases cause ALTEs (Table 28–2). Respiratory abnormalities are often associated with an infectious etiology. Respiratory syncytial virus (RSV) infections (including bronchiolitis), viral upper respiratory tract infections, and pertussis are the most frequently reported infectious causes of ALTEs.[8,10-16] The symptoms for both RSV infections and pertussis are variable and may be subtle, particularly in young infants. Patients with RSV infections may present with rhinorrhea or apnea as the sole symptom, without wheezing as seen in cases of RSV bronchiolitis (see Chapter 57, Bronchiolitis). Young infants with pertussis may present with periods of apnea as the sole complaint. Cough may be a minor component of the clinical scenario or absent.

These young infants do not manifest the characteristic "whoop" of pertussis infections. Bacterial meningitis, perhaps the most feared infectious disease of infancy, has been reported in patients with an ALTE.[12,14] Studies of ALTEs may not include any infants with bacterial meningitis simply due to sample size and the relative rarity of bacterial meningitis.[10,11,13,15,16]

Accidental and nonaccidental trauma are important causes of ALTEs. In one case series, 2.5% of the infants presenting for evaluation of ALTEs harbored nonaccidental head injuries.[12] These infants tended to present with cardiorespiratory instability, signs of trauma on physical examination, or both. It has been suggested that all infants presenting with ALTEs have a funduscopic evaluation for retinal hemorrhages.[17] Given the inherent difficulties in performing funduscopic examinations in infants in the ED, this is probably not a realistic expectation for emergency physicians. However, infants who have experienced an ALTE are typically admitted to the hospital. A funduscopic examination can be performed during the infant's inpatient stay. Intentional suffocation and Munchausen syndrome by proxy may also be the cause of ALTEs. Although perhaps suspected at the time of the ED evaluation, these diagnoses are usually made during the inpatient stay.[18,19]

The role of cardiac abnormalities as the underlying cause of ALTEs is unclear. In the largest reported series of patients evaluated for cardiac abnormalities after an ALTE, 62% had one or more dysrhythmias. These dysrhythmias included prolonged corrected QT intervals (30%), premature ventricular depolarizations (25%), and premature atrial beats (15%).[20] Most of these dysrhythmias are not clinically important or diagnostic. Other studies, however, have reported the incidence of dysrhythmias and structural cardiac abnormalities to be less than 1%.[8,10,12-16]

The role of gastroesphageal reflux in ALTE is controversial. Gastroesophageal reflux symptoms are common in infancy.

Table 28–2	Differential Diagnosis for Apparent Life-Threatening Events
Cardiac	Atrial and ventricular septal defect
	Cardiomyopathy
	Double aortic arch
	Dysrhythmia
	Fibroelastosis
	Hypoplastic left ventricle
	Myocarditis
	Patent ductus arteriosus
Gastrointestinal	Gastroesophageal reflux
	Strangulated hernia
	Upper gastrointestinal bleed
Infectious	Bronchiolitis
	Croup
	Encephalitis
	Gastroenteritis
	Lower respiratory tract infection
	Meningitis
	Pertussis
	Pneumonia
	Sepsis
	Upper respiratory tract infection
	Urinary tract infection
Metabolic	β-Ketothiolase deficiency
	Carnitine deficiency
	Galactosemia
	Glutaric aciduria type II
	Hyperammonemia, undetermined disorders
	Hypocalcemia
	Hypoglycemia
	Hypomagnesemia
	Lactic acidosis, undetermined disorders
	Menkes' syndrome
	Mitochondrial fatty acid oxidation disorders
	Nesidioblastosis
	Reye's syndrome
	Urea cycle defects
Neurologic	Brain tumor
	Central apnea
	Cerebral artery infarct
	Craniosynostosis
	Epilepsy
	Febrile seizure
	Head injury
	Hydrocephalus
	Infantile spasm
	Intraventricular hemorrhage
	Seizure
	Subarachnoid hemorrhage
	Ventriculoperitoneal shunt malfunction
	Werdnig-Hoffmann disease
Respiratory	Accidental smothering/asphyxia
	Anatomic airway obstruction/abnormalities
	Aspiration pneumonia
	Asthma
	Choking episode
	Foreign body aspiration
	Laryngomalacia
	Laryngostenosis
Other	Anemia
	Breath-holding spells
	Developmental delay
	Feeding difficulty/overfeeding
	Medications/toxins
	Munchausen syndrome by proxy
	Trauma
	Vaccine reaction
	Vagal reaction

Even though gastroesophageal reflux is diagnosed in an infant who has experienced an ALTE, this does not establish a causal relationship.[21]

Identifying risk factors for recurrent ALTEs or serious underlying etiologies is problematic. Definitional problems, heterogeneity of study populations, and small sample sizes lead to problems with reproducibility and external validity. Factors identified as being associated with a repeat ALTE or an identifiable cause include an abnormal physical examination, age greater than 2 months, low serum bicarbonate, high serum lactate, and a history of prematurity.[11,12]

Management

The history and physical examination may suggest an underlying cause for an ALTE. When this is the case, an appropriate evaluation directed toward the presumptive cause is indicated. When the etiology is not clear based on the history and physical examination, a laboratory evaluation, radiographic evaluation, or both is likely indicated. The components of the most appropriate ED diagnostic evaluation of infants who have experienced an ALTE remain controversial. The differential diagnosis is large, and therefore the ED diagnostic evaluation is often extensive. Components of the "ALTE workup" may include cultures of blood, urine, and cerebrospinal fluid, a complete blood count, electrolytes (including a serum glucose), a catheterized urinalysis, and cerebrospinal fluid cell counts, glucose, and protein. If respiratory symptoms are present, a chest radiograph and tests for RSV and pertussis may be added. If the infant has an abnormal cardiac examination, a history of sweating with feeds, hepatomegaly on physical examination, or a murmur, an electrocardiogram, chest radiograph, and perhaps an echocardiogram may be added. If the history or physical examination is suspicious for nonaccidental trauma, a computed tomography scan of the head and a skeletal survey may be added. Metabolic etiologies are rare, but frozen samples of blood and urine obtained near the time of the event may help identify a metabolic disorder.

Unfortunately, in cases in which the history and physical examination fail to guide further evaluation, the yield of any particular diagnostic test is low. In the absence of an evidence-based approach for the diagnostic evaluation of these patients, several authors have presented their own recommendations (Table 28–3). These recommendations may be clinically useful. However, the differences suggest further research is needed to determine the optimal ED workup.[8,10-13,22,23] In 2003, the European Society for the Study and Prevention of Infant Death published a consensus document titled "Recommended Clinical Evaluation of Infants with an Apparent Life-Threatening Event."[24] This document states there is no standard minimal workup for infants who have experienced an ALTE. The history and physical examination should direct the diagnostic evaluation.[24]

Summary

Evaluating infants who have experienced ALTEs is challenging. In many cases, an underlying etiology can be determined. However, this etiology may not be identified while the patient is in the ED. Diagnostic testing may identify abnormalities such as gastroesophageal reflux that are present, but not the underlying etiology of the ALTE. The utility of the

Table 28–3   Varying Recommendations for Diagnostic Testing for Infants Who Have Experienced Apparent Life-Threatening Events

Recommendations	Comments
Hemoglobin, glucose, lactate; chest radiograph; ECG; pertussis swab; urinalysis; hold (freeze) samples of blood and urine for metabolic and toxicologic studies[11]	Physical examination to include funduscopy for retinal hemorrhages
Glucose; hold (freeze) samples of blood and urine for metabolic and toxicologic studies[6]	Authors recommend "considering" blood gases, lactate, and, in all patients under 28 days, CBC and bacteriologic cultures.
CBC, C-reactive protein, sodium, potassium, urea, calcium, magnesium, glucose, blood gas, ammonia, lactate, pyruvate, blood culture; urinalysis, urine culture, urine toxicology screen; hold (freeze) urine sample for metabolic studies; investigations for lower respiratory tract infection (chest radiograph, pertussis and RSV swabs); ECG; ultrasound of brain[19]	Recommendations not specific to the ED. Authors recommend "considering" child abuse. No comment regarding timing or urgency to perform an ultrasound of the brain.

Abbreviations: CBC, complete blood count; ECG, electrocardiogram; ED, emergency department; RSV, respiratory syncytial virus.

components of the history and physician examination is variable. The yield of any individual diagnostic test is low. Hospital admission is typically indicated. Further research is needed to identify the most appropriate ED evaluation.

REFERENCES

1. National Institutes of Health Consensus Development Conference on Infantile Apnea and Home Monitoring, Sept 29 to Oct 1, 1986.
2. Maffei FA, Powers KS, van der Jagt EW: Apparent life-threatening events as an indicator of occult abuse. Arch Pediatr Adolesc Med 158:402, 2004.
3. Poets CF, Samuels MP, Noyes JP, et al: Home event recordings of oxygenation, breathing movements, and heart rate and rhythm in infants with recurrent life-threatening events. J Pediatr 123:693–701, 1993.
4. Tirosh E, Haddad F, Lanir A, et al: Relationship of sweat electrolytes to apparent life-threatening events (ALTE): a case control study. Acta Paediatr 83:1268–1271, 1994.
5. Wennergren G, Milerad J, Lagercrantz H, et al: The epidemiology of sudden infant death syndrome and attacks of lifelessness in Sweden. Acta Paediatr Scand 76:898–906, 1987.
6. Gibb SM, Waite AJ: The management of apparent life-threatening events. Curr Paediatr 8:152–156, 1998.
7. Kiechl-Kohlendorfer U, Hof D, Pupp Peglow U, et al: Epidemiology of apparent life threatening events. Arch Dis Child 90:297–300, 2005.
8. Kurz R, Kerbl R, Reiterer F, et al: The role of triggers in apparent life-threatening events (ALTE). J Sudden Infant Death Syndr Infant Mortal 2:3–12, 1997.
9. Gershan WM, Besch NS, Franciosi RA: A comparison of apparent life-threatening events before and after the back to sleep campaign. West Med J 101: 39–45, 2002.
10. Gray C, Davies F, Molyneux E: Apparent life-threatening events presenting to a pediatric emergency department. Pediatr Emerg Care 15:195–199, 1999.
*11. Davies F, Gupta R: Apparent life threatening events in infants presenting to an emergency department. Emerg Med J 19:11–16, 2002.

*12. Altman RL, Brand DA, Forman S, et al: Abusive head injury as a cause of apparent life-threatening events in infancy. Arch Pediatr Adolesc Med 157:1011–1015, 2003.
13. De Piero AD, Teach SJ, Chamberlain JM: ED evaluation of infants after an apparent life-threatening event. Am J Emerg Med 22:83–86, 2004.
14. Veereman-Wauters G, Bochner A, Van Caillie-Bertrand M: Gastroesophageal reflux in infants with a history of near-miss sudden infant death. J Pediatr Gastroenterol Nutr 12:319–323, 1991.
15. Sheikh S, Stephen T, Frazer A, et al: Apparent life-threatening events in infants. Clin Pulm Med 7:81–84, 2000.
16. Tsukada K, Kosuge N, Hosokawa M, et al: Etiology of 19 infants with apparent life-threatening events: relationship between apnea and esophageal dysfunction. Acta Paediatr Jpn 35:306–310, 1993.
17. Pitetti RD, Maffei F, Chang K, et al: Prevalence of retinal hemorrhages and child abuse in children who present with an apparent life-threatening event. Pediatrics 110:557–562, 2002.
18. Southall DP, Janczynski RE, Alexander JR, et al: Cardiorespiratory patterns in infants presenting with apparent life-threatening episodes. Biol Neonate 57:77–87, 1990.
19. Kravitz RM, Wilmott RW: Munchausen syndrome by proxy presenting as factitious apnea. Clin Pediatr 29:587–592, 1990.
20. Woolf PK, Gewitz MH, Preminger T, et al: Infants with apparent life threatening events: cardiac rhythm and conduction. Clin Pediatr 28:517–520, 1989.
21. Arad-Cohen N, Cohen A, Tirosh E: The relationship between gastroesophageal reflux and apnea in infants. J Pediatr 137:321–326, 2000.
*22. McGovern MC, Smith MB: Causes of apparent life threatening events in infants: a systematic review. Arch Dis Child 89:1043–1048, 2004.
23. Lewis JM, Ganick DJ: Initial laboratory evaluation of infants with 'presumed near-miss' sudden infant death syndrome. Am J Dis Child 140:484–486, 1986.
*24. Kahn A, European Society for the Study and Prevention of Infant Death: Recommended clinical evaluation of infants with an apparent life-threatening event: consensus document of the European Society for the Study and Prevention of Infant Death, 2003. Eur J Pediatr 163:108–111, 2004.

*Selected readings.

Chapter 29

Inborn Errors of Metabolism

T. Kent Denmark, MD

Key Points

Children with known and previously undiagnosed inborn errors of metabolism present to emergency departments more commonly than is generally recognized.

An elevated ammonia level is useful for identifying children with previously undiagnosed inborn errors of metabolism presenting to the emergency department.

Of acute metabolic derangements resulting from exacerbations of inborn errors of metabolism, hypoglycemia has some of the most serious sequelae, but is easily diagnosed and treated in the emergency department.

Inborn errors of metabolism are caused by single gene defects.

Although older infants, children, and adolescents may develop abnormalities evident on physical examination due to the consequences of their inborn errors of metabolism, most of these children are not inherently dysmorphic.

Introduction and Background

Children with inborn errors of metabolism probably present to emergency departments more commonly than generally recognized. There are four main reasons the incidence of inborn errors of metabolism is likely underestimated in the emergency department. First, inborn errors of metabolism are caused by a single gene defect. As opposed to children with chromosomal disorders (e.g., Down syndrome), children with inborn errors of metabolism will have a normal phenotypic appearance and not manifest dysmorphism.[1,2] Second, common emergency department presentations for children with previously undiagnosed inborn errors of metabolism include extreme presentations such as profound shock, fatal coma, and cardiopulmonary arrest.[3] These children may not live long enough for a detailed differential diagnosis to be entertained. Emergency physicians are likely to mentally classify these children as having "sepsis" or "full arrest" and never identify or acknowledge the underlying metabolic derangement even if identified at autopsy. Third, some children will have very mild manifestations of their inborn errors of metabolism.[4] These children may become somewhat sicker than other children during common illnesses such as gastroenteritis, but harbor an undiagnosed inborn error of metabolism with relatively mild clinical features.[5] In one study, more than 25% of children diagnosed with an inborn error of metabolism had presented to an emergency department for an acute complaint prior to the diagnosis being made.[3] Some of these patients are identified in adulthood.[6] It is likely that a substantial proportion of the population, especially in the subpopulation of developmentally delayed individuals,[7] lives with undiagnosed inborn errors of metabolism. Fourth, even though there are currently more than 9000 recognized inborn errors of metabolism, more continue to be discovered.[4] This suggests not all inborn errors of metabolism have been identified. Particularly in cases with milder manifestations, children may harbor inborn errors of metabolism that cannot be diagnosed yet.

Recognition and Approach

Each state in the United States screens newborns for inborn errors of metabolism.[8] The first widely adopted screening test was developed in the early 1960s by Guthrie and Susi to identify phenylketonuria.[9] According to the Centers for Disease Control and Prevention, each year 4 million newborns are screened for metabolic disorders.[10] Severe disorders are detected in about 3000 (0.075%).[10] In a population-based study from Italy, a similar incidence (0.04%) was reported.[11] There are problems with newborn screening that impact emergency department care. First, the infant is usually discharged from the nursery prior to the results of the screening tests being known. Clinical symptoms may appear and the infant may present to the emergency department before positive results return. Second, few inborn errors of metabolism are included in the mandated screening programs. The list of metabolic disorders for which each state screens is not uniform, and the number of disorders for which testing is mandated is relatively small.[8] Although it is rare to find an older infant or toddler with undiagnosed phenylketonuria in the United States, the same cannot be said of many other inborn errors of metabolism. Third, as testing becomes more sophisticated, physicians' familiarity with these disorders increases, and therapeutic interventions for affected individuals improve, it is likely that the prevalence of adolescents and young adults with recently diagnosed inborn errors of metabolism will rise. In one study, 11% of patients with an inborn error of metabolism survived beyond their 18th birthday.[11] Fourth, as with all tests, the test characteristics are imperfect. False-negative tests occur.[4] For these reasons, the newborn screening tests provide an imperfect safety net for identifying inborn errors of metabolism.

Clinical Presentation

History

In many cases of exacerbations of inborn errors of metabolism, the history is frustratingly nonspecific (Table 29–1) (see Chapter 7, The Critically Ill Neonate). Reports of poor tone, lethargy, vomiting, or episodes of apnea are common to many serious disorders of infancy and early childhood. The rapidity and age of symptom onset are highly variable. The blocked metabolic pathways of inborn errors of metabolism may result in a rapid accumulation of devastating toxins, a slow accumulation of less injurious toxins, a cellular energy deficiency, or the inability to appropriately respond to changes in nutrition or nutritional status.[12] This heterogeneity results in signs and symptoms being identified in early infancy, later infancy, childhood, or adolescence; during intercurrent illnesses such as gastroenteritis; and at times when the schedule or composition of feedings change.[1] Because inborn errors of metabolism are genetic, the family history may be somewhat revealing. In particular, a history of unexplained deaths in the family and parental consanguinity are supportive of a diagnosis of an inborn error of metabolism. Of course, the family history would be expected to be unrevealing in cases arising from new genetic mutations.[13]

One relatively specific finding seen in some inborn errors of metabolism is a characteristic odor (Table 29–2). These odors are due to the accumulation of toxins. Characteristic odors have been described as arising from urine, stool, perspiration, cerumen, and saliva.[14] The parents may report the unusual odor, or the clinician may identify it upon examination of a fresh specimen at the bedside.[14] Another technique

for evaluating body fluids for characteristic odors is to place a small amount of the liquid specimen on filter paper, place this into a urine container, and allow the specimen to sit for several minutes at room temperature before an olfactory examination is undertaken.[15]

Physical Examination

Although older infants, children, and adolescents may develop abnormalities evident on physical examination due to the consequences of their inborn errors of metabolism, most of these children are not inherently dysmorphic. The physical examination is usually nonspecific. Failure to thrive as evidenced by poor weight gain may be apparent. Developmental delay may be recognized. In acute exacerbations, the child may present with clinically evident dehydration, lethargy, coma, weak muscle tone, hypothermia, or fever[2,13] (see Table 29–1). Other serious but relatively nonspecific physical findings include seizures, jaundice, hepatomegaly or hepatosplenomegaly, cataracts, and dysrhythmias.[16] Unfortunately, some children do not present until they are in cardiopulmonary arrest.[2,13]

Ancillary Studies

The most helpful studies in evaluating children specifically for inborn errors of metabolism are a blood glucose measurement and an ammonia level. These tests are likely to fall within the context of a more generalized evaluation. There are two main reasons for this. First, in cases of previously undiagnosed inborn errors of metabolism, there is a broad differential diagnosis for the presenting signs and symptoms of an acute exacerbation of an inborn error of metabolism (Table 29–3). In most of these cases, it would be imprudent to dismiss alternative diagnoses without ancillary studies being performed during the emergency department course. Second, intercurrent illnesses may exacerbate known inborn errors of metabolism or cause previously undiagnosed inborn errors of metabolism to become clinically evident. In both instances, the intercurrent illness will need to be identified and treated in addition to the inborn error of metabolism. The ancillary studies needed to evaluate these children typically encompass a wide range of laboratory studies, including cultures and radiologic studies (see Chapter 7, The Critically Ill Neonate; Chapter 8, Circulatory Emergencies: Shock; and Chapter 11, Altered Mental Status/Coma).

Of the acute metabolic derangements resulting from exacerbations of inborn errors of metabolism, both acidosis and

Table 29–1	Frequency of Emergency Department Signs and Symptoms in Children with Previously Undiagnosed Inborn Errors of Metabolism
55%	Abnormal muscle tone
51%	Lethargy or coma
41%	Seizures
34%	Vomiting
31%	Psychomotor delay
31%	Hepatic dysfunction
21%	Failure to thrive
15%	Apnea
11%	Cardiopulmonary arrest
6%	Fever
4%	Hypothermia

Adapted from Calvo M, Artuch R, Macia E, et al: Diagnostic approach to inborn errors of metabolism in an emergency unit. Pediatr Emerg Care 16:405–408, 2000.

Table 29–2	Odors Associated with Individual Inborn Errors of Metabolism
Inborn Error of Metabolism	**Characteristic Odor**
Phenylketonuria	Musty or mousy
Isovaleric academia	Sweaty feet
Oasthouse urine disease	Brewery odor
Maple syrup urine	Caramelized sugar
Tyrosinemia type I	Cabbage-like odor
Glutaric acidemia type II	Sweaty feet
Trimethylaminuria	Fishy odor

Adapted from Berry GT, Bennett MJ: A focused approach to diagnosing inborn errors of metabolism. Contemp Pediatr 15(11):79–102, 1998; and Rizzo WB, Roth KS: On "Being led by the nose": rapid detection of inborn errors of metabolism. Arch Pediatr Adolesc Med 148:869–872, 1994.

Table 29-3	Differential Diagnosis of Signs and Symptoms of Acute Exacerbations of Inborn Errors of Metabolism

Congenital heart disease
Congenital herpes
Encephalitis
Gastroenteritis with dehydration
Hyponatremia due to incorrect formula preparation
Idiopathic ketotic hypoglycemia
Incarcerated inguinal hernia
Increased intracranial pressure
Infant botulism
Malrotation with midgut volvulus
Meningitis
Methemoglobinemia
Nonaccidental trauma
Seizure
Sepsis
Shaken infant
Supraventricular tachycardia

hypoglycemia have some of the most serious sequelae. Fortunately, hypoglycemia is easily diagnosed and treated in the emergency department (see Chapter 106, Hypoglycemia). For young infants, there continues to be some debate regarding the numeric interventional threshold for hypoglycemia.[17,18] This debate is peripheral to the treatment of ill-appearing infants in the emergency department who may harbor an inborn error of metabolism. Many of these infants require the administration of a continuous infusion of dextrose, typically administered as dextrose 10% in water ($D_{10}W$), whether or not they are hypoglycemic. Acidosis is treated by reversing catabolism with IV fluids plus dextrose, liberal use of bicarbonate, as well as the addition of specific substances (e.g., vitamins and amino acids) based on the specific deficiency (see also Chapter 7, The Critically Ill Neonate).[11]

An elevated ammonia level may be the first and most helpful test in identifying infants with inborn errors of metabolism. Although not all inborn errors of metabolism will manifest an elevated ammonia level, many do. These include organic acidurias (e.g., methylmalonic acidemia, propionic acidemia, isovaleric acidemia) and urea cycle defects. Mild to moderate hyperammonemia may occur in acutely ill neonates, particularly premature neonates, without an underlying inborn error of metabolism.[19] However, an elevation of serum ammonia greater than 120 µmol/L (200 µg/dL) in an infant outside of the neonatal intensive care unit who is not manifesting liver failure is strongly suggestive of an inborn error of metabolism.[12,19] Ammonia collection requires immediate placement of the specimen on ice and rapid transport to the laboratory to avoid false-positive results.

A urinary test for reducing substances may be performed routinely in some clinical laboratories on specimens from infants and toddlers. The utility of these tests in the emergency department has not been explored. A urinary test for reducing substances will detect lactose, fructose, galactose, and pentose in addition to the more common glucose. In the absence of urinary glucose, a positive test is suggestive of an inborn error of metabolism affecting the metabolism of one of these other sugars. However, other signs and symptoms of liver failure typically lead to the diagnosis, rather than a positive test for reducing substances obtained in the emergency department.[16]

Important Clinical Features and Considerations

Idiopathic ketotic hypoglycemia and glutaric aciduria type I are two conditions associated with inborn errors of metabolism that might lead to substantial confusion.

Idiopathic Ketotic Hypoglycemia

The most common cause of hypoglycemia in toddlers and preschoolers between 1 and 5 years of age is idiopathic ketotic hypoglycemia.[20] This condition is not seen in school-age children or adolescents due to their greater muscle mass and larger glycogen stores. Toddlers and preschoolers presenting with idiopathic ketotic hypoglycemia usually present with lethargy or unresponsiveness following a period of fasting.[20] A reasonable scenario in which this occurs is a toddler who develops vomiting in the evening and presents the next morning hypoglycemic and unresponsive. These children are expected to have a history of normal growth, have no history of an acute ingestion, and have a prompt return to normal following administration of intravenous dextrose. Most of these children require no further workup for their hypoglycemic episode. Patients who have recurrent episodes, hepatomegaly, or growth retardation require further investigation.[20]

Glutaric Aciduria Type I

One inborn error of metabolism deserving special attention for emergency physicians is glutaric aciduria type I. This disorder may mimic nonaccidental trauma manifesting chronic subdural hemorrhages and retinal hemorrhages. Glutaric aciduria type I does not present with a metabolic or lactic acidosis, hyperammonemia, or hypoglycemia. There are obvious challenges in considering an inborn error of metabolism in this setting. The indications for testing for glutaric aciduria type I in the emergency department are unclear. Glutaric aciduria type I can be identified from a positive test for urine organic acids with confirmation by an enzyme assay.[21,22]

Management

The management of a child with an inborn error of metabolism follows the generalized approach appropriate for all seriously ill infants and children (see Chapter 7, The Critically Ill Neonate). Particularly in cases of undiagnosed inborn errors of metabolism, emergency physicians should expect to perform a "septic workup," evaluate serum electrolytes, administer empirical antibiotics, identify and treat hypoglycemia, support the blood pressure, manage the airway, and address other serious problems as they do with other patients. There are, however, some management features that are relatively specific for children with inborn errors of metabolism.

Since many inborn errors of metabolism involve the accumulation of toxic metabolites from a component of feedings, the child should be kept *nil per os* (NPO) during the emergency department course. In general, critically ill children receive intravenous dextrose with maintenance fluids and are too ill to feed. Therefore, withholding feeds is seldom an issue in the emergency department.

In many instances, intravenous dextrose by continuous infusion is indicated. Like other serious illnesses in infants and children, hypoglycemia needs to be identified and treated promptly. For infants, this is typically accomplished by administering a $D_{10}W$ bolus of 5 to 10 ml/kg. For children, this is typically accomplished by administering a $D_{25}W$ bolus of 2 to 4 ml/kg. In contrast to other serious illnesses, infants and children with inborn errors of metabolism may need a continuous infusion of dextrose both to avoid recurrent hypoglycemia and reverse a catabolic state. This is usually accomplished by adding 10% dextrose to the maintenance fluids.

The treatment of hyperammonemia is often guided by a conversation with a pediatric metabolic specialist. Treatment options include the administration of sodium benzoate, sodium phenylbutyrate, and hemodialysis.[23,24]

Seizures in infants are distinct from febrile seizures and idiopathic seizures seen in older children (see Chapter 40, Seizures). In one study based in an emergency department, 42% of infants younger than 6 months of age presenting with a seizure had an underlying syndrome, malformation, or inborn error of metabolism.[25] Some children with acute exacerbations of inborn errors of metabolism will present to the emergency department with refractory seizures. These children characteristically have a normal blood glucose and serum sodium. In addition to standard treatment (e.g., the administration of an intravenous benzodiazepine), the administration of intravenous pyridoxine and folinic acid may be needed to stop the seizures in children whose inborn error of metabolism involve pyridoxine or folinic acid.[23]

The greatest resources in treating children with known inborn errors of metabolism are the parents and the child's metabolic specialist. In general, parents are much more sensitive to the early "glazed" encephalopathic appearance in their children than physicians unfamiliar with the child.[26] Parents may carry specific instructions and information about their child with them to the emergency department. This information can be extremely helpful in guiding the child's management. A phone consultation with the child's metabolic specialist can also provide important guidance with respect to complications to anticipate and specific treatment. The child's metabolic specialist may also play a key role in getting the child transferred to a tertiary care pediatric facility.

In the unfortunate circumstances in which a resuscitation is coming to a fatal conclusion, sending some specimens to the laboratory prior to conclusion of the resuscitation may help the family. This may be the only opportunity to obtain useful evidence to answer questions and to counsel the family regarding future family planning.[13,15] Several milliliters of urine should be collected and frozen, a tube of plasma separated from whole blood and frozen, and a snip of skin stored at room temperature.[27]

Summary

Inborn errors of metabolism are "individually rare and collectively numerous."[16] The prevalence of children, adolescents, and young adults with recognized inborn errors of metabolism is rising, and those with known and previously undiagnosed inborn errors of metabolism will present to the emergency department with increasing frequency. The addition of a serum ammonia level to the laboratory evaluation of these patients will identify many children with inborn errors of metabolism. For children with a known inborn error of metabolism, the parents and the child's metabolic specialist are extremely valuable resources for guiding management decisions.

REFERENCES

1. Roth KS: Inborn errors of metabolism: the essentials of clinical diagnosis. Clin Pediatr 30:183–190, 1991.
2. Allanson JE: Pitfalls of genetic diagnosis in the adolescent: the changing face. Adolesc Med 13:257–268, 2002.
*3. Calvo M, Artuch R, Macia E, et al: Diagnostic approach to inborn errors of metabolism in an emergency unit. Pediatr Emerg Care 16:405–408, 2000.
4. Berry GT, Bennett MJ: A focused approach to diagnosing inborn errors of metabolism. Contemp Pediatr 15(11):79–102, 1998.
5. Pien K, van Vlem B, van Coster R, et al: An inherited metabolic disorder presenting as ethylene glycol intoxication in a young adult. Am J Forensic Med Pathol 23:96–100, 2002.
6. Gaspani R, Arcangeli A, Mensi S, et al: Late-onset presentation of ornithine transcarbamylase deficiency in a young woman with hyperammonemic coma. Ann Emerg Med 41:104–109, 2003.
7. Kahler SG, Fahey MC: Metabolic disorders and mental retardation. Am J Med Genet Part C Semin Med Genet 117:31–41, 2003.
8. About Newborn Screening: Current newborn screening by state. October, 2006. Available at *http://www.AboutNewbornScreening.com/ stats.htm*
9. Guthrie R, Susi A: A simple phenylalanine method for detecting phenylketonuria in large populations of newborn infants. Pediatrics 32:338–343, 1963.
10. Division of Laboratory Sciences, National Center for Environmental Health: Quality assurance and proficiency testing for newborn screening. Centers for Disease Control and Prevention, October 2006. Available at *http://www.cdc.gov/nceh/dls/newborn_screening.htm*
11. Dionisi-Vici C, Rizzo C, Burlina AB, et al: Inborn errors of metabolism in the Italian pediatric population: a national retrospective survey. J Pediatr 140:321–327, 2002.
12. Goodman SI, Greene CL: Metabolic disorders of the newborn. Pediatr Rev 15:359–365, 1994.
13. Greene CL, Goodman SI: Catastrophic metabolic encephalopathies in the newborn period. Clin Perinatol 24:773–786, 1997.
14. Rizzo WB, Roth KS: On "Being led by the nose": rapid detection of inborn errors of metabolism. Arch Pediatr Adolesc Med 148:869–872, 1994.
15. Saudubray JM, Ogier H: Clinical approach to inherited metabolic diseases in the neonatal period: a 20-year survey. J Inherit Med Dis 12(Suppl 1):1–17, 1989.
16. Saudubray JM, Nassogne MC, de Lonlay P, et al: Clinical approach to inherited metabolic disorders in neonates: an overview. Semin Neonatol 7:3–15, 2002.
17. Cornblath M, Hawdon JM, Williams AF, et al: Controversies regarding definition of neonatal hypoglycemia: suggested operational thresholds. Pediatrics 105:1141–1145, 2000.
18. Alkalay AL, Sarnat HB, Flores-Sarnat L, et al: Population meta-analysis of low plasma glucose thresholds in full-term normal newborns. Am J Perinatol 23:115–119, 2006.
19. Chow SL, Gandhi V, Krywawych S, et al: The significance of a high plasma ammonia value. Arch Dis Child 89:585–586, 2004.
20. Pershad J, Monroe K, Atchison J: Childhood hypoglycemia in an urban emergency department: epidemiology and a diagnostic approach to the problem. Pediatr Emerg Care 14:268–271, 1998.
21. Hartley LM, Khwaja OS, Verity CM: Glutaric aciduria type 1 and nonaccidental head injury. Pediatrics 107:174–176, 2001.
22. Kyllerman M, Skjeldal OH, Lundberg M, et al: Dystonia and dykinesia in glutaric aciduria type I: clinical heterogeneity and therapeutic considerations. Mov Disord 9:22–30, 1994.
23. Prietsch V, Lindner M, Zschocke J, et al: Emergency management of inherited metabolic diseases. J Inherit Metab Dis 25:531–546, 2002.
*24. Ogier de Baulny H: Management and emergency treatments of neonates with a suspicion of inborn errors of metabolism. Semin Neonatol 7:17–26, 2002.
25. Bui T, Delgado CA, Simon HK: Infantile seizures are not so infantile: first-time seizures in children under six months of age presenting to the emergency department. Am J Emerg Med 20:518–520, 2002.
*26. Dixon MA, Leonard JV: Intercurrent illness in inborn errors of intermediary metabolism. Arch Dis Child 67:1387–1391, 2002.
*27. Burton BK: Inborn errors of metabolism in infancy: a guide to diagnosis. Pediatrics 102:e69, 1998.

*Selected readings.

Chapter 30

Congenital Heart Disease

Alson S. Inaba, MD

Key Points

Infants with undiagnosed congenital heart disease generally present to the emergency department with congestive heart failure (left-to-right shunts), unresponsive cyanosis (right-to-left shunts), or profound shock (congenital obstructive left heart lesions). Discriminating between these major categories will aid in the initial evaluation and management.

Always consider the possibility of an undiagnosed congenital heart defect in the differential diagnosis of an infant who presents in severe cardiopulmonary distress.

The hyperoxia test may serve as a useful bedside diagnostic tool to differentiate between cardiac and pulmonary etiologies for central cyanosis in infants. When obtaining blood for the hyperoxia test, use the right upper extremity to avoid falsely depressed values cause by a right-to-left ductal shunt.

Suspect ductal-dependent cardiac lesions in infants who present with sudden onset of cyanosis or cardiovascular collapse within the first 3 weeks of life. Prostaglandin E_1 infusion may be life saving in these infants.

Introduction and Background

The incidence of congenital heart disease in the United States is approximately 8 to 10 cases per 1000 live births.[1-3] Currently about 1 million people in the United States have some form of congenital heart defect (CHD), and each year another 32,000 to 35,000 infants are born with some form of CHD. Heart disorders are the most common birth defect and are the leading cause of birth defect–related deaths during the first year of life. One third of all patients born with a CHD become critically ill during the first year of life, often within the first month of life.[4]

Despite newborn and prenatal screening, infants with undiagnosed CHDs can present to the emergency department (ED) with cardiopulmonary distress secondary to acute decompensation. Physicians must be able to manage a wide array of problems in these infants, including congestive heart failure (CHF), cyanosis, cardiovascular collapse, and multiple infections.

Recognition and Approach

Fetal Circulation and Circulatory Changes that Occur after Birth

The three major anatomic features of the fetal circulation are the presence of the ductus venosus, the ductus arteriosus, and a patent foramen ovale (Fig. 30–1). During fetal development, oxygenation of the fetal circulation bypasses the fetal lungs and is accomplished via the placenta. Blood that is oxygenated by the placenta is carried to the fetus via the umbilical vein, bypasses the fetal liver via the ductus venosus, and is delivered to the fetal heart via the inferior vena cava. Oxygenated blood entering the right atrium is preferentially shunted to the left atrium through the foramen ovale and then into aorta via the left ventricle (LV). This oxygenated blood is preferentially directed to the fetal coronary and cerebral circulations. In contrast, deoxygenated blood that returns to the fetal right atrium via the superior vena cava (SVC) is preferentially directed through the tricuspid valve and into the right ventricle (RV). This blood is ejected out of the RV via the pulmonary artery and bypasses the fetal lungs because of the higher vascular resistance in the fetal pulmonary circuit. This deoxygenated blood that bypasses the fetal lungs is shunted into the descending aorta via the ductus arteriosus. Therefore, the blood in the fetal descending aorta contains a mixture of both placentally oxygenated blood and deoxygenated blood from the fetal SVC.

After delivery, expansion and aeration of the infant's lungs causes a decrease in the pulmonary vascular resistance (PVR) with a concomitant increase in pulmonary blood flow. This increased oxygenation causes a physiologic closure of the umbilical arteries, umbilical vein, ductus venosus, and ductus arteriosus. An increase in blood flow to the infant's left atrium also promotes the closure of the foramen ovale. Although the ductus arteriosus functionally closes at about 10 to 15 hours of life, complete anatomic closure does not occur until about 2 to 3 weeks of life. Up until that time,

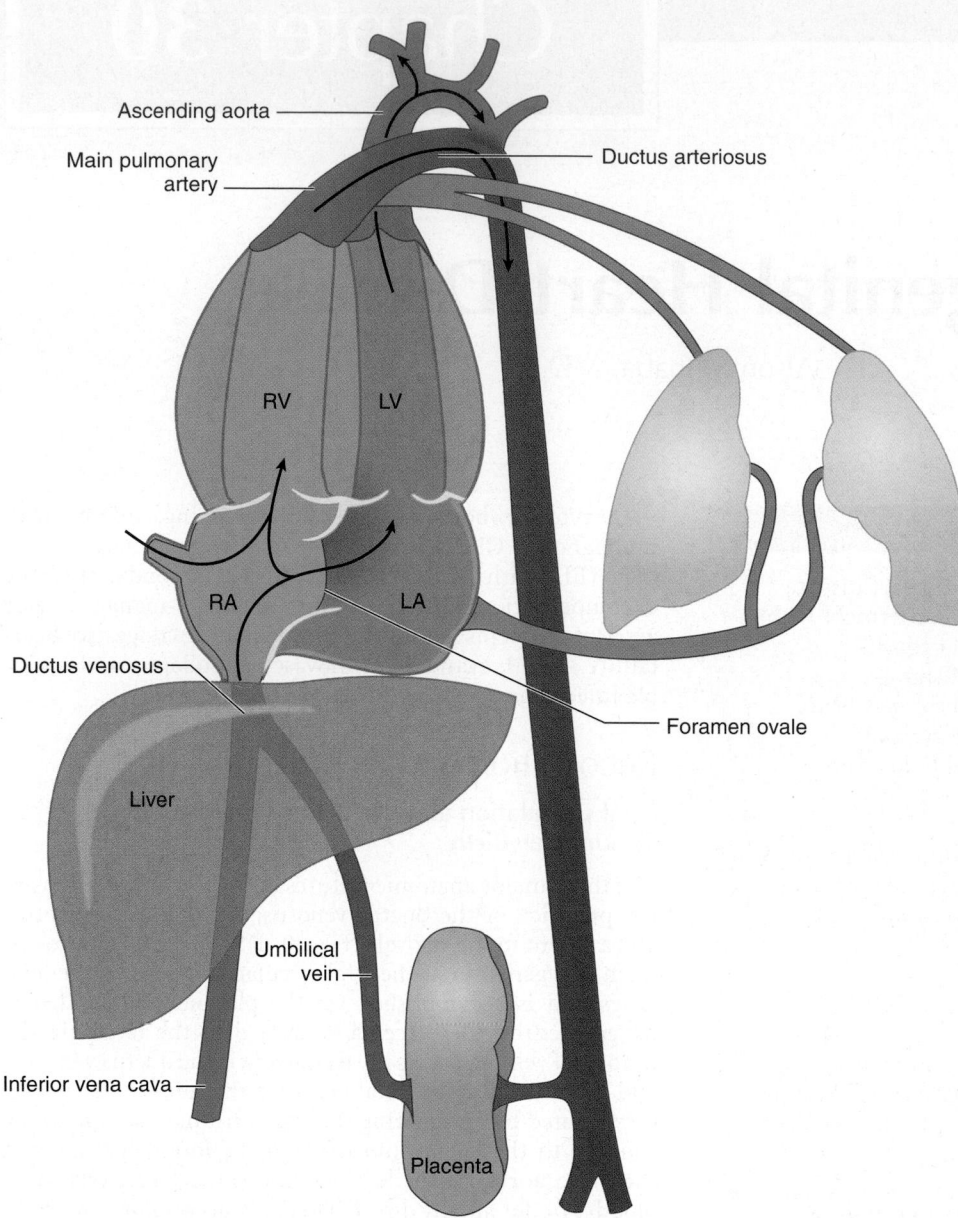

Ascending aorta

Main pulmonary artery

Ductus arteriosus

RV   LV

RA   LA

Ductus venosus

Foramen ovale

Liver

Umbilical vein

Inferior vena cava

Placenta

FIGURE 30–1. The fetal circulation, with *arrows* indicating the directions of flow. A fraction of umbilical venous blood enters the ductus venosus and bypasses the liver. This relatively highly oxygenated blood flows across the foramen ovale to the left side of the heart, preferentially perfusing the coronary arteries, head, and upper trunk. The output of the right ventricle flows preferentially across the ductus arteriosus and circulates to the placenta, as well as to the abdominal viscera and lower trunk. (From Zipes: Braunwald's Heart Disease: A Textbook of Cardiovascular Medicine, 7th ed. Philadelphia: WB Saunders, 2005, p 1493. Copyright © 2005 Saunders, An Imprint of Elsevier.)

prostaglandin E_1 (PGE$_1$) has the potential to reopen the ductus arteriosus and improve cardiopulmonary hemodynamics in critically ill infants with certain CHDs.

In the absence of any CHD, transitional circulatory changes pose no physiologic problems to the infant. However, complete anatomic closure of the ductus arteriosus may pose acute life-threatening complications in infants with CHDs who are dependent upon the patency of the ductus arteriosus for survival. Infants with ductal-dependent CHDs typically present to the ED with acute circulatory collapse or acute cyanosis within the first 3 weeks of life.

Physiology of Major Congenital Cardiac Disorders

A few major underlying mechanisms are responsible for most congenital cardiac defects. These include left-to-right shunt lesions, right-to-left shunts, and lesions that obstruction the outflow from the right or left ventricle.

Left-to-Right Shunts

Left-to-right shunt lesions occur when there is an abnormal connection between the right and left side of the heart (atrial septal defect [ASD], ventricular septal defect [VSD], patent ductus arteriosis [PDA], and more complex endocardial cushion defects involving the atrial and ventricular septa). Since left heart pressures are generally higher than right-sided pressures, blood preferentially flows to the lower pressure right side of the heart across defects (i.e., ASD, VSD, PDA). The combination of normal venous return to the right side of the heart via the vena cava in addition to the excess flow from the left side of the heart tends to overload the lungs with excess blood (Figs. 30–2 and 30–3).

Eventually, excess flow leads to CHF. As the right atrium, RV, and pulmonary artery receive excess flow, they may dilate with time resulting in electrocardiographic (ECG) and radiographic changes of right atrial, right ventricular, and pulmonary artery enlargement (see Figs. 30–2 and 30–3). With an

Atrial Septal Defect

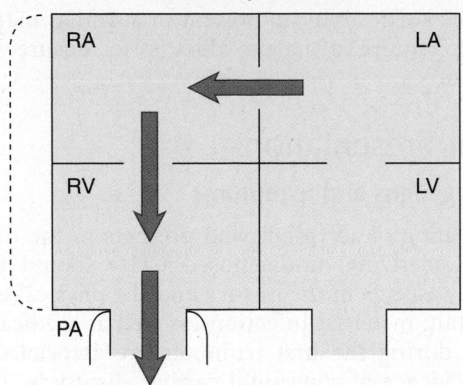

FIGURE 30–2. Atrial septal defect (ASD). Flow from higher to lower pressure chamber (left to right atrium) across an ASD can lead to dilation of right heart chambers and excess flow to lungs over a prolonged time, with occasional congestive heart failure in adults or teenagers. Abbreviations: LA, left atrium; LV, left ventricle; PA, pulmonary artery; RA, right atrium; RV, right ventricle. *Red arrow* signifies oxygenated blood; *blue arrow,* deoxygenated blood; *pink arrow,* partially oxygenated blood.

Moderate to Large Ventricular Septal Defect

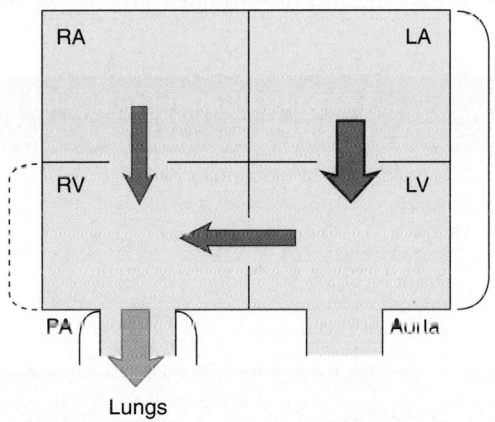

FIGURE 30–3. Ventricular septal defect (VSD). If large enough, blood flow across a VSD will cause chamber enlargement (*dotted arrows*) and provide excess flow to the lungs, with resulting congestive heart failure. Abbreviations: LA, left atrium; LV, left ventricle; PA, pulmonary artery; RA, right atrium; RV, right ventricle. *Red arrow* signifies oxygenated blood; *blue arrow,* deoxygenated blood; *pink arrow,* partially oxygenated blood.

ASD, the gradient between chambers is small and the excess flow provided to the lungs is minimal, and symptoms may take decades to occur. With VSDs, excess blood flow to the lungs depends upon the PVR and the size of the defect. Chambers that receive excess flow dilate, with resulting ECG and chest radiograph (CXR) changes. After delivery, PVR is normally elevated, and it may take weeks for the excess blood flow from left to right to overload the lungs and cause symptoms.

Hemodynamic consequences of a PDA mimic those of a VSD, with enlarged ventricles and pulmonary artery on ECG and radiography and delayed presentations due to the normal drop in PVR in the first few weeks to months following birth.

Right-to-Left Shunts

Right-to-left shunt lesions result in deoxygenated blood bypassing the lungs and being sent directly to the systemic

Tetralogy of Fallot

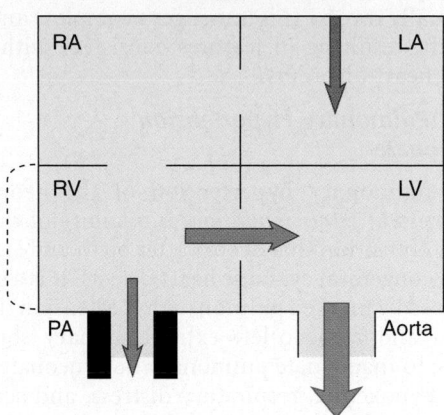

FIGURE 30–4. Tetralogy of Fallot. Pulmonary stenosis limits flow to the lungs via the pulmonary arteries, increasing right ventricular pressures and shunting deoxygenated blood (*blue arrow*) through the ventricular septal defect to the left ventricle (LV) and into the systemic circulation. In tetralogy, an overriding aorta is also present (not depicted in figure). Abbreviations: LA, left atrium; PA, pulmonary artery; RA, right atrium; RV, right ventricle. *Red arrow* signifies oxygenated blood; *blue arrow,* deoxygenated blood; *pink arrow,* partially oxygenated blood.

circulation. Pulmonary flow can be diminished (e.g., tetralogy of Fallot) or increased (e.g., D-transposition of the great arteries). Tetralogy of Fallot consists of a VSD and pulmonary stenosis with associated right ventricular hypertrophy and an overriding aorta. In this disorder, there is obstruction of flow to the lungs (pulmonary stenosis). Desaturated blood bypasses the lungs, traverses the VSD to the left side of the heart, and is sent into the systemic circulation (Fig. 30–4).

In D-transposition of the great arteries, the aorta and pulmonary arteries no longer connected to the left and right ventricles. Instead, the aorta arises from the RV and the pulmonary artery arises from the LV. The only way that blood can intermix with saturated blood reaching the systemic circulation is via an ASD or VSD. Because excess blood is supplied to the right side of the heart and pulmonary artery, right atrial enlargement, right ventricular hypertrophy, pulmonary artery dilation, and CHF occur.

Right Ventricular Outflow Obstruction

Right ventricular outflow obstruction can cause profound hypoxia. Disorders often involve a defect in the pulmonary valve, the infundibulum (the area below the pulmonic valve), or the peripheral pulmonary artery. In isolated pulmonary valve stenosis with an intact ventricular septum, valve cusps are deformed resulting in incomplete opening during systole. The obstruction to outflow from the RV to the pulmonary artery results in increased systolic pressures and right ventricular hypertrophy. Right-to-left shunting may occur through the patent foramen ovale in neonates with critical pulmonic stenosis. If this occurs, cyanosis is often present. Signs of right-sided CHF (e.g., hepatic enlargement) may occur. If an ASD or VSD is present, either right-to-left or left-to-right shunting may occur depending upon the degree of pulmonary stenosis and the subsequent increase in right ventricular pressures. High-grade stenosis will increase right ventricular pressures and cause a right-to-left shunt with cyanosis. Minimal stenosis with an ASD or VSD will lead to left-to-right shunt symptoms (i.e., CHF). However, with time, pulmonary stenosis will worsen and the shunt may eventually reverse (Eisenmenger's complex) and become right to left, resulting in features consistent with cyanotic congenital heart disorders.

Persistent Pulmonary Hypertension of the Neonate

Persistent pulmonary hypertension of the neonate, also termed *persistent fetal circulation,* is a failure of the normal circulatory transition that occurs after birth and can be confused with congenital cyanotic heart defects. It is a syndrome characterized by marked pulmonary hypertension that causes hypoxemia and right-to-left extrapulmonary shunting of blood. Due to inadequate pulmonary flow, neonates develop refractory hypoxemia, respiratory distress, and acidosis. By definition, these infants have no evidence of a cardiac lesion. The most common causes include perinatal asphyxia and hypoventilation, although some cases are due to congenital disorders (e.g., hypoplasia of pulmonary vessels) while others are idiopathic. These neonates present with hypoxia and may develop right-to-left shunts with clinical features consistent with a cyanotic CHD. Management consists of assisting ventilation, providing oxygen, correcting acidosis, and administering inhaled nitric oxide (which relaxes the vascular smooth muscle in pulmonary vessels).

Left Ventricular Outflow Obstruction

Left ventricular outflow obstruction occurs due to defects in the left ventricle or aorta. These defects can cause profound shock and acidosis. In hypoplastic left heart syndrome, the left ventricle is malformed and unable to supply a pressure head to the systemic circulation. A patent ductus is required to supply right ventricular blood flow to restore systemic circulation. In addition, an ASD can help shunt oxygenated blood to the right heart as it, in turn, supplies blood to the systemic circulation (Fig. 30–5). Closure of the ductus can result in abrupt worsening of circulation, profound shock,

and acidosis. Infants with coarctation of the aorta and an interrupted aortic arch can present in a similar manner and also may require a patent ductus to ensure systemic circulation.

Clinical Presentations

Presenting Signs and Symptoms

The evaluation of an infant who presents to the ED with a possible underlying, undiagnosed CHD should focus on several key aspects in the history and the physical examination. Certain maternal infections as well as medication and drug use during the first trimester are associated with a higher incidence of congenital cardiac disorders. The presence of certain maternal medical conditions have also been associated with a higher incidence of cardiac disorders. For example, congenital heart blocks have been associated with maternal systemic lupus erythematosus and other collagen vascular disorders. Infants of diabetic mothers have a higher incidence of cardiomyopathy.

Infants with complex and severe underlying CHDs generally present to the ED in one of three manners: (1) with CHF that is responsive to oxygen, (2) with cyanosis that is unresponsive to oxygen with or without CHF, or (3) with pro-

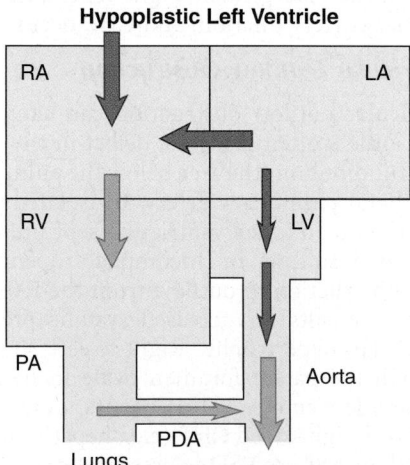

Hypoplastic Left Ventricle

FIGURE 30–5. Example of hypoplastic left heart syndrome. Oxygenated blood (*red arrow*) returning from the lungs to the left atrium (LA) or left ventricle (LV) mixes with deoxygenated blood (*blue arrow*) returning from the systemic circulation (right atrium [RA] and right ventricle [RV]). The right ventricle supplies a pressure head and partially oxygenated blood (*pink arrow*) to reach the systemic circulation via a patent ductus arteriosus (PDA). Abbreviation: PA, pulmonary artery.

Table 30–1	Categorization of Congenital Heart Disease*

CYANOSIS and Diminished Pulmonary Flow

Tetralogy of Fallot
Tricuspid atresia
Ebstein's anomaly of the tricuspid valve
Pulmonary atresia (with VSD or PDA)
Severe pulmonary stenosis
Hypoplastic right heart syndrome
Double-outlet right ventricle with pulmonary stenosis
Eisenmenger's complex (large VSD with eventual development of pulmonary hypertension and reversal of flow; due to pulmonary obstruction, blood flows from right to left through VSD)
D-Transposition of the great arteries with pulmonary stenosis

CYANOSIS and Increased Pulmonary Flow (CHF) Unresponsive to Oxygen

Transposition of the great arteries
Total anomalous pulmonary venous return
Persistent truncus arteriosus
Double-outlet right ventricle (without pulmonary stenosis)
Single ventricle
Hypoplastic left heart syndrome

SHOCK

Hypoplastic right heart syndrome
Coarctation of the aorta
Interrupted aortic arch
Critical aortic stenosis

CHF (May Be Cyanotic but Are Responsive to Oxygen)

Ventricular septal defects
Atrial septal defect
Patent ductus arteriosus
Endocardial cushion defects
Coarctation of the aorta
Critical aortic stenosis

*Many disorders can present in varied fashion depending upon the specific associated defect and exact anatomic abnormality. Abbreviations: CHF, congestive heart failure; PDA, patent ductus arteriosus; VSD, ventricular septal defect.

Table 30–2		Most Common Congenital Cardiac Defects Diagnosed at Different Neonatal Ages			
0–6 Days		**7–13 Days**		**14–28 Days**	
D-Transposition of great arteries	19%	Coarctation of aorta	16%	VSD	16%
Hypoplastic LH	14%	VSD	14%	Coarctation of aorta	12%
Tetralogy of Fallot	8%	Hypoplastic LH	8%	Tetralogy of Fallot	7%
Coarctation of aorta	7%	D-Transposition of great arteries	7%	D-Transposition of great arteries	7%
VSD	3%	Tetralogy of Fallot	7%	Patent ductus	5%
Other defects	49%	Other defects	48%	Other defects	53%

Abbreviations: LH, left heart; VSD, ventricular septal defect.
From Marino BS, Bird GL, Wernovsky G: Diagnosis and management of the newborn with suspected congenital heart disease. Clin Perinatol 28:91–136, 2001.

found shock (Table 30–1). The age and time of presentation in addition to the severity of presenting symptoms in an infant with an underlying CHD will vary depending upon the specific defect, the complexity and severity of the defect, and the timing of normal physiologic changes that occur as the fetal circulation transitions to that of the neonate (Table 30–2).[5] In one study, 63% of infants with undiagnosed CHDs who presented to the ED had pulmonary edema.[6] In general, the more severe defects with compromised pulmonary or systemic blood flow tend to present earlier during infancy, while less severe defects may not become clinically apparent until early childhood.

Congestive Heart Failure Responsive to Oxygen

Infants with CHD lesions with large left-to-right shunts (e.g., VSD) may initially go undetected in the first few weeks of life due to the relatively high PVR that persists immediately after birth. However, PVR diminishes rapidly in the first few months of life. This results in increased left-to-right shunting, resulting in excessive pulmonary blood flow. These infants present with progressive respiratory distress, wheezing, diaphoresis with feedings, poor weight gain, and failure to thrive.[7] Due to the nonspecificity of their symptoms, they easily can be misdiagnosed as having viral respiratory infections or acute bronchospasm. Clinical features of CHF in infants bear no resemblance to those of their adult counterparts. On examination, diaphoresis, wheezing, and a gallop rhythm may predominate. With time, the liver enlarges. In contrast, infants rarely manifest jugular venous distention, basilar rales, or peripheral edema.

Cyanosis Unresponsive to Oxygen (with or without CHF)

The age of onset, associated symptoms, and location of an infant's cyanosis may provide valuable clues as to the etiology (i.e., cardiac, pulmonary, or hematologic etiologies). Central cyanosis involves tissues that receives blood from an internal carotid artery branch (tongue and mucus membranes), while peripheral cyanosis (acrocyanosis) involves tissues with an external carotid artery source (the lips, hands, and feet). Acrocyanosis is a common phenomenon in neonates secondary to cold stress and peripheral vasoconstriction. Central cyanosis always reflects a pathologic etiology and is therefore a more ominous sign compared to peripheral cyanosis. Infants with cyanosis secondary to CHDs may not exhibit as much respiratory distress as infants with cyanosis solely due to a pulmonary etiology. Thus, in a child who appears "comfortably blue," a cardiac etiology as the cause for central cyanosis may be more likely than a purely pulmonary etiology. Another important clinical clue as to the etiology of central cyanosis is that the cardiac etiologies of cyanosis usually worsen with crying, while cyanosis due to pulmonary etiologies may improve when the infant cries.[5]

The response to administration of 100% oxygen for 10 minutes (also known as the hyperoxia test) can help differentiate between cardiac and pulmonary etiologies of central cyanosis. If the patient's oxygen saturation increases by more than 10% or the arterial partial pressure of oxygen (Pao_2) rises by more than 20% to 30%, then the most likely etiology is pulmonary.[5] The measured Pao_2 in patients with a pulmonary etiology for cyanosis should rise well above 100 mm Hg unless the degree of pulmonary disease that is present is severe. A Pao_2 that remains less than 50 mm Hg despite 100% oxygen is suggestive of a CHD with decreased pulmonary blood flow or right-to-left shunting. Infants with CHDs with an increased pulmonary blood flow due to left-to-right shunt lesions may exhibit a rise in their Pao_2 (up to 150 mm Hg) in response to 100% oxygen.[5] Importantly, when obtaining blood for the hyperoxia test, the right upper extremity should be used. This will avoid misinterpretation due to falsely depressed values caused by a right-to-left ductal shunt.

Profound Shock or Congenital Obstructive Left Heart Syndromes

Infants with disorders that obstruct the left ventricular outflow tract or congenital obstructive left heart syndromes usually present early in life. These disorders consist of hypoplastic left heart syndrome, critical aortic stenosis, coarctation of the aorta, and an interrupted aortic arch. Infants with these anomalies generally present within a few days of birth with profound shock. In fact, they are often misdiagnosed as being in septic shock.[8] Prominent features overlap with sepsis and include respiratory distress, feeding difficulty, and irritability. Physical examination often reveals cyanosis (55%), diminished upper extremity (32%) and lower extremity (70%) pulses with a pulse differential, and a murmur (53%). Radiography shows cardiomegaly in up to 85% of cases, while ECG abnormalities are noted in 80% of cases.[8]

Diagnostic Tests: Chest Radiographs, Electrocardiograms, and Various Laboratory Studies

A CXR is an essential component in the evaluation of any infant with a suspected CHD. Three important radiographic features requiring assessment are (1) the cardiac size (cardiothoracic ratio), (2) the shape of the cardiac silhouette, and

(3) the degree of pulmonary vascular markings. The easiest method of determining the heart size in children is to determine the cardiothoracic ratio, which is obtained by relating the largest transverse diameter of the cardiac shadow on the posterior-anterior view of the CXR to the widest internal diameter of the chest. The normal cardiothoracic ratio in neonates is up to 65%; this ratio drops to 55% in older children.[9] However, the cardiothoracic ratio may not be accurate in the newly born and small infants, in whom a good inspiratory view is difficult to obtain. In addition, the presence of a large overlying thymic shadow may also make if difficult to accurately assess the cardiac size in infants. An enlarged heart shadow on a CXR more reliably reflects a problem with volume overload than a problem with pressure overload. Problems with pressure overload are better represented by electrocardiography.

The degree of pulmonary vascular markings is one of the key factors to consider when working through the differential diagnosis of CHDs. An increase in pulmonary vascularity is present when the pulmonary arteries appear enlarged and extend into the lateral third of the lung fields, or if there is an increased vascularity to the lung apices.[10] Another criterion that suggests an increased pulmonary vascularity is if the diameter of the right pulmonary artery in the right hilum on the posterior-anterior view of the chest is wider than the internal diameter of the trachea.[10] Categorization into cyanotic versus acyanotic disease and assessment of pulmonary blood flow can help differentiate among CHDs (Table 30–3). Three classic cardiac silhouettes that can be seen in CHDs are (1) the "boot-shaped" silhouette of tetralogy of Fallot (Fig. 30–6); (2) the "egg-on-a-string" silhouette of D-transposition of the great arteries (Fig. 30–7); and (3) the "snowman" or "figure-of-8" silhouette of total anomalous pulmonary venous return (TAPVR) (Fig. 30–8).

In a normal left-sided aortic arch, the aorta descends to the left of the midline and displaces the tracheal air shadow slightly toward the right of midline above the level of the carina. In contrast, the tracheal air shadow may be midline or deviated toward the left in the presence of a right-sided aortic arch.[5] This finding is important to note since a right-sided aortic arch may be present in up to 25% of the children with tetralogy of Fallot.[10] Rib notching secondary to increased collateral blood flow along the intercostal vessels may sometimes be appreciated between the fourth and eighth ribs in older children with undiagnosed coarctation of the aorta. However, this rib notching is rarely visualized in children who are less than 5 years old.[10]

An ECG is another useful diagnostic tool in the evaluation of an infant with a suspected underlying CHD. However,

Table 30–3	Chest Radiography in Congenital Heart Disease
Acyanotic Congenital Heart Disease	
Normal pulmonary flow	PS, MS or MR, AS, coarctation of the aorta
↑ Pulmonary flow	ASD, VSD, PDA, left-to-right shunts with pulmonary hypertension, atrioventricular canal
Cyanotic Congenital Heart Disease	
↓ Pulmonary flow	Severe PS, pulmonary atresia, tetralogy of Fallot (normal or boot-shaped heart), L-TGA with PS, tricuspid atresia, Ebstein's anomaly (massive heart), Eisenmenger's complex
↑ Pulmonary flow	TAPVR (snowman sign [late finding], supracardiac venous return via dilated right & left superior vena cava), hypoplastic left heart, TGA (egg-shaped heart tilted on its side with a narrow mediastinum: "egg-on-a-string") ± VSD, truncus arteriosus

Abbreviations: AS, aortic stenosis; ASD, atrial septal defect; MR, mitral regurgitation; MS, mitral stenosis; PDA, patent ductus arteriosus; PS, pulmonary stenosis; TAPVR, total anomalous pulmonary venous return; TGA, transposition of the great arteries; VSD, ventricular septal defect.

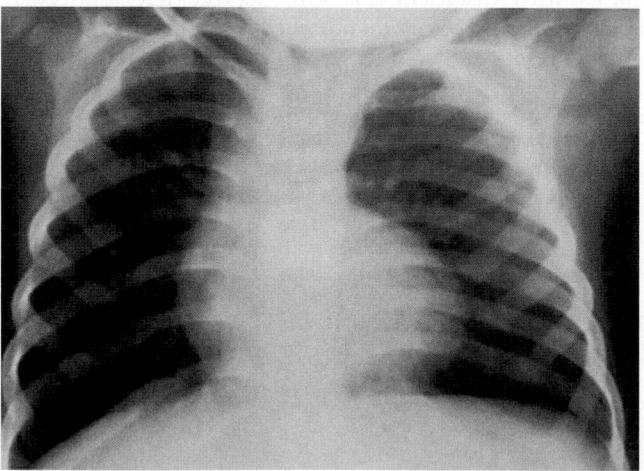

FIGURE 30–6. "Boot-shaped heart" of tetralogy of Fallot. The apex appears elevated due to right ventricular hypertrophy, the main pulmonary artery segment is missing, and there is diminished pulmonary blood flow. (From Park MK: Cyanotic congenital heart defects. In Park MK: Pediatric Cardiology for Practitioners, 4th ed. St. Louis: Mosby, 2002, p 191.)

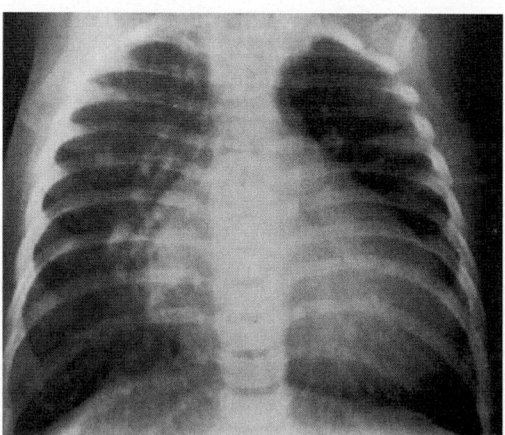

FIGURE 30–7. "Egg-on-a-string" appearance of D-transposition of the great arteries. The cardiac silhouette is enlarged (egg shaped) while the mediastinum is narrow (stringlike) due to overlapping aorta and pulmonary trunk. Note the prominent pulmonary vascular congestion characteristic of this disorder. (From Park MK: Cyanotic congenital heart defects. In Park MK: Pediatric Cardiology for Practitioners, 4th ed. St. Louis: Mosby, 2002, p 176.)

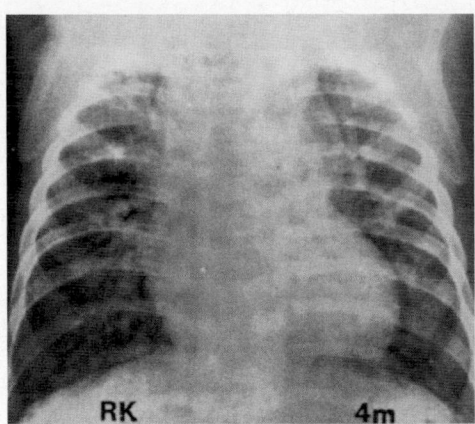

FIGURE 30–8. "Snowman sign" or "figure-of-8" sign in total anomalous pulmonary venous return. In the supracardiac type of this disorder, there are prominent venous structures returning blood to the right side of the heart, including right and left superior vena cava, and prominent left innominate vein. (From Park MK: Cyanotic congenital heart defects. In Park MK: Pediatric Cardiology for Practitioners, 4th ed. St. Louis: Mosby, 2002, p 204.)

Table 30–4	Ductal-Dependent Congenital Heart Defects (CHDs)

CHD that requires a patent ductus arteriosus to PRESERVE PULMONARY BLOOD FLOW (i.e., blood flow from the aorta to the main pulmonary artery):
- Tetralogy of Fallot
- Ebstein's anomaly
- Critical pulmonary stenosis
- Tricuspid atresia
- Pulmonary atresia
- Hypoplastic right heart syndrome
- D-Transposition of the great vessels
- Infracardiac (subdiaphragmatic) total anomalous pulmonary venous return (TAPVR)*

CHDs that require a patent ductus arteriosus to PRESERVE SYSTEMIC BLOOD FLOW (i.e., blood flow from the main pulmonary artery to the aorta):
- Severe coarctation of the aorta
- Critical aortic stenosis
- Hypoplastic left heart syndrome
- Interrupted aortic arch

*Opening the ductus arteriosus can worsen hypoxia in patients with supracardiac TAPVR.

ECG findings in infants and children can sometimes be problematic because various components of the ECG change according to the child's age. At birth, the muscle mass of the RV is greater than that of the LV. However, by the end of the first month of life the LV assumes dominance. By 6 months of age, the LV-to-RV mass ratio is 2 : 1, which then reaches the adult ratio of 2.5 : 1 by adolescence. The durations of the PR interval, QRS complex, and QT interval all increase with age (see Chapter 63, Dysrhythmias).

A hemoglobin and hematocrit level may reveal a compensatory physiologic elevation (i.e., polycythemia) in infants with underlying cyanotic CHDs. Any concurrent medical illness or blood loss that produces an acute anemia in infants with underlying cyanotic CHD can precipitate an acute deterioration by compromising their oxygen carrying capacity. A hematocrit level also is helpful in evaluating whether an infant's pallor is due to CHF-induced shock or anemia.

Limited studies have evaluated the utility and clinical accuracy of cardiac biochemical markers such as creatinine phosphokinase MB and cardiac troponin T in the pediatric population. Brain natriuretic peptide hormone (BNP) mediates arterial and venous vasodilation in response to ventricular wall tension and left ventricular filling pressures and is secreted by the ventricular myocytes. In children with CHF, BNP is elevated and correlates with the ejection fraction of the failing heart. Although studies are limited, measurement of BNP appears to be useful for diagnosing CHF in infants and children and for monitoring the effects of various treatments in children with CHF.[11,12] When interpreting BNP results, clinicians must be aware that, during the first week of life, the mean plasma concentration of BNP in healthy newborn infants is 232 pg/ml and decreases to 48 pg/ml by the end of the first week. By 2 weeks of age, normal BNP levels are less than 33 pg/ml.[13,14] In contrast, 85% of infants with a clinically significant VSD and nearly 100% with persistant pulmonary hypertension of the neonate will have a BNP greater than 40 pg/ml.[15,16] Moreover, premature infants with a PDA almost always have a BNP value greater than 100 pg/ml.[15,16] Importantly, normal BNP reference ranges may vary depending on infants' degree of prematurity, their sex, and the specific immunoassay used. Limited studies also show elevated troponin I in infants with hypoplastic left heart syndrome (mean 1.5 ng/ml) and VSD (mean 0.6 ng/ml) who required cardiac surgery.[17] However, use of this test in many other congenital defects and specific cutoffs for clinical decision making in the ED have not been defined.

Ideally, bedside echocardiography is required to define most congenital cardiac lesions. However, bedside echocardiography is not available in many EDs, and clinicians must rely upon the clinical examination, ECG, CXR, and limited beside tests (e.g., arterial blood gases) to initiate treatment in these patients.

Important Clinical Features and Considerations

Ductal-Dependant Congenital Heart Disease

Infants with CHDs who present within the first 3 weeks of life with a sudden onset of cyanosis or cardiovascular collapse may have ductal-dependent cardiac lesions that respond to prostaglandin E_1 (PGE$_1$) administration.[5,18] Closure of the ductus arteriosus in infants with certain defects causes life-threatening interruption of blood flow to the lungs, resulting in cyanosis (i.e., tricuspid atresia), or disrupted flow to the systemic circulation, producing shock (i.e., hypoplastic left heart syndrome)[5] (Table 30–4). Measurements of oxygen saturations or Pao$_2$ values from the right upper extremity compared to values from the lower extremity in an infant with a suspected ductal-dependent lesion may further aid in the diagnosis. If the oxygenation in the lower extremity is significantly lower than that in the right upper extremity, coarctation of the aorta or an interrupted aortic arch should be suspected. However, if oxygenation is higher in the lower extremities as compared to the infant's upper extremities, transposition of the great arteries should be suspected.[19]

Clinical Features of Hypercyanotic Spells in Tetralogy of Fallot

Tetralogy of Fallot accounts for approximately 10% of all CHDs and is the most common cause of cyanotic CHDs beyond infancy. Tetralogy of Fallot arises from a single embryologic defect in which the subpulmonic conus fails to expand, resulting in the four classic abnormalities: (1) right ventricular outflow tract obstruction; (2) a large, unrestrictive, malaligned VSD; (3) an overriding aorta that receives blood flow from both ventricles; and (4) right ventricular hypertrophy due to the high pressure load from the right ventricular outflow tract obstruction. These anatomic defects collectively result in decreased pulmonary blood flow and varying degrees of right-to-left shunting of deoxygenated blood across the VSD.

The degree of cyanosis and the age of presentation are directly dependent upon the degree of right ventricular outflow tract obstruction. Infants with tetralogy of Fallot typically have worsening of their cyanosis during crying and feeding. Older children with tetralogy of Fallot may have cyanotic exacerbations during periods of physical exertion. Infants who have milder forms of right ventricular outflow tract obstruction may be acyanotic, and are sometimes referred to as "pink tets." However, the majority of cases of tetralogy of Fallot will exhibit some degree of cyanosis. Infants with severe right ventricular outflow tract obstruction may exhibit profound cyanosis within the first few days of life and may even require a PGE_1 infusion to preserve pulmonary blood flow via left-to-right shunting from the aorta into the main pulmonary artery via a PDA.

A potentially life-threatening complication of tetralogy of Fallot is an acute hypoxic episode, also known as a "tet spell" or "hypercyanotic spell." These episodes occur most commonly in infants between 2 and 4 months of age and may occur in other cyanotic cardiac disorders.[20]

During a hypoxic spell, an event such as crying or defecation suddenly lowers the systemic vascular resistance (SVR), producing a large right-to-left shunt across the VSD and increased flow of deoxygenated blood into the systemic circulation. The decrease in the SVR with increased right-to-left shunting of deoxygenated blood across the VSD begins the cycle of a hypoxic spell. Acute hypovolemia and tachycardia can also precipitate these tet spells. The large right-to-left shunt through the VSD bypasses the lungs, which then causes a decrease in the Pao_2, an increase in the partial pressure of carbon dioxide (Pco_2), and a fall in the arterial pH. These metabolic changes then stimulate the respiratory centers in the brain to produce hyperpnea (deep and rapid respirations). This hyperpnea then increases the negative intrathoracic pressure during inspiration, which then causes an increase in the systemic venous blood return to the right side of the heart. This increased volume of blood in the RV is then shunted to the LV through the VSD due to the combination of the existing right ventricular outflow tract obstruction and the acute decrease in the SVR. This in turn further decreases the arterial oxygen saturation, which then further perpetuates the hypoxic spell (Fig. 30–9). Clinically these hypoxic spells are characterized by periods of hyperpnea (rapid and deep respirations), uncontrollable crying, and worsening cyanosis. The deep quality of the respirations in addition to the increase in the respiratory rate are what distinguishes

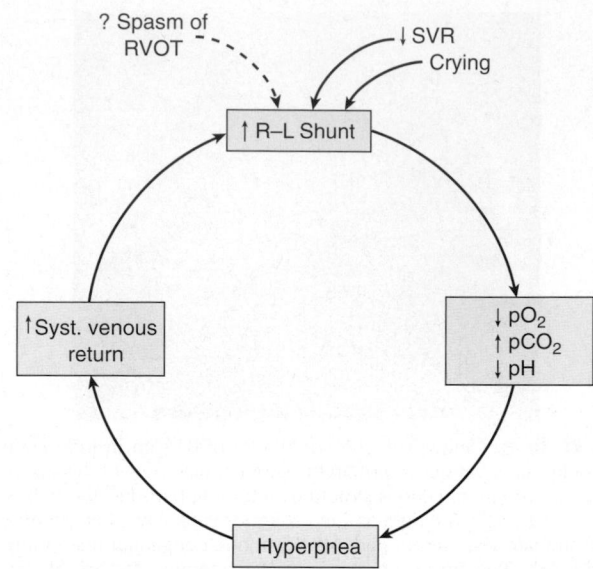

FIGURE 30–9. Mechanism of hypoxic spell. An event such as crying, defecation, or increased physical activity suddenly lowers the systemic vascular resistance (SVR), increasing the right-to-left ventricular shunt and worsening hypoxia. The decrease in the arterial partial pressure of oxygen (PO_2) stimulates the respiratory center, causing hyperventilation, which increases systemic venous return. Increased systemic venous return results in increased right-to-left (R-L) shunt, worsening cyanosis. (From Park MK: Pathophysiology of cyanotic congenital heart defects. In Park MK: Pediatric Cardiology for Practitioners, 4th ed. St. Louis: Mosby, 2002, p 122.)

the hyperpnea of a tet spell from the tachypnea due to other respiratory problems such as respiratory tract infections, which more commonly cause rapid but shallow respirations. Limpness, seizures, cerebrovascular accidents, and even death have been reported with more severe tet spells. During a tet spell, the intensity of the murmur decreases due to a decrease in blood flow through the right ventricular outflow tract obstruction and more blood being shunted from the RV to the LV through the VSD.

Respiratory Syncytial Virus Infections in Infants and Children with CHD

Infants with CHDs who develop respiratory syncytial virus (RSV) infections tend to have a higher rate of intensive care unit admissions and require mechanical ventilation more frequently than other infants with RSV infections.[21] Children with CHDs who require hospitalization for RSV have a fatality rate that is two to six times greater than children without CHDs.[22] In fact, the mortality rate from RSV is as high as 40% in infants with CHDs and 70% infants with CHDs plus pulmonary hypertension.

When evaluating infants with CHDs and respiratory symptoms, it is important to determine whether or not they have received prophylaxis (palizivumab) to decrease the probability of developing RSV infection and severity of disease.[23] Treatment of RSV bronchiolitis consists primarily of supportive measures such as providing supplemental oxygen, ensuring adequate hydration, use of bronchodilators (i.e., albuterol) in those children who seem to respond to such agents, and deep tracheal suction in more severe cases. Admission with continuous cardiopulmonary monitoring is required.

Management

Initial Stabilization and Management of Shock

The majority of the children who present to the ED with shock due to dehydration and hypovolemia are given intravenous (IV) fluids in 20-ml/kg boluses. However, this standard approach to hypovolemia cannot be routinely applied to infants with suspected CHDs who present with hypovolemic shock. Smaller (10-ml/kg) boluses should be considered in order to prevent fluid overload.[5] Frequent reassessment is crucial in determining whether the infant's shock is solely due to hypovolemia or is due to a cardiac defect.

PGE$_1$ (alprostadil) can be potentially life saving in infants with CHDs and ductal-dependent systemic blood flow (e.g., hypoplastic left heart, coarctation of the aorta, critical aortic stenosis, or an interrupted aortic arch) or ductal-dependent pulmonary flow (tetralogy of Fallot, Ebstein's anomaly, critical pulmonary stenosis, pulmonary valve atresia, tricuspid atresia, D-transposition of the great arteries) (see Table 30–4).[24] PGE$_1$ is a potent vasodilator that acts to maintain the patency of the ductus arteriosus. PGE$_1$ can also maintain patency of the ductus venosus, aiding infants with TAPVR who have abnormal infradiaphragmatic obstructions or connections to the inferior vena cava. However, worsening hypoxia following its administration may also indicate that TAPVR (supradiaphragmatic form) is present and that PGE$_1$ should be discontinued. Although it is ideal to have echocardiographic confirmation of CHDs prior to initiating a prostaglandin infusion, this potentially life-saving therapy should be started immediately in any critically ill neonate with a suspected ductal-dependent CHD who presents in acute shock or cyanosis (e.g., failed hyperoxia test).[6] The PGE$_1$ infusion is typically started at 0.05 to 0.1 mcg/kg/min. If there is no clinical response, the infusion rate may be increased to a maximum of 0.4 mcg/kg/min.[25]

The effects of the prostaglandin infusion are usually seen within 15 minutes.[19] Response to therapy is determined by assessing for improvements in systemic perfusion and pulmonary blood flow.[6] Since one of the adverse reactions to a PGE$_1$ infusion is apnea, it may be worthwhile to intubate these infants prior to the initiation. Intubation will provide a secured airway, and controlled ventilations will help to decrease the infant's work of breathing.[19] Other adverse reactions to a PGE$_1$ infusion include fever, seizures, bradycardia, hypotension, flushing, and decreased platelet aggregation.[26] Because sepsis should always be considered in the differential diagnosis of any critically ill infant, a full sepsis workup and appropriate empirical antibiotics should be considered in these infants if the diagnosis is uncertain.

Treatment of CHF

Although a wide array of disorders can cause CHF in pediatric patients, the primary etiology is an underlying CHD in infants, while myocarditis predominates in older children. The defects that are most likely to cause heart failure include left-to-right shunts (e.g., VSD, PDA, common atrioventricular canal, and truncus arteriosus), right-to-left shunts (e.g., D-transposition of the great arteries, TAPVR), and left heart obstructive lesions (e.g., hyoplastic left heart, severe aortic coarctation, critical aortic stenosis).[27] The specific treatment of CHF in any given case will depend upon whether there is

volume overload (left-to-right shunts), excess afterload (left heart obstructive lesions), rhythm abnormalities, or decreased contractility (e.g., cardiomyopathy). For example, inotropic agents and diuretics may be required in an infant with volume overload and decreased cardiac contractility, while vasodilating agents may be required in an infant with CHF due to increased afterload.

Acute stabilization of any infant who presents with CHF includes the administration of supplemental oxygen and administering agents to augment cardiac contractility and improve the cardiac output. Infants who present with severe respiratory distress may require intubation to support adequate oxygenation and ventilation. They also may benefit from elevation of the head and upper torso in addition to morphine sulfate (0.1 to 0.15 mg/kg per dose) administration.

Diuretics and other inotropic agents have been the mainstay of treatment for the majority of infants with CHF. Furosemide (Lasix) in a dose of 1 mg/kg per dose is the most common loop diuretic used to decrease preload. Although digoxin has remained as the most widely used inotropic agent to treat chronic CHF in infants and children, its acute use in decompensated CHF may be detrimental, increasing ischemia and worsening CHF.[28,29] *Inotropes* are used to increase cardiac output and are particularly useful in infants with a depressed cardiac output. Inotropic agents include dopamine (5 to 10 mcg/kg/min), dobutamine, and epinephrine (<0.3 mcg/kg/min or > 0.3 mcg/kg/min when combined with a vasodilator). Importantly, vasopressors do not affect the neonatal cardiac system in a manner similar to older children and adults. Only one third of a neonate's heart is composed of contractile tissue, compared to two thirds of an adult heart. For this reason, neonates cannot alter their cardiac output by increasing contractility well. Myocardial norepinephrine stores are also immature and become rapidly depleted, making dopamine less effective in neonates and infants. Changes in adrenergic receptor expression during critical illness and production of local vasodilators during shock also can make neonates appear unresponsive to dopamine. In neonates, dobutamine is less effective than dopamine in raising blood pressure.[30] *Vasodilators* (e.g., nitroprusside) are used to decrease the pressure head against which the heart must pump blood to the body. Nesiritide (synthetic BNP) is an arterial and venous vasodilator with modest diuretic and natriuretic properties that has been shown useful in treating CHF in infants in limited studies, although its use is not yet routine.[31] Amrinone and milrinone (phosphodiesterase inhibitors) have combined inotropic and vasodilating properties. Importantly, many other agents also have inotropic, vasodilator, or vasopressors effects at different doses (see Chapter 8, Circulatory Emergencies: Shock).

Management of Cyanotic Heart Disease

Most infants with cyanotic heart disease have either diminished pulmonary circulation, limiting the amount of oxygenated blood that reaches the systemic circulation, or increased pulmonary flow with a shunt that allows for deoxygenated blood to traverse from the right side of the heart to the left side of the heart and into the systemic circulation. PGE$_1$ can improve oxygenation in most of these patients. For infants with limited pulmonary circulation (e.g., pulmonary stenosis, tetralogy of Fallot), opening the ductus arteriosus directly increases pulmonary flow, and thus more oxygenated blood returns to the systemic circulation. For disorders in which pulmonary hypertension plays a significant role, inhaled nitric oxide can reduce the hypertension and improve pulmonary flow.[32] Low doses of magnesium sulfate (20 mg/kg/hr) may also diminish pulmonary hypertension by releasing endogenous nitric oxide and by directly reducing pulmonary and systemic vascular resistance.

For infants with increased pulmonary flow and CHF, opening the ductus allows oxygenated blood to traverse from the pulmonary arteries to the aorta (e.g., D-transposition of the great arteries). In TAPVR, PGE₁ can either improve or worsen cyanosis. With a subdiaphragmatic connection, PGE₁ can help dilate the ductus venosus and improve pulmonary venous flow. In supradiaphragmatic TAPVR, this agent dilates the ductus arteriosus, increasing right-to-left shunting and worsening cyanosis.

Any infant with a cyanotic CHD may develop a hypercyanotic spell from events that decrease SVR (e.g., crying, pain, defecation). This decrease in SVR increases right-to-left shunting, causing acidosis, worsened hypoxia, hypercarbia, and spasm of the right ventricular outflow tract. This further increases venous return to the right side of the heart, which leads to an increase in the right-to-left shunt. The overall treatment goals in the treatment of hypercyanotic spells are aimed at increasing the SVR, abolishing hyperpnea, and correcting the metabolic acidosis.[33] Although supplemental oxygen should be provided, oxygen alone will not reverse a hypercyanotic spell since there is a decrease in the amount of pulmonary blood flow and an increase in the amount of right-to-left shunting across the VSD. The infant should be picked up and placed in a knee-to-chest position.[34] Older children can be placed in the squatting position. Both of these maneuvers decrease the venous return to the heart and increase SVR, which in turn decreases the degree of right-to-left shunting through the VSD and increases the pulmonary blood flow. An IV fluid bolus in addition to vasoconstrictor administration (phenylephrine) will increase systemic blood pressure and SVR, which decreases shunting. Morphine (0.1 to 0.15 mg/kg) theoretically suppresses the respiratory center, and thereby abolishes the hyperpnea that is associated with a hypercyanotic episode. One potential adverse affect of morphine is that it may cause systemic vasodilation, further decreasing SVR. Although there are no current studies evaluating the use of other medications that may also suppress the respiratory centers, fentanyl and midazolam could be utilized for the same effect without the potential risk of endogenous histamine release seen with morphine. Ketamine (1 to 2 mg/kg IV or intramuscularly) has also been suggested for its sedative effect as well as for its effect on increasing the SVR.[20] Sodium bicarbonate may also be given to correct metabolic acidosis, reducing respiratory center stimulation. Most infants will respond to these measures and exhibit an improvement in their oxygenation and a decrease in their degree of cyanosis. Infants who do not improve may require a vasopressor such as phenylephrine (5 to 20 mcg/kg per dose by IV bolus) to increase the SVR and thereby decrease the degree of right-to-left shunting across the VSD.[35] Propranolol (0.02 mg/kg) has also been used as an adjunct to break the cycle in refractory hypercyanotic episodes.[33] Although the exact pharmacophyiologic mechanisms by which it accomplishes this is uncertain, propranolol is thought to increase the SVR and perhaps promote an increase in the pulmonary blood flow by reducing spasms of the right ventricular outflow tract obstruction.

Patients with repaired CHDs comprise a population of infants at risk for unique disorders and complications requiring specialized treatment (see Chapter 66, Postsurgical Cardiac Conditions and Transplantation).

Summary

Infants and children who present to the ED with undiagnosed or untreated congenital heart disease can pose a myriad of challenges. The possibility of an undiagnosed CHD must always be considered in the differential diagnosis of any infant who presents to the ED with recurrent or persistent respiratory infections, respiratory distress, cyanosis, or shock. Ongoing advances in the technology of bedside echocardiography may provide the ED physician with the opportunity to more accurately confirm CHDs within the ED.

While it may not be possible to identify the exact defect present in each patient, clinicians usually can categorize patients into major categories of disease (e.g., cyanotic lesions, acyanotic lesions, ventricular outflow tract obstruction). Based on these categories, management can be initiated. Importantly, ductal-dependent lesions must be suspected early so that administration of PGE₁ can begin promptly. Those infants with profound shock or a failed hyperoxia should be considered candidates for this agent.

Timely consultation with a pediatric cardiologist or a pediatric cardiovascular surgeon is also an essential component in the ongoing management of any infant or child with a suspected or known CHD.

REFERENCES

*1. Hoffman JI, Kaplan S, Liberthson RR: Prevalence of congenital heart disease. Am Heart J 147:425–439, 2004.

2. Hoffman JI, Kaplan S: The incidence of congenital heart disease. J Am Coll Cardiol 39:1890–1900, 2002.

*3. Wren C: Presentation of congenital heart disease in infancy: implications for routine examination. Arch Dis Child Fetal Neonatal Ed 80:49–53, 1999.

4. Collins-Nakai RL: When to consult a pediatric cardiologist: 2002. Indian J Pediatr 69:315–319, 2002.

5. Marino BS, Bird GL, Wernovsky G: Diagnosis and management of the newborn with suspected congenital heart disease. Clin Perinatol 28:91–136, 2001.

*6. Savitsky E, Alejos J, Votey S: Emergency department presentations of pediatric congenital heart disease. J Emerg Med 24:239–245, 2003.

7. Ackerman IL, Karn CA, Denne SC, et al: Total but not resting energy expenditure is increased in infants with ventricular septal defects. Pediatrics 102:1172–1177, 1998.

8. Pickert CB, Moss MM, Fiser DH: Differentiation of systemic infection and congenital obstructive left heart disease in the very young infant. Pediatr Emerg Care 14:263–267, 1998.

9. Dahlstrom A, Ringertz HG: Normal radiographic heart volume in the neonate: 3—comparison with the cardiothoracic ratio. Pediatr Radiol 15:25–28, 1985.

10. Park MK: Chest roentgenography. In Park MK: Pediatric Cardiology for Practitioners, 4th ed. St. Louis: Mosby, 2002, pp 52–59.

11. Westlind A, Wahlander H, Lindstedt G, et al: Clinical signs of heart failure are associated with increased levels of natriuretic peptide types B and A in children with congenital heart defects or cardiomyopathy. Acta Paediatr 93:340–345, 2004.

*Selected readings.

12. Mir TS, Marohn S, Laer, et al: Plasma concentrations of N-terminal pro-brain natriuretic peptide in control children from the neonatal to adolescent periods and children with congestive heart failure. Pediatrics 110:e76, 2002.

13. Rauh M, Koch A: Plasma N-terminal pro-b-type natriuretic peptide concentrations in a control population in infants and children. Clin Chem 49:1563–1564, 2003.

14. Koch A, Singer H: Normal values of B-type natriuretic peptide in infants, children and adolescents. Heart 89:875–878, 2003.

15. Law YM, Keller BB, Feingold BM, Boyle GJ: Usefulness of plasma B-type natriuretic peptide to identify ventricular dysfunction in pediatric and adult patients with congenital heart disease. Am J Cardiol 15:474–478, 2005.

16. Puddy VF, Amirmansour C, Williams AF, et al: Plasma brain natriuretic peptide as a predictor of haemodynamically significant patent ductus arteriosus in preterm infants. Clin Sci (Lond) 103:75–77, 2002.

17. Montgomery VL, Sullivan JE, Buchino JJ: Prognostic value of pre and postoperative cardiac troponin I measurement in children having cardiac surgery. Pediatr Dev Pathol 3:53–60, 2000.

18. Woodard GA, Mahle WT, Forkey HC: Sepsis, septic shock, acute abdomen? The ability of cardiac disorders to mimic other medical illnesses. Pediatr Emerg Care 12:317–324, 1996.

19. Sharieff GQ, Wylie TW: Pediatric cardiac disorders. J Emerg Med 26:65–79, 2004.

20. Park MK: Cyanotic congenital heart defects. In Park MK: Pediatric Cardiology for Practitioners, 4th ed. St. Louis: Mosby, 2002, pp 174–240.

21. Shay DK, Holman RC, Roosevelt GE, et al: Bronchiolitis-associated mortality and estimates of respiratory syncytial virus-associated deaths among US children, 1979–1999. J Infect Dis 183:16–22, 2001.

22. Shay DK, Holman RC, Newman RD, et al: Bronchiolitis-associated hospitalizations among US children, 1980–1996. JAMA 282:1440–1446, 1999.

23. Pickering LK, Baker CJ, Overturf GD, et al: Respiratory syncytial virus. In American Academy of Pediatrics Red Book: 2003 Report of the Committee on Infectious Diseases, 26th ed. Elk Grove Village, IL: American Academy of Pediatrics, 2003, pp 523–528.

24. Freed MD, Heyman AB, Lewis SL, et al: Protaglandin E1 in infants with ductus arteriosus dependent congenital heart disease. Circulation 64:899–905, 1981.

25. Park MK: Appendix D: Pediatric cardiovascular drug dosages. In Park MK: Pediatric Cardiology for Practitioners, 4th ed. St. Louis: Mosby, 2002, pp 489–504.

26. Hallidie-Smith KA: Prostaglandin E1 in suspected ductus dependent cardiac malformation. Arch Dis Child 59:1020–1026, 1984.

27. Kay J, Colan S, Graham T: Congestive heart failure in pediatric patients. Am Heart J 142:923–928, 2001.

28. Seguchi M, Nakazawa M, Momma K: Further evidence suggesting a limited role of digitalis in infants with circulatory congestion secondary to large ventricular septal defect. Am J Cardiol 831:408–411, 1999.

29. Digitalis Investigation Group: The effect of digoxin on mortality and morbidity in patients with heart failure. N Engl J Med 336:525–533, 1997.

30. Subhedar NV, Shaw NJ: Dopmamine versus dobutamine for hypotensive preterm infants. Cochrane Database Syst Rev (3):CD001242, 2003.

31. Mahle WT, Cuadrado AR, Kirshbom PM, et al: Nesiritide in infants and children with congestive heart failure. Pediatr Crit Care Med 6:543–546, 2003.

32. Rimensberger PC, Spahr-Schopfer I, Berner M, et al: Inhaled nitric oxide versus aerosolized iloprost in secondary pulmonary hypertension in children with congenital heart disease: vasodilator capacity and cellular mechanisms. Circulation 103:544–548, 2001.

33. Van Roekens CN, Zuckerberg AL: Emergency management of hypercyanotic crises in tetralogy of Fallot. Ann Emerg Med 25:256–258, 1995.

34. Guntheroth WG, Morgan BC, Mullins GL, et al: Venous return with knee-chest position and squatting in tetralogy of Fallot. Am Heart J 75:313–318, 1968.

35. Shaddy RE, Viney J, Judd VE, et al: Continuous intravenous phenylephrine infusion for treatment of hypoxemic spells in tetralogy of Fallot. J Pediatr 114:468–470, 1989.

Chapter 31

Excessive Crying

Marilyn P. Hicks, MD and Lance Brown, MD, MPH

Key Points

There are no evidenced-based guidelines for the emergency department evaluation of the infant with persistent, excessive crying.

There is a substantial subset of infants with persistent, excessive crying who harbor a serious illness.

Colic is a diagnosis of exclusion.

Introduction and Background

Infant crying occurs as a response to physiologic needs, such as hunger, cold, or discomfort. As such, crying is the primary form of nonverbal communication between an infant and his or her caregiver. As the demands of crying are met, conditioning occurs and infant-parent bonding is established. In 1962, Brazelton studied daily crying records of 80 infants during the first 12 weeks of life and described an escalation of normal crying from a median of 1.75 hours at age 2 weeks to a peak of 2.75 hours at 6 weeks, followed by a gradual decrease in total daily crying to approximately 1 hour daily at age 12 weeks.[1] Excessive crying occurs outside the normal cycle of infant demand and parental response.[1-5] Brazelton identified a subset of infants whom he referred to as "heavy fussers" who cried on average 1 hour more per day than the "light" fussers, who exhibited "normal patterns" of crying.[1]

Some infants with acute, excessive crying harbor serious illnesses (Table 31–1). Differentiating infants at high risk for harboring a serious illness from others is a key task for emergency physicians. The body of medical literature addressing acute, excessive crying secondary to organic disease consists of Poole's study of 56 healthy, afebrile infants presenting to an emergency department,[6] a small case series,[7] and case reports.[8-11] Poole's study is significant in that nearly two thirds of the infants who presented with acute, unexplained, excessive crying had a serious etiology. In this study, neither the duration nor the intensity of the crying were related to the seriousness of the underlying condition.

Recognition and Approach

The definition of excessive crying is highly variable and largely dependent upon parental perception and assessment.[12] The majority of studies of excessive crying are concerned with the prevalence, etiology, and treatment of colic or the behavioral aspects of crying. The relevance of these studies to the practice of emergency medicine is minimal. Based on these studies and inherent definitional problems, the incidence of excessive crying is between 1.5% and 43% of infants.[5,12-14] The epidemiology of serious illnesses in infants who present to the emergency department with a chief complaint of excessive crying is unknown. Parental misperception may account for some complaints of excessive crying. Clinical experience suggests new parents may present to the emergency department because they are uncertain how much crying is normal.

Clinical Presentation

The differential diagnosis of the infant with excessive crying is very broad and encompasses life-threatening as well as benign conditions (see Table 31–1). The differential diagnosis is to a certain degree age-based, specifically in reference to the very young infant in the first 2 months of life.

The history may identify "red flags" suggesting an increased likelihood of a serious condition being present (Table 31–2). Certain features of the history may require special attention. Breastfeeding mothers may be unaware that medications they are taking might be transmitted to their infant during feeds.[15-17] Although present, use of illicit drugs or parental alcoholism may lead to false histories in an attempt to hide culturally stigmatized behavior. In Poole's study, the history provided clues to the diagnosis in only 20% of infants.[6]

The physical examination may suggest the etiology of the excessive crying. In Poole's study, the physical examination revealed the diagnosis in 41% of cases and provided clues to the diagnosis in another 13%.[6] Therefore, a rather detailed physical examination directed at specific findings has good utility. While at the examination room doorway, the clinician should take note of the infant's overall appearance, mental status, and parental interaction. The quality of the cry should be noted. A shrill or high-pitched cry suggests a central nervous system abnormality, and a weak and feeble cry is common to many serious illnesses. Vital signs should be evaluated, including blood pressure and pulse oximetry.

Table 31–1	Differential Diagnosis of Excessive Crying

Infectious

Meningoencephalitis
Sepsis
Urinary tract infection
Osteomyelitis, septic arthritis, diskitis
Pneumonia, bronchiolitis
Otitis media
Gingivostomatitis, pharyngitis, thrush
Retropharyngeal cellulitis/abscess

Trauma

Nonaccidental injury
Accidental fracture, dislocation
Corneal abrasion or foreign body

Gastrointestinal

Malrotation with midgut volvulus
Intussusception
Gastroesophageal reflux disease
Constipation
Anal fissure
Milk protein allergy
Gastroenteritis
Appendicitis

Genitourinary

Incarcerated inguinal hernia
Testicular torsion, hydrocele

Cardiovascular

Supraventricular tachycardia
Myocarditis
Congestive heart failure
Coronary ischemia

Hematologic

Sickle cell disease
Iron deficiency anemia

Neurologic

Increased intracranial pressure
Hydrocephalus
Pseudotumor cerebri

Toxic-Metabolic

Neonatal drug withdrawal syndrome
Breast milk drug transmission
Immunizations
Ingestion
Electrolyte abnormalities
Inborn errors of metabolism
Hypoglycemia

Dermatologic

Eczema
Diaper dermatitis
Cellulitis, abscess
Hair tourniquet
Insect bites and stings

Table 31–2	"Red Flags" for Serious Etiologies Presenting with Excessive Crying

History

Maternal drug use
Premature rupture of membranes
Perinatal maternal fever or infection
History of fever (particularly in the first 2 months of life)
Vomiting (particularly if bilious)
History of bloody stools
Decreased feeding or activity
Increased somnolence
Abnormal behavior or "spells"
Difficulty feeding, sweating with feeds, or poor weight gain
Recent antibiotic use
Recent trauma, unexplained bruising, or inconsistent history
Delay in seeking care
Caregiver intoxication
Caregiver mental illness

Physical Examination

Abnormal vital signs
Ill appearance
Persistent, unexplained tachycardia or tachypnea
Paradoxical irritability
Pseudoparalysis
Jitteriness
Abnormal muscle tone
Blood in the diaper
Low weight

The infant's weight should be measured and compared to the birth weight (see Chapter 36, Failure to Thrive). The infant should be evaluated for paradoxical irritability. Normally, infants are soothed and calmed by being held and rocked gently in a caregiver's arms. Paradoxical irritability is present when an infant appears to be more comfortable when lying still than when gently rocked. Conditions such as meningitis may present with paradoxical irritability as the infant's inflamed meninges are aggravated by motion. In cases of pseudoparalysis of an extremity, an infant will fail to move an injured extremity such that it appears paralyzed. Inflammatory processes such as osteomyelitis and septic arthritis may present with pseudoparalysis.

Fluorescein staining of the eyes may reveal a corneal abrasion.[10] Infants have rapidly growing fingernails and poor hand control, putting them at risk for corneal abrasions. Scleral injection is less likely to be present in young infants than in older children. If a topical ophthalmic anesthetic is instilled into the eyes in preparation for the fluorescein staining, the infant with a corneal abrasion may abruptly stop crying and resume normal activity. The ears should be examined for otitis media. If the ipsilateral tympanic membrane is intact and otitis media appears to be contributing to the crying, instillation of two to four drops of benzocaine/antipyrine (i.e., Auralgan) into the ear canal may be diagnostic if the infant abruptly stops crying and resumes normal activity. If the infant presents a quiet moment, the fontanelles should be evaluated for size and fullness, and the neck examined for evidence of trauma, adenopathy, or masses and for range of motion.

The clinician should assess the infant's work of breathing and auscultate the lungs. Abnormal breath sounds may be suggestive of pneumonia, bronchiolitis, or congestive heart failure. The heart should be auscultated for abnormal tones. The presence of a murmur, ventricular heave, or thrill suggests congenital cardiac disease. The clavicles should be palpated, assessing for fracture. In addition to observation of the chest for increased work of breathing and auscultation of the lungs and heart, the chest wall, ribs, and clavicles should be palpated for tenderness or deformity. Examination of the abdomen of the crying infant is exceedingly difficult and may require repeat assessments over time. The anal area should be examined for rash, signs of trauma, and fissures. Each finger and toe and the genitalia should be examined for hair tourniquets (see Chapter 37, Minor Infant Problems). The scrotum should be examined for swelling, which may be suggestive of a hernia, a hydrocele, or testicular torsion (see Chapter 87, Testicular Torsion). The skin should be examined for bruises, abrasions, abscesses, burns, and scars. Bruising in young infants is uncommon and more likely to be a manifestation of abuse than in older children.[18]

Important Clinical Features and Considerations

Although the main objective of the emergency department visit for an infant with excessive crying is to identify serious illnesses, there are several benign causes amenable to treatment in the emergency department. These include corneal abrasions, hair tourniquets, oral thrush, nasal congestion, anal fissure, eczema, diaper dermatitis, constricting clothing, and overbundling (see Chapter 37, Minor Infant Problems). Although relatively common, colic is a diagnosis of exclusion.

Management

There is no specific treatment for excessive crying. There are no practice guidelines, and very limited evidence exists on which to base a management plan. If an infant can demonstrate an awake, calm period in the emergency department and has no "red flags" on history or physical examination, the infant is very unlikely to harbor a serious disease. Therefore, discharge home with follow-up the next day with the pediatrician or in the emergency department (e.g., on weekends and holidays) is probably a reasonable plan in these cases. If there is uncertainty as to the adequacy of the duration of the calm period, further observation in the emergency department is prudent. Simple causes of excessive crying such as constrictive clothing, overbundling, corneal abrasions, anal fissures, oral thrush, and hair tourniquets should have been identified and treatment should have been initiated following the physical examination. If a simple cause has been identified and the infant can demonstrate an awake, calm period after the simple cause has been addressed, it is reasonable to discharge the infant home with primary care follow-up.

Infants who cannot show a period during which they are awake, calm, and acting normally after simple causes have been ruled out pose a diagnostic dilemma. These infants have a relatively high likelihood of harboring a serious condition, but the differential diagnosis is extremely broad (see Table 31–1). To evaluate each infant for all of these conditions is not intuitively appealing. Clinical experience suggests one reasonable approach is to perform a septic workup, including a complete blood count, blood culture, catheterized urinalysis, urine culture, and cerebrospinal fluid studies (cell count, glucose, protein, and culture), and obtain a set of electrolytes, including glucose measurement. If nonaccidental trauma is suspected, a head computed tomography scan and skeletal survey of plain radiographs may be included in the workup. Other studies that may be rather simply added to the

workup include a serum ammonia level and venous pH (see Chapter 29, Inborn Errors of Metabolism) and an electrocardiogram to evaluate the infant for supraventricular tachycardia.

Summary

There are no evidenced-based guidelines specific to the infant with excessive crying. Crying episodes may resolve without any specific intervention on the part of the parents or health care providers. These infants are at a very low risk of harboring a serious illness. Colic is a diagnosis of exclusion. There is a subset of infants presenting to emergency departments with acute, unexplained, excessive crying who have serious organic disease. Infants who persist in having excessive crying after benign causes have been ruled out are at relatively high risk for harboring a serious illness. An extensive laboratory workup and admission to the hospital are indicated for these infants.

REFERENCES

1. Brazelton TB: Crying in infancy. Pediatrics 29:579–588, 1962.
2. St. James-Roberts I, Halil T: Infant crying patterns in the first year; normal community and clinicial findings. J Child Psychol Psychiatry 32:951–968, 1991.
3. Wessel M, Cobb J, Jackson E, et al: Paroxysmal fussing in infancy, sometimes called "colic." Pediatrics 14:421–434, 1954.
4. Illingsworth RS: "Three months" colic. Arch Dis Child 29:165–174, 1954.
5. Barr RG: Management of clinical problems in emotional care: colic and crying syndromes in infants. Pediatrics 102:1282–1286, 1998.
*6. Poole SR: The infant with acute, unexplained, excessive crying. Pediatrics 88:450–455, 1991.
7. Ruiz-Contreras J, Urquia L, Bastero R: Persistent crying as predominant manifestation of sepsis in infants and newborns. Pediatr Emerg Care 15:113–115, 1999.
*8. Brown L, Hicks M: Subclinical mastitis presenting as acute unexplained, excessive crying in an afebrile 31-day-old female. Pediatr Emerg Care 17:189–190, 2001.
9. Singer JI, Rosenberg NM: A fatal case of colic. Pediatr Emerg Care 8:171–172, 1992.
10. Harkness MJ: Corneal abrasion in infancy as a cause of inconsolable crying. Pediatr Emerg Care 5:242–244, 1989.
11. Mahle WT: A dangerous case of colic: anomalous left coronary artery presenting with paroxysms of irritability. Pediatr Emerg Care 14:24–27, 1998.
12. Reijneveld SA, Brugman E, Hirasing R: Excessive infant crying: the impact of varying definitions. Pediatrics 108:893–897, 2001.
*13. Wade S, Kilgour T: Infantile colic. Extracts from "Clinical Evidence". BMJ 323:437–440, 2001.
14. Garrison MM, Christakis DA: Early childhood. Colic, child development and poisoning prevention: a systematic review of treatments for infant colic. Pediatrics 106:184–190, 2000.
15. Curet LB, His AC: Drug abuse during pregnancy. Clin Obstet Gynecol 45:73–88, 2002.
16. Mitchell JL: Use of cough and cold preparations during breastfeeding. J Hum Lact 15:347–349, 1999.
17. Gunn VL, Taha SH, Liebelt EL, et al: Toxicity of over-the-counter cough and cold medicines. Pediatrics108:e52, 2001.
*18. Sugar NF, Taylor JA, Feldman KW: Bruises in infants and toddlers: those who don't cruise rarely bruise. Puget Sound Pediatric Research Network. Arch Pediatr Adolesc Med 153:399–403, 1999.

*Selected reading.

Chapter 32

Fever in the Well-Appearing Young Infant

Kristine G. Williams, MD, MPH and David M. Jaffe, MD

Key Points

Febrile illnesses account for 10% to 20% of pediatric visits to emergency departments.

Due to immunologic deficiencies, neonates and infants (<3 months) are particularly susceptible to infections by certain organisms.

The clinical detection of serious infection is more challenging in the young infant than in other age groups because of a more limited behavioral repertoire.

A well appearing young infant may still have a serious bacterial illness.

Judicious use of antibiotics and hospitalization continue to be goals in the evaluation and treatment of febrile infants.

Introduction and Background

Fever is one of the most common reasons for sick children to visit the emergency department, and it accounts for 10% to 20% of pediatric visits. Two thirds of all children will have visited a physician for the evaluation of fever by 2 years of age. Because of maturational immunologic deficiencies and a limited behavioral repertoire, febrile infants younger than 3 months of age are a distinct subset of this population. The unique characteristics of the young infant must be considered during evaluation and treatment.

By convention, fever in a young infant is defined as a rectal temperature of 38° C (100.4° F) or above.[1] Although axillary and tympanic thermometers are convenient, they are not reliable in young infants. In any case, temperature should not be the only factor used to make a management decision. This is particularly important if the infant is afebrile but has a history of irritability, poor feeding, lethargy, or any other behavioral change that is of concern to the parent. Although the predictive value of hyperpyrexia (temperature > 40° C/ 104° F) is low for individual infants, there is a correlation between height of temperature and rate of serious bacterial illness (SBI). According to one study, SBI is found in approximately 26% of 4- to 8-week old infants with temperatures over 40° C.[2] The clinician needs to appreciate, however, that serious illness may also be present in infants with normal or below-normal body temperatures.

Serious bacterial infection is defined as the growth of a bacterial pathogen in cultures of specimens of the blood, urine, cerebrospinal fluid (CSF), bone, joint fluid, or stool. The most common bacterial pathogens causing SBI vary by age. In the first month of life, *Escherichia coli* and group B streptococcus (GBS) are the usual sources. From 1 to 3 months, SBI is still predominantly caused by GBS and *E. coli*, but other organisms such as *Listeria monocytogenes, Streptococcus pneumoniae, Neisseria meningococcemia, Salmonella,* and *Haemophilus influenzae* are also found.[3] Young infants are also at risk for serious infection from viruses, such as herpes simplex virus (HSV) and enterovirus. HSV is more common in infants born to mothers with primary rather than secondary HSV infection. Within the United States, enteroviruses are the most common cause of childhood aseptic meningitis and nonspecific febrile illness.[4] Both HSV and enterovirus can cause life-threatening meningitis or encephalitis.

The young infant is particularly susceptible to infection because of an immature immune system. Neonates have definable deficiencies in specific antibody, complement, and other opsonins, and in phagocyte number and function.[5] These deficiencies contribute to their increased susceptibility to GBS and other pyogenic bacteria. Serious infection from intracellular organisms is likely due to reduced attraction of macrophages to the site of infection because of insufficient generation of lymphokines and interleukins in those infants with an immature immune system. The neonate's susceptibility to HSV infection is thought to be due to a lack of passively acquired antibodies and the decreased activity of nonimmune and immune cellular cytotoxic mechanisms. The exact age at which most of the immune system reaches maturity is unknown, though the risk of severe infection with most of these pathogens seems to wane by 2 to 3 months of age.[5]

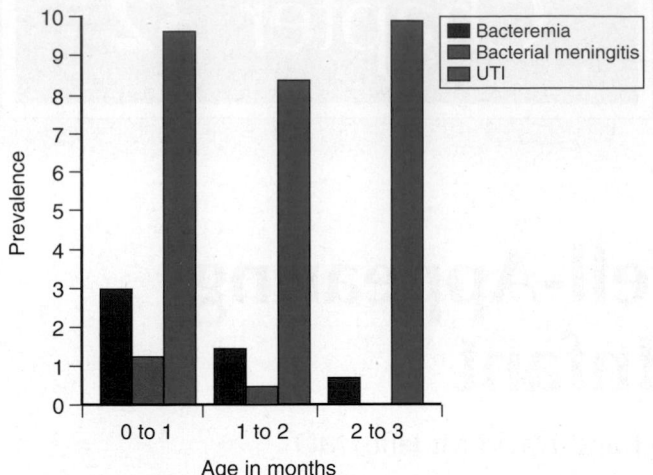

FIGURE 32–1. Prevalence of bacteremia, bacterial meningitis, and urinary tract infection (UTI) in febrile infants. (Data from Newman TB, Bernzweig J, Takayama J, et al: Urine testing and urinary tract infections in febrile infants seen in office settings: the Pediatric Research in Office Settings' Febrile Infant Study. Arch Pediatr Adolesc Med, 156:44–54, 2002; and Pantell RH, Newman T, Bernzweig J, et al: Management and outcomes of care of fever in early infancy. JAMA 291:1203–1212, 2004.)

Recognition and Approach

Based on data from a nationwide prospective cohort study conducted by the Pediatric Research in Office Settings (PROS) Network of the American Academy of Pediatrics, the rate of bacteremia and bacterial meningitis in febrile young infants appears to decrease with age.[6] In a consecutive sample of 3066 infants ages 3 months or younger with temperatures of at least 38° C seen by office practitioners, the overall rates of bacteremia and bacterial meningitis were 1.8% and 0.5%, respectively. For infants up to 1 month of age, the rate of bacteremia was 3%, that of bacterial meningitis was 1.2%, and that of bacteremia with bacterial meningitis was 4.1%. As the infants matured, the rates decreased. By 1 to 2 months of age, the risk of bacteremia was 1.5%, that of bacterial meningitis was 0.4% and that of bacteremia/bacterial meningitis was 1.9%. Infants 2 to 3 months had rates of 0.7% for bacteremia, 0% for bacterial meningitis, and 0.7% for bacteremia/bacterial meningitis (Fig. 32–1). Age less than 30 days, higher temperatures, ill appearance, abnormal cry, and abnormal white blood cell (WBC) count (<5000 or >15,000 WBC/mm³) were associated with a high risk of bacteremia/bacterial meningitis. A low risk of bacteremia/bacterial meningitis (0.4%) was found in those who were well-appearing, 25 days of age or older, and with a temperature below 38.6° C.[6] The overall prevalence of urinary tract infection (UTI) was 5% for the entire cohort and 9% for those tested for UTI.[7] The rate was highest for girls (11.9%) and uncircumcised boys (19.5%). Infants younger than 30 days with a UTI had a rate of 17% for associated bacteremia. The risk of UTI-associated bacteremia decreased with age, with a rate of 8% for 1- to 2-month-old infants and 6% for 2- to 3-month-old infants.[7] It is important to note that all laboratory testing was performed at the discretion of the practitioner after recording signs and symptoms and an overall assessment of clinical appearance. This practical approach worked well in this study setting, where over half

of the 1975 infants treated as outpatients were examined on more than one occasion. However, in the emergency setting, where infants are evaluated during a single visit, a more cautious approach is warranted.

A complete sepsis evaluation is recommended in a febrile infant ≤28 days of age.[1,8-10] The sepsis evaluation should include a complete blood count (CBC) with differential count; a urinalysis; examination of the cerebrospinal fluid (CSF) for cells, glucose, and protein; and cultures of blood, urine, and CSF. If there are respiratory symptoms or diarrhea, a chest radiograph and a stool culture, respectively, should also be obtained. Hospitalization and administration of a parenteral antibiotic combination such as ampicillin and either cefotaxime or gentamicin is generally indicated until culture results are available.

While the approach to the infant ≤28 days of age is straightforward based on current data, controversy and variation exist regarding the evaluation and management of infants 29 to 60 days of age with fever. Many of these infants have self-limited viral infections. Routine hospitalization and administration of intravenous antibiotics may not be optimal as this practice is costly and associated with iatrogenic complications.[11] Prospective research on this population has resulted in criteria to help distinguish patients at low risk for bacterial disease from patients at high risk.[12] The purpose of defining these groups is to help identify which patients should be hospitalized and which patients can be treated as outpatients either with or without antibiotics. The Boston, Rochester, and Philadelphia strategies are results of this research. Although each approach is slightly different in terms of patient age, evaluation components, and management, any of them is a suitable guideline for helping the clinician identify infants at low risk for SBI (Table 32–1).

The study conducted in Boston tested the safety and efficacy of outpatient management of 503 one- to three-month-old infants judged to be low-risk for bacterial disease by screening criteria[13] (see Table 32–1). All infants received intramuscular ceftriaxone, 50 mg/kg, at 24 and 48 hours and had close follow-up. Although 5% of the population initially judged to be low risk had bacterial disease, including bacteremia, UTI, and gastroenteritis, all recovered without incident and had no complications attributable to their initial outpatient management. The authors concluded that, although the clinical screening criteria did not satisfactorily discriminate between infants with and without SBI, all infants with SBI received appropriate therapy and were well at follow-up.[13] After full evaluation for sepsis, outpatient management of low-risk febrile infants with intramuscular ceftriaxone seems to be a safe alternative to hospitalization. It is important that patients managed this way receive a full evaluation for sepsis, including a lumbar puncture, and close follow-up until final culture results are available.

Investigators in Philadelphia initially studied 747 infants 29 through 56 days of age to evaluate the efficacy of managing fever without routine hospitalization and antibiotic therapy.[14] Infants not meeting all the low-risk criteria were hospitalized for parenteral antimicrobial therapy. Those judged to be low risk were assigned to either inpatient observation without antibiotics or outpatient care without antibiotics but with reexamination after 24 and 48 hours. There were no serious illnesses in the outpatient group who were observed without antibiotics.[14] A follow-up study done to

Table 32–1	Summary of Low-Risk Criteria for Serious Bacterial Illness: The Boston, Philadelphia and Rochester Criteria		
	Boston	**Philadelphia**	**Rochester**
Age	1–3 months	1–2 months	Birth–3 months
History	No antibiotics No immunizations past 48 hr	No immune deficiency	Term (>37 wk) No antibiotics Never hospitalized No unexplained hyperbilirubinemia No chronic or underlying illness Not hospitalized longer than mother
Physical Examination	Nontoxic No focal infection	Infant observation score ≤ 10 No sign of bacterial infection	Appears generally well No focal infection
Labs	WBC < 20,000 U/A: < 10 WBC/hpf or negative leukocyte esterase	WBC < 15,000 Band/neutrophil ratio < 0.2 Spun U/A: < 10 WBC/hpf, no bacteria CSF: < 8 WBC/hpf, negative Gram stain Stool (if diarrhea): < 5 WBC/hpf	WBC 5000–15,000 Absolute band count < 1500 Spun urine: < 10 WBC/hpf Stool (if diarrhea): < 5 WBC/hpf
CXR	(if obtained): No focal infiltrate	No focal infiltrate	

Abbreviations: CSF, cerebrospinal fluid; CXR, chest radiograph; hpf, high-power field; U/A, urinalysis; WBC, white blood cells.

evaluate the efficacy of this strategy 18 months after it was introduced found that none of 43 febrile infants 29 to 60 days old with SBI were identified as low risk. Thus the Philadelphia protocol for outpatient management without antibiotics for low-risk febrile infants 29 to 60 days of age was shown to be practical, reliable, and safe.[15] However, when the criteria were applied retrospectively to 254 febrile infants less than 28 days of age, 109 (42.9%) of them would have been identified as at low risk for bacterial disease. Of these 109 infants classified as low risk for SBI, 5 had bacterial diseases (2 UTI, 2 bacteremia, 1 bacterial gastroenteritis). The authors concluded that the Philadelphia protocol does not adequately predict SBI in febrile neonates.[8]

The Rochester criteria, based on data from 233 infants birth to 60 days of age, were developed to identify which infants are at low risk for SBI. Only one of the infants classified as low risk was found to have SBI (*Salmonella* gastroenteritis without bacteremia), compared to 25% of the infants in the high-risk group.[16] Unlike the Boston and Philadelphia studies, however, this study does not address the issue of hospitalization or antibiotic therapy. The Rochester criteria were evaluated prospectively in a sample of 931 well-appearing infants. SBI (all UTIs) occurred in 1% of the 511 infants who met all of the low-risk criteria.[17] More than one third of the low risk infants were managed initially without antimicrobial therapy and experienced no untoward effects. The negative predictive value of the criteria was found to be 98.9% for SBI and 99.5% for bacteremia. The authors recommended that febrile infants less than 60 days of age who met all of the low-risk criteria could be managed as inpatients or outpatients by observation without antibiotics or with a single dose of intramuscular ceftriaxone after blood, urine, and CSF samples had been obtained for culture.[17]

Both the Boston and the Philadelphia management protocols have been applied retrospectively to infants in the first month of life. Within this age group, these strategies have a 97% negative predictive value. In other words, when the strategies were applied to infants birth to 28 days, 3% of the infants who fulfilled all the low-risk criteria were found to have SBI.[9] Since infants less than 28 days of age have the

Table 32–2	Signs and Symptoms Associated with Neonatal Infection

Signs

Fever
Tachypnea
Full or bulging fontanelle
Joint swelling
Soft tissue swelling
Abdominal distention
Rash
Lethargy
Agitation

Symptoms

History of fever
Abnormal sleep patterns
Decreased feeding
Vomiting
Diarrhea
Irritability
Respiratory distress
Agitation
Lethargy
Seizure
Rash
Joint swelling

highest risk of SBI and the most limited behavioral repertoire, this suggests that all infants younger than 28 days of age should be managed with a complete sepsis evaluation and hospitalization.

Clinical Presentation

The young infant presenting with fever is a diagnostic challenge. The clinician must have a low threshold for concern because of the broad range of signs and symptoms associated with neonatal infection (Table 32–2). Since the scope of presentation ranges from well-appearing to toxic-appearing, the history and laboratory evaluation become extremely important in guiding the clinician's decisions.

The differential diagnosis for fever in the first few months of life includes bacterial infection acquired in utero, at delivery, in the nursery, at home, or because of an underlying anatomic abnormality (e.g., vesicoureteral reflux, posterior urethral valves, ureteropelvic junction obstruction). Viral infections are also a consideration. In particular, one should consider viruses acquired at birth, such as HSV, and those commonly spread by contact, such as enterovirus, respiratory syncytial virus (RSV), and influenza virus. The immunizations given at the 2-month check up, diptheria/tetanus/acellular pertussis (DTaP) and *H. influenzae* type b (Hib), may cause fever for 24 to 48 hours after inoculation. However, immunizations should not be considered the cause of fever in a toxic-appearing infant. Although it is extremely rare that fever in this age group is caused by noninfectious causes, overbundling a young infant can cause temporary elevations in body temperature. If an infant is well-appearing, it is reasonable to unbundle the infant for 15 to 30 minutes and reassess the temperature prior to making management decisions. If the temperature normalizes, the infant still appears healthy and has not received an antipyretic, the infant can be considered to be afebrile.

A young infant with fever should first be evaluated for a toxic appearance. A toxic-appearing infant is one with a clinical picture of the sepsis syndrome—lethargy, signs of poor perfusion, hypoventilation, hyperventilation, or cyanosis. Because toxic-appearing infants under 12 weeks of age have a 17% chance of having bacterial infection, rapid evaluation and treatment are vital in these infants.[18] After obtaining cultures of blood, urine and CSF, parenteral antibiotics should be administered. A broad-spectrum antibiotic such as ceftriaxone is effective against most organisms that cause sepsis. Ampicillin is recommended to cover *L. monocytogenes*. Acyclovir should be added if there is concern for herpes or herpes meningitis. Therapy should not be delayed if specimen collection is prolonged.

The rapid assessment of appearance is complex. Observation scales have been developed in an attempt to quickly identify serious illness in febrile children. One such scale, the Infant Observation Score (IOS), was created based on data from febrile children under 24 months.[19] Patients were scored for quality of cry, reaction to parental stimulation, state variation, color, hydration, and response to social overtures. In children under 24 months of age, the score was reliable, predictive, specific, and sensitive for identifying serious illness in children.[19] Subsequently, it was tested on febrile infants 4

to 8 weeks old, whose neurologic immaturity and limited behavioral range make scoring difficult and imprecise. In this age group, 22% of those with a score classifying them as low risk had serious illness.[20] This suggests that the IOS alone is not sufficient to identify serious illness in the 4- to 8-week-old infant. However, when it is used in combination with other examination and laboratory screening criteria, as it is in the Philadelphia criteria, it may be helpful in defining a low-risk population.

After the initial assessment, a thorough history and a detailed physical examination should be completed. Key historical questions focus on changes in the infant's behavior: increased or decreased sleeping, decreased feeding, irritability, respiratory distress, agitation, or lethargy. Since these infants are often only a few days or weeks old, the behavioral changes may be difficult for new parents to appreciate unless they are asked about them specifically. An infant with a history of documented fever at home who is afebrile in the emergency unit should be managed as if fever is present.[21,22]

Very young infants with febrile illness have an inconsistent presentation. The neurologic and behavioral immaturity during the first few months of life may also confound the presentation. In the first month of life, most newborns sleep approximately 16 to 18 hours a day. The amount of time spent in sleep may make it difficult to assess whether an infant is more sleepy than usual. As the brain matures, the amount of time spent in a wakeful state increases, making some of the behavioral changes associated with illness more apparent. An understanding of the timing of some developmental milestones may help the clinician assess behavioral change, adding another dimension to the evaluation of the newborn infant[23] (Table 32–3). Older infants and children have a more established sleep/wake cycle and more complex social interaction, making deviations from normal more apparent.

The choice of diagnostic tests should be guided by the infant's age and presentation. A toxic-appearing infant or an infant under the age of 1 month should receive a full sepsis evaluation with a chest radiograph and stool culture, if indicated. Well-appearing infants and those older than 1 month may receive any combination of tests in the sepsis evaluation based on presentation. There is no single laboratory test that entirely predicts a bacterial disease, nor is there one that entirely rules out a bacterial disease.

A CBC should be obtained for all infants receiving a sepsis evaluation. In older infants and children, a high absolute neutrophil count (>10,000/mm^3) is associated with higher

Table 32–3	Developmental Changes during the First 3 Months of Life*				
Age (mo)	Sleep (hr/day)	Social	Movement	Vision	Hearing
0–1	16–18	None	Startles easily with loud noise or sudden movement Jerky arm and leg movement Strong reflex movements	Eyes wander, cross Able to focus 8–12 inches away	May turn to familiar sound/voice
1–2	16–18†	Responsive social smile (6–8 wk)	Increasing head control	Coordinated eye movement Tracks object to midline	Turns head to sound May coo
2–3	14	Laughs Spontaneous smile	Brings hands together at midline	Tracks objects past midline	Squeals in delight

*Ages are approximate and information is a sample of some developmental changes.
†Beginning to develop more regular sleep pattern.

risk of bacteremia.[24] Although this has not been reproduced in young infants, the outcomes of the studies done in Rochester and Philadelphia suggest that a normal WBC count (between 5000 and 15,000/mm[3]) and a low band count can help stratify patients as being at low risk for SBI.[14,16] Specifically, the investigators in Philadelphia were able to achieve 100% accuracy when prospectively identifying infants 1 to 2 months old at low risk for bacterial disease by incorporating a band-to-neutrophil ratio of less than 0.2.[14]

Blood cultures are the "gold standard" for determination of bacteremia. Although blood culture results are not available immediately, most true pathogens are detected by 24 hours. In the well-appearing infant, nonpathogenic organisms may be considered contaminants, especially if recovered after 48 hours.

Lumbar puncture (LP) is indicated if sepsis or meningitis is suspected, if the infant is 28 days of age or less, or if the clinician plans to administer antibiotics. Evaluation of the CSF should include cell count, differential, protein and glucose measurement, and Gram stain and culture. As normal values for serum WBC counts vary slightly by age (Table 32–4), so do normal values for spinal fluid[25] (Table 32–5). Since the CSF does not normally contain red blood cells, their presence indicates a traumatic LP or central nervous system (CNS) hemorrhage. The latter is more likely if the red blood cells do not diminish between the first and the last specimen tube. CNS hemorrhage may be a result of trauma or infection, particularly with HSV. In the healthy neonate, it is not unusual to see 8 to 10 WBC/mm[3]. There is typically a predominance of neutrophils in the CSF of patients with bacterial meningitis. Infants with bacterial meningitis will often have an elevated protein (>100 mg/dl) and a low glucose (<30 mg/dl) level. However, early in the course of meningitis, parameters also may be normal. If indicated by history or physical examination, the spinal fluid should also be sent for herpes and enterovirus polymerase chain reaction (PCR) studies.

The decision to order a chest radiograph should be based on the infant's symptoms. Routine ordering of chest radiographs is not indicated in the absence of respiratory signs.[26] However, the presence of retractions, rales, rhonchi, and isolated tachypnea or the presence of cough with another respiratory sign, such as tachypnea or retractions, is predictive of focal changes on a chest radiograph.

Stool samples are not indicated for all febrile infants. However, if the infant presents with watery or bloody diarrhea, a stool sample should be obtained for microscopic examination and culture. Bacterial enteritis is indicated by the presence of blood or greater than 5 WBCs per high-power field. Blood in the stool is associated with bacterial gastroenteritis, but it is a nonspecific finding also seen with rotavirus and other viral causes of diarrhea. Although WBCs may be present on stool smear in those infants with bacterial gastroenteritis, absence of WBCs does not indicate absence of bacterial disease.

UTIs are the most common of the serious bacterial illnesses in the well-appearing febrile young infant, occurring in approximately 7.5% of febrile infants under 8 weeks of age. Uncircumcised males and white girls are at highest risk.[7,27] UTI should be considered in all febrile neonates because of associated bacteremia and sepsis. Although urinalysis alone has been shown to be a sensitive and independent indicator of the presence of UTI in older children, it is not so in infants. Appropriate evaluation for a UTI in infants includes a urinalysis and urine culture on a specimen obtained by catheter or suprapubic aspiration.[28]

Viruses are a common cause of fever in the neonatal period. A nasopharyngeal swab for fluorescent antibody stain and culture should be considered in an infant with fever and wheezing, cough, tachypnea, or other respiratory symptoms, particularly during the winter months. The sample should be tested for RSV; influenza A and B viruses; parainfluenza 1, 2, and 3 viruses; and adenovirus. Enterovirus is the most common cause of aseptic meningitis. Detection of enterovirus by culture is limited by a sensitivity of only 65% to 75% and a processing time of 3 to 10 days. Compared with viral culture, the CSF PCR was 100% sensitive and 90% specific for the diagnosis of enteroviral meningitis in a study of febrile infants less than 3 months of age.[4] PCR assays of serum and urine are also more sensitive than culture, but for the detection of enteroviral meningitis, CSF PCR is adequate.[29] Although concurrent viral and bacterial disease can occur, the detection of enterovirus by PCR in an otherwise well-appearing infant with normal laboratory results may help the clinician be judicious about using antibiotics. Herpes simplex virus PCR or culture should be obtained in infants with a concerning history or with seizures; signs of sepsis; characteristic skin, eye, or mouth lesions; or CSF findings suggestive of CNS hemorrhage. If the clinician suspects HSV, acyclovir should be started empirically.

Important Clinical Features and Considerations

Approximately 7% of febrile infants younger than 3 months of age have SBI, and the remainder are presumed to have a

Table 32–4	Infant Laboratory Reference Values: Hematology	
	WBC (1000/mm[3])	
Age	**Mean**	**95% CI**
1–3 days	18.9	9.4–34.0
2 wk	11.4	5.0–20.0
1–3 mo	10.8	5.0–19.5

From Rowe P: Laboratory values. *In* Oski F, DeAngelis C, Feigin R, et al: Principles and Practice of Pediatrics, 2nd ed. Philadelphia: JB Lippincott, pp 2168–2169, 1994.

Table 32–5	Infant Laboratory Reference Values for Cerebrospinal Fluid			
	WBC (cells/mm[3])			
Age	**Mean**	**Range**	**Glucose (mg/dl)**	**Protein (mg/dl)**
Preterm	9.0	0–25	24–63	65–150
Term	8.2	0–22	34–119	20–170

From Rowe P: Laboratory values. *In* From Oski F, DeAngelis C, Feigin R, et al: Principles and Practice of Pediatrics, 2nd ed. Philadelphia: JB Lippincott, 1994, pp 2168–2169.

self-limited viral cause for fever. It is important to consider whether infants with a self-limited viral illness have coexisting bacterial disease. It is generally believed that infants with objective evidence of a viral infection do not need a complete sepsis evaluation. RSV is a common cause of lower respiratory disease in infants. Patients typically present with symptoms such as wheezing, tachypnea, respiratory distress, apnea, and fever. Studies of older infants (>28 days) and children suggest that the risk of bacteremia in non–toxic-appearing patients with documented RSV infection is rare enough that routine cultures of blood and spinal fluid are not indicated.[30] In most of the studies, UTI was the most common concurrent SBI.[31-35] In a prospective study of 1248 infants under 2 months of age, the rate of SBI in RSV-negative infants was 12.5% as compared to 7% in patients with RSV. A subanalysis of the data by age revealed that the overall rate of SBI in infants 28 days or younger did not differ significantly between those who were and those who were not infected with RSV (10.1% vs. 14.2%). In RSV-positive infants, the overall rate of UTI was 5.4% as compared to 10.1% in those without RSV.[31] Although there is wide variability in diagnostic testing of young infants with bronchiolitis, the risks of bacteremia and meningitis in this population seem to be low if the infant is non–toxic appearing and older than 28 days. However, there continues to be a risk of UTI similar to that of a well-appearing febrile young infant without RSV. Thus it is prudent to obtain a urinalysis and urine culture of a catheterized urine specimen from the infant with fever. Despite the reassuring data about the risk of bacteremia and meningitis in infants under 90 days of age with RSV infection, in those 28 days or younger, it is best to assume that the risk of SBI is not changed by the presence of RSV and to perform a full sepsis evaluation.

Acute otitis media is the most common bacterial infection in children. Bacterial organisms are identified in 60% to 70% of cases when tympanocentesis is performed as part of a study protocol. *S. pneumoniae, H. influenzae,* and *Moraxella catarrhalis* are the predominant organisms in all age groups, though gram-negative enteric bacilli and *Staphylococcus aureus* may also be found in the first month of life. Few studies specifically address the risk of bacteremia associated with otitis media. In developing the Rochester criteria, the authors noted that a diagnosis of otitis media was the only reason for considering nine infants to be at high risk, and none had SBI.[16] However, a study of febrile infants younger than 8 weeks reported bacteremia in 1 of 24 patients with otitis media.[27] Although it is not common, infants with otitis media on examination are still at risk for invasive disease. A diagnosis of otitis media in a febrile infant 28 days or younger should not influence the patient's evaluation or management. It is reasonable to obtain a CBC, blood culture, urinalysis, and urine culture prior to initiating appropriate oral antibiotic therapy in febrile infants 29 to 60 days of age with otitis media. An LP is not necessary if the infant is well-appearing, has reliable follow-up, meets all other low-risk criteria, and will not be receiving parenteral antibiotics. Well-appearing infants 2 to 3 months of age with an unequivocal diagnosis of otitis media may be treated with appropriate oral antibiotic therapy without a laboratory evaluation. It is important to note that otitis media is a difficult diagnosis to make in very young infants since they often have narrow ear canals and indistinct landmarks. If the clinician is unsure about the diagnosis of otitis media, it is best to approach the patient as a febrile infant without a source.

The introduction of the heptavalent pneumococcal vaccine has decreased the risk of serious infection with *S. pneumoniae.*[36,37] The vaccine is given at 2, 4, 6, and 12 to 15 months of age. The four-dose regimen is highly efficacious against invasive disease and somewhat efficacious against otitis media and pneumonia. In particular, the rate of SBI in the African American population has decreased dramatically. However, the risk of invasive infection with *S. pneumoniae* in the infant less than 3 months of age has not changed significantly, likely due to the fact that only one vaccination is given during this time frame. Therefore, even if the infant has received a pneumococcal vaccination, it is prudent to consider that the infant is, in effect, not vaccinated.

Management

Although in the first 28 days of life, the risk of SBI in low-risk infants is small, most experts recommend an evaluation for sepsis.[38] This conservative approach is rooted in the difficulty in evaluating the behavioral state of neonates, the immature neonatal immune system, the rapid evolution of bacterial infections in this age group, and the possibility of life-threatening enteroviral or herpes meningoencephalitis. Based on current data, febrile infants ≤ 28 days of age should receive a full septic evaluation, admission to the hospital, and administration of parenteral antibiotics. Although the risk of infection with *L. monocytogenes* is low, it is still a possibility and ampicillin is indicated. The choice of a second antibiotic may vary. Gentamicin is a good choice for most patients ≤ 28 days of age, unless there is a concern for meningitis or for an unusual pathogen. Cefotaxime may be a better choice if meningitis is suspected (Table 32–6).

A combination of clinical evaluation and laboratory studies can be used to define a specific population of infants 29 to 60 days of age who appear well and are at low risk for SBI. The probability of having an SBI in a febrile young infant who meets all of the low-risk criteria is approximately 0.2% to 0.7%. Most experts agree that low-risk infants 28 to 90 days of age with reliable parents and good follow-up can be managed as outpatients with reevaluation in 24 hours. The infants should meet all the low-risk historical, clinical, and laboratory criteria except that infants with otitis media can be included in this category.[10,16,17] Empirical outpatient therapy with ceftriaxone should be considered if an LP has been completed. It is optional to give a second dose of intramuscular ceftriaxone. If a child receives antimicrobials before a CSF specimen is obtained, it may be difficult to distinguish whether CSF pleocytosis with negative culture results on subsequent examinations is due to a virus or to partially treated meningitis. If it is unclear, a full course of parenteral antibiotic therapy is indicated.

As the rate of SBI in the low-risk 4- to 8-week-old infant is approximately 0.2% to 0.7%, an alternate strategy for low-risk febrile infants without an obvious source of infection is outpatient observation without antibiotics.[10,17,18] Children managed in this way should have blood and urine cultures, but do not necessarily need spinal fluid collection. All of the patients should be reevaluated within 24 hours. Those who deteriorate should receive the remainder of the septic evaluation, be hospitalized, and receive antimicrobial therapy.

Table 32–6	Evaluation and Management of Infants 0 to 3 months with T > 38°C	

Age	Evaluation	Management

0–28 d	1. **Detailed history and complete physical exam**
	2. **Laboratory evaluation for sepsis:**
	  • Blood: CBC w/ diff and culture
	  • Urine: cath urinalysis and culture
	  • CSF: cell count, protein, glucose, gram stain, culture
	  • Chest radiograph (if indicated)
	  • Stool for heme test and culture (if indicated)
	  • Consider HSV and enteroviral PCR for CSF
		1. **Admit for IV/IM antibiotics until culture results available:**
		Ampicillin:
		  <1 wk, 100 mg/kg/dose, Q 12 h
		  >1 wk, 50 mg/kg/dose, Q 6 h
		Plus cefotaxime:
		  <1 wk, 50 mg/kg/dose, Q 8 h
		  1–4 wk, 50 mg/kg/dose, Q 6 h
		Or plus gentamycin:
		  5 mg/kg/day, Q 24 h
		If herpes suspected, acyclovir: 20 mg/kg/dose, Q 8 h

29–60 d	1. **Detailed history and complete physical exam**
	2. **Laboratory evaluation for sepsis:** as for ≤28 d
	3. **Determine if patient is low-risk for SBI by meeting ALL criteria listed here:**
	  • Non-toxic appearance
	  • No focus of infection on exam (except OM)
	  • No known immunodeficiency
	  • WBC <15,000/mm³
	  • BNR <0.2
	  • Normal urinalysis
	  • *CSF: <8 WBC/mm³, negative gram stain, normal glucose and protein
	  • Normal chest radiograph (if done)
		1. **If toxic-appearing, hosp. for IV/IM antibiotics until culture results available:**
		Ampicillin:
		  50 mg/kg/dose, Q 6 h
		Plus cefotaxime:
		  50 mg/kg/dose, Q 6 h (meningitic dose)
		  (Or plus gentamycin 2.5 mg/kg/dose, Q 8 h if meningitis not suspected)
		If herpes suspected, acyclovir: 20 mg/kg/dose, Q 8 h
		2. **If high-risk, hospitalize for IV/IM antibiotics until culture results available:**
		Ampicillin:
		  50 mg/kg/dose, Q 6 h
		Plus cefotaxime:
		  50 mg/kg/dose, Q 6 h (meningitic dose)
		  (Or plus gentamycin 2.5 mg/kg/dose, Q 8 h if meningitis not suspected)
		3. **If low-risk, choose option:**
		  A. 50 mg/kg ceftriaxone IM, reexamination at 24 & 48 h (<u>Must have LP</u>)
		  B. No antibiotics and reexamination at 24 & 48 h (May consider deferring LP)

61–90 d	1. **Detailed history and complete physical exam**
	2. **Limited laboratory evaluation for sepsis:**
	  • Blood: CBC w/ diff and culture
	  • Urine: cath urinalysis and culture
	  • LP if clinical concern for meningitis
	  • Chest radiograph (if indicated)
	  • Stool for heme test and culture (if indicated)
		1. **If toxic-appearing, perform LP and hospitalize for IV/IM antibiotics until culture results available:**
		Ceftriaxone:
		  50 mg/kg/dose, Q 12 h
		2. **If not toxic-appearing:**
		  No antibiotics and reexamination at 24 and 48 h

*Although the default is to obtain CSF for evaluation in febrile infants 29–60 days of age, in some cases LP may be deferred.
Abbreviations: BNR, band to neutrophil ratio; CBC, complete blood count; CSF, cerebrospinal fluid; hpf, high power field; IM, intramuscular; IV, intravenous; LP, lumbar puncture; OM, otitis media; WBC, white blood cells.

Infants ages 29 to 60 days with otitis media should receive appropriate oral antibiotic therapy. A well-appearing infant with a UTI without bacteremia who is afebrile at reevaluation can be treated as an outpatient with a 10-day course of oral antibiotics chosen based on local sensitivity patterns. Infants who are ill appearing at reevaluation or who have positive blood or CSF cultures should be admitted for observation and antibiotic therapy.

Summary

Fever in the young infant is a common occurrence, and it has been established that a well-appearing young infant may have an SBI. The immunologic immaturity of infants makes them especially vulnerable to certain bacterial and viral organisms that can cause life-threatening disease. The limited range of behaviors of young infants makes diagnosing illness by physical examination challenging. It is necessary to have both a clear understanding of the risk of SBI and a practical and prudent approach to evaluation and management. The overall risk of SBI drops from 7% for all febrile infants 1 to 3 months of age to 0.2% to 0.7% if the infant meets all low-risk criteria

proposed by any of the Boston, Philadelphia, or Rochester strategies.

There is strong agreement among experts regarding the approach to infants ≤28 days of age. These infants should receive a full evaluation for sepsis, be admitted to the hospital, and receive parenteral antimicrobials. Acyclovir should be considered for any infant with a concerning history or with seizures; signs of sepsis; characteristic skin, eye, or mouth lesions; or CSF findings suggestive of CNS hemorrhage.

Infants ages 29 to 60 days should also receive a complete sepsis evaluation. Patients meeting all of the low-risk criteria of any of the prospectively evaluated studies mentioned previously may be treated as outpatients with intramuscular ceftriaxone and reexamination in 24 and 48 hours. Low-risk infants in this age category may also be observed as outpatients without antibiotics but with reevaluation in 24 and 48 hours. It is acceptable to defer LP in low-risk patients greater than 60 days of age who will not receive antibiotics. Non–toxic-appearing febrile infants 61 to 90 days of age should receive a complete history and physical examination and a limited laboratory evaluation. If they meet the low-risk criteria, they can be observed as outpatients without antibiotics, but with reexamination at 24 and 48 hours.

This approach to infants between the ages of 1 and 3 months has been found to be safe and reliable in prospective research. Although the populations that present to the emergency department versus the clinician's office may be different, the PROS study suggests that there may be a subset of infants, even in the first month of life, for whom outpatient observation and close follow-up might be a reasonable option. This approach has not been proven for these youngest patients, but future research may help clarify this.

REFERENCES

*1. Baraff L, Bass J, Fleisher G, et al: Practice guideline for the management of infants and children 0 to 36 months of age with fever without a source. Pediatrics 92:1–12, 1993.

2. Bonadio W, McElroy K, Jacoby P, et al: Relationship of fever magnitude to rate of serious bacterial infections in infants aged 4–8 weeks. Clin Pediatr (Phila) 30:478–480, 1991.

*3. Baskin M: The prevalence of serious bacterial infections by age in febrile infants during the first 3 months of life. Pediatr Ann 22:462–466, 1993.

4. Rotbart H, Ahmed A, Hickey S, et al: Diagnosis of enterovirus infection by polymerase chain reaction of multiple specimen types. Pediatr Infect Dis J 16:409–411, 1997.

5. Wilson C: Immunologic basis for increased susceptibility of the neonate to infection. J Pediatr 108:1–12, 1986.

6. Pantell R, Newman T, Bernzweig J, et al: Management and outcomes of care of fever in early infancy. JAMA 291:1203–1212, 2004.

7. Newman T, Bernzweig J, Takayama J, et al: Urine testing and urinary tract infections in febrile infants seen in office settings: the Pediatric Research in Office Settings' Febrile Infant Study. Arch Pediatr Adolesc Med 156:44–54, 2002.

*8. Baker M, Bell L: Unpredictability of serious bacterial illness in febrile infants from birth to 1 month of age. Arch Pediatr Adolesc Med 153:508–511, 1999.

9. Kadish H, Loveridge B, Tobey J, et al: Applying outpatient protocols in febrile infants 1–28 days of age: can the threshold be lowered? Clin Pediatr (Phila) 39:81–88, 2000.

*10. Baraff L: Management of fever without a source in infants and children. Ann Emerg Med 36:602–614, 2000.

11. DeAngelis C, Joffe A, Wilson M, et al: Iatrogenic risks and financial costs of hospitalizing febrile infants. Am J Dis Child 137:1146–1149.

*12. Baker M: Evaluation and management of infants with fever. Pediatr Clin North Am 46:1061–1071.

*13. Baskin M, O'Rourke E, Fleisher G: Outpatient treatment of febrile infants 28–89 days of age with intramuscular administration of ceftriaxone. J Pediatr 120:22–27, 1992.

*14. Baker M, Bell L, Avner J: Outpatient management without antibiotics of fever in selected patients. N Engl J Med 329:1437–1441, 1993.

*15. Baker M, Bell L, Avner J: The efficacy of routine outpatient management without antibiotics of fever in selected infants. Pediatrics 103:627–631, 1999.

16. Dagan R, Powell K, Hall C, et al: Identification of infants unlikely to have serious bacterial infection although hospitalized for suspected sepsis. J Pediatr 107:855–860, 1985.

17. Jaskiewicz J, McCarthy C, Richardson A, et al: Febrile infants at low risk for serious bacterial infection: an appraisal of the Rochester criteria and implications for management. Pediatrics 94:390–396, 1994.

*18. Baraff L, Oslund S, Schriger D, et al: Probability of bacterial infections in febrile infants less than three months of age: a meta-analysis. Pediatr Infect Dis J 11:257–265, 1992.

19. McCarthy P, Sharpe M, Spiesel S, et al: Observation scales to identify serious illness in febrile children. Pediatrics 70:802–809, 1982.

20. Baker M, Avner J, Bell L: Failure of infant observation scales in detecting serious illness in febrile, 4- to 8-week old infants. Pediatrics 85:1040–1043, 1990.

21. Bonadio W: Incidence of serious infections in afebrile neonates with a history of fever. Pediatr Infect Dis J 6:911–914, 1987.

22. Bonadio W, Hegenbarth M, Zachariason M: Correlating reported fever in young infants with subsequent temperature patterns and rate of serious bacterial infections. Pediatr Infect Dis J 9:158–160, 1990

23. Fishman M: Evaluation of the child with neurologic disease. *In* Oski F, DeAngelis C, Feigin R, et al (eds): Principles and Practice of Pediatrics, 2nd ed. Philadelphia: JB Lippincott, 1994, p 2011.

24. Kupperman N, Fleisher GR, Jaffe DM: Predictors of occult pneumococcal bacteremia in young febrile children. Ann Emerg Med 31:679–687, 1998.

25. Rowe P: Laboratory values. *In* Oski F, DeAngelis C, Feigin R, et al (eds): Principles and Practice of Pediatrics, 2nd ed. Philadelphia: JB Lippincott, 1994, pp 2168–2169.

*26. Crain E, Bulas D, Bijur P, et al: Is a chest radiograph necessary in the evaluation of every febrile infant less than 8 weeks of age? Pediatrics 88:821–824, 1991.

27. Crain E, Shelov S: Febrile infants: predictors of bacteremia. J Pediatr 101:686–689, 1982.

*28. Crain E, Gershel J: Urinary tract infections in febrile infants younger than 8 weeks of age. Pediatrics 86:363–367, 1990.

29. Ahmed A, Brito F, Goto C, et al: Clinical utility of the polymerase chain reaction for diagnosis of enteroviral meningitis in infancy. J Pediatr 131:393–397, 1997.

30. Purcell K, Fergie J: Concurrent serious bacterial infections in 912 infants and children hospitalized for treatment of respiratory syncytial virus lower respiratory tract infection. Pediatr Infect Dis J 23:267–269, 2004.

*31. Levine D, Platt S, Dayan P, et al: Risk of serious bacterial infection in young febrile infants with respiratory syncytial virus infections. Pediatrics 113:1728–1734, 2004.

32. Liebelt E, Qi K, Harvey K: Diagnostic testing for serious bacterial infections in infants aged 90 days or younger with bronchiolitis. Arch Pediatr Adolesc Med 153:525–530, 1999.

33. Melendez E, Harper M: Utility of sepsis evaluation in infants 90 days of age or younger with fever and clinical bronchiolitis. Pediatr Infect Dis J 22:1053–1056, 2003.

*34. Byington D, Enriquez R, Hoff C, et al: Serious bacterial infections in febrile infants 1 to 90 days old with and without viral infections. Pediatrics 113:1662–1666, 2004.

*35. Titus M, Wright S: Prevalence of serious bacterial infections in febrile infants with respiratory syncytial virus infection. Pediatrics 112:282–284, 2003.

36. Klein J: Management of the febrile child without a focus of infection in the era of universal pneumococcal immunization. Pediatr Infect Dis J 21:584–588, 2002.

37. Black S, Shinefield H, Fireman B, et al: Efficacy, safety and immunogenicity of heptavalent pneumococcal conjugate vaccine in children. Pediatr Infect Dis J 19:187–195, 2000.

*38. American College of Emergency Physicians: Clinical policy for children younger than three years presenting to the emergency department with fever. Ann Emerg Med 42:530–545, 2003.

*Selected readings.

Chapter 33

Urinary Tract Infection in Infants

Rakesh D. Mistry, MD, MS and Marc H. Gorelick, MD, MSCE

Key Points

The classic triad of urinary tract infection (UTI)—fever, frequency, and dysuria—are rarely all present in infants and children; symptoms are often nonspecific.

UTI should be suspected in infants younger than 12 months of age with fever without source, especially if other risk factors are present, such as female sex, Caucasian race, >39°C, fever greater than 2 days, and, for males, being uncircumcised.

In children who are not toilet trained, urine specimen for culture should be obtained by urethral catheterization or suprapubic aspiration.

The majority of infants and children with UTI can safely be managed as outpatients.

Prompt identification and treatment of UTI can prevent potentially serious sequelae, including renal scarring and chronic renal failure.

Introduction and Background

Urinary tract infection (UTI) results when microorganisms infect usually sterile sites within the urinary tract. Bacterial pathogens are responsible for the majority of cases, and are the focus of this chapter; however, viruses, fungi, and, rarely, parasites may also infect the urinary tract. Infection may occur in the lower urinary tract (cystitis), or ascend into the upper tract to include the ureters and kidney (pyelonephritis). The presentation in infants and young children with UTI is often nonspecific, making the diagnosis challenging. Differentiation of upper versus lower tract infection can be especially difficult. Moreover, failure to diagnose UTI may result in significant long-term complications. Therefore, an astute approach to diagnosis and treatment of UTI in the pediatric population is of great importance to emergency physicians.

Recognition and Approach

Epidemiology

Acute UTI is the most commonly occurring serious bacterial illness in infants and young children. Rates of infection vary greatly with respect to age, gender, and race. Peak incidence is in infants less than 12 months of age, with UTI rates of approximately 40 per 1000 patients, after which the incidence decreases until adolescence. The incidence of UTI is equivalent in males and females until the age of 3 months, at which point the infection rate for males drops. From 3 to 12 months of age, there is a fourfold increased risk of UTI in females compared to males; between the ages of 1 and 3 years, females are 10 times more likely to have a UTI. Of note, males less than 12 months of age are 10 times more likely to develop UTI if they are uncircumcised.[1]

The overall prevalence of UTI in febrile infants less than 12 months of age evaluated in emergency departments has been estimated at 5%.[2,3] In addition to female gender, there is a higher prevalence in whites, patients with fever of ≥39°C, and absence of an alternative source of fever.

Pathophysiology

Bacterial invasion of the urinary tract primarily occurs via ascending infection. Enteric pathogens present in the stool, or flora present on the skin, enter the urinary tract via the urethral opening. Pathogens then ascend via the urethra into the bladder, where they multiply and produce a local infection of the lower urinary tract, known as cystitis. The offending pathogen may continue to ascend into the upper urinary tract and kidney via the ureters, leading to pyelonephritis. Although the overwhelming majority of UTI develops via the ascending route, infants may also develop infection via hematogenous spread.

Several host properties increase the likelihood of an ascending infection. The shorter urethra in females provides a more direct route for ascending infection. Uncircumcised males often have colonization of the prepuce, increasing the chance of entry of pathogens via the urethral meatus.[4] Decreased effectiveness of bladder emptying may also contribute to development of UTI. Patients with dysfunctional voiding, from neurogenic bladder or voluntary retention (e.g., in constipation) or from obstructive uropathies (e.g., posterior urethral valves), have impaired ability to clear bacteria that have ascended into the bladder. In addition, overdistention and increased bladder pressure facilitate movement of pathogens into the ureters, increasing the propensity for upper tract infection. Children with special needs, such as frequent self-catheterization, or with indwelling urinary catheters and hardware, are also more prone to UTI.

Etiology

Similar to adults, the most common pathogens isolated in pediatric UTI are gram-negative enteric organisms of the family Enterobacteriaceae. Of these, *Escherichia coli* accounts for approximately 80% of all UTIs in children. Other gram-negatives commonly isolated include *Klebsiella, Proteus, Serratia,* and *Enterobacter. Pseudomonas* species are a rare cause of UTI, usually found in patients that are immunosuppressed or frequently catheterized. Virulence factors that facilitate adherence to the urinary epithelium, produce local inflammation, and impair host phagocytosis and cell lysis are common in gram-negative pathogens, enhancing their ability to produce UTI. Gram-positive organisms less frequently produce UTI. Of these, *Enterococcus* species are the most frequent, while group A and B streptococci and *Staphylococcus* species are rare causes. It is important to note that patients with recurrent UTI may develop multidrug-resistant strains of any of the aforementioned pathogens.

Clinical Presentation

The clinical presentation of UTI can be quite variable in the pediatric age group, ranging from the so-called occult UTI to the classic presentations of cystitis and pyelonephritis. Children who are preverbal or have yet to develop urinary continence pose a unique challenge, since classic historical and physical findings often present in adults are not easily identified. Furthermore, infants and young children with UTI often manifest nonspecific symptoms that mimic other common viral illnesses. Irritability and poor feeding are common complaints, and vomiting and/or diarrhea is present in one third of infants with UTI.[5,6] Rarely, young infants may present with evidence of failure to thrive or jaundice.[7] Although a common complaint, parental report of malodorous urine has been found to be of questionable historical value.[5,8]

Fever is the most common presenting symptom of UTI in infants. Moreover, fever is increasingly being recognized as the lone symptom of UTI in infants. An estimated 5.9% to 7.5% of infants under the age of 12 months, presenting with fever without source, have a UTI.[2,3,9] Additionally, UTI is frequently found in infants presenting with other distinct clinical illnesses; in a prospective study by Shaw et al., physicians attributed fever to other sources of infection in 64% of infants prior to diagnosis of UTI.[3] More often than not the physical examination is unrevealing, further adding to the diagnostic challenge. Therefore, in these infants, consideration of UTI should be given in the presence of fever, with or without demonstrable source of infection.

The absence of clinical findings in infants and toddlers makes the distinction between cystitis and pyelonephritis difficult. Renal scintigraphy has demonstrated that up to 70% of children with febrile UTI have involvement of the kidney, leading to an increased incidence of renal scarring.[10] Therefore, all patients with UTI in this age group should be presumed to have pyelonephritis, and treated accordingly.

As the child becomes toilet-trained, the clinical presentation of UTI becomes less problematic. Urinary frequency, hesitancy, dysuria, suprapubic abdominal pain, and low-grade temperature are common complaints in preschool- and school-age children with cystitis. Secondary enuresis (bedwetting after the child has fully developed bladder control) may also be a subtle sign of UTI in this age group. The physical examination is generally unremarkable in simple cystitis, but may reveal tenderness over the suprapubic region of the abdomen. In contrast, older children with pyelonephritis often complain of fever, rigors, and flank pain in the region of the affected kidney, in addition to urinary symptoms of lower tract disease. Physical examination may reveal an ill appearance, fever, abdominal tenderness, and profound tenderness over the costovertebral angle of the affected kidney.

In children with suspected UTI, history and examination for potential predisposing conditions should be sought. Frequent UTI is common in patients with neurogenic bladder, dysfunctional voiding, and intermittent bladder catheterization. History should include assessment for known anatomic abnormalities of the genitourinary tract, such as obstruction of the ureteropelvic junction, hydronephrosis, and vesicoureteral reflux, all of which increase risk of UTI. Inquiry about the path and flow of the urine stream may be helpful. Typically, infants with posterior urethral valves have slow emptying and dribbling while urinating, as opposed to a constant urine stream. A history of poor hygiene should be sought in recently toilet-trained females, who often acquire UTI as a result of incorrect hygienic techniques. Constipation and encopresis are frequent cause of UTI in children, as a result of voluntary retention and bladder neck obstruction.

On physical examination, careful attention should be given to the abdomen and perineum. Examination may reveal an overdistended bladder or presence of a stool mass from fecal impaction. Additionally, identification of a flank mass may be a sign of ureteropelvic junction obstruction or hydronephrosis. Examination of the genitalia and urethra may reveal important clues, such as a meatal stenosis, circumcision status in males, and labial adhesions in females.

Differential Diagnosis

Because many signs and symptoms in infants and children are neither sensitive nor specific, the differential diagnosis of UTI is broad. Infants may have vomiting and diarrhea, similar to gastroenteritis. Irritability should elicit consideration of meningitis. Dysuria and urinary frequency are often present with UTI, yet may be present in several other conditions. In females, vulvovaginitis and retained vaginal foreign bodies may present with dysuria. Erythema and inflammation of the introitus and labia, the presence of vaginal discharge, and a history of poor hygiene or bubble baths may provide important clues for these conditions. Exclusion of potential sexual abuse is also appropriate, as these children may present with urinary complaints. Young males with epididymitis may also complain of dysuria, and have sterile pyuria. For both genders, inflammatory processes of the abdomen, such as appendicitis, may produce irritability, vomiting, and pyuria on urine analysis, and should be considered and appropriately excluded. Urinary frequency also should prompt consideration of metabolic conditions such as diabetes mellitus, diabetes insipidus, and hypercalcemia, although these diseases are rare. Impaired bladder distention from constipation, abdominal mass, or pregnancy may also produce urinary frequency.

Diagnosis and Testing

In older children and adolescents, the presence of signs and symptoms suggestive of UTI make the decision to perform tests to investigate for UTI relatively straightforward. The diagnosis of UTI in children under 2 years of age is less obvious. The inability to verbalize symptoms, lack of reliability of the physical examination, and high prevalence of UTI presenting as fever alone illustrate the need for accurate and reliable diagnostic testing strategies.

Physicians must have a reasonable index of suspicion but be selective in testing for possible UTI in febrile children less than 2 years of age. The results of large, emergency department–based studies have determined several risk factors for UTI in this subset of children. Female infants carry an increased risk of UTI with age ≤ 12 months, Caucasian race, ill appearance, fever ≥ 39°C, duration of fever ≥ 2 days, and absence of an alternative source of fever.[2,3,11,12] White females without ascertainable source of their fever incur the highest risk of occult UTI, estimated at 15% to 20%. Using these risk factors, a clinical decision rule has been developed and validated to optimize testing strategies for febrile young females.[12,13] The presence of three or more of these risk factors has a sensitivity of 88% and specificity of 30% in identifying UTI. This allows the physician to effectively identify a select population of febrile female infants for which testing is indicated, thereby decreasing the need for unnecessary tests and minimizing missed cases of UTI. For febrile male infants, no valid clinical decision rule for detection of UTI currently exists. Risk factors for UTI in male infants have been clearly identified, including age ≤ 6 months, absence of alternative source of fever,[2,3] and being uncircumcised.[1,3,9,14] Therefore, testing should be strongly considered in febrile male infants with the presence of these characteristics. The threshold for testing should be lower in children with a history of recurrent UTI, urogenital abnormality, recent bladder catheterization, or prolonged, unexplained fevers.

Isolation of pathogenic bacteria from the normally sterile urine is the "gold standard" for diagnosis of UTI. Therefore, growth of a pathogenic organism in urine culture indicates the presence of UTI. The difficulty in obtaining sterile urine for culture remains problematic, as a result of contamination. Clinicians need to be aware of the variation in interpretation of urine culture based on the method of collection.

Urine may be obtained via the midstream clean-catch method in cooperative children, and the results are quite accurate[15] if appropriately done. Unfortunately, contamination rates of urine obtained via clean catch may approach 30%, depending on technique.[16-18] As a result of potential contamination, permissive definitions of a positive culture are used. Growth of ≥ 10^5 colony-forming units (CFU) of a urinary tract pathogen in culture is considered definitive for UTI using the clean-catch method. If there is a question as to the results of the culture, because of either mixed pathogens or isolation of an unusual urinary pathogen, the culture should be repeated.

In infants and young children, the clean-catch method is not feasible, and urine must be collected directly by urethral catheterization or suprapubic aspiration. Because it is safe, rapid, and easily performed, urethral catheterization is currently the preferred urine collection method for infants and young children in the emergency department. Although better than the clean-catch method, contamination may still occur, and the classification of a positive urine culture is still not absolute. Using urethral catheterization, growth of ≥ 10^4 CFU of a pathogen is considered definitely positive; 10^3 to 10^4 CFU of a single pathogen is considered suspicious for UTI and should be correlated with the clinical picture. Suprapubic aspiration remains the most specific method of collection of urine for culture. When performed correctly, there is virtually no risk of contamination. Therefore, presence of any bacteria in culture obtained via suprapubic aspiration is considered a UTI. The suprapubic method is rarely used due to technical demands, invasiveness, and relatively equivalent performance to urethral catheterization.[19] Culture of urine via the bag collection method is not recommended; urine samples collected via the bag method are frequently contaminated, with rates as high as 87%.[9,20,21]

Unfortunately for the emergency physician, results of urine culture are not available for 24 to 48 hours. Therefore, several rapid screening techniques have been developed to identify children at risk for UTI. The urine dipstick is inexpensive and can be performed at the bedside. Two components of the dipstick are useful for diagnosis of UTI: nitrites, which are formed by common urinary tract pathogens, and leukocyte esterase (LE), a product of urinary leukocytes. Nitrites are assessed as positive or negative, and LE is typically scored from trace to 4+. When used in combination, nitrites and LE perform very well as a screening method for UTI. The presence of any nitrites *or* LE has a sensitivity of 80% to 88%.[22-26] When used individually, nitrites have a specificity of 98%, and 2+ or greater LE has a specificity of 84%; when used in combination, the specificity of nitrite *and* 2+ or greater LE is 96% to 99%.[23,26] Microscopic urinalysis of centrifuged and uncentrifuged urine are common methods used to detect pyuria (≥10 white blood cells per high-power field or per cubic millimeter, respectively). However, both methods of microscopic urinalysis have consistently demonstrated specificity and sensitivity inferior to the urine dipstick in infants.[23,26] Identification of any bacteria via Gram stain of uncentrifuged urine has a high sensitivity and specificity, similar to that of the urine dipstick,[23,27] but is more expensive, technically difficult, and operator dependent. Recent investigations have cited superior sensitivity of enhanced urinalysis, which combines properties of conventional microscopic analysis and Gram stain. False-positive rates are higher than that of the urine dipstick,[23,26,28,29] and enhanced urinalysis is the most expensive and least available method of screening. In summary, the urine dipstick appears to be the most useful of all screening tests. The false-negative rates for all screening tests preclude ruling out UTI based on their results; urine cultures should be sent for on any patient with suspected UTI.

Use of serum tests, such as complete blood count, C-reactive protein, and erythrocyte sedimentation rate, are nonspecific for UTI, and may only provide adjunctive evidence in the setting of the clinical presentation. Blood cultures are more likely to be positive in infants less than 6 months of age,[30] although the clinical course of UTI appears to be unaffected by the presence of bacteremia.[31,32]

Imaging

Several imaging modalities are available for evaluation of the kidneys and urinary tract, including renal cortical scintigraphy with technetium-99m–labled dimercaptosuccinic acid ("renal scan"), renal ultrasound, and voiding cystourethrogram (VCUG). Regardless of clinical symptoms, renal scans have demonstrated that between 70% and 80% of infants with UTI have pyelonephritis[10,33,34]; however, this does not appear to affect subsequent management or outcome. Although imaging may assist in diagnosis of pyelonephritis, the use of imaging in the emergency department setting is of limited value. Renal scanning in the emergency department may be of value when the diagnosis of UTI is unclear. Emergency department renal ultrasound or CT scan is helpful when considering the presence of an abscess.

Although imaging studies are rarely indicated in the emergency department, they do have an important role in the subsequent evaluation of children with UTI. It is estimated that 20% to 49% of infants with first-time UTI will have an abnormality detected by renal ultrasound or VCUG, including vesicoureteral reflux, duplicated collecting systems, and obstructive uropathies, such as posterior urethral valves or ureteropelvic junction obstruction.[5,35,36] As a result, the American Academy of Pediatrics published guidelines in 1999 recommending routine performance of renal ultrasound and VCUG for all children 2 to 24 months of age after first-time UTI.[37] The findings of a recent prospective trial of infants and young children with UTI suggest that the presence of urinary tract abnormalities does not significantly influence patient management or outcome.[38] Further studies will be needed to determine the usefulness of imaging after UTI. In addition, the issue of optimal timing for these imaging studies—during the acute UTI or after resolution of inflammation—has yet to be resolved.

Important Clinical Features and Considerations

Clinical Pearls

Maintenance of a high index of suspicion by the emergency physician is essential for diagnosis of UTI in the infants and young children. When cases of UTI are missed in infants, it is usually a result of nonspecific presentations or failure to perform screening tests as indicated.

As mentioned earlier, fever may be the only evidence of UTI in infants and young children, and is the most common presenting symptom. In addition, the physical examination is most notable for the lack of physical findings. Therefore, detection of UTI is highly dependent on the clinician's knowledge of risk factors for occult UTI.

Lack of screening, secondary to the presence of a potential source of fever, is another common pitfall. It is important to recall that, among patients less than 1 year of age, UTI still occurs at greater than baseline risk, even in the setting of an upper respiratory infection, gastroenteritis, or otitis media. Attributing fever to other concurrent illnesses, without consideration of other risk factors, can lead to missed diagnosis of UTI.

Common childhood illnesses can easily confound the clinical picture of UTI in infants. Vomiting and diarrhea are common symptoms of UTI as well, and misdiagnosis of gastroenteritis is possible. Diarrhea occurs in UTI from the local inflammation of the bowel by an infected bladder and/or kidney. Irritability may lead the physician to the diagnosis of meningitis; in fact, cerebrospinal fluid pleocytosis has been reported in infants with UTI.[39]

Potential Complications

The primary complication of UTI is renal scarring, which may lead to hypertension, impaired renal function, and end-stage renal failure. Renal scarring is described even after a single, first-time UTI, and is increased with presence of urinary tract abnormalities. The risk of complications from renal scarring is significantly increased with recurrent episodes of UTI and pyelonephritis.[4,40] Recurrence of UTI is not uncommon, occurring in 20% to 40% of patients after first-time infection, usually within the first 6 months after the initial UTI.[41-44] Reinfection rates are highest in patients under 1 year of age, especially females. Patients with anatomic abnormality of the urinary tract, such as high-grade vesicoureteral reflux,[45,46] are at increased risk for reinfection, although recurrences may occur in the setting of normal anatomy.[43] Recurrent UTI also significantly increases the risk of renal scarring and sequelae, further emphasizing the importance of accurate diagnosis early in life. Fortunately, renal function is generally preserved with adequate treatment of the UTI and underlying abnormalities.[47,48]

Management

The majority of infants and children with UTI will not be acutely ill. Nevertheless, because of the nonspecific clinical picture of UTI, infants and young children may present to the emergency department late in their illness, and appear quite ill or toxic from concomitant sepsis or dehydration. Therefore, initial management should focus on stabilization of the "ABCs." Intravenous fluid resuscitation may be necessary, especially if there is a history of frequent emesis or fluid losses. Once the patient is physiologically stable, attention can be turned to more specific therapies.

Prompt recognition and early treatment of UTI reduces the risk of renal scarring and associated sequelae[44,49]; its importance cannot be overemphasized. Emergency physicians must maintain a high index of suspicion, and have an astute, systematic approach to identify infants and young children at high risk for UTI. A clinically sensible strategy, using current knowledge of risk factors and performance of available screening tests, is presented in Figure 33–1. This approach identifies patients at high risk for UTI, allowing for empirical therapy with minimal overtreatment. Despite fair sensitivity of screening tests, a urine culture should still be obtained in all cases of suspected UTI.

Antibiotic therapy should be guided by local resistance patterns of known urinary tract pathogens. Fortunately, the majority of known pathogens are sensitive to commonly available antibiotics (Table 33–1). Importantly, despite frequent resistance of urinary pathogens, the kidneys concentrate the majority of antibiotics, resulting in urinary concentration. In the clinical setting, these high concentrations often overcome pathogen resistance. Duration of antibiotic therapy is 10 to 14 days; short-course regimens are not recommended for infants and young children since effectiveness of shorter regimens has not been established in children.[50]

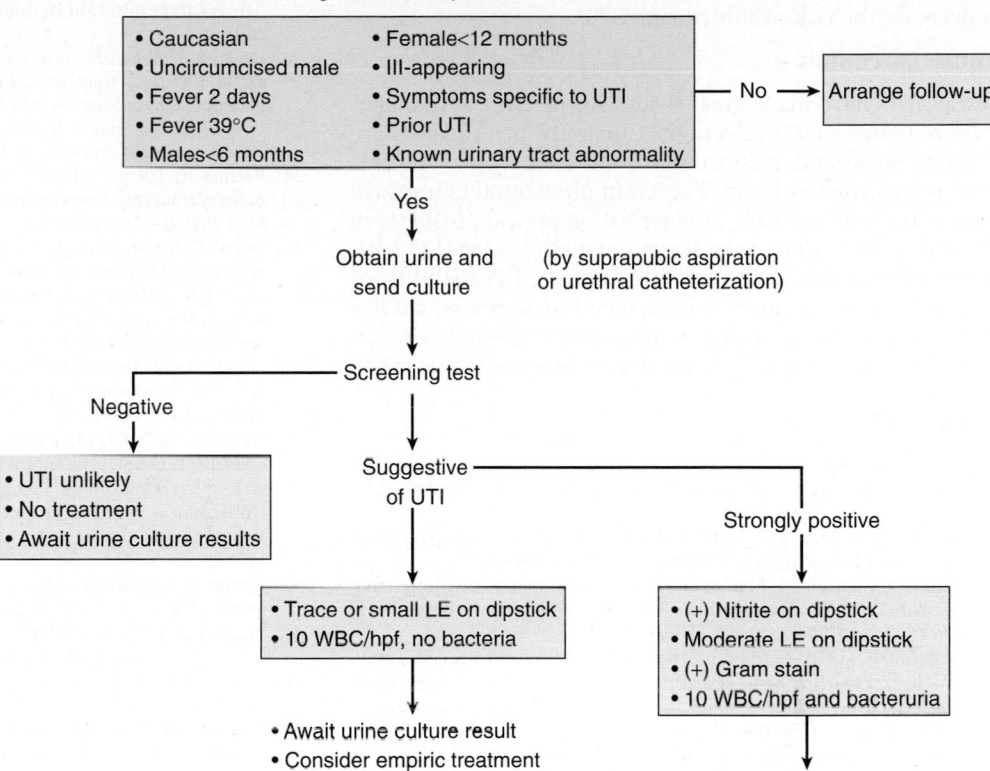

FIGURE 33–1. Screening for urinary tract infection (UTI) in febrile children ages 2 to 23 months in the emergency department. Abbreviations: hpf, high-power field; LE, leukocyte esterase; WBC, white blood cells. (Modified from Shaw KN, Gorelick MH: Urinary tract infection in the pediatric patient. Pediatr Clin North Am 46:1119, 1999.)

Table 33–1	Commonly Prescribed Antibiotics for Urinary Tract Infection
Drug	**Usual Dosage (per day)**
Oral	
cotrimoxazole	8–10 mg/kg of trimethoprim divided bid
nitrofurantoin	5–7 mg/kg divided qid
sulfisoxazole	120–150 mg/kg divided qid
cefixime	8 mg/kg once daily
cefdinir	14 mg/kg once daily
cephalexin	25–50 mg/kg divided qid
Parenteral	
ampicillin	100 mg/kg divided qid
gentamicin	7.5 mg/kg divided tid
ceftriaxone	50–100 mg/kg once daily
cefotaxime	150 mg/kg divided tid

Abbreviations: bid, two times a day; tid, three times a day; qid, four times a day.
From Shaw KN, Gorelick MH: Urinary tract infection in the pediatric patient. Pediatr Clin North Am 46:1120, 1999.

The decision to treat infants with pyelonephritis with parenteral antibiotics is debatable. Previously, the most children with pyelonephritis were admitted for intravenous antibiotic therapy. Recent studies using cefixime now suggest that infants over 2 months of age may be safely managed as outpatients, without affecting the natural course of the illness or increasing the risk of recurrence and renal scarring.[51] Inpatient therapy is still recommended for infants under 2 months of age, as there is a paucity of evidence supporting outpatient therapy. Inpatient therapy should be also considered for patients who are ill appearing, dehydrated, vomiting, or unable to tolerate oral antibiotics, have known urologic abnormality, are at risk for poor compliance, or have failed outpatient therapy. Supportive therapy includes hydration, fever control, and pain management. Acetaminophen and/or ibuprofen is adequate for pain and fever in most cases. Phenazopyridine is an effective urinary analgesic; however, its usefulness is limited to older children, since it is only available in tablet form.

Summary

Prognosis

With treatment, the outcome of pediatric UTI is uniformly excellent. UTI generally follows a benign clinical course, with defervescence usually occurring within 24 to 48 hours. The urine usually becomes sterile within 48 hours after onset of treatment, although test of cure is not necessary if the patient is clinically improved.[52]

The importance of follow-up for infants and children with UTI cannot be understated. During follow-up, those at high risk for future UTI can be identified and appropriately managed, decreasing the potential complications associated with renal scarring. After the emergency department visit, routine follow-up will ensure resolution of symptoms, hydration status, and compliance with therapy. At this time, physicians may elect to perform imaging studies on patients with first-time UTI. In the setting of a detected urinary tract abnormality, many physicians institute antibiotic prophylaxis until definitive repair is completed, in an effort to decrease the risk of subsequent UTI.

Future Directions

Researchers have made great strides in the clinical management of urinary tract infections. Currently, investigators are focusing on several areas to improve the emergency department management of UTI. The use of ultrasound to improve success rates of urethral catheterization appears to be very promising. Development of screening methods for UTI with improved sensitivity, and possible increased availability of enhanced urinalysis are still necessary. Furthermore, studies are already being conducted to determine the safety of outpatient management of UTI for infants less than 2 months.

REFERENCES

1. Wiswell TE, Roscelli JD: Corroborative evidence for the decreased incidence of urinary tract infections in circumcised male infants. Pediatrics 78:96–99, 1986.
*2. Hoberman A, Chao HP, Keller DM, et al: Prevalence of urinary tract infection in febrile infants. J Pediatr 123:17–23, 1993.
*3. Shaw KN, Gorelick M, McGowan KL, et al: Prevalence of urinary tract infection in febrile young children in the emergency department. Pediatrics 102:e16, 1998.
*4. Rushton HG: Urinary tract infections in children: epidemiology, evaluation, and management. Pediatr Clin North Am 44:1133–1169, 1997.
5. Ginsburg CM, McCracken GH Jr: Urinary tract infections in young infants. Pediatrics 69:409–412, 1982.
6. McCracken GH Jr: Diagnosis and management of acute urinary tract infections in infants and children. Pediatr Infect Dis J 6:107–112, 1987.
7. Garcia FJ, Nager AL: Jaundice as an early diagnostic sign of urinary tract infection in infancy. Pediatrics 109:846–851, 2002.
8. Struthers S, Scanlon J, Parker K, et al: Parental reporting of smelly urine and urinary tract infection. Arch Dis Child 88:250–252, 2003.
9. Crain EF, Gershel JC: Urinary tract infections in febrile infants younger than 8 weeks of age. Pediatrics 86:363–367, 1990.
10. Benador D, Benador N, Slosman DO, et al: Cortical scintigraphy in the evaluation of renal parenchymal changes in children with pyelonephritis. J Pediatr 124:17–20, 1994.
11. Newman TB, Bernzweig JA, Takayama JI, et al: Urine testing and urinary tract infections in febrile infants seen in office settings: the Pediatric Research in Office Settings' Febrile Infant Study. Arch Pediatr Adolesc Med 156:44–54, 2002.
*12. Gorelick MH, Shaw KN: Clinical decision rule to identify febrile young girls at risk for urinary tract infection. Arch Pediatr Adolesc Med 154:386–390, 2000.
*13. Gorelick MH, Hoberman A, Kearney D, et al: Validation of a decision rule identifying febrile young girls at high risk for urinary tract infection. Pediatr Emerg Care 19:162–164, 2003.
14. To T, Agha M, Dick PT, Feldman W: Cohort study on circumcision of newborn boys and subsequent risk of urinary-tract infection. Lancet 352:1813–1816, 1998.
15. Aronson AS, Gustafson B, Svenningsen NW: Combined suprapubic aspiration and clean-voided urine examination in infants and children. Acta Paediatr Scand 62:396–400, 1973.
16. Lohr JA, Donowitz LG, Dudley SM: Bacterial contamination rates in voided urine collections in girls. J Pediatr 114:91–93, 1989.
17. Saez-Llorens X, Umana MA, Odio CM, Lohr JA: Bacterial contamination rates for non-clean-catch and clean-catch midstream urine collections in uncircumcised boys. J Pediatr 114:93–95, 1989.
18. Ramage IJ, Chapman JP, Hollman AS, et al: Accuracy of clean-catch urine collection in infancy. J Pediatr 135:765–767, 1999.
19. Pollack CV Jr, Pollack ES, Andrew ME: Suprapubic bladder aspiration versus urethral catheterization in ill infants: success, efficiency and complication rates. Ann Emerg Med 23:225–230, 1994.
20. Bonadio WA: Urine culturing technique in febrile infants. Pediatr Emerg Care 3:75–78, 1987.

21. Li PS, Ma LC, Wong SN: Is bag urine culture useful in monitoring urinary tract infection in infants? J Paediatr Child Health 38:377–381, 2002.
22. Doley A, Nelligan M: Is a negative dipstick urinalysis good enough to exclude urinary tract infection in paediatric emergency department patients? Emerg Med (Fremantle) 15(1):77–80, 2003.
*23. Gorelick MH, Shaw KN: Screening tests for urinary tract infection in children: a meta-analysis. Pediatrics 104:e54, 1999.
24. Bachur R, Harper MB: Reliability of the urinalysis for predicting urinary tract infections in young febrile children. Arch Pediatr Adolesc Med 155:60–65, 2001.
25. Craver RD, Abermanis JG: Dipstick only urinalysis screen for the pediatric emergency room. Pediatr Nephrol 11:331–333, 1997.
26. Shaw KN, McGowan KL, Gorelick MH, Schwartz JS: Screening for urinary tract infection in the emergency department: which test is best? Pediatrics 101:e1, 1998.
27. Lockhart GR, Lewander WJ, Cimini DM, et al: Use of urinary Gram stain for detection of urinary tract infection in infants. Ann Emerg Med 25:31–35, 1995.
28. Herr SM, Wald ER, Pitetti RD, Choi SS: Enhanced urinalysis improves identification of febrile infants ages 60 days and younger at low risk for serious bacterial illness. Pediatrics 108:866–871, 2001.
29. Hoberman A, Wald ER, Penchansky L, et al: Enhanced urinalysis as a screening test for urinary tract infection. Pediatrics 91:1196–1199, 1993.
30. Bachur R, Caputo GL: Bacteremia and meningitis among infants with urinary tract infections. Pediatr Emerg Care 11:280–284, 1995.
31. Pitetti RD, Choi S: Utility of blood cultures in febrile children with UTI. Am J Emerg Med 20:271–274, 2002.
32. Honkinen O, Jahnukainen T, Mertsola J, et al: Bacteremic urinary tract infection in children. Pediatr Infect Dis J 19:630–634, 2000.
33. Andrich MP, Majd M: Diagnostic imaging in the evaluation of the first urinary tract infection in infants and young children. Pediatrics 90:436–441, 1992.
34. Majd M, Rushton HG, Jantausch B, Wiedermann BL: Relationship among vesicoureteral reflux, P-fimbriated *Escherichia coli,* and acute pyelonephritis in children with febrile urinary tract infection. J Pediatr 119:578–585, 1991.
35. Goldman M, Lahat E, Strauss S, et al: Imaging after urinary tract infection in male neonates. Pediatrics 105:1232–1235, 2000.
36. Dick PT, Feldman W: Routine diagnostic imaging for childhood urinary tract infections: a systematic overview. J Pediatr 128:15–22, 1996.
*37. Practice parameter: the diagnosis, treatment, and evaluation of the initial urinary tract infection in febrile infants and young children. American Academy of Pediatrics, Committee on Quality Improvement, Subcommittee on Urinary Tract Infection. Pediatrics 103(4 Pt 1):843–852, 1999.
38. Hoberman A, Charron M, Hickey RW, et al: Imaging studies after a first febrile urinary tract infection in young children. N Engl J Med 348:195–202, 2003.
39. Syrogiannopoulos GA, Grivea IN, Anastassiou ED, et al: Sterile cerebrospinal fluid pleocytosis in young infants with urinary tract infection. Pediatr Infect Dis J 20:927–930, 2001.
40. Winberg J, Bergstrom T, Jacobsson B: Morbidity, age and sex distribution, recurrences and renal scarring in symptomatic urinary tract infection in childhood. Kidney Int Suppl 4:S101–S106, 1975.
41. Hellerstein S: Recurrent urinary tract infections in children. Pediatr Infect Dis 1:271–281, 1982.
42. Mingin GC, Hinds A, Nguyen HT, Baskin LS: Children with a febrile urinary tract infection and a negative radiologic workup: factors predictive of recurrence. Urology 63:562–565; discussion 565, 2004.
43. Bratslavsky G, Feustel PJ, Aslan AR, Kogan BA: Recurrence risk in infants with urinary tract infections and a negative radiographic evaluation. J Urol 172(4 Pt 2):1610–1613; discussion 1613, 2004.
44. Winberg J, Bollgren I, Kallenius G, et al: Clinical pyelonephritis and focal renal scarring: a selected review of pathogenesis, prevention, and prognosis. Pediatr Clin North Am 29:801–814, 1982.
45. Cascio S, Chertin B, Colhoun E, Puri P: Renal parenchymal damage in male infants with high grade vesicoureteral reflux diagnosed after the first urinary tract infection. J Urol 168(4 Pt 2):1708–1710; discussion 1710, 2002.
46. Nuutinen M, Uhari M: Recurrence and follow-up after urinary tract infection under the age of 1 year. Pediatr Nephrol 16:69–72, 2001.

*Selected readings.

47. Rushton HG, Majd M, Jantausch B, et al: Renal scarring following reflux and nonreflux pyelonephritis in children: evaluation with ^{99m}technetium-dimercaptosuccinic acid scintigraphy. J Urol 147:1327–1332, 1992.

48. Wennerstrom M, Hansson S, Jodal U, et al: Renal function 16 to 26 years after the first urinary tract infection in childhood. Arch Pediatr Adolesc Med 154:339–345, 2000.

49. Bartkowski DP: Recognizing UTIs in infants and children: early treatment prevents permanent damage. Postgrad Med 109:171–172, 177–181, 2001.

50. Keren R, Chan E: A meta-analysis of randomized, controlled trials comparing short- and long-course antibiotic therapy for urinary tract infections in children. Pediatrics 109:e70, 2002.

51. Hoberman A, Wald ER, Hickey RW, et al: Oral versus initial intravenous therapy for urinary tract infections in young febrile children. Pediatrics 104(1 Pt 1):79–86, 1999.

52. Currie ML, Mitz L, Raasch CS, Greenbaum LA: Follow-up urine cultures and fever in children with urinary tract infection. Arch Pediatr Adolesc Med 157:1237–1240, 2003.

Stridor in Infancy

Antonio E. Muñiz, MD

Introduction and Background

Stridor is an audible harsh, high-pitched musical sound produced by turbulent airflow through a partially obstructed upper airway. During inspiration, areas of the airway that are easily collapsible (e.g., supraglottic region) are "suctioned" closed due to negative intraluminal pressure generated during inspiration. These same areas are forced open during expiration. For this reason, disorders causing supraglottic obstruction (e.g., epiglottis) cause stridor that is mostly heard on inspiration. The glottic and subglottic airway extends from the vocal cords to the extrathoracic trachea. This part of the airway has firmer cartilaginous support and does not collapse, and its shape does not easily change with inspiration. Stridor that occurs due to glottic (e.g., croup) and tracheal (e.g., tracheitis) disorders is often biphasic or heard during both inspiration and expiration. The intrathoracic airway is composed of the trachea, which lies within the thorax, and the mainstem bronchi. Obstruction at these sites causes stridor that is loudest on expiration since intrathoracic pressure rises on expiration and tends to collapse airway structures.

Important characteristics of airway disorders have been used to differentiate between disorders causing stridor in infants and children.

Age

Congenital disorders (e.g., tracheomalacia, laryngomalacia) present in the first few weeks of life. By 6 months of age, infants begin to explore their environment and place objects in their mouth. The ability to grasp objects improves until a distinct pincer grasp is present in most 1-year-old infants. These developmental aspects contribute to foreign body aspiration that peaks by 2 to 3 years of age. Croup also occurs mostly in infants under the age of 3 years. Retropharyngeal abscesses are most common in those under age 4 since retropharyngeal lymph nodes are present at this age, often disappearing by age 4 to 5 years. Prior to introduction of an effective *Haemophilus influenzae* type b vaccine, epiglottis generally occurred in children 2 to 7 years old. Since the introduction of this vaccine, the overall incidence of epiglottis has dropped substantially.

Acuity

An immediate onset of stridor in an appropriately aged child suggests foreign body ingestion or angioedema. Epiglottitis can produce an acute onset of stridor, although children often have a 1- to 2-day prodrome prior to development of airway obstruction.

Infants with stridor due to or preceded by viral infections (croup, tracheitis, retropharyngeal abscess) often have several days to 1 week of cough, congestion, and rhinorrhea prior to development of stridor.

Appearance

Serious bacterial infections (e.g., epiglottitis, airway abscesses, diphtheria, tracheitis) are a likely cause of stridor in infants and children who are toxic appearing, with apprehension, air hunger, and tripoding (holding self up with extended arms). Children with viral infections such as croup are usually not toxic appearing, although airway edema may become severe enough to cause hypoxia and a more toxic appearance.

Associated Symptoms

Serious bacterial infections are associated with the presence of a fever, while foreign bodies and congenital disorders do not cause a temperature elevation. However, temperature alone cannot be used to discriminate between serious and mild infections. Up to 25% of children with epiglottis and airway abscess are not febrile on initial presentation to a physician, while a significant number of children with croup have an elevated temperature.

Supraglottic obstructions block sounds exiting the glottis and the opening to the esophagus. For this reason, these obstructions (e.g., airway abscess, epiglottitis) can cause a muffled voice and drooling. Hyoid pain and tenderness are present in most cases of epiglottitis. Aspirated foreign bodies are one type of subglottic obstruction that can lead to drooling due to direct compression of the esophagus. Hoarseness is due to inflammation of the vocal cords and is associated with glottic and subglottic disorders. A cough also is associated with glottic and subglottic disorders, while its presence makes epiglottitis less likely.

Acoustics

Stridor during inspiration implicates supraglottic obstruction, biphasic stridor[1] implies glottic or subglottic obstruction, and expiratory stridor is often due to intrathoracic obstruction. Stridor that changes its pattern and timing may be due to an obstruction that is migrating (e.g., foreign body). While some experts state that pitch and frequency are useful in locating the source or cause of stridor, pitch has not been found to be a discriminator.

Air-Shadow Interface—Radiography

Infants and children with stridor who have the potential to develop obstruction of their airway require portable radiography. Alternately, they must be accompanied by appropriate resuscitation equipment (e.g., bag-valve mask) and personnel who can manage an obstructed airway while being transported to the radiology department. An appropriate soft tissue lateral film of the neck requires neck extension during the terminal phase of inspiration. Clinicians must realize that this position can obstruct an already compromised obstructed airway.

Classic plain radiographic findings of epiglottis include an enlarged epiglottis with the appearance of a thumb, enlarged aryepiglottic folds, and a ballooned hypopharynx. However, these findings are subjective and may not be noted on initial plain films in up to 50% of patients. Objective findings that may be more accurate in diagnosing epiglottitis on lateral radiography include an epiglottite width–to–third cervical vertebral width ratio greater than 0.5, or an aryepiglottic width–to–third cervical vertebral body width ratio greater than 0.35.

Radiographic findings described with retropharyngeal abscesses include a retropharyngeal space greater than 7 mm anterior to the inferior border of the second vertebral body and a retrotracheal space greater than 14 mm anterior to the inferior border of the sixth cervical vertebral body. Other plain radiographic findings include soft tissue air-fluid levels and cervical retroflexion. Computed tomography is more accurate than plain films in identifying abscesses but requires patient stability and the ability to maintain a supine position.

Soft tissue radiography is often used to evaluate children with croup, with up to 50% of pediatricians routinely obtaining plain films in infants and children with this disorder. However, plain films are often misleading or nondiagnostic in this disorder. One study that examined radiologists' interpretations of plain films found that 24% to 28% of children with croup had plain films interpreted as possible epiglottis, while only 33% to 38% of plain films were called croup.[2] Thus plain films should not be relied upon to diagnose this disorder.

A final important use for plain films is to detect aspirated foreign bodies. Unfortunately, less than 10% of aspirated foreign bodies are radiopaque. Therefore, the clinician should not rely on normal plain films to exclude an airway foreign body when there is a strong clinical suspicion.

Airway Visualization

In the past, it was taught that direct visualization of the pharynx and use of a tongue blade or mirror to examine the airway were hazardous techniques to be avoided in children with stridor, especially if epiglottitis was a possibility. Laryngospasm involving children with epiglottitis was rare, and only occurred in children who were in extremis and already required immediate airway management.[3] Moreover, there has never been a case of laryngospasm in over 1000 adult cases of epiglottis who underwent direct visualization.[4] Two series with more than 120 children with epiglottis showed that no complications occurred during direct laryngoscope visualization with care taken not to touch the epiglottis and hypopharynx.[5] Importantly, these series indicate that the majority of stable children will tolerate careful laryngoscopy or application of a tongue blade to the middle or anterior tongue. Only clinicians who are skilled with pediatric airway management should perform these techniques. Importantly, it is best to only consider using direct visualization in children with a moderate to low suspicion of epiglottis who are deemed clinically stable.

Stridor may occur in a wide variety of disease processes (Table 34–1). It is also important to categorize the differential to exclude those that are life-threatening when evaluating any infant who presents with stridor (Table 34–2).

This chapter presents the causes of stridor in infancy and provides a practical approach to their diagnoses and management.

Croup (Laryngotracheobronchitis)

Recognition and Approach

Croup is an acute viral infection characterized by a barklike cough, hoarseness, inspiratory stridor, and respiratory distress that can range from mild to severe respiratory failure. This infection involves primarily the larynx and may extend into the trachea and bronchi. It is the most common etiology for stridor in the febrile infant. Although the disease is most often self-limited, it may lead to severe airway obstruction and death.

Croup typically occurs in children ages 6 months to 3 years, with a mean age of 18 months. There is a male predominance with a ratio of 2 : 1. This syndrome typically occurs in late fall and early winter.

The most common organism causing croup is parainfluenza virus type 1 which is recovered in 60 % of cases.[6] Mild sporadic cases are caused by parainfluenza type 2 and 3, influenza A, adenoviruses, measles, rhinovirus, echovirus, reovirus, coxsackievirus, respiratory syncytial virus, metapneumovirus, and *micoplasma pneumoniae*.[7,8] Influenza A has been implicated in children with severe respiratory compromise.

Transmission of the causative virus is by the respiratory route. The initial port of entry is the nose and nasopharynx. The infection spreads to the larynx and trachea, and their

Table 34–1	Differential Diagnoses of Stridor
Location	**Etiology**
Nose and Pharynx	
Congenital anomalies	Lingual thyroid, choanal atresia, craniofacial anomalies (Apert's, Down syndrome, Pierre Robin syndrome), cysts (dermoid, thyroglossal)
Inflammatory/infectious	Abscess (peritonsillar, retropharyngeal, parapharyngeal), allergic polyps, diphtheria, uvulitis, infectious mononucleosis
Other	Adenotonsillar hyperplasia, foreign body, decreased muscle coordination from neurologic syndrome
Larynx	
Congenital anomalies	Laryngomalacia, laryngeal web, laryngeal cyst, laryngocele, cartilage dystrophy, subglottic stenosis, cleft larynx, hemangioma
Inflammatory/infectious	Croup, epiglottitis, tracheitis, angioneurotic edema, tuberculosis, diphtheria, sarcoidosis
Vocal cord paralysis	Congenital or traumatic
Neoplasm	Subglottic hemangioma, laryngeal papilloma, cystic hygroma, malignant (rhabdomyosarcoma), neurofibromas
Laryngospasm	Hypocalcemic tetany, irritant, drug effect, spasmodic croup
Foreign body	Laryngeal or upper esophageal
Trauma	Laryngeal fracture or dislocation, hematoma, inhalation injury
Trachea and Bronchi	
Congenital	Vascular anomalies, webs, cysts, tracheal stenosis, tracheoesophageal fistula
Neoplasm	Tracheal, compression from adjacent tumors (thyroid, thymus, esophageal)
Inflammatory/infectious	Bacterial tracheitis
Foreign body	Tracheal or esophageal
Other	
	Psychogenic stridor Hemophilia (hematoma) Cervical spinal trauma Caustic ingestion

Table 34–2	Life-Threatening Causes of Stridor
Croup Epiglottitis Tracheitis Foreign body Angioneurotic edema Neck trauma Laryngeal, tracheal or bronchial trauma Neoplasm (compressing trachea) Thermal or caustic burns	

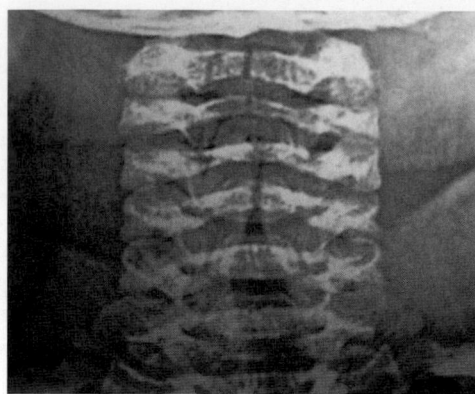

FIGURE 34–1. "Steeple sign" in croup.

mise due to an already narrowed diameter of the airway, especially in the region of the cricoid cartilage. Hypoxemia may occur from progressive luminal narrowing, and impaired alveolar ventilation and ventilation-perfusion mismatch.

Clinical Presentation

The prodrome lasts a few days and consists of a mild upper respiratory infection with fever, coryza, and cough. It is followed by the development of a hoarse voice and harsh, brassy "seal's bark" cough. Stridor usually develops at night, often awakening the child from sleep and frightening the parents.

The patient's symptoms range from minimal inspiratory stridor to severe respiratory failure secondary to airway obstruction. In mild cases, respiratory sounds at rest are normal; however, mild expiratory wheezing may be heard. Children with more severe cases have inspiratory and expiratory stridor at rest with suprasternal, intercostal, and subcostal retractions. Air entry may be poor. Lethargy or agitation may be a result of hypoxemia. Other warning signs of severe respiratory disease are tachypnea, tachycardia out of proportion to fever, and hypotonia. Children may be unable to maintain adequate oral intake, which results in dehydration. Cyanosis is often a late ominous sign. In uncomplicated cases the illness lasts 4 to 7 days.

The white blood cell count is generally normal; however, lymphocytosis may occur. In mild cases, transcutaneous oximetry is usually normal, but hypoxemia exists with severe disease. Arterial blood gases are unnecessary and show neither hypoxia nor hypercarbia unless respiratory fatigue ensues.

In typical cases, radiographs are not required for the diagnosis of croup, unless the diagnosis is in question. Lateral soft tissue radiographs of the neck may show subglottic narrowing from soft tissue edema in severe disease, but most are normal or may show overdistention (ballooning) of the hypopharynx during inspiration. The anteroposterior view of the neck will show narrowing of the laryngeal air column for about 5 to 10 mm below the level of the vocal cord ("steeple sign") in 50% to 60% of cases[9] (Fig. 34–1).

Complications in croup occur in only a small minority of patients. The most common is worsening airway obstruction, which is seen in infants or young children. The inflammation may extend into the lower airway, causing wheezing and tachypnea. Pneumonia is uncommon and usually associated with bacterial tracheitis.[10] Other complications include

walls become erythematous and edematous. There is endothelial damage and loss of ciliary function. A fibrinous exudate partially occludes the lumen of the trachea. In addition to luminal narrowing, edema of the vocal cords and subglottic larynx leads to stridor, hoarseness, and the characteristic barklike cough. The edema formation in young children and infants will lead to a significant airway compro-

lymphadenitis and otitis media. Inability to maintain adequate oral intake may lead to dehydration.

Management

Any infant who presents with respiratory complaints must have a good evaluation to ensure the patency of the airway and maintenance of effective oxygenation and ventilation. Infants with severe respiratory distress or compromise require 100% oxygenation with ventilation support using a bag-valve-mask device. If the airway and breathing require continued maintenance, the patient should be intubated with an endotracheal tube.

Most children with croup have no stridor at rest and can be managed as outpatients. Gentle handling and avoidance of unnecessary painful procedures should be the rule since persistent crying increases oxygen demands and respiratory muscle fatigue, and makes the obstruction worse. Careful monitoring of the heart rate, respiratory rate, respiratory mechanics, and pulse oximetry are important to detect early hypoxia. Use of a croup score may aid in management[11-13] (Table 34-3).

Providing high humidity has not been proven clinically to be effective but seems to be beneficial in most children.[14-18] It works by providing water droplets that penetrate the area of inflammation and deliver moisture to the mucosa. Increasing humidity will decrease the viscosity of the secretions in the trachea, which facilitates clearance from the airways. Cool mist may activate mechanoreceptors in the larynx that produce a reflex slowing of respiratory flow rate. Methods used to deliver high humidity include a croup tent, croupettes, masks, and blow-by oxygen. However, methods that separate the child from the parents may increase anxiety, making blow-by oxygen the preferred method. The use of hot steam should be avoided since there are reports of scalds.[19]

In children with stridor at rest or more severe symptoms not responding to humidified oxygen, racemic epinephrine (Vaponefrin) has been effective in improving clinical outcome.[20-24] It is a mixture of the *d*- and *l*-isomers of epinephrine. It works by adrenergic stimulation, which causes constriction of the precapillary arterioles, thereby decreasing capillary hydrostatic pressure. This leads to fluid resorption from the interstitium and improvement in the laryngeal mucosal edema. Its β_2-adrenergic activity leads to bronchial smooth muscle relaxation and bronchodilation. The dose ranges from 0.25 to 1 ml of a 2.25% solution in 3 ml saline given via a nebulizer. The dose can be gauged by weight: less than 20 kg, 0.25 ml; 20 to 40 kg, 0.5 ml; and greater than 40 kg, 0.75 ml of a 2.25% solution. Multiple doses may be required for children in severe respiratory distress. It may be repeated at 1- to 2-hours intervals. Its clinical effect last about 2 hours. Previously feared rebound phenomenon appears quite uncommon, although some patients do return to their baseline status after the effect of the drug wears off. Most patients sustain their improvement after racemic epinephrine, particularly if steroids are begun early, and may be safely discharged after at least a 3-hour observation. This period of observation is suggested for all children who receive racemic epinephrine.[25,26] Those who were initially severely ill, responded incompletely, relapsed during the observation period, or required multiple doses must be hospitalized. L-Epinephrine in equal doses of the active *l*-isomer has been shown to have the same beneficial effects as racemic epinephrine.[27] This finding is important since racemic epinephrine is not readily available outside of the United States and is less expensive. The dose is 5 ml of a 1:1000 solution diluted in 2 ml of saline.

After several decades of controversy, the use of corticosteroids has been shown to be beneficial in the management of severe, moderate, and even mild croup.[28-35] Several studies have shown improvement in clinical symptoms and a decrease in return visits for medical care.[29,32,36-39] Corticosteroids exert their beneficial effect by means of their anti-inflammatory action, whereby laryngeal mucosal edema is decreased. They also decrease the amount of racemic epinephrine needed.[40,41] A single dose of oral or intramuscular dexamethasone (0.6 mg/kg) has been shown to be useful in reducing the overall severity of croup if given within the first 4 to 24 hours after onset of illness. The long half-life of dexamethasone (54 hours) makes only one injection usually necessary. Dexamethasone 0.15 mg/kg is as effective as 0.3 mg/kg or 0.6 mg/kg in relieving the symptoms of mild to moderate croup.[30,38,42] In addition, oral dexamethasone (0.6 mg/kg) has been shown to be equally effective when compared to placebo, and as effective as intramuscular administration.[38,43-49] Oral administration

Table 34-3	Croup Score and Implications			
	Croup Score			
	0	**1**	**2**	**3**
Stridor	Normal	Only with agitation	Mild at rest	Severe at rest
Retractions	Normal	Mild	Moderate	Severe
Air entry	Normal	Mild decrease	Moderate decrease	Marked decrease
Color	Normal	Normal	Normal	Cyanotic
LOC	Normal	Restless when disturbed	Restless when disturbed	Lethargic

Management Implications

Score	Degree	Management
≤4	Mild	Outpatient; mist therapy
5–6	Mild to moderate	Outpatient if child improves in ED after mist and steroids, >6 months old, reliable family
7–8	Moderate	Admit; racemic epinephrine, steroids
≥9	Severe	Admit; racemic epinephrine, steroids, oxygen, ICU

Abbreviations: ED, emergency department; ICU, intensive care unit; LOC, level of consciousness.

is easier and cheaper. Recently, a smaller dose of dexamethasone (0.15 mg/kg) and even a single dose of a shorter acting corticosteroid, prednisolone (1 mg/kg) has been shown to be as effective as the higher dose of dexamethasone.[38,41,50] However, one study did show more returns to the emergency department in children treated with prednisolone.[51] Corticosteroids should not be administered to children with varicella or untreated tuberculosis.

The use of inhaled corticosteroids, especially budesonide, has been shown to be effective.[43,52] Budesonide is a synthetic glucocorticoid with strong topical anti-inflammatory effects and low systemic activity. Administration of 2 to 4 mg of nebulized budesonide has been shown to decrease the croup score substantially, and to decrease emergency department length of stay and hospitalization, when compared to nebulized saline.[53-57] Nebulized corticosteroids are as effective as oral or intramuscular corticosteroids for croup.[52] However, they are more expensive than dexamethasone, and one study with oral dexamethasone showed better improvement than with nebulized budesonide.[39]

Less than 2% of those patients with severe croup will be unresponsive to therapy and will require intubation.[58,59] Intubation should be accomplished with an endotracheal tube that is 0.5 to 1.0 mm smaller than predicted. Others have used a Heliox (helium 60% to 80%) mixture in order to prevent intubation. Heliox is a metabolically inert, nontoxic gas that is combined with oxygen. It has low viscosity and low specific gravity, which allows for greater laminar airflow through the respiratory tract.[60] Helium will decrease the force necessary to move the gas through the airways and decrease the mechanical work of respiratory muscles. Heliox has been shown to improve symptoms with severe croup that fails to improve with racemic epinephrine.[61] It has been shown to be equally effective in moderate to severe croup when compared to racemic epinephrine.[62]

Epiglottitis

Recognition and Approach

Acute epiglottitis is a potentially life-threatening bacterial infection with significant morbidity and mortality. Epiglottitis, or more correctly supraglottitis, is an inflammation of the structures above the site of insertion of the glottis, including the epiglottis, the aryepiglottic folds, the arytenoidal soft tissue, and occasionally the uvula. The upper airway obstruction can evolve rapidly and may lead to respiratory arrest and death.

Fortunately, the prevalence has declined due to the availability of the *H. influenzae* vaccine.[63] However, mortality can be as high as 6% to 10% in children without intubation, while mortality is reduced to less than 1% when intubation is performed. Historically, the most common bacterial cause in children was *H. influenzae* type b (>90%). Other bacterial causes include *Streptococcus pneumoniae*, groups A, B, and C streptococcus, and *Staphylococcus aureus*. Unusual causes include *Moraxella catarrhalis, Haemophilus parainfluenzae,* Pseudomonas, *Neisseria meningitidis, Candida albicans, Klebsiella pneumoniae,* and *Pasteurella multocida.* Viral agents implicated in epiglottitis have included herpes simplex, parainfluenza, varicella-zoster, and Epstein-Barr viruses. Other

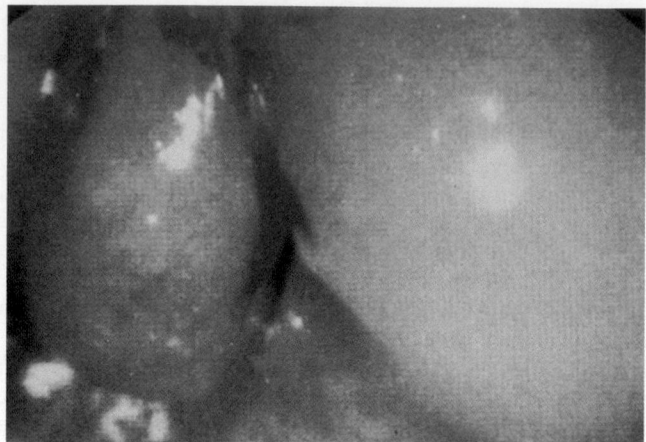

FIGURE 34–2. Epiglottitis.

noninfectious etiologies have included thermal or caustic injuries, traumatic blind finger sweep to remove a pharyngeal foreign body, inhaled foreign bodies, angioneurotic edema, and acute leukemia.[64-66]

Epiglottitis may be acquired by respiratory transmission from an intimate contact or from bacteria that have colonized the pharynx of normal children. These bacteria may penetrate the mucosal barrier and invade the bloodstream. During the bacteremia, seeding of the epiglottis and surrounding tissues may occur. Other places of potential seeding, especially with *H. influenzae,* include the meninges, facial skin, lung, and joints.

Acute onset of inflammatory edema ensues, beginning on the lingual surface of the epiglottis where the submucosa is loosely attached. The swelling leads to considerable reduction in the aperture of the airway. This swelling progresses rapidly to involve the aryepiglottic folds, the arytenoids, and the entire supraglottic larynx (supraglottitis) (Fig. 34–2). The tightly bound epithelium on the vocal cords halts the spread at this level. Respiratory arrest can occur with aspiration of oropharyngeal secretions or mucous plugging.

Clinical Presentation

Epiglottitis is characterized by an abrupt, explosive onset of symptoms that may progress rapidly to respiratory obstruction and death in a matter of hours in the absence of airway control and medical management. The first symptoms include fever, often reaching 40° C. Shortly afterward, the child develops stridor and labored breathing. Other common signs and symptoms include dysphagia, muffled (guttural) or hoarse voice, refusal to eat, and sore throat. Less commonly occurring symptoms are cough and ear pain.

The child has a toxic appearance, and shock may occur early in the course of the disease. Marked restlessness, irritability, and extreme anxiety are common. The child assumes a sitting position with the chin hyperextended and the body leaning forward (tripod position) in order to maximize air entry past the swollen epiglottis and improve diaphragmatic excursion. The mouth is wide open and the tongue protruding. Frequently the child will drool because of the difficulty or pain in swallowing secretions.

The pulmonary findings include stridor with marked suprasternal, subcostal, and intercostal retractions. The ante-

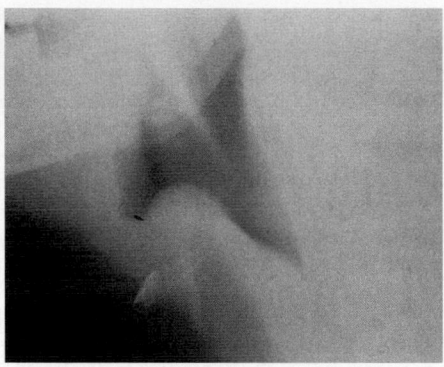

FIGURE 34-3. "Thumbprint sign" of epiglottitis.

Table 34-4	Antimicrobial Agents Effective against Common Epiglottitis Organisms
Antimicrobial	**Dose**
Ceftriaxone	75–100 mg/kg per day IV/IM once or divided q12h
Cefotaxime	50–75 mg/kg per day IV/IM divided q6 8h
Cefuroxime	50–100 mg/kg per day IV/IM divided q6–8h
Ampicillin	100–400 mg/kg per day IV divided q4–6h

Abbreviations: IM, intramuscularly; IV, intravenously.

rior neck examination may reveal tender adenopathy. An erythematous and swollen epiglottis can often be seen by a careful examination of the oropharynx. Cyanosis is a late finding, indicating poor prognosis.

The laboratory evaluation is nonspecific and should be performed once the airway is secured. The white blood cell count may be elevated from 15,000 to 45,000/mm[3] with a predominance of bands occurring. The blood cultures may recover the organism 12% to 90% of the time, especially with *H. influenzae*.[63,67-69] The epiglottic cultures are positive in half the cases.

Radiographic evaluation is not needed in classic cases of epiglottitis; however, it may be needed in certain cases to establish the diagnosis and to exclude other potential causes of acute airway obstruction. Since epiglottitis is a disease of acute deterioration, and since sudden airway obstruction has been described in children with epiglottitis during radiographic manipulation, the child should never be sent to radiology without personnel capable of establishing an airway if such acute deterioration occurs. It is best to have a portable radiograph performed in the emergency department. In addition, the lateral neck radiograph should never delay definitive airway control in children who need it immediately.

The lateral soft tissue radiograph of the neck classically reveals a swollen epiglottis ("thumbprint sign"), thickened aryepiglottic folds, obliteration of the vallecula, and dilation of the hypopharynx (Fig. 34-3). A chest radiograph may reveal a concomitant pneumonia in up to 25% of patients.[70]

Complications associated with a swollen epiglottis and surrounding tissues include airway obstruction, which can lead to respiratory arrest and death from hypoxia. The respiratory arrest that may occur with epiglottitis does not appear to occur because of total airway obstruction, but rather seems to result from fatigue. Other complications may include epiglottic abscess, adenitis, cervical cellulitis, and rarely pulmonary edema. Historically with the bacteremia from *H. influenzae*, other concomitant infectious processes occur, such as meningitis, pneumonia, septicemia, cellulitis, septic arthritis, and rarely pericarditis.[71]

Management

Treatment is directed toward relief of the airway obstruction and eradication of the infectious agent. These children generally present to the emergency department in marked respiratory distress and are very anxious. Procedures that are normally performed on infants in acute respiratory distress may not apply to infants with acute epiglottitis. For example, blood venipunctures and establishing an intravenous access, although appropriate in most cases of acutely ill infants, may heighten the anxiety and precipitate airway compromise in infants with epiglottitis.

As with every acute resuscitation, the airway, breathing, and circulation are the first aspects to evaluate. Providing supplemental oxygen by a nonthreatening and less anxiety-provoking method is the initial step. This is best accomplished easily with blow-by oxygen administered by the parent. Equipment for emergent airway management is placed at the bedside, and the patient remains in the view of the physician at all times. If acute respiratory arrest occurs, the infant should be ventilated with a bag-valve-mask device using 100% supplemental oxygen until arrangements for intubation are made.[72] In cases in which the appropriate personnel are not available and the infant has a respiratory arrest, attempts to intubate may be performed. Other alternative methods to gain immediate control of the airway include a needle cricothyrotomy. This procedure is a temporizing method used until a more permanent procedure, such as a tracheostomy, can be performed. The use of racemic epinephrine plays little role in the management of infectious or thermal epiglottitis.

The next crucial step is mobilization of the appropriate team to establish an appropriate airway. The patient is taken to the operating room, where equipment for tracheostomy and bronchoscopy are prepared. Laryngoscopy is performed under general anesthesia and an orotracheal tube (0.5 to 1.0 mm smaller than predicted for the child) inserted. After placement of the endotracheal tube, the supraglottic structures are examined by direct laryngoscopy and appropriate surface cultures of the epiglottis are done.

Eradication of the bacterial organism may be accomplished by using antibiotics effective against the more common organisms (Table 34-4). This may include ceftriaxone, cefotaxime, cefuroxime, or ampicillin, and chloramphenicol. It is recommended that chemoprophylaxis with rifampin be given to close contacts in children under 4 years of age. Intravenous hydration should be initiated and the child hospitalized in a pediatric intensive care unit (ICU) setting.

The use of corticosteroids, which has been advocated in the past based on anecdotal reports, remains controversial and has not been shown to be efficacious in the acute setting of epiglottitis.

Bacterial Tracheitis (Membranous Laryngotracheobronchitis, Pseudomembranous Croup)

Recognition and Approach

Bacterial tracheitis is a disease caused by a bacterial infection of the subglottic area that complicates patients with croup. It is more common than epiglottitis but less common than croup. There is a 2 : 1 male : female ratio. A preponderance of infections occur in fall and winter. It may occur at any age, but the average age is 3 years. Mortality has been between 4% and 20%.

Bacterial tracheitis is characterized by subglottic edema and inflammation of the larynx, trachea, bronchi, and sometimes the lung. There are copious purulent secretions and semiadherent mucopurulent pseudomembrane formation in the trachea and bronchi, which increases luminal narrowing and may cause severe respiratory distress.[73] Extension of the disease into the bronchi and alveoli is common.

The infection is polymicrobial, but the primary organism responsible for this disease is *S. aureus*. Other organisms include *S. pneumoniae, H. influenzae,* α-hemolytic streptococcus, group A β-hemolytic streptococcus, Klebsiella, Pseudomonas species, *Escherichia coli, Moraxella catarrhalis, Corynebacterium diphtheriae, Bacillus cereus,* parainfluenza and influenza, measles, respiratory syncytial virus, anaerobes (*Peptostreptococcus, Bacteroides, Prevotella*), and *Aspergillus.*[74-78]

Clinical Presentation

The illness begins with a prodrome of an upper respiratory illness, lasting 1 to 2 weeks, followed by several days of mild to moderate crouplike illness. Soon afterward, a rapid deterioration occurs over several hours. Once acute respiratory distress occurs, it is indistinguishable from epiglottitis; however, the history of a slower onset will make bacterial tracheitis more likely. At this time there is a high fever and toxicity, and the infant may be quite anxious or may be lethargic. There are obvious signs of severe upper airway obstruction, such as significant stridor, tachypnea, suprasternal retractions, poor air entry, and brassy or barky cough.[79] Late signs include cyanosis. On occasion there may be evidence of wheezing. The respiratory distress tends to be severe and unresponsive to croup therapy. On radiographs, there is subglottic and tracheal narrowing on the anteroposterior view and there may be a pseudomembrane (auspicated secretion) visible within the tracheal lumen. The supraglottic region is normal in appearance. The chest radiograph may reveal a concomitant pneumonia in 50% of cases. Laryngotracheobronchoscopy is the definitive means of diagnosis, showing the purulent tracheal secretions.

The laboratory evaluation may reveal leukocytosis with a left shift. Positive blood cultures are unusual; however, tracheal cultures are usually positive.

The main complication is the risk of upper and lower airway obstruction, with its attendant risk of hypoxemia, respiratory arrest, and death. Pneumonia often occurs and may progress to acute respiratory distress syndrome (ARDS), and a rare association with toxic shock syndrome exists.[73] Other complications include postobstructive pulmonary edema and subglottic stenosis.[78]

Table 34-5	Antimicrobial Agents Effective against Common Bacterial Tracheitis and RPA Organisms
Antimicrobial	**Dose**
Nafcillin	50–100 mg/kg per day IV/IM divided q6–12h
Cefuroxime	50–100 mg/kg per day IV/IM divided q6–8h
Ceftriaxone	75–100 mg/kg per day IV/IM qd or divided q12h
Cefotaxime	50–75 mg/kg per day IV/IM divided q6–8h
Clindamycin	25–40 mg/kg per day IV/IM divided q6–8h
Piperacillin/tazobactam	240–400 mg/kg per day IV divided q6–8h
Ampicillin/sulbactam	100–400 mg/kg per day IV/IM divided q6h
Ticarcillin/clavulanate	200–300 mg/kg per day IV divided q4–6h
Vancomycin	10–15 mg/kg per day IV divided q8–12h

Abbreviations: IM, intramuscularly; IV, intravenously; RPA, retropharyngeal abscess.

Management

Emergent intubation is usually required. An endotracheal tube 0.5 to 1.0 mm smaller than expected should be used in order to minimize trauma in the inflamed subglottic area. Aggressive pulmonary toilet is quintessential to relieve the obstruction caused by the thick and tenacious secretions. Antibiotic therapy should be initiated with agents effective against the usual organisms (Table 34-5). This may be accomplished with nafcillin and cefuroxime or ceftriaxone or cefotaxime. Clindamycin may be added for anaerobic coverage. Other agents include piperacillin/tazobactam, ampicillin/sulbactam, and ticarcillin/clavulanate. Patients allergic to penicillin may require chloramphenicol and clindamycin. Intravenous hydration should be initiated and the child hospitalized in a pediatric ICU setting.

Retropharyngeal Abscess

Recognition and Approach

Retropharyngeal abscess (RPA) is a deep neck infection filling the potential space between the prevertebral fascia of the cervical vertebrae and the posterior wall of the pharynx. It has the potential for airway compromise.[80] It occurs most often in young children less than 6 years of age, with a peak at 6 to 12 months of age.

The retropharyngeal space can become infected by either spread of an infection from a contiguous area or direct inoculation of the space secondary to penetrating trauma. Typically an upper respiratory infection spreads to the retropharyngeal lymph nodes. Other sources of infection can include pharyngitis, tonsillitis, adenitis, otitis media, parotitis, sinusitis, and dental infection. Osteomyelitis of the spine can also spread anteriorly from the prevertebral space. Penetrating trauma typically occurs from objects in the mouth forced posteriorly during a fall or from impacted foreign bodies, such as fish bones or chicken bones.[81,82] Iatrogenic causes include laryngoscopy, endotracheal intubation, surgery, endoscopy, feeding or nasogastric tube placement, and dental procedures.[83] The lymphadenitis can form a cellulitis that then can suppurate as an abscess. The progressive swelling and the relatively higher larynx and narrow airway in infants make airway obstruction a significant early complication.

Usual organisms include group A β-hemolytic streptococcus, *S. aureus,* viridans streptococci, S. epidermis, and occasionally *E. coli, H. influenzae, Neisseria,* Klebsiella, Salmonella, Eikenella, corynebacterium, anaerobes (*Bacteroides,* Peptostreptococcus, Fusobacterium), *Mycobacterium tuberculosis,* Blastomyces, and Coccidioides.[84-87]

Clinical Presentation

Presentation is similar to epiglottitis, but onset is less abrupt. A prodrome of nasopharyngitis or pharyngitis occurs. It is followed by abrupt onset of high fever, chills, toxic appearance, pain with neck movement, stridor, drooling, odynophagia, trismus, sore throat, dysphagia, refusal to eat, anorexia, torticollis, and muffled ("hot potato") voice or voice that sounds like a duck quack (*cri du canard*).[88-90] There is usually unilateral cervical lymphadenopathy. A "tracheal rock sign" occurs when pain is elicited while gently moving the larynx and trachea from side to side. Meningismus may be present from irritation of the paravertebral ligaments. RPA must be considered in an infant with nuchal rigidity but no pleocytosis in cerebrospinal fluid. Rarely, the examination shows an obvious midline swelling of the pharynx.

The laboratory evaluation is nonspecific, with leukocytosis and a left shift. The lateral neck radiograph may show an increase in width of the soft tissues anterior to the vertebrae, and on occasion an air-fluid level may be noted (Fig. 34–4). A plain radiograph, however, may miss up to 30% of RPAs. Ultrasound can be used to visualize an abscess. Dynamic fluoroscopy may show widening of the retropharyngeal space. However, computed tomography scan of the neck is the imaging modality of choice and has been used to assess the extent of the infection.[89,91] It may not, however, be as accurate in differentiating cellulites from abscess.[92]

Complications are due to mass effect, rupture of abscess, or spread of infection. These include airway compromise, aspiration pneumonia, sepsis, ARDS, spontaneous perforation, reformation of retropharyngeal abscess, mediastinitis, purulent pericarditis, tamponade, pyopneumothorax, pleuritis, empyema, bronchial erosion, osteomyelitis of the spinal column, necrotizing fasciitis, carotid artery rupture, jugular vein thrombosis, or atlanto-occipital dislocation.[91]

Management

As with any infection that can compromise the airway, a thorough assessment of the patency of the airway and adequacy of oxygenation and ventilation must be performed. Less than a third of infants will require endotracheal intubation. Eradication of the bacterial organism may be accomplished by using antibiotics effective against the more common organisms.[86,93] This may be accomplished with nafcillin and cefuroxime or ceftriaxone or cefotaxime. Clindamycin may be added for anaerobic coverage. Other agents include piperacillin/tazobactam, ampicillin/sulbactam, and ticarcillin/clavulanate. Patients allergic to penicillin may require chloramphenicol and clindamycin. Intravenous

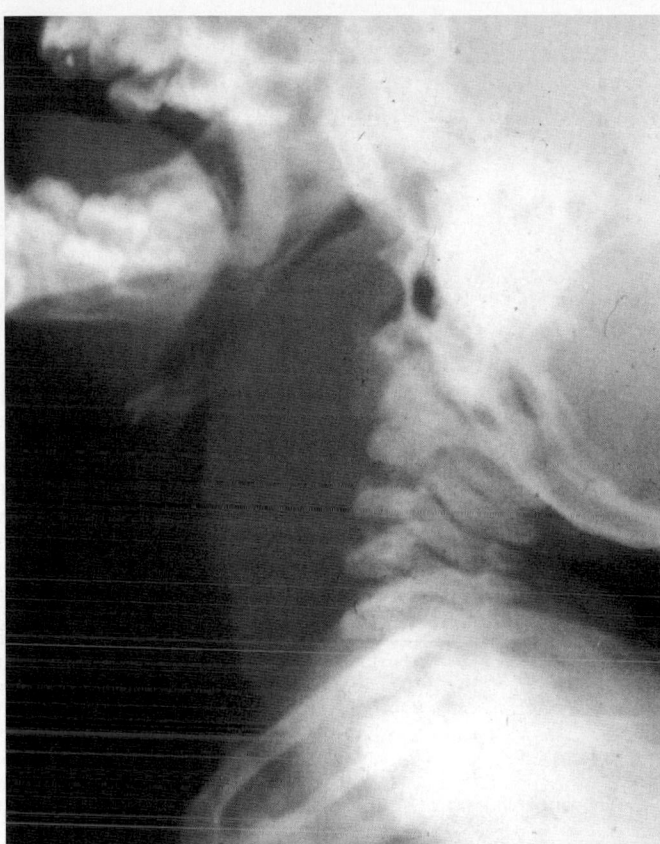

FIGURE 34–4. Widening of the retropharyngeal space.

hydration should be initiated and the child hospitalized in a pediatric ICU setting.

Treatment without surgical drainage can be successful in a select group of infants.[76] Failure of medical management or the presence of a large abscess requires drainage, and the intraoral route is preferred.[77]

Congenital Anomalies

The onset of stridor shortly after birth is most likely caused by a structural defect. This type of stridor tends to worsen slowly and is severe only when the infant is stressed, such as during crying or a respiratory illness. The causes of congenital stridor are shown in Tables 34–6 and 34–7.[94-102]

Foreign Body Aspiration

Recognition and Approach

Foreign body aspiration can cause stridor in infants. Through play, oral curiosity, or normal daily activities, infants are likely to place foreign bodies just about anywhere. In addition, the lack of fully developed dentition and oral protective reflexes places the infant at increased risk for the object to lodge in the respiratory tree.

Aspirated foreign bodies can be found in any segment of the respiratory tree. The size and shape of the object and the forcefulness of inspiration determine where in the airway a foreign body lodges. Most are in the mainstem bronchi or distal trachea near the carina, though smaller objects can

Table 34–6	Laryngeal Causes of Congenital Stridor
Laryngomalacia	Most common cause of congenital stridor (75%). It may be caused by an enlarged epiglottis that prolapses posteriorly on inspiration, short aryepiglottic folds, or bulky arytenoid cartilage that prolapses anteriorly over the larynx on inspiration. Symptoms are present at birth or within the first 4–6 weeks. Infants typically have high-pitched inspiratory stridor that increases with crying and when supine. Stridor is positional and is relieved by placing the infant in the prone position with head extended. It rarely interferes with feeding or is associated with dyspnea. Radiographic evaluation may show downward and inferior displacement and bowing of aryepiglottic folds. Diagnosis is by laryngoscopy. It usually resolves on its own by 12–24 months of age. Infants with respiratory distress, cor pulmonale, apnea, or failure to thrive may require epiglottoplasty, laryngoplasty, and/or tracheotomy.[94,95]
Vocal cord paralysis	The second most common cause of neonatal stridor.[96] Most cases are diagnosed within first 12 hours of life. Neonates usually have a weak or absent cry, respiratory distress (bilateral vocal cord paralysis), and difficulty feeding. The stridor is biphasic. If unilateral, it improves with lying down on the affected side. Unilateral vocal cord paralysis can be congenital or due to trauma at birth or at the time of cardiac or intrathoracic surgery. Unilateral vocal cord paralysis may improve spontaneously or with vocal cord reinnervation procedures.[97] Bilateral vocal cord paralysis has been associated with malformations of the central nervous system, such as Arnold-Chiari malformation.[98] Bilateral paralysis is a life-threatening emergency. These neonates present with a high-pitched biphasic stridor that may progress to severe respiratory distress. Treatment is tracheostomy.
Subglottic stenosis	Can be congenital or acquired. Congenital types occur from an incomplete canalization of the subglottic and cricoid ring causing a narrowing of the subglottic lumen. Acquired form arises from prolonged endotracheal intubation or infections (diphtheria, tuberculosis). Infants present with stridor, cough, and recurrent croup. Stridor is usually biphasic or inspiratory. If not present at birth, it may be mistaken for asthma. Tracheostomy, laryngeal dilation, endoscopic scar excision, or laryngeal reconstruction may be required.[99]
Laryngeal web	Caused by incomplete recanalization of the laryngeal lumen during embryogenesis. Most are in the glottic area. Infants present with a weak cry and biphasic stridor. Treatment is surgical.
Laryngeal cyst	Found in the supraglottic region in the epiglottic folds. Infants present with stridor, cough, hoarse voice, or aphonia.[100] If the cyst is large, it may cause respiratory obstruction and require surgical excision.
Layngeal hemangioma	Approximately 50% of cases are accompanied by hemangiomas in the head and neck region. Infants have inspiratory or biphasic stridor that worsen as the hemangioma enlarges. Hemagioma usually regresses by 12–18 months of age. May require surgical resection or laser therapy if respiratory symptoms occur. Medical management may include oral corticosteroids or intralesional corticosteroids.
Laryngeal papilloma	Most common laryngeal tumor. Occurs from vertical transmission of the human papilloma virus in maternal condylomata or infected vaginal cells to the larynx or pharynx of the infant during delivery. Infants present with stridor and hoarseness. Treatment requires recurrent surgical excisions.

Table 34–7	Tracheal Causes of Congenital Stridor
Extrinsic compression	Anomalies that may lead to stridor include double aortic arch, right aortic arch, inominate artery compression, aberrant right subclavian vein, and pulmonary artery sling.[101]
Bronchogenic cysts	Can cause extrinsic compression of the trachea and require surgical excision.
Tracheomalacia	The most common cause of expiratory stridor. It is caused by a defect in the cartilage resulting in loss of rigidity necessary to maintain the tracheal lumen patent or by extrinsic compression of the trachea (vascular ring or sling). It leads to tracheal collapse on inspiration. It can be primary or secondary to vascular abnormalities, tracheoesophageal fistula, relapsing polychondritis, or Ehlers-Danlos syndrome, or acquired after intubation or tracheotomy. It may occur with laryngomalacia and gastroesophageal reflux. It has been mistaken for asthma or prolonged bronchiolitis. Symptoms usually subside by the age of 3 years. Definitive diagnosis is with bronchoscopy. Infants with respiratory distress or failure to thrive may require a tracheostomy.[102]
Tracheal stenosis	Can be congenital or due to extrinsic compression. Congenital stenosis is usually related to complete tracheal rings, is characterized by persistent stridor, and requires surgery based on severity of symptoms. The most common extrinsic causes include vascular rings, slings, and a double aortic arch that encircles the trachea and esophagus. Infants present during the first year of life with noisy breathing, intercostal retractions, and a prolonged expiratory phase. Treatment is with dilation or surgical correction.

lodge more peripherally. The most serious sequela of foreign body airway aspiration is complete obstruction of the airway. In such cases, the foreign body becomes lodged in the larynx or trachea, leaving little room peripherally for air exchange. If the object lodges in the glottis and stimulates spasm, the infant may die before aid is available. Fortunately, the foreign body more often passes into the bronchi, resulting in unilateral obstructive emphysema.

Clinical Presentation

An accurate history and a strong suspicion are of paramount importance in diagnosing foreign body aspiration in infants, because in 33% to 64% of cases nothing in the initial history indicates aspiration.[103,104] Certainly, new-onset bronchopulmonary symptoms in an otherwise healthy infant must alert the physician to the possibility of airway foreign body aspiration. When an infant has unexplained, recurrent, or persistent respiratory illness that does not respond to adequate medical therapy, aspiration, as well as atypical asthma, should be part of the differential diagnosis. Foreign body aspiration can mimic other disease processes, leading to a misdiagnosis of croup, pneumonia, bronchiolitis, or asthma.

Physical examination may reveal wheezing, stridor, crackles, dyspnea, retractions, decreased air entry, tachypnea, rhonchi, hoarseness, cyanosis, fever, and apnea.[103-105] One fourth of infants may be asymptomatic at the time of presentation, and 39% may have no helpful physical examination findings.[106] The complete triad of coughing, wheezing, and decreased breath sounds is present in only 40% of cases.[106]

Specific manifestations of aspirated foreign bodies depend on whether the object is located in the trachea or bronchi and on the size of the object, which relates to the degree of obstruction. Although most patients are seen within a day of aspiration, some have symptoms that last weeks or months before the proper diagnosis is made.[103,105] Signs and symptoms associated with foreign body aspiration occur in three stages. In the initial stage, there is a history of a choking episode, followed by violent paroxysms of coughing, gagging, and occasionally complete airway obstruction. An asymptomatic interval generally follows the aspiration, during which the foreign body becomes lodged, the reflexes become fatigued, and the immediate irritating symptoms subside. This stage is the most treacherous and accounts for a large percentage of delayed diagnoses or overlooked foreign bodies. The third stage is characterized by symptoms of complications caused by the foreign body, such as obstruction, erosion, or infection. Chronic cough, hemoptysis, pneumonia, lung abscess, unexplained fever, and malaise are common presentations of chronic airway foreign bodies.

Although only 6% to 17% of aspirated foreign bodies are radiopaque, the lung abnormalities caused by aspirated objects are generally detectable.[107-109] Radiographic evaluation should start with anteroposterior and lateral views of the chest and neck. Lateral soft tissue radiographs may reveal the foreign object in the hypopharynx, glottis, subglottis, or cervical esophagus or embedded in the posterior pharyngeal wall. Ballooning of the hypopharynx may indicate subglottic obstruction. Widening of the retropharyngeal soft tissues or air in the soft tissues, or both, are signs of perforation with abscess formation. Coins lodged in the trachea generally appear to be aligned in the sagittal plane on an anteroposterior or posteroanterior chest radiograph.

The effect of an airway foreign body on the lung depends on the object's location and how it obstructs the flow of air. The intrathoracic airways tend to dilate on inspiration and contract on expiration, causing most bronchial foreign bodies to act as check valves. During inspiration, air can bypass the foreign body, but during expiration the bronchus narrows and is occluded, causing obstructive emphysema and sometimes pneumothorax or pneumomediastinum.

Routine radiographs are normal in 25% of children who have aspirated foreign bodies, especially when the object is not radiopaque and is located in the trachea. When the object is in the bronchus, radiographic findings include hyperlucency or obstructive emphysema (38% to 52%), atelectasis (10% to 20%), pneumonia (16% to 27%), opaque foreign body (4% to 19%), pneumomediastinum (6%), consolidation (5%), effusion (2%), pneumothorax (1%), abscess (<1%), and bronchiectasis (<1%).[102-105] Foreign bodies may

completely occlude the airway as a result of edema and granulation tissue, acting as a stop valve. Air beyond the obstruction is resorbed, resulting in atelectasis of the affected lobe.

Radiographs often detect hyperaeration of the affected lung or lobe. Differential inflation and deflation of the affected lung may be documented by fluoroscopy, lateral decubitus radiographs, or an assisted expiratory film when suspicion persists despite normal routine radiographs[104-107] (Fig. 34–5). In a recent review, decubitus radiographs had

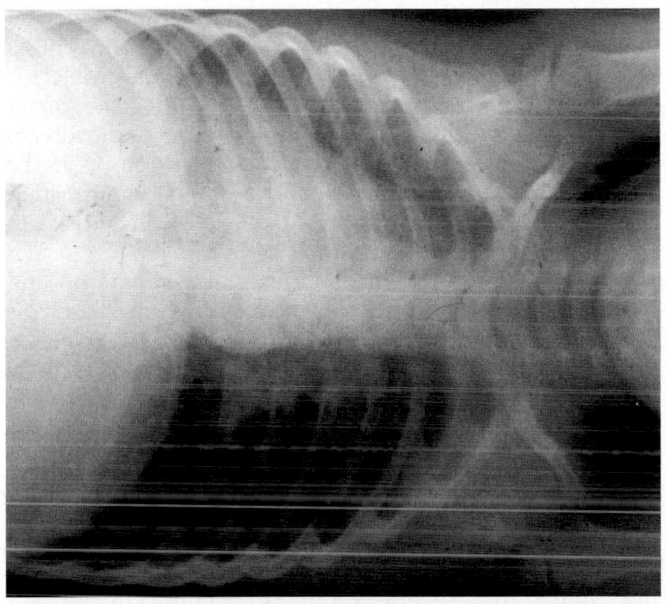

A

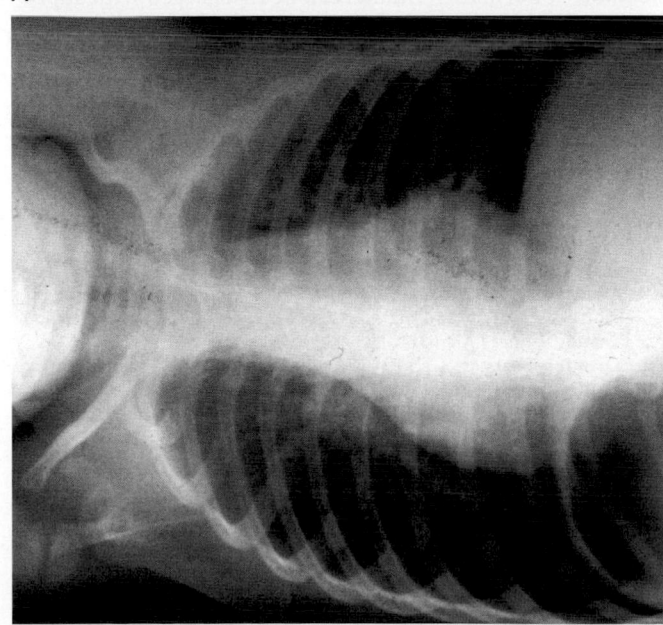

B

FIGURE 34–5. **A,** Left decubitus film showing normal deflation of the left lung. **B,** Right decubitus film showing hyperaeration of the right lung with a foreign body suspected in the right bronchus.

only a sensitivity of 27% for children with foreign body aspiration.[110] Aluminum and plastic foreign bodies may sometimes be seen when radiographs are exposed with more than the usual amount of x-ray energy (overpenetrated views). Recently, low-dose multidetector computed tomography (MDCT) and virtual bronchoscopy has been shown to be accurate in detecting suspected foreign body aspiration.[111]

Management

Initial management must focus on establishment of adequate oxygenation and ventilation. Recognition of the infant whose airway is completely obstructed is critical to the success of first aid efforts. If an infant can cough or talk, obstruction is not yet complete, and the infant should be allowed to cough without interference. Delivering first aid to such an infant is unnecessary and potentially dangerous. Complete airway obstruction in the conscious infant may be recognized by sudden respiratory distress, followed by an inability to speak or cough. When the airway is completely obstructed, first aid must be delivered promptly. This consists of delivering a sequence of back blows and chest thrusts until the object is dislodged. Emergency strategies may also include direct laryngoscopy, which may permit visualization of the foreign body, allowing for removal with McGill forceps.[112] If the object is in the subglottic trachea, orotracheal intubation may be life saving, dislodging the object into a mainstem bronchus and converting a complete obstruction to a partial obstruction. If the foreign body cannot be removed and endotracheal intubation cannot be achieved, needle cricothyrotomy can bypass the obstruction and deliver oxygen to the patient. In stable children, removal of the foreign body can be performed with rigid bronchoscopy or flexible bronchoscopy.[111,112]

Summary

Stridor in infants can occur from a variety of causes, such as inflammatory or infectious diseases, congenital anomalies, and trauma. After excluding a life-threatening etiology or a treatable abnormality, infants can be discharged with appropriate otolaryngologic or pulmonary follow-up.

REFERENCES

1. Holinger LD: Etiology of stridor in the neonate, infant and child. Ann Otol Rhinol Laryngol 89:397–400, 1980.
2. Stankiewicz JA, Bowes AK: Croup and epiglottitis: a radiologic study. Laryngoscope 95:1159–1160, 1985.
3. Andreassen UK, Baer S, Nielsen TG: Acute epiglottitis—25 years experience with nasotracheal intubation, current management policy and future trends. J Laryngol Otol 106:1072–1075, 1992.
4. MayoSmith MF, Hirsch PJ, Wodzinski SF, Schiffman FJ: Acute epiglottitis in adults: an eight-year experience in the state of Rhode Island. N Engl J Med 314:1133–1139, 1986.
5. Diaz JH, Lockhart CH: Early diagnosis and airway management of acute epiglottitis in children. South Med J 75:399–403, 1982.
6. Denny FW, Murphy TF, Clyde Jr WA, et al: Croup: an 11-year study in a pediatric practice. Pediatrics 71:871–876, 1983.
7. Chapman R, Henderson F, Cleyde W, et al: The epidemiology of tracheobronchitis in pediatric practice. Am J Epidemiol 114:786–797, 1981.
8. Williams J, Harris P, Tollefson S, et al: Human metapneumovirus and lower respiratory tract disease in otherwise healthy infants and children. N Engl J Med 350:443–450, 2004.
9. Salour M: The steeple sign. Radiology 216:428–429, 2000.
10. Britto J, Habibi P, Walters S, et al: Systemic complications associated with bacterial tracheitis. Arch Dis Child 74:249–250, 1996.
11. Taussig LM, Castro O, Beaudry PH, et al: Treatment of laryngotracheobronchitis (croup): use of intermittent positive-pressure breathing and racemic epinephrine. Am J Dis Child 129:790–793, 1975.
*12. Jacobs S, Shortland G, Warner J, et al: Validation of a croup score and its use in triaging children with croup. Anaesthesia 49:903–906, 1994.
13. Westley C, Cotton E, Brooks J: Nebulized racemic epinephrine by IPPB for the treatment of croup. Am J Dis Child 132:484–487, 1978.
14. Bourchier D, Dawson KP, Fergusson DM: Humidification in viral croup: a controlled trial. Aust Paediatr J 20:289–291, 1984.
15. Neto GM, Kentab O, Klassen TP, Osmond MH: A randomized controlled trial of mist in the acute treatment of moderate croup. Acad Emerg Med 9:873–879, 2002.
16. Colletti JE: Myth: Cool mist is an effective therapy in the management of croup. Can J Emerg Med 6:357–358, 2004.
17. Scolnik D, Coates AL, Stephens D, et al: Controlled delivery of high vs low humidity vs mist therapy for croup in emergency department: a randomized control trial. JAMA 295:1274–1280, 2006.
18. Moore M, Little P: Humidified air inhalation for treating croup (Review). Cochrane Database Systemic Reviews.
19. Greally P, Cheng K, Tanner MS, Field DJ: Children with croup presenting with scalds. BMJ 301:113, 1990.
20. Gardner HG, Powell KR, Roden VJ, Cherry JD: The evaluation of racemic epinephrine in the treatment of infectious croup. Pediatrics 52:52–55, 1973.
21. Kristjansson S, Berg-Kelly K, Winso E: Inhalation of racemic adrenaline in the treatment of mild and moderately severe croup: clinical symptom score and oxygen saturation measurements for evaluation of treatment effects. Acta Paediatr 83:1156–1160, 1994.
22. McDonogh AJ: The use of steroids and nebulized adrenaline in the treatment of viral croup over a seven year period at a district hospital. Anaesth Intensive Care 22:175–178, 1994.
23. Martinez Fernandez A, Sanchez Gonzalez E, Rica Etxebarria I, et al: Estudio randomizado doble ciego del tratamiento del crup en la infancia con adrenalina y/o dexametasona. [Randomized double-blind study of treatment of croup with adrenaline and/or dexamethasone in children]. An Esp Pediatr 38:29–32, 1993.
24. Kuusela A, Vesikari T: A randomized, double-blind, placebo-controlled trial of dexamethasone and racemic epinephrine in the treatment of croup. Acta Paediatr Scand 77:99–104, 1988.
25. Rizos JD, DiGravio BE, Sehl MJ, Talloon JM: The disposition of children with croup treated with racemic epinephrine and dexamethasone in the emergency department. J Emerg Med 16:535–539, 1998.
26. Kunkel NC, Baker MD: Use of racemic epinephrine, dexamethasone, and mist in the outpatient management of croup. Pediatr Emerg Care 12:156–159, 1996.
27. Waisman Y, Klein BL, Boenning DA, et al: Prospective randomized double-blind study comparing L-epinephrine with racemic epinephrine aerosols in the treatment of laryngotracheitis (croup). Pediatrics 89:302–306, 1992.
28. Geelhoed GC: Croup. Pediatr Pulmonol 23:370–374, 1997.
29. Kairy SW, Olmstead EM, O'Connor GT: Steroid treatment of laryngotracheitis: a meta-analysis of the evidence from randomized trials. Pediatr 83:683–693, 1989.
*30. Ausejo MP, Saenz AM, Pham BM, et al: Glucocorticoids for croup. Cochrane Database Syst Rev (2):CD001955, 2000.
31. Ausejo MP, Saenz AM, Pham BM, et al: The effectiveness of glucocorticoids in treating croup: meta-analysis. BMJ 319:595–600, 1999.
32. Geelhoed GC: Sixteen years of croup in a Western Australian teaching hospital: effects of routine steroid treatment. Ann Emerg Med 28:621–626, 1996.
33. Bjornson CL, Klassen TP, Williamson J, et al: A randomized trial of a single dose of oral dexamethasone for mild croup. N Engl J Med 351:1306–1313, 2004.
34. Parker R, Powell CV, Kelly AM: How long does stridor at rest persist in croup after the administration of oral prednisolone? Emerg Med Australas 16:135–138, 2004.
35. Russell K, Wiebe N, Saenz A, et al: Glucocorticoids for croup. Cochrane Database Syst Rev (1):CD001955, 2004.
36. Tibballs J, Shann FA, Landau LI: Placebo-controlled trial of prednisolone in children intubated for croup. Lancet 340:745–748, 1992.

*Selected readings.

37. Cruz MN, Stewart G, Rosenberg N: Use of dexamethasone in the outpatient management of acute laryngotracheitis. Pediatrics 96:220–223, 1995.
38. Geelhoed GC, Turner J, Macdonald WB: Efficacy of a small single dose of oral dexamethasone for outpatient croup: a double blind placebo controlled clinical trial. BMJ 313:140–142, 1996.
39. Luria JW, Gonzalez-del-Rey JA, DiGiulio GA, et al: Effectiveness of oral or nebulized dexamethasone for children with mild croup. Arch Pediatr Adolesc Med 155:1340–1345, 2001.
40. Super DM, Cartelli NA, Brooks LJ, et al: A prospective randomized double-blind study to evaluate the effect of dexamethasone in acute laryngotraacheitis. J Pediatr 115:323–329, 1989.
41. Fifoot AA, Ting JY: Comparison between single-dose oral prednisone and oral dexamethasone in the treatment of croup: A randomized, double-blinded clinical trial. Emerg Med Australas 19:51–58, 2007.
42. Geelhoed GC, Macdonald WB: Oral dexamethasone in the treatment of croup: 0.15 mg/kg versus 0.3 mg/kg versus 0.6 mg/kg. Pediatr Pulmonol 20:362–368, 1995.
43. Geelhoed G, MacDonald W: Oral and inhaled steroids in croup: a randomized, placebo-controlled trial. Pediatr Pulmonol 20:355–361, 1995.
44. Tibbals J, Shann F Landau L: Placebo-controlled trial of prednisolone in children intubated for croup. Lancet 340:745–748, 1992.
45. Novick A: Corticosteroid treatment of non-diphtheritic croup. Acta Otolaryngol 158:20, 1960.
46. Muhlendahl K, Kahn D, Spohr H: Steroid treatment in pseudo-croup. Helv Paediatr Acta 37:431, 1982.
47. Martensson B, Nilson G, Torbjar J: The effect of corticosteroids in the treatment of pseudo-croup. Acta Otolaryngol 158:20, 1960.
48. Donaldson D, Poleski D, Knipple E, et al: Intramuscular versus oral dexamethasone for the treatment of moderate-to-severe croup: a randomized, double-blind trial. Acad Emerg Med 10:16–21, 2003.
49. Rittichier KK, Ledwith CA: Outpatient treatment of moderate croup with dexamethasone: intramuscular versus oral dosing. Pediatrics 106:1344–1348, 2000.
50. Chub-Uppakarn S, Sangsupawanich P: A randomized comparison of dexamethasone 0.15 mg/kg versus 0.6 mg/kg for the treatment of moderate to severe croup. Int J Pediatr Otorhinolaryngol 71:473–477, 2007.
51. Sparrow A, Geelhoed G: Prednisolone versus dexamethasone in croup: a randomized equivalence trial. Arch Dis Child 91:580–583, 2006.
*52. Cetinkaya F, Tufekci BS, Kutluk G: A comparison of nebulized budesonide, and intramuscular, and oral dexamethasone for treatment of croup. Int J Pediatr Otorhinolaryngol 68:453–456, 2004.
*53. Klassen TP, Craig WAR, Moher D, Osmond MH: Nebulized budesonide and oral dexamethasone for treatment of croup: a randomized controlled trial. JAMA 279:1629–1632, 1998.
54. Husby S, Agertoft L, Mortensen S, Pedersen S: Treatment of croup with nebulized steroid (budesonide): a double blind, placebo controlled study. Arch Dis Child 68:352–355, 1993.
55. Godden CW, Campbell MJ, Hussey M, Gogswell JJ: Double blind placebo controlled trial of nebulized budesonide for croup. Arch Dis Child 76:155–158, 1997.
56. Klassen TP, Feldman ME, Watters LK, et al: Nebulized budesonide for children with mild-to-moderate croup. N Engl J Med 331:285–289, 1994.
57. Johnson DW, Jacobson S, Edney PC, et al: A comparison of nebulized budesonide, intramuscular dexamethasone, and placebo for moderately severe croup. N Engl J Med 339:498–503, 1998.
*58. Yates RW, Doull IJ: A risk-benefit assessment of corticosteroids in the management of croup. Drug Safety 16:48–55, 1997.
59. Osmond M: Croup. Clin Evidence 8:319–328, 2002.
60. McGee DL, Wald DA, Hinchliffe S: Helium-oxygen therapy in the emergency department. J Emerg Med 15:291–296, 1997.
61. Nelson DS, McClellan L: Helium-oxygen mixtures as adjunctive support for refractory viral croup. Ohio State Med J 78:729–730, 1982.
62. Weber JE, Chudnofsky CR, Younger JG, et al: A randomized comparison of helium-oxygen mixture (Heliox) and racemic epinephrine for the treatment of moderate to severe croup. Pediatrics 107:e96, 2001.
63. McEwan J, Giridharan W, Clarke RW, Shears P: Paediatric acute epiglottitis: not a disappearing entity. Int J Pediatr Otorhinolaryngol 67:317–321, 2003.
64. Yen K, Flanary V, Estel C, et al: Traumatic epiglottitis. Pediatr Emerg Care 19:27–28, 2003.
65. Kabbani M, Goodwin SR: Traumatic epiglottitis following blind finger sweep to remove a pharyngeal foreign body. Clin Pediatr 34:495–497, 1995.
66. O'Bier A, Muñiz AE, Foster RL: Hereditary angioedema presenting as epiglottitis. Pediatr Emerg Care 21:27–30, 2005.
67. Trollfors B, Nylen O, Strangert K: Acute epiglottitis in children and adults in Sweden 1981–3. Arch Dis Child 65:491–494, 1990.
68. Wong EY, Berkowitz RG: Acute epiglottitis in adults: the Royal Melbourne Hospital experience. Aust N Z J Surg 71:740–743, 2001.
69. Berg S, Trollfors B, Nylen O, et al: Incidence, aetiology, and prognosis of acute epiglottitis in children and adults in Sweden. Scand J Infect Dis 28:261–264, 1996.
70. Mayo-Smith MF, Spinale JW, Donskey CJ, et al: Acute epiglottitis. An 18-year experience in Rhode Island. Chest 108:1640–1647, 1995.
71. Abdullah AM, Chowdhury MN, Al Mazrou A, et al: Spectrum of *Haemophilus influenzae* type b disease in children: a university hospital in Riyadh, Saudi Arabia. J Trop Pediatr 43:10–12, 1997.
72. Ghirga G, Ghirga P, Palazzi C, et al: Bag-mask ventilation as a temporizing measure in acute infectious upper-airway obstruction: does it really work? Pediatr Emerge Care 17:444–446, 2001.
73. Donnelly BW, McMillan JA, Weiner LB: Bacterial tracheitis: report of eight new cases and review. Rev Infect Dis 12:729–735, 1990.
74. Strauss R, Mueller A, Wehler M, et al: Pseudomembranous tracheobronchitis due to *Bacillus cereus*. Clin Infect Dis 33:E39–E41, 2001.
75. Barnes C, Berkowitz R, Curtis N, Waters K: *Aspergillus* laryngotrachoebronchial infection in a 6-year-old girl following bone marrow transplantation. Int J Pediatr Otorhinolaryngol 31:59–62, 2001.
76. Berner R, Leititis JU, Furste HO, Brandis M: Bacterial tracheitis caused by *Corynebacterium diphtheriae*. Eur J Pediatr 156:207–208, 1997.
*77. Brook I: Aerobic and anaerobic microbiology of bacterial tracheitis in children. Pediatr Emerg Care 13:16–18, 1997.
78. Hopkins A, Lahiri T, Salerno R, et al: Changing epidemiology of life-threatening upper airway infections: The reemergence of bacterial tracheitis. Pediatrics 118:1418–1421, 2006.
79. Berstein T, Brilli R, Jacobs B: Is bacterial tracheitis changing? A 14 month experience in a pediatric intensive care unit. Clin Infect Dis 27:458–462, 1998.
80. Hari MS, Nirvala KD: Retropharyngeal abscess presenting with upper airway obstruction. Anaesthesia 58.714–715, 2003.
81. Etchevarren V, Bello O: Retropharyngeal abscess secondary to traumatic injury. Pediatr Emerge Care 18:189–191, 2002.
82. Poluri A, Singh B, Sperling N, et al: Retropharyngeal abscess secondary to penetrating foreign bodies. J Craniomaxillofac Surg 28:243–246, 2000.
*83. Furst I, Ellis D, Winton T: Unusual complication of endotracheal intubation: retropharyngeal space abscess, mediastinitis, and empyema. J Otolaryngol 29:309–311, 2000.
84. Hansen K, Maani C: Blastomycosis presenting as a retropharyngeal abscess. Otolaryngol Head Neck Surg 130:635–658, 2004.
85. Ungkanont K, Yellon RF, Weissman JL, et al: Head and neck space infections in infants and children. Otolaryngol Head Neck Surg 112:375–382, 1995.
86. Abdel-Haq NA, Harahsheh A, Asmar BI: Retropharyngeal abscess in children: the emerging role of group A beta hemolytic streptococcus. S Med J 99:927–931, 2006.
87. Philpott CM, Selvadurai D, Banerjee AR: Paediatric retropharyngeal abscess. J Laryngol Otol 118:919–926, 2004.
88. Harries PG: Retropharyngeal abscess and acute torticollis. J Laryngol Otol 111:1183–1185, 1997.
89. Craig FW, Schunk JE: Retropharyngeal abscess in children: clinical presentation, utility of imaging, and current management. Pediatrics 111:1394–1398, 2003.
90. Coulthard M, Isaacs D: Retropharyngeal abscess. Arch Dis Child 66:1227–1230, 1991.
*91. Lalakea M, Messner AH: Retropharyngeal abscess management in children: current practices. Otolaryngol Head Neck Surg 121:398–405, 1999.
*92. Vural C, Gungor A, Comerci S: Accuracy of computerized tomography in deep neck infection in the pediatric population. Am J Otolaryngol 24:143–148, 2003.
93. Plaza Mayor G, Martinez-San Millan J, Martinez-Vidal A: Is conservative treatment of deep space infections appropriate? Head Neck 23:126–133, 2001.

94. McSwiney PF, Cavanagh NP, Languth P: Outcome in congenital stridor (laryngomalacia). Arch Dis Child 52:215–218, 1977.

95. Zalzal GH, Anon JB, Cotton RT: Epiglottoplasty for the treatment of laryngomalacia. Ann Otol Rhinol Laryngol 96:72–76, 1987.

96. De Jong AL, Kuppersmith RB, Sulek M, Friedman EM: Vocal cord paralysis in infants and children. Otolaryngol Clin North Am 33:131–149, 2000.

97. Tucker HM: Human laryngeal reinnervation in laryngeal reinnervation: long term experience with nerve-muscle pedicle technique. Laryngoscope 88:598, 1987.

98. Parnell FW, Brandenburg JH: Vocal cord paralysis: a review of 100 cases. Laryngoscope 80:1036–1045, 1970.

99. Cotton RT: Mangement of laryngotracheal stenosis and tracheal lesions including single laryngotracheoplasty. Int J Pediatr Otorhinolaryngol 32(Suppl):S89–S91, 1995.

100. Marien S, Jespers A, Vidts G, Schmelzer B: Congenital laryngeal cyst: a case report. Acta Otorhinolaryngol Belg 57:119–121, 2003.

*101. Yilmaz M, Ozkan M, Dogan R, et al: Vascular anomalies causing tracheoesophageal compression: a 20-year experience in diagnosis and management. Heart Surg Forum 6:149–152, 2003.

*102. Austin J, Ali T: Tracheomalacia and bronchomalacia in children: pathophysiology, assessment, treatment and anesthesia management. Paediatr Anaesth 13:3–11, 2003.

103. Burton EM, Brick WG, Hall JD, et al: Tracheobronchial foreign body aspiration in children. South Med J 89:195–198, 1996.

104. Laks Y, Barzilay Z: Foreign body aspiration in childhood. Pediatr Emerg Care 4:102–106, 1988.

105. Mantel K, Butenandt I: Tracheobronchial foreign body aspiration in childhood: a report on 224 cases. Eur J Pediatr 145:211–216, 1986.

106. McGuirt WF, Holmes KD, Feehs R, Browne JD: Tracheobronchial foreign bodies. Laryngoscope 98:615–618, 1988.

107. Wiseman NE: The diagnosis of foreign body aspiration in childhood. J Pediatr Surg 19:532–555, 1984.

108. Taylor RB: Esophageal foreign bodies. Emerg Med Clin North Am 5:301–311, 1987.

109. Svedstrom E, Puhakka H, Kero P: How accurate is chest radiography in the diagnosis of tracheobronchial foreign bodies in children? Pediatr Radiol 19:520–522, 1989.

110. Assefa D, Amin N, Stringel G, et al: Use of decubitus radiographs in the diagnosis of foreign body aspiration in young children. Pediatr Emerg Care 23:154–157, 2007.

111. Heyer CM, Bollmeier ME, Rossler L, et al: Evaluation of clinical, radiologic, and laboratory prebronchoscy findings in children with suspected foreign body aspiration. J Pediatr Surg 41:1882–1888, 2006.

*112. Muñiz AE, Joffe M: Foreign body: aspirated or ingested. Contemp Pediatr 14:78–103, 1997.

Chapter 35

Vomiting, Spitting Up, and Feeding Disorders

Barbara E. McDevitt, MD

Key Points

The significance of vomiting encompasses a spectrum of problems ranging from the trivial (mild gastroesophageal reflux) to the catastrophic (small bowel obstruction).[1]

Acute vomiting of an underlying critical nature must be distinguished from regurgitation or spitting up.

Regurgitation is the passive, nonforceful expulsion of gastric contents up the esophagus, and commonly into the oropharynx, during and between feeds.

Bilious vomiting etiologies must be distinguished from those entities associated with nonbilious etiologies, such as esophageal atresia, tracheoesophageal fistula, pyloric stenosis, and gastroenteritis.

Contributing to feeding disorders may be a wide range of psychosocial and behavioral problems. These may be exacerbated by the current mobility of our society, frequently leaving young parents with a limited family support system.[4-6]

Introduction and Background

Emergency department (ED) visits for vomiting and feeding complaints are common in infancy. The differential diagnosis is quite extensive. These visits to the ED may be precipitated by a wide spectrum of symptoms, including crying, recurrent emesis, inadequate nutritional intake, and the parental perception of inadequate intake.[1-7] The vast majority of children with vomiting who visit the ED will have self-limited gastroenteritis or simple reflux. The clinician must be able to differentiate serious life-threatening disorders from simple spit-ups in an emergent yet thorough manner.

Recognition and Approach

The evaluation of the infant with vomiting begins by obtaining a history from the caregiver. Many caregivers consider feeding to be the primary means of assessing their ability to appropriately care for their child.[8] They may be concerned that the newborn's intake is inadequate, as reflected by crying or irritability. In today's society, fewer parents/caregivers have extended family to provide experience and reassurance. In addition, it is now the norm to discharge both mother and infant within 48 hours of delivery.[9] This may leave parents unprepared to recognize what is or is not normal behavior for a neonate.[7,10]

Neonatal conditions that in the past would have been recognized prior to discharge may not present until the newborn is at home, unsupervised by medical personnel. For example, infants lose up to 10% of their birth weight in the first week of life. They then regain their birth weight by 2 weeks. After the first 2 weeks, expected weight gain is approximately $1/2$ to 1 ounce a week.[10] Thus, obtaining the birth weight and present weight in the ED is valuable in recognizing an infant with an underlying disorder.[7]

Approximately 85% of all infants will have some vomiting or "spitting up" in the first 9 months of life and, in particular, during their first weeks at home. This generally resolves by the age of 1 year. Between birth and 3 months of age, 40% to 65% will vomit at least an ounce daily.[10,11] Combined, these normal patterns of feeding and reflux may create great anxiety, especially among new parents.

Infants differ from adults in that they have a short, narrow esophagus that allows passive regurgitation of stomach contents into the esophagus and then into the oropharynx. Contributing factors also include delayed gastric emptying, relaxed lower esophageal sphincter tone, overfeeding, or poor positioning of an infant after feeds.[11,12]

Pathogenic gastroesophogeal reflux disease is distinguished by the number and severity of the reflux episodes and the presence of complications, including esophagitis, weight loss or inadequate weight gain, and respiratory problems. Secondary aspiration, pneumonia, and wheezing with recurrent cough are currently believed to play a significant role in apparent life-threatening events.[11,13]

Vomiting is the forceful expulsion of gastric contents through the mouth and nose. It is caused by coordinated diaphragmatic and abdominal contractions in conjunction with the relaxation of the gastroesophageal sphincter.[2] An infant with true forceful recurrent vomiting requires an expedient and thorough evaluation to rule out a potentially lethal disorder.[1]

Less emergent are the infants who present to the ED with a wide range of disorders such as congenital heart disease, neurologic impairments, or congenital syndromes. These infants have difficulty coordinating their suck-gag reflex,[4] which places them at risk for aspiration. They may chronically aspirate both their formula and their own secretions. They may also have impairments secondary to the technology they depend on for nutrition.[14]

Clinical Presentation

The clinical presentations of vomiting may be grouped by the age of the patient, by medical or surgical etiology, or by the nature of the emesis.[15,16] Bilious and forceful vomiting are of particular concern as they suggest an obstruction beyond the part of the duodenum where the ampulla of Vater connects.[17-19] This is a significant symptom in young babies as it may indicate malrotation, volvulus, duodenal atresia, or meconium ileus.[7,20] Many other conditions associated with the gastrointestinal (GI) tract in infants also require urgent recognition and intervention due to their potentially catastrophic outcome if not diagnosed promptly.

Two of the most common causes of vomiting in infants are overfeeding and physiologic gastroesophageal reflux (GER).[11] However, vomiting can also be a symptom of more systemic entities, including metabolic disorders, infectious disease, intracranial pathology, and renal disease and, in current times, it may be seen in association with neonatal narcotic withdrawal secondary to maternal addiction. Table 35–1 lists common causes of pediatric vomiting.

The history should ascertain whether the infant is in pain, the amount and the frequency of the emesis, the timing of the emesis with respect to recent feeding or coughing paroxysm, recent bowel movements, and fever.[19] The family history should cover any relatives with metabolic disorders, trisomy 21, cystic fibrosis, or Hirschsprung's disease.[21,22]

Table 35–1	Important Causes of Vomiting in Infancy

Feeding problems, including overfeeding/gastroesophageal reflux
Infection—including otitis media, pneumonia, sepsis, urinary tract infections, meningitis, enteritis, and pertussis
Gastrointestinal tract obstructions—including esophageal atresia, duodenal atresia, malrotation/volvulus, Hirschsprung's disease
Neurologic—raised intracranial pressure or brain subdural hematoma, hydrocephalus, meningitis
Incarcerated hernia
Metabolic—congenital adrenal hyperplasia, hypothyroidism, phenylketonuria
Cow's milk intolerance or malabsorption
Narcotic withdrawal due to maternal addiction

Formula Issues

Overfeeding and Underfeeding

Full-term, healthy neonates typically require 105 to 115 cal/kg per day of nutrition. Most formulas contain 20 calories per ounce (30 ml) unless they are fortified with extra calories. Using these numbers, clinicians can determine if formula-fed neonates and young infants are receiving inadequate nutrition or if they are being overfed. Moreover, infants who are overfed (e.g., >150 cal/kg per day) have more frequent stools and may have more frequent regurgitation, spitting up, and vomiting. These symptoms typically occur soon after feeding and are exacerbated when infants are placed in a recumbent position. If any of these symptoms occur in an overfed young infant, decreasing the amount of feeds, decreasing the volume of each feed, and increasing the frequency of feeding may decrease vomiting.

Inappropriate Feeding

A gradual introduction of solid foods (e.g., cereals) to an infant's diet should not occur until the age of 4 to 6 months. Too early use of solid foods may lead to increased regurgitation or spitting up.

Formula Intolerance and Allergy

Infants may develop intolerance or allergy to components of formula. Nearly 3% of infants are allergic to cow's milk protein, while over 1% have soy protein allergies. Reactions to these proteins are often immunoglobulin E mediated, with prominent GI symptoms (vomiting, diarrhea [often heme positive], chronic constipation, and colic). Respiratory symptoms (wheezing, rhinitis) and cutaneous manifestations (atopy, urticaria, angioedema) may also occur. Laboratory testing occasionally reveals an eosinophilia. Infants with true formula intolerance may benefit from use of hypoallergenic formulas (e.g., extensively hydrolyzed or free amino acids). For infants above the age of 6 months who have cow's milk intolerance, a soy formula may also be tried.

Breast Milk Issues

Breast-feeding is recommended by the American Academy of Pediatrics, the World Health Organization, and UNICEF as the ideal route for providing nutrition to neonates and young infants.[23] In general, breast-fed infants have less constipation and colic and fewer GI symptoms than bottle-fed infants.[23,24] However, an altered maternal diet or maternal medication or drug ingestion may lead to GI symptoms, including vomiting and spitting up. Maternal ingestion of illicit drugs (e.g., heroin, cocaine) can lead to vomiting and spitting up, in addition to multiple other toxic effects. Additionally, prenatal maternal ingestion of heroin or narcotics may cause severe withdrawal symptoms in neonates, including seizures, jitteriness, vomiting, and diarrhea. While maternal ingestion of medications is often safe for breast-fed infants, the list of drugs that might be responsible for GI symptoms or other more toxic effects is extensive.[25] Clinicians should consult authoritative references to determine the possible impact of maternal medications on symptoms in breast-fed infants. For most herbal supplements, levels within human milk and effects on breast-fed infants have not been studied. For this reason, they should be avoided by breast-feeding mothers.[24]

Although a food allergy is uncommon in breast-fed infants compared to formula-fed infants, rare cases of anaphylaxis to cow's milk proteins have been reported in breast-fed infants, as well as more frequent cases of cow's milk–induced proctocolitis. Importantly, immunologically recognizable proteins from the maternal diet can be found in breast milk. Elimination of cow's milk, eggs, fish, peanuts and tree nuts, and other foods from the maternal diet may lead to resolution of allergic symptoms in the nursing infant.[26] Gastrointestinal complaints other than allergy (e.g., spitting up, gas, diarrhea) can be due to ingestion by the mother of specific foods (e.g., onions, cruciferous vegetables such as cabbage, tomatoes, berries, chocolate, and spices).[26] If a reaction to any of these foods is highly suspected, the mother consider removing them from her diet.

Gastroesophageal Reflux

GER is defined as the passive movement of gastric contents into the esophagus and higher. Relaxation of the lower esophageal sphincter is the most common cause. Other important causes include increased intra-abdominal pressure, excessive crying (with air swallowing), delayed gastric emptying, and sluggish esophageal motility. Neonates who are premature or stressed (especially due to respiratory illness) are most at risk for developing GER. Importantly, GER is not always a benign disorder. When a fluid comes into contact with the mucosal surface, nerve endings are stimulated, resulting in a laryngeal chemoreflex.[27] These receptors mediate several aspiration preventive reflex responses, which include swallowing, airway constriction or closure, and coughing. Cessation of breathing or apnea also may occur.[27]

Symptoms of GER include postprandial spitting up and coughing or choking during feeding. Aspiration may cause recurrent pneumonitis, laryngospasm, and bronchospasm. Esophageal irritation may lead to food aversion, weight loss, and failure to thrive.

Management consists of decreasing the volume of each feed while increasing the frequency of feeding. For formula-fed infants, thickening of formula (1 tablespoon of cereal for each 1 to 2 ounces of formula) may decrease regurgitation. Parents should be instructed to maintain infants in an upright position for at least 15 to 20 minutes after feeding. The seated position should be avoided as this may increase abdominal pressure and worsen regurgitation. If cow's milk or soy protein allergy is a possibility, the parents should consider changing to a hypoallergenic formula.

Medications that may be useful include histamine$_2$-receptor antagonists (cimetidine, famotidine, nizatidine, and ranitidine), and proton pump inhibitors (omeprazole, lansoprazole, pantoprazole, rabeprazole, and esomeprazole) to decrease acidity of stomach contents and lessen esophageal and laryngeal symptoms. Prokinetic agents (e.g., metoclopromide, bethanecol, erythromycin) increase lower esophageal sphincter pressure and may increase the clearance of esophageal and gastric contents. As a final resort, surgical procedures can be used to decrease or eliminate regurgitation via the esophagus.

Infants with severe symptoms (e.g., apnea, aspiration pneumonitis, failure to thrive) require admission, inpatient confirmation of diagnosis, monitoring, and initiation of therapy.

Mild Systemic Illness

Neonates are obligate nose breathers until they reach the age of 4 to 6 months. The presence of upper respiratory infections may lead to difficulty with feeding and breathing. Excess air may be swallowed as young infants attempt to feed, leading to abdominal distention and vomiting. Vomiting may be a symptom of minor illness, minor upper respiratory infection, or gastroenteritis. With this in mind, it is important to exclude major systemic illness and surgical disorders as a cause of vomiting in neonates and infants.

Major Systemic Illness

Metabolic disorders may cause vomiting, but many are now detected during newborn screenings.[1,9] However, though rare, urea cycle defects may present early after discharge from the nursery with vomiting and elevated ammonia levels.[28] The adrenogenital syndrome commonly presents with vomiting as the presenting event in males. Symptoms begin at the 7th to 10th day, or earlier if the infant is stressed. Diagnosis is easier in girls as virilization of the external genitalia may have been noticed at birth. Diagnosis is supported by the finding of hyperkalemia, hyponatremia, and hypoglycemia and by an infant who may then rapidly progress into shock[1,28] (see Chapter 29, Inborn Errors of Metabolism; and Chapter 108, Addisonian Crisis).

Neurologic disorders typically lead to vomiting associated with an altered mental status or abnormal neurologic examination. Any suspicion for intracranial disease requires a cranial computed tomography (CT) scan. This is necessary to rule out a subdural hemorrhage secondary to accidental trauma or abuse, an intracranial tumor, or increased intracerebral pressure secondary to congenital hydrocephalus.[1,28]

Infants who have had shunts placed at birth for congenital hydrocephalus or status post intraventricular hemorrhage or meningitis may develop vomiting as the first symptom of increasing hydrocephalus from a malfunctioning shunt. In addition, the shunt's tubing, which empties into the peritoneal cavity, may in itself cause a volvulus or form adhesions. Finally, the lumen itself may become blocked by debris and stop draining spinal fluid in an appropriate manner, leading to hydrocephalus.[29]

Serious bacterial and viral infections must be considered and excluded in neonates and infants with vomiting. Findings on examination are particularly subtle at younger ages, and fever is often absent in the setting of a serious bacterial infection. Simple viral enteritis may present with vomiting and fever. However due to the low reserves for hydration and limited glucose storage in neonates and very young infants, a lower threshold for intravenous rehydration should be established, and clinicians should consider and exclude congenital, metabolic, and surgical disorders.[10] An infant with meningitis may present with vomiting, but fever, altered mental status, and sepsis will predominate.[1,10]

Emesis may be the presenting symptom in an infant with otitis media or a urinary tract infection. A practitioner may be fooled by erythematous tympanic membranes, which are often associated with fever and crying in the young infant. This can lead to the inadvertently attribution of all the infant's symptoms to an ear infection. Therefore, a urinalysis and culture of a specimen obtained by catheterization should always be included in an ED evaluation.[1]

Pertussis is having a resurgence in this country due to parental resistance to immunizations. Parents may bring their infant to the ED because of their concern about the post-tussive emesis associated with the disease's paroxysms of coughing.[2]

Renal stones or ureteropelvic junction obstruction may manifest through cyclic vomiting. Vomiting associated with colicky pain and hematuria is suggestive of this diagnosis.[30,31]

Narcotic withdrawal in an infant may be manifested by vomiting or irritability. This diagnosis will involve urine tests, as well as skillful questioning of the mother.[1,10]

Surgical Disorders

Esophageal Atresia and Tracheoesophageal Fistula

Infants with esophageal atresia may be diagnosed in utero, or when they fail to tolerate their first feed or are unable to swallow their own secretions. A history of maternal polyhydramnios and prematurity is common.[22] A plain radiograph will show a soft nasogastric tube passed into the esophagus coiling back on itself, unable to pass into the stomach. Further confirmation can be obtained by injecting a small quantity of air down this catheter; this will distend the proximal esophageal pouch. Contrast material should not be used as it could lead to aspiration.[22]

Esophageal atresia is associated with a tracheoesophageal fistula (TEF) in 85% of the cases, and 64% of infants with esophageal atresia had associated anomalies, including vertebral, renal, and anal anomalies as well as duodenal atresia and congenital heart disease.[32,33] If a TEF is present, the radiograph will show gas in the intestine. The abdomen is gasless in those infants without a fistula.[34] An infant with isolated TEF may present to the ED in respiratory distress due to recurrent aspiration, or with a history of choking and coughing with all feeds.[32,35]

Proximal Gastrointestinal Surgical Disorders

PYLORIC STENOSIS

Pyloric stenosis is the most common pediatric surgical condition that causes emesis (nonbilious) in young infants. It is the most common condition requiring surgery in the first few months of life. Pyloric stenosis is an idiopathic hypertrophy of the pyloric muscle whose etiology is not well understood. It is characterized by elongation and narrowing of the pyloric lumen, secondary gastritis, and mucosal edema that will eventually result in almost complete obstruction.[36]

Infants with pyloric stenosis are usually healthy the first few weeks of life. They have successfully established their feeding regimen and regained their birth weight.[7] By the third to fourth week of life, these infants typically will begin to vomit intermittently with feeds, with progressively increasing force, volume, and frequency. Throughout the progression of these symptoms, these infants are hungry, eager to take the breast or bottle, but then vomit within 30 minutes of feeding.[36,37] The emesis will not contain bile but may be blood-tinged from associated esophagitis/gastritis.

If symptoms have been present for several days, the infant will present with dehydration, projectile nonbilious vomiting, and a hypochloremic, hypokalemic metabolic alkalosis. This metabolic state is unique to infants with pyloric steno-sis. That is because the gastric fluid loss from these infants is associated with the loss of H^+ and Cl^-, unlike fluid losses in conditions caused by vomiting with an open pylorus, which involves loss of gastric, pancreatic, biliary, and/or intestinal fluids.[38,39]

On physical examination, these infants may have a palpable "olive" mass, as well as peristaltic waves across the abdomen, though in reality neither is commonly palpated.[37] A radiograph of the abdomen may show a large gastric bubble secondary to gastric outlet obstruction.[36] Ultrasound is the diagnostic modality of choice. It is both highly sensitive and specific for pyloric stenosis,[40] and clearly demonstrates hypertrophied muscle whose length and thickness can be measured to confirm the diagnosis. Pyloric stenosis is present if the muscle thickness exceeds 4 mm.[39,41] In cases in which ultrasound is inconclusive, an upper GI series may be done to evaluate for possible GER, duodenal atresia, or malrotation[39,42] (see Chapter 76, Pyloric Stenosis).

DUODENAL ATRESIA

Duodenal atresia, duodenal webs, and duodenal stenosis can lead to intestinal narrowing or to a complete blockage of the intestinal lumen. The blockage may also be secondary to extrinsic causes, including an annular pancreas or a midgut volvulus with Ladd bands.[32] The etiology of duodenal atresia is unknown. It may be secondary to a failure of recanalization of the duodenal lumen during the early gestational stage of the embryo.[32]

The primary symptom of duodenal atresia is vomiting, which may or may not be bilious depending on the level of the obstruction. In 85% of the infants, the obstruction is distal to the ampulla of Vater. Therefore, the papilla of Vater opens into the proximal duodenum, accounting for the bilious nature of the emesis.[22,32] If the obstruction is proximal to the ampulla, then the infant may vomit clear material. If it is only a partial stenosis, the diagnosis may not be made until well beyond the newborn period. At that time, the infant may present with dehydration, weight loss, and constipation in addition to intermittent vomiting.

In atresia, the classic diagnostic sign is the double bubble sign on abdominal radiography. The double bubble sign is two air-filled structures in the upper abdomen with little or no air distally.[34] The proximal left-sided bubble is the air- and fluid-filled stomach. The proximal duodenum represents the second bubble to the right of the midline. When there is gas distal to the dilated proximal duodenum, malrotation must be distinguished from duodenal stenosis by ultrasound or an upper GI study.[15,43] However, even in the neonate with the classic appearance of a "double bubble" without distal air, intrinsic causes of obstruction, especially malrotation, must be considered.[19] If surgical intervention is delayed or if there are additional symptoms on physical examination suggestive of acute obstruction, further radiologic investigation is mandatory.[20] A neonate with bilious vomiting has malrotation with midgut volvulus until proven otherwise.[22]

MALROTATION WITH MIDGUT VOLVULUS

Malrotation with midgut volvulus occurs when there is failure of the developing bowel to undergo the usual counterclockwise rotation during embryogenesis. Peritoneal bands (which normally attach the bowel to the abdominal wall) can compress the duodenum, partially obstructing it.[41]

Additionally, as the mesentery is not well attached, patients are at risk for developing a midgut volvulus. Volvulus refers to the complete twisting of a loop of bowel around its mesenteric attachment, leading to intestinal obstruction. The superior mesenteric artery can be compressed, leading to ischemia of the small bowel from the duodenal-jejunal junction to the midtransverse colon.[17,20]

Unless recognized and treated promptly, bowel ischemia progresses to infarction and necrosis, fever, peritonitis, abdominal distention, hypovolemia, and septic shock. This anomaly may be a difficult diagnostic problem. Clinical presentations may include intermittent vomiting, distention, and constipation that may become more constant, or progress to full-blown obstruction with peritonitis. The hallmark symptom of bilious emesis is present in 75% to 100% of the cases of midgut volvulus.[44]

In a review of 22 patients undergoing surgery for malrotation, 50% had normal abdominal examinations and 32% had abnormal distention without tenderness.[45] The obstruction on midgut volvulus is usually high, and abdominal distention may not be present. The newborn may only present with crying and bilious vomiting and then rapidly progress to abdominal distention. As midgut ischemia progresses, the infant may rapidly dehydrate and develop metabolic acidosis.[17,39]

Infants with bilious vomiting require emergent imaging. Plain abdominal films may show a distended stomach and a proximal duodenal bulb with little or no intestinal air, and ultrasound may detect an abnormal relationship between the superior mesenteric artery and vein, also referred to as the whirlpool sign.[39] The definitive study is the upper GI series with small bowel follow-through. It can conclusively differentiate a midgut volvulus from duodenal atresia/stenosis.[31,46] The barium enema is now less frequently used due to frequent false-negative studies.

Laboratory analyses are of little benefit in early presentation, but as bowel compromise progresses, they will reflect increasing hypovolemia and the beginning of extensive ischemic bowel and intestinal necrosis.[39] All bilious vomiting in the neonate should be considered a malrotation with midgut volvulus until proven otherwise. An emergency upper GI series must be performed as the patient is being evaluated.[18,19] All patients require aggressive fluid resuscitation, placement of a nasogastric tube, parenteral antibiotics effective against enteric organisms, and surgical consultation (see Chapter 83, Malrotation and Midgut Volvulus).

Distal Surgical Disorders

JEJUNAL ATRESIA

Jejunal atresia is classified into four types, but the symptoms and signs are identical regardless of the type of lesion. It is more common than duodenal atresia, occurring in 1 in 1500 births, and is also associated with polyhydramnios and premature birth.[47] It is not associated with chromosomal anomalies or with anomalies of systems outside of the GI tract.[32] Infants may present with a varied complex of symptoms including bilious vomiting, abdominal distention, and failure to pass meconium.[32] The acuteness of the symptoms may also vary. Vomiting may be only bile stained, abdominal distention may be minimal, and small amounts of meconium may be passed. Five percent of the lesions may involve only partial obstruction or stenosis caused by incomplete intraluminal

occlusion.[19] Diagnosis may be aided by obtaining an obstructive radiographic series, which would show multiple dilated loops of intestine with air-fluid levels.[18] The small bowel close to the atresia may become grossly distended.[18,19,31,32,48]

MECONIUM ILEUS

Meconium ileus is actually a mechanical obstruction. As a result of pancreatic enzyme deficiency, the distal ileum is plugged by thick meconium, leading to a functional obstruction. Ninety percent to 95% of these infants have cystic fibrosis, and thus a deficit of pancreatic enzymes in the intestines.[36] Fifteen percent of infants with cystic fibrosis are born with meconium ileus.[45] This entity should be detected in the neonatal period prior to discharge from the hospital. In approximately 50% of the patients the bowel is intact and its continuity preserved. However, the emergency physician should be aware that an ileus can reoccur at any time in a patient with cystic fibrosis.

Infants with a meconium ileus will present with bilious vomiting and a distended, tender abdomen with palpable thickened loops of bowel. Plain abdominal films show distended loops of intestine with thickened bowel walls. Meconium mixed with swallowed air will give a characteristic ground-glass appearance without air-fluid levels. Treatment of meconium ileus involves evacuation of the meconium, preferably by nonsurgical management. Contrast enemas (using Gastrograffin) may be used with careful ongoing hydration and observation of the patient, as the risk of perforation reportedly is 3% to 10%.[19,32] A meconium ileus may lead to peritonitis if a volvulus or perforation of the bowel occurs. Calcifications, free air, or very large air-fluid levels are consistent with bowel perforation, which require urgent surgical intervention.[22]

MECONIUM PLUG SYNDROME

Meconium plug syndrome occurs when plugs of meconium obstruct the colon. It is associated with conditions that predispose to dysmotility of the neonatal bowel. Conditions predisposing to meconium plugs are prematurity and or low birth weight in the neonate. Also at risk are infants born to mothers with hypothyroidism or diabetes or those whose mothers received magnesium sulfate during delivery.[19] While it is not associated with cystic fibrosis, a small percentage of these infants have associated Hirschsprung's disease. Infants may not develop symptoms until several days after birth.

Infants may present with bilious vomiting, abdominal distention, and no passage of meconium.[32] Usually the abdomen is nontender early in presentation. This disorder can resemble small bowel obstruction. In this condition, the colon is believed to be normally innervated but functionally immature. The radiograph may be consistent with low small bowel obstruction or large bowel obstruction.[31,39,41] A simple rectal examination may allow the plug to pass. A water-contrast enema is usually both diagnostic and curative, with passage of the plug. The GI tract is decompressed and normal GI function established. However, 10% to 15% of these infants may have agangliosis of the colon and need close follow-up to rule out Hirschsprung's disease.[32,49]

COLONIC ATRESIA

Colonic atresia is rare. It accounts for less than 15% of all distal intestinal atresias.[49] Patients present with abdominal distention, failure to pass stool, and vomiting. It may occur in conjunction with small bowel atresia or Hirschsprung's disease. It is diagnosed via a contrast enema to distinguish it from distal ileal atresia and Hirschsprung's disease.[19,29]

HIRSCHSPRUNG'S DISEASE

Hirschsprung's disease is a common form of distal bowel obstruction in the newborn. It is defined by the absence of ganglion cells in a variable length of distal bowel (in 80% cases it involves only the rectosigmoid colon). It affects 1 in 5000 infants, and is increased in cases of trisomy 21.[22,39] A lack of ganglion cells in the colon leads to a failure of parasympathetic-mediated relaxation in the involved segment. An aganglionic colon cannot maintain normal peristalsis, the internal sphincter does not relax, and a functional intestinal obstruction occurs.[19]

Clinical manifestations in the neonate include bilious vomiting, failure to pass meconium, abdominal distention, constipation, anorexia, and no stool in the rectum on digital examination.[22] Vomiting may be bilious or feculent due to the distal site of obstruction. Although most infants present in the first month of life with bowel obstruction, a minority of infants present later with chronic constipation. A plain film may show distended bowel loops, air-fluid levels, and stool in the proximal colon, making this condition difficult to distinguish from a small bowel obstruction.[22,39] In Hirschprung's disease a barium enema will, 80% of the time, show a transitional zone at the junction between the aganglionic and ganglionic intestine.[49] Diagnosis is confirmed by rectal biopsy[16,49] (see Chapter 77, Constipation).

Hirschsprung's enterocolitis may occur when the diagnosis of Hirschsprung's disease is delayed or when an extremely large length of aganglionic segment is involved. Symptoms include abdominal distention, vomiting, explosive diarrhea, and sepsis. This is believed to occur when the mucosal integrity of the massively dilated proximal colon is compromised, allowing for the bacterial invasion of the epithelium with impaired mucosal or neuronal immunity.[19] The physical examination will be consistent with peritonitis and sepsis. Radiographs may show distended loops of bowel along the left flank with an abrupt termination in the pelvis (intestinal cutoff sign).[22] These infants will require rapid and aggressive intervention, including volume resuscitation, antibiotics, and possibly urgent colonic decompression or a colostomy.

ANORECTAL MALFORMATIONS

Anorectal malformations range from a slight anterior displacement of the anal opening to a completely imperforate anus. All of these should be picked up on neonatal examination, but low lesions with perineal fistulas or an anterior ectopic anus may be difficult to discern.[50] Infants with imperforate anus may have several associated problems: vertebral anomalies, anal atresia, cardiac anomalies (tetralogy of Fallot, ventricular septal defects), TEF, and various renal, urologic, and GI anomalies. The morbidity and mortality in these infants may be related to the severity of their associated lesions. Therefore, an initial evaluation plan should include a chest radiograph, electrocardiogram, echocardiogram, and appropriate urologic and orthopedic studies as indicated.[50]

NECROTIZING ENTEROCOLITIS

Necrotizing enterocolitis is commonly associated with premature infants, but also with full-term infants who had a hypoxic insult at birth.[51,52] It is a rapidly progressive disease producing hemorrhagic necrosis of the intestines, leading to peritonitis and sepsis. Its etiology is unknown but is believed to be related to the inability of the immature GI tract and an infant's immune system to deal with postnatal stresses, especially perinatal hypoxia.[53] It may affect any part of the GI tract but has a predilection for the ileocecal region.[52] It will usually present in the immediate newborn period, but some infants do not manifest symptoms until 10 to 12 days of age.[52]

The infant may present to the ED with bilious vomiting, bloody stools, abdominal distention, and ileus. More insidiously, the infant's symptoms may be very nonspecific, including lethargy, apnea, anorexia, and full-blown sepsis and shock. The kidney-ureter-bladder film may be pathognomonic for necrotizing enterocolitis, with pneumatosis intestinalis or gas within the bowel wall, as well as air in the portal vein; free air will be noted with perforation. Sequential films that show fixed loops of bowel and/or an ileus may indicate bowel ischemia.[22] Laboratory values consistent with sepsis and shock, especially thrombocytopenia, indicate the need for urgent surgical intervention along with ongoing resuscitation and stabilization.[18,52]

INCARCERATED INGUINAL HERNIAS

Incarcerated inguinal hernias are an important and easily overlooked cause of bowel obstruction in infants. A hernia is defined as the protrusion of a portion of tissue through the wall normally containing it. Inguinal hernias result from the incomplete obliteration of a small diverticulum of the peritoneal sac, the processus vaginalis, in the lower abdomen. This can lead to the development of hernia that may also involve the testes in the male or the ovaries in the female. There is a 6:1 male:female predominance, but females have higher rate of incarceration.[54] Its incidence increases with premature birth as well as with conditions associated with increased intra-abdominal pressure. These include, among other less common causes, ventriculoperitoneal shunts, peritoneal dialysis, or ascites.[55] Most infants are asymptomatic unless incarceration develops. Incarceration is defined as the inability to reduce the contents of the hernia back into the inguinal cavity. Fifty percent of incarcerations present at less than 6 months of age. These are almost always indirect inguinal hernias.[55]

Parents commonly bring their infants to the ED because of a swelling or bulge noted in the inguinal or umbilical area. Other symptoms may include vomiting, constipation, abdominal distention, and poor feeding.[55,56] Nearly 95% of these inguinal hernias can be reduced by constant, gentle upward pressure on the hernia sac.[36] Undescended testes can appear to be hernias. The physician should be sure to palpate both testicles in the scrotum prior to diagnosing an inguinal hernia.

It is appropriate as well as therapeutic to first treat the infant with an agent to reduce pain and anxiety before attempting reduction. If the infant's hernia is easily and successfully reduced, the infant may be referred to a pediatric surgeon for close follow-up and further evaluation.[21] However, infants may also present with a toxic appearance secondary to strangulation of the bowel. These infants may present with an erythematous, firm, immobile mass, and manual reduction should not be attempted. Intestinal obstruction due to strangulation of the bowel may present with bilious vomiting, abdominal distention and tenderness, bloody stools, and a hypovolemic state.[36,55] These symptoms necessitate emergent intervention, including fluid resuscitation, placement of a nasogastric tube, laboratory assessments for sepsis and degree of hypovolemia, the initiation of appropriate antibiotics, and immediate surgical consultation. Plain films are generally not necessary and would simply confirm bowel obstruction[22,56] (see Chapter 84, Abdominal Hernias).

APPENDICITIS

Appendicitis is rare in infancy. If it occurs, the diagnosis is usually delayed. Almost all cases are perforated upon presentation, and the typical symptom duration prior to diagnosis is more than 3 days. Vomiting is present in nearly all infants. Common symptoms include abdominal pain, fever, and diarrhea. Nonspecific symptoms include irritability, difficulty breathing or grunting, and right hip stiffness or pain. Nearly all infants have diffuse abdominal tenderness, while localized right lower quadrant tenderness is noted in only a few cases. Other described features include lethargy due to sepsis, abdominal rigidity or distention, and an abdominal or rectal mass due to abscess formation[2,36,57] (see Chapter 73, Appendicitis).

INTUSSUSCEPTION

Intussusception can lead to vomiting in infancy.[28,58] The incidence of this disorder peaks at 10 months of age, with a range of 3 months to 2 years, although 10% of children are older than 2 years at the time of presentation.[36,59] In this entity, a segment of bowel telescopes into the lumen of the portion of intestine just distal to it. This occurs most commonly at the ileocolic junction. As the distal ileum invaginates and advances into the ascending colon, the prolapsed segment compresses mesenteric vessels, thereby limiting blood flow, leading to obstruction, strangulation, and, if unrecognized and allowed to progress, bowel necrosis.[59]

The classic textbook triad of colicky abdominal pain, vomiting and bloody stools with mucus ("currant jelly stools") is seen in less than one third of cases.[59] More commonly infants present with the sudden onset of cramping, intermittent abdominal pain (83% to 92% of patients) that recurs at frequent intervals, accompanied by crying and frequently flexing of the legs as the child attempts to find a position of relief. Nonbilious vomiting occurs in 85% of cases, but the vomitus may eventually become bile stained as the obstruction progresses.[58,59] Hematochezia is both a late, as well as an infrequent, sign (<8% of infants) associated with high morbidity and mortality.[56] A more recently recognized set of behavioral symptoms in infants has been well documented in association with intussusception, though their exact etiology has yet to be delineated. An infant with an altered mental status, or lethargy, on presentation to the ED must have intussusception included prominently in the differential diagnosis.[36] A right upper quadrant mass may be palpated and, when combined with a schaphoid right lower quadrant (Dance's sign), is highly suggestive of intussusception.

Diagnosis is primarily by history and observation of the child. Radiographs may rarely show "target signs," or a paucity of gas in the distal colon. Ultrasound is very sensitive (98% to 100%), though less specific than an enema. Water, contrast, or air enema may be diagnostic as well as curative, allowing for nonoperative intervention.[60,61] However, prior to attempting reduction, the infant's metabolic and volume status must be stabilized and pediatric surgery must be readily available in anticipation of possible perforation of the bowel during the attempted reduction. Absolute contraindications for nonoperative reduction are peritonitis, high-grade bowel obstruction, and perforation. Rates of perforation associated with barium enema are estimated to be 0.7%, and those with an air enema, 2.8%.[58] Any infant who presents with signs of peritonitis, pneumoperitoneum, or associated shock is a candidate for surgical reduction only after stabilization. There is a 5% to 8% recurrence rate, regardless of the method of reduction[62] (see Chapter 74, Intussusception).

Nonaccidental Trauma

Nonaccidental trauma can be an important cause of vomiting in infants with intracranial and abdominal injuries. The recognition of nonaccidental abdominal injury may be difficult because of subtle abdominal findings or minimal histories.

Risk factors include the caregiver's delay in seeking treatment for prolonged vomiting or for emesis stained by blood or bile. There may also be inconsistencies in the history and duration of the infant's symptoms, as given by the family members.[46,63] Infants with duodenal hematomas may present initially with emesis, consistent with a viral gastroenteritis. As the hematoma causes increasing obstruction or even rupture of the viscus, symptoms of peritonitis or septic or hypovolemic shock may develop. Trauma must always be part of the differential diagnosis of the young infant with emesis that is bilious or blood tinged or suggestive in any way of an abdominal injury.

Abdominal CT is the diagnostic modality of choice and, if positive, should be followed by a complete evaluation for evidence of abuse.[64,65]

Important Clinical Features and Considerations

Vomiting is a common presenting complaint among young infants presenting to the ED. Its etiologies range from the manifestation of a systemic illness to a congenital anatomic or metabolic anomaly, to an infectious entity or simple overfeeding. As it is a common presenting symptom in childhood, the majority of infants do not require any imaging.[41]

The diagnosis of disorders that cause vomiting must center on a careful history and physical examination, as well as a period of observation with repeat examinations in the ED.[7,10] Surgically correctable causes of vomiting in the young infant are less common than medical ones. As etiologies that can be treated by surgical intervention are rarely seen in the ED, the physician must always be aware of the symptoms and signs of bowel obstruction. Importantly, clinicians must realize that plain abdominal radiographs are normal in half of all infants with surgical abdominal disorders.[66] They must be aware of appropriate diagnostic techniques for each disease.

Rapid diagnosis of an anatomic anomaly of the GI tract can mean the difference between complete recovery and the catastrophic loss of bowel, with its associated morbidity and mortality.

Bilious vomiting in an infant indicates obstruction beyond the level of the second part of the duodenum.[19] This is of great significance in a newborn as it may indicate malrotation and possible volvulus. The infant may also present with hypovolemic shock and appear septic. Stabilizing a potentially septic infant, who also has symptoms suggestive of a bowel obstruction, should not preclude his or her management as having a malrotation and possible volvulus until proven otherwise. A surgical consultant should be involved in the infant's care immediately, with appropriate imaging (a rapid ultrasound or a definitive upper GI series with bowel follow-through) ordered simultaneously. However, bowel obstruction may present with more subtle symptoms, including nonbilious vomiting or a distended abdomen. Diarrhea may also be present.

The infant with intussusception may be inconsolable secondary to pain or may be lethargic.[21,59] The "classic" three findings of vomiting, intermittent abdominal pain, and currant jelly stools actually occur concomitantly in less than 10% of all cases. The presence of blood and mucus in the stool is suggestive of an intussusception that has already led to bowel necrosis.[59]

Management

Management of infants with vomiting and spitting up requires an initial determination of hydration, cardiopulmonary status, and likelihood of serious medical or surgical disorders. If symptoms suggest the presence of intestinal obstruction (bilious vomiting, abdominal distention or tenderness, bloody stool, a hypovolemic state or an altered mental status lacking a clear neurologic basis), the physician should proceed aggressively with preparation for surgical intervention.[36] A nasogastric tube is placed if bowel obstruction or perforation is present, and any drainage is replaced with appropriate isotonic intravenous fluids.[21,38,53] Hypoglycemia and electrolyte abnormalities should be corrected during hydration. Appropriate imaging studies, if time allows, should be ordered. Intravenous access should be established for rapid isotonic fluid resuscitation. Cardiopulmonary monitoring is required, with frequent reassessment of volume status, vital signs, and mental status.

Infants with gastroenteritis or minor illness and mild to moderate dehydration potentially can be orally dehydrated. For infants, a rehydration solution is used that contains 50 mEq of sodium and 25 g/L of glucose (e.g., Pedialyte). The infant is given 1 to 2 teaspoons every 5 to 15 minutes over the first hour, and the hydration status is reassessed. The volume is doubled every hour afterward until the infant tolerates 2 ounces every 20 minutes. If the infant looks well, he or she can be discharged home with instructions on how to advance the diet. If the infant vomits at home, the caregiver should wait an hour and repeat the process of introducing rehydration solution at 1 teaspoon every 15 minutes. If the infant vomits again, he or she must be brought back to the ED for reassessment.[62] Once the infant can tolerate oral rehydration liquids, the caregiver should give breast milk or full-strength formula. A clear liquid diet should not be continued for more than 24 hours. Breast-feeding may be attempted throughout the hydration process.

The use of antiemetics in infants remains controversial. In a 1996 position statement, the American Academy of Pediatrics recommended that the use of antiemetics be avoided because of questionable side effects.[67] There is also the potential of masking a more serious condition. Promethazine has recently received a black box from the Food and Drug Administration (FDA), secondary to its association with respiratory failure in infants less than 2 years of age. The FDA also recommended using caution in children above age 2 with this agent due to multiple potential side effects. However, many EDs are now using 5-hydroxytryptamine$_3$ antagonists in dehydrated children. Two recent studies have shown that oral and intravenous ondansetron therapy is safe in children and reduces hospital admission rates.[68,69] However, much larger evidence-based studies are still needed to demonstrate their efficacy, and their use in infants younger than 6 months may obscure a more potentially serious underlying cause for these infants' emesis.

Summary

Vomiting in infancy is quite common. Determining which infants have serious medical and surgical disorders can be difficult. The practitioner must be able to distinguish between benign, non–life-threatening conditions and true surgical emergencies. Knowledge of presenting features, typical and atypical signs and symptoms, and appropriate diagnostic adjuncts will aid in diagnosing serious disorders in a timely manner. For infants who are not ill, caregivers must be comforted and instructed in how to rehydrate their infant at home and when they should bring the infant back to the emergency department for further evaluation.

REFERENCES

1. Gurry DL: Vomiting in the newborn. Br Med J 2:241–243, 1972.
2. Valman HB: Vomiting in the newborn. Br Med J 1:620–624, 1980.
3. Catto-Smith T: Gastroesophageal reflux in infants and children. Pediatr Gastroenterol 4:451–457, 2001.
*4. Lifschitz C: Feeding problems in infants and children. Curr Treat Options Gastroenterol 4:451–457, 2001.
5. Forsyth BW, Leventhal JM, McCarthy PL: Mothers' perceptions of feeding and crying behaviors: a prospective study. Am J Dis Child 139:269–272, 1985.
6. Forsyth BW, McCarthy PL, Leventhal JM: Problems of early infancy, formula changes and mothers' beliefs about their infants. J Pediatr 106:1012–1017, 1985.
7. Osborne MR, Marco C: Is it normal or abnormal? Approaching neonates in the emergency department. Pediatr Emerg Med Rep 206:911–912, 2004.
8. Finney JW: Preventing common feeding problems in infants and young children. Pediatr Clin North Am 33:775–788, 1986.
9. Soskolne EL, Schumacher R, Fyock C, et al: The effect of early discharge and other factors on readmission rates of newborns. Arch Pediatr Adolesc Med 150:373–379, 1996.
*10. McCollough M, Sharieff GQ: Common complaints in the first thirty days of life. Emerg Med Clin North Am 20:27–48, 2002.
11. Nelson SP, Chen EH, Syniar GM, Christoffel KK: Prevalence of symptoms of gastroesophageal reflux during infancy. Arch Pediatr Adolesc Med 151:569–572, 1997.
*12. Henry SM: Discerning differences: gastroesophageal reflux and gastroesophageal disease in infants. Adv Neonatal Care 4:235–247, 2004.

---

*Selected readings.

13. Badriul H, Vandenplas Y: Gastro-oesophageal reflux in infancy. J Gastroenterol Hepatol 14:13–19, 1999.

14. Tech DL: Tricks of the Trade. Assessment of the high tech gear in special needs children. Clin Pediatr Emerg Med 3:62–75, 2002.

*15. Sadow K, Atabak S, Teach S, et al: Bilious emesis in the pediatric emergency department: etiology and outcome. Clin Pediatr (Phila) 41:475–479, 2002.

16. Coran AG, Teitelbaum DH: Recent advances in the management of Hirschsprung's disease. Am J Surg 180:383–387, 2000.

17. Ford EG, Senac NO, Srikanth MS, et al: Malrotation of the intestine in children. Arch Surg 215:172, 1992.

18. Kimura K, Loening-Baucke V: Bilious vomiting in the newborn: rapid diagnosis of intestinal obstruction. Am Fam Physician 61:2791–2798, 2000.

19. Adamson W, Hebra A: Bowel obstruction in the newborn. E-medicine web site, 2004. Available at *http://www.emedicine.com/ped/topic2857.htm*

20. Bonadia WA, Clarkson T, Naus J: The clinical features of children with malrotation of the intestine. Pediatr Emerg Care 7:348, 1991.

21. Garcia EA: Intestinal obstruction in infants and children. Clin Pediatr Emerg Med 3:14–20, 2002.

22. O'Kada PS, Hicks B: Neonatal surgical emergencies. Clin Pediatr Emerg Med 3:3–13, 2002.

23. Lawrence RM, Lawrence RA: The evidence for breastfeeding: given the benefits of breastfeeding, what contraindications exist? Pediatr Clin North Am 48:235–251, 2001.

24. Ostrea EM, Mantaring JB, Silvestre MA: Drugs that affect the fetus and newborn infant via the placenta or breast milk. Pediatr Clin North Am 51:539–579, 2004.

25. American Academy of Pediatrics, Committee on Drugs: Transfer of drugs and other chemicals into human milk. Pediatrics 108:776–789, 2001.

26. American Academy of Pediatrics, Committee on Nutrition Pediatrics: Hyoallergenic infant formulas. Pediatrics 106:346–349, 2000.

27. Thach B: Reflux associated apnea in infants: evidence for a laryngeal chemoreflex. Am J Med 103:120S–124S, 1997.

28. Squires RH: Intracranial tumors: vomiting as a presenting sign. A gastroenterologist's perspective. Clin Pediatr (Phila) 28:351–354, 1989.

29. Leung A, Wong A, Lemay J: Alimentary tract atresias. Consult Pediatr 391–396, 2004.

*30. Orenstein SR: Vomiting and regurgitation. In Kliegman RM, Neider I, Super DM (eds): Practical Strategies in Pediatric Diagnosis and Therapy. Philadelphia: WB Saunders, 1996, pp 301–331.

*31. Cohen HL, Babcock DS, et al: Vomiting in infants up to three months of age. ACR Appropriateness Criteria, American College of Radiology web site, 2005. Available at *http://www.acr.org/s_acr?departments/appropriateness_criteria/pdf/0779-786_vomiting_ac.pdf*

32. Firor HV: Surgical emergencies in newborns and infants. Surg Clin North Am 52:77–99, 1971.

33. Noblett HR: Treatment of uncomplicated meconium ileus by Gastrogaffin enema: a preliminary report. J Pediatr Surg 4:190–197, 1969.

34. Traubici J: The double-bubble sign. Radiology 220:463–464, 2001.

35. Mandell G: Duodenal atresia. E-medicine web site, 2004. Available at *http://www.emedicine.com/ped/topic2776.htm*

*36. D'Agostino JD: Common abdominal emergencies in children. Emerg Med Clin North Am 20:139–153, 2002.

37. Macdessi J, Oates RK: Clinical diagnosis of pyloric stenosis: a declining art. BMJ 306:553–555, 1993.

38. Liebelt EL: Clinical and laboratory evaluation and management of children with vomiting, diarrhea, and dehydration. Curr Opin Pediatr 19:461–469, 1998.

39. Pearl RH, Irish MS, Caty MG, Glick PL: The approach to common abdominal diagnoses in infants and children, Part II. Pediatr Clin North Am 45:1287–1326, 1998.

40. Rollins MD, Shields MD, Quinn RJM, et al: Value of US in differentiating causes of persistent vomiting in infants. Gut 32:612–614, 1991.

41. Pollack ES: Pediatric abdominal surgical emergencies. Pediatr Ann 25:448–457, 1996.

42. Mandell G, Wolfson P, Adins E, et al: Cost-effective imaging approach to the nonbilious vomiting infant. Pediatrics 103:1198, 1999.

43. Kao H-A: Bilious vomiting during the first week of life. Zhonghua Min Guo Xiao Er Ke Yi Xue Hui Za Zhi 35:202–207, 1994.

44. Anfrassy RJ, Mahou GH: Malrotation of the midgut in infants and children. Arch Surg 16:158–160, 1981.

45. Allan JL, Robbie M, Phelan PD: Familial occurrence of meconium ileus. Eur J Pediatr 135:291–292, 1981.

46. Heller RM, Hernanz-Schulman M: Applications of new imaging modalities to the evaluation of common pediatric conditions. J Pediatr 135:632–639, 1999.

47. Lillien LD, Srinivasan G, Pyati SP, et al: Green vomiting in the first 72 hours in normal infants. Am J Dis Child 140:662–664, 1986.

*48. Swischuk LE: Imaging techniques for abdominal emergencies. Clin Pediatr Emerg Med 3:45–54, 2002.

49. Davenport M: ABCs of general surgery in correctable causes of vomiting in infants. BMJ 312:236–239, 1996.

50. Beals D: Imperforate anus. E-medicine web site, 2004. Available at *http://www.emedicine.com/ped/topic1171.htm*

51. Ng S: Necrotizing enterocolitis in the full-term neonate. J Paediatr Child Health 37:1–4, 2001.

52. Coit AK: Necrotizing enterocolitis. J Perinat Neonatal Nurs 12(4):53–68, 1999.

53. Irish MS, Pearl RH, Caty MG, Glick PL: The approach to common abdominal diagnoses in infants and children, Part 1. Pediatr Clin North Am 45:729–765, 1998.

54. Kapur P, Caty MG: Pediatric hernias and hydrocoeles. Pediatr Clin North Am 45:773–788, 1998.

55. Weber P, Von Lengerke HJ, Oleszczuk-Rascke K: Internal abdominal hernias in childhood. J Pediatr Gastroenterol Nutr 25:358–362, 1997.

56. Rowe MI, Clatworth HW: Incarcerated and strangulated hernias in children. Arch Surg 101:136–139, 1970.

57. Rothrock SG, Pagane J: Acute appendicitis in children: emergency department diagnosis and management. Ann Emerg Med 36:39–51, 2000.

58. Stringer MD, Pablot SM, Brereton RJ: Paediatric intussusception. Br J Surg 79:867–876, 1992.

59. Garcia EA, Wiebe RA: Intussusception in childhood. Pediatr Emerg Med Rep 5:93–100, 2000.

60. Stanley A, Logan H, Bate TW, Nicholson AJ: Ultrasound in the diagnosis and exclusion of intussusception. Ir Med J 90:64–65, 1997.

61. Bruce J, Huh YS, Cooney DR, et al: Intussusception: evolution of current management. J Pediatr Gastroenterol Nutr 6:663–674, 1987.

*62. American Academy of Pediatrics: Practice Parameter: the management of acute gastroenteritis in young children. Available at *http://aap.org/policy/gastro.htm*

63. Seashore JH, Touloukian RJ: Midgut volvulus: an ever-present threat. Arch Pediatr Adolesc Med 148:43–46, 1994.

64. Sadow KB, Atabacki SM, Johns CM, et al: Bilious emesis in the pediatric emergency department: etiology and outcome. Clin Pediatr (Phila) 41:475–479, 2002.

65. Orenstein S: Vomiting and regurgitation. In Kliegman et al (eds): Practical Strategies in Pediatric Diagnosis and Therapy. Philadelphia: WB Saunders, 1996, pp 401–431.

66. Rothrock SG, Green SM, Hummel CB: Plain abdominal radiography in the detection of major disease in children: a prospective analysis. Ann Emerg Med 21:1423–1429, 1992.

67. Practice parameter: The management of acute gastroenteritis in young children. Subcommittee on acute gastroenteritis and provisional committee on quality improvement. Pediatrics 97:424–435, 1996.

68. Ramsook C, Sahagun-Carreon I, Kozinetz CA, Moro-Sutherland D: A randomized clinical trial comparing oral ondansetron with placebo in children with vomiting and acute gastroenteritis. Ann Emerg Med 39:397–400, 2002.

69. Reeves JJ, Shannon MW, Fleischer GR: Ondansetron decreases vomiting from gastroenteritis: a randomized controlled trial. Pediatrics 109:e62, 2002.

Chapter 36

Failure to Thrive

Todd A. Mastrovitch, MD

Key Points

Knowledge of normal growth and development patterns is necessary to evaluate a patient with failure to thrive.

Failure to thrive is a multifactorial process.

The differential diagnosis must include both organic and nonorganic causes of failure to thrive.

Introduction and Background

The evaluation of failure to thrive presents a unique challenge for the emergency practitioner. Weight loss in an infant or child presenting to the emergency department (ED) is an infrequent chief complaint but one for which there are many causes. The term *failure to thrive* is a description for a process in an infant or child whose weight and growth has been interrupted by an organic or nonorganic process. Numerous conditions have been described that lead an infant or child to begin and continue to lose weight. Diseases of medical, nutritional, psychological, behavioral, and environmental origin have all been implicated in leading to failure to thrive.

Recognition and Approach

Normal Pediatric Growth, Development, and Feeding

It is important for practitioners in the ED to have an understanding of normal infant and childhood growth in order to determine which children are failing to thrive. For healthy term newborn infants, a loss of 5% to 10% from their birth weight is seen initially. Infants should have regained their birth weight by 2 weeks of age. Infants should then double their birth weight by 4 to 5 months and triple their birth weight by 1 year of age.

During the first 3 months of life, an infant should have a steady gain of 30 g (1 ounce) per day. The amount gained will decrease to 20 g/day at 3 to 6 months, 12 g/day at 6 to 12 months, and 8 g/day at 12 to 18 months. The child's height should double within the first 4 years of life. As a general rule,

exclusively breast-fed infants are smaller than comparable formula-fed infants at 1 year of age.[1]

The American Academy of Pediatrics suggests exclusive breast-feeding as the feeding of choice for the infant under 1 year of age. Questions must be asked of the caregiver regarding the type, frequency, volume, and tolerance of the breast or formula feedings to help determine the nutritional adequacy provided.[2] Infants do not require water supplementation under normal circumstances. Excessive fruit juice consumption is associated with failure to thrive and should be limited in older infants. Solid foods are usually started between 4 and 6 months, when the infant's oral-motor and gastrointestinal mechanisms have matured.[3]

The standard method of evaluating growth in a child is by plotting serial weight, height, and head circumference measurements on the revised growth charts for children published by the Centers for Disease Control and Prevention. These growth charts take into account different sexes, ethnicities, and feeding types. It is important in the ED to contact the patient's primary care practitioner to obtain more data points in time to evaluate a child's true growth. Failure to thrive should be considered if the weight of the infant is less than the 3rd percentile or the infant's weight drops and crosses over two percentile lines in a few months' time (usually less than 6 months) (Figs. 36–1 and 36–2).

Clinical Presentation

Causes of failure to thrive can be divided into two categories: organic and nonorganic (Table 36–1). Organic causes affect the infant's ability to intake, absorb, and utilize the nutrition provided for growth. Nonorganic causes disrupt the normal psychosocial/behavioral elements of feeding between the infant and caregiver, which then results in malnutrition of the infant.[3,4]

By gathering historical data during the interview of the caregivers, the clinician may begin to piece together the reasons for the infant's growth failure (Table 36–2). The infant's history usually provides key reasons for growth disturbance. Reasons such as inadequate breast-feeding or formula intake, increased vomiting with feedings, or absorption problems with frequent diarrhea may be found to be causing the growth difficulty.[5] It is essential that, during the physical examination, the infant or child is carefully weighed and the length and head circumference are measured. The

Text continued on p. 333.

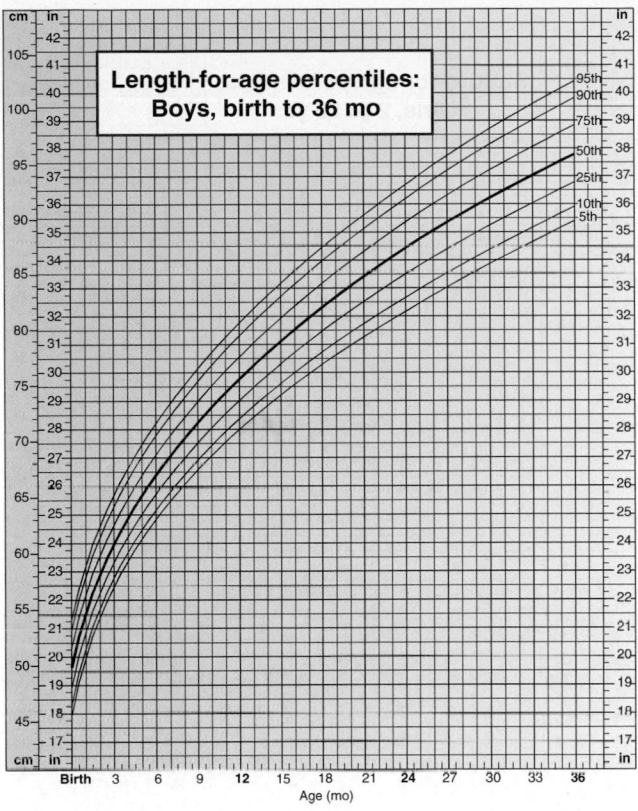

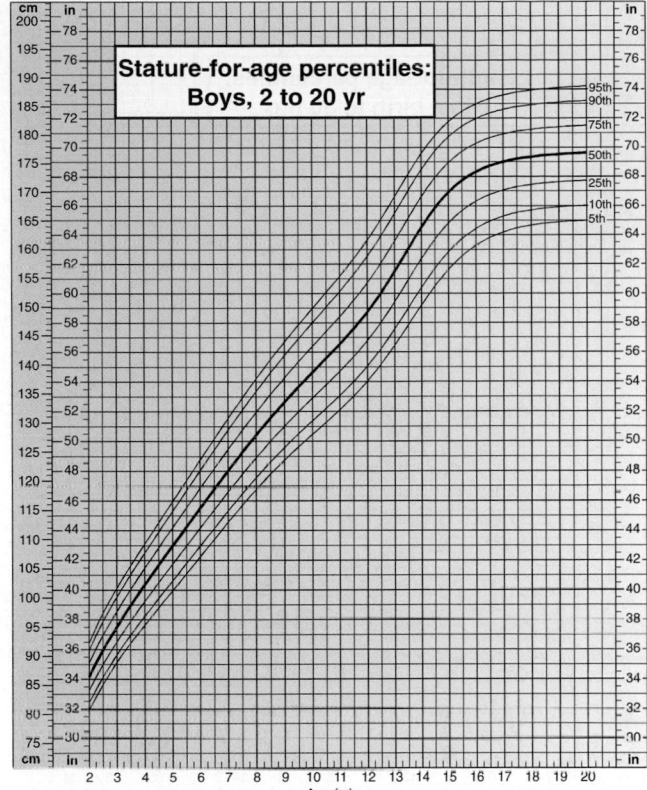

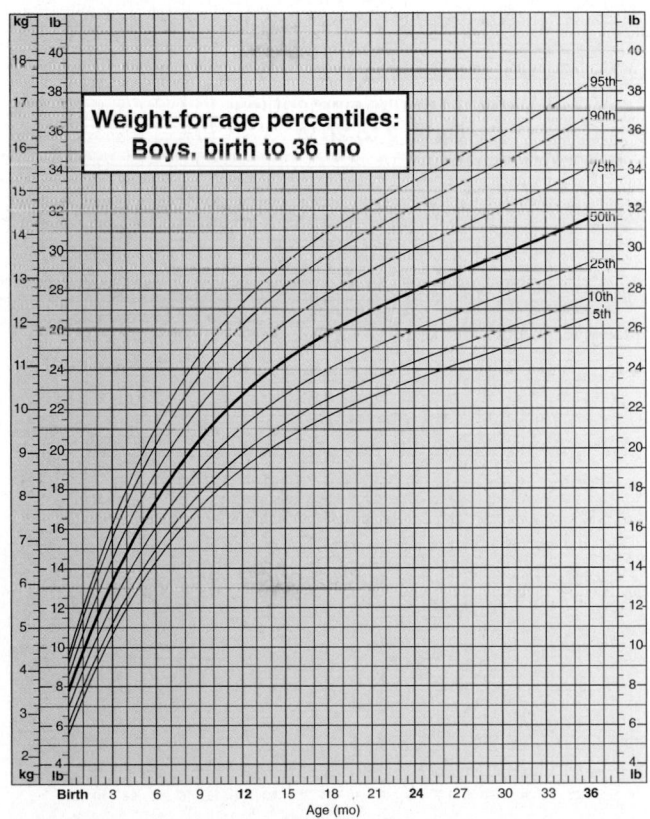

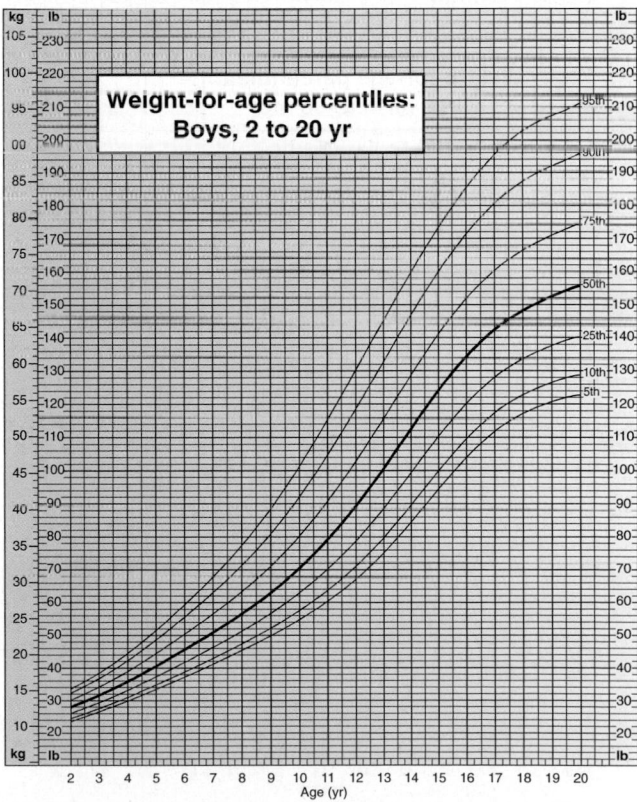

A

FIGURE 36–1. Percentile curves for weight and length/stature by age for boys **(A)** and girls **(B)** from birth to 20 years. (Official 2000 Centers for Disease Control and Prevention [CDC] growth charts, created by the National Center for Health Statistics [NCHS]. Infant length was measured supine; older children's stature was measured standing. Additional information and technical reports are available at *http://www.cdc.gov/nchs.*)

Continued

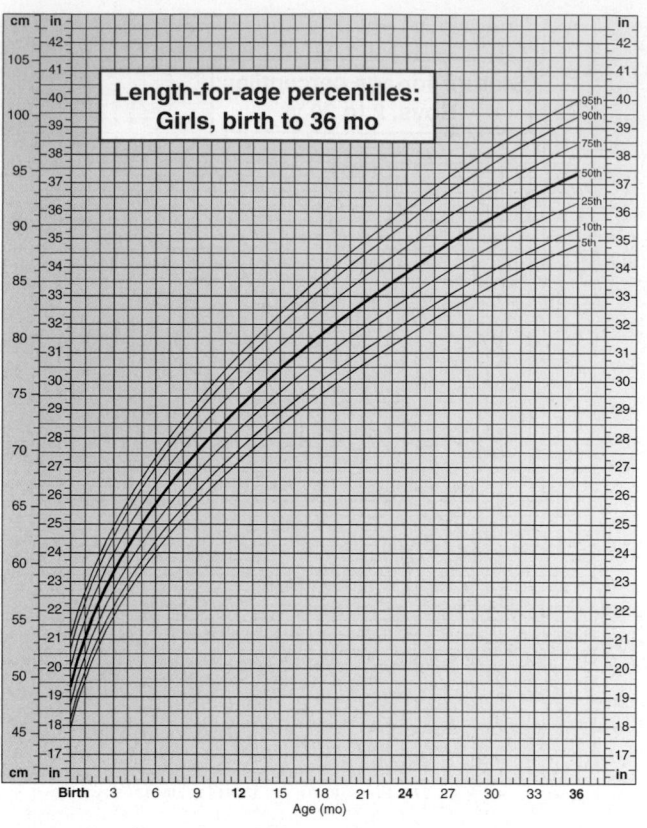

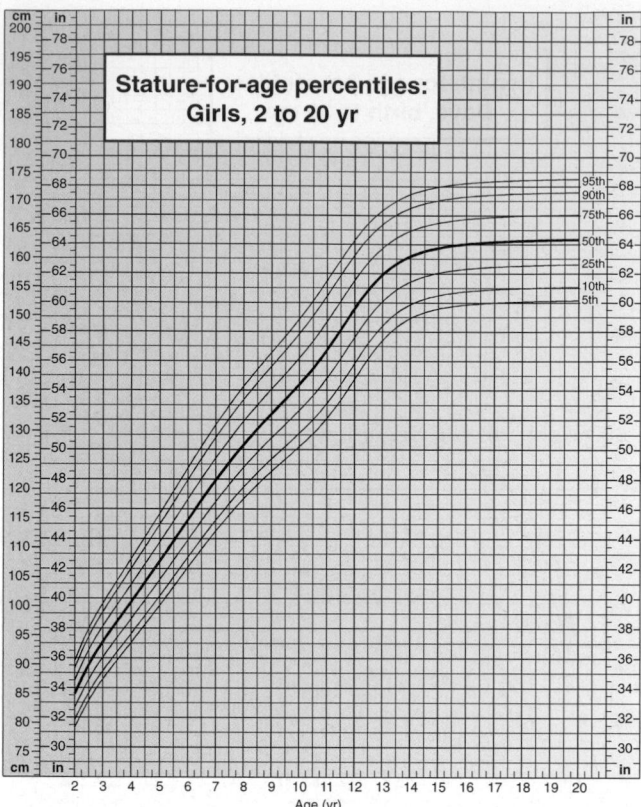

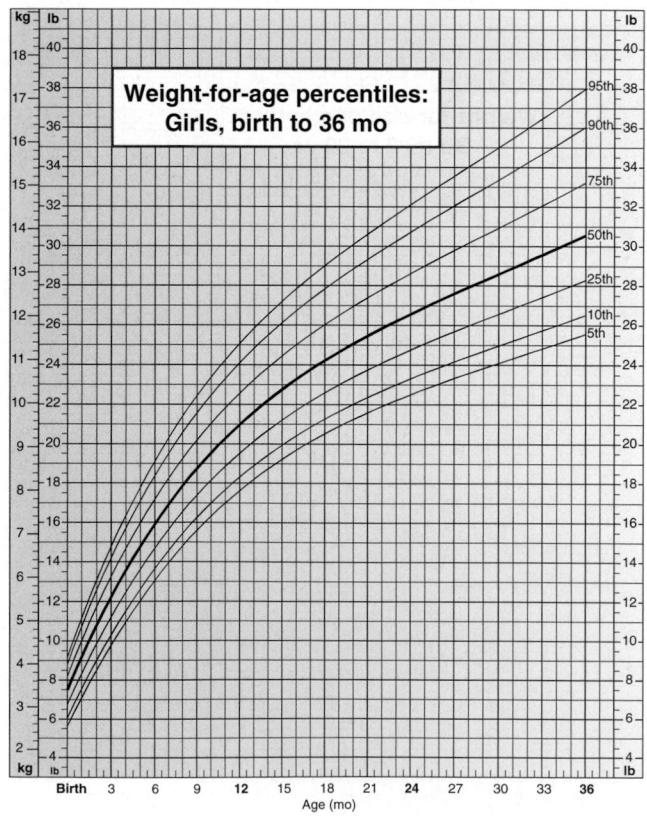

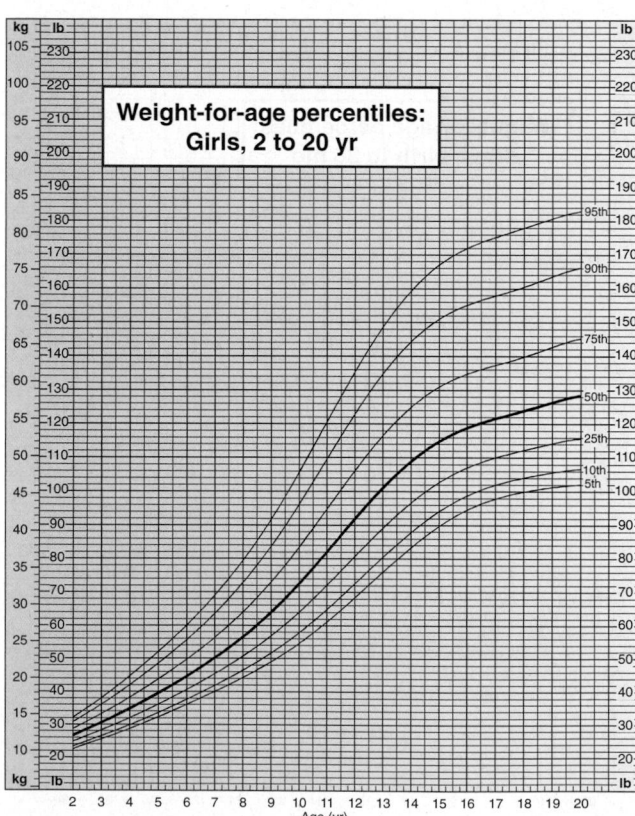

B

FIGURE 36–1, cont'd

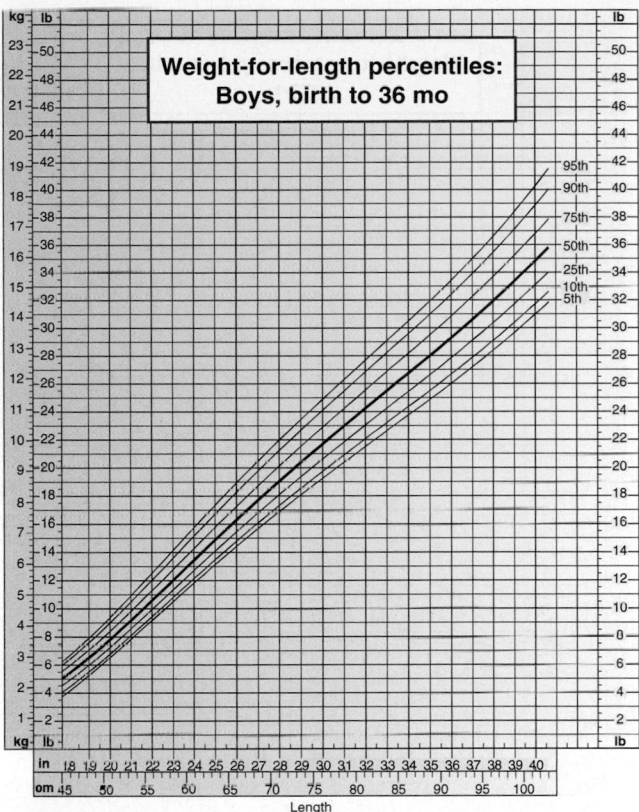

Weight-for-length percentiles:
Boys, birth to 36 mo

Length

Revised and corrected June 8, 2000.

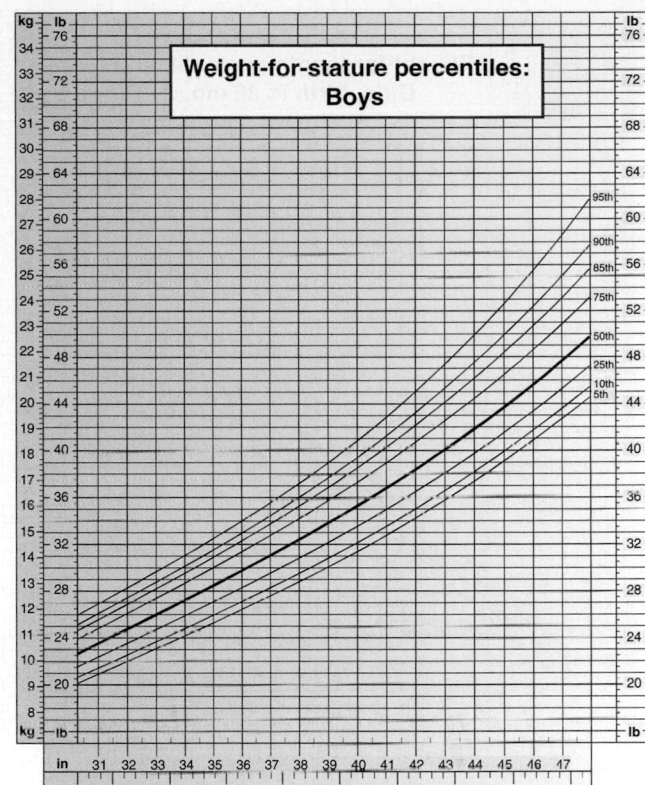

Weight-for-stature percentiles:
Boys

Stature

Revised and corrected November 21, 2000.

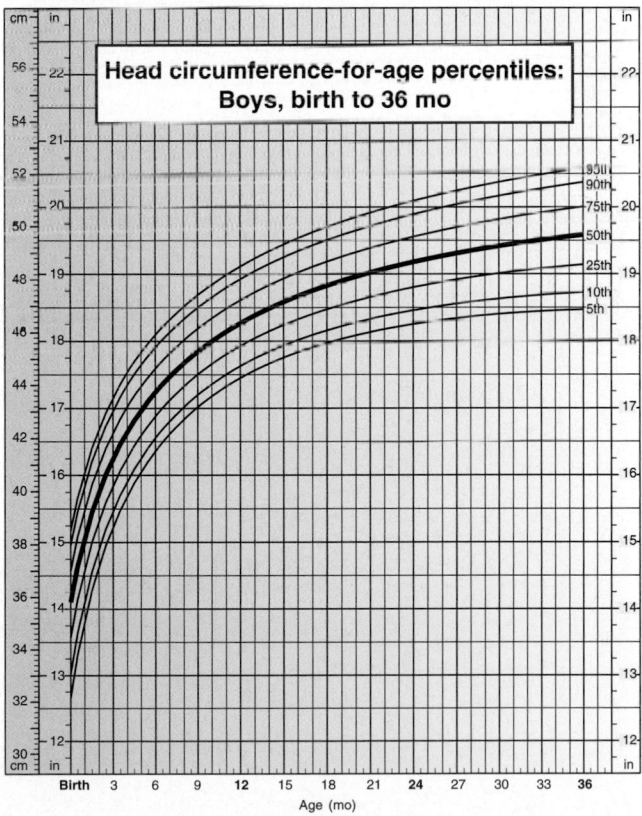

Head circumference-for-age percentiles:
Boys, birth to 36 mo

Age (mo)

A

FIGURE 36–2. Head circumference and length/stature by weight for boys **(A)** and girls **(B).** (Official 2000 Centers for Disease Control and Prevention [CDC] growth charts, created by the National Center for Health Statistics [NCHS]. Additional information and technical reports are available at *http://www.cdc.gov/nchs.*)   *Continued*

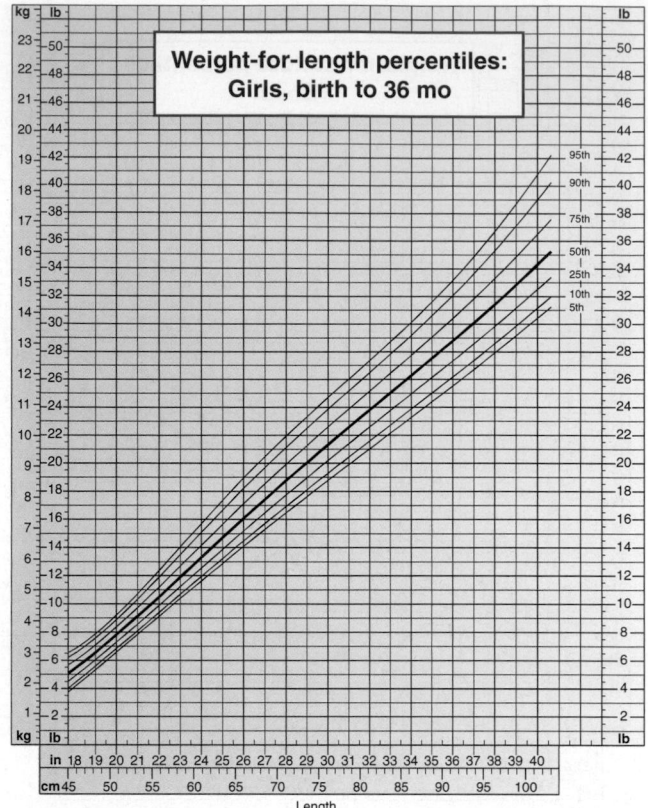

Revised and corrected June 8, 2000.

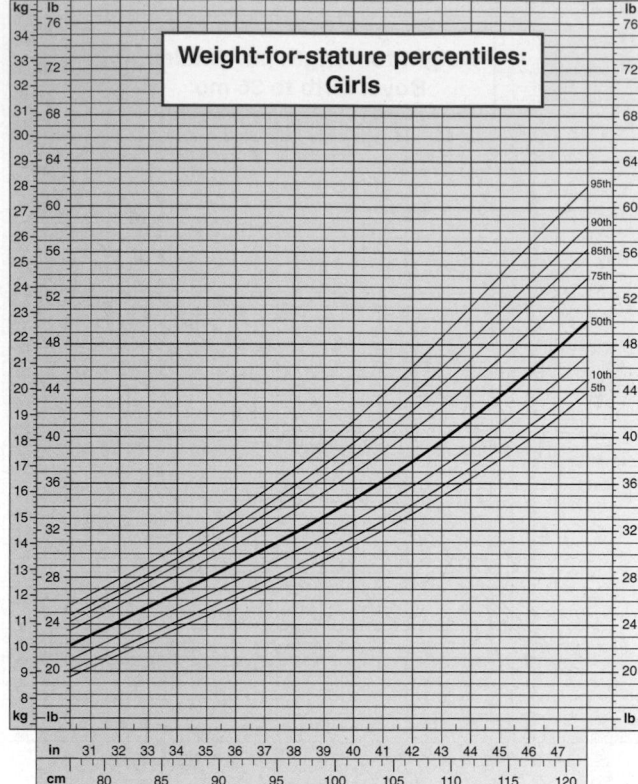

Revised and corrected November 21, 2000.

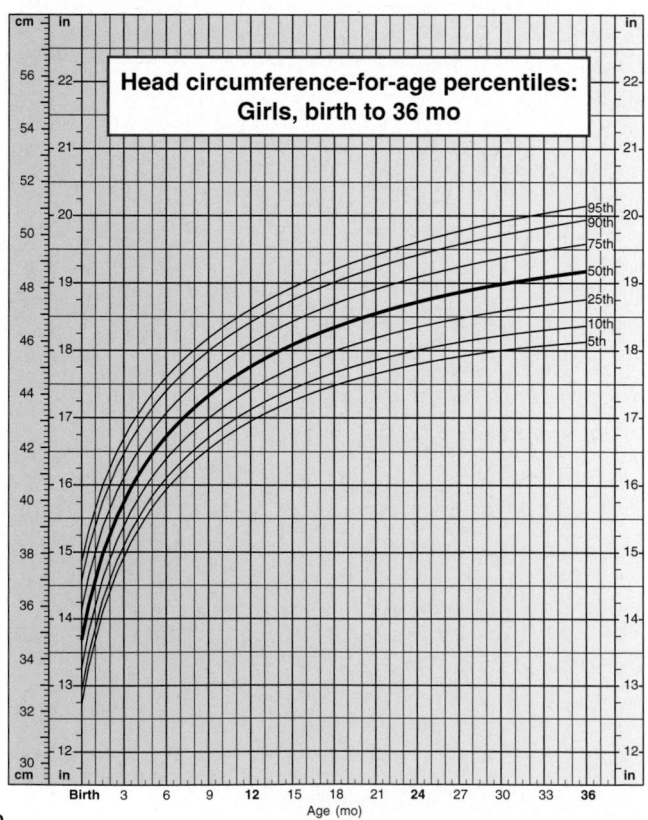

B

FIGURE 36–2, cont'd

Table 36–1	Conditions Associated with Failure to Thrive
Organic Causes	
Cardiopulmonary	Congenital heart disease, cystic fibrosis, bronchopulmonary dysplasia, severe reactive airway disease, chronic inflammation of tonsils and adenoids
Congenital	Chromosomal abnormalities (e.g., Noonan's, Turner's, Williams syndromes), cleft palate
Endocrinologic	Diabetes, Addison's disease, hyperthyroidism, hypothyroidism, congenital adrenal hyperplasia, growth hormone deficiency
Gastrointestinal	Oral/esophageal anatomic abnormalities, pyloric stenosis, gastroesophageal reflux, parasites/chronic enteric infections, biliary disease, pancreatic insufficiency, liver disease, celiac disease, milk allergy
Hematologic	Lead toxicity, iron deficiency anemia
Immunologic	Chronic immunodeficiency, HIV/AIDS, TB, chronic UTI, recurrent infection, malignancy, rheumatologic disease
Metabolic	Inborn errors of metabolism
Neurologic	Cerebral palsy, developmental disabilities, CNS neuromuscular/esophageal motility problems, anosmia, blindness
Nutritional	Insufficient lactation in mother
Perinatal factors	Prematurity, very-low-birth-weight infants, intrauterine growth retardation
Renal	Renal insufficiency, renal tubular acidosis, Bartter's syndrome
Nonorganic Causes	
Inappropriate feeding technique	
Disturbed mother-child relationship (e.g., bonding and feeding difficulty)	
Socioeconomic factors	
Psychosocial factors/apathy	
Insufficient family support/family discord	
Chronic disease states with increased support needs by the caregivers	
Child abuse/neglect	

Abbreviations: CNS, central nervous system; HIV/AIDS, human immunodeficiency virus/acquired immunodeficiency syndrome; TB, tuberculosis; UTI, urinary tract infection.

Table 36–2	Historical Considerations

History of Present Illness

Was the pregnancy, delivery, or newborn period difficult?
Do the parents note a problem with the infant?
Exactly what is the infant/child being fed?
Any cultural factors affecting the child's intake?
What support system is in place for the caregivers of the infant?

Family History

History of the parents' growth as an infant
Any fetal losses or infantile deaths in the family?
What are the parents' and siblings' height, weight, and head circumferences?
Any family history of mental illness, abuse, neglect, extreme dieting, or eating disorders?

Social History

Evaluation of maternal coping mechanisms/maternal depression
Adequacy of financial support for food
Who makes up the infant's/child's support system?
What are the major events in the child's life? (e.g., frequent moves, recent homelessness, family instability)

Breast-Fed Infants

What are the length and frequency of the feeds?
How is the infant's suck mechanism?
What are the maternal attitudes toward breast-feeding?
Is there adequate milk production and let-down?
Is there spitting up, vomiting, or coughing during feeding?

Bottle-Fed Infants

How is the formula prepared?
How many ounces are taken per feed or per day?
Who feeds the infant?
Is there spitting up, vomiting, or coughing during feeding?

Toddlers

How many meals per day?
What is a normal meal composed of for the child?
Who feeds the child?
How long do mealtimes last?

Initial routine laboratory testing of electrolyte levels, blood urea nitrogen and creatinine, calcium, complete blood count, liver function tests with protein and albumin, urinalysis and urine culture, chest radiograph, and Mantoux tuberculin testing is appropriate. Further testing and radiographic and imaging studies may be indicated on the basis of the clinical examination.

Management

In patients who are less severely growth impaired, not ill appearing, and clinically and psychologically stable, a trial of outpatient management is instituted, with close monitoring by the primary care provider.

In cases in which the clinical and psychological status of the patient is more severely affected, hospitalization plays a key role in helping to improve the patient's nutritional status. Hospitalization is also helpful for those patients who need correction of fluid and electrolyte imbalance. While in the hospital, more information is gathered over time as to how the infant feeds, the interaction between the infant and caregiver, and the daily physiologic functions of the child (i.e., stools, sleep/wake periods, general disposition). By examining this information, the medical team will then be able to help the family unit understand and treat the causes of failure

scale used for weighing should be frequently zeroed and calibrated, and attention should be paid to the way in which the infant was weighed last (e.g., clothed/unclothed, diaper/no diaper), with the standard being a completely undressed/undiapered infant or child. These data points should then be plotted on the standardized growth charts, hopefully with a previous growth point for comparison. If head circumference, weight, and length are all decreased compared to normal percentiles, genetic and prenatal disorders should be suspected. If weight and height growth are delayed and head circumference is normal, endocrine disorders and constitutional delay are possible causes. Children with normal head circumference and low weight relative to height often have inadequate nutrition as the cause. In cases of nonorganic failure to thrive, the only physical finding is usually growth failure (e.g., a thin, cachectic appearing infant or child with minimal subcutaneous tissue).[6] Typically a child with an organic failure to thrive will have a specific finding (e.g., metabolic or renal abnormality)[7] that helps guide the practitioner in the diagnosis.

to thrive.[8] The desired result of hospitalization for the growth-impaired infant is weight gain and improvement in social interaction with caregivers.[9]

Infants and children who have physical findings of systemic disease or who fail to gain weight while under care in the hospital setting should be further evaluated for organic causes of failure to thrive. More extensive testing and consultation with pediatric subspecialists in gastroenterology, endocrinology, infectious diseases, neurology, or psychiatry may be necessary to elucidate a cause for the growth failure. It is also often helpful to seek the assistance of social workers, nutritionists, physical/occupational therapists, and behavioral pediatricians due to the multifactorial nature of this disease process.[10] In working together, the treatment team often will be able to identify the issues leading to the infant's or child's poor growth status.[11]

Summary

Failure to thrive is a multifactorial disorder resulting from malnutrition in infants and children. Medical, psychological, nutritional, behavioral, abusive, environmental, and congenital factors have been implicated. The emergency physician must be able to begin to sort out the organic versus the nonorganic causes of failure to thrive, and to identify those patients who require hospitalization in order to stabilize their clinical status. Diagnosing failure to thrive and identifying which patients need laboratory and/or radiologic testing depends on the key findings in the history and physical examination. To treat failure to thrive, the emergency physician must focus on the correction of the underlying causes and enlistment of the multidisciplinary team to improve the nutritional and psychological status of the patient.

REFERENCES

1. Krugman SD, Dubowitz H: Failure to thrive. Am Fam Physician 68:879–884, 2003.
*2. Liternick R: Accurate feeding history key to failure to thrive. Pediatr Ann 33:161–166, 2004.
3. Black MM, Cutts DB, Frank DA, et al; Children's Sentinel Nutritional Assessment Program Study Group: Special Supplemental Nutritional Program fro Women, Infants, and Children participation and infants' growth and health: a multisite surveillance study. Pediatrics 114:169–176, 2004.
4. Rahman A, Iqbal Z, Bunn J, et al: Impact of maternal depression on infant nutritional status and illness: a cohort study. Arch Gen Psychiatry 61:946–952, 2004.
5. Orenstein SR, Izadnia F, Khan S: Gastroesophageal reflux disease in children. Gastroenterol Clin 28:947–980, 1999.
6. Homer C, Ludwig S: Categorization of etiology of failure to thrive. Am J Dis Child 135:848, 1981.
7. Adedoyin O, Gottlieb B, Frank R, et al: Evaluation of failure to thrive: diagnostic yield of testing for renal tubular acidosis. Pediatrics 112(6 Pt 1):e463, 2003.
8. Singer LT, Song LY, Hill BP, Jaffe AC: Stress and depression in mothers of failure-to-thrive children. J Pediatr Psychol 15:711–720, 1990.
9. Fryer GE: The efficacy of hospitalization of non-organic failure to thrive children: a meta-analysis. Child Abuse Negl 12:375, 1988.
10. Stewart KB, Meyer L: Parent-child interactions and everyday routines in young children with failure to thrive. Am J Occup Ther 58:342–346, 2004.
11. Casey PH, Kelleher KJ, Bradley RH, et al: A multifaceted intervention for infants with failure to thrive: a prospective study. Arch Pediatr Adolesc Med 148:1071–1077, 1994.

---

*Selected readings.

Minor Infant Problems

Jonathan H. Valente, MD

Selected Diagnoses

Breath-holding spells
Hair-thread tourniquets
Congenital muscular torticollis
Oral thrush
Neonatal vaginal bleeding

Discussion of Individual Diagnoses

Breath-holding Spells

The use of the term *breath-holding spell* is actually a misnomer as these episodes occur involuntarily and during the exhalation phase. The typical spell begins after an event that is frightening, startling, painful, or upsetting to a child. This is followed by a brief period of crying that leads to a stage of apnea and silent, noiseless expiration. During this period, the child's skin may become either pale or cyanotic. This has led to the classic description and classification of these episodes as being either pallid or cyanotic spells. In mild spells, the episode resolves without loss of motor tone or syncope. This is followed by a loud inspiratory response and a fairly prompt return to normal activity. However, in more severe spells, the child may experience loss of motor tone or syncope as well as other symptoms such as loss of consciousness, myoclonic jerks, incontinence, or stiffness. Drowsiness is common following a more severe spell, but a return to normal consciousness is usually fairly prompt. The typical breath holding spell lasts from a few seconds to a few minutes depending upon the severity of the episode.[1] Pallid spells are thought to result from a vagally mediated cardiac inhibitory pathway, whereas cyanotic spells are believed to result from a more complex mechanism involving a hyperventilatory-Valsalva pathway.[2] In some cases, breath-holding spells defy classification as either pallid or cyanotic and are classified as "mixed." Approximately 60% are cyanotic, 20% are pallid, and 20% are mixed.[1]

Recognition and Approach

Breath-holding spells are relatively common. Severe spells occur in 0.1% to 4.6% of healthy children. Simple spells occur in up to 27% of healthy children.[1,3,4] The age at onset is as follows: neonatal in 5%, in the first 6 months of life in 12%, in the first year in 66%, and in the first 2 years in 94%.[1,3,5] Virtually all children who will manifest breath-holding spells will have their first spell before their third birthday.

The frequency with which infants and young children have breath-holding spells is quite variable. Spells may occur as a weekly or even daily event in more severe cases. The peak frequency typically occurs at about 18 months of age. In more severe cases, up to one third of these children have more than one spell each day at the age of peak frequency.[5] Children outgrow breath-holding spells. By age 4 years, about half of children experiencing breath-holding spells will stop having them. By age 6 years, 90% have stopped having breath-holding spells. Nearly all children stop having breath-holding spells by age 8 years.[1,3,6]

Clinical Presentation

A detailed description of the event is the key to making the diagnosis. For example, a breath-holding spell never occurs in the sleeping child. The differential diagnosis for similar events includes seizures, cardiac disturbances, orthostasis, brain tumors, and developmental disorders. Unlike many of these other diagnoses, breath-holding spells are almost always immediately preceded by a painful or emotionally provocative event. In addition, the cyanosis or pallor presents *prior* to the loss of motor tone or syncope. Family history may be helpful as 20% to 30% of children with severe breath-holding spells will have a family history of breath-holding spells.[1,7]

Management

The evaluation of a child suspected of having had a breath-holding spell does not involve extensive testing or imaging. The physical examination is focused on the cardiac and neurologic status of the child. An electrocardiogram (ECG) may be performed to look for abnormalities such as prolonged QT syndrome. A bedside hemoglobin may be obtained to identify anemia.[8] In cases in which the diagnosis is not clearly a breath-holding spell, ECG monitoring during an ocular compression test may elicit episodes of asystole consistent with pallid breath-holding spells.[9] Although rarely indicated, an electroencephalogram may help rule out seizures.[2,9]

Medications to treat breath-holding spells are seldom, if ever, indicated in the emergency department. On occasion, a child who is being treated for repeated episodes of breath-holding spells will present to the emergency department. Such children may be taking oral atropine, oral theophylline, iron supplements, or have a transdermal scopolamine patch.[1,8,10-15] A prospective double-blind study showed that iron therapy was beneficial in the treatment of breath-holding spells. More than 50% of the treatment group showed a complete response to therapy with iron compared with none in the placebo group.[11] Other researchers have reported similar outcomes with iron therapy and even studied blood transfusion therapy in children with breath-holding spells.[8,12-15] For severe refractory cases, permanent pacemaker therapy has been utilized and been shown to have some efficacy in these rare instances.[16,17]

Parental reassurance is an important feature in successfully treating children with breath-holding spells. Recurrent breath-holding spells cause a significant amount of stress in the mothers of these children—twice as much as in mothers of children with a seizure disorder.[18] Breath-holding spells are benign. In otherwise healthy children, there is no evidence to suggest any increased risk of epilepsy or serious long-term sequelae except, perhaps, a slightly increased risk of syncope later in life.[3] Parents should be careful not to succumb to their child's every wish just to avert a breath-holding spell. Doing so may lead to behavioral problems and parental manipulation by the child. Parents should be instructed to simply observe the child and take measures to protect him or her from injury during a breath-holding spell. Children diagnosed with breath-holding spells may be discharged home from the emergency department with primary care follow-up.

Hair-Thread Tourniquets

The hair-thread tourniquet syndrome is caused by a hair or thread encircling a finger, toe, penis, clitoris, or uvula (Fig. 37–1).[19-21] The circumferential strangulation of the digit leads to decreased venous and lymphatic drainage with the subsequent formation of edema distal to the tourniquet. Arterial insufficiency may follow due to inflammation and edema. In more prolonged or severe cases, the surrounding tissues may even epithelialize over the hair or thread, making visualization extremely difficult or impossible. Ultimately, tissue necrosis may develop and lead to autoamputation or the need for surgical amputation.[22] A physical property of human hair is that it stretches when wet and shrinks when dried. This most likely contributes to the constrictive phenomenon observed with this syndrome.[21] The time course to recogni-

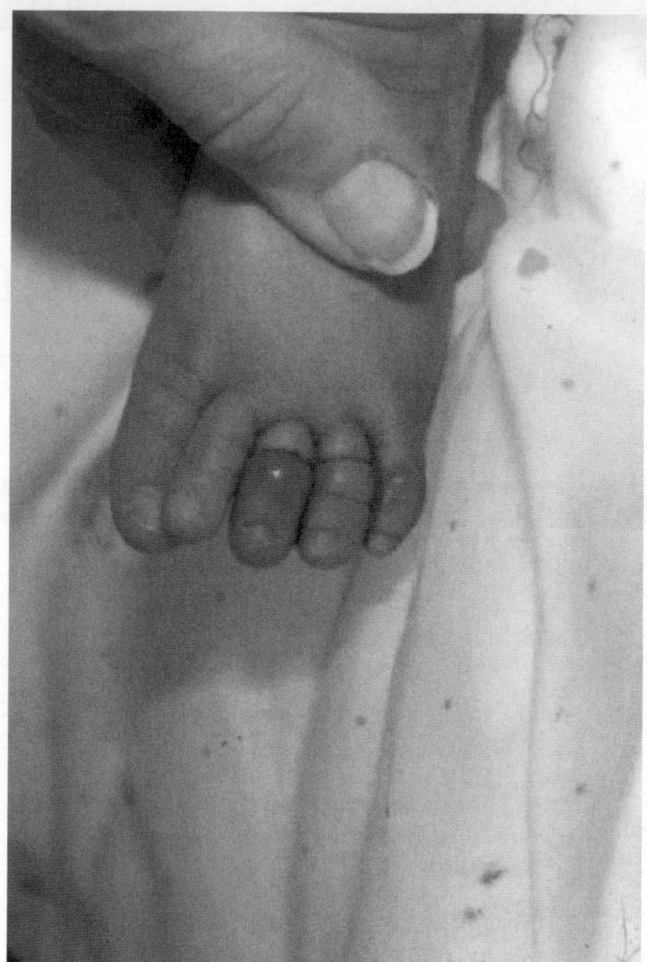

FIGURE 37–1. Toe hair tourniquet. (Photo courtesy of Robert Acosta, MD, Jacobi Medical Center, Bronx, NY.)

tion and presentation has been reported to range from hours to months following the initial constriction.[23]

Clinical Presentation

The majority of toe and genital tourniquets are caused by hair, while most finger tourniquets are caused by strings or thread (e.g., from mittens). Infants at highest risk for hair tourniquets are typically younger than 6 months of age and infants of mothers with long hair. This coincides with the period of greatest maternal hair loss following delivery. This period of postpartum hair loss is termed *telogen effluvium* and affects up to 90% of otherwise healthy mothers.[24] In a review of 66 cases of hair and thread tourniquets, 43% involved toes, 24% involved fingers, and 33% involved the genitalia. The hair-thread tourniquet syndrome may involve multiple digits, but more often involves only one. On the hand, the middle finger and index fingers are reported to be at higher risk for strangulation. Similarly, on the foot, the middle and second toes are most frequently involved.[25]

The hair-thread tourniquet syndrome is a cause of excessive crying (see Chapter 31, Excessive Crying). The syndrome is most frequently accidental and not due to abuse.[26] In the rare cases in which it has been associated with child abuse, the genitals are often involved (e.g., tourniquets created by caregivers to prevent nocturnal enuresis).[26-28] Poor public and clinician awareness that this syndrome is not often associated with abuse has been highlighted by a 1994 survey by Biehler et al.[29] In this study, more than half of the respondents claimed that they would report a classic case of the toe tourniquet syndrome to the child protective service. The group that responded included 42 physicians, 19 child welfare workers, and 23 nurses.[29]

Management

The most effective treatment is expedient removal of the tourniquet. Often the tourniquet can be removed by using a probe to lift up the fiber and then cut the fiber with scissors or a scalpel blade. Another technique is to use a short, deep dorsal longitudinal incision over the area of strangulation in toes.[30] The incision is made down to the bone. The retrospective study supporting this technique suggested that this approach may decrease the risk of injury to the digital nerves and vascular structures. However, injury to the extensor tendon is possible, and there are no prospective studies evaluating the potential complication rates or long-term functional deficits associated with this technique. If this technique is used, splinting of the digit is prudent to promote healing of the extensor tendon. Other well-documented surgical techniques involve longitudinal incisions made at the lateral and medial aspects (3-o'clock and 9-o'clock positions) of the toe or finger. These incision locations are selected to avoid neurovascular and tendon structures.[31] For tourniquets involving the genitals, emergent urologic consultation is generally indicated for surgical removal, unless the tourniquet is superficial. The use of depilatory agents has been suggested, but this chemical approach may lead to tissue toxicity, since the epithelium and soft tissues are already damaged, and would be ineffective for tourniquets made of material other than hair.[31] Following removal of the thread or hair, patients should be followed on a regular basis for at least 1 month to evaluate for retention of tourniquet remnants or epithelialized fibrous connective tissue bands.[73] Surgical exploration under magnification may ultimately be needed when doubt exists as to the complete removal of the hair or thread.

Anticipatory guidance for parents, especially in the first few months of life, may help to better recognize this clinical entity. Careful inspection of the baby's fingers, toes, and genitalia are important aspects of routine care. Washing clothing turned inside out and turning clothing inside out to look for and remove loose hairs or threads also may be helpful in preventing this syndrome.[24]

Congenital Muscular Torticollis

Congenital muscular torticollis is a term used to describe a painless clinical condition of neonates and young infants manifested by unilateral tightening or shortening of a sternocleidomastoid muscle.[32] Related terms include *neonatal torticollis, pseudotumor of infancy, sternocleidomastoid tumor of infancy,* and *fibromatosis colli.*[32-35] Due to definitional problems, it is not clear if these are different names for the same conditions, names for findings along the clinical spectrum of a single condition, or distinct clinical entities. There is no predilection for gender or sidedness.[36] Bilateral torticollis is extremely rare.[37] Congenital muscular torticollis is the most common cause of infantile torticollis, with an incidence of 0.3% to 1.9%.[32,34,35]

Clinical Presentation

Patients present within the first few weeks of life with their heads tilted to the side of the affected sternocleidomastoid muscle and their chins turned toward the contralateral side.[34,35] This clinical presentation has been referred to as a "cock robin" or "wryneck" deformity.[38] These infants exhibit a limited range of motion of their necks. Some infants may have a palpable, firm, fibrous mass within the sternocleidomastoid muscle.[32,38]

There are many theories regarding the cause of congenital muscular torticollis, but the true etiology remains unknown. Some theories include birth trauma to the sternocleidomastoid muscle with hematoma formation leading to localized fibrous scar formation, ischemia due to venous occlusion, intrauterine malposition, hereditary factors, neurogenic causes, infections, and a form of compartment syndrome during the intrauterine period.[35] Infants with congenital muscular torticollis have a higher incidence of difficult births, breech presentations, and congenital hip dysplasia than other infants.[34,38] Long-term complications associated with this disorder include possible functional and cosmetic abnormalities such as facial asymmetry, plagiocephaly (i.e., a parallelogram-shaped head or a flattened area on one side of the head), and scoliosis.[32,39,40]

In most cases, the diagnosis is evident based on the history and physical examination. Testing and radiography are reserved for those cases in which initial therapy fails or the infant's condition changes to suggest an alternative diagnosis. Other categories of disorders that may cause torticollis in infants include traumatic, ocular, gastrointestinal (e.g., Sandifer's syndrome), aplastic, infectious, neoplastic, inflammatory, or congenital osseous conditions (e.g., cervical vertebral abnormalities).[38,41] Of note, most neurologic causes of torticollis will present after infancy.[38] Potentially useful diagnostic studies include fine-needle biopsy, radiographs, ultrasound, computed tomograph, and magnetic resonance imaging.[33,34,40]

Management

Significant controversy surrounds the optimal treatment for congenital muscular torticollis. About 95% of these infants will respond to conservative therapy such as exercise and stretching performed by the parents at home, manual stretching by a therapist, and observation.[39,42,43] Patients with a palpable mass, an initial head rotation deficit of greater than 15 degrees, and a delay of initial treatment to after the first birthday tend to have worse outcomes and may require surgical intervention.[39] The optimal age for surgical intervention is between 1 and 4 years.[44] Other treatment options include simple observation, orthotic devices, and botulinum toxin.[38,44]

Oral Thrush

Thrush, also known as oral mucocandidiasis, is most frequently caused by *Candida albicans*. Thrush presents with discrete whitish plaques on an erythematous background on the buccal mucosa, tongue, and gingiva (Fig. 37–2). Lesions may also present on the tonsils and palate. These plaques are quite adherent and a little bleeding may occur if they are scraped with a tongue blade. Infants may have a history of irritability and poor feeding or be asymptomatic.

There is a high prevalence of oral colonization in infants due in part to the direct contact of the infant's mouth with

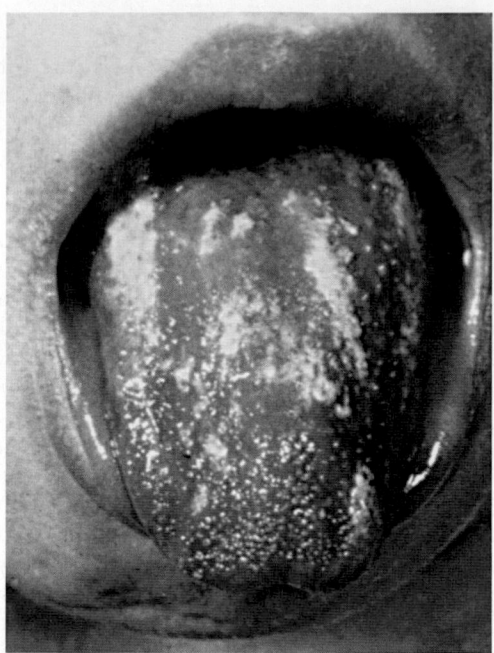

FIGURE 37–2. Oral thrush. (Photo courtesy of Deirdre Fearon, MD, Hasbro Children's Hospital, Providence, RI.)

the birth canal. During pregnancy, the prevalence of vaginal *Candida* increases up to 40% compared to about 15% in nonpregnant, asymptomatic women.[45,46] Both breast-fed and bottle-fed infants may develop thrush, but bottle-fed infants are at increased risk.[46-49] Risk factors for developing thrush include pacifier use, being admitted to a special care unit in a hospital, and maternal symptomatic vaginal candidiasis around the time of delivery.[46,47,50-52]

Nystatin is the standard topical drug of choice to treat infantile thrush due to its low cost and high safety profile. Nystatin is used topically on the lesions four times per day for 10 to 14 days. However, its use has been associated with high recurrence rates attributed to limited duration of contact of the medicine with the thrush and the difficulty in administration leading to poor compliance.[53] A recent study reported only a 54% clinical cure rate at day 12 in healthy infants treated with nystatin suspension as compared with a 99% cure rate in infants treated with miconazole gel. Relapse rates were similar between the two groups.[54] However, a miconazole gel formulation is currently not available in the United States. One small pilot study of 47 infants showed superior efficacy of oral fluconazole compared with nystatin for the treatment of infants ages 1 to 12 months.[53] Clinical cure rates were 29% for nystatin at day 10 and 100% for fluconazole at day 7. Patients in this study received a dose of fluconazole of 3 mg/kg per day for 7 days.[53] However, in the healthy host, thrush is not a life-threatening disease and the added cost and potential side effects with systemic therapy may outweigh the risk of treatment failure.

Maternal Nipple Candidiasis

In breast-fed infants, recurrence is especially common in mothers who develop nipple candidiasis. A clear correlation has been established between nipple candidiasis and vaginal candidiasis, previous antibiotic use, and nipple trauma.[55] In such cases, both maternal and infant treatment is advised. Fluconazole can be used to treat maternal nipple candidiasis.

It is excreted in small amounts in the breast milk and there are limited safety data regarding its use in the breast-feeding infant. However, the amount excreted in the breast milk is less than the normal infant dose if the infant were to be treated systemically with oral fluconazole for thrush. A recent survey of 312 members of the Academy for Breastfeeding Medicine evaluating the treatment of thrush in the breast-feeding infant showed that the majority recommended treatment of the infant and mother, even if the mother was asymptomatic.[56] Of those surveyed, 47% recommended the use of oral nystatin for the infant and nystatin cream for the mother, 3% recommended oral nystatin for the infant and oral fluconazole for the mother, and 2% recommended oral fluconazole for both as the initial therapy. In cases with symptomatic maternal nipple candidiasis and oral infantile thrush, 56% recommended oral nystatin for the infant and cream for the mother, 13% recommended oral nystatin for the infant and oral fluconazole for the mother, and 4% recommended oral fluconazole for both as initial therapy. Of those surveyed, oral fluconazole for both the infant and the mother was recommended by 21% in recurrent cases and by 33% in persistent cases. Alternatively, miconazole cream may also be applied to the affected nipples four times per day. The cream will need to be applied until 48 hours after the resolution of symptoms. The cream is applied after breast-feeding, and the nipples should be cleaned prior to the next feeding. When administering antifungals or other medications, medication droppers or spoons should not be reused without boiling or sterilizing. Alternatively, application of the antifungal can be via disposable cotton-tip swabs. Breast pumps, bottles, and toys will require thorough cleaning and sterilization. Strict hand washing may prevent reexposure.[57]

Neonatal Vaginal Bleeding

Vaginal bleeding in neonates may occur within the first few weeks of life and is usually due to the withdrawal of maternal estrogen. Bleeding may last a few days. No treatment is necessary for such cases. Reassurance is very important as this can be a very worrisome experience for caregivers.[58] Other causes of vaginal bleeding in the neonate should be considered in the atypical cases with prolonged or excessive bleeding, an abnormal external genital examination, or an unusual history. The differential diagnosis includes but is not limited to abuse, vaginitis, urethral prolapse, and tumor.

Literature regarding neonatal vaginal bleeding is very limited. A study published in 1978 covering 15 years of experience at one institution reported on 51 girls being evaluated for vaginal bleeding.[59] This study included a neonate ultimately diagnosed with McCune-Albright syndrome and a 1-month-old with cyclical vaginal bleeding who, at 3-year follow-up, appeared to be developing normally and had no secondary sexual characteristics. About 80% of children with urethral prolapse will present with bleeding as a complaint. However, most of these children will be toddlers and young school-age girls. In a study of 192 cases of urethral prolapse, the mean age was 5.4 years and the range of ages at presentation was 1.5 months to 16 years.[60] In another study of 55 girls under the age of 10 years evaluated for vaginal bleeding, hormonal withdrawal bleeding in the neonate accounted for 6 cases (11%).[58] Aside from withdrawal bleeding in the neonate, other causes of vaginal bleeding in the neonate are uncommon.

REFERENCES

1. DiMario FJ Jr: Breath-holding spells in childhood. Am J Dis Child 146:125–131, 1992.
2. Breningstall GN: Breath-holding spells. Pediatr Neurol 14:91–97, 1996.
*3. Lombroso CT, Lerman P: Breath-holding spells (cyanotic and pallid infantile syncope). Pediatrics 39:563–581, 1967.
4. Linder CW: Breath-holding spells in children. Clin Pediatr 7:88–90, 1968.
*5. DiMario FJ Jr: Prospective study of children with cyanotic and pallid breath-holding spells. Pediatrics 107:265–269, 2001.
6. Goraya JS, Virdi VS: Persistence of breath-holding spells into late childhood. J Child Neurol 16:697–698, 2001.
7. DiMario FJ Jr, Sarfarazi M: Family pedigree analysis of children with severe breath-holding spells. J Pediatr 130:647–651, 1997.
8. Colina KF, Abelson HT: Resolution of breath-holding spells with treatment of concomitant anemia. J Pediatr 126:395–397, 1995.
9. Stephenson JB: Reflex anoxic seizures ("white breath-holding"): non-epileptic vagal attacks. Arch Dis Child 53:193–200, 1978.
10. Yager JY, Hartfield DS: Neurologic manifestations of iron deficiency in childhood. Pediatr Neurol 27:85–92, 2002.
*11. Daoud AS, Batieha A, al-Sheyyab M, et al: Effectiveness of iron therapy on breath-holding spells. J Pediatr 130:547–550, 1997.
12. Tam DA, Rash FC: Breath-holding spells in a patient with transient erythroblastopenia of childhood. J Pediatr 130:651–653, 1997.
13. Bhatia MS, Singhal PK, Dhar NK, et al: Breath holding spells: an analysis of 50 cases. Indian Pediatr 27:1073–1079, 1990.
14. Orii KE, Kato Z, Osamu F, et al: Changes of autonomic nervous system function in patients with breath-holding spells treated with iron. J Child Neurol 17:337–340, 2002.
15. Mocan H, Yildiran A, Orhan F, et al: Breath holding spells in 91 children and response to treatment with iron. Arch Dis Child 81:261–262, 1999.
16. DiMario FJ Jr: Breath-holding spells and pacemaker implantation. Pediatrics 108:765–766, 2001.
17. Kelly AM, Porter CJ, McGoon MD, et al: Breath-holding spells associated with significant bradycardia: successful treatment with permanent pacemaker implantation. Pediatrics 108:698–702, 2001.
18. Mattie-Luksic M, Javornisky G, DiMario FJ Jr: Assessment of stress in mothers of children with severe breath-holding spells. Pediatrics 106:1–5, 2000.
19. Krishna S, Paul RI: Hair tourniquet of the uvula. J Emerg Med 24:325–326, 2003.
20. Rich MA, Keating MA: Hair tourniquet syndrome of the clitoris. J Urol 162:190–191, 1999.
21. Kuo JH, Smith LM, Berkowitz CD: A hair tourniquet resulting in strangulation and amputation of the clitoris. Obstet Gynecol 99:939–941, 2002.
22. Liow RYL, Budny P, Regan PJ: Hair thread tourniquet syndrome. J Accid Emerg Med 13:138–139, 1996.
23. Sunil TM: The hair-thread-tourniquet syndrome—report of an unusual presentation of this rare condition. Hand Surg 6:231–233, 2001.
24. Strahlman RS: Toe tourniquet syndrome in association with maternal hair loss. Pediatrics 111:685–687, 2003.
25. Barton DJ, Sloan GM, Nichter LS, et al: Hair-thread tourniquet syndrome. Pediatrics 82:925–928, 1988.
*26. Biehler JL, Sieck C, Bonner B, et al: A survey of health care and child protective services provider knowledge regarding the toe tourniquet syndrome. Child Abuse Negl 18:987–993, 1994.
27. Kerry RL, Chapman DD: Strangulation of appendages by hair and thread. J Pediatr Surg 8:23–27, 1973.
28. Garty BZ, Mimouni MM, Varsano I: Penile tourniquet syndrome. Cutis 31:431–432, 1983.
29. Klusmann A, Lenard HG: Tourniquet syndrome—accident or abuse? Eur J Pediatr 163:495–498, 2004
*30. Serour F, Gorenstein A: Treatment of the toe tourniquet syndrome in infants. Pediatr Surg Int 19:598–600, 2003.
31. Harris EJ: Acute digital ischemia in infants: the hair-thread tourniquet syndrome—a report of two cases. J Foot Ankle Surg 41:112–116, 2002.

*32. Wei JL, Schwartz KM, Weaver AL, et al: Pseudotumor of infancy and congenital muscular torticollis: 170 cases. Laryngoscope 111:688–695, 2001.
33. Parikh SN Crawford AH, Choudhury S: Magnetic resonance imaging in the evaluation of infantile torticollis. Orthopedics 27:509–515, 2004.
34. Cheng JCY, Metreweli C, Chen TMK, et al: Correlation of ultrasonographic imaging of congenital muscular torticollis with clinical assessment in infants. Ultrasound Med Biol 26:1237–1241, 2000.
*35. Cheng JCY, Tang SP, Chen TMK, et al: The clinical presentation and outcome of treatment of congenital muscular torticollis in infants—a study of 1,086 cases. J Pediatr Surg 35:1091–1096, 2000.
36. Blyth WR, Logan TC, Holmes DK, et al: Fibromatosis colli: a common cause of neonatal torticollis. Am Fam Physician 54:1965–1967, 1996.
37. Kumar V, Prabhu BV, Chattopadhayay A, et al: Bilateral sternocleidomastoid tumor of infancy. Int J Pediatr Otorhinolaryngol 67:673–675, 2003.
*38. Luther BL: Congenital muscular torticollis. Orthop Nurs 21:21–27, 2002.
39. Cheng JCY, Wong MWN, Tang SP, et al: Clinical determinants of the outcome of manual stretching in the treatment of congenital muscular torticollis in infants: a prospective study of eight hundred and twenty-one cases. J Bone Joint Surg Am 83:679–687, 2001.
40. Porter SB, Blount BW: Pseudotumor of infancy and congenital muscular torticollis. Am Fam Physician 52:1731–1736, 1995.
41. Adams SB, Flynn JM, Halsikar H, et al: Torticollis in an infant caused by hereditary muscle aplasia. Am J Orthop 32:556–558, 2003.
42. Cheng JCY, Tang SP, Chen TMK: Sternocleidomastoid pseudotumor and congenital muscular torticollis in infants: a prospective study of 510 cases. J Pediatr 134:712–716, 1999.
43. Cheng JCY, Chen TMK, Tang SP, et al: Snapping during manual stretching in congenital muscular torticollis. Clin Orthop 384:237–244, 2001.
44. Cheng JCY, Tang SP: Outcome of surgical treatment of congenital muscular torticollis. Clin Orthop 362:190–200, 1999.
45. Rowen JL: Mucocutaneous candidiasis. Semin Perinatol 27:406–413, 2003.
*46. Hoppe JE: Treatment of oropharyngeal candidiasis and candidal diaper dermatitis in neonates and infants: review and reappraisal. Pediatr Infect Dis J 16:885–894, 1997.
47. Daftary SS, Desai SV, Shah MV, et al: Oral thrush in the newborn. Indian Pediatr 17:287–288, 1980.
48. Zollner MSA, Jorge AOC: Candida spp.: occurrence in oral cavities of breastfeeding infants and their mother's mouths and breasts. Pesqui Odontol Bras 17:151–155, 2003.
49. Darwazeh AM, al-Bashir A: Oral candida flora in healthy infants. J Oral Pathol Med 24:361–364, 1995.
50. Mattos-Graner RO, de Moraes AB, Rontani RM, et al: Relation of oral yeast infection in Brazilian infants and use of a pacifier. ASDC J Dent Child 68:33–36, 2001.
51. Lay KM, Russell C: Candida species and yeasts in mouths of infants from a special care unit of a maternity hospital. Arch Dis Child 52:794–796, 1977.
52. Prachniak GK: Common breastfeeding problems. Obstet Gyncol Clin North Am 29:77–88, 2002.
*53. Goins RA, Ascher D, Waecker N, et al: Comparison of fluconazole and nystatin oral suspensions for treatment of oral candidiasis in infants. Pediatr Infect Dis J 21:1165–1167, 2002.
54. Hoppe JE: Treatment of oropharyngeal candidiasis in immunocompetent infants: a randomized multicenter study of miconazole gel vs. nystatin suspension. The Antifungals Study Group. Pediatr Infect Dis J 16:288–293, 1997.
55. Tanguay KE, McBean MR, Jain E: Nipple candidiasis among breastfeeding mothers: case-control study of predisposing factors. Can Fam Physician 40:1407–1413, 1994.
56. Brent NB: Thrush in the breastfeeding dyad: results of a survey on diagnosis and treatment. Clin Pediatr 40:503–506, 2001.
57. Shepherd J: Thrush and breastfeeding. Pract Midwife 5:24–27, 2002.
*58. Aribarg A, Phupong V: Vaginal bleeding in young children. Southeast Asian J Trop Med Public Health 34:208–212, 2003.
59. Heller ME, Savage MO, Dewhurst J: Vaginal bleeding in childhood: a review of 51 patients. Br J Obstet Gynaecol 85:721–725, 1978.
60. Anveden-Hertzberg L, Gauderer MWL, Elder JS: Urethral prolapse: an often misdiagnosed cause of urogenital bleeding in girls. Pediatr Emerg Care 11:212–214, 1995.

---

*Selected readings.

Chapter 38

Jaundice

Niranjan Kissoon, MD

Introduction and Background

Jaundice is a yellowish pigmentation of the skin, tissues, and body fluids caused by the deposition of bile pigments. In most cases in which the infant is born at term, newborn jaundice arising during the first few days of life is of little clinical significance.[1] However, severe jaundice is associated with permanent brain damage.[1-4] Managing neonates with jaundice may be challenging for emergency physicians as these cases are relatively uncommon in most emergency departments and yet are occasionally fatal.[5]

Brain injury is the predominant factor in the morbidity and mortality directly attributable to neonatal jaundice.[1,6-9] Since the early 20th century, the term *kernicterus* has been somewhat loosely used to describe any brain injuries associated with severe hyperbilirubinemia.[6,10,11] In the last few years, organizations such as the American Academy of Pediatrics Subcommittee on Hyperbilirubinemia have proposed language to describe neurologic damage associated with neonatal jaundice more precisely.[12] The term *kernicterus* is used for cases of "chronic and permanent clinical sequelae of bilirubin toxicity."[12] The term *acute bilirubin encephalopathy* is used for the acute manifestations of bilirubin toxicity seen in the first few weeks of life. Acute bilirubin encephalopathy has also been referred to as "early bilirubin toxicity."[13]

Recognition and Approach

While jaundice is common, acute bilirubin encephalopathy and kernicterus are not. Approximately 60% of the 3.5 million healthy infants born each year in the United States will develop jaundice during the first week of life.[14] Of jaundiced newborns, approximately 25% will develop "severe hyperbilirubinemia," which corresponds to a total serum bilirubin level above the 95th percentile based on age (in hours).[14] For low-risk, full-term neonates, the 95th percentile corresponds to a total serum bilirubin level of approximately 17 mg/dl (291 μmol/L).[15] Extreme elevations of total serum bilirubin are rare. For example, for total serum bilirubin levels greater than 20, 25, and 30 mg/dl (342, 428, and 513 μmol/L), the corresponding incidences are approximately 2%, 0.2%, and 0.02% respectively.[16] While jaundice is common, demonstrable brain injury due to severe hyperbilirubinemia is not. There is no mandatory reporting mechanism for cases of kernicterus. This results in incomplete epidemiologic data. However, by one estimate approximately 125 cases of kernicterus were identified in the United States from 1984 to 2002.[17] This represents fewer than 10 cases per year in the United States.

Neonatal hyperbilirubinemia results from a buildup of bilirubin in newborn infants who have a limited ability to excrete it.[18] Neonates and young infants have high rates of bilirubin production due to rapid turnover of their red blood cells.[19] The strongest predictors of hyperbilirubinemia or early jaundice are a family history of jaundice in a newborn, exclusive breast-feeding with some difficulties encountered, bruising or cephalohematoma development during delivery, Asian race, maternal age greater than 25 years, and lower gestational age at birth[20,21] (Table 38–1).

Clinical Presentation

There are two main presentations of jaundice during early infancy. Infants may be brought to the emergency department primarily for a chief complaint of jaundice. These infants are typically robust and doing well. At times, however, infants may be brought to the emergency department for complaints in addition to jaundice. In the context of other potentially serious signs and symptoms, an evaluation for the underlying etiology is indicated[21,22] (Table 38–2) (see Chapter 7, The Critically Ill Neonate).

Table 38–1 Factors That Place Infants at Increased Risk for Severe Hyperbilirubinemia

Gestational age < 38 wk
Sibling received phototherapy
Cephalohematoma
Bruising sustained during delivery
Exclusive breast-feeding that is not going well
East Asian race
Maternal age ≥ 25 yr
Macrosomia and maternal diabetes
Glucose-6-phosphate dehydrogenase (G6PD) deficiency
Serum albumin < 3.0 g/dl
Temperature instability
Acidosis
Isoimmune hemolytic disease
Lethargy or sepsis

Adapted from American Academy of Pediatrics, Subcommittee on Hyperbilirubinemia: Management of hyperbilirubinemia in the newborn infant 35 or more weeks of gestation. Pediatrics 114:297–316, 2004.

Table 38–2 Signs and Symptoms in Jaundiced Neonates Consistent with a Serious Comorbid Illness

Apneic episodes
Decreased urine output
Distended abdomen
Ill appearance
Irritability
Lethargy
Poor tone
Respiratory distress
Temperature instability
Vomiting

History

Several historical features can assist in risk-stratifying jaundiced neonates (see Table 38–1). In particular, gestational age is an important risk factor for hyperbilirubinemia.[23] In most circumstances, there is little difference in the home care or medical management of healthy-appearing, appropriate-weight neonates born between 35 and 40 weeks' gestation. There is, however, an inverse relationship between gestational age and risk for severe hyperbilirubinemia.[12,23] Full-term neonates are at much lower risk for developing severe hyperbilirubinemia than those born preterm. Knowing whether the infant is breast-fed, bottle-fed, or both is helpful. Particularly if the mother and her neonate are having difficulties with feedings, exclusively breast-fed infants are at increased risk for severe hyperbilirubinemia.[12] Exclusive bottle feeding decreases the risk.[12]

Infants whose jaundice is due to hemolytic disease are at a higher risk for acute bilirubin encephalopathy. Historical factors suggestive of hemolytic disease include a family history of significant hemolytic disease, the onset of jaundice within the first 24 hours of life, a mother who is Rh negative (especially if the mother has not received Rh immune globulin), and a complaint of pallor.[20] On occasion, a prior bilirubin level will be available either from testing in the newborn nursery or from a check in the doctor's office. If this information is available, a rise in total serum bilirubin by more than 0.5 mg/dl per hour is also suggestive of hemolytic disease.[20]

Occasionally a neonate or young infant will present with a history consistent with cholestatic jaundice. These infants may have biliary atresia or other serious causes of cholestasis. In particular, a history of dark urine or dark urine stains in the diaper and very light-colored stools is suggestive of cholestatic jaundice. A history of prolonged jaundice, particularly if lasting more than 3 weeks, is suggestive of cholestatic jaundice. If infants with cholestatic jaundice have had bilirubin testing from another hospital or doctor's office prior to presentation in the emergency department, these infants will have an elevation of direct bilirubin that may prompt the visit.

For several decades, clinicians have recognized that the timing of the onset of jaundice appears to risk-stratify infants for severe hyperbilirubinemia and identify infants at risk for underlying comorbid illnesses.[24] Clinical experience supports this concept, although no evaluation of this framework has been performed using contemporary methodology. It is clear that jaundice with an onset within the first 24 hours of life is likely to be associated with a serious underlying illness.[12,20] Unless the child is the product of a home delivery, it is unlikely these infants will be discharged from the newborn nursery prior to the jaundice being recognized and addressed. Therefore, these infants are unlikely to present to the emergency department. Benign jaundice typically becomes evident during the second or third day of life, peaks at the fifth day and resolves by day 10.[25] A later onset of jaundice raises the likelihood of a comorbid illness, particularly sepsis.

Physical Examination

Fortunately, discoloration of the dermis and body fluids is fairly obvious to the naked eye. Some cases of jaundice are obvious to the mother, the triage nurse, and the physician. In more subtle cases, appreciating jaundice can be enhanced by blanching the skin with digital pressure to reveal the underlying color of the skin and subcutaneous tissue. Dermal icterus is first seen in the face and progresses caudally to the trunk and extremities.[26] As the total serum bilirubin level rises, the extent of cephalocaudad color progression parallels the degree of jaundice.[27] Unfortunately, estimating the total serum bilirubin based solely on the physical examination is not reliable.[12] After the identification of jaundice, the next step in the evaluation of these neonates is to determine their risk for severe hyperbilirubinemia and concurrent illnesses.

Besides the presence of jaundice, some physical examination findings are helpful in identifying infants at increased risk for severe hyperbilirubinemia. In particular, the presence of pallor and hepatosplenomegaly suggests hemolytic disease and a higher risk for severe hyperbilirubinemia. Excessive weight loss in the setting of exclusive breast-feeding places the infant at higher risk for severe hyperbilirubinemia. Determining if weight loss is excessive during the first week or two of life may be challenging if few infants are seen in an emergency physician's usual practice. It is assumed that infants will lose some weight during the first week of life. An appropriate weight loss for most infants is probably less than 10% of the birth weight. After the first week, a neonate is expected to gain about 1 ounce per day throughout the first month or two of life. By about 4 months of age, the infant should weigh approximately twice the birth weight.

So, excessive weight loss during the first week of life would be the loss of more than approximately 10% of the birth weight. Comparing birth weight, which is usually verbally provided by the parents, with a weight measured in the emergency department is inherently inaccurate, but is the only information typically available and provides a rough estimate of weight change. Physical examination findings suggestive of a serious underlying comorbid illness include poor tone, a weak suck, irritability, lethargy, temperature instability or fever, a distended abdomen, respiratory distress, ill appearance, a sunken fontanelle, and delayed capillary refill (see Chapter 7, The Critically Ill Neonate). Neonates who harbor comorbid illnesses have clinical features similar to neonates experiencing acute bilirubin encephalopathy, with severe jaundice, lethargy, and hypotonia with a poor suck.[12]

Diagnostic Tests

Laboratory testing is fundamental in risk-stratifying neonates for severe hyperbilirubinemia. Fortunately, the initial evaluation of hyperbilirubinemia requires tests readily available in emergency departments (Table 38–3). The measurements of total and direct serum bilirubin are the foundation of this evaluation.[28] Treatment recommendations are typically based on the assumption that a neonate has an unconjugated hyperbilirubinemia. Unfortunately, there is not a universally accepted definition of what constitutes an "unconjugated" or a "conjugated" hyperbilirubinemia. In general, a conjugated hyperbilirubinemia is present when the direct serum bilirubin level is greater than 20% of the total serum bilirubin level.[29] In the future, measurement of free bilirubin (i.e., bilirubin not bound to proteins) may play an important role in risk-stratifying jaundiced neonates.[13]

In addition to measuring bilirubin levels, one goal of laboratory testing is to assess the neonate for hemolysis. Test results suggestive of hemolysis include a positive Coombs' test, a peripheral blood smear revealing red cell destruction, and ABO or Rh incompatibility between the neonate and the mother (see Table 38–3). A serum albumin below 3 g/dl (30 g/L) is a risk factor for severe hyperbilirubinemia. Urine reducing substances may be helpful in identifying inborn errors of metabolism, which, if present, place the neonate at increased risk for severe hyperbilirubinemia and comorbid

Table 38–3	Laboratory Tests for the Evaluation of Jaundice in a Newborn Presenting to the Emergency Department*

Total serum bilirubin
Direct serum bilirubin
Blood type and Rh
Direct antibody test (Coombs')
Complete blood count with peripheral smear
Reticulocyte count
Serum albumin
Urine for reducing substances

*These tests are specifically for the evaluation of jaundice. If a comorbid illness such as dehydration or sepsis is suspected, additional tests (e.g., electrolytes, cultures) are indicated.
Adapted from American Academy of Pediatrics, Subcommittee on Hyperbilirubinemia: Management of hyperbilirubinemia in the newborn infant 35 or more weeks of gestation. Pediatrics 114:297–316, 2004.

illnesses (see Chapter 29 Inborn Errors of Metabolism). Additional testing is indicated if the neonate demonstrates signs or symptoms consistent with a comorbid illness (see Table 38–2).

Important Clinical Features and Considerations

One promising technology is the use of transcutaneous bilirubin measurement devices,[26,27,30,31] which noninvasively measure total serum bilirubin.[12] The use of these devices in the emergency department has not been evaluated. The quality of the output is sufficiently accurate that the American Academy of Pediatrics recommends against ordering a confirmatory serum bilirubin measurement before starting treatment.[12]

One concern in the emergency department is intravenous access in neonates (see Chapter 161, Vascular Access). If there is concern over obtaining intravenous access or performing a successful venipuncture, capillary blood from a heel stick is an acceptable specimen for the measurement of bilirubin, pH, hematocrit, hemoglobin, sodium, calcium, glucose, serum bicarbonate, and lactate.[28,32] Capillary specimens are not accurate for the measurement of serum potassium.[32]

Exhaled carbon monoxide has been shown to be effective in accurately identifying infants who are experiencing hemolysis.[33] The measurement most often cited is the end-tidal carbon monoxide level corrected for ambient carbon monoxide ($ETCO_c$).[12] The $ETCO_c$ has been shown to have better test characteristics than the Coombs' test.[34] However, the $ETCO_c$ is not currently used in emergency departments.

Management

In 1994 and again in 2004, the American Academy of Pediatrics published recommendations for the identification, evaluation, and treatment of hyperbilirubinemia.[12,20] In general, these recommendations are evidence based. Not all of the recommendations are relevant to emergency department care. Distilling the relevant information from these documents is challenging as multiple caveats for each recommendation and algorithms containing as many as 27 text boxes are presented. In general, young gestational age is the greatest risk factor for severe hyperbilirubinemia. Infants younger than 36 weeks' gestation are considered to be at much higher risk than those who were born at ≥ 38 weeks' gestation. Second, the traditional treatment threshold of 20 mg/dl (342 μmol/L) has been replaced with treatment thresholds based on the age of the neonate in hours[6,11,12] (Table 38–4). For healthy neonates born after 38 weeks' gestation who are at least 96 hours old, the treatment threshold remains 20 mg/dl (342 μmol). The three basic management plans for hyperbilirubinemia are observation and monitoring, phototherapy, and exchange transfusion.

Observation and Monitoring

Observation and monitoring is appropriate for neonates who do not meet treatment thresholds, but may develop further increases in serum bilirubin. The most common scenario is a jaundiced neonate who presents to the emergency department, does not demonstrate signs or symptoms of a serious comorbid illness, does not have a conjugated hyperbilirubi-

Table 38-4	Age- and Risk-Based Phototherapy Thresholds for Jaundiced Newborns	
	Total Serum Bilirubin, mg/dL (μmol/L)	
Age (hr)	**Higher Risk Infants**	**Lower Risk Infants**
24	8 (137)	12 (205)
36	9 (154)	14 (239)
48	11 (188)	15 (257)
60	12 (205)	17 (291)
72	13 (222)	18 (308)
84	14 (239)	19 (325)
≥96	15 (257)	20 (342)

Adapted from American Academy of Pediatrics, Subcommittee on Hyperbilirubinemia: Management of hyperbilirubinemia in the newborn infant 35 or more weeks of gestation. Pediatrics 114:297–316, 2004.

nemia, does not demonstrate historical, examination, or laboratory evidence of hemolysis, lacks high risk factors (see Table 38–1) and has a total serum bilirubin level below the treatment threshold (see Table 38–4). If the neonate has reliable caregivers, it is reasonable to discharge these children home from the emergency department and arrange a recheck of the total serum bilirubin as an outpatient. There is no evidence upon which to base the decision as to when follow-up should occur. Factors impacting this decision include availability of the neonate's primary care physician, the distance the family must travel to receive care, reliability of the parents, how close the total serum bilirubin level is to the treatment threshold, and the presence of vague complaints such as "just a little fussy," which may represent an early manifestation of a serious comorbid illness but probably does not. For many of these neonates, a conservative plan would be to have them return to the emergency department or their doctor's office in 12 hours for a repeat physical examination and total serum bilirubin measurement. Of course, the neonate should return to the emergency department sooner if worrisome signs or symptoms arise in the interim. For the neonate being discharged from the emergency department, there are no evidence-based guidelines regarding the continuance of breast-feeding. For infants unlikely to cross the threshold for phototherapy, continuing breast-feeding is probably reasonable. For infants at higher risk, decisions will need to be made on an individual basis.

Phototherapy

Phototherapy is the most commonly performed treatment specifically designed for hyperbilirubinemia. Phototherapy is generally safe and inexpensive. Phototherapy was introduced into clinical practice in 1958, but did not play a significant role in the treatment of jaundiced neonates until the late 1960s and 1970s.[35] Clinical experience suggests that phototherapy is very rarely initiated in the emergency department and, when it is, it is a temporary situation arising because of hospital overcrowding. Initiating phototherapy is based on the neonate's risk of severe hyperbilirubinemia, the age of the infant (in hours), and the total serum bilirubin level (see Tables 38–1 and 38–4). Coordinating care with the patient's primary care physician, the on-call pediatrician, or a neona-

tologist at a hospital to which the infant may be transferred is indicated.

Exchange Transfusion

For more than 50 years, exchange transfusion has been recognized as a treatment for hyperbilirubinemia.[36,37] Exchange transfusion was originally developed to treat severe hemolytic hyperbilirubinemia from Rhesus isoimmunization.[38] Prior to the introduction and acceptance of phototherapy, exchange transfusion was the treatment of choice for neonates with severe hyperbilirubinemia.[11] Now, exchange transfusion is primarily used in very high-risk situations and when phototherapy fails.[12]

Pharmacologic Therapy

In the future, pharmacologic treatment for severe hyperbilirubinemia may play a substantial role in the management of these neonates. In particular, laboratory experiments and case reports suggest the metalloporphyrins, particularly tin mesoporphyrin, are effective in dramatically lowering serum bilirubin levels.[39] Tin mesoporphyrin is appealing as a potential treatment in the emergency department because it is administered subcutaneously.[39] Currently, the metalloporphyrins have no role in the emergency department management of hyperbilirubinemia and have not been approved by the Food and Drug Administration.

Fluid Administration

The administration of intravenous normal saline is common in the management of jaundiced neonates seen in the emergency department. In general, exclusively breast-fed neonates who have jaundice also have dehydration. Treating this dehydration is prudent. The results of a small randomized, controlled trial suggested that both oral and intravenous rehydration may be effective.[40] Continuing feeds with a milk-based formula will inhibit enterohepatic circulation of bilirubin.[12] Clinical experience suggests that, if intravenous access has been established, an initial fluid bolus of 20 ml/kg of normal saline is reasonable during the initial evaluation and management of jaundiced neonates seen in the emergency department. Excessive hydration is not recommended.[12]

Summary

In most cases the healthy neonate with jaundice has a very good outcome.[41-43] However, hyperbilirubinemia in apparently healthy infants continues to hold the potential threat of acute bilirubin encephalopathy and kernicterus. Admission to the hospital is necessary if the phototherapy treatment threshold is approached or surpassed. Phototherapy is the treatment of choice for most cases of severe hyperbilirubinemia. Neonates who exhibit signs and symptoms of comorbid illnesses or cholestasis require approaches different from standard hyperbilirubinemia treatment pathways.

REFERENCES

1. Newman TB, Klebanoff MA: Neonatal hyperbilirubinemia and long-term outcome: another look at the Collaborative Perinatal Project. Pediatrics 92:651–657, 1993.
2. Groenendaal F, van der Grond J, Vries LS: Cerebral metabolism in severe neonatal hyperbilirubinemia. Pediatrics 114:291–294, 2004.
3. Britton JR, Britton HL, Beebe SA: Early discharge of the term newborn: a continued dilemma. Pediatrics 94:291–295, 1994.

4. Centers for Disease Control and Prevention: Kernicterus in full-term infants—United States, 1994–1998. MMWR Morb Mortal Wkly Rep 50:491–494, 2001.

*5. Mollen TJ, Scarfone R, Harris MC: Acute, severe bilirubin encephalopathy in a newborn. Pediatr Emerg Care 20:599–601, 2004.

*6. Watchko JF: Vigintiphobia revisited. Pediatrics 115:1747–1753, 2005.

*7. Newman TB, Liljestrand P, Jeremy RJ, et al: Outcomes among newborns with total serum bilirubin levels of 25 mg per deciliter or more. N Engl J Med 354:1889–1900, 2006.

*8. Newman TB, Liljestaran P, Escobar GJ: Infants with bilirubin levels of 30 mg/dL or more in a large managed care organization. Pediatrics 111:1303–1311, 2003.

9. Bhutani VK, Donn SM, Johnson LH: Risk management of severe neonatal hyperbilirubinemia to prevent kernicterus. Clin Perinatol 32:125–139, 2005.

10. Schmorl CG: Zur Kenntnis des Ikterus neonatorum, insbesondere der dabei auftretenden Gehirnveränderungen. Verh Dtsch Pathol Ges 6:109–115, 1904.

11. Watchko JF, Oski FA: Bilirubin 20 mg/dL = vigintiphobia. Pediatrics 71:660–663, 1983.

*12. American Academy of Pediatrics, Subcommittee on Hyperbilirubinemia: Management of hyperbilirubinemia in the newborn infant 35 or more weeks of gestation. Pediatrics 114:297–316, 2004.

13. Wennberg RP, Ahlfors CE, Bhutani VK, et al: Toward understanding kernicterus: a challenge to improve the management of jaundiced newborns. Pediatrics 117:474–485, 2006.

14. Bhutani VK, Johnson LH, Keren R: Diagnosis and management of hyperbilirubinemia in the term neonate: for a safer first week. Pediatr Clin North Am 51:843–861, 2004.

15. Halamek LP, Stevenson DK: Neonatal jaundice and liver disease. In Fanaroff AA, Martin RJ (eds): Neonatal-Perinatal Medicine, Vol 2: Diseases of the Fetus and Infant, 6th ed. St. Louis: Mosby–Year Book, 1997, pp 1345–1389.

16. Newman TB, Escobar GJ, Gonzales VM, et al: Frequency of neonatal bilirubin testing and hyperbilirubinemia in a large health maintenance organization. Pediatrics 104:1198–1203, 1999.

17. Schwoebel A, Gennaro S: Neonatal hyperbilirubinemia. J Perinat Neonatal Nurs 20:103–107, 2006.

*18. Dennery PA, Seidman DS, Stevenson DK: Neonatal hyperbilirubinemia. N Engl J Med 344:581–590, 2001.

19. Johnson L: Yet another expert opinion on bilirubin toxicity! Pediatrics 89:827–828, 1992.

20. American Academy of Pediatrics, Provisional Committee for Quality Improvement and Subcommittee on Hyperbilirubinemia: Practice parameter: Management of hyperbilirubinemia in the healthy term newborn. Pediatrics 94:558–56l, 1994.

21. Newman TB, Xiong B, Gonzales VM, et al: Prediction and prevention of extreme neonatal hyperbilirubinemia in a mature health maintenance organization. Arch Pediatr Adolesc Med 154:1140–1147, 2000.

22. Garcia FJ, Nager AL: Jaundice as an early diagnostic sign of urinary tract infection in infancy. Pediatrics 109:846–851, 2002.

23. Bhutani VK, Johnson L: Kernicterus in late preterm infants cared for as term healthy infants. Semin Perinatol 30:89–97, 2006.

24. Brown AK: Neonatal jaundice. Pediatr Clin North Am 9:575–603, 1962.

25. Smitherman H, Stark AR, Bhutani VK: Early recognition of neonatal hyperbilirubinemia and its emergent management. Semin Fetal Neonatal Med 11:214–224, 2006.

26. Kramer LI: Advancement of dermal icterus in the jaundiced newborn. Am J Dis Child 118:454, 1969.

27. Ebbesen F: The relationship between the cephalopedal progress of clinical icterus and the serum bilirubin concentration in newborn infants without blood type sensitization. Obstet Gynecol Scand 54:329–332, 1975.

28. Dale JC, Hamrick HJ: Neonatal bilirubin testing practices: reports from 312 laboratories enrolled in the College of American Pathologists Excel Proficiency Testing Program. Arch Pathol Lab Med 124:1425–1428, 2000.

*29. Moyer V, Freese DK, Whitington PF, et al: Guideline for the evaluation of cholestatic jaundice in infants: recommendations of the North American Society for Pediatric Gastroenterology, Hepatology and Nutrition. J Pediatr Gastroenterol Nutr 39:115–128, 2004.

30. Schumacher RE: Noninvasive measurements of bilirubin in the newborn. Clin Perinatol 17:417–435, 1990.

31. Madlon-Kay DJ: Home health nurse clinical assessment of neonatal jaundice. Arch Pediatr Adolesc Med 155:583–586, 2001.

32. Yang KC, Su BH, Tsai FJ, et al: The comparison between capillary blood sampling and arterial blood sampling in an NICU. Acta Paediatr Taiwan 43:124–126, 2002.

33. Vreman HF, Stevenson DK, Oh W, et al: Semiportable electrochemical instruments for determining carbon monoxide in breath. Clin Chem 40:1927–1933, 1994.

34. Herschel M, Karrison T, Wen M, et al: Evaluation of the direct antiglobulin (Coombs') test for identifying newborns at risk for hemolysis as determined by end-tidal carbon monoxide concentration ($ETCO_c$) for detecting significant jaundice. J Perinatol 22:341–347, 2002.

35. Lucey J, Ferreiro M, Hewitt J: Prevention of hyperbilirubinemia of prematurity by phototherapy. Pediatrics 41:1047–1054, 1968.

36. Mollison PL, Cutbush M: A method of measuring the severity of a series of cases of hemolytic disease of the newborn. Blood 6:777–788, 1951.

37. Hsia DY, Allen FH, Gellis SS, et al: Erythroblastosis fetalis. VIII. Studies of serum bilirubin in relation to kernicterus. N Engl J Med 247:668–671, 1952.

38. Shapiro SM, Bhutani VK, Johnson L: Hyperbilirubinemia and kernicterus. Clin Perinatol 33:387–410, 2006.

39. Dennery PA: Metalloporphyrins for the treatment of neonatal jaundice. Curr Opin Pediatr 17:167–169, 2005.

40. Boo NY, Lee HT: Randomized controlled trial of oral versus intravenous fluid supplementation on serum bilirubin level during phototherapy or term infant with severe hyperbilirubinemia. J Pediatr Child Health 38:151–155, 2002.

41. Bhutani VK, Johnson L, Sivieri EM: Predictive ability of discharge hour-specific serum bilirubin for subsequent significant hyperbilirubinemia in healthy term and near-term newborns. Pediatrics 103:6–14, 1999.

42. Stevenson, DK, Avroy AF, Maisels JM, et al: Prediction of hyperbilirubinemia in near-term and term infants. Pediatrics 108:31–39, 2001.

43. Harris MC, Bernbaum JC, Polin JR, et al: Developmental follow-up of breastfed term and near-term infants with marked hyperbilirubinemia. Pediatrics 107:1075–1079, 2001.

*Selected readings.

Chapter 39

Neonatal Skin Disorders

Antonio E. Muñiz, MD

Key Points

Most neonatal rashes are benign in nature.

Erythema toxicum neonatorum must be differentiated from pustules that result from bacterial infections or sepsis.

Omphalitis is a serious infection that requires antibiotics and occasionally surgical débridement

Selected Diagnoses

Milia
Miliaria rubra
Sebaceous gland hyperplasia
Cutis marmorata
Erythema toxicum neonatorum
Transient neonatal pustular melanosis
Acne neonatorum
Omphalitis

Introduction and Background

Skin lesions appearing in the first month of life usually prompt parents to seek medical advice. The skin of the neonate differs from that of an adult in that it is thinner, has less hair and weaker intercellular attachments, and produces fewer sweat and sebaceous gland secretions. The normal full-term newborn's skin feels soft and smooth. The skin of a postmature neonate often appears dry and cracked because the stratum corneum, which has accumulated in utero, has not yet been shed. Fissures and bleeding may be seen on the ankles and wrists.

The skin at birth usually has a purplish red hue that is most pronounced over the extremities, known as acrocyanosis. This occurs because of increased tone of the peripheral arterioles, which creates vasospasm, secondary dilation, and pooling of blood in the venous plexuses, and results in cyanosis of the distal extremities. Skin care should involve gentle cleansing with a nontoxic, nonabrasive neutral material, and moisturizers should be applied frequently to hydrate the skin.[1]

Discussion of Individual Diagnoses

Milia

Milia are benign, keratin-filled cysts that occur in 40% to 50% of newborns. They usually appear 1 to 2 days after birth, but on occasion develop weeks after birth.[2] Milia result from retention of keratin and sebaceous material within the pilosebaceous apparatus of the newborn. The skin lesions consist of multiple, pearly white or yellow papules, 1 to 2 mm in diameter, located over the forehead, cheeks, nose, and chin (Fig. 39–1). Occasionally they may occur on the upper trunk, limbs, penis, or mucous membranes. These cystic spheres rupture onto the skin surface and exfoliate their contents within weeks of birth.

A discrete round, pearly white or yellow, freely movable mass, 2 to 3 mm in diameter, on the midline of the hard palate (Epstein's pearl) or gum margins (Bohn's nodule) is the counterpart of facial milia.

Lesions that may mimic milia include molluscum contagiosum, sebaceous gland hyperplasia, erythema toxicum neonatorum (ETN), herpes simplex virus (HSV) infection, transient neonatal pustular melanosis, and neonatal acne.

No treatment is necessary for this rash. It usually disappears during the first 3 to 4 weeks of life but occasionally may persist until 3 months of age. Milia is a benign disorder that should not be confused with other more serious rashes, such as HSV infection.

Miliaria Rubra

Miliaria rubra is characterized by an erythematous papular or vesicular eruption in areas of skinfolds. It is seen more commonly in conditions of high heat and humidity that lead to excessive sweating.[3] Lesions are exacerbated by wearing tightly fitted clothes. Miliaria rubra is caused by blockage of eccrine ducts by keratinous plugs at the level of the stratum corneum. Maceration of the ducts and escape of eccrine sweat into the dermis creates a localized inflammatory response resulting in the skin eruption.[4]

It rarely is present at birth and usually develops during the first week of life, especially in association with warming of the infant by an incubator, occlusive clothing or dressings, or fever.

Lesions are small, discrete, erythematous papules, vesicles, or papulovesicles surrounded by a thin, erythematous rim (Fig. 39–2). They occur in the neck, groin, and axilla and may be pruritic. The diagnosis is based upon clinical features.

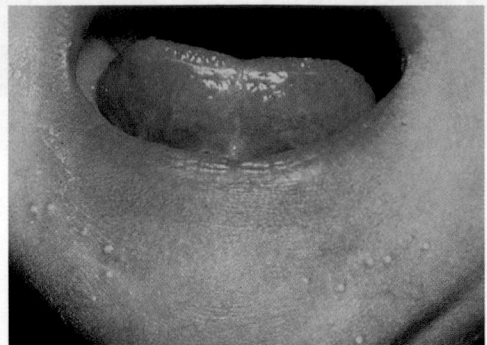

FIGURE 39–1. Milia.

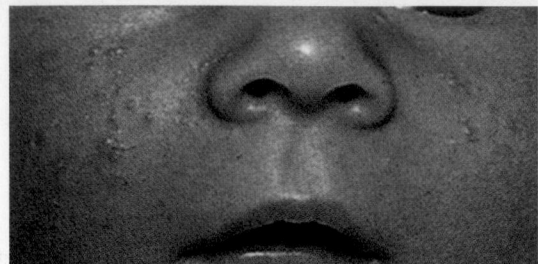

FIGURE 39–3. Sebaceous gland hyperplasia.

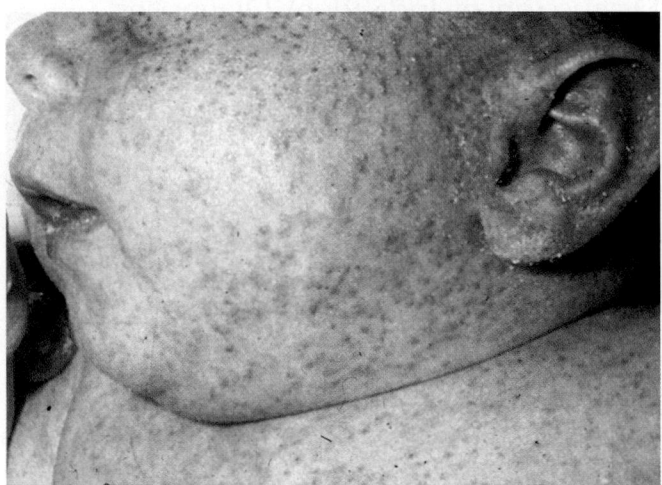

FIGURE 39–2. Miliaria rubra.

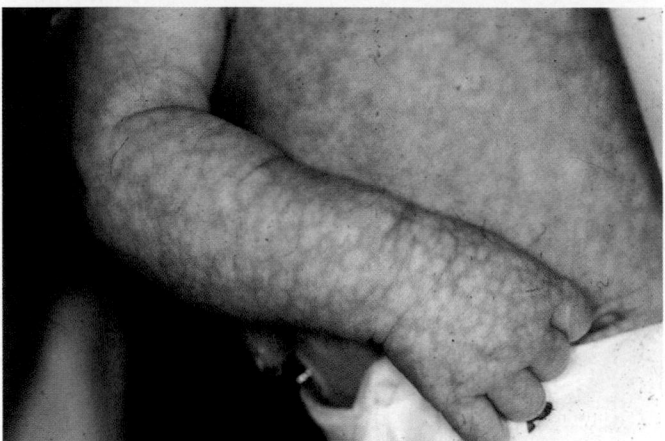

FIGURE 39–4. Cutis marmorata.

Sparse squamous cells and lymphocytes are seen on Wright-stained smear of the vesicular content. Differential diagnosis includes cutaneous candidiasis, varicella, ETN, folliculitis, HSV infection, and neonatal acne.

Treatment is directed toward avoidance of excessive heat and humidity. Lightweight clothing, cool baths, and air conditioning are useful in ameliorating the lesions.

Sebaceous Gland Hyperplasia

Sebaceous gland hyperplasia occurs in about 50% of newborns.[2] Maternal androgenic stimulation is responsible for the increase in sebaceous gland volume and size. Lesions consist of multiple small, yellow to flesh-colored macules or papules, 1 mm in diameter, that are seen at the opening of each pilosebaceous follicle over the nose, upper lips, and cheeks (Fig. 39–3). The lesions of sebaceous gland hyperplasia can be easily confused with milia.

There is no treatment for these lesions, and they usually resolve spontaneously within 1 week of life, but occasionally may persist up to 4 to 6 months of age. If treatment is deemed necessary, cryotherapy, cauterization, topical chemicals, or surgical excision may be tried. The major disadvantage of these therapeutic strategies is a considerable risk of posttraumatic scarring or dyspigmentation. Recently, pulsed dye laser has been shown to be effective without scarring.[5]

Cutis Marmorata (Mottling)

Cutis marmorata is a normal, reticulated, bluish mottling of the skin seen in the trunk and extremities caused by exposure to a cold ambient environment.[6] It is caused by the immature nature of the autonomic control of the dermal plexus with constriction of the deeper plexus and vasodilation of the superficial plexus. It occurs in response to hypothermia and disappears as the infant is rewarmed.

The skin exhibits a lacelike pattern of dusky erythema over the extremities and trunk when the neonate is exposed to cold ambient temperature (Fig. 39–4). In some neonates, cutis marmorata may recur until early childhood or remain persistent, as in cases of Down syndrome, trisomy 18, and Cornelia de Lange's syndrome. Mottling that persists beyond 6 months of age may be a sign of hypothyroidism, vascular malformation, or cutis marmorata telangiectasia congenita, all of which can be associated with musculoskeletal or vascular abnormalities.[7] Other mimickers may include livedo reticularis, which is seen in neonatal lupus erythematosus.

No treatment is required except rewarming the infant and maintaining a normal skin temperature.

Erythema Toxicum Neonatorum

ETN is a benign, self-limited, transient rash characterized by vesicles or pustules that are surrounded by blotchy, red macules. The eruption occurs by day 3 or 4 day of life, but may be seen at birth or may be noted as late as 2 weeks after birth.[8,9] It occurs in about 30% to 50% of full-term infants and in only 5% of preterm infants.[10,11]

ETN is of unknown etiology but may be due to an allergic reaction to substances passed transplacentally or a result of

FIGURE 39–5. Erythema toxicum neonatorum.

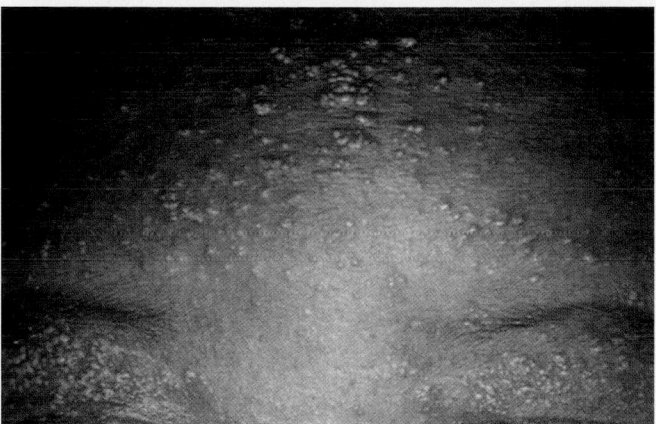

FIGURE 39–6. Transient neonatal pustular melanosis.

an acute graft-versus-host reaction induced by the maternal-fetal transfer of lymphocytes before or during delivery.[12]

The lesions begin as blotchy, erythematous macules, 2 to 3 cm in diameter, with small (1- to 4-mm) vesicles or pustules in the center of the macules ("flea-bitten" appearance).[13] They occur on the chest, back, face, and proximal extremities, sparing the palms and soles, and may vary from a few to several hundred lesions[14] (Fig. 39–5). The individual lesions clear in 4 to 5 days, and new lesions may appear up to the second week of life.

A smear of the fluid from the vesicle or pustule will reveal numerous eosinophils on Wright- or Giemsa-stained preparations. A peripheral blood eosinophilia may also occur.[15] The differential diagnosis may include HSV infection, impetigo, varicella, neonatal sepsis, miliaria rubra, folliculitis, milia, transient neonatal pustular melanosis, and cutaneous candidiasis.

ETN is a benign disorder requiring no treatment, but is extremely important to distinguish from other conditions with a worse prognosis, such as bacterial infection or sepsis, in which systemic symptoms are usually present.

Transient Neonatal Pustular Melanosis

Transient neonatal pustular melanosis is a benign, self-limited disorder of unknown etiology characterized by vesiculopustular lesions that rupture easily and evolve into evanescent hyperpigmented macules.[16] Seen in 0.2% to 4% of neonates, it is more common in African Americans.[17,18]

The lesions occur at birth as vesicles, pustules, or ruptured vesicles or pustules with a collarette of surrounding fine white scales[19] (Fig. 39–6). The lesions are located on the chin, forehead, neck, lower back, and shins, and occasionally can be found on the cheeks, trunk, and extremities. Intact vesicles and pustules rupture and leave behind brown, hyperpigmented macules (Fig. 39–7).[20]

Smears of the fluid in the vesicles or pustules show numerous neutrophils and occasionally eosinophils on Wright-stained preparations, while Gram staining reveals no organisms. Transient neonatal pustular melanosis may be misdiagnosed as ETN, HSV infection, milia, miliaria rubra, or acropustulosis of infancy.

FIGURE 39–7. Hyperpigmented macules in transient neonatal pustular melanosis.

There is no recommended treatment for this disorder. The vesicles and macules disappear by day 5 of life, while the brown hyperpigmented macules resolve over 3 weeks to 3 months.[21] The most important entity to exclude is bacterial infection or sepsis, which also may manifest a pustular eruption. Bacterial infection and sepsis are often associated with other signs of illness or a history of prolonged rupture of amniotic membranes; infants with transient neonatal pustular melanosis are well appearing.

Acne Neonatorum

Neonatal acne is characterized by a facial eruption of inflammatory and noninflammatory lesions. It rarely presents at birth and generally appears after the second week of life. It may persist up to the eighth month of life. It occurs in up to 20% of neonates and is more common in males.[22]

This condition appears to develop as a result of androgen hormonal stimulation of sebaceous glands.[22] Multiple, discrete papules on the face, chest, back, and groin are characteristic. Papules evolve into pustules after a few weeks (Fig. 39–8). Closed comedones are more common, but open comedones as well as inflammatory lesions, such as papules and pustules, may be seen.[23] The differential diagnosis includes neonatal pustules from sepsis, ETN, transient neonatal pustular melanosis, cutaneous candidiasis, infantile acropustulosis, nevus comedonicus, psoriasis, and sebaceous gland hyperplasia.

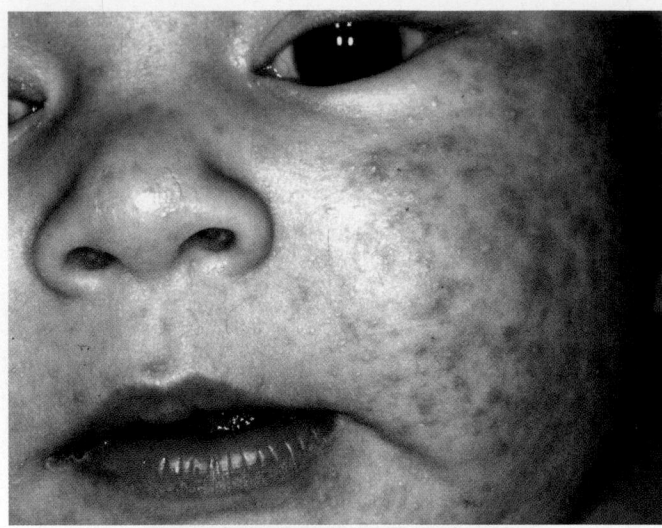

FIGURE 39–8. Acne neonatorum.

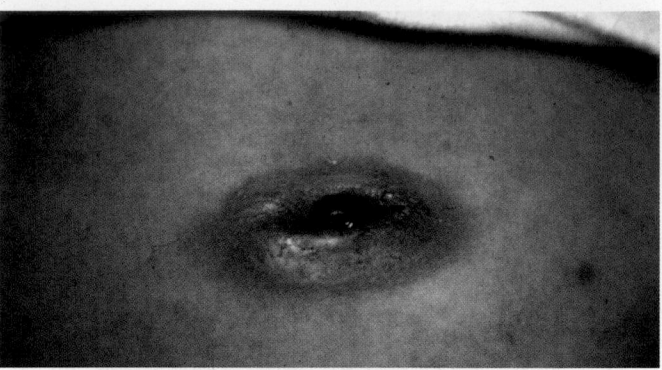

FIGURE 39–9. Omphalitis.

Acne neonatorum usually resolves spontaneously without treatment within 4 months, with therapy required only for cosmetic improvement. In mild cases, daily cleansing with soap and water may help. For comedonal acne neonatorum, azelaic acid (20%) topical or mild tretinoin preparation (0.025% to 0.05%) may be used.[24] Topical salicylic acid (1%) is another alternative.[24] For inflammatory lesions, topical erythromycin (2%) or benzoyl peroxide (2.5%) gel can be applied.[24,25]

Omphalitis

Omphalitis, or umbilical sepsis, is a bacterial infection of the umbilical stump and surrounding tissues. Widespread aseptic umbilical cord care has greatly reduced its occurrence.[26,27] Risk factors for the development of omphalitis include low birth weight (<2500 g), prior umbilical catheterization, and premature rupture or prolonged rupture of amniotic membranes.[28]

A bacterial infection through an open wound of the umbilical cord or surrounding tissue is the usual cause, although primary bacteremia with seeding of the umbilical stump can occur. Most infections are polymicrobial. The primary organisms responsible for omphalitis include *Staphylococcus aureus,* group A streptococcus, *Escherichia coli, Kliebsiella pneumoniae, Proteus mirabilis,* and anaerobes such as *Bacteroides fragilis* and *Clostridium perfringens.*[29-31]

Initial findings include a purulent discharge from the umbilical stump, followed by periumbilical erythema, edema, induration, and tenderness (Fig. 39–9). Late in the course of infection, neonates manifest signs of sepsis, including lethargy, irritability, and hypothermia or hyperthermia. If the infection is left untreated, it can progress to superficial abscess, necrotizing fasciitis, myonecrosis, portal vein thrombosis, peritonitis, bowel evisceration, hepatic abscess, endocarditis, sepsis, and death.[32-34] An irritant dermatitis produced by treatment of the umbilicus may mimic omphalitis.

Omphalitis is treated with antibiotics directed toward the more common causative organisms. These may include nafcillin and cefotaxime. Metronidazole can be added for anaerobic coverage, especially if necrotizing fasciitis or myonecrosis is suspected. Surgical débridement may be required for complications.[35-37] Omphalitis is a potentially life-threatening infection.

REFERENCES

1. Wallach D: Diagnosis of common, benign neonatal dermatoses. Clin Dermatol 21:264–268, 2003.
2. Rivers JK, Frederiksen PC, Dibdin C: A prevalence survey of dermatoses in the Australian neonate. J Am Acad Dermatol 23:77–81, 1990.
3. Feng E, Janniger CK: Miliaria. Cutis 55:213–216, 1995.
4. Nedwich JA: Summer and skin. Aust Fam Physician 21:35–41, 1992.
5. Schonermark MP, Schmidt C, Raulin C: Treatment of sebaceous gland hyperplasia with pulsed dye laser. Lasers Surg Med 21:313–316, 1997.
6. Verbov J: Common skin conditions in the newborn. Semin Neonatol 5:303–310, 2000.
7. Amitai DB, Fichman S, Merlob P, et al: Cutis marmorata telangiectasia congenital: clinical findings in 85 patients. Pediatr Dermatol 17:100–104, 2000.
8. Levy HL, Cothran F: Erythema toxicum neonatorum present at birth. Am J Dis Child 103:617–619, 1962.
9. Marino LJ: Toxic erythema at birth. Arch Dermatol 92:402–403, 1965.
10. Carr JA, Hodgman JE, Freedman RI, Levan NE: Relationship between toxic erythema and infant maturity. Am J Dis Child 112:129–134, 1966.
11. Taylor WB, Bondurant CP Jr: Erythema neonatorum allergicum: a study of the incidence in two hundred newborn infants and a review of the literature. Arch Dermatol 76:591–594, 1957.
12. Bassukas ID: Is erythema toxicum neonatorum a mild self-limited acute cutaneous graft-versus-host reaction from maternal-to-fetal lymphocyte transfer? Med Hypotheses 38:334–338, 1992.
13. Wagner A: Distinguishing vesicular and pustular disorders in the neonate. Curr Opin Pediatr 9:396–405, 1997.
14. Schwartz RA, Janniger CK: Erythema toxicum neonatorum. Cutis 58:153–155, 1996.
15. Berg FJ, Solomon LM: Erythema neonatorum toxicum. Arch Dis Child 62:327–328, 1987.
16. Simon MW: Transient neonatal pustular melanosis: an uncommon rash. Am Fam Physician 51:1401, 1995.
17. Barr RJ, Globerman LM, Werber FA: Transient neonatal pustular melanosis. Int J Dermatol 18:636–638, 1979.
18. Merlob P, Metzker A, Reisner SH: Transient neonatal pustular melanosis. Am J Dis Child 136:521–522, 1982.
19. Wrye HW Jr, Murphy MO: Transient neonatal pustular melanosis. Arch Dermatol 115:458, 1979.
20. Treadwell PA: Dermatoses in newborns. Am Fam Physician 56:443–450, 1997.
21. Ramamurthy RS, Reveri M, Esterly NB, et al: Transient neonatal pustular melanosis. J Pediatr 88:831–835, 1976.
22. Katsambas AD, Katoulis AC, Stavropoulos P: Acne neonatorum: a study of 22 cases. Int J Dermatol 38:128–130, 1999.
23. Jansen T, Burgdorf WH, Plewig G: Pathogenesis and treatment of acne in childhood. Pediatr Dermatol 14:17–21, 1997.
24. Kaminer MS, Gilchrest BA: The many faces of acne. J Am Acad Dermatol 32:S6–S14, 1995.
25. Van Praag MC, Rooji RW, Folkers E, et al: Diagnosis and treatment of pustular disorders in the neonate. Pediatr Dermatol 14:131–143, 1997.
26. Panyavudhikrai S, Danchaivijitr S, Vantanasiri C, et al: Antiseptics for preventing omphalitis. J Med Assoc Thai 85:229–234, 2002.

27. Pezzati M, Biagioli EC, Martelli E, et al: Umbilical cord care: the effects of eight different cord-care regimens on cord separation time and other outcomes. Biol Neonate 81:38–44, 2002.

28. Guvenc H, Guvenc M, Yenioglu H, et al: Neonatal omphalitis is still common in eastern Turkey. Scand J Infect Dis 23:613–616, 1991.

29. Airede AI: Pathogens in neonatal omphalitis. J Trop Pediatr 38:129–131, 1992.

30. Cushing AH: Omphalitis: a review. Pediatr Infect Dis 4:282–285, 1985.

*31. Sawardekar KP: Changing spectrum of neonatal omphalitis. Pediatr Infect Dis J 23:22–26, 2004.

_____

*Selected readings.

32. Brook I: Microbiology of necrotizing fasciitis associated with omphalitis in the newborn infant. J Perinatol 18:28–30, 1998.

33. Gormley D: Neonatal anaerobic (clostridial) cellulitis and omphalitis. Arch Dermatol 113:683–684, 1977.

34. Ameh EA, Nmadu PT: Major complications of omphalitis in neonates and infants. Pediatr Surg Int 18:413–416, 2002.

35. Kosloske AM, Bartow SA: Debridement of periumbilical necrotizing fasciitis: importance of excision of the umbilical vessels and urachal remnant. J Pediatr Surg 26:808–810, 1991.

36. Samuel M, Freeman NV, Vaishnav A, et al: Necrotizing fasciitis: a serious complication of omphalitis in neonates. J Pediatr Surg 29:1414–1416, 1994.

37. Stunden RJ, Brown RA, Rode H, et al: Umbilical gangrene in the newborn. J Pediatr Surg 23:130–134, 1988.

Approach to the Acutely Ill Patient

Chapter 40

Seizures

Jonathan Marr, MD and Pamela J. Okada, MD

Key Points

Febrile seizures are unique to young children, commonly lead to an emergency department visit, and are generally managed the same way as fever without a seizure.

Neonatal seizures may have subtle manifestations and require a different approach than seizures in older infants and children.

Benzodiazepines are the first-line pharmacologic agents for treating ongoing seizures.

Stable doses of anticonvulsants in growing children will tend to become subtherapeutic over time.

There are quite a few conditions that share some presenting features with seizures, but are not seizures.

Introduction and Background

Shaking, odd behaviors, unusual movements, or eye rolling commonly leads to pediatric visits in the emergency department. These events may be called "fits," "spells," "convulsions," or "seizures" by the family. Clinical experience suggests it is common for families to want to know if their child actually had a seizure. One accepted definition of a seizure is a sudden change in behavior due to unregulated electrical activity in the brain.[1] Unfortunately, definitions such as this are not helpful when evaluating children presenting to the emergency department because the electrical activity of the brain is not routinely evaluated in our clinical setting. Over the last few decades, multiple categorization schemes have been developed for pediatric seizures.[2-6] Although these categorization schemes may be useful in the development of standardized research, they have limited utility in the emergency department as they tend not to guide acute management. However, several relatively simple clinical features are helpful in the emergency department evaluation of these children. These include the age of the child

(Table 40–1), the presence or absence of fever, whether the body movements were generalized or focal, whether the child has a known past history of seizures, whether the postseizure neurologic examination is normal or not, and whether the child is continuing to seize or not. One additional feature that is important to elicit is whether known trauma was associated with the seizure (see Chapter 17, Head Trauma). With these simple clinical features used as a basic framework, emergency physicians can develop a rational approach to managing these children in the emergency department.

Recognition and Approach

In the United States, approximately 120,000 children per year seek medical attention for a newly recognized seizure.[7] Some of these children will go on to have lifelong seizures, while others will have either a single event or a small number of seizures during a limited time in their lives.

Given the complexity of the human nervous system, there are nearly limitless ways in which seizures and seizure-like events may present to the emergency department. Fortunately, there are a few broad categories into which many of these events fit. To at least some extent, each of these categories has been defined and studied. This structure allows for the development of some evidence upon which to base diagnostic and management decisions. These categories include status epilepticus, febrile seizures, first-time afebrile seizures, neonatal seizures, seizures occurring in children with known seizure disorders, and seizure-like events.

Status Epilepticus

Status epilepticus can be defined as "a continuous series of generalized tonic-clonic seizures without return to consciousness" or "any prolonged series of similar seizures without return to full consciousness between them."[8] Clinical research on status epilepticus typically includes the caveat that the combination of seizures and abnormal consciousness has lasted at least 30 minutes.[6,9-11] Based on data from the North London Status Epilepticus in Childhood Surveillance Study, the incidence of status epilepticus is estimated to be 20 episodes per 100,000 children per year.[10] In this population-based study, more than half of the children were neurologically healthy before experiencing their first episode of status epilepticus. Of these previously neurologically healthy children, half were febrile on presentation, 10% were diagnosed with bacterial meningitis, and 3% died.[10]

Table 40–1	Age-Based Causes of Pediatric Seizures

Neonatal

Congenital brain abnormalities
Drug intoxication or withdrawal
Encephalitis
Hypocalcemia
Hypoglycemia
Hypomagnesemia
Inborn error of metabolism
Infarction
Intracranial hemorrhage
Meningitis
Nonaccidental brain injury
Perinatal hypoxic brain injury

Infants and Toddlers

Accidental head injury
Brain tumor
Encephalitis
Febrile seizure
Hyponatremia
Meningitis
Nonaccidental head injury
Shigella gastroenteritis
Toxic ingestion

Children

Accidental head injury
Brain tumor
Inborn error of metabolism

Adolescents

Accidental head injury
Brain tumor
Epilepsy
Hypertensive encephalopathy
Toxic ingestion

Febrile Seizures

The term *febrile seizure* has a specific meaning to clinicians. A commonly accepted formal definition is a seizure occurring in a child between 6 months and 5 years of age who has a temperature greater than 38° C (100.4° F) or a history of recent fever, without a prior history of seizures or other neurologic disorders.[12,13] Febrile seizures are very common, occurring in as many as 5% of all children.[12] Since the mid-1970s, febrile seizures have been subclassified as either simple or complex.[14] Simple febrile seizures are defined as generalized seizures lasting less than 15 minutes and occurring only once within a 24-hour period.[12] Simple febrile seizures are common, benign events. Complex febrile seizures include any combination of being focal, lasting longer than 15 minutes, or recurring within 24 hours. A subset of children with complex febrile seizures harbors serious diseases, including bacterial meningitis.[10,11] Clinical experience suggests two important points about febrile seizures. First, regardless of the formal definition, in the vernacular used among pediatricians and emergency physicians, the term *febrile seizure* is synonymous with "simple febrile seizure." Second, there is a wide spectrum of disorders that fall within the formal definition of a "complex febrile seizure." This spectrum ranges from a well-appearing, febrile toddler who has experienced two 30-second seizures within 24 hours to a

critically ill febrile young child in status epilepticus. This heterogeneity makes generalizations about complex febrile seizures problematic.

A term coined in 1997, febrile seizures plus, has appeared in the literature and may lead to confusion. Febrile seizures plus refers to "children suffering febrile seizures extending beyond 6 years, with or without associated afebrile generalized tonic-clonic seizures, who do not have one of the recognized [seizure] syndromes."[15] Most emergency physicians would categorize these children as simply having a known seizure disorder whether or not this disorder has an official name. These children do not fit the common use of the term *febrile seizure*.

First-Time Afebrile Seizures

Each year in the United States, approximately 30,000 previously neurologically healthy children older than 1 month of age experience their first afebrile seizure.[16] Although such cases are not as common as febrile seizures, these children commonly present to emergency departments for evaluation.

Neonatal Seizures

It is difficult to determine the epidemiology of neonatal seizures relevant to the practice of emergency medicine. This is because much of the literature and study involve neonates in intensive care units and may include electroencephalographic data in the definitions and classification schemes. About 65% of clinically apparent neonatal "seizures" are not associated with electroencephalographic seizure activity.[17] Prematurity is a risk factor for clinically defined seizures. Preterm infants are more than 40 times more likely to have clinically evident seizures than term infants.[18] Since many preterm infants will be diagnosed with seizures prior to their initial discharge from the hospital, these infants are typically considered to have a known seizure disorder by the time they present to an emergency department. In addition, the presentation of a seizure in neonates may be subtle and includes staring episodes, rhythmic blinking, eyes rolling back, or lip smacking.[19] Alternatively, the initial clinical picture may be best classified as an apparent life-threatening event (ALTE) rather than as a seizure[20] (see Chapter 28, Apparently Life-Threatening Events). Approximately 10% of infants presenting to the emergency department with ALTEs are ultimately diagnosed with a seizure as the cause.[20]

Children with a Known Seizure Disorder

Although these are perhaps the most commonly seen seizure presentations in the emergency department, there are no epidemiologic data on these children. The wide variability in causes, presentations, chronic medications prescribed, and ages makes generalized statements about this diverse group of children problematic.

Seizure-like Events

There are quite a few conditions that can mimic or be mistaken for seizures (Table 40–2). Familiarity with these conditions may lead to a correct, alternative diagnosis. Benign conditions such as breath-holding spells, if mistaken for a seizure, may lead to unnecessary diagnostic testing and worry in the parents (see Chapter 37, Minor Infant Problems).

Table 40–2	Conditions That Share Clinical Features with Seizures

Benign paroxysmal vertigo
Breath-holding spell
Cataplexy*
Chills
Choreoathetosis
Dystonia
Infantile torticollis
Masturbation
Migraine
Narcolepsy
Night terrors
Pseudoseizures
Rage attacks
Sandifer's syndrome[†]
Shuddering attacks
Sleepwalking
Spasmus nutans[†]
Syncope
Tics

*Cataplexy is characterized by abrupt attacks of weakness and decreased tone associated with strong emotions.
[†]Sandifer's syndrome is characterized by intermittent torticollis due to gastroesophageal reflux.
[‡]Spasmus nutans is characterized by nodding of the head accompanied by nystagmus.

Clinical Presentation

A few features are particularly helpful in developing a diagnostic and management plan for children who present to the emergency department for evaluation of one or more seizures.

Age

The age of the child determines the initial differential diagnosis (see Table 40–1). For example, simple febrile seizures only occur in children between the ages of 6 months and 5 years.

Fever

The presence of fever also modifies the differential diagnosis. Outside the age group for simple febrile seizures, infectious etiologies increase in likelihood if a fever is present. These infections may include relatively benign conditions such as viral meningitis or life-threatening conditions such as bacterial meningitis or encephalitis (see Chapter 43, Central Nervous System Infections). Fever in a child with a known seizure disorder may suggest an acute infection that has lowered that child's seizure threshold and led to either an increase in seizure frequency or a seizure after a fairly long seizure-free period.

Generalized or Focal Body Movements

Focal refers to a seizure whose initial symptomatology indicates initial activation of only part of one cerebral hemisphere. An example of a focal seizure would be a child who shakes only one arm during the first part of a seizure. In some instances, the seizure may then generalize. *Generalized* refers to a seizure whose initial symptomatology indicates involvement of both cerebral hemispheres. Typically, generalized seizures start with whole body stiffening or shaking. In one study of 500 children with a first-time seizure, those who were younger than 33 months and had a focal seizure were more likely to have an abnormal finding on neuroimaging than other children.[21]

Known Prior History of Seizures

Clinical experience suggests that children with known prior seizures are the most common presenters to the emergency department with a chief complaint of seizure. These children have frequently already had neuroimaging and undergone electroencephalographic studies. They frequently have a pediatric neurologist who either coordinates their seizure care with a primary care pediatrician or manages their seizure disorder primarily. Most of these children are expected to have occasional seizures without apparent provocation. Assessing them for an acute infection may reveal a suspected viral or bacterial infection that has lowered the seizure threshold. One situation unique to these children is "outgrowing" their antiepileptic medications. Eliciting a history that the child has been on the same dose of an antiepileptic drug for a prolonged period during which the child grew can be very helpful. During this time, although the same dose of medication was administered the same way, the child is now larger and heavier. This leads to a smaller dose based on milligrams per kilogram since the kilograms are now greater. These children may also have a ventriculoperitoneal shunt for hydrocephalus that may impact on decision making (see Chapter 42, Conditions Causing Increased Intracranial Pressure). These children may also have vagal nerve stimulators in place. They are often selected for vagal nerve stimulation when they have an exceedingly large number of seizures each day that are not adequately controlled with medications.[22] Vagal nerve stimulators are implanted devices that allow for electrical stimulation of the left vagus nerve. Coordinated care with a pediatric neurologist or pediatric neurosurgeon is typically indicated when these children have uncontrolled seizures.

Postseizure Examination

Physical examination findings may be suggestive of syndromes with increased risk for seizures. A facial vascular nevus (port-wine stain) involving the cutaneous distribution of the ophthalmic division of the trigeminal nerve suggests Sturge-Weber syndrome. Hypomelanotic macules with irregular borders (ash-leaf spots) at birth or erythematous papules distributed over the nose and malar region of the face (adenoma sebaceum) of a child are characteristic of tuberous sclerosis. Multiple hyperpigmented skin macules (café-au-lait spots) becoming prominent at puberty, axillary or inguinal freckling, skin fibromas, and iris hamartomas (Lisch nodules) suggests neurofibromatosis. Iris colobomas in infant girls are suggestive of Acardi's syndrome. A young infant with bruising may have sustained nonaccidental head trauma (see Chapter 119, Physical Abuse and Child Neglect).

If the child awakens following a postictal period and has an abnormal neurologic examination, the likelihood of a benign cause for the seizure decreases. For children with an unremarkable prior neurologic history, the differential diagnosis includes rupture of an intracranial arteriovenous malformation, a stroke, a brain tumor, meningitis, and encephalitis (see Chapter 43, Central Nervous System Infections; Chapter 44, Central Nervous System Vascular Disorders; and Chapter 45, Brain Tumor). In particular, a simple febrile seizure is ruled out by an abnormal postseizure physical examination.

Continuing Seizure Activity

A child in status epilepticus may have frequent seizures without a lucid interval between them or continuous seizure activity. Although making a specific diagnosis is desirable, and a preliminary differential diagnosis guides diagnostic and management decisions, the primary goal during episodes of status epilepticus is to stop the seizure activity.

Important Clinical Features and Considerations

A long and diverse list of diagnoses can mimic seizures in children (see Table 40–2). Breath-holding is a common event occurring in young children (see Chapter 37, Minor Infant Problems). Stiffness may occur as part of an ALTE (see Chapter 28, Apparent Life-Threatening Events). Syncope and the resultant transient ischemia of the brain cortex may lead to brief twitching or stiffening that can be mistaken for a seizure (see Chapter 61, Syncope). Night terrors, events typically occurring in younger children in the middle of the night, manifest as a sudden awakening with screaming, diaphoresis, hyperventilation, dilated pupils, and irrational speech.[23] Depending on the characteristics exhibited by a particular child, parents or prehospital care providers may suspect a seizure as the cause of these events.[24] Sleepwalking may be confused with a complex partial seizure since the child appears to walk around in a trancelike state.[23] Tics are stereotyped, patterned sequences involving nonrhythmic movement of multiple muscles and may be mistaken for seizures.[24] Spasmus nutans affects children between the ages of 4 and 12 months; the characteristic symptoms include a head tilt, head nodding, and asymmetric nystagmus. This condition may be initially assumed to be a seizure, but is a self-limited condition that typically resolves in later childhood. It is exceedingly unlikely that this diagnosis will be made during an emergency department visit.[25,26] Chills associated with fever may be mistaken for seizures. Sandifer's syndrome or gastroesophageal reflux may be confused with tonic seizures since tonic posturing occurs with these conditions.[27]

Pseudoseizures are nonepileptic events resembling epileptic seizures as they both present with paroxysmal, involuntary, time-limited alteration in behavior, motor activity, autonomic function, consciousness, and sensation.[28] Other names that have been used in the past include hysterical epilepsy, hysterical seizures, psychogenic seizures, factitious seizures, functional seizures, conversion fits, pseudo-attacks, paroxysmal somatoform disorder, and pseudo–status epilepticus.[29] There is no epileptogenic pathology or epileptiform electroencephalographic ictal pattern in cases of pseudoseizure. Clinically, children with pseudoseizures have bizarre postures, verbalizations, thrashing movements, reactive pupils, and rigid-appearing posture with "waxy" flexibility, and they lack cyanosis, tongue biting, or injury during the attack, and do not occur during sleep.[24]

Management

There is no standard approach to all pediatric seizures. For many children, particularly those with known seizure disorders or who have experienced an event that is unlikely to be a seizure, care will necessarily need to be individualized. Factors impacting these decisions include a description of the event prompting the emergency department visit, family dynamics, availability of prompt follow-up, and the child's physical examination in the emergency department. Fortunately, management follows the few broad categories into which many of these events fit.

Status Epilepticus

Status epilepticus encompasses a fairly wide range of events, from a single seizure lasting just a bit longer than 30 minutes that has resolved upon presentation to the emergency department to continuous seizure activity in the emergency department. The most concerning are those children who have ongoing seizure activity on presentation, since neurologic morbidity is directly related to the duration of the seizure activity.[30,31] A bedside glucose check may reveal hypoglycemia requiring treatment (see Chapter 106, Hypoglycemia). If hypoglycemia is not the cause of the seizure activity, the administration of a benzodiazepine is the accepted first-line therapy. While intravenous administration is probably best, vascular access is particularly difficult in continuously shaking children. If initial attempts at peripheral venous access are unsuccessful, options include administering rectal diazepam or lorazepam[32,33] (Table 40–3) or obtaining intraosseous access[34] (see Chapter 161, Vascular Access). The intramuscular route is notorious for its variability in absorption and pharmacokinetics and may account for the paucity of prospective studies. The intramuscular route, however, may have a role in the prehospital setting for children with difficult intravenous access, as one study has found that intramuscularly administered midazolam results in more rapid cessation of seizures when compared to intravenous diazepam.[35] Midazolam is also an accepted benzodiazepine for the treatment of status epilepticus.[36] Midazolam has the advantages of a short half-life, faster clearance, and fewer venous complications than seen with other benzodiazepines.[37] A small number of subjects have been studied evaluating the delivery of midazolam through buccal and nasal mucosa for pharmacologic control of seizures in children, and the results have been generally favorable.[38-40] Before widespread use of these routes, more research is probably needed. Adverse effects of benzodiazepines include respiratory depression, hypotension, and impaired consciousness. If successive doses of benzodiazepines are required to stop the seizure activity, it is prudent for the emergency physician to be prepared to promptly manage apnea in these children (see Chapter 3, Rapid Sequence Intubation).

If successive doses of benzodiazepines are ineffective, a second-line agent is indicated.[9] Choices typically include phenytoin and phenobarbital (see Table 40–3). Phenytoin is an efficacious, long-acting agent that has been widely used for more than 30 years in the acute and chronic treatment of seizures in children.[41] It has been used as initial therapy for the termination of status epilepticus and when benzodiazepines fail.[42] Side effects of phenytoin include hypotension, arrhythmias, asystole, and renal and hepatic damage.[41] The manner in which phenytoin is prepared leads to the administration of propylene glycol along with the phenytoin. Because of this, phenytoin should be given no faster than 1 mg/kg per minute (up to 50 mg/min) to avoid cardiac

Table 40-3 Selected Antiepileptic Drugs Used to Treat Pediatric Seizures in the Emergency Department

Drug	Route	Initial Dose	Repeat Dose	Frequency	Maximum Single Dose
Lorazepam	IV	Neonate: 0.05 mg/kg	Same	10–15 min	4 mg
		Child: 0.1 mg/kg	0.05 mg/kg		
		Adolescent: 0.07 mg/kg	Same		
Diazepam	IV	Child: 0.05–0.3 mg/kg	0.05 mg/kg	15–30 min	5 mg (<5 yr old)
					10 mg (>5 yr old)
	PR	Child > 2 yr: 0.5 mg/kg	Same	4–12 hr	Round to nearest 2.5, 5, 10, 15, or 20 mg per dose
		Child 6–11 yr: 0.3 mg/kg			
		>12 yr: 0.2 mg/kg			
Phenytoin	IV	Neonate: 15–20 mg/kg loading dose	None	Once	
		Child: 15–18 mg/kg loading dose			
Fosphenytoin	IV/IM	Child: 10–20 mg/kg of Phenytoin Equivalents	10 mg/kg	Once	
Phenobarbital	IV	Neonate: 15–20 mg/kg	5 mg/kg	Twice	30 mg/kg
		Child: 15–18 mg/kg			

Abbreviations: IM, intramuscularly; IV, intravenously; PR, per rectum.

complications. Phenytoin should not be given intramuscularly as the drug is poorly absorbed and causes hemorrhagic necrosis of the soft tissues at the injection site. Fosphenytoin is a water-soluble prodrug of phenytoin that is rapidly converted to phenytoin by serum phosphatases. Dosages are expressed as phenytoin equivalents, which are the amounts of phenytoin released from the prodrug. The advantages of fosphenytoin include predictable pharmacokinetics via the intramuscular route and faster delivery to therapeutic concentrations without the cardiovascular complications seen with phenytoin, as well as less common phlebitis and soft tissue damage.[34,42] The cost of fosphenytoin compared with phenytoin remains the main disadvantage.[43]

Phenobarbital is a long-acting, potent antiepileptic agent that is typically used to treat status epilepticus after benzodiazepines fail to control the seizures. Phenobarbital has potent respiratory depressant and sedative properties, especially when administered after a benzodiazepine. Phenobarbital remains the standard for the treatment of persistent neonatal seizures after failure of benzodiazepines.[44] Studies have demonstrated that phenobarbital and phenytoin are equivalent but incompletely effective in controlling neonatal seizures.[45,46]

If seizure activity continues despite the administration of a benzodiazepine, phenytoin (or fosphenytoin), and phenobarbital, transfer to a pediatric intensive care unit should be anticipated. For most of these children, endotracheal intubation will be indicated at this point if it has not occurred earlier in the management. A short-acting muscle relaxant or "paralytic" (e.g., succinylcholine) is recommended to allow for the continued monitoring of the patient for seizure activity when electroencephalographic monitoring has not yet been established. Further history may reveal specific toxicologic agents responsible for the ongoing seizures. For example, an inappropriate ingestion of isoniazid may require the administration of pyridoxine to stop the seizure activity. Transfer to a setting in which ongoing electroencephalographic monitoring can be accomplished while the patient is given pentobarbital to the point of suppression of all brain electrical activity (i.e., a "pentobarbital coma") is indicated. Children who reach this point in management typically have a poor neurologic outcome.[47]

Approaches currently under study include the use of propofol and intravenous valproic acid.[34,42,48-50] Further research is needed before these agents can be recommended in the routine management of status epilepticus.

Simple Febrile Seizures

In 1996, the American Academy of Pediatrics created practice parameters for the evaluation of children with simple febrile seizures.[12] Recommendations include that a lumbar puncture be "strongly considered" for the first febrile seizure in infants younger than 12 months, and that a lumbar puncture should be "considered" for infants between 12 and 18 months of age. The American College of Emergency Physicians refined this concept in 2003 and suggested that a lumbar puncture be "strongly considered" in a child younger than 18 months of age who has had a febrile seizure with any of the following features: a history of irritability, decreased feeding, or lethargy; an abnormal appearance or mental status on observation after the postictal period; any physical signs of meningitis, such as a bulging fontanelle; any complex features; a slow postictal recovery of mentation; or pretreatment with antibiotics.[13] If these factors are absent, a lumbar puncture can be safely deferred.[13] In general, a child with a simple febrile seizure is treated no differently that a child of the same age and gender who presents with fever without having had a seizure (see Chapter 33, Urinary Tract Infection). Blood tests and neuroimaging are not indicated for well-appearing children.

First-Time Afebrile Seizures

For children with a normal postictal neurologic examination, the management of a single afebrile seizure in a young child is rather straightforward. In 2000, the American Academy of Neurology, the Child Neurology Society, and the American Epilepsy Society published a practice parameter for first afebrile seizures in children.[16] In general, the ordering of tests should be made on a case-by-case basis. This includes the option of ordering of laboratory tests if dehydration is present. Lumbar puncture should be reserved for those instances in which there is a concern for possible meningitis or encephalitis based on criteria other than a single seizure (see Chapter 43, Central Nervous System Infections).

Toxicologic screening is indicated if an ingestion is suspected. Emergent neuroimaging is only indicated if the postictal physical examination reveals a focal deficit or the child does not return to baseline within several hours after the seizure. The recommended study is magnetic resonance imaging of the brain. Subsequent research supports this selective approach in emergent neuroimaging.[21] The only standard test required is an electroencephalogram, which can be obtained on an outpatient basis.[16]

Neonatal Seizures

The approach to neonatal seizures is similar to that of the approach to a critically ill neonate or an ALTE (see Chapter 7, The Critically Ill Neonate; and Chapter 28, Apparent Life-Threatening Events). If the infant is not in status epilepticus, a "septic workup," including a lumbar puncture with cerebrospinal fluid studies, is indicated (see Chapter 171, Lumbar Puncture). One condition of particular concern is encephalitis due to herpes simplex virus. It is currently controversial whether the administration of intravenous acyclovir should be standard therapy for neonates who undergo a "septic workup." The most effective test for herpes simplex virus is the polymerase chain reaction study performed on cerebrospinal fluid.

Children with a Known Seizure Disorder

These children typically require individualized care. Assessing these children for common infections, including urinary tract infections in those not toilet trained and pneumonia in those who are ventilator dependent, is usually prudent. Taking guidance from experienced parents is a key to successfully managing these cases. If the dosages of the child's antiepileptic medications can be adjusted to achieve therapeutic levels in a reasonable time frame, it is usually prudent to obtain these levels. Adjusting medications in coordination with the child's primary care physician or neurologist may be all that is needed in some instances.

Seizure-like Events

If the event can be confidently diagnosed as something other than a seizure, management is guided by this alternative diagnosis. Well-appearing, active, playful children who have experienced a brief event can often be discharged home with prompt follow-up. An outpatient electroencephalogram may be indicated and can be arranged by the primary care physician.

Summary

Seizures are a common occurrence in pediatrics, with diverse etiologies, multiple diagnostic decisions, and assorted treatment modalities. Determining disposition can be challenging for both physicians and families, particularly when the event does not readily fall into one of the known broad categories of seizures. Factors such as test results, physician judgment, family reliability, and proximity and access to health services are all integral components to the disposition decision. Discharge criteria include return to baseline neurologic status, no focus of serious infection, therapeutic drug levels, and family comfort with caring for the child at home. Close follow-up with the child's pediatrician or neurologist is prudent in many of these cases.

REFERENCES

1. National Library of Medicine and National Institutes of Health: Seizures. *In* Medical Encyclopedia. Available at *http://www.nlm.nih.gov/medlineplus/ency/article/003200.htm* (last accessed August 26, 2006).
2. Gastaut H: Clinical and electroencephalographical classification of epileptic seizures. Epilepsia 11:102–113, 1970.
3. Luders H, Acharya J, Bumgartner C, et al: Seminologic seizure classification. Epilepsia 39:1006–1013, 1998.
4. Commission on Classification and Terminology of the International League Against Epilepsy: Proposal for revised clinical and electroencephalographic classification of epileptic seizures. Epilepsia 22:489–501, 1981.
5. Commission on Classification and Terminology of the International League Against Epilepsy: Proposal for revised clinical and electroencephalographic classification of epileptic seizures. Epilepsia 22:489–501, 1989.
6. Commission on Epidemiology and Prognosis, International League Against Epilepsy: Guidelines for epidemiologic studies of epilepsy. Epilepsia 34:592–596, 1993.
7. Shinnar S, Pellock JM: Update on the epidemiology and prognosis of pediatric epilepsy. J Child Neurol 17:S4–S17, 2002.
8. Anderson DM, Novak PD, Keith J, et al: Dorland's Illustrated Medical Dictionary, 30th ed. Philadelphia: WB Saunders, 2003, p 1756.
*9. Lewena S, Young S: When benzodiazepines fail: how effective is second line therapy for status epilepticus in children? Emerg Med Australas 18:45–50, 2006.
*10. Chin RFM, Neville BGR, Peckham C, et al: Incidence, cause, and short-term outcome of convulsive status epilepticus in childhood: prospective population based study. Lancet 368:222–229, 2006.
11. Asadi-Pooya AA, Poordast A: Etiologies and outcomes of status epilepticus in children. Epilepsy Behav 7:502–505, 2005.
12. American Academy of Pediatrics Provisional Committee on Quality Improvement, Subcommittee on Febrile Seizures: Practice parameter: the neurodiagnostic evaluation of the child with first simple febrile seizure. Pediatrics 97:769–775, 1996.
13. Warden CR, Zibulewsky J, Mace S, et al: Evaluation and management of febrile seizures in the out-of-hospital and emergency department settings. Ann Emerg Med 41:215–222, 2003.
14. Nelson KB, Ellenberg JH: Predictors of epilepsy in children who have experienced febrile seizures. N Engl J Med 295:1029–1033, 1976.
15. Scheffer IE, Berkovic SF: Generalized epilepsy with febrile seizures plus: a genetic disorder with heterogeneous clinical phenotypes. Brain 120:479–490, 1997.
16. Hirtz D, Ashwal S, Berg A, et al: Practice parameter: evaluating a first nonfebrile seizure in children. Report of the Quality Standards Subcommittee of the American Academy of Neurology, The Child Neurology Society, and The American Epilepsy Society. Neurology 55:616–623, 2000.
17. Mizrahi EM, Kellaway P: Characterization and classification of neonatal seizures. Neurology 37:1837–1844, 1987.
18. Scher MS: Neonatal seizure classification: a fetal perspective concerning childhood epilepsy. Epilepsy Res 70S:S41–S57, 2006.
19. Bui TT, Delgado CA, Simon HK: Infant seizures not so infantile: first-time seizures in children under six months of age presenting to the ED. Am J Emerg Med 20:518–520, 2002.
20. Davies F, Gupta R: Apparent life threatening events in infants presenting to an emergency department. Emerg Med J 19:11–16, 2002.
*21. Sharma S, Riviello JJ, Harper MB, et al: The role of emergent neuroimaging in children with new-onset afebrile seizures. Pediatrics 111:1–5, 2003.
22. Patwardhan RV, Stong B, Bebin EM, et al: Efficacy of vagal nerve stimulation in children with medically refractory epilepsy. Neurosurgery 47:1353–1358, 2000.
23. Derry CP, Davey M, Johns M, et al: Distinguishing sleep disorders from seizures: diagnosing bumps in the night. Arch Neurol 63:705–709, 2006.
24. Vining EP: Pediatric seizures. Emerg Med Clin North Am 12:973–988, 1994.
25. Gottlob I, Wizov SS, Reinecke RD: Spasmus nutans: a long-term follow-up. Invest Ophthalmol Vis Sci 36:2768–2771, 1995.
26. Aung T, Yap SK, Yap EY, et al: Spasmus nutans. Ann Acad Med Singapore 25:596–598, 1996.

*Selected readings.

27. Bray PF, Herbst JJ, Johnson DG, et al: Childhood esophageal reflux: neurologic and psychiatric syndromes mimicked. JAMA 237:1342, 1977.

28. LaFrance WC Jr, Devinsky O: The treatment of nonepileptic seizures: historical perspectives and future directions. Epilepsia 45(Suppl 2):15–21, 2004.

29. Wood BL, Haque S, Weinstock A, et al: Pediatric stress related seizures: conceptualization, evaluation, and treatment of nonepileptic seizures in children and adolescents. Curr Opin Pediatr 16:523–531, 2004.

30. Hauser WA: Status epilepticus: epidemiologic considerations. Neurology 40(Suppl 2):9–13, 1990.

31. DeLorenzo RJ, Towne AR, Pellock JM, et al: Status epilepticus in children, adults, and the elderly. Epilepsia 33:S15–S25, 1992.

32. Appleton R, Sweeney A, Choonara I, et al: Lorazepam versus diazepam in the acute treatment of epileptic seizures and status epilepticus. Dev Med Child Neurol 37:682–688, 1995.

33. Graves NM, Kriel RL: Rectal administration of antiepileptic drugs in children. Pediatr Neurol 3:321–326, 1987.

34. Hanhan US, Fiallos MR, Orlowski JP: Status epilepticus. Pediatr Clin North Am 48:683–694, 2001.

35. Chamberlain JM, Altieri MA, Futterman C, et al: A prospective, randomized study comparing intramuscular midazolam with intravenous diazepam for the treatment of seizures in children. Pediatr Emerg Care 13:92–94, 1997.

36. Singhi S, Murthy A, Singhi P, et al: Continuous midazolam versus diazepam infusion for refractory convulsive status epilepticus. J Child Neurol 17:106–110, 2002.

37. Pellock JM: Use of midazolam for refractory status epilepticus in pediatric patients. J Child Neurol 13:581–587, 1998.

38. Fisgin T, Gurer Y, Tezic T, et al: Effects of intranasal midazolam and rectal diazepam on acute convulsions in children: prospective randomized study. J Child Neurol 17:123–126, 2002.

39. Mahmoudian T, Zadeh NM: Comparison of intranasal midazolam with intravenous diazepam for treating acute seizures in children. Epilepsy Behav 5:253–255, 2004.

40. Kutlu NO, Dogrul M, Yakinci C: Buccal midazolam for treatment of prolonged seizures in children. Brain Dev 25:275–278, 2003.

41. Wheless JW: Pediatric use of intravenous and intramuscular phenytoin: lessons learned. J Child Neurol 13(Suppl 1):S11–S14, 1998.

42. Lowenstein DH, Alldredge BK: Status epilepticus. N Engl J Med 338: 970–976, 1998.

43. Rudis MI, Touchette DR, Swadron SP, et al: Cost-effectiveness of oral phenytoin, intravenous phenytoin, and intravenous fosphenytoin in the emergency department. Ann Emerg Med 43:386–397, 2004.

44. Zupanc ML: Neonatal seizures. Pediatr Clin North Am 51:961–978, 2004.

45. Painter MJ, Scher MS, Stein AD, et al: Phenobarbital compared with phenytoin for the treatment of neonatal seizures. N Engl J Med 341:485–489, 1999.

46. Booth D, Evans DJ: Anticonvulsants for neonates with seizures. Cochrane Database Syst Rev (4):CD004218, 2004.

47. Kim SJ, Lee DY, Kim JS: Neurologic outcomes of pediatric epileptic patients with pentobarbital coma. Pediatr Neurol 25:217–220, 2001.

48. Yamamoto LG, Yim GK: The role of intravenous valproic acid in status epilepticus. Pediatr Emerg Care 16:296–298, 2000.

49. Yu KT, Mills S, Thompson N, et al: Intravenous valproate for pediatric status epilepticus. Epilepsia 44:724–726, 2003.

50. Hodges BM, Mazur JE: Intravenous valproate in status epilepticus. Ann Pharmacother 35:1465–1470, 2001.

Chapter 41

Headaches

Tommy Y. Kim, MD and Tonya M. Thompson, MD

Key Points

Pediatric headaches are often a part of a constellation of symptoms and are usually benign.

The key to the diagnosis of migraine headaches is the presence of associated disability.

Loss of previously acquired developmental milestones is concerning for a secondary cause of pediatric headaches.

Laboratory and imaging studies are rarely needed in the emergency department evaluation of pediatric headaches.

Most headaches are managed with nonsteroidal anti-inflammatory medications.

Introduction and Background

Headache is a common complaint encountered in the pediatric emergency department, accounting for approximately 1% of all visits.[1,2] The emergency medicine physician's role in the management of pediatric headaches is to rule out organic causes of headache, manage headache symptoms, and, when appropriate, give reassurance. It is helpful to categorize headaches according to standardized terminology. This permits clearer communication between the emergency physician and the child's neurologist or primary care pediatrician. Appropriate classification allows for the selection of treatment with the highest likelihood of success. Fortunately, most children with headaches who present to the emergency department harbor benign conditions, and their headaches are a part of a constellation of symptoms associated with minor viral illnesses.[1,2]

Recognition and Approach

Confusingly, there are two overlapping categorization schemes for headaches. One scheme is based on whether or not there is an identifiable cause for the headache. In this scheme, headaches for which a "cause" cannot be identified are termed *primary*. An example of a primary headache would be a classic migraine headache. Headaches for which a "cause" can be identified are termed *secondary*. Examples of secondary headaches include those due to brain tumors, meningitis, a subdural hematoma, or fever. A key task for emergency physicians is identifying secondary headaches. The other classification scheme is based on the temporal pattern of the headaches. This scheme consists of five general types of headaches: acute, acute recurrent, chronic progressive, chronic nonprogressive, and mixed. The overlap in these two schemes leads to dual designations applying to a single child. Primary headaches are usually either acute recurrent or chronic nonprogressive headaches. New-onset acute headaches are usually secondary headaches. Accurate classification of pediatric headaches can be difficult or impossible in a single emergency department visit.

Clinical Presentation

Acute Headaches

Acute headaches are usually a manifestation of a secondary illness (Table 41–1). The causes are diverse. The evaluation is guided by the dominant clinical features.

Acute Recurrent Headaches

The most common acute recurrent headaches are migraine headaches, migraine variants, tension headaches, and cluster headaches.

Migraine Headaches

Migraines and migraine variants are increasingly recognized as conditions of childhood.[3] Migraine headaches can be further subdivied into those without aura and those with aura (Table 41–2). Migraine headaches without auras are probably underdiagnosed and underappreciated in children. The prevalence of migraine headaches increases with age.[4,5] At a younger age, migraines are more prevalent in boys, but in adolescence girls are more likely to suffer from migraine headaches. Girls are less likely to have auras than boys. Children younger than 15 years do not usually have associated aura. Headache attacks in children can be variable, and attacks can last less than an hour.[6] Without appropriate treatment, central sensitization may occur and lead to chronic daily headaches. Migraine headaches with auras can be associated with transient focal deficits prior to or during the onset of the headache. Transient focal deficits can be visual, motor,

Table 41–1	Secondary Causes of Acute Headaches

Systemic illness or inflammatory process
  Systemic lupus erythematosus
  Meningitis and encephalitis
  Epstein-Barr virus infection
  Fever
Trauma and posttraumatic headache
Intracranial hemorrhage
Subarachnoid hemorrhage
Increased intracranial pressure
Hypoxia
Dental problems
  Caries or abscess
  Cracked tooth syndrome
  Temporomandibular joint pain
  Phantom tooth pain
Exertional headaches
Endocrine causes
  Hyperparathyroidism
  Hypoglycemia
  Hyperprolactinemia
Otitis media and sinusitis
Pharyngitis
Ocular disorders
  Phantom eye pain
  Optic neuritis
  Orbital myositis
  Eye strain
  Narrow-angle glaucoma
Substance abuse
  Cocaine
  Methamphetamines
  Marijuana
  Caffeine
Toxicology
  Carbon monoxide
  Lead
Diet
  Nitrates
  Monosodium gluconate
  Ice cream headaches

or sensory. Visual deficits can consist of scotomas, fortification, visual field deficits, and photopsia. Motor deficits can consist of weakness and ataxia, and sensory deficits can consist of parethesias.

There are three specific types of migraine headaches with characteristic and dramatic features: hemiplegic, basilar-type, and confusional migraines. Hemiplegic migraines have an initial phase of transient focal deficits, including hemisensory deficits, visual field deficits, and speech disturbances.[7] Deficits usually precede the headaches but may continue even after the onset of headache. Hemiplegic migraines may have a genetic basis.[8] Basilar-type migraines are present in about 15% of all migraines, and the age of onset is usually 7 years. There is usually an associated dizziness and vertigo that lasts from 5 to 60 minutes and is followed by an occipital headache. Other initial symptoms can include nausea, vomiting, ataxia, tinnitus, diplopia, weakness, confusion, and visual defects. It is advisable to obtain magnetic resonance imaging (MRI) of the brain and magnetic resonance angiography to rule out a posterior fossa tumor or compromise of the basilar circulation. Confusional migraines are associated with acute confusional or delirium states and also with transient global amnesia of childhood. Agitation, disorientation, dysarthria, and dysphasia are common during an attack, but the headache phase may be mild. Confusional migraines are often triggered by trauma, so a computed tomographic (CT) scanning of the head is indicated (see Chapter 17, Head Trauma).

Migraine Variants

Other childhood syndromes associated with headaches include benign paroxysmal vertigo, cyclic vomiting syndrome, and abdominal migraine. These syndromes are usually a diagnosis of exclusion. Benign paroxysmal vertigo typically occurs in toddlers.[9] This form of vertigo is characterized by abrupt attacks of ataxia and vomiting without a loss of consciousness. The spells last minutes and can occur in clusters. The differential diagnosis includes epilepsy, posterior fossa tumors, Meniere's disease, positional vertigo, and vestibular neuronitis.

Table 41–2	International Headache Society Diagnostic Criteria for Migraines

Migraine Without Aura	Migraine With Aura
At least 5 attacks of headache lasting 4–72 hr* **PLUS** At least 2 of the following: Unilateral location Pulsating quality Moderate or severe pain intensity Aggravation by or causing avoidance of routine physical activity **AND** During headache at least 1 of the following: Nausea and/or vomiting Photophobia and phonophobia (may be inferred from behavior)	At least 2 attacks of headache **PLUS** Aura consisting of at least 1 of the following: Fully reversible visual symptoms Fully reversible sensory symptoms Fully reversible dysphasic disturbance **AND** At least 2 of the following: Homonymous visual symptoms and/or unilateral symptoms Aura symptom develops over ≥ 5 min Each symptom last ≥ 5 min and ≤ 60 min **AND** Headache fulfilling criteria for migraine without aura that begins during the aura or follows within 60 min

*Attacks in children last from 1 to 72 hours.
Adapted from the Headache Classification Committee of the International Headache Society.[48]

Cyclic vomiting syndrome is associated with recurrent episodes of intense but otherwise unexplained nausea and vomiting.[3] These episodes can last 1 hour to 5 days in children. Vomiting occurs at least 4 times in an hour, but can be as high as 13 times per hour. The age of onset of symptoms is around 5 years, and most children have resolution of symptoms by 10 years of age. Only 40% of children with cyclic vomiting syndrome will complain of headaches. Since vomiting is common in childhood, these children may undergo extensive gastrointestinal testing prior to the diagnosis being made.

Abdominal migraines were first described by Symon and Russell in 1986.[10] Abdominal migraines are estimated to have a prevalence of approximately 4% in children.[11] The abdominal pain is severe enough to interfere with normal daily activities and can last from 1 to 72 hours. The pain is usually described as midline, periumbilical, dull, and colicky. The diagnosis of abdominal migraine requires at least two of the following four symptoms: anorexia, nausea, vomiting, and pallor. Between attacks of abdominal pain, there is complete resolution of symptoms. There is no requirement for headache to make the diagnosis of abdominal migraine.

Tension Headaches

Tension headaches are characterized by their intermittent nature and the absence of nausea or vomiting. Episodic tension headaches are further divided into frequent and infrequent types (Table 41–3). Tension headaches are the most frequent type of headache encountered. Most data regarding tension headaches are extrapolated from the adult literature. Tension headaches can have an onset during adolescence with a slight female predominance. Unlike migraines (which are based on positive features), the diagnosis of tension headaches is predominantly based on the absence of certain clinical features. To appropriately make the diagnosis, the headache must lack photophobia, phonophobia, nausea, and vomiting, and must not worsen with activity. The pain is often described as vicelike or a squeezing steady pain and is often associated with neck or upper back pain.

Tension headaches are more common during the week and usually begin during the daytime, with gradual progression through the course of the day. The headaches may be precipitated by stress, lack of sleep, poor posture, or "stress letdown" (e.g., following an important examination in school).

Cluster Headaches

Cluster headaches are very rare in children (Table 41–4). Although the peak age of onset is 20 to 50 years, cluster headaches may occur during adolescence. These headaches affect less than 1% of the population and have a male predominance. The pain is unilateral, severe, and located either retro-orbitally, periorbitally, or frontally. The intensity peaks about 5 minutes after the onset of pain. The key to the diagnosis is the presence of associated unilateral autonomic features such as lacrimation, nasal congestion, and conjunctival injection that occur in a predictable time cycle. Because the headache is most likely to occur during periods of relaxation rather than intense activity, most patients prefer to be moving during the headache episode and may pace the examination room. The headache episodes may be clustered into time blocks lasting from 6 to 8 weeks in duration and are more common during the spring and fall. The headaches may regularly awaken the patient at the same time each night.

Chronic Progressive Headaches

Chronic progressive headaches usually have an organic etiology. The most common causes of chronic progressive headaches include idiopathic intracranial hypertension (formerly known as pseudotumor cerebri), tumors, masses, and intracranial abscesses. Idiopathic intracranial hypertension presents with a chronic, progressive headache with or without associated vomiting. The headache can manifests with transient visual obscuration and palsy of the sixth cranial nerve. There is a slight female predominance, with risk factors including obesity, hyperthyroidism, hypoparathyroidism, hypervitaminosis A, and tetracycline use. The exact cause is unknown, but etiologic factors could include cerebral edema, high cerebral fluid outflow resistance, and high cerebral venous pressure.

Tumors, masses, and abscesses have a more insidious onset and are frequently associated with vomiting. Neurologic

Table 41–3	International Headache Society Diagnostic Criteria for Tension Headaches

Infrequent episodic—at least 10 episodes occurring on <1 day/mo on average (<12 days/yr)
OR
Frequent episodic—at least 10 episodes occurring on ≥1 but <15 days/mo for at least 3 mo (≥12 and < 180 days/yr)
PLUS
Headache lasting from 30 min to 7 days
AND
At least 2 of the following characteristics:
  Bilateral location
  Pressing or tightening quality
  Mild or moderate intensity
  Not aggravated by routine physical activity
AND
Both of the following:
  No nausea or vomiting
  No more than one of photophobia or phonophobia

Adapted from the Headache Classification Committee of the International Headache Society.[48]

Table 41–4	International Headache Society Diagnostic Criteria for Cluster Headaches

At least 5 attacks with a frequency of one every other day to 8/day
PLUS
Severe or very severe unilateral orbital, supraorbital, and/or temporal pain lasting 15–180 min if untreated
AND
Headache accompanied by at least one of the following:
  Ipsilateral conjunctival injection and/or lacrimation
  Ipsilateral nasal congestion and/or rhinorrhea
  Ipsilateral eyelid edema
  Ipsilateral forehead and facial sweating
  Ipsilateral miosis and/or ptosis
  A sense of restlessness or agitation

Adapted from the Headache Classification Committee of the International Headache Society.[48]

signs and symptoms may include gait abnormalities, vision changes, and behavioral problems. The headaches may initially be rather mild, but progressively worsen. A history of polydipsia and polyuria suggests a craniopharyngioma. The physical examination may be normal in the early phase of the illness. Classically, a mass above the tentorium is associated with a frontal headache, a mass below the tentorium is associated with a neck or occipital headache, and with a chiasmal mass the pain is referred to the vertex. The location of the headache correlates with the tumor site only about one third of the time.

Chronic Nonprogressive Headaches

Chronic nonprogressive headaches occur daily to almost daily without associated neurologic symptoms. These can be difficult and frustrating to manage. The headache generally lasts approximately 4 hours and occurs greater than 15 days per month. Comorbidities include depression, anxiety, panic disorders, and psychopathologic sleep disturbances.

Characteristic chronic nonprogressive headaches include medication rebound headaches and caffeine-induced headaches. Rebound headaches occur in patients with preexisting headaches.[12,13] These are self-sustaining and predictable. Eighty percent of patients are using acute agents daily.[14] Refractory headaches are, by definition, refractory to otherwise appropriate symptomatic and preventative treatments. Medication withdrawal results in escalation of headache intensity. Another type of recurrent nonprogressive headache is caffeine-induced headaches. Caffeine has been used to treat headaches and is included in over-the-counter migraine preparations, but the overconsumption of caffeine can lead to chronic headaches. Consumption of cola drinks is a prominent and common risk factor. In a study of 36 children and adolescents with caffeine-induced headaches, the average consumption of caffeine was found to be 1.5 L of cola drinks per day. With the gradual withdrawal of caffeine, sustained resolution of the headaches is likely.[15]

Mixed Headaches

Mixed headaches exhibit features of more than one type of headache. The heterogeneity of these cases makes research very difficult and leaves us without a generalizable evaluation and management plan for these children. Coordinated care with the patient's primary physician or pediatric neurologist is prudent.

Emergency Department Evaluation

The first and most important step in the evaluation of headaches is obtaining an appropriately directed history and physical examination. Family history of headaches or a previous history of similar headache suggests a primary headache disorder. A history of recent trauma alters the differential diagnosis and increases the likelihood of an intracranial injury being present. The location, quality, intensity, duration, and associated symptoms help classify headaches. Provoking and relieving factors, including response to medications, are useful for assessing the severity of the child's condition. A loss of previously acquired milestones or failure to achieve developmental milestones is concerning for a secondary cause of headache.

The physical examination provides further clues to the etiology of headaches. Identifying fever supports a secondary cause for the headache. Unless the child has known confusional migraines, abnormal mental status suggests a secondary cause. A focused and detailed neurologic examination has a high sensitivity for intracranial pathology. In children with brain tumors, up to 98% of neurologic abnormalities are found on a focused examination of mental status, coordination, deep tendon reflexes, sensation, motor function, and examination of the eyes.[16] The skin may reveal characteristic findings such as petechiae associated with meningococcemia, café-au-lait spots associated with neurofibromatosis I, or ash-leaf spots associated with tuberous sclerosis.

No standard set of laboratory tests is indicated when a child presents to the emergency department complaining of headache. In general, laboratory tests are selected to confirm or rule out suspected diagnoses in cases of secondary headaches. No routine laboratory tests have been shown to be of clinical use in the evaluation of headache.[17,18]

Most children with headaches do not require neuroimaging during their emergency department visit. The indications for neuroimaging are few (Table 41–5). In the limited studies in children with headaches, there is a low incidence of positive findings on neuroimaging in those children who had a normal physical examination.[19-24] In an acute situation, CT scanning of the head is the preferred imaging modality to evaluate for intracranial bleeds or brain edema. Brain MRI is preferred for the evaluation of a brain tumor or if an abnormality in the posterior fossa or brainstem is suspected.

Lumbar puncture (LP) is useful for the evaluation of suspected meningitis, subarachnoid hemorrhage, or idiopathic intracranial hypertension (see Chapter 171, Lumbar Puncture). Previously, for children with a closed anterior fontanelle, a head CT prior to LP was recommended. It is currently thought that the physical examination is more sensitive in detecting impending herniation that a CT scan.[25] The American College of Emergency Physicians has recommended that a head CT be performed prior to LP only if papilledema, altered mental status, a focal finding on neurologic examination, or a clinical impression of impending herniation is present.[26] Although relatively rare in children, a post-LP headache may arise. This risk can be minimized by using the smallest needle possible, inserting the needle such that the bevel is perpendicular to the longitudinal fibers of the dura,

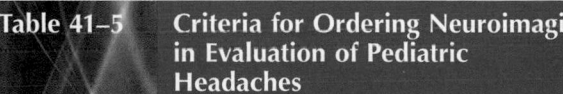

Table 41–5	Criteria for Ordering Neuroimaging in Evaluation of Pediatric Headaches

Suspicion of intracranial hemorrhage or infarct
Stroke evolution
Acute signs of increased ICP
Blunt head trauma with signs of increased ICP
Penetrating head injury
Suspected skull fracture
Suspicion of mass lesion
First or worst headache of life
Altered mental status
New symptom complex
Abnormal neurologic examination

Abbreviation: ICP, intracranial pressure.

and replacing the stylet before withdrawing the needle from the patient.[19] Prophylactic bed rest following LP is of no benefit.[27]

Important Clinical Features and Considerations

A potential pitfall to avoid in the emergency department is confusing a tension headache with a tumor, pseudotumor cerebri, or hydrocephalus. Certain "red flags," if present, may alert the emergency physician to a higher likelihood of a serious secondary cause being present (Table 41–6). In particular, headaches occurring upon awakening in the morning are associated with brain tumors (see Chapter 45, Brain Tumor). Headaches that occur simultaneously in multiple family members suggest carbon monoxide exposure.

Management

Most headaches in children are treated symptomatically by parents and primary caregivers, usually with acetaminophen or ibuprofen. By the time the child presents to the emergency department, most outpatient therapies have failed and parents have a fear of a more serious underlying disorder. Once secondary causes of the headache have been excluded, the role of the emergency physician is to provide reassurance about the benign nature of the headache and to treat the acute attack.

The first-line therapy in pharmacologic management of migraine headaches is oral analgesics. Acetaminophen, ibuprofen, naproxen, and ketorolac are the most commonly used oral analgesics. Appropriate doses of ibuprofen (10 mg/kg) or acetaminophen (15 mg/kg) have been found to be more effective in relieving migraine headaches in children when compared to placebo, and ibuprofen was twice as likely to abort migraines compared to acetaminophen.[28] In the presence of nausea and vomiting, ketorolac (Toradol), a nonsteroidal

anti-inflammatory agent, is available for use either intramuscularly or intravenously (IV).

The antiemetics prochlorperazine, droperidol, and metaclopramide have also been recommended for use in the management of migraine headaches due to their dopaminergic effects. These agents not only provide relief of nausea and vomiting but also have been found to provide headache relief.[29-31] Unfortunately, the side effect profile includes the potential for extrapyramidal reactions.

Most data on the pediatric emergency management of headaches are largely based on adult studies. The only study to evaluate the emergency department management of pediatric migraine compares the use of IV ketorolac with IV prochlorperazine.[32] After 60 minutes, 55% of those receiving ketorolac and 85% of those receiving prochlorperazine had improvement of their headaches, as shown by a reduction in a Nine Faces Pain Scale score. Both treatment groups were discharged with naproxen, and both groups had an approximately 30% recurrence rate at telephone follow-up.

Other drugs, such as butalbitols and isometheptene, have limited use in the management of childhood migraines. Butalbitols (Fiorinal, Fioricet, and Esgic) are very addictive and have the potential for analgesic rebound. No single trial indicates that these are effective in treating migraine headaches,[33] and some feel that it should be banned.[34] There is also no evidence that isometheptene (Midrin) has use in the management of childhood migraines.

Triptans (serotonin receptor agonists) are gaining increased use in the management of pediatric migraines. Oral sumatriptan has been shown to be effective in the treatment of adult migraines,[35] but has not been shown to be useful in children.[36] However, sumatriptan nasal spray has been shown to be effective in treating migraine headaches in adolescents and children and has been used by pediatric neurologists down to the age of 5 years with no reported morbidity or mortality.[37-40] Subcutaneous sumatriptan showed a reduction in headache severity in 78% of pediatric patients from a pediatric neurology clinic.[41] Other oral triptans, including zolmitriptan, naratriptan, rizatriptan, and almotriptan, are not currently approved by the Food and Drug Administration for use in children. Studies on rizatriptan have not shown any significant improvement compared to placebo in adolescents.[42]

The side effects of triptans are usually transient and consist of flushing, chest tightness or pain, tingling, abdominal discomfort, neck pain, metallic taste in the mouth, and a feeling of heaviness. These side effects are often better tolerated in children than adults. Although there is a fear of rare cardiac complications, no cardiac events have been reported in children. Patients develop a tolerance to the side effects with time. The use of triptans should be avoided with hemiplegic migraines, basilar artery migraine, hypertension, congenital heart disease, or pregnancy. Multiple types and routes are available and are chosen based on the side effect profile.

Narcotics are indicated when abortive treatment fails. It is important to avoid narcotics in the presence of chronic abuse, and they are contraindicated with pregnancy, breastfeeding, or allergy. When using narcotics for rescue, it is best to use long-acting agents with appropriate dosing. The key for any analgesic use is to give the maximum allowable

Table 41–6	**Red Flags and Comfort Signs in Evaluation of Headaches**
Red Flags in Headache	**Comfort Signs in Headache**
New severe headache	Stable pattern
First or worse headache ever	Long-standing headache history
Headache when less than 5 yr of age	Family history of similar headaches
Fundamental change in headache pattern	Normal physical examination
Headache with fever or stiff neck	Consistently triggered by Hormonal cycles Specific foods Specific sensory inputs Lights/glare, odors, or weather changes
Headache with neurologic signs or symptoms	
Headache with nocturnal awakening	
Worsening headache over time	
History of trauma	
History of cancer or immunosuppression	

dose, give it early (within 30 minutes), make prescriptions available for school use, and save narcotics for use as a last resort.

Prophylaxis is not the purview of emergency medicine, but clinicians should keep the following in mind. It is generally recommended in the presence of more than three headaches a month. Less than 30% of patients with headaches need daily prophylactic medications.[43] Prophylaxis demonstrates an improvement in headache frequency and severity in up to 89% of patients.[44] Commonly used agents are periactin and tricyclic antidepressants in children less than 12 years of age. The most common tricyclic antidepressant used is amitriptyline. Adolescents are given propranolol, calcium channel blockers, anticonvulsants (e.g., valproate, topiramate, gabapentin), or selective serotonin reuptake inhibitors. The majority of young headache patients, including those with migraines, are managed with as-needed analgesics plus or minus antiemetics.[2]

Cluster headaches and tension headaches are managed similarly to migraine headaches. With cluster headaches, oral therapy is not indicated due to the rapidity of the headache. Intramuscular sumatriptan and inhaled high-flow oxygen are given for the acute management of cluster headaches. Tension headaches usually respond well to first-line oral analgesics as described for the treatment of migraines. With chronic tension headaches, it is helpful to identify "stressors" and make lifestyle changes as needed. For refractory tension headaches, treatment can include central-acting muscle relaxants or benzodiazepines.

Nonpharmacologic strategies for management of chronic headaches include behavioral therapy,[45] such as stress management, relaxation programs,[46] cognitive control, and biofeedback. These measures have been shown to reduce headache frequency by as much as 80% to 85%.[47] If children are missing more than 15 days of school because of headaches, psychological evaluation for stress, social, or psychological disorders should be considered.

Education for the family is paramount at the disposition of the child from the emergency department. It is important to keep a headache diary, follow a regular schedule, not skip meals (especially breakfast), avoid caffeinated beverages, and get 8 hours of sleep a night. Patients should have good follow-up with their primary care physician when dealing with chronic headaches. The parents should initiate nonpharmacologic strategies and give the maximum allowable dosage of medication at the earliest sign of headaches. They should be advised to limit the use of over-the-counter medications to no more than 2 days per week. If there is more frequent use, then prophylaxis should be considered with the primary care physician or a subspecialist.

Summary

Most headaches in children are benign unless red flags are involved. Most are quick in onset and short in duration. Most headaches respond to analgesics with or without antiemetics. If a child can get to sleep, most benign headaches are relieved. Pediatric migraine is real and often underdiagnosed. Treatment includes using medications quickly and using the maximum allowable dosage based on the patient's age and weight. Nonpharmacologic measures should be employed in conjunction with medications whenever possible. The emergency physician should refer the patient or involve subspecialists in nonresponders or in red flag cases.

REFERENCES

1. Burton LJ, Quinn B, Pratt-Cheney JL, et al: Headache etiology in the pediatric emergency department. Pediatr Emerg Care 13:1–4, 1997.
2. Kan L, Nagelberg J, Maytal J: Headaches in the pediatric emergency department: etiology, imaging, and treatment. Headache 40:25–29, 2000.
3. Lipton RB, Bigal ME, Steiner TJ, et al: Classification of primary headaches. Neurology 63:427–435, 2004.
4. Lipton RB, Silberstein SD, Stewart WF: An update on the epidemiology of migraine. Headache 34:319–328, 1994.
5. Stewart WF, Linet MS, Celentano DD, et al: Age and specific incidence rates of migraine with and without visual aura. Am J Epidemiol 34:1111–1120, 1991.
6. Abu-Arafeh I, Callaghan M: Short migraine attacks of less than 2 hours duration in children and adolescents. Cephalalgia 24:333–338, 2004.
7. Ducros A, Denier C, Joutel A, et al: The clinical spectrum of familial hemiplegic migraine associated with mutations in a neuronal calcium channel. N Engl J Med 345:17–24, 2001.
8. May A, Ophoff RA, Terwindt GM, et al: Familial hemiplegic migraine locus on chromosome 19p13 is involved in the common forms of migraine with and without aura. Hum Genet 96:604–608, 1995.
9. Drigo P, Carli G, Laverda AM: Benign paroxysmal vertigo of childhood. Brain Dev 23:38–41, 2001.
10. Symon DNK, Russell G: Abdominal migraine: a syndrome defined. Cephalgia 6:223–228, 1986.
11. Abu-Arafeh I, Russel G: Prevalence and clinical features of abdominal migraine compared with those of migraine headache. Arch Dis Child 72: 413–417, 1995.
12. Hering-Hanit R, Gadoth N, Cohen A, et al: Successful withdrawal from analgesic abuse in a group of youngsters with chronic daily headache. J Child Neurol 16:448–449, 2001.
13. Mathew NT: Drug induced headache. Neurol Clin 8:903–912, 1990.
14. Zed PJ, Loewen PS, Robinson G: Medication induced headache: overview and systemic review of therapeutic approaches. Ann Pharmacother 33:61–72, 1999.
15. Hering-Hanit R, Gadoth N: Caffeine-induced headache in children and adolescents. Cephalgia 23:332–335, 2003.
16. The Childhood Brain Tumor Consortium: The epidemiology of headache among children with brain tumor. J Neurooncol 10:31–46, 1991.
*17. Lewis DW, Ashwal S, Dahl G, et al: Practice parameter: evaluation of children and adolescent with recurrent headaches. Report of the Quality Standards Subcommittee of the American Academy of Neurology and the Practice Committee of the Child Neurology Society. Neurology 59:490–498, 2002.
18. Sugarman JM, Rodgers GC, Paul RI: Utility of toxicologic screening in pediatric emergency department. Pediatr Emerg Care 13:194–197, 1997.
19. Chu ML, Shinnar S: Headaches in children younger than 7 years of age. Arch Neurol 49:79–82, 1992.
20. Dooley JM, Camfield PR, O'Neill M, et al: The value of CT scans for children with headaches. Can J Neurol Sci 17:309–310, 1990.
21. Lewis DW, Dorbad D: The utility of neuroimaging in the evaluation of children with migraine or chronic daily headache who have normal neurological examinations. Headache 40:629–632, 2000.
22. Maytal J, Bienkowski RS, Patel M, et al: The value of brain imaging in children with headaches. Pediatrics 96:413–416, 1995.
23. Medina LS, Pinter JD, Zurakowski D, et al: Children with headache: clinical predictors of the surgical space-occupying lesions and the role of neuroimaging. Radiology 202:819–824, 1997.
24. Wober-Bingol C, Wober C, Prayer D, et al: Magnetic resonance imaging for recurrent headache in childhood and adolescence. Headache 36:83–90, 1996.
25. Gopal AK, Whitehouse JD, Simel DL, et al: Cranial computed tomography before lumbar puncture: a prospective clinical evaluation. Arch Intern Med 159:2681–2685, 1999.
26. American College of Emergency Physicians: Clinical policy: critical issues in the evaluation and management of patients presenting to the

*Selected readings.

emergency department with acute headache. Ann Emerg Med 39:108–122, 2002.

*27. Ebinger F, Kosel C, Pietz J, et al: Strict bed rest following lumbar puncture in children and adolescents is of no benefit. Neurology 62:1003–1005, 2004.

*28. Hamlainen ML, Hoppu K, Valkeila E, et al: Ibuprofen or acetaminophen for the acute treatment of migraine in children: a double-blind, randomized, placebo-controlled, crossover study. Neurology 48:103–107, 1997.

29. Kabbouche MA, Vockell AB, LeCates SL, et al: Tolerability and effectiveness of prochlorperazine for intractable migraine in children. Pediatrics 107:e62, 2001.

30. Silberstein SD, Young WB, Mendizabal JE, et al: Acute migraine treatment with droperidol: a randomized, double-blind, placebo-controlled trial. Neurology 60:315–321, 2003.

31. Tek DS, McClellan DS, Olshaker JS, et al: A prospective, double-blind study of metoclopramide hydrochloride for the control of migraine in the emergency department. Ann Emerg Med 19:1083–1087, 1990.

*32. Brousseau DC, Duffy SJ, Anderson AC, et al: Treatment of pediatric migraine headaches: a randomized, double-blind trial of prochlorperazine versus ketorolac. Ann Emerg Med 43:256–262, 2004.

33. Wenzel R, Sarvis C: Do butalbatol-containing products have a role in the management of migraine? Pharmacotherapy 22:1029–1035, 2002.

34. Young WB, Chiang-Siow H: Should butalbital-containing analgesics be banned? Yes. Curr Pain Headache Rep 6:151–155, 2002.

35. Lipton RB, Stewart WF, Cady R, et al: Sumatriptan for the range of headaches in migraine sufferers: results of the Spectrum Study. Headache 40:783–791, 2000.

36. Hamalainen ML, Hoppu K, Sanavuori P: Sumatriptan for migraine attacks in children: a randomized placebo-controlled study. Neurology 48:1100–1103, 1997.

37. Ahonen K, Hamalainen ML, Rantala H, et al: Nasal sumatriptan is effective in treatment of migraine attacks in children: a randomized trial. Neurology 62:883–887, 2004.

38. Ueberall M, Wenzel D: Intranasal sumatriptan for the acute treatment of migraine in children. Neurology 52:1507–1510, 1999.

*39. Winner P, Rothner AD, Saper J, et al: A randomized, double-blind, placebo-controlled study of sumatriptan nasal spray in the treatment of acute migraine in adolescents. Pediatrics 106:989–997, 2000.

40. Pakalnis A, Krig D, Paolicchi J: Parental satisfaction with sumatriptan nasal spray in childhood migraine. J Child Neurol 18:772–775, 2003.

41. Linder SL: Subcutaneous sumatriptan in the clinical setting: the first 50 consecutive patients with acute migraine in a pediatric neurology office practice. Headache 36:419–422, 1996.

42. Winner P, Lewis D, Visser WH, et al: Rizatriptan 5mg for the acute treatment of migraine in adolescents: a randomized, double-blind, placebo-controlled study. Headache 42:49–55, 2002.

43. Wasiewski WW: Preventive therapy in pediatric migraine. J Child Neurol 16:71–78, 2001.

*44. Lewis DW, Diamond S, Scott D, et al: Prophylactic treatment of pediatric migraine. Headache 44:230–237, 2004.

45. Baumann RJ: Behavioral treatment of migraine in children and adolescents. Paediatr Drugs 4(9):55–61, 2002.

46. Fichtel A, Larsson B: Does relaxation treatment have differential effects on migraine and tension type headache in adolescents? Headache 41:290–296, 2001.

47. Larson B, Melin L: Follow-up on behavioral treatment of recurrent headache in adolescents. Headache 29:250–254, 1989.

*48. Headache Classification Committee of the International Headache Society: The International Classification of Headache Disorders. Cephalgia 24:1–160, 2004.

Conditions Causing Increased Intracranial Pressure

Gail M. Stewart, DO, Tommy Y. Kim, MD, and Alexander Zouros, MD

Key Points

The number of children who require intracranial shunting for hydrocephalus has increased in recent decades.

Early signs and symptoms of increased intracranial pressure are nonspecific and can be subtle, overlapping with those of other, more common childhood illnesses.

A missed or delayed diagnosis of increased intracranial pressure can result in permanent neurologic damage or death.

When shunt malfunction is suspected, early consultation with a neurosurgeon experienced in the management of pediatric shunts can be life saving.

Introduction and Background

Increased intracranial pressure in children is often due to hydrocephalus, which is not rare. The prevalence of children with hydrocephalus is rising because of improved treatments leading to improved survival. Prior to the mid-20th century, there were no successful treatments for hydrocephalus, and many of these children died in infancy or early childhood. Now, with the use of intracranial shunting, many of these children are surviving and thriving. There are multiple causes of increased intracranial pressure in children (see Chapter 9, Cerebral Resuscitation; Chapter 17, Head Trauma; Chapter 43, Central Nervous System Infections; Chapter 44, Central Nervous System Vascular Disorders; and Chapter 45, Brain Tumor). Some of these conditions are associated with hydrocephalus and others are not. This chapter focuses on conditions associated with hydrocephalus (Table 42–1) and intracranial shunt complications, including shunt malfunction.

Recognition and Approach

Hydrocephalus is caused by impeded cerebrospinal fluid flow or resorption. Cerebrospinal fluid is produced primarily in the choroid plexus of the lateral third and fourth ventricles at a rate of approximately 20 ml/hr in adults. Cerebrospinal fluid can freely flow into the third ventricle, pass through the aqueduct of Sylvius into the fourth ventricle, and circulate in the subarachnoid spaces of the brain, spinal nerve roots, and cranial basal cisterns (Fig. 42–1). Cerebrospinal fluid is resorbed into the venous circulation at these sites through active transport as well as pressure gradient–driven flow. Impairment of cerebrospinal fluid resorption at the interface with the venous circulation is termed *communicating hydrocephalus*. Impairment of cerebrospinal fluid flow through the ventricular system or subarachnoid spaces is termed *obstructive hydrocephalus*. The net accumulation of intracranial cerebrospinal fluid results in expansion of the ventricles (i.e., ventriculomegaly). If the volume of cerebrospinal fluid increases to the point that the brain's compliance is exceeded, intracranial pressure will rise.[1]

Intracranial shunts were developed in the mid-20th century to divert the excess accumulation of cerebrospinal fluid and avert or reverse the development of hydrocephalus. Shunts are composed of proximal tubing, which is placed into the ventricle; a one-way valve; and a distal tube that drains fluid to an extracranial location (see Chapter 167, Ventriculoperitoneal and Other Intracranial Shunts). The most common extracranial location is the peritoneal cavity, but others include the right atrium, pleural cavity, gallbladder, urinary bladder, ureter, stomach, fallopian tube, bone marrow, mastoid, and thoracic duct.[1,2]

Although life saving, intracranial shunts are prone to malfunction and failure. Of the approximately 18,000 shunts placed annually in the United States, up to 25% to 40% will fail in the first year after placement.[3-8] Fifty-six percent to 80% of patients will experience at least one episode of malfunction in the 10 years following insertion, and the annual rate of shunt malfunction is estimated to be 2% to 5%.[1,8] The mortality from a shunt malfunction is as high as 1% to 2%.[3,7,8] The number of children requiring intracranial shunts has increased more in the past decade than previously. This is due to the improved survival of the smallest premature infants. Hydrocephalus develops from intraventricular hemorrhages in these neonates.[9] Once shunted, these neonates are at a higher risk for shunt malfunction than children who were not born prematurely.[9-11]

The most common causes for malfunction are obstruction, overdrainage, loculation, and infection.[4] Less common causes include disconnection and migration. Some causes of malfunction are relatively specific to the extracranial location to which the shunt drains (Table 42–2). Obstruction is the most common cause of malfunction and can occur anywhere along the shunt tubing. The proximal catheter can become wedged against the ventricular walls, embedded in the brain parenchyma, or occluded with choroid plexus.[12] Failure of the distal catheter seems to be time dependent. As the distal catheter ages, it can calcify and become fibrotic. It can also accumulate intraluminal debris, leading to fracture, occlusion, or degradation.[13,14] Overdrainage occurs when too much cerebrospinal fluid is siphoned from the ventricles, leading to intracranial hypotension. With overdrainage, brain shrinking away from the dura can tear the bridging vessels and cause a subdural hematoma.[1] Loculation occurs when the proximal tube is trapped in a small pocket within a ventricle, thereby failing to communicate with the rest of the ventricular system. This leads to a buildup of cerebrospinal fluid in all locations outside of the small loculated area.

Shunt infections most often result from contamination at the time of surgery. Ninety percent of shunt infections are diagnosed within 6 months of initial shunt placement or revision.[1,12] Shunts can also become secondarily infected in the presence of septicemia or abdominal infections such as appendicitis or abscess. Disconnection occurs when the shunt tubing disconnects from the valve. Migration occurs when the distal tubing finds its way into unintended anatomic locations. Shunts have been reported to perforate the intestine and extrude through the anus, migrate through the fallopian tube and out the vagina, coil up in the scrotal sac, perforate the gallbladder, and protrude through the nipple, neck, umbilicus, knee, or other sites.[15-22]

Clinical Presentation

The clinical presentation of a shunt malfunction is varied and dependent on multiple factors, including the presumed

Table 42–1	Conditions Associated with Hydrocephalus

Aqueductal stenosis
Arnold-Chiari malformation
Bacterial meningitis
Congenital hydrocephalus
Craniosynostosis
Cyst
Dandy-Walker malformation
Developmental skull anomalies
Encephalocele
Intraventricular hemorrhage
Meningocele
Myelomeningocele
Posttraumatic hemorrhage
Spina bifida
Tumor
Vascular malformation

Table 42–2	Causes of Shunt Malfunction by Initial Distal Tube Anatomic Location
Type of Shunt	**Relatively Specific Causes of Malfunction**
Ventriculoperitoneal	Peritonitis
	Intestinal volvulus
	Obstruction by omentum
	Intra-abdominal adhesion formation
	Abdominal pseudocyst
Ventriculoatrial	Pulmonary embolism
	Pulmonary hypertension
	Endocarditis
	Cor pulmonale
	Cardiac arrhythmias
	Immune-mediated nephritis
	Immune-mediated renal failure
Ventriculopleural	Tension hydrothorax
	Pneumothorax
	Fibrothorax
	Pleural empyema
	Cerebrospinal fluid overdrainage

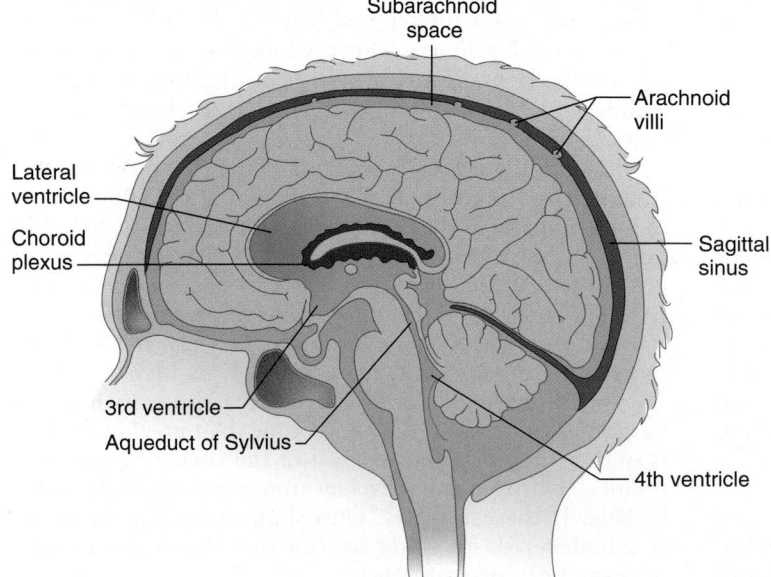

FIGURE 42–1. Cerebrospinal fluid circulation.

Table 42–3	Signs and Symptoms Reported to be Associated with Intracranial Shunt Malfunction

Abdominal pain
Anorexia
Apnea
Ataxia
Cranial nerve palsy
Distended head veins
Dizziness
Fever
Fluid tracking around shunt
Headache
Hemiparesis
Increased head circumference
Irritability
Lethargy*
Loss of developmental milestones
Muscle rigidity
Neck pain
Nuchal rigidity
Papilledema
Peritonitis
Personality change
Poor head control
Seizure
Shunt pain
Shunt site swelling*
Slurred speech
Suture diastases
Tense fontanel
Vision change
Vomiting
Weakness
Worsening school performance

*Identified as statistically associated with shunt malfunction in a population of children presenting to an emergency department.
From Kim TY, Stewart G, Voth M, et al: Signs and symptoms of cerebrospinal fluid shunt malfunction in the pediatric emergency department. Pediatr Emerg Care 22:20–24, 2006.

rate in the rise in intracranial pressure, age of the child, timing of the most recent shunt placement or revision, location of the distal tip of the tubing, and underlying comorbid conditions. The progression of shunt malfunction may be slow. In these cases, the initial signs and symptoms are often nonspecific, vague, and subtle (Table 42–3). These children are easily misdiagnosed as having common childhood illnesses due to the substantial overlap in presentation of early shunt malfunction with these illnesses. Some of these children are sent to the emergency department from the pediatrician's office for the evaluation of increasing head circumference, loss of developmental milestones, or increasing difficulty in school. If shunt malfunction is identified under these circumstances, these children are often deemed to have "chronic" shunt malfunction. In other cases, the shunt malfunction is more acute. In these cases, signs and symptoms will have a shorter duration before presentation and are likely to appear more serious. Finally, if the child either has a very rapid rise in intracranial pressure or has a delayed diagnosis, the presentation may be hyperacute. These children are typically critically ill appearing and may be unresponsive with dilated pupils, papilledema, respiratory failure, posturing, hypertension, and bradycardia. Interestingly, clinical experience suggests parents whose children have had

prior shunt malfunctions seem to be adept at identifying subsequent episodes of shunt malfunction. In the single study available evaluating the signs and symptoms associated with shunt malfunction in a population of children presenting to the emergency department, only lethargy and shunt site swelling were statistically significantly associated with shunt malfunction.[23]

The age of the child also impacts on the presenting signs and symptoms. Neonates and young infants might present with a bulging fontanelle, widened cranial sutures, prominent scalp veins, poor head control, or an upward gaze palsy. These findings are relatively specific to this age group. Unfortunately, neonates and young infants with early and slowly progressing hydrocephalus may also present with nonspecific signs and symptoms similar to other illnesses in this age group (see Chapter 7, The Critically Ill Neonate). In addition, children younger than 1 year are at a higher risk for shunt infections than are older children.

The timing of the most recent shunt placement or revision helps risk-stratify these children for shunt infections. Shunt infection is the second most common cause of shunt-related complications. The epidemiologic data regarding shunt malfunction suggest wide variability, with reported rates of infection ranging from 2% to 30%.[2] A shunt infection can occur on the equipment itself, at the wound site, in the cerebrospinal fluid, or at the site of the distal tube. The most common pathogens causing shunt infection are *Staphylococcus epidermidis* and *Staphylococcus aureus*.[1,2,12,24] The clinical presentation for shunt infection is variable. Children might present with low-grade temperature elevations and nonspecific complaints or with irritability and meningeal signs. If the surgical wound becomes infected, erythema, swelling, cellulitis, or purulent discharge is likely to be seen. When the infection site is primarily in the cerebrospinal fluid, the classic signs of meningitis may be absent. Fever is present in most patients with shunt infection but is an unreliable predictor. Approximately 50% of infected shunts will become obstructed with bacteria and inflammatory cells, so these children may also present with signs and symptoms of shunt malfunction.[2]

One way to categorize shunts is by the initial location of the tip of the distal tubing. There are certain clinical syndromes and conditions associated with each type of shunt (see Table 42–2). For example, children with ventriculopleural shunts may develop chest pain, shortness of breath, or respiratory failure if excess fluid accumulates in the pleural cavity. A child with a ventriculoatrial shunt may present with complaints of chest pain or shortness of breath due to a pulmonary embolus or cardiac arrhythmia. Patients with ventriculoatrial shunts who develop shunt nephritis will have persistent low-grade fevers, proteinuria, and hematuria.[12]

The presence of comorbid illnesses also impacts on the presentation of shunt malfunction. The presentation of shunt malfunction in children with spina bifida or myelodysplasia can be insidious. Staring spells are a common presentation in these patients, as well as neck pain, lower cranial nerve palsy, and myelopathy. These signs may be due to an associated type II Chiari's malformation and worsening brainstem compression. This association puts patients with spina bifida at a particularly high risk for rapid and critical deterioration with shunt malfunctions. For patients with myelomeningocele, the clinical signs of a urinary tract infection, including lethargy, headache, and abdominal pain, might mimic shunt malfunction. Children with myelomeningocele may also be more susceptible to bowel perforation from the distal catheter due to insufficient innervation causing weakness of the bowel wall.[25-27]

The ability to diagnose a malfunction by assessing the shunt pumping mechanism is unreliable. It is intuitively appealing to think that if the valve depresses easily, the distal tube is patent. Similarly, if the valve refills quickly after being depressed, the proximal tube should be functional. Unfortunately, the sensitivity for predicting shunt malfunction by this method is only 19%.[1]

The primary imaging studies for evaluating children with possible shunt malfunction are a computed tomographic scan of the head and a series of plain radiographs covering the entire course of the shunt tubing (i.e., a shunt series). Children who have undergone shunting often have abnormal underlying brain architecture and will likely have abnormally large ventricles even after successful shunting. Therefore, obtaining images from prior, relatively recent computed tomographic scans of the head is very valuable for determining if ventricular enlargement is present for that particular child. If they are available, it is important to know whether the prior images were obtained during a prior episode of shunt malfunction or during an asymptomatic period. Unfortunately, computed tomographic scanning of the brain is known to produce a substantial number of false-negative scans. In approximately 11% to 16% of shunt failures, the imaging demonstrates small to normal-sized ventricles.[28,29] A shunt series may reveal disruption, fracture, migration, or kinking of the tubing.

The definitive test for diagnosing a shunt infection is analysis of the cerebrospinal fluid. The fluid is usually obtained by "tapping" the shunt rather than by performing a standard lumbar puncture. Whether the emergency physician taps the shunt or defers to a neurosurgeon depends on factors such as the geographic location of the hospital, the urgency with which the fluid needs to be obtained, and the availability of a neurosurgeon. Nonetheless, performing a shunt tap in consultation with a neurosurgeon seems prudent. Once obtained, cerebrospinal fluid is typically analyzed for cell count, Gram stain, cultures, glucose, and protein levels[24] (see Chapter 171, Lumbar Puncture). Cerebrospinal fluid results consistent with infection include a positive Gram stain, pleocytosis, low glucose, high protein, or a positive culture. There appears to be an association of cerebrospinal fluid eosinophilia and shunt complications, including infections and malfunctions.[30]

Important Clinical Features and Considerations

Slit Ventricle Syndrome

Children with slit ventricle syndrome typically present with a constellation of findings consistent with shunt malfunction despite having small ventricles on computed tomographic scanning of the head. The etiology of slit ventricle syndrome is unknown. The peak occurrence is 5 to 10 years after the initial insertion of the shunt.[31] Intermittent proximal catheter obstruction is a common problem for children with slit ventricle syndrome.[25] Patients with slit ventricle syndrome

may present with chronic, cyclic headaches, nausea and vomiting, or acutely with signs of increased intracranial pressure. Some children have postural headaches. Overdrainage occurs in the upright position, causing a headache that is relieved by lying down and allowing the ventricle to re-expand.[25] Treatment options for slit ventricle syndrome include medications commonly used to treat migraines and neurosurgical procedures, including shunt revision.[2,32]

Management

Management of infants and children suspected of having shunt malfunction is typically directed by a neurosurgeon familiar with the management of pediatric shunts. The available management options include tapping the shunt, inserting an intracranial pressure monitor, observing the child for progression of symptoms in a pediatric intensive care unit, invasive shunt patency studies, or operative shunt revision. If shunt infection is confirmed or strongly suspected, the best treatment is operative removal of the shunt and placement of an external ventricular drain.[33] In general, intravenous antibiotics are administered postoperatively rather than empirically in the emergency department.

Treatment of the patient presenting in extremis from shunt failure is similar to managing other critically ill children (see Chapter 1, Approach to Resuscitation and Advanced Life Support for Infants and Children). The single unique aspect of such a resuscitation is the performance of an emergently performed shunt tap. This procedure is not without risk of complications, but may be life saving. If the emergency physician determines that the child's condition is such that death is likely to occur before the arrival of a neurosurgeon or before a child can be transferred to an appropriate tertiary care facility, the emergency physician should proceed with the shunt tap.[2] By removing cerebrospinal fluid, the decrease in intracranial pressure may be sufficient to stabilize a child until a more definitive neurosurgical evaluation and intervention can be performed. Potential complications associated with a emergent shunt tapping include damage to the shunt tubing or valve, persistent cerebrospinal fluid leakage, infection, and intracranial bleeding if cerebrospinal fluid is removed too rapidly.[12]

Summary

Shunt-related complications are not negligible and can result in neurologic impairment or death. Studies show that patients who experience one shunt failure are at risk for subsequent failures. The incidence of epilepsy increases significantly following each shunt revision.[8] Furthermore, each revision carries a 5% risk of infection.[3] The morbidity of shunt infection is significant. Studies have documented a marked decline in children's IQ scores following shunt infection, reflecting its devastating effect on a maturing central nervous system.[7] Mortality rates of 1% to 2% have been observed with shunt failure.[3,7,8] Approximately 20% of children treated with shunts die from causes related to the original disease or its treatment. Most deaths occur during the first 2 years after shunt placement and are due to complications of the surgery or progression of the underlying disease.[7] The most common causes of shunt-related mortality are obstruction, infection, and pulmonary embolism.[7] Children with suspected or confirmed shunt complications are typically admitted to a neurosurgeon familiar with the management of pediatric shunts at a hospital that has a pediatric intensive care unit.

In addition, there is no way to measure the considerable psychological impact on families of shunted children, who must remain ever watchful for subtle signs of malfunction. Oftentimes numerous, and time-consuming, trips to the office or emergency department are required to evaluate for shunt malfunction. Understanding the difficulties these families face is helpful in coordinating care with them.

Despite ongoing research and exploration of alternative methods for the treatment of hydrocephalus, the shunting system is likely to remain the principle means of cerebrospinal fluid diversion for the near future. Even with their associated problems and complications, shunts have saved many children with hydrocephalus.

REFERENCES

*1. Madikians A, Conway E: Cerebrospinal fluid shunt problems in pediatric patients. Pediatr Ann 26:613–620, 1997.

2. Teoh DL: Pediatric surgical emergencies—tricks of the trade: assessment of high tech gear in special needs children. Clin Pediatr Emerg Med 3:62–75, 2002.

3. Drake JM, Kestle J; The Pediatric Hydrocephalus Treatment Evaluation Group: Rationale and methodology of the multicenter pediatric cerebrospinal fluid shunt design trial. Childs Nerv Syst 12:434–447, 1996.

*4. Kestle J, Drake J, Milner R, et al: Long-term follow-up data from the shunt design trial. Pediatr Neurosurg 33:230–236, 2000.

5. Vernet O, Rilliet B: Late complications of ventriculoatrial or ventriculoperitoneal shunts. Lancet 358:1569–1570, 2001.

*6. Bondurant CP, Jimenez DF: Epidemiology of CSF shunting. Pediatr Neurosurg 23:253–258, 1995.

7. Kang, JK, Lee IW: Long-term follow-up of shunting therapy. Childs Nerv Syst 15:711–717, 1999.

8. Sainte-Rose C, Piatt JH, Renier D: Mechanical complications in shunts. Pediatr Neurosurg 17:2–9, 1991-92.

9. Reinprecht A, Dietrich W, Berger A, et al: Posthemorrhagic hydrocephalus in preterm infants: long-term follow-up and shunt-related complications. Childs Nerv Syst 17:663–669, 2001.

10. Lazareff JA, Peacock W, Holly L, et al: Multiple shunt failures: an analysis of relevant factors. Childs Nerv Syst 14:271–275, 1998.

11. Korinth MC, Gilsbach JM: What is the ideal initial valve pressure setting in neonates with ventriculoperitoneal shunts? Pediatr Neurosurg 36:169–174, 2002.

12. Naradzay JF, Browne BJ, Rolnick MA, et al: Cerebral ventricular shunts. J Emerg Med 17:311–322, 1999.

13. McGirt MJ, Wellons JC, Nimjee SM, et al: Comparison of total versus partial revision of initial ventriculoperitoneal shunt failures. Pediatr Neurosurg 38:34–40, 2002.

14. Yamamoto S, Ohno K, Aoyagi M, et al: Calcific deposits on degraded shunt catheters: long-term follow-up of V-P shunts and late complications in three cases. Childs Nerv Syst 18:19–25, 2002.

15. Bal RK: Intestinal volvulus—a rare complication of ventriculoperitoneal shunt. Pediatr Surg Int 15:577–578, 1999.

16. Jindal A: Unusual complication—VP shunt coming out per rectum and brain abscess. Indian J Pediatr 66:463–465, 1999.

17. Wani AA: Protrusion of a peritoneal catheter through the umbilicus: an unusual complication of a ventriculoperitoneal shunt. Pediatr Surg Int 18:171–172, 2003.

18. Karla N: Cerebrospinal fluid pseudocyst of the breast. Australas Radiol 46:76–79, 2002.

19. Nourisamie K: Two unusual complications of ventriculoperitoneal shunts in the same infant. Pediatr Radiol 31:814–816, 2001.

20. Silver RI: A ventriculoperitoneal shunt masquerading as a paratesticular tumor. J Pediatr Surg 35:1407–1408, 2000.

21. Washington EC: Ventriculoperitoneal shunt migration presenting with vaginal discharge and hydrosalpinx in a 16-year-old patient. Pediatr Emerg Care 18:28–30, 2002.

22. Byard RW, Koszyca B, Qiao M: Unexpected childhood death due to a rare complication of ventriculoperitoneal shunting. Am J Forensic Med Pathol 22:207–210, 2001.

*23. Kim TY, Stewart G, Voth M, et al: Signs and symptoms of cerebrospinal fluid shunt malfunction in the pediatric emergency department. Pediatr Emerg Care 22:28–34, 2006.

24. Brook I: Meningitis and shunt infection caused by anaerobic bacteria in children. Pediatr Neurol 26:99–105, 2002.

25. Kestle JRW: Pediatric hydrocephalus: current management. Neurol Clin 21:883–895, 2003.

26. Rekate HL: Shunt revision: complications and their prevention. Pediatr Neurosurg 92:155–162, 1991.

27. Sathyanarayana S, Wylen EL, Baskaya MK, et al: Spontaneous bowel perforation after ventriculoperitoneal shunt surgery: case report and a review of 45 cases. Surg Neurol 54:388–396, 2000.

*28. Iskandar BJ, McLaughlin C, Mapstone TB, et al: Pitfalls in the diagnosis of ventricular shunt dysfunction: radiology reports and ventricular size. Pediatrics 101:1031–1036, 1998.

29. Barnes NP, Jones SJ, Hayward RD, et al: Ventriculoperitoneal shunt block: what are the best predictive clinical indicators? Arch Dis Child 87:198–201, 2002.

30. McClinton D, Carraccio C, Englander R: Predictors of ventriculoperitoneal shunt pathology. Pediatr Infect Dis J 20:593–597, 2001.

31. Del Bigio MR: Neuropathological findings in a child with slit ventricle syndrome. Pediatr Neurosurg 37:148–151, 2002.

32. Le H, Yamini B, Frim DM: Lumboperitoneal shunting as a treatment for slit ventricle syndrome. Pediatr Neurosurg 36:178–182, 2002.

33. Schreffler RT, Schreffler AJ, Sittler RR: Treatment of cerebrospinal fluid shunt infections: a decision analysis. Pediatr Infect Dis J 21:632–636, 2002.

*Selected readings.

Chapter 43

Central Nervous System Infections

James A. Wilde, MD

Bacterial meningitis is relatively rare in the United States outside of the neonatal period.

Viral meningitis due to enteroviruses is the most common central nervous system infection in the pediatric emergency department setting.

Bacterial and viral meningitis are different diseases with overlapping signs and symptoms.

While infection with West Nile virus is now common in the United States, overt encephalitis with severe neurologic sequelae due to West Nile virus is not.

Brain abscess should be considered in febrile patients who present with new focal neurologic abnormalities.

Introduction and Background

Emergency physicians manage many infectious diseases in the course of their duties. One study in an academic pediatric emergency department estimated that 50% to 60% of these diseases were self-limited viral infections primarily affecting the respiratory or gastrointestinal tract, and another 30% were minor bacterial infections such as acute otitis media or sinusitis.[1] Less than 5% of children had a serious bacterial infection. An even smaller subset of febrile illnesses target the central nervous system (CNS), but they have the potential to cause severe morbidity and mortality. For this reason, emergency physicians must be vigilant when managing a child with fever so that these more dangerous CNS infections may be diagnosed in a timely fashion. Unfortunately, the signs and symptoms of these infections can be quite subtle, making early recognition difficult despite the best efforts of clinicians.

One of the most feared CNS infections among clinicians is bacterial meningitis. In some cases, the course of the illness from symptom onset to death may be less than 24 hours, particularly if the infection is due to *Neisseria meningitidis,* also known as meningococcus. Fortunately, bacterial meningitis has become a rare diagnosis in the United States since the introduction of conjugate vaccines for *Haemophilus influenzae* type b (Hib) in 1991 and *Streptococcus pneumoniae* in 2000. As a result of the Hib vaccine alone, cases of bacterial meningitis dropped by 87% nationwide.[2] A smaller but still significant drop can be expected after use of the pneumococcal vaccine becomes widespread.[3,4] Just prior to the introduction of the pneumococcal vaccine, total bacterial meningitis cases in children under 18 years of age in the United States were estimated to be less than 2800 per year, or approximately one case for every 22,000 children.[2] The incidence is higher in younger children, particularly neonates, for whom effective vaccines have not yet been developed (Table 43–1). The most common causative organisms vary by age: in neonates, group B streptococcus and *Listeria monocytogenes* predominate, although gram-negative enteric organisms such as *Escherichia coli,* Klebsiella, and Enterobacter species also play a role; in children between 1 and 23 months, *S. pneumoniae* and *N. meningitidis* cause most cases; and in children 2 to 18 years, *N. meningitidis, S. pneumoniae,* and *H. influenzae* type b predominate.

Viral meningitis is a related disease that is quite common in the United States, causing more than 75,000 symptomatic infections per year.[5] The ratio of viral meningitis to bacterial meningitis in U.S. children is at least 20 : 1. The causative organism in all but a small percentage of cases is Enterovirus, a group of viruses that circulate primarily in the warm months of the year from April to September. Over 70 distinct serotypes of Enterovirus have been described, most classified as either echoviruses or coxsackieviruses. Many different serotypes of ECHO and Coxsackie have been implicated in outbreaks of meningitis. Viral meningitis tends to be most common in children, who account for up to 96% of cases in some reports.[6] Unlike bacterial meningitis, viral meningitis due to Enterovirus rarely causes significant sequelae in children, and death is rare.[7]

Encephalitis is an infection that includes direct brain parenchymal invasion, whereas meningitis is an infection of the cerebrospinal fluid (CSF) and tissues that surround the brain. Many cases of enteroviral meningitis actually represent a combination of both, a syndrome referred to as meningoencephalitis. Prior to 1999, herpes simplex virus (HSV) was the most common cause of nonepidemic, acute focal encephalitis in the United States.[8] The most common cause of encephalitis in the United States in 2005 is West Nile virus, a newly imported infectious agent that has spread throughout the country with amazing rapidity since the first case was

Table 43–1	Bacterial Meningitis in Children in the United States*	
Age	Estimated Cases per Year[†]	Rate per 100,000
<1 mo	529	182
1–23 mo	948	13.5
2–18 yr	1316	2.3
All children birth to 18 yr	2793	4.4

*Based on estimated 3.5 million children per birth cohort in the United States.
[†]Based on data from Schuchat A, Robinson D, Wenger JD, et al: Bacterial meningitis in the United States in 1995. N Engl J Med 337:970–976, 1997.

documented in New York in 1999. In 2003, there were 9000 cases reported in the United States, with 220 deaths.[9] West Nile virus is a flavivirus spread by mosquitoes; birds are the primary reservoir. Other less common causes of encephalitis in the United States include arboviruses such as the La Crosse strain of California encephalitis virus, St. Louis encephalitis virus, western equine encephalomyelitis virus, and eastern equine encephalomyelitis virus. Infections due to arboviruses generally occur during the warm months of the year and tend to parallel mosquito activity. HSV encephalitis can occur during any time of the year and at any age, although the most severe form tends to occur in neonates in the first 2 to 3 weeks of life.

Brain abscess is rare in children. Even with prompt diagnosis and treatment, the mortality rate is 25% or more. Aerobic and anaerobic streptococci cause about half of all brain abscesses in children, followed by staphylococci (10% to 30%) and enteric bacteria such as Enterobacteriaceae (10% to 25%). Mixed infections are found in 30%.[10]

Recognition and Approach

Any child who develops a fever and headache may have a CNS infection, but most do not. Due to the subtlety of the symptoms, it can be very difficult to detect all CNS infections on the initial presentation. In addition, some patients may be at the beginning stage of a series of events that will lead eventually to CNS infection, such as patients with bacteremia (Fig. 43–1). This series of events may occur over several hours or several days. In the clinical setting, it is not possible to precisely determine the point at which CNS invasion has occurred. Several authors have suggested guidelines to identify children with occult bacteremia in an effort to interrupt the progression to meningitis.[11] Even with the use of laboratory screens as suggested in these guidelines, more than one third of children with occult bacteremia will not be identified, and a small proportion of them will go on to develop meningitis (see Chapter 68, Bacteremia). Thus it is inevitable that some febrile children without meningitis who are seen early in the course of their illness will develop bacterial meningitis later in the illness despite the best efforts of physicians to detect the disease.

Two different presentations for bacterial meningitis have been described. These include a fulminant form and an insidious form. Patients with fulminant meningitis have rapid progression of their disease with obvious signs and

symptoms pointing to the severity of their illness, such as altered mental status, shock, and nuchal rigidity. Recognition of fulminant meningitis is relatively easy early in the course if these signs and symptoms are present. The insidious form develops more slowly, often over several days, and recognition early in the course is difficult since the more specific signs and symptoms develop later. Despite potential delay in making the diagnosis in the case of the insidious form, patients are generally not as ill at the point of diagnosis, and the outcome is better than in patients with fulminant meningitis.[12-14] Given the pathophysiology of bacterial meningitis, one explanation for these differences is that, in those with the insidious course, bacterial invasion of the CNS is a late event. For example, patients who present with the insidious form may not have had meningitis at all if evaluated for fever 2 days before meningitis is eventually recognized. The reason for this delayed invasion is unclear; it may be related to the virulence of the organism,[15] or it may be related to variations in host response to infection. This helps explain an apparent paradox in patients with meningococcal infections, in whom the presence of meningitis at the time of diagnosis is actually associated with a better outcome.[16] Highly virulent meningococcal strains may be so lethal that progression to sepsis and multiorgan failure occurs before significant invasion of the CNS can occur. Less virulent strains have more time to invade the CNS and produce typical symptoms of meningitis. Conversely, recent data indicate that the systemic response to infection shows profound genetic variation and that patients with variations in cytokine production may be at increased risk for morbidity and mortality due to bacterial pathogens such as N. meningitidis.[17,18] In these patients, the outcome may depend more on the patient's own innate immune response than on the invading organism.

One fourth of all brain abscesses are diagnosed in children under 15 years of age.[10] The most common predisposing conditions are cyanotic congenital heart disease, usually with hematogenous spread of bacteria, or direct invasion from a contiguous site such as infected sinuses or middle ear infection. Immunosuppression has also emerged as a leading predisposing factor over the last 25 years, as has premature birth.[19] Brain abscess is an unusual complication of bacterial meningitis. Brain abscess after head trauma also is unusual, and tends to lag well behind the initial injury. Physicians should have a heightened level of suspicion for brain abscess if a child with one of these risk factors develops symptoms suggestive of CNS infection, particularly if new neurologic deficits are noted.

Up to 80% of infections with West Nile virus are asymptomatic, and less than 1% of infected patients develop severe neurologic illness such as meningitis, encephalitis, or flaccid paralysis.[9] Viral encephalitis should be considered in the differential diagnosis of patients who present with these neurologic manifestations during the summer months. West Nile virus infection is 10 times more common in patients over age 50 than in children, and illness in children tends to be milder. West Nile fever is the term given to patients who are symptomatic with West Nile infection but who have no neurologic disease.[20] Patients with West Nile fever have an acute febrile illness lasting 3 to 6 days in addition to headache, vomiting, myalgia, and rash. The most severe form of viral encephalitis in the United States is eastern equine encephalitis. Encephalitis due to other arboviruses in the United States have much

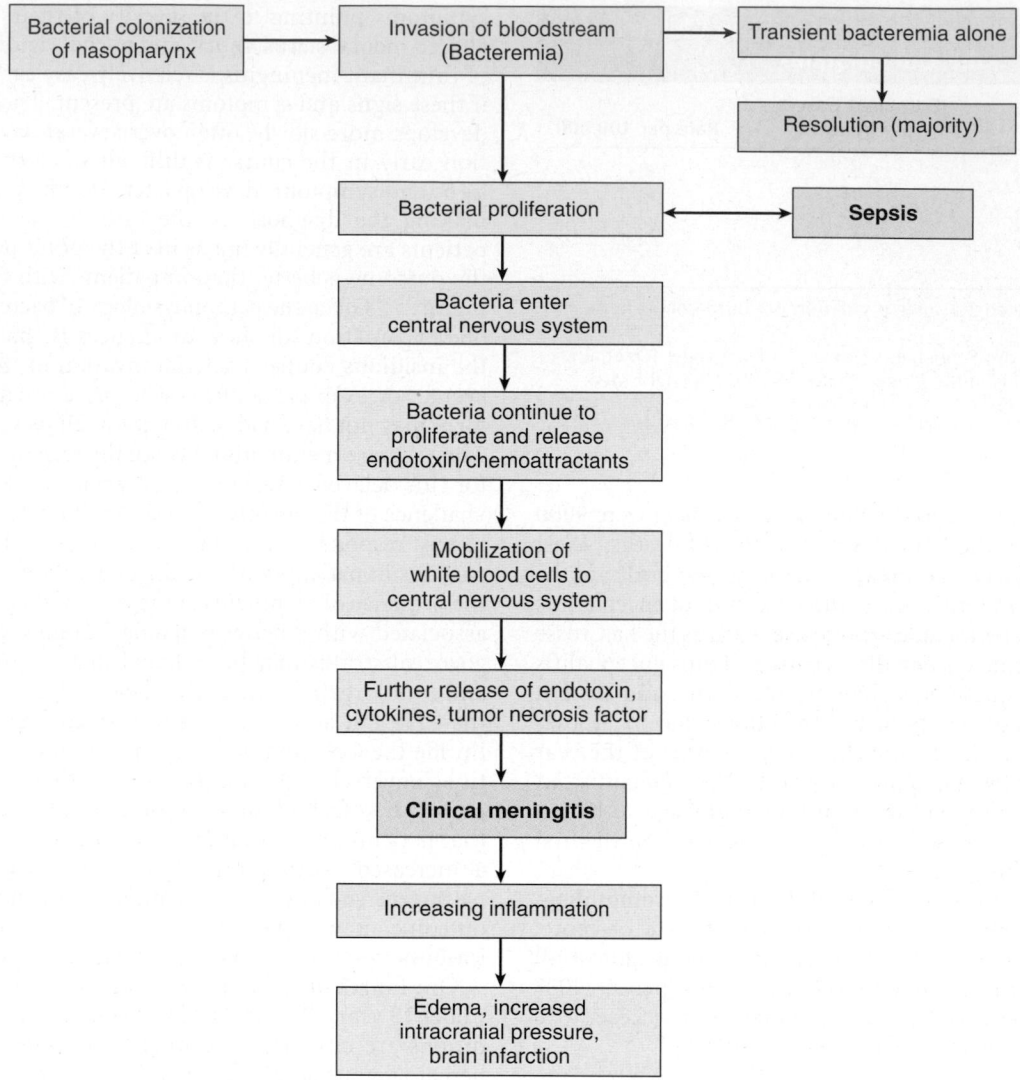

FIGURE 43–1. Steps in the development of bacterial meningitis.

lower rates of morbidity and mortality, and many infections remain subclinical. Arboviruses are maintained in nature through a cycle involving transmission from mosquitoes to birds and small mammals. Humans are considered "dead-end hosts" for arboviruses such as West Nile due to low levels of viremia; person-to-person spread does not occur.

Clinical Presentation

Nonspecific signs and symptoms that are generally present with CNS infections include fever, headache, and vomiting. In the absence of more specific signs or symptoms, further workup outside the newborn period is generally not warranted and symptomatic therapy alone is appropriate, since the overwhelming majority of these patients will not have a CNS infection. Inflammation of the meninges may lead to more specific signs or symptoms such as increased pain on flexion of the neck, stiff neck (nuchal rigidity), photophobia, altered mental status, or irritability. Seizures, focal neurologic abnormalities, petechial or purpuric rash, and hypoten-

sion may suggest meningitis, encephalitis, or brain abscess. Patients who present with fever, headache, and vomiting in addition to one or more of these other signs and symptoms, and patients with unusually severe symptoms, generally require further evaluation for meningitis. Patients with risk factors for CNS infection, such as those with ventriculoperitoneal shunts, cyanotic congenital heart disease, recent CNS surgery or head trauma, or immunocompromised states, may also require a more aggressive workup even in the absence of these additional signs and symptoms.

Another subset of patients that requires more aggressive evaluation is the newly born, in whom specific signs and symptoms often do not develop until very late in the course of their CNS infection. In this population, clinical signs and symptoms of meningitis may be very subtle, including poor oral intake, increased sleep, irritability, respiratory distress, or jaundice. Many neonates with meningitis are afebrile at presentation,[21] and most have no meningeal signs.[22]

One of the most important signs of bacterial meningitis is a change in the child's affect or state of alertness. In one study, 36% to 60% of children older than 3 months with this diagnosis were described as toxic or moribund, and 73% to 100% were described as lethargic or comatose.[22] Physicians should be careful to document the presence of lethargy based on clinical findings rather than on a parent's report. Children who are febrile for any reason tend to show decreased activity and an increased desire for sleep. This does not necessarily indicate that they are lethargic. "Lethargy" in the medical sense refers to an inappropriately decreased response to external stimuli. For example, children can be expected to cry and resist attempts at examination by medical personnel, particularly in the younger age groups. They should react similarly to venipuncture and other painful procedures. Children who do not respond vigorously to these stimuli may be truly lethargic. Lethargy is an ominous finding that should prompt further investigation. On the other hand, most patients with fever and headache who are active, alert, playful, or smiling are unlikely to have a serious CNS infection in the absence of more specific signs or symptoms.

Up to 30% of children with acute bacterial meningitis have seizures on initial presentation.[23] Most of these children are profoundly ill at presentation. A study focusing on seizures as the initial presenting symptom in bacterial meningitis revealed that almost all of these children have marked alterations in their sensorium; over 90% were either comatose or semicomatose.[24] It is important to note that most children who have seizures and fever do not have acute bacterial meningitis. Children who meet the case definition for a simple febrile seizure and who return to a normal level of alertness shortly thereafter are at low risk for bacterial meningitis; except in those under 12 months of age, further laboratory investigation for meningitis is not recommended.[25]

Meningismus is a term that refers to irritation of the meninges, usually from bacterial or viral meningitis. Meningismus can be assessed in a number of ways. The prime method is to examine the patient for nuchal rigidity, or a stiff neck. Flexing the neck causes the meninges to stretch, so the neck muscles tend to resist flexion as an involuntary protective mechanism in the presence of inflamed meninges. Many medical students are taught to test for nuchal rigidity by pulling up on the back of the supine patient's head. This method may be less helpful in very young children, who tend to resist examination and manipulation of any sort. A simpler method that can be used in any age group is to assess the patient from a sitting position, asking the child to look down toward his or her umbilicus. In younger children, the physician may simply place something of interest such as a toy or light in the region of the umbilicus. A child who readily looks down by flexing the neck so that the chin touches the chest does not have nuchal rigidity. Two other helpful signs to assess for meningismus are Kernig's and Brudzinski's signs. Kernig's sign is positive if the patient actively flexes the neck in response to a maneuver that includes passive flexion at the hip followed by passive extension at the knee. Brudzinski's sign is positive if passive flexion of the neck by the examiner causes an involuntary active flexion at the hip. Meningismus is almost always present in children who present with bacterial meningitis beyond 13 months of age, but it is usually absent in children under 6 months.[22]

Children with brain abscess usually present with headache, fever, and vomiting, but the classic triad of headache,

fever, and focal deficits occurs in less than one third. Up to half will have seizures, altered mental status, or focal neurologic signs, but more than half have none of these additional signs or symptoms.

Patients who present with signs and symptoms that suggest acute CNS infection warrant further evaluation. This includes all children with meningismus or photophobia, even if the child presents with a nontoxic appearance that suggests viral meningitis. Central to that evaluation is an examination of CSF after performance of a lumbar puncture (LP)[26] (see Chapter 171, Lumbar Puncture). In uncomplicated bacterial meningitis, LP can be performed safely without a prior head computed tomography (CT) scan. The practice of routinely ordering a head CT scan before the LP is performed in these patients can lead to unnecessary delays in administration of antibiotics and should be discouraged.[27,28]

It may be appropriate to delay the LP in some patients with suspected CNS infection. For instance, CSF findings are nonspecific in patients with brain abscesses, and bacteria are rarely isolated from culture. Thus for patients in whom brain abscess is suspected, LP is of marginal value. It may be more appropriate to first order a head CT scan to determine if an abscess is present. If an abscess is found, LP is not required. If no abscess is found, the LP can be done to search for evidence of meningitis. Due to the risk of cerebral herniation, LP should also be delayed in patients with focal neurologic abnormalities or focal neurologic symptoms that suggest a CNS mass lesion. LP in patients with papilledema or a limited neurologic examination due to a decreased level of consciousness should also be delayed for the same reason. In each of these cases, CT of the head should be ordered first to assess for a space-occupying lesion. If a space-occupying lesion is not present, LP can be performed in the absence of any other contraindications. Other reasons to delay performance of an LP include the presence of thrombocytopenia or uncorrected coagulopathy; cellulitis overlying the lumbar vertebra; or an unstable patient who would be at risk for acute clinical deterioration from the procedure itself. If the LP is to be delayed for any reason, blood should be collected for bacterial culture prior to administration of antibiotics. Bacterial pathogens can be isolated from blood culture in up to 80% of patients with bacterial meningitis.[29,30]

Examination of the CSF can provide clues to the presence or absence of inflammation. Normal CSF in the neonatal period contains less than 26 white blood cells (WBCs)/mm^3. Beyond the neonatal period, there should be fewer than 7 WBCs/mm^3.[31] Pleocytosis is present if the number of WBCs in the CSF is above those limits. CSF pleocytosis is indirect evidence for inflammation. An elevated level of CSF protein or a decreased level of CSF glucose also indicates the presence of inflammation. The results of these three tests provide useful clues about the underlying diagnosis (Table 43–2). However, there is a considerable degree of variability in these tests. For example, up to 10% of children with viral meningitis have been reported to have CSF WBC counts greater than 1000/mm^3,[5] and 1% of children with bacterial meningitis have a normal CSF WBC count on initial examination.[32]

The rapid test that is most helpful and practical in assessing for the presence of bacterial meningitis is the CSF Gram stain. The Gram stain will reveal bacteria in up to 90% of patients with bacterial meningitis.[33,34] It is important to note also that appropriate antibiotic therapy does little to

Table 43–2	Typical Cerebrospinal Fluid Characteristics in Central Nervous System Infections			
	Bacterial Meningitis	**Viral Meningitis**	**Encephalitis**	**Brain Abscess**
WBC/mm³	>1000	<500	<200	Variable
Protein	Markedly elevated	Normal	Elevated	Variable
Glucose	Markedly decreased	Normal	Normal	Variable
Gram stain	Bacteria	No bacteria	No bacteria	Bacteria rarely present
	Polymorphonuclear cells	Mononuclear cells and polymorphonuclear cells	Mononuclear cells	

Abbreviation: WBC, white blood cells.

diminish the inflammatory response in the first few days of treatment. It is not unusual to find an increased degree of pleocytosis 1 to 2 days after starting antibiotic therapy, and CSF pleocytosis persists for at least 7 to 10 days.[35]

Important Clinical Features and Considerations

The diagnosis of bacterial meningitis does not depend on the measurement of a peripheral WBC count. Even in clinically apparent meningitis, the WBC count often is not elevated significantly; more than 50% of patients with meningitis due to *N. meningitidis* have WBC counts under 15,000/mm³.[36] The diagnosis of bacterial meningitis is based on clinical criteria, examination of CSF for evidence of inflammation, and isolation of bacteria from CSF. Patients outside of the neonatal period who do not have specific signs or symptoms pointing to meningitis are highly unlikely to have the disease. Physicians who choose to use the peripheral WBC count as a screen to detect occult bacteremia in an effort to "prevent" a case of meningitis, or as a means to diagnose clinically inapparent bacterial meningitis, should be aware of the significant limitations and pitfalls of that strategy.

A particularly vexing problem for clinicians is how to distinguish viral meningitis from the early stage of bacterial meningitis, when the degree of CSF pleocytosis may still be mild. Although viral meningitis typically is associated with mononuclear cell predominance in the CSF, early in the course of infection polymorphonuclear cells often predominate. Some authors have devised a clinical "scoring system" to determine which patients with CSF pleocytosis are likely to have viral meningitis and which are likely to have bacterial meningitis.[37,38] The only validated prediction model in the era after the Hib vaccine was introduced was found to have a high sensitivity for detecting a case of bacterial meningitis as well as a high negative predictive value for this diagnosis.[38] The authors concluded that patients who had a bacterial meningitis score of zero were highly unlikely to have bacterial meningitis and may be managed as outpatients (Table 43–3). A subsequent multicenter retrospective validation study showed that the risk of bacterial meningitis is less than 0.1% in patients with a score of zero.[39]

Another dilemma for clinicians is how to decide who requires an LP and who does not. Some physicians take the approach that any child with possible meningitis requires an LP, without regard to whether viral or bacterial meningitis is suspected. Viral meningitis and bacterial meningitis are two different diseases, with different pathophysiology, management, and prognosis. If a patient's symptoms include meningismus or photophobia, an LP should be performed even in

Table 43–3	Predictors for Bacterial versus Viral Meningitis

- Positive Gram stain
- CSF protein ≥ 80 mg/dL
- Peripheral ANC ≥ 10,000 cells/mm³ (10 × 10⁹ cells/L)
- Seizure at or before presentation
- CSF ANC ≥ 1000 cells/mm³ (1 × 10⁹ cells/L)

Scoring: Two points for positive Gram stain, one point for all other items.
All negative: likely viral meningitis; negative predictive value for bacterial meningitis 97%–100%
Positive Gram stain or any two other items positive: likely bacterial meningitis; sensitivity 87%

Abbreviations: ANC, absolute neutrophil count; CSF, cerebrospinal fluid.
Adapted from Nigrovic LE, Kuppermann N, Malley R: Development and validation of a multivariable predictive model to distinguish bacterial from aseptic meningitis in the post-*Haemophilus influenzae* era. Pediatrics 110:712–719, 2002.

the nontoxic patient. However, physicians in the United States should keep in mind that it is not imperative to search for evidence of viral meningitis in a patient if symptoms are not severe, since virtually all patients recover without specific therapy. It is imperative to search for evidence of bacterial meningitis, since appropriate antibiotic therapy can be life saving. Thus, a nontoxic child who presents with fever and headache in the absence of meningismus or photophobia does not *require* an LP even if a sibling was diagnosed with viral meningitis 3 days earlier.

In light of the fact that bacteria are rarely isolated from the CSF in patients with brain abscess, the CSF profile in these patients may be similar to that seen in viral meningitis or encephalitis. Once again, a high level of suspicion for this infection should be maintained for children at increased risk for brain abscess since many of them do not present with seizures or new focal neurologic deficits on physical examination.[19]

The hallmark of viral encephalitis is CNS dysfunction. This dysfunction may be manifested by an altered level of consciousness, focal neurologic abnormalities, seizures, or unprovoked emotional outbursts. Encephalitis should be considered in patients with headache and fever who present with these additional features.

Management

Expeditious diagnostic studies and therapeutic interventions are important in patients with signs and symptoms of CNS infection who present to the emergency department (Table

Table 43–4	Suggested Steps in the Management of Bacterial Meningitis in the Emergency Department

Rapid evaluation to include:
- Head computed tomography in selected cases
- Blood culture *before* administration of antibiotics
- Serum chemistry panel
- Lumbar puncture (in the absence of contraindications)
- Cerebrospinal fluid culture and Gram stain
- Cerebrospinal fluid protein and glucose
- Cerebrospinal fluid cell count and differential

Rapid administration of antibiotics targeted against suspected pathogens

Fluid resuscitation to maintain adequate blood pressure (fluid restriction is **not** recommended)

Vasopressor agents as needed if blood pressure does not improve with fluid boluses

Dexamethasone as adjunctive therapy if infection due to *Haemophilus influenzae* type b is suspected

Transfer to a pediatric intensive care unit for definitive care

Antibiotic prophylaxis for selected close contacts if disease due to *H. influenzae* type b or *Neisseria meningitidis* is suspected

Table 43–5	Suggested Empirical Antibiotic Regimen for Bacterial Meningitis	
Age	**Suggested Antibiotic Regimen**
<1 mo	Gentamicin 2.5 mg/kg **OR** cefotaxime 50 mg/kg **Plus** Ampicillin 50 mg/kg. Use vancomycin if staphylococcus species or *Pneumococcus* is suspected
>1 mo	Ceftriaxone 75 mg/kg **OR** cefotaxime 100 mg/kg **Plus** Vancomycin 10–15 mg/kg

43–4). All of these emergency department evaluations should include blood culture, most should include LP, and some may include head CT scan. If the patient is likely to have bacterial meningitis or brain abscess, antibiotics should be administered quickly. Dogmatic pronouncements that the antibiotics must be given within a specified time frame, such as within 30 minutes of the patient's arrival in the emergency department, should be avoided. These time intervals are based more on opinion than on solid evidence; there are no data that conclusively show a better outcome if antibiotics are administered within the first 30 minutes compared with 1 or 2 hours.[13] In addition, a 30-minute time interval may be impractical for many cases, particularly if the diagnosis is not obvious. One retrospective study of bacterial meningitis in a general emergency department showed that the average duration from arrival in the emergency department to administration of antibiotics was more than 2 hours.[40] The authors of this study correctly pointed out that, since the standard of care is based on the actual practice in the community, this is a more realistic "standard." Since randomized studies examining various intervals between presentation and treatment of established bacterial meningitis would be unethical, it may not be possible to prove that one interval provides a better outcome than another. If bacterial meningitis is likely, a reasonable recommendation is to administer the antibiotics immediately after collecting blood for culture, or immediately after completion of the LP if there is no delay in performing the procedure. The yield for CSF culture declines within 1 to 2 hours of third-generation cephalosporin administration in patients with meningococcal meningitis, within 4 hours with pneumococcal meningitis, and within 8 hours with meningitis due to group B streptococcus.[30]

The proper antibiotic choice for bacterial meningitis in the United States depends on the age of the patient, the presence or absence of risk factors for unusual organisms, and information gained from the Gram stain. A patient with CNS hardware such as a ventriculoperitoneal shunt, a history of recent CNS surgery, or recent head trauma is at higher risk for staphylococcus or streptococcus species than is a patient without these conditions. If either *Staphylococcus aureus* or *Staphylococcus epidermidis* is likely, the antibiotic regimen should include vancomycin. A patient with sickle cell disease and gram-negative rods on Gram stain should be given an antibiotic that targets salmonella, such as a third-generation cephalosporin. A patient over the age of 1 month with an unremarkable past medical history and gram-positive organisms on Gram stain should be given antibiotics that are active against *S. pneumoniae*, such as third-generation cephalosporins. Given the current rate of penicillin-resistant pneumococcus in the United States, empirical therapy with ampicillin or penicillin should no longer be considered adequate therapy, although penicillin is still the drug of choice if the isolate is determined to be sensitive to penicillin. Some authors have shown equivalent benefit from carbapenems such as meropenem when compared with cephalosporins; these agents should be considered in the cephalosporin-allergic patient.[41] In light of recent trends toward increased levels of penicillin resistance among pneumococci, the addition of vancomycin to any regimen chosen is now recommended if this pathogen is suspected[12] (Table 43–5).

The adjunctive use of dexamethasone in bacterial meningitis is controversial.[42,43] Early studies examining the use of dexamethasone showed no clear benefit. However, these studies focused on mortality as the outcome measure. More recent studies that evaluated the effect of dexamethasone on both mortality and morbidity appeared to show less hearing loss in the group treated with dexamethasone.[44] Upon closer inspection, the benefit appeared to be confined to patients with meningitis due to *H. influenzae* type b. Multiple studies have been undertaken since then to determine if that benefit extends to patients with meningitis due to *S. pneumoniae* or *N. meningitidis*. Unfortunately, the data for these pathogens have been less clear. One meta-analysis performed in 1989 showed benefit only for *H. influenzae* type b.[45] Another meta-analysis performed in 1997 concluded that there is benefit in patients with *H. influenzae* type b, and possible benefit in patients with *S. pneumoniae*.[46] The definitive answer to this question may never be known. Most of the data from these two meta-analyses relied on studies done before vancomycin and third-generation cephalosporins were recommended in combination as the initial antibiotic regimen. In light of the fact that vancomycin appears to provide a synergistic effect against these pathogens, the question today should ideally be answered using study designs including both antibiotics.[43] Only two such studies have been performed, and they came to conflicting conclusions. In an era in which meningitis due to *S. pneumoniae* has become increasingly rare due to vaccination, randomized studies designed to settle the issue will be difficult to perform. Dexamethasone has not been shown to reduce hearing loss in meningococcal meningitis.

The Committee on Infectious Diseases of the American Academy of Pediatrics (AAP) stated that the use of adjunctive dexamethasone "may be beneficial" in patients over the age of 2 months if they are suspected to have meningitis due to *H influenzae* type b.[47] This panel of experts suggested only that dexamethasone be "considered" for bacterial meningitis due to pneumococcus because "data are not sufficient to demonstrate a clear benefit in children."[48] Given the available literature and this recommendation from the AAP panel, the use of dexamethasone should not be considered the standard of care in the management of bacterial meningitis in children; physicians may reasonably decide not to use dexamethasone in the early management of this infection. If dexamethasone is to be used, it should be given in a dosage of 0.15 mg/kg per dose intravenously before or concurrently with the first dose of an antimicrobial agent. Dexamethasone should not be used in aseptic meningitis or in children with bacterial meningitis who are less than 6 weeks of age.[43]

For many years clinicians were advised to restrict fluids to two thirds of maintenance requirements in patients with bacterial meningitis. The reason given was that the syndrome of inappropriate secretion of antidiuretic syndrome (SIADH) commonly occurred during the acute stages of bacterial meningitis, and too much fluid during a period of SIADH could potentially cause increased brain edema with concomitant increased intracranial pressure. However, recent studies have shown that SIADH may actually provide a protective effect during early meningitis by maintaining a blood pressure sufficient to overcome some of the impedance to cerebral perfusion brought about by brain edema.[49-51] The gathering consensus among experts is that fluid restriction is no longer warranted in the treatment of bacterial meningitis. Fluids should be provided as needed to support blood pressure and cover maintenance requirements.

Invasive infections due to *H. influenzae* type b and *N. meningitidis* pose a risk to some close contacts of the index patient.[47,52] For this reason, prophylaxis of some close contacts is recommended to prevent further spread of the infection. However, care must be taken to avoid alarm in hospital staff, families, and the community in general. The risk is significant only for close contacts, but even in those cases the risk is not as high as anxious hospital personnel and families might imagine. For disease due to *H. influenzae* type b, the risk is primarily confined to unimmunized children under 4 years of age; hospital personnel are not at risk. For *H. influenzae* type b prophylaxis, rifampin is given orally once daily for 4 days at a dose of 20 mg/kg (maximum dose 600 mg). For disease due to meningococcus, while the risk for secondary meningococcal infection among household contacts is at least 1000-fold greater than for the public at large, secondary infections occur in less than 5% of cases.[53] Prophylaxis against *H. influenzae* type b and meningococcus should be offered to family contacts and close social contacts such as day care or school classmates, but extending the "net" of prophylaxis beyond that point is rarely indicated. Among hospital personnel, prophylaxis against meningococcus should be offered to health care workers involved in direct contact with the index patient, particularly if the contact

involved tracheal intubation, deep suctioning of the airway, or other direct exposure to the patient's oral secretions.[51] Recommended regimens include rifampin 600 mg every 12 hours for 2 days (5 mg/kg for children < 1 month), a single 500-mg dose of ciprofloxacin, or a single 250-mg dose of intramuscular ceftriaxone (125 mg for children < 15 years). Prophylaxis is not warranted for health care personnel without direct contact with oral secretions. Consultation with public health authorities or an infectious disease expert is recommended to coordinate decisions regarding prophylaxis.

If clinical findings and laboratory data suggest viral meningitis as the diagnosis, further management will depend primarily on the severity of the symptoms. Enterovirus can be isolated in viral culture from CSF in 50% to 70% of patients, but in most cases has little impact on patient management.[54] Polymerase chain reaction has also been described for definitive diagnosis.[55] This diagnostic technique may have more impact on patient management since it can be performed more rapidly. Admission of a patient who is suspected to have viral meningitis is not mandatory. Patients who have mild to moderate symptoms and who are not dehydrated may be candidates for discharge from the emergency department and supportive care at home. Children who are under 1 year of age, children whose diagnosis is uncertain, and children with severe symptoms should be managed as inpatients until preliminary culture data are available. The decision to administer antibiotics to a child with suspected viral meningitis depends on the clinical situation and the likelihood of the diagnosis. If there is significant doubt about the diagnosis, antibiotic therapy should be begun. For particularly severe meningoencephalitis due to Enterovirus, recent studies have shown some benefit from the antiviral agent pleconaril, although it is not yet widely available.[56]

Patients with suspected encephalitis should always be managed as inpatients. Even with optimal management, significant morbidity and mortality do occur, particularly with infections due to eastern equine encephalomyelitis virus and HSV encephalitis. Neurodiagnostic tests such as head CT scanning, magnetic resonance imaging (MRI), and electroencephalography may be helpful in the evaluation of a patient with suspected encephalitis, particularly if the infection is due to HSV.[8] HSV can be isolated from CSF in 50% of cases of neonatal HSV encephalitis but is rarely isolated from older children or adults.[54] Arboviruses are rarely isolated in culture; arboviral encephalitis is diagnosed on the basis of arbovirus-specific immunoglobulin M in spinal fluid. Acyclovir has been shown to improve survival in patients with HSV encephalitis. For this reason, intravenous acyclovir should be considered in patients with a clinical syndrome suggestive of encephalitis. For most cases of encephalitis due to arboviruses, specific antiviral therapy has not been shown to be beneficial, although in vitro data suggest a possible role for ribavirin in West Nile encephalitis and interferon-alfa in both West Nile and St. Louis encephalitis.[9]

Evaluation for brain abscess should include CT or MRI with contrast, which typically shows a ring-enhancing hypodense lesion. Surgical drainage is required in most cases, so neurosurgical consultation should be sought as soon as the diagnosis is confirmed.[19] For brain abscesses associated with sinusits, otitis media, or cyanotic congenital heart disease, the recommended antibiotic regimen is a third-generation cephalosporin plus metronidazole. Alternatives include meropenem and ampicillin/sulbactam. Vancomycin should be added in cases associated with penetrating head trauma, ventriculoperitoneal shunts, endocarditis, and meningitis.[10]

Summary

Children with bacterial meningitis, encephalitis, and brain abscess should all be admitted, preferably to a tertiary care pediatric hospital that can manage complications. Selected patients with viral meningitis may be candidates for outpatient management, but close follow-up should be arranged within 24 hours. Most CNS infections can be diagnosed on the patient's initial presentation. Some, however, present with nonspecific signs and symptoms due to an early stage of disease evolution. In the latter category, "missed" diagnoses are inevitable no matter how astute the physician may be. Physicians can protect themselves from allegations of substandard care in these cases by careful documentation of the visit and by providing thorough discharge instructions.

REFERENCES

1. McCarthy PL: Fever in infants and children. *In* Mackowiak PA (ed): Fever: Basic Mechanisms and Management, 2nd ed. Philadelphia: Lippincott Raven, 1997, pp 351–362.
*2. Schuchat A, Robinson D, Wenger JD, et al: Bacterial meningitis in the United States in 1995. N Engl J Med 337:970–976, 1997.
3. Kaplan SL, Mason EO, Wald ER, et al: Decrease in invasive pneumococcal infections. Pediatrics 113(3 Pt 1):443–449, 2004.
*4. Whitney CG, Farley MM, Hadler J, et al: Decline in invasive pneumococcal disease after the introduction of protein-polysaccharide conjugate vaccine. N Engl J Med 348:1737–1746, 2003.
5. Sawyer MH: Enterovirus infections: diagnosis and treatment. Curr Opin Ped 13:65–69, 2001.
6. Centers for Disease Control and Prevention: Echovirus type 13—United States, 2001. MMWR Morb Mortal Wkly Rep 50:777–780, 2001.
7. Rorabaugh ML, Berlin LE, Heldrich F, et al: Aseptic meningitis in infants younger than 2 years of age: acute illness and neurologic complications. Pediatrics 92:206–211, 1993.
8. Whitley RJ, Gnann JW: Viral encephalitis: familiar infections and emerging pathogens. Lancet 359:507–514, 2002.
9. Gea-Banacloche J, Johnson RT, Bagic A, et al: West Nile virus: pathogenesis and therapeutic options. Ann Intern Med 140:545–553, 2004.
*10. Yogev R, Bar-Meir M: Management of brain abscesses in children. Pediatr Infect Dis J 23:157–159, 2004.
11. Baraff LJ, Bass JS, Fleisher GR, et al: Practice guideline for the management of infants and children 0 to 36 months of age with fever without source. Pediatrics 92:1–12, 1993.
12. Kallio MJT, Kilpi T, Anttila M, et al: The effect of a recent previous visit to a physician on outcome after childhood bacterial meningitis. JAMA 272:787–791, 1994.
13. Kilpi T, Anttila M, Kallio M, et al: Severity of childhood bacterial meningitis and duration of illness before diagnosis. Lancet 338:406–409, 1991.
14. Radetsky M: Duration of symptoms and outcome in bacterial meningitis: an analysis of causation and the implications of a delay in diagnosis. Pediatr Infect Dis J 11:694–698, 1992.
15. Trotter CL, Fox AJ, Ramsay ME, et al: Fatal outcome from meningococcal disease—an association with meningococcal phenotype but not with reduced susceptibility to benzylpenicillin. J Med Microbiol 51:855–860, 2002.
16. Malley R, Inkelis SH, Coelho P, et al: Cerebrospinal fluid pleocytosis and prognosis in invasive meningococcal disease in children. Pediatr Infect Dis J 17:855–859, 1998.
17. Sparling PF: A plethora of host factors that determine the outcome of meningococcal infection. Am J Med 112:72–74, 2002.
18. Read RC, Cannings C, Naylor SC, et al: Variation within genes encoding interleukin-1 and the interleukin-1 receptor antagonist influence the severity of meningococcal disease. Ann Intern Med 138:534–541, 2003.
19. Goodkin HP, Harper MB, Pomeroy SL: Intracerebral abscess in children: historical trends at Children's Hospital Boston. Pediatrics 113:1765–1770, 2004.
20. Watson JT, Gerber SI: West Nile virus: a brief review. Pediatr Infect Dis J 23:357–358, 2004.
21. Bell AH, Brown D, Halliday HL, et al: Meningitis in the newborn—a 14 year review. Arch Dis Child 64:873–874, 1989.
22. Walsh-Kelly C, Nelson DB, Smith DS, et al: Clinical predictors of bacterial versus aseptic meningitis in childhood. Ann Emerg Med 21:910–914, 1992.
23. Rosman NP, Peterson DB, Kaye EM, et al: Seizures in bacterial meningitis: prevalence, patterns, pathogenesis, and prognosis. Pediatr Neurol 1:278–285, 1985.
*24. Green SM, Rothrock SG, Clem KJ, et al: Can seizures be the sole manifestation of meningitis in febrile children? Pediatrics 92:527–534, 1993.
25. American Academy of Pediatrics, Provisional Committee on Quality Improvement: Practice parameter: The neurodiagnostic evaluation of the child with a first simple febrile seizure. Pediatrics 97:769–771, 1996.
26. Cronan KM, Wiley JF: Lumbar puncture. *In* Henretig FM, King C (eds): Textbook of Pediatric Emergency Procedures. Baltimore: Williams & Wilkins, 1997, pp 541–551.
*27. Archer BD: Computed tomography before lumbar puncture in acute meningitis: a review of the risks and benefits. Can Med Assoc J 148:961–965, 1993.
28. Mellor DH: The place of computed tomography and lumbar puncture in suspected bacterial meningitis. Arch Dis Child 67:1417–1419, 1992.
29. Bohr V, Rasmussen N, Hansen B, et al: Eight hundred seventy-five cases of bacterial meningitis: diagnostic procedures and the impact of preadmission antibiotic therapy. J Infect 7:193–202, 1983.
30. Kanegaye JT, Soliemanzadeh P, Bradley JS: Lumbar puncture in pediatric bacterial meningitis: defining the time interval for recovery of cerebrospinal fluid pathogens after parenteral antibiotic pretreatment. Pediatrics 108:1169–1174, 2001.
31. Nechyba C: Blood chemistry and body fluids. *In* Gunn VL, Nechyba C (eds): Harriet Lane Handbook, 16th ed. St. Louis: Mosby–Year Book, 2002, p 557.
32. Sivakmaran M: Meningococcal meningitis revisited: normocellular CSF. Clin Pediatr 36:258–262, 1997.
33. Marton KI, Gean AD: The spinal tap: a new look at an old test. Ann Intern Med 104:840–848, 1986.
34. Hristeva L, Bowler I, Booy R, et al: Value of cerebrospinal fluid examination in the diagnosis of meningitis of the newborn. Arch Dis Child 69:514–517, 1993.
35. Blazer S, Berant M, Alon U: Bacterial meningitis: effect of antibiotic treatment on CSF. Am J Clin Pathol 80:386, 1983.
*36. Wang VJ, Kuppermann N, Malley R, et al: Meningococcal disease among children who live in a large metropolitan area, 1981–1996. Clin Infect Dis 32:1004–1009, 2001.
37. Freedman SB, Marrocco A, Pirie J, et al: Predictors of bacterial meningitis in the era after *Haemophilus influenzae*. Arch Pediatr Adolesc Med 155:1301–1310, 2001.
*38. Nigrovic LE, Kuppermann N, Malley R: Development and validation of a multivariable predictive model to distinguish bacterial from aseptic meningitis in the post-*Haemophilus influenzae* era. Pediatrics 110:712–719, 2002.
39. Nigrovic LE, Kupperman N, Macias CG, et al: Clinical prediction rule for identifying children with cerebrospinal fluid pleocytosis at very low risk of bacterial meningitis. JAMA 297:52–60, 2007.
40. Meadow WL, Lantos J, Tanz R, et al: Ought 'standard care' be 'standard of care'? Am J Dis Child 147:40–43, 1993.
41. Odio CM, Puig JR, Feris JM, et al: Prospective, randomized, investigator-blinded study of the efficacy and safety of meropenem vs. cefotaxime therapy in bacterial meningitis in children. Pediatr Infect Dis J 18:581–590, 1999.
42. Kaplan SL: Management of pneumococcal meningitis. Pediatr Infect Dis J 21:589–592, 2002.

*Selected readings.

43. Feigin RD: Use of corticosteroids in bacterial meningitis. Pediatr Infect Dis J 23:355–357, 2004.
44. Lebel MH, Freij BJ, Syrogiannopoulos GA, et al: Dexamethasone therapy for bacterial meningitis: results of two double-blind, placebo-controlled trials. N Engl J Med 319:964, 1988.
45. Havens PL, Wendelberger KJ, Hoffman GM, et al: Corticosteroids as adjunctive therapy in bacterial meningitis. Am J Dis Child 143:1051–1055, 1989.
46. McIntyre PB, Berkey CS, King SM, et al: Dexamethasone as adjunctive therapy in bacterial meningitis. JAMA 278:925–931, 1997.
47. American Academy of Pediatrics: *Haemophilus influenzae* infections. *In* Pickering LK (ed): 2003 Red Book: Report of the Committee on Infectious Diseases, 26th ed. Elk Grove Village, IL: American Academy of Pediatrics, 2006, pp 310–318.
48. American Academy of Pediatrics: Pneumococcal infections. *In* Pickering LK (ed): 2003 Red Book: Report of the Committee on Infectious Diseases, 26th ed. Elk Grove Village, IL: American Academy of Pediatrics, 2006, pp 525–537.
*49. Singhi SC, Singhi PD, Srinivas B, et al: Fluid restriction does not improve the outcome of acute meningitis. Pediatr Infect Dis J 14:495–503, 1995.
50. Duke T: Fluid management of bacterial meningitis in developing countries. Arch Dis Child 79:181–185, 1998.
51. Powell KR, Sugarman LI, Eskenazi AE, et al: Normalization of plasma arginine vasopressin concentrations when children with meningitis are given maintenance plus replacement fluid therapy. J Pediatr 117:515–522, 1990.
52. American Academy of Pediatrics: Meningococcal infections. *In* Pickering LK (ed): 2003 Red Book: Report of the Committee on Infectious Diseases, 26th ed. Elk Grove Village, IL: American Academy of Pediatrics, 2003, pp 430–436.
53. Anderson MS, Glode MP, Smith AL: Meningococcal disease. *In* Feigin RD, Cherry JD, Demmler GJ, Kaplan SL (eds): Textbook of Pediatric Infectious Diseases. Philadelphia: Elsevier, 2004, pp 1265–1280.
54. Gutierrez KM, Prober CG: Encephalitis. Postgrad Med 103:123–143, 1998.
55. Lukeman FD, Whitley RJ, for the National Institute of Allergy and Infectious Diseases Collaborative Antiviral Study Group: Diagnosis of herpes simplex encephalitis: application of polymerase chain reaction to cerebrospinal fluid from brain-biopsied patients and correlation with disease. J Infect Dis 171:857, 1995.
56. Rotbart, HA, Webster AD, for the Pleconaril Treatment Registry Group: Treatment of potentially life-threatening enterovirus infections with pleconaril. Clin Infect Dis 32:228–235, 2001.

Chapter 44

Central Nervous System Vascular Disorders

Stuart Lewena, MBBS and Franz E. Babl, MD, MPH

Key Points

Failure to recognize the signs and symptoms of strokes in children leads to a delay in diagnosis.

The disease and conditions predisposing children to strokes are numerous and diverse.

For most cases of pediatric stroke, there is no evidence-based treatment.

Introduction and Background

A stroke is "a condition with sudden onset caused by acute vascular lesions of the brain."[1] These brain lesions can be broadly classified as either ischemic or hemorrhagic. While the vast majority of strokes in adults are ischemic and due to atherosclerosis,[7] strokes in children are more evenly divided between ischemic and hemorrhagic types and are due to a wide range of causes.[3,4] Unfortunately, due to the relative rarity of strokes in children and clinical presentations that frequently differ from those of most adults with stroke, the diagnosis is often delayed in children.[5] Increased awareness and understanding of pediatric strokes could lead to more prompt diagnoses and improved emergency department care.

Recognition and Approach

The overall incidence of pediatric stroke is between 2 and 8 cases per 100,000 population per year.[3,4,6-8] Neonates and infants account for about one third of all pediatric strokes.[8,9] There are specific risk factors that place children at risk for strokes (Table 44–1).

Ischemic Strokes

Risk factors that place infants and children at risk for ischemic stroke include congenital cardiac diseases, sickle cell disease, arteriopathies, traumatic arterial dissections, and prothrombotic disorders. Approximately 20% to 30% of children with ischemic stroke have a congenital cardiac disease.[8-10] Complex cardiac anomalies constitute the greatest risk, but almost any lesion may be implicated. The nature of the lesion is usually known prior to the diagnosis of stroke. Children rarely present with stroke due to previously undiagnosed congenital heart disease. Cardiogenic emboli and polycythemia of cyanotic heart disease predispose to both embolic and thrombotic strokes.

Sickle cell disease is an extremely common cause of pediatric stroke in communities where this condition is prevalent, accounting for up to one third of cases in some studies.[11] Approximately 10% of children with sickle cell disease will suffer a stroke at some time before 20 years of age.[12] While the exact pathophysiology remains unclear, anemia, microvascular occlusion, and endothelial damage from sickled cells are all likely to play a role. There is much interest in identifying which children with sickle cell disease are most at risk. The Childhood Arterial Stroke Guideline,[13] developed by the British Paediatric Neurology Association, recommends annual screening from the age of 3 years for changes in internal carotid artery or middle cerebral artery flow velocity. Approximately 8% of children with sickle cell disease have velocities greater than 200 cm/sec, and children in this group have only a 60% probability of remaining stroke free over the next 40 months.[14] Other risk factors in sickle cell disease are thought to include nocturnal hypoxemia and depressed protein C and protein S levels[15,16] (see Chapter 127, Sickle Cell Disease).

An increasing number of children with ischemic stroke are identified as having preexisting vascular disease on the basis of conventional or magnetic angiographic studies.[17,18] In one study of arterial stroke using contrast angiography, 53% of children had arteriopathies.[19] These arteriopathies included arterial dissections and progressive vasculopathies, including moyamoya disease, and a significant number were classified as idiopathic intracranial arterial disease. An episode of preceding cerebral vasculitis is thought to explain some of these cases. It is through this mechanism that varicella-zoster virus is thought to predispose to stroke in the year following chickenpox infection.

Approximately 10% of ischemic strokes in children can be attributed to arterial dissection and subsequent thromboembolism. Intracranial and extracranial vessels may be affected, with trauma more likely to be implicated in extracranial

Table 44–1	Underlying Conditions That Place Children at Increased Risk for Stroke

Cardiac Disorders

Congenital heart disease
Endocarditis
Cardiomyopathies
Arrhythmias

Central Nervous System Vasculopathies

Congenital lesions
Vasculitis
Traumatic vascular injuries
Idiopathic

Hematologic Conditions

Sickle cell disease
Leukemia
Platelet disorders
Hemophilia
Factor V Leiden
Protein C deficiency
Protein S deficiency
Activated protein C resistance
Prothrombin disorders
Increased lipoprotein (a)
Hypercholesterolemia syndromes

Infectious Diseases

Sepsis
Intracranial infections

Metabolic Conditions

Homocystinuria
Organic acidemias
"Metabolic stroke"*

*The term *metabolic stroke* refers to a range of mitochondrial disorders that produce stroke through disrupting neuronal cellular metabolism directly rather than via a vascular event.

dissections. Trauma-associated dissections most frequently follow trivial head and neck trauma resulting in small intimal tears. The time from traumatic event until onset of neurologic symptoms is highly variable, with the peak risk period being 1 to 7 days.[20,21] There is a significant male predominance that cannot be explained by trauma alone, suggesting a sex-linked vascular predisposition. In contrast to adults, children with cerebrovascular dissection rarely present with warning symptoms of headache or neck pain in the absence of neurologic deficit. Hemiparesis at presentation is the most common clinical finding.

In addition to nonspecific prothrombotic states associated with conditions including malignancy and hematologic disorders, an increasing number of specific prothrombotic disorders are being recognized.[22-24] Several factors predispose to sinovenous thrombosis in the neonatal period. Severe birth asphyxia and maternal preeclampsia are common associations. Prothrombotic abnormalities are said to occur in 20% of neonates with sinovenous thrombosis, although the precise role these conditions play in this disorder is uncertain.[25]

Causes of sinovenous thrombosis beyond the neonatal period are more relevant to the emergency physician. Head and neck infections and systemic illness with dehydration or bacterial sepsis would remove risk factors. Frequent presentations include headache, papilledema, seizures, sixth nerve palsies, and visual disturbances.

Hemorrhagic Stroke

Arteriovenous malformation is the most common cause of hemorrhagic stroke in childhood beyond the neonatal period.[10] Other frequent causes of nontraumatic intracranial hemorrhage include aneurysms, bleeding into tumors, and coagulopathies, including various causes of thrombocytopenia, hemophilia, and von Willebrand's disease (see Chapter 45, Brain Tumor; and Chapter 130, Disorders of Coagulation). Previously, about 25% of spontaneous intracranial hemorrhages were idiopathic; however, the utilization of better and more extensive investigation has decreased this number to approximately 10%.[3,26] Small arteriovenous malformations have a greater risk of hemorrhage than large ones, and preceding warning symptoms are less frequently recognized than in the adult population.

Clinical Presentation

Children with stroke are less likely to present with a well-defined neurologic deficit than adults. Subtle isolated single limb weakness, incoordination, and sensory disturbances are often initially attributed to causes other than stroke in young children. Frequently cited alternative diagnoses include presumed soft tissue injury, normal "clumsiness," and behavioral problems.[5] Up to a third of children who have had a stroke will have a history of recent events consistent with transient ischemic attacks.[9] The younger the child, the more likely gross neurologic deficits will be present at the time of diagnosis and earlier subtler signs and symptoms will have been missed.

To some extent, the presentation of pediatric stroke is age dependent. An understanding of the developmental abilities of children at different ages is quite helpful in evaluating children for stroke. Neonates and young infants frequently present with lethargy, coma, and seizures. Older infants and children more often present with hemiparesis or a gross, focal motor deficit. Subtle signs at presentation are generally only appreciated in older children and adolescents.[9]

Diagnostic tests, including imaging studies, are helpful for narrowing the differential diagnosis, confirming the diagnosis of stroke, differentiating hemorrhagic stroke from ischemic stroke, and guiding the emergency department management. By far the most useful tests for establishing the diagnosis of stroke are imaging studies. Particularly useful for identifying hemorrhagic stroke is computed tomography (CT) scanning of the head. In most emergency departments, CT scanning of these children can be performed promptly, especially with the aid of procedural sedation (see Chapter 159, Procedural Sedation and Analgesia). For ischemic strokes, magnetic resonance imaging (MRI) of the brain is usually indicated when CT scanning does not reveal acute hemorrhage. Further imaging, including standard or magnetic resonance angiography, may be helpful to neurosurgical consultants for their management plans.[27,28] Once a pediatric stroke has been identified, multiple studies may be helpful for the ongoing inpatient evaluation and management of these children.[23] However, for most cases, the results of these studies will not have an impact on emergency department care.

Important Clinical Features and Considerations

Migraine is a condition that warrants specific consideration. Complicated migraines in which the patient presents with focal neurologic abnormalities may initially be diagnosed as stroke. A classic history with aura or other migraine-associated symptoms is frequently absent in children with migrane headaches.[29] The neurologic deficit may last from hours to days and can vary from subtle abnormalities to dense hemiplegia. In cases in which this is suspected, early neuroimaging is still required to exclude a central nervous system vascular event or other intracranial pathology before expectant management may be safely pursued. Further complicating this entity is the possibility of migraine actually causing an ischemic stroke. While accepted in the adult population,[30,31] the development of cerebral infarction as a consequence of migraine in childhood has not been definitively described. Several small studies, however, support the concept.[29,32]

Management

For many children suspected of having a stroke, the initial treatment and resuscitation follow the same basic principles as those for other serious medical conditions (see Chapter 9, Cerebral Resuscitation; Chapter 11, Altered Mental Status/Coma; and Chapter 40, Seizures). For children with sickle cell disease and stroke, exchange transfusion is the treatment of choice (see Chapter 127, Sickle Cell Disease). For arteriovenous malformations and leaking intracranial aneurysms, specific treatments such as coil embolization and aneurysmal clipping are performed by pediatric neurosurgeons.[33,34] For other children, specific acute stroke interventions have not been adequately studied. The use of antiplatelet agents, heparin, low-molecular-weight heparin, anticoagulants, and thrombolytics is not supported by adequate evidence to make any general recommendations.[35-37] The small case series that do suggest benefit with these therapies tend to focus on prevention of further stroke rather than acute benefits. The conditions with consensus statements supporting the use of anticoagulation are ischemic stroke secondary to arterial dissection and cerebral venous sinus thrombosis.[13,20] In the absence of any prospective trials, the decision regarding use of any form of anticoagulation needs to be made on a case-by-case basis.

Summary

The delay in recognition and diagnosis of stroke in children contributes to the significant neurologic deficits that are established by the time of presentation. Although the majority of patients experience some improvement, some permanent disability occurs in 50% to 80% of children who experience strokes.[8,10] Overall mortality is 5% to 10%. Mortality is as high as 21% in cases of hemorrhagic stroke secondary to arteriovenous malformations.[8,38] Stroke recurrence occurs in 8% of children with a single risk factor and in up to 42% of those with multiple risk factors.[39] For most cases of pediatric stroke, there is no evidence-based treatment.

REFERENCES

1. Anderson DM, Novak PD, Keith J, et al (eds): Dorland's Illustrated Medical Dictionary, 30th ed. Philadelphia: WB Saunders, 2003, p 1833.
2. Truelsen T, Piechowski-Jozwiak B, Bonita R, et al: Stroke incidence and prevalence in Europe: a review of available data. Eur J Neurol 13:581–598, 2006.
3. Schoenberg B, Mellinger J, Schoenberg D: Cerebrovascular disease in infants and children: a study of incidence, clinical features and survival. Neurology 28:763–768, 1978.
4. Giroud M, Lemesle M, Gouyon JB, et al: Cerebrovascular disease in children under 16 years of age in the city of Dijon, France: a study of incidence and clinical features from 1985 to 1993. J Clin Epidemiol 48:1343–1348, 1995.
5. Gabis L, Yangala R, Lenn N: Time lag to diagnosis of stroke in children. Pediatrics 110:924–928, 2002.
*6. Fullerton H, Wu Y, Zhao S, et al: Risk of stroke in children. Neurology 61:189–194, 2003.
7. Broderick J, Talbot TG, Prenger E, et al: Stroke in children within a major metropolitan area: the surprising importance of intracerebral hemorrhage. J Child Neurol 8:250–255, 1993.
*8. Barnes C, Newall F, Furmedge J, et al: Arterial ischemic stroke in children. J Paediatr Child Health 40:384–387, 2004.
9. De Veber G: Stroke and the child's brain: an overview of epidemiology, syndromes and risk factors. Neurology 15:133–138, 2002.
*10. Calder K, Kokorowski P, Tran T, et al: Emergency department presentation of pediatric stroke. Pediatr Emerg Care 19:320–328, 2003.
11. Obama MT, Dongmo L, Nkemayim C, et al: Stroke in children in Yaounde, Cameroon. Indian Pediatr 31:791–795, 1994.
12. Powars D, Wilson B, Imbus C, et al: The natural history of stroke in sickle cell disease. Am J Med 65:467–471, 1978.
13. Baumer JH: Childhood arterial stroke. Arch Dis Child Educ Pract Ed 89:ep50–ep53, 2004.
14. Adams RJ, McKie VC, Carl EM, et al: Long-term stroke risk in children with sickle cell disease screened with transcranial Doppler. Ann Neurol 42:699–704, 1997.
15. Kirkham FJ, Hewes DK, Prengler M, et al: Nocturnal hypoxaemia and central nervous system events in sickle cell disease. Lancet 357:1656–1659, 2001.
16. Tam DA: Protein C and protein S activity in sickle cell disease and stroke. J Child Neurol 12:19–21, 1997.
17. Shirane R, Sato S, Yoshimoto T: Angiographic findings of ischemic stroke in children. Childs Nerv Syst 8:432–436, 1992.
18. Chabrier S, Rodesch G, Lasjaunias P: Transient cerebral arteriopathy: a disorder recognized by serial angiograms in children with stroke. J Child Neurol 13:27–32, 1998.
19. Chabrier S, Husson B, Lasjaunias P, et al: Stroke in childhood: outcome and recurrence risk by mechanism in 59 patients. J Child Neurol 15:290–294, 2000.
20. Fullerton H, Johnstone C, Smith W: Arterial dissection and stroke in children. Neurology 57:1155–1160, 2001.
21. Payton TF, Siddiqui KM, Sole DP, et al: Traumatic dissection of the internal carotid artery. Pediatr Emerg Care 20:27–29, 2004.
22. Kirkham F: Is there a genetic basis for pediatric stroke? Curr Opin Pediatr 15:547–558, 2003.
23. Barreirinho S, Ferro A, Santos M, et al: Inherited and acquired risk factors and their combined effects in pediatric stroke. Pediatr Neurol 28:134–138, 2003.
24. Ganesan V, Prengler M, McShane M, et al: Investigation of risk factors in children with arterial ischemic stroke. Ann Neurol 53:167–173, 2003.
25. De Veber G, Andrew M, Canadian Pediatric Ischemic Stroke Study Group: Cerebral sinovenous thrombosis in children. N Engl J Med 345:417–423, 2001.
26. Al-Jarallah A, Al-Rifai M, Riela A, et al: Non traumatic brain hemorrhage in children: etiology and presentation. J Child Neurol 15:284–289, 2000.
27. Hunter JV: Magnetic resonance imaging in pediatric stroke. Top Magn Reson Imaging 13:23–28, 2002.
28. Husson B, Rodesch G, Lasjaunias P, et al: Magnetic resonance angiography in childhood arterial brain infarcts. Stroke 33:1280–1285, 2002.
29. Ebinger F, Boor R, Gawehn J, et al: Ischemic stroke and migraine in childhood: coincidence or causal relation? J Child Neurol 14:451–455, 1999.
30. Broderick JP, Swanson JW: Migraine-related strokes. Arch Neurol 44:868–871, 1987.
31. Rothrock JF, Walicke P, Swenson MR, et al: Migrainous stroke. Arch Neurol 45:63–67, 1988.

*Selected readings.

32. Wober-Bingol C, Wober C, Karwautz A, et al: Migraine and stroke in childhood and adolescence. Cephalalgia 15:26–30, 1995.
33. Blount JP, Oakes WJ, Tubbs RS, et al: History of surgery for cerebrovascular disease in children, Part 1. Intracranial arterial aneurysms. Neursurg Focus 2:E9, 2006.
34. Blount JP, Oakes WJ, Tubbs RS, et al: History of surgery for cerebrovascular disease in children, Part III. Arteriovenous malformations. Neurosurg Focus 20:E11, 2006.
35. Nowak-Gottl U, Straeter R, Sebire G, et al: Antithrombotic drug treatment of pediatric patients with ischemic stroke. Pediatr Drugs 5:167–175, 2003.
36. Adams H: Emergent use of anticoagulation for treatment of patients with ischemic stroke. Stroke 33:856–861, 2002.
*37. Burak C, Bowen M, Barron T: The use of enoxaparin in children with acute, nonhemorrhagic stroke. Pediatr Neurol 29:295–298, 2003.
38. Celli P, Ferrante L, Palma L, et al: Cerebral arteriovenous malformations in children: clinical features and outcome of treatment in children and adults. Surg Neurol 22:43–49, 1984.
39. Lanthier S, Carmant L, David M, et al: Stroke in children: the coexistence of multiple risk factors predicts poor outcome. Neurology 54:371–378, 2000.

Chapter 45

Brain Tumor

Ann Klasner, MD, MPH

Key Points

Brain tumors are the most common solid tumors of childhood.

The diagnosis of a pediatric brain tumor is often delayed due to the insidious onset of symptoms.

A computed tomographic scan of the head without contrast is a useful screening tool for identifying brain tumors in children presenting to the emergency department.

Prompt and early consultation with a pediatric neurosurgeon is indicated once the diagnosis of a pediatric brain tumor has been made.

Introduction and Background

Brain tumors are the most common solid tumors identified in children.[1,2] Of all cancers, only leukemia is more common than brain tumors. Unfortunately, the presentation of these tumors is often insidious. This frequently leads to a delay in diagnosis.

Recognition and Approach

Pediatric brain tumors represent 16% to 20% of all childhood cancers. Incidence rates range between 2.8 and 4.3 cases per 100,000 children per year.[1,2] Brain tumors are classified by histology and location within the cranium. Five major histologic categories represent 80% of all pediatric brain tumors: juvenile pilocytic astrocytoma (20%), diffuse astrocytoma (22%), medulloblastoma/primitive neuroectodermal tumor (23%), ependymoma (8%), and craniopharyngioma (7%).[2] Notably, nearly half of all pediatric brain tumors are astrocytomas. In general, pediatric brain tumors are nearly evenly divided between infratentorial and supratentorial locations, with a small percentage involving multiple locations within the central nervous system. The location of pediatric brain tumors varies by age. More tumors are located in the supratentorial space in the first year of life and in children older than 10 years.[3 6] The location of the tumor is helpful in predicting and explaining the signs and symptoms with which a child may present.

Clinical Presentation

The clinical signs and symptoms of pediatric brain tumors are dependent on the age of the child, the location of the tumor, and the size of the tumor. In infants, the signs and symptoms are nonspecific and mimic other disorders. The most common presenting signs and symptoms in infants include irritability, listlessness, vomiting, a bulging fontanelle, increased head circumference, head tilt, and behavioral changes.[3,4] As children age, the signs and symptoms generally become more specific and localizing. Younger children will have bouts of nausea and vomiting, and may complain of headaches. In school-age children and adolescents, the dominant presenting signs and symptoms include seizures, focal neurologic deficits, and ataxia.[7,8] Supratentorial tumors may compress adjacent structures and produce signs such as vision changes or abnormal eye movements, personality changes, aphasia, and seizures. Children with infratentorial tumors are likely to display signs such as ataxia, hemiparesis, and neck pain due to cerebellar tonsil herniation. Any intracranial tumor may obstruct cerebrospinal fluid flow and cause increased intracranial pressure. These children are likely to present with headache and vomiting early in the course and depressed mental status as the obstruction progresses (see Chapter 42, Conditions Causing Increased Intracranial Pressure).

Specific syndromes associated with brain tumors have been described. For example, a common presentation of pineal tumors is Parinaud's syndrome.[9] This syndrome is characterized by paralysis of upward gaze, eyelid retraction, convergence-retraction nystagmus, and pupils reactive to accommodation but not to light directly. Another example seen in infants with suprasellar tumors is diencephalic syndrome characterized by failure to thrive, emaciation, increased appetite, and a euphoric affect.[10] This syndrome may also be referred to as Russell's syndrome.[11] Diabetes insipidus may arise from suprasellar and third ventricle tumors.[12]

Adult and pediatric brain tumors have several major differences. Adults are more likely to have intracranial metastases from a distant primary cancer. The histologic types of tumors found in children and adults are different. The most common primary brain tumors in adults are gliomas and central nervous system lymphoma.[13] The location of the tumors also differs, with posterior fossa tumors being much more common in children. Children derive greater benefit from resection and have increased survival rates with chemotherapy.[5]

The key to evaluating a child suspected of having a brain tumor is neuroimaging. In the emergency department, a noncontrast computed tomographic scan of the head is helpful in identifying ventricular enlargement suggestive of cerebrospinal fluid obstruction. Mass effect with edema may also be identified even if the tumor itself is poorly visualized on the scan. Although not typically obtained during the emergency department evaluation of children suspected of having a brain tumor, a magnetic resonance image of the brain is indicated early in the hospital course.

Important Clinical Features and Considerations

Given the vague, nonspecific, and varied presentations of pediatric brain tumors, the number of conditions on the initial differential diagnosis for these children is long. These conditions include meningitis, failure to thrive, abusive head injury, the ingestion of drugs or toxins, adverse effects from vaccinations, postviral illness, gastroesophageal reflux, subarachnoid hemorrhage, and vascular headache.[3,14-18] Only one third of pediatric brain tumors are diagnosed in the first month after the onset of signs and symptoms. On average, there is a 30- to 60-day delay in diagnosis from the onset of symptoms.[1,7,19,20] Two symptoms that are very confusing are headache and vomiting.

Although children with brain tumors may complain of headaches, headaches are seldom due to brain tumors. One study of pediatric headaches found that 7% of cases harbored a serious neurologic diagnosis, but most of these were cases of viral meningitis.[21] These researchers did not identify any children with brain tumors. In another study of 104 children younger than 7 years with headaches as their main complaint, no brain tumors were identified.[22] It may be the case that headaches with a normal neurologic examination are extremely unlikely to be associated with a brain tumor. In a study of 72 children who had headaches and brain tumors, 69 (96%) exhibited focal neurologic or ocular findings.[23] In the setting of a child with a headache, findings suggestive of a brain tumor include a change in the quality or location of the pain, an abnormal oculomotor examination, and an abnormal neurologic examination.[8,21,23,24]

Just like headaches, many children with brain tumors will exhibit vomiting, but few vomiting children have brain tumors. At the time of initial presentation, 60% to 80% of children with brain tumors will have a history of vomiting.[1,7,23,25] Unfortunately, vomiting is common throughout childhood and is a feature in many illnesses, including atypical migraines headaches.[25] The signs and symptoms associated with vomiting that raise the likelihood of a brain tumor being present include the absence of fever and diarrhea, lethargy that does not improve or worsens with rehydration, a head tilt, and an abnormal neurologic examination.[17,23]

Lumbar puncture has no role in the initial diagnosis of pediatric brain tumors. However, prior to the correct diagnosis being made, a lumbar puncture may be performed during an effort to rule out other diagnoses such as meningitis or a subarachnoid hemorrhage. No definitive information exists regarding the risk of brain herniation in the setting of a lumbar puncture being performed on a child with an undiagnosed brain tumor.[18,26-29] It may be the case that, for children who are stable and have an abnormal neurologic examination, a noncontrast computed tomographic scan of the head prior to lumbar puncture is indicated.[30]

Management

There is no specific emergency department treatment for pediatric brain tumors. Critically ill children with brain tumors are managed similarly to other critically ill children (see Chapter 11, Altered Mental Status/Coma; and Chapter 42, Conditions Causing Increased Intracranial Pressure). Consultation with a pediatric neurosurgeon is indicated for all newly identified brain tumors. The urgency of the consultation is related to the severity of the child's overall clinical condition. Awake and stable children may require a phone conversation between the emergency physician and the pediatric neurosurgeon to arrange outpatient follow-up. Obtunded children typically require prompt transport to a tertiary care pediatric facility and emergent consultation.

Treatment of pediatric brain tumors includes surgical resection, radiation, and chemotherapy. Treatment choices depend on location of tumor, age of the child, and type of tumor. Surgery provides and may also be either palliative or curative depending on the type of tumor. With the advent of stereotactic biopsy and endoscopy, minimally invasive surgery is now possible. The effectiveness of radiation therapy and chemotherapy to treat pediatric brain tumors has dramatically improved in the last decade. Radiation therapy has witnessed improvements in delivery with focal irradiation and lower dosing options. Chemotherapy is playing an increasingly import role in the care of children with brain tumors as it avoids the risk of radiation injury to the developing nervous system. On average, 25% of patients undergo surgical resection alone, 40% require surgery plus radiation, and 30% require surgery, radiation, and chemotherapy.[31]

The emergency physician may see children with brain tumors at nearly any stage in the disease from making the initial diagnosis to managing serious complications near the end of life. The overall 5-year survival rate for all pediatric brain tumors is approximately 70%. However, there is considerable variation depending on the type of tumor, completeness of excision, and patient age.[32,33] Up to 50% of survivors have long-term sequelae from either the tumor, the treatment, or both. Almost 45% of patients have one or more endocrine issues, including hypothyroidism, growth failure, delayed puberty, and osteoporosis. These children may be on hormone replacement therapy. Late cardiovascular complications are seen in 18% of survivors, including blood clots, strokes, and angina.[33] Whole-brain radiation has been shown to have deleterious effects on cognitive functioning, with younger children being the most profoundly affected.[4,31,33-35] Steroid use is fairly routine in the perioperative period. Steroids decrease brain edema, which may exacerbate the neurologic impairment resulting from surgical resection or from the presence of the tumor. The most commonly used steroid is dexamethasone[5,36] (see Chapter 107, The Steroid-Dependent Child). These children may be on antiepileptic drugs. They may also have a ventriculoperitoneal shunt (see Chapter 42, Conditions Causing Increased Intracranial Pressure).

Summary

Brain tumors are the most common solid tumor in children. The overall 5-year survival rate is 70%, but there is wide variation in survival based type of tumor, completeness of excision, and patient age. Morbidity from pediatric brain tumors is quite high, with half of the survivors having long-term effects from the tumor, the treatment, or both. Early consultation with a pediatric neurosurgeon is indicated in all cases of newly discovered pediatric brain tumors.

REFERENCES

*1. Mehta V, Chapman A, McNeely PD, et al: Latency between symptom onset and diagnosis of pediatric brain tumors: an eastern Canadian geographic study. Neurosurgery 51:365–373, 2002.

2. Bunin G: What causes childhood brain tumors? Limited knowledge, many clues. Pediatr Neurosurg 32:321–326, 2000.

3. Gordon GS, Wallace SJ, Neal JW: Intracranial tumours during the first two years of life: presenting features. Arch Dis Child 73:345–347, 1995.

*4. Reed UC, Rosemberg S, Gherpelli JL, et al: Brain tumors in the first two years of life: a review of forty cases. Pediatr Neurosurg 19:180–185, 1993.

*5. Pollack IF: Pediatric brain tumors. Semin Surg Oncol 16:73–90, 1999.

*6. Albright AL: Pediatric brain tumors. CA Cancer J Clin 43:272–288, 1993.

7. Halperin EC, Watson DM, George SL: Duration of symptoms prior to diagnosis is related inversely to presenting disease stage in children with medulloblastoma. Cancer 91:1444–1450, 2001.

8. Gilles FH, Sobel E, Leviton A, et al: Epidemiology of seizures in children with brain tumors. The Childhood Brain Tumor Consortium. J Neurooncol 12:53–68, 1992.

9. Kageyama N, Kobayashi T, Kida Y, et al: Intracranial germinal tumors. Prog Exp Tumor Res 30:255–267, 1987.

10. Fleischman A, Brue C, Poussaint TY, et al: Diencephalic syndrome: a cause of failure to thrive and a model of partial growth hormone resistance. Pediatrics 115: 742–748, 2005.

11. Russell A: A diencephalic syndrome of emaciation in infancy and childhood. Arch Dis Child 26: 274, 1951.

12. Imura H, Kato Y, Nakai Y: Endocrine aspects of tumors arising from suprasellar, third ventricular regions. Prog Exp Tumor Res 30:313–324, 1987.

13. Behin A, Hoang-Xuan K, Carpentier AF, et al: Primary brain tumours in adults. Lancet 361:323–331, 2003.

14. Shemie S, Jay V, Rutka J, et al: Acute obstructive hydrocephalus and sudden death in children. Ann Emerg Med 29:524–528, 1997.

15. Davis DP, Marino A: Acute cerebellar ataxia in a toddler: case report and literature review. J Emerg Med 24:281–284, 2003.

16. Cupini LM, Santorelli FM, Iani C, et al: Cyclic vomiting syndrome, migraine, and epilepsy: a common underlying disorder? Headache 43:407–409, 2003.

17. Squires RH: Intracranial tumors: vomiting as a presenting sign. A gastroenterologist's perspective. Clin Pediatr 28:351–354, 1989.

18. Opeskin K, Anderson RM, Lee KA: Colloid cyst of the 3rd ventricle as a cause of acute neurological deterioration and sudden death. J Paediatr Child Health 29:476–477, 1993.

19. Dobrovoljac M, Hengartner H, Boltshauser E, et al: Delay in the diagnosis of paediatric brain tumours. Eur J Pediatr 161:663–667, 2002.

20. Flores LE, Williams DL, Bell BA, et al: Delay in the diagnosis of pediatric brain tumors. Am J Dis Child 140:684–686, 1986.

*21. Burton LJ, Quinn B, Pratt-Cheney JL, et al: Headache etiology in a pediatric emergency department. Pediatr Emerg Care 13:1–4, 1997.

*22. Chu ML, Shinnar S: Headaches in children younger than 7 years of age. Arch Neurol 49:79–82, 1992.

*23. Honig PJ, Charney EB: Children with brain tumor headaches: distinguishing features. Am J Dis Child 136:121–124, 1982.

24. Pfund Z, Szapáry L, Jászberényi O, et al: Headache in intracranial tumors. Cephalagia 19:787–790, 1999.

*25. Edgeworth J, Bullock P, Bailey A, et al: Why are brain tumours still being missed? Arch Dis Child 74:148–151, 1996.

26. Evan RW: Complications of lumbar puncture. Neurol Clin 16:83–105, 1998.

27. Zisfein J, Tuchman AJ: Risks of lumbar puncture in the presence of intracranial mass lesions. Mt Sinai J Med 55:283–287, 1988.

28. Duffy GP: Lumbar puncture in the presence of raised intracranial pressure. BMJ 1:407–409, 1969.

29. Duffy GP: Lumbar puncture in the spontaneous subarachnoid hemorrhage. BMJ 285:1163–1164, 1982.

*30. Silvers SM, Simmons B, Wall S, et al: Clinical Policy: critical issues in the evaluation and management of patients presenting to the emergency department with acute headache. Ann Emerg Med 39:108–121, 2002.

*31. Spiegler BJ, Bouffer E, Greenberg ML, et al: Change in neurocognitive functioning after treatment with cranial radiation in childhood. J Clin Oncol 22:706–713, 2004.

*32. Gurney JG, Kadan-Lottick NS, Packer RJ, et al: Endocrine and cardiovascular late effects among adult survivors of childhood brain tumors: Childhood Cancer Survivor Study. Cancer 97:663–673, 2003.

33. Packer RJ, Gurney JG, Punyko JA, et al: Long-term neurologic and neurosensory sequelae in adult survivors of a childhood brain tumor: Childhood Cancer Survivor Study. J Clin Oncol 21:255–261, 2003.

34. Glaser AW, Buxton N, Walker D: Corticosteroids in the management of central nervous system tumours. Arch Dis Child 76:76–78, 1997.

35. Radcliffe J, Packer RJ, Atkins TE, et al: Three- and four-year cognitive outcome in children with noncortical brain tumors treated with whole-brain radiation. Ann Neurol 32:551–554, 1992.

*36. Mulhern RK, Merchant TE, Gajjar A, et al: Late neurocognitive sequelae in survivors of brain tumor in childhood. Lancet Oncol 5:399–408, 2004.

*Selected readings.

Chapter 46

Disorders of Movement

Martin I. Herman, MD and Barry G. Gilmore, MD

Key Points

Disorders of movement can present to the emergency department as new complaints or as an exacerbation of a known condition.

Without a prior diagnosis, the etiologies of movement disorders are difficult to differentiate.

For children with disorders of movement, the gait is often the most revealing part of the physical examination.

The etiologies of movement disorders in children are diverse.

Selected Diagnoses

Postinfectious acute cerebellar ataxia
Acute disseminated encephalomyelitis
Acute dystonia
Huntington's disease
Sydenham's chorea
Tourette's syndrome

Discussion of Individual Diagnoses

Postinfectious Acute Cerebellar Ataxia

Postinfectious acute cerebellar ataxia is the most common cause of acute ataxia in children.[1] Most cases occur in the second year of life.[2] Seventy-five percent of patients report an antecedent febrile illness within the 3 weeks preceding the onset of ataxia. About half of the patients will have nystagmus. A staggering gait, dysarthria, and truncal ataxia are the characteristic features.[2] Peripheral white blood cell counts are expected to be normal. Cerebrospinal fluid studies typically yield a mild pleocytosis with normal protein. A computed tomographic scan of the head will typically be normal. In contrast, magnetic resonance imaging of the head typically shows abnormal signal intensity in the cerebellum, cerebral white matter, or globus pallidus.[3] The pathophysiology of postinfectious acute cerebellar ataxia is poorly understood. The offending agent may produce the ataxia via direct invasion of the cerebellar tissues or via an autoimmune-mediated effect.[4] Cerebral and cerebellar antibodies have been found after varicella infections.[5] Parvovirus B19 has been associated with cerebellar vascular injuries.[6] Single-photon emission computed tomography of the head may demonstrate reduced regional cerebellar blood flow.[7]

Treatment is controversial and predominantly supportive. For severe or persistent cases, glucocorticoids and intravenous immune globulin have been used with some success.[4] Fortunately, most children experience a benign course and recover fully.

Acute Disseminated Encephalomyelitis

Acute disseminated encephalomyelitis, also know as parainfectious encephalitis, is the most common demyelinating condition in children.[8] This demyelinating disease of childhood has an acute onset, and children with acute disseminated encephalomyelitis typically present with ataxia, abnormal motor control, and altered mental status. This condition is typically considered a self-limited, monophasic disorder that is thought to be immune mediated[9] (Table 46–1). The incidence of acute disseminated encephalomyelitis is estimated to be as high as 5 in 10,000 hospital admissions. The association with an antecedent viral infection is reported to be between 54% and 77%. However, the true cause-and-effect relationship has not been definitively established due to the high background frequency of viral illnesses in children.[8,10-12] The average age of onset is 8 years, with a reported age range of 3 months to 18 years of age. A common reported prodrome is headache, fever, nausea, vomiting, and malaise. There are no clinical, laboratory, or computed tomographic findings pathognomonic for acute disseminated encephalomyelitis. The diagnosis is made based on the neurologic examination and the presence of large, multifocal, hyperdense areas in the brain and spinal cord on T2-weighted magnetic resonance imaging. Electroencephalograms typically reveal nonspecific findings and are not diagnostic. Cerebrospinal fluid findings are also nondiagnostic and may reveal mild pleocytosis.

Acute disseminated encephalomyelitis is thought to be due to an immune-mediated process. Treatment is primarily aimed at modulating the immune response and includes the use of glucocorticoids, intravenous immune globulin, and plasmapheresis. To date there have been no clinical trials that compare the effectiveness of these modalities to each other

Table 46–1	Known Causes of Acute Disseminated Encephalomyelitis	
Viral	**Bacterial**	**Immunizations**
Hepatitis A virus	*Clostridium tetani*	Influenza (killed)
Herpes simplex virus	β-Hemolytic	Measles (live)
HIV	streptococci	Meningococcal
Human herpesvirus 6	*Legionella*	A and C
Cytomegalovirus	*Mycoplasma*	Rabies (killed)
Coronavirus	Rickettsiae	Rubella (live)
Mumps virus		
Varicella-zoster virus		

Abbreviation: HIV, human immunodeficiency virus.

Table 46–2	Causes of Dystonia by Rapidity of Symptom Onset	
Acute		**Gradual**
Carbon monoxide		Ataxia-telangiectasia
Cerebral abscess		Brain tumor
Cerebrovascular accidents		Glutaric aciduria type I
Cisapride		Hallervorden-Spatz disease
Dextromethorphan		Leigh disease
Disulfram		Mitochondrial disorders
Droperidol		Neonatal hypoxia
Encephalitis		Wilson's disease
Hemolytic-uremic syndrome		
Infantile bilateral striatal necrosis		
Methanol		
Metoclopramide		
Promethazine		

or to placebo. This is mostly due to the relative rarity of these cases. Treatment recommendations are usually based on small case series.[10] Response to these interventions has been reported to be rapid and dramatic in many cases, with complete recovery in 57% to 81% of patients.[8] In general, the clinical outcome is good, with complications mainly involving mild cognitive deficits. Unfortunately, relapses may occur in as many as one third of patients.

Acute Dystonia

Dystonic reactions are characterized by opisthotonus, lateral neck flexion, oculogyric spasm, tightening of the extremities, and pain.[13] Onset of dystonia may occur acutely or gradually, and the causes are heterogeneous (Table 46–2). Because the causes of dystonia are varied, there is not a single overall approach that is appropriate to these children. The evaluation and management is typically guided by the likely cause based on the history and physical examination. Although clinical experience suggests acute dystonia is relatively rare in children, one of the more common causes is exposure to medications. Commonly implicated medications include dextromethorphan, cisapride, and metoclopramide. Treatment for medication-induced acute dystonia is often accomplished by administering 1.25 mg/kg (up to 50 mg) of intravenous or intramuscular diphenhydramine. Unless there are other extenuating circumstances, children who respond well to the diphenhydramine can usually be dis-

charged home from the emergency department after a short period of observation. Continuing oral diphenhydramine at home for a few days is probably prudent. Coordinating the discontinuance of the inciting medication with the prescribing physician is a reasonable courtesy in many cases.

Huntington's Disease

Huntington's disease is an inherited neurodegenerative disorder that is characterized by movement, cognitive, and behavioral problems. Huntington's disease is autosomal dominant and affects 1 in 10,000 people.[14] Huntington's disease is primarily a disease of middle-aged adults; fewer than 10% of cases are diagnosed in children younger than 20 years of age. The term *juvenile Huntington's disease* is sometimes used to designate these early-onset cases. While adults will often have uncontrolled choreic movements, children are much more likely to manifest rigid akinetic symptoms.[15] The initial presentation of juvenile Huntington's disease is often very subtle and nonspecific, making early diagnosis difficult. Common early symptoms include personality changes, school performance problems, rigidity, slowness, stiffness, an awkward gait, clumsiness, speech difficulties, drooling, frequent choking episodes, and seizures.[16-19]

There is no specific emergency department evaluation for children suspected of having juvenile Huntington's disease. If suspected, the decision to pursue an inpatient or outpatient diagnostic evaluation for children with suspected juvenile Huntington's disease is made on a case-by-case basis. Because Huntington's disease is a progressive disorder, patients may present for a variety of issues over the course of their disease. Seizures, poorly controllable myoclonus, increased rigidity, feeding difficulties, deteriorating mental status, and complications associated with medications are a few of the reasons a child with known Huntington's disease may present to the emergency department. Coordinating care with the family and the child's neurologist is usually prudent.

Sydenham's Chorea

First described by Thomas Sydenham, MD, in 1685, Sydenham's chorea is a hypotonic, hyperkinetic syndrome, characterized by spontaneous involuntary and uncoordinated movements. Other features may include muscular weakness, frequent falls, dysarthria, difficulty concentrating, impaired writing, slurred speech, and emotional lability.[20,21] In particular, Sydenham's chorea has been shown to be associated with neuropsychiatric disorders.[20-22] Sydenham's chorea is currently thought to be part of a somewhat controversial grouping of disorders known as "pediatric autoimmune neuropsychiatric disorders associated with streptococcal infections" (PANDAS).[23,24] The disorders of movement in Sydenham's chorea are usually bilateral, but hemichorea may be seen in as many as 20% of these patients.[21] There is a clear relationship between Sydenham's chorea and rheumatic fever. The presence of Sydenham's chorea is one of the major criteria used to clinically diagnose rheumatic fever. Sydenham's chorea is seen in as many as 25% of patients diagnosed with rheumatic fever. School-age children are the pediatric group most commonly affected. A single episode of chorea can last 2 to 6 months.[22,25,26] If performed, magnetic resonance imaging of the brain typically reveals injury to the caudate nucleus.[20] The etiology of Sydenham's chorea is unknown, but an immune-mediated process is likely.[20]

A variety of treatments for Sydenham's chorea have been tried over the years, including haloperidol, barbiturates, chlorpromazine, benzodiazepines, and valproic acid.[27,28] Immune modulators such as corticosteroids and intravenous immune globulin have also been tried with variable success. Currently, the most promising treatment is valproic acid, which has been shown to be safe and relatively effective.[25] Valproic acid has been shown to both control the motor movements and stabilize mood swings.[25]

Tourette's Syndrome

Tourette's syndrome is the most common and well-known tic disorder.[29] The onset is usually between 2 and 28 years of age, with the peak around 11 years. Tourette's syndrome is characterized by repetitive, stereotypical tics that are intermittent and have a compulsive quality to them. The range of symptoms can be divided between vocal, motor, and behavioral. Boys tend to manifest motor and vocal symptoms, while girls tend to manifest more behavioral symptoms. The most well-known and dramatic of the vocal manifestations is coprolalia, the expression of "dirty" words or phrases. Most patients do not demonstrate this feature. Between 5% and 30% of patients with Tourette's syndrome manifest coprolalia. The vocal tics range from simple sounds to complex phrases or speech patterns such as echolalia (repetition of words) or palilalia (rapid repetition of words or phrases). The motor manifestations may be simple, fast, meaningless muscle movements or they may be slower, stereotyped movements that look purposeful. The behavioral symptoms include those labeled attention-deficit/hyperactivity disorder, obsessive-compulsive disorder, self-mutilation, aggression, and various learning disabilities.[30-33]

There is no specific emergent treatment for the manifestations of Tourette's syndrome. Coordinated care with the child's neurologist is prudent. Most children essentially "outgrow" their tics, but about 10% of children have persistence and worsening symptoms into adulthood.[29,34,35]

REFERENCES

1. Gieron-Korthals MA, Westberry KR, Emmanuel PJ: Acute childhood ataxia: 10-year experience. J Child Neurol 9:381–384, 1994.
2. Nussinovitch M, Prais D, Volovitz B, et al: Post-infectious acute cerebellar ataxia in children. Clin Pediatr (Phila) 42:581–584, 2003.
3. Sunaga Y, Hikima A, Ostuka T, et al: Acute cerebellar ataxia with abnormal MRI lesions after varicella vaccination. Pediatr Neurol 13:340–342, 1995.
*4. Go T: Intravenous immunoglobulin therapy for acute cerebellar ataxia. Acta Paediatr 92:504–506, 2003.
5. Adams C, Diadori P, Schoenroth L, et al: Autoantibodies in childhood post-varicella acute cerebellar ataxia. Can J Neurol Sci 27:316–320, 2000.
6. Shimizu Y, Ueno T, Komatsu H, et al: Acute cerebellar ataxia with human parvovirus B19 infection. Arch Dis Child 80:72–73, 1999.
7. Nagamitsu S, Matsuishi T, Ishibashi M, et al: Decreased cerebellar blood flow in postinfectious acute cerebellar ataxia. J Neurol Neurosurg Psychiatry 67:109–112, 1999.
*8. Anlar B, Basaran C, Kase G, et al: Acute disseminated encephalomyelitis in children: outcome and prognosis. Neuropediatrics 34:194–199, 2003.
9. Gupte G, Stonehouse M, Wasserman E, et al: Acute disseminated encephalomyelitis: a review of 18 cases in childhood. J Paediatr Child Health 39:336–342, 2003.
10. Dale R, Church A, Cardoso F, et al: Poststreptococcal acute disseminated encephalomyelitis with basal ganglia involvement and autoreactive antibasal ganglia antibodies. Ann Neurol 50:588–595, 2001.
11. Hynson J, Kornberg A, Coleman L, et al: Clinical and neuroradiologic features of acute disseminated encephalomyelitis in children. Neurology 56:1308–1312, 2001.
12. Murthy S, Faden H, Cohen M, et al: Acute disseminated encephalomyelitis in children. Pediatrics 110:e21, 2002.
13. Park CK, Choi HY, Oh IY, et al: Acute dystonia by droperidol during intravenous patient-controlled analgesia in young patients. J Korean Med Sci 17:715–717, 2002.
14. Wexler N, Lorimer J, Porter J, et al: Venezuelan kindreds reveal that genetic and environmental factors modulate Huntington's disease age of onset. Proc Natl Acad Sci U S A 101:3498–3503, 2004.
15. Siesling S, Vegter-van der Vils M, Roos R: Juvenile Huntington disease in the Netherlands. Pediatr Neurol 17:37–43, 1997.
16. Nance M, Myers RH: Juvenile onset Huntington's disease—clinical and research perspectives. Ment Retard Dev Disabil Res Rev 7:153–157, 2001.
17. Gordon N: Huntington's disease of early onset or juvenile Huntington's disease. Hosp Med 64:576–580, 2003.
18. Gabardella A, Muglia M, Labate A, et al: Juvenile Huntington's disease presenting as progressive myoclonic epilepsy. Neurology 57:708–711, 2001.
19. Landau M, Cannard K: EEG characteristics in juvenile Huntington's disease: a case report and review of the literature. Epileptic Disord 5:145–148, 2003.
*20. Faustino PC, Terreri MT, da Rocha AJ, et al: Clinical, laboratory, psychiatric and magnetic resonance findings in patients with Sydenham chorea. Neuroradiology 45:456–462, 2003.
21. Rotstein M, Harel S: Sydenham's chorea—an entity in progress. Isr Med Assoc J 6:492–493, 2004.
22. Cardoso F, Eduardo C, Silva AP, et al: Chorea in fifty consecutive patients with rheumatic fever. Mov Disord 12:701–703, 1997.
23. Swedo SE, Leonard HL, Garvey M, et al: Pediatric autoimmune neuropsychiatric disorders associated with streptococcal infections: clinical description of the first 50 cases. Am J Psychiatry 155:264–271, 1998.
*24. Kurlan R, Kaplan R: The pediatric autoimmune neuropsychiatric disorders associated with streptococcal infection (PANDAS) etiology for tics and obsessive-compulsive symptoms: hypothesis or entity? Practical considerations for the clinician. Pediatrics 113:883–886, 2004.
25. Daoud AS, Zaki M, Shakir R, et al: Effectiveness of sodium valproate in the treatment of Sydenham's chorea. Neurology 40:1140–1141, 1990.
26. Davutoglu V, Kilinc M, Dinckal H, et al: Sydenham's chorea—clinical characteristics of nine patients. Int J Cardiol 96:483–484, 2004.
27. Polizzi A, Incorpora G, Ruggieri M: Dystonia as acute adverse reaction to cough suppressant in a 3-year-old girl. Eur J Paediatr Neurol 5:167–168, 2001.
28. Carapetis JR, Currie BJ: Rheumatic chorea in northern Australia: a clinical and epidemiological study. Arch Dis Child 80:353–358, 1999.
29. Leckman J: Phenomenology of tics and natural history of tic disorders. Brain Dev 25(Suppl 1):S24–S28, 2003.
30. Chang H, Tu M, Wang H: Tourette's syndrome: psychopathology in adolescents. Psychiatry Clin Neurosci 58:353–358, 2004.
31. Kano Y, Ohta M, Nagai Y, et al: Obsessive-compulsive symptoms in parents of Tourette syndrome proband and autism spectrum disorder probands. Psychiatry Clin Nurosci 58:348–352, 2004.
32. Mathews C, Waller J, Glidden D, et al: Self injurious behavior in Tourette syndrome: correlates with impulsivity and impulse control. J Neurol Neurosurg Psychiatry 75:1149–1155, 2004.
33. Tan H, Buyukavci M, Arik A: Tourette's syndrome manifests as chronic persistent cough. Yonsei Med J 45:145–149, 2004.
34. O'Quinn A, Thompson R Jr: Tourette's syndrome: an expanded view. Pediatrics 66:420–424, 1980.
35. Romano A, Cundari G, Bruni O, et al: Tic disorders and arousal dysfunction: clinical evaluation of 49 children and adolescents. Minerva Pediatr 56:327–344, 2004.

*Selected readings.

Chapter 47

Peripheral Neuromuscular Disorders

Jay Pershad, MD and Kelly L. Kriwanek, MD

Key Points

Patients with acute-onset neuropathic weakness require a prompt assessment and frequent re-evaluations to determine the risk of developing respiratory failure.

Guillain-Barré syndrome is the most commonly acquired peripheral polyneuropathy seen in children.

The most common peripheral mononeuropathy seen in children involves the seventh cranial nerve (e.g., Bell's palsy).

Neuromuscular blocking agents should be avoided in children with muscular dystrophy if possible.

Selected Diagnoses

Guillain-Barré syndrome
Myasthenia gravis
Mitochondrial disorders
Complications of muscular dystrophy
Benign paroxysmal vertigo
Peripheral seventh cranial nerve palsies
Optic neuritis
Spinal muscular atrophy
Channelopathies

Discussion of Individual Diagnoses

Guillain-Barré Syndrome

Guillain-Barré syndrome is an acute inflammatory demyelinating polyneuropathy that typically appears as symmetric ascending flaccid paralysis with loss of deep tendon reflexes and variable sensory changes. Guillain-Barré syndrome affects children of all ages, but is rarely seen in infants. Guillain-Barré syndrome is the most common cause of acute flaccid paralysis in developed countries. The annual incidence is 0.5 to 1.5 cases per 100,000 persons younger than 18 years.[1,2] An acute, seemingly minor infection often occurs 1 to 2 weeks before the onset of Guillain-Barré syndrome.[1,2] Viruses, Mycoplasma, and Campylobacter are some of the most commonly reported organisms associated with Guillain-Barré syndrome.[3] The pathophysiology is thought to primarily involve autoimmune-mediated neuronal tissue injury.

Clinical Presentation

There are two primary types of Guillain-Barré syndrome. The first type is generally referred to simply as Guillain-Barré syndrome or "classic" Guillain-Barré syndrome. Children with this syndrome present with ascending, symmetric weakness that begins in the lower extremities and progresses cephalad. The condition of most patients reaches a nadir within 2 to 4 weeks after the onset of symptoms.[4] Pain and ataxia can be prominent symptoms of childhood Guillain-Barré syndrome.[2,5] The hallmark of the disease is depressed or absent deep tendon reflexes. The absence of such reflexes helps to identify early Guillain-Barré syndrome, especially in preverbal children whose symptoms can be mistakenly attributed to a musculoskeletal disorder or a primary cerebellar disorder. Paresthesias, dysautonomia, bilateral involvement of facial nerves, and rapid progression to respiratory failure may be observed early in the course of the illness. The second type is generally referred to as the Miller Fisher syndrome, the Fisher syndrome, or the one-and-a-half syndrome. This syndrome is characterized by areflexia, ataxia, and external ophthalmoplegia without motor weakness. In children with this syndrome, the symptoms may begin with the cranial nerves and progress caudally.

Autonomic dysfunction is commonly seen in children with Guillain-Barré syndrome. The typical manifestations of this condition include orthostatic hypotension, urinary retention, paroxysmal hypertension, and arrhythmias. Specific therapeutic intervention is only required for hypertension in the presence of end-organ damage. Respiratory insufficiency requiring airway management may result from three underlying pathophysiologic processes: inadequate inspiratory effort due to weakness of intercostal muscles and the diaphragm; bulbar paralysis; and hypoxemia due to ineffective cough, atelectasis, or poor clearance of secretions from the airways. Peripheral muscle strength may not correlate with diaphragmatic weakness. If endotracheal intubation is undertaken, dysautonomia and bradyarrhythmias may be encountered during airway manipulation. Hypotension may be exaggerated by the use of conventional sedative-hypnotic agents. Generous application of topical anesthesia, preemptive use of vagolytic agents (e.g., atropine) and titration of benzodiazepines may be the most appropriate adjunctive measures to facilitate endotracheal intubation in these children (see Chapter 3, Rapid Sequence Intubation). Judicious use of opiate analgesics for ongoing pain is also beneficial.

The differential diagnosis of rapid ascending peripheral motor weakness includes tick paralysis, food-borne botulism, and ciguatera. Tick paralysis results from inoculation with toxin from a tick's salivary glands during its blood meal. Signs observed during neurologic examination mimic those of Guillain-Barré syndrome, including the progression to respiratory failure. Constitutional symptoms are rare in tick paralysis. Removal of the attached tick results in prompt reversal of the paralysis. Food-borne botulism is commonly characterized by nausea and emesis that precede acute neuropathic weakness. Unlike classic Guillain-Barré syndrome, botulism is associated with oculobulbar weakness, a descending pattern of paralysis, dilated and poorly responsive pupils, and prominent autonomic involvement (e.g., dry mouth, constipation, urinary retention). Mentation is typically normal in cases of botulism. Ciguatera is caused by the consumption of fish containing ciguatoxin in their tissues. Commonly implicated fish include grouper and snapper. Vomiting and diarrhea typically ensue several hours after ingestion of the contaminated fish, and the condition progresses to generalized itching, myalgias, weakness, and dysesthesias of the perioral area and the lower extremities. Ciguatera is a self-limited illness that does not typically lead to respiratory failure. There is no known specific therapy for ciguatera.

The diagnosis of Guillain-Barré syndrome is based on the presence of the typical clinical features of weakness, areflexia, and sensory disturbances. Cerebrospinal fluid studies and electromyography may be helpful in supporting the diagnosis. The cerebrospinal fluid protein concentration is typically elevated in the absence of pleocytosis.

Management

All patients with suspected Guillain-Barré syndrome require hospital admission until the maximum degree of disability has occurred. Dysautonomia and impending or actual respiratory failure warrant intensive care monitoring. There is currently insufficient evidence concerning treatment modalities for childhood Guillain-Barré syndrome to warrant any evidence-based recommendations. Data extrapolated from adult studies suggest that plasma exchange and intravenous immune globulin therapy are effective treatment for severe disease. When initiated within 2 to 4 weeks of symptom onset, intravenous immune globulin therapy and plasma exchange seem to have equivalent efficacy.[6,7] Corticosteroids do not appear to be effective in treating Guillain-Barré syndrome.[8]

Mortality due to childhood Guillain-Barré syndrome is rare. It is a self-limited illness in which spontaneous recovery usually begins within 3 to 4 weeks after symptom progression ceases. Most children (90% to 95%) achieve a complete functional recovery within 6 to 12 months.[2] Factors associated with a poor prognosis include rapid progression of symptoms, the need for ventilatory support, severely reduced action potential of muscle on an electromyogram, recent *Campylobacter jejuni* enteritis, recent cytomegalovirus infection, and poor recovery of motor function at 8 weeks after diagnosis.[9] There is an increased risk of long-term deficits in children younger than 9 years of age and those who have progression to maximal weakness within 10 days of disease onset.[10]

Myasthenia Gravis

Myasthenia gravis is an autoimmune disorder of the neuromuscular junction caused by circulating antibodies directed against the acetylcholine receptor (Table 47–1). This leads to a deficiency of acetylcholine at postsynaptic neuromuscular junctions. The clinical hallmark of myasthenia gravis is fluctuating, painless, asymmetric weakness that most often affects ocular, lower bulbar or proximal limb musculature. Fatigability of voluntary muscles with repetitive motion is essentially diagnostic. Mentation, sensation, pupillary response, and tendon reflexes are characteristically spared. Weakness of neck flexors parallels bulbar and respiratory muscle weakness.

Clinical Presentation

The three forms of myasthenia gravis affecting children are the juvenile form, neonatal form, and congenital form. Juvenile myasthenia gravis accounts for 10% to 15% of all myasthenia gravis cases and is the most common form in children.[11] Juvenile myasthenia gravis occurs in children older than 12 months. Unlike the adult form, which more commonly affects women, prepubertal boys and girls are equally affected. The clinical course of juvenile myasthenia gravis is variable

Table 47–1	Anatomic Site of Derangement in Peripheral Neuromuscular Disorders
Anatomic Site	**Condition**
Anterior Horn Cell	Paralytic poliomyelitis*
	Spinal muscular atrophy†
Motor Root	Traumatic plexopathy
Peripheral Nerve	Guillain-Barré syndrome*
	Tick paralysis*
	Bell's palsy
	Acute intermittent porphyria*
	Organophosphate poisoning*
	Heavy metal poisoning*
	Ciguatera poisoning*
	Diphtheria*
Neuromuscular Junction	Myasthenia gravis*‡
	Botulism*
	Hypophosphatemia*
Muscle	Benign childhood viral myositis
	Polymyositis*†
	Dermatomyositis
	Hypokalemic periodic paralysis*‡
	Muscular dystrophies†
	Metabolic myopathy*†‡
	Tetanus*

*May present as rapidly progressive weakness.
†Preexisting symptoms or chronic disease.
‡Fluctuating weakness.

and is characterized by exacerbations and remissions. As many as 14% to 30% of children diagnosed with myasthenia gravis will experience a spontaneous remission.[12,13] The younger the child is at the time of diagnosis, the higher the likelihood that complete, lifelong remission will occur. Adolescents are likely to have symptoms continue into adulthood.

Neonatal myasthenia gravis occurs in approximately 20% of infants born to mothers with myasthenia gravis.[14] The pathophysiology is based on passive transfer of maternal antibodies across the placenta. The typical presentation is in the first 72 hours of life, with nonspecific signs and symptoms including hypotonia, poor suck, a weak cry, facial weakness, and respiratory difficulties. Neonatal myasthenia gravis is a self-limited disorder. Weakness usually resolves within the first 2 to 3 weeks of life, but may last as long as 12 weeks.[11] Treatment with cholinesterase inhibitors (e.g., pyridostigmine bromide) may be required while awaiting full recovery.

Congenital myasthenia gravis is a heterogeneous group of nonimmune, hereditary illnesses arising from presynaptic, synaptic, and postsynaptic molecular defects. Symptom onset occurs in the neonatal period or early childhood, and symptoms persist throughout life. Common presenting signs are ophthalmoplegia, ptosis, myopathic facies, and mild generalized weakness. Patients with congenital myasthenia gravis do not experience myasthenic crises. Diagnosis is made by a response to cholinesterase inhibitors or a decremental response to repetitive nerve stimulation in limb muscles. It is difficult to differentiate congenital myasthenia gravis from the juvenile form.[15,16] Children with congenital myasthenia gravis show a more variable response to cholinesterase inhibitors than do children with juvenile myasthenia gravis.

The most dangerous complication of myasthenia gravis is a myasthenic crisis leading to respiratory failure. Precipitating factors include medication changes, infections, surgery, stress, aspiration, hypokalemia, and pregnancy.[17,18] The most common cause of a myasthenic crisis is a change in medications. Children demonstrating weakness of the bulbar or respiratory muscles require admission to an intensive care unit in anticipation of respiratory failure if it has not occurred already. Differentiating a myasthenic crisis from a cholinergic crisis due to excessive dosing of cholinesterase inhibitors is often difficult. During a myasthenic crisis, it is prudent to discontinue all medications and treat precipitating factors if possible. Certain classes of medications that affect neuromuscular transmission require cautious use in children with myasthenia gravis. These include aminoglycosides, lidocaine, β-blockers, and neuromuscular blocking agents. Increased airway secretions from cholinergic excess may complicate rapid sequence intubation.

The definitive diagnosis of myasthenia gravis is based on the typical clinical features, a positive edrophonium or neostigmine test, repetitive nerve stimulation, single fiber electromyography, and an acetylcholine receptor antibody assay. The edrophonium test is commonly called a "Tensilon test" based on a brand name preparation of edrophonium. In this test, edrophonium, a short-acting cholinesterase inhibitor, is administered intravenously (0.2 mg/kg to a maximum of 10 mg) after a small test dose (0.04 mg/kg). Atropine must be immediately available to treat a potential cholinergic crisis. Muscle strength is evaluated before and after injection. If weakness is transiently improved, the edrophonium test is considered positive and consistent with the diagnosis of myasthenia gravis.

Management

Treatment of myasthenia gravis is initiated with a cholinesterase inhibitor. Although this treatment will provide symptomatic relief, the course of the disease is not altered. Pyridostigmine is the preferred cholinesterase inhibitor due to its relatively long duration of action and muscarinic side effect profile. Although thymomas are less commonly seen in children compared with adults, thymectomy is widely used as a treatment option for myasthenia gravis. An evidence-based review concluded that thymectomy offers an increased likelihood of remission or improvement.[19] The greatest effect is seen when the thymectomy is performed within the first 2 years of symptom onset.[20] Clinical improvement may be delayed for months to years after the surgery. In prepubertal-onset disease, thymectomy is recommended as second-line therapy if cholinesterase inhibitors fail. Other medications that may be used in patients with myasthenia gravis include corticosteroids, azathioprine, cyclophosphamide, cyclosporin A, and mycophenolate mofetil.[21-23] Immunosuppressive therapy is less frequently used for children with onset of disease before puberty. For adolescents and young adults, corticosteroids induce remissions in 50% to 80% of cases.[21] Symptom exacerbation is frequently noted after starting treatment with corticosteroids, and this may prompt an emergency department visit. Azathioprine, cyclophosphamide, cyclosporin A, and mycophenolate mofetil have been used as adjunctive, steroid-sparing agents.[22,23] For short-term therapy in patients with acutely worsening symptoms of myasthenia gravis or refractory myasthenia gravis, or as preoperative preparation, plasma exchange and intravenous immune globulin have been shown to provide improvement within a week. Effects from these treatments may last as long as 2 months. Randomized, controlled trials comparing plasma exchange with intravenous immune globulin demonstrate equal efficacy, but intravenous immune globulin has fewer side effects.[24,25]

Mitochondrial Disorders

Mitochondrial encephalomyopathies are a group of clinically, genetically, and biochemically heterogeneous disorders caused by a defect in the oxidative phosphorylation pathway of the respiratory chain. In general, organs that consume relatively large amounts of oxygen, such as the skeletal muscle, brain, and heart, are dominantly affected. The worldwide incidence is one case in 10,000 live births.[26] Mitochondrial disorders are in the differential diagnosis of encephalopathy, failure to thrive, neurodevelopmental delay, hypotonia, apparent life-threatening events, seizures, unexplained lactic acidosis, and cardiomyopathy. Although the clinical features of mitochondrial disorders vary, their predominant signs are cardiomyopathy and nonspecific encephalopathy.

Classic phenotypic syndromes associated with mitochondrial DNA mutation have been described but are uncommon in pediatric mitochondrial diseases. Most pediatric mitochondrial diseases fall outside of these well-described syndromes. These syndromes are best known by their abbreviations and include MELAS (*m*itochondrial *e*ncephalopathy with *l*actic *a*cidosis and *s*troke-like episodes); MERRF (*m*yoclonic *e*pilepsy with *r*agged *r*ed *f*ibers); LIMD (*l*ethal *i*nfantile *m*itochondrial *d*isease); NARP (*n*europathy, *a*taxia, and *r*etinitis *p*igmentosa); and MNGIE (*m*itochondrial *n*eurogastro*i*ntestinal *e*ncephalomyopathy). Other named mitochondrial disorders emergency physicians may encounter include Leber's hereditary optic neuropathy, Kearns-Sayre syndrome, necrotizing subacute encephalomyelopathy (Leigh disease), and Pearson's syndrome. Definitive diagnosis requires an integrated approach incorporating clinical, pathologic, enzymatic, molecular, and metabolic criteria.[27] Life expectancy for most patients with a classic mitochondrial syndrome is 5 years or less. Patients with noncardiac phenotypes have somewhat better survival rates.[28]

Complications of Muscular Dystrophy

Muscular dystrophies are a group of chronic, progressive, genetically determined disorders characterized by cellular degeneration of muscle. These disorders are characterized by muscle atrophy without nervous system derangements. There are a number of muscular dystrophies, including Duchenne's muscular dystrophy, Becker's muscular dystrophy, Emery-Dreifuss muscular dystrophy, limb-girdle muscular dystrophy, facioscapulohumeral muscular dystrophy, myotonic dystrophy, oculopharyngeal dystrophy, distal muscular dystrophy, and congenital muscular dystrophy. These disorders differ in the age of onset, the order in which muscle groups are affected, the degree to which cardiac involvement is expected, the rate of symptom progression, and life expectancy.

There are four major clinical "pearls" associated with the emergency department management of children with muscular dystrophy. First, glucocorticoids are used to treat children with muscular dystrophy. For those children on chronic steroid treatment, adrenal suppression and an overall immunocompromised state should be assumed (see Chapter 107, The Steroid-Dependent Child). Second, when respiratory failure occurs, the use of neuromuscular blocking (i.e., paralytic) agents should be avoided. If used, prolonged neuromuscular blockade may occur. Succinylcholine, in particular, should be avoided in these children due to the increased risk of malignant hyperthermia.[29] Third, rhabdomyolysis with myoglobinuria may be present and suggests an intercurrent infection or excessive physical exertion.[30] Fourth, cardiomyopathies are associated with many of the muscular dystrophies. Cardiomyopathy associated with tachyarrhythmias, congestive heart failure, and cardiomegaly occurs in 50% to 80% of these children at some time during their disease course.[31] Supportive care in an intensive care setting is indicated. The overall clinical course of the muscular dystrophies is generally slow but progressive. The cause of death in these children is often intractable congestive heart failure or an overwhelming infection.

Benign Paroxysmal Vertigo

Benign paroxysmal vertigo typically develops in children between 1 and 3 years of age. This disorder is characterized by a sudden onset of unsteadiness, pallor, and anxiety. These may manifest as the child falling or refusing to walk or sit. The verbal child may describe a spinning sensation. Throughout the episode, consciousness is preserved. The physical examination often reveals no abnormalities except the horizontal nystagmus that occurs during an attack of vertigo.

Episodes are brief, typically lasting between 1 and 5 minutes.[32] Symptoms are expected to recur and may occur daily or monthly, but typically resolve within 2 years of the onset of symptoms. Between episodes, these children are asymptomatic. Benign paroxysmal vertigo is thought to be a migraine equivalent[33] (see Chapter 41, Headaches). Many children with benign paroxysmal vertigo have a family history of migraine headaches and are thought to be at high risk for migraine headaches later in life. Benign paroxysmal vertigo is a diagnosis of exclusion and has a benign, self-limited course. Treatment is supportive.

Peripheral Seventh Cranial Nerve Palsies

Peripheral cranial nerve VII palsies are caused by lesions in the facial nerve nucleus in the brainstem or in the extra-axial portion of the nerve. The result is partial or complete paralysis of the forehead and lower facial musculature. Because of this innervation, cranial nerve VII is also known as the facial nerve. Peripheral cranial nerve VII palsies can be clinically differentiated from a cortical lesion in the brain by the weakness or paralysis in the forehead. A brain lesion would spare the forehead. The first step in the emergency department evaluation of a child with a suspected peripheral cranial nerve VII palsy is to evaluation the motor function of the forehead. If the forehead musculature is weak or paralyzed, peripheral nerve palsy is confirmed. If the forehead musculature appears normal, a central process is likely and the child should be evaluated for stroke (see Chapter 44, Central Nervous System Vascular Disorders).

The facial nerve has motor, sensory, and autonomic components. The motor component controls the muscles involved in facial expression and the stapedius muscle (which protects the middle ear from damage due to loud noises). The sensory branches provide cutaneous sensation to the auricular canal. The autonomic component consists of the parasympathetic afferents that innervate the lacrimal and salivary glands and the efferent fibers that innervate the anterior two thirds of the tongue. Depending on the portion of the facial nerve that is affected, varying degrees of sound sensitivity and dysfunction in lacrimation, salivation, or taste may be noted. The most common type of isolated peripheral mononeuropathy of cranial nerve VII is idiopathic and is commonly referred to as "Bell's palsy" named after Sir Charles Bell who first described this clinical entity in the early 19th century. The incidence of Bell's palsy is 2.7 cases per 100,000 in children younger than 10 years and 10.1 cases per 100,000 in children who are 10 to 20 years old.[34]

The history and physical examination should focus on assessing the risk of a secondary cause for the nerve palsy. Unfortunately, high-quality pediatric-specific epidemiologic data are not available regarding Bell's palsy. Some general features are applicable in the study of all age groups who experience Bell's palsy. Although classic Bell's palsy is a mononeuropathy, one third of patients have associated involvement of cranial nerves V, IX, or XII. Systemic illnesses and infections that can cause facial palsy include acute otitis media, mastoiditis, cholesteatoma, Epstein-Barr viral infection, herpes simplex viral infection, Lyme disease, herpes zoster (Ramsay Hunt syndrome), mycoplasma infection, tuberculosis, Guillain-Barré syndrome, myasthenia gravis, lymphoma, leukemia, hypertension, diabetes, and sarcoidosis. In rare circumstances, Bell's palsy can be bilateral, although one side is usually more involved than the other. The utility of additional testing in cases of an uncomplicated mononeuropathy is probably very limited. Additional testing such as nerve conduction studies and cranial magnetic resonance imaging should be reserved for atypical cases or those in which recovery is not achieved within 4 to 6 weeks of diagnosis. Urgent imaging is probably indicated for those children who have a recent history of head trauma, a systemic illness, recurrent palsies, hypertension, acute otitis media, a parotid mass, bilateral facial nerve weakness, and multiple cranial nerves involved. Recurrent unilateral facial paralysis suggests the presence of a vascular malformation, neoplasia, or Melkersson-Rosenthal syndrome (a rare genetic syndrome occurring in patients younger than 16 years of age and characterized by a fissured tongue and recurrent orofacial edema).

The treatment of Bell's palsy in children is, for the most part, controversial. The least controversial component of care is the associated eye care. Incomplete lid closure can predispose patients to desiccant keratitis, corneal abrasions, and an ectropion (an everted eyelid). The use of artificial tears during the day and the application of a moisturizing ophthalmic ointment in conjunction with eye patching at bedtime are considered helpful in preventing ophthalmologic complications. If eye redness or irritation occurs, ophthalmologic consultation is prudent. In one trial conducted exclusively in children 2 to 6 years old, no benefit from corticosteroid therapy was noted.[35] In trials that enrolled adults and children, steroids were effective when treatment was initiated during the first 2 weeks of symptoms.[36] Recent data suggest a possible benefit when antiviral drugs (e.g., acyclovir, valacyclovir) are combined with prednisone.[37] There are insufficient data about the effectiveness of surgical facial nerve decompression therapy in treating typical Bell's palsy. The prognosis of Bell's palsy in children is thought to be good, as most patients fully recover within 6 months to a year from the onset of symptoms.[38]

Optic Neuritis

Optic neuritis in childhood presents as an acute loss of central visual acuity, an afferent pupillary defect, and a funduscopic appearance that resembles papilledema and hemorrhage. Some patients have headache and pain that are associated with extraocular movement. Optic neuritis is bilateral in 60% of pediatric patients. Prior to widespread routine immunizations, optic neuritis was seen following acute infections including mumps, measles, or varicella. The visual prognosis of pediatric patients with optic neuritis is better than that of adults with the same type of neuritis.[39] The mean age of children at the time of onset is 9.4 years, with a reported age range of 2.5 to 16 years. Multiple sclerosis may eventually be diagnosed in up to one third of patients with uncomplicated optic neuritis.[40] Ancillary diagnostic tests include visual evoked response testing and magnetic resonance imaging. Most patients with bilateral disease recover complete visual function. The role of corticosteroid therapy is controversial because it is unknown whether this treatment alters the natural course of optic neuritis.[41]

Spinal Muscular Atrophy

Spinal muscular atrophy (SMA) is an autosomal recessive disorder caused by degeneration of anterior horn cells in the spinal cord and brainstem. SMA is the second most common neuromuscular disease of childhood, with an incidence of 1 in 10,000 live births.[42] The clinical features of SMA include progressive, symmetric weakness and atrophy affecting the proximal muscle groups more than the distal groups, loss of deep tendon reflexes, preservation of sensation, and normal intelligence. Fasciculations, especially of the tongue, are frequently seen. SMA is classified into three types according to age of onset and clinical severity. Type I SMA (Werdnig-Hoffmann disease) is the most severe form and presents within the first 6 months of life with profound generalized muscle weakness, hypotonia, and areflexia. Most patients die within the first 2 years of life from respiratory failure. Type II SMA is the intermediate form, with disease onset before 18 months of age. With supportive care, patients can survive into adulthood. Type III (Kugelberg-Welander syndrome) is the juvenile form of the disease, with onset of symptoms after 18 months of age. These patients may have a near-normal life expectancy. Confirmatory diagnosis requires genetic testing. Electromyography, nerve conduction studies, and muscle biopsy are also helpful for confirming the diagnosis. There is no known cure for SMA. Treatment is supportive. In severe cases, life span may be prolonged with the aid of noninvasive respiratory support or tracheostomy[43] (see Chapter 164, Tracheostomy Tubes; and Chapter 165, Noninvasive and Mechanical Ventilation).

Channelopathies

The channelopathies are a heterogeneous group of disorders involving specific ion channel dysfunctions. Many of these disorders occur episodically and affect otherwise healthy, active people.[44] Diverse clinical entities including migraine headaches, some forms of epilepsy, and cardiac conduction disturbances, such as seen in cases of a prolonged QT interval, are thought to be due, at least in part, to channelopathies.[44] A subset of these disorders, primarily those involving potassium channels, clinically manifest with episodes of profound muscle weakness followed by complete resolution.[45]

Hypokalemic periodic paralysis is the most common periodic paralysis, having a prevalence of about 1 in 100,000.[46] The first clinical symptoms typically occur in the first 2 decades of life and are characterized by the onset of muscular weakness usually sparing the facial and respiratory muscles.[46] Symptoms typically last several hours and resolve gradually. Precipitating factors include prolonged rest after vigorous exercise, ingestion of a carbohydrate-rich meal the day prior to the onset of symptoms, fatigue, stress, and intercurrent viral illnesses.[46] Medications known to precipitate symptoms include β-agonists, corticosteroids, and insulin.[46] A low serum potassium level is characteristically identified during periods of weakness. Aggressive intravenous potassium replacement should be avoided in these patients as marked hyperkalemia may develop as the attack resolves. Oral replacement of potassium in the emergency department is often effective in normalizing the patient's serum potassium which, in turn, leads to symptom resolution.[46]

Less common is hyperkalemic periodic paralysis. These children typically develop symptoms earlier in life and may exhibit muscle stiffness or weakness. These children more commonly have facial involvement and may develop respiratory compromise. The continuance of mild activity, the ingestion of sweets, and the use of inhaled β-agonists may minimize the effects of attacks in these children.[46]

REFERENCES

1. Jansen PW, Perkin RM, Ashwal S: Guillain-Barre syndrome in childhood: natural course and efficacy of plasmapheresis. Pediatr Neurol 9:16–20, 1993.
2. Sladky JT: Guillain-Barre syndrome in children. J Child Neurol 19:191–200, 2004.
3. Jacobs BC, Rothbarth PH, van der Meche FG, et al: The spectrum of antecedent infections in Guillain-Barré syndrome: a case-control study. Neurology 51:1110–1115, 1998.
4. Korinthenberg R, Monting JS: Natural history and treatment effects in Guillain-Barre syndrome: a multicentre study. Arch Dis Child 74:281–287, 1996.
5. Jones HR: Childhood Guillain-Barré syndrome: clinical presentation, diagnosis, and therapy. J Child Neurol 11:4–12, 1996.
*6. Hughes RA, Wijdicks EF, Barohn R, et al: Practice parameter: immunotherapy for Guillain-Barré syndrome: report of the Quality Standards Subcommittee of the American Academy of Neurology. Neurology 61:736–740, 2003.
7. Kanra G, Ozon A, Vajsar J, et al: Intravenous immunoglobulin treatment in children with Guillain-Barré syndrome. Eur J Paediatr Neurol 1:7–12, 1997.
8. van Koningsveld R, Schmitz PI, Meche FG, et al: Effect of methylprednisolone when added to standard treatment with intravenous immunoglobulin for Guillain-Barré syndrome: randomized trial. Lancet 363:192–196, 2004.
9. Visser LH, Schmitz PI, Meulstee J, et al: Prognostic factors of Guillain-Barré syndrome after intravenous immunoglobulin or plasma exchange. Dutch Guillain-Barré Study Group. Neurology 53:598–604, 1999.
*10. Vajsar J, Fehlings D, Stephens D: Long-term outcome in children with Guillain-Barré syndrome. J Pediatr 142:305–309, 2003.
11. Andersson P-B, Rando TA: Neuromuscular disorders of childhood. Curr Opin Pediatr 11:497–503, 1999.
12. Rodriguez M, Gomez MR, Howard FM, et al: Myasthenia gravis in children: long-term follow-up. Ann Neurol 13:504–510, 1983
13. Adams C, Theodorescu D, Murphy EG, et al: Thymectomy in juvenile myasthenia gravis. J Child Neurol 5:215–218, 1990
14. Papazian O: Transient neonatal myasthenia gravis. J Child Neurol 7:135–141, 1992.
15. Harper CM, Engel AG: Quinidine sulfate therapy for the slow channel congenital myasthenic syndrome. Ann Neurol 43:480–484, 1998.
16. Jaison SG, Abraham AP: Childhood myasthenia gravis in a toddler. Indian J Ophthalmol 43:136–137, 1995.
17. Thomas CE, Mayer SA, Gungor Y, et al: Myasthenic crisis: clinical features, mortality, complications, and risk factors for prolonged intubation. Neurology 48:1253–1260, 1997
18. Werneck LC, Scola RH, Branco FM, et al: Myasthenic crisis: report of 24 cases. Arq Neuropsiquiatr 60:519–526, 2002.
19. Gronseth GS, Barohn RJ: Practice parameter: thymectomy for autoimmune myasthenia gravis (an evidence-based review): report of the Quality Standards Subcommittee of the American Academy of Neurology. Neurology 55:7–15, 2000.
20. DeFilippi VJ, Richman DP, Ferguson MK: Transcervical thymectomy for myasthenia gravis. Ann Thorac Surg 57:194–197, 1994
21. Richman DP, Aguis MA: Treatment of autoimmune myasthenia gravis. Neurology 61:1652–1661, 2003.
22. Palace J, Newsome-Davis J, Lecky B: A randomized double-blind trial of prednisolone alone or with azathioprine in myasthenia gravis. Myasthenia Gravis Study Group. Neurology 50:1778–1783, 1998.
23. Meriggioli MN, Ciafaloni E, Al-Hayk KA, et al: Mycophenolate mofetil for myasthenia gravis: an analysis of efficacy, safety, and tolerability. Neurology 61:1438–1440, 2003.
24. Gajdos P, Chevret S, Clair B, et al: Clinical trial of plasma exchange and high-dose intravenous immunoglobulin in myasthenia gravis. Myasthenia Gravis Clinical Study Group. Ann Neurol 41:789–796, 1997.
25. Ronager J, Ravenborg M, Hermansen I, et al: Immunoglobulin treatment versus plasma exchange in patients with chronic moderate to severe myasthenia gravis. Artif Organs 25:967–973, 2001.
*26. Skladal D, Sudmeier C, Konstantopoulou V, et al: The clinical spectrum of mitochondrial disease in 75 pediatric patients. Clin Pediatr 42:703–710, 2003.
27. Bernier FP, Boneh A, Dennett X, et al: Diagnostic criteria for respiratory chain disorders in adults and children. Neurology 59:1406–1411, 2002.
28. Scaglia F, Towbin JA, Craigen WJ, et al: Clinical spectrum, morbidity, and mortality in 113 pediatric patients with mitochondrial disease. Pediatrics 114:925–931, 2004.
29. Kleopa KA, Rosenberg H, Heiman-Patterson T: Malignant hyperthermia-like episode in Becker muscular dystrophy. Anesthesiology 93:1535–1537, 2000.
30. Mackay MT, Kornberg AJ, Shield LK, et al: Benign acute childhood myositis: laboratory and clinical features. Neurology 53:2127–2131, 1999.
31. Muntoni F: Cardiac complications of childhood myopathies. J Child Neurol 18:191–202, 2003.
32. Al-Twaijri WA, Shevell MI: Pediatric migraine equivalents: occurrence and clinical features in practice. Pediatr Neurol 26:365–368, 2002.
33. Ravid S, Bienkowski R, Eviatar L: A simplified diagnostic approach to dizziness in children. Pediatr Neurol 29:317–320, 2003.
34. Rowlands S, Hooper R, Hughes R, et al: The epidemiology and treatment of Bell's palsy in the UK. Eur J Neurol 9:63–67, 2002.
*35. Unuvar E, Oguz F, Sidal M, et al: Corticosteroid treatment of childhood Bell's palsy. Pediatr Neurol 21:814–816, 1999.
36. Gilden DH: Clinical practice: Bell's palsy. N Engl J Med 351:1323–1331, 2004.
37. Hato N, Matsumoto S, Kisaki H, et al: Efficacy of early treatment of Bell's palsy with oral acyclovir and prednisolone. Otol Neurotol 24:948–951, 2003.
38. Singhi P, Jain V: Bell's palsy in children. Semin Pediatr Neurol 10:289–297, 2003.
39. Tekavcic-Pompe M, Stirn-Kranjc B, Brecelj J: Optic neuritis in children—clinical and electrophysiological follow-up. Doc Ophthalmol 107:261–270, 2003.
40. Boiko AN, Guseva ME, Guseva MR, et al: Clinico-immunogenetic characteristics of multiple sclerosis with optic neuritis in children. J Neurovirol 6(Suppl 2):S152–S155, 2000.
41. Mizota A, Niimura M, Adachi-Usami E: Clinical characteristics of Japanese children with optic neuritis. Pediatr Neurol 31:42–45, 2004.
42. Ogino S, Leonard DGB, Rennert H, et al: Genetic risk assessment in carrier testing for spinal muscular atrophy. Am J Med Genet 110:301–307, 2002.
43. Bach JR, Baird JS, Plosky D, et al: Spinal muscular atrophy type 1: management and outcomes. Pediatr Pulmonol 34:16–22, 2002.
44. Ptácek LJ: Channelopathies: ion channel disorders of muscle as a paradigm for paroxysmal disorders of the nervous system. Neuromuscul Disord 7:250–255, 1997.
45. Bond EF: Channelopathies: potassium-related periodic paralyses and similar disorders. AACN Clin Issues 11:261–270, 2000.
*46. Venance SL, Cannon SC, Fialho D, et al: The primary periodic paralyses: diagnosis, pathogenesis and treatment. Brain 129:8–17, 2006.

*Selected readings.

Eye Disorders

Michael C. Bachman, MD, MBA and Neil Schamban, MD

Key Points

Evaluation of the patient with a red eye requires a thorough history and physical examination, including lid eversion and slit-lamp examination when age appropriate.

The physician must differentiate between orbital and preseptal cellulitis by presence of proptosis, limited range of extraocular movements, chemosis, and decreased visual acuity.

Age of patient and presenting symptoms will help determine the etiology of conjunctivitis.

Immediate irrigation is the cornerstone of the management of chemical eye injuries.

Selected Diagnoses

The red eye
Iritis
Lacrimal duct pathology
Periorbital and orbital cellulitis
Hordeolum (stye) and chalazion
Conjunctivitis
Chemical injury
Contact lens complications
Traumatic eye injuries

Discussion of Individual Diagnoses

The Red Eye

In evaluating a patient with a red eye, a detailed history must be taken, including the onset, presence of pain, photophobia, visual changes, presence of discharge, history of trauma, prior episodes and ophthalmologic history, whether symptoms are unilateral or bilateral, and the use of contact lenses. The physical examination must include testing of visual acuity; extraocular movements; pupil size, shape, and reactivity; presence of photophobia; slit-lamp examination (age appropriate); eyelid inspection with lid eversion; and intra-ocular pressure measurement. The differential diagnosis of the red eye is summarized in Table 48–1.

Iritis

Inflammation of the iris can occur as a result of blunt trauma to the eye. Nontraumatic iritis is associated with certain diseases, such as ankylosing spondylitis, Reiter's syndrome, sarcoidosis, inflammatory bowel disease, and psoriasis. Infectious causes may include Lyme disease, tuberculosis, toxoplasmosis, syphilis, and herpes simplex and herpes zoster viruses. Iritis has a rapid onset and typically affects only one eye. Signs and symptoms of irtis include pain in the eye, photophobia, tearing, and blurred vision.

Diagnosis is based on slit-lamp examination findings of keratitic precipitates (white blood cells on the endothelium) and detection of an increase in the protein content of the aqueous humor evident by flare.[1] Treatment includes cycloplegic drops and ophthalmology consultation.

Lacrimal Duct Pathology

Lacrimal duct inflammation, know as canaliculitis, is uncommon in children. Canaliculitis usually presents with induration and erythema in the medial eyelid and is often coupled with discharge from the involved puncta. The cause is often *Actinomyces israelii*, and the condition may result in stone formation within the lacrimal ducts. In cases without dacryoliths, topical or systemic antibiotics may be adequate treatment. In cases in which stones have formed, punctual dilation, canaliculoplasty, curettage, and antibiotic irrigation become necessary to cure the disease.[2]

Dacrocystitis results from the obstruction of the flow of tears from the eye through the nasolacrimal duct. Lack of tear drainage results in stasis and accumulation of bacteria and toxins, thus promoting more inflammation. The nasolacrimal system becomes more stenotic, and an abscess forms in the nasolacrimal sac. The mainstay of treatment for dacryoadenitis is application of warm compresses for 15 minutes four times per day to promote drainage and prevent the spread of infection. If the condition does not improve with conservative management, the patient should be referred to an ophthalmologist for incision and drainage.

Periorbital Cellulitis

Periorbital or preseptal cellulitis is an infection of the eyelid and periorbital soft tissues anterior to the orbital septum, a fibrous tissue that arises from the periosteum of the skull and

Table 48–1	Differential Diagnosis of the Red Eye
Diagnosis	**Clinical Findings**
Blepharitis	Eyelid margin inflammation with erythema, crusting, or scaling. Symptoms include irritation, burning, and itching. Usually bilateral. Two main types are staphylococcal and seborrheic.
Canaliculitis	Mild red eye, usually unilateral. Discharge can be expressed from the canaliculus.
Conjunctivitis	Presence of vascular dilation, cellular infiltration, and exudation. May be allergic, viral, bacterial, or chemical.
Corneal inflammation	May have decreased visual acuity and photophobia, severe eye pain. Fluorescein staining may detect an epithelial defect.
Dacrocystis	Inflammation of the lacrimal duct resulting in localized pain, edema, and erythema.
Episcleritis	Inflammation tends to be limited to an isolated patch.
Foreign body	Detect abrasions with fluorescein, exclude globe injury by slit limp, and always evert eyelids to exclude retained foreign body.
Iritis	Presence of perilimbic flush, cells, and flare noted in the anterior chamber during slit-lamp examination; may be decreased visual acuity and photophobia. Usually is unilateral.
Hordeolum	Infection of glands of the lid; can be internal or external.
Subconjunctival hemorrhage	Bright or dark red patches in the bulbar conjunctiva, secondary to injury or inflammation.

continues into the eyelids. Periorbital cellulitis can be secondary to spread from adjacent infectious sinusitis and upper respiratory tract infections (usually children < 5 years of age) or local spread from adjacent facial infections (usually children ≥ 5 years of age), or can result from primary bacteremia (usually children < 1 year of age). *Streptococcus pneumoniae* is currently the primary causative agent of bacteremia resulting in periorbital cellulitis. Other organisms responsible include *Staphylococcus aureus, Staphylococcus epidermidis,* and group A streptococcus.[3]

The patient typically presents with erythema, edema, induration, and tenderness or warmth of the periorbital tissues, but often shows no signs of systemic illness such as fever or leukocytosis. A break in the skin or an insect bite may be noted. It is important to rule out conditions that can simulate periorbital cellulitis, including allergic reactions, severe conjunctivitis, and orbital cellulitis. While preseptal cellulitis is confined to the tissues anterior to the septum, the infection may spread beyond the septum to the subperiosteal tissue and create an intraorbital infection.

Well-appearing children beyond infancy with no systemic signs and mild periorbital cellulitis can be treated with oral antibiotics against gram-positive bacteria (cephalexin, dicloxacillin, clindamycin).[4] Clinical improvement should be seen within 24 to 48 hours. If the patient deteriorates, orbital cellulitis must be ruled out.

Orbital Cellulitis

Orbital cellulitis is an infection of the orbit itself. Orbital cellulitis occurs

1. As a complication of sinusitis with extension of the infection to the orbit
2. Secondary to penetrating trauma
3. As an extension of a nearby facial infection

Infectious agents include *S. pneumoniae,* nontypeable *Haemophilus influenzae, Moraxella catarrhalis,* group A streptococcus, *S. aureus,* and anaerobes. Patients present with signs of periorbital cellulitis and decreased eye movement, proptosis, chemosis, decreased visual acuity, and papilledema. Local complications include abscess formation, optic neuritis, retinal vein thrombosis, and panophthalmitis. Resulting septic thrombophlebitis can lead to meningitis, epidural and subdural abscesses and cavernous sinus thrombosis.

If orbital cellulitis is suspected, a computed tomography (CT) scan of the orbit is indicated. Signs of orbital cellulitis

on CT scan include proptosis, inflammation of the ocular muscles, subperiosteal abscess, or frank orbital abscess (Fig. 48–1). Ophthalmologic consultation is indicated for suspected orbital cellulitis, and an otorhinolaryngology consultation may be necessary when associated with sinusitis.

Patients with orbital cellulitis must receive prompt treatment with intravenous antibiotics. Third-generation cephalosporins and ampicillin/sulbactam are the antibiotics of choice. If the child is penicillin allergic, vancomycin is an appropriate choice.[5] Inpatient admission is required for frequent monitoring and observation for progression of the infection. When an abscess is present, surgical drainage is indicated.[6]

Hordeolum (Stye) and Chalazion

An external hordeolum or stye is an infection involving the gland of Zeis at the base of the cilia on the eyelid. Patients present with localized lid edema, erythema, and tenderness, and purulent drainage may be noted along the lid margin (Fig. 48–2). A chalazion is an internal hordeolum that results in a chronic granulomatous inflammation of the meibomian glands within the tarsal plate. Patients present with painful swelling and erythema in the body of the eyelid. The chalazion may rupture to the conjunctival surface (Fig. 48–3) or externally to the skin, or become chronic and develop into a nontender, noninflamed mass in the eyelid body. It is essential to perform a thorough eye examination to rule out a foreign body under eyelid.

Management of both styes and chalazions consists of eyelash scrubs with baby shampoo once or twice daily and warm compresses applied for 15 minutes four times daily.[7] The use of topical antibiotics remains controversial and is not recommended by the American Academy of Ophthalmology.[8] If a chalazion has not resolved after 4 weeks, ophthalmologic consultation should be sought.

Conjunctivitis

Inflammation of the conjunctiva can be due to various etiologies. The age at presentation and type of symptoms can help in differentiating between the various etiologies (Table 48–2). Special attention must be paid to the presence and quality of eye discharge and the presence of pruritis and pain. The physical examination should include a complete eye examination, visual acuity testing, fluorescein staining, and, if indicated, slit-lamp examination and tonometry. Conjunc-

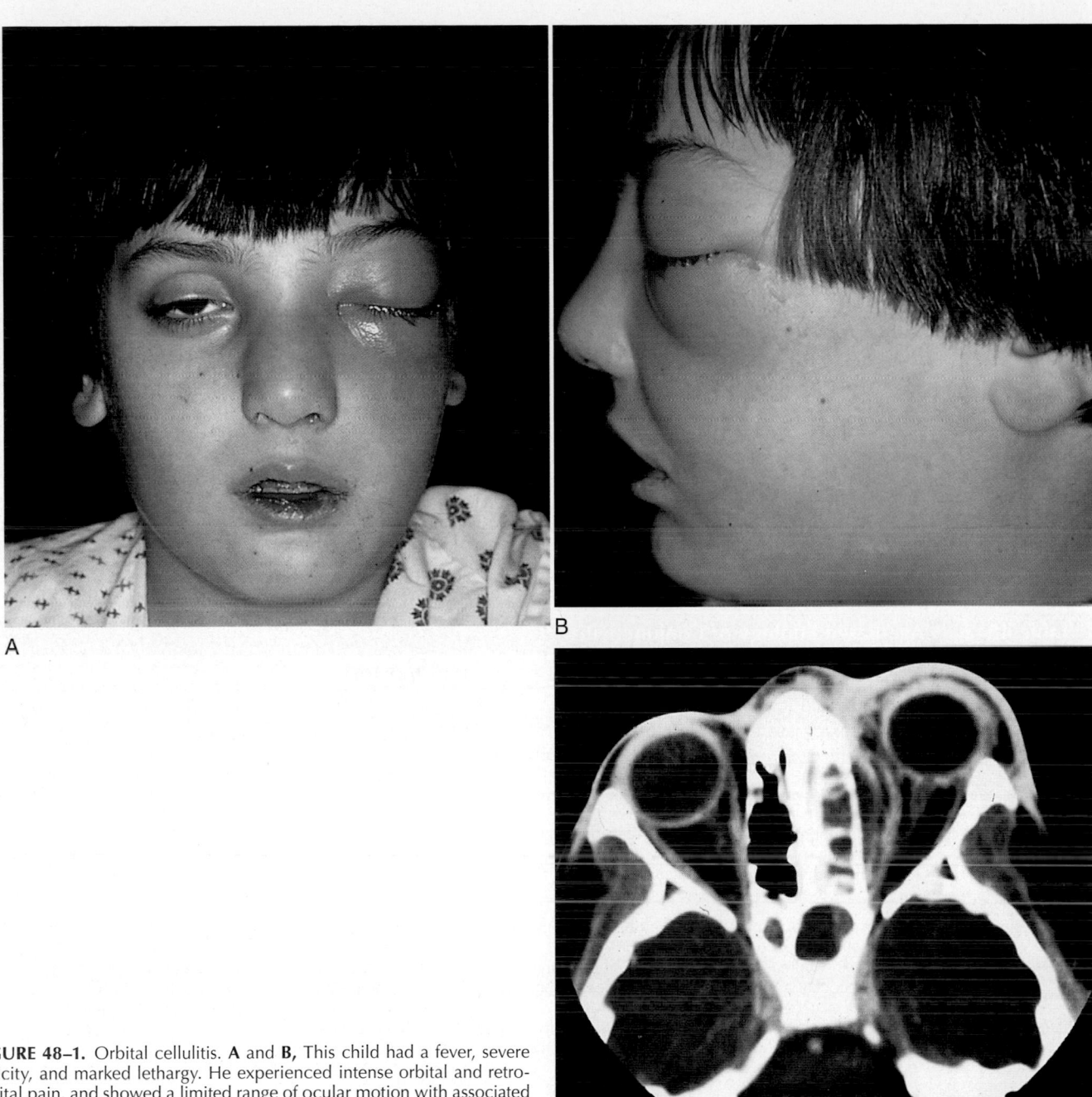

FIGURE 48–1. Orbital cellulitis. **A** and **B,** This child had a fever, severe toxicity, and marked lethargy. He experienced intense orbital and retro-orbital pain, and showed a limited range of ocular motion with associated exacerbation of pain. **C,** Computed tomography scan showing preseptal swelling, proptosis, and lateral displacement of the globe and orbital contents by a subperiosteal abscess.

tivitis is usually diagnosed clinically by history and physical examination. Culture and Gram stain are indicated for those patients with persistent symptoms despite treatment, in all neonates, and when gonorrheal infection is suspected. Chlamydial etiology can be proven with immunofluorescent antibody testing of conjunctival discharge.[9,10] Treatment is based on etiology of the inflammation[11] (see Table 48–2).

Chemical Injury

A chemical injury to the eye is an ophthalmic emergency and must be treated promptly to prevent permanent damage. The severity of the injury is based on the pH of the chemical, the duration of the exposure, and the concentration of the chem-ical in the involved solution. It is of utmost importance to differentiate between acid and alkali burns. Acid burns tend to be less severe and cause conjunctival erythema, edema, and small hemorrhages. Alkalis, including lime, lye, and ammonia, cause more severe injury than acids. They can destroy the conjunctiva and penetrate the cornea, anterior chamber, and retina. Due to their rapid penetration of the ocular tissue, damage continues long after the injury. A chemical conjunctivitis may also be caused by smoke from house fires. Other common irritants that can cause discomfort include household detergents and pepper spray.[12]

Patients with a chemical eye injury may present with pain, erythema, tearing, difficulty keeping the eye open, a

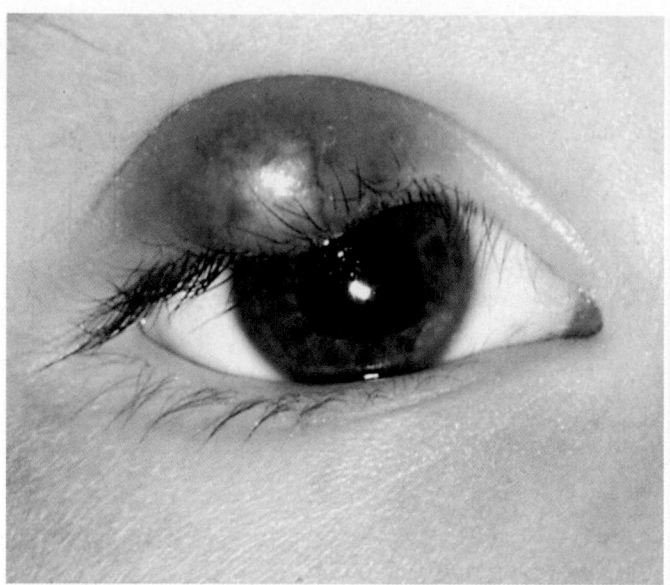

FIGURE 48-2. Acute hordeolum of the eyelid (pointing externally) with swelling, induration, and purulent contents.

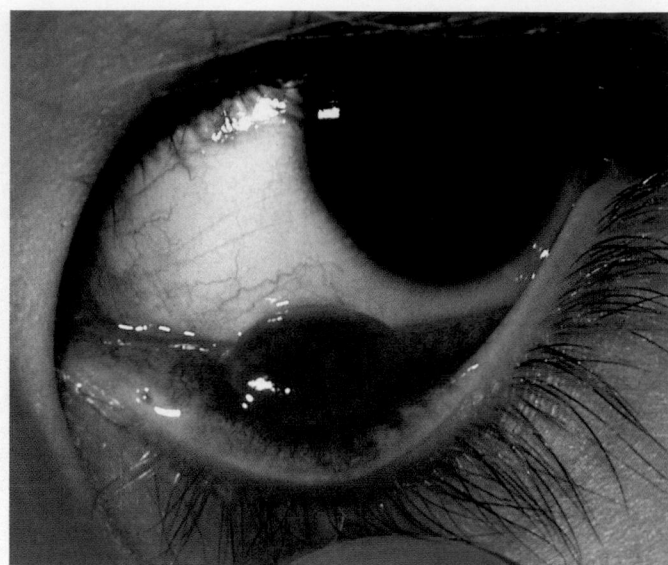

FIGURE 48-3. Chalazion of the left lower lid pointed internally. A pyogenic granuloma consisting of a vascularized mound of conjuctival tissue has developed over the chalazion because of spontaneous rupture of the chalazion under the palpebral conjunctiva.

Table 48–2	Age-Based Etiology of Conjunctivitis	
Etiology	**Clinical Findings**	**Treatment**
Neonates		
Silver nitrate	6–12 hours after birth. Erythema, chemosis, eyelid edema, and purulent exudates.	Spontaneous resolution by 24–48 hr
Neisseria gonorrhoeae	2–5 days of life. Thick mucopurulent drainage, tense lid edema.	Ceftriaxone 25–50 mg/kg IV given once; frequent eye irrigation until discharge is eliminated
Chlamydia	5–14 days of life. Mild inflammation to severe swelling with purulent exudates.	Oral erythromycin 50 mg/kg per day in 4 divided doses for 14 days
Herpesvirus	5–15 days of life. Diffuse hyperemia, watery drainage.	Steroids are contraindicated. Immediate ophthalmology consultation for further examination and treatment.
Children		
Viral	Acute or subacute. Thin, seropurulent discharge; marked conjunctival injection. Pruritis is common.	Self-limited but highly contagious. No treatment necessary. Artificial tears may alleviate symptoms.
Bacterial	Acute onset. Minimal pain; thick, purulent discharge. Staphylococcal and streptococcal are most common.	Ointment is better for infants and young children. Choices include bacitracin/polymyxin B, trimethoprim, erythromycin, and ofloxacin.
Chlamydia	Chronic with exacerbations and remissions. History of STD. Minimal discharge and moderate conjunctival injection.	Doxycycline 100 mg twice a day for 10 days *or* azithromycin 1 g in a single dose.
Gonococcal	Copious mucopurulent drainage.	Ceftriaxone 50 mg/kg (maximum 1 g) IM in a single dose.
Allergic	Acute or subacute. Painless, with moderate injection, clear watery drainage, and significant pruritis.	Cool compresses, lubricants, decongestants (naphazoline), and mast cell stabilizers (cromolyn).

Abbreviations: IM, intramuscularly; IV, intravenously; STD, sexually transmitted disease.

sensation of something in the eye, eyelid edema, and blurred vision. Immediate irrigation is the cornerstone of the management of chemical eye injuries. Irrigation should commence immediately after a patient has been triaged with a steady stream of eye irrigation solution, normal saline, or lactated Ringer's solution for 15 to 20 minutes. If readily available, topical anesthetic drops should be used prior to and during irrigation. Conjunctival pH should be checked periodically with litmus paper, and irrigation continued until the pH normalizes to 7.0. After completing irrigation, patients should be referred to an ophthalmologist for evaluation and ongoing treatment.[13]

Contact Lens Complications

Contact lens wearers can experience complications affecting the lids, conjunctiva, and cornea. The most prevalent complication is a hypersensitivity reaction to the contact lens solution. This can cause corneal staining and conjunctival injection. Treatment involves removal of the lens, cold compresses, and follow-up with an ophthalmologist. Contact lens wearers can also develop giant papillary conjunctivitis and present with conjunctival injection, mucoid discharge, itching, and blurred vision. Corneal abrasions are common among contact lens wearers. A severe infectious complication in contact lens wearers is bacterial infectious keratitis. Patients present acutely with pain, photophobia, tearing, purulent discharge, and blurry vision. The most common causative agents are *Pseudomonas aeuruginosa, S. aureus,* and *S. epidermidis.* Prompt treatment with topical antibiotics is indicated. Use of disposable contact lenses and reduced wearing time have decreased the incidence of these complications.[14]

Traumatic Eye Injuries

Conjunctival and Corneal Foreign Bodies

Conjunctival and corneal foreign bodies must be removed. Local anesthetics are useful for detecting the foreign body during a thorough eye examination and allows for removal of the foreign body. However, they should never be given to the patients to use themselves because they slow healing, and the patients may cause further damage rubbing the anesthetized eye.

Small, loose conjunctival foreign bodies can be removed with a cotton-wool bud or irrigated with saline. It is important to evert the upper lid to exclude a subtarsal foreign body, especially if the patient reports the sensation that a foreign body is still present. Lid eversion should not be performed if a penetrating injury is suspected.[15] Corneal foreign bodies may be more difficult to remove. If they are metallic, they may have formed a rust ring that may permanently stain the cornea. They should be removed with a needle tip or rotary drill.[16] These procedures require meticulous care, and these patients should be evaluated by an ophthalmologist.

Corneal Abrasions and Corneal Ulcers

Corneal abrasion, the most common eye injury in children, occurs because of a disruption in the integrity of the corneal epithelium.[17] While corneal epithelial abrasions usually will heal without serious sequelae, deeper corneal involvement may result in epithelial facet formation or stromal scar formation. Symptoms range from mild foreign body sensation with small abrasions to severe pain with larger abrasions. Pain typically starts immediately after the trauma and can last for days, and may be accompanied by photophobia and excessive tearing. Typically conjunctival injection and occasionally eyelid swelling are present. In cases of a significant abrasion, slit-lamp examination reveals a defect in the corneal epithelium. This defect can be confirmed by placing a drop of fluorescein in the inferior fornix. The defect takes up the fluorescein and appears to glow under the blue cobalt light of the slit lamp.

Topical antibiotics are recommended for all corneal abrasion as prophylaxis from developing a bacterial corneal ulcer. Topical fluoroquinolones, ciprofloxacin drops, polymyxin B/trimethoprim drops, erythromycin ointment, bacitracin ointment, and bacitracin/polymyxin B ointment are appropriate choices. Close follow-up care of corneal abrasions is necessary because of possible progression to an ulcer.[12] Patients with abrasions should receive follow-up care until healing is complete and no staining with fluorescein occurs. Patching has not been found to increase the rate of healing and is not routinely recommended for use in children.[18]

Subconjunctival Hemorrhage

Generally, this condition is painless. Vision is not affected. The eye will have a red spot of blood on the sclera (the white part of the eye). This occurs when there is a rupture of a small blood vessel on the surface of the eye. The area of redness may be fairly large, and its appearance is sometimes alarming. It is not dangerous and generally goes away slowly with no treatment.

REFERENCES

1. Zierhut M, Michels H, Stubiger N, et al: Uveitis and related ocular inflammations: a global perspective from the International Uveitis Study Group. Int Ophthalmol Clin 45:135–156, 2005.
2. Park A, Morgenstern K, Kahwash S, et al: Pediatric canaliculitis and stone formation. Ophthalmic Plast Reconstr Surg 20:243–246, May 2004.
3. Shwartz G, Wright S: Changing bacteriology of periorbital cellulitis. Ann Emerg Med 28:617–620, 1996.
*4. Givner LB: Periorbital versus orbital cellulitis. Pediatr Infect Dis J 21:1157–1158, 2002.
5. Gilbert DN, Moellering RC, Elipoulos GM, Sande MA: The Sandford Guide to Antimicrobial Therapy, 34th ed. Hyde Park, VT: Antimicrobial Therapy Inc, 2004.
6. Starkey C, Steele R: Medical management of orbital cellulitis. Pediatr Infect Dis J 20:1002–1005, 2001.
*7. Smythe D, Hurwitz JJ, Tayfour F: The management of chalazion: a survey of Ontario ophthalmologists. Can J Ophthalmol 25:252–255, 1990.
8. Jackson, TL, Beun L: A prospective study of cost, patient satisfaction, and outcome of treatment of chalazion by medical and nursing staff. Br J Ophthalmol 84:782–785, 2000.
9. de Toledo AR, Chandler JW: Conjunctivitis of the newborn. Infect Dis Clin North Am 6:807–813, 1992.
10. Gigliotti F, Williams W, Hayden F, et al: Etiology of acute conjunctivitis in children. J Pediatr 98:531–536, 1981.
*11. Teoh DL, Reynolds S: Diagnosis and management of pediatric conjunctivitis. Pediatr Emerg Care 19:48–55, 2003.
12. Levin A: Eye emergencies: acute management in the pediatric ambulatory care setting. Pediatr Emerg Care 7:367–377, 1991.
*13. Wagoner MD: Chemical injuries of the eye: current concepts in pathophysiology and therapy. Surv Ophthalmol 41:275–313, 1997.
14. American Optometric Association: Care of the Contact Lens Patient. St. Louis: American Optometric Association, 2000.
15. Khaw P, Shah P, Elkington AR: ABC of eyes: injury to the eye [Authors' reply]. BMJ 328:644, 2004.
16. Lit ES, Young LHY: Anterior and posterior segment intraocular foreign bodies. Int Ophthalmol Clin 42:107–120, 2002.
*17. Nelson LB, Wilson TW, Jeffers JB: Eye injuries in childhood: demography, etiology, and prevention. Pediatrics 84:438–441, 1989.
18. Patterson J, Fetzer D, Krall J: Eye patch treatment for the pain of corneal abrasion. South Med J 89:227–229, 1996.

*Selected readings.

Chapter 49

Epistaxis

Kenneth B. Briskin, MD

Key Points

Blood supply to the septum is from both the internal and external carotid systems, which affects the approach to management.

Most episodes of epistaxis are anterior and can be controlled with 5 to 10 minutes of direct pressure.

Management of epistaxis in children needs to proceed in a stepwise, organized fashion from local measures to packing to surgical intervention.

Control of significant bleeding should take precedence over a lengthy history.

Universal precautions must be observed at all times, with protective eyewear, gowns, mask, and gloves for all caregivers.

Introduction and Background

Epistaxis is an anxiety-provoking occurrence that affects both patients and parents. Children with acute hemorrhage from the nasal cavity or nasopharynx present with varying degrees of blood loss.[1] Patients may present with intermittent blood streaking or life-threatening hemorrhage. Fortunately, severe epistaxis is rare in children, and in most cases only simple measures are necessary to control the bleeding.[2] The emergency physician must be ready to quickly evaluate and treat these children in an orderly fashion. He or she needs knowledge of the procedures to control epistaxis and when a referral to an otolaryngologist is indicated. Having an organized, systematic approach will allay the fears of the patient and parents.

Recognition and Approach

Epistaxis can occur at almost any age, but generally first appears at about 3 years of age. Its frequency increases from ages 2 to 10 years and levels off by adolescence.[1] Epistaxis most commonly occurs from the nasal septum, where superficial vessels can become easily exposed with minimal trauma.

The nasal mucosa is adherent to the periosteum and perichondrium on the inside of the nose and provides little support and protection to the overlying plexus of vessels. The most common site of bleeding is in Little's area in the superior area of the anterior septum. Bleeding occurs here in a confluence of richly supplied vessels known as Kiesselbach's plexus.

Epistaxis in children can be very different than in adults. Both children and parents are generally very anxious, making diagnosis and treatment difficult. It is more difficult in children to gauge the amount of blood loss, which tends to be exaggerated. The significantly smaller nasal airway in children makes identification of the bleeding site much more difficult.[2,3]

Clinical Presentation

Patients with epistaxis present with varying degrees of acuity. Most patients present to the emergency department with active bleeding that does not stop quickly at home. Patients who present early on do so most commonly with anterior, unilateral bleeding. These patients are otherwise normal in appearance, with normal vital signs and laboratory values. Bleeding is most commonly unilateral from the Kiesselbach plexus area of the anterior septum.[4]

Late presentation can include changes in mental status, color, and vital signs.[3,4] Bleeding from a posterior site must be considered in these cases. Fortunately, posterior epistaxis is rare in children. If bleeding is seen bilaterally, a posterior bleed must be considered. This could be coming from a nasopharyngeal mass, such as a juvenile nasopharyngeal angiofibroma, seen most commonly in adolescent males.[4] If the patient has a septal perforation, bilateral bleeding may also be present.

Patients with posterior bleeding may present with little anterior bleeding from the nares. There may be significant blood loss that is swallowed, and these patients may only present to the emergency department after vomiting a large amount of blood. A posterior source of bleeding is likely in these cases, and the oropharynx must be examined for blood streaming down from above.[4,5]

Children most commonly present with a history of local irritation.[4] This may come from digital trauma. A recent upper respiratory infection or exacerbation of allergic symptoms can cause vasodilation of the nasal mucosa, making this more susceptible to bleeding.

Table 49–1	Etiology of Epistaxis

Local Factors

Trauma, picking
Local inflammation: allergic rhinitis, viral upper respiratory
  infection, mononucleosis, measles, furuncle
Foreign body
Rhinitis sicca

Masses

Polyps
Juvenile nasopharyngeal angiofibroma
Malignant neoplasms (rare)

Systemic Factors

Platelet disorders: leukemia, idiopathic thrombocytopenic
  purpura, von Willebrand's disease, uremia
Hereditary hemorrhagic telangiectasia (Osler-Weber-Rendu
  syndrome)
Hepatic disease
Vitamin K deficiency
AIDS
Drugs: aspirin, NSAIDs, warfarin
Hypertension

Abbreviations: AIDS, acquired immunodeficiency syndrome;
NSAIDs, nonsteroidal anti-inflammatory drugs.

Table 49–2	Management of Epistaxis

Local Measures

Pressure for 5–10 min to lower third of nose
Anesthetic-vasoconstrictor placed into nasal cavity
Cauterization with silver nitrate

Packing

Anterior packing
  Self-expanding packs
  Petrolatum-soaked gauze
Posterior packing
  Nasal balloons
  Posterior gauze/Foley balloon catheter

Surgical Intervention

Nasal endoscopy with electrocauterization
Endoscopic ligation of sphenopalatine artery
Transantral ligation of internal maxillary artery
Ligation of ethmoid arteries

Interventional Radiology

Embolization of external carotid system

Important Clinical Features and Considerations

Patients presenting with epistaxis are very anxious, as are their parents. Many parents have already tried to stop the bleeding with pressure or ice. Parents often try home methods unsuccessfully or put pressure on an ineffective area, such as over the nasal bones. Patients frequently position their heads with the neck extended, swallowing a great deal of blood. Patients will be more comfortable sitting up with their head forward to avoid more blood going down the back of their throat. It is unlikely that a dangerous amount of blood has been lost in an acute bleed; however, hypovolemia must be a concern if the history of when the bleeding started is unclear.

Management

Management of epistaxis should be approached in an orderly fashion (Table 49–2). The initial assessment and physical examination should be performed as described earlier. Immediate management involves positioning the patient in an upright position and providing gauze pads and possible suction for the oral cavity. The obvious initial treatment maneuver is local compression. The thumb and index finger are used to compress the lower third of the nose for 5 to 10 minutes. This will likely slow and possibly stop the bleeding, allowing formation of a hemostatic plug over the bleeding vessel. It also allows the physician time to set up for the next step in management[9,10] (see Chapter 174, Epistaxis Control).

Cauterization is the next step if bleeding is not controlled or if the bleeding has been recurrent. Topical anesthetic with 2% lidocaine can be combined with a local vasoconstrictor. Cotton pledgets can be soaked in this solution and placed into the nose for 5 minutes. Accurate identification of the bleeding site and a good head light are necessary to successfully control epistaxis by cauterization. Silver nitrate sticks are used to control the bleeding sites. Pressure is applied to the bleeding site with the stick for 10 to 15 seconds. Following this, further pressure can be held on the site with

Laboratory studies in cases of epistaxis are dependent on the history and presentation. Often a recent onset of mild acute bleeding requires no blood work at all. However, a history of persistent, intermittent bleeding warrants a complete blood count with platelets and type and screen. If there is any suspicion of bleeding disorders through a history of other unusual bleeding or bruising, tests for coagulopathies and platelet disorders should be included. Initial studies include prothrombin time, partial thromboplastin time, international normalized ratio, and platelet function analyzer (PFA). Radiologic studies are rarely necessary unless a neoplasm is suspected[1,4-6] (see Chapter 129, Acute Childhood Immune Thrombocytopenic Purpura and Related Platelet Disorders; and Chapter 130, Disorders of Coagulation).

There are many causes of nose bleeds (Table 49–1). Local causes (e.g., nose picking) are the most common. Other causes include facial trauma, neoplasms, foreign bodies, chemical irritants, and inhalation of dry air. Local infections and inflammation (i.e., rhinitis, sinusitis) can lead to epistaxis, but generally only lead to blood-tinged mucus. Foreign bodies can cause unilateral bleeding with a foul-smelling discharge. Iatrogenic causes include nasogastric and nasotracheal tubes.

Episodes of epistaxis can be associated with systemic causes. Coagulopathies, platelet disorders, hereditary hemorrhagic telangiectasia (Osler-Weber-Rendu syndrome), and renal disease are possible causes. Neoplasms associated with epistaxis include intranasal arteriovenous malformations. Juvenile nasopharyngeal angiofibromas are benign neoplasms seen in adolescent males and must be considered in this population.[7,8]

Many medications can cause epistaxis. Nonsteroidal anti-inflammatory agents, aspirin, and warfarin are commonly associated with epistaxis. Allergy medications, including antihistamines, can dry mucosa, and topical nasal decongestants can irritate mucosa, inducing bleeding. Topical nasal steroid sprays can cause irritation from the medication as well as trauma to the septum from the tip of the dispenser.[4]

a cotton-tipped applicator. If silver nitrate gets on the patient's skin, it will leave a black mark that will remain for 2 to 3 days.

When bleeding continues following cauterization, nasal packing is needed. Packing can be very uncomfortable; therefore, topical anesthetic with lidocaine and intravenous sedation may be necessary prior to placement. Many different materials for anterior packing are currently available. They include synthetic sponges that expand when moist and balloons that are filled with saline, putting pressure on the bleeding point. These are quick and easy to insert and can be used for bilateral epistaxis if necessary. The success rate of these packs is over 90% regardless of the extent of experience of the physician.[11] A more traditional type of packing is with petrolatum-soaked gauze. Placement of this packing is technically more difficult, but it can provide more pressure than the sponges. After placement of this packing, the oropharynx should be examined for blood trickling down from the nasopharynx. If this occurs, either the packing is inadequate or the bleeding is posterior.

Posterior epistaxis in pediatric patients, fortunately, is uncommon. Packing in the posterior aspect of the nasal cavity can fall into the nasopharynx. Therefore, a pack must be placed against the nasopharynx in such a manner that it will not unravel. Alternatively, balloon catheters are inserted into the nasopharynx via the nostril and filled with saline. Posterior packing is an unpleasant experience for the patient while in place. These patients require admission with cardiopulmonary monitoring and sedation. Packing should be left in place 48 to 72 hours.

Complications with nasal packing exist, but can be easily avoided if anticipated. Infection and toxic shock syndrome are uncommon in the pediatric population, but antibiotics should be used when the packing is in place. The packing can become dislodged or aspirated. Septal perforation and alar necrosis can occur. Nasal-vagal response has been reported with bradycardia, hypotension, hypoxia, and apnea. Therefore, sedation should be kept to a minimum.[11]

When packing is ineffective, an otolaryngologist should be consulted for surgical intervention. Initial surgical intervention includes nasal endoscopy with direct visualization of bleeding and electrocautery. This is extremely effective in controlling bleeding and can also help when packing is removed, especially in patients with recurrent epistaxis. The sphenopalatine artery can also be identified endoscopically and clipped, controlling most bleeding.[12] More traditional surgical interventions, such as transantral ligation of the internal maxillary artery and clipping of the ethmoid artery, are also possible but rarely necessary.

Interventional radiology has a growing role in the control of persistent epistaxis. The external carotid artery branches can be embolized. This technique, however, is currently used in adults who are at high risk for general anesthesia. The success rate is high, and the procedure can avoid the need for posterior packing.[13,14]

Summary

Epistaxis is a common clinical problem. Management of nosebleeds in an organized fashion has a high success rate. With proper treatment, the prognosis for these patients is excellent. Patients discharged with packing in place should see an otolaryngologist for removal in 48 to 72 hours. Patients need to be aware that the greatest risk is recurrent bleeding. These cases should be referred to an otolaryngologist for a complete nasal and nasopharyngeal examination.

REFERENCES

1. Katsanis E, Luke KH, Hsu E, et al: Prevalence and significance of mild bleeding disorders in children with recurrent epistaxis. J Pediatr 113:73–76, 1998.
*2. Viducich RA, Blanda MP, Gerson LW: Posterior epistaxis: clinical features and acute complications. Ann Emerg Med 25:592–596, 1995.
*3. Wuman LH, Sack JG, Flannery JV, et al: The management of epistaxis. Am J Otolaryngol 13:193–209, 1992.
*4. Tan LK, Calhoun KH: Epistaxis. Med Clin North Am 83:43–56, 1999.
*5. Alvi A, Joyner-Triplett N: Acute epistaxis: how to spot the source and stop the flow. Postgrad Med 99:83–96, 1996.
6. Jackson KR, Jackson RT: Factors associated with active, refractory epistaxis. Arch Otolaryngol Head Neck Surg 114:862–865, 1988.
7. Herkner H, Laggner AN, Mullner M, et al: Hypertension in patients presenting with epistaxis. Ann Emerg Med 35:126–130, 2000.
8. Lubianca-Neto JF, Fuchs FD, Facco SR, et al: Is epistaxis evidence of end-organ damage in patients with hypertension? Laryngoscope 109:1111–1115, 1999.
9. Mcgarry GW, Moulton C: Epistaxis first aid. Arch Emerg Med 10:298–300, 1993.
10. Shaw CB, Wax MK, Wetmore SJ: Epistaxis: a comparison of treatment. Otolaryngol Head Neck Surg 109:60–65, 1993.
11. Pollice PA, Yoder MG: Epistaxis: a retrospective review of hospitalized patients. Otolaryngol Head Neck Surg 117:49–53, 1997.
12. El-Guindy A: Endoscopic transeptal sphenopalatine artery ligation for intractable posterior epistaxis. Ann Otol Rhinol Laryngol 107:1033–1037, 1998.
13. Scaramuzzi N, Walsh RM, Brennan P, et al: Treatment of intractable epistaxis using arterial embolization. Clin Otolaryngol 26:307–309, 2001.
14. Siniluoto TM, Leinonen AS, Karttunen AI, et al: Embolization for the treatment of posterior epistaxis: an analysis of 31 cases. Arch Otolaryngol Head Neck Surg 119:837–841, 1993.

*Selected readings.

Rhinosinusitis

Robert Acosta, MD

Introduction and Background

Sinusitis is the inflammation of one or more of the paranasal sinuses, which include the ethmoid, maxillary, sphenoid, and frontal sinuses. This inflammation can be due to infection, allergy, or anatomic obstruction. The obstruction of the sinus ostia, whether due to infection, allergy, or anatomic malformations (Fig. 50–1), is the common pathway leading to the symptoms and pathology of sinusitis.[1,7] The term *rhinosinusitis* is considered by many experts to be a more accurate term since the nasal mucosa is almost always involved in sinus infections.[3] Rhinosinusitis, based on the duration of symptoms, is further subdivided into acute rhinosinusitis, chronic rhinosinusitis, and recurrent rhinosinusitis.[1,2] It has been estimated that between 5% and 10% of children with an upper respiratory infection will go on to develop rhinosinusitis.[2,4]

The etiology of rhinosinusitis can be divided into the following categories: infectious and allergic. Among infectious etiologies, viral causes of rhinosinusitis include rhinovirus, influenza virus, and coronavirus.[3] Viral infections cause local inflammation and blockage of the sinus ostia. Additionally, they can disrupt the ciliary function of the sinuses, leading to stasis and subsequent bacterial colonization. Cultures obtained from individuals presenting to an outpatient clinic with signs and symptoms consistent with acute bacterial rhinosinusitis revealed a number of organisms, as reported by the Respiratory Surveillance Program.[4] The most common bacterial organisms causing rhinosinusitis are listed in Table 50–1.

There is a strong association between rhinosinusitis and allergy. Children with a family history of allergy are at a higher risk of developing rhinosinusitis.[1] Some authors have considered whether rhinosinusitis and asthma are variations of the same disease.[5] When an allergen is identified and exposure to that allergen reduced or eliminated, there is a marked decrease in rhinosinusitis symptoms.[5,6]

Recognition and Approach

The maxillary and ethmoid sinuses form in utero and are present at birth. The sphenoid sinus forms at approximately 5 years of age and the frontal sinuses at 7 to 8 years. This timeline becomes important when considering the clinical symptoms and complications that accompany rhinosinusitis at various ages. Maxillary sinusitis, for example, is more common in younger children than sphenoid or frontal sinusitis.

Clinical Presentation

Acute Bacterial Rhinosinusitis

According to the American Academy of Pediatrics clinical practice guideline on sinusitis, acute bacterial sinusitis is defined as a bacterial infection of the paranasal sinuses that persists less than 30 days.[1] Goldsmith and Rosenfeld defined acute rhinosinusitis as an upper respiratory infection that persists beyond 10 days.[3] Ueda and Yoto used the same definition for rhinosinusitis in his study group and was able to demonstrate radiographic proof of sinusitis in 92.5% of patients.[7] Acute bacterial sinusitis can also be further divided by the severity of the presenting symptoms. Severe symptoms include illness duration of more than 10 to 14 days, fever $\geq 102°$ F, and purulent nasal discharge in an ill-appearing child.[1]

The symptoms of an acute rhinosinusitis include nasal discharge, cough, fever, and halitosis. Nasal discharge can be clear or mucopurulent and does not correlate with the severity of disease. Cough is the most common complaint and is classically worse at night. The cough is described as persistent and may be dry or accompanied by copious nasal secretions. Fever is more indicative of a bacterial rhinosinusitis infection, especially when it lasts longer than 3 days and accompanies the rhinitis.[3] Children with maxillary sinusitis can present with pain to the upper posterior teeth. Rhinosinusitis can be differentiated from an upper respiratory tract infection (URI) by the worsening of symptoms

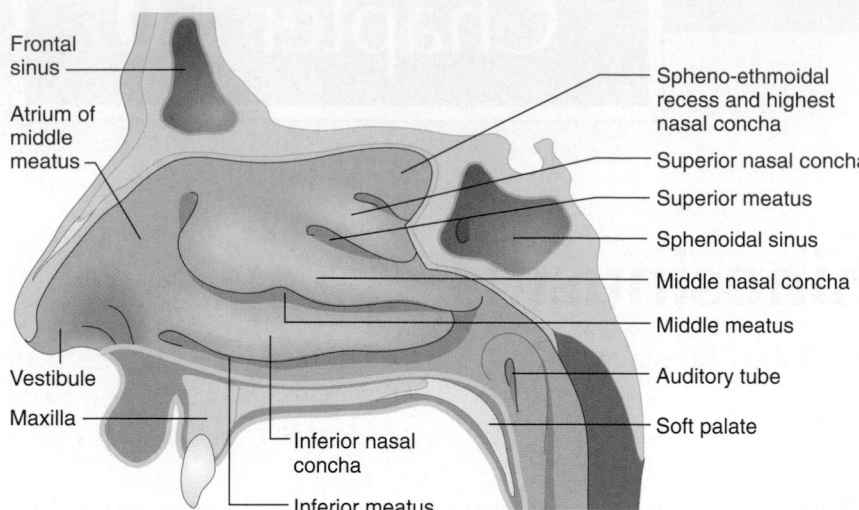

Frontal sinus
Atrium of middle meatus
Vestibule
Maxilla
Inferior nasal concha
Inferior meatus

Spheno-ethmoidal recess and highest nasal concha
Superior nasal concha
Superior meatus
Sphenoidal sinus
Middle nasal concha
Middle meatus
Auditory tube
Soft palate

FIGURE 50–1. Lateral view of the nasal passages. (From Williams PL, Warwick R: Gray's Anatomy, 36th ed. London: Churchill Livingstone, 1980.)

Table 50–1	Frequency of Organisms in Acute Pediatric Sinusitis	
		Frequency (%)
*Streptococcus pneumoniae**		30–66
Haemophilus influenzae non–type b		20–30
Moraxella catarrhalis		12–28
Staphylococcus aureus		<10

*Seventy percent penicillin resistance.
From Anon JB: Acute bacterial rhinosinusitis in pediatric medicine: current issues in diagnosis and management. Paediatric Drugs 5(Suppl):25–33, 2003.

over time. URI symptoms will usually improve after a week. Most viral URIs have a fever that peaks early in the disease.[1,3,8]

The physical examination often is of limited value because the clinical findings mimic those of a viral URI. The use of an otoscope to examine the nose is recommended.[3] The nasal mucosa should be examined for edematous turbinates, polyps, and foreign bodies. Reproducible facial tenderness on percussion or pressure over the sinuses may be indicative of sinusitis, although complaints of facial pain are not consistent in children.[1]

Chronic Bacterial Rhinosinusitis

Chronic bacterial rhinosinusitis is described as an infection of the sinuses that lasts more than 90 days. Symptoms include persistent nasal congestion, cough, nasal discharge, and halitosis. Headache is a more common symptom in chronic rhinosinusitis, and a history of behavioral changes may also be present.[3]

Important Clinical Features and Considerations

Children with asthma who continue to have persistent symptoms of cough and rhinorrhea despite appropriate asthma therapy may benefit from antibiotic treatment for rhinosi-nusitis. Resolution of rhinosinusitis in these patients may decrease the number of asthma exacerbations.[5,6]

Intubated patients or patients with a recent history of intubation are at a higher risk of developing rhinosinusitis. Antimicrobial therapy should be aimed at treating *Pseudomonas aeruginosa*, Acinetobacter species, Escherichia species, Enterobacter species, Streptococcus species, and *Staphylococcus aureus*.[9]

Differential Diagnosis

The differential diagnosis for rhinosinusitis includes URI, allergic rhinitis, pneumonia, asthma, nasal foreign bodies and tumors, and immune deficiency (common with human immunodeficiency virus).

Complications

- Frontal sinusitis can result in several complications, including osteomyelitis, intracranial abscesses, meningitis, orbital complications, and dural sinus thrombophlebitis.[10]
- Maxillary sinusitis complications include intracranial abscesses, meningitis, and oral abscesses.
- Sphenoid sinusitis may cause complications as a result of compression or bacterial infiltration and involve the internal carotid artery, cavernous sinus, cranial nerve palsy, ocular disease, intracranial abscess, and meningitis.[11]
- Ethmoid sinusitis has been reported to cause intracranial abscesses, orbital cellulitis, and osteomyelitis.

Imaging Studies

Although rare, children with severe acute and chronic rhinosinusitis are at risk for intracranial pathology. Any child presenting with an abnormal neurologic examination should undergo brain imaging with computed tomography (CT) or magnetic resonance imaging (MRI).[10-12]

Plain Radiography/Sinus Series

These studies have a poor correlation with CT scanning; as many as 75% of them either underestimate or overestimate disease. Plain radiography is a fairly inaccurate screening method for maxillary sinus disease. Inaccuracies are compounded by mucosal tears, asymmetric facial or sinus development, overlying soft tissue, multiple septal walls, sinus overlap, improper exposure, and head rotation.

Computed Tomography

Thin-cut axial and coronal images of the paranasal sinuses are optimal. A limited number of coronal images alone are used by some as a screening method. Contrast is not necessary for routine sinus evaluation, but it is necessary when a complication such as orbital or intracranial abscess is suspected. The best images for chronic sinusitis are taken at the point of maximal wellness, usually during the last week of a 4 week course of maximal medical therapy. Maximal medical therapy includes appropriate antibiotics and possibly nasal saline irrigations, topical nasal steroids, or decongestants.

A 45% occurrence of incidental sinusitis/opacification has been found on pediatric facial CT scans taken for other reasons. In an asymptomatic patient, no treatment or further workup is necessary. In children younger than 12 years, mucosal thickening or sinus opacification is associated with only a 50% chance of actual sinusitis. During an acute viral URI, the sinuses are routinely opacified on CT scan. In the early stages, URIs do not require treatment with antibiotics.

Anatomic abnormalities, hypoplastic maxillary sinuses, concha bullosa, and changes consistent with cystic fibrosis (e.g., medial displacement of the lateral nasal wall) should be noted on review of CT scans. A thinning of the surrounding bone with wispy areas of calcium density may be observed in patients with allergic fungal sinusitis.

Management

Antimicrobial therapy continues to be the mainstay of the treatment of rhinosinusitis. Because of increasing resistance of bacteria to antibiotics, it is important that treating physicians understand the local resistance patterns in their communities. When used judiciously, antibiotics can decrease the number of symptom days in rhinosinusitis.[13] First-line drugs for acute bacterial rhinosinusitis are listed in Table 50–2. The duration of treatment is from 10 to 14 days or for 7 days after symptoms resolve.[1,3,13]

Adjunctive therapy, such as antihistamines, decongestants, and steroids, is controversial, and there are no definitive data concerning their use. Saline drops may help clear the nasal passages and give some comfort to the patient but do not hasten clinical cure.

Overall, imaging has no role in the diagnosis of uncomplicated acute bacterial rhinosinusitis. It may be useful in cases of chronic rhinosinusitis and in those patients who failed medical therapy and for whom surgery is a possibility (Figs. 50–2 and 50–3). Proper positioning of children for radiographs is difficult, and some children may require sedation for CT or MRI.

All patients require re-evaluation after 72 hours to ensure that the antimicrobial therapy is adequate, and that there is no worsening in the patient's condition. Any deterioration in the patient's condition may necessitate a change in the antibiotic regimen.

Table 50–2	First-Line Drugs for Acute Bacterial Rhinosinusitis	
Mild to Moderate Rhinosinusitis	**Severe Rhinosinusitis or Nonresponder to Initial Antibiotic Treatment**
First Line	
Amoxicillin 45 mg/kg *or*	Amoxicillin/clavulanate 90 mg/kg (amoxicillin component) divided bid
Amoxicillin 90 mg/kg divided bid	
Amoxicillin Allergy	
Cefdinir 7 mg/kg q12h or 14 mg/kg daily	Consider ceftriaxone for those patients unable to tolerate drug by mouth.
Cefuroxime 30 mg/kg divided bid	
Cefpodoxime 5 mg/kg q12h	
Severe Amoxicillin Allergy	
Azithromycin	If hospitalized, the patient should have a computed tomography scan of the sinuses. Obtain otorhinolaryngology consult and consider starting the patient on vancomycin.
Clarithromycin Clindomycin	

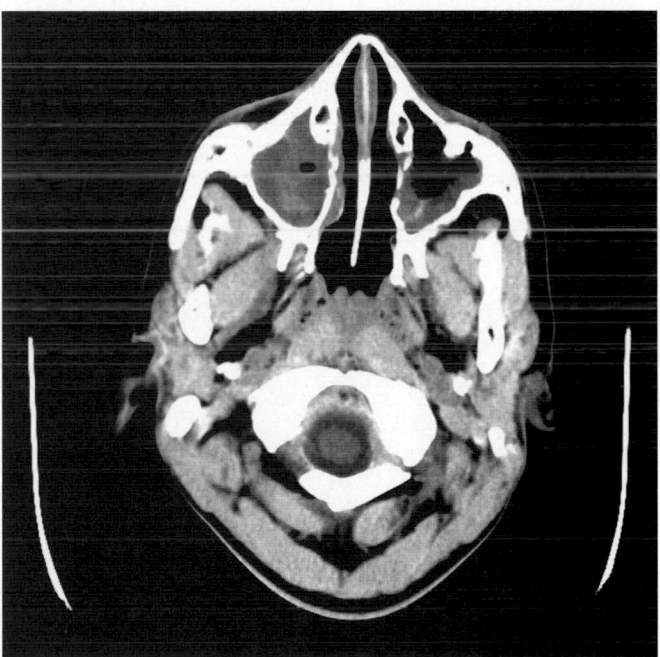

FIGURE 50–2. Computed tomography scan demonstrating maxillary sinusitis (opacified right maxillary sinus).

Summary

Rhinosinusitis affects a large number of children every year. As a result, it is important that clinical criteria be used to decide who has the disease and when to treat. This will decrease the unnecessary use of radiographs and CT scans and allow the appropriate use of antibiotics.

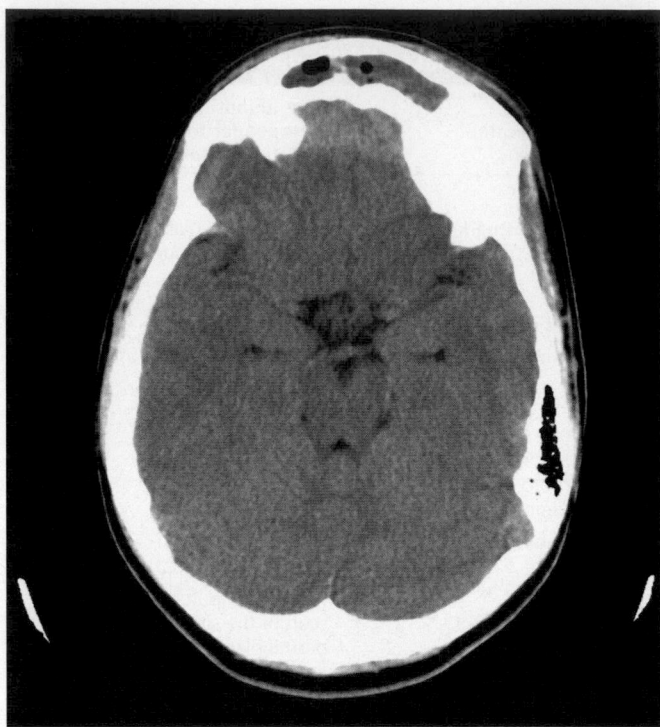

FIGURE 50–3. Computed tomography scan of a child with frontal sinusitis (opacified frontal sinus).

REFERENCES

*1. American Academy of Pediatrics, Subcommittee on Management of Sinusitis and Committee on Quality Improvement: Clinical practice guideline: management of sinusitis. Pediatrics 108:798–808, 2001.

*Selected readings.

2. Lasley MV, Shapiro GG: Rhinitis and sinusitis in children. Immunol Allergy Clin North Am 19:437–452, 1999.
*3. Goldsmith AJ, Rosenfeld RM: Treatment of pediatric sinusitis. Pediatr Clin North Am 50:413–426, 2003.
4. Sokol W: Epidemiology of sinusitis in the primary care setting: results from the 1999–2000 respiratory surveillance program. Am J Med 111(9A):19s–24s, 2001.
*5. Bachert, C, Vignola AM, Gevaert P, et al: Allergic rhinitis, rhinosinusitis, and asthma: one airway disease. Immunol Allergy Clin North Am 24:19–43, 2004.
6. Tsao C, Chen L, Yeh K, et al: Concomitant chronic sinusitis treatment in children with mild asthma. Chest 123:757–764, 2003.
7. Ueda D, Yoto Y: The ten-day mark as a practical diagnostic approach for acute paranasal sinusitis in children. Pediatr Infect Dis J 15(7):576–579, 1996.
8. Clement PAR, Bluestone CD, Gordts F, et al: Management of rhinosinusitis in children. Int J Pediatr Otorhinolaryngol 49(Suppl 1):S95–S100, 1999.
9. McCormick JT, O'Mara MS, Wakefield W, et al: Effect of diagnosis and treatment of sinusitis in critically ill burn victims. Burns 29:79–81, 2003.
10. Goldberg AN, Oroszlan G, Anderson TD: Current concepts in the surgical management of frontal sinus disease: complications of frontal sinusitis and their management. Otolaryngol Clin North Am 34:211–225, 2001.
11. Cannon ML, Antonio BL, McCloskey JJ, et al: cavernous sinus thrombosis complicating sinusitis. Pediatr Crit Care Med 5:86–88, 2004.
12. Awaida JS, Woods SE, Doerzbacher M: Four-cut sinus computed tomographic scanning in screening for sinus disease. South Med J 97:18–20, 2004.
13. Morris P, Leach A: Antibiotics for persistent nasal discharge (rhinosinusitis) in children. Cochrane Database Syst Rev (4):CD001094, 2002.

Chapter 51

Ear Diseases

Irene Tien, MD, MSc and Miriam Aschkenasy, MD, MPH

Key Points

A healthy child age 6 months to 2 years with a mild illness (fever < 39° C, mild otalgia) and an unclear diagnosis, or a child over the age of 2 without severe symptoms or with an uncertain diagnosis, can be observed for 48 to 72 hours without antibiotic therapy.

Otitis externa is generally a localized disease that responds well to appropriate outpatient, topical antibiotic therapy.

The most common causes of vertigo in children are migraine and benign paroxysmal vertigo. Treatment should be directed at the underlying cause.

Facial palsy associated with a vesicular eruption on the ear is diagnostic of Ramsay Hunt syndrome. Treatment with acyclovir is recommended to improve prognosis.

Selected Diagnoses

Acute otitis media
Acute mastoiditis
Cholesteatoma
Otitis externa
Vertigo
Ramsay Hunt syndrome
Other ear disorders
    Impacted cerumen
    Cauliflower ear
    Barotrauma
    Complications of ear piercings

Discussion of Individual Diagnoses

Acute Otitis Media

Approximately 90% of children have had acute otitis media (AOM) by the age of 7.[1] Peak incidence occurs during the first 24 months of life, and the prevalence of infection as well as recurrent infection are increasing.[2-4] AOM is an infection of the middle ear that leads to an acute inflammatory response that may extend to include the tympanic membrane (myringitis). The most common pathogens are viruses, *Streptococcus pneumoniae*, *Moraxella catarrhalis*, and *Haemophilus influenzae* non–type b.[5,6]

Clinical Presentation

Symptoms can vary slightly with different pathogens but are not predictive of a bacterial versus a viral cause.[5] In general, older children will complain of ear pain and possibly fever and hearing loss. Vertigo, fullness in the ear, or symptoms of an upper respiratory tract infection may also be associated. Symptoms in young children can be vague, including irritability, inability to sleep, crying, feeding problems, ear pulling, eye discharge, vomiting, diarrhea, and upper respiratory tract symptoms. In infants less than 2 months of age, the most common presenting symptoms are fever, conjunctivitis, and upper respiratory tract symptoms.[7]

Risk factors for AOM include a preceding upper respiratory tract infection or exposure to tobacco smoke; day care exposure, sibling history or history of adenoidectomy for children 6 to 24 months old; history of tonsillectomy if the child is 12 to 24 months old; history of tympanostomy tubes, or if the first attack of AOM occurred at less than 1 year of age.[8] Findings upon examination of the ear can be variable depending on the age of the child and the course of the infection. The hallmark finding is that of a red, bulging, nonmoving tympanic membrane (TM). In an early infection the only sign may be a red eardrum. The light reflex of the anterior inferior quadrant may disappear, and exudate may be visible behind the TM. Late infection may reveal a ruptured eardrum with draining exudate.

Management

The current management of AOM is controversial.[9-12] A meta-analysis of the natural history of AOM found that 70% of children had complete resolution of symptoms in 7 to 14 days, with no significant change in the rate of suppurative complications.[11] Management of AOM must balance considerations for antibiotic resistance with optimal treatment. The American Academy of Pediatrics (AAP) and American Academy of Family Physicians (AAFP) published clinical practice guidelines that suggest that a healthy child aged 6 months to 2 years with mild illness (fever < 39° C, mild otalgia) and an unclear diagnosis, or a child over the age of 2 without severe symptoms or with an uncertain diagnosis, can be observed for 48 to 72 hours without antibiotic

Table 51–1	Treatment Options for Acute Otitis Media (AOM)
Clinical AOM Scenario	**Treatment Options**
No systemic systems, healthy child, and no recurrence in last 30 days	Observation for 48 hr
Systemic symptoms (e.g., fever)	Amoxicillin • low dose (40–45 mg/kg/day divided tid) if low local resistance rates • high dose (80–90 mg/kg/day divided tid) if unknown or high local resistance rates
Severe illness	Amoxicillin/clavulanate (90/6.4 mg/kg/day divided bid)
Systemic symptoms, amoxicillin allergic	Azithromycin (10 mg/kg/day on day 1 then 5 mg/kg/d × 4 days) Cefdinir (14 mg/kg/day divided qd or bid), cefpodoxime (10 mg/kg/day qd), or cefuroxime (30 mg/kg/day divided bid); if more severe illness, consider ceftriaxone 50 mg/kg/day qd for 1–3 days.
Treatment failure (no improvement after 48–72 hr of antibiotics)	Amoxicillin/clavulanate (90/6.4 mg/kg/day divided bid), ceftriaxone (50 mg/kg/day divided qd), or clindamycin Consider tympanocentesis
Tympanostomy tubes	Topical 0.3% ciprofloxacin/0.1% dexamethasone otic suspension (4 drops bid for 7 days)
Cochlear implants	No special considerations
Otitis media with effusion without symptoms of AOM	Watchful waiting, close follow-up, early referral

therapy.[12] If this option is chosen, the child should be re-evaluated within 48 to 72 hours so that antibiotic therapy may begin if needed.[12]

If management with antibiotics is chosen, AAP/AAFP guidelines recommend amoxicillin at 45 or 90 mg/kg per day as first-line therapy in the majority of cases. However, recent studies have shown that local prevalence of nonsusceptible *S. pneumoniae* can help to dictate therapy. Standard-dose amoxicillin is sufficient to treat the majority of cases of AOM.[13] In cases of high fever (39° C or higher), in which more broad-spectrum coverage is desired, high-dose amoxicillin/clavulanate can be used (Table 51–1).[12]

Therapy for AOM should include pain management. Options include topical anesthetics containing benzocaine or antipyrine or oral agents such as acetaminophen, ibuprofen, or even narcotic analgesia in moderate to severe cases. There is no role for antihistamine or corticosteroid use in the treatment of AOM. Both of these classes of drugs have been shown to increase the duration of middle ear effusion and should be avoided.[14] Children with AOM can be selectively referred for otolaryngology follow-up if they have persistent symptoms or infections or if they are at high risk for recurrence (age < 15 months, prior history of failure of AOM treatment, family history).[15]

Important Clinical Features and Considerations

AOM IN THE PRESENCE OF TYMPANOSTOMY TUBES

Children with AOM may present differently if they have tympanostomy tubes in place. The TM is not intact, and the hallmark of infection is usually an acute purulent otorrhea rather than fever, otalgia, or hearing loss. Pathogens also differ in this patient subset, with *Pseudomonas aeruginosa* and *Staphylococcus aureus* becoming more common. Topical ciprofloxacin with dexamethasone otic suspension (4 drops of 0.3% ciprofloxacin with 0.1% dexamethasone twice daily for 7 days) is an effective therapy for AOM in patients with tympanostomy tubes. This approach has been demonstrated to have better cure rates than oral antibiotics or topical ofloxacin alone.[16-19]

AOM WITH COCHLEAR IMPLANT

Children with cochlear implants are not at higher risk for AOM, nor do these patients have more severe infections or higher complication rates. Conventional antibiotic therapy has been shown to be effective in these patients.[20]

SEROUS OM WITH EFFUSION

It can be difficult to distinguish AOM from serous otitis media with effusion (OME). "Otitis media with effusion" refers to a presence of fluid in the middle ear without signs or symptoms of an acute infection. OME can be persistent and result in short- and long-term hearing loss due to decreased movement of the TM and conduction delay.

Diagnosis of OME is best made with pneumatic otoscopy. A cloudy TM with impaired mobility and possibly an air-fluid level in the middle ear, without a history of acute inflammatory symptoms, is suggestive of OME. Redness of the TM alone is not enough to distinguish between AOM and OME.

OME tends to be self-limited and should be watched without intervention for 3 months. Spontaneous resolution is the most likely outcome. OME in children at risk for learning or speech difficulties should receive early referral for evaluation and intervention. There is no role for antihistamines, decongestants, or corticosteroids in the treatment of OME.[21,22]

Acute Mastoiditis

Acute mastoiditis (AM) is an infectious and inflammatory process of the posterior portion of the temporal bone that can result in osteolysis of the bony trabeculae. This process is often preceded by AOM. The use of sulfa antibiotics decreased the incidence of AM from 0.4% in 1959 to 0.0004% in the 1980s.[23,24] Because of a recent decline in the use of antibiotics for AOM, there is now evidence of a small rise in the incidence of AM.[25,26]

AM has presenting symptoms similar to those of AOM, the most common being pain, irritability, and fever. Signs include an abnormal TM, retroauricular tenderness and swelling, protrusion of the auricle, and retroauricular erythema. The organisms commonly involved in AM are *S. pneumoniae, S. aureus,* and *Streptococcus pyogenes,* with *P. aeruginosa* being the most common cause of chronic mastoiditis.[26,27] Diagnosis can be made with clinical findings and computed tomography demonstrating coalescence of mastoid air cells, subperiosteal abscess, osteitis, or clouding of the mastoid.

Management includes hospital admission and administration of an intravenous cephalosporin (ceftriaxone, cefuroxime, or cefotaxime). Myringotomy, tympanostomy tube placement, and simple or radical mastoidectomy are possible treatment options for complicated cases. Complications from AM can include osteomyelitis, subperiosteal abscess, sinus thrombosis, bacteremia, meningitis, epidural and intracerebral abscesses, cholesteatoma formation, and facial nerve palsy.

Cholesteatoma

The term *cholesteatoma* refers to a sac of stratified squamous epithelium that is filled with exfoliated keratin. This sac grows in the middle ear space and can result in local destruction of the ossicles and conductive hearing loss. Cholesteatomas can occur at any age but tend to be more aggressive in children. Acquired cholesteatomas are the most common type and result from retraction pockets that form in the TM in patients with long-term eustachian tube dysfunction. Otoscopic examination will reveal a white, round, pearly mass behind an intact TM, usually in the anterior superior quadrant of the middle ear. At initial diagnosis, hearing loss is generally not a problem. These patients should be referred to an otolaryngologist for further evaluation as the intervention of choice is surgical.[28-30]

Otitis Externa

Otitis externa (OE), also known as "swimmer's ear" or "tropical ear," is an infection or inflammation of the external ear canal. It is caused by a break in the skin in the external ear canal and changes in the canal environment leading to increased moisture and transition from an acidic to a basic pH.[31] OE occurs commonly in situations of high humidity and warm temperature. Multiple bacterial and a few fungal organisms have been documented to cause OE.[32]

Clinical Presentation

OE begins with itching, followed by pain and discharge. Cases may range from simply a painful, edematous canal without discharge to an erythematous and edematous canal associated with a clear odorless secretion, a seropurulent or debris-laden discharge.[31] The infection also may rarely spread beyond the canal and into surrounding tissues. This is known as malignant OE. This is more common in the elderly and very rare in the healthy child. Pain from OE may also be accompanied by a feeling of fullness in the ear and reduced hearing secondary to canal swelling.

On clinical examination, generally no changes are visible external to the ear, except for discharge. Tender periauricular and preauricular lymph nodes may be palpable. If the child has malignant OE, erythema and edema of the skin adjacent to the affected ear may be visible.[31] Rarely, facial paralysis, other cranial nerve abnormalities, vertigo, or sensorineural hearing loss may occur.

Pulling the pinna of the affected ear may produce increased pain because the canal skin is closely adherent to the underlying perichondrium and periosteum. Direct visualization of the canal will reveal an edematous, erythematous ear canal with thick, clumpy otorrhea. Cerumen will often appear white as opposed to its normal yellow color. The tympanic membrane is often not visible because of canal debris and swelling, but should appear normal.

Important Clinical Features and Considerations

It is important to differentiate OE from furunculosis, AOM with a ruptured TM, and mastoiditis. Furuncles of the ear canal present with a localized swelling originating from the hair-bearing portion of the canal. The swelling associated with a furuncle is localized to a single quadrant, whereas OE is concentric and involves the entire length of the canal.

It may be difficult to differentiate OE from AOM with a ruptured TM because the TM is often not visible due to pain, swelling, and debris associated with OE. Purulent secretions from AOM with a ruptured TM may also cause canal irritation and pain similar to OE. This should be kept in mind when choosing therapy (see "Management" section).

Children with mastoiditis may present with an obliterated postauricular fold, which may help in differentiation from OE. Tenderness over the mastoid bone as opposed to pain with pulling of the pinna may also be helpful in making the diagnosis of mastoiditis.

Complications of OE include ear canal stenosis, cellulitis, chondritis, parotiditis, persistent disease (chronic OE), and necrotizing or malignant OE. This is usually the result of systemic invasion by *P. aeruginosa,* and is very rare in healthy children.

Management

OE is caused by bacteria in a vast majority of cases. In one study of 2240 diseased ears, bacteria were cultured from 98.3% of adults and children with otitis externa.[32] Of these, 53% were gram-negative, and 45.3% were gram-positive bacteria (38% *P. aeruginosa,* 9.1% *Staphylococcus epidermidis,* 7.8% *S. aureus,* 6.6% *Microbacterium otitidis,* 2.9% *Microbacterium alconae*). Fungi were isolated in only 1.7% of cases and included only *Aspergillus* and *Candida.*

Topical acetic acid has been used for several centuries to treat OE. Its efficacy is based upon its ability to reduce the pH of the canal environment, which restricts the growth of bacteria and fungi.[33] Acetic acid–containing solutions for treatment of OE are discouraged for many reasons: (1) they are painful to the patient because they irritate inflamed skin, (2) they have been shown to damage cochlear outer hair cells if they come into contact with the inner ear, and (3) treatment for up to 3 weeks may be required for them to be effective.[33]

Topical antibiotics are the most common and preferred approach to the treatment of OE. Advantages include the high concentration of antibiotic delivered to the infection site and negligible systemic absorption of antibiotic when applied topically to the ear canal. Maintenance of antibiotic concentrations well over minimum inhibitory concentrations needed for pathogen eradication has been documented for up to 8 hours.[33]

The oldest and most common topical antibiotic treatment for OE is a combination drug containing hydrocortisone, neomycin sulfate, and polymyxin B. Clinical studies have documented a clinical cure rate of 87% to 97%, which has remained consistent over the last 20 years.[34,35] Despite its proven efficacy, this treatment is associated with a high number of adverse effects, including hypersensitivity to neomycin, hydrocortisone, and thimerosal (a preservative found in one version of this drug) and irritation from propylene glycol (a solvent commonly used in this drug formulation). Eighteen percent to 35% of children who were patch tested have been shown to be hypersensitive to neomycin or thimerosal.[36] The redness, pain, and pruritis associated with hypersensitivity or irritation are easily mistaken for treatment failure.

The development of topical formulations of fluoroquinolones has allowed for effective single-drug treatment of OE. In the late 1990s, otic suspension and solution formulations of ofloxacin and ciprofloxacin/hydrocortisone became available. Direct comparisons with the older neomycin-polymyxin-hydrocortisone formulation have demonstrated equivalent efficacy. Clinical studies have shown cures of almost 100% in children treated with ofloxacin or ciprofloxacin twice a day or neomycin-polymyxin-hydrocortisone four times a day.[34,35] Topical ofloxacin and ciprofloxacin also have the advantage of rarely causing hypersensitivity and being non-ototoxic.

The theoretical benefit of topical hydrocortisone in reducing symptoms associated with inflammation is not well established for OE. One study found that the addition of hydrocortisone to ciprofloxacin reduced the time to resolution of ear pain by only 0.8 day.[35] The only OE antibiotic formulation currently available without hydrocortisone is ofloxacin.

Gentle removal of canal debris and insertion of an ear wick prior to instillation of antibiotic drops may improve delivery of the medication. Necrotizing or malignant OE requires treatment with 2 to 3 weeks of intravenous antipseudomonal antibiotics.[31]

Pain management with ibuprofen, acetaminophen, or narcotics is an important part of OE management.

Summary

OE is generally a localized disease that responds well to appropriate outpatient, topical antibiotic therapy. A topical fluoroquinolone is the preferred method of treatment. Topical ofloxacin is preferred when there is the possibility of a TM rupture. OE can result in systemic infection in immunosuppressed children, requiring hospital admission and prolonged intravenous antibiotic therapy. Maintenance of a dry ear canal may prevent OE.

Vertigo

Vertigo is described as a hallucination of motion.[37] It is uncommon in children, and the differential diagnosis is broad (Table 51–2).[38] Vertigo can originate from central (neurologic) or peripheral (otologic, ophthalmologic) lesions.

Clinical Presentation

The most common causes of vertigo in children are migraine and benign paroxysmal vertigo (BPV).[39] It is important to obtain a detailed description of the patient's experience of dizziness in order to correctly classify it as vertigo. In younger children, it may be necessary to base the diagnosis of vertigo on parental description of the child's behavior during the

Table 51–2	Differential Diagnosis of Vertigo in Children

Central Lesions

Seizures
Trauma
Neoplasm
Infection
Demyelinization (multiple sclerosis)
Familial ataxia
Anemia
Migraine
Transient ischemic attack, cerebrovascular accident
Hydrocephalus
Dandy-Walker syndrome
Arnold-Chiari malformation

Peripheral Lesions

Otologic
Otitis media
Cholesteatoma
Tympanic membrane perforation
Placement of pressure equalization tubes
Perilymph fisula
Endolymphatic hydrops
Labrynthitis
Retrocochlear tumor or trauma
Benign paroxysmal vertigo of children
Vestibular neuronitis
Benign paroxysmal positional vertigo
Ophthalmologic
Refractive errors (ametropia)
Amblyopia
Latent strabismus
Convergence insufficiency

Other

Drugs
Thyroid dysfunction
Hypoglycemia
Functional
Addison's disease
Heart disease/arrhythmia
Hypoperfusion
Vasculitis

episodes. For example, the child may suddenly stop and cling to a nearby object with a frightened look on his or her face and then cry to be picked up. Older children may simply state something like "I'm falling." Children may become pale or diaphoretic during these episodes. They do not experience a sleepy period after the episodes, nor do they become incontinent or unconscious. Vertigo may last anywhere from a few seconds to a few days.

CENTRAL ORIGIN

Vertigo of central origin is often associated with serious disease.[37] Basilar migraines may present with sudden onset of headache, vertigo, and cerebellar signs, including ataxia. A family history of migraines may be helpful in making this diagnosis. Cerebrospinal fluid obstruction by brainstem and posterior fossa lesions may result in hydrocephalus and symptoms associated with increased intracranial pressure in addition to cerebellar symptoms such ataxia. Neurofibromatosis II is an autosomal dominant disorder characterized by various posterior fossa tumors. These children have sensorineural hearing loss or impaired speech discrimination.

PERIPHERAL ORIGIN

Vertigo of peripheral origin is commonly accompanied by horizontal nystagmus and may be associated with concomitant auditory symptoms. BPV "is a paroxysmal, non-epileptic, recurrent event characterized by subjective or objective vertigo that occurs in neurologically intact children" and accounted for 30.9% of cases of childhood vertigo in one series of 55 children.[40,41] Age of onset is generally between 2 and 4 years, and BPV presents with a sudden episode of visible anxiety or fear followed by grasping of nearby people or objects for support. Children often ask to be picked up or refuse to stand. Older children may complain that they feel as if they will fall. These episodes may be associated with pallor, nausea, sweating, and sometimes unusual head postures. BPV is thought to fall on the continuum of migraine headache syndromes.[40] Benign paroxysmal positional vertigo (BPPV), however, is characterized by vertigo resulting from turning the head to a particular position. BPPV most commonly occurs after head injury in children and is believed to be due to displacement of free-floating otoconia into the posterior semicircular canal.[42] Spontaneous resolution after a few months to years is likely.[40]

Perilymphatic fistulas from disruption of the oval or round window, causing a connection between the middle and inner ear, may also form after head trauma or barotrauma. This generally presents with vertigo followed by progressive hearing loss and may be associated with a temporal bone fracture. Traumatic perilymphatic fistulas are difficult to demonstrate on imaging studies and are often identified on surgical exploration, and require surgical repair.[43]

Ménière's disease is an idiopathic condition of excessive endolymph. It presents with spontaneous attacks of prolonged vertigo, fluctuating hearing loss, and tinnitus. It is treated with a low-sodium diet, sometimes a diuretic, and occasionally surgery. Vestibular neuronitis is caused by a viral infection of a ganglion of the vestibular nerve. It presents with sudden onset of severe vertigo, made worse with head movement preceded or accompanied by an obvious viral infection. "Labyrinthitis" refers to an infection and/or inflammation of the labyrinth and cochlea. Children present with vertigo and sudden sensorineural hearing loss.

Management

Treatment of vertigo in children should be directed at its underlying cause.[38] The key is to not mistake central for peripheral vertigo. Referral to an otolaryngologist, neurologist, or ophthalmologist for cases in which there is no clear cause of a child's vertigo is prudent.

Ramsay Hunt Syndrome

Ramsay Hunt syndrome (RHS) refers to an acute facial palsy associated with a herpetic eruption on the auricle. It is frequently complicated by vestibulocochlear dysfunction.[44] It is caused by reactivation of latent varicella-zoster infection in the geniculate ganglion. RHS is rare in children under 6 years, but older children have an incidence similar to adults. Chickenpox in children under 1 year is an important risk factor for development of RHS.[44] There is some evidence that the varicella vaccination may be protective against the development of RHS.[44,45]

Presentation

Children with RHS generally present with milder symptoms than in adults.[44] Facial palsy may occur without associated herpetic lesions or with development of lesions several days later. In one study, approximately 88.3% of children developed herpetic lesions, half of which appeared simultaneously with the palsy.[44] RHS may cause hearing loss (24.4%), tinnitus (11.1%), vertigo (17.4%), and paralysis of cranial nerves (CNs) IX and X (extremely rare in children).[44]

Important Clinical Features and Considerations

Differentiation of RHS without vesicular lesions from herpes simplex virus (HSV)–related Bell's palsy may be difficult. Because HSV is believed to affect only the peripheral CN VII, whereas RHS arises from inflammation of the geniculate ganglion, there is some evidence to suggest that more severe cases of what appear to be Bell's palsy may be RHS without the associated vesicular eruption.[45] The prognosis of RHS in children is better than for adults. Complete or near-complete resolution of the facial palsy and of hearing loss occurred in 78.6% and in 83.3% of cases, respectively, in one series of children.[44]

Management

Acyclovir (80 mg/kg per day orally, or 45 mg/kg per day intravenously if the patient is unable to tolerate oral medications) has been shown to improve resolution of the facial palsy and hearing loss associated with RHS.[44,45] In cases of apparent Bell's palsy in which RHS is suspected, vigilance must be maintained in watching for the development of vesicles so that acyclovir may be initiated if necessary. The addition of prednisone to the treatment regimen may be beneficial only in severe cases of RHS.

Summary

Facial palsy associated with a vesicular eruption on the ear is diagnostic of RHS. RHS may be mistaken for Bell's palsy because of delay in the appearance of vesicles or failure of the vesicles to appear. Treatment with acyclovir is recommended to improve prognosis.

Other Ear Disorders

Impacted Cerumen

Cerumen impaction occurs when the normal self-cleansing mechanism of epithelial migration is disrupted. When cotton-tipped devices are used to clean the ear canal, protective layers of keratin are rubbed away, exposing the underlying delicate skin cells. When these cells are exposed to minor trauma, an infection may result, which produces debris that can form the nidus of a wax plug.[46]

Symptomatic impacted cerumen is an indication for removal. Instillation of ceruminolytics to soften the wax prior to removal is generally helpful. Cerumenex, Cerumol, benzocaine otic, aluminum acetate topical, alcohol, and oils may take more than 18 hours to disintegrate cerumen versus 90 minutes for the sodium bicarbonate solutions.[47] Hydrogen peroxide is another commonly used ceruminolytic, but its use has not been systemically studied. One study found that the liquid preparation of the stool softener docusate sodium (Colace) was much more effective as a ceruminolytic than Cerumenex.[48] Irrigation of the ear canal after instillation of a ceruminolytic results in successful removal of cerumen in most cases. Some cases in which cerumen cannot be removed with the use of ceruminolytics or in which the child cannot cooperate adequately for safe removal may require referral to an otolaryngologist for treatment.

Cauliflower Ear

"Cauliflower ear" refers to a disfiguration of the cartilage of the ear generally following infection of a traumatic hematoma of the pinna.[49] Prompt evacuation of a hematoma of the pinna and prevention of infection is key to avoiding cauliflower ear.

Barotrauma

Barotrauma causes ear injury when the pressure in the middle ear is unable to adequately equalize with pressure external to the ear. This may happen when there is cerumen or a foreign body in the ear canal, although this is uncommon. More commonly, it occurs when there is a dysfunction of the eustachian tube.

Barotrauma to the ear can result in pain, reduced hearing, and vertigo. Rarely, it may result in facial nerve palsy, ossicle fracture or dislocation, or round window rupture.

Management of barotrauma of the ear may include use of vasoconstrictor nasal drops, prevention of pressure changes during an upper respiratory tract infection, use of Valsalva maneuvers to open eustachian tubes, and placement of myringotomy tubes. Traumatic TM rupture generally resolves after 10 to 14 days. If round or oval window rupture is suspected, referral to otolaryngology for surgical correction is recommended.

Complications of Ear Piercing

Infection is one of the most common complications of ear piercing. Although skin organisms are the most likely culprits, *P. aeruginosa* infection should be kept in mind for cases that do not respond promptly to antibiotics. Auricular chondritis can be slow to heal and may require aggressive therapy, including surgical débridement and drainage.[50] Empirical therapy should include coverage for *P. aeruginosa*.

Differentiation of infection from metal sensitivity may be challenging.[50] Itching is more likely to predominate over pain when a patient presents with a red ear following piercing. Removal of the stud is recommended.

Summary

Overuse of antibiotics in otherwise healthy children with ambiguous signs and symptoms of AOM/AOE should be avoided. Vertigo in children is uncommon. Peripheral vertigo is usually of a benign cause, whereas central vertigo is more often associated with a serious disease.[51] An appropriate history and physical examination, a logical approach to antibiotic use, and follow-up medical care are three of the most important ingredients for the management of ear disease.

REFERENCES

1. Teele D, Klein J, Rosner B: Epidemiology of acute otitis media in Boston children from birth to seven years of age: a prospective cohort study. J Infect Dis 160:83–94, 1989.
*2. Schappert S: National Ambulatory Medical Care Survey: 1994 summary. Advance data from Vital and Health Statistics of the Centers for Disease Control and Prevention National Center for Health Statistics (DHHS Publication No 273). Washington, DC: US Department of Health and Human Services, 1996.
3. Schappert S: Office visits for otitis media: United States, 1975–1990. Advance data from Vital and Health Statistics of the Centers for Disease Control and Prevention National Center for Health Statistics (DHHS Publication No 214). Washington, DC: US Department of Health and Human Services, 1992.
4. Lanphear B, Byrd R, Auinger P, et al: Increasing prevalence of recurrent otitis media among children in the United States. Pediatrics 99:e1–e7, 1997.
*5. Palmu A, Herva E, Savolainene J, et al: Association of clinical signs and symptoms with bacterial findings in acute otitis media. Clin Infect Dis 38:234–242, 2004.
6. Barnett E, Klein J: The problem of resistant bacteria for the management of acute otitis media. Pediatr Clin North Am 42:509–517, 1995.
*7. Turner D, Leibovitz E, Aran A, et al: Acute otitis media in infants younger then two months of age: microbiology, clinical presentation and therapeutic approach. Pediatr Infect Dis J 21:669–674, 2002.
8. Froom J, Culpepper L, Green LA, et al: A cross-national study of acute otitis media: risk factors, severity, and treatment at initial visit. Report from the International Primary Care Network (IPCN) and the Ambulatory Sentinel Practice Network (ASPN). J Am Board Fam Pract 14:406–417, 2001.
9. Eskin B: Should children with otitis media be treated with antibiotics? Ann Emerg Med 44:537–539, 2004.
10. Culpepper L, Froom J: Routine antimicrobial treatment of acute otitis media: is it necessary? JAMA 278:1643–1645,1997.
11. Rosenfeld R, David K. Natural history of untreated otitis media. Laryngoscope 113:1645–1657, 2003.
*12. American Academy of Pediatrics, Subcommittee on Management of Acute Otitis Media: Diagnosis and management of acute otitis media. Pediatrics 113:1451–1465, 2004.
*13. Garbutt J, Beme J, May A, et al: Developing community-specific recommendations for first line treatment of acute otitis media: is high dose amoxicillin necessary? Pediatrics 114:342–347, 2004.
14. Chonmaitree T, Saeed K, Tatsuo U, et al: A randomized, placebo-controlled trial of the effect of antihistamine or corticosteroid treatment in acute otitis media. J Pediatr 143:377–385, 2003.
15. Hathaway T, Katz H, Dershewitz R, et al: Acute otitis media: who needs post treatment follow-up? Pediatrics 94:143–147, 1994.
16. Dohar J, Garner E, Nielsen R, et al: Topical ofloxacin treatment of otorrhea in children with tympanostomy tubes. Arch Otolaryngol Head Neck Surg 125:537–545, 1999.
17. Simpson K, Markham A: Ofloxacin otic solution: a review of its use in the management of ear infections. Drugs 58:509–531, 1999.
18. Goldblatt E, Dohar J, Nozza R, et al: Topical ofloxacin versus systemic amoxicillin/clavulanate in purulent otorrhea in children with tympanostomy tubes. Int J Pediatr Otorhinolaryngol 46:91–101, 1998.
*19. Roland P, Kreisler L, Reese B, et al: Topical ciprofloxacin/dexamethasone otic suspension is superior to ofloxacin otic solution in the treatment of children with acute otitis media with otorrhea through tympanostomy tubes. Pediatrics 113:40–46, 2004.
20. Luntz M, Hodges A, Balkany T, et al: Otitis media in children with cochlear implants. Laryngoscope 106:1403–1405, 1996.
*21. Rosenfeld R, Culpepper L, Doyle K, et al: Clinical practice guideline: otitis media with effusion. Otolaryngol Head Neck Surg 130:595–5118, 2004.
*22. Subcommittee on Otitis Media with Effusion, American Academy of Family Physicians, American Academy of Pediatrics, and American Academy of Otolaryngology–Head and Neck Surgery: Otitis media with effusion. Pediatrics 113:1412–1429, 2004.
23. Palva T, Pulkkinen K: Mastoiditis. J Laryngol Otol 73:573–588, 1959.
24. Lund F: Acute and latent mastoiditis. J Laryngol Otol 103:1158–1160, 1989.
25. Van Zuijlen D, Schlider A, Van Balen F, et al: National differences in incidence of acute mastoiditis: relationship to prescribing patterns of antibiotics for acute otitis media? Pediatr Infect Dis J 30:140–144, 2001.
26. Ghaffar F, Wordermann M, McCracken G: Acute mastoiditis in children: a seventeen-year experience in Dallas, Texas. Pediatr Infect Dis J 20:376–380, 2001.

*Selected readings.

27. Bitar C, Kluka E, Steele R: Mastoiditis in children. Clin Pediatr 35:391–395, 1996.
28. Swartz J: Cholesteatomas of the middle ear: diagnosis, etiology, and complications. Radiol Clin North Am 22:15–35, 1984.
29. Prescott C: Cholesteatoma in children—the experience at the Red Cross War Memorial Children's Hospital in South Africa 1988–1996. Int J Pediatr Otorhinolaryngol 49:15–19, 1999.
30. Nelson M, Roger G, Koltai P, et al: Congenital cholesteatoma classification, management, and outcome. Arch Otolaryngol Head Neck Surg 128:810–814, 2002.
*31. Beers SL, Abramo TJ: Otitis externa review. Pediatr Emerg Care 20:250–256, 2004.
32. Roland PS, Stroman DW: Microbiology of acute otitis externa. Laryngoscope 112:1166–1177, 2002.
33. Dohar JE: Evolution of management approaches for otitis externa. Pediatr Infect Dis J 22(4):299–305, 2003.
34. Jones RN, Milazzo J, Seidlin M: Ofloxacin otic solution for treatment of otitis externa in children and adults. Arch Otolaryngol Head Neck Surg 123:1193–1200, 1997.
35. Pistorius B, Westberry K, Drehobl M: Prospective, randomized, comparative trial of ciprofloxacin otic drops, with or without hydrocortisone, vs. polymyxin B-neomycin-hydrocortisone otic suspension in the treatment of acute diffuse otitis externa. Infect Dis Clin Pract 8:387–395, 1999.
36. Barros MA, Baptista A, Correia RM, Azevedo F: Patch testing in children: a study of 562 schoolchildren. Contact Dermatitis 25:156–159, 1991.
37. Miyamoto RC, Miyamoto RT: Pediatric neurotology. Semin Pediatr Neurotol 10:298–303, 2003.
38. Bower CM, Cotton RT: The spectrum of vertigo in children. Arch Otolaryngol Head Neck Surg 121:911–915, 1995.
39. Ravid S, Bienkowski R, Eviatar L: A simplified diagnostic approach to dizziness in children. Pediatr Neurol 29:317–320, 2003.
40. Drigo P, Carli G, Laverda AM: Benign paroxysmal vertigo of childhood. Brain Dev 23:38–41, 2001.
41. Choung YH, Park K, Moon SK, et al: Various causes and clinical characteristics in vertigo in children with normal eardrums. Int J Pediatr Otorhinolaryngol 67:889–894, 2003.
42. Baloh RW, Honrubia V: Childhood onset of benign positional vertigo. Neurology 50:1494–1496, 1998.
43. Megerian DA, Hadlock RA: Weekly clinicopathological exercises. Case 40-2001: an eight-year-old boy with fever, headache, and vertigo two days after aural trauma. N Engl J Med 345:1901–1907, 2001.
44. Hato N, Kisaki H, Honda N, et al: Ramsay Hunt syndrome in children. Ann Neurol 48:254–256, 2000.
45. Grose C, Bonthius D, Adel F: Chickenpox and the geniculate ganglion: facial nerve palsy, Ramsay Hunt syndrome and acyclovir treatment. Pediatr Infect Dis J 21:615–617, 2002.
46. Warwick-Brown NP: Wax impaction in the ear. Practitioner 230:301, 1986.
47. Robinson AC, Hawke M: The efficacy of ceruminolytic: everything old is new again. J Otolaryngol 18:263, 1989.
48. Singer AJ, Sauris E, Viccellio AW: Ceruminolytic effects of docusate sodium: a randomized, controlled trial. Am J Emerg Med 36:228, 2000.
49. Khalak R, Roberts JK: Cauliflower ear. N Engl J Med 335:399, 1996.
50. Keene WE, Markum AC, Samadpour M: Outbreak of *Pseudomonas aeruginosa* infections caused by commercial piercing of upper ear cartilage. JAMA 291:981–985, 2004.
51. Anoh-Tanon MJ, Bremond-Gignac D, Wiener-Vacher SR: Vertigo is an underestimated symptom of ocular disorders: dizzy children do not always need MRI. Pediatr Neurol 23:49–53, 2000.

Oral Lesions

Esther Maria Sampayo, MD

Selected Diagnoses

Congenital lesions
    Alveolar and palatal cysts
    Natal teeth
    Epulis
    Lymphangiomas, hemangiomas, and vascular malformations
    Lingual thyroid
Infectious lesions
    Candidiasis
    Herpes simplex infections
    Coxsackievirus infections
    Other infections
Tumors
    Pyogenic granuloma
    Fibroma
    Mucocele and ranula
    Rhabdomyosarcoma
Idiopathic lesions
    Miscellaneous lesions
    Recurrent oral ulcers
    Lesions associated with systemic diseases

Discussion of Individual Diagnoses

Congenital Lesions

Alveolar and Palatal Cysts

Cysts are by far the most common of the congenital oral lesions (Table 52–1). They are caused by epithelial remnants on the palate or gums and are found in over 80% of newborns. Palatal cysts such as Epstein's or epithelial pearls appear as white or yellow keratin-containing cysts in the midline at the junction of the soft and hard palate As many as three to six lesions measuring less than 3 mm in size can be seen. Alveolar cysts, also known as Bohn's nodules, dental lamina, or gingival cysts, appear on the mandibular or maxillary gingiva and alveolar dental ridges.[1] Palatal cysts are usually larger and less numerous than alveolar cysts; however, the two entities are otherwise clinically identical. The terms *Epstein's pearls* and *Bohn's nodules* are used interchangeably for both palatal and alveolar cysts of the newly borns. These congenital lesions are asymptomatic and regress spontaneously within a few weeks or months.[2]

Natal Teeth

Teeth are classified as natal if they are present at birth or as neonatal if found within the first month of life. This premature eruption of primary teeth is most commonly found in the lower incisor alveolar ridge. Since only 1% to 10% are supernumerary, they only require extraction when there is poor crown formation or they are loose and tooth aspiration is a concern.[3]

Epulis

Epulis is a firm, fibrous, sarcomatous benign tumor that is usually pedunculated and arises from the alveolar ridge of the mandible or maxilla. Lesions may regress spontaneously; however, they require excision if they are associated with feeding or breathing difficulties or are cosmetically unappealing.[4]

Lymphangiomas, Hemangiomas, and Vascular Malformations

Lymphangiomas are congenital benign tumors of the lymphatic vessels. The most common intraoral site is the tongue. Lesions may also appear on the lips or buccal mucosa. They appear as soft, fluctuant, smooth masses with the color of surrounding tissues.

Table 52–1   Differential Diagnosis of Lesions of the Oral Mucosa

Congenital	Infectious	Tumor	Idiopathic
Alveolar cysts 　Bohn's nodules 　Dental lamina cysts 　Gingival cysts	Acute necrotizing ulcerative 　gingivitis (trench mouth, 　Vincent's angina)	Eruption cyst	Apthous stomatitis
Epulis	Candidiasis	Fibroma	Benign migratory glossitis 　(geographic tongue)
Hemangioma	Coxsackievirus 　Hand, foot, and mouth disease 　Herpangina	Lipoma	Fordyce's granules
Lingual thyroid Lymphangioma	Hairy tongue Herpes simplex 　Gingivostomatitis 　Labialis	Mucocele Pyogenic granuloma	Gingival hyperplasia Leukoplakia
Natal teeth Palatal cysts 　Bohn's nodules 　Epithelial pearls 　Epstein's pearls	HIV Measles	Ranula Rhabdomyosarcoma	Retrocuspid papillae
	Odontogenic cysts Papilloma Parulis (periapical abscess) Pericoronitis Scarlet fever Syphilis Varicella		

Abbreviation: HIV, human immunodeficiency virus.

Hemangiomas and vascular malformations may appear anywhere in the head and neck area, including the mouth. Clinically, hemangiomas are soft, purplish lesions that blanch with application of pressure and are usually associated with other vascular lesions throughout the body, especially on the skin. Vascular malformations have a bluish hue and should be auscultated for a thrill or a bruit. Hemangiomas are not present at birth. They manifest within the first month of life, exhibit a rapid proliferative phase, and slowly involute to near-complete resolution. Vascular malformations are more stable and fail to regress.

Treatment of lymphangiomas, hemangiomas, and vascular malformations is necessary if lesions cause cosmetic disfigurement, masticatory problems, or respiratory, speech, or swallowing difficulties. Treatment includes steroids, cryotherapy, embolization, sclerotherapy, surgery, and laser therapy.[5] Furthermore, they may be associated with syndromes such as Rendu-Osler-Weber syndrome, Sturge-Weber syndrome, and Kasabach-Merritt syndrome.

Lingual Thyroid

Of all ectopic thyroids, 90% are found on the lingual dorsum, where they are referred to as lingual thyroid or ectopic lingual thyroid. A lingual thyroid is an asymptomatic nodular mass of the posterior lingual midline, usually less than 1 cm in size but sometimes reaching more than 4 cm. Surgical excision or radioiodine therapy are effective treatments for lingual thyroid, but no treatment should be attempted until an iodine radioisotope scan has determined that there is adequate thyroid tissue in the neck. In those patients lacking thyroid tissue in the neck, the lingual thyroid can be excised and autotransplanted to the muscles of the neck.[6]

Infectious Lesions

Inflammation of the soft tissues in the mouth resulting in mouth sores, otherwise known as stomatitis, is common

in childhood. Viral infections are by far the most common causes of stomatitis—in particular, infections with herpes simplex, Coxsackie, varicella-zoster, and Epstein-Barr viruses. Bacterial infections are rare and mostly secondary to the viral infections. In infants, oral candidiasis (thrush) is a common cause of stomatitis and is treated with nystatin. Most infections have a self-limiting course, and reassurance to the parents is essential. Treatment is supportive. Dehydration is a common complication that can be prevented by analgesics and hydration to avoid hospitalization.

Superficial ulcerations of the oral mucosa may present a diagnostic challenge to the emergency physician because of

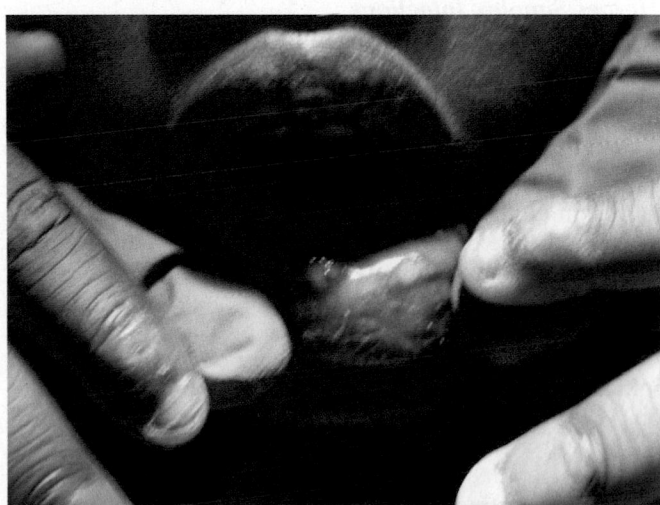

FIGURE 52–1. Herpetic gingivostomatitis.

Table 52–2	Oral Ulcerations		
Type	**Location**	**Fever**	**Recurrence**
Apthous ulcers	Buccal/labial	No	Yes
Coxsackie herpangina	Posterior pharynx, buccal, tongue, soft/hard palate	Yes	No
Herpes gingivostomatitis	Anterior pharynx, gingiva/hard palate, buccal/labial	Yes	No
Herpes labialis	Labial	Yes	Yes
Vincent's angina (ANUG)	Interdental papillae	Yes	No

Abbreviation: ANUG, acute necrotizing ulcerative gingivitis.

the similarity of one ulcer to another. Many features might help in the differential diagnosis. The age of the patient, time of onset, course of disease, and other associated symptoms are important components of the history (Table 52–2). Furthermore, the physical examination must take into consideration the lesion type (mass, ulcer, or vesicle), location, size grouping, and involvement of other organ systems of the body.[7] Oral lesions associated with a toxic-appearing child could represent toxic shock syndrome or Stevens-Johnson syndrome.

Candidiasis

Candidiasis is the most common infection of the oral cavity. Candidiasis, also known as thrush, is caused by *Candida albicans* and appears as white plaque on the buccal mucosa, gingiva, palate, and tongue that typically does not scrap off with a tongue blade. When these patches are scraped or rubbed, pinpoint areas of bleeding can be seen underneath. Candidiasis occurs commonly in infants less than 1 year of age; if it occurs at a later age, the immunologic status of the child must be taken into account. Topical antifungal treatment with nystatin suspension or miconazole gel is the treatment of choice. Miconazole oral gel has been studied and found to be more effective than nystatin suspension. Miconazole also has a superior cure rate and a lower rate of recurrence.[8]

Herpes Simplex Infections

PRIMARY HERPETIC GINGIVOSTOMATITIS

Primary herpetic gingivostomatitis (Fig. 52–1) usually occurs in infants and young children. Intraoral infection with herpes simplex virus 1 initially presents with a prodrome of fever, pain, headache, malaise, and odynophagia as the predominant symptoms. Regional cervical adenopathy is also characteristic in the prodrome stage. Subsequently, diffuse pain in the oral cavity and lips may occur, followed by the development of yellowish fluid–filled vesicles located throughout the oral cavity on both mobile mucosa (buccal and labial) and mucosa attached to bone (gingiva and hard palate).[9] These initial vesicles are rarely seen because they rupture spontaneously and progress to multiple groups of shallow, painful ulcers that are prone to superinfection. Treatment is supportive with analgesics and antipyretics. Topical application of "magic mouthwash," which consists of diphenhydramine

and magnesium hydroxide, has also been advocated, although evidence does not indicate that it causes faster resolution.[10,11] Mixtures with lidocaine added have demonstrated toxicity.[12] Acyclovir can shorten the duration of herpetic gingivostomatitis symptoms as compared to placebo. Treatment should be started within the first 3 days of disease onset. The dosage is 15 mg/kg 5 times daily for 5 to 7 days.[13,14] Lesions usually heal in 1 to 2 weeks. The most common complication is dehydration.

SECONDARY HERPES LABIALIS

Recurrent infections may be expected in 30% to 40 % of affected children secondary to latent herpes simplex virus in the trigeminal ganglion. This is manifested by stomatitis in the oral cavity or herpes labialis on the lips, which may recur in less severe form and resolve in 1 to 2 weeks as well. Fever, stress, sunlight, trauma, or fatigue may act as potential triggers. Treatment consists of acyclovir.

Coxsackievirus Infections

HAND, FOOT, AND MOUTH DISEASE

Hand, foot, and mouth disease is caused by enteroviruses and is most commonly associated with coxsackievirus A-16 or enterovirus 71.[15] It primarily affects children under 10 years of age. It is usually seen during late summer and early autumn. This disease is highly communicable and is spread by oral-oral and fecal-oral routes. A brief prodrome of low-grade fever, malaise, cough, anorexia, and abdominal pain may occur.

Ulceration may occur anywhere in the oral cavity, but is most common on the hard palate, tongue, and buccal mucosa. The ulcer evolves from a small erythematous macule, through a papulovesicular stage to a yellow-gray ulcer with an erythematous border. These ulcers may coalesce, the tongue may become red and edematous, and the pain may interfere with oral intake; thus dehydration is the most common complication of this disease.

These lesions are self-limited and resolve without treatment in less than a week. Soon after the oral lesions, an exanthem may develop characterized by small erythematous macules or papules with a central gray vesicle on the hands more commonly than the feet, and on the sides of the fingers and dorsal surfaces of the foot more commonly than the palms and soles. The lesions may be asymptomatic or painful and resolve over 5 to 10 days without scarring.

Although most cases are benign and self-limiting, there are case reports of complications including myocarditis, meningoencephalitis, pulmonary edema, and even death. The Taiwan epidemic of 1998 secondary to enterovirus 71 caused significant morbidity and mortality secondary to neurogenic pulmonary edema.[16]

There is no specific treatment for hand, foot, and mouth disease. Current strategies are aimed at providing relief of painful oral lesions to ensure proper fluid intake. Topical anesthetics and analgesics composed of viscous lidocaine, diphenhydramine, and magnesium hydroxide, such as magic mouthwash, have traditionally been used for symptomatic relief, although studies have not demonstrated significant differences in time for the cessation of the signs and symptoms in cancer patients suffering from mucositis.[10,11] Furthermore some studies have demonstrated toxicity with topical lidocaine.[12] One study of children treated with acyclovir showed symptomatic relief and involution of lesions with 24 hours.[17]

HERPANGINA

Herpangina is typically caused by coxsackievirus group A1-6, -8, -10, and -22 serotypes during the late summer and early autumn months. Herpangina affects any age group but is most commonly seen in younger children less than 5 years of age. The prodrome is associated with fever and malaise. Presenting complaints often include anorexia, dysphagia, sore throat, headache, and neck and back pain. Characteristic lesions evolve from papulovesicular lesions to gray-based ulcers with an erythematous border. These are usually found on the soft palate, anterior tonsillar pillars, uvula, and tongue. There is no associated exanthem. These ulcers heal spontaneously in less than a week, and treatment is symptomatic.

Other Infections

Varicella-zoster virus, otherwise known as chickenpox, may have oral manifestations characterized by small bullae along the mucosal surface that rupture easily and become ulcerations that may become superinfected. These lesions also resolve spontaneously with the course of the disease.

Epstein-Barr virus, the etiologic agent of infectious mononucleosis, may also cause an ulcerative stomatitis or gingivitis and soft palatal petechial hemorrhages. These may be seen with the characteristic symptoms of sore throat, malaise, fever, fatigue, and lymphadenopathy.

Scarlet fever, caused by group B streptococcus, may have intraoral manifestations that precede the characteristic sandpaper-textured rash by 1 to 2 days. Exudative tonsillitis is often accompanied by erythematous oral mucous membranes, along with petechiae and punctate red macules on the hard and soft palate and uvula. The most classic presentation is that of a "strawberry tongue" caused by hyperemia and edema of the fungiform papillae, which project above the surface of the tongue. Circumoral pallor is also associated with this disease.

Hairy tongue results from overgrowth of the filiform papillae on the dorsum of the tongue. A yellow to black, discolored, thick layer of accumulated keratin on the tongue is characteristic. Multiple bacterial as well as fungal organisms may be cultured from the tongue. Treatment is empirical with oral rinses and débridement with a toothbrush.

Acute necrotizing ulcerative gingivitis, otherwise known as Vincent's angina or trench mouth, is caused by an imbalance in the normal flora of the gingival sulcus with predominant presence of the spirochete *Borrelia vincentii* and the gram-negative bacillus *Fusiformis fusiform*. Clinically, patients present with a sore mouth, and on physical examination, the interdental papillae are seen to be affected, which differentiates this condition from gingivostomatitis and apthous ulcers. Treatment includes hydrogen peroxide mouthwash, débridement, and antibiotics such as penicillin or doxycycline (if >8 years old).

Koplik's spots are pathognomonic for measles. These irregular bluish white lesions surrounded by an erythematous halo appear on the buccal mucosa opposite the second molars 2 to 3 days before the cutaneous rash of rubeola emerges. These lesions resolve spontaneously and are significant only in the early identification of the disease in a child who has been exposed.

Oral manifestations of primary, secondary, and tertiary syphilis may be characterized by *chancres, mucous patches,* or *gummas,* respectively. Hutchinson's teeth, which are pointed, lateral incisors and notched central incisors, are also characteristic of syphilis.

Oral disease is frequently associated with human immunodeficiency virus (HIV). Many HIV-associated oral disorders occur early in HIV infection and therefore may be a presenting sign or symptom. The most common HIV-associated oral diseases are candidiasis, herpes simplex ulceration, oral hairy leukoplakia, and Kaposi's sarcoma.[18]

A *parulis* or gum boil is a sessile nodule at the site where a draining sinus tract reaches the surface. An *odontogenic cyst,* such as a periapical cyst or abscess, is a soft, fluctuant gingival mass on the facial or lingual area of a carious or traumatized tooth that has undergone pulp necrosis and is thus nonvital. Antibiotics and management of the nonvital tooth via incision and drainage, root canal, or extraction is the treatment. *Pericoronitis* refers to the inflamed or infected tissue over erupting teeth.

A *papilloma* is a benign sessile or pedunculated exophytic papillary growth of stratified squamous epithelium anywhere in the mouth that may be white or pink in color. It is caused by human papillomavirus. Treatment is via excision.

Tumors

Pyogenic Granuloma

Pyogenic granulomas are a fast-growing reactive proliferation of endothelial cells, commonly on the gingiva and usually in response to chronic irritation. The lesions may be sessile or pedunculated with a smooth or verrucose surface that has a reddish hue due to vascularity of the tissue, with a gray pseudomembrane over the surface. They are painless and are prone to bleeding with trauma or manipulation. Treatment consists of complete local surgical excision. Recurrence is common.[3]

Fibroma

Fibroma is the most common benign soft tissue tumor. Frequently located on the gingiva, buccal mucosa, tongue, lips, or palates, it is soft or firm with a sessile or pedunculated base and usually less than 1 cm in size. It is usually secondary to chronic irritation.

Mucocele and Ranula

Mucocele and *ranula* are clinical terms for a pseudocyst that is associated with mucus extravasation into the surrounding soft tissues. These lesions occur as the result of trauma or obstruction to the salivary gland excretory duct. A mucocele originates from the minor salivary glands and presents as a painless, asymptomatic swelling that has a relatively rapid onset and fluctuates in size. It is commonly found in the labial mucosa of the lower lip. Treatment is surgical excision, yet occasionally the cyst may recur.

Ranula originates from the major salivary glands and presents as a painless, blue (if superficial) or translucent, unilateral swelling of the floor of the mouth. However, the lesion may cross the midline if large. The ranula may interfere with speech, mastication, respiration, and swallowing because of the upward and medial displacement of the tongue. Treatment is surgical via excision or marsupialization, and the lesion also may recur.

Rhabdomyosarcoma

Rhabdomyosarcoma is a rare, rapidly growing malignant neoplasm of striated muscle. It is characterized by a painless, infiltrative, ulcerated, fixed, rapidly growing mass that occurs in the first decade of life. Treatment is via excision and chemotherapy. It has a very poor prognosis.

Idiopathic Lesions

Miscellaneous Lesions

Fordyce's granules are asymptomatic, multifocal, benign, small yellow papules that are present in 80% to 90% of adults and represent ectopic sebaceous glands that may coalesce to form plaques. They are bilaterally symmetric and are most commonly found on the buccal mucosa of the cheeks and mandibular molars as well as the vermilion of the upper lip. These developmental lesions appear around the age of 10 and increase in size and number around puberty. No treatment is required for Fordyce's granules, except for cosmetic removal of labial lesions.

"Geographic tongue" or *benign migratory glossitis* occurs secondary to desquamation of the filiform papillae in several patchy, irregular areas on the dorsum of the tongue. These areas heal over and new ones appear. Patients may complain of pain while eating spicy or salty foods. The etiology is not known, and reassurance that this is a benign condition is the recommended treatment.

Gingival hyperplasia is caused by gingival overgrowth, most commonly secondary to drugs such as dilantin, cyclosporine, and nifedipine. Studies have demonstrated that the interaction of these drugs with epithelial keratinocytes, fibroblasts, and collagen can lead to an overgrowth of gingival tissue in susceptible individuals. Gingival enlargement occurs primarily on the labial gingival mucosa and in between the teeth (interdental papillae area).

An *eruption cyst* is a soft, fluctuant, blue to dark red, well-demarcated odontogenic cyst that surrounds an erupting tooth (molar or canine) on the alveolar ridges. No treatment is necessary as the cyst often ruptures spontaneously.

Leukoplakia is a precancerous disease of the mouth that presents as painless, white plaques or patches on the tongue or buccal mucosa and is differentiated from candidiasis in that it does not scrape off. It is associated with smokeless tobacco use and may precede carcinoma.

Retrocuspid papillae are sessile nodules on the gingival margin of the lingual aspect of the mandibular cuspids and are a normal variant in children.

Recurrent Oral Ulcers

Recurrent oral ulcerations are usually categorized as either aphthous ulcers (canker sores) or recurrent herpes labialis (cold sores/fever blisters). The clinical appearance of these entities has frequently confused practitioners secondary to their similar characteristics. They both last 7 to 14 days; have a history of reoccurrence; and have similar

triggering factors, such as stress, mechanical irritation, and illness. However, they have different etiologies and therefore different treatments, thus correct identification is paramount.

Recurrent aphthous stomatitis (RAS) is a common condition that typically starts in childhood or adolescence as recurrent small, round, or ovoid ulcers with circumscribed margins, erythematous haloes, and a white to yellow or gray membrane floor. Most apthous ulcers heal in 1 to 2 weeks and are associated with pain and interference with eating. RAS is classified as minor, major, and herpetiform on the basis of ulcer size and number. The principle differential diagnosis for RAS is recurrent herpes simplex infection.

The etiology of RAS is not entirely clear, and it is therefore termed idiopathic. RAS may be the manifestation of a group of disorders of quite different etiology, rather than a single entity. Immune mechanisms appear to play a role in persons with a genetic predisposition to oral ulceration. Deficiencies of iron, folate, and vitamin B_{12} have also been implicated, as well as the association with immune deficiencies, stress, trauma, and food allergies.

The primary goals of therapy for RAS are relief of pain, reduction of ulcer duration, and restoration of normal oral function. Secondary goals include reduction in the frequency and severity of recurrences and maintenance of remission. Immunosuppressants currently appear to be the most effective in the management of RAS. Topical mixtures of corticosteroids and antibiotic and/or peroxide mouthwashes remain the mainstays of treatment. At best, they can reduce the number of painful ulcer days compared with controls, but they have no consistent effect on the incidence of ulceration. Systemic treatment with oral corticosteroids and immunomodulators may be utilized for more severe, intractable lesions, although the evidence so far has not demonstrated that their efficacy outweighs their toxic effects.[19]

Lesions Associated with Systemic Diseases

Systemic diseases associated with oral mucosa manifestations include gastrointestinal disorders such as Crohn's disease, ulcerative colitis, malabsorption disorders such as gluten-sensitive enteropathy, HIV infection, Behçet's syndrome, Kawasaki disease, toxic shock syndrome, malignancy (leukemia), immune-mediated disorders (agranulocytosis, cyclic neutropenia), trauma, Stevens-Johnson syndrome, epidermolysis bullosa, and lichen planus (Table 52–3).

Summary

The differential diagnosis of oral lesions is vast, and knowledge pertaining to the patient's age, general appearance, and associated symptoms, such as fever, pain, recurrence, or rash, is an important component of classification. During physical examination, attention to hyperemia of the oral mucosa and the type (mass, ulcer, or vesicle), color, size, and location of the lesion further guide the clinician to the correct diagnosis. The most common oral lesions in pediatrics are infectious in etiology and self-limiting. However, rapid recognition of oral mucosa manifestations in the toxic-appearing child is crucial in life-threatening conditions such as toxic shock syndrome and Stevens-Johnson syndrome.

Table 52–3 Oral Lesions Associated with Systemic Disease

Disease	Oral Mucosa	Systemic Findings
Behçet's syndrome	Ulcers	Uveitis, skin and genital ulcers
Crohn's disease	Ulcers, hyperplastic mucosa	Gastrointestinal symptoms, weight loss
Epidermolysis bullosa	Vesicles/bullae of teeth and mucous membranes	Vesiculobullous disorder of skin, Koebner's phenomenon
Kawasaki disease	Hyperemia, cracked lips, strawberry tongue	Fever > 5 days, exanthem, bilateral nonexudative limbic-sparing conjunctivitis, edema/erythema leading to desquamation of hands and feet, single anterior lymph node, arthritis, coronary aneurysm
Lichen planus	White papules or streaks	Violaceous pruritic rash, Wickham's striae (white cross-hatching), Koebner's phenomenon, pitted nails
Mucositis	Ulcers, exudates, pseudomembrane	Associated with neutropenia/chemotherapy
Scarlet fever	Hyperemia, strawberry tongue, circumoral pallor, pharyngitis	Diffuse cervical lymphadenopathy, sandpaper rash, Pastia's lines
Stevens-Johnson syndrome	Erythematous or hemorrhagic plaques, vesicles or bullae, pseudomembrane	Target lesions, exudative conjunctivitis, arthralgia, urethritis
Toxic shock syndrome	Hyperemia, strawberry tongue	Fever, vomiting, erythroderma, shock, coagulopathy

REFERENCES

1. Jorgenson RJ, Shapiro SD, Salinas CD, Levin LS: Intraoral findings and anomalies in neonates. Pediatrics 69:577–582, 1982.
2. Balciunas BA, Kelly M, Siegal MA: Clinical management of common oral lesions. Cutis 47:31, 1991.
*3. Dilley DC, Siegal MA, Budnick S: Diagnosing and treating common oral pathologies. Pediatr Clin North Am 38:1227–1264, 1991.
4. Welbury RR: Congenital epulis of the newborn. Br J Oral Surg 18:238–243, 1980.
5. Fishman SJ, Mulliken JB: Hemangiomas and vascular malformations of infancy and childhood. Pediatr Surg 40:1177–1200, 1993.
6. Kansal P, Sakati N, Rifai A, Woodhouse N: Lingual thyroid: diagnosis and treatment. Arch Intern Med 147:2046–2048, 1987.
7. Chole RA, Domb GH: Differential diagnosis of superficial ulcerations of the oral mucosa. Otolaryngol Head Neck Surg 87:734–740, 1979.
8. Hoppe JE: Treatment of oropharyngeal candidiasis and candidal diaper dermatitis in neonates and infants: review and reappraisal. Pediatr Infect Dis J 16:885–894, 1997.
9. Scott LA, Stone MS: Viral exanthems. Dermatol Online J 9(3):4, 2003.

*10. Worthington HV, Clarkson JE, Eden OB: Interventions for treating oral mucositis for patients with cancer receiving treatment. Cochrane Database Syst Rev (2):CD001973, 2004.
11. Dodd MJ, Dibble SL, Miaskowski C, et al: Randomized clinical trial of the effectiveness of 3 commonly used mouthwashes to treat chemotherapy-induce mucositis. Oral Surg Oral Med Oral Pathol Oral Radiol Endod 90:39–47, 2000.
12. Hess GP, Walson PD: Seizures secondary to oral viscous lidocaine. Ann Emerg Med 17:725–727, 1988.
13. Amir J: Clinical aspects and antiviral therapy in primary herpetic gingivostomatitis. Paediatr Drugs 3:593–597, 2001.
14. Amir J, Harel L, Smetana Z, Varsano I: Treatment of herpes simplex gingivostomatitis with acyclovir in children: a randomized double blind placebo controlled study. BMJ 314:1800–1803, 1997.
*15. Graham B: Hand, foot, and mouth disease. E-medicine J 3(2):1–10, 2002.
16. Liu C, Tseng HW, Wang SM, et al: An outbreak of enterovirus 71 infection in Taiwan, 1998: epidemiologic and clinical manifestations. J Clin Virol 17:23–30, 2000.
*17. Shelley WB, Hashim M, Shelley ED: Acyclovir in the treatment of hand-foot-and-mouth disease. Cutis 57:232–234, 1996.
18. Sirois D: Oral manifestations of HIV disease. Mt Sinai J Med 65:322–332, 1998.
19. Barrons RW: Treatment strategies for recurrent oral aphthous ulcers. Am J Health Syst Pharm 58:41–50, 2001.

*Selected readings.

Chapter 53

Dental Disorders

Linda L. Brown, MD, MSCE

Key Points

There are over 400,000 pediatric emergency department visits a year secondary to dental-related complaints.

The management of dental injuries in children depends on whether the tooth is a primary or permanent tooth.

The urgency of treatment of a dental injury is dependent on the type of injury.

Selected Diagnoses

Traumatic injuries
  Crown fractures
  Root fractures
  Luxation injuries
  Alveolar ridge fractures
Nontraumatic disorders
  Dental caries
  Dentoalveolar abscess
  Pericoronitis

Introduction and Background

Patients with dental-related complaints are seen commonly in emergency departments across the United States, with an estimated 2.95 million emergency department visits from 1997 to 2000 attributed to such complaints.[1] Children comprise about 15% of these visits, the majority (60% to 70%) of which are reported as nontraumatic in origin.[2,3]

Prior to and during the evaluation of pediatric patients with dental-related complaints, it is important to remember the normal anatomy of the tooth. The tooth is divided into the crown, which is visible beyond the gingiva, and the root, which is buried beneath. The crown is composed of a hard covering of enamel over a layer of dentin, which acts to hydrate and cushion, and connects to the pulp, which acts as the neurovascular supply of the tooth. The periodontal ligament is a connective tissue hammock that anchors the tooth

in its socket, and also functions as a "double periosteum," laying down cementum on one side and alveolar bone on the other.

A unique consideration in children is the need to understand normal dental development, as proper identification of primary versus permanent dentition may affect diagnosis and treatment. Tables 53–1 and 53–2 show the most commonly observed pattern and ranges of eruption and exfoliation, although normal variations may occur.[4,5] Inspection of the affected tooth may also give clues to the practitioner. Primary teeth tend to be smaller, shorter, and milky white or opalescent in color, with a smooth occlusal surface, while permanent teeth are wider and white to gray in color, with a ridged occlusal surface.

Discussion of Individual Diagnoses

Traumatic Injuries

Pediatric dental trauma has a bimodal incidence, with a peak from ages 2 to 4 years and another from ages 8 to 10 years. Boys and girls are equally affected during this time period. However, in older school-age children and adolescents, boys are more frequently injured and sports-related trauma and altercations are often reported as the cause.[6,7] Dental injuries may be classified as crown and root fractures, luxation injuries, and alveolar ridge fractures.

Each patient with dental trauma should foremost be considered a trauma patient. Evaluation should proceed with special attention given to the airway, as patients with dental trauma may also have other maxillofacial injuries that could result in blood and soft tissues occluding the airway. Subsequently, a careful history should be taken to include specifics about the mechanism of injury, symptoms (including pain, hot/cold sensitivity), and change in occlusion. With nonverbal children, asking the parent if the child's teeth and occlusion appear "normal" may give added information. The oral cavity should then be examined to assess for damage to dentition, as well as for any soft tissue injury. Foreign debris and dental fragments may be embedded in the surrounding tissues. Finally, the teeth should be examined to assess for any change in their location, pain with percussion, presence of mobility, or swelling along the alveolar ridge.[8] It is also important to examine the mandible by palpating along the temporomandibular joint and evaluating for normal, full, symmetric jaw opening.

Table 53-1	Typical Pattern of Eruption and Exfoliation of Primary Teeth	
	Age at Eruption of Primary Teeth (mo)	Age at Exfoliation (yr)
Maxillary		
Central incisor	7–12	6–8
Lateral incisor	9–13	7–8
Canine	16–22	10–12
First molar	13–19	9–11
Second molar	25–33	10–12
Mandibular		
Central incisor	6–10	6–8
Lateral incisor	7–16	7–8
Canine	17–23	9–12
First molar	12–18	9–12
Second molar	20–31	10–12

Table 53-2	Typical Pattern of Eruption of Permanent Teeth	
	Age at Eruption of Permanent Teeth (yr)	
	Maxillary	Mandibular
Central incisor	7–8	6–6.5
Lateral incisor	8–8.5	7–8
Canine	11–12	9–10.5
First premolar	10–11	10–11
Second premolar	10–11.5	10.5–11.5
First molar	6–6.5	6–6.5
Second molar	12–13	11–12
Third molar	17–21	17–21

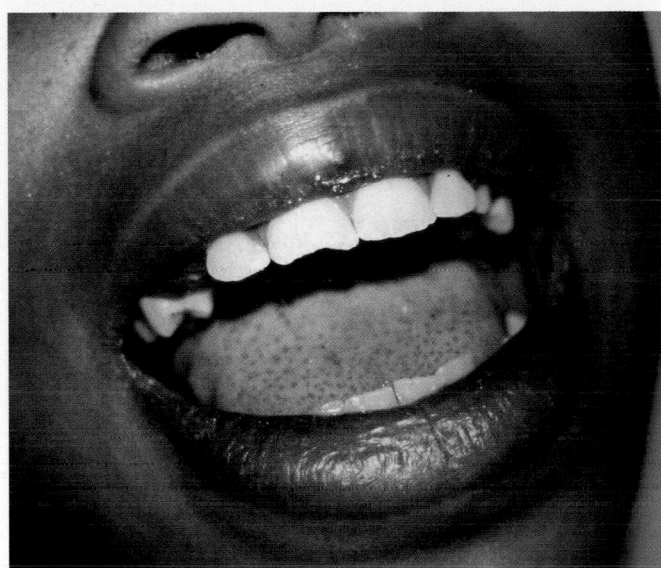

FIGURE 53-1. Uncomplicated dental fracture.

Table 53-3	Treatment Guidelines
Type of Injury	Treatment Urgency*
Crown and crown + root fractures	Acute, subacute or delayed
Root fractures	Acute or subacute
Alveolar fractures	Acute[†]
Concussion and subluxation	Subacute
Extrusion and lateral luxation	Acute or subacute[†]
Intrusion	Subacute[†]
Avulsion	
Tooth not replanted at time of injury	Acute
Tooth replanted	Subacute
Primary tooth injury	
Primary with occlusal problems	Acute
Displaced into follicle of permanent tooth	Acute

*Acute, within a few hours; subacute, within the first 24 hours; delayed, after the first 24 hours.
[†]Evidence questionable.
From Andreasen JO, Andreasen M, Skele A, et al: Effect of treatment delay upon pulp and periodontal healing of traumatic dental injuries—a review article. Dent Traumatol 18:116–128, 2002.

Crown Fractures

Crown fractures are seen commonly in children, and it is important to correctly identify the exposed components, as treatment options and long-term outcome may depend upon this classification. These fractures are usually referred to as uncomplicated (involving enamel, dentin, cementum) versus complicated (with pulp involvement) fractures.

Patients with uncomplicated dental fractures (Fig. 53-1) rarely have pain without manipulation. Pain may be elicited with mastication as well as with exposure to hot or cold. The loss of the enamel and dentin layers may allow bacterial and chemical irritants access to the pulp.[9] Treatment is therefore primarily aimed at protection of the pulp, with placement of a calcium hydroxide or glass ionomer coating, even without obvious exposure. Overall, the risk of long-term complications, including pulp necrosis, is low (<10%), and published guidelines from the American Association of Endodontists (AAE) state that referral for treatment within the next 24 hours is appropriate.[10] A recent review looked at the effect that treatment delay of traumatic dental injuries had upon pulp and periodontal healing and, although evidence was limited, recommendations were made for treatment guidelines (Table 53-3).[11,12]

Complicated fractures involve the pulp and can be identified by the presence of blood at the tooth core. Patients may present with pain, as the neurovascular supply of the tooth is exposed. It is also important to remember that dental fragments may become lodged in soft tissues or, less commonly, aspirated. Therefore, evaluation of soft tissue lacerations must be complete, utilizing radiographs if needed. Chest radiographs may also be considered if large fragments are unaccounted for and a history of possible aspiration is obtained. These injuries are at a higher risk of pulp necrosis than uncomplicated fractures, although guidelines state that treatment, which may include pulp capping or pulpectomy, within 24 hours is still appropriate.[10,11] Dental radiographs will also be needed on follow-up to evaluate for root fracture, which may not be clinically evident on presentation.

Root Fractures

Classified by their location along the root, these fractures are identified as coronal, midroot, or apical, and are seen most commonly in teeth with complete root formation, approximately 2 to 3 years after eruption.[13] Coronal fractures may be associated with crown displacement and, therefore, are usually the easiest to diagnose. Fractures with displacement

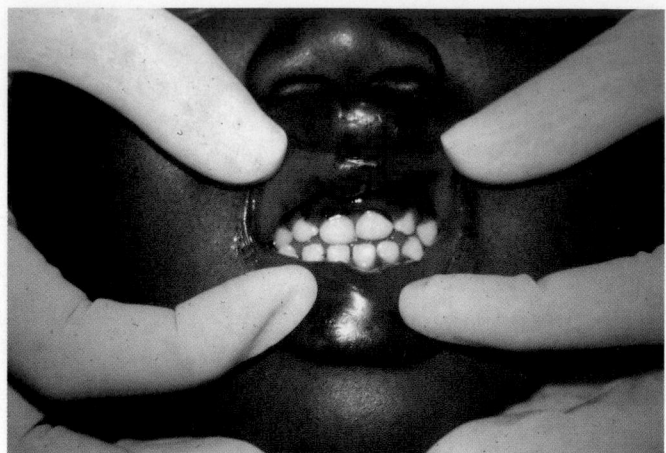

FIGURE 53–2. Visible blood in the gingival sulcus.

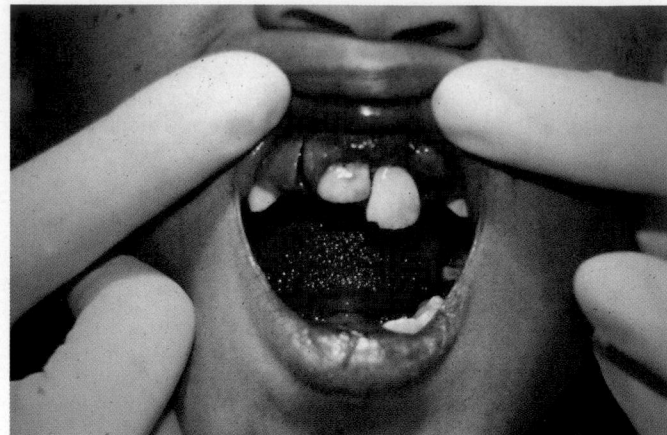

FIGURE 53–3. Intrusion injury.

often require immediate dental consultation for splinting. Midroot and apical fractures, however, may only be suspected by the presence of bleeding from the gingival sulcus after a traumatic event, and require follow-up intraoral dental radiographs for confirmation and evaluation for further treatment interventions.

Luxation Injuries

Luxation injuries may be classified as concussion, subluxation, intrusion, extrusion, lateral luxation, or avulsion injuries. Dental concussion injuries are seen commonly after trauma, when children may present with complaints of tenderness with biting pressure or with percussion of the tooth. The tooth remains immobile in the socket, however, which differentiates the injury from a subluxation injury, in which the tooth is loosened and mobile with palpation, although not displaced. Blood may also be visible in the gingival sulcus, as shown in Figure 53–2. With both concussion and subluxation injuries, the long-term risk to the primary and permanent tooth is low, although eventual pulp necrosis is possible, and the need for immediate intervention is usually limited. In the event of a subluxed tooth with significant mobility, a dental consultation should be obtained to assess the need for splinting or potential extraction, if primary dentition is involved. All other patients should have outpatient dental follow-up arranged to assess the need for radiographs and further intervention.[11,12]

Intrusion injuries involve displacement of the tooth into the alveolar bone and crushing of the periodontal ligament (Fig. 53–3). They can result in significant long-term damage to the dentition. Although seen more frequently in primary teeth, intrusion of the permanent teeth can occur with significant trauma. On examination, the tooth will often be immobile and minimally tender to percussion. Occasionally it will not be visible beyond the gingiva, mimicking the look of an avulsed tooth. When the injury involves a primary tooth, the main concern is for the effect upon the underlying permanent dentition, with an estimated 50% to 75% damage rate.[10,13] Since the damage occurs at the time of trauma, immediate intervention, including extraction, results in little improvement in outcome. Therefore, published treatment guidelines from the International Association of Dental Traumatology (IADT) state that, if the primary tooth is

intruded into the developing tooth germ, extraction is required. Otherwise, the tooth may be allowed to re-erupt spontaneously.[14,15] It is important to note that allowing the tooth to re-erupt leads to unpredictable results, and practice variation is still possible between dental consultants.

When the intruded tooth is a permanent tooth, the most important factor in outcome has been found to be the amount of intrusion present. Several studies have reported that intrusions of less than 3 mm have an excellent prognosis, while those of greater than 6 mm have a universally poor outcome secondary to inflammatory root resorption and pulp necrosis.[16,17] Guidelines published by the Royal College of Surgeons of England utilize the amount of intrusion to determine treatment regimens. The IADT and the AAE suggest that spontaneous re-eruption may be possible for teeth with incomplete root formation, whereas orthodontic or surgical repositioning is needed for teeth with complete root formation. Close dental follow-up within 24 hours, with the potential for future endodontic therapy, is also required.

Extrusion injuries are diagnosed when the tooth is partially displaced out of the socket and into the oral cavity. Similarly, in lateral luxation injuries, which constitute the largest proportion of all dental displacement injuries, the involved tooth or teeth are displaced relative to the other teeth. The direction of this movement can be buccal, labial, or lingual (Fig. 53–4), and the tooth when palpated will usually be mobile within the socket. Soft tissue injuries, including gingival lacerations, and root fractures will often be seen in association with these injuries. Emergent dental consultation is required for injuries with significant mobility or malocclusion, as immediate splinting may be required. When primary dentition is involved, extraction may be performed if exfoliation is predicted in the near future. As with most dental trauma, follow-up radiographs by a dentist are required to evaluate for further injury.

Avulsion injuries, also referred to as complete luxation injuries, are one of the most urgent dental injuries. The prognosis for the affected tooth is time dependent, and management is aimed at maintaining the viability of the periodontal ligament (PDL). Several published studies have reported that, after dry storage time of more than 15 to 30 minutes, almost all PDL cells have died, making successful reimplantation unlikely.[14] Therefore, it is important to inform parents, teachers, and other caregivers of the appropriate steps to reimplant an

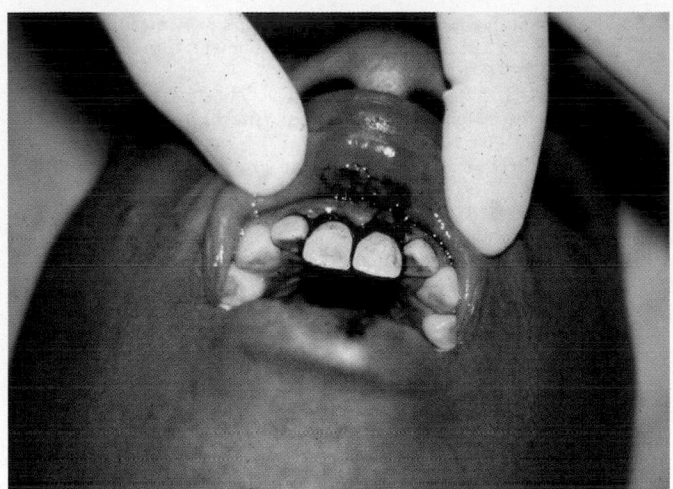

FIGURE 53–4. Lingual luxation injury.

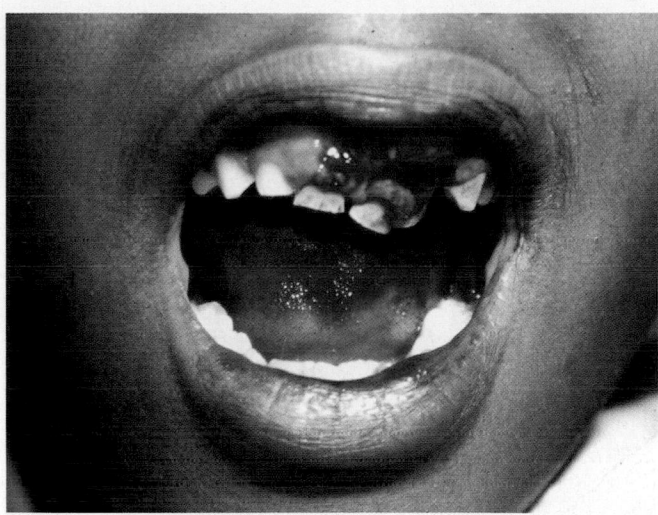

FIGURE 53–5. Alveolar ridge fracture.

avulsed tooth. After an injury, the tooth should immediately be identified as a primary versus permanent tooth. It is generally accepted that primary teeth should not be reimplanted to prevent further damage to the underlying permanent tooth secondary to inflammation or ankylosis. Once a permanent tooth is identified, it should be cleaned of debris by rinsing it briefly with saline (or water, if saline is unavailable). The tooth should not be scrubbed, as this will further damage PDL cells. The socket should then be examined for debris or significant damage and irrigated if necessary. The tooth can then be held by the crown and placed into the socket with slow, steady pressure. If immediate reimplantation is not possible, then the tooth should be placed in a liquid medium to help maintain viability of the PDL cells. Acceptable solutions include cell culture media such as Viaspan or Hank's Balanced Salt Solution. Milk, especially chilled milk, has also been found to be an excellent, and readily available, transport medium.[18] Saline or the patient's own saliva are not ideal substitutes, but are more acceptable than dry storage. After the tooth has been reimplanted, emergent dental consultation is required for splinting, and close dental follow-up is required for an optimal outcome. Treatment guidelines from the IADT and AAE also state that these patients should receive a course of oral antibiotics (penicillin VK for 7 days or doxycycline if patients are penicillin allergic and > 8 years old), as several studies have suggested that antibiotics decrease the risk of inflammatory root resorption and may improve outcome.[19,20] Tetanus status should also be assessed if significant debris was found contaminating the wound.

Alveolar Ridge Fractures

Alveolar ridge fractures occur in 5% to 9% of all dentoalveolar injuries.[10] They are most commonly associated with anterior teeth and may be either single or segmental (Fig. 53–5). Identification of subtle fractures may be possible with palpation of the gingiva, looking for any evidence of crepitus or step-offs. The most important management strategy involves repositioning and splinting of the affected area, and therefore immediate dental consultation is often necessary. Oral antibiotics (penicillin VK or doxycycline) may also be utilized, although little evidence is available regarding the effectiveness of this strategy.

Nontraumatic Disorders

Dental Caries

Between 50% and 75% of pediatric, nontraumatic, dental-related complaints seen in the emergency department are secondary to caries, with 18% due to "baby bottle" caries.[2,3,21] Beginning with the fermentation of carbohydrates by oral bacteria and the production of acid, the enamel and dentin layers of the tooth are demineralized. Without intervention, decay erodes to the pulp, and inflammation, referred to as pulpitis, occurs.[22] Patients may complain of pain as well as hot/cold insensitivity. On examination, dental caries appear as brownish cavitations in the tooth surface. With more advanced inflammation of the pulp, pain may be severe and may worsen with percussion of the tooth. Emergency department management should center on analgesia and appropriate referral to a dentist for removal of the affected area and placement of a filling.

Dentoalveolar Abscess

When inflammation of the pulp is left untreated, the localized collection of purulent fluid results in a dentoalveolar abscess. Patients complain of severe pain, and on examination have significant tenderness with percussion. The gingivae around the affected tooth often appear erythematous and swollen, and occasionally areas of fluctuance are palpated. Associated regional lymphadenopathy and facial swelling may also be present. When an apical or "periapical" abscess develops, fistula formation to the gingiva (Fig. 53–6) or, less commonly, to the face may occur. Often when this drainage occurs, the pain is less severe. Management in the emergency department focuses again on analgesia. Complications with dental abscess, including localized cellulitis and more severe extension into the soft tissues of the head and neck, require the addition of antibiotics. Oral penicillin, or erythromycin or clindamycin for patients with true penicillin allergy, are most commonly used for this purpose. Emergent otorhinolaryngology consultation should be obtained for patients requiring incision and drainage due to severe pain or with extension of infection into the deeper tissues of the head and neck. Close dental follow-up should be obtained for all patients who require more definitive treatment.

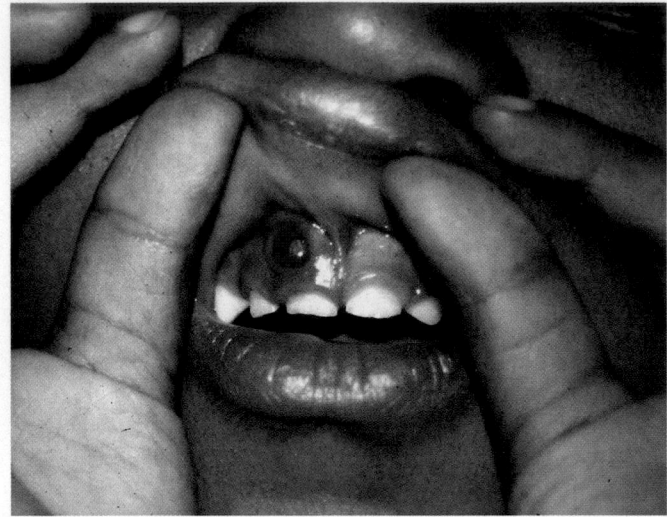

FIGURE 53–6. Fistula formation to the gingiva from a periapical abscess.

Pericoronitis

Pericoronitis refers to an inflammation of the soft tissues surrounding the crown of an erupting tooth. Food debris and bacteria become trapped under the gum overlying the tooth, and localized infection can result. This is most commonly associated with erupting wisdom teeth, and children often present with pain. In more severe cases, extension of this inflammation and secondary infection can result in cellulitis with regional lymphadenopathy and trismus. Primary treatment involves local irrigation with mouthwashes. If increased swelling and significant pain is present or if cellulitis is diagnosed, then treatment with oral antibiotic therapy may also be indicated. Appropriate follow-up with a dentist should be arranged to confirm improvement of patient symptoms or, if symptoms worsen, to evaluate the potential need for surgical removal of the flap.

REFERENCES

*1. Lewis C, Lynch H, Johnston B: Dental complaints in emergency departments: a national perspective. Ann Emerg Med 42:93–99, 2003.

---

*Selected readings.

*2. Wilson S, Smith GA, Preisch J, Casamassimo PS: Nontraumatic dental emergencies in a pediatric emergency department. Clin Pediatr (Phila) 36:333–337, 1997.
3. Dorfman DH, Kastner B, Vinci RJ: Dental concerns unrelated to trauma in the pediatric emergency department. Arch Pediatr Adolesc Med 155:699–703, 2001.
4. Dock M, Creedon RL: The teeth and oral cavity. In Rudolph CD, Rudolph AM, Hostetter MK, et al (eds): Rudolph's Pediatrics. New York: McGraw Hill, 2003, pp 1283–1304.
5. Rousset MM, Boualam N, Delfosse C, Roberts WE: Emergence of permanent teeth: secular trends and variance in a modern sample. J Dent Child (Chic) 70:208–214, 2003.
6. McTigue DJ: Diagnosis and management of dental injuries in children. Pediatr Clin North Am 47:1067–1084, 2000.
7. Wilson S, Smith GA, Preisch J, Casamassimo PS: Epidemiology of dental trauma treated in an urban pediatric emergency department. Pediatr Emerg Care 13:12–15, 1997.
8. Kenny DJ, Barrett EJ: Recent developments in dental traumatology. Pediatr Dent 23:464–468, 2001.
9. Dewhurst SN, Mason C, Roberts GJ: Emergency treatment of orodental injuries: a review. Br J Oral Maxillofac Surg 36:165–175, 1998.
10. Dale RA: Dentoalveolar trauma. Emerg Med Clin North Am 18:521–538, 2000.
*11. Andreasen JO, Andreasen M, Skele A, et al: Effect of treatment delay upon pulp and periodontal healing of traumatic dental injuries—a review article. Dent Traumatol 18:116–128, 2002.
12. American Association of Endodontists: Recommended Guidelines of the American Association of Endodontists for Traumatic Dental Injuries. 2004. Available at http://www.aae.org/dentalpro/guidelines.htm
*13. Flores MT: Traumatic injuries in the primary dentition. Dent Traumatol 18:287–298, 2002.
14. Kenny DJ, Barrett EJ, Casas MJ: Avulsions and intrusions: the controversial displacement injuries. J Can Dent Assoc 69:308–313, 2003.
15. Flores MT, Andreasen JO, Bakland LK, et al; International Association of Dental Traumatology: Guidelines for the management of traumatic dental injuries. Dent Traumatol 17:145–148, 2001.
16. Al-Badri S, Kinirons M, Cole B, Welbury R: Factors affecting resorption in traumatically intruded permanent incisors in children. Dent Traumatol 18:73–76, 2002.
17. Kinirons MJ, Sutcliffe J: Traumatically intruded permanent incisors: a study of treatment and outcome. Br Dent J 170:144–146, 1991.
*18. Sigales E, Regan JD, Kramer PR, et al: Survival of human periodontal ligament cells in media proposed for transport of avulsed teeth. Dent Traumatol 20:21–28, 2004.
19. Finucane D, Kinirons MJ: External inflammatory and replacement resorption of luxated and avulsed replanted permanent incisors: a review and case presentation. Dent Traumatol 19:170–174, 2003.
*20. Trope M: Clinical management of the avulsed tooth: present strategies and future directions. Dent Traumatol 18:1–11, 2002.
21. Graham DB, Webb MD, Seale NS: Pediatric emergency room visits for nontraumatic dental disease. Pediatr Dent 22:134–140, 2000.
22. Douglass AB, Douglass JM: Common dental emergencies. Am Fam Physician 67:511–516, 2003.

Neck Infections

Amy L. Puchalski, MD

Introduction and Background

Children commonly develop infections of the soft tissues of the neck due in part to their propensity for upper respiratory tract infections (URIs) and in part to their relatively large amount of lymphoid tissue compared to adults. Over half of all children have palpable cervical lymph nodes, and this number increases to 80% to 90% among 4- to 8-year-olds.[1] Viral lymphadenitis is the most common neck infection. It is important to follow these patients clinically for development of a secondary suppurative infection, which can lead to more serious morbidity. In addition, a directed history and physical examination is invaluable to help differentiate a suspected infectious process from either congenital neck masses or neoplasms.

Selected Diagnoses

Lymphadenitis
Retropharyngeal and parapharyngeal abscesses
Lemierre syndrome
Ludwig's angina
Parotitis

Discussion of Individual Diagnoses

Lymphadenitis

Lymphadenitis from various causes is by far the most common neck infection in the pediatric population, and a thorough history and physical examination is imperative to help identify the likely etiology as well as the nidus for infection. Table 54–1 includes some key points on which to focus in obtaining the history of a patient presenting with enlarged neck lymph nodes. Lymph nodes are considered enlarged if they are cervical nodes greater than 10 mm or supraclavicular nodes of any size.[2] Other physical examination features may help differentiate the cause of lymphadenitis. Nodes in viral disease tend to be small, discrete, mobile, bilateral, and minimally tender. Bacterial infection is characterized by large, warm, tender, often unilateral, and sometimes fluctuant nodes. More chronic infectious lymph nodes are minimally tender, discrete, and adherent to underlying tissue, and lack signs of inflammation.[2] Often the emergency physician is faced with the decision of when to obtain surgical consultation for potential biopsy of an enlarged lymph node. A retrospective study in children sought to identify which patients undergoing lymph node biopsy were more likely to have significant disease. Table 54–2 summarizes some of those findings and gives suggestions for which children warrant biopsy. Of the patients in this study, over half had reactive hyperplasia, one third had granulomatous disease, 13% had a malignancy, and 3% had chronic lymphadenopathy.[3]

Viral Lymphadenitis

Viral infection is the most common cause of lymphadenitis in infants and children. Lymph node enlargement is most often a result of reactive hyperplasia of the lymphoid tissue in response to a URI, but the nodes can also be directly infected by the virus. The list of viral pathogens is lengthy and includes rhinovirus, adenovirus, enterovirus, measles, mumps, rubella, Epstein-Barr virus (EBV), cytomegalovirus (CMV), and human immunodeficiency virus (HIV). EBV infection classically presents with fever, exudative tonsillitis, fatigue, malaise, and often hepatosplenomegaly, along with enlarged bilateral cervical nodes. The lymphadenopathy may be more extensive and enlarged than with many other URIs and at times raises concerns for malignancy. Children with CMV infection clinically present similarly to those with EBV and can be differentiated with serologic testing. Up to 95% of children with EBV infection and 75% with CMV infection

Table 54–1	History in Children with Lymphadenitis

Symptom onset
Duration
Rate of enlargement
Exposure to animals
HIV risk factors
Possible TB contact
Recent antibiotic use
Travel outside the United States
Weight loss
Presence, duration and severity of fever
History of rash

Abbreviations: HIV, human immunodeficiency virus; TB, tuberculosis.

Table 54–2	Indications for Lymph Node Biopsy

Supraclavicular lymph nodes
Fixed or matted nodes
Incomplete or no response to antibiotics
Signs of airway, neurologic, or cardiovascular impingement
Persistent fever, weight loss, night sweats
Abnormal chest radiograph
Rapidly enlarging nodes

From Knight PJ, Mulne AF, Vassy LE: When is a lymph node biopsy indicated in children with enlarged peripheral nodes? Pediatrics 69:391–396, 1982.

have cervical lymphadenopathy.[2] Adenovirus may cause conjunctivitis, pharyngitis, and a rash in addition to cervical lymphadenopathy and classic URI symptoms. Features of acute HIV infection are similar to other acute viral URIs with similar degrees of lymphadenopathy. Chronic HIV infection often causes large, soft nodes in the posterior triangle of the neck as well as generalized mild lymphadenopathy. It is important to question adolescent patients with cervical lymphadenitis about sexual activity to help in recommendations for possible outpatient HIV testing. Questioning about prolonged fever, weight loss, duration of lymphadenopathy, and malaise is important with suspected viral infection to help differentiate those patients who may have a more chronic or malignant process.

The need for testing with suspected viral lymphadenitis is usually minimal, and in the vast majority of cases no testing is needed. Serology for EBV and CMV may be considered in appropriate clinical scenarios. Recommendation for appropriate outpatient HIV testing should be considered for sexually active adolescents and children with failure to thrive or a history of recurrent infections. In rare instances, patients with significant or prolonged lymphadenopathy or with systemic symptoms out of proportion to those of a typical viral URI may require contrast computed tomography (CT) imaging of the neck to differentiate malignancy or suppurative lymphadenitis. In addition, fine-needle aspiration or open biopsy may be performed by consultants to rule out a malignant process, if one is suspected. Care of patients with viral lymphadenitis is largely supportive with the exception of those with HIV infection.[4]

Bacterial Lymphadenitis

Bacterial suppurative lymphadenitis is the most common cause of sudden onset of rapidly enlarging cervical lymph nodes.[5] The bacterial pathogens responsible for the majority of these infections are streptococcus and staphylococcus species, but also include *Neisseria* species, *Bacteroides, Fusobacterium*, and other oral anaerobes. Infections are often polymicrobial, and up to 38% of bacterial lymphadenitis in children 2 to 16 years of age may include anaerobes.[5] Children ages 1 to 4 years more commonly develop streptococcal and staphylococcal lymphadenitis, whereas older children and adolescents more often develop anaerobic and group A streptococcal infection.[2] Pathophysiologically, bacterial lymphadenitis is generally preceded by a pharyngeal infection, either viral or bacterial, which leads to superinfection of the cervical lymph nodes draining those regions. Impetigo on the face or scalp may also precede a bacterial cervical lymphadenitis.

Patients typically present with tender, warm, erythematous cervical and submandibular nodes following pharyngitis. Nodes may or may not feel fluctuant at the time of presentation. Overall, about 25% of bacterial lymphadenitis will progress to suppuration, more commonly occurring with staphylococcal infections. Generally, suppuration will occur within 2 weeks of initial cervical node enlargement.[2] Adjuvant testing is determined primarily by the initial history and physical examination. A complete blood count and blood culture in febrile patients should be considered. CT with contrast is the imaging study of choice if there is clinical concern for a focal abscess or need for surgical drainage, as it can differentiate cellulitis, phlegmon, and abscess. This study should be obtained on initial presentation in children with palpable areas of fluctuance, airway or vascular compromise, ill appearance, or any concern for a malignancy. Ultrasound may have a role in evaluating for the presence of fluid pockets, but will not provide sufficient information to determine need for surgical intervention.

Treatment of bacterial lymphadenitis includes antibiotics, either oral or intravenous, warm compresses, and analgesia if needed. The majority of children may be treated and followed in the outpatient setting as long as follow-up within 24 to 48 hours of initial presentation can be established to evaluate response to oral antibiotics. Potential choices for oral therapy include amoxicillin/clavulanate, clindamycin, and the cephalosporins. Inpatient treatment with intravenous antibiotics is reserved for children who have not responded adequately to oral antibiotics (persistent fever, increasing lymph node size or tenderness, developing fluctuance), and those who are ill appearing, have significant swelling or nodal involvement, or have a potential complication such as bacteremia, cellulitis, or development of a deep neck space abscess. Surgical consultation for incision and drainage should be obtained for children with abscess identified on CT.

MYCOBACTERIAL LYMPHADENITIS

Mycobacterial lymphadenitis falls into two groups: tuberculous and atypical mycobacterial infections. In infants and children, up to 90% of mycobacterial lymphadenitis is caused by atypical pathogens, with *Mycobacterium avium-intracellulare* and *Mycobacterium scrofulaceum* being the most common.[2,6,7] Atypical mycobacteria are the most common cause of granulomatous lymphadenitis and account for 7% to 8% of chronic lymphadenitis in children.[1,6] In contrast, cases of tuberculous lymphadenitis outnumber atypical infection in the adult population.[7] Lymphadenitis with atypical pathogens typically affects otherwise healthy children ages 1 to 5 years, more often from rural areas, who come in contact with and ingest contaminated soil, dust, eggs, and unpasteurized dairy products.[2,6,7] Breaks in the gingiva from erupting teeth serve as a route by which atypical mycobacteria may then infect submandibular and cervical lymph nodes.[1] There is no documentation of human-to-human transmission of these pathogens.

Children with mycobacterial lymphadenitis will present with unilateral preauricular, submandibular, or upper cervical lymph nodes that enlarge over several weeks. These nodes are painless or only minimally tender and classically develop a violaceous color of the overlying skin. If untreated, the nodes may liquefy and eventually spontaneously drain through the skin, often resulting in significant cosmetic deformity. Patients are generally afebrile and lack significant systemic symptoms.[2,6,8] Among 105 cases, the mean age of patients was 3 years, and most presented in the winter and spring with cervical or facial lymphadenitis (91%).[9]

Evaluation of children with suspected atypical mycobacterial lymphadenitis often includes purified protein derivative (PPD) testing, chest radiography, and possible contrast CT. Approximately half of the patients have a positive PPD skin test, with a typical area of induration between 5 and 15 mm.[2,9] Chest radiography should be obtained to help differentiate from tuberculous infections, and should be negative in those with atypical disease.[2] An enhanced CT scan of the chest and neck is useful to establish the extent of involvement and development of suppuration. CT findings include a rim-enhancing mass with central lucency but minimal surrounding inflammation or fat stranding.[6,8] The optimal treatment for atypical infection is resection to minimize the scarring and cosmetic deformity that occurs once nodes suppurate and drain, though there is still some controversy over surgical management. Initial therapy with oral macrolide antibiotics may be another option, particularly in children who are poor surgical candidates. In one review including 10 children who were initially treated with macrolide antibiotics, half were cured and half still required later surgical resection.[8] Early surgical consultation for suspected atypical mycobacterial lymphadenitis should always be a part of the care of these children in the emergency department.

Tuberculous lymphadenitis is rare in infants and children and differs from atypical infection in presentation and treatment. Epidemiologically, it is seen more often in urban and immigrant populations or in immunocompromised children.[2,6] Patients generally have systemic disease and constitutional symptoms at the time of presentation, and up to 20% will have generalized lymphadenopathy.[2] The route of infection is an extension from either the apical pleural or paratracheal nodes and typically affecting supraclavicular and lower cervical nodes.[2] Tuberculous disease will more often suppurate and drain through sinus tracts in the skin than will atypical mycobacterial lymphadenitis.[2] In addition to surgical consultation for biopsy or resection to aid in diagnosis and treatment, it is important to involve infectious disease specialists in initiating antituberculosis medication therapy

Table 54–3	Atypical Mycobacterial vs. Tuberculous Lymphadenitis
Atypical Mycobacterial	**Mycobacterial**
Healthy children	Immunocompromised
Rural populations	Urban and immigrant populations
Family PPD negative	PPD-positive contact, usually family
Age 1–5 yr	More common in adults
Minimal constitutional symptoms	Systemic symptoms, pulmonary disease
PPD negative or <15 mm	PPD positive, usually >15 mm
CXR negative	CXR usually positive
Resection to treat	Resection + TB medications to treat

Abbreviations: CXR, chest radiograph; PPD, purified protein derivative (of tuberculin); TB, tuberculosis.

as well as investigating the child's environment to establish the index case, who most often is a family member.[10] A variety of social factors, clinical features, and diagnostic studies can be used to discriminate between atypical and tuberculous lymphadenitis (Table 54–3)

CAT-SCRATCH LYMPHADENITIS

This disease is most often seen in children and is caused by *Bartonella henslae*, a slow growing gram negative bacillus. It usually causes regional lymphadenopathy in immunocompetent patients. Transmission to humans is via a scratch from an infected young cat, though other animals such as dogs, rabbits, and monkeys have been implicated as well.[6] Transmission between cats occurs through flea bites. Cervical nodes are the third most common lymph node region affected by this disease, with axillary and inguinal nodes being more commonly infected. Clinically, a granuloma may be seen half the time at the site of the initial inoculation, usually on the face or extremity, and it heals in about 1 week. Lymphadenitis develops 1 to 4 weeks after the initial inoculation, so this granuloma may not be evident at presentation. Enlarged lymph nodes may persist for 2 to 3 months before complete resolution. About half of the patients will have mild systemic symptoms such as low-grade fever or malaise. While this is generally a self-limited disease process, 10% to 35% of cases will progress to suppuration, possibly requiring incision and drainage or needle aspiration. A distinct clinical entity of cat-scratch disease is Parinaud's oculoglandular syndrome, consisting of a conjunctival granuloma and preauricular lymphadenopathy. Rarely children have other systemic complications, including encephalitis, rash, hepatosplenomegaly, thrombocytopenic purpura, erythema nodosum, and bacillary angiomatosis, though immunocompromised patients are usually those at risk for these complications.[2,6,11]

Diagnosis generally relies on clinical suspicion with confirmatory serologic testing. The organism is very difficult to culture, but polymerase chain reaction tests from nodal tissue may be helpful. Uncomplicated lymphadenitis is usually self-limited, and treatment with oral antibiotics is not routinely recommended. One recent, small, placebo-controlled study in children and adults concluded, however, that azithromycin may provide a substantial decrease in lymph node volume.[11] Surgical consultation for incision and drainage or needle aspiration may be required for patients with very tender, fluctuant nodes.

TULAREMIA LYMPHADENITIS

One form of infection by the gram-negative rod *Francisella tularensis* is ulceroglandular, characterized by ulceration at the site of inoculation and painful regional lymphadenopathy.[6,12] Exposure is through contact with infected animals, such as rabbits, or bites of infected ticks and mosquitoes.[6] After a 2- to 6-day period of incubation, children with tularemia frequently develop constitutional symptoms such as fever, chills, malaise and arthralgias, pharyngitis, nausea and vomiting.[12] It typically affects children under the age of 10 years from May to September, when they are outdoors.[6] While most children develop constitutional symptoms, adult patients do so less frequently. Another clinical form of tularemia is the oropharyngeal form, when exposure to contaminated water or milk results in oral ulcers, fever, pharyngitis, and cervical lymphadenopathy.[12] The most common complication of tularemia infection is pneumonia, which can affect up to 15% of children with lymphadenitis, although pericarditis and hepatitis have been seen as well.[6]

Diagnosis of tularemia depends primarily on serologic testing in the appropriate clinical setting. Either a fourfold increase in titers over a 2-week period or a single titer of 1 : 160 at the end of the second week of symptoms is diagnostic. The causative agent can be cultured from infected lymph nodes, though it may be difficult to isolate the organism. Treatment for tularemia lymphadenitis ideally consists of a 10-day course of streptomycin, gentamicin, or amikacin, though tetracycline, doxycycline, and ciprofloxacin are alternative choices.[6,12]

OTHER CAUSES OF BACTERIAL LYMPHADENITIS

Actinomyces israelii is a gram-positive organism that is a rare cause of lymphadenitis in children in the United States. Half of all infections with this organism involve the neck and face and usually follow a dental procedure or oral trauma. Children present with a slowly growing, painless mass near the mandible; 10% of the time it will directly infect cervical nodes as well. Some patients will have chronic drainage through sinus tracts. Treatment consists of surgical resection plus a 6-month course of penicillin, clindamycin, erythromycin, or tetracycline.[4]

Brucellosis can cause mild cervical lymphadenitis along with nonspecific symptoms such as fever, malaise, fatigue, and anorexia. Disease is generally mild in children as opposed to adults, who can suffer more severe systemic complications. Patients are exposed through infected livestock and unpasturized dairy products. Diagnosis can be made with serology, blood culture, or culture from lymph node tissue. A prolonged course of treatment with rifampin or streptomycin is required to prevent relapse.[4] Finally, primary syphilis is a rare cause of cervical lymphadenopathy in patients with an oral chancre.

Histoplasmosis Lymphadenitis

Histoplasmosis is the most common fungal cause of lymphadenitis in the pediatric population. It is most commonly seen in the central United States and Ohio River valley, where infection occurs from inhalation of spores, often found in bat or bird droppings. Primary pulmonary infection is the most common manifestation, though young children and immunocompromised patients are at risk for disseminated disease that includes generalized lymphadenopathy as one clinical finding. Fever, pneumonia, hepatosplenomegaly, disseminated intravascular coagulation, and failure to thrive are part of disseminated infection as well. Culture of infected lymph nodes or other tissue is the best way to diagnose this infection. Treatment of young children with disseminated disease or significant lymphadenitis consists of antifungal therapy such as amphotericin B along with excision of infected nodes. For the majority of patients, the disease is self-limited and requires only outpatient follow-up. Candida and Aspergillus can rarely cause lymphadenitis in immunocompromised patients as well.[4,6,13]

Toxoplasmosis Lymphadenitis

Toxoplasmosis gondii is the most common cause of lymphadenitis due to a parasitic infection. Cervical lymphadenitis is the most frequent manifestation of infection acquired neonatally, though only 3% to 7% of cases in children involve cervical lymphadenitis. Most patients infected with toxoplasmosis remain asymptomatic. Of those with clinical manifestations, up to 90% will have cervical lymphadenitis. Immunocompromised children may suffer more serious consequences, such as blindness and central nervous system disease. Infection occurs through exposure to cats, cat litter, uncooked meat, or unpasturized milk. Diagnosis is usually made with serum titers. Patients often undergo excisional biopsy of cervical nodes, as this infection is frequently confused with lymphoma or other malignancies. Otherwise healthy patients do not require additional systemic therapy for toxoplasmosis lymphadenitis.[4,13]

Retropharyngeal and Parapharyngeal Abscesses

Deep neck space infections, including retropharyngeal and parapharyngeal abscesses, are polymicrobial infections that arise from lymphoid tissue in those spaces. Retropharyngeal abscesses (RPAs) most often affect children less than 6 years of age as they have lymph nodes in that space that can act as a nidus for infections that spread from the paranasal sinuses, middle ear, and nasopharynx. These lymph nodes involute by age 5 or 6 years. Older children and adolescents still suffer from deep neck space infections, though they are more often a result of direct trauma, spread from superficial cervical lymphadenitis, or spread from dental infection. These infections are typically polymicrobial, and commonly include streptococcal species, staphylococcal species, non-typable *Haemophilus influenzae,* Neisseria species, Veillonella, Peptostreptococcus, Bacteroides, and Fusobacterium.[14] One retrospective review of both children and adults with deep neck space infections reported that 62% of the cultured abscess were polymicrobial infections, with *Streptococcus viridans* an etiologic agent in 39%, *Staphylococcus epidermidis* present in 21%, and anaerobes growing in 35%.[5] In a study of 20 children who had cultures obtained intraoperatively, 13 were positive for group A streptococcus, 2 for *Staphylococcus aureus,* 1 for *H. influenzae,* and 1 for anaerobes.[15]

The clinical course of an RPA often begins with a preceding URI days to weeks prior to the abscess. Symptoms of the abscess may include fever, drooling, torticollis, pain with neck movement, poor oral intake, irritability, and trismus. Physical examination may reveal signs consistent with meningitis, such as nuchal rigidity, limited neck movement, ill appearance, drooling, and dehydration. Lateral neck swelling and/or a bulge in the posterior oropharynx are physical signs of a possible RPA. Signs and symptoms are often nonspecific, and this disease entity largely affects preverbal children. Older children with parapharyngeal abscesses are likely to complain of a worsening sore throat, difficulty swallowing, pain with neck movement, palpable cervical lymphadenopathy, or neck swelling.

The mean age of children with RPA is 36 months, with 75% of patients less than 5 years of age. The primary chief complaint is neck pain, in 38% of cases, followed by fever (17%), sore throat (17%), neck mass (16%), and stridor (5%). The most common clinical finding documented is limited neck extension, seen in 45% of children. Torticollis is reported in 36.5% of children. Interestingly, few patients have respiratory compromise, with only 1.5% having stridor and 1.5% wheezing. Respiratory distress and compromise, while certainly a potential threat to these patients, may not be as common as once thought with RPA.[15] Other concerning potential complications of deep neck space abscesses include sepsis, septic venous thrombosis, mediastinitis, and aspiration pneumonia if the abscess ruptures and purulent material is inadvertently inhaled.[14] Children who have had recurrent deep neck space infections require evaluation for possible congenital neck lesions predisposing to infection in that space.[16] The differential diagnosis in a child with a suspected RPA includes hematoma trauma, perforation from a foreign body or trauma, neoplasm involving retropharyngeal lymphoid tissue, hemangioma, a branchial cleft cyst, ectopic thyroid tissue, or myxedema.[4]

The diagnosis of a retropharyngeal or parapharyngeal abscess relies mainly on imaging studies as well as repeated clinical examination. A lateral neck radiograph is generally the best starting point, and it is important that those performing the radiography realize that optimal information is gained when the film is a true lateral with the neck in slight extension and the patient in the inspiratory phase of respiration. Otherwise, the retropharyngeal space in a child may appear falsely enlarged. As a rule of thumb, the width of the retropharyngeal space is normally <50% of the width of C2 and a retropharyngeal space greater than 14 mm is abnormal[17] (Fig. 54–1). In one study, 93% of patients with RPA had abnormal lateral neck radiographs while only 7% had normal radiographs.[15] CT with contrast is best obtained in those patients with abnormal radiographs or symptoms that support the diagnosis of an RPA, and is generally useful in differentiating cellulitis, phlegmon, and focal abscess. Up to 97% of those with an RPA will have an abnormal CT, though some studies suggest a false-negative rate of up to 13% for identifying the presence of a focal collection of fluid.[18] Airway fluoroscopy is another alternative in detecting retropharyngeal swelling, though it cannot differentiate cellulitis from abscess.

Treatment options include antibiotic therapy and, in some cases, surgical intervention. The decision to surgically drain an abscess depends on various factors, including CT findings of focal abscess, response to initial antibiotic therapy, and clinical toxicity. Some children with documented abscess may respond just as well to antibiotic therapy alone as to surgical drainage along with antibiotics.[15] Early surgical consultation is helpful in following patients and determining the point at which operative intervention is necessary. All patients with retropharyngeal or parapharyngeal abscess require admission for intravenous antibiotics and monitoring for progression of symptoms and complications, such as upper airway obstruction. Progressive symptoms of airway obstruction may require endotracheal intubation or, as some data suggest, nasal continuous positive airway pressure for respiratory support.[19] Intravenous antibiotic therapies to

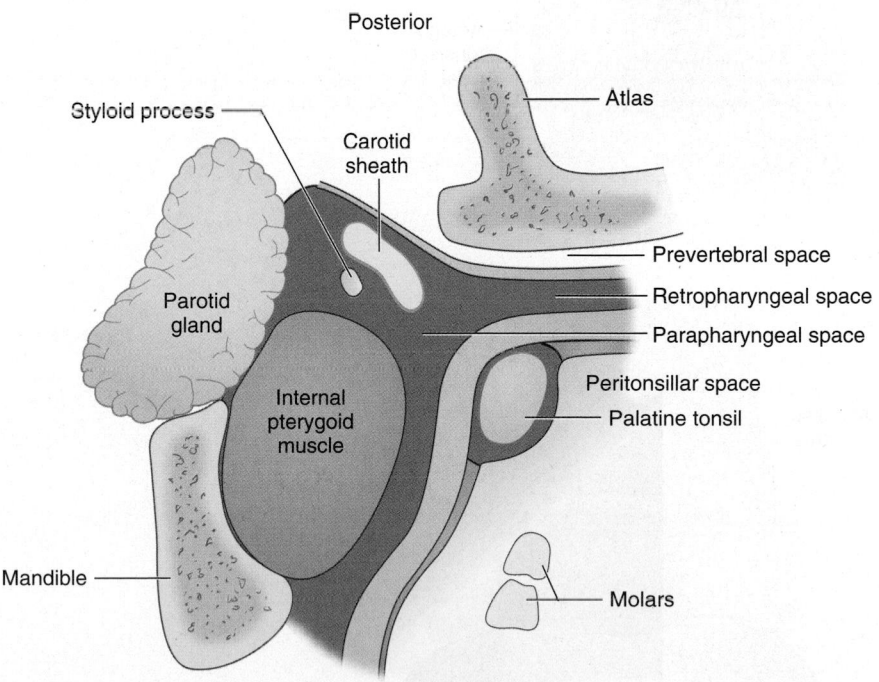

FIGURE 54–1. Anatomy of the retropharyngeal space.

consider include clindamycin, ampicillin/sulbactam, a third-generation cephalosporin, or a combination of penicillin and oxacillin or nafcillin.

Other Airway Abscesses

Other airway abscess include peritonsillar, lateral or parapharyngeal, and pterygoid abscesses.[20,21] The most common airway/neck abscesses requiring hospital admission include peritonsillar (45% to 49%), submandibular (10% to 22%), retropharyngeal (14% to 22%) buccal/masticator (0 to 11%), superficial (21%), and lateral or parapharyngeal (3% to 5%) abscesses.

Knowledge of surrounding structures (Fig. 54–2) and the resulting clinical features can be used to discriminate between abscesses (Table 54–4). Importantly, peritonsillar abscesses are an extension of tonsillar infection. The development of pus in this area leads to loss of landmark structures around the tonsils (tonsillar pillar effacement), bulging of the lateral pharyngeal wall and soft palate, and deviation of the uvula away from the infected side. While patients often have pain on chewing and mouth opening, true trismus is usually absent since masticator and pterygoid muscles are not affected. Parapharyngeal abscesses are deeper infections (see Fig. 54–2B) and do not disrupt the anatomy of the tonsillar pillars. Due to their location, they can involve muscles of mastication, causing trismus, swelling of the medial wall of the pharynx, and swelling along the angle of the mandible. Systemic toxicity is often prominent. Ptery-

Table 54–4	Comparison of Clinical Features in Deep Space Infection of the Neck				
Space/Abscess	**Pain**	**Trismus**	**Swelling Sites**	**Dysphagia**	**Dyspnea**
Peritonsillar	++	+	Lateral pharynx	++	−
Parapharyngeal					
anterior	++++	++++	Lateral pharynx and neck	++	+
posterior	+	+	Posterior pharynx	++	+++
Retropharyngeal	++	+	Posterior pharynx	++	++
Submandibular	++	−	Floor mouth	++	++
Masticator	++	++++	Hidden, face	−	−

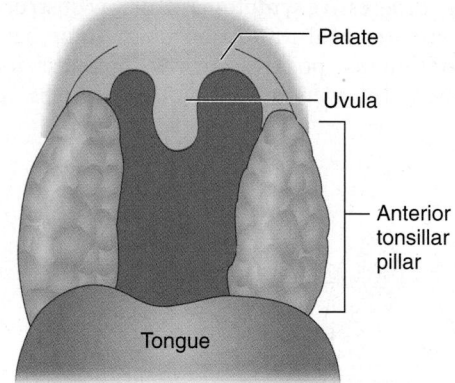

A

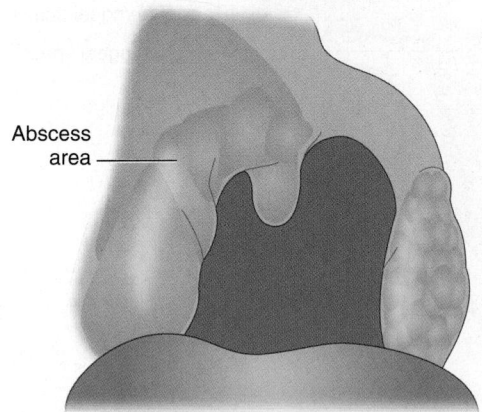

B

FIGURE 54–2. A, Normal location of peritonsillar structures. **B,** Distortion of surrounding structures resulting from peritonsillar abscess.

goid abscesses, due to their location (see Fig. 54–1), also can cause true trismus. In addition to the clinical examination, differentiation between these infections often involves CT scanning. Peritonsillar abscesses are also easily identified by ultrasonography.

Guidelines for managing peritonsillar abscess support the use of bedside needle aspiration performed by non-otorhinolaryngology surgeons.[22] A meta-analysis of 10 reports showed this technique to be 94% effective at relieving symptoms with few complications.[23] Most other abscesses (other than superficial abscess) require admission, intravenous antibiotics, and possible surgical draininage.

Lemierre Syndrome

Lemierre syndrome is a rare but serious constellation of symptoms caused by *Fusobacterium necrophorum*, a gram-negative obligate intracellular anaerobe that is part of normal oral flora. After initial tonsillitis or dental infection with the organism, patients develop bacteremia, venous thrombophlebitis, and septic emboli, most often to the pulmonary vasculature. High spiking fevers start about 1 week after onset of pharyngitis or dental infection, along with other nonspecific symptoms such as vomiting, fatigue, and weight loss. Often one side of the neck is swollen and tender to palpation, and patients who have already suffered from pulmonary emboli may complain of chest pain or dyspnea. Patients usually present to the emergency department in shock, and without appropriate therapy, mortality from sepsis is around 90%.[4] Some cases of peritonsillar abscess caused by Fusobacterium do not necessarily progress to sepsis and thrombophlebitis. Laboratory findings are often consistent with sepsis, including leukocytosis with a left shift, thrombocytopenia, and prolonged coagulation times. Contrast CT of the neck and Doppler study of the jugular venous system are options for imaging modalities to diagnose venous thrombosis. A review at a single pediatric institution from 1996 to 2002 showed an increase in children admitted with clinical Lemierre syndrome as well as blood cultures positive for Fusobacterium.[24] Along with the respiratory and cardiovascular supportive measures required by these patients, options for intravenous antibiotic therapy include ticarcillin/clavulanate, ampicillin/sulbactam, clindamycin, and flagyl.[24] Certainly, very broad coverage should be initiated in any febrile child with signs of sepsis, but consideration should be given to including anaerobic coverage initially when a child has complaints of a severe sore throat or prominent neck swelling and tenderness. Anticoagulation is a controversial treatment considered in patients with documented jugular venous thrombophlebitis.[24]

Ludwig's Angina

Though more often seen in the adult population, older children and adolescents may present to the emergency department with this infection of the sublingual space in the floor of the mouth. This is a polymicrobial oral flora infection that is often associated with poor oral hygiene or a recent dental procedure. Patients often present with fever, trismus, and difficulty swallowing due to elevation of the base of the tongue, and are at risk for airway obstruction. Progression of infection to cause mediastinitis is another life-threatening complication in addition to airway obstruction. Many patients require a tracheostomy to protect their airway until the infection resolves. A subset of one study that examined 36 cases of Ludwig's angina showed that 75% required a tracheostomy as part of their therapy. One half of the patients underwent awake, elective tracheostomy while half attempted endotracheal intubation. Of the latter group, over half of these attempts were unsuccessful and required emergent tracheostomy.[5] Therefore, elective awake tracheostomy is the best option for airway protection when time allows. Treatment consists of surgical drainage as well as antimicrobial therapy aimed at covering oral flora.

Parotitis

While the bulk of the parotid gland is preauricular in location, the tail of the parotid extends below the mandible. Thus, infection or swelling of this gland can present as neck swelling. Parotitis in children is most often viral in etiology, although bacterial infection or obstruction of Stensen's duct by stones can also result in parotid swelling. Typical viral etiologies of parotitis include enterovirus, CMV, influenza, parainfluenza, and HIV. Mumps should also be considered, particularly in unimmunized children or those with signs and symptoms of orchitis. *Staphylococcus aureus* is the most common bacterial cause of parotitis, and atypical mycobacterial infections of the gland can occur as well. Viral parotitis usually presents with bilateral parotid swelling following low-grade fever and malaise. Treatment is supportive, consisting of pain control and a bland diet. Consideration should be given to sending acute mumps titers with the intention of outpatient convalescent titers to be sent by the primary care provider. Children with bacterial parotitis may be more ill appearing, and have more significant pain and fever than those with viral infection. It is vital to look for expressed purulent material from Stensen's duct in children with parotitis to help differentiate viral from bacterial etiologies. Choices for outpatient antibiotic therapy include clindamycin and amoxicillin/clavulanate to provide coverage for *Staphylococcus, Streptococcus,* and oral flora. Warm compresses, massaging the gland, and use of sialagogues, such as lemon drops, provide symptomatic relief as well. Children with HIV or a past history of mumps parotitis maybe more susceptible to recurrent parotitis.[4]

Summary

Emergency physicians frequently encounter children with infectious lesions of the neck in their clinical practice. While many of these are viral, bacterial infections must be excluded as their progression can lead to deep neck space abscesses, mediastinitis, or airway compromise.[25] Contrast CT of the neck is indicated if the patient fails to respond to initial antibiotic therapy. Surgical consultation for possible biopsy or incision and drainage should be obtained for children with deep space infections, airway compromise, or those who are not responding to initial therapy or conservative management.

REFERENCES

*1. Brown RL, Azizkhan RG: Pediatric head and neck lesions. Pediatr Clin North Am 45:889–905, 1998.
2. Kelly CS, Kelly RE: Lymphadenopathy in children. Pediatr Clin North Am 45:875–888, 1998.

---

*Selected readings.

3. Knight PJ, Mulne AF, Vassy LE: When is a lymph node biopsy indicated in children with enlarged peripheral nodes? Pediatrics 69:391–396, 1982.

4. Wetmore RF, Muntz HR, McGill TJ, et al (eds): Pediatric Otolaryngology: Principles and Practice. New York: Thieme, 2000.

5. Parhiscar A, Har-El G: Deep neck abscess: a retrospective review of 210 cases. Ann Otol Rhinol Laryngol 110:1051–1054, 2001.

6. Robson CD: Imaging of granulomatous lesions of the neck in children. Radiol Clin North Am 38:99–977, 2000.

7. Albright JT, Pransky SM: Nontuberculous mycobacterial infections of the head and neck. Pediatr Clin North Am 50:503–514, 2003.

8. Hazra R, Robson CD, Perez-Atayde AR, Husson RN: Lymphadenitis due to nontuberculous mycobacteria in children: presentation and response to therapy. Clin Infect Dis 28:123–129, 1999.

9. Wolinsky E: Mycobacterial lymphadenitis in children: a prospective study of 105 nontuberculous cases with long-term follow-up. Clin Infect Dis 20:954–964, 1995.

10. McMaster P, Isaacs D: Critical review of evidence for short course therapy for tuberculous adenitis in children. Pediatr Infect Dis J 19:401–404, 2000.

11. Bass JW, Freitas BC, Freitas AD, et al: Prospective randomized double blind placebo-controlled evaluation of azithromycin for treatment of cat-scratch disease. Pediatr Infect Dis J 17:447–452, 1998.

12. Bryant KA: Tularemia: lymphadenitis with a twist. Pediatr Ann 31:187–190, 2002.

*13. Pickering LK (ed): Red Book: 2003 Report of the Committee on Infectious Diseases. Elk Grove Village, IL: American Academy of Pediatrics, 2003.

14. Su F, Shen P, Chiu Y, Chen J: Salmonella retropharyngeal abscess in a child: case report and literature review. Pediatr Infect Dis J 22:833–836, 2003.

15. Craig FW, Schunk JE: Retropharyngeal abscess in children: clinical presentation, utility of imaging, and current management. Pediatrics 111:1394–1398, 2003.

16. Nusbaum AO, Som PM, Rothschild MA, Shugar JMA: Recurrence of a deep neck infection. Arch Otolaryngol Head Neck Surg 125:1379–1382, 1999.

17. Barratt GE, Koopmann CF Jr, Coulthard SW: Retropharyngeal abscess, a ten-year experience. Laryngoscope 94:455–463, 1984.

18. Lazor JB, Cunningham MJ, Eavey RD, Weber AL: Comparison of computed tomography and surgical findings in deep neck infections. Otolaryngol Head Neck Surg 111:746–750, 1994.

19. Soong W, Jeng M, Hwang B: Respiratory support of children with a retropharyngeal abscess with nasal CPAP. Clin Pediatr (Phila) 40:55–56, 2001.

20. Ungkanont K, Yellon RF, Weissman JL, et al: Head and neck space infections in infants and children. Otolaryngol Head Neck Surg 112:375–382, 1995.

21. Dodds B, Maniglia AJ: Peritonsilar and neck abscesses in the pediatric age group. Laryngoscope 98:956–959, 1988.

22. Herzon FS, Nicklaus P: Pediatric peritonsilar abscess: management guidelines. Curr Probl Pediatr 26:270–278, 1996.

23. Herzon FS, Harris P: Mosher Award thesis. Peritonsilar abscess: Incidence, current management practices, and a proposal for treatment guidelines. Laryngoscope 105(8 Pt 3 suppl 74):1–17, 1995.

24. Ramirez S, Hild TG, Rudolph CN, et al: Increased diagnosis of Lemierre syndrome and other *Fusobacterium necrophorum* infections at a children's hospital. Pediatrics 112:e380–e385, 2003.

*25. Peters TR, Edwards KM: Cervical lymphadenopathy and adenitis. Pediatr Rev 21:399–405, 2000.

Chapter 55

Neck Masses

Amy L. Puchalski, MD

Key Points

Most pediatric neck masses are benign.

Palpable lymph nodes in a neonate are not normal.

Malignancy of a mass or node should be considered if it is supraclavicular, enlarges over 6 weeks, is greater than 4 cm, is associated with constitutional symptoms, or causes central nervous system, airway, or vascular symptoms.

Congenital neck lesions should be considered in patients with a history of recurrent neck infections.

Introduction and Background

When faced with a child with a neck mass, the emergency physician should consider an infectious etiology, a congenital lesion, or a neoplasm. This chapter focuses on congenital lesions, benign neoplasms, and malignant neoplasms (see Chapter 54, Neck Infections, for information on lesions caused by neck infections). Fortunately, the majority of neck masses in children are benign. A thorough history and physical examination along with close follow-up will aid in differentiating those pediatric patients who require evaluation for possible malignancy.

Selected Diagnoses

Congenital masses presenting in the neonatal period
    Cystic hygroma
    Hemangioma
    Cervical teratoma
    Congenital muscular torticollis
Congenital masses presenting in infancy and childhood
    Branchial cleft anomalies
    Thyroglossal duct cyst
    Dermoid cyst
Acquired benign masses
    Laryngocele
    Ranula

Benign neoplasms
    Thyroid nodules
    Salivary tumors
    Neurofibromas
Malignant neoplasms
    Lymphoma
    Neuroblastoma
    Thyroid carcinoma
    Rhabdomyosarcoma
    Ewing's sarcoma
    Langerhans' cell histiocytosis
    Posttransplantation lymphoproliferative disorder

Discussion of Individual Diagnoses

Congenital Masses Presenting in the Neonatal Period (Table 55-1)

Cystic Hygroma

This multiloculated cystic proliferation of lymphatic tissue is present at birth in 50% to 65% of cases, with nearly all others presenting by the end of the second year of life.[1] About 70% of these lesions are in the neck, usually on the left side.[1] On physical examination, cystic hygromas are large, compressible, soft mobile masses that are nontender and located in the posterior triangle of the neck.[1,2] They can be transilluminated and in some instances are confused with hemangiomas if hemorrhage occurs with minor trauma. They grow in proportion to the infant and can become acutely larger with an upper respiratory tract infection, superinfection, or trauma. Larger lesions may cause stridor, dysphagia, failure to thrive, or airway compromise. Diagnosis is based on computed tomography (CT) scan with contrast or ultrasound, though the latter imaging modality may not give information required to plan surgical resection. Sometimes needle decompression may be used to temporarily relieve acute airway obstruction. Lesions rarely regress spontaneously, thus treatment requires total surgical resection, and recurrence of cystic hygromas is possible if resection is incomplete.[1,2]

Hemangiomas

Hemangiomas are the most common head and neck lesion of infancy, affecting 2.5% of newborns. About one third of lesions are present at birth, with the remainder generally presenting by age 1 month. They grow in size over the first year of life, and then begin to involute. Approximately 80%

Table 55–1	**Congenital Neck Masses**		
Lesion	**Location**	**Age at Presentation**	**Physical Examination**
Cystic hygroma	Posterior triangle	~½ at birth, remainder by 2 yr	Soft, compressible, cystic, transilluminates
Thyroglossal duct cyst	Midline anterior neck	2–10 yr	Soft, nontender, moves with tongue movement
Branchial cleft anomalies	Preauricular to supraclavicular area, anterior to SCM	Various	Tags, fistulas, sinus tracts, cystic lesions
Dermoid cyst	Usually midline	Birth–2 yr	Nontender, mobile, does not move with tongue
Hemangioma	Various	By age 1 mo	Soft, mobile, nontender, vascular appearance; deep lesions may be flesh colored

Abbreviation: SCM, sternocleidomastoid muscle.

Table 55–2	**Branchial Cleft Anomalies**		
Branchial Arch	**Resultant Structures**	**Location of Anomalies**	**End Point**
First	Eustachian tube, tympanic cavity, mastoid air cells	Preauricular anomalies, parotid cyst	External auditory canal
Second (most common)	Palatine tonsil, tonsillar fossa, hyoid bone	Mid to lower neck, anterior to SCM	Tonsillar fossa
Third (rare)	Thymus, inferior parathyroids	Lower 1/3 of neck, anterior to SCM	Piriform sinus
Fourth (extremely rare)	Superior parathyroids	Lower neck	

Abbreviation: SCM, sternocleidomastoid muscle.

to 90% will resolve completely by age 5 years without any intervention. Those that involve deeper structures and organs are less likely to regress without any intervention. On physical examination, hemangiomas are soft, mobile, nontender, and bluish or red in color, though very deep lesions may not cause any cutaneous discoloration and have a rubbery consistency. Complications of hemangiomas include hemorrhage, ulceration, necrosis, and superinfection. Hemangiomas in the head and neck region may cause airway obstruction, and very large lesions can lead to high-output cardiac failure and consumptive coagulopathy or thrombocytopenia (Kasabach-Merritt syndrome). Treatment of extensive lesions, those involving vital structures, or those with residual cosmetic defect includes therapy with steroids, sclerotic agents, laser treatments, or, rarely, radiation therapy.[1,2]

Cervical Teratomas

Teratomas are masses consisting of differentiated ectoderm, mesoderm, and endoderm that can present in various locations. Between 2% and 9% involve the head and neck region, with the majority of those being cervical. Most cervical teratomas are present at birth, and they very rarely present after age 2 years. Neonatal teratomas are benign lesions, unlike those presenting in adulthood, which generally are malignant. These lesions most commonly present with some degree of airway or esophageal obstruction in the neonatal period. They often have palpable cystic areas, are about 5 to 10 cm in size at presentation, do not transilluminate, and are usually fixed to deep cervical fascia or the hyoid.[3] The differential diagnosis of cervical teratomas includes thyroglossal duct cyst, cystic hygroma, goiter, branchial cleft cyst, lymphangioma, hemangioma, laryngocele, and lipoma. Teratomas are treated by surgical resection.[4]

Congenital Muscular Torticollis

Congenital muscular torticollis, or sternocleidomastoid tumor of infancy, is a focal area of fibrosis and shortening within the sternocleidomastoid muscle identifiable within a few weeks of birth, most often a result of birth trauma. Clinically, shortening of the sternocleidomastoid muscle causes the head to tilt toward that side while the chin points away from the affected side. A firm mass can be palpated and sometimes seen within the muscle. Treatment rests on physical therapy with range of motion and stretching exercises. In rare cases in which the lesion does not resolve by age 6 months, facial and cranial anomalies, such as hemihyperplasia, may result. In such extreme cases, surgical correction may be required.[1]

Congenital Masses Presenting in Infancy and Childhood

Branchial Cleft Anomalies

Remnants of branchial arches, pouches, and grooves can present clinically as sinus tracts, fistulas, cystic lesions, or skin tags.[5] Remnants of the second branchial groove, which result in lesions anterior to the midportion of the sternocleidomastoid, are the most common. Table 55–2 shows the embryology and locations of anomalies associated with each of the four branchial arches. Cystic lesions resulting from these anomalies often present with recurrent infections[6] or increase in size during upper respiratory tract infections. While lesions often present in infancy, some are diagnosed later in childhood or even adulthood. Contrast CT and magnetic resonance imaging (MRI) are the imaging modalities used to diagnose these lesions when clinical suspicion arises. Lesions are treated with resection once any concomitant infection has been treated.[1,2]

Thyroglossal Duct Cyst

These lesions arise when the tract by which the thyroid descends from the foramen cecum in the tongue to the neck does not close. They are the most common congenital neck mass in children and usually present between ages 2 and

10 years.[1] On physical examination, thyroglossal duct cysts are midline, soft, smooth, nontender lesions that move with swallowing or tongue protrusion.[7] These lesions often come to attention when they become secondarily infected. They can be confused with dermoid cysts, sebaceous cysts, submental lymphadenopathy, ectopic thyroid or neoplasm, lipomas, and cervical lymphadenopathy. Twenty-five percent to 35% of these lesions contain ectopic thyroid tissue, so thyroid scan or ultrasound prior to surgical resection is necessary to document the location of active thyroid tissue. Complications are generally limited to secondary infection of the cyst, hypothyroidism following surgical treatment, and development of thyroid adenocarcinoma in adulthood, which occurs in about 10% of patients with thyroglossal duct cysts.[1] Children with a history of resection, especially of previously infected lesions, have a 10% rate of recurrence.[1]

Dermoid Cysts

Dermoid cysts are lesions consisting of ectodermal tissue that is buried beneath the skin surface. They can potentially contain sebaceous glands, hair follicles, and connective tissue. Their location is generally midline, and they are nontender and mobile, unless they become infected. They are often confused with thyroglossal duct cysts given their location, and can be differentiated by the fact that they do not move with tongue movement. Dermoid cysts rarely undergo malignant transformation, and treatment of these benign lesions consists of surgical excision.[2]

Acquired Benign Masses

Laryngocele

These rare lesions consist of a dilated laryngeal saccule that becomes filled with air and mucus, causing it to extend laterally from the airway. They cause a soft tissue mass lateral to the thyroid cartilage with associated hoarseness due to airway compression. Laryngoceles can be diagnosed with CT, MRI, or laryngoscopy and require surgical intervention for treatment.[2]

Ranula

A ranula is a mucocele of a salivary gland, usually the submandibular gland, caused by partial obstruction of the salivary duct. It initially presents as a mass on the floor of the mouth, but can progress to rupture into the anterior neck muscles, forming a pseudocyst. This latter entity is referred to as a *plunging ranula* and is treated with surgical excision. Patients usually undergo imaging with CT or MRI to establish the diagnosis prior to definitive treatment.[2]

Benign Neoplasms

Thyroid Nodules

Thyroid nodules are less common in children than adults, with a prevalence of 0.2% in 9- to 16-year-olds and 1.8% in 11- to 18-year-olds.[8] However, palpable thyroid nodules are more likely malignant in children than adults, with 25% to 55% of pediatric thyroid nodules representing malignant disease. Benign lesions are generally asymptomatic, presenting as nontender lesions in the thyroid. Less commonly, benign nodules may be slightly tender or inflamed if they are cystic in nature and become hemorrhagic or infected. Some patients may suffer from hoarseness or dysphagia, though this may indicate a malignancy. The differential diagnosis for a palpable thyroid nodule or adenoma includes cervical lymphadenopathy, an asymmetric thyroid lobe, Hashimoto's thyroiditis, thyroglossal duct cyst, and dermoid cyst.[9] Evaluation should include measurement of thyroid function and a thyroid nuclear scan, ultrasound of the thyroid, and surgical consultation for possible biopsy or excision. Fine-needle aspiration is well documented to be a reliable method of evaluation of thyroid nodules in adults, but given the high rate of malignancy in the pediatric population, some advocate excisional biopsy as an alternative.[9]

Salivary Tumors

Salivary tumors are rare and usually involve either the parotid or submandibular gland. Hemangiomas are the most common benign lesion of salivary glands and present as previously discussed. Pleomorphic adenomas are the next most common, usually occurring in children after the age of 1 year. Lymphangiomas are the third most common benign salivary tumor. CT and MRI are used to assist in diagnosis and plan for surgical resection in lesions other than hemangiomas. A thorough physical examination in a child with a parotid mass should include assessment for facial nerve involvement.[2]

Neurofibromas

These benign lesions of neural tissue components are seen in children with neurofibromatosis, usually type 1, for which neurofibromas are one of the diagnostic criteria. Occasionally solitary lesions develop in otherwise normal patients. Neurofibromas are usually either cutaneous or plexiform, and have the potential of becoming very extensive and involving deep structures of the neck. The cutaneous lesions are usually small, soft, and flesh colored, sometimes being confused with lipomas or hemangiomas. A small percentage of lesions can undergo malignant transformation to neurofibrosarcomas. Treatment may consist of observation of lesions with resection when symptoms of neurologic impairment or significant cosmetic deformity become issues.[7]

Malignant Neoplasms

Approximately 5% of pediatric malignancies involve the head and neck, with lymphomas and rhabdomyosarcoma comprising 50% of the diagnoses.[1] Among children under age 6 years, the most common head and neck malignancy is neuroblastoma, followed by non-Hodgkin's lymphoma, rhabdomyosarcoma and Hodgkin's lymphoma. In the 7- to 13-year-old group, lymphomas predominate, followed by thyroid malignancy and rhabdomyosarcoma. In the adolescent population, Hodgkin's lymphoma is by far the most common malignancy of the neck.[1] Malignant lesions are generally painless, firm, and adherent to underlying tissue, often with a matted feeling.[1] It is important to maintain a high degree of suspicion for malignancy in children presenting with neck masses in order to appropriately evaluate and refer those who require biopsy for evaluation.[10]

Lymphoma

Overall, about 11% of childhood malignancies are lymphomas. In the pediatric population, lymphomas usually cause a mediastinal or abdominal mass, but, in general, lymphomas of the neck occur as enlarged lymph nodes.[11] Both Hodgkin's and non-Hodgkin's lymphoma occur in children, with non-Hodgkin's being slightly more common and having a peak incidence between ages 7 and 11 years.[12] In contrast, Hodgkin's lymphoma is seen later in adolescence.[2,12] Certain pediatric populations are more at risk for lymphoma, including those with congenital immunodeficiencies or human immunodeficiency virus infection, or recipients of organ and bone marrow transplants.[12] Clinically, children present with painless cervical lymphadenopathy[13] that feels rubbery, matted, and fixed to underlying tissue. Constitutional symptoms such as fever, weight loss, and night sweats may be present. Physical examination may reveal more diffuse lymphadenopathy, hepatosplenomegaly, or signs of a mediastinal mass, including respiratory compromise and superior vena cava syndrome.[12] Initial evaluation in a patient with suspected lymphoma includes a contrast CT to evaluate the extent of disease, a chest raiograph to evaluate for mediastinal involvement, and laboratory work to evaluate for bone marrow involvement and tumor burden, including electrolytes, complete blood count, calcium, phosphorus, magnesium, lactate dehydrogenase, and urinalysis.[12] Ultimately, diagnosis rests on biopsy of involved lymph nodes. In the emergency department, patients with concern for tumor lysis syndrome may require hydration and alkalinization, while those with airway compromise may require intubation or arrangement for emergent radiation therapy or chemotherapy to reduce airway compression.

Neuroblastoma

Neuroblastoma is the second most common solid tumor in pediatrics, usually occurring in children under age 5 years. Cervical disease is the third most common location for neuroblastoma, following disease within the abdomen and chest. Neuroblastoma of the head and neck region may present with a cervical mass or enlarged cervical nodes, Horner's syndrome, proptosis, periorbital ecchymosis, nasal obstruction, and epistaxis. Prognosis is generally better in children less than 1 year of age. Treatment is dependent on the stage of the disease and involves many modalities, including resection, radiation, chemotherapy, and peripheral stem cell transplantation.[2]

Thyroid Carcinoma

About 2% of pediatric malignancies are thyroid carcinoma, and almost all cases are papillary thyroid carcinomas.[8,14] Most pediatric patients are in mid to late adolescence, and the disease is two to three times more common in girls.[9] Important historical factors in patients presenting with a thyroid nodule include a history of radiation therapy to the neck, family history of multiple endocrine neoplasia type II (MEN II), history of autoimmune thyroiditis, and complaints of hoarseness or dysphagia, as these all put patients at increased likelihood of a malignant process.[9] Thyroid nodules in children are more likely to be malignant than nodules in adults. On physical examination, 70% of children with thyroid carcinoma have cervical lymphadenopathy at presentation.[9] Most patients are euthyroid, though thyroid function tests, calcitonin, and antithyroid antibodies should remain part of the initial laboratory evaluation.[2] Treatment of papillary thyroid carcinoma with thyroidectomy, lymph node dissection, and radioactive iodine generally yields excellent survival rates. Lung metastasis are not uncommon, so obtaining a chest radiograph is an important part of the evaluation of a child presenting with a thyroid mass. Medullary thyroid carcinoma is rare in pediatrics and generally limited to cases of MEN IIa (medullary thyroid carcinoma, hyperparathyroidism, pheochromocytoma) or MEN IIb (medullary thyroid carcinoma, pheochromocytoma, mucosal neuromas, marfanoid habitus). It usually occurs in adolescence and is a more aggressive tumor than papillary carcinoma.[5] An elevated serum calcitonin raises concern for this disease.

Rhabdomyosarcoma

This is the most common soft tissue malignancy of the head and neck in the pediatric population, though it usually presents with disease in the nasopharynx or oropharynx. Some children will develop tumors of the neck musculature primarily and may have symptoms such as dysphagia or hoarseness. Only about 10% of cases develop cervical lymph node metastatic disease; however, because of the potential for malignant cervical lymphadenopathy, a prompt and thorough examination of the oral cavity and nose must be completed. Multimodal therapy yields the best outcomes, and children with this disease generally have better survival than adults.[2]

Ewing's Sarcoma

This disease is one of the primitive neuroectodermal tumors seen in children, and while it most commonly presents as long bone disease, patients can have a primary neck lesion or metastatic disease in cervical lymph nodes. Primary head and neck tumors have a better prognosis than primaries of the pelvis and proximal extremities. Almost all patients have some metastatic disease at presentation, usually to lung or bone. Prognosis is best in those who undergo multimodal therapy and do not have gross metastatic disease at presentation.[2]

Langerhans' Cell Histiocytosis

This disease entity has an unclear etiology, representing perhaps either a malignant process or an immune response, and has a wide array of clinical presentations. Up to 20% of the patients will have cervical or generalized lymphadenopathy, and other manifestations include chronic seborrheic rashes, chronic otitis media, lytic skull and other bony lesions, failure to thrive, diarrhea, hepatosplenomegaly, pancytopenia, and interstitial pneumonitis. It is important for emergency physicians to be aware of this clinical entity when evaluating infants and children with cervical lymphadenopathy in order to ask about these other associated symptoms and refer for biopsy.[2]

Posttransplantation Lymphoproliferative Disorder

Approximately 2% of transplant patients develop this proliferation of B cells, which is thought to be associated with Epstein-Barr virus (EBV) infection. Cervical lymphadenopathy and tonsillar hypertrophy are manifestations of the disease seen in the neck, though generalized lymphadenopathy and hepatosplenomegaly should be assessed in the physical examination. Treatment consists of decreasing immunosuppression as well as starting gancyclovir to potentially treat EBV.[2]

Summary

Neck masses in children are due to a wide array of etiologies.[15] Diagnosing a congenital lesion is important so that consideration can be given to possible surgical intervention. Differentiating a benign lesion from a malignant lesion is clearly vital in determining the course of treatment. Historically, suspicion for malignancy should be raised when a mass is painless, rapidly enlarging, associated with constitutional symptoms, supraclavicular in location, or causing central nervous system, airway, or vascular compromise. Any suspicion of malignancy warrants imaging studies[16] and surgical referral for possible biopsy to establish a definitive diagnosis.

REFERENCES

1. Brown RL, Azizkhan RG: Pediatric head and neck lesions. Pediatr Clin North Am 45:889–905, 1998.
*2. Wetmore RF, Muntz HR, McGill TJ, et al (eds): Pediatric Otolaryngology: Principles and Practice. New York: Thieme, 2000.
3. Carr MM, Thorner P, Phillips JH: Congenital teratomas of the head and neck. J Otolaryngol 26:246–252, 1997.

4. Ward RF, April M: Teratomas of the head and neck. Pediatr Otolaryngol Clin North Am 22:621–629, 1989.
5. Rea PA, Hartley BE, Bailey CM: Third and fourth branchial pouch anomalies. J Laryngol Otol 118:19–24, 2004.
*6. Nusbaum AO, Som PM, Rothschild MA, Shugar JM: Recurrence of a deep neck infection: a clinical indication of an underlying congenital lesion. Arch Otolaryngol Head Neck Surg 125:1379–1382, 1999.
7. Brousseau VJ, Solares CA, Xu M, et al: Thyroglossal duct cysts: presentation and management in children versus adults. Int J Pediatr Otorhinolaryngol 67:1285–1290, 2003.
8. Bentley AA, Gillespie C, Malis D: Evaluation and management of a solitary thyroid nodule in a child. Otolaryngol Clin North Am 36:117–128, 2003.
9. Geiger JD, Thompson NW: Thyroid tumors in children. Otolaryngol Clin North Am 29:711–719, 1996.
*10. Knight PJ, Mulne AF, Vassy LE: When is lymph node biopsy indicated in children with enlarged peripheral nodes? Pediatrics 69:391–396, 1982.
11. Weisberger EC, Davidson DD: Unusual presentations of lymphoma of the head and neck in childhood. Laryngoscope 100:337–342, 1990.
12. Sandlund JT, Downing JR, Crist WM: Non-Hodgkin's lymphoma in childhood. N Engl J Med 334:1238–1249, 1996.
*13. Kelly CS, Kelly RE: Lymphadenopathy in children. Pediatr Clin North Am 45:875–888, 1998.
14. Flannery TK, Kirkland JL, Copeland KC, et al: Papillary thyroid cancer: a pediatric perspective. Pediatrics 98:464–466, 1996.
*15. Connolly AA, MacKenzie K: Pediatric neck masses—a diagnostic dilemma. J Laryngol Otol 111:541–545, 1997.
*16. Koch BL: Imaging extracranial masses of the pediatric head and neck. Neuroimaging Clin N Am 10:193–214, 2000.

*Selected readings.

Chapter 56

Management of Acute Asthma

Sharon R. Smith, MD

Key Points

Any asthma patient can present with a sudden, severe exacerbation regardless of baseline asthma severity.

The vast majority of asthma patients will require bronchodilators *and* anti-inflammatory agents to control exacerbation symptoms.

Recurrent wheezing in very young infants may not be asthma; a cardiac etiology should at least be considered during the evaluation.

Introduction and Background

Asthma is the most common chronic disease of childhood, and accounts for approximately 1.8 million pediatric emergency visits annually.[1] The National Health Interview Survey completed in 2001 estimates that over 6 million children in the Untied States have asthma. The highest prevalence rates are noted in children 5 to 14 years of age, boys, and African Americans. Making the diagnosis of asthma in the emergency department (ED) may be difficult. For the purposes of this chapter, an asthma patient is defined as any child who presents with a history of asthma by report of parents, or has had two or more wheezing episodes without another reason (or chronic illness). The *National Asthma Education Program Expert Panel Report 2: Guidelines for the Diagnosis and Management of Asthma* from the National Institutes of Health defines asthma as "a chronic inflammatory disorder of the airways. In susceptible individuals, this inflammation causes recurrent episodes of wheezing, breathlessness, chest tightness, and cough, particularly at night and in the early morning. These episodes are usually associated with widespread but variable airflow obstruction that is often reversible either spontaneously or with treatment."[2]

There are many reasons a child can develop wheezing. The first episode of wheezing may be a symptom of a chronic illness, such as asthma or cystic fibrosis, or caused by a number of other etiologies. The differential diagnoses for asthma are listed in Table 56–1. Bronchiolitis is an acute infectious disease of the lower respiratory tract, proceeded by fever, rhinitis, or both, and characterized by tachypnea, wheezing, hyperinflation, and increased respiratory effort (see Chapter 57, Bronchiolitis). Bronchiolitis is typically seen in children younger than 12 months and rarely in those older than 2 years. Young children who develop infection with respiratory syncytial virus (RSV) are more likely to have wheezing illnesses during the toddler and early school years.[3] Treatment of RSV does not affect subsequent development of wheezing or asthma. Children sometimes wheeze in association with other viral upper respiratory infections (URIs).[4] Those who wheeze with almost every URI have "recurrent wheezing." Some of these patients continue to have wheezing and other asthma symptoms as they get older, while others do not. Although it may not be possible to diagnose asthma in young children, those with recurrent wheezing who respond to asthma therapy should be managed similarly to any child with a formal diagnosis of asthma.[4,5]

Confounding Diagnoses

Vocal cord dysfunction (VCD) is a clinical condition characterized by abnormal adduction of the vocal cords or spasm in a partially closed position. Children with VCD may present with wheezing and dyspnea.[6-8] These children typically have normal or near-normal respiratory rate and oxygen saturation, unlike children with asthma. The spasm typically resolves in minutes to hours without treatment. On rare occasion the spasm is so severe that it requires airway management, such as intubation. Causes of VCD include gastroesophageal reflux, sinusitis, allergens, and psychogenic factors. Some children have both asthma and VCD, and the VCD may cause an asthma exacerbation to appear more severe. A definitive diagnosis of VCD is made by evaluating the symptomatic patient with direct laryngoscopy to visualize the vocal cords. Therapies that may be helpful include relaxation techniques, helium-oxygen (heliox) therapy, or panting, which increases the glottic aperture and may decrease symptoms. Children with only VCD usually do not respond to β-agonists or steroids.

Infants with cardiac disease may present with intermittent wheezing or unexplained tachypnea. Cardiac conditions that may cause wheezing include vascular rings (often with right aortic arch); abnormalities with large left-to-right shunts, such as ventricular septal defects or patent ductus arteriosus; or any abnormality that can cause pulmonary edema. Otherwise healthy infants (no history of prematurity, bronchopulmonary displasia, or infection) are unlikely to have asthma or a primary pulmonary etiology for wheezing in the first few weeks of life. A cardiac evaluation should at least be considered for any infant younger than 12 weeks of age who presents with recurrent wheezing not suggestive of any other etiology.[9]

History

Key information must be obtained when a child presents with an acute asthma exacerbation. With respect to the current exacerbation, the clinician should ask about triggers (typical and potential), infectious symptoms, duration of asthma symptoms, frequency of rescue medications, chronic medications, time of last medication doses, and peak flow rates. Questions regarding past exacerbations should cover the last ED visit, number of ED visits within the past year, last hospital admission, number of hospital admissions, intensive care unit admissions, and prior intubations.

Potential triggers, such as animal dander and cigarette smoke, should be identified, and the caregivers educated about the importance of avoiding triggers whenever possible. Continued exposure to triggers may decrease response to therapy. Other possible triggers include infection, allergies, dust mites, exercise, and a change in weather. The patient should be evaluated for URIs, such as otitis media and sinusitis, and appropriately treated. Children with allergic rhinitis may benefit from chronic therapy, which may prevent future acute exacerbations.[10]

Frequent ED visits or hospital admissions suggest poor control of asthma or underlying severe disease. These children should be closely monitored in the ED. It is also important to ask about intensive care admissions and intubations for asthma. These children are more likely to have a severe course and are prone to fatal asthma. Risk factors for fatal asthma include intensive care unit admission, prior intubation, two or more admissions or more than three ED visits within a year, and either an ED visit or admission within the previous month.[11-14] Children with fatality-prone asthma may be discharged from the ED if they respond well to therapy, but extreme caution should be used if there is any concern about access to medications, ability to return to the ED, follow-up, or if the child or parent reports uncertainty about being discharged.

Clinical Presentation

Infants and toddlers with asthma or recurrent wheezing present with cough and wheezing that has a high-pitched, squeaky, expiratory sound and is more musical sounding than wheezing in older children and adults. Parents may report that the infant is breathing faster than normal, is having "trouble" breathing, or is not drinking as well as usual. Toddlers may be irritable, and are not able to communicate that they are short of breath. School-age children and adolescents present similarly to adults, with cough, wheezing, shortness of breath, and chest tightness. Children with asthma typically cough before they wheeze. Fever may accompany wheezing due to atelectasis, URIs (otitis media, sinusitis, pharyngitis), and, infrequently, bacterial pneumonia. Children with asthma who present with minimal aeration or difficult-to-hear breath sounds are likely to have significant airway obstruction and warrant immediate therapy.

Severity of Asthma

Assessment of the severity of an asthma exacerbation helps to determine management, evaluate the response to treatment, and communicate with other medical providers.[15] A global sense of severity can be obtained using the information in Table 56–2.[2] The best objective measure of severity is spirometry or pulmonary function testing, such as forced expiratory volume in 1 second (FEV_1) or forced vital capacity (FVC). However, most EDs do not have the equipment or trained staff to perform pulmonary function testing. Therefore, peak expiratory flow rate (PEFR) is commonly used as an alternative objective measure of airway obstruction and asthma severity. PEFR reflects the caliber of the airways and

Table 56–1	Differential Diagnosis of Asthma in Children

Chronic illnesses/diseases
  Cystic fibrosis
  Bronchopulmonary dysplasia
  Gastroesophageal reflux
  Cardiac disease (e.g., vascular ring)
Infections
  Bronchiolitis
  Respiratory syncytial virus infection
  Viral upper respiratory infections
Foreign body
Vocal cord dysfunction
Laryngeal web
Tracheastenosis
Laryngomalacia
Enlarged nodes or tumor

Table 56–2	Severity of Asthma Exacerbations		
	Mild	**Moderate**	**Severe**
PEFR	>80%	50–80%	<50%
Oxygen saturation	>95%	91–95%	<91%
Respiratory rate			
<6 yr old	<30/min	31–60/min	>60/min
≥6 yr old	<20/min	21–50/min	>50/min
Wheezing	End expiratory	Entire expiratory	Inspiratory and expiratory *or* None due to minimal air exchange
Accessory muscle use	None/mild	Increased	Significantly increased
Speech/infant cry	Normal/normal	Phrases/softer cry	Single words/grunting or no crying

Abbreviation: PEFR, peak expiratory flow rate.

the degree of obstruction. It can be easily obtained in most EDs and correctly performed by the majority of children 5 years of age or older. In order for the test to be valid, the child must stand, take a deep breath, and blow quickly and forcefully through the PEFR tube.[16] Traditionally, the best of three attempts is used as the PEFR. A height-based chart can be used to determine the predicted PEFR for an individual child (Table 56–3). PEFR classification of severity is as follows: mild, greater than 80% of predicted; moderate, 50 to 80% of predicted; and severe, less than 50% of predicted.[2]

A validated scoring system should be used to assess obstruction for younger children, sicker children, or those who are unable to correctly perform spirometry or PEFR. There are numerous examples of scoring systems for asthma.[17,18] A classic scoring system is the Pulmonary Index Score (PIS).[17] The PIS is the aggregate of four measures: respiratory rate, wheezing, inspiratory/expiratory ratio, and accessory muscle use; each is rated on a 3-point scale. The PIS correlates well with pulmonary function tests, but the inspiratory/expiratory ratio makes this score difficult to use. Another example of an asthma scoring system is the Pulmonary Score (PS), which is derived from the PIS and has been shown to correlate with PEFR, FEV_1, and FVC. The PS does not include the inspiratory/expiratory ratio and uses an age-dependent respiratory rate (Table 56–4). The PS correlates well with PEFR in children with mild to severe asthma exacerbations.[19] PS ≤ 3 suggests mild, PS 4–6 moderate, and PS > 6, severe exacerbation.

Chronic severity of the underlying disease state is difficult to determine in the ED, and does not always correlate with the severity of the current exacerbation. For instance, a child with mild asthma that is poorly controlled may present with a severe exacerbation. However, the chronic management of asthma is determined by severity of the underlying disease, and knowing the severity may help determine discharge medications. Chronic asthma is defined as mild intermittent, mild persistent, moderate persistent, and severe persistent disease.[2] Persistent asthma is thought to occur in children because of chronic underlying inflammation. Symptoms of persistent asthma (when the child is not acutely ill) include coughing, wheeze, or shortness of breath 2 or more days a week during the daytime, 2 or more days a week at night, and/or 2 or more times a week during moderate exercise or play. Treating children with persistent asthma early in life (younger than 3 or 4 years of age) with anti-inflammatory agents may improve the inflammation and prevent long-term changes in lung function.[21,22] Children with persistent asthma should be treated with inhaled steroids.[23] Starting a child on inhaled steroids in the ED should be done in consultation with the primary care physician whenever possible.

Assessment of Oxygenation/Ventilation

Oxygenation and ventilation should be evaluated for all children presenting with an asthma exacerbation.[15] Few pediatric studies specifically address the need for arterial blood gas determinations in children with asthma, but in general they

Table 56–3	Predicted Peak Expiratory Flow Rate (PEFR) by Height		
	PEFR		
Height (cm)	**100%**	**80%**	**50%**
92	90	72	45
94	96	77	48
96	104	83	52
98	112	90	56
100	121	97	60
102	130	104	65
104	140	112	70
106	149	119	75
108	158	126	79
110	168	134	84
112	177	141	89
114	186	149	93
116	195	156	98
118	205	164	103
120	214	171	107
122	223	178	112
124	233	186	117
126	242	194	121
128	251	201	126
130	260	208	130
132	270	216	135
134	279	223	140
136	288	230	144
138	298	238	149
140	307	246	157
142	316	253	158
144	326	261	163
146	335	268	168
148	344	275	172
150	354	283	177
152	363	290	182
154	372	298	186
156	381	305	191
158	391	313	196
160	400	320	200
162	409	327	205
164	419	335	210
166	428	342	214
168	437	350	219
170	447	358	224
172	456	365	228
174	465	372	233
176	474	379	237
178	484	387	242
180	493	395	247

Table 56–4	Pulmonary Score (PS)			
	Respiratory Rate			
Score	**<6 yr**	**≥6 yr**	**Wheezing***	**Accessory Muscle Use**
0	<30	<20	None	No apparent activity
1	31–45	21–35	Terminal expiration	Mild increase
2	46–60	36–50	Entire expiration	Increase apparent
3	>60	>50	Inspiration and expiration	Maximal activity

*If no wheezing due to minimal air exchange, score as 3.

are considered painful, invasive, and unnecessary. Noninvasive measures of oxygenation and ventilation are readily available. The arterial partial pressure of oxygen (Pao_2) is commonly estimated using pulse oximetry. For most children, an O_2 saturation of 90% correlates with a Pao_2 of 60 mm Hg. The pulse oximeter probe can be placed on a finger or toe; placing a sock over a toe probe may help warm the foot and prevent removal by the child. True ventilation can only be assessed by measurement of the arterial partial pressure of carbon dioxide ($Paco_2$), but noninvasive measurements may still provide important information despite their inherent limitations. The partial pressure of CO_2 from a capillary blood gas sample is often higher than the $Paco_2$, especially in a sick child with poor perfusion. End-tidal CO_2 is not accurate because significant airway obstruction with a rapid respiratory rate prevents movement of CO_2 into peripheral air spaces (nose and mouth), and underrepresents the $Paco_2$. Measuring of $Paco_2$ in a well-appearing child with oxygen saturation above 90% is not necessary. Studies suggest that children with oxygen saturations above 90% to 92% and PEFRs greater than 25% to 30% are unlikely to have an elevated $Paco_2$.[15,24,25]

Management

Initial assessment for children with asthma includes respiratory rate, room air oxygen saturation, heart rate, blood pressure, auscultation for breath sounds, assessment of respiratory effort and accessory muscle use, level of consciousness, and a measure of severity (PEFR or severity score). Children with a severe exacerbation should be placed on continuous pulse oximetry and cardiac monitoring. Treatment pathways have the potential to improve efficiency of care, improve quality of care, and lower costs. Developing evidence-based pathways that reflect local and institutional practices may be helpful (Table 56–5).[15] The three basic components of asthma therapy are oxygen, bronchodilators, and corticosteroids, with specific medications, dosing, and options for each (Table 56–6).

Oxygen

Oxygen should be provided to any child who presents with respiratory difficulty and oxygen saturation below 95%.[2] Humidified oxygen is more comfortable and less drying to the nasal and airway mucosa than oxygen alone, and should be used whenever possible.

Bronchodilators

Bronchodilators are used to relax bronchial smooth muscle, and inhibit the release of inflammatory mediators. β_2-Agonists are the drugs of choice for treating acute bronchoconstriction. β_2-Agonists work by attaching to the β receptors on bronchial smooth muscle, resulting in activation of cyclic

---

Table 56–5   Asthma Treatment Algorithm

	β-Agonists	Corticosteroids	Monitors

Mild Exacerbation
PEFR > 80% or PS ≤ 3
RAO$_2$ sat ≥ 95%
	MDI with spacer q15min × 3
	  ≤30 kg: 4 puffs
	  >30 kg: 8 puffs
	or
	Albuterol nebulized q15min × 3
	Assess after each treatment.
	If worsening or no improvement, move to moderate exacerbation pathway.
	Discharge: PEFR > 80% or PS ≤ 3
		2 mg/kg prednisone or equivalent (max. 60 mg)
		Give ASAP
			Pulse oximeter

Moderate Exacerbation PEFR 50–80% or PS 4–6	Intermittent albuterol treatment with ipratropium (500–750 μg), then continuous albuterol treatment(s) or For children < 24 mo of age: albuterol with ipratropium (250 μg) q15min × 3 If worsening or no improvement, move to severe exacerbation pathway. If improving but not ready for discharge, consider admission. May attempt another continuous treatment or series of 3 nebulized treatments. Discharge: PEFR > 80% or PS ≤ 3	2 mg/kg prednisone or equivalent (max. 60 mg) Give ASAP	Pulse oximeter
Severe Exacerbation PEFR < 50% or PS > 6	Intermittent albuterol treatment with ipratropium (500–750 μg), then continuous albuterol treatment(s) or For children < 24 mo of age: albuterol with ipratropium (250 μg) q15min × 3 Consider ancillary medications If worsening clinical condition or no improvement, admit to intensive care unit. Give continuous nebulized albuterol until admission or transfer. Consider starting an intravenous line.	2 mg/kg prednisone or equivalent (max. 60 mg) Give ASAP	Pulse oximeter Cardiac monitor

Abbreviations: ASAP, as soon as possible; MDI, metered-dose inhaler; RAO$_2$ sat, room air oxygen saturation; PEFR, peak expiratory flow rate; PS, Pulmonary Score.

AMP. This leads to bronchodilation, enhanced mucociliary clearance and vascular integrity, and inhibition of inflammatory mediator release. Albuterol is the most commonly used bronchodilator. Other bronchodilators include levalbuterol, terbutaline, and salmeterol (a long-acting agent not used in emergency management).

Albuterol is delivered by nebulization or metered-dose inhaler (MDI) (see Table 56–6).[26-28] Oral albuterol is not appropriate because it has variable absorption from the gas-

trointestinal tract, and has significantly less efficacy compared to the inhaled route. Nebulized albuterol delivered via face mask can be given as a series of small doses with patient assessment between doses, or continuously with frequent assessments.[29-32] Typically, a series of one to three smaller doses are used for younger children (under 24 months) who have difficulty tolerating longer treatments or for children with mild exacerbations. Continuous albuterol is a combination of three or four smaller doses given over 45 to 60 minutes.

Table 56–6	Emergency Department Medications		
Medication	**Dose**	**Route**	**Details**
Corticosteroids (Choose one)			
Prednisolone (Orapred)	2 mg/kg (max. 60 mg)	PO	Preferred for children unable to swallow pills (palatable). Give once as soon as possible.
Prednisone	2 mg/kg (max. 60 mg)	PO	Appropriate for children able to swallow pills. Give once as soon as possible.
Methylprednisolone (Solu-Medrol)	2 mg/kg (max. 80 mg)	IV/IM	For critically ill children who cannot safely take oral medications. Consider giving if significant vomiting. Give once as soon as possible.
Dexamethasone (Decadron)	0.6 mg/kg (max. 10 mg)	PO/IM	Consider using highly concentrated parenteral formulation (10 mg/ml).
β-Agonists (Choose one)			
Albuterol (may switch route if desired)	2.5 mg (children < 30 kg) 5.0 mg (children ≥ 30 kg)	Nebulized	Repeat q15–20min as needed. Add normal saline (dilute to minimal volume [4 ml], flow [6–8 L/min]). Consider this option for mild exacerbations, children < 24 mo of age.
	or 10 mg (children < 30 kg) 20 mg (children ≥ 30 kg)	Nebulized	Continuous treatment (lasts 45–60 min). Add normal saline (dilute to minimal volume [4 ml], flow [6–8 L/min]). Repeat as needed for moderate to severe exacerbations. Consider admission if > one continuous treatment required.
	or 4 puffs (children <30 kg) 8 puffs (children ≥ 30 kg)	MDI/spacer	Repeat q15–20min as needed. Child should breathe 6–8 times between each puff.
L-Albuterol (levalbuterol) (Xopenex)	1.25–2.5 mg	Nebulized	Repeat q15–20min as needed. Continuous dosing not well studied.
Anticholinergic			
Ipratropium bromide (Atrovent)	250 mcg (max. 750 μg)	Nebulized	Give ONLY with albuterol, q15–20min. Recommended for moderate to severe exacerbations. Safety/efficacy not studied when used with continuous albuterol.
Ancillary Medications			
Consider using ONLY if severe exacerbation, or moderate exacerbation with no response to above medications. These have no proven advantage over combined β-agonist and corticosteroid therapy. Add cardiac monitoring.			
Epinephrine (1 : 1000)	0.01 mg/kg (max. 0.3 mg)	SubQ	Consider for life-threatening exacerbations. May repeat q15–20min × 3 if needed.
Terbutaline	0.01 mg/Kg (max. 0.25 mg)	SubQ	Consider if very poor aeration. May repeat q15–20min × 3 if needed.
	or 10 μg (over 20 min) *and*	IV bolus	Bolus is followed by a continuous drip.
	0.1–0.2 μg/kg/min	IV drip	Increase drip as needed in 0.1-μg/kg/min increments. STOP immediately if ventricular dysrythmias or hypotension develops.
Magnesium sulfate	25–50 mg/kg (over 30 min) (max. 3 g)	IV bolus	Consider if intensive care unit admission anticipated.
Heliox	70 : 30 (helium : oxygen) 80 : 20 (helium : oxygen)	Face mask or Ventilator	Consider if significant hypoxia (if oxygen saturations 80–85% with maximal O$_2$ therapy). May give albuterol at same time.
Ketamine	0.5–1.0 mg/kg	IV	Use as sedative for intubation. Use atropine or glycopyrrolate as premedication. Consider adding benzodiazepine prior to intubation.

Abbreviations: IM, intramuscular; IV, intravenous; MDI, metered-dose inhaler; PO, oral; SubQ, subcutaneous.

Continuous albuterol is used for children with moderate to severe exacerbations. Blow-by nebulization (not using a face mask) is not an effective method to deliver albuterol. An MDI can be used to deliver albuterol to children of any age. A mask with a spacer device is appropriate for children younger than 5 years of age, and a mouthpiece with a spacer device is appropriate for older children. The child should breathe six to eight times between each puff. The exact number of puffs required has not been well studied. Some children and parents will know the correct number of puffs needed from prior experience. MDIs can even be used for children with severe exacerbations.[33] Levalbuterol is the *R*-isomer of albuterol. Some studies suggest that levalbuterol may be more efficacious for some children with asthma; however, it is also more expensive than albuterol.[34,35] Levalbuterol should be considered for children who use it at home or have a history of improved benefit over albuterol (see Table 56–6). More studies are needed to support universal use of levalbuterol for all children with an acute asthma exacerbation.

Anticholinergics

The anticholinergic agent ipratropium bromide (Atrovent) is useful in the management of children with moderate to severe asthma exacerbations.[36-39] Ipratropium is similar to atropine, but contains an ammonium group, which prevents systemic absorption. It blocks acetylcholine receptors at the neuromuscular junction of bronchial smooth muscle, resulting in bronchodilation. Studies in children with moderate to severe asthma have shown improved bronchodilation when ipratropium and albuterol are used in combination compared to albuterol alone. This benefit is not seen in children with mild exacerbations. A series of two to three albuterol treatments with 250 mcg of ipratropium with each (total 500 to 750 mcg of ipratropium) is more beneficial than one treatment. Doses larger than 750 mcg have not been studied. Ipratropium causes bronchodilation, but is not as effective as albuterol and is not used as monotherapy. Combination MDIs with both albuterol and ipratropium have not been well studied in children with asthma.

Corticosteroids

Corticosteroids are the only therapy directly aimed at reducing inflammation, and play a vital role in the treatment of children with acute asthma exacerbations (see Table 56–6).[40,41] Corticosteroids decrease production of inflammatory mediators, and increase production of β receptors. Inflammatory mediators cause increased secretions, mucosal edema, and spasm of smooth muscle in the bronchial tree. Corticosteroids should be given as early as possible in the course of an exacerbation. Improvement in lung function begins within an hour, although clinical benefit may not be apparent for 2 to 4 hours after administration. When possible, the oral route is preferred because it obviates the need for intravenous catheter placement, is well tolerated, and is as efficacious as the intravenous route. Palatable formulations of methylprednisolone are available that enhance compliance among children. All children who present with an acute exacerbation should be treated with corticosteroids except those with a mild exacerbation who have not received any β-agonist therapy prior to arrival. If these children do not improve after one β-agonist treatment, the clinician should consider starting corticosteroids. Dexamethasone, not typically used for asthma, has been shown to be effective and is also a reasonable choice (see Table 56–6). Although inhaled corticosteroids (ICS) may provide some benefit to children with an acute exacerbation, parenteral corticosteroids remain the mainstay of acute asthma management.[42-44]

Ancillary Therapies

Administration of albuterol and corticosteroids is adequate treatment for the majority of children with asthma. Children with moderate to severe exacerbations may benefit from the addition of ipratropium. Additional medications may provide benefit to some children who do not initially respond to basic therapy, but there is limited evidence to support any significant improvement in outcome.[15,45,46] Commonly used adjuncts for children with moderate or severe exacerbations include subcutaneous epinephrine, intravenous or subcutaneous terbutaline, intravenous magnesium sulfate, heliox, ketamine, and aminophylline (see Table 56–6).[47,48] These are all second- or third-line therapies, and necessitate the addition of cardiac monitoring because of potential side effects. Addition of ancillary therapies can be considered for children with severe exacerbations or those with moderate exacerbations not responding to conventional therapies.

Epinephrine stimulates α receptors and nonspecific β receptors and causes bronchodilation.[47,48] It can be given subcutaneously or nebulized via face mask. Racemic epinephrine offers no advantages over nebulized albuterol, and there are increased side effects related to a receptor activity (vasoconstriction, pallor). Subcutaneous epinephrine was the drug of choice for acute asthma before the development of inhaled β-agonists, but now is rarely used. Subcutaneous epinephrine, along with continuous nebulized albuterol, may be considered for children with a life-threatening exacerbation or those deteriorating rapidly (see Table 56–6).

Terbutaline is a β2-agonist, and can be given intravenously or via MDI (see Table 56–6).[15,47,48] Although terbutaline is an effective bronchodilator, albuterol is the β-agonist of choice for acute exacerbations. Intravenous terbutaline may be considered for a severe exacerbation that is not responding to continuous nebulized albuterol and corticosteroids. Typically, terbutaline is administered intravenously as a bolus and followed by a continuous drip. There is some evidence to suggest that intravenous terbutaline may decrease the length of stay for children admitted to an intensive care unit. There is a small risk of ventricular dysrhythmias, so all children on intravenous terbutaline must have continuous cardiac monitoring. Terbutaline should be stopped immediately if dysrhythmias or hypotension develops.

Magnesium sulfate causes bronchodilation and stimulates calcium channels on mast cells, which results in decreased release of histamine. It is given as an intravenous bolus (see Table 56–6); it is not effective as an inhaled agent. The use of magnesium is controversial.[15,47,48] Some studies suggest improved bronchodilation when added to inhaled albuterol, whereas other studies do not support these findings. Magnesium may be considered for children with a severe exacerbation not responding to other therapies. Side effects include flushing, tachycardia, bradycardia, hypotension, and muscle weakness.

Heliox is an inhaled combination of helium and oxygen, often in 70 : 30 or 80 : 20 mixtures.[49-51] The lower density of helium allows the mixture to pass through narrow airways with less turbulence than oxygen alone, and can improve distal oxygen delivery. This may improve hypoxia and gain time for other therapies to work. Helium is an inert gas with no direct therapeutic benefit.

Ketamine is used primarily as an induction agent for children with asthma who require intubation. There are limited pediatric studies evaluating its use for asthma therapy, and is it not routinely used (see Table 56–6).[52] Theophylline or intravenous aminophylline are rarely used in asthma management. If a child takes theophylline for chronic asthma, a serum theophylline level should be measured in the ED, and the result used to guide therapy. Theophylline is unlikely to improve bronchodilation when continuous albuterol is used, and there are numerous side effects, including nausea, vomiting, and cardiac dysrythmias.

Potential Complications

Pneumothorax and pneumomediastinum are rare complications of asthma.[24,25] Pneumothorax often presents with sudden onset of chest pain with shortness of breath. A pneumomediastinum should be suspected in children who develop pain in the neck or shoulder or crepitus. Specific treatment is usually not required. Maintaining oxygen saturation above 95% with high-flow oxygen may be helpful for both conditions because it facilitates the reabsorption of nitrogen from the surrounding tissues. A thoracostomy tube should be considered if the pneumothorax is greater than 25% or is enlarging, the patient requires positive pressure ventilation (PPV), or oxygen saturation remains below 90% despite maximal oxygen therapy. A tension pneumothorax or pneumomediastinum from asthma is extremely rare, but requires immediate decompression with needle thoracostomy or needle pericardiocentesis (see Chapter 168, Thoracostomy; and Chapter 180, Pericardiocentesis).

Respiratory Failure

Children with asthma may develop respiratory compromise or failure. The most common cause of respiratory failure is ineffective ventilation from a combination of severe obstruction and muscle fatigue. Infants and young children initially will be tachypneic, fussy, and irritable. As respiratory failure ensues, infants and younger children become sleepier, do not interact with parents, may be cyanotic, and can develop paradoxical breathing. Older children may have decreased level of consciousness and tachypnea. Elevated $Paco_2$ (>60 mm Hg), rapidly increasing $Paco_2$, and tachypnea are signs of muscle fatigue and impending respiratory failure.[15,24] A sudden decrease in level of consciousness or drop in respiratory rate is an ominous sign. Supplying high-flow oxygen can maintain oxygen saturation above 90% but may be falsely reassuring, leading to underrecognition of hypoventilation and early respiratory failure. An arterial blood gas measurement should be considered in a child with continued oxygen saturation less than 90% on maximal oxygen therapy, no improvement despite aggressive treatment, and mental status changes.

Intubation

Most children with asthma do not require intubation, and are able to oxygenate and ventilate even with significant bronchconstriction. Any child with apnea, respiratory failure, or progressively deteriorating mental status should be intu-

bated.[15,24,25] The emergency physician should consider planning for intubation in children with increasing hypercarbia, inability to maintain oxygen saturation above 80% to 85% on maximal supplemental oxygen, or significant fatigue (decreasing respiratory rate without accompanying improvement in oxygenation or ventilation) (see Chapter 3, Rapid Sequence Intubation). Ketamine is a good induction agent under these circumstances and can be used along with an anticholinergic agent (atropine or glycopyrrolate) to decrease oral secretions, and a benzodiazepine to decrease dysphoria or emergence reactions.

Positive pressure ventilation (PPV) may be useful instead of intubation for some children.[53-55] PPV is a noninvasive way to decrease the work of breathing, improve oxygenation and ventilation, and re-expand atelectasis. PPV allows the child to control respiratory rate, tidal volume, and inspiratory and expiratory time. A tight-fitting face or nasal mask is used to deliver continuous positive airway pressures between 2 and 6 mm H_2O. Younger children may not tolerate the tight-fitting mask because of fear or anxiety. Some sedation may be required to utilize this technology, but is often less than what is required for intubation. This modality has not been well studied in children and should be viewed is a short-term measure for respiratory support.

Outpatient Treatment Versus Admission

Primary care physicians will successfully manage most asthma patients as outpatients. Any child seen in the ED for an acute asthma exacerbation should have follow-up with their primary provider within 7 days of the ED visit to evaluate recovery from the acute event, discuss reasons for the ED visit, and update the action plan to prevent future ED visits.[2,15] Consultation with a pulmonologist or allergist should be considered for children with life-threatening exacerbations, frequent ED visits, frequent hospitalizations, poor control, or lack of ongoing primary care.[56]

Almost 30% of children treated for asthma in the ED are admitted.[57,58] It is difficult to predict who will require admission early in the course of therapy. After initial therapy, children should be considered for discharge to home if the following are true:

- PEFR is greater than 70% to 80% of predicted
- There is minimal to no wheezing
- There is little or no work of breathing
- Medications can be filled
- Follow-up can be obtained
- Return to ED is feasible if needed

Admission should be considered if any of these conditions cannot be met or there are social issues that raise concern about the ability of the caregiver to adequately care for the child at home. Other reasons that may influence the decision to admit include hospital or ED standards, cost of care, or the availability of a short-stay or observation unit. Consideration should be given to transferring a child to a facility with pediatric critical care capability if he or she requires intubation, requires continuous albuterol therapy for 2 or more hours, is worsening, is not improving with conventional therapy, or cannot be closely monitored in the current facility.

All children discharged to home must be given prescriptions for their acute medications and have the ability to fill them. Albuterol should be prescribed, either as a nebulized solution premixed with normal saline or with a prescription

Table 56-7	Discharge-to-Home Medications			

Medication	Dose	Route	Details	
Corticosteroids (Choose one)				
Prednisolone (Orapred)	2 mg/kg/day (max. 60 mg)	PO	Preferred for children unable to swallow pills (palatable). Once-a-day dosing preferred, but may divide and give bid. Give for a total of 3–5 days.	
Prednisone	2 mg/kg/day (max. 60 mg)	PO	Appropriate for children able to swallow pills. Once-a-day dosing preferred, but may divide and give bid. Give for a total of 3–5 days.	
Dexamethasone (Decadron)	0.6 mg/kg (max. 10 mg)	PO	One dose given in ED. Second dose given at home the following day.	
β-Agonists (Choose one)				
Albuterol (may use either/ both routes if desired)	2.5–5.0 mg	Nebulized	Add normal saline (dilute to minimum 4 ml) with each treatment. Give q3–4h at home, AND space to q5–6h as tolerated.	
	or 4 puffs (children < 30 kg) 8 puffs (children ≥ 30 kg)	MDI/spacer	Give q3–4h at home, AND space to q5–6h as tolerated. Child should breath 6–8 times between each puff.	
L-Albuterol (levalbuterol) (Xopenex)	1.25–2.5 mg	Nebulized	Give q3–4h at home, AND space to q5–6h as tolerated.	
Inhaled Corticosteroids (Choose one)				
Consider doubling the dose for children currently taking an inhaled corticosteroid (use corticosteroid child is currently taking). Consider starting an inhaled corticosteroid for children with persistent asthma: any child with 2 or more days per week of coughing, wheezing, and shortness of breath at night, during the day, or with exercise. Consult with PCP when possible before starting. Use fluticasone for children discharged to home with an MDI and spacer, and budesonide for children discharged to home with nebulizer.				
Fluticasone (Flovent)	44 µg/actuation (children < 12 yr)	MDI with face mask *or* MDI/ mouthpiece	2 puffs bid if never taken before. Double dose if currently taking. PCP will determine length of therapy.	
	or 110 µg/actuation (children ≥ 12 yr)	MDI/mouthpiece	2 puffs bid if never taken before. Double the dose if currently taking. PCP will determine length of therapy.	
Budesonide (Pulmicort Respules)	0.5 mg/day (max. 1.0 mg/day)	Nebulized	May divide and give bid. Double the dose if currently taking. PCP will determine length of therapy	

Abbreviations: bid, twice daily; ED, emergency department; MDI, metered-dose inhaler; PCP, primary care provider.

for normal saline, or in the form of an MDI with a spacer device. Training on proper use of the nebulizer or the technique for an MDI should be provided to the family in the ED if they are previously uneducated in asthma medication administration. Albuterol is typically given every 4 to 6 hours depending on need, and the family should be educated about how to decrease the frequency as the exacerbation resolves. Oral prednisone solution or tablets should be continued for 3 to 5 days, given once daily or divided and given twice daily (Table 56–7).[40]

Children who are categorized with any level of persistent asthma should be discharged to home with ICS. Although several studies suggest that ICS given during an acute exacerbation are beneficial, most show that ICS alone are less efficacious than parenteral corticosteroids. However, chronic ICS has clear benefit and no significant side effects. If ICS are already being used, doubling the dose during the acute exacerbation should be considered.[42] The primary provider should be consulted before initiating ICS whenever possible. If the primary provider cannot be reached, ICS should be started, and adjustments in dosing can be done during follow-up (see Table 56–7).

It is important to discuss reasons for the ED visit with the family. These may include lack of understanding about how and when to use medications, lack of appropriate medica-tions, uncertainty about when or how to contact the primary provider, or lack of an asthma action plan. There may be other reasons for the ED visit, such as parental anxiety or inability to fill medication prescriptions. It is also important to emphasize the need for follow-up with the primary provider within a week of the ED visit.

The role of newer medications, such as leukotriene inhibitors, in the acute management of asthma has yet to be determined. One study of adult ED patients showed modest benefit from adding intravenous montelukast, a leukotriene inhibitor, to standard acute management.[59] No studies have been published showing similar results in children.

Another challenge for asthma care is linking children seen in the ED with their primary providers, and finding ways to establish regular asthma care. Regular care may improve adherence to medical and preventive management plans and should improve the relationship between the family and primary provider. Teaching families early recognition of an acute exacerbation, and how and when to start or escalate therapy, may prevent future ED visits.

REFERENCES

1. Mannino DM, Homa DM, Akinbami LJ, et al: Surveillance for asthma—United States, 1980–1999. MMWR Surveill Summ 51:1–13, 2002.

*2. National Heart, Lung and Blood Institute: National Asthma Education Program Expert Panel Report 2: Guidelines for Diagnosis and Management of Asthma. Washington, DC: National Institutes of Health, 1997.

3. Martinez FD: Respiratory syncytial virus bronchiolitis and the pathogenesis of childhood asthma. Pediatr Infect Dis J 22(2Suppl):S76–S82, 2003.

4. Weinberger M: Consensus statement from a conference on treatment of viral respiratory infection-induced asthma in young children. J Pediatr 142(2 Suppl):S45–S46, 2003.

5. Weinberger M: Treatment strategies for viral respiratory infection-induced asthma. J Pediatr 142(2 Suppl):S34–S38; discussion S38–S39, 2003.

*6. Landwehr L, Wood R, Blager F, et al: Vocal cord dysfunction mimicking exercise-induced bronchospasm in adolescents. Pediatrics 98:971–974, 1996.

7. Poirier M, Pancioli A, DiGiulio G: Vocal cord dysfunction presenting as acute asthma in a pediatric patient. Pediatr Emerg Care 12:213–214, 1996.

8. Weir M, Ehl L: Vocal cord dysfunction mimicking exercise-induced bronchospasm in adolescents [Letter; Comment]. Pediatrics 99:923–924, 1997.

9. Hederos CA, Janson S, Andersson H, Hedlin G: Chest x-ray investigation in newly discovered asthma. Pediatr Allergy Immunol 15:163–165, 2004.

10. Corren J, Manning BE, Thompson SF, et al: Rhinitis therapy and the prevention of hospital care for asthma: a case-control study. J Allergy Clin Immunol 113:415–419, 2004.

*11. Jenkins HA, Cherniack R, Szefler SJ, et al: A comparison of the clinical characteristics of children and adults with severe asthma. Chest 124:1318–1324, 2003.

12. Lang D, Polansky M: Patterns of asthma mortality in Philadelphia for 1969–1991. N Engl J Med 331:1542–1554, 1994.

13. LeSon S, Gershwin E: Risk factors for asthmatic patients requiring intubation. I. Observations in children. J Asthma 32:285–294, 1995.

14. LeSon S, Gershwin E: Risk factors for asthmatic patients requiring intubation. II. Observations in teenagers. J Asthma 32:379–389, 1995.

15. Smith S, Strunk RC: Acute asthma in the pediatric emergency department. Pediatr Clin North Am 46:1145–1165, 1999.

16. Gorelick MH, Stevens MW, Schultz T, Scribano PV: Difficulty in obtaining peak expiratory flow measurements in children with acute asthma. Pediatr Emerg Care 20:22–26, 2004.

17. Becker A, Nelson N, Simons F: The Pulmonary Index: assessment of a clinical score for asthma. Am J Dis Child 138:574–576, 1984.

18. Wood D, Downes J, Lecks H: A clinical scoring system for the diagnosis of respiratory failure: preliminary report on childhood status asthmaticus. Am J Dis Child 123:227–228, 1972.

19. Smith S, Hodge D, Baty J: The Pulmonary Score: an asthma severity measure for children in the emergency department. Acad Emerg Med 5:383, 1998.

20. Baker KM, Brand DA, Hen J Jr: Classifying asthma: disagreement among specialists. Chest 124:2156–2163, 2003.

*21. Perng DW, Huang HY, Lee YC, Perng RP: Leukotriene modifier vs inhaled corticosteroid in mild-to-moderate asthma: clinical and anti-inflammatory effects. Chest 125:1693–1699, 2004.

22. Thi TN, Le Bourgeois M, Scheinmann P, de Blic J: Airway inflammation and asthma treatment modalities. Pediatr Pulmonol Suppl 26:229–233, 2004.

*23. Ververeli K, Chipps B: Oral corticosteroid-sparing effects of inhaled corticosteroids in the treatment of persistent and acute asthma. Ann Allergy Asthma Immunol 92:512–522, 2004.

24. Levy B, Kitch B, Fanta C: Medical and ventilatory management of status asthmaticus. Intensive Care Med 24:105–117, 1998.

25. Paret G, Kornecki A, Szeinberg A, et al: Severe acute asthma in a community hospital pediatric intensive care unit: a ten years' experience. Ann Allergy Asthma Immunol 80:339–344, 1998.

*26. Delgado A, Chou KJ, Silver EJ, Crain EF: Nebulizers vs metered-dose inhalers with spacers for bronchodilator therapy to treat wheezing in children aged 2 to 24 months in a pediatric emergency department. Arch Pediatr Adolesc Med 157:76–80, 2003.

*27. Iqbal S, Ritson S, Prince I, et al: Drug delivery and adherence in young children. Pediatr Pulmonol 37:311–317, 2004.

28. Karpel J, Aldrich T, Prezant D, et al: Emergency treatment of acute asthma with albuterol metered-dose inhaler plus holding chamber. Chest 112:348–356, 1997.

*29. Katz R, Kelly W, Crowley M, et al: Safety of continuous nebulized albuterol for bronchospasm in infants and children. Pediatrics 92:666–669, 1993.

30. Kelly HW, Keim KA, McWilliams BC: Comparison of two methods of delivering continuously nebulized albuterol. Ann Pharmacother 37:23–26, 2003.

31. Khine H, Fuchs S, Saville A: Continuous vs intermittent nebulized albuterol for emergency management of asthma. Acad Emerg Med 3:1019–1024, 1996.

32. Rudnitsky G, Eberlain R, Schoffstall J, et al: Comparison of intermittent and continuously nebulized albuterol for treatment of asthma in an urban emergency department. Ann Emerg Med 22:1842–1846, 1993.

*33. Mandhane P, Zuberbuhler P, Lange CF, Finlay WH: Albuterol aerosol delivered via metered-dose inhaler to intubated pediatric models of 3 ages, with 4 spacer designs. Respir Care 48:948–955, 2003.

*34. Carl JC, Myers TR, Kirchner HL, Kercsmar CM: Comparison of racemic albuterol and levalbuterol for treatment of acute asthma. J Pediatr 143:731–736, 2003.

*35. Kattan M: Mirror images: is levalbuterol the fairest of them all? J Pediatr 143:702–704, 2003.

36. Brophy C, Ahmed B, Bayson S, et al: How long should atrovent be given in acute asthma? Thorax 53:363–367, 1998.

37. Karpel J, Schacter N, Fanta C, et al: A comparison of ipratropium and albuterol vs albuterol alone for the treatment of acute asthma. Chest 110:611–616, 1996.

38. Qureshi F, Pestian J, Davis P, et al: Effect of nebulized ipratropium on the hospitalization rates of children with asthma. N Engl J Med 339:1030–1035, 1998.

39. Zorc J, Ogborn J, Pulsic M: Ipratropium bromide: What role does it have in asthma therapy? Contemp Pediatr 4:81–94, 1998.

*40. Scarfone RJ, Friedlaender E: Corticosteroids in acute asthma: past, present, and future. Pediatr Emerg Care 19:355–361, 2003.

41. Kayani S, Shannon DC: Adverse behavioral effects of treatment for acute exacerbation of asthma in children: a comparison of two doses of oral steroids. Chest 122:624–628, 2002.

*42. FitzGerald JM, Becker A, Sears MR, et al: Doubling the dose of budesonide versus maintenance treatment in asthma exacerbations. Thorax 59:550–556, 2004.

43. Hendeles L, Sherman J: Are inhaled corticosteroids effective for acute exacerbations of asthma in children? J Pediatr 142(2 Suppl):S26–S32, 2003.

44. Nakanishi AK, Klasner AK, Rubin BK: A randomized controlled trial of inhaled flunisolide in the management of acute asthma in children. Chest 124:790–794, 2003.

45. Lanski SL, Greenwald M, Perkins A, Simon HK: Herbal therapy use in a pediatric emergency department population: expect the unexpected. Pediatrics 111(5 Pt 1):981–985, 2003.

46. Hunt LW, Frigas E, Butterfield JH, et al: Treatment of asthma with nebulized lidocaine: a randomized, placebo-controlled study. J Allergy Clin Immunol 113:853–859, 2004.

47. South M: Second line treatment for severe acute childhood asthma, Thorax 58:284–285, 2003.

48. Niven AS, Argyros G: Alternate treatments in asthma. Chest123:1254–1265, 2003.

49. Kudukis T, Manthous C, Schmidt G, et al: Inhaled helium-oxygen revisited: effect of inhaled helium-oxygen during the treatment of status asthmaticus in children. J Pediatr 130:217–224, 1997.

50. Manthous C, Hall J, Melmed A, et al: Heliox improves pulsus paradoxus and peak expiratory flow in nonintubated patients with severe asthma. Am J Respir Crit Care Med 151:310–314, 1995.

51. Rodrigo G, Pollack C, Rodrigo C, Rowe BH: Heliox for nonintubated acute asthma patients. Cochrane Database Syst Rev (4):CD002884, 2003.

52. Howton J, Rose J, Duffy S, et al: Randomized, double-blind, placebo-controlled trial of intravenous ketamine in acute asthma. Ann Emerg Med 27:170–175, 1996.

53. Birnbaumer D: Noninvasive ventilatory support—saving a life without intubation. West J Med 168:182–183, 1998.

54. Meduri G, Cook T, Turner R, et al: Noninvasive positive pressure ventilation in status asthmaticus. Chest 110:767–774, 1996.

---

*Selected readings.

55. Soroksky A, Stav D, Shpirer I: A pilot prospective, randomized, placebo-controlled trial of bilevel positive airway pressure in acute asthmatic attack. Chest 123:1018–1025, 2003.

56. Sly R, O'Donnell R: Stabilization of asthma mortality. Ann Allergy Asthma Immunol 78:347–354, 1997.

57. Brenner B, Kohn M: The acute asthmatic patient in the ED: to admit or discharge. Am J Emerg Med 16:69–75, 1998.

58. Wilson MM, Irwin RS, Connolly AE, et al: A prospective evaluation of the 1-hour decision point for admission versus discharge in acute asthma. J Intensive Care Med 18:275–285, 2003.

59. Camargo CA Jr, Smithline HA, Malice MP, et al: A randomized controlled trial of intravenous montelukast in acute asthma. Am J Respir Crit Care Med 167:528–533, 2003.

Chapter 57

Bronchiolitis

Deborah A. Levine, MD

Key Points

Bronchiolitis is the most common lower respiratory infection in children less than 2 years of age.

There is a risk of apnea and dehydration, especially in the youngest infants.

Infants with prematurity, chronic lung disease, and congenital heart disease are at risk for severe disease.

Diagnostic tests are not useful in management of bronchiolitis.

Introduction and Background

Bronchiolitis is an acute viral-induced inflammation of the airways of the lower respiratory tract resulting in airway obstruction. It is the most common lower respiratory tract infection in children under 2 years of age, with a peak age between 2 and 6 months.[1] Reinfection can occur at any age. Each year approximately 12% of infants develop bronchiolitis.[2] Between 1997 and 2000, there were over 700,000 emergency department (ED) visits (22.8 per 1000) by infants less than 1 year of age for a lower respiratory infection. Approximately half of these visits occurred during January and February.[3] Thirty percent of these ED patients were hospitalized, and 68% of these hospitalized patients were under 1 year of age. Respiratory syncytial virus (RSV) bronchiolitis was the leading cause of infant hospitalization each year during 1997 through 2000.[3] Hospitalizations continue to rise compared to prior years' data.[4] The total medical expenses for ED patients with lower respiratory infection were approximately $200 million during that time period.[3] Bronchiolitis-associated deaths occur in approximately 95 children a year.[5] Three fourths of the deaths are in infants less than 1 year of age.[5]

Recognition and Approach

Bronchiolitis is a common cause for hospitalization and can result in severe morbidity and mortality. RSV causes the majority of cases of bronchiolitis, especially during the winter and early spring months.[6] Other etiologic pathogens causing bronchiolitis are parainfluenza virus, human metapneumovirus, influenza virus, adenovirus, rhinovirus, enterovirus, and herpes simplex virus.

The viral etiologic agent invades the respiratory tract, causing necrosis and sloughing of the respiratory epithelium of the smaller airways, and initiates an immune response with inflammatory infiltration and edema. The bronchioles become narrowed from this cellular infiltrate, edema, and mucus, leading to air trapping and atelectasis. The infant's airway is smaller than its adult counterpart, which drastically further limits airflow. This leads to an increased work of breathing with respiratory distress. If severe airway obstruction ensues, ventilation-perfusion mismatch, hypoxemia, and respiratory muscle fatigue and failure may subsequently develop.

Clinical Presentation

Bronchiolitis usually presents with symptoms of an upper respiratory infection, such as coryza for 1 to 2 days. These symptoms progress to wheezing, cough, and tachypnea. Patients can be febrile as well. Respiratory symptoms in infants often cause post-tussive emesis, irritability, and difficulty with feeding (Table 57–1). Infants with a mild form of bronchiolitis can appear playful and have adequate hydration with mild wheezing. More significant presentations of bronchiolitis include lethargy, signs of dehydration, and significant respiratory accessory muscle use (intercostal and supraclavicular retractions), head bobbing, and/or nasal flaring. Apnea can occur in up to 20% of hospitalized infants and may be the initial manifestation of bronchiolitis, before respiratory symptoms begin.[7] The risk of apnea is usually abated by the third day of infection. Younger age (<2 months), prematurity, or radiographic findings such as infiltrates or atelectasis have been described as risk factors for apnea in patients with bronchiolitis.[8,9]

Premature infants, those with congenital heart disease, those with chronic lung disease (e.g., cystic fibrosis, bronchopulmonary dysplasia, congenital pulmonary anomaly), those who are immunocompromised, and infants younger than 3 months of age are at risk for a severe course of bronchiolitis.[10] Complications from bronchiolitis, such as intensive care unit admission, mechanical ventilation, and death, were highest in children with cardiac disease, chronic lung disease, immunocompromised status, gestation less than 37 weeks or age less than 6 weeks.[10] Patients age 13 months and younger who

Table 57-1	Clinical Manifestations of Bronchiolitis by Age
Neonate	**Infant/Young Child**
Lethargy	Coryza
Irritability	Wheezing
Poor feeding	Retractions
Apnea	Flaring
Fever	Tachypnea

Table 57-2	Differential Diagnosis of Bronchiolitis
Asthma	
Pneumonia	
Cystic fibrosis	
Foreign body	
Congestive heart failure and congenital heart disease	
Acquired heart disease, such as myocarditis	
Tracheoesophageal fistula	
Gastroesophageal reflux	
Mycoplasma pneumoniae infection	
Chlamydia trachomatis infection	
Congenital rings, webs	
Pulmonary sequestration	
Toxins, poisonings (organophosphates)	

present to an ED are more likely to have severe illness if they have a toxic appearance, oxygen saturation less than 95%, gestational age less than 34 weeks, respiratory rate greater than 70 breaths/min, atelectasis on chest radiograph and are younger than 3 months.[11] Death rates from bronchiolitis are highest in infants ages 1 to 3 months and infants weighing less than 1500 grams at birth.[12]

Bronchiolitis is a clinical diagnosis based on signs and symptoms from the history and physical examination. Since there is no confirmatory test or "gold standard" for diagnosing bronchiolitis, laboratory testing is not helpful. Pulse oximetry is helpful in the identification of infants with moderate to severe hypoxemia associated with bronchiolitis. No study has demonstrated the utility of a complete blood count in diagnosing bronchiolitis or directing therapy.[13] Elevated white blood cell counts have limited usefulness in diagnosing bacterial disease as well.[13]

Because RSV is the most common etiology in bronchiolitis, virology testing is frequently performed. Rapid viral antigen detection tests on nasopharyngeal specimens are 80% to 90% sensitive compared to viral cultures.[14] These have limited usefulness except for epidemiologic surveillance, cohorting inpatients to reduce nosocomial spread, and perhaps designating a patient at lower risk for concurrent serious bacterial infection.[15,16]

Chest radiographs are not indicated for making the diagnosis of bronchiolitis, but can exclude other disease processes that may present with wheezing, such as foreign body or congestive heart failure. Some studies have reported a more severe clinical course in patients with atelectasis on chest radiographs.[10,11] Other studies have found an increased rate of treatment with antibiotics in bronchiolitis patients with lobar infiltrates, but equal recovery times, compared to those with normal radiographs.[17] Radiologic findings suggestive of bronchiolitis are hyperinflation, flattened diaphragm, atelectasis, and peribronchial cuffing. Infiltrates may be present as well.[18] There is limited evidence to support the routine use of diagnostic testing in most children with bronchiolitis since no studies have addressed the impact of testing on patient outcomes. Patients who are severely ill or toxic in appearance or those with an unusual clinical course may be good candidates for laboratory and radiographic testing. Differential diagnosis of bronchiolitis includes other infectious, inflammatory, anatomic, and systemic conditions (Table 57–2).

Important Clinical Features and Considerations

Infants with bronchopulmonary dysplasia can have episodes of wheezing that may mimic respiratory infections such as bronchiolitis, but these infants are also at risk for respiratory infections.[1] Patients with pneumonia can present with wheezing, especially with an interstitial processes due to viral etiologies. The clinician should look for systemic signs of congestive heart failure in patients with undiagnosed congenital or acquired heart disease. These infants can present acutely with respiratory distress and wheezing but may have accompanying organomegaly, cardiac murmur, peripheral edema, and abnormal chest radiograph and/or electrocardiogram.

Fever can be a presenting sign of bronchiolitis. The decision to adequately exclude other sources of infection such as meningitis, bacteremia, urinary tract infection, or bacterial enteritis in the febrile infant with bronchiolitis is a difficult one for the emergency physician, who must ask the question, does every febrile infant with bronchiolitis warrant a complete fever evaluation, including lumbar puncture? A recent large, prospective, multicenter study of febrile infants less than 60 days of age with fever greater than 100.3° C studied the risk of serious bacterial infection in infants with RSV and bronchiolitis. Although the infants with bronchiolitis had a lower rate of serious bacterial infections compared to infants without bronchiolitis (7.1% vs. 12.5%, $P = 0.069$), this was not statistically significant. Both groups of infants had substantial rates of urinary tract infection. There were too few patients in the study with either meningitis or bacteremia to draw meaningful conclusions about these two types of infection.[19] Other studies have reported low rates of serious bacterial infections in infants with bronchiolitis but also lack sufficient sample sizes to adequately compare rates of the most severe infections.[15,16,20-23] Studies examining the rates of concomitant bacterial infection in older infants and children with bronchiolitis show low rates of such infection, though the prevalence of urinary tract infection may still merit screening in these patients.[20,24] The incidence of serious bacterial infections in febrile infants with bronchiolitis remains low but not negligible. Until larger studies are completed, febrile infants with bronchiolitis may still be at risk for concomitant bacterial infections. Emergency physicians must plan the evaluation of the febrile infant based on this information.

Acutely, approximately 10% to 20% of infants with bronchiolitis require hospitalization. Potential morbidity and mortality may occur due to respiratory failure, dehydration, and apnea. Aspiration and bacterial superinfection are uncommon.[25,26] Otitis media is a common secondary infection, occurring in up to two thirds of infants with bronchiolitis.[27] Approximately 15% to 25% of patients with bronchiolitis will develop asthma.[28] In children followed for 18 to 20 years, bronchiolitis in infancy was a significant predictor of asthma in early adulthood (odds ratio, 3.37; 95% confidence interval, 1.12–10.10).[29] Another large prospective study of children found that a history of RSV bronchiolitis within the first year of life was a significant risk factor for wheezing at age 6, but this risk decreased with age.[30]

Management

There remains considerable controversy over the management of bronchiolitis. Historically, bronchiolitis is a self-limited illness, requiring only supportive care such as adequate oxygenation and hydration until the disease abates.[14] Nasal suctioning is commonly employed to reduce secretions. Occasionally, mechanical ventilation is necessary to maintain gas exchange.

Pharmacologic therapy has been commonly employed in the treatment of infants and children with bronchiolitis.[31] β-Agonists, bronchodilators, corticosteroids, antivirals, and immunoglobulins have been studied in infants with bronchiolitis. Many of these are small studies in varied populations (different clinical severity) and settings (hospitalized vs. outpatients) using nonstandardized definitions of bronchiolitis (such as the inclusion of infants with recurrent wheezing) and heterogeneity of outcome measures (various respiratory scores, admission criteria). Therefore, the evidence base for the treatment of bronchiolitis is not particularly strong.

Epinephrine

Epinephrine contains α- and β-adrenergic properties resulting in vasoconstriction, which has been postulated to reduce the airway edema associated with bronchiolitis, decreasing airway obstruction.[32] Acutely wheezing patients who received 0.01 mg/kg of subcutaneous epinephrine versus placebo had a significantly better clinical appearance.[33] A meta-analysis of 14 studies of children treated with nebulized epinephrine versus placebo or salbutamol showed no overall difference in admission rates among outpatients or length of stay among inpatients.[34,35] There was evidence supporting the use of epinephrine among outpatients based on short-term benefits such as clinical score, oxygen saturation, heart rate, and respiratory rate during the first 90 minutes of drug administration. A recent multicenter, randomized, double-blind controlled trial comparing nebulized epinephrine to placebo in 194 hospitalized infants with bronchiolitis showed no difference in length of hospital stay or time until discharge between the groups.[36] The more severely affected patients in this study who received epinephrine had a longer length of stay than those who received placebo. Adverse effects reported included pallor and tachycardia, but these were well tolerated without sequelae.[37] Overall, there may be some benefit from nebulized epinephrine, but larger, well-designed studies are warranted to evaluate its use in bronchiolitis.

Bronchodilators (Including Anticholinergics)

Bronchodilators are the mainstay of therapy for bronchiolitis. This is due to the belief that the pathophysiology of bronchiolitis may be similar to that of asthma (reversible bronchospasm). A meta-analysis of prospective, randomized, controlled trials involving over 900 patients ages 24 months or younger who received bronchodilators (albuterol, salbutamol, or ipratropium bromide) revealed a statistically significant improvement in clinical score compared to placebo-treated infants, though the magnitude of the difference was of questionable clinical significance.[38] No improvement in oxygenation, rate of hospitalization, or length of hospital stay was found in the bronchodilator-treated infants.[38] Although there was a modest improvement in clinical respiratory score in bronchodilator-treated infants, patients with a history of wheezing who may respond better to bronchodilators were included. A meta-analysis of five outpatient randomized controlled trials of inhaled β-agonists in over 250 patients revealed no difference in hospital admissions or respiratory rate. There was a statistically significant increase in oxygen saturation and heart rate in the infants treated with β-agonists, but this was clinically insignificant.[2] Nebulized ipratropium bromide was evaluated in four studies included in a systematic review. No differences in hospitalization rates or clinical scores were noted in patients who received this drug as either as a single agent or when used in combination with other bronchodilators.[39] Based on the literature, the use of nebulized bronchodilators does not alter clinical course or hospitalization rates in patients with bronchiolitis.

Corticosteroids

The similarity between the clinical presentation of bronchiolitis and asthma has encouraged clinicians to utilize common therapies such as bronchodilators and corticosteroids. Corticosteroids have been thought to help in the early phase of bronchiolitis, moderating bronchiolar inflammation and the production of inflammatory mediators such as leukotrienes and cytokines.[40-43] However, most studies contain few patients, differing clinical scoring systems, various dosages and routes of medication delivery, and nonstandardized outcome measures.[44,45]

A meta-analysis of six clinical trials of corticosteroid therapy in the treatment of over 300 hospitalized infants with bronchiolitis showed that infants treated with corticosteroids (either parenteral or oral) had a lower mean length of stay than those patients in the placebo group. The mean clinical score (including wheezing, oxygen saturation, accessory muscle use, and respiratory rate) at 24 hours after initial therapy was lower in those infants who received steroids compared to the placebo group.[46] Based on these results, steroids may improve the course of bronchiolitis but probably only when applied to a more severely affected, hospitalized population. Also, the clinical importance of these results are questionable since the benefit of reducing hospitalization by less than half a day may be clinically insignificant. A systematic review of 14 studies of over 900 patients with bronchiolitis treated with oral, parenteral, or inhaled steroid showed conflicting results among studies with regard to hospitalization rate or duration of inpatient stay. Collectively, these studies failed to show significant improvements in clinical scores or hospitalization rates in infants treated with corticosteroids.[37]

Few studies have examined the role of steroids in the management of patients with bronchiolitis in the ED until recently.

Two studies found beneficial effects of corticosteroids given to bronchiolitic patients in the ED, rather than later in their hospital courses.[44,45] One study that enrolled only patients with the first episode of wheezing and utilized a higher dose of oral dexamethasone in the ED found a significantly decreased rate of hospitalization (19% vs. 44%) and a greater improvement in clinical score at 4 hours in the steroid-treated group.[45]

Preliminary results of a recently completed multicenter, randomized, controlled trial of the effectiveness and safety of the administration of oral dexamethasone for acute moderate to severe outpatient bronchiolitis indicated no difference between groups with regard to the need for hospitalization.[47] In conclusion, there are no data to support the use of steroids in ED patients with bronchiolitis at the current time.

Ribavirin

Ribavirin is the only Food and Drug Administration–approved antiviral medication for RSV disease. It is administered as a continuous aerosol. Initially, a series of randomized controlled trials found ribavirin to decrease the severity of RSV bronchiolitis, and thus it was recommended as a standard therapy.[48,49] Subsequently, a systematic review of 10 randomized, controlled trials of ribavirin found that it reduced the duration of mechanical ventilation and may reduce the length of hospital stay, but has not been shown to reduce mortality or respiratory deterioration. No adverse effects have been reported.[50] Due to conflicting reports in the literature, high costs, and potential teratogenicity to health care personnel, ribavirin is currently not recommended.[14]

Immunoglobulin Therapy

RSV intravenous immune globulin and monoclonal antibody (palivizumab) administered intramuscularly given in monthly doses prophylactically during RSV season have been shown to reduce RSV-related hospitalizations in high-risk infants.[39,51] RSV immune globulin was studied as a treatment for acute bronchiolitis and found not to alter the days of hospitalization or mechanical ventilation, but did show a trend toward shorter stays in the intensive care ward.[52,53] Currently there is evidence only to support the use of palivizumab in the prevention of RSV bronchiolitis in high-risk populations; it is not indicated in the treatment of active disease.[14]

Additional Therapies

Other novel treatment modalities have been studied in patients with bronchiolitis. Heliox is a helium-oxygen mixture that has a lower density than regular air. This lower density lowers air resistance, especially in obstructed bronchioles, improves airflow and ventilation, and decreases the work of breathing. Two small studies of nonintubated infants with bronchiolitis treated with Heliox showed improvements in clinical scores.[54,55] Intramuscular interferon alfa-2, herbal treatments, antibiotics, surfactant, aerosolized furosemide, nebulized recombinant human deoxyribonuclease, and hypertonic saline have also been studied in small numbers of infants with bronchiolitis, but none has conclusively been shown to be effective, and these therapies are therefore not routinely recommended.[56-61]

Summary

The following are indications for admission in a patient with bronchiolitis: hypoxia (defined as oxygen saturation less than 90% to 95% depending on elevation), dehydration, poor feeding, lethargy, severe respiratory distress (respiratory rate > 60 breaths/min, retractions, flaring, head bobbing, poor air entry), or an unreliable caregiver. Very high-risk infants include those with a history of prematurity, heart disease, lung disease, or young age (<3 months), and all should be strongly considered for admission.

Infants with severe nasal congestion or tachypnea may not be able to feed sufficiently and may be at risk for dehydration and/or aspiration. Patients with hypoxia need supplemental oxygen. Cautious practice patterns should to be exercised with the youngest infants (<3 months) with bronchiolitis and those with comorbidities who may develop a more severe course and have the highest risk for apnea. Infants with severe hypoxia or CO_2 retention require intensive care management for possible mechanical ventilation. Infants with a history of apnea require intensive care monitoring since recurrence of apnea is common. Intravenous access is indicated for infants who have apnea and those with dehydration. Empirical therapy with antibiotics is not warranted unless bacterial infection is suspected. Infants and children who are discharged need close follow-up (within 1 to 2 days). Parents must be made aware of possible complications of the disease and should be assessed for telephone access and available transportation if the clinical condition worsens.

Prevention

Vigilant hand washing and contact isolation of affected patients can prevent spread of the viral pathogens causing bronchiolitis. The monoclonal antibody palivizumab, given intramuscularly on a monthly basis during RSV season, is the currently indicated prophylactic therapy for infants at high risk for RSV disease. Purified fusion protein vaccines against the most common etiologic viral causes of bronchiolitis are currently under development and appear promising.

REFERENCES

1. La Via WV, Marks MI, Stutman HR: Respiratory syncytial virus puzzle: clinical features, pathophysiology, treatment, and prevention. J Pediatr 121:503–510, 1992.
2. Flores G, Horwitz RI: Efficacy of beta₂-agonists in bronchiolitis: a reappraisal and meta-analysis. Pediatrics 100(2 Pt 1):233–239, 1997.
3. Leader S, Kohlhase K: Recent trends in severe respiratory syncytial virus (RSV) among US infants, 1997 to 2000. J Pediatr 143(5 Suppl): S127–S132, 2003.
4. Centers for Disease Control and Prevention: Bronchiolitis-associated outpatient visits and hospitalizations among American Indian and Alaska Native children—United States, 1990–2000. MMWR Morb Mortal Wkly Rep 52:707–710, 2003.
5. Shay DK, Holman RC, Roosevelt GE, et al: Bronchiolitis-associated mortality and estimates of respiratory syncytial virus-associated deaths among US children, 1979–1997. J Infect Dis 183:16–22, 2001.
*6. Shay DK, Holman RC, Newman RD, et al: Bronchiolitis-associated hospitalizations among US children, 1980–1996. JAMA 282:1440–1446, 1999.
7. Hall CB: Respiratory syncytial virus: a continuing culprit and conundrum. J Pediatr 135(2 Pt 2):2–7, 1999.

*Selected readings.

8. Kneyber MC, Brandenburg AH, de Groot R, et al: Risk factors for respiratory syncytial virus associated apnoea. Eur J Pediatr 157:331–335, 1998.

9. Bruhn FW, Mokrohisky ST, McIntosh K: Apnea associated with respiratory syncytial virus infection in young infants. J Pediatr 90:382–386, 1977.

*10. Wang EE, Law BJ, Stephens D: Pediatric Investigators Collaborative Network on Infections in Canada (PICNIC) prospective study of risk factors and outcomes in patients hospitalized with respiratory syncytial viral lower respiratory tract infection. J Pediatr 126:212–219, 1995.

*11. Shaw KN, Bell LM, Sherman NH: Outpatient assessment of infants with bronchiolitis. Am J Dis Child 145:151–155, 1991.

*12. Holman RC, Shay DK, Curns AT, et al: Risk factors for bronchiolitis-associated deaths among infants in the United States. Pediatr Infect Dis J 22:483–490, 2003.

13. Bordley WC, Viswanathan M, King VJ, et al: Diagnosis and testing in bronchiolitis: a systematic review. Arch Pediatr Adolesc Med 158:119–126, 2004.

14. Pickering LK, Baker CJ, Long SS, et al (eds): 2003 Red Book: Report of the Committee on Infectious Diseases, 26 ed. Elk Grove Village, IL: American Academy of Pediatrics, 2003.

15. Antonow JA, Hansen K, McKinstry CA, Byington CL: Sepsis evaluations in hospitalized infants with bronchiolitis. Pediatr Infect Dis J 17:231–236, 1998.

*16. Byington CL, Enriquez FR, Hoff C, et al: Serious bacterial infections in febrile infants 1 to 90 days old with and without viral infections. Pediatrics 113:1662–1666, 2004.

17. Swingler GH, Hussey GD, Zwarenstein M: Randomised controlled trial of clinical outcome after chest radiograph in ambulatory acute lower-respiratory infection in children. Lancet 351:404–408, 1998.

18. Gadomski AM, Aref GH, el Din OB, et al: Oral versus nebulized albuterol in the management of bronchiolitis in Egypt. J Pediatr 124:131–138, 1994.

19. Levine DA, Platt SL, Dayan PS, et al: Risk of serious bacterial infection in young febrile infants with respiratory syncytial virus infections. Pediatrics 113:1728–1734, 2004.

20. Kuppermann N, Bank DE, Walton EA, et al: Risks for bacteremia and urinary tract infections in young febrile children with bronchiolitis. Arch Pediatr Adolesc Med 151:1207–1214, 1997.

21. Titus MO, Wright SW: Prevalence of serious bacterial infections in febrile infants with respiratory syncytial virus infection. Pediatrics 112:282–284, 2003.

22. Liebelt EL, Qi K, Harvey K: Diagnostic testing for serious bacterial infections in infants aged 90 days or younger with bronchiolitis. Arch Pediatr Adolesc Med 153:525–530, 1999.

23. Melendez E, Harper MB: Utility of sepsis evaluation in infants 90 days of age or younger with fever and clinical bronchiolitis. Pediatr Infect Dis J 22:1053–1056, 2003.

24. Purcell K, Fergie J: Concurrent serious bacterial infections in 2396 infants and children hospitalized with respiratory syncytial virus lower respiratory tract infections. Arch Pediatr Adolesc Med 156:322–324, 2002.

25. Khoshoo V, Edell D: Previously healthy infants may have increased risk of aspiration during respiratory syncytial viral bronchiolitis. Pediatrics 104:1389–1390, 1999.

26. Hall CB, Powell KR, Schnabel KC, et al: Risk of secondary bacterial infection in infants hospitalized with respiratory syncytial viral infection. J Pediatr 113:266–271, 1988.

27. Andrade MA, Hoberman A, Glustein J, et al: Acute otitis media in children with bronchiolitis. Pediatrics 101(4 Pt 1):617–619, 1998.

28. Perlstein PH, Kotagal UR, Bolling C, et al: Evaluation of an evidence-based guideline for bronchiolitis. Pediatrics 104:1334–1341, 1999.

29. Piippo-Savolainen E, Remes S, Kannisto S, et al: Asthma and lung function 20 years after wheezing in infancy: results from a prospective follow-up study. Arch Pediatr Adolesc Med 158:1070–1076, 2004.

30. Stein RT, Sherrill D, Morgan WJ, et al: Respiratory syncytial virus in early life and risk of wheeze and allergy by age 13 years. Lancet 354:541–545, 1999.

31. Plint AC, Johnson DW, Wiebe N, et al: Practice variation among pediatric emergency departments in the treatment of bronchiolitis. Acad Emerg Med 11:353–360, 2004.

32. Wohl ME, Chernick V: State of the art: bronchiolitis. Am Rev Respir Dis 118:759–781, 1978.

33. Lowell DI, Lister G, Von Koss H, McCarthy P: Wheezing in infants: the response to epinephrine. Pediatrics 79:939–945, 1987.

34. Hartling L, Wiebe N, Russell K, et al: Epinephrine for bronchiolitis. Cochrane Database Syst Rev (1):CD003123, 2004.

*35. Hartling L, Wiebe N, Russell K, et al: A meta-analysis of randomized controlled trials evaluating the efficacy of epinephrine for the treatment of acute viral bronchiolitis. Arch Pediatr Adolesc Med 157:957–964, 2003.

36. Wainwright C, Altamirano L, Cheney M, et al: A multicenter, randomized, double-blind, controlled trial of nebulized epinephrine in infants with acute bronchiolitis. N Engl J Med 349:27–35, 2003.

37. King VJ, Viswanathan M, Bordley WC, et al: Pharmacologic treatment of bronchiolitis in infants and children: a systematic review. Arch Pediatr Adolesc Med 158:127–137, 2004.

38. Kellner JD, Ohlsson A, Gadomski AM, Wang EE: Bronchodilators for bronchiolitis. Cochrane Database Syst Rev (2):CD001266, 2000.

39. Palivizumab, a humanized respiratory syncytial virus monoclonal antibody, reduces hospitalization from respiratory syncytial virus infection in high-risk infants. The IMpact-RSV Study Group. Pediatrics 102(3 Pt 1):531–537, 1998.

40. Lugo RA, Nahata MC: Pathogenesis and treatment of bronchiolitis. Clin Pharm 12:95–116, 1993.

41. Sheeran P, Jafri H, Carubelli C, et al: Elevated cytokine concentrations in the nasopharyngeal and tracheal secretions of children with respiratory syncytial virus disease. Pediatr Infect Dis J 18:115–122, 1999.

42. Volovitz B, Welliver RC, De Castro G, et al: The release of leukotrienes in the respiratory tract during infection with respiratory syncytial virus: role in obstructive airway disease. Pediatr Res 24:504–507, 1988.

43. Noah TL, Becker S: Respiratory syncytial virus-induced cytokine production by a human bronchial epithelial cell line. Am J Physiol 265(5 Pt 1):L472–L478, 1993.

44. Csonka P, Kaila M, Laippala P, et al: Oral prednisolone in the acute management of children age 6 to 35 months with viral respiratory infection-induced lower airway disease: a randomized, placebo-controlled trial. J Pediatr 143:725–730, 2003.

45. Schuh S, Coates AL, Binnie R, et al: Efficacy of oral dexamethasone in outpatients with acute bronchiolitis. J Pediatr 140:27–32, 2002.

46. Garrison MM, Christakis DA, Harvey E, et al: Systemic corticosteroids in infant bronchiolitis: a meta-analysis. Pediatrics 105(4):e44, 2000.

47. Corneli HM, Mahajan P, Shaw KN, et al; Pediatric Emergency Care Applied Research Network: Oral dexamethasone in bronchiolitis: a multi-center randomized controlled trial. Paper presented at the American Academy of Pediatrics National Convention and Exhibition, Atlanta, October 2006.

48. Groothuis JR, Woodin KA, Katz R, et al: Early ribavirin treatment of respiratory syncytial viral infection in high-risk children. J Pediatr 117:792–798, 1990.

49. Smith DW, Frankel LR, Mathers LH, et al: A controlled trial of aerosolized ribavirin in infants receiving mechanical ventilation for severe respiratory syncytial virus infection. N Engl J Med 325:24–29, 1991.

50. Ventre K, Randolph A: Ribavirin for respiratory syncytial virus infection of the lower respiratory tract in infants and young children. Cochrane Database Syst Rev (4):CD000181, 2004.

51. Reduction of respiratory syncytial virus hospitalization among premature infants and infants with bronchopulmonary dysplasia using respiratory syncytial virus immune globulin prophylaxis. The PREVENT Study Group. Pediatrics 99:93–99, 1997.

52. Rodriguez WJ, Gruber WC, Groothuis JR, et al: Respiratory syncytial virus immune globulin treatment of RSV lower respiratory tract infection in previously healthy children. Pediatrics 100:937–942, 1997.

53. Rodriguez WJ, Gruber WC, Welliver RC, et al: Respiratory syncytial virus (RSV) immune globulin intravenous therapy for RSV lower respiratory tract infection in infants and young children at high risk for severe RSV infections. Respiratory Syncytial Virus Immune Globulin Study Group. Pediatrics 99:454–461, 1997.

54. Hollman G, Shen G, Zeng L, et al: Helium-oxygen improves Clinical Asthma Scores in children with acute bronchiolitis. Crit Care Med 26:1731–1736, 1998.

55. Martinon-Torres F, Rodriguez-Nunez A, Martinon-Sanchez JM: Heliox therapy in infants with acute bronchiolitis. Pediatrics 109:68–73, 2002.

56. Chipps BE, Sullivan WF, Portnoy JM: Alpha-2$_A$-interferon for treatment of bronchiolitis caused by respiratory syncytial virus. Pediatr Infect Dis J 12:653–658, 1993.
57. Kong XT, Fang HT, Jiang GQ, et al: Treatment of acute bronchiolitis with Chinese herbs. Arch Dis Child 68:468–471, 1993.
58. Luchetti M, Casiraghi G, Valsecchi R, et al: Porcine-derived surfactant treatment of severe bronchiolitis. Acta Anaesthesiol Scand 42:805–810, 1998.
59. Van Bever HP, Desager KN, Pauwels JH, et al: Aerosolized furosemide in wheezy infants: a negative report. Pediatr Pulmonol 20:16–20, 1995.
60. Nasr SZ, Strouse PJ, Soskolne E, et al: Efficacy of recombinant human deoxyribonuclease I in the hospital management of respiratory syncytial virus bronchiolitis. Chest 120:203–208, 2001.
61. Mandelberg A, Tal G, Witzling M, et al: Nebulized 3% hypertonic saline solution treatment in hospitalized infants with viral bronchiolitis. Chest 123:481–487, 2003.

Chapter 58

Pneumonia

Shari L. Platt, MD

Key Points

Causative pathogens of pneumonia in children can be difficult to identify.

Streptococcus pneumoniae is the most common bacterial cause of pneumonia in children.

Viral causes of pneumonia in children vary based on age and season.

Tachypnea is the most reliable clinical predictor of pneumonia in children.

Laboratory and radiologic testing offers limited diagnostic benefit.

Introduction and Background

Community-acquired pneumonia (CAP) is one of the most common infections in children and is the leading cause of mortality in children worldwide. Acute respiratory illnesses are responsible for more than 5 million fatalities each year in children less than 5 years of age in developing countries. The annual incidence in children less than age 5 is approximately 35 to 40 cases per 1000 in Europe and North America.[1] The mortality rate from pneumonia in children in the United States has declined by 97% from 1939 to 1996.[2] This decline is primarily attributable to the introduction of penicillin in the 1940s. Availability of the measles vaccine and improved access to medical care for poor children, primarily as a result of the Medicaid program, have contributed to further reduction in mortality rates recorded from 1963 to 1985. The rate of pneumonia remains high in developing countries. The World Health Organization (WHO) reported a global annual incidence of clinical pneumonia in children less than 5 years of age estimated to be 146.5 million new cases in developing countries and 2.1 million new cases in developed countries.[3] The definition of clinical pneumonia for the purpose of the WHO estimates encompasses pneumonia, bronchiolitis, and reactive airways disease associated with respiratory infections.

Recognition and Approach

Probably the greatest challenge in the approach to children with pneumonia is that the microbiologic etiology is difficult to identify. This is primarily due to limitations of diagnostic testing modalities: blood cultures, antigen testing and antibody titers, and the need for invasive means to retrieve specimens.[1,4] Two studies illustrate our limited ability to diagnose the etiology of pneumonia in children. In a prospective study of 168 *ambulatory* children with CAP, an etiologic agent was identified in only 43% of cases.[5] These included *Streptococcus pneumoniae* (27%), *Mycoplasma pneumoniae* (7%) and *Chlamydia pneumoniae* (6%). Patients with *S. pneumoniae* frequently had a mixed infection (40%). Of 157 patients tested for viral infection, 20% were positive by culture and/or direct fluorescent antibody test. Viral etiologies identified included respiratory syncytial virus (RSV), influenza viruses A and B, parainfluenza viruses 1 and 3, adenovirus, enterovirus, cytomegalovirus, and herpes simplex virus. All viral isolates were identified in children less than 8 years of age.[5] A similar study, in 254 *hospitalized* children with CAP, identified a potential causative agent in 85% of cases.[6] Extensive diagnostic testing accounted for the relatively high yield in this study. Similar etiologies identified, in decreasing frequency of occurrence, included *S. pneumoniae, Haemophilus influenzae, M. pneumoniae, Moraxella catarrhalis, C. pneumoniae, Streptococcus pyogenes,* and *Chlamydia trachomatis.* Viral etiologies included (most common to least common) RSV, rhinovirus, parainfluenza viruses 1 through 3, adenovirus, influenza virus A and B, coronavirus, human herpesvirus 6, Epstein-Barr virus, and varicella-zoster virus. Mixed viral-bacterial infections were detected in 30% of patients, and 41% of patients had more than one microbiologic agent identified. Of interest, of 93 patients with *S. pneumoniae,* only one had a positive blood culture. The remaining 92 patients were diagnosed based solely on serologic evidence.[6]

A prospective analysis seeking to identify etiologic agents via a pneumolysin-based polymerase chain reaction assay identified a respiratory pathogen in 79% of 154 pediatric patients with lower respiratory tract infection. The most common etiologic agent was *S. pneumoniae* (44%). Of 68 patients with *S. pneumoniae* infection, 18% had a co-infection with another bacteria and 31% had a co-infection with a virus. Atypical agents (*M. pneumoniae* and *C. pneumoniae*) accounted for 22% of all infections (14% and 9%, respectively). The most common viral etiologies included influenza viruses A and B, RSV, parainfluenza viruses 1 through 3, and adenovirus.[7] While *S. pneumoniae* remains the most common bacterial cause for pneumonia in children, atypical infections are emerging as a common respiratory pathogen, particularly in adolescents.[8] In developing countries, aspiration from the upper respiratory tract accounts for nonserotypable *H. influenzae* as a cause of pneumonia in children.[9]

Published data reveal the limitations of diagnostic testing in pneumonia, with nearly 30% to 40% of cases unidentified. To aid management decisions, common patterns of infectious agents exist that help to guide diagnosis and therapy. Age is the most helpful marker for the cause of pediatric pneumonia. When considering age as a factor, *S. pneumoniae* remains the most common agent for all ages, and is reported as a causative agent in 15% to 35% of all childhood pneumonias. The atypical agents *M. pneumoniae* and *C. pneumoniae* are less common in children less than 5 years of age (<10%) and occur in increasing proportions in adolescents, reported as high as 50% in some studies. Viral etiologies, most commonly RSV, adenovirus, and influenza viruses A and B, are most common in infants and children less than 2 years of age (30%). The incidence of viral infection reduces dramatically with age.[1,4,10]

Other factors that aid in identifying the etiology of pneumonia include season and vaccine status. Viral infections, specifically RSV and influenza virus, peak in late fall and winter, though there is little seasonal influence on bacterial causes. Immunization status is also a helpful indicator of disease potential. Influenza infection is less likely if a child has received the influenza vaccine during the same season. *Haemophilus influenzae* type B vaccination eliminates the potential for this infection in children. The conjugated pneumococcal vaccine imparts partial protection from this pathogen as the causative agent.[4,10]

Clinical Presentation

Children with pneumonia present with a variety of clinical findings. Early findings are varied, and most cases present initially with symptoms of an upper respiratory infection. These may include low-grade fevers and rhinorrhea. Intermediate and late findings include fever, tachypnea, and cough. Several studies have sought to identify pneumonia based solely on clinical findings. These studies define the "gold standard" for pneumonia diagnosis as the chest radiograph.[11,12] Tachypnea was defined based on the WHO definition, as follows: in children less than 2 months old, respiratory rate (RR) greater than 60 breaths/min; in children 2 to 12 months old, RR greater than 50 breaths/min; and children older than 12 months, RR greater than 40 breaths/min.[13,14] In 1997, a Canadian task force developed an evidence-based guideline to diagnose pneumonia in children. This guideline states that, although no single clinical finding may accurately diagnose pneumonia, the absence of a cluster of signs, specifically respiratory distress, tachypnea, crackles, and decreased breath sounds, excludes the presence of pneumonia with a sensitivity of 100%.[1] These findings were applied to a cohort of 319 children who had a chest radiograph for possible pneumonia, 20% of whom had radiologic findings consistent with pneumonia. The Canadian guideline had a 45% sensitivity and 66% specificity for the diagnosis of pneumonia when applied to this patient cohort. Additionally, tachypnea was only 10% sensitive and 5% specific in this study.[15]

Despite these findings, several other studies have identified tachypnea as the best clinical indicator. A report on 572 children less than 2 years old, 7% with radiologic signs of pneumonia, defined tachypnea as having a 74% sensitivity and 76% specificity to identify pneumonia.[16] In a trial comparing clinical data to chest radiographs in 110 children, of 59 patients diagnosed with pneumonia, 35 had positive findings on chest radiograph. Of all clinical findings, the sensitivity to diagnose pneumonia was best for tachypnea (74%; specificity 67%), followed by retractions (71%) and rales (46%). Combinations of these improved specificity slightly, but did not improve sensitivity to recognize pneumonia. When the cohort was stratified by age, tachypnea was most sensitive: 83% in the youngest infants (<6 months old).[17] In a prospective study examining RR cutoffs for pediatric patients hospitalized with pneumonia, a RR greater than 57 in infants 2 to 11 months old, a RR greater than 48 in children 1 to 5 years old, and a RR greater than 36 in children more than 5 years old identified severe pneumonia requiring hospitalization.[18] These findings closely parallel the WHO definitions for tachypnea.

A prospective study of 570 children ages 1 to 16 years identified the following risk factors to be statistically significant in predicting pneumonia: history of fever, decreased breath sounds, crackles, retractions, grunting, fever, and tachypnea. A multivariate prediction model including fever, decreased breath sounds, crackles, and tachypnea had a sensitivity of 98%, but only an 8% specificity. Of note, fever and tachypnea alone were 93% sensitive for identifying pneumonia in this study.[19] This highlights the difficulty in predicting pneumonia based solely on clinical evaluation, though fever and tachypnea seem to strongly suggest the potential for lower respiratory infection and warrant further evaluation.

Pulse oximetry has also been examined as a predictor of pneumonia in children. Of 803 children less than 2 years of age who had a chest radiograph performed for respiratory symptoms, 80 (11%) had an opacity suggesting pneumonia. Mean pulse oximetry was not predictive of pneumonia in this cohort.[20] The addition of laboratory studies to aid diagnosis has been evaluated in several ways. A study of 154 hospitalized children with CAP, of whom 79% had an identifiable etiology, compared etiologies of pneumonia with respect to clinical and laboratory findings. This analysis revealed that wheezing was most commonly seen in patients with either a viral or an atypical bacterial etiology (41%) compared to patients who had a bacterial etiology (14%). Laboratory studies showed that bacterial etiologies were more likely to be associated with bandemia and elevated serum procalcitonin compared to viral or atypical causes. A multivariate logistic analysis of all variables identified two predictors of bacterial pneumonia: elevated temperature (>38.4° C) less than 72 hours after admission and presence of a pleural effusion, with a sensitivity of 79% and specificity of 59%.[7] Of 1248 febrile infants less than 60 days of age, three simple variables—rales, RR greater than 60 breaths/min, and absolute band count less than 1500/mm^3—identified 85% of infants with lobar pneumonia (85% sensitivity and 59% specificity).[21] It has been reported that, in a cohort of febrile children, leukocytosis as a sole diagnostic finding may indicate pneumonia, despite a lack of supportive clinical findings. A prospective cohort study of 278 febrile (temperature > 39.0° C) children less than 5 years of age with a white blood count (WBC) greater than 20,000/mm³ identified a lobar infiltrate in 26% of patients (36 of 146) who had a radiograph performed and no signs of pneumonia.[22]

Important Clinical Features and Considerations

Differentiating bacterial and viral causes of pediatric pneumonia remains a challenge to the emergency physician. Since treatment guidelines may be directly influenced by microbiologic causes, identifying bacterial pneumonia is an important goal. As already mentioned, the most helpful differentiating epidemiologic factor is age, since viral causes are more likely in children less than age 2 years; however, there is much overlap. The only clinical finding that correlates with viral infection is wheezing, yet specificity is low.[7] Laboratory evaluation has been used as an adjunct to help differentiate the cause of pneumonia. Serum procalcitonin, C-reactive protein (CRP), and interleukin-6 (IL-6) were measured in 126 children hospitalized for pneumonia. Children with bacterial pneumonia had higher serum procalcitonin and CRP concentrations than children with viral infections, though the specificity was low. If all three markers were elevated, the specificity for bacterial pneumonia was greater than 80%.[23] In a similar study, procalcitonin was found to be more sensitive and specific than CRP, IL-6, or WBC count for differentiating bacterial and viral causes of pneumonia in hospitalized children.[24] Despite these studies, procalcitonin has not become a widely used test in the evaluation of a child with pneumonia.

Radiographs have not been traditionally thought to be helpful in distinguishing viral from bacterial pneumonia, though alveolar infiltrates are suggestive of a bacterial etiology.[25-27] A systematic literature review of five studies examined this relationship and reported a low sensitivity and specificity of chest radiography in the identification of a bacterial etiology.[28] These studies are limited since there is no reliable reference standard. As mentioned previously, identifying the microbiologic etiology of childhood pneumonia is difficult, and therefore it is problematic to assess the diagnostic capability of a radiograph related to the microbiologic etiology; as a result, the test accuracy estimate of the radiograph may be falsely low.[28] A prospective report examined the influence of laboratory tests, specifically the WBC count, erythrocyte sedimentation rate, and serum CRP, in combination with the radiograph to aid in diagnostic capability.[29] In 254 children admitted to the hospital with pneumonia, a bacterial etiology was identified in 53%. Of these, 72% had an alveolar infiltrate (most commonly lobar) compared to 49% of patients with a viral infection. There was no difference between etiologies in patients with an interstitial infiltrate; 50% identified a bacterial etiology. Though there remains a fair amount of overlap, this study supports the finding that a lobar alveolar pattern is more likely to represent a bacterial etiology while an interstitial pattern does not differentiate between viral and bacterial infections. An elevated CRP (>80 mg/dl) suggested a bacterial cause (72% sensitivity and 52% specificity); however, laboratory findings did not significantly enhance the sensitivity of the radiograph in identifying a cause for pneumonia.[29]

Radiographic findings of focal consolidation suggest a bacterial etiology for pneumonia, although an atypical pneumonia (*Mycoplasma*) may also be represented, illustrating the lack of specificity to differentiate cause by radiograph findings alone. This overlap is exemplified when looking at a diffuse interstitial pattern. Given the proper clinical setting, atelectasis due to reactive airways disease may be indistinguishable from a viral or atypical process manifesting as a diffuse interstitial pattern. A unique finding that strongly supports a bacterial etiology is a "round pneumonia," which appears as a circular lesion in the retrocardiac area. A round pneumonia is most commonly caused by *S. pneumoniae* in children. Other possible infections include *H. influenzae, M. tuberculosis,* and *Klebsiella.* In the case of occult pneumonia in febrile children with leukocytosis,[22] round pneumonia is often discovered, despite few clinical respiratory findings.

In an effort to reduce radiation exposure and cost, the utility of the lateral chest radiograph was recently examined. In a review of 1268 children who had a chest radiograph, 19% with pneumonia, radiologists found the frontal view alone to have a sensitivity of 85% and specificity of 98% to diagnose pneumonia.[30] Pediatric emergency physicians found no difference in the sensitivity or specificity for identifying pneumonia on radiograph with or without the lateral view (91% vs. 87% sensitivity and 58% vs. 57% specificity, respectively).[31] The lateral view adds little diagnostic information for patients with lobar infiltrates; however, it may aid in diagnosing pneumonia in a small number of patients with a nonlobar infiltrate seen on the frontal view.

A systematic review identified a single trial examining the utility of the chest radiograph in diagnosing pneumonia in children. In 522 ambulatory children less than 5 years of age with a clinical diagnosis of pneumonia, there was no difference in outcome (time to recovery) when comparing children who had and did not have a chest radiograph performed.[32,33] Children who had a chest radiograph performed were more likely to receive antibiotic therapy and to be admitted to the hospital. When considering cost, inconvenience, and potential adverse effects associated with the chest radiograph, routine use of the chest radiograph in a child with suspected pneumonia is discouraged if the clinical presentation and management issues are straightforward.

While there are no reported studies examining clinical signs and symptoms of pneumonia and a negative chest radiograph in children, there is one report in the adult literature. A cohort of 2706 patients with clinically suspected CAP found only 1795 (66%) with radiographic confirmation of disease. Of the 34% of patients with a normal radiograph, only 7% developed a consolidation within 72 hours of presentation. There were no differences in pulmonary symptoms, laboratory testing, or mortality risk. The patients with a confirmed consolidation were more likely to have *S. pneumoniae* bacteremia (64%) compared to 14% of patients with no consolidation. Of patients with a consolidation, 92% of these were in the lower lobe and 25% also had a pleural effusion.[34] In children, the presence of tachypnea, rales, and fever suggests pneumonia, regardless of radiographic findings, but there are no well-established studies to support a diagnosis of clinical pneumonia in children. Management options may be based on clinical severity and reliability of the patient for follow-up. If a patient is only mildly ill and will reliably follow up, no antibiotic therapy is recommended. At follow-up, a repeat radiograph may be performed or antibiotic treatment initiated if clinically indicated. If at the initial visit the patient is moderate to severely ill and/or follow-up is not guaranteed, then appropriate antibiotic therapy may be initiated based on the age of the patient and pattern of infection.

The most common impersonator of pneumonia in children is atelectasis associated with reactive airways disease, asthma, and/or bronchiolitis. Fever or markers of inflammation do not help to differentiate pneumonia, since patients with reactive airways disease may have fever and/or inflammation due to atelectasis or upper respiratory tract infection. As reported previously, wheezing is unlikely in patients with typical bacterial infections; however, atypical causes such as M. pneumoniae or C. pneumoniae should be considered. Foreign bodies may also mimic pneumonia; however, a high suspicion for aspiration or history of choking, unilateral hyperaeration, or asymmetric breath sounds may suggest the need for further investigation.[35]

The risk of bacteremia remains a consideration in children with pneumonia. In 86 patients with findings suggestive of a bacterial process (temperature > 40° C, lobar infiltrate on chest radiograph, WBC count > 20,000/mm[3] or absolute band count > 2000/mm[3], ill appearance, tachypnea, tachycardia, or otitis media), only 1 had a bacterial pathogen (H. influenzae) isolated by blood culture.[36] These findings are supported in additional studies with similarly low rates of bacteremia in pediatric patients with pneumonia. These studies support the lack of utility of blood cultures in patients with pneumonia, and suggest that they be reserved for the child who is toxic and/or ill appearing, is immunocompromised, has an underlying illness, or has not responded to conventional therapy.

The most common complications of pneumonia in children include necrosis, empyema, parapneumonic effusion, and lung abscess. A multicenter, retrospective study involving eight children's hospitals in the United States examined 368 hospitalized children with pneumococcal pneumonia. Of these, 133 were complicated cases and required thoracostomy drainage. The frequency of complicated cases increased during the study period from 23% in 1994 to 53% in 1999. Patients with complicated pneumonia were older (mean age 45 vs. 27 months) and more likely to be of white race and to present with chest pain. Ninety-eight percent of all patients recovered completely from the pneumonia. Antibiotic resistance was not more prevalent in the complicated patients; however, pneumococcal serotype 1 was responsible for 24% of the complicated cases and only 4% of the noncomplicated cases.[37] Pneumococcal serotype 1 is not included in the heptavalent pneumococcal conjugate vaccine, and therefore the vaccine may have a smaller impact upon the incidence of complicated pneumonia than anticipated. The issue of serotype surveillance, particularly in complicated pneumonia, remains an important component of future preventive measures.

Management

The British Thoracic Society has published an evidence-based guideline for treatment of childhood pneumonia.[38,39] Their consensus confirms a lack of good supporting evidence for management decisions. Treatment studies have small patient numbers, high recovery rates for both therapy modalities, and do not examine harm. Furthermore, the strategy to study nontreatment of a child with pneumonia is challenging.

Currently, the treatment of a child with CAP is based upon the clinical presentation and the presumed etiologic agent. Since identification of the etiologic agent remains difficult, antibiotic therapy is empirical in most cases and certainly most often in the emergency department. The reported use of antibiotics ranges from 10% to 45% to treat undifferentiated lower respiratory tract infections despite a likely viral etiology.[40-44] The issue of overuse of antibiotics is concerning, and antibiotic resistance continues to rise. Observation and close follow-up without antibiotic treatment is strongly recommended in children with a presumed viral etiology or who are relatively well appearing with only mild respiratory symptoms, as long as there is reliable follow-up.

In children who are moderately ill and/or have a presumed bacterial source of infection, antibiotics may be initiated. Since the causative pathogen is rarely known, and radiologic features do not distinguish etiology, the choice of antibiotics is based on established patterns of infection related to age and clinical findings. Several studies have found little difference in outcome when comparing different treatment modalities. One study of 88 children less than 5 years of age with pneumonia compared treatment with azithromycin and amoxicillin-clavulanate and found no difference in effectiveness. The same study compared treatment with azithromycin to erythromycin estolate in 59 children older than 5 years with pneumonia and also found no difference in outcome. Four children failed treatment, but there was no difference in failure rates among the different antibiotic regimens. Adverse events were recorded in 67% of patients who received amoxicillin-clavulanate, 25% who received erythromycin, and in 14% who received azithromycin. The most common adverse events were diarrhea and rash.[5] Another study supports the use of azithromycin for pediatric bacterial pneumonia, both classic and atypical patterns.[45] Oral azithromycin is found to be well tolerated with very few treatment-related adverse events.[46,47]

The choice of an antibiotic regimen is guided by age, severity of illness, and likelihood of a bacterial pathogen (Table 58–1).[1,5,37,39,48,49] Parenteral therapy is indicated for children who require hospitalization and who are unable to tolerate oral medication. In these cases, ampicillin or a second-generation cephalosporin (e.g., cefuroxime) is recommended. In hospitalized children 5 years and older, the addition of an oral macrolide is recommended. Replacement by an appropriate oral agent may be initiated after 2 to 4 days of clinical improvement, with resolution of fever and the ability to tolerate oral medication.[1]

Since empirical antibiotic therapy is so commonly initiated, the role for extensive microbiologic testing is of questionable value. In a prospective study of 153 hospitalized children with acquired pneumonia, only 9% had fever lasting more than 48 hours after onset of antibiotic treatment. Of these, most had RSV and H. influenzae infection, with more than half identified as mixed viral-bacterial etiologies. At follow-up, 94% of all patients showed no pneumonia-related symptoms. There is no role for expensive microbiologic testing in otherwise healthy children with CAP since most make a rapid, uneventful recovery after a brief hospital stay and short course of antibiotics, regardless of etiology.[50]

Table 58-1	Guidelines for Antibiotic Regimen for Community-Acquired Pneumonia in Children		
Age	Most Common Bacterial Pathogen	First-Line Therapy	Second-Line Therapy
<5 yr	Streptococcus pneumoniae	Amoxicillin (high dose: 80–90 mg/kg/day)	Second- or third-generation cephalosporin Amoxicillin-clavulanate Macrolide*
5 yr and older	Mycoplasma pneumoniae, Chlamydia pneumoniae	Macrolide	Second- or third-generation cephalosporin
All ages			
	Staphylococcus aureus	Macrolide Nafcillin	Vancomycin
	Penicillin-resistant S. pneumoniae	Amoxicillin Amoxicillin-clavulanate	Nafcillin
Hospitalized children			
<5 yr		Ampicillin IV	Second- or third-generation cephalosporin IV
5 yr and older		Ampicillin IV Add oral or IV macrolide	Second- or third-generation cephalosporin IV Add oral or IV macrolide

*Azithromycin, clarithromycin, or erythromycin.

The heptavalent pneumococcal vaccine was introduced in 2000, and showed 97% effectiveness in reducing invasive pneumococcal disease in children less than 5 years of age based on results from the Kaiser Permanente effectiveness trial of over 36,000 children.[51] Utilizing the same patient database, the overall incidence of positive radiographic pneumococcal pneumonia in children was reported to be reduced by 18% in immunized children, with a 32% reduction in children less than 1 year of age and a 23% reduction in children less than 2 years of age. There was no difference in children older than 2 years of age.[52]

Children with the following clinical signs and symptoms should be considered for hospital admission regardless of the decision to initiate antibiotic therapy as they may require more intensive monitoring[1]: age less than 6 months, toxic appearance, severe respiratory distress, need for supplemental oxygen, dehydration, vomiting, no response to appropriate oral antimicrobial therapy, immunocompromised status, noncompliant caregiver, and presence of bilobar pneumonia.

Summary

Despite how commonly it occurs, childhood pneumonia continues to challenge the practitioner. Diagnostic testing and identification of the causative agent are limited. Routine blood tests and/or cultures are not recommended since they provide little information. Radiologic testing does not differentiate between viral and bacterial causes of pneumonia. A clinical diagnostic approach is applied for most patients, with tachypnea as the most reliable predictor of pneumonia. Wheezing suggests an atypical or viral etiology. Empirical therapy is discouraged for mildly ill children with pneumonia due to the concern for antibiotic resistance. Antimicrobial therapy is recommended for children in whom a bacterial etiology is strongly suspected or who are moderately to severely ill.

REFERENCES

*1. Jadavji T, Law B, Lebel M, et al: A practical guide for the diagnosis and treatment of pediatric pneumonia. CMAJ 156(Suppl):S703–S711, 1997.

*Selected readings.

2. Dowell SF, Kupronis BA, Zell ER, Shay DK: Mortality from pneumonia in children in the United States, 1939 through 1996. N Engl J Med 342:1399–1407, 2000.
3. Rudan I, Tomaskovic L, Boschi-Pinto C, Campbell H; WHO Child Health Epidemiology Reference Group: Global estimate of the incidence of clinical pneumonia among children under five years of age. Bull World Health Organ 82:895–903, 2004.
*4. McCracken GH: Etiology and treatment of pneumonia. Pediatr Infect Dis J 19:373–377, 2000.
*5. Wubbell L, Muniz L, Ahmed A, et al: Etiology and treatment of community-acquired pneumonia in ambulatory children. Pediatr Infect Dis J 18:98–104, 1999.
6. Juven T, Mertsola J, Waris M, et al: Etiology of community-acquired pneumonia in 254 hospitalized children. Pediatr Infect Dis J 19:293–298, 2000.
*7. Michelow I, Olsen K, Lozano J, et al: Epidemiology and clinical characteristics of community-acquired pneumonia in hospitalized children. Pediatrics 113:701–707, 2004.
8. Hammerschlag MR: Pneumonia due to Chlamydia pneumoniae in children: epidemiology, diagnosis and treatment. Pediatr Pulmonol 36:384–390, 2003.
9. Shann F: Haemophilus influenzae pneumonia: type b or non-type b? Lancet 354:1488–1490, 1999.
10. Nelson JD: Community-acquired pneumonia in children: guidelines for treatment. Pediatr Infect Dis J 19:251–253, 2000.
*11. McCracken GH: Diagnosis and management of pneumonia in children. Pediatr Infect Dis J 19:924–928, 2000.
12. Ruuskanen O, Mertsola J: Childhood community-acquired pneumonia. Semin Respir Infect 14:163–172, 1999.
13. Programme for the Control of Acute Respiratory Infections: Case Management of Acute Respiratory Infections in Children in Developing Countries: Report of a Working Group Meeting (WHO/RSD/85.15). Geneva: World Health Organization, 1984.
14. The WHO Young Infants Study Group: Serious infection in young infants in developing countries: rationale for a multi-center study. Pediatr Infect Dis J 18(10 Suppl):S4–S7, 1999.
15. Rothrock SG, Green SM, Fanelli JM, et al: Do published guidelines predict pneumonia in children presenting to an urban ED? Pediatr Emerg Care 17:240–243, 2001.
16. Taylor JA, Del Beccaro M, Done S, Winters W: Establishing clinically relevant standards for tachypnea in febrile children younger than 2 years. Arch Pediatr Adolesc Med 149:283–287, 1995.
17. Palafox M, Guiscafre H, Reyes H, et al: Diagnostic value of tachypnea in pneumonia defined radiologically. Arch Dis Child 82:41–45, 2000.
18. Nascimento-Carvalho CM, Benguigui Y: Evaluation of the degree of tachypnea for hospitalizing children with pneumonia. Indian Pediatr 41:175–179, 2004.
*19. Lynch T, Platt R, Gouin S, et al: Can we predict which children with clinically suspected pneumonia will have the presence of focal infiltrates on chest radiographs? Pediatrics 113:e186–e189, 2004.

20. Tanen DA, Trocinski DR: The use of pulse oximetry to exclude pneumonia in children. Am J Emerg Med 20:521–523, 2002.

21. Platt SL, Levine DA, Fefferman N, et al: Predictors of pneumonia in young febrile infants [Abstract]. Acad Emerg Med 11:437–438, 2004.

22. Bachur R, Perry H, Harper MB: Occult pneumonias: empiric chest radiographs in febrile children with leukocytosis. Ann Emerg Med 33:166–173, 1999.

23. Toikka P, Irjala K, Juven T, et al: Serum procalcitonin, C-reactive protein and interleukin-6 for distinguishing bacterial and viral pneumonia in children. Pediatr Infect Dis J 19:598–602, 2000.

24. Moulin F, Raymond J, Lorrot M, et al: Procalcitonin in children admitted to hospital with community acquired pneumonia. Arch Dis Child 84:332–336, 2001.

25. Korppi M, Kiekara O, Heiskanen-Kosma T, Soimakallio S: Comparison of radiological findings and microbial aetiology of childhood pneumonia. Acta Paediatr 82:360–363, 1993.

26. Wahlgren H, Mortensson W, Eriksson M, et al: Radiographic patterns and viral studies in childhood pneumonia at various ages. Pediatr Radiol 25:627–630, 1995.

27. Kauppinen MT, Lahde S, Syrjala H: Roentgenographic findings of pneumonia caused by *Chlamydia pneumoniae*: a comparison with *Streptococcus* pneumonia. Arch Intern Med 156:1851–1856, 1996.

28. Swigler GH: Radiologic differentiation between bacterial and viral lower respiratory infection in children: a systematic literature review. Clin Pediatr 39:627–633, 2000.

29. Virkki R, Juven T, Rikalainen H, et al: Differentiation of bacterial and viral pneumonia in children. Thorax 57:438–441, 2002.

30. Rigsby CK, Strife JL, Johnson ND, et al: Is the frontal radiograph alone sufficient to evaluate for pneumonia in children? Pediatr Radiol 34:379–383, 2004.

31. Lynch T, Gouin S, Larson C, Patenaude Y: Does the lateral chest radiograph help pediatric emergency physicians diagnose pneumonia? A randomized clinical trial. Acad Emerg Med 11:625–629, 2004.

32. Swigler GH, Hussey GD, Zwarenstein M: Randomised controlled trial of clinical outcome after chest radiograph in ambulatory acute lower respiratory infection in children. Lancet 351:404–408, 1998.

33. Swigler GH, Zwarenstein M: Chest radiograph in acute respiratory infections in children. Cochrane Database Syst Rev (2):CD001268, 2000.

34. Basi SK, Marrie TJ, Huang JQ, et al: Patients admitted to hospital with suspected pneumonia and normal chest radiographs: epidemiology, microbiology and outcomes. Am J Med 117:305–311, 2004.

35. Zerella JT, Dimler M, McGill LC, Pippus KJ: Foreign body aspiration in children: value of radiography and complications of bronchoscopy. J Pediatr Surg 33:1651–1654, 1998.

36. Bonadio WA: Bacteremia in febrile children with lobar pneumonia and leukocytosis. Pediatr Emerg Care 4:241–242, 1988.

*37. Tan TQ, Mason EO, Wald ER, et al: Clinical characteristics of children with complicated pneumonia caused by *Streptococcus pneumoniae*. Pediatrics 110:1–6, 2002.

*38. BTS guidelines for the management of community acquired pneumonia in childhood. Thorax 57(Suppl 1):1–24, 2002.

39. Kumar P, McKean MC: Evidence based paediatrics: review of BTS guidelines for the management of community acquired pneumonia in children. J Infect 48:134–138, 2004.

40. Davy T, Dick PT, Munk P: Self-reported prescribing of antibiotics for children with undifferentiated acute respiratory tract infections with cough. Pediatr Infect Dis J 17:457–462, 1998.

41. Le Saux N, Bjornson C, Pitters C: Antimicrobial use in febrile children diagnosed with respiratory tract illness in an emergency department. Pediatr Infect Dis J 18:1078–1080, 1999.

42. Arnold SR, Allen UD, Al-Zahrani M, et al: Antibiotic prescribing by pediatricians for respiratory tract infection in children. Clin Infect Dis 29:312–317, 1999.

43. Kozyrskyj AL, Dahl ME, Chateau DG, et al: Evidence-based prescribing of antibiotics for children: role of socioeconomic status and physician characteristics. CMAJ 171:139–145, 2004.

44. Kozyrskyj AL, Carrie AG, Mazowita GB, et al: Decrease in antibiotic use among children in the 1990s: not all antibiotics, not all children. CMAJ 171:133–138, 2004.

45. Kogan R, Martinez AM, Rubilar LF, et al: Comparative randomized trial of azithromycin versus erythromycin and amoxicillin for treatment of community acquired pneumonia in children. Pediatr Pulmonol 35:91–98, 2003.

46. Ruuskanen O: Safety and tolerability of azithromycin in pediatric infectious diseases: 20 year update. Pediatr Infect Dis J 23(2 Suppl):s135–s139, 2004.

47. Langley JM, Halperin SA, Boucher FD, Smith B; Pediatric Investigators Collaborative Network on Infections in Canada (PICNIC): Azithromycin is as effective as and better tolerated than erythromycin estolate for the treatment of pertussis. Pediatrics 114:e96–e101, 2004.

48. Harris JA, Kolokathis A, Campbell M, et al: Safety and efficacy of azithromycin in the treatment of community-acquired pneumonia in children. Pediatr Infect Dis J 17:865–871, 1998.

49. Russell G: Community-acquired pneumonia. Arch Dis Child 85:445–446, 2001.

50. Juven T, Mertsola J, Waris M, et al: Clinical response to antibiotic therapy for community acquired pneumonia. Eur J Pediatr 163:140–144, 2004.

51. Black S, Shinefield H, Ray P, et al: Efficacy of heptavalent conjugate pneumococcal vaccine (Wyeth-Lederle) in 37,000 infants and children: impact on pneumonia, otitis media, and an update on invasive disease. Results of the Northern California Kaiser Permanente Efficacy Trial [Abstract 1398]. Presented at the 39th ICAAC, San Francisco, September 1999.

*52. Black SB, Shinefield HR, Ling S, et al: Effectiveness of heptavalent pneumococcal conjugate vaccine in children younger than five years of age for prevention of pneumonia. Pediatr Infect Dis J 21:810–815, 2002.

Chapter 59

Cystic Fibrosis

Eron Y. Friedlaender, MD, MPH

Key Points

Emergency physicians must be prepared both to manage acute complications of disease and to recognize signs and symptoms of undiagnosed disease in cystic fibrosis patients.

Given that cystic fibrosis is a progressive disease, signs and symptoms change with age.

Complications of cystic fibrosis are potentially life threatening; early identification and aggressive interventions in the acute care setting are essential for improving outcome.

Introduction and Background

Prompt recognition of complications and timely institution of aggressive treatment is essential for decreasing morbidity and mortality in cystic fibrosis (CF) patients. While investigation into correction of the underlying genetic defects responsible for the expression of disease holds promise,[1] current management of patients with CF in acute care settings must focus on relief of symptoms and correction of organ dysfunction. The emergency physician must appreciate the spectrum of multiorgan dysfunction and be familiar with available interventions.

Recognition and Approach

CF is the most common inherited lethal condition among whites in most Western countries. In the United States, the estimated frequency is 1 in 3200 white live births.[2] Most cases represent transmission of an autosomal recessive disorder in which a single gene mutation on the long arm of chromosome 7, where the cystic fibrosis transmembrane conductance regulator (CFTR) is encoded, is responsible for expression of the disease.[3-5]

Patients with CF experience generalized dysfunction of all exocrine gland secretions. This results in viscous mucoid secretions that obstruct normal functioning of the respira-

tory and gastrointestinal tracts. In addition, identification of the characteristic electrolyte losses (predominantly sodium and chloride) from altered absorption within sweat glands, especially in the context of well-described clinical features, allows for diagnosis of CF in affected individuals. The manifestations and severity of disease vary significantly from individual to individual,[6] posing challenges to practitioners in recognition of the disease and predicting complications.

Clinical Presentation

The diagnosis of CF is largely based on clinical criteria rather than genetic testing (Table 59–1). The Cystic Fibrosis Foundation Consensus Panel issued guidelines, later supported by recommendations from the World Health Organization, on which to base the clinical diagnosis of CF. They also provide guidance on the appropriate use and interpretation of laboratory tests to confirm CFTR dysfunction.[7-10] Despite the availability of prenatal and neonatal screening,[11,12] only a minority of affected individuals are identified through these programs; most are recognized upon presentation with defining clinical features.[8,13-15]

Although many clinical presentations are consistent with the diagnosis of CF, the classic triad is defined as chronic pulmonary disease, malabsorption due to pancreatic insufficiency, and elevated concentrations of sweat electrolytes.[6,14] However, few undiagnosed patients present acutely with this constellation of findings. Furthermore, emergency medicine physicians are not positioned to make a definitive diagnosis of cystic fibrosis given the nature of confirmatory testing, but should be familiar with the clinical features that would prompt referral for ultimate definitive diagnosis. In the pediatric population, commonly associated, although nonspecific, signs and symptoms of undiagnosed CF include failure to thrive despite adequate caloric intake, persistent cough, chronic pneumonia, jaundice or conjugated hyperbilirubinemeia, hypochloremic alkalosis, rectal prolapse (Fig. 59–1), nasal polyposis (Fig. 59–2), unexplained cirrhosis, and malabsorption manifested by either chronic diarrhea, milk allergy, or vitamin K deficiency.[8,13,14] In patients with known disease, familiarity with complications of CF and initiation of management is expected knowledge for emergency physicians as many of these processes are potentially life-threatening or disabling without intervention.

Table 59–1	Clinical Features of Cystic Fibrosis (CF)

Chronic Sinopulmonary Disease
Persistent cough
Airway colonization or infection with *Staphylococcus aureus* or *Pseudomonas aeruginosa*
Endobronchial disease
Pansinusitis
Nasal polyposis
Gastrointestinal/Nutritional Disease
Meconium ileus
Distal intestinal obstruction syndrome
Pancreatic insufficiency
   Malabsorption (exocrine dysfunction)
   CF-related diabetes (endocrine dysfunction)
Recurrent pancreatitis
Rectal prolapse
Biliary cirrhosis
Failure to thrive (protein-calorie malnutrition)
Deficiency of vitamins A, D, E, and K
Metabolic Disease
Hypochloremia
Hyponatremia
Metabolic alkalosis
Musculoskeletal Disease
Pathologic bone fractures
Kyphosis
Infertility/Obstructive Azoospermia

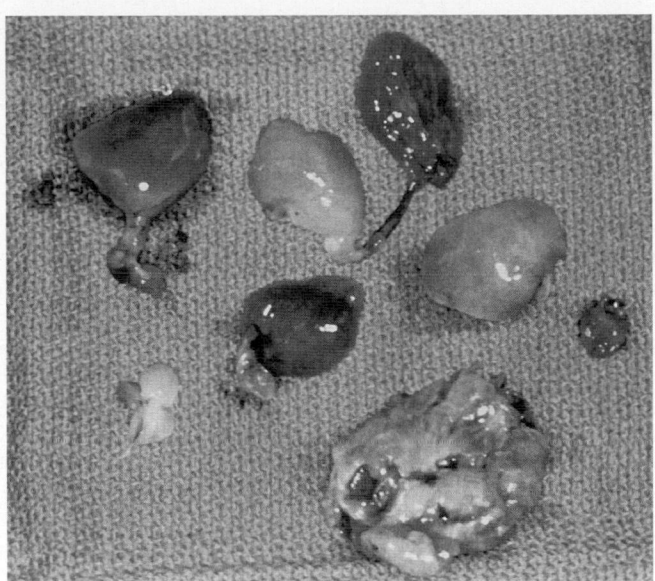

FIGURE 59–2. Nasal polyp.

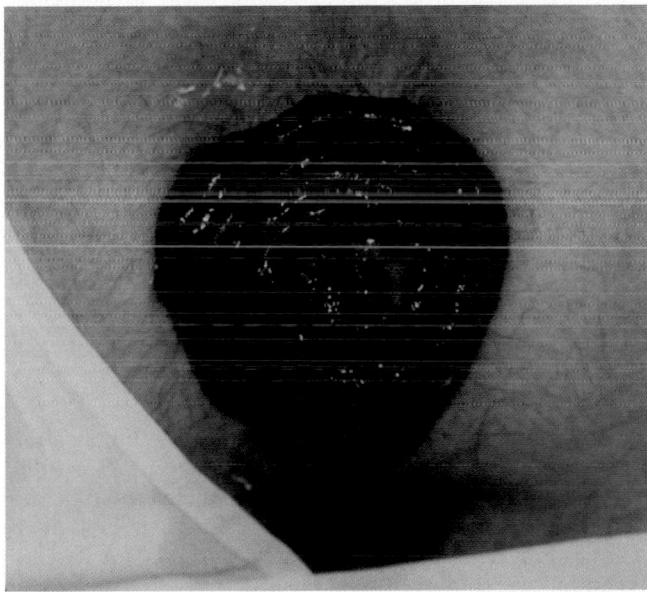

FIGURE 59–1. Rectal prolapse.

Important Clinical Features and Considerations

Emergency management of patients with CF largely revolves around disease complications rather than diagnosis. Many of these complications are age specific and share management techniques applicable to a number of different disease states. Most conditions requiring emergency intervention relate to either pulmonary or sinus disease, gastrointestinal disorders, metabolic derangements, or musculoskeletal complaints.

Pulmonary or Sinus Disease

The predominant pulmonary conditions acutely compromising the health of CF patients include pneumothorax, pulmonary hemorrhage, pulmonary exacerbations, cor pulmonale, and respiratory failure. Pneumothorax, resulting from either a pleural tear or rupture of a subpleural bleb during an acute increase in intra-airway or intrapleural pressure, typically presents with the sudden onset of chest pain that may be referred to the shoulder, dyspnea, and cyanosis. It typically occurs in CF patients with advanced pulmonary disease.[16] Hemoptysis results from erosion of an inflamed or infected area of bronchiectatic lung into a bronchial vessel.[14,17] Life-threatening pulmonary hemorrhage occurs with expectoration of more than 300 to 500 ml of fresh blood in 24 hours.[14,18]

Pulmonary exacerbations are characterized by an acute or subacute worsening of obstructive airway disease from bacterial infection and subsequent local inflammatory reactions. Patients may present with increased cough productive of sputum, dyspnea, tachypnea, fever, fatigue, anorexia, weight loss, or hemoptysis.[14] Examination may demonstrate reduced pulmonary function and possibly rales, rhonchi, decreased aeration, and accessory muscle use.[14] Chest radiographs have limited utility in defining pathophysiology of acute disease in CF patients; the airways and submucosal glands rather than the interstitium and alveolar spaces of the lung are predominantly affected.[8] During pulmonary exacerbations, however, peribronchial thickening, patchy infiltrates, or hyperinflation above baseline may be appreciated on plain films.

Patients with advanced lung disease from CF may present with complications related to cor pulmonale[19-21] or respiratory failure.[22] The majority of mortality related to CF is due to respiratory decompensation,[6,23] precipitated by overwhelming bacterial infection, right-sided heart failure, or irreversible obstructive disease compromising oxygenation and ventilation. Pulmonary hypertension develops from long-standing respiratory insufficiency and associated hypoxemia, with subsequent right ventricular hypertrophy. Acute stressors such as pulmonary exacerbations may precipitate congestive heart failure, seen clinically as cyanosis, increased respiratory effort, tachycardia, a gallop rhythm, hepatic congestion, peripheral edema, and ascites. Chest radiography demonstrates cardiomegaly with prominent pulmonary vasculature. Respiratory insufficiency from CF may also require emergent intervention. Patients present with distress related to inability to sufficiently ventilate, defined by hypercarbia and hypoxemia. This may represent the natural progression of disease in end-stage patients or may result from an aggressive infectious process in an individual with otherwise stable disease. Recent evidence has also documented metabolic alkalosis as a precipitant of respiratory failure in adults with CF, and should be considered in the fluid and ventilatory requirements of these patients.[24]

Sinusitis is a common infection of the upper airways of patients with CF. Symptomatic disease presents with facial pain or swelling and air-fluid levels on radiographs.

Gastrointestinal Disorders

Gastrointestinal complications of CF that may require emergent care include meconium ileus, distal intestinal obstruction syndrome (DIOS), rectal prolapse, pancreatic insufficiency, and hepatobiliary disease. Meconium ileus is exclusively a disease of the neonate, typically resulting in intestinal obstruction in the first 48 hours of life. Exceptionally dense intestinal contents resulting from both a failure to secrete water into the intestinal lumen and abnormally viscous mucus cause the impaction, typically at the terminal ileum. Patients present with vomiting, abdominal distention after feeding, visible peristaltic waves across the abdomen, and failure to pass meconium after birth.[25] Abdominal radiographs may show dilated loops of bowel, granular material or calcifications within the intestinal lumen, and an absence of air-fluid levels.[25] A contrast enema may further demonstrate the site of impaction and the resulting microcolon of disuse associated with this condition.[25] Early recognition of meconium ileus is imperative to preventing potential life-threatening complications, including intestinal perforation and volvulus.[25]

DIOS, formerly referred to as meconium ileus equivalent, occurs in older patients (beyond childhood) with CF. This complication is similarly characterized by impaction of abnormally dessicated stool at or near the ileocecal junction.[5,14] Crampy abdominal pain and a mass in the right lower quadrant are suggestive of this process.[5] An obstruction series will demonstrate air-fluid levels and dilated loops of bowel.[5] Complications of DIOS have included intussusception and volvulus.

Rectal prolapse (see Fig. 59–1) may present in young patients with CF suffering from malnutrition and overall poor tissue integrity.[14] In undiagnosed patients, the finding of rectal prolapse, especially when recurrent, warrants outpatient screening for CF given the strong association between the two conditions. Rectal prolapse most often affects children 3 years of age and younger.[5]

Metabolic Derangements

Pancreatic insufficiency manifests as both exocrine and endocrine dysfunction. Given the progressive nature of pancreatic disease in CF, older patients tend to have more severe complications related to abnormal pancreatic function. The majority of patients have some degree of malabsorption due to compromised pancreatic enzyme activity. The loss of exocrine function has been associated with recurrent pancreatitis. Of note, young children who present with failure to thrive and malabsorptive symptoms ought to be evaluated for CF. Endocrine dysfunction, resulting in CF-related diabetes (CFRD), tends to affect an older population: 9% of children with CF, 26% of adolescents, and 35% of individuals 20 to 29 years of age.[26,27] Typical age of onset is 18 to 21 years. CFRD is distinct from both types 1 and 2 diabetes mellitus as both insulin and glucagon secretion are impaired.[26,28] Therefore, ketoacidosis rarely accompanies hyperglycemia.[14,28]

Hepatobiliary disease in CF results in a high frequency of gallstones. In addition, 1% to 3% of patients develop hepatic cirrhosis with associated biliary obstruction and portal hypertension. Uncommonly, esophageal varicies and hepatic failure ensue.

Acute metabolic derangements in patients with CF may develop under conditions in which an individual experiences increased sweating, poor oral intake, or during physical stress, including intercurrent illnesses. Most commonly, hypochloremia, hyponatremia, and a metabolic alkalosis develop.[14,29-32]

Musculoskeletal Problems

Finally, older patients with CF universally suffer from osteopenia and osteoporosis, predisposing them to pathologic bone fractures.[26,28,33] Chronic malnutrition, gonadal dysfunction, physical inactivity, frequent glucocorticoid use during episodes of pulmonary insufficiency, and long-standing respiratory acidosis contribute to the reduced bone density. Specifically, patients with CF have been shown to have significantly higher rates of rib and vertebral fractures.[28,33,34] Kyphosis is a second musculoskeletal complication of CF that results in back pain and disability in a majority of older patients.[26,33]

Management

Pulmonary and Sinus Complications

Immediate management of pulmonary-related complications of CF begins with stabilization of the airway and breathing. In patients with pneumothoraces, this may require tube thoracostomy if the air leak involves greater than 10% of the volume of the hemithorax, or needle decompression if hemodynamics are compromised. Pleural sclerosis (surgical or chemical) or parietal pleurectomy may ultimately be indicated in the inpatient setting as definitive therapy.[17,35,36] Patients with pulmonary hemorrhage require constant monitoring of hemodynamic parameters with aggressive intervention to correct tachycardia or hypotension. Parenteral antibiotics with coverage against staphylococcal and pseudomonal disease must be initiated early as pulmonary hemorrhage may be an indication of bacterial infection.[17,18] In addition, vitamin K at a dose of 5 mg should be administered if the prothrombin time is prolonged, and blood products should be replaced if blood losses are ongoing. Surgical ligation of the bleeding vessel or bronchial artery embolization may be required to manage massive pulmonary hemorrhage.[18,37]

Treatment of pulmonary exacerbations entails antibiotic therapy and aggressive chest physiotherapy.[38] CF patients have characteristic bacterial pathogens acquired in a predicatable, age-dependent sequence.[8] Young children with CF typically are infected with *Haemophilus influenzae, Staphylococcus aureus,* and *Pseudomonas aeruginosa.*[14,39] *Haemophilus influenzae* is most prevalent at ages 2 to 5 years, while *S. aureus* reaches maximum prevalence at ages 6 to 17 years.[8,14] Symptomatic infection with these organisms is best treated on an outpatient basis with trimethoprim-sulfamethoxazole or amoxicillin-clavulanate, or with either a parenteral penicillin (nafcillin or oxacillin) or a first-generation cephalosporin (cefazolin) in patients with severe infection or worsening of symptoms on an outpatient regimen.[8,39] Vancomycin is indicated for patients with suspected or confirmed methicillin-resistant species of *S. aureus. Pseudomonas aeruginosa* reaches 80% prevalence by age 18 years and responds to treatment with an oral quinolone (ciprofloxicin) or, if inpatient care is indicated due to degree of illness, a parenteral β-lactam (ticarcillin) combined with an aminoglycoside (tobramycin or gentamicin).[8,39-41] Of note, many patients with CF have increased renal clearance of antibiotics and thus require more frequent dosing intervals.[14,39] Late-emerging pathogens include *Pseudomonas cepacia, Pseudomonas maltophilia, Alcaligenes xylosoxidans, Aspergillus,* and nontuberculous mycobacteria.[8] Similar pathogens cause sinus infections in patients with CF; therapy should be broad spectrum and include coverage of *Pseudomonas.*[14]

Cor pulmonale and respiratory failure typically present in patients with end-stage disease. Management of the former includes provision of oxygen, diuretics (furosemide),[42] and possibly digitalis. Respiratory failure may respond to initiation of supplemental oxygen and chest physiotherapy with a combination of parenteral antibiotics, bronchodilators, subcutaneous epinephrine, and/or aerosolized recombinant human deoxyribonuclease (rhDNase).[43] Aerosolized hypertonic saline has been promoted as an alternative to the rhDNase, but must be used with caution as it may cause paradoxical bronchospasm.[44] In the event these measures fail to reverse hypoxia and work of breathing, mechanical ventilation must be considered with the knowledge that patients with a history of significant pulmonary insufficiency prior to an acute decompensation have poor outcomes from such interventions.[45]

Gastrointestinal Complications

Gastrointestinal complications of CF may also require emergent management. Meconium ileus rarely presents outside of the newborn nursery; however, with early discharge following delivery, exceptions may occur. These patients should be treated with a diatrizoate methylglucamine enema to break up the impacted fecal material and release the obstruction. If these measures fail, emergent laparotomy is indicated.[46] Similarly, patients with DIOS should be initially managed with a barium, diatrizoate methylglucamine, or saline enema.[14,47] Oral or rectal mineral oil and *N*-acetylcysteine, or the addition of a balanced electrolyte lavage solution containing polyethylene glycol, may also help to relieve the impaction.[5,25] For patients unable to tolerate the large volume required (5 to 6 L for adults), administration through a nasogastric tube at a rate of 20 to 40 ml/kg (maximum 1 L/hr)

may be necessary.[5] Aggressive intravenous hydration must be maintained, with close monitoring of electrolytes, during therapy with serial enemas given the potential for dramatic fluid shifts from the high osmotic load. The enema should be repeated several times prior to resorting to laparotomy given the added morbidity of a surgical procedure. If the patient exhibits signs of peritoneal irritation, however, enemas are contraindicated and surgical consultation should not be delayed.

Rectal prolaspe usually responds to simple manual reduction. The clinician should assess the need for sedation in the young child who resists the maneuver, then place the patient in the knee-chest position, lubricate the prolapsed tissue, and apply firm pressure to the edges of the prolapse, with one finger in the central orifice guiding the reduction until it resolves. Petrolatum gauze should be taped over the anus as a pressure dressing to help prevent recurrence, which is common. Pulmonary consultation as an outpatient is required to adjust pancreatic enzyme replacement and assess nutritional status, with the goal of improving stool bulk and maximizing tissue integrity. Surgical intervention is rarely indicated, unless manual reduction fails or prolapse recurs with such frequency that it is disabling.

Hepatobiliary disease, manifesting usually as gallstones and infrequently as hepatic failure,[14] requires accurate confirmation of the acute process with ultrasound and evidence of biliary obstruction on liver function studies in the former condition and signs of coagulopathy or abnormal synthetic function of albumin in the latter process. Both require supportive care. Patients with gallstones typically require pain control and a low-fat diet, with ultimate surgical consultation as an outpatient for definitive management. In the event the patient has cholecystitis, parenteral antibiotic therapy is necessary. Liver failure represents end-stage disease, and emergency department management is largely supportive in terms of treating coagulopathy and encephalopathy until inpatient care can be arranged.

Metabolic Complications

Exocrine dysfunction from pancreatic insufficiency rarely causes acute issues and may be treated on an outpatient basis with adjustment of pancreatic enzyme replacements and fat-soluble vitamins. Pancreatitis, which may complicate exocrine dysfunction, requires bowel rest and pain control with close monitoring as an inpatient. CFRD requires insulin therapy, either chronically or intermittently if symptoms occur exclusively during periods of physical stress. Often, insulin requirements are significant as many patients with CF exhibit some degree of insulin resistance.[26]

Hypoelectrolytemia requires targeted correction of the specific metabolic derangement with frequent monitoring of serum electrolytes.

Musculoskeletal Complications

Musculoskeletal disease, including discomfort from kyphosis or pathologic bone fractures, requires pain control, splinting if practical, and follow-up with both orthopedic surgery and pulmonary consultants to optimize nutrition, investigate the severity of hypogonadism, initiate an exercise regimen, and consider use of antiresorptive medications such as calcitonin and etidronate.

Summary

Improved outcomes and life expectancies for patients with CF have largely been attributed to early recognition of affected individuals, allowing for timely maintenance care as well as aggressive management of disease complications to be initiated. Familiarity with the signs and symptoms of CF and the most common urgent and emergent complications is essential to reducing the burden of disease imposed by this debilitating condition.

REFERENCES

1. Jaffe A, Bush A, Geddes D, et al: Prospects for gene therapy in cystic fibrosis. Arch Dis Child 80:286–289, 1999.
2. Hamosh A, FitzSimmons S, Macek M, et al: Comparison of the clinical manifestations of cystic fibrosis in black and white patients. J Pediatr 132:255–259, 1998.
3. Collins F: Cystic fibrosis: molecular biology and therapeutic implications. Science 256:774–779, 1992.
4. Kerem B, Rommens J, Buchanan J, et al: Identification of the cystic fibrosis gene: genetic analysis. Science 245:1073–1080, 1989.
5. Shalon L, Adelson J: Cystic fibrosis. Pediatr Clin North Am 43:157–196, 1996.
6. Witt H: Chronic pancreatitis and cystic fibrosis. Gut 52(Suppl II): ii31–ii41, 2003.
*7. Rosenstein BJ, Cutting GR, Cystic Fibrosis Foundation Consensus Panel: The diagnosis of cystic fibrosis: a consensus statement. J Pediatr 132:589–595, 1998.
*8. Gibson R, Burns J, Ramsey B: Pathophysiology and management of pulmonary infections in cystic fibrosis. Am J Respir Crit Care Med 168:918–951, 2003.
9. World Health Organization: Classification of Cystic Fibrosis and Related Disorders (Report No. WHO/CF/HGN/00.2). Stockholm: World Health Organization, 2000.
10. Cystic Fibrosis Foundation Patient Registry: 2001 Annual Data Report to the Center Directors. Bethesda, MD: Cystic Fibrosis Foundation, 2002.
11. Wagener J, Sontag M, Accurso F: Newborn screening for cystic fibrosis. Curr Opin Pediatr 15:309–315, 2003.
12. Farrell M, Farrell P: Newborn screening for cystic fibrosis: ensuring more good than harm. J Pediatr 143:707–712, 2003.
13. Ratjen F, Doring G: Cystic fibrosis. Lancet 361:681–689, 2003.
*14. Davis P: Cystic fibrosis. Pediatr Rev 22:257–264, 2002.
15. Robinson P: Cystic fibrosis. Thorax 56:237–241, 2001.
16. Flume P: Pneumothorax in cystic fibrosis. Chest 1:217–221, 2003.
17. Batra J, Holinger L: Etiology and management of pediatric hemoptysis. Arch Otolaryngol Head Neck Surg 127:377–382, 2001.
18. Stern R, Wood R, Boat T, et al: Treatment and prognosis of massive hemoptysis in cystic fibrosis. Am Rev Respir Dis 117:825–828, 1978.
19. Stern R, Borkat G, Hirschfeld S, et al: Heart failure in cystic fibrosis. Am J Dis Child 134:267–272, 1980.
20. Vizza C, Lynch J, Ochoa L, et al: Right and left ventricular dysfunction in patients with severe pulmonary disease. Chest 113:576–583, 1998.
21. Moss A: The cardiovascular system in cystic fibrosis. Pediatrics 70:728–741, 1982.
22. Berlinski A, Fan L, Kozinetz C, et al: Invasive mechanical ventilation for acute respiratory failure in children with cystic fibrosis: outcome analysis and case-control study. Pediatr Pulmonol 34:297–303, 2002.
23. Ramsey B: Management of pulmonary disease in patients with cystic fibrosis. N Engl J Med 335:179–188, 1996.
24. Holland A, Wilson J, Kotsimbos T, et al: Metabolic alkalosis contributes to acute hypercapnic respiratory failure in adult cystic fibrosis. Chest 124:490–493, 2003.
25. Lewis T, Casey S, Kapur R: Clinical pathologic correlation: a 3-year-old boy with cystic fibrosis and intestinal obstruction. J Pediatr 134:514–519, 1999.
26. Moran A: Endocrine complications of cystic fibrosis. Adolesc Med 13:145–159, 2002.
27. Moran A, Doherty L, Wang X, et al: Abnormal glucose metabolism in cystic fibrosis. J Pediatr 133:10–16, 1998.
28. Nasr S: Cystic fibrosis in adolescents and young adults. Adolesc Med 11:589–603, 2000.
29. Ruddy R, Anolik R, Scanlin T: Hypoelectrolytemia as a presentation and complication of cystic fibrosis. Clin Pediatr 21:367–369, 1983.
30. Mauri S, Pedroli G, Rudeberg A, et al: Acute metabolic alkalosis in cystic fibrosis: prospective study and review of the literature. Miner Electrolyte Metab 23:33–37, 1997.
31. Sojo A, Rodriguez-Soriano J, Vitoria J, et al: Chloride deficiency as a presentation or complication of cystic fibrosis. Eur J Pediatr 153:825–828, 1994.
32. Beckerman R, Taussig L: Hypoelectrolytemia and metabolic alkalosis in infants with cystic fibrosis. Pediatrics 63:580–583, 1979.
33. Aris RM, Renner JB, Winders AD, et al: Increased rate of fractures and severe kyphosis: sequelae of living into adulthood with cystic fibrosis. Ann Intern Med 128:186–193, 1998.
34. Henderson RC, Specter BB: Kyphosis and fractures in children and young adults with cystic fibrosis. J Pediatr 125:208–212, 1994.
35. McLaughlin F, Matthews W, Strieder D: Pneumothorax in cystic fibrosis: management and outcome. J Pediatr 100:863–869, 1982.
36. Spector M, Stern R: Pneumothorax in cystic fibrosis: a 26-year experience. Ann Thorac Surg 47:204–207, 1989.
37. Fellows K, Khaw K, Schuster S, et al: Bronchial artery embolization in cystic fibrosis: technique and long-term results. J Pediatr 95:959–963, 1979.
38. Davidson K: Airway clearance strategies for the pediatric patient. Respir Care 47:823–828, 2002.
*39. Weiner D: Respiratory tract infections in cystic fibrosis. Pediatr Ann 31:116–123, 2002.
40. Hoiby N: New antimicrobials in the management of cystic fibrosis. J Antimicrob Chemother 49:235–238, 2002.
41. Ramsey B: Management of pulmonary disease in patients with cystic fibrosis. N Engl J Med 335:179–188, 1996.
42. Whitman V, Stern R, Doershuk C, et al: Studies on cor pulmonale in cystic fibrosis: I. Effects of diuresis. Pediatrics 55:83–85, 1975.
43. Robinson P: Cystic fibrosis. Thorax 56:237–241, 2001.
44. Doull I: Recent advances in cystic fibrosis. Arch Dis Child 85:62–66, 2001.
45. Davis P, di Sant'Agnese P: Assisted ventilation for patients with cystic fibrosis. JAMA 239:1851–1854, 1978.
46. Del Pin C, Czyrko C, Ziegler M, et al: Management and survival of meconium ileus. Ann Surg 215:179–185, 1992.
47. Shidrawi R, Murugan N, Westaby D, et al: Emergency colonoscopy for distal intestinal obstruction syndrome in cystic fibrosis patients. Gut 51:285–286, 2002.

*Selected readings.

Chapter 60

Upper Airway Disorders

Robert Bruce Wright, MD and Terry P. Klassen, MD

Introduction and Background

Differences in the anatomy of the pediatric airway render children more susceptible to acute airway compromise than adults (see Chapter 2, Respiratory Distress and Respiratory Failure). The narrowed subglottic area of a child's upper airway is completely encircled by cricoid cartilage and restricted in its ability to expand. The subglottic connective tissue can become rapidly edematous, causing further reduction in the airway caliber. Upper airway disorders include infectious, inflammatory, and mechanical conditions that can exacerbate these differences. Many upper airway disorders have similar presenting signs and symptoms and can be diagnosed clinically. The need to differentiate rapidly between various upper airway disorders is paramount to begin definitive therapy, and in some cases may be life saving. For this reason, knowledge of advanced pediatric airway management is a significant part of management (see Chapter 3,

Rapid Sequence Intubation; and Chapter 4, Intubation, Rescue Devices, and Airway Adjuncts).

Selected Diagnoses

Croup
Bacterial tracheitis
Retropharyngeal abscess
Epiglottitis
Foreign bodies

Discussion of Individual Diagnoses

Croup

Croup, otherwise known as laryngotracheobronchitis, is one of the most common causes of infectious upper airway obstruction in children. It primarily affects children between the ages of 6 months and 6 years and is rare after that.[1] Peak occurrence is around age 2, but recurrences are possible. Males are slightly more affected than females (1.4 : 1).[1] The most common etiologic agents are viral, with parainfluenza (types 1 and 3) and respiratory syncytial virus being the most frequent.[1] The estimated health care costs of emergency department (ED) visits and hospitalizations for croup caused by parainfluenza virus are between $20 and $56 million.[2]

Clinical Presentation

Croup can begin as an upper respiratory tract infection (URI) with symptoms of coryza and cough. Fever may or may not be present during the illness, and if present usually ranges from 38° C to 39° C. Approximately 1 to 2 days after URI symptoms have begun, edema in the subglottic area increases and the symptoms of a hoarse voice and barky, "seal-like" cough become predominant. Symptoms usually peak on day 3 or 4 of the illness. Symptoms of croup have traditionally been classified as mild, moderate, or severe according to the Westley Croup Score, devised in 1978.[3] The Westley Croup Score is an aggregate number based on the presence or degree of severity of the following: stridor, retractions, air entry, cyanosis, and level of consciousness; it is used primarily as a research tool. Symptoms of croup are traditionally worse at night and when the child is agitated. Severe cases will have suprasternal and intercostal retractions plus biphasic stridor upon auscultation. Cyanosis is rare in

Table 60–1	Differential Diagnosis of Upper Airway Disorders

Croup
Epiglottitis
Peritonsilar abscess
Uvulitis
Hemangioma
Bacterial tracheitis
Retropharyngeal abscess
Obstruction caused by foreign body
Neoplasms

children even with severe croup. In contrast to children with epiglottitis, the child with croup is not toxic appearing and is usually not drooling. The differential diagnosis of croup and other disorders affecting the upper airway is presented in Table 60–1.

The diagnosis of croup is primarily a clinical one. Additional tests for diagnosis are generally not necessary or recommended. The most common ancillary tool is a radiograph of the soft tissues of the neck when the clinician suspects other diagnostic possibilities, such as foreign body or epiglottitis. The classic presentation of croup on radiograph is the "steeple sign" that results from subglottic edema in moderate to severe disease (Fig. 60–1).

Management

Many children with croup present to the ED, but many are also managed at home without seeking medical attention or are seen in the outpatient setting. Of those who present to the ED, most can be treated briefly and then managed as outpatients. Patients are admitted if they have ongoing symptoms of stridor at rest after appropriate ED management, or the social situation is not safe to allow the child to return home with the current caregivers. This can include poor access to transportation or lack of communication to call for assistance if needed.

The child who presents to the ED has often had cold air exposure, which often improves symptoms. Parents will also mention that they have tried some form of mist therapy prior to arriving in the ED. It is thought that the mist may soothe the inflamed airway, and the comfort of being held by a caregiver while the mist is being given may decrease anxiety and prevent hyperventilation.[4] Three randomized controlled trials have looked at the benefit of mist therapy in the ED.[5-7] The most recent study, by Neto et al.,[7] showed that there was no statistical difference in clinical symptoms when children who were given dexamethasone received mist or no mist therapy in the ED. The authors concluded that mist therapy is of no benefit in the ED.[7]

A systemic review from the Cochrane Library has clearly demonstrated the effectiveness of corticosteroids for the treatment of croup.[8] The most common steroid studied is dexamethasone, but budesonide, methylprednisolone, and fluticasone have also been used in trials. Dexamethasone given at a dose of 0.6 mg/kg results in improvement of croup symptoms within 6 hours and decreases return ED visits and admissions to hospital. Studies have shown no differences between the route of delivery (inhaled, oral, and intramuscular) or type of steroid (dexamethasone, budesonide, or fluticasone) used.

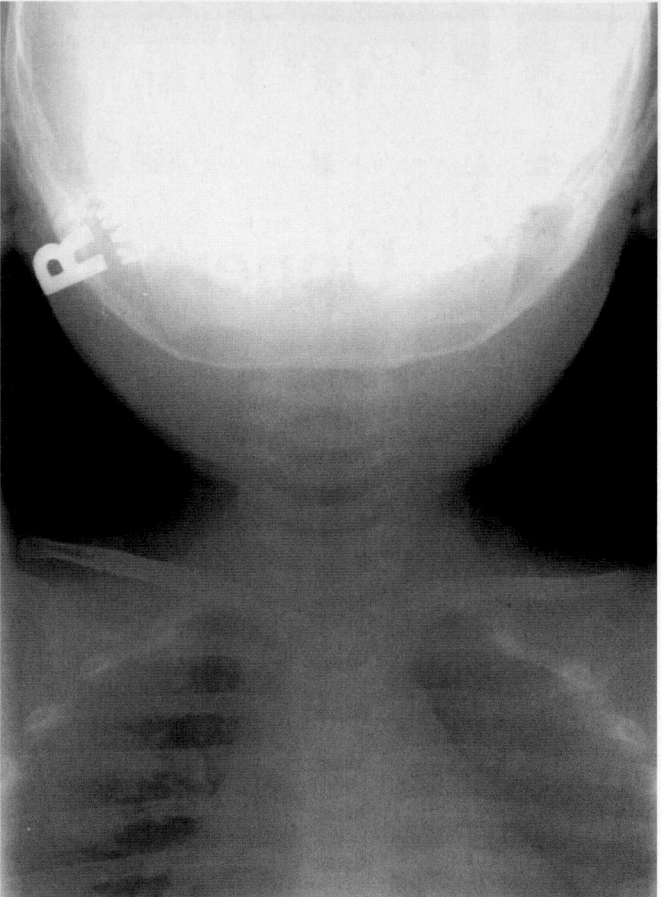

FIGURE 60–1. Soft tissue radiograph of the neck in a patient with croup showing typical subglottic narrowing ("steeple sign").

For mild croup, a recent study[9] demonstrated that those children who received a single dose of dexamethasone (0.6 mg/kg) had a significantly lower chance of returning to medical care. In addition, there was a faster resolution of symptoms and decreased parental anxiety. Based on all of these findings, children who present to the ED with croup symptoms of any severity (mild, moderate, or severe) should receive dexamethasone unless otherwise contraindicated. The dose of dexamethasone has been debated. The majority of studies used a dose of 0.6 mg/kg with a maximum of 10 mg, but some authors have demonstrated effectiveness using doses of 0.15 and 0.3 mg/kg as well.[10]

For children who present with symptoms of moderate to severe croup, racemic epinephrine (2.25%) has been used since 1971.[11] It is postulated that the local vasoconstriction caused by the epinephrine relieves symptoms. A nebulized dose of 0.5 ml of racemic epinephrine mixed with 2.5 ml of normal saline is given over 5 to 10 minutes. Alternatively if racemic epinephrine is not available, 5 ml of L-epinephrine (1 : 1000) may also be nebulized.[12,13] As the effect of either form of epinephrine has been estimated to last approximately 2 hours, the child must be observed in the ED for this time period before discharge. If there is no worsening of symptoms within 2 to 3 hours, and the patient has received steroids, he or she may be safely discharged.[14] For those patients who continue to have stridor or who need repeat treatment

Table 60–2	Suggested Management Plan for Croup	
Mild (Croup Score ≤ 2)	**Moderate (Croup Score 3–8)** **Severe (Croup Score > 8)**	
Oral dexamethasone in a dose of 0.15–0.6 mg/kg (max 12 mg)	Racemic epinephrine (2.25%)	
	Dexamethasone	
Responds to Treatment		
YES		
>2 hr	**<2 hr**	**NO**
Discharge home with reliable caregivers	Repeat racemic epinephrine	Repeat racemic epinephrine Consider other diagnosis
	Consider admission	Admit for airway management and monitoring

with racemic epinephrine, continued observation or admission is necessary (Table 60–2).

Bacterial Tracheitis

First described prior to the 1940s, and again in the postantibiotic era by Jones et al. in 1979,[15] bacterial tracheitis is an infectious illness of the upper airway with subglottic edema and purulent tracheal secretions. Cases have been reported in children ages 3 weeks to 13 years, with presentation in the winter months being the most common.[16,17] The overall mortality has been estimated at approximately 4%.[16] The most common bacterial agents responsible for bacterial tracheitis are *Staphylococcus aureus*, *Streptococcus pneumoniae*, α-hemolytic streptococcus, and *Moraxella catarrhalis*. Rarely in this day, due to current immunization practices, *Haemophilus influenzae* has also been found in respiratory cultures of patients with bacterial tracheitis.[15,16,18] It is not clear whether bacterial tracheitis is an entity in itself or represents overcolonization of bacteria in children with croup.

Clinical Presentation

Bacterial tracheitis shares common presentations with both croup and epiglottitis. In comparison to croup, bacterial tracheitis usually presents with a high fever and a systemically toxic-appearing child. The patient has a poor response to treatment with racemic epinephrine and steroids. The illness usually presents with a longer duration of symptoms than croup. In contrast to epiglottitis, the patient with bacterial tracheitis usually has an insidious onset of symptoms, and patients can exhibit both inspiratory and expiratory stridor. The patient with bacterial tracheitis is comfortable lying flat and will not drool.[16] Patients with bacterial tracheitis usually have an elevated white blood cell count. Recent studies have suggested that bacterial tracheitis is becoming less severe, with lower morbidity and a decrease in the need for intubation.[17]

The use of lateral neck radiographs as a tool for diagnosis is controversial. Although not reliable for diagnosis, some authors suggest that irregularities of the tracheal mucosa and a partially detached membrane may serve as additional clues[18]

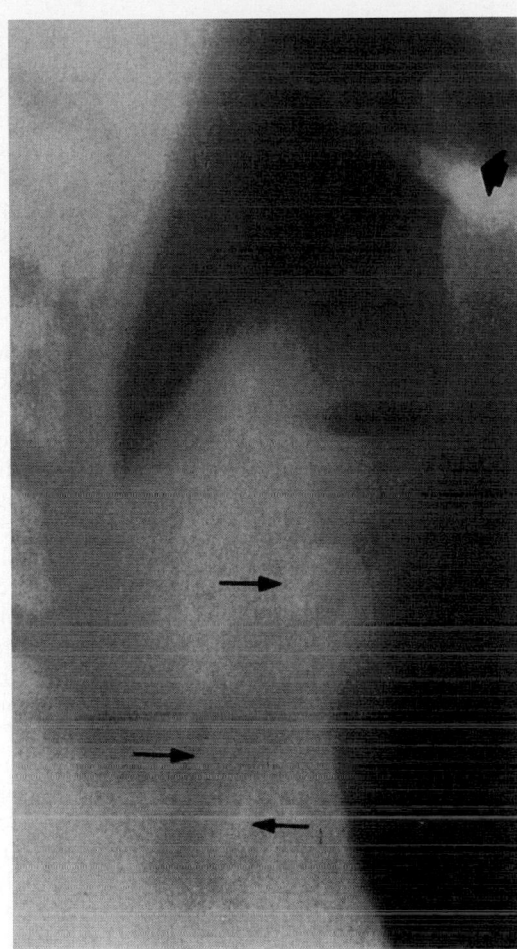

FIGURE 60–2. Bacterial tracheitis in a lateral soft tissue radiograph with obscured tracheal airway caused by sloughed mucosa (*arrows*). The epiglottis (*arrowhead*) is normal. (From Cummings CW (ed): Otolaryngology—Head & Neck Surgery, 4th ed. Philadelphia: Elsevier Mosby, 2005, p. 4364.)

(Fig. 60–2). In order to make a confirmatory diagnosis, direct visualization of the upper airway is necessary. One will see purulent material and secretions, which may form a pseudomembrane that is easily removed with minimal bleeding.[16]

Management

The first priority in managing the patient with bacterial tracheitis is securing the airway. In addition to intubation, secretions and debris can be removed from the airway with the use of suction and lavage. Treatment should include broad-spectrum antibiotics to cover the most common pathogens. Patients usually remain intubated until respiratory secretions and debris are minimal and fever has subsided. Pediatric intensive care specialists and otolaryngologists should be consulted early and for ongoing management beyond the ED.

Retropharyngeal Abscess

Retropharyngeal abscess (RPA) is a potentially serious deep space infection in the otherwise sterile retropharyngeal space. RPA usually results from lymphatic spread of infection, although hematologic spread is also possible. Trauma from direct invasion of the retropharyngeal space or by foreign bodies can also be potential etiologies for RPA. The majority of cases of RPA occur in children less than 6 years of age, with cases reported in children as young as 2.5 months.[20,21] This may be due to the high concentration of lymph nodes in younger patients.[20,22,23] Several bacterial agents are responsible for RPA. Those that have been found on aspiration are *Staphylococcal aureus*, *Klebsiella* species, and group A β-hemolytic streptococci as well as several anaerobes.[24,25]

Clinical Presentation

The presentation of RPA is often subtle and nonspecific. The same symptoms as croup, epiglottitis, and bacterial tracheitis are seen, which can make the diagnosis difficult. In a recent review, the most common presenting symptoms were neck pain, fever, sore throat, and neck mass.[26] Respiratory distress and stridor were seen in only 5% of patients presenting with RPA and are more common in the younger child.[27] The complaints of neck stiffness and torticollis help distinguish RPA from other upper respiratory infections, including croup, epiglottitis, and bacterial tracheitis.[28] The majority of children will be febrile with an elevated white blood cell count.[29,30] Common physical findings include a child who has limited neck movement, including neck extension and rotation.[26]

Diagnosis can be confirmed by a combination of plain radiographs and computed tomography (CT). The inspiratory lateral soft tissue radiograph in full extension that shows increased thickness of the prevertebral soft tissue space can have a sensitivity as high as 90%.[28] The presence of air-fluid levels or gas within the retropharyngeal space strongly suggests the diagnosis of RPA. Once RPA is suspected on plain radiographs, CT with enhancement may be used for confirmation and to help in determining the whether the observed swelling is cellulitis or phlegmon or has evolved to an abscess in need of immediate surgical drainage. CT also aids in identifying the anatomic location for surgical incision and drainage.

Management

In the unstable child with significant respiratory distress, achieving a secure airway is the first priority. In the stable patient without airway compromise, elective intubation is not recommended. Procedural sedation for imaging studies needs to be used with caution in children with upper airway lesions, as sedation may convert a child with a stable airway to one with an unstable airway. Once the airway is secure, antibiotic treatment is commenced and directed toward eliminating the common bacteria responsible for RPA. Success rates for antibiotic treatment alone have ranged from 25% to 50%.[30,31] If antibiotic therapy has failed, surgical drainage or CT-guided aspiration are other possibilities. Overall mortality from RPA is relatively low.[31]

Epiglottitis

Epiglottitis is a serious and possibly life-threatening infection of the epiglottis and surrounding tissue. If left untreated, it can progress rapidly to complete airway obstruction and death. The most common organism responsible for epiglottitis is *H. influenzae* type b, but due to current immunization practices, the incidence has dropped significantly.[32] In children less than 5 years of age, the incidence of *H. influenzae* epiglottitis decreased from 41 cases per 100,000 in 1987 to 1.3 per 100,000 in 1997.[32] Other organisms, including *Streptococcus pneumoniae*, *Staphylococcus aureus*, *Pseudomonas* species, *Klebsiella pneumoniae*, *Pasturella multocida*, and *Neisseria* species, are replacing *H. influenzae* as the primary causative agents.[33]

Clinical Presentation

A recent study demonstrated that the epidemiology of patients with epiglottitis has shifted toward older patients and those who have not been immunized against *H. influenzae*.[33] Symptoms regardless of age remain the same. These can include high fever, "hot potato" voice, drooling, and positioning of the head and neck to maintain airway patency. The patient is usually described as appearing toxic or anxious and can be found sitting in a tripod position. In patients who present with classic symptoms, including older children, the physician must take steps to exclude this diagnosis in order to not miss a potentially fatal disease. Laboratory findings typically include a high white blood cell count but are not necessary to make the diagnosis.

Diagnosis of epiglottitis is based primarily upon the constellation of symptoms noted previously. When the diagnosis is suspected, a physician competent in managing the difficult pediatric airway should accompany the patient at all times (Table 60–3). This should include all stages of investigation that occur in and outside of the ED. Direct visualization of the posterior pharynx and epiglottis is strongly discouraged as there is a high chance that complete airway obstruction may occur due to further local trauma or increasing anxiety and distress in the patient.[20] If the patient is stable and radiographs can be performed without causing further distress, they may aid in confirming epiglottitis or diagnosing other entities such as croup or RPA. The lateral neck radiograph (Fig. 60–3) will demonstrate a round, thickened epiglottis ("thumbprint" sign) along with a loss of the valecular air space and thickening of the aryepiglottic folds. Direct visualization of the supraglottic area should be performed under controlled and optimal conditions in the pediatric operating

Table 60–3	Suggested Management Plan for Epiglottitis		
Definite		**Suspected**	
Unstable	**Stable**	**Stable**	**Unstable**
Notify ear, nose, and throat (ENT) and anesthesia consultants immediately	Place in position of comfort (POC)		Place in POC
Attempt bag-valve-mask ventilation	Minimal handling and investigations		Minimal handling
Intubate if in respiratory failure	Notify ENT and anesthesia consultants for direct visualization of airway in operating room		Notify ENT and anesthesia consultants Intubate if in respiratory failure

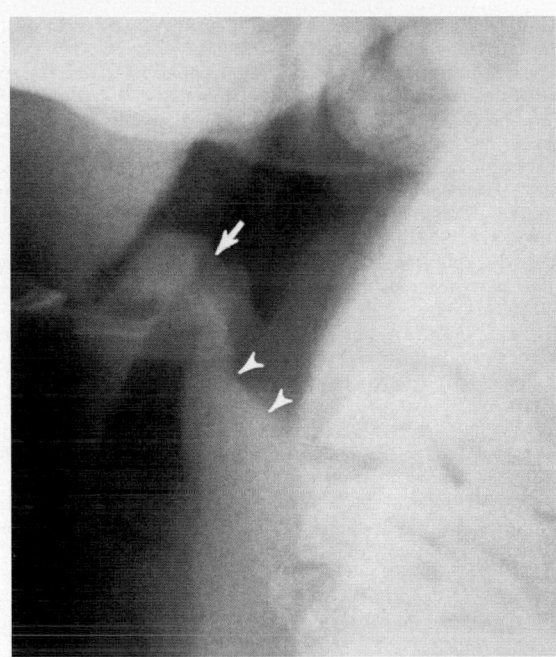

FIGURE 60–3. Epiglottitis. Marked thickening of the epiglottis (*arrow*) and aryepiglottic folds (*arrowheads*) is seen. Mild hypopharyngeal overdistention is also present. (From Cummings CW (ed): Otolaryngology—Head & Neck Surgery, 4th ed. Philadelphia: Elsevier Mosby, 2005, p. 4362.)

room with proper airway equipment. An otolaryngologist should be present should the need for a surgical airway arise.

Management

Once the airway is secure, the goal of therapy is to eradicate the offending bacterial organisms. Single therapy with ampicillin-sulbactam or ceftriaxone was found to be used most commonly in a recent review and was effective.[33] Patients usually remain intubated in the pediatric intensive care unit until there is evidence of an air leak around the endotracheal tube. Direct visualization of the supraglottic area may also be performed to assess clinical progress.

Foreign Bodies

Foreign body aspiration is a common pediatric problem that has the potential to lead to a partial or complete airway obstruction. Suspecting the diagnosis is the most important step in making the diagnosis, as patients can be asymptomatic prior to and after the aspiration. The majority of events will occur in the toddler age group but can happen at any age. Common foods that are aspirated are peanuts, hot dogs, candy, popcorn, and grapes.[34,35] Other items can include pieces of rubber balloons, coins, toys, or other nonorganic objects that are found commonly in the child's environment.

Clinical Presentation

Usually a coughing episode precedes symptoms of ensuing respiratory distress, but this may not always happen. Drooling, respiratory distress with accessory muscle use, stridor, and wheezing may be present as the degree of obstruction worsens. Depending on the location of the foreign body,

symptoms will vary. For example, an extrathoracic foreign body may cause inspiratory and expiratory stridor, whereas an intrathoracic foreign body may be associated with expiratory wheezing.

Investigations with radiographs are helpful if the aspirated object is radiopaque. Radiographs may also be useful if the aspirated agent is in a bronchus and "air trapping" has occurred. This is indicated by hyperinflation of the affected lung on the side in which the foreign body is present. If the history is suggestive, a normal chest radiograph does not rule out the possibility of foreign body aspiration, and bronchoscopy must be performed to confirm or refute the diagnosis.

Management

There are several techniques for removal of foreign bodies. These can include the use of rigid esophagoscopy, flexible endoscopy, or balloon-tipped (Foley) catheters with fluoroscopic guidance[36] (see Chapter 162, Foreign Body Removal). These methods all have high success rates. For aspirated foreign bodies, bronchoscopy is the method of choice with a very high success rate.[37]

REFERENCES

1. Denny FW, Murphy TF, Clyde WA Jr, et al: Croup: an 11 year study in pediatric practice. Pediatrics 71:871–876, 1983.
2. Henrickson KJ, Kuhn SM, Savatski LL: Epidemiology and cost of infection with human parainfluenza virus types 1 and 2 in young children. Clin Infect Dis 18:770–779, 1994.
3. Westley CR, Cotton EK, Brooks JG: Nebulized racemic epinephrine by IPPB for the treatment of croup. Am J Dis Child 132:484, 1978.
4. Kaditis AG, Wald ER: Viral croup: current diagnosis and treatment. Pediatr Infect Dis J 17:827–834, 1998.
5. Kristjansson S, Berg-Kelly K, Winso E: Inhalation of racemic adrenaline in the treatment of mild and moderately severe croup: clinical symptom score and oxygen saturation measurements for the evaluation of treatment effects. Acta Paediatr 83:1156, 1994.
6. Bourchier D, Dawson KP, Fergusson DM: Humidification in viral croup: a controlled trial. Aust Paediatr J 20:289–291, 1984.
7. Neto GM, Kentab O, Klassen TP, Osmond MH: A randomized controlled trial of mist in the acute treatment of moderate croup. Acad Emerg Med 9:873–879, 2002.
8. Russell K, Wiebe N, Saenz A, et al: Glucocorticoids for croup (Cochrane Review). Cochrane Database Syst Dis (1):CD001955, 2004.
9. Bjornson CL, Klassen TP, Williamson J, et al; Pediatric Emergency Research Canada Network: A randomized trial of a single dose of oral dexamethasone for mild croup. N Engl J Med 351:1306–1313, 2004.
10. Geelhoed GC, Macdonald WBG: Oral dexamethasone in the treatment of croup: 0.15 mg/kg versus 0.3 mg/kg versus 0.6 mg/kg. Pediatr Pulmonol 20:362–368, 1995.
11. Adair JC, Ring WH, Jordan WS, Elwyn RA: Ten year experience with IPPB in the treatment of acute laryngotracheobronchiolitis. Anesth Analg 50:649, 1971.
12. Fraser B: Nebulized levo-epinephrine as an alternative to racemic epinephrine in pediatrics. Can J Hosp Pharm 48:303, 1995.
13. Waisman Y, Klein BL, Boenning DA, et al: Prospective randomized double blind study comparing L-epinephrine and racemic epinephrine aerosols in the treatment of laryngotracheitis (croup). Pediatrics 89:302–306, 1992.
14. Kelley PB, Simon JE: Racemic epinephrine use in croup and disposition. Am J Emerg Med 10:181–183, 1992.
15. Jones R, Santos JI, Overall JC Jr: Bacterial tracheitis. JAMA 242:721–726, 1979.
16. Donaldson JD, Maltby CC: Bacterial tracheitis in children. J Otolaryngol 18:101–104, 1989.
17. Bernstein T, Brilli R, Jacobs B: Is bacterial tracheitis changing? A 14 month experience in a pediatric intensive care unit. Clin Infect Dis 27:458–462, 1998.
18. Liston SL, Gehrz RC, Siegel LG, Tilelli J: Bacterial tracheitis. Am J Dis Child 137:764–767, 1983.

19. Han BK, Dunbar JS, Striker TW: Membranous laryngotracheobronchitis (membranous croup). AJR Am J Roentgenol 133:53–58, 1979.

20. Rotta AT, Wiryawan B: Respiratory emergencies in children. Respir Care 48:248–258, 2003.

21. Cmejrek RC, Coticchia JM, Arnold JE: Presentation, diagnosis and management of deep-neck abscesses in infants. Arch Otolaryngol Head Neck Surg 128:1361–1364, 2002.

22. Thompson JW, Cohen SR, Peddix P: Retropharyngeal abscess in children: a retrospective and historical analysis. Laryngoscope 98:589–592, 1988.

23. Goldenberg D, Golz A, Joachims HZ: Retropharyngeal abscess: a clinical review. J Laryngol Otol 511:546–550, 1997.

24. Asmar BL: Bacteriology of retropharyngeal abscess in children. Pediatr Infect Dis J 9:595–596, 1990.

25. Brook I: Microbiology of retropharyngeal abscess in children. Am J Dis Child 141:202–204, 1987.

26. Craig FW, Schunk JE: Retropharyngeal abscess in children: clinical presentation, utility of imaging, and current management. Pediatrics 111(6 Pt 1):1394–1398, 2003.

27. Bank DE, Krug SE: New approaches to upper airway disease. Emerg Med Clin North Am 13:473–487, 1995.

28. Coulthard M: Retropharyngeal abscess. Arch Dis Child 66:1227–1230, 1991.

29. DeLorenzoR, Singer J, Matre W: Retropharyngeal abscess in an afebrile child. Am J Emerg Med 11:151–154, 1993.

30. Lee SS, Schwartz RH, Bahadori RS: Retropharyngeal abscess: epiglottitis of the new millennium. J Pediatr 138:435–437, 2001.

31. Morrison JE Jr, Pahley NR: Retropharyngeal abscess in children: a 10 year review. Pediatr Emerg Care 4:9–11, 1988.

32. Centers for Disease Control and Prevention: Progress towards eliminating *Haemophilus influenzae* type b disease among infants and children—United States, 1987–1997. MMRW Morb Mortal Wkly Rep 47:993–998, 1998.

33. Shah RK, Roberson DW, Jones DT: Epiglottitis in the *Haemophilus influenzae* type b vaccine era: changing trends. Laryngoscope 114:557–560, 2004.

34. Wiseman N: The diagnosis of fereign body aspiration in childhood. J Pediatr Surg 19:531–535, 1984.

35. Freidman EM: Foreign bodies in the pediatric aerodigestive tract. Pediatr Ann 17:640, 642, 644–647, 1988.

36. Morrow SE, Bickler SW, Kennedy AP, et al: Balloon extraction of esophageal foreign bodies in children. J Pediatr Surg 33:266–270, 1998.

37. Zerella JT, Dimler M, McGill LC, Pippus KJ: Foreign body aspiration in children: value of radiography and complications of bronchoscopy. J Pediatr Surg 33:1651–1654, 1998.

Syncope

Theodore E. Glynn, MD and Earl J. Reisdorff, MD

Key Points

Most children with syncope can be effectively assessed by history, physical examination, and 12-lead electrocardiogram.

Most syncopal events result from benign causes.

Despite the low incidence, physicians must reasonably exclude serious cardiac disorders as a cause of syncope.

Pregnancy-related causes of syncope should be considered in adolescent women.

Introduction and Background

Syncope is defined as a transient loss of consciousness and postural tone with spontaneous recovery.[1] Between 15% and 50% of children will have at least one episode of syncope before reaching adulthood.[2,3] Children with syncope typically have a rapid return to normal mental status without any residual deficit.[4] The terms *presyncope* and *near syncope* are used to describe the feeling that a patient is about to pass out and can precede a true syncopal attack.[1,5] Etiology and outcome are similar to that in children with syncope. Most children and adolescents with syncope have an excellent prognosis, with long-term survival that parallels the general population.[6] Nonetheless, some children will have an underlying life-threatening disorder.

Recognition and Approach

Causes of syncope can be divided into cardiac and noncardiac disorders (Table 61–1). Some experts further delineate a third cause of syncope termed *neurocardiogenic syncope*.[7] The causes of syncope are numerous, and serious life-threatening disorders fall into each category. Individual children with syncope can have cardiac and noncardiac derangements that contribute to causing syncope. Neurocardiogenic (vasovagal) syncope is the most common cause in adolescents and adults.[3,5,8-10] Under the age of 6 years, breath-holding, sei-

zures, and arrhythmias are more likely to be the cause of syncope than are the case in older children.

Since a child with syncope has a normal physical examination up to 96% of the time, a detailed history of events surrounding the syncopal episode is essential in guiding the diagnostic evaluation.[10] Performing extensive diagnostic testing for all patients has a poor diagnostic yield and is not cost effective.[2] Determining the cause of syncope requires attention to certain historical factors, a focused physical examination, minimal laboratory evaluation, and electrocardiographic (ECG) analysis. With these basic diagnostic elements, the clinician can identify those children who require a more detailed assessment, looking for more concerning causes.

Clinical Presentation

Distinguishing "benign" syncope from a rare yet life-threatening entity does not require an extensive diagnostic evaluation in most cases.[2,10] In fact, defining the absolute cause of syncope in every case in the emergency department (ED) is impractical and simply impossible. The patient and parents should be cautioned that finding a definitive cause is often not possible. Nonetheless, it is the obligation of the emergency physician to reasonably exclude serious conditions within the diagnostic limitations of the ED.

A screening process involving a focused history, a symptom-specific physical examination, and a 12-lead ECG identifies patients requiring a more intensive diagnostic evaluation and subspecialty referral, usually as an outpatient.[2,10] The presence of certain features that are typical for serious causes of syncope indicate that a more detailed workup may be indicated, to include laboratory tests, echocardiogram, stress test, tilt-table testing, electrophysiologic testing, cardiac catheterization, electroencephalography, and advanced imaging of the head or chest (e.g., magnetic resonance imaging, computed tomography [CT]).

History

The history and physical examination are sufficient to determine the cause of syncope in 25% to 77% of cases.[11,12] The circumstances preceding a syncopal episode provide clues to the underlying cause. For example, if a diaphoretic, weak, and tachycardic child has missed meals, hypoglycemia is a consideration. Dieting, diuretic use, and exertional activity can lead to orthostatic hypotension. The activity and

Table 61–1	Causes of Syncope*

Cardiac

Structural Defect
Aortic stenosis
Hypertrophic cardiomyopathy
Primary pulmonary hypertension
Congenital heart defects
Eisenmenger's syndrome
Hypoplastic left heart syndrome
Interrupted aortic arch
Postoperative repair of:
  Tetralogy of Fallot
  Transposition of the great arteries (after Mustard/Senning operation)
  Transposition of the great arteries (after arterial switch operation)
  Hypoplastic right ventricle
  Hypoplastic left heart syndrome (Fontan operation or Norwood palliation and cavopulmonary anastomosis)
  Coarctation of aorta (after patch angioplasty, aneurysm at repair site)
Cardiac transplantation
Atrial myxoma

Myocardial Dysfunction
Dilated cardiomyopathy
Myocarditis
Ischemia (e.g., anomalous coronary artery, Kawasaki disease)
Neuromuscular disease (e.g., muscular dystrophy)
Metabolic diseases
Cardiac tamponade
Constrictive pericarditis

Arrhythmias
Ventricular tachycardia (VT)
  Primary VT with structurally normal heart
  Congenital heart disease
  Long QT syndrome
  Arrhythmogenic right ventricular cardiomyopathy (dysplasias)
Supraventricular tachycardia
  Wolff-Parkinson-White syndrome
Bradycardia
  Sinus node dysfunction
  Atrioventricular block

Noncardiac

Neurally Mediated
Vasovagal (also known as vasodepressor and neurocardiogenic)
Cough syncope
Micturation syncope
Gastrointestinal origin (defecation, swallow syncope)
Breath-holding spells (suspected etiology is autonomic dysregulation)

Orthostatic or Altered Blood Pressure Control
Idiopathic
Dehydration or blood loss
Drug-induced vasodilation

Cerebrovascular, Neurologic, Pulmonary, and Psychiatric
Intracranial hemorrhage
Seizure
Hypoglycemia
Migraine—vertebrobasilar vascular spasm
Toxin/drug exposure
Pulmonary embolism
Psychogenic
Hyperventilation

*Individual patients may have coexisting cardiac and noncardiac underlying etiologies for their syncope.

Table 61–2	Clinical Features Suggestive of Serious Cardiovascular Causes of Syncope*

History of rapid onset without prodrome (e.g., "face plant," or no warning symptoms and inability to protect face from fall)
Syncope onset while recumbent
Syncope preceded by chest pain or palpitations
Syncope during exercise
Recurrent syncope, especially over hours or days
Congenital deafness
History of congenital heart disease or any structural heart defect
History of use of medications or illicit drugs with cardiac side effects (see Chapter 137, Cardiovascular Agents)
Marfanoid appearance or family history of collagen vascular disease
Family history of cardiomyopathy or sudden death (especially at young age)
Abnormal cardiovascular examination (e.g., murmur)

*List is not all inclusive.

position of the child at the time of the event also provide hints. If, at the onset of the event, the child was crying, urinating, defecating, or coughing, a vagally-mediated syncopal event is probable. Changing positions from lying to standing just prior to syncope indicates orthostatic hypotension. Syncope that occurs when a child is sitting is more likely to be a cardiac arrhythmia. Typical vagally-mediated (neurocardiogenic) episodes are preceded by nausea, lightheadedness, and a slow visual loss.

Witnesses can provide information as to the duration of the event as well as any concomitant seizure activity (e.g., abnormal eye movement or urinary incontinence). A slow recovery or mental confusion following the event suggests a seizure.[13] Severe pallor or cyanosis suggests a cardiac origin. A menstrual history should be taken, since both the physiologic intravascular volume changes of pregnancy as well as bleeding from an ectopic pregnancy can lead to syncope. The use of any over-the-counter or prescription drugs (especially those that prolong the QT interval) should be determined. Illicit drugs (including volatile substances) or ethanol misuse can cause syncope. Historical factors that can indicate more serious causes of syncope include the lack of any prodromal symptoms, syncope during exertion, a supine position at onset of symptoms, and recurrent episodes over a short time period (Table 61–2).

Key elements in a family history include sudden death, heart disease, hypercholesterolemia, diabetes, epilepsy, or recurrent syncope. The family history is most relevant in cases in which the cause of syncope is uncertain. Family members with a history of sudden cardiac death, arrhythmias, seizures, congenital deafness, or early-onset myocardial infarction further raise the consideration of a potential cardiac condition.

Physical Examination

A rapid assessment of the airway, breathing, and circulation is axiomatic for the emergency physician. Review of the temperature, pulse, respiratory rate, orthostatic blood pressure, and pulse oximetry is additionally helpful in this regard. In adolescents, a standing blood pressure of less than 80 mm Hg is abnormal, and a decrease in the systolic blood pressure of

≥ 30 mm Hg or an increase in heart rate ≥ 25 to 30 beats per minute on standing is diagnostic of orthostatic hypotension, especially when accompanied by a feeling of lightheadedness.[14,15] Orthostatic testing may further identify children who have abnormal autonomic reflex mechanisms. Beyond a general assessment and attention to all vital signs, the physical examination must focus on the cardiovascular and neurologic systems.

The cardiovascular system is closely examined, including auscultation for murmurs, gallop rhythms, irregularity, and extracardiac sounds suggesting valvular disease or left ventricular dysfunction. It is important to listen for murmur characteristics suggestive of ventricular outflow obstruction (i.e., hypertrophic cardiomyopathy [HCM]). Auscultatory findings of HCM include a fourth heart sound (S_4) as well as a murmur of turbulence or obstruction emanating from the left ventricular outflow track. This murmur classically increases in intensity during performance of the Valsalva maneuver or other activities that decrease venous return (standing). The murmur of HCM decreases with maneuvers that increase venous return (squatting).

A midsystolic click is heard with mitral valve prolapse. The presence of any heaves or thrills on chest palpation may indicate valvular disease or a cardiomyopathy. Auscultation over the carotid arteries (primarily for translated cardiac murmurs) must be performed.

A focused neurologic examination is performed, beginning with the child's mental status. Persistent or focal neurologic findings suggest brain injury (e.g., leakage from an arteriovenous malformation, shaken infant syndrome) or a seizure. The value of carotid sinus massage as a diagnostic maneuver in children is limited.[16] Other physical features associated with cardiovascular disease are an abnormal facies, marfanoid habitus, deafness, and ataxia. Neurogenic etiologies are suspected in the presence of ash-leaf spots, café-au-lait spots, or cleft palate.

Diagnostic Evaluation

Most children with syncope require limited laboratory evaluation. If bleeding or anemia is suspected, a complete blood count is indicated. Patients with seizures, an altered mental status, or a history of diabetes require testing of blood glucose. In menstruating adolescents, a pregnancy test should be obtained. Serum electrolytes (including magnesium, calcium, and phosphorus) are measured if the history suggests an electrolyte disturbance, dehydration, endocrine abnormality, or malnutrition. Electrolytes are also measured if there are abnormalities on the ECG. A urinalysis can reveal dehydration and malnutrition if there is an elevated specific gravity or ketonuria. Ketonuria with an elevated urine glucose may indicate hypovolemia from diabetic ketoacidosis. Toxicologic screens and arterial blood gas analyses are performed only as indicated by the history and physical examination.

Electrocardiography and cardiac rhythm monitoring are the most important diagnostic studies for excluding life-threatening cardiac conditions. Attention is paid to the heart rate, rhythm, conduction intervals (PR interval, QRS complex duration, and QT interval) and chamber hypertrophy (Table 61–3). Moreover, the ECG can provide information on heart chamber size, thereby revealing the presence of structural heart disease.

Advanced outpatient studies (e.g., echocardiography, tilt-table testing) should be coordinated with specialists. Subsequent outpatient advanced studies can include Holter monitoring, angiography, electroencephalography, and cardiac electrophysiology studies. Heart rate and blood pressure responses to formal tilt table testing can often define the physiologic causes of syncope.[17,18] In summary, children with

---

Table 61-3   Electrocardiography (ECG) Features Associated with Disorders Causing Syncope*

Disorder	ECG Abnormality
Arrhythmogenic right ventricular cardiomyopathy (dysplasia)	Right bundle branch block or prolonged QRS > 111 msec in leads V_1 to V_3 in absence of right bundle branch block with T-wave inversion in V_2 and V_3 (if older that 12 yr)
	Left bundle branch configuration to ectopic beats
Brugada syndrome	Right bundle branch block with ST segment elevation in V_1 to V_3
	Incomplete right bundle branch block with ST segment elevation in V_1 and V_2
Conduction defects from multiple diseases (e.g., Lyme disease, myocarditis, rheumatic fever)	Type II second- or third-degree atrioventricular block
Hyperkalemia	Early narrow and peaked T waves with short QT interval, later widening of QRS complex with P-wave amplitude diminishing
	Eventual loss of P waves, high-degree atrioventricular block, sine wave pattern, and asystole
Hypocalcemia	Prolonged QT interval
Hypokalemia	ST segment depression with flat T waves and prominent U wave
Idiopathic subaortic stenosis (hypertrophic cardiomyopathy)	Nonspecific ST segment and T-wave abnormalities
	Left ventricular hypertrophy with QRS complexes that are tallest in the mid-precordial leads
	Prominent Q waves in the inferior (II, III, aV_F) or precordial (V_2 to V_6) leads, or both
Ischemia (e.g., arteritis or anomalous coronary artery)	With anomalous coronary arteries, resting ECG is often normal
	Focal ST segment elevation or depression, Q waves, T-wave inversion
	Reciprocal changes may be present
Long QT syndrome	QT interval > 0.46–0.50 msec, although may need stress test to uncover prolongation of QT
Pericarditis	Diffuse ST segment elevation, PR interval depression
Wolff-Parkinson-White syndrome	Delta wave, short PR interval with wide QRS complex

*The list is not all inclusive and only describes common ECG findings for listed diseases. Other ECG findings can occur with listed diseases.
Adapted from Rothrock SG (ed): Pediatric Emergency Medicine Pocketbook, 5th ed. Lompoc, CA: Tarascon Publishing, 2006.

syncope who are seen in the emergency department are most often adequately evaluated by review of the vital signs, including orthostatic changes, a complete blood count, a glucose level, a 12-lead ECG, and continuous cardiac rhythm monitoring. A urine pregnancy test is performed on postmenarcheal females.

Differential Diagnosis

Most children seen in the ED with transient loss of consciousness have neurocardiogenic (vasovagal) syncope. This can involve as many as 80% of cases, followed by neurologic disorders such as seizures (9%).[10] About 5% of children seen in the ED for syncope have a cardiac cause for the event.[4,10,19]

Neurally Mediated Syncope

Neurocardiogenic syncope is caused by the vasovagal reflex. It is the most common cause of syncope in healthy children and adolescents.[9] This phenomenon accounts for 50% to 80% of infants and children presenting to pediatric EDs with syncope.[10,20,21] Neurocardiogenic syncope and other neurally mediated disorders causing syncope (e.g., cough syncope, micturation syncope, swallow syncope) are thought to share a similar underlying mechanism.[7] There is a triggering event that stimulates sympathetic activity, followed by a clinical prodrome of parasympathetic or vagal hyperactivation (e.g., nausea, vomiting). Then, there is an abrupt withdrawal of sympathetic activity with persistence of parasympathetic activity. Resulting hypotension or bradycardia result in syncope unless the patient lies down and the causative stimulus is removed.[7,22] Fluid shifts with decreased thoracic blood volume and increased splanchnic, pelvic, and leg blood volumes contribute to hypotension.[23] In some patients, autonomic nervous system–mediated alterations in cerebral blood flow may be the cause of syncope.[24]

The three main clinical variants of neurocardiogenic syncope are vasodepressor (marked hypotension), cardioinhibitory (profound bradycardia), and mixed (combined hypotension-bradycardia).[8,9] Children often report prodromal feelings of nausea, diaphoresis, and light-headedness prior to passing out. These symptoms often give them the time to sit or lie down, accounting for the fact that patients with neurocardiogenic syncope rarely hurt themselves during their episodes. Emotional or physical stressors frequently incite episodes. The associated loss of consciousness is brief, especially if the patient is allowed to assume a recumbent position. There is a rapid return to baseline mental status. Short-term recurrence is rare unless the patient is allowed to stand soon thereafter. Multiple episodes within a short period of time are more likely associated with structural cardiac disease or a neurologic disorder.

While a typical history with a normal examination is all that is required to diagnose neurocardiogenic syncope, the role of adjunct testing is controversial. Tilt-table testing is used to diagnose this disorder in adults; however, use of this test in children is controversial.[7] In children and adolescents, this test has 43% to 57% sensitivity and 83% to 100% specificity for diagnosing neurocardiogenic syncope.[7] Interestingly, tilt-table testing leads to a marked decrease in the frequency and magnitude of symptoms in patients with neurocardiogenic syncope. Use of this test allows patients to identify prodromal symptoms that they may not have previously recognized, institute preventative measures (i.e., sitting down), and prevent syncope.[7] The prognosis for all forms of neurally-mediated syncope is excellent. The risk of recurrent events diminishes over time.

Cardiac Syncope

Cardiac causes of syncope are important to identify. The 1-year mortality of all patients (adults and children) with a cardiac cause of syncope is 18% to 33%.[25,26] Cardiac disease must be considered in children with a variety of clinical features, including exertional syncope, absence of a prodrome, recurrent episodes, onset while recumbent, and associated chest pain or palpitations (see Table 61–2). Cardiac disease causes syncope due to low cardiac outflow (due to either obstruction or low-output conditions) or arrhythmias (see Chapter 63, Dysrhythmias). Structural heart disease resulting in outflow obstruction–related syncope includes valvular heart disease (e.g., congenital or acquired aortic stenosis) and HCM. Conditions that depress myocardial function include both inflammatory processes (e.g., myocarditis) and ischemia (e.g., anomalous origin of a coronary artery). Arrhythmogenic syncope can occur in patients with congenital heart disease as well as those with "structurally normal" hearts (see Chapter 30, Congenital Heart Disease; and Chapter 66, Postsurgical Cardiac Conditions and Transplantation). Reentrant tachyarrhythmic syndromes (e.g., Wolff-Parkinson-White [WPW]), as well as prolonged QT and Brugada syndromes can cause malignant dysrhythmias leading to sudden cardiac death. Intermittent atrioventricular (AV) block (sometimes referred to as a "Stokes-Adam attack") can cause syncope that is accompanied by tonic-clonic seizure activity occurring 10 to 20 seconds after the onset of asystole. These events are usually short-lived, with a rapid return to normal mentation. Patients suffering from this life-threatening disorder may be misdiagnosed as having a seizure disorder.[8,27]

STRUCTURAL HEART DISEASE

HCM is the most common cause of sudden cardiac death in young athletes.[28,29] HCM may initially present as syncope or seizure during or immediately after exertion due to decreased cerebral perfusion. HCM causes syncope due to a low cardiac output. This usually occurs when the patient develops tachycardia in the presence of a structurally reducing filling volume. Atrial fibrillation associated with HCM results from secondary atrial enlargement. Atrial fibrillation further decreases ventricular filling, increasing the risk of syncope. The physical findings of HCM can be subtle. A fourth heart sound (S_4) is usually audible. The murmur usually increases with increased Valsalva maneuvers. The ECG may reveal left ventricular hypertrophy with a strain pattern or may be normal in up to 25% of cases.[30-32]

In familial right ventricular dysplasia, the myocardium is composed of abnormal fatty cells and degenerated myocardial cells. This erratic architecture can lead to ventricular dysrhythmias that cause syncope.[33,34] Mitral valve prolapse rarely causes syncope.[35] However, some patients with mitral valve prolapse have an elevated adrenergic tone that predisposes them to arrhythmia.[36]

Severe aortic stenosis causes syncope from a cardiac outflow obstruction. The murmur of aortic stenosis is a systolic murmur at the middle and upper parasternal areas associated with a palpable thrill at the base of the heart. Peripheral pulses can be diminished. With coarctation of the aorta, infants can develop syncope, elevated systolic and diastolic blood pressures, and decreased or absent femoral pulses. Anomalous coronary arteries cause syncope, dysrhythmias, and sudden cardiac death during exercise. Ischemia-induced arrhythmia presumably results from compression or kinking of the aberrantly coursing vessel. Subclavian steal syndrome causes syncope by diverting blood from the cerebral basilar circulation. Congenital heart disease raises concerns about life-threatening ventricular arrhythmias. There is an increased incidence of ventricular tachycardia following repair of tetralogy of Fallot, presumably because of elevated right ventricular pressures from persistent obstruction in the right ventricular outflow track. Atrial and ventricular arrhythmias and AV block resulting in syncope and sudden death are associated with specific procedures for repairing many congenital cardiac defects (see Table 61–3; also see Chapter 66, Postsurgical Cardiac Conditions and Transplantation). Adolescents with primary pulmonary hypertension usually experience dyspnea on exertion. Syncope from pulmonary hypertension results from an inadequate cardiac output through a progressively narrowing and constricting pulmonary vascular bed. There is no murmur until pulmonary hypertension becomes extremely advanced.[26,37,38]

RHYTHM ABNORMALITIES

Cardiac rhythm and conduction disturbances can cause syncope by decreasing cardiac output and reducing cerebral perfusion (see Chapter 63, Dysrhythmias). Bradyarrhythmias can result from excess vagal tone or sick sinus syndrome. Bradycardia or asystole can be seen with neurocardiogenic (vasovagal) syncope. Congenital heart block presents as marked bradycardia and complete AV dissociation in the fetus or neonate. Unfortunately, congenital heart block can go undetected for years. Lyme disease can cause complete heart block that is transient and usually does not require a cardiac pacemaker.[9,39,40] In addition, other forms of infectious as well as noninfectious myocarditis can cause arrhythmogenic syncope.

Supraventricular and ventricular tachycardia can cause syncope.[41,42] In sick sinus syndrome, an episode of atrial tachycardia or atrial flutter may spontaneously terminate without the prompt return of normal sinus rhythm or a junctional escape rhythm. Thus a period of asystole follows immediately after spontaneous termination of the aforementioned tachycardia, resulting in syncope. Syncope after pacemaker insertion in a patient with sick sinus syndrome ("tachy-brady" syndrome) suggests that a tachyarrhythmia is the underlying cause. Though sick sinus syndrome is more common following corrective surgery for congenital heart disease, it can also occur in an otherwise "normal" heart.[43]

WPW syndrome is associated with a shortened PR interval, an abnormal QRS complex that is often slurred in its initial portion (delta wave), and tachycardia owing to a reentrant accessory pathway (bundle of Kent) between the atria and the ventricles. The most common arrhythmia associated with WPW syndrome is a reciprocating or reentrant loop supraventricular tachycardia. Tachycardia rarely causes syncope by itself.[44,45] Atrial fibrillation with transmission of the impulses across both the AV node and accessory pathway results in ventricular rates as high as 300 to 400 beats per

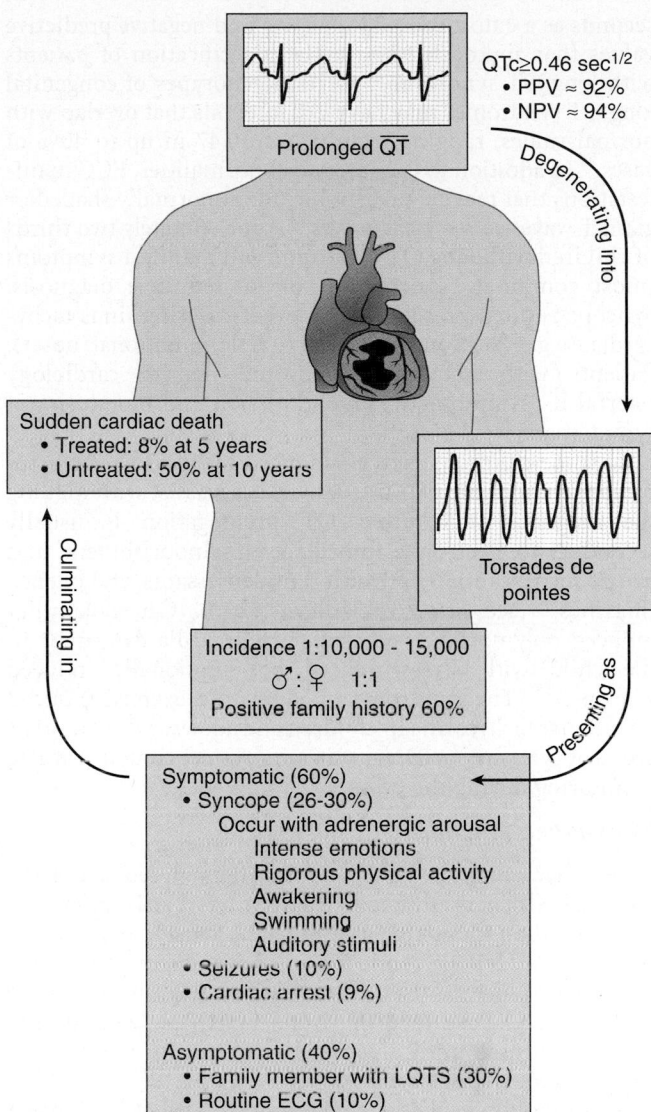

FIGURE 61–1. Key clinical characteristics of inherited long QT syndrome (LQTS), including prolongation of QT interval on electrocardiogram (ECG), commonly associated arrhythmia (torsades de pointes), clinical manifestation, and long-term outcomes. Abbreviations: NPV, negative predictive value; PPV, positive predictive value; QTc, corrected QT interval.

minute. This can rapidly lead to hemodynamic instability and syncope.

Congenital long QT syndrome is a rare inherited condition resulting from delayed ventricular repolarization (Fig. 61–1). There is an increased risk of fatal ventricular arrhythmias, most commonly polymorphic ventricular tachycardia (torsades de pointes). Patients have a 50% ten-year mortality if untreated, and 9% of children with long QT syndrome suffer sudden cardiac death as their initial presentation.[46,47] This syndrome can be associated with congenital deafness. Patients with long QT syndrome typically manifest a corrected QT interval (QT_c) greater than 0.46 seconds on ECG, although this may be difficult to assess when the patient is in normal sinus rhythm. Because the QT interval varies with the heart rate, the QT_c (QT interval ÷ square root of R-R interval) must be used to determine prolongation. Using a QT_c of 0.46

seconds as a cutoff provides positive and negative predictive values that approach 95% in the identification of patients with long QT syndrome.[46] Certain genotypes of congenital long QT syndromes may have QT intervals that overlap with normal values, ranging from 0.42 to 0.47 in up to 40% of cases.[48] In addition to QT interval abnormalities, ECG manifestations that may be present include abnormally shaped or giant T waves as well as U waves.[46] Approximately two thirds of children with long QT syndrome will manifest symptoms (most commonly syncope) prior to definitive diagnosis. Syncope is often precipitated by events causing sinus tachycardia (e.g., exertion, a sudden startle, emotional upset). Patients with long QT syndrome require cardiology referral if asymptomatic, and admission and monitoring if symptomatic.

In some children, exercise-induced tachycardia increases prolongation of the QT_c interval and can assist with making the diagnosis.[49] Acquired QT prolongation is usually secondary to electrolyte imbalances, malnourishment, and drugs, such as antiarrhythmics, antidepressants, and phenothiazines[40] (see *http://www.qtdrugs.org/*). Catecholamine-induced polymorphic ventricular tachycardia can occur in the child with stress-induced or emotionally induced syncope.[50,51] The syndrome of idiopathic exercise-induced ventricular tachycardia in children and adolescents is another cause of syncope.[52,53] Diagnosis requires continuous cardiac monitoring during the event.

Noncardiac Syncope

Noncardiac causes of syncope include hypoglycemia, breath-holding spells, neurally-mediated disorders, basilar migraine, toxins (carbon monoxide and inhalant abuse), and psychogenic illness. Hypoglycemic patients have a history of diminished oral intake or use of medications (e.g., insulin) that cause their glucose to drop. Importantly, patients usually remain confused until glucose levels return to normal (see Chapter 106, Hypoglycemia).

Breath-holding spells are a common cause of syncope in infants, although an exact physiologic cause and description can only be inferred from limited case series.[54,55] Severe breath-holding spells are associated with a loss of consciousness, whereas simple spells are not. Severe breath-holding spells have been reported in 1.7% to 4.6% of healthy children.[55,56] The typical age of onset is 6 to 24 months, with up to 15% of affected children having an onset within the first 6 months of life.[54,56] Most infants and children have frequent spells (more than once per week), and most have resolution of symptoms by the age of 4 years.[56] While the etiology is unknown, many experts believe this disorder is due to autonomic dysregulation, which leads to cerebral anoxia through a variety of mechanisms.[55,57] Many patients have iron deficiency anemia, and up to 88% of patients having improved symptoms following iron therapy regardless of whether or not they are anemic.[58] Inheritance of breath-holding spells is autosomal dominant, with up to 27% of parents and 21% of siblings having a history of breath-holding spells.[59]

There is a distinctive sequence of events in breath-holding spells. Initially, there is provocation resulting in crying or emotional upset that leads to a noiseless state of expiration accompanied by color change and ultimately loss of consciousness and postural tone.[56] Occasionally, brief jerking or urinary incontinence occurs. The event usually terminates with an inspiratory gasp or spontaneous resumption of quiet breathing.[54] Recovery of normal tone and mental status may take a few minutes, making the differentiation of this disorder from seizures difficult.[54] The color change is used to differentiate between the more common cyanotic spells (52% to 62% of cases), less common pallid spells (19% to 28%), and spells with mixed or unclassifiable features (19% to 20%).[54,56] Cyanotic spells are believed to be due to hypersympathetic effects, with more prolonged crying, intrapulmonary shunting, hypoxia, and cerebral anoxia leading to loss of consciousness.[55] Pallid breath-holders have hyperparasympathetic effects with associated asystole or bradycardia causing cerebral hypoperfusion and anoxia.[55] Iron is the only therapy that has been shown to decrease the frequency of breath-holding spells.[58] Rarely, anoxic episodes and seizures are so frequent that pacemaker implantation is required in children with breath-holding spells.[60]

Tussive syncope or post-tussive syncope is provoked by severe coughing paroxysms. These episodes can be associated with respiratory illnesses, including bronchospasm from an acute infection, asthma, pertussis, or cystic fibrosis. Presumably, severe paroxysms of coughing result in reduced cardiac output owing to the high intrathoracic pressures.

An atypical migraine headache can cause syncope. These patients usually have other symptoms atypical for syncope, including visual changes, ataxia, and vertigo. Other neurologic causes of syncope include central nervous system trauma, tumors, and cerebrovascular accidents involving arteriovenous malformations (see Chapter 41, Headaches).

Many drugs can cause syncope, including both prescription and nonprescription medications, even when used as recommended. Certain drugs can cause QT prolongation (e.g., droperidol) with resultant torsades de pointes (see *http://www.qtdrugs.org/*). Prolongation of the QT_c is exacerbated with the concurrent use of macrolides (e.g., erythromycin) and ketoconazole. Substances of abuse such as cocaine, alcohol, marijuana, inhalants, and opiates can all cause an acute loss of consciousness (usually as a consequence of intoxication or inebriation). Inhalant abuse (especially freons) can result in ventricular tachycardia and death. There is an increased frequency of sudden death in preadolescent boys taking tricyclic antidepressants for attention-deficit/hyperactivity disorder.[61]

Important Clinical Features and Considerations

Differentiating Syncope from Other Events

Seizures and breath-holding spells share characteristics with true syncope that makes differentiating these entities difficult. Obviously, an appropriate disposition and treatment decision are based on an accurate diagnosis. Misdiagnosing a patient as having a tonic-clonic seizure can have unfavorable consequences if the underlying cause of the event is actually a malignant dysrhythmia. Patients with congenital heart block or long QT syndrome frequently develop tonic-clonic activity or posturing that is easily misinterpreted as seizure activity. The lack of postictal confusion is one important factor that can differentiate most cases of syncope from seizure episodes. Breath-holding spells, although generally benign and self-limited, can often be incorrectly suspected of being a seizure due to the common occurrence of cyanosis and myoclonic jerking. Hypoglycemia is typified by a gradual onset of depressed mental status. Moreover, hypoglycemia is associated with hyperadrenergic symptoms without hemodynamic compromise. In summary, a detailed history surrounding an episode supplemented by an ECG may allow the clinician to successfully determine the exact etiology.

Syncope can be readily confused with a seizure. Seizures are the most common mimic for a syncopal event. Given the variety of presentations of syncope as well as seizures, it can be extremely difficult to ultimately define the episode. Complicating this yet further, a brief seizure can follow a vasovagal episode. Yet one more confounding factor is that cardiac dysrhythmias can accompany status epilepticus. For this reason, patients who have a first-time, nonfebrile seizure require an ECG to assess for QT prolongation or other important abnormalities[62] (see Table 61–3).

Patients with seizures commonly have a prodromal aura; this is uncommon with syncope. Facial cyanosis, frothing at the mouth, tongue biting, postictal drowsiness, and prolonged mental status changes after the event suggest a seizure. When the cause of the patient's symptoms is unclear, evaluation for both syncope and seizure is required. Electroencephalography may differentiate between syncope and seizure. Seizures may present with atypical findings; for example, temporal lobe epilepsy may demonstrate only simple motor activity, which often appears semipurposeful.

Syncope and the Athlete

Exertional or exercise-induced syncope is associated with a significant risk of sudden cardiac death, and thus referral for a complete noninvasive cardiac evaluation is indicated. HCM is the most common cause of sudden death in young competitors, followed by anomalous origin of a coronary artery. Other causes of sudden death in the athlete are arrhythmogenic right ventricular cardiomyopathy, myocarditis, and dilated cardiomyopathy.[29] Unfortunately, sudden cardiac death is often the first manifestation of disease in such patients. However, up to one third of patients will suffer exertional syncope or chest pain prior to sudden cardiac death.[29,63] The physical examination of patients with HCM may reveal an S_4 due to impaired ventricular relaxation as well as a systolic ejection murmur that is elicited or accentuated by Valsalva maneuver. Typical ECG changes may be present (see Table 61–3). Athletes with sickle cell trait have up to a 21-fold higher risk of sudden death during exertion compared to nonsicklers. The reasons for this remain unclear. Since malignant arrhythmias may play a role in athletes with sudden death, liberal distribution of automated externa defibrillators to sporting events and training sites may improve outcome from syncope in this population.[64]

Management

When treating the child with syncope, assessing the airway, breathing, and circulation is important. Orthostatic vital signs are taken. However, most children presenting with syncope will be asymptomatic in the ED. Treatment must be specific to any identifiable cause. A complaint-focused history and physical examination, as well as an ECG, should guide management. A rapid bedside glucose measurement is obtained and pulse oximetry is performed. Further laboratory assessment is of limited use unless there evidence of a specific metabolic derangement (e.g., dehydration with orthostasis).[2] Children with persistent alterations in mental status or focal neurologic deficits require a CT scan, electrolyte measurements, and toxicologic screens (including carbon monoxide). Unstable tachyarrhythmias are treated by pediatric advanced life support guidelines. If a tachycardia is toxin-induced, therapy focuses on the underlying cause. For example, sodium bicarbonate is used for cocaine- and tricyclic-induced wide-complex tachycardia. Likewise, diazepam or lorazepam may slow a cocaine-induced narrow-complex tachycardia. Initially, hypotension is treated with a bolus of isotonic fluid (20 ml/kg). If this is ineffective, inotropic agents may be required. If all diagnostic studies are normal, the child does not require immediate therapeutic intervention in the ED, and a serious cause for syncope is not suspected, the child should be sent home under the care of a responsible adult who can observe the child and ensure follow-up with the primary care provider. A key task remains the identification of that minority of patients who require a further, more sophisticated cardiac evaluation or specialty referral.

Summary

Most infants, children, and adolescents with syncope have a benign cause for their complaints. A directed history, physical examination, and ECG can identify children requiring more intensive testing. Clinicians must be able to identify clinical and ECG features signifying that a serious disorder may be causing syncope. Knowledge of the presentation of common and serious disorders causing syncope can improve the efficiency of the ED diagnostic evaluation and help identify serious and life-threatening disorders.

REFERENCES

1. Benditt DG, Lurie KG, Fabian WH: Clinical approach to diagnosis of syncope. Cardiol Clin 15:165–176, 1997.
*2. Steinberg LA, Knilans TK: Syncope in children: diagnostic tests have a high cost and low yield. J Pediatr 146:355–358, 2005.
3. Narchi H: The child who passes out. Pediatr Rev 21:384–388, 2000,.
4. Ritter S, Tani LY, Etheridge SP, et al: What is the yield of screening echocardiography in pediatric syncope? Pediatrics 105:e58, 2000.
5. Feinberg AN, Lane-Davies A: Syncope in the adolescent. Adolescent Med 13:553–567, 2002.
6. Driscoll DJ, Jacobsenn SJ, Porter CJ, Wollan PC: Syncope in children and adolescents. J Am Coll Cardiol 29:1039–1045, 1996.
7. Tanel RE, Walsh EP: Syncope in the pediatric patient. Cardiol Clin 15:277–294, 1997.
8. Lewis DA, Dhala A: Syncope in the pediatric patient: the cardiologist's perspective. Pediatr Clin North Am 46:205–219, 1999.
9. Tanel RE: Putting the bite into the pediatric syncope evaluation. Pediatr Case Rev 1:3–18, 2001.
10. Massin MM, Bourguignont A, Coremans C, et al: Syncope in pediatric patients presenting to an emergency department. J Pediatr 145:223–228, 2004.
11. Kapoor WN, Karpf M, Wieand S, et al: A prospective evaluation and follow-up of patients with syncope. N Engl J Med 309:197–204, 1983.
12. Lerman-Sagie T, Lerman P, Mukamel M, et al: A prospective evaluation of pediatric patients with syncope. Clin Pediatr (Phila) 33:67–70, 1994.
13. Hoefnagels WA, Padberg GW, Overweg J, et al: Transient loss of consciousness: the value of the history for distinguishing seizure from syncope. J Neurol 238:39–43, 1991.

---

*Selected readings.

14. Ross BA, Hughes S, Anderson E, Gillette PC: Abnormal responses to orthostatic testing in children and adolescents with recurrent unexplained syncope. Am Heart J 122(3 Pt 1):748–754, 1991.

*15. Fuchs SM, Jaffe DM: Evaluation of the "tilt test" in children. Ann Emerg Med 16:386–390, 1987.

16. Brignole M, Menozzi C, Gianfranchi L, et al: Carotid sinus massage, eyeball compression, and head-up tilt test in patients with syncope of uncertain origin and in healthy control subjects. Am Heart J 122:1644–1651, 1991.

17. Massin M: Neurocardiogenic syncope in children: current concepts in diagnosis and management. Paediatr Drugs 5:327–334, 2003.

*18. Ozme S, Alehan D, Yalaz K, et al: Causes of syncope in children: a prospective study. Int J Cardiol 40:111–114, 1993.

19. Geggel RL: Conditions leading to pediatric cardiology consultation in a tertiary academic hospital. Pediatrics 114:e409–e417, 2004.

20. Nienaber CA, Hiller S, Spielmann RP, et al: Syncope in hypertrophic cardiomyopathy: multivariate analysis of prognostic determinants. J Am Coll Cardiol 15:948–955, 1990.

21. Pongiglione G, Fish FA, Strasburger JF, Benson DW Jr: Heart rate and blood pressure response to upright tilt in young patients with unexplained syncope. J Am Coll Cardiol 16:165–170, 1990.

22. Morillo CA, Ellenbogen KA, Pava LF: Pathophysiologic basis for vasodepressor syncope. Cardiol Clin 15:233–243, 1997.

23. Stewart JM, McLeod KJ, Sanyal S, et al: Relation of postural vasovagal syncope to splanchnic hypervolemia in adolescents. Circulation 110:2575–2581, 2004.

24. Rodriquez-Nunez A, Fernandez-Cebrian S, Perez-Munuzuri A, et al: Cerebral syncope in children. J Pediatr 136:542–544, 2000.

25. Kapoor WN: Evaluation and outcome of patients with syncope. Medicine (Baltimore) 69:160–175, 1990.

*26. Wren C: Cardiac causes for syncope or sudden death in childhood. Arch Dis Child 81:289–291, 1999.

27. Harbison J, Newton JL, Seifer C, Kenny RA: Stokes Adams attacks and cardiovascular syncope. Lancet 359:158–160, 2002.

28. Maron BJ, Epstein SE, Roberts WC: Causes of sudden death in competitive athletes. J Am Coll Cardiol 7:204–214, 1986.

29. Cook S, Franklin WH: Evaluation of the athlete who 'goes to ground'. Prog Pediatr Cardiol 13:91–100, 2001.

30. Corrado D, Basso C, Schiavon M, et al: Screening for hypertrophic cardiomyopathy in young athletes [Abstract]. N Engl J Med 339:364–369, 1998.

31. Maron BJ: The electrocardiogram as a diagnostic tool for hypertrophic cardiomyopathy: revisited. Ann Noninvas Electrocardiol 6:277–279, 2001.

32. Montgomery JV, Gohman TE, Harris KM, et al: Electrocardiogram in hypertrophic cardiomyopathy revisited: does ECG pattern predict phenotypic expression and left ventricular hypertrophy or sudden death? J Am Coll Cardiol 39(Suppl A):161A, 2002.

33. Dungan WT, Garson A, Jr., Gillette PC: Arrhythmogenic right ventricular dysplasia: a cause of ventricular tachycardia in children with apparently normal hearts. Am Heart J 102:745–750, 1981.

34. Gemayel C, Pelliccia A, Thompson PD: Arrhythmogenic right ventricular cardiomyopathy. J Am Coll Cardiol 38:1773–1781, 2001.

35. Kavey RE, Blackman MS, Sondheimer HM, Byrum CJ: Ventricular arrhythmias and mitral valve prolapse in childhood. J Pediatr 105:885–890, 1984.

36. Boudoulas H, Reynolds JC, Mazzaferri E, Wooley CF: Metabolic studies in mitral valve prolapse syndrome. A neuroendocrine–cardiovascular process. Circulation 61(6):1200-1205, 1980.

37. Kerstein D, Levy PS, Hsu DT, et al: Blade balloon atrial septostomy in patients with severe primary pulmonary hypertension. Circulation 91:2028–2035, 1995.

38. Hannon DW, Knilans TK: Syncope in children and adolescents. Curr Probl Pediatr 23:358–384, 1993.

39. Steere AC, Batsford WP, Weinberg M, et al: Lyme carditis: cardiac abnormalities of Lyme disease. Ann Intern Med 93:8–16, 1980.

40. Scott WA: Evaluating the child with syncope. Pediatr Ann 20:350–351, 354–356, 359, 1991.

41. von Bernuth G, Bernsau U, Gutheil H, et al: Tachyarrhythmic syncopes in children with structurally normal hearts with and without QT-prolongation in the electrocardiogram. Eur J Pediatr 138:206–210, 1982.

42. Kilic A, Ozer S, Turanli G, et al: Dysrhythmia as a cause of syncope in children without neurological or cardiac morphological abnormalities. Pediatr Int 44:358–362, 2002.

43. Pratt JL, Fleisher GR: Syncope in children and adolescents. Pediatr Emerg Care 5:80–82, 1989.

44. Benson DW Jr, Dunnigan A, Benditt DG, et al: Transesophageal study of infant supraventricular tachycardia: electrophysiologic characteristics. Am J Cardiol 52:1002–1006, 1983.

45. Garson A Jr: Sudden death in the young. Hosp Pract (Off Ed) 26(6):51–60, 1991.

46. Ackerman MJ: The long QT syndrome: ion channel diseases of the heart. Mayo Clin Proc 73:250–269, 1998.

47. Garson A Jr, Dick M 2nd, Fournier A, et al: The long QT syndrome in children: an international study of 287 patients. Circulation 87:1866–1872, 1993.

48. Khositseth A, Martinez MW, Driscoll DJ, Ackerman MJ: Syncope in children and adolescents and the congenital long QT syndrome. Am J Cardiol 92:746–749, 2003.

49. Wang YS, Scheinman MM, Chien WW, et al: Patients with supraventricular tachycardia presenting with aborted sudden death: incidence, mechanism and long-term follow-up. J Am Coll Cardiol 18:1711–1719, 1991.

50. De Rosa G, Delogu AB, Piastra M, et al: Catecholaminergic polymorphic ventricular tachycardia: successful emergency treatment with intravenous propranolol. Pediatr Emerg Care 20:175–177, 2004.

51. Leenhardt A, Lucet V, Denjoy I, et al: Catecholaminergic polymorphic ventricular tachycardia in children: a 7-year follow-up of 21 patients. Circulation 91:1512–1519, 1995.

52. Alexander ME, Berul CI: Ventricular arrhythmias: when to worry. Pediatr Cardiol 21:532–541, 2000.

53. Bricker JT, Traweek MS, Smith RT, et al: Exercise-related ventricular tachycardia in children. Am Heart J 112:186–188, 1986.

54. DiMario FJ: Breath holding spells in childhood. Am J Dis Child 146:125–131, 1992.

55. DiMario FJ: Increased QT dispersion in breath holding spells. Acta Paediatr 93:728–730, 2004.

*56. DiMario FJ: Prospective study of children with cyanotic and pallid breath holding spells. Pediatrics 110:265–269, 2001.

57. Akalin F, Turan S, Guran T, et al: Increased QT dispersion in breath-holding spells. Acta Paediatr 93:770–774, 2004.

58. Daoud AS, Batieha A, al-Sheyyab M, et al: Effectiveness of iron therapy on breath-holding spells. J Pediatr 130:547–550, 1997.

59. DiMario FJ Jr, Sarfarazi M: Family pedigree analysis of children with severe breath-holding spells. J Pediatr 130:647–651, 1997.

60. Kelly AM, Porter CJ, McGoon MD, et al: Breath-holding spells associated with significant bradycardia: successful treatment with permanent pacemaker implantation. Pediatrics 108:698–702, 2001.

61. Riddle MA, Nelson JC, Kleinman CS, et al: Sudden death in children receiving Norpramin: a review of three reported cases and commentary. J Am Acad Child Adolesc Psychiatry 30:104–108, 1991.

62. Garson A Jr: Medicolegal problems in the management of cardiac arrhythmias in children. Pediatrics 79:84–88, 1987.

63. Basso C, Maron BJ, Corrado D, Thiene G: Clinical profile of congenital coronary artery anomalies with origin from the wrong aortic sinus leading to sudden death in young competitive athletes. J Am Coll Cardiol 35:1493–1501, 2000.

64. Berger S, Utech L, Hazinski MF: Sudden death in children and adolescents. Pediatr Clin North Am 51:1653–1677, 2004.

Chapter 62

Chest Pain

Stephen R. Knazik, DO, MBA and Earl J. Reisdorff, MD

Introduction and Background

Chest pain is a fairly infrequent complaint among pediatric emergency department (ED) patients. At Children's Hospital of Michigan, of 68,260 children seen in 2002, 219 patients (0.32% of patients without sickle cell disease) had a chief complaint of chest pain (S. Knazik, unpublished data, January 2005). This is similar to the experience in a pediatric hospital in Spain, where 0.34% of patients younger than 14 years complained of chest pain as part of their ED presentation.[1] Chest pain causes considerable anxiety among patients and parents often due to concern about cardiac disease. Unlike adults, cardiac disease (especially atherosclerotic disease) rarely causes chest pain in children. Most often, chest discomfort is caused by relatively benign processes (e.g., musculoskeletal disease), even in children with serious underlying conditions. Notable exceptions include children with sickle cell disease who develop acute chest syndrome, children with cancer or central venous catheters who develop pulmonary emboli (PEs), and children with collagen vascular disorders who develop aortic dissection. Fortunately, the medical history, physical examination, and, when needed, simple diagnostic testing usually can exclude serious causes of chest pain.

Recognition and Approach

Musculoskeletal pain (including costochondral pain) is the most common cause of pain among children referred to pediatric cardiology clinics (76% to 89%).[2,3] Other causes include exercise-induced asthma (4% to 12%), gastrointestinal causes (8%), and psychogenic causes (4%). In one study of 50 children referred to a cardiology clinic, no patient had a cardiac cause of discomfort.[2] Another study reported that 7% of children had a supraventricular tachyarrhythmia as the cause of the chest pain.[3]

Among ED patients, common causes of chest pain include musculoskeletal (64%) and idiopathic (21%).[4] Cardiac problems are found in only 4% to 5%. Other causes include pulmonary (13%), psychological (9%), and trauma (5%).[3] Younger children are more likely to have cardiac or respiratory problems, while children older than 12 years have a higher incidence of psychogenic pain. Although electrocardiograms (ECGs) are frequently obtained (nearly one half of all patients), only 16% of ECGs are "abnormal." However, only 2% of all ECGs demonstrate abnormalities that are related to the final diagnosis.

Clinical Presentation

Chest pain is a symptom, not a diagnosis. Since chest pain is a symptom, discussion about chest pain in the preverbal child is problematic. Preverbal children are usually brought to the ED for respiratory symptoms or changes in general appearance and not chest pain. Treatment and symptomatic relief are based on the presumed cause of the chest pain (Table 62–1). The exact etiology is often not identified during a single ED visit.

Despite the generally benign nature of most cases of chest pain, certain conditions require prompt medical attention. Many of these causes are readily apparent, such as penetrating trauma or acute chest syndrome, while others (e.g., myocarditis) can present in a subtle fashion. Inflammatory cardiac disease and congenital disorders are particularly concerning due to the potential for fatal arrhythmias, heart failure, and cardiogenic shock[5] (see Chapter 64, Pericarditis, Myocarditis, and Endocarditis; and Chapter 30, Congenital Heart Disease).

Table 62–1	Differential Diagnosis of Chest Pain

Musculoskeletal

Chest wall contusion
Costochondritis
Malignancy
Muscle strain
Rib fracture
Slipping rib

Pulmonary

Acute chest syndrome (sickle cell disease)
Acute sickle cell vaso-occlusive crisis
Asthma
Bronchitis
Malignancy
Pleurisy
Pneumomediastinum
Pneumonia
Pneumothorax
Pulmonary embolism

Gastrointestinal

Achalasia
Cholecystitis
Colonic flexure syndrome
Esophageal foreign body
Esophageal spasm
Esophagitis
Fitz-Hugh–Curtis syndrome
Gastritis
Gastroesophageal reflux
Hepatitis
Pancreatitis
Peptic ulcer disease
Splenomegaly

Cardiovascular

Aortic dissection
Arrhythmia (especially tachycardias)
Congenital vascular anomalies
Coronary angiitis (Kawasaki disease)
Mitral valve prolapse
Myopericarditis
Pericarditis
Pneumopericardium

Other

Child abuse
Hyperventilation
Idiopathic
Psychogenic
Pyelonephritis
Toxins (cocaine, amphetamines, volatile substance abuse)

Pneumomediastinum or pneumothorax can occur in patients who have status asthmaticus or pertussis. Any condition requiring a pronounced increase in the work of breathing (e.g., diabetic ketoacidosis) can result in musculoskeletal discomfort from chest wall inflammation. Inflammatory cardiac disease (pericarditis, myocarditis) must be considered in any ill-appearing child with chest pain or congestive heart failure. Lyme disease is an important cause of myocarditis in the Northeast during seasons when children are outdoors (April to September). The late summer months are also associated with an increase in the incidence of Coxsackie virus infection with a resultant increase in viral pericarditis.

Chest trauma can result in rib fractures, pulmonary trauma, and abdominal trauma that can cause pain that refers to the chest and shoulder girdle (Kehr's sign). Importantly, intrathoracic injuries may occur following trauma with minimal to no external evidence (see Chapter 24, Thoracic Trauma; and Chapter 25, Abdominal Trauma).

Esophageal injury (e.g., Boerhaave's syndrome) can occur in children and can be notoriously difficult to diagnose. Congenital or acquired abnormalities of the coronary arteries (e.g., coronary angiitis from Kawasaki disease) may also produce chest discomfort. Aortic dissection must be excluded in children with Down or Marfan syndrome who present with chest or back pain.[6] Aortic dissection is also associated with invasive medical procedures performed on children with congenital heart disease.[6]

Differences between Pediatric and Adult Chest Pain Complaint

Unlike adults, myocardial ischemia from atherosclerotic coronary artery disease is extremely rare in children. Nonetheless, in rare cases of extreme familial hyperlipidemias, atherosclerotic disease can appear in childhood. Children can develop coronary artery occlusion from trauma or congenital coronary artery anomalies such as coronary artery fistulas, severe myocardial bridging (coronary artery compression during systole by overlying myocardial muscle), or anomalous origin of the coronary arteries. Chest pain often occurs during or immediately after exercise. A coronary artery embolus with subsequent myocardial infarction can occur as a consequence of hypercoagulability due to malignancy or due to emboli from endocarditis, a prosthetic valve, or a patent foramen ovale.[7] In addition, nephrotic syndrome can cause hypercoagulopathy resulting in coronary artery occlusion.[8] Finally, sickle cell disease can cause microvascular cardiac ischemia. In older children with severe sickle cell disease and chest pain, nuclear medicine cardiac stress testing is abnormal in 64% of cases.[9] Adolescents who use cocaine and amphetamines may develop arrhythmias, aortic dissection, and ischemia that all can be felt as chest pain or discomfort.

When compared to adolescents, younger children tend to have more cardiorespiratory disease and less psychogenic disease.[4] Adolescents can have chest pain from trauma or as a consequence of exertion, coronary artery vasospasm from cocaine abuse, or pulmonary barotrauma. Inhalant abuse through the act of "huffing" can cause chest pain as a result of barotrauma or pulmonary atelectasis. Pulmonary barotrauma (bilateral pneumothoraces and pneumomediastinum) has also been reported in association with "ecstasy" abuse.[10]

The child with sickle cell disease may have chest pain on the basis of vaso-occlusive ischemia, osseous infarction, pulmonary infarction, or acute chest syndrome. Acute chest syndrome is characterized by a pulmonary infiltrate in a child with difficulty breathing, pain, cough, and frequently fever.[11] The pathophysiology of acute chest syndrome is incompletely understood. However, it almost certainly involves microvascular occlusion within the lungs, ribs, and bony thorax from sickling erythrocytes with a resulting parenchymal lung infiltration. Frequently, the radiographic findings associated with acute chest syndrome mimic pneumonia. Additionally, concurrent pneumonia occurs in up to one third of children[11] (see Chapter 127, Sickle Cell Disease).

Children with a PE differ in several important repects from adults. While 70% of adults have an underlying risk factor, nearly 95% of children have a major risk factor for PE.[12] The most common risk factors include the presence of a central venous catheter, underlying cancer, congenital heart disease, sepsis, trauma, and acquired or genetic prothrombotic defects (e.g., factor V Leiden, antithrombin deficiency, antiphospholipid antibodies, nephrotic syndrome, proteins S and C deficiency, hyperhomocystinemia).[12] Unlike in adults, upper extremity deep venous thrombi are a common source for emboli since central venous catheters often involve veins in the proximal upper extremity, or the central chest or neck[13] (see Chapter 130, Disorders of Coagulation).

History

The medical history should focus on the usual elements used to assess any person with pain, including the pain character, onset, duration, progression, intensity, radiation, and ameliorating factors. Other potentially important symptoms include fever, fatigue, dyspnea, diaphoresis, orthopnea, and syncope (or near syncope). A brief appetite and dietary history and assessment of elimination patterns may help to determine if a gastrointestinal disorder is causing pain. Current prescription medication use should be noted. Certain medications (e.g., tetracycline, metronidazole, nonsteroidal anti-inflammatory agents) can produce chest pain as a consequence of gastrointestinal irritation, esophagitis, or reflux.[14]

If a psychogenic basis for chest pain is suspected, the clinician should inquire about potential stressors. These include schoolwork, family problems, peer pressure, chronic disease or disability in parents, family moves, psychiatric disorder in parents, and poor coping abilities.[15]

A past medical and family history to exclude hemoglobinopathies is important regardless of ethnicity. Pulmonary embolism should be considered in children with central venous catheters, underlying cancer, sepsis, recent trauma, or other disorders that promote development of thrombi. Sudden death in young relatives increases the suspicion that a congenital cardiac defect is present. An inquiry regarding recent illness, trauma, and any hospitalizations or surgeries should also be included. A comment on the approximate developmental stage is helpful to provide a context for the quality of the information self-reported by the child.

Physical Examination

The physical examination should focus on a global constitutional assessment, a pulmonary examination, and a cardiovascular examination. The child's general constitution can be gauged by noting his or her general appearance, including weight, hydration status, temperature, pulse, respiratory rate, and blood pressure. When coarctation or dissection of the aorta is a diagnostic consideration, four-extremity blood pressures are performed. Orthostatic vital signs may reveal a rise in pulse of greater than 20 to 25 beats per minute with standing if there is volume depletion.[16]

The head and neck examination focuses on detecting additional infectious disease processes as well as detecting lymphadenopathy. The chest wall is first observed for signs of increased work of breathing (e.g., retractions). The chest wall is palpated to identify areas of point tenderness or reproducible pain along the ribs, costochondral junction, and spine. Pulmonary auscultation focuses on the detection of wheezing, rhonchi, diminished breath sounds, or a pleural friction rub. Hyperresonance to percussion may indicate a pneumothorax, while dullness to percussion is found with effusions and infiltrates. Wheezing can be extremely faint or nonexistent in the child with severe bronchospasm.

The cardiac examination should include an evaluation for the point of maximal impulse, as well as auscultation for murmurs and quality of the heart sounds. Hemic or flow murmurs may be present simply as a function of physiologically appropriate tachycardia. A cardiac rub or Ewart's sign suggests pericarditis. Ewart's sign is an area of dullness with bronchial breathing and bronchophony below the angle of the left scapula due to compression of the left lung by pericardial effusion. If pneumomediastinum is suspected, auscultation over the sternum may detect Hamman's crunch, which is heard in a minority of patients with pneumomediastinum.[17]

Although the abdominal examination involves the entire abdomen, it should carefully focus on the upper half of the abdomen. The abdominal examination specifically seeks any masses, tenderness, guarding, or potential foci for referred pain. Importantly, chest pain and epigastric pain can be concurrent. Right-sided abdominal tenderness can be the result of gallbladder disease in the obese adolescent or the patient with sickle cell disease, liver disease, or peptic ulcer disease. Epigastric tenderness may indicate esophageal, pancreatic, stomach, or intestinal pathology as the cause of chest pain. Left-sided abdominal tenderness may indicate pancreatic, splenic, or gastric disorders as the underlying cause of chest pain.

Diagnostic Testing

If the history and physical examination are sufficient to exclude serious causes, no further diagnostic tests are indicated. Ancillary diagnostic testing has an extremely low diagnostic yield in children with chest pain.[3] Although it is frequently impossible to establish an absolute cause of the chest discomfort, the physician must reasonably exclude life-threatening pathology. A sensitive and thoughtful discussion with the child and parents explaining the unlikelihood of a cardiac cause is sufficient for establishing reassurance. This instructive discussion should mention the pathophysiologic differences between chest pain in children and in adults as well as the diagnostic limitations of an ED evaluation.

The chest radiograph provides additional information about the cardiovascular and pulmonary systems. The chest film can detect barotrauma, pneumonia, pleural-based processes, and osseous abnormalities, including malignancies. The cardiac and vascular silhouettes are clearly seen, and the area behind the heart can be inspected for retrocardiac infiltrates. Special attention is paid to the apices for small pneumothoraces. In pneumomediastinum, radiographically apparent subcutaneous emphysema (especially about the neck) is a common finding, as is pneumomediastinal air that commonly appears parallel to the left heart border.[17] Plain radiographs in pulmonary embolism may be normal or reveal atelectasis, small infiltrates, a wedge-shaped defect, absence of pulmonary vasculature, or a pleural effusion.[18]

The ECG and echocardiogram are usually of limited assistance in defining the cause of chest pain in children.[4] A rational approach is to reserve these tests for children who have other concomitant conditions or symptoms that increase the likelihood of a life-threatening or cardiac causes of pain. Certain ECG patterns suggest serious underlying cardiac disease that can cause chest discomfort due to ischemia, inflammation, or palpations due to arrhythmias. A baseline ECG in Wolff-Parkinson-White syndrome usually manifests with a short PR interval and a delta wave that widens the appearance of the QRS complex. Long QT syndrome is associated with polymorphic ventricular tachycardia. ST segment elevation or depression occurs during acute ischemia, with eventual development of Q waves and T-wave inversion during a myocardial infarction. Pericarditis often causes diffuse ST segment elevation and PR interval depression. Arrhythmogenic right ventricular cardiomyopathy (or dysplasia) is associated with T-wave inversion in V_2 and V_3 with a right bundle branch block, or a prolonged QRS (>110 msec) in leads V_1 to V_3 in the absence of right bundle branch block. A left bundle branch configuration to ectopic beats is present. Patients with this disorder are at risk for developing ventricular tachycardia. The ECG in idiopathic hypetrophic subaortic stenosis often shows nonspecific ST-segment and T-wave abnormalities, left ventricular hypertrophy with QRS complexes that are tallest in the midprecordial leads, and prominent Q waves in the inferior (II, III, aV_F) or precordial (V_2 to V_6) leads (see Chapter 61, Syncope). Children with this disorder are at risk for chest pain or sudden death during or immediate after exertion.

Computed tomography (CT) of the chest may be required to exclude certain life-threatening disorders. A chest CT can accurately detect an otherwise occult pulmonary contusion, pneumothorax, subtle pneumonia, pleural effusions, pneumomediastinum, esophageal rupture, aortic aneurysm, and aortic dissection. Newer multidetector CT scans with thin columnation (0.6 to 1.25 mm), rapid data acquisition, improved resolution and quality of images, diminished motion artifact, and accurate depiction of subsegmental pulmonary arteries are as accurate as pulmonary angiography for detecting pulmonary emboli.[19,20] However, accuracy of ventilation-perfusion scanning, angiography, and CT scanning for diagnosis of PE in children has been extrapolated from adult studies; there have been no individual large series or direct comparisons of these tests in children.

Nuclear medicine imaging for cardiac ischemia is performed at the discretion of a pediatric cardiologist. Recently, positron emission tomography has also been shown to be effective is assessing myocardial perfusion.[21]

Finally, other laboratory testing is used selectively, based on the presumed differential diagnoses. A complete blood count is useful to assess for hemoglobinopathies, anemia, or malignancies. Other serum assays are rarely helpful in determining the cause of chest pain. Serum troponin is elevated in 55% to 71% of children with myocarditis who have had symptoms for less than 1 month, and in nearly half of all children with pericarditis.[22-26] Lyme titers can be obtained in children with presumed pericarditis. Brain natriuretic peptide (BNP) may be a useful marker for Kawasaki myocarditis, with most cases manifesting a level greater than 50 pg/ml.[27] Use of BNP in other disorders associated with myocarditis is undefined. Nonspecific indices for inflammatory processes (e.g., erythrocyte sedimentation rate and C-reactive protein) rarely assist in determining an exact cause of chest pain, although elevations in these parameters increase the probability that an organic disease is present. Fecal occult blood testing, as well as measurement of liver and pancreatic enzymes, may help to identify abdominal causes of chest pain. Blood cultures are often recommended in patients with pneumonia, although the yield is low in children who are healthy with no underlying disease. Blood cultures may be of use in children at risk for serious disease or abnormal pathogens (e.g., sickle cell disease, neutropenia, cancer).

Oxygen saturation is an important measurement in patients with chest pain or shortness of breath. During vaso-occlusive episodes, this number may be falsely depres-sed by up to 10% if pulse oximetry is used instead of the traditional co-oximetry used during arterial blood gas analysis.[28]

Important Clinical Features and Considerations

Children with chest pain can be sorted into categories with a high and low risk of serious disease based on their history, physical examination, and oxygen saturation augmented by an ECG and chest radiograph if indicated (Table 62–2). Abnormal vital signs, hypoxia, dyspnea, diaphoresis, and syncope are indicators of the need for further diagnostic testing. Any abnormal vital signs should be repeat-tested and warrant an explanation prior to discharging the child with chest pain. The general impression of an experienced physician is helpful in garnering a "global sense" for whether or not the patient has a life-threatening condition. Finally, the failure to have symptomatic improvement during the ED course should also lead the physician to consider potentially serious conditions (see Table 62–2).

Clinical Pearls and Pitfalls

Children with sickle cell disease and a new infiltrate with cough, fever, or respiratory complaints are defined as having

Table 62–2	Select Features Associated with Serious Cause of Chest Pain
Historical Features	**Examination and Diagnostic Features**
Pain associated with:	Marfanoid appearance
Exertion	Respiratory distress
Dyspnea	Abnormal vital signs:
Syncope	Tachycardia
Illicit drug use	Bradycardia
Trauma	Hypotension
Family history of:	Tachypnea
Sudden death in young	Friction rub or pathologic murmur
family members	Abnormal lower extremity pulses
Marfan's syndrome	Abnormal lung examination
Sickle cell disease	Presence of a central venous
Past medical history of:	access catheter
Sickle cell disease	Hypoxemia
Congenital heart disease	Abnormal electrocardiogram (see
Cancer	Chapter 61, Syncope)
Congenital deafness	Evidence of specific medical
Medications/drugs with	diseases associated with serious
cardiac side effects:	cardiac effects (e.g., Kawasaki,
Antihypertensives	Lyme diseases)
Antiarrhythmics	Appearance or odor of toxic
Phenothiazines	inhalation agents
Anticholinergics	
Sympathomimetics (legal	
and illegal)	

acute chest syndrome. All patients with this diagnosis require hospital admission. Admission should be strongly considered for sickle cell patients with acute chest pain or difficulty breating even if no infiltrate is seen on chest radiograph. One prospective study of children with acute chest syndrome found that nearly half of all patients were admitted with an alternate diagnosis. While fever (80%) and cough (62%) were the most common symptoms in children less than 10 years old, 44% had chest pain, 41% complained of shortness of breath, a third complained of pain in the abdomen or extremities, and 45% were tachypneic on admission.[11] Importantly, radiographic and clinical findings appeared a mean 2.5 days after hospital admission.[11] For this reason, clinicians should consider the diagnosis of acute chest syndrome in children with severe vaso-occlusive crises, any respiratory symptoms including cough or shortness of breath, or tachypnea on admission even if the initial radiograph is normal. Even if acute chest syndrome is not initially present, these symptoms may identify a group of patients at risk for developing this disorder.

PE is often missed in children. One study found that only 50% of children who died from a PE had suggestive symptoms, and the diagnosis was only suspected in 15% prior to death.[29] Most children have serious underlying disorders with signs and symptoms that overlap with PE (e.g., cancer, sepsis). Unlike adults, there are no studies that have detailed the typical presentation or developed scoring systems for stratifying children into categories of high or low risk for thromboemboli. For this reason, clinicians must consider the diagnosis of PE in any child with risk factors (e.g., central venous catheter, cancer, sepsis, recent trauma) who has any acute cardiac or respiratory complaint or change in vital signs, oxygen saturation, or chest radiography (see Chapter 130, Disorders of Coagulation).

Pulmonary barotrauma is a consideration in every patient with bronchospasm and chest pain. The chest film must be closely inspected along the left cardiac border and in the cervical soft tissue for extrapulmonary air. The lateral radiograph may be more sensitive than a frontal view for detecting pneumomediastinum.[30]

Potential Complications

Undiagnosed congenital lesions may progress to heart failure. Myocarditis can produce malignant arrhythmias or cardiogenic shock. Children suspected of having myocarditis should be monitored for hemodynamically unstable cardiac arrhythmias.

Pneumothorax can progress to hemodynamically compromising tension pneumothorax. Rarely, pneumomediastinum can progress to pneumomediastinum with hypotension due to compression of the heart and inadequate cardiac contraction. For this reason, any child with pulmonary barotrauma who is discharged requires a mandatory recheck in the ED or physician's office, including a repeat chest radiograph, to determine any progression of disease. Any worsening of symptoms requires hospitalization.

Management

Immediate Therapeutic Interventions

The management of the child with chest pain is determined both by symptoms and by presumptive diagnosis. If a serious cardiopulmonary disorder is suspected, oxygen is supplied and intravenous access is obtained. Cardiac rhythm monitoring and continuous oxygen saturation monitoring are appropriate in the patient with abnormal vital signs, especially hypoxia. Patients who must leave the department for additional testing (e.g., CT, echocardiography) require continuous cardiac and oxygen saturation monitoring. Personnel who can intervene acutely must accompany the child.

Secondary Therapeutic Interventions

During the ED evaluation, analgesics should be administered to children with significant pain. Children with musculoskeletal disease are often best treated with acetaminophen or a nonsteroidal anti-inflammatory agent. Parenteral narcotics are administered if pain is severe or immediate analgesia is desired. If there is bronchospasm, aerosolized β agonists and systemic steroids are given. For gastrointestinal disease (e.g., epigastric discomfort) antacids, proton pump inhibitors, or histamine$_2$-receptor blockers are appropriate. In children with acute chest syndrome, exchange transfusion is recommended for severe symptoms, severe anemia, or hypoxia, or for patients who do not improve with administration of intravenous fluids, antibiotics, and pain medications.[11,31] Patients with pulmonary emboli require anticoagulation, with consideration of thrombolytic therapy if severe hypoxia or persistent hypotension is present.

Summary

Most cases of chest pain in children are caused by benign conditions. Prognoses are further stratified based on the underlying cause of the pain and coexisting medical conditions. The clinical course of each disorder causing chest pain is varied. Chest wall pain may disappear in days, while pain from rib fractures may take 4 to 6 weeks to completely resolve. The reassessment of pulmonary barotrauma, including a repeat chest radiograph, is indicated in all cases. Patients with chest disorders (and their parents) should be encouraged to return to the ED or see their physician immediately if pain or breathing worsens, if symptoms of infection develop, or if any new concerning symptoms (e.g., syncope) occur.

The decision to admit each patient is based on the requirement for inpatient care or intervention, continuous cardiac and respiratory monitoring for deterioration, or inpatient diagnostic evaluation. Most suspected serious cardiovascular conditions require admission to the hospital or ED cardiology consultation with an expedited outpatient evaluation. Serious noncardiac disorders requiring admission include severe pneumonia, pulmonary embolism, pulmonary barotrauma (unless minor), pulmonary contusion, acute chest syndrome in sickle cell disease, and serious intra-abdominal disorders causing chest pain.

REFERENCES

1. Gastesi-Larranaga M, Fernandez-Landaluce A, Mintegi-Raso S, et al: Dolor toracico en urgencias de pediatria: un proceso habitualmente benigno. [Chest pain in pediatric emergency departments: a usually benign process.] An Pediatr (Barc) 59:234–238, 2003.
*2. Evangelista JA, Parsons M, Renneburg AK: Chest pain in children: diagnosis through history and physical examination. J Pediatr Health Care 14:3–8, 2000.

*Selected readings.

3. Massin MM, Bourguignont A, Coremans C, et al: Chest pain in pediatric patients presenting to an emergency department or to a cardiac clinic. Clin Pediatr (Phila) 43:231–238, 2004.

*4. Selbst SM, Ruddy RM, Clark BJ, et al: Pediatric chest pain: a prospective study. Pediatrics 82:319–323, 1988.

5. Hallagan LF, Dawson PA, Eljaiek F Jr: Pediatric chest pain: case report of a malignant cause. Am J Emerg Med 10:43–45, 1992.

*6. Zalzstein E, Hamilton R, Zucker N, et al: Aortic dissection in children and young adults: diagnosis, patients at risk, and outcomes. Cardiol Young 13:341–344, 2003.

7. Aragon J: A rare noncardiac cause for acute myocardial infarction in a 13-year-old patient. Cardiol Rev 12:31–36, 2004.

*8. Osula S, Bell GM, Hornung RS: Acute myocardial infarction in young adults: causes and management. Postgrad Med J 78:27–30, 2002.

9. de Montalembert M, Maunoury C, Acar P, et al: Myocardial ischaemia in children with sickle cell disease. Arch Dis Child 89:359–362, 2004.

10. Mazur S, Hitchcock T: Spontaneous pneumomediastinum, pneumothorax and ecstasy abuse. Emerg Med (Fremantle) 13:121–123, 2001.

11. Vichinsky EP, Neumayr LD, Earles AN, et al: Causes and outcomes of the acute chest syndrome in sickle cell disease. N Engl J Med 342:1855–1865, 2000.

12. Andrews M, David M, Adams M, et al: Venous thromboembolic complications (VTE) in children: first analysis of the Canadian Registry of VTE. Blood 83:1251–1257, 1994.

13. Kuhle S, Massicotte P, Chan A, et al: Systemic thromboembolism in children. Thromb Haemost 92:722–728, 2004.

14. Palmer KM, Selbst SM, Shaffer S, Proujansky R: Pediatric chest pain induced by tetracycline ingestion. Pediatr Emerg Care 15:200–201, 1999.

15. Brill SR, Patel DR, MacDonald E: Psychosomatic disorders in pediatrics. Indian J Pediatr 68:597–603, 2001.

16. Fuchs SM, Jaffe DM: Evaluation of the tilt test in children. Ann Emerg Med 16:386–390, 1987.

17. Miura H, Taira O, Hiraguri S, et al: Clinical features of medical pneumomediastinum. Ann Thorac Cardiovasc Surg 9:188–191, 2003.

18. Babyn PS, Gahunia HK, Massicotte P: Pulmonary thromboembolism in children. Pediatr Radiol 35:258–274, 2005.

19. Gulsun M, Goodman LR, Washington L: Venous thromboembolic disease: where does multidetector computed tomography fit? Cardiol Clin 21:631–638, 2003.

20. Quiroz R, Kucher N, Zou KH, et al: Clinical validity of a negative computed tomography scan in patients with suspected pulmonary embolism: a systematic review. JAMA 293:2012–2017, 2005.

21. Singh TP, Muzik O, Forbes TF, Di Carli MF: Positron emission tomography myocardial perfusion imaging in children with suspected coronary abnormalities. Pediatr Cardiol 24:138–144, 2003.

22. Bonnefoy E, Godon P, Kirkorian G, et al: Serum cardiac troponin I and ST-segment elevation in patients with acute pericarditis. Eur Heart J 21:798, 2000.

23. Brandt RR, Filzmaier K, Hanrath P: Circulating cardiac troponin I in acute pericarditis. Am J Cardiol 87:1326, 2001.

24. Imazio M: Cardiac troponin I in acute pericarditis. J Am Coll Cardiol 42:2144–2148, 2003.

25. Smith SC, Ladenson JH, Mason JW, et al: Elevations of cardiac troponin I associated with myocarditis: experimental and clinical correlates. Circulation 95:163–168, 1997.

26. Soongswang J, Durongpisitkul K, Nana A, et al: Cardiac troponin T: a marker in the diagnosis of acute myocarditis in children. Pediatr Cardiol 26:45–49, 2005.

27. Kawamura T, Wago M: Brain natriuretic peptide can be a useful biochemical marker for myocarditis in patients with Kawasaki disease. Cardiol Young 12:153–158, 2002.

28. Ahmed S: Hemoglobin oxygen saturation discrepancy using various methods in patients with sickle cell vaso-occlusive painful crisis. Eur J Haematol 7:309–314, 2005.

29. Derish MT, Smith DW, Frankel LR: Venous catheter thrombus formation and pulmonary embolism in children. Pediatr Pulmonol 20:349–354, 1995.

30. Shanmuganathan K: Imaging diagnosis of nonaortic thoracic injury. Radiol Clin North Am 37:533–551, 1999.

31. Liem RI, O'Gorman MR, Brown DL: Effect of red cell exchange transfusion on plasma levels of inflammatory mediators in sickle cell patients with acute chest syndrome. Am J Hematol 76:19–25, 2004.

Chapter 63

Dysrhythmias

Stephanie J. Doniger, MD and Ghazala Q. Sharieff, MD

Key Points

Paroxysmal supraventricular tachycardia is the most common symptomatic dysrhythmia.

Arrhythmia treatment depends on whether the patient has a pulse, hemodynamic stability, and the presenting rhythm.

Atrial flutter and atrial fibrillation in children are largely attributed to structural heart disease (i.e., repaired and unrepaired congenital heart disease).

Bradycardias are defined as a heart rate less than the lower limit of normal for a child's age. The most common cause is sinus bradycardia, which is for the most part benign. Other causes include first-, second-, and third-degree (complete) heart blocks.

Long QT syndrome may be either hereditary or acquired, and may manifest as syncope or sudden death. On electrocardiogram, the most accurate determination of the QT interval is calculated using the Bazett formula ($QT_c = QT/\sqrt{RR}$), with a QT_c greater than 460 ms as prolonged.

Introduction and Background

Pediatric dysrhythmias are much less common than dysrhythmias that occur in adults. However, with the advent of life-saving procedures to repair congenital heart diseases, there has been a notable increase in postoperative dysrhythmias, thereby increasing the overall incidence of dysrhythmias in the pediatric population. The overall incidence of arrhythmias is 13.9 per 100,000 emergency department (ED) visits and 55.1 per 100,000 pediatric ED visits (children under 18 years of age).[1] Among children with arrhythmias, the most common are sinus tachycardia (50%), supraventricular

The authors would like to acknowledge CDR Jonathan T. Fleenor, MD in the division of Pediatric Cardiology at the Naval Medical Center San Diego for his electrocardiogram contributions.

tachycardia (13%), bradycardia (6%), and atrial fibrillation (4.6%).[1]

The presentation of dysrhythmias can serve as a diagnostic challenge to clinicians, in that most children present with vague and nonspecific symptoms such as "fussiness" or "difficulty feeding." Despite the infrequency and vague presenting symptoms, it is critical to identify and appropriately manage these disorders. When left unrecognized and untreated, dysrhythmias can lead to further decompensation.

The Electrocardiogram in Pediatrics

A review of pediatric emergency department utilization of electrocardiograms (ECGs) revealed that the most common reasons for obtaining ECGs in children are chest pain, suspected dysrhythmias, seizures, syncope, drug exposure, electrical burns, electrolyte abnormalities, and abnormal physical examination findings. The most life threatening are dysrhythmias, either primary or caused by electrolyte disturbances, drug exposure, and burns.[2] Patients presenting with dysrhythmias should have an immediate ECG in order to expeditiously identify the underlying disorder and facilitate appropriate therapy.

When evaluating ECGs, it is advisable to use a systematic approach with special attention to rate, rhythm, axis, ventricular and atrial hypertrophy, and the presence of any ischemia or repolarization abnormalities. It is essential to interpret pediatric ECGs based on age-specific rates and intervals[3-5] (Table 63–1). In children, the cardiac output is mostly determined by heart rate and not stroke volume. For this reason, age- and activity-appropriate heart rates must be recognized. Average resting heart rate varies with age: newborns can have a heart rate ranging from 90 to 160 beats per minute (bpm) and adolescents from 50 to 120 bpm.[3] Heart rates grossly outside the normal range for age should be closely scrutinized for dysrhythmias. Using the heart rate, dysrhythmias can be further classified into two categories: tachydysrhythmias (rate greater than the upper limit of normal for age), and bradydysrhythmias (rate less than the lower limit of normal for age). Once the rate has been established, the rhythm must be determined. Normal sinus rhythm is characterized by P waves preceding each QRS complex, a regular PR interval, and a normal P wave axis (0 to +90 degrees).

Next, it is useful to measure intervals—the PR interval, the QRS duration, and the QT interval. The PR interval, which is measured as the time from the onset of the P wave to the onset of the QRS complex, also varies with age as the

Table 63–1	Pediatric Electrocardiogram Normal Heart Rate (HR) and Intervals by Age		
Age	HR	PR Interval (sec)	QRS Interval (sec)
1st wk	90–160	0.08–0.15	0.03–0.08
1–3 wk	100–180	0.08–0.15	0.03–0.08
1–2 mo	120–180	0.08–0.15	0.03–0.08
3–5 mo	105–185	0.08–0.15	0.03–0.08
6–11 mo	110–170	0.07–0.16	0.03–0.08
1–2 yr	90–165	0.08–0.16	0.03–0.08
3–4 yr	70–140	0.09–0.17	0.04–0.08
5–7 yr	65–140	0.09–0.17	0.04–0.08
8–11 yr	60–130	0.09–0.17	0.04–0.09
12–15 yr	65–130	0.09–0.18	0.04–0.09
≥16 yr	50–120	0.12–0.20	0.05–0.10

Courtesy of Ra'id Abdullah, MD, University of Chicago, Illinois.

heart matures. In neonates, it ranges from 80 to 150 msec and in adolescents from 120 to 200 msec (see Table 63–1).[3-5] A prolonged PR interval suggests a type I atrioventricular (AV) heart block. The QT interval represents the time from onset of depolarization to completion of repolarization. It is measured from the onset of the QRS complex to the end of the T wave, where it returns to the baseline. For greatest accuracy, the QT and preceding R-R intervals should be measured for three consecutive beats and averaged. Due to wide variability in heart rates, the QT interval must be corrected for the heart rate by utilizing the Bazett formula ($QT_c = QT \div$ square root of the RR interval).[6] A prolonged QT interval is defined as a QT_c greater than or equal to 460 msec. A QT_c within the range of 420 to 460 msec is considered borderline, and warrants further assessment.[7-9]

Once normal intervals are evaluated, the ECG can then be scrutinized for chamber size and T-wave morphology. The P-wave height and width can be used to determine if there is right atrial enlargement and left atrial enlargement, respectively. Ventricular hypertrophy can be identified by determining whether the voltages in the precordial leads are greater than the upper limit of normal for the age group. Unlike the adult population, children tend to have nonspecific T-wave changes. This is often a source of great controversy. What is agreed upon is that flat, inverted T waves are normal in the newly born, while upright T waves in V_1 after 3 days of age are a sign of right ventricular hypertrophy.[10]

Selected Diagnoses

Tachydysrhythmias
  Sinus tachycardia
  Supraventricular tachycardia
  Atrial flutter
  Atrial fibrillation
  Premature atrial contractions
  Premature ventricular contractions
  Ventricular tachycardia
  Ventricular fibrillation
Bradydysrhythmias
  Sinus bradycardia
  Conduction abnormalities
Sinus arrhythmia
Long QT syndrome

Discussion of Individual Diagnoses

Tachydysrhythmias

Tachycardia is defined as a heart rate beyond the upper limit of normal for the patient's age. Tachycardias can be classified broadly into those that originate above the AV node (i.e., supraventricular), those that originate from the AV node (AV node reentrant tachycardias), and those that originate from the ventricle. The vast majority of tachycardias are supraventricular in origin. Those that are ventricular in origin are typically associated with hemodynamic compromise.[4] Upon recognition of a tachycardia, stepwise questioning can help evaluate the ECG tracing. Is the rhythm regular or irregular? Is the QRS complex narrow or wide? Does every P wave result in a single QRS complex? Once this is established, treatment options are considered according to whether or not the patient has a pulse, and the presenting rhythm on ECG[11] (Fig. 63–1).

Sinus Tachycardia

Sinus tachycardia can be differentiated from other tachycardias by a narrow QRS complex and a P wave that precedes every QRS complex. The rate is usually greater than 140 bpm in children, and greater than 160 bpm in infants. Sinus tachycardia is benign. It can be seen in normal healthy individuals during anxiety, pain, or exercise or with fevers. Pulse rate has been shown to increase linearly with temperature in children greater than 2 months of age. For every 1° C (1.8° F) increase in body temperature, pulse rate increases an average of 9.6 bpm.[12] Sinus tachycardia can also be associated with such underlying conditions as hypoxia, anemia, hypovolemia, shock, myocardial ischemia, pulmonary edema, hyperthyroidism, medications (catecholamines), hypocalcemia, and illicit drug use. Most commonly, it is a result of dehydration and hypovolemia.[1,4] Since children augment cardiac output by increasing heart rate rather than stroke volume, heart rate increases appear early, while hypotension is a late sign of dehydration. Treatment aimed at correcting the heart rate alone may be harmful to the patient, since the tachycardia is a compensatory response to sustain adequate cardiac output. For this reason, treatment of sinus tachycardia is largely targeted at treating the underlying disorder, rather than treating the tachycardia itself.

Supraventricular Tachycardia

Paroxysmal supraventricular tachycardia (SVT) is the most common symptomatic dysrhythmia in infants and children. In neonates and infants with SVT, the heart rate is greater than 220 bpm. In older children, SVT is defined as having a heart rate of more than 180 bpm.[13] The ECG shows a narrow QRS complex tachycardia, either without discernible P waves or with retrograde P waves with an abnormal axis (Fig. 63–2). The QRS duration is usually normal but is occasionally increased with aberrancy.

RECOGNITION AND APPROACH

There are three types of SVT. The most common is AV reentrant tachycardia. In addition to the normal conduction from the sinoatrial (SA) node to the AV node, to the bundle of His, and then to the Purkinje fibers, there is an accessory "bypass" pathway in conjunction with the AV node. This pathway is

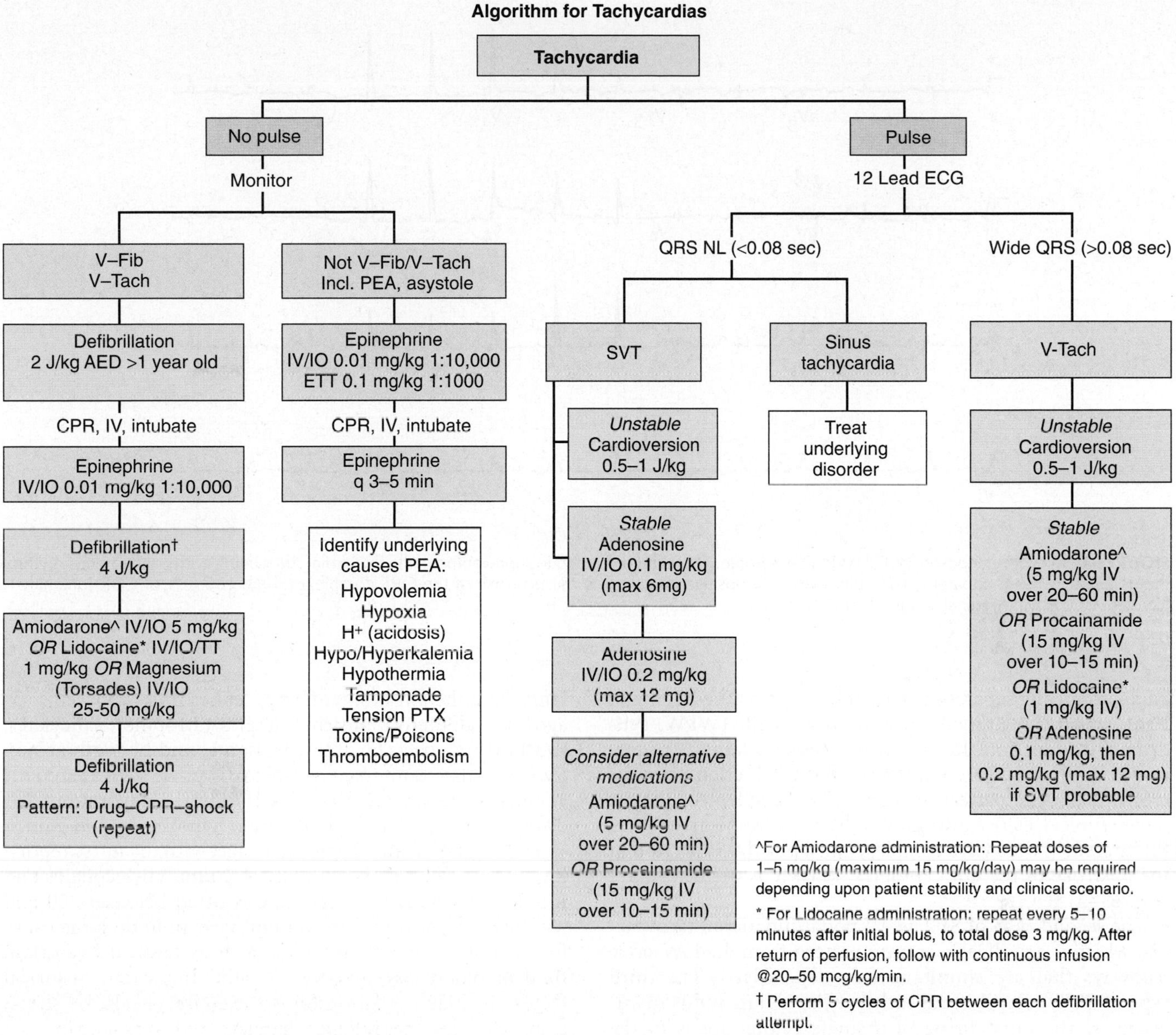

Algorithm for Tachycardias

Tachycardia

- **No pulse**
  - Monitor
- **Pulse**
  - 12 Lead ECG

No pulse branch:

V–Fib / V–Tach

Defibrillation
2 J/kg AED >1 year old

CPR, IV, intubate

Epinephrine
IV/IO 0.01 mg/kg 1:10,000

Defibrillation†
4 J/kg

Amiodarone^ IV/IO 5 mg/kg
OR Lidocaine* IV/IO/TT
1 mg/kg *OR* Magnesium
(Torsades) IV/IO
25-50 mg/kg

Defibrillation
4 J/kg
Pattern: Drug–CPR–shock
(repeat)

Not V–Fib/V–Tach Incl. PEA, asystole

Epinephrine
IV/IO 0.01 mg/kg 1:10,000
ETT 0.1 mg/kg 1:1000

CPR, IV, intubate

Epinephrine
q 3–5 min

Identify underlying
causes PEA:
Hypovolemia
Hypoxia
H+ (acidosis)
Hypo/Hyperkalemia
Hypothermia
Tamponade
Tension PTX
Toxins/Poisons
Thromboembolism

Pulse branch:

- **QRS NL (<0.08 sec)**
- **Wide QRS (>0.08 sec)**

SVT

Unstable
Cardioversion
0.5–1 J/kg

Stable
Adenosine
IV/IO 0.1 mg/kg
(max 6mg)

Adenosine
IV/IO 0.2 mg/kg
(max 12 mg)

*Consider alternative
medications*
Amiodarone^
(5 mg/kg IV
over 20–60 min)
OR Procainamide
(15 mg/kg IV
over 10–15 min)

**Sinus
tachycardia**

Treat
underlying
disorder

V-Tach

Unstable
Cardioversion
0.5–1 J/kg

Stable
Amiodarone^
(5 mg/kg IV
over 20–60 min)
OR Procainamide
(15 mg/kg IV
over 10–15 min)
OR Lidocaine*
(1 mg/kg IV)
OR Adenosine
0.1 mg/kg, then
0.2 mg/kg (max 12 mg)
if SVT probable

^For Amiodarone administration: Repeat doses of
1–5 mg/kg (maximum 15 mg/kg/day) may be required
depending upon patient stability and clinical scenario.

* For Lidocaine administration: repeat every 5–10
minutes after initial bolus, to total dose 3 mg/kg. After
return of perfusion, follow with continuous infusion
@20–50 mcg/kg/min.

† Perform 5 cycles of CPR between each defibrillation
attempt.

FIGURE 63–1. Approach to managing infants and children with tachycardia. Abbreviations: CPR, cardiopulmonary resuscitation; ETT, endotracheal tube; IO, intraosseously; IV, intravenously; NL, normal; PEA, pulseless electrical activity; PTX, pneumothorax; SVT, supraventricular tachycardia; TT, transtracheal; V-Fib, ventricular fibrillation; V-Tach, ventricular tachycardia.

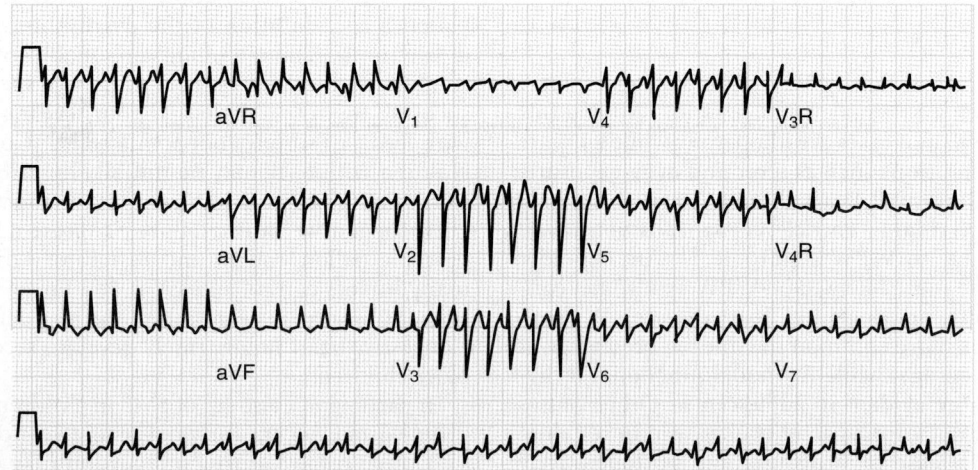

FIGURE 63–2. Supraventricular tachycardia. This 13-year-old male had no previous cardiac history. After playing football, he began having palpitations and difficulty breathing. After a delay in treatment of approximately 48 hours, he presented with this rhythm and congestive heart failure. The patient had subsequent episodes, prompting radioablation treatment. (Photo courtesy of Stephanie Doniger, MD, Children's Hospital, San Diego.)

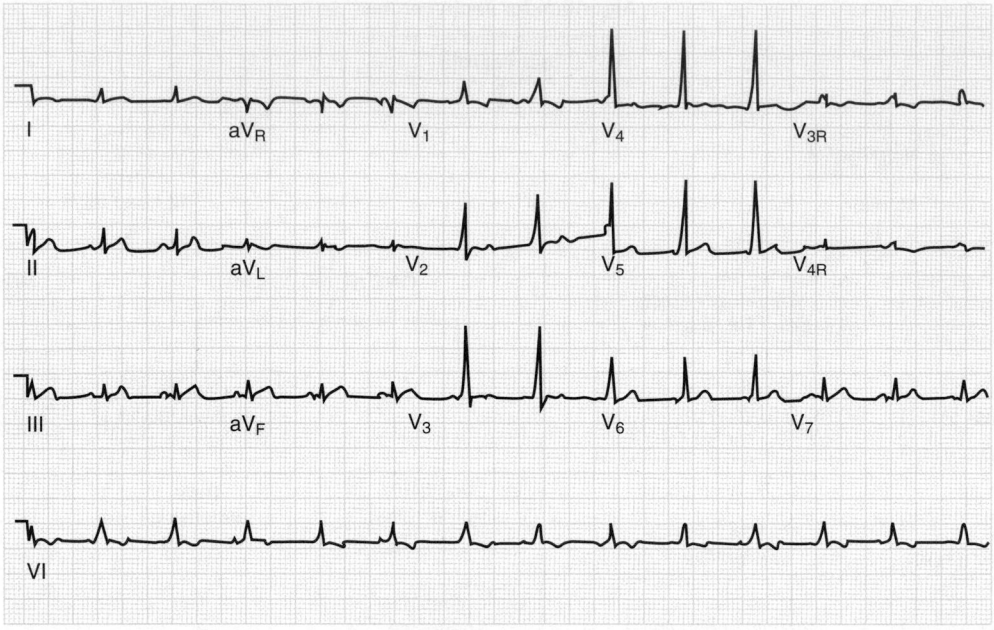

FIGURE 63–3. Wolff-Parkinson-White (WPW) syndrome. This child presented in supraventricular tachycardia. After being converted to sinus rhythm, the delta waves were apparent. The delta wave is a positive inflection in the upstroke of the QRS complex. (Photo courtesy of CDR Jonathan T. Fleenor, MD, Naval Medical Center, San Diego.)

an anatomically separate bypass tract, such as the bundle of Kent, which is seen in Wolff-Parkinson-White (WPW) syndrome. Conduction through this accessory pathway occurs more rapidly than through the normal conduction pathway, creating a cyclic pattern of reentry independent of the SA node. Typical ECG findings of WPW syndrome are a short PR interval, a wide QRS complex, and a positive inflection in the upstroke of the QRS complex, known as the delta wave (Fig. 63–3).

The second type of SVT is AV nodal/junctional tachycardia, which is a cyclical reentrant pattern from dual AV node pathways that are simultaneously depolarized. The third type of SVT, ectopic atrial tachycardia, is rare and is manifested by the rapid firing of a single ectopic focus in the atrium. The hallmark of ectopic atrial tachycardia is the presence of different P wave morphologies. Each P wave is conducted to the ventricle and, since the ectopic atrial focus is faster than the SA node, it takes over rate determination.

CLINICAL PRESENTATION

The majority of infants with SVT present at less than 4 months of age, with a 3 : 2 male : female ratio.[14] Among this group, almost one half of cases are idiopathic, while 24% are associated with conditions such as fever and drug exposure, 23% are due to congenital heart disease (most commonly Ebstein's anomaly, single ventricle, L-transposition), and 10% to 22% are due to WPW syndrome.[13,15] Among older children, causes are more likely to be WPW syndrome, concealed bypass tracts, or congenital heart disease. AV reentrant tachycardia is more common in children presenting at less than 12 years of age, while AV nodal/junctional tachycardia becomes more evident in adolescents.[5] Other causes include hyperdynamic cardiac activity as is seen in response to catecholamine release or drug use, and postoperatively following cardiac repair. Toxic causes of SVT include stimu-

lants (amphetamines, caffeine, ephedrine, tobacco), β-agonists (albuterol), anticholinergics (atropine), salicylates, theophylline, tricyclic antidepressants, and phenothiazines. SVT may also result from nontoxic disorders such as anxiety, anemia, sedative and ethanol withdrawal, dehydration, acidosis, exercise, fever, hypoglycemia, hypoxemia, and pain.

The diagnosis often begins in triage, with the nurse reporting a heart rate that is "too fast to count." In neonates and infants with SVT, the heart rate is often between 220 and 280 bpm.[11,13] Most patients do not have an underlying cause to account for the tachycardia, such as fever, dehydration, fluid or blood loss, anxiety, or pain. Important historical factors include a relationship to exercise, meals, or stress; color changes; neurologic changes; and syncope. A past medical history significant for cardiac problems, current medications, allergies, or a family history of sudden death or cardiac disease should be investigated.

The clinical presentation of SVT is dependent on the patient's age, duration of the dysrhythmia, and rate of the dysrhythmia. Though infants are unable to verbally describe symptoms, the history may elicit nonspecific complaints, such as "fussiness," lethargy, poor feeding, pallor, sweating with feeds, or simply "not acting right." Complaints of older children with SVT may be initially described as "pounding in the chest," chest pain, dizziness, or shortness of breath.

If congestive heart failure is present, caregivers may describe pallor, cough, and respiratory distress. Although many infants can tolerate SVT well for 24 hours, within 48 hours 50% develop heart failure and may deteriorate rapidly.[13] Congestive heart failure rarely develops secondary to SVT in older children.

In particular, episodes of SVT in children with WPW syndrome usually occur early in the first year of life. Episodes of SVT often resolve during infancy but may recur later in life, usually between 6 and 8 years of age.[16] The characteristic finding of delta waves is not present during an episode of tachydysrhythmia. It is not until the patient returns to sinus rhythm that these waves become evident. In addition, children with WPW syndrome, especially those older than 12 years of age, are predisposed to developing atrial fibrillation.

MANAGEMENT

Management of SVT always begins with ensuring that the patient is maintaining good airway, breathing, and cardiovascular status. It is important to promptly administer oxygen, and to obtain a 12-lead ECG with rhythm strip. Clinicians must expeditiously differentiate between infants and children who are stable and those who are unstable. In children with asymptomatic SVT or with mild heart failure, vagal maneuvers such applying as ice to the face of an infant or having an older child blowing through a straw may be attempted. If these are unsuccessful, adenosine is administered through an intravenous (IV) line that is preferably close to the heart. Due to its extremely short half-life, adenosine must be pushed at the most proximal port and flushed (with 5 ml normal saline) quickly in order to be effective. The initial dose of adenosine is 0.1 mg/kg (up to 6 mg), and it can be increased to 0.2 mg/kg per dose (up to 12 mg) if the first dose is ineffective. An effective response is a brief period of asystole on ECG, with the return of a normal sinus rhythm. Failure to terminate the dysrhythmia after the second dose of adenosine in a stable patient should prompt consultation with a pediatric cardiologist. Alternatives include procainamide (10 to 15 mg/kg IV over 30 to 45 minutes, followed by a continuous infusion at 20 to 80 mcg/kg per minute if needed, up to 2 g/day) and amiodarone (5 mg/kg over 20 to 60 minutes, with a maximum single dose of 150 mg followed by bolus dosing of 1 to 5 mg/kg if needed, and a maximum daily dose of 15 mg/kg).[17] Continuous infusions of amiodarone should be avoided as this route causes leaching of toxic metabolites from IV tubing. Amiodarone must not be used in neonates (birth to 30 days old) as it may cause a gasping syndrome (respiratory distress, metabolic acidosis, followed by cardiac arrest). Importantly, amiodarone is not approved by the Food and Drug Administration for use in children, although the American Heart Association recognizes that this is an important agent whose therapeutic benefit outweighs theoretical risks in certain pediatric dysrhythmias (see *http://www.americanheart.org/*). β-Blockers such as propranolol or esmolol may be used for SVT, but with caution, as propranolol may cause hypotension. Digoxin is effective in converting SVT; however, the onset of action is slow. β-Blockers, calcium channel blockers, and digoxin should be avoided in SVT or atrial fibrillation/flutter with a wide QRS complex (i.e., WPW syndrome) as these agents can increase the transmission through the bypass tract and induce ventricular tachycardia or ventricular fibrillation. If the SVT has a narrow QRS complex, a bypass tract is not conducting beats via an accessory pathway and these agents should not increase the ventricular rate. In addition, calcium channel blockers (e.g., verapamil, diltiazem) should be avoided in children less than 1 year of age and used cautiously in older infants and children (1 to 8 years old), as cardiovascular collapse and death can occur due to electromechanical dissociation.[13,18]

Alternatively, immediate synchronized cardioversion is warranted in a child with unstable SVT with severe heart failure and poor perfusion. Cardioversion is initiated at 0.5 joules/kg, and can be increased up to 1 joule/kg. Adenosine may be given prior to cardioversion if intravenous access has already been established. In unstable patients, cardioversion should not be delayed for attempts at IV access or sedation.

Adenosine has negative chronotropic, dromotropic, and ionotropic actions of short duration. Its action is in blocking AV conduction and sinus pacemaker activity, terminating almost all SVTs in which the AV node forms a reentry circuit. Adenosine can be both diagnostic and therapeutic. If the diagnosis of SVT is in question, adenosine can be administered to stable patients who have a regular tachycardia, to monitor for a response. Adenosine is not effective with nonreciprocating atrial tachycardia, atrial flutter, atrial fibrillation, or ventricular tachycardia. There are minimal hemodynamic consequences associated with adenosine administration.[19] Contraindications include a denervated heart (transplant) and second- or third-degree heart block unless a pacemaker is present. Additionally, adenosine can worsen bronchospasm in asthmatics and increase heart block or precipitate ventricular arrhythmias in patients taking carbamazepine, verapamil, or digoxin.

The evaluation of SVT includes attempts at determining the etiology of SVT in order to prevent future episodes. Laboratory studies may include electrolytes (especially potassium, calcium, magnesium, and glucose), complete blood count, toxicology screen, blood gases, and thyroid function tests. Additionally, creatine kinase and troponins may be added if myocarditis is suspected. Imaging studies can include a chest radiograph (including anteroposterior and lateral views) and echocardiogram. Once stabilized, the majority of patients with new-onset SVT require hospital admission to investigate the underlying cause of SVT, and the potential for long-term medical management or radiofrequency ablation.[20] Clinicians can safely discharge patients with a history of SVT, minor symptoms such as palpitations, and a clear precipitant.

SUMMARY

Supraventricular tachycardia is the most common type of tachyarrhythmia in childhood. The most common type of SVT is reentrant tachycardia, one cause of which is WPW syndrome. In patients presenting with SVT, symptoms can vary from nonspecific to florid heart failure. Upon their presentation to the ED, it is crucial to quickly distinguish stable from unstable patients. Unstable patients require more aggressive, immediate cardioversion, while vagal maneuvers and adenosine are first-line treatments for stable patients. Collaboration with cardiology can help discover the underlying cause of the SVT, and determine the most appropriate prophylactic regimen for the child in preventing future episodes.

Atrial Flutter

Atrial flutter is an uncommon rhythm in the pediatric population. Atrial rates may range from 240 to 450 bpm,[4] with the ventricular response depending on the AV nodal conduction. The pacemaker lies in an ectopic focus.

Causes of atrial flutter in children are largely attributed to structural heart disease, including dilated atria, myocarditis, or acute infection. It is most notably associated with postoperative complications of congenital heart disease repairs,

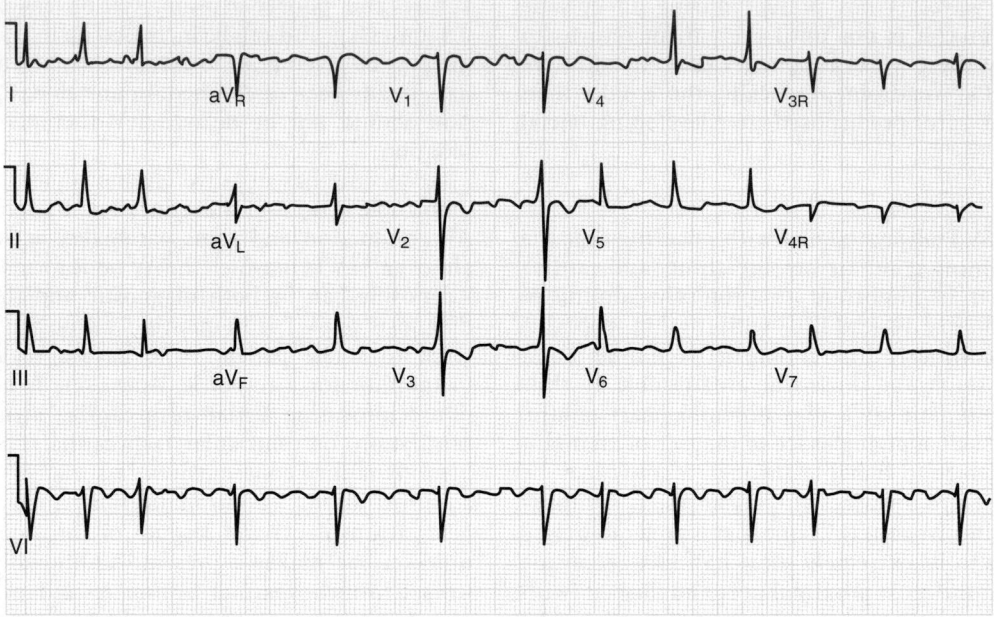

FIGURE 63–4. Atrial flutter. This electrocardiogram is from a child who had a Fontan repair for hypoplastic left heart. (Photo courtesy of CDR Jonathan T. Fleenor, MD, Naval Medical Center, San Diego.)

such as atrial septal defect (ASD) repairs, the Mustard operation for D-transposition of the great arteries, or the Fontan procedure for single ventricle. These procedures cause atrial flutter via disruption in the conduction system, such as when there is suturing through the atrial septum. Occasionally, patients who have had ventricular surgeries, such as tetralogy of Fallot repair, may present with atrial arrhythmias. Atrial flutter is also seen in such conditions as Duchenne's muscular dystrophy and central nervous system injury.

CLINICAL PRESENTATION

On ECG, the hallmark pattern is "saw-toothed" flutter waves, which are best viewed in leads II, III, and V_1. The atrial rate is on average approximately 300 atrial bpm.[3] Since the AV node cannot respond this quickly, there is an AV block that can present as a 2 : 1, 3 : 1, or 4 : 1 block. The QRS complex is generally normal in configuration (Fig. 63–4).

Significant cardiac pathology usually accompanies atrial flutter. Since cardiac output is determined by the ventricular rate, with atrial flutter, the ventricular rate is too fast to maintain an efficient cardiac output. Atrial arrhythmias are an important cause of morbidity and mortality in patients with congenital heart disease.

MANAGEMENT

Initially, the clinician must recognize whether the patient is hemodynamically stable. An unstable patient may require electrical cardioversion, with consideration given to adding heparin to prevent embolization.[4,21] In patients receiving digoxin, it is advisable to avoid electrical cardioversion, unless the condition is life-threatening, since the combination is associated with malignant ventricular arrhythmias.[22,23] Alternatives in those receiving digoxin are rapid atrial pacing with catheterization or cardioversion with lower current settings.[21] For patients who are hemodynamically stable, digoxin is administered to increase AV blockade, thereby slowing the ventricular rate. Propranolol (1.0 to 4.0 mg/kg

per day PO, divided three to four times per day) may also be added. Recurrences are then prevented by administering quinidine.

SUMMARY

Although atrial flutter is an uncommon dysrhythmia in children, its presence can suggest an underlying cardiac problem. In those who have underlying congenital heart disease, atrial flutter is an especially important cause of morbidity and mortality. The mainstay of treatment lies in cardioversion for hemodynamically unstable patients, while stable patients receive digoxin with or without propranolol.

Atrial Fibrillation

Atrial fibrillation is another rare rhythm in children. It is defined as disorganized, rapid atrial activity with atrial rates ranging from 350 to 600 bpm.[15] The ventricular rate is variable, and is dependent upon a varying AV block. Children at increased risk of developing atrial fibrillation include patients with an underlying structural heart defect (e.g., congenital mitral valve disease), those with hyperthyroidism, and those who have had an intra-atrial operative procedure.

CLINICAL PRESENTATION

The rhythm of atrial fibrillation is described as being irregularly irregular, alternating between fast and slow rates. On ECG, hallmark features are irregular atrial waves, with beat-to-beat variability of the waves' size and shape. This is best recognized in lead V_1. The atrial rate may range from 350 to 600 atrial bpm, with a variable ventricular response. The QRS complexes appear normal.

As with atrial flutter, atrial fibrillation is associated with decreased cardiac output. With a significantly increased ventricular rate, incoordination between the atria and ventricles occurs, thereby decreasing cardiac output. A patient presenting with atrial fibrillation generally has significant underlying cardiac pathology.

MANAGEMENT

Upon presentation to the emergency department, hemodynamically unstable patients warrant immediate cardioversion. However, in patients who are hemodynamical stable, digoxin can be administered for ventricular rate control, allowing for a 24-hour time period in order to assess its efficacy. After that time period elapses, should digoxin prove to be ineffective, a second medication may be added, such as propranolol, esmolol, or procainamide. Alternatively, calcium channel blockers such as verapamil may be considered for rate control in children. It is important to note that IV verapamil (0.1 to 0.3 mg/kg per dose, with a maximum of 10 mg/dose) should not be used in children younger than 1 year of age, and should be used with caution in those between 1 and 8 years of age, due to the risks of apnea, bradycardia, hypotension, and cardiac arrest.[24] In patients who have undergone cardioversion, recurrence is common. During admission, cardioverted patients are often started on an agent to keep them in normal sinus rhythm (e.g., amiodarone, procainamide, quinidine, or a β-blocker).[25]

SUMMARY

Atrial fibrillation is an irregularly irregular rhythm, with rapid atrial rates and beat-to-beat variability. Its presence usually suggests an underlying cardiac pathology in the pediatric population. Those patients who are stable may receive digoxin, while those who are hemodynamically unstable require cardioversion. Admission is warranted for patients who are newly diagnosed with atrial fibrillation or are diagnosed with chronic atrial fibrillation with rapid ventricular rate, or with cardiovascular compromise.

Premature Atrial Contractions

Premature atrial contractions (PACs) are common in children, and are defined as premature P waves with premature QRS complexes. There is an incomplete compensatory pause, making the premature beat less than two normal cycles. While most P waves have a subsequent QRS wave, rarely are PACs nonconducted.

The majority of children presenting with PACs are healthy children and neonates. Others include postoperative cardiac surgery patients and those with hypoxia, use of sympathomimetic drugs, hyperthyroidism, and digoxin toxicity. With the exception of treating the underlying disease or drug toxicity, no treatment is necessary for PACs.

Premature Ventricular Contractions

A premature ventricular contraction (PVC) is a premature wide QRS complex that has a distinct configuration and is not preceded by a P wave. They may appear in patterns of two consecutive PVCs (couplet), alternating PVC with normal QRS complex (bigeminy), or a PVC every third beat (trigeminy). The SA node maintains a normal conduction pace, and the PVC replaces a normal QRS complex while maintaining a rhythm. Three or more consecutive PVCs is considered ventricular tachycardia. The morphology of PVCs may be further classified into unifocal PVCs and multifocal PVCs. Unifocal PVCs have the same configuration in a single lead, and originate from a single focus. Alternatively, multifocal PVCs have an abnormal, inconsistent configuration in a single lead, and originate from different foci.

Although most children who have PVCs are healthy, PVCs can be associated with congenital heart disease, mitral valve prolapse, long QT syndrome (LQTS), and cardiomyopathies (dilated and hypertrophic). Malignant etiologies further include electrolyte imbalances, drug toxicities (general anesthesia, digoxin, catecholamines, amphetamines, sympathomimetics, phenothiazines), cardiac injury, cardiac tumors, myocarditis (Lyme and viral), hypoxia, and an intraventricular catheter.

CLINICAL PRESENTATION

For the most part, patients with PVCs are asymptomatic. When examined, 50% to 75% of otherwise normal children may have PVCs on Holter monitoring.[4] It is crucial to determine whether or not the heart has underlying pathology. This can be accomplished by history and physical examination, 12-lead ECG, and chest radiograph. If all of these are normal, no further investigation is necessary. For couplets and multiform PVCs, referral to a pediatric cardiologist and further investigation is indicated.

Though PVCs are for the most part benign, when left unrecognized and untreated, there is a risk of developing ventricular tachycardia in those patients with a serious underlying cause. PVCs are considered malignant if they are associated with underlying heart disease, if there is a history of syncope or family history of sudden death, if they are precipitated or increased with activity, if they have multiform morphology, or if there are symptomatic runs of PVCs or frequent episodes of paroxysmal ventricular tachycardia.

MANAGEMENT

Children presenting with PVCs require evaluation and possibly treatment of conditions that are likely to cause cardiopulmonary compromise. Evaluation is required when there are two or more PVCs in a row, they are multifocal in origin, there is an "R-on-T phenomenon," or there is underlying heart disease. The R-on-T phenomenon is when a PVC occurs on the T wave, which is considered a "vulnerable period" for stimulating abnormal rhythms. This can be seen with hypoxia or hypokalemia, and may result in life-threatening arrhythmias.[26] For patients with an underlying cause (e.g., electrolyte abnormality, hypoxia, severe acidosis), treatment consists of managing the underlying cause. Treatment is with IV lidocaine (1 mg/kg per dose), followed by a lidocaine drip (20 to 50 mcg/kg per minute). Amiodarone, procainamide, and β-blockers are reserved for those patients who are refractory to lidocaine.[15]

Asymptomatic patients presenting with isolated PVCs and normal cardiac structure and function require no treatment. Those who have frequent PVCs should have an evaluation to rule out myocarditis. Use of 24-hour Holter monitoring may be necessary to distinguish isolated PVCs from SVT. Patients with PVCs should avoid stimulants such as caffeine, theophylline, and pseudoephedrine since they may precipitate more frequent PVCs. While most patients with coupled PVCs or bigeminy may not require therapy, a pediatric cardiologist should be consulted.

Ventricular Tachycardia

Although rare in children, ventricular tachycardia is an important rhythm to recognize and promptly treat. Nonperfusing ventricular rhythms are seen in up to 19% of pediatric

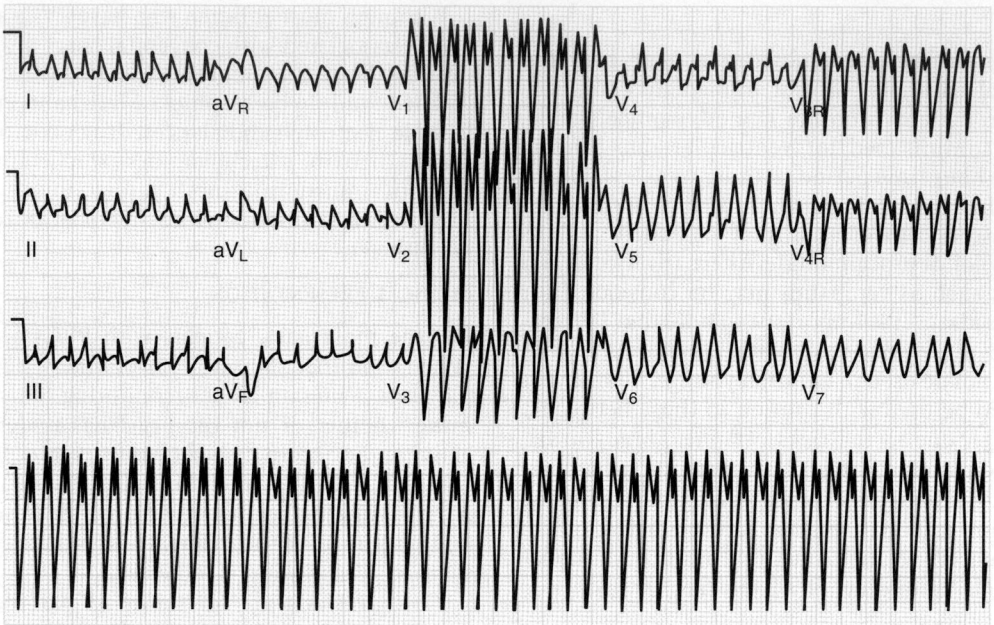

FIGURE 63–5. Ventricular tachycardia. This is an example of an extraordinarily fast ventricular tachycardia with a heart rate of almost 300 bpm. (Photo courtesy of CDR Jonathan T. Fleenor, MD, Naval Medical Center, San Diego.)

cardiac arrests, when sudden infant death syndrome (SIDS) cases are excluded.[27] By definition, ventricular tachycardia is three or more consecutive PVCs, with heart rates ranging from 120 to 200 bpm. The rate may be as rapid as 400 or 500 bpm.[28]

Ventricular tachycardia may result from electrolyte disturbances (hyperkalemia, hypokalemia, hypocalcemia), metabolic abnormalities, congenital heart disorders, myocarditis, or drug toxicity. Other causes include cardiomyopathies, cardiac tumors, acquired heart disease, LQTS, and idiopathic causes.

CLINICAL PRESENTATION

On ECG, the QRS complexes have a wide configuration. The QRS duration is prolonged, ranging from 0.06 to 0.14 seconds. Complexes may appear monomorphic, with a uniform contour and absent or retrograde P waves. Alternatively, the QRS complexes may appear polymorphic, or vary randomly as is seen in torsades de pointes. Electrocardiogram findings that further support the presence of ventricular tachycardia include the presence of AV dissociation with the ventricular rate exceeding the atrial rate (Fig. 63–5).

Children can generally tolerate rapid ventricular rhythms for a few hours. However, decreased cardiac output and hypotension can quickly follow. Though the heart may be contracting and pulses palpable in some patients with ventricular tachycardia, those contractions are hemodynamically inefficient and can ultimately lead to syncope and death if left untreated. Ventricular tachycardia can also decompensate into ventricular fibrillation, which is a nonperfusing, terminal arrhythmia.

MANAGEMENT

In a patient with ventricular tachycardia, the urgency of treatment depends on the patient's clinical status. Initially, it must be determined whether or not the patient has a pulse and is hemodynamically stable. The American Heart Asso-

ciation has set forth treatment algorithms[11] in order to facilitate prompt treatment for this potentially fatal rhythm (see Fig. 63–1).

Ventricular tachycardia with a pulse in an unstable patient warrants immediate synchronized cardioversion at 0.5 to 1 joule/kg. It is important to pretreat conscious patients with light sedation (i.e., IV midazolam 0.1 mg/kg). Pharmacologic interventions include amiodarone (see dosing recommendations/cautions in the section on SVT), procainamide (10 to 15 mg/kg IV over 30 to 45 minutes), and lidocaine (1 mg/kg IV bolus, repeated every 5 to 10 minutes, with a maximum total dose of 3 mg/kg). When using procainamide, the infusion is stopped once the arrhythmia resolved, if the QRS widens more than 50% over the baseline, or if hypotension develops.

Pulseless ventricular tachycardia should be treated as ventricular fibrillation. Amiodarone has been studied extensively in adults as a treatment modality for hemodynamically unstable ventricular tachycardia and recurrent ventricular fibrillation.[29] It is a class III antidysrhythmic agent that results in potassium channel blockade. It also has some properties of class I (sodium channel blockade), class II (β-blockade), and class IV (calcium channel blockade) agents. Therefore, it is useful in treating both supraventricular and ventricular tachyarrhythmias.[30] Amiodarone is considered a class Ib recommendation for ventricular tachycardia with a pulse, secondary to the paucity of directly relevant published information on the safety profile in children.[31]

After cardioversion, the return to normal sinus rhythm is usually transient. If lidocaine or procainamide is used to achieve sinus rhythm, it should be continued: lidocaine at 20 to 50 mcg/kg per minute, procainamide at 20 to 80 mcg/kg per minute (maximum dose of 2 g/day). However, a continuous infusion of amiodarone leads to leaching of toxic metabolites, requiring bolus dosing of 1 to 5 mg/kg as needed (maximum of 15 mg/kg per day). In polymorphic ventricular tachycardia, temporary atrial or ventricular pacing may be required.

Overall, the treatment goal is to keep the heart rate less than 150 bpm in infants and less than 130 bpm in older children.

Ventricular Fibrillation

Ventricular fibrillation is an uncommon rhythm in the pediatric population, but is certainly life-threatening. The hallmark is chaotic, irregular ventricular contractions without circulation to the body. Causes of ventricular fibrillation include postoperative complications from congenital heart disease repair, severe hypoxemia, hyperkalemia, medications (digitalis, quinidine, catecholamines, anesthesia), myocarditis, and myocardial infarction.

CLINICAL PRESENTATION

On ECG, the rhythm is one of bizarre QRS complexes with varying sizes and configurations. It is characterized by a rapid, irregular rate.

MANAGEMENT

Ventricular fibrillation is an uncommon cause of cardiac arrest in infants less than 1 year of age, but the incidence increases with increasing age.[27] With the increased use and efficacy of automatic external defibrillators (AEDs) in the adult setting, controversy has arisen regarding the use of AEDs in prehospital treatment of children in cardiac arrest. Many adult AEDs deliver high energy settings for defibrillation. In addition, some rhythms presenting in children, such as sinus tachycardia and SVT, may be misinterpreted by the AED as "shockable rhythms." Currently AEDs are approved for children older than 8 years of age.[27] However, according to the American Heart Association International Liaison Committee on Resuscitation, AEDs may be used in children 1 to 8 years of age without signs of circulation, ideally with the pediatric energy setting. For a lone rescuer responding to a child without signs of circulation, cardiopulmonary resuscitation (CPR) for 1 minute is recommended prior to attaching an AED or activating the Emergency Management System. For documented ventricular fibrillation or pulseless ventricular tachycardia, defibrillation is recommended.[11]

Ventricular fibrillation is a nonperfusing rhythm. Therefore, CPR must be initiated immediately. Ventricular fibrillation is treated the same as ventricular tachycardia without a pulse. Defibrillation is initiated at 2 joules/kg, and then increased to 2 to 4 joules/kg, then to 4 joules/kg. Perform 5 cycles of CPR between each individual defibrillation attempt. If defibrillation is unsuccessful, epinephrine (0.01 mg/kg 1 : 10,000 solution) should be given, and repeated every 3 to 5 minutes as necessary.

If pulseless ventricular tachycardia is refractory to defibrillation, antiarrhythmics are indicated: amiodarone (5 mg/kg IV bolus) or lidocaine (1 mg/kg IV bolus, repeated to a maximum of 3 mg/kg) may be used. Although the pediatric dosing of amiodarone has not been clearly established, the recommended loading dose is 5 mg/kg IV and may be given over minutes to 1 hour. If rate control is not achieved, the dose may be repeated in 5-mg/kg IV increments, to a maximum of 15 mg/kg per day IV.[17] Clinicians should be aware that higher doses are associated with immediate side effects (e.g., prolonged QT, bradydysrhythmias, AV blocks). For polymorphic ventricular tachycardia (torsades de pointes), the mainstay of treatment is magnesium (20 to 50 mg/kg IV to a maximum of 2 g) administered slowly.

SUMMARY

Though uncommon in the pediatric population, ventricular fibrillation is a nonperfusing, potentially lethal dysrhythmia. Defibrillation is the mainstay of therapy, with epinephrine as an adjunct when defibrillation is unsuccessful.

Bradydysrhythmias

Bradycardia is defined as a heart rate slower than the lower limit of normal for the patient's age (see Table 63–1), while in adults it is defined as a heart rate less than 60 bpm. Mechanisms of bradycardia include depression of the pacemaker in the sinus node and conduction system blocks. Complete heart block is a common cause of significant bradycardia in pediatric patients and may be acquired or congenital.

Bradycardia in children may be attributable to vagal stimulation, hypoxemia, acidosis, or an acute elevation of intracranial pressure. The most common cause of bradycardia in the pediatric population is hypoxemia. It is important to correct hypoxemia prior to increasing the heart rate with medicines in children.

Sinus Bradycardia

Sinus bradycardia includes a heart rate less than the lower limit of normal for the patient's age (see Table 63–1), while maintaining P waves preceding each QRS complex. Usually, the heart rate is less than 80 bpm in infants and less than 60 bpm in older children.[32] Sinus bradycardia is predominantly a benign entity, most often seen in athletes and during sleep.

However, sinus bradycardia can also be associated with underlying causes. One such ominous cause is an acute onset of increased intracranial pressure as part of Cushing's triad of bradycardia, hypertension, and irregular respirations. It can also be associated with hyperkalemia, hypercalcemia, hypoxia, hypothermia, hypothyroidism, and medications (digitalis, β-blockers). Just as with sinus tachycardia, the treatment of sinus bradycardia is targeted at the treatment of the underlying cause.

An important distinction must be made between sinus bradycardia and junctional (nodal) bradycardia. On ECG, junctional bradycardia has either no P waves or inverted P waves after QRS complexes. QRS complexes have normal configuration, and generally have rates between 40 and 60 bpm. Junctional bradycardia may occur in an otherwise normal heart, postoperatively, with digitalis toxicity, or with increased vagal tone. If the patient is asymptomatic, no acute treatment is indicated. However, if the patient has signs of decreased cardiac output, atropine or pacing may be indicated.[4]

Conduction Abnormalities

RECOGNITION AND APPROACH

First-degree AV block is an abnormal delay in conduction through the AV node. This type of AV block is a disturbance in the conduction between the normal sinus impulse and its eventual ventricular response. This manifests as a prolonged PR interval on ECG. Meanwhile, the heart is maintained in sinus rhythm, with a normal QRS configuration. There are no dropped beats. First-degree heart block can be an incidental finding on an otherwise normal ECG. Common causes include an infectious disease in an otherwise healthy child.

It may also be associated with myocarditis (e.g., rheumatic fever, Lyme disease), cardiomyopathies, and congenital heart disease (ASD, Ebstein's anomaly).

There are two types of second-degree AV block: Mobitz type I (Wenckebach) and Mobitz type II. In *Mobitz type I or Wenckebach phenomenon*, the PR interval progressively lengthens until a QRS complex is dropped. This usually occurs over three to six cardiac cycles, followed by a long diastolic pause, and then resumption of the cycle. There are occasional and frequent P waves that conduct, and the QRS configuration is normal. The block is due to an increased refractory period at the level of the AV node. Though this can be seen in otherwise healthy individuals, it can also be seen in patients with myocarditis, myocardial infarction, cardiomyopathies, congenital heart disease, and digoxin toxicity, and postoperatively following cardiac repairs.

Mobitz type II second-degree heart block is known as the "all or none" phenomenon. There is either normal AV conduction with a normal PR interval, or completely blocked conduction. The failure of conduction is at the level of the bundle of His, with a prolongation of the refractory period in the His-Purkinje system. Since some of the atrial impulses are not conducted to the ventricle, the ventricular rate depends on the number of conducted atrial impulses.

Third-degree heart block, otherwise known as complete heart block, occurs when none of the atrial impulses is conducted to the ventricles. There is a complete loss of rhythm conduction from a working atrial pacemaker, thereby allowing the ventricular pacemaker to take over. On ECG, the P waves are completely dissociated from the QRS complexes. Even though they are dissociated, both the atrial and ventricular rhythms are regular, maintaining regular P-P intervals and R-R intervals, respectively. The QRS duration is usually normal if the block is proximal to the bundle of His, while a wide QRS complex indicates that the block is most likely in the bundle branches (e.g., surgically induced complete heart block). Oftentimes, the ventricular rhythm is slower than normal (Fig. 63–6).

Complete heart block may be an isolated anomaly. It may also be congenital, and is associated with structural lesions such as L-transposition of the great arteries and maternal connective tissue disorders. Acquired heart block may result from cardiac surgery, especially when there is suturing in the atrium. This effect can either be transient, resolving within 8 days postoperatively, or permanent. Other etiologies include infectious causes such as myocarditis, Lyme disease, rheumatic fever, and diphtheria, and inflammatory disorders such as Kawasaki disease and lupus. Complete heart block is also associated with myocardial infarction, cardiac tumors, muscular dystrophies, hypocalcemia, and drug overdoses.

CLINICAL PRESENTATION

Children presenting with first-degree heart block are largely asymptomatic, but have the potential to progress to further heart block, including second- and third-degree heart blocks. Those with second-degree, type I (Wenckeback) block rarely progress to complete heart block, while those with type II second-degree block frequently progress to complete heart block.[4] Children with complete heart block, most notably in infancy, may present with signs of congestive heart failure. Older children may present with syncopal attacks, otherwise known as Stokes-Adams attacks, with heart rates less than 40 to 45 bpm, or even sudden death.

Patients presenting with complete heart block may have symptoms related to hypoperfusion, including fatigue, dizziness, impaired exercise tolerance, syncope, confusion, and sudden death.[33] Acquired or surgically induced heart block generally has a slower ventricular rate, between 40 and 50 bpm, than is common with congenital complete heart block, which generally manifests with a rate of 50 to 80 bpm.[4]

Management

Management of bradycardia includes identification of the etiology and appropriate cardiopulmonary resuscitation, with assisted ventilation, oxygenation, and chest compressions as indicated. If symptomatic bradycardia persists despite

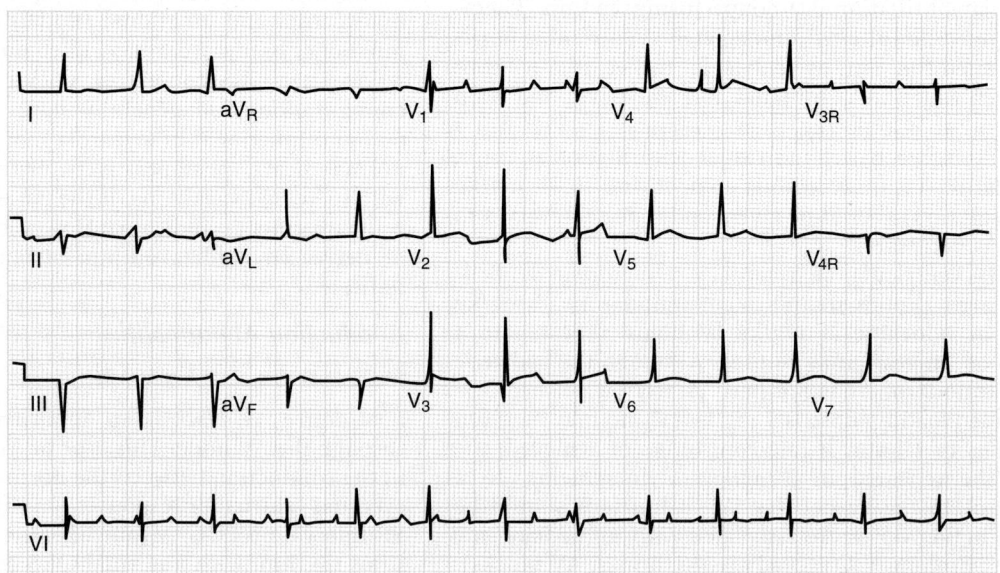

FIGURE 63–6. Complete heart block. This electrocardiogram is of an infant presenting at birth; notice the complete dissociation of P waves from QRS complexes. The child's mother had systemic lupus erythematosus, which is commonly associated with complete heart block. (Photo courtesy of CDR Jonathan T. Fleenor, MD, Naval Medical Center, San Diego.)

initial resuscitative measures, pharmacologic intervention is initiated with epinephrine at 0.01 mg/kg IV or atropine at 0.02 mg/kg IV (minimum 0.1 mg, maximum single dose is 0.5 mg in children and 1 mg in adolescents). Chest compressions are indicated for neonates or infants with heart rates less than 60 bpm with hemodynamic compromise.[11]

No treatment is indicated for a first-degree heart block. However, if suspicious features are present, patients may require evaluation for underlying disease (i.e., Lyme disease, rheumatic fever). For second-degree heart block, treatment is directed at the underlying cause. In patients with Mobitz type II second-degree heart block, a prophylactic pacemaker may be warranted, since there is a risk of progressing to complete heart block. For complete heart block, the mainstay of therapy is a pacemaker. While the patient is awaiting pacemaker insertion, it may be necessary to administer atropine or isoproterenol, which temporarily increases the heart rate, or to apply an external pacemaker.

Sinus Arrhythmia

A frequent finding on ECG assessment is sinus arrhythmia, which is the normal phasic variation in the heart rate. By definition, a P wave is present prior to each QRS complex. This can be best demonstrated on a long rhythm strip, when the heart rate varies with the cycle of respiration. As the heart rate increases with inspiration, the R-R interval consequently decreases. Conversely, the heart rate decreases with expiration while the R-R interval increases. Since this is a benign entity, no treatment is necessary.

Long QT Syndrome

LQTS, otherwise referred to as prolonged QT syndrome, is a disorder of delayed ventricular repolarization, characterized by prolongation of the QT interval on ECG. Prolongation of the QT interval may be either hereditary or acquired. Jervell and Lange-Nielsen syndrome is an autosomal recessive form of LQTS associated with congenital deafness, whereas Romano-Ward syndrome is an autosomal dominant form that is not associated with deafness. Congenital LQTS has an estimated incidence of 1 in 10,000 to 15,000 and is responsible for 3000 to 4000 cases of sudden death each year in the United States.[7] While congenital forms of LQTS present in childhood, patients with the acquired type of LQTS usually present in their fifth or sixth decades of life.[7] There are many causes of acquired LQTS, with medications among the most common (Table 63-2). It is also seen with electrolyte abnormalities, such as hypokalemia, hypocalcemia, and hypomagnesemia.

Table 63-2	Drugs That Prolong the QT Interval
Antiarrhythmics (classes IA and III)	
Antiemetics: droperidol	
Antifungals: ketoconazole	
Antihistamines: astemizole, terfenadine	
Antimicrobials: erythromycin, trimethoprim-sulfamethoxazole	
Antipsychotics: haloperidol, risperidone	
Organophosphate insecticides	
Phenothiazines: thioridazine	
Promotility agents: cisapride	
Tricyclic antidepressants: amitryptyline	

Clinical Presentation

Patients with LQTS commonly present between the ages of 9 and 15 years with recurrent episodes of syncope.[34] Of the patients with acquired LQTS, 60% of affected individuals are symptomatic at diagnosis.[7,35] Syncopal episodes are often precipitated by intense emotion, vigorous physical activity, or loud noises. Syncopal episodes may be mistaken for seizures as they can result in loss of consciousness, tonic-clonic movements, and temporary residual disorientation following the event.

Spontaneous return of consciousness usually follows a syncopal episode, but the dysrhythmia has the potential to degenerate into ventricular fibrillation and sudden death. Approximately 10% of children with LQTS present with sudden death. Age at presentation is related to death, with younger children more likely to die suddenly.[36] LQTS may present in infancy as SIDS, or later in life as near drowning. Children may also present with milder symptoms such as diaphoresis, palpitations, or light-headedness.

When a patient presents with syncope, there are a number of historical factors that should be viewed as warning signs of potential cardiac disease and sudden death. Syncope that occurs with exertion is almost always an ominous sign. The strongest risk factors for developing malignant dysrhythmias or sudden death include a prior history of syncope, documented ventricular tachydysrhythmias, and a history of resuscitated cardiac arrest. Furthermore, a history of congenital deafness and the female gender are both independently associated with an increased likelihood of recurrent cardiac events.

The hallmark dysrhythmia of LQTS is a polymorphic ventricular tachycardia known as *torsades de pointes* ("twisting of the points"), a French term first used in 1966 by Dessertenne to describe a QRS axis shifting back and forth around the baseline[37] (Fig. 63-7). During this dysrhythmic episode, cardiac output is markedly impaired, often resulting in syncope or seizures. Although many of these events are self-limiting, with the spontaneous return of consciousness, the dysrhythmia has the potential to degenerate into ventricular fibrillation and sudden death. With the potential for fatal consequences in undiagnosed affected individuals, the recognition of LQTS is of paramount importance.

LQTS should be considered, and an ECG obtained, in any patient presenting with a suggestive history, including first-degree relatives of a known LQTS carrier; family history of syncope, seizures, or sudden death; a sibling with SIDS; seizure of unknown etiology; and unexplained near drowning. Other risk factors include congenital deafness, and bradycardia in infants. Suggestive features of syncopal episodes include those that are triggered by emotion, exertion, or stress and those that are associated with chest pain or palpitations.

On ECG, the QT interval is manually measured, with lead II generally accepted as being most accurate. To account for the normal physiologic shortening of the QT interval that occurs with increasing heart rate, the QT_c is calculated using the Bazett formula[6]: $QT_c = (QT/\sqrt{RR})$.

Current practice identifies a QT_c of 460 msec as prolonged in infants and children and a QT_c of 500 msec as prolonged in neonates. A QT_c value between 420 and 460 msec is borderline and warrants additional assessment.[8,9] Though ECG

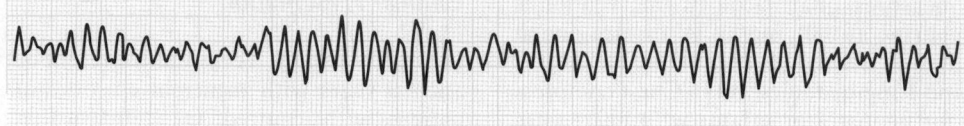

FIGURE 63–7. Rhythm strip showing torsades de pointes. This child had a history of dilated cardiomyopathy, and returned to sinus rhythm after defibrillation. (Photo courtesy of CDR Jonathan T. Fleenor, MD, Naval Medical Center, San Diego.)

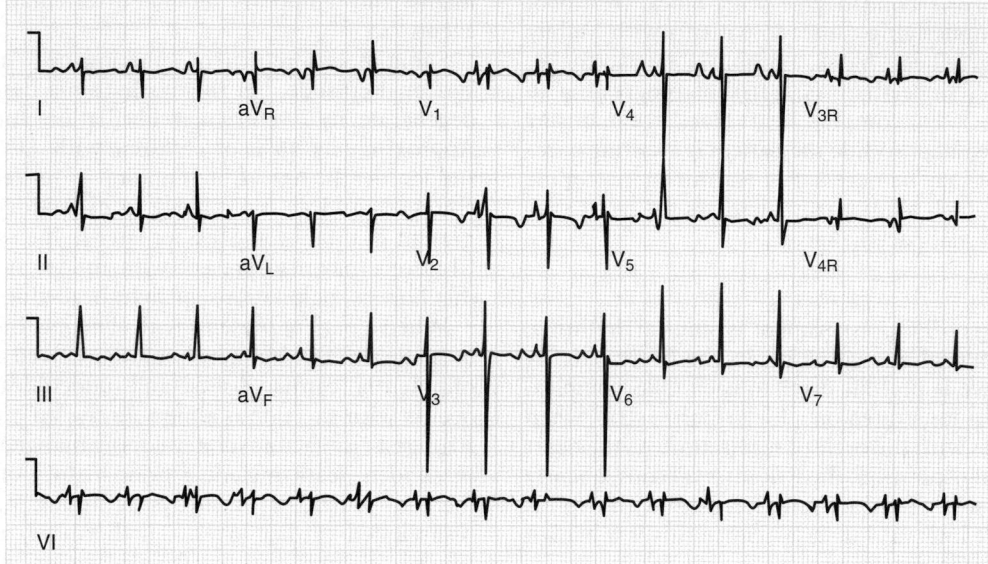

FIGURE 63–8. Long QT syndrome without associated heart block. A markedly prolonged QT interval is calculated with the Bazett formula[6]: QT_c = QT ÷ square root of the preceding R-R interval. Thus

$$QT_c = 0.452/\sqrt{0.612}$$
$$= 578 \text{ msec}$$

Of note, for improved accuracy three consecutive R-R intervals and QT intervals are averaged, where each small box = 0.04 msec. (Photo courtesy of CDR Jonathan T. Fleenor, MD, Naval Medical Center, San Diego.)

equipment automatically calculates the QT and QT_c, in those patients with suggestive history an ECG with manual calculation of the QT_c should be performed, as the computer calculation often is inaccurate. If the diagnosis of LQTS is suspected but the screening ECG is not diagnostic, increasing sympathetic activity such as with vagal maneuvers may trigger abnormalities on ECG. These abnormalities include QT interval prolongation, prominent U waves, T-wave alternans, and ventricular dysrhythmias (Fig. 63–8).

Management

Patients presenting with LQTS may require emergency intervention. Patients presenting with an episode of polymorphic ventricular tachycardia or torsades de pointes of unknown etiology should receive IV magnesium (25 to 50 mg/kg to a maximum of 2 g). Serum electrolytes and a toxicology screen should be obtained. β-Blockers may be useful in suppressing catecholamine surges and further dysrhythmic activity. In patients with torsades due to prolonged QT interval, β-blockers may worsen the blood pressure, whereas they improve the hemodynamic status of patients with a normal QT interval associated with polymorphic ventricular tachycardia. Patients with recurrent ventricular tachycardia may require temporary transcutaneous ventricular pacing.

Any patient with a compatible history, borderline prolongation of the QT interval with symptoms, or identified LQTS should be referred to a cardiologist for further management. Admission is limited to those who are symptomatic or have cardiovascular compromise. Holter monitoring may be helpful in capturing a prolonged QT interval not apparent on a resting ECG. Therapy is aimed at reducing sympathetic activity of the heart, either pharmacologically or surgically. Long-term β-blocker use is generally recommended as the initial therapy of choice as these drugs effectively eradicate dysrhythmias in 60% of patients, and decrease mortality from 71% in untreated patients to 6% in those who are treated.[38,39] Alternative therapies include left-sided cervicothoracic sympathetic ganglionectomy and implantation of automatic implantable cardiac defibrillators.

Once a patient is diagnosed with LQTS, an ECG should be performed on all other family members. All affected individuals, regardless of age, should be restricted from competitive sports but not necessarily recreational sports. Patients should be educated to avoid triggering factors, such as certain medications, loud noises, emotionally stressful situations, and dehydration. Because of the high risk of unexpected cardiac events, family members and close friends should be instructed in CPR and consider purchasing a home AED.

Summary

Due to the potentially severe consequences of untreated disease, the recognition of LQTS is of utmost importance. Physicians must always consider this diagnosis in patients presenting with syncope. A personal and family history of syncope, seizures, congenital deafness, or sudden death should be noted. Syncope that is recurrent or associated with exercise, emotion, chest pain, or difficulty breathing is worrisome. Identification of a patient with LQTS necessitates further assessment of all first-degree relatives. With appropriate treatment of affected individuals, the significant morbidity and mortality associated with LQTS is greatly reduced.

REFERENCES

*1. Sacchetti A, Moyer V, Baricella R, et al: Primary cardiac arrhythmias in children. Pediatr Emerg Care 15:95–98, 1999.

2. Horton L, Mosee S, Brenner J: Use of the electrocardiogram in a pediatric emergency department. Arch Pediatr Adolesc Med 148:184–188, 1994.

3. Park MK, Guntheroth WG: How to Read Pediatric ECGs, 3rd ed. St. Louis: Mosby–Year Book, 1992.

4. Park MK, George R: Pediatric Cardiology for Practitioners, 4th ed. St. Louis: Mosby, 2002, pp 34–51.

5. Robinson B, Anisman P, Eshagh E: A primer on pediatric ECGs. Contemp Pediatr 11:69, 1994.

6. Bazett HC: An analysis of the time-relations of electrocardiograms. Heart 7:353–370, 1920.

*7. Ackerman MJ: The long QT syndrome: ion channel diseases of the heart. Mayo Clin Proc 73:250–269, 1998.

8. Miller MD, Porter CJ, Ackerman MJ: Diagnostic accuracy of screening electrocardiograms in long QT syndrome I. Pediatrics 108:8–12, 2001.

9. Schwartz PJ, Moss AJ, Vincent GM, Crampton RS: Diagnostic criteria for the long QT syndrome: an update. Circulation 88:782–784, 1993.

10. Sharieff GQ, Rao SO: The pediatric ECG. Emerg Med Clin North Am 24:195–208, 2006.

11. Hazinski MF, Zaritsky AL, Nadkarini VM, et al (eds): PALS Provider Manual. Dallas, TX: American Heart Association, 2002.

12. Hanna CM, Greenes DS: How much tachycardia in infants can be attributed to fever? Ann Emerg Med 43:699–705, 2004.

13. Perry JC: Supraventricular tachycardia. In Garson A Jr, Bricker JT, Fisher DJ, Neish SR (eds): The Science and Practice of Pediatric Cardiology, 2nd ed. Baltimore: Williams & Wilkins, 1998.

14. Chauhan VS, Krahn AD, Klein GJ, et al: Cardiac arrhythmias: supraventricular tachycardia. Med Clin North Am 85:193–223, 2001.

*15. Garson A, Gillette PC, McNamara DG: Supraventricular tachycardia in children: clinical features, response to treatment and long term followup in 217 patients. J Pediatr 98:875–882, 1981.

*16. Perry JC, Garson A Jr: Supraventricular tachycardia due to Wolff Parkinson White syndrome in children: early disappearance and late recurrence. J Am Coll Cardiol 16:1215–1220, 1990.

17. Etheridge SP, Craig JE, Compton SJ: Amiodarone is safe and highly effective therapy for supraventricular tachycardia in infants. Am Heart J 141:105–110, 2001.

18. American Heart Association: Circulation 102:112–128, 291–342, 2000.

19. Losek JD, Endom E, Dietrich A, et al: Adenosine and pediatric supraventricular tachycardia in the emergency department: multicenter study and review. Ann Emerg Med 33:185–191, 1999.

20. Danford D, Kugler J, Deal B, et al: The learning curve for radiofrequency ablation of tachyarrhythmias in pediatric patients. Am J Cardiol 18:356–365, 1991.

21. Cummins RO, Field JM, Hazinski MF, et al (eds): ACLS Provider Manual. Dallas, TX: American Heart Association, 2003.

22. Ditchey RV, Karliner JS: Safety of electrical cardioversion in patients without digitalis toxicity. Ann Intern Med 95:676–679, 1981.

23. Ali N, Dais K, Banks T, Sheikh M: Titrated electrical cardioversion in patients on digoxin. Clin Cardiol 5:417–419, 1982.

24. Taketomo C: Pediatric Dosing Handbook and Formulary, Childrens Hospital Los Angeles edition. Hudson, OH: Lexi-Comp, 2003–2004.

25. Balaji SB, Harris L: Atrial arrhythmias in congenital heart disease. Cardiol Clin 20:459–468, 2002.

26. Dubin D: Rapid Interpretation of EKG's: An Interactive Course, 6th ed. Tampa, FL: Cover Publishing Co., 2000.

27. Samson R, Berg R, Bingham R: Use of automated external defibrillators for children: an update. An advisory statement from the Pediatric Advanced Life Support Task Force, International Liaison Committee on Resuscitation. Resuscitation 57:237–243, 2003.

28. Garson A: Abnormalities of cardiac rate and rhythm. In McMillan JA, Deangelis CD, Feigin RD, et al (eds): Oski's Pediatrics: Principles and Practice, 13th ed. Philadelphia: Lippincott Williams & Wilkins, 1999, pp 1428–1433.

29. Field JM: Update on cardiac resuscitation for sudden death: International Guidelines 2000 on Resuscitation and Emergency Cardiac Care. Curr Opin Cardiol 18:14–25, 2003.

30. McEvoy GK: Cardiovascular drugs: antiarrhythmic agents. In AHFS Drug Information 2004. Bethesda, MD: American Society of Health-System Pharmacists, 2004, pp 24:04.04.04–24.04.04.92.

31. McKee MR: Amiodarone—an "old" drug with new recommendations. Curr Opin Pediatr 15:193–199, 2003.

32. Behrman RE, Kliegman RM, Jenson HB: Cardiac arrhythmias. In Behrman RE (ed): Nelson Textbook of Pediatrics, 16th ed. Philadelphia: WB Saunders, 2000, pp 1413–1424.

33. Gomes JA, El-Sherif N: Atrioventricular block: mechanism, clinical presentation, and therapy. Med Clin North Am 68:955–967, 1984.

34. Garson AJ, Dick MI, Fournier A, et al: The long QT syndrome in children: an international study of 287 patients. Circulation 87:1866–1872, 1993.

35. Salen P, Nadkarni V: Congenital long QT syndrome: a case report illustrating diagnostic pitfalls. J Emerg Med 17:859–864, 1999.

36. Moss AJ: Prolonged QT interval syndromes. JAMA 256:2985–2987, 1986.

37. Dessertenne F: La tachycardia ventriculaire a deux foyers opposes variables. Arch Mal Coeur 59:263–272, 1966.

38. Schwartz PJ, Periti M, Malliani A: The long QT syndrome. Am Heart J 89:378–390, 1975.

39. Schwartz PJ: Idiopathic long QT syndrome: progress and questions. Am Heart J 109:399–411, 1985.

---

*Selected readings.

Chapter 64

Pericarditis, Myocarditis, and Endocarditis

Ghazala Q. Sharieff, MD and Todd Wylie, MD, MPH

Key Points

Pericarditis and myocarditis may occur simultaneously.

Pleuritic chest pain that is relieved by sitting upright and increased with the supine position suggests pericarditis.

Pericardiocentesis can be life-saving in patients with cardiac tamponade.

Clinicians must not rely on a normal echocardiogram to exclude endocarditis.

Endocarditis prophylaxis is mandatory in patients with prosthetic valves, a history of previous bacterial endocarditis, complex cyanotic heart disease, or surgical systemic pulmonary shunts or conduits.

Selected Diagnoses

Pericarditis
Myocarditis
Infective endocarditis

Discussion of Individual Diagnoses

Pericarditis

Pericarditis is an inflammatory condition of the pericardial lining of the heart. Pericarditis alone may not cause significant hemodynamic compromise; however, the complications of pericardial effusion and cardiac tamponade can result in shock, cardiac arrest, and death. Both infectious and noninfectious etiologies of pericarditis exist[1] (Table 64–1). Among infectious causes, viral etiologies (coxsackievirus A and B, echoviruses, influenza viruses) are most common. Bacterial organisms most commonly associated with pericarditis include *Staphylococcus aureus*, *Streptococcus pneumoniae*, *Neisseria meningitidis*, *Borrelia burgdorferi* (Lyme disease), and *Mycobacterium tuberculosis*.[1]

The pericardium consists of two layers, the visceral layer and the parietal layer. In a healthy person, a small amount (10 to 15 ml in a child) of serous fluid normally exists between the visceral and parietal pericardial layers. When inflammation of the pericardium occurs, fluid accumulates between the two layers of the pericardium and forms a pericardial effusion. Normally, the pericardium does not affect filling of the heart. However, a significant pericardial effusion may limit the filling capacity of the heart chambers, resulting in increased end-diastolic filling pressures and decreased cardiac output. Large effusions may lead to cardiac tamponade. Acute development of an effusion is more likely to result in tamponade because the pericardium does not have the capacity to accommodate an abruptly increased volume.

Clinical Presentation

Symptoms vary depending on the etiology and how rapidly a pericardial effusion develops. Common presenting symptoms include respiratory difficulty, fever, and substernal chest pain that may radiate to the left shoulder, scapula, or trapezius. Chest pain is often accentuated by lying flat or respiratory motion, and improved with sitting forward. Patients with a viral etiology may have a recent history of a viral illness, including upper respiratory tract symptoms and fever. Physical findings vary depending on the severity of disease. With a small effusion, the only sign on physical examination may be a friction rub. With more serious disease, tachypnea and tachycardia develop. The lungs are generally clear to auscultation. Signs of cardiac tamponade include distended neck veins, clear lungs, weak peripheral pulses, tachycardia, distant heart tones with auscultation, and a pulsus paradoxus. Beck's triad (hypotension, distended neck veins, and muffled heart tones) is present in less than half of all patients with cardiac tamponade.

Laboratory evaluation of a patient with suspected pericarditis includes a complete blood count (CBC), electrolytes, glucose, blood urea nitrogen, and creatinine. The CBC may reveal an elevated white blood cell count in the presence of bacterial pericarditis or normocytic, normochromic anemia associated with chronic disease. The CBC may be normal with other etiologies. Appropriate cultures including blood, urine, and viral serology should also be obtained depending upon the suspected etiology. An erythrocyte sedimentation

Table 64–1   Causes of Pericarditis

Idiopathic*
Infectious
  Viral* (echovirus, coxsackievirus, adenovirus, cytomegalovirus,
    hepatitis B, infectious mononucleosis, HIV/AIDS)
  Bacterial* (*Pneumococcus, Staphylococcus, Streptococcus,
    Mycoplasma*, Lyme disease, *Haemophilus influenzae,
    Neisseria meningitidis*)
  Mycobacteria* (*Mycobacterium tuberculosis, Mycobacterium
    avium-intracellulare*)
  Fungal (histoplasmosis, coccidioidomycosis)
  Protozoal
Immune-inflammatory
  Connective tissue disease* (systemic lupus erythematosus,
    rheumatoid arthritis, scleroderma, mixed)
  Arteritis (polyarteritis nodosa, temporal arteritis)
Early post–myocardial infarction
Late post–myocardial infarction (Dressler syndrome),* late post-
  cardiotomy/thoracotomy,* late posttrauma*
Drug induced* (e.g., procainamide, hydralazine, isoniazid,
  cyclosporine)
Neoplastic disease
  Primary: mesothelioma, fibrosarcoma, lipoma, and the like
  Secondary*: breast and lung carcinoma, lymphomas, leukemias
Radiation induced*
Early post–cardiac surgery
Device and procedure related: Coronary angioplasty, implantable
  defibrillators, pacemakers
Trauma: Blunt and penetrating,* post–cardiopulmonary resuscitation*
Congenital
Cysts, congenital absence
Miscellaneous
  Chronic renal failure, dialysis related
  Hypothyroidism
  Amyloidosis
  Aortic dissection

*Etiologies that manifest as acute pericarditis.
Abbreviations: AIDS, acquired immunodeficiency syndrome; HIV,
human immunodeficiency virus.
From LeWinter MM, Kabbani S: Pericardial diseases. In Zipes DP
(ed): Braunwald's Heart Disease: A Textbook of Cardiovascular
Medicine, 7th ed. Philadelphia: WB Saunders, 2005, pp
1757–1781.

rate may be elevated, with high values (>50 to 60 mm/hr) seen in tuberculosis, Kawasaki disease, and autoimmune diseases.[2] Cardiac troponins are elevated in nearly half of all cases of pericarditis, with nearly one quarter meeting the threshold for myocardial infarction.[3,4] These cardiac tests may be a marker for subclinical involvement of the myocardium.

The electrocardiogram (ECG) typically shows diffuse ST-segment elevation in both the limb and precordial leads with associated upright T waves (leads I, V_5, and V_6). ST-segment depression in aV_R and PR-segment depression in leads II, aV_F, and V_4 to V_6 may also be present (Fig. 64–1). With chronic pericarditis, the ST-segment elevation resolves and widespread T-wave inversion develops. A large effusion can cause generalized ECG low voltage and electrical alternans (alternate-beat variation in the direction, amplitude, and duration of any component of the ECG waveform), although this is an uncommon finding.

The initial chest radiograph usually demonstrates clear lung fields. An effusion may be mistaken as cardiomegaly. A large effusion may give the appearance of a "water-bottle"–shaped heart. An echocardiogram is the diagnostic study of choice. It can reveal an effusion, quantify the effusion, and demonstrate the thickness of the pericardium. An echocar-

diogram also allows evaluation of cardiac hemodynamic function.

Advanced techniques of nonsurgical percutaneous pericardial biopsy, pericardioscopy, cytologic analysis of pericardial fluid, and molecular techniques such as polymerase chain reaction and fluorescent in situ hybridization are currently available for diagnostic purposes.[5-7] Such techniques significantly improve diagnosis of specific etiologies, but are not immediately available in the emergency department (ED).

Management

In an unstable patient with cardiac tamponade, a pericardiocentesis should be performed expeditiously (see Chapter 180, Pericardiocentesis). An initial normal saline fluid bolus (20 ml/kg) is administered if hypotension is present. Antibiotics should be initiated until a bacterial source can be excluded. Recommended antibiotics include nafcillin (150 mg/kg per 24 hours intravenously [IV], divided every 4 to 6 hours) and cefotaxime (100 to 150 mg/kg per 24 hours IV, divided every 6 hours).[8] A pediatric cardiology consult is obtained, and the patient is admitted to a pediatric intensive care unit for further management.

Pericardiocentesis may be safely deferred in stable patients with no evidence of decompensation, particularly if removal of fluid is for diagnostic purposes only. Stable patients should be admitted to the hospital for further evaluation, bed rest, and initiation of antibiotics and anti-inflammatory agents. The clinician should consider administration of salicylates (50 to 75 mg/kg per 24 hours PO, divided every 6 hours) or ibuprofen (10 mg/kg PO, divided every 6 hours).[8] Corticosteroids have only been found effective with certain etiologies of pericarditis (i.e., autoreactive).[9] However, they should not be used until a bacterial etiology can be excluded. Corticosteroids are also not recommended in acute viral pericarditis.

Myocarditis

Myocarditis is an inflammation of the heart muscle resulting from infectious and noninfectious causes. It may occur in conjunction with pericarditis or in isolation. The most common etiology in North America is viral (coxsackievirus A and B, echoviruses, and influenza viruses),[10,11] while parasites (e.g., Chagas' disease) are most common in underdeveloped countries. There are numerous other causes, including nonviral infections, drugs, endocrine disorders, radiation, and collagen vascular diseases.

Clinical Presentation

Multiple factors, including the etiology and patient age, influence the clinical presentation. Neonates and infants may present with lethargy, poor feeding, irritability, pallor, fever, or failure to thrive.[12] Wheezing is an important physical examination finding that is often mistakenly attributed to a viral syndrome.[13] Symptoms suggestive of heart failure, such as diaphoresis with feeding, rapid breathing, or respiratory distress, may be present.[12] Older children and adolescents can present with similar features. In addition, they may complain of weakness, fatigue, chest pain, and shortness of breath.[12] With viral myocarditis, there may be a recent history of a nonspecific viral syndrome. Potential findings on physical examination include tachypnea, tachycardia, hyperthermia or hypothermia, hypotension, and wheezing or rales due to congestive heart failure. Signs of poor

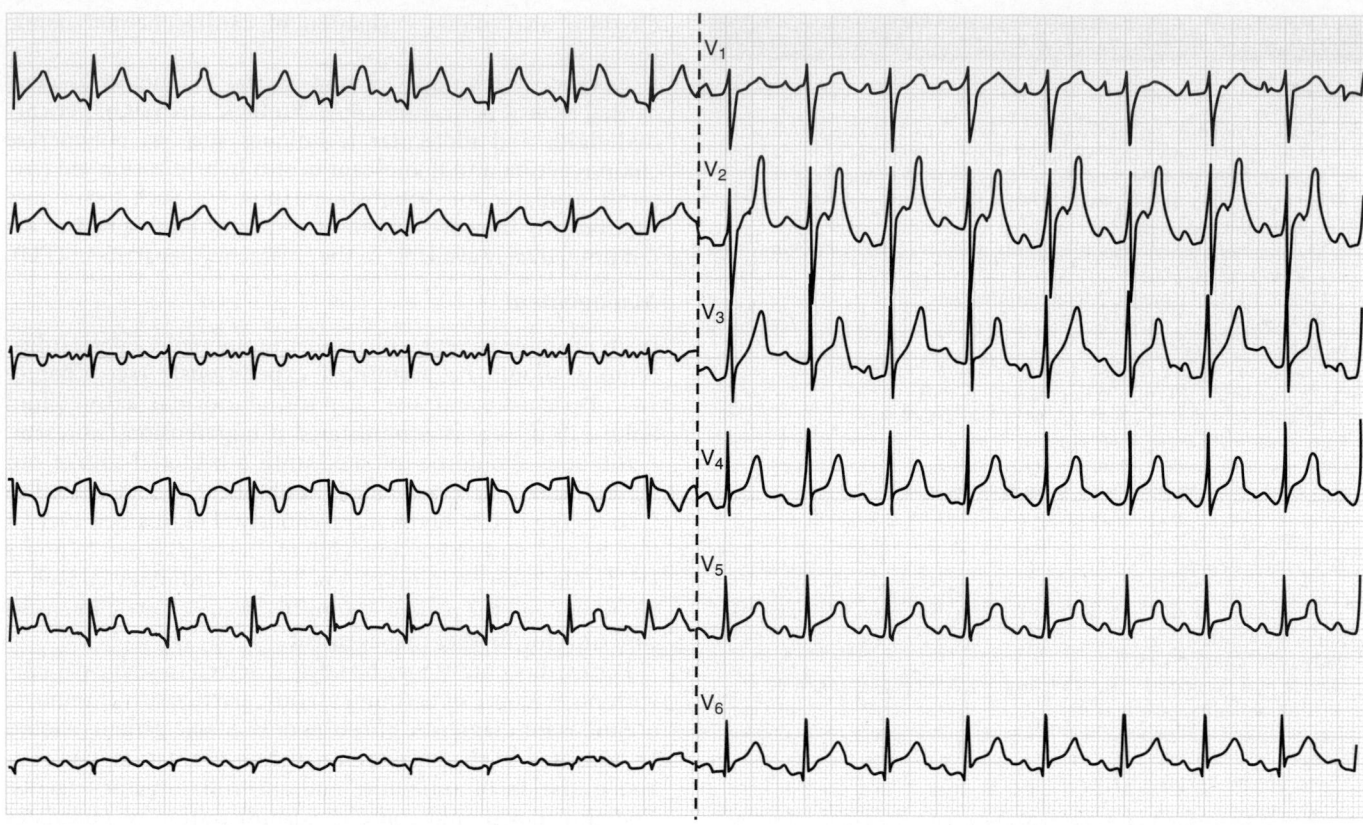

FIGURE 64–1. Typical electrocardiogram in pericarditis with PR segment depression and diffuse ST segment elevation. (Photo courtesy of Amal Mattu, MD, Program Director, Emergency Medicine Residency, University of Maryland School of Medicine, Baltimore, Maryland.)

perfusion and heart failure, including tachycardia, weak pulses, decreased capillary refill time, cool mottled extremities, jugular venous distention, hepatomegaly, and lower extremity edema, may be present. Heart tones may include an S_3, and may be muffled if pericarditis is present. Although several types of dysrhythmias occur, the most common dysrhythmia is sinus tachycardia. Sinus tachycardia that is faster than expected for the degree of fever (an average of 9.6 beats/min for every 1° C increase in body temperature) may indicate myocarditis.[14]

A CBC, electrolytes, glucose, blood urea nitrogen, creatinine, sedimentation rate, C-reactive protein, and cardiac enzymes may occasionally provide information in patients with myocarditis. While an elevated white blood cell count may be present in many cases, a lymphocytic predominance on the differential suggests a viral etiology. The sedimentation rate and C-reactive protein are usually elevated, but normal values do not rule out myocarditis. Elevation of creatine kinase MB and lactate dehydrogenase can occur. Cardiac troponins are elevated in 35% to 71% of cases.[15,16] Brain natriuretic peptide may be a useful marker, with most cases of Kawasaki myocarditis manifesting a level greater than 50 pg/ml.[17] Accuracy of this test for diagnosing other types of myocarditis has not been studied well. Blood samples as well as throat, nasopharyngeal, stool, and urine specimens should be sent for culture to identify bacterial or viral pathogens. Endomyocardial biopsy is the gold standard for diagnosis of myocarditis.

Of the multiple ECG abnormalities that may occur, sinus tachycardia is the most common dysrhythmia. Other abnor-malities such as premature ventricular beats, junctional tachycardias, ventricular tachycardias, and even second- and third-degree atrioventricular blocks may also be present. A low-voltage QRS complex, less than 5 mm in all limb leads, suggests myocarditis or tamponade. As pericarditis may occur simultaneously, the ECG may show ST-segment elevation and PR-interval depression.[12]

Radiologic evaluation should include a chest radiograph and an echocardiogram. The chest radiograph may show cardiomegaly and pulmonary edema. An echocardiogram can demonstrate changes in myocardial function. If heart failure is present, an echocardiogram will show increased left ventricular end-diastolic and systolic dimensions. Other potential echocardiogram findings include left ventricular wall dysfunction, decreased ejection fraction, segmental wall motion abnormalities, or global hypokinesis.

Management

Initial management should focus on respiratory and circulatory status. All patients in respiratory distress are placed on supplemental oxygen and cardiac monitoring and pulse oximetry are initiated. If the patient continues to deteriorate, or is in cardiogenic shock, endotracheal intubation and ventilatory support may be necessary. Vascular access should be obtained immediately.

Goals for managing patients with myocarditis-induced heart failure include reduction of high ventricular filling pressures, a decrease in systemic vascular resistance, and improvement in oxygen delivery and oxygen consumption. Toward this goal, diuretics, inotropes, and afterload reducing agents are administered. Intravenous furosemide is used to decrease fluid overload and preload. Digoxin is not recommended in myocarditis since it is ineffective acutely, and there is evidence that this agent increases production of cytokines and increases mortality in myocarditis.[12] Inotropic agents such as dopamine or dobutamine may be necessary if cardiogenic shock is present. Afterload reducing agents help reduce the workload of a poorly functioning myocardium, and if hypotension is not present, an easily titrated IV agent such as nitroprusside may be used to decrease systemic vascular resistance (see Chapter 8, Circulatory Emergencies: Shock).

High-dose intravenous gamma globulin (2 g/kg given over the first 24 hours) in the setting of acute myocarditis may improve ventricular function and survival.[18] The use of immunosuppressive agents such as steroids or cyclosporine in acute myocarditis is controversial, and therefore should not be initiated in the ED. All patients with myocarditis should be admitted to an intensive care unit for further management and observation. The diagnosis of myocarditis often cannot be confirmed in the ED as many patients present with a seemingly benign viral illness with weakness, fever, and emesis; however, it is more important to recognize that the child is critically ill, initiate treatment, and admit the patient.

Infective Endocarditis

The incidence of infective endocarditis in children is approximately 1 case per 1000 hospital admissions.[19,20] The majority of infective endocarditis cases in the Western world are now associated with congenital heart disease. Up to 69% to 87% of all childhood endocarditis cases occur in children with congenital heart defects.[19 21] Central venous catheters are also a risk factor for infective endocarditis.[22] Other risk factors include immunodeficiency states and intravenous drug abuse.

Clinical Presentation

Clinical signs and symptoms of infective endocarditis can vary. Subacute endocarditis has an insidious onset over several weeks with nonspecific signs and symptoms. Flulike symptoms with low-grade fever, cough, decreased appetite, nausea, weight loss, generalized myalgias, and joint pains may all be present. Physical examination often reveals a fever and a heart murmur. Acute endocarditis develops rapidly over several days to weeks with high fevers, malaise, a toxic appearance, and congestive heart failure. A new or changing murmur is more common with acute endocarditis due to the larger size of vegetations associated with it. However, as few as one quarter of children with endocarditis have a new murmur noted on examination.[23,24] Physical findings of embolic phenomena (arterial clot, stroke) are also more common in acute endocarditis.

Embolization of infected vegetations can involve any organ system of the body, but most commonly involves the brain, spleen, and kidneys. Emboli may cause infarction or abscess development in these organs. Diffuse or focal glomerulonephritis, nephrotic syndrome, and renal failure may result from emboli to the kidneys. Infective endocarditis involving the right side of the heart may result in emboli to the lungs, causing pneumonia, abscesses, and pulmonary emboli. Cardiac complications may include perforation of valve leaflets, leading to valve insufficiency and congestive heart failure. Conduction disorders may develop secondary to

myocardial abscesses. Splenomegaly is present in nearly a third of all cases, while petechiae are present in one quarter of cases.[23,24] Other uncommon peripheral signs of infectious endocarditis include Osler's nodes (pea-sized subcutaneous nodules on the palms, soles, and digits), Janeway lesions (painless palmar macules), and splinter hemorrhages.

Streptococci and staphylococci, particularly *S. aureus*, are the most commonly identified infectious organisms. *Staphylococcus aureus* was identified in 39% of cases in one study.[19] More recent studies have identified *Streptococcus viridans* in 26% to 32% of cases and *S. aureus* in 27% to 29% of cases.[23,24] Staphylococci are also common causative organisms in neonates, as are fungal organisms such as *Candida* species.[22] Gram-negative organisms have been identified but are much less common. Fungal organisms are more likely to occur in neonates and IV drug abusers.[22]

Unfortunately, no single test is definitive for endocarditis. The CBC generally shows a normocytic and normochromic anemia, and the white blood cell count may be elevated. Both the erythrocyte sedimentation rate and serum C-reactive protein are usually elevated. In prolonged cases, the rheumatoid factor is positive approximately half the time. The urinalysis may show proteinuria, microscopic hematuria, and white or red blood cell casts. Blood cultures are the most important laboratory test for identifying infective endocarditis. Three sets should be drawn within the first 24 hours.[25] The echocardiogram is the radiologic study of choice, as it is helpful for identifying presence, size, and location of vegetations. However, it is important to note that the echocardiogram may appear normal in as many as 21% to 54% of cases.[23,24] The Duke criteria are a combination of diagnostic parameters and echocardiographic findings used to identify infective endocarditis[26] (Table 64–2).

Management

Initial management depends on the patient's presenting condition. Unstable patients require aggressive initial interventions. Maintaining a patent airway, adequate oxygenation and ventilation, and circulatory support are the primary objectives. If patients present with signs of embolic phenomena (e.g., stroke, arterial clot) or other complications, therapy should be directed toward those problems until the patient is stabilized. All patients diagnosed with infective endocarditis, or suspected of having infective endocarditis, require hospitalization. This should include all patients with fever and high-risk congenital heart disease (see Table 64–2), those with indwelling central venous access catheters, IV drug users, and patients with physical examination findings suspicious for endocarditis regardless of underlying disease.

Medical treatment consists of parenteral antibiotics, generally at least two agents, for 6 weeks. Since multiple organisms cause infective endocarditis, antibiotic therapy needs to be directed by culture results and sensitivities. Initial empirical antibiotic combinations should cover common infecting organisms (*S. viridans*, *Streptococcus bovis*, and enterococci) and should include the following IV drugs: (1a) penicillin G 150,000 units/kg per day, divided every 4 to 6 hours (maximum 24 million units/day), or (1b) ampicillin 200 mg/kg per day, divided every 4 hours (maximum 12 g/day), PLUS either (2) nafcillin or oxacillin 100 to 200 mg/kg per day, divided every 6 hours (maximum 12 g/day), PLUS (3) gentamicin 6 to 7.5 mg/kg per day, divided every 8 hours. If the patient is allergic to penicillin, vancomycin in a dose of 30 mg/kg per day, divided every 12 hours (maximum of 2 g/ day) can be used in combination with gentamicin. Patients with staphylococcal infection should be started on nafcillin and gentamicin. Patients with methicillin-resistant strains of staphylococcus or prosthetic heart valves should be started

on vancomycin, rifampin, and gentamicin.[27] Indications for surgical intervention include heart failure, an obstructed valve, perivalvular abscess, fungal endocarditis, and large vegetations (>10 mm).

Prophylaxis

Stratifying people in to high-, moderate-, and negligible-risk categories is helpful in order to identify which individuals need prophylaxis for endocarditis[20] (Table 64–3). Patients in the negligible-risk category have no greater risk of developing infective endocarditis than the general public, and therefore prophylactic antibiotics are not necessary. Individuals in the moderate and high risk categories require prophylaxis for various medical and dental procedures[28] (Tables 64–4 and 64–5).

Table 64–2	Dukes Criteria for Infective Endocarditis*

Major Criteria

1. Isolation of organisms from 2 blood cultures: must be typical organisms (viridans streptococci, *Streptococcus bovis*, HACEK group, or *Staphylococcus aureus*) or enterococci in absence of primary focus
2. Persistently positive blood culture: 2 or more positive blood cultures for same organism separated by 12 hr, *or* ≥3 positive blood cultures for same organism with 1 hr between first and last culture
3. Positive echocardiogram for oscillating intracardiac mass at sites where vegetations typically occur
4. Intracardiac abscess identified by echocardiogram
5. New partial dehiscence of prosthetic valve as identified by echocardiogram
6. New regurgitant murmur

Minor Criteria

1. Fever greater than 38° C
2. Predisposing heart condition or IV drug use
3. Vascular phenomena: Includes major arterial emboli, mycotic aneurysms, CNS hemorrhages, Janeway lesions, conjunctival hemorrhages, peripheral necrotic skin lesions
4. Immunologic phenomena: includes elevated rheumatoid factor, immune complex glomerulonephritis, Osler's nodes
5. Echocardiogram findings consistent with endocarditis but not meeting major criterion: nonoscillating masses, nodular valve thickening

*Clinical diagnosis of definite infective endocarditis requires 2 major criteria, 1 major with 3 minor criteria, or 5 minor criteria. Abbreviations: CNS, central nervous system; HACEK, *Haemophilus parainfluenzae, Haemophilus aphrophilus, Actinobacillus actinomycetemcomitans, Cardiobacterium hominis, Eikenella corrodens,* and *Kingella kingae*; IV, intravenous.

Table 64–3	Cardiac Conditions Requiring Prophylaxis against Endocarditis

Endocarditis Prophylaxis Recommended

High-risk category
Presence of prosthetic valves
Previous bacterial endocarditis
Complex cyanotic heart disease
Surgical systemic pulmonary shunts or conduits
Moderate-risk category
Other congenital heart malformations
Acquired valve dysfunction
Hypertrophic cardiomyopathy
Mitral valve prolapse with regurgitation or thickened leaflets

Endocarditis Prophylaxis Not Recommended

Negligible-risk category
Isolated secundum atrial septal defect
Surgically repaired atrial septal defect, ventricular septal defect, or patent ductus arteriosus
History of coronary bypass graft surgery
Mitral valve prolapse without regurgitation
Physiologic, functional, or innocent murmurs
History of Kawasaki disease without valve dysfunction
History of rheumatic fever without valve dysfunction
Cardiac pacemakers and implanted defibrillators

Table 64–4	Prophylaxis for Dental, Oral, Respiratory Tract, or Esophageal Procedures	
Situation	**Recommended Antibiotic**	**Dosing Regimen**
Standard prophylaxis	Amoxicillin	50 mg/kg PO 1 hr prior to procedure, not to exceed 2 g
Unable to take oral medications	Ampicillin	50 mg/kg IM or IV within 30 min prior to procedure, not to exceed 2 g
Allergic to penicillin	Clindamycin	20 mg/kg PO 1 hr prior to procedure, not to exceed 600 mg
	Azithromycin or clarithromycin	15 mg/kg PO 1 hr prior to procedure, not to exceed 500 mg
Allergic to penicillin and unable to take oral medications	Clindamycin	20 mg/kg IV within 30 min before procedure, not to exceed 600 mg

Table 63–5	Endocarditis Prophylaxis for Genitourinary and Gastrointestinal Procedures	
Situation	**Recommended Antibiotic**	**Dosing Regimen**
High-risk patients	Ampicillin and gentamicin	Ampicillin 50 mg/kg IM or IV, not to exceed 2 g, plus gentamicin 1.5 mg/kg IV, not to exceed 120 mg; 6 hr later, ampicillin 25 mg/kg IM/IV or amoxicillin 25 mg/kg PO
High-risk patients with penicillin allergy	Vancomycin and gentamicin	Vancomycin 20 mg/kg IV over 1–2 hours, not to exceed 1 g, plus gentamicin as above
Moderate-risk patients	Amoxicillin or ampicillin	Amoxicillin 50 mg/kg PO 1 hr prior to procedure, not to exceed 2 g; *or* ampicillin 50 mg/kg IV/IM within 30 min of procedure, not to exceed 2 g
Moderate-risk patients with penicillin allergy	Vancomycin	Vancomycin 20 mg/kg IV over 1–2 hours, complete within 30 min of procedure, not to exceed 1 g

REFERENCES

1. LeWinter MM, Kabbani S: Pericardial diseases. In Zipes DP (ed): Braunwald's Heart Disease: A Textbook of Cardiovascular Disease, 7th ed. Philadelphia: WB Saunders, 2005, pp 1757–1781.

2. Hara KS, Ballard DJ, Ilstrup DM, et al: Rheumatoid pericarditis: clinical features and survival. Medicine (Baltimore) 69:81–91, 1990.

3. Bonnefoy E, Godon P, Kirkorian G, et al: Serum cardiac troponin I and ST-segment elevation in patients with acute pericarditis. Eur Heart J 21:798, 2000.

4. Brandt RR, Filzmaier K, Hanrath P: Circulating cardiac troponin I in acute pericarditis. Am J Cardiol 87:1326, 2001.

5. Maisch B: Pericardial diseases, with a focus on etiology, pathogenesis, pathophysiology, new diagnostic imaging methods, and treatment. Curr Opin Cardiol 9:379–388, 1994.

6. Uthaman B, Endrys J, Abushaban L, et al: Percutaneous pericardial biopsy: technique, efficacy, safety, and value in the management of pericardial effusion in children and adolescents. Pediatr Cardiol 18:414–418, 1997.

7. Maisch B, Ristic AD, Seferovic PM: New directions in diagnosis and treatment of pericardial disease: a project of the Taskforce on Pericardial Disease of the World Heart Federation. Herz 25:769–780, 2000.

*8. Troughton RW, Asher CR, Klein AL: Pericarditis. Lancet 363:717–726, 2004.

9. Maisch B, Ristic AD: The classification of pericardial disease in the age of modern medicine. Curr Cardiol Rep 4:13–21, 2002.

*10. Kopeck SL, Gersh BJ: Dilated cardiomyopathy and myocarditis: natural history, etiology, clinical manifestations, and management. Curr Probl Cardiol 12:569–647, 1987.

11. Cotran RS, Kumar V, Robbins SL (eds): Robbins Pathologic Basis of Disease, 4th ed. Philadelphia: WB Saunders, 1989.

12. Wheeler DS, Kooy NW: A formidable challenge: the diagnosis and treatment of viral myocarditis in children. Cardiol Clin 19:365–391, 2003.

13. Singer JI, Isaacman DJ, Bell LM: The wheezer that wasn't. Pediatr Emerg Care 8:107–109, 1992.

14. Hanna CM, Greenes DS: How much tachycardia in infants can be attributed to fever? Ann Emerg Med 43:699–705, 2004.

15. Smith SC, Ladenson JH, Mason JW, et al: Elevations of cardiac troponin I associated with myocarditis: experimental and clinical correlates. Circulation 95:163–168, 1997.

16. Soongswang J, Durongpisitkul K, Nana A, et al: Cardiac troponin T: a marker in the diagnosis of acute myocarditis in children. Pediatr Cardiol 26:45–49, 2005.

17. Kawamura T, Wago M: Brain natriuretic peptide can be a useful biochemical marker for myocarditis in patients with Kawasaki disease. Cardiol Young 12:153–158, 2002.

18. Drucker NA, Colan SD, Lewis AB, et al: Gamma-globulin treatment of acute myocarditis in the pediatric population. Circulation 89:252–257, 1994.

19. Saiman L, Prince A, Gersony WM: Pediatric infective endocarditis in the modern era. J Pediatr 122:847–853, 1993.

20. Parras F, Bouza E, Romero J, et al: Infectious endocarditis in children. Pediatr Cardiol 11:77–81, 1990.

21. Johnson CM, Rhodes KH: Pediatric endocarditis. Mayo Clin Proc 57:86–94, 1982.

22. Daher AH, Berkowitz FE: Infective endocarditis in neonates. Clin Pediatr 34:198–206, 1995.

23. Stockheim JA, Chadwick EG, Kessler S, et al: Are the Duke criteria superior to the Beth Israel criteria for the diagnosis of infective endocarditis in children? Clin Infect Dis 27:1451–1456, 1998.

24. Del Pont JM, De Cicco LT, Vartalitis C, et al: Infective endocarditis in children: clinical analyses and evaluation of two diagnostic criteria. Pediatr Infect Dis J 14:1079–1086, 1995.

25. Werner AS, Cobbs CG, Kaye D, Hook EW: Studies on the bacteremia of bacterial endocarditis. JAMA 202:199–203, 1967.

26. Durack DT, Lukes AS, Bright DK: New criteria for diagnosis of infective endocarditis: utilization of specific echocardiographic findings. Duke Endocarditis Service. Am J Med 96:200–209, 1994.

*27. Stock JH, Sahn DJ: Endocarditis in the pediatric population. Curr Treat Options Cardiovasc Med 2:481–488, 2000.

*28. Dajani AS, Taubert KA, Wilson W, et al: Prevention of Bacterial Endocarditis Recommendations by the American Heart Association. JAMA 277:1794–1801, 1997.

---

*Selected readings.

Chapter 65

Hypertensive Emergencies

Todd Wylie, MD, MPH and Nazeema Khan, MD

Introduction and Background

The prevalence of hypertension in the pediatric population ranges from 1% to 3%.[1] The prevalence varies based on age, genetic background, and body weight. Hypertension can be diagnosed by comparing the patient's blood pressure to standard values for age and gender (Tables 65–1 and 65–2). A normal blood pressure is defined as a systolic and diastolic blood pressure (SBP and DBP, respectively) less than the 90th percentile for age, gender, and height.[2] An SBP or DBP equal to the 90th percentile but less than the 95th percentile is designated as prehypertension.[2] An SBP or DBP level ranging from the 95th percentile to 5 mm Hg above the 99th percentile is defined as stage 1 hypertension, and SBP or DBP levels greater than 5 mm Hg above the 99th percentile are defined as stage 2 hypertension.[2]

Although the discovery of hypertension may not require immediate treatment in the ED, hypertensive emergencies in children demand rapid recognition and intervention to prevent further morbidity or even mortality. Importantly, a hypertensive emergency is not defined by the degree of elevation of the blood pressure, but rather by the presence of end-organ damage in the setting of an elevated blood pressure. Involved organ systems may include the renal, cardiac, visual, neurologic, or pulmonary systems. Examples of end-organ damage include congestive heart failure, hypertensive encephalopathy, acute nontraumatic intracranial hemorrhage, acute renal failure, and retinopathy.

Recognition and Approach

Adolescents more commonly have essential hypertension (no identifiable cause) compared to younger children.[3,4] Hypertension in the first decade of life may be due to essential hypertension, but is more likely to have an underlying cause (secondary hypertension).[3] Renal disorders, such as glomerulonephritis, renal artery stenosis, systemic lupus erythematosus, renal transplantation, polycystic kidney disease, or reflux nephropathy, are the most common causes of hypertension in children[5] (Table 65–3). A hypertensive emergency can be an acceleration of preexisting hypertension or can occur suddenly. Hypertensive emergencies commonly occur secondary to underlying renal disorders.[6] Extrarenal causes of hypertensive emergencies include coarctation of the aorta, neuroblastoma, pheochromocytoma, and increased intracranial pressure.[5,6] Drug ingestions such as corticosteroids, sympathomimetics, cocaine, or theophylline may also precipitate hypertensive crises.[5]

The pathophysiology of hypertensive emergencies is not completely understood. It is known that the vascular endothelium has a role in blood pressure homeostasis through the release of vasodilatory substances such as nitric oxide and prostacyclin.[7] Generally, these substances are released by the endothelium as a compensatory mechanism to decrease vascular resistance in reaction to an initial increase in blood pressure. When the increase in blood pressure is prolonged, or of sufficient severity, these vasodilatory substances can no longer compensate, and increased vascular resistance and endothelial damage result. This leads to increased vascular resistance, increased blood pressure, and, ultimately, end-organ damage.

Clinical Presentation

Children with hypertension may be asymptomatic or present with nonspecific symptoms. Most adolescents with

Table 65–1   Blood Pressure for Females by Age and Height Percentiles

Age (yr)	BP Percentile	Systolic Blood Pressure (mm Hg) Percentile of Height			Diastolic Blood Pressure (mm Hg) Percentile of Height		
		10th	50th	90th	10th	50th	90th
1	90th	97	100	102	53	54	55
	95th	101	104	106	57	58	59
	99th	108	111	113	64	65	67
2	90th	99	101	104	58	59	61
	95th	103	105	108	62	63	65
	99th	110	112	115	69	70	72
3	90th	100	103	106	62	63	64
	95th	104	107	109	66	67	68
	99th	111	114	116	73	74	76
4	90th	102	104	107	64	66	67
	95th	106	108	111	68	70	71
	99th	113	115	118	76	77	79
5	90th	103	106	109	67	68	69
	95th	107	110	112	71	72	73
	99th	114	117	120	78	79	81
6	90th	105	108	110	68	70	71
	95th	109	111	114	72	74	75
	99th	116	119	121	80	81	83
7	90th	107	109	112	70	71	72
	95th	111	113	116	74	75	76
	99th	118	120	123	81	82	84
8	90th	109	111	114	71	72	74
	95th	112	115	118	75	76	78
	99th	120	122	125	82	83	85
9	90th	110	113	116	72	73	75
	95th	114	117	119	76	77	79
	99th	121	124	127	83	84	86
10	90th	112	115	118	73	74	76
	95th	116	119	121	77	78	80
	99th	123	126	129	84	86	87
11	90th	114	117	119	74	75	77
	95th	118	121	123	78	79	81
	99th	125	128	130	85	87	88
12	90th	116	119	121	75	76	78
	95th	120	123	125	79	80	82
	99th	127	130	132	86	88	89
13	90th	118	121	123	76	77	79
	95th	122	124	127	80	81	83
	99th	129	132	134	87	89	90
14	90th	120	122	125	77	78	80
	95th	123	126	129	81	82	84
	99th	131	133	136	88	90	91
15	90th	121	123	126	78	79	81
	95th	125	127	130	82	83	85
	99th	132	134	137	89	91	92
16	90th	122	124	127	78	80	81
	95th	126	128	131	82	84	85
	99th	133	135	138	90	91	93
17	90th	122	125	127	79	80	81
	95th	126	129	131	83	84	85
	99th	133	136	138	90	91	93

Reproduced with permission from National High Blood Pressure Education Program Working Group on High Blood Pressure in Children and Adolescents: The Fourth Report on the diagnosis, evaluation, and treatment of high blood pressure in children and adolescents. Pediatrics 114:555–576, 2004.

hypertension are asymptomatic.[4] Young children, infants, and neonates with chronic hypertension often have nonspecific signs and symptoms such as feeding difficulties, polydipsia, polyuria, nocturia, growth failure, irritability, listlessness, and confusion.[4,8] Multiple other findings on the history and physical examination may exist and may be indicative of the underlying disorder causing hypertension. For example, tachycardia with thyromegaly may suggest hyperthyroidism as a secondary cause of hypertension. A drop in the blood pressure from the upper to lower extremities may indicate coarctation of the aorta. Truncal obesity, moon facies, acne, and hirsutism may all indicate Cushing's syndrome. Tachycardia along with pallor, flushing, and diaphoresis may suggest pheochromocytoma. A malar rash in addition to joint swelling suggests systemic lupus erythematosus. Café-au-lait spots are found with neurofibromatosis. A bruit detected in the epigastric or flank area may indicate renal artery stenosis. An abdominal mass may be found with

Table 65–2   Blood Pressure for Males by Age and Height Percentiles

Age (yr)	BP Percentile	Systolic Blood Pressure (mm Hg) Percentile of Height			Diastolic Blood Pressure (mm Hg) Percentile of Height		
		10th	50th	90th	10th	50th	90th
1	90th	95	99	102	50	52	53
	95th	99	103	106	54	56	58
	99th	106	110	113	62	64	66
2	90th	99	102	105	55	57	58
	95th	102	106	109	59	61	63
	99th	110	113	117	67	69	71
3	90th	101	105	108	59	61	63
	95th	105	109	112	63	65	67
	99th	112	116	119	71	73	75
4	90th	103	107	110	63	65	66
	95th	107	111	114	67	69	71
	99th	114	118	121	75	77	78
5	90th	105	108	111	66	68	69
	95th	109	112	115	70	72	74
	99th	116	120	123	78	80	81
6	90th	106	110	113	68	70	72
	95th	110	114	117	72	74	76
	99th	117	121	124	80	82	84
7	90th	107	111	114	70	72	74
	95th	111	115	118	74	76	78
	99th	118	122	125	82	84	86
8	90th	109	112	115	72	73	75
	95th	112	116	119	76	78	79
	99th	120	123	127	84	86	87
9	90th	110	114	117	73	75	76
	95th	114	118	121	77	79	81
	99th	121	125	128	85	87	88
10	90th	112	115	119	73	75	77
	95th	116	119	122	78	80	81
	99th	123	127	130	86	88	89
11	90th	114	117	120	74	76	78
	95th	118	121	124	78	80	82
	99th	125	129	132	86	88	90
12	90th	116	120	123	75	76	78
	95th	120	123	127	79	81	82
	99th	127	131	134	87	89	90
13	90th	118	122	125	75	77	79
	95th	122	126	129	79	81	83
	99th	130	133	136	87	89	91
14	90th	121	125	128	76	78	79
	95th	125	128	132	80	82	84
	99th	132	136	139	88	90	92
15	90th	124	127	130	77	79	80
	95th	127	131	134	81	83	85
	99th	135	138	142	89	91	93
16	90th	126	130	133	78	80	82
	95th	130	134	137	83	84	86
	99th	137	141	144	90	92	94
17	90th	128	132	135	80	82	84
	95th	132	136	139	85	87	88
	99th	140	143	146	93	94	96

Reproduced with permission from National High Blood Pressure Education Program Working Group on High Blood Pressure in Children and Adolescents: The Fourth Report on the diagnosis, evaluation, and treatment of high blood pressure in children and adolescents. Pediatrics 114:555–576, 2004.

polycystic kidney disease, Wilms' tumor, or neuroblastoma. Ambiguous genitalia or virilization should make one think of adrenal hyperplasia.

Signs and symptoms of a hypertensive emergency vary considerably. Clinical manifestations generally reflect the end-organs damaged. The most commonly affected organs include the eyes, the central nervous system, the heart, and the kidneys.[9] In one study of children with hypertensive emergencies, the most common presenting complications included hypertensive retinopathy, hypertensive encephalopathy, convulsions, left ventricular hypertrophy, facial palsy, visual symptoms, and hemiplegia.[10]

Hypertensive encephalopathy describes the transient cerebral dysfunction that ensues when blood pressure rapidly increases.[11] It is characterized by the triad of severe hypertension, altered mental status, and papilledema.[12] Headache, visual disorders, and seizures may occur. Hypertensive encephalopathy is more likely to occur in individuals with

Table 65–3	Etiology of Hypertension at Different Ages		
Neonates (0–30 days)	**Infants–6 yr**	**6–10 yr**	**10-yr–Adolescence**

Renal Disorders:
  Renal artery thrombosis
  Renal venous thrombosis
  Renal dysplasia
  Polycystic kidney disease
  Obstructive uropathy
Neoplasia:
  Neuroblastoma
  Mesoblastic nephroma
Cardiovascular disorders:
  Coarctation of the aorta
Endocrine disorders:
  Hyperthyroidism
  Adrenogenital syndrome
Drugs:
  Corticosteroids
  Phenylephrine eye-drops
  Theophylline
  Caffeine
  Maternal cocaine use
Miscellaneous:
  Bronchopulmonary dysplasia
  Intracranial hemorrhage
  Seizures
  ECMO
  Volume overload
  Abdominal wall defect closure
	Renal disorders:
	  Pyelonephritis
	  Glomerulonephritis
	  Hemolytic-uremic syndrome
	  Renal dysplasia
	  Polycystic kidney disease
	  Obstructive uropathy
	Neoplasia:
	  Wilms' tumor
	Essential hypertension
	Cardiovascular disorders:
	  Coarctation of the aorta
	Endocrine disorders:
	  Corticosteroid excess
	  Pheochromocytoma
	Central nervous system disorders:
	  Space occupying lesions
	Drugs:
	  Amphetamines
	  Glucocorticoids
	  Mineralocorticoids
	Toxins:
	  Lead
	  Mercury
		Renal disorders:
		  Renal artery stenosis
		  Glomerulonephritis
		  Reflux nephropathy
		  Pyelonephritis
		Vasculitis
		Endocrine disorders:
		  Corticosteroid excess
		  Hyperaldosteronism
		  Pheochromocytoma
		Essential hypertension
			Essential hypertension
			Renal disorders:
			  Glomerulonephritis
			  Pyelonephritis
			  End-stage renal disease
			Pregnancy:
			  Eclampsia

Adapted from Miller K: Pharmacological management of hypertension in paediatric patients. A comprehensive review of the efficacy, safety and dosage guidelines of the available agents. Drugs 48:868–887, 1994.

previously normal blood pressures who suffer rapid onset of severe hypertension, such as children with acute glomerulonephritis or pregnant adolescents with preeclampsia or eclampsia.[12]

Congestive heart failure as the initial complication of a hypertensive emergency may have relatively nonspecific signs and symptoms depending on the age of the child. Common symptoms in infants include prolonged feeding times, poor feeding, excessive sweating, and increased respiratory rate and effort.[13,14] The infant may also be described as fussy or irritable. Physical examination findings may include pallor, tachycardia, tachypnea, diaphoresis, hepatomegaly, and an S_3 gallop rhythm. Rales are not always heard on auscultation. Peripheral edema is uncommon in infants. Older children may present with poor exercise tolerance, fatigue, poor appetite, growth failure, and increased respiratory rate and effort.[15] Signs of congestive heart failure in older children include tachycardia, tachypnea, rales, hepatomegaly, jugular venous distention, and peripheral edema.

Children with acute renal failure often have decreased urine output. There may also be a history of hematuria or edema. If there is significant solute retention, signs and symptoms of uremia may be present, such as vomiting, fetid odor, pruritus, fatigue, psychiatric disturbances, seizures, and coma.

Diagnostic Tests

The diagnostic evaluation of a child with a hypertensive crisis to some extent will be dictated by the presenting signs and symptoms. However, certain studies should be obtained in all cases of suspected hypertensive emergency. An electrocardiogram is helpful in detecting hyperkalemia, dysrhythmias, and left ventricular hypertrophy. An echocardiogram is the recommended study to evaluate for left ventricular hypertrophy in hypertensive children,[2] but is generally not necessary in the initial ED evaluation of the patient. A complete blood count should be obtained in all suspected cases. Findings may include evidence of a microangiopathic hemolytic anemia, with schistocytes and other fragmented erythrocyte forms found on the peripheral smear. If the child has a history of chronic hypertension, an anemia consistent with chronic renal insufficiency may be present. A basic chemistry profile including electrolytes, blood urea nitrogen, creatinine, glucose, and calcium is mandatory. It is important to note that the blood urea nitrogen and creatinine levels may not reflect mild to moderate degrees of renal damage.[16] Specifically, creatinine does not generally increase until the glomerular filtration rate has reached approximately 30% of the baseline value.[16] A urinalysis is always indicated, and may show hyaline and granular casts, red cell casts, trace proteinuria, and microalbuminuria. Urine should also be sent for culture to evaluate for evidence of chronic infection. A urine drug screen may be useful in some instances. Other laboratory studies that may help identify secondary causes of hypertension include plasma and urine catecholamine studies, a plasma renin determination, thyroid function studies, or serum cortisol levels.

Radiologic studies in the ED should include a chest radiograph. A computed tomography (CT) scan of the head is indicated if there are any neurologic deficits, seizures, or change in mental status. If coarctation of the aorta or aortic dissection is suspected, a spiral CT scan of the chest or transesophageal echocardiogram is indicated. A renal ultrasound is helpful to identify congenital renal anomalies or scarring, but is not needed in the ED in most cases. Renovascular imaging with techniques such as magnetic resonance angiography, intra-arterial angiography, digital subtraction angiography, or scintigraphy is helpful in identifying possible renovascular lesions.

Important Clinical Features and Considerations

Proper measurement of blood pressure is important in order to avoid incorrectly high or low results. Accurate measurement of a child's blood pressure requires an appropriately sized cuff for the upper arm. The cuff should have an inflatable bladder width that is at least 40% of the arm circumference at a point midway between the olecranon and the acromion.[2] The bladder length of the cuff should cover 80% to 100% of the circumference of the arm.[2] Confirmation of an elevated blood pressure in a child requires measurement of the blood pressure with a standard clinical sphygmomanometer, and a stethoscope placed over the brachial artery.[2] Noninvasive oscillometric (automated) blood pressure measurements are as accurate as auscultatory measurements with less interobserver variability in children.[17] However, SBP can average as much as 10 mm Hg above that obtained by auscultation, while DBP measurements are 5 mm Hg higher in children.[18] For this reason, standard blood pressure tables that define normal values for children may not apply to blood pressure measurements obtained by oscillometric methods.[18]

Management

Management of hypertensive emergencies in children requires prompt recognition and appropriate management to prevent further complications. Initial efforts should focus on the airway, breathing, and circulation as in other emergent situations. Vascular access should be obtained and the patient should be placed on continuous cardiac monitoring with frequent blood pressure measurements. The blood pressure and neurologic status of the patient must be monitored carefully and frequently throughout the duration of therapy. An arterial line may be indicated in children on certain potent intravenous antihypertensives requiring frequent monitoring and titration.

It is important to realize that the goal of treatment is not to rapidly reduce the blood pressure to a "normal" level. Such actions can result in hypoperfusion of end organs and subsequent renal failure, blindness, and permanent neurologic deficits.[10,19,20] The presumed mechanism of action for these complications is a loss of vascular auto-regulation secondary to severe hypertension.[6] Vessels are unable to accommodate rapid reductions in blood pressure, and end-organ perfusion is compromised.

To avoid complications, blood pressure should be gradually reduced in a controlled manner using an intravenous infusion of an antihypertensive medication under carefully monitored conditions. The goal is to reduce the mean arterial pressure (MAP) by less than 25% over the first 2 to 8 hours and gradually normalize the blood pressure over the next 24 to 48 hours.[2,5] There are several available agents, and choice of a specific agent depends on the clinical presentation and current medical condition of the patient (Table 65–4).

Sodium Nitroprusside

Sodium nitroprusside is a rapidly acting parenteral agent with proven efficacy in children.[10,21] It is contraindicated in pregnancy and should be used only with caution in patients with renal disorders. Nitroprusside is metabolized to nitric oxide, which causes both arterial and venous dilation. This effect is immediate and results in a decrease in both preload and afterload. This decrease in systemic vascular resistance generally results in a reflex tachycardia. Control of tachycardia with a β-blocker (e.g., esmolol) may be required in specific aortic hypertensive emergencies (e.g., dissection). Sodium nitroprusside has a very short half-life, and blood pressure will return to previous levels within 30 to 60 seconds of discontinuing the infusion.[3,6]

The recommended dose range for nitroprusside is 0.5 to 10 mcg/kg per minute.[2] Nitroprusside is started at the lowest dose (0.5 mcg/kg per minute) and titrated to achieve the desired blood pressure.

A significant concern with the use of nitroprusside is the associated potential toxicity of its metabolites. Nitroprusside is initially metabolized to cyanide, which is then metabolized in the liver to thiocyanate, and finally cleared by the kidneys.[22] Hepatic or renal impairment, or long-term infusions of nitroprusside, may lead to accumulation of these toxic

Table 65–4	Antihypertensive Medications for Use in Hypertensive Emergencies in Pediatric Patients			
Medication	**Drug Class**	**Dose**	**Onset of Action**	**Duration of Action**
Sodium nitroprusside	Vasodilator	0.5–10 mcg/kg/min IV infusion	Immediate	30–60 sec
Esmolol	β-blocker	Initial loading dose of 100–500 mcg/kg over 1 min, then 25–200 mcg/kg/min IV infusion	Immediate	9–30 min
Nicardipine	Calcium channel blocker	0.5–3 mcg/kg/min IV infusion	<1 min	30–60 min
Labetalol	α- and β-blocker	0.2–1.5 mg/kg/hr IV infusion, *or* 0.2–1 mg/kg IV bolus (max. 20 mg single dose)	2–4 min	Up to 4 hr
Fenoldopam	Dopamine receptor agonist	0.2–2 mcg/kg/min IV infusion	5–15 min	8–10 min
Enalaprilat	Angiotensin-converting enzyme inhibitor	5–10 mcg/kg IV bolus (max. 1.25 mg/dose)	Up to 60 min	4–6 hr
Phentolamine	Competitive α-adrenergic blocker	0.05–0.1 mg/kg/dose (max. 5 mg/dose)	Immediate	30–60 min

metabolites. Signs of cyanide toxicity include an odor of bitter almonds, tachypnea, mydriasis, cardiac dysrhythmias, hypotension, seizures, apnea, and coma. An elevated serum lactic acid level and elevated anion gap metabolic acidosis are present. Signs and symptoms of thiocyanate toxicity include tinnitus, blurred vision, nausea, altered mental status, seizures, and coma.[5,23]

Nicardipine

Nicardipine is a dihydropyridine calcium channel blocker that reduces blood pressure and peripheral vascular resistance by selectively dilating peripheral arteries. Multiple studies and case reports have shown nicardipine to be safe and effective in a variety of patients, including neonates, children with postoperative hypertension, and children with hypertensive crises.[24-31] It has also been used effectively in children with renal disease.[74] The onset of action is 1 to 2 minutes and the half-life is approximately 40 minutes.[5,6] Nicardipine is metabolized in the liver.

Nicardipine can be started at a dose of 0.5 to 1 mcg/kg per minute and titrated to a maximum infusion rate of 3 mcg/kg per minute.[25-28] Some studies have shown it to be safe at doses as high as 5 mcg/kg per minute.[24,29,31]

Nicardipine can be given through a central venous or peripheral intravenous catheter, although superficial thrombophlebitis may occur following infusion through peripheral intravenous lines.[24,25] Other side effects of intravenous nicardipine include tachycardia, palpitations, and flushing.[27,29] Nicardipine is not recommended in the presence of space-occupying intracranial lesions due to the vasodilatory effects, which can increase intracranial pressure.[32]

Esmolol

Esmolol is an easily titratable, ultra-short-acting cardioselective β-blocking agent given as an intravenous infusion. It has an elimination half-life of approximately 2 to 4 minutes in children.[33] Esmolol is metabolized by erythrocyte esterases to an inactive acid metabolite.[34,35]

Esmolol is first given as a loading dose of 100 to 500 mcg/kg over 1 minute.[2,5,36] This is followed by a continuous infusion of 25 to 200 mcg/kg per minute.[8] Although higher infusion doses have been reported (to a mean dose of 700 mcg/kg per minute),[37] they have only been used in a small number of patients, and the safety of these higher doses cannot be confirmed.

Esmolol should be used cautiously in patients with asthma, high-degree heart block, bradycardia, and decreased left ventricular function. Side effects include nausea, vomiting, bronchospasm, and bradycardia.

Labetalol

Labetalol is a nonselective β-blocker as well as an α_1-adrenergic receptor blocker. It reduces the blood pressure by decreasing both systemic vascular resistance and cardiac output. A parenteral infusion produces effects within 5 to 10 minutes. It is metabolized entirely in the liver via glucuronide metabolites, thus clearance is not affected by renal failure.[38]

Labetalol can be given in a continuous infusion or as intermittent bolus doses. The recommended dose for a continuous infusion ranges from 0.2 to 1.5 mg/kg per hour.[5,6,38] Alternately, an initial intravenous bolus dose of 0.2 mg/kg

per dose can be given. If ineffective, this dose can be doubled every 15 to 30 minutes to a maximum of 1 mg/kg per dose, with a maximum single dose of 20 mg.[38]

Due to its β-blocking effects, labetalol should not be used in patients with asthma or obstructive lung disease. It should also be avoided in patients with decreased ventricular function or high-degree heart block. Other reported side effects include fatigue, nausea, vomiting, itching, rash, hepatotoxicity, and possibly hyperkalemia in renal transplant patients.[5,38] Hypoglycemia may also occur in association with labetalol.

Fenoldopam

Fenoldopam is a direct vasodilator that acts at dopamine$_1$ receptors in the kidneys, mesentery, coronary system, and skeletal muscle, resulting in a decrease of MAP.[39,40] It increases renal plasma flow, glomerular filtration rate, and urinary sodium excretion.[41] Fenoldopam is primarily cleared through hepatic conjugation. Therefore, the dose need not be adjusted if renal pathology is present.[39] Its efficacy in controlling blood pressure in adults with hypertensive crisis has been demonstrated in several studies.[42-44] Its effects have been compared to sodium nitroprusside without adverse renal effects, cyanide toxicity, or light sensitivity.[45] Infusion rates for pediatric patients range from 0.2 to 2 mcg/kg per minute.[39,42] Side effects of fenoldopam include tachycardia, headache, dizziness, and skin flushing.[39,40] Increased intraocular pressure has been reported.[46] Although fenoldopam appears to be safe in pediatric patients, experience is limited in this population. Its use should be restricted primarily to patients requiring potent titratable intravenous agents who have contraindications to the use of sodium nitroprusside.

Enalaprilat

Enalaprilat is an intravenous angiotensin-converting enzyme inhibitor. The recommended dose is 5 to 10 mcg/kg to a maximum of 1.25 mg per dose, given as an intravenous bolus every 8 to 24 hours as needed. It has been used safely for blood pressure control in pediatric patients.[47,48] However, the effects can be variable, and individuals most likely to respond are those with high renin levels, renal artery stenosis, or a mass lesion of the kidney. In addition, enalaprilat may cause significant hypotension in volume-contracted patients, or may cause acute renal failure in patients with bilateral renal artery stenosis. Due to these potential side effects, the inability to titrate, and the potential for a delayed onset of action (up to 60 minutes), other medications are preferable to enalaprilat in the setting of a hypertensive emergency.

Phentolamine

Phentolamine is a competitive α-adrenergic blocking agent that has direct relaxant effects on vascular smooth muscle. It is only indicated in the specific setting of acute hypertensive crises secondary to excess circulating catecholamines from a pheochromocytoma, or reactions involving a monoamine oxidase inhibitor. The dose is 0.05 to 0.1 mg/kg intravenously up to a maximum of 5 mg per dose every 1 to 4 hours as indicated. Phentolamine should be used with caution if cerebral ischemia, renal impairment, arrhythmias, or significant cardiac disease is present. Adverse reactions include tachycardia, dysrhythmias, and hypotension.

Other Medications

Diazoxide and hydralazine have been used to treat hypertensive emergencies as bolus intravenous injections. However, bolus injection of these drugs has been reported to result in abrupt hypotension and irreversible neurologic damage.[10] Multiple other intravenous medications that are easily titrated and more appropriate for treating most hypertensive emergencies are available. Hydralazine is still recommended for treating hypertension in patients with preeclampsia or eclampsia. Magnesium is used for seizure prophylaxis and treatment of seizures associated with eclampsia, but only temporarily decreases blood pressure during bolus injection. The dose of hydralazine for the treatment of hypertension associated with preeclampsia or eclampsia is 5 mg intravenously as an initial dose. This dose may be repeated every 30 minutes as needed to a maximum of 20 mg every 4 to 6 hours.

Nifedipine is a calcium channel blocker that can be administered orally or sublingually. This agent is not approved by the Food and Drug Administration for use in children, although many pediatric nephrologists use nifedipine routinely for severe hypertension.[49-51] In severe pediatric hypertension, retrospective studies show that up to 10% of patients develop hypoxia and 4% develop neurologic events, including stroke, seizures, and altered consciousness, following use of this agent.[51] Moreover, dosing errors can easily occur since 10-mg capsules (29 mg/ml) and 20-mg capsules (44 mg/ml) require puncture and measurement of minute amounts to ensure administration of 0.25 to 0.5 mg/kg orally or sublingually.[49] The response to typical dosing is erratic, with an SBP drop of up to 63% and a DBP drop of up to 89% noted in some series.[49-51] Finally, management of hypertensive emergencies requires use of short-acting, easily titratable, reversible agents with predictable onset and peak effects, none of which is a feature of orally or sublingually administered nifedipine.

Summary

The goal of therapy for hypertensive emergencies is to reduce the MAP by less than 25% over the first 2 to 8 hours. Rapid reduction of the blood pressure can lead to cerebral hypoperfusion and neurologic complications. While multiple medications are available for treating hypertensive crises, other therapeutic interventions should be used to address specific end-organ damage. For instance, furosemide will improve pulmonary mechanics in patients with pulmonary edema, dialysis may be required for acute renal failure, magnesium will prevent seizures in preeclampsia, and pain management may diminish the requirement for antihypertensives in patients with severe pain. All children diagnosed with a hypertensive emergency should be admitted to a pediatric intensive care unit (PICU). If one is not available in the hospital in which the child is initially evaluated, the patient should be transferred to the nearest available hospital with a PICU after appropriate stabilization has been completed.

REFERENCES

1. Lieberman E: Pediatric hypertension: clinical perspective. Mayo Clin Proc 69:1098–1107, 1994.
2. National High Blood Pressure Education Program Working Group on High Blood Pressure in Children and Adolescents: The fourth report on the diagnosis, evaluation, and treatment of high blood pressure in children and adolescents. Pediatrics 114:555–576, 2004.
3. Temple ME, Nahata MC: Treatment of pediatric hypertension. Pharmacotherapy 20:140–150, 2000.
4. Miller K: Pharmacological management of hypertension in paediatric patients: a comprehensive review of the efficacy, safety and dosage guidelines of the available agents. Drugs 48:868–887,1994.
5. Porto I: Hypertensive emergencies in children. Pediatr Pharmacol 14:312–319, 2000.
6. Groshong T: Hypertensive crisis in children. Pediatr Ann 25:368–371, 375–376, 1996.
7. Vaughn CJ, Delanty N: Hypertensive emergencies. Lancet 356:411–417, 2000.
8. Hackman AE, Bricker JT: Preventive cardiology, hypertension, and dyslipidemia. In Garson A, Bricker JT, Fisher DJ, Neish SR (eds): The Science and Practice of Pediatric Cardiology. Baltimore: Williams & Wilkins, 1998, pp 2243–2259.
9. Adelman RD, Coppo R, Dillon MJ: The emergency management of severe hypertension. Pediatr Nephrol 14:422–427, 2000.
10. Deal JE, Barratt TM, Dillon MJ: Management of hypertensive emergencies. Arch Dis Child 67:1089–1092, 1992.
11. van Vught AJ, Troost J, Willemse J: Hypertensive encephalopathy in childhood: diagnostic problems. Neuropadiatrie 7:92–100, 1976.
12. Shayne PH, Pitts SR: Severely increased blood pressure in the emergency department. Ann Emerg Med 41:513–529, 2003.
13. Ross RD, Bollinger RO, Pinsky WW: Grading the severity of congestive heart failure in infants. Pediatr Cardiol 13:72–75, 1992.
14. Clark BJ 3rd: Treatment of heart failure in infants and children. Heart Dis 2:354–361, 2000.
15. Kay JD, Colan SD, Graham TP: Congestive heart failure in pediatric patients. Am Heart J 142:923–928, 2001.
16. Mensah GA, Croft JB, Giles WH: The heart, kidney, and brain as target organs in hypertension. Cardiol Clin 20:225–247, 2002.
17. Mattu GS, Heran BS, Wright JM: Comparison of the automated non-invasive oscillometric blood pressure monitor (BpTRU) with the auscultatory mercury sphygmanometer in a paediatric population. Blood Press Monit 9:39–45, 2004.
18. Park MK, Menard SW, Yuan C: Comparision of auscultatory and oscillometric blood pressures. Arch Pediatr Adolesc Med 155:50–53, 2001.
19. Green TP, Nevins TE, Houser MT, et al: Renal failure as a complication of acute antihypertension therapy. Pediatrics 67:850–854, 1981.
20. Taylor D, Ramsay J, Day S, Dillon M: Infarction of the optic nerve head in children with accelerated hypertension. Br J Ophthalmol 65:153–160, 1981.
21. Gordillo-Panigua G, Velasquez-Jones L, Martini R, Valdez-Bolanos E: Sodium nitroprusside treatment of severe arterial hypertension in children. J Pediatr 87:799–802, 1975.
22. Linakis JG, Lacouture PG, Woolf A: Monitoring cyanide and thiocyanate concentration during infusion of sodium nitroprusside in children. Pediatr Cardiol 12:214–218, 1991.
23. DiPalma JR: Antihypertensive drugs. In DiPalma JR, DiGregorio JG (eds): Basic Pharmacology in Medicine, 3rd ed. New York: McGraw-Hill, 1990, pp 421–435.
24. Michael J, Groshong T, Tobias JD: Nicardipine for hypertensive emergencies in children with renal disease. Pediatr Nephrol 12:40–42, 1998.
25. Tenney F, Sakarcan A: Nicardipine is a safe and effective agent in pediatric hypertensive emergencies. Am J Kidney Dis 35:e20, 2000.
26. Milou C, Debuche-Benouachkou V, Semama DS, et al: Intravenous nicardipine as a first-line antihypertensive drug in neonates. Intensive Care Med 26:956–958, 2000.
27. Flynn JT, Mottes TA, Brophy PD, et al: Intravenous nicardipine for treatment of severe hypertension in children. J Pediatr 139:38–43, 2001.
28. Treyuler JM, Hubert P, Jouvet P, et al: Intravenous nicardipine in hypertensive children. Eur J Pediatr 152:712–714, 1993.
29. Tobias JD: Nicardipine to control mean arterial pressure after cardiothoracic surgery in infants and children. Am J Ther 8:3–6, 2001.
30. Tobias JD, Lowe S, Deshpande JK: Nicardipine: perioperative applications in children. Paediatr Anaesth 5:171–176, 1995.
31. Tobias JD, Pietsch JB, Lynch A: Nicardipine to control mean arterial pressure during extracorporeal membrane oxygenation. Paediatr Anaesth 6:57–60, 1996.

32. Nishikawa T, Omote K, Namiki A, Takahashi T: The effects of nicardipine on cerebrospinal fluid pressure in humans. Anesth Analg 65:507–510, 1986.
33. Wiest DB, Trippel DL, Gillette PC, Garner SS: Pharmacokinetics of esmolol in children. Clin Pharmacol Ther 49:618–623, 1991.
34. Sum CY, Yacobi A, Kartzinel R, et al: Kinetics of esmolol, an ultrashort-acting beta blocker, and of its major metabolite. Clin Pharmacol Ther 34:427–434, 1983.
35. Turlapaty P, Laddu A, Murthy S, et al: Esmolol: a titratable short-acting intravenous beta blocker for acute critical care settings. Am Heart J 114:866–885, 1987.
36. Fivush B, Neu A, Furth S: Acute hypertensive crises in children: emergencies and urgencies. Curr Opin Pediatr 9:233–236, 1997.
37. Wiest DB, Garner SS, Uber WE, Sade RM: Esmolol for the management of pediatric hypertension after cardiac operations. J Thorac Cardiovasc Surg 115:890–897, 1998.
38. Bunchman TE, Lynch RE, Wood EG: Intravenously administered labetalol for treatment of hypertension in children. J Pediatr 120:140–144, 1992.
39. Strauser LM, Pruitt RD, Tobias JD: Initial experience with fenoldopam in children. Am J Ther 6:283–288, 1999.
40. Tobias JD: Fenoldopam for controlled hypotension during spinal fusion in children and adolescents. Paediatr Anaesth 10:261–266, 2000.
41. Shusterman NH, Elliott WJ, White WB: Fenoldopam, but not nitroprusside, improves renal function in severely hypertensive patients with impaired renal function. Am J Med 95:161–168, 1993.
42. Bednarczyk EM, White WB, Munger MA, et al: Comparative acute blood pressure reduction from intravenous fenoldopam mesylate versus sodium nitroprusside in severe hypertension. Am J Cardiol 63:993–996, 1989.
43. Pilmer BL, Green JA, Panacek EA, et al: Fenoldopam mesylate versus sodium nitroprusside in the acute management of severe systemic hypertension. J Clin Pharmacol 33:959–965, 1993.
44. Panacek EA, Bednarczyk EM, Dunbar LM, et al: Randomized, prospective trial of fenoldopam versus sodium nitroprusside in the treatment of acute severe hypertension. Acad Emerg Med 2:959–965, 1995.
45. Post JB, Frishman WH: Fenoldopam: a new dopamine agonist for the treatment of hypertensive urgencies and emergencies. J Clin Pharmacol 38:2–13, 1998.
46. Everitt DE, Boike SC, Piltz-Seymour JR, et al: Effect of intravenous fenoldopam on intraocular pressure in ocular hypertension. J Clin Pharmacol 37:312–320, 1997.
47. Rouine-Rapp K, Mello DM, Hanley FL, et al: Effect of enalaprilat on postoperative hypertension after surgical repair of coarctation of the aorta. Pediatr Crit Care Med 4:327–332, 2003.
48. Schneeweiss A: Cardiovascular drugs in children II: angiotensin-converting enzyme inhibitors in pediatric patients. Pediatr Cardiol 11:199–207, 1990.
49. Blaszack RT, Savage JA, Ellis EN: The use of short acting nifedipine in pediatric patients with hypertension. J Pediatr 139:34–37, 2001.
50. Egger DW, Deming DD, Hamada N, et al: Evaluation of the safety of short acting nifedipine in children with hypertension. Pediatr Nephrol 17:35–40, 2002.
51. Yiu V, Orrbine E, Rosychuk RJ, et al: The safety and use of short acting nifedipine in hospitalized hypertensive children. Pediatr Nephrol 19:644–650, 2004.

Postsurgical Cardiac Conditions and Transplantation

Grace J. Kim, MD and Richard E. Chinnock, MD

Key Points

The typical presenting symptoms of congestive heart failure in children are dyspnea, tachypnea, tachycardia, sweating with feeding, and a palpable, enlarged liver edge on physical examination. Peripheral edema and rales are usually absent.

For children with intrathoracic cardiovascular shunts, dehydration can rapidly become life threatening as the shunt may begin to clot and fail.

Cardiac allograft vasculopathy is a leading cause of death in patients greater than 3 years posttransplantation.

Thrombolytic therapy and acute percutaneous angioplasty are not indicated for heart transplant recipients who are having acute myocardial infarctions.

Introduction and Background

Since the mid-20th century, children with complicated heart conditions who would have died in the past are now living with the use of life-saving medications and with the advent of multiple palliative and definitive surgeries, including heart transplantation. Because of the increasing survival of these patients, all emergency physicians need to be familiar with these conditions.

Recognition and Approach

It is estimated that 1% of live-born infants have isolated congenital heart disease (CHD). The incidence increases if the heart defect is a characteristic of a syndrome or is associated with chromosomal abnormality.[1] Since most data are usually collected by a tertiary cardiology center, the reported incidence varies depending on the study methods. The incidence is 0.75% for all forms of CHD and 0.2% for moderate to severe CHD.[2] Care of infants and children with CHD is dependent on the abnormal heart lesions and their hemodynamic effects on the patient. Treatments can vary from expectant waiting for trivial lesions to maintenance of relatively normal hemodynamics with medication, to palliative or definitive corrective cardiac surgery, including heart transplantation. When evaluating patients with a history of cardiac surgery, asking about each patient's baseline status (energy, oxygenation, feeding, weight) is imperative. Although emergency physicians do not need to know all possible complications from cardiac surgery and transplantation, knowledge about common and important postsurgical complications can aid in expediting the emergency department care of these patients (Table 66–1).

Clinical Presentation

Congestive Heart Failure

The term *congestive heart failure* (CHF) implies a physiologic condition in which there is decreased perfusion so that the blood flow is unable to meet the metabolic demands of the body. In infants, the signs and symptoms are nonspecific and include poor feeding, tachypnea, abnormal respiratory pattern, diastolic filling sound, and hepatomegaly. With increasing severity, hepatomegaly is more pronounced and perfusion decreases. In contrast to adults, children are less likely to have ventricular dysfunction as the pathophysiology of heart failure. Patients are more likely to be symptomatic on the basis of pulmonary congestion and volume overload resulting from a left-to-right cardiac shunt.[3] However, the view of heart failure as purely a hemodynamic disorder is incorrect. There is a body of evidence suggesting neurohormonal mechanisms regulate CHF. Brain natriuretic peptide hormone (BNP) mediates arterial and venous vasodilation in response to ventricular wall tension and left ventricular filling pressures and is secreted by the ventricular myocytes. In children with CHF, the BNP level is elevated and correlates with the ejection fraction of the failing heart. Although studies are limited, measurement of BNP appears to be useful for diagnosing CHF in infants and children.[4]

With the chronic abnormal hemodynamic state, the renin-angiotensin system is activated and catecholamine levels are elevated.[5] Traditional treatment of CHF in adults consists of furosemide and digoxin. Conflicting evidence suggests that

Table 66–1	Specific Defect Repairs and Associated Complications	
Disorder	**Repair**	**Selected Complications**
Atrial septal defect (ASD)	Patching or suturing ASD	Obstructed vena cava or pulmonary vein leading to pulmonary edema/hepatic congestion, atrial arrhythmias (especially atrial fibrillation/flutter)
Ventricular septal defect (VSD)	Patching or suturing VSD	Right bundle branch block
Atrioventricular (AV) septal (canal) defects	Multiple depending upon defects	Heart block, atrial arrhythmias, heart failure, residual VSD, AV valvular regurgitation, pulmonary hypertension
Cyanotic lesion (with ↓ pulmonary flow) temporizing for tetralogy of Fallot, tricuspid or pulmonary atresia	*Blalock Taussig (B-T) shunt* connecting subclavian artery and pulmonary artery (PA) *Potts and Watterson anastomosis—* aorta to PA	If shunt is too small, residual cyanosis may be present; if shunt is too large, pulmonary edema may result (up to 28% of B-T shunts) Thrombosis of shunt due to dehydration (especially with respiratory syncytial virus or rotavirus infection) with ↑ cyanosis Aneurysm of shunt
Left-to-right shunts (ASD, VSD, AV canal)	Pulmonary band to prevent pulmonary hypertension	Branch pulmonary artery stenosis or impingement with hypoxia Coronary artery compression, band loosening with CHF development
Tetralogy of Fallot	Patching VSD plus surgery to decrease pulmonary outflow tract obstruction (e.g., infundibulotomy)	Bundle of His injury with residual right bundle branch, bifascicular or complete AV block, sudden death, congestive heart failure, right ventricular dysfunction, pulmonary hypertension, pulmonary regurgitation
Coarctation of aorta	Resection with anastomosis, subclavian flap aortoplasty or synthetic aortoplasty	Acute postoperative hypertension, restenosis (up to 60% with direct anastomosis), sudden death from arrhythmias, left ventricular hypertrophy on electrocardiogram
Transposition of the great arteries (TGA)	*Mustard and Senning operations—* baffle is placed across atria to redirect flow into correct ventricle	Syncope, atrial/junctional arrhythmias (sudden death), thrombosis of pulmonary/systemic flow with superior/inferior vena cava syndrome, ascites, protein-losing enteropathy, and edema
TGA	*Arterial switch—*aorta and coronary arteries are switched to the left ventricle (LV) and the PA is switched to the right ventricle (RV)	Sudden death, pulmonary artery stenosis, left ventricular failure, inferior or superior vena cava thrombosis (syndrome), coronary artery stenosis and myocardial infarction, stenosis of anastomoses (PA to RV and aorta to LV)
TGA—if complexed with subpulmonary stenosis with VSD	*Rastelli procedure—*patch to shunt blood from LV across VSD and out aorta; ligate proximal PA with conduit from RV to PA	Right ventricular hypertension, ventricular arrhythmias and cardiac conduction abnormalities
Single-ventricle physiology (e.g., severe Ebstein's anomaly, hypoplastic left heart syndrome)	*Fontan procedure—*bypass RV to provide pulmonary blood flow (e.g., superior vena cava to right PA + inferior vena cava to RA, then into left PA)	Sudden death, thromboembolism, thrombosis, anastomotic stenosis, fluid retention, atrial arrhythmias, pulmonary effusions, pericardial effusions, protein-losing enteropathy, peripheral edema
Hypoplastic left heart syndrome (Tricuspid atresia)	1. *Norwood procedure—*create neoaorta: disconnect branch pulmonary artery stenosis and perform B-T shunt; main PA used to contruct aortic arch 2. *Glenn (hemi-Fontan) procedure—* connect superior vena cava to PA 3. (at 18 mo) Complete Fontan procedure so systemic venous blood drains directly to pulmonary system	See Fontan procedure complications above; increased cyanosis due to venovenous collaterals

digoxin is beneficial in some children with CHF and potentially detrimental in others depending upon baseline systemic and pulmonary resistence.[6-8] In children with chronic CHF, β-blockers (e.g., propranolol and carvedilol) may improve symptoms.[9-12]

Cardiac Shunt Thrombosis

The *Blalock-Taussig (B-T) shunt* is one of the most common pulmonary-to-systemic shunt procedures performed in children with cyanotic heart disease as a palliative therapy before a definitive correction is performed. The B-T shunt consists of an anastomosis of the subclavian artery to the ipsilateral pulmonary artery (Fig. 66–1). The classic B-T shunt sacrificed the subclavian artery for the procedure. The modified B-T utilizes a Gore-Tex conduit between the subclavian and

pulmonary artery. This procedure is performed in patients with tetralogy of Fallot (TOF), tricuspid atresia, pulmonary atresia, and right ventricular hypoplasia.[13,14] Although the B-T shunt is generally well tolerated, it is not without complications. The presentation of B-T shunt complications is due to too much or too little flow to the pulmonary vasculature and results in a worsening of the patient's baseline oxygenation. Excessive pulmonary blood flow through the shunt is the most common complication, and causes pulmonary edema and liver congestion, while too little flow through the shunt will result in decreased pulmonary blood flow.[14] Dehydration has been implicated as a probable cause for development of thrombosis in patients with synthetic conduits. Patients with inborn clotting disorders are also at increased risk for shunt thrombosis.[15,16] Another complication, albeit uncommon, is pseudoaneurysm of the shunt. Patients present with cough, fever, and cyanosis, with chest radiographs revealing right upper lobe consolidation ("shadowing").[17-19] Diagnosis of shunt occlusion can be made by transthoracic echocardiography, transesophageal echocardiography, and angiogram.

A *Fontan procedure* is performed in patients who have a single functional ventricle, such as those with tricuspid atresia, hypoplastic left heart syndrome, and pulmonary atresia with intact ventricular septum. The Fontan and its modification provides an atriopulmonary or cavopulmonary anastomosis so the systemic venous return can reach the pulmonary circulation, bypassing the ventricle[20] (Fig. 66–2). The complications of the Fontan procedure are thrombosis and thromboembolism (i.e., cerebrovascular accidents, systemic venous obstructive symptoms such as superior vena cava syndrome, pulmonary embolism, and emboli to extremities),[21-23] especially in the face of dehydration. Arrhythmias also may lead to thrombus formation.[21] Hepatic congestion resulting in abnormalities in prothrombin time and galactose elimination are also noted following the Fontan procedure.[24] Protein-losing enteropathy occurs, possibly due to the chronically elevated systemic venous pressure. Infants and children present with peripheral edema and ascites, hypoproteinemia, lymphocytopenia, hypocalcemia, and low immunoglobulin concentrations.[25,26]

Post-pericardiotomy Syndrome

Pericardial effusions develop in 23% to 53% of patients who undergo pericardiotomy, with 23% to 45% of these patients developing post-pericardiotomy syndrome (PPS).[27,28] This disorder occurs due to an immune-mediated response to pericardial or direct myocardial injury.[29] PPS syndrome consists of fever, irritability, and poor feeding. The cardiac examination can reveal a friction rub and hepatomegaly. Other findings include chest pain, vomiting, and signs of cardiac tamponade with tachypnea, tachycardia, and hypotension.[28,30] Chest radiographs may reveal an enlarged cardiac shadow, but the ultimate diagnosis is made by an echocardiogram that shows a pericardial effusion.[27,28,30] PPS is typically a self-limiting condition and can be managed

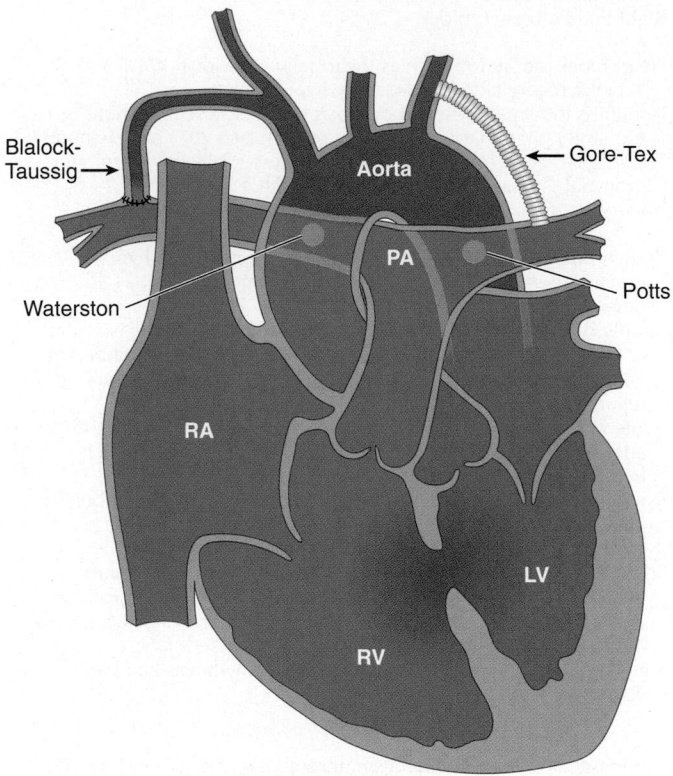

FIGURE 66–1. Pulmonary-to-systemic shunts with the classic and current Blalock-Taussig shunt. (From Park M: Pediatric Cardiology for Practitioners, 4th ed. St. Louis: Mosby, 2002.)

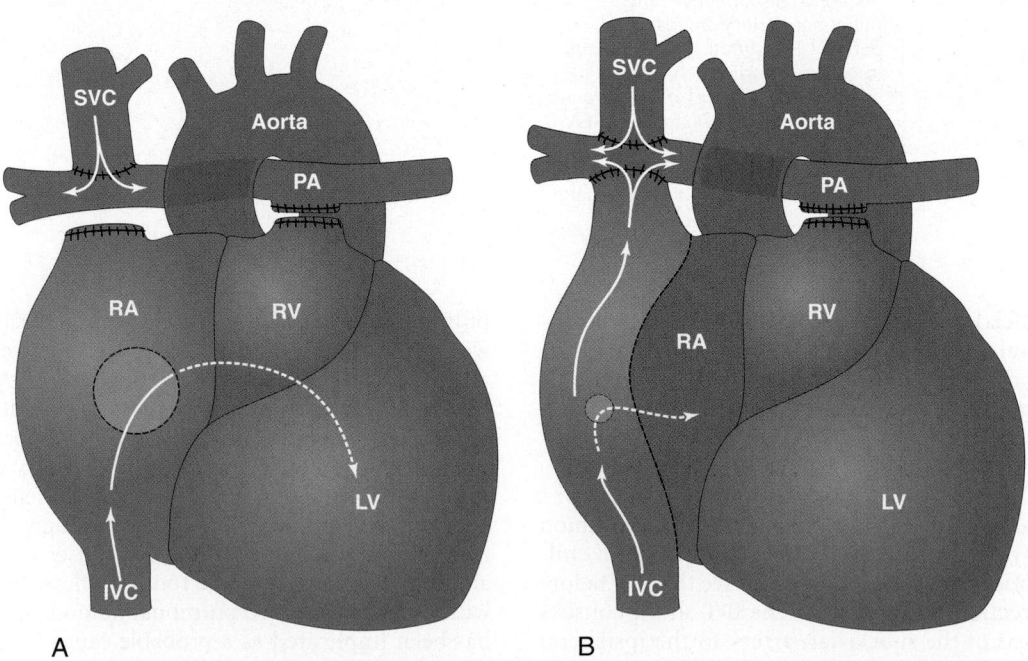

FIGURE 66–2. Modified Fontan operation. **A,** Bidirectional Glenn operation or superior vena cava (SVC)–to–right pulmonary artery anastomosis. **B,** Cavocaval baffle-to–pulmonary artery (PA) connection, with or without fenestration. (See text for description of these procedures.) Abbreviations: IVC, inferior vena cava; LV, left ventricle; RA, right atrium; RV, right ventricle.

medically with fluid restriction, diuretics (e.g., furosemide 1 mg/kg per dose), and nonsteroidal anti-inflammatory medications or glucocorticoids for severe or recurrent pericardial effusion. Glucocorticoids may contribute to faster resolution of symptoms but not to earlier hospital discharge. The recommended dose of prednisone is 2 mg/kg per day tapered over 14 days.[31] Aspirin has been used widely but has not been proven effective.[27] Occasionally, this condition will progresses to cardiac tamponade. If this complication occurs, pericardiocentesis in the emergency department will be required.[32]

Viral Infections

Respiratory syncytial virus (RSV) infections are an important cause of morbidity in infants with congenital heart disease, postsurgical cardiac disorders, and cardiac transplants. Risk factors for severe disease include young age of patient, history of prematurity, chronic lung disease, CHD, and metabolic disorders.[33] High-risk patients have increased incidence of arrhythmias, hypotension or shock, and respiratory failure when infected with RSV.[34] Therefore, patients with risk factors for severe disease who have pneumonia, hypoxia, respiratory distress, or tachypnea will require admission. RSV testing can be obtained by any of the commercially available antigen detection kits, allowing for rapid diagnosis.[35] Multiple studies have evaluated the use of ribavirin in high-risk patients. Thus far, there is no significant difference in patients treated with ribavirin. Currently, the American Academy of Pediatrics states that ribavirin "may be considered in patients at high risk for complicated disease."[36] For heart transplantation patients, high-risk factors for severe disease with RSV include age less than 1 year, increased immunosuppressive therapy (i.e., shortly after transplantation or recent allograft failure), or underlying lung disease. In patients with isolated upper respiratory infection who have no risk factors, only supportive care is recommended. If the posttransplantation patient has upper respiratory infection with risk factors or lower respiratory illness, treatment options to consider include aerosolized ribavirin in conjunction with RSV intravenous immune globulin *(Respi-Gam)* or palivizumab *(Synagis)*.[37]

Influenza A and B virus infection in the heart transplantation patient should prompt treatment with zanamivir or oseltamivir. Amantadine and rimantadine are not currently recommended due to high resistance. Patients who have respiratory symptoms such as tachypnea or hypoxia require admission. For severe lower respiratory illness, aerosolized ribavirin is an option.[38]

Post–Cardiac Surgery Arrhythmias

Post–cardiac surgery arrhythmias occur in nearly half of all patients, especially in the early postoperative period spent in the intensive care unit.[39] Arrhythmias that occur weeks to years after cardiac surgery are attributed to multiple factors: scarring of the myocardium, the type of surgery performed, the natural history of the specific cardiac defect, history of preexisting arrhythmias, and the patient's postoperative hemodynamic status (Table 66–2).[40] Intra-atrial reentrant tachycardias (IARTs) are seen in patients who have had atrial surgery and are thought to be due to the variable location of the suture lines. IATR is an atrial tachycardia (like atrial flutter) that uses a reentry circuit that does not involve the

Table 66–2	Post–Cardiac Surgery Arrhythmias
Arrhythmia	**Heart Defect/Procedure**
Sinus bradycardia	Transposition of the great arteries (TGA)
Right bundle branch block	Tetralogy of Fallot (TOF)
Complete heart block	TOF, TGA, aortic stenosis (AS)/Fontan procedure
Junctional rhythm	TGA/Fontan procedure
Atrial flutter	Atrial septal defect (ASD), TOF,
IART	TGA/Fontan procedure
Atrial fibrillation	
Supraventricular tachycardia	ASD, TGA/Fontan procedure
Ventricular tachycardia	TOF, AS/Fontan procedure, AV canal repair

Abbreviations: AV, atrioventricular; IART, intra-atrial reentrant tachycardia.

atrioventricular node.[40-42] Isolated ventricular septal defect repair is not highly associated with arrhythmias, although reports of atrioventricular conduction defects exist. However, when the ventricular septal defect is a part of TOF, the incidence of arrhythmias is markedly increased. Surgery in patients with TOF ranges from palliation with B-T shunt to complete repair of the defects. Right bundle branch block, atrial fibrillation/flutter, ventricular arrhythmias, and complete heart block are associated with these repairs. The greatest risks for late morbidity and mortality are unpaced complete heart block and ventricular tachycardia.[40,43] Correction of transposition of the great arteries has evolved over the years. The common surgeries, which involve an intra-atrial switch or intra-atrial baffle, are the Mustard and Senning repairs. Because of the extensive manipulation of the atrial muscle and sinus node, these repairs result in a high propensity for arrhythmias.[44] However, with arterial switch procedures, there is a significantly lowered incidence of arrhythmias, with 96% of patients manifesting sinus rhythm at follow-up to 8.5 years.[45] Catheter ablation therapy is used for patients who have life-threatening or drug-resistant arrhythmias, adverse drug reactions, or tachycardia-induced cardiomyopathy. It has also been performed on IART with good success.[46,47] Implantable cardioverter-defibrillators can effectively manage dangerous, refractory ventricular arrhythmias in selected patients.[48] Management of dysrhythmias is discussed in Chapter 63 (Dysrhythmias). Importantly, adenosine should be avoided post-transplant as it can lead to permanent asystole.

Endocarditis

Endocarditis is a relatively uncommon disease that has high morbidity and mortality despite advances in antimicrobial therapies, diagnostic capabilities, and treatments. Patients at high risk for endocarditis include those with palliative shunts, conduit procedures, prosthetic valves, and indwelling catheters.[49] Those who are at moderate risk are patients with uncorrected ventricular septal defect, patent ductus arteriosus, primum atrial septal defect, coarctation of the aorta and bicuspid aortic valve, and mitral valve prolapse. Six months after successful surgical correction of congenital heart defects in the moderate-risk category, the patients are considered to have negligible risk for developing endocarditis, and do not need prophylactic antibiotics prior to invasive procedures.[50,51] Patients with endocarditis present with indolent fevers lasting from days to weeks. There are also nonspecific complaints of malaise, myalgia, arthralgia, weight loss, rigors, and diaphoresis. Development of CHF as a complication of endocarditis is a grave prognostic factor. It may develop acutely with valve perforation (aortic, mitral, or tricuspid), chordae rupture, valve obstruction from large vegetations, or development of intracardiac shunts from fistulous tracts or prosthetic dehiscence. It may also develop insidiously as a result of progressive worsening of the valvular insufficiency and resultant ventricular dysfunction.[52] Occasionally, infants and children with endocarditis will present acutely with high fevers and rapid development of symptoms. Conditions that require cardiovascular surgical intervention include worsening CHF, valvular obstruction, perivalvular extension of infection, fungal endocarditis, and persistent bacteremia despite appropriate antibiotic therapy.[49] Antibiotics for endocarditis need to cover the gram-positive organisms that are the causative organisms. Antibiotic recommendations for native and prosthetic valve endocarditis are discussed in Chapter 64 (Pericarditis, Myocarditis, and Endocarditis). In general, antibiotic regimens for repaired cardiac defects should mirror these recommendations.

Heart Transplantation

In 2002, 359 pediatric patients received a heart transplant, with approximately 80 centers performing this procedure.[53] These patients are followed closely initially by the transplanting centers, then return home with scheduled follow-ups with decreasing frequency depending upon complications.

Posttransplantation Infection

Fever is a common reason for a heart transplantation patient to present to the emergency department. Infection following transplantation has three phases. During the first phase, in the first month after transplantation, the causes of infection are most commonly the underlying disease the recipient had prior to the transplantation, a contaminated allograft introducing infection, or the usual postoperative infections that can be found in all patients, although in an individual receiving a transplant, the episodes are accentuated.[54] Bacterial infections are the most common type of infection immediately posttransplantation, especially in infants younger than 6 months of age.[55] The majority of infections are in the blood and lungs.[54] The second phase is 1 to 6 months after transplantation. The major classes of infection are viral (cytomegalovirus [CMV], Epstein-Barr virus [EBV], hepatitis virus, and herpesvirus), and opportunistic infections such as *Listeria monocytogenes, Aspergillus fumigatus,* and *Pneumocystis jiroveci.* Greater than 6 months posttransplantation, the majority of patients who are stable in their maintenance immunosuppression are at the greatest risk from community-acquired viruses such as influenza virus, RSV, and parainfluenza virus.[54] Patients with CMV infection present with a "viral syndrome." Patients may present with fever, malaise, hepatitis, pneumonitis, retinitis, or gastrointestinal disease. Leukopenia and thrombocytopenia may also be present. CMV infection is a risk factor for development of bacteremia or invasive fungal disease, and it has been implicated in posttransplantation lymphoproliferative disorder (PTLD) and cardiac allograft vasculopathy (CAV). Treatment is with ganciclovir 5 mg/kg per dose IV twice daily for 2 to 4 weeks.[54,56] Patients with EBV infection can present similarly to those

with CMV infection. Primary EBV infection has been implicated in the development of PTLD.[57,58] This is a lymphoproliferative disorder that ranges in severity from a relatively benign condition that improves with adjustment of immunosuppressive medication to lymphoma.[54]

Acute Transplant Rejection

Acute transplant rejection occurs most frequently within the first year after heart transplantation. Presenting symptoms include poor feeding, irritability, low-grade fever, ileus, and dyspnea. Clinically, the patient may display tachycardia, tachypnea, hepatomegaly, gallop, or ventricular ectopy.[59] Thirty-eight percent of patients with heart transplants require therapy for arrhythmias. The most common arrhythmias are sinus bradycardia and atrial tachyarrhythmias.

The new onset of Wenckebach periodicity is associated with either rejection or coronary artery disease.[60] However, any new arrhythmia requires evaluation for rejection. Endomyocardial biopsy is the "gold standard" for diagnosing acute rejection.[61] Because of its invasiveness, cost, and labor intensity, other less invasive methods for diagnosing rejection have been explored. In cardiac transplantation patients, initially the belief was that a decrease in the electrocardiogram (ECG) QRS voltages could be related to acute rejection.[62] Studies in animals and humans suggest that there is great variability in voltage even in normal hearts, and that the ECG finding of decreasing voltage is not specific for rejection.[63,64] However, ECG abnormalities that have been known to precede onset of cardiac failure include a decrease in voltage, axis deviation, arrhythmias, and conduction abnormalities.[65] Echocardiography of patients with acute rejection may show increased ventricular mass, decreased ventricular volume, or ventricular dysfunction. These findings do not correlate well with endomyocardial biopsies; therefore, they cannot be used solely to predict rejection.[66,67] However, the positive predictive value (of these tests) is increased when patients are evaluated for change from baseline.[68] The BNP level is elevated in adult patients during acute cardiac allograft rejection,[69] but studies in children have not been definitive. Although BNP is elevated during graft rejection, levels cannot be used to gauge the severity of the episode.[70-72] Objective evaluation of patients in the emergency department with suspected acute rejection may include the combination of BNP level, ECG, and echocardiogram, then admission for further evaluation and management.

Cardiac Allograft Vasculopathy

CAV is one of the major limitations to long-term graft survival. It is the leading single cause of death in patients greater than 3 years posttransplantation.[53] It is a progressive form of atherosclerosis that is unique to the transplantation patient. CAV is caused by both immunologic and nonimmunologic mechanisms. Immunologic mechanisms include frequent and late (>1 year posttransplantation) acute rejection episodes.[73] Nonimmunologic mechanisms are those relating to the transplant itself or the recipient (donor age, smoking, obesity, history of diabetes, hyperlipidemia, or hypertension) and to side effects from immune suppression, such as CMV infection, which may impair endothelial function[74]; nephrotoxicity; and new-onset diabetes.[56] CAV is different from atherosclerosis in that the narrowing of the arteries caused by proliferation of the intima is concentric, and involves the length of the coronary arteries. This process involves vessels of all sizes. Ischemia often involves very small, patchy areas of the myocardium. Therefore, treatment with angioplasty or bypass surgery will not be as successful as it is in conventional atherosclerotic heart disease.[75,76] There is some evidence that myocardial infarction and ischemia are usually silent and devoid of chest pain due to de-innervation of the heart. However, some re-innervation may occur posttransplant. In fact, the first clinical manifestations of myocardial infarction may be congestive heart failure, ventricular arrhythmias, or sudden death.[77,78] A small number of transplantation patients may require pacemakers for arrhythmias. These patients present with dizziness and syncope. If these symptoms are present, an evaluation for CAV is required.[79] CAV is diagnosed by coronary angiography; however, intravascular ultrasound is even more sensitive at detecting early stages of coronary endothelial dysfunction, which leads to CAV.[80] The only current treatment for CAV is a new heart transplant.[56] However, there is evidence of vasculopathy regression after introducing sirolimus to the immunosuppressive regimen.[81] Further trials are needed to determine the efficacy of this agent.

Posttransplantation Lymphoproliferative Disorder

PTLD is a heterogeneous entity found more frequently in children than in adults.[57] It is due to an abnormal proliferation of lymphoid cells. Severity of the disease may range from local, isolated lymphadenopathy to lymphoma. Symptoms vary, depending on the location of the lesions, from cough, dyspnea, or respiratory difficulty, including upper airway obstruction, with lung nodules, to gastrointestinal symptoms that include diarrhea, bleeding, abdominal pain, or masses. Constitutional symptoms such as fever, fatigue, and weight loss are also common.[82] There are multiple risk factors for developing PTLD, including recurrent rejection episodes and primary infection with EBV after transplantation.[83] Diagnosis is confirmed by histopathologic evaluation of the involved tissues. Treatment ranges from withdrawal of immunosuppressive therapy to chemotherapy. There is a report of complete resolution of PTLD in a child treated with rituximab (an anti-CD20 monoclonal antibody) along with reduced immunosuppression, and treatment for an active EBV hepatitis with ganciclovir.[84]

Transplantation Medication Side Effects

Several important side effects are associated with medications used to treat post–cardiac transplantation patients.[85-93] These effects are listed by the affected organ systems in Table 66–3.

Important Clinical Features and Considerations

Nonspecific symptoms of poor feeding, irritability, lethargy, and tachypnea are common in children with post–cardiac surgery conditions, including CHF and acute rejection in heart transplantation patients. Patients with congenital heart disease who present with complaints of chest pain, dizziness, or syncope should be evaluated for arrhythmias with an ECG or Holter monitoring.

Dehydration in patients with intrathoracic cardiovascular shunts can be life-threatening if thrombosis ensues with

Table 66–3	Side Effects of Medications Used to Treat Posttransplantation Patients
Medication	**Side Effects**
Glucocorticoids	*Neurologic:* steroid psychosis, memory or cognitive dysfunction *Ocular:* cataracts, glaucoma *Endocrine:* decreased growth hormone, hypogonadism, osteopenia, diabetes, mellitus, Cushing's syndrome *Cardiovascular:* hypertension, dyslipidemia
Cyclosporin A (CSA) Tacrolimus	*Renal:* nephrotoxicity *Neurologic:* seizure, tremors, paresthesias, peripheral neuropathies *Cardiovascular:* hypertension, hyperlipidemia *Hepatic:* hepatotoxicity (CSA) *Endocrine:* Glucose intolerance and diabetes mellitus (tacrolimus)
Mycophenolate mofetil (MMF)	*Gastrointestinal:* discomfort, diarrhea *Hematologic:* leukopenia

resulting shunt failure. Patients will present with worsening baseline oxygen saturation, tachypnea, and malaise.

Cardiac troponins are elevated in CAV; however, this test is less useful as a predictor of acute transplant rejection. Creatine kinase is not useful for detecting acute rejection.[92]

Management

Chronic management of CHF may include furosemide, digoxin, angiotensin-converting enzyme inhibitors or β-blockers. However, acute management is supportive, with semi-upright positioning, supplemental oxygen, and furosemide 1 mg/kg per dose for pulmonary edema. Inotropic support with dopamine or dobutamine is administered for severe low-output states in CHF or cardiogenic shock.[93]

Shunt thrombosis can be evaluated and diagnosed (with increasing sensitivity) by transthoracic echocardiography, transesophageal echocardiography, or angiography.[20] Initial therapy includes correction of dehydration with intravenous fluids. Treatment of the thrombus can be accomplished through administration of heparin, balloon angioplasty,[94] catheter-directed infusion of low-dose alteplase[23] or stent replacement. Because of the choices available for treatment, a cardiologist should be consulted prior to starting heparin therapy.

Acute rejection is treated with methylprednisolone at 20 mg/kg per dose twice daily for eight doses. This agent should be given in consultation with a transplant team.

Therapy for specific infections (e.g., PTLD; bacterial, viral, and parasitic infections) may be required following evaluation for fever or nonspecific complaints.

Summary

Survival of patients with complex congenital heart disease is markedly improved by better surgical techniques and heart transplantation. Evaluating patients with these disorders can be challenging due to their intricate underlying physiology, complex past medical history, and unique medical regimens. Recognizing the many disorders that can occur in these patients is difficult and requires knowledge of common and important complications, awareness of the utility of various diagnostic adjuncts, and an understanding of unique medications. When there is uncertainty about the management of a patient, the patient's transplant coordinator or the on-call cardiologist should be contacted.

REFERENCES

1. Brennan P, Young I: Congenital heart malformations: aetiology and associations. Semin Neonatol 6:17–25, 2001.
2. Hoffman J, Kaplan S: The incidence of congenital heart disease. J Am Coll Cardiol 34:1890–1900, 2004.
*3. Ross R, Bollinger R, Pinsky W: Grading the severity of congestive heart failure in infants. Pediatr Cardiol 13:72–75, 1992.
4. Mir T, Marohn S, Laer S, et al: Plasma concentrations of N-terminal pro-brain natriuretic peptide in control children from the neonatal to adolescent period and in children with congestive heart failure. Pediatrics 110:e76–e86, 2002.
5. Buchhorn R, Bartmus D, Siekmeyer W, et al: Beta-blocker therapy of severe congestive heart failure in infants with left to right shunts. Am J Cardiol 81:1366–1368, 1998.
6. Berman W Jr, Yabek S, Dillon T, et al: Effects of digoxin in infants with congested circulatory state due to a ventricular septal defect. N Engl J Med 308:363–366, 1983.
7. Seguchi M, Nakazawa M, Momma K: Further evidence suggesting a limited role of digitalis in infants with circulatory congestion secondary to large ventricular septal defect. Am J Cardiol 83:1408–1411, 1999.
8. Kimball T, Daniels S, Meyer R, et al: Effect of digoxin on contractility and symptoms in infants with a large ventricular septal defect. Am J Cardiol 68:1377–1382, 1991.
9. Bruns L, Chrisant M, Lamour J, et al: Carvedilol as therapy in pediatric heart failure: an initial multicenter experience. J Pediatr 138:505–511, 2001.
10. Bucchorn R, Hulpke-Wette M, Hilgers R, et al: Propranolol treatment of congestive heart failure in infants with congenital heart disease: the CHF-PRO-INFANT Trial. Int J Cardiol 79:167–173, 2001.
11. Laer S, Mir T, Behn F, et al: Carvedilol therapy in pediatric patients with congestive heart failure: a study investigating clinical and pharmacokinetic parameters. Am Heart J 143:916–922, 2002.
12. Williams R, Tani L, Shaddy R: Intermediate effects of treatment with metoprolol or carvedilol in children with left ventricular systolic dysfunction. J Heart Lung Transplant 21:906–909, 2002.
13. Woods W, Schutte D, McCulloch M: Care of children who have had surgery for congenital heart disease. Am J Emerg Med 21:318–327, 2003.
14. Gladman G, McCrindle B, Williams W, et al: The modified Blalock-Taussig shunt: clinical impact and morbidity in Fallot's tetralogy in the current era. J Thorac Cardiovasc Surg 114:25–30, 1997.
15. Tireli E, Basaran M: Early Blalock-Taussig shunt thrombosis in a neonate with protein C deficiency. Ann Thorac Surg 77:2260–2261, 2004.
16. Simsic J, Uber W, Lazarchick J, et al: Systemic-to-pulmonary artery shunt thrombosis in a neonate with factor V Leiden mutation. Ann Thorac Surg 74:2179–2181, 2002.
*17. Coren M, Green C, Yates R, et al: Complications of modified Blalock-Taussig shunts mimicking pulmonary disease. Arch Dis Child 79:361–362, 1998.
18. Sundararaghavan S, Khalid O, Suarez W, et al: Single-stage repair of tetralogy of Fallot with pseudoaneurysm: a unique approach. Ann Thorac Surg 77:2184–2186, 2004.
19. Pongprot Y, Silvilairat S, Woragidpoonpol S, et al: Pseudoaneurysm following modified Blalock-Taussig shunt: a rare complication mimicking pulmonary disease. J Med Assoc Thai 86:365–368, 2003.
20. Jahangiri M, Ross D, Redington A, et al: Thromboembolism after the Fontan procedure and its modifications. Ann Thorac Surg 58:1409–1414, 1994.
21. Rosenthal D, Friedman A, Kleinman C, et al: Thromboembolic complications after Fontan operations. Circulations 92:287–293, 1995.
22. Wilson W, Greer G, Tobias J: Cerebral venous thrombosis after the Fontan procedure. J Thorac Cardiovasc Surg 116:661–663, 1998.
23. Ruud E, Holmstrom H, Aagenaes I, et al: Successful thrombolysis by prolonged low-dose alteplase in catheter-directed infusion. Acta Paediatr 92:973–976, 2003.
24. Narkewicz M, Sondheimer H, Ziegler J, et al: Hepatic dysfunction following the Fontan procedure. J Pediatr Gastroenterol Nutr 36:352–357, 2003.
*25. Kaulitz R, Luhmer I, Bergmann F, et al: Sequelae after modified Fontan operation: postoperative haemodynamic data and organ function. Heart 78:154–159, 1997.
26. Kim S, Park I, Song J, et al: Reversal of protein-losing enteropathy with calcium replacement in a patient after Fontan operation. Ann Thorac Surg 77:1456–1457, 2004.
27. Cheung E, Ho S, Tang K: Pericardial effusion after open heart surgery for congenital heart disease. Heart 89:780–784, 2003.
28. Hoffman M: Anti-heart antibodies an epiphenomenon? A prospective, longitudinal pilot study. Autoimmunity 35:241–245, 2002.
29. Clapp S, Garson A, Gutgesell H, et al: Postoperative pericardial effusion and its relation to postpericardiotomy syndrome. Pediatrics 66:585–588, 1980.
30. Tsang T, Barnes M, Hayes S, et al: Clinical and echocardiographic characteristics of significant pericardial effusions following cardiothoracic surgery and outcomes of echo-guided pericardiocentesis for management. Chest 116:322–331, 1999.
31. Wilson N, Webber S, Patterson M, et al: Double-blind placebo-controlled trial of corticosteroids in children with postpericardiotomy syndrome. Pediatr Cardiol 15:62–65, 1994.
32. Scarfone R. Donoghue A, Alessandrini E: Cardiac tamponade complicating postpericardiotomy syndrome. Pediatr Emerg Care 19:268–271, 2003.
33. Law B, Wang E, MacDonald N, et al: Does ribavirin impact on the hospital course of children with respiratory syncytial virus (RSV) infection? An analysis using the Pediatric Investigators Collaborative Network on Infections in Canada (PICNIC) RSV database. Pediatrics 99:e7, 1997.
34. Wilson D, Landrigan C, Horn S, et al: Complications in infants hospitalized for bronchiolitis or respiratory syncytial virus pneumonia. J Pediatr 143:s143–s149, 2003.
35. Michaels MG, Serdy C, Barbadora K, et al: Respiratory syncytial virus: a comparision of diagnostic modalities. Pediatr Infect Dis J 11:613–616, 1992.
36. Committee on Infectious Diseases, American Academy of Pediatrics: Reassessment of the indications for ribavirin therapy in respiratory syncytial virus infections. Pediatrics 97:137–140, 1996.
37. Englund J, Piedra P, Whimbey E: Prevention and treatment of respiratory syncytial virus and parainfluenza viruses in immunocompromised patients. Am J Med 102:61–70, 1997.
38. Uyeki T: Influenza diagnosis and treatment in children: a review of studies on clinically useful tests and antiviral treatment for influenza. Pediatr Infect Dis J 22:164–177, 2003.
39. Valsangiacomo E, Schmid E, Schupbach R, et al: Early postoperative arrhythmias after cardiac operation in children. Ann Thorac Surg 74:792–796, 2002.
40. Vetter V: What every pediatrician needs to know about arrhythmias in children who have had cardiac surgery. Pediatr Ann 20:378–385, 1991.
41. Lan Y, Lee J, Wetzel G: Postoperative arrhythmia. Curr Opin Cardiol 18:73–78, 2003.
42. Wei L, Somerville J: Atrial flutter in grown-up congenital heart (GUCH) patients: clinical characteristics of affected population. Int J Cardiol 75:129–137, 2000.
43. Nakazawa M, Shinohara T, Sasaki A, et al: Arrhythmias late after repair of tetralogy of Fallot: a Japanese multicenter study. Circ J 68:126–130, 2004.
44. Weindling S, Saul J, Gamble W, et al: Duration of complete atrioventricular block after congenital heart disease surgery. Am J Cardiol 82:525–527, 1998.
45. Rhodes L, Wernovsky G, Keane J, et al: Arrhythmias and intracardiac conduction after the arterial switch operation. J Thorac Cardiovasc Surg 109:303–310, 1995.
46. Weipert J, Noebauer C, Schreiber C, et al: Occurrence and management of atrial arrhythmia after long-term Fontan circulation. J Thorac Cardiovasc Surg 127:457–464, 2004.
47. Friedman R, Walsh E, Silka M, et al; NASPE Expert Consensus Conference: Radiofrequency catheter ablation in children with and without congenital heart disease: report of the writing committee. Pacing Clin Electrophysiol 25:1000–1017, 2002.

---

*Selected readings.

48. Alexander M, Cecchin F, Walsh E, et al: Implications of implantable cardioverter defibrillator therapy in congenital heart disease and pediatrics. J Cardiovasc Electrophysiol 15:72–79, 2004.

49. Ferrieri P, Gewitz M, Gerber M, et al: Unique features of infective endocarditis in childhood. Circulation 105:2115–2127, 2002.

50. Dajani A, Taubert K, Wilson W, et al: Prevention of bacterial endocarditis: recommendations by the American Heart Association. JAMA 277:1794–1801, 1997.

51. Choi M, Mailman T: Pneumococcal endocarditis in infants and children. Pediatr Infect Dis J 23:166–171, 2004.

52. Bayer A, Bolger A, Taubert K, et al: Diagnosis and management of infective endocarditis and its complications. Circulation 98:2936–2948, 1998.

53. Boucek M, Edwards L, Keck B, et al: Registry for the International Society for Heart and Lung Transplantation: seventh official pediatric report—2004. J Heart Lung Transplant 23:933–947, 2004.

54. Fishman J, Rubin R: Infection in organ-transplant recipients. N Engl J Med 338:1741–1751, 1998.

55. Schowengerdt K, Naftel D, Seib P, et al: Infection after heart transplantation: results of a multiinstitutional study. The Pediatric Heart Transplant Study Group. J Heart Lung Transplant 16:1207–1216, 1997.

*56. Valantine H: Cardiac allograft vasculopathy after heart transplantation: risk factors and management. J Heart Lung Transplant 23:s187–s193, 2004.

57. Boyle G, Michaels M, Webber S, et al: Posttransplantation lymphoproliferative disorders in pediatric thoracic organ recipients. J Pediatr 131:309–313, 1997.

58. Zangwill S, Hsu D, Kichuk M, et al: Incidence and outcome of primary Epstein-Barr virus infection and lymphoproliferative disease in pediatric heart transplant recipients. J Heart Lung Transplant 17:1161–1166, 1998.

59. Chinnock R, Sherwin T, Robie S, et al: Emergency department presentation and management of pediatric heart transplant recipients. Pediatr Emerg Care 11:355–360, 1995.

60. Kertesz N, Towbin J, Clunie S, et al: Long term follow up of arrhythmias in pediatric orthotopic heart transplant recipients: incidence and correlation with rejection. J Heart Lung Transplant 22:889–893, 2003.

61. Caves P, Stinson E, Billingham M, et al: Diagnosis of human cardiac allograft rejection by serial cardiac biopsy. J Thorac Cardiovasc Surg 66:461–466, 1973.

62. Stinson E, Dong E Jr, Bieber C, et al: Cardiac transplantation in man. 1: early rejection. JAMA 207:2233–2242, 1969.

63. Nakhleh R, Bolman R 3rd, Shumway S, et al: Correlation of endomyocardial biopsy findings with electrocardiogram voltage in pediatric cardiac allografts. Clin Transplant 6:114–118, 1992.

64. Haberl R, Manz P, Steinbigler J, et al: Can ECG spectral analysis improve the noninvasive surveillance of acute rejection? Transplant Proc 30:900–903, 1998.

65. Cooper D, Charles R, Rose A, et al: Does the electrocardiogram detect early acute heart rejection? J Heart Transplant 4:546–549, 1985.

66. Boucek M, Mathis C, Kanakriyeh M, et al: Serial echocardiographic evaluation of cardiac graft rejection after infant heart transplantation. J Heart Lung Transplant 12:824–831, 1993.

67. Rosenthal D, Chin C, Nishimura K, et al: Identifying cardiac transplant rejection in children: diagnostic utility of echocardiography, right heart catheterization and endomyocardial biopsy data. J Heart Lung Transplant 23:323–329, 2004.

68. Putzer G, Cooper D, Keehn C, et al: An improved echocardiographic rejection-surveillance strategy following pediatric heart transplantation. J Heart Lung Transplant 19:1166–1174, 2000.

69. Masters R, Davies R, Veinot J, et al: Discoordinate modulation of natriuretic peptides during acute cardiac allograft rejection in humans. Circulation 100:287–291, 1999.

70. Arnau-Vives M, Almenar L, Hervas I, et al: Predictive value of brain natriuretic peptide in the diagnosis of heart transplant rejection. J Heart Lung Transplant 23:850–856, 2004.

71. Hervas I, Arnau M, Almenar L, et al: Ventricular natriuretic peptide (BNP) in heart transplantation: BNP correlation with endomyocardial biopsy, laboratory and hemodynamic measures. Lab Invest 84:138–145, 2004.

72. Claudius I, Lan Y, Chang R, et al: Usefulness of B-type natriuretic peptide as a noninvasive screening tool for cardiac allograft pathology in pediatric heart transplant recipients. Am J Cardiol 92:1368–1370, 2003.

73. Mulla N, Johnston J, Dussen L, et al: Late rejection is a predictor of transplant coronary artery disease in children. J Am Coll Cardiol 37:243–250, 2001.

74. Petrakopoulou P, Kubrich M, Pehlivanli S, et al: Cytomegalovirus infection in heart transplant recipients is associated with impaired endothelial function. Circulation 110(Suppl II):II-207–II-212, 2004.

75. Billingham M: Histopathology of graft coronary disease. J Heart Lung Transplant 11:s38–s44, 1992.

76. Billingham M: Pathology and etiology of chronic rejection of the heart. Clin Transplant 8:289–292, 1994.

77. Halpert I, Goldberg A, Levine A, et al: Reinnervation of the transplanted human heart as evidenced from heart rate variability studies. Am J Cardiol 77:180–183, 1996.

78. Wilson R, McGinn A, Johnson T, et al: Sympathetic reinnervation after heart transplantation in human beings. J Heart Lung Transplant 11:s88–s89, 1992.

79. Cannon B, Denfield S, Friedman R, et al: Late pacemaker requirement after pediatric orthotopic heart transplantation may predict the presence of transplant coronary artery disease. J Heart Lung Transplant 23:67–71, 2004.

80. Hollenberg S, Klein L, Parrillo J, et al: Coronary endothelial dysfunction after heart transplantation predicts allograft vasculopathy and cardiac death. Circulation 104:3091–3096, 2001.

81. Ruygrok P, Webber B, Faddy S, et al: Angiographic regression of cardiac allograft vasculopathy after introducing sirolimus immunosuppression. J Heart Lung Transplant 22:1276–1279, 2003.

82. Lim G, Newman B, Kurland G, et al: Posttransplantation lymphoproliferative disorder: manifestations in pediatric thoracic organ recipients. Radiology 222:699–708, 2002.

83. Gao S, Chaparro S, Perlroth M, et al: Post-transplantation lymphoproliferative disease in heart and heart-lung transplant recipients: 30-year experience at Stanford University. J Heart Lung Transplant 22:505–514, 2003.

84. Herman J, Vandenberghe P, van den Heuvel I, et al: Successful treatment with rituximab of lymphoproliferative disorder in a child after cardiac transplantation. J Heart Lung Transplant 21:1304–1309, 2002.

85. Schacke H, Docke W, Asadullah K: Mechanisms involved in the side effects of glucocorticoids. Pharmacol Ther 96:23–43, 2002.

86. Hathout E: Growth after heart transplantation. Pediatr Transplant 8:97–100, 2004.

87. Braith R, Howard C, Fricker J, et al: Glucocorticoid-induced osteopenia in adolescent heart transplant recipients. J Heart Lung Transplant 19:840–845, 2000.

88. Keogh A: Calcineurin inhibitors in heart transplantation. J Heart Lung Transplant 23:s202–s206, 2004.

89. Chand D, Southerland S, Cunningham R III: Tacrolimus: the good, the bad, and the ugly. Pediatr Transplant 5:32–36, 2001.

90. Patel J, Kobashigawa J: Cardiac transplant experience with cyclosporine. Curr Opin Cardiol 19:162–165, 2004.

91. Dipchand A, Benson L, McCrindle B, et al: Mycophenolate mofetil in pediatric heart transplant recipients: a single-center experience. Pediatr Transplant 5:112–118, 2001.

92. Moran, A, Lipshultz S, Rifai N, et al: Non-invasive assessment of rejection in pediatric transplant patients: serologic and echocardiographic prediction of biopsy-proven myocardial rejection. J Heart Lung Transplant 19:756–764, 2000.

93. Talner N, McGovern J, Carboni M: Congestive heart failure. In Moller J, Hoffman J (eds): Pediatric Cardiovascular Medicine. Philadelphia: Churchill Livingstone, 2000, pp 823–826.

94. Wang J, Wu M, Chang C, et al: Balloon angioplasty for obstructed modified systemic-pulmonary artery shunts and pulmonary artery stenoses. J Am Coll Cardiol 37:948–950, 2001.

Chapter 67

Valvular Heart Disease

Mark S. McIntosh, MD, MPH and Nazeema Khan, MD

Key Points

Asymptomatic children with murmurs that are not clearly innocent require nonemergent consultation by a pediatric cardiologist who will guide further testing (i.e., echocardiography).

Symptomatic children with pathologic murmurs require management of acute symptoms and emergent consultation.

The need for endocarditis prophylaxis must be evaluated in all patients with suspected valvular heart disease.

The clinician should confirm that children with a history of rheumatic fever are on antibiotic prophylaxis.

Introduction and Background

Valvular cardiac lesions of congenital or acquired causes are classified as valvular stenosis or valvular regurgitation. Valvular stenosis is characterized by mild or moderate obstruction of blood flow. Complete obstruction is termed *atresia* and is usually part of a complex structural cardiac defect. Valvular regurgitation occurs when blood leaks across the pathologically affected valve from a high-pressure region to one of low pressure. Patients with valvular heart disease often present with major systemic symptom complexes, including congestive heart failure, chest pain, palpitations, syncope, and acute neurologic deficits. However, patients with endocarditis or rheumatic heart disease may present with a more obscure clinical syndrome not immediately recognized as being due to valvular heart disease.

Recognition and Approach

Up to 72% of children will have a murmur noted at some point during their childhood.[1] Most of these children have innocent or benign murmurs rather than murmurs caused by structural cardiac disease. A stepwise approach can be

used to assess, diagnose, and plan treatment for patients presenting to the emergency department with signs and symptoms that may be indicative of valvular heart disease. Following the history and physical examination, the severity of the patient's condition and the murmur's grade (Table 67–1) and characteristics will dictate the need for supplemental data obtained from an electrocardiogram (ECG) and chest radiograph. At this point, the clinician will have acquired sufficient information to decide if the patient's condition suggests structural heart disease or is more likely due to an innocent murmur. This conclusion will guide plans for treatment, consultation, and final disposition.

Innocent and Pathologic Murmurs

Distinguishing innocent murmurs from pathologic murmurs resulting from significant structural heart disease is important for children with murmurs newly diagnosed in the emergency department (Table 67–2).

A *prenatal history* suggestive of exposure to infections (e.g., maternal rubella in the first trimester), medications known to have teratogenic cardiac effects (e.g., anticonvulsants, amphetamines), or maternal conditions with higher incidence of congenital heart disease (e.g., diabetes, collagen vascular disease) may alert the clinician to consider a cardiac lesion. *Family histories* of congenital heart disease, rheumatic fever, sudden death, or inherited disease are important to identify. *Signs or symptoms* of reduced cardiac output and pulmonary edema suggest a pathologic origin of a heart murmur. Shortness of breath, failure to thrive, easy fatigability, syncope, neurologic deficits, and chest pain are alarming in the context of a newly identified murmur.[2] Furthermore, physical examination findings suggestive of valvular pathology include obvious syndromal or chromosomal abnormalities, tachypnea, tachycardia, hyperdynamic precordium, cyanosis, clubbing caused by hypoxia, abnormal pulses, and hepatomegaly. A thorough, step-by-step auscultation evaluating heart sounds and systolic and diastolic murmurs is critical for distinguishing the innocent from the pathologic murmur[3,4] (Table 67–3). Murmur location is an important determinant of the specific cardiac lesion present (Fig. 67–1).

The heart sounds in innocent murmurs are normal. Any abnormality of the first or second heart sound (S_1/S_2), including quality, abnormal splitting, or extra heart sound (click), is indicative of pathology. Innocent murmurs are typically grade I or II in intensity but rarely grade III. Innocent

Table 67–1	Grading of Murmurs

Grade	Characteristics
I	Very soft murmur only heard with careful auscultation
II	Soft murmur that is readily evident
III	Moderately intense murmur that is not associated with a palpable precordial thrill (vibration)
IV	Loud murmur with an associated precordial thrill
V	Loud murmur heard with a stethoscope partially placed on chest and a palpable precordial thrill
VI	Loud murmur that is audible when the stethoscope is lifted off of the chest and a palpable precordial thrill

Table 67–2	Key Risk Factors for Pathologic Murmurs[2,3]

Historical Facts

Prenatal
Maternal health history during pregnancy
Maternal exposure to infections, medications, illicit drug/tobacco/ alcohol use
Postnatal or Past/Immediate History
Delivery complications, birth weight
Inappropriate development
Reported history of murmur
Genetic or chromosomal disorders
Cyanosis
Change in feeding pattern/respiratory pattern
Exercise intolerance
Chest pain
Syncope
Palpitations
Neurologic deficits or congestive heart failure
Family History
Congenital heart disease
Rheumatic fever
Sudden death
Hereditary disease

Physical Examination Findings

General appearance (note dysmorphic facial features suggesting syndromal abnormalities)
Signs of malnutrition
Observation of cyanosis/pallor
Precordial activity (thrills)
Respiratory activity (rate/retractions)
Clubbing
Hepatomegaly
Abnormal blood pressure
Character of pulse: Narrow pulse pressure (aortic valve stenosis), wide pulse pressure (aortic regurgitation)
Auscultation: Heart rate and regularity, cardiac heart sounds, murmurs

Table 67–3	Characteristics of Pathologic Murmurs[3,4]

Symptomatic presentation, including exertional chest pain, syncope, shortness of breath
Abnormal pulses (diminished or bounding)
Pan-systolic murmur
Diastolic murmur
Systolic murmur that is grade III–VI, or midsystolic or holosystolic
Cyanosis
Abnormal heart sounds (e.g., early/midsystolic click)
Harsh, loud murmur ≥ grade III or thrill
Increase in murmur with standing
Abnormal chest radiograph
Abnormal electrocardiogram

present.[9] Therefore, an emergency department ECG and chest radiograph are warranted when the clinician continues to consider underlying cardiac pathology as the source of the murmur.

Echocardiography is the primary test used for the diagnosis of structural heart disease and is the modality of choice for evaluating heart murmurs of uncertain etiology. Cardiac pathology will not always be evident by clinical examination even to the pediatric cardiologist.[10] If there is any diagnostic uncertainty in the evaluation of an asymptomatic murmur, then prompt referral should be arranged for pediatric cardiology consultation or performance and interpretation of an echocardiogram by a laboratory with expertise in pediatric heart disease. Cost analysis studies suggest that most cases of innocent murmurs will be diagnosed without echocardiography by the pediatric cardiologist, resulting in an overall cost savings.[11,12] However, the higher sensitivity for pathology achieved with a strategy of echocardiography in all cases of suspected pathologic murmur warrants a low threshold for using this test, especially in patients with any concerning clinical features.[13]

Clinical Presentation (Table 67–5)

Obstructive Cardiac Lesions to Ventricular Outflow

Obstructive valvular lesions to ventricular outflow include aortic stenosis (AS) and pulmonary stenosis (PS). As the outflow tract pressure gradient across the stenotic valve increases and becomes hemodynamically significant, the respective ventricle undergoes severe concentric hypertrophy. Ultimately, progression of this process results in ventricular dilation and decreased stroke volume and cardiac output. The reduction in cardiac output results from a combination of obstruction and impaired function. These patients will present with a combination of compromised ventricular function and pulmonary venous or systemic vascular congestion.

Aortic Stenosis

AS accounts for 3% to 6% of all congenital heart defects. Up to 85% of these stenotic valves are bicuspid. The stenosis is valvular, supravalvular, or subvalvular, depending on its position in relation to the aortic valve. Infants with severe aortic stenosis generally present within the first few weeks to months of life. With critical AS, systemic blood flow

murmurs are characterized as systolic, or occasionally as continuous (venous hum), but never as isolated diastolic (Fig. 67–2). Patients with innocent murmurs should have a normal history and physical examination and be free of symptoms or signs suggestive of congenital or acquired heart disease[3,5,6] (Table 67–4).

Electrocardiograms and radiographs are insensitive and nonspecific and rarely enhance the diagnostic accuracy of the clinician who needs to distinguish between pathologic and innocent murmurs of asymptomatic children.[7,8] However there are classic ECGs and chest radiography findings that enhance the diagnostic accuracy when heart lesions are

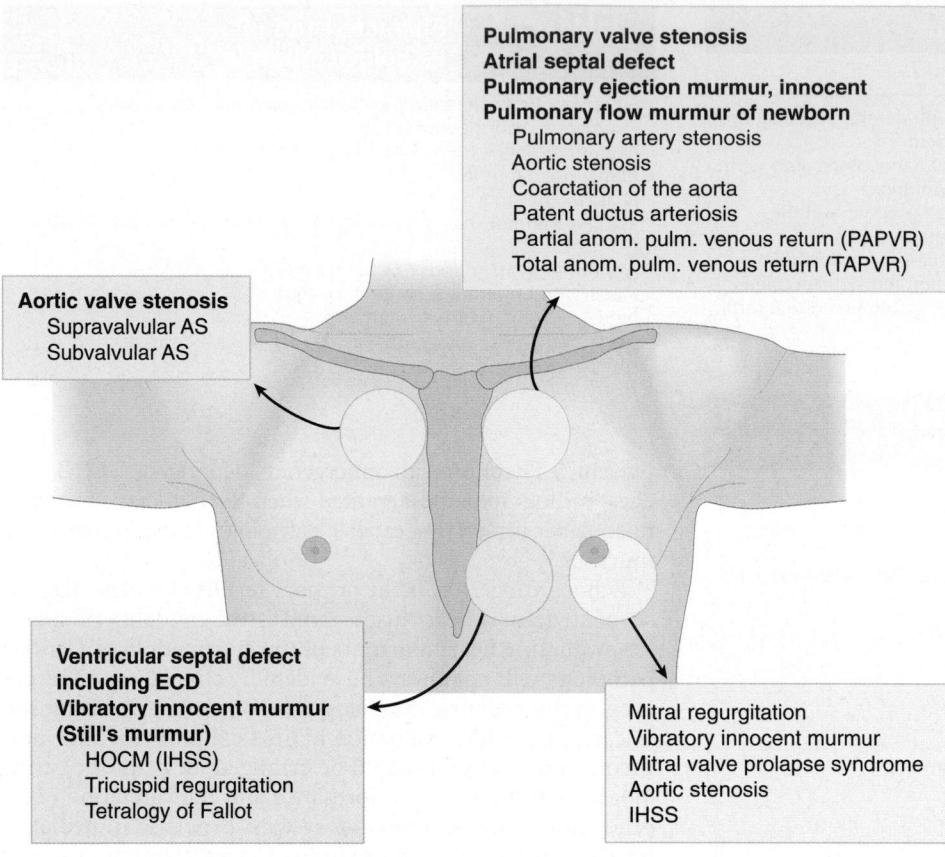

Pulmonary valve stenosis
Atrial septal defect
Pulmonary ejection murmur, innocent
Pulmonary flow murmur of newborn
    Pulmonary artery stenosis
    Aortic stenosis
    Coarctation of the aorta
    Patent ductus arteriosis
    Partial anom. pulm. venous return (PAPVR)
    Total anom. pulm. venous return (TAPVR)

Aortic valve stenosis
    Supravalvular AS
    Subvalvular AS

Ventricular septal defect
including ECD
Vibratory innocent murmur
(Still's murmur)
    HOCM (IHSS)
    Tricuspid regurgitation
    Tetralogy of Fallot

Mitral regurgitation
Vibratory innocent murmur
Mitral valve prolapse syndrome
Aortic stenosis
IHSS

FIGURE 67–1 Diagram showing systolic murmurs audible at various locations. Less common conditions are shown in smaller type. Abbreviations: AS, aortic stenosis; ECD, endocardial cushion defect; HOCM, hypertrophic obstructive cardiomyopathy; IHSS, idiopathic hypertrophic subaortic stenosis. (From Park M: Basic tools in routine evaluation of cardiac patients: physical examination. *In* Pediatric Cardiology for Practitioners, 4th ed. St. Louis: Mosby, 2002, pp 19–23.)

Table 67–4   Pediatric Innocent Heart Murmurs[3,5,6]

Innocent Heart Murmur	Description	Characteristics of Murmur	Child's Age at Diagnosis
Vibratory Still's murmur	Origin: pulmonary valves vibrate, resonance of flow across ventricular outflow tract and ascending aorta produces murmur	*Timing:* Systolic *Quality:* Vibratory, musical; low pitch *Location:* Left mid or lower sternal border	2–6 yr; can also hear as early as infancy and late as adolescence
Physiologic peripheral pulmonic stenosis murmur	Turbulent flow from main to branch pulmonary arteries Peripheral branch arteries are smaller and come off at sharp angles	*Timing:* Systolic *Quality:* Blowing, high pitch *Location:* Axillae, back, upper left sternal border	Birth–9 mo
Pulmonary flow murmur of newborn	Turbulent flow through relatively hypoplastic left and right pulmonary arteries at birth	*Timing:* Systolic *Quality:* Blowing, high pitch *Location:* Upper left sternal border, transmits to the left and right chest, axillae, and back	Neonates, especially low birth weight; disappears by 3–6 mo
Pulmonary flow murmur of childhood	Flow across pulmonary outflow tract	*Timing:* Systolic *Quality:* Blowing, high pitch *Location:* Upper left sternal border, transmits to chest, axillae, and back	8–14 yr
Supraclavicular murmur	Turbulent flow in the subclavian and carotid arteries	*Timing:* Systolic, very short and early *Quality:* Blowing, medium pitch *Location:* Over clavicle, neck and varies with extension of shoulders	Children, young adults
Venous hum	Turbulent flow from drainage of the internal jugular and subclavian veins into the intrathoracic veins	*Timing:* Continuous *Quality:* "hum" *Location:* Neck/clavicles; absent if supine, changes with rotation of neck	3–6 yr

Evaluation of Undiagnosed Cardiac Murmurs

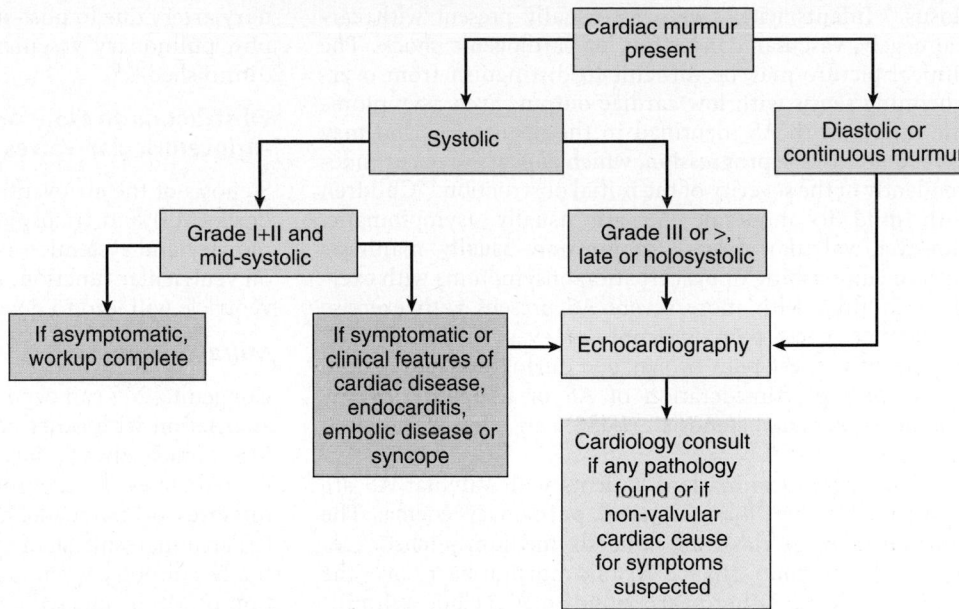

FIGURE 67–2 Evaluation of undiagnosed cardiac murmurs. (Adapted from Braunwald E, Perloff JK: Physical examination of the heart and circulation. *In* Zipes DP [ed]: Braunwald's Heart Disease: A Textbook of Cardiovascular Medicine, 7th ed. Philadelphia: Elsevier, 2005, p 103.)

Table 67–5   Pathologic Murmurs[17-19,21-23,26]

Valvular Lesion	Clinical Presentation	Physical Examination	Auscultation	ECG/CXR
Aortic stenosis	History of bicuspid valve *Infants:* CHF, shock *Older children:* Syncope, chest pain, sudden death, exercise intolerance	Acyanotic, pulmonary edema	Harsh, medium-pitched, crescendo-decrescendo systolic murmur; paradoxically split S_2, ejection click and S_4 gallop	*ECG:* Left ventricular hypertrophy *CXR:* Dilated ascending aorta, cardiomegaly
Pulmonary stenosis	*Infants:* Cyanosis, poor feeding, tachypnea, cardiac shock *Children:* Exertional dyspnea, exercise intolerance, chest pain, right-sided heart failure	Cyanosis, tachypnea, dependent edema, and organomegaly (spleen, liver)	Harsh crescendo-decrescendo ejection systolic murmur heard best at the upper left sternal border, radiates to back or left infraclavicular area; ejection click, split S_2	*ECG:* Right axis deviation, right ventricular hypertrophy *CXR:* cardiomegaly, prominence of the main and left pulmonary artery
Mitral stenosis	Dyspnea, rarely hemoptysis	Pulmonary edema	Low-pitched, rumbling, diastolic murmur over apex; opening snap	*ECG:* Left atrial enlargement, right ventricular hypertrophy *CXR:* Left atrial enlargement, prominent pulmonary vasculature, pulmonary congestion
Aortic regurgitation	Exercise intolerance, CHF, chest pain	Wide pulse pressure, bounding arterial pulses	Decrescendo mid-diastolic high-pitched murmur over the 3rd or 4th ICS; S_1 diminished	*ECG:* Left ventricular hypertrophy in severe AR; PVCs *CXR:* Cardiomegaly, dilation of ascending aorta, pulmonary congestion
Mitral regurgitation	History of rheumatic fever	*Acute MR:* acute pulmonary edema and evidence of right-sided heart failure *Chronic MR:* minimal symptoms	High-pitched, blowing, pan-systolic murmur at the apex and radiating to left axilla; widely split S_2	*ECG:* Left ventricular hypertrophy, left atrial enlargement *CXR:* Left ventricular hypertrophy, left atrial enlargement
Mitral valve prolapse	*Adolescents:* Palpitations, chest pain, syncope	Healthy appearing	Midsystolic click, late systolic murmur	*ECG:* Dysrhythmias—SVT, premature atrial or ventricular contractions

Abbreviations: AR, aortic regurgitation; CHF, congestive heart failure; CXR, chest radiography; ECG, electrocardiogram; ICS, intercostal space; MR, mitral regurgitation; PVCs, premature ventricular contractions; SVT, supraventricular tachycardia.

often depends on a left-to-right shunt across a patent foramen ovale and a right-to-left shunt across the patent ductus arteriosus.[14] Infants with severe AS usually present with cardiomegaly, vascular congestion, or cardiogenic shock. The clinical picture may be difficult to distinguish from overwhelming sepsis with low cardiac output. Even asymptomatic infants with AS identified in the neonatal period may have rapid disease progression, which appears to occur independently of the severity of the initial obstruction.[15] Children with mild to moderate AS are usually asymptomatic. However, valvular disease progression usually manifests with the unmasking or exacerbation of symptoms with exercise. Children with more severe AS present with exercise intolerance, chest pain, syncope, or even sudden death.[16] Importantly, chest pain or syncope during exertion should always prompt consideration of AS or idiopathic hypertrophic subaortic stenosis (IHSS) in the differential diagnosis.

On physical examination, patients with valvular AS are acyanotic but may have signs of pulmonary edema. The murmur of AS is classically a harsh, medium-pitched, crescendo-decrescendo–shaped systolic murmur heard over the aortic valve area. Other heart sounds may include a diminished, paradoxically split S_2, an ejection click, and an S_4 gallop. The ECG can be normal or may reveal left ventricular hypertrophy. Chest radiography occasionally may show cardiomegaly, but the only abnormal finding may be dilation of the ascending aorta. As the child grows and cardiac output increases, the pressure gradient across the valve increases. This natural progression of disease eventually leads to ventricular dysfunction and congestive heart failure.[17,18]

Supravalvular and subvalvular aortic stenosis are less prevalent. Patients with the idiopathic form of diffuse subaortic stenosis, also referred to as IHSS, will present with many symptoms similar to those with valvular aortic stenosis. Clinical and echocardiographic findings will distinguish these entities.

Pulmonary Stenosis

Lesions that cause PS also may be valvular, supravalvular, or subvalvular. Abnormalities of the pulmonary leaflets are the cause of valvular PS. Supravalvular PS is characterized by stenosis of the main pulmonary artery, while subvalvular PS involves the infundibulum and is often associated with tetralogy of Fallot. Infants with critical PS will depend on a patent ductus to provide pulmonary blood flow and an interatrial shunt to direct most of the systemic venous return. Clinically, during the postnatal period these infants will have varying degrees of cyanosis depending on the blood flow through the patent ductus and the interatrial shunt. They may have symptoms of poor feeding and tachypnea that can progress to cardiac shock as the ductus closes. Children with mild PS are generally asymptomatic, but as stenosis progresses, they may develop exertional dyspnea and increased exercise intolerance. Children with severe PS can have chest pain and heart failure. The harsh, medium-pitched, crescendo-decrescendo ejection-type systolic murmur of PS, best heard over the upper left sternal border, may be associated with an ejection click and split S_2. It radiates to the back or to the left infraclavicular area. The ECG may be normal in patients with mild PS, but with increased severity of stenosis, right axis deviation and right ventricular hypertrophy

develop. With progression of PS, chest radiography will reveal cardiomegaly and prominence of the main and left pulmonary artery due to post-stenotic dilation. On chest radiography, pulmonary vascular markings are normal or slightly diminished.[18,19]

Obstruction to Flow Across the Atrioventricular Valves

Stenosis of the atrioventricular valves, as seen in mitral stenosis (MS) and tricuspid stenosis (TS), causes passive pulmonary and systemic vascular congestion without an effect on ventricular function. However, impaired filling of the left ventricle will lead to decreased cardiac output.

Mitral Stenosis

Congenital MS can occur as an isolated valvular lesion or in association with other congenital cardiac defects. Acquired MS, almost always due to rheumatic fever, is rare in the United States. Thickening of the leaflets, fusion of the commissures, or "parachute mitral valve" obstructs flow from the left atrium, resulting in increases in atrial pressure and eventually pulmonary venous congestion. The clinical presentation of MS includes the signs and symptoms of pulmonary edema and pulmonary hypertension, which reflect the severity of stenosis. Congenital MS is usually severe, presenting in early infancy. On physical examination, patients have a low-pitched, rumbling, diastolic murmur appreciated over the apex. A diastolic opening snap may rarely be heard. The ECG demonstrates left atrial enlargement and right ventricular hypertrophy. Atrial fibrillation as a manifestation of left atrial dilation and hypertrophy is rare in children. The chest radiograph shows left atrial enlargement and prominent pulmonary vasculature and interstitial edema reflective of pulmonary congestion.[20-22]

Tricuspid Stenosis

Congenital tricuspid valve disease is usually due to valvular atresia or Ebstein's anomaly. Isolated congenital TS is rare. Tricuspid stenosis is almost always rheumatic in origin, and symptoms rarely present in childhood. Signs and symptoms of systemic venous obstruction due to TS include peripheral edema with passive congestion and enlargement of organs such as the liver and spleen.[23]

Regurgitant Flow Across the Cardiac Valves

Cardiac valves that allow retrograde or regurgitant flow across the valve result in volume overload and dilation of the cardiac chamber or great vessel on either side of the valve. Significant chronic regurgitation or acutely developing regurgitation manifests clinically as congestive heart failure. Commonly recognized valvular regurgitant lesions are mitral regurgitation (MR) and aortic regurgitation (AR). Hemodynamically significant pulmonary and tricuspid regurgitation are much rarer clinical entities. Patients with late-stage obstructive or regurgitant valvular dysfunction will present to the emergency department with shock or pulmonary edema.

Aortic Regurgitation

AR in childhood is most commonly associated with a bicuspid valve. Incomplete closure or prolapse of the bicuspid valve may lead to isolated regurgitation or a combination of stenosis and regurgitation.[24] AR is associated with many clinical entities, including dilation of the aortic root as seen in Marfan syndrome, destruction of the semilunar cusps due to endocarditis, ventricular septal defects, and rheumatic fever. Mild AR is generally asymptomatic, but disease progression can result in exercise intolerance and eventual congestive heart failure. Chest pain, multiple premature ventricular contractions, and congestive heart failure are ominous signs. However, these symptoms are usually not evident until well into adulthood. Acute AR, as seen in infectious endocarditis or trauma, presents with rapid onset of heart failure symptoms and even sudden cardiovascular collapse. The murmur of AR is a decrescendo, mid-diastolic, high-pitched murmur best heard at the third or fourth left intercostal space. S_1 is abnormally diminished. A wide pulse pressure and bounding arterial pulses are often present with severe chronic AR. In more severe AR, the ECG will show left ventricular hypertrophy. Chest radiographs may reveal left ventricular cardiomegaly, dilation of the ascending aorta, and pulmonary venous congestion.[21,23]

Mitral Regurgitation

Congenital MR is most frequently diagnosed in the context of other congenital heart defects. Isolated congenital MR is extremely rare. MR is the common manifestation of valvular dysfunction in children with rheumatic heart disease.[25] Other major causes of MR include infectious endocarditis, collagen vascular disorders, primary abnormalities of the valve, myocardial ischemia (e.g., anomalous left coronary artery, Kawasaki disease), and cardiomyopathy. Patients with chronic MR are relatively asymptomatic until adulthood, when progression of disease leads to decreased cardiac output and eventually heart failure. Patients with acute MR, as seen in infectious endocarditis, acute dysfunction of the papillary muscle, or chordae tendineae, present with symptoms of acute pulmonary edema and right-sided heart failure. A regurgitant, high-pitched, blowing pan-systolic murmur is appreciated at the apex and radiates to the left axilla. The S_2 is widely split because the aortic valves close early, with the decreased stroke volume ejected from the left ventricle. The ECG may show left ventricular and left atrial hypertrophy. The chest radiograph may reveal left ventricular hypertrophy and left atrial enlargement in chronic MR and pulmonary edema in acute MR.[21,23,26]

Mitral Valve Prolapse

Mitral valve prolapse (MVP) is the most common valvular problem seen in practice and is the most common cause of MR in the United States. It is more commonly seen in adolescents. Most cases of MVP are considered a normal variant whereby the posterior or anterior leaflet bulges into the left atrium. MVP is often recognized in children with congenital heart defects, Marfan syndrome, or other connective tissue disorders. Children are usually asymptomatic but may present with palpitations, chest pain, or rarely syncope. The natural history of uncomplicated MVP is not well understood, and cardiovascular complication of arrhythmias, progression of MR, overt congestive heart failure, chordae tendineae rupture, and even sudden death have been described.[16,27] On auscultation, patients with mitral regurgitation may have a midsystolic click followed by a late systolic murmur (click-murmur syndrome). ECG rarely may reveal

arrhythmias such as supraventricular tachycardias or premature atrial or ventricular contractions.[21]

Cardinal Systemic Manifestations of Valvular Heart Disease

Patients with valvular heart disease present with a constellation of systems determined by age and progression of valvular disease pathology. The cardinal symptoms of valvular heart disease include congestive heart failure, chest pain, palpitations, syncope, and neurologic deficits.

Congestive heart failure results from volume or pressure overload. Time of onset of congestive heart failure due to congenital heart disease can be reliably predicted. Severe pulmonary or tricuspid atresia will result in symptoms of volume overload at birth. Patients with critical AS or PS will likely become symptomatic during the first few weeks of life. However, complex congenital heart disease, episodes of supraventricular tachycardia, congenital heart block, hydrops fetalis, and bonchopulmonary dysplasia also cause congestive heart failure in the neonatal period and must be distinguished from isolated critical AS/PS. AR, MS, and MR leading to congestive heart failure will have highly variable presentations ranging from early childhood to late adulthood. The onset of acquired valvular heart disease will be less predictable and must be distinguished from other disease processes such as sepsis, viral myocarditis, infiltrative or hypertrophic cardiomyopathy, and recurrent bouts of "pneumonia."[28]

Children who present to the emergency department with *chest pain* rarely have serious valvular disease.[29] However, patients with severe valvular pathology (e.g., AS, IHSS) occasionally develop chest pain due to ventricular hypertrophy, increased wall stress, and resultant unmet oxygen demand. Similar to angina pectoris, patients may develop exertional chest pain that usually resolves with rest. Other conditions causing chest pain must be considered, including coronary artery anomalies, arrhythmias, cardiovascular disease, hypertrophic obstructive cardiomyopathy, cocaine abuse, pericarditis, and myocarditis[30] (see Chapter 62, Chest Pain).

Cardiac arrhythmias clinically perceived as *palpitations* are associated with all cardiac valvular lesions. Supraventricular rhythms (e.g., paroxysmal supraventricular tachycardia, atrial fibrillation, and atrial flutter) are frequently associated with MS and MR. In all patients presenting with palpitations, thorough evaluation for valvular causes is warranted. Specifically, MVP has been associated with atrial and ventricular premature contractions, paroxysmal supraventricular tachycardias, and ventricular tachyarrhythmias.[31]

Patients with severe obstructive cardiac lesions such as AS, PS, or IHSS may have *syncope* (see Chapter 61, Syncope). Clinically, these patients often present with exercise-induced syncope. The demand for cardiac output is not met, resulting in decreased cerebral perfusion and syncope. Furthermore, patients with valvular disease may experience syncope due to arrhythmias resulting from the underlying valve pathology.[32-35]

In the absence of signs and symptoms consistent with endocarditis, systemic embolization manifested as an acute *neurologic deficit* in a young patient warrants thorough investigation for left-sided valvular lesions or right-sided lesions associated with an interatrial communication[36] (see Chapter 44, Central Nervous System Vascular Disorders).

Important Clinical Features and Considerations

Endocarditis and Antibiotic Prophylaxis

Valvular heart disease causes significant pressure gradients and turbulent blood flow, which predispose to endothelial damage and thrombus formation. This environment of vascular damage and overlying thrombus formation produces a nidus for bacterial growth. Any focal infection (e.g., pyelonephritis, pneumonia, skin abscess) or procedures performed on patients can lead to bacteremia. This combination of factors produces the milieu for development of endocarditis. The onset of illness is usually insidious and is suspected when there are signs and symptoms of fever, chills, sweats, malaise, fatigue, and cardiac murmur. Endocarditis can be life-threatening. The emergency physician must be cognizant of the patient's underlying valve disease because special considerations need to be exercised to prevent development of infectious endocarditis. Recommended antibiotic prophylaxis regimens for endocarditis developed by the American Heart Association depend on the level of risk associated with the procedure and the cardiac lesions (see Chapter 64, Pericarditis, Myocarditis, and Endocarditis).[37,38]

Rheumatic Heart Disease

Acute rheumatic fever is a common cause of heart disease in underdeveloped countries, but is rarely seen in the United States except for occasional localized outbreaks.[39] Valvular lesions are believed to be caused by antibodies against the group A streptococcus that cross-react with antigen in various components of the heart. The revised Jones criteria are used to diagnose acute rheumatic fever (see Chapter 95, Musculoskeletal Disorders in Systemic Diseases). Carditis occurs in 50% of patients and invariably is associated with the murmurs of valvulitis (MR or AR).[40] Permanent damage to heart valves often results from the carditis, leading to chronic valvular disease affecting predominantly the aortic and mitral valves. Recurrent episodes of rheumatic fever increase the valvular pathology. Patients with a history of rheumatic fever must receive antibiotic prophylaxis.[41]

Management

The initial stabilization and management of the newborn with cardiac valvular disease is dictated by the underlying valvular pathology and severity of symptoms. The critically ill infant or child will require emergent medical treatment and coordination of management with the pediatric cardiac specialist (see Chapter 7, The Critically Ill Neonate; and Chapter 30, Congenital Heart Disease). Newborns with critical right-sided obstruction to pulmonary outflow, causing cyanosis, or left-sided obstruction to systemic outflow, causing shock, benefit temporarily from prostaglandin E_1 infusion, which reopens the ductus arteriosus. Vasodilators should be avoided in the treatment of ventricular failure due to AS, but their use should be considered in the treatment of MR to maintain the forward flow state. Symptoms of pulmonary venous congestion due to severe MS are treated with diuretics. The pediatric cardiologist will help coordinate further diagnostic procedures as indicated, including echocardiography (M-mode, two-dimensional, and Doppler studies) and catherization, the results of which will direct further management to include medical therapy, valvuloplasty, or surgery.

The asymptomatic child with potential cardiac valvular pathology requires referral to a pediatric cardiologist. The child with symptoms such as chest pain and syncope or symptoms suggestive of congestive heart failure will require an expedited evaluation. Indications and timing of interventions such as balloon valvuloplasty or surgery are based on the symptoms of the patient and evaluation of Doppler gradients across the affected valve, peak systolic pressure gradients, and calculated effective area of the valve orifice determined during echocardiography and catheterization.

Patients with valvular heart disease may experience complications resulting from their medical management. Drug interactions and potential toxicities of cardiac medications warrant consideration. Patients presenting to the emergency department with problems unrelated to their valvular disease may need endocarditis prophylaxis for conditions or procedures that may cause bacteremia (see Chapter 64, Pericarditis, Myocarditis, and Endocarditis). These patients may also be more susceptible to other illnesses such as gastrointestinal bleeding or pulmonary infections.[18,21,42]

Summary

One of the most important roles of the emergency physician in caring for pediatric patients with valvular heart disease is to first consider the diagnosis. A thorough history and physical examination with minimal testing will enable the physician to guide management and disposition. Patients with findings consistent with innocent murmurs can appropriately be followed by the primary physician. Asymptomatic patients who potentially have a pathologic murmur can usually be referred for outpatient evaluation by the pediatric cardiologist. Symptomatic patients will require acute management and disposition by the emergency physician augmented by a pediatric cardiologist. If an infant or child with known valvular heart disease presents to the emergency department, the clinician must consider whether symptoms are suggestive of complications of the valvular disease or if antibiotic prophylaxis is needed to prevent complications such as endocarditis.

REFERENCES

1. McLaren M, Lachman A, Pocock WA, Barlow JB: Innocent murmurs and third heard sounds in black school children. Br Heart J 43:67–73, 1980.
2. Park M: Basic tools in routine evaluation of cardiac patients: history taking. *In* Pediatric Cardiology for Practitioners, 4th ed. St. Louis: Mosby, 2002, pp 3–9.
3. Park M: Basic tools in routine evaluation of cardiac patients: physical examination. *In* Pediatric Cardiology for Practitioners, 4th ed. St. Louis: Mosby, 2002, pp 10–33.
4. McCrindle B, Shaffer K, Kan JS, et al: Cardinal clinical signs in the differentiation of heart murmurs in children. Arch Pediatr Adolesc Med 150:169–174, 1996.
5. Pelech A: The cardiac murmur: when to refer? Pediatr Clin North Am 45:107–122, 1998.
6. Braunwald E, Perloff JK: Physical examination of the heart and circulation. *In* Zipes DP (ed): Braunwald's Heart Disease: A Textbook of Cardiovascular Medicine, 7th ed. Philadelphia: Elsevier, 2005, pp 77–106.
7. Danford D: Decision analysis in pediatric cardiology outcomes research. Prog Pediatr Cardiol 7:67–75, 1997.

8. Birkebaek N, Hansen LK, Elle B, et al: Chest roentgenogram in the evaluation of heart defects in asymptomatic infants and children with a cardiac murmur: reproducibility and accuracy. Pediatrics 103:e15, 1999.

9. Danford D, Gumbiner C, Martin AB, et al: Effects of electrocardiography and chest radiograph on the accuracy of preliminary diagnosis of common congenital cardiac defects. Pediatr Cardiol 21:334–340, 2000.

10. Smythe J, Teixeira OH, Vlad P, et al: Initial evaluation of heart murmurs: are laboratory tests necessary? Pediatrics 86:497–500, 1990.

11. Danford D, Nasir A, Gumbiner C: Cost assessment of the evaluation of heart murmurs in childhood. Pediatrics 91:365–368, 1993.

12. Yi M, Kimball TR, Rsevat J, et al: Evaluation of heart murmurs in children: cost-effectiveness and practical implications. J Pediatr 141:504–511, 2002.

13. Danford D, Martin AB, Fletcher SE, Gumbiner CH: Echocardiographic yield in children when innocent murmur seems likely but doubts linger. Pediatr Cardiol 23:410–414, 2002.

14. Westmoreland D: Critical congenital cardiac defects in the newborn. J Perinat Neonatal Nurs 12(4):67–87, 1999.

15. Yetman A, Rosenberg H, Joubert G: Progression of asymptomatic aortic stenosis identified in the neonatal period. Am J Cardiol 75:636–637, 1995.

16. Basso C, Corrado D, Thiene G: Cardiovascular causes of sudden death in young individuals including athletes. Cardiol Rev 7:127–135, 1999.

17. Freed M: Aortic stenosis. In Allen H, Clark E, Gutgesell H, Driscoll D (eds): Moss and Adams' Heart Disease in Infants, Children and Adolescents, Including the Fetus and Young Adult, 6th ed. Philadelphia: Lippincott Williams & Williams, 2001, pp 970–987.

18. Park M: Obstructive lesions. In Pediatric Cardiology for Practitioners, 4th ed. St. Louis: Mosby, 2002, pp 155–165.

19. Latson L, Priesto L: Pulmonary stenosis. In Allen H, Clark E, Gutgesell H, Driscoll D (eds): Moss and Adams' Heart Disease in Infants, Children and Adolescents, Including the Fetus and Young Adult, 6th ed. Philadelphia: Lippincott Williams & Williams, 2001, pp 820–844, 2002.

20. Okubo S, Nagata S, Masuda Y, et al: Clinical features of rheumatic heart disease in Bangladesh. Jpn Circ J 48:1345–1349, 1984.

21. Park M: Valvular heart disease. In Pediatric Cardiology for Practitioners, 4th ed. St. Louis: Mosby, 2002, pp 311–320.

22. Baylen B: Mitral inflow obstruction. In Allen H, Clark E, Gutgesell H, Driscoll D (eds): Moss and Adams' Heart Disease in Infants, Children and Adolescents, Including the Fetus and Young Adult, 6th ed. Philadelphia: Lippincott Williams & Williams, 2001, pp 924–937.

23. Bonow RO, Braunwald E: Valvular heart disease. In Zipes ZD (ed): Braunwald's Heart Disease: A Textbook of Cardiovascular Medicine, 7th ed. Philadelphia: Elsevier, 2005, pp 1553–1615.

24. Roberts W, Morrow A, McIntosh C, et al: Congenitally bicuspid aortic valve causing severe, pure aortic regurgitation without superimposed infective endocarditis. Am J Cardiol 47:206–209, 1981.

25. Marcus R, Sareli P, Pocock WA, Barlow JB: The spectrum of severe rheumatic mitral valve disease in a developing country: correlations among clinical presentation, surgical pathologic findings, and hemodynamic sequelae. Ann Intern Med 120:177–183, 1994.

26. Boudoulasa H, Wooley C: The floppy mitral valve, mitral valve prolapse and mitral valvular regurgitation. In Allen H, Clark E, Gutgesell H, Driscoll D (eds): Moss and Adams' Heart Disease in Infants, Children and Adolescents, Including the Fetus and Young Adult, 6th ed. Philadelphia: Lippincott Williams & Wilkins, 2001, pp 947–969.

27. Kamei F, Nakaharan N, Yuda S, et al: Long-term site-related differences in the progression and regression of the idiopathic mitral valve prolapse syndrome. Cardiology 91:161–168, 1999.

28. Park M: Congestive heart failure. In Pediatric Cardiology for Practitioners, 4th ed. St. Louis: Mosby, 2002, pp 399–401.

29. Selbst S, Rudy R, Clark B: Chest pain in children: follow-up of patients previously reported. Clin Pediatr (Phila) 29:374–377, 1990.

30. Park M: Child with chest pain. In Pediatric Cardiology for Practitioners, 4th ed. St. Louis: Mosby, 2002, pp 441–448.

31. Boudoulas H, Kolibash A Jr, Baker P, et al: Mitral valve prolapse and the mitral valve prolapse syndrome: a diagnostic classification and pathogenesis of symptoms. Am Heart J 118:796–818, 1989.

32. Park M: Syncope. In Pediatric Cardiology for Practitioners, 4th ed. St. Louis: Mosby, 2002, pp 449–459.

33. Benditt D, Lurie K, Fabian W: Clinical approach to diagnosis of syncope: an overview. Cardiol Clin 15:165–176, 1997.

34. Linzer M, Yang E, Estes N III, et al: Diagnosing syncope, Part 1. Value of history, physical examination, and electrocardiography. Clinical Efficacy Assessment Project of the American College of Physicians. Ann Intern Med 126:989–996, 1997.

35. Linzer M, Yang E, Estes N III, et al: Diagnosing syncope, Part 2. Unexplained syncope. Clinical Efficacy Assessment Project of the American College of Physicians. Ann Intern Med 127:76–86, 1997.

36. Cerrato P, Grasso M, Imperiale D, et al: Stroke in young patients: etiopathogenesis and risk factors in different age classes. Cerebrovasc Dis 18:154–159, 2004.

37. Karchmer AW: Infectious endocarditis. In Zipes DP (ed): Braunwald's Heart Disease: A Textbook of Cardiovascular Medicine, 7th ed. Philadelphia: Elsevier, 2005, pp 1633–1658.

*38. Dajani AS, Taubert KA, Wilson W, et al: Prevention of bacterial endocarditis: recommendations by the American Heart Association. JAMA 277:1794–1801, 1997.

39. Centers for Disease Control: Acute rheumatic fever—Utah. MMWR Morb Mortal Wkly Rep 36:108–110, 115, 1987.

40. Stollerman GH: Rheumatic fever. Lancet 349:935–942, 1997.

41. Park M: Acute rheumatic fever. In Pediatric Cardiology for Practitioners, 4th ed. St. Louis: Mosby, 2002, pp 304–310.

*42. Bonow R, Carabello B, de Leon A Jr, et al: ACC/AHA guidelines for the management of patients with valvular heart disease: executive summary. A report of the American College of Cardiology/American Heart Association Task Force on Practice Guidelines. Circulation 98:1949–1984, 1998.

---

*Selected readings.

Chapter 68

Bacteremia

Elizabeth R. Alpern, MD, MSCE

Introduction and Background

Occult bacteremia is the presence of pathogenic bacteria in the blood of a well-appearing febrile child who lacks a focal bacterial source of infection. Occult bacteremia carries a risk of progressing to focal infection, meningitis, or sepsis; therefore, a patient's risk, methods for early identification, and treatment options for this entity have been widely studied. The population at risk has been identified as those children 2 to 24 months of age (some studies included children up to 36 months of age) with fever. It is an important concept for the emergency physician to differentiate children at risk for occult bacteremia from those children at risk for "nonoccult" bacteremia. Certainly young children with signs or symptoms of invasive disease, underlying immunodeficiencies, or evidence of systemic infection stemming from focal bacterial infections have an important and known risk of bacteremia. This bacteremia is not *occult* and therefore is a different entity from that described in this chapter.

Recognition and Approach

As with every clinical entity, identification of the at-risk population is the first step to diagnosis and treatment. Occult

bacteremia, by definition, affects healthy, well-appearing children from 2 to 24 or 36 months of age.[1-8] This chapter is thus limited to those healthy children considered immunocompetent hosts. In most cases, the patient's medical history will establish this prerequisite condition, which is vitally important to ascertain. The patient should not have a known underlying oncologic process, acquired or inborn immunodeficiency, sickle cell anemia, congenital heart disease, or indwelling medical device. Children who fall into those categories are certainly at risk for bacteremia; however, this is not the population that comprises those at risk for occult bacteremia. In addition, immunization status and concurrent antibiotic use may influence the risk of occult bacteremia (as discussed later in detail), and therefore should be identified. Although fever is typically recognized as a temperature above 38.5° C, for purposes of population definition, most studies use 39° C as a cutoff for fever in children at risk for occult bacteremia.[2-5,7,8]

Another prerequisite condition for considering the diagnosis of occult bacteremia is a well-appearing child without evidence of focal bacterial infection (other than otitis media) that may predispose to bacteremia, such as pneumonia or urinary tract infections (see Chapter 33, Urinary Tract Infection in Infants; Chapter 58, Pneumonia/Pneumonitis; and Chapter 86, Urinary Tract Infections in Children and Adolescents). Some researchers believe that, if a child appears ill enough to warrant assessment with a lumbar puncture based on physical examination at initial evaluation, then he or she should not be included in the at-risk population for occult bacteremia, though he or she may certainly be at risk for nonoccult bacteremia.[3]

Historically, the most common etiologic organisms for occult bacteremia were *Streptococcus pneumoniae* and *Haemophilus influenzae* type b.[2,4,6,7] Other common causative organisms included Salmonella species, *H. influenzae* nontype b, group A streptococci, Enterococcus species, and *Neisseria meningitidis*.[3,5] Recent innovations in childhood immunizations have had the opportunity to dramatically change the prevalence and causative organisms of occult bacteremia. The *H. influenzae* type b (Hib) vaccine was introduced in 1987. Since that time, in the population at large, there has been a 94% decrease in the incidence of Hib meningitis and a shift in the median age of Hib meningitis from 15 months to 25 years of age.[9,10] Prior to the licensure of the Hib vaccine, studies reported the prevalence of occult bacteremia to be between 3% and 11%.[2,4,6,11,12] However, since the widespread use of the Hib vaccine, two studies have reported the overall rate of occult bacteremia to be between 1.6% and 1.9%.[3,5] The conjugate pneumococcal vaccine was licensed in 2000, with subsequent impressive declines in invasive pneumococcal disease.[13-16] There are 90 pneumococcal serotypes, and the current conjugate pneumoccocal vaccine licensed in the United States is a heptavalent vaccine. The seven serotypes covered by the current vaccine, however, accounted for 98% of cases of occult pneumococcal bacteremia in a recent study.[17] The results of a single study since the introduction of the conjugate pneumoccocal vaccine indicate that the overall prevalence of the disease has decreased to less than 1% of children at risk.[8]

Occult bacteremia is of concern to the clinician due to the risk of possible progression from bacteremia to sepsis or death via hematogenously spread focal infection. This risk of invasive disease associated with occult bacteremia is dependent on the causative organism of the bacteremia. Prior to the Hib vaccine era, the risk of invasive disease associated with identified *H. influenzae* type b bacteremia was 25% to 44%.[2,18] However, occult pneumococcal bacteremia is associated with a significantly decreased risk of invasive disease, estimated at less than 1%.[2,18] Subsequent to the use of Hib vaccine, but prior to the introduction of the conjugate pneumococcal vaccine, the risk of meningitis or death in children considered to be at risk for occult bacteremia was approximately 0.03%.[3]

Clinical Presentation

The diagnosis of occult bacteremia is dependent upon a complete history, including immunization status, and a thorough physical examination. There are several findings on the physical examination of the at-risk child that influence the probability that the patient has occult bacteremia. The incidence of occult bacteremia remains constant between 6 and 24 months of age.[3,5,19] There is a lower incidence from 3 to 6 months of age hypothesized to be due to presence of maternal antibody after birth. However, selection bias in the studies performed (i.e., younger children may have undergone more invasive evaluations, and focal infections were identified at a higher rate) may have influenced results. The risk of occult bacteremia increases with increasing temperature and is more than two times the risk once temperature rises above 40° C.[3,19] However, a patient's response to antipyretics does not reflect the risk of underlying occult bacteremia; a patient whose appearance improves after antipyretics does not have a lowered risk of bacteremia.[20-22]

The risk of occult bacteremia with certain concomitant diseases has also been studied. Children with identified otitis media have the same overall risk of occult bacteremia as those without ear infections.[3,18] Children presenting with simple febrile seizures without focal identifiable infections also have rates of occult bacteremia comparable to those of all children at risk.[23] Children with particular viral illnesses, such as bronchiolitis, croup, and stomatitis, however, have a lower risk of occult bacteremia associated with those febrile illnesses.[7,24,25]

The final diagnosis of occult bacteremia is contingent upon a positive blood culture. However, an inherent limitation of this test is the delay until growth of the organism indicating a positive culture. In a continuously monitored carbon dioxide detection pediatric blood culture system, approximately 94% of pathogenic cultures became positive within 18 hours.[3,26] The majority of contaminated cultures are not positive until after that time point. As the rate of occult bacteremia declines due to improved immunization practices, the rate of truly positive pathogenic cultures approximates that of contaminated cultures.[3,8]

Many laboratory studies have been evaluated as screening tools for the identification of occult bacteremia. However, due to the overall low rate of occult bacteremia, their usefulness for the emergency medicine physician is limited by their positive predictive value. The complete blood count is the most widely studied laboratory screening test for occult bacteremia.[2,5,6,8,12,19,27] If a white blood cell count of 15,000/mm^3 or greater is used for a "positive" screen for occult bacteremia, the current positive predictive value of that test is between 3% and 5%.[5,8] In other words, approximately 3% of children with white blood cell counts ≥ 15,000/mm^3 will have occult bacteremia. An absolute neutrophil count of ≥ 10,000/mm^3 has predicted approximately 8% of patients with occult bacteremia.[19] Therefore, although an increased white blood cell count or neutrophil count is associated with an increased risk of occult bacteremia, the vast majority of patients with a "positive" screen will not have occult bacteremia. The emergency physician must balance the risk of not identifying a small percentage of cases of occult bacteremia with the ubiquitous use of screening tests that add time and invasive testing to the emergency department (ED) visit of a young child.

C-reactive protein has also been studied as a screen for serious bacterial infections, including pneumonia, urinary tract infections, and occult bacteremia.[28,29] The positive predictive value of C-reactive protein, depending on the cutoff for positivity, is between 30% and 65% for identification of all patients at risk for "serious bacterial infections."[29,30] However, when applied solely to patients with occult bacteremia, approximately 3% of at-risk children with a C-reactive protein level ≥ 4.4 have occult bacteremia. Thus the same considerations apply to the use of C-reactive protein as a screening tool for occult bacteremia.

The risk of occult urinary tract infection far outweighs the risk of occult bacteremia in some at-risk children, especially febrile well-appearing boys under 6 months of age and uncircumcised boys or any girls prior to toilet training. Therefore, assessment for occult urinary tract infections is extremely important (see Chapter 33, Urinary Tract Infection in Infants; and Chapter 86, Urinary Tract Infections in Children and Adolescents).

Important Clinical Features and Considerations

There are several important misconceptions or problem areas regarding the evaluation and treatment of occult bacteremia. Emergency physicians must be aware of these issues so the correct strategy is applied to febrile children who are at risk for both occult and nonoccult bacteremia (Table 68–1).

The evaluation and treatment of young, febrile, well-appearing children at risk for occult bacteremia has long been a topic of controversy in pediatrics and emergency medicine. In response to one of the many studies of occult

| Table 68–1 | Misconceptions or Problem Areas Regarding the Evaluation and Treatment of Occult Bacteremia in Children |

Misconception/Problem Area	Clarification/Appropriate Action
Applying the approach to the wrong population (i.e., those who are not at risk for occult bacteremia)	Identify host factors and exclude those children with oncologic process, immune disorders, sickle cell disease, congenital heart disease, or indwelling medical device.
Performing a lumbar puncture on an ill-appearing child and, if normal, considering the child to be at risk for occult bacteremia	If a child appears ill enough to warrant a lumbar puncture, then he or she should not be included in the at-risk population for occult bacteremia; however, he or she may still be at risk for nonoccult bacteremia.
Believing that screening tests will be able to identify patients at greater risk of occult bacteremia	Due to the overall low prevalence of occult bacteremia, screening tests have been shown to have a very low positive predictive value in these patients.
Failure to appreciate the risk or prevalence of occult urinary tract infection	The risk of occult urinary tract infection far outweighs the risk of occult bacteremia in selected populations; therefore, screening for urinary tract infection in young febrile children is extremely important.
Failure to arrange close outpatient follow-up	Follow-up care is imperative for any child with persistent fever or other symptoms regardless of emergency department evaluation as focal bacterial sources may become evident at a later date.
Failure to understand the laboratory methods used to identify positive blood cultures and their impact on the interpretation of the culture result	In a continuously monitored system, the vast majority of pathogenic blood cultures will turn positive within 18 hr; the vast majority of contaminants will turn positive after that time point.

infections in young children, an insightful editorial summarized this controversy as follows.[30] Physicians typically approach the workup and treatment of the young child at risk for occult bacteremia in one of two basic ways: as a "risk-minimizer" or a "test-minimizer."[30] If the physician leans more toward minimizing any possible risk of adverse outcome, then a "structured, methodical, laboratory intensive" strategy, including obtaining a blood culture, is often used to identify and treat all patients at risk for occult bacteremia (risk minimizer).[30] Alternatively, if the physician leans toward "careful clinical examination, close follow-up, and avoiding invasive testing" (test minimizer), then he or she likely believes that the risk of adverse outcome is so low as to not justify broad-spectrum antibiotics in all possible patients at risk.[30] Physicians in this group are likely to avoid ordering blood cultures on patients at risk for occult bacteremia. Recognition of where one stands on this continuum at different points in one's career as a physician is as important as understanding the studies of possible evaluation and treatment strategies of children at risk for occult bacteremia.

Management

Due to the difficult nature of the process of diagnosing occult bacteremia without some delay in test results, expectant antibiotic use has been advocated by some to decrease the risk of adverse outcomes such as meningitis or sepsis. However, as the risk of occult bacteremia and subsequent adverse sequelae have changed due to immunization innovations, with resultant changes is causative organisms, many advocate treating only patients identified to have documented bacteremia, not all those at risk. There are also risks associated with expectant antibiotic therapy, including adverse and allergic reactions and increasing the prevalence of drug-resistant organisms.

Several large studies have evaluating the benefits of expectant antibiotics. In the pre-Hib vaccine era, three studies evaluated antibiotic treatment of patients at risk for occult bacteremia.[2,4,12] In a trial of amoxicillin versus placebo, there

was no statistical difference between the antibiotic group and the placebo group in the incidence of major infectious morbidity.[4] In a study of amoxicillin/clavulanate versus ceftriaxone, there was no difference in serious adverse outcomes in patients treated with either drug.[12] The third study examined the difference in risk of focal infections of patients treated with ceftriaxone versus amoxicillin.[2] Ceftriaxone was noted to decrease the risk of "definite" focal infections but was not effective in decreasing the risk of acquiring a "definite or probable" focal infection.[2,31] In this particular study, *H. influenzae* and Salmonella species were the only causes of subsequent meningitis in patients with occult bacteremia. Several meta-analyses have also evaluated expectant antibiotic treatment of patients at risk for occult bacteremia.[32-34] These studies concluded that expectant antibiotics do not prevent serious bacterial infections in all children at risk for occult bacteremia, especially in light of the extremely low risk of meningitis or death associated with pneumococcal bacteremia.[32-34]

A review of the risk of serious bacterial illness associated with occult bacteremia when antibiotics are reserved for only culture-proven bacteremia showed that the risk of adverse outcome associated with reserved treatment was exactly the same as the risk associated with treatment with expectant antibiotics published in prior literature.[35] In addition, a cost-effectiveness analysis indicated that, as the rates of occult bacteremia and meningitis decline with epidemiologic changes, empirical testing with complete blood counts and use of expectant antibiotic will become significantly less cost effective.[36] Whichever treatment plan is instituted for an individual patient, follow-up within 24 to 36 hours with the child's primary care provider or alternative site of care is imperative for any child with persistent fever or other symptoms as focal bacterial infections may become evident after the ED visit.

The emergency physician is likely to see children return or referred to the ED for evaluation and treatment following a "positive" blood culture obtained at a prior visit to the ED or primary care provider. If the blood culture becomes

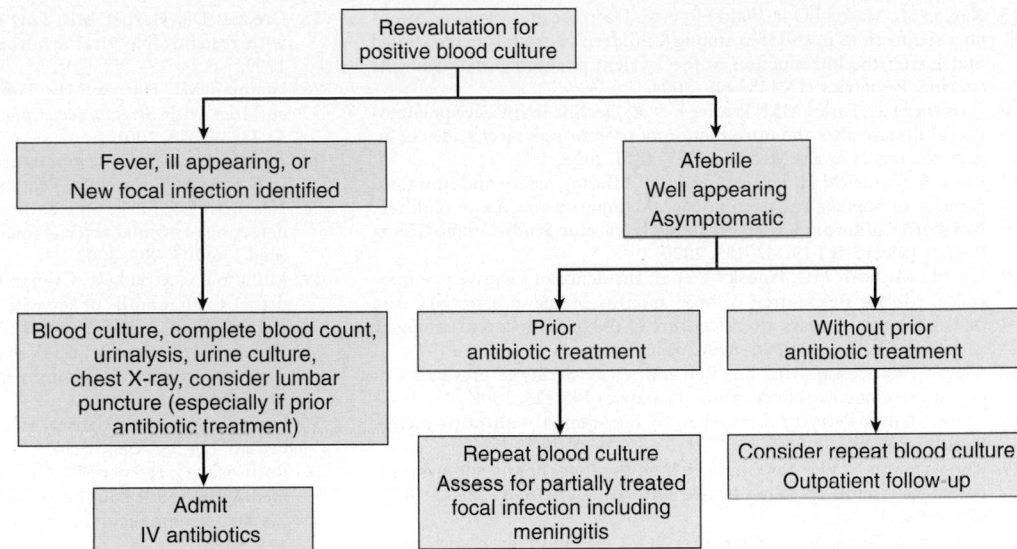

FIGURE 68–1. Reevaluation for positive blood culture.

positive within 18 to 24 hours utilizing a continuously monitored carbon dioxide detection system, the risk that this represents a true pathogenic culture is high.[3,26] Cultures that become positive after this time period are most probably contaminants; however, they still have a small risk of representing more uncommon pathogens. Although *S. pneumoniae* is currently the most common causative organism of occult bacteremia and has a very high spontaneous resolution rate, there is still a risk of seeding deep infection. Therefore, a systematic approach to the patient who returns or is "recalled" due to a positive blood culture is recommended.[37]

Patients with a positive blood culture and resolution of fever and lack of signs or symptoms of focal infection on reevaluation can be safely treated as outpatients after a repeat blood culture is obtained (Fig. 68–1). However, patients with positive cultures who are persistently febrile and/or ill appearing need a full evaluation to assess for new focal infections, including meningitis. If no prior antibiotics have been prescribed, physical examination by an experienced practitioner may reliably indicate the presence or absence of a focal infection. Complete blood count, urinalysis and culture, chest radiograph, and lumbar puncture should all be considered in the ill-appearing febrile child with known occult bacteremia. Admission and broad-spectrum intravenous antibiotic treatment are indicated.

Summary

Occult bacteremia is an entity that affects well-appearing febrile children without an identifiable focus of infection. The prevalence of and risks associated with occult bacteremia have changed significantly over the past decades as immunizations have targeted the most common etiologic organisms. Although there is a risk of serious bacterial illness associated with occult bacteremia, now that *S. pneumoniae* is the most common cause, this risk has greatly decreased. The impact of the pneumococcal conjugate vaccine is yet to be fully determined. Due to the decreasing prevalence of the disease, evaluation of children at risk for occult bacteremia with complete blood counts and treatment with

expectant antibiotics now has limited impact. Outpatient follow-up for all persistently febrile children is also a crucial step in the management of patients at risk for occult bacteremia.

REFERENCES

*1. American College of Emergency Physicians Clinical Policies Subcommittee on Pediatric Fever: Clinical policy for children younger than three years presenting to the emergency department with fever. Ann Emerg Med 42:530–545, 2003.
2. Fleisher GR, Rosenberg N, Vinci R, et al: Intramuscular versus oral antibiotic therapy for the prevention of meningitis and other bacterial sequelae in young, febrile children at risk for occult bacteremia. J Pediatr 124:504–512, 1994.
*3. Alpern ER, Alessandrini EA, Bell LM, et al: Occult bacteremia from a pediatric emergency department: current prevalence, time to detection, and outcome. Pediatrics 106:505–511, 2000.
4. Jaffe D, Tanz R, Davis T, et al: Antibiotic administration to treat possible occult bacteremia in febrile children. N Engl J Med 317:1175–1180, 1987.
5. Lee GM, Harper MB: Risk of bacteremia for febrile young children in the post-*Haemophilus influenzae* type B era. Arch Pediatr Adolesc Med 152:624–628, 1998.
6. McGowan J, Bratton L, Klein J, Finland M: Bacteremia in febrile children seen in a "walk-in" pediatric clinic. N Engl J Med 288:1309–1312, 1973.
7. Kuppermann N, Bank DE, Walton EA, et al: Risks for bacteremia and urinary tract infections in young febrile children with bronchiolitis. Arch Pediatr Adolesc Med 151:1207–1214, 1997.
*8. Stoll ML, Rubin LG: Incidence of occult bacteremia among highly febrile young children in the era of the pneumococcal conjugate vaccine. Arch Pediatr Adolesc Med 158:671–675, 2004.
9. Centers for Disease Control and Prevention: Progress toward elimination of *Haemophilus influenzae* type B disease among infants and children—United States, 1987–1995. MMWR Morb Mortal Wkly Rep 45:901–906, 1996.
10. Schuchat A, Robinson K, Wenger J, et al: Bacterial meningitis in the United States in 1995. N Engl J Med 337:970–976, 1997.
11. Teele DW, Pelton SI, Grant MJ, et al: Bacteremia in febrile children under 2 years of age: results of cultures of blood of 600 consecutive febrile children seen in a "walk-in" clinic. J Pediatr 87:227–230, 1975.
12. Bass J, Steele R, Wittler R, et al: Antimicrobial treatment of occult bacteremia: A multicenter cooperative study. Pediatr Infect Dis J 12:466–473, 1993.

---

*Selected readings.

13. Kaplan SL, Mason EO Jr, Wald ER, et al: Decrease of invasive pneumococcal infections in children among 8 children's hospitals in the United States after the introduction of the 7-valent pneumococcal conjugate vaccine. Pediatrics 113:443–449, 2004.

*14. Whitney CG, Farley MM, Hadler J, et al: Decline in invasive pneumococcal disease after the introduction of protein-polysaccharide conjugate vaccine. N Engl J Med 348:1737–1746, 2003.

15. Black S, Shinefield H, Fireman B, et al: Efficacy, safety and immunogenicity of heptavalent pneumococcal conjugate vaccine in children. Northern California Kaiser Permanente Vaccine Study Center Group. Pediatr Infect Dis J 19:187–195, 2000.

16. Lin PL, Michaels MG, Janosky J, et al: Incidence of invasive pneumococcal disease in children 3 to 36 months of age at a tertiary care pediatric center 2 years after licensure of the pneumococcal conjugate vaccine. Pediatrics 111:896–899, 2003.

17. Alpern ER, Alessandrini EA, Bell LM, et al: Serotype prevalence of occult pneumococcal bacteremia. Pediatrics 108:e23, 2001.

18. Schutzman S, Petrycki S, Fleisher G: Bacteremia with otitis media. Pediatrics 87:48–53, 1991.

19. Kuppermann N, Fleisher GR, Jaffe DM: Predictors of occult pneumococcal bacteremia in young febrile children. Ann Emerg Med 31:679–687, 1998.

20. Baker MD, Fosarelli PD, Carpenter RO: Childhood fever: correlation of diagnosis with temperature response to acetaminophen. Pediatrics 80:315–318, 1987.

21. Bonadio WA, Bellomo T, Brady W, Smith D: Correlating changes in body temperature with infectious outcome in febrile children who receive acetaminophen. Clin Pediatr (Phila) 32:343–346, 1993.

22. Torrey SB, Henretig F, Fleisher G, et al: Temperature response to antipyretic therapy in children: relationship to occult bacteremia. Am J Emerg Med 3:190–192, 1985.

23. Shah SS, Alpern ER, Zwerling L, et al: Low risk of bacteremia in children with febrile seizures. Arch Pediatr Adolesc Med 156:469–472, 2002.

*24. Levine D, Platt S, Dayan P, et al; Multicenter RSV-SBI Study Group for the Pediatric Emergency Medicine Collaborative Research Committee of the American Academy of Pediatrics: The risk of serious bacterial infection in young febrile infants with respiratory syncytial virus infections. Pediatrics 113:1728–1734, 2004.

25. Greenes DS, Harper MB: Low risk of bacteremia in febrile children with recognizable viral syndromes. Pediatr Infect Dis J 18:258–261, 1999.

26. Neuman MI, Harper MB: Time to positivity of blood cultures for children with *Streptococcus pneumoniae* bacteremia. Clin Infect Dis 33:1324–1328, 2001.

27. Jaffe D, Fleisher G: Temperature and total white blood cell count as indicators of bacteremia. Pediatrics 87:670–674, 1991.

28. Isaacman DJ, Burke BL: Utility of the serum C-reactive protein for detection of occult bacterial infection in children. Arch Pediatr Adolesc Med 156:905–909, 2002.

29. Pulliam PN, Attia MW, Cronan KM: C-reactive protein in febrile children 1 to 36 months of age with clinically undetectable serious bacterial infection. Pediatrics 108:1275–1279, 2001.

*30. Green SM, Rothrock SG: Evaluation styles for well-appearing febrile children: are you a "risk minimizer" or a "test minimizer"? Ann Emerg Med 33:211–214, 1999.

31. Long SS: Antibiotic therapy in febrile children: "best-laid schemes." J Pediatr 124:585–588, 1994.

32. Rothrock SG, Harper MB, Green SM, et al: Do oral antibiotics prevent meningitis and serious bacterial infections in children with *Streptococcus pneumoniae* occult bacteremia? A meta-analysis. Pediatrics 99:438–444, 1997.

33. Bulloch B, Craig WR, Klassen TP: The use of antibiotics to prevent serious sequelae in children at risk for occult bacteremia: a meta-analysis. Acad Emerg Med 4:679–683, 1997.

34. Rothrock SG, Green SM, Harper MB, et al: Parenteral vs oral antibiotics in the prevention of serious bacterial infections in children with *Streptococcus pneumoniae* occult bacteremia: a meta-analysis. Acad Emerg Med 5:599–606, 1998.

35. Bandyopadhyay S, Bergholte J, Blackwell CD: Risk of serious bacterial infection in children with fever without a source in the post-*Haemophilus influenzae* era when antibiotics are reserved for culture-proven bacteremia. Arch Pediatr Adolesc Med 156:512–517, 2002.

36. Lee GM, Fleisher GR, Harper MB: Management of febrile children in the age of the conjugate pneumococcal vaccine: a cost-effectiveness analysis. Pediatrics 108:835–844, 2001.

37. Bachur R, Harper MB: Reevaluation of outpatients with *Streptococcus pneumoniae* bacteremia. Pediatrics 105:502–509, 2000.

Human Immunodeficiency Virus Infection and Other Immunosuppressive Conditions

Marina Catallozzi, MD

Key Points

Human immunodeficiency virus infection and acquired immunodeficiency syndrome have different manifestations in children and adults.

Early anticipation and aggressive management of overwhelming postsplenectomy infection are vital to outcome.

Patients with asplenia of any etiology should be considered at high risk for invasive and life-threatening bacterial and parasitic infection and should be managed aggressively.

Neutropenic patients can present with severe infections without localizing signs or symptoms.

Since it is not possible to determine which immunocompromised patients are or are not infected on presentation to the emergency department, empirical antibiotics should be given to all such patients.

Selected Diagnoses

Human immunodeficiency virus and acquired immunodeficiency syndrome
Asplenia: congenital, splenectomy, and functional
Primary immunodeficiencies
Immunosuppression

Discussion of Individual Diagnoses

Human Immunodeficiency Virus/Acquired Immunodeficiency Syndrome

The perinatally acquired human immunodeficiency virus (HIV) epidemic peaked in the 1980s and 1990s. The United States has seen a dramatic decrease in the number of new cases of perinatal HIV transmission since 1995, when voluntary HIV testing in pregnant women and antiretroviral therapy for HIV-positive women during pregnancy and delivery became routine. Reducing mother-to-child HIV transmission, institution of appropriate prophylaxis of opportunistic infections (OIs), and offering antiretroviral therapy when indicated have all contributed to decreases in OIs in children with HIV and/or acquired immunodeficiency syndrome (AIDS).[1] However, in 2005 there were still an estimated 68 cases of AIDS reported in children under age 13, and 9112 estimated cumulative cases of AIDS in children under 13.[2] Thus, OIs are still a cause for concern in the pediatric HIV-infected population. Additionally, HIV-positive women with OIs are more likely to transmit infections congenitally to both HIV-exposed but uninfected children and those with HIV infection.[3] In contrast to OIs in adults, children do not have reactivation of latent pathogens, but primary infection with pathogens. Thus clinicians should be aware that the clinical manifestations and treatment differ from that in adults with OIs.

The Centers for Disease Control and Prevention estimates that approximately half of all new HIV infections in the United States are among people less than 25 years of age.[2] A disproportionate number of 13- to 24-year-olds with newly diagnosed HIV infection are racial and ethnic minorities, and most are infected sexually, either young men who have sex with men or young women who have sex with men. In 2005, there were an estimated 2546 new cases of AIDS and a cumulative estimated 41,311 cases of AIDS in 13- to 24-year-olds.[2] In seeing patients in this age group, clinicians must be aware of the acute seroconversion syndrome in people at risk for acquiring HIV, and presentations of illness in those who do and do not know their HIV status. Many 13- to 24-year-olds infected with HIV are unaware of their status. Additionally, not all patients who are prescribed antiretroviral therapy have a good response to therapy. Reasons for this include poor adherence to regimens, drug toxicity, drug interactions, and initial infection with resistant HIV. Thus OIs in the HIV-infected adolescent must be considered.[4]

Clinical Presentation

Children and adolescents with HIV with signs and symptoms of acute illness will most commonly have OIs. These infections cause a varied array of clinical findings, including most commonly fever, respiratory distress, gastrointestinal symptoms, mucocutaneous manifestations, and neurologic syndromes. Table 69–1 presents the differential diagnosis to consider, clinical manifestations to recognize, and diagnostic tests to order when approaching these patients.

For children and adolescents on antiretroviral therapy, drug toxicity must also be considered, with the most common presentations including rash, gastrointestinal symptoms, and fever. Additionally, pain is a common complaint in children

Table 69–1	Differential Diagnosis of Acute Illness in Children and Adolescents with HIV/AIDS	
Diagnosis	**Clinical Presentation**	**Diagnostic Tests**
Bacterial infections, invasive	*Children:* febrile illness, pneumonia, meningitis, sepsis, UTI, sinusitis, otitis osteomyelitis, septic arthritis, abscess	Blood culture, urine culture, CBC, CXR, LP if indicated; radiologic testing based on localizing signs
	Adolescents: pneumonia with fever, chest pain, productive cough	Blood culture, CXR, sputum culture
Candida infections	*Children:* oral thrush, diaper dermatitis, esophagitis; rarely invasive but more common in those with advanced disease, central lines	Physical exam, KOH prep, fungal culture, barium swallow or endoscopy, blood culture; if fungemic, retinal exam, abdominal CT or US, bone scan if osteomyelitis suspected
	Adolescents: oral thrush, esophagitis, vulvovaginitis	
Coccidiomycosis	*Children:* fever, respiratory distress, lymphadenopathy, headache, wasting	Blood culture, sputum culture, LP for CSF culture, serum antibody testing
	Adolescents: disseminated disease (fever, lymphadenopathy, skin manifestations), meningitis	
Cryptococcosis	*Children:* meningoencephalitis (fever, headache, altered mental status more common than meningismus, photophobia, focal neurologic signs), disseminated cryptococcosis (cutaneous lesions resembling molluscum), pulmonary cryptococcosis (fever, nonproductive cough, mediastinal lymphadenopathy)	Cryptococcal antigen (serum and CSF), LP (for cell count, glucose, protein, opening pressure); fungal cultures of CSF, sputum, and blood; BAL; biopsy of pulmonary or skin lesions
	Adolescents: meningitis (can see clinical presentation of meningitis), meningoencephalitis	
Cryptosporidiosis/ Microsporidiosis	*Children:* fever and vomiting, nonbloody watery diarrhea, dehydration, weight loss; presents as any other acute gastroenteritis; can present with fever, right upper quadrant pain if infects the bile duct	Stool for ova and parasites; endoscopy if indicated
	Adolescents: watery diarrhea, abdominal cramping; can see nausea & vomiting; cholangitis, and pancreatitis; in rare cases, microsporidia can cause eye infections, encephalitis, and disseminated infection	
Cytomegalovirus (CMV)	*Children:* febrile illness, retinitis, mono-like illness, colitis, pneumonitis, encephalitis, congenital manifestations	Dependent on presentation, CMV serum and urine antigen, CMV antibody titers, CMV PCR, endoscopy, CXR, LP, head imaging, eye exam
	Adolescents: retinitis, colitis, esophagitis	
Hepatitis B and C	*Children:* asymptomatic or clinical hepatitis	Hepatitis B surface antigen, hepatitis C virus PCR, LFTs
	Adolescents: asymptomatic or clinical hepatitis (fever, nausea, vomiting, jaundice)	
Herpes simplex virus (HSV)	*Congenital:* disseminated multiorgan disease; localized CNS, skin, eye, or mouth disease	Clinical diagnosis based on seeing vesicles and ulcers, viral culture from lesions, direct immunofluorescence for HSV antigen from lesions; Tzanck preparation from lesions no longer recommended because nonspecific; CSF for HSV PCR if indicated
	Children: orolabial disease with dissemination and visceral involvement in severely immunocompromised; esophagitis, genital	
	Adolescents: skin, eye, or mouth disease, genital lesions	
Histoplasmosis	*Children:* fever, fatigue, weight loss, nonproductive cough, cutaneous nodules	Blood culture (takes up to 6 wk to grow); antigen in serum, urine, CSF, BAL
	Adolescents: interstitial pneumonitis, meningitis	
Mycobacterium avium complex disease	*Children:* recurrent fever, weight loss, night sweats, diarrhea, abdominal pain, lymphadenopathy	Blood culture (for AFB, can take up to 6 wk to grow), biopsy specimens, CBC (neutropenia, anemia, thrombocytopenia), LFTs (evidence of infiltrative liver disease)
	Adolescents: usually disseminated disease with fever, night sweats, weight loss, diarrhea	
Mycobacterium tuberculosis	*Neonates:* congenital, nonspecific, failure to thrive, symptoms, pneumonia, meningitis	CXR, skin testing (anergy testing not indicated), history of contact with infected adult, AFB stain of morning gastric aspirate (children), sputum, or BAL
	Children: no symptoms or nonspecific, fever, failure to thrive, acute pneumonia, extrapulmonary disease	
	Adolescents: fever, cough, wasting, lymphadenopathy	
Pneumocystis jiroveci	*Children:* fever, respiratory distress, cough, hypoxia	Low alveolar-arterial oxygen gradient on arterial blood culture, elevated lactate dehydrogenase; CXR can appear normal (early on) or have diffuse parenchymal infiltrates; visualization of the organism on histopathology or direct fluorescent antibody of BAL or sputum (in adolescents)
	Adolescents: fever, SOB, cough, hypoxia	

Table 69-1	Differential Diagnosis of Acute Illness in Children and Adolescents with HIV/AIDS (Continued)	
Diagnosis	**Clinical Presentation**	**Diagnostic Tests**
Progressive multifocal leukoencephalopathy	Focal neurologic signs, seizures, cognitive dysfunction	Radiographic findings (demyelination) on CT or MRI, CSF, or PCR for JC virus support diagnosis; brain biopsy may be indicated
Syphilis	*Congenital:* if no symptoms at birth, can see symptoms within the first 6 mo of life; organomegaly, jaundice, rash, nasal discharge, mucocutaneous lesions, anemia, pseudoparalysis	In infants, cannot rely on antibody testing because reflects mother's immunoglobulins; diagnosis made by combination of physical, radiologic, serologic, and direct microscopic exam; CBC, CSF for VDRL; if indicated can check CXR, long bone radiograph, eye exam
	Adolescents: primary (painless genital ulcer), secondary (skin lesions— generalized and on palms and soles, lymphadenopathy, fever, HA, aseptic meningitis), late syphilis (dementia, aortitis)	Nontreponemal antibody tests (VDRL or RPR), treponemal tests if former are positive (DFA-TP or FTA-ABS). LP should be considered in HIV-positive patients with serologic evidence of syphilis to rule out neurosyphilis; consider diagnosis if high-risk sexual activity (MSM, other STDs)
Toxoplasmosis	*Congenital:* maculopapular rash, lymphadenopathy, organomegaly, jaundice, pancytopenia, CNS disease (seizures, microcephaly, hydrocephalus)	Toxo-specific serum IgM, IgA, IgE, IgG (after 6 mo), head imaging (CT with multiple ring-enhancing lesions)
	Children: fatigue, fever, sore throat, mono-like syndrome, rash, cervical lymphadenopathy	
	Adolescents: fever, headache, confusion, seizures, encephalitis	
Varicella-zoster virus (VZV)	*Congenital:* skin scarring, lymph hypoplasia, neurologic manifestations (seizures, microcephaly, etc.)	Clinical diagnosis based on typical appearance of generalized vesicular rash and fever or painful vesicular rash in dermatomal pattern; direct immunofluorescence for VZV antigen on cells collected from skin, conjunctiva, or mucosa. Tzanck preparation is nonspecific (see giant cells with HSV as well). VZV isolation from culture of vesicular fluid; eye exam
	Children: generalized pruritic vesicular rash, fever; zoster with typical dermatomal distribution, but can see more disseminated rash; retinitis; encephalitis	
	Adolescents: zoster/shingles (dermatomal, rarely disseminated if immunocompromised); retinal necrosis	

Abbreviations: AFB, acid-fast bacilli; BAL, bronchoalveolar lavage; CBC, complete blood count; CNS, central nervous system; CSF, cerebrospinal fluid; CT, computed tomography; CXR, chest radiograph; DFA-TP, direct fluorescent antibody–treponemal test; FTA-ABS, fluorescent treponemal antibody absorption test; HA, headache; HIV, human immunodeficiency virus; Ig, immunoglobulin; KOH, potassium hydroxide; LFTs, liver function tests; LP, lumbar puncture; MRI, magnetic resonance imaging; MSM, men who have sex with men; PCR, polymerase chain reaction; RPR, rapid plasma reagent test; SOB, shortness of breath; STDs, sexually transmitted diseases; US, ultrasound; UTI, urinary tract infection; VDRL, Venereal Disease Research Laboratory test.

Adapted from Mofenson LM, Oleske J, Serchuck L, et al [3] and Benson CA, Kaplan JE, Masur H, et al [4]

with HIV infection secondary to systemic manifestations such as cardiomyopathy, myositis, drug reactions, and other secondary infections.[5]

In adolescents engaging in high-risk behaviors (unprotected sex, young men who have sex with men, history of a sexually transmitted disease, known HIV-positive sexual contact or forced sex within the 4 weeks prior to presentation), a diagnosis of acute HIV seroconversion must be considered when patients present with symptoms such as fever, fatigue, lymphadenopathy, pharyngitis, generalized rash, or, in general, a mononucleosis-like syndrome. While HIV antibody testing is not helpful in this acute setting, a baseline test should be obtained. Diagnostic testing should include a measurement of plasma viremia (by HIV polymerase chain reaction), with viral loads of greater than 50,000 copies/ml diagnostic of HIV seroconversion in the setting of a negative HIV antibody test.[6-8]

In the acute setting, the most common diagnoses to recognize in HIV-infected children and adolescents include invasive bacterial infections (bacteremia and pneumonia in particular), *Pneumocystis jiroveci* (PCP; formerly *Pneumocystis carinii*) pneumonia, herpes zoster, esophageal candidiasis, and disseminated *Mycobacterium avium* complex. Studies of opportunistic infections in perinatally infected children prior to antiretroviral therapy showed that bacterial infec-

tions were the most common infections, with pneumonia, bacteremia, and urinary tract infections the most common manifestations.[3] One explanation for this finding is that, in children, infection with HIV occurs before primary immune function against common bacterial infections develops (specifically B-cell and humoral responses). While *Streptococcus pneumoniae* was found to be the most important bacterial pathogen in this group, this pattern may change given the institution of pneumococcal conjugate vaccinations as part of the primary vaccine series. While bacteremia with gram-positive organisms is more common than gram-negative bacteremia, gram-negative bacteremia is observed in children with advanced diseased, those with central lines, and those less than 5 years of age with less severe immunosuppression.[9] Typical gram-negative organisms include *Pseudomonas aeruginosa*, nontyphoidal salmonellae, *Escherichia coli*, and *Haemophilus influenzae*.

In the absence of bacteremia, acute pneumonia is presumed to be bacterial in the setting of a febrile child with pulmonary symptoms and an abnormal chest radiograph. Lymphoid interstitial pneumonitis (LIP) is common in pediatric AIDS. LIP or any underlying chronic lung disease makes development of acute pneumonia more likely.[10] The clinical presentation of bacterial infections is based on the type of infection, as HIV-infected children will most likely present with signs and symptoms similar to those of children without HIV (fever, increased white blood cell count). However, severely immunocompromised patients may not be able to produce either fever or an elevated white blood cell count.

PCP is still the most common AIDS-defining disease in the pediatric population, with the incidence peaking in the first year of life, between 3 and 6 months. In contrast to children over 1 year of age and to adults, in whom PCP occurs when CD4 cell counts are less than 200/mm³, low CD4 cell counts are not a risk factor for disease in infants as many infected with PCP have CD4 counts over 1500/mm³. This is why PCP prophylaxis is recommended in infants of HIV-positive mothers until the absence of HIV infection is proven. As in adults, the presentation of PCP can be either sudden, with classic symptoms of fever, tachypnea, and cough, or more subtle, with mild cough, dyspnea, and poor feeding.[3,11]

Mucocutaneous manifestations and infections that are rare in immunocompetent children are more common in perinatally infected HIV-positive children with moderate (defined as CD4 percentage of 15 to 24) and severe (defined as CD4 percentage of 1 to 14) immunosuppression. One study found that fungal infections were most common, notably oral candidiasis with *Candida albicans*. Viral infections were the second most common. As in HIV-infected adults, herpes zoster is more common in children with AIDS than in uninfected children. Herpes simplex virus (HSV) stomatitis occurs with greater frequency and severity. Presentations can be atypical, and more than one mucocutaneous manifestation can present in the same patient.[12]

Management

When invasive bacterial infection is suspected in the emergency department (ED), treatment regimens should take into consideration local resistance patterns to common infectious agents (e.g., penicillin-resistant *S. pneumoniae* or methicillin-resistant *S. aureus*) and any recent use of prophylactic or therapeutic medications by the patient. HIV-infected children who are severely immunocompromised require broad-spectrum antibiotic treatment for a range of organisms (resistant and nonresistant); those who are neither immunocompromised nor neutropenic can be treated as HIV-negative patients. An HIV-infected pediatric patient (non-neonatal) with suspected bacteremia, bacterial pneumonia, or meningitis should be treated with broad-spectrum cephalosporins such as ceftriaxone (80 to 100 mg/kg in one or two divided doses with a maximum dose of 4 g daily) or cefotaxime (200 mg/kg divivded in three or four doses with a maximum dose of 8 to 10 g daily) until an organism can be identified. In HIV-infected pediatric patients with fever and an indwelling catheter, both gram-negative and gram-positive organisms should be treated with a regimen with pseudomonal and methicillin-resistant *S. aureus* coverage, such as ceftazidime and vancomycin.[3,4]

Treatment for PCP should be initiated if the diagnosis is suspected, and not withheld pending the diagnosis. Bronchoalveolar lavage is positive for at least 72 hours after PCP treatment has been initiated. In the absence of allergy, trimethoprim-sulfamethoxazole (TMP-SMX) can be started at 15 to 20 mg/kg of body weight per day (TMP component; 75 to 100 mg/kg of SMX) in three to four divided doses for patients older than 2 months of age and adults. It should be given

intravenously (IV) over 1 hour. Once the acute phase has passed, the TMP-SMX can be administered orally in the same dose to complete the 21-day course of treatment. If patients are not able to take TMP-SMX, pentamidine may be given (4 mg/kg as a single daily dose given IV over 60 to 90 minutes for 14 to 21 days). If pentamidine cannot be used, alternative oral regimens can be initiated, but are poorly studied in children.

Early initiation of corticosteroids (within 72 hours of diagnosis) can be beneficial in moderate or severe cases of PCP. This is usually defined as the presence of hypoxemia with a partial pressure of arterial oxygen less than 70 mm Hg or an alveolar-arterial gradient greater than 35 mm Hg. Recommended initial doses include prednisone 40 mg twice a day, prednisone or IV methylprednisolone 1 mg/kg twice a day, or IV methylprednisolone 1 mg/kg every 6 hours.[3,4,11]

Uncomplicated oropharyngeal candidiasis can usually be treated with topical therapy such as clotrimazole troches used at 10 mg orally four to five times a day for 14 days or regimens utilizing nystatin suspension at 400,000 to 600,000 U/ml four times daily for 7 to 14 days. Since many of the topical therapies fail, some providers choose to begin therapy with an oral azole in severe cases, either fluconazole (best tolerated and most effective; 3 to 6 mg/kg by mouth once a day for 14 days), itraconazole, or ketoconazole. The patient's liver function should be assessed prior to beginning this therapy. Interactions with other medications (particularly antiretrovirals) that utilize the cytochrome P-450 system should also be considered.[3,4]

Acyclovir is the first-line treatment for HIV-infected children with primary varicella and zoster. With primary varicella, IV acyclovir is recommended because of the risk of disseminated and life-threatening illness (fever, numerous or deep and hemorrhagic skin lesions, moderate or severe immunosuppression). Neonatal HSV disease should be treated with high-dose IV acyclovir (20 mg/kg of body weight per dose three times daily) administered for 21 days for central nervous system and disseminated disease and for 14 days for skin, eye, and mouth disease. The dose for children less than 1 year of age is 10 mg/kg over 1 hour every 8 hours for 21 days. Oral acyclovir at 20 mg/kg per dose given four times a day should be reserved for children with normal CD4 counts or for those with very mild disease. Acyclovir is also first-line treatment for HIV-infected children with zoster. Intravenous acyclovir should be used in children who are very immunosuppressed if there is risk of eye involvement (trigeminal nerve distribution), or multidermatomal distribution. Renal function should be checked with a baseline serum creatinine so the dose can be adjusted for renal impairment if necessary.[3]

Asplenia: Congenital, Splenectomy, and Functional

Patients without a spleen or with functional hyposplenism are at risk for life-threatening infection. Congenital asplenia is associated with very low survival rates past 1 year of age and usually seen in conjunction with cardiac abnormalities and biliary atresia. Surgical splenectomies are performed secondary to trauma, cysts, malignancy, or other hematologic conditions (Hodgkin's disease, hemolytic anemia, and idiopathic thrombocytopenic purpura).[13] While some surgeons attempt to retain splenic tissue or autotransplant splenic tissue, there is no good evidence that this helps to preserve splenic function. Functional asplenia occurs from other primary medical conditions that result in degrees of hyposplenism: sickle cell disease (hemoglobin SC, hemoglobin SE, β-thalassemia), thrombocytopenia, malignant histiocytosis, gastrointestinal causes (celiac disease, dermatitis herpetiformis, ulcerative colitis), liver disease (portal hypertension), immunologic disorders (systemic lupus erythematosus, rheumatoid arthritis, Graves' disease, polyarteritis nodosum), infiltrative diseases (amyloidosis, sarcoidosis), and other miscellaneous causes (Bartonella infection, HIV infection, graft-versus-host disease, post–bone marrow transplantation, total parenteral nutrition, cancer therapy that includes either high-dose steroids or splenic irradiation).[13]

Important Clinical Features and Considerations

The spleen plays a critical role in responding to antigens both by antigen clearance and antibody production, as well as through filtering, phagocytosis, and opsonization of cells. This places asplenic patients at higher risk for sepsis caused by bacteria, particularly encapsulated organisms such as *Strep. pneumoniae*, *H. influenzae*, and *Neisseria meningitidis*. While *Strep. pneumoniae* is the most common pathogen, other important causes of infection include gram-negative bacteria (associated with high mortality rates) such as *E. coli* and *P. aeruginosa*. Other bacteria include group B stretococcus, *Staphylococcus aureus*, Salmonella species, Enterococcus species, Bacteroides species, Bartonella, and Plesiomonas. Unusual organisms such as *Capnocytophaga carnimorsus* (also implicated after dog bites) and protozoa (e.g., those causing babesiosis, malaria, and ehrlichiosis) have also been implicated in asplenic patients. These infections must be considered in patients with asplenia with recent travel.[14,15]

Overwhelming postsplenectomy infection (OPSI) risk is thought to be highest in children, people undergoing splenectomy for hematologic conditions, and patients who are immunosuppressed for other reasons. While the risk of infection has been found to be highest in the first 2 years after splenectomy, lifetime risk of OPSI remains at 5% and carries a mortality rate of 38% to 69%.[15] Despite preventive measures to reduce the risk of OPSI—immunization again *Strep. pneumoniae*, *H. influenzae* type b, and *N. meningitides*; prophylactic antibiotics; standby antibiotics (to be used if the patient becomes acutely febrile or ill and does not have quick access to a medical center)—asplenic patients remain at risk for OPSI, and no studies have specifically shown the efficacy of these measures. Also, it cannot be assumed that asplenic patients have been counseled regarding the risk of infection or the importance of compliance with daily prophylaxis.[14]

Streptococcus pneumoniae is the most important pathogen in asplenic pediatric patients, and has been implicated in over 50% of invasive infections.[14] Prior to the institution of vaccination with conjugate pneumococcal vaccine, the median time to come to medical attention was 24 hours. Presenting signs and symptoms include fever, shock, petechiae or purpura, disseminated intravascular coagulopathy, and respiratory distress. Types of illnesses in these children include bacteremia (with or without other focal infections), meningitis, and osteomyelitis. While there are studies to support an overall decline in invasive pneumococcal disease after the introduction of the conjugate vaccine, approximately 19% of invasive pneumococcal disease has been caused by serotypes not included in the conjugate pneumococcal vaccine. Thus protection against pneumococcus cannot be presumed.[16,17]

OPSI does not always have a focus of infection. One possible explanation for the lack of localizing findings is that nasal carriage and colonization may lead to later invasive infection.[13] Patients may present with septic shock, but often the presentation is more protean—viral-type symptoms such as fever, fatigue, headache, vomiting, and abdominal pain. OPSI must be suspected and therapy must be instituted very early as the disease can progress very quickly. The overall mortality rate of OPSI is between 50% and 70%. Other morbidities can include hearing loss, gangrene, skin grafts, and amputations. Early anticipation of OPSI and aggressive management are vital.[13,16]

Management

The best way to improve survival is to recognize the risk for the illness before the full clinical picture of sepsis emerges. Sepsis should be aggressively treated, and empirical therapy should take precedence over any diagnostic testing. Ideally, blood cultures would be drawn prior to the administration of antibiotics, but should never delay treatment. Even though Pneumococcus is the most common pathogen, IV antibiotics should be administered that cover the spectrum of possible bacterial etiologies. Combination antibiotics should cover penicillin-resistant pneumococci, gram-negative organisms, β-lactamase–resistant organisms, and any other local resistance issues. Consultation should be sought with infectious disease specialists in areas where both penicillin and cephalosporin resistance is known, or when patients have multiple allergies. Proposed regimens include ceftriaxone (50 to 75 mg/kg IV per dose every 12 hours; adult dose 2 g IV per dose every 12 to 24 hours) *or* cefotaxime (25 to 50 mg/kg IV per dose every 6 hours; adult dose 2 g IV per dose every 8 hours) *plus* gentamycin (2.5 mg/kg IV per dose every 8 hours; adult dose 5 to 7 mg/kg IV per dose every 24 hours) *or* vancomycin (10 to 15 mg/kg per dose every 6 hours; adult dose 2 to 3 g per day in divided doses every 6 to 12 hours). Some authors also suggest the addition of rifampin in initial management.[13,14] While some authors suggest steroids or immunoglobulin, there are no clear recommendations or data to support these measures. Patients with asplenia or splenectomy are at high risk for OPSI after animal or bite wounds and should be treated with prophylactic antibiotics, either ampicillin-sulbactam or amoxicillin–clavulinic acid by mouth depending on the severity of the wound. Particular attention to the possibility of malaria (whether or not the patient was on prophylaxis), babesiosis, or ehrlichiosis should be considered in asplenic patients who travel to endemic regions.[14]

Diagnostic workup (before or after the initiation of IV antibiotics), depending on the clinical scenario, should include blood culture, urine culture, sputum culture (in older children and adolescents), lumbar puncture if indicated, complete blood count, chemistry, and chest radiograph.

Primary Immunodeficiencies

Primary immunodeficiencies (PIs) are a group of disorders in which the primary defect is intrinsic to one or more of the four components of the immune system: B lymphocytes, T lymphocytes, phagocytes, and complement. The World Health Organization classifies PIs on a molecular basis as T- and B-cell immunodeficiencies; predominantly antibody deficiencies; other well-defined immunodeficiency syndromes; diseases of immune dysregulation; congenital defects of phagocyte number, function, or both; defects in innate immunity; autoinflammatory disorders; and complement deficiencies. For the purposes of this chapter, PIs are discussed in terms of the components of the immune system affected.[18,19]

Clinical Presentation

In the ED, children with PIs may present with known diagnoses, as overwhelming infections representing the first sign of a PI, or with recurrent infections indicating an underlying PI. It is helpful to approach the disorders in terms of types of infections with which they are likely to present.[18,19]

B-lymphocyte defects are the most common PIs (approximately 70%) and manifest as an impaired antibody response.[20-22] Those patients affected are more susceptible to bacterial infections, particularly encapsulated pyogenic bacteria such as *H. influenzae*, *Strep. pneumoniae*, and staphylococci, but also infections with other bacteria (*P. aeruginosa*, *Mycoplasma hominis*, and *Ureaplasma urealyticum*) as well as enteroviruses. Most of the B-lymphocyte defects (except common variable immunodeficiency, which presents between 20 and 30 years of age) present after 3 to 6 months when maternal antibodies wane. Types of bacterial infection include pneumonia, otitis, sinusitis, and bacteremia.[20-22]

T-lymphocyte defects usually present at birth or in early infancy. While T-cell disorders are thought of as cellular immunodeficiencies, these patients are also at risk for pneumococcal disease because of impaired antibody responses.[20,21,23] Patients with T-cell defects are primary thought to be at high risk for OIs secondary to viruses (severe respiratory infections caused by parainfluenza or respiratory syncytial virus; herpesvirus infections such as HSV, varicella-zoster virus, or cytomegalovirus), and PCP. They may also be at risk for infections with bacterial pathogens as seen in B-lymphocyte defects. These children are also more prone to fungal and mycobacterial disease.[20,21,23]

Phagocyte defects (affecting neutrophils and macrophages) present in early childhood and display very specific infections with pyogenic bacteria (Pseudomonas, *Serratia marcescans*, *Staph. aureus*) and fungi (*Aspergillus fumigatus* and Candida). They do not typically cause infection with PCP, pneumococcus, or viruses. Infections of the skin and reticuloendothelial system frequently occur.[21,24]

Complement defects are rare, but can occur in nearly every component of the complement system—the classical pathway, alternative pathway, and membrane attack complex. This defect predisposes patients to encapsulated bacterial infections, most notably pneumococcal infections. Clinical presentations include bacteremia or meningitis. Defects of the terminal components (C5 to C9) predispose to infection with *Neisseria* species.[20,21] Table 69–2 contains examples of primary immunodeficiencies in each part of the immune system.

Management

Whether or not the underlying immunologic defect is known, acute management should be guided by the patient's clinical situation. In the ED, supportive and resuscitative management and coverage with broad-spectrum antibiotic therapy are always appropriate until further diagnostic workup can be pursued. PIs are an important group of disorders in the pediatric population. Careful attention to overwhelming or recurrent infection is the key to guiding diagnosis and man-

Table 69–2	Examples of Primary Immunodeficiencies[20-23]	
Affected Part of the Immune System	**Examples**	**Typical Presentation**
B lymphocytes	X-linked agammaglobulinemia Autosomal recessive agammaglobulinemia Hyper-IgM syndrome IgA deficiency Common variable immunodeficiency IgG subclass deficiencies Selective antipolysaccharide antibody deficiencies	First year of life with infection from encapsulated bacteria such as *Pneumococcus, Giardia,* or enteroviruses
T lymphocytes	DiGeorge syndrome Purine nucleoside phosphorylase deficiency	Thymic hypoplasia, hypocalcemia secondary to hypoparathyroidism, and congenital cardiac anomalies; classic facies associated
Combined B and T lymphocytes	Severe combined immunodeficiency Wiskott-Aldrich syndrome (X-linked recessive) Ataxia-telangiectasia (autosomal recessive) Progressive cerebellar ataxia Oculocutaneous telangiectasia Recurrent lung infections	Failure to thrive, chronic diarrhea, oral thrush, skin rash, pneumonia, sepsis, PCP, severe pneumonias due to several possible etiologies; fatal without intervention, bone marrow transplantation Eczema, thrombocytopenia, and recurrent infections
Phagocytes	Chronic granulomatous disease (defect of the nicotinamide adenine dinucleotide phosphatase oxidase pathway) Leukocyte adhesion defect Chédiak-Higashi syndrome	Recurrent and often life-threatening infection with catalase-positive bacteria and fungi most often in the skin, lung, lymph nodes, and liver; excessive granuloma formation

Abbreviations: Ig, immunoglobulin; PCP, *Pneumocystis jiroveci* pneumonia.

agement. Knowledge of an already diagnosed PI also helps to guide therapy.

Immunosuppression

Immunodeficiencies can be either primary or secondary and can affect any component of the immune system. Causes of secondary immunosuppression include cancer and transplantation (bone marrow or solid organ). Risk of infection in cancer is high because of the underlying disease process or organ involved, chemotherapeutic agents utilized in treatment, degree of neutropenia, alteration of mucosal immunity, and frequent need for an indwelling catheter. Infection risk in bone marrow transplantation is high for the reasons mentioned, and because of the need for immunosuppressive medications, risk of infection with cytomegalovirus, and graft-versus-host disease. Solid organ transplantation is associated with infection risk at the site of the transplanted organ, an underlying disease process for which the patient received the transplant, poor nutritional status of the patient prior to transplantation due to chronic disease, and the need for immunosuppressive medications. All of these factors make the initial evaluation and treatment of the immunosuppressed patient crucial to outcome.[25]

Clinical Presentation

Fever can often be the only sign of a serious infection in an immunocompromised patient. Half of febrile neutropenic patients with cancer have an occult infection.[25] The Infectious Diseases Society of America Fever and Neutropenia Guidelines Panel defines fever as a single oral temperature of greater than 38.3° C (101° F) or a temperature of greater than 38.0° C (100.4° F) for more than 1 hour. They define neutropenia as a neutrophil count of less than 500 cells/mm³ or a count of less than 1000 cells/mm³ with the likelihood that the count will decrease to less than 500 cells/mm³. Increased risk of infection is associated with lower neutrophil count, prolonged neutropenia, and a low nadir of neutrophil count.[25,26]

If pathogens are able to be isolated, bacteria are most common and include gram-positive, gram-negative, and anaerobic organisms. Fungi are common in patients with a history of exposure to broad-spectrum antibiotics. Neutropenic patients can present with severe infections without localizing signs or symptoms (i.e., induration, erythema) due to lack of ability to mount a local inflammatory response. Body fluids may not always reflect a pleocytosis.[25,26]

A careful history and physical examination is paramount, and attention should be focused on common sites of infection—the oral cavity, including the teeth, gums, and oropharynx; the lungs; the gastrointestinal tract (with special attention to the perineum and anus); the eyes and fundi; the skin (focus on any access sites, bone marrow aspirate sites), and soft tissue (particularly around the nails).[25,26]

If the patient is hemodynamically stable, the following diagnostic evaluation should be obtained prior to empirical treatment with antibiotics: blood culture (from both the peripheral vein and catheter lumen) for bacterial and fungal culture; Gram stain and culture (for bacteria, fungi and, if the lesion is chronic, mycobacteria) of any fluid draining from the indwelling catheter site; urinalysis and urine culture; and chest radiograph. Other studies (such as cerebrospinal fluid) are dependent on the patient's clinical status.

A complete blood count and serum chemistry (electrolytes, blood urea nitrogen, creatinine, liver function tests) should also be obtained. Workup for fungal infection can be pursued at a later date or if the patient does not respond to initial antimicrobial therapy.[25,26]

Management

As with patients with asplenia, infection in neutropenic patients can progress rapidly, and all febrile and neutropenic patients should be presumed to have an invasive infection until proven otherwise. Empirical therapy should include coverage for both gram-positive and gram-negative bacteria. The antibiotic choice should be dependent on the susceptibility and resistance patterns of a given institution as well as the patient's allergies or organ impairment. Suggested management can include monotherapy with a third- or fourth-generation cephalosporin (cefepime, ceftazidime), or carbapenem, or two-drug therapy (an aminoglycoside *and* either an antipseudomonal penicillin *or* cefepime, ceftazidime, or carbapenem).[25,26] Vancomycin should be added if local rates of gram-positive infections are high, if the infection is suspected to be catheter related, if the patient is know to be colonized with resistant bacteria, if the patient was recently treated for gram-positive bacteremia, if the patient received chemotherapy that is known to cause severe mucosal impairment, or the patient is hypotensive or clinically unstable.[25,26] Other coverage should be based on the patient's clinical examination and findings. Empirical antifungal coverage is almost never initiated in the ED unless the patient is known to have fungal disease. Central indwelling catheters should stay in place unless there is a clear indication for removal (tunnel infection, recurrent infections), and that decision is usually not made in the ED. For well-appearing low-risk patients, some institutions manage fever and neutropenia in the outpatient setting with oral antibiotics, but this must be in consultation with the oncologist and with assurance that the patient has a reliable social situation, ability to return to the hospital for worsening status, and prearranged close follow-up.[25,26]

Fever is a common presenting symptom in immunocompromised, neutropenic patients and is usually indicative of an underlying infection. Since it is not possible to determine which patients are or are not infected on presentation to the ED, empirical antibiotics should be given to all such patients.

REFERENCES

1. Graham SM: HIV and respiratory infections in children. Curr Opin Pulm Med 9:215–220, 2003.
*2. Centers for Disease Control and Prevention: HIV/AIDS Surveillance Report, 2005 (Vol. 17). Atlanta: Centers for Disease Control and Prevention, 2007. http://www.cdc.gov/hiv/topics/surveillance/resources/reports
*3. Mofenson LM, Oleske J, Serchuck L, et al: Treating opportunistic infections among HIV-exposed and infected children: recommendations from CDC, the National Institutes of Health, and the Infectious Diseases Society of America. MMWR Recomm Rep 53(RR-14):1–100, 2004.
4. Benson CA, Kaplan JE, Masur H, et al: Treating opportunistic infections among HIV-infected adults and adolescents: recommendations from CDC, the National Institutes of Health, and the HIV Medicine Association/Infectious Diseases Society of America. MMWR Recomm Rep 53(RR-15):1–120, 2004.

*Selected readings.

5. National Institutes of Health: Guidelines for the Use of Antiretroviral Agents in Pediatric HIV Infection. Supplement II: Managing Complications of HIV Infection in HIV-Infected Children on Antiretroviral Therapy. Bethesda, MD: National Institutes of Health, 2006.

6. Bisno AL: Acute pharyngitis. N Engl J Med 344:205–211, 2001.

7. Vanhems P, Dassa C, Lambert J, et al: Comprehensive classification of symptoms and signs reported among 218 patients with acute HIV-1 infection. J Acquir Immune Defic Syndr 21:99–106, 1999.

8. Kahn JO, Walker BD: Acute human immunodeficiency virus type 1 infection. N Engl J Med 339:33–39, 1998.

9. Dankner WM, Lindsey JC, Levin MJ; Pediatric AIDS Clinical Trials Group Protocol Teams: Correlates of opportunistic infections in children infected with the human immunodeficiency virus managed before highly active antiretroviral therapy. Pediatr Infect Dis J 20:40–48, 2001.

10. Gonzalez CE, Samakoses R, Boler AM, et al: Lymphoid interstitial pneumonitis in pediatric AIDS: natural history of the disease. Ann N Y Acad Sci 918:358–361, 2000.

*11. Thomas CF, Limper AH: Pneumocystic pneumonia. N Engl J Med 350:2487–2498, 2004.

12. Wananukul S, Deekajorndech T, Panchareon C, Thisyakorn U: Mucocutaneous findings in pediatric AIDS related to degree of immunosuppression. Pediatr Dermatol 20:289–294, 2003.

*13. Bridgen ML, Patullo AL: Prevention and management of overwhelming postsplenectomy infection—an update. Crit Care Med 27:836–842, 1999.

14. Davidson RN, Wall RA: Prevention and management of infections in patients without a spleen. Clin Microbiol Infect 7:657–660, 2001.

15. Bisharat N, Omari H, Lavi I, Raz R: Risk of infection and death among post-splenectomy patients. J Infect 43:182–186, 2001.

16. Schutze GE, Mason, EO Jr, Barson WJ, et al: Invasive pneumococcal infections in children with asplenia. Pediatr Infect Dis J 21:278–282, 2002.

17. Whitney CG, Farley MM, Hadler J, et al; Active Bacterial Core Surveillance of the Emerging Infections Program Network: Decline in invasive pneumococcal disease after the introduction of protein-polysaccharide conjugate vaccine. N Engl J Med 348:1737–1746, 2003.

*18. Notarangelo L, Casanova JL, Fischer A, et al; International Union of Immunological Societies Primary Immunodeficiency Diseases Classification Committee: Primary immunodeficiency diseases: an update. J Allergy Clin Immunol 114:677–687, 2004.

19. Bonilla FA, Geha RS: Primary immunodeficiency diseases. J Allergy Clin Immunol 111(Suppl):S571–S581, 2001.

20. Picard C, Puel A, Bustamante J, et al: Primary immunodeficiencies associated with pneumococcal disease. Curr Opin Allergy Clin Immunol 3:451–459, 2003.

21. Buckley RH: Pulmonary complications of primary immunodeficiencies. Paediatr Respir Rev 5(Suppl A):S225–S233, 2004.

22. Ballow M: Primary immunodeficiency disorders: antibody deficiency. J Allergy Clin Immunol 109:581–591, 2002.

23. Buckley RH: Primary cellular immunodeficiencies. J Allergy Clin Immunol 109:747–757, 2002.

24. Rosenzweig SD, Holland SM: Phagocyte immunodeficiencies and their infections. J Allergy Clin Immunol 113:620–626, 2004.

*25. Pizzo PA: Fever in immunocompromised patients. N Engl J Med 341:893–900, 1999.

*26. Hughes WT, Armstrong D, Bodey GP, et al: 2002 guidelines for the use of antimicrobial agents in neutropenic patients with cancer. Clin Infect Dis 34:730–751, 2002.

Chapter 70

Sexually Transmitted Infections

Cynthia J. Mollen, MD, MSCE

Key Points

Evaluation for sexually transmitted diseases in adolescent females can often be done without the speculum examination, if nucleic acid amplification techniques are available for organism identification

Empirical treatment is generally recommended when suspicion of a sexually transmitted infection (STI) is high, in order to reduce the risk of complications and shorten infectivity.

Confidentiality and consent issues should be considered for all adolescent patients presenting for evaluation of a possible STI.

Selected Diagnoses

Pelvic inflammatory disease
Cervicitis
Vaginitis
Genital ulcers
    Herpes genitalis
    Syphilis
    Lymphogranuloma venereum
    Chancroid
Genital growths
    Human papillomavirus
    Molluscum contagiosum
Urethritis and epididymitis
Neonatal infections

Discussion of Individual Diagnoses

The rates of many sexually transmitted infections (STIs) are highest among adolescents, due at least in part to increased frequency of unprotected intercourse when compared to adults. In addition, adolescents are biologically more susceptible to infection, often have short-term serial relationships, and may have barriers to access to health care. Clinicians can make an impact on future acquisition of STIs by discussing risk factors and healthy sexual behaviors with the adolescent patient. Of paramount importance is obtaining an accurate sexual history in private, in a nonjudgmental fashion, in order to assess risk for the infections discussed in this chapter.

Pelvic Inflammatory Disease

Pelvic inflammatory disease (PID) is a polymicrobial infection of the upper genital tract, and is one of the most common infections in sexually active young women. A range of inflammatory disorders can be classified as PID, including endometritis, salpingitis, oophoritis, perihepatitis, and tubo-ovarian abscess (TOA). Adolescents are at approximately 10-fold higher risk for acquiring PID when compared to adult women (women under 25 years old account for 70% of cases); this increased risk is due to a number of factors, including lower levels of secretory immunoglobulin A in adolescents and differences in the epithelial cells of young women when compared to adults, which allow pathogens to cause infection more easily. In addition, adolescents may be more likely to be exposed to bacterial and viral causes of STIs as they tend to have short-term serial intimate relationships and most likely are less effective users of condoms than adults.[1,2]

PID usually begins as an STI, often caused by *Neisseria gonorrhoeae* or *Chlamydia trachomatis*. However, PID is a polymicrobial infection that often involves other organisms as well, including anaerobes. Once the lower genital tract is infected, bacteria ascend to the upper genital tract and cause symptoms of PID.[1] In addition to age, other risk factors for PID include previous episodes of PID, use of an intrauterine device, vaginal douching, and bacterial vaginosis. The use of condoms and oral contraceptives is a protective factor; oral contraceptives cause thickening of the cervical mucus and decrease cervical dilation, uterine contraction, and blood flow during menses, all of which are mechanisms that support ascension of bacteria to the upper genital tract.[2]

Clinical Presentation

Patients can present with a wide variety of symptoms and signs, and the presentation can be subtle, particularly with mild disease. Therefore, it is important to consider PID in the differential of any young women presenting to the emergency department (ED) with the complaint of abdominal pain. The clinical diagnosis of PID is imprecise; studies suggest that the clinical diagnosis of symptomatic PID has a positive predictive value for salpingitis of only 65% to 90% when compared to laparoscopy, which is considered to be the best diagnostic tool for PID.[3,4] Clearly laparoscopy is not

Table 70–1	Diagnosis of Pelvic Inflammatory Disease
Minimum Criteria (at least one)	**Additional Supporting Criteria**
Uterine tenderness Adnexal tenderness Cervical motion tenderness	Oral temperature >101° F (38.3° C) Abnormal cervical or vaginal mucopurulent discharge Elevated erythrocyte sedimentation rate Elevated C-reactive protein Laboratory documentation of cervical infection with *N. gonorrhoeae* or *C. trachomatis* Presence of abundant numbers of WBC on saline microscopy of vaginal secretions

From Centers for Disease Control and Prevention: Sexually transmitted diseases treatment guidelines—2006. MMWR Recomm Rep 55(RR-11):1–100, 2006.

indicated for the majority of patients with suspected PID, so a clinical diagnosis is usually necessary (Table 70–1).

Most patients presenting with PID will complain of abdominal pain, abnormal vaginal bleeding, or vaginal discharge. Patients may report a history of fever, and may complain of nausea and vomiting, although gastrointestinal symptoms are usually not the primary complaint. Major diagnoses to consider in adolescent patients presenting with abdominal pain, in addition to PID, include appendicitis, constipation, cholecystitis, ovarian torsion, ovarian tumor, pregnancy and associated complications, pyelonephritis, and nephrolithiasis.

When assessing an adolescent for the possibility of PID, it is crucial to obtain an accurate social history. This is best obtained by interviewing the patient alone. One approach is to establish a practice of interviewing all adolescents without a parent present, in order to maintain consistency and limit the possibility of missing important information. This approach will also minimize the possibility of missing the diagnosis of PID in a patient who "seems" unlikely to be sexually active, such as the patient with a chronic medical condition or special health care needs. It is important to outline the limits of confidentiality for both the parent and the patient (suicidal or homicidal ideation, or an indication of abuse) (see also Chapter 151, Issues of Consent, Confidentiality, and Minor Status).

Because there is no laboratory or radiologic test that can make a definitive diagnosis of PID, the physical examination is of the utmost importance. In addition to a general physical examination, the pelvic examination provides key information. The pelvic examination, which consists of three traditional components (external inspection, speculum examination, and bimanual examination), is generally associated with a significant amount of anxiety for the adolescent patient.[5] According to the Centers for Disease Control and Prevention (CDC) 2006 Sexually Transmitted Diseases Treatment Guidelines, the diagnosis of PID should be considered in all patients at risk for an STI who have either uterine *or* adnexal *or* cervical motion tenderness on physical examination, if no other explanation for the findings can be found.[3] Furthermore, a recent study suggests that the most sensitive physical examination finding for diagnosing PID is adnexal tenderness.[6] Both of these physical examination criteria can

be assessed through the bimanual examination, without the use of a speculum. In addition, recent advances in diagnostic testing techniques for *N. gonorrhoeae* and *C. trachomatis* have helped pave the way for a reduction in the use of the speculum.[7] Urine-based and vaginal swab nucleic acid amplification techniques have been shown to be at least as sensitive as endocervical culture. Cervical culture for gonorrhea has a sensitivity of 87% to 94%, compared with a sensitivity of 92% to 96% for urine-based tests and up to 100% for vaginal swab–based tests. Similarly, while cervical culture for chlamydia has a sensitivity of only 77% to 84%, urine-based tests have a sensitivity of 88% to 95%, and vaginal swab–based tests have a sensitivity of 91% to 93%. Furthermore, urine-based and vaginal swab–based tests for both organisms have specificities of 100%.[8-16] Therefore, in healthy, nonpregnant adolescents being evaluated in the ED for possible PID, a speculum examination can be avoided in most cases. A key exception to this is the patient with profuse vaginal bleeding.

A variety of symptoms, signs, and laboratory values support the diagnosis of PID (see Table 70–1). None of these criteria requires the use of a speculum. The presence of a cervical discharge is not necessary for the diagnosis; the presence of a mucopurulent discharge in the vagina, whether originating from the cervix or the vagina, is an adequate supportive finding. Most patients with PID have either a mucopurulent discharge or evidence of white blood cells (WBCs) on microscopic evaluation of a saline preparation of vaginal fluid; if neither of these findings is present, another explanation for the patient's findings should be sought. Transvaginal ultrasound may be helpful in diagnosing some patients.[17]

Patients with suspected PID should have urine or vaginal swabs sent for detection of *N. gonorrhoeae* or *C. trachomatis*. Vaginal swabs should be sent for a wet preparation to evaluate for *Trichomonas vaginalis* and a Gram stain. To obtain adequate specimens, two Dacron-tipped specimen swabs should be simultaneously inserted about 1 inch into the vagina, and remain for approximately 30 seconds. In addition, a complete blood count, erythrocyte sedimentation rate, and C-reactive protein level can all be helpful in making the diagnosis. Depending on the local prevalence of syphilis, a rapid plasma reagin test may be done as well.

Important Clinical Features and Considerations

An important consideration for the patient diagnosed with PID is the concern for the presence of a TOA, which is the most serious acute complication of PID. Studies suggest that the prevalence of TOA among hospitalized patients may approach 20%, and that it is difficult to assess clinically whether or not a patient has a TOA.[18-20] Based on these findings, some adolescent experts recommend pelvic ultrasound (the most specific and sensitive test for TOA) for all patients diagnosed with PID. To date, there are no clear guidelines to indicate which patients are at highest risk of TOA. A review of the literature suggests that, at a minimum, ultrasound should be obtained on patients in whom other diagnoses cannot be excluded (such as appendicitis), patients who are ill appearing or have elevated inflammatory markers, or patients who are not responding to therapy. Decisions about imaging should be based on the individual patient, and should take into account the patient's ability to follow up with a health care provider within a few days.

Perihepatitis (Fitz-Hugh–Curtis syndrome) is another complication of salpingitis. Signs and symptoms include right upper quadrant pain and tenderness, fever, nausea, and vomiting. Signs and symptoms of salpingitis are usually present, but not in all cases.

The ED physician should remember to keep PID on the differential diagnosis list of any adolescent female presenting with abdominal pain; it is important to treat mild disease, so therapy should be instituted even if the diagnosis is not certain. One common misperception is that patients with cervicitis (discussed later) can have abdominal pain; this is generally not the case, so if a patient with vaginal discharge also has abdominal pain that is not explained by an additional diagnosis, the patient should be treated for PID rather than cervicitis. Other complications of PID include ectopic pregnancy, infertility, recurrent and chronic PID, chronic abdominal pain, and pelvic adhesions.

Management

Any patient meeting the minimum criteria for the diagnosis of PID (see Table 70–1), if no other diagnosis is apparent, should be treated empirically (Table 70–2). Up-to-date treatment recommendations can be found on the CDC website (*http://www.cdc.gov/STD/*). Of note, single-dose therapy of azithromycin has not been shown to be adequate treatment for PID.[3] The decision about whether or not to admit a patient for inpatient therapy can be difficult. The CDC recommends inpatient treatment for patients in whom surgical emergen-

cies cannot be excluded; for pregnant patients; for patients not responding to oral therapy or who are unable to follow or tolerate an outpatient oral regimen; for patients with severe illness, nausea and vomiting, or high fever; and for patients with TOA. In addition, many adolescent experts recommend hospitalizing patients who are 14 years old or younger and patients for whom follow-up within 72 hours cannot be arranged. One randomized, controlled trial comparing inpatient to outpatient therapy for mild to moderate PID has been performed,[21] which concluded that there was no difference in reproductive outcomes between women treated as inpatients compared with those treated as outpatients. However, that trial did not involve many adolescents, making it difficult to generalize the results to that population. Any patient treated as an outpatient should have clinical follow up 3 days after beginning treatment. For adolescents, who may have issues with particular compliance or access to health care, it is important to ensure that the prescribed regimen will be completed and that follow-up can be arranged. In addition, male sex partners should be treated if they have had sexual contact with the patient within 60 days of the onset of symptoms. Options for partner treatment include self-referral and patient-delivered treatment.

When determining the best treatment strategy for the adolescent with PID, it is important to keep issues of confidentiality in mind. Patients under the age of 18 years are able to seek care for treatment of sexually transmitted diseases without parental consent.[22] It is important to engage the adolescent in a discussion about disclosing the diagnosis, and, whenever possible, it is helpful to involve the parent in treatment plans in order to improve compliance and follow-up. However, the patient has the right to confidential treatment, although some states allow the physician to notify the patient's parents.[23] If the patient chooses not to inform a parent, it can be helpful to obtain private numbers (such as a cell phone or beeper number) in order to communicate culture results or to follow up the patient's clinical status.

Summary

PID is a difficult clinical diagnosis. It is important to consider the diagnosis of PID in any adolescent patient at risk for an STI in whom the minimum clinical criteria are met. All patients diagnosed with PID who are treated on an outpatient basis should have follow-up arranged within 72 hours. Adolescents may require more intensive education and follow-up than adult patients. Therefore, treatment decisions should be individualized and should take into account follow-up options, support systems at home, and the resources available on an outpatient or inpatient basis.

Cervicitis

Gonorrhea and chlamydia are among the most frequently reported infectious diseases in the United States. In fact, chlamydia is the most commonly reported bacterial STI, with 834,555 cases reported in 2002[24]; because patients are often not tested before being treated, and because underreporting remains a problem, the CDC estimates that 2.8 million Americans are infected with chlamydia each year. The CDC estimates that there are approximately 700,000 people newly infected with gonorrhea yearly.[25] While both of these infections are often asymptomatic, they can both present with mucopurulent cervicitis (MPC).

Table 70–2	Treatment of Pelvic Inflammatory Disease
Parenteral Regimen A*	**Outpatient Regimen A**
Cefotetan 2 g IV q12h *or*	Ofloxacin[†] 400 mg orally bid × 14 days *or*
Cefoxitin 2 g IV q6h	Levofloxacin[†] 500 mg orally qd × 14 days
Plus	*With or without*
Doxycycline 100 mg orally q12h	Metronidazole 500 mg orally bid × 14 days
Parenteral Regimen B	**Outpatient Regimen B**
Clindamycin 900 mg IV q8h	Ceftriaxone 250 mg IM once *or*
Plus	Cefoxitin 2 g IM once *and* probenecid 1 g orally once
Gentamicin loading dose IV or IM (2 mg/kg) followed by a maintenance dose (1.5 mg/kg) q8h	*Plus* Doxycycline 100 mg orally bid × 14 days
	With or without Metronidazole 500 mg orally bid × 14 days

*Parenteral therapy can be discontinued 24 hours after clinical improvement, and the patient should complete a 14-day course of doxycycline (100 mg twice daily). When tubo-ovarian abscess is present, clindamycin or metronidazole is used with doxycyline to provide more effective anaerobic coverage.
†Fluoroquinolones are not recommended for use in patients younger than 18 years old; however, no joint damage has been observed in patients treated with prolonged courses of ciprofloxacin, so the CDC has stated that children who weigh more than 45 kg can be treated with any regimen.
Abbreviations: IM, intramuscularly; IV, intravenously.
From Centers for Disease Control and Prevention: Sexually transmitted diseases treatment guidelines—2006. MMWR Recomm Rep 55(RR-11):1–100, 2006.

Clinical Presentation

MPC is characterized by a purulent endocervical discharge, which is often noted by the patient as a thick vaginal discharge. Patients with uncomplicated lower genital tract infection will not have abdominal pain or adnexal or cervical motion tenderness; conversely, patients who present only with vaginal discharge may have subclinical upper genital tract infection.[26,27] Patients may complain of dyspareunia or postcoital spotting. Differential diagnoses to consider for the patient presenting with vaginal discharge include vaginitis (described later); cervicitis due to organisms other than *N. gonorrhoeae* and *C. trachomatis,* such as Candida species or herpes simplex virus; foreign body; and physiologic discharge. Laboratory testing for patients with vaginal discharge should include testing for *N. gonorrhoeae* and *C. trachomatis.* As mentioned earlier, vaginal swab–based and urine-based tests are sensitive and specific, and may obviate the need for a speculum examination in the adolescent patient. Additional testing includes vaginal swabs for Gram stain and wet preparation, as described previously. Recent studies suggest that women with vaginal polymorphonuclear cells (PMNs) noted on examination of their vaginal discharge are more likely to have subclinical PID; therefore, the finding of many PMNs on Gram stain may alter treatment.[26,27] However, there are no clear guidelines as to whether or not these women need to be treated similarly to patients with clinical PID.

The diagnosis of cervicitis is fairly straightforward, and should be considered in any patient with an abnormal vaginal discharge. Although it can be difficult to distinguish with certainty between cervicitis and vaginitis without a speculum examination, because most etiologies of vaginitis can be diagnosed quickly with laboratory tests (as described later) the clinician can usually determine which patients are likely to benefit from empirical treatment for infection with *N. gonorrhoeae* and *C. trachomatis.* In many cases of MPC, neither organism is identified.

Other infections in females caused by *N. gonorrhoeae* include urethritis, which is characterized by dysuria, urinary frequency, exudate from the urethra or periurethral glands, and suprapubic pain; bartholinitis and bartholin gland abscess; pharyngitis, which usually resolves spontaneously; rectal infection; conjunctivitis; and otitis externa. Although pharyngeal infection is generally self-limited, patients should be treated to limit the spread of the organism and to limit the possibility of dissemination.[28] Patients with gonorrheal infection can also develop disseminated disease, characterized by arthritis/arthralgia, tenosynovitis, and dermatitis. Other sites of disseminated disease include perihepatitis, meningitis, myopericarditis, endocarditis, osteomyelitis, and pneumonia. *C. trachomatis* can also cause urethritis, which is often asymptomatic but can be associated with dysuria. Newborns of infected mothers are at risk for ophthalmia neonatorum, scalp abscess at the site of fetal monitors, rhinitis, pneumonia, and anorectal infections.

Management

The CDC recommends that patients suspected of being infected with *N. gonorrhoeae* and *C. trachomatis* should be treated empirically if the prevalence of these infections is high in the patient population, and if the patient might be difficult to locate for treatment after test results are available.

Table 70–3	Treatment of Cervicitis
Chlamydial Infection	**Gonococcal Infection**
Azithromycin 1 g orally once *or* Doxycycline 100 mg orally bid × 7 days	Cefixime 400 mg orally once *or* Ceftriaxone 125 mg intramuscularly once *or* Ofloxacin 400 mg orally once *or* Levofloxacin 250 mg orally once
Erythromycin base 500 mg orally qid × 7 days Erythromycin ethylsuccinate 800 mg orally qid × 7 days Ofloxacin* 300 mg orally bid × 7 days Levofloxacin* 500 mg orally qd × 7 days	Treatment for chlamydia if chlamydia infection not ruled out

*For quinolones, children who weigh more than 45 kg can be treated with any regimen recommended for adults.
From Centers for Disease Control and Prevention: Sexually transmitted diseases treatment guidelines—2006. MMWR Recomm Rep 55(RR-11):1–100, 2006.

For most adolescents, empirical treatment is warranted because of the difficulty with locating teenagers after an ED visit combined with potential problems with maintaining confidentiality once the patient has left the ED.

Patients should be treated for both gonorrhea and chlamydia infections (Table 70–3). For chlamydial infection, single-dose azithromycin therapy has been shown in randomized, controlled trials to be equally efficacious when compared with 7 days of doxycycline.[29] Although treatment with azithromycin is more expensive, this should be weighed against the benefit of providing complete treatment during the ED visit. Ofloxacin is also efficacious, but is not recommended as first-line therapy because of increased cost. Although erythromycin is an alternative treatment, it is not as effective as the others and the gastrointestinal side effects can affect compliance. In order to maximize compliance, particularly with the adolescent population, it can be useful to dispense the entire treatment course at the time of the ED visit and to observe the first dose. All sex partners within 60 days should be treated, and the most recent sex partner should be evaluated even if the most recent contact was more than 60 days prior to the patient's presentation. Patients should abstain from sexual intercourse until 7 days after the onset of treatment. Currently, there is no need for a patient to be retested once therapy is complete. For pregnant patients, azithromycin is thought to be safe and effective.

The preferred treatment for gonococcal infection is ceftriaxone.[30] Strains of *N. gonorrhoeae* resistant to quinolones are becoming more common. In fact, the CDC recommends that patients with gonorrhea who live in Hawaii and California not be treated with a quinolone; in addition, there have been recent increases in fluoroquinolone-resistant gonococci in Massachusetts, Michigan, New York City, and Seattle.[31] In areas where resistance is a concern, ceftriaxone should be used as primary therapy. With the exception of cefixime, which at present is available sporadically and only as an oral suspension, other oral cephalosporin regimens have not been shown to be effective for the treatment of *N. gonorrhoeae.* Similarly, a 1-g dose of azithromycin is also not effective;

although a 2-g dose of azithromycin is effective, due to cost and a high frequency of gastrointestinal side effects it is also not a recommended treatment.[3] Pregnant patients can be treated with ceftriaxone or spectinomycin intramuscularly (a single 2-g dose).

Patients with isolated cervicitis can be treated as outpatients, with follow-up within 5 to 7 days to assess for resolution of symptoms. Patients being treated for cervicitis should be counseled about the signs and symptoms of PID. In addition, patients with persistent symptoms after appropriate therapy should be rescreened for infection, as in most situations this represents a new infection rather than treatment failure. Some experts recommend that adolescents be screened every 3 to 4 months, even if asymptomatic, because of the risk of acquiring a new chlamydia infection. For the treatment of sex partners, one study suggests that patient-delivered treatment is comparable to self-referral, and so should be considered for some patients.[32]

Vaginitis

The three most common infectious causes of vaginitis are *Candida albicans, Trichomonas vaginalis,* and bacterial vaginosis (BV). Herpes simplex virus can also cause vaginitis; it is discussed in detail later. It is estimated that up to 75% of women will experience at least one episode of vulvovaginal candidiasis (VVC) in their lifetimes.[33] Patients at particularly high risk include pregnant women, patients using corticosteroids or broad-spectrum antibiotics, and patients with diabetes mellitus. Although VVC is generally due to overgrowth of a patient's own organisms, the infection can be sexually transmitted. Approximately 15% of asymptomatic women may harbor Candida species during their reproductive years.[34] *T. vaginalis* is the most common treatable STI. The CDC estimates there are approximately 7.4 million new cases of trichomoniasis diagnosed each year in women and men.[35] Women can contract trichomoniasis from penis-vagina contact or from vulva-vulva contact; men usually contract trichomoniasis from infected women.[36]

BV is the most common cause of vaginal discharge in women of childbearing age, and is diagnosed in approximately 15% of pregnant women in the United States.[37] The infection is characterized by an overgrowth of predominantly anaerobic organisms (*Gardnerella vaginalis, Mycoplasma hominis,* and Prevotella and Mobiluncus species), which replace the normal lactobacilli and increase the vaginal pH from less than 4.5 to as high as 7.0. It is more common in black women, in those who smoke, and in those who use intrauterine devices. Although sexual activity, particularly with multiple partners, is a risk factor for BV, it is unclear what role sexual activity plays in acquiring the infection. Studies suggest that exposure to a new sexual partner is a more important risk factor than frequency of sexual encounters[38,39]; however, questions remain about the role of sexual activity in the acquisition of BV, particularly because partner treatment shows no benefit. It is thought that frequent episodes of BV are more likely to be relapsed infections rather than reinfection.[39]

Clinical Presentation

Women with vaginitis generally present with some combination of vulvar irritation and itching, edema or erythema of the genitalia, and excessive or malodorous vaginal discharge. VVC, trichomoniasis, and BV all have specific clinical characteristics that can help narrow the differential diagnosis and guide laboratory evaluation (Table 70–4). Thick, curdy discharge, the classic description of vaginal discharge caused by VVC, is a specific but not very sensitive finding.[33] The classic frothy yellow discharge occurs in approximately 10% to 30% of women with Trichomonas.[36] Studies suggest that trichomoniasis infection is generally not associated with lower abdominal pain and dysuria.[40] BV is asymptomatic in up to 50% of infected women; symptomatic women generally present with a homogeneous white discharge without signs of inflammation.[37]

Adolescents presenting with an abnormal vaginal discharge should have a Gram stain of the vaginal discharge as

Table 70–4	Common Causes of Vaginitis		
Etiology	**Vulvovaginal Candidiasis**	**Trichomoniasis**	**Bacterial Vaginosis**
Symptoms/Signs	Vulvar itching and soreness Vaginal discharge Superficial dyspareunia Vulvar erythema, edema Fissures, excoriations Satellite lesions	Yellow or purulent vaginal discharge Vulvar itching Vulvar erythema Vaginal erythema	Vaginal discharge No signs of inflammation
Diagnosis	Saline microscopy 10% KOH microscopy Gram stain Culture if previously treated, question about species	Saline microscopy Rapid test (some labs) Culture pH > 4.5	Amsel criteria (at least 3) • homogeneous, white d/c • clue cells • fishy odor with 10% KOH • pH > 4.5
Treatment	Fluconazole 150 mg orally once (not in pregnant patients) *or* Multiple topical azoles; 1-, 3-, and 7-day treatment options	Metronidazole 2 g once *or* Metronidazole 500 mg bid × 7 days	Metronidazole 500 mg orally bid × 7 days *or* Metronidazole gel 0.75%, one full applicator (5 g) intravaginally qd × 5 days *or* Clindamycin cream 2%, one full applicator (5 g) intravaginally at bedtime for 7 days
Partner Treatment	No, unless partner symptomatic	Yes	No

well as microscopy to help distinguish between the likely causative agents. Symptoms alone should not be used to guide therapy.[41] Gram stain has a sensitivity of 65% for detecting pseudohyphae; microscopy with 10% potassium hydroxide (KOH) has a sensitivity of 70%.[34] Of note, KOH is toxic to *T. vaginalis*, so additional microscopy with saline is necessary to detect trichomonads. The saline wet preparation has a sensitivity of 60% to 80% for detecting trichomoniasis. The use of spun urine can improve the detection of *T. vaginalis* in patients with suspected trichomoniasis who have negative wet preparations,[42] and some laboratories can perform a rapid nucleic acid detection test. If necessary, culture for *T. vaginalis* can be performed, which has a sensitivity of approximately 95%.[36] Determining the pH of the vaginal fluid can also be helpful, as both trichomoniasis and BV are associated with a pH greater than 4.5. Culture of vaginal discharge is generally not helpful, with the exception of cases of recurrent VVC or to definitively diagnose a suspected case of trichomoniasis in the setting of a negative wet preparation.

BV can be diagnosed using clinical criteria (proposed by Amsel et al.)[43] or by Gram stain (using a scoring system introduced by Nugent et al.).[44] The two diagnostic methods have been shown to be relatively similar; in a multicenter study comparing Gram stains of vaginal smears to the standard criteria of Amsel et al. for the diagnosis of BV, the sensitivity of the Gram stain method was 89%, with a specificity of 83%.[45] Although the Gram stain method is more objective, the clinical criteria are more practical in many settings. The clinical criteria require three of the following: (1) a homogeneous, white, noninflammatory discharge that smoothly coats the vaginal walls, (2) the presence of clue cells on microscopic examination (clue cells are irregularly bordered squamous epithelial cells whose cell outlines are obliterated by sheets of small bacteria; they are seen in saline, not KOH, preparations), (3) a vaginal fluid pH of greater than 4.5, and (4) a fishy odor of vaginal discharge before or after addition of 10% KOH. Definitive diagnosis can be made by Gram stain demonstrating few or no lactobacilli with a predominance of *Gardnerella vaginalis* plus other organisms resembling gram-negative Bacteroides species, anaerobic gram-positive cocci, or curved rods.

The differential diagnosis for patients with vaginitis includes urinary tract infection and cervicitis, as well as noninfectious irritation of the vulva (e.g., mechanical, chemical, or allergic). In patients at risk for an STI who are diagnosed with vaginitis, it is important to consider concomitant treatment for cervicitis after specimens are sent for *N. gonorrhoeae* and *C. trachomatis*. If these specimens can be obtained without a speculum examination (i.e., urine or vaginal swab), there is generally no indication for a speculum examination in adolescents with vaginitis.[46]

Important Clinical Features and Considerations

It is important to consider the diagnosis of VVC in any patient with vaginal discharge and irritation, even if the discharge is not described as the "classic" thick, curdy discharge. Patients who have four or more episodes of VVC a year are defined as having recurrent VVC; the pathogenesis of this is not well understood, and most women with recurrent VVC do not have an apparent predisposing condition. Vaginal cultures should be obtained in these patients to identify unusual

species.[3,34] Patients can also present with severe VVC, characterized by extensive vulvar erythema, edema, excoriation, and fissure formation.[3] VVC during pregnancy is associated with an increased risk of neonatal oral thrush. Other potential complications of vaginitis include recurrent infections as well as pregnancy-related complications, such as chorioamnionitis, particularly with trichomonas and BV. BV is also associated with premature rupture of membranes, preterm labor, and postpartum endometritis. Finally, BV is associated with an increased risk of infection with *N. gonorrhoeae* and *C. trachomatis*, as well as upper genital tract infection.[47,48]

Patients who are at risk for an STI can present with more than one infection, so all causes of vaginitis should be considered for every sexually active adolescent. It is possible for patients to be diagnosed with any combination of VVC, trichomoniasis, and BV; therefore, regardless of the characteristics of the vaginal discharge, laboratory evaluation for all three infections should be included as standard workup for the sexually active adolescent presenting with vaginal discharge.

Management

Patients with VVC can be treated either orally, with a single dose of fluconazole,[49] or with a variety of topical azole therapies (see Table 70–4). For patients with recurrent VVC, although each individual episode usually responds well to short-term azole therapy, experts generally recommend a longer course of topical therapy (7 to 14 days) or, if treating orally, repeating a 150-mg dose of fluconozole on day 3. Patients with recurrent VVC benefit from suppressive maintenance therapy, which is usually continued for 6 months. Similarly, patients with severe VVC should also be treated with a 7- to 14-day course of topical therapy or two doses of oral fluconazole, 72 hours apart.

Infection with *T. vaginalis* is treated with metronidazole, either as a single dose or a 7-day course. Because of compliance issues, most adolescents should be treated with the single dose. Metronidazole gel is not recommended because, as a topical preparation, it is unlikely to achieve therapeutic levels in the urethra or perivaginal glands.[3] Some strains of *T. vaginalis* have decreased susceptibility to metronidazole; however, these strains usually respond to higher doses, so patients who remain symptomatic after either regimen should be treated with 500 mg twice a day for 7 days. A third course of antibiotics, using 2 g daily for 3 to 5 days, can also be used. If the patient remains symptomatic after three courses of metronidazole, the CDC recommends consultation with a specialist; CDC specialists can be reached by telephone (770-488-4115).

All women with symptomatic BV should be treated, with the goal of relieving vaginal symptoms and signs of infection and to reduce the risk for other infections, such as human immunodeficiency virus (HIV) and PID.[38] In the pregnant patient, treatment of BV is particularly important. Recommended treatment for BV is with oral metronidazole for 7 days, intravaginal metronidazole gel, or intravaginal clindamycin cream; the clindamycin cream is thought to be less effective than the metronidazole regimens. Other alternative treatments include metronidazole in a single 2-g dose and oral clindamycin for 7 days; these regimens are also less effective than the other metronidazole regimens. Intravaginal preparations are not recommended for pregnant patients.

Patients with isolated vaginitis generally do very well with appropriate therapy. Follow-up for uncomplicated VVC, trichomonas, and BV is unnecessary for patients unless symptoms persist. Nucleic acid amplification tests are under development for *Trichomonas,* which may in the future aid in diagnosis. BV is a difficult diagnosis, particularly in the acute care setting; if uncertainty about the diagnosis exists and the patient is not pregnant, it is appropriate to arrange follow-up without providing treatment.

Genital Ulcers

Herpes Genitalis

Genital herpes, caused by either herpes simplex virus type 1 (HSV-1) or type 2 (HSV-2), is the second most prevalent STD in the United States, affecting at least 50 million people.[50] HSV-2 is believed to be the most common cause of genital herpes, although recent studies suggest that HSV-1 may account for more than the 30% of infections previously attributed to HSV-2, particularly in certain populations. Specifically, sexually acquired HSV-1 is more common in younger age groups, in women, and in men who have sex with men.[51] The two strains of herpesvirus have very different natural histories, so determining the particular type of infection can be important for treatment and counseling.[52] HSV initially causes epithelial infection, and then establishes latency in sacral neuronal ganglia. Once latency is established, there is no cure for the disease, and reactivation of the virus causes recurrent disease.

CLINICAL PRESENTATION

Patients with either type of HSV usually present with multiple painful 1- to 2-mm vesicles on an erythematous base. The eruption of ulcers is often preceded by paresthesias or burning sensations in the genital area. The early lesions then erode to become shallow ulcers, and may coalesce. Patients are at risk for secondary infection as well. Primary infections tend to be more severe than recurrences, and patients with a primary infection can also present with systemic symptoms such as fever, malaise, and myalgias. In addition, patients may complain of dysuria, urinary retention, and dyspareunia. Systemic symptoms peak within 3 to 4 days and then improve; pain and irritation are maximal between days 7 and 11, and lesions can persist for about 2 weeks. The total duration of a primary episode, including healing, is about 3 weeks. In contrast, recurrent infections generally present with fewer lesions that are smaller in size, with a total duration from onset to resolution of about 1 week. After the first year, recurrences tend to decrease in frequency, and recurrence of disease caused by HSV-1 is much less common than recurrence of disease caused by HSV-2. In fact, some studies suggest that the recurrence rate of HSV-1 is just 20% of the rate of HSV-2, and that recurrence after the first year with HSV-1 is very uncommon.[52]

The differential diagnosis of patients presenting with genital ulcers includes early syphilis, chancroid, lymphogranuloma venereum (LGV), contact dermatitis, molluscum contagiosum, and genital lesions of Behçet's syndrome.

Because the prognoses for infection with HSV-1 and HSV-2 differ dramatically, most experts recommend testing both to confirm the diagnosis of herpes genitalis and to identify the viral serotype. Multiple testing strategies for HSV exist.[53,54]

Isolation of HSV in cell culture is the preferred test, although the sensitivity of culture declines as lesions begin to heal. A culture specimen can be obtained when intact vesicles are present by aspirating the vesicle fluid using a fine-gauge needle, or unroofing a vesicle and swabbing the fluid using a cotton or Dacron swab. If pustules are present, a specimen can be obtained by unroofing the pustule, washing away purulent material with sterile saline, and swabbing the base of the lesion. For ruptured vesicles or ulcers, or for crusted lesions, a specimen can be obtained by washing away any necrotic material with sterile saline and swabbing the base of the lesion. Cervical Papanicolaou smears and Tzanck tests of genital lesions are both insensitive (30% to 70%) and nonspecific, and so should not be used routinely. Immunfluorescence techniques can differentiate between the two serotypes, and are very sensitive and specific, and rapid. Because of the possibility of false-positive tests, repeat or confirmatory testing (with an immunoblot assay) may be indicated in some patients.[53]

Although the classic presentation of herpes genitalis is unmistakable, many patients present with less classic symptoms. Therefore, it is important to consider other causes of genital ulcers in most patients. Complications of infection with HSV include significant psychological distress; local complications such as secondary bacterial infection, phimosis, labial adhesions, urinary retention, and constipation; proctitis, particularly in men who have sex with men; herpes keratitis; and encephalitis and meningitis. Furthermore, infants born to women with genital herpes infection are at risk for neonatal infection.

MANAGEMENT

Sitz baths or tap water compresses can provide some symptomatic relief, and petroleum jelly may also relieve some discomfort from crusting and fissuring. Three systemic antiviral medications have been shown in randomized, controlled trials to provide clinical benefit for first clinical episodes, for recurrent episodes, and as suppressive therapy: acyclovir, valacyclovir, and famciclovir.[55-58] Topical antiviral therapy has little proven benefit and is not recommended.[3] For the first clinical episode, antivirals used within 6 days of the onset of lesions have been shown to shorten viral shedding by 10 days, to dramatically reduce the number of new lesions, to decrease pain by about 25%, and to reduce time to healing by 4 to 9 days. Episodic therapy for recurrences reduces viral shedding and healing time by about 1 day; a more dramatic effect in healing time has been noted when patients initiate therapy early in the recurrence. In order to be effective, therapy should begin within 1 day of lesion onset. Suppressive therapy can reduce the frequency of recurrent infections by more than 75% in patients with six or more recurrences per year.[59,60] All three medications have an excellent safety profile and are well tolerated. For patients with severe disease or complications that require hospitalization, such as disseminated infection, pneumonitis, hepatitis, encephalitis, or meningitis, intravenous acyclovir should be used[3] (Table 70–5).

The safety of systemic acyclovir, valacyclovir, and famciclovir therapy in pregnant patients has not been well established, although studies suggest that there is not an increased risk for major birth defects compared with the general population for women exposed to acyclovir during the first

Table 70–5	Treatment for Herpes Genitalis
First Clinical Episode Treat for 7–10 days, longer if healing incomplete	Acyclovir 400 mg orally tid *or* Acyclovir 200 mg orally 5 times a day *or* Famciclovir 250 mg orally tid *or* Valacyclovir 1 g orally bid
Recurrent Episodes Treat for 5 days, unless using valacyclovir 500 mg orally twice a day; then 3 days is sufficient	Acyclovir 400 mg orally tid *or* Acyclovir 200 mg orally 5 times a day *or* Acyclovir 800 mg orally bid *or* Famciclovir 125 mg orally bid *or* Valacyclovir 500 mg orally bid *or* Valacyclovir 1 g orally qd
Suppressive Therapy Valacyclovir 500 mg regimen may be less effective than the other regimens in patients with ≥10 episodes per year	Acyclovir 400 mg orally bid *or* Famciclovir 250 mg orally bid *or* Valacyclovir 500 mg orally qd *or* Valacyclovir 1 g orally qd

From Centers for Disease Control and Prevention: Sexually transmitted diseases treatment guidelines—2006. MMWR Recomm Rep 55(RR-11):1–100, 2006.

trimester. Some experts recommend acyclovir therapy, particularly late in pregnancy, in order to reduce the risk of recurrences.

Approximately 90% of patients with HSV-2 will experience at least one recurrence; up to 40% can have at least six recurrences in the first year. Recurrence with HSV-1 infection is much less likely. Patients should refrain from sexual intercourse until the lesions are healed, and should be counseled that transmission can occur even in the absence of symptoms. Counseling about the disease is an important aspect of treatment, although many patients benefit more from counseling once the acute episode has resolved. The CDC has a National STD/HIV Hotline (800-227-8922), and a useful website is *http://www.ashastd.org*. Follow-up in 1 week is recommended, particularly to reinforce the implications of the diagnosis and to address psychological concerns. Vaccines for HSV are currently under development.[61]

Syphilis

Syphilis, a systemic disease caused by *Treponema pallidum*, is becoming much less common in the United States, due at least in part to the fact that in 1998 the CDC launched a national plan to eliminate the disease. However, despite an 80% decrease in the number of cases of syphilis reported to the CDC since 1990, syphilis continues to be among the top 10 reportable diseases, and in 2000 affected almost 6000 people.[62] In adolescents, syphilis is more common among females. The disease in adolescents has been linked to cocaine use and drug-related sexual behavior. Real and perceived barriers to health care access likely also contribute to the rate of syphilis in this population due to delayed treatment and prolonged infectivity.[63]

CLINICAL PRESENTATION

Syphilis can be divided into three stages: primary, secondary, and tertiary. In addition, latent infections (which can be early or late) are detected by serology in the absence of clinical symptoms. Primary syphilis presents with an ulcer or chancre at the infection site. The site of infection is usually the ano-

genital area or the mouth; breasts and fingers are less common sites. In fact, 95% of chancres are located on the external genitalia. Single lesions are common, but multiple lesions do occur; lesions that touch each other across folds of skin are referred to as "kissing lesions." The chancre is usually 1 to 2 cm in diameter, and begins as a painless papule that erodes into an indurated, painless ulcer. Regional firm, nontender lymphadenopathy can accompany the lesion.

Secondary syphilis develops about 4 to 10 weeks after the chancre, and is characterized most commonly by a general skin eruption with a predilection for the palms and soles. The eruption involves mucous membranes, is bilateral and symmetric, and tends to follow lines of cleavage. Individual lesions are sharply demarcated, up to 2 cm in diameter, and have a reddish brown hue. The rash is usually macular, papular, or papulosquamous; vesicular and pustular rashes are rare. The eruption may last anywhere from several weeks to up to a year. Other manifestations of secondary syphilis include general or regional lymphadenopathy (nonpainful, rubbery, discrete nodes) and a flulike syndrome, most often with sore throat and malaise but also with headaches, lacrimation, nasal discharge, arthralgias, weight loss, and fever. Other rare manifestations of secondary syphilis include syphilis alopecia (moth-eaten appearance of the scalp and eyebrows), arthritis or bursitis, hepatitis, iritis and anterior uveitis, and glomerulonephritis.

Tertiary syphilis, which occurs 2 to 10 years after initial exposure in untreated patients, is rare in adolescents. Tertiary syphilis presents with cardiovascular symptoms (usually 10 to 30 years after exposure) and with gummas, which are granulomatous lesions that involve skin, soft tissue, viscera, or bones. The lesions are few in number, asymmetric, and not contagious.

Neurosyphilis is also rare in adolescents; most cases in this age group are asymptomatic or present as acute syphilitic meningitis. Acute syphilitic meningitis has signs and symptoms similar to those of other causes of acute meningitis, including fever, headache, photophobia, and meningismus. Cranial nerve palsies are present in about 40% of cases.

DIAGNOSIS

The differential diagnosis of primary syphilis includes sexually transmitted causes of genital ulcers, such as herpes, chancroid, and LGV, as well as non–sexually transmitted causes of ulcers, including traumatic lesions, fixed drug reaction, Candida, Behçet's syndrome, psoriasis, lichen planus, and erythema multiforme. Also in the differential diagnosis is cancer, which is very rare in adolescents. Other etiologies with presentations similar to secondary syphilis include pityriasis rosea, drug eruptions, tinea versicolor, lupus erythematosus, scabies, pediculosis, rosacea, infectious mononucleosis, and condyloma acuminatum. Although the clinical history and appearance of the lesions can often distinguish these etiologies, serology tests for syphilis should be performed if there is any doubt about the diagnosis.

Darkfield microscopic examination and direct fluorescent antibody (DFA) tests of lesion exudate or tissue are the definitive methods for diagnosing primary syphilis, according to the CDC. Darkfield examination is simple and fairly reliable, with a sensitivity of 73% to 79%.[64] Some experts recommend repeating the examination on 3 separate days before determining that the test is negative. Failure to detect the organism using this technique does not ensure that the patient does not have syphilis; in addition, technical factors, such as too little or too much fluid on the slide, can affect the results. Darkfield microscopy should not be performed on samples of lesions on the mouth or anus, areas where nonpathogenic treponemes are often present. DFA is performed at some reference laboratories and some state health departments, and has a slightly better sensitivity than darkfield microscopy (73% to 100%).[64]

A presumptive diagnosis of syphilis can be made using two types of serologic tests: (1) nontreponemal tests, including the Venereal Disease Research Laboratory (VDRL) and the rapid plasma reagin (RPR) tests; and (2) treponemal tests, including the fluorescent treponemal antibody, absorbed (FTA-Abs) and the *T. palladium* particle agglutination (TP-PA) tests.[64,65] Nontreponemal tests are used for screening and to monitor therapy. The VDRL is the test of choice for evaluating for neurosyphilis, and has a slightly higher specificity when compared to the RPR (96% to 99% compared to 93% to 99%), resulting in fewer false-positive tests. However, the RPR has a slightly better sensitivity (86% compared to 78% for primary syphilis), and so is most often used for screening. Both tests have 100% sensitivity for secondary syphilis; the RPR is slightly more sensitive than the VDRL for detecting tertiary syphilis (73% vs. 71%) and latent syphilis (98% vs. 95%). Many disorders can result in false-positive nontreponemal tests, including acute infections (such as viral infections, chlamydial infections, Lyme disease, *Mycoplasma* infections, and nonsyphilitic spirochetal infections), autoimmune diseases, narcotic addiction, sarcoidosis, lymphoma, cirrhosis, and aging. Therefore, all positive nontreponemal tests need to be confirmed with a treponemal test.

Presumptive diagnosis of primary or secondary syphilis can be made based on a positive nontreponemal test with a titer of at least 1:8 (for primary syphilis) or a titer that rises more than two dilutions, combined with a positive treponemal test. Adolescents with a positive darkfield examination should be treated, as well as adolescents with a typical lesion and a positive serologic test. Routine lumbar puncture is not indicated for patients with primary syphilis; this test should be limited to patients with clinical signs and symptoms of neurologic involvement. Adolescents suspected of having secondary syphilis who have atypical findings or a nontreponemal titer of less than 1:16 should have a second nontreponemal test and a treponemal test performed. The titer results of an RPR and a VDRL cannot be compared.

The diagnosis of neurosyphilis can be difficult, because although the cerebrospinal fluid (CSF) VDRL is highly specific, it is somewhat insensitive (60% to 70%).[3,64] Other laboratory findings in neurosyphilis include an elevated CSF leukocyte count (>5 WBCs/mm^3) and increased CSF protein. The CSF FTA-Abs is less specific than the CSF VDRL, but is much more sensitive; some experts believe that a negative CSF FTA-Abs excludes neurosyphilis. In addition to patients with neurologic symptoms, evaluation for neurosyphilis should be performed in patients with ophthalmologic symptoms (e.g., uveitis), in patients who have treatment failure, in patients who have serum nontreponemal test titers of ≥1:32 unless disease duration is known to be less than 1 year, and in patients in whom nonpenicillin therapy is planned, unless disease duration is known to be less than 1 year.

If latent syphilis is a concern, both an RPR/VDRL and an FTA-Abs test should be performed, because the nontreponemal tests have a sensitivity of about 70%. The adolescent should be treated if the FTA-Abs is positive and there is no documentation of prior treatment.

The diagnosis of syphilis should be considered in any sexually active patient with a genital ulcer or a generalized rash. The clinical presentation of syphilis can manifest in many different ways, and can mimic other diagnoses such as pityriasis rosea. One of the most difficult aspects of diagnosing syphilis is interpreting the various serologic tests. As mentioned earlier, many other disorders can result in a false-positive nontreponemal test. False-negative nontreponemal tests can occur in early or late syphilis. False-negative and false-positive treponemal tests are rare. However, both types of tests can be negative if sexual contact with an infected individual occurred within the preceding 90 days. Most treated patients continue to have positive treponemal tests for life; persistently positive nontreponemal tests usually indicate inadequately treated disease. The complications of syphilis, which result from untreated early disease, can be prevented with timely therapy.

MANAGEMENT

The treatment of choice for syphilis is penicillin G, administered parenterally (Table 70-6). Penicillin is the only proven therapy for neurosyphilis and syphilis during pregnancy. Penicillin-allergic patients in these categories should undergo desensitization prior to treatment. Although there are some data indicating that oral azithromycin may prove to be an effective therapy, currently that drug is not recommended.[66]

The Jarisch-Herxheimer reaction occurs within 2 hours after treatment in 50% of patients with primary syphilis, 90% of patients with secondary syphilis, and 25% of patients with early latent syphilis. Fever and chills, myalgias, headache, elevated neutrophil count, and tachycardia characterize the reaction. The symptoms last 12 to 24 hours, and treatment is reassurance, bed rest, and antipyretics. The reaction can produce uterine contractions in pregnant women; however, this is not a contraindication to treatment.[3]

Syphilis is spread from person to person only when mucocutaneous lesions are present, which are rare after 1 year of infection. However, anyone who has been exposed sexually to a patient with syphilis should be evaluated. Patients exposed to someone with primary, secondary, or latent syphilis within the last 90 days should be treated presumptively; if exposure occurred more than 90 days ago but follow-up is uncertain, the patient should also be treated presumptively. For the purposes of partner notification and presumptive treatment, patients with syphilis of unknown duration who have high nontreponemal serologic test titers (i.e., at least 1:32) can be considered to have early syphilis. However, the titer should not be used to differentiate early from late latent syphilis for the purposes of treatment. Long-term sex partners of patients with latent syphilis should be evaluated clinically and serologically; treatment can be based on the results of this evaluation.

Adolescents diagnosed with syphilis require close follow-up to monitor the results of therapy. Some experts recommend HIV testing for all patients diagnosed with syphilis. Consultation with an infectious disease expert should be considered.

Table 70–6	Treatment for Syphilis				
	Primary/Secondary	**Early Latent**	**Late Latent**	**Tertiary**	**Neurosyphilis**
Recommended	Benzathine PCN G 2.4 million units IM once	Benzathine PCN G 2.4 million units IM once	Benzathine PCN G 2.4 million units IM weekly × 3 doses	Benzathine PCN G 2.4 million units IM weekly × 3 doses	Aqueous PCN G 3–4 million units IV q4h × 10–14 days *or* Procaine PCN 2.4 units IM qd *plus* probenecid 500 mg orally qid × 10–14 days
Possible alternatives (nonpregnant patients)	Doxycycline 100 mg orally bid × 14 days *or* Tetracycline 500 mg qid × 14 days	Doxycycline 100 mg orally bid × 14 days *or* Tetracycline 500 mg qid × 14 days	Doxycycline 100 mg orally bid × 14 days *or* Tetracycline 500 mg qid × 14 days		Ceftriaxone 2 g qd × 10–14 days
Potentially effective (close follow-up necessary)	Ceftriaxone 1 g qd IM or IV × 10 days *or* Azithromycin 2 g orally once				

Abbreviations: IM, intramuscularly; IV, intravenously; PCN, penicillin.
From Centers for Disease Control and Prevention: Sexually transmitted diseases treatment guidelines—2006. MMWR Recomm Rep 55(RR-11):1–100, 2006.

Lymphogranuloma Venereum

LGV is rare in the United States; there were 113 known cases in 1997, although this number likely represents a falsely low prevalence due to underreporting and misdiagnosis. LGV is caused by serovars L1, L2, and L3 of *C. trachomatis*. The peak incidence of the disease is in people ages 15 to 40 years, and males account for about 75% of cases.

CLINICAL PRESENTATION

After an incubation period of 3 to 30 days, the primary stage of LGV is characterized by a small, painless papule at the site of the inoculation. The lesion may ulcerate, and is self-limiting. It is often not noticed by the patient. An associated mucopurulent discharge of the urethra or cervix can also be present. The secondary stage occurs several weeks later, and chiefly involves the inguinal lymph nodes; the anus or rectum can also be involved, particularly in women or in men who have sex with men. In women, the deep iliac or perirectal nodes can be involved, which may result in low back pain or abdominal pain. Painful regional adenopathy is the most common manifestation of secondary disease; nodes are typically enlarged and unilateral, and can become infected and develop necrotic abscesses. The characteristic bubo is produced when the lymph nodes become matted and fluctuant. The buboes may rupture in as many as one third of patients, but most buboes heal without problems. Most men present during this phase, but only one third of women do, since women tend not to develop inguinal lymphadenopthy. Patients may also complain of constitutional symptoms such as headache, fever, chills, and myalgias. The third phase is a genitoanorectal syndrome, which is uncommon but occurs more commonly in women who were asymptomatic earlier in the disease.[67]

Differential diagnosis considerations for a genital-inguinal lesion include syphilis, HSV, chancroid, granuloma inguinale, pyogenic infection, and cat-scratch fever. For patients with rectal fistulas, inflammatory bowel disease, chronic rectal infections such as gonorrhea and amebiasis, and granuloma inguinale should be considered. The diagnosis of LGV is made serologically and by excluding other causes of inguinal lymphadenopathy or genital ulcers.

Clinically, it can be difficult to distinguish LGV from chancroid. It is important to keep LGV in the differential diagnosis for patients presenting with genital ulcers or inguinal adenopathy, particularly if the patient has had sexual contact with a person in or from Asia or Africa, where the disease is much more common. Late-stage disease can be complicated by elephantiasis of the genitalia, rectal strictures, and rectal fissures.

MANAGEMENT

The preferred treatment is doxycycline 100 mg orally twice a day for 21 days. Alternatively, erythromycin base, 500 mg orally four times a day for 21 days, can be used. Buboes may require aspiration or incision and drainage to prevent the formation of inguinal/femoral ulcerations. Sexual contacts within 30 days before the onset of the patient's symptoms should be examined, tested for urethral or cervical chlamydial infection, and treated. Pregnant women should be treated with erythromycin.[3,67]

Treatment cures the infection and prevents ongoing tissue damage, although scarring can result from tissue reaction. Rectovaginal fistulas, bowel obstruction, and extensive genital destruction require surgical treatment. Patients should be followed clinically until signs and symptoms have resolved.

Chancroid

Chancroid is a genital ulcer infection caused by *Haemophilus ducreyi*. It is endemic in some parts of the United States, and occurs in discrete outbreaks as well. In 2000, 78 cases of chancroid were reported to the CDC; like LGV, however, chancroid is likely very underreported because of the difficulty of culturing the organism as well as the fact that the diagnosis is not often considered.[68] Using new DNA amplification methods, the CDC has identified this infection in cities where it was previously not diagnosed. About 10% of patients in the United States with chancroid are co-infected with *T. pallidum* or HSV, and chancroid is a cofactor for transmission of HIV.[3]

CLINICAL PRESENTATION

After an incubation period of 3 days to 2 weeks, a small inflammatory papule or pustule develops at the inoculation site. Within days the papule erodes to form a very painful, deep ulceration, usually 3 to 20 mm in diameter, that is soft, friable, and nonindurated. A foul-smelling, yellow-gray exudative covering is usually present, along with surrounding erythema. Men often have a single ulcer, while women often have several. Within several weeks, up to 60% of patients will develop unilateral, painful inguinal lymphadenopathy, which can develop into a suppurative bubo. Fever and malaise may occur. Extragenital sites are rare. Other forms include transient chancroid, which consists of an ulcer that rapidly resolves in less than a week and is followed by suppurative inguinal lymphadenitis; follicular chancroid, which has ulcerations in hair-bearing areas; the dwarf variety, which manifests as one or more herpetiform ulcerations; and giant chancroid, which consists of multiple small ulcerations that rapidly expand and coalesce to form a single large ulceration. A painful ulcer and tender inguinal adenopathy, combined with suppurative inguinal adenopathy, is almost pathognomonic for chancroid.[69]

The differential diagnosis is similar to that for LGV: herpes genitalis, primary syphilis, Behçet's syndrome, traumatic lesions, or fixed drug eruptions. In adolescents, the most common causes of ulcerative lesions are, in descending order, herpes, nonspecific trauma, syphilis, and chancroid. A definitive diagnosis of chancroid can be made using a special culture medium for *H. ducreyi*; however, this medium is not widely available, and culture has a sensitivity of only 80%.[70] A probable diagnosis can be made if all of the following criteria are met[69]: (1) the patient has one or more painful genital ulcers, (2) the patient has no laboratory evidence of syphilis at least 7 days after the onset of the ulcers, (3) the clinical presentation is consistent with chancroid, and (4) a test for HSV performed on ulcer exudate is negative. It is important to keep chancroid in the differential for patients with genital ulcers; the diagnosis can be easily missed because it is not very common.

MANAGEMENT

Recommended treatments are azithromycin 1 g orally in a single dose; ceftriaxone 250 mg intramuscularly (IM) in a single dose; ciprofloxacin 500 mg orally twice a day for 3 days; or erythromycin base 500 mg orally three times a day for 7 days. Ciprofloxacin should not be used in pregnant or lactating women.[69,71]

Treatment cures the infection, leads to resolution of clinical symptoms, and prevents transmission to others. Patients who are uncircumcised or who have HIV infection may not respond as well as other patients to therapy. The CDC recommends that all patients diagnosed with chancroid be tested for HIV, and retested for syphilis and HIV 3 months after the

diagnosis if initial tests are negative. Patients should be reexamined 3 to 7 days after initiation of therapy; ulcers generally improve symptomatically within 3 days and objectively within 7 days. Sex partners should be examined and treated if they had contact with the patient within the 10 days preceding the onset of symptoms.

Genital Growths

Human Papillomavirus

Human papillomavirus (HPV) is the most prevalent STI in the United States among adolescent and young adult women. More than 30 types of HPV can infect the genital tract; most infections are asymptomatic, subclinical, or go unrecognized. HPV types 6 and 11 are the usual etiologies for visible genital warts and can cause respiratory papillomatosis in infants and children, although the risk is less than 0.04%.

Major risk factors are related to sexual behavior, and include multiple sex partners, first intercourse within 18 months after menarche, increased frequency of sexual intercourse, and, for men, failure to use a condom.[72,73] The relationship between condom use and the acquisition of HPV by women is less clear.

CLINICAL PRESENTATION

There are four major types of warts caused by HPV. Condylomata acuminatum is the classic cauliflower-shaped growth with a granular surface. Papular warts are flesh-colored, smooth, dome-shaped papules that are 1 to 4 mm in size. Keratotic warts have a thick, crustlike layer, and resemble common skin warts. Flat-topped warts are macular or slightly raised and are invisible to the naked eye. The lesions occur most commonly on the cervix of women (70%) and the inner surface of the prepuce of men (70%); circumcised males are more likely to have involvement of the shaft of the penis. Other sites include the vulva (25%), the anus (20%), the vagina (10%), and the urethra (5%) for women. Up to 25% of males can have involvement of the urethral meatus. Lesions are usually asymptomatic, but can cause itching, burning, fissuring, pain, or bleeding.

The differential diagnosis for HPV includes condylomata lata (secondary syphilis), molluscum contagiosum, granuloma inguinale, seborrheic keratosis, neoplasia, and, in males, pink pearly papules (parallel rows of lesions at the corona of the penis that are normally present in about 15% of the population).

In most cases, external genital warts can be diagnosed clinically. If the diagnosis is uncertain, if the lesions do not respond to therapy, or if the disease worsens during therapy, biopsy can be used to confirm the diagnosis. All women with external genital warts should undergo a speculum examination to look for the presence of disease internally.

Although genital HPV is sexually transmitted, it is possible to contract external condylomata by autoinoculation or inoculation with HPV from skin warts. In addition, virus can be passed to an infant during delivery. The HPV types that cause skin warts can be transmitted by fomites, and virus has been recovered from sauna benches, underwear, examination gloves, and tanning couches. It is unclear whether or not fomites are an important source of infection for transmission of genital HPV. Any pediatric patient presenting with genital warts should be evaluated for evidence of sexual abuse.

MANAGEMENT

The primary goal of treating visible warts is symptomatic treatment, although some patients with asymptomatic lesions will want to be treated for cosmetic or psychological reasons. If left untreated, some warts will resolve spontaneously, although there is no way to predict which patients will experience spontaneous resolution. Some patients may choose to wait and see how the lesions progress prior to initiating therapy. Current data suggest that treating warts may reduce infectivity, but probably does not completely eliminate it. There are quite a few acceptable treatment regimens; selection of treatment should be based on the preference of the patient, the available resources, and the experience of the health care provider (Table 70–7).

All therapies are cytodestructive, except for topical 5% imiquimod cream and intralesional interferons, which are immunotherapies. Treatments are rarely administered in the ED. Patients should be referred to a gynecologist or primary care physician for definitive therapy. Complications from therapy are rare when the treatments are employed properly. Persistent hypo- or hyperpigmentation is common after ablation. Other complications include depressed or hypertrophic scars or, rarely, chronic pain syndromes. Local inflammatory reactions are common with the use of podofilox and imiquimod. Pain and sometimes necrosis and blistering can occur after application of liquid nitrogen. Imiquimod, podophyllin, and podofilox should not be used during pregnancy.

Patients should be counseled that recurrences, particularly within the first 3 months, might occur. Sex partners of patients with genital warts should be examined, because self- or partner examination has not been evaluated as a diagnostic method, and patients may miss lesions. However, there is no indication for treating in order to prevent future transmission, since the role of treatment in affecting infectivity is unknown. In addition, there is no indication that reinfection plays a role in recurrences. Many young women will become negative for HPV within 24 months of diagnosis.[73] There is no evidence that the presence of external genital warts is associated with the development of cervical cancer.

Molluscum Contagiosum

Molluscum contagiosum is a viral infection that is becoming increasingly common in sexually active adolescents. In adolescents and adults, molluscum is most commonly transmitted by sexual contact, although it can be transmitted by casual contact, fomites, or self-inoculation.[74] In sexually active adolescents, the lesions are commonly seen on the genital and pubic areas. The lesions are firm, flesh-colored, waxy, dome-shaped, globular nodules with central umbilication. There are usually between 1 and 20 lesions between 3 and 7 mm in diameter, which occur in clusters. The lesions are usually asymptomatic, although inflammatory changes can occur. Some patients may experience pruritis or tenderness.

Differential diagnosis includes condylomata acuminata and vulvar syringoma for multiple small lesions, and squamous or basal cell carcinoma for large, solitary lesions. The diagnosis is usually made clinically, although several techniques can aid in the diagnosis. For example, spraying the lesion with ethyl chloride produces a distinct central area of darkness that is not found in warts, and unroofing the lesion with a 27-gauge needle reveals the presence of a white "pearl." Biopsy is rarely necessary.

Most molluscum lesions will resolve spontaneously, although this process can take 6 months to 5 years. Many experts recommend treatment of genital molluscum lesions to reduce the risk of transmission and to prevent autoinoculation, as well as to improve the patient's quality of life. Treatment modalities are similar to those for external genital warts, and include physician-administered (electrosurgery, curettage, cryosurgery, trichloroacetic acid [TCA] application, and podophyllin) and patient-administered (podofilox, retinoic acid, and imiquimod 1% or 5% cream) modalities. The physical and chemical ablation techniques are associated with pain, irritation, and mild scarring; because of the caustic nature of TCA and podophyllin, only a small area can be treated at one time. Several open-label and randomized, controlled trials indicate that imiquimod cream is well tolerated and effective for the treatment of molluscum lesions, providing a novel treatment, particularly for patients who do not tolerate other therapies or in whom other therapies are not effective.[3,74-76]

Patients should be followed up in 30 days in order to assess for new lesions that may have been incubating at the time of treatment. Sex partners require treatment only if lesions are present.

Table 70–7	Treatment of Genital Warts	
Patient Administered	**Provider Administered**
Podofilox 0.5% solution or gel, applied with a cotton swab (solution) or finger (gel) to warts twice a day for 3 days, then no therapy for 4 days. Can repeat for up to 4 cycles. Limit to 10 cm² of area and 0.5 ml of podofilox.	Cryotherapy; can repeat every 1–2 wk.
Imiquimod 5% cream, applied once daily at bedtime, 3 times a week for up to 16 weeks.	Podophyllin resin 10%–25% in a compound tincture of benzoin, applied to each wart and allowed to air dry. Can repeat weekly. Limit to 10 cm² of area and ≤0.5 ml of podophyllin. BCA/TCA 80%–90%, with a small amount applied only to warts. A white "frosting" will develop. If excess acid is applied, remove with talc, baking soda, or liquid soap. Can repeat weekly.
The treatment area should be washed 6–10 hr after the application.	Surgical removal with tangential scissor excision, tangential shave excision, curettage, or electrosurgery.

Abbreviations: BCA, bichloroacetic acid; TCA, trichloroacetic acid.
From Centers for Disease Control and Prevention: Sexually transmitted diseases treatment guidelines—2006. MMWR Recomm Rep 55(RR-11):1–100, 2006.

Urethritis and Epididymitis

STIs in males include urethritis, epididymitis, and orchitis. Orchitis is discussed in Chapter 89 (Penile/Testicular Disorders). Urethritis is the most common manifestation of *N. gonorrhoeae* and *C. trachomatis* infection in males. Other etiologies of nongonococcal urethritis include *Ureaplasma urealyticum* and *Mycoplasma genitalium,* as well as *T. vaginalis* and HSV.

Clinical Presentation

Urethritis presents with urethral discharge and inflammation. Spontaneous discharge is often noted in the morning, after holding urine overnight. Dysuria and pruritis can also be present. Infection with *C. trachomatis* is often asymptomatic; when symptoms are present, they tend to be more mild than those associated with gonococcal infection. Even without symptoms, however, males infected with *C. trachomatis* usually have evidence of urethral inflammation on laboratory evaluation of secretions or urine.[77-79]

The presence of mucopurulent urethral discharge is adequate to make the diagnosis of urethritis; if in doubt, a Gram stain of the urethral secretions demonstrating ≥5 WBCs per oil immersion field can confirm the diagnosis. Gram stain is the preferred diagnostic test, because it has high sensitivity and specificity, and can also identify gonococcal infection by the presence of intracellular diplococci. Alternatively, a positive leukocyte esterase test on first-void urine or microscopic examination of first-void urine demonstrating ≥10 WBCs per high-power field supports the diagnosis. Definitive tests for *N. gonorrhoeae* and *C. trachomatis* should also be sent; either cultures from the urethra or nucleic acid amplification tests, using a urine specimen, are appropriate.[80] Testing for *T. vaginalis* is generally reserved for patients who do not respond to therapy, or to patients with a known infected contact. The differential diagnosis of urethritis includes the infectious etiologies noted previously, as well as allergic inflammation, trauma, and foreign body.

Gonococcal infection can spread and cause prostatitis, epididymitis, seminal vesiculitis, and infection of Cowper's and Tyson's glands. Epididymitis is characterized by urethral discharge, dysuria, scrotal pain and tenderness that is usually unilateral, scrotal swelling and erythema, pain/tenderness/swelling of the lower pole of the epididymis, and swelling and pain of the spermatic cord. Prostatitis can be asymptomatic; when symptoms are present, they include chills, fever, malaise, rectal pain, lower back pain, lower abdominal pain, and urinary symptoms such as dysuria, frequency, and acute urinary retention. Like females, males are also at risk for pharyngitis, rectal infection, conjunctivitis, otitis externa, and disseminated disease. Proctitis has become much less common over the last decade, but is still important to consider in the differential of any sexually active patient with gastrointestinal symptoms.

Chlamydial infection can also cause epididymitis, which is often a more indolent infection than that caused by *N. gonorrhoeae.* Other complications include proctitis as well as Reiter's syndrome, which is characterized by conjunctivitis, dermatitis, urethritis, and arthritis. Some patients can have isolated arthritis or reactive tenosynovitis without the other characteristics of Reiter's syndrome. The role of *C. trachomatis* in prostatitis is unclear.

Management

Patients with confirmed uncomplicated gonococcal infection of the urethra or rectum should be treated with ceftriaxone or a fluoroquinolone, preferably administered during the ED visit (Table 70–8). Although there has been some concern about the use of fluoroquinolones in children younger than 18 years, the CDC has stated that, because no joint injury has been documented in children treated with prolonged

Table 70–8	Treatment for Other Gonococcal* and Chlamydial Infections
Infection	**Treatment[†]**
Uncomplicated gonococcal infection of the urethra or rectum	Ceftriaxone 125 mg IM once *or* Ciprofloxacin 500 mg orally once *or* Ofloxacin 400 mg orally once *or* Levofloxacin 250 mg orally once
Nongonococcal urethritis	Azithromycin 1 g orally once *or* Doxycycline 100 mg orally bid × 7 days
Recurrent/persistent urethritis	Metronidazole 2 g orally once *plus* erythromycin base 500 mg orally qid for 10 days
Epididymitis	Ceftriaxone 250 mg IM once *plus* doxycycline 100 mg orally bid × 10 days *Or, if allergy* Ofloxacin 300 mg orally bid × 10 days *or* Levofloxacin 500 mg orally qd × 10 days
Uncomplicated gonococcal infections of the pharynx	Ceftriaxone 125 mg IM once *or* Ciprofloxacin 500 mg orally once
Gonococcal conjunctivitis	Ceftriaxone 1 g IM once; saline lavage of the affected eye(s)
Disseminated gonococcal infection: therapy should continue for 24–48 hr after improvement; then be switched to oral therapy to complete 7 days treatment	Ceftriaxone 1 g IM q24h *or* Ciprofloxacin 400 mg IV q12h *or* Levofloxacin 250 mg IV daily
Gonococcal meningitis or endocarditis	Ceftriaxone 1–2 g q12h for 10–14 days (meningitis) or at least 4 wk (endocarditis)

*Patients with gonococcal infections should generally be treated for concomitant chlamydial infection.
[†]The reader is referred to the CDC Sexually Transmitted Diseases web site *(http://www.cdc.gov/STD/)* for additional regimens.
Abbreviation: IM, intramuscularly.
From Centers for Disease Control and Prevention: Sexually transmitted diseases treatment guidelines—2006. MMWR Recomm Rep 55(RR-11):1–100, 2006.

ciprofloxacin regimens, any patient weighing over 45 kg can be treated with any of the recommended regimens. Treatment for gonococcal pharyngitis is either ceftriaxone 125 mg IM in a single dose, or ciprofloxacin 500 mg orally in a single dose. Patients with gonococcal conjunctivitis should be treated with ceftriaxone 1 g IM once, as well as one lavage of the eye with normal saline. Patients with epididymitis can usually be treated as outpatients, although hospitalization is recommended when severe pain suggests other diagnoses, such as torsion, or if the patient is febrile. For all infections, if chlamydial infection is not ruled out, dual therapy is recommended.[3] Patients with disseminated gonococcal infection should be hospitalized for treatment, particularly if compliance is questionable, the diagnosis is uncertain, or purulent synovial effusions or other complications are present.

Cure rates for uncomplicated gonococcal and chlamydial infections are high. If symptoms recur, patients should be re-treated with the original regimen if compliance is in doubt or if the patient has been reexposed to an infected partner. Patients with nongonococcal urethritis that is not due to *C. trachomatis* have relapse rates of up to 50% after 2 months; some cases are caused by tetracycline-resistant *U. urealyticum*. Patients with gonococcal infection who have persistent symptoms after treatment should be evaluated by culture in order to assess sensitivities of the organism.[3] Patients with epididymitis who do not improve after 3 days of therapy should be re-evaluated to assess for other causes, such as tumor, abscess, infarction, tuberculosis, and fungal infection. All sex partners within 60 days, as well as the patient's most recent sex partner if more than 60 days ago, should be treated whether or not they are symptomatic. Patients should refrain from sexual intercourse for 7 days after treatment is completed and until symptoms have resolved.

Neonatal Infections[3,81,82]

Both *N. gonorrhoeae* and *C. trachomatis* can cause ophthalmia neonatorum, which generally presents in patients less than 30 days old. Prophylaxis with erythromycin eye drops helps prevent gonococcal disease, but does not affect the incidence of chlamydia.[3] Therefore, gonococcal ophthalmia should be considered in patients who did not receive prophylaxis and in children of mothers who did not receive prenatal care or who have a history of STIs. Other gonococcal infections include scalp abscess and disseminated disease with bacteremia, arthritis, or meningitis. *C. trachomatis* can also cause pneumonia.

Clinical Presentation

Infants born to mothers with a history of HSV can present with a variety of clinical syndromes; in addition, neonatal herpes can be present in infants born to mothers without a clear history of HSV, as well as in infants born via cesarean section. Infections have been documented despite presumed intact membranes. The risk to an infant born to a mother with a primary HSV infection is 33% to 50%; risk to infants of mothers with reactivated infection is less than 5%.[83] Infections usually present within the first 4 weeks of life. Most cases of congenital syphilis are diagnosed through routine prenatal and antenatal screening of the mother. However, a small number of patients may present to the ED during the neonatal period.

Infants with gonococcal ophthalmia generally present with a hyperpurulent eye discharge and very injected conjunctivae, although symptoms can be more subtle. Other causes of conjunctivitis in this age group include chemical conjunctivitis (often from prophylactic eyedrops, which presents in the first 3 days of life), other bacterial causes, and viral causes. Any infant with a purulent eye discharge should have a Gram stain of the discharge to evaluate for intracellular diplococci, as well as a viral culture of conjunctival cells (obtained via conjunctival scraping with a Dacron-tipped swab) to evaluate for Chlamydia. Culture of the eye discharge alone is not adequate to diagnose chlamydial infection. A limited number of nonculture tests are licensed by the Food and Drug Administration for conjunctival specimens.[84] Patients with intracellular diplococci on Gram stain should be treated presumptively for gonococcal infection until culture results are available. Culture is important for definitive diagnosis because other species of Neisseria can be indistinguishable from *N. gonorrhoeae* on Gram stain. Blood cultures and lumbar puncture can be reserved for patients with other signs of systemic disease, such as fever.

Infants with chlamydia pneumonia generally present with a staccato cough, tachypnea, and hyperinflation and bilateral diffuse infiltrates on chest radiograph. Specimens for Chlamydia testing should be obtained from the nasopharynx.

Neonatal HSV can present with disseminated disease, most often involving the lung and the liver; with localized central nervous system disease, with meningitis and focal seizures; or with disease localized to the skin, eyes, and mouth. Infants with HSV often present without skin lesions. Lesions can be evaluated for HSV as described earlier; if CSF is obtained, an HSV polymerase chain reaction test is available in many laboratories. In addition, serum can be sent for culture for the systemically ill infant.

Infants with congenital syphilis who are symptomatic can present with hepatosplenomegaly, snuffles, lymphadenopathy, mucocutaneous lesions, edema, rash, hemolytic anemia, or thrombocytopenia. Testing for syphilis in the neonate is similar to that described earlier; diagnosis is likely if the patient has clinical features consistent with syphilis and either a serum quantitative nontreponemal serologic titer that is fourfold greater than the mother's titer, or a positive darkfield or FTA-Abs test of body fluids. Patients with proven or highly probable disease should have a lumbar puncture and a complete blood count, and other tests, such as long-bone radiographs and liver function tests, as clinically indicated.

Important Clinical Features and Considerations

Because of the severe sequelae of gonococcal ophthalmia, infants with eye discharge should be assumed to have this infection until proven otherwise. Untreated, the infection can progress to corneal ulceration and to globe rupture within 24 hours of infection. Topical therapy is not adequate for either gonococcal or chlamydial ophthalmia neonatorum.

Given the high morbidity and mortality of neonatal herpes infection, this should be considered in any neonate with fever, irritability, and abnormal CSF results. A careful physical examination is necessary to identify skin lesions, particularly in the scalp and near the eyebrows.

Evaluation for congenital syphilis in the ED setting is limited to patients with clinical symptoms. There is no indication for routine screening in this setting.

Management

Patients with presumed gonococcal ophthalmia should be treated with ceftriaxone, 25 to 50 mg/kg intravenously (IV) or IM in a single dose (maximum 125 mg), and should be admitted to the hospital for frequent saline lavage of the eye until the discharge clears. These patients should be evaluated by an ophthalmologist. Patients with scalp abscesses or disseminated infection should be treated for 7 days, or for 10 to 14 days if meningitis is present. Patients with chlamydial ophthalmia neonatorum or pneumonia should be treated with erythromycin base or ethylsuccinate 50 mg/kg per day orally, in four divided doses, for 14 days. Infants treated with erythromycin for chlamydial infection should be followed up to determine treatment effectiveness; about 20% of these patients fail initial therapy and require a second course.

Infants with HSV should be treated with acyclovir 20 mg/kg IV every 8 hours for 14 days for skin disease, and for 21 days for meningitis. Infants with ocular involvement should also receive a topical ophthalmic drug, such as 1% to 2% trifluridine, and be evaluated by an ophthalmologist.

Infants with symptomatic congenital syphilis should be treated with aqueous penicillin G 50,000 units/kg per dose IV every 12 hours for the first 7 days of life and every 8 hours thereafter, for a total of 10 days, or procaine penicillin G 50,000 units/kg per dose IM daily for 10 days. All infants with congenital syphilis require close follow-up and repeat testing.

REFERENCES

1. Brook I: Microbiology and management of polymicrobial female genital tract infections in adolescents. J Pediatr Adolesc Gynecol 15:217–226, 2002.
2. Washington AE, Aral SO, Wolner-Hanssen P: Assessing risks for pelvic inflammatory disease and its sequelae. JAMA 266:2581–2586, 1991.
*3. Centers for Disease Control and Prevention: Sexually transmitted diseases treatment guidelines—2006. MMWR Recomm Rep 55(RR-11):1–100, 2006.
4. Simms I, Warburton F, Westrom L: Diagnosis of pelvic inflammatory disease: time for a rethink. Sex Transm Infect 79:491–494, 2003.
5. Millstein SG, Adler NE, Irwin CE Jr: Sources of anxiety about pelvic examinations among adolescent females. J Adolesc Health Care 5:105–111, 1984.
*6. Peipert JF, Ness RB, Blume J, et al: Clinical predictors of endometritis in women with symptoms and signs of pelvic inflammatory disease. Am J Obstet Gynecol 184:856–864, 2001.
7. Blake DR, Fletcher K, Joshi N, Emans SJ: Identification of symptoms that indicate a pelvic examination is necessary to exclude PID in adolescent women. J Pediatr Adolesc Gynecol 16:25–30, 2003.
8. Bryant DK, Fox AS, Spigland I, et al: Comparison of rapid diagnostic methodologies for chlamydia and gonorrhea in an urban adolescent population: a pilot study. J Adolesc Health 16:324–327, 1995.
9. Carroll KC, Aldeen WE, Morrison M, et al: Evaluation of the Abbott LCx ligase chain reaction assay for detection of Chlamydia trachomatis and Neisseria gonorrhoeae in urine and genital swab specimens from a sexually transmitted disease clinic population. J Clin Microbiol 36:1630–1633, 1998.
10. Hook EW 3rd, Ching SF, Stephens J, et al: Diagnosis of Neisseria gonorrhoeae infections in women by using the ligase chain reaction on patient-obtained vaginal swabs. J Clin Microbiol 35:2129–2132, 1997.
11. Hook EW 3rd, Smith K, Mullen C, et al: Diagnosis of genitourinary Chlamydia trachomatis infections by using the ligase chain reaction on patient-obtained vaginal swabs. J Clin Microbiol 35:2133–2135, 1997.
12. Johnson RE, Newhall WJ, Papp JR, et al: Screening tests to detect Chlamydia trachomatis and Neisseria gonorrhoeae infections—2002. MMWR Recomm Rep 51(RR-15):1–38, 2002.
13. Lee HH, Chernesky MA, Schachter J, et al: Diagnosis of Chlamydia trachomatis genitourinary infection in women by ligase chain reaction assay of urine. Lancet 345:213–216, 1995.
14. Thomas BJ, Pierpoint T, Taylor-Robinson D, et al: Sensitivity of the ligase chain reaction assay for detecting Chlamydia trachomatis in vaginal swabs from women who are infected at other sites. Sex Transm Infect 74:140–141, 1998.
15. Newhall WJ, Johnson RE, DeLisle S, et al: Head-to-head evaluation of five chlamydia tests relative to a quality-assured culture standard. J Clin Microbiol 37:681–685, 1999.
16. Van Dyck E, Leven M, Pattyn S, et al: Detection of Chlamydia trachomatis and Neisseria gonorrhoeae by enzyme immunoassay, culture, and three nucleic acid amplification tests. J Clin Microbiol 39:1751–1756, 2001.
17. Molander P, Sjoberg J, Paavonen J, et al: Transvaginal power Doppler findings in laparoscopically proven acute pelvic inflammatory disease. Ultrasound Obstet Gynecol 17:233–238, 2001.
18. Golden N, Cohen H, Gennari G, et al: The use of pelvic ultrasonography in the evaluation of adolescents with pelvic inflammatory disease. Am J Dis Child 141:1235–1238, 1987.
19. Golden N, Neuhoff S, Cohen H: Pelvic inflammatory disease in adolescents. J Pediatr 114:138–143, 1989.
20. Slap GB, Forke CM, Cnaan A, et al: Recognition of tubo-ovarian abscess in adolescents with pelvic inflammatory disease. J Adolesc Health 18:397–403, 1996.
*21. Ness RB, Soper DE, Holley RL, et al: Effectiveness of inpatient and outpatient treatment strategies for women with pelvic inflammatory disease: results from the Pelvic Inflammatory Disease Evaluation and Clinical Health (PEACH) Randomized Trial. Am J Obstet Gynecol 186:929–937, 2002.
22. English A: Understanding legal aspects of care. In Neinstein LS (ed): Adolescent Health Care: A Practical Guide, 4th ed. Philadelphia: Lippincott Williams & Wilkins, 2002, pp 186–198.
23. Guttmacher Institute State Center: State Policies in Brief: Minors' Access to STD Services, 2006. Available at http://www.guttmacher.org/statecenter/spibs/spib_MASS.pdf
24. Centers for Disease Control and Prevention: Chlamydia—CDC Fact Sheet, 2006. Available at http://www.cdc.gov/STD/Chlamydia/STDFact-Chlamydia.htm
25. Centers for Disease Control and Prevention: Gonorrhea—CDC Fact Sheet, 2006. Available at http://www.cdc.gov/STD/Gonorrhea/STDFact-gonorrhea.htm
26. Wiesenfeld HC, Hillier SL, Krohn MA, et al: Lower genital tract infection and endometritis: insight into subclinical pelvic inflammatory disease. Obstet Gynecol 100:456–463, 2002.
27. Yudin MH, Hillier SL, Wiesenfeld HC, et al: Vaginal polymorphonuclear leukocytes and bacterial vaginosis as markers for histologic endometritis among women without symptoms of pelvic inflammatory disease. Am J Obstet Gynecol 188:318–323, 2003.
28. Hutt DM, Judson FN: Epidemiology and treatment of oropharyngeal gonorrhea. Ann Intern Med 104:655–658, 1986.
29. Martin DH, Mroczkowski TF, Dalu ZA, et al; The Azithromycin for Chlamydial Infections Study Group: A controlled trial of a single dose of azithromycin for the treatment of chlamydial urethritis and cervicitis. N Engl J Med 327:921–925, 1992.
30. Moran JS, Levine WC: Drugs of choice for the treatment of uncomplicated gonococcal infections. Clin Infect Dis 20:S47–S65, 1995.
31. Centers for Disease Control and Prevention: Fluoroquinolone resistance in Neisseria gonorrhoeae, Hawaii, 1999, and decreased susceptibility to azithromycin in N. gonorrhoeae, Missouri, 1999. MMWR Morb Mortal Wkly Rep 49:833–837, 2000.
32. Schillinger JA, Kissinger P, Calvet H, et al: Patient-delivered partner treatment with azithromycin to prevent repeated Chlamydia trachomatis infection among women: a randomized, controlled trial. Sex Transm Dis 30:49–56, 2003.
33. Eckert LO, Hawes SE, Stevens CE, et al: Vulvovaginal candidiasis: clinical manifestations, risk factors, management algorithm. Obstetr Gynecol 92:757–765, 1998.

---

*Selected readings.

34. Association of Genitourinary Medicine and the Medical Society for the Study of Venereal Diseases, Clinical Effectiveness Group: National guideline for the management of vulvovaginal candidiasis. Sex Transm Infect 75:S19–S20, 1999.

35. Centers for Disease Control and Prevention: Trichomoniasis—CDC Fact Sheet, 2004. Available at *http://www.cdc.gov/STD/Trichomonas/STDFact-Trichomoniasis.htm*

36. Association of Genitourinary Medicine and the Medical Society for the Study of Venereal Diseases, Clinical Effectiveness Group: National guidelines for the management of *Trichomonas* vaginalis. Sex Transm Infect 75:S21–S23, 1999.

37. Association of Genitourinary Medicine and the Medical Society for the Study of Venereal Diseases, Clinical Effectiveness Group: National guideline for the management of bacterial vaginosis. Sex Transm Infect 75:S16–S18, 1999.

38. Joesoef MR, Schmid GP, Hillier SL: Bacterial vaginosis: review of treatment options and potential clinical indications for therapy. Clin Infect Dis 28(Suppl 1):S57–S65, 1999.

39. Wilson J: Managing recurrent bacterial vaginosis. Sex Transm Dis 80:8–11, 2004.

40. Wolner-Hanssen P, Krieger JN, Stevens CE, et al: Clinical manifestations of vaginal trichomoniasis. JAMA 261:571–576, 1989.

41. Landers DV, Wiesenfeld HC, Heine RP, et al: Predictive value of the clinical diagnosis of lower genital tract infection in women. Am J Obstet Gynecol 190:1004–1010, 2004.

42. Blake DR, Duggan A, Joffe A: Use of spun urine to enhance detection of *Trichomonas* vaginalis in adolescent women. Arch Pediatr Adolesc Med 153:1222–1225, 1999.

43. Amsel R, Totten PA, Spiegel CA, et al: Nonspecific vaginitis: diagnostic criteria and microbial and epidemiologic associations. Am J Med 74:14–22, 1983.

44. Nugent RP, Krohn MA, Hillier SL: The reliability of diagnosing bacterial vaginosis is improved by a standardized method of Gram stain interpretation. J Clin Microbiol 29:297–301, 1991.

45. Schwebke JR, Hillier SL, Sobel JD, et al: Validity of the vaginal Gram stain for the diagnosis of bacterial vaginosis. Obstet Gynceol 88:573–576, 1996.

*46. Blake DR, Duggan A, Quinn T, et al: Evaluation of vaginal infections in adolescent women: can it be done without a speculum? Pediatrics 102:939–944, 1998.

47. Peipert JF, Montagno AB, Cooper AS, Sung CJ: Bacterial vaginosis as a risk factor for upper genital tract infection. Am J Obstet Gynecol 177:1184–1187, 1997.

48. Wiesenfeld HC, Hillier SL, Krohn MA, et al: Bacterial vaginosis is a strong predictor of *Neisseria gonorrhoeae* and *Chlamydia trachomatis* infection. Clin Infect Dis 36:663–668, 2003.

49. Sobel JD, Brooker D, Stein GE, et al; Fluconazole Vaginitis Study Group: Single oral dose fluconazole compared with conventional clotrimazole topical therapy of *Candida* vaginitis. Am J Obstet Gynecol 172:1263–1268, 1995.

50. Centers for Disease Control and Prevention: Herpes—CDC Fact Sheet, 2004. Available at *http://www.cdc.gov/STD/Herpes/STDFact-Herpes.htm*

51. Roberts CM, Pfister JR, Spear SJ: Increasing proportion of herpes simplex virus type 1 as a cause of genital herpes infection in college students. Sex Transm Dis 30:797–800, 2003.

52. Engelberg R, Carrell D, Krantz E, et al: Natural history of genital herpes simplex virus type 1 infection. Sex Transm Dis 30:174–177, 2003.

*53. Ashley RL: Sorting out the new HSV type specific antibody tests. Sex Transm Infect 77:232–237, 2001.

54. Turner KR, Wong EH, Kent CK, Klausner JD: Serologic herpes testing in the real world: validation of new type-specific serologic herpes simplex virus tests in a public health laboratory. Sex Transm Dis 29:422–425, 2002.

55. Bryson YJ, Dillon M, Lovett M, et al: Treatment of first episodes of genital herpes simplex virus infection with oral acyclovir: a randomized double-blind controlled trial in normal subjects. N Engl J Med 308:916–921, 1983.

56. Corey L, Wald A, Patel R, et al; Valacyclovir HSV Transmission Study Group: Once-daily valacyclovir to reduce the risk of transmission of genital herpes. N Engl J Med 350:11–20, 2004.

57. Strand A, Patel R, Wulf HC, Coates KM; International Valacyclovir HSV Study Group: Aborted genital herpes simplex virus lesions: findings from a randomized controlled trial with valacyclovir. Sex Transm Infect 78:435–439, 2002.

58. Wald A: New therapies and prevention strategies for genital herpes. Clin Infect Dis 28(Suppl 1):S4–S13, 1999.

59. Douglas JM, Critchlow C, Benedetti J, et al: A double-blind study of oral acyclovir for suppression of recurrences of genital herpes simplex virus infection. N Engl J Med 310:1551–1556, 1984.

60. Mertz GJ, Jones CC, Mills J, et al: Long-term acyclovir suppression of frequently recurring genital herpes simplex virus infection: a multicenter double-blind trial. JAMA 260:201–206, 1988.

61. Stanberry LR, Cunningham AL, Mindel A, et al: Prospects for control of herpes simplex virus disease through immunization. Clin Infect Dis 30:549–566, 2000.

62. Centers for Disease Control and Prevention: Syphilis Elimination Key Facts, November 28, 2001. Available at *http://www.cdc.gov/std/media/SyphElimKeyFacts.htm*

63. Shew ML, Fortenberry JD: Syphilis screening in adolescents. J Adolesc Health 13:303–305, 1992.

*64. Wicher K, Horowitz HW, Wicher V: Laboratory methods of diagnosis of syphilis for the beginning of the third millennium. Microbes Infect 1:1035–1049, 1999.

65. Augenbraun M, Rolfs R, Johnson R, et al; Syphilis and HIV Study Group: Treponemal specific tests for the serodiagnosis of syphilis. Sex Transm Dis 25:549–552, 1998.

66. Hook EW 3rd, Martin DH, Stephens J, et al: A randomized, comparative pilot study of azithromycin versus benzathine penicillin G for treatment of early syphilis. Sex Transm Dis 29:486–490, 2002.

67. Mabey D, Peeling RW: Lymphogranuloma venereum. Sex Transm Infect 78:90–92, 2002.

68. Centers for Disease Control and Prevention: Other sexually transmitted diseases. *In* STD Surveillance 2000: National Profile, 2001. Available at *http://www.cdc.gov/std/stats00/2000OtherSTDs.htm*

69. Lewis DA: Chancroid: clinical manifestations, diagnosis, and management. Sex Transm Infect 79:68–71, 2003.

70. Lewis DA: Diagnostic tests for chancroid. Sex Transm Infect 76:137–141, 2000.

71. Schmid GP: Treatment of chancroid, 1997. Clin Infect Dis 28(Suppl 1):S14–S20, 1999.

72. Gunter J: Genital and perianal warts: new treatment opportunities for human papillomavirus infection. Am J Obstet Gynecol 189:S3–S11, 2003.

73. Moscicki AB, Shiboski S, Broering J, et al: The natural history of human papillomavirus infection as measured by repeated DNA testing in adolescent and young women. J Pediatr 132:277–284, 1998.

*74. Ting PT, Dytoc MT: Therapy of external anogenital warts and molluscum contagiosum: a literature review. Dermatol Ther 17:68–101, 2004.

75. Tyring SK: Molluscum contagiosum: the importance of early diagnosis and treatment. Am J Obstet Gynecol 189:S12–S16, 2003.

76. Syed TA, Goswami J, Ahmadpour OA, Ahmad SA: Treatment of molluscum contagiosum in males with an analog of imiquimod 1% in cream: a placebo-controlled, double-blind study. J Dermatol 25:309–313, 1998.

*77. Richens J: Main presentations of sexually transmitted infections in men. BMJ 328:1251–1253, 2004.

78. Sherrard J, Barlow D: Gonorrhoea in men: clinical and diagnostic aspects. Genitourin Med 72:422–426, 1996.

79. Burstein GR, Zenilman JM: Nongonococcal urethritis—a new paradigm. Clin Infect Dis 28:S66–S73, 1999.

80. Palladino S, Pearman JW, Kay ID, et al: Diagnosis of *Chlamydia trachomatis* and *Neisseria gonorrhoeae* genitourinary infections in males by the Amplicor PCR assay of urine. Diagn Microbiol Infect Dis 33:141–146, 1999.

81. Pickering LK (ed): Red Book: 2006 Report of the Committee on Infectious Diseases, 27th ed. Elk Grove Village, IL: American Academy of Pediatrics, 2006.

82. O'Hara MA: Ophthalmia neonatorum. Pediatr Clin North Am 40:715–725, 1993.

83. American Academy of Pediatrics: *In* Pickering LK (ed): Red Book: 2006 Report of the Committee on Infectious Diseases, 27th ed. Elk Grove Village, IL: American Academy of Pediatrics, 2006, pp 301–309.

84. American Academy of Pediatrics: *In* Pickering LK (ed): Red Book: 2006 Report of the Committee on Infectious Diseases, 27th ed. Elk Grove Village, IL: American Academy of Pediatrics, 2006, pp 361–371.

USEFUL WEBSITES

The American Academy of Pediatrics Committee on Infectious Diseases Red Book: *http://aapredbook.aappublications.org/*

The Centers for Disease Control and Prevention Sexually Transmitted Diseases Treatment Guidelines: *http://www.cdc.gov/std/treatment/*

The Centers for Disease Control and Prevention website (for information on any sexually transmitted infection): *http://www.cdc.gov/std*

The American Social Health Association home page, with information and hotline access: *http://www.ashastd.org*

Chapter 71

Selected Infectious Diseases

Robert P. Olympia, MD

Selected Diagnoses

Tick-borne illnesses
  Lyme disease
  Ehrlichiosis
Food-borne illness
Diseases associated with foreign travel
Infectious mononucleosis
Severe acute respiratory syndrome

Discussion of Individual Diagnoses

Tick-borne Illnesses

Lyme Disease

Lyme disease is the leading cause of vector-borne infectious illness in the United States, with 23,000 cases reported in

2002. It is caused by the spiral-shaped bacterium *Borrelia burgdorferi*. The bacterium is transmitted to humans via the bite of an infected deer tick, of which there are two types: the western black-legged tick (*Ixodes pacificus*), causing disease on the Pacific coast, and the black-legged tick (*Ixodes scapularis*), causing disease in the northeastern and north-central United States. The reservoirs for these ticks are the white-footed mouse and deer. Transmission is based on the length of attachment of the tick, with low risk of transmission associated with less than 24 to 48 hours of attachment. Lyme disease is commonly found in the northeastern mid-Atlantic and midwestern portions of the United States, as well as several counties in northwestern California. Outside the United States, the disease can be found in Spain, France, Austria, Germany, Russia, and Japan. Clinical manifestations of Lyme disease may present year-round, with a higher incidence during late spring to summer (May to August).

CLINICAL PRESENTATION

Lyme disease is associated with three distinct clinical stages: early localized, early disseminated, and late disseminated (Table 71–1). Clinical findings are based on time from the initial exposure (bite of the infected tick). The classic rash of Lyme disease is erythema migrans (EM), commonly found on the head or neck in young children or the extremities of older children. The lesion begins as a small red maculae or papule at or adjacent to the site of the bite, which enlarges in an annular centrifugal fashion to approximately 10 to 15 cm in diameter, resembling a "bull's eye." EM is commonly associated with nonspecific symptoms such as fever, fatigue, malaise, headache, myalgias, and arthralgias. EM, found in only two thirds of humans bitten by an infected tick, appears typically 14 days after the initial exposure. The rash and constitutional symptoms are typically self-limited and not dependent on treatment with antibiotics.

If untreated, early disseminated Lyme disease may occur weeks to months following initial exposure. Of those cases that progress, 20% develop neurologic manifestations (cranial neuropathy, radiculoneuropathy, aseptic meningitis/encephalitis),[1] 10% develop cardiac manifestations (myopericarditis, atrioventricular [AV] block, or cardiomyopathy), and 20% develop multiple EM. The most common cranial neuropathy associated with Lyme disease is Bell's palsy (peripheral VII nerve palsy), which may be unilateral or bilateral. While commonly confused with viral meningitis, Lyme meningitis is more often associated with Bell's palsy,

Table 71–1   Clinical Findings and Treatment* in Lyme Disease

Stage (Time from Initial Exposure)	Treatment[†]
Early Localized (7–14 days)	
Erythema migrans	Amoxicillin 50 mg/kg/day divided bid *or* Doxycycline[‡] 100 mg bid × 14–21 days
Early Disseminated (days to weeks)	
Multiple erythema migrans	Amoxicillin (as above) × 21–28 days
Neurologic	
Cranial neuropathy (Bell's palsy)	Amoxicillin (as above) × 21–28 days
Radiculoneuritis	Amoxicillin (as above) × 21–28 days
Aseptic meningitis/ encephalitis	Ceftriaxone 75–100 mg/kg/day × 14–28 days or 30–60 days depending on clinical response
Cardiac	
Myopericarditis	Ceftriaxone (as above) × 14–21 days
Atrioventricular block	Cardiology consult
Cardiomegaly	Cardiology consult
Musculoskeletal	
Arthralgias	Supportive care
Myalgias	Supportive care
Late Disseminated (weeks to months)	
Arthritis	Amoxicillin (as above) × 28 days
Chronic polyneuropathy	Supportive care
Chronic encephalopathy[§]	Supportive care

*Treatment for Lyme disease may have different recommendations from different sources; consultation with an infectious disease expert should be considered.
[†]Cefuroxime axetil or erythromycin can be used for penicillin-allergic patients.
[‡]Only in children 8 years or older.
[§]Sleep disturbance, fatigue, mood changes, concentration difficulty, and memory loss.

Table 71–2   Diagnosis of Lyme Disease

Erythema migrans *or* at least one manifestation (arthritis, cranial neuropathy, AV block, aseptic meningitis, radiculoneuritis) and isolation or serologic evidence of *Borellia burgdorferi* infection
Serologic evidence
  Perform enzyme-linked immunosorbent assay (ELISA) first
  If positive, confirm with Western immunoblot
Polymerase chain reaction (PCR)   may be used on blood, CSF fluid, or synovial fluid
Supportive
  Elevated WBC count, sedimentation rate, AST, complement C3/C4
  Joint fluid with 25,000–125,000 WBCs/mm³ with polymorphonuclear predominance
  CSF with mild pleocytosis (<1000 cells) and neutrophil predominance

Abbreviations: AST, aspartate aminotransferase; AV, atrioventricular; CSF, cerebrospinal fluid; WBC, white blood cell.

Table 71–3   Differential Diagnosis of Lyme Disease

Musculoskeletal

Fibromyalgia
Chronic fatigue syndrome
Viral illness (infectious mononucleosis)

Bell's Palsy

Trauma
Ramsay Hunt syndrome
Local invasion from suppurative mastoiditis or otitis media
Mumps, varicella, or enterovirus neuritis
Guillain-Barré syndrome
Brainstem tumor
Sarcoidosis

Aseptic Meningitis

Coxsackievirus
Enterovirus
Echovirus
Poliovirus

Arthritis

Septic
Reactive
Juvenile rheumatoid
Parvovirus
Traumatic
Rheumatic fever

papilledema, longer duration of symptoms prior to lumbar puncture, lack of fever at time of diagnosis, and cerebrospinal fluid (CSF) pleocytosis (especially neutrophils).[2]

Late disseminated Lyme disease is associated with oligoarthritis (most common manifestation), chronic polyneuropathy, and chronic encephalopathy (commonly manifesting as sleep disturbance, fatigue, mood changes, concentration difficulty, memory loss).[3] The arthritis associated with late disseminated disease is often limited to large weight-bearing joints.[4]

The diagnosis of Lyme disease can be made clinically, serologically, or by polymerase chain reaction (PCR) (Table 71–2). The clinical diagnosis can be made simply by identifying the classic EM rash, or by identifying one clinical manifestation (arthritis, cranial neuropathy, AV block, aseptic meningitis, or radiculoneuritis) and isolation of or serologic evidence of *B. burgdorferi* infection. Enzyme-linked immunosorbent assay (ELISA) or Western blot techniques, both of which detect immunoglobulin M (IgM) and immunoglobulin G (IgG), are serologic tests that can confirm the diagnosis. In Lyme disease, IgM peaks approximately 4 weeks and IgG approximately 6 weeks after initial exposure. The Centers for Disease Control and Prevention recommends the use of ELISA as the initial screening test, and confirmation with the Western blot if the ELISA is positive (due to cross reactivity

on ELISA of Epstein-Barr virus [EBV], parvovirus, syphilis, systemic lupus erythematosus, and juvenile rheumatoid arthritis).[5] PCR may also be used to amplify DNA of *Borrelia burgdorferi* in blood, CSF fluid, and synovial fluid. Other laboratory tests, such as complete blood count, erythrocyte sedimentation rate, aspartate aminotransferase (AST), and complement factors (C3/C4), may help to support the diagnosis of Lyme disease. The differential diagnosis of Lyme disease can be found in Table 71–3.

MANAGEMENT

Early localized Lyme (EM) can be treated with oral antibiotics for 14 to 21 days (see Table 71–1). Children from an endemic area presenting with constitutional symptoms without EM and a documented tick bite may be tested for Lyme and treated prophylactically. While most experts do not recommend performing a lumbar puncture on children with Bell's palsy and suspected Lyme disease who are otherwise well appearing, clinical evidence of meningitis or encephalitis does warrant a lumbar puncture, with cerebrospinal fluid sent for PCR analysis, hospitalization of the child, and intravenous antibiotics for 30 to 60 days. Cardiac manifestations of Lyme disease require hospitalization of the child, intravenous antibiotics, and cardiology consultation. Oligoarthritis associated with Lyme disease should be confirmed by either serologic or PCR analysis and treated with oral antibiotics for 28 days. Chronic polyneuropathy and chronic encephalopathy require neurologic consultation. It is recommended that all complicated cases of Lyme disease be referred to either a pediatric infectious disease or rheumatology specialist.

Children presenting with a deer tick attached to the skin should have it removed promptly. Ticks should be removed with either tweezers or fingers shielded with rubber gloves, grasping the tick as close to the skin as possible and pulling with steady, even pressure without squeezing or crushing the body of the tick. Prophylactic antibiotic treatment has not traditionally been recommended in the case of an attached tick since the transmission rate is low (<10%), but a recent prospective study found that 200 mg of doxycycline was effective in preventing EM in adults living in hyperendemic areas who had removed an attached deer tick within the prior 72 hours. However, this regimen is unproven in children and has the potential for significant side effects in those less than 8 years of age. Therefore, it cannot be routinely recommended.[6,7]

Ehrlichiosis

Human ehrlichiosis is caused by the bite of an infected tick. In the United States, the lone star tick (*Amblyonmma americanum*), the black-legged tick (*Ixodes scapularis*), and the western black-legged tick (*Ixodes pacificus*) are known vectors. The four species known to cause disease in humans are *Ehrlichia chaffeensis, phagocytophila, equi,* and, most recently, *ewingii.*[8] Erlichiae are small, gram-negative bacteria that invade leukocytes, causing two clinically similar illnesses: human monocytic ehrlichiosis (reported from the southeastern and south-central United States) and human granulocytic ehrlichiosis (reported from Wisconsin and Minnesota).[8-10]

CLINICAL PRESENTATION

Disease caused by *Ehrlichia* species occurs more frequently in the spring and summer months, especially between April and September. Although rates of ehrlichiosis increase with age, there have been reported cases of severe and fatal infections in children and young adults. The incubation of *Ehrlichia* is 5 to 10 days after the initial tick bite. Infected humans may be asymptomatic, or may exhibit constitutional symptoms such as fever (>38°C), headache, malaise, myalgias, nausea, vomiting, diarrhea, cough, photophobia, arthralgias, confusion, and rash. The rash associated with ehrlichiosis occurs in 60% of infected children, and can be described as macular, maculopapular, or petechial, occurring on the face, trunk, and extremities, or rarely (<10%) on the palms or soles. If untreated, ehrlichiosis may progress to more severe illness: meningoencephalitis, seizure, coma, cardiomyopathy, adult respiratory distress syndrome, respiratory failure, disseminated intravascular coagulation, and renal failure. The mortality rate is 2% to 3%.[8-10]

The diagnosis of human ehrlichiosis can be made on clinical suspicion, but is confirmed by blood smear (demonstrating the organisms by Giemsa staining or Diff-Quick methods), serologic testing (indirect immunofluorescence), PCR, or blood culture. Serologic testing may not be useful in the first week as IgM and IgG levels increase during the second week of illness. Laboratory findings associated with ehrlichiosis include leukopenia (60%), thrombocytopenia (70%), elevated liver enzymes (85%), and hyponatremia less than 130 mEq/L (40%). Differential diagnosis of ehrlichiosis includes Rocky Mountain Spotted Fever, meningococcal infection, subacute bacterial endocarditis, secondary syphilis, idiopathic thrombocytopenic purpura, gonococcemia, and neoplastic disease.[8-10]

MANAGEMENT

Antibiotics should not be withheld pending diagnostic studies in children with clinical suspicion for human ehrlichiosis. Doxycycline (4.4 mg/kg per day divided twice a day, maximum daily dose 200 mg) for children ages 8 years or older should be given by either the oral or the intravenous route and continued for at least 3 days after the defervescence of the fever, for a minimum of 5 to 10 days. The use of doxycycline may be considered in children less than 8 years of age in consultation with an infectious disease expert, recognizing the potential for significant side effects. Children who are toxic appearing, have severe constitutional symptoms, or have severe illness (adult respiratory distress syndrome, meningoencephalitis, renal failure, disseminated intravascular coagulation, coma, cardiomyopathy) should be admitted to the hospital for supportive care. Consultation with pediatric infectious disease and critical care specialists should be considered.

Food-borne Illness

"Food-borne illness" refers to an acute onset of symptoms caused by the ingestion of contaminated food. The etiology of contamination in food may be infectious agents such as bacteria, bacterial toxins, or viruses, or noninfectious causes, such as poisons or chemicals. Onset and duration of symptoms vary, depending on the specific cause.[11]

CLINICAL PRESENTATION

The clinical manifestations of food-borne illness caused by infections depend on whether an enterotoxin or cytotoxin is released by the etiologic organism.[12] Enterotoxins, which can be formed prior to ingestion or while in the intestine, cause symptoms without penetrating the intestinal mucosa, leading to watery diarrhea, usually without leukocytes (Table 71–4). Cytotoxins cause destruction of the lining of the intestinal mucosa, resulting in bloody diarrhea with leukocytes, and may invade lymphatic tissue, causing systemic symptoms (Table 71–5). An infectious etiology not caused by either an enterotoxin or cytotoxin is *Clostridium botulinum*. Symptoms include descending weakness and paralysis within 4 days of the ingestion of contaminated canned foods, such as mushrooms, smoked fish, or vegetables. Symptoms result from the absorption of botulinum toxin by the intestine,

Table 71–4   Enterotoxins Causing Food-borne Illness

Agent	Source	Incubation (hr)	Clinical Manifestations*	Treatment
Staphylococci	Improperly stored meats, bakery, dairy	2–6	Intense vomiting and watery diarrhea, abdominal cramps, low-grade fever	Supportive
Bacillus cereus	Contaminated grains, meats, vegetables	1–6	Intense vomiting, abdominal cramps	Supportive; vancomycin or ciprofloxacin if invasive
		8–16	Diarrhea and abdominal cramps	
Clostridium perfringens	Inadequately cooked meats and poultry	8–20	Abdominal cramps and diarrhea; vomiting and fever are rare	Supportive
Vibrio cholerae	Contaminated water and food (shellfish)	8–24	Profuse "rice" watery diarrhea for 3–5 days without abdominal cramps or fever	Tetracycline or doxycycline (shortens duration of symptoms)
Vibrio parahaemolyticus	Raw or improperly cooked seafood	8–24	Profuse watery diarrhea for 3–5 days	Tetracycline or doxycycline (shortens duration of symptoms)
Enterotoxic Escherichia coli	Contaminated meats, cheese, salads	8–18	Watery diarrhea ± vomiting or abdominal cramping	Supportive
Giardia lamblia	Contaminated water	2–3 days	Mild bloody diarrhea ± abdominal cramping for possibly more than 1 wk, ± anorexia	Metronidazole

*Clinical manifestations for less than 2 days unless noted.

Table 71–5   Cytotoxins Causing Food-borne Illness

Agent	Source	Incubation (hr)	Clinical Manifestations	Treatment
Salmonella	Beef, poultry, dairy, eggs, fish, reptiles	12–30	Abrupt onset of moderate to large amount of diarrhea becoming bloody ± abdominal pain or vomiting or low-grade fever	Intravenous cephalosporin if bacteremic, <3 mo of age, or immunosuppressed
Shigella	Potato, egg salad, lettuce, raw vegetables	12–30	Abrupt onset of bloody diarrhea, tenesmus, abdominal cramps lasting 3–7 days	Bactrim or ampicillin if severe disease, dysentery, or immunosuppressed
Campylobacter jejuni	Undercooked chicken or cattle	3–5 days	Foul-smelling, watery then bloody diarrhea ± abdominal cramps for 5–8 days, ± fever	Azithromycin or erythromycin (shortens duration of symptoms)
Yersinia enterocolitica	Contaminated pork or milk	4–6 days	Acute abdominal pain, fever, diarrhea	Bactrim or gentamycin (decreases duration of fecal excretion)
Escherichia coli O157:H7	Food or water contaminated with cow feces	3–5 days	Severe bloody diarrhea with painful abdominal cramps and low-grade fever; hemolytic-uremic syndrome in 3%–5%	Supportive
Entamoeba histolytica	Contaminated food or water	12–24	Sudden onset of bloody diarrhea with vomiting or abdominal cramps possibly lasting for more than a week	Metronidazole

which blocks the release of acetylcholine at the neuromuscular junction. Treatment may require respiratory support in an intensive care setting.

Enterotoxins, which produce symptoms within 4 to 6 hours of ingestion, include *Staphylococcus aureus* and *Bacillus cereus*. Cytotoxin-induced illness requires ingestion of organisms that must then multiply and invade the mucosa of the gastrointestinal tract. For this reason, patients often develop symptoms more than 6 to 12 hours after the food is ingested. Cytotoxins are more likely to produce fever, bloody diarrhea, and severe systemic symptoms.

For the most part, diagnosis is made clinically. However, a majority of food-borne illness can be diagnosed by routine stool culture or specialized staining, microscopic analysis for ova and parasites, or detection of toxin in the stool. Prior to laboratory results, history, such as onset and duration of symptoms, frequency and consistency of vomiting and/or diarrhea, presence of abdominal cramping, or systemic symptoms, will provide some clues to the etiology of the illness in the emergency department. Also important is the type of food ingested prior to symptoms, recent travel history, and similar symptoms in close contacts.

Physical examination should focus on the state of hydration as well as other potential life-threatening complications, such as neurologic, respiratory, hepatic, and renal failure. Laboratory studies, such as complete blood count, blood culture, or serum electrolyte analysis, may be helpful to determine the extent of systemic involvement. Stool cultures should be reserved for cases of bloody diarrhea, severe abdominal pain, immunocompromised or very young hosts, or toxic-appearing infants and children. Stool analysis for ova and parasites should be considered in cases of prolonged incubation or duration of symptoms. Some infectious causes, such as *Yersinia*, may mimic appendicitis, and therefore radiologic studies may be required to rule out an acute abdomen. In pediatric patients, two potential complications that should be looked for are Guillain-Barré syndrome (associated with Campylobacter infection) and hemolytic-uremic syndrome (associated with *Escherichia coli* O157:H7) (see Chapter 47, Peripheral and Neuromuscular Disorders; and Chapter 88, Renal Disorders).[13]

MANAGEMENT

While a majority of cases of food-borne illness can be managed at home without any specific therapy, some children require hospitalization, intravenous hydration therapy, and antibiotics (see Tables 71–4 and 71–5; see also Chapter 72, Vomiting and Diarrhea, for additional information on food-borne illness).

Diseases Associated with Foreign Travel

Distinguishing between diseases associated with foreign travel can be difficult since many present with fever associated with constitutional symptoms such as headache, myalgias, malaise, anorexia, and vomiting/diarrhea. Therefore, history of recent travel to endemic areas should point to a possible diagnosis.

Typhoid fever, caused by ingestion of contaminated water or food with *Salmonella typhi*, is endemic to India and Africa. Malaria, caused by the bite of an infected mosquito transmitting a species of Plasmodium, is endemic to sub-Saharan Africa, Southeast Asia, and India. Dengue fever, caused by the bite of an infected mosquito (*Aedes aegypti*), is endemic to the Caribbean and Central and South America.

The clinical features and complications associated with these selected diseases are varied and often overlap (Table 71–6). Management includes diagnosis by clinical suspicion, followed by supportive care and antibiotics if indicated. Intensive care hospitalization is necessary if complications are present. Consultation with a pediatric infectious disease specialist is also suggested.[14-17]

Infectious Mononucleosis

Clinical Presentation

Infectious mononucleosis is caused by Epstein-Barr virus (EBV), a member of the herpesvirus family. Infection is transmitted via contact with oropharyngeal secretions. While commonly asymptomatic in young children, adolescents and young adults often pre-sent with low-grade fever, pharyngitis, lymphadenopathy, and splenomegaly after an incubation of 4 to 6 weeks. Other constitutional symptoms associated with EBV include malaise, rash, headache, anorexia, nausea, chills, and myalgias. Rare complications of EBV infections include pancreatitis, cholecystitis, myocarditis, myositis, glomerulonephritis, encephalitis, transverse myelitis, and cranial nerve palsies (Table 71–7). Spontaneous splenic rupture occurs in 1% to 2% of cases of infectious mononucleosis. The differential diagnosis of infectious mononucleosis includes rubella, *Toxoplasma gondii*, adenovirus, human immunodeficiency virus, cytomegalovirus, human herpesvirus-6, and Stevens-Johnson syndrome.

The diagnosis of infectious mononucleosis can be made either by clinical suspicion or serologic testing.[18] Heterophile antibodies are typically present in 75% of older children and adolescents by the end of the first week of symptoms, and in 90% by the third week of symptoms. In children younger than 10 years, there is a 10% to 15% false-negative rate for detecting heterophile antibodies. EBV antigens can also be detected to determine stage of illness. Laboratory

Table 71–6	Selected Infections Associated with Foreign Travel			
Disease	**Initial Symptoms**	**Complications**	**Diagnosis**	**Treatment**
Typhoid fever	Fever increase over 2–3 days, headache, malaise, cough, rose spots. After 1st week: coma, abdominal distention, "pea soup" diarrhea, respiratory distress	Intestinal hemorrhage, intestinal perforation, acute renal failure, myocarditis, DIC	Stool culture for Salmonella; serologic tests (ELISA); elevated ESR, PT/PTT, LFTs; hyponatremia, hypokalemia, anemia	Ciprofloxacin, chloramphenicol, cefotaxime, ampicillin
Malaria	Paroxysms of fever, chills, sweats; flulike symptoms, vomiting and diarrhea, febrile seizures, meningitis, anemia, jaundice	Toxicity, high fever, dehydration, severe anemia, seizure/coma, pulmonary edema, renal failure, shock, bleeding diathesis	Blood smear (thick/thin); serologic tests (ELISA)	Chloroquine, quinine, quinidine, mefloquine, halofantrine
Dengue fever	Fever, headache (frontal/retro-orbital), generalized macular rash, bone pain, nausea/vomiting, anorexia, cutaneous hyperesthesias	Dehydration, bleeding diathesis, DIC, shock, myocarditis, encephalopathy, liver failure	Serologic tests (ELISA); leukopenia, thrombocytopenia; elevated BUN, LFTs	Supportive care

Abbreviations: BUN, blood urea nitrogen; DIC, disseminated intravascular coagulation; ELISA, enzyme-linked immunosorbent assay; ESR, erythrocyte sedimentation rate; LFTs, liver function tests; PT, prothrombin time; PTT, partial thromboplastin time.

Table 71–7	Clinical Manifestations of Infectious Mononucleosis

Early Findings

Classic triad
  Fever
  Pharyngitis (exudative or nonexudative)
  Lymphadenopathy (bilateral posterior cervical)
Rash (generalized maculopapular)

Late Findings

Hepatomegaly/splenomegaly
Jaundice
Palatal petechiae
Chronic fatigue

Rare Findings

Pancreatitis
Cholecystitis
Myocarditis
Myositis
Glomerulonephritis
Encephalitis
Transverse myelitis
Cranial nerve palsies

Unique to EBV

Bilateral upper lid edema
Uvular edema

studies supportive of EBV include elevated transaminase levels, relative lymphocytosis (>60%) with greater than 10% atypical lymphocytes, mild to moderate leukocytosis (12,000 to 20,000 cells/μl), mild thrombocytopenia, and elevated erythrocyte sedimentation rate.

Management

Treatment of infectious mononucleosis is supportive. Several studies have demonstrated some effectiveness of corticosteroids in reducing the pain associated with pharyngitis.[19,20] In children and young adults with splenomegaly, close follow-up (at least 3 weeks from the beginning of symptoms) is required with their primary care physician. Those who participate in contact sports or extreme activities should refrain over this time period.[21]

Severe Acute Respiratory Syndrome

Severe acute respiratory syndrome (SARS), caused by a member of the Coronaviridae virus family, produces a flulike illness that may progress to life-threatening complications, such as pneumonia, respiratory failure, or death.[22] Thought to be originally from the Guangdong providence in southern China when 305 cases of atypical pneumonia occurred there in February 2003, subsequent outbreaks have seen the illness spread to Asia, Canada, and the United States. The mortality rate has been estimated at 10%. A detailed clinical case definition of SARS may be found at *www.cdc.gov/ncidod/sars/*.

Clinical Presentation

After an incubation period of 2 to 10 days, patients present with constitutional symptoms such as fever (>100.4°F), headache, myalgias, fatigue, chills, anorexia, and diarrhea, followed in 2 to 7 days with nonproductive cough, dyspnea, and progressive hypoxemia. Mechanical ventilation may be nec-

essary in patients with respiratory failure. Chest radiographs demonstrate pneumonia (focal interstitial or generalized patchy infiltrates) after a week of symptoms. Lymphopenia develops in 70% to 90% of infected patients. Other laboratory findings associated with SARS include leukopenia, thrombocytopenia, mild hyponatremia and hypokalemia, elevated liver enzymes, and elevated creatine kinase.

The diagnosis of SARS can be made in patients with both (1) radiologic confirmation of pneumonia or acute respiratory distress syndrome of unknown etiology and (2) one of the following risk factors 10 days before onset of illness: travel to mainland China, Hong Kong, or Taiwan or close contact with an ill person with history of recent travel to those areas; health care or laboratory worker in close contact with patient with suspected SARS; or involvement in cluster of cases of atypical pneumonia. Other serologic testing is necessary, but should be at the recommendation of local and state health departments.

Management

Patients with a suspicion of SARS should be admitted to a critical care unit for supportive care. Respiratory droplet precautions should be instituted. Controversy exists regarding the efficacy of corticosteroids or ribavirin in the treatment of patients with SARS.[23]

REFERENCES

1. Bingham PM, Galetta SL, Athreya B: Neurologic manifestations in children with Lyme disease. Pediatrics 96:1053–1056, 1995.
2. Eppes SC: Characterization of Lyme meningitis and comparison with viral meningitis. Pediatrics 103:957–960, 1999.
3. Bujak DI, Weinstein A, Dornbush RL: Clinical and neurocognitive features of the post Lyme syndrome. J Rheumatol 23:1392–1397, 1996.
4. Gerber MA, Zemel LS, Shapiro ED: Lyme arthritis in children: clinical epidemiology and long term outcomes. Pediatrics 102:905–908, 1998.
5. Johnson BJ, Robbins KE, Bailey RE, et al: Serodiagnosis of Lyme disease: accuracy of a two-step approach using a flagella-based ELISA and immunoblotting. J Infect Dis 174:346–353, 1996.
6. Halsey NA, Abramson JS, Chesney PJ; American Academy of Pediatrics, Committee on Infectious Diseases: Prevention of Lyme disease. Pediatrics 105:142–147, 2000.
7. Nadelman RB: Prophylaxis with single dose doxycycline for the prevention of Lyme disease after an *Ixodes scapularis* tick bite. N Engl J Med 354:79–82, 2001.
8. Buller RS, Arens M, Hmiel SP, et al: *Ehrlichia ewingii*, a newly recognized agent of human ehrlichiosis. N Engl J Med 341:148–155, 1999.
*9. Dumler JS, Bakken JS: Ehrlichial diseases of humans: emerging tick-borne infections. Clin Infect Dis 20:1102–1110, 1995.
*10. Jacobs RF, Schutze GE: Ehrlichiosis in children. J Pediatr 131:184–192, 1997
11. Lacey RW: Food-borne bacterial infections. Parasitology 107:S75–S93, 1993.
*12. Caeiro JP, Mathewson JJ, Smith MA, et al: Etiology of outpatient pediatric nondysenteric diarrhea: a multicenter study in the United States. Pediatr Infect Dis J 18:94–97, 1999.
13. Wong CS, Jelacic S, Habeeb RL, et al: The risk of the hemolytic-uremic syndrome after antibiotic treatment of *Escherichia coli* O157:H7 infections. N Engl J Med 342:1930–1936, 2000.
14. Frenck RW, Nakhla I, Sultan Y, et al: Azithromycin versus ceftriaxone for the treatment of uncomplicated typhoid fever in children. Clin Infect Dis 31:1134–1138, 2000.
15. Gupta A: Multidrug-resistant typhoid fever in children: epidemiology and therapeutic approach. Pediatr Infect Dis J 13:134–140, 1994.
16. Emanuel B, Aronson N, Shulman S: Malaria in children in Chicago. Pediatrics 92:83–85, 1993.

*Selected readings.

17. Williams HA, Roberts J, Kachur SP: Malaria surveillance—United States, 1995. MMWR Morb Mortal Wkly Rep 48:1–23, 1999.

*18. Cohen JI: Epstein-Barr virus infection. N Engl J Med 343:481–492, 2000.

19. Bulloch B, Kabani A, Tenenbein M: Oral dexamethasone for the treatment of pain in children with acute pharyngitis: a randomized, double-blind, placebo-controlled trial. Ann Emerg Med 41:601–608, 2003.

20. Roy M, Bailey B, Amre DK, et al: Dexamethasone for the treatment of sore throat in children with suspected infectious mononucleosis. Arch Pediatr Adolesc Med 158:250–254, 2004.

21. Konvolinka CW, Wyatt DB: Splenic rupture and infectious mononucleosis. J Emerg Med 7:471–475, 1989.

22. Centers for Disease Control and Prevention: Update: outbreak of severe acute respiratory syndrome—worldwide, 2003. MMWR Morb Mortal Wkly Rep 52:269–272, 2003.

*23. Ho W: Guideline on management of severe acute respiratory syndrome (SARS). Lancet 361:1313–1315, 2003

*24. Centers for Disease Control and Prevention: Notice to readers: Final 2002 reports of notifiable diseases. MMWR Morb Mortal Wkly Rep 52:741–750, 2003.

Vomiting and Diarrhea

Courtney H. Mann, MD

Points

The differential diagnosis and workup of the patient with *isolated* vomiting are different from those for a patient with vomiting *and* diarrhea.

The differential diagnosis for vomiting is age specific.

To be confident of the diagnosis of gastroenteritis, vomiting *and* diarrhea must be present.

Assessment for dehydration must incorporate historical, physical, and laboratory findings, as no one finding alone can sufficiently predict the degree of fluid deficit present.

Oral rehydration and new antiemetics are proving to have a role in treating pediatric vomiting and diarrhea.

Introduction and Background

Vomiting is an extremely common complaint in infants and children who present to the emergency department (ED). A large percentage of infants and children with vomiting have a viral etiology for their symptoms and have a self-limiting, vomiting disease process. However, vomiting may be the presenting symptom for several life-threatening conditions. The child who presents to the ED with vomiting may not require multiple laboratory analyses and extensive testing; however, a complete history and physical examination tailored to identify serious conditions is essential.

"Diarrhea" is defined as an increase in the quantity of stools. Children frequently have an occasional "loose" stool; however, an increase in stool volume separates children with true diarrhea from those with normal stool patterns. While vomiting may be caused by a viral illness, *gastroenteritis*, as a diagnosis, must include both vomiting and diarrhea. Gastroenteritis accounts for significant illness in young children; estimates suggest that the average child younger than 5 years old in the United States has between 1.3 and 2.3 episodes of gastroenteritis per year.[1] Gastroenteritis is a common cause of mortality for children in developing countries, accounting for over 2 million deaths annually, and also results in over

1.5 million outpatient visits, 200,000 hospitalizations, and 300 deaths per year in the United States.[2,3]

Recognition and Approach

Generally, it is not difficult to recognize the child who presents with vomiting and diarrhea; however, the history is often as important as the physical examination in determining the underlying etiology and the potential for dehydration. Depending on the underlying etiology and severity of illness, clinical presentations vary widely.

The pathophysiology of nausea and vomiting is complex and not completely understood. There are multiple different input triggers to the brain for vomiting; however, the actual coordination of vomiting by the brain occurs in the same area of the medulla oblongata regardless of the type of input. Input areas include receptors in the gastrointestinal (GI) tract, chemoreceptors in the area postrema of the brainstem that monitor emetic agents in the blood and cerebrospinal fluid, and vestibular and visual afferents.[4] Because there are many different neurotransmitters involved in vomiting, not all therapies will abolish all types of vomiting. In general, serotonin receptor antagonism has been the target of pharmacologic therapies for vomiting.

The pathophysiology of diarrhea is also multifactorial. The average adult intestinal epithelium must handle 6500 ml of fluids per day, and this volume is reduced to less than 250 ml/day of stool output. During diarrhea, fluid output overwhelms the capacity of the GI tract to reabsorb fluids.[2,5] Diarrheal illness may result from a great number of causes. From an infectious standpoint, however, there are two types of pathogens that cause a diarrheal illness: inflammatory and noninflammatory. Inflammatory illness is usually caused by invasion of the intestinal border and cytotoxin production by certain types of bacteria. In contrast, the pathogens that cause noninflammatory diarrhea produce endotoxins and cause local destruction of the intestinal border.

Clinical Presentation

Clinical features of a child who presents to the ED with vomiting or diarrhea depend on the severity of the illness and the underlying etiology. Diagnostically, it is convenient to consider the child who presents with isolated vomiting separately from the child who presents with vomiting and diarrhea. The differential diagnosis of isolated vomiting is extraordinarily broad and age specific. Possible etiologies include toxicologic, infectious, metabolic, neurologic, and pregnancy, as well as psychological and behavioral issues (Table 72–1).

Disorders Causing Vomiting or Diarrhea

Gastroesophageal Reflux

In the young infant, gastroesophageal reflux (GER) is often a cause of recurrent vomiting or "spitting up"; however, reflux is a diagnosis of exclusion in the ED. Physiologically, GER is distinct from vomiting. GER results from effortless regurgitation of gastric contents and is attributed to a motility disturbance affecting the esophagus and lower esophageal sphincter.[6] GER is common during infancy, with as many as 50% of infants having recurrent regurgitation during the first 4 months of life[7] (see Chapter 35, Vomiting, Spitting Up, and Feeding Disorders). Formula changes are largely unnecessary and can become expensive and frustrating for parents. Basic reflux precautions such as smaller, more frequent feeds and allowing the infant to remain upright for 30 minutes after feeds can be helpful. Reassuring the family that most children spontaneously outgrow GER by the age of 1 usually helps alleviate parental anxiety.

Once more life-threatening conditions are excluded, the healthy newborn with suspected reflux, who is well appearing and gaining weight, may be safely discharged with close follow-up by the primary physician. Pharmacologic intervention and specific diagnostic testing for GER are reserved for children with serious disease manifesting as respiratory symptoms or poor weight gain. There are no current data to suggest that pharmacologic therapy affects the natural history of uncomplicated GER.[7] Symptomatic GER that persists past the first year of life should be further investigated on an outpatient basis with possible referral to a pediatric gastroenterologist.

Pyloric Stenosis and Malrotation with Volvulus

In contrast to GER, two causes of life-threatening vomiting in the newborn period are pyloric stenosis and malrotation with volvulus. It is important to consider the diagnosis of pyloric stenosis in the newborn child with progressively worsening vomiting (see Chapter 76, Pyloric Stenosis). The classically taught "projectile" vomiting may not be present; however, the progressively worsening nature of the emesis usually helps distinguish it from simple reflux. Although infants may appear quite well early in the illness, they often seem frustrated and hungry. Both an upper GI tract series and ultrasound are useful in establishing the definitive diagnosis. Surgical pyloromyotomy is curative.

Another life-threatening consideration in the newborn period is malrotation with volvulus (see Chapter 83, Malrotation and Midgut Volvulus). These infants have bowel that congenitally was not positioned or attached properly, allowing for the possibility of twisting of this bowel onto itself and the formation of a volvulus. These infants are often well appearing and present with bilious emesis and a distended abdomen. An upper GI series is the diagnostic test of choice, and surgical correction is the treatment.

Age-Specific Causes

Determining the presence of diarrhea in the young infant based on a parent's history may be difficult given the broad

Table 72–1	Differential Diagnosis of Vomiting by Age

Newborn

Reflux
Pyloric stenosis
Sepsis
Meningitis
Viral illness, gastroenteritis
Urinary tract infection
Inborn errors of metabolism
Congenital adrenal hyperplasia
Milk allergy
Malrotation with/without volvulus
Ileus
Incarcerated hernia
Hirschsprung's disease
Esophageal atresia/stenosis
Hydrocephalus
Intracranial bleed/mass
Renal insufficiency

Infant

Viral illness
Gastroenteritis
Urinary tract infection
Meningitis
Sepsis
Post-tussive
Nonspecific & other infections (otitis, pneumonia)
Reflux
Intussusception
Incarcerated hernia
Intracranial bleed/mass
Hirschsprung's disease
Renal insufficiency/obstructive uropathy

Toddler, Older Child

Viral illness
Gastroenteritis
Nonspecific symptom of other infections (i.e., strep throat, otitis, pneumonia)
Meningitis
Urinary tract infection
Sepsis
Post-tussive
Appendicitis
Postconcussive from head trauma
Intussusception
Incarcerated hernia
Intracranial bleed/mass
Ingestion
Foreign body aspiration/ingestion
Diabetes mellitus
Pancreatitis
Obstructive uropathy
Migraines
Behavioral

Adolescent

Viral illness
Gastroenteritis
Meningitis
Urinary tract infection/pyelonephritis
Sepsis
Appendicitis
Postconcussive from head trauma
Intracranial bleed/mass
Ingestion/overdose
Diabetes mellitus
Pancreatitis
Hepatitis
Obstructive uropathy
Migraines
Pregnancy
Psychological (bulimia/anorexia)

range of normal stool patterns. Infants who are breast-fed may normally have several loose stools a day. These stools tend to be poorly formed, with a yellow or green tint, and may be mistaken by parents as diarrhea. Stool frequency must be considered abnormal if there is a significant change from the child's normal pattern. Young infants may become infected with viral or bacterial gastroenteritis, and because they lack the fluid reserves of older children, are more likely to become significantly dehydrated.

Another age-specific cause of vomiting and diarrhea in the young infant is a food allergy. Although true food allergies in infants are not as common as the formula changes initiated to address them, the most common food hypersensitivity reactions in infants are to cow's milk or soy protein. The most prominent symptom is typically diarrhea, which may be Hemoccult positive. A leukocytosis with eosinophilia may be present. Vomiting is common, although most vomiting in this age group is related to GER and not to a milk allergy. Children with a severe allergy also may develop anemia and hypoproteinemia. Treatment consists of removal of the offending agent from the diet; a trial of hypoallergenic formula is also reasonable.[8,9] Resolution of symptoms usually occurs in the first few days after dietary change. Symptoms that do not resolve in the first 2 weeks may be related to GER or another etiology. Allergy to human milk is very rare; however, breast-fed infants may develop symptoms in response to foods in the mother's diet. Therefore, it is important to remove cow's milk from the mother's diet as well as from the infant's. Unlike allergies to peanuts, shellfish, and eggs, children usually outgrow their sensitivity to cow's milk before the age of 3 years.[10]

Bacteria, Viruses, and Parasites

Most older infants and young children who present with diarrhea and vomiting have an infectious etiology as the cause for their symptoms. Bacteria, viruses, and parasites all may cause acute gastroenteritis in children; however, viruses are the most common offending agent. The most frequent causes of viral gastroenteritis are rotaviruses, adenoviruses, *Astrovirus,* and *Calicivirus.* Rotaviruses account for a large majority of the cases and contribute to significant hospitalization of children annually, as well as 20 to 40 deaths per year in the United States. Attempts at developing a rotavirus vaccine continue despite difficulty with earlier trials, which showed an increased rate of intussusception in children who received the vaccine.[11-13]

Bacterial causes of diarrhea include *Aeromonas, Campylobacter jejuni, Clostridium difficile,* and enteroinvasive, enterohemorrhagic, enteroaggregative, enteropathogenic, and enterotoxigenic strains of *Escherichia coli,* as well as *Salmonella, Shigella,* and *Vibrio cholerae.* Specific bacterial pathogens have important clinical manifestations and epidemiologic considerations that may impact treatment and the aggressiveness with which the specific bacterial species is investigated. *Shigella* species include over 40 serotypes of gram-negative bacilli that cause inflammatory colitis. In the United States, the majority of infections are caused by *Shigella sonnei* and typically result in a watery diarrhea without gross blood or severe systemic symptoms. However, complications from *Shigella* can include bacteremia, Reiter's syndrome, hemolytic-uremic syndrome (HUS), and encephalopathy. *Shigella* infections have been associated with

seizures and may represent an important cause of febrile seizures. The mode of transmission is the fecal-oral route, and risk factors include living in or travel to areas with poor sanitation, crowded living situations, and day care center attendance. The illness is typically self-limited, resolving within 72 hours of illness onset, and treatment is generally not indicated unless children are immunocompromised, develop severe dysentery, or manifest severe systemic symptoms (Table 72–2). Outbreaks in child care centers require treatment of all symptomatic persons to limit the duration of the carrier state and prevent further spread of the disease.

Clostridium difficile is a gram-positive bacillus that is commonly present in the environment. Infections typically cause a colitis termed *pseudomembranous colitis* with bloody or heme-positive diarrhea. Systemic symptoms are common, and the disease can be severe and even fatal in immunocompromised children. Acute infection is usually the result of recent prolonged antimicrobial therapy. Colonization of healthy newborns and children less than 2 years old is common and does not typically warrant treatment unless these children are symptomatic. However, discontinuation of antibiotics is reasonable in this age group. Diagnosis of the disease occurs by detection of the *C. difficile* toxin in the stool using laboratory enzyme assays.

Salmonella organisms are gram-negative bacilli with more than 2460 serotypes. The primary sources of *Salmonella* include direct contact with animals such as poultry, livestock, and reptiles as well as contact with or ingestion of contaminated food sources such as beef, poultry, fish, eggs, and dairy products. Other foods and objects may become cross contaminated after coming in contact with infected foods and serve as a vector for transmission. Infections with *Salmonella* generally causes a watery diarrhea with mild fever and abdominal cramping. The illness is typically self-limited, and antibiotic treatment is unnecessary in healthy patients. However, *Salmonella* can cause serious illness, such as meningitis and osteomyelitis, and can cause invasive infections that result in bacteremia. Mortality from invasive disease is higher in young infants, children with hemoglobinopathies such as sickle cell disease, and immunocompromised children. Antimicrobial therapy is generally indicated those children considered at increased risk for invasive disease (see Table 72–2).

In addition to perinatal and newborn sepsis, *Listeria* may also cause diarrhea and fever, and rarely meningitis and encephalitis, in otherwise healthy children and young adults. Exposure generally occurs from contact with contaminated foods such as unpasteurized milk and cheeses, hot dogs, deli meats, undercooked poultry, and raw vegetables. Antibiotics are indicated in neonates with sepsis and in infants and children with severe systemic symptoms and extraintestinal manifestations.

Giardia lamblia is a flagellate protozoan that typically causes an asymptomatic infection. Both humans and animals serve as reservoirs, and infection can occur from contact with contaminated water or food, or directly from hand-to-mouth transfer of cysts from an infected person. Infection generally results in diffuse, watery, foul smelling, mucoid diarrhea, as well as abdominal pain and flatulence. Because the illness may be protracted with diarrhea that is intermittent, diagnosis may be delayed. Weight loss, anemia, and

Table 72–2	Management of Organisms Causing Diarrhea	
Organism	**Indications for Treatment**	**Medications**
Aeromonas	More than mild symptoms	Third-generation cephalosporins (e.g., cefixime)
Campylobacter	More than mild symptoms, those who have a relapse of illness, immunocompromised	Erythromycin, azithromycin, doxycycline (if ≥8 yr old) for total of 5–7 days If bacteremia, administer aminoglycoside, meropenem, or imipenem
Clostridium difficile	More than mild symptoms or mild disease	Discontinue causative antibiotics Oral metronidazole or vancomycin
Listeria	Infection identified during pregnancy, severe symptoms, meningitis, encephalitis	Ampicillin and aminoglycoside together Trimethoprim-sulfamethoxazole if penicillin allergic
Giardia lamblia	Symptomatic patients, household contacts of high-risk patients such as those with hypogammaglobulinemia, cystic fibrosis, pregnant women with toddlers	Metronidazole, albendazole, nitazoxanide In pregnant women use paromomycin
*Salmonella**	Age <3 mo, chronic GI tract disease, malignancy, hemoglobinopathies, HIV, immunosuppressive therapy, severe colitis, bacteremia, or sepsis	Ampicillin, amoxicillin, trimethoprim-sulfamethaxazole, cefotaxime, ceftriaxone
*Shigella**	Antibiotics are recommended for all patients except those with mild or resolving disease	Sulfamethoxazole-trimethoprim (resistance is rising) *or* cefixime *or* azithromycin for 5 days *or* ceftriaxone
Yersinia	Sepsis, non-GI infections, immunocompromised patients.	Trimethoprim-sulfamethoxazole, aminoglycosides, cefotaxime, doxycycline (if ≥8 yr old)
Vibrio	Patients with severe symptoms, immunocompromised, liver disease ? carriers	Doxycycline or tetracycline if ≥8 yr old Cefotaxime, gentamicin, chloramphenicol

*NOTE: There is currently high ampicillin, amoxicillin, and sulfa resistance in *Salmonella* and *Shigella* infections.
Abbreviations: GI, gastrointestinal; HIV, human immunodeficiency virus.
From Pickering LK (ed): Red Book: 2003 Report of the Committee on Infectious Disease, 26th ed. Elk Grove Village, IL: American Academy of Pediatrics, 2003.

anorexia are common by the time of final diagnosis. Trophozoites may be identified by direct smear examination of diarrheal stools. Treatment is indicated for all symptomatic patients and for asymptomatic carriers exposed to high-risk people such as those with hypogammaglobulinemia and cystic fibrosis.

Campylobacter species are gram-negative bacilli that cause diarrhea, abdominal pain, and fever. Stool may contain blood, especially in neonates and young infants. Although most infections are self-limited, 20% of patients may have a relapse of symptoms of a prolonged illness. Immunoreactive complications, including arthritis, erythema nodosum, and polyneuritis (e.g., Guillain-Barré syndrome), may occur during the convalescent period. Infection generally occurs from contact with or ingestion of contaminated water, improperly cooked poultry, or unpasteurized milk. Pets such as dogs, cats, hamsters, and birds are also potential sources of infection. Treatment can prevent relapses if given early in the illness.

Yersinia is a gram-negative bacillus that can cause diarrhea, fever, and abdominal pains. The diarrhea is often bloody with mucus. Older children infected with *Yersinia* may develop a pseudoappendicitis syndrome with fever, right lower quadrant abdominal pain, and an elevated white blood cell count. *Yersina* bacteremia occurs most frequently in the very young child and those who are immunosuppressed or have a condition with excessive iron storage, such as desferrioxamine use, sickle cell anemia, or thalassemias.

Routine stool culturing and testing is unnecessary in the healthy child who presents with an acute onset of illness and a short duration of symptoms. Antibiotic treatment of bacterial pathogens is only recommended in subsets of patients at risk for complications who also might benefit from treatment (see Table 72–2). Generally, supportive care and close follow up are the most essential treatments. Diarrhea that appears bloody, suggesting acute dysentery, or that is chronic in nature requires additional testing. During outbreaks of specific bacterial pathogens, more aggressive surveillance testing may be warranted and will usually be coordinated by local health authorities.

Minor Head Injury

Another frequent presentation associated with vomiting is minor head injury. The toddler age group is highly mobile, and minor head injuries are common. Children frequently present with vomiting after a minor head injury and, although parents are often warned to watch for vomiting, there is no clear association between the severity of head injury and vomiting.[14] There is evidence to suggest that vomiting after a minor head injury may be related to intrinsic patient factors rather than the severity of the injury. There appears to be a subset of children who are more likely to vomit and who have a higher incidence of motion sickness, migraines, family history of migraines, and prior unexplained vomiting episodes.[15] Vomiting that is persistent or latent in onset may be more likely to signify head injury.

Diagnostic Considerations in the Adolescent Patient

There are some unique diagnostic considerations in the adolescent patient who presents to the emergency department with vomiting. Isolated vomiting in a postmenarche adolescent female should always raise the suspicion of pregnancy, and ED testing can ensure proper follow-up and counseling. In addition, psychological disorders such as bulimia and anorexia may also present as recurring episodes of vomiting and diarrhea. Adolescents are also more likely to take intentional overdoses or abuse recreational drugs and then have vomiting as a symptom of toxicity or withdrawal. Migraines also become more common in older children and adolescents, and vomiting is typically a predominant feature of presentation.

Dehydration

Although the differential diagnosis for vomiting and diarrhea is exhaustive, fluid loss is a common consequence, regardless of etiology. The terms *volume depletion* and *dehydration* are used interchangeably daily on a clinical basis; however, it is important to remember that "dehydration" specifically refers to a state of hypertonicity and cannot be truly determined without laboratory analysis.[16] Fortunately, most children in the United States have only mild to moderate hypovolemia from their illness. One of the most important clinical indicators in determining the degree of hypovolemia is a documented weight loss. Previous visits to the ED or a private physician during the same illness can provide a source of weights for comparison. A parental report of history and observations of clinical symptoms in their child is highly sensitive, although not very specific, for predicting dehydration. A parental report of normal fluid intake and urine output significantly reduces the likelihood of significant dehydration.[17] Conventionally used clinical signs of dehydration are important and have fair interobserver reliability; however, individually they lack sufficient sensitivity in determining the degree of dehydration.[18,19]

Diagnosis of clinically significant dehydration must be based on the presence of a constellation of clinical findings as well as historical features (Table 72–3). Conventional teaching of the clinical signs and their estimated degree of dehydration are included for consideration; however, the provider is cautioned to remember that there has not been any systematic validation of these signs. The presence or absence of these signs must be considered in the context of the child's history, ongoing fluid losses, comorbid conditions, and severity of possible underlying etiology. Analyzing these classic parameters, one author found that all features were associated with dehydration, although there were only four independent predictors of dehydration: capillary refill greater than 2 seconds, absent tears, dry mucous membranes, and general ill appearance.[19] The presence of two of these four features predicted 5% dehydration with 79% sensitivity and 87% specificity, while the presence of three of the four features predicted 10% dehydration with 82% sensitivity and

83% specificity.[19] Severely dehydrated children with fluid deficits over 10% are much more likely to have a significant clinical finding; however, clinical findings tend to overestimate the degree of dehydration in patients with mild to moderate dehydration.

Diagnostic Testing

Diagnostic testing in the patient who presents with vomiting or diarrhea includes both laboratory and radiographic evaluation. Most patients who present with symptoms of vomiting and/or diarrhea will need only a thorough history and physical examination. As with physical findings, conventionally used serum electrolyte studies have poor predictive value in determining the degree of dehydration.[20-23] Routine laboratory testing is not essential and, given the trend of oral rehydration in these children, venipuncture to obtain a specimen for laboratory analysis is not clinically necessary and often traumatic for the child. In addition, serum electrolyte testing has been shown to be the 12th most costly contributor to hospital costs.[24] Although laboratory analysis may not prove useful by itself in determining the degree of dehydration in a child, the question of whether or not laboratory testing identifies clinically significant abnormalities that alter management and change outcome is a separate one. In one study, investigators found that all children with a clinically significant electrolyte abnormality had at least one of the following features: age less than 6 months, vomiting, delayed capillary refill, dry mucous membranes, tachycardia, or the presence of diabetes mellitus.[24] Ultimately, the provider is left to use clinical judgment when deciding to obtain serum electrolytes. In general, it is probably prudent to check serum electrolytes in children who are ill appearing, have a history inconsistent with simple gastroenteritis or viral-induced illness, have a history to support new-onset diabetes, have underlying comorbid conditions, require intravenous (IV) hydration, or are not clinically improving as expected.

Further laboratory testing in the patient with gastroenteritis is generally not indicated. Most episodes of gastroenteritis are viral induced and self-limited, and routine stool studies are not indicated.[25] Available tests include fecal leukocytes, occult blood testing, bacterial cultures, and *C. difficile* toxin, *Giardia* antigen, and rotavirus antigen detection. Fecal leukocytes may be present when the infecting pathogen causes a diffuse, invasive colitis; however, it is important to remember that the lack of fecal leukocytes does not exclude the

Table 72–3	Clinical Signs and Estimated Degree of Dehydration		
	Signs of Dehydration		
	Minimal or None	**Moderate**	**Severe**
General appearance	Well/alert	Fatigued/irritable	Lethargic
Eyes	Normal	Sunken	Very sunken
Tears	Present	Absent	Absent
Mucous membranes	Moist	Somewhat dry	Very dry
Thirst	Not thirsty	Drinks	Will not drink
Skin pinch	Retracts immediately	Slow	Very slow
Capillary refill	Normal	Prolonged	Prolonged
Pulses	Normal	Normal	Weak/thready
Heart rate	Normal	Increased	Increased
Urine output	Normal	Decreased	Minimal
Blood pressure	Normal	Normal	Normal/low

diagnosis of infectious diarrhea or the possibility of significant illness. For example, patients infected with the causative agent of HUS, enterohemorrhagic *E. coli*, generally have minimal to no white blood cells on stool smears.

Radiographic studies may be a valuable adjunct to the evaluation of the child who presents with isolated vomiting, especially when the diagnosis is in question and the history does not support the diagnosis of a straightforward viral illness. Radiographic testing should be tailored to answer a specific diagnostic question and refine the differential, and should never replace a complete history and physical examination. Indiscriminate use of higher radiation content studies such as computed tomography scans should be discouraged given recent concerns over radiation exposure in children with growing tissues and organs.[26] It is important to appreciate the limitations of certain frequently obtained studies, such as plain radiographs of the abdomen. Findings on plain films of the abdomen, for example, are extremely nonspecific and cannot exclude diagnoses such as intussusception, appendicitis, or malrotation.[27] Plain abdominal radiographs are most useful in detecting bowel obstructions, foreign bodies, and catastrophic events such as bowel perforation or volvulus. Investigators have shown that limiting radiographs to patients with prior abdominal surgery, suspected foreign body ingestions, abnormal bowel sounds, abdominal distention, or peritoneal signs can identify all patients with a radiographic diagnosis of a major disease and could have eliminated 48% of all studies ordered.[28] Plain films of the chest to rule out pneumonia as a cause for vomiting and referred abdominal pain may also be considered if clinically indicated.

Important Clinical Features and Considerations

Several important clinical signs should raise the suspicion for certain specific etiologies. Bilious emesis suggests obstruction or pathology distal to the ampulla of Vater and has classically been considered a herald sign for surgical disease. While this may certainly be the case in the neonate with bilious emesis, the importance of bilious emesis in older infants and children is less clear.[29] Studies have shown that between 20% and 50% of infants presenting with bilious emesis within the first week of life have a surgical condition.[30,31] For example, it is the classic common presentation in infants who have malrotation with volvulus (see Chapter 83, Malrotation and Midgut Volvulus).

Bloody emesis is another clinical symptoms that will frequently panic parents and lead them to seek medical care. Hematemesis may result from trauma to the nasopharynx or from the GI tract. Most upper GI bleeds due to vomiting in children are self-limited (see Chapter 75, Gastrointestinal Bleeding). Reports of endocsopy findings in children with hematemesis after vomiting suggest that Mallory-Weiss tears are rare and that another postemetic condition called prolapse gastropathy syndrome may be a more likely cause for the hematemesis.[32] Prolapse gastropathy syndrome describes a small gastric mucosal hemorrhage occurring in the proximal stomach resulting in hematemesis. Whether the infrequent incidence of Mallory-Weiss tears is a result of pediatric physiology or is related to underdiagnosis, the management of hematemesis in children is largely supportive and endoscopy is rarely indicated.

Bloody diarrhea is another symptom that requires the consideration of specific etiologies. Bloody diarrhea may be due to dysentery from infections, while any concern for enterohemorrhagic *E. coli* O157:H7 requires additional work up given its potential for causing HUS. If a child has a history of diarrhea for several days that suddenly becomes bloody, the diagnosis of HUS should be considered (see Chapter 131, Hemolytic-Uremic Syndrome). HUS is characterized by bloody diarrhea, hemolysis, and renal insufficiency. Laboratory testing to evaluate for anemia, renal failure, and the presence of *E.coli* O157:H7 is indicated. Another important consideration in the child with bloody stools is intussusception. The history may be complicated by the presence of a recent gastroenteritis illness. Bowel edema and inflammation from a recent gastroenteritis can make bowel more likely to intussuscept. Recurrent episodes of abdominal pain may not be prominent, requiring the provider to maintain a high degree of clinical suspicion to avoid missing this clinical entity (see Chapter 74, Intussusception).

Abdominal pain is a frequent complaint in the patient with frequent vomiting. However, persistent, reproducible abdominal tenderness on clinical examination suggests a diagnosis beyond a simple viral illness (e.g., appendicitis). Pain associated with gastroenteritis frequently resolves with hydration therapy and is typically described as crampy in nature and ill-localized. In addition, abdominal distention is not frequently associated with a routine vial illness and is more likely to be present in the child who has additional pathology, such as intestinal obstruction, mass, or ascites.

The child with chronic medical conditions or special health care needs requires additional consideration of unique etiologies. Children with central nervous system ventricular shunts may present with vomiting as a sign of shunt malfunction (see Chapter 42, Conditions Causing Increased Intracranial Pressure). Although drowsiness has been shown to be the best clinical predictor of ventriculoperitoneal shunt malfunction, vomiting is also common, affecting as many as 73% of patients.[33] Children with a history of malignancy may present with vomiting related to chemotherapy or secondary to recurrent disease (see Chapter 45, Brain Tumor). Neurologically impaired children also have an oversensitive emetic reflex and are more likely to have frequent vomiting episodes. These children may also have subtle findings such as isolated vomiting with a volvulus. Vomiting may be a sign of bladder perforation in children who have received bladder augmentation for a small or neurogenic bladder. Rupture may occur even years after a repair, and symptoms may be subtle, particularly in children with spina bifida.[34,35] Following fundoplication, children may still have activation of the emetic reflex, resulting in retching symptoms without frank emesis.[6] Vomiting in children with metabolic disorders such as diabetes may signal underlying infections and diseases as well as contribute to significant morbidity in these children if it is not rapidly addressed.

Management

Management of presumed viral-induced isolated vomiting or gastroenteritis focuses on fluid therapy. Since its inception in the 1960s, the use of oral rehydration therapy (ORT) with oral glucose-electrolyte solutions has directly contributed to a decrease in mortality from acute gastroenteritis worldwide.[2]

Table 72–4	Sample Protocol for Oral Rehydration Therapy (ORT)

- Obtain current weight and estimate percentage dehydration
- Consider ondansetron 0.2 mg/kg per dose (max. 4 mg) orally 20 min prior to start of therapy
- Administer 20 ml/kg per hour of Rehydralyte/Pedialyte for 2–4 hr via syringe, or consider continuous nasogastric feeds through a 5-French feeding tube
- Add additional 10 ml/kg for each diarrheal stool
- If child tolerates 2 hr of ORT and is clinically improving, may continue ORT at home for next 2 hr of therapy
- Resume age-appropriate diet in 4–6 hr
- If more than 2 episodes of vomiting during ORT, may change to intravenous fluid therapy

Contraindications to ORT:

- Severe dehydration (oral rehydration may still proceed cautiously if no other contraindications exist)
- Shock
- Altered mental status
- Child < 3 mo of age
- Concerns for abdominal pathology
- Abdominal distention or ileus
- Significant comorbid conditions (congenital heart problems, prior abdominal surgeries, metabolic diseases, diabetes)

With ORT, pediatric mortality from diarrheal illness has declined from an estimated 5 million deaths per year in 1982 to 3 million in 1992 and 1.5 to 2.5 million per year currently.[2] Despite its worldwide success, the use of the technically more simple ORT has lagged behind in the United States. Research has shown that ORT leads to shorter length of stay in the ED, increased parental satisfaction with the visit, decreased hospital admission rates, and rapid improvement in symptoms.[36-40] ORT not only encompasses the rehydration phase, as the term implies, but also refers to the replacement of ongoing losses and early enteral feeding.

In the patient with minimal or no evidence of dehydration who has symptoms of gastroenteritis, the treatment goal is to provide compensation for ongoing losses. Parents should continue normal feedings and supplement each diarrheal stool or emesis with an additional 10 ml/kg of a commercially available pediatric electrolyte replacement solution. In children with mild to moderate dehydration, the fluid deficit is replaced rapidly over 4 hours, with subsequent return to normal enteral feedings and continuing replacement for ongoing losses (Table 72–4). Children with signs of severe dehydration or shock require immediate resuscitation with rapid initiation of IV fluids. An initial IV fluid bolus of 20 ml/kg over 30 minutes using normal saline or lactated Ringer's solution is appropriate and may be repeated in boluses of 20 ml/kg as needed, to a typical maximum of 60 ml/kg. Failure to respond to treatment with IV fluids must raise the suspicion of other illnesses such as cardiac, metabolic, or neurologic disorders.

Pharmacologic therapy for gastroenteritis includes medications marketed for vomiting and diarrhea. In general, antidiarrheal medications are not recommended. In particular, antimotility agents containing ingredients such as loperamide, diphenoxylate, and atropine are not intended for use in children, and there is no clinically significant evidence that they change outcomes.[1,2] These medications have significant side effects, including ileus, sedation, respiratory depression, paradoxical agitation, and increased nausea. Deaths

have also been reported with loperamide use.[41] Agents such as bismuth subsalicylate have shown limited efficacy in acute gastroenteritis, and toxicity from the salicylate component is a concern. Until recently, experience with antiemetic treatment was limited to phenothiazines, most frequently promethazine. Because children are particularly sensitive to the side effects of promethazine, the Food and Drug Administration (FDA) recently added warnings to its label stating that it should not be used in children less than 2 years of age and should be used with caution in children if used at all. Side effects include agitation and dystonic reactions; however, more commonly, phenothiazines cause significant sedation. This extreme sedation is problematic for two reasons. First, a profoundly sedated child will be unable to participate in aggressive ORT either at home or in the ED. Second, sedation caused by phenothiazines makes it difficult to assess a child and determine clinical improvement or deterioration.

Fortunately, newer antiemetic medications have emerged over the last several years. Studies have recently demonstrated benefit from the use of the serotonin antagonist ondansetron in the treatment of pediatric gastroenteritis.[42-45] Ondansetron has been used extensively for the management of vomiting in the pediatric postoperative and oncology settings; however, its application to the patient with gastroenteritis is a relatively new development. A single dose of ondansetron administered either IV or orally in the ED can decrease the frequency of vomiting and hospital admission rates.[42,43] Oral ondansetron also decreases the need for IV fluid therapy in the ED setting and can be a valuable adjunct in the management of gastroenteritis with ORT. The oral dose is typically 0.2 mg/kg per dose and the IV dose is typically 0.15 mg/kg per dose, with a maximum of 4 mg per dose. Use is generally limited to children over the age of 6 months. The routine practice of sending patients home with a prescription for ondansetron is generally unnecessary and not likely to be currently cost effective. In addition, although the diarrhea component of gastroenteritis may persist for days, the vomiting is typically self-limited and occurs early in the illness. Parents who receive a prescription for an antiemetic could theoretically be more likely to wait out a progressively worsening illness at home, when the actual etiology of persistent vomiting may be more severe than a viral acute gastroenteritis.

Zinc supplementation is associated with improved intestinal permeability and in developing countries has been shown to decrease number of stools per day and number of days of illness, and to be a cost-effective adjunct to ORT.[2,46,47] Further research is needed before zinc supplements can be recommended as a standard adjunct to therapy in developed countries. The addition of probiotics, defined as live microorganisms in fermented foods that improve balance in intestinal microflora, has also been the topic of research in acute gastroenteritis. The Lactobacillus species has been shown to be effective as a treatment for children with acute gastroenteritis; however, specific supplements marketed for this use are not subject to regulation by the FDA and therefore are not routinely recommended.[2,48]

Recommendations for the timing and composition of feeding during acute gastroenteritis have changed significantly in recent years. The "refeeding syndrome," described as severe fluid and electrolyte shifts that occur when malnourished or starved patients begin enteral feeds, has not been described in children with simple gastroenteritis who begin enteral feeds. The syndrome is an uncommon yet potential problem in the severely malnourished, and was classically described in adult survivors of concentration camps.[49] Children should be allowed to resume a normal diet as soon as the rehydration phase of ORT or IV fluid therapy is completed.

The availability of over-the-counter rehydration solutions may also lead parents to think they are superior to a normal diet for their child with diarrhea. Severe malnutrition and deprivation stools can result from the prolonged, inappropriate use of these solutions. Parents need to be reminded that they should never be used as a substitute for more nutritious foods. Breast-fed infants should be encouraged to breast-feed even during the rehydration phase, while formula-fed infants should resume their normal formula as soon as rehydration is completed. Early refeeding improves weight gain after rehydration and is not associated with a significant increase in diarrhea.[49] True lactose intolerance following acute viral gastroenteritis is uncommon, and changing an infant to a lactose-free formula is unnecessary. If diarrhea worsens after introduction of lactose-containing formulas, a temporary trial of a lactose-free formula is reasonable. There is evidence that soy formulas may provide additional bulk to the stools; however, overall stool output remains unchanged.[50] Soy formula is therefore not recommended, although it may provide some relief from the irritant diaper dermatitis that results from liquid stools. Formula is not superior to a normal mixed diet in children who are taking solid foods.[51] These children should be encouraged to resume a nonrestricted diet with a focus on foods high in complex carbohydrates such as fruits, lean meats, vegetables, and yogurt. Foods high in simple sugars, such as juices and sodas, should be consumed sparingly. The classically recommended BRAT (bananas, rice, applesauce, and toast) diet is considered too restrictive and does not supply the nutrition needed for optimal recovery.[2]

Summary

The prognosis for an infant or child with vomiting and diarrhea depends on the specific etiology. Clinicians must diligently evaluate these children for serious abdominal and extra-abdominal disorders that can cause vomiting. Children with gastroenteritis typically recover with appropriate supportive care and treatment. Those with mild to moderate dehydration should begin to improve in the ED a couple of hours after the initiation of fluid therapy. They generally become more alert and interested in their surroundings, such as toys, and express the desire to drink or eat. Admission should be considered for any child who is not responding to appropriate fluid therapy, has abdominal pain that remains vague and requires serial examinations, or requires the services of a consultant such as a surgeon. Transfer to a pediatric hospital for evaluation by pediatric subspecialists may be required in areas where the local medical staff is uncomfortable caring for children or when the etiology requires subspecialists found only at a children's center.

REFERENCES

1. American Academy of Pediatrics, Provisional Committee on Quality Improvement, Subcommittee on Acute Gastroenteritis: Practice parameter: the management of acute gastroenteritis in young children. Pediatrics 97:424–435, 1996.
*2. King C, Glass R, Bresce J, et al: Managing acute gastroenteritis among children. MMWR Recomm Rep 52(RR-16):1–16, 2003.
3. Black R, Morris S, Bryce J: Where and why are 10 million children dying every year? Lancet 361:2226–2234, 2003.
4. Miller A: Central mechanisms of vomiting. Dig Dis Sci 44(8 Suppl):39S–43S, 1999.
5. Acra SA, Ghishan GK: Electrolyte fluxes in the gut and oral rehydration solutions. Pediatric Clin North Am 43:433–439, 1996.
6. Richards CA, Milla PJ, Andrews PL, Spitz L: Retching and vomiting in neurologically impaired children after fundoplication: predictive preoperative factors. J Pediatr Surg 36:1401–1404, 2001.
7. Rudolph CD, Mazur LJ, Liptak GS, et al; North American Society for Pediatric Gastroenterology and Nutrition: Guidelines for evaluation and treatment of gastroesophageal reflux in infants and children: recommendations of the North American Society for Pediatric Gastroenterology and Nutrition. J Pediatar Gastroenterol Nutr 32(Suppl 2), 2001.
8. Steffen R: Vomiting and gastric motility in infants with cow's milk allergy. Clin Pediatr (Phila) 40:469, 2001.
9. Ravelli A, Tobanelli P, Volpi S, et al: Vomiting and gastric motility in infants with cow's milk allergy. J Pediatr Gastroenterol Nutr 32:59–64, 2001.
10. Host A: Frequency of cow's milk allergy in childhood. Ann Allergy Asthma Immunol 89(6 Suppl 1):33–37, 2002.
11. Ford-Jones E, Wang E, Petric M, et al; Greater Toronto Area/Peel Region PRESI Study Group; Pediatric Rotavirus Epidemiology Study for Immunization: Hospitalization for community-acquired, rotavirus-associated diarrhea: a prospective, longitudinal, population-based study during the seasonal outbreak. Arch Pediatr Adolesc Med 154:578–585, 2000
12. Parashar UD, Holman RC, Clarke MJ: Hospitalization associated with rotavirus infection in the United States. J Infect Dis 177:13–17, 1998.
13. Suzuki H, Katsushima N, Konno T: Rotavirus vaccine put on hold. Lancet 354:1390, 1999.
14. Dunning J, Batchelor J, Stratford-Smith P, et al: A meta-analysis of variables that predict significant intracranial injury in minor head trauma. Arch Dis Child 89:593–594, 2004.
15. Brown F, Brown J, Beattie T: Why do children vomit after minor head injury? J Accid Emerg Med 17:268–271, 2000.
16. Mange K, Matsuura D, Cizman B, et al: Language guiding therapy: the case of dehydration versus volume depletion. Ann Intern Med 127:848–853, 1997.
17. Porter S, Fleisher G, Kohane I, et al: The value of parental report for diagnosis and management of dehydration in the emergency department. Ann Emerg Med 41:196–205, 2003.
18. Steiner MJ, DeWalt DA, Byerly JS, et al: Is this child dehydrated? JAMA 291:2746–2754, 2004.
19. Gorelick M, Shaw K, Murphy K: Validity and reliability of clinical signs in the diagnosis of dehydration in children. Pediatrics 99:e6, 1997.
20. Teach S, Yates E, Feld L: Laboratory predictors of fluid deficit in acutely dehydrated children. Clin Pediatr (Phila) 36:395–400, 1997.
21. Shaoul R, Okev N, Tamir A, et al: Value of laboratory studies in assessment of dehydration in children. Ann Clin Biochem 41(Pt 3):192–196, 2004.
22. Narchi H: Serum bicarbonate and dehydration severity in gastroenteritis. Arch Dis Child 79:379–380, 1998.
23. Duggan C, Refat M, Hashem M, et al: How valid are clinical signs of dehydration in infants? J Pediatr Gastroenterol Nutr 22:56–61, 1996.
24. Rothrock SG, Green SM, McArthur CL, et al: Detection of electrolyte abnormalities in children presenting to the emergency department: a multicenter, prospective analysis. Acad Emerg Med 4:1025–1031, 1997.
25. Zaidi AK, Macone A, Goldmann AD: Impact of simple screening criteria on utilization of low-yield bacterial stool cultures in a children's hospital. Pediatrics 103(6 Pt 1):1189–1192, 1999.
26. Brenner D, Ellisston C, Hall E, et al: Estimated risks of radiation-induced fatal cancer from pediatric CT. AJR Am J Roentgenol 176:289–296, 2001.

---

*Selected readings.

27. Lilien LD, Srinivasan G, Pyati SP, et al: Green vomiting in the first 72 hours in normal infants. Am J Dis Child 140:662–664, 1986.

*28. Rothrock SG, Green SM, Harding M, et al: Plain abdominal radiography in the detection of acute medical and surgical disease in children: a retrospective analysis. Pediatr Emerg Care 7:281–285, 1991.

29. Sadow K, Atabaki S, Johns C, et al: Bilious emesis in the pediatric emergency department: etiology and outcome. Clin Pediatr (Phila) 41:475–479, 2002.

30. Dawson KP, Graham D: The assessment of dehydration in congenital pyloric stenosis. N Z Med J 104:162–163, 1991.

31. Kao H-A: Bilious vomiting during the first week of life. Acta Paediatr Sin 35:202–207, 1994.

32. Bishop P, Nowicki M, Parker P: Vomiting-induced hematemesis in children: Mallory-Weiss tear or prolapse gastropathy? J Pediatr Gastroenterol Nutr 30:436–441, 2000.

33. Barnes N, Jones S, Hayward R, et al: Ventriculoperitoneal shunt block: what are the best predictive clinical indicators? Arch Dis Child 87:198–201, 2002.

34. Rushton HG, Woodard JR, Parrott TS: Delayed bladder rupture after augmentation enterocystoplasty. J Urol 140:344–346, 1988.

35. Glass RB, Rushton HG: Delayed spontaneous rupture of augmented bladder in children: diagnosis with sonography and CT. AJR Am J Roentgenol 158:833–835, 1992.

36. Santosham M, Keenan E, Tulloch J, et al: Oral rehydration therapy for diarrhea: an example of reverse transfer of technology. Pediatrics 100:e10, 1997.

*37. Atherly-John YC, Cunningham SJ, Crain EF: A randomized trial of oral vs intravenous rehydration in a pediatric emergency department. Arch Pediatr Adolesc Med 156:1240–1243, 2002.

*38. Fonesecca BK, Holdgate A, Craig JC: Enteral vs intravenous rehydration therapy for children with gastroenteritis. Arch Pediatr Adolesc Med 158:483–490, 2004.

39. Nager AL, Wang VJ: Comparison of nsaogastric and intravenous methods of rehydration in pediatric patients with acute dehydration. Pediatrics 109:566–572, 2002.

40. Bender BJ, Ozuah PO: Intravenous rehydration for gastroenteritis: how long does it really take? Pediatr Emerg Care 20:215–218, 2004.

41. Bhutta TI, Tahir KI: Loperamide poisoning in children. Lancet 335:363, 1990.

42. Scuderi P: Pharmacology of antiemetics. Int Anesthesiol Clin 41:41–66, 2003.

43. Reeves J, Shannon M, Fleisher G: Ondansetron decreases vomiting associated with acute gastroenteritis: a randomized, controlled trial. Pediatrics 109:e62, 2002.

*44. Ramsook C, Sahagun-Carreon I, Kozinetz C, et al: A randomized clinical trial comparing oral ondansetron with placebo in children with vomiting from acute gastroenteritis. Ann Emerg Med 39:397–403, 2002.

45. Cubeddu LX, Trujillo LM, Taqlmaciu I, et al: Antiemetic activity of ondansetron in acute gastroenteritis. Aliment Pharmacol Ther 11:185–189, 1997.

46. Bhatnagar S, Bahl R, Sharma PK, et al: Zinc with oral rehydration therapy reduces stool output and duration of diarrhea in hospitalized children: a randomized controlled trial. J Pediatr Gastroenterol Nutr 38:34–40, 2004.

47. Robberstad B, Strand T, Blace RE, et al: Cost-effectiveness of zinc as adjunct therapy for acute childhood diarrhoea in developing countries. Bull World Health Organ 82:523–531, 2004.

48. Huang J, Bousvaros A, Lee J, et al: Efficacy of probiotic use in acute diarrhea in children: a meta-analysis. Dig Dis Sci 47:2625–2634, 2002.

49. Sandhu BK; European Society of Paediatric Gastroenterology, Hepatology and Nutrition Working Group on Acute Diarrhoea: Rationale for early feeding in childhood gastroenteritis. J Pediatr Gastroenterol Nutr 33:S13–S16, 2001.

50. Brown KH, Perez F, Peerson J, et al: Effect of dietary fiber on the severity, duration, and nutritional outcome of acute, watery diarrhea in children. Pediatrics 92:241–247, 1993.

51. Maulen-Radovan I, Brown KH, Acosta MA, et al: Comparison of a rice-based, mixed diet versus a lactose-free, soy-protein isolate formula for young children with acute diarrhea. J Pediatr 125(5 Pt 1):699–706, 1994.

52. American Academy of Pediatrics: Red Book Online, 2006. Available at *http://aapredbook.aappublications.org/*

Chapter 73

Appendicitis

Steven G. Rothrock, MD

Key Points

Infants and young children frequently present with atypical clinical features (e.g., vomiting that precedes pain, diarrhea, genitourinary features, and diffuse tenderness).

Clinicians should not rely exclusively on normal serum parameters (e.g., white blood cell count, C-reactive protein) to rule out appendicitis.

Computed tomography (CT) can be an accurate test if proper techniques are used (spiral CT, thin collimation, thin reconstructed images, rectal contrast with or without intravenous contrast).

Performance of a rectal examination to elicit tenderness does not add useful information to the clinical evaluation of children with possible appendicitis.

Introduction and Background

Appendicitis is the most common surgical abdominal disorder in children ages 2 and older.[1] While abdominal pain is a common symptom in children presenting to the emergency department, only 1% to 8% with this complaint will have appendicitis.[2-4] As features of appendicitis (e.g., fever, vomiting) frequently overlap with those of more common diseases (e.g., gastroenteritis, viral syndromes), identifying this disorder can be difficult. This overlap of clinical features, in part, accounts for misdiagnosis rates of nearly 70% to 100% in infants, up to 57% for toddlers, 12% to 28% for school-age children, and nearly 15% for adolescents.[1]

Recognition and Approach

To accurately diagnose appendicitis, clinicians must be aware of the age-specific variations in anatomy and development that affect presenting features (Table 73–1).

In neonates and infants, the appendix is funnel shaped and not easily obstructed. This accounts for an extremely low rate of appendicitis in infancy. The thin-walled appendix is prone to perforation, and the cecum is less able to distend and decompress the appendix when it expands. As children age, lymphatic tissue increases within the gastrointestinal tract, increasing the propensity for appendiceal luminal obstruction and development of appendicitis. Lymphatic tissue proliferation peaks in the late teen years, the age at which appendicitis is most common.[1,5]

Appendices of infants and young children have greater mobility and are less likely to be fixed to mesentery compared to older children. Moreover, an underdeveloped omentum often cannot contain purulent material following perforation. These features account for a lower rate of contained abscesses and a higher rate of diffuse peritonitis in infants and children ≤ 5 years old compared to older children.[1]

Communication skills play an important role in describing onset, quality, and characteristics of pain. As infants less than 2 years old cannot describe pain, the median time from symptom onset to diagnosis is 3 to 4 days. Most cases are perforated at diagnosis, and most are evaluated by a physician and incorrectly diagnosed before appendicitis is detected.[1] Preschool-aged children usually cannot describe their symptoms well, and the classic sequence of abdominal pain followed by vomiting is often not appreciated. In fact, vomiting is often the first symptom noted by parents, while pain is often not noted until after the onset of vomiting.[6] Moreover, diagnosis usually occurs after perforation, with symptoms of pain, fever, and vomiting predominating. In school-age children and adolescents, the history and physical examination are generally more reliable. Older children more accurately relay descriptors including onset of centrally located pain that later migrates to the right lower quadrant, quality of pain, and features that aggravate pain.

Advanced appendicitis (e.g., perforation, gangrenous appendix) is more common in younger age groups. This advanced disease state is reflected in radiologic examinations. Compared to adults, bowel obstruction and ileus are more common with perforation, while ultrasonography (US) may be less able to visualize an increased wall-to-wall diameter following appendiceal perforation. Diminished mesenteric and intra-abdominal fat have the potential to obscure typical computed tomography (CT) findings of inflammation in uncomplicated appendicitis, while intra-abdominal abscess formation is more common in younger children (especially those < 10 years old).[7]

Table 73-1	Frequency of Age Specific Presenting Features of Appendicitis		
	Age		
Presenting Feature	**<2 years**	**2 to 5 years**	**6 to 12 years**
Pain	35% to 77%	89% to 100%	98% to 100%
Vomiting	85% to 90%	66% to 100%	68% to 95%
Fever	40% to 60%	80% to 87%	4% to 64%*
Diarrhea	18% to 46%	33%	9% to 16%
RLQ tenderness	<50%	58% to 85%	>80% to 95%
Diffuse tenderness	55% to 92%	19% to 28%	15% to 83%†

*The percentage of school-aged children with fever varies with the duration of symptoms. Only 4% are expected to have fever within the first 24 hours of symptoms.
†The percentage of school-aged children with diffuse abdominal tenderness varies with the presence of perforation. Without perforation, the rate is 15%. With perforation, the rate is 83%.
Abbreviation: RLQ, right lower quadrant.
Adapted from Rothrock SG, Pagane J: Acute appendicitis in children: emergency department diagnosis and management. Ann Emerg Med 36:39–51, 2000.

Clinical Presentation

Presenting Features

Presenting clinical features of appendicitis differ depending upon the child's age (see Table 73–1).

Neonates

Cases of neonatal appendicitis are rare, occur primarily in premature neonates, and are due to distal colonic obstruction (e.g., Hirschsprung's disease), cardiac emboli, incarcerated hernias, or a localized form of necrotizing enterocolitis and not appendiceal lumen obstruction.[8-11] Due to difficulty with diagnosis and rarity of this disorder in neonates, mortality exceeds 80% and most cases are diagnosed at autopsy.[9,10] Abdominal distention and vomiting are the most common symptoms present in the majority of cases. Other features include irritability or lethargy, a palpable mass, abdominal wall cellulites, hypotension, hypothermia, and respiratory distress.[1]

Infants and Toddlers

Appendicitis is a rare disease in children younger than 2 years, with initial misdiagnosis rates of nearly 100%.[12-15] Typical symptom duration prior to diagnosis is greater than 3 days, with perforation rates that approach 100%.[12] The most common symptoms are vomiting, abdominal pain, fever, and diarrhea[5,12-16] (see Table 73–1). Other nonspecific presenting symptoms include irritability in one third of cases, difficulty breathing or grunting in 8% to 23%, upper respiratory infection symptoms in 40%, and right hip pain/stiffness in 3% to 23%.[13-15,17,18] Diffuse abdominal tenderness is present in most cases, while localized right lower quadrant tenderness is noted in few cases.[12-14,16,18] Other features include lethargy due to sepsis, abdominal rigidity or distention, and an abdominal or rectal mass due to abscess formation.[5,13,14,18]

Preschoolers

Diagnosis of appendicitis in preschool-age children is difficult. Most preschool-age children have symptoms for 2 or more days before presenting, and nearly half are initially misdiagnosed.[19,20] Abdominal pain, vomiting, and a complaint of fever are present in most cases.[16,19-23] Parents often report that vomiting preceded the onset of pain.[6] This atypical sequence of events may be due to the fact that parents may only notice their child is ill after vomiting begins. Anorexia, a symptom common to older children and adults, may be difficult to elicit in younger children. Guarding, rebound tenderness, and a documented temperature above 37.5° C (99.5° F) are variably present.[16,19-23] Unlike younger infants, right lower quadrant tenderness is more common than diffuse tenderness as a result of a more well-formed omentum with more localized peritonitis following perforation.[22,24]

School-Age Children

The incidence of appendicitis increases and the clinical evaluation becomes more reliable in school-age children. Nearly one third of children at this age relay that their pain began centrally and later migrated to the right lower quadrant.[1,25] In those without this sequence, pain usually begins and remains in the right lower quadrant or begins and remains diffuse.[25] Pain is described as steady and worse with movement in most cases, while it is described as colicky in 11% to 35%.[25,26] Pain with jumping or with coughing is present in 93%.[27] Vomiting is present in 68% to 95% of cases and may precede or begin simultaneously with the pain in 18%.[25,26] Anorexia occurs in 47% to 75%, diarrhea in 9% to 16%, constipation in 5% to 28%, and dysuria in 4% to 20% of school-age children with appendicitis.[6,25] Prior episodes of similar pain are found in up to one third of cases.[25] Family history is often overlooked when considering the diagnosis of appendicitis. However, having a first-degree relative who has had appendicitis (especially under the age of 11) increases a child's risk for developing appendicitis 3- to 10-fold.[28-31]

Physical examination findings differ depending upon the timing and stage of presentation. If symptoms have been present for less than 24 hours, 4% of patients will have a temperature ≥ 38° C (100.4° F). If symptoms have been present for 24 to 48 hours, 64% of patients will have a temperature elevation, while even more are febrile if symptoms have been present for 48 hours or more.[32] Right lower quadrant tenderness is present in almost all school-age children with appendicitis. However, tenderness may extend to the entire lower abdomen in 15% without perforation, and in up to 83% with perforation.[25] Bowel sounds are normal or hyperactive in 93% of children with appendicitis and may not be hypoactive or absent unless diffuse peritonitis or bowel obstruction is present.[33] Guarding is present in 51% of cases, and rebound in 41% without perforation, while these features are present in 91% and 85% of cases with perforation, respectively.[25,26] Importantly, assessing for peritoneal signs is more difficult in children than in adults. Rebound tenderness should not be elicited in children as many without appendicitis will have some degree of tenderness with this maneuver. Instead, percussion tenderness is considered to be a more reliable means of assessing for peritonitis.[27] Finally, performance of a rectal examination to elicit tenderness does not add useful information to the clinical evaluation of children with possible appendicitis.[1]

Adolescents

The peak incidence of appendicitis is during adolescence and early adulthood. While the history and physical examination become more reliable, pelvic pathology becomes more common in females, potentially obscuring the diagnosis. Adnexal tenderness and cervical motion tenderness are often present in these cases. In fact, one third of females ages 15 and older with appendicitis are initially misdiagnosed as having pelvic disorders, gastroenteritis, or urinary infections.[34]

Ancillary Studies

The only required test for children with possible appendicitis is a serum or urine β-human chorionic gonadotropin test (i.e., a pregnancy test) in adolescent girls (see Chapter 90, Ectopic Pregnancy). Other tests, including serum markers, urinalysis, and imaging adjuncts, have variable utility for either excluding or diagnosing appendicitis. Knowing the utility and limitations of each of these studies is useful for emergency physicians.

While many authors have recommended a serum white blood cell (WBC) count in children with suspected appendicitis, this test has only limited utility for diagnosing this disorder. Sensitivity of an elevated WBC count (>10 to 12×10^9 cells per liter) ranges from 51% to 91%.[1] Sensitivity falls even further (18% in one study) if symptoms have been present less than 24 hours.[1] In contrast, an elevated neutrophil percentage (i.e., a left shift) is present in the majority of cases in the first 24 hours after symptom onset.[1] Either the WBC count or neutrophil percentage is elevated in most children with appendicitis who have had symptoms for more than 24 hours.[1] These tests also are elevated in nearly half of all patients with gastroenteritis, mesenteric adenitis, pelvic inflammatory disease, and many other infectious disorders that must be differentiated from appendicitis. The WBC count cannot differentiate between cases of perforated and nonperforated appendicitis. Moreover, it is unclear if following serial WBC counts in suspected appendicitis is useful. Conflicting studies (primarily limited to adult patients) have found serial WBC counts will fall,[35-37] rise,[38] or remain unchanged[39] in cases of appendicitis.

Another inflammatory mediator, C-reactive protein (CRP), has been used widely to stratify the risk of appendicitis. An elevated CRP is 43% to 92% sensitive and 33% to 95% specific for diagnosing appendicitis in children.[1] These wide ranges are due to the varied upper thresholds used for defining an abnormal CRP (0.9 to 5.0 mg/dl). CRP level has been shown to be superior to the WBC upper thresholds at detecting appendiceal perforation and abscess formation (disorders that are more common in pediatric appendicitis).[1]

In a study that included adults, one author found sequential CRP levels useful at diagnosing appendicitis. Initial CRP was 60% sensitive, with sensitivity rising to 86% by 4 hours, 95% by 8 hours, and 100% by 12 hours after admission.[36]

Seven percent to 14% of children with appendicitis have greater than 5 WBCs per high-power field or greater than 5 red blood cells per high-power field on microscopic urinalysis.[6] These findings can lead to an erroneous diagnosis of a urinary tract infection or nephrolithiasis. In fact, 17% of children with appendicitis have bacteriuria, a finding that becomes even more common in advanced disease states (e. g., perforation, abscess formation).[40] Proposed mechanisms for these abnormalities include direct spread of bacteria from the inflamed appendix to the urinary tract and inflammatory changes due to a proximate inflamed appendix.[40]

Scoring Systems

Numerical scoring systems that combine clinical features and serum markers can stratify the risk that a child has appendicitis. One of the simplest and most widely studied clinical appendicitis scores is the MANTRELS or Alvarado score. This score assigns points for clinical features and serum WBC count and neutrophil percentage (Table 73–2). The MANTRELS score, while originally derived in adults, has shown utility at stratifying appendicitis risk in adolescents, although reliance solely on this test to make the diagnosis of appendicitis has limitations.[41] Studies have shown a score of ≥ 7 to be 86% to 90% sensitive and 72% to 86% specific for diagnosing appendicitis in children, while a score ≥ 5 is 93% to 100% sensitive.[41-43] Other authors have modified the MANTRELS score in children by dropping the neutrophil percentage and found a modified score ≥ 7 to be 76% to 90% sensitive for detecting appendicitis.[1] One prospective study modified the MANTRELS score further, by substituting rebound tender-

Table 73–2	Clinical Appendicitis Scores	
Feature	**MANTRELS Score**	**Pediatric Appendicitis Score (PAS)**
Migration of pain from central to right lower quadrant area	1	1
Anorexia or acetonuria	1	1
Nausea with vomiting	1	1
Tender right lower quadrant	2	2
Rebound tenderness	1	—
(Rebound equivalent—pain with hopping or coughing, or percussion tenderness)	—	2
Elevated temperature ≥ 38° C (100.4° F)	1	1
Leukocytosis	2	1
Shifted white blood cell count (>75% neutrophils)	1	1

Total Score	**Interpretation**
MANTRELS	
≤4	Low likelihood of appendicitis
5–6	Possible appendicitis
≥7	Probable appendicitis
PAS	
≤6	Low likelihood of appendicitis
≥6	Possible or probable appendicitis

ness with an alternate test for peritonitis (pain with cough, pain with jumping, or percussion tenderness) and assigning 2 points to this feature while removing 1 point from the leukocyte count[27] (see Table 73–2). The authors found this modified Pediatric Appendicitis Score had 100% sensitivity and 92% specificity for diagnosing appendicitis if a cutoff of ≥ 6 was used to diagnose appendicitis.[27] However, the prevalence of appendicitis was high (>60% of cases), children may have been seen late in their disease course, and it is uncertain if the Pediatric Appendicitis Score's test characteristics will be as accurate if applied to a less ill emergency department population.

Imaging Studies

In general, plain abdominal radiographs are not helpful for diagnosing uncomplicated appendicitis in children. Commonly cited findings of rightward scoliosis, soft tissue changes, localized ileus, and "free peritoneal fluid" occur in children with and without appendicitis.[44] Radiographs in children with appendiceal perforation may show bowel obstruction, a right lower quadrant mass, or a calcified appendicolith.[12,45] Of these radiographic findings, a calcified appendicolith is the most specific for appendicitis, present in 10% to 20% of young children with perforated appendicitis, in less than 10% with uncomplicated appendicitis, and in only 1% to 2% of children without appendicitis.[45-47] However, plain radiographs are normal or nonspecific in over three quarters of children with appendicitis, and this modality, in general, should not be used to exclude or diagnose this disorder.[46-48]

Ultrasonography has been studied extensively in children with suspected appendicitis. Experienced centers have found ultrasound to be nearly 90% sensitive and greater than 95% specific for diagnosing appendicitis, while others have reported a sensitivity as low as 44% to 48%.[49-52] Ultrasonographic findings diagnostic of nonperforated appendicitis include an appendiceal diameter greater than 6 mm, a "target sign" with five concentric layers, distention or obstruction of the appendiceal lumen, and muscular wall thickness greater than 2 mm. Ultrasonographic accuracy is diminished in perforated cases as the appendix may no longer be enlarged, and nonspecific features of absent peristalsis or a pericecal or perivesical mass may be the only findings. The primary advantages of ultrasound are noninvasiveness, lack of radiation exposure, and high specificity. Retrospective studies have found its use to be associated with increased cost, increased time to surgery, and increased length of hospitalization without altering complication rates.[53] Due to limited experience and reported poor sensitivity, many centers do not perform ultrasound on children with suspected appendicitis. For those sites performing ultrasound, a negative examination should not be relied upon to exclude appendicitis due to its limited sensitivity.

CT is an accurate test for diagnosing appendicitis. CT has superior sensitivity to ultrasonography.[51,52,54,55] Moreover, radiologists are more confident in their interpretation of CT for appendicitis compared to ultrasound.[56] The most accurate CT studies have employed a standardized, focused helical technique with narrow collimation (3 to 5 mm) and narrow reconstructed images (every 1 to 3 mm) starting at the top of L3 or the iliac crest and extending distally to the acetabular roof or pubic symphysis. Using these techniques, sensitivities ≥ 95% have been achieved in children.[51,52,54,57-60] Some experts recommend rectal contrast for improved visualization of the cecum and pericecal structures, and to opacify the lumen of uninflamed, unobstructed appendices.[7,51,58-60] Administration of rectal contrast requires a cooperative patient who can retain the material (e.g., age > 3 to 4 years, no mental disability, and absent diarrhea). Others recommend intravenous contrast to improve bowel wall visualization. A single study found unenhanced CT to be accurate in children.[52,54,57] Sensitivity of CT is substantially lower (53% to 84%) when nonstandarzied techniques are used, CT is not helical, or narrow collimation and narrow reconstructed images are not employed.[55,61,62] False-negative CT scans also may be related to diminished pericecal fat at in children less than 10 years old, use of adult diagnostic criteria (e.g., 6 mm wall to wall appendiceal diameter), and lack of radiologic experience.[7,63] The most common CT abnormalities, found in more than 90% of appendicitis cases, are an appendiceal wall-to-wall diameter greater than 6 mm and periappendiceal fat stranding.[7,63,64] Other less common findings include focal cecal wall thickening adjacent to an inflamed appendix, an abscess, adenopathy, and right lower quadrant or pelvic fluid.[7,63,64] An appendicolith is identified on CT in 65% of children with appendicitis and in 14% of nondiseased appendices.[65] Alternate diagnoses in children without appendicitis are found in 30% to 34% of cases (e.g., nephrolithiasis, pyelonephritis, ovarian cyst or mass, ovarian torsion, inflammatory bowel disease, Meckel's diverticulum).[59,66] The main concern with CT scanning is radiation exposure.

Important Clinical Features and Considerations

An important reason that it is difficult to diagnose appendicitis at younger ages is the multitude of more common nonsurgical disorders that cause similar symptoms. In fact, gastroenteritis and upper respiratory tract infections are the most common misdiagnoses in infants and children ultimately diagnosed with appendicitis[6] (Table 73–3).

Management

During evaluation, it is appropriate to control pain with short-acting intravenous analgesics. Providing analgesics to children with acute abdominal pain does not affect diagnostic accuracy or alter the clinical outcome of these children.[67-69] Pediatric surgeons are significantly less likely to provide analgesia before definitive diagnosis compared to emergency physicians.[70] To address their concerns, it may be appropriate to devise a policy whereby the surgeons are given a short window of opportunity to evaluate the patient. After their evaluation or if they are unable to see the patient in an expeditious manner, analgesics are administered. A reasonable initial medication is 0.05 mg/kg of intravenous morphine sulfate.[68]

Intravenous volume replacement should be administered to all children with suspected appendicitis and evidence of dehydration or sepsis. Maintenance fluids are indicated because children suspected of having appendicitis should be kept nil per os (NPO). Children with sepsis or evidence of perforation (e.g., temperature > 100.4° F, diffuse peritonitis,

Table 73-3	Most Common Misdiagnoses in Children with Appendicitis
Initial Misdiagnosis	**Percentage of Cases**
Gastroenteritis	42
Upper respiratory tract infection*	18
Pneumonia	4
Sepsis	4
Urinary tract infection	4
Encephalitis/encephalopathy	2
Febrile seizure	2
Blunt abdominal trauma	2
Unknown	22

*Includes otitis media, sinusitis, pharyngitis, and upper respiratory tract infection.
From Rothrock SG, Skeoch G, Rush JJ, et al: Clinical features of misdiagnosed appendicitis in children. Ann Emerg Med 20:45–50, 1991.

ill appearance, symptoms duration > 36 to 48 hours) require broad-spectrum intravenous antibiotics. A single study found that use of ticarcillin/clavulanate plus gentamicin was associated with quicker defervesence and fewer infectious complications compared to traditional therapy of ampicillin and gentamicin plus clindamycin.[71] Small studies have shown that monotherapy with cefoxitin, piperacillin/tazobactam, imipenem/cilastin, or ampicillin/sulbactam is equivalent to traditional multiple-drug therapy in preventing infectious complications from ruptured appendicitis.[72] A meta-analysis also suggests that antibiotics are effective in preventing postoperative complications in children with uncomplicated appendicitis.[73] However, antibiotics were effective whether they were given pre- or postoperatively in uncomplicated appendicitis.[73] For this reason, antibiotic decisions in uncomplicated appendicitis can be deferred to the admitting surgeon.

Definitive therapy of acute appendicitis is appendectomy prior to perforation. Unfortunately, a large of number of children develop perforation prior to diagnosis. For these patients, immediate fluid resuscitation and antibiotic therapy are required. A subset of children with perforated appendicitis and an appendiceal abscess may undergo delayed (interval) appendectomy 4 to 8 weeks following an initial course of intravenous antibiotics, depending upon the clinical presentation and initial response to intravenous antibiotics.[74,75]

Summary

Most children who receive appropriate treatment for appendicitis do well. While a retrospective audit of adult patients with appendicitis who underwent interhospital transfer concluded no harm came to low-risk patients, no such studies have been performed in children.[76] Children with appendicitis suffer more morbidity than adults, and transferring for economic reasons alone is inappropriate. Children with complicated appendicitis have a better outcome when cared for by pediatric surgeons.[77] With this in mind, it may be appropriate to transfer a subset of complicated cases that do not require immediate surgery in addition to cases in which the general surgeon is inexperienced with children and unable to provide appropriate care (see Chapter 150, Emergency Medical Treatment and Labor Act [EMTALA]).

REFERENCES

*1. Rothrock SG, Pagane J: Acute appendicitis in children: emergency department diagnosis and management. Ann Emerg Med 36:39–51, 2000.
2. Reynolds SL, Jaffe DM: Children with abdominal pain in a pediatric emergency department. Pediatr Emerg Care 6:8–12, 1990.
3. Reynolds SL, Jaffe DM: Diagnosing abdominal pain in a pediatric emergency department. Pediatr Emerg Care 8:126–128, 1992.
4. Scholer SJ, Pituch K, Orr DP, et al: Clinical outcomes of children with acute abdominal pain. Pediatrics 98:680–685, 1996.
5. Lin Y, Lee C: Appendicitis in infancy. Pediatr Surg Int 19:1–3, 2003.
6. Rothrock SG, Skeoch G, Rush JJ, et al: Clinical features of misdiagnosed appendicitis in children. Ann Emerg Med 20:45–50, 1991.
7. Grayson DE, Wettlaufer JR, Dalrymple NC, et al: Appendiceal CT in pediatric patients: relationship of visualization to amount of peritoneal fat. AJR Am J Roentgenol 176:497–500, 2001.
8. Bax NM, Pearse RG, Dommering N, et al: Perforation of the appendix in the neonatal period. J Pediatr Surg 15:200–202, 1980.
9. Bryant LR, Trinkle JK, Noon JA, et al: Appendicitis and appendiceal perforation in neonates. Am Surg 36:523–525, 1970.
10. Buntain WL, Krempe RE, Kraft JW: Neonatal appendicitis. Alabama J Med Sci 21:295–298, 1984.
11. Shaul WL: Clues to the early diagnosis of neonatal appendicitis. J Pediatr 98:473–476, 1981.
12. Alloo J, Gerstle T, Shilyansky J, Ein SH: Appendicitis in children less than 3 years of age: a 28-year review. Pediatr Surg Int 19:777–779, 2004.
13. Barker AP, Davey RB: Appendicitis in the first three years of life. Aust N Z J Surg 58:491–494, 1988.
14. Bartlett RH, Eraklis AJ, Wilkinson RH: Appendicitis in infancy. Surg Gynecol Obstet 130:99–105, 1970.
15. Grosfeld JL, Weinberger M, Clatworthy HW: Acute appendicitis in the first two years of life. J Pediatr Surg 8:285–292, 1973.
16. Horwitz JR, Gursoy M, Jaksic T, et al: Importance of diarrhea as a presenting symptom of appendicitis in very young children. Am J Surg 173:80–82, 1997.
17. Puri P, O'Donnell B: Appendicitis in infancy. J Pediatr Surg 13:173–174, 1978.
18. Daehlin L: Acute appendicitis during the first three years of life. Acta Chir Scand 148:291–294, 1982.
19. Graham JM, Pokorny WJ, Harbery FJ: Acute appendicitis in preschool age children. Am J Surg 139:247–250, 1980.
20. Golladay ES, Sarrett JR: Delayed diagnosis in pediatric appendices. South Med J 81:38–41, 1988.
21. Williams N, Kapila L: Acute appendicitis in the under five year old. J R Coll Surg Edinb 39:168–170, 1994.
22. Williams N, Kapila L: Acute appendicitis in the preschool child. Arch Dis Child 66:1270–1272, 1991.
23. Siegal B, Hyman E, Lahat E, et al: Acute appendicitis in early childhood. Helv Paediatr Acta 37:215–219, 1982.
24. Wilson D, Sinclair S, McCallion WA, et al: Acute appendicitis in young children in the Belfast urban area: 1985–1992. Ulster Med J 63:3–7, 1994.
25. Rasmussen OO, Hoffman J: Assessment of the reliability of the symptoms and signs of acute appendicitis. R Coll Surg Edinb 36:372–377, 1991.
26. Williams NM, Johnstone JM, Everson NW: The diagnostic value of symptoms and signs in childhood abdominal pain. J R Colle Surg Edinb 43:390–392, 1998.
*27. Samuel M: Pediatric appendicitis score. J Pediatr Surg 37:877–881, 2002.
28. Gauderer MWL, Crane MM, Green JA, et al: Acute appendicitis in children: the importance of family history. J Pediatr Surg 36:1214–1217, 2001.
29. Basta M, Morton NE, Mulvhill JJ, et al: Inheritance of acute appendicitis: familial aggregation in the United States. Am J Epidemiol 132:910–924, 1990.
30. Brender JD, Marcuse EK, Weiss NS, et al: Is childhood appendicitis familial? Am J Dis Child 139:338–340, 1985.
31. Andersson N, Griffith H, Murphy J, et al: Is appendicitis familial? Br Med J 2:697–698, 1979.

---

*Selected readings.

32. Doriaswamy NW: Pregress of acute appendicitis: a study in children. Br J Surg 65:877–879, 1978.
33. Dickson JA, Jones A, Telfer S, et al: Acute abdominal pain in children. Scand J Gastroenterol Suppl 144:43–46, 1988.
34. Rothrock SG, Green SM, Dobson M, et al: Misdiagnosis of appendicitis in non-pregnant women of child bearing age. J Emerg Med 24:1–9, 1995.
35. Eriksson S, Granstrom L, Olander B, Wretlind B: Sensitivity of interleukin-6 and C-reactive protein concentrations in the diagnosis of acute appendicitis. Eur J Surg 161:41–45, 1995.
36. Eriksson S, Granstrom L, Carlstrom A: The diagnostic value of repetitive preoperative analysis of C-reactive protein and total leucocyte count in patients with suspected appendicitis. Scand J Gastroenterol 29:1145–1149, 1994.
37. Anderson RE, Hugander A, Ravn H, et al: Repeated clinical and laboratory examinations in patients with equivocal diagnosis of appendicitis. World J Surg 24:479–485, 2000.
38. Thompson MM, Underwood MJ, Dookeran KA, et al: Role of sequential leucocyte counts and C-reactive protein measurements in acute appendicitis. Br J Surg 79:822–824, 1992.
39. Lyons D, Waldron R, Ryan T, et al: An evaluation of the clinical value of the leucocyte count and sequential counts in suspected acute appendicitis. Br J Clin Pract 41:794–796, 1987.
40. Arnbjornsson E: Bacturia in appendicitis. Am J Surg 155:356–358, 1988.
41. Bond GR, Tully SG, Chan LS, Bradley RL: Use of the MANTRELS score in childhood appendicitis: a prospective study of 187 children with abdominal pain. Ann Emerg Med 19:1014–1018, 1990.
42. Owen TD, Williams H, Stiff G, et al: Evaluation of the the Alvarado score in acute appendicitis. J R Soc Med 85:87–88, 1992.
43. Gwynn LK: The diagnosis of acute appendicitis: clinical assessment versus computed tomography evaluation. J Emerg Med 21:119–123, 2001.
44. Bakha RK, McNair MM: Useful radiologic signs in acute appendicitis in children. Clin Radiol 28.193–196, 1977.
45. Johnson JF, Coughlin WF, Stark P: The sensitivity of plain films for detecting perforation in children with appendicitis. ROFO Fortschr Geb Rontgenstr Nuklearmed 149:619–623, 1988.
46. Rothrock SG, Green SM, Harding M, et al: Plain abdominal radiography in the detection of acute medical and surgical disease in children: a retrospective analysis. Pediatr Emerg Care 7:281–285, 1991.
47. Rothrock SG, Green SM, Hummel CB: Plain abdominal radiography in the detection of major disease in children. Ann Emerg Med 21:1423–1429, 1992.
48. Boleslawski E, Panis Y, Benoist S, et al: Plain abdominal radiography as a routine procedure for acute abdominal pain of the right lower quadrant: prospective evaluation. World J Surg 23:264–266, 1999.
49. Hahn HB, Hoepner FU, Kalle T, et al: Sonography of acute appendicitis in children: 7 years experience. Pediatr Radiol 28:147–151, 1998.
50. Schulte B, Beyer D, Kaiser C, et al: Ultrasonography in suspected acute appendicitis in childhood—report of 1285 cases. Eur J Ultrasound 8:177–182, 1998.
*51. Garcia Pena BM, Mandl KD, Kraus SJ, et al: Ultrasonography and limited computed tomography in the diagnosis and management of appendicitis in children. JAMA 282:1041–1046, 1999.
52. Sivit CJ, Applegate KE, Stallion A, et al: Imaging evaluation of suspected appendicitis in a pediatric population: effectiveness of sonography versus CT. AJR Am J Roentgenol 175:977–981, 2000.
53. Roosevelt GE, Reynolds SL: Does the use of ultrasonography improve the outcome of children with appendicitis? Acad Emerg Med 5:1071–1075, 1998.
54. Kaiser S, Frenckner B, Jourlf HK: Suspected appendicitis in children: US and CT—a prospective randomized study. Radiology 223:633–638, 2002.
55. Karakas SP, Guelfuat M, Leonidas JC, et al: Acute appendicitis in children: comparison of clinical diagnosis with US and CT imaging. Pediatr Radiol 30:94–98, 2000.
56. Garcia Pena BM, Taylor GA: Radiologists' confidence in interpretation of sonography and CT in suspected pediatric appendicitis. AJR Am J Roentgenol 175:71–74, 2000.
57. Lowe LH, Penney MW, Stein SM, et al: Unenhanced limited CT of the abdomen in the diagnosis of appendicitis in children: comparison with sonography. AJR Am J Roentgenol 176:31–35, 2001.
58. Mullins ME, Kircher MF, Ryan DP, et al: Evaluation of suspected appendicitis in children using limited helical CT and colonic contrast material. AJR Am J Roentgenol 176:37–41, 2001.
59. Sivit CJ, Dudgeon DL, Applegate KE, et al: Evaluation of suspected appendicitis in children and young adults: helical CT. Radiology 216:430–433, 2000.
60. Stephen AE, Segev DL, Ryan DP, et al: The diagnosis of acute appendicitis in a pediatric population: to CT or not to CT. J Pediatr Surg 38:367–371, 2003.
61. Patrick DA, Janik JE, Janik JS, et al: Increased CT scan utilization does not improve the diagnostic accuracy of appendicitis in children. J Pediatr Surg 38:659–662, 2003.
62. Reich JK, Brogdon B, Ray WE, et al: Use of CT scan in the diagnosis of pediatric acute appendicitis. Pediatr Emerg Care 16:241–243, 2000.
63. Callahan MJ, Rodriguez DP, Taylor GA: CT of appendicitis in children. Radiology 224:325–332, 2002.
64. Friedland JA, Siegel MJ: CT appearance of acute appendicitis in childhood. AJR Am J Roentgenol 168:439–442, 1997.
65. Lowe LH, Penney MW, Scheker LE, et al: Appendicolith revealed on CT in children with suspected appendicitis: how specific is it in the diagnosis of appendicitis? AJR Am J Roentgenol 175:981–984, 2000.
66. Lowe LH, Perez R, Scheker LE, et al: Appendicitis and alternate diagnoses in children: findings on unenhanced limited helical CT. Pediatr Radiol 31:569–577, 2001.
67. Kim MK, Strait RT, Sato TT, Hennes IIM: A randomized clinical trial of analgesia in children with acute abdominal pain. Acad Emerg Med 9:281–287, 2002.
68. Green R, Bulloch B, Kabani A, et al: Early analgesia for children with acute abdominal pain. Pediatrics 116:978–983, 2005.
69. Goldman RD, Crum D, Bromberg R, et al: Analgesia administration for acute abdominal pain in the pediatric emergency department. Pediatr Emerg Care 22:18–21, 2006.
70. Kim MK, Galustyan S, Sato TT, et al: Analgesia for children with acute abdominal pain: a survey of pediatric emergency physicians and pediatric surgeons. Pediatrics 112:1122–1126, 2003.
71. Rodriguez JC, Buckner D, Schoenike S, et al: Comparison of two antibiotic regimens in the treatment of perforated appendicitis in pediatric patients. Int J Clin Pharmacol Ther 38:492–499, 2000.
72. Kaplan S: Antibiotic usage in appendicitis in children. Pediatr Infect Dis J 17:1047–1048, 1998.
*73. Andersen BR, Kallehave FL, Andersen HK: Antibiotics versus placebo for prevention of postoperative infection after appendicectomy. Cochrane Database Syst Rev (2):CD001439, 2003.
74. Gillick J, Velayudham M, Puri P: Conservative management of appendix mass in children. Br J Surg 88:1539–1542, 2001.
75. Weber TR, Keller MA, Bower RJ, et al: Is delayed operative treatment worth the trouble with perforated appendicitis in children? Am J Surg 186:685–688, 2003.
76. Norton VC. Schriger DL: Effect of transfer on outcome of patients with appendicitis. Ann Emerg Med 29:467–473, 1997.
77. Alexander F, Magnusion D, DiFiore J, et al: Specialty versus generalist care of children with appendicitis: an outcome comparison. J Pediatr Surg 36:1510–1513, 2001.

Chapter 74

Intussusception

Jonathan I. Singer, MD

Key Points

The diagnosis of intussusception should be considered in any infant or child with severe, episodic abdominal pain.

The combination of rhythmic abdominal pain, vomiting, blood in the stool, and an abdominal mass is absent in most patients with intussusception.

An atypical clinical pattern (e.g., atypical age, absence of pain, nonbloody diarrhea, altered mental status) is common in intussusception.

Prolonged history, in the face of a normal examination, should not exclude the diagnosis of intussusception.

A normal plain abdominal radiograph cannot exclude the diagnosis of intussusception.

Introduction and Background

Intussusception is an invagination (or telescoping) of one segment of the intestinal tract into another. The invagination may be within the same portion of gastrointestinal (GI) tract (intragastric, jejunojejunal, colocolic), or a proximal portion of the intestine can invaginate into a distal adjacent part (duodenal-jejunal, ileocolic, sigmoid-rectal). More than 90% of cases of intussusception that occur in infants and children are ileocolic.[1] The telescoped bowel causes bowel wall ischemia and edema and leads to abdominal pain and other associated features of intussusception.[2]

Recognition and Approach

Intussusception may occur at any age (Fig. 74–1). Cases have been described in preterm infants, throughout childhood, and into adulthood.[3] Neonates constitute less than 1% of all reported pediatric cases. In large series, most intussusceptions occur prior to age 2. A majority of this subgroup have occurred between the fifth and ninth month of life. Of late, more cases have been depicted in children beyond the fifth

year of age. Intussusception historically has been described in well-nourished children, but institutional reviews from the past decades have substantiated encounters in undernourished children.[4] Intussusception affects males two times more frequently than females. While most cases are sporadic, occasional familial associations have been reported.[5,6]

The cause of intussusception is unknown in 90% of pediatric cases. There is no recognized etiology for an abnormal peristaltic wave that leads to the invagination. Venous and lymphatic flow from the intussuscepted segment is interrupted. Obstructed venous drainage produces edema of the bowel wall. Epithelium may be sloughed and mixed with stool, leading to bloody, mucus-filled stools. If the intussusception is undiagnosed, compromised arterial blood flow may lead to bowel necrosis with bowel perforation.

In 10% of cases an identifiable cause for intussusception is found.[7] Intussusceptions that occur within the first month of life are more often associated with an abnormal congenital malformation.[8,9] An abnormal "lead point" (pathologic lesion) for intussusception is common in children older than 4 years, and may be due to various infections, inflammatory disease states, posttraumatic events, and surgical procedures (Table 74–1). Beyond the 14th year of life, intussusception is uniformly associated with a lead point.[7]

The tempo of intussusception may be variable. Most children have an abrupt onset of symptoms, and parents seek medical attention within 24 hours of onset. This acute presentation results from complete intestinal obstruction or release of neuroactive GI tract hormones.[10] Some children have symptoms that are prolonged from days to weeks (chronic intussusception).[11] A longer duration of symptoms is more characteristic of patients beyond 2 years of age and in those who have an incomplete (nonstrangulating, nonischemic) intussusception.

Clinical Presentation

The pain of intussusception can produce a sudden screaming fit in a child, with doubling of the thighs onto the abdomen. Pain may last several minutes. After an asymptomatic interval, repeated paroxysms will cause the child to cry out again. The child may be inconsolable or may seem comfortable in a knee-chest position in the arms of the caregiver. Vomiting tends to occur shortly after the initial painful episode. Children typically vomit only gastric contents. Occasionally, the emesis may be bilious, fecal, or bloody. Bowel movements

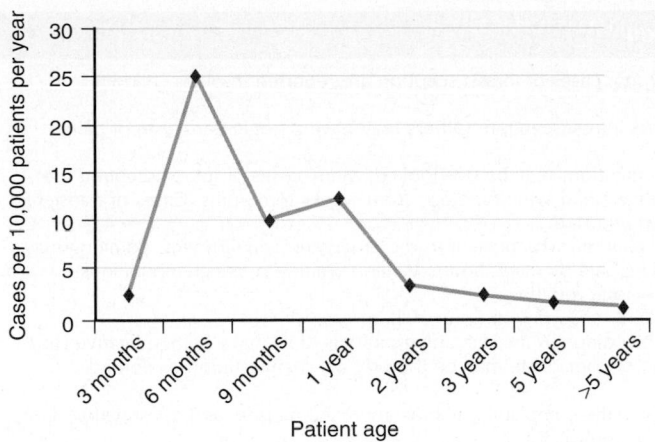

FIGURE 74–1. Annual incidence of intussusception at different ages.[2,42-45]

Table 74–1	Risk Factors and Pathologic Lead Points for Intussusception

Cystic fibrosis
Foreign body ingestion
Gastrojejunal feeding tube
Hemangiomas
Hemophilia
Henoch-Schönlein purpura (intussusception develops in 3–5% with this disorder)
Intestinal duplications
Intestinal lymphoma
Intestinal polyps (e.g., juvenile polyps, Peutz-Jeghers syndrome)
Meckel's diverticulum
Neurofibromatosis
Peyer's patch hypertrophy (postviral or parasitic enteritis)
Rotavirus vaccine
Surgical procedures (especially retroperitoneal surgery, as in Wilms' tumor removal)
Trauma with bowel wall edema or hemorrhage

vary from formed to liquid. Within 3 to 24 hours, stool is passed that has a gelatinous, mucus-like consistency. The presence of blood in fecal material may be trace to copious.[12]

While the classic triad of intussusception is colicky, intermittent severe abdominal pain, vomiting, and rectal bleeding, this combination of features is found in less than one third of all patients.[13] Between 85% and 92% of children manifest colicky abdominal pain, while 60% to 80% of patients experience vomiting.[1,4] Gross blood is present in the stools of 40% to 50% of patients.[12,14] "Current jelly" stools, which are mucoid, bloody, and maroon in color, account for a minority of bloody stools.[12] Of those children without gross blood in the stool, 75% have occult blood on rectal examination.[14]

The child with intussusception is often well perfused, hydrated, and alert despite apparent discomfort.[13] The abdomen is flat, nondistended, and occasionally scaphoid. The abdomen is typically soft and nontender except in the region of the intussusception, where voluntary guarding may be seen. A sausage-shaped, sometimes ill-defined, and variably tender mass may be present on palpation of the right upper quadrant or right midabdomen. The combination of a right upper quadrant mass and a scaphoid right lower

abdomen is termed *Dance's sign* and is highly suggestive of an intussusception. In some cases, rectal examination may reveal a mass. Classic signs are often absent in infants and children with intussusception, and no single or combination of examination features can reliably exclude this disorder.[13,15]

Atypical symptoms and signs may lead to misdiagnosis or a delay in diagnosis.[16-18] Clinicians need to be aware of the broad range of atypical presentations that occur in intussusception (Table 74–2). When patients present with typical clinical features (e.g., intermittent severe pain, an abdominal mass, and bloody stool), the diagnosis is readily apparent. When the picture is less complete, and atypical manifestations dominate, other diagnoses may be entertained.[19] The differential diagnosis is broad and based on the wide variety of pediatric disorders causing pain, vomiting, an abdominal mass, and rectal bleeding (Table 74–3).

Diagnostic Evaluation

Several laboratory tests should be undertaken when there is suspicion of intussusception. Following a rectal examination, the stool should be tested for occult blood. A negative guaiac test does not exclude the diagnosis, but decreases the likelihood that intussusception is present.[14] When the duration of symptoms is brief, and the child is without dehydration, hyperthermia, or peritoneal irritation, blood chemistries and complete blood count are not useful diagnostically. However, these tests are of utility in the face of significant bleeding, shock, or dehydration. Cultures of blood, urine, and stool are appropriate for the septic-appearing child.[20] The child with altered mental status requires a bedside estimate of blood sugar.

One of several imaging procedures should be undertaken when there is a suspicion of intussusception. Diagnostic emergency imaging may take the form of plain abdominal radiography, ultrasonography (US), or computed tomography (CT).

Plain abdominal radiographs usually constitute the first imaging test when intussusception is suspected. A supine and upright or supine and left lateral decubitus film of the abdomen can be obtained. The most important role of plain abdominal radiography is to uncover contraindications to contrast enema. Patients with radiographic evidence of a high-grade bowel obstruction, intraperitoneal air, or pneumatosis intestinalis should not be subjected to contrast enema. The secondary function of plain radiographs is to see if intussusception is likely. The radiographic findings suggestive of intussusception include minimal intestinal gas, minimal fecal content in the colon, mass lesion, inability to visualize the liver tip, localized air-fluid levels, and dilated small bowel loops.[21] In fact, intussusception may be the most common cause of bowel obstruction under the age of 2 years.[22] The diagnosis can be confirmed only when plain film shows the head of the intussusception within the bowel lumen.[22] It is important to recognize that films may be normal in up to 25% to 26% of cases, with another 53% of plain films having nonspecific or equivocal findings.[23,24] Due to nonspecificity of plain films, radiologists agree on the radiographic findings in as few as 12% of cases.[24]

Ultrasonography may also be useful in establishing the diagnosis of intussusception and, when it is discovered, may dictate the optimum mode of reduction. Ultrasonography tends to be of greater utility in patients with a nonspecific

Table 74–2	Atypical Clinical Features in Intussusception[1,11,13,15,17,40,46-52]
Age	While the most common age range is 5–9 mo, cases of intussusception are reported in older children, adolescents, and even adults.
Absent pain	8–18% of infants and children have painless intussusception. Others may have a single paroxysm of pain without rhythmic, periodic pain.
Chronic and transitory pain	Individuals with subacute and chronic presentations may be overlooked. Many cases of intussusception are ultimately diagnosed in individuals who have had symptomology from weeks to months. Cases of transient (self-reducing) intussusception have been reported.
Vomiting	Vomiting is the chief complaint in 40% of children who present to the emergency department. Vomiting may be the first identified complaint, preceding pain by many hours. While vomiting is usually nonbilious, occasional infants have presented with bilious vomiting.
Diarrhea	Nonbloody diarrhea is a prominent complaint, occurring in up to 19% of cases.
Nonbloody stool	Only half of all patients have gross rectal bleeding. Of the remaining patients, 25% have heme-negative stool.
Altered mental status	Depressed consciousness with obtundation or coma state may be the primary manifestation or dominant concern of the caregiver.
Nonspecific prodrome	Respiratory manifestations, fever, and nonspecific complaints such as anorexia, nausea, and constipation may precede the readily diagnosed symptom complex.
Prior surgery	Previous abdominal surgery, particularly retroperitoneal dissection (e.g., Wilms' tumor removal), is a risk factor for intussusception. Intussusception of the appendiceal stump is a known complication of appendectomy. The interval from operation to onset of intussusception may be as long as 5 years. Gastrojejunal tubes predispose to intussusception.
Vital signs	Tachycardia, fever, hypertension, or apnea may be seen early in the course of intussusception. Hypotension, poor perfusion with pallor, and diaphoresis may be seen in the context of prolonged symptomology, excessive blood loss, and ischemic bowel with secondary sepsis.
Neurologic findings	Apathy, miosis, decreased motor tone, seizure, or opisthotonic posturing may occur as the initial indication of illness or well after gastrointestinal signs are present.
Abdominal mass	Between bouts of invagination, an abdominal mass may be absent. During invagination, the mass may pass into the hepatic flexure and may be difficult or impossible to feel.
Rectal examination	Despite only a brief history of illness, the intussusception may protrude through the anus.

Table 74–3	Differential Diagnosis of Intussusception					
	Prominent Symptoms			**Physical Features**		
				Abdominal Mass		
Abdominal Pain	**Vomiting or Diarrhea**	**Altered Mental Status**	**Congenital**	**Acquired**	**Rectal Bleeding**
Appendicitis	Malrotation with midgut volvulus	Metabolic derangement	Teratoma	Wilms' tumor	Ischemic bowel due to shock
Epiploic appendicitis	Appendicitis	Endocrinopathy	Dysgerminoma	Pheochromocytoma	Rectal prolapse
Primary peritonitis	Bowel obstruction	Diabetic ketoacidosis	Yolk sac tumor	Lymphoma*	Meckel's diverticulum*
Torsion, ovary/testicle	Incarcerated hernia	Drug intoxication	Embryonal carcinoma		Juvenile polyp*
Mesenteric ischemia	Infectious enterocolitis Pseudomembranous colitis or invasive bacterial enteritis	Closed head injury		Adenocarcinoma	Fissure

*These disorders can also serve as a lead point and cause intussusception.

history, normal physical examination, or atypical clinical pattern. Sonographic findings of intussusception are a large sonolucent target, a bull's-eye or donut sign on the transverse (cross) section, and a sleeve or pseudo–kidney sign on the longitudinal section.[25] When either plain films or US exhibits positive findings that are nonspecific or highly suggestive, an air or barium contrast enema should be undertaken to reduce the intussusception if no contraindications exist.

A contrast enema with barium or air under fluoroscopic or sonographic guidance is the procedure of choice for diagnosing intussusception. Moreover, these techniques can successfully reduce the intussusception in 65% to 90% of cases.[26-28] Success rates are highest for individuals who have had symptoms for less than 24 hours.[13] Neonates and patients beyond age 4 are less likely to experience reduction and more likely to require surgical exploration. Rare complications of

air and barium contrast studies include bleeding and perforation.[29] Additional risks include the reduction of necrotic bowel or reduction without detecting a pathologic lead point.[7,30]

Spiral CT has occasionally been employed to diagnose equivocal cases, although this technique is not routinely recommended. CT findings include a distended bowel loop with a thickened, edematous wall and an eccentric, crescentic or wedge-shaped, low-density intraluminal mass that represents the invaginated mesentery.[11]

Important Clinical Features and Considerations

An unusual type of intussusception is a small bowel intussusception (SBI), accounting for less than 2% of all cases.[31]

Children with this variant are older than typical cases (mean age 4 to 4.5 years) and have a longer duration of symptoms prior to initial presentation (mean 76 hours).[31,32] In contrast to typical ileocolic cases, an SBI can be located in the left side of the abdomen. Ultrasound may miss this disease in up to 24% of cases since the outer diameter of the intussusception is smaller than for ileocolic cases and the location is often atypical.[31,32] Due to its proximal location, air contrast and barium enema are not useful for diagnosis or reduction of SBI.[32] Diagnosis is often made by CT or during laparotomy when other surgical disorders are suspected.[31,32]

Controversy exists as to the exact sequence of radiologic procedures needed in suspected intussusception. Some centers with extensive US experience rely on a normal scan to exclude the diagnose in patients with a moderate to low clinical suspicion, only obtaining contrast studies if the US is positive or equivocal.[33] Since US misses up to 5% of ileocolic cases (and 24% of SBI cases), close observation is required for patients with a negative US. If a high clinical suspicion is present, contrast enema is still required.[33-35] Use of US in this manner can decrease the radiation risk and exposure to an invasive procedure. Moreover, US can be used to direct the hydrostatic reduction and improve the reduction rates with contrast enemas.[36,37] Ultrasound-guided hydrostatic reduction is less successful if the intussusception is left sided or contains entrapped fluid (edema). One study of US-guided reduction analyzed the thickness of the hypoechogenic external layer of the intussusceptum to determine its association with successful reduction. The authors found that reduction was 100% successful if this layer was less than 7.2 mm thick, 68% successful if it was 7.5 to 12 mm thick, and never successful if the bowel wall was greater than 14 mm thick.[38]

During evaluation or reduction of intussusception, clinicians may be tempted to administer sedatives. However, infants and children must be able to perform a Valsalva maneuver during contrast studies, and administration of these medications may reduce the successful reduction rates.[33]

Management

The uncomplicated patient does not require airway intervention or either respiratory or circulatory support. Monitoring that is appropriate for the degree of patient instability should be initiated. Intravenous lines are inserted in all patients, and a fluid bolus is administered to all individuals with either excessive diarrhea or blood loss from ischemia or frank hemorrhage. A normal saline bolus is administered at a rate of 20 ml/kg over a brief time frame and repeated until the patient becomes hemodynamically stable. All patients should be placed on "nothing by mouth" status. Although not universally performed, pending surgical consultation and imaging procedures, a nasogastric tube is recommended.

Following resuscitation, a decision must be made concerning whether there are contraindications to nonoperative attempts at reduction of the intussusception. For patients without contraindications, the radiologist and surgical consultant can determine whether air insufflation or barium reduction is employed.[29] If pneumatic or hydrostatic pressure techniques fail to reduce the intussusception, a repeated effort at nonoperative reduction from 30 minutes to 24 hours later is an option.[26,39] With failure of reduction, operative therapy must be employed. About 60% of cases that could not be reduced nonoperatively are successfully reduced at surgery without resection.[26]

Summary

Patients who require surgical reduction of intussusception generally have an uncomplicated postoperative course. Those who undergo surgical reduction experience a recurrence rate between 2% and 5%.[25] Individuals who have successful nonoperative reduction who had been stabilized before undergoing the contrast enema have prompt return of intestinal function. Their vital signs, if altered, return to normal within hours. Patients who have presented with altered mental status have abrupt return to alertness following reduction.[40] Patients who have had nonoperative reduction have a 2% to 20% rate of recurrence.[30] Recurrence may occur up to 1 year following the initial intussusception. However, most cases occur within 1 to 3 days following pneumatic or hydrostatic reduction. It is not possible to establish which patients are likely to have recurrent intussusception based on presenting signs and symptoms, age, or sex.[41] Some facilities admit the child to the hospital for a 24-hour time frame. Other institutions observe the child in the emergency department for less than a 24-hour time frame prior to discharge home.[27] Otherwise healthy children who have a successful enema reduction suffer no adverse outcomes when discharged from the emergency department.[39] If observation within the emergency department is carried out, at discharge the emergency physician must ascertain if parents understand the indications that warrant a return for further medical attention (i.e., recurrent symptoms, vomiting, new or different pain, or GI bleeding).

REFERENCES

1. Bergdahl S, Hugosson C, Lauren T, Soderlund S: Atypical intussusception. J Pediatr Surg 7:700–705, 1972.
2. O'Ryan M, Lucero Y, Pena A, Valenzuela MT: Two year review of intestinal intussusception in six large public hospitals of Santiago, Chile. Pediatr Infect Dis J 22:717 721, 2003.
3. Martinez Biarge M, Garcia-Alix A, Luisa del Hoyo M, et al: Intussusception in a preterm neonate: a very rare, major intestinal problem— systematic review of cases. J Perinat Med 32:190–194, 2004.
4. Luks FI, Yazbeck S, Perreault G, Desjardins JG: Changes in the presentation of intussusception. Am J Emerg Med 10:574–576, 1992.
5. Stringer MD, Holmes SJ: Familial intussusception. J Pediatr Surg 27:1436–1437, 1992.
6. McGovern CM: Intussusception in twins. Am J Emerg Med 18:742–743, 2000.
7. Blakelock RT, Beasley SW: The clinical implications of non-idiopathic intussusception. Pediatr Surg Int 14:163–167, 1998.
8. Patriquin HB, Afshani E, Effman E, et al: Neonatal intussusception: report of 12 cases. Radiology 125:463–466, 1977.
9. Wang NL, Yeh ML, Chang PY, et al: Prenatal and neonatal intussusception. Pediatr Surg Int 13:232–236, 1998.
*10. Conway EE Jr: Central nervous system findings and intussusception: how are they related? Pediatr Emerg Care 9:15–18, 1993.
11. Schulman H, Laufer L, Kurzbert E, et al: Chronic intussusception in childhood. Eur Radiol 8:1455–1456, 1998.
*12. Yamamoto LG, Morita SY, Boychuk RB, et al: Stool appearance in intussusception: assessing the value of the term "currant jelly." Am J Emerg Med 15:293–298, 1997.
13. Fanconi S, Berger D, Rickham PP: Acute intussusception: a classic clinical picture? Helv Paediatr Acta 37:345–352, 1982.

*Selected readings.

*14. Losek JD, Fiete RL: Intussusception and the diagnostic value of testing stool for occult blood. Am J Emerg Med 9:1–3, 1991.

15. Ravitch M: Considerations of errors in the diagnosis of intussusception. Am J Dis Child 84:17, 1952.

16. Teitelbaum JE, Fishman SJ, Leichtner AM, Tunnessen WW: "Read my lips": abdominal pain in a 14-year-old. Contemp Pediatr 16:31–41, 1999.

17. Shteyer E, Koplewitz BZ, Gross E, Granot E: Medical treatment of recurrent intussusception associated with intestinal lymphoid hyperplasia. Pediatrics 111:682–685, 2003.

18. Pollack CV Jr, Pender ES: Unusual cases of intussusception. J Emerg Med 9:347–355, 1991.

19. Case records of the Massachusetts General Hospital. Weekly clinicopathological exercises. Case 24-1997: a six-year-old boy with bouts of abdominal pain, vomiting, and a left-sided abdominal mass. N Engl J Med 337:329–336, 1997.

20. McCabe JB, Singer JI, Love T, Roth R: Intussusception: a supplement to the mnemonic for coma. Pediatr Emerg Care 3:118–119, 1987.

21. Daneman A, Alton DJ: Intussusception: issues and controversies related to diagnosis and reduction. Radiol Clin North Am 34:743–756, 1996.

22. Lazar L, Rathaus V, Erez I, Katz S: Interrupted air column in the large bowel on plain abdominal film: a new radiological sign of intussusception. J Pediatr Surg 30:1551–1553, 1995.

23. Eklof O, Hartelius H: Reliability of the abdominal plain film diagnosis in pediatric patients with suspected intussusception. Pediatr Radiol 9:199–206, 1980.

24. Sargent MA, Babyn P, Alton DJ: Plain abdominal radiography in suspected intussusception: a reassessment. Pediatr Radiol 24:17–20, 1994.

25. Harrington L, Connolly B, Hu X, et al: Ultrasonographic and clinical predictors of intussusception. J Pediatr 132:836–839, 1998.

26. Sandler AD, Ein SH, Connolly B, et al: Unsuccessful air-enema reduction of intussusception: is a second attempt worthwhile? Pediatr Surg Int 15:214–216, 1999.

27. Le Masne A, Lortat-Jacob S, Sayegh N, et al: Intussusception in infants and children: feasibility of ambulatory management. Eur J Pediatr 158:707–710, 1999.

28. Peh WC, Khong PL, Lam C, et al: Reduction of intussusception in children using sonographic guidance. AJR Am J Roentgenol 173:985–988, 1999.

29. Daneman A, Navarro O: Intussusception, Part 2: an update on the evolution of management. Pediatr Radiol 34:97–108, 2004.

30. Eshel G, Barr J, Heiman E, et al: Incidence of recurrent intussusception following barium versus air enema. Acta Paediatr 86:545–546, 1997.

31. Ko SF, Lee TY, Ng SH, et al: Small bowel intussusception in symptomatic pediatric patients: experiences with 19 surgically proven cases. World J Surg 26:438–443, 2002.

32. Kim JH: US features of transient small bowel intussusception in pediatric patients. Kor J Radiol 5:178–184, 2004.

33. Henrikson S, Blane CE, Koujok K, et al: The effect of screening sonography on the positive rate of enemas for intussusception. Pediatr Radiol 33:190–193, 2003.

34. Rohrschneider WK, Troger J: Hydrostatic reduction of intussusception under US guidance. Pediatr Radiol 25:530–534, 1995.

35. del-Pozo G, Albillos JC, Tejedor D, et al: Intussusception in children: current concepts in diagnosis and enema reduction. Radiographics 19:299–319, 1999.

36. Crystal P, Hertzanu Y, Farber B, et al: Radiographically guided hydrostatic reduction of intussusception in children. J Clin Ultrasound 30:343–348, 2002.

37. Grant RL, Piotto L: Benefits of sonographic hydrostatic reduction as opposed to air reduction in a case of intussusception due to lymphoma. Australas Radiol 48:264–266, 2004.

38. Mirilas P, Koumanidou C, Vakaki M, et al: Sonographic features indicative of hydrostatic reducibility of intestinal intussusception in infancy and early childhood. Eur Radiol 11:2576–2580, 2001.

39. Gonzalez-Spinola J, Del Pozo G, Tejedor D, Blanco A: Intussusception: the accuracy of ultrasound-guided saline enema and the usefulness of a delayed attempt at reduction. J Pediatr Surg 34:1016–1020, 1999.

40. Singer J: Altered consciousness as an early manifestation of intussusception. Pediatrics 64:93–95, 1979.

41. Champoux AN, Del Beccaro MA, Nazar-Stewart V: Recurrent intussusception: risks and features. Arch Pediatr Adolesc Med 148:474–478, 1994.

*42. Bajaj L, Roback MG: Postreduction management of intussusception in a children's hospital emergency department. Pediatrics 112(6 Pt 1):1302–1307, 2003.

43. Parashar UD, Holman RC, Cummings KC, et al: Trends in intussusception association hospitalizations and deaths among US infants. Pediatrics 106:1413–1421, 2000.

44. Perez-Schael I, Escalona M, Salinas B, et al: Intussusception associated hospitalization among Venezuelan infants during 1998 through 2001: anticipating rotavirus vaccines. Pediatr Infect Dis J 22:234–239, 2003.

*45. Fischer TK, Bihrmann K, Perch M, et al: Intussusception in early childhood: a cohort study of 1.7 million children. Pediatrics 114:782–785, 2004.

46. Birkhahn R, Fiorini M, Gaeta TJ: Painless intussusception and altered mental status. Am J Emerg Med 17:345–347, 1999.

47. Losek JD: Intussusception: don't miss the diagnosis! Pediatr Emerg Care 9:46–51, 1993.

48. Orenstein J: Update on intussusception. Contemp Pediatr 17:180–191, 2000.

49. Ein SH, Stephens CA: Intussusception: 354 cases in 10 years. J Pediatr Surg 6:16–27, 1971.

50. La Salle AJ, Andrassy RJ, Page CP, et al: Intussusception of the appendiceal stump. Clin Pediatr (Phila) 19:432–435, 1980.

51. Barton LL, Chundu K: Intussusception associated with transient hypertension. Pediatr Emerg Care 4:249–250, 1988.

52. Goetting MG, Tiznado-Garcia E, Bakdash TF: Intussusception encephalopathy: an underrecognized cause of coma in children. Pediatr Neurol 6:419–421, 1990.

Chapter 75

Gastrointestinal Bleeding

Jeffrey S. Blake, MD and Stephen J. Teach, MD, MPH

Key Points

Most gastrointestinal bleeding in children is self-limited and not life threatening.

The presence of significant gastrointestinal bleeding usually can be identified clinically.

Emergency department evaluation should prioritize early recognition and management of active bleeding and hemorrhagic shock.

Severe gastrointestinal bleeding requires rapid volume resuscitation and consultation with a gastroenterologist or surgeon to identify and control the source of hemorrhage.

Establishing a definitive diagnosis in the emergency department is not always possible, but making a presumptive diagnosis may be acceptable once life-threatening disorders are excluded.

Introduction and Background

Many causes of gastrointestinal (GI) bleeding are unique to infants and children (e.g., necrotizing enterocolitis, formula intolerance, midgut volvulus). The frequency of specific causes depends on both the age of the patient and the location of bleeding[1] (Tables 75–1 and 75–2). Fortunately, mortality is low in infants and children with GI bleeding since most causes are benign and comorbid conditions (e.g., atherosclerosis, coronary artery disease) are rare.

Recognition and Approach

While GI bleeding in children occurs frequently in the intensive care setting,[2] this complaint is not commonly seen in infants and children presenting to an emergency department (ED). In fact, GI bleeding only accounts for 0.3% of children presenting to a pediatric ED.[3] Moreover, only 4% of these cases have a serious cause for their disorder, and mortality is less than 1%.[3]

Bleeding from the GI tract is never normal and can signify serious disease or common benign disorders. At any age, swallowed blood may be misinterpreted as gastrointestinal bleeding. Neonates can ingest blood at the time of birth or may ingest blood while nursing from a nipple that has nearby maternal bleeding. Swallowed blood from a nosebleed or intraoral source can be mistaken for GI bleeding, especially if bleeding is heavy and triggers hematemesis that consists of swallowed blood. Food and drinks may contain red dye that turns the stool, red but the stool will be heme negative when tested for occult blood. Clinicians must be able to differentiate between disorders that mimic bleeding, benign causes of bleeding, serious causes of bleeding, and surgical disorders that require acute intervention.

Clinical Presentation

Initial evaluation is directed at assessing the hemodynamic stability of infants and children with GI bleeding. Assessment is also directed at determining whether or not there is ongoing bleeding (Table 75–3). This assessment is based on heart rate, palpation of central and peripheral pulses, blood pressure, mental status, respiratory rate and pattern, and signs of cutaneous perfusion. Although tachycardia is a sensitive indicator of acute, significant GI bleeding in children, children have an impressive ability to increase their systemic vascular resistance and to maintain a normal blood pressure in response to hypovolemia (compensated shock). Therefore, hypotension is considered a late finding in progression of shock (decompensated shock). Quantifying the amount of bleeding requires visual inspection or a historical description of the bleeding. Importantly, children may present with fatigue, syncope, weakness or other alteration in mental status without any bleeding noted from the GI tract.[4]

Confirming the presence of bleeding is an important evaluation step since true GI bleeding can easily be confused with hemoptysis, hematuria, vaginal bleeding, or swallowed blood from the nose, mouth, or oropharynx. Several "mimickers" of true GI bleeding include foods and medications that make vomitus appear red (food coloring, tomatoes, fruit juices), stools appear red (food coloring, beets, ampicillin), or stools appear black (licorice, spinach, iron supplements). Testing stool and emesis or gastric aspirates for occult blood is usually sufficient to confirm or rule out true GI bleeding in these cases. There are a large number of reasons for false positive and false negative stool testing[5] (Tables 75–4 and 75–5).

Table 75–1	Causes of Acute Upper Intestinal Bleeding*	
	Common	**Uncommon**
Newborn and Infant		
	Swallowed maternal blood	Gastric ulcer
	Human milk	Bleeding diathesis
	During delivery	
	Esophagitis	
Older Child		
Esophagus	Esophagitis	Esophagitis
	Acid reflux	Viral (herpes, cytomegalovirus)
	Pill induced	Allergic
	Mallory-Weiss tear	Fungal
		Caustic ingestion
		Varices
		Dieulafoy lesion
		Foreign body
		Duplication cyst
Stomach	Gastritis	Gastritis
	Prolapse gastropathy	Crohn's disease
	Aspirin	Portal hypertension
	Nonsteroidal anti-inflammatory drug	*Helicobacter pylori* infection
	Stress ulcer/gastritis	Ulcer
		Zollinger-Ellison syndrome
		Cushing's ulcer
		Leiomyoma
		Varices
		Vascular malformation
		Dieulafoy disease
Duodenum	Duodenitis	Ulcer
	Crohn disease	*Helicobacter pylori* infection
		Curling's ulcer
		Vascular malformation
		Foreign body
		Lymphoid hyperplasia
		Varices
		Dieulafoy disease
		Duplication cyst
		Hemobilia
Other	Swallowed blood	Swallowed blood
	Oral/nasal pharynx	Munchausen syndrome by proxy
		Pulmonary hemorrhage

*From Squires R Jr: Gastrointestinal bleeding. Pediatr Rev 20: 95–101, 1999. Copyright 1999.

Table 75–2	Causes of Lower Intestinal Bleeding*	
	Common	**Uncommon**
Newborn and Infant		
	Allergic colitis	Juvenile polyp
	Anal fissure	Vascular lesions
	Milk protein intolerance	Hirschsprung's enterocolitis
	Necrotizing enterocolitis (premature)	Meckel's diverticulum
		Intestinal duplication
	Swallowed maternal blood	Intussusception
	Infectious diarrhea	Infectious enterocolitis
Older Child		
	Anal fissure	Inflammatory bowel disease (<4 yr of age)
	Intussusception	Vascular malformations
	Infectious enterocolitis	Intestinal duplication
	Salmonella	Henoch-Schönlein purpura
	Shigella	Cecitis
	Campylobacter	Infectious diarrhea
	Escherichia coli O157:H7	Cytomegalovirus colitis
	Yersinia enterocolitica	Amebiasis
	Clostridium difficile	Hemorrhoids
	Inflammatory bowel disease (>4 yr of age)	Colonic or rectal varices
	Meckel's diverticulum	Ulcer at surgical anastomosis
	Perianal streptococcal cellulites	Solitary ulcer of the rectum
	Juvenile/inflammatory polyp	Nodular lymphoid hyperplasia
		Sexual abuse
		Rectal trauma

*From Squires R Jr: Gastrointestinal bleeding. Pediatr Rev 20: 95–101, 1999. Copyright 1999.

Table 75–3	Important Questions during Evaluation of Gastrointestinal (GI) Bleeding

Does this patient have severe bleeding or signs of hemorrhagic shock?
Does this patient have true bleeding or a mimicker?
Is the blood coming from the GI tract, nasopharynx, or vagina?
Is it an upper or lower GI tract source of bleeding?
Does this patient have a potentially life-threatening condition associated with the GI bleeding?
Is there an associated coagulopathy or platelet disorder?
Does this patient need emergent endoscopy or emergent surgery?

Clues to help distinguish upper from lower GI tract bleeding sources include the appearance of the stools and emesis. Vomited blood, or hematemesis, typically comes from an upper GI source (proximal to the ligament of Treitz). Blood may appear bright red if it is fresh blood or resemble dark "coffee grounds" if it is older blood that has been exposed to gastric acid for a period of time. Melena is described as dark, black or maroon, tarlike stools that usually also come from an upper GI source unless the bleeding is abrupt. Lower GI bleeding with a slow transit time may occasionally present as melena as well. Hematochezia is bright red blood coming from the rectum and usually comes from the lower GI tract (distal to the ligament of Treitz). However, upper GI bleeding in large amounts or in the presence of a rapid intestinal transit time also can cause hematochezia. Streaks of blood on the outside of a stool, as opposed to being mixed together with the stool, point to an anorectal source of bleeding such as hemorrhoids or rectal fissures.

Although definitively identifying the source of GI bleeding may not be possible in the ED, clinical features can be used to discriminate between benign and life-threatening causes.

Historical Features

Age is an important determinant of likely causes of GI bleeding (see Tables 75–1 and 75–2). A description of the bleeding (color, quality, location, and quantity) can aid in distinguishing between an upper and a lower GI tract source. The presence of light-headnesss or syncope suggest significant volume loss and the need for rapid assessment and management.

Abdominal pain associated with bilious emesis and abdominal distention should alert clinicians to the possibility of intestinal obstruction as seen with volvulus (see Chapter

Table 75–4	Causes of False-Positive Guaiac Card Testing

Bromides
Chlorophyll
Cupric sulfate
Hypochlorites
Iodide
Iron supplements
Peroxidase-rich vegetables (turnips, horseradish, artichokes, mushrooms, radishes, broccoli, bean sprouts, cauliflower, oranges, bananas, cantaloupes, grapes)

Data from Gogel HK, Tandberg D, Strickland RG: Substances that interfere with guaiac card tests: implications for gastric aspirate testing. Am J Emerg Med 7:474–480, 1989.

Table 75–5	Causes of False-Negative Guaiac Card Testing

Antacids
Barium sulfate
Bile
Charcoal
Chili sauce
Cocoa
Dimethylaminoethanol (health food additive)
Jello
N-acetylcysteine
Orange juice
Pepto-Bismol
Peaches
Raisins
Red bell peppers
Red chili powder
Red wines
Rifampin
Simethicone
Spaghetti sauce
Sucralfate
Tomato paste
Vitamin C

Data from Gogel HK, Tandberg D, Strickland RG: Substances that interfere with guaiac card tests: implications for gastric aspirate testing. Am J Emerg Med 7:474–480, 1989.

83, Malrotation and Midgut Volvulus) or intussusception (see Chapter 74, Intussusception). Both volvulus and intussusception can cause intermittent, or "colicky," abdominal pain and bloody, mucoid stools. An abdominal mass or tenderness is not always present with intussusception and stools are often not characterized as resembling "current jelly." Stools may range from bright red blood to melena or they may be Hemoccult negative.[6] Another unique condition is necrotizing enterocolitis, which occurs most often in premature infants but can also be seen in full-term infants during the first few weeks of life. Patients often present with abdominal distention and feeding intolerance, and, in more severe cases, they develop septic shock or an acute abdomen from ischemia, peritonitis, or a perforated bowel.

Focal epigastric abdominal pain suggests esophagitis, gastritis, or peptic ulcer disease, all of which are common causes of GI bleeding in children.[7] Mild, diffuse abdominal pain associated with bloody, mucus-containing diarrhea and fever suggests infectious enteritis (see Chapter 72, Vomiting and

Diarrhea). Hemolytic-uremic syndrome (see Chapter 131, Hemolytic-Uremic Syndrome) can cause bloody diarrhea, most often due to *Escherichia coli* O157:H7, and has a classic triad of hemolytic anemia, thrombocytopenia, and renal failure.

Painless rectal bleeding is often related to structural lesions, including juvenile polyps, Meckel's diverticulum, and arteriovenous malformations. Juvenile polyps, also known as inflammatory polyps, are present in up to 3% of children, with most children remaining asymptomatic or presenting after the age of 1 to 2 years.[8] Symptoms include bright red, painless, rectal bleeding during or immediately after defecation.[8] Bleeding usually stops on its own, and severe bleeding or hemorrhage is rare. Up to 30% of children have iron deficiency anemia. Rarely, polyps can act as an intussusception, causing abdominal pain or prolapse through the rectum, resulting in pruritis and a bloody discharge. A Meckel's diverticulum is a remant of the embryonic yolk sac found in 2% of the population.[9] Two thirds of the time it is lined with gastric mucosa, which can lead to painless intermittent rectal bleeding due to ulceration of the adjacent bowel. The mean age at presentation is 8 to 10 years, although symptoms can develop at any age.[9] Arteriovenous malformations of the GI tract are rare lesions that lead to painless bleeding. The cecum and proximal small intestine are the most common bleeding sites.[10] Diagnosis can be difficult, and many of these lesions are detected during evaluation for other disorders (e.g., Meckel's diverticulum).

A known history of constipation or new description of infrequent, hard stools or pain with passage of stools (tenesmus) suggests anal fissures, one of the most common cause of lower GI bleeding in children[3] Severe constipation in a toxic-appearing infant could represent Hirschsprung's enterocolitis and is a surgical emergency (see Chapter 77, Constipation).

Infants and children may have recurrent bleeding from inflammatory bowel disease, peptic ulcers, severe gastroesophageal reflux disease (GERD), and, less commonly, bleeding esophageal varices from portal hypertension caused by cirrhosis or extrinsic etiologies.[7] Chronic use of steroids and nonsteroidal anti-inflammatory agents can cause peptic ulcer bleeding.[11] While gastritis and peptic ulcers may be due to stress from trauma, burns, surgery, systemic illness, or mechanical trauma from a gastrostomy tube,[12] they are often associated with *Helicobacter pylori* infection in children.[13] *Helicobacter pylori* can cause chronic, intermittent epigastric pain with emesis, hematemesis, and occult bloody stools.[13] Other uncommon, but important, causes of GI bleeding include caustic ingestions and foreign body ingestions.

A history of cutaneous vascular malformation or problems with easy bruising or bleeding from other sites suggest a bleeding diathesis. Other inherited causes of bleeding include familial polyposis, coagulopathies, and inflammatory bowel disease.

A dietary history may indicate ingestion of specific foods that mimic true GI bleeding. Formula-fed infants may develop allergies to milk or soy proteins, which are found in most standard infant formulas.[14] Breast-fed infants occasionally have allergic colitis since food antigens can be passed through breast milk[14] (see Chapter 35, Vomiting, Spitting Up, and Feeding Disorders). Besides bleeding, infants may present with irritability, vomiting, diarrhea, poor feeding, or failure to thrive.[14] Infants commonly have "physiologic" gastroesophageal reflux, which is usually asymptomatic.

Occasionally, however, reflux can be complicated by esophagitis and may be difficult to distinguish clinically from allergic colitis, although infants with reflux esophagitis are more likely to have a prominent vomiting history without diarrhea.[7]

Finally, acute-onset vomiting or retching from any etiology followed by brisk hematemesis may be due to a Mallory-Weiss tear, a mechanical injury of the esophagus.[15]

Physical Examination

An immediate first step is to check the vital signs for the presence of fever or evidence of hypovolemia. Then, the nose should be inspected for epistaxis, the oropharynx for signs of trauma, and the maternal nipples (of breast-fed infants) for lacerations since all of those situations can lead to swallowed blood that may then be perceived as intestinal bleeding. Mucosal pigmentation of the lips and gums may point to Peutz-Jeghers syndrome, a rare condition associated with hamartomas of the stomach and intestines that are predisposed to bleeding.

An abdominal examination is performed to elicit tenderness, signs of an acute abdomen or bowel obstruction, masses, or features of liver disease such as hepatomegaly, splenomegaly, ascites, or caput medusa. If a gastrostomy tube is present, aspiration of the contents may reveal gross or occult blood.

Visual inspection of the anus may reveal anal fissures, surrounding erythema suggesting a perianal group A β-hemolytic streptococcal infection, perianal fistulas, or hemorrhoids. A digital rectal examination is required after visual inspection to look for hard, impacted stool in the rectal vault, a mass or polyps, or an empty rectal vault (Hirschprung's disease) and to test stool for gross or occult blood. An examination of the external genitalia is performed to identify vaginal bleeding or a prolapsed urethra in females. Finally, skin breakdown from contact or infectious diaper dermatitis also can be a source of bleeding.

Inspection of the dermis may reveal pale, mottled, cool skin, with weak or absent peripheral pulses and delayed capillary refill, which would indicate hypovolemia. Bruising or petechiae suggests a coagulopathy, thrombocytopenia, or Henoch-Schönlein purpura, a vasculitis characterized by diffuse abdominal pain, arthralgias, and palpable purpura of the lower extremities and buttocks.

Important Clinical Features and Considerations

Gastrc Aspiration and Lavage

Aspiration of blood from a nasogastric (NG) tube indicates a high risk that a serious upper GI bleed is present. However, in adults, this technique does not reveal blood in 21% to 31% of patients with endoscopically proven upper GI bleeding.[16,17] Furthermore, blood is obtained from NG aspiration in a significant number of patients without a GI bleeding source; in these cases the blood is possibly due to trauma associated with NG tube placement.[16,17] Therefore, clinicians should not rely soley on this test to diagnose or exclude upper GI bleeding.

In the past, gastric lavage with iced saline was recommended for treating upper GI bleeding. It was thought that the saline caused vasoconstriction at the bleeding site and diminished bleeding. However, studies have failed to demonstrate diminished bleeding or improved outcome with this technique, and it can no longer be recommended.[18–20]

Laboratory Testing

In general, routine laboratory testing is of limited utility in the evaluation of GI bleeding, and the need for testing can be guided by findings on the history or physical examination. A complete blood cell count and a type and crossmatch are indicated in suspected anemia due to acute or chronic blood loss. However, the hematocrit may be normal in acute bleeding since sufficient time may not have passed for extravascular fluid reaccumulation, which lowers the hematocrit. Thrombocytopenia may be present in leukemia, platelet disorders (e.g., idiopathic thrombocytopenic purpura), or disseminated intravascular coagulopathy. Although eosinophilia in peripheral blood or stool is associated with allergic colitis, the diagnosis of this disorder is largely clinical. Coagulation studies (prothrombin time, partial thromboplastin time) are used to indirectly assess hepatic function and confirm a coagulopathy that may be causing or contributing to GI bleeding. A blood urea nitrogen–creatinine ratio greater than 30 is 98% to 100% specific for an upper GI bleeding source, although this cutoff is only 68% sensitive.[21,22]

Other optional tests include a serum bilirubin level to further assess liver function, serum transaminase levels to look for hepatocellular injury, serum H. pylori titer to guide treatment in suspected peptic ulcer disease, serum creatinine level to assess renal function, and stool cultures in patients with possible bacterial enteritis.

An Apt test may be useful in breast-feeding infants suspected of swallowing maternal blood when the mother has dry, cracked, bleeding nipples. This test uses sodium hydroxide solution to distinguish maternal from fetal blood since fetal blood remains stable in an alkaline environment and retains its pink color, whereas maternal blood reduces and takes on a yellow color. The Apt test is designed for bright red blood, not that which has already been denatured such as coffee grounds–colored emesis or melena.

Imaging

Radiologic imaging may be helpful in specific clinical scenarios. For example, plain abdominal radiographs can confirm intestinal obstruction (volvulus, intussusception), mass effect, perforated bowel (peptic ulcer disease), enterocolitis (necrotizing or Hirschsprung's) or a foreign body. Plain radiographic findings in necrotizing enterocolitis include pneumatosis intestinalis and thickened bowel walls containing multiple small air collections. Plain radiographic findings in intussusception include a small bowel obstruction, sparse large bowel gas, a soft tissue mass, or a crescent sign (soft tissue mass projecting into the transverse colon), or the plain film may be completely normal.[23,24] Ultrasonography is used to diagnose intussusception, while a barium or air enema is used to diagnose and reduce intussuscepted segments of bowel.[23,24] An upper GI series can confirm cases of intestinal malrotation with intermittent volvulus. Abdominal computed tomography may be helpful if mass lesions or vascular malformations are suspected or in the evaluation of the acute abdomen. Technetium-labeled nuclear medicine scans may be helpful in diagnosing a bleeding Meckel's diverticulum ("Meckel's scan") or in identifying a bleeding source where diffuse bleeding does not permit endoscopy. Angiography may also be useful in localizing a site of bleeding when a focal source is suspected.

Endoscopy

Endoscopy is often the most reliable and definitive method of diagnosing certain conditions in patients with significant or chronic upper or lower GI bleeding. It is most useful in cases of active bleeding with focal lesions such as esophagitis, Mallory-Weiss tears, gastritis, gastric and duodenal ulcers, polyps, and vascular malformations.[7] Endoscopy can be performed electively or emergently depending on the severity and cause of the GI bleeding.

Management

Immediate Management of Severe GI Bleeding

Initial management includes rapid establishment of intravenous (IV) access (two large-bore IV lines, of at least 20 g in a child and 22 g in infants), administration of supplemental oxygen, and assessment of the patient's hemodynamic status. For patients with signs of hypovolemic shock, rapid bolus infusion of crystalloid solution (20 ml/kg of either normal saline or lactated Ringer's solution) is indicated, followed by an immediate reassessment of intravascular volume status. For persistent signs of hypovolemia, the child should receive repeated fluid boluses and an infusion of packed red blood cells. Existing coagulopathies are treated with fresh frozen plasma or specific factor products, and platelet disorders with platelet transfusions. If bleeding appears to come from an upper GI source, a histamine$_2$ (H$_2$)-receptor antagonist or proton pump inhibitor can be administered to help decrease gastric acidity. Octreotide, vasopressin, or somatostatin is administered IV in patients with variceal bleeding.[7] Desmopressin (DDAVP) 0.3 mcg/kg IV will reverse bleeding diatheses associated with renal failure.[25]

Patients with significant ongoing upper GI bleeding (e.g., shock, hypotension, anemia) require emergent endoscopy to identify the source and control the bleeding. Gastroenterologists can employ several techniques to control bleeding: electrocoagulation, laser photocoagulation, injection of sclerosing agents or epinephrine, and application of elastic bands or mechanical clips to bleeding vessels.[7] Surgery consultation is indicated for patients with suspected surgical disorders (Hirschsprung's enterocolitis, intussusception, volvulus, perforation), persistent bleeding despite attempted endoscopic intervention, complicated esophageal varices, or bleeding from large vascular anomalies.

Patients with a suspected serious cause for their bleeding (e.g., surgical disorder, varices, ulcer) or with hypotension, persistent tachycardia, or signs of hypovolemia require admission. If the cause of bleeding is unknown, vital signs are normal, the amount of blood loss is minimal, and no serious disorder is suspected, closely coordinated follow-up in 1 to 2 days with a primary care physician or gastroenterologist may be appropriate.

Disease-Specific Treatments

Allergic Colitis

Treatment of allergic colitis consists of eliminating the offending antigen from the diet. Many patients who are allergic to cow's milk protein will also have an allergy to soy milk protein.[26] If allergic colitis seems very likely, then a trial of protein hydrolysate formula could be helpful since these formulas have smaller peptides with fewer antigens. In persistent cases, amino acid–based formulas may be necessary. Breast-fed infants may also have allergic colitis from antigens transmitted through breast milk; therefore, the mother may also need to eliminate soy and milk, or even other typical allergenic foods (peanuts, seafood, etc.), from her diet. Symptoms of allergic colitis usually resolve within several days of removing the offending antigen.

Anal Fissures

Since anal fissures are most often a consequence of constipation, treatment focuses on treatment of constipation which, in uncomplicated cases, includes increased fluid intake, increased dietary fiber, decreased dietary fat, and the use of stool softeners.

Esophagitis, Gastritis, and Peptic Ulcer Disease

Empirical use of acid-suppressive medications (H$_2$-receptor blockers or proton pump inhibitors) may be all that is needed for managing esophagitis secondary to GERD. In infants, GERD is a common and mostly benign condition. For this reason, medications are usually reserved for infants with complications such as GI bleeding, respiratory complaints (stridor, aspiration), or failure to thrive. If severe or complicated GERD is suspected, acid-suppressive medications should be administered. For patients with insignificant GI bleeding, outpatient referral to a gastroenterologist is acceptable for confirmation of diagnosis and further management, such as testing and treatment for *H. pylori*. Eradication of *H. pylori* with antibiotics can dramatically reduce relapse rates of duodenal ulcers. Severe bleeding from a peptic ulcer requires immediate consultation with a gastroenterologist since endoscopic control of bleeding may be needed.

Esophageal Varices

Endoscopic band ligation and sclerotherapy as well as vasoactive therapies (vasopressin, octreotide) have successfully been used in children to treat bleeding esophageal varices.[27] If time permits, a gastroenterologist should be consulted when using these agents. In rare cases in which endoscopic and medical management fail, surgical control of bleeding may be required.

Summary

GI bleeding in children is usually benign and self-limited. However, the list of potential causes is extensive. The clinical examination can exclude most life-threatening causes. Early recognition and management of hypovolemic shock and prompt identification of disorders requiring surgical intervention are required to ensure a good outcome for patients with serious causes of bleeding.

REFERENCES

1. Squires R Jr: Gastrointestinal bleeding. Pediatr Rev 20:95–101, 1999.
2. Chaibou M, Tucci M, Dugas MA, et al: Clinically significant upper gastrointestinal bleeding acquired in a pediatric intensive care unit: a prospective study. Pediatrics 102:933–938, 1998.

3. Teach SJ, Fleisher GR: Rectal bleeding in the pediatric emergency department. Ann Emerg Med 23:1252–1258, 1994.
4. Blecker U, Renders F, Lanciers S, Vandenplas Y: Syncope leading to the diagnosis of *Helicobacter pylori* positive chronic active haemorrhagic gastritis. Eur J Pediatr 150:560–561, 1991.
5. Gogel HK, Tandberg D, Strickland RG: Substances that interfere with guaiac card tests: implications for gastric aspirate testing. Am J Emerg Med 7:474–480, 1989.
6. Yamamoto LG: Stool appearance in intussusception: assessing the value of the term "currant jelly." Am J Emerg Med 15:293–298, 1997.
7. Fox VL: High risk, under appreciated, obscure, or preventable causes of GI bleeding in infancy. Gastroenterol Clin North Am 29:37–66, 2000.
8. Desai DC, Neal KJ, Talbot IC, et al: Juvenile polyposis. Br J Surg 82:14–17, 1995.
9. Yahchouchy EK, Marano AF, Etienne JC, Fingerhut AL: Meckel's diverticulum. J Am Coll Surg 192:658–662, 2001.
10. Tokawi K, Iwai N, Michihata T, Kinugasa A: Arteriovernous malformation of the jejunum in a child. J Pediatr Surg 24:311–312, 1989.
*11. Li Voti G, Acierno C, Tulone V, et al: Relationship between upper gastrointestinal bleeding and non steroidal anti-inflammatory drugs in children. Pediatr Surg Int 12:264–265, 1997.
12. Weiss B: Upper gastrointestinal bleeding due to gastric ulcers in children with gastrostomy tubes. J Clin Gastroenterol 29:48–50, 1999.
13. Drumm B: Helicobacter pylori and peptic ulcer: Working Group Report of the second World Congress of Pediatric Gastroenterology, Hepatology, and Nutrition. J Pediatr Gastroenterol Nutr 39 Suppl 2: S626–31, 2004.
14. Heldenberg D, Abudy Z, Keren S, et al: Cow's milk-induced hematemesis in an infant. J Pediatr Gastroenterol Nutr 17:450–452, 1993.

———————

*Selected readings.

15. Bak-Romaniszyn L: Mallory-Weiss syndrome in children. Dis Esophagus 12:65–67, 1999.
16. Cuellar RE, Gavaler JS, Alexander JA, et al: Gastrointestinal tract hemorrhage: the value of a nasogastric aspirate. Arch Intern Med 150:1379–1380, 1990.
*17. Witting MD, Magder L, Heins AE, et al: Usefulness and validity of diagnostic nasogastric aspiration in patients without hematemesis. Ann Emerg Med 43:525–532, 2004.
18. Gilbert DA, Saunders D: Iced saline lavage does not slow bleeding from experimental canine gastric ulcers. Dig Dis Sci 26:1065–1068, 1981.
19. Andrus C, Ponsky J: The effects of irrigant temperature in upper gastrointestinal hemorrhage: a requiem for iced saline lavage. Am J Gastroenterol 82:1062–1064, 1987.
20. Ponsky J, Hoffman M, Swayngim D: Saline irrigation in gastric hemorrhage: the effect of temperature. J Surg Res 28:204–205, 1980.
21. Urashima M: BUN/Cr ratio as an index of gastrointestinal bleeding mass in children. J Pediatr Gastroenterol Nutr 15:89–92, 1992.
22. Felber S: The BUN/creatinine ratio in localizing gastrointestinal bleeding in pediatric patients. J Pediatr Gastroenterol Nutr 7:685–687, 1998.
23. Ratcliffe JF, Fong S, Cheong L, O'Connell P: The plain abdominal film in intussusception: the accuracy and incidence of radiologic signs. Pediatr Radiol 22:110–111, 1992.
24. Sargent MA, Babyn P, Alton DJ: Plain abdominal radiography in suspected intussusception: a reassessment. Pediatr Radiol 24:17–20, 1994.
25. Sutor AH: Desmopressin (DDAVP) in bleeding disorders of childhood. Semin Thromb Hemost 24:555–566, 1998.
26. Felber S, Zeiger RS, Sampson HA, et al: Soy allergy in infants and children with IgE-associated cow's milk allergy. J Pediatr 134:614–622, 1999.
27. Molleston JP: Variceal bleeding in children. J Pediatr Gastroenterol Nutr 37:538–545, 2003.

Chapter 76

Pyloric Stenosis

David D. Cassidy, MD

Key Points

Pyloric stenosis is most commonly seen in previously healthy white male infants, 2 to 8 weeks of age, who present with progressively worsening vomiting that eventually becomes projectile.

The classic presentation of pyloric stenosis is of a dehydrated-appearing infant, 2 to 8 weeks old, who presents with nonbilious projectile vomiting. On physical examination, the infant may have visible peristaltic waves in the left upper abdomen and a palpable olive-shaped mass in the epigastrium, which is the hypertrophied pylorus.

If the hypertrophied pylorus is palpated in the appropriate clinical setting, no further workup is necessary.

If the presentation is atypical and the physical examination is not conclusive, either ultrasound or upper gastrointestinal imaging contrast studies are needed to confirm or exclude the diagnosis.

Introduction and Background

Pyloric stenosis, also known as infantile hypertrophic pyloric stenosis (IHPS), is the most common cause of gastric outlet obstruction in infancy and the most common abdominal condition requiring surgery in the first few months of life. Pyloric stenosis occurs because of hypertrophy and hyperplasia of the circular musculature surrounding the pylorus and antrum of the stomach. This results in constriction and obstruction of the antral region of the stomach and pyloric channel by compression of the longitudinal folds of the mucosa with subsequent gastric outlet obstruction and hyperperistalsis of the stomach. As a result of the obstruction and hyperperistalsis, gastric musculature hypertrophy and dilation occurs. Gastritis with hematemesis may result from prolonged stasis.

Recognition and Approach

Pyloric stenosis occurs in approximately 2 to 5 cases per 1000 live births and is most common in white males.[1,2] The male : female incidence ratio ranges from 2.5 : 1 to 5.5 : 1, with the highest incidence occurring in first-born males. There appears to be a genetic predisposition, with a greater than fivefold increased risk in first-degree relatives.[3] Recent data suggest that the incidence of IHPS is increasing in the United States and abroad.[4]

It is now thought that pyloric stenosis is not a result of a developmental defect of the pylorus present at birth.[5,6] Biochemical, hormonal, and environmental theories have been proposed as to why pyloric stenosis develops in some infants.[7-13] Numerous reports have suggested the association between early postnatal exposure to macrolide antibiotics (erythromycin) and pyloric stenosis in infants.[14-18] Experts have proposed that early exposure (between 3 and 13 days of life) is associated with an eightfold increased risk of pyloric stenosis.[18]

Clinical Presentation

Pyloric stenosis typically occurs in infants 2 to 8 weeks old, with a peak incidence at 3 to 5 weeks, but has been seen in infants as early as 1 day of age[19,20] and as old as 5 months.[21] Initially, the infant's vomiting may be unpredictable and infrequent, but later it occurs with almost every feeding. Misdiagnosis of pyloric stenosis is usually due to early presentations of the disease in which the infant appears well and the vomiting history seems more consistent with gastroesophageal reflux or a viral syndrome. As the disease progresses, the intensity of the vomiting increases until projectile vomiting ensues. Observation of the child after oral fluid challenges and serial examinations in the emergency department may reveal persistent or projectile vomiting that will help lead to the diagnosis. Emesis is nonbilious with stomach contents but may contain old or new blood if gastritis is also present. Constipation may be present because the infant is dehydrated. Some infants may have diarrhea, referred to as "starvation stools," which further confuses the clinical picture.

On physical examination, the infant will appear hungry and readily accept a bottle but will subsequently vomit, usually within 5 to 10 minutes of feeding. Early in the disease the infant may appear healthy, but prolonged vomiting leads to dehydration, metabolic alterations, lethargy, and malnutrition. Obtaining a birth weight and comparing it to the current weight is crucial. Infants with pyloric stenosis should have no weight gain or even a weight loss, whereas an infant with reflux regurgitation typically continues to gain weight. One interesting physical finding that has been described in the literature is a hypoplastic or absent mandibular frenulum found in 92% of infants with pyloric stenosis compared to only 1.6% of controls.[22]

In the past, experts have stated that a definitive diagnosis can be made in up to 87% of infants with IHPS by performing a careful physical examination of the upper abdomen and palpating the enlarged pylorus.[23,24] However, more recent prospective studies have shown that physical examination reveals a pyloric olive in only 23% to 55% of cases.[25-27] Palpation of an enlarged pylorus, commonly referred to as an "olive" because of its shape, is an important skill for emergency practitioners. In many cases, palpation of a pyloric olive is all that is needed to confirm the diagnosis of IHPS and no further studies are indicated. The combination of the classic history of vomiting in the appropriate age group with the identification of the pyloric olive has a positive predictive value of nearly 100%.[28-30] In order to facilitate the palpation of the pylorus, the infant must be calm and cooperative. This can be accomplished using a blanket for warmth and a pacifier or gauze soaked with a small amount of dextrose water for sucking. If the stomach is distended, it will hamper the examination unless aspirated by nasogastric tube. Most experts recommend that the infant be in the supine position during examination, but others have found better success at identifying the olive by placing the infant in the left lateral decubitus position[31] or in the prone position.[32] Bringing the infant's knees up to the abdomen helps relax the abdominal musculature, which aids in palpation of the olive. Once positioned, the examiner identifies the edge of the liver with his or her fingertips just to the right of the xiphoid process. Gentle pressure deep to the liver and progressing downward or caudally should reveal a palpable 2-cm pyloric olive just on or to the right of the midline (Fig. 76–1). To confirm the diagnosis, the pylorus should be rolled under the examiner's fingertips. In the later stages of the disease, visible peristalsis of the stomach from left to right in the upper quadrant of the abdomen is sometimes seen just prior to vomiting. This peristalisis occurs in response to vigorous contractions of the stomach against the obstruction in the pylorus but may not be present if the stomach is empty.

The differential diagnosis for the vomiting infant is extremely broad (see Chapter 35, Vomiting, Spitting Up, and Feeding Disorders; and Chapter 72, Vomiting and Diarrhea). The most common conditions that are confused with pyloric stenosis include gastroesophageal reflux, improper feeding techniques, gastroenteritis, and pylorospasm. Helpful information in determining the etiology of the vomiting includes the age of the child and the timing, frequency, consistency, and volume of emesis. Infants with gastroesophageal reflux typically present shortly after birth with nonprojectile, low-volume regurgitation that occurs after most feedings and remains fairly constant. In pyloric stenosis, the vomiting does not begin until 2 to 3 weeks of age and becomes progressively worse and later projectile. Obstructive causes usually present with an abrupt presentation of vomiting that can be bilious in certain cases. Bilious vomiting in the neonate

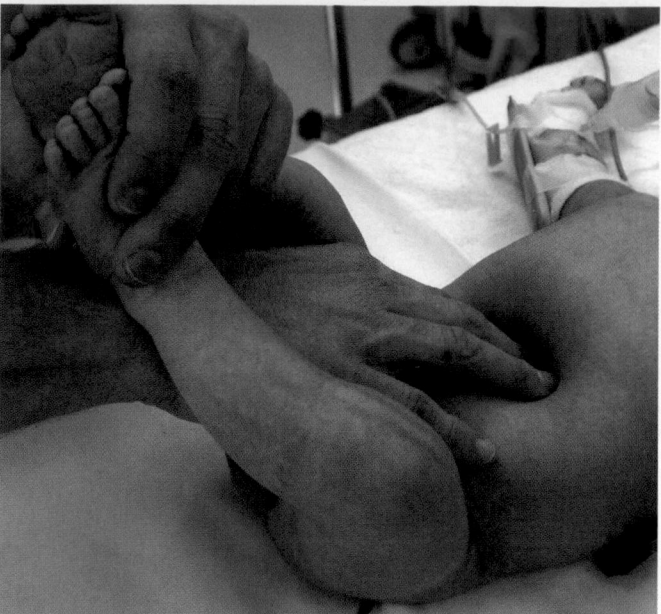

FIGURE 76–1. Examination of an infant for an enlarged pylorus.

should always prompt an aggressive workup to rule out malrotation and midgut volvulus (see Chapter 83, Malrotation and Midgut Volvulus). Nongastrointestinal causes of vomiting should also be considered, including sepsis, urinary tract infections, increased intracranial pressure, inborn errors of metabolism, pain, toxins, and medications (see Chapter 35, Vomiting).

Infants with severe and prolonged vomiting may become profoundly dehydrated with associated metabolic derangements. Persistent vomiting results in loss of hydrogen and chloride ions as well as compensatory renal sodium conservation and potassium wasting in response to volume loss. Laboratory analysis in patients who have been ill for a prolonged period may reveal varying degrees of a hypochloremic, hypokalemic metabolic alkalosis. Despite only being seen in delayed presentations, the presence of hypochloremic metabolic alkalosis significantly increases the likelihood that the cause of the infant's symptoms is pyloric stenosis.[33,34] If the infant remains dehydrated for a prolonged period of time, a metabolic acidosis may ensue, indicating the need for aggressive resuscitation.

If a pyloric mass is not palpated, further diagnostic imaging studies are warranted. Plain abdominal radiographs may reveal gastric dilation, which is suggestive of but not pathognomic for pyloric stenosis. The two main diagnostic studies that are used for pyloric stenosis are ultrasound and an upper gastrointestinal tract (UGI) series. Both studies have a similar accuracy with sensitivity of 90% to 100%.[28,35] Despite this, ultrasound is more commonly recommended over UGI studies as the initial imaging modality of choice, mainly due to its rapid noninvasive nature, its lack of radiation, and the elimination of the risk of contrast aspiration that may be associated with UGI studies. Ultrasound allows for direct visualization and measurement of the hypertrophied pyloric muscle, whereas a UGI series does not see the muscle, although hypertrophy is inferred by the demonstration of thinning and elongation of barium in the region of the

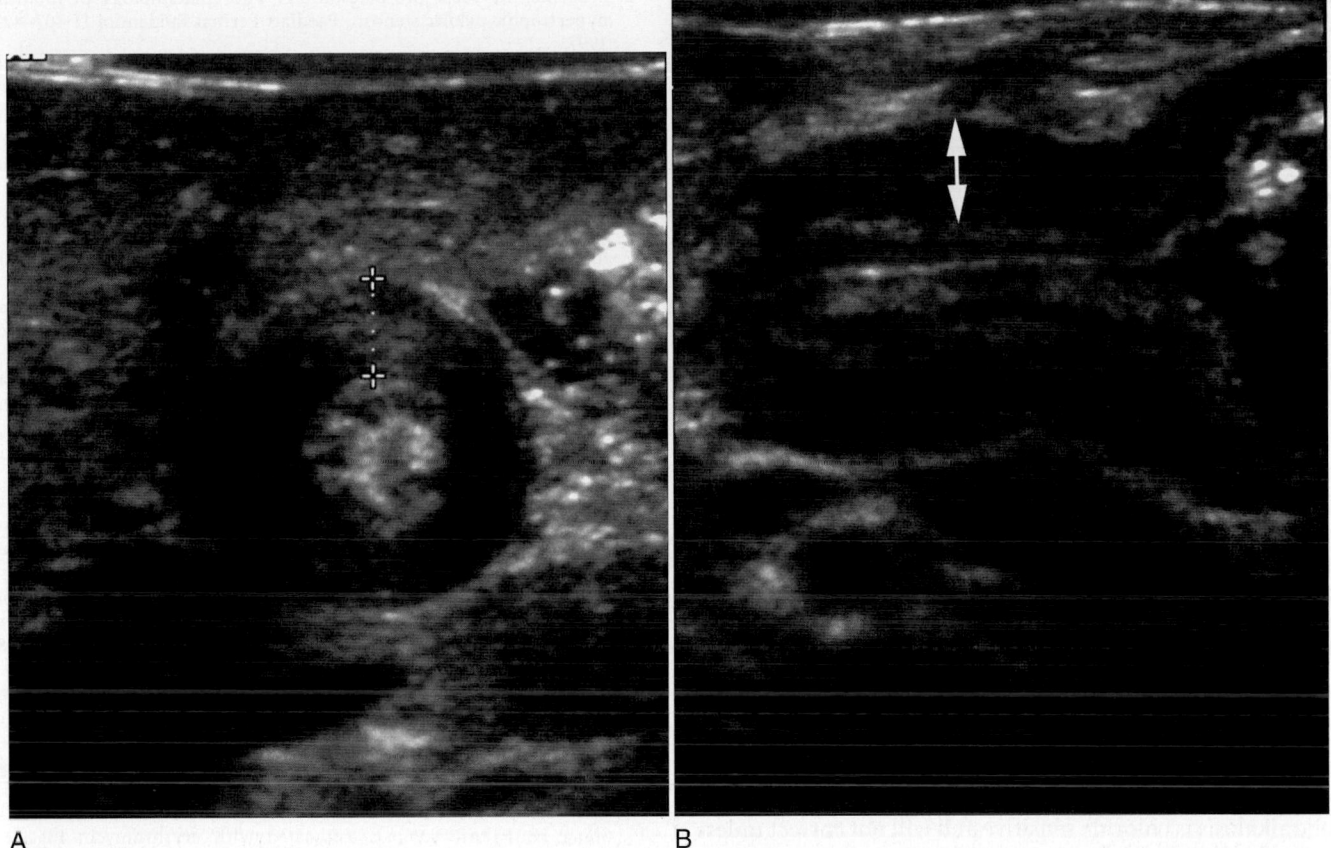

A   B

FIGURE 76–2. A, Cross-sectional or transverse sonogram of an infant revealing the classic "target sign" as well as an abnormally thickened hypoechoic muscle (cursor marks) measuring 4.4 mm (>3.0 mm is diagnostic for pyloric stenosis). **B,** Longitudinal sonogram of an infant revealing an abnormally thickened hypoechoic muscle (*arrows*).

pylorus. The accuracy of ultrasound for pyloric stenosis is operator dependent and therefore ultrasound should only be performed by experienced sonographers. Ultrasound diagnostic criteria for pyloric stenosis vary and include a pyloric muscular thickness (serosa to mucosa) greater than 3 to 4 mm, a pyloric canal length of more than 14 to 16 mm, and pyloric thickness or diameter (serosa to serosa) of 11 mm or greater (Fig. 76–2). Using these criteria, sensitivities of 91% to 100% and specificities of 99% to 100% have been reported.[36-38] Pyloric muscular thickness greater than 3 mm is the most widely accepted diagnostic criterion for pyloric stenosis (see Fig. 76–2). Ultrasound is more accurate than UGI in differentiating pylorospasm from pyloric stenosis. Both cause canal narrowing and delayed gastric emptying, but on ultrasound the entire pyloric muscle can be seen and the thickness of the muscle measured. To avoid a false-positive result, the thickened pylorus should be observed by ultrasound for at least 5 minutes to differentiate pyloric stenosis from the transient thickening of the pylorus seen with pylorospasm. False-negative studies are usually a result of improper technique and measurement errors. Pyloric muscle thickness correlates with the size of the infant and increases as the disease progresses; therefore, false-negative studies may also be seen with premature or extremely small infants as well as early presentations of pyloric stenosis.[39]

In most cases, a UGI imaging study is indicated if ultrasonography is unavailable or if the ultrasound examination is inconclusive. It is the preferred and most cost-effective study

in atypical presentations or if an alternative diagnosis such as gastroesophageal reflux or malrotation is more likely.[28,29] In a study in which a UGI series was used as the first imaging study over ultrasound, only 6% of infants required an ultrasound as second study to complete their evaluation. In contrast, 25% of infants required a UGI series to complete their workup when ultrasound was the initial test.[28] The UGI contrast study will reveal an elongated pyloric channel (the "string sign") and a bulge of the pyloric muscle into the gastric antrum (the shoulder or nipple sign) best seen on oblique views. The classic "railroad" or "double track" sign of two thin parallel streams of barium traversing the pylorus, caused by redundant mucosa in a narrowed pyloric lumen, is pathognomonic. The barium should be evacuated from the infant's stomach after the procedure is completed.

One proposed algorithm to determine which study to order in atypical cases is based on gastric aspirate volume. After at least a 1-hour fast, gastric contents are removed from the infant and quantified. If the aspirate is ≥5 ml, gastric outlet obstruction is suspected and an ultrasound should be the initial test, followed by a UGI series if necessary. If the aspirate is less than 5 ml, a medical cause for the emesis is suggested and a UGI series should be ordered first. Using this approach saves time and cost and has a sensitivity of 91%, a specificity of 88%, and an accuracy of 89%. The accuracy is greatly increased if the infant has fasted at least 3 to 4 hours.[27] Others have used volumes of 10 ml and the 3- to 4-hour fast with similar accuracy.[40] Another less common yet very accurate diagnostic tool that has been used in pyloric stenosis is endoscopy. It is sometimes used if other diagnostic modalities have failed to confirm or exclude the diagnosis of pyloric stenosis.[41,42]

Important Clinical Features and Considerations

It is important to realize that a significant number of infants with pyloric stenosis will present early in their course and therefore have less of these typical features. Infants may only have postprandial vomiting as their chief complaint and lack a palpable pyloric olive. Although the presence of hypochloremic, hypokalemic metabolic alkalosis significantly increases the likelihood of pyloric stenosis, these metabolic derangements are becoming rarer because of earlier recognition of the disease. Recent studies have revealed that only 10% to 22% of patients presenting with pyloric stenosis have electrolyte abnormalities.[43,44] Premature infants commonly present atypically. They present later than term infants, have less vomiting that is usually not projectile, and are less likely to have the diagnostic physical examination finding of a palpable hypertrophied pylorus.[39,45]

Management

Before surgery is performed, the infant must be adequately hydrated and electrolyte disturbances corrected. The metabolic alkalosis is chloride sensitive and will not correct unless excess chloride in the form of sodium chloride is given. After initial fluid resuscitation of normal saline with 20 ml/kg is complete, 5% dextrose with one-half normal saline at a rate of 1.5 times maintenance is used.[46,47] Potassium is replaced as needed after urine output has been established. Because correction of pyloric stenosis is not a surgical emergency, correction of dehydration and metabolic derangements may be performed over a 12- to 48-hour period prior to surgery. Ramstedt pyloromyotomy is the most common procedure used to correct pyloric stenosis. Some surgeons prefer laparoscopic pyloromyotomy repair because of its shorter recovery time, but open pyloromyotomy appears to have fewer complications and a higher efficacy.[48] Two small patient series with 33 total cases studied the effect of atropine administered intravenously initially and then orally for several weeks. Over 90% percent of infants had successful normalization of pyloric muscle hypertrophy with resolution of symptoms, thus avoiding operative management.[49,50]

Summary

With early recognition, preoperative management, and operative management, morbidity and mortality from pyloric stenosis is extremely low. Knowing the classic features of the disease, early and atypical presentations, and laboratory and radiologic features will assure prompt diagnosis and appropriate surgical referral.

REFERENCES

1. Applegate MS, Druschel CM: The epidemiology of infantile hypertrophic pyloric stenosis in New York State, 1983 to 1990. Arch Pediatr Adolesc Med 149:1123–1129, 1995.

*2. Schechter R, Torfs CP, Bateson TF: The epidemiology of infantile hypertrophic pyloric stenosis. Paediatr Perinat Epidemiol 11:407–427, 1997.

3. Mitchell LE, Risch N: The genetics of infantile hypertrophic pyloric stenosis: a reanalysis. Am J Dis Child 147:1203–1211, 1993.

4. Tam PK, Chan J: Increasing incidence of hypertrophic pyloric stenosis. Arch Dis Child 66:530–531, 1991.

5. Wallgren A: Preclinical stage of infantile hypertrophic pyloric stenosis. Am J Dis Child 72:371, 1946.

6. Rollins MD, Shields MD, Quinn RJ, Wooldridge MA: Pyloric stenosis: congenital or acquired. Arch Dis Child 64:138–139, 1989.

7. Jona J: Electron microscopic observation in infantile hypertrophic pyloric stenosis (IHPS). J Pediatr Surg 13:17–20, 1978.

8. Langer JC, Berezin I, Daniel EE: Hypertrophic pyloric stenosis: ultrastructural abnormalities of enteric nerves and the interstitial cells of Cajal. J Pediatr Surg 30:1535–1543, 1995.

9. Kobayashi H, Wester T, Puri P: Age-related changes in innervation in hypertrophic pyloric stenosis. J Pediatr Surg 32:1704–1707, 1997.

10. Spitz L, Zail S: Serum gastrin levels in congenital hypertrophic pyloric stenosis. J Pediatr Surg 11:33–35, 1976.

11. Tam PK: Observation and perspectives of the pathology and possible aetiology of infantile hypertrophic pyloric stenosis: a histological, biochemical, histochemical, and immunocytochemical study. Ann Acad Med Singapore 14:523–529, 1985.

12. Hernanz-Schulman M, Lowe L, Johnson J, et al: In vivo visualization of pyloric mucosal hypertrophy in infants with hypertrophic pyloric stenosis: is there an etiologic role? AJR Am J Roentgenol 177:843–848, 2001.

13. Kusafuka T, Puri P: Altered messenger RNA expression of the neuronal nitric oxide synthase gene in infantile hypertrophic pyloric stenosis. Pediatr Surg Int 12:576–579, 1997.

14. SanFilippo JA: Infantile hypertrophic pyloric stenosis related to ingestion of erythromycin estolate: a report of five cases. J Pediatr Surg 11:177–180, 1976.

15. Stang H: Pyloric stenosis associated with erythromycin ingested through breast milk. Minn Med 69:669–670, 682, 1986.

16. Mahon BE, Rosenman MB, Kleiman MB: Maternal and infant use of erythromycin and other macrolide antibiotics as risk factors for infantile hypertrophic pyloric stenosis. J Pediatr 139:380–384, 2001.

17. Hauben M, Amsden GW: The association of erythromycin and infantile hypertrophic pyloric stenosis. Drug Safety 25:929–942, 2002.

18. Cooper WO, Griffin MR, Arbogast P, et al: Very early exposure to erythromycin and infantile hypertrophic pyloric stenosis. Arch Pediatr Adolesc Med 156:647–650, 2002.

19. Tashjian DB, Konefal SH: Hypertrophic pyloric stenosis in utero. Pediatr Surg Int 18:539–540, 2002.

20. Zenn MR, Redo SF: Hypertrophic pyloric stenosis in the newborn. J Pediatr Surg 28:1577–1578, 1993.

21. Tiao MM, Huang HC, Shieh CS, et al: Infantile hypertrophic pyloric stenosis in a 5-month-old baby: case report. Changgeng Yi Xue Za Zhi 23:442–445, 2000.

22. De Felice C, Di Maggio G, Zagordo L, et al: Hypoplastic or absent mandibular frenulum: a predictive sign of infantile hypertrophic pyloric stenosis. J Pediatr 136:408–410, 2000.

23. Macdessi J, Oates RK: Clinical diagnosis of pyloric stenosis: a declining art. BMJ 306:1065–1066, 1993.

24. Formann HP, Leonidas JC, Kronfeld GD: A rational approach to the diagnosis of hypertrophic pyloric stenosis: do the results match the claims? J Pediatr Surg 25:262–266, 1990.

*25. Hulka F, Campbell TJ, Campbell JR, Harrison MW: Evolution in the recognition of infantile hypertrophic pyloric stenosis. Pediatrics 100: e9, 1997.

26. Ozsvath RR, Poustchi-Amin M, Leonidas JC, Elkowitz SS: Pyloric volume: an important factor in the surgeon's ability to palpate the pyloric "olive" in hypertrophic pyloric stenosis. Pediatric Radiology 27:175–177, 1997.

27. Mandell GA, Wolfson PJ, Adkins ES, et al: Cost-effective imaging approach to the nonbilious vomiting infant. Pediatrics 103:1198–1202, 1999.

*Selected readings.

28. Hulka F, Campbell JR, Harrison MW, Campbell TJ: Cost-effectiveness in diagnosing infantile hypertrophic pyloric stenosis. J Pediatr Surg 32:1604–1608, 1997.

29. Olson AD, Hernandez R, Hirschl RB: The role of ultrasonography in the diagnosis of pyloric stenosis: a decision analysis. J Pediatr Surg 33:676–681, 1998.

30. White MC, Langer JC, Don S, DeBaun MR: Sensitivity and cost minimization analysis of radiology versus olive palpation for the diagnosis of hypertrophic pyloric stenosis. J Pediatr Surg 33:913–917, 1998.

31. Senquiz AL: Use of decubitus position for finding the "olive" of pyloric stenosis. Pediatrics 87:266, 1991.

32. Gellis SS: Ancient technique of olive detection [letter]. Pediatrics 88:655–656, 1991.

33. Breaux CW, Hood JS, Georgeson KE: The significance of alkalosis and hypochloraemia in hypertrophic pyloric stenosis. J Paediatric Surg 24:1250–1252, 1989.

*34. Oakley EA, Barnett PLJ: Is acid base determination an accurate predictor of pyloric stenosis? J Paediatr Child Health 36:587–589, 2000.

35. Leonidas JC: The role of ultrasonography in the diagnosis of pyloric stenosis: a decision analysis. J Pediatr Surg 34:1583–1584, 1999.

36. Keller H, Waldmann D, Greiner P: Comparison of preoperative sonography with intraoperative findings in congenital hypertrophic pyloric stenosis. J Pediatr Surg 22:950–952, 1987.

37. Hernanz-Schulman M, Sells LL, Ambrosino MM, et al: Hypertrophic pyloric stenosis in the infant without a palpable olive: accuracy of sonographic diagnosis. Radiology 193:771–776, 1994.

38. Neilson D, Hollman AS: The ultrasonic diagnosis of infantile hypertrophic pyloric stenosis: technique and accuracy. Clin Radiol 49:246–247, 1994.

39. Janik JS, Wayne ER, Janik JP: Pyloric stenosis in premature infants. Arch Pediatr Adolesc Med 150:223–224, 1996.

40. Finkelstein MS, Mandell GA, Tarbell KV: Hypertrophic pyloric stenosis: volumetric measurement of nasogastric aspirate to determine the imaging modality. Radiology 177:759–761, 1990.

41. De Backer A, Bove T, Vandenplas Y, et al: Contribution of endoscopy to early diagnosis of hypertrophic pyloric stenosis. J Pediatr Gastoenterol Nutr 18:78–81, 1994.

42. Donovan GK, Yazdi AJ: The endoscopic diagnosis of pyloric stenosis. J Okla State Med Assoc 89:58–59, 1996.

*43. Papadakis K, Chen EA, Luks FI, et al: The changing presentation of pyloric stenosis. Am J Emerg Med 17:67–69, 1999.

*44. Chen EA, Luks FI, Gilchrist BF, et al: Pyloric stenosis in the age of ultrasonography: fading skills, better patients? J Pediatr Surg 31:829–830, 1996.

45. Tack ED, Perlman JM, Bower RJ, McAlister WH: Pyloric stenosis in the sick premature infant: clinical and radiological findings. Am J Dis Child 142:68–70, 1988.

46. Letton RW: Pyloric stenosis. Pediatr Ann 30:745–750, 2001.

47. Miozzari HH, Tonz M, von Vigier RO, Bianchetti MG: Fluid resuscitation in infantile hypertrophic pyloric stenosis. Acta Paediatr 90:511–514, 2001.

48. Hall NJ, Van Der Zee J, Tan HL, Pierro A: Meta-analysis of laparoscopic versus open pyloromyotomy. Ann Surg 240:774–778, 2004.

49. Yamataka A, Tsukada K, Yokoyama-Laws Y, et al: Pyloromyotomy versus atropine sulfate for infantile hypertrophic pyloric stenosis. J Pediatr Surg 35:338–341, 2000.

50. Nagita A, Yamaguchi J, Amemoto K, et al: Management and ultrasonographic appearance of infantile hypertrophic pyloric stenosis with atropine sulfate. J Pediatr Gastroenterol Nutr 23:172–177, 1996.

Chapter 77

Constipation

David D. Cassidy, MD and Aaron Wohl, MD

Key Points

Ninety-five percent of children with constipation have no serious underlying pathology.

Emergency physicians and families of children with chronic functional constipation must initiate treatment with the understanding that success requires 6 to 24 months for most children.

Treatment consists of child and family education, evacuation of stool impaction, and a maintenance stage that needs to be closely followed in the primary care setting.

Introduction and Background

Constipation, though rarely an emergent condition, is a very common complaint in children presenting to the emergency department. In one study, it was found to be the third most common medical etiology for abdominal pain in children presenting to a pediatric emergency department.[1] Constipation accounts for up to 3% of all general pediatric outpatient visits and 25% of pediatric gastroenterology consultations.[2,3] This condition is extremely unpleasant for both the patient and the parents and, if chronic, can completely disrupt the family's normal lifestyle. It is therefore extremely important for the emergency physician to be well versed in the evaluation and treatment options for this very common condition.

In children, constipation can be defined by many different diagnostic criteria but can be broadly labeled as infrequent bowel movements with one or more associated symptoms. These associated symptoms include a change in a usual non-problematic bowel pattern, painful defecation, hard stools that cause abdominal pain, purposeful withholding of stool, fecal retention, rectal prolapse, fecal soiling, and encopresis. *Soiling* is used to describe fecal material leakage around a buildup of stool impaction. *Encopresis* is defined as the involuntary, or voluntary, passage of formed, semi-formed, or liquid stool into a place other than a toilet after 4 years of age for at least once a month for 6 months.[4] Many use the two terms interchangeably. Some base the definition of constipation on the history of fewer than two to three bowel movements per week.[2,5] Confirming the diagnosis of constipation based on bowel patterns is a very difficult task. There is a large variation in the frequency of bowel movements in individual children depending on their age as well as their diet.[6]

Recognition and Approach

Functional or idiopathic constipation is the most common cause and is responsible for 90% to 95% of all defecation difficulties in children.[7] The peak incidence occurs between 2 and 4 years of age, which corresponds with the typical time of toilet training.[2] Constipation is equally distributed by gender in the toddler-age child but becomes more prevalent in males by school age, with an approximate ratio of 3 : 1. Many factors have been proposed as precipitants of constipation during early childhood, including the initiation of toilet training, dietary transitions from breast milk to formula, starting school or day care, and lack of fiber intake. In adults, an increase in fiber intake can be an appropriate treatment for constipation. For children, though, the role of dietary fiber is controversial, as evidence from controlled studies indicating that dietary modification is beneficial does not exist.[8]

The most common cause of constipation is an acquired behavior brought on by a painful or unpleasant episode of defecation that leads to stool withholding by the child in order to avoid further painful bowel movements. In one study, 63% of children with constipation and soiling had painful defecation that began before 3 years of age.[9] This withholding of stool then leads to incomplete rectal emptying, which leads to stool impaction. The impacted stool becomes more firm as the reabsorption of fluids continues. The retention of stool in the rectum leads to an increased volume of the colon and distention of the rectum. Distention causes the sensory threshold to increase, and the signal for the need to defecate now arises only with significantly more stool in the rectum than normal. Experts suggest that increased distention leads to rectal and sphincter muscle weakening, leading to more chances of incomplete evacuation and soiling accidents in between stool attempts.[6] When the child finally defecates, it is even more unpleasant, which results in further withholding, thus perpetuating the problem. Leakage of loose stool around the fecal impaction in the rectum is the mechanism for soiling and encopresis.

These factors underscore the importance of early recognition and treatment of constipation in order to prevent this worsening cascade of events. Early, effective treatment of painful defecation in infancy and early childhood might reduce the incidence of chronic fecal impaction and fecal soiling in school-age children.

Clinical Presentation

Parents may bring in their infants with the complaint of grunting, screaming, and straining prior to what appears to be normal bowel movements and a normal bowel pattern. This is usually not a sign of constipation but is a result of immature coordination between the contraction of the infant's abdominal muscles and the relaxation of the pelvic floor muscles and is termed *infant dyschezia*. Parents should be reassured that, with time and practice, this process becomes coordinated and the symptoms resolve.[10] Infants usually do not have formed stools, and if formula fed may only have one to two stools per week. If the infant is passing hard, pellet-like stools, this will result in inappropriate contraction of the anal sphincter while straining to defecate. This leads to the pain and withholding cycle described previously and constipation in infants.

The older child will typically present with abdominal pain, abdominal distention, nausea and vomiting, anorexia, and irritability.[10] There may not be a history of decreased frequency of stools because neither the parent nor the child pays close attention to bowel patterns once the child is toilet trained. There may be a history of previous episodes of transient colicky abdominal pain relieved with passage of a large bowel movement. Occasionally, the chief complaint is constipation. The parent may describe the child squirming, performing rhythmic movements, standing on the toes, or assuming the fetal position, all of which are attempts to withhold stool by tightening of the gluteal muscles and anal sphincter. Children with a long-standing problem will also have symptoms of painful defecation, very hard and large stools, stool withholding, soiling, and encopresis. A recent study found that some children with unrecognized constipation may present with upper gastrointestinal symptoms, including recurrent vomiting and gastroesophageal reflux.[11]

There is a clear link between constipation and optimal functioning of the urinary system. Constipated children may present with a history of urinary incontinence, urinary frequency, poorly emptying bladder, and recurrent urinary tract infections.[12,13] The frequently full, dilated rectum pushes on the bladder, causing frequent urination and improper emptying of the bladder, which may lead to stasis and infection. Soiling, especially in girls, leads to increased incidence of urinary tract infections from fecal flora.

The differential diagnosis for functional constipation is extensive and varies with age (Table 77–1). It is imperative that the emergency physician conduct a thorough history and physical examination to aid in ruling out an organic cause of constipation. Delay of passage of meconium stool or constipation in the newborn should always be considered organic in nature. Hirschsprung's disease, anal anatomic abnormalities, and intestinal obstruction should be considered as possible causes.

Hirschsprung's disease is a rare condition resulting from the lack of ganglion cells in the rectosigmoid colon, which

Table 77–1	Differential Diagnosis of Constipation

Functional Causes of Constipation

Fecal retention
Depression
Harsh toilet training, toilet phobia
Avoidance of public/school bathrooms
Anorexia nervosa
Sexual abuse
Developmental and behavior disorders

Organic Causes of Constipation

Anatomic/Obstructive
Anal fissure, anal stricture, anal stenosis
Imperforate anus, anteriorly displaced anus
Pelvic masses
Rectal abscess, rectal polyps
Acquired strictures from inflammatory bowel disease or
    necrotizing enterocolitis
Foreign body

Metabolic/Endocrine
Dehydration
Malnutrition
Hypomagnesemia, hypokalemia, hypercalcemia,
    hypophosphatemia
Cystic fibrosis
Meconium ileus
Celiac disease
Hypothyroidism, hyperparathyroidism
Diabetes mellitus and insipidus
Renal tubular acidosis
Multiple endocrine neoplasia type IIb
Acute illness
Cow's milk intolerance

Neurologic
Hirschsprung's disease
Cerebral palsy
Spina bifida
Myelomeningocele
Neurofibromatosis
Intestinal neuronal dysplasia
Spinal cord lesions
Werdnig-Hoffmann disease and hypotonia
Botulism

Connective Tissue Disorders
Scleroderma
Systemic lupus erythematosus
Ehlers-Danlos syndrome

Drugs
Anticholinergics
Opiates
Phenobarbital
Antidepressants
Sympathomimetics
Antihypertensives
Sucralfate
Antacids
Iron, lead
Vitamin D intoxication

leads to a nonfunctioning, dilated rectum. Less than 10% of neonates with Hirschsprung's disease pass meconium in the first 48 hours; therefore, a delay of defecation in a full-term infant should raise the suspicion for this diagnosis.[14] Most infants with Hirschsprung's disease are symptomatic during the first month of life and may present with signs and symptoms of an intestinal obstruction. Bilious vomiting, abdominal distention, decreased bowel movements, and reluctance to feed are the most common symptoms. Other presentations include failure to thrive, malnutrition, or intermittent vomiting with abdominal distension. A fecal mass may be palpated in the left lower abdomen. Rectal examination reveals an empty, nondilated vault. Life-threatening complications of Hirschsprung's disease include toxic megacolon and enterocolitis. Abdominal distention (83%), explosive diarrhea (69%), vomiting (51%), fever (34%), lethargy (27%), rectal bleeding (5%), and colonic perforation (2.5%) are seen with Hirschsprung's enterocolitis, with the mortality rate being as high as 20%.[15] Plain film findings may reveal colonic distention with a 90% sensitivity but only 24% specificity. The identification of the intestinal "cutoff sign" (gaseous intestinal distention with an abrupt cutoff air-fluid level at the pelvic brim) has a sensitivity of 74% and a specificity of 86% for Hirschsprung's enterocolitis.[15] After the first year of life, Hirschsprung's disease is found in less than 1% of children with constipation.[14]

After a few weeks of life, the most common causes of constipation are dietary factors and anal fissures. Organic causes can be divided into metabolic, endocrine, neurologic, anatomic (obstructive), connective tissue disorders, and medication/drug-induced constipation (see Table 77–1). Beyond infancy, the most common cause is functional.[5]

Historical factors that aid in the diagnosis of functional constipation are meconium passage within 48 hours of birth, decrease in the usual frequency of bowel movements, pain or discomfort with stool passage, hiding with defecation during toilet training, a small amount of blood on stools associated with anal fissures, and abdominal pain that appears to be relieved with stool passage. Families may also report a low-fiber, high-dairy diet.

Historical factors that suggest an organic cause for constipation are first meconium passage greater than 48 hours after birth, constipation since birth, the passage of pencil-thin stools, bloody diarrhea, significant abdominal distention, fatigue, fever, bilious vomiting, weight loss, abnormal child development, development of constipation prior to initiation of toilet training, and absence of encopresis. Specific medications and supplements can lead to constipation (see Table 77–1).

Important features of the physical examination include a thorough abdominal examination looking for tenderness and a fecal mass in the suprapubic or left lower quadrant of the abdomen. A digital rectal examination is recommended, as well as an external examination of the perineum and perianal area. This allows for assessment of anal location and permits the examiner to evaluate for the presence or absence of anal fissures and hemorrhoids, to test for occult blood in the stool, to evaluate for the presence of an anal wink and a cremasteric reflex, to assess anal sphincter tone, and to assess the size and contents of the rectal vault.[16] Organic disorders are associated with absent of anal wink, clinical dehydration and muscle wasting, pilonidal dimples and hair tufts, a flat buttocks, an anteriorly displaced anus, an empty rectal vault, and diminished or absent deep tendon reflexes, an absent cremasteric reflex, and decreased lower extremity strength and tone. A rectal examination is an important part of the clinical examination that is often overlooked. One study found that only 77% of children who were referred to pediatric gastroenterologists had a prior rectal examination.[17] Firm, packed stool is found in the rectum in most children who have functional constipation and correlates highly with the objective findings of constipation on abdominal radiographs.[18,19]

No specific laboratory assessments are recommended in the evaluation for constipation in children unless particular organic causes are suspected. There is also no strong evidence to support the routine use of abdominal radiographs to aid in the diagnosis of constipation. However, fecal impaction of the rectum and colon can be accurately assessed objectively from a plain abdominal radiograph.[18-21] In order to limit exposure to ionizing radiation, plain abdominal radiographs should be reserved for ruling out more serious underlying pathology, when the history and physical do not strongly support the diagnosis of simple functional constipation, and in cases of severe intractable constipation.

Important Clinical Features and Considerations

Misdiagnosis of this condition is common in children because of difficulty in properly assessing the frightened child and a frequent lack of a good history of infrequent bowel movements. Parents are usually not knowledgeable about the bowel habits of their toilet-trained children, and the child is usually too young to reliably describe his or her habits. Encopresis or soiling might be misinterpreted by some parents as diarrhea, leading to confusion as to the real problem of constipation. The key to diagnosing functional constipation is a suggestive history and examination that excludes serious pathology in a child who has undergone or is currently undergoing toilet training. It is essential that the emergency physician carefully evaluate young infants with the complaint of constipation to exclude organic causes and to initiate appropriate treatment for functional constipation. Organic causes of constipation are more common in infants and, if not recognized, can result in significant morbidity and mortality.

Management

Management options for constipation vary with the age of the child, the underlying cause of the problem, and the degree of constipation. In infants, treatment should be limited to mild osmotic agents such as malt soup extract, corn syrup, or the addition of a small amount of sugar to the infant's formula. Providing one of these options in cases of anal fissures will result in soft stools while the fissure heals. In toddlers and older children with mild constipation, addressing psychosocial issues surrounding toilet training and dietary advice may be all that is needed to remedy the problem. Treatment of moderate to severe constipation involves a three-step process: disimpaction, maintenance therapy, and monitoring (Fig. 77–1).[22]

Disimpaction options include oral agents, rectal agents, or both, and disimpaction should be performed over 3 to 5 days depending on the severity of the problem. Recommended oral agents for disimpaction include mineral oil, magnesium citrate, lactulose, senna, and polyethylene glycol solutions either alone or in combination[6] (see Fig. 77–1). Caution is necessary when selecting magnesium citrate as an oral agent in the very young because of the possibility of magnesium toxicity and electrolyte disturbances.[22] Rectal disimpaction using phosphate and mineral oil enemas is very effective and

Diagnosis/Management
Idiopathic Constipation/Soiling In Children

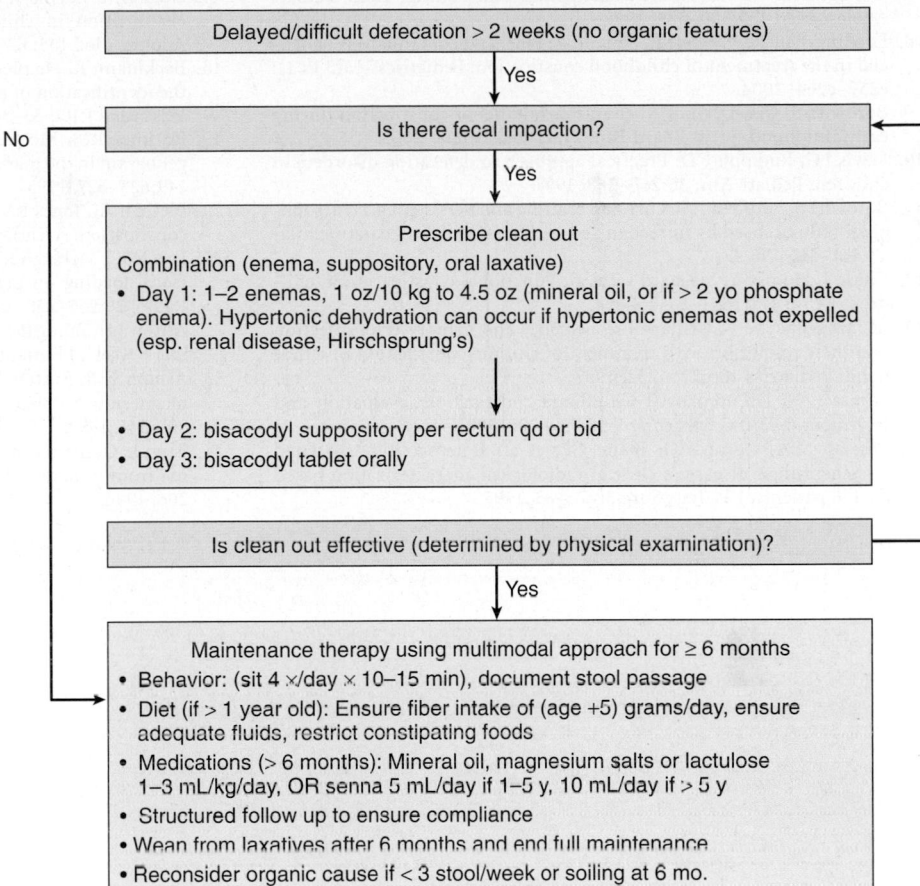

Delayed/difficult defecation > 2 weeks (no organic features)

Yes

No ← Is there fecal impaction?

Yes

Prescribe clean out
Combination (enema, suppository, oral laxative)
- Day 1: 1–2 enemas, 1 oz/10 kg to 4.5 oz (mineral oil, or if > 2 yo phosphate enema). Hypertonic dehydration can occur if hypertonic enemas not expelled (esp. renal disease, Hirschsprung's)

- Day 2: bisacodyl suppository per rectum qd or bid
- Day 3: bisacodyl tablet orally

Is clean out effective (determined by physical examination)?

Yes

Maintenance therapy using multimodal approach for ≥ 6 months
- Behavior: (sit 4 ×/day × 10–15 min), document stool passage
- Diet (if > 1 year old): Ensure fiber intake of (age +5) grams/day, ensure adequate fluids, restrict constipating foods
- Medications (> 6 months): Mineral oil, magnesium salts or lactulose 1–3 mL/kg/day, OR senna 5 mL/day if 1–5 y, 10 mL/day if > 5 y
- Structured follow up to ensure compliance
- Wean from laxatives after 6 months and end full maintenance
- Reconsider organic cause if < 3 stool/week or soiling at 6 mo.

FIGURE 77–1. Diagnosis and management of idiopathic constipation in children.

provides results more rapidly but is invasive and can be unpleasant for the child and family. Enemas should be avoided in children less than 3 years old and in young children with severe neurologic disabilities. These children are at a higher risk of prolonged retention of the enema, leading to absorption of the solution and subsequent toxicity due to magnesium and phosphate content in the most widely used enemas.[23] Soap suds enemas have also been reported to cause bowel necrosis with perforation, and tap water enemas may cause water intoxication, hypervolemia, and dilution of electrolytes, thus leading to seizures.[2,5] Choosing between the oral route, the rectal route, or both is based on the degree of constipation and a discussion with the parents and child.

Once disimpaction is accomplished, the goal of treatment is to prevent recurrence of constipation. Education on the mechanism of constipation as well as fecal soiling helps with the overall treatment plan. Dietary modification, pharmacologic interventions, and behavior modifications are crucial in the maintenance stage. Increasing fiber in the diet and the increasing the child's fluid intake are helpful in maintaining normal bowel patterns (see Fig. 77–1). A short course of stimulant laxative followed by a long-term lubricant is needed in most cases. Mineral oil is an excellent maintenance agent but should not be used if there is an apparent aspiration risk due to young age or severe disability.[24] Follow-up with the patient's primary care physician is essential to assist with long-term care.

Summary

Constipation is commonly seen in the emergency department and a frequent cause of abdominal pain in young children. A careful history and physical examination are usually all that is needed to make the diagnosis. Initiating proper therapy as well as educating the child and parents is essential for long-term success in this sometimes chronic and complex condition.

REFERENCES

1. Reynolds SL, Jaffe DM: Children with abdominal pain: evaluation in the emergency department. Pediatr Emerg Care 6:8–12, 1990.
2. Loening-Baucke V: Chronic constipation in children. Gastroenterology 105:1557–1564, 1993.
3. Molnar D, Taitz LS, Urwin OM, Wales JK: Anorectal manometry results in defecation disorders. Arch Dis Child 58:257–261, 1983.
4. American Psychiatric Association: Diagnostic and Statistical Manual of Mental Disorders, 4th ed. Washington, DC: American Psychiatric Association, 1994.
5. Bulloch B, Tenenbein M: Constipation: diagnosis and management in the pediatric emergency department. Pediatr Emerg Care 18:254–258, 2002.
*6. Baker SS, Liptak GS, Colletti RB, et al: Constipation in infants and children: evaluation and treatment. A medical position statement of the North American Society for Pediatric Gastroenterology and Nutrition. J Pediatr Gastroenterol Nutr 29:612–626, 1999.

———————
*Selected readings.

7. Felt B, Wise CG, Olson A, et al: Multidisciplinary team from the University of Michigan Medical Center in Ann Arbor: Guideline for the management of idiopathic constipation and soiling. Arch Pediatr Adolesc Med 153:380–385, 1999.

8. Loening-Baucke V, Miele E, Staiano A: Fiber (glucomannan) is beneficial in the treatment of childhood constipation. Pediatrics 113(3 Pt 1): e259–e264, 2004.

9. Borowitz S, Cox D, Tam A, et al: Precipitants of constipation during early childhood. J Am Board Fam Pract 16:213–218, 2003.

10. Lewis LG, Rudolph CD: Practical approach to defecation disorders in children. Pediatr Ann 26:260–268, 1997.

11. Borowitz S, Sutphen J: Recurrent vomiting and persistent gastroesophageal reflux caused by unrecognized constipation. Clin Pediatr (Phila) 43:461–466, 2004.

12. Chase J, Homsy Y, Siggaard C, et al: Functional constipation in children. J Urol 171:2641–2643, 2004.

13. Loening-Baucke V: Urinary incontinence and urinary tract infection and their resolution with treatment of chronic constipation of childhood. Pediatrics 100:228–232, 1997.

*14. Youssef, N, DiLorenzo C: Childhood constipation: evaluation and treatment. J Clin Gastroenterol 33:199–205, 2001.

15. Elhalaby EA, Coran AG, Blane CE, et al: Enterocolitis associated Hirschsprung's disease: a clinical-radiological characterization based on 168 patients. J Pediatr Surg 30:76–83, 1995.

16. Loening-Baucke V: Encopresis. Curr Opin Pediatr 14:570–575, 2002.

17. Gold DM, Levine J, Weinstein TA, et al: Frequency of digital rectal examination in children with chronic constipation. Arch Pediatr Adolesc Med 153:377–379, 1999.

18. Beckmann K, Hennes H, Sty J, et al: Accuracy of clinical variables in the identification of radiographically proven constipation in children. Wisc Med J 100:33–36, 2001.

19. Rockney RM, McQuade WH, Days AL: The plain abdominal roentgenogram in the management of encopresis. Arch Pediatr Adolesc Med 149:623–627, 1995.

20. Blethyn AJ, Jones KV, Newcombe R, et al: Radiological assessment of constipation. Arch Dis Child 73:532–533, 1995.

21. Leech SC, McHugh K, Sullivan PB: Evaluation of a method of assessing faecal loading on plain abdominal radiographs in children. Pediatr Radiol 29:255–258, 1999.

22. Alison LH, Bulugahapitiya D: Laxative induced magnesium poisoning in a 6 week old infant. BMJ 300:125, 1990.

23. Ashton MR, Sutton D, Nielson M: Severe magnesium toxicity after magnesium sulphate enema in a chronically constipated child. BMJ 300:541, 1990.

24. Fan LL, Graham LM: Radiological cases of the month: lipoid pneumonia from mineral oil aspiration. Arch Pediatr Adolesc Med 148:205–206, 1994.

Chapter 78

Gastrointestinal Foreign Bodies

Craig A. Kizewic, DO and Madeline Matar Joseph, MD

Key Points

Consider the diagnosis of an esophageal foreign body in any child with a history of choking with or without vomiting, excessive salivation, dysphagia, or odynophagia.

Eighty percent to 90% of all objects, sharp or smooth, reaching the stomach will pass spontaneously over a 4- to 10-day period.

Esophageal button batteries can produce injury in as little as 2 hours and perforation in as little 6 hours. Therefore, immediate removal is advised.

Asymptomatic patients with esophageal coins can be observed for up to 24 hours with little risk of esophageal injury or aspiration.

Introduction and Background

Foreign body ingestion is a common, emergent problem in infants and children. Small children have a natural tendency to put objects in their mouths due to their oral orientation. The majority of ingestions occur between 6 months and 6 years of age, with 65% to 85% occurring in children less than 3 years of age.[1-6]

Historically, esophageal foreign bodies have been considered less serious than bronchial foreign bodies. However, the prognosis of an untreated or unsuspected esophageal foreign body can be devastating. Unrecognized esophageal foreign bodies can cause a myriad of complications such as esophageal perforation, abscess formation, mediastinitis, or fistula formation, some cases of which have been fatal. Annually, 1500 children die from complications of esophageal foreign bodies. Recognition becomes even more challenging when dealing with developmentally delayed, emotionally disturbed, or very young children as they communicate less effectively and can ingest a wide variety of objects. Fortunately, the majority of foreign bodies reaching the stomach will pass through the gastrointestinal system without any major complications. For the 10% to 20% of foreign bodies that do not pass, endoscopic removal is advised.[1,4,6-8]

Many types of foreign bodies are ingested, such as nails, pins, thumbtacks, keys, jewels, toys, bones, various metal objects, and clothes holders. Of interest, variations with ethnicity occur. In Western cultures, up to 89% of gastrointestinal foreign body ingestions are coins and up to one third become impacted in the esophagus. In Asia, up to 90% of gastrointestinal foreign body ingestions are fish bones. Fish bones, however, represent up to 90% of sharp foreign bodies ingested in either culture. If the bone impacts in the esophagus, immediate removal is necessary to prevent esophageal perforation, mediastinitis, and abscess formation. Safety pins lodged in the esophagus pose this same risk.[8-10]

Button battery ingestion is becoming more frequent in the pediatric population as our technology advances and smaller batteries are used in cameras, hearing aids, flashlights, and games. The concern with button batteries is their tendency to cause esophageal erosion and perforation. All types of batteries can cause gastrointestinal trauma.

Magnets are found less frequently in the gastrointestinal tract, but pose a significant problem if more than one magnet is ingested. Multiple magnets are especially hazardous after separating from each other as they pass from the stomach to the duodenum through the pylorus. The individual magnets can then attract each other through the bowel wall and cause pressure necrosis, fistula formation, and/or bowel perforation.[1,3,4,10-18]

Food impactions are rare in infants and children unless there is an anatomic or acquired stricture or a gastrointestinal motility disorder. When seen, they occur primarily in males and appear related to immature behavior or eating too quickly without adequately chewing the food. Even though this is rare, erythema and bleeding of the esophagus can be seen after removal of the food bolus. Bleeding is secondary to the actual food impaction or trauma to the esophageal wall during removal.[19]

Bezoars are concretions of incompletely digested particles such as hair, vegetable fiber, or milk products. Patients with gastrointestinal bezoars may present with a myriad of complaints ranging from subtle presentations such as epigastric pain, nausea, and vomiting to serious complications such as weight loss, gastric outlet obstruction, gastric ulceration, peritonitis, gastrointestinal bleeding, intussusception, obstruction, or perforation. Bezoars may appear as a food-filled stomach or fecal matter in the colon and are easily missed on plain radiography. They can cause chronic abdominal pain in children as well as adults.[20,21] The two most common types seen in the pediatric population are trichobezoars (hair) and lactobezoars (milk curds). In adults, phytobezoars (vegetable matter) predominate and most commonly affect adults with prior gastric surgery, gastroparesis, or decreased gastric acidity.[21]

Trichobezoars most commonly occur in young females 10 to 19 years of age with psychiatric disorders such as trichotillomania, mental retardation, or pica. Caregivers report trichophagia (eating or chewing on hair) in up to half of all cases. The trichobezoar starts from the intake of small quantities of hair that eventually do not pass the pylorus. The hair then mixes with other food particles to become a semisolid mass. Air trapped within the trichobezoar may be evident on plain films. A rare condition termed *Rapunzel syndrome* may occur if strands of swallowed hair extend from the trichobezoar past the pylorus into to intestine. This condition may lead to bowel obstruction.[20-23]

Lactobezoars are concretions of undigested milk products that occur in infants and toddlers and do not appear to affect children past 3 years of age. They can affect any child but are found mostly in premature infants, full-term breast-fed infants, and infants receiving concentrated formulas. Almost all types of milk products, including breast milk and soy-based formulas, can lead to the formation of lactobezoars. Similar to the presentation of other bezoars, lactobezoars may mimic a variety of medical and surgical conditions related to gastric outlet obstruction.[20,24]

In children, the majority of foreign bodies lodge at the usual sites of anatomic narrowing. This includes locations such as the level of the cervical esophagus just inferior to the cricopharyngeus muscle, the aortic arch, the esophagogastric junction, the curvature of the duodenum, and the ileocecal valve. Up to 95% of fish bone ingestions lodge in the palatine tonsils, base of the tongue, vallecula, or pyriform sinus.[1,2,8,10,25,26]

Recognition and Approach

Obtaining a history of foreign body ingestion in infants and small children can be difficult. Children less than 5 years of age cannot provide a reliable history, convey their degree of discomfort or distress, or indicate the presence of a foreign body. As such, their histories are often vague. The foreign body ingestion may not have been witnessed or may have occurred long before the patient presents to the physician. Children may have a history of choking, but symptoms are usually transient and not witnessed. These symptoms may not arouse concern in the caregiver and may have resolved before arrival at the emergency department.[1,10]

Signs and symptoms such as refusal to eat, blood-tinged saliva, drooling, or crying can represent a myriad of other diagnoses; nevertheless, the two most sensitive indicators of an impacted foreign body are refusal to eat and blood-tinged saliva.[10,14] The diagnosis of gastrointestinal foreign bodies is even more challenging in children who are developmentally delayed. They may have excess drooling and lack the ability to communicate any swallowing difficulty. Symptoms can persist for weeks before the discovery of an ingested foreign body.[1,25]

A history of esophageal instrumentation or surgery should be elicited. Five clinical symptoms that should raise suspicion that acute foreign body ingestion has occurred are vomiting, dysphagia, odynophagia, choking, and excessive salivation.

Clinical Presentation

Patients with foreign body ingestion often present within the first 24 to 36 hours of ingestion, while the vast majority present within the first 6 hours of ingestion. Children less than 5 years of age may present with vague symptoms of refusal to eat, blood-tinged sputum, drooling, or vomiting. They are usually uncomfortable and crying. Children older than 5 years of age are usually able to provide a more detailed history of the ingestion and are able to communicate some degree of discomfort associated with a foreign body. If there is a history of ingestion coupled with vomiting, a foreign body sensation, and odynophagia, an esophageal foreign body is likely.[1,17] A majority of patients will present with more than one symptom. However, 50% of children who swallow a coin are asymptomatic and present because the caregiver witnessed the ingestion.[7,10,19,25]

Up to 76% of patients with chronic esophageal foreign bodies (1 week or greater after ingestion) present with respiratory distress, a cough, wheezing, or respiratory tract infection. Symptoms result from extension of esophageal wall edema to the highly compliant soft tissue separating the esophagus from the trachea. This can lead to partial tracheal or bronchial compression. The population most affected by chronic esophageal bodies includes children who are less than 5 years old or who are developmentally delayed.[1,6]

Although rare, children with psychiatric disorders who present with the following symptoms should be evaluated for a bezoar: chronic abdominal pain, early satiety, weight loss, alteration in normal stool patterns, or passage of hair fragments in vomitus or stool. The symptoms have an insidious onset, and the diagnosis is often delayed. If undiagnosed, bezoars may lead to gastrointestinal bleeding, obstruction, or perforation. Although not reported in children, the mortality rates in adults are as high as 30%.[20]

Patients can also present with complications from their esophageal foreign body, including fever, dysphagia, odynophagia, cough, dyspnea, pneumonia, or bilious vomiting. The presence of nonspecific or vague symptoms tends to obscure the diagnosis over hours to weeks in some instances. Rare complications, including vascular hemorrhage or mediastinitis, can occur. Rarely, children may develop hemoptysis or hematemesis due to vascular injury from migration or erosion of the esophageal foreign body through the aorta or another major blood vessel and require aggressive management. Mediastinitis has occurred up to 12 weeks or later from the initial ingestion. Patients present with fever, tachycardia, respiratory distress, stridor, retractions, and hypoxia.[13,16,18,27]

Body packing is a recently reported phenomenon as smugglers are now using children as couriers. Both heroin and cocaine are the typical drugs that are smuggled in this fashion. The packets of drugs are wrapped and sealed in waterproof vehicles such as condoms or examination gloves. They are then swallowed or packed in the rectum or vagina. A single individual may transport as many as 200 individual packets internally. Patients may present with drug toxicity due to complications from ruptured or leaking packets, intestinal obstruction, or perforation, or with rectal or vaginal bleeding due to retrograde packing, or they may be asymptomatic.[28]

Important Clinical Features and Considerations

Several risk factors predict complications of ingested esophageal foreign bodies. Objects impacted for 2 or more days prior to presentation, foreign bodies lodged in the upper esophagus at the level of the cricopharyngeus muscle, or those visualized on a lateral cervical radiograph have higher complication rates. Sharp objects are the most dangerous and difficult to remove. As time passes, perforation rates increase to as high as 15% to 30%. Since the likelihood of hemorrhage and mucosal damage is higher, removal should occur within 4 to 6 hours.[7,14,29] Some authors also state that rigid, irregular, wide (>2 cm), or long (>3 to 6 cm) objects should be removed since they are more likely to become impacted.[7,23]

Delayed presentation of an ingested disk battery frequently occurs in children. Their symptoms consist of dysphagia, retrosternal chest pain, choking, odynophagia, and pneumonia. Complications resulting in burns to the trachea or esophagus have led to fatal tracheoesophageal fistulas. Batteries may cause damage in several ways. Leakage of caustic material causes liquefaction necrosis. Pressure from the battery itself causes necrosis of the esophageal wall, and completion of an electrical circuit leads to current injury. One study proved batteries immersed in saline release their toxic contents almost immediately. Another study showed leakage of potentially toxic materials after 4 hours of gastric acid exposure. Almost 50% of batteries recovered in stool show dissolution or fragmentation. Minor histologic changes occur as early as 2 hours postingestion, esophageal erosion from the epithelium to the muscle layer within 4 hours, and frank perforation in as little as 6 hours. Consequently, esophageal button batteries require expeditious removal. Mercuric oxide batteries can contain lethal doses of toxins; however, most of the toxin converts to a nontoxic substance after ingestion. For those batteries containing more than the lethal dose, elevated mercury levels and symptoms of toxicity can occur. Other batteries using heavy metals such as lithium and magnesium do not cause toxicity. All types of button batteries can cause a similar amount of esophageal damage. In general, larger batteries cause more damage. Batteries greater than 15 mm are more likely to become impacted and cause damage to the esophagus.[13,18,30]

Ingestion of multiple magnets can cause severe damage. If multiple magnets are discovered in the stomach, they should be removed immediately. If allowed to pass through the pylorus, they can separate into groups and be attracted to each other through the bowel wall. This can lead to bowel wall necrosis with subsequent perforation or enteric-enteric fistula formation. If multiple magnets have already passed through the pylorus, the child must be monitored for signs and symptoms of intestinal obstruction or perforation. Should the child show any signs or symptoms of perforation or obstruction, emergent exploratory laparoscopy or laparotomy is mandated.[3,4]

Patients with open safety pins or fish bones impacted in the upper esophagus usually are more symptomatic than those with lower esophageal foreign bodies. Symptoms of sharp esophageal foreign body ingestion include coughing, dysphagia, odynophagia, drooling, and blood-tinged sputum. Complications resulting from safety pins and fish bones lodged lower in the esophagus include perforation, paraesophageal or retroesophageal abscess, mediastinitis, or, rarely, esophagocarotid or esophagoaortic fistula.[2,8,26]

Other pitfalls include failure to recognize a sharp foreign body or a second foreign body, or foreign body impaction in an asymptomatic patient (which occurs in 35% to 50% of patients), and relying on plain radiographic studies to exclude a foreign body. A negative plain film study does not rule out the presence of a foreign body.[1,14]

Management

Imaging Studies

Multiple diagnostic tests exist to help aid in the detection of gastrointestinal foreign bodies (Fig. 78–1). Plain radiographs have been the gold standard and are almost 100% sensitive in detecting safety pins, batteries, coins, and other metallic objects. Depending upon the site of the foreign body, anterior-posterior cervical, lateral cervical, posterior-anterior chest, and abdominal films may be required in patients with button battery, coin, or multiple magnet ingestions. A lateral cervical radiograph is one of the most important radiographs for identifying all objects. Button batteries show a step-off on lateral view and double density on the posterior-anterior view. While subcutaneous glass is visible on 100% of plain radiographs, ingested glass may not be visible on plain films. Moreover, nearly three quarters of fish bones and chicken bones cannot be seen on plain films. Thus, routine radiographs cannot be recommended for many foreign bodies.[9,18,25,26,31]

Metal detectors are another viable option to localize metallic foreign bodies. They have a 98% sensitivity in determining whether coin ingestion has occurred and whether the coin is impacted in the esophagus. Even in the hands of inexperienced operators, metal detectors are an accurate screening test.[31]

Since Gastrografin is relatively contraindicated due to the risk of aspiration and chemical pneumonitis, a barium swallow study can be used to detect radiolucent foreign bodies lodged in the esophagus. This study not only provides useful information on the anatomy of the gastrointestinal system, such as anomalies and presence or absence of strictures, diverticulae, or congenital abnormalities, but also can identify bezoars, which appear as freely mobile, intraluminal masses.[1,11,20] However, barium should be avoided if a perforation is suspected.

Computed tomography (CT) is underutilized for the detection of foreign bodies. CT is easy to perform and interpret and can clearly visualize multiple foreign bodies, bezoars, points of obstruction, radiolucent foreign bodies, and abscesses as well as associated inflammatory changes. CT scans using 2- to 5-mm thick cuts have 100% sensitivity and 94% specificity in detecting esophageal fish bones not visualized on plain radiographs.[9,26,27,32]

Magnetic resonance imaging (MRI), like CT, is able to detect radiolucent gastrointestinal foreign bodies. However, the exact role for using MRI for managing patients with suspected foreign body ingestions is not defined.[1]

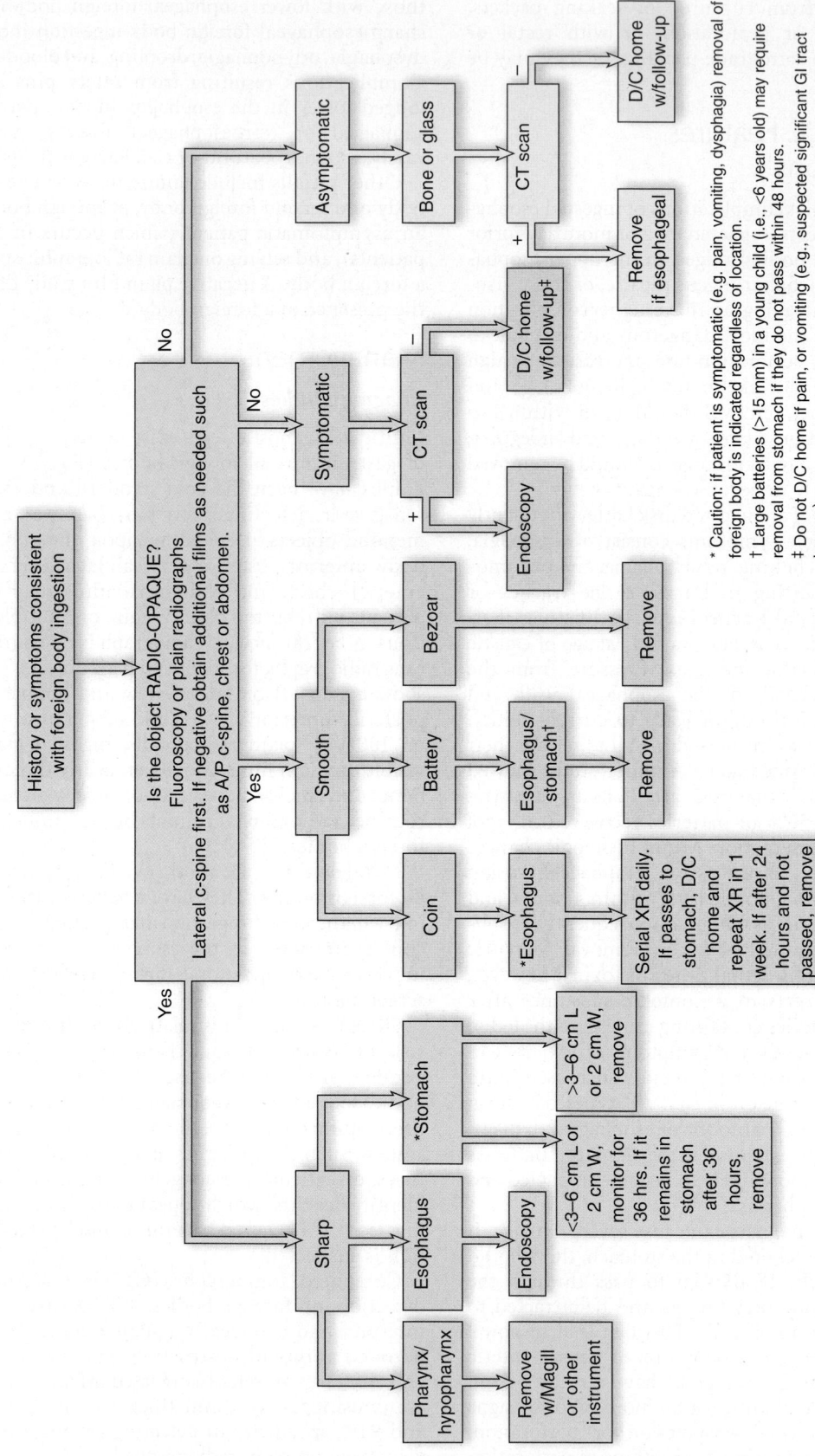

FIGURE 78–1. General approach to foreign body ingestion. (*Caution: If patient is symptomatic (e.g., pain, vomiting, dysphagia), removal of foreign body is indicated regardless of location.) Abbreviations: A/P, anterior-posterior; CT, computed tomography; D/C, discharge; L, long; W, wide; XR, radiograph.

Foreign Body Removal

The most acceptable technique to remove a gastrointestinal foreign body remains controversial. If the patient is symptomatic because of the ingestion, regardless of where the foreign body is, it should be removed as soon as possible.[1]

Rigid endoscopy offers the major advantage of visualizing the esophageal lumen and determining the degree of esophageal injury. Multiple foreign bodies can be detected, and the mortality and perforation rate are almost nonexistent. This technique is indicated for patients whose symptoms have persisted for 12 hours, not improved, or deteriorated, or if there are positive radiographic findings and retrosternal symptoms.[1,2,10,14]

Flexible endoscopy has an overall success rate of 99% for removing foreign bodies in the esophagus and stomach and is useful for sharp or smooth objects. It is safe, it offers the advantage of visualizing the patient's nasopharynx, pharynx, and larynx, and it is effective at removing foreign bodies that have failed to pass out of the stomach.[11,12,25]

In the emergency department, Magill forceps can be used to remove occasional foreign bodies lodged in the oropharynx, hypopharynx, and upper esophagus. The greatest success rates with this technique are when fish bones, safety pins, or coins are visualized. If visualization of the foreign body fails, direct laryngoscopy under general anesthesia may be required.[5,10,14]

One study looked at upper esophageal coin removal by emergency physicians using Magill forceps following rapid sequence intubation. Of 13 patients, 10 had coins successfully removed in this manner. The other 3 patients' coins were not visualized using laryngoscope and were successfully removed by using a Foley catheter. All patients were successfully treated in the emergency department, extubated, and discharged home within 5 hours.[33]

In asymptomatic patients, Foley catheters or magnet probes with fluoroscopic guidance can be used to remove coins or magnetic objects such as batteries, needles, and pins. The success rate is as high as 94%. Depending upon the type of object, location, associated symptoms, and duration of ingestion, endoscopy to evaluate for esophageal trauma may be required following this technique.[14,18,25,31]

Glucagon, a rapid, short-acting enteric smooth muscle relaxant, is successful in 75% of adults with impacted food in the esophagus. However, it has the potential to induce vomiting and possibly cause aspiration if given too rapidly. Moreover, in infants and children, attempts at coin removal with glucagon have proven unsuccessful and cannot be recommended.[19,34]

Watchful waiting for coins or a single magnet impacted in the esophagus for less than 24 hours in the asymptomatic patient is successful if there is no history of esophageal disease or esophageal surgery. The majority of objects will pass into the stomach. Once in the stomach, the majority of objects will pass spontaneously within a week to 10 days.[16] If the object fails to pass into the stomach after 24 hours or if symptoms (e.g., pain, vomiting, dysphagia) develop, endoscopic removal will be necessary.[16,31,33,35] Safety pin management depends on where the safety pin is located in the gastrointestinal tract and whether the safety pin is open or closed. An open safety pin in the esophagus must be removed immediately due to the risk of perforation. If it has passed into the stomach, daily radiographs may be obtained to monitor its movement as long as the patient remains asymptomatic. If the patient becomes symptomatic, immediate removal is necessary. If an open safety pin is lodged anywhere in the gastrointestinal tract for 2 days, surgical intervention is required.

Closed safety pins located in the esophagus may be treated as a smooth foreign body. Daily radiographs should be obtained to monitor the safety pin progress. If the patient becomes symptomatic or if it remains in the esophagus after 24 hours, it must be removed. For closed safety pins that pass into the stomach, serial radiographs may be taken on a daily basis to monitor the progress. If the safety pin has not passed after 7 days or the patient becomes symptomatic at any time, immediate surgical intervention is required. Once past the ligament of Treitz, the safety pin has a high likelihood of being eliminated without difficulty.[2,5,8,25]

Summary

Gastrointestinal foreign body ingestion is a common problem in children presenting to the emergency department. Although esophageal foreign bodies have been historically viewed as less serious than bronchial foreign bodies, deaths from impacted esophageal foreign bodies do occur. An untreated or unsuspected foreign body can result in devastating complications such as esophageal perforation, abscess formation, mediastinitis, and fistula formation. While coins and smooth objects are relatively benign ingestions, some objects are more dangerous, including button batteries, fish bones, small chicken bones, and sharp objects.

Although signs of esophageal foreign body ingestion include coughing, dysphagia, odynophagia, drooling, and blood-tinged sputum, eliciting the history from a developmentally delayed child or a child younger than 5 years of age is challenging. Refusal to eat and blood-tinged sputum in the child younger than 5 and a history of ingestion coupled with vomiting, vague sensation of foreign body, and odynophagia in the child older than 5 indicates an ingested foreign body until proven otherwise.

Some pitfalls to avoid are failure to recognize a sharp foreign body, the presence of a second foreign body, or a foreign body impaction in the asymptomatic patient, and relying on negative plain films, which do not rule out the possibility of a foreign body. If a plain film is positive and the object is in the stomach, such as a single magnet, an open or closed safety pin, a coin, or an object less than 2 cm wide and less than 3 to 6 cm long, a short watch-and-wait approach has been used successfully with a good outcome.

REFERENCES

1. Al-Qudah A, Daradkeh S, Abu-Khalaf M: Esophageal foreign bodies. Eur J Cardiothorac Surg 13:494–499, 1998.
2. Gun F, Salman T, Abbasoglu L, et al: Safety-pin ingestion in children: a cultural fact. Pediatr Surg Int 19:482–484, 2003.
3. Cauchi JA, Shawis RN: Multiple magnet ingestion and gastrointestinal morbidity. Arch Dis Child 87:539–540, 2002.
4. Chung J, Kim J, Song Y: Small bowel complication caused by magnetic foreign body ingestion of children: two case reports. J Pediatr Surg 38:1548–1550, 2003.
5. Karaman A, Cavusoglu Y, Karaman I, et al: Magill forceps technique for removal of safety pins in upper esophagus: a preliminary report. Int J Pediatr Otorhinolaryngol 68:1189–1191, 2004.

*6. Mohiuddin S, Siddiqui M, Mayhew J, et al: Esophageal foreign body aspiration presenting as asthma in the pediatric patient. South Med J 97:93–95, 2004.

7. Jeen Y, Chun H, Song C, et al: Endoscopic removal of sharp foreign bodies impacted in the esophagus. Endoscopy 33:518–522, 2001.

*8. Sarihan H, Kaklikkaya I, Ozcan F: Pediatric safety pin ingestion. J Cardiovasc Surg 39:515–518, 1998.

9. Eliashar R, Dano I, Dangoor E, et al: Computed tomography diagnosis of esophageal bone impaction: a prospective study. Ann Otol Rhinol Laryngol 108:708–711, 1999.

10. Pak M, Lee W, Fung H, et al: A prospective study of foreign-body ingestion in 311 children. Int J Pediat Otorhinolaryngol 58:37–45, 2001.

11. Kim J, Kim S, Kim J, et al: Management of foreign bodies in the gastrointestinal tract: an analysis of 104 cases in children. Endoscopy 31:302–304, 1999.

12. Higo R, Matsumoto Y, Ichimura K, et al: Foreign bodies in the aerodigestive tract in pediatric patients. Auris Nasus Larynx 30:397–401, 2003.

13. Okuyama J, Kubota A, Oue T, et al: Primary repair of tracheoesophageal fistula secondary to disc battery ingestion: a case report. J Pediar Surg 39:243–244, 2004.

*14. Arana A, Hauser B, Hachimi-Idrissi S, et al: Management of ingested foreign bodies in childhood. Eur J Pediatr 160:468–472, 2001.

15. Lai AT, Chow TL, Lee DT, et al: Risk factors predicting the development of complications after foreign body ingestion. Br J Surg 90:1531–1535, 2003.

16. Sharieff GQ, Brousseau TJ, Bradshaw JA, et al: Acute esophageal coin ingestion: is immediate removal necessary? Pediatr Radiol 33:859–863, 2003.

17. Shinhar S, Strabbing R, Madgy D: Esophagoscopy for removal of foreign bodies in the pediatric population. Int J Pediat Otorhinolaryngology 67:977–999, 2003.

*18. Yardeni D, Yardeni H, Coran AG, et al: Severe esophageal damage due to button battery ingestion: can it be prevented? Pediatr Surg Int 207:496–501, 2004.

19. Lao J, Bostwick H, Berezin S, et al: Esophageal food impaction in children. Pediatr Emerg Care 19:402–407, 2003.

20. Lynch KA, Feola PG, Guenther E: Gastric trichobezoar: an important cause of abdominal pain presenting to the pediatric emergency department. Pediatr Emerg Care 19:343–347, 2003.

21. Memon S, Mandhan P, Qureshi JN, Shairani AJ: Recurrent Rapunzel syndrome—a case report. Med Sci Monit 9:CS92–CS94, 2003.

22. Faria, A, Silva I, Santos A, et al: [The Rapunzel syndrome—a case report: trichobezoar as a cause of intestinal perforation.] J Pediatr (Rio J) 76:83–86, 2003.

23. Singla SL, Rattan KN, Kaushik N, Pandit SK: Rapunzel syndrome—a case report. Am J Gastroenterol 94:1970–1971, 1999.

24. DuBose TM, Southgate WM, Hill JG: Lactobezoars: a patient series and literature review. Clin Pediatr (Phila) 40:603–606, 2001.

*25. Cheng W, Tam PH: Foreign-body ingestion in children: experience with 1,265 cases. J Pediatr Surg 34:1472–1476, 1999.

26. Watanabe K, Kikuchi T, Katori Y, et al: The usefulness of computed tomography in the diagnosis of impacted fish bones in the oesophagus. J Laryngol Otol 112:360–364, 1998.

27. Kerscher JE, Beste DJ, Conley SF, et al: Mediastinitis associated with foreign body erosion of the esophagus in children. Int J Pediatr Otorhinolaryngol 59:89–97, 2001.

*28. Traub S, Kohn G, Hoffman R, et al: Pediatric "body packing." Arch Pediatr Adolesc Med 157:174–177, 2003.

29. Schalamon J, Haxhija EQ, Ainoedhofer H, et al: The use of a hand-held metal detector for localization of ingested metallic foreign bodies—a critical investigation. Eur J Pediatr 163:257–259, 2004.

*30. Rebhandl W, Steffan I, Schramel P, et al: Release of toxic metals from button batteries retained in the stomach: an in vitro study. J Pediatr Surg 37:87–92, 2002.

31. Bassett K, Schunk J, Logan L: Localizing ingested coins with a metal detector. Am J Emerg Med 17:338–341, 1999.

32. Ripolles T, Garcia-Aguayo J, Martinez MJ, Gil P: Gastrointestinal bezoars: sonographic and CT characteristics. AJR Am J Roentgenol 177:65–69, 2001.

*33. Vargas E, Mody A, Kim T, et al: The removal of coins from the upper esophageal tract of children by emergency physicians: a pilot study. Can J Emerg Med 6:434–440, 2004.

34. Mehta D, Attia M, Quintana E, et al: Glucagon use for esophageal coin dislodgement in children. Acad Emerg Med 8:200–203, 2001.

35. Conners G, Cobaugh D, Feinberg R, et al: Home observation for asymptomatic coin ingestion. Acad Emerg Med 6:213–217, 1999.

*Selected readings.

Chapter 79

Hepatitis

Evan J. Weiner, MD and Madeline Matar Joseph, MD

Key Points

Mild hepatitis is common, self-limited, and usually due to a generalized viral syndrome.

Vaccination has dramatically reduced the incidence of hepatitis B.

Hepatitis C remains underrecognized in children.

Half of acute liver failure cases are of unknown etiology. Liver transplantation teams should be involved early in the management of these cases.

New treatments are improving the outcomes of chronic hepatitis in children.

Introduction and Background

Hepatitis, defined as inflammation of the liver, encompasses a wide array of acute and chronic liver diseases from many etiologies. In the pediatric population, most hepatitis is related to a viral infection.

The overall incidence of hepatitis in children has changed dramatically over the past few decades due to many factors. Widespread hepatitis B vaccination has substantially decreased the incidence of hepatitis B in children.[1] In 1990, there were 3.0 cases of hepatitis B per 100,000 population among children ages birth to 19. By 2002, that rate decreased to 0.3 per 100,000.[1] Perinatal surveillance has decreased transmission of hepatitis B from mother to baby.[2] The prevalence of hepatitis C in children has been reported as 0.2% (ages 6 to 11 years) and 0.4% (ages 12 to 19 years).[3,4] The identification of the hepatitis C virus has led to increased recognition of its role in chronic disease in children.[3] Blood product screening for viral hepatitis has markedly decreased its iatrogenic transmission.[3] New medical treatments for chronic hepatitis, specifically hepatitis C, offer hope for preventing end-stage liver disease.[3] In addition, the success of pediatric liver transplantation programs has significantly improved outcomes in liver failure.[5]

Hepatitis A is widespread, with one third of the general U.S. population showing evidence of prior infection. Children ages 5 to 14 years have the highest reported incidence of hepatitis A; however, it is postulated that children under 5 have the actual highest incidence but they remain either undetected or asymptomatic.[6] The overall incidence of hepatitis A has steadily been decreasing in the United States.[7] Besides A, B, and C, other hepatitis viruses exist such as D (delta), E, and G. Hepatitis D can cause fulminant hepatitis in children with hepatitis B; however, it is rare in the United States.[2] Hepatitis E is also rare in the United States, but causes epidemics in the developing world.[2] Hepatitis G virus has been detected in U.S. children, especially those who have received blood products, but studies suggest it is not virulent.[2]

Recognition and Approach

The different hepatitis viruses are each distinct in their virology, transmission, and complications (Table 79–1). Hepatitis A virus infects the gastrointestinal tract and the liver, replicates in the liver, and sheds virus in bile and stool. A patient is most contagious 2 weeks prior to and 1 week after the onset of symptoms.[7] Children are at risk of contracting hepatitis A if they ingest infected stool. Inadequate hygiene at home, child-care centers, and places of food preparation can contribute to infection. Foreign travel, contact with foreign travelers, or contact with those at occupational risk (e.g., food handlers) also can place a child at risk.[7] Hepatitis A vaccination plays an important role in the prevention of hepatitis A, although routine vaccination is not yet recommended in nonendemic areas.[6,8]

Hepatitis B virus infects the liver and causes a brisk viremia. It is readily found in all body fluids, such as saliva, semen, vaginal fluid, and breast milk. Chronic infection rates vary by age, with neonates and younger children having a higher risk. Complications of chronic hepatitis B include cirrhosis and hepatocellular carcinoma. Hepatitis C virus initially infects the liver, leading to a mild systemic illness. However, unlike hepatitis B, chronic infection rates are very high. This is primarily due to the rapid mutation rate of the virus, and its success in evading host defenses. Perinatal transmission occurs in 5% of babies born to an infected mother; however, this is increased if the mother is co-infected with human immunodeficiency virus (HIV).[3] Injection drug use accounts for most cases of hepatitis C, now that there is universal screening of transfused blood products.

Table 79–1	Comparison of Clinical Features of Hepatitis A, B, and C				
Virus	**Family**	**Transmission**	**Incubation**	**Risk factors**	**Complications**
Hepatitis A	Picornavirus	Fecal-oral	28 days	Poor hygiene Travel Endemic areas Occupational Male homosexual sex	Self-limited Fulminant hepatic failure (rare)
Hepatitis B	Hepadnavirus (DNA virus)	Percutaneous— blood exposure Perinatal Sexual	45–160 days	Baby of infected mother Unimmunized Sexual contacts Injection drugs Needle sticks	Chronic infection Hepatocellular carcinoma Fulminant hepatic failure Papular acrodermatitis Glomerulonephritis
Hepatitis C	Flavivirus (RNA virus)	Percutaneous— blood exposure Perinatal Sexual	2 wk–6 mo	Blood product recipient Baby of infected mother HIV Injection drugs Tattoos Sexual contacts	Chronic infection Cirrhosis Hepatocellular carcinoma

Abbreviation: HIV, human immunodeficiency virus.
Data from References 2, 3, and 7.

Clinical Presentation

Children with acute hepatitis often present with many nonspecific symptoms such as fever, nausea, vomiting, and malaise. More specific signs and symptoms include jaundice, icterus, right upper quadrant pain, and hepatosplenomegaly.[3,6] More severe hepatic and extrahepatic complications may also be seen. Gastrointestinal bleeding can occur with cirrhosis. Encephalopathy and coagulopathy can occur in cases of hepatic failure. Chronic liver disease can also manifest as angiomas, anasarca, ascites, and growth retardation.[9]

Viral infections account for the majority of hepatitis cases in children. In addition to hepatitis A through E and non–A-E hepatitis, other viral syndromes such as Epstein-Barr virus, cytomegalovirus (CMV), adenovirus, enteroviruses, parvovirus B19, varicella-zoster virus, and herpes simplex virus can cause a degree of liver injury and inflammation.[10-13] There have also been reports of cat-scratch disease causing granulomatous hepatitis.[14] Genetic diseases such as Wilson's disease, α_1-antitrypsin deficiency, and hemochromatosis may also be considered.[15] Autoimmune diseases such as autoimmune hepatitis and systemic lupus erythematosus are other noninfectious causes of hepatic inflammation.[16] Toxins and drugs such as acetaminophen, isoniazid, minocycline, nitrofurantoin, propylthiouracil, alcohol, and inhalants can cause significant liver injury.[17,18] Although rare, Reye's syndrome may also be considered in cases of hepatitis and encephalopathy.[19] Pregnancy, specifically HELLP syndrome (hemolysis, elevated liver enzymes, and low platelet count), can be associated with elevated transaminases. In neonates, considerations include sepsis, inborn errors of metabolism, structural liver disease, and maternally acquired infections (syphilis, CMV, and HIV).[5]

An appropriate laboratory evaluation is very helpful and typically includes a complete blood count with platelets and reticulocytes, electrolytes, blood urea nitrogen, creatinine, transaminases, γ-glutamyl transpeptidase, total and direct bilirubin, alkaline phosphatase, albumin, prothrombin time, and activated partial thromboplastin time to rule out coagulopathy. If viral hepatitis is likely, a hepatitis antibody/antigen panel may be assessed. This includes hepatitis A antibody immunoglobulin M (IgM) and immunoglobulin G (IgG) (anti-HA), hepatitis B surface antigen (HBsAg) and antibody (anti-HBs), hepatitis B core antibody IgM and IgG (anti-HBc), hepatitis C antibody (anti-HC), and hepatitis B e antigen (HBeAg) and antibody (anti-HBe) (Table 79–2). Hepatitis B and C virus polymerase chain reaction can quantify viremia in chronic patients and also diagnose patients in very early stages of acute disease before the appearance of antibodies.[3] Other antibody tests include titers for Epstein-Barr virus, CMV, and parvovirus B19.[10] Rapid viral testing (e.g., adenovirus) may provide a quick diagnostic tool in mild viral hepatitis.[13] As clinically indicated, other tests may include an ammonia level, erythrocyte sedimentation rate, immunoglobulins, direct Coombs' test, tests for sexually transmitted diseases (gonorrhea/chlamydia, syphilis, HIV) (see Chapter 70, Sexually Transmitted Diseases), acetaminophen/drug levels (see Chapter 133, Classic Pediatric Ingestions), ceruloplasmin, copper, and α_1-antitrypsin. In neonates, sepsis evaluation, titers for maternally acquired infection, and tests for inborn errors of metabolism may be considered[15-17] (see Chapter 29, Inborn Errors of Metabolism).

Diagnostic imaging is usually not necessary in most cases of acute viral hepatitis. In cases of cholestatic or suspected structural liver disease, imaging options include ultrasonography, magnetic resonance imaging, and cholescintigraphy. Liver biopsy is indicated in acute liver failure, unclear diagnoses, cholestasis, neoplasm, chronic disease, and infiltrative disorders.

Important Clinical Features and Considerations

Viral hepatitis can be associated with many serious complications, ranging from chronic disease to hepatocellular carcinoma to fulminant liver failure and death. Chronic disease is caused by chronic hepatitis B and C infection, with hepatitis C causing the majority of cases in recent years. Chronic

Table 79–2	Interpretation of Hepatitis B Testing Results	
Tests	**Results**	**Interpretation**
HBsAg	Negative	Susceptible
anti-HBc	Negative	
anti-HBs	Negative	
HBsAg	Negative	Immune due to natural infection
anti-HBc	Positive	
anti-HBs	Positive	
HBsAg	Negative	Immune due to hepatitis B vaccination
anti-HBc	Negative	
anti-HBs	Positive	
HBsAg	Positive	Acutely infected
anti-HBc	Positive	
IgM anti-HBc	Positive	
anti-HBs	Negative	
HBsAg	Positive	Chronically infected
anti-HBc	Positive	
IgM anti-HBc	Negative	
anti-HBs	Negative	
HBsAg	Negative	Four interpretations possible*
anti-HBc	Positive	
anti-HBs	Negative	

*1. Might be recovering from acute HBV infection.
2. Might be distantly immune and test not sensitive enough to detect very low level of anti-HBs in serum.
3. Might be susceptible with a false-positive anti-HBc.
4. Might be undetectable level of HBsAg present in the serum and the person is actually chronically infected.
Abbreviations: anti-HBc, hepatitis B core antibody; anti-HBs, hepatitis B surface antibody; HBsAg, hepatitis B surface antigen; IgM anti-HBc, hepatitis B core antigen immunoglobulin M.
Adapted from Centers for Disease Control and Prevention: Guidelines for Viral Hepatitis Surveillance and Case Management. Atlanta: Centers for Disease Control and Prevention, 2004.

liver inflammation from these viruses can cause progressive fibrosis and cirrhosis. Fortunately, unlike adults, most children with hepatitis C demonstrate only mild fibrosis, and many even clear the virus.[3] Patients with hepatitis C are frequently co-infected with HIV. The additional presence of HIV may increase the chances of progression of chronic liver disease from hepatitis C. However hepatitis C may or may not cause the progression of HIV disease.[20]

Hepatocellular carcinoma is a recognized long-term complication of chronic hepatitis B infection. Unfortunately, survival with pediatric hepatocellular carcinoma is poor. Any child with evidence of chronic hepatitis B infection requires close surveillance with α-fetoprotein levels and ultrasonography.[21] In adults, chronic hepatitis C infection has also been linked to hepatocellular carcioma; however, this relationship has not been established in children.[2]

Fulminant liver failure is defined as the onset of hepatic encephalopathy and failure of vital liver function within 8 weeks of new-onset acute liver disease. Of interest, most cases of fulminant liver failure are caused by an unidentified (seronegative) hepatitis. Of the identified cases, most are due to hepatitis A and B, and rare cases are caused by hepatitis C.[22] It is postulated that a yet-to-be-identified virus is the etiology for the remainder of cases.[9] Aplastic anemia develops in a significant portion of these cases, some of which show evidence of parvovirus B19 infection.[23] A large proportion of patients with fulminant liver failure will require liver transplantation.[9]

Management

Since most cases of acute viral hepatitis are self-limited, supportive care is the mainstay of treatment. For patients with chronic hepatitis, medical therapy improves outcome. The antiviral drug lamivudine has been shown to produce a significant virologic response in patients with chronic hepatitis B.[24] In patients with hepatitis C, courses of injected interferon alfa combined with oral ribavirin have been effective in viral clearance.[25] Interferon alfa and ribavirin therapy are cost effective and reduce the incidence of cirrhosis, hepatocellular carcinoma, and the need for liver transplantation in patients with hepatitis C.[26] Interferon alfa has also been used successfully to treat chronic hepatitis B, and interferon beta can be an effective option in patients unresponsive to interferon alfa.[27] Side effects of interferon alfa therapy include influenza-like syndrome, neutropenia, and behavioral changes.[28]

There is a wide range of diagnoses that may cause hepatitis. Each diagnosis carries with it specific principles of management. Examples include chelation therapy in Wilson's disease and N-acetylcysteine in acetaminophen toxicity. In autoimmune hepatitis, anti-inflammatory drugs (e.g., prednisone) are the primary treatment. Other drugs such as cyclosporine, tacrolimus, mycophenolate mofetil, methotrexate, and cyclophosphamide remain options for treatment failures.[16]

The breakthrough of pediatric orthotopic liver transplantation has significantly improved outcomes in acute liver failure. Without transplantation, acute liver failure carries a greater than 70% mortality rate. One-year survival rates for acute liver failure patients following liver transplantation range from 65% to 92%. Unfortunately, in the neonate and infant, survival rates are much lower. To maximize outcome, orthotopic liver transplantation should be considered early in cases of fulminant liver failure.[5]

Summary

Most children with mild acute viral hepatitis can be followed as outpatients. Depending on their degree of illness severity, patients may need hospital admission for supportive care. Evidence of acute liver failure or impending liver failure requires admission to an intensive care unit. A pediatric gastroenterologist typically manages cases of acute and chronic hepatitis B and C, autoimmune hepatitis, and fulminant liver failure. Early involvement of a pediatric liver transplantation team is vital in the management of acute liver failure (see Chapter 81, Post–Liver Transplantation Complications). All cases of acute hepatitis A through G and unspecified hepatitis (including fulminant liver failure) should be reported to public health officials.[29]

All patients with hepatitis should have appropriate follow-up with their primary care physician and consultant specialists. Measures to prevent the spread of hepatitis should be implemented, such as inpatient precautions, public health measures, and patient education. All susceptible children should ne referred to their primary care physician for vaccination against hepatitis B. Susceptible children living in or traveling to endemic areas, patients with chronic liver disease, men who have sex with men, patients with clotting factor disorders, users of illegal drugs (injection and noninjection), and people at occupational risk should be vaccinated against hepatitis A. Postexposure immunoprophylaxis should be administered to healthy patients exposed to hepatitis A or B. All pregnant women require hepatitis B surface antigen surveillance[30] (see Chapter 156, Postexposure Prophylaxis).

REFERENCES

1. Centers for Disease Control and Prevention: Incidence of acute hepatitis B—United States, 1990–2002. MMWR Morb Mortal Wkly Rep 52:1252–1254, 2004.
2. Schwarz K, Balistreri W: Viral hepatitis. J Pediatr Gastroenterol Nutr 35:S29–S32, 2002.
3. Hochman J, Balistreri W: Chronic viral hepatitis. Pediatr Rev 24:399–403, 2003.
4. Alter M, Kruszon-Moran D, Nainan O, et al: The prevalence of hepatitis C virus infection in the United States, 1988 through 1994. N Engl J Med 341:556–562, 1999.
*5. Durand P, Debray D, Mandel R, et al: Acute liver failure in infancy: a 14-year experience of a pediatric liver transplantation center. J Pediatr 139:871–876, 2001.
6. Armstrong G, Bell B: Hepatitis A virus infections in the United States: model-based estimates and implications for childhood immunization. Pediatrics 109:839–845, 2002.
7. Fiore A: Hepatitis A transmitted by food. Clin Infect Dis 38:705–715, 2004.
8. Averhoff F, Shapiro C, Bell B, et al: Control of hepatitis A through routine vaccination of children. JAMA 286:2968–2973, 2001.
*9. Whitington PF, Alonso EM: Fulminant hepatitis in children: evidence for an unidentified hepatitis virus. J Pediatr Gastroenterol Nutr 33:529–536, 2001.
10. Rajwal S, Davison S, Wyatt J, McClean P: Primary Epstein-Barr virus hepatitis complicated by ascites with Epstein-Barr virus reactivation during primary cytomegalovirus infection. J Pediatr Gastroenterol Nutr 37:87–90, 2003.
11. Yuge A, Kinoshita E, Moriuchi M, et al: Persistant hepatitis associated with chronic active Epstein-Barr virus infection. Pediatr Infect Dis J 23:74–76, 2004..
12. Kawashima H, Ryou S, Nishimata N, et al: Enteroviral hepatitis in children. Pediatr Int 46:130–134, 2004.
*13. Rocholl C, Gerber K, Daly J, et al: Adenoviral infections in children: the impact of rapid diagnosis. Pediatrics 113:e51–e56, 2004.
14. Malatack J, Jaffe R: Granulomatous hepatitis in three children due to cat-scratch disease without peripheral adenopathy: an unrecognized cause of fever of unknown origin. Am J Dis Child 147:949–953, 1993.
15. Wilson DC Phillips J, Cox D, Roberts E: Severe hepatic Wilson's disease in preschool-aged children. J Pediatr 137:719–722, 2000.
16. Li DY, Schwartz KB: Autoimmune hepatitis. Adolesc Med Clin 15:131–143, 2004.
*17. Tenenbein M: Acetaminophen: the 150 mg/kg myth. J Toxicol 42:145–148, 2004.
18. Teitelbaum JE, Perez-Atayde AR, Cohen M, et al: Minocycline-related autoimmune hepatitis. Arch Pediatrc Adolesc Med 152:1132–1136, 1998.
19. Chow E, Cherry J: Reassessing Reye syndrome. Arch Pediatr Adolesc Med 157:1241–1242, 2003.
20. Sulkowski M, Moore R, Mehta S, et al: Hepatitis C and progression of HIV disease. JAMA 288:199–206, 2002.
21. Wen WH, Chang MH, Hsu HY, et al: The development of hepatocellular carcinoma among prospectively followed children with chronic hepatitis B virus infection. J Pediatr 144:397–399, 2004.
22. Farci P, Alter H, Shimoda A, et al: Hepatitis C virus-associated fulminant hepatic failure. N Engl J Med 335:631–634, 1996.
23. Tung J, Hadzic N, Layton M, et al: Bone marrow failure in children with acute liver failure. J Pediatr Gastroenterol Nutr 31:557–561, 2000.
24. Jonas M, Kelley D, Mizerski J, et al: Clinical trial of lamivudine in children with chronic hepatitis B. N Engl J Med 346:1706–1713, 2002.
25. Lackner H, Moser A, Deutsch J, et al: Interferon-alpha and ribavirin in treating children and young adults with chronic hepatitis C after malignancy. Pediatrics 106:e53, 2000.
26. Sinha M, Das A: Cost effectiveness analysis of different strategies of management of chronic hepatitis C infection in children. Pediatr Infect Dis J 19:23–30, 2000.
27. Ruiz-Moreno M: Pilot interferon-beta trial in children with chronic hepatitis B who had previously not responded to interferon-alpha therapy. Pediatrics 99:222–225, 1997.
28. Broderick A, Jonas M: Management of hepatitis B in children. Clin Liver Dis 8:387, 2004.
*29. Centers for Disease Control and Prevention: Guidelines for Viral Hepatitis Surveillance and Case Management. Atlanta: Centers for Disease Control and Prevention, 2004.
30. American Academy of Pediatrics: Hepatitis A and B. *In* Pickering LK (ed): Red Book: 2003 Report of the Committee on Infectious Diseases, 26th ed. Elk Grove Village, IL: American Academy of Pediatrics, 2003, pp 309–336.

*Selected readings.

Chapter 80

Pancreatitis

Mardi Steere, MBBS and Madeline Matar Joseph, MD

Key Points

Clinical signs of pancreatitis may be less distinct in children than in adults, with the absence of abdominal pain occurring in up to 13% of children.

A significant number of children with pancreatitis have an underlying etiology that may predispose them to recurrence or complications of pancreatitis.

Management in the acute setting is usually nonoperative, with a focus on bowel rest and narcotic analgesia.

Amylase and lipase can be normal in patients with pancreatitis (especially due to trauma).

Introduction and Background

Acute pancreatitis, while uncommon in children, is an important disease due to the potential complications and the frequent presence of a serious underlying etiology. Inappropriately activated and circulating pancreatic enzymes and antigens result in an inflammatory response and cause local pancreatic injury due to direct enzyme damage. This causes microvascular ischemia and pancreatic acinar obstruction,[1] which can result in peritoneal inflammation and a systemic inflammatory response. Other complications, such as pseudocyst and, rarely, exocrine insufficiency, also may occur.

While pancreatitis occurs less frequently in children than in adults, this disorder can occur as early as infancy and can be more difficult to recognize.[1] In this age group, complications are rare, although acute recurrent pancreatitis and chronic pancreatitis can occur. Recurrent and chronic inflammation lead to progressive destruction of the pancreatic parenchyma and ultimately to pancreatic insufficiency.

Recognition and Approach

Many etiologies of acute pancreatitis in children exist[2-4] (Table 80–1). The most common cause is multisystem disease. This includes malignancies (such as acute lymphoblastic and myeloblastic leukemias), systemic lupus erythematosus (SLE), hemolytic-uremic syndrome, and Crohn's disease.[3] Blunt trauma is an important cause of acute pancreatitis, most commonly from bicycle handlebar injuries, although the diagnosis may be delayed due to associated injuries and hemodynamic instability.[5] Specific drugs are strongly associated with the development of pancreatitis, including valproic acid (which may account for 60% of drug-related occurrences), azathioprine, L-asparaginase, acetaminophen, metronidazole, and multiple other medications. Although idiopathic disease occurs in 8% to 23% of cases, it is rare in children less than 3 years of age. An underlying etiology can be found in nearly 100% of children with pancreatitis who are younger than 3 years old.[4]

Recurrent pancreatitis occurs in some children, and chronic pancreatitis may occur in up to 10% of those with acute pancreatitis.[2,3] Most cases of recurrent or chronic pancreatitis are due to an underlying disorder or anomaly of the pancreas. Recurrent or chronic pancreatitis may be due to hereditary illnesses that predispose children to pancreatic dysfunction, with the most common being cystic fibrosis.[6] Hereditary pancreatitis, while rare, is an autosomal dominant mutation in the cationic trypsinogen gene, which results in progressive pancreatic inflammation and destruction, usually beginning in childhood or adolescence.[7] This is a debilitating condition with a high risk of pancreatic insufficiency and a 40% lifetime risk of pancreatic cancer. Recurrent pancreatitis can also be due to congenital and acquired abnormalities of the pancreas such as traumatic stricture, pancreas divisum (in which the ventral and dorsal ducts fail to fuse embryonically), congenital sphincter of Oddi abnormality, choledochal cyst, duodenal duplication, and annular pancreas.[6]

Clinical Presentation

The most common symptoms and signs of pancreatitis in children are similar to those in adults, and include abdominal pain, vomiting, and abdominal tenderness and distention. Abdominal pain, however, may have a different pattern than in adults, occurring more commonly in the epigastrium, right upper quadrant, or left upper quadrant. Pain that radiates to the back is less common in children compared to adults.[3,4] Of note, abdominal pain may be completely absent in up to 13% of children. Less common signs and symptoms include fever, tachycardia, hypotension, jaundice, and signs of acute abdomen such as guarding, rebound tenderness, and decreased bowel sounds (Table 80–2).

Laboratory investigations most often reveal an elevated serum amylase and lipase. These parameters are elevated up to three times normal in 63% to 83% of children with pancreatitis.[2,3] Unfortunately, an elevated amylase is not specific for pancreatitis and can be found in many abdominal and nonabdominal disorders (Table 80–3). An elevated lipase is more specific than hyperamylasemia for pancreatitis, although elevated levels can be found in renal failure, biliary tract disease, hypertriglyceridemia, and alcohol abuse. Less reliable diagnostic tests include trypsin and amylase to creatinine clearance, which have not been studied well in children.

In pancreatitis, imaging can help determine the etiology of the disease. Ultrasonography (US) is 62% to 95% sensitive in detecting acute pancreatitis, while the sensitivity of computed tomography (CT) is 80% to 95%.[8] Pancreatic size and pancreatic duct diameter measured by US are increased in pancreatitis[9] (Table 80–4). These measurements can help identify biliary obstruction in jaundiced patients and other anatomic abnormalities with acute pancreatitis.[9] Ultrasonog-

raphy is also able to identify gallstones with near-100% sensitivity.[8] Abdominal CT may be more sensitive than US in diagnosing pancreatitis, with sensitivities greater than 94% for diagnosing severe disease. On CT, most patients with acute pancreatitis have an enlarged pancreas, surrounding inflammation, and peripancreatic fluid collections.[10,11] CT can identify abscesses, pancreatic necrosis, and pseudocysts.[10,11] Moreover, CT can be used to grade disease severity and establish prognosis.[10]

Endoscopic retrograde cholangiopancreatography (ERCP) enables the measurement of biliary and pancreatic sphincter manometry and may help to identify morphologic changes of the pancreatic duct and branches. It is most helpful in children with acute recurrent or chronic pancreatitis, in whom the pancreatic duct may be abnormal in up to 56% of cases.[12] It may also be useful in cases of acute pancreatitis when ultrasound is nondiagnostic. Therapeutic ERCP at the time of imaging is also possible, and includes biliary or pancreatic sphincterotomy, stone extraction, and balloon dilation or stenting of the duct.[12,13]

Magnetic resonance cholangiopancreatography (MRCP) is a noninvasive test that can visualize the pancreatic duct, bile duct, and stones. MRCP does not cause pancreatitis and has the advantage over ERCP of visualization of pseudocysts and of the dorsal pancreatic duct in the case of pancreas divisum.[14,15] It does, however, have lower resolution than ERCP and lacks the option of therapeutic intervention at the time of imaging.

The differential diagnosis of pancreatitis can be extensive depending on the presentation. Abdominal pain and vomiting may be due to myriad causes, both intra-abdominal and extra-abdominal.[1] Fever and jaundice should prompt the clinician to investigate hepatic and biliary etiologies in addition to pancreatic causes. A family history of peptic ulcer disease or chronic abdominal pain may be misleading, as cases of hereditary pancreatitis may have been undiagnosed, or misdiagnosed, in other family members.

Table 80–1	Etiologies of Pancreatitis in Children
Etiology	**Percentage**
Multisystem	25–53
Idiopathic	8–23
Trauma	14–22
Structural	10–15
Drugs/toxins	12
Infectious	8–10
Hereditary	2
Metabolic	2
Data from references 2–4.	

Table 80–2	Diagnostic Features of Pancreatitis			
Physical Examination	**Location**	**Symptoms**		**Signs**
	Systemic			Elevated temperature
				Jaundice (uncommon)
	Abdominal	Pain: epigastrium, right or left upper quadrant (87%); radiating to back (1%)		Tenderness (77%)
				Distention (18%)
		Vomiting (64%)		Guarding, rebound, decreased bowel sounds (uncommon)
	Cardiovascular			Tachycardia, hypotension (uncommon)
Laboratory	**Analyte**	**Finding**		
	Amylase	Elevated		
	Lipase	Elevated		
Imaging	**Modality**	**Uses**		
	Ultrasound	Determines pancreatic size, duct size		
		May identify structural anomalies, stones		
	CT	May identify necrosis		
	ERCP	Useful for duct and anatomic abnormalities, stones		
		Therapeutic		
	MRCP	May identify areas not visible with ERCP		
Abbreviations: CT, computed tomography; ERCP, endoscopic retrograde cholangiopancreatography; MRCP, magnetic resonance cholangiopancreatography.				

Table 80–3	Nonpancreatic Causes of an Elevated Amylase Level	

Gastrointestinal/ Gynecologic Disorders	Medical Disorders
Appendicitis	Acidosis (e.g., diabetic ketoacidosis)
Bowel obstruction	Alcoholism
Bowel perforation	Anorexia/bulimia
Celiac disease	Burns
Cholecystitis	Diabetic ketoacidosis
Crohn's disease	Elevated triglycerides
Ectopic pregnancy	Head injury
Liver disease	Parotitis (mumps)
Ovarian cyst	Pneumonia
Peritonitis	Renal failure
Salpingitis	Toxins/drugs (e.g., organophosphates)
Surgery (abdominal and nonabdominal)	Trauma (maxillofacial)

Table 80–4	Ultrasound Measurement of Pancreatic Duct Size Consistent with Pancreatitis		

	Age (yr)		
	1–6	7–12	13–18
Abnormal duct size (mm)	>1.5	>1.9	>2.2

Adapted from Chao HC, Lin SJ, Kong MS, et al: Sonographic evaluation of the pancreatic duct in normal children and children with pancreatitis. J Ultrasound Med 19:757 763, 2000.

Important Clinical Features and Considerations

The absence of abdominal pain does not preclude the diagnosis of acute pancreatitis in children. In patients with vomiting, abdominal distention, or fever, a history of risk factors for pancreatic disease should be obtained. Important historical features include recent medications or drugs, recent infections, symptoms of systemic disease, and family history of pancreatic disorders or inflammatory disorders such as Crohn's disease, SLE, or diabetes mellitus. A family history of nonspecific recurrent abdominal pain should raise suspicion of a hereditary cause.

Complications of acute pancreatitis, while uncommon, have important and sometimes debilitating sequelae. Pancreatic pseudocysts are the most common complication, especially in the setting of trauma or chronic pancreatitis.[2] Conservative management and bowel rest results in spontaneous resolution of pseudocysts more frequently in children than in adults. Up to 25% completely resolve, although endoscopic, percutaneous, or surgical drainage may be required if a pseudocyst is persistent or causes symptoms.[16] Complications of pseudocysts, while rare in children, include pseudocyst rupture, abscess formation, hemorrhage, and fistula formation. Pancreatic necrosis is very rare but is associated with infection of pancreatic tissue with gram-positive or gram-negative bacteria or with fungal organisms in up to 30% to 70%. Such infection of necrotic pancreatic tissue is the major risk factor for multiorgan failure and has a mortality of 2% to 24%. Treatment of pancreatic necrosis includes intravenous antibiotics, with surgical intervention often indicated.[1] Pancreatic failure with exocrine insufficiency is an exceptionally rare complication of chronic pancreatitis in children, but results in malabsorption and diabetes mellitus.[17] Death is rare in children and is usually due to multisystem failure resulting from underlying systemic disease.[3]

Potential pitfalls exist in the diagnosis of acute pancreatitis. Importantly, abdominal pain may be absent. Serum amylase and lipase may be normal in over 10% to 30% of affected children; conversely, they may be elevated in nonpancreatic disease (see Table 80–3). Plain radiographs of the abdomen usually appear normal in pancreatitis, as plain radiography is a poor imaging modality for this diagnosis. Ultrasonography has a high specificity and sensitivity for diagnosing pancreatitis, but if the pancreatic duct is not well visualized, the clinician may be falsely reassured that pancreatitis is absent.[2] CT may also be normal in early and mild pancreatitis.

Amylase and lipase elevations are common in patients with blunt abdominal trauma with no evidence of pancreatic trauma. Amylase and lipase also have poor sensitivity, with elevations reported in only 13% to 77% of CT-proven or laparoscopically proven cases of traumatic pancreatitis.[18-24] Repeat values over time may increase the sensitivity of these tests in detecting significant pancreatic injury.[22] Amylase and lipase levels cannot discriminate between pancreatic and nonpancreatic trauma. One study found than only 2% of patients with an elevated amylase or lipase actually had pancreatic injury.[21] Moreover, as few as 13% with pancreatic trauma have elevated pancreatic enzymes.[24] For this reason, serum amylase and lipase should not be relied upon to diagnose or exclude pancreatic injury. Unfortunately, CT is also inaccurate for diagnosing pancreatic trauma, with normal scans in 33% to 53% of patients with laparoscopically proven pancreatic trauma.[20,22,23,25] However, since there are no good studies for identifying pancreatic trauma (including CT), patients with a suspicious mechanism (e.g., significant handlebar trauma to the abdomen) may require admission, repeated pancreatic enzyme measurements, and observation (Fig. 80–1).

Management

Initial treatment of pancreatitis is primarily supportive. This includes complete bowel rest and intravenous fluids as ileus and third spacing of fluids can be significant. Placement of a nasogastric (NG) tube has been traditionally recommended; however, its use has not been shown to alter outcome of patients with mild to moderate pancreatitis. Patients with peritonitis, intractable vomiting, or severe systemic illness may require an NG tube.[26] Narcotic analgesia is often required for pain management and should be instituted early.[2,3] In the past, meperidine was recommended for treating the pain of pancreatitis based on animal studies. However, all narcotics increase sphincter of Oddi contractions and interfere with peristalsis, and studies have never directly compared the effects of meperidine and morphine on sphincter of Oddi pressures. No outcome-based studies comparing these drugs have been performed in patients with acute pancreatitis. Morphine may be of more benefit than meperidine by offering longer pain relief with less risk of seizures. Experts now recommend morphine and other narcotics rather than meperidine for treating pain due to pancreatitis.[27]

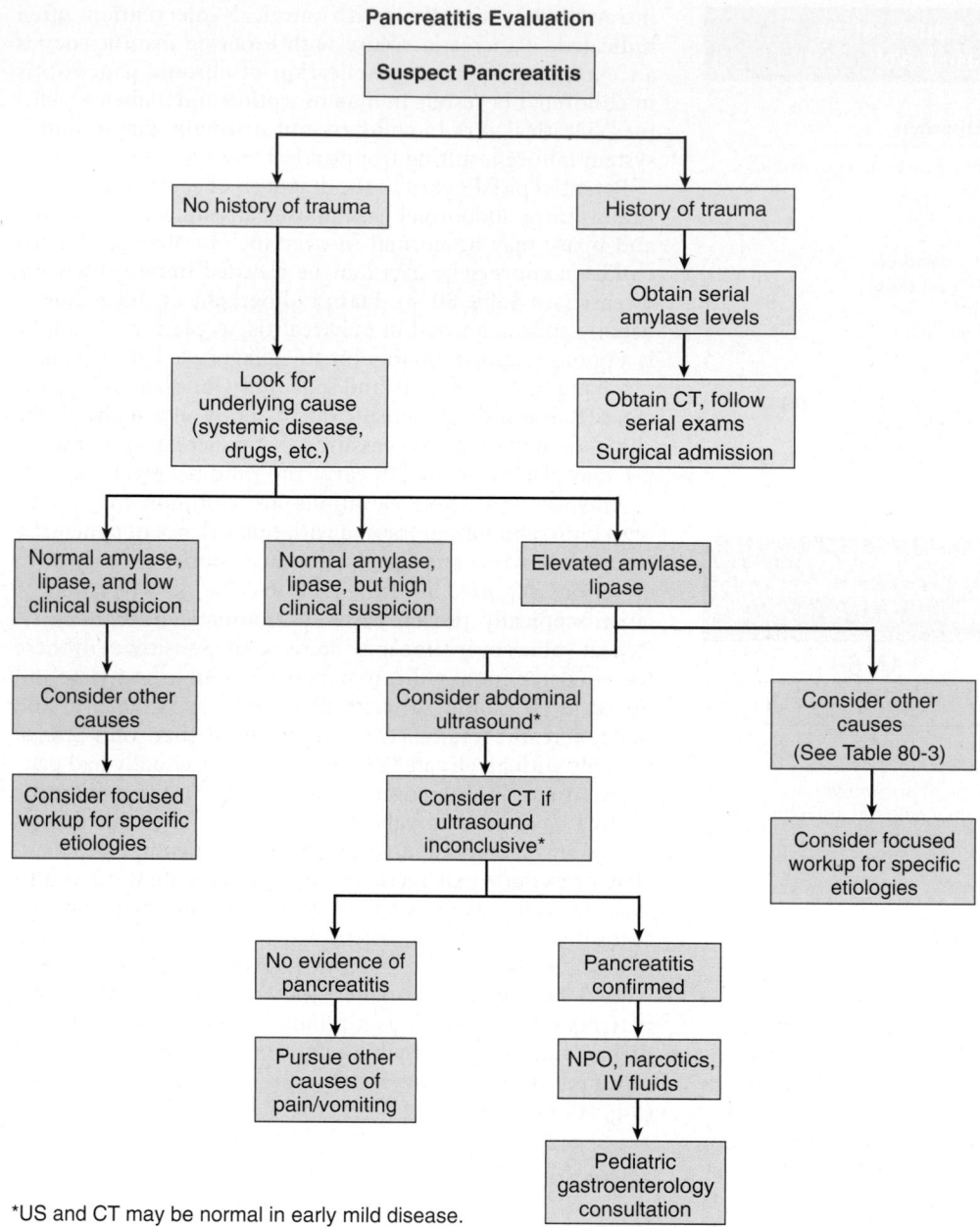

Pancreatitis Evaluation

FIGURE 80–1. Pancreatitis evaluation. (*Ultrasound and CT may be normal in early mild disease.) Abbreviations: CT, computed tomography; IV, intravenous; NPO, nothing by mouth.

Antibiotic prophylaxis is only indicated if there are signs of concurrent infection or if a phlegmon, abscess, or necrosis develops. Total parenteral nutrition may be required if the illness is severe or prolonged, as the length of an acute episode of pancreatitis can last from 8 to 24 days, with a mean hospital stay of 13 days.[2]

Therapeutic ERCP with biliary sphincterotomy may be helpful in acute, recurrent, and chronic pancreatitis in children if manometry reveals abnormalities. This modality may have beneficial long-term effects, reducing frequency and severity of painful episodes.[13]

The indications for surgical intervention remain controversial. Laparotomy may be indicated in blunt trauma, during which acute pancreatitis may be discovered and treated surgically with external drainage.[13] In severe acute pancreatitis with pancreatic necrosis, surgery may be indicated especially if infection of necrotic pancreatic tissue is suspected or confirmed by needle biopsy.[1] Pseudocyst formation may necessitate surgical drainage, marsupialization, or complete resection, although observation for spontaneous resorption, followed by percutaneous drainage if the cyst persists, may be reasonable first-line options.[28]

Due to the high potential for complications, consultation with a gastroenterologist should be initiated following admission. Surgical consultation is required in cases that are unresponsive to nonoperative management or for patients with phlegmon, hemorrhagic pancreatitis (to provide hemostasis), abscess formation, large pseudocysts, or necrosis. Patients with biliary tract disease also may require cholecystectomy or removal of biliary duct stones.

Complex surgical intervention may be indicated for chronic pancreatitis, particularly if the pancreatic duct is abnormal and therapeutic ERCP is unsuccessful.[29,30] If patients experience persistent pain despite fat restriction, enzyme replace-

Table 80–5 Ranson Criteria in Pancreatitis*

On Admission	Within 48 Hr
Age > 55 yr	Hematocrit decrease > 10%
WBC > 16,000/mm³	BUN rise > 5 mg/dl
Glucose > 200 mg/dl	Calcium < 8 mg/dl
LDH > 350 IU/L	Arterial P_{O_2} < 60 mm Hg
AST > 250 IU/L	Base deficit > 4 mEq/L
	Fluid deficit > 6 L

*Three or more criteria predict a complicated clinical course; mortality rises when 4 or more criteria are met.
Abbreviations: AST, aspartate transaminase; BUN, blood urea nitrogen; LDH, lactate dehydrogenase; P_{O_2}, partial pressure of oxygen; WBC, white blood cell count.
Adapted from Di Magno EP, Chari S: Acute pancreatitis. In Feldman M, Friedman LS, Sleisenger MH (eds): Sleisenger & Fordtran's Gastrointestinal and Liver Disease, 7th ed. Philadelphia, WB Saunders, 2002, pp 914–928.

Table 80–6 Pediatric Criteria for Severe Pancreatitis*

On Admission	Within 48 Hr
Age < 7 yr	48-hr trough Ca²⁺ (<8.3 mg/dl)
Weight < 23 kg	48-hr trough albumin (<2.6 g/dl)
WBC > 18,500/mm³	48-hr fluid sequestration (>75 ml/kg in 48 hr)
LDH > 2000 IU/L	Rise in BUN (>5 mg/dl)

*Three criteria predict a severe outcome.
Abbreviations: BUN, blood urea nitrogen; LDH, lactate dehydrogenase; WBC, white blood cell count.
Adapted from DeBanto JR, Goday PS, Pedroso MR, et al; Midwest Multicenter Pancreatic Study Group: Acute pancreatitis in children. Am J Gastroenterol 97:1726–1731, 2002.

ment, and non-narcotic analgesia, or a complication of chronic pancreatitis has occurred, the goal of surgery is to open the pancreatic duct, enabling its direct drainage into a loop of bowel.[31,32]

Complications of therapy include acute pancreatitis, which may occur after therapeutic ERCP.[28] Surgical intervention may result in pancreatic insufficiency, peptic ulcer, or anastamotic ulcer.[33] For this reason, a trial of conservative treatment is usually recommended prior to any surgical intervention.

Severity of illness in adults can be predicted using scoring systems such as the Glasgow score or Ranson score, which identifies 11 criteria[34] (Table 80–5). These systems have not been widely validated in children, although one study has shown them to have 30% to 35% sensitivity and a specificity of 94% for diagnosing pancreatitis.[29] A pediatric scoring system developed by De Banto found that the presence of any 3 of 8 criteria predicted severe pancreatitis in children with a sensitivity of 70% and specificity of 79%[29] (Table 80–6). Evaluation for complications of pancreatitis should be ongoing, with monitoring of renal and respiratory function as well as close observation for signs of infection, necrosis, or hemorrhage.

Summary

Pancreatitis is an uncommon disease that is difficult to diagnose in children. Serum lipase and amylase may be normal while US and CT may not reveal abnormalities in uncomplicated or early disease. Prognosis and likelihood of recurrence depend upon the etiology of the disease and vary depending on the underlying pancreatic abnormality. Diagnostic and therapeutic options continue to remain under investigation, with the roles of ERCP and MRCP still being refined in this population. To accurately diagnose this disease, clinicians must be aware of the myriad of risk factors and accuracy of the clinical examination and diagnostic adjuncts. Early diagnosis, close observation, appropriate resuscitation, and selective intervention may improve outcome for this serious disease.

REFERENCES

*1. Jackson WD: Pancreatitis: etiology, diagnosis and management. Curr Opin Pediatr 13:447–451, 2001.
*2. Benifla M, Weizman Z: Acute pancreatitis in childhood: analysis of literature data. J Clin Gastroenterol 37:169–172, 2003.
3. Werlin SL, Kugathasan S, Frautschy BC: Pancreatitis in children. J Pediatr Gastroenterol Nutr 37:591–595, 2003.
4. Lopez MJ: The changing incidence of acute pancreatitis in children: a single institution perspective. J Pediatr 140:622–624, 2002.
5. Kao LS, Bulger EM, Parks DL: Predictors of morbidity after traumatic pancreatic injury. J Trauma 55:898–905, 2003.
6. Durie PR: Pancreatic aspects of cystic fibrosis and other inherited causes of pancreatic dysfunction. Med Clin North Am 84:609–620, 2000.
7. Charnley RM: Hereditary pancreatitis. World J Gastroenterol 9:1–4, 2003.
8. Turner MA: The role of US and CT in pancreatitis. Gastrointest Endosc 56(6 Suppl):S241–S245, 2003.
9. Chao HC, Lin SJ, Kong MS, et al: Sonographic evaluation of the pancreatic duct in normal children and children with pancreatitis. J Ultrasound Med 19:757–763, 2000.
10. Balthazar EJ, Robinson DL, Megibow AJ, et al: Acute pancreatitis: value of CT in establishing prognosis. Radiology 174:331–336, 1990.
11. Paulson EK, Vitellas KM, Keogan MT, et al: Acute pancreatitis complicated by gland necrosis: spectrum of findings on contrast enhanced CT. AJR Am J Roentgenol 172:609–613, 1999.
12. Graham KS, Ingram JD, Steinberg SE, Narkewicz MR: ERCP in the management of pediatric pancreatitis. Gastrointest Endosc 47:492–495, 1998.
13. Hsu RK, Draganov P, Leung JW, et al: Therapeutic ERCP in the management of pancreatitis in children. Gastrointest Endosc 51:396–400, 2000.
14. Barish MA, Yucel EK, Ferucci JT: Magnetic resonance cholangiopancreatography. N Engl J Med 341:258–264, 1999.
15. MacEneaney P, Mitchell MT, McDermott R: Update on magnetic resonance cholangiopancreatography. Gastroenterol Clin North Am 31:731–746, 2002.
16. Ford EG, Hardin WD Jr, Mahour GH, Woolley MM: Psuedocysts of the pancreas in children. Am Surg 56:384–387, 1990.
17. Little JM, Tait N, Richardson A, Dubois R: Chronic pancreatitis beginning in childhood and adolescence. Arch Surg 127:90–92, 1992.
18. Akhrass R, Kim K, Brandt C: Computed tomography: an unreliable indicator of pancreatic trauma. Am Surg 62:647–651, 1996.
19. Gorenstein A, O'Halpin D, Wesson DE, et al: Blunt injury to the pancreas in children: selective management based on ultrasound. J Pediatr Surg 22:1110–1118, 1987.
20. Smith SD, Nakayama DK, Gantt N, et al: Pancreatic injuries in children due to blunt trauma. J Pediatr Surg 23:610–614, 1988.
21. Buechter KJ, Arnold M, Steele B, et al: The use of serum amylase and lipase in evaluating and managing blunt abdominal trauma. Am Surg 56:204–208, 1990.
22. Shilyansky J, Sena LM, Kreller M, et al: Nonoperative management of pancreatic injuries in children. J Pediatr Surg 33:343–349, 1998.
23. Sivit CJ, Eichelberger MR, Taylor GA, et al: Blunt pancreatic trauma in children: CT diagnosis. AJR Am J Roentgenol 158:1097–1100, 1992.

*Selected readings.

24. Simon HK, Muehlberg A, Linakis JG: Serum amylase determinations in pediatric patients presenting to the ED with acute abdominal pain or trauma. Am J Emerg Med 12:292–295, 1994.

25. Nakayama DK, Copes WS, Sacco W: Differences in trauma care among pediatric and non-pediatric trauma centers. J Pediatr Surg 27:427–431, 1992.

26. Sarr MG, Sanfey H, Cameron JL: Prospective randomized trial of naso-gastric suction in patients with acute pancreatitis. Surgery 100:500–504, 1986.

27. Thompson DR: Narcotic analgesic effects on the sphincter of Oddi: a review of the data and therapeutic implications in treating pancreatitis. Am J Gastroenterol 96:1266–1272, 2001.

28. Usatoff V, Brancatisano R, Williamson RC: Operative treatment of pseudocysts in patients with chronic pancreatitis. Br J Surg 87:1494–1499, 2000.

29. DeBanto JR, Goday PS, Pedroso MR, et al; Midwest Multicenter Pancreatic Study Group: Acute pancreatitis in children. Am J Gastroenterol 97:1726–1731, 2002.

30. Rollins MD, Meyers RL: Frey procedure for surgical management of chronic pancreatitis in children. J Pediatr Surg 39:817–820, 2004.

31. Peterson C, Goetz A, Burger D, Mildenberger H: Surgical therapy and follow-up of pancreatitis in children. J Pediatr Gastroenterol Nutr 25:204–209, 1997.

32. Sakorafas GH, Farnell MB, Farley DR, et al: Long-term results after surgery for chronic pancreatitis. Int J Pancreatol 27:131–142, 2000.

33. Soergel KH: Pancreatitis. In Goldman L, Bennett JC (eds): Cecil Textbook of Medicine, 21st ed. Philadelphia: WB Saunders, 2000, pp 752–759.

34. Di Magno EP, Chari S: Acute pancreatitis. In Feldman M, Friedman LS, Sleisenger MH (eds): Sleisenger & Fordtran's Gastrointestinal and Liver Disease, 7th ed. Philadelphia, WB Saunders, 2002, pp 914–928.

Chapter 81

Post–Liver Transplantation Complications

Samir S. Shah, MD

Introduction and Background

Given the rarity of pediatric solid organ transplantations, most emergency physicians had little chance of seeing any of these children during their careers in the past. However, advances in the care of these children has led to greater longevity and therefore greater prevalence of these children in many communities[1] (see Chapter 66, Postsurgical Cardiac Conditions and Transplantation). One institution has reported that nearly two thirds of their pediatric liver transplant recipients live for 15 years or more after undergoing transplantation.[2] With more children undergoing liver transplantation and with their greater longevity, the likelihood that an emergency physician will see one of these children in the emergency department for a problem related or unrelated to their transplant increases. Given this fact, it is prudent to have some familiarity with the problems these children encounter posttransplantation.

Recognition and Approach

Identifying children who have undergone liver transplantation is typically straightforward. There are multiple indications for liver transplantation, and occasionally the indication is relevant to the presenting complaint. This is particularly true if the indication involves a systemic disease not cured by liver transplantation. Common indications for liver transplantation include cholestatic liver disease (e.g., biliary atresia, sclerosing cholangitis), acute fulminant liver failure (e.g., viral- or toxin-mediated destruction), chronic active hepatitis (e.g., autoimmune, chronic hepatitis B or C), metabolic disorders (e.g., Wilson's disease, urea cycle defects, disorders of bile acid metabolism), neoplasia (e.g., hepatoblastoma), and other conditions causing severe liver impairment (e.g., cystic fibrosis, chronic parenteral nutrition).

There are three basic types of liver transplantations based on how the liver was procured.[3-5] One type is reduced-size transplantation. For these cases, a cadaveric liver is reduced in size until it is appropriate to fit the recipient. A second type is split-liver transplantation. In these cases, a cadaveric liver is divided into two separate functioning allografts. The third type is living-related donor transplantation. In these cases, a relative of the child donates part of his or her liver to be used for transplantation.

Clinical Presentation

Although children who have undergone liver transplantation can present to the emergency department with unrelated problems, there are well described complications related to transplantation and maintenance therapy. These complications most commonly arise from infections, the ongoing use of immunosuppressive agents, and graft rejection.

Infections

Post–liver transplantation infections can be related to donor-associated infections, seasonal variations, and posttransplantation-related immune suppression. Donor-associated infections are transmitted from the donor to the new host via the graft or accompanying blood cells, or from blood product transfusions. Infectious agents that can be transmitted from an asymptomatic donor to the new host include viruses, parasites, and endemic fungi (Table 81–1). Respiratory viruses might be seasonal (e.g., respiratory syncytial virus, influenza, human metapneumovirus) or endemic (e.g., parainfluenza virus type 3, adenovirus) and either community or

Table 81–1	Differential Diagnosis of Post–Liver Transplantation Infections by Site and Relative Frequency
Infection Site	**Potential Causes (in Order of Frequency)**
Central Nervous System	Herpes simplex virus
	Enteroviruses
	Streptococcus pneumoniae
	Cryptococcus neoformans
	Cytomegalovirus
	JC virus
	Human herpesvirus 6
	Varicella-zoster virus
	Epstein-Barr virus
	Endemic mycoses*
Gastrointestinal Tract	Cytomegalovirus
	Clostridium difficile
	Giardia lamblia
	Cryptosporidium species
	Rotavirus
	Adenoviruses
Hepatobiliary Tract	Cytomegalovirus
	Herpes simplex virus
	Enteric gram-negative bacilli
	Varicella-zoster virus
	Epstein-Barr virus
	Human herpesviruses 6, 7, and 8
	Adenovirus
	Hepatitis B virus
	Hepatitis C virus
	Candida species
	Aspergillus species
	Cryptococcus neoformans
	Endemic mycoses*
	Toxoplasma gondii
	Cryptosporidium species
	Bartonella henselae
	Candida species
Lower Respiratory Tract	Respiratory viruses†
	Staphylococcus aureus
	Klebsiella pneumoniae
	Streptococcus pneumoniae
	Pseudomonas aeruginosa
	Legionella pneumophila
	Cytomegalovirus
	Candida species
	Aspergillus species
	Pneumocystis jiroveci
	Cryptococcus neoformans
	Coccidioides immitis
	Epstein-Barr virus
	Mycobacterium tuberculosis
	Atypical mycobacteria
Central Venous Catheter	Coagulase-negative staphylococci
	Enterococcus faecalis
	Escherichia coli
	Klebsiella species
	Pseudomonas aeruginosa
	Candida species
	Staphylococcus aureus
	Other gram-negative bacilli

*Endemic mycoses include *Histoplasma capsulatum, Coccidioides immitis,* and *Blastomyces dermatitidis.*
†Respiratory viruses include respiratory syncytial virus, influenza viruses, parainfluenza viruses, adenovirus, and human meta-*Pneumovirus.*

nosocomially acquired. Respiratory viral infections are most severe if acquired early after transplantation. Opportunistic infections arise due to immunosuppression, especially with agents that affect T-cell function. The causative organisms vary by site of infection (see Table 81–1).

The posttransplantation period is often categorized as "early," "middle," and "late," which is useful for risk-stratifying children for specific infections.[6,7] The early period is defined as the first month posttransplantation. The middle period is from 1 to 6 months posttransplantation. The late period is defined as greater than 6 months posttransplantation. Early-period infections commonly include surgical site infections, invasive device–related infections (e.g., central venous and urinary catheter-related infections), and nosocomially transmitted infections.[8] The offending organisms are usually enteric and skin flora, including Enterococcus species, *Escherichia coli,* Klebsiella species, *Pseudomonas aeruginosa, Staphylococcus aureus,* and Candida species.[9] Risk factors for invasive candidiasis include antibiotic prophylaxis for spontaneous bacterial peritonitis, posttransplantation dialysis, and repeat transplantation.[10] Herpes simplex virus (HSV) infections occur 2 to 3 weeks following transplantation in those recipients not receiving antiviral prophylaxis with acyclovir.[11-13] HSV mainly occurs through viral reactivation in seropositive individuals, though primary infection may also cause fulminant disease. Common manifestations of HSV infection include orolabial or mucocutaneous infections, esophagitis, and hepatitis. Middle-period infections include donor-associated and opportunistic infections such as cytomegalovirus (CMV), Epstein-Barr virus (EBV), *Pneumocystis jiroveci* (formerly *Pneumocystis carinii*) pneumonia, *Nocardia* species, and *Toxoplasma gondii.* Late-period infections include community-acquired respiratory and skin infections as well as infections associated with immunosuppression. Fungal infections, including those caused by Aspergillus species, and infections with EBV cause late infections that occur as a consequence of prolonged immunosuppression. The late period is also a time during which posttransplantation lymphoproliferative disorder (PTLD) is seen.[14] It is thought that infections with organisms such as EBV contribute to this form of lymphoma. Unlike other lymphomas, PTLD frequently fails to respond to chemotherapy.

Immunosuppressive Agents

Agents used for immunosuppression after transplantation can be divided into the following categories: corticosteroids, cytotoxic agents, calcineurin inhibitors, antilymphocytic agents, and monoclonal antibodies. Though the risk and types of infection vary with drug category, most patients receive immunosuppressive agents from more than one category.[15] Besides placing the child at risk for severe and unusual infections, these medications also have significant side effects that may lead to an emergency department visit (Table 81–2). Side effects often occur as a consequence of drug interactions rather than as adverse effects of single agents in isolation.[6] Three common types of drug interactions may occur in transplant recipients. First, up-regulation of cyclosporine or tacrolimus metabolism due to rifampin, isoniazid, phenytoin, and nafcillin may lead to lower blood levels for a given dose of immunosuppressive agent. Second, down-regulation of cyclosporine, tacrolimus, and rapamycin metabolism due to macrolide antibiotics and azole antifungal agents results in higher blood

Table 81–2	Immunosuppressive Agents, Mechanism of Action, and Potential Side Effects		
Agent Category	**Examples**	**Mechanism of action**	**Important adverse effects**
Corticosteroids	Prednisone, methylprednisolone	Inhibit T-cell activation, proliferation, and function	Hyperglycemia, hypertension, gastritis, central nervous system changes (euphoria, depression, and rarely psychosis)
Cytotoxic agents	Azathioprine, cyclophosphamide, mycophenylate mofetil	Decrease number of functional T and B cells	Bone marrow suppression, diarrhea, emesis, hepatotoxicity (azathioprine)
Calcineurin inhibitors	Cyclosporine, tacrolimus, rapamycin, sirolimus	Inhibit T-cell activation, proliferation, and function	Hyperglycemia, nephrotoxicity, hepatotoxicity, hypertension, seizures
Antilymphocyte agents	OKT3	Monoclonal lymphocyte–depleting antibody	Aseptic meningitis, seizures, bone marrow suppression, diarrhea, pulmonary edema
Monoclonal antibodies*	Daclizumab, basiliximab	Anti–interleukin-2 receptor-specific antibody prevents T-cell proliferation and activation of the effector arms of the immune system	Nephrotoxicity, diarrhea, hyperglycemia

*All reported events for this class of drugs were similar in treatment and placebo recipients.

levels for a given dose of an immunosuppressive agent.[16] Third, cyclosporine- and tacrolimus-associated nephrotoxicity can be exacerbated with high, but not low, doses of fluoroquinolones and trimethoprim-sulfamethoxazole. Patients receiving agents that may interact with their immunosuppressive medications require frequent monitoring of medication blood levels and tests of liver and renal function.

Graft Rejection

Acute graft rejection occurs in 60% of liver transplant recipients, and most episodes of rejection occur within the first 3 months following transplantation.[17] Initial symptoms include fever, lethargy, jaundice, dark urine, light stools, pruritus, and occasionally anorexia. Ascites may be noted on physical examination. Chronic rejection occurs in 5% to 10% of patients undergoing transplantation. The primary clinical manifestations of chronic rejection include progressive jaundice and pruritus.

Important Clinical Features and Considerations

Phone Consultation

For physicians unfamiliar with pediatric liver transplant recipients, phone consultation with the transplant physician, a pediatric gastroenterologist, or a pediatric infectious disease specialist is usually indicated. At large pediatric tertiary care centers, there may be an on-call pediatric transplant coordinator who can be very helpful in connecting the emergency physician with the proper consultant. This arrangement can minimize frustration and expedite obtaining the information needed to appropriately care for the child in the emergency department. Once reached by phone, the consultant may request information that is not a typical part of an emergency department history. This is particularly true if the on-call specialist is unfamiliar with this particular child or if the consultation hospital is different from the hospital in which the child underwent transplantation. If possible, it is helpful to have the following information in hand while on the phone with the consultant. Consultants often find it helpful to know:

- Type of transplant: reduced-size, split-liver, or living-related transplant
- The time after transplant: to stratify the patient's risk for early, middle or late period infectious pathogens
- Candidate status at transplantation for varicella, HSV, measles, and mumps
- Candidate *and* donor status at transplantation for CMV, EBV, and hepatitis C virus
- Current antimicrobial prophylaxis, which reduces the risk of certain pathogens as follows: gancyclovir (CMV), acyclovir (HSV), nystatin or fluconazole (*Candida* species), and trimethoprim-sulfamethoxazole (*P. jiroveci, T. gondii*)
- Date of catheter placement and prior infections in the existing catheter

Obviously, not all of this information will be readily available to the emergency physician. However, it is helpful for the emergency physician to have some insight into what information the consultant will likely use to guide his or her decision making.

Blunted Presenting Signs and Symptoms

Fever is the most common reason for the emergency department evaluation of a liver transplant recipient. Fever can be the initial manifestation of a spectrum of illnesses that range from systemic viral or bacterial infection to acute organ rejection or hepatic artery thrombosis. However, fever does not accompany 40% of infections among liver transplant recipients; fever is less likely to accompany fungal infections than either viral or bacterial infections.[18] Immunosuppressive medications also blunt other manifestations of severe disease (see Chapter 69, Human Immunodeficiency Virus Infection and Other Immunosuppressive Conditions; and Chapter 107, The Steroid-Dependent Child). Therefore, transplant recipients with subtle signs and symptoms typically warrant a more extensive evaluation than other children. Abdominal pain may represent a surgical emergency, even when relatively mild. Steroid therapy may dull the inflammatory response in a transplantation patient such that typical peritoneal signs may not accompany visceral perforation, bile leak, or infectious peritonitis. Central nervous system complaints also warrant aggressive evaluation. For example, mild persistent headache or intermittent photophobia may be the only complaint in an immunosuppressed patient with cryptococcal or tuberculous meningitis.

Management

Initial Approach

The initial approach to the child who has undergone liver transplantation follows the same general principles used to evaluate any child presenting to the emergency department (see Chapter 1, Approach to Resuscitation and Advanced Life Support for Infants and Children; Chapter 5, Monitoring in Critically Ill Children; and Chapter 13, Sepsis). Because these children may have subtle presentations of serious conditions, they must be given a higher triage category than warranted by their chief complaint alone (see Chapter 155, Triage).

Laboratory Evaluation

The specific laboratory evaluation differs based on the presenting complaint. The following laboratory studies may be useful: hepatic function panel, electrolytes, creatinine, and prothrombin time. Elevated transaminases are usually seen with acute rejection, systemic viral syndromes (e.g., HSV, varicella), and viral hepatitis, and occasionally with chronic rejection and ascending cholangitis. Elevated conjugated bilirubin and alkaline phosphatase levels are usually seen with acute and chronic rejection and ascending cholangitis. The prothrombin time may be elevated with acute rejection, fat malabsorption (vitamin K deficiency), disseminated intravascular coagulation, and severe liver disease. In patients in the middle period posttransplantation, serum viral studies should be performed to detect CMV and EBV (Table 81–3).[19,20] In patients with fever or with suspected infection, cultures of blood (including from a central venous catheter, if present) and urine should be performed. Patients with altered mental status may have elevated ammonia levels that suggest hepatic encephalopathy. In patients undergoing lumbar puncture, routine testing should include bacterial and fungal cultures of the cerebrospinal fluid (CSF), Gram stain, and protein and glucose levels. When possible, HSV polymerase chain reaction (PCR) and cryptococcal antigen testing should be performed on CSF specimens since early treatment of these conditions improves outcome. It is prudent to send additional CSF to the laboratory in case additional testing is required. Specific laboratory evaluation depends on the presenting symptoms (see Table 81–3).

Radiologic Evaluation

Children presenting with fever, respiratory complaints, or hypoxia require chest radiography. Pneumonia develops in up to 20% of liver transplant recipients within the early and middle periods posttransplantation.[21] Diffuse alveolar or interstitial infiltrates suggest viral (e.g., CMV) and atypical bacterial pathogens. In these children, *Mycoplasma pneumoniae* infection may also manifest with lobar involvement. Perihilar infiltrates are often seen with *P. jiroveci* pneumonia. The bilateral alveolar infiltrates first appear in the perihilar areas and then progress peripherally. These patients often present with significant hypoxia despite minimal auscultatory abnormalities. Nodular infiltrates (defined as one or

Table 81–3	Pathogen-Specific Tests
Infection Location	**Specimens and Potential Laboratory Tests**
Central Nervous System	**Cerebrospinal Fluid**
	Cryptococcus neoformans polysaccharide antigen
	Histoplasma capsulatum polysaccharide antigen
	Coccidioides immitis complement fixation antibodies
	Herpes simplex virus PCR
	Enterovirus PCR
	Varicella-zoster virus DNA PCR
	Epstein-Barr virus PCR
	Cytomegalovirus PCR
	JC virus PCR*
	Toxoplasma gondii PCR*
	India ink stain
	Bacterial culture
	Fungal culture
	Viral culture
	Acid-fast smear and culture
Gastrointestinal Tract	**Stool**
	Clostridium difficile toxins A and B ELISA
	Giardia lamblia ELISA
	Rotavirus ELISA
	Bacterial culture
	Ova and parasite examination
	Blood
	Cytomegalovirus pp65 antigen detection in leukocytes (antigenemia) or by PCR
Hepatobiliary Tract	**Blood**
	Blood culture
	Cytomegalovirus pp65 antigen detection in leukocytes (antigenemia) or by PCR
	Epstein-Barr virus antibodies or quantative PCR
	Toxoplasma gondii PCR*
	Bartonella henselae antibodies and PCR
	Adenovirus PCR
	Hepatitis B serology and PCR
	Hepatitis C serology and PCR
	Human herpesviruses 6, 7, and 8 PCR*
	Urine
	Adenovirus PCR
	Skin Vesicle Scraping
	Herpes simplex virus direct fluorescent antibody or PCR
	Varicella-zoster virus direct fluorescent antibody or PCR
Lower Respiratory Tract	**Blood**
	Blood culture
	Sputum
	Bacterial culture
	Fungal culture
	Viral culture
	Gomori methenamine-silver stain (*Pneumocystis jiroveci*)
	Acid-fast bacilli staining
	Legionella culture
	Immunofluorescence (RSV, influenza, parainfluenza, adenovirus)†
	Respiratory virus PCR (adenovirus, human meta-*Pneumovirus*, influenza)†
	Bacterial PCR (mycoplasma)†
Central Venous Catheter	**Blood**
	Blood culture (central and peripheral)
	Skin
	Catheter insertion site discharge Gram stain and bacterial culture

*Not widely available.
†Tests can be reliably performed on nasal aspirate specimens.
Abbreviations: ELISA, enzyme-linked immunosorbent assay; PCR, polymerase chain reaction; RSV, respiratory syncytial virus.

more focal defects at least 1 cm in diameter with well-defined borders, surrounded by aerated lung) more commonly suggest *Legionella pneumophila*, Candida species, and *Nocardia asteroides* and occasionally represent Aspergillus species, *Mycobacterium tuberculosis*, and *P. jiroveci*. Micronodular infiltrates are seen with CMV and varicella pneumonitis.[22] Segmental or lobar consolidation or pleural effusions (frequently bilateral) might be seen with bacterial causes, including gram-negative bacilli and *L. pneumophila*. Specific diagnostic testing is usually indicated (see Table 81–3) since detection of a specific pathogen may alter therapy. Definitive diagnosis of *P. jiroveci* penumonia requires detection of the organism by silver stain in a properly obtained induced sputum or bronchoscopy sample. Those children with respiratory complaints or fever without a source and normal or nonspecific findings on radiography, as well as those with mediastinal or hilar lymphadenopathy, should undergo computed tomography (CT) of the chest for a more detailed evaluation.

Abdominal radiographs and CT is usually indicated for patients with fever or with gastrointestinal complaints. Fever without a source in liver transplant recipients may indicate the presence of an occult intra-abdominal abscess. Other potential intra-abdominal complications include intestinal perforation, intussusception, or luminal obstruction as a result of enlarged abdominal lymph nodes caused by PTLD. CMV colitis has also been associated with bowel perforation. Doppler ultrasound of the abdomen is useful for evaluating patients with suspected hepatobiliary complications. Potential hepatobiliary complications include stenosis, leaks, infectious cholangitis, and vascular complications (i.e., hepatic artery thrombosis, portal vein thrombosis, and venous outflow tract obstruction). Vascular complications are most common within the first 3 months following transplantation.[23] Hepatic artery thrombosis may present insidiously with impaired hepatobiliary perfusion leading to gradual biliary necrosis with strictures and, ultimately, allograft failure.

Empirical therapy for suspected bacteremia or cholangitis includes piperacillin-tazobactam, ticarcillin-clavulanate, imipenem, or a combination of ampicillin-sulbactam and gentamicin or ceftriaxone and metronidazole. Vancomycin should be added in patients with cardiovascular instability or a central access port. Patients with lobar consolidation should receive therapy with cefotaxime or ampicillin-sulbactam. Azithromycin should be added if atypical bacterial disease is suspected. Patients with suspected central nervous system infections should receive a combination of vancomycin and cefotaxime. The empirical initiation of antiviral and antifungal agents depends on the patient's presenting symptoms and initial laboratory studies. Patients with meningoencephalitis or lymphocytic CSF pleocytosis should empirically receive intravenous acyclovir. The HSV genome can be detected by CSF PCR for up to 7 days after the initiation of acyclovir.[24] Decisions to begin other empirical antiviral therapy or antifungal therapy should be made in consultation with infectious disease or liver transplantation experts. Agents for suspected viral infections include acyclovir for HSV, gancyclovir for EBV and CMV,[25] and oseltamivir for influenza. Potential antifungal agents include amphotericin B, fluconazole, caspofungin, and voriconazole.

Conditions that impair the patient's ability to ingest or absorb medications (e.g., vomiting, diarrhea) necessitate hospital admission for parenteral administration of immunosuppressive medications and careful monitoring of immunosuppressive medication levels. Inadequate immunosuppression levels place the patient at high risk for acute rejection and graft loss.[26]

Summary

Liver transplant recipients are at high risk for infectious and graft-related complications. The infecting organisms can be predicted to some extent by the time period following transplantation; however, any organism can cause disease during any given period posttransplantation. The clinical manifestations of illness can be subtle due to the anti-inflammatory and immunosuppressive effects of transplant-related medications. The transplant center and infectious disease specialists can assist in the management of these complex patients.

REFERENCES

1. McDiarmid SV, Anand R; SPLIT Research Group: Studies of Pediatric Liver Transplantation (SPLIT): A summary of the 2003 Annual Report. Clin Transpl 119–130, 2003.
2. Busuttil RW, Farmer DG, Yersi ZH, et al: Analysis of long-term outcomes of 3200 liver transplantations over two decades: a single center experience. Ann Surg 241:905–916, 2005.
*3. Otte JB, de Ville de Goyet J, Reding R, et al: Pediatric liver transplantation: from full-size liver graft to reduced, split, and living related liver transplantation. Pediatr Surg Int 13:308–318, 1998.
4. Broering DC, Topp S, Schaefer U, et al: Split liver transplantation and risk to the adult recipient: analysis using matched pairs. J Am Coll Surg 195:648–657, 2002.
5. Borenstein S, Diamond IR, Grant DR, et al: Outcome of pediatric live-donor transplantation: the Toronto experience. J Pediatr Surg 38:668–671, 2003.
*6. Fishman JA, Rubin RH: Infection in organ transplant recipients. N Engl J Med 338:1741–1751, 1998.
7. Kusne S, Dummer JS, Singh N, et al: Infections after liver transplantation: an analysis of 101 consecutive cases. Medicine 67:132–143, 1998.
*8. Garcia S, Roque J, Ruza F, et al: Infection and associated risk factors in the immediate postoperative period of pediatric liver transplantation: a study of 176 transplants. Clin Transplant 12:190–197, 1998.
9. George DL, Arnow PM, Fox A, et al: Patterns of infection after pediatric liver transplantation. Am J Dis Child 146:924–929, 1992.
10. Husain S, Tollemar J, Dominguez EA, et al: Changes in the spectrum and risk factors for invasive candidiasis in liver transplant recipients: prospective, multicenter, case-control study. Transplantation 75:2023–2029, 2003.
11. Kusne S, Schwartz M, Breinig MK, et al: Herpes simplex virus hepatitis after solid organ transplantation in adults. J Infect Dis 163:1001–1007, 1991.
12. Breinig MK, Zitelli B, Starzl TE, Ho M: Epstein-Barr virus, cytomegalovirus, and other viral infections in children after liver transplantation. J Infect Dis 156:273–279, 1987.
13. Gold D, Corey L: Acyclovir prophylaxis for herpes simplex virus infection. Antimicrob Agents Chemother 31:361–367, 1987.
14. Newell KA, Alonso EM, Whitington PF, et al: Posttransplant lymphoproliferative disease in pediatric liver transplantation: interplay between primary Epstein-Barr virus infection and immunosuppression. Transplantation 62:370–375, 1996.
15. Husain S, Singh N: The impact of novel immunosuppressive agents on infections in organ transplant recipients and the interactions of these agents with antimicrobials. Clin Infect Dis 35:53–61, 2002.
16. Amacher DE, Schomaker SJ, Retsema JA: Comparison of the effects of the new azalide antibiotic, azithromycin, and erythromycin estolate on rat liver cytochrome P-450. Antimicrob Agents Chemother 35:1186–1190, 1991.

---

*Selected readings.

17. Winston DJ, Pakrasi A, Busuttil RW: Prophylactic fluconazole in liver transplant recipients: a randomized, double-blind, placebo-controlled trial. Ann Intern Med 131:729–737, 1999.

*18. Chang FY, Singh N, Gayowski T, et al: Fever in liver transplant recipients: changing spectrum of etiologic agents. Clin Infect Dis 26:59–65, 1998.

19. Mendez J, Espy M, Smith TF, et al: Clinical significance of viral load in the diagnosis of cytomegalovirus disease after liver transplantation. Transplantation 65:1477–1481, 1998.

20. Green M, Cacciarelli TV, Mazariegos GV, et al: Serial measurement of Epstein-Barr viral load in peripheral blood in pediatric liver transplant recipients during treatment for posttransplant lymphoproliferative disease. Transplantation 66:1641–1644, 1998.

21. Mack CL, Millis JM, Whitington PG, et al: Pulmonary complications following liver transplantation. Pediatr Transplant 4:39–44, 2000.

22. Golfieri R, Giampalma E, Morselli Labate AM, et al: Pulmonary complications of liver transplantation: radiological appearance and statisti-

cal evaluation of risk factors in 300 cases. Eur Radiol 10:1169–1183, 2000.

23. Sieders E, Peeters PMJG, Ten Vergert EM, et al: Early vascular complications after pediatric liver transplantation. Liver Transpl 6:326–332, 2000.

24. Lakeman FD, Whitley RJ: Diagnosis of herpes simplex encephalitis: application of polymerase chain reaction to cerebrospinal fluid from brain-biopsied patients and correlation with disease. J Infect Dis 171:857–863, 1995.

25. Paya CV, Wilson JA, Espy MJ, et al: Preemptive use of oral ganciclovir to prevent cytomegalovirus infection in liver transplant patients: a randomized, placebo-controlled trial. J Infect Dis 185:854–860, 2002.

*26. Martin SR, Atkison P, Anand R, et al: Studies of pediatric liver transplantation 2002: patient and graft survival and rejection in pediatric recipients of a first liver transplant in the United States and Canada. Pediatr Transplant 8:273–283, 2004.

Chapter 82

Inflammatory Bowel Disease

Barbara M. Garcia Peña, MD, MPH

Key Points

The use of steroids and other immunosuppressants can mask complications (e.g., perforation) in patients with inflammatory bowel disease.

Stress-dose steroids should be considered in ill-appearing patients who are already taking prednisone.

Clinicians should not rely on plain films to exclude most serious intra-abdominal complications such as bowel perforation, abscess formation, and biliary and pancreatic disorders.

Introduction and Background

Inflammatory bowel disease (IBD) is a chronic, remitting condition characterized by inflammation of the gastrointestinal (GI) tract. The two most common types of IBD are Crohn's disease and ulcerative colitis (UC). Crohn's disease is characterized by transmural segmental inflammation and granulomas affecting any segment of the GI tract. UC manifests as inflammation of the mucosal lining of the colon and rectum. Both diagnoses are relatively common in the pediatric population since up to 40% of patients who have Crohn's disease and 20% of patients who have UC come to medical attention before 20 years of age.[1,2] The majority of children with IBD can be managed as outpatients on chronic pharmacotherapy. Despite their chronicity, these disorders can present to the emergency department as acute and potentially life-threatening GI emergencies.

Recognition and Approach

The cause of IBD is believed to be inappropriate activation of the mucosal immune system driven by normal GI flora. This abnormal response is facilitated by defects in the barrier function of the GI epithelium and the mucosal immune system.[3] Although the cause of IBD continues to be unknown, genetic factors, environmental precipitants, and disease cofactors are thought to be the major etiologic agents. The aggregate effect of genetic, environmental, and a myriad of other processes is the continual activation of mucosal immune responses with the resultant clinical manifestation of IBD.[3-5]

The inflammation in UC is typically limited to the colon and rectum and is seen primarily in the mucosal layer. It consists of continuous involvement along the bowel length with areas of inflammation, ulceration, hemorrhage, and edema. In severe cases, the inflammation may extend into the submucosa. Intervening areas of granulation tissue and regenerating epithelium may form islands of tissue called "pseudopolyps." Unlike Crohn's disease, there are no granulomas and little fibrosis is present.[6]

The incidence of UC in children has been gradually increasing, with the prevalence currently 41.1 to 80 cases per 100,000 population. The disease is more prevalent with white ethnicity and occurs more commonly in Northern Europe and North America. Females outnumber males by 50%. The age of onset is typically bimodal, with the major peak in the second and third decades and a second peak in the fifth and sixth decades.[7,8]

Crohn's disease is a transmural inflammatory disorder that may affect any segment of the GI tract from mouth to anus and most often is discontinuous. Anal involvement, composed of skin tags, anal fissures, abscesses, and fistulas, occurs in approximately 25% of patients. Approximately 40% of patients with Crohn's disease have involvement of the terminal ileum. The inflammation is commonly transmural and manifests as mesenteric inflammation, fibrotic stiffening of the small bowel loops, adhesions, stricture formation, and fistulas to bowel, bladder, skin, or vagina. Histology reveals noncaseating granulomas in as many as 50% of patients.[6]

The incidence of Crohn's disease is approximately 3.5 per 100,000 population per year, making Crohn's disease more common than UC in pediatric patients. The epidemiology is similar to that of UC, with an increased prevalence among whites and a bimodal age of onset. There is approximately equal female:male representation.[8,9]

Clinical Presentation

Patients with Crohn's disease and UC may present to the emergency department with similar symptoms. Fluctuating symptoms of diarrhea, crampy abdominal pain, and variable amounts of GI bleeding may be seen. In addition, systemic symptoms such as fever, weight loss, and fatigue, seen with any chronic inflammatory process, are commonly manifested in patients with IBD. A variety of extraintestinal signs and symptoms, such as arthritis, uveitis, aphthous stomatitis, and pyoderma gangrenosum, are also often seen in these patients and may even be the sole presenting symptoms.[6]

Fortunately, true abdominal catastrophes occur only rarely. However, the emergency physician should be aware of these grave complications.

Ulcerative Colitis Complications

Fulminant Colitis

Fulminant colitis is a severe form of UC that affects approximately 5% to 15% of patients and has been shown to represent the initial presentation of the disease in up to one third of patients. Recent mortality rates have been described to be 10% or less.[6] A several-week history of worsening GI symptoms accompanied by weight loss often precedes the presentation. These signs may be subtle or even absent in patients taking immunosuppressant medications or high-dose steroids.

Physical examination findings usually include a child who is pale, tachycardic, and febrile with postural changes in pulse and blood pressure. Clinical features of fulminant colitis include diffuse abdominal tenderness with signs of peritoneal irritation, fever, distention, and absent bowel sounds. Laboratory findings may include leukocytosis with a shift to the left, anemia, hypoalbuminemia, hypokalemia, and azotemia.[10] Abdominal radiographs, including left lateral decubitus views, should be obtained to look for free air in the peritoneum. The radiograph may also show loss of colonic haustra, classic "thumbprinting," which represents bowel wall edema and inflammation or dilation, seen most prominently in the transverse colon[10] (Fig. 82–1).

Toxic Megacolon

Toxic megacolon is the persistent dilation of the colon in the setting of fulminant colitis, which occurs in 1.6% to 18% of patients with UC.[11-13] Possible triggering events include recent colonoscopy, barium enema, hypokalemia, and the use of opiates or anticholinergic drugs. Reported mortality rates vary between zero and 50%, with the higher numbers resulting from colonic perforation and sepsis.[12,14]

Clinical features include an ill-appearing patient who may have changes in mentation with fever, toxicity, and dehydration. Tachycardia and hypotension are often present. Patients with toxic megacolon may actually show a decline in the frequency of bowel movements, reflecting increased colonic dilation instead of improvement. On abdominal examination, there is distention and tympany particularly in the region of the left and transverse colon. If peritoneal signs are present, they often signal perforation.[6] Plain films usually show a nonobstructed, dilated large bowel with loss of haustra or thumbprinting. Computed tomography (CT) scans may be more accurate than plain films and also aid in excluding other disorders causing abdominal pain.

Bowel Perforation

Bowel perforation is a serious and lethal complication of UC that occurs in up to one third of patients with toxic megacolon.[12,13] Clinical features include a patient with signs of sepsis with high fever, leukocytosis with left shift, and increasing abdominal pain with guarding. However, these signs and symptoms may be diminished or absent in patients taking

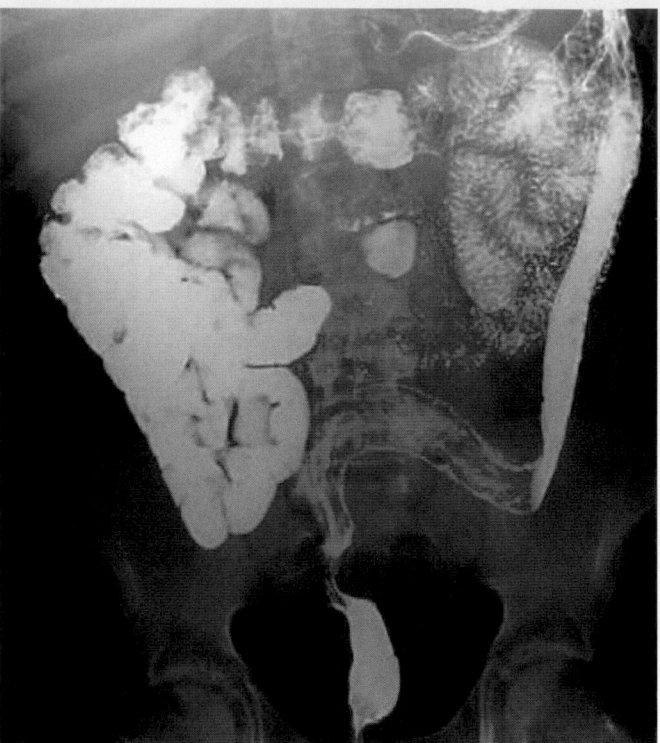

FIGURE 82–1. Barium study demonstrating fulminant ulcerative colitis. Note the pipelike colon on the left with no houstral markings identified.

high-dose steroids, those on immunosuppressants, and those who are malnourished. While abdominal radiographs may be helpful to demonstrate free air in the peritoneal cavity, CT may be required to make the diagnosis.[10]

Gastrointestinal Bleeding

Although *bloody diarrhea* is the hallmark of ulcerative colitis and occurs in over 95% of patients, *severe gastrointestinal bleeding*, although uncommon, also may be seen in these patients. Hemorrhage accounts for only 6% to 10% of all urgent colectomies in ulcerative colitis.[14,15] Patients with pancolitis as well as those with toxic megacolon are more prone to hemorrhage.[16]

Crohn's Disease Complications

Bowel Obstruction

Patients with Crohn's disease involving the gastroduodenum can mimic the presentation of peptic ulcer disease with epigastric pain, postprandial vomiting, and hematemesis and melena. These patients may also present acutely with *gastric outlet obstruction* with a several-week history of epigastric pain, worsening postprandial vomiting, and progressive weight loss. Physical examination may reveal a dehydrated, tachycardic patient with hypoactive bowel sounds.[10,17]

Patients with Crohn's disease involving the small bowel most often have right lower quadrant pain and diarrhea. As the fibrosing process progresses, *small bowel obstruction* may occur. Patients usually present with a history of low-grade symptoms prior to the onset of the acute episode, which is usually a partial obstruction. Rarely, a patient may present more urgently with a high-grade obstruction without prior premonitory symptoms. Small bowel adhesions should also be considered in the patient with prior abdominal surgical history, and present in an abrupt fashion. This type of obstruction can rapidly progress to strangulation and bowel necrosis.[10] The diagnosis of bowel obstruction can usually be made by plain abdominal radiograph. If plain films are normal and bowel obstruction still suspected, CT is indicated.

Patients with disease involving the large bowel rarely manifest complications of obstruction. When it occurs, it is usually secondary to a stricture, giant pseudopolyposis, or an underlying malignancy.[10,18]

Abscesses and Fistulas

Abscesses and fistula formation are common complications due to the invasive nature of Crohn's disease. Abscesses can be seen in the peritoneum, retroperitoneum, pelvis, and liver. Abscesses occur in 12% to 25% of patients with Crohn's disease and occur most often in those with ileocolitis.[10,19,20] Patients commonly present with fever and a right lower quadrant mass. The mass may be a phlegmon with inflamed loops of bowel and mesentery or a frank abscess, in which case the patient appears toxic with high fever and leukocytosis with left shift. A history of fistulas predisposes to abscess formation.[10] The diagnosis of intra-abdominal abscess can usually be made by abdominal ultrasonography or CT (Fig. 82–2).

An abscess in the psoas muscle is a rare complication of Crohn's disease and is caused by a fistula into the retroperitoneum. The patient commonly presents with fever in association with groin or hip pain. It may be the first presentation of IBD. On examination, a palpable flank mass or a flexion contracture of the hip may be seen.[10]

Another urgent presentation is perianal fistula complicated by abscess in patients with Crohn's disease. Perianal disease is more commonly associated with disease of the large bowel than the small bowel.[10]

Liver abscesses occur with greater frequency in patients with Crohn's disease than in the general population. The pathogenesis seems to be direct extension from an intraabdominal abscess and portal bacteremia. *Streptococcus milleri* is the organism frequently found on culture. Patients present with fever, right upper quadrant pain and tenderness, jaundice, and weight loss.[19,21]

Perforation

Patients with Crohn's disease, like those with UC, can present urgently with peritonitis secondary to perforation, which is usually microperforation. This often occurs in the right lower quadrant, and features may mimic appendicitis. Free perforation with peritonitis is rare in patients with Crohn's disease. It may occur spontaneously or be due to a ruptured abscess. Patients appear toxic and often have a high fever, worsening abdominal pain, tenderness, and peritoneal signs. These signs may be muted in those patients who are immunosuppressed, malnourished, or taking steroids.[10]

Other Presentations

Significant *hemorrhage*, although uncommon (published prevalence of 1.3%), can also been seen in patients with Crohn's disease. Those patients with ileocolitis have the greatest frequency of severe hemorrhage (see Chapter 75, Gastrointestinal Bleeding).[22]

Fulminant colitis and *toxic megacolon* can also be seen in patients with Crohn's disease, but are much less common than in ulcerative colitis.[10] Patients' presenting features are similar to those with ulcerative colitis.

Extraintestinal Complications

Pancreatitis is a common cause of abdominal pain in patients with IBD. The diagnosis must be considered in any patient with abdominal pain and the underlying diagnosis of IBD. Many of the drugs used to treat IBD, such as azathioprine,[23] 6-mercaptopurine,[24] sulfasalazine,[25] mesalamine,[26] and metronidozole,[27] can cause acute pancreatitis. Elevated serum amylase and lipase and abdominal ultrasonography or CT scan confirm the diagnosis (see Chapter 80, Pancreatitis).

Biliary tract disease is common in Crohn's disease due to an increased risk of gallstone formation. Extensive disease of the ileum or ileal resection causes a decreased bile acid pool, which makes bile lithogenic. Patients may present with biliary colic, acute cholecystitis, or cholangitis (see Chapter 85, Gallbladder Disorders).[10]

Patients with IBD are at an increased risk for *thromboemboli* due to their intrinsic hypercoagulable state. IBD patients have increased factor V and VIII levels, thrombocytosis, abnormal platelet activity, and decreased antithrombin III levels.[28-30] They may present with deep venous thrombosis or pulmonary emboli. Rarely, patients with IBD may even present with cerebrovascular accidents caused by arterial thrombosis (see Chapter 130, Disorders of Coagulation).

IBD is associated with both central and peripheral *arthritis*. Sacroiliitis and spondylitis are the most common types of central arthropathy and are independent of IBD intestinal exacerbations. The peripheral arthritis is often oligoarticular and migratory, usually involving the wrists, fingers, knees, and ankles. Peripheral arthritis usually follows exacerbations of intestinal disease. Treatment is directed at controlling the IBD either with steroids or sulfasalazine. Nonsteroidal anti-inflammatory drugs should be used with caution since they have been shown to exacerbate the symptoms of IBD.[10]

Ocular emergencies consist of episcleritis and anterior uveitis. The episcleritis parallels the course of the intestinal disease, while the anterior uveitis typically does not. Anterior

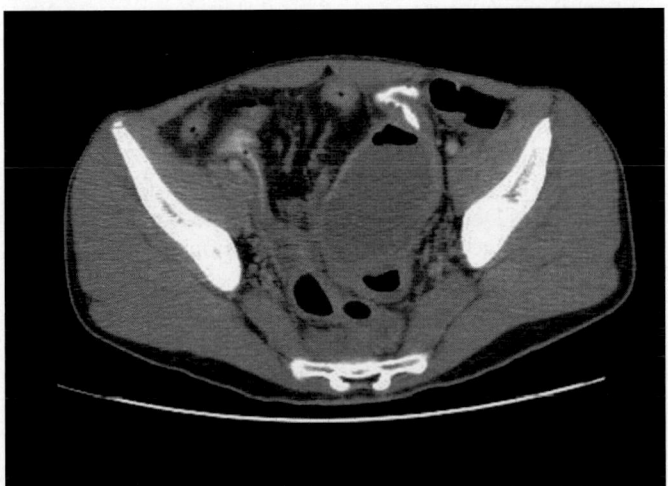

FIGURE 82–2. Intra-abdominal abscess diagnosed in a patient with Crohn's disease.

uveitis presents rapidly with photophobia, blurred vision, and pain. On examination, one can distinguish anterior uveitis from conjunctivitis by the involvement of the perilimbic area. Treatment is with topical steroids and closely coordinated ophthalmology follow-up (see Chapter 48, Eye Disorders).[10]

IBD patients have an increased frequency of *urolithiasis*. Chronic dehydration, metabolic acidosis induced by diarrhea, and a hypercatabolic state associated with IBD cause uric acid stones. In addition, patients with Crohn's disease who have extensive ileal disease and steatorrhea are at greater risk for calcium oxalate stones (see Chapter 88, Renal Disorders).[10]

Urosepsis is a second urologic condition complicating patients with Crohn's disease. Infection may result from an enterovesical fistula that subsequently leads to cystitis and pyelonephritis. Pyelonephritis can also be caused by an obstructive nephropathy. Patients with Crohn's disease may form fistulas posteriorly that involve the ureter, most often on the right. This leads to hydroureter and hydronephrosis with resulting urosepsis (see Chapter 86, Urinary Tract Infections in Children and Adolescents).[10]

Important Clinical Features and Considerations

Infants and children with IBD are often prescribed strong immunosuppressant agents, including steroids, aminosalicylates (e.g., sulfasalazine, mesalamine), infliximab (tumor necrosis factor monoclonal antibody), methotrexate, cyclosporine, and azathioprine. These agents can mask serious underlying infections and GI complications such as bowel perforation, while making treatment of these complications difficult. Importantly, steroids can suppress endogenous production of adrenocortocoid hormones, making treatment of infections and sepsis difficult (see Chapter 107, The Steroid-Dependent Child).

Management

For patients with IBD who present with abdominal pain or vomiting, clinicians must initiate resuscitation while performing an expedited evaluation to determine if specific GI complications are present. Patients should be resuscitated with normal saline and administered intravenous (IV) antibiotics if bowel perforation is suspected. For patients on chronic steroids, a stress dose of hydrocortisone may be required. While plain films may reveal complications of obstruction or perforation, CT scan may be required to make these diagnoses. Surgical consultation for immediate surgery (e.g., perforation) or close monitoring (toxic megacolon, significant bleeding, intra-abdominal abscess) will be required in many cases.

Management of fulminant colitis necessitates aggressive therapy due to the possibility of impending perforation. Deaths occur because the severity of the colitis is not diagnosed early enough and appropriate therapy is begun too late.[31] The clinician should immediately administer IV fluids with concomitant correction of any electrolyte abnormalities. Abdominal radiographs should be taken and stool cultures performed to exclude bacterial pathogens, ova and parasites, and *Clostridum difficile*. Early gastroenterology or surgical consultation with a limited flexible sigmoidoscopy will help confirm the diagnosis and evaluate for peudomembranous colitis. More extensive endoscopic evaluation and barium studies are contraindicated since they could potentially precipitate toxic megacolon or perforation.[32] All patients should be placed on bowel rest. Narcotic analgesics, antidiarrheal medications, and nonsteroidal anti-inflammatory medications are contraindicated due to the risk of precipitating toxic megacolon.[10,32-36] The mainstay of therapy for fulminant colitis is systemic steroids. Hydrocortisone (1 to 5 mg/kg per 24 hours divided every 8 to 12 hours, to a maximum of 250 mg), prednisone (2 mg/kg IV every 8 hours, to a maximum of 80 mg/day), or methylprednisolone (0.5 to 1.7 mg/kg per 24 hours divided every 6 to 12 hours) should be started as soon as possible. Antibiotics are not indicated in fulminant colitis unless the patient appears toxic and exhibits fever, leukocytosis with left shift, and abdominal tenderness. If there is not a significant improvement within 2 weeks, surgical intervention is indicated.[10,32]

Treatment for toxic megacolon requires close monitoring. In addition to the therapy for fulminant colitis mentioned previously, broad-spectrum antibiotics such as metronidazole, in addition to a third-generation cephalosporin (or ampicillin and gentamicin), should be initiated.[10,37] A nasogastric tube is placed to decompress the bowel. If there is no evidence for perforation, an initial trial of aggressive medical therapy should be initiated.[31] If there is no improvement within 48 to 72 hours, surgery is indicated.[10,37]

Due to the high morbidity and mortality seen with bowel perforation, the slightest evidence suggesting perforation in patients with IBD mandates immediate surgical consultation. Immediate IV antibiotics effective against enteric organisms are indicated.

Severe GI bleeding is uncommon in patients with IBD. However, in those who are hemodynamically unstable and present with GI hemorrhage, aggressive IV fluids and early transfusion of blood are indicated. Surgery is the definitive, and often life-saving, treatment (see Chapter 75, Gastrointestinal Bleeding).[10]

Treatment for bowel obstruction is initially conservative and includes bowel rest, nasogastric suction, intravenous fluid and electrolyte replacement, intravenous corticosteroids, and parenteral nutrition. If patients do not respond to medical therapy, surgery is indicated.[10]

Management of intra-abdominal abscesses initially includes bowel rest, parenteral nutrition, and antibiotics providing both aerobic and anaerobic coverage. Single-drug regimens, including imipenem or cefipime, or multiple-drug regimens, such as metronidazole plus a third- or fourth-generation cephalosporin or aztreonam plus metronidazole, can be used.[38] Definitive therapy involves a percutaneous or surgical drainage procedure and resection of the diseased bowel that harbors the fistulous tract.[39]

Summary

UC and Crohn's disease are usually characterized by a chronic, relapsing course. Despite the protracted nature of these diseases, patients can also present acutely with GI emergencies. Urgent manifestations may include intestinal and extraintestinal disease. Intestinal emergencies, such as obstruction, perforation, abscess formation, and hemorrhage, are often more severe and can be life-threatening. Extraintestinal emergencies include rheumatologic, ocular, urologic, and hematologic complications. Successful management of the complications associated with IBD depends on early diagnosis and expedient treatment involving both medical and surgical options.

REFERENCES

*1. Grand RJ, Ramakrishna J, Calenda KA: Inflammatory bowel disease in the pediatric patient. Gastroenterol Clin North Am 24:613–632, 1995.

2. Aideyan UO, Smith WL: Inflammatory bowel disease in children. Radiol Clin North Am 34:885–902, 1996.

*3. Podolsky DK: Inflammatory bowel disease. N Engl J Med 347:417–429, 2002.

4. Mashimo H, Wu DC, Podolsky DK, Fishman MC: Impaired defense of intestinal mucosa in mice lacking intestinal trefoil factor. Science 274:262–265, 1996.

5. Schmitz H, Barmeyer C, Fromm M, et al: Altered tight junction structure contributes to the impaired epithelial barrier function in ulcerative colitis. Gastroenterology 115:301–309, 1998.

*6. Roy MA: Inflammatory bowel disease. Surg Clin North Am 77:1419–1431, 1997.

7. Fish D, Kugathasan S: Inflammatory bowel disease. Adolesc Med Clin 15:67–90, 2004.

8. Russel MG: Changes in the incidence of inflammatory bowel disease: what does it mean? Eur J Intern Med 11:191–196, 2000.

9. Montgomery SM, Wakefield AJ, Ekbom A: Sex specific risks for pediatric onset among patients with Crohn's disease. Clin Gastroenterol Hepatol 1:303–309, 2003.

*10. Bitton A, Peppercorn MA: Emergencies in inflammatory bowel disease. Crit Care Clin 11:513–529, 1995.

11. Edwards FC, Truelove SC: The course and prognosis of ulcerative colitis. Part I. Gut 4:299–308, 1963.

12. Strauss RJ, Flint GW, Platt N, et al: The surgical management of toxic dilatation of the colon: a report of 28 cases and review of the literature. Ann Surg 184:682–688, 1976.

13. Greenstein AJ, Sachar DB, Gibas A, et al: Outcome of toxic dilatation in ulcerative colitis and Crohn's colitis. J Clin Gastroenterol 7:137–144, 1985.

14. Caprilli R, Vernia P, Latella G, et al: Early recognition of toxic megacolon. J Clin Gastroenterol 9:160–164, 1987.

15. Binder SC, Miller HH, Deterling RA: Emergency and urgent operations for ulcerative colitis. Arch Surg 110:284–289, 1975.

16. Robert JH, Sachar DB, Aufses AH, et al: Management of severe hemorrhage in ulcerative colitis. Am J Surg 19:550–555, 1990.

17. Levine MS: Crohn's disease of the upper gastrointestinal tract. Radiol Clin North Am 25:79–91, 1987.

18. Di Febo GF, Gizzi G, Cappello IP: Unusual case of colonic sub-obstruction by giant pseudopolyposis in Crohn's colitis. Endoscopy 13:90–92, 1981.

19. Greenstein AJ, Sachar DB, Greenstein RJ, et al: Intraabdominal abscess in Crohn's (ileo)colitis. Am J Gastroenterol 143:727–730, 1982.

20. Nagler SM, Poticha SM: Intra-abdominal abscess in regional enteritis. Am J Surg 137:350–354, 1979.

21. Mir-Madjlessi SH, McHenry MC, Farmer RG: Liver abscess in Crohn's disease: report of four cases and review of the literature. Gastroenterology 91:987–993, 1986.

22. Robert JR, Sachar DB, Greenstein AJ: Severe gastrointestinal hemorrhage in Crohn's disease. Ann Surg 213:207–211, 1991.

23. Sturdevant RA, Singleton JW, Deren JL, et al: Azathioprine-related pancreatitis in patients with Crohn's disease. Gastroenterology 4:883–886, 1979.

24. Bank L, Wright JP: 6-Mercaptopurine-related pancreatitis in two patients with inflammatory bowel disease. Dig Dis Sci 29:357–359, 1984.

25. Block MB, Genant HK, Kirsner JB: Pancreatitis as an adverse reaction to salicylazosulfapyridine. N Engl J Med 282:380–382, 1970.

26. Fiorentini MT, Fracchia M, Galatola G, et al: Acute pancreatitis during oral 5-aminosalicylic acid therapy. Dig Dis Sci 35:1480–1182, 1990.

27. Corey WA, Doebbeling BN, Dejong KJ, et al: Metronidazole-induced acute pancreatitis. Rev Infect Dis 13:1213–1215, 1991.

28. Lam A, Borda I, Inwood M: Coagulation studies in ulcerative colitis and Crohn's disease. Gastroenterology 68:245–251, 1975.

29. Webberly MJ, Hart MT, Melikian V: Thromboembolism in inflammatory bowel disease: role of platelets. Gut 34:247–251, 1993.

30. Koutroubakis ID: Role of thrombotic vascular risk factors in inflammatory bowel disease. Dig Dis 18:161–167, 2000.

31. Farthing M: Severe inflammatory bowel disease: medical management. Dig Dis 21:46–53, 2003.

*32. Cheung O, Regueiro MD: Inflammatory bowel disease emergencies. Gastroenterol Clin North Am 32:1269–1288, 2003.

33. Berg DF, Bahadursingh AM, Kaminski DL, Longo WE: Acute surgical emergencies in inflammatory bowel disease. Am J Surg 184:45–51, 2002.

34. Sheth SG, LaMont JT: Toxic megacolon. Lancet 351:509–512, 1998.

35. Evans JM, McMahon AD, Murray FE, et al: Non-steroidal anti-inflammatory drugs are associated with emergency admission to hospital for colitis due to inflammatory bowel disease. Gut 40:619–622, 1997.

36. Zenilman ME, Becker JM: Emergencies in inflammatory bowel disease. Gastroenterol Clin North Am 2:387–408, 1988.

37. Bharucha AE, Phillips SF: Megacolon: acute, toxic and chronic. Curr Treat Options Gastroenterol 2:517–523, 1999.

38. Solomkin, J, Mazuski JE, Baron EJ, et al: Guidelines for the selection of anti-infective agents for complicated intra-abdominal infections. Clin Infect Dis 37:997, 2003.

39. Lambiase RE, Cronan JJ, Dorman GS, et al: Percutaneous drainage of abscesses in patients with Crohn's disease. AJR Am J Roentgenol 150:1043–1045, 1988.

---

*Selected readings.

Chapter 83

Malrotation and Midgut Volvulus

James D'Agostino, MD

Key Points

Infants and children with malrotation may be asymptomatic or present with duodenal obstruction, internal hernias, or an acute volvulus.

Bilious emesis in a young infant is a midgut volvulus until proven otherwise.

Infants with midgut volvulus are usually well appearing and often have few abnormal physical findings.

An upper gastrointestinal tract series is the diagnostic study of choice in patients suspected of having midgut volvulus.

Introduction and Background

During embryologic development, the intestinal tract is a linear tube that extends from the stomach to the anus. The proximal (duodenojejunal) midgut is initially situated above and the distal (cecocolic) midgut is situated below the superior mesenteric artery (SMA). During the 4th and 5th week of gestation, the midgut grows rapidly and normally herniates out of the peritoneal cavity into the umbilical cord.[1] Each section returns to the abdominal cavity and rotates 270 degrees counterclockwise, leaving the duodenojejunal section to the anatomic right of the SMA and the cecocolic loop to the anatomic left of the SMA. Following rotation, the intestines fix to the posterior abdominal wall, with the cecum attaching to the right iliac fossa and the duodenojejunal junction fixating in the left upper quadrant at the ligament of Treitz, and the connecting midgut mesentery extending between these two points and adhering to the posterior abdominal wall.

Malrotation results from either absent (nonrotation) or incomplete rotation about the SMA. Incomplete fixation of the mesentery is often associated with malrotation. When nonrotation occurs, the bowel lengthens at the site of the SMA. The mesentery does not enlarge and forms a narrow base that can easily twist about the SMA. When nonrotation or malrotation occurs, the bowel can twist upon itself, causing

a volvulus with bowel obstruction and vascular compromise[2,3] (Fig. 83–1). Other complications can occur when obstructing fibrous bands (Ladd's bands) directly cause proximal intestinal obstruction (especially at the duodenum) or when incomplete fixation of the mesentery leads to an internal hernia. A small percentage of patients with malrotation may be asymptomatic, with anatomic abnormalities only noted during surgery for other disorders.[1]

Recognition and Approach

In the first week of life, up to one half of all neonates with bilious vomiting have a surgical cause for their symptoms. Intestinal obstruction due to malrotation and midgut volvulus, followed by intestinal atresia and meconium ileus, are the most common disorders found at this age.[4,5] Importantly, most neonates with these surgical lesions have normal or nonspecific findings on abdominal radiographs, and few have abnormal physical examination findings.[6] Beyond the first 1 to 2 months of life, midgut volvulus is a rare cause of bilious vomiting. In infants and children older than 2 months, gastroenteritis is the most common cause of bilious vomiting,[7] while intussusception is the most common pathologic cause in children 3 months to 2 years old.[8]

The incidence of malrotation is 1 in 500 births.[8] Nearly half of all patients present in the first week of life, two thirds present in the first month of life, and more than three quarters present by 1 year.[8,9] A small number of patients with complications from malrotation present beyond 1 year of age, with occasional cases documented in adults.[3,10,11]

Nearly half of all patients with malrotation have associated congenital anomalies. Common associations include intestinal atresia, duodenal webs, imperforate anus, cardiac anomalies, Meckel's diverticulum, and trisomy 21. Gastroschisis, omphaloceles, congenital diaphragmatic hernias, Hirschsprung's disease, gastroesophageal reflux, intussusception, and extrahepatic anomalies are also associated with malrotation.[1,12]

Clinical Presentation

Infants and children born with malrotation may present with symptoms related to an acute or chronic midgut volvulus, duodenal obstruction, or complications of an internal hernia, or they may be completely asymptomatic, with anatomic abnormalities found during evaluation for unrelated disorders.

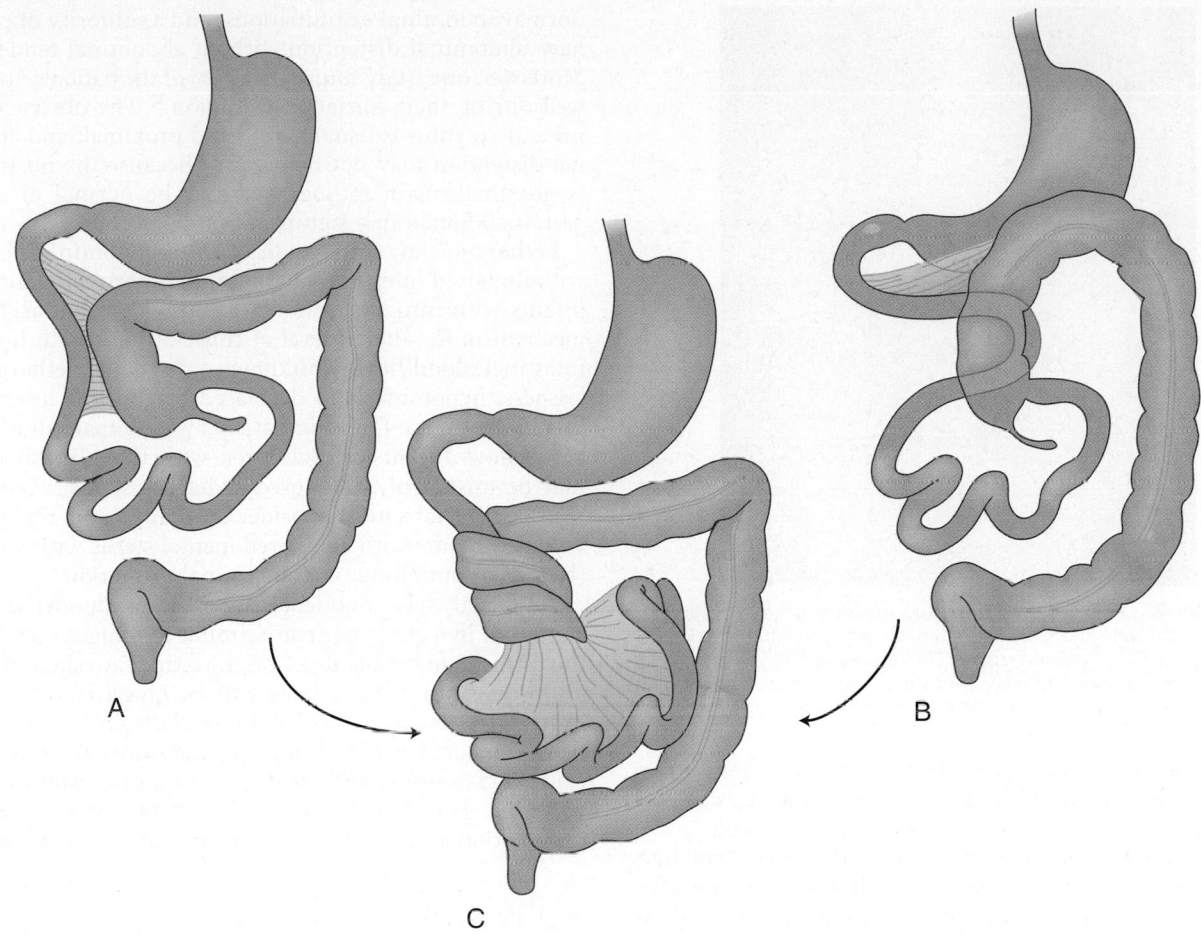

FIGURE 83–1. Incomplete mesenteric attachment in nonrotation (**A**) and in incomplete rotation (**B**) below can lead to volvulus (**C**).

Midgut Volvulus

Infants with an acute midgut volvulus typically have an onset of bilious vomiting and abdominal distention with eventual dehydration and shock due to bowel obstruction and intestinal ischemia. In infants less than 2 months old, bilious vomiting is present in 71% to 97% of cases.[3,13,14] Constipation is variably present, and rectal bleeding is noted in a minority of patients.[13,14] Physical examination abnormalities are uncommon in midgut volvulus. Most young infants are well appearing, while nearly three quarters have a normal abdominal examination. Abdominal distention, a palpable mass, and tenderness are occasionally present.[13]

Infants older than 2 months and children with an acute midgut volvulus often present with less classic features than younger infants. In one series, bilious emesis was present in only half of all cases.[14] Older children may have symptoms of chronic intermittent vomiting, crampy abdominal pain, failure to thrive, constipation, bloody diarrhea, and hematemesis.[15,16] Chronic diarrhea and failure to thrive due to malabsorption have been documented in children with malrotation and chronic midgut volvulus.[17]

With acute midgut volvulus, intestinal ischemia progresses to gangrene, and virtually all patients will develop abdominal pain and peritoneal signs. At this stage, tachycardia and hypovolemia are present. After bowel infarction, peritonitis, abdominal distension, profound dehydration, and shock occur.[8] When the diagnosis is delayed, the patient may be pale and grunting.[18]

Duodenal Obstruction

Obstructing Ladd's bands may compress the duodenum, causing obstruction in infants with malrotation. Vomiting may or may not be bilious depending upon the location of the obstruction. Infants may have progressively forceful vomiting similar to patients with pyloric stenosis (see Chapter 76, Pyloric Stenosis). Unlike with midgut volvulus, abdominal distention does not occur due to the proximal nature of the obstruction. Many infants with malrotation and duodenal obstruction have failure to thrive and chronic vomiting, with the obstruction only noted after patients have been evaluated for presumptive gastroesophageal reflux.[12]

Internal Hernias

Infants and children with malrotation-associated internal hernias have chronic recurrent abdominal pain. Intermittent vomiting and constipation are present. Due to the chronicity of symptoms, older children are often diagnosed with psychosocial behavioral abnormalities prior to being correctly diagnosed.

Diagnostic Studies in Malrotation

A complete blood cell count, electrolytes, blood urea nitrogen, creatinine, and type and crossmatch are usually obtained

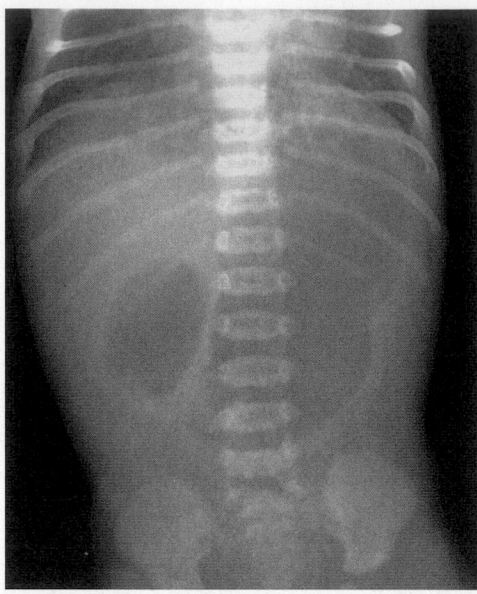

FIGURE 83–2. Double bubble sign due to duodenal obstruction by Ladd's bands. Note the gas-filled stomach and proximal duodenum. (From Warner BW: Pediatric surgery. *In* Townsend CM Jr, Beauchamp RD, Evers BM, Mattox KL (eds): Sabiston's Textbook of Surgery, 17th ed. Philadelphia: WB Saunders, 2004, p 2108.)

in these patients and may reveal dehydration, acidosis, or an elevated white blood cell count. However, these tests are not useful in diagnosing malrotation and midgut volvulus.

Radiographic findings in patients with midgut volvulus are variable. Plain radiography of the abdomen may demonstrate a small bowel obstruction or a paucity of gas.[11] A duodenal obstruction may cause a "double bubble" sign, with a gas-filled stomach and proximal duodenum with a paucity of gas distal to the duodenal obstruction (Fig. 83–2). At times, a normal bowel gas pattern can be seen because the obstruction is usually in the proximal bowel.[9]

In patients suspected of having malrotation with midgut volvulus or duodenal obstruction, the diagnostic study of choice is an upper gastrointestinal tract (UGI) series.[8,9] Malrotation with midgut volvulus is suspected when the duodenojejunal junction is in an abnormal location (i.e., not to the left of the vertebral column) and the contrast material either ends abruptly or tapers in a corkscrew fashion, indicating abdominal proximal intestinal obstruction.[8,19] Alternately, a UGI series may reveal the site of blockage with duodenal obstruction.

Ultrasonography is an alternate study that may reveal an abnormal anatomic relationship between the superior mesenteric artery and vein in malrotation.[9] Ultrasonographic examination below the head of the pancreas may reveal a circle of vascularity representing the superior mesenteric vein twisting around the SMA, forming the "whirlpool" sign.[19,20] This sign may be absent in one tenth to one third of malrotation cases.[21,22]

Important Clinical Features and Considerations

Infants and children with malrotation and even early volvulus have few, if any, abnormal physical findings.[13,23] The majority of infants and children with this disorder have normal abdominal examinations, and a minority of patients have abdominal distention without abdominal tenderness.[3] Moreover, one study found that 95% of the patients appeared well during their initial examination.[13] The obstruction in midgut volvulus is usually high and proximal, and abdominal distention may not be present. Because the obstruction is proximal, plain radiographs may be normal or show a gasless abdomen in a significant number of cases.[12]

Lethargy as an initial sign of intra-abdominal disorders with impaired intestinal blood flow has been documented in infants with intussusception[24-26] and with volvulus.[14,27] The mechanism for altered level of consciousness with impaired intestinal blood flow is unknown.[24,28] Apathy, lethargy, listlessness, hypotonia, and decreased reaction to intravenous line insertion are found in patients with impaired intestinal blood flow. Infants and children with this clinical picture may be mistakenly diagnosed as having sepsis.[26,28] For this reason, clinicians must consider the diagnosis of midgut volvulus in infants with an altered mental status with vomiting (bilious or nonbilious) or abdominal distention.

Duodenal webs, duodenal stenosis, and duodenal atresia can result in a clinical picture similar to midgut volvulus. In the immediate neonatal period, intestinal atresia and meconium ileus can cause bilious emesis. Lower intestinal tract obstruction usually causes abdominal distention. Adynamic ileus, duodenal reflux of bile into the stomach from benign causes of vomiting, and intussusception can result in bilious vomiting. However, bilious vomiting in a young infant is malrotation and midgut volvulus until proven otherwise.

Management

When midgut volvulus is suspected, surgical consultation for immediate laparotomy is required. Intravenous fluids are begun and, if vascular collapse is present, rapid normal saline boluses are given until adequate perfusion is attained. A nasogastric tube is inserted into the stomach. Intravenous antibiotics effective against enteric organisms are administered to all septic-appearing infants, and all infants with peritonitis. While plain film findings can be suggestive, normal films should not dissuade clinicians from considering the diagnosis. A UGI series should be coordinated with the consulting surgeon to ensure that prompt surgical repair takes place if volvulus is proven.

Summary

Malrotation represents absent or incomplete rotation of the intestine during fetal development. The most serious consequence of malrotation is the development of a midgut volvulus. Infants with this disorder usually present in the first few months of life with bilious vomiting. However, most infants are well appearing and physical examination findings are often absent. Suspicion for this disorder requires simultaneous initiation of resuscitation, radiologic confirmation, and surgical consultation. Clinicians must be aware of the utility and limitations of plain radiography, ultrasonography, and a UGI series in diagnosing this disorder.

REFERENCES

1. Ford EG, Senac MO, Srikanth MS, Weitzman JJ: Malrotation of the intestine in children. Ann Surg 215:172–178, 1992.

2. Felter RA: Non-traumatic surgical emergencies in children. Emerg Med Clin North Am 9:589–610, 1991.

*3. Torres AM, Ziegler MM: Malrotation of the intestine. World J Surg 17:326–331, 1993.

4. Murray K, Christie D: Vomiting. Pediatr Rev 19:337–341, 1998.

5. Vitale P, O'dea T, Sharieff G: Rare cause of bilious emesis in a 7 month old. Pediatr Emerg Care 18:290–291, 2002.

*6. Lillien LD, Srinivasan G, Pyati SP, et al: Green vomiting in the first 72 hours in normal infants. Am J Dis Child 140:662–664, 1986.

7. Sadow KB, Atabaki SM, Johns CM, et al: Bilious emesis in the pediatric emergency department: etiology and outcome. Clin Pediatr 41:475–479, 2002.

8. Irish MS, Pearl RH, Caty MG, et al: The approach to common abdominal diagnoses in infants and children. Pediatr Clin North Am 45:729–772, 1998.

9. Weinberger E, Winters W: Abdominal pain and vomiting in infants and children: imaging evaluation. Comp Ther 23:679–686, 1997.

10. Bernstein SM, Russ PD: Midgut volvulus: a rare cause of acute abdomen in an adult patient. AJR Am J Roentgenol 171:639–641, 1998.

11. Swischuk LE: Volvulus. In Swischuk LE (ed): Emergency Radiology of the Acutely Ill or Injured Child. Baltimore: Williams & Wilkins, 1994, pp 289–321.

12. Rescola FJ, Shedd FJ, Grosfeld JI, et al: Anomalies of intestinal rotation in childhood: analysis of 447 cases. Surgery 108:710–716, 1990.

*13. Bonadio WA, Clarkson T, Naus J: The clinical features of children with malrotation of the intestine. Pediatr Emerg Care 7:348, 1991.

*14. Powell DM, Othersen B, Smith CD: Malrotation of the intestines in children: the effect of age on presentation and therapy. J Pediatr Surg 24:777–780, 1989.

15. Maxson RT, Franklin PA, Wagner CW: Malrotation in the older child: surgical management, treatment and outcome. Am Surg 61:135, 1995.

—————

*Selected readings.

16. Samuel M, Boddy SA, Nichols E, et al: Large bowel volvulus in childhood. Aust N Z J Surg 70:258–262, 2000.

17. Imamoglu M, Cay A, Sarihan H, et al: Rare clinical presentation mode of intestinal malrotation after neonatal period: malabsorption-like symptoms due to chronic midgut volvulus. Pediatr Int 46:167–170, 2004.

18. Pool SR: Grunting respirations in infants and children. Pediatr Emerg Care 11:158–161, 1995.

19. Patino MO, Munden MM: Utility of the sonographic whirlpool sign in diagnosing midgut volvulus in patients with atypical clinical presentations. J Ultrasound Med 23:397–401, 2004.

20. Pacros SP, Sann L, Genin G, et al: Ultrasound diagnosis of midgut volvulus: the 'whirlpool' sign. Pediatr Radiol 22:18–20, 1992.

21. Chao HC, Kong MS, Chen JY, et al: Sonographic features related to volvulus in neonatal intestinal malrotation. J Ultrasound Med 19:371–376, 2000.

22. Zerin JM, DiPietro MA: Superior mesenteric vascular anatomy at US in patients with surgically proved malrotation of the midgut. Radiology 183:693–694, 1992.

23. Seashore JH, Touloukian RJ: Midgut volvulus: an ever-present threat. Arch Pediatr Adolesc Med 148:43, 1994.

24. Godbole A, Concannon P, Glasson M: Intussusception presenting as profound lethargy. J Pediatr Child Health 36:392–394, 2000.

25. Goetting MG, Tiznado-Garcia E, Bakdash TF: Intussusception encephalopathy: an underrecognized cause of coma in children. Pediatr Neurol 6:419–421, 1990.

26. Singer J: Altered consciousness as an early manifestation of intussusception. Pediatrics 64:93–94, 1979.

27. Pumberger W, Dinhobl I, Dremsek P: Altered consciousness and lethargy from compromised intestinal blood flow in children. Am J Emerg Med 22:307 309, 2004.

28. Heldrich FJ: Lethargy as a presenting symptom in patients with intussusception. Clin Pediatr 25:363, 1986.

Chapter 84

Abdominal Hernias

Michael Witt, MD, MPH and John C. Brancato, MD

Introduction and Background

A hernia is an abnormal protrusion from one anatomic space into another. Each type of abdominal hernia has its own underlying cause, frequency, diagnosis, and indications for acute and elective repair; however, the management is similar for each. The hernia sac is usually lined with parietal peritoneum, although the bowel wall can occasionally comprise one wall. Contents of the sac can include intestines, omentum, appendix (including acute appendicitis), ovaries, fallopian tubes, Meckel's diverticuli, or even ventriculoperitoneal shunt catheters.[1,2]

Recognition and Approach

Inguinal Hernia

Inguinal hernias are the most frequent type of abdominal hernia in children. They are six times more frequent in males than females. At least 5% of all males develop a hernia in their lifetime. Inguinal hernias are most frequent in the first year of life, manifesting in up to 30% of premature infants.[3,4] They occur equally among ethnicities. They are located on the right side in 60% of cases and on the left side in 30% of cases, and are bilateral in 10%.

In males, the processus vaginalis is a portion of the peritoneum that follows the path of the descending testicle and becomes a component of the inguinal canal together with connective tissue and muscle. In females, the processus vaginalis follows the round ligament as it travels through the inguinal ring into the labia. Typically the layers of the processus vaginalis fuse. However, in some infants the structure remains patent and the possibility exists for abdominal contents to enter. The processus vaginalis is patent in 60% of infants less than 12 months old, 40% of infants less than 24 months old, and up to 20% of adults.[5]

"Direct" hernias are defined as an inguinal canal defect medial to the inferior epigastric vessels. This hernia sac travels through the internal inguinal ring, within the cremasteric fascia, and down the spermatic cord. "Indirect" hernias are present when the inguinal canal defect is lateral to the inferior epigastric vessels, and the hernia sac travels through the posterior wall of the canal into the scrotum. Indirect hernias are far more common in children, because in infancy the canal is short and the external ring lies almost directly over the internal ring.[4]

Risk factors for hernias include prematurity, low birth weight, urologic conditions (exstrophy of the bladder, cryptorchidism, hypospadias and epispadias), abdominal wall defects (prune-belly syndrome, patent processus vaginalis), and a family history. Other risk factors include ventriculoperitoneal shunts and peritoneal dialysis catheters, severe ascites, connective tissue disorders (Ehlers-Danlos or Marfan syndrome), cystic fibrosis, meconium peritonitis, intersex syndromes (testicular feminization, hermaphrodism), mucopolysaccharidoses (Hunter's or Hurler's syndromes), hepatosplenomegaly, abdominal masses such as Wilms' tumor, and congenital dislocation of the hips.[6]

Umbilical Hernia

Umbilical hernias are also extremely common, occurring in 1 in 6 Americans. Unlike other types of hernias, they are 6 to 10 times more common in African Americans. Because they frequently resolve on their own, their frequency drops rapidly beyond toddlerhood.

Closure of the umbilical ring usually occurs around the end of the first trimester of gestation. If the ring does not close, this may lead to an umbilical hernia varying in size from undetectable to "giant" (>2.5 cm). These hernias generally contain omentum and not intestine. Specific risk factors include Beckwith-Wiedemann and Down syndromes, ascites, peritoneal dialysis, or a history of abdominal laparoscopy.[7]

Less Common Pediatric Hernias

Femoral hernias are uncommon, with less than 500 cases reported in all age groups. They are especially rare under the age of 15 years.[8] They are equally common in males and females across all pediatric ages. They are thought to be due to enlarged femoral rings. The contents of the hernia sac may include intestine, appendix, ovary, fallopian tube, or ectopic testis.[8] Because these hernias are rare and difficult to diagnose, they are often diagnosed as lymphadenopathy or inguinal hernias. In fact, many patients have inguinal herniorrhaphies prior to the final diagnosis. Difficulty with diagnosis leads to prolonged incarceration periods and a high risk of strangulation.[4,9]

Spigelian hernias are even less common in children (<30 reports in the pediatric literature), although they closely resemble traumatic anterior abdominal wall hernias.[10,11] They occur along the lateral border of the rectus muscle at the junction of the semilunar line and the semicircular line of Douglas. The defect is generally 1 to 3 cm and usually contains fat or bowel. These hernias may sit under the external oblique muscle, making them difficult to diagnose.[10,11] Children with spigelian hernias present with pain, abdominal tenderness, or signs of incarceration. To further complicate the diagnosis, these hernias may coexist with inguinal hernias, or they may even contain an acutely inflamed appendix.[12]

Sliding hernias occur when one wall of the hernia sac is formed by the wall of the intestine. *Richter's hernias* occur when only the antimesenteric surface of the bowel, nearly always the lower ileum, protrudes through an abdominal wall defect and obstruction or strangulation occurs.[13] Richter's hernias can occur in children as young as 8 years old, although the average presenting age is 70 years. The location of the hernia is most frequently femoral, followed by ventral abdominal wall defects. Symptoms generally include nausea and vomiting, abdominal distention, and occasionally a palpable mass. Because only part of the bowel circumference is involved, these hernias may not cause an obstruction as they progress to incarceration. This may delay correct diagnosis and result in poor outcomes. In contrast, hernias with complete obstruction manifest with signs and symptoms such as vomiting and distention, leading to earlier exploration and diagnosis.[14]

Obturator hernias are most common in elderly debilitated women, but occur rarely in children. Patients tend to present with symptoms similar to those with other types of hernias. The hernia mass is generally hidden beneath the thigh adductor muscles and is generally not diagnosed until surgery for a bowel obstruction.[15]

Epigastric hernias occur midline just superior to the umbilicus, and the defect arises where the blood vessels penetrate the linea alba. The hernia sac generally contains incarcerated but not strangulated epigastric fat. Patients with these hernias usually can wait for elective surgical intervention, but occasionally strangulation occurs.[3,4]

Lumbar hernias are also quite uncommon. These are often associated with the lumbocostovertebral syndrome, which consists of a lumbar hernia and associated skeletal abnormalities such as hypoplastic or absent ribs, scoliosis, and hemivertibrae. They are most frequently noted in infancy, and patients generally present with prominent lumbar swelling. These hernias require early operation to avoid complications, and large defects often need prosthetic graft material.[16]

Incarceration and Strangulation

At any given time, the majority of infants and children with hernias are asymptomatic. Many children are undiagnosed until signs or symptoms of incarceration or strangulation occur. A *reducible hernia* is one in which the hernia sac and contents can be replaced into the abdominal cavity, either spontaneously or with methods described later (see Chapter 169, Hernia Reduction). *Incarceration* occurs when the abdominal contents are trapped through the wall defect and are unable to spontaneously reduce. This results in edema and subsequent blockage of the regional lymphatics and venous blood flow. Further increasing edema compromises the arterial blood supply to the herniating tissue, resulting in ischemia, necrosis, and gangrene. This complication is termed *strangulation*.

Clinical Presentation

In the emergency department, patients often present with the first occurrence of a hernia after noting a bulge at the inguinal rings, within the scrotum or labia, or within the abdominal wall (Fig. 84–1). While this is often concerning to the parents, it is usually not painful. The mass can appear intermittently and often evades detection, making diagnosis difficult. The swelling may protrude with straining or crying, and resolve with relaxation and the supine position. This often results in a history of crying associated with the lump and the subsequent erroneous conclusion that the hernia is causing pain. By increasing intra-abdominal pressure, clinicians may be able to identify a hernia that has reduced. Techniques for identifying the hernia include having the patient cough, growl, blow bubbles, or lean posteriorly. For inguinal hernias, the mass may be identified by direct visualization or by palpating the superficial inguinal ring and feeling the mass protrude during one of the previously noted maneuvers. The "silk glove sign" describes a physical examination technique used to identify the presence of a hernia sac within the inguinal canal. It is elicited by laying a finger over the inguinal structures and lightly rubbing perpendicularly along the superior-inferior axis at the level of the pubic tubercle. A feeling similar to rubbing two pieces of silk together may represent thicker cord structures in the canal, such as a hernia sac.[3]

Patients with new or previously identified hernias may present to the emergency department with an abrupt change in symptoms due to incarceration or strangulation. These symptoms can be nonspecific, and include pain, irritability, crying, decreased feeding, nausea and vomiting, or abdominal distention.[17,18] The swelling may be discolored, irreducible (incarcerated), erythematous, or tender.

If herniation is allowed to continue, progression to incarceration and strangulation can occur. This change can occur in as little as 2 hours.[3] Patients who present during late incarceration or strangulation may display increasing pain and irritability and signs of systemic toxicity. Specifically, dehydration, peritonitis, abdominal distention, bilious vomiting, and hemodynamic compromise may be present.

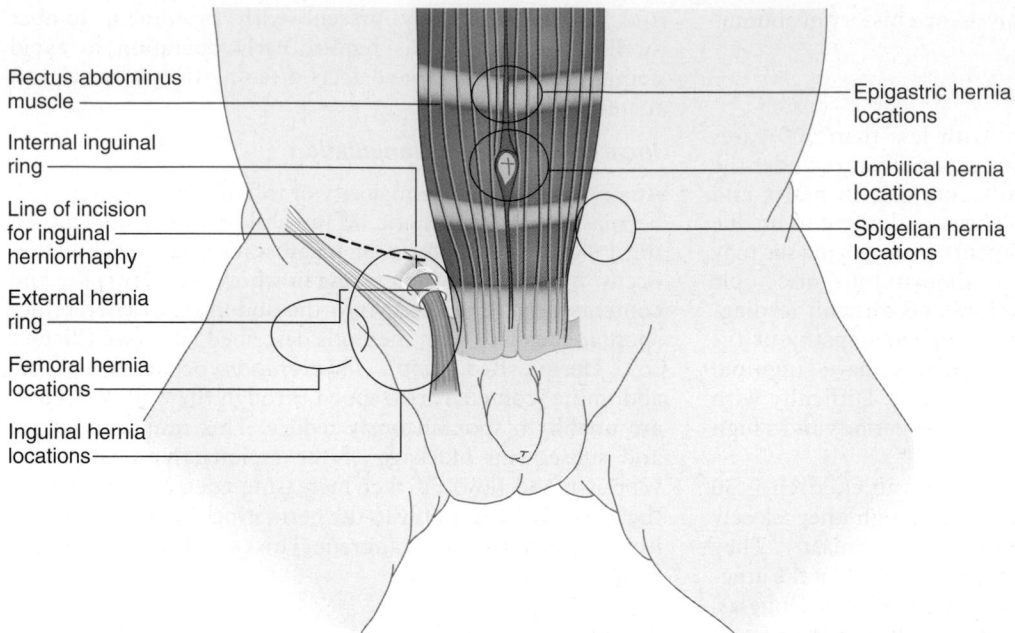

Rectus abdominus muscle

Internal inguinal ring

Line of incision for inguinal herniorrhaphy

External hernia ring

Femoral hernia locations

Inguinal hernia locations

Epigastric hernia locations

Umbilical hernia locations

Spigelian hernia locations

FIGURE 84–1. Anatomic location of various abdominal hernias.

Clinicians needs to be aware of unusual presentations of abdominal hernias as these are easily misdiagnosed and can result in significant morbidity. Irritability may be the only indication that there is a problem. An acute abdomen may misdirect the physician toward other intra-abdominal pathology before a hernia is recognized. Importantly, all infants and children with irritability or any gastrointestinal-related complaints require a genitourinary examination to exclude a hernia or associated scrotal pathology. The presence of an acute scrotum may indicate acute testicular pathology or an incarcerated or strangulated hernia.[19] Furthermore, it is possible to have an inguinal hernia with a concomitant testicular strangulation.

Infants who are unable to communicate may present with increasing fussiness, crying, decreased oral intake, or fever. Younger children can also be a diagnostic challenge because they may not disclose concerns about their genitalia, such as a lump or pain.

Children with special health care needs are a population with a greater incidence of hernias due to their frequent prematurity, low birth weight, and coexisting disease (e.g., ventriculoperitoneal shunts, mucopolysaccharidoses, connective tissue diseases).

While the diagnosis is often obvious, an abdominal wall hernia may be difficult to diagnose (Table 84–1).[2,3,17,20] Most cases can be diagnosed clinically, and adjunctive diagnostic studies are primarily reserved for questionable cases. Plain films of the abdomen are not useful unless intestinal obstruction is suspected. Transillumination of the scrotum is a simple diagnostic method that may help to differentiate hydrocele from hernia. While an otoscope may be effective for transillumination, the head can become prohibitively warm; a true transilluminator used for intravenous line placement provides better illumination. Transillumination can identify the homogeneous bright-light transmission of a hydrocele versus a more varied appearance or even peristalsis seen with intestinal contents of a hernia sac.

Table 84–1	Differential Diagnosis of Abdominal Wall Hernias

Inguinal lymphadenopathy
Hydroceles
Undescended or retracted testicles
Testicular torsion
Torsion of the appendix testis
Testicular neoplasm (seminoma, cystic lymphangioma, gonadoblastoma)
Diastasis recti abdominus
Other abdominal wall hernias (especially femoral)
Traumatic abdominal wall defect

Ultrasound can help identify the contents of a hernia sac. An ultrasound scan also can identify the size of the abdominal wall defect and can be used in cases of acute scrotum to differentiate and diagnose testicular versus scrotal pathology.[1,21] In many centers, ultrasonography is used to identify contralateral wall defects opposite to the known hernia rather than exploring the opposite side during surgery.[22]

Important Clinical Features and Considerations

While many hernias are obvious, some patients require several physician visits to confirm a spontaneously reducing hernia, with much frustration and concern on the part of both parents and clinicians. Simultaneously, the physician should be aware of the other possible diagnoses, particularly testicular disorders (see Chapter 87, Testicular Torsion and Chapter 89, Penile and Testicular Disorders). The most frequent alternate diagnoses in patients initially suspected of having an inguinal hernia are hydroceles, retracted or undescended testicles, and lymphadenopathy. Separation of testis and epididymis also can result in both an inguinal mass and a full scrotum.[23] Patients may have multiple simultaneous hernias, potentially confusing the clinical picture.

The vast majority of patients with hernias do not present with acute complications. However, intestinal obstruction or infarction can occur rapidly with few initial symptoms. If allowed to continue, infarction of bowel or omentum, testicular or ovarian necrosis, or sepsis can follow and result in significant morbidity or even death.

Management

Immediate therapeutic management is based on the clinical condition of the child. Ill-appearing or septic children require fluid hydration, antibiotics with gastrointestinal flora coverage, gastric decompression, prompt surgical evaluation, and possible operative intervention.[17] Well-appearing children with a hernia require evaluation for incarceration and strangulation. In the non–toxic-appearing child, reduction of the hernia should be attempted to identify incarceration. If the hernia is easily reducible and not incarcerated, further efforts are directed toward surgical evaluation and elective repair as an outpatient.

Hernias that cannot be reduced (e.g., incarcerated hernias) will eventually become strangulated if not promptly treated. Approximately 70% of inguinal hernias resulting in incarceration occur in infants less than 12 months old. The question of whether to reduce a hernia in the emergency department in a relatively well-appearing child is an important one, as there is a possibility of reducing infarcted and gangrenous hernia contents into the abdominal cavity. A hernia should not be reduced if there is suspicion of peritonitis or if the hernia has been incarcerated for a prolonged period, the length of which is not established but at maximum is likely 4 to 6 hours.[24] If an incarcerated hernia is reduced in the emergency department, surgical consultation, serial examinations, or admission for close observation may be warranted. For discharged children, parents should be instructed to return if an irreducible mass returns, or if pain, swelling, or gastrointestinal symptoms (e.g., vomiting) occur.

Reduction is most likely to be successful by using a combination of methods. Calming the child with parents and distraction will help decrease the intra-abdominal pressure during crying or screaming. Placing the child in the Trendelenburg position may allow gravity to pull the hernia contents back into the abdominal cavity. Local application of ice may decrease localized edema.[17] Detailed directions for manual reduction techniques are described in Chapter 169 (Hernia Reduction).

Frequently, a hernia is difficult to reduce due to pain or guarding, which increases intra-abdominal pressure. This obstacle can be overcome by administering intravenous pain medication or sedation to relax the abdominal muscles. Urgent surgical reduction is mandated if manual reduction of the hernia is not successful, as incarceration will progress to strangulation, potentially with bowel necrosis, sepsis, or death.

Prompt repair of abdominal wall hernias is indicated (except umbilical hernias) to avoid the majority of surgical complications, preferably within 1 to 4 weeks of diagnosis due to the common occurrence of incarceration (~10%).[25] Admission for early repair of other hernias may be mandated

in some situations, such as prematurity, difficulty with reduction, or coexisting medical conditions. In one study, over 15% of children scheduled for elective repair after reduction of an incarceration had an incarceration recurrence prior to surgery.[26] Exploration of the contralateral inguinal region during surgical repair, a previously common practice, may not be necessary except in known bilateral hernias or in children at higher risk for bilaterality, such as those with a left-sided hernia, boys less than 1 year of age, and all females (who have a higher incarceration rate).[27] Furthermore, ultrasound is increasingly being used to identify the presence of an inguinal defect on the opposite side, negating the need for contralateral exploration.[28-30]

Complications from surgical hernia repair are as high as 7% to 8%. This risk rises dramatically when the repair is performed emergently.[7,31] The most common complications of surgery are hernia recurrence, bladder injury, infection, injury to several pelvic nerves (ilioinguinal, iliohypogastric, genitofemoral), fallopian tube injury, testicular atrophy, and vas deferens injury that can lead to serum antisperm antibodies.[7,32] Up to 6% of repaired hernias may recur, although these hernias may actually be direct inguinal or femoral hernias that were not repaired initially.[7] The greatest risk of complications is in the most extremely premature infants. In this population, impaired healing, spermatic cord injury, hernia recurrence, and postoperative respiratory failure may occur.[2,6]

Most umbilical hernias close spontaneously by 3 to 5 years of age, and those that require surgical intervention are not generally repaired until after 4 years of age. Complications rarely occur and include incarceration (1 in 1500 cases) and strangulation.[2,33] The primary pediatrician can follow these defects until closer to the age of repair. Simple closure is used for defects 1.5 to 2 cm, and for those greater than 2.5 cm, an umbilicoplasty is performed.[4,34] Wound infection, seroma, and hematoma are the most frequent complications of repair.

Summary

Abdominal wall hernias are a frequent surgical problem seen in the emergency department. Although they rarely result in serious complications, accurate and prompt identification of incarceration or strangulation is mandatory. Abdominal wall hernias should be considered in the differential diagnosis of all children with abdominal or scrotal pain, vomiting, fussiness or inconsolability, fever, or decreased oral intake. A thorough examination is mandated, with prompt attention required to hernias that are not easily reducible. Because many subtypes of abdominal wall hernias are uncommon in children, knowledge of their incidence and unique presentation may result in earlier diagnosis and successful treatment.

Prompt surgical consultation is required in suspected cases of incarceration or strangulation. Early intervention is necessary to improve outcomes and decrease the risk of complications.

REFERENCES

1. Celik A, Ergun O, Ozbek SS, et al: Sliding appendiceal inguinal hernia: preoperative sonographic diagnosis. J Clin Ultrasound 31:156–158, 2003.

2. Katz DA: Evaluation and management of inguinal and umbilical hernias. Pediatr Ann 30:729–735, 2001.

3. Kapur P, Caty MG, Glick PL: Pediatric hernias and hydroceles. Pediatr Clin North Am 45:773–789, 1998.

4. Graf JL, Caty MG, Martin DJ, et al: Pediatric hernias. Semin Ultrasound CT MR 23:197–200, 2002.

5. Klein BL, Ochsenschlager DW: Scrotal masses in children and adolescents: a review for the emergency physician. Pediatr Emerg Care 9:351–361, 1993.

6. Scherer LR 3rd, Grosfeld JL: Inguinal hernia and umbilical anomalies. Pediatr Clin North Am 40:1121–1131, 1993.

7. Meier AH, Ricketts RR: Surgical complications of inguinal and abdominal wall hernias. Semin Pediatr Surg 12:83–88, 2003.

8. Nayeem N: Femoral hernia in children. Br J Clin Pract 44:383, 1990.

*9. Chapman WH, Barcia PJ: Femoral hernia in children: an infrequent problem revisited. Mil Med 156:631–633, 1991.

*10. Toms AP, Dixon AK, Murphy JM, et al: Illustrated review of new imaging techniques in the diagnosis of abdominal wall hernias. Br J Surg 86:1243–1249, 1999.

11. White JJ: Concomitant spigelian and inguinal hernias in a neonate. J Pediatr Surg 37:659–660, 2002.

*12. Losanoff JE, Richman BW, Jones JW: Spigelian hernia in a child: case report and review of the literature. Hernia 6:e191–e193, 2002.

13. Steinke W, Zellweger R: Richter's hernia and Sir Frederick Treves: an original clinical experience, review, and historical overview. Ann Surg 232:710–718, 2000.

14. Gillespie RW, Glas WW, Mertz GH, et al: Richter's hernia; its etiology, recognition, and management. AMA Arch Surg 73:590–594, 1956.

15. Bergstein JM, Condon RE: Obturator hernia: current diagnosis and treatment. Surgery 119:133–136, 1996.

16. Wakhlu A, Wakhlu AK: Congenital lumbar hernia. Pediatr Surg Int 16:146-8, 2000.

17. D'Agostino J: Common abdominal emergencies in children. Emerg Med Clin North Am 20:139–153, 2002.

18. Sheldon CA: The pediatric genitourinary examination: inguinal, urethral, and genital diseases. Pediatr Clin North Am 48:1339–1380, 2001.

19. Myers JB, Lovell MA, Lee RS, et al: Torsion of an indirect hernia sac causing acute scrotum. J Pediatr Surg 39:122–123, 2004.

20. Abantanga FA: Groin and scrotal swellings in children aged 5 years and below: a review of 535 cases. Pediatr Surg Int 19:446–450, 2003.

21. Chen KC, Chu CC, Chou TY, et al: Ultrasonography for inguinal hernias in boys. J Pediatr Surg 33:1784–1787, 1998.

22. Toki A, Watanabe Y, Sasaki K, et al: Ultrasonographic diagnosis for potential contralateral inguinal hernia in children. J Pediatr Surg 38:224–226, 2003.

23. Al-Arfaj AA, Al-Saflan AA: Complete separation of the testis and epididymis presenting as inguinal hernia. Saudi Med J 23:1275–1277, 2002.

24. Strauch ED, Voigt RW, Hill JL: Gangrenous intestine in a hernia can be reduced. J Pediatr Surg 37:919–920, 2002.

25. Niedzielski J, Brancato JC, Gawlowska A: Could incarceration of inguinal hernia in children be prevented? Med Sci Monit 9:CR16–CR18, 2003.

*26. Gahukamble DB, Khamage AS: Early versus delayed repair of reduced incarcerated inguinal hernias in the pediatric population. J Pediatr Surg 31:1218–1220, 1996.

27. Skinner MA, Grosfeld JL: Inguinal and umbilical hernia repair in infants and children. Surg Clin North Am 73:439–449, 1993.

28. Lotan G, Efrati Y, Stolero S, et al: Transinguinal laparoscopic examination: an end to the controversy on repair of inguinal hernia in children. Isr Med Assoc J 6:339–341, 2004.

29. Miltenburg DM, Nuchtern JG, Jaksic T, et al: Laparoscopic evaluation of the pediatric inguinal hernia—a meta-analysis. J Pediatr Surg 33:874–879, 1998.

30. Nassiri SJ: Contralateral exploration is not mandatory in unilateral inguinal hernia in children: a prospective 6-year study. Pediatr Surg Int 18:470–471, 2002.

31. Primatesta P, Goldacre MJ: Inguinal hernia repair: incidence of elective and emergency surgery, readmission and mortality. Int J Epidemiol 25:835–839, 1996.

32. Matsuda T, Muguruma K, Horii Y, et al: Serum antisperm antibodies in men with vas deferens obstruction caused by childhood inguinal herniorrhaphy. Fertil Steril 59:1095–1097, 1993.

33. Okada T, Yoshida H, Iwai J, et al: Strangulated umbilical hernia in a child: report of a case. Surg Today 31:546–549, 2001.

34. Billmire DF: A technique for the repair of giant umbilical hernia in children. J Am Coll Surg 194:677–680, 2002.

*Selected readings.

Chapter 85

Gallbladder Disorders

Marc Y. R. Linares, MD and Nestor Martinez, MD

Introduction and Background

Gallbladder disorders are uncommon during childhood and often associated with predisposing conditions. During infancy, gallstones predominantly appear as a result of sepsis or the use of parenteral nutrition. Hemolytic diseases and diseases with rapid red blood cell turnover (e.g., sickle cell disease, hereditary spherocytosis, thalassemia, pernicious anemia) are the most commonly associated factors during early childhood and remain so during adolescence. Obesity and pregnancy during adolescence increase the risk of gallstone formation. There has been a recent increase in the recognition of pediatric cholelithiasis. Whether this represents a true increase in the incidence of cholelithiasis or simply better use of diagnostic tools in abdominal illnesses is impossible to determine at the present time. The prevalence of gallstones in the pediatric population varies according to age and geographic location and can only be estimated. Prevalence rates ranging as high as 0.2% have been reported.[1,2]

Recognition and Approach

Infants and children with gallbladder disorders can present with (1) stones in the gallbladder (cholelithiasis), cystic duct, or common bile duct (choledocholithiasis); (2) inflammation of the gallbladder with (calculous cholecystitis); or (3) bacterial infection of the biliary tree (cholangitis). Gallstones are absent in acalculous cholecystitis, biliary dyskinesis, and some cases of cholangitis.

The two main types of gallstones are cholesterol and bile-pigmented stones. Gallstone composition in children differs from that in the adult population. Cholesterol stones account for 10% of all gallstones in children compared to 70% to 90% in the adult population.[3] The majority of gallstones in children are black pigmented stones (50%), while the prevalence of this type of gallstone varies from 4% to 40% in adults.[3] These stones are associated with hemolytic diseases and parenteral nutrition. Diseases associated with hemolysis (e.g., sickle cell anemia, thalassemia, hereditary spherocytosis, pernicious anemia) constitute the most common predisposing factor in pediatrics and are seen in almost 60% of children younger than 12, but rarely before 5 years old.[4-6] Diagnosis of gallstones follows a bimodal distribution; a small peak in infancy is followed by a steady increase until adolescence. The mean age at presentation is 12.2 years. Female predominance becomes noticeable after 14 years of age.[4,7]

Clinical Presentation

Cholelithiasis

Pediatric cholelithiasis can occur at any age, from the neonatal period to adolescence. Fetal gallstones have been reported.[8] Neonatal gallstones have a male preponderance, tend to resolve spontaneously within a few months, and are not associated with any known predisposing factors.[9] Neonates are frequently asymptomatic. In the neonatal period, cholelithiasis is discovered incidentally or during evaluation of a risk factor such as parenteral nutrition or sepsis, or following surgery. Of note, parenteral nutrition is more often associated with sludge of the gallbladder than cholelithiasis.[4] When cholelithiasis is uncomplicated, the physical examination is usually unremarkable and laboratory tests are normal. Ultrasound of the gallbladder is diagnostic in 96% to 100% of cases. Typical findings on ultrasound are a calculus with an acoustic shadow.

Gallbladder pseudolithiasis can mimic cholelithiasis. It has been associated with the prolonged use of ceftriaxone, a third-generation cephalosporin. In a prospective study, 11 of 44 children treated with ceftriaxone developed gallbladder pseudolithiasis.[10] Only 2 of the 11 patients complained of right upper quadrant pain. Ultrasonography of pseudolithiasis was indistinguishable from that of cholelithiasis. All pseudolithiasis cases resolved within 7 to 23 days after cessation of the drug.

Calculous Cholecystitis

Older children with calculous cholecystitis may have biliary symptoms (e.g., dyspepsia, nausea, fatty food intolerance), acute abdominal pain and fever, or nonspecific abdominal pain, or they may be relatively asymptomatic.[4] Pain is often located in the right upper quadrant, is colicky in nature, and is associated with nausea and vomiting. Jaundice is present in 7% to 94% of cases depending upon the underlying etiology.[4,11,12] Patients with cholecystitis due to hemolytic disease are more likely to have jaundice, while older patients with no underlying disease are less likely to have associated jaundice.[4,11,12] The physical examination may reveal right upper quadrant abdominal tenderness with guarding, and an elevated temperature. Epigastric tenderness is reported in one third of patients. Patients less than 6 years old tend to present with nonspecific symptoms, such as poorly localized abdominal pain, nausea, and chest pain.[7] Fatty food intolerance is usually seen in children 6 years and older.[4,7] Laboratory tests often reveal an elevated white blood cell count. Elevation of alkaline phosphatase and γ-glutamyl transpeptidase (GGT) may indicate common bile duct lithiasis.[13] Since this disorder is associated with pancreatitis, clinicians should obtain a serum amylase or lipase level when evaluating patients for possible cholecystitis. Ultrasound will reveal stones within the gallbladder or cystic duct in nearly 100% of cases, while a thickened gallbladder wall or pericholecystic fluid is present in 85% to 100% of children with calculous cholecystitis.

Acalculous Cholecystitis

Acalculous cholecystitis is rarely seen in children, and is usually associated with infectious or systemic illness. Coagulase-negative *Staphylococcus* species, *Brucella* species, *Escherichia coli,* and *Salmonella typhii* are some of the pathogens recovered from gallbladder bile cultures.[14] It is more often seen in males, in the immediate postoperative period, and following abdominal trauma, systemic illness, or infection.[15,16] The classic presentation includes acute onset of fever, right upper quadrant abdominal pain, and vomiting.[16] Jaundice is present in about 40% of cases.[15,16] The physical examination reveals right upper quadrant tenderness with guarding. In 25% of cases, the gallbladder is palpable and tender.[15] Laboratory evaluation often shows an elevated white blood cell count and abnormal liver function tests. The diagnosis is confirmed by ultrasound of the gallbladder. Ultrasonographic criteria for diagnosis of acalculous cholecystitis include the following: gallbladder distention (diameter ≥ 1.5 to 2 cm longitudinally or ≥ 4 to 6 cm transversely), gallbladder thickening (wall thickness ≥ 3.5 mm), nonshadowing echogenic material or sludge in the gallbladder, and pericholecystic fluid collection.[15] A combination of at least two of these criteria establishes the diagnosis.

Biliary Dyskinesia

Biliary dyskinesia is a disorder that involves motility abnormality of the biliary tract; it includes sphincter of Oddi dysfunction, cystic duct syndrome, and gallbladder hypokinesia. This disorder has been recognized as a cause of chronic abdominal pain, nausea, and vomiting in children and adolescents. Gallbladder hypokinesia is associated with obesity (39%) and a family history of cholelithiasis (43%).[17] The pain is reported as right upper quadrant in 48% and epigastric in 29% of cases. Nausea, vomiting, and fatty food intolerance are other predominant complaints. The diagnosis can be ascertained by measurement of ultrasonographic contractility of the gallbladder before and after injection of cholecystokinin (CCK). Ultrasonographic gallbladder contractility of less than 50% is present in all patients with this disorder. Gallbladder hypokinesia can also be diagnosed by determining a gallbladder ejection fraction of less than 35% using hepatobiliary [99m]technetium-labeled iminodiacetic acid (HIDA) scanning prior to and after CCK stimulation.

Hydrops

Hydrops of the gallbladder occurs when there is acute distention of the gallbladder without cholelithiasis or inflammation. Hydrops of the gallbladder has been associated with several infections, including ascariasis, staphylococcus, streptococcus, and Epstein-Barr virus infections.[18] It has also been reported in conjunction with sepsis, trauma, Henoch-Schönlein purpura, and Kawasaki disease.[19] Affected children typically present to the emergency department with acute onset of crampy abdominal pain, nausea, and vomiting associated with fever and jaundice. A right upper quadrant mass can be palpated in more than 75% of patients. Ultrasonography of the gallbladder confirms the diagnosis by showing an enlarged, acalculous gallbladder.

Acute Cholangitis

Acute cholangitis is rarely seen in children and is almost always associated with biliary tract surgery. The child usually presents with right upper quadrant pain associated with jaundice, high fever (≥39° C), and shaking chills (Charcot's triad). Overwhelming gram-negative sepsis and shock can complicate the presentation.

Other Complications

Other complications of gallbladder disease include common bile duct stones, emphysematous cholecystitis, and gallbladder perforation. Common bile duct stones are rare in infants and children, while gallbladder perforation and emphysematous cholecystitis are primarily complications found in elderly, diabetic adults with vascular disease.

Differential Diagnosis

The differential diagnosis of cholelithiasis, acalculous cholecystitis, and hydrops of the gallbladder includes hepatitis, Fitz-Hugh–Curtis syndrome, gastritis, peptic ulcer disease, pancreatitis, renal lithiasis, pyelonephritis, atypical appendicitis, and right lower lobe pneumonia. Physical examination and ancillary data will help guide the diagnostic evaluation.

Important Clinical Features and Considerations

Laboratory tests are rarely helpful in diagnosing gallbladder disease. A pregnancy test is mandatory in females of childbearing age. Since pancreatitis occurs in up to 8% of patients with symptomatic cholelithiasis, a serum amylase or lipase level should be obtained in cases of suspected symptomatic disease[7] (see Chapter 80, Pancreatitis). Serum electrolytes, blood urea nitrogen, and creatinine levels should be obtained in patients with vomiting and dehydration. Liver function tests are unreliable for diagnosing biliary tract disease. If the alkaline phosphatase or GGT level is elevated, a common bile duct stone should be considered. Jaundice is associated with the development of cholangitis, the most serious pediatric complication of gallbladder disease.

Some controversy exists regarding the most appropriate diagnostic test for symptomatic biliary tract disease. While ultrasonography is nearly 100% sensitive at detecting cholelithiasis, this test is only 60% to 85% sensitive at diagnosing cholecystitis (e.g., thickened wall, pericholecystic fluid, stone obstructing cystic duct).[13] A HIDA scan has greater sensitivity for the diagnosis of acute cholecystitis than ultrasound and has been recommended by some experts as the initial diagnostic test in suspected cholecystitis.[20] However, ultrasound is the preferred diagnostic test for most types of biliary disease in the emergency department setting since it is easier to perform, is less invasive, and can be performed rapidly.

Management

A surgical consultation should be obtained early in the course of the management of symptomatic gallbladder disease in children. Patients with symptomatic biliary disease should be admitted to the hospital and placed on "nothing by mouth" status. Patients with protracted vomiting require placement of a nasogastric tube connected to suction or gravity drainage. The clinician should administer intravenous fluids and correct electrolyte imbalances. Narcotics should be used for pain relief. It is a widely held misconception that meperidine should be used instead of morphine to avoid sphincter of Oddi constriction and pressure elevation, since meperidine has anticholinergic properties. Meperidine raises the common bile duct pressure 14% more than morphine, and anticholinergics have little to no effect on pain due to biliary tract disease.[21,22] Moreover, pain is related to inflammation and not biliary pressures in most patients with symptomatic cholelithiasis.[22] The duration of analgesic action of morphine is almost twice as long as meperidine, and its use in acute cholecystitis is appropriate. Nonsteroidal analgesics also have proven effective in adults, although their use for symptomatic biliary disease is limited in children.[23,24] Antibiotics are indicated in cases of cholecystitis and cholangitis, and in febrile or ill-appearing patients. A blood specimen for culture should be obtained prior to their use. Therapeutic regimens vary, but are usually geared toward broad-spectrum coverage. Enteric organisms tend to predominate in gallbladder infections, and antibiotics are selected accordingly[25-28] (Table 85–1).

Asymptomatic cholelithiasis and hydrops of the gallbladder may be managed by observation coupled with dietary restriction of fatty foods.[29] In patients with sickle cell or hemolytic disease, prophylactic cholecystectomy may be indicated if the patient is undergoing abdominal surgery for another reason.[30] In asymptomatic neonates and infants with gallstones, observation is the most appropriate management since the gallstones tend to spontaneously resolve.[31] If an infant becomes symptomatic, placement of a cholecystotomy tube with biliary irrigation is the next approach. If this treatment is unsuccessful, cholecystectomy is performed.[32]

Table 85–1	Antibiotic Choices in Childhood Cholecystitis
Single Drug Regimens	
Ampicillin/sulbactam* or ticarcillin/clavulanate* or Cefepime[†] or Imepenem/cilastatin[†] or meropenem[†]	
Multiple Drug Regimens	
Mezlocillin plus gentamicin[†,*] or (Cefazolin or cefuroxime) plus metronidazole* or (Third-/fourth-generation cephalosporin) plus metronidazole[†] or Aztreonam plus metronidazole[†]	

*Mild to moderate infection choices.
[†]Severe infection choices.
[‡]Mezlocillin is available in Europe but not in the United States.
Data from references 25–28.

Symptomatic cholelithiasis, acute cholecystitis, and acute cholangitis will require a combination of medical and surgical management. For calculous cholecystitis, early surgical therapy, within 7 days of diagnosis, is associated with a lower perioperative complication rate and avoids the risks of recurrent and complicated disease (e.g., cholangitis, pancreatitis, choledocholithiasis).[33] Laparoscopic cholecystectomy has become the treatment of choice, replacing open cholecystectomy. The laparoscopic procedure results in less postoperative discomfort for the patient and decreased length of hospitalization.[34-36] However, laparoscopic surgery is associated with an increased risk of bile duct trauma and retained common duct stones, which may prompt patients to return to the ED with increasing pain, jaundice, or fever. In the presence of acute cholangitis, surgery may need to be delayed until the infection is under control. Broad-spectrum antibiotics are used to provide coverage for enteric organisms, most commonly Enterococcus or E. coli[37] (see Table 85–1). Once the patient has responded to antibiotic treatment, endoscopic drainage of the biliary system is performed.[38] Open surgical drainage can also be used, although it carries a higher rate of mortality and morbidity.[39] Initial nonoperative treatment is the best approach for acalculous cholecystitis.[15] Close follow-up with serial gallbladder ultrasonographic examination is safe and effective in most cases. If the condition persists or worsens, cholecystectomy is performed. For patients with biliary dyskinesia, cholecystectomy will lead to complete relief of symptoms in up to 90% of cases, although 10% will have continued gastrointestinal complaints on follow-up.

Summary

With few exceptions, the approach to gallbladder disease in children does not differ from that in adults. The tendency for gallstones to resolve spontaneously in infancy should be kept in mind. Symptomatic patients should be admitted to a pediatric surgical service. If the hospital lacks one, the patient should be transferred to a tertiary pediatric hospital if possible. Ideally, all infants and children with biliary tract disease should be managed by a pediatric surgeon. However, logistics, local expertise, pediatric surgical availability, and patient characteristics (age, stability, and disease state) dictate when children should be transferred to a hospital with pediatric surgical expertise. If acute cholangitis is suspected, aggressive treatment should be performed. This includes immediate fluid resuscitation, blood cultures, and antibiotic therapy. Pain control is an integral part of the initial treatment. If the patient is asymptomatic, referral to a pediatric surgical service and, in most cases, discharge home with surgical follow-up is appropriate.

REFERENCES

1. Toscano E, Trivellini V, Andria G: Cholelithiasis in Down syndrome. Arch Dis Child 85:242–243, 2001.
2. Nomura H, Kashiwagi S, Hayashi J, et al: Prevalence of gallstone disease in a general population of Okinawa, Japan. Am J Epidemiol 128:598–605, 1988.
3. Stringer M, Taylor D, Soloway R: Gallstone composition: are children different? J Pediatr 142:435–440, 2003.
4. Wesdorp I, Bosman D, de Graaff A, et al: Clinical presentations and predisposing factors of cholelithiasis and sludge in children. J Pediatr Gastroenterol Nutr 31:411–417, 2000.
5. Tamary H, Aviner S, Freud E, et al: High incidence of early cholelithiasis detected by ultrasonography in children and young adults with hereditary spherocytosis. J Pediatr Hematol Oncol 25:952–954, 2003.
6. Walker T, Hambleton I, Serjeant G: Gallstones in sickle cell disease: observations from the Jamaican Cohort study. J Pediatr 136:80–85, 2000.
7. Reif S, Sloven D, Lebenthal E: Gallstones in children: characterization by age, etiology, and outcome. Am J Dis Child 145:105–108, 1991.
8. Stringer M, Lim P, Cave M, et al: Fetal gallstones. J Pediatr Surg 31:1589–1591, 1996.
9. Brown D, Teele R, Doubilet P, et al: Echogenic material in the fetal gallbladder: sonographic and clinical observations. Radiology 182:73–76, 1992.
10. Papadopoulou F, Efremidis S, Karyda S, et al: Incidence of ceftriaxone-associated gallbladder pseudolithiasis. Acta Paediatr 88:1352–1355, 1999.
*11. Lugo-Vicente HL: Trends in the management of gallbladder disorders in children. Pediatr Surg Int 12:348–352, 1997.
12. Ruibal FJ, Aleo LE, Alvarez MA, Pinero ME: [Childhood cholelithiasis: analysis of 24 patients diagnosed in our department and review of 123 cases published in Spain.] An Esp Pediatr 54:120–125, 2001.
13. Rescorla F: Cholelithiasis, cholecystitis, and common bile duct stones. Curr Opin Pediatr 9:276–282, 1997.
14. Ternberg J, Keating J: Acute acalculous cholecystitis: complication of other illnesses in childhood. Arch Surg 110:543–547, 1975.
*15. Imamoglu M, Sarihan H, Sari A, et al: Acute acalculous cholecystitis in children: diagnosis and treatment. J Pediatr Surg 37:36–39, 2002.
16. Tsakayannis D, Kozakewich H, Lillehei C: Acalculous cholecystitis in children. J Pediatr Surg 31:127–130; discussion 130–131, 1996.
17. Dumont R, Caniano D: Hypokinetic gallbladder disease: a cause of chronic abdominal pain in children and adolescents. J Pediatr Surg 34:858–861; discussion 861–862, 1999.
18. Barton L, Luisiri A, Dawson J: Hydrops of the gallbladder in childhood infections. Pediatr Infect Dis J 14:163–164, 1995.

19. Coskun Y, Bayraktaroglu Z, Gökalp A, et al: Kawasaki disease associated with gallbladder hydrops. Turk J Pediatr 37:269–273, 1995.
20. Alobaidi M, Gupta R, Jafri SZ, Fink-Bennet DM: Current trends in imaging evaluation of acute cholecystitis. Emerg Radiol 10:256–258, 2004.
21. Radnay P, Brodman E, Mankikar D, et al: The effect of equi-analgesic doses of fentanyl, morphine, meperidine and pentazocine on common bile duct pressure. Anaesthesist 29:26–29, 1980.
22. Rothrock SG, Green SM, Gorton E: Atropine for the treatment of biliary tract pain: a double blind placebo controlled trial. Ann Emerg Med 22:1234–1237, 1993.
23. Goldman G, Kahn P, Alon R, et al: Biliary colic treatment and acute cholecystitis prevention by prostaglandin inhibitor. Dig Dis Sci 34:809, 1989.
24. Thornell E, Nilsson B, Jansson R, et al: Effect of short-term indomethacin treatment on the clinical course of acute obstructive cholecystitis. Eur J Surg 15:127, 1991.
25. Yellin A, Berne T, Appleman M, et al: A randomized study of cefepime versus the combination of gentamicin and mezlocillin as an adjunct to surgical treatment in patients with acute cholecystitis. Surg Gynecol Obstet 177(Suppl):23–29; discussion 35–40, 1993.
26. Ohdan H, Oshiro H, Yamamoto Y, et al: Bacteriological investigation of bile in patients with cholelithiasis. Surg Today 23:390–395, 1993.
27. Leung J, Ling T, Chan R, et al: Antibiotics, biliary sepsis, and bile duct stones. Gastrointest Endosc 40:716–721, 1994.
*28. Solomkin JS, Mazuski JE, Baron EJ, et al: Guidelines for the selection of anti-infective agents for complicated intra-abdominal infections. Clin Infect Dis 37:997–1005, 2003.
29. Ransohoff D, Gracie W, Wolfensen L, et al: Prophylactic cholecystectomy or expectant management for silent gallstones. Ann Intern Med 99:199, 1983.
30. Bragg L, Thompson J: Concomitant cholecystectomy for asymptomatic cholelithiasis. Arch Surg 124:460, 1989.
31. Jacir N, Anderson K, Eichelberger M, et al: Cholelithiasis in infancy: resolution of gallstones in three of four infants. J Pediatr Surg 21:567–569, 1986.
32. Ishitani M, Shaul D, Padua E, et al: Choledocholithiasis in a premature neonate. J Pediatr 128:853–855, 1996.
33. Papi C, Catarci M, D'Ambrosio L, et al: Timing of cholecystectomy for acute calculous cholecystitis: a meta-analysis. Am J Gastroenterol 99:147–155, 2004.
34. Kiviluoto T, Siren J, Luukkonen P, et al: Randomised trial of laparoscopic versus open cholecystectomy for acute and gangrenous cholecystitis. Lancet 351:321–325, 1998.
35. Kim P, Wesson D, Superina R, et al: Laparoscopic cholecystectomy versus open cholecystectomy in children: which is better? J Pediatr Surg 30:971–973, 1995.
36. Lo C, Fan S, Liu C, et al: Early decision for conversion of laparoscopic to open cholecystectomy for treatment of acute cholecystitis. Am J Surg 173:513–517, 1997.
37. van den Hazel S, Speelman P, Tytgat G, et al: Role of antibiotics in the treatment and prevention of acute and recurrent cholangitis. Clin Infect Dis 19:279–286, 1994.
38. Lai E, Mok F, Tan E, et al: Endoscopic biliary drainage for severe acute cholangitis. N Engl J Med 326:1582–1586, 1992.
39. Lai E, Tam P, Paterson I, et al: Emergency surgery for severe acute cholangitis: the high-risk patients. Ann Surg 211:55–59, 1990.

*Selected readings.

Urinary Tract Infections in Children and Adolescents

Francis Mencl, MD and Daan Biesbroeck, MD

Key Points

Throughout childhood and adolescence, girls are more likely than boys to experience urinary tract infections.

The signs and symptoms of urinary tract infections are age dependent.

Escherichia coli causes the vast majority of pediatric urinary tract infections.

Most children with pyelonephritis can be treated as outpatients.

Introduction and Background

The urinary tract is a common site of infection for toddlers, school-age children, and adolescents (see Chapter 33, Urinary Tract Infection). Urinary tract infections can occur in any location within the urinary system from the kidney to the distal urethra. It is useful to discuss the urinary system as consisting of an upper tract (i.e., the kidneys and ureters) and a lower tract (i.e., the bladder and urethra). The clinical presentation, evaluation, and management of upper and lower tract infections differ somewhat.

When discussing urinary tract infections, one term that may cause confusion is *pyelonephritis*. The basic definition is rather straightforward. Pyelonephritis is simply inflammation of the kidney and renal pelvis from a bacterial infection.[1] In clinical practice, however, emergency physicians do not typically perform scintigraphy or other tests that can confirm kidney inflammation.[2-5] In older children and adolescents, we assume pyelonephritis is present in the setting of fever, unilateral flank pain, and urinalysis findings consistent with infection. In younger children, flank pain is seldom recognized. It seems that this has led to the use of terms such as *febrile urinary tract infection* for younger children.[6-9] When scintigraphy is performed, renal lesions are seen in 70% to 80% of children with febrile urinary tract infections.[3] From

studies like this, it would appear that most children with concurrent fever and a urinalysis consistent with infection have renal involvement and could properly be categorized as having pyelonephritis. The inconsistent application of the term *pyelonephritis* to young children with febrile urinary tract infections makes reading the relevant literature confusing at times.

Recognition and Approach

Clinical experience suggests that urinary tract infections are common. Remarkably few studies address the epidemiology of these common infections. This is probably because urinary tract infections are not reportable diseases, and most children have uneventful clinical courses. From the available data, it seems quite clear that, outside early infancy, urinary tract infections are substantially more common in girls than boys.[6,7,10-16] From Swedish population-based studies, the cumulative incidence of urinary tract infections during the first 6 to 10 years of life is 3% to 8% for girls and 1% to 2% for boys.[17-19] Although immunocompromised children are more likely than other children to have unusual organisms such as fungi as the etiologic agents for clinically important urinary tract infections,[20-23] *Escherichia coli* is the most common cause of urinary tract infections in all groups of children.[6,10,12-14,24-28] The most common ages to see urinary tract infections in girls are during the toddler years, around the time of toilet training, and adolescence, when sexual activity begins.[25] Recurrent urinary tract infections also appear to be relatively common.[7,25,26]

The anatomic features of the urinary tract make this a site likely to develop relatively frequent infections. The urinary tract is lined with transitional cells that usually form an impermeable lining and create a sterile space. Infection occurs when bacteria enter this space, adhere to the lining, and cause an inflammatory response. The virulence of the bacteria is directly related to their ability to attach and adhere to this lining. It is assumed that host susceptibility plays a role in the development of clinically important infections as well. In particular, girls are thought to be prone to urinary tract infections due to the presence of a relatively short urethra that resides in close proximity to the anus. Although bacteria may frequently enter the bladder, normal voiding is thought to clear these potential pathogens out of the bladder with each episode of voiding. Underlying conditions that disrupt the normal flow of urine out of the bladder place the child at increased risk for a urinary tract infection.

Besides gender, risk factors for urinary tract infections include urinary stasis, diabetes, and race. Conditions that cause urinary stasis include vesicoureteral reflux, posterior ureteral valves, pelvic tumors, bladder diverticuli, urethral strictures or stenosis, phimosis, congenital megaureter and other anatomic abnormalities of the ureter, urethral foreign bodies, renal calculi, renal scarring, and various voiding disorders that require frequent bladder catheterization (e.g., spina bifida).[29,30] Diabetes mellitus increases the risk of urinary tract infections in all age groups, and this may be increasingly important as the prevalence of pediatric diabetes is rising.[31] It would appear that white children are at a higher risk for urinary tract infections than black children.[8,32,33] The reasons for this are unclear.

Clinical Presentation

Signs and Symptoms

Signs and symptoms of urinary tract infections in children can be variable and nonspecific. This is especially true in children who are difficult to assess, including preverbal, developmentally delayed, and technology-dependent children. For all age groups, the exact frequency of various symptoms is unknown. This is most likely because these signs and symptoms are inconsistently reported in studies, have inconsistent definitions, or are used to define inclusion criteria for studies. Malodorous urine may prompt an emergency department visit. Although it is prudent to evaluate these children for urinary tract infections, malodorous urine poorly correlates with urinary tract infections.[24,34]

The overall clinical presentation is age dependent. A nonspecific or sepsis-like presentation is a common manifestation of urinary tract infections in infants (see Chapter 33, Urinary Tract Infection in Infants). Fever appears to be commonly associated with urinary tract infections, particularly in infants and toddlers.[6,7,10,15-17,26,28,35] Toddlers commonly exhibit a "gastrointestinal" presentation that may or may not include fever. Vomiting, diarrhea, or both are often the stated reason for the emergency department visit.[36] Lower abdominal pain with or without vomiting and diarrhea may also be the dominant complaint associated with urinary tract infections in toddlers. In children who have already been successfully toilet trained, enuresis might be the dominant manifestation of a urinary tract infection. School-age children and adolescents most often present with typical "adult" symptoms, including dysuria, hematuria, urinary frequency, and urinary urgency.

Physical Examination

In general, children and adolescents with urinary tract infections have normal physical examinations. At times, however, the physical examination may reveal clinically important findings. For example, palpation of the abdomen might reveal a mass that is partially obstructing normal urinary flow. One such "mass" that might be revealed in this manner is fecal impaction. Visual inspection of the genitalia is useful. In girls, the presence of labial adhesions, clinically appreciable

vulvovaginitis, or visible foreign bodies might reveal secondary causes of urinary tract infections.[37,38]

Urine Testing

Growth of a single urinary pathogen from a culture of an appropriately obtained urine specimen is the criterion standard for making the diagnosis of a urinary tract infection. However, the results of a urine culture are not available during a routine emergency department visit. Therefore, the emergency physician must use alternative, suboptimal, available information to diagnose children with urinary tract infections. This process is imperfect. At best, emergency physicians can identify children highly likely to have clinically important urinary tract infections. Although the history and physical examination may suggest a urinary tract infection, testing of the urine is the primary tool used by emergency physicians to make the diagnosis of urinary tract infections in children. There are two main aspects of urine testing that greatly impact the results. The first is specimen collection. The second is the interpretation of the findings on urine testing.

There are several ways in which a urine specimen can be collected. For children and adolescents, these include using a perineal bag, clean-catch technique, or a urinary catheter. Suprapubic aspiration is another technique used to obtain urine, but is typically only used in young infants[39,40] (see Chapter 33, Urinary Tract Infection in Infants). Commercially available perineal bags are conceptually simple, noninvasive, and inexpensive. A perineal bag is simply a relatively small plastic bag with a circumferential area of adhesive at the top around the opening. The bag can be placed with the opening around the genitalia of a child who is not yet toilet trained. Then, when the child spontaneously voids, the urine is collected in the bag and retrieved at the clinician's convenience. The greatest problem with using urinary bags is that the specimen cannot be used for culture due to perineal contamination.[9,41,42] Some clinicians consider a urinary bag specimen appropriate as a screening tool. It is probably true that, if the urine from a bag specimen shows no evidence of infection on the initial testing available in the emergency department, then a child is very unlikely to have a urinary tract infection. However, if the bag specimen shows any evidence of a urinary tract infection or is inconclusive, then another urine specimen must be obtained for a confirmatory urine culture. This can lead to very inefficient emergency department care and a frustrating experience as it may take quite a long time for a young child to have enough urine accumulate in the bladder for additional testing. Clean-catch urine specimens involve the simple collection of voided urine after appropriate cleaning of the distal urethral opening. Contamination is likely if proper cleaning is not performed. This is the most common technique used for collecting urine from toilet-trained children, adolescent boys, and adolescent girls who are not menstruating. Catheterized urine specimens are most appropriate for infants and toddlers who are not toilet trained, medically complicated children who cannot spontaneously void on command, and menstruating adolescent girls.

Several urinary tests can return useful results during the emergency department visit. These include leukocyte esterase and nitrate tests on the urinary dipstick, the white blood cell count from a microscopic urinalysis of centrifuged sediment, and a Gram stain on a centrifuged specimen. These tests have been studied for predicting a positive urine culture.

The leukocyte esterase test has a sensitivity and specificity of about 80% each.[9] The sensitivity in the emergency department may be somewhat lower.[43-47] The nitrate test is less sensitive (about 50%) but has excellent specificity (about 98%).[9] The presence of white blood cells on microscopic urinalysis has a sensitivity of about 75% and a specificity of about 80%.[9] Detection of bacteria on microscopic urinalysis has a sensitivity and specificity of about 80% each.[9] When leukocyte esterase, nitrate, white blood cells, and bacteria tests are combined such that the overall urinary testing is considered positive for infection if any of them are positive, the sensitivity is nearly 100% and the specificity is about 70%.[9] The tests that provide results during the emergency department visit are imperfect surrogates for a properly collected urine culture.

Blood Tests

Blood testing has a very limited role in the emergency department evaluation of children for urinary tract infections. In particular, blood cultures are frequently negative and, when positive, simply reflect the organism that can be easily identified from the urine culture.[6,35,48-50] The indications for testing renal function and electrolytes are not entirely clear, but clinical dehydration or concerns over impaired renal function are probably reasonable (see Chapter 88, Renal Disorders; and Chapter 110, Dehydration and Disorders of Sodium Balance). One test that recently received substantial attention is a serum procalcitonin level to detect renal parenchymal involvement in children who have urinary tract infections.[51-55] There is no current role for serum procalcitonin levels in children with urinary tract infections in the emergency department.

Pregnancy Testing

For adolescent females, pregnancy testing plays an important role in the evaluation of urinary tract infections. In general, the treatment is more aggressive for the pregnant girl than it would be otherwise. As examples, asymptomatic bacteriuria is often treated with antibiotics and pyelonephritis usually is treated with parenteral antibiotics and admission to the hospital (see Chapter 91, Pregnancy-Related Complications).

Imaging

Imaging studies are rarely indicated in the emergency department. Guidelines published by the American Academy of Pediatrics suggest that a radiographic evaluation is indicated in young children with recurrent or persistent urinary tract infections, to rule out structural anomalies and find sources of infections.[9] However, the timing and type of imaging are controversial. There are no controlled studies properly evaluating or comparing different management strategies, nor do any studies properly address the different age groups. Most studies are descriptive in design and the majority sample children through referral or hospitalization, or with recurrent urinary tract infections. Very few use prospective recruitment.[2]

Important Clinical Features and Considerations

Bubble Bath Urethritis

Despite numerous references to bubble bath urethritis, cystitis, or vaginitis in review articles, textbooks, and the lay press and on the Internet, we found no epidemiologic information in the peer-reviewed literature. This condition appears to be uncommon, with one study of 54 premenarcheal girls with vulvovaginitis reporting a single case attributed to bubble bath use.[56] More cases were attributed to poor hygiene, and one girl had pinworms.[56] It is not clear if bubble baths actually cause dysuria. It is conceivable that this diagnosis is just a convenient term for transient dysuria that would have resolved on its own regardless of whether or not these girls stopped taking bubble baths.

Labial Adhesions

On occasion, an infant girl will have labial adhesions that impede the passage of a urinary catheter to obtain a specimen for testing. Clinical experience suggests that gentle lateral traction can often atraumatically separate these adhesions. If this is unsuccessful, the risks and benefits of obtaining a urine specimen through suprapubic aspiration or interpreting a bag urine specimen during the current emergency department visit will need to be weighed (see Chapter 33, Urinary Tract Infection in Infants). Treatment of the labial adhesions with topical estrogen appears to be effective.[57] The use of topical estrogen will take several days or weeks to release the adhesions.

Sexually Transmitted Diseases

In sexually active adolescents, acute uncomplicated urinary tract infection needs to be differentiated from urethritis, cervicitis, and vaginitis (see Chapter 70, Sexually Transmitted Diseases). Urethritis symptoms are generally milder than those seen with urinary tract infections, demonstrate a more gradual onset, and test positive for *Chlamydia trachomatis*, *Neisseria gonorrhoeae*, or herpes simplex virus. Patients with vaginitis generally complain of vaginal discharge, dyspareunia, and pruritus. *Candida* or *Trichomonas vaginalis* are frequently responsible. These findings in a young child or in an adolescent who has not yet initiated sexual activity should raise suspicion of sexual abuse (see Chapter 118, Sexual Abuse).[58]

Missed Appendicitis

A low-grade pyuria may be seen in cases of appendicitis. Children who have abdominal tenderness and a few white cells in their urine on microscopic urinalysis may have appendicitis. Familiarity with identifying these children is very helpful in avoiding mistakenly diagnosing a child who has appendicitis with a urinary tract infection (see Chapter 73, Appendicitis).[59,60]

Management

The management of acute pediatric urinary tract infections is generally straightforward. The primary decisions that have to be made are determining if the child should be admitted to the hospital and selecting an appropriate empirical antibiotic. Based on clinical experience, the most common reason to admit a previously healthy child with an acute urinary tract infection to the hospital is concurrent, intractable vomiting (Table 86-1). Pyelonephritis is not an indication for admission in most children.

Antibiotic selection is primarily based on the local resistance patterns and cost. Antibiotic resistance is a continuing

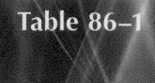

Table 86–1	Admission Criteria for Children with Proven or Suspected Urinary Tract Infections

Associated kidney stone with ureteral obstruction
Concurrent illness requiring admission
Diabetes mellitus
Documented severe reflux
Family challenges precluding successful outpatient therapy
Immunocompromised state
Intractable vomiting
Outpatient treatment failure
Pregnancy and fever (with or without flank pain)
Renal failure
Severe and frequent recurrent infections
Shock
Solitary kidney or single functioning kidney
Transplant recipient

concern.[11,13,61,62] Since urine culture results are not available during the first emergency department visit, antibiotics will have to be selected empirically. Commonly selected antibiotics include cephalexin (25 mg/kg per dose given 3 or 4 times per day), nitrofurantoin (5 mg/kg per dose given twice a day), and trimethoprim-sulfamethoxazole (5 mg/kg per dose given twice daily with dosing based on the trimethoprim component). For children selected for outpatient treatment, the addition of a dose of parenteral antibiotics in the emergency department prior to discharge does not improve the clinical outcome.[6,15,26,63,64] The duration of outpatient therapy for acute urinary tract infections in children is controversial.[63-65] The traditional approach is to have a young child with a urinary tract infection be prescribed at least 7 days of oral antibiotics. During this week, the child is to follow up with the primary care physician, who will arrange for imaging studies of the urinary tract. If the child has abnormal anatomy, he or she is typically placed on prophylactic antibiotics until a pediatric urologist evaluates him or her for surgical repair of the abnormal anatomy. There have been no new practice guidelines to suggest an alternative course of action, but the utility of this approach for first urinary tract infections has been questioned.[5] Older school-age girls and adolescents are often treated with short, 3- to 5-day courses of oral antibiotics in a manner similar to adult women.

Summary

Pediatric urinary tract infections can be difficult to diagnose. The symptoms in the very young, developmentally delayed, medically complicated, immunocompromised, or technology-dependent child might be vague or suggestive of alternative, incorrect diagnoses. The tools available to diagnose urinary tract infections in the emergency department are imperfect. Although multiple antibiotics are effective for treating acute urinary tract infections, antibiotic resistance is a continuing concern.[11,13,61,62] Most patients can be treated as outpatients with appropriate follow-up with their primary care physician. Recurrent infections are common, but the clinical significance and long-term sequelae of untreated or recurrent urinary tract infections are unknown. The prognosis for children with urinary tract infections is usually excellent.

REFERENCES

1. Anderson DM, Novak PD, Keith J, et al: Dorland's Illustrated Medical Dictionary, 30th ed. Philadelphia: WB Saunders, 2003, p 1549.
2. Dick PT, Feldman W: Routine diagnostic imaging for childhood urinary tract infections: a systematic overview. J Pediatr 128:15–22, 1996.
3. Benador D, Benador N, Slosman D, et al: Are younger children at highest risk of renal sequelae after pyelonephritis? Lancet 349:17–19, 1997.
4. Zamir G, Sakran W, Horowitz Y, et al: Urinary tract infection: is there a need for routine renal ultrasonography? Arch Dis Child 89:398–399, 2004.
*5. Hoberman A, Charron M, Hickey RW, et al: Imaging studies after a first febrile urinary tract infection in young children. N Engl J Med 348:195–202, 2003.
6. Nelson DS, Gurr MB, Schunck JE: Management of febrile children with urinary tract infections. Am J Emerg Med 16:643–647, 1998.
7. Mingin GC, Hinds A, Nguyen HT, et al: Children with a febrile urinary tract infection and a negative radiologic workup: factors predictive of recurrence. Urology 63:562–565, 2004.
*8. Shaw KN, Gorelick M, McGowan KL, et al: Prevalence of urinary tract infections in febrile young children in the emergency department. Pediatrics 102:e16, 1998.
*9. Practice parameter: The diagnosis, treatment, and evaluation of the initial urinary tract infection in febrile infants and young children. American Academy of Pediatrics, Committee on Quality Improvement, Subcommittee on Urinary Tract Infection. Pediatrics 103(4 Pt 1):843–852, 1999. [Published errata in Pediatrics 105(1 Pt 1):141, 2000; Pediatrics 103(5 Pt 1):1052, 1999; and Pediatrics 104(1 Pt 1):118, 1999.]
10. Halevy R, Smolkin V, Bykov S, et al: Power Doppler ultrasonography in the diagnosis of acute childhood pyelonephritis. Pediatr Nephrol 19:987–991, 2004.
11. Haller M, Brandis M, Berner R: Antibiotic resistance of urinary tract pathogens and rationale for empirical intravenous therapy. Pediatr Nephrol 19:982–986, 2004.
12. Pape L, Gunzer F, Ziesing S, et al: Bacterial pathogens, resistance patterns and treatment options in community acquired pediatric urinary tract infection [German]. Klin Padiatr 216:83–86, 2004.
13. McLoughlin TG, Joseph MM: Antibiotic resistance patterns of uropathogens in pediatric emergency department patients. Acad Emerg Med 10:347–351, 2003.
14. Sakran W, Miron D, Halavy R, et al: Community acquired urinary tract infection among hospitalized children in Northern Israel: pathogens, susceptibility patterns and urinary tract anomalies [Hebrew]. Harefuah 142:269–271, 2003.
15. Baker PC, Nelson DS, Schunk JE: The addition of ceftriaxone to oral therapy does not improve outcome in febrile children with urinary tract infections. Arch Pediatr Adolesc Med 155:135–139, 2001.
16. Wennerstrom M, Hanson S, Jodal U, et al: Primary and acquired renal scarring in boys and girls with urinary tract infection. J Pediatr 136:50–54, 2000.
17. Marild S, Jodal U: Incidence rate of first-time symptomatic urinary tract infection in children under 6 years of age. Acta Paediatr 87:549–552, 1998.
18. Hellstrom A-L, Hanson E, Hanson S, et al: Association between urinary symptoms at 7 years old and previous urinary tract infection. Arch Dis Child 66:232–234, 1991.
19. Winburg J, Anderson H, Bergstrom T, et al: Epidemiology of symptomatic urinary tract infection in childhood. Acta Paediatr Scand 63(Suppl 252):1–20, 1974.
20. Ashram K, Bhimma R, Adhikari M: Human immunodeficiency virus and urinary tract infections in children. Ann Trop Paediatr 23:273–277, 2003.
21. Rongkavilit C, Rodriguez ZM, Gomez-Marin O, et al: Gram-negative bacillary bacteremia in human immunodeficiency virus type 1-infected children. Pediatr Infect Dis J 19:122–128, 2000.
22. Ruiz-Contreras J, Ramos JT, Hernandez-Sampelayo TH, et al: Sepsis in children with human immunodeficiency virus infection. Pediatr Infect Dis J 14:522–526, 1995.

*Selected readings.

23. Langley JM, Hanakowski M, LeBlanc JC: Unique epidemiology of nosocomial urinary tract infection in children. Am J Infect Control 29:94–98, 2001.

24. Struthers S, Scanlon J, Parker K, et al: Parental reporting of smelly urine and urinary tract infection. Arch Dis Child 88:250–252, 2003.

25. Nguyen H, Weir M: Urinary tract infection as a possible marker for teenage sex. South Med J 95:867–869, 2002.

26. Benadour D, Neuhaus TJ, Papazyan J-P, et al: Randomized controlled trial of three day versus 10 day intravenous antibiotics in acute pyelonephritis: effect on renal scarring. Arch Dis Child 84:241–246, 2001.

27. Nuutinen M, Uhari M: Recurrence and follow-up after urinary tract infection under the age of 1. Pediatr Nephrol 16:69–72, 2001.

*28. Craig JC, Knight JF, Sureshkumar P, et al: Effect of circumcision on incidence of urinary tract infection in preschool boys. J Pediatr 128:23–27, 1996.

29. Altieri IMF, Camarca MA, Bock GH: Pediatric urinary tract infections. Emerg Med Rep 19:1–8, 1998.

30. Shapiro E, Elder JS: The office management of recurrent urinary tract infection and vesicoureteral reflux in children. Pediatr Clin North Am 25:725–734, 1998.

31. Libman I, Arslanian SA: Type II diabetes mellitus: no longer just adults. Pediatr Ann 28:589–593, 1999.

32. Chand DH, Rhoades T, Poe SA, et al: Incidence and severity of vesicoureteral reflux in children related to age gender, race and diagnosis. J Urol 170(4 Pt 2):1548–1550, 2003.

33. Keeton JE, Hillis RS: Urinary tract infections in black female children. Urology 6:39–42, 1975.

34. Nayir A: Circumcision for the prevention of significant bacteriuria in boys. Pediatr Nephrol 16:1129–1134, 2001.

35. Pitetti RD, Choi S: Utility of blood cultures in febrile children with UTI. Am J Emerg Med 20:271–274, 2002.

36. Buchta RM, Dunn M: Urinary tract infection due to *Salmonella* species in children/adolescents. Clin Pediatr (Phila) 42:647–648, 2003.

37. Stricker T, Navratil F, Sennhauser FH: Vaginal foreign bodies. J Paediatr Child Health 40:205–207, 2004.

38. Smith YR, Berman DR, Quint EH: Premenarchal vaginal discharge: findings of procedures to rule out foreign bodies. J Pediatr Adolesc Gynecol 15:227–230, 2002.

39. Munir V, Barnett P, South M: Does the use of volumetric bladder ultrasound improve the success rate of supraapubic aspiration of urine? Pediatr Emerg Care 18:346–349, 2002.

40. Chu RW, Wong YC, Luk SH, et al: Comparing suprapubic urine aspiration under real-time ultrasound guidance with conventional blind aspiration. Acta Paediatr 91:512–516, 2002.

41. Li PS, Ma LC, Wong SN: Is bag urine culture useful in monitoring urinary tract infection infants? J Paediatr Child Health 38:377–381, 2003.

42. Al-Orifi F, McGillivray D, Tangs S, et al: Urine culture from bag specimens in young children: are the risks too high? J Pediatr 137:221–226, 2000.

43. Novak R, Powell K, Christopher N: Optimal diagnostic testing for urinary tract infection in young children. Pediatr Dev Pathol 7:226–230, 2004.

44. Pugia MJ, Sommer R, Corey P, et al: The Uristatin dipstick is useful in distinguishing upper respiratory from urinary tract infections. Clin Chim Acta 341:73–81, 2004.

45. Leman P: Validity of urinalysis and microscopy for detecting urinary tract infection in the emergency department. Eur J Emerg Med 9:141–147, 2002.

46. Huicho L, Campos-Sanchez M, Alamos C, et al: Metaanalysis of urine screening tests for determining the risk of urinary tract infection in children. Pediatr Infect Dis J 21:1–11, 2002.

47. Armengol CE, Hendley JO, Schlager TA: Should we abandon standard microscopy when screening for urinary tract infections in young children? Pediatr Infect Dis J 20:1176–1177, 2001.

48. Velasco M, Martinez JA, Moreno-Martinez A, et al: Blood cultures for women with uncomplicated acute pyelonephritis: are they necessary? Clin Infect Dis 37:1127–1130, 2003.

49. Pasternak EL, Topinka MA: Blood cultures in pyelonephritis: do results change therapy? Acad Emerg Med 7:1170, 2000.

50. McMurray BR, Wrenn KD, Wright SW: Usefulness of blood cultures in pyelonephritis. Am J Emerg Med 15:137–140, 1997.

51. Smolkin V, Koren A, Raz R, et al: Procalcitonin as a marker of acute pyelonephritis in infants and children. Pediatr Nephrol 17:409–412, 2002.

52. Gervaix A, Galetto-Lacour A, Gueron T, et al: Usefulness of procalcitonin and C-reactive protein rapid tests for the management of children with urinary tract infection. Pediatr Infect Dis J 20:507–511, 2001.

53. Pecile P, Miorin E, Romanello C, et al: Procalcitonin: a marker of severity of acute pyelonephritis among children. Pediatrics 114:e249–e254, 2004.

54. Prat C, Dominguez J, Rodrigo C, et al: Elevated serum procalcitonin values correlate with renal scarring in children with urinary tract infection. Pediatr Infect Dis J 22:438–442, 2003.

55. Benador N, Siegrist CA, Gendrel D, et al: Procalcitonin is a marker of severity of renal lesions in pyelonephritis. Pediatrics 102:1422–1425, 1998.

56. Paradise JE, Campos JM, Friedman HM, et al: Vulvovaginitis in premenarchal girls: clinical features and diagnostic evaluation. Pediatrics 70:193–198, 1982.

57. Leung AK, Robinson WL, Kao CP, et al: Treatment of labial fusion with topical estrogen therapy. Clin Pediatr (Phila) 44:245–247, 2005.

58. Siegel RM, Schubert CJ, Myers PA, et al: The prevalence of sexually transmitted diseases in children and adolescents evaluated for sexual abuse in Cincinnati: rationale for limited STD testing in prepubertal girls. Pediatrics 96:1090–1094, 1995.

59. Puskar D, Bedalov G, Fridrith S, et al: Urinalysis, ultrasound analysis, and renal dynamic scintigraphy in acute appendicitis. Urology 45:108–112, 1995.

60. Scott JH, Amin M, Harty JI: Abnormal urinalysis in appendicitis. J Urol 129:1015, 1983.

61. Karlowsky JA, Kelly LJ, Thornsberry C, et al: Trends in antimicrobial resistance among urinary tract infection isolates of *Escherichia coli* from female outpatients in the United States. Antimicrob Agents Chemother 46:2540–2545, 2002.

62. Kahlmeter G: The ECO-SENS project: a prospective, multinational, multicentre epidemiological survey of the prevalence of urinary tract pathogens—interim report. J Antimicrob Chemother 46(Suppl 1):15–22, 2000.

*63. Tran D, Muchant DG, Aronoff SC: Short-course versus conventional therapy for uncomplicated lower urinary tract infections in children: a meta-analysis of 1279 patients. J Pediatr 139:93–99, 2001.

64. Keren R, Chan E: A meta-analysis of randomized controlled trials comparing short- and long-course antibiotic therapy for urinary tract infection in children. Pediatrics 109:e70, 2002.

65. Michael M, Hodson EM, Craig JC, et al: Short versus standard duration oral antibiotic therapy for acute urinary tract infection in children. Cochrane Database Syst Rev (1):CD003966, 2003.

Chapter 87

Testicular Torsion

Martin I. Herman, MD

Key Points

Early recognition of testicular torsion is important to a successful outcome as testicular viability may be lost within hours of the onset of torsion.

Manual or surgical detorsion is required to relieve testicular torsion.

Testicular torsion is one of several causes of the "acute scrotum," and ultrasound is currently the preferred imaging modality for making a definitive diagnosis.

Although most boys with testicular torsion presenting to the emergency department are adolescents, torsion may occur at any age.

Introduction and Background

Testicular torsion (i.e., twisting of the spermatic cord) is one of the three most common causes of the "acute scrotum."[1] In prior decades, testicular torsion commonly led to testicular necrosis. Orchiectomy rates as high as 90% were common prior to the 1960s. By the 1980s, testicular loss due to torsion dropped to 33% of identified cases.[2] Unfortunately, as of the late 1990s, the rate of orchiectomy following testicular torsion has remained at approximately 33%.[3] A key role for emergency physicians is to expeditiously recognize boys with testicular torsion so that prompt treatment may be rendered. As in other conditions involving ischemia, "time is tissue."

Recognition and Approach

The epidemiology of testicular torsion can be somewhat confusing. This is especially true when cases of testicular torsion involving an undescended testis and cases in very young infants are included. Testicular torsion is not a reportable diagnosis and does not lead to a publicly visible problem, debilitating morbidity, or mortality if untreated. Because of this, there may be cases of testicular torsion that go unrecognized. Reported rates range from 1 in 4000 males younger than 25 years[2] to 1 in more than 22,000 males between 1 and 25 years of age.[3] The age distribution of cases of testicular torsion is bimodal, with peaks in early infancy and in adolescence. More than half of all cases of testicular torsion occur in adolescents.[2]

During embryonic development, the testes descend from the abdomen and enter the scrotum through the inguinal canal. The peritoneum invaginates into the scrotum and forms a sac, the tunica vaginalis. The tunica vaginalis envelops the testicle and epididymis partially or completely. Normally, the tunica surrounds only part of the testicle and epididymis, leaving the posterior aspect of the epididymis and the superior pole of the testis able to attach to the posterior wall of the scrotum. If the tunica surrounds the entire complex and attaches higher up on the cord structures, the testicle does not become fixed to the posterior scrotal wall and is left free to twist upon its vertical axis. This twisting disrupts the blood supply to the testis.

Several risk factors have been identified for testicular torsion. These include spasm of the cremaster muscle and increased gonad size due to a surge in testosterone level, cold weather,[4] scrotal trauma,[5] or bicycling.[6] In a recent study, age was the sole identifiable risk factor for orchiectomy in cases of testicular torsion.[3]

Clinical Presentation

Infants with torsion usually present with a painless, swollen scrotum that does not transilluminate. Typically, the testicle has already necrosed and orchiectomy is indicated. Adolescent boys typically present with a history of sudden, severe scrotal and lower abdominal pain. A history of heavy exercise or seemingly minor blunt trauma is often elicited. In the setting of an acute scrotum, nausea and vomiting have been reported to have a high positive predictive value for testicular torsion, but only modest sensitivity.[7] Fever is uncommon. Many adolescent boys diagnosed with testicular torsion will admit to having had prior similar pain episodes that resolved without treatment.[8]

In addition to testicular tenderness, emergency physicians may find an elevated testicle with a palpable twist, an abnormal axis of the testicle, an abnormal scrotal position of the epididymis, or an abnormal testicular axis when compared to the contralateral testis. The presence of any of these findings is highly suggestive of testicular torsion.[8] Absence of the cremasteric reflex is also suggestive of testicular torsion, but it is normal for this reflex to be absent in boys younger than

30 months.[9-11] Unfortunately, physical examination findings may be unreliable as the position of the epididymis may seem normal if the torsion involves 360 or 720 degrees of rotation. The epididymis-testis interface can be obscured by pain or swelling. Relief of pain by elevating the scrotum (i.e., Prehn's sign), indicative of epididymitis, is unreliable. Pyuria, also suggestive of epididymitis, may be present in 30% of males with testicular torsion. Clinical experience suggests the only reliable sign ruling out testicular torsion is the presence of a cremaster reflex.

When the diagnosis cannot confidently be made on the basis of history and physical examination, urgent scintigraphy, ultrasound, or magnetic resonance imaging (MRI) of the scrotum is typically indicated. In fact, in one study, up to 50% of patients with an acute scrotum were misdiagnosed when the examiners relied solely on the physical examination to make their diagnosis.[12] Since it was first advocated in 1973, scintigraphy has been the preferred imaging procedure for the acute scrotum. Scintigraphy provides high sensitivity and specificity in detecting testicular torsion.[13] However, exposure to radionuclides, poor after-hours availability, equipment complexity, and length of examination times has limited the usefulness of this technique for emergency department patients with suspected testicular torsion. In contrast, ultrasound poses no exposure to ionizing radiation, is more widely available, allows the sonographer to obtain fairly detailed images of scrotal anatomy, and also has high sensitivity and specificity.[14-17] Color Doppler ultrasound is used to detect blood flow to the testes. Unfortunately, color Doppler ultrasound is quite user dependent. In one study of asymptomatic boys, bilateral blood flow, although almost certainly present in all of them, was detected in only 58%.[10] Color Doppler ultrasound is now more commonly used than scintigraphy.[16,19] The factors most likely to determine the selection of imaging study are the time frame in which the study can be performed and the experience of the examiner in interpreting the results.[16] Emergency physicians are increasingly performing bedside ultrasound in the emergency department (see Chapter 179, Ultrasonography). Although described in the literature,[20,21] the performance of bedside ultrasound by emergency physicians to evaluate patients for testicular torsion is not a standard procedure. MRI can be used to quantify testicular perfusion and evaluate the scrotal contents.[22,23] The use of MRI to evaluate children with an acute scrotum is uncommon. This is most likely due to limited availability, the common need for sedation, and prolonged scanning times.[24]

Important Clinical Features and Considerations

Pitfalls to the diagnosis occur because not all patients have the typical history or findings on examination. Testicular torsion may be painless in as many as 10% of cases, particularly in young infants. Intermittent torsion may occur, resulting in intermittent episodes of pain and a normal ultrasound and physical examination at the time of presentation to the emergency department. Location of the pain may be abdominal rather than scrotal. This is particularly true in cases of undescended testes.[25] A history of sexual activity or significant pyuria, more typically seen with epididymitis, may be seen in cases of testicular torsion. Any or all of these may mislead the examiner, leading to a delayed or missed diagnosis.[26]

Delaying a diagnosis or missing the diagnosis of testicular torsion can result in decreased spermatogenesis and testicular atrophy with complete resorption of the testis later in life.[2,27-31] Spermatogenesis can be impaired after as little as an hour of ischemia.[31] Semen and endocrine function may be preserved if blood flow is returned to the testis within about 12 hours.[27] Although not intuitively obvious, testicular torsion may affect the contralateral testis. The etiology of this deleterious effect is unknown but is currently being pursued through animal studies.[32] One theory is that antispermatozoa antibodies are developed and affect spermatogenesis in the contralateral testis.[30,33] This can limit future fertility. Medical malpractice issues also arise in the setting of a delayed or missed diagnosis of testicular torsion. An analysis of medical liability insurance data from New Jersey revealed a mean indemnity payment of $60,191 in cases of missed testicular torsion.[34] Unfortunately, many adolescent boys present too late for gonadal salvage.[28,35]

Management

Detorsion (i.e., physical untwisting of the spermatic cord) is the only way to return blood flow to a testis involved in testicular torsion. Most other causes of an acute scrotum are readily treatable with analgesics or antibiotics (see Chapter 89, Penile and Testicular Disorders). The main diagnosis to identify or exclude is testicular torsion. Once torsion is identified, testis survival is dependent on two primary factors, the duration of the torsion and the tightness of the twist.[30,36]

Manual detorsion is an important intervention for emergency physicians to be able to perform. If a twist in the cord can be felt on examination or the testicular axis is clearly abnormal and the boy has had pain for fewer than 12 hours, manual detorsion by the emergency physician is indicated.[3,20,30,36,37] Manual detorsion can provide immediate relief of pain, increase the chance for testicular survival, and minimize the risk of immunologic injury to the contralateral testis.[38-40] Torsions typically twist medially. Hence, rotating the testicle laterally will untwist the cord and bring pain relief. If the clinician is standing at the foot of the bed, facing the boy, the right testis would undergo detorsion by twisting it counterclockwise. The left testis would undergo detorsion by twisting it clockwise. It may be necessary to repeat the derotation procedure as spermatic cords twist as many as three times around. Detorsion should be repeated until pain is relieved and the testis returns to a normal anatomic position. On occasion, a testicular torsion will twist laterally. In these instances, the usual detorsion technique will result in increased resistance and pain. Obviously, attempts at detorsion in the opposite direction are indicated.[41] If available at the bedside, ultrasound can be used to monitor detorsion efforts, documenting the return of blood flow to the testis.[38,42] Surgical confirmation should follow immediately as testicular infarctions have been noted after manual detorsion was performed.[43] For patients with pain for more than 12 hours, observation and symptomatic treatment may be all that is needed, but this decision must be made after surgical consultation since intermittent torsion is always a possibility.[37,44] Color Doppler ultrasound may be prudent in these cases to investigate alternative diagnoses.

Adjunctive therapy to minimize reperfusion injury or immunologic damage to the salvaged testicle and contralateral testicle has been studied. When allopurinol, dexamethasone, or free radical scavengers have been given prior to detorsion, each has demonstrated some protective effect.[45-48] However, more study is needed before incorporating pharmaceutical adjuncts into the emergency department management of testicular torsion.

Summary

Emergent urologic consultation to assess the need for scrotal exploration is indicated when the history and physical examination strongly suggest testicular torsion. Manual detorsion may provide immediate relief of pain and restore blood flow at least temporarily. Imaging studies should be reserved for cases for which there is diagnostic uncertainty. Delaying the surgeon's evaluation or impeding the patient's transport to the operating room by waiting for results of imaging studies in cases with a high probability of the child having testicular torsion should be avoided. Testicular salvage and potential future fertility depend on a timely restoration of blood flow to the involved testis.

REFERENCES

1. McAndrew HF, Pemberton R, Kikiros CS, et al: The incidence and investigation of acute scrotal problems in children. Pediatr Surg Int 18:435–437, 2002.
*2. Anderson JB, Williamson RC: Testicular torsion in Bristol: a 25-year review. Br J Surg 75:988–992, 1988.
3. Mansbach JM, Forbes P, Peters C: Testicular torsion and risk factors for orchiectomy. Arch Pediatr Adolesc Med 159:1167–1171, 2005.
4. Shukla RB, Kelly DG, Daly L, et al: Association of cold weather with testicular torsion. Br Med J 285:1459–1460, 1982.
5. Elsaharty S, Pranikoff K, Magoss IV, et al: Traumatic torsion of the testis. J Urol 132:1155–1156, 1984.
6. Cos LR, Rabinowitz R: Trauma-induced testicular torsion in children. J Trauma 22:244–246, 1982.
7. Jefferson RH, Perez LM, Joseph DB: Critical analysis of the clinical presentation of acute scrotum: a 9-year experience at a single institution. J Urol 158:1198–1200, 1997.
8. Knight PJ, Vassy LE: The diagnosis and treatment of the acute scrotum in children and adolescents. Ann Surg 200:664–673, 1984.
*9. Rabinowitz R: The importance of the cremasteric reflex in acute scrotal swelling in children. J Urol 132:89–90, 1984.
10. Caldamone AA, Valvo JR, Altebarmakian VK, et al: Acute scrotal swelling in children. J Pediatr Surg 19:581–584, 1984.
11. Caesar RE, Kaplan GW: The incidence of the cremasteric reflex in normal boys. J Urol 152:779–780, 1994.
12. Melekos MD, Asbach HW, Markou SA: Etiology of acute scrotum in 100 boys with regard to age distribution. J Urol 139:1023–1025, 1988.
13. Valvo JR, Caldamone AA, O'Mara R, et al: Nuclear imaging in the pediatric acute scrotum. Am J Dis Child 136:831–835, 1982.
14. Middleton WD, Middleton MA, Dierks M, et al: Sonographic prediction of viability in testicular torsion: preliminary observations. J Ultrasound Med 16:23–27, 1997.
*15. Atkinson GO Jr, Patrick LE, Ball TI Jr, et al: The normal and abnormal scrotum in children: evaluation with color Doppler sonography. AJR Am J Roentgenol 158:613–617, 1992.
16. Middleton WD, Siegel BA, Melson GL, et al: Acute scrotal disorders: prospective comparison of color Doppler US and testicular scintigraphy. Radiology 177:177–181, 1990.
17. Lerner RM, Mevorach RA, Hulbert WC, et al: Color Doppler US in the evaluation of acute scrotal disease. Radiology 176:355–358, 1990.
18. Ingram S, Hollman AS: Colour Doppler sonography of the normal paediatric testis. Clin Radiol 49:266–267, 1994.
19. Nussbaum Blask AR, Bulas D, Shalaby-Rana E, et al: Color Doppler sonography and scintigraphy of the testis: a prospective, comparative

analysis in children with acute scrotal pain. Pediatr Emerg Care 18:67–71, 2002.
20. Blaivas M, Batts M, Lambert M: Ultrasonographic diagnosis of testicular torsion by emergency physicians. Am J Emerg Med 18:198–200, 2000.
*21. Blaivas M, Sierzenski P, Lambert M: Emergency evaluation of patients presenting with acute scrotum using bedside ultrasonography. Acad Emerg Med 8:90–93, 2001.
22. Costabile RA, Choyke PL, Frank JA, et al: Dynamic enhanced magnetic resonance imaging of testicular perfusion in the rat. J Urol 149:1195–1197, 1993.
23. Landa HM, Gylys-Morin V, Mattery RF, et al: Detection of testicular torsion by magnetic resonance imaging in a rat model. J Urol 140:1178–1180, 1988.
24. Sidhu PS: Clinical and imaging features of testicular torsion: role of ultrasound. Clin Radiol 54:343–352, 1999.
25. Assassa GS, Siegel ME, Chen D, et al: Missed torsion of an undescended testicle detected by testicular scintigraphy. Clin Nucl Med 18:1024–1025, 1993.
26. Lewis AG, Bukowski TP, Jarvis PD, et al: Evaluation of acute scrotum in the emergency department. J Pediatr Surg 30:277–282, 1995.
27. Anderson MJ, Dunn JK, Lipshultz LI, et al: Semen quality and endocrine parameters after acute testicular torsion. J Urol 147:1545–1550, 1992.
*28. Barada JH, Weingarten JL, Cromie WJ: Testicular salvage and age-related delay in the presentation of testicular torsion. J Urol 142:746–748, 1989.
29. Thomas WE, Williamson RC: Diagnosis and outcome of testicular torsion. Br J Surg 70:213–216, 1983.
30. Tryfonas G, Violaki A, Tsikopoulos G, et al: Late postoperative results in males treated for testicular torsion during childhood. J Pediatr Surg 29:553–556, 1994.
31. Turner TT, Brown KJ: Spermatic cord torsion: loss of spermatogenesis despite return of blood flow. Biol Reprod 49:401–407, 1993.
32. Ozkan KU, Kucukaydin M, Muhtaroglu S, et al: Evaluation of contralateral testicular damage after unilateral testicular torsion by serum inhibin B levels. J Pediatr Surg 36:1050–1053, 2001.
33. Kosar A, Kupeli B, Alcigir G, et al: Immunologic aspect of testicular torsion: detection of antisperm antibodies in contralateral testicle. Eur Urol 36:640–644, 1999.
34. Matteson JR, Stock JA, Hanna MK, et al: Medicolegal aspects of testicular torsion. Urology 57:783–787, 2001.
35. Bennett S, Nicholson MS, Little TM: Torsion of the testis: why is the prognosis so poor? Br Med J 294:824, 1987.
36. Cummings JM, Boullier JA, Sekhon D, et al: Adult testicular torsion. J Urol 167:2109–2110, 2002.
*37. Hastie KJ, Charlton CAC: Indications for conservative management of acute scrotal pain in children. Br J Surg 77:309–311, 1990.
38. Garel L, Dubois J, Azzie G, et al: Preoperative manual detorsion of the spermatic cord with Doppler ultrasound monitoring in patients with intravaginal acute testicular torsion. Pediatr Radiol 30:41–44, 2000.
39. Cattolica EV: Preoperative manual detorsion of the torsed spermatic cord. J Urol 133:803–805, 1985.
40. Cornel EB, Karthaus HFM: Manual derotation of the twisted spermatic cord. BJU Int 83:672–674, 1999.
*41. Sessions AE, Rabinowitz R, Hulbert WC, et al: Testicular torsion: direction, degree, duration and disinformation. J Urol 169:663–665, 2003.
42. Betts JM, Norris M, Cromie WJ, et al: Testicular detorsion using Doppler ultrasound monitoring. J Pediatr Surg 18:607–610, 1983.
43. Haynes BE, Haynes VE: Manipulative detorsion: beware the twist that does not turn. J Urol 137:118–119, 1987.
44. Kass EJ, Stone KT, Cacciarelli AA, et al: Do all children with an acute scrotum require exploration? J Urol 150:667–669, 1993.
45. Akgur FM, Kilinc K, Aktug T, et al: The effect of allopurinol pretreatment before detorsing testicular torsion. J Urol 151:1715–1717, 1994.
46. Bozlu M, Coskun B, Cayan S, et al: Inhibition of poly(adenosine diphosphate-ribose) polymerase decreases long-term histologic damage in testicular ischemia-reperfusion injury. Urology 63:791–795, 2004.
47. Can C, Tore F, Tuncel N, et al: Protective effect of vasoactive intestinal peptide on testicular torsion-detorsion injury: association with heparin-containing mast cells. Urology 63:195–200, 2004.
48. Yazawa H, Sasagawa I, Suzuki Y, et al: Glucocorticoid hormone can suppress apoptosis of rat testicular germ cells induced by testicular ischemia. Fertil Steril 75:980–985, 2001.

---

*Selected readings.

Chapter 88

Renal Disorders

Suzanne M. Beno, MD

Key Points

Kidney stones are uncommon in children and do not typically present with dramatic renal colic.

Glomerulonephritis leads to hypertension, while nephrotic syndrome leads to hypotension.

Renal tubular acidosis is a rare but well-described cause of a non–anion gap acidosis in children.

Selected Diagnoses

Acute renal failure
Chronic renal failure
Poststreptococcal glomerulonephritis
Nephrotic syndrome
Kidney stones
Human immunodeficiency virus–associated nephropathy
Renal tubular acidosis
Hypertension
Renal transplantation

Discussion of Individual Diagnoses

Acute Renal Failure

Acute renal failure is an acute reduction in renal function characterized by an increase in creatinine and nitrogenous waste products, as well as a reduced ability to appropriately regulate fluid and electrolyte homeostasis. Acute renal failure can appear de novo or can arise in the setting of preexisting renal dysfunction. Advances in technology and improvement of care have shifted the epidemiology of acute renal failure. Previously, the most common etiologies of acute renal failure were hemolytic-uremic syndrome, intrinsic renal disease, burns, and sepsis.[1] More recently, acute renal failure is most commonly a comorbidity of underlying or systemic disease[1] (Table 88–1). The incidence of acute renal failure is highest in critically ill neonates, infants with congenital heart disease, and recipients of bone marrow or solid organ transplants.[2] Oncologic complications are now a more frequent cause of acute renal failure than sepsis.

Clinical Presentation

The clinical presentation of acute renal failure is variable, somewhat age dependent, and strongly influenced by the underlying comorbid disorder. The variable presentation can typically be intuited from the general pathophysiologic processes the child is experiencing. When a hypertensive emergency develops, the dominant presentation may be that of congestive heart failure or encephalopathy with altered mental status or seizures (see Chapter 65, Hypertensive Emergencies). Due to fluid and electrolyte disturbances, cardiac dysrhythmias from hyperkalemia or seizures from hyponatremia may be prominent components of the clinical presentation. Children with acute renal failure are at increased risk of serious infections, and the presentation may be dominated by a comorbid infection. Anemia may lead to weakness and pallor. In addition, the likelihood of various specific diagnoses is somewhat age dependent. Urinary obstruction from posterior urethral valves is seen in neonates. Cortical necrosis and renal vein thrombosis occur more commonly in neonates. Hemolytic-uremic syndrome is most often seen in young children. Rapidly progressive glomerulonephritis generally occurs in older children and adolescents. Compared to adults, children frequently develop severe multiorgan system failure early in their course of illness.[3]

Various diagnostic tests are used in the diagnosis and management of acute renal failure. If the child still produces urine, a urinalysis provides useful information regarding urinary casts, can identify coexisting urinary tract infection or hematuria, and provides a specimen for additional testing (e.g., urinary electrolytes). Obviously, blood tests such as a serum blood urea nitrogen (BUN) and creatinine are useful in assessing overall renal function. Serum electrolytes can identify hyperkalemia and hyponatremia, which are commonly seen in acute renal failure. A complete blood count can determine the degree to which the child is anemic. A chest radiograph is useful for identifying pulmonary edema and assessing the size of the cardiac silhouette. An electrocardiogram may be useful for definitively characterizing cardiac dysrythmias. Although infrequently obtained in the emergency department, an echocardiogram is useful for identifying pericardial effusions and assessing overall cardiac pump function. A renal ultrasound is a quick, noninvasive study that can assess kidney size and identify hydronephrosis. Other imaging studies, including a dimercaptosuccinic acid scan, voiding cystouretethrogram, technetium-99m–labeled mercaptoacetyltriglycine scan, and intravenous

Table 88–1	Etiologies of Acute Renal Failure in Infants and Children

Acute tubular necrosis
Glomerulonephritis
Hemolytic-uremic syndrome
Postoperative complication (particularly cardiac surgery)
Oncologic complications
Sepsis
Nephrotoxin ingestion
Transplantation complication
Urinary obstruction

pyelogram, are seldom indicated as part of the emergency department evaluation of children with acute renal failure.

Management

The basic principles of emergency department management include identification of life-threatening complications, restoration of fluid and electrolyte balance, the initiation of prompt dialysis when indicated, and restoration of renal function when possible. Identifying the exact cause of acute renal failure may require renal biopsy and therefore is seldom done in the emergency department. Fortunately, the emergency department management of these children does not require knowing the exact diagnosis.

Prerenal acute renal failure is defined by clinically important fluid deficits and should be managed with bolus infusions of isotonic crystalloid, and is confirmed with restoration of normal urine flow and a decrease in solute retention with establishment of euvolemia. Failure to establish urine flow can mean that volume losses have been underestimated, urinary obstruction exists, or irreversible parenchymal or tubular injury has already occurred. If cardiac pump function is compromised, overly aggressive fluid administration can lead to worsening fluid overload and respiratory compromise from pulmonary edema. The combination of intravenous normal saline and medication to increase urine output may be needed. Mannitol, furosemide, dopamine, and fenoldopam have all been used to treat children with prerenal acute renal failure and maximize their urine flow. Hyperkalemia is an urgent concern and is managed with resins such as sodium polystyrene sulfonate (i.e., Kayexalate), calcium gluconate for cardiac stabilization, a combination of intravenous insulin and glucose, and sodium bicarbonate to drive potassium into the intracellular compartment, which can be a life-saving, temporizing measure (see Chapter 114, Hyperkalemia). Gross fluid overload and life-threatening hyperkalemia are indications for emergent hemodialysis.[2] Other electrolyte and metabolic derangements may require specific treatment (see Chapter 111, Metabolic Acidosis; and Chapter 115, Hypocalcemia).

Mortality from acute renal failure is related to the etiology, the need for renal replacement therapy, and the degree of multiorgan system failure.[3] The highest mortality remains in children who develop acute renal failure following cardiopulmonary bypass surgery.[3] Critically ill children have a survival rate of about 50%.[2] Infants with acute renal failure have a somewhat better survival rate of about one third.[2] Survival rates for children undergoing hemodialysis are higher than those receiving peritoneal dialysis or continuous

renal replacement therapy. Vasopressor use and hypoalbuminemia have emerged as markers for poor outcome.[3] Patients with severe electrolyte or hemodynamic instability require hospitalization in a pediatric intensive care setting. Stable patients can be managed on the floor with pediatric nephrology consultation. Early identification and management of children developing multisystem organ failure currently holds the most promise for improving pediatric outcomes.[3]

Chronic Renal Failure

Chronic renal failure is the progressive decline in renal function that can ultimately lead to end-stage renal disease, a condition currently affecting 5 to 10 children per million each year in the United States.[3] Various etiologies account for chronic renal failure in children, including hereditary diseases, glomerulopathies, obstructive uropathy, reflux nephropathy, renal dysplasias, and complications of multisystem diseases.[4]

Clinical Presentation

Signs and symptoms of renal failure do not appear until the glomerular filtration rate falls below 20% of normal.[5] The signs and symptoms of chronic renal failure are typically nonspecific. Children experiencing chronic renal failure may present with excessive fatigue, anorexia, vomiting, short stature, skeletal pain, polyuria, and polydipsia.[4] Signs of anemia, including congestive heart failure, fetid breath, chronic sequelae of hypertension, asterixis, peripheral neuropathies, growth retardation, abnormal neurocognitive development, pubertal delay, and disordered psychosocial maturation, may also be present.[4] Infants may simply present with failure to thrive (see Chapter 36, Failure to Thrive).

The diagnostic evaluation of children with chronic renal failure depends on whether the condition is previously known or not. For those children not known to harbor chronic renal failure, the emergency physician will typically focus the evaluation on identifying the child's overall diagnosis. For example, an infant with poor weight gain may undergo an evaluation including tests specifically directed at assessing renal function in addition to others that address alternative diagnoses in the differential diagnosis of failure to thrive. For children with known chronic renal failure, the workup is typically focused on assessing current renal function, identifying a decline in renal function, identifying concurrent illnesses, and assessing the child for relatively common complications of chronic renal failure. Frequently indicated tests include a serum BUN and creatinine to assess the degree of azotemia in children not yet dialysis dependent. Electrolytes (specifically looking for clinically significant hyponatremia, hyperkalemia, hypocalcemia, and hypophosphatemia) and a complete blood count to assess for anemia are also useful. If obtained, a renal ultrasound typically reveals small kidneys. Radiographs usually demonstrate diffuse osteomalacia. Children undergoing peritoneal dialysis may require testing of the dialysate for peritonitis.

Management

Immediate therapeutic interventions are directed at correcting electrolyte, fluid, and acid-base balance in addition to supporting cardiovascular function. Congestive heart failure can be managed with diuresis (typically with intravenous furosemide) and judicious transfusion with packed red blood cells to increase the oxygen-carrying capacity of the blood. Immediate hemodialysis is not often indicated in children with chronic renal failure, but is indicated if life-threatening fluid overload or clinically significant hyperkalemia are present.[6]

Disposition and follow-up depend upon the degree of azotemia, the severity of uremic symptoms, the severity of fluid and electrolyte imbalances, and the presence of concurrent illnesses or complications. Coordinating care with a child's nephrologist is prudent.

Poststreptococcal Glomerulonephritis

The term *glomerulonephritis* refers to kidney inflammation accompanied by inflammation of the capillary loops in the renal glomeruli.[7] Given this definition, renal biopsy is required to definitively identify glomerulonephritis. Thus this diagnosis is not formally made in the emergency department. Instead, a constellation of clinical and laboratory findings is used to support a presumptive diagnosis. Of the myriad causes of the acute forms of disease, the most common is poststreptococcal glomerulonephritis. Since the exact cause of acute glomerulonephritis is not identified in the emergency department, understanding the paradigm of poststreptococcal glomerulonephritis offers insight into this and other causes of acute glomerulonephritis.

Clinical Presentation

Poststreptococcal glomerulonephritis is caused by immune complexes becoming lodged in the glomeruli of the kidneys.[8] These immune complexes are typically composed of streptococcal antigens (from group A β-hemolytic *Streptococcus pyogenes*), antibodies, and complement.[8] The presence of these immune complexes leads to glomerular inflammation, which in turn results in the loss of blood and protein in the urine, azotemia (i.e., a rise in serum BUN and creatinine), fluid retention, and systemic hypertension. The clinical presentation can be predicted from this pathophysiologic process. The typical presentation is of a child between 3 and 15 years of age with edema, hypertension, hematuria, and proteinuria.[8] The urine may be the color of tea or cola due to the presence of blood. These children will often have a history of untreated pharyngitis 1 to 2 weeks prior or an untreated skin infection 2 to 4 weeks prior to the onset of symptoms.[8] Nonspecific symptoms such as malaise, lethargy, anorexia, abdominal pain, headache and low-grade fever can also be present.[8]

The evaluation of these children typically involves testing blood and urine. Useful blood tests include a BUN and creatinine to assess for azotemia, a set of electrolytes to assess for gross disturbances, and a complete blood count to assess for anemia or thrombocytopenia. Serum tests useful in identifying a prior streptococcal infection include the anti–streptolysin O titer, the anti–deoxyribonuclease B titer, and the streptozyme test.[8] Urinalysis typically reveals hematuria, proteinuria, a degree of pyuria, and cellular casts. Other tests such as complement levels are usually ordered in coordination with a pediatric nephrologist.

Management

Immediate therapeutic interventions include restriction of fluid intake, correction of electrolyte abnormalities, and management of hypertension. Traditional treatment of poststreptococcal glomerulonephritis is directed toward eradication of the infectious source with penicillin, amoxicillin, or erythromycin and symptomatic relief. The utility of antibiotics has recently been questioned.[9] Children with postinfectious glomerulonephritis have more than a 95% chance of complete recovery resulting in normal renal function and normal blood pressure, denoted by return of blood pressure and renal function to baseline.[8]

The disposition of a child with suspected poststreptococcal glomerulonephritis is controversial. Universal hospitalization is advocated by some, while selective hospitalization is advocated by others. Coordinating care with the pediatric nephrologist who will be caring for the child after the emergency department visit is prudent and can provide guidance as to local practice styles and expectations.

Nephrotic Syndrome

The term *nephrotic syndrome* refers to a group of diseases involving defective glomeruli whereby marked proteinuria and lipiduria occur.[10] More than 85% of cases of nephrotic syndrome in children are idiopathic. When these children undergo renal biopsy, the biopsies are normal or near normal and these children are referred to as having "minimal change disease." Nephrotic syndrome is relatively rare. Emergency physicians are more likely to encounter children experiencing complications from a known diagnosis of nephrotic syndrome than to identify a new case. Although children of any age can develop nephrotic syndrome, toddlers are the most commonly affected group.[11]

Clinical Presentation

The initial clinical presentation of nephrotic syndrome usually includes edema that can be most easily appreciated in the hands and face but may be present elsewhere, such as in the scrotum or vulva.[11] For children with known nephrotic syndrome, complications may include recurrent edema, ascites with or without spontaneous bacterial peritonitis, and pleural effusions.[12] Children with nephrotic syndrome are thought to be in a hypercoagulable state and are at an increased risk for thromboembolic events such as deep venous thromboses and stroke.[13] Because children with nephrotic syndrome are treated with relatively long-term corticosteroids, they are at increased risk for serious or life-threatening infections (see Chapter 107, The Steroid-Dependent Child). If relatively severe disease occurs, these children may present with edema and dehydration or hypotension.

Urine and blood tests are useful in assessing children with known or suspected nephrotic syndrome. The presence of abundant protein in the urine can be the first clue to diagnosing children who manifest subtle clinical symptoms. A simple dipstick urine test is usually sufficient in the emergency department. A low serum albumin supports the diagnosis of nephrotic syndrome and can be used, to some extent, to assess the severity of disease. Serum albumin may be as low as 5 g/L (0.5 g/dl). Electrolyte abnormalities are seldom clinically significant, but minor abnormalities are expected given the dehydration and fluid shifts occurring in cases of nephrotic syndrome. Other tests are not typically indicated for the emergency department management of children with nephrotic syndrome unless they are part of working through a differential diagnosis or evaluating complications such as infections.

Management

The emergency department management of children with nephrotic syndrome is relatively straightforward. For stable toddlers with edema, proteinuria, and hypoalbuminemia, specific treatment can await phone consultation with a pediatric nephrologist to coordinate the next phase in the diagnostic and management plan. For unstable children who are markedly dehydrated and intravascularly depleted, the administration of intravenous albumin is indicated.[11] These children are at risk for fluid overload, and intravenous furosemide may be needed to avoid or treat pulmonary edema during fluid resuscitation. Central venous pressure monitoring in these children is likely indicated. The mainstay of subacute management in children with nephrotic syndrome is the administration of oral corticosteroids. The initiation of steroids is seldom emergent. One exception to this is in children who are on chronic steroids to treat their nephrotic syndrome who become acutely ill or traumatized. These children are adrenally suppressed and require supplemental steroids during these acute physiologic challenges. In the emergency department, a single dose of intravenous hydrocortisone is indicated in these acutely ill or injured steroid-dependent children (see Chapter 107, The Steroid-Dependent Child).

The disposition of children with nephrotic syndrome depends on whether the diagnosis is previously known, disease severity, and the likelihood of a concurrent illness. Known cases with mild symptoms and an adequate serum albumin may be treated as outpatients with care coordinated with the child's pediatric nephrologist. An increase in the dose of oral steroids or reinitiating a course of oral steroids may be the primary intervention in these cases. Newly diagnosed toddlers, children outside toddlerhood (i.e., infants, school-aged children, and adolescents), children with known nephrotic syndrome suspected of having a complication or infection, and otherwise medically complicated children typically require admission to a hospital with a pediatric nephrologist. Children in shock or experiencing hemodynamic compromise and those experiencing serious neurologic sequelae typically require admission or transfer to a pediatric intensive care unit.

Fortunately, the prognosis for toddlers with nephrotic syndrome is good. About 90% of these children will achieve remission with standard treatment. However, many will relapse several times throughout childhood prior to becoming persistently symptom free. Steroid-resistant forms (e.g., focal segmental glomerulosclerosis) have a much worse prognosis; one third of these children will progress to end-stage renal disease and require dialysis within 5 years of their diagnosis.[13]

Kidney Stones

Kidney stones are uncommon in children. Incidence is equal among boys and girls. The cause of pediatric kidney stones is usually a metabolic abnormality, a structural abnormality, or a chronic urinary tract infection. When analyzed, the majority of pediatric kidney stones are either calcium oxalate (about 50%) or calcium phosphate (about 25%). Struvite, cystine, uric acid, and other types of stones are individually uncommon. Children on ketogenic diets and those with metabolic conditions such as cystic fibrosis are at increased risk for developing kidney stones.[14]

Clinical Presentation

Children rarely have the classic adult presentation of dramatic flank pain with stone passage.[14] The younger the child, the lower the likelihood the child will have adult-like symptoms. Abdominal, flank, or pelvic pain occurs in about half of children, while infants may present with acute crying episodes.[14] Like many other pediatric conditions, kidney stones may present with nonspecific signs and symptoms, including abdominal pain with vomiting. Identifying the rare case of a kidney stone in the context of many children with gastroenteritis, acute cystitis or pyelonephritis, intussusception, and appendicitis is challenging.

The emergency department evaluation of a child with a suspected kidney stone includes laboratory tests and imaging. Serum tests assessing the BUN and creatinine will identify children with renal insufficiency and renal failure. Examining urine may reveal gross hematuria, and a urinalysis may reveal microscopic hematuria and a few white blood cells per high-powered field. The presence of many white blood cells per high-powered field suggests pyelonephritis or an infected kidney stone. A kidney-ureter-bladder plain radiograph may reveal a kidney stone in the renal pelvis or ureter. In cases of a suspected kidney stone, renal ultrasound is indicated; the expected finding is unilateral hydronephrosis. The utility of a noncontrast computed tomography scan of the abdomen looking specifically for hydronephrosis and the stone is limited by concerns over radiation exposure and the sensitivity of the scan for detecting kidney stones in children.[15] Half of children younger than 10 years of age with kidney stones have an identifiable metabolic disorder.[16] Therefore, unlike most adults, children diagnosed with kidney stones warrant a metabolic workup at some point. Although this practice has been de-emphasized in the care of adults with kidney stones, straining the urine (from a bagged specimen or a spontaneous void) through cheesecloth may yield a stone that can be sent to the laboratory for analysis. This may assist the follow-up physician in making a specific diagnosis.

Management

The emergency department management of children diagnosed with kidney stones is much more straightforward than making the diagnosis. Analgesia is clearly indicated in those children experiencing pain. The administration of intravenous fluids is usually indicated, particularly if the child is dehydrated from vomiting or able to maintain adequate oral intake. Children with fever, hydronephrosis, and pyuria may harbor an infected kidney stone. These children require prompt pediatric nephrology and urology consultations. Prompt percutaneous drainage of the involved ureter may be indicated.

The disposition of a child with a newly diagnosed kidney stone depends on several factors. Admission is clearly indicated when persistent vomiting is present, the child is suspected of having an infected kidney stone, the child has uncontrollable pain, the diagnosis is unclear, or adequate follow-up is unlikely to occur, or for medically complicated children with kidney stones. Selected older children with known stones and an episode of renal colic who have their pain controlled may be appropriate for discharge home provided that ongoing care can be coordinated with their pediatric nephrologist.

Human Immunodeficiency Virus–Associated Nephropathy

The term *HIV–associated nephropathy* is used for a fulminant form of focal sclerosing glomerulosclerosis seen in children (and adults) infected with the human immunodeficiency virus (HIV).[17-19] As of 2001, there were only 60 cases of HIV-associated nephropathy identified in children younger than 21 years of age in the United States.[17] These children develop severe protenuria without edema. Advanced renal disease is usually present at the time of diagnosis, and rapid progression to end-stage renal disease is expected. The earliest sign or symptom of HIV-associated nephropathy is usually proteinuria. Providing highly active antiretroviral therapy (HAART) seems to be the most effective treatment approach in these children. Given that these children are typically immunocompromised, an overall assessment for comorbid illnesses is prudent (see Chapter 69, Human Immunodeficiency Virus and Other Immunosuppressive Conditions). Coordinated care with a pediatric nephrologists and a pediatric infectious disease specialist are indicated.

Renal Tubular Acidosis

Renal tubular acidosis is a rare condition characterized by a hyperchloremic, non–anion gap metabolic acidosis in which bicarbonate handling by the kidney is deranged. Confusingly, there are three types of renal tubular acidosis designated types 1, 2, and 4. What was previously called "type 3 renal tubular acidosis" is now thought to be a mixed form of types 1 and 2, thus the term is no longer used.[20] The classic presentation is of an infant who is failing to thrive.[21] The most common cause of a hyperchloremic, non–anion gap metabolic acidosis is diarrheal disease. This may obscure the diagnosis in children who have both renal tubular acidosis and diarrhea. However, one presentation of renal tubular acidosis is the very slow resolution of a hyperchloremic, non–anion gap metabolic acidosis following a diarrheal illness.[20]

Diagnostic tests specifically useful in identifying and classifying children with renal tubular acidosis include a venous blood gas to assess the bicarbonate level and blood pH, serum electrolytes to determine if hyperkalemia is present and calculate the anion gap, a urinalysis to assess the urinary pH, and urinary electrolytes to calculate the urinary anion gap.[20,21] In general, these diagnostic studies are undertaken as part of a workup for failure to thrive, and renal tubular acidosis is identified secondarily. If a normal urinary anion gap is present, the diagnosis of type 2 renal tubular acidosis is supported.[20] If the urinary anion gap is elevated and the patient is hypokalemic, the diagnosis of type 1 renal tubular acidosis is supported.[20] If the urinary anion gap is elevated and the patient is hyperkalemic, the diagnosis of type 4 renal tubular acidosis is supported.[20]

Emergency department management is directed at treating the metabolic acidosis. For seriously ill children, treatment with intravenous sodium bicarbonate is reasonable. For stable children, coordinated care with a pediatric nephrologist is prudent. Oral treatment with citrate is a reasonable option for stable children.[20] Severe abnormalities in the serum potassium may require specific treatment (see Chapter 113, Hypokalemia; and Chapter 114, Hyperkalemia). Disposition is usually determined by the overall presentation of the child. Children who require a more extensive workup for failure to thrive often benefit from inpatient evaluation and treatment.[21]

Hypertension

In the emergency department, elevated blood pressure readings range from clinically insignificant numbers to life-threatening emergencies (see Chapter 65, Hypertensive Emergencies). Besides life-threatening emergencies, there are a few key issues regarding pediatric hypertension in the emergency department. These include defining hypertension, the appropriateness of screening for pediatric hypertension, and the evaluation and management of a child thought to have hypertension.

In order to diagnose a child with hypertension, an agreed-upon standard against which to compare blood pressure readings needs to exist. The most widely recognized standard has been written by the National High Blood Pressure Education Program Working Group on High Blood Pressure in Children and Adolescents, organized by the National Heart, Lung, and Blood Institute.[22] This group has developed tables of both systolic and diastolic blood pressure measurements based on age, gender, and height. Based on these tables, a blood pressure measurement can be compared with the 50th, 90th, 95th, and 99th percentiles. With this data set as a standard, the working group defined hypertension as "average systolic blood pressure and/or diastolic blood pressure that is ≥ 95th percentile on ≥ 3 occasions." In addition, children were defined as having "prehypertension" or "high normal" blood pressure if "average systolic blood pressure or diastolic blood pressure levels are ≥ 90th percentile but less than < 95th percentile." Adolescents with blood pressure levels are ≥ 120/80 mm Hg should be considered "prehypertensive." Although these definitions seem rather straightforward, the tables used for these determinations contain over 1900 individual blood pressure values. The complexity of these tables limits their utility. The working group also states, "Elevated blood pressure must be confirmed on repeated visits before characterizing a child as having hypertension."[22] Since three visits are required to define hypertension, it would seem unlikely that hypertension, particularly in otherwise asymptomatic children, could be identified in the emergency department.

Screening children for hypertension is an area of interest for those focusing on the public health of children. The working group even suggests "children > 3 years old who are seen in a medical setting should have their blood pressure measured."[22] As laudable as this seems, it is unlikely that the working group considered emergency department visits included in this "medical setting." It is not intuitive that a child who is highly febrile or has just had a seizure or has sustained a fracture after falling off a bicycle should have his or her blood pressure measurements used as part of universal screening for pediatric hypertension.[23] In one study of those children who had their blood pressure measured, more than half had blood pressures greater than the 90th percentile.[24] It is unlikely this represents the prevalence of prehypertension in children. It is likely these children had elevated blood pressures due to fear, pain, fever, or some other confounding factors.

If a child in the emergency department is thought to have clinically significant hypertension, an evaluation is indicated. Compared with adults, who predominantly have essential hypertension, children are more likely to have secondary hypertension.[25] Of these secondary causes, renal causes predominate. Therefore, if consultation is needed for a child with hypertension, a pediatric nephrologist (instead of a cardiologist) is preferred. A first approach is to obtain blood pressures in all four extremities; if coarctation of the aorta is present, the blood pressure in the legs may be higher than that in the arms.[22] In obese adolescents, essential hypertension is probably the most likely diagnosis, and primary care follow-up may be all that is required. For younger children with markedly elevated blood pressures on repeated measurements during the emergency department visit and in those children with known renal disease, serum BUN and creatinine, a microscopic urinalysis looking for hematuria and casts, a chest radiograph looking for an abnormal cardiac silhouette or pulmonary edema, and an electrocardiogram evaluating age-adjusted voltage as a marker for left ventricular hypertrophy are indicated.[26] In certain circumstances, other studies may be useful, including a renal ultrasound, an echocardiogram, thyroid studies, or a urinary drug screen. Initiating pharmacologic treatment for children with asymptomatic hypertension cannot be advocated because multiple blood pressure measurements in a setting other than the emergency department are needed to appropriately make the diagnosis. Close follow-up with a primary care provider is the most prudent course of action in the vast majority of these cases.

Renal Transplantation

Renal transplantation is considered the treatment of choice for end-stage renal disease in children.[27] Better psychomotor development, psychosocial outcome, rehabilitation, and quality of life are expected when renal transplantation is compared to long-term dialysis. The general care of children following solid organ transplantation is a balance between optimizing patient growth rates and maintaining allograft function with adequate immunosuppression and minimal drug complications. Transplant recipients are at risk for rejection of the allograft, complications from their immunosuppressive therapy, and specific transplant-related conditions such as posttransplantation lymphoproliferative disease. Transplant recipients may present to the emergency department with a variety of surgical issues, including wound complications and problems involving urine leak and ureteral stenosis or obstruction. They will often present with decreased urine output, increased serum creatinine, and lower abdominal or suprapubic discomfort. A renal ultrasound might identify hydronephrosis. Lymphoceles can develop and cause compression of the iliac vessels resulting in leg swelling and discomfort. After transplantation, these children are at risk for hypertension, hyperlipidemia, metabolic bone disease, and chronic allograft nephropathy.

Surveillance for signs and symptoms of renal allograft dysfunction is a priority for these children. The most sensitive indicator of renal dysfunction is an elevated serum creatinine.[27] Urine output may not be a useful clinical indicator because of decreased concentrating ability. Volume depletion

should be treated aggressively as it both hinders graft survival and increases immunosuppressive-related nephrotoxicity. Fever in these children must be investigated as it can be a manifestation of many different infections, rejection, or sepsis. Renal imaging studies and further workup should be performed in consultation with a pediatric nephrologist, the child's transplant surgeon, or both. The prognosis for these children continues to improve, and future directives involve increasing numbers of renal transplantations while new induction therapies and augmentation of tolerance in immunosuppression are advanced.

REFERENCES

*1. Williams DM, Sreedhar SS, Mickell JJ, et al: Acute kidney failure: a pediatric experience over 20 years. Arch Pediatr Adolesc Med 156:893–900, 2002.
2. Hoschek JC, Dreyer P, Dahal S, et al: Rapidly progressive renal failure in childhood. Am J Kidney Dis 40:1342–1347, 2002.
3. McDonald SP, Craig JC: Long-term survival of children with end-stage renal disease. N Engl J Med 350:2654–2662, 2004.
4. Derakhshan A, Hashemi GH, Fallahzadeh MH: Chronic renal failure in children. Transplant Proc 35:2590–2591, 2003.
5. Milliner DS: Pediatric renal-replacement therapy—coming of age. N Engl J Med 350:2637–2639, 2004.
6. Leonard MB, Donaldson LA, Martin H, et al: A prospective cohort study of incident maintenance dialysis in children: an NAPRTC study. Kidney Int 63:744–755, 2003.
7. Anderson DM, Novak PD, Keith J, et al: Dorland's Illustrated Medical Dictionary, 30th ed. Philadelphia: WB Saunders, 2003, p 779.
8. Kasahara T, Hayakawa H, Okubo S, et al: Prognosis of acute poststreptococcal glomerulonephritis (APSGN) is excellent in children, when adequately diagnosed. Pediatr Int 43:364–367, 2001.
9. Coppo R, Amore A: New perspectives in treatment of glomerulonephritis. Pediatr Nephrol 19:256–265, 2004.
10. Anderson DM, Novak PD, Keith J, et al: Dorland's Illustrated Medical Dictionary, 30th ed. Philadelphia: WB Saunders, 2003, p 1826.
11. Hogg RJ, Portman RJ, Milliner D, et al: Evaluation and management of proteinuria and nephrotic syndrome in children: Recommendations from a pediatric nephrology panel established at the National Kidney Foundation Conference on Proteinuria, Albuminuria, Risk, Assessment, Detection, and Elimination (PARADE). Pediatrics 105:1242–1249, 2000.
12. Filler G: Treatment of nephrotic syndrome in children and controlled trials. Nephrol Dial Transplant 18(vi):75–78, 2003.
13. Cavagnaro F, Lagomarsino E: Peritonitis as a risk factor of acute renal failure in nephrotic children. Pediatr Nephrol 15:248–251, 2000.
14. Fisher JD, Reeves JJ: Presentation variability of acute urolithiasis in school-aged children. Am J Emerg Med 22:108–110, 2004.
15. Strouse PJ, Bates DG, Bloom DA, et al: Non-contrast thin-section helical CT of urinary tract calculi in children. Pediatr Radiol 32:326–332, 2002.
16. Butani L, Kalia A: Idiopathic hypercalciuria in children—how valid are the existing diagnostic criteria? Pediatr Nephrol 19:577–582, 2004.
17. Ahuja TS, Abbott KC, Pack L, et al: HIV-associated nephropathy and end-stage renal disease in children in the United States. Pediatr Nephrol 19:808–811, 2004.
18. Ray PE, Xu L, Rakusan T, et al: A 20-year history of childhood HIV-associated nephropathy. Pediatr Nephrol 19:1075–1092, 2004.
19. Ross MJ, Klotman PE: HIV-associated nephropathy. AIDS 18:1089–1099, 2004.
*20. Roth KS, Chan JCM: Renal tubular acidosis: a new look at an old problem. Cin Pediatr (Phila) 40:533–543, 2001.
21. Adedoyin O, Gottlieb B, Frank R, et al: Evaluation of failure to thrive: diagnostic yield of testing for renal tubular acidosis. Pediatrics 112: e463–e466, 2003.
*22. National High Blood Pressure Education Program Working Group on High Blood Pressure in Children and Adolescents: The fourth report

*Selected readings.

on the diagnosis, evaluation, and treatment of high blood pressure in children and adolescents. Pediatrics 114:555–576, 2004.

23. Gilhotra Y, Willis F: Blood pressure measurements on children in the emergency department. Emerg Med Australas 18:148–154, 2006.

24. Silverman MA, Walker AR, Nicolaou DD, et al: The frequency of blood pressure measurements in children in four EDs. Am J Emerg Med 18:784–788, 2000.

25. Flynn JT: Differentiation between primary and secondary hypertension in children using ambulatory blood pressure monitoring. Pediatrics 110:89–93, 2002.

26. Fernandes E, McCrindle BW: Diagnosis and treatment of hypertension in children and adolescents. Can J Cardiol 16:801–811, 2000.

27. Samsonov D, Briscoe DM: Long-term care of pediatric renal transplant patients: from bench to bedside. Curr Opin Pediatr 14:205–210, 2002.

Chapter 89

Penile and Testicular Disorders

Roger A. Band, MD

Key Points

Epididymitis is being recognized with increasing frequency in prepubertal boys.

Paraphimosis is a time-sensitive emergency requiring prompt reduction.

Ultrasonography is a noninvasive, accurate, and readily available modality for the evaluation of the acute scrotum.

Selected Diagnoses

Epididymitis and epididymo-orchitis
Balanitis and balanoposthitis
Torsion of the appendix testis
Hydroceles, inguinal hernias, and varicoceles
Testicular masses
Priapism
Hemospermia
Paraphimosis
Minor genital injuries

Discussion of Individual Diagnoses

Epididymitis and Epididymo-orchitis

Epididymitis is inflammation of the epididymis and is commonly thought to be due to an infection. *Epididymo-orchitis* is inflammation of the epididymis and testis and is along the same continuum of disease as epididymitis. These conditions are being recognized with increasing frequency in prepubescent boys. Previously, epididymitis was thought to be a condition limited to sexually active adolescents and adults. Urinary pathogens have traditionally been thought to be the cause of epididymitis in prepubertal boys. Some recent evidence suggests that epididymitis either is a post-infectious phenomenon or is due to the combination of a minor anatomic abnormality and chemical irritation by urine.[1-3] In sexually active adolescents, epididymitis is usually caused by pathogenic, sexually transmitted bacteria. The most common are *Chlamydia trachomatis* and *Neisseria gonorrhoeae*.[3,4]

The classic manifestations of epididymitis are testicular pain, scrotal swelling, an intact cremasteric reflex, and a normal testicular orientation within the scrotum.[3] With the exception of an intact cremasteric reflex, testicular torsion may share many of these features. Testicular torsion and torsion of the appendix testis are thought to occur with greater frequency than epididymitis in the prepubertal age group.[5] The currently accepted diagnostic approach in these boys typically involves obtaining a color Doppler ultrasound to rule out testicular torsion[6] (see Chapter 87, Testicular Torsion). The expected ultrasonographic finding in cases of epididymitis and epididymo-orchitis is unilateral increased blood flow to the involved testis.[6] The utility of a urinalysis is unclear. Serum studies are nonspecific and of no utility in differentiating causes of the acute scrotum.

The generally accepted management of epididymitis and epididymo-orchitis is supportive care and antibiotics. Supportive care includes analgesics (e.g., acetaminophen with codeine), anti-inflammatory agents (e.g., ibuprofen), and bed rest with scrotal elevation. Appropriate antibiotics are determined by the boy's age. The American Urologic Association has suggested that most cases of epididymitis and epididymo-orchitis can be treated on an outpatient basis with oral antibiotics.[7] Appropriate antibiotics for prepubertal children include azithromycin and trimethoprim-sulfamethoxazole.[7] Sexually active adolescents should be treated for presumptive *C. trachomatis* and *N. gonorrhoeae*. Appropriate antibiotic selections for adolescent boys with epididymitis or epididymo-orchitis include the combination of a single oral dose of cefixime 400 mg plus a single oral dose of azithromycin 1 g. The American Urologic Association suggests inpatient admission and parenteral antibiotics if the boy has intractable pain, vomiting, very high fever, or overall severe illness.[7] As new data emerge in support of noninfectious causes, the recommendation that all patients receive antibiotics has been challenged. In one study of 44 boys ages 2 to 14 years, 38 (86%) had immunologic studies suggesting recent infections with viruses or *Mycoplasma pneumoniae*.[1] Only 3 of the boys received antibiotics, and all 44 were without testicular abnormalities or symptom recurrence on follow-up. Current practice suggests against withholding antibiotics from boys with epididymitis. However, larger studies, if performed, may lead to a change in the management of epididymitis and epididymo-orchitis in the future.

Balanitis and Balanoposthitis

Balanitis is inflammation of the glans penis. *Balanoposthitis* is inflammation of the glans penis and the foreskin. Balanitis and balanoposthitis can have irritant, infectious, or traumatic etiologies and represent a continuum of the same disease process.[8,9] Although balanoposthitis may occur in sexually active adolescents and young men, the most common presentation in the pediatric emergency department is of an uncircumcised preschool-age boy who presents with a red, swollen foreskin and a complaint of localized pain. Discharge, if present, is scant. Clinical experience suggests difficulty with urination is rare in these cases.

Little has been written about this clinical condition in prepubertal children. In a single study of 100 boys with balanitis or balanoposthitis, 3 boys were younger than 2 years, 76 were 2 to 5 years, 15 were 6 or 7 years, and 6 were 8 or 9 years of age.[10] Only 5% of the boys in this study were not yet toilet trained. The most common signs and symptoms reported in this study were redness (100%), swelling (91%), and discharge (73%). Dysuria was seen in only 13%. Of these 100 boys, 32 presented acutely and had cultures of their penile discharge obtained. Of these, 15 (47%) showed no growth on culturing, 7 (22%) revealed mixed growth, 5 (16%) grew *Staphylococcus aureus,* 4 (13%) grew *Proteus vulgaris,* and one (3%) grew *Morganella morgagni.* The authors of this small study concluded that balanitis and balanoposthitis are self-limited and can be managed expectantly (i.e., without antibiotics).[10]

The only published guidelines for the treatment of balanitis focus on sexually active adults.[11] There are no evidence-based treatment options. Oral analgesia and rest seem prudent. For intense inflammation, the use of topical 1% hydrocortisone cream may be beneficial. Based on the available microbiologic epidemiology, the reasonable options include expectant care without antibiotics, prescribing an oral antistaphylococcal antibiotic (e.g., cephalexin 25 mg/kg per dose administered four times per day) for 7 to 10 days, or prescribing an extended-coverage oral antibiotic that is antistaphylococcal and also is active against *P. vulgaris* and *M. morgagni* (e.g., amoxicillin/clavulanic acid 10 mg/kg per dose based on the amoxicillin component, administered 3 times per day) for 7 to 10 days.

Torsion of the Appendix Testis

Torsion of the appendix testis is a common, benign, self-limited cause of acute scrotal pain and swelling in the prepubertal age group, accounting for approximately 25% to 50% of all acute scrotal complaints.[2] Caused by torsion of an embryologic remnant, torsion of the appendix testis typically involves a gradual onset of unilateral scrotal pain associated with an intact cremasteric reflex and a normal testicular orientation within the scrotum.[12] Focal tenderness can be elicited at the superior lateral testicular pole. Early in the process, a focal area of echymotic or blue discoloration, referred to as the "blue dot sign," may be visible.[2,3] Aside from the focal area of tenderness, the remainder of the testis examination is normal. Boys with torsion of the appendix testis generally have fewer associated systemic complaints, such as nausea and vomiting, than boys with testicular torsion.[2] In cases of presumed torsion of the appendix testis, it is difficult to definitively rule out testicular torsion (see Chapter 87, Testicular Torsion), and therefore an ultrasonographic evaluation is generally recommended.[6,13] Once a definitive diagnosis of torsion of the appendix testis has been made, supportive care including oral analgesics, bed rest, and scrotal elevation are the mainstays of therapy.

Hydroceles, Inguinal Hernias, and Varicoceles

The broad rubric of painless scrotal masses includes hydroceles, indirect inguinal hernias, and varicoceles. A *hydrocele* is an accumulation of fluid within the tunica vaginalis that remains after closure of the processus vaginalis during infancy or occurs secondary to a patent processus vaginalis.[14] This process can occur secondary to epididymitis, orchitis, torsion of the appendix testis, and testicular torsion.[15,16] An *indirect inguinal hernia,* like a hydrocele, results from a patent processus vaginalis. This allows bowel to escapes from the pelvis into the scrotum via the inguinal canal, which can sometimes be difficult to distinguish clinically from a hydrocele. An attempt should be made to reduce the herniated mass as soon as possible so long as the child appears well. If reducible in the emergency department, children with these hernias can be referred to a pediatric surgeon for an outpatient evaluation. However, the herniated contents may become entrapped or incarcerated distal to the inguinal rings. Consultation with a pediatric surgeon or transfer to a facility with a pediatric surgeon is indicated in these cases (see Chapter 84, Abdominal Hernias; and Chapter 169, Hernia Reduction).

Varicoceles are uncommon in young children. Varicoceles have been described as having a "bag of worms" feel within the scrotum on physical examination and are most prominent on standing, with near resolution of the "mass" upon lying down. Varicoceles involve dilation of the testicular vein and the associated pampiniform plexus of veins that are within the spermatic cord. Adolescent boys with varicoceles may experience stunted testicular growth and subsequent infertility. If a varicocele is diagnosed in the emergency department, referral to a urologist for an outpatient evaluation is prudent.[13,16,17]

Testicular Masses

A painless scrotal mass is the most common presentation of testicular cancer.[18] Although rare in children, testicular tumors occur in all age groups. Testicular tumors have a bimodal age distribution, with peak incidence between 2 and 4 years of age and in young adult men. Often, young boys give a history of minor groin trauma, which leads them to identify the unrelated painless testicular mass.[19] Testicular tumors are generally firm, irregular, and inseparable from the testicle.[2,3] Urgent urologic referral and ultrasonography are prudent in these cases.[2,18] The anticipated tests needed to begin the workup of a testicular mass include a chest radiograph, a complete blood cell count, a serum β-human chorionic gonadotropin level, and a serum α-fetoprotein level.[19] Obtaining these tests in coordination with the urologist who will follow up with the patient may expedite the diagnosis.

Priapism

Priapism refers to a sustained erection that is painful and occurs in the absence of sexual stimulation. This condition primarily involves engorgement of the corpora cavernosa and is relatively uncommon in children.[20] Priapism is seen in the setting of poor venous outflow as occurs with the sludging associated with sickle cell disease, leukemic infiltration, and polycythemia of the newborn.[5,20,21] For boys with sickle cell disease, as many as one third may experience priapism in their lifetime.[21] Due to the marked pain and potential for ischemic changes, fibrosis, and impotence that are associated with priapism, this process should be addressed emergently. Management is directed at treating the underlying cause. In children, the most common cause of priapism is vaso-occlusive crisis associated with sickle cell disease (see Chapter 127, Sickle Cell Disease). If conservative measures (e.g., oxygen, hydration, analgesia) fail to relieve the priapism, transfusion and corporal irrigation with saline and vasoconstrictive agents, including phenylephrine, may be necessary.[5,20] Invasive management of priapism in children is typically undertaken by pediatric urologists if available.

Hemospermia

Hemospermia is the presence of blood in the ejaculate. Although potentially morbid conditions may underlie this surprising and angst-provoking sign, hemospermia is most often a benign condition in adolescent boys. The most common history is that of an adolescent boy who notices blood-tinged semen either after masturbation or upon removing a condom after sexual intercourse.[22-24] The differential diagnosis of hemospermia includes genitourinary infections, inflammatory disorders (primarily younger patients), genitourinary tuberculosis, blood dyscrasias, supratherapeutic anticoagulant therapy, and malignancy.[25,26] Nonetheless, hemospermia in otherwise healthy adolescent boys is overwhelmingly idiopathic, self-limited, and benign.[24-26] Reassurance and primary care or urologic follow-up are typically all that is indicated.

Paraphimosis

Paraphimosis is a time-sensitive emergency seen after retraction of the foreskin without return of the foreskin over the glans. This constriction of the glans by the swollen, retracted foreskin leads to venous congestion and edema of the glans and the foreskin. As swelling increases, reduction of the foreskin becomes increasingly difficult and painful. This is a relatively uncommon condition that only occurs in uncircumcised boys.[5,27] Manual reduction of the foreskin should be attempted after adequate regional anesthesia with a dorsal nerve ring block, topical anesthesia, oral analgesics, or parenteral procedural sedation. Reduction can be accomplished by compressing the foreskin to mechanically reduce the swelling and then placing direct pressure on the glans to reduce it through the phimotic ring of tissue[5,14,27] (see Chapter 177, Paraphimosis Reduction). Inability to manually reduce the foreskin will necessitate an urgent dorsal slit procedure or circumcision. These invasive procedures are typically performed by a urologist.

Minor Genital Injuries

Accidental injury to the scrotum is fairly common during childhood.[5] These injuries generally result from straddle injuries or a direct blow to the groin. Testicular injuries exist along a continuum of severity from mild contusions to testicular rupture.[28] Scrotal hematomas arise from bleeding that occurs within the scrotal wall and are characterized by pain, swelling, and ecchymosis. Scrotal hematomas typically obscure injuries to the scrotal contents, making ultrasonographic evaluation particularly valuable in this setting.[28] Penetrating injuries to the male genitalia are uncommon in children.[28,29] Surgical exploration by a surgeon or urologist familiar with the pediatric scrotum is typically indicated. Testicular torsion can present with a history of pain that is temporally related to a coincident, apparently minor blunt scrotal injury (see Chapter 87, Testicular Torsion). The pain associated with testicular torsion can be mistakenly attributed to the trauma, leading to a delay in diagnosis that can result in loss of testicular viability, orchiectomy, and infertility.[28]

Zipper injuries involving the penile foreskin are relatively common in boys between 2 and 6 years of age. A hurried attempt to zip the pants after urinating is a common history.[5,30] The two most commonly accepted modalities for freeing the entrapped skin include soaking the penis in mineral oil before trying to loosen the zipper, and cutting the median bar of the zipper with wire cutters. This allows the zipper mechanism to fall apart, in turn freeing the foreskin. Clinical experience suggests that procedural sedation is very helpful in facilitating the release of the boy's foreskin from the zipper. Warm soaks and oral analgesia are usually the only care necessary after releasing the zipper.[5,30]

REFERENCES

1. Somekh E, Gorenstein A, Serour F: Acute epidiymitis: evidence of a post-infectious etiology. J Urol 171:391–394, 2004.
2. Marcozzi D, Suner S: Genitourinary emergencies. Emerg Med Clin North Am 19:547–568, 2001.
3. Kadish H: Pediatric Surgical emergencies: the tender scrotum. Clin Pediatr Emerg Med 3:5–61, 2002.
4. Simpson T, Oh KM: Urethritis and cervicitis in adolescents. Adolesc Med Clin 15:253–271, 2004.
5. Gausche M: Genitourinary surgical emergencies. Pediatr Ann 25:458–464, 1996.
6. Schalamon J, Ainoedhofer H, Schleef J, et al: Management of acute scrotum in children—the impact of Doppler ultrasound. J Pediatr Surg 41:1377–1380, 2006.
7. American Urological Association: Epididymitis and orchitis. Available at http://www.urologyhealth.org/ (accessed August 24, 2006).
8. Vohra S, Gopal Badlani: Balanitis and balanoposthitis. Urol Clin North Am 19:143–147, 1992.
9. Waugh MA: Balanitis. Dermatol Clin North Am 16:757–762, 1998.
10. Escala JM, Rickwood AMK: Balanitis. Br J Urol 63:196–197, 1989.
11. National guideline for the management of balanitis. Clinical Effectiveness Group (Association of Genitourinary Medicine and the Medical Society for the Study of Venereal Diseases). Sex Transm Infect 75(Suppl 1):S85–S88, 1999.
12. Edwards S: Balanitis and balanoposthitis: a review. Genitourin Med 72:155–159, 1996.
13. Pillai SB, Besner GE: Pediatric testicular problems. Pediatr Clin North Am 45:813–830, 1998.
14. Rosenstein D, McAninch JW: Urologic emergencies. Med Clin North Am 88:495–518, 2004.
15. Skoog SJ, Conlin MJ: Pediatric hernias and hydroceles. Urol Clin North Am 22:119–130, 1995.
16. Skoog SJ: Benign and malignant scrotal masses. Pediatr Clin North Am 44:1229–1250, 1997.
17. Bong GW, Koo HP: The adolescent varicocele: to treat or not to treat. Urol Clin North Am 31:509–515, 2004.
18. Metcalfe PD, Farivar-Mohseni H, Farhat W: Pediatric testicular tumors: contemporary incidence and efficacy of testicular preserving surgery. J Urol 170:2412–2416, 2003.
19. Wu H, Snyder HM: Pediatric urologic oncology. Urol Clin North Am 31:619–627, 2004.
*20. Adeyoju AB, Olujohungbe J, Morris A: Priapism in sickle-cell disease: incidence, risk factors and complications—an international multicentre study. Br J Urol 90:898–902, 2002.

---

*Selected readings.

21. Bruno D, Wigfall D, Delbert R: Genitourinary complications of sickle cell disease. J Urol 166:803–811, 2001.

22. Mulhall JP, Albertsen PC: Hematospoermia: diagnosis and management. Urology 46:463–467, 1995.

23. Ferrari ND: Hematospermia in the adolescent. J Adolesc Health Care 10:561–563, 1989.

24. Murphy NJ, Weiss BD: Hematospermia. Am Fam Pract 32:167–171, 1985.

25. Papp GK, Kopa Z, Szabo KF, et al: Aetiology of haemospermia. Andrologia 35:317–320, 2003.

26. Leary FJ: Hematospermia. J Fam Pract 2:185–186, 1975.

27. Choe JM: Paraphimosis: current treatment options. Am Fam Physician 62:2623–2626, 2628, 2000.

28. Dreitlein DA, Suner S, Basler J: Genitourinary trauma. Emerg Med Clin North Am 19:569–590, 2001.

29. El-Bahnasawy MS, El-Sherbiny MT: Paediatric penile trauma. BJU Int 90:92–96, 2002.

*30. Mydlo JH, Harris CF, Brown JG: Blunt, penetrating and ischemic injuries to the penis. J Urol 168:1433–1435, 2002.

Chapter 90

Ectopic Pregnancy

Daniel F. Brennan, MD

Key Points

Ectopic pregnancy should be considered in any menstruating female with abdominal pain or vaginal bleeding.

β-Human chorionic gonadotropin (βhCG) testing (qualitative urine or serum) is a reliable starting point in diagnosis.

Transvaginal sonography can "rule in" intrauterine pregnancy at 4 to 5 weeks, when βhCG levels are 1000 to 1400 IU/L, essentially "ruling out" ectopic pregnancy.

Sonography often reveals signs diagnostic of or suspicious for an ectopic pregnancy. Even an indeterminate sonogram is highly suggestive of ectopic pregnancy when the quantitative βhCG exceeds the discriminatory zone.

Therapy with laparoscopy or methotrexate is not 100% effective in eliminating ectopic pregnancy.

Introduction and Background

Ectopic pregnancy is the extrauterine implantation of an ovum, most commonly (95%) within the fallopian tube, and usually in the ampulla (73%).[1] Over the past 35 years, ectopic pregnancy has become increasingly common, exceeding 100,000 cases per year in the United States.[2-4] Much of this increase occurred in the 1970s and 1980s, mirroring a similar increase in risk factors (notably pelvic inflammatory disease [PID]), but the relatively larger increase in absolute numbers also reflects improved detection. Adolescents have increased behavioral and perhaps physiologic susceptibility to sexually transmitted infections (STIs),[5] especially *Chlamydia*, which predisposes them to an increased risk of ectopic pregnancy. Although ectopic pregnancy rates seem to have stabilized over the past 10 to 15 years, tubal pregnancy still carries significant morbidity. Delay in presentation or diagnosis

can result in tubal rupture, hemoperitoneum, and maternal death.

Enhanced patient and physician awareness of this disease will allow existing and developing diagnostic tools to be used to detect ectopic pregnancy earlier, improving maternal health and future fertility. The use of sensitive β-human chorionic gonadotropin (βhCG) assays in combination with ultrasonography has become the mainstay of diagnosis, reducing the need for invasive testing. Additionally, earlier diagnosis allows noninvasive treatment options to be used more commonly.

Recognition and Approach

Since 1970, the frequency of ectopic pregnancy has increased to now represent about 2% of all pregnancies.[2-4] Given the likelihood of acquiring risk factors (prior ectopic pregnancy, PID, intrauterine device, tubal surgery, infertility) with increased sexual maturity, it is not surprising younger women are at lower risk. Indeed, women ages 15 to 24 years have a 0.66% ectopic pregnancy rate, while women ages 25 to 34 years and 35 to 44 years have two- (1.54%) and threefold (2.15%) this risk.[2] With more recent trends toward outpatient therapy of ectopic pregnancy in the 1990s, reliable data on incidence has been more difficult to obtain.[3,5] Encouragingly, a significant reduction in PID has occurred over this later time period, with possible stabilization of the ectopic pregnancy rate.[6] Although rates of *Gonorrhea* and *Chlamydia* infections in women less than 19 years old have fallen by nearly 50% since the 1980s, prevalence remains highest in this age group.[7] Increased cervical ectopy makes adolescent women particularly susceptible to *Chlamydia* infection,[7] now the most frequent STI in the United States, with adolescent women leading all groups (see Chapter 70, Sexually Transmitted Infections).[8] With an often indolent course and predisposition for ascending infection and tubal damage, it is a major cause of ectopic pregnancy.[8] Frequent unprotected sex and high fertility rates make ectopic pregnancy an important diagnostic consideration in any young woman with abdominal pain or vaginal bleeding.

During the same era, case fatality rates have declined 90% due to improved and earlier diagnosis.[2] Improved pregnancy testing (βhCG), sonography, and laparoscopy permit diagnosis of ectopic pregnancy before tubal rupture in 60% to 90% of cases.[9] Despite enhanced diagnostic techniques, misdiagnosis is still problematic. Ectopic pregnancy continues to be the most common cause of pregnancy-related first trimester maternal death, nearly always due to hemorrhage.[10] Mortality rates are highest in young women less than 19 years old, markedly in nonwhites.[2]

Clinical Presentation

Clinically, ectopic pregnancy is primarily a disease of the first trimester, with most cases presenting in the first 8 weeks of gestation with abdominal pain or abnormal vaginal bleeding.[11,12] Given the physiologic similarity of adolescent and older but generally healthy menstruating women, one would expect the clinical presentation to be very similar. An abrupt, life-threatening illness with tubal rupture and hemoperitoneum was more common in the past, manifesting as signs of peritoneal or diaphragmatic irritation, orthostasis, syncope, tachycardia, or shock. A more benign and insidious presentation is more common currently, although adolescents lacking access to care may present later with a greater degree of illness.

The early manifestations of pregnancy are primarily related to the evolving hormonal milieu, regardless of site of implantation. Later, as the conceptus outstrips the limited decidual reaction afforded it by the fallopian tube, declining hormonal levels may mimic those of failing intrauterine pregnancies (IUPs). Endometrial decline with vaginal bleeding is common. Consequently, early ectopic pregnancies may be difficult to distinguish clinically from normal or abnormal IUPs. Invasion into submucosal vessels can produce pain from a tubal hematoma, and bleeding with or without frank rupture. Common clinical findings are summarized in Table 90–1.[11-19] The differential diagnosis is broad, including a host of abdominal and pelvic conditions (Table 90–2).[20] Commonly the diagnostic challenge is to differentiate ectopic pregnancy from viable or nonviable IUP.

Standard history and physical examination are insufficiently sensitive to detect unruptured ectopic pregnancies, since there are no significant differences in symptoms between ectopic and intrauterine pregnancy patients.[14] Clinical diagnosis is only 55.3% sensitive and 49% accurate for detecting ectopic pregnancy on initial visit.[14,21] Common pitfalls in diagnosis include overlooking risk factors (25%) or subtle signs of blood loss (36%).[22] Delays in diagnosis have often occurred when pain was "atypical" and examination benign.[22] Tubal rupture is likewise poorly predicted by clinical features,[17] although shock index may have some predictive value.[23]

Thus, history and physical examination value lies primarily in identifying risk factors and physical findings to heighten suspicion.[24,25] As a consequence, the clinician should pursue the diagnosis in all women of reproductive age who present with abdominal or pelvic pain, or abnormal vaginal bleeding. Given the unreliability of menstrual and sexual history in establishing pregnancy status,[26] liberal βhCG pregnancy testing is warranted.

Diagnosis

Diagnosis of ectopic pregnancy initially relies upon βhCG testing to confirm pregnancy status, and ultrasonography to attempt to determine location. Early detection reduces maternal morbidity and mortality and allows more conservative treatment options, including medical therapy.

Table 90–1	Clinical Manifestations of Ectopic Pregnancy[11-19]

History

Risk factors (past history of infertility, PID, IUD, tubal surgery, prior ectopic): 51–56%
"Classic" history (amenorrhea followed by abdominal pain, vaginal bleeding): 69% (but this more often represents threatened abortion)
Abdominal pain: >90–100%
   Variable character, intensity, location
   Absence of pain does predict absence of tubal rupture
Menstrual history
   Normal menstrual history: 15–30% or more
   Amenorrhea < 4 wk: 15%
   Amenorrhea > 12 wk: 15%
   Rupture before missed menses: 15%
Abnormal vaginal bleeding: 50–80%
   Usually scant, dark; heavier favors miscarriage
Symptoms of pregnancy (breast tenderness, morning sickness, "feeling pregnant")
Shoulder pain (infrequent)

Physical Examination

"Classic": shock & adnexal mass ("rarity")
Hemodynamic status
   Shock: <5%
   Parasympathetic response to hemoperitoneum (paradoxically low pulse)
Abdominal examination
   Tenderness: 50%
   Peritoneal signs (less common)
Pelvic examination
   Adnexal mass: 25–33%
   Adnexal tenderness/cervical motion tenderness: 50%
   Uterine size
      Normal: 71%
      6–8 wk size: 26%
      9–12 wk size: 3%
   Normal pelvic examination: 10%

Abbreviations: IUD, intrauterine device; PID, pelvic inflammatory disease.

Table 90–2	Differential Diagnosis of Ectopic Pregnancy[20]

Normal intrauterine pregnancy
Spontaneous abortion
Corpus luteum cyst, hemorrhage
Ovarian cysts/torsion
Appendicitis
Pelvic inflammatory disease
Renal colic/pyelonephritis
Endometriosis
Diverticulitis
Ileitis

Laboratory Diagnosis: Pregnancy Testing

The detection of human chorionic gonadotropin (hCG) produced by trophoblasts in early pregnancy is the key to pregnancy diagnosis. Furthermore, the predictable rise of this hormone with normal IUP growth can help identify abnormal gestations—both by serial measurement of quantitative βhCG levels over time and by correlation of ultrasound findings with βhCG levels.[27,28]

QUALITATIVE URINE OR SERUM βHCG TESTING

Although the time of implantation has been found to be variable with respect to the expected menses,[29] by the time of missed menses (13 to 14 days after conception), the smaller than 1-mm zygote produces serum βhCG levels of 50 to 300 IU/L. A variable but similar range of βhCG concentrations in urine and serum has been noted in early pregnancy: in the fourth week, serum concentrations range from 11 to 3476 IU/L (median 254 IU/L) and urine concentrations from 12 to 2548 IU/L (median 210 IU/L).[30] Butler et al. found even a variety of home urine pregnancy tests, with manufacturers' reported sensitivities of 25 to 100 IU/L, to reliably detect hCG at 50 IU/L concentration (15 of 15 kits tested).[31] Also, although many office or emergency department (ED) point-of-care urine tests are sensitive to 25 IU/L, significant variability has been reported in the ability of home, point-of-care, and laboratory βhCG tests to detect hyperglycosylated hCG, which may be the predominant form of hCG initially.[29,30] Despite variation in assay performance, hCG secretion, and urine concentration, all qualitative tests reliably detect pregnancy, although the time at which they do so varies.[30] Clinically, qualitative urine tests have performed well when compared to qualitative serum tests, with 100% sensitivity and 99% specificity.[32] Similarly, as compared to serum quantitative tests (sensitivity 5 IU/L), urine assays with sensitivity of 20 IU/L had a 1% false-negative rate.[33] Urine "false-positives" may actually represent detection of βhCG in early pregnancy losses.[32] Serum false-positive hCG up to 900 IU/L can occur in 1 in 3300 women due to the presence of heterophilic antibodies, a problem not encountered with urine testing.[30] Various investigators have found urine βhCG tests to be 95% to 100% sensitive and specific for pregnancy when compared to serum assays.[32,34] In the detection of ectopic pregnancies, qualitative assays with a threshold βhCG of 10 IU/L would have a sensitivity of 99.5% and tests with a threshold βhCG of 25 to 50 IU/L would detect 91% to 96%.[35,36] The convenience of obtaining urine samples and comparable performance makes urine βhCG testing the preferred method in many EDs. In the event that clinical suspicion of pregnancy persists despite a negative qualitative test, quantitative serum immunoassays are sensitive to 5 IU/L or less and can rule out pregnancy in virtually 100% of cases.[36-38]

QUANTITATIVE SERUM βHCG TESTING

Although ectopic pregnancies tend to produce less βhCG than IUPs of comparable gestational age,[39,40] the range and variation of βhCG produced by both (0 to 100,000 IU/L)[35] makes a single level nondiagnostic.[40,41] Quantitative βhCG may be low or high in both ectopic pregnancy and IUP. Similarly, quantitative βhCG is not diagnostic in predicting tubal status. Both ruptured and unruptured ectopic pregnancies are seen in the βhCG less than 100 and greater than 50,000 IU/L ranges.[35,42] Although one can be *somewhat* reassured that tubal rupture is less likely at low βhCG levels, rupture can certainly be seen at low levels. In one series, 10% of ectopic pregnancies with βhCG less than 100 IU/L were ruptured, and 7% of ruptures occurred at βhCG less than 100 IU/L.[35] In summary, single quantitative βhCG levels are poor predictors of ectopic pregnancy size and tubal rupture risk.[35] Additionally, quantitative βhCG poorly predicts utility of sonography. However, quantitative values are useful serially (βhCG dynamics) and to interpret the results of indeterminate sonography (discriminatory zone).

Sonography

Pelvic ultrasonography has become the key diagnostic test to ascertain pregnancy location in symptomatic first trimester pregnancy.[43] Endovaginal ultrasonography by emergency resident and attending physicians was successfully incorporated into protocols for the diagnosis of ectopic pregnancy as early as 1996,[44,45] and has become part of the core curriculum of emergency medicine residencies.[46]

The goal of imaging is to ascertain whether the pregnancy is intrauterine or not. The presumption is that, if an IUP exists, an ectopic pregnancy is extremely unlikely. Parenthetically, this same assumption is used in evaluating uterine curettage specimens. The incidence of coexisting intrauterine and ectopic pregnancies is traditionally reported as 1 : 30,000 pregnancies.[47,48] More current estimates of heterotopic pregnancy (simultaneous intrauterine and extrauterine pregnancies) are 1 : 1500 to 1 : 3900,[9] 1 : 4000,[47] and 1 : 2600.[48] In women undergoing ovulation induction, risk is much greater, up to 1 : 35 (2.9%).[47,48] In these high-risk patients, proof of an IUP may not exclude ectopic pregnancy, but in most women it does with a very high degree of confidence.

Results of sonography require careful interpretation (Fig. 90–1 and Table 90–3).[28,40,43,49-75] Pregnancy location is not definitely established until fetal heart activity is localized, but uterine or adnexal signs are suggestive. Definite or probable

Text continued on p. 669.

Table 90–3	Timing and Frequency of Sonographic Findings in Intrauterine and Ectopic Pregnancies[28,40,43,49-75]	
Intrauterine Pregnancy		
Finding	**Time**	**βhCG Value**
Decidual reaction		
Gestational sac (double decidual sign, intradecidual sign)		
Transvaginal	$4^1/_2$–5 wk	>1,000–1,400 IU/L
Transabdominal	6 wk	>6,500 IU/L
Yolk sac	5–6 wk	>7,200 IU/L
Fetal pole/fetal heart tones	$5^1/_2$–7 wk	>10,800–17,200 IU/L
Ectopic Pregnancy		
Finding		**Frequency**
Uterus		
Decidual reaction		
Empty uterus, or pseudosac		10–20%
Pelvis—cul-de-sac		
Free fluid		24–63%
Echogenic (bloody)		20–26%
Adnexal masses		
Cystic or complex		60–90%
Tubal ring		26–68%
Corpus luteum cyst		
Fetal heart activity		
Transabdominal		4–10%
Transvaginal		8–23%

Abbreviation: βhCG, β-human chorionic gonadotropin.

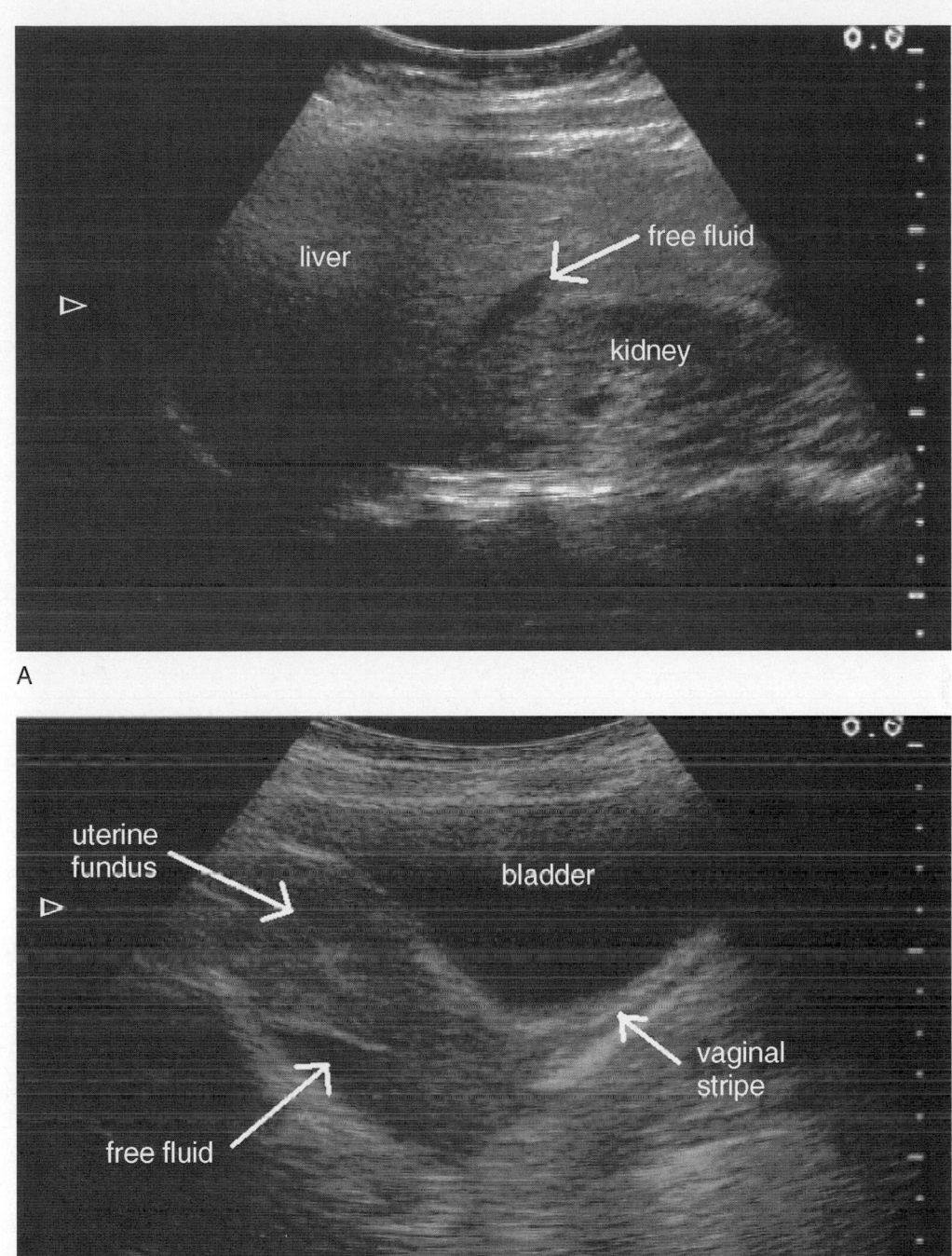

FIGURE 90–1A. Free fluid in the abdomen. Morrison's pouch (hepatorenal space) shows an area of anechogenicity (blackness), indicating free fluid in the abdomen between the kidneys and liver. This case was a ruptured cornual pregnancy that went to the operating room shortly after this scan. **B.** Large amount of free fluid in the pelvis. Transabdominal sagittal scan showing free fluid posterior to the uterus in the pouch of Douglas (recto-uterine space).

Continued

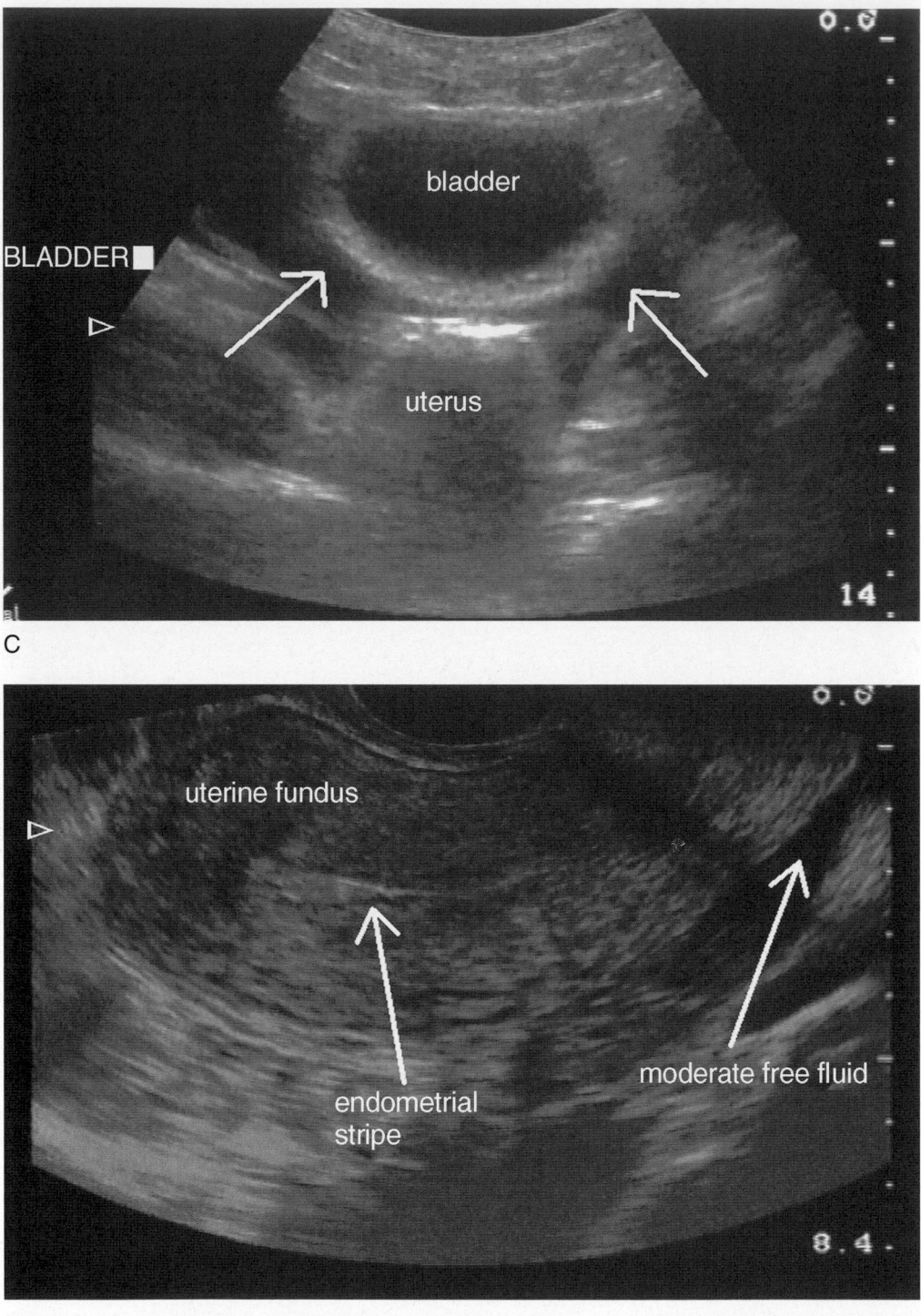

FIGURE 90–1C. Pelvic free fluid. Transverse abdominal view of the pelvis with a large amount of free fluid *(arrows)*. Bladder is anterior, with uterus posterior. **D.** Moderate pelvic fluid. Transvaginal sagittal scan with empty uterus and moderate free fluid in the pouch of Douglas.

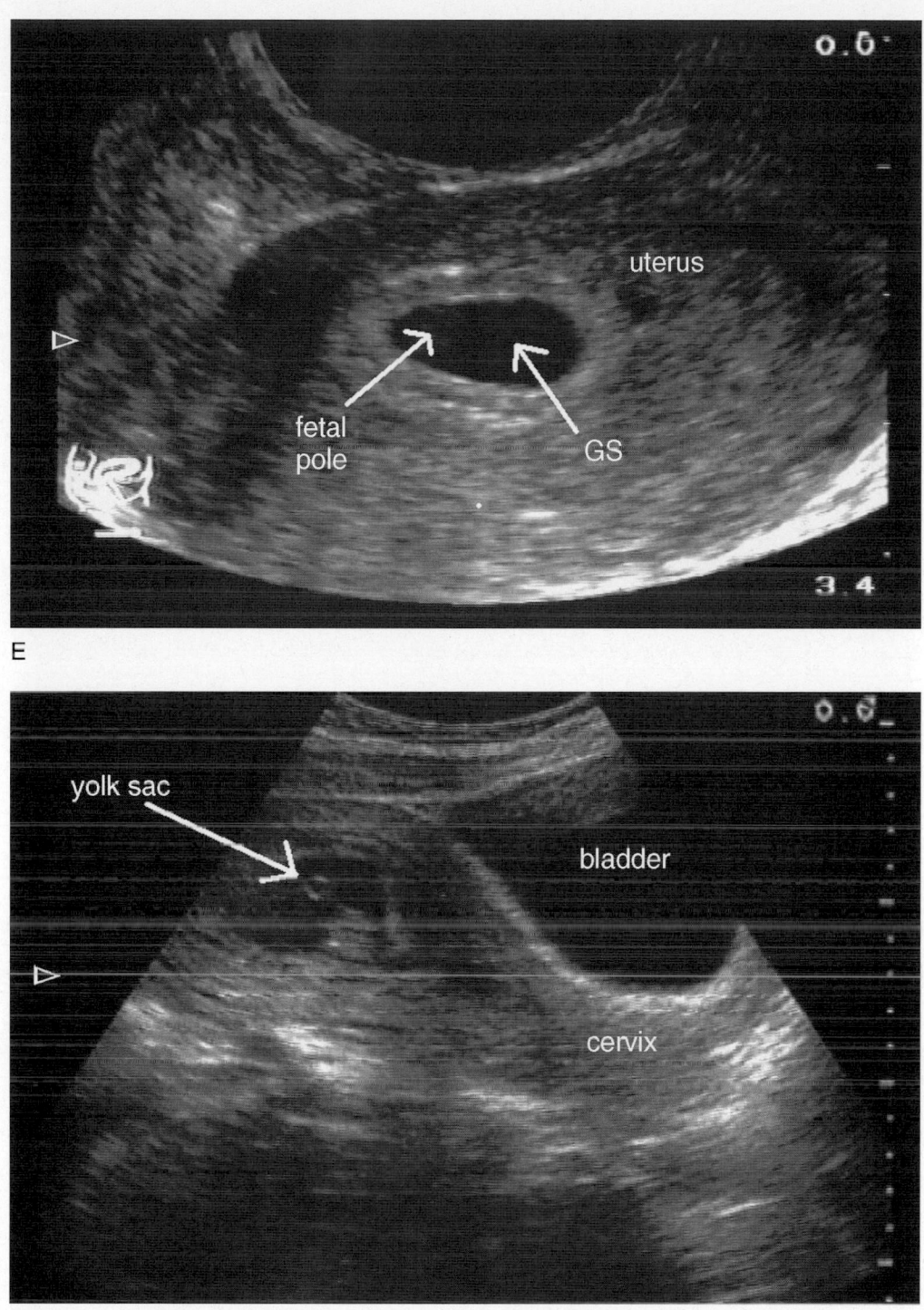

FIGURE 90–1E. Transvaginal coronal scan of the uterus showing gestational sac (GS) with faint image of the fetal pole. Notice the characteristic hyperechoic double decidual sac sign surrounding the anechoic sac. **F.** Intrauterine pregnancy. Transabdominal sagittal scan shows the uterus superior to the bladder, with an intrauterine gestational sac, and yolk sac. Notice the regular circular size of the yolk sac.

Continued

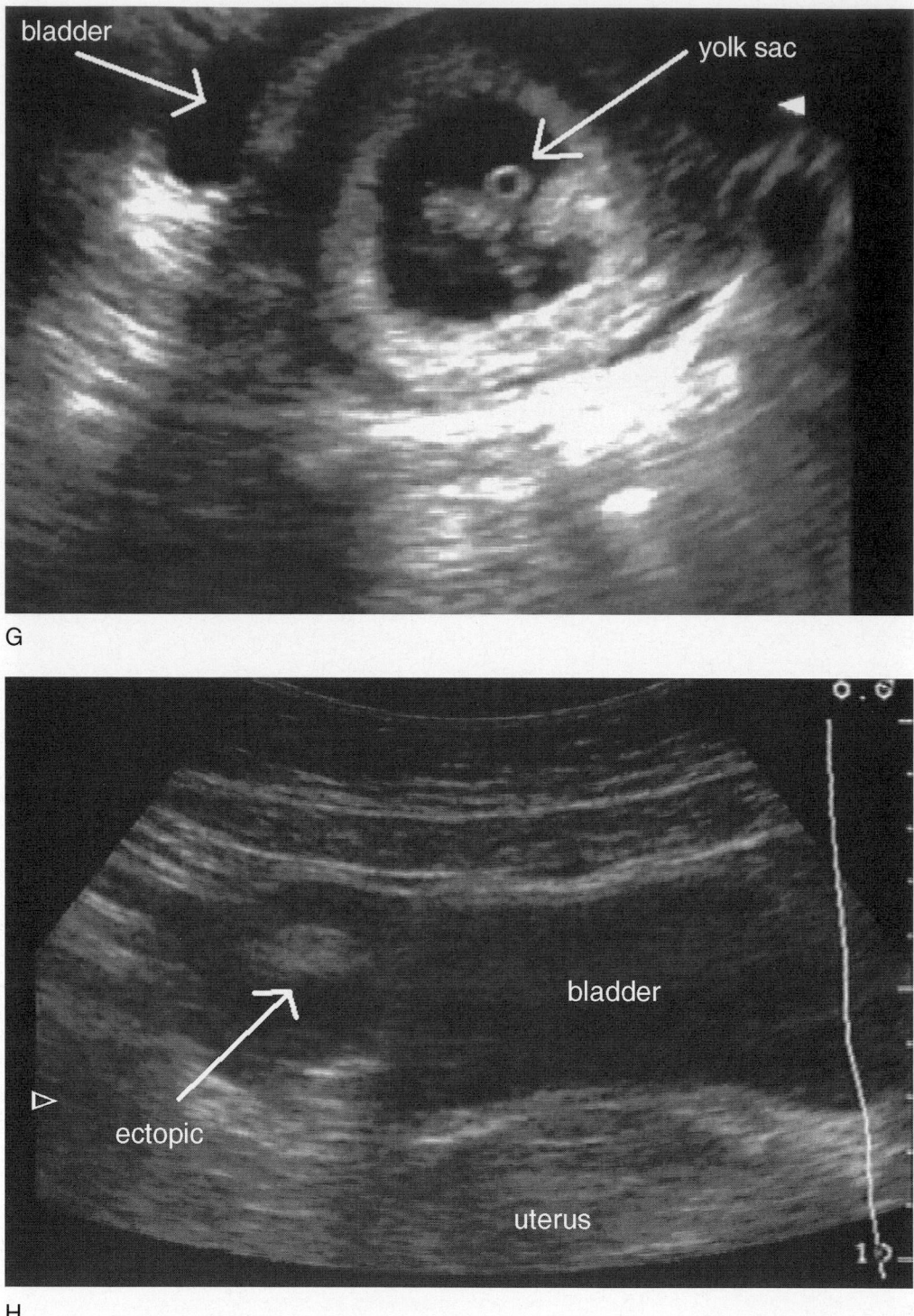

G

H

FIGURE 90–1G. Intrauterine pregnancy. Transvaginal coronal scan shows the bladder anteriorly and an intrauterine fetal pole with yolk sac. **H.** Extrauterine gestation. Transabdominal scan showing the bladder anteriorly and the uterus posteriorly, with an adnexal mass on the right side.

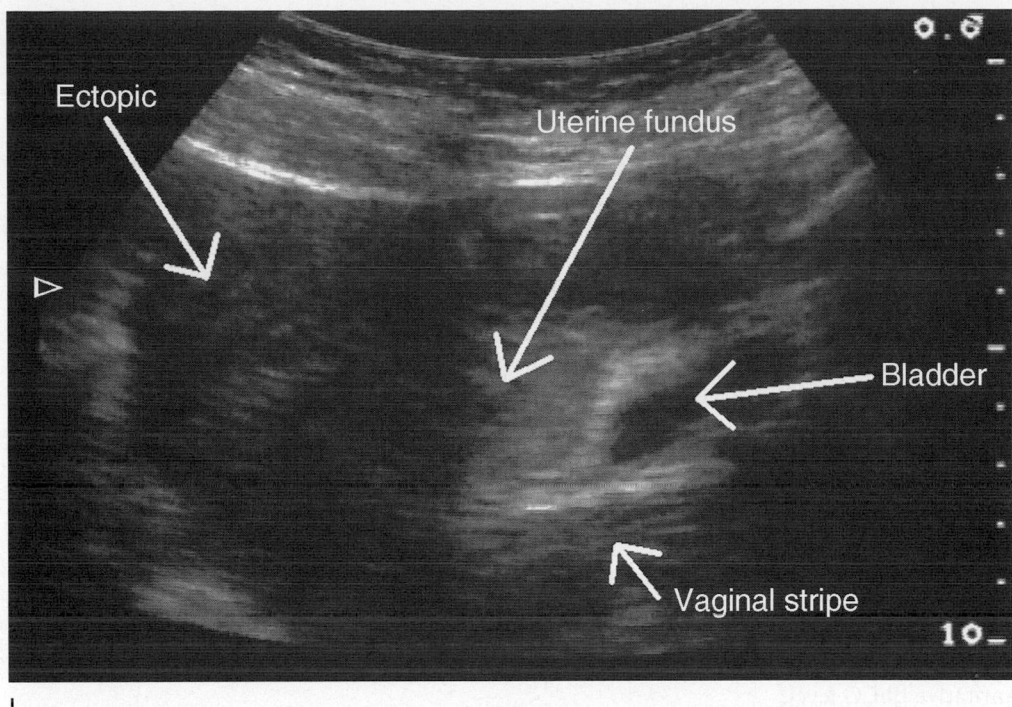

FIGURE 90–1I. Ectopic gestation. Sagittal transabdominal view with ectopic gestation (later shown to be cornual) at the upper edge of the uterine fundus.

diagnosis of intrauterine or ectopic pregnancy can usually be made by vaginal sonography.[40] The presence of a true gestational sac (intradecidual, double sac sign), yolk sac, and fetal pole infers a greater degree of certainty to the probable diagnosis of IUP. Cystic masses, cul-de-sac fluid (simple, particulate), tubal rings, and complex adnexal masses likewise make the tentative diagnosis of ectopic pregnancy more likely. Doppler may be helpful in further defining adnexal masses.[76-78] However, not uncommonly the sonogram of a pregnant woman with abdominal pain or vaginal bleeding will be normal and yield none of these signs. Such "nondiagnostic" sonograms could represent early IUP, blighted ovum, threatened or missed abortion, or ectopic pregnancy.[52] It is here that use of quantitative βhCG levels may be helpful (Table 90–4).[9,18,28,40,52-57,79-83]

Combination of Sonography with Quantitative βhCG: The Discriminatory Zone

Kadar and colleagues developed the concept of the *discriminatory zone* to help interpret transabdominal sonograms when an IUP was not seen.[54] The discriminatory zone is the level of βhCG at which almost all viable IUPs should be seen.[54] As such, it is dependent upon ultrasound resolution, operator skill, and hCG assay used. An empty uterus in combination with a βhCG level above the discriminatory zone is often diagnostic of ectopic pregnancy.[54] The zone will vary from institution to institution; however, advances in transvaginal sonography have reduced the discriminatory zone to as low as the βhCG range of 1200 to 1500 IU/L.[58,80]

"Nondiagnostic" ultrasounds (i.e., no IUP) are, in fact, abnormal when βhCG *exceeds* the discriminatory zone. This combination implies abnormal gestation, and is highly specific for ectopic gestation (86% to 100%).[9,81,83] Further diag-

Table 90–4	Performance of Sonography in Possible Ectopic Pregnancy[9,18,28,40,52-7,79-83]

Transvaginal Sonography

Diagnostic in 80–90% of "possible ectopic pregnancy" patients at 5–7 weeks' gestation
    Intrauterine pregnancy (IUP) visualized in most (76–98%)
    Ectopic pregnancy (EP) visualized in many (20–62%)
    Failure to visualize EP never rules it out: 20% of EP patients have normal sonograms
Indeterminate sonograms (10–20%)

Use of Quantitative βhCG to Interpret Indeterminate Sonogram

Discriminatory zone of βhCG (DZ): βhCG level above which all viable IUPs should be seen
If βhCG > DZ: abnormal
    86–100% are EP → pursue diagnosis
If βhCG < DZ: truly nondiagnostic
    Early IUP, nonviable IUP, EP

Abbreviation: βhCG, β-human chorionic gonadotropin.

nostic efforts are justified (e.g., diagnostic laparoscopy, dilation and curettage [D&C]).[79] However, a normal sonogram combined with a βhCG level *below* the discriminatory zone is truly nondiagnostic. This scenario could represent early viable IUP, nonviable IUP, or ectopic pregnancy. A thin endometrial stripe, likely correlated with low serum progesterone levels, has been found to be predictive of ectopic pregnancy risk.[84,85] In the stable patient, observation with serial quantitative βhCG levels is reasonable; repeat sonography when βhCG exceeds the discriminatory zone is suggested.[79] Regardless of βhCG level, indeterminate sonography will require further diagnostic efforts in coordination with gynecology.

Why is sonography recommended on the basis of a positive qualitative βhCG, that is, before a quantitative βhCG? As sonography has improved, the "window" between positive βhCG pregnancy testing and sonographic evidence of pregnancy has narrowed. Currently βhCG tests become positive at about $3^1/_2$ weeks from the last menstrual period (LMP)[81,86,87] and vaginal sonography at about $4^1/_2$ weeks.[52,63,88] In a prospective study of 200 potential ectopic pregnancy patients, vaginal sonograms were diagnostic in 91% of patients without quantitative βhCG data.[55] Quantitative βhCG levels do not assist in the diagnosis in the great majority of cases, but they play a helpful role in the minority with nondiagnostic sonograms.[40,55]

Sonography may often demonstrate an IUP when βhCG is less than the discriminatory zone, and has made the definitive diagnosis of ectopic pregnancy with quantitative βhCG levels as low as 30 to 60 IU/L.[64] One study found that 89% of ectopic pregnancy patients with βhCG less than 1000 IU/L had suggestive sonographic signs such as cul-de-sac fluid or adnexal masses. In fact, 25% of all patients diagnosed with ectopic gestations had low βhCG and suggestive ultrasounds.[89] This suggests that βhCG level cannot predict the utility of sonography and thus sonography should be pursued regardless of quantitative βhCG level.

Improved imaging combined with quantitative βhCG data allows more ectopic pregnancy patients to reach a definite diagnosis at the first visit, often by 35 to 37 days post LMP, and before significant risk of tubal rupture.[50] The diagnostic accuracy of the combination of sonography with the βhCG discriminatory zone is excellent. The best diagnostic criteria, based on literature evidence, are the absence of an intrauterine sac when βhCG is greater than 1000 IU/L and/or the presence of an adnexal mass.[55] This criteria set has a sensitivity of 97%, a specificity of 98%, a positive predictive value of 98%, and a negative predictive value of 98%. Similar results have been obtained in other studies.[80,83] Thus the need for serial βhCG monitoring has diminished and other diagnostic procedures have assumed more of a confirmatory role.

Additional Laboratory Diagnostic Tests

SERIAL βHCG TESTING: βHCG DYNAMICS

Normally βhCG rises from about 100 IU/L at 4 weeks to greater than 100,000 IU/L at the end of the first trimester (Table 90–5).[27,50,90-104] Early concentrations of βhCG increase exponentially, reflecting trophoblastic proliferation. The early exponential increase in βhCG in healthy IUPs is fairly predictable, with levels doubling approximately every 2 days. Mean doubling time for normal IUPs is 1.9 ± 0.5 days, with an upper 95% confidence level of 2.8 days when initial βhCG is less than 10,000 IU/L.[91] An increase in βhCG of greater than 66% over 48 hours has been found to be the minimum seen at the 85% confidence level for normal IUPs.[93]

The value of βhCG dynamics is in differentiating normal from abnormal gestations, including ectopic pregnancy.[105,106] In ectopic pregnancy, inadequate tubal decidual reaction results in stunted trophoblastic tissue growth, and βhCG production lags. Subnormal increases in βhCG are seen in 85% of ectopic pregnancies.[93] When βhCG rises less than 66% over 48 hours, the pregnancy is often abnormal.[93] Thus an abnormal rise in βhCG *could* be a normal IUP (15%), but one must suspect an abnormal pregnancy, such as ectopic

Table 90–5	βhCG Dynamics[27,50,90-104]
Normal Intrauterine Pregnancies (IUP)	
50–100 IU/L at 4 wk from last menstrual period	
Reach maximum of 100,000 IU/L at 12 wk	
Doubling times 1.9 ± 0.5 days when βhCG < 10,000 IU/L	
Normal Dynamics	
≥66% increase in βhCG over 48 hr	
Occurs in 85% of normal IUPs	
May occur in early, asymptomatic ectopic pregnancy	
Abnormal Dynamics	
<66% rise in βhCG over 48 hr	
May occur in 15% of normal IUPs	
Suggests abnormal gestation	
75% sensitive, 93% specific	
Occurs in 85% of ectopic pregnancy patients (especially if symptomatic)	
May be nonviable IUP	
Declining βhCG Values	
Indicate nonviability	
Spontaneous intrauterine abortion	
Tubal regression/abortion	
May be useful in monitoring success of therapy	

Abbreviation: βhCG, β-human chorionic gonadotropin.

pregnancy, impending miscarriage, or blighted ovum. However, ectopic pregnancies may initially have normal βhCG dynamics,[91,93] especially in asymptomatic patients.[50,94] Ultimately, 85% of ectopic pregnancy patients do manifest abnormal βhCG dynamics.[94]

Declining βhCG values indicate nonviability of the pregnancy, either intra- or extrauterine. In these patients, D&C may be helpful by documenting the presence of a blighted IUP rather than ectopic pregnancy. Declining βhCG values may represent complete abortion or tubal regression/abortion; thus observation alone may be reasonable in the asymptomatic patient.[96] However, tubal hematoma rupture remains possible, and clinical symptoms must be heeded.[107] After therapy, lack of decline in βhCG can be helpful in monitoring for treatment failure and persistent ectopic pregnancy.[108,109]

PROGESTERONE

Progesterone is often low in abnormal pregnancies.[90,110-113] Low levels of this hormone may reflect decreased production by abnormal trophoblastic tissue, or decreased corpus luteal function.[90] Normal corpus luteal function early in abnormal pregnancies may account for low sensitivities of these assays.[90] Most nonviable pregnancies have progesterone less than 10 ng/ml.[110] Progesterone values greater than 25 ng/ml imply a 97% chance of normal IUP.[111-113] However, no single cutoff value can predict ectopic pregnancy.[39,41,110,114-116] One cannot rely on progesterone levels to diagnose ectopic pregnancy, but low values should heighten suspicion for an abnormal pregnancy. Progesterone probably has more value in settings in which sonography is less available,[117] or in selected patients when diagnosis is uncertain after sonography and quantitative βhCG have been performed.[112,118,119]

Diagnostic Procedures

Dilation and Curettage

D&C is helpful in establishing the presence of an IUP and, thus, virtually excluding ectopic pregnancy. If products of conception are present, this makes ectopic pregnancy doubtful, given the rarity of heterotopic pregnancy in most populations. D&C should only be undertaken to establish the location of a pregnancy when nonviability is assured, unless the patient desires termination of the pregnancy. Nonviability may be established by stable or decreasing serial βhCG levels or suggested by very low progesterone values (<5.0 ng/ml).[120]

Laparoscopy

This technique provides the opportunity for the definitive diagnosis and treatment of ectopic pregnancy.[79,121] Due to advances in noninvasive diagnostic (transvaginal sonography) and pharmacologic methods for treating ectopic pregnancy, the role of laparoscopy has diminished somewhat.[51,80] However, diagnostic laparoscopy remains the procedure of choice in the patient with uncertain diagnosis despite thorough evaluation.[79]

With ectopic pregnancy, laparoscopy usually reveals a characteristic bluish swelling of the tube, but can be falsely negative early[122] in about 3% to 4% of cases.[15] False positives reportedly occur in 5% of cases.[15]

Important Clinical Features and Considerations

Common pitfalls in making the diagnosis of ectopic pregnancy generally arise from failure to consider the diagnosis or misinterpretation of diagnostic tests[22] (Table 90–6).

Management

Emergency physician therapy of ectopic pregnancy consists of stabilization. Resuscitation of the unstable patient follows the usual guidelines: securing airway, breathing, and circulation; establishing intravenous lines (large bore); providing fluid resuscitation with crystalloid and red blood cell transfusions; and initiating prompt definitive therapy (gynecologic consultation for surgical management). Rh immuno-

Table 90–6	Clinical Pitfalls

Failure to Consider the Diagnosis

Ignorance of the clinical spectrum of presentation (minimal or atypical symptoms)

Failure to consider diagnosis when risk factors are present, or if pain or bleeding exists

Misinterpretation of Diagnostic Tests

Failure to understand the limitations of various tests

Failure to pursue additional diagnostic testing

Dismissing low βhCG level
  Does not preclude EP or rupture: symptomatic patients with low βhCG are at increased risk of EP[123]
  Does not predict utility of sonography: many scans show IUP or signs of EP even with low βhCG values

Sonography
  Pseudosacs, nonspecific intrauterine fluid collections: occur in up to 20% of EPs
  Should not exclude EP until more definitive signs of IUP are present (double decidual sac sign, yolk sac, fetal pole)

Abbreviation: βhCG, β-human chorionic gonadotropin; EP, ectopic pregnancy; IUP, intrauterine pregnancy.

prophylaxis (50 μg anti-D immune globulin intramuscularly) is generally recommended in the Rh-negative woman with ectopic pregnancy or spontaneous abortion, although use of $Rh_o(D)$ immune globulin is currently without clear-cut justification in threatened miscarriages of less than 7 weeks.[48,109,124,125]

Stable patients allow for a more sequential evaluation. Therapeutic options are more varied, and decisions may be influenced by the methods necessary for diagnosis as well as the preferences of the gynecologist.[126-150] Many gynecologists still prefer surgery, although laparoscopy now supplants laparotomy in most centers.[151-154] With improved anesthesia and laparoscopy skills, this has become an option even in unstable patients.[155-157] Surgeons may prefer laparotomy in patients with tubal rupture and larger volumes of intraperitoneal blood.[157]

Medical therapy of early ectopic pregnancy with the folate antagonist methotrexate has expanded greatly given its efficacy and cost effectiveness.[152,153,158-160] In a randomized trial of methotrexate versus laparoscopy, no significant differences were seen in primary treatment success, tubal preservation, or patency.[161] Although methotrexate involved more side effects[161] and outpatient follow-up,[158] significant savings in terms of hospitalization and overall cost can be achieved.[152,158,159] Contraindications to medical management are unstable vital signs or active bleeding, tubal rupture, or contraindications to methotrexate (liver, renal, or hematologic disease). Various relative exclusions, including larger tubal size, higher βhCG level, and fetal heart activity, have been applied since failure rates are higher with these signs of more advanced disease.[109,126,162] Methotrexate achieves successful resolution in 92% of cases (range 78% to 96%).[162] Tubal patency is preserved in 78% of cases, with subsequent pregnancy rates (65%) and ectopic rates (13%) similar to those in laparoscopically treated groups.[162] Although regimens involving oral, intravenous, multiple dose, and local injection are possible, methotrexate is most commonly given by single-dose intramuscular injection (50 mg/m²), with repeat doses as needed based upon close observation of βhCG patterns. About 8% to 20% of patients will need repeat methotrexate, often when βhCG levels at posttreatment day 7 fail to fall below day 4 levels.[126,163] The emergency physician must be aware of the potential for methotrexate failure, continued growth of the ectopic pregnancy or hematoma, and tubal rupture; thus close follow-up with the treating physician is imperative. βhCG levels often need to be followed for weeks until resolution, with reliability an issue to consider in adolescents.

Outcome is measured in terms of morbidity/mortality, success in eradicating ectopic pregnancy (i.e., persistent ectopic pregnancy rate), complications (bleeding), rapidity of convalescence, and future fertility (IUP rate, recurrent ectopic pregnancy rate). In general, conservative laparoscopic surgery (linear salpingostomy) is the current standard, although medical management (methotrexate) is being utilized with increasing frequency.

Summary

Ectopic pregnancy is an increasingly common and potentially catastrophic condition that often presents to the ED with abdominal pain or vaginal bleeding. Recent

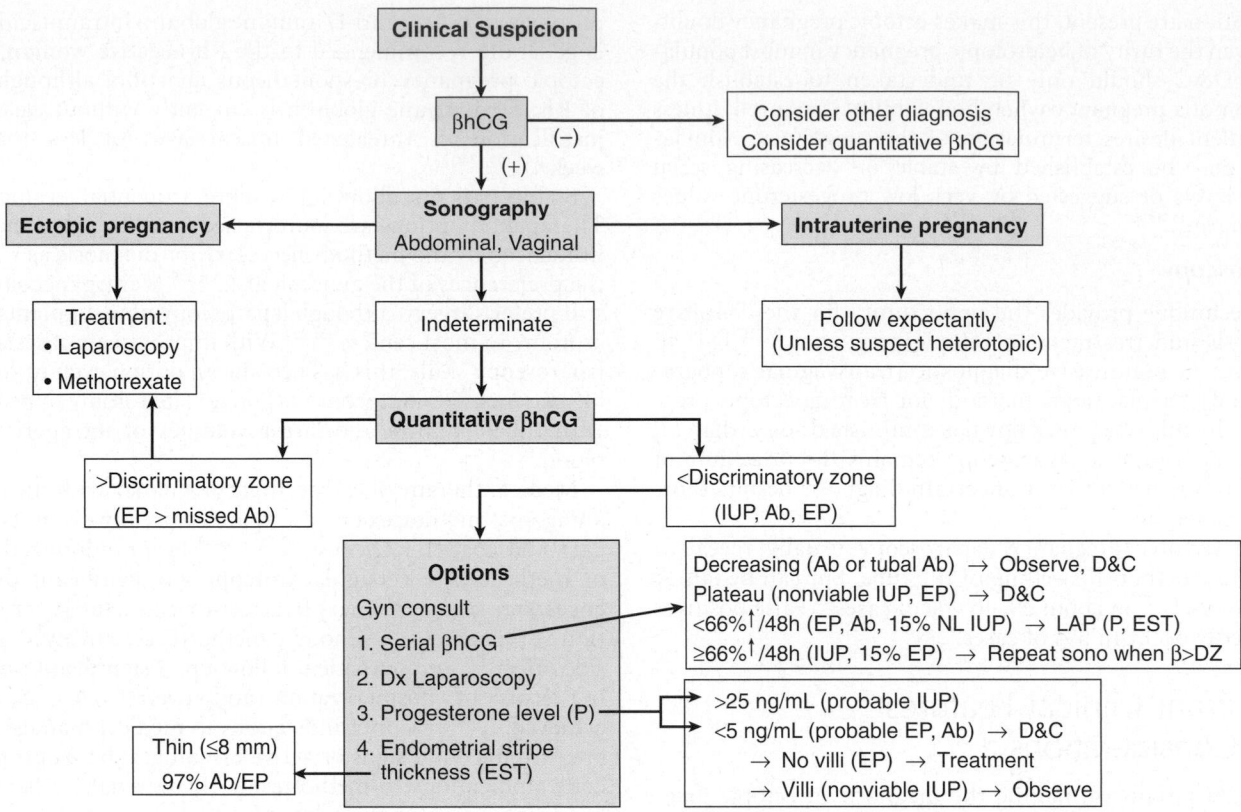

FIGURE 90–2. Diagnostic algorithm for ectopic pregnancy. NOTE: If the patient is unstable, resuscitation and immediate gynecology consultation for laparoscopy are recommended. Abbreviations: Ab, abortion; βhCG/β, β-human chorionic gonadotropin; D&C, dilation and curettage; Dx, diagnostic; DZ, discriminatory zone; EP, ectopic pregnancy; LAP, laparoscopy; IUP, intrauterine pregnancy; NL, normal; SONO, sonography.

developments in the laboratory (sensitive βhCG and progesterone assays), in ultrasonography (transvaginal probes, Doppler ultrasound), and in the combination of modalities (discriminatory zone of hCG for ultrasonographic evidence of IUP) have allowed the earlier diagnosis of ectopic pregnancy. Conservative laparoscopic surgery and medical treatment options have evolved, making maternal mortality rare (<0.04%)[2] and future fertility more viable.

Understanding the strengths and limitations of the variety of diagnostic modalities available will allow the clinician to formulate a rational strategy for the early diagnosis of ectopic pregnancy. Numerous algorithms have been developed.[9,28,48,51,52,79,80,111,122,164] All begin with high clinical suspicion in women of reproductive age with abdominal/pelvic pain or vaginal bleeding. Pregnancy testing with a sensitive βhCG qualitative test is next. In stable patients found to be pregnant, sonography follows, first transabdominally and then transvaginally. Unstable patients require immediate resuscitation and gynecology consultation; invasive diagnostic methods may supplant laboratory tests and sonography. Unclear cases may require the use of quantitative βhCG (discriminatory zone), other pregnancy hormones (progesterone), invasive procedures (laparoscopy, culdocentesis, D&C), or observation (serial βhCG levels). A suggested algorithm incorporating these elements is presented in Figure 90–2.

Collaboration of emergency physicians and obstetrician-gynecologists is essential for patients with possible ectopic pregnancy. In the unstable patient, the transition of care from the ED resuscitation and stabilization phase to the gynecologist for subsequent evaluation and therapy best serves the patient when well planned and coordinated. Local resources such as bedside sonography will make the details site specific. More commonly, stable patients are being evaluated for possible ectopic pregnancy, which increasingly can be diagnosed within the initial ED visit. In children's facilities without gynecology services, transfer agreements will facilitate the coordination of care for both groups. Finally, many patients will remain with ectopic pregnancy as a diagnostic consideration after indeterminate ED sonography and low quantitative βhCG level. This last group, if stable, are candidates for further evaluation as outpatients. Often this entails arranging follow-up in 48 hours for serial βhCG determination and gynecologic examination. Patients should also receive threatened abortion and ectopic pregnancy precautions, with instructions to return to the ED for increased pain or signs of increased bleeding.

REFERENCES

1. Bouyer J, Coste J, Fernandez H, et al: Sites of ectopic pregnancy: a 10 year population-based study of 1800 cases. Hum Reprod 17:3224–3230, 2002.
2. Centers for Disease Control and Prevention: Surveillance for ectopic pregnancy—United States, 1970–1989. Morb Mortal Wkly Rep CDC Surveill Summ 42(SS-6):73–85, 1993.
3. Centers for Disease Control and Prevention: Ectopic pregnancy—United States, 1990–92. MMWR Morb Mortal Wkly Rep 44:46–48, 1995.
4. Centers for Disease Control and Prevention: Ectopic pregnancy—hospitalization of women 15–44 years of age: United States, 1980–2000. In National Hospital Discharge Survey, National Center for Health Statistics. Available at *http://www.cdc.gov/std/stats01/Women&Infants/sld009.htm* (accessed January 20, 2005).

5. Zane SB, Kieke Jr BA, Kendrick JS, Bruce C: Surveillance in a time of changing health care practices: estimating ectopic pregnancy incidence in the United States. Matern Child Health J 6:227–236, 2002.

6. Centers for Disease Control and Prevention: STDs in women and infants. *In* Sexually Transmitted Disease Surveillance, 2003. Atlanta: Centers for Disease Control and Prevention, 2004, pp 43–51.

7. Centers for Disease Control and Prevention. STDs in adolescents and young adults. *In* Sexually Transmitted Disease Surveillance, 2003. Atlanta: Centers for Disease Control and Prevention, 2004, pp 53–62.

8. Centers for Disease Control and Prevention. Chlamydia. *In* Sexually Transmitted Disease Surveillance, 2003. Atlanta: Centers for Disease Control and Prevention, 2004, pp 7–14.

9. Maymon R, Shulman A, Maymon BB, et al: Ectopic pregnancy, the new gynecological epidemic disease: review of the modern work-up and the nonsurgical treatment option. Int J Fertil 37:146–164, 1992.

*10. Centers for Disease Control and Prevention: Pregnancy-related mortality surveillance—United States, 1991–1999. Morb Mortal Wkly Rep CDC Surveill Summ 52(SS-2):1–8, 2003.

11. Cartwright PS: Diagnosis of ectopic pregnancy. Obstet Gynecol Clin North Am 18:19–37, 1991.

12. Burry KA, Thurmond AS, Suby-Long TD, et al: Transvaginal ultrasonographic findings in surgically verfied ectopic pregnancy. Am J Obstet Gynecol 168:1796–1802, 1993.

13. Dwyer BJ: Ectopic pregnancy requires precise diagnosis and prompt intervention. Emerg Med Rep 13:113–120, 1992.

14. Stovall TG, Kellerman AL, Ling FW, et al: Emergency department diagnosis of ectopic pregnancy. Ann Emerg Med 19:1098–1103, 1990.

15. Weckstein LN: Current perspective on ectopic pregnancy. Obstet Gynecol Surv 40:259–272, 1985.

16. Quan MA, Johnson RA, Puffer JC: The diagnosis of ectopic pregnancy. Am Fam Physician 31:201–207, 1985.

17. Hirata AJ, Soper DE, Bump RC, et al: Ectopic pregnancy in an urban teaching hospital: can tubal rupture be predicted? South Med J 84:1467–1469, 1991.

18. Hebertson RM, Storey ND: Ectopic pregnancy. Crit Care Clin 7:899–915, 1991.

19. Krantz SC, Gray RH, Damewood MD, Wallach EE: Time trends in risk factors and clinical outcome of ectopic pregnancy. Fertil Steril 54:42–46, 1990.

20. Jones EE: Ectopic pregnancy: common and some uncommon misdiagnoses. Obstet Gynecol Clin North Am 18:55–72, 1991.

21. Weckstein LN, Boucher AR, Tucker H, et al: Accurate diagnosis of early ectopic pregnancy. Obstet Gynecol 65:393–397, 1985.

22. Abbott J, Emmans LS, Lowenstein SR: Ectopic pregnancy: ten common pitfalls in diagnosis. Am J Emerg Med 8:515–522, 1990.

23. Birkhahn RH, Gaeta TJ, Bei R, Bove JJ: Shock index in the first trimester of pregnancy and its relationship to ruptured ectopic pregnancy. Acad Emerg Med 9:115–119, 2002.

24. Buckley RG, King KJ, Disney JD, et al: History and physical examination to estimate the risk of ectopic pregnancy: validation of a clinical prediction model. Ann Emerg Med 34:589–594, 1999.

25. Dart RG, Kaplan B, Varaklis K: Predictive value of history and physical examination in patients with suspected ectopic pregnancy. Ann Emerg Med 33:283–290, 1999.

26. Ramoska EA, Sacchetti AD, Nepp M: Reliability of patient history in determining the possibility of pregnancy. Ann Emerg Med 18:48–50, 1989.

*27. Brennan DF: Ectopic pregnancy—part I: clinical & laboratory diagnosis. Acad Emerg Med 2:1081–1089, 1995.

*28. Brennan DF: Ectopic pregnancy—part II: diagnostic procedures & imaging. Acad Emerg Med 2:1090–1097, 1995.

29. Wilcox AJ, Baird DD, Dunson D, et al: Natural limits of pregnancy testing in relation to the expected menstrual period. JAMA 286:1759–1761, 2001.

30. Davies S, Byrn F, Cole LA: Human chorionic gonadotropin testing for early pregnancy viability and complications. Clin Lab Med 23:257–264, 2003.

31. Butler SA, Khanlian SA, Cole LA: Detection of early pregancy forms of human chorionic gonadotropin by home pregacy testing devices. Clin Chem 47:2131–2136, 2001.

32. O'Connor RE, Bibro CM, Pegg PJ, Bouzoukis JK: The comparative sensitivity and specificity of serum and urine HCG determinations in the ED [Letter]. Am J Emerg Med 11:434–436, 1993.

33. Fritz K, Kristal SL: High false-negative rate of urine HCG pregnancy testing [Abstract]. Ann Emerg Med 38:S70, 2001.

34. Kingdom JC, Kelly T, MacLean AB, et al: Rapid one step urine test for human chorionic gonadotropin in evaluating suspected complications of early pregnancy. BMJ 302:1308–1311, 1991.

*35. DiMarchi JM, Kosasa TS, Hale RW: What is the significance of the human chorionic gonadotropin value in ectopic pregnancy? Obstet Gynecol 74:851–855, 1989.

36. Olson CM, Holt JA, Alenghat E, et al: Limitations of qualitative serum beta-HCG assays in the diagnosis of ectopic pregnancy. J Reprod Med 12:838–842, 1983.

37. Maccato ML, Estrada R, Faro S: Ectopic pregnancy with undetectable serum and urine β-hCG levels and detection of β-hCG in the ectopic trophoblast by immunocytochemical evaluation. Obstet Gynecol 81:878–880, 1993.

38. Lonky NM, Sauer MV: Ectopic pregnancy with shock and undetectable β-human chorionic gonadotropin: a case report. J Reprod Med 32:559–560, 1987.

39. Kuscu E, Vicdan K, Turhan NO, et al: The hormonal profile in ectopic pregnancies. JMPA J Pak Med Assoc 44:45–47, 1994.

40. Popp LW, Colditz A, Gaetje R: Diagnosis of intrauterine and ectopic pregnancy at 5–7 postmenstrual weeks. Int J Gynaecol Obstet 44:33–38, 1993.

41. Ledger WL, Sweeting VM, Chatterjee S: Rapid diagnosis of early ectopic pregnancy in an emergency gynaecology service—are measurements of progesterone, intact and free β human chorionic gonadotropin helpful? Hum Reprod 9:157–160, 1994.

42. Dart RG, Kaplan B, Cox C: Transvaginal ultrasound in patients with low β-human chorionic gonadotropin values: how often is the study diagnostic? Ann Emerg Med 30:135–140, 1997.

*43. Dart R: Role of pelvic ultrasonography in evaluation of symptomatic first-trimester pregnancy. Ann Emerg Med 33:310–320, 1999.

44. Mateer JR, Valley VT, Aiman EJ, et al: Outcome analysis of a protocol including bedside endovaginal sonography in patients at risk for ectopic pregnancy. Ann Emerg Med 27:283–289, 1996.

45. Durham B, Lane B, Burbridge L, et al: Pelvic ultrasound performed by emergency physicians for the detection of ectopic pregnancy in complicated first-trimester pregnancies. Ann Emerg Med 29:338–347, 1997.

46. Walsh GA, Isenhour JL, Seth NB: Analysis of current emergency medicine ultrasound training [Abstract]. Ann Emerg Med 38:S27, 2001.

47. Ory SJ: New options for diagnosis and treatment of ectopic pregnancy. JAMA 267:534–537, 1992.

48. Sanfilippo JS, Woodworth SH: Ectopic pregnancy. Telindes Oper Gynecol Updates 1(4):1–14, 1992.

49. Emerson DS, McCord ML: Clinician's approach to ectopic pregnancy. Clin Obstet Gynecol 39:199–222, 1996.

50. Cacciatore B, Stenman UH: Early screening for ectopic pregnancy in high-risk symptom-free women. Lancet 343:517–518, 1994.

51. Stovall TG, Ling FW: Ectopic pregnancy: diagnostic and therapeutic algorithms minimizing surgical intervention. J Reprod Med 38:807–812, 1993.

52. Anandakumar C, Lee CS, Wong YC, et al: Accuracy in diagnosis of ectopic pregnancy by transvaginal ultrasonography. Asia Oceanic J Obstet Gynaecol 18:107–113, 1992.

53. Russell SA, Filly RA, Damato N: Sonographic diagnosis of ectopic pregnancy with endovaginal probes: what really has changed? J Ultrasound Med 3:145–151, 1993.

*54. Kadar N, DeVore G, Romero R: Discriminatory HCG zone: its use in the sonographic evaluation for ectopic pregnancy. Br Obstet Gynaecol 58:156–161, 1981.

*55. Cacciatore B, Stenman UH, Ylostalo P: Diagnosis of ectopic pregnancy by vaginal ultrasonography in combination with a discriminatory serum HCG level of 1000 IU/l (IRP). Br J Obstet Gynaecol 97:904–908, 1990.

56. Ackerman TE, Levi CS, Lyons EA, et al: Decidual cyst: endovaginal sonographic sign of ectopic pregnancy. Radiology 189:727–731, 1993.

57. Braffman BH, Coleman BG, Ramchandani P, et al: Emergency department screening for ectopic pregnancy: a prospective US study. Radiology 190:797–802, 1994.

*Selected readings.

58. Stiller RJ, de Regt RH, Blair E: Transvaginal ultrasonography in patients at risk for ectopic pregnancy. Am J Obstet Gynecol 161:930–933, 1989.

59. Penzias AS, Huang PL: Imaging in ectopic pregnancy. J Reprod Med 37:47–53, 1992.

60. Kivikoski AI, Martin CM, Smeltzer JS: Transabdominal and transvaginal ultrasonography in the diagnosis of ectopic pregnancy: a comparative study. Am J Obstet Gynecol 163:123–128, 1990.

61. Thorsen MK, Lawson TL, Aiman EJ, et al: Diagnosis of ectopic pregnancy: endovaginal versus transabdominal sonography. AJR Am J Roentgenol 155:307–310, 1990.

62. Cacciatore B, Stenman UH, Ylostalo P: Comparison of abdominal and vaginal sonography in suspected ectopic pregnancy. Obstet Gynecol 73:770–774, 1989.

63. Timor-Tritsch IE, Yeh MN, Peisner DB, et al: The use of transvaginal ultrasonography in the diagnosis of ectopic pregnancy. Obstet Gynecol 161:157–161, 1989.

64. Fleischer AC, Pennell RG, McKee MS, et al: Ectopic pregnancy: features at transvaginal sonography. Radiology 174:375–378, 1990.

65. Bateman BG, Nunley WC, Kolp LA, et al: Vaginal sonography findings and HCG dynamics of early intrauterine and tubal pregnancies. Obstet Gynecol 75:421–427, 1990.

66. Fossum G, Davajan V, Kletzky O: Early detection of pregnancy with transvaginal ultrasound. Fertil Steril 49:788–791, 1988.

67. Ghorashi B, Gottesfeld KR: The gray scale appearance of the normal pregnancy from 4 to 16 weeks of gestation. J Clin Ultrasound 5:195–201, 1977.

68. Batzer FR, Weiner SW, Corson SL, et al: Landmarks during the first forty-two days of gestation demonstrated by the β-subunit of human chorionic gonadotropin and ultrasound. Am J Obstet Gynecol 146:973–979, 1983.

69. DeCherney AH, Romero R, Polan ML: Ultrasound in reproductive endocrinology. Fertil Steril 37:323–333, 1982.

70. Bree RL, Edwards M, Bohm-Velez M, et al: Transvaginal sonography in the evaluation of normal early pregnancy: correlation with hCG level. AJR Am J Roentgenol 153:75–79, 1989.

71. Sherer DM, Abramowicz JS, Kogut PL, et al: Use of endovaginal color Doppler ultrasound to document fetal heart motion in a 5-week ectopic gestation. J Diagn Med Sonogr 8:266–268, 1992.

72. Burry KA, Thurmond AS, Suby-Long TD, et al: Transvaginal ultrasonographic findings in surgically verfied ectopic pregnancy. Am J Obstet Gynecol 168:1796–1802, 1993.

73. Frates MC, Brown DL, Doubilet PM, Hornstein MD: Tubal rupture in patients with ectopic pregnancy: diagnosis with transvaginal US. Radiology 191:769–772, 1994.

74. Nyberg DA, Mack LA, Jeffrey RB, Laing FC: Endovaginal sonographic evaluation of ectopic pregnancy: a prospective study. AJR Am J Roentgenol 149:1181–1186, 1987.

75. Romero R, Kadar N, Castro D, et al: The value of adnexal sonographic findings in the diagnosis of ectopic pregnancy. Am J Obstet Gynecol 158:52–55, 1988.

76. Blaivas M: Color Doppler in the diagnosis of ectopic pregnancy in the emergency department: is there anything beyond a mass and fluid? J Emerg Med 22:379–384, 2002.

77. Megier P, Desroches A: [Color and pulsed Doppler ultrasonography imaging of tubal ectopic pregnancy: study of 100 cases]. J Radiol 84:1753–1756, 2003.

78. Atri M: Ectopic pregnancy versus corpus luteum cyst revisited: best Doppler predictors. J Ultrasound Med 22:1181–1184, 2003.

79. Nager CW, Murphy AA: Ectopic pregnancy. Clin Obstet Gynecol 34:403–411, 1991.

80. Ankum WM, Van der Veen, Hamerlynck JV, Lammes FB: Transvaginal sonography and human chorionic gonadotropin measurements in suspected ectopic pregnancy: a detailed analysis of a diagnostic approach. Hum Reprod 8:1307–1311, 1993.

81. Chambers SE, Muir BB, Haddad NG: Ultrasound evaluation of ectopic pregnancy including correlation with human chorionic gonadotropin levels. Br J Radiol 63:246–250, 1990.

82. Parvey HR, Maklad N: Pitfalls in the transvaginal sonographic diagnosis of ectopic pregnancy. J Ultrasound Med 3:139–144, 1993.

83. Soussis I, Dimitry ES, Oskarsson T, et al: Diagnosis of ectopic pregnancy by vaginal ultrasonography in combination with a discriminatory serum HCG level of 1000 IU/l (IRP) [Comment]. Br J Obstet Gynaecol 98:233, 1991.

84. Dart RG, Dart L, Mitchell P, Berty C: The predictive value of endometrial stripe thickness in patients with suspected ectopic pregnancy who have an empty uterus at ultrasonography. Acad Emerg Med 6:602–608, 1999.

85. Spandorfer SD, Barnhart KT: Endometrial stripe thickness as a predictor of ectopic pregnancy. Fertil Steril 66:474–477, 1996.

86. Mishell DR Jr, Nakamura RM, Barberia JM, Thorneycroft IH: Initial detection of human chorionic gonadotropin in serum in normal human gestation. Am J Obstet Gynecol 118:990–991, 1974.

87. Wilcox AJ, Weinberg CR, O'Connor JF, et al: Incidence of early loss of pregnancy. N Engl J Med 319:189–194, 1988.

88. Hill LM, Kislak S, Martin JG: Transvaginal sonographic detection of the pseudogestational sac associated with ectopic pregnancy. Obstet Gynecol 75:986–988, 1990.

89. Counselman FL, Shaar GS, Heller RA, King DK: Quantitative β-hCG levels less than 1000 IU/L in patients with ectopic pregnancy: pelvic ultrasound still useful. J Emerg Med 16:699–703, 1998.

90. Buyalos RP, Glassman LM, Rifka SM, et al: Serum β-human chorionic gonadotropin, estradiol and progesterone as early predictors of pathologic pregnancy. J Reprod Med 37:261–266, 1992.

91. Pittaway DE: βhCG dynamics in ectopic pregnancy. Clin Obstet Gynecol 30:129–135, 1987.

92. Kadar N: Use of serial human chorionic gonadotropin measurements to differentiate between intrauterine and ectopic pregnancies [Letter]. Am J Obstet Gynecol 163:259–260, 1990.

*93. Kadar N, Caldwell BV, Romero R: A method of screening for ectopic pregnancy and its indications. Obstet Gynecol 58:162–166, 1981.

94. Shepherd RW, Patton PE, Novy MJ, et al: Serial βhCG measurements in the early detection of ectopic pregnancy. Obstet Gynecol 75:417–420, 1990.

95. Tinga DJ, van Lier JJ, de Bruijn HW: Doubling time and hCG score for the early diagnosis of ectopic pregnancy in asymptomatic women. Acta Obstet Gynecol Scand 69:505–509, 1990.

96. Korhonen J, Stenman UH, Ylostalo P: Serum human chorionic gonadotropin dynamics during spontaneous resolution of ectopic pregnancy. Fertil Steril 62:632–636, 1994.

97. Kadar N, Romero R: Further observations on serial human chorionic gonadotropin patterns in ectopic pregnancies and spontaneous abortions. Fertil Steril 50:367, 1988.

98. Popp LW, Colditz A, Gaetje R: Management of early ectopic pregnancy. Int J Gynaecol Obstet 44:239–244, 1994.

99. Peisner DB, Timor-Tritsch IE: The discriminatory zone of βhCG for vaginal probes. J Clin Ultrasound 18:280–285, 1990.

100. Hellemans P, Gerris J, Joostens M, et al: Serum hCG decline following salpingotomy or salpingectomy for extrauterine pregnancy. Eur J Obstet Gynecol Reprod Biol 53:59–64, 1994.

101. Tulandi T: "Resolution" and "success" of medical treatment of ectopic pregnancy [Editorial]. Fertil Steril 57:963–964, 1992.

102. Ory SJ: Chemotherapy for ectopic pregnancy. Obstet Gynecol Clin North Am 18:123–134, 1991.

103. Bengtsson G, Bryman I, Thornburn J: Low dose oral methotrexate as second line therapy for persistent trophoblast after conservative treatment of ectopic pregnancy. Obstet Gynecol 79:589–591, 1992.

104. Thompson GR, O'Shea RT, Harding A: Beta HCG levels after conservative treatment of ectopic pregnancy: is a plateau normal? Aust N Z J Obstet Gynaecol 34:96–98, 1994.

105. Dart RG, Mitterando J, Dart LM: Rate of change of serial beta-human chorionic gonadotropin values as a predictor of ectopic pregnancy in patients with indeterminate transvaginal ultrasound findings. Ann Emerg Med 34:703–710, 1999.

106. Mol BWJ, Hajenius PJ, Engelsbel S, et al: Serum human chorionic gonadotropin measurement in the diagnosis of ectopic pregnancy when transvaginal ultrasound is inconclusive. Fertil Steril 70:972–981, 1998.

107. Lurie S, Katz Z, Weissman A, et al: Declining β-human chorionic gonadotropin level may provide false security that tubal pregnancy will not rupture. Eur J Obstet Gynecol Reprod Biol 53:72–73, 1994.

108. Billieux MH, Petignat P, Anguenot JL, et al: Early and late half-life of human chorionic gonadotropin as a predictor of persistent trophoblast after laparoscopic conservative surgery for tubal pregnancy. Acta Obstet Gynecol Scand 82:550–555, 2003.

109. American College of Obstetricians and Gynecologists: Medical Management of Tubal Pregnancy (ACOG Practice Bulletin 3). Washington, DC: Amercan College of Obstetricians and Gynecologists, 1998.

110. Long CA, Lincoln SR, Whitworth NS, Cowan BD: Serum progesterone predicts abnormal gestations in clomiphene citrate conception cycles as well as in spontaneous conception cycles. Fertil Steril 61:838–842, 1994.

111. Carson SA, Buster JE: Ectopic Pregnancy. N Engl J Med 329:1174–1181, 1993.

112. Williams RS, Gaines IL, Fossom GT: Progesterone in diagnosis of ectopic pregnancy. J Fla Med Assoc 79:237–239, 1992.

113. Stovall TG: Discussion. Am J Obstet Gynecol 166:1729–1737, 1992.

114. Grosskinsky CM, Hage ML, Tyrey L, et al: hCG, progesterone, alpha-fetoprotein, and estradiol in the identification of ectopic pregnancy. Obstet Gynecol 81:705–709, 1993.

115. Gelder MS, Boots LR, Younger JB: Use of a single random serum progesterone value as a diagnostic aid for ectopic pregnancy. Fertil Steril 55:497–500, 1991.

116. Buckley RG, King KJ, Disney JD, et al: Serum progesterone testing to predict ectopic pregnancy in symptomatic first-trimester patients. Ann Emerg Med 36:95–100, 2000.

117. Peterson CM, Kreger D, Delgado P, et al: Laboratory and clinical comparison of a rapid versus a classic progesterone radioimmunoassay for use in determining abnormal and ectopic pregnancies. Am J Obstet Gynecol 166:562–566, 1992.

118. Hahlin M, Wallin A, Sjoblom P, et al: Single progesterone assay for early recognition of abnormal pregnancy. Hum Reprod 5:622–626, 1990.

119. Dart R, Ramanujam P, Dart L: Progesterone as a predictor of ectopic pregancy when ultrasound is indeterminate. Am J Emerg Med 20:575–579, 2002.

*120. Stovall TG, Ling FW, Carson SA, et al: Serum progesterone and uterine curettage in differential diagnosis of ectopic pregnancy. Fertil Steril 57:456–458, 1992.

121. Maruri F, Azziz R: Laparoscopic surgery for ectopic pregnancies: technology assessment and public health implications. Fertil Steril 59:487–498, 1993.

122. Zorn JR, Risquez F, Cedard L: Ectopic pregnancy. Curr Opin Obstet Gynecol 4:238–245, 1992.

123. Kohn MA, Kerr K, Malkevich D, et al: Beta-human chorionic gonadotropin levels and the likelihood of ectopic pregnancy in emergency department patients with abdominal pain or vaginal bleeding. Acad Emerg Med 10:119–126, 2003.

124. American College of Obstetricians and Gynecologists: Prevention of Rh D Alloimmunization (ACOG Practice Bulletin 4). Washington, DC; American College of Obstetricians and Gynecologists, 1999.

125. American College of Emergency Physicians: Clinical policy: critical issues in the initial evaluation and management of patients presenting to the emergency department in early pregnancy. Ann Emerg Med 41:123–133, 2003.

*126. Lipscomb GH, Stovall TG, Ling FW: Nonsurgical treatment of ectopic pregnancy. N Engl J Med 343:1325–1329, 2000.

127. Stovall TG, Ling FW: Expectant management of ectopic pregnancy. Obstet Gynecol Clin North Am 18:135–144, 1991.

128. Risquez F, Pennehouat G, Foulot H, et al: Transcervical tubal cannulation and falloposcopy for the management of tubal pregnancy. Hum Reprod 7:274–275, 1992.

129. Thornton KL: Linear salpingostomy for ectopic pregnancy. Obstet Gynecol Clin North Am 18:95–109, 1991.

130. Lindblom B: Ectopic pregnancy: laparoscopic and medical treatment. Curr Opin Obstet Gynecol 4:400–405, 1992.

131. Lang PF, Tamussino K, Honingl W, et al: Treatment of unruptured tubal pregnancy by laparoscopic instillation of hyperosmolar glucose solution. Am J Obstet Gynecol 166:1378–1381, 1992.

132. Saunders NJ: Non-surgical treatment of ectopic pregnancy. Br J Obstet Gynaecol 97:972–973, 1990.

133. Stovall TG, Ling FW, Gray LA: Single dose methotrexate for treatment of ectopic pregnancy. Obstet Gynecol 77:754–757, 1991.

134. Prevost RR, Stovall TG, Ling FW: Methotrexate for treatment of unruptured ectopic pregnancy. Clin Pharm 11:529–532, 1992.

135. Stovall TG, Ling FW, Buster JE: Reproductive performance after methotrexate treatment of ectopic pregnancy. Am J Obstet Gynecol 162:1620–1624, 1990.

136. Rose PG, Cohen SM: Methotrexate therapy for persistent ectopic pregnancy after conservative laparoscopic management. Obstet Gynecol 76:947–949, 1990.

137. Domesic DA, Hafez GR: Delayed hemorrhage of a persistent ectopic pregnancy following laparoscopy salpingostomy and methotrexate therapy. Obstet Gynecol 78:960–962, 1991.

138. Lubowski TJ, Rozek SL: Methotrexate in ectopic pregnancy. DICP 24:387–388, 1990.

139. Leach RE, Ory SJ: Management of ectopic pregnancy. Am Fam Physician 41:1215–1222, 1990.

140. Lundorff P: Modern management of ectopic pregnancy. Acta Obstet Gynecol Scand 71:158–159, 1992.

141. Torp VA: Therapeutic options for ectopic pregnancy [Letter]. West J Med 156:651–652, 1992.

142. Baumann R, Magos AL, Turnbull A: Prospective comparison of videopelviscopy with laparotomy for ectopic pregnancy. Br J Obstet Gynaecol 98:765–771, 1991.

143. Koninckx PR, Witters K, Brosens J, et al: Conservative laparoscopic treatment of ectopic pregnancies using the CO_2-laser. Br J Obstet Gynaecol 98:1254–1259, 1991.

144. Seifer DB, Gutman JN, Doyle MB, et al: Persistent ectopic pregnancy following linear salpingostomy. Obstet Gynecol 76:1121–1125, 1990.

145. Lundorff P, Thornburn J, Lindblom B: Fertility outcome after conservative surgical treatment of ectopic pregnancy evaluated in a randomized trial. Fertil Steril 57:998–1002, 1992.

146. Levin JH, Lacarra M, d'Ablaing G, et al: Mifepristone (RU 486) failure in an ovarian heterotopic pregnancy. Am J Obstet Gynecol 163:543–544, 1990.

147. Egarter C: Methotrexate treatment of ectopic gestation and reproductive outcome [Letter]. Am J Obstet Gynecol 164:698–699, 1991.

148. Segna RA, Mitchell DR, Misas JE: Successful treatment of cervical pregnancy with oral etoposide. Obstet Gynecol 76:945–947, 1990.

149. Lang PF, Honigl W: Hyperosmolar glucose solution or prostaglandin F2 for ectopic pregnancy [Letter]. Lancet 336:685, 1990.

150. Koike H, Chuganji Y, Hiroyuki W, et al: Conservative treatment of ovarian pregnancy by local prostaglandin F2 injection [Letter]. Am J Obstet Gynecol 162:696, 1990.

151. Odejinmi F, Madhuvrata P, Naftalin A, et al: Enthusiasm and teamwork—the basis for increase in laparoscopic surgery for ectopic pregnancy: an Inner London district hospital experience. J Obstet Gynaecol 23:645–647, 2003.

152. Vaissade L, Gerbaud L, Pouly JL, et al: Cost effectiveness analysis of laparoscopic surgery versus methotrexate: comparison of data recorded in an ectopic pregnancy registry. J Gynecol Obstet Biol Reprod (Paris) 32:447–458, 2003.

153. Cooray H, Harilall M, Farquhar CM: A six year audit of the management of ectopic pregnancy. Aust N Z J Obstet Gynaecol 42:598–542, 2002.

154. Jedrzejczak P, Kubiaczyk B, Pisarski T, et al: Comparison of the frequency of selected gynecologic operations conducted as laparotomy and laparoscopy during 1993–1997. Ginekol Pol 72:228–235, 2001.

155. Sagiv R, Debby A, Sadan O, et al: Laparoscopic surgery for extrauterine pregnancy in hemodynamically unstable patients. J Am Assoc Gynecol Laparoscopists 8:529–532, 2001.

156. Li Z, Leng J, Lang J, et al: Laparoscopic surgery in patients with hypovolemic shock due to ectopic pregnancy. Chung Hua Fu Chan Ko Tsa Chih [Chin J Obstet Gynecol] 37:653–655, 2002.

157. Akhan SE, Baysal B: Laparotomy or laparoscopic surgery? Factors affecting the surgeon's choice for the treatment of ectopic pregnancy. Arch Gynecol Obstet 266:79–82, 2002.

158. Lecuru F, Camatte S, Viens-Bitker C, et al: Hospital resources used for ectopic pregnancy treatment by laparoscopy and methotrexate. J Soc Laparoendosc Surg 5:117–122, 2001.

159. Sowter MC, Farquhar CM, Gudex G: An economic evaluation of single dose systemic methotrexate and laparoscopic surgery for the treatment of unruptured ectopic pregnancy. BJOG 108:204–212, 2001.

160. Alshimmiri MM, Al-Saleh EA, Al-Harmi JA, et al: Treatment of ectopic pregnancy with a single intramuscular dose of methotrexate. Arch Gynecol Obstet 268:181–183, 2003.

161. Hajenius PJ, Engelsbel S, Mol BW, et al: Randomised trial of systemic methotrexate versus laparoscopic salpingostomy in tubal pregnancy. Lancet 350:774–779, 1997.

162. Namnoum AB: Medical management of ectopic pregnancy. Clin Obstet Gynecol 41:382–386, 1998.

163. Buster JE, Pisarska MD: Medical management of ectopic pregnancy. Clin Obstet Gynecol 42:23–30, 1999.

164. Sauer MV, Rodi IA: Utility of an algorithm to diagnose ectopic pregnancy. Int J Gynaecol Obstet 31:29–34, 1990.

Chapter 91

Pregnancy-Related Complications

Angela M. Mills, MD and Elizabeth M. Datner, MD

Key Points

All adolescent females should be tested for pregnancy; social support and appropriate referrals should be provided to all pregnant teenagers.

Vaginal bleeding in the first trimester should be evaluated with the focus to rule out ectopic pregnancy and stabilize the patient hemodynamically.

Seizures in the setting of pregnancy should be considered as possible eclampsia.

Futile resuscitation of a gravid patient with a potentially viable fetus should prompt consideration of emergency cesarean section.

All pregnant patients should be screened for domestic violence and offered referral resources and safe housing.

Introduction and Background

Teenage pregnancy is an important public health concern, accounting for over 10% of all births in the United States in 2003.[1] Even with recent declines in adolescent birth rates, approximately 800,000 to 900,000 adolescents become pregnant yearly.[2] This population has unique issues and requires a distinct understanding of both their medical and psychosocial circumstances. In comparison to pregnancies in adult women, teenage pregnancies have been associated with an increased risk of adverse outcomes, including preterm deliveries, low birth weight, and higher neonatal mortality.[3-5] Younger adolescents may be at even higher risk. One study demonstrated that teenage mothers under 15 years of age are less likely than older adolescents to have adequate prenatal care.[6] In addition to inadequate utilization of prenatal care, pregnant adolescents are also more likely to have poor health habits and engage in health risk behaviors such as smoking, which is one of the strongest risk factors for adverse perinatal outcomes.[7] The psychosocial concerns of pregnant teenagers are myriad and are equally important as the medical issues,

if not more so. They may include but are certainly not limited to an unstable home life, lost educational opportunities, poor employability, and welfare dependence.[5]

Because of the high-risk nature of teen pregnancy, all female adolescents who seek care in emergency departments should be tested for pregnancy in order to identify patients who may need referral for early prenatal care. In addition, those who present with abdominal pain, vaginal bleeding, syncope, altered mental status, or hypotension and are pregnant will require further detailed evaluation specifically addressing potential pregnancy-related complications. The clinician must maintain a high suspicion for pregnancy, and especially ectopic pregnancy, when treating adolescents (see Chapter 90, Ectopic Preganancy). This chapter focuses on other pregnancy-related complications in the adolescent patient.

Selected Diagnoses

First trimester bleeding
Complications of induced abortion
Amniotic fluid embolus
Molar pregnancy
Nausea and vomiting of pregnancy and hyperemesis gravidarum
Pregnancy-induced hypertension
Vaginal bleeding in the second half of pregnancy
Trauma in pregnancy
Rh immunization
Medication use in pregnancy

Discussion of Individual Diagnoses

First Trimester Bleeding

First trimester vaginal bleeding is common, occurring in up to 25% of all pregnancies, with spontaneous abortion (SAb) resulting in over half of cases prior to sonographic evaluation.[8,9] Spontaneous abortion (also termed *miscarriage*) occurs in several stages, with *threatened abortion* defined as vaginal bleeding during the first half of pregnancy with a closed cervical os. If cervical dilation is present, the term *inevitable abortion* is used. *Incomplete abortion* occurs with partial passage of the gestational products. When all fetal tissue is passed and the cervical os is closed, a *complete abortion* has occurred. This may be difficult to distinguish

Table 91-1	Definitions of Terms for Vaginal Bleeding at Less Than 20 Weeks of Pregnancy	
Cervix Examination	**Products of Conception**	**Abortion Term**
Closed	Present	Threatened
Closed	Absent	Complete
Open	Present	Inevitable
Open	Partially passed	Incomplete

from an incomplete abortion and may require diagnosis with pathologic confirmation of the products of conception. A SAb is defined as any unintentional fetal loss prior to 20 weeks' gestation (Table 91-1). A *missed abortion* is the term for a fetal death at less than 20 weeks' gestation when the products of conception have not been passed for more than 4 weeks.

Patients with the diagnosis of threatened abortion at any time in the first trimester are at increased risk for spontaneous loss prior to 24 weeks' gestation. The risk of pregnancy loss is directly proportional to the amount of vaginal bleeding experienced by the patient.[8] The risk rises with increasing maternal age, multiparity, and history of prior vaginal bleeding. Although SAb is more common in older women, approximately 12% occur in women less than 20 years of age. Women with heavy vaginal bleeding in the first trimester are also at increased risk for preterm delivery, intrauterine growth retardation, placental abruption, premature rupture of the membranes, and cesarean delivery. If a viable fetus is diagnosed by ultrasound when first trimester bleeding has occurred, greater than 95% of these pregnancies will continue to the second half of pregnancy.[8]

The history of patients with bleeding in the first trimester should include the date of the last menstrual period, quantity of bleeding, and passage of clots or tissue. Pelvic examination is necessary to determine the status of the cervical os, the amount of bleeding, and whether fetal tissue is evident. Products of conception at the os should be gently removed using a ring forceps to decrease bleeding and discomfort. However, if any resistance to removal is encountered, the tissue should be left in place until obstetric evaluation is possible. Ancillary testing should include a quantitative serum β-human chorionic gonadotropin (βhCG) level, blood type with Rh factor, and pelvic ultrasound (US). Rh-negative women require immune globulin as discussed later.

β-hCG is a hormone secreted by the placenta that doubles approximately every 48 hours in early pregnancy. This hormone may be correlated with US by use of the discriminatory zone, which is the β-hCG level above which an intrauterine pregnancy (IUP) may be visualized using US with near-100% sensitivity. This level varies by institution and is approximately 1200 to 1500 mIU/ml when using transvaginal US and between 4000 and 6500 mIU/ml with transabdominal US. If the level is above the discriminatory zone and an IUP is not visualized, ectopic or abnormal pregnancy must be considered.[10-12] In one study, the group of patients with a β-hCG level below the discriminatory zone with an indeterminate US was found to have a fourfold higher relative risk of ectopic pregnancy than patients with higher β-hCG levels.[13] Other studies have found lower rates of ectopic pregnancies in this subgroup.[11] The differential diagnosis in this group of patients includes ectopic pregnancy, early viable IUP, and nonviable IUP. An accepted protocol in the stable patient who is not bleeding excessively is following serial β-hCG levels with repeat US on an outpatient basis. Gynecologic consultation for follow-up is necessary in patients with indeterminate US (see Chapter 90, Ectopic Pregnancy).

Patients who are bleeding heavily or have an open cervical os require gynecologic consultation, as dilation and evacuation may be necessary. Stable patients with the diagnosis of threatened abortion may be discharged with close follow-up. Precautions should be given for prompt return if there is heavy bleeding (soaking more than one pad per hour), symptomatic anemia, fever, or significant pain.

Complications of Induced Abortion

Approximately 2% of all women of reproductive age in the United States elect to have an induced abortion each year, and in 2001, teenagers accounted for 18% of all abortions. Adolescents under 15 years had the highest abortion ratio at 744 per 1000 live births.[14] Induced abortion may be performed either medically or surgically. Legal abortion is one of the safest surgical procedures with a relatively low complication rate. In a large case series of over 170,000 first trimester abortions, complications requiring hospitalization comprised 0.7 per 1000 abortions and included suspected perforation, sepsis, ectopic pregnancy, hemorrhage, and incomplete abortion. Less serious complications, defined as those not requiring referral to a hospital, included mild infection, retained tissue or clots requiring resuctioning, cervical tear, and underestimation of gestational age. These accounted for 8.46 per 1000 abortions, with an overall complication rate of 9.05 per 1000 abortions.[15]

Adolescents are more likely than older women to have abortions later in pregnancy. Approximately 15% of abortions in patients less than 15 years old, and 10% of those in patients between 15 and 19 years of age, occur later than 15 weeks' gestation, higher than any other age group.[16] Therefore, teens are less often candidates for medical abortion and may require surgical abortion instead. One study showed greater than a third of mortality risk in teenagers was due to having an induced abortion at a later gestational age when compared to women over 30 years of age.[17] The risk factor that continues to be most strongly related to mortality from legal abortion is gestational age at the time of abortion.

The most common complications of induced abortion include hemorrhage, retained products of conception, hematometra, and infection. Hemorrhage is commonly due to uterine atony, retained tissue, and, less often, traumatic injury. Patients with retained tissue usually present with vaginal bleeding and abdominal cramping within the first few days after surgical abortion. Ultrasound may aid in diagnosis. Hematometra, or the accumulation of blood clots in the uterus, may occur after surgical abortion. Symptoms include pelvic or rectal pressure with a tense and tender uterus on examination. Acutely, vaginal bleeding is often minimal while dark clots may be passed with delayed hematometra. Sonography may demonstrate heterogeneous echoes within the uterus.

Perforation is a less common complication of induced abortion and may range from a simple puncture of the uterine wall to injury to the blood vessels or intra-abdominal contents. Practitioners must be concerned about perforation when patients present with atypical or refractory abdominal pain or persistent bleeding after an induced abortion. Infection after abortion is often characterized by endometritis with uterine tenderness with or without fever. Less common infectious complications include salpingitis, peritonitis, pelvic abscess, and sepsis.[18] Prophylactic antibiotics have been shown to decrease infection and are routinely prescribed after elective abortions.[19] Complications of induced abortion necessitate gynecologic consultation. Care of the adolescent in the emergency department may also provide an opportune time to offer contraceptive and sexually transmitted infection counseling.

Amniotic Fluid Embolus

Amniotic fluid embolus is a rare and rapidly progressive complication of pregnancy with high maternal morbidity and mortality. Historically mortality rates were over 60%, although more recent studies suggest mortality rates of less than 30%.[20] Patients often present with sudden cardiovascular collapse, disseminated intravascular coagulation, and death. Amniotic fluid embolus is most common during labor but may also occur during induced and spontaneous abortions. It is thought that this disease process is consistent with an allergic or anaphylactic reaction rather than a true embolism, and the term *anaphylactoid syndrome of pregnancy* has been proposed.[21] Diagnosis is based on the clinical setting with a high index of suspicion. Treatment involves prompt resuscitation with airway and hemodynamic support. Emergent cesarean section may be required.

Molar Pregnancy

Gestational trophoblastic disease (GTD) consists of a spectrum of conditions originating from the placenta and is characterized by disordered proliferation of chorionic villi. The spectrum includes complete hydatidiform mole, where there is an absence of fetal tissue; incomplete mole, when fetal tissue is present; and invasive moles, gestational choriocarcinomas, and placental site trophoblastic tumors. Molar pregnancies occur in approximately 1 in 1500 pregnancies in the United States. Risk factors include extremes of maternal age (<15 years and >45 years), prior GTD, and Asian race.[22-24] Metastatic disease may occur, requiring chemotherapy and oncologic management.

Patients may present with vaginal bleeding or hyperemesis gravidarum (HG), and are found to have uterine enlargement greater than expected for dates, absent fetal heart tones, and an abnormally high level of βhCG for gestational age.[25] Patients with GTD may also develop pregnancy-induced hypertension (PIH) or preeclampsia. Diagnosis of molar pregnancy may be established using US. As some molar pregnancies are not detected by sonography, histologic examination of abortion specimens should occur. Patients with suspected GTD should have immediate gynecologic consultation.

Nausea and Vomiting of Pregnancy and Hyperemesis Gravidarum

Nausea and vomiting are very common in early pregnancy, occurring in up to 80% of all pregnant women, with 10% to 20% requiring medications.[26] Nausea and vomiting of pregnancy (NVP) may begin shortly after the first missed menses and usually resolves by the 16th to 20th week of gestation.

Symptoms are often worse in the morning but may continue throughout the day. Vomiting has been shown to be more common in younger women, primigravidas, obese women, and nonsmokers.[26] NVP may be quite disruptive and may greatly affect utilization of health care resources, lost time from work, and quality of life.[27] HG is a more severe form of NVP, occurring in approximately 1% to 2% of pregnancies, and is often defined as nausea and vomiting leading to dehydration, weight loss, ketosis, and electrolyte abnormalities.[27] Up to 1.5% of all pregnancies may require hospitalization due to HG.[28]

The cause of NVP is unclear, but various etiologies have been suggested, including increasing estrogen and human chorionic gonadotropin levels, other maternal hormone levels, thyroid hormones, genetic factors, and lifestyle factors, including tobacco and caffeine use.[29] One study found a significantly increased female:male infant sex ratio in those patients requiring hospitalization for HG, which may in part be due to increased estrogen levels.[28] Nausea and vomiting accompanied by abdominal pain, or severe vomiting occurring after the first trimester, may be due to other underlying diseases and requires further evaluation.

Initial management of NVP includes rehydration with intravenous fluids and antiemetics (Table 91–2). Intravenous isotonic fluids containing 5% glucose may be used for volume repletion and to reverse ketonuria. A number of medications and nondrug therapies have been used with various success rates and side effects, including pyridoxine (vitamin B_6), acupuncture or acupressure, ginger, antihistamines, phenothiazines, and corticosteroids.[30] Most standard antiemetics are classified as category C in the Food and Drug Administration (FDA) classification of teratogenic risk of medications but have been used successfully for the treatment of NVP. In severe cases, enteral nutrition may be necessary.[27] For discharge, patients should demonstrate ability to tolerate oral hydration and may require outpatient antiemetic therapy.

Pregnancy-Induced Hypertension

Hypertension is the most common medical condition affecting pregnancy, occurring in approximately 10% to 20% of pregnancies worldwide.[31] Several syndromes with hypertension as the key element should be considered in the hypertensive pregnant patient. PIH, or gestational hypertension, is defined as a systolic blood pressure (BP) of greater than 140 mm Hg and/or a diastolic BP of greater than 90 mm Hg diagnosed after the 20th week of gestation, which resolves postpartum.[32,33] It can also occur before the 20th week of gestation in women with a molar pregnancy. This is distinct from a pregnant patient with preexisting chronic hypertension; however, these patients may also develop the associated hypertension related complications. Preeclampsia is defined as PIH with proteinuria (>300 mg/24-hour period or >30 mg/dl on dipstick on two occasions at least 6 hours apart) and is the second leading cause of maternal death in the United States.[32] Preeclampsia may occur in up to 7% of healthy primigravid women. In addition to nulliparity, other risk factors for preeclampsia include prior history of preeclampsia, extremes of maternal age, twin or molar pregnancies, obesity or high body mass index, and family history of preeclampsia.[34,35] Severe PIH and preeclampsia are defined as a systolic BP of greater than 170 mm Hg and/or a diastolic BP greater than 110 mm Hg. Symptoms of PIH may include

Table 91–2	Medications Commonly Used for Complications of Pregnancy		
	Medication	**Dosage/Administration**	**FDA Category***
Vaginal bleeding in Rh-negative mother	Anti-D immune globulin (RhoGAM)	50 mcg IM <12 wk 300 mcg IM >12 wk	C
Nausea and vomiting/ hyperemesis gravidarum	Promethazine (Phenergan)	25–50 mg IV/IM push or over 2 hr 25 mg PO q4h 25 mg PR q4h	C
	Prochlorperazine (Compazine)	5–10 mg IV over 10 min (max 40 mg/day) 25 mg PR q12h 10 mg PO q6–8h	C
	Chlorpromazine (Thorazine)	25 mg in 500 ml 0.9% NS at 250 ml/hr IV 10–25 mg PO q4–6h 100 mg PR q6–8h	C
	Metoclopramide (Reglan)	10 mg IV over 1–2 min or 10 mg PO qid	B
	Ondansetron (Zofran)	4–8 mg IV over 15 min q12h 8 mg PO q12h	B
Eclampsia or severe preeclampsia	Magnesium sulfate	2–6 g IV over 15 min, followed by 2 g/hr	A
Hypertension	Labetalol	20 mg slow IV, then 40–80 mg IV q10min (max 300 mg)	C
	Hydralazine	Initial dose 5 mg IV, then maintenance dose of 5–10 mg IV q20min	C

*Food and Drug Administration categories for medications used in pregnancy are as follows:
A: Adequate, well-controlled studies in pregnant women have not shown an increased risk of fetal abnormalities.
B: Animal studies have revealed no evidence of harm to the fetus, however, there are no adequate and well-controlled studies in pregnant women OR animal studies have shown an adverse effect, but adequate and well-controlled studies in pregnant women have failed to demonstrate a risk to the fetus.
C: Animal studies have shown an adverse effect and there are no adequate and well-controlled studies in pregnant women OR no animal studies have been conducted and there are no adequate and well-controlled studies in pregnant women.
D: Studies, adequate well-controlled or observational, in pregnant women have demonstrated a risk to the fetus. However, the benefits of therapy may outweigh the potential risk.
X: Studies, adequate well-controlled or observational, in animals or pregnant women have demonstrated positive evidence of fetal abnormalities. The use of the product is contraindicated in women who are or may become pregnant.
Abbreviations: IM, intramuscularly; IV, intravenously; NS, normal saline; PO, orally; PR, rectally.

nausea, vomiting, midepigastric abdominal pain, and headache. The HELLP syndrome (*h*emolysis, *e*levated *l*iver enzymes, and *l*ow *p*latelets) is a particularly severe form of PIH complicating up to 10% of patients with preeclampsia. The presence of HELLP syndrome is associated with an increased risk of both maternal and fetal morbidity and mortality. Diagnosis, management, and outcome remain controversial for this syndrome.[36,37]

The cause of preeclampsia remains unknown, with multiple etiologies proposed. Some potential causes include immunologic intolerance of fetoplacental tissue, genetic factors, dietary deficiencies, uterine blood vessel invasion by abnormal trophoblasts, and maladaptation to the changes of pregnancy.[34] Currently there are no screening tests to predict preeclampsia or methods to prevent the disease. There have been various conflicting trials examining calcium for the prevention of preeclampsia. A large randomized, prospective trial of almost 4600 healthy nulliparous women showed no reduction in the rate of preeclampsia with calcium supplementation.[38] Low-dose aspirin has also been studied for preeclampsia prevention. A large multicenter trial with over 2500 high-risk women with chronic hypertension, multifetal gestations, history of preeclampsia, or pregestational diabetes showed no benefit from low-dose aspirin.[39] Eight other large trials including a total of over 30,000 patients showed minimal to no benefit in preventing preeclampsia with low-dose aspirin.[34,40,41]

Eclampsia is the new onset of seizures, not attributable to other causes, in a woman with preeclampsia. Eclampsia occurs in approximately 1 in 2000 births in developed countries, and the incidence may be higher in developing countries.[42,43] Patients with severe preeclampsia have the highest risk, but less than 1% of preeclampsia patients develop eclampsia.[44] Seizures attributable to eclampsia may occur in patients without warning signs of preeclampsia; in one study, seizures were the first sign of preeclampsia 60% of the time.[45] Caution when evaluating patients with pre-eclampsia as digital examination may precipitate eclampsia. Eclampsia may lead to maternal death, stillbirth, or neonatal demise.

Definitive treatment for eclampsia and severe preeclampsia is delivery of the fetus, with the ultimate goal of maternal and fetal safety by preventing seizures and minimizing end-organ damage. Intravenous magnesium sulfate is the drug of choice for the treatment of seizures in eclampsia and the prevention of seizures in preeclampsia.[42,43] The dosage of magnesium is 2 to 6 g intravenously over 15 minutes followed by a maintenance drip of 2 g/hr. A large randomized, placebo-controlled trial showed magnesium to halve the risk of eclampsia and to reduce maternal mortality.[43] Magnesium toxicity is characterized by slurred speech, areflexia, and neuromuscular depression leading to respiratory and cardiac depression and arrest. Deep tendon reflexes, respiratory rate, and urine output should be monitored in those patients receiving magnesium infusions. Loss of deep tendon reflexes precedes respiratory arrest. Serum levels between 4 and 7 mEq/L are desired for therapeutic effect; toxic side affects are typically seen at levels greater than 8 mEq/L. Magnesium excretion is impaired by renal insufficiency. If toxicity is present, the infusion should be stopped, and 1 g of calcium gluconate (10 ml of a 10% solution administered intravenously over 2 minutes) may be used as an antidote. For continued seizures despite magnesium, consider alternate diagnoses and seizure management (see Chapter 40, Seizures). BP control may be achieved using labetalol or hydralazine. Antihypertensives are indicated for diastolic BP $\geq$ 105 mmHg with the goal of decreasing to 90–95 mmHg or lower if baseline is <75 mmHg. Some studies have shown a benefit to using labetalol in preference to hydralazine. Labetalol may be given as a dose of 10 to 20 mg intravenously followed by repeat doses if needed to a maximum of 80 mg. Hydralazine may be dosed initially as 5 mg intravenously followed by 5 to 10 mg every 20 minutes as needed to keep diastolic blood pressure below 110 mm Hg.[31,46,47] Fetal heart rate should also be monitored, and obstetric consultation should be obtained immediately. Steroids are recommended to reduce neonatal complications in pregnancies less than 34 weeks' gestation with severe preeclampsia.[48]

Vaginal Bleeding in the Second Half of Pregnancy

Vaginal bleeding in the second half of pregnancy is relatively uncommon, yet it is responsible for a significant amount of maternal and fetal morbidity and mortality. The differential diagnosis includes abruptio placentae, placenta previa, preterm labor, and bleeding lesions from the lower genital tract. In the emergency department, patients should be stabilized with two large-bore intravenous catheters, fluid resuscitation with crystalloid and packed red blood cells if needed, and fetal monitoring. Obstetric consultation and transfer to a facility with obstetric and pediatric capabilities should be initiated early.

Abruptio placentae (or placental abruption), a premature separation of the placenta from the uterine wall, accounts for about 30% of bleeding during the latter half of pregnancy. Approximately 1 in 120 births is complicated by abruption, which is responsible for approximately 20% of perinatal mortality.[49,50] Hemorrhage may be concealed as the blood can be contained between the uterus and the detached placenta, or it may dissect along the uterine wall and through the cervix and present as vaginal bleeding.[50] Placental abruption should be suspected in women who present with unexplained vaginal bleeding after the 20th week of gestation, spontaneous preterm labor, premature rupture of membranes, abdominal pain, uterine tenderness, excessive contractions, or fetal distress.[51] Absence of any of these signs or symptoms does not rule out the diagnosis as vaginal bleeding occurs in approximately 80% and uterine pain or tenderness in 66% of patients with abruption.[50]

Risk factors for abruption include maternal hypertension, multiparity, cigarette smoking, drug abuse (specifically cocaine), advanced maternal age, unmarried status, and previous SAb.[51-53] One study that examined the increasing trends in abruption showed the greatest increase among women under the age of 25, unmarried mothers, and those women on Medicaid.[54] Another study showed no association between placental abruption and eclampsia, proteinuria, or blood pressure, but abruption was associated with platelet count less than 60,000/mm³ and bleeding.[49] Although various risk factors may lead to abruption, approximately 70% of cases occur in low-risk pregnancies as a sudden, unpredictable

emergency.[52] Abruption may also occur secondary to trauma. Placental abruption is responsible for significant complications, including preterm delivery, low birth weight, intrauterine growth retardation, stillbirth, and perinatal death.[51,52] Unlike placenta previa, abruption is not easily identified with US, which diagnoses only half of all cases. Patients with placental abruptions require continuous fetal monitoring and hospitalization and may need early delivery. Treatment varies with gestational age and maternal and fetal condition.[50] Maternal hemodynamic instability and coagulopathies can result in cases of severe placental abruptions.

Placenta previa, or implantation of the placenta over the cervical os, accounts for approximately 20% of bleeding in the latter half of pregnancy and results in significant maternal and fetal morbidity and mortality. Risk factors include multiparity, advanced maternal age, history of prior cesarean section, and increasing number of previous abortions.[55-57] The most common presenting symptom is sudden, painless, bright red vaginal bleeding. Pregnancies complicated by placenta previa are at risk for preterm delivery and hemorrhage that may require transfusion and even hysterectomy.[57]

Digital examination may precipitate severe hemorrhage with placenta previa and is therefore contraindicated. Ultrasound localization of the placenta is thus necessary and has a diagnostic accuracy of 90% to 95%.[58] Transvaginal sonography is a safe and accurate method of diagnosing placenta previa and is superior to the transabdominal approach.[59,60] If ultrasound is inconclusive, vaginal examination (if necessary) should be performed in an operating room in case of hemorrhage. Expectant management is the treatment of choice in those preterm patients who are not actively hemorrhaging, while cesarean section is indicated for severe bleeding.[50]

Trauma in Pregnancy

Trauma affects approximately 7% of all pregnancies and is the leading cause of nonobstetric maternal mortality. Severe or nonsevere, trauma has been associated with an increased risk of spontaneous abortion, preterm labor, placental abruption, uterine rupture, stillbirth, and maternal death. Even minor traumas can lead to significant adverse outcomes in pregnancy. Motor vehicle crashes, falls, and assaults, including domestic violence, account for the majority of trauma.[61,62] While domestic violence is known to be common during pregnancy, it is even more prevalent in the pregnant adolescent population. One study noted that as many as 21% of pregnant adolescents were abused and thus at greater risk for vaginal bleeding, poor weight gain, smoking, and alcohol or drug abuse.[63] Various studies have shown an increased risk of injury and adverse outcomes in pregnant adolescents when compared with older pregnant women who have been abused.[61,64] Screening for domestic violence in all pregnant patients is necessary as domestic abuse is a significant risk factor for repeated injury during pregnancy, with resultant morbidity and mortality.[62]

Maternal stabilization is the most important aspect in the management of the pregnant patient sustaining trauma. Thus all initial resuscitation efforts should be directed at maternal evaluation and hemodynamic support. The normal physiologic changes of pregnancy—increased blood volume, relative hypotension, tachycardia, tachypnea, respiratory alkalosis, and decreased hematocrit—may make the diagnosis of shock more difficult. These changes may allow for a greater loss of blood volume before the clinical signs of hypovolemia are evident. Oxygen and blood volume reconstitution should be provided to patients with even minor trauma. The enlarging uterus of pregnancy compresses the retroperitoneal vasculature when the patient is supine, decreasing venous return. As a result of this recumbent position, cardiac output may be decreased by 25% in the latter portion of pregnancy.[65] While resuscitating the critically ill patient beyond approximately 20 weeks' gestation, left lateral displacement of the uterus or a 30-degree left lateral tilt should be performed to limit aortocaval compression and optimize venous return. When maternal resuscitation is futile and a viable fetus is present, emergent cesarean section should be considered and performed.

As transplacental hemorrhage (also called fetomaternal hemorrhage) may occur with trauma, the Kleihauer-Betke test is recommended for hemorrhage quantification in patients with abdominal trauma. Some authors suggest the Kleihauer-Betke test is not indicated in the Rh-positive patient.[62,66] This test has traditionally been used to detect subclinical volumes of hemorrhage to determine the need for prophylaxis against Rh sensitization. The Kleihauer-Betke test has also been studied as an independent predictor of preterm labor in 71 pregnant trauma patients.[67] Forty-four of 46 women with a positive test also had contractions while none of the 25 patients without contractions had a positive test.[67] We recommend use of the Kleihauer-Betke test in all cases of suspected transplacental hemorrhage in pregnant trauma patients.

Disposition after maternal trauma varies with the severity of injury and the resulting signs and symptoms. It is recommended that patients beyond 20 weeks' gestation with blunt abdominal trauma be closely monitored with continuous cardiotocography for 4 to 6 hours in the absence of and for 24 hours in the presence of uterine tenderness, preterm labor, abnormal fetal heart rate tracings, vaginal bleeding, and/or significant injury to the mother.[62,66,68] Development of fetal distress in these situations may necessitate emergency cesarean section.

Rh Immunization

Rh immunization occurs when an Rh-negative mother is exposed to Rh-positive fetal blood during pregnancy or delivery secondary to fetomaternal hemorrhage. When the mother and fetus are ABO compatible, the risk of Rh immunization is 16%, whereas it is only 2% if they are ABO incompatible. This risk of sensitization also occurs with spontaneous and therapeutic abortion, and therefore anti-D immune globulin (RhoGAM) is indicated in all Rh-negative mothers with bleeding during pregnancy. A dose of 50 mcg intramuscularly prior to 12 weeks' gestation, and 300 mcg after 12 weeks' gestation, is indicated.[69]

Medications in Pregnancy

The FDA classifies the teratogenic risk of medications used during pregnancy. Acetaminophen, standard asthma treatments, penicillins, and cardiopulmonary resuscitation drugs are considered safe in pregnancy. For a complete listing, consult a Physician's Desk Reference or the Internet site maintained by the Food and Drug Administration (*http://www.fda.gov*) and the Center for the Evaluation of Risks to Human Reproduction (*http://cerhr.niehs.nih.gov*). Medications that are commonly used for the complications of pregnancy discussed in this chapter, and their FDA classifications, are listed in Table 91–2.

Summary

Teenage pregnancy presents a unique set of circumstances to the emergency department physician and is often associated with unfavorable pregnancy and birth outcomes. Pregnancy in adolescents is common in all social, economic, and racial groups, although adolescent mothers are more likely to be psychosocially disadvantaged and biologically immature. Both the medical complications and psychosocial concerns should be attended to and addressed, with appropriate social support and referrals provided.

REFERENCES

1. Hamilton BE, Martin JA, Sutton PD: Births: preliminary data for 2003. Natl Vital Stat Rep 53:1–17, 2004.
2. Centers for Disease Control and Prevention: National and state-specific pregnancy rates among adolescents—United States, 1995–1997. MMWR Morb Mortal Wkly Rep 49:605–611, 2000. [Published erratum appears in MMWR Morb Mortal Wkly Rep 49:672, 2000].
3. Abu-Heija A, Ali AM, Al-Dakheil S: Obstetrics and perinatal outcome of adolescent nulliparous pregnant women. Gynecol Obstet Invest 53:90–92, 2002.
4. Treffers PE, Olukoya AA, Ferguson BJ, et al: Care for adolescent pregnancy and childbirth. Int J Gynaecol Obstet 75:111–121, 2001.
5. Satin AJ, Leveno KJ, Sherman ML, et al: Maternal youth and pregnancy outcomes: middle school versus high school age groups compared with women beyond the teen years. Am J Obstet Gynecol 171:184–187, 1994.
6. Chang SC, O'Brien KO, Nathanson MS, et al: Characteristics and risk factors for adverse birth outcomes in pregnant black adolescents. J Pediatr 143:250–257, 2003.
7. Smith GC, Pell JP: Teenage pregnancy and risk of adverse perinatal outcomes associated with first and second births: population based retrospective cohort study. BMJ 323:476, 2001.
8. Weiss JL, Malone FD, Vidaver J, et al: Threatened abortion: a risk factor for poor pregnancy outcome, a population-based screening study. Am J Obstet Gynecol 190:745–750, 2004.
9. Everett C: Incidence and outcome of bleeding before the 20th week of pregnancy: prospective study from general practice. BMJ 315:32–34, 1997.
10. Kadar N, Bohrer M, Kemmann E, et al: The discriminatory human chorionic gonadotropin zone for endovaginal sonography: a prospective, randomized study. Fertil Steril 61:1016–1020, 1994.
11. Cacciatore B, Tiitinen A, Stenman UH, et al: Normal early pregnancy: serum hCG levels and vaginal ultrasonography findings. [see comment]. Br J Obstet Gynaecol 97:899–903, 1990.
12. Dart RG, Kaplan B, Cox C: Transvaginal ultrasound in patients with low beta-human chorionic gonadotropin values: how often is the study diagnostic? Ann Emerg Med 30:135–140, 1997.
13. Kaplan BC, Dart RG, Moskos M, et al: Ectopic pregnancy: prospective study with improved diagnostic accuracy. Ann Emerg Med 28:10–17, 1996.
14. Strauss LT, Herndon J, Chang J, et al: Abortion surveillance—United States, 2001. Mor Mortal Wkly Rep CDC Surveill Summ 53(SS-9):1–32, 2004.
15. Hakim-Elahi E, Tovell HM, Burnhill MS: Complications of first-trimester abortion: a report of 170,000 cases. Obstet Gynecol 76:129–135, 1990.
16. Ludmer PI, Nucci-Sack A, Diaz A: Adolescent abortion: trends and techniques. Curr Womens Health Rep 3:438–444, 2003.
17. Bartlett LA, Berg CJ, Shulman HB, et al: Risk factors for legal induced abortion-related mortality in the United States. Obstet Gynecol 103:729–737, 2004.
18. Paul M: Office management of early induced abortion. Clin Obstet Gynecol 42:290–305, 1999.

19. Sawaya GF, Grady D, Kerlikowske K, et al: Antibiotics at the time of induced abortion: the case for universal prophylaxis based on a meta-analysis. Obstet Gynecol 87:884–890, 1996.

20. Gilbert WM, Danielsen B: Amniotic fluid embolism: decreased mortality in a population-based study. Obstet Gynecol 93:973–977, 1999.

21. Aurangzeb I, George L, Raoof S: Amniotic fluid embolism. Crit Care Clin 20:643–650, 2004.

22. Sebire NJ, Fisher RA, Foskett M, et al: Risk of recurrent hydatidiform mole and subsequent pregnancy outcome following complete or partial hydatidiform molar pregnancy. BJOG 110:22–26, 2003.

23. Matsui H, Iitsuka Y, Yamazawa K, et al: Changes in the incidence of molar pregnancies: a population-based study in Chiba Prefecture and Japan between 1974 and 2000. Hum Reprod 18:172–175, 2003.

24. Sebire NJ, Foskett M, Fisher RA, et al: Risk of partial and complete hydatidiform molar pregnancy in relation to maternal age. BJOG 109:99–102, 2002.

25. Soper JT, Mutch DG, Schink JC, et al: Diagnosis and treatment of gestational trophoblastic disease: ACOG Practice Bulletin No. 53. Gynecol Oncol 93:575–585, 2004.

26. Klebanoff MA, Koslowe PA, Kaslow R, et al: Epidemiology of vomiting in early pregnancy. Obstet Gynecol 66:612–616, 1985.

*27. Attard CL, Kohli MA, Coleman S, et al: The burden of illness of severe nausea and vomiting of pregnancy in the United States. Am J Obstet Gynecol 186:S220–S227, 2002.

28. Schiff MA, Reed SD, Daling JR: The sex ratio of pregnancies complicated by hospitalisation for hyperemesis gravidarum. BJOG 111:27–30, 2004.

29. Lagiou P, Tamimi R, Mucci LA, et al: Nausea and vomiting in pregnancy in relation to prolactin, estrogens, and progesterone: a prospective study. Obstet Gynecol 101:639–644, 2003.

*30. Jewell D, Young G: Interventions for nausea and vomiting in early pregnancy. Cochrane Database Syst Rev (4):CD000145, 2003.

31. Henry CS, Biedermann SA, Campbell MF, et al: Spectrum of hypertensive emergencies in pregnancy. Crit Care Clin 20:697–712, 2004.

32. Report of the National High Blood Pressure Education Program Working Group on High Blood Pressure in Pregnancy. Am J Obstet Gynecol 183:S1–S22, 2000.

33. Ramin KD: The prevention and management of eclampsia. Obstet Gynecol Clin North Am 26:489–503, 1999.

*34. Sibai BM: Diagnosis and management of gestational hypertension and preeclampsia. Obstet Gynecol 102:181–192, 2003.

35. Sibai BM, Ewell M, Levine RJ, et al: Risk factors associated with preeclampsia in healthy nulliparous women: the Calcium for Preeclampsia Prevention (CPEP) Study Group. Am J Obstet Gynecol 177:1003–1010, 1997.

36. Martin JN Jr, Rinehart BK, May WL, et al: The spectrum of severe preeclampsia: comparative analysis by HELLP (hemolysis, elevated liver enzyme levels, and low platelet count) syndrome classification. Am J Obstet Gynecol 180:1373–1384, 1999.

37. Sibai BM: Diagnosis, controversies, and management of the syndrome of hemolysis, elevated liver enzymes, and low platelet count. Obstet Gynecol 103:981–991, 2004.

38. Levine RJ, Hauth JC, Curet LB, et al: Trial of calcium to prevent preeclampsia. N Engl J Med 337:69–76, 1997.

39. Caritis S, Sibai B, Hauth J, et al: Low-dose aspirin to prevent preeclampsia in women at high risk. National Institute of Child Health and Human Development Network of Maternal-Fetal Medicine Units. N Engl J Med 338:701–705, 1998.

40. Duley L, Henderson-Smart D, Knight M, et al: Antiplatelet drugs for prevention of pre-eclampsia and its consequences: systematic review. BMJ 322:329–333, 2001.

41. Sibai BM: Prevention of preeclampsia: a big disappointment. Am J Obstet Gynecol 179:1275–1278, 1998.

42. Which anticonvulsant for women with eclampsia? Evidence from the Collaborative Eclampsia Trial. Lancet 345:1455–1463, 1995.

43. Altman D, Carroli G, Duley L, et al: Do women with pre-eclampsia, and their babies, benefit from magnesium sulphate? The Magpie Trial: a randomised placebo-controlled trial. Lancet 359:1877–1890, 2002.

44. Witlin AG, Sibai BM: Magnesium sulfate therapy in preeclampsia and eclampsia. Obstet Gynecol 92:883–889, 1998.

*45. Katz VL, Farmer R, Kuller JA: Preeclampsia into eclampsia: toward a new paradigm. Am J Obstet Gynecol 182:1389–1396, 2000.

46. Magee LA, Elran E, Bull SB, et al: Risks and benefits of beta-receptor blockers for pregnancy hypertension: overview of the randomized trials. Eur J Obstet Gynecol Reprod Biol 88:15–26, 2000.

47. Mabie WC, Gonzalez AR, Sibai BM, et al: A comparative trial of labetalol and hydralazine in the acute management of severe hypertension complicating pregnancy. Obstet Gynecol 70:328–333, 1987.

48. Amorim MM, Santos LC, Faundes A: Corticosteroid therapy for prevention of respiratory distress syndrome in severe preeclampsia. Am J Obstet Gynecol 180:1283–1288, 1999.

49. Witlin AG, Saade GR, Mattar F, et al: Risk factors for abruptio placentae and eclampsia: analysis of 445 consecutively managed women with severe preeclampsia and eclampsia. Am J Obstet Gynecol 180:1322–1329, 1999.

50. Baron F, Hill WC: Placenta previa, placenta abruptio. Clin Obstet Gynecol 41:527–532, 1998.

51. Ananth CV, Berkowitz GS, Savitz DA, et al: Placental abruption and adverse perinatal outcomes. JAMA 282:1646–1651, 1999.

52. Toivonen S, Heinonen S, Anttila M, et al: Reproductive risk factors, Doppler findings, and outcome of affected births in placental abruption: a population-based analysis. Am J Perinatol 19:451–460, 2002.

53. Kramer MS, Usher RH, Pollack R, et al: Etiologic determinants of abruptio placentae. Obstet Gynecol 89:221–226, 1997.

54. Saftlas AF, Olson DR, Atrash HK, et al: National trends in the incidence of abruptio placentae, 1979–1987. Obstet Gynecol 78:1081–1086, 1991.

55. Miller DA, Chollet JA, Goodwin TM: Clinical risk factors for placenta previa–placenta accreta. Am J Obstet Gynecol 177:210–214, 1997.

56. Tuzovic L, Djelmis J, Ilijic M: Obstetric risk factors associated with placenta previa development: case-control study. Croat Med J 44:728–733, 2003.

57. Dola CP, Garite TJ, Dowling DD, et al: Placenta previa: does its type affect pregnancy outcome? Am J Perinatol 20:353–360, 2003.

58. Kuhlmann RS, Warsof S: Ultrasound of the placenta. Clin Obstet Gynecol 39:519–534, 1996.

59. Timor-Tritsch IE, Yunis RA: Confirming the safety of transvaginal sonography in patients suspected of placenta previa. Obstet Gynecol 81:742–744, 1993.

60. Farine D, Peisner DB, Timor-Tritsch IE: Placenta previa—is the traditional diagnostic approach satisfactory? J Clin Ultrasound 18:328–330, 1990.

*61. El-Kady D, Gilbert WM, Anderson J, et al: Trauma during pregnancy: an analysis of maternal and fetal outcomes in a large population. Am J Obstet Gynecol 190:1661–1668, 2004.

62. Pak LL, Reece EA, Chan L: Is adverse pregnancy outcome predictable after blunt abdominal trauma? Am J Obstet Gynecol 179:1140–1144, 1998.

63. Parker B, McFarlane J, Soeken K: Abuse during pregnancy: effects on maternal complications and birth weight in adult and teenage women. Obstet Gynecol 84:323–328, 1994.

64. Weiss HB: Pregnancy-associated injury hospitalizations in Pennsylvania, 1995. Ann Emerg Med 34:626–636, 1999.

*65. Corsi PR, Rasslan S, de Oliveira LB, et al: Trauma in pregnant women: analysis of maternal and fetal mortality. Injury 30:239–243, 1999.

66. Connolly AM, Katz VL, Bash KL, et al: Trauma and pregnancy. Am J Perinatol 14:331–336, 1997.

67. Muench MV, Baschat AA, Reddy UM, et al: Kleihauer-Betke testing is important in all cases of maternal trauma. J Trauma Injury Infect Crit Care 57:1094–1098, 2004.

68. Curet MJ, Schermer CR, Demarest GB, et al: Predictors of outcome in trauma during pregnancy: identification of patients who can be monitored for less than 6 hours. J Trauma 49:18–24; discussion 24–15, 2000.

69. Bowman J: Thirty-five years of Rh prophylaxis. Transfusion 43:1661–1666, 2003.

*Selected readings.

Chapter 92

Menstrual Disorders

Sandra H. Schwab, MD and Jill C. Posner, MD, MSCE

Introduction and Background

In order to understand and diagnose menstrual disorders, a basic understanding of normal pubertal development and the menstrual cycle is essential. The classic method of describing pubertal development is by Sexual Maturity Rating (SMR) or Tanner staging[1] (Table 92–1). There is wide variation in timing of individual development through the stages, but the physiologic changes and physical signs of puberty are predictable at the various stages. Females generally attain menarche at SMR 3 to 4, with 90% menstruating by SMR 4. The average age of menarche in the United States is 12 to 13 years. The normal menstrual cycle lasts 21 to 35 days and with adolescents may be as long as 45 days, with the first day of menstruation marking the beginning of each cycle. Bleeding occurs for 3 to 7 days on average. A normal cycle has between 20 and 40 ml of blood loss, and greater than 80 ml is considered abnormal. In general, changing three to six pads per day without soiling from oversaturation suggests normal flow.[2] Menstrual disorders and irregular cycles are common in adolescents, especially in the first few years after menarche. The later a female experiences menarche, the longer it takes to achieve normal ovulatory cycles. Menstrual irregularities constitute a large proportion of female health concerns, beginning in adolescence.[3]

In addition to the medical aspects of the encounter, the physician should be sensitive to the various emotional and psychosocial stresses that the patient may be facing. This may be the first encounter with a medical professional dealing with the physical and sexual changes that adolescence brings. The clinician must also keep an open mind and allow the patient to express any concerns in a confidential manner. Some adolescents may use menstrual complaints as a way to approach subjects of sexual activity and preference, pregnancy, contraception, fear of sexually transmitted infections (STIs), assault, and various other sensitive topics.

Recognition and Approach

Any patient presenting with menstrual complaints requires a complete menstrual and sexual history. This is best accomplished in private so the patient will feel at ease to disclose any pertinent information (Table 92–2). Most parents will leave the examination room willingly when this is requested by the clinician. In addition, pregnancy testing should be routine for all adolescents with menstrual complaints, even if sexual activity is denied.

Once a history is obtained, the physician can tailor the physical examination to each patient and chief complaint. In addition to the general examination, an examination of the genital area is essential for patients with a menstrual complaint. This may or may not include a speculum examination depending on the individual needs of each patient. A pelvic examination consists of three components: the external genital examination, the bimanual examination, and the speculum examination. Every patient with a menstrual complaint should have an external genital examination. This allows for SMR staging, recognition of external genital abnormalities, and evaluation of the genital tract as the source of the bleeding. The bimanual examination is tolerated by most pubertal females and should be done in the majority of cases. A bimanual examination is indicated in patients with abdominal pain, abdominal mass, vaginal discharge, menorrhagia, suspected foreign body, or known sexual activity. The speculum examination is the most anxiety-provoking portion of the examination for young females. The speculum examination is indicated when it is essential to visualize the cervical os, for example, in patients with an unclear source of bleeding or suspected pregnancy.

Table 92–1	Classification by Sexual Maturity Rating (SMR)	
	Breasts	**Pubic Hair**
SMR 1	No development	Vellous hair
SMR 2	Small buds	Sparse, straight, downy hair
SMR 3	Areolas and breasts enlarged, no separation	Sparse, dark, coarse hair
SMR 4	Elevation of areolas, secondary mounds	Dark, coarse, adult-type hair but decreased
SMR 5	Mature female breasts	Inverse triangle, spread to medial thighs

Table 92–2	Adolescent Menstrual and Sexual History

History of Present Illness

Last menstrual period
Irregular bleeding
Amount of bleeding
   Number of pads
   Soiling clothing
Abdominal pain
Vaginal discharge
Dysuria
Sexual activity
Contraception (Depo-Provera, IUD, or OCPs)

Past History

Age at menarche
Length of cycles
Regular cycles
Menstrual cramps
Previous pregnancy
History of sexually transmitted infections
Sexual assault or rape
Systemic diseases
Abdominal/pelvic surgeries
Eating habits
Exercise habits
Growth history

Review of Systems

Headaches
Visual changes
Fevers
Weight changes
Hirsuitism

Abbreviations: IUD, intrauterine device; OCPs, oral contraceptive pills.

Table 92–3	Differential Diagnosis of Amenorrhea

Genetic Abnormalities

Turner syndrome
Gonadal dysgenesis
Androgen insensivity
Intersex disorders
Premature ovarian failure
Kallmann's syndrome

Structural and Developmental Disorders

Imperforate hymen
Transverse vaginal septum
Müllerian agenesis (Rokitansky-Küster-Hauser syndrome)
Vaginal agenesis
Intrauterine adhesions (Asherman's syndrome)
Uterine scarring

Alterations in Normal Hormonal Axes

Pregnancy
Lactation
Severe emotional or physical stress
Systemic disease
   Crohn's disease
   Thyroid disorders
   Cushing's syndrome
   MEN I and II
Drugs and medications
CNS tumor
   Pituitary tumor
   Hypothalamic tumor
   Craniopharyngioma
Eating disorders
Polycystic ovarian syndrome
Destruction of pituitary gland
   Autoimmune
   Radiation induced
Androgen-secreting tumor

Abbreviations: CNS, central nervous system; MEN, multiple endocrine neoplasia.

Selected Diagnoses

Primary amenorrhea
Secondary amenorrhea
Oligomenorrhea
Dysmenorrhea
Metorrhagia
Menorrhagia
Premenstrual syndrome

Discussion of Individual Diagnoses

Primary Amenorrhea

Primary amenorrhea is defined as failure to reach menarche by age 16 when development of secondary sexual characteristics is evident, or by age 14 when no secondary sexual characteristics are present. There are three broad categories to describe causes of amenorrhea: genetic etiologies, structural and developmental abnormalities, and alteration of growth and sexual hormonal axes (Table 92–3). It is estimated that genetic and developmental disorders account for 60% of primary amenorrhea cases, while the remaining 40% are due to endocrine and hormonal causes.[4]

After exclusion of pregnancy and pregnancy-related disorders, a detailed history and physical will guide additional

It is also indicated if cervical cultures are needed to rule out STIs. Recent advances in the ability to detect chlamydia and gonorrhea in the urine via nucleic acid testing negate the need for the speculum examination in a majority of patients with abnormal vaginal bleeding. Therefore, a clinician may opt to defer this examination if no additional information will be gained from direct visualization of the vaginal walls or cervix. It is imperative that a speculum examination be performed for pregnant adolescents and children with vaginal bleeding, but the clinician should consider obtaining an ultrasound prior to a speculum examination, especially in patients suspected of being beyond the first trimester of pregnancy.

diagnostic and therapeutic interventions. Constitutional delay is hereditary, and a family history with otherwise negative findings is suggestive. Long-standing problems with growth and development suggest a genetic abnormality such as Turner's syndrome or hypothalamic or pituitary pathology. A history of cyclic abdominal pain would suggest a vaginal outlet obstruction such as imperforate hymen or vaginal septum, especially if there is a discrepancy between the patient's advanced pubertal development (i.e., SMR staging) and the apparent absence of menarche. The general physical examination provides information about body habitus and growth. Eating disorders affect as many as 1% of young women in developing countries, and often present with menstrual irregularity or amenorrhea in adolescence.[5] Hirsuitism, severe acne, and signs of systemic disease such as acanthosis nigricans or thyroid enlargement should be noted. A thorough neurologic examination might reveal central nervous system (CNS) pathology. Development of secondary sexual characteristics and/or signs of virilization should be noted on the external genital examination.

The emergency physician should ensure that serious or life-threatening causes or complications of an underlying disorder are not present. Laboratory tests such as blood glucose, serum chemistries, complete blood count, and thyroid studies should be considered. An electrocardiogram should be performed for patients with suspected anorexia nervosa because of the potential for arrhythmias related to electrolyte disturbances. Imaging such as a computed tomography (CT) scan of the head or magnetic resonance imaging (MRI) should be done if a CNS tumor is suspected. A pelvic ultrasound or MRI will aid in diagnosis and treatment of underlying structural or developmental abnormalities. Physicians should consider hospital admission for further workup in patients with abnormal screening tests.

Many of the causes of primary amenorrhea require a comprehensive diagnostic evaluation that may involve subspecialists and a multidisciplinary team approach. This is best coordinated by a primary care physician, and can be done in the outpatient setting. Appropriate follow-up should be arranged prior to discharge from the emergency department.

Secondary Amenorrhea

Secondary amenorrhea is strictly defined as absence of menstruation for greater than 6 months after menarche. Some practitioners use absence of menstruation for three cycle lengths in the setting of oligomenorrhea, 6 months after establishing regular menses, or by 18 months after menarche as a working clinical definition.[6] Excluding the genetic and developmental etiologies, many of the causes of primary amenorrhea can also present as secondary amenorrhea. Again, pregnancy should be excluded at the onset of evaluation. Unlike adults, in whom the most common cause of secondary amenorrhea is pregnancy, immaturity or disruption of the normal hypothalamic-pituitary-ovarian axis is the most common cause in adolescents. Many adolescent girls have anovulatory cycles due to this physiologic immaturity of the hypothalamic-pituitary-ovarian axis. Most girls with anovulatory cycles experience an absence of regular monthly bleeding or irregular periods, though some will develop menorrhagia (see section on menorrhagia for details). Polycystic ovarian syndrome is another common cause of secondary amenorrhea and may account for up to a third of menstrual irregularities in young females.[7] The clinical manifestations, such as obesity, hirsuitism, acne, and irregular menstrual cycles, are a result of the hyperandrogenic state and ovarian dysfunction that are hallmarks of the disease. Specific questions addressing eating habits, current medications, and contraception can narrow the differential diagnosis in females with previously normal cycles.

The physical examination and diagnostic workup can be tailored to each individual case. As with primary amenorrhea, the emergency physician should ensure that any serious or life-threatening causes or complications are identified. The remainder of the workup, such as a progesterone challenge and measurement of the various sex hormone levels, should be done on an outpatient basis with the primary physician coordinating care with any necessary subspecialists.

Oligomenorrhea

Oligomenorrhea is defined as menstrual cycle length of greater than 35 days. The various causes of secondary amenorrhea may first present as oligomenorrhea. Like secondary amenorrhea, a common cause of oligomenorrhea in adolescents is a hyperandrogenic state secondary to polycystic ovarian disease.[8] The approach to the patient with oligomenorrhea is the same as with secondary amenorrhea. After ruling out pregnancy and other serious and life-threatening causes and complications, the emergency physician should ensure proper follow up. The majority of the diagnostic workup and treatment are best done in the outpatient setting with a primary physician coordinating care.

Dysmenorrhea

Dysmenorrhea is defined as cyclic abdominal pain and uterine cramping associated with ovulatory menstrual cycles. It is the most common gynecologic complaint and the leading cause of school and work absenteeism among young women.[9,10] In the absence of underlying organic pathology, it is considered primary dysmenorrhea. If pelvic pathology such as endometriosis is present, secondary dysmenorrhea is diagnosed. Nausea, vomiting, back pain, headaches, and leg pain are common associated symptoms. The vast majority of adolescents with dysmenorrhea have primary dysmenorrhea, with prevalence rates greater than 90% in some studies.[11,12]

Primary dysmenorrhea varies widely among females and ranges from mild, without any disruption of daily living, to severe, causing absence from school or work. Symptoms begin just prior to or at the onset of menstruation and typically last 1 to 2 days. The pain is bilateral and colicky in nature, and resolves with the end of menstruation. If the patient's presentation is consistent with primary dysmenorrhea, little additional workup needs to be done. The complete pelvic examination may be deferred, and no laboratory studies are required. If the presentation is atypical, the physician should consider other causes of abdominal pain and vaginal bleeding, especially potentially life-threatening disorders related to pregnancy, such as ectopic pregnancy, spontaneous abortion, or placenta previa/abruption. Other possibilities to consider include ovarian cysts, endometriosis, pelvic neoplasms, and gastrointestinal disease.[13,14] Sexual assault and its lasting physical and emotional consequences should also be considered, as gynecologic complaints such as dysmenorrhea are more common among victims with such a history.[15]

Nonpharmacologic alternative and traditional medical therapies are commonly used by patients. Adolescents report using a wide range of nonpharmacologic treatments such as rest, heat, exercise, and even alcohol or illegal drugs for relief of symptoms.[12] Other reported treatments include acupuncture, spinal manipulation, electromagnetic therapy, vitamin and herbal supplements, and dietary changes. Many of these treatments are based on anecdotal accounts and have not been shown to consistently relieve dysmenorrhea in randomized clinical trials.[16]

The first line of medical therapy for treatment of dysmenorrhea is the use of analgesic and anti-inflammatory medications such as nonsteroidal anti-inflammatory drugs (NSAIDs). Multiple studies have shown the effectiveness and safety of this group as a whole, even with over-the-counter dosing. Naproxen may provide faster, more effective relief of symptoms than ibuprofen or acetaminophen.[17] For patients with more severe symptoms, oral contraceptives, taken for at least 3 months, have shown significant reduction in incidence and severity of symptoms.[18] Topical glyceryl trinitrate ointment has shown some promising results, but continues to be under investigation.[19]

Metrorrhagia

Metrorrhagia is abnormal bleeding between regular menstrual periods. Few data exist on the prevalence of metrorrhagia in adolescents. Common causes of metrorrhagia include pregnancy, use of certain contraceptives (especially Depo-Provera) and intrauterine devices, and STIs. Other causes include coagulation disorders, genital trauma, neoplasms, and infections such as tuberculosis. The history should include questions focusing on these etiologies, specifically addressing accompanying symptoms such as abdominal pain and vaginal discharge. A complete pelvic examination, including a speculum examination, should be considered when other symptoms are present.

Diagnostic testing and treatment depend on the etiology of the metrorrhagia. As with any other menstrual complaint, pregnancy should be ruled out at the onset of evaluation. Breakthrough bleeding with initiation of Depo-Provera is common, and reassurance is sufficient in the absence of other symptoms. The clinician should consider screening tests for STIs even if sexual activity is denied due to the potential for serious lifelong complications if untreated. Other tests, such as coagulation studies, pelvic ultrasound, or abdominal/pelvic CT scan, should be considered on an individual basis.

Menorrhagia

Menorrhagia is defined as excessive bleeding (>80 ml) or prolonged bleeding (>7 days) during the menstrual cycle. Menorrhagia is more common among adolescents than adults and is frequently diagnosed in the first few years after menarche. The most common causes of menorrhagia in adolescents are anovulatory cycles and cervicitis due to STIs. Other causes of menorrhagia include pregnancy-related disorders, hematologic disorders, trauma, systemic disease, and, rarely, neoplasms[20] (Table 92–4). Dysfunctional uterine

Table 92–4	Causes of Abnormal Vaginal Bleeding

Anovulation

Hypothalamic dysfunction
Polycystic ovarian syndrome
Breakthrough bleeding secondary to hormonal contraception
Physiologic immaturity of the hypothalamic-pituitary-ovarian axis

Infectious Causes

Pelvic inflammatory disease
Vaginitis
Cervicitis

Pregnancy-Related Conditions

Ectopic pregnancy
Threatened or spontaneous abortion
Complications of termination procedures

Coagulation Disorders

Thrombocytopenia (idiopathic thrombocytopenic purpura, leukemia)
Platelet function disorders (von Willebrand's disease)
Clotting factor abnormalities
Anticoagulation medications

Trauma

Accidental injury
Coital trauma
Sexual abuse
Foreign body

Neoplasms

Vaginal tumor
Cervical carcinoma
Uterine myoma
Ovarian tumor
Uterine carcinoma
Polyps

Systemic Diseases

Hepatic dysfunction
Renal dysfunction
Diabetes mellitus

Endocrine Causes

Thyroid disease
Prolactinoma
Adrenal disease

bleeding (DUB) is a specific type of menorrhagia defined as excessive bleeding in the absence of organic pathology or systemic disease. DUB is a diagnosis of exclusion, and the clinician should use this term only if other causes have been ruled out.

Anovulatory cycles are most common in the first years after menarche and are due to immaturity of the hypothalamic-pituitary-ovarian hormonal axis. In anovulatory cycles, the second half of the normal menstrual cycle (i.e., the luteal phase) does not occur. As a result, the follicular phase continues and the uterine lining is subjected to unopposed estrogen stimulation. When unopposed by luteal-phase progesterone, estrogen overstimulation causes the uterine lining to proliferate beyond the supporting capabilities of the stroma. Eventually, erratic sloughing of the lining occurs and, in some areas, the basal arterioles are exposed, resulting in heavy bleeding.

Coagulation disorders account for 3% to 33% of hospitalized adolescents with abnormal vaginal bleeding.[21-23] In one series, 50% of patients with newly diagnosed coagulation disorders presented at menarche.[21] A case-control study in one center revealed that 5 of 38 patients (13%) given an initial diagnosis of DUB were later diagnosed with von Willebrand's disease.[24]

Although exact amounts of blood loss are difficult to assess, patients may give a history of soaking through multiple pads, clothing, and bedding. In addition to excessive bleeding, patients may present with symptoms and signs of anemia such as fatigue, shortness of breath, and pallor. In extreme cases, patients may present in hypovolemic shock with hypotension and severe anemia secondary to blood loss.

The physical examination, laboratory evaluation, and treatment depend on the etiology and severity of the bleeding. For unstable, actively bleeding patients, resuscitation should begin immediately with securing the airway, breathing, and circulation; establishing vascular access; and providing volume resuscitation as well as transfusion of blood products if necessary. Packing the vagina with sterile gauze may be necessary to stop acute hemorrhage. A pregnancy test is again essential. Serum specimens for a complete blood count, coagulation studies, and type and crossmatch should be sent. After stabilization, a complete pelvic examination, including speculum examination, to evaluate the origin of the bleeding is necessary. Further evaluation, such as ultrasound, STI testing and hematologic workup, may be necessary. Immediate consultation with a gynecologist, preferably one with experience treating adolescent patients, is recommended. Other consultants who may be required for definitive care, depending on the situation, are endocrinologists, adolescent medicine specialists, and pediatric surgeons. If these resources are unavailable, the patient should be transported to a facility that can provide such services after stabilization. For hemodynamically stable patients, a tailored physical examination, pregnancy test, complete blood count, and STI screening should be included in the initial evaluation.

Treatment should be directed at the underlying cause of vaginal bleeding. If no cause is identified, a diagnosis of DUB is made. Treatment of DUB depends on the severity of bleeding and whether the patient is symptomatic. For asymptomatic patients with mild DUB and normal hemoglobin (Hb), high-dose NSAIDs and iron supplementation can be initiated. Reassurance and follow-up should be emphasized.

For those patients who are symptomatic or anemic (Hb < 12), or have active hemorrhage, hormonal therapy is indicated. Treatment is directed at restoring a normal uterine lining, including the denuded areas of exposed basal arterioles, and requires both estrogen and progesterone in most cases. Oral and intravenous regimens are effective in stopping acute bleeding.[25,26] Intravenous conjugated estrogen (20 to 25 mg every 4 to 6 hours, maximum of six doses) can be used as initial therapy for unstable patients requiring inpatient treatment. Low dose oral contraceptive pills (OCPs) with combined norethindrone/ethinyl estradiol (30 mcg/0.3 mg) may be used alternatively, and should be initiated as soon as possible in patients receiving intravenous therapy. A simple regimen to remember is 1 pill every 6 hours until bleeding stops, followed by a taper of 1 pill four times daily for 4 days, then 1 pill three times daily for 3 days, and 1 pill twice daily for weeks. Then, after a 7-day OCP-free period

(placebo pills) and withdrawal bleeding, 1 pill daily on a normal OCP schedule for an additional six cycles is recommended.[27] It is important to prescribe antiemetics for patients taking more than one OCP per day due to the high incidence of nausea and vomiting with this regimen. For patients in whom estrogen is contraindicated, cyclic oral medroxyprogesterone (10 mg daily for 10 days, repeated monthly for three to six cycles starting on day 14 of the cycle) can be used. Admission should be considered for symptomatic patients, those with active heavy bleeding, and those with moderate to severe anemia (Hb < 9). Re-evaluation with a primary care provider is necessary to determine if additional therapy is needed.

Premenstrual Syndrome

Premenstrual syndrome (PMS) is a collection of physical and emotional changes that occur in the luteal phase (second half) of the menstrual cycle. Eighty percent of women have some premenstrual symptoms, although most do not have alterations in their daily living. There is now recognition of a wide clinical spectrum of these premenstrual symptoms, with the most severe symptoms being classified as premenstrual dysphoric disorder (PMDD). PMDD is considered a "Depressive Disorder Not Otherwise Specified" in the *Diagnostic and Statistical Manual of Mental Disorders, Fourth Edition* (DSM-IV). Severe PMS and PMDD affect 3% to 8% of menstruating women.[28-30]

Symptoms begin after ovulation, around day 14 of an average cycle, and continue until menstruation. There is a symptom-free period during the follicular phase of the cycle. PMS includes physical changes such as breast tenderness, bloating, headaches, and extremity edema. In addition, most affected females report significant emotional changes such as irritability, mood swings, anxiety, social withdrawal, and, in most severe cases, major depression.

In order to diagnose PMS or PMDD, it is recommended that a prospective symptom diary be completed by the patient.[31] This will allow the clinician to determine if a symptom-free period exists after menstruation. If there are continued symptoms throughout the entire menstrual cycle, a mood disorder exacerbated by hormonal changes is more likely.

Selective serotonin reuptake inhibitors are the mainstay of treatment for moderate to severe PMS and PMDD. Treatment may be continuous or intermittent depending on tolerance of the medications and severity of symptoms. Patients with PMS and PMDD usually begin to note changes within 3 days of starting medication, unlike patients with mood disorders, in whom 4 to 6 weeks are needed to see effects. These medications are more appropriately instituted by a continuing care physician, with prompt referral made at the time of emergency department disposition.

For minor symptoms, a variety of therapies ranging from herbal and complementary treatments to vitamin supplements and OCPs have been tried. Many of these are based on anecdotal evidence and show conflicting results in scientific trials.[32,33] Some studies have shown benefits of daily vitamin B_6 (50 to 100 mg) and calcium carbonate (1200 mg) supplementation.[30] Some therapies such as exercise, dietary changes, and weight control have not been shown to unequivocally help with PMS symptoms, but are recommended for good general health and are relatively risk free.[32]

REFERENCES

1. Marshall WA, Tanner JM: Variations in patterns of pubertal changes in girls. Arch Dis Child 44:291,1969.
*2. Hillard PJA: Menstruation in young girls: a clinical perspective. Obstet Gynecol 99:655–662, 2002.
3. Balen AH, Fleming C, Robinson A: Health needs of adolescents in secondary gynaecological care: results of a questionnaire survey and a review of current issues. Hum Fertil (Camb) 5:127–132, 2002.
4. Nelson LM, Bakalov V, Pastor C: Amenorrhea. eMedicine, May 17, 2005. Available at *http://www.emedicine.com/med/topic117.htm* (accessed August 8, 2005).
5. Tamburrino MB, McGinnis RA: Anorexia nervosa: a review. Panminerva Med 44:301–311, 2002.
*6. Pletcher JR, Slap GB: Menstrual disorders: amenorrhea. Pediatr Clin North Am 46:505–518, 1999.
7. Venturoli S, Porcu E, Fabbri R, et al: Menstrual irregularities in adolescents: hormonal pattern and ovarian morphology. Horm Res 24:269–279, 1986.
*8. Hickey M, Balen A: Menstrual disorders in adolescence: investigation and management. Hum Reprod Update 9:493–504, 2003.
9. Klein JR, Litt IF: Epidemiology of adolescent dysmenorrhea. Pediatrics 68:661, 1981.
10. Harlow SD, Park M: A longitudinal study of risk factors for occurrence, duration and severity of menstrual cramps in a cohort of college women. Br J Obstet Gynaecol 103:1134–1142, 1996.
11. Jamieson DJ, Steege JF: The prevalence of dysmenorrhea, dyspareunia, pelvic pain and irritable bowel syndrome in primary care practices. Obstet Gynecol 87:55–58, 1996.
12. Campbell MA, McGrath PJ: Non-pharmacologic strategies used by adolescents for the management of menstrual discomfort. Clin J Pain 15:313–320, 1999.
13. Porpora MG, Picarelli A, Prospero Porta R, et al: Celiac disease as a cause of chronic pelvic pain, dysmenorrhea, and deep dyspareunia. Obstet Gynecol 99(5 Pt 2):937–939, 2002.
14. Durain D: Primary dysmenorrhea: assessment and management update. J Midwifery Womens Health 49:520–528, 2004.
15. Golding JM, Wilsnack SC, Learman LA: Prevalence of sexual assault history among women with common gynecological symptoms. Am J Obstet Gynecol 179:1013–1019, 1998.
16. Wilson MI, Murphy PA: Herbal and dietary therapies for primary and secondary dysmenorrhea. Cochrane Database Syst Rev (3):CD002124, 2001.

17. Milsom I, Minic M, Dawood MY, et al: Comparison of the efficacy and safety of nonprescription doses of naproxen and naproxen sodium with ibuprofen, acetaminophen, and placebo in the treatment of primary dysmenorrhea: a pooled analysis of five studies. Clin Ther 24:1384–1400, 2002.
18. Callejo J, Diaz J, Ruiz A, Garcia RM: Effect of a low-dose oral contraceptive containing 20 μg ethinylestradiol and 150 μg desogestrel on dysmenorrhea. Contraception 68:183–188, 2003.
19. Ghazizadeh S, Dadkhah T, Modarres M: Local application of glyceril trinitrate ointment for primary dysmenorrhea. Int J Gynecol Obstet 79:43–44, 2002.
20. Ferrera PC, Whitman MCW: Ovarian small cell carcinoma: a rare neoplasm in a 15-year-old female. Pediatr Emerg Care 16:170–172, 2000.
21. Claessens EA, Cowell CA: Acute adolescent menorrhagia. Am J Obstet Gynecol 139:277–280, 1981.
22. Falcone T, Desjardins C, Bourque J, et al: Dysfunctional uterine bleeding in adolescents. J Reprod Med 39:761–764, 1994.
23. Smith YR, Quint EH, Hertzberg RB: Menorrhagia in adolescents requiring hospitalization. J Pediatr Adolesc Gynecol 11:13–15, 1998.
24. Woo YL, White B, Corbally R, et al: von Willebrand's disease: an important cause of dysfunctional uterine bleeding. Blood Coagul Fibrinolysis 13:89–93, 2002.
25. DeVore GR, Owens O, Kase N: Use of intravenous Premarin® in the treatment of dysfunctional uterine bleeding—a double-blind randomized control study. Obstet Gynecol 59:285–291, 1982.
26. Agarwal N, Kriplani A: Medical management of dysfunctional uterine bleeding. Int J Gynecol Obstet 75:199–201, 2001.
*27. Levine LJ, Catallozzi M, Schwarz D: An adolescent with vaginal bleeding. Pediatr Case Rev 3:83–90, 2003.
28. Mortola J: Premenstrual syndrome—pathophysiologic considerations. N Engl J Med 338:256–257, 1998
29. Steiner M: Recognition of premenstrual dysphoric disorder and its treatment. Lancet 356:1126–1127, 2000.
30. Grady-Weliky TA: Premenstrual dysphoric disorder. N Engl J Med 348:433–438, 2003.
*31. Dell DL: Premenstrual syndrome, premenstrual dysphoric disorder and premenstrual exacerbation of another disorder. Clin Obstet Gynecol 47:568–575, 2004.
32. Stevinson C, Ernst E: Complementary/alternative therapies for premenstrual syndrome: a systematic review of randomized controlled trials. Am J Obstet Gynecol 185:227–235, 2001.
33. Joffe H, Cohen LS, Harlow BL: Impact of oral contraceptive pill use on premenstrual mood: predictors of improvement and deterioration. Am J Obstet Gynecol 189:1523–1530, 2003.

*Selected readings.

Chapter 93

Ovarian Disorders

Beverly H. Bauman, MD and Robert L. Cloutier, MD

Selected Diagnoses

Ovarian cysts
Mittelschmerz
Ovarian neoplasm
Ovarian and adnexal torsion
Polycystic ovarian syndrome

Discussion of Individual Diagnoses

Ovarian Cysts

Ovarian cysts may occur in all age groups and are very frequently seen in adolescents after the onset of menarche. Most neonates also have small cysts, which develop in response to maternal hormones.[1,2] The majority of ovarian cysts are painless and are incidental findings when patients undergo an ultrasound of the abdomen or pelvis for the evaluation of another condition. However, large functional ovarian cysts may also be the source of pain or hemorrhage that can prompt

a child or adolescent to present to the emergency department for evaluation and treatment. Ovarian cysts also predispose to ovarian torsion, an important surgical emergency.[3,4]

There are two types of physiologic or functional ovarian cysts: follicular and corpus luteum cysts. Follicular cysts are the result of a functioning hypothalamic-pituitary-ovarian axis. During the menstrual cycle, when primordial follicles are stimulated by follicle-stimulating hormone, one primordial follicle develops into a dominant follicle prior to ovulation. This dominant follicle is normally a small simple fluid-filled follicular cyst. Once ovulation occurs, the dominant follicle becomes a corpus luteum cyst. Occasionally the follicular cyst will grow excessively large in response to hormonal stimulation and will fail to quickly involute after ovulation. This large follicular cyst can produce symptoms of unilateral pelvic pain or heaviness. The corpus luteum cyst may likewise become symptomatic if it becomes a larger mass and hemorrhages into the cyst.

In the emergency department, ovarian cysts are frequently diagnosed by ultrasound imaging (Fig. 93–1). When a large follicular cyst is diagnosed, it should be followed over several weeks to ensure that it resolves and does not enlarge further.[5] The majority of these cysts will resolve without sequelae. Oral contraceptives may be prescribed to prevent ovulation and the formation of further new cysts while the cyst in question is being monitored. Oral contraceptives will not cause resorption or resolution of the current cyst.

When a large follicular or corpus luteum cyst ruptures acutely into the peritoneal cavity, it may cause considerable pain from transient irritation and peritonitis. Free fluid will be seen on ultrasound of the pelvis. Rarely the rupture of a cyst may cause considerable intraperitoneal bleeding if the rupturing cyst crosses a large vessel. If the hemorrhage is significant, serial hemotocrits and monitoring for hemodynamic instability may be necessary. Rarely, severe hemorrhage from a ruptured cyst necessitates surgical intervention.

Ovarian cysts predisposing to torsion in younger children do occur and require vigilance on the part of practitioners due to the wide variability of clinical presentations; this is discussed later.

Mittelschmerz

During ovulation, the follicular cyst ruptures and can release a small amount of free intraperitoneal fluid. This fluid may be irritating to the peritoneum and cause acute unilateral

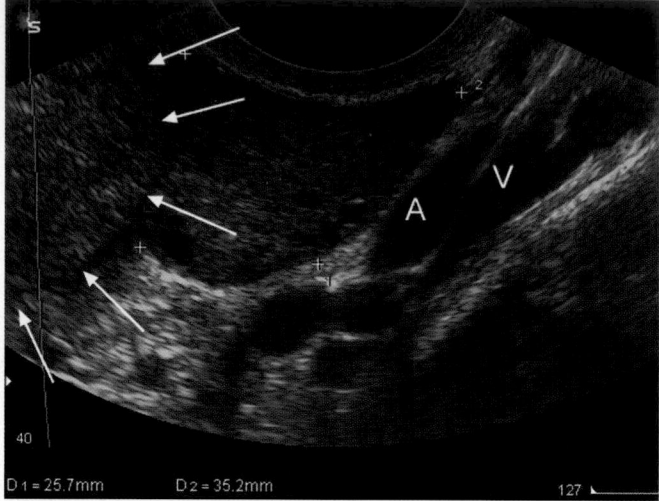

A

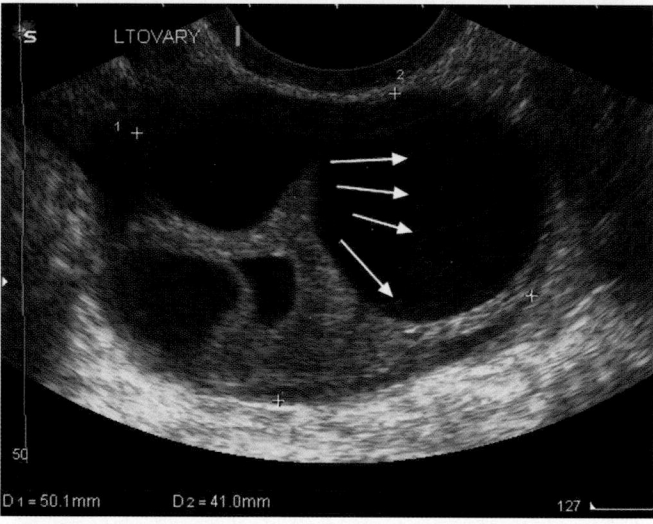

B

FIGURE 93–1. Endovaginal images of a normal ovary (**A**) and one with several abnormally large cysts (**B**) (calipers in both cases). **A,** The ovarian parenchyma is typically slightly less echodense (darker) than the adjacent uterus (outlined by *arrows*). The ovary is often found between the uterus and the internal iliac vessels (A and V). Normal ovarian follicles are usually defined as being less than 10 mm in diameter; when larger than this, they are referred to as "cysts." Many larger cysts are part of the normal ovulatory cycle. More than 14, and up to more than 30, follicles in an ovary have been advocated as the criterion for polycystic ovarian syndrome. The follicles are often arrayed around the periphery of the ovary with the appearance of a "string of pearls" (not shown). **B,** An ovary with multiple large cysts, including one with internal hemorrhage as suggested by a fluid-fluid level (*arrows*), is shown. The reticular heterogeneity of the clot suggests that it has been present for long enough to be partially organized. Cysts can cause acute pain from internal hemorrhage, external hemorrhage, or torsion.

lower abdominal or pelvic pain, which is called mittelschmerz. This condition is benign, and treatment is directed at control of symptoms. However, emergency providers will need to consider other more serious causes of acute pelvic pain prior to making the diagnosis of mittelschmerz. Mittelschmerz pain is a postmenarchal phenomenon and presents in a fashion similar to that in adult females.

Ovarian Neoplasms

Benign or malignant ovarian neoplasms are uncommon in the pediatric age range, yet an ovarian tumor may occasionally explain signs and symptoms for which a patient presents to the emergency department.[5] Complaints may be acute or chronic abdominal pain, abdominal distention, anorexia, weight change, back pain, or bowel or bladder dysfunction. Because ovarian tumors may be large, the physical appearance of an adolescent with an ovarian tumor may resemble pregnancy. Some hormonally active ovarian tumors can cause signs of precocious puberty in a child.[5,6] If the neoplasm is complicated by ovarian torsion, the pain may be acute and severe.[3]

The ovary consists of three types of cells: oocytes, follicular cells, and the supporting stromal cells. Benign or malignant ovarian tumors may arise from any of these three cell types. While there are numerous classification schemes for ovarian tumors, fundamentally there exist three general types: (1) epithelial cell tumors, (2) germ cell tumors, and (3) metastatic tumors. The vast majority of pediatric ovarian masses are germ cell tumors, which include dermoid tumors (which fall under the subclassification of teratomas), yolk sac tumors, and choriocarcinoma. Dermoid tumors tend to be benign and are characterized by multiple tissue types within the tumor, and frequently include calcified tissues that show up on abdominal plain films.[6]

Ultrasound findings that indicate the possibility of an ovarian tumor include a solid mass, a complex mass, or a large cyst that does not resolve under surveillance over 6 to 10 weeks. If the emergency physician identifies an ovarian mass, prompt consultation with a gynecologist or pediatric surgeon is indicated for further workup and treatment of a suspected ovarian neoplasm.

Ovarian and Adnexal Torsion

Ovarian and adnexal torsion is the twisting of the ovary on its pedicle. Ovarian enlargement with cysts or benign or malignant masses, predisposes to ovarian torsion, yet torsion has also been described in normal-appearing ovaries.[7] With torsion, the ovarian blood supply is compromised by the twisted vascular pedicle, and this results in acute pain from ovarian ischemia. This constitutes a surgical emergency to promptly relieve the pain and attempt to preserve ovarian perfusion and prevent ovarian necrosis.[8] Therefore, immediate consultation with gynecologic or surgical colleagues is essential when the diagnosis is made or highly suspected.

Although ovarian torsion is rare in infants and children, it may occur in females of all ages and has even been described in female fetuses antenatally.[7] However, torsion is much more common after menarche because large ovarian cysts produced during the menstrual cycle can predispose to torsion. Diagnosis can be challenging because the presenting signs and symptoms mimic other more common causes of abdominal pain.[9-11] The classic presentation is the sudden onset of severe, focal, constant, unilateral lower abdominal and pelvic pain, which may be associated with nausea, vomiting, or urinary tract symptoms. However, the pain may also be described as a dull ache and radiate to the flank or leg. The pain may have intermittent exacerbations if the ovary torses and then detorses spontaneously.[8] Physical examination may reveal a palpable painful pelvic or abdominal mass if the torsion is associated with a large ovarian mass. In prepubertal females, the ovarian mass associated with torsion is frequently located within the abdominal cavity, but in pubertal females, the ovarian mass is typically within the pelvis. The white blood cell count is commonly elevated in pediatric patients with ovarian torsion, and this can confuse the clinician when considering other causes of abdominal and pelvic pain related to infections, such as appendicitis, tubo-ovarian abscess, or pelvic inflammatory disease.[8,9,12]

Color flow Doppler ultrasound is a very useful test to evaluate for an ovarian mass and to visualize blood flow to the ovary and adnexa. If blood flow is abnormal within the vascular pedicle, then perfusion to the ovary is decreased, yet even this test can produce false-negative results.[13-15] If the clinician continues to suspect ovarian torsion after color flow Doppler ultrasound, surgical consultation for laparoscopic visualization may still be needed to diagnose torsion. With laparoscopy, surgeons may attempt to salvage the ovary through detorsion or perform salpingoophorectomy if necrosis has already occurred.[16] Recent data suggest that salvage rates may be as high as 27% and that ovaries may be salvageable up to 24 hours after onset of symptoms.[17]

Polycystic Ovarian Syndrome

Polycystic ovarian syndrome is a common chronic endocrine disorder that causes menstrual irregularities in adolescents. Increased ovarian androgen production results in hirsuitism. Most of these adolescents are obese and have oligomenorrhea. Ultrasound reveals multiple small follicles on the ovarian periphery, which is often described as the appearance of a "string of pearls." While patients are not likely to present to the emergency department with acute symptoms related to polycystic ovarian syndrome, emergency providers should be aware of this common condition that may be discovered during the evaluation of other conditions.

REFERENCES

1. Hamrick H: Ovarian cyst and torsion in a young infant [Letter to the Editor]. Arch Pediatr Adolesc Med 152:1245–1246, 1998.
2. Schmahmann S, Haller J: Neonatal ovarian cysts: pathogenesis, diagnosis and management. Pediatr Radiol 27:101–105, 1997.
3. Kokoska E, Keller M, Weber T: Acute ovarian torsion in children. Am J Surg 180:462–465, 2000.
4. Dolgin S: Acute ovarian torsion in children [Letter to the Editor]. Am J Surg 183:95, 2002.
5. Pomeranz A, Sabnis S: Misdiagnosis of ovarian masses in children and adolescents. Pediatr Emerg Care 20:172–174, 2004.
6. Brown M, Hebra A, McGeehin K, et al: Ovarian masses in children: a review of 91 cases of malignant and benign masses. J Pediatr Surg 28:930–932, 1993.
7. Mordehai J, Mares A, Barki Y, et al: Torsion of uterine adnexa in neonates and children: a report of 20 cases. J Pediatr Surg 26:1195–1199, 1991.
8. Houry D, Abbott J: Ovarian torsion: a fifteen-year review. Ann Emerg Med 38:156–159, 2001.
9. Rothrock S, Pagane J: Acute appendicitis in children: emergency department diagnosis and management. Ann Emerg Med 36:39–51, 2000.
10. Legome E, Belton A, Murray R, et al: Epiploic appendagitis: the emergency department presentation. J Emerg Med 22:9–13, 2002.
11. Helmrath M, Dorfman S, Minifee P, et al: Right lower quadrant pain in children caused by omental infarction. Am J Surg 182:729–732, 2001.
12. Meyer J, Harmon C, Harty P, et al: Ovarian torsion: clinical and imaging presentation in children. J Pediatr Surg 30:1433–1436, 1995.
13. Pena J, Ufberg D, Cooney N, et al: Usefulness of Doppler sonography in the diagnosis of ovarian torsion. Fertil Steril 73:1047–1050, 2000.
14. Lee E, Kwon H, Joo H, et al: Diagnosis of ovarian torsion with color Doppler sonography: depiction of twisted vascular pedicle. J Ultrasound Med 17:83–89, 1998.
15. Albayram F, Hamper U: Ovarian and adnexal torsion: spectrum of sonographic findings with pathologic correlation. J Ultrasound Med 20:1083–1089, 2001.
16. Shalev E, Mann S, Romano S: Laparoscopic detorsion of adnexa in childhood: a case report. J Pediatr Surg 26:1193–1194, 1991.
17. Anders JF, Powell EC: Urgency of evaluation and outcome of acute ovarian torsion in pediatric patients. Arch Pediatr Adolesc Med 159:532–535, 2005.

Chapter 94

Vaginal and Urethral Disorders

Beverly H. Bauman, MD, and Robert L. Cloutier, MD

Selected Diagnoses

Vaginal discharge and vaginitis
Vaginal foreign body
Labial adhesion (labial agglutination)
Vaginal outflow obstruction
Bartholin's duct cyst and abscess
Urethral prolapse
Urethritis

Discussion of Individual Diagnoses

Vaginal Discharge and Vaginitis

Staining discovered on the undergarments or diapers of infants and children presumed to be from vaginal discharge or bleeding may prompt an emergency department evaluation. However, in neonates and premenarchal young adolescents, not all types of vaginal discharge are pathologic. Estrogen effects on the vagina cause physiologic leukorrhea, a white or clear mucoid discharge. A newborn acquires maternal estrogen transplacentally prior to birth, and for several weeks after delivery her hymen and vagina will show the effects of estrogen. The hymen appears pale, thickened, and redundant and the vagina secretes a normal mucoid discharge. The endometrium in the uterus of a neonate also responds to maternal estrogen, and after birth a small amount of vaginal bleeding can sometimes be seen from estrogen withdrawal. Six to 12 months prior to the onset of menarche, physiologic leukorrhea will again appear in response to the young adolescent's increased levels of estrogen. No treatment except reassurance is needed for physiologic leukorrhea and neonatal withdrawal bleeding.

Pathologic vaginal discharge and inflammation (vaginitis) is much more common in postmenarchal adolescents and adults than in the pediatric age range (see Chapter 70, Sexually Transmitted Infections). If the inflammation includes the vulva, it is termed *vulvovaginitis*. Pediatric patients may complain of pruritis, perineal pain, and dysuria.[1,2] Reduced levels of estrogen and the more alkaline pH of the vagina in premenarchal girls are two important reasons why the prevalence, etiology, and presentation of vaginitis is different in premenarcheal girls than postmenarchal adolescents and adults. After puberty, the vagina changes in response to estrogen and the normal flora has a greater amount of *Lactobacillus* species.

In premenarchal girls, the etiology of vaginitis and vulvovaginitis may be local irritation, poor hygiene, and a variety of bacterial, viral, helmenthic, or protozoal infections. The majority of cases of premenarchal vulvovaginitis are not caused by an infection, yet when the patient has a visible vaginal discharge, there is a higher likelihood of a specific infectious cause.[1,2] Workup includes a careful history and physical examination with consideration for the risk of a sexually transmitted infection (from sexual abuse). If a discharge is present, workup includes culture, wet mount, and potassium hydroxide preparation. These studies will help guide specific therapy when it is indicated and help avoid unnecessary antibiotics for nonspecific vaginitis. Nonspecific vaginitis and vulvovaginitis may be precipitated by poor local hygiene or spread of enteric organisms from the rectum to the vulvar and vaginal areas. Irritation from bubble baths or soaps, vaginal foreign bodies, and viruses and bacteria from upper respiratory tract infections can also cause nonspecific vaginitis. Based on the findings from history and physical examination, treatment for nonspecific vaginitis may include removal of a vaginal foreign body, improved perineal hygiene, teaching a child to wipe her perineum from the front to the back after using the toilet, avoidance of irritating bubble bath products and soaps, and avoidance of tight-fitting pants.

Candidal vaginitis is common in adolescents and adults, yet uncommon in children. Diagnosis is by microscopy of the discharge with potassium hydroxide preparation. If candidal vaginitis is seen in a child, it may be related to recent broad-spectrum antibiotic use, immunosuppression, or diabetes. Treatment is with topical or oral antifungal agents.[3] Common causes of bacterial vaginitis in children include several types of streptococcus and *Staphylococcus aureus* and coagulase-negative staphylococci. Gram-negative organisms have also been cultured from children with vaginitis.[1,2,4] Pinworms (*Enterobius vermicularis*) can migrate from the rectum to the vagina, also resulting in vaginitis. These parasites lay their ova at night on the perirectal skin, which can be detected using the "tape test" (cellophane tape pressed to the perineum) to collect the ova for diagnosis by microscopy. One study found a significant number of unsuspected cases of *Neisseria gonorrhoeae* in children with a vaginal discharge and concluded that cultures for gonococcus should be included in routine bacterial cultures for children with a discharge[2] (see Chapter 70, Sexually Transmitted Infections; and Chapter 118, Sexual Abuse).

After the first few weeks of life, when a neonate may have estrogen withdrawal bleeding, vaginal bleeding in prepubertal children mandates a thorough evaluation to rule out potentially serious causes such as a malignant tumor or trauma. Less worrisome causes of bleeding from the genital area that may present as vaginal bleeding include precocious puberty, vulvovaginitis, hemangioma, vaginal foreign body, urethral prolapse, hematuria, and lichen sclerosis, which is an uncommon chronic pruritic inflammatory skin disease of the perineum and perianal area.[5] The examination to determine the source of the vaginal bleeding may require monitored sedation or general anesthesia because the hymen of a prepubertal child is very sensitive.

Vaginal Foreign Body

A vaginal foreign body should be considered in the differential diagnosis of a child presenting with persistent vaginal drainage or bleeding, although it is an uncommon finding.[1,6] A wad of toilet paper is one of the most common vaginal foreign bodies in children,[6] while a retained tampon is a common vaginal foreign body in adolescents. Visualization of the vaginal foreign body may be easiest with the child in the knee-chest position. If the foreign body is large, it might be palpable with a rectal examination. Techniques to remove the foreign body include gentle irrigation with saline using a small catheter and gentle extraction with forceps. Monitored sedation or general anesthesia may be needed in prepubertal girls when attempting vaginal foreign body removal.[6]

Labial Adhesions (Labial Agglutination)

Fusion of the labia minora is a common condition in infants and toddlers that may be found incidentally on examination or during attempts to perform urinary catheterization.[7] The delicate skin of the labia minora can be easily irritated and inflamed from mild local trauma, harsh soaps, or soiled diaper contents. Upon healing, the labial surfaces may become fused to one another, resulting in labial agglutina-

tion. Usually the adhesions start in the area of the posterior forchette and slowly advance towards the clitoris. This fusion may prevent visualization of the hymen and urethral opening (Fig. 94–1).

Most young children are asymptomatic with labial adhesions, and therefore treatment is not routinely necessary. The adhesions may spontaneously resolve or resolve later around puberty with endogenous estrogen. However, if the patient has dysuria or if the parents have a preference to treat the condition, it can be managed with a several-week course of once- or twice-daily application of topical 0.1% conjugated estrogen cream (Premarin cream). Potential side effects from systemic absorption of topical estrogen cream include breast tenderness. Therefore, parents should be cautioned to avoid excessive use of the topical estrogen cream and discontinue its use after the adhesions have resolved. Following successful labial separation, the application of petrolatum jelly to the labial area at night for several weeks can help prevent recurrence of adhesions. Routine rapid forceful separation of the adhesions is discouraged because it is painful and will likely result in bleeding. If the labial adhesions cause urinary obstruction, topical lidocaine may be used to decrease the pain of manual separation in the emergency department, yet the procedure is still likely to be painful, so systemic analgesics are advised.[7,8]

Vaginal Outflow Obstruction

Several congenital anomalies may cause obstruction to vaginal outflow. The most common causes of vaginal outflow

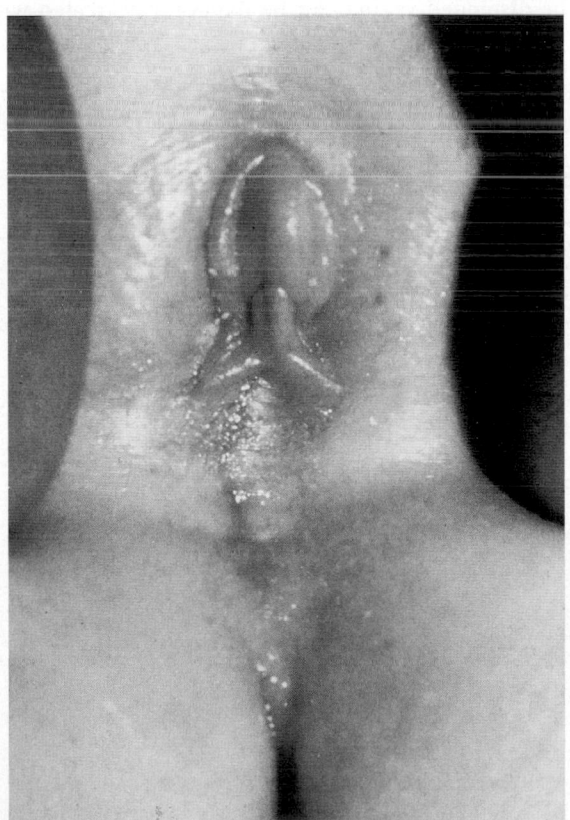

FIGURE 94–1. Labial adhesions. (From Rink R, Kaefer M: Surgical management of intersexuality, cloacal malformation, and other abnormalities of the genitalia in girls. *In* Wein A (ed): Campbell-Walsh Urology, 9th ed. Philadelphia: WB Saunders, 2007.)

obstruction are imperforate hymen and a transverse vaginal septum. Although these conditions are present at birth, the diagnosis may be easily missed during the newborn examination because of the small size of the newborn perineum and the thick and redundant state of the newborn hymen under the effect of maternal estrogen. A female infant may present to the emergency department with mucocolpos (the distention of the vagina from the collection of vaginal secretions) or hematocolpos (the distention of the vagina from endometrial blood) related to withdrawal from maternal estrogen. If the diagnosis of vaginal obstruction is not made in the newborn period, the fluid will be reabsorbed and the patient usually remains asymptomatic until puberty, when menstrual blood accumulates proximal to the obstruction. Family history may be helpful in arriving at the diagnosis of imperforate hymen because some families demonstrate an inheritance pattern consistent with either a dominant or recessive mode of genetic transmission.[9]

Signs and symptoms related to vaginal outflow obstruction in postmenarchal girls include primary amenorrhea, pelvic or abdominal pain that may or may not be cyclical, and difficulties with urination or defecation related to distention of the vagina. Physical examination may reveal a lower abdominal or pelvic mass (hydrometrocolpos). The hymen may be bulging and have a bluish discoloration if the etiology of obstruction is an imperforate hymen (Fig. 94–2). If the cause of the vaginal outflow obstruction is located higher in the vagina, such as from a high transverse vaginal septum, the hymen may have a normal appearance.

In the emergency department, urinary retention caused by the distended vagina can be temporarily treated with a

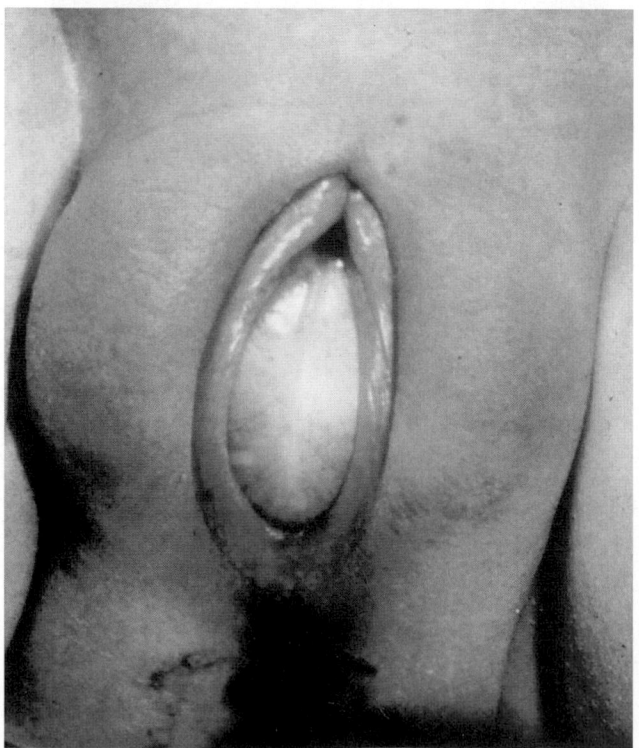

FIGURE 94–2. Imperforate hymen. (From Rink R, Kaefer M: Surgical management of intersexuality, cloacal malformation, and other abnormalities of the genitalia in girls. *In* Wein A (ed): Campbell-Walsh Urology, 9th ed. Philadelphia: WB Saunders, 2007.)

urinary catheter. Definitive treatment of the vaginal outflow obstruction will require surgical repair by a consulting gynecologist or pediatric surgeon. Transabdominal ultrasound provides useful anatomic information to aid in specific diagnosis and assist the surgeon or gynecologist in preoperative evaluation.[10]

Bartholin's Duct Cyst and Abscess

Disorders related to Bartholin's duct and glands may present at puberty when the gland starts secreting fluid into the vaginal vestibule. The two Bartholin's glands are located at approximately the 4 o'clock and 8 o'clock positions of the labia minora when a female is examined in the dorsal lithotomy position. These pea-sized glands drain through ducts into the vaginal vestibule, near the hymenal ring. Cysts and abscesses of the duct and glands may develop if secretions or infection occlude the duct. Small cysts (1 to 3 cm) that are not infected are typically asymptomatic and do not require drainage. Larger cysts and abscesses cause pain with sitting, walking, or sexual intercourse and will require incision and drainage for treatment. This simple procedure can be performed in the emergency department under local anesthesia with an incision through the mucosa using a number 11 scalpel blade. After incision and drainage, an inflatable Word catheter is placed to allow ongoing drainage and the formation of an epithelialized tract. The Word catheter is left in place for 2 to 4 weeks or as needed prior to removal. Alternatively, the abscess cavity may be packed with sterile gauze. Recurrent Bartholin's cysts may require marsupialization of the cyst cavity or excision of the gland by a gynecologist. Bartholin's duct abscesses are typically polymicrobial and should be treated with empirical broad-spectrum antibiotics directed against *N. gonorrhoeae* and *Chlamydia trachomatis* in sexually active patients, as well as against skin flora.[11]

Urethritis

Urethritis is an inflammation of the urethra, which has many possible etiologies: chemical irritation, trauma, foreign body, systemic inflammatory disease, allergic reaction, or infection. In comparison to adults, pediatric patients with urethritis are much less likely to have an infection as the source of the inflammation. The history of the presenting illness may include contact with irritants such as soaps or bubble bath, trauma from catheter placement or other foreign body, systemic illness and rash, or concern of sexual assault in small children or history of sexual activity in adolescents. Catheters made of latex are more likely to cause an allergic reaction in the urethra than are silicon catheters.[12]

Presenting signs and symptoms may include discomfort with urination, urinary frequency and urgency, itching and pain in the genital area, and hematuria or blood seen on the underpants. The urethral inflammation may be also associated with vaginitis or vulvovaginitis. Kawasaki disease, a pediatric multisystem vasculitis, is also associated with sterile pyuria and urethritis.[13]

A urine specimen should be obtained to look for white blood cells and red blood cells on microscopy and a culture sent to evaluate for infection. If sexually transmitted infections are suspected by history, studies to detect *C. trachomatis* and *N. gonorrhoeae* should be specifically obtained since

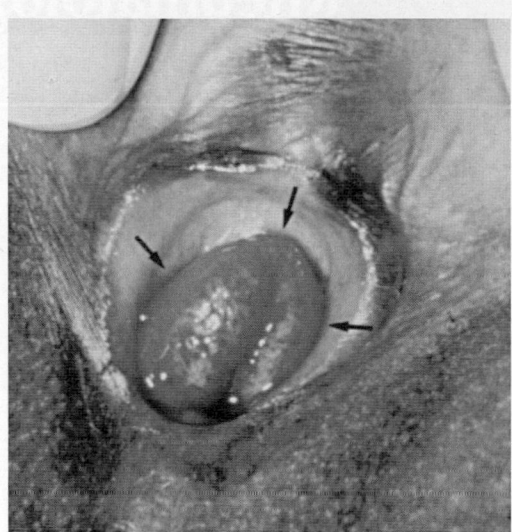

FIGURE 94–3. Urethral prolapse. (From Elder JS: Urologic disorders in infants and children: abnormalities of the penis and urethra. *In* Behrman RE, Kliegman RM, Jenson HB (eds): Nelson Textbook of Pediatrics, 17th ed. Philadelphia: WB Saunders, 2004.)

routine bacterial urine cultures will not detect those infections.

Urethral Prolapse

Urethral prolapse is an uncommon pediatric condition. It is the protrusion of distal urethral mucosa through the urethral meatus. Although it is usually asymptomatic and found incidentally on examination, it may also present as blood stained diapers or undergarmets, dysuria, urinary frequency, or urinary obstruction. Urethral prolapse typically appears as a red circular mass around the end of the urethra (Fig. 94–3). The exact etiology of this condition is not known, but it is most commonly seen in African American infants, tod-

dlers, and young girls. Conservative treatment is a trial of topical estrogen cream and gentle hygiene to prevent infection. Children should have follow-up for this condition as conservative measures frequently fail, and it may require surgical resection by a urologist for definitive repair.[5,14]

REFERENCES

1. Jacquiery A, Stylianopoulos A, Hogg G, Grover S: Vulvovaginitis: clinical features, aetiology, and microbiology of the genital tract. Arch Dis Child 81:64–67, 1999.
2. Shapiro R, Schubert C, Siegel R: *Neisseria gonorrhea* infections in girls younger than 12 years of age evaluated for vaginitis. Pediatrics 104:e72, 1999.
3. Pickering LK (ed): 2003 Red Book: Report of the Committee on Infectious Diseases, 26th ed. Elk Grove Village, IL: American Academy of Pediatrics, 2003.
4. Dhar V, Roker K, Adhami Z, et al: Streptococcal vulvovaginitis in girls. Pediatr Dermatol 10:366–367, 1993.
5. Anvenden-Hertzberg L, Guaderer M, Elder J: Urethral prolapse: an often misdiagnosed cause of urogenital bleeding in girls. Pediatr Emerg Care 11:212–214, 1995.
6. Herman-Giddens M: Vaginal foreign bodies and child sexual abuse. Arch Pediatr Adolesc Med 148:195–200, 1994.
7. Bacon J: Prepubertal labial adhesions: evaluation of a referral population. Am J Obstet Gynecol 187:327–331; discussion 332, 2002.
8. Nurzia M, Eickhortst K, Ankem M, et al: The surgical treatment of labial adhesions in pre-pubertal girls. J Pediatr Adolesc Gynecol 16:21–23, 2003.
9. Stelling J, Gray M, Davis A, et al: Dominant transmission of imperforate hymen. Fertil Steril 74:1241–1244, 2000.
10. Blask A, Sanders R, Rock J: Obstructed uterovaginal anomalies: demonstration with sonography. Part II. Teenagers. Radiology 179:84–88, 1991.
11. Aghajanian A, Bernstein L, Grimes D: Bartholin's duct abscess and cyst: a case-control study. South Med J 87:26–29, 1994.
12. Nacey J, Tulloch A, Ferguson A: Catheter-induced urethritis: a comparison between latex and silicone catheter in a prospective clinical trial. Br J Urol 57:325–328, 1985.
13. Dajani A, Taubert K, Gerber M, et al: Diagnosis and therapy of Kawasaki disease in children. Circulation 87:1776–1780, 1993.
14. Valerie E, Gilchrist B, Firscher J, et al: Diagnosis and treatment of urethral prolapse in children. Urology 54:1082–1084, 1999.

Musculoskeletal Disorders in Systemic Disease

Blake Spirko, MD and Allison V. Brewer, MD

Key Points

Kawasaki disease should be considered in the differential diagnosis of all children with a prolonged fever.

Since the earlier manifestations of Lyme disease are easier to treat than the later stages, early diagnosis and treatment are particularly important.

Acute rheumatic fever is characterized by nonsuppurative manifestations weeks after a preceding group A streptococcus pharyngeal infection.

The diagnosis of juvenile rheumatoid arthritis encompasses a heterogeneous group of chronic arthritic conditions and is made by exclusion.

Selected Diagnoses

Kawasaki disease
Lyme disease
Acute rheumatic fever
Juvenile rheumatoid arthritis

Discussion of Individual Diagnoses

Kawasaki Disease

Kawasaki disease is the most frequent pediatric vasculitis, and, more importantly, it is the most common cause of acquired heart disease in children.[1] Kawasaki disease is a systemic vasculitis with significant complications from coronary vessel involvement. Development of coronary artery ectasia and aneurysms can lead to myocardial ischemia, infarction, and sudden death. Although the etiology of this condition is uncertain, early treatment decreases the incidence of coronary artery aneurysms and thrombosis. Early treatment of Kawasaki disease (within the first 10 days of fever) decreases the appearance of coronary artery aneu-

rysms and ectasia from 20% to less than 5%.[2] The vascular inflammation is slowly replaced by fibrinous tissue, and, although usually not clinically significant, there is evidence of abnormal endothelial function years after disease onset.[3] Eighty-five percent of cases develop in children less than 5 years old, with the average age being approximately 2 years.[4]

Clinical Presentation

Kawasaki disease requires a clinical diagnosis, as there is no definitive diagnostic test. The original diagnostic criteria include fever for 5 days plus four out of five principal clinical criteria: (1) nonexudative conjunctival injection, (2) oropharyngeal mucosa abnormalities, (3) changes in the peripheral extremities, (4) polymorphous rash, (5) cervical lymphadenopathy greater than 1.5 cm[5] (Table 95–1). Conjunctival injection typically is painless and spares the limbus (Fig. 95–1). Uveitis may occur in a large number of cases. The pharynx and lips typically become red within 1 to 3 days of the onset of disease. The lips are often dry, crusted, and fissured and may become secondarily infected (see Fig. 95–1). Hypertrophy of tongue papillae gives rise to a strawberry appearance. The hands and feet become edematous while the palms and soles become red within 3 days of onset (Fig. 95–2). Edema is nonpitting and lasts approximately 1 week. Peeling of the hands and feet begins at the nail margins and occurs 10 to 14 days after onset. The rash is most commonly a diffuse, deep red, maculopapular eruption. The rash may resemble erythema multiforme, scarlet fever, or erythema marginatum. Dermatitis in the diaper area is also common. With time, macules and papules become confluent. Desquamation occurs within 1 week, with onset of perineal desquamation 2 to 6 days before desquamation of the fingertips and toes. Lymphadenopathy is usually nontender and nonsuppurative and is often limited to a single lymph node.

While 5 days of fever is typically required to make the diagnosis, the American Heart Association recommends making the diagnosis with only 4 days of fever if four or more principal criteria are present.[2] The diagnosis can also be made with less than four principal criteria if echocardiography demonstrates coronary artery features consistent with Kawasaki disease. Infants are less likely to meet the original diagnostic criteria compared to older children.[6] Some experts

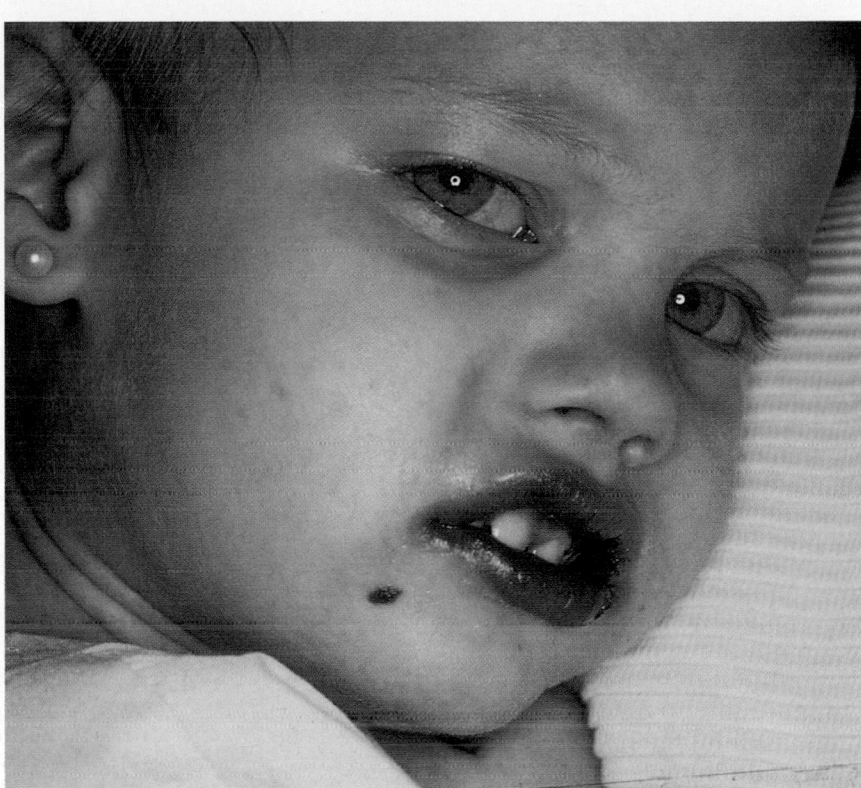

FIGURE 95–1. Nonpurulent conjunctival injection and "cherry-red" lips with fissuring and crusting are early signs of Kawasaki disease. (From Habif TP: Clinical Dermatology: A Color Guide to Diagnosis and Therapy, 4th ed. St. Louis: Mosby, 2004, p 475.)

Table 95–1	Principal Criteria of Kawasaki Disease

Fever persisting at least 5 days PLUS
Presence of at least 4 of 5 principal features:
1. Bilateral nonexudative bulbar conjunctival injection
   Typically appears shortly after fever onset
2. Mucosal changes
   Red, fissured, perhaps bleeding lips
   Strawberry tongue (identical to that of streptococcal scarlet fever)
   Oral/pharyngeal mucosal injection
3. Altered appearance of extremities
   Erythema of palm and soles
   Edema of hands and feet
4. Polymorphous rash
   Most commonly diffuse maculopapular eruption
   May be scarlitiniform or erythema multiforme–like
   Usually extensive
5. Cervical lymphadenopathy > 1.5 cm
   Least common of principal features
   Usually unilateral and within the anterior triangle

Adapted from Newburger J, Takahashi M, Gerber M, et al: Diagnosis, treatment, and long-term management of Kawasaki disease: a statement for health professionals from the Committee on Rheumatic Fever, Endocarditis and Kawasaki Disease, Council on Cardiovascular Disease in the Young, American Heart Association. Circulation 110:2747–2771, 2004.

recommend that infants less than 6 months old with fever for 7 days and an undetermined etiology should have laboratory testing (erythrocyte sedimentation rate [ESR] or C-reactive protein [CRP]) looking for a systemic inflammatory process. If laboratory tests indicate an inflammatory process, echocardiography should be performed even if there are no other signs of Kawasaki disease.[2]

Although not part of the original diagnostic criteria, other clinical and diagnostic features can aid in the diagnosis. Irritability is characteristically seen in young children. Aseptic meningitis develops in approximately 50% of patients.[7] Periungual desquamation typically occurs in the second and third week of illness, thus limiting its usefulness as a diagnostic clue in the emergency department. A vesicular rash is rare. Cervical lymphadenopathy is the least common principal feature and usually is not diffuse in nature. Children also may develop hydrops of the gallbladder. Laboratory values that aid but do not confirm the diagnosis include increased ESR and CRP values, pyuria from urethritis, anemia, and slightly increased transaminase values.[8] Obtaining both an ESR and a CRP level will increase the sensitivity for diagnosing this disorder.[9] A reactive thrombosis tends to develop after the first week of illness. The majority of electrocardiograms are normal; however, approximately 35% show some abnormalities consistent with myocarditis, such as T-wave flattening and ST-segment changes. Children with Kawasaki disease and a brain naturetic peptide level greater than 50 pg/ml usually have acute myocarditis.[10]

An incomplete form of the disease occurs and can make the diagnosis even more challenging. Patients with incomplete Kawasaki disease have a fever for 5 days but have less than four diagnostic criteria. The clinical features that develop are still typical. Unfortunately, patients with incomplete Kawasaki disease also have a propensity for coronary artery aneurysms.[11] The American Heart Association has provided guidelines for the evaluation of suspected incomplete Kawasaki disease. Patients with two or three principal criteria and fever for 5 or more days should be assessed clinically for Kawasaki disease. CRP and ESR levels are recommended if an alternate diagnosis is not suspected. If the CRP

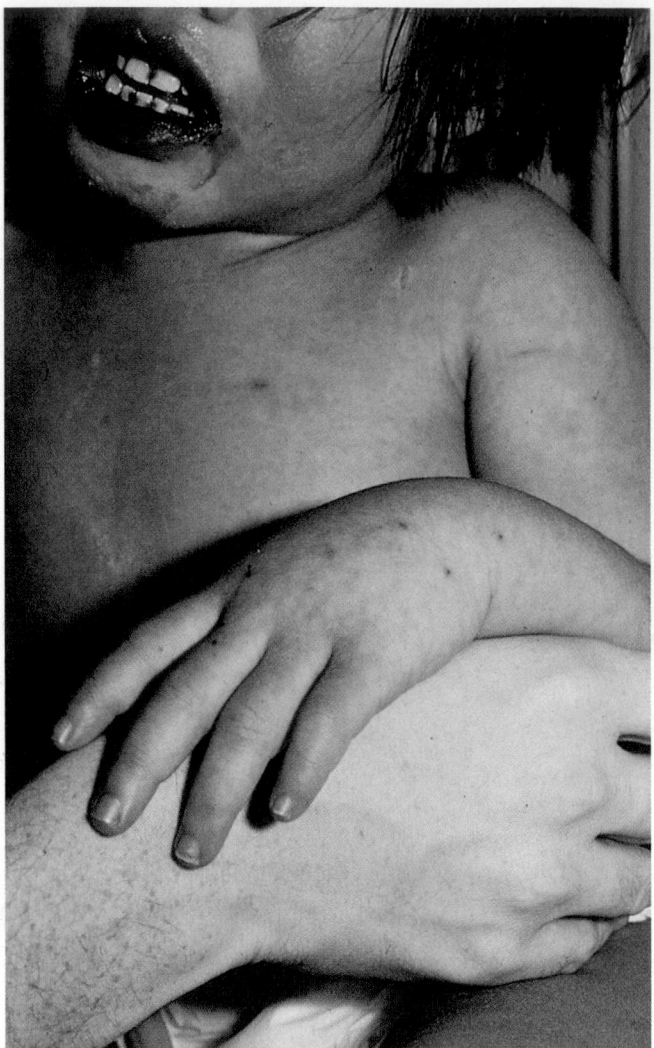

FIGURE 95–2. Hand and foot edema typically occurs within the first 3 days of illness in Kawasaki disease. (From Habif TP: Clinical Dermatology: A Color Guide to Diagnosis and Therapy, 4th ed. St. Louis: Mosby, 2004, p 475.)

is 3.0 mg/dl or greater or the ESR is 40 mm/hr or greater, treatment should be instituted in patients with three clinical criteria. Patients with only two criteria who meet these laboratory cutoff values require an echocardiogram. If the echocardiogram shows evidence of Kawasaki disease, these patients should also be treated. Echocardiographic evaluation focuses on measurement of coronary artery diameter for evidence of ectasia and aneurysm formation. Other possible echocardiographic signs include perivascular echogenicity, depressed ventricular contractility, aortic root dilation, pericardial effusion, and valvular regurgitation.[2] Small studies indicate that multidetector computed tomography may be as accurate as echocardiography at detecting coronary aneurysms and may detect the stenoses and occlusions in most adolescents.[12] If verified in larger studies, this technique may augment echocardiography in the future.

The differential diagnosis varies with the clinical presentation but includes adenovirus and other viral infections. Other considerations include drug reactions, scarlet fever, staphylococcal scalded skin syndrome, and bacterial cervical lymphadenitis (see Chapter 120, Skin and Soft Tissue Infec-

tions; Chapter 123, Classic Viral Exanthems; and Chapter 126, Other Important Rashes). Clinical subjectivity of the principal diagnostic criteria often makes the diagnosis challenging. Depending upon the institution, pediatric cardiologists, rheumatologists, and infectious disease physicians often have expertise in diagnosing and treating Kawasaki disease and may be a helpful resource.

Management

The emergency physician's main role is to formulate a timely diagnosis and admit patients with Kawasaki disease to the hospital for intravenous gamma globulin (IVIG) and high-dose salicylate treatment. IVIG is administered by a slow infusion at a dose of 2 g/kg.[13] IVIG treatment has better efficacy if given before day 10 of illness, and ideally should be administered before the seventh day.[2] Treatment prior to the fifth day is effective but is also associated with an increased need for IVIG retreatment.[14] High-dose aspirin therapy (80 to 100 mg/kg per day) is instituted during the acute phase of illness. Typically, a few days after defervescence, aspirin therapy is converted to a lower dose (3 to 5 mg/kg per day). Low-dose salicylate treatment is continued during a prolonged follow-up period that includes repeat echocardiograms. Debate exists as to the utility of steroids in Kawasaki disease. One meta-analysis concluded that adding corticosteroids to standard aspirin and IVIG regimens significantly reduces the incidence of coronary aneurysms.[15] A more recent randomized, double-blinded, placebo-controlled trial did not support the use of single pulse dose steroids.[15a]

Although coronary artery aneurysms develop later in the disease course, baseline coronary artery evaluation by echocardiography is recommended early in the management of the disease. Occasionally, children may present with myocardial ischemia or infarction secondary to coronary artery thrombus formation, which differs from atherosclerotic plaque rupture as seen in adults. In general, modified adult acute coronary syndrome protocols are used in the treatment of children presenting with a myocardial infarction, including such therapies as aspirin, heparin, and thrombolytic therapy. As there are no randomized controlled trials for pediatric patients, the American Heart Association extrapolated adult data and recommends using either thrombolytic or mechanical reperfusion therapy for acute ischemia depending upon available expertise and time constraints.[2]

Summary

Kawasaki disease should be considered in the differential diagnosis of all children with persistent fever. The diagnosis of this systemic inflammatory condition must be made clinically, with incomplete presentations making the diagnosis more challenging. Specialists with expertise in Kawasaki disease, such as pediatric infectious disease clinicians or pediatric cardiologists, may help confirm the diagnosis. Patients with Kawasaki disease require admission for treatment with both IVIG and high-dose salicylates in addition to cardiac evaluation. Early treatment significantly reduces coronary artery aneurysm and ectasia formation and possible subsequent thrombosis.

Lyme Disease

The spirochete *Borrelia burgdorferi* causes Lyme disease. Since the earlier manifestations of Lyme disease are easier to treat than the later stages, early diagnosis and treatment are particularly important. The spirochete is transmitted by *Ixodes* tick bites, most commonly in the Northeast and Midwest, although most states have reported the disease. In 2002, 95% of Lyme cases came from the following 12 states: Connecticut, Delaware, Rhode Island, Maine, Maryland, Massachusetts, Minnesota, New Jersey, New Hampshire, New York, Pennsylvania, and Wisconsin.[16] Among children, the incidence is highest among those between 5 and 14 years.[17] The incidence within different regions of a state is also highly variable. Patients who spend time outdoors in these endemic regions are the most susceptible. The *Ixodes* ticks transmit Lyme disease mostly during the late spring and summer while in their smaller lymph stage, although the larger adult tick can transmit the disease. Lymph ticks are 1 to 2 mm in size, and most patients do not recall a tick bite. Spirochete transmission generally requires tick attachment for a minimum of 24 hours; however, periods greater than 48 to 72 hours of tick attachment may be required.[18,19] Even in endemic regions only about 1.4% of patients bitten by *Ixodes* ticks develop Lyme disease, because most of the ticks are not infected with the spirochete and there is a need for a prolonged tick attachment period.[20]

Clinical Presentation

Lyme disease is classified into three stages. The first stage is the erythema migrans or early localized stage. Erythema migrans occurs in approximately 80% of cases[21] and usually develops 7 to 10 days after the tick bite, although the range is 1 to 36 days.[22] The erythematous macular or papular rash generally expands over a period of days to an average diameter of 16 cm[23] (Fig. 95–3). Erythema migrans can take various shapes, and often does not have a classic central clearing. Associated flulike symptoms may accompany this first stage, including mild myalgias, fever, chills, fatigue, lymphadenopathy, and stiff neck.[22] Patients with erythema migrans present most often during the summer months.

The early disseminated stage or second stage of Lyme disease develops weeks to months after the tick bite. This stage has a vast array of presentations as the disease may involve most organ systems, including cutaneous, neuro-logic, cardiac, ophthalmologic, and musculoskeletal. Skin lesions called secondary erythema migrans may develop. These lesions are similar in appearance to erythema migrans but tend to be smaller and develop in multiple locations. Cardiac involvement may include pericarditis, myocarditis, and various degrees of atrioventricular blocks[24] (see Chapter 47, Peripheral Neuromuscular Disorders; and Chapter 64, Pericarditis, Myocarditis, and Endocarditis). Neurologic involvement may include lymphocytic meningitis and facial nerve palsies. Approximately 50% of facial nerve palsies in children living in endemic areas are due to Lyme disease.[25] Bilateral seventh nerve palsy occurs approximately one third of the time.[26] Arthritis can also develop during the second or third stage of the disease. Lyme arthritis tends to be mono-articular or oligoarticular and has a propensity for larger joints, especially the knee.[27] Arthritis tends to be transient, brief, and minimally painful, although large effusions may develop. Late Lyme disease includes chronic recurrent or persistent arthritis as well as chronic neurologic syndromes. Neurologic syndromes include such entities as neuropathies, subtle encephalopathies, and fatigue syndromes.

The diagnosis of erythema migrans or stage one Lyme disease should be made clinically as two thirds of erythema migrans patients have false-negative results by serologic testing. Furthermore, serologic testing at the time of a tick bite is not recommended.[28] The likelihood of spirochete exposure by means of outdoor activities in endemic regions should be considered when making the diagnosis. The peak incidence of erythema migrans is from May through August. Unlike stage one, patients thought to have early disseminated Lyme disease should have serologic testing. Testing should include an enzyme-linked immunosorbent assay, with positive results confirmed by a Western blot as recommended by the Centers for Disease Control and Prevention.[29] Clinic judgment is important when ordering serologic testing as false-negative and false-positive results are common. Other laboratory tests have limited roles in making the diagnosis of Lyme disease, although they may aid in making other diagnoses. The complete blood count and ESR are generally normal in Lyme disease.[30] Cerebrospinal fluid (CSF) and synovial joint fluid analyses are more helpful in their ability

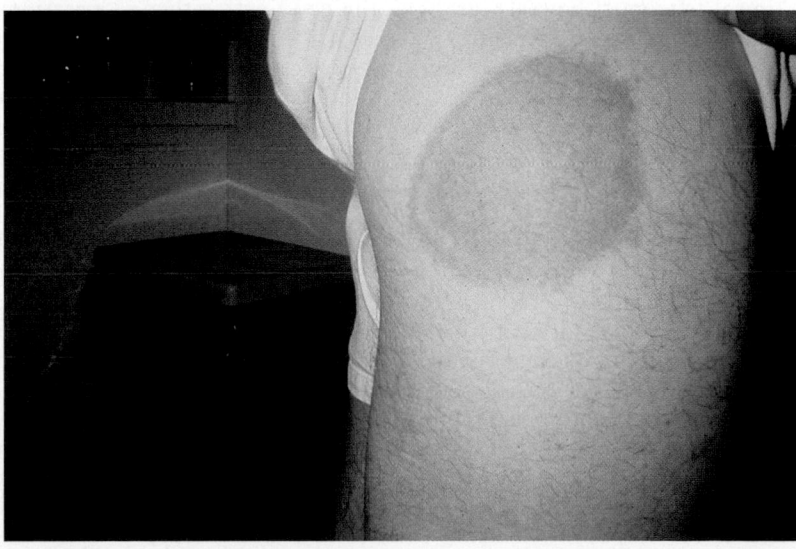

FIGURE 95–3. Erythema migrans: enlarging macular rash with central clearing and target appearance. (From Cohen J, Powderly WG (eds): Infectious Diseases, 2nd ed. St. Louis: Mosby, 2004, p 594.)

to exclude bacterial causes rather than confirm Lyme disease. Lyme CSF typically has a lymphocytic pleocytosis with less than a few hundred cells. Synovial fluid from Lyme arthritis typically has between a few hundred and 50,000 white blood cells with a predominance of polymorphonuclear cells.[31]

The differential diagnosis varies depending upon the stage of disease and the predominant organ systems involved. Spider bites and cellulitis can present similarly to erythema migrans but are generally more tender (see Chapter 120, Skin and Soft Tissue Infections; and Chapter 141, Snake and Spider Envenomations). Target lesions of erythema multiforme and viral exanthems can be confused with secondary erythema migrans (see Chapter 121, Erythema Multiforme Major and Minor; and Chapter 123, Classic Viral Exanthems). The neurologic manifestations of Lyme disease can also be consistent with the diagnoses of idiopathic Bell's palsy or aseptic meningitis. Juvenile rheumatoid arthritis (JRA) and septic arthritis are considered in the differential with Lyme arthritis, yet Lyme arthritis tends to cause less discomfort than a septic joint.

Management

All stages of Lyme disease are treated with antibiotics. Erythema migrans is treated orally with doxycycline 1 to 2 mg/kg twice a day (maximum, 100 mg/dose) for 14 to 21 days in children 8 years old or greater. As doxycycline is relatively contraindicated in children less than 8 years old, amoxicillin 50 mg/kg per day (maximum of 500 mg/dose three times a day) or cefuroxime 30 mg/kg per day (maximum of 500 mg/dose twice a day) for 14 to 21 days is used at this age. Patients with mild early disseminated Lyme disease, including mild cardiac involvement and isolated facial nerve palsy, can be treated with the same regimen as used for erythema migrans. Lyme arthritis can be treated with either oral or intravenous antibiotics. Doxycycline and amoxicillin can be administered in the doses mentioned previously, but the duration should be for 28 days. Severe cardiac involvement, meningitis, and severe arthritis are treated with ceftriaxone 75 to 100 mg/kg per day (maximum, 2 g) by intravenous administration for 14 to 28 days.[32] Because the CSF analysis is usually abnormal, some experts urge CSF analysis in all children with a seventh cranial nerve palsy in endemic areas.[33] Clinical outcomes, however, are typically good with either oral or intravenous treatment.[34]

Prophylactic antibiotics for *Ixodes* tick bites can be considered in highly endemic areas. In one study, a single 200-mg dose of doxycycline decreased the risk of Lyme disease from 3.2% to 0.4%.[35] The study showing this benefit occurred where the prevalence of infected *Ixodes* ticks is high, ticks were determined to be *Ixodes scapularis* by entomologists, and patients less than 12 years old were not included.[35,36] Although pediatric antimicrobial prophylaxis for *Ixodes* tick bites is not routinely recommended,[20] it can be supported in highly endemic areas for patients 12 years old or greater who are bitten by partially engorged nymphal deer ticks.

In general, the emergency management of Lyme disease consists of making a proper diagnosis and initiating antimicrobial therapy. Serologic testing is indicated for cases of suspected early disseminated and late Lyme disease. Although most patients with Lyme disease are treated with oral antibiotics as an outpatient, patients with complicated disease manifestations will require hospital admission and antibiotics administered intravenously.

Acute Rheumatic Fever

Acute rheumatic fever (ARF) is characterized by nonsuppurative manifestations (arthritis, carditis, subcutaneous nodules, chorea, erythema marginatum) that occur between 2 and 3 weeks after a group A streptococcus (GAS) pharyngeal infection.[37] While the exact pathophysiology of ARF is still unknown, there is strong evidence that a preceding streptococcal pharyngeal infection is required for manifestation of the disease. Pharyngitis is the only streptococcal infection known to be associated with ARF in industrially developed regions of the world. The severity and mortality of the disease have declined since the initiation of antibiotics in developed countries, but still remain a serious problem in undeveloped countries where the majority of the world population resides.[37]

Clinical Presentation

ARF presents as an acute febrile illness associated with any combination of the following symptoms: migratory polyarthritis primarily involving the large joints, erythema marginatum, chorea, carditis, and/or subcutaneous nodules. The disease usually first presents in patients between 5 and 15 years of age, with approximately 5% of cases presenting before the age of 5.[38,39] While the majority of the clinical manifestations resolve without sequelae, patients with cardiac involvement can have progressive deterioration, including death, secondary to congestive heart failure and dysrhythmias.[37]

Arthritis occurs in three fourths of patients with ARF and is usually the first manifestation of disease. Inflammation is migratory, and several large joints are usually involved (e.g., knee, ankle, elbow, wrist). Joint fluid analysis usually reveals 2000 to 50,000 white blood cells per milliliter with a predominance of neutrophils. Rheumatic heart disease due to carditis is the most serious manifestation of rheumatic fever and occurs in 50% to 60% of cases. Inflammation can affect the myocardium, pericardium, and endocardium (valves). Signs and symptoms of myocarditis or pericarditis may occur (see Chapter 64, Pericarditis, Myocarditis, and Endocarditis). Acute valvular involvement manifests as a murmur and occasionally congestive heart failure due to aortic or mitral regurgitation. Over time, progressive valvular deterioration can occur necessitating replacement. Sydenham's chorea is uncommon in rheumatic fever, occurring in only 10% to 15% of cases. Clinical features include involuntary spontaneous movements, lack of coordination of voluntary movements, and muscular weakness. Involvement may be unilateral.[40] The face tongue, and upper extremities are most commonly involved. Emotional lability, dysarthria, restlessness, and facial grimacing occur. Neurologic manifestations increase with stress and disappear with sleeping. Clinical maneuvers that elicit chorea include asking the patient to squeeze the examiner's fingers, which causes irregular contractions of the muscles of the hands (milkmaid's grip); arm extension, which leads to spooning and pronation of the hands; tongue protrusion with uncontrolled darting movements; and drawing and writing, which reveal loss of fine motor skills. Neurologic abnormalities usually resolve within 2 to 3 months.[41] Erythema marginatum occurs in a small

Table 95–2	Diagnostic Requirements for Acute Rheumatic Fever

Diagnosis requires evidence of group A streptococcal (GAS) infection PLUS fulfillment of the Revised Jones Criteria*

Evidence of GAS Infection (confirmed by one of these criteria)†

Positive throat culture for GAS
Increased streptolysin O or other streptococcal antibodies
Positive rapid direct GAS carbohydrate antigen test
Recent scarlet fever

Jones Criteria (Revised)

Diagnosis requires that 2 major, or 1 major and 2 minor, criteria are met

Major Criteria	Minor Criteria
Carditis	Fever
Polyarthritis	Arthralgia
Chorea	Previous rheumatic fever or heart disease
Subcutaneous nodules	Elevated acute-phase reactant levels
Erythema marginatum	Leukocytosis
	Prolonged PR interval

*Patients with latent manifestations of chorea or carditis are the exceptions to this rule and do not have to have evidence of GAS infection to be diagnosed with ARF.
†Antibodies are the test of choice, as throat cultures are often negative by the time of onset of ARF, and do not distinguish between active infection and carrier state.
Adapted from Gibofsky A: Rheumatic fever: the relationships between host, microbe, and genetics. Rheum Dis Clinic North Am 24:237–259, 1998.

number of patients with rheumatic fever. The rash is nonpruritic, red, serpiginous, and macular with a pale center in the macules. It occurs on the trunk and extremities, spares the face, and is accentuated by warming the skin. Subcutaneous nodules are the least common major manifestion of rheumatic fever. They are firm nodules that are located along the extensor surfaces of tendons near bony protuberances.[40]

The diagnosis of ARF is often difficult to make. A diagnosis of ARF requires both evidence of recent streptococcal infection and appropriate application of the revised Jones criteria.[37,42,43] Evidence of GAS infection can be confirmed by one of the following: positive throat culture for GAS, increased antistreptolysin O or other streptococcal antibodies, positive rapid direct GAS carbohydrate antigen test, or recent scarlet fever.[37,42] Serum antibodies are the test of choice, as throat cultures are often negative by the time of onset of ARF, and do not distinguish between active infection and carrier state.[37] Patients with latent manifestations of chorea or carditis are the exceptions to this rule, and are not required to have evidence of GAS infection to be diagnosed with ARF. The revised Jones Criteria are used to help with the diagnosis of ARF, and require that two major or one major and two minor criteria are met (Table 95–2).[37,42,43]

Acute-phase reactants (ESR, CRP), while nonspecific, are usually elevated with acute disease unless chorea is the only presenting symptom. In addition to supporting the diagnosis of ARF, acute-phase reactants also serve as markers for resolution as well as recurrence of the disease.[37] While chest radiographs and an electrocardiogram should be obtained as basic screening tests, a complete echocardiogram should also be performed for more specific evaluation and assessment of cardiac function and valvular lesions that may not be clinically apparent.[42]

Management

The management of ARF is directed at accomplishing three major goals: symptomatic and supportive treatment of acute disease processes, antibiotics to ensure eradication of GAS, and prophylaxis for prevention of future disease. Emergency department management of patient care is directed at recognition of the disease, as well as initial treatment with antibiotics, salicylates, and supportive treatment depending on the severity of symptom manifestation. All patients should be admitted to the hospital for complete evaluation and treatment. Transfer to an appropriate intensive care facility should be arranged for patients with acute life-threatening carditis.

All patients with ARF are treated with antibiotics to eliminate streptococcal organisms and bacterial antigens. Penicillin is the drug of choice and is recommended orally for a 10-day course or as a one-time intramuscular dose of benzathine penicillin G (600,000 units for children <27 kg, or 1.2 million units for those >27 kg) to ensure compliance. If patients are penicillin allergic, narrow-spectrum cephalosporins, clindamycin, azithromycin, or clarithromycin are also acceptable choices. Family members should be cultured, and treated if they are GAS positive. Antibiotics do not alter the course, frequency, or severity of cardiac involvement of ARF.[37]

High-dose salicylates (80 to 100 mg/kg per day in children, up to 4 to 8 g/day) are most commonly used for symptomatic relief of arthritis and fever, often producing dramatic results soon after initiation of therapy. If no contraindications exist, treatment is continued until symptom resolution and normalization of acute phase reactants.[37] All other clinical manifestations of ARF are treated individually depending on symptom severity.

Cardiac manifestations of ARF are the most severe sequelae, and must be recognized and treated promptly. Valvular and muscular damage result in a variety of clinical signs, including murmurs, cardiomegaly, atrioventricular blocks, pericarditis, and congestive heart failure.[37] While corticosteroids and intravenous immunoglobulins have frequently been implemented in the treatment of carditis, current evidence has shown that there is no risk reduction or alteration of the natural history or course of heart disease with either of these agents.[44,45] Unfortunately, no known current therapy that has been shown to alter the course of heart disease in ARF.[45] Patients with carditis and severe heart failure should be treated supportively and conventionally with digoxin, vasodilators, and diuretics as appropriate, and with prompt involvement of a cardiology specialist. It is currently believed that severe connective tissue destruction rather than myocyte damage leads to the valvular incompetence that causes the heart failure associated with ARF.[46] Surgery, including valve replacement or balloon mitral commissurotomy, may be necessary if heart failure is refractory to medical treatment. Rheumatic heart disease (RHD), the most devastating sequela of ARF, is still the most commonly acquired heart disease in the world. RHD most often presents 10 to 20 years after the initial attack of ARF, secondary to severe mitral valve stenosis from valvular calcification.[37]

Chorea often responds to haloperidol and sedation to achieve complete physical and mental rest. Arthritic pain is best treated with aspirin as well as bed rest until symptoms resolve to prevent joint damage. Both the rash and subcutaneous nodules often resolve spontaneously during the course of the disease and do not need specific treatment.

Prevention of further infection and attacks is accomplished by long-term antimicrobial prophylaxis, which should be started immediately after the resolution of an acute exacerbation of ARF. Most commonly, recurrences of ARF occur within the first 2 to 5 years after the initial attack, but they can present at any time. Therefore, prophylaxis is recommended for 10 years after the last episode of ARF, or until patients are well into adulthood. However, patients with documented RHD, or those at risk for frequent exposure, may benefit from continuous, indefinite prophylaxis. This can be accomplished by the use of either oral penicillin, sulfadiazine, or penicillin G intramuscularly every 4 weeks.[47]

The prognosis of ARF is highly variable. Ninety percent of patients have resolution of the episode within 3 months with adequate treatment and rest. All patients require period follow-up as outpatients to ensure complete resolution of symptoms and to ensure compliance with prophylactic treatment. Extended antibiotic courses are usually due to unremitting carditis or prolonged chorea. Although patients with underlying heart disease are at higher risk for a more severe course of carditis, 65% to 70% of all patients will not have sequelae. Those that have recurrence are at high risk of severe cardiac failure, which may lead to death.[37] Future advancements in the prevention and treatment of ARF lie in vaccine development aimed at the eradication of GAS,[37,48] as well as in advancements of echocardiography.[42]

Juvenile Rheumatoid Arthritis

JRA is defined as an arthritic process lasting a minimum of 6 weeks, affecting at least one joint, and presenting in a child less than 16 years of age. It is a diagnosis of exclusion.[49,50] The prevalence of JRA, also known as juvenile idiopathic arthritis, ranges between 0.16 : 1000 and 1.1 : 1000.[51] The incidence varies among different ethnic and geographic regions of the world.[49] JRA is further classified into one of three main categories: pauciarticular, polyarticular, and systemic.

Clinical Presentation

Pauciarticular JRA is not associated with systemic symptoms and affects fewer than five joints.[50] A monoarticular presentation is seen in 50% of cases. Asymptomatic uveitis is the only associated extra-articular presenting sign.[49,51] Pauciarticular JRA can be further subdivided into type 1 and type 2, both of which are rheumatoid factor negative. Type 1 predominately affects girls ages 2 to 5, most commonly involving knee and ankle joints, followed by elbows and wrists, and rarely involving the hips. Affected joints are typically warm yet without erythema, and parents often bring the child to medical attention with complaints of a limp.[51] Type 2 typically occurs in children 8 years and older and tends to involve the lower extremities (tarsal, ankle, knee, and hip joints), often causing an enthesis of the Achilles, plantar, and patellar tendons. Most laboratory values are normal with the exception of a positive antinuclear antibody (ANA), which is present 85% of the time.[50] The prognosis of pauciarticular JRA is relatively good, with spontaneous resolution often seen within 6 months. Recurrences of pauciarticular JRA occur in 20% of those affected, most commonly within the first year after initial onset. Patients who develop extended pauciarticular JRA often have destructive disease that lasts well into adulthood, and require aggressive treatment, similar to those with polyarticular JRA. The most severe and common sequela of pauciarticular JRA is uveitis, and routine ophthalmologic screening must be performed every 4 to 6 months in any child with the diagnosis of JRA for prevention of ocular complications.[52,53]

Polyarticular JRA involves five or more joints but often begins insidiously, leading to multiple joint involvement over a period of 6 months. It is subdivided into rheumatoid factor negative and positive subgroups. Rheumatoid factor–negative patients are typically girls less than 6 years old, while the rheumatoid factor–positive patients are generally early adolescents. Extra-articular manifestations such as vasculitis, lung disease, and rheumatoid nodules can develop in rheumatoid factor–positive patients. Laboratory values often show a positive ANA, anemia, and elevated acute-phase reactant levels.[49-51] Polyarticular JRA has a guarded prognosis, with 50% of cases leading to disabilities.[54]

Systemic JRA is associated with high intermittent fevers, rash, lymphadenopathy, hepatosplenomegaly, anemia, leukocytosis, pericarditis, peritonitis, pleuritis, and arthritis affecting any number of joints at a time. Children often present acutely and are ill appearing, making this subset of JRA the most difficult to both treat and diagnose. Systemic JRA has no gender preference, may occur at any age under 16, and is the only subset of JRA that involves the hips.[49-51] The diagnosis of systemic JRA is one of exclusion and requires the combination of arthritis and daily fevers greater than 38.5° C that are present for at least 6 weeks.[55] Many of the following laboratory abnormalities are suggestive of the disease and can help with diagnosis: profound leukocytosis, thrombocytosis, anemia, and elevated ESR and CRP. Rheumatoid factor and a positive ANA are not present. Systemic JRA has a highly variable course and prognosis. Nearly three quarters of patients will have remission of their articular erosions at 5 years after disease onset. Approximately one third will have a prolonged course and commonly have significant morbidity due to destructive arthritis, persistent systemic manifestations, medication side effects, and growth retardation.[56]

Management

Nonsteroidal anti-inflammatory agents (NSAIDs) are the initial treatment of choice for all subtypes of JRA. Children with refractory disease or failure to respond to NSAID use alone require prompt consultation with a pediatric rheumatologist for the initiation of appropriate second-line immunosuppressive agents with the intention of preventing permanent joint destruction. Risk:benefit ratios should always be considered when initiating any new therapeutic modalities.[49-51,56] JRA is a diagnosis of exclusion, with a complex differential including connective tissue diseases, malignancy, malaria, infective or reactive arthritis, postinfectious arthritis, systemic lupus erythematosus, systemic inflammatory conditions, orthopedic disorders, pain syndromes, immunodeficiencies, and other rheumatic diseases. Patients presenting with acutely inflamed joints, systemic signs of illness, or hip involvement are more likely to have an alternate diagnosis.

Emergency physicians may encounter patients with various complications due to JRA. Pericarditis occurs in 10% to 36% of JRA patients, while myocarditis develops much less frequently.[57] JRA patients may present with respiratory distress due to rare causes such as cardiac tamponade, pleural effusions,[57] and cricoarytenoiditis.[58,59] Emergency treatment of these complications requires steroids as well as potentially requiring specific cardiopulmonary resuscitation measures such as pericardiocentesis for cardiac tamponade[57] and endotracheal intubation for cricoarytenoiditis.[58] JRA may cause joint disease of the upper cervical spine in which atlantoaxial instability may develop.[60] Understanding this potential instability is particularly important for patients requiring endotracheal intubation and those presenting secondary to trauma. In summary, emergency physicians are more likely to treat complications of JRA than to make the initial diagnosis. Understanding of the varied presentations of this disease and its associated complications will serve to improve the outcome for these children.

REFERENCES

1. Taubert K, Rowley A, Shulman S: Nationwide survey of Kawasaki disease and acute rheumatic fever. J Pediatr 119:279–282, 1991.
*2. Newburger J, Takahashi M, Gerber M, et al: Diagnosis, treatment, and long-term management of Kawasaki disease: a statement for health professionals from the Committee on Rheumatic Fever, Endocarditis and Kawasaki Disease, Council on Cardiovascular Disease in the Young, American Heart Association. Circulation 110:2747–2771, 2004.
3. Dhillon R, Clarkson P, Donald A, et al: Endothelial dysfunction late after Kawasaki disease. Circulation 94:2103–2106, 1996.
4. Sundel R, Szer I: Vasculitis in childhood. Rheum Dis Clin North Am 28:625–654, 2002.
5. Kawasaki T: Acute febrile mucocutaneous syndrome with lymphoid involvement with specific desquamation of the fingers and toes in children [in Japanese]. Arerugi 16:178, 1967.
6. Rosenfeld E, Corydon K, Shulman S, et al: Kawasaki disease in infants less than one year of age. J Pediatr 126:524–529, 1995.
7. Dengler L, Capparelli E, Bastian J, et al: Cerebrospinal fluid profile in patients with acute Kawasaki disease. Pediatr Infect Dis J 17:478–481, 1998.
8. Burns J, Mason W, Glode M, et al: Clinical and epidemiologic characteristics of patients referred for evaluation of possible Kawasaki disease. United States Multicenter Kawasaki Disease Study Group. J Pediatr 118:680–686, 1991.
9. Anderson MS, Burns J, Treadwell TA, et al: Erythrocyte sedimentation rate and C-reactive protein discrepancy and high prevalence of coronary artery abnormalities in Kawasaki disease. Pediatr Infect Dis J 20:698–702, 2001.
10. Kawamura T, Wago M: Brain natriuretic peptide can be a useful biochemical marker for myocarditis in patients with Kawasaki disease. Cardiol Young 12:153–158, 2002.
11. Rowley A: Incomplete (atypical) Kawasaki disease. Pediatr Infect Dis J 21:563–565, 2002.
12. Kanamaru H, Sato Y, Takayama T, et al: Assessment of coronary artery abnormalities by multislice spiral computed tomography in adolescents and young adults with Kawasaki disease. Am J Cardiol 95:522–525, 2005.
13. Dajani A, Taubert K, Gerber M, et al: Diagnosis and therapy of Kawasaki disease in children. Circulation 87:1776–1780, 1993.
14. Fong N, Hui Y, Li C, Chiu M: Evaluation of the efficacy of treatment of Kawasaki disease before day 5 of illness. Pediatr Cardiol 25:31–34, 2004.
15. Wooditch AC, Aronoff SC: Effect of initial corticosteroid therapy on coronary artery aneurysm formation in Kawasaki disease: a meta-analysis of 862 children. Pediatrics 116:989–995.
15a. Newburger J, Sleeper L, McCrindle B, et al: Randomized trial of pulsed corticosteroid therapy for primary treatment of Kawasaki disease. N Engl J Med 356:663–675, 2007.
16. Centers for Disease Control and Prevention: Notice to readers: final 2002 reports of notifiable diseases. MMWR Morb Mortal Wkly Rep 52:741–750, 2003.
17. Centers for Disease Control and Prevention: Lyme disease—United States, 2001–2002. MMWR Morb Mortal Wkly Rep 53:365–369, 2004.
18. Piesman J: Dynamics of Borrelia burgdorferi transmission by nymphal Ixodes dammini ticks. J Infect Dis 167:1082–1085, 1993.
19. Sood S, Salzman M, Johnson B, et al: Duration of tick attachment as a predictor of the risk of Lyme disease in an area in which Lyme disease is endemic. J Infect Dis 175:996–999, 1997.
20. Halsey N, Abramson J, Chesney P, et al; American Academy of Pediatrics: Prevention of Lyme disease. Pediatrics 105:142–147, 2000.
21. Rahn D, Felz M: Lyme disease update: current approach to early, disseminated, and late disease. Postgrad Med 103:51–54, 57–59, 63–64, 1998.
22. Nadelman R, Wormser G: Lyme borreliosis. Lancet 352:557–565, 1998.
23. Nadelman R, Norwakoski J, Forester G, et al: The clinical spectrum of early Lyme borreliosis in patients with culture-confirmed erythema migrans. Am J Med 100:502–508, 1996.
24. Steere A: Lyme disease. N Engl J Med 345:115–125, 2001.
25. Cook S, Macartney K, Rose C, et al: Lyme disease and seventh nerve paralysis in children. Am J Otolaryngol 18:320–323, 1997.
26. Coyle P, Schutzer S: Neurologic aspects of Lyme disease. Med Clin North Am 33:680–693, 1999.
27. Massarotti E: Lyme arthritis. Med Clin North Am 86:297–309, 2002.
28. Fix A, Strickland G, Grant J: Tick bites and Lyme disease in an endemic setting: problematic use of serologic testing and prophylactic antibiotic therapy. JAMA 279:206–210, 1998.
29. Centers for Disease Control and Prevention: Recommendations for test performance and interpretation from the Second National Conference on Serologic Diagnosis of Lyme Disease. MMWR Morb Mortal Wkly Rep 44:590–591, 1995.
30. Edlow J: Lyme disease and related tick-borne illnesses. Ann Emerg Med 33:680–693, 1999.
31. Sivadas R, Rahn D, Luft B: Lyme disease. In Cohn J, Powderly W (eds): Infectious Diseases. Philadelphia, Mosby, 2004, pp 591–602.
*32. Wormser G, Nadelman R, Dattwyler R, et al: Practice guidelines for the treatment of Lyme disease. The Infectious Disease Society of America. Clin Infect Dis 31:S1–S14, 2000.
33. Belman A, Reynolds L, Preston T, et al: Cerebrospinal fluid findings in children with Lyme disease-associated facial nerve palsy. Arch Pediatr Adolesc Med 151:1224, 1997.
34. Vázquez M, Sparrow S, Shapiro E: Long-term neuropsychologic and health outcomes of children with facial nerve palsy attributed to Lyme disease. Pediatrics 112:e93–e97, 2003.
35. Nadelman R, Nowakowski J, Fish D, et al: Prophylaxis with single-dose doxycycline for prevention of Lyme disease after Ixodes scapularis tick bite. N Engl J Med 345:79–84, 2001.
36. Shapiro E: Doxycycline for tick bites: not for everyone. N Engl J Med 345:133–134, 2001.
*37. Gibofsky A: Rheumatic fever: the relationships between host, microbe, and genetics. Rheum Dis Clinic North Am 24:237–259, 1998.
38. El-Said G: Rheumatic fever. In McMillan J, DeAngelis C, Feigin R, et al (eds): Oski's Pediatrics: Principles and Practice. Philadelphia: Lippincott Williams & Wilkins, 1999, p 1417.
39. Lloyd T, Veasy G, Minich L, Shaddy R: Rheumatic fever in children younger than 5 years: is the presentation different? Pediatrics 112:1065–1068, 2003.
40. Hahn RG: Evaluation of post streptococcal illness. Am Fam Physician 71:1949–1954, 2005.
41. McMahon WM, Filloux FM, Ashworth JC, Jensen J: Movement disorders in children and adolescents. Neurol Clin 20:1101–1124, 2002.
42. Saxena A: Diagnosis of rheumatic fever: current status of Jones criteria and role of echocardiography. Indian J Pediatr 67:283–286, 2000.
*43. Digenea A, Ayoub E: Guidelines for the diagnosis of rheumatic fever: Jones criteria updates 1992. Circulation 87:302–307, 1993.
44. Cilliers A: Anti-inflammatory treatment for carditis in acute rheumatic fever. Cochrane Database Syst Rev (2):CD003176, 2003.
45. Voss L: Intravenous immunoglobulin in acute rheumatic fever: a randomized control trial. Circulation 103:401–406, 2001.

*Selected readings.

46. Gupta M, Lent RW, Kaplan EL, Zabriskie JB: Serum cardiac troponin I in acute rheumatic fever. Am J Cardiology 89:779–782, 2002.

47. Dajani A, Taubert K, Ferrieri P, et al: Treatment of acute streptococcal pharyngitis and prevention of rheumatic fever: a statement for health professionals. Pediatrics 96:758–764, 1995.

48. McDonald M, Currie BJ, Carapetis JR: Acute rheumatic fever: a chink in the chain that links the heart to the throat? Lancet Infect Dis 4:240–245, 2004.

*49. Schneider R, Passo M: Juvenile rheumatoid arthritis. Rheum Dis Clinics North Am 28:503–530, 2002.

50. Rheumatology and miscellaneous clinical conditions. In Joffe A, Blythe MJ (eds): Handbook of Adolescent Medicine. Adolesc Med 14:499–524, 2003.

51. Emery HM: Juvenile rheumatoid arthritis and the spondyloarthropathies. Adolesc Med 9:45–58, 1998.

52. Paroli M: Prognosis of juvenile rheumatoid arthritis-associated uveitis. Eur J Ophthamol 13:616–621, 2003.

53. Friedman L, Kaufman L: Guidelines for pediatrician referrals to the ophthamologist. Pediatr Clin North Am 50:41–53, 2003.

54. Emery H: Pediatric rheumatology: what does the future hold? Arch Phys Med Rehabil 85:1382–1384, 2004.

55. Brewer E, Bass J, et al: Criteria for the classification of juvenile rheumatoid arthritis. Bull Rheum Dis 23:712–719, 1972.

56. Ilowite N: Current treatment of juvenile rheumatoid arthritis. Pediatrics 109:109–115, 2002.

57. Yancey C, Doughty R, Cohlan B, Athreya B: Pericarditis and cardiac tamponade in juvenile rheumatoid arthritis. Pediatrics 68:369–373, 1981.

58. Goldhagen J: Cricoarytenoiditis as a cause of acute airway obstruction in children. Ann Emerg Med 17:532–533, 1988.

59. Jacobs J: Cricoarytenoid arthritis and airway obstruction in juvenile rheumatoid arthritis. Pediatrics 59:292–294, 1977.

60. Cassidy JT, Petty RE: Juvenile rheumatoid arthritis. *In* Cassidy JT, Petty RE (eds): Textbook of Pediatric Rheumatology, 3rd ed. Philadelphia: WB Saunders, 1995, pp 181–182.

Chapter 96

Bone, Joint, and Spine Infections

Charles G. Macias, MD, MPH and Coburn Allen, MD

Key Points

A history of trauma or upper respiratory infection occurs in a significant number of children with septic arthritis and may lead to misdiagnosis of this disorder.

Acute-phase reactants (erythrocyte sedimentation rate and C-reactive protein) are more likely to be elevated than a white blood cell count in septic arthritis and osteomyelitis.

Bone scans are helpful in detecting subtle evidence of osteomyelitis or multiple bone involvement. Magnetic resonance imaging is helpful in detecting subtle changes in osteomyelitis and is the preferred imaging modality for identifying infections of the spine.

Antimicrobial treatment strategies for bone and joint infections should consider community resistance patterns, which vary between geographic regions.

Selected Diagnoses

Acute hematogenous osteomyelitis
Other forms of osteomyelitis
Septic arthritis
Spine infections

Discussion of Individual Diagnoses

Acute Hematogenous Osteomyelitis

Osteomyelitis, or bone infection, is a rare condition in children. However, it is a disorder that must be recognized early and treated adequately in order to prevent chronic sequelae. In recent years, the emergence of community-acquired methicillin-resistant *Staphylococcus aureus* (CA-MRSA) has added another level of complexity to managing pediatric osteomyelitis. The most common form of osteomyelitis in children is acute hematogenous osteomyelitis, which occurs when bone (usually the metaphysis) is seeded with pathogens from the bloodstream.

Clinical Presentation

CA-MRSA osteomyelitis, the most common cause of bone infections in children, is characterized by increasing extremity pain often associated with systemic signs and symptoms of infection. Infection of the bone usually occurs following bacterial seeding from bacteremia related to a distant source. Infection often begins where sludging of blood flow occurs within the distal metaphysis. Other, less common variants of osteomyelitis include posttraumatic or postsurgical (via direct inoculation of bone) osteomyelitis, and chronic wound—or chronic ulcer—associated osteomyelitis.

Other diseases that may present similarly to acute hematogenous osteomyelitis include septic arthritis; toxic synovitis; skin and soft tissue infections; fractures and sprains; bone pain or infarct secondary to hemoglobinopathies; osteosarcoma and Ewing's sarcoma; and autoimmune processes such as juvenile rheumatoid arthritis, lupus, mixed connective tissue disease, and rheumatic fever. Often the diagnosis of acute hematogenous osteomyelitis cannot be made by clinical findings alone and requires ancillary studies (e.g., blood and tissue cultures), imaging, and pathology studies.

Multiple clinical, laboratory, and radiographic predictors of acute hematogenous osteomyelitis in children exist (Table 96–1).[1-3] Classically, this disease is associated with fever and point tenderness in the metaphyseal regions of long bones (most commonly the femur, tibia, or humerus, although any bone can become infected).[1,2] A history of recent trauma to the involved bone is obtained in more than a third of patients and may be explained by increased blood flow to the damaged area boosting the likelihood of bacterial seeding.[1,2] The majority of cases in children occur in those less than 10 years of age, with almost half of the cases in children less than 5. Males have twice the risk of developing osteomyelitis compared to females, perhaps secondary to increased trauma and associated skin scrapes and insect bites acting as portals of entry.[1-3] These factors may also explain why more episodes occur during warmer times of the year than during cooler seasons.

Specific underlying diseases entities increase the risk of an atypical pathogen-related osteomyelitis. Most notable is the association between hemoglobinopathies and *Salmonella* species. Additonal relationships exist between recent varicella infection and *Streptococcus pyogenes* (group A streptococci); intravenous drug abuse and *Pseudomonas aeruginosa*; vertebral/sacral involvement and *Brucella* species; and

Table 96–1	Features of Acute Hematogenous Osteomyelitis[1-5]
Findings	**% Present**
History of fever	40–92
History of extremity pain	84
History of recent trauma	35
Point tenderness	84
Adjacent arthritis	16–35
Chills	9
Malaise	12
ESR > 15–20 mm/hr	86–100 (mean 47–70 mm/hr)
CRP > 1 mg/dl	90–97
WBC > 15,000/mm³	32–33
Initial radiographic bony changes	19–21
Bone scan abnormal	94

Abbreviations: CRP, C-reactive protein; ESR, erythrocyte sedimentation rate; WBC, white blood cell count.

chronic granulomatous disease and *Mycobacterium tuberculosis, Aspergillus,* and *Serratia.*[6]

Most children with acute hematogenous osteomyelitis have a normal white blood cell count; however, the erythrocyte sedimentation rate (ESR) and C-reactive protein (CRP) are almost always elevated.[1-3,7] Blood cultures are positive in approximately a third of patients, while bone aspirate or open bone cultures are diagnostic in most cases.[1,3] Children with culture-negative acute hematogenous osteomyelitis tend to have delayed presentations, are older, and are less likely to report prior trauma or localizing soft tissue changes.[2] Pathologic examination of bone obtained by biopsy (needle aspiration or open) is particularly useful in confirming the diagnosis of osteomyelitis and providing information about the chronicity of the condition.

Plain films are usually normal in children with acute hematogenous osteomyelitis at the time they present for medical evaluation. Radiographic changes begin to appear 1 week after symptom onset since up to 50% demineralization of the affected bone must occur before changes are visualized.[8] Soft tissue swelling and periosteal elevation at the metaphyseal region of the affected extremity is usually the first radiographic finding on plain films (Fig. 96–1).[1,3] Magnetic resonance imaging (MRI) may detect bone marrow changes consistent with osteomyelitis early in the course of the illness, and has a high sensitivity and specificity as a diagnostic tool (Fig. 96–2). A bone scan is less sensitive and specific than MRI; however, it can prove helpful in cases in which the location of the infection is uncertain (i.e., toddler with a limp and fever), or if multiple bones appear to be involved (e.g., neonates).[8]

Management

A small percentage of children presenting with osteomyelitis will require rapid stabilization, generally secondary to associated bacteremia and sepsis. Specifically, antibiotics and fluid resuscitation should not be delayed in order to further evaluate the presence of a bone infection. In children who are not systemically ill, empirical antibiotics may be withheld for a minimal period of time while microbiologic and pathologic studies are obtained to maximize the chance of a specific etiologic diagnosis.

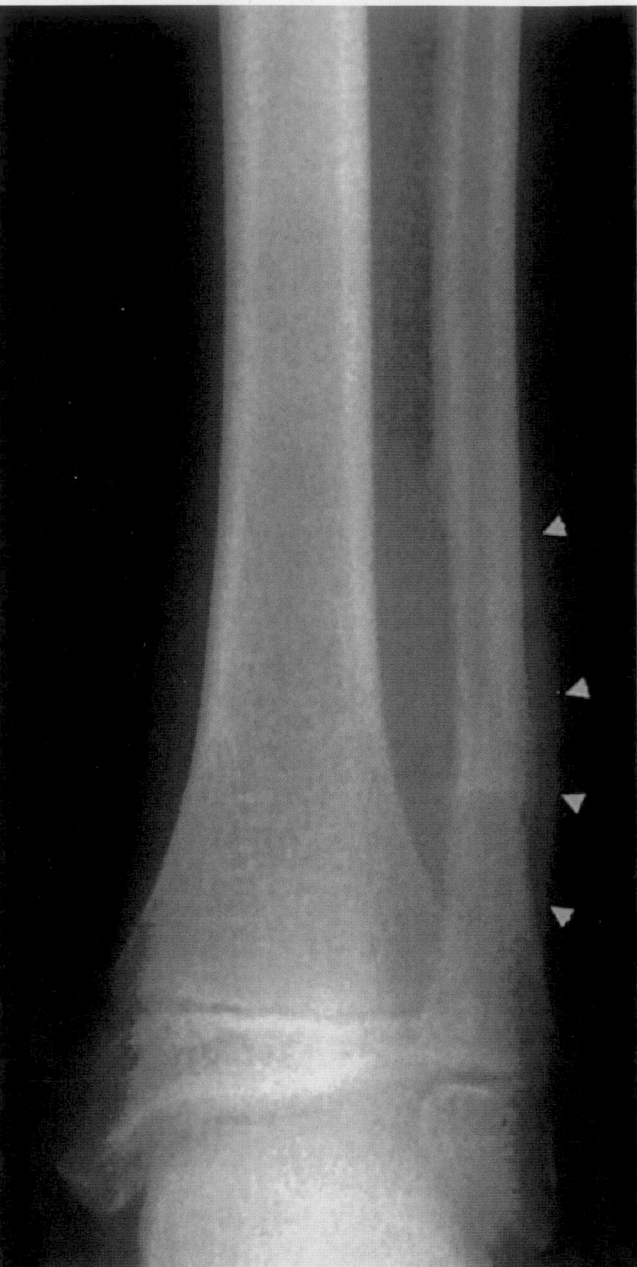

FIGURE 96–1. Osteomyelitis of the distal fibula in a 15-year-old male. Note the periosteal elevation (*arrowheads*), an early finding in osteomyelitis. (From Perron AD: Orthopedic pitfalls in the ED. Am J Emerg Med 21:61–67, 2003.)

The management of acute hematogenous osteomyelitis optimally involves medical and surgical therapy. Generally, empirical parenteral antimicrobial therapy should cover the most likely organisms involved. *Staphylococcus aureus* accounts for 70% to 90% of recovered organisms. Other less common pathogens include group A streptococci, coagulase-negative staphylococci, and gram-negative organisms such as *P. aeruginosa, Escherichia coli,* and *Salmonella* species, especially if specific risk factors exist. In younger children, *S. aureus* is less commonly recovered, although in all age groups it remains the most common pathogen.[1-3,6,7,9-11]

With the advent of CA-MRSA, it is important to know the local prevalence of this pathogen. In areas where CA-MRSA

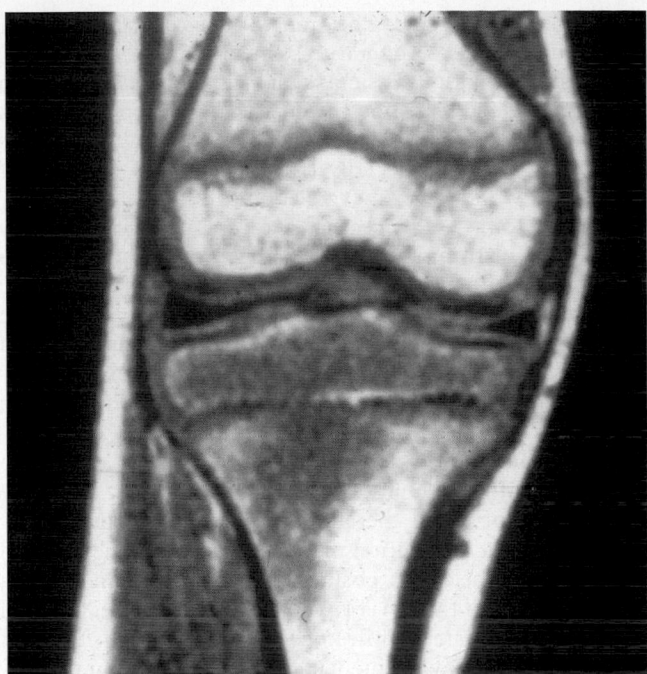

FIGURE 96–2. MRI of fifteen-year-old male with knee pain and acute osteomyelitis. Coronal T1 weighted image of the knee demonstrates low signal in the proximal epiphysis extending through the growth plate into the metaphysis of the tibia. (From Santiago Restrepo C, Gimenez CR, McCarthy K: Imaging of osteomyelitis and musculoskeletal soft tissue infections: current concepts. Rheum Dis Clin North Am 29:89–109, 2003.)

is common, empirical therapy for acute hematogenous osteomyelitis should include clindamycin, vancomycin, or linezolid.[13,17] If CA-MRSA is unlikely, clindamycin, nafcillin, or oxacillin has traditionally afforded excellent results for methicillin-susceptible *S. aureus* (MSSA). In septic-appearing children with suspected staphylococcal disease, published recommendations from the American Academy of Pediatrics include the use of empirical vancomycin plus nafcillin (or oxacillin) plus gentamicin.[14] Children with historical predictors associated with atypical organisms should receive broadened empirical therapy (i.e., additional gram-negative coverage) until antimicrobial sensitivities become available.

The need for surgical therapy for routine cases of acute hematogenous osteomyelitis is controversial. Most cases do not require an open drainage procedure.[4] However, the decision to operate is left to consulting orthopedic surgeons. From a diagnostic standpoint, an orthopedic procedure doubles the chance of recovering an organism either by simple needle aspiration of subperiostial pus, or by open biopsy and cultures of tissue.[1] Findings more likely to require surgical intervention include involvement of the adjacent joint, a subacute (≥2 weeks) to chronic presentation, atypical organisms, and the presence of an abscess within the bone marrow (Brodie's abscess).[15]

Occasionally, acute hematogenous osteomyelitis will occur in nontubular bones such as the calcaneus, pelvis, or vertebrae. In one series, the calcaneus was the third most common bone involved (13% of cases) and was not associated with puncture wounds in any patient, as had been reported in prior studies.[3] A recent review of pelvic osteomyelitis in 146

children reported that these children, compared to children with tubular bone involvement, were younger (2 to 5 vs. 8.1 years), had less prior trauma (17% vs. 35%), more commonly were males than females but to a lesser degree (1.5 : 1 vs. 2 : 1 male:female ratio), and had a more subacute or atypical presentation. This led to a delayed diagnosis in most cases (12 days vs. 5 to 7 days). This delay is likely due to the fact that these children are younger and have fewer "classic" signs and symptoms. Often, the pain of pelvic osteomyelitis will refer to the hip or thigh, leading to an incorrect initial diagnosis in up to 66% of cases. Of interest, the right side of the pelvis was twice as likely to be involved as the left, and the most common area involved was the ilium in nearly half of the cases. *Staphylococcus aureus* was recovered in 92% of cases with an etiology identified.[16] In a series of 14 children with vertebral osteomyelitis, unique features included prolonged symptoms prior to diagnosis (average 33 days), refusal to walk in young children, and localized back pain in older children. Although *S. aureus* was the most common etiologic agent, atypical organisms such as *Bartonella henselae* (cat-scratch disease), *Salmonella*, and *Propionibacterium* species were recovered more often than expected (4 of 10 cases with known etiology). MRI was found to be helpful in making the diagnosis, as only half of the cases had abnormal radiographs on presentation.[17]

The initial management of acute hematogenous osteomyelitis requires hospital admission with administration of parenteral antibiotics. Most patients require at least a week of antibiotics in the hospital while clinical and laboratory improvement is documented. Children are discharged once fever resolves, extremity pain improves, pus is drained, and inflammatory markers (ESR and CRP) approach normal. Children can be switched to suitable oral antibiotics once such improvement occurs, and complete a prolonged (typically 3 to 6 weeks) course at home with stringent follow up to detect recurrence of infection or complications of disease or therapy.[4,5]

Complications or sequelae of acute hematogenous osteomyelitis (e.g., growth delay, arthritis, recurrence of infection) occur in fewer than 10% of affected children. While the goal of aggressive therapy is to prevent all of these problems, complications still occur with appropriate therapy.[1-3,16,18,19]

Other Forms of Osteomyelitis in Children

The two most common traumatic mechanisms associated with osteomyelitis in children are plantar puncture wounds and open fractures, especially of the tibia. A disproportionately high percentage of plantar puncture wound osteomyelitis is due to *P. aeruginosa* (especially if puncture occurs through a rubber-soled shoe), while staphylococcal, streptococcal, and mixed infections are not unusual.[20-22] Plain films of the foot are abnormal in more than half of cases, but when no changes are noted, MRI can prove diagnostic accuracy.[22,23] Surgical débridement is usually required, and empirical antibiotics should cover the wide range of possible pathogens (i.e., vancomycin *or* clindamycin *plus* ceftazidime *or* cefipime *or* ticarcillin *or* piperacillin).[24] Children with open fractures of the lower leg develop osteomyelitis in up to 3% of cases.[25-27] It may take a week to several months postinjury for these patients to present for care. The likelihood of polymicrobial infection (including skin flora, soil organisms, and anaerobes) in these contaminated wounds is high, and they require extensive débridement and broad-spectrum empirical antibiotics.[28,29]

Children rarely develop diabetes-related ulcers, but may develop pressure sores that predispose them to this form of osteomyelitis. Children with cerebral palsy, spina bifida, and neurodegenerative disorders are especially vulnerable. Pressure sores tend to be superficial to the greater trochanter, sacrum, ischium, and calcaneus. Lack of improvement with local therapy is associated with a prolonged duration of healing, deep sores (especially if bone is exposed), and abnormal plain radiography. Bacteria colonizing or infecting soft tissue may not be responsible for the underlying bone infection. Most cases of confirmed osteomyelitis due to soft tissue infection grow more than one species of bacteria from bone biopsy cultures. Typically, cultures grow gram-negative (including *P. aeruginosa*) and gram-positive aerobes combined with anaerobes. Bone scans, although sensitive, are nonspecific in this population, as many patients have false-positive scans due to pathologic bone. The best method for confirming the diagnosis is bone biopsy for culture (anaerobic and aerobic) and pathology. Empirical antibiotic selection should be broad, and can be withheld in non–toxic-appearing patients until deep cultures and débridement have been obtained.[30]

Septic Arthritis

The terms *septic arthritis, infectious arthritis,* and *pyogenic arthritis* are often used interchangeably. They refer to microbial invasion and subsequent inflammation of the joint space. Early recognition is essential as a delay in diagnosis can lead to cartilaginous destruction. Septic arthritis is a medical and surgical emergency requiring prompt action.

Septic arthritis is primarily a disease of children[31,32] and occurs most frequently in children less than 2 years old.[33-35] It appears to be more common in males.[35-38] Several mechanisms have been proposed to explain how organisms enter into the joint. The most common mechanism is hematogenous spread.[39] Other mechanisms include local spread from a contiguous osteomyelitis or cellulitis rupturing into the joint; direct inoculation from trauma, such as from a penetrating wound; and infection acquired as a complication of a surgical procedure, such as an intra-articular steroid infection.[36,38,39] Over 90% of cases are monoarticular.[33,37,38] Most involve the lower extremity, with the knee and hip being the most common sites.[31-34,37]

Clinical Presentation

Pain is the most common and earliest symptom of septic arthritis.[31,33,35,40] In contrast to adults, children may not be able to verbalize or localize their pain. They may present with nonspecific clues of discomfort such as limp, inability to ambulate, or simply not using the affected extremity. Children often have referred pain. For example, children with a septic hip may present with thigh or knee pain. Infants with pain due to a septic arthritis may present with even more nonspecific findings such as poor feeding, irritability, or pseudoparalysis of the affected extremity.

Most patients with septic arthritis have systemic symptoms such as fever, malaise, or poor appetite within the first few days of infection. Children with septic arthritis are more likely to demonstrate a history of fever (>38.5° C)[41] during the week before the initial evaluation than those with transient synovitis. Children with septic arthritis have significantly higher temperatures (mean 37.7° C to 38.7° C) than children with transient synovitis (mean 36.6° C to 37.4° C).[42-44] However, one third of the children have peak temperatures less than 38.3° C.[33,38] Thus fever may not always be present. This is especially true in neonates with septic arthritis, in whom fever may be absent in most cases.[45,46]

There is some evidence that a recent upper respiratory infection[33,37] or traumatic injury[37] may predispose a child to septic arthritis. A history of immune deficiency or systemic disease may also predispose children to developing septic arthritis. Recent antibiotic use may make the diagnosis of septic arthritis a more difficult task. In one series, approximately one third of the patients had received an antibiotic in the week prior to admission.[33]

The infected joint is usually swollen, warm, and tender to palpation. Both active and passive motion of the joint are extremely painful and therefore limited.[31] An effusion may be present. Joint dislocation may be observed.[36] The affected joint is usually held in a position that allows for maximum joint distention. If the hip is involved, the leg may be abducted and externally rotated, while knee involvement leads to slight flexion, and ankle involvement manifests with plantar flexion. There is a wide range of possible presentations, from the child with septic arthritis who presents moribund in septic shock, to the well-appearing child with a limp who is afebrile.

As there is no single diagnostic test that can diagnose septic arthritis, clinical evaluation in combination with test results can help guide management. The peripheral leukocyte count may be elevated in septic arthritis (mean 13,200/mm^3 vs. mean 11,200/mm^3 in transient synovitis),[37,43] thereby providing a means to differentiate septic arthritis from transient synovitis of the hip.[42-44] Other studies have described a white blood cell count of greater than 11,000/mm^3 to 12,000/mm^3 to be an independent predictor of acute septic arthritis.[43,44] However, the peripheral leukocyte counts are not reliable indicators. In one series,[46] only 23% of patients had a leukocyte count greater than 15,000/mm^3. Similarly, another described only one third of the septic arthritis cohort with leukocytosis.[7]

The ESR is a nonspecific marker of inflammation or infection that has been used to aid in the diagnosis of septic arthritis and in monitoring response to treatment. The ESR is elevated (>20 mm/hr) in 85% to 90% of children with septic arthritis at the time of admission.[33,38,47] It has also been recommended as a tool in combination with other factors to differentiate septic arthritis of the hip from toxic synovitis,[42-44] and is a more sensitive indicator of septic arthritis of the hip than temperature or leukocyte count.[46] It does not appear to correlate with the duration, severity, or final outcome of the disease. Furthermore, the ESR does not rise until 24 to 48 hours after the onset of symptoms or signs of infection and stays elevated 3 to 4 weeks after resolution of the infection.[48,49]

CRP, another acute-phase reactant, has gained favor because it is a rapid indicator of inflammation, rising within 6 hours of the triggering stimulus.[40,50] Therefore, it has been recommended as a more accurate independent predictor of septic arthritis than the ESR.[51] In one study, only 13% of children with suspected joint infection and a CRP of less than 1.0 mg/dl had septic arthritis.[51] It has also been recommended as an adjunct screening test with the ESR in septic arthritis because it increases and decreases much more quickly than the ESR.[52] It may also be useful in detecting potential complications sooner than other laboratory indices (e.g., ESR).[52] In this regard, it has been shown to be useful in the identification of concurrent septic arthritis in children who have acute osteomyelitis.[49] Lastly, it may be of greater value than the ESR in determining resolution of inflammation.[40,49,50]

Although many studies have attempted to incorporate several of these combined variables into predication models that distinguish septic arthritis of the hip from transient or toxic synovitis,[41-44,51,53] (Table 96–2) most clinical prediction models have failed to demonstrate sufficient validity outside of the originating institution.[53]

Septic arthritis must be differentiated from other causes of limb pain in children, including fractures, sprain, strains, neoplasms (metastatic disease, Ewing's and osteogenic sarcoma), ischemia or infarction from hemoglobinopathies, slipped capital femoral epiphysis, Legg-Calvé-Perthes disease, transient synovitis, cellulitis, myositis, bursitis, and osteomyelitis. In general, these disorders do not cause the same degree of joint pain, joint swelling, and limited joint range of motion compared to septic arthritis. It also must be distinguished from other causes of arthritis, including reactive arthritis, rheumatic fever, juvenile rheumatoid arthritis, Lyme disease, serum sickness, lupus erythematosus, Henoch-Schönlein purpura, parvovirus, mumps, rubella, hepatitis B, and fungal causes. The presence of specific diagnostic features and arthrocentesis are required to differentiate these disorders from septic arthritis.

Blood cultures should be obtained on all patients with possible septic arthritis. They are positive in 30% to 40% of patients.[33,34,38,54] Although the yield may be relatively low, the ease of obtaining the culture can be instrumental in isolating an etiologic organism and enabling the most effective treatment. Furthermore, in as many as 20% of cases of septic arthritis, there is a positive blood culture in the presence of a negative synovial fluid culture.[33-35]

The most important diagnostic test is direct aspiration of the joint and subsequent fluid analysis. Others have provided extensive detail regarding the techniques for aspiration of specific joints for diagnostic purposes (Table 96–3).[54a] Gram stain should always be performed and will yield a presumptive diagnosis in about one third of patients.[34] A joint fluid leukocyte count greater than 80,000 to 100,000/ml with greater than 70% to 75% polymorphonuclear neutrophils is consistent with a septic joint. However, one study of 126 cases with a known bacterial etiology[34] demonstrated that 55% had joint cell counts $\leq$ 50,000 cells/mm^3 and 34% had counts $\leq$ 25,000 cells/mm^3. A low glucose (less than one third of serum value) is also consistent with a septic joint, yet in that same study of 126 children with proven bacterial septic arthritis, glucose levels were above 40 mg/dl in 44 specimens and reduced in only 41 specimens.[34] The confirmatory study is a positive synovial fluid culture, present in 50% to 70% of patients.[33-36,54] A significant number of children with septic arthritis have persistently negative cultures even without receiving antibiotics prior to diagnosis. Culture-negative cases have been shown to have clinical and synovial similarities to those with positive cultures. Therefore, the same aggressive therapy is recommended in those cases with or without identification of a causative organism.[55]

In septic arthritis, plain radiography may show joint space widening, disruption of the normal fat planes (which may

Table 96–2	Predictors of Septic Arthritis of the Hip in Children				
		Operator Characteristics of Predictors			
Author	**Predictors**	**Sensitivity***	**Specificity†**	**PPV**	**NPV**
Del Beccaro et al[43]	ESR > 20 mm/hr Temperature > 37.5° C	97%	86%	46%	2%
	ESR > 30 mm/hr	71%	86%	68%	12%
Jung et al[42]	Temperature > 37° C ESR > 20 mm/hr CRP > 1.0 mg/dl WBC > 11,000 cells/mm^3 Joint space distance > 2 mm on radiograph	NR	NR	99.1%	0.1%
Kocher et al[44]	History of fever Non–weight bearing ESR > 40 mm/hr WBC > 12,000 cells/mm^3	NR	NR	99.8%	0.1%
Kunnamo et al[41]	CRP > 2 mg/dl Temperature >38.5° C	100%	87%	46%	100%
Levine et al[54]	CRP $\geq$ 1.0 mg/dl	90%	29%	34%	87%
	ESR $\geq$ 25 mm/hr	92%	22%	35%	86%
Luhmann et al[53]	History of fever Non–weight bearing ESR > 40 mm/hr WBC > 12,000 cells/mm^3	NR	NR	59%	NR

*Sensitivity if any one of the listed features was present.
†Specificity if any one of the listed features was present.
Abbreviations: CRP, C-reactive protein; ESR, erythrocyte sedimentation rate; NPV, negative predictive value, or probability of disease if none of features is present; NR, not reported; PPV, positive predictive value, or probability of disease if all features are present; WBC, white blood cell count.

Table 96-3	Analysis of Joint Fluid			
	Noninflammatory	**Inflammatory**	**Septic**	**Hemorrhagic**
Clarity	Clear	Cloudy	Purulent/turbid	Bloody
Color	Yellow	Yellow	Yellow	Red/brown
WBC count/ml	<200–2000	200–100,000	>50,000	<200[†]
PMNs (%)	<25%	>75%	>75%	<25%
Glucose*	95–100%	80–100%	<50%	100%
Culture	Negative	Negative	Positive in > 50%	Negative
Disease	Arthritis, trauma, rheumatic fever, osteochondritis	Spondyloarthropathy, Lyme disease, Reiter's syndrome, Kawasaki disease, tuberculosis, fungal or viral infection, rheumatoid arthritis, crystals (gout, pseudogout)	Septic arthritis	Trauma, bleeding diathesis, neoplasm

*(Joint glucose/serum glucose) × 100%.
[†]Pure blood, joint fluid WBC count = serum WBC count.
Abbreviations: PMNs, polymorphonuclear leukocytes; WBC, white blood cell.

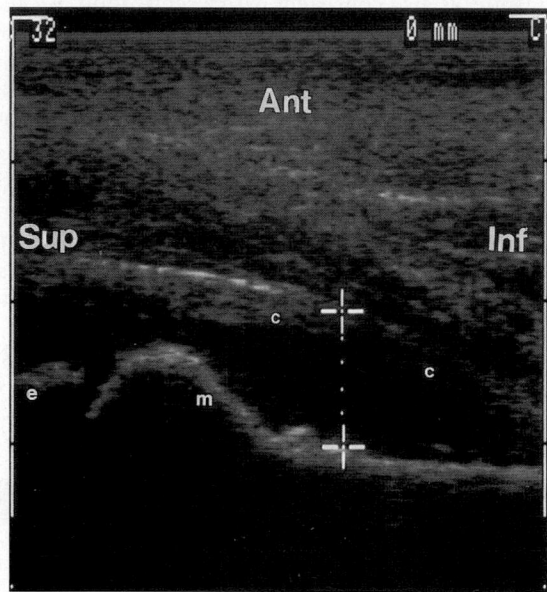

FIGURE 96–3. An effusion is diagnosed on ultrasound (US) when the joint capsule bows anteriorly or distends 3 mm or more with fluid, or when the distention of the capsule is 2 mm more than the contralateral asymptomatic side. This US shows joint effusion within the hip of an infant found to have septic arthritis. (From Bellah R: Ultrasound in pediatric musculoskeletal disease: techniques and applications. Radiol Clin North Am 39:597–618, 2001.)

require contralateral films for comparison), or soft tissue swelling. Neonates with septic arthritis of the hip have a higher incidence of subluxation with hip infection, and therefore should have plain films obtained as part of their diagnostic workup.[56] Another role for plain films in the pediatric population is to rule out other causes of pain such as fractures, slipped capital femoral epiphyses, or avascular necrosis of the femoral head.

Ultrasound may be useful in detecting early fluid collections and can provide guidance for aspiration of an effusion (Fig. 96-3). However, ultrasound cannot differentiate infectious from noninfectious effusions and cannot reliably detect osteomyelitis.[57] Bone scans and computed tomography (CT) scans are less sensitive for identifying joint effusions but may demonstrate areas of adjacent osteomyelitis.[58] MRI is highly

sensitive in detecting even a small joint effusion[58] and is superior to CT for delineating soft tissue structures that can aid in diagnosing adjacent osteomyelitis. No radiographic study should delay definitive care of a patient with septic arthritis. Only those studies that are absolutely necessary to establish a diagnosis and can be obtained expeditiously should be performed. Antibiotics should never be withheld because of delays in obtaining imaging studies.

Management

The management of infants and children with septic arthritis begins with establishing the diagnosis as quickly as possible. Aspiration of synovial fluid should be performed promptly once a septic joint is suspected. This is especially important in the hip, where the blood supply to the epiphyseal plate and femoral head may be compromised.[34] Depending on the level of suspicion, intravenous antibiotics should be administered. Gram stain may guide the antibiotic choice; otherwise, empirical antibiotic choice should be based on the pathogens common to the patient's age group and the known antibiotic resistance patterns in the demographic area. Since the introduction of *Haemophilus influenzae* type B immunization, *S. aureus* has become the predominant isolate in young children with septic arthritis.[59] *Kingella kingae* has also become especially common in children below the age of 4 years.[60] A reasonable empirical approach would include a third-generation cephalosporin and coverage for *S. aureus* (e.g., vancomycin). Patients with acute septic arthritis should be admitted to the hospital.

Established indications for surgical drainage in children with septic arthritis include (1) involvement of the hip joint; (2) presence of large amounts of pus, fibrin, or loculation within the joint space; and (3) lack of clinical improvement noted within 3 days of appropriate therapy.[36]

Delay in diagnosis and treatment is the single most important factor affecting prognosis of septic arthritis in children.[47]

Spine Infections

Diskitis

Although children have a fairly high incidence of back pain, they seldom seek medical attention for minor symptoms. Thus the incidence of organic causes in children who seek medical attention is high.[61] Several mechanisms are postulated to cause diskitis and other spinal infections: direct inoculation after accidental trauma or surgical procedures, contiguous spread from an adjacent infection, or hematogenous spread of pathogens (presumed to be the most common cause). The relative avascularity of the intervertebral disks facilitate the growth of bacteria.

CLINICAL PRESENTATION

The clinical presentation of diskitis is variable, owing to the child's developmental level and ability to localize symptoms, and the variable nature of growth of the child and the spine.[62,63] A concurrent or recent illness, or a history of trauma that may be unrelated to the anatomic location of the disease, may be described.[63] Symptom duration may be from days to weeks, but a median duration of 14 days has been described.[64] The chief complaint is influenced by the child's level of development: one study described 67% of children 3 years and older as presenting with back pain, whereas 78% of children less than 3 years old had gait-related presenting symptoms (difficulty walking/refusal to walk or bear weight, limp, or unsteady gait).[63]

Acute toxicity is rarely described in children with diskitis.[60,61] Fewer than 26% to 28% of children may present with a temperature of greater than 100.3° F.[63,65] Any loss of normal and fluid spinal motion with walking or playing, or a history of abnormal gait, should alert the examining physician to conduct a more thorough spinal examination.[60,63] Approximately 78% to 83% of children with diskitis have involvement of the lumbar or lumbosacral area.[63,65] Infants and children may have generalized back, buttock, or leg pain from nerve root irritation.[62] Neurologic findings (e.g., decreased muscle tone, muscle weakness, decreased tendon reflexes) are dependent on the degree of inflammation and infection that extends from the intervertebral disk. Consequently, neurologic impairment should not exclude a diagnosis of diskitis, but should alert the clinician to the need for imaging studies to exclude intraspinal involvement.[64]

The mean white blood cell count at admission in one of the larger cohorts of children was 10,900/mm³ with a range of 7500 to 25,400.[63] In one study, only 10% of children with diskitis had an elevated white blood cell count and only 5% had a mild left shift.[64] In this same study, 94% had an elevated ESR.[63] Unfortunately, these indicators are nonspecific. CRP has been suggested to test for early infection, but its predictive value for diskitis in children has not been described.

Blood cultures seldom yield pathogens[63] and may confound the picture if contaminants are responsible for positive blood cultures, but continue to be recommended by many authors. *Kingella kingae* is one organism that has been increasingly isolated on blood culture.[64] In most studies, disk aspiration seldom yields positive cultures, but when positive, *S. aureus* and *K. kingae* are most commonly isolated.[66-68] Biopsy should be reserved for intravenous antibiotic treatment failures and not for routine diagnosis.[62]

Radiographs may be abnormal in 76% to 82% of children with diskitis.[62,69] Four phases of radiologic findings have been described for diskitis[70]:

1. Normal radiograph shortly after onset of symptoms (latent phase)
2. Narrowed isolated intervertebral disk space, decreased vertebral height, and demineralized adjacent vertebral margins 2 to 4 weeks later in the acute phase (Fig. 96–4)
3. Distinct vertebral margins from remineralization 2 to 3 months after onset in the healing phase
4. Flat vertebral bodies with narrow involved disk space and marginal irregularities (with variable reconstitution of the disk) in the late phase and long-term follow-up.

In general, the most commonly described plain radiographic finding among children with diskitis is decreased height of the disk space and erosion of adjacent vertebral end plates[63] (see Fig. 96–4). Technetium-99m–labeled bone scan can confirm a diagnosis where clinical suspicion persists despite negative plain radiograph. Technetium scanning abnormalities usually preceed changes on plain radiographs, with abnormalities occurring as early as 3 to 5 days after the onset of symptoms[62,63] (see Fig. 96–4). However, bone scans may be more useful in the patient with poorly localized findings (i.e., younger patients). In contrast, MRI is more sensitive than nuclear studies or CT scan and can help differentiate diskitis from vertebral osteomyelitis or paraspinal or epidural abscesses.[62] MRI can define vertebral osseous involvement and inflammatory lesions in adjacent structures, making it

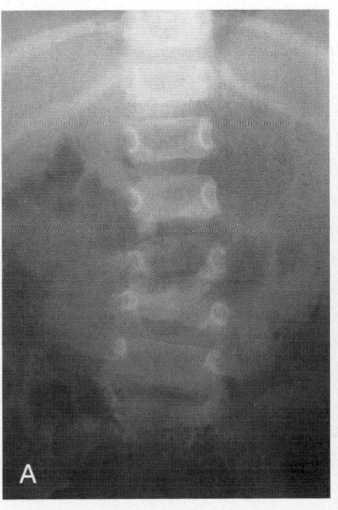
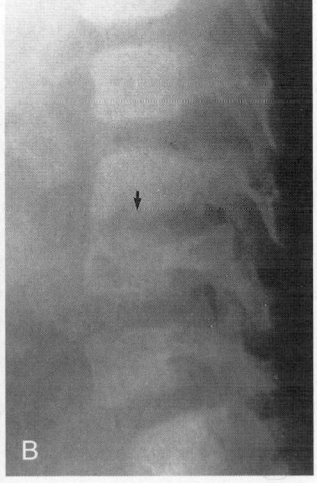
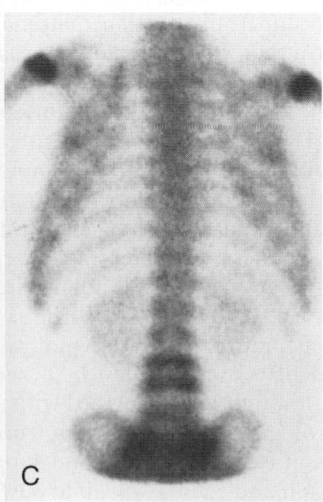

FIGURE 96–4. Diskitis in a 9-month-old girl with a history of refusing to sit up and bear weight, mild fever, and increased sedimentation rate for 2 weeks. Frontal **(A)** and lateral **(B)** radiographs of the lumbar spine show narrowing of the L3-4 intervertebral disk space with irregularity of the adjacent vertebral end plate *(arrow)*. **C,** Radioisotope bone scan shows increased activity at L3 and L4 levels. (From Mahboubi S, Morris MC: Imaging of spinal infections in children. Radiol Clin North Am 39:215–222, 2001.)

the study of choice for diskitis among children with negative plain radiographs.[71]

MANAGEMENT

Management goals are directed at the presumption that the disease is infectious despite the lack of comprehensive controlled trials to guide therapy. Prior retrospective studies have concluded that treatment with antibiotic therapy is more likely to result in symptom relief without recurrence of disease, regardless of the use of immobilization.[65] Empirical therapy should be directed against *S. aureus* (the most commonly described causative agent), with a recommended duration of intravenous antibiotics of 1 to 8 weeks, while oral antibiotics may be continued for as long as 3 to 6 months.[62,66,72,73] The duration of therapy is uncertain; therefore, some experts base treatment duration on changes of CRP and ESR levels. Relative rest and immobilization with an orthotic device may help reduce pain.[62]

Inpatient observation is indicated to initiate intravenous antimicrobial therapy and to help coordinate care. Transfer to a tertiary pediatric center from institutions with limited access to pediatric subspecialty services is warranted for nonemergent consultation with pediatric infectious disease and pediatric orthopedics. Surgical intervention is rarely necessary, but should be considered if clinical improvement does not occur in a patient with a documented abscess who is systemically ill or has neurologic deficits.[62,66,74]

Spinal Epidural Abscess

A spinal epidural abscess (SEA) is a collection of pus in the epidural space; it may arise secondary to pyogenic infection of the spine (described as a secondary epidural abscess), or as an entity independent of spondylodiskitis (described as a primary epidural abscess).[75] The incidence has been described as less than 0.2 to 1.2 per 10,000 hospital admissions.[76] SEA occurs more frequently in adults than in children; one review of spinal epidural abscesses in children described fewer than 90 cases reported in the literature from 1945 to 1994.[77]

CLINICAL PRESENTATION

The history may reveal a distant focus of infection in 25% of cases, including skin infections, urinary tract infections, pneumonia, or pharyngitis.[77,78] A history of back trauma may precede SEA in 17% of patients. SEA is speculated to occur from a small hematoma that may have developed from trauma in the epidural space and created a focus for bacteria.[77]

The clinical presentation has been described in four phases: (1) back pain and fever result from a growing spinal epidural abscess; (2) neurologic symptoms that may include root pain that mimics sciatic/hip pain, extremity pain or acute abdomen, and changes in reflexes that can precede motor weakness; (3) increasing muscle weakness and bowel/bladder symptoms; and (4) total paralysis.[77,79-82] These phases may vary and develop in as little as a few hours.[77,81] In the presence of epidural abscess or epidural granulation tissue, neurologic deficits may manifest in 37% of adults (primarily paralysis), although 18% recovered with surgery.[75] The concern for neurologic morbidity comes from direct pressure on the cord and ischemia from blood supply compromise by inflammation and edema.[77,83] Up to 80% of children have some neuro-

logic compromise prior to surgical intervention.[77] In the adult population, the most common site for secondary epidural abscess is the lumbar spine (39%); however, the rate of epidural abscess complicating spondylodiskitis is increased when more cephalad regions of the spine are involved (e.g., 90% of cervical spine epidural abscesses have a preceding spondylodiskitis).[75]

Laboratory evaluation is most significant for elevated white blood cell count and ESR (sensitivity of 90% and 100%, respectively).[75] *Staphylococcus aureus* (with methicillin resistance becoming increasingly important) has been described as the most common pathogen (79% to 86%). Other pathogens include *Streptococcus viridans, Streptococcus pneumoniae, Salmonella enteritidis, Pseudomonas,* and *E. coli.*[76,77,84] Patients may have normal lumbar punctures (10%) or may manifest purulent cerebrospinal fluid (52%), mild leukocytosis or low glucose levels (26%), and increased protein (12% to 53%).[76,85] If frank pus is aspirated during lumbar puncture, the abscess is usually dorsal to the cord.[77]

Plain radiographs are usually negative (unless osteomyelitis is present). Thus, MRI is the imaging modality of choice.[77,82] MRI of the entire spine should be obtained when there is suspicion of a SEA, as multiple abscesses may be present.[77,80,86]

MANAGEMENT

Disease lasting for more than 2 weeks may be self-contained and result in epidural granulation tissue rather than frank purulent abscess.[77,87] The mortality rate in children has been reported at 12%, and 41% of children will manifest neurologic deficits at follow-up.[77] Although treatment with antibiotic therapy alone is often successful in adults, evidence of success with this approach in children is lacking. Given the absence of evidence for a definitive approach, most authors recommend surgical drainage (typically by laminectomy) and antibiotic therapy, while cases without neurologic deficits may be considered for management with antibiotics alone.[76,77,82,85]

Immediate stabilization efforts are directed to the patient's individual presentation. An extensive physical examination looking for an infectious source with a thorough neurologic evaluation should be performed. While laboratory tests are often suggestive (e.g., elevated ESR and CRP), MRI is performed to confirm the diagnosis. If MRI is unavailable, contrast CT can reveal adjacent bone destruction and fluid collections. Inpatient management for antibiotic therapy and surgical consultation and intervention is required. Transfer to a tertiary care facility should be considered if pediatric orthopedic, pediatric neurology, and pediatric neurosurgery consultants are unavailable.

Summary

Young children with bone and joint infections often present with irritability, pain, and fever. Tenderness to palpation of the extremity in the absence of a skin lesion may suggest osteomyelitis, whereas refusal to use the extremity or complaint of joint pain may suggest a septic arthritis. Back pain (especially lumbosacral pain) with refusal to walk, with or without localized back tenderness, may indicate diskitis, vertebral osteomyelitis, or spinal epidural abscess. Radiographs may aid in the diagnosis of most bone and joint infections

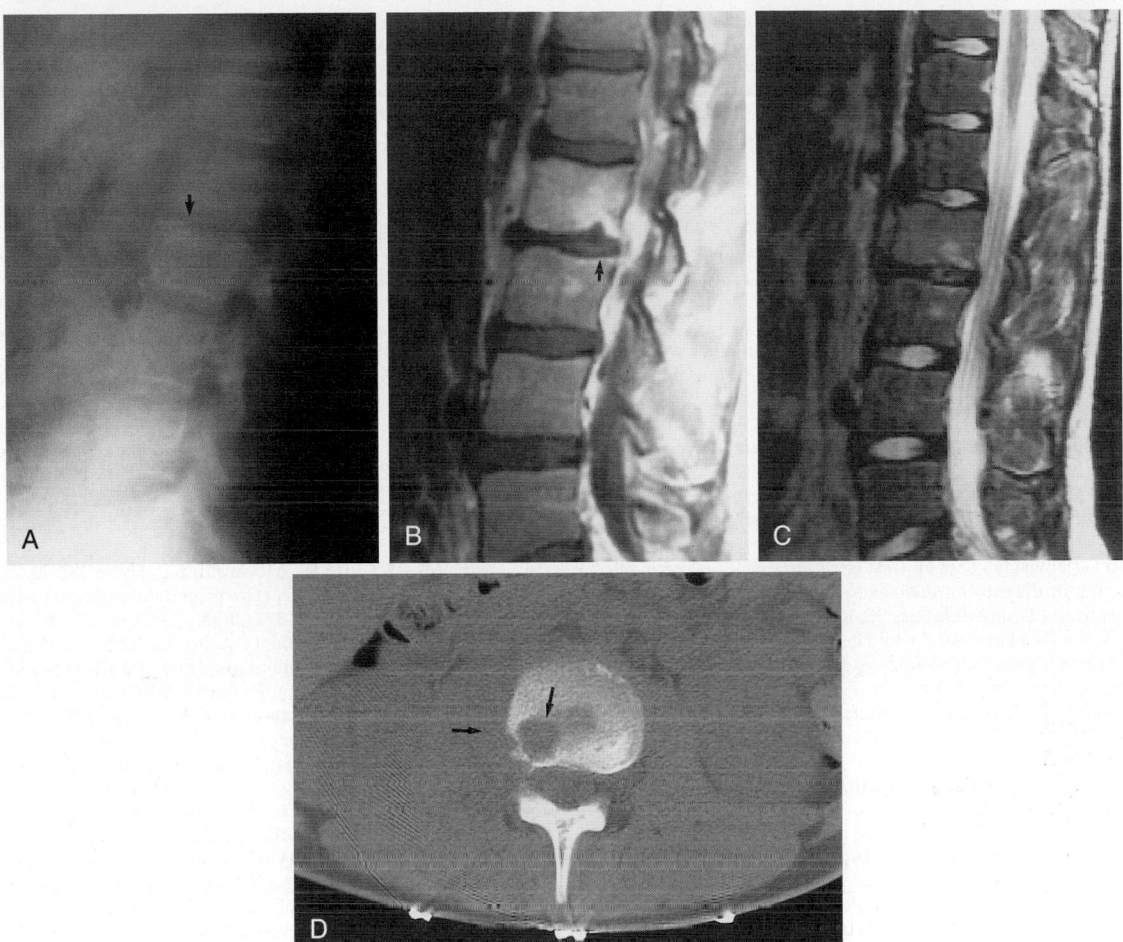

FIGURE 96–5. Spinal staphylococcus osteomyelitis in a 15-year-old boy. **A,** The lateral radiograph of the spine shows loss of a distinct cortical margin of the adjacent L2 and L3 end plates *(arrow)*. **B,** Sagittal T1-weighted image (TR 566, TE 16) after intravenous administration of gadolinium diethylene-triamine pentaacetic acid (DTPA) shows enhancement of the affected vertebrae at L2-3 with loss of disk height *(arrow)*. **C,** Sagittal T2-weighted image (TR 4000, TE 102) shows focal area of increased signal in the inferior part of the body of L2 and decreased signal within the intervertebral disk at L2-3. **D,** Prone axial CT scan before biopsy of L2 shows lytic lesion with destruction of the overlying cortex in the vertebral body and right paraspinal soft tissue mass *(arrows)*. (From Mahboubi S, Morris MC: Imaging of spinal infections in children. Radiol Clin North Am 39:215–222, 2001.)

and help to rule out fractures. Bone scans may be helpful to detect early osteomyelitis and spinal infections (in young children without localizing signs). MRI is the test of choice for subtle osteomyelitis or spinal infections (to describe the extent of involvement) (Fig. 96–5). *Staphylococcus aureus* (including methicillin-resistant forms) has emerged as one of the most common pathogens in bone and joint infections in children.

REFERENCES

1. Dich QV, Nelson JD, Haltalin KC: Osteomyelitis in infants and children. Infect Dis J 129:1273–1278, 1975.
2. Floyed RL, Steele RW: Culture-negative osteomyelitis. Pediatr Infect Dis J 22:731–736, 2003.
3. Karwowska A, Davies DH, Jadavji T: Epidemiology and outcome of osteomyelitis in the era of sequential intravenous-oral therapy. Pediatr Infect Dis J 17:1021–1026, 1998.
4. Peltola H, Unkila-Kallio L, Kallio MJT: Simplified treatment of acute staphylococcal osteomyelitis of childhood. Pediatrics 99:846–850, 1997.
5. Roine I, Faingezicht I, Arguedas A, et al: Serial serum C-reactive protein to monitor recovery from acute hematogenous osteomyelitis in children. Pediatr Infect Dis J 14:40–44, 1995.
6. Krogstad P: Osteomyelitis and septic arthritis. *In* Feigin RD, Cherry J, Demmter G, et al (eds): Textbook of Pediatric Infectious Diseases, 5th ed. Philadelphia: WB Saunders, 2004, pp 713–729.
7. Unkila-Kallio L, Kallio MJ, Eskola J, Peltola H: CRP, ESR and WBC count in acute hematogenous osteomyelitis of children. Pediatrics 93:59–62, 1994.
8. Kothari NA, Pelchovitz DJ, Meyer JS: Imaging of musculoskeletal infections. Radiol Clin North Am 39:653–671, 2001.
9. Ibia EO, Imoisili M, Pikis A: Group A beta-hemolytic streptococcal osteomyelitis in children. Pediatrics 112(1 Pt 1):e22–e26, 2003.
10. Asmar BI: Osteomyelitis in the neonate. Infect Dis Clin North Am 6:117–132, 1992.
11. Baevsky RH: Neonatal group B beta-hemolytic streptococcus osteomyelitis. Am J Emerg Med 17:619–622, 1999.
12. Martinez-Aguilar G, Hammerman WA, Mason EO, Kaplan SL: Clindamycin treatment of invasive infections caused by community-acquired, methicillin-resistant and methicillin-susceptible *Staphylococcus aureus* in children. Pediatr Infect Dis J 22:593–598, 2003.
13. Kaplan SL, Afghani B, Lopez P, et al: Linezolid for the treatment of methicillin-resistant *Staphylococcus aureus* infections in children. Pediatr Infect Dis J 22:S178–S185, 2003.
14. Committee on Infectious Diseases: Staphylococcal infection. *In* Pickering LK (ed): 2003 Red Book: Report of the Committee on Infectious Diseases, 26th ed. Elk Grove Village, IL: American Academy of Pediatrics, 2003, pp 561–573.

15. Lindenbaum S, Alexander H: Infections simulating bone tumors: a review of subacute osteomyelitis. Clin Orthop 184:193–203, 1984.
16. Zvulunov A, Gal N, Segev Z: Acute hematogenous osteomyelitis of the pelvis in childhood: diagnostic clues and pitfalls. Pediatr Emerg Care 19:29–31, 2003.
17. Fernandez M, Carrol CL, Baker CJ: Discitis and vertebral osteomyelitis in children: an 18 year review. Pediatrics 105:1299–1304, 2000.
18. Roine I, Arguedas A, Faingezicht I, Rodriguez F: Early detection of sequela-prone osteomyelitis in children with use of simple clinical and laboratory criteria. Clin Infect Dis 24:849–853, 1997.
19. Martinez-Aguilar G, Avalos-Mishaan A, Hulten K, et al: Community-acquired, methicillin-resistant and methicillin-susceptible *Staphylococcua aureus* musculoskeletal infections in children. Pediatr Infect Dis J 23:701–706, 2004.
20. Eidelman M, Bialik V, Miller Y, Kassis I: Plantar puncture wounds in children: analysis of 80 hospitalized patients and late sequelae. Isr Med Assoc J 5:268–271, 2003.
21. Laughlin TJ, Armstrong DG, Caporusso J, Lavery LA: Soft tissue and bone infections from puncture wounds in children. West J Med 166:126–128, 1997.
22. Puffenbarger WR, Gruel CR, Herndon WA, Sullivan JA: Osteomyelitis of the calcaneus in children. J Pediatr Orthop 16:224–230, 1996.
23. Lau LS, Bin G, Jaovisidua S, et al: Cost effectiveness of magnetic resonance imaging in diagnosing *Pseudomonas aeroginosa* infection after puncture wound. J Foot Ankle Surg 36:36–43, 1997.
24. Inaba AS, Zukin DD, Perro M: An update on the evaluation and management of plantar puncture wounds and *Pseudomonas* osteomyelitis. Pediatr Emerg Care 8:38–44, 1992.
25. Khatod M, Botte MJ, Hoyt DB, et al: Outcomes in open tibia fractures: relationship between delay in treatment and infection. J Trauma 55:949–954, 2003.
26. Jones BG, Duncan RD: Open tibial fractures in children under 13 years of age: 10 year experience. Injury 34:776–780, 2003.
27. Cramer KE, Limbird TJ, Green NE: Open fractures of the diaphysis of the lower extremity in children: treatment, results, and complications. J Bone Joint Surg Am 74:218–232, 1992.
28. Brook I: Aerobic and anaerobic microbiology of infections after trauma in children. J Accid Emerg Med 15:162–167, 1998.
29. Hall BB, Fitzgerald RH, Rosenblatt JE: Anaerobic osteomyelitis. J Bone Joint Surg Am 65:30–35, 1983.
30. Sugarman B, Hawes S, Musher DM, et al: Osteomyelitis beneath pressure sores. Arch Intern Med 143:683–688, 1983.
31. Griffin PP: Bone and joint infections in children. Pediatr Clin North Am 14:533–548, 1967.
32. Heberling JA: A review of two hundred and one cases of suppurative arthritis. Bone Joint Surgery 23:917–921, 1941.
33. Welkon CJ, Long SS, Fisher MC, Alburger PD: Pyogenic arthritis in infants and children: a review of 95 cases. Pediatr Infect Dis 5:669–676, 1986.
34. Fink CW, Nelson JD: Septic arthritis and osteomyelitis in children. Clin Rheum Dis 12:423–435, 1986.
35. Bonhoeffer J, Haeberle B, Schaad UB, Heininger U: Diagnosis of acute haematogenous osteomyelitis and septic arthritis: 20 years experience at the University Children's Hospital Basel. Swiss Med Wkly 131:575–581, 2001.
36. Shetty AK, Gedalia A: Septic arthritis in children. Rheum Dis Clin North Am 24:287–304, 1998.
37. Nelson JD, Koontz WC: Septic arthritis in infants and children: a review of 117 cases. Pediatrics 38:966–971, 1966.
38. Yagupsky P, Bar-Ziv Y, Howard CB, Dagan R: Epidemiology, etiology, and clinical features of septic arthritis in children younger than 24 months. Arch Pediatr Adolesc Med 149:537–540, 1995.
39. Goldenberg DL, Reed JI: Bacterial arthritis. N Engl J Med 312:764–771, 1985.
40. Morrissy RT: Bone and joint sepsis. *In* Morrissy RT, Weinstein SL (eds): Lovell & Winter's Pediatric Orthopaedics, 4th ed. Philadelphia: Lippincott–Raven, 1996, pp 579–624.
41. Kunnamo I, Kallio P, Pelkonen P, Hovi T: Clinical signs and laboratory tests in the differential diagnosis of arthritis in children. Am J Dis Child 141:34–40, 1987.
42. Jung ST, Rowe SM, Moon ES, et al: Significance of laboratory and radiologic findings for differentiating between septic arthritis and transient synovitis of the hip. J Pediatr Orthop 23:368–372, 2003.

43. Del Beccaro MA, Champoux AN, Bockers T, Mendelman PM: Septic arthritis versus transient synovitis of the hip: the value of screening laboratory tests. Ann Emerg Med 21:14–18, 1992.
44. Kocher MS, Zurakowski D, Kasser JR: Differentiating between septic arthritis and transient synovitis of the hip in children: an evidence-based clinical prediction algorithm. J Bone Joint Surg Am 81:1662–1670, 1999.
45. Frederiksen B, Christiansen P, Knudsen FU: Acute osteomyelitis and septic arthritis in the neonate: risk factors and outcome. Eur J Pediatr 152:577–580, 1993.
46. Klein DM, Barbera C, Gray ST, et al: Sensitivity of objective parameters in the diagnosis of pediatric septic hips. Clin Orthop Relat Res 338:153–159, 1997.
47. Morrey BF, Bianco AJ, Rhodes KH: Septic arthritis in children. Orthop Clin North Am 6:923–934, 1975.
48. Tetzlaff TR, McCracken GH, Nelson JD: Oral antibiotic therapy for skeletal infections of children. J Pediatr 3:485–490, 1978.
49. Unkila-Kallio L, Kallio MJT, Peltola H: The usefulness of C-reactive protein levels in the identification of concurrent septic arthritis in children who have acute hematogenous osteomyelitis. J Bone Joint Surg Am 76:848–853, 1994.
50. Pepys MB: C-reactive protein fifty years on. Lancet 1:653–656, 1981.
51. Levine MJ, McGuire KJ, McGowan KL, Flynn JM: Assessment of the test characteristics of C-reactive protein for septic arthritis in children. J Pediatr Orthop 23:373–377, 2003.
52. Kallio MJT, Unkila-Kallio L, Aalto K, Peltola H: Serum C-reactive protein, erythrocye sedimentation rate and white blood cell count in septic arthritis of children. Pediatr Infect Dis J 16:411–413, 1997.
53. Luhmann SJ, Jones A, Schootman M, et al: Differentiation between septic arthritis and transient synovitis of the hip in children with clinical prediction algorithms. J Bone Joint Surg Am Am 86:956–962, 2004.
54. Nelson JD: The bacterial etiology and antibiotic management of septic arthritis in infants and children. Pediatrics 50:437–440, 1972.
54a. Parillo SJ, Fisher J. Arthrocentesis. In Roberts JR, Hedges JR, Chanmugan AS, et al (eds): Clinical Procedures in Emergency Medicine, 4th ed. St. Louis: WB Saunders, 2004, pp 1042–1106.
55. Lyon RM, Evanich JD: Culture-negative septic arthritis in children. J Pediatr Orthop 19:655–659, 1999.
56. Volberg FM, Sumner TE, Abramson JS, Winchester PH: Unreliability of radiographic diagnosis of septic hip in children. Pediatrics 74:118–120, 1984.
57. Zawin JK, Hoffer FA, Rand FF, Teele RL: Joint effusion in children with an irritable hip: US diagnosis and aspiration. Radiology 187:459–463, 1993.
58. Kothari NA, Pelchovitz DJ, Meyer JS: Imaging of musculoskeletal infections. Radiol Clin North Am 39:653–671, 2001.
59. Luhmann JD, Luhmann SJ: Etiology of septic arthritis in children: an update for the 1990s. Pediatr Emergy Care 15:40–42, 1999.
60. Yagupsky P: *Kingella kingae*: from medical rarity to an emerging pediatric pathogen. Lancet 4:358–367, 2004.
61. King HA: Back pain in children. Orthop Clin North Am 30:467–474, 1999.
62. Early SD, Kay RM, Tolo VT: Childhood diskitis. J Am Acad Orthop Surg 11:413–420, 2003.
63. Fernandez M, Carrol CL, Baker CJ: Discitis and vertebral osteomyelitis in children: an 18-year review. Pediatrics 105:1299–1304, 2000.
64. Nussinovitch M, Sokolover N, Volovitz B, Amir J: Neurologic abnormalities in children presenting with discitis. Arch Pediatr Adolesc Med 156:1052–1054, 2002.
65. Ring D, Johnston CE, Wenger DR: Pyogenic infectious spondylitis in children: the convergence of discitis and vertebral osteomyelitis. J Pediatr Orthop 15:652–660, 1995.
66. Brown R, Hussain M, McHugh K, et al: Discitis in young children. J Bone Joint Surg Br 83:106–111, 2001.
67. Cushing AH: Diskitis in children. Clin Infect Dis 17:1–6, 1993.
68. Amir J, Shockelford PG: *Kingella kingae* intervertebral disk infection. J Clin Microbiol 29:1083–1086, 1991.
69. Crawford AH, Kucharzyk DW, Ruda R, Smitherman HC: Diskitis in children. Clin Orthop 266:70–79, 1991.
70. Mahboubi S, Morris MC: Imaging of spinal infections in children. Radiol Clin North Am 39:215–222, 2001.
71. Rothman SL: The diagnosis of infections of the spine by modern imaging techniques. Orthop Clin North Am 27:15–31, 1996.

72. Song KS, Ogden JA, Ganey T, Guidera TJ: Contiguous discitis and osteomyelitis in children. J Pediatr Orthop 17:470–477, 1997.

73. Glazer PA, Hu SS: Pediatric spinal infections. Orthop Clin North Am 27:111–123, 1996.

74. Garron E, Viehweger E, Launay F, et al: Nontuberculous spondylodiscitis in children. J Pediatr Orthop 22:321–328, 2002.

75. Hadjipavlou AG, Mader JT, Necessary JT, Muffoletto AJ: Hematogenous pyogenic spinal infections and their surgical management. Spine 25:1668–1679, 2000.

76. Rubin G, Shalom M, Ashenasi A, et al: Spinal epidural abscess in the pediatric age group: case report and review of the literature. Pediatr Infect Dis J 12:1007–1011, 1993.

77. Jacobsen FS, Sullivan B: Spinal epidural abscesses in children. Orthopedics 17:1131–1138, 1994.

78. Quanch C, Tapiero B, Noya F: Group A streptococcus spinal epidural abscess during varicella. Pediatrics 109:e14, 2002.

79. Heusner AP: Nontuberculous spinal epidural infections. N Engl J Med 239:845–854, 1948.

80. Gasul BM, Jaffe RH: Acute epidural spinal abscess—a clinical entity: report of three cases in children with a complete review of the literature. Arch Pediatr 52:361–390, 1935.

81. Koppel BS, Tuchman AJ, Mangiardi JR, et al: Epidural spinal infection in intravenous drug abusers. Arch Neurol 45:1331–1337, 1988.

82. Bair-Merritt MH, Chung C, Collier A: Spinal epidural abscess in a young child. Pediatrics 106:e39, 2000.

83. Hlavin ML, Kaminski HJ, Ross JS, Ganz E: Spinal epidural abscess: a ten-year perspective. Neurosurgery 27:177–184, 1990.

84. Auletta JJ, John CJ: Spinal epidural abscesses in children: a 15-year experience and review of the literature. Clin Infect Dis 32:9–16, 2001.

85. Rockney R, Ryan R, Knucky N: Spinal epidural abscess: an infectious emergency. Clin Pediatr 28:332–334, 1989.

86. Yu L, Emans JB: Epidural abscess associated with spondylolysis. J Bone Joint Surg Am 70:444–447, 1988.

87. Baker AS, Ojemann RG, Swartz MN, Richardson EP: Spinal epidural abscess. N Engl J Med 293:463–468, 1975.

Chapter 97

Muscle and Connective Tissue Disorders

Vivian Hwang, MD

Connective tissue disorders and inflammatory myopathies are uncommon in children.

Most of these disorders have prominent clinical manifestations that the emergency physician should be familiar with. It is important to note, however, that some of the classic findings associated with these diseases may be age dependent.

Patients may present with life-threatening complications related to their underlying disease, and young patients without a known diagnosis who present to the emergency department with an atypical illness can be truly challenging both diagnostically and therapeutically.

Selected Diagnoses

Marfan syndrome
Ehlers-Danlos syndrome
Scleroderma
Juvenile dermatomyositis

Discussion of Individual Diagnoses

Marfan Syndrome

Marfan syndrome is a variable, autosomal dominant connective tissue disorder that primarily involves the skeletal, ocular, and cardiovascular systems (Table 97–1). Diagnosis is based on clinical manifestations, some of which are age dependent. Progressive dilation of the aortic root and ascending aorta is the major life-threatening complication of this disorder, and patients may present to the emergency department (ED) with aortic valve incompetence or aortic dissection.

Marfan syndrome occurs in approximately 1 in 10,000 births.[1] All ethnic groups are affected. It is an autosomal dominant disorder that results from a mutation involving the fibrillin 1 gene on chromosome 15. Fibrillin is a glycoprotein

that is the main component of the microfibril found in tissues such as the aorta, ciliary zonules in the eye, bone periosteum, and tendon.[1] Within the aorta, the abnormal fibrillin results in elastic fiber fragmentation and disarray, paucity of smooth muscle cells, and deposition of collagen and mucopolysaccharide between the cells of the media, also described as "cystic medial degeneration."[2] This leads to reduced distensibility in response to the pulse pressure wave and gradual dilation of the aorta.

Clinical Presentation

It is important to be able to recognize patients with clinical manifestations of Marfan syndrome as patients may present to the ED without a known diagnosis. The Ghent nosology is a recently revised set of diagnostic criteria that require a patient to have at least one major criterion in two organ systems and involvement of a third[3] (Table 97–2). Echocardiography is indicated to evaluate for aortic root dilation and other cardiac abnormalities in these patients. Slit-lamp examination should be performed to evaluate for ocular abnormalities such as lens dislocation.

Marfan syndrome may be more difficult to recognize in younger patients because many features are age dependent in their occurrence. For example, the development of scoliosis and protrusio acetabuli occurs following periods of rapid growth. In one series of children less than 16 years old with established Marfan syndrome, tall stature with a height greater than the 97th percentile was the most common presenting feature.[4]

Neonatal Marfan syndrome is typically a more severe disease and may present with hypotonia and clinical findings suggestive of failure to thrive. Physical examination may reveal arachnodactyly, joint laxity and dislocations, flexion contractures, heart murmurs, and ocular abnormalities. Young patients who either have a family history of Marfan syndrome or have a marfanoid appearance without a family history and do not completely fulfill the diagnostic criteria often will require repeat evaluations to assess for age-dependent features.

The skeletal features of patients with Marfan syndrome are unique and include an elongated facies; a tall, slender body habitus; disproportionately long extremities (dolichostenomelia); and arachnodactyly (Fig. 97–1). Objectively, adult

Table 97–1   Manifestations of Select Collagen Vascular and Muscular Disorders

Disorder	Etiology	Female : Male Ratio	Prominent Clinical Features	Important Complications
Marfan syndrome	Defect in gene that encodes glycoprotein fibrillin, a major building block for structural components of the suspensory ligament of the lens and substrate for connective tissues	1 : 1	• Height >97th percentile for age • Long thin face, narrow maxilla • Ectopic lentis, myopia, blue sclera • Pectus excavatum or carinatum • Long, thin fingers that are hyperextensible • Steinberg thumb sign (see Fig. 97–2) • Walker-Murdoch wrist sign	• Aorta and aortic root dilation with aortic valve disorder and aortic dissection • Lens dislocation • Spontaneous pneumothorax • Pulmonary blebs • Scoliosis • Recurrent temporomandibular joint dislocations • Dental caries
Ehlers-Danlos syndrome	Quantitative defect in collagen and connective tissue synthesis and structure (>10 different variants exist)	1 : 1	• Skin hyperelasticity • Fragile skin (scarring and poor healing) • Fragile blood vessels (easily bruised) • Joint hypermobility • Muscle weakness, hypotonia • Short stature • Abnormal facies	• Arterial aneurysms • Mitral valve prolapse • Spontaneous pneumothorax • Joint dislocations • Visceral perforations • Spontaneous vessel ruptures (abdominal and splenic)
Scleroderma	Unknown cause that may be related to endothelial cell injury, fibroblast activation, or immunologic derangement	5 : 1	• Skin hyperpigmentation • Skin thickening/tightness • Myalgias, fatigue, weight loss • Raynaud's phenomenon • Pulmonary fibrosis • Cardiomyopathy, pericardial effusion • Reflux, esophagitis, malabsorption	• Accelerated hypertension • Renal failure • Pulmonary hypertension and respiratory failure
Juvenile dermatomyositis	Unknown cause with nonsuppurative inflammation of skeletal muscle and skin lesions	2 : 1	• Proximal > distal muscle weakness with high CPK, LDH and abnormal electromyogram • Stiff and sore muscles • Arthralgias, dysphagia, dysphonia • Nonpitting edema • Heliotrope (violaceous erythematous) rash—especially eyelids • Scaly, red, atrophic skin over extensor surface of joints • Subcutaneous calcinosis	• Gastrointestinal bleeding or perforation • Respiratory infection/failure • Extremity contractures

Abbreviations: CPK, creatine phosphokinase; LDH, lactate dehydrogenase.

patients have an upper segment–to–lower segment ratio of less than 0.86 (with the lower segment measured from the symphysis pubis to the floor) or an armspan-to-height ratio of greater than 1.05.[2] Arachnodactyly can be identified by the Steinberg thumb sign, in which the entire thumbnail projects beyond the ulnar border of the hand, and the Walker-Murdock wrist sign, in which the thumb and fifth finger overlap around the wrist.[2] Other skeletal abnormalities that may be evident on physical examination include pectus excavatum or pectus carinatum and scoliosis. Diagnostic imaging may be required to evaluate for protrusio acetabuli and dural ectasia.

The major ocular abnormality that occurs in patients with Marfan syndrome is lens dislocation. This can occur as early as infancy, and clinical findings of megalocornea or iridodonesis may be helpful clues. Slit-lamp examination aids in the diagnosis. Other complications include retinal detachment and acute glaucoma.

The cardiovascular manifestations that occur contribute to both morbidity and mortality. Progressive mitral valve prolapse can cause substantial morbidity with the development of arrhythmias, heart failure, thromboemboli, or endocarditis. Mitral regurgitation is common, with approximately 50% of patients younger than 20 years of age affected. Dilation of the aortic valve and ascending aorta leading to aortic valve incompetence typically occurs as the patient ages, with 90% of patients having some aortic root dilation by age 20 years. Aortic dissection is a life-threatening complication of

Table 97–2	Ghent Criteria for Diagnosis of Marfan Syndrome

Skeletal System

A major skeletal criterion is assigned when at least four of the following are present:
- Pectus carinatum
- Pectus excavatum requiring surgery
- Upper segment–to–lower segment ratio < 0.86 or armspan-to-height ratio >1.05
- Wrist and thumb signs: both signs should be present to diagnose arachnodactyly according to the Ghent criteria
- Scoliosis > 20 degrees or spondylolisthesis
- Reduced elbow extension (<170 degrees)
- Pes planus
- Protrusio acetabuli

Involvement of the skeletal system is diagnosed when two of the major features above, or one major feature and two of the following, are present:
- Pectus excavatum of mild severity
- Joint hypermobility
- High palate with dental crowding
- Characteristic facies (dolicocephaly, malar hypoplasia, enophthalmos, retrognathia, down-slanting palpebral fissures)

Cardiovascular System

Major:
- Aortic root dilation
- Dissection of the ascending aorta

Involvement:
- Mitral valve prolapse
- Dilation of the pulmonary artery
- Calcified mitral annulus in individuals < 40 years of age
- Other dilation or dissection of the aorta

Ocular System

Major: Lens dislocation (ectopia lentis)

Involvement:
- Flat cornea
- Increased axial length of globe (causing myopia)
- Hypoplastic iris or ciliary muscle (causing decreased miosis)

Skin/Integument System

Major: None

Involvement:
- Striae atrophicae
- Recurrent or incisional hernia

Pulmonary System

Major: none

Minor:
- Spontaneous pneumothorax
- Apical blebs

Nervous System

Major: lumbosacral dural ectasia

Minor: none

Genetic Criteria

Major:
- Parent, child, or sibling meets the criteria independently
- *FBN1* mutations known to cause Marfan syndrome
- Inheritance of DNA marker haplotype linked to Marfan syndrome in the family

Minor: none

Marfan syndrome, with pain being the most common presenting complaint. It is usually described as an acute onset of sharp, excruciating pain either in the chest, neck and jaw, interscapular area, or lumbar area depending on the site of the dissection. Physical examination may reveal hypertension or hypotension, aortic regurgitation, findings suggestive of cardiac tamponade, pulse deficits, and blood pressure dis-

crepancies between limbs. Diagnostic imaging is necessary to make a definitive diagnosis of aortic dissection. Chest radiography is often abnormal in patients with aortic dissection; however, the findings are typically nonspecific. Noninvasive imaging modalities that are highly sensitive for detection of aortic dissection include computed tomography (CT), magnetic resonance imaging, and transesophageal echocardiography.[5]

Management

Once aortic dissection is suspected, medical therapy must be initiated immediately with the goal of stabilizing the dissection and preventing rupture. Blood pressure and heart rate control can be achieved with labetalol, an α- and β-adrenergic antagonist, or a combination of a β-blocker such as esmolol or propranolol and a vasodilating agent such as sodium nitroprusside. It is important to start the β-blocker before the vasodilating agent to prevent tachycardia.[6] With Marfan syndrome, dilation is usually confined to the proximal ascending aorta, and patients will ultimately require surgery for definitive repair.

Patients are at risk for recurrent spontaneous pneumothoraces as a result of increased distensibility of the lung parenchyma. Management includes chest tube thoracostomy.

The cardiovascular complications that occur with Marfan syndrome primarily determine life expectancy in these patients. Recent studies, including a randomized clinical trial involving adult and adolescent patients with Marfan syndrome, have shown that β-blocker treatment reduces the rate of aortic dilation and aortic complications.[7] Although the exact mechanism is not fully understood, it is believed that long-term treatment with β-adrenergic blockade reduces the impulse of left ventricular ejection (dP/dt) and the heart rate, consequently reducing repeated strain on the aortic root.[7]

The long-term survival for patients with Marfan syndrome has certainly increased because of effective medical therapy with the use of β-adrenergic blockade and prophylactic aortic root surgery. Unfortunately, there are patients without a known diagnosis who present with a catastrophic cardiovascular event, and it is important for the emergency physician to be able to recognize patients who may have this condition.

Patients with a known diagnosis of Marfan syndrome may present to the ED with a complication related to their condition. If an ocular abnormality is suspected, appropriate consultation and close follow-up with an ophthalmologist are warranted. Patients who present with a cardiovascular complication and require blood pressure control with intravenous titratable agents must be admitted to an intensive care unit, and will likely require a multidisciplinary approach by a team of specialists for appropriate treatment. Patients without a known diagnosis of Marfan syndrome who present to the ED for other reasons and are found to have features suggestive of Marfan should be queried about a family history of the disease and be referred to their primary care physician for additional testing.

Ehlers-Danlos Syndrome

Ehlers-Danlos syndrome (EDS) is a heterogeneous, hereditary soft connective tissue disease characterized by excessive skin elasticity, joint hypermobility, and easy bruising. There are many different types, as well as variations within each type, of EDS. The basic underlying defect is an abnormality

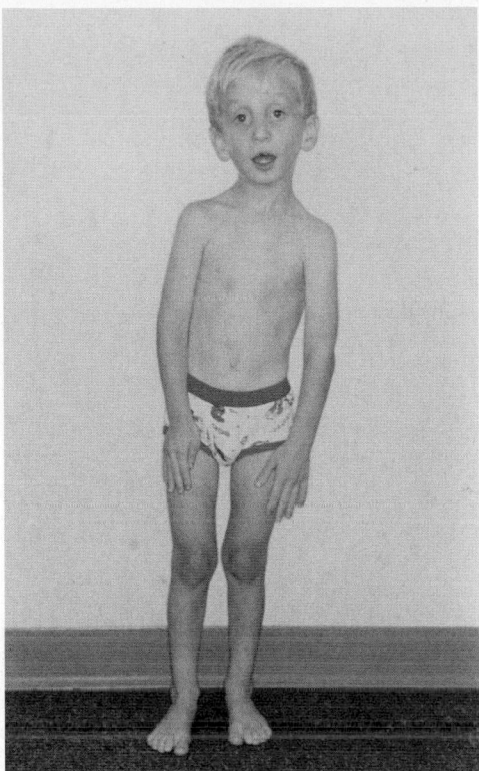

FIGURE 97–1. A young child with Marfan syndrome. Skeletal features include an elongated facies, long extremities (dolichostenomelia), and mild scoliosis. (From Robinson I: Marfan syndrome. *In* Behrman R, Kliegman R, Jenson H [eds]: Nelson Textbook of Pediatrics, 17th ed. Philadelphia: WB Saunders, 2004, p 2339.)

of collagen synthesis and metabolism. Life-threatening complications, including vascular catastrophes, occur with EDS type IV. EDS is a rare disorder with a reported incidence of one in 150,000.[8] It is now recognized that patients with EDS can have variable clinical manifestations with symptoms so mild that they often go unrecognized. Thus the incidence is probably much greater than previously reported.

Over eight different kinds of collagen have been identified in connective tissues. Abnormalities of type I or III collagen are associated with the different forms of EDS.[9] Currently, there are 10 recognized types of EDS of which most are autosomal dominant. Each type depends on the type of collagen affected, the structural integrity, and quantity produced. There is considerable variability within each type as well as overlap of different types, with approximately half of patients not meeting the criteria for any one specific type.[10] Type IV, ecchymotic (arterial) type, involves a defect in type III procollagen, which is found in arteries, skin, peritoneum, and intestines. Among the different types, it occurs in approximately 4% of all EDS cases.[10] However, it is most commonly associated with life-threatening complications, including rupture of large vessels and hollow organs.

Clinical Presentation

Children with EDS often appear normal at birth. Some types of EDS, including type IV, are associated with premature birth and low birth weight. These infants often exhibit hypotonia. Short stature may be recognized as these patients age. Other characteristics include a unique facies with midface flattening, floppy ears, thin lips, broad or thin nose, and

widely spaced eyes. Not all patients with type IV EDS exhibit these abnormal features. A biochemical diagnosis is the preferred way of establishing EDS and relies on the use of molecular probes on protein extracts or RNA obtained from cultured skin fibroblast or other tissues rich in type III collagen.

It is common for patients with EDS to have benign clinical manifestations, including mild skin elasticity and hypermobile joints, that are unrecognized. Unfortunately, there are case reports of young patients with the more severe type IV EDS who are diagnosed at autopsy after presenting with a vascular catastrophe.[10] It is often found in retrospect that these patients have had a history of joint hypermobility and easy bruisability. Thus the emergency physician should keep in mind the possibility of a life-threatening problem when encountering a young patient with an atypical chief complaint and a history causing concern for EDS.

Joint hypermobility is one of the hallmark characteristics found with EDS. Objective scoring methods using maneuvers shown in Figure 97–2 are used to define joint hypermobility in these patients.[11] Other musculoskeletal findings include joint dislocation, scoliosis, broad clavicles, occipital horns, carpal bone fusion, and arthritis.[10]

EDS is characterized by skin elasticity and skin fragility. Gorlin's sign, in which a patient is able to touch the tip of the tongue to the nose, may be demonstrated. Patients tend to bruise easily, and skin lesions often heal slowly after injury or surgery. Patients are prone to the development of "cigarette paper" scars in which the skin on the forehead, chin, and lower extremities appears thin, atrophic, and hyperpigmented.[11] The connective tissue defects with EDS may also lead to the development of ocular fragility, periodontitis, hernias, and striae distensae.

Patients with type IV EDS typically die before the fifth decade of life.[10] The most important complication is spontaneous rupture of the great vessels, although aneurysms have also been reported in other large vessels. Resuscitative procedures and surgical repair are often met with difficulty because of the fragility of these tissues. Other serious complications include colon perforation, pneumothorax, and splenic and uterine rupture. Pregnancy is not recommended in patients with EDS type IV; the reported maternal death rate is 25%.[8]

Management

Currently, there is no cure for EDS. The goals are to recognize patients with this disease and its complications as well as to prevent further injury. Because EDS is uncommon, a young, otherwise healthy patient presenting to the ED with an atypical illness can truly be a diagnostic challenge. Patients in whom a vascular or visceral complication is suspected require an approach similar to that for other patients who require emergent resuscitation. Two large-bore peripheral intravenous lines are preferred over central venous access because of the tissue friability that occurs with EDS. Potential complications include hematoma formation, persistent bleeding, and thrombosis. If central venous access becomes necessary, a compressible site is preferred.

Noninvasive diagnostic modalities such as CT, magnetic resonance imaging, ultrasound, and transesophageal echocardiography are preferred for the detection of aneurysms and/or dissection because of the possibility of complications

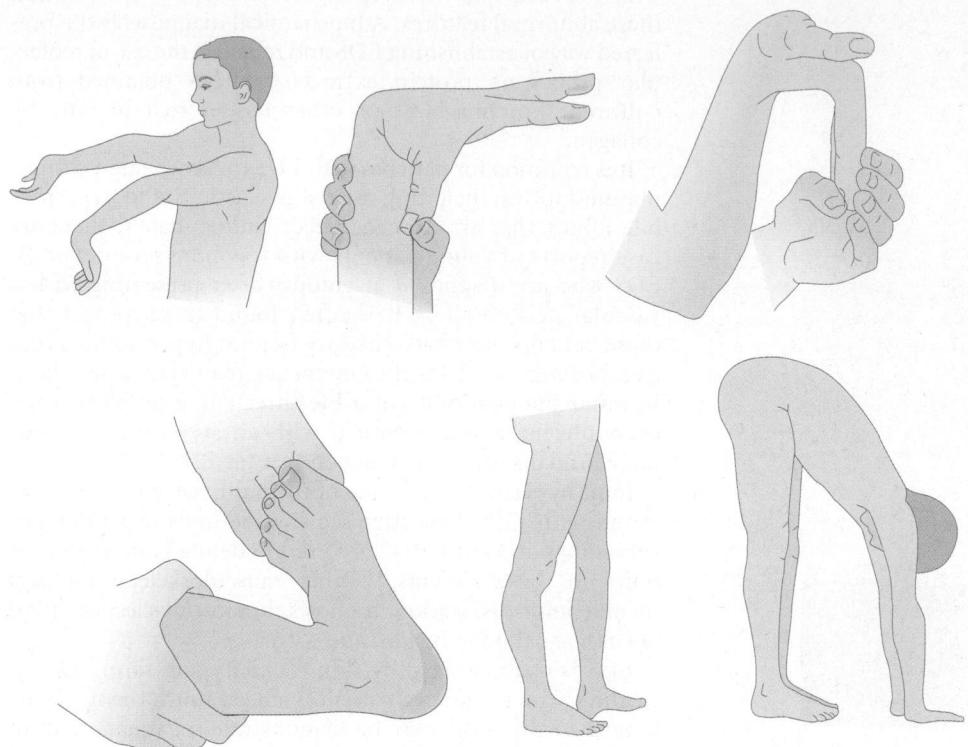

FIGURE 97–2. Maneuvers demonstrating joint laxity in Ehlers-Danlos syndrome. (From Shapiro J, Rowe D, Sponseller P: Heritable disorders of structural proteins. *In* Harris E, Budd R, Firestein G, et al [eds]: Kelley's Textbook of Rheumatology, 7th ed. Philadelphia: Elsevier Saunders, 2005, p 1561.)

associated with invasive procedures such as arteriography. In fact, arteriography has a 67% complication rate in these patients.[12]

Early surgical consultation and evaluation is extremely important if vascular or intra-abdominal pathology is suspected in these patients. It is imperative to communicate to the surgeon that a patient has known or suspected EDS as it may impact the choice of surgery, instruments, and materials used.[13] Patients requiring emergent surgery for either vascular or intra-abdominal pathology require admission to an intensive care unit. Patients who come to the ED for concerns unrelated to EDS but have features causing concern for EDS should be referred to their primary care physician for further evaluation.

Scleroderma

Scleroderma, or systemic sclerosis (SSc), is an autoimmune connective tissue disease that has variable effects on several organ systems, including the skin, gastrointestinal (GI) tract, lungs, kidney, and heart. It is characterized by fibrosis and vascular obliteration of these organs with debilitating and life-threatening complications.

Scleroderma is rare, with an annual incidence of 0.6 to 19.1 in 1 million per year.[14] The incidence is higher in African Americans with females more commonly affected.[14] Children make up fewer than 10% of all cases. It is common for patients with scleroderma to have first-degree relatives with another autoimmune disorder such as systemic lupus or rheumatoid arthritis.[14]

The cause of scleroderma is largely unknown, but it seems to have an immunologic basis involving both cellular and humoral immunity.[15] Other implicated factors include genetic, toxic, and infectious factors.[14] Fibrosis occurs primarily in small arteries, microvessels, and the diffuse connective tissue. Histologically, there are increased amounts of the usual components of connective tissue in both the interstitium and the intima of small arteries.[16] This leads to significant vascular and microvascular lesions.[16]

Clinical Presentation

Scleroderma is classified as either localized or generalized. Localized disease does not involve visceral organs. Generalized scleroderma is subdivided into diffuse (dSSc) or limited scleroderma (lSSc) depending on the extent of skin involvement.[16] Localized scleroderma occurs in three forms depending on the involved area: morphea, linear scleroderma, and generalized morphea. Although limited to skin, this disease can have cosmetic and debilitating manifestations including contractures and growth failure.[17] Patients with lSSc, previously referred to as CREST syndrome (*c*alcinosis, *R*aynaud's phenomenon, *e*sophageal dismotility, *s*clerodactyly, and *t*elangiectasias), represent the majority of patients with generalized scleroderma. It is a more stable disease in which complications tend to develop later in life. Patients with dSSc tend to be young or middle-aged females with more rapidly progressive disease resulting in early and significant organ failure.[16] Both localized and generalized scleroderma occur in children, with the loca-lized form being more common. There may be a delay in diagnosis of dSSc due to the subtle early manifestations of the disease.[18] Children have clinical findings similar to those in adults.

Patients with SSc require routine evaluation for the development of cardiac, pulmonary, and esophageal complications. Testing may include echocardiography, pulmonary function testing, radiography, CT scan, and esophageal motility studies.

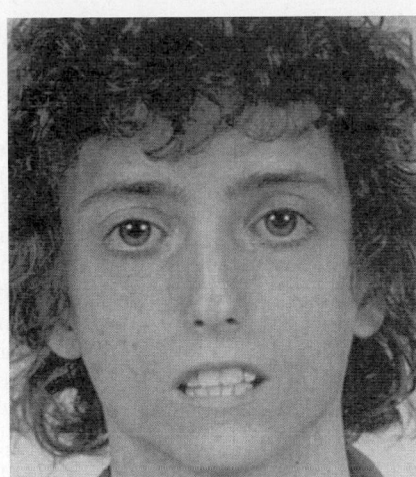

FIGURE 97–3. Typical facies of scleroderma, characterized by tightening of the skin, loss of subcutaneous tissue in the face, and small mouth. (From Uziel Y, Miller M, Laxer R: Scleroderma in children. Pediatr Clin North Am 42:1777, 1995.)

Skin changes are characteristic of scleroderma, with edema occurring in the early stages of the disease followed by tightening and atrophy of the skin as a result of fibrosis. The skin often has a shiny, waxy appearance (Fig. 97–3). Skin ulceration and calcinosis may develop over pressure points (e.g., elbows). Sclerodactyly develops as skin tightens over the fingers, giving them a tapered appearance. Telangiectasias are also characteristic.

Raynaud's phenomenon is one of the hallmark features of the disease and is often the earliest manifestation, preceding other involvement by months to years. It is characterized by episodic digital ischemia provoked by cold and emotion. It is important to recall that it can occur in isolation or with conditions other than SSc.

Complications of SSc are related to progressive organ failure. Lungs are affected as fibrosis causes interstitial lung disease and eventually pulmonary hypertension. Myocardial fibrosis can develop and lead to a cardiomyopathy. Pericarditis as a primary disease has also been reported.[19] Other complications include esophageal dysmotility manifesting as dysphagia, renal hypertensive crisis and oliguric renal failure, and biliary cirrhosis.

Management

ED management consists of recognition and treatment of disease complications (e.g., acute hypertension, renal failure, cardiac or respiratory compromise) and medication side effects (e.g., infection, nephrotoxicity). Long-term therapy of SSc includes vasodilators (e.g., calcium channel blockers, angiotensin II receptor blockers, and prostaglandins); antiplatelet aggregation drugs; immunosuppressants (e.g., methotrexate, cyclosporine); and antifibrotic agents (D-penicillamine, colchicines, interferon-gamma, and relaxin).[15] Corticosteroids are not useful in improving or preventing the progression of skin involvement.[15]

Scleroderma can have a variable course depending on the extent of organ involvement. Ten-year survival rates are roughly 60% to 70% for patients with lSSc and 20% for patients with dSSc. The prognosis for children with dSSc is especially poor.[18] Patients with the generalized form of scleroderma are often managed by a multidisciplinary team of specialists including a rheumatologist, pulmonologist, and gastroenterologist. Patients with dSSc will inevitably develop complications related to progressive organ failure necessitating inpatient care.

Juvenile Dermatomyositis

Dermatomyositis is an autoimmune, multisystemic disorder most commonly involving the skin and muscles. It is characterized by an inflammatory myopathy as well as cutaneous manifestations. Juvenile dermatomyositis is considered to be a subset of the idiopathic inflammatory myopathies, which include dermatomyositis, polymyositis, myositis with cancer, and myositis overlapping with another collagen vascular disorder. The childhood form is frequently complicated by calcinosis, which can be both painful and debilitating.

Juvenile dermatomyositis (JDM) is a rare disorder in which the etiology is largely unknown. It accounts for approximately 6% of children with a major connective tissue disease in pediatric rheumatology clinics.[18] Onset typically occurs between 4 and 10 years of age and occurs more frequently in girls.[18] JDM has been demonstrated to have an immunologic basis and has been shown to be associated with particular human leukocyte antigen class I and II antigens as well as specific autoantibodies.[20] Infectious agents such as group A streptococcus have also been implicated as potential precipitants.[21]

Clinical Presentation

The inflammatory myopathy is caused by a complement-mediated microangiopathy that leads to loss of capillaries, muscle ischemia, muscle fiber necrosis, and perifascicular atrophy.[22] Clinically, this results in muscle weakness that occurs primarily in the proximal muscles. This disease is usually suspected based on the clinical manifestations. Diagnostic criteria for dermatomyositis include symmetric proximal muscle weakness, elevated muscle enzyme levels, abnormal findings on electromyogram, abnormal findings from muscle biopsy, and typical cutaneous findings. Dermatomyositis is considered *definite* with the presence of three of four criteria, *probable* with two, and *possible* with one; all cases are associated with the characteristic skin rash.[23]

The onset of JDM is usually indolent, but a fulminant course is possible. Children often present with a dermatitis, proximal muscle weakness, and constitutional symptoms including low-grade fever, fatigue, weight loss, and anorexia. There is a greater potential for calcinosis in children, with a reported rate of up to 40%.[24]

This disease is usually suspected based on the clinical manifestations; however, muscle involvement can be identified with the use of enzymatic testing. Characteristically, there is an increase in concentrations of creatine kinase, lactate dehydrogenase, aldolase, or alanine aminotransferase.[18] Patients have characteristic electromyogram abnormalities and muscle biopsy findings.

The heliotrope rash (Fig. 97–4) and Gottron's papules are pathognomonic cutaneous manifestations of dermatomyositis. The heliotrope rash is a violaceous to dusky erythematous rash, with or without edema, that involves the periorbital tissues in a symmetric distribution. Gottron's papules are slightly raised violaceous papules and plaques found

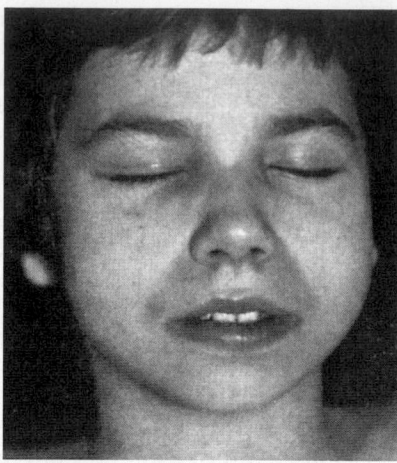

FIGURE 97–4. Heliotrope rash on upper eyelids and facial erythema demonstrated in a child with juvenile dermatomyositis. (From Pachman L: Juvenile dermatomyositis. *In* Behrman R, Kliegman, Jenson H [eds]: Nelson Textbook of Pediatrics, 17th ed. Philadelphia: WB Saunders, 2004, p 814.)

most commonly on bony prominences, particularly on the hands.[24]

Calcinosis, which develops more often in children, is associated with increased morbidity and mortality.[21] Calcium deposits are found mainly in the subcutaneous tissue and fascia and around joints. They may not only be painful and debilitating, but can serve as a nidus for infection, leading to sepsis and death. Hypercalcemia can occur as calcinosis resolves.[25] Other cutaneous manifestations include cuticular changes with hypertrophy of the cuticle, malar erythema, poikiloderma, and scaly alopecia. Both localized and generalized edema can occur, with anasarca usually associated with severe disease activity.[26]

The myopathy that occurs with JDM primarily affects the proximal muscles in a symmetric distribution. Symptoms occur over a period of weeks to months and include myalgias, fatigue, and weakness. Patients may complain of difficulty walking up stairs or raising their arms to brush their hair. Gowers' sign, in which patients attempting to stand from the ground begin with both hands and feet on the floor and then work up the legs with the hands, may be demonstrated. Esophageal involvement may manifest as dysphagia or dysphonia. It is associated with a poor prognosis as patients are at risk for sudden aspiration.[18]

JDM is a multisystem disorder that can involve other organ systems, leading to complications involving the lungs, heart, and GI tract. Although the association of dermatomyositis with malignancy at disease onset has clearly been established in adults, this does not appear to be the case for children.[27]

All patients with respiratory symptoms require evaluation for pneumonia due to aspiration or opportunistic infections. All patients with pneumonia should be admitted as respiratory failure can occur due to weakened respiratory muscles. Gastrointestinal complications can also be life threatening. Since most patients are on some type of immunosuppressant, presenting features may be masked. Moreover, 17% to 21% of patients with GI perforation may have normal plain film findings, and CT may be required to make the diagnosis. Suspicion of carditis requires electrocardiography, chest

radiography, cardiac enzyme tests, echocardiography, and inpatient management.

Management

The mainstay of chronic treatment for JDM is systemic corticosteroids. However, there are patients who are resistant to steroids or are dependent on high doses, making this disease often difficult to treat. For refractory cases, immunosuppression with azathioprine and cyclosporine has been used with success.[24] In addition, recent trials in adults have shown high-dose intravenous immune globulin to be a safe and effective treatment for refractory dermatomyositis.[22] Plasmapheresis has also been used but may not offer increased benefit.[28] Hydroxychloroquine is used for patients with only mild cutaneous findings and appears to be steroid sparing.[18,21]

Calcinosis may not respond to steroids and immunosuppressant therapy used to treat the myositis. The use of diltiazem, a calcium channel blocker, has anecdotally been shown to cause regression of calcinosis.[29] Other treatments for calcinosis, including low-dose warfarin, aluminum hydroxide, and probenicid, have met with mixed success.[18] Spontaneous remission can occur.

In contrast to adults, children with dermatomyositis have a fairly good prognosis, with an overall mortality rate of about 1%. The course can be variable, but patients typically have myositis and dermatitis for 1 to 2 years followed by functional recovery with residual muscle atrophy and contractures with or without calcinosis.[18] Children with JDM are typically followed closely by a pediatric rheumatologist. Patients may come to the ED with complications such as aspiration pneumonia and sepsis, necessitating aggressive inpatient care.

REFERENCES

1. Braverman A: Exercise and the Marfan syndrome. Med Sci Sports Exerc 30:S387–S395, 1998.
2. Dean J: Management of Marfan syndrome. Heart 88:97–103, 2002.
3. De Paepe A, Devereux R, Dietz H, et al: Revised diagnostic criteria for the Marfan syndrome. Am J Med Genet 62:417–426, 1996.
4. Lipscomb K: Evolving phenotype of Marfan's syndrome. Arch Dis Child 76:41–46, 1997.
5. Neinaber C, von Kodolitsch Y, Nicolas V, et al: The diagnosis of thoracic aortic dissection by noninvasive imaging procedures. N Engl J Med 328:1–9, 1993.
6. Khan I, Nair C: Clinical, diagnostic and management perspectives of aortic dissection. Chest 12:311–328, 2002.
7. Shores J, Berger K, Murphy E, et al: Progression of aortic dilatation and the benefit of long-term beta-adrenergic blockade in Marfan's syndrome. N Engl J Med 330:1335–1341, 1994.
8. Peaceman A, Cruishank D: Ehlers-Danlos syndrome and pregnancy: association of type IV with maternal death. Obstet Gynecol 69:428–436, 1987.
9. Prockop D, Kivirikko K: Heritable diseases of collagen. N Engl J Med 6:376–386, 1984.
10. Wimmer P, Howes D, Rumoro D, et al: Fatal vascular catastrophe in Ehlers-Danlos syndrome: a case report and review. J Emerg Med 14:25–31, 1996.
11. Shapiro J, Rowe D, Sponseller P: Heritable disorders of structural proteins. *In* Harris E, Budd R, Firestein G, et al (eds): Kelley's Textbook of Rheumatology, 7th ed. Philadelphia: Elsevier Saunders, 2005, pp 1547–1578.
12. Mattar S, Kumar A, Lumsden A: Vascular complications in Ehlers-Danlos syndrome. Am Surg 60:827–831, 1994.
13. Hamano K, Minami Y, Fujimura Y, et al: Emergency operation for thoracic aortic aneurysm caused by the Ehlers-Danlos syndrome. Ann Thorac Surg 58:1180–1182, 1994.

14. Ferri C, Valentini G, Cozzi F, et al: Systemic sclerosis: demographic, clinical, and serologic features and survival in 1,012 Italian patients. Medicine 81:139–153, 2002.

15. Sapadin A, Fleischmajer R: Treatment of scleroderma. Arch Dermatol 138:99–105, 2002.

16. Leroy E, Black C: Scleroderma (systemic sclerosis) classification, subsets and pathogenesis. J Rheumatol 15:202–205, 1988.

17. Uziel Y, Feldman B, Krafchik B, et al: Methotrexate and corticosteroid therapy for pediatric localized scleroderma. J Pediatr 136:91–95, 2000.

18. Cassidy J: Systemic lupus erythematosus, juvenile dermatomyositis, scleroderma and vasculitis. *In* Harris E, Budd R, Genovese M, et al (eds): Kelley's Textbook of Rheumatology, 7th ed. Philadelphia, Elsevier Saunders, 2005, pp 1547–1578.

19. Byers R, Marshall D, Freemont A: Pericardial involvement in systemic sclerosis. Ann Rheum Dis 56:393–394, 1997.

20. Sansome A, Dubowitz V: Intravenous immunogobulin in juvenile dermatomyositis—four year review of nine cases. Arch Dis Child 72:25–28, 1995.

21. Pachman L: An update on juvenile dermatomyositis. Curr Opin Rheumatol 7:437–441, 1995.

22. Dalakas M, Illa I, Dambrosia M, et al: A controlled trial of high-dose intravenous immune globulin infusions as treatment for dermatomyositis. N Engl J Med 329:1993–2000, 1993.

23. Bohan A, Peter B: Polymyositis and dermatomyositis. N Engl J Med 292:344–347, 403–407, 1975.

24. Siguregeirsson B, Lindelof B, Edhag O, et al: Risk of cancer in patients with dermatomyositis or polymyositis. N Engl J Med 325:363–367, 1992.

25. Wilsher M, Holdaway J, North J: Hypercalcemia during resolution of calcinosis in juvenile dermatomyositis. BMJ 288:1345, 1984.

26. Mitchell J, Dennis G, Rider, L: Juvenile dermatomyositis presenting with anasarca: a possible indicator of severe disease activity. J Pediatr 138:942–945, 2001.

27. Airio A, Pukkala E, Isomaki H: Elevated cancer incidence in patients with dermatomyositis: a population based study. J Rheumatol 22:1300–1303, 1995.

28. Miller F, Leitman S, Cronin M, et al: Controlled trial of plasma exchange and leukapharesis in polymyositis and dermatomyositis. N Engl J Med 326:1380–1384, 1992.

29. Oliveri M, Palermo R, Mautalen C, et al: Regression of calcinosis during diltiazem treatment of juvenile dermatomyositis. J Rheumatol 23:2152–2155, 1996.

Overuse Syndromes and Inflammatory Conditions

Charles G. Macias, MD, MPH and Victoria S. Gregg, MD

Selected Diagnoses

Specific overuse syndromes of the upper extremity
  Rotator cuff tendonitis
  Little League shoulder (proximal humeral epiphysitis)
  Little League elbow (proximal epicondylar apophysitis)
Specific overuse syndromes of the lower extremity
  Osteochondral injuries
  Osgood-Schlatter disease (tibial tubercle apophysitis)
  Sinding-Larsen-Johansson disease and jumper's knee
  Iliotibial band syndrome
  Sever's disease (calcaneal apophysitis)
  Plantar fasciitis
  Medial tibial stress syndrome (periostitis)
  Köhler's disease
Spine injuries
  Spondylolysis
  Juvenile kyphosis (Scheuermann's disease)

Discussion of Individual Diagnoses

Specific Overuse Syndromes of the Upper Extremity

Athletes who play sports such as baseball, softball, tennis, and swimming are at risk for developing overuse injuries of the shoulder and arm due to the repetitive overhead motions required by these activities (Table 98–1). In one report of patients evaluated for sports injury, 20% were less than 16 years of age, and 15% of these injuries involved the upper extremity (with shoulder injuries comprising 45% of upper extremity injuries).[1]

Rotator Cuff Tendonitis

Tendonitis refers to injury of the tendon or tendon sheath almost always due to overuse. It is uncommon in children because the structures adjacent to tendons are weaker and more likely to fail. However, chronic injury (typically from overuse) can lead to tissue injury and repair that ultimately results in a weakened tensile strength as compared to that of healthy tendon. The rotator cuff includes four muscles and their conjoined tendons (supraspinatus, infraspinatus, teres minor, and subscapularis muscles). They control internal and external rotation of the shoulder and keep the humeral head in place during upward elevation of the arm. Shoulder laxity and muscle imbalance places younger athletes at greater risk for rotator cuff tendonitis than older athletes, who are more prone to impingement of the tendons along the cora-coacromial arch.

Patients with rotator cuff tendonitis typically complain of dull localized pain or pain referred to the lateral arm with overhead activity. The diagnosis is based on shoulder examination by demonstrating weakness of the rotator cuff muscles. In the drop arm test, the examiner passively abducts the patient's shoulders to 90 degrees with the thumbs pointed downward. If the patient is unable to hold this position, a complete tear of the rotator cuff should be suspected.[2] Radiographs may be helpful in young children to rule out an avulsion fracture at the site of tendon attachment. Acute treatment involves ice, nonsteroidal analgesics, and rest from the offending activity for 2 to 6 weeks. Additionally, physical therapy should be considered to strengthen shoulder and

Table 98–1	**Common Sporting Activity Associated with Overuse Injuries**	
Location	**Overuse Injury**	**Associated sport**
Shoulder	Rotator cuff tendonitis	Swimming, softball, tennis, racquetball
	Little League shoulder	Baseball
Elbow	Little League elbow, Panner's disease	Baseball, softball, tennis, golf
Back	Spondylolysis	Gymnastics
	Juvenile kyphosis	Football, weightlifting, skating, dancing
Patella	Sinding-Larsen-Johansson syndrome, jumper's knee	Volleyball, basketball
Tibia	Medial tibial stress syndrome, Osgood-Schlatter disease	Basketball, track and field
Heel	Sever's disease, plantar fasciitis, Köhler's disease	Soccer, track and field

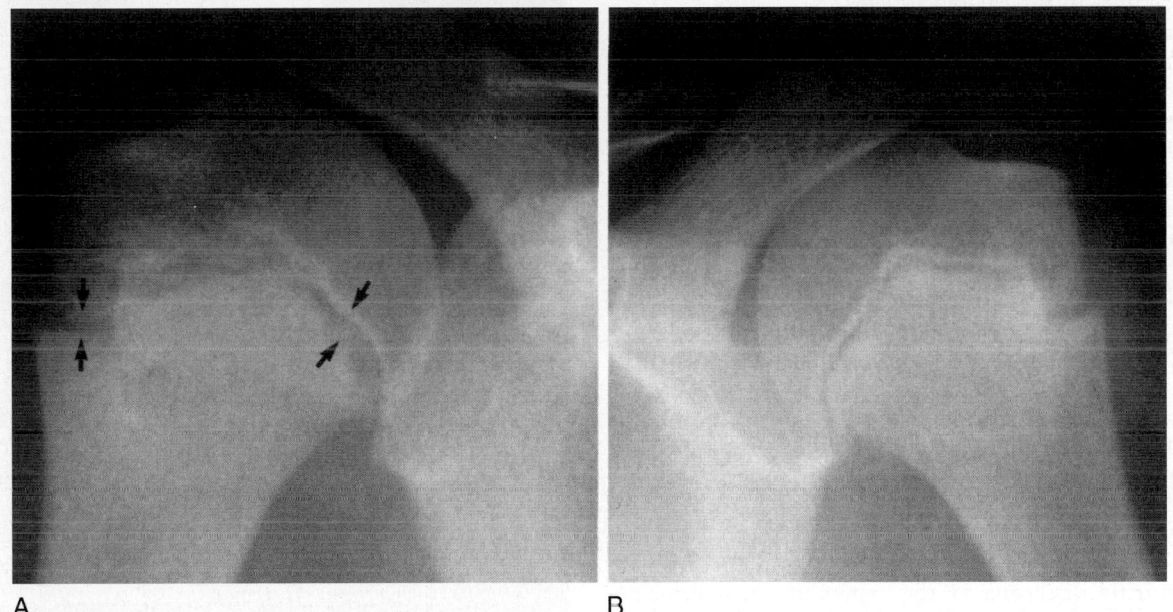

A   B

FIGURE 98–1. Left, A normal shoulder without widening of the physis. **Right,** "Little League shoulder" with widening of proximal humeral physis consistent with a stress fracture. (From DeLee J, Drez D [eds]: DeLee & Drez's Orthopaedic Sports Medicine, 2nd ed. Philadelphia: WB Saunders, 2003, p 1136.)

rotator cuff muscles.[3] Surgical intervention is typically reserved for complete tears.[4]

Little League Shoulder (Proximal Humeral Epiphysitis)

The demand of large rotational forces necessary to throw a ball causes repetitive microtrauma to the skeletally immature athlete. However, it is unclear whether "Little League shoulder" is due to inflammation or a Salter I fracture of the proximal humeral physis.[4,5] Children ages 11 to 16 years are typically more at risk for Little League shoulder than more skeletally mature adolescents.[6] Children who throw repetitively for longer durations (i.e., a pitcher or a catcher) are prone to overuse throwing injuries. The chief complaint is pain in the lateral aspect of the proximal humerus while throwing. The onset of symptoms is gradual, as is the case in most overuse injuries. Athletes may notice a loss of speed and/or control of pitches.

The physical examination may be unremarkable. In one series, 87% of patients had tenderness to palpation over the proximal humerus and 70% had tenderness over the lateral aspect of the proximal humerus.[6] Decreased active and passive range of motion at the shoulder joint also may be present. Cervical spine pathology should be excluded by

evaluating for referred pain from the neck. Radiographs can help confirm the diagnosis by demonstrating a widening of the proximal humeral physis (Fig. 98–1). Associated lateral fragmentation or calcification, sclerosis, demineralization, or cystic changes also may be present.[6] As physeal widening may be subtle, comparison views may be helpful. Magnetic resonance imaging (MRI) and computed tomography are usually not necessary.

Acute treatment involves anti-inflammatory medications. Treatment should also include rest (for at least 3 months) and physical therapy programs to enhance strength and flexibility of the rotator cuff.[3,6] Little League shoulder is usually a self-limited injury, with a return of full strength and full range of motion and no apprehension or discomfort while throwing. Although concerns for complications such as avascular necrosis, growth plate injuries, and permanent loss of speed and accuracy while throwing have been described, there appear to be no significant growth disturbances in long-term follow-up among patients with appropriate treatment.[6]

Little League Elbow (Medial Epicondylar Apophysitis)

Apophyses are attachment sites of muscles and tendons to bone that develop as accessory ossification centers. In younger children, apophyseal inflammation and microtrauma are more common then tendon injuries. Sports involving jumping motions, such as basketball, volleyball, or track and field events such as the long jump or hurdles, may predispose a young athlete to traction injuries to the apophysis.[4] "Little League elbow" is a common apophyseal injury. The term describes a spectrum of etiologies that include hypertrophy of the ulna, osteochondritis dissecans of the capitellum, fragmentation of the medial epicondyle, and medial epicondylitis.[7] The medial epicondyle of the humerus is the weakest structure in the skeletally immature elbow and can easily be damaged by the forces generated with throwing and racket sports. It is most commonly seen in 8- to 15-year-old athletes.[5]

The chief complaint is typically pain in the medial elbow and proximal forearm while throwing, or prolonged pain for 24 hours after throwing. The physical examination may be normal, but may also reveal pain over the medial epicondyle. Pain may also be elicited with resisted wrist flexion and pronation, and with valgus stress to a 20- to 30-degree flexed elbow.[4] Signs and symptoms of advanced pathology include pain when performing any task that requires rotational movement. Sensory abnormalities following the ulnar nerve distribution suggest more extensive involvement.[4] Apophysitis may often be accompanied by avulsion fractures; thus radiographs may be important in the initial evaluation of this injury.

Osteochondrosis of the capitellum, or Panner's disease, occurs in children 6 to 12 years old, almost exclusively in baseball pitchers.[8] *Osteochondrosis* refers to the degeneration, then reossification, of one of the ossification centers in children. Panner's disease is a benign process that causes pain over the lateral elbow and resolves with rest. In contrast, osteochondritis dissecans of the capitellum also presents with pain over the lateral elbow, but this disease can be debilitating with resultant vascular insufficiency and avascular necrosis.[9]

Although radiographs are usually normal in Little League elbow, widening of the medial epicondylar physis and sclerosis and fragmentation of the lateral epicondyle apophysis may be seen. A comparison view of the other elbow may be helpful.

Acute treatment includes ice, anti-inflammatory medications, and rest. Physical therapy to include wrist flexor strengthening is also warranted. Return to play is advised when the patient experiences full range of motion without pain.

Specific Overuse Syndromes of the Lower Extremities

Osteochondral Injuries

Osteochondral injuries are characterized by injury to cartilage and bone at the joint surfaces with resultant fragmentation and sclerosis. Osteochondritis dissecans is one type of osteochondral injury in which a segment of subchondral bone and articular cartilage separates from the underlying bone. In the lower extremity, the usual areas of involvment are the medial or lateral epicondyle of the knee or the patella, while the capitellum, radial head, trochlea, and olecranon are the most commonly affected sites in the upper extremity (Fig. 98–2).

Although marginal vascularity and coagulopathies may predispose athletes to this type of injury, the etiology of

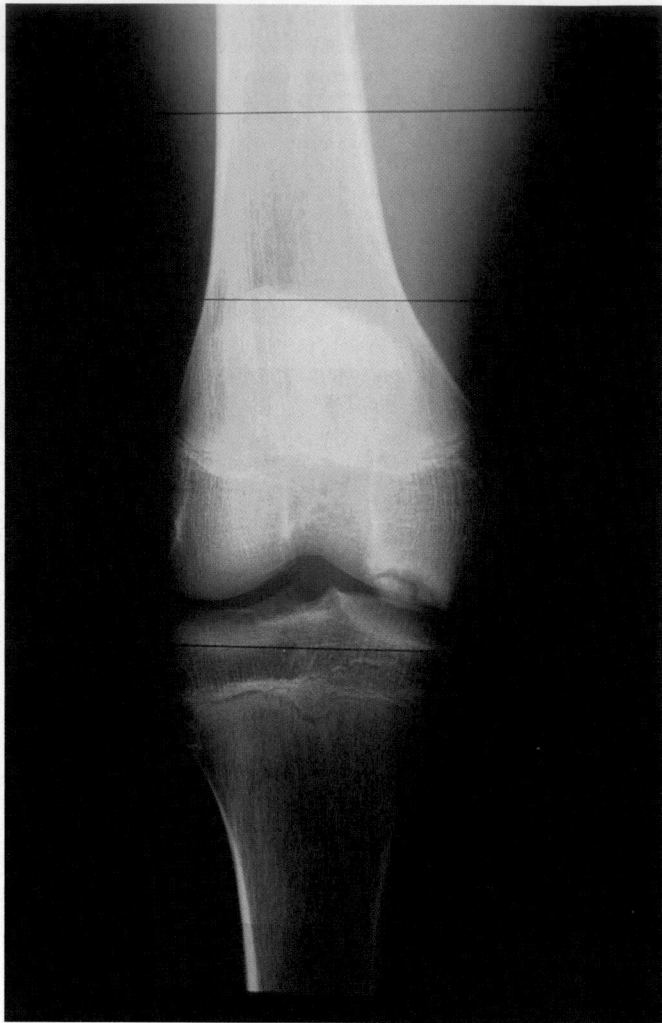

FIGURE 98–2. Osteochondritis dissecans in a 12-year-old male with recurrent knee pain while training for football. Note the well-circumscribed crescent-shaped area of radiolucency above an area of subchondral bone, separated from the femoral condyle.

osteochondritis dissecans is thought to involve repetitive microtrauma.[10] The lesions are most commonly seen during adolescence at the end of growth and in early adulthood. Symptoms may include pain and a mild effusion. Classification schemas describe stages of disease in which a progression to instability and finally separation of the lesion ensue, with the development of a loose body of bone. Osteochondritis dissecans lesions can often be appreciated on plain radiographs, but MRI may be needed to help determine the classification of injury and appropriate management (i.e., conservative vs. operative). Dynamic bone scans in younger patients can help assess activity and healing potential.

Acute therapy involves symptomatic treatment, but bracing and physical therapy may also be necessary. Activity restriction is also warranted because this injury often has a poor outcome with the potential to cause permanent disability. Athletes should not return to play until they have pain-free range of motion. In multicenter studies of osteochondritis dissecans of the knee, preadolescent children tended to have a more favorable prognosis than older children.[11] Smaller lesions, earlier onset, and a more favorable location (classic

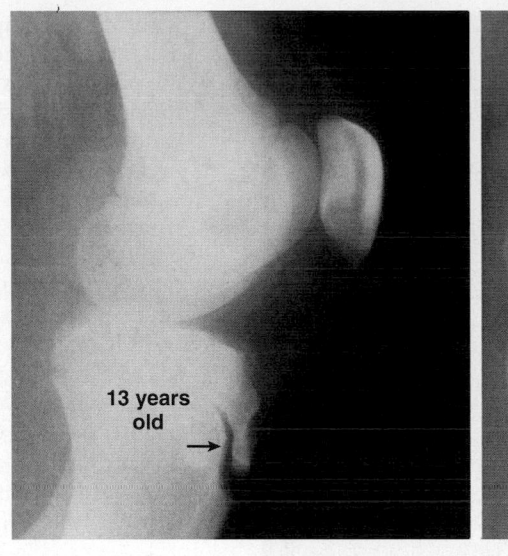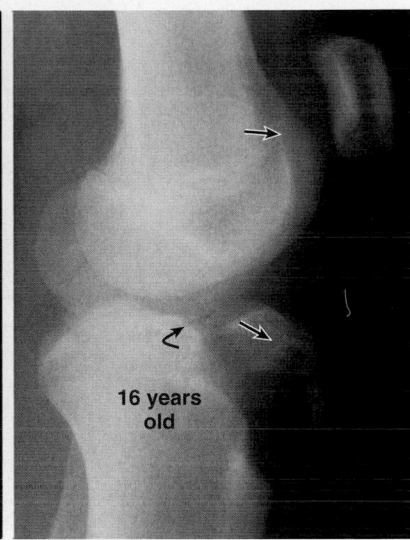

FIGURE 98–3. A, Osgood-Schlatter changes (*arrow*) in a 13-year-old male. **B,** Acute tibial tubercle avulsion fracture 3 years later in the same patient, predisposed to fracture due to Osgood-Schlatter history. *Top arrow* shows patella alta; *curved arrows* show fragment displacement and patellar tendon avulsion fragment. (From DeLee J, Drez D [eds]: DeLee & Drez's Orthopaedic Sports Medicine, 2nd ed. Philadelphia: WB Saunders, 2003, p 1768.)

13 years old

16 years old

A

B

Osgood-Schlatter Disease (Tibial Tubercle Apophysitis)

Osgood-Schlatter disease or tibial tubercle apophysitis is one of the most frequently diagnosed overuse injuries in children. Repeated contraction of the quadriceps muscle results in injury of the tibial tubercle.[7] It occurs in children 10 to 15 years old, with onset in girls preceding that of boys by approximately 2 years.[4,12] Signs and symptoms include pain, tenderness, and swelling over the tibial tubercle. Pain may worsen with jumping sports, climbing stairs, or rising from a seated position.[7] Radiographs are not needed but may show soft tissue swelling or fragmentation of the tibial tubercle (Fig. 98–3).

Treatment includes local pressure, anti-inflammatory medications, ice, and rest. Severe pain may require a 1- to 2-week period of knee immobilization. Resolution may be slow, often taking 12 to 18 months.[12] Once the growth plate is closed, persistent pain may indicate a residual ossicle. Surgical excision of the tubercle may relieve pain.[13] Although the disease is generally self-limited, patients with the disease may go on to experience some level of disability with sports activity later in life.[14]

Sinding-Larsen-Johansson Disease and Jumper's Knee

Sinding-Larsen-Johansson (SLJ) disease is an apophysitis that typically occurs in children 10 to 13 years old. Its cause is repetitive tensile stress at the junction of the patella and patellar tendon with subsequent calcification and ossification of the inferior aspect of the patella. Patients may describe a subtle onset of pain and demonstrate palpable pain isolated to the inferior pole of the patella (allowing it to be easily distinguished from Osgood-Schlatter disease). Pain occurs during jumping, climbing, or kneeling or with direct trauma to the area. Radiographs may show fragmentation of the distal pole of the patella, but imaging is not needed for diagnosis. Treatment includes rest, anti-inflammatory medica-

tions, and quadriceps flexibility exercises.[15] Resolution typically occurs in 6 to 12 months.[12]

Although commonly combined in the category of SLJ, patellar tendonitis or "jumper's knee" is thought to occur from partial thickness tears of the patella tendon.[4] It is characterized by proximal patellar tendon pain and tenderness on palpation. This entity may result in long-lasting symptoms.[16] A progressive exercise plan for drop squats and quadricep extension and hamstring exercises has been reported to successfully reduce pain at 12 weeks.[17] Occasionally, surgical repair may be necessary to relieve symptoms.[18]

Illiotibial Band Syndrome

The illiotibial band extends from the tensor fascia lata and inserts on the lateral aspect of the proximal tibia. This band changes position during knee extension, snapping forward over the lateral condyle from its posterior location behind the lateral epicondyle when the knee is flexed. The movement is only detectable when there is inflammation. Running with a high step (e.g., up and down stairs) elicits pain. A positive Noble test is diagnostic: the physician places a thumb over the lateral femoral epicondyle and actively flexes and extends the knee with the patient supine. Pain over the epicondyle is reproduced when the knee is in 20 to 30 degrees of flexion.[2] Radiographs are generally not necessary. Treatment includes rest, anti-inflammatory medications, and reduction of all activities that involve heavy weight bearing. Local corticosteroid injection has been described in adults with recent onset of symptoms, but is not well described in children.[19]

Sever's Disease (Calcaneal Apophysitis)

This overuse injury occurs at the insertion of the Achilles tendon into the secondary ossification center of the calcaneus from repetitive traction, subsequent inflammation, and fragmentation. Whether the injury represents a true metaphyseal trabecular stress fracture or an apophysitis is controversial.[20] The patient typically complains of heel pain that worsens during activity. Physical examination is remarkable for pain that is elicited by lateral and medial pressure on the calcaneus. Radiographs often show fragmentation and sclerosis

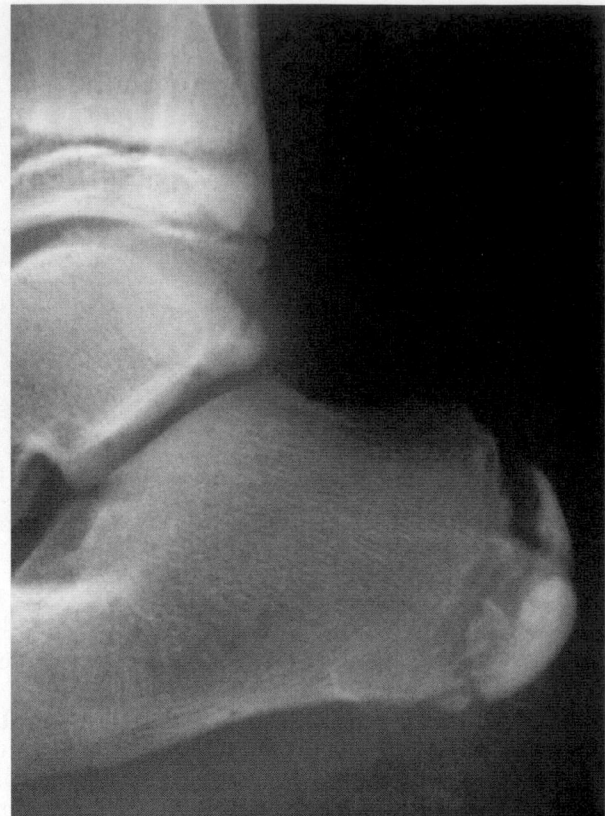

FIGURE 98–4. Sever's disease in an 11-year-old male with fragmentation of the calcaneal apophysis. (From Green NE, Swiontkowski MF [eds]: Skeletal Trauma in Children, 3rd ed. Philadelphia: WB Saunders, 2003, p 540.)

of the secondary ossification center (Fig. 98–4). A return to sports can be expected in approximately 2 months if patients adhere to a treatment regimen that includes rest, anti-inflammatory medications, Achilles tendon stretching exercises, and orthotics.[21]

Plantar Fasciitis

Pain at the insertion of the plantar fascia into the calcaneus is suggestive of plantar fasciitis. Patients often complain of heel pain after a period of inactivity that gradually subsides with increased activity (e.g., inactivity at bedtime with pain on awakening). However, the pain will become continuous when untreated. If the pain becomes acutely severe, a partial or complete disruption of the plantar fascia or nerve entrapment may have occurred.[7] With the ankle stabilized, pain with dorsiflexion of the first metatarsophalangeal joint is a highly specific but low-sensitivity test for plantar fasciitis.[22] Radiographs are usually normal. Treatment primarily involves ice, anti-inflammatory medications, rest, and gradual reintroduction of activity. Non–weight-bearing stretching exercise specific to the plantar fascia has been shown to improve symptoms in patients with chronic pain within 8 weeks.[23]

Medial Tibial Stress Syndrome (Periostitis)

Medial tibial stress syndrome (MTSS) is a common cause of shin pain. It results from repetitive forceful pronation and plantar flexion of the foot leading to periosteal inflammation along the tibia at the insertion of the soleus muscle. Patients with MTSS complain of diffuse pain along the middle and distal third of the posteromedial aspect of the tibia. Initially the pain resolves with exercise and returns with rest, but, as the problem persists, the pain will increase with activity. Pain can be elicited with ankle plantar flexion against resistance, by having the patient stand on the toes, or by asking the patient to jump in place. The pain of MTSS is diffuse in contrast to that of stress fractures, which is localized with point tenderness over the bone. The location of pain in addition to the adjunct of normal radiographs and a normal neurovascular examination assure the diagnosis. Treatment includes ice and rest (generally for a 3- to 4-week period).[24] MTSS can progress to a stress fracture, so athletes should not be allowed to "work through the pain." Many variables contribute to the development of MTSS; therefore, preventative measures, including proper shoes, evaluation of running surfaces, and stretching and strengthening exercises, are useful in preventing further injury.[7]

Köhler's Disease

Also known as tarsal navicular osteochondritis, this disease affects younger children (<9 years old). Pain occurs in the midfoot, and physical examination is remarkable for point tenderness overlying the navicular bone. Radiographic changes, depending on the stage of the disease, may show initial collapse of bone, patchy deossification, or a reconstituted navicular bone.[12] The disease is self-limited and responds to rest, ice, and anti-inflammatory medications. Application of a cast that allows weight bearing for a brief period may be required for patients with severe symptoms.[25]

Spine Injuries

Pediatric athletes presenting with back pain are more likely than adult patients to have a pathologic cause for their symptoms.[26] Athletes who participate in sports with axial stresses are susceptible to injuries of the spine and may commonly experience back pain.

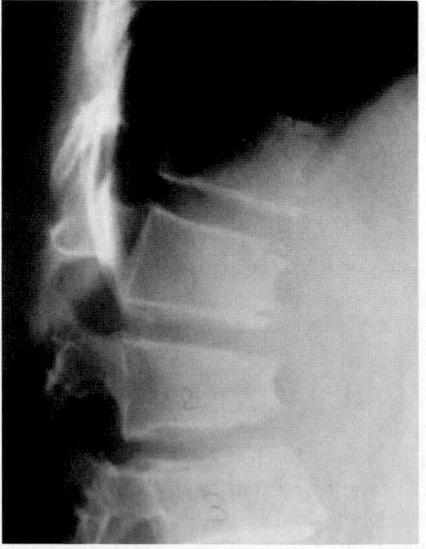

FIGURE 98–5. Scheuermann's disease in a 12-year-old female gymnast with chronic back pain. Note anterior wedging of three adjacent vertebrate (T12, L1, and L2). (From Green NE, Swiontkowski MF [eds]: Skeletal Trauma in Children, 3rd ed. Philadelphia: WB Saunders, 2003, p 51.)

Spondylolysis

Spondylolysis results from repetitive loading of the lumbar spine with a resultant stress reaction and defects of the pars interarticularis. The stress fracture of the pars interarticularis is usually at the level of L5. Although many hereditary risk factors may contribute to the development of the lesion, it is believed that repetitive hyperextension and lateral flexion of the spine during strenuous exercises and torsion against resistance contribute to this injury.[27] During a period of rapid adolescent growth, patients complain of dull back pain. Physical examination reveals pain overlying the lumbar paraspinal region. Rest alleviates pain except in progressive disease. The pars fracture may be seen on oblique radiographs, but a bone scan offers a definitive diagnosis.

Longitudinal studies demonstrate that early diagnosis is essential to the complete resolution of symptoms as conservative measures alone allow young athletes to regain full function in 4 to 6 weeks.[28,29] If under-arm bracing and limitation of movement do not improve symptoms, or if the disease is identified too late in its progression, surgical intervention may be needed.[30,31] Abdominal and hamstring strengthening exercises provide spinal support and can sometimes prevent progression of disease.

Juvenile Kyphosis (Scheuermann's Disease)

Repetitive axial loading (e.g., weight lifting) produces trauma that injures the apophyses of the involved vertebrae, causing an increase in the normal thoracic kyphosis or a decrease in the normal lumbar lordosis of the spine. Most patients are asymptomatic or have mild pain, but a progressive deformity of the spine causes them to seek medical attention. The diagnosis is confirmed by classic radiographic findings that include anterior wedging of three or more adjacent vertebrae (Fig. 98–5). Treatment regimens for the patient who is experiencing pain should include flexibility and strengthening exercises, and bracing for severe kyphosis (>50 degrees).[32] Operative spinal correction is only necessary with progressive thoracic kyphosis.

Summary

Musculoskeletal pain in the young athlete should never be overlooked. The diagnosis of most overuse injuries is suggested by the history of the offending activity and the risk factors associated with various sports activities. Conservative management with rest, ice, and nonsteroidal analgesia is adequate acute treatment for most overuse injuries in children. A plan for initial rest with gradual return of activity, and educating families on developmentally appropriate training programs, equipment, and facilities, should be addressed with all overuse injuries. The earlier most overuse injuries are diagnosed and treated, the better the prognosis.

REFERENCES

*1. Andrish JT: Upper extremity injuries in the skeletally immature athlete. *In* Nicholas JA, Hershman EB (eds): The Upper Extremity in Sports Medicine. St. Louis: Mosby, 1990, pp 676–678.

2. Dugan S, Weber K: Selected topics in sports medicine. Dis Mon 48:572–616, 2002.

3. Gómez JE: Upper extremity injuries in youth sports. Pediatr Clin North Am 49:593–626, 2002.

*4. Hogan KA, Gross RH: Overuse injuries in pediatric athletes. Orthop Clin North Am 34:405–415, 2003.

5. Walter KD, Congeni JA: Don't let Little League shoulder or elbow sideline your patient permanently. Contemp Pediatr 21:69–88, 2004.

6. Carson WG Jr, Gasser SI: Little Leaguer's shoulder: a report of 23 cases. Am J Sports Med 26:575–580, 1998.

7. Christopher NC, Congeni J: Overuse injuries in the pediatric athlete: evaluation, initial management, and strategies for prevention. Clin Pediatr Emerg Med 3:118–128, 2002.

8. Singer KM, Roy SP: Osteochondrosis of the humeral capitellum. Am J Sports Med 12:351–360, 1984.

9. Kobayashi K, Burton KJ, Rodner C, et al: Lateral compression injuries in the pediatric elbow: Panner's disease and osteochondritis dissecans of the capitellum. J Am Acad Orthop Surg 12:246–254, 2004.

10. Carr KE: Musculoskeletal injuries in young athletes. Clin Fam Pract 5(2):1–21, 2003.

11. Hefti F, Bequiristain J, Krauspe R, et al: Osteochondritis dissecans: a multicenter study of the European Pediatric Orthopedic Society. J Pediatr Orthop B 8:231–245, 1999.

12. Staheli LT: Fundamentals of Pediatric Orthopedics, 3rd ed. Philadelphia: Lippincott Williams & Wilkins, 2003, pp 58–70.

13. Flowers MJ, Bhadreshwar DR: Tibial tuberosity excision for symptomatic Osgood-Schlatter disease. J Pediatr Orthop 15:292–297, 1995.

14. Ross MD, Villard D: Disability levels of college-aged men with a history of Osgood-Schlatter disease. J Strength Cond Res 17:659–663, 2003.

15. Medlar RC, Lyne ED: Sinding-Larsen-Johansson disease: its etiology and natural history. J Bone Joint Surg Am 60:1113–1116, 1978.

16. Kettunen JA, Kvist M, Alanen E, Kujala UM: Long-term prognosis for jumper's knee in male athletes: a prospective follow-up study. Am J Sports Med 30:689–692, 2002.

17. Cannell LJ, Taunton JE, Clement DB, et al: A randomised clinical trial of the efficacy of drop squats or leg extension/leg curl exercises to treat clinically diagnosed jumper's knee in athletes: pilot study. Br J Sport Med 35:60–64, 2001.

18. Ferretti A, Conteduca F, Camerucci E, Morelli F: Patellar tendinosis: a follow-up study of surgical treatment. J Bone Joint Surg Am 84:2179–2185, 2002.

19. Gunter P, Schwellnus MP: Local corticosteroid injection in iliotibial band friction syndrome in runners: a randomised controlled trial. Br J Sports Med 38:269–272, 2004.

20. Ogden JA, Ganey TM, Hill JD, Jaakkola JI: Sever's injury: a stress fracture of the immature calcaneal metaphysis. J Pediatr Orthop 24:488–492, 2004.

21. Micheli LF, Ireland ML: Prevention and management of calcaneal apophysitis in children: an overuse syndrome. J Pediatr Orthop 7:34–38, 1987.

22. De Garceau D, Dean D, Requejo SM, Thordarson DB: The association between diagnosis of plantar fasciitis and Windlass test results. Foot Ankle Int 24:251–255, 2003.

23. DiGiovanni BF, Nawoczenski DA, Lintal ME, et al: Tissue-specific plantar fascia-stretching exercise enhances outcomes in patients with chronic heel pain: a prospective, randomized study. J Bone Joint Surg Am 85:1270–1277, 2003.

24. Metzl JD, Metzl JA: Shin pain in an adolescent soccer player: a case based look at shin splints. Contemp Pediatr 21:36–48, 2004.

25. Borges JL, Guille JT, Bowen JR: Köhler's bone disease of the tarsal navicular. J Pediatr Orthop 15:596–598, 1995.

*26. Waicus KM, Smith BW: Back injuries in the pediatric athlete. Curr Sports Med Rep 1(1):52–58, 2002.

27. Soler T, Calderon C: The prevalence of spondylolysis in the Spanish elite athlete. Am J Sports Med 28:57–62, 2000.

28. Miller SF, Congeni J, Swanson K: Long-term functional and anatomical follow-up of early detected spondylolysis in young athletes. Am J Sports Med 32:928–933, 2004.

29. d'Hemecourt PA, Zurakowski D, Kriemler S, Micheli LJ: Spondylolysis: returning the athlete to sports participation with brace treatment. Orthopedics 25:653–657, 2002.

30. Reitman CA, Esses SI: Direct repair of spondylolytic defects in young competitive athletes. Spine J 2:142–144, 2002.

31. Lim MR, Yoon SC, Green DW: Symptomatic spondylolysis: diagnosis and treatment. Curr Opin Pediatr 16:37–46, 2004.

32. Riddle EC, Bowen JR, Shah SA, et al: The duPont kyphosis brace for the treatment of adolescent Scheuermann kyphosis. J South Orthop Assoc 12:135–140, 2003.

*Selected readings.

Chapter 99

Rhabdomyolysis

Nicole S. Sroufe, MD, MPH and Rachel M. Stanley, MD, MHSA

Key Points

The classic triad of rhabdomyolysis includes myalgias, muscle weakness, and dark urine (myoglobinuria).

Elevations in creatine kinase are diagnostic of rhabdomyolysis, but are not prognostic.

A urinalysis positive for blood with the absence of red blood cells occurs in rhabdomyolysis.

The mainstay of therapy for rhabdomyolysis is aggressive hydration, alkalinization of the urine, and adequate diuresis to prevent the development of acute renal failure.

Introduction and Background

Rhabdomyolysis is a potentially lethal syndrome that occurs after skeletal muscle injury with release of intracellular myocyte contents into extracellular fluid, resulting in elevations of serum myoglobin, creatine kinase (CK), lactate dehydrogenase (LDH), aldolase, aspartate aminotransferase, and alanine aminotransferase.[1-7] Rhabdomyolysis was defined by Gabow as any condition resulting in a fivefold or greater rise in serum CK (in the absence of brain or heart disease).[1,8] However, others have defined rhabdomyolysis by elevations of CK from at least 3- to more than 100-fold, the upper limit of normal.[8]

As a result of skeletal muscle injury with loss of integrity of the myocyte, several physiologic alterations occur, including hyperkalemia, hyperphosphatemia, hyperuricemia, hypocalcemia, metabolic acidosis, hypoalbuminemia, and myoglobinuria.[1,2,8,9] These electrolyte derangements contribute to the multiple complications that occur in patients with rhabdomyolysis. Many complications may arise in patients with rhabdomyolysis, including acute renal tubular necrosis, myoglobinuric renal failure, severe muscle necrosis, cardiac arrhythmias resulting in arrest, disseminated intravascular coagulation (DIC), lactic acidosis, and compartment syndrome.[2,5,9-13]

Recognition and Approach

Epidemiologic information regarding rhabdomyolysis in the pediatric population is limited given that no large case series have been reported. The list of disorders causing rhabdomyolysis is extensive (Table 99–1).

Rhabdomyolysis may occur in isolation, or in combination with other features diagnostic of specific syndromes. Heat stroke is defined by altered mental status in patients with core temperatures of 39.5° C or more, leading to multisystem organ failure, including circulatory collapse, liver failure, neurologic dysfunction, DIC, renal failure, and rhabdomyolysis.[14] In malignant hyperthermia, an autosomal dominant disorder of skeletal muscle, susceptible patients develop a potentially fatal hypermetabolic reaction with hyperthermia, muscle rigidity, tachycardia, metabolic acidosis, and rhabdomyolysis when exposed to depolarizing muscle relaxants and inhalation anesthetics, as well as extreme stress in the form of heat or exercise.[15-17] When neuroleptic malignant syndrome develops as an adverse effect of antipsychotic medication, patients experience muscle rigidity, hyperthermia, altered mental status, autonomic dysfunction, and rhabdomyolysis.[18] Rhabdomyolysis may also develop in patients with propofol infusion syndrome, characterized by the sudden onset of refractory bradycardia progressing to asystole, lipemia, fatty infiltration of the liver with hepatomegaly, and severe metabolic acidosis.[19,20]

Rhabdomyolysis may develop acutely in otherwise healthy children, or intermittently in children affected by myopathies, muscular dystrophies, and metabolic derangements.[10] Many acquired illnesses, including infections secondary to viral or bacterial agents, have resulted in the development of rhabdomyolysis.[3,4,11,12,21-25] Medications, exposure to toxins, and the use of drugs of abuse have also resulted in the development of rhabdomyolysis.[7,9,15-20,26-38] Traumatic injury with insult to muscle tissue secondary to nonaccidental trauma, immobilization, crush injury, electrical injury, burns, and ischemic injury may also result in rhabdomyolysis[10,13,39-42] (see Chapter 26, Burns; Chapter 119, Physical Abuse and Child Neglect; and Chapter 142, Electrical Injury). Conditions resulting in hyperthermia predispose patients to the development of rhabdomyolysis, as does exertion in the untrained/unconditioned athlete or in individuals with sickle cell trait.[2,14-18,43,44] Metabolic derangements, including diabetic ketoacidosis, nonketotic hyperosmolar coma, hypothyroidism/

Table 99–1	Nonexhaustive List of Precipitating Factors of Rhabdomyolysis in Children

Viral Infections

Coxsackie virus
Echovirus
Epstein-Barr virus
Influenza virus types A and B
Varicella-zoster virus

Bacterial Infections

Clostridium tetani
Coxiella burnetti
Group B streptococcus
Mycoplasma pneumoniae
Neisseria meningitides
Salmonella enteritidis
Staphylococcus aureus

Medications

Acetaminophen
Amoxapine
Amphotericin B
Anticholinergics
Antipsychotics
Barbiturates
Benzodiazepines
Colchicine
Corticosteroids
Cyclosporine
Diphenhydramine
Diuretics
Haloperidol
Inhalation anesthetics
Isoniazid
Ketamine
Lithium
Loxapine
Narcotics
Pemoline
Phenytoin
Propofol
Serotonin antagonists
Statins
Succinylcholine
Suxamethonium
Sympathomimetics
Tacrolimus
Theophylline
Tricyclic antidepressants
Trimethoprim-sulfamethoxazole

Drugs of Abuse

Caffeine
Cocaine
Ecstasy
Ethanol
Heroin
Methamphetamine
Phencyclidine

Withdrawal Syndromes

Alcohol
Intrathecal baclofen
Sedative-hypnotics

Toxic Substances

Barium
Carbon monoxide poisoning
Cyanide
Hydrogen sulfide
Rattlesnake venom
Strychnine

Trauma

Crush injury
Electrical injury/lightning strikes
Immobilization
Ischemic injury
Nonaccidental trauma/child abuse
Third-degree burns
Traumatic positioning

Hyperthermia

Heatstroke
Malignant hyperthermia
Neuroleptic malignant syndrome

Exertion

Exercise-induced (running or weight training)
Exertion in patients with sickle cell trait

Metabolic/Endocrine

Diabetic ketoacidosis
Electrolyte imbalances (hypernatremia/hyponatremia, hypokalemia, hypophosphatemia, hypocalcemia)
Hyperthyroidism/hypothyroidism
Nonketotic hyperosmolar coma

Genetic

Disorders of carbohydrate metabolism
Disorders of fatty acid metabolism (carnitine palmitoyltransferase I or II deficiency, very-long-chain acyl-coenzyme A dehydrogenase deficiency, medium-chain acyl-coenzyme A dehydrogenase deficiency)
Muscular dystrophies

Miscellaneous

Adrenoleukodystrophy
Dermatomyositis
Hypothermia
Idiopathic
Polymyositis

hyperthyroidism, and electrolyte imbalances, may also precipitate rhabdomyolysis[10,41,42,45,46] (see Chapter 105, Diabetic Ketoacidosis; Chapter 109, Thyrotoxicosis; Chapter 110, Dehydration and Disorders of Sodium Balance; Chapter 111, Metabolic Acidosis; and Chapter 114, Hyperkalemia). Children with disorders of metabolism and myopathies often present with intermittent rhabdomyolysis and myoglobinuria.[1,5,11,15,35,41,45,47]

A 3-year retrospective study of neurology consultations at the University of California, San Diego, demonstrated an incidence of childhood rhabdomyolysis of 0.26% of hospital admissions.[11] A retrospective review of children admitted to the Medical College of Virginia during an 8-year period identified 19 cases of rhabdomyolysis (excluding intermittent/relapsing rhabdomyolysis) with causes ranging from trauma (5 cases), nonketotic hyperosmolar coma (2 cases), viral myositis (2 cases), dystonia (2 cases) and malignant hyperthermia–related conditions (2 cases), and additional cases resulting from hypernatremia, polymyositis, hypothermia, and muscle exertion.[10]

Clinical Presentation

Rhabdomyolysis is characterized by the classic triad of myalgias, muscle weakness, and darkened urine, although a broad spectrum of symptoms and disease severity can occur.[5,7,43] Myoglobin released from myocytes after cell injury is partially excreted by the kidneys, resulting in the dark brown pigmentation of the urine.[7,8] Patients may report localized or diffuse muscle tenderness, weakness, and stiffness, and may develop muscle edema, skin changes consistent with pressure necrosis, or compartment syndrome.[2,5,10,12,19,43] Systemic symptoms including fever, malaise, nausea, and vomiting may be present, dependent on the underlying cause of muscle injury.[10,19]

Early in the disease course, patients may present only with myalgias and weakness without darkened urine, given that 100 g of muscle tissue must be injured before serum proteins become saturated and patients develop myoglobinuria.[7,8] As additional muscle is injured, serum myoglobin increases and myoglobinuria develops. Therefore, patients may be misdiagnosed as having merely a viral syndrome with myalgias. Conversely, patients presenting late in the disease course may present in acute, fulminant renal failure.[7] Patients presenting with lethargy or coma or as victims of severe trauma may be diagnosed with rhabdomyolysis much further into their disease course.[7,10]

Serum CK is the most sensitive biochemical indicator of myocyte injury, and should be measured to assess for rhabdomyolysis.[1,5,43,48] The MM fraction of CK reflects skeletal muscle injury; CK begins to rise within 2 hours of myocyte injury, peaks within 12 to 36 hours, and decreases by 40% each day after the insult to muscle tissue ceases.[1,5,7,43] Rhabdomyolysis may be present with elevations of CK from as little as 3- to more than 100-fold the upper limit of normal.[8] Although CK is highly sensitive for identifying myocyte injury, elevations of CK are not predictive of disease severity, or of progression to myoglobinuric renal failure.[1,10,48]

Additional laboratory studies provide support for the diagnosis of rhabdomyolysis, but are not diagnostic. Careful evaluation of the dipstick urinalysis can provide valuable clues indicative of myocyte injury. A positive urine dipstick for blood with no, or very few, red blood cells visualized with microscopy is suggestive of myoglobinuria, and should prompt an investigation for the presence of rhabdomyolysis.[7,10,12,43] Myoglobinuria can be confirmed with direct measurement of myoglobin in the urine. Myoglobin may also be quantitated in serum, increasing quickly after myocyte injury, and normalizing within 1 to 6 hours of the cessation of cellular injury.[10] Given the short half-life of myoglobin, it is not reliable in confirming the diagnosis of rhabdomyolysis. In fact, nearly 50% of patients with rhabdomyolysis do not have myoglobinuria on presentation.[5,7] Myoglobinuria may be the only feature that cues the clinician to consider the diagnosis of rhabdomyolysis. However, myoglobinuria is not predictive of the development of renal failure.[1]

Serum electrolytes, LDH, aminotransferases, and creatinine should be assessed in the evaluation for rhabdomyolysis, as myocyte injury results in the release of potassium, phosphorus, purines, and LDH from muscle tissue.[7,8,12,19,43] Serum aldolase is also elevated.[7,8,12] Additionally, renal function should be evaluated, given that myoglobinuria results in acute tubular necrosis with potential for renal failure.[3,5,9-11,43]

Additional disorders of muscle tissue may present with myalgias and weakness, including autoimmune disorders, genetic defects of metabolism, and dermatomyositis, requiring further investigation based on clinical suspicion[5] (see Chapter 95, Musculoskeletal Disorders in Systemic Disease; and Chapter 97, Muscle and Connective Tissue Disorders). Additionally, inflammatory conditions in localized muscle tissue may present with muscle pain. Myositis, inflammation of muscle secondary to infection of deep fascial and muscle planes, and pyomyositis, a bacterial infection of skeletal muscle resulting in abscess formation, should be differentiated from rhabdomyolysis, which is a noninflammatory condition.[3,49]

Important Clinical Features and Considerations

Early recognition of rhabdomyolysis is paramount to prevent potentially fatal complications. The most common and potentially devastating complication of rhabdomyolysis is acute renal failure. The incidence of acute renal failure in children ranges from 5–42%.[1,10,50] A recent retrospective review of 191 children with rhabdomyolysis reported that the risk of acute renal failure in this series was much less than the risk reported for adults.[50] Renal failure develops as a result of myoglobin casts obstructing renal tubules, decreased glomerular filtration rate, and the direct nephrotoxic effects of myoglobin by-products.[3,5,7,9-11,43] In an acidic milieu, with a pH less than 5.6, myoglobin dissociates into ferrihemate and globin.[5] Ferrihemate is directly nephrotoxic, impairs renal tubular transport, and produces additional renal injury secondary to the production of free hydroxyl radicals.[7,43] Patients with urinary pH less than 5.6, hypovolemia, and metabolic acidosis are at greater risk for the development of renal failure.

The release of intracellular potassium from myocytes results in hyperkalemia. Hypocalcemia develops due to the deposition of calcium in injured tissues and is exaggerated by the formation of calcium-phosphorus precipitants resulting from hyperphosphatemia.[2,5,7,11,43] These electrolyte imbalances place patients at risk for cardiac arrhythmias and arrest.[2,5,7,10,43,50] Interestingly, patients with rhabdomyolysis secondary to heatstroke are less likely to develop hyperkalemia given the presence of a respiratory alkalosis, increased sweating, and overproduction of aldosterone.[14] These patients commonly present with normal serum potassium levels or hypokalemia.[14]

DIC may develop in patients with rhabdomyolysis, further complicating their course and management.[2,5,7] Compartment syndrome also may develop as a result of fluid accumulation in muscle tissue secondary to intracellular fluid shifts.[7]

Management

Standard protocols for the management of rhabdomyolysis do not exist, and no randomized controlled trials have been carried out to evaluate the efficacy of current recommended therapies. Attention should be focused on primary resuscitation efforts, ensuring adequate ventilation and circulation.[5,7,43] All patients require continuous cardiac monitoring, frequent assessment of vital signs, and monitoring of urine output. An appropriate evaluation to determine the cause of muscle injury must be completed to identify and treat potential causes of myocyte destruction (hyperthermia/hypothermia, electrolyte abnormalities, metabolic derangements, toxins, hypovolemia)[5,7,43] (see Chapter 111, Metabolic Acidosis; Chapter 114, Hyperkalemia; and Chapter 139, Hyperthermia).

The mainstay of therapy for rhabdomyolysis is aggressive hydration with isotonic saline to restore intravascular volume, induce diuresis, and prevent renal failure.[5,9,11,43] Urine output must be closely monitored and adequate urine output maintained (>2 to 3 ml/kg per hour) to reduce the risk of acute tubular necrosis. Sodium bicarbonate administration is recommended to alkalinize the urine to a pH greater than 6.0 to prevent the breakdown of myoglobin into ferrihemate, preventing ferrihemate precipitation in the renal tubules.[7-9,14,43,50] To further induce diuresis and prevent oliguric renal failure, osmotic agents are recommended.[9,11,14,43] Mannitol (0.5 to 1 g/kg intravenously [IV] initially, followed by 0.25 to 0.5 g/kg IV every 4 to 6 hours) and furosemide (1 mg/kg IV every 6 hours) have been used successfully to induce diuresis in patients with rhabdomyolysis.[9,11,14,43]

In addition to ensuring adequate hydration and renal perfusion, electrolyte disturbances that occur secondary to muscle injury must be aggressively treated. Treatment of hyperkalemia must be a priority, and appropriate therapy should be instituted promptly (see Chapter 114, Hyperkalemia).[5,11,43] If oliguric renal failure or persistent electrolyte disturbances develop, dialysis may be required.[43] However, dialysis does not prevent acute renal failure as myoglobin is not a dialyzable substance.[11] Early consultation with a pediatric nephrologist is encouraged when managing rhabdomyolysis in patients with renal insufficiency and failure.

Additional therapy may be required, specific to the complications that develop from rhabdomyolysis. DIC must be treated aggressively with platelets, coagulation factors, and other blood products to prevent further complications,[5] and the development of compartment syndrome will require appropriate surgical consultation with the potential need for fasciotomy.[7] If malignant hyperthermia (autosomal dominant patients with muscle rigidity after succinylcholine or anesthetic) or neuroleptic malignant syndrome are considerations, dantrolene (2 to 3 mg/kg IV) should be administered (see Chapter 139, Hyperthermia).

Summary

Rhabdomyolysis results from various insults to skeletal muscle via direct or indirect means. Given the potentially fatal complications, patients with rhabdomyolysis require aggressive treatment in an inpatient setting. The primary treatment goal is to prevent further skeletal muscle breakdown and the development of acute renal failure.[11] Additional data are needed in the pediatric population to better define the most appropriate approach to the management and care of children with rhabdomyolysis.

Given the limited data available in pediatric populations, the mortality secondary to rhabdomyolysis is not well defined. However, patients with myoglobinuric renal failure tend to have a better prognosis if hypotension is minimized and cortical necrosis avoided.[5] Some authors report a return of full muscle mass and function within 1 to 6 weeks of the initial insult, with variable degrees of residual weakness observed.[11]

REFERENCES

*1. Gabow P, Kaehny W, Kelleher S: The spectrum of rhabdomyolysis. Medicine 61:141–152, 1982.

2. Walsworth M, Kessler T: Diagnosing exertional rhabdomyolysis: a brief review and report of two cases. Mil Med 166:275–277, 2001.

3. Singh U, Scheld W: Infectious etiologies of rhabdomyolysis: three case reports and review. Clin Infect Dis 22:642–649, 1996.

4. Minami K, Maeda H, Yanagawa T, et al: Rhabdomyolysis associated with *Mycoplasma pneumoniae* infection. Pediatr Infect Dis J 22:291–293, 2003.

5. Will M, Hecker R, Wathen P: Primary varicella-zoster induced rhabdomyolysis. South Med J 89:915–920, 1996.

6. Osamah H, Finkelstein R, Brook J: Rhabdomyolysis complicating acute Epstein-Barr virus infection. Infection 23:119–120, 1995.

7. Coco T, Klasner A: Drug-induced rhabdomyolysis. Curr Opin Pediatr 16:206–210, 2004.

*8. Ng Y, Johnston H: Clinical rhabdomyolysis. J Paediatr Child Health 36:397–400, 2000.

9. Bush S, Jansen P: Severe rattlesnake envenomation with anaphylaxis and rhabdomyolysis. Ann Emerg Med 25:845–848, 1995.

*10. Watemberg N, Leshner R, Armstrong B, et al: Acute pediatric rhabdomyolysis. J Child Neurol 15:222–227, 2000.

*11. Chamberlain M: Rhabdomyolysis in children: a 3 year retrospective study. Ped Neurol 7:226–228, 1991.

12. Swaringen J, Seiler J, Bruce R: Influenza A induced rhabdomyolysis resulting in extensive compartment syndrome. Clin Orthop Relat Res 375:243–249, 2000.

13. Malinoski D, Slater M, Mullins R: Crush injury and rhabdomyolysis. Crit Care Clin 20:171–192, 2004.

14. Wang A, Li P, Lui S, et al: Renal failure and heatstroke. Ren Fail 17:171–179, 1995.

15. Pedrozzi N, Ramelli G, Tomasetti R, et al: Rhabdomyolysis and anesthesia: a report of two cases and review of the literature. Pediatr Neurol 15:254–257, 1996.

16. Kozack J, MacIntyre D: Malignant hyperthermia. Phys Ther 81:945–952, 2001.

17. Wappler F, Fiege M, Steinfath M, et al: Evidence for susceptibility to malignant hyperthermia in patients with exercise induced rhabdomyolysis. Anesthesiology 94:95–100, 2001.

18. Yoshikawa H, Watanabe T, Abe T, et al: Haloperidol-induced rhabdomyolysis without neuroleptic malignant syndrome in a handicapped child. Brain Dev 22:256–258, 2000.

19. Kang T: Propofol infusion syndrome in critically ill patients. Ann Pharmacother 36:1453–1456, 2002.

20. Hanna J, Ramundo M: Rhabdomyolysis and hypoxia associated with prolonged propofol infusion in children. Neurology 50:301–303, 1998.

21. Goebel J, Harter H, Boineau F, et al: Acute renal failure from rhabdomyolysis following influenza A in a child. Clin Pediatr 36:479–481, 1997.

22. Brook I: Tetanus in children. Pediatr Emerg Care 20:48–52, 2004.

23. Carrascosa M, Pascual F, Victoria M, et al: Rhabdomyolysis associated with acute Q fever. Clin Infect Dis 25:1243–1244, 1997.

24. Berger R, Wadowksy R: Rhabdomyolysis associated with infection by *Mycoplasma pneumoniae*: a case report. Pediatrics 105:433–436, 2000.

25. Karis C, Triantafyllidis G: Index of suspicion. Pediatr Rev 23:25, 27–28, 2002.

26. Stucka K, Mycyk M, Leikin J, et al: Rhabdomyolysis associated with unintentional antihistamine overdose in a child. Pediatr Emerg Care 19:25–26, 2003.

27. Cassidy J, Bolton D, Haynes S, et al: Acute rhabdomyolysis after cardiac transplantation: a diagnostic conundrum. Paediatr Anaesth 12:729–732, 2002.

28. Nakamura H, Blumer J, Reed M: Pemoline ingestion in children: a report of five cases and review of the literature. J Clin Pharmacol 42:275–282, 2002.

29. Panganiban L, Makalinao I, Cortes-Maramba N: Rhabdomyolysis in isoniazid poisoning. J Toxicol Clin Toxicol 39:143–151, 2001.

_____

*Selected readings.

30. Chattopadhyay I, Shetty H, Routledge P, et al: Colchicine induced rhabdomyolysis. Postgrad Med J 77:191–192, 2001.

31. Kalaria D, Wassenaar W: Rhabdomyolysis and cerivastatin: was it a problem of dose? CMAJ 167:737, 2002.

32. Halachanova V, Sansone R, McDonald S: Delayed rhabdomyolysis after ecstasy use. Mayo Clin Proc 76:112–113, 2001.

33. McCann B, Hunter R, McCann J: Cocaine/heroin induced rhabdomyolysis and ventricular fibrillation. Emerg Med J 19:264, 2002.

34. Johnson C, VanTassell V: Acute barium poisoning with respiratory failure and rhabdomyolysis. Ann Emerg Med 20:1138–1142, 1991.

35. Frankowski G, Johnson J, Tobias J: Rapacuronium administration to two children with Duchenne's muscular dystrophy. Pediatr Anesth 91:27–28, 2000.

36. Gronert G: Cardiac arrest after succinylcholine: mortality greater with rhabdomyolysis than receptor upregulation. Anesthesiology 94:523–529, 2001.

37. Hibi S, Misawa A, Tamai M, et al: Severe rhabdomyolysis associated with tacrolimus. Lancet 346:702, 1995.

38. Carroll R, Hall E, Kitchens C: Canebrake rattlesnake envenomation. Ann Emerg Med 30:45–48, 1997.

39. DiGiacomo J, Frankel H, Haskell R: Unsuspected child abuse revealed by delayed presentation of periportal tracking and myoglobinuria. J Trauma Injury Infect Crit Care 49:348–350, 2000.

40. Schwengel D, Ludwig S: Rhabdomyolysis and myoglobinuria as manifestations of child abuse. Pediatr Emerg Care 1:194–197, 1985.

41. Sauret J, Marinides G, Wang G: Rhabdomyolysis. Am Fam Physician 65:907–912, 2002.

42. Alshanti M, Eledrisis M, Jones E: Rhabdomyolysis associated with hyperthyroidism. Am J Emerg Med 19:317, 2001.

43. Moghtader J, Brady W, Bonadio W: Exertional rhabdomyolysis in an adolescent athlete. Pediatr Emerg Care 13:382–385, 1997.

44. Sherry P: Sickle cell trait and rhabdomyolysis: case report and review of the literature. Mil Med 155:59–61, 1990.

45. Hollander A, Olney R, Blackett P, et al: Fatal malignant hyperthermia-like syndrome with rhabdomyolysis complicating the presentation of diabetes mellitus in adolescent males. Pediatrics 111:1447–1452, 2003.

46. Pena D, Vaccarello M, Neiberger R: Severe hemolytic uremic syndrome associated with rhabdomyolysis and insulin-dependent diabetes mellitus. Child Nephrol Urol 11:223–227, 1991.

47. Straussberg R, Harel L, Varsano I, et al: Recurrent myoglobinuria as a presenting manifestation of very long chain acyl coenzyme A dehydrogenase deficiency. Pediatrics 99:894–896, 1997.

48. Lappalainen H, Tiula E, Uotila L, et al: Elimination kinetics of myoglobin and creatine kinase in rhabdomyolysis: implications for follow-up. Crit Care Med 30:2212–2215, 2002.

49. Falasca G, Reginato A: The spectrum of myositis and rhabdomyolysis associated with bacterial infection. J Rheumatol 21:1932–1937.

50. Mannix R, Tan ML, Wright R, Baskin M: Acute pediatric rhabdomyolysis: causes and rates of renal failure. Pediatrics 118:2119–2125, 2006.

51. Savage D, Forbes M, Pearce G: Idiopathic rhabdomyolysis. Arch Dis Child 46:594–607, 1971.

Diseases of the Hip

Ronald I. Paul, MD

Selected Diagnoses

Developmental dysplasia of the hip
Legg-Calvé-Perthes disease
Slipped capital femoral epiphysis
Transient synovitis of the hip

Discussion of Individual Diagnoses

Developmental Dyspasia of the Hip

Developmental dysplasia of the hip (DDH) describes a spectrum of diseases that result from abnormal formation of the hip joint during fetal development and the first few months of life. The term replaces the older and more traditional designation, "congenital dislocation of the hip," which was too narrow in its description. Many cases are not dislocated at the time of diagnosis, and not all cases are congenital. Although most cases are detected during routine newborn and early infancy examinations by a primary care physician, some cases either are not discovered early or have a delayed presentation.

Clinical Presentation

DDH is variable in its presentation, depending on the severity and age at diagnosis. Some newborn hip joints are simply loose or slide in the acetabulum and are referred to as being subluxatable. Other hip joints lie within the acetabulum, but are dislocatable as they can be manually displaced with an audible "click" or palpable "clunk." The least common but more severe form of DDH includes hips that are dislocated while at rest. They may or may not be able to be reduced with simple measures.

The incidence of hip dysplasia in neonates is thought to be 1%, with 0.1% dislocated.[1] However, routine ultrasonography of babies in England has shown up to a 6% incidence of abnormal hips, although 90% of these return to normal by 9 weeks of age.[2] DDH is found more often in white and less often in African American infants.[1] Female gender and family history of DDH are risk factors, and up to 25% of DDH infants are born breech.[2,3]

Because of the variability in presentation of DDH, clinical findings and appropriate diagnostic tests depend on the severity of dysplasia and patient age. Initially, parents may report difficulty in diapering an infant whose hips resist abduction. If not detected prior to walking, parents may notice gait asymmetry due to leg length differences. Eventually, pain in the hips and increasing limp will be noticed by the parent, patient, or physician.

The Ortolani and Barlow maneuvers have been the standard examination techniques used by physicians[4] (Fig. 100-1). Both techniques should be performed on calm infants as a crying infant's muscle tone may inhibit the subtle changes in DDH. In the Barlow maneuver, each hip should be flexed to 90 degrees while one hand stabilizes the other hip or pelvis. The thumb is placed on the medial thigh and the index and middle fingers are placed on the greater trochanter. The thigh is adducted and then pressure is applied longitudinally in a posterior direction in an attempt to dislocate the hip. A palpable clunk or audible click may occur with dislocation. The Ortolani maneuver is used to detect a hip that is dislocated by trying to reduce the dislocation. The thigh is flexed and abducted and the femoral head is lifted anteriorly into the acetabulum. If reduction is possible, the relocation will be felt as a clunk, not heard as a click. Loose hips may be detected by increased laxity in the hip joint.

Ortolani or Barlow maneuvers become more difficult to detect as the infant ages beyond 4 to 6 months because soft tissue contractures develop as the hip becomes more fixed in place. After this time, the infant may have a hip dislocation with severe limitations of abduction along with other signs, including leg-length discrepancy and asymmetric thigh skinfolds.

Although most cases are diagnosed clinically, radiographs and ultrasonography (US) have been helpful in confirming the diagnosis.[5] Some centers recommend routine US of all

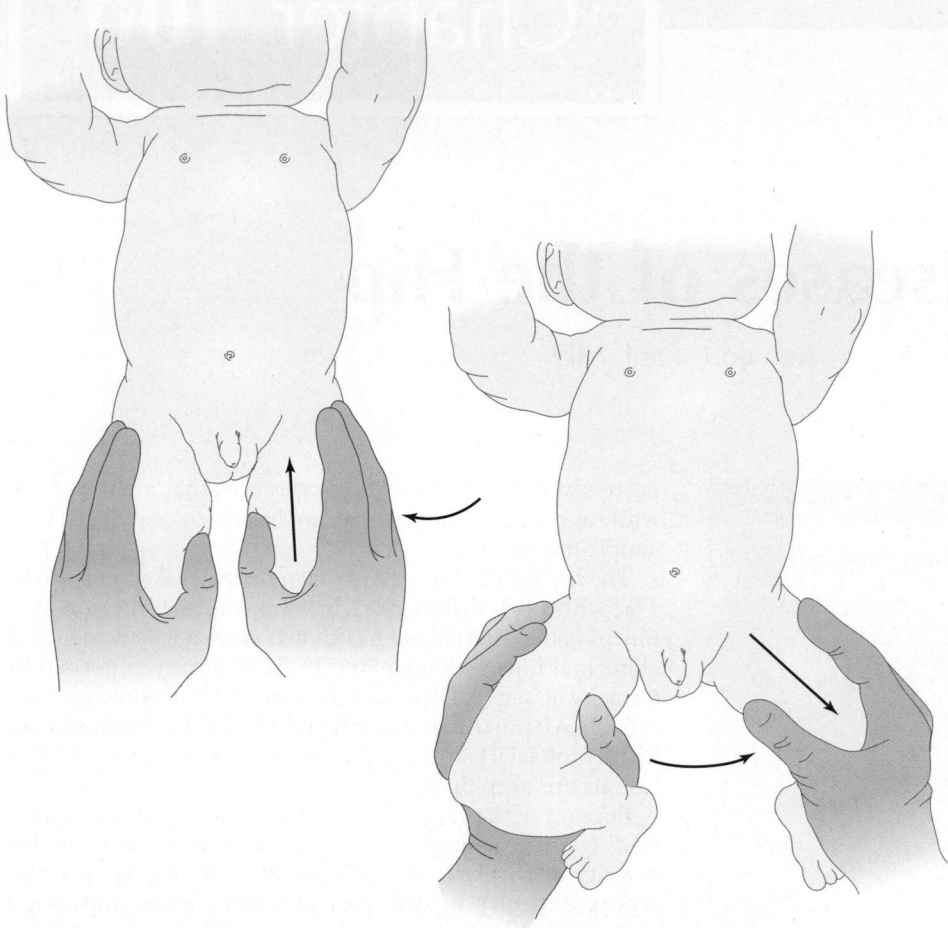

FIGURE 100–1. Ortolani **(right)** and Barlow **(left)** tests for detecting development dysplasia of the hip.

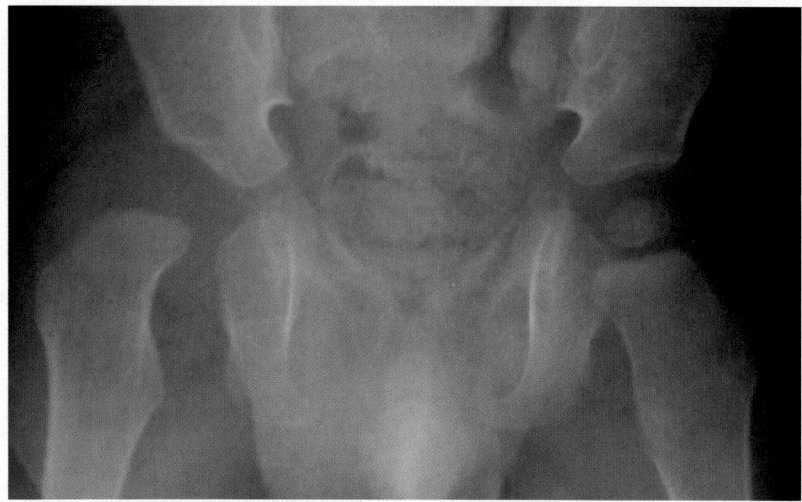

FIGURE 100–2. Radiograph of a 17-month-old infant with congenital dislocation of the right hip. There is delayed ossification of the femoral epiphysis and an abnormal position of the femoral metaphysis.

infants for DDH. However, US is not routinely performed in the United States since it may be too sensitive for mild hip dyplasia, and many cases will resolve spontaneously.[1,2,5] Therefore, clinical examination is the primary method of diagnosis until 4 to 6 weeks of age. Ultrasound may be helpful at that time if clinical examination results warrant it. Plain radiographs of the pelvis are helpful, but only after the femoral head starts to ossify at about 4 months of age.[5] Prior to 4 months of age, plain radiographs may be difficult to interpret and falsely reassuring. Abnormal position or delayed ossification of the femoral head may be seen in older patients with DDH (Fig. 100–2).

The differential diagnosis of DDH is broad. Consideration should be given to causes of abnormal hip movement or abnormal resting position of hips. The list includes trauma, septic joints, and contractures caused by cerebral palsy (see Chapter 20, Lower Extremity Trauma; Chapter 21, Pelvic and Genitourinary Trauma; Chapter 46, Disorders of Movement; and Chapter 47, Peripheral Neuromuscular Disorders). An older child who presents with unrecognized DDH and a limp should be investigated for metatarsus adduction, internal tibial torsion, Legg-Calvé-Perthes (LCP) disease, slipped capital femoral epiphysis, and transient synovitis of the hip. The workup will depend on patient age and other associated symptoms and physical findings.

Management

Once the diagnosis is made, management is directed by orthopedic consultants. Treatment is more successful when DDH is recognized earlier in its course. Mild laxity that is recognized in the first few days of life may not need therapy if the follow-up examination becomes normal. If symptoms persist, the main therapy is a Pavlik harness, which splints the leg in flexion and abduction. The splint prevents hip extension and limits adduction. If unsuccessful, a hip spica cast may be necessary. Infants older than 6 months may need closed reduction of a dislocated hip under general anesthesia. If unsuccessful, open reduction or femoral osteotomies may be needed. Prognosis is excellent if diagnosed early in the newborn period. Untreated patients are at risk for osteoarthritis, gait disturbances, leg length discrepancies, and chronic pain.

Legg-Calvé-Perthes Disease

LCP disease, named after the three physicians who first described this disorder in the early 1900s, is a sequence of events that includes ischemic hip degeneration and subsequent regeneration that takes place in young children over several years. Although the disease is self limited and usually has a benign outcome during childhood and adolescence, many patients develop significant osteoarthritis later in life. The etiology of LCP disease is unclear, and the disease may have a hormonal or an abnormal blood viscosity or clotting origin.[6,7] The end result is an ischemic insult to the developing femoral head resulting in necrosis.

The disease occurs in a young age group, with 80% of patients between 4 and 9 years of age, and an outer range of 2 to 13 years of age.[8] The disease is more common in males than females and there is an increased incidence in siblings.[7] Birth weight below 2.5 kg, short stature, and delayed skeletal maturation have also been shown to be risk factors. About 10% of patients will develop bilateral disease.

Clinical Presentation

Children with this disease generally present with pain or a limp. Pain may be localized to the hip, groin, thigh, or knee. Parents may relate the pain or limp to minor trauma. Pain onset is usually not abrupt, but develops over days to months. Physical examination may show a limp (antalgic gait) secondary to either pain or a leg-length discrepancy. The length of both legs should be measured and compared in the supine position by measuring from the anterior superior iliac spine to the medial malleolus. The patient may also have pain with external hip rotation, and limited internal rotation and abduction.

Radiographs are the most common method for confirming a diagnosis. The diseased hip joint will progress through several stages, and radiographs will demonstrate different findings. Initially, anteroposterior and frog-leg lateral pelvic radiographs will demonstrate a smaller femoral head compared to the contralateral normal hip. A widened joint space may also be apparent. Within several months, a crescent-shaped radiolucent line may appear in the femoral head as it becomes more radiopaque. Following this, the epiphysis becomes fragmented (Fig. 100–3). Finally, reossification takes place, which may leave a residual deformity in both the femoral head and corresponding acetabulum. The entire process may take 2 to 4 years. Magnetic resonance imaging (MRI) has been used to evaluate children with LCP disease. With MRI, cartilaginous and metaphyseal abnormalities can be seen. The thickness of the articular cartilage of the femoral head has been shown to be increased in LCP disease and may be associated with loss of containment of the femoral head. Importantly, MRI has been shown to be more sensitive than radiography for the determination of subluxation of the femoral head during the active phase of LCP disease.[9]

The differential diagnosis of patients with LCP disease is large and includes inflammatory disorders, trauma, neoplasias, and congenital abnormalities. DDH also may occur in this age group, especially if it is unrecognized in infancy.

Management

Since the disease is self-limiting and resolves in 2 to 4 years, initial treatment is aimed at reducing pain. This may be

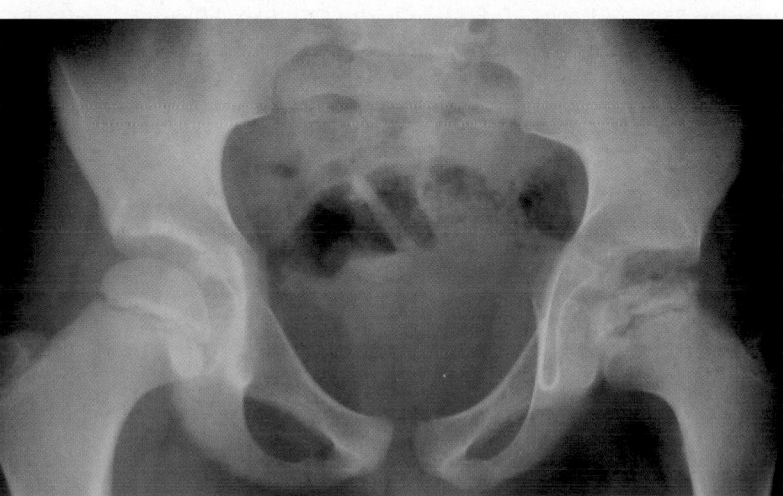

FIGURE 100–3. Radiograph of an 8-year-old boy with left hip pain. There is fragmentation of the left femoral head demonstrating Legg-Calvé-Perthes disease.

accomplished with nonsteroidal anti-inflammatory drugs and reduction of activity. Occasionally, non–weight-bearing, braces, casting, and osteotomies are utilized to decrease pain and improve femoral head reossification in a normal spherical shape.[10] Orthopedic outpatient referral is appropriate for most cases.

Long-term outcome studies show that most patients are active and pain free for 20 to 40 years postdiagnosis. However, beyond 40 to 50 years, over 50% of patients develop degenerative joint disease and osteoarthritis.[6,10] The largest prognostic risk factors for long-term morbidity are age at diagnosis and the extent of residual femoral head deformity.[6] Patients who are diagnosed at an earlier age (under 6 years of age) do better than older children. Patients with more residual deformity in the femoral head are at risk for earlier onset of degenerative joint disease.

Slipped Capital Femoral Epiphysis

Slipped capital femoral epiphysis (SCFE) is defined as displacement of the femoral epiphysis (femoral head) on the femoral metaphysis (femoral neck). The slippage initially occurs in a posterior and medial direction, and occurs most frequently during adolescent growth spurts. Due to the potential for damage to the tenuous vascular supply of the femoral head, the process is an important one to diagnose as delays in implementing treatment can lead to further slippage and increased morbidity.

Most practitioners now classify SCFE into two categories, stable and unstable.[11,12] Clinically, a stable SCFE is one in which the patient can bear weight with or without crutches and an unstable SCFE is when the child cannot walk, even with crutches. An older classification based on duration of symptoms (chronic vs. acute) is no longer recommended as it has less prognostic capabilities. The vast majority of patients present with a stable SCFE, which carries a better prognosis if recognized early.

Although SCFE is usually associated with overweight children, it can also occur in nonobese patients. It is thought that obesity causes increased shear forces across an already weak and vertically oriented physis, resulting in slippage.[12] It occurs more often in African Americans compared to whites, and 60% of patients are male.[13] SCFE usually occurs in adolescents during prepubescent growth. Therefore, it occurs earlier in females (average 12 years) than males (average 13.5 years) and rarely occurs after menarche in females.[12,14] Between 25% and 40% of children with SCFE have bilateral involvement, with 50% of these presenting with simultaneous involvement and the others develop symptoms on the contralateral side within 18 months of initial diagnosis.[12]

Clinical Presentation

Children present with a variety of symptoms, including a limp and pain. Symptoms are usually present for several weeks before diagnosis and may be initially attributed to minor injuries or "growing pains." Patients may have pain in the hip, thigh, groin, or knee. The absence of hip pain and the presence of thigh pain have been associated with a missed diagnosis.[15] Errant diagnoses by physicians have included Osgood-Schlatter disease, bursitis, growing pains, chondromalacia, thigh contusions, muscle strains, stress fractures, and tendonitis. Because delayed diagnosis can result in further slippage, it is important for practitioners to include

SCFE in their differential diagnosis whenever evaluating patients with thigh, groin, or knee pain. In addition to pain, children may have an antalgic gait or loss of internal rotation of the hip. As slippage increases, there will be a worsening gait abnormality and decreased internal rotation of the hip. Unstable SCFE presents with extreme pain and can be thought of as an acute Salter-Harris type I fracture.[16] Minor trauma, as in slipping off a curb edge or simply twisting in bed, may immediately precede an unstable SCFE. In addition to severe pain, patients with an unstable SCFE will resist any motion at the hip. The hip is usually held in flexion and external rotation. Gentle passive hip flexion usually leads to external rotation of the hip. No attempts at reduction should be made in the emergency department as this can cause further damage to the femoral head's vascular supply.[17]

All patients with symptoms compatible with a stable SCFE should have anteroposterior and frog-leg lateral pelvic radiographs. Because early slippage is posterior and inferior, initial radiographic findings may only be seen on the lateral radiographs, revealing minimum posterior step-off at the physeal plate. Klein's line represents a line drawn along the femoral neck on an anteroposterior film that should bisect the lateral portion of the femoral head. In patients with mild slippage, the line will be flush with or lateral to the lateral edge of the epiphysis (Fig. 100–4). As the slippage continues, there is further inferior and posterior movement of the epiphysis relative to the metaphysis, and radiographs will eventually show the typical picture similar to a scoop of ice cream slipping off a cone.

Patients suspected of having an unstable SCFE should not be forced into a frog-leg lateral position, but should have a lateral hip radiograph taken instead. A lateral view or frog-leg lateral view of the opposing leg should be taken for comparison and to detect mild slippage in bilateral cases.

The differential diagnosis for patients with SCFE includes other processes that can cause pain in the hip and lower leg. LCP disease usually occurs in younger children, but there is overlap in the age distribution. Patients with transient synovitis, septic hip, osteomyelitis, and muscle or ligamentous injuries of the thigh or hip may also present with similar symptoms (see Chapter 20, Lower Extremity Trauma; Chapter 21, Pelvic and Genitourinary Trauma; Chapter 95, Musculoskeletal Disorders in Systemic Disease; and Chapter 96, Bone, Joint, and Spine Infections). Because hip pathology often presents with knee pain, acute or chronic injuries of the knee, including Osgood-Schlatter disease and chondromalacia, should be considered. However, the knee examination is usually normal in patients with SCFE.

Management

All patients with SCFE need orthopedic referral as surgery is needed in all cases. Patients with unstable SCFE will need immediate orthopedic referral. Children with stable SCFE can be made non–weight bearing with crutches and seen promptly as outpatients. The most common surgical procedure for stable SCFE is a single central screw to maintain the femoral head in its current location until the physis is closed.[12] No attempts are made to reduce the slippage. Once physeal closure occurs, the patient is able to return to running and contact sports. Surgical treatment for unstable SCFE is controversial and may involve closed reduction, single or multiple screws, or osteotomies, and will depend on the degree of slippage and the preference of the orthopedic surgeon.[18]

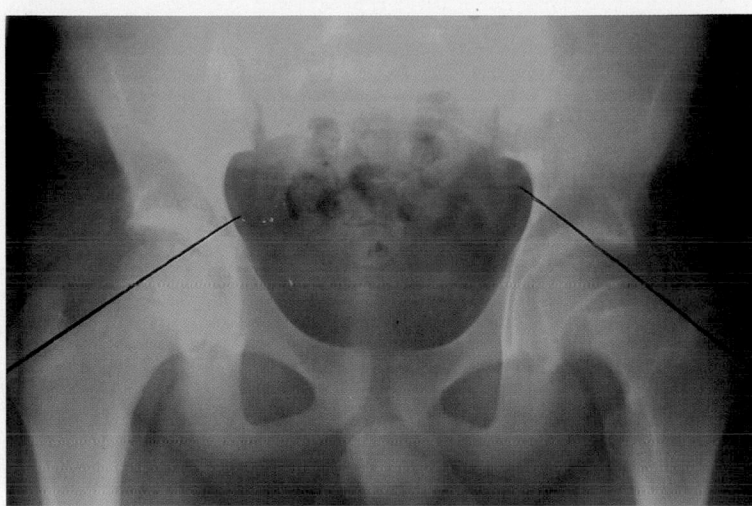

FIGURE 100–4. Radiograph of a 12-year-old with left hip pain. There is mild slippage of the left femoral epiphysis. Klein's line, drawn along the femoral neck, does not bisect the left femoral epiphysis as it does on the normal right hip.

Patients with stable SCFE usually do very well with minimal complications or morbidity, especially when diagnosed early. Complications of unstable SCFE include avascular necrosis of the femoral head, occurring in up to 35% of cases, and chondrolysis or loss of cartilage in the femoral head and acetabulum.[10,15,17] Chondrolysis also develops more often as the degree of slippage increases and underscores the need to avoid missed or delayed diagnoses.

Transient Synovitis of the Hip

The most common cause of painful hips in children is transient synovitis of the hip (TSH). While the etiology of TSH is unknown, there is usually no long-term morbidity from this disorder. Importantly, clinicians must be able to differentiate this disorder from serious disorders causing a painful hip, including septic hip, osteomyelitis, LCP disease, SCFE, and neoplasias.

Although cases have been described in infants as young as 9 months and children as old as 18 years, the average age of children with TSH is 6 years, with a typical range of 3 to 10 years.[19,20] This range overlaps with other causes of hip disease, including LCP disease and SCFE. The disorder is found more often in males, with a male:female ratio of between 1.5 : 1 and 2.6 : 1.[19,21,22] Over 95% of children present with unilateral involvement, with an even distribution between right and left hips.[20]

Clinical Presentation

Many patients have pain or limp for less than 24 hours, and two thirds have symptoms for less than 1 week.[20] Most others have symptoms for less than 1 month. A preceding or concurrent respiratory infection is found in 50% of patients with TSH, leading some to believe there is an infectious or postinfectious etiology. Most patients will either be afebrile or have a low temperature elevation,[20,22] although temperatures as high as 40° C have been reported.[20] Patients may report pain of the hip, thigh, or knee, and have a mild limp or refuse to bear weight. Infants and children are not ill appearing and have a varying degree of restriction of hip movement and pain elicited at extremes of rotation.

The evaluation of patients suspected of having TSH should include a white blood cell (WBC) count, erythrocyte sedimentation rate (ESR), and C-reactive protein (CRP) level,

and a blood culture to differentiate this disorder from septic arthritis.[21-25] The WBC count is usually normal to mildly elevated, with a mean count between 8600/mm³ and 11,200/ mm³.[20,21] However, some patients may have a WBC count greater than 20,000/mm³. The mean ESR is less than 20 mm/ hr but may be greater than 20 mm/hr in as many as 25% of cases.[22] CRP is usually less than 1 mg/dl but may be greater than 2 mg/dl in up to 14% of cases.[22]

Radiographs may be normal or may show signs consistent with a joint effusion, with widening of the joint space or displacement or obliteration of periarticular fat planes. All patients with TSH will have an abnormal US showing mild or moderate effusion, with a small percentage showing severe effusion[22,26,27] (Fig. 100–5). Joint aspiration is performed by orthopedic consultants and is reserved for patients in whom septic arthritis is still considered as a possible diagnosis after review of the clinical examination findings and other less invasive laboratory studies. Joint fluid should be sterile in TSH, with no bacteria seen on Gram stain and negative synovial fluid culture.

Although many etiologies have to be considered in the differential diagnosis of a child with a painful hip, radiographs can usually reveal abnormalities associated with LCP disease, SCFE, and trauma. Clinicians must be able to differentiate TSH from a septic hip. Several studies have found that the historical features and diagnostic adjuncts differ statistically between the two diseases: mean WBC count, ESR, CRP, temperature, joint space differences, history of fever, and an inability to bear weight.[21-25] A combination of several factors, including temperature greater than 37° C to 38° C, WBC count greater than 11,000/mm³, ESR greater than 20 mm/hr, CRP greater than 1 mg/dl, joint space difference of greater than 2 mm on radiographs, and a history of fever or non–weight bearing, is more predictive of patients at increased risk of septic hip and therefore in need of a hip aspiration. If none of these features is present, the probability of septic arthritis is less than 1%[22-25] (see Chapter 96, Bone, Joint, and Spine Infections). The more abnormal factors present, the greater likelihood the patient has a septic hip and not TSH.[22-25] Limited studies have found MRI to be helpful in differentiating between the two entities, although there should be no delay in confirming the diagnosis of septic hip.[28] If septic arthritis is suspected after initial imaging and

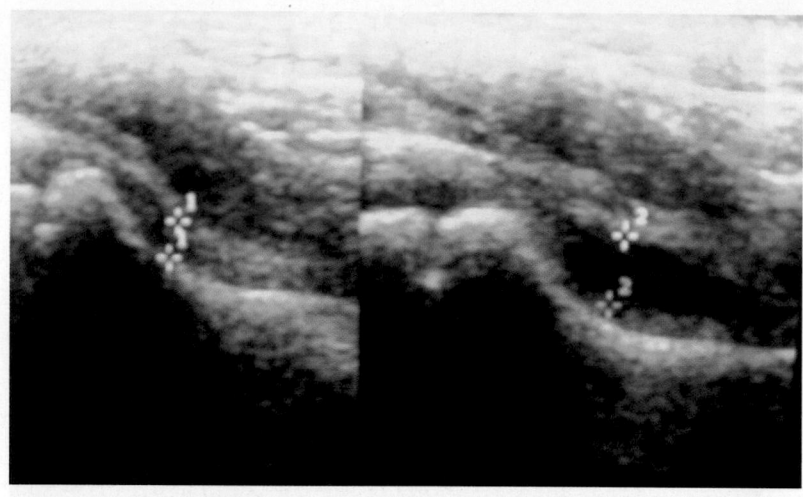

FIGURE 100–5. Ultrasound of a 5-year-old with right hip pain. Hip effusion is demonstrated with widening of the intracapsular space, especially when compared with normal left hip.

laboratory evaluation, orthopedic specialists should be consulted for hip joint aspiration.

Management

Most patients with TSH have rapid resolution of symptoms with bed rest. While most patients can be treated at home, some with more severe symptoms are treated in the hospital with traction for pain management. Recurrence of symptoms after initial resolution is unusual but may occur in 4% of cases.[19] Follow-up US examinations or radiographs in 6 months may reveal a small number of patients who develop LCP disease,[19,20,22] although it is unclear if TSH increases the risk for LCP disease, or the LCP cases were simply not recognized during the initial presentation. Because of the reported association with LCP disease, patients with TSH should be considered for repeat US examinations or radiographs if recurrent symptoms develop several months later. Unlike septic arthritis and SCFE, no long-term complications or morbidity is associated with TSH.

REFERENCES

1. French LM, Dietz FR: Screening for developmental dysplasia of the hip. Am Fam Physician 60:177–184, 1999.
2. Marks DS, Clegg J, al-Chalabi AN: Routine ultrasound screening for neonatal hip instability: can it abolish late-presenting congenital dislocation? J Bone Joint Surg Br 76:534–538, 1994.
3. Barlow TG: Early diagnosis and treatment of congenital dislocation of the hip. J Bone Joint Surg Br 44:292–301, 1962.
4. Novacheck TF: Developmental dysplasia of the hip. Pediatr Clin North Am 43:829–848, 1996.
5. Donaldson JS, Feinstein KA: Imaging of developmental dysplasia of the hip. Pediatr Clin North Am 44:591–614, 1997.
6. Weinstein SL: Natural history and treatment outcomes of childhood hip disorders. Clin Orthop 344:227–242, 1997.
7. Wenger DR, Ward WT, Herring JA: Current concepts review. Legg-Calvé-Perthes disease. J Bone Joint Surg Am 73:778–788, 1991.
8. Koop S, Quanbeck D: Three common causes of childhood hip pain. Pediatr Clin North Am 43:1053–1066, 1996.
9. Hubbard AM: Imaging of pediatric hip disorders. Radiol Clin North Am 39: 721–732, 2001.
10. Herring JA: Current concepts review. The treatment of Legg-Calvé-Perthes disease: a critical review of the literature. J Bone Joint Surg Am 76:448–458, 1994.
11. Loder RT: Unstable slipped capital femoral epiphysis. J Pediatr Orthop 21:694–699, 2001.
12. Loder RT: Slipped capital femoral epiphysis. Am Fam Physician 57:2135–2142, 1998.
13. Loder RT: The demographics of slipped capital femoral epiphysis: an international multicenter study. Clin Orthop Relat Res 322:8–27, 1996.
14. Swiontkowski MF, Gill EA: Slipped capital femoral epiphysis. Am Fam Physician 33:167–171, 1986.
15. Ledwith CA, Fleisher GR: Slipped capital femoral epiphysis without hip pain leads to missed diagnosis. Pediatrics 89:660–662, 1992.
16. Stanitski CL: Acute slipped capital femoral epiphysis. J Am Acad Orthop Surg 2:96–106, 1994.
17. Maeda S, Kita A, Funayama K, Kokubun S: Vascular supply to slipped capital femoral epiphysis. J Pediatr Orthop 21:664–667, 2001.
18. Rattey T, Piehl F, Wright JG: Acute slipped capital femoral epiphysis: review of outcomes and rates of avascular necrosis. J Bone Joint Surg Am 78:398–402, 1996.
19. Landin LA, Damielsson LG, Wattsgard C: Transient synovitis of the hip: its incidence, epidemiology and relation to Perthes' disease. J Bone Joint Surg Br 69:238–242, 1987.
20. Haueisen DC, Weiner DS, Weiner S: The characterization of "trans-ient synovitis of the hip" in children. J Pediatr Orthop 6:11–17, 1986.
21. Del Beccro MA, Champoux AN, Bockers T, Mendelman PM: Septic arthritis versus transient synovitis of the hip: the value of screening laboratory tests. Ann Emerg Med 21:1419–1422, 1992.
22. Eich GF, Superti-Furga A, Umbricht FS, Willi UV: The painful hip: evaluation of criteria for clinical decision making. Eur J Pediatr 158:923–928, 1999.
23. Kocher MS, Zurakowski D, Kasser JR: Differentiating between septic arthritis and transient synovitis of the hip in children: an evidence-based clinical prediction algorithm. J Bone Joint Surg Am 81:1662–1670, 1999.
24. Kocher, MS, Mandiga R, Zurakowski D, et al: Validation of a clinical prediction rule for the differentiation between septic arthritis and transient synovitis of the hip in children. J Bone Joint Surg Am 86:1629–1635, 2004.
25. Jung ST, Rowe SM, Moon EU, et al: Significance of laboratory and radiologic findings for differential between septic arthritis and transient synovitis of the hip. J Pediatr Orthop 23:368–372, 2003.
26. Terjesen T, Osthus P: Ultrasound in the diagnosis and follow-up of transient synovitis of the hip. J Pediatr Orthop 11:608–613, 1991.
27. Eggl H, Drekonja T, Kaiser B, Dorn U: Ultrasonography in the diagnosis of transient synovitis of the hip and Legg-Calvé-Perthes disease. J Pediatr Orthop 8:177–180, 1999.
28. Lee SK, Suh JK, Ryeom HK, et al: Septic arthritis versus transient synovitis at MR imaging: preliminary assessment with signal intensity alterations in bone marrow. Radiology 211:459–465, 1999.

Serum Sickness

Lee S. Benjamin, MD

Introduction and Background

Serum sickness is an uncommon clinical syndrome associated with exposure to animal serum. The typical symptoms include fever, arthralgias, skin eruptions that can include palpable purpura or urticaria, lymphadenopathy, nephritis, edema, and neuritis.[1,2] Historically, antisera derived from horse serum were the most common causes of serum sickness. These antisera were used to treat snake bites, botulism, and pneumococcal, meningococcal, and streptococcal infections, and to immunize patients against diphtheria, tetanus, and rabies.[3-7] Refinements and advances in treatments for these conditions have substantially mitigated the risk of serum sickness for patients in recent years.

Serum sickness–like reactions are more common than cases of serum sickness. Serum sickness–like reactions have some clinical signs and symptoms in common with serum sickness. These include rash and joint pains.[8-11] The rash may include urticaria or erythema multiforme, or be morbilliform. The child may exhibit arthralgias or clinically appreciable arthritis. The presence of fever or lymphadenopathy is variable. Unlike serum sickness, serum sickness–like reactions are not associated with circulating immune complexes. Therefore, palpable purpura, nephritis, edema, and neuritis are not expected in cases of serum sickness–like reactions. Oral antibiotics are currently the most common cause of serum sickness–like reactions.[9] Even though they share some clinical features, it is unknown if serum sickness–like reactions and serum sickness are different points along a single continuum. Unfortunately, the term *serum sickness* is sometimes applied to cases of serum sickness–like reactions.[12] This intermingling of terms likely leads to confusion.

Recognition and Approach

There are no recent epidemiologic studies reporting the incidence, but clinical experience suggests serum sickness presenting to the emergency department is rare. Serum sickness is a type III hypersensitivity reaction to foreign proteins that leads to the development of circulating immune complexes that deposit in small vessels, activation of complement, and recruitment of granulocytes.[1,3,13-15] The deposition of the circulating immune complexes is thought to be the dominant pathophysiologic derangement.

Children with serum sickness–like reactions are rare, but relatively more common than those with serum sickness. Population-based epidemiologic data are not available. The pathophysiology of serum sickness–like reactions remains elusive.[8,10,16] Circulating immune complexes are inconsistently identified. The vast majority of cases of serum sickness–like reactions occur in children younger than 5 years.[10-12] A history of taking a new antibiotic or other medication is nearly universal[12] (Table 101–1). In particular, the use of oral cefaclor has been implicated in cases of serum sickness–like reactions.[8,9,12] Prior sensitization to medication is not a prerequisite.[8,10]

Clinical Presentation

Children may present to the emergency department for evaluation of possible serum sickness or a serum sickness–like reaction. A history of exposure to horse serum makes the

Table 101–1	Medications Associated with Serum Sickness–like Reactions

Bupropion
Carbamazepine
Cephalosporins
Ciprofloxacin
Fluoxetine
Griseofulvin
Metronidazole
NSAIDs
Penicillins
Phenytoin
Propranolol
Rifampin
Streptomycin
Sulfa medications
Tetracyclines
Thiouracil

Abbreviation: NSAIDs, nonsteroidal anti-inflammatory drugs.

diagnosis of serum sickness quite likely. However, the history is seldom so straightforward. It is more likely to include some vague symptoms arising after treatment with a new medication has begun. The temporal relationship between starting the new medication and symptom onset is sometimes helpful. For both serum sickness and serum sickness–like reactions, the onset of symptoms is usually delayed several days from the exposure to the inciting antigen. The exact time span is not known. Rough estimates based on limited data suggest the symptoms of serum sickness arise 1 to 2 weeks after antigenic exposure and the symptoms of serum sickness–like reactions arise 2 to 17 days after drug exposure.[10,13,14] The most common symptoms include rash and arthralgia.[8,9,11,12,17] A history of neurologic symptoms or dark urine is most consistent with a diagnosis of serum sickness. A history of recently beginning a course of oral cefaclor suggests a serum sickness–like reaction.[8,9,12,18,19]

Physical examination findings in cases of serum sickness and serum sickness–like reactions are often nonspecific. In both conditions, a rash is expected. In both conditions, the rash may be urticarial or morbilliform.[8,9,11] In cases of serum sickness, but not serum sickness–like reactions, the rash may include petechiae and palpable purpura. In both conditions, the physical examination may reveal swollen, tender joints consistent with an acute arthritis. Fever and lymphadenopathy are characteristic of serum sickness, but variably seen in cases of serum sickness–like reactions.[8,9,12-14] Facial edema and an abnormal neurologic examination may be seen in cases of serum sickness, but not cases of serum sickness–like reactions.[20] A child with acute nephritis associated with serum sickness may be hypertensive.

Laboratory tests have modest utility in the evaluation of a child with possible serum sickness or a serum sickness–like reaction. For cases suggestive of serum sickness–like reactions, no routine laboratory tests are indicated. The history of initiating a new medication, particularly an antibiotic, 2 to 17 days prior to presentation and the presence of a nonpetechial rash and joint pains with or without fever are likely diagnostic. For cases in which serum sickness is likely, testing is generally directed at the overall differential diagnosis. For example, for children with a petechial rash or purpura, a

measurement of platelets (usually obtained as part of a complete blood count) and a prothrombin time are probably indicated. A microscopic urinalysis is helpful for identifying acute nephritis. A measurement of blood urea nitrogen and creatinine is also indicated if serum sickness is suspected. Other laboratory tests are indicated on a case-by-case basis, guided by signs and symptoms. The child's primary care physician may request other tests to guide him or her in the outpatient management of serum sickness.

Important Clinical Features and Considerations

The differential diagnosis of the signs and symptoms associated with children suspected of having serum sickness or serum sickness–like reactions is broad. The differential diagnosis includes conditions such as bacterial, viral, and parasitic infections, as well as vasculitis, connective tissue disease, syphilis, atopic disease, inflammatory bowel disease, sarcoidosis, cystic fibrosis, Behçet's syndrome, pemphigus, bullous pemphigoid, and allergic vasculitis.[21]

Management

Discontinuation of the offending agent is the mainstay of treatment and is usually curative.[17] There is no evidence on which to base management decisions. Although systemic steroids have been recommended, their utility is uncertain, particularly given that the vast majority of children will have spontaneous resolution of their symptoms with the removal of the offending agent as the sole intervention.[11,17] Other treatments are supportive and symptomatic. These include acetaminophen for fever and analgesia, antihistamines for allergic-type symptoms such as urticaria, and nonsteroidal anti-inflammatory medications such as ibuprofen for joint inflammation and pain. In general, children with serum sickness or serum sickness–like reactions can be managed as outpatients. Uncertainty in the diagnosis may warrant hospital admission or transfer to a tertiary pediatric center to work through the differential diagnosis. The most common reason for admission to the hospital in cases of serum sickness–like reactions is for uncontrollable joint pains.[11]

In general, the emergency physician should recommend that the family avoid giving the offending agent to the child in the future. One pair of authors recommends avoiding the entire class of medications to which the offending agent belongs.[22] There is no evidence to support this recommendation. Others have noted no significant cross reactivity within the same class of medications.[11,23]

Summary

A history of antigen exposure is very helpful in evaluating a child suspected of possibly harboring serum sickness or a serum sickness–like reaction to a new medication. The presence of palpable purpura, nephritis, edema, and neuritis helps differentiate serum sickness from a serum sickness–like reaction. Removing the offending agent is the mainstay of treatment. Most children do well with symptomatic treatment and recover uneventfully. Avoidance of the offending agent in the future is prudent.

REFERENCES

*1. Roujeau JC, Stern RS: Severe adverse cutaneous reactions to drugs. N Engl J Med 331:1272–1285, 1994.

2. Parker CW: Drug allergy. N Engl J Med 292:511–514, 1975.

3. von Pirquet CF, Schick B: Serum Sickness. Baltimore: Williams & Wilkins, 1951.

4. Bielory L, Kemeny DM, Richards D, et al: IgG subclass antibody production in human serum sickness. J Allergy Clin Immunol 85:573–577, 1990.

5. Corrigan P, Russell FE, Wainschel J: Clinical reactions to antivenin. Toxicon 16(1 Suppl):457–465, 1978.

6. Karliner JS, Belaval GS: Incidence of reactions following administration of antirabies serum; study of 526 cases. JAMA 193:359–362, 1965.

7. Moynihan NH: Serum-sickness and local reactions in tetanus prophylaxis: a study of 400 cases. Lancet 269:264–267, 1955.

8. Levine LR: Quantitative comparison of adverse reactions to cefaclor vs. amoxicillin in a surveillance study. Pediatr Infect Dis 4:358–361, 1985.

*9. Parshuram CS, Phillips RJ, Nash MC: Serum sickness in a paediatric emergency department: the role of cefaclor. J Paediatr Child Health 35:223–224, 1999.

10. Kearns GL, Wheeler JG, Childress SH, et al: Serum sickness-like reactions to cefaclor: role of hepatic metabolism and individual susceptibility. J Pediatr 125:805–811, 1994.

11. Vial T, Pont J, Pham E, et al: Cefaclor-associated serum sickness-like disease: eight cases and review of the literature. Ann Pharmacother 26:910–914, 1992.

12. Heckbert SR, Stryker WS, Coltin KL, et al: Serum sickness in children after antibiotic exposure: estimates of occurrence and morbidity in a health maintenance organization population. Am J Epidemiol 132:336–342, 1990.

13. Bielory L, Gascon P, Lawley TJ, et al: Human serum sickness: a prospective analysis of 35 patients treated with equine anti-thymocyte globulin for bone marrow failure. Medicine 67:40–47, 1988.

14. Lawley TJ, Bielory L, Gascon P, et al: A prospective clinical and immunologic analysis of patients with serum sickness. N Engl J Med 311:1407–1413, 1984.

15. Lawley TJ, Bielory L, Gascon P, et al: A study of human serum sickness. J Invest Dermatol 85(1 Suppl):129s 132s, 1985.

*16. King BA, Geelhoed GC: Adverse skin and joint reactions associated with oral antibiotics in children: the role of cefaclor in serum sickness-like reactions. J Paediatr Child Health 39:677–681, 2003.

17. Hebert AA, Sigman ES, Levy ML: Serum sickness-like reactions from cefaclor in children. J Am Acad Dermatol 25:805–808, 1991.

18. Parshuram CS, Phillips RJ: Retrospective review of antibiotic-associated serum sickness in children presenting to a paediatric emergency department. Med J Aust 169:116, 1998.

19. Platt R, Dreis MW, Kennedy DL, et al: Serum sickness-like reactions to amoxicillin, cefaclor, cephalexin and trimethoprim-sulfamethoxazole. J Infect Dis 158:474–477, 1988.

20. Tatum AJ, Ditto AM, Patterson R, et al: Severe serum sickness-like reaction to oral penicillin drugs: three case reports. Ann Allergy Asthma Immunol 86:330–334, 2001.

21. Van Es LA, Daha MR, Valentijn RM, et al: The pathogenetic significance of circulating immune complexes. Neth J Med 27:350–358, 1984.

22. McCullough H, Grammar LC: Cefaclor serum sickness. JAMA 275:1152–1153, 1996.

23. Ackley AM Jr, Felsher J: Adverse reactions to cefaclor. South Med J 74:1550, 1981.

*Selected readings.

Chapter 102

Vaccination-Related Complaints and Side Effects

Franz E. Babl, MD, MPH and Stuart Lewena, MBBS

Key Points

Most vaccination-related complaints are mild and self-limited.

The probability that a given problem is related to a recent vaccination can be predicted by knowing which vaccines were given and the timing of the administration of the vaccines in relation to the emergency department visit.

Knowledge of the immunization schedule is useful for determining which vaccines a child is likely to have received. This is particularly helpful when the parents cannot reliably identify which vaccines were given during a recent office visit.

Due to the low incidence of some events and the high rate of vaccination in the developed world, it is difficult or impossible to determine if some very rare adverse events are causally related to immunizations or merely temporally associated with them.

Selected Diagnoses

Allergic reactions and anaphylaxis
Rash
Fever
Encephalitis and encephalopathy
Generalized weakness
Seizures
Syncope
Hypotonic-hyporesponsive episodes (shocklike state)
Protracted, inconsolable crying
Arthralgias and arthritis
Extensive limb swelling
Thrombocytopenia

Discussion of Individual Diagnoses

Allergic Reactions and Anaphylaxis

Vaccine-related allergic reactions, particularly serious reactions such as anaphylaxis, are rare.[1] The measles vaccine, diphtheria and tetanus toxoids and pertussis vaccine (DTP) and hepatitis B vaccine (HepB) are the most commonly identified vaccine-related causes of anaphylaxis.[2] The rates of anaphylaxis are 1.8 per 1 million doses for measles vaccine (0.00018%) and 1.6 per 1 million doses for HepB (0.00016%).[1,3] Serious allergic reactions due to other vaccines are even rarer.[4]

Vaccines contain various additives and other components that may cause allergic reactions in children sensitive to these agents. The measles and mumps vaccines (most commonly combined in the measles-mumps-rubella vaccine [MMR]) are derived from chick embryo fibroblast tissue and contain very small amounts of egg protein. Children with an egg allergy are at increased risk of having an allergic reaction to these immunizations, but the risk is exceedingly small. In contrast, the influenza vaccine contains a greater amount of egg protein and places children at such a great risk for allergic reactions that it is recommended that this vaccine be withheld from children with egg allergies.[5] Inactivated poliovirus vaccine (IPV) contains trace quantities of neomycin, streptomycin, and polymyxin B. Children with allergies to any of these antimicrobials are at risk for allergic reactions to IPV. The MMR and varicella vaccines contain trace amounts of neomycin and gelatin. Children allergic to neomycin or gelatin can develop allergic reactions, including delayed-type local reactions manifesting as erythematous, pruritic papules 48 to 96 hours after vaccination.[3,6,7] Yeast protein is present in HepB, and children with yeast allergies can have reactions to this vaccine.[6]

The timing of allergic reactions, including anaphylaxis, in relation to vaccine administration is an important factor in determining whether or not the vaccine could be the cause. Parents may not be able to list the vaccines given during a recent office visit or may provide inaccurate information.[8] Because of this, it is helpful for emergency physicians to have some familiarity with the recommended schedule of immunizations to allow for a reasoned guess as to what vaccinations were likely given based on the child's age (Table 102–1).

Table 102–1   Simplified Pediatric Immunization Schedule

| | Vaccines | | | | | | | | | | | |
Age	HepB	DTaP	Tdap	Hib	IPV	PCV	Influenza*	MMR	Varicella	Rota	MCV4	HPV†
Birth	✓											
2 mo	✓	✓		✓	✓	✓				✓		
4 mo		✓		✓	✓	✓				✓		
6 mo	✓	✓		✓	✓	✓	✓			✓		
12 mo				✓		✓		✓	✓			
15 mo		✓										
4–6 yr		✓			✓			✓	✓			
11–12 yr			✓								✓	✓

*Influenza vaccine is given yearly thereafter up to age 5 years.
†HPV is administered as a series of 3 immunizations given over 6 months.
Abbreviations: DTaP, diphtheria and tetanus toxoids and acellular pertussis vaccine; HepB, hepatitis B vaccine; Hib, *Haemophilus influenzae* type b conjugate vaccine; HPV, human papillomavirus vaccine; IPV, inactivated poliovirus vaccine; MCV4, meningococcal conjugate vaccine; MMR, measles-mumps-rubella vaccine; PCV, pneumococcal conjugate vaccine; Rota, rotavirus vaccine; Tdap, tetanus and diphtheria toxoids and acellular pertussis vaccine.
Adapted from American Academy of Pediatrics Committee on Infectious Diseases. Recommended immunization schedules for children and adolescents—United States, 2007. Pediatrics 119:207–208, 3 p following 208, 2007.

In general, anaphylaxis, if it develops, does so shortly after immunization. In a review of 366 patients with adverse reactions to DTaP, 34 patients developed anaphylaxis and 76 developed urticaria.[7] Most cases of anaphylaxis manifested within 15 minutes of vaccine administration, and none occurred after 60 minutes. In contrast, urticaria developed up to 24 hours after immunization. In another study of adverse events after 3 million MMR vaccinations, 30 (0.001%) anaphylaxis-like reactions appeared, 29 within 20 minutes of immunization.[9] None of these cases was fatal. The management of vaccine-related allergic reactions and anaphylaxis does not differ from that for cases due to other causes (see Chapter 14, Anaphylaxis/Allergic Reactions).

Rash

The vaccines most commonly associated with rashes are the varicella and MMR vaccines. A localized injection site rash develops in 4% of children receiving the varicella vaccine.[10] Most varicella vaccine–related rashes become apparent 9 to 16 days after immunization. Most of these cases involve mild, localized, papular lesions. Some children manifest what appears to be a mild case of varicella with a handful of the characteristic vesicular lesions and crusting in approximately the same time frame as the papular rashes. Based on the virology, at least some of these cases are due to varicella infection and not the varicella vaccination. In a polymerase chain reaction analysis of 70 post–varicella vaccine rashes, 61% of cases had the wild-type varicella virus strain and 31% showed the Oka-type vaccine strain.[11] Disseminated varicella due to the vaccine strain may occur in previously undiagnosed immune-compromised patients.[12] MMR is associated with transient rashes in 5% of those vaccinated. This rash is fairly nonspecific in appearance and typically occurs 7 to 10 days after immunization.[4,13] This MMR-associated rash is associated with transient lymphadenopathy in some cases.

Fever

Many childhood vaccines have been associated with causing fever after vaccination.[6] Febrile episodes occur at low rates, and within the first 1 to 2 days postvaccination, after admin-

istration of HepB, influenza virus vaccine, *Haemophilus influenzae* type b conjugate vaccine, and pneumococcal conjugate vaccine (PCV). Fever due to MMR, however, usually occurs 7 to 12 days after immunization. Approximately 5% of children develop a fever of ≥39.4° C (103° F) after MMR vaccination.[13,14] In some ways, fever is so common in children that most are expected to develop fever *at some point* after an immunization. Attributing fever to an immunization is fraught with problems if the time course is drawn out. For example, the incidence of fever within 42 days after the first dose of varicella vaccine is 15%, which is similar to the incidence seen in children who received placebo.[10,15] Very high fevers may be seen within 48 hours of the administration of DTP.[6] Temperatures ≥40.5° C (104.8° F) are seen in 0.3% of children receiving DTP.[6] Following the introduction of the acellular pertussis vaccine into DTP (designated as DTaP), the incidence of fever has been much lower.[6] It is prudent to consider alternative diagnoses in children who manifest fever that is temporally associated with vaccines. In one study, 80% of children who experienced fever after receiving the varicella vaccine harbored another illness[10] (see Chapter 32, Fever in the Well-Appearing Young Infant).

Encephalitis and Encephalopathy

Encephalopathy refers to any acute or chronic acquired abnormality of the function of the brain. *Encephalitis* refers to an encephalopathy caused by an inflammatory response in the brain usually manifested by pleocytosis (i.e., white blood cells in the cerebrospinal fluid).[2] Encephalitis with resultant residual permanent encephalopathy develops in approximately 1 in 1000 people (0.1%) infected with the measles virus.[13] There is not enough evidence to accept or reject a causal relationship between immunization with live measles vaccine virus and encephalitis or encephalopathy.[2] In the United States, 166 cases of encephalopathy occurring 6 to 15 days after measles vaccine were identified over 30 years through a number of passive surveillance systems.[13,16] In other words, the incidence of encephalopathy possibly due to measles vaccines is approximately 1 in 2 million (0.00005%). This incidence is so low and the percentage of the population who receives vaccinations is so high, it is essentially impossible to perform a study to determine if encephalitis can be caused by the measles component of MMR. So, although measles (the disease) can cause encephalitis, it is not clear if the measles vaccine can cause encephalitis. A 10-year follow-up of a study from the United Kingdom on vaccination-related encephalopathy showed no evidence of a risk of long-term neurological damage associated with measles vaccine.[17] Some strains of the mumps component of MMR can cause aseptic meningitis. However, the strain used in the United States does not.[2,13] DPT might cause acute encephalopathy, but with an incidence of 0 to 10 cases per million vaccinations (0 to 0.001%).[1,18] There is no difference in the management of children presenting with acute encephalopathy or acute encephalitis temporally associated with vaccines and that of other children with a similar presentation (see Chapter 11, Altered Mental Status/Coma).

Generalized Weakness

The two main types of weakness associated with vaccines are paralytic poliomyelitis and the Guillain-Barré syndrome. The oral poliovirus vaccine (OPV) has been causally linked with paralytic poliomyelitis.[2] The case definition of vaccine-associated poliomyelitis is acute flaccid paralysis in a vaccine recipient 7 to 30 days after receiving OPV, with no sensory or cognitive loss, and with paralysis still present 60 days after the onset of symptoms. The risk is low at 1 case per 2.4 million doses (0.00004%).[19] In the United States, the routine childhood immunization schedule has replaced OPV with IPV which is not associated with paralytic poliomyelitis. However, outside the United States, OPV is still widely used. The Guillain-Barré syndrome has been associated with a number of vaccines, but there are inadequate data to determine if a causal relationship exists.[2,4,19] This is another example of a very rare event occurring in the context of a very high incidence of vaccination.

Seizures

The two vaccines associated with high fevers, MMR and DTP, are also associated with febrile seizures. The available data are difficult to reconcile. For example, the risk of febrile seizures following MMR vaccination has been reported to range from 1 in 100,000 (0.001%) up to 1 in 3000 (0.03%).[9,20] Case definitions likely cause these differences. The timing of the febrile seizures correlates with the timing of peak post-vaccination temperatures.[21] There is no evidence that MMR is associated with an increased risk of epilepsy.[2] The change from DTP (with the whole-cell pertussis adsorbed component, also referred to as DTwP) to DTaP (with an acellular pertussis component) vaccine has dramatically decreased the risk of fever and also febrile seizures. The incidence of febrile seizures associated with DTaP is 0.5 events per 100,000 vaccinations (0.0005%).[22] The treatment of febrile seizures associated with vaccinations is no different than that of children with febrile seizures thought to be due to other causes (see Chapter 40, Seizures).

Syncope

Syncope can occur after any of the routine childhood vaccinations.[23] Syncope can be preceded by symptoms such as light-headedness, dizziness, diaphoresis, and visual changes. Syncope associated with vaccinations is typically brief. Adolescent girls are the most common population to experience syncope following vaccination.[23,24] In a review of 697 cases of syncope after vaccination, 57% occurred within 5 minutes of administration, 80% occurred within 15 minutes, and 88% within 30 minutes. Like other causes of syncope, 24% of the children experiencing syncope manifested some brief seizure-like movements.[23] In most cases, postvaccination syncope is neurocardiogenic. The approach to children who experience syncope following vaccination is the same as that of other children who experience syncope (see Chapter 61, Syncope).

Hypotonic-Hyporesponsive Episodes (Shocklike State)

Hypotonic-hyporesponsive episodes have been associated with DTP vaccines. Although the highest rates occur after immunization with the older DTwP, episodes may occur after DTaP administration.[25] These events occur with an incidence of 0 to 140 cases per 100,000 doses (0 to 0.14%).[4,18,26] Hypotonic-hyporesponsive episodes have been defined as limpness or hypotonia, reduced responsiveness, and pallor or cyanosis occurring within 48 hours of immunization and lasting from 1 minute to 48 hours in children younger than 10 years of age.[27] The etiology and pathophysiology of these events is unknown. By the time patients present for medical attention, symptoms have often resolved. In a series of 215 cases of hypotonic-hyporesponsive episodes, the median age was 4 months (range, 1 month to 8.9 years) and the median interval from the time of vaccination to onset of symptoms was 3.5 hours (range, 1 minute to 2 days).[28] None of the events was fatal, and 99% of children returned to their pre-vaccination state with a median time to return of 6 hours (range, 1 minute to 4 months). The three children reported as not returning to baseline were diagnosed with conditions not known to be causally associated with immunizations.

Assessment of a child with a possible hypotonic-hyporesponsive episode should exclude other known causes of sudden onset of hypotonia, hyporesponsiveness, or pallor. Evidence of preceding seizure activity or a postictal state, or evidence of urticaria, wheezing, or other signs and symptoms of anaphylaxis should be assessed. Other considerations in the setting of immunizations that are painful are syncope and breath-holding spells. There are no known residual effects from having a hypotonic-hyporesponsive episode.[27,28]

Protracted, Inconsolable Crying

Protracted, inconsolable crying has been recognized as an adverse event causally related to DTP.[18] It has been defined as persistent, severe, inconsolable screaming or crying for 3 or more hours observed within 48 hours of DTP vaccination.[6] The incidence of this syndrome is 1 in 100 (1%) doses administered for DTP vaccines containing the whole-cell pertussis component (DTwP) and significantly less with newer acellular pertussis vaccines (DTaP).[6,17,29] The significance or cause of protracted inconsolable crying is unknown.[6] There are no specific management recommendations for children with protracted inconsolable crying following immunization. Serious sequelae have not been described (see Chapter 31, Excessive Crying).

Arthralgias and Arthritis

Joint symptoms such as arthralgias (i.e., joint pains) and arthritis (i.e., joint redness and swelling) are associated with the rubella component of MMR. Acute arthralgia or arthritis after vaccination with the rubella vaccine strain used in the United States occurs rarely in children. In contrast, 26% of young women develop acute arthralgias and 11% develop acute arthritis after rubella vaccination.[30-32] Joint symptoms generally begin 1 to 3 weeks after vaccination, persist for 1 day to 3 weeks, and rarely recur. Although many different joints can be involved in the reaction to rubella vaccines, knees and fingers are the most common. The hips are seldom involved. The question of whether rubella vaccine can cause chronic arthritis in adult women is controversial.[18] Recent data from a prospective, randomized, placebo-controlled trial of 546 seronegative women receiving rubella vaccine show a small excess risk of developing chronic joint pain.[33] There is no evidence that vaccine-related joint problems should be managed differently from non–vaccine-related arthralgias or arthritis (see Chapter 95, Musculoskeletal Disorders in Systemic Diseases).

Extensive Limb Swelling

Extensive limb swelling is defined as edema extending at least to the elbow or knee in a vaccinated limb. In a 13-year review of reports to the Vaccine Adverse Events Reporting System (VAERS), 418 cases of extensive limb swelling were identified.[34] A broad range of vaccines have been implicated, with those most frequently cited being the PCV, DTaP, and adult tetanus and diphtheria toxoids (Td) vaccines. In most cases the swelling develops within 24 hours after vaccination and is limited to the proximal half of the extremity. Associated erythema, warmth, or pain was reported in more than 70% of cases, and constitutional symptoms such as fever were reported in 20% to 25%. Children younger than 2 years had associated agitation or crying in 32% of cases of extensive limb swelling. Adolescents and adults had influenza-like symptoms in 10% to 18% of cases.[31] Extensive limb swelling has been associated with booster doses of DTaP.[35] Extensive thigh swelling was reported in 2% of patients after the fourth dose of this vaccine; most cases were associated with erythema and pain. The etiology of extensive limb swelling is unknown.[34,35] Extensive limb swelling after vaccination appears to be self-limited and resolves without sequelae. There are no specific management recommendations for patients with extensive limb swelling.

Thrombocytopenia

MMR is associated with thrombocytopenia. The risk of thrombocytopenia is estimated to be 1 in 35,000 doses (0.003%).[2] It is unknown which vaccine component is responsible for the development of thrombocytopenia. The presentation is similar to cases of idiopathic thrombocytopenic purpura (ITP)[36,37] (see Chapter 122, Petechiae and Purpura). Vaccine-associated thrombocytopenia typically presents within 6 weeks of MMR immunization, with the highest incidence between 15 and 28 days after vaccination.[38] Compared to cases of ITP that are not temporally associated with vaccine administration, vaccine-associated cases tend to be milder and have higher platelet counts.[37] There is no evidence to suggest that vaccine-associated thrombocytopenia should be evaluated and managed differently from other cases of thrombocytopenia.

REFERENCES

1. Centers for Disease Control and Prevention: Update: vaccine side effects, adverse reactions, contraindications, and precautions. Recommendations of the Advisory Committee on Immunization Practices (ACIP). MMWR Recomm Rep 45(RR-12):1–35, 1996.
2. Stratton KR, Howe CJ, Johnston RB (eds): Adverse Events Associated with Childhood Vaccines: Evidence Bearing on Causality. Washington, DC: National Academy Press, 1994.
3. Pool V, Braun MM, Kelso JM, et al: Prevalence of anti-gelatin IgE antibodies in people with anaphylaxis after measles-mumps-rubella vaccine in the United States. Pediatrics 110:e71, 2002.
*4. Chen RT, Mootrey G, DeStefano F: Safety of routine childhood vaccinations: an epidemiological review. Paediatr Drugs 2:273–290, 2000.
5. Centers for Disease Control and Prevention: Key facts about influenza (flu) vaccine. Available at *www.cdc.gov/flu/protect/keyfacts.htm* (Accessed December 20, 2006).
6. Pickering LK, Baker CJ, Long SS, et al (eds): Red Book: 2006 Report of the Committee on Infectious Disease, 27th ed. Elk Grove Village, IL: American Academy of Pediatrics, 2006.
7. Nakayama T, Aizawa C, Kuno-Sakai H: A clinical analysis of gelatin allergy and determination of its causal relationship to the previous administration of gelatin-containing acellular pertussis vaccine combined with diptheria and tetanus toxoid. J Allergy Clin Immunol 103:321–325, 1993.
8. Goldstein KP, Kviz FJ, Daum RS: Accuracy of immunization histories provided by adults accompanying preschool children to a pediatric emergency department. JAMA 270:2190–2194, 1993.
9. Patja A, Davidkin I, Kurki T, et al: Serious adverse events after measles-mumps-rubella vaccination during a fourteen year prospective follow-up. Pediatr Infect Dis J 19:1127–1134, 2000.
10. Ngai A, Staehle BO, Kuter BJ, et al: Safety and immunogenicity of one vs. two injections of Oka/Merck varicella vaccine in healthy children. Pediatr Infect Dis J 15:49–54, 1996.
11. Wise RP, Salive ME, Braun M, et al: Postlicensure safety surveillance for varicella vaccine. JAMA 284:1271–1279, 2000.
12. Kramer JM, LaRussa P, Tsai W et al: Disseminated vaccine strain varicella as the acquired immune deficiency syndrome defining illness in a previously undiagnosed child. Pediatrics 108:e39, 2001.
13. Centers for Disease Control and Prevention: Measles, mumps, and rubella vaccine use and strategies for elimination of measles, rubella and congenital rubella syndrome and control of mumps: recommendations of the Advisory Committee on Immunization Practices (ACIP). MMWR Recomm Rep 47(RR-8):1–57, 1998.
14. Peltola H, Heinonen OP: Frequency of true adverse reactions to measles-mumps-rubella vaccine: a double blind placebo controlled trial in twins. Lancet 1:939–940, 1986.
15. Weibel RE, Neff BJ, Kuter BJ, et al: Live attenuated varicella virus vaccine: efficacy trial in healthy children. N Engl J Med 310:1409–1415, 1984.
16. Weibel RE, Caserta V, Benor DE, et al: Acute encephalopathy followed by permanent brain injury or death associated with further attenuated measles vaccines: a review of claims submitted to the National Vaccine Injury Compensation program. Pediatrics 101:383–387, 1998.
17. Miller D, Wadsworth J, Diamond J, et al: Measles vaccination and neurological events. Lancet 349:729–730, 1997.
18. Howson CP, Howe CJ, Finberg HV (eds): Adverse Events of Pertussis and Rubella Vaccines. Washington, DC: National Academy Press, 1991.
19. Centers for Disease Control and Prevention: Poliomyelitis prevention in the United States: introduction of a sequential vaccination schedule of inactivated polio virus vaccine followed by oral polio virus vaccine. MMWR Recomm Rep 46(RR-3):1–25, 1997.
20. Farrington CP, Pugh S, Colville A, et al: A new method for active surveillance of adverse events from diptheria/tetatus/pertussis and measles/mumps/rubella vaccines. Lancet 345:567–569, 1995.
21. Griffin MR, Ray WA, Mortimer EA, et al: Risk of seizures after measles-mumps-rubella immunization. Pediatrics 88:881–885, 1991.
22. Rosenthal S, Chen R, Hadler S: The safety of acellular pertussis vaccine vs whole-cell pertussis vaccine: a postmarketing assessment. Arch Pediatr Adolesc Med 150:457–460, 1996.

*Selected readings.

*23. Braun MM, Patriarca PA, Ellenberg SS: Syncope after immunization. Arch Pediatr Adolesc Med 151:255–259, 1997.

24. Centers for Disease Control and Prevention: General recommendations on immunizations. MMWR Recomm Rep 51(RR-02):1–36, 2002.

25. LeSaux N, Barrowman NJ, Moore DL, et al: Decrease in hospital admissions for febrile seizures and reports of hypotonic-hyporesponsive episodes presenting to hospital emergency departments since switching to acellular pertussis vaccine in Canada: a report from IMPACT. Pediatrics 112:e348, 2003.

26. Brown F, Greco D, Mastrantonio P, et al: Pertussis vaccine trials. Dev Biol Stand 89:1–407, 1997.

27. Braun MM, Teracciano G, Salive ME, et al: Report of a US Public Health Service Workshop on hypotonic-hyporesponsive episode (HHE) after pertussis immunization. Pediatrics 102:e1201, 1998.

28. DuVernoy TS, Braun MM; the VAERS Working Group: Hypotonic-hyporesponsive episodes reported to the Vaccine Adverse Events Reporting System (VAERS), 1996–1998. Pediatrics 106:e52, 2000.

29. Decker MD, Edwards KM, Steinhoff MC, et al: Comparison of 13 acellular pertussis vaccines: adverse reactions. Pediatrics 96:557–566, 1995.

30. Freestone DS, Prydie J, Smith SG, et al: Vaccination of adults with Wistar RA 27/3 rubella vaccine. J Hygiene 69:471–477, 1971.

31. Polk BF, Modlin JF, White JA, et al: A controlled comparison of joint reactions among women receiving one of two rubella vaccines. Am J Epidemiol 115:19–25, 1982.

32. Centers for Disease Control and Prevention: Epidemiology and Prevention of Vaccine Preventable Diseases, 7th ed. Atlanta: Centers for Disease Control and Prevention, 2002.

33. Tingle A, Mitchell L, Grace M, et al: Randomized, double-blind placebo-controlled study of adverse events of rubella immunization in seronegative women. Lancet 349:1277–1281, 1996.

34. Woo EJ, Burwen DR, Gatumu SN, et al: Extensive limb swelling after immunization: reports to the Vaccine Adverse Event Reporting System. Clin Infect Dis 37:351–358, 2003.

*35. Rennels MB, Deloria MA, Pichichero ME, et al: Extensive swelling after booster doses of acellular pertussis-tetanus-diphtheria vaccines. Pediatrics 105:e12, 2000.

36. Vlacha V, Forman EN, Miron D: Recurrent thrombocytopenic purpura after repeated measles-mumps-rubella vaccination. Pediatrics 97:738–739, 1996.

37. Drachtman RA, Murphy S, Ettinger LJ: Exacerbation of chronic idiopathic thrombocytopenic purpura following measles-mumps-rubella immunization. Arch Pediatr Adolesc Med 148:326–327, 1994.

38. Miller E, Waight P, Farrington CP, et al: Idiopathic thrombocytopenic purpura and MMR vaccine. Arch Dis Child 84:227–229, 2001.

Chapter 103

Tetanus Prophylaxis

Fredrick M. Abrahamian, DO and David A. Talan, MD

Key Points

Tetanus in children in the United States is rare.

Children at higher risk for developing tetanus in the United States include those who are not completely vaccinated (including those children whose parents choose not to immunize them), adolescent injection-drug users, and immigrants from outside North America or Western Europe.

The decision to initiate postexposure prophylaxis is dependent on the wound characteristics and the child's vaccination history.

Wounds at higher risk for tetanus include contaminated wounds (e.g., with dirt, feces, soil, or saliva), puncture wounds, avulsions, wounds resulting from missiles, crush injuries, burns, frostbite, and those with neurovascular compromise.

The two important factors to determine about a patient's vaccination history are whether or not the patient has had a primary immunization series (i.e., at least three doses of adsorbed tetanus toxoid) and the elapsed time period since the last vaccination dose.

Introduction and Background

Although the global incidence of tetanus is high and continues worldwide to claim thousand of lives annually, it remains a rare disease in the United States and other developed countries.[1] Implementation of large-scale tetanus immunization programs, widespread availability of tetanus toxoid vaccine and immune globulin, and improved wound care management and childbirth practices have all contributed to the dramatic decline in the incidence of tetanus in developed countries. Although no active immunization practice is considered 100% effective, tetanus immunization has shown to be one of the most effective immunization practices ever developed.[2,3]

Recognition and Approach

In the United States, tetanus occurs primarily in adults, although internationally, neonatal tetanus accounts for the majority of cases.[1] During 1998–2000, a total of 130 cases of tetanus were reported to the Centers for Disease Control and Prevention (CDC).[4] The majority were males (60%) between the ages of 20 and 59 years (55%). Twelve (9%) of the cases involved children younger than 20 years of age, including one neonate. Of the 130 cases identified, the outcome was known for only 113 patients. Twenty of these patients died. None of the deaths occurred in children or adults younger than 30 years of age.

From a review of tetanus cases reported to the CDC from 1987 to 2000, the majority of the cases had an acute injury identified prior to the onset of illness.[4-8] Puncture wounds were the most frequent type of acute injury, followed by lacerations and abrasions. A common circumstance for a puncture wound was stepping on a nail. Other puncture wounds included splinters, tattooing, and animal bites. The sites of antecedent injury were, in order of decreasing frequency, a lower extremity, an upper extremity, the head, and the trunk.

Tetanus surveillance reports indicate that the populations relevant to pediatric emergency medicine that are at highest risk for developing tetanus in the United States are children who are not completely vaccinated, adolescent injection-drug users,[4-9] and immigrants from outside North America or Western Europe.[10-12]

Parental objections to immunizations are a key risk factor for children who develop tetanus in the United States. Neonates born to parents who object to and do not receive vaccinations, due to either religious or philosophical reasons, are at higher risk of developing tetanus. During 1992–2000, 13 cases of non-neonatal tetanus in children younger than 15 years were reported. Of those, 11 (85%) were not protected due to parental objections to immunizations.[13] Similarly, the three reported neonatal tetanus cases in the United States during 1989–2000 were associated with absent or incomplete maternal vaccination.[5,7,13,14]

Evaluation

The decision to initiate postexposure prophylaxis is dependent on the wound characteristics and the patient's vaccination history. Regarding tetanus postexposure prophylaxis, the Advisory Committee on Immunization Practices (ACIP) of the CDC categorizes wounds as either clean, minor wounds, or "all other wounds." Examples of "all other wounds" include contaminated wounds (e.g., with dirt, feces, soil, or saliva), puncture wounds, avulsions, wounds resulting from missiles, crush injuries, burns, and frostbite. These wounds are at higher risk for harboring *Clostridium tetani* since they have occurred in an environment in which *C. tetani* spores are prevalent or they are the type of tissue injury that provides low oxygen tension conducive for anaerobic conditions allowing *C. tetani* spore germination and proliferation.[15,16] Children who have not received at least three doses of adsorbed tetanus toxoid are also at increased risk for tetanus.[13]

In clinical practice, some parents are uncertain if their child has received a complete primary immunization series.[17] Current tetanus prophylaxis guidelines recommend considering a child as not having had any previous tetanus vaccinations if the history of past immunizations is unknown or uncertain.[15,16] Fortunately, young adults who have served in the military and children who have attended public schools in North America or Western Europe are likely to have completed a primary immunization series. Immigrants from outside North America or Western Europe and adults who do not have an education level beyond grade school are more likely to lack primary immunization.[10]

Management

The primary immunization series ensures adequate baseline levels of tetanus antibody and future anamnestic response to booster injections. Since immunity to tetanus with vaccination declines with time, booster doses are required to keep the antitoxin levels in a protective range. Periodic injections of tetanus toxoid result in sequentially higher peak responses, higher residual antitoxin levels, and longer periods during which antibodies are detected.[2] Primary immunization is

recommended beginning in infancy with intramuscular (IM) injections of diphtheria and tetanus toxoids and acellular pertussis vaccine (DTaP)[18-20] (Table 103–1). A catch-up tetanus immunization schedule and minimum intervals between doses for children and adolescents who start late or who are more than 1 month behind is also available[18] (Table 103–2). At age 19 and greater, a booster dose of tetanus and diphtheria toxoids vaccine (adult) (Td) administered every 10 years provides adequate protection for clean, minor, uncontaminated wounds. For all high-risk wounds that are also associated with a shorter tetanus incubating period, to make certain there is rapid attainment of adequate antibody levels, a booster dose is recommended if the preceding tetanus toxoid was given greater than 5 years prior[15,16,21] (Table 103–3). Since the ACIP regularly updates the recommended childhood and adolescent immunization schedules, we recommend reviewing the latest immunization recommendation by contacting local or state health departments, by accessing the CDC's National Immunization Program web site at *http://www.cdc.gov/nip*, or by calling the National Immunization Information Hotline at 800-232-2522 (English) or 800-232-0233 (Spanish).

Active Immunization

Active immunization is provided by the administration of tetanus toxoid, which is provided in various preparations[22] (Table 103–4). DTaP is indicated for primary and booster vaccinations against diphtheria, tetanus, and pertussis for children 6 weeks to 7 years (i.e., prior to the seventh birthday). DTaP is preferred over diphtheria and tetanus toxoids and whole-cell pertussis vaccine adsorbed (DTwP) due to its lower incidence of local and systemic adverse reactions and improved efficacy.[23] DTaP is given as a 0.5-ml IM injection into the anterolateral aspect of the thigh (for infants) or the deltoid muscle of the upper arm (for children). The most frequently encountered adverse events include local reactions such as injection site tenderness, redness, induration, and

Table 103–1	Routine Diphtheria, Tetanus, and Pertussis Vaccination Schedule Summary for Children and Adolescents		
Dose	**Customary Age**	**Age/Interval***	**Product**
Primary 1	2 mo	6 wk old or older	DTaP[†]
Primary 2	4 mo	4–8 wk after first dose	DTaP[†]
Primary 3	6 mo	4–8 wk after second dose	DTaP[†]
First booster	15–18 mo[‡]	6–12 mo after third dose	DTaP[†]
Second booster	4–6 yr old, before entering kindergarten or elementary school (not necessary if fourth dose [first booster] is administered after fourth birthday)		DTaP[†]
Additional boosters	Recommended at age 11–12 yr if at least 5 yr have elapsed since the last dose of tetanus and diphtheria toxoid–containing vaccine. Ages 13–18 yr should serve as a catch-up interval for those who were not immunized at ages 11–12 yr. Subsequent routine Td boosters are recommended every 10 yr		Tdap

*Prolonging the interval does not require restarting the series.
[†]Use diphtheria and tetanus toxoids vaccine adsorbed (pediatric) (DT) if encephalopathy has occurred after administration of a previous dose of pertussis-containing vaccine. If the child is ≥1 year of age at the time that primary dose three is due, a third dose 6 to 12 months after the second dose completes primary vaccination with DT.
[‡]The fourth dose of DTaP may be administered at age 12 months provided that 6 months have elapsed since the third dose and the child is unlikely to return at age 15 to 18 months. The final dose in the series should be given at age 4–6 years.
Abbreviations: DTaP, diphtheria and tetanus toxoids and acellular pertussis vaccine adsorbed; Tdap, tetanus and diphtheria toxoids and acellular pertussis vaccine adsorbed formulated for use in adolescents and adults ≤64 years of age (Boostrix® approved for use in persons aged 10–18 years; Adacel™ approved for use in persons aged 11–64 years); Td, tetanus and diphtheria toxoids vaccine adsorbed (minimum age: 7 years).
This immunization schedule is based on information in references 18, 19, 20, and 34.

Table 103–2   Catch-up Tetanus Immunization Schedule and Minimum Intervals between Doses for Children and Adolescents Who Start Late or Who Are More Than or Equal to 1 Month Behind—United Sates, 2007

Catch-up Schedule for Children Ages 4 mo–6 yr Minimum Interval between Doses				
Dose 1 (Minimum Age)	Dose 1 to Dose 2	Dose 2 to Dose 3	Dose 3 to Dose 4	Dose 4 to Dose 5
DTaP (6 wk)	4 wk	4 wk	6 mo	6 mo*

Catch-up Schedule for Children Ages 7–18 yr[†] Minimum Interval between Doses		
Dose 1 to Dose 2	Dose 2 to Dose 3	Dose 3 to Dose 4
4 wk	8 wk: If first dose administered at age < 12 mo. 6 mo: If first dose administered at age > 12 mo.	6 mo: If first dose administered at age < 12 mo.

Note: There is no need to restart a vaccine series regardless of the time that has elapsed between doses.
*The fifth dose is not necessary if the fourth dose was given after the fourth birthday. Minimum age for DTaP administration is 6 weeks and maximum age is 6 years.
†Tdap should be substituted for a single dose of Td in the primary catch-up series or as a booster if age appropriate. Td should be used for all other doses. A 5-year interval from the last Td dose is encouraged when Tdap is used as a booster dose.
Abbreviations: DTaP, diphtheria and tetanus toxoids and acellular pertussis vaccine adsorbed; Tdap, tetanus and diphtheria toxoids and acellular pertussis vaccine adsorbed formulated for use in adolescents and adults ≤ 64 years of age; Td, tetanus and diphtheria toxoids vaccine adsorbed.
Data from Centers for Disease Control and Prevention: Recommended immunization schedules for persons aged 0–18 years—US, 2007. MMWR Morb Mortal Wkly Rep 55(51&52):1–4, 2007.

Table 103–3   Current Summary Guide to Tetanus Prophylaxis in Routine Wound Management

History of Adsorbed Tetanus Toxoid (Doses)	Clean, Minor Wounds		All Other Wounds*	
	Td or Tdap[†]	TIG	Td or Tdap[†]	TIG
Unknown or <3	Yes	No	Yes	Yes
3 or more	No[‡]	No	No[§]	No

*Such as, but not limited to, wounds contaminated with dirt, feces, soil, or saliva; puncture wounds; avulsions; and wounds resulting from missiles, crushing, burns, or frostbite.
†Tdap is preferred to Td for adolescents aged 11–18 years and adults aged 19–64 years who have never received Tdap. The preferred tetanus toxoid-containing vaccine for children aged < 7 years is DTaP. Minimum age for DTaP administration is 6 weeks and maximum age is 6 years. Minimum age for Td is 7 years.
‡Yes, if ≥10 years have elapsed since the last tetanus toxoid-containing vaccine dose.
§Yes, if ≥5 years have elapsed since the last tetanus toxoid-containing vaccine dose.
Abbreviations: Tdap, tetanus-diphtheria-acellular pertussis vaccine adsorbed formulated for use in adolescents and adults ≤64 years of age (Boostrix® approved for use in persons aged 10–18 years; Adacel™ approved for use in persons aged 11–64 years); Td, tetanus and diphtheria toxoids vaccine adsorbed; DTaP, diphtheria and tetanus toxoids and acellular pertussis vaccines; TIG, human tetanus immunoglobulin.
Data from references 15, 16, 35, and 36.

swelling[16,24] (see Chapter 102, Vaccination-Related Complaints and Side Effects).

Absolute contraindications to further vaccination with DTP include immediate anaphylactic reaction and encephalopathy, in the absence of other identifiable etiologies, occurring within 7 days following previous DTP vaccination. Precautions to further DTP vaccinations include occurrence of fever ≥40.5° C (105° F) within 48 hours (not due to another identifiable cause), collapse or shocklike state (hypotonic-hyporesponsive episode) within 48 hours, convulsions with or without fever within 3 days, and persistent inconsolable crying lasting ≥3 hours within 48 hours.[20,24] Children with a personal or family history of seizures are at higher risk for developing seizures following DTP immunizations. We recommend giving these children 15 mg/kg of acetaminophen at the time of vaccination and every 4 hours for the ensuing 24 hours to reduce the possibility of postvaccination fever.[25,26]

Td is indicated for primary and booster vaccination against diphtheria and tetanus for adolescents, adults, and children 7 years of age or older. Tdap (tetanus and diphtheria toxoids and acellular pertussis vaccine adsorbed formulated for use in adolescents and adults ≤64 years of age) should be substituted for a single dose of Td in the primary catch-up series or as a booster if age appropriate. Td should be used for all other doses. A 5-year interval from the last Td dose is encouraged when Tdap is used as a booster dose. The Tdap or Td is given as a 0.5-ml IM injection into the anterolateral aspect of the upper thigh (preferred site for small children) or the deltoid muscle. A history of a neurologic reaction (e.g., encephalopathy) or an immediate anaphylactic reaction is a contraindication to further Td and Tdap vaccinations. Patients who have experienced an Arthus-type hypersensitivity reaction following a prior dose of tetanus toxoid often have high serum tetanus antitoxin levels due to inadequately spaced booster injections. These individuals should not be given further routine or even emergency booster doses of Td or Tdap more frequently than every 10 years.[16]

Immunosuppressed children such as those afflicted with the human immunodeficiency virus, patients undergoing radiation therapy, or those receiving antineoplastic or immunosuppressive agents (e.g., long-term corticosteroid use) may

Table 103–4	Various Forms of Tetanus Toxoid Preparations	
Preparation (Abbreviation)	**Route (0.5 ml)**	**Indication**
Diphtheria and tetanus toxoids and pertussis vaccine adsorbed (DTP)	IM	Preferred agent for children <7 yr old; the pertussis component of DTP can be either whole cell (DTwP) or acellular (DTaP). The acellular version is the preferred preparation.
Diphtheria and tetanus toxoids vaccine adsorbed (pediatric) (DT)	IM	Use in children <7 yr old if pertussis vaccine is contraindicated.
Tetanus and diphtheria toxoids and acellular pertussis vaccine adsorbed (adolescents and adults ≤64 years of age) (Tdap)	IM	Boostrix® approved for use in persons aged 10–18 years; Adacel™ approved for use in persons aged 11–64 years.
Diphtheria and tetanus toxoids vaccine adsorbed (adult) (Td)	IM	Use in adults and children ≥7 yr old.
Tetanus toxoid adsorbed (TTA)	IM	Use in patients who have a contraindication to combined antigens. It is the preferred single-agent formulation due to its greater antigenic effects.
Tetanus toxoid fluid (TT)	IM or SC	Use in patients who have a contraindication to combined antigens or those who are hypersensitive to the aluminum adjuvant in the adsorbed toxoid.

Abbreviations: IM, intramuscularly; SC, subcutaneously.
Adapted from Abrahamian FM: Tetanus—an update on an ancient disease. Infect Dis Clin Pract 9:228–235, 2000.

receive tetanus toxoid. However, due to their disease state, these children may not mount an adequate immunologic response to the vaccination. Although there is no evidence to suggest Td (classified in U.S. Food and Drug Administration Pregnancy Category C) has any teratogenic effects, as a precaution, the ACIP recommends withholding the Td until the second trimester of pregnancy based on the balance between risks and benefits.[16,24] Due to lack of safety data, currently Tdap is not recommended for administration in pregnant patients.

Passive Immunization

Passive immunization is provided by the administration of human tetanus immune globulin (HTIG). The dosage for postexposure tetanus prophylaxis is 250 international units (IU) IM into the anterolateral muscles of the lateral thigh (for infants) or the deltoid muscle in the upper arm (for older children). Theoretically, the prophylactic dose of HTIG may be calculated by body weight and administered at a dose of 4 IU/kg. However, we recommend administering the entire contents of the vial (250 IU) regardless of the child's size. This recommendation is based on the concept that the amount of toxin produced by the organism is independent of the child's body size. The 250-IU dose will provide adequate antitoxin levels about 2 to 3 days after administration and for a period lasting at least 4 weeks, with a half-life of 23 days.[27]

The route of administration of HTIG should be IM. HTIG should not be given intravenously due to an increased risk of developing an anaphylactic reaction. Although intrathecal administration of HTIG has been investigated for therapy of active tetanus, this route is not recommended for prophylactic therapy.[28,29] Otherwise, there are no specific contraindications to HTIG administration. HTIG is categorized as a Pregnancy Category C drug, and when indicated can be given to a pregnant adolescent. No dosage adjustment is necessary in patients with renal impairment.

Although the concurrent administration of HTIG with tetanus toxoid may result in some period of delay in the induction of active immunity, the ACIP tetanus prophylaxis guidelines recommend HTIG and tetanus toxoid be given at the same time for patients with tetanus-prone wounds who are uncertain about their primary immunization history or have received fewer than three prior tetanus toxoid doses in the past.[15,16,27,30-32] (see Table 103–3). However, HTIG and tetanus toxoid should not be administered at the same anatomic site or given by the same syringe. Similarly, immunologic response may diminish with simultaneous administration of HTIG with other live virus vaccines (e.g., measles, mumps, rubella, oral polio). To avoid this interaction, live virus vaccination should be delayed for 3 months after HTIG is given. If simultaneous injections are necessary, administration should occur at different sites. Such patients need to be assessed for seroconversion at a later time and may require revaccination.[33]

Summary

Tetanus immunization is one of the most effective immunization practices ever developed. In the United States, tetanus occurs primarily in adults, and the majority of the cases had an acute injury identified prior to the onset of illness. Puncture wounds were the most frequent type of acute injury associated with clinical tetanus, followed by lacerations and abrasions.

Children at higher risk of developing tetanus are those who are not completely vaccinated, adolescent injection-drug users, immigrants from outside North America or Western Europe, and young adults uneducated beyond grade school. Neonates born to parents who object to and do not receive vaccinations are also at higher risk of developing tetanus.

The decision to initiate postexposure prophylaxis is dependent on the characteristics of the wound and the patient's vaccination history. Wounds at higher risk for tetanus include contaminated wounds (e.g., with dirt, feces, soil, or saliva), puncture wounds, avulsions, wounds resulting from missiles, crush injuries, burns, frostbite, and neurovascularly compromised wounds. HTIG and tetanus toxoid should be given at the same time for children with tetanus-prone wounds who are uncertain about their primary immunization history or have received fewer than three prior tetanus toxoid doses in the past.

REFERENCES

1. Vandelaer J, Birmingham M, Gasse F, et al: Tetanus in developing countries: an update on the maternal and neonatal tetanus elimination initiative. Vaccine 21:3442–3445, 2003.
2. Edsall G: Specific prophylaxis of tetanus. JAMA 171:417–427, 1959.
3. Wassilak SGF, Roper MH, Murphy TV, et al: Tetanus toxoid. *In* Plotkin SA, Orenstein WA (eds): Vaccines. Philadelphia: WB Saunders, 2004, pp 745–781.
4. Pascual FB, McGinley EL, Zanardi LR, et al: Tetanus surveillance—United States, 1998–2000. Morb Mortal Wkly Rep Surveill Summ 52(SS 3):1–8, 2003.
5. Bardenheier B, Prevots DR, Khetsuriani N, et al: Tetanus surveillance—United States, 1995–1997. Morb Mortal Wkly Rep Surveill Summ 47(SS-2):1–13, 1998.
6. Izurieta HS, Sutter RW, Strebel PM, et al: Tetanus surveillance—United States, 1991–1994. Morb Mortal Wkly Rep Surveill Summ 46(SS-2):15–25, 1997.
7. Prevots R, Sutter RW, Strebel PM, et al: Tetanus surveillance—United States, 1989–1990. Morb Mortal Wkly Rep Surveill Summ 41(SS-8):1–9, 1992.
8. Centers for Disease Control and Prevention: Current trends tetanus—United States, 1987 and 1988. MMWR Morb Mortal Wkly Rep 39:37–41, 1990.
9. Scher KS, Baldera A, Wheeler WE, et al: Inadequate tetanus protection among the rural elderly. South Med J 78:153–156, 1985.
*10. Talan DA, Abrahamian FM, Moran GJ, et al: Tetanus immunity and physician compliance with tetanus prophylaxis practices among emergency department patients presenting with wounds. Ann Emerg Med 43:305–314, 2004.
11. Gergen PJ, McQuillan GM, Kiely M, et al: Population-based serologic survey of immunity to tetanus in the United States. N Engl J Med 332:761–766, 1995.
12. McQuillan GM, Kruszon Moran D, Deforest A, et al: Serologic immunity to diphtheria and tetanus in the United States. Ann Intern Med 136:660–666, 2002.
13. Fair E, Murphy TV, Golaz A, et al: Philosophic objection to vaccination as a risk for tetanus among children younger than 15 years. Pediatrics 109:e2, 2002.
14. Centers for Disease Control and Prevention: Neonatal tetanus—Montana, 1998. MMWR Morb Mortal Wkly Rep 47(43):928–930, 1998.
15. Centers for Disease Control and Prevention: Diphtheria, tetanus, and pertussis: recommendations for vaccine use and other preventive measures. Recommendations of the Immunization Practices Advisory Committee (ACIP). MMWR Recomm Rep 40(RR-10):1–28, 1991.
16. Centers for Disease Control and Prevention: Update on adult immunization—recommendations of the Immunization Practices Advisory Committee (ACIP). MMWR Recomm Rep 40(RR-12):1–94, 1991.
17. Callahan JM, Reed D, Meguid V, et al: Utility of an immunization registry in a pediatric emergency department. Pediatr Emerg Care 20:297–301, 2004.
18. Centers for Disease Control and Prevention: Recommended childhood and adolescent immunization schedule—United States, July–December 2004. MMWR Morb Mortal Wkly Rep 53:Q1–Q3, 2004.

19. Centers for Disease Control and Prevention: Recommended childhood and adolescent immunization schedule—United States, January–June 2004. MMWR Morb Mortal Wkly Rep 53:Q1–Q4, 2004.
20. Centers for Disease Control and Prevention: Pertussis vaccination: use of acellular pertussis vaccines among infants and young children. Recommendations of the Advisory Committee on Immunization Practices (ACIP). MMWR Recomm Rep 46(RR-7):1–25, 1997.
21. Centers for Disease Control and Prevention: Recommended adult immunization schedule—United States, 2003–2004. MMWR Morb Mortal Wkly Rep 52:965–969, 2003.
*22. Abrahamian FM: Tetanus—an update on an ancient disease. Infect Dis Clin Pract 9:228–235, 2000.
23. Greco D, Salmaso S, Mastrantonio P, et al: A controlled trial of two acellular vaccines and one whole-cell vaccine against pertussis. N Engl J Med 334:341–348, 1996.
24. Centers for Disease Control and Prevention: Update: vaccine side effects, adverse reactions, contraindications, and precautions. Recommendations of the Advisory Committee on Immunization Practices (ACIP). MMWR Recomm Rep 45(RR-12):1–35, 1996.
25. Ipp MM, Gold R, Greenberg S, et al: Acetaminophen prophylaxis of adverse reactions following vaccination of infants with diphtheria-pertussis-tetanus toxoids-polio vaccine. Pediatr Infect Dis J 6:721–725, 1987.
26. Lewis K, Cherry JD, Sachs MH, et al: The effect of prophylactic acetaminophen administration on reactions to DTP vaccination. Am J Dis Child 142:62–65, 1988.
27. Levine L, McComb JA, Dwyer RC, et al: Active-passive tetanus immunization: choice of toxoid, dose of tetanus immune globulin and timing of injections. N Engl J Med 274:186–190, 1966.
28. Miranda-Filho D de B, Ximenes RA, Barone AA, et al: Randomized controlled trial of tetanus treatment with antitetanus immunoglobulin by the intrathecal or intramuscular route. BMJ 328:615, 2004.
29. Gupta PS, Kapoor R, Goyal S, et al: Intrathecal human tetanus immunoglobulin in early tetanus. Lancet 2:439–440, 1980.
30. Porter JD, Perkin MA, Corbel MJ, et al: Lack of early antitoxin response to tetanus booster. Vaccine 10:334–336, 1992.
31. Mahoney LJ, Aprile MA, Moloney PJ: Combined active-passive immunization against tetanus in man. Can Med Assoc J 96:1401–1404, 1967.
32. Dal-Ré R, Gil A, González A, et al: Does tetanus immune globulin interfere with the immune response to simultaneous administration of tetanus-diphtheria vaccine? A comparative clinical trial in adults. J Clin Pharmacol 35:420–425, 1995.
33. Centers for Disease Control and Prevention: General recommendations on immunization: recommendations of the Advisory Committee on Immunization Practices (ACIP) and the American Academy of Family Physicians (AAFP). MMWR Recomm Rep 51(RR-2):1–36, 2002.
*34. Centers for Disease Control and Prevention: Recommended immunization schedules for persons aged 0–18 years—US, 2007. MMWR Morb Mortal Wkly Rep 55(51&52):1–4, 2007.
*35. Centers for Disease Control and Prevention: Preventing tetanus, diphtheria, and pertussis among adults: use of tetanus toxoid, reduced diphtheria toxoid and acellular pertussis vaccine. MMWR Morb Mortal Wkly Rep 55(RR-17):1–37, 2006.
*36. Centers for Disease Control and Prevention: Preventing tetanus, diphtheria, and pertussis among adolescents: use of tetanus toxoid, reduced diphtheria toxoid and acellular pertussis vaccine. MMWR Morb Mortal Wkly Rep 55(early release):1–43, 2006.

*Selected readings.

Chapter 104

Rabies Postexposure Prophylaxis

Fredrick M. Abrahamian, DO and David A. Talan, MD

Key Points

In the United States, bites from raccoons, skunks, bats, foxes, bobcats, coyotes, and mongooses are considered high risk for rabies transmission.

Domestic animal bites (from dogs, cats, ferrets, and livestock) are generally considered low risk; however, dogs along the U.S.-Mexico border and cats that roam freely in endemic areas pose a higher risk.

Rabies postexposure prophylaxis is not warranted for bites from smaller mammals (e.g., mice, squirrels, rabbits, chipmunks, rats, hamsters, gerbils, guinea pigs).

The decision to initiate rabies postexposure prophylaxis is dependent on the animal species; a detailed account of the animal contact, including whether the attack was provoked; local rabies epidemiology for the animal species involved (information typically available from local health officials); and the availability of the animal for observation or euthanasia for rabies brain testing.

Rabies postexposure prophylaxis consists of the administration of human rabies immune globulin and rabies vaccine.

Introduction and Background

Rabies exerts a considerable public health impact worldwide, especially in developing countries.[1] Globally, the annual number of rabies-associated deaths is predicted to be between 40,000 and 70,000.[2,3] However, in the United States and other developed countries, human rabies remains a rare disease. From 1980 to 1996, only 32 laboratory-confirmed cases of human rabies were diagnosed in the United States, and 1 to 5 cases of rabies each year in humans were reported to the Centers for Disease Control and Prevention (CDC) during 2000–2003.[4-8] The decline is attributed to the control of rabies in domestic animal populations and effective pre- and post-exposure vaccination programs.

Worldwide, an estimated 10 million people receive rabies postexposure prophylaxis (RPEP) annually, and although human rabies is rare in the United States, approximately 16,000 to 39,000 U.S. patients per year receive RPEP.[2,9] A multicenter, prospective study of patients presenting to the emergency department with an animal exposure demonstrated that RPEP is at times used inappropriately.[10] Since children who have sustained animal bites commonly present to the emergency department, the emergency department is a common location for RPEP to be initiated. Emergency physicians will best help their patients if they have a clear understanding of the guidelines published by the Advisory Committee on Immunization Practices (ACIP) on rabies prevention that direct the use of RPEP.[11]

During 2000–2003, approximately 7000 to 8000 cases of animal rabies were reported to the CDC.[5-8] In the United States, raccoons, mostly reported from the eastern states, continue to be the most frequently encountered rabid wildlife species. In addition to raccoons, other wild animals most often infected with rabies in the United States, in order of decreasing frequency, include skunks, bats, and foxes.[5-8] Bites from bobcats, coyotes, and mongooses are also considered high risk for rabies transmission.[12]

Recognition and Approach

Rabies is a deadly disease and surviving it is exceedingly rare. A case report published in 2005 of a 15-year-old girl who survived rabies, albeit with substantial neurologic damage, highlights the rarity of this devastating disease in the United States.[13] When a child has come into contact with an animal and rabies is a consideration, diagnosing rabies is not the key task of emergency physicians. Instead, prevention of the development of rabies through the selection of appropriate patients for the initiation of RPEP is the main concern for emergency physicians.

Evaluation

The transmission of rabies occurs when the virus is introduced from animal saliva into an open wound from a bite, or when the virus comes in contact with an open wound or mucous membrane. One of the first steps in evaluating a child who has come into contact with an animal is whether or not there is a reasonable likelihood that clinically significant exposure to the virus has occurred.

Exposures versus Nonexposure Contact

Exposures can be categorized as bites and nonbites. Bites are the predominant type of exposure. Regardless of the severity, bites are always considered potential exposures. Bats, due to their small, thin, and sharp teeth, often leave minimal external signs of a bite, and as a result, their bites may go unnoticed. This circumstance is most likely in preverbal toddlers, minimally verbal developmentally delayed children, and intoxicated adolescents. In the United States, the majority of the human rabies cases are caused by bat-associated rabies virus variant and, in most of these cases, no knowledge of a bite existed.[4,14,15]

Nonbite exposures include contamination of open wounds (e.g., abrasions, scratches) or mucous membranes with the saliva or neuronal tissue of a potentially rabid animal. In comparison to a bite, exposure via this mechanism carries a lower risk for acquiring the disease. Other reported nonbite modes of transmission include exposure to large amounts of aerosolized rabies virus (e.g., inhaling bat guano in a cave) and organ transplantation from infected donors.[16-21] The risk of disease transmission to a recipient of an organ from an infected donor is high.[22] Apart from transplants, there is no evidence of laboratory-confirmed cases of human-to-human transmission of rabies either among household contacts or in the health care setting.[11,23]

Activities such as petting a rabid animal are not thought to place the patient at risk for contracting rabies. Similarly, contact with blood, urine, or feces of a rabid animal is also not considered a clinically significant exposure.[11]

Animal Species

Domesticated Animals

The prevalence of rabies among domestic animals (e.g., dog, cat, ferret, and livestock) has declined dramatically over the past century due to effective rabies vaccination practices. Although bites from domestic animals are generally considered low risk, dogs along the U.S.-Mexico border and cats that roam freely through areas in which animal rabies is endemic are considered to pose a higher risk. In developing countries, dogs are the main reservoir for disease transmission and the principle source of human rabies.[24] State or local health officials should be consulted when there is a question regarding the prevalence of rabies in a specific species and region.

Bats

Unlike the varied geographic prevalence of rabies in wild terrestrial mammals, rabies in bats has remained widely distributed throughout the United States. RPEP should be initiated for patients in whom there is apparent or reasonable probability of a bat bite, scratch, or mucous membrane exposure. Postexposure prophylaxis is also warranted if a bat is found in the room of an individual who is incapable of attesting to absence of direct contact. Examples of this situation are when a sleeping person awakens to find a bat in the room or a bat is found in a room occupied by an unattended child, a person with mental disability, or an intoxicated individual. The only exceptions when RPEP could be withheld are if the bat is captured and immediate brain testing is available, or if the individual is certain that contact has not occurred.[11]

Wild Rodents

Although all mammals are susceptible to rabies virus, smaller mammals (e.g., mice, squirrels, rabbits, chipmunks, rats, hamsters, gerbils, guinea pigs) are often not able to survive an attack from another animal with the potential to transmit rabies. Consequently, these smaller mammals are not thought to be likely to be infected with rabies virus. Larger rodents such as woodchucks and beavers are an exception, and have been reported to be rabid in areas where terrestrial rabies is enzootic.[12,25]

Wild Terrestrial Carnivores and Hybrids

The prevalence of rabies in wild terrestrial carnivores varies geographically. In most instances, a clinically significant exposure is assumed to have occurred with a bite from a wild terrestrial carnivore (e.g., raccoons, skunks, foxes, coyotes, bobcats, mongoose) or a hybrid resulting from breeding of a wild terrestrial carnivore with a domestic animal (e.g., a wolf-dog hybrid). Patients and their families should not be encouraged to capture the suspected animal since this might result in additional risk of exposure.

Birds, Reptiles, and Sea Creatures

Rabies is exclusively seen in mammals. Nonmammalian bites do not pose a risk of rabies transmission.

Attack Provocation

With the exception of bats, an animal's behavior and the circumstances of an attack are also factors to assess the likelihood of rabies virus exposure. Rabid animals tend to act agitated and attack indiscriminately. Normal behavior in an animal makes the possibility of rabies less likely, although an assessment of "normal" behavior in wild terrestrial carnivores is difficult. Typically, most animals avoid humans and bites are commonly provoked. Feeding, handling, taunting, or surprising animals are considered provocative actions. For exposures involving normally behaving domestic animals (e.g., dogs, cats), in areas where rabies is not endemic, attacks are considered provoked and the animal is unlikely to be rabid.

Local Epidemiology

Local health officials are the best sources of information for the local epidemiology of animal reservoirs of rabies. If an emergency physician is unfamiliar with the local epidemiology, contacting a local health official can clarify many concerns of the health care providers, the patients, and their families.

Management

The three main components of managing a child who has come into contact with an animal and for whom concern about rabies exposure has arisen are local wound care, the decision on whether or not to initiate RPEP, and the implementation of RPEP when indicated.

Local Wound Care

Local wound care should include cleansing the wound with a solution of soap and water, which has been shown to potentially reduce the risk of acquiring rabies.[26-28] Irrigating the wound with a virucidal cleansing solution based in iodine (e.g., diluted povidone-iodine solution) is also advised.[11,24] Concentrated forms of povidone-iodine solution, detergents, and hydrogen peroxide are toxic to tissues and should not be used to irrigate wounds.[29,30] Other basic measures of wound care include débridement of necrotic and devitalized tissues, tetanus prophylaxis, assessment for and management of concurrent injuries (e.g., fractures), and initiation of antibiotics, as indicated (see Chapter 160, Wound Management).

Deciding on Initiating Rabies Prophylaxis

The decision to initiate RPEP is dependent on several key factors that include: animal type and its behavior, type of exposure (e.g., bite vs. nonbite), circumstances of the attack (e.g., provoked vs. unprovoked), local rabies epidemiology for the species involved, and availability of the animal for brain testing or observation (Fig. 104–1).

Animal Observation

Observation allows beloved family pets to be spared immediate death for brain testing. Dogs, cats, and ferrets are the only animal species suitable for observation. Wild animal hybrids (e.g., wild animal crossbred to domestic dogs or cats) are not suitable for observation and they should be regarded as wild animals.[11] The observation period is 10 days and is best done by animal control authorities. Rabies vaccination should not be given to the animal during this observation period. Any abnormal behavior or illness developing within this observation period necessitates evaluation by a veterinarian. If rabies is suggested, the animal should immediately be euthanized and undergo brain testing. Although a history of prior rabies vaccination of an animal makes the possibility of rabies infection and transmission unlikely, it should not deter entertaining animal observation, or if necessary, euthanasia and brain testing.[11,12] Diagnostic testing should be completed within 24 to 48 hours in order to avoid further delay in initiating RPEP. If the diagnosis cannot be made within this time frame, it is best to initiate RPEP pending the results of brain testing.

Active and Passive Immunization

RPEP should always include administration of both active and passive immunization, except in individuals who have previously been immunized. Active immunization is commonly achieved by human diploid cell vaccine. Other licensed preparations include rabies vaccine adsorbed (RVA) and purified chick embryo cell vaccine. RVA is not currently available in the United States.[12] All three types of vaccine are equally safe and efficacious when used properly.[11] The development of antibodies by active immunization takes about 7 to 10 days and usually persists for ≥2 years. For the purpose of postexposure prophylaxis, a regimen of five 1.0-ml doses of any of the vaccines should be given intramuscularly (IM). The first dose is given as soon as possible after exposure (day 0), with the remaining four doses administered on days 3, 7, 14, and 28 after the first vaccination. Patients with a prior history of vaccination should only receive vaccine on days 0 and 3. The preferred site for IM injection in adolescents and adults is the deltoid area and in children is the anterolateral aspect of the thigh. The gluteal region should be avoided for rabies vaccine injections due to a diminished antibody response.[31]

Passive immunization is achieved by the administration of human rabies immune globulin (RIG). It provides rapid protection with a serum half-life of 21 days.[32] Two human RIG products are available in the United States (BayRab and Imogam Rabies-HT) with equal efficacy and safety profiles.[11,12] The recommended dosage for both immune globulins is 20 IU/kg body weight and it applies to all age groups, including children. Adherence to this dosage is important since higher doses have the potential for suppressing active antibody production.[33] A full dose should be infiltrated into and around the wounds if anatomically possible.[34] If not (e.g., finger wound), following infiltration of the wound area, the remaining dose should be administered IM in the deltoid or quadriceps muscle. To avoid antigen-antibody antagonism, RIG and rabies vaccine should not be administered at the same site or by the same syringe. Repeated injections of RIG are not necessary and should not be administered to individuals with a prior history of rabies immunization. If the administration of rabies vaccine and RIG were not on the same day, RIG may be given up to the seventh day after the first dose of vaccine. Beyond this period, RIG is no longer indicated since active immunization has taken effect.[11,35]

Humans Previously Immunized Against Rabies

Some animal workers and laboratory assistants who work with the rabies virus routinely get immunized against rabies. These previously immunized individuals should not receive RIG.

Vaccination-Related Complaints

Injection-site reactions (e.g., local tenderness, erythema, swelling) are the most common adverse reactions following vaccination. Systemic reactions are less common and can include headache, myalgias, abdominal pain, and dizziness (see Chapter 102, Vaccination-Related Complaints and Side Effects). There are no contraindications to the administration of rabies biologics during pregnancy.[36] Response to active immunization may not be adequate in individuals who are considered immunocompromised or those on immunosuppressive agents (e.g., corticosteroids). In such situations, it is important to assess antibody levels 2 to 4 weeks after postexposure prophylaxis to ensure an acceptable antibody response.[11] With the exception of yellow fever and oral Ty21a typhoid vaccines, simultaneous administration of live vaccines (e.g., measles, mumps, rubella, varicella) and human RIG should be avoided for a duration of at least 4 months.[37,38] If simultaneous administration of measles- or varicella-containing vaccine is necessary, administer the vaccine and human RIG at different sites and revaccinate or test for seroconversion after a period of 4 months. Human RIG and inactivated vaccines or toxoids (e.g., tetanus toxoid) can be administered simultaneously at different sites or at any time between doses.[38]

Summary

Rabies is rare. Emergency department evaluation of children who have come into contact with an animal is not rare. Familiarity with the overall decision-making strategies for

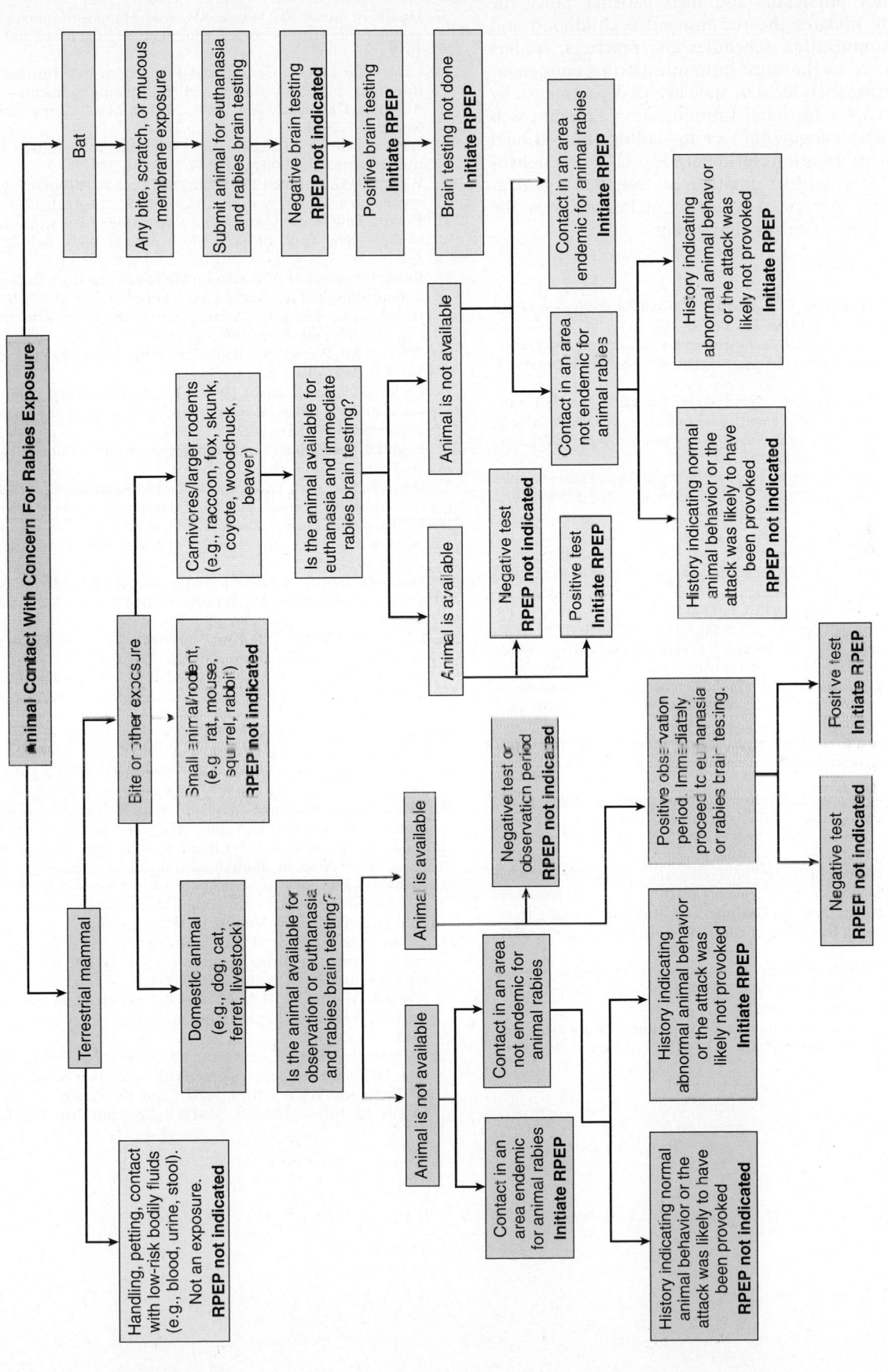

FIGURE 104–1. Algorithm for initiating rabies postexposure prophylaxis (RPEP).

*RPEP=rabies postexposure prophylaxis

evaluating these children for their risk of exposure to rabies helps emergency physicians and their patients. Since the ACIP regularly updates the recommended childhood and adolescent immunization schedules and practices, readers are advised to review the latest immunization recommendation by contacting their local or state health departments, by accessing the CDC's National Immunization Program web site at *http://www.cdc.gov/nip/*, or by calling the National Immunization Information Hotline at 800-232-2522 (English) or 800-232-0233 (Spanish) or other professional organizations such as the American Academy of Pediatrics or the American Academy of Family Physicians.

REFERENCES

1. Coleman PG, Fèvre EM, Cleaveland S: Estimating the public health impact of rabies. Emerg Infect Dis 10:140–142, 2004.
2. World Health Organization: Fact sheet No. 99. Available at *http://www.who.int/entity/mediacentre/factsheets/fs099/en/* (Accessed February 15, 2005).
3. World Health Organization: World Survey for Rabies No. 35 for the Year 1999. Geneva: World Health Organization, 2002. Available at *http://www.who.int/emc-documents/rabies/whocdscsreph200210.html* (Accessed February 15, 2005).
4. Noah DL, Drenzek CL, Smith JS, et al: Epidemiology of human rabies in the United States, 1980 to 1996. Ann Intern Med 128:922–930, 1998.
5. Krebs JW, Mandel EJ, Swerdlow DL, et al: Rabies surveillance in the United States during 2003. J Am Vet Med Assoc 225:1837–1849, 2004.
6. Krebs JW, Wheeling JT, Childs JE: Rabies surveillance in the United States during 2002. J Am Vet Med Assoc 223:1736–1748, 2003.
7. Krebs JW, Noll HR, Rupprecht CE, et al: Rabies surveillance in the United States during 2001. J Am Vet Med Assoc 221:1690–1701, 2002.
8. Krebs JW, Mondul AM, Rupprecht CE, et al: Rabies surveillance in the United States during 2000. J Am Vet Med Assoc 219:1687–1699, 2001.
9. Krebs JW, Long-Martin SC, Childs JE: Causes, costs and estimates of rabies postexposure prophylaxis treatments in the United States. J Public Health Manage Pract 4:56–62, 1998.
*10. Moran GJ, Talan DA, Mower W, et al: Appropriateness of rabies postexposure prophylaxis treatment for animal exposures. JAMA 284:1001–1007, 2000.
*11. Centers for Disease Control and Prevention: Human rabies prevention—United States, 1999: recommendations of the Advisory Committee on Immunization Practices (ACIP). MMWR Recomm Rep 48(RR-1):1–21, 1999.
*12. Rupprecht CE, Gibbons RV: Prophylaxis against rabies. N Engl J Med 351:2626–2635, 2004.
*13. Willoughby RE Jr, Tieves KS, Hoffman GM, et al: Survival after treatment of rabies with induction of coma. N Engl J Med 352:2508–2514, 2005.
14. Messenger SL, Smith JS, Rupprecht CE: Emerging epidemiology of bat-associated cryptic cases of rabies in humans in the United States. Clin Infect Dis 35:738–747, 2002.
15. Centers for Disease Control and Prevention: Human death associated with bat rabies—California, 2003. MMWR Morb Mortal Wkly Rep 53:33–35, 2004.
16. Javadi MA, Fayaz A, Mirdehghan SA, et al: Transmission of rabies by corneal graft. Cornea 15:431–433, 1996.
17. Houff SA, Burton RC, Wilson RW, et al: Human-to-human transmission of rabies virus by corneal transplant. N Engl J Med 300:603–604, 1979.
18. Centers for Disease Control and Prevention: Investigation of rabies infections in organ donor and transplant recipients—Alabama, Arkansas, Oklahoma, and Texas, 2004. MMWR Morb Mortal Wkly Rep 53:1–3, 2004.
19. Gibbons RV: Cryptogenic rabies, bats, and the question of aerosol transmission. Ann Emerg Med 39:528–536, 2002.
20. Winkler WG, Fashinell TR, Leffingwell L, et al: Airborne rabies transmission in a laboratory worker. JAMA 226:1219–1221, 1973.
21. Centers for Disease Control and Prevention: Rabies in a laboratory worker—New York. MMWR Morb Mortal Wkly Rep 26:183–184, 1977.
22. Kusne S, Smilack J: Transmission of rabies virus from an organ donor to four transplant recipients. Liver Transpl 11:1295–1297, 2005.
23. Helmick CG, Tauxe RV, Vernon AA: Is there a risk to contacts of patients with rabies? Rev Infect Dis 9:511–518, 1987.
*24. Warrell MJ, Warrell DA: Rabies and other lyssavirus diseases. Lancet 363:959–969, 2004.
25. Childs JE, Colby L, Krebs JW, et al: Surveillance and spatiotemporal associations of rabies in rodents and lagomorphs in the United States, 1985–1994. J Wild Dis 33:20–27, 1997.
26. Dean DJ: Pathogenesis and prophylaxis of rabies in man. N Y State J Med 63:3507–3513, 1963.
27. Dean DJ, Baer GM, Thompson WR: Studies on the local treatment of rabies-infected wounds. Bull World Health Organ 28:477–486, 1963.
28. Kaplan MM, Cohen D, Koprowski H, et al: Studies on the local treatment of wounds for the prevention of rabies. Bull World Health Organ 26:765–775, 1962.
29. Faddis D, Daniel D, Boyer J: Tissue toxicity of antiseptic solutions: a study of rabbit articular and periarticular tissues. J Trauma 17:895–897, 1977.
30. Oberg MS, Lindsey D: Do not put hydrogen peroxide or povidone iodine into wounds. J Trauma 20:323–324, 1980.
31. Fishbein DB, Sawyer LA, Reid Sanden FL, et al: Administration of human diploid-cell rabies vaccine in the gluteal area. N Engl J Med 318:124–125, 1988.
32. Cabasso VJ, Loofbourow JC, Roby RE, et al: Rabies immune globulin of human origin: preparation and dosage determination in nonexposed volunteer subjects. Bull World Health Organ 45:303–315, 1971.
33. Helmick CG, Johnstone C, Sumner J, et al: A clinical study of Merieux human rabies immune globulin. J Biol Stand 10:357–367, 1982.
34. Wilde H, Sirikawin S, Sabcharoen A, et al: Failure of postexposure treatment of rabies in children. Clin Infect Dis 22:228–232, 1996.
35. Khawplod P, Wilde H, Chomchey P, et al: What is an acceptable delay in rabies immune globulin administration when vaccine alone had been given previously? Vaccine 14:389–391, 1996.
36. Chutivongse S, Wilde H, Benjavongkulchai M, et al: Postexposure rabies vaccination during pregnancy: effect on 202 women and their infants. Clin Infect Dis 20:818–820, 1995.
37. Siber GR, Werner BC, Halsey NA, et al: Interference of immune globulin with measles and rubella immunization. J Pediatr 122:204–211, 1993.
*38. Centers for Disease Control and Prevention: General recommendations on immunization: recommendations of the Advisory Committee on Immunization Practices (ACIP) and the American Academy of Family Physicians (AAFP). MMWR Recomm Rep 51(RR-2):1–36, 2002.

---

*Selected readings.

Diabetic Ketoacidosis

Nicole Glaser, MD and Nathan Kuppermann, MD, MPH

Key Points

Classic symptoms of diabetic ketoacidosis (DKA) include polyuria, polydipsia, weight loss, vomiting, abdominal pain, and signs of dehydration

New onset of diabetes or missed insulin injections are the most frequent causes of DKA in children. Infections or other intercurrent illnesses are uncommon in children seen in the emergency department for DKA.

Dehydration, acidosis, and electrolyte depletion are the main physiologic and biochemical abnormalities in children with DKA. These abnormalities can be corrected with insulin, intravenous fluids, and electrolyte replacement.

Bicarbonate should not be routinely administered to children with DKA.

Cerebral edema is the most frequent serious complication of DKA in children.

Introduction and Background

Diabetic ketoacidosis (DKA) is a common presentation of type 1 diabetes mellitus in children. Twenty five percent to 40% of children with a new diagnosis of type 1 diabetes present in DKA.[1,2] Reports have also documented DKA in children with new diagnoses of type 2 diabetes.[3,4] In children with established diabetes, DKA episodes occur at a rate of 1% to 8% per year, and most often result from missed insulin injections.[2,5-7] In contrast to adults, in whom infections or other illnesses are frequently triggers of DKA, intercurrent illness is uncommon in children presenting to the emergency department with DKA.[8] Although most children with DKA recover uneventfully from the episode, DKA remains the most frequent diabetes-related cause of death in children.[9,10] The majority of these DKA-related deaths in children result from cerebral edema.

Recognition and Approach

DKA develops in children with diabetes when serum concentrations of insulin are low in relation to those of counter-regulatory hormones (glucagon, cortisol, growth hormone, and catecholamines) (Fig. 105–1). This hormonal imbalance causes hyperglycemia, resulting in osmotic diuresis, as well as hepatic ketone production, resulting in acidosis with an elevated anion gap. Osmotic diuresis leads both to dehydration and to electrolyte depletion with loss of sodium, potassium, calcium, phosphate, and magnesium. Vomiting and increased insensible fluid losses exacerbate this process. Physiologic and biochemical abnormalities in children with DKA thus include hyperglycemia, dehydration, acidosis, and electrolyte depletion.

Classic presenting symptoms of diabetes and DKA include polyuria, polydipsia, and weight loss. Nausea, vomiting, and abdominal pain are also frequently present in DKA. Abdominal pain may be severe and can be mistaken for an acute abdomen. In this regard, the history of persistently increased urine output despite vomiting and signs of dehydration should alert the clinician to the diagnosis of DKA. A fruity breath odor, caused by acetone, may also be present and can be helpful in alerting the clinician to the likelihood of DKA.

Clinical Presentation

Children with DKA typically present with an ill appearance, tachypnea in response to metabolic acidosis, tachycardia, and signs of dehydration. Tachypnea may be extreme and may give the appearance of respiratory distress, initially suggesting a diagnosis of pneumonia or other respiratory disease. A history of polyuria and polydipsia is an important distinguishing factor. Tachycardia is also typically present, along with signs of dehydration such as cool extremities and delayed capillary refill time. Even in the setting of severe acidosis and dehydration, children rarely develop hypotension or cardiovascular instability due to DKA. The presence of hypotension in a child with DKA suggests profound dehydration or the presence of sepsis or another associated illness.

The diagnosis of DKA can be confirmed when laboratory studies demonstrate a serum glucose concentration above 200 mg/dl, a venous pH below 7.30 (or serum bicarbonate concentration below 15 mmol/L), and ketonuria. The severity of DKA is classified according to the severity of acidosis, with mild DKA corresponding to a venous pH less than 7.30

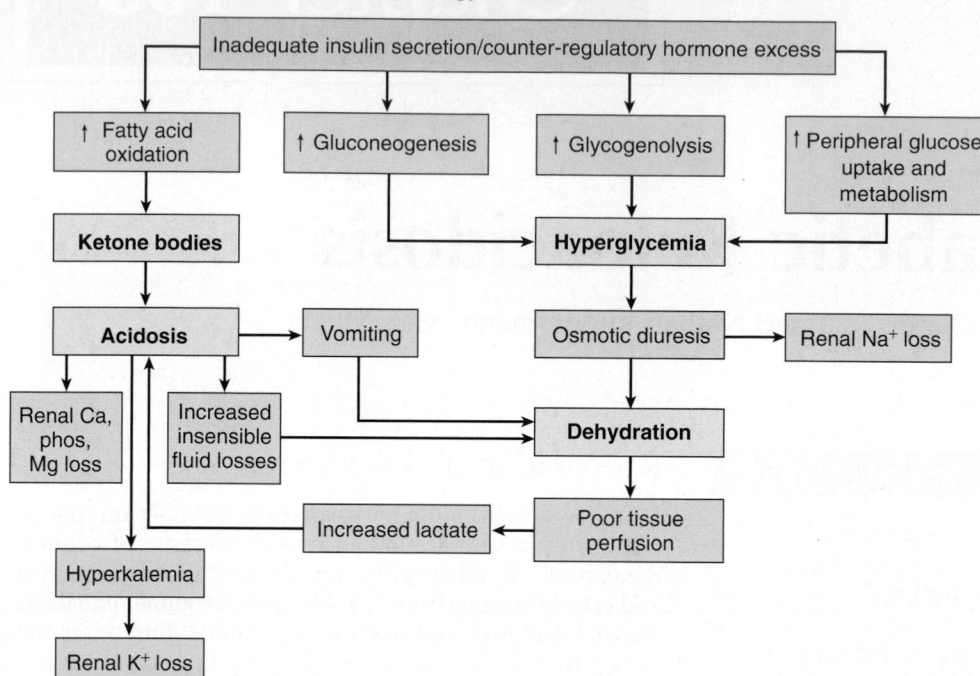

Pathophysiology of Diabetic Ketoacidosis

FIGURE 105–1. Pathophysiology of diabetic ketoacidosis. (From Styne DM, Glaser NS: Endocrine disorders. *In* Behrman R, Kliegman R [eds]: Nelson Essentials of Pediatrics, 4th ed. Philadelphia: WB Saunders, 1997, pp 711–766.)

(or serum bicarbonate concentration <15 mmol/L); moderate DKA to a pH less than 7.2 (or serum bicarbonate <10 mmol/L); and severe DKA to a pH less than 7.1 (or serum bicarbonate <5 mmol/L).[2,11] Infrequently, DKA can be present in patients with near-normal serum glucose concentrations. "Euglycemic DKA" has been described most frequently in pregnant women,[12] but can also occur in children with known diabetes, typically when additional insulin is administered at home in response to hyperglycemia. In this setting, insulin administration may correct hyperglycemia prior to correction of ketosis and acidosis.

In DKA, an elevated anion gap is present and the partial pressure of CO_2 (PCO_2) is low, reflecting respiratory compensation for metabolic acidosis. Elevated lactic acid concentrations may be present due to poor tissue perfusion and may contribute to acidosis (in addition to the ketosis). Serum sodium concentrations are typically low as a result of the osmotic effect of hyperglycemia. The serum sodium concentration decreases by approximately 1.6 mEq/L for every 100-mg/dl increase in serum glucose concentration above a concentration of 100 mg/dl.[13] Although serum potassium concentrations are typically normal or elevated at the time of presentation of DKA, total body potassium stores are usually profoundly depleted. Elevated serum potassium concentrations at presentation generally are a reflection of acidosis, and potassium concentrations typically decrease rapidly after the initiation of treatment. This is an important consideration in therapy of DKA.

Dehydration may result in prerenal azotemia with elevated blood urea nitrogen (BUN) and creatinine concentrations. Age-based standards for BUN and creatinine concentrations should be used because the normal ranges for these values increase with age.[14] The serum glucose concentration also may be viewed as an indicator of the adequacy of renal perfusion because serum glucose concentrations generally do not rise above 500 to 600 mg/dl in patients who maintain adequate renal perfusion. Blood glucose concentrations above 600 mg/dl in a child without preexisting renal disease likely reflect diminished renal perfusion resulting in a decreased glomerular filtration rate.

Important Clinical Features and Considerations

In infants and very young children, recognition of DKA may be difficult because polyuria, polydipsia, and abdominal pain are more difficult to detect in preverbal and non–toilet trained children. In young children who present with vomiting and signs of dehydration without diarrhea or other obvious cause, it is therefore advisable to obtain a bedside serum glucose measurement and/or urinalysis to rule out DKA.

While it is important to diagnose DKA and initiate appropriate treatment, clinicians must also attempt to identify the precipitant. New-onset of diabetes and noncompliance are the most common causes of DKA in children.[1,2,5-7] Insulin pump failure may also result in DKA, if not recognized promptly. Bacterial infections are a cause in only 13% and viral infections in 18% of all cases.[8] Infection is more likely to be a cause of DKA in children 3 years old and younger compared to older children.[8] Importantly, the serum white blood cell count is not generally helpful in discriminating between infected and uninfected patients.[8] In fact, white blood cell count elevations are common in children with DKA and are primarily a reflection of low pH and disease severity, rather than infection.

Management

Initial Management

An initial bolus of isotonic intravenous fluids (10 to 20 ml/kg of 0.9% saline or other isotonic fluid) is often needed to restore adequate perfusion. Additional boluses are necessary if the patient is severely dehydrated or if hemodynamic instability is present. An initial fluid bolus may not be necessary, however, for patients who are well perfused and hemodynamically stable on presentation. Initial rehydration alone often results in a substantial decrease in the serum glucose concentration through restoration of renal perfusion and a decrease in the levels of counter-regulatory hormones. Rehydration is continued to restore fluid deficits over a 48-hour period. Simultaneous with initiation of intravenous fluids, blood should be obtained for measurement of electrolytes, venous pH, magnesium, calcium, and phosphate. All patients should be placed on a cardiac monitor; an electrocardiogram is also recommended, particularly for children with suspected hyperkalemia.

Treatment with bicarbonate is rarely indicated as children are generally able to tolerate even severe acidosis without hemodynamic instability. Bicarbonate administration does not result in more rapid recovery from DKA, may lead to hypokalemia, and is associated with a fourfold increase in the risk of cerebral edema.[15-19] Therefore, bicarbonate should

not routinely be used in children with DKA. In rare clinical circumstances such as symptomatic hyperkalemia or hemodynamic instability due to extreme acidosis, bicarbonate therapy may be necessary.

Ongoing Management (Table 105–1)

Fluids and Insulin

International consensus guidelines for treatment of DKA have recently been published.[20,21] Following an initial fluid bolus, an intravenous insulin infusion is initiated at a rate of 0.1 units/kg/hr.[22] An initial bolus or loading dosage of insulin is not necessary, provided that a continuous infusion is begun promptly. Intravenous rehydration should be given along with the insulin infusion. The rate of fluid infusion should be calculated to replace the fluid deficit (typically 7% to 10% of body weight[23]) evenly over 48 hours. The sodium concentration of the intravenous fluids should be 0.45% saline or greater. Higher concentrations of sodium chloride (up to 0.9% saline) are also acceptable, although the high chloride

---

Table 105–1	Suggested Approach to DKA Management in Children

Fluid and Sodium Replacement

- Begin fluid replacement immediately.
- Base the volume of initial fluid bolus on the patient's circulatory status. Administer 10 to 20 ml/kg of isotonic fluids (0.9% saline or lactated Ringer's solution) for the fluid bolus(es). Repeat the bolus if necessary to restore perfusion. Some children may not require an initial fluid bolus if they are well perfused at presentation.
- Calculate subsequent fluid replacement rates to replace the fluid deficit (typically ~70 ml/kg), in addition to maintenance fluids, evenly over 48 hours. Use fluids with a tonicity between 0.45% and 0.9% saline.

Insulin

- Administer insulin intravenously at a rate of 0.1 units/kg/hr.
- An initial bolus or loading dose of insulin is not necessary.
- Continue insulin at 0.1 units/kg/hr until ketoacidosis has resolved (pH > 7.30, HCO_3 > 15, normalization of anion gap).
- To prevent hypoglycemia during treatment, add glucose to the intravenous fluids when the plasma glucose concentration falls below ~250 to 300 mg/dl.

Potassium, Phosphate, and Other Electrolyte Replacement

- Potassium replacement is required, and should be based on measurements of serum potassium.
- Begin potassium replacement immediately in patients with hypokalemia, and concurrent with insulin treatment in all others. For patients with hyperkalemia, base potassium replacement on the serum potassium measurement and administer potassium only after adequate urine output has been established.
- The initial potassium concentration in the intravenous fluids should be 30–40 mEq/L, except in rare circumstances in which the patient presents with substantial hyperkalemia. Adjust subsequent potassium administration according to serum potassium concentrations.
- Monitor calcium, magnesium, and phosphate concentrations during therapy. Phosphate concentrations typically decrease during treatment, and replacement of phosphate by using potassium phosphate in combination with potassium chloride can be considered. Replacement of calcium and magnesium is rarely required.

Use of Bicarbonate

- Do not routinely administer bicarbonate.
- Bicarbonate is only indicated in rare circumstances (symptomatic hyperkalemia, cardiovascular instability caused by severe acidosis).

Monitoring

- Assess vital signs hourly. Cardiac monitoring is recommended.
- Record fluid intake and output hourly.
- Measure blood glucose concentrations hourly. Measure electrolytes, serum urea nitrogen, creatinine, venous pH and PCO_2 every 2 to 4 hours. Calcium, magnesium, and phosphate should be monitored approximately every 6 hours. More frequent electrolyte measurements may be necessary in patients with abnormal or rapidly changing electrolyte concentrations.
- Assess mental status hourly. More frequent assessment may be necessary for patients with symptoms or signs of intracranial complications of DKA. The following signs and symptoms should raise concern about the possibility of cerebral edema: headache, inappropriate slowing of heart rate, rising blood pressure, recurrence of vomiting, mental status changes (e.g., irritability, lethargy), and specific neurologic signs (e.g., cranial nerve palsies, diminished pupillary reactivity).

Complications

- Hypokalemia and hypoglycemia occur frequently during DKA treatment, but are usually mild and easily corrected.
- Cerebral edema is the most frequent serious complication of DKA. If cerebral edema is suspected, promptly administer mannitol (0.25 to 1 g/kg).

Data from references 20 and 21.

content of these solutions increases the likelihood of developing hyperchloremic acidosis during therapy.

Typically, hyperglycemia resolves before the resolution of acidosis. For this reason, it is necessary to add dextrose to the intravenous fluids to prevent hypoglycemia during continued insulin infusion. When the serum glucose concentration decreases below approximately 250 to 300 mg/dl, dextrose is added to the intravenous fluids. A "two-bag system" allows more efficient and cost-effective administration of dextrose to children with DKA than traditional methods.[24] This system employs two bags of intravenous fluids with different dextrose concentrations (0 and 10%), but identical electrolyte content, administered simultaneously. The relative rates of administration of the two fluids are adjusted to increase or decrease the dextrose concentration while keeping fluid and electrolyte replacement constant. The insulin infusion should not be decreased or discontinued until acidosis has resolved and the serum bicarbonate concentration is above 15 to 18 mmol/L.[20]

Electrolyte Replacement

Serum potassium concentrations often decrease precipitously after the initiation of insulin therapy; therefore, replacement of potassium is mandatory. With the exception of children who present with significant hyperkalemia, replacement of potassium can be initiated as soon as adequate urine output is verified. Potassium chloride, or a combination of potassium chloride plus potassium phosphate or potassium acetate, is added to the intravenous fluids at a concentration of 30 to 40 mEq/L.

Whether or not phosphate replacement should be given routinely is controversial. Case reports have described rare episodes of severe hypophosphatemia during DKA treatment that resulted in hemolytic anemia and rhabdomyolysis.[25,26] Phosphate replacement, however, increases the likelihood of hypocalcemia during treatment, particularly if phosphate is infused rapidly. Hypocalcemia is infrequent when phosphate replacement is given in modest dosages.[27] Regardless of whether or not phosphate is administered, serum phosphate concentrations, along with calcium and magnesium concentrations, should be monitored during therapy as serum concentrations of these electrolytes tend to decrease during DKA treatment, which may occasionally necessitate replacement.

Monitoring

Monitoring of a child with DKA usually requires a pediatric intensive care unit or a hospital unit with similar capabilities for monitoring and managing such children. Continuous cardiac monitoring should be instituted, and vital signs and neurologic status are assessed hourly, or more frequently if there is concern about possible intracranial complications. Fluid intake and output should be recorded hourly. Glucose concentrations are measured on an hourly basis and electrolyte concentrations every 2 to 4 hours, depending on the degree of initial abnormality and rapidity of change during treatment. Calcium, phosphate, and magnesium concentrations can be measured less frequently, but a minimum of every 6 hours is recommended.

Complications

With appropriate treatment, most children recover uneventfully from DKA. The most frequent complications are hypo-

glycemia and mild hypokalemia, but these are generally easily detected and treated, provided that laboratory studies are measured according to schedule. Hypocalcemia, hypomagnesemia, and hypophosphatemia may occur during treatment but are rarely symptomatic. More serious complications of DKA are rare, but can have devastating consequences. These complications include cerebral edema,[19] pulmonary edema,[28-30] central nervous system (CNS) hemorrhage or thrombosis,[31] other large vessel thromboses,[32] cardiac arrhythmias,[19] pancreatitis,[33] renal failure,[34] intestinal necrosis,[35-37] and rhinocerebral mucormycosis.[38] Several reports have documented a prothrombotic state in both children and adults with DKA.[32,39] Children who are more severely hyperosmolar at presentation may be at greater risk for thrombotic complications. Femoral venous catheter use is associated with an increased risk for deep venous thrombosis, and should only be used when alternate venous access cannot be obtained.[32]

Although most serious complications of DKA are rare, cerebral edema is the most common, occurring in approximately 1% of pediatric DKA episodes.[19,40,41] The cause of this complication has been the subject of substantial debate. Initial hypotheses attributed cerebral edema to fluid influx into brain cells caused by rapid declines in serum osmolality and rapid fluid infusion. This hypothesis, however, has not been supported by data from clinical investigations. Symptomatic and even fatal cerebral edema can occur before hospital treatment for DKA is initiated. Asymptomatic or subclinical cerebral edema is present frequently, if not uniformly, at presentation.[10,42-44] In addition, studies that have adjusted for differences in DKA severity among patients have not found statistical associations between fluid or sodium infusion rates, or the rate of change in serum glucose concentration, and risk for cerebral edema.[19,45] More recent evidence suggests that cerebral edema during DKA may be predominantly vasogenic, and that cerebral ischemia during DKA or other factors may be more important determinants than osmolar changes.[46,47] Children at greatest risk for cerebral edema are those who present with higher BUN concentrations[19] and more severe hypocapnia.[19,45] A lesser rise in the measured serum sodium concentration during treatment (as the serum glucose concentration falls) also indicates increased risk for cerebral edema.[19,48] Finally, bicarbonate therapy, even after adjusting for acid-base status and other markers of severe DKA, has been found to be associated with cerebral edema.[19] Signs and symptoms that should prompt the clinician to consider evaluation for cerebral edema include inappropriate slowing of heart rate, hypertension, headache, recurrent vomiting, and irritability, lethargy, or other mental status changes.

Outcomes of DKA-related cerebral edema are poor, with 21% to 24% mortality and 21% to 26% permanent neurologic deficits.[19,41] Because DKA-related cerebral edema is relatively rare, few studies have been done to assess the effectiveness of pharmacologic interventions to treat this condition. To date, no pharmacologic agents have been clearly demonstrated to be effective for this condition. Several case reports suggest that treatment with mannitol (0.25 to 1 g/kg) may be beneficial.[49,50] Therefore, mannitol should be promptly administered if cerebral edema is suspected. Mannitol treatment should not be withheld until cerebral edema is confirmed radiographically, particularly because initial imaging studies in children with DKA-related cerebral edema may be normal.[51] While intubation may be required due to severe alterations in mental status and impaired airway reflexes, hyperventilation in intubated patients has been associated with poorer outcomes of DKA-related cerebral edema.[52] Therefore, therapeutic hyperventilation, which attempts to decrease PCO_2 below the patient's own compensation for metabolic acidosis in intubated children with DKA, should be avoided except where absolutely necessary to treat impending cerebral herniation. A reasonable approach would be to initially maintain the patient's current PCO_2 level and then gradually allow the PCO_2 to increase as acidosis corrects. Cranial computed tomography or magnetic resonance imaging is recommended to exclude other etiologies of altered mental status, such as CNS thromboses in children with suspected cerebral edema. Treatment should not be withheld while awaiting imaging results.

Disposition

Most children with DKA require monitoring in a pediatric intensive care unit or other unit with similar capacities because of the requirement for hourly laboratory studies and vital signs and frequent careful assessments of mental status. Transfer to a tertiary care pediatric facility is advisable for children who are very young or who have severe acidosis (pH < 7.1), extreme hyperosmolality, risk factors for cerebral edema (e.g., substantially depressed PCO_2 or substantially elevated BUN), or altered mental status, severe headache, or other symptoms or signs of complications of DKA.

Summary

DKA occurs frequently in children with new onset of type 1 diabetes. In children with established diabetes, DKA episodes are most often caused by missed insulin injections. A history of polydipsia and persistent polyuria despite signs of dehydration is an important clue to the diagnosis. Once the diagnosis of DKA is established, therapy should be promptly instituted with intravenous rehydration, intravenous insulin infusion, and replacement of electrolytes, particularly potassium. Treatment of acidosis with bicarbonate is rarely indicated and may contribute to the development of cerebral edema. Cerebral edema remains the most frequent serious complication of DKA, and the cause and appropriate treatment of this complication are topics of continued investigation.

REFERENCES

1. Faich G, Fishbein H, Ellis E: The epidemiology of diabetic acidosis: a population-based study. Am J Epidemiol 117:551, 1983
2. Pinkney J, Bingley P, Sawtell P: Presentation and progress of childhood diabetes mellitus: a prospective population-based study. Diabetologia 37:70–74, 1994.
3. Banerji M: Diabetes in African Americans: unique pathophysiologic features. Curr Diabetes Rep 4:219–223, 2004.
4. Matthews D, Wallace T: Children with type 2 diabetes: the risks of complications. Horm Res 57:34–39, 2002.
5. Rewers A, Chase H, Mackenzie T, et al: Predictors of acute complications in children with type 1 diabetes. JAMA 287:2511–2518, 2002.
6. Rosilio M, Cotton J, Wieliczko M, et al: Factors associated with glycemic control: a cross-sectional nationwide study in 2,579 French children with type 1 diabetes. The French Pediatric Diabetes Group. Diabetes Care 21:1146–1153, 1998.
7. Norfeldt S, Ludvigsson J: Adverse events in intensively treated children and adolescents with type 1 diabetes. Acta Paediatr 88:1184–1193, 1999.
8. Flood R, Chiang V: Rate and prediction of infection in children with diabetic ketoacidosis. Am J Emerg Med 19:270–273, 2001.
9. Scibilia J, Finegold D, Dorman J, et al: Why do children with diabetes die? Acta Endocrinol Suppl 279:326–333, 1986.
10. Edge J, Ford-Adams M, Dunger D: Causes of death in children with insulin-dependent diabetes 1990–96. Arch Dis Child 81:318–323, 1999.
11. Chase H, Garg S, Jelley D: Diabetic ketoacidosis in children and the role of outpatient management. Pediatr Rev 11:297–304, 1990.
12. Cullen M, Reece E, Homko C, Sivan E: The changing presentations of diabetic ketoacidosis during pregnancy. Am J Perinatol 13:449–451, 1996.
13. Katz M: Hyperglycemia-induced hyponatremia—calculation of expected serum sodium depression. N Engl J Med 289:843–844, 1973.
14. Davis ID, Avneer ED: Introduction to glomerular disease. *In* Behrman R, Kliegman R, Arvin A (eds): Nelson Textbook of Pediatrics, 17th ed. Philadelphia: Elsevier Saunders, 2004, pp 1731–1734.
15. Soler N, Bennet M, Dixon K, et al: Potassium balance during treatment of diabetic ketoacidosis with special reference to the use of bicarbonate. Lancet 30:665–667, 1972.
16. Green S, Rothrock S, Ho J, et al: Failure of adjunctive bicarbonate to improve outcome in severe pediatric diabetic ketoacidosis. Ann Emerg Med 31:41–48, 1998.
17. Lever E, Jaspan J: Sodium bicarbonate therapy in severe diabetic ketoacidosis. Am J Med 75:263–268, 1983.
18. Morris L, Murphy M, Kitabchi A: Bicarbonate therapy in severe diabetic ketoacidosis. Ann Intern Med 105:836–840, 1986.
*19. Glaser N, Barnett P, McCaslin I, et al: Risk factors for cerebral edema in children with diabetic ketoacidosis. N Engl J Med 344:264–269, 2001.
*20. Sperling M, Dunger D, Acerini C, et al: ESPE/LWPES consensus statement on diabetic ketoacidosis in children and adolescents. Pediatrics 113:e133–e140, 2003.
21. Dunger D, Sperling M, Acerini C, et al: ESPE/LWPES consensus statement on diabetic ketoacidosis in children and adolescents. Arch Dis Child 89:188–194, 2003.
22. Burghen G, Etteldorf J, Fisher J, Kitabchi A: Comparison of high-dose and low-dose insulin by continuous intravenous infusion in the treatment of diabetic ketoacidosis in children. Diabetes Care 3:15–20, 1980.
23. Smith L, Rotta A: Accuracy of clinical estimates of dehydration in pediatric patients with diabetic ketoacidosis. Pediatr Emerg Care 18.395–396, 2002.
24. Grimberg A, Cerri R, Satin-Smith M, Cohen P: The "two bag system" for variable intravenous dextrose and fluid administration: benefits in diabetic ketoacidosis management. J Pediatr 134:376–378, 1999.
25. Lord G, Scott J, Pusey C, et al: Diabetes and rhabdomyolysis: a rare complication of a common disease. BMJ 307:1126–1128, 1993.
26. Shilo S, Werner D, Hershko C: Acute hemolytic anemia caused by severe hypophosphatemia in diabetic ketoacidosis. Acta Haematol 73:55–57, 1985.
27. Becker D, Brown D, Steranka B, Drash A: Phosphate replacement during treatment of diabetic ketoacidosis. Am J Dis Child 137:241–246, 1983.
28. Young M: Simultaneous acute cerebral and pulmonary edema complicating diabetic ketoacidosis. Diabetes Care 18:1288–1290, 1995.
29. Hoffman W, Locksmith J, Burton E, et al: Interstitial pulmonary edema in children and adolescents with diabetic ketoacidosis. J Diabetes Complications 12:314–320, 1998.
30. Breidbart S, Singer L, St.Louis Y, Saenger P: Adult respiratory distress syndrome in an adolescent with diabetic ketoacidosis. J Pediatr 111: 736–737, 1987.
31. Rosenbloom A: Intracerebral crises during treatment of diabetic ketoacidosis. Diabetes Care 13:22–33, 1990.
32. Gutierrez J, Bagatell R, Sampson M, et al: Femoral central venous catheter-associated deep venous thrombosis in children with diabetic ketoacidosis. Crit Care Med 31:80–83, 2003.
33. Slyper A, Wyatt D, Brown C: Clinical and/or biochemical pancreatitis in diabetic ketoacidosis. J Pediatr Endocrinol 7:261–264, 1994.
34. Murdoch I, Pryor D, Haycock G, Cameron S. Acute renal failure complicating diabetic ketoacidosis. Acta Paediatr 82:498–500, 1993.
35. Todani T, Sato Y, Watanabe Y, et al: Ischemic jejunal stricture developing after diabetic coma in a girl: a case report. Eur J Pediatr Surg 3:115–117, 1993.

—————————————
*Selected readings.

36. Chan-Cua S, Jones K, Lynch F, Friedenberg G: Necrosis of the ileum in a diabetic adolescent. J Pediatr Surg 27:1236–1238, 1992.

37. Dimeglio L, Chaet M, Quigley C, Grosfled J: Massive ischemic intestinal necrosis at the onset of diabetes mellitus with ketoacidosis in a three-year old girl. J Pediatr Surg 38:1537–1539, 2003.

38. Khanna S, Soumekh B, Bradley J, et al: A case of fatal rhinocerebral mucormycosis with new onset diabetic ketoacidosis. J Diabetes Complications 12:224–227, 1998.

39. Carl G, Hoffman W, Passmore G, et al: Diabetic ketoacidosis promotes a prothrombotic state. Endocr Res 29:73–82, 2003.

40. Bello F, Sotos J: Cerebral oedema in diabetic ketoacidosis in children. Lancet 336:64, 1990.

*41. Edge J, Hawkins M, Winter D, Dunger D: The risk and outcome of cerebral oedema developing during diabetic ketoacidosis. Arch Dis Child 85:16–22, 2001.

42. Hoffman W, Steinhart C, El Gammal T, et al: Cranial CT in children and adolescents with diabetic ketoacidosis. AJNR Am J Neuroradiol 9:733–739, 1988.

43. Glasgow A: Devastating cerebral edema in diabetic ketoacidosis before therapy. Diabetes Care 14:77–78, 1991.

44. Krane E, Rockoff M, Wallman J, Wolfsdorf J: Subclinical brain swelling in children during treatment of diabetic ketoacidosis. N Engl J Med 312:1147–1151, 1985.

45. Mahoney C, Vlcek B, Del Aguila M: Risk factors for developing brain herniation during diabetic ketoacidosis. Pediatr Neurol 21:721–727, 1999.

46. Glaser NS, Wootton-Gorges SL, Marcin JP, et al: Mechanism of cerebral edema in children with diabetic ketoacidosis. J Pediatr 145:164–171, 2004.

47. Lam T, Anderson S, Glaser N, O'Donnell M: Bumetanide reduces cerebral edema formation in rats with diabetic ketoacidosis. FASEB J 17: A76, 2003.

48. Harris G, Fiordalisi I, Harris W, et al: Minimizing the risk of brain herniation during treatment of diabetic ketoacidemia: a retrospective and prospective study. J Pediatr 117:22–31, 1990.

49. Roberts M, Slover R, Chase H: Diabetic ketoacidosis with intracerebral complications. Pediatr Diabetes 2:103–114, 2001.

50. Franklin B, Liu J, Ginsberg-Fellner F: Cerebral edema and ophthalmoplegia reversed by mannitol in a new case of insulin-dependent diabetes mellitus. Pediatrics 69:87–90, 1982.

51. Muir A, Rosenbloom A, Williams L, et al: Cerebral edema in childhood diabetic ketoacidosis: natural history, radiographic findings and early identification. Diabetes Care 27:1541–1546, 2004.

*52. Marcin J, Glaser N, Barnett P, et al: Clinical and therapeutic factors associated with adverse outcomes in children with DKA-related cerebral edema. J Pediatr 141:793–797, 2003.

Chapter 106

Hypoglycemia

Nicole Glaser, MD and Gregory M. Enns, MB, ChB

Hypoglycemia should be considered in any child who presents with unexplained lethargy, shock, seizures, or an altered mental status.

Bedside glucose measurements can be used as an initial screening test. If screening shows hypoglycemia, treatment should be initiated without waiting for confirmatory tests.

Hormonal and biochemical studies must be measured *at the time of hypoglycemia, prior to glucose or glucocorticoid administration,* to determine the cause of the episode. Whenever possible, blood should be drawn and saved in a serum-separator tube as well as EDTA, heparin, and sodium fluoride/potassium oxalate tubes on ice.

Hypoglycemia should be treated with rapid intravenous infusion of dextrose (D): 5 ml/kg of D_{10} in infants under 1 year old, 2 ml/kg of D_{25} in the 1- to 5-year-old, or 1 ml/kg of D_{50} in the child greater than 5 years old.

Introduction and Background

The precise blood glucose concentration that should be considered pathologic is a subject of controversy, particularly in neonates. Conservative guidelines suggest that blood glucose concentrations below 40 mg/dl should be considered abnormal at any age, blood glucose concentrations between 40 and 50 mg/dl require further evaluation at any age but may possibly be normal in neonates, and blood glucose concentrations below 60 mg/dl beyond early infancy should be considered borderline, with further evaluation required. Inaccuracies of bedside glucose meters should be taken into account in determining whether to undertake further evaluation and treatment for hypoglycemia. In children with diabetes, hypoglycemic symptoms, including mental status changes, may occur at glucose concentrations above those previously mentioned, particularly in children with chronic poor glycemic control. In this setting, treatment should be considered even if blood glucose concentrations are in the low-normal range.

Hypoglycemia in Children with Diabetes

Children with type 1 diabetes frequently experience mild episodes of hypoglycemia. These episodes are not associated with significant alterations in mental status and are treated easily with oral glucose. Rarely, children with type 1 diabetes may have episodes of hypoglycemia of sufficient severity to result in mental status changes, loss of consciousness, or seizures. These severe hypoglycemic events occur at a rate of approximately 5 to 19 events per 100 patient-years.[1-3] Errors in insulin dosing, inadequate carbohydrate intake, or exercise may cause these severe hypoglycemic episodes, but in almost 40% of episodes, no cause can be determined.[3] Severe hypoglycemic events occur more frequently in younger children, those with lower hemoglobin A_{1c} values, underinsured populations, and patients using higher daily insulin dosages.[1,3]

Hypoglycemia in Children without Diabetes

In children without diabetes mellitus, hypoglycemia may result from a variety of causes, including hormonal excess or deficiency states, sepsis, inborn errors of metabolism, or toxic ingestions. The most frequent causes of hypoglycemia vary according to the patient's age (Table 106–1).

Recognition and Approach

Hypoglycemia in Infants

In infancy, severe hypoglycemia is often the result of hyperinsulinism. Transient hyperinsulinism occurs frequently in neonates born to mothers with poorly controlled diabetes. This disorder, however, is generally recognized at the time of birth and usually resolves before the infant is discharged from the newborn nursery. Persistent hyperinsulinism in infants may be caused by a variety of genetic mutations, most commonly those affecting the sulfonylurea receptor and related proteins.[4-8] An additional rare cause of neonatal hypoglycemia is the hyperinsulinism-hyperammonemia syndrome, an autosomal dominant condition caused by hyperactivity of hepatic glutamate dehydrogenase. These disorders vary in severity, and less severe forms may present after the neonatal period. Presentation after the first year of life, however, is rare.

Table 106–1	Causes of Non–Diabetes-Related Hypoglycemia According to Age of Patient
Patient Age	**Notable Features**
Neonatal–Early Infancy	
Hyperinsulinism	May be large for gestational age
	High glucose infusion rate required to maintain normal serum glucose
Hypopituitarism/growth hormone deficiency	Microphallus in males, midline craniofacial anomalies
	Nystagmus/optic nerve hypoplasia
Congenital adrenal hyperplasia	Ambiguous genitalia in females, hyperpigmentation
	Hyperkalemia, hyponatremia
Galactosemia	Liver disease, renal Fanconi's syndrome, gram-negative sepsis
Hereditary fructose intolerance	Liver disease, poor feeding, vomiting
	Renal Fanconi's sydrome
Glycogen storage disease type I	Hepatomegaly, enlarged kidneys, lactic acidemia
	Hypertriglyceridemia, hyperuricemia
Gluconeogenic disorders (fructose-1,6-bisphosphatase deficiency, phosphoenolpyruvate carboxykinase deficiency)	Hepatomegaly, lactic acidosis
Organic acidemias (propionic acidemia, methylmalonic acidemia, isovaleric acidemia)	Overwhelming illness
	Metabolic acidosis, ketosis
Maple syrup urine disease	Feeding difficulty, vomiting, neurologic deterioration; acidosis is uncommon
Fatty acid oxidation disorders (VLCAD deficiency, MCAD deficiency)	Reye-like syndrome, hypoketosis, cardiomyopathy
Mitochondrial disorders	Lactic acidosis, multiorgan system involvement
Congenital disorders of glycosylation	Hyperinsulinism, abnormal fat distribution, strabismus, pericardial effusion
	Liver disease, protein-losing enteropathy
Late Infancy–Early Childhood	
Ketotic hypoglycemia	Thin child, typically presents in early morning after moderate (10–16-hr) fast
Toxic ingestions	Sulfonylureas, β-blockers, ethanol, salicylates
Hypopituitarism/growth hormone deficiency	(as above)
Hereditary fructose intolerance	(as above)
Glycogen storage disease type I	(as above)
Gluconeogenic disorders (fructose-1,6-bisphosphatase deficiency, phosphoenolpyruvate carboxykinase deficiency)	(as above)
Organic acidemias	(as above)
Maple syrup urine disease	(as above)
Fatty acid oxidation disorders (VLCAD deficiency, MCAD deficiency)	(as above)
Mitochondrial disorders	(as above)
Congenital disorders of glycosylation	(as above)
Late Childhood–Adolescence	
Acquired hypopituitarism or adrenal suppression	Acquired (associated with CNS tumors/CNS trauma)
	Adrenal suppression due to prior glucocorticoid treatment
Addison's disease	Hyperpigmentation, weight loss, abdominal pain
Ethanol ingestion	
Insulinoma	Hypoglycemia in the absence of significant fasting
Fatty acid oxidation disorders (especially MCAD deficiency)	(as above)

Abbreviations: CNS, central nervous system; VLCAD, very long-chain acyl-coenzyme A dehydrogenase deficiency; MCAD, medium-chain acyl-coenzyme A dehydrogenase deficiency.

Hypoglycemia in infants and toddlers may also be caused by deficiencies in counter-regulatory hormones, mainly growth hormone and cortisol.[9] Hypoglycemia may occur in infants with isolated growth hormone deficiency or with hypopituitarism (in which both growth hormone and cortisol are deficient). Congenital adrenal hyperplasia also results in cortisol deficiency, and this deficiency may be of sufficient severity to cause hypoglycemia[10] (see Chapter 108, Addisonian Crisis).

Although inborn errors of metabolism may present at any age, these patients usually present during infancy. Gluconeogenic disorders (fructose-1,6-bisphosphatase deficiency and phosphoenolpyruvate carboxykinase deficiency) are often first noted in the neonatal period[11] (see Chapter 29, Inborn Errors of Metabolism). Infants with glycogen storage disorders typically present in later infancy, when feedings become less frequent, but they may present as early as the first week of life.[12] Fatty acid oxidation disorders also typically manifest in later infancy (6 to 24 months).[13] Hereditary fructose intolerance is first noted after the introduction of fructose and sucrose into the diet, usually between 4 and 8 months. These infants often have associated hepatic dysfunction and a renal Fanconi's syndrome.[14] Hypoglycemia also may occur in organic acidemias (e.g., methylmalonic, propionic, and isovaleric acidemias), but metabolic acidemia and ketosis are more prominent features of these disorders.[15,16] Hypoglycemia and ketosis may occur in maple syrup urine disease, although ketosis is usually not a prominent early finding. Rare enzymatic defects (succinyl-coenzyme A [CoA]:oxoacid transferase deficiency, glycogen synthetase deficiency [glycogen storage disease type 0], β-ketothiolase deficiency, and short-chain 3-hydroxyacyl-CoA dehydrogenase deficiency) may present with ketosis and hypoglycemia.[17,18] Hypoglycemia may also be present in galactosemia and tyrosinemia, but liver disease is usually the primary clinical manifestation.[19] Finally, mitochondrial disorders may first be noted in this age group, although presentation at any age is possible.[20,21] These disorders typically feature striking neurologic or systemic involvement, but hypoglycemia occasionally may be a feature (see Chapter 29, Inborn Errors of Metabolism).

Hypoglycemia in Toddlers

In toddlers, toxic ingestions are among the more common causes of hypoglycemia (Table 106–2). Important agents that may cause hypoglycemia include sulfonylureas, β-blockers, ethanol, and salicylates[22-26] (see Chapter 133, Common Pediatric Overdoses; Chapter 134, Toxic Alcohols; and Chapter 137, Cardiovascular Agents). Plant toxins that contain hypoglycin, such as the Ackee tree found in south Florida and the Caribbean, can cause hypoglycemia.

Table 106–2	Drugs and Toxins That Cause Hypoglycemia

6-Mercaptopurine
Ackee fruit (unripe fruit from Jamaican Ackee tree found in South Florida and Caribbean)
Alcohols (ethanol, methanol, isopropanol, ethylene glycol)
Angiotensin-converting enzyme inhibitors
β-Blockers
Bishydroxycoumarin (rat poison)
Bitter melon gourds
Chlorpromazine
Climbing ivory gourd
Clofibrate
Didanosine
Disodium ethylenediaminetetra-acetic acid
Disopyramide
Fenfluramine
Fenugreek herb
Fluoxetine
Ginseng plant (American, Asian, Siberian)
Haloperidol
Hypoglycemic agents (sulfonylureas, biguanides, α glucosidase inhibitors, thiazolidinediones, benzoic acid derivatives)
Insecticides (carbamates and organophosphates)
Insulin (exogenous)
Isoniazid
Lithium
Mamijava plant
Methotrexate
Monoamine oxidase inhibitors
Nonsteroidal anti-inflammatory agents
Para-aminobenzoic acid
Pentamidine
Phenylbutazone
Phenytoin
Pomegranate tree
Probenicid
Quinine
Ritodrine
Salicylates
Sertraline
Steroids (anabolic: stanazol)
Sulfonamides
Thiazide diuretics
Thioglycolate
Thyroid hormone
Tremetol
Tricyclic antidepressants
Trimethoprim

Ketotic hypoglycemia is also a common cause of hypoglycemic episodes in children over 6 months and under 5 years of age. In one series, ketotic hypoglycemia accounted for 24% of all non–diabetes-related episodes of hypoglycemia presenting to the emergency department in children over 6 months old, and 31% of episodes in children who were previously healthy.[27] Most children were less than 5 years old, with a median age of 31 months; two thirds were male, three quarters were white, and 70% weighed below the 25th percentile for their age.[27] Most children with this disorder present with symptomatic hypoglycemia during the morning hours after a moderate fast of 10 to 16 hours. Many have a coexisting illness (e.g., gastroenteritis) that contributes to hypoglycemia. Ketotic hypoglycemia is thought to be caused by deficient release of alanine to fuel gluconeogenesis. Symptoms usually disappear by 8 to 9 years of age when a child's muscle mass and glycogen stores increase. Because there is no specific diagnostic test to detect this condition, ketotic hypoglycemia is generally a diagnosis of exclusion that can be made only after ruling out other endocrine and metabolic conditions.

Other metabolic disorders should also be considered in toddlers presenting with hypoglycemia. Many of these conditions require prolonged fasting to provoke hypoglycemia and therefore may not have any manifestations during infancy. Fatty acid oxidation defects, especially medium-chain acyl-CoA dehydrogenase deficiency, are among the most common of these disorders. Fatty acid oxidation defects may present with Reye's syndrome–like features in a child with no past history of illness or other problems. *Hypo*ketotic hypoglycemia is characteristic because of the role the fatty acid oxidation cycle plays in generating ketone bodies.[13]

Hypoglycemia in Older Children

In older children and adolescents, hypoglycemia occurs infrequently outside of the setting of diabetes. Disorders that cause hypoglycemia in this age group include acquired hypopituitarism due to central nervous system (CNS) tumors or other brain injury, Addison's disease, and insulinoma (see Chapter 42, Conditions Causing Increased Intracranial Pressure; and Chapter 108, Addisonian Crisis). Ethanol intoxication can also cause hypoglycemia in older children and adolescents. Patients treated for prolonged periods with glucocorticoids (oral or inhaled) may also present with hypoglycemia due to adrenal insufficiency if glucocorticoid preparations are abruptly discontinued or the dosage dramatically decreased[28,29] (see Chapter 107, The Steroid-Dependent Child). Adolescents with inborn errors of metabolism may also present with hypoglycemia if they are noncompliant with special diets or other measures necessary to control their disorders.[30]

Unsuspected Hypoglycemia

On occasion, unsuspected hypoglycemia may be encountered in patients who present to the emergency department for evaluation of other disorders. Of children evaluated in the emergency department with an incidental blood glucose concentration below 50 mg/dl, 28% had previously undiagnosed fatty acid oxidation defects and 19% had previously undiagnosed endocrine disorders.[31] Thus, further evaluation (see later) should always be considered when an incidental blood glucose concentration below 50 mg/dl is detected.

Clinical Presentation

Clinical Manifestations

The manifestations of hypoglycemia in infants differ from those in older children. In infants, symptoms and signs of hypoglycemia are less specific than those in older children and include lethargy or jitteriness, poor feeding, hypotonia, hypothermia, apnea, and seizures.[4] Such nonspecific findings are often mistaken for sepsis. In older children, manifestations of hypoglycemia are similar to those seen in adults. These manifestations include neuroglycopenic symptoms such as headaches, confusion, lethargy, irritability, and seizures, and adrenergic symptoms such as tremulousness, tachycardia, and sweating.

Diagnostic Clues

Additional findings in the history or physical examination may provide clues to the cause of the hypoglycemic episode. A history of recent introduction of new foods into the diet of an infant (e.g., fructose, sucrose), weaning, or a history of poor oral intake prior to the hypoglycemic episode suggests the possibility of metabolic disorders. The family history may be significant for similarly affected children or other clues to the presence of an inherited metabolic disorder (e.g., sudden infant death syndrome). Significant hepatomegaly is often encountered in glycogen storage disorders, disorders of gluconeogenesis, and hereditary fructose intolerance. More moderate hepatomegaly can be present during acute decompensation in fatty acid oxidation disorders.[19] Congenital disorders of glycosylation are frequently associated with other systemic manifestations, including dysmorphic features, strabismus, cerebellar hypoplasia, unusual body fat distribution, pericardial effusion, and protein-losing enteropathy.[8]

Hyperpigmentation is a helpful clue to the presence of primary adrenal insufficiency, but is absent in patients with secondary adrenal insufficiency (adrenocorticotropic hormone deficiency) (see Chapter 108, Addisonian Crisis). A history of recent discontinuation of glucocorticoids (including inhaled corticosteroids) suggests the possibility of secondary adrenal insufficiency (see Chapter 107, The Steroid-Dependent Child). Infants with hypopituitarism may have microphallus, optic nerve hypoplasia with nystagmus, or midline craniofacial defects. Ketotic hypoglycemia is most common in boys under 5 years of age who have low body weight.[27] Patients with ketotic hypoglycemia typically give a history of hypoglycemic episodes occurring on awakening in the morning after a modest (10- to 16-hour) fast. An anion gap acidosis as well as serum and urine ketones are usually present. Finally, the presence of oral hypoglycemic agents, salicylates, or β-blockers in the home of a toddler suggests the possibility of a toxic ingestion (see Chapter 133, Common Pediatric Overdoses; Chapter 134, Toxic Alcohols; and Chapter 137, Cardiovascular Agents).

Important Clinical Features and Considerations

While the diagnosis of hypoglycemia is straightforward in a child with diabetes who cannot ingest carbohydrates due to vomiting, clinical features in other patients can be subtle or misleading. Rapid bedside glucose testing should be considered in a wide range of ill infants and children, including those with apnea, sepsis, cyanosis, hypothermia, vomiting, poor feeding, hypotonia, or any neurologic complaint or those who are undergoing resuscitation.[32] In fact, any time venous access or venipuncture is undertaken, the clinician should consider whether or not hypoglycemia is a potential cause for a patient's symptoms. If hypoglycemia is a possibility, rapid beside testing for glucose is mandatory.

Management

Whenever bedside testing reveals hypoglycemia, treatment should be initiated; however, additional evaluation should be performed concurrently. Bedside glucose meters may be inaccurate,[33] and a confirmatory glucose measurement on a venous sample is essential. Venous samples for measurement of glucose should be transported promptly to the laboratory to avoid metabolism of glucose by blood cells, resulting in a falsely low glucose measurement. In addition, at the time of the hypoglycemic episode, a venous sample should be obtained for possible measurement of hormone concentrations and other biochemical measures, including serum insulin, cortisol, growth hormone, ketone, lactate, ammonia, and free fatty acid concentrations[34] (Fig. 106–1). A urine sample should also be tested for ketones and reducing substances. Without the diagnostic information gained from these samples, the cause of the hypoglycemic episode generally cannot be determined.

If an inborn error of metabolism is suspected, additional studies should be considered, including plasma quantitative amino acids, carnitine levels, acylcarnitine profile, and urine organic acids. It is essential to obtain metabolic laboratory tests at the time of the hypoglycemic episode, because diagnostic metabolites can disappear or become less apparent after treatment has started.[35]

Many metabolic disorders are associated with high mortality and may present as apparent life-threatening events or cardiac arrest. Specimens of blood (5 ml in heparinized plasma and 10 ml collected in an ethylenediaminetetra-acetic acid [EDTA] tube) and urine (10 to 20 ml) should be obtained and stored frozen at −20° C for metabolic and genetic testing in all children who die unexpectedly from unknown causes.

If there is a suspicious clinical history, toxicologic screening for ethanol, salicylates, propranolol, and oral hypoglycemic agents should also be considered. In rare cases in which insulin administration to a nondiabetic child is suspected (suicide attempts in adolescents or child abuse), simultaneous measurement of insulin and C-peptide concentrations may be used to distinguish endogenous insulin production from exogenous insulin administration.

Immediate Intervention

Hypoglycemia must be corrected as rapidly as possible with an intravenous infusion of 0.5 g/kg of dextrose. In infants, the typical dosage is 5 ml/kg of 10% dextrose (D_{10}). In toddlers, 2 ml/kg of 25% dextrose (D_{25}) is typically used, and in older children, 1 ml/kg of 50% dextrose (D_{50}). The product of the number of milliliters per kilogram and the dextrose percentage should equal 50. In children with diabetes or known hyperinsulinism of any cause, glucagon (1 mg via intramuscular injection) can be administered if intravenous access cannot be established rapidly. Hypoglycemia caused

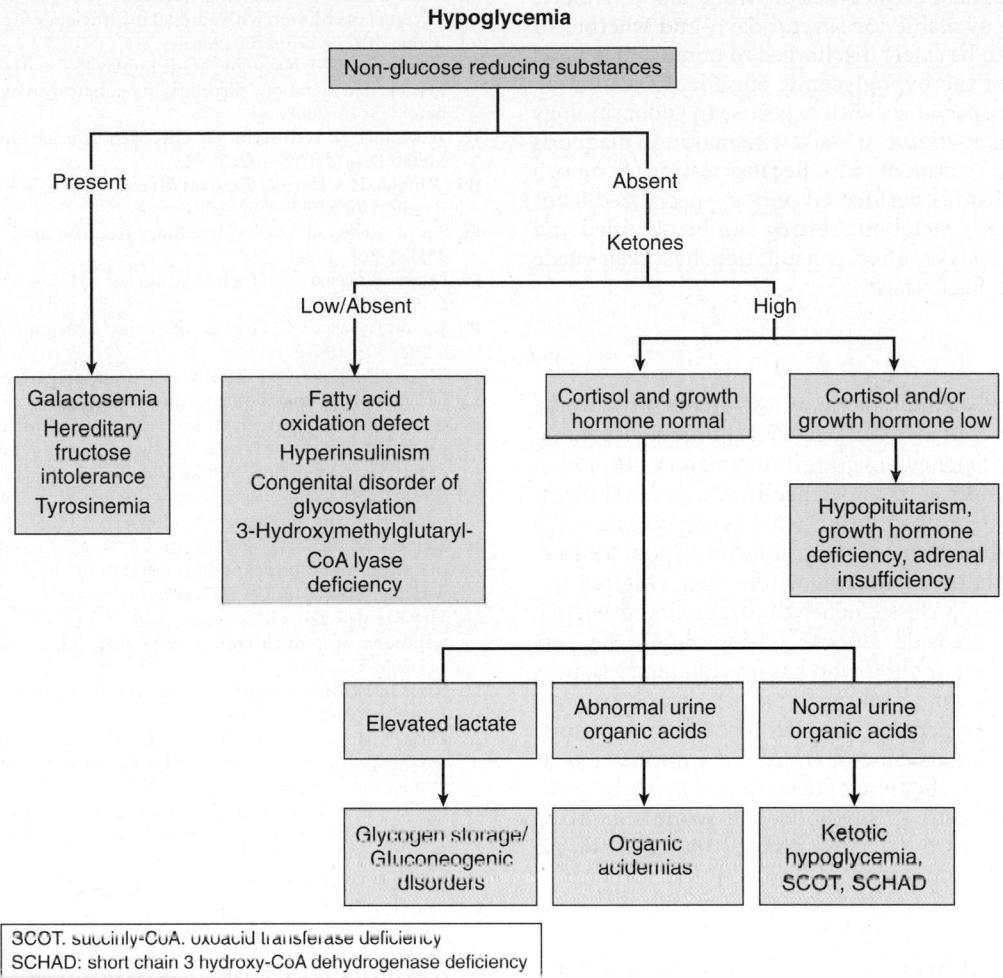

FIGURE 106–1. Algorithm for determining the cause of hypoglycemia. For an episode of hypoglycemia, urine reducing substances and urine ketones along with serum insulin, cortisol, growth hormone, ketone, lactate, ammonia, and free fatty acid concentrations are measured. The algorithm can then be used to determine the most likely cause.

by disorders other than hyperinsulinism, however, generally will not respond to glucagon. If adrenal insufficiency is known or strongly suspected, intravenous hydrocortisone should be administered at a dose of 50 mg for children under 4 years of age and 100 mg for children over 4 years of age.

Definitive Therapy

In children with diabetes, hypoglycemia generally corrects after the initial dextrose infusion, and additional intravenous administration of dextrose is rarely necessary. Despite return of the serum glucose concentration to the normal range, however, alterations in mental status such as irritability, combativeness, lethargy, or disorientation occasionally may persist for prolonged periods. Other neurologic deficits, such as hemiplegia or aphasia, may also occur following such episodes and may likewise persist for many hours.[36] Although persistent neurologic abnormalities after severe hypoglycemic events in children with diabetes have been described, additional toxicological studies and CNS imaging should be considered to rule out other possible causes.

In children without diabetes, the initial intravenous bolus of dextrose is followed with a continuous intravenous dextrose infusion sufficient to reverse the catabolic state. This can generally be accomplished with 10% dextrose in normal saline infused at 1.5 times the maintenance rate. Hypoglycemia caused by an inborn error of metabolism may respond poorly to therapy. These children may require intravenous glucose supplementation at higher than expected levels, and it may be difficult to wean the infusion. Additional treatment may be necessary depending on the cause of the hypoglycemic episode. Details of treatment for toxic ingestions, adrenal insufficiency, and other specific causes of hypoglycemia are beyond the scope of this chapter, but can be found in Chapter 108 (Addisonian Crisis), Chapter 133 (Classic Pediatric Ingestions), and Chapter 134 (Toxic Alcohols).

Disposition

Most children with hypoglycemia in the setting of type 1 diabetes can be safely discharged to home from the emergency department after serum glucose levels have normalized and mental status has returned to normal. Clinicians should ensure that the cause for hypoglycemia is corrected, such as resolution of vomiting, adequate oral intake, or correction of insulin dose. Most children with hypoglycemia of other etiologies, however, require a period of observation in the hospital. Diagnostic information from blood samples often will not be available for several days, and whether or not the patient can be safely discharged to home will depend on the etiology of the hypoglycemic episode. Consultation with pediatric subspecialists with expertise in endocrinology and metabolism is advisable to assist with making a diagnosis and formulating a treatment plan. Because testing for inborn errors of metabolism is performed only in specialized laboratories, samples for metabolic testing can be obtained and stored for later analysis after consultation has been made with a biochemical geneticist.

Summary

Childhood hypoglycemia occurs most frequently in the setting of diabetes, but also can occur in children with metabolic disorders, deficiencies of counter-regulatory hormones, genetic defects resulting in hyperinsulinism, or toxic ingestions. Infants and young children with hypoglycemia often present with variable symptoms (e.g., jitteriness, poor feeding, hypotonia, hypothermia, apnea), while older children are more likely to develop classic neuroglycopenic or adrenergic symptoms. Rapid bedside glucose testing should be performed for any infant or child who has unexplained lethargy, other mental status abnormalities, or shock or who requires resuscitation in the emergency department. If hypoglycemia is detected, intravenous glucose must be administered as rapidly as possible. At the time of detection of hypoglycemia, critical diagnostic samples of blood and urine should be obtained so that future determination of the cause of the hypoglycemic event is possible.

REFERENCES

1. Rewers A, Chase HP, Mackenzie T, et al: Predictors of acute complications in children with type 1 diabetes. JAMA 287:2511–2518, 2002.
2. Levine B, Anderson B, Butler D, et al: Predictors of glycemic control and short-term adverse outcomes in youth with type 1 diabetes. J Pediatr 139:197–203, 2001.
3. Davis E, Keating B, Byrne G, et al: Hypoglycemia: incidence and clinical predictors in a large population-based sample of children and adolescents with IDDM. Diabetes Care 20:22–25, 1997.
*4. Sperling M, Menon R: Differential diagnosis and management of neonatal hypoglycemia. Pediatr Clin North Am 51:703–723, 2004.
5. Stanley C, Baker L: The causes of neonatal hypoglycemia. N Engl J Med 340:1200–1201, 1999.
6. Stanley C: Advances in diagnosis and treatment of hyperinsulinism in infants and children. J Clin Endocrinol Metab 87:4857–4859, 2002.
7. Stanley C, Lieu Y, Hsu B, et al: Hyperinsulinism and hyperammonemia in infants with regulatory mutations of the glutamate dehydrogenase gene. N Engl J Med 338:1352–1357, 1998.
8. Jaeken J, Matthijs G: Congenital disorders of glycosylation. Annu Rev Genomics Hum Genet 2:129–151, 2001.
9. Ogilvy-Stuart A: Growth hormone deficiency (GHD) from birth to 2 years of age: diagnostic specifics of GHD during the early phase of life. Horm Res 60(Suppl 1):2–9, 2003.
10. Artavia-Loria E, Chaussain J, Bougneres P, Job J: Frequency of hypoglycemia in children with adrenal insufficiency. Acta Endocrinol Suppl (Copenh) 279:275–278, 1986.
*11. Saudubray J-M, Nassogne M, de Lonlay P, Touati G: Clinical approach to inherited metabolic disorders in neonates: an overview. Semin Neonatol 7:3–15, 2002.
12. Wolfsdorf J, Weinstein D: Glycogen storage diseases. Rev Endocr Metab Disord 4:95–102, 2003.
*13. Rinaldo P, Matern D, Bennett M: Fatty acid oxidation disorders. Annu Rev Physiol 64:477–502, 2002.
14. Ali M, Rellos P, Cox T: Hereditary fructose intolerance. J Med Genet 35:353–365, 1998.
15. Ozand P, Gascon G: Organic acidurias: a review. Part 1. J Child Neurol 6:196–219, 1991.
16. Ozand P, Gascon G: Organic acidurias: a review. Part 2. J Child Neurol 6:288–303, 1991.
17. Mitchell G, Kassovska-Bratinova S, Boukaftane Y, et al: Medical aspects of ketone body metabolism. Clin Invest Med 18:192–216, 1995.
18. Bennett M, Weinberger M, Kobori J, et al: Mitochondrial short-chain L-3-hydroxyacyl-coenzyme A dehydrogenase deficiency: a new defect of fatty acid oxidation. Pediatr Res 39:185–188, 1996.
*19. Enns G, Packman S: Diagnosing inborn errors of metabolism in the newborn: clinical features. NeoReviews 2:e183–e191, 2001.
20. Jackson M, Schaefer J, Johnson M, et al: Presentation and clinical investigation of mitochondrial respiratory chain disease: a study of 51 patients. Brain 118:339–357, 1995.
21. Von Kleist-Retzow J, Cormier-Daire V, Viot G, et al: Antenatal manifestations of mitochondrial respiratory chain deficiency. J Pediatr 143:208–212, 2004.
22. Ricci L, Hoffman S: Ethanol-induced hypoglycemic coma in a child. Ann Emerg Med 11:202–204, 1982.
23. Ernst A, Jones K, Nick T, Sanchez J: Ethanol ingestion and related hypoglycemia in a pediatric and adolescent emergency department population. Acad Emerg Med 3:46–49, 1996.
24. Spiller H, Villalobos D, Krenaelok E, et al: Prospective multicenter study of sulfonylurea ingestion in children. J Pediatr 131:141–146, 1997.
25. Spiller H: Management of sulfonylurea ingestions. Pediatr Emerg Care 15:227–230, 1999.
26. Love J, Sikka N: Are 1-2 tablets dangerous? Beta-blocker exposure in toddlers. J Emerg Med 26:309–314, 2004.
27. Daly L, Osterhoudt K, Weinzimer S: Presenting features of idiopathic ketotic hypoglycemia. J Emerg Med 25:39–43, 2003.
28. Todd G, Acerini C, Ross-Russell R, et al: Survey of adrenal crisis associated with inhaled corticosteroids in the United Kingdom. Arch Dis Child 87:457–461, 2002.
29. Drake A, Howells R, Shield J, et al: Symptomatic adrenal insufficiency presenting with hypoglycaemia in children with asthma receiving high dose inhaled fluticasone propionate. BMJ 324:1081–1083, 2002.
30. Enns G, Packman W: The adolescent with an inborn error of metabolism: medical issues and transition to adulthood. Adolesc Med 13:315–329, 2002.
31. Weinstein D, Butte A, Raymond K, et al: High incidence of unrecognized metabolic and endocrinologic disorders in acutely ill children with hypoglycemia. Pediatr Res 49:88A, 2001.
32. Losek J: Hypoglycemia and the ABC'S (Sugar) of pediatric resuscitation. Ann Emerg Med 35:43–46, 2000.
33. Ho H, Yeung W, Young B: Evaluation of "point of care" devices in the measurement of low blood glucose in neonatal practice. Arch Dis Child Fetal Neonatal Ed 89:F356–F359, 2004.
*34. Lteif A, Schwenk W: Hypoglycemia in infants and children. Endocrinol Metab Clin 28:620–646, 1999.
35. Enns G, Packman S: Diagnosing inborn errors of metabolism in the newborn: laboratory investigations. NeoReviews 2:e192–e200, 2001.
36. Pocecco M, Ronfani L: Transient focal neurologic deficits associated with hypoglycaemia in children with insulin-dependent diabetes mellitus. Acta Paediatr 87:542–544, 1998.

*Selected readings.

The Steroid-Dependent Child

Ameer P. Mody, MD, MPH

Introduction and Background

The language of "steroids" can be very confusing. The general term *steroid* is defined chemically and therefore includes such disparate substances as progesterone, androgenic and anabolic steroids, cardiac aglycones, bile acids, cholesterol, saponins, toad poisons, carcinogenic hydrocarbons, and corticosteroids.[1] From a medical standpoint, the "steroid-dependent child" is dependent on corticosteroids. Unfortunately, there are multiple synonyms for the word "corticosteroid," including "adrenocorticoid steroid," "corticoid steroid," "adrenal cortical steroid," "adrenocortical steroid," "adrenocortical hormone," and "cortical hormone."[2]

Corticosteroids are generally referred to as either glucocorticoids or mineralocorticoids. Glucocorticoids influence carbohydrate, fat, and protein metabolism, and the predominant clinical effect is anti-inflammatory.[2,3] Mineralocorticoids affect electrolyte and water balance, and the predominant clinical effect is sodium retention.[2,3] A single corticosteroid may impact both carbohydrate, fat, and protein metabolism and electrolyte and water balance, but be classified only by the term that best fits its predominant action. This leads to the unfortunate situation wherein "glucocorticoids" can have substantial mineralocorticoid effects or none at all. For example, the glucocorticoid methylprednisolone has five times as much glucocorticoid activity as hydrocortisone, but only half as much mineralocorticoid activity.[3] In contrast, another drug also deemed a "corticosteroid," dexamethasone, has 25 times as much glucocorticoid activity as hydrocortisone, but essentially no mineralocorticoid effects.[3] Being aware of the potential confusion that can arise when "steroids" are discussed is useful in understanding the proper care for the "steroid-dependent child."

Recognition and Approach

Corticosteroids are commonly prescribed to children. Steroids are effective in treating a wide range of diseases mostly because of their anti-inflammatory effects (Table 107–1). There are several commonly employed dosing patterns for corticosteroids. For example, patients who have received solid organ transplants may require continuous low-dose steroid therapy (see Chapter 66, Postsurgical Cardiac Conditions and Transplantation; Chapter 81, Post–Liver Transplantation Complications; and Chapter 88, Renal Disorders). Patients with rheumatologic disease may require relatively frequent, intermittent high-dose steroid therapy. Similarly, patients with leukemia or lymphoma receive pulses of steroids at high doses to initiate tumor lysis and then lower dose steroids as maintenance chemotherapy (see Chapter 128, Cancer and Cancer-Related Complications). There are also children who have had adrenalectomies or have congenital adrenal hyperplasia who receive total steroid replacement therapy for the rest of their lives. Historically, patients with symptoms of moderate or severe asthma have been given systemic steroid therapy for control of symptoms (see Chapter 56, Acute Asthma). The introduction of inhaled corticosteroids has reduced the number of children who require systemic corticosteroid therapy.[4,5] Inhaled steroids have few systemic effects, and those that occur are mild.[6] Children taking inhaled corticosteroids are not considered "steroid dependent."[6]

Long-term and high-dose synthetic corticosteroid therapy can have numerous adverse effects. One well-known effect of exogenous corticosteroids is the suppression of endogenous cortisol release from the adrenal gland via a negative feedback loop on the hypothalamic-pituitary axis. A child on 2 consecutive weeks of systemic corticosteroid therapy may undergo significant suppression of the hypothalamic-pituitary-adrenal axis.[4,7] Children who have a suppressed

Table 107–1	Conditions Commonly Associated with Long-Term Steroid Treatment

Pulmonary

Asthma
Bronchopulmonary dysplasia or chronic lung disease
Cystic fibrosis
Laryngeal papillomas

Neurologic

Seizures
Panhypopituitarism
Multiple sclerosis
Nephrotic syndrome

Renal

Glomerulosclerosis
Goodpasture's syndrome
Nephrotic syndrome

Oncology

Leukemia
Lymphoma
Brain tumors

Immune

Solid organ transplantation patients
Bone marrow transplantation patients

Rheumatologic

Juvenile rheumatoid arthritis
Systemic lupus erythematosus
Henoch-Schönlein purpura

Gastrointestinal

Inflammatory bowel disease

Hematologic

Idiopathic thrombocytopenic purpura
Diamond-Blackfan anemia

Endocrine

Addison's disease
Congenital adrenal hyperplasia

Allergic

Allergies
Eczema

Table 107–2	Complications of Long-Term Steroid Treatment

Endocrine and Metabolic

Suppression of hypothalamic-pituitary-adrenal axis
Growth retardation in children
Hyperinsulinemia/insulin resistance/diabetes
Hyperglycemia
Hyperlipidemia

Dermatologic

Subcutaneous fat accumulation (cushingoid features)
Poor wound healing
Glucocorticoid-induced acne
Thin and fragile skin
Striae

Gastrointestinal

Gastric irritation
Peptic ulcer
Acute pancreatitis
Fatty infiltration of liver

Immune

Leukocytosis
Neutrophilia
Lymphopenia
Eosinopenia
Monocytopenia

Hematopoietic

Suppression of delayed (type IV) hypersensitivity
Inhibition of leukocyte and tissue macrophage migration
Inhibition of cytokine secretion/action
Suppression of the primary antigen response

Musculoskeletal

Osteoporosis, spontaneous fractures
Avascular necrosis of femoral and humoral heads and other bones
Myopathy (particularly of the proximal muscles)

Ophthalmologic

Posterior subcapsular cataracts
Elevated intraocular pressure/glaucoma

Cardiovascular

Hypertension
Congestive heart failure in predisposed patients

Central Nervous System

Sleep disturbances, insomnia
Euphoria
Depression
Mania
Psychosis
Obsessive behaviors
Idiopathic intracranial hypertension

hypothalamic-pituitary-adrenal axis do not make sufficient endogenous corticosteroids and are at risk for adrenal crisis if their long-term steroid therapy is abruptly ended without replacement. In addition, children on chronic corticosteroid therapy do not generate the additional corticosteroids that are normally made during physiologic stressors such as acute illnesses, injuries, or surgical procedures. These children will require additional or increased doses of corticosteroids during acute illnesses or injuries to simulate the normal physiologic response. Without the administration of these "stress-dose steroids," they may have great difficulty recovering from these acute events, or may die.

There are many other documented effects of corticosteroid therapy (Table 107–2). Most of the studies that have evaluated the effects of corticosteroid therapy have included only adults. The incidence of these complications in children is not known. The extent of the hypothalamic-pituitary axis suppression and the incidence of the other side effects correlate with the potency of the corticosteroid drug, dosage, and timing of administration. In many instances, the exact mechanisms by which corticosteroids cause these detrimen-

tal effects are unknown. Pediatric-specific complications, aside from growth retardation, have not been detailed in the literature. However, with the increasing use of steroids in many pediatric conditions, complications are bound to occur, and some of these conditions may cause a patient to present to the emergency department. For example, fractures may arise more commonly due decreased bone mineral density that has been reported in children on long-term glucocorticoids for treatment of nephrotic syndrome, arthritis, Crohn's disease, systemic lupus erythematosus, and cancer.[8-12]

Multiple drug interactions are associated with steroid therapy.[13] These interactions may involve the effect of the steroid or of the other medications. Drug effectiveness or toxicity may be impacted. For example, steroid doses may need to be increased with the coadministration of antacids, barbiturates, phenobarbitol, phenytoin, or rifampin. Toxicity associated with cyclosporine or digitalis may occur more often in the steroid-dependent child than in other children. Conversely, chronic steroid therapy may reduce the effectiveness of salicylates.

Clinical Presentation

Steroid-dependent children may present to the emergency department with exacerbations of their underlying illness, complications from their underlying illness, unrelated problems, or complications related to their chronic corticosteroid therapy. Clinical experience suggests it is common for these children to present with some combination of these. The symptoms can range from mild, such as agitation and restlessness, to life-threatening, such as adrenal crisis. It is important to obtain information regarding the length of therapy, dosages, and indication for the patient's treatment. Patients on long-term therapy may manifest the clinical features of Cushing's syndrome: short stature, central obesity, moon facies, hirsutism, and abdominal striae. For patients who are severely ill or injured, steroid dependence may lead to the inability to produce an appropriate stress response, resulting in adrenal crisis with refractory hypotension, hyponatremia, and hyperkalemia.[14]

The immunosuppressive and anti-inflammatory effects of corticosteroids contribute to the increased risk of opportunistic infections such as tuberculosis, *Listeria monocytogenes*, Staphylococcus species, gram-negative bacteria, varicella virus, herpes simplex virus, cytomegalovirus, *Candida albicans*, Aspergillus species, and *Crytococcus neoformans*.[15] These infections are more common with higher dosages and longer durations of therapy.[15] In addition, many chronic diseases that require corticosteroid treatment further increase the risk of infection. The immunomodulation associated with corticosteroids may diminish the clinical findings associated with acute infection. For example, cellulitis or otitis media may not develop the same degree of inflammation and erythema as normally expected.

The laboratory data necessary to evaluate a steroid-dependent child depend on the presenting clinical situation. Hyperglycemia may be present in any child receiving glucocorticoid therapy. A nonspecific leukocytosis is commonly seen in steroid-dependent children and is not necessarily a marker for infection. Routine cultures of blood and urine may be obtained if there is concern for an infectious process. Serum electrolytes may demonstrate hyponatremia and hyperkalemia with mineralocorticoid deficiency. A serum cortisol level obtained prior to administering corticosteroids to patients suspected of having acute adrenal insufficiency may help with the inpatient management of these children.

Important Clinical Features and Considerations

A variety of conditions are associated with chronic corticosteroid use. Knowledge of the increased likelihood of these conditions may assist the emergency physician in making the

correct diagnosis. Patients on corticosteroid therapy presenting with headache, visual impairment, and nausea may have idiopathic intracranial hypertension (see Chapter 41, Headaches). Proximal, symmetric weakness may be a symptom of steroid-induced myopathy (see Chapter 97, Muscle and Connective Tissue Disorders). Myopathies may occur after any glucocorticoid therapy, but more frequently follow the administration of 9-α-fluorine preparations such as triamcinolone. Additionally, the diagnosis of avascular necrosis of the femoral head should be considered in patients presenting with limp (see Chapter 100, Diseases of the Hip; and Chapter 188, A Quick Look at Limp). Symptoms such as nausea and abdominal pain in a steroid-dependent child may indicate peptic ulcers or pancreatitis (see Chapter 75, Gastrointestinal Bleeding; and Chapter 80, Pancreatitis). Impaired wound healing from inhibited fibroblast function in steroid-dependent children is an important consideration as well (see Chapter 160, Wound Management).

Management

There are four main principles to the emergency department management of the steroid-dependent child. These principles highlight the differences between these children and others who are not steroid dependent. These main principles involve the requirement for stress-dose steroids, the increased risk of common and uncommon infections, the muted signs and symptoms of inflammation, and modifications to wound management.

Stress-Dose Steroids

When a steroid-dependent child is under physiologic stress due to an acute illness or injury, stress-dose steroids should be administered. The dose of hydrocortisone can be calculated based on body surface area, but this is uncommonly done in the emergency department. One suggested approach is to administer 50 mg of hydrocortisone to children younger than 4 years of age and 100 mg of hydrocortisone to children 4 years of age and older.[16] Alternatively, 1 to 2 mg/kg of hydrocortisone may also be a reasonable, as well as simple, dosing regimen (see Table 108–1). The administration of hydrocortisone may be life saving in steroid-dependent children who are in refractory shock.

Increased Risk for Common and Uncommon Infections

Steroid-dependent children are immunocompromised and at increased risk for serious infections. In particular, organisms that rarely, if ever, cause disease in other children may cause steroid-dependent children to become critically ill. Steroid-dependent children are also at increased risk for disseminated infections.[17]

Muted Signs and Symptoms of Inflammation

Steroid-dependent children may have muted signs and symptoms of inflammation. This is particularly problematic when diagnosing conditions dependent on pain, erythema, or fever for making the diagnosis. Therefore, common diagnoses such as cellulitis, otitis media, and appendicitis may be missed because the usual features of the disease are muted. This places steroid-dependent children at increased risk for disease progression and resultant complications.

Modified Wound Management

The management of wounds may need to be modified for the steroid-dependent child. The wounds of steroid-dependent children may require a longer time to heal, may occur in skin that has decreased tensile strength, are more likely to become infected and more likely to have relatively subtle signs of infection. Controlling the length of time sutures remain in place to avoid wound dehiscence is an important part of managing wounds in steroid-dependent children. Therefore, it is probably prudent to use nonabsorbable sutures, keep the sutures in place longer than usual, and have frequent rechecks of the wound for these children.

Summary

The broad spectrum of activity of glucocorticoids has made their use common in pediatric medicine. Steroid-dependent children may present to the emergency department with complaints related to the side effects of chronic steroid therapy or with unrelated complaints. Steroid-dependent children are at increased risk for a wide range of complications that may affect nearly every system in the body. Awareness of these risks helps the emergency physician manage these children when they present to the emergency department.

REFERENCES

1. Dorland's illustrated medical dictionary, 30th ed. Philadelphia: WB Saunders, 2003, p 1760.
2. Dorland's illustrated medical dictionary, 30th ed. Philadelphia: WB Saunders, 2003, p 425.
3. Keyes C: Endocrine principles. *In* Goldfrank LR, Flomenbaum NE, Lewin NA, et al (eds): Goldfrank's Toxicologic Emergencies, 6th ed. Stamford, CT: Appleton & Lange, 1998, pp 431–445.
4. Payne DN, Balfour-Lynn IM: Children with difficult asthma: a practical approach. J Asthma 38:189–203, 2001.
5. Allen DB: Growth suppression by glucocorticoid therapy. Endocrinol Metab Clin North Am 25:699–717, 1996.
6. Irani AM, Cruz-Rivera M, Fitzpatrick S, et al: Effects of budesonide inhalation suspension on hypothalamic-pituitary-adrenal axis function in infants and young children with persistent asthma. Ann Allergy Asthma Immunol 88:306–312, 2002.
7. Linder BL, Esteban NV, Yergey AL, et al: Cortisol production rate in childhood and adolescence. J Pediatr 117:892–896, 1990.
8. Gulati S, Godbole M, Singh U, et al: Are children with idiopathic nephrotic syndrome at risk for metabolic bone disease? Am J Kidney Dis 41:1163–1169, 2003.
9. Celiker R, Bal S, Bakkaloglu A, et al: Factors playing a role in the development of decreased bone mineral density in juvenile chronic arthritis. Rheumatol Int 23:127–129, 2003.
10. Thearle M, Horlick M, Bilezikian JP, et al: Osteoporosis: an unusual presentation of childhood Crohn's disease. J Clin Endocrinol Metab 85:2122–2126, 2000.
11. Trapani S, Civinini R, Ermini M, et al: Osteoporosis in juvenile systemic lupus erythematosus: a longitudinal study on the effect of steroids on bone mineral density. Rheumatol Int 18:45–49, 1998.
12. Henderson RC, Madsen CD, Davis C, et al: Longitudinal evaluation of bone mineral density in children receiving chemotherapy. J Pediatr Hematol Oncol 20:322–326, 1998.
*13. Lester RS, Knowles SR, Shear NH: The risks of systemic corticosteroid use. Dermatol Clin 16:277–288, 1998.
*14. Arnaldi G, Angeli A, Atkinson AB, et al: Diagnosis and complications of Cushing's syndrome: a consensus statement. J Clin Endocrinol Metab 88:5593–5602, 2003.
*15. Truhan AP, Ahmed AR: Corticosteroids: a review with emphasis on complications of prolonged systemic therapy. Ann Allergy 62:375–390, 1989.
16. Glaser N, Enns GM, Kuppermann N: Metabolic disease. *In* Gausche-Hill M, Fuchs S, Yamamoto L (eds): APLS: The Pediatric Emergency Medicine Resource. Boston: Jones & Bartlett, 2004, p 196.
17. Pickering LK, Baker CJ, Long SS, et al (eds): Varicella-zoster infections. *In* Red Book: 2003 Report of the Committee on Infectious Diseases, 26th ed. Elk Grove Village, IL: American Academy of Pediatrics, 2003, p 679.

*Selected readings.

Chapter 108

Addisonian Crisis

Ameer P. Mody, MD, MPH

Key Points

Addisonian crisis is caused by the adrenal cortex releasing insufficient cortisol to meet physiologic needs.

Congenital adrenal hyperplasia is a form of primary adrenal insufficiency.

Chronic glucocorticoid use is a common cause of secondary adrenal insufficiency.

The characteristic features of addisonian crisis are altered mental status, hypotension, and hypoglycemia.

The critical, specific intervention in cases of suspected addisonian crisis is the administration of parenteral steroids.

Introduction and Background

Addisonian crisis is named for Thomas Addison, a London doctor who practiced in the mid-19th century.[1] Addison was the first to associate specific clinical features with diseases of the adrenal glands. This original description involved chronic cases of adrenal insufficiency due to tuberculous adrenalitis. In the 20th century, the incidence of tuberculosis fell due to the widespread use of antibiotics, and other causes of adrenal insufficiency and failure were identified.[2] Even though the importance of the functioning of the adrenal cortex has been recognized for more than 150 years, addisonian crisis remains a life-threatening condition requiring prompt recognition and treatment to avoid death.

Recognition and Approach

A few features of the normal physiology of the adrenal gland are helpful for understanding addisonian crisis. The adrenal gland has two main anatomic divisions, the medulla and the cortex. The adrenal medulla releases catecholamines such as epinephrine and norepinephrine and is not directly involved in addisonian crises. The adrenal cortex releases cortisol, a key endogenous steroid hormone. The adrenal cortex is under the control of corticotropin, a hormone released from the pituitary gland (Fig. 108–1A). Corticotropin is also known as adrenocorticotropic hormone. Addisonian crisis may arise from failure of the intrinsic function of the adrenal cortex (Fig. 108–1B). This is typically referred to as "primary" addisonian crisis or "primary adrenal insufficiency." Alternatively, addisonian crisis may arise from a failure in the hypothalamic-pituitary-adrenal axis leading to inappropriately low corticotropin stimulation of the adrenal cortex (Fig. 108–1C and 108–1D). This is typically referred to as "secondary" addisonian crisis or "secondary adrenal insufficiency." Occasionally, authors will refer to adrenal insufficiency due to malfunction at the level of the hypothalamus as "tertiary adrenal insufficiency."[3,4] When acute deterioration occurs, the terms *addisonian crisis* and *acute adrenal failure* are appropriate. When chronic symptoms are present, the terms *Addison's disease* and *adrenal insufficiency* are appropriate. Adrenal insufficiency and adrenal failure occur along the same clinical continuum.

The causes of primary addisonian crisis and Addison's disease are few and pathophysiologically varied. One group of conditions frequently implicated in addisonian crises are the congenital adrenal hyperplasias. This is a group of disorders involving autosomal recessive defects in adrenal steroid production.[5-7] Addisonian crisis associated with congenital adrenal hyperplasia typically occurs in early infancy.[8,9] Another cause of primary addisonian crises is sepsis, particularly in the setting of meningococcal disease. Since the 1950s, the syndrome of meningitis, fever, coma, cyanosis, petechial hemorrhages of the skin, and adrenal hemorrhages accompanied by adrenal insufficiency has been referred to as the Waterhouse-Friderichsen syndrome.[10] More recent work suggests adrenal insufficiency may arise in the setting of any serious illness.[11] It may be the case that the underlying pathophysiologic derangements seen in cases of meningococcemia are responsible for the accompanying adrenal insufficiency and are not a feature unique to meningococcal infections.[12-14] In 2005, methicillin-resistant *Staphylococcus aureus* was implicated in pediatric cases of Waterhouse-Friderichsen syndrome.[15] Tuberculous adrenalitis may still cause primary addisonian crisis, but is unlikely to be seen in children from developed countries. Bilateral traumatic adrenal hemorrhages may cause adrenal insufficiency, and this has been described in adults.[16] Traumatic adrenal hemorrhages are usually unilateral children.[17-20] Even if present, traumatic

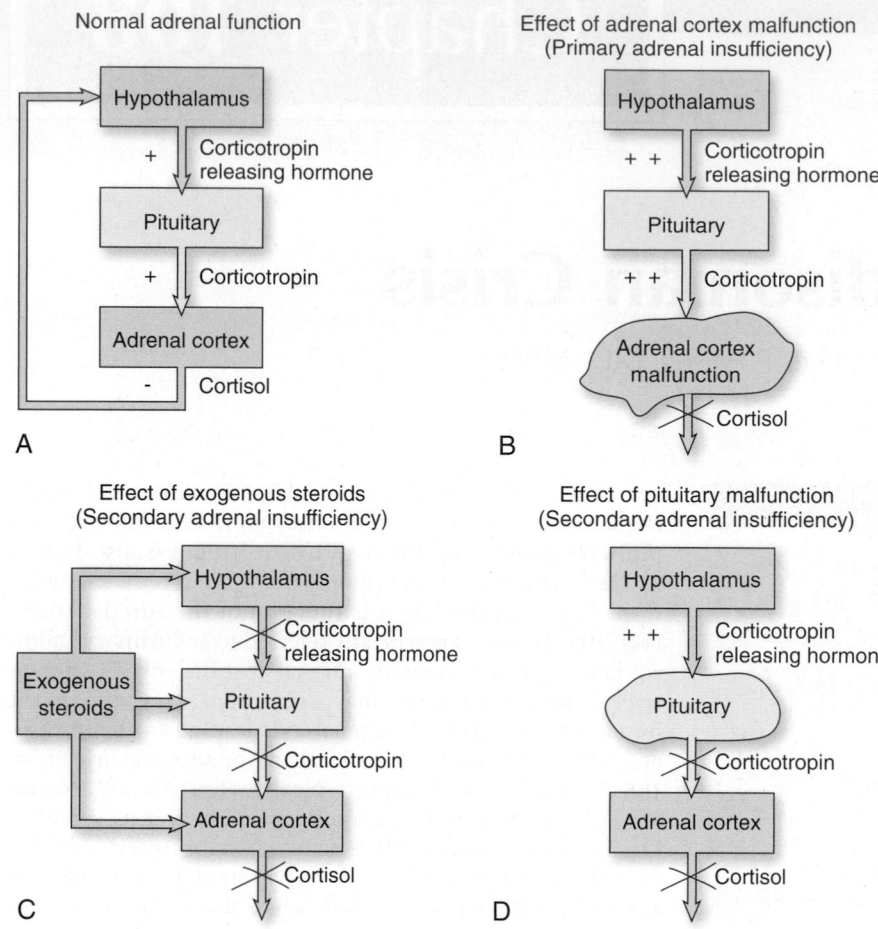

Normal adrenal function

Effect of adrenal cortex malfunction
(Primary adrenal insufficiency)

Effect of exogenous steroids
(Secondary adrenal insufficiency)

Effect of pituitary malfunction
(Secondary adrenal insufficiency)

FIGURE 108–1. Simplified schematic representation of the effects of primary and secondary adrenal insufficiency on cortisol production.

bilateral adrenal hemorrhages may not lead to clinically significant adrenal insufficiency in children.[17] Addisonian crisis may occur from an exacerbation of chronic autoimmune adrenal insufficiency.[8,21] This group of disorders may be the most common cause of adrenal insufficiency in school-age children and adolescents. Another cause of primary adrenal insufficiency are the adrenoleukodystrophies.[22] This group of disorders is most prominently characterized by central nervous system dysfunction and adrenal insufficiency.

Secondary addisonian crisis and Addison's disease is due to disruption of stimulation to the adrenal cortex. Although solid epidemiologic data are not available, it is likely that chronic steroid use is the most common contributing factor to the onset of secondary addisonian crisis. Glucocorticoids are administered for a wide range of conditions (see Chapter 107, The Steroid-Dependent Child). Systemic steroids (e.g., prednisolone, prednisone, dexamethasone) suppress the hypothalamic-pituitary-adrenal axis[4,23,24] (see Fig. 108–1C). These exogenous steroids inhibit the usual release of corticotropin from the pituitary. This leads to an inappropriately diminished release of steroids by the adrenal cortex. If a chronically administered steroid is abruptly withdrawn, the hypothalamic-pituitary-adrenal axis cannot recover sufficiently quickly to meet physiologic demands for cortisol. The paradigm for this is the child taking chronic steroids who develops gastroenteritis and repeatedly vomits his or her medications. This leaves the child vulnerable to developing addisonian crisis.[25] Similarly, if a child on chronically administered steroids experiences an acute physiologic stress such

as occurs in an acute infection, during an operation, or because of traumatic injuries, the child's adrenal cortex will not appropriately release cortisol. Addisonian crisis may ensue. In addition, problems with the pituitary gland and hypothalamus may lead to secondary addisonian crisis. These problems may arise from central nervous system tumors), traumatic brain injury, or pituitary irradiation.

Clinical Presentation

Children experiencing an addisonian crisis characteristically present in extremis with depressed mentation, hypotension, hypoglycemia, and shock. Patients with chronic adrenal insufficiency will have a slowly progressive, indolent course with a variety of nonspecific constitutional symptoms.

Neonates and Young Infants

Neonates and young infants with primary adrenal insufficiency are likely to have congenital adrenal hyperplasia. In the emergency department, this is most likely to be seen in boys. Girls with congenital adrenal hyperplasia are more likely than boys to be identified in the nursery because of ambiguous genitalia. Male infants may not have genitourinary anomalies, but may exhibit darkly pigmented scrotal skin. The earliest signs and symptoms in infants with primary adrenal insufficiency are nonspecific and include poor feeding, poor weight gain, and lethargy.[26] Infants with sepsis and secondary adrenal insufficiency will present in a similar fashion. Many critically ill appearing neonates and young infants will require a generalized approach due to the non-specific features of addisonian crisis in this age group (see Chapter 7, The Critically Ill Neonate).

Older Infants and Children

Older infants and children with adrenal insufficiency may also present with acute, severe symptoms or with more indolent, chronic symptoms. Primary adrenal insufficiency in this age group is commonly due to an autoimmune or degenerative process with an indolent progression of symptoms. Constitutional symptoms prevail, including developmental delay or poor school performance, weakness, abdominal pain, and failure to thrive.[8] Skin hyperpigmentation, a result of excessive corticotropin secretion, is not uniformly present, but might be found in areas seldom exposed to the sun and on the oral mucosa.[27] Patients with addisonian crisis most commonly present with an altered level of consciousness, hypotension, vomiting, and dehydration.[8] In this setting, a history of chronic steroid therapy suggests secondary adrenal insufficiency. These children may exhibit cushingoid features such as moon facies, central adiposity, and abdominal striae (see Chapter 107, The Steroid-Dependent Child).

Laboratory Evaluation

The laboratory evaluation of children experiencing addisonian crisis is approached similarly to the evaluation of other seriously ill children (see Chapter 8, Circulatory Emergencies: Shock). Hypoglycemia is common in addisonian crisis and is easily identified with bedside glucose testing (see Chapter 106, Hypoglycemia). Serum electrolytes may reveal hyponatremia and hyperkalemia, particularly in cases of primary addisonian crisis. This finding may be particularly pronounced in young infants with an acute salt-wasting crisis associated with congenital adrenal hyperplasia. A mild metabolic acidosis, evident by a low serum bicarbonate or a low venous pH, is expected in most cases. In cases of suspected, but previously undiagnosed primary addisonian crisis, serum cortisol and corticotropin levels should be obtained prior to the administration of exogenous steroids if this can be done without delaying treatment. This may help with establishing a diagnosis during the inpatient hospital stay.[28,29]

Important Clinical Features and Considerations

At times, children with known adrenal insufficiency will present to the emergency department with an apparent minor illness or injury. In these cases, in addition to treating the minor illness or injury, the child's steroid dosing will need to be temporarily increased to mimic a normal stress response. Although a rough guide is that the patient's usual steroid dosing will need to be doubled or tripled for a few days,[26] coordinating care with the child's pediatric endocrinologist prior to discharge from the emergency department is prudent in these cases.

Management

Initial management of patients suspected of being in addisonian crisis is similar to that for other critical illnesses (see Chapter 8, Circulatory Emergencies: Shock). An evaluation

for a comorbid illness, particularly sepsis is prudent. Initiating empirical therapy for sepsis is also reasonable in most cases (see Chapter 13, Sepsis). Hypoglycemia, substantial dehydration, and a mild metabolic acidosis are common and require prompt treatment. The administration of normal saline to treat dehydration is usually also an effective treatment for hyponatremia if present. Hyperkalemia associated with addisonian crisis seldom requires specific treatment. It is appropriate to treat hyperkalemia if cardiac dysrhythmias are present (see Chapter 114, Hyperkalemia). A reasonable choice for an initial maintenance fluid is 10% dextrose in normal saline ($D_{10}NS$). Hypotonic fluids and fluids containing potassium should be avoided until serum electrolyte results are available.

For children with a known risk for addisonian crisis, the prompt administration of parenteral steroids may be life saving. For children in refractory shock with hypotension unresponsive to isotonic fluids and vasopressors, the administration of intravenous hydrocortisone may lead to the prompt resolution of shock.[13] Given the rarity of these conditions, the optimal dosing in children has not been investigated. The recommended dosing for adults is the rapid intravenous administration of 100 mg of hydrocortisone.[2,3] Unfortunately, recommended dosing for hydrocortisone is sometimes provided as milligrams per square meter of body surface area, units generally unfamiliar to emergency physicians.[30] There are accepted calculations for estimating surface area based on body weight[31] (Table 108–1). There is little downside to administering a slightly larger dose of hydrocortisone than absolutely necessary, but inadequate dosing places the child at great risk. When in doubt, the physician should err on the side of a somewhat higher dose. Both hydrocortisone and methylprednisolone provide some

Table 108–1	Weight-Based Estimated Body Surface Area and Hydrocortisone Dosing for Children Experiencing an Addisonian Crisis	
Weight (kg)	Body Surface Area* (m^2)	Hydrocortisone Dosing† (mg)
3	0.21	10
5	0.30	15
7	0.38	19
10	0.49	25
15	0.65	33
20	0.79	40
25	0.92	46
30	1.10	55
35	1.2	60
40	1.3	65
45	1.4	70
50	1.5	75
55	1.6	80
60	1.7	85
70	1.9	95
>70	N/A	100

*Body surface area estimations adapted from Sharkey I, Boddy AV, Wallace H, et al: Body surface area estimation in children using weight alone: application in paediatric oncology. Br J Cancer 85:23–28, 2001.
†Hydrocortisone dosing based on 50 mg/m^2.

mineralocorticoid activity at high doses. Dexamethasone does not provide mineralocorticoid activity, but may be the preferred agent in children with suspected, but undiagnosed secondary adrenal insufficiency because it does not interfere with subsequent diagnostic laboratory testing.[28]

Summary

Untreated addisonian crisis is fatal. There is little downside to the empirical administration of a single dose of hydrocortisone to a critically ill child who may harbor adrenal insufficiency. Admission or transfer to a tertiary pediatric facility for intensive care and evaluation by a pediatric endocrinologist is nearly always the best disposition when addisonian crisis is the likely diagnosis.

REFERENCES

1. Eknoyan G: Emergnce of the concept of endocrine function and endocrinology. Adv Chronic Kidney Dis 11:371–376, 2004.
*2. Arlt W, Allolio B: Adrenal insufficiency. Lancet 361:1881–1893, 2003.
3. de Herder WW, van der Lely AJ: Addisonian crisis and relative adrenal failure. Rev Endocr Metab Disord 4:143–147, 2003.
4. Coursin DB, Wood KE: Corticosteroid supplementation for adrenal insufficiency. JAMA 287:236–240, 2002.
5. Warinner SA, Zimmerman D, Thompson GB, et al: Study of three patients with congenital adrenal hyperplasia treated by bilateral adrenalectomy. World J Surg 24:1347–1352, 2000.
6. Speiser PW: Toward better treatment of congenital adrenal hyperplasia. Clin Endocrinol 51:273–274, 1999.
7. Irony I, Cutler GB: Effect of carbenoxolone on the plasma renin activity and hypothalamic-pituitary adrenal axis in congenital adrenal hyperplasia due to 21-hydroxylase deficiency. Clin Endocrinol 51:285–291, 1999.
*8. Simm PJ, McDonnell CM, Zacharin MR: Primary adrenal insufficiency in childhood and adolescence: advances in diagnosis and management. J Paediatr Child Health 40:596–599, 2004.
9. Eugster EA, DiMeglio LA, Wright JC, et al: Height outcome in congenital adrenal hyperplasia caused by 21-hydroxylase deficiency: a meta-analysis. J Pediatr 138:26–32, 2001.
10. Friderichsen C: Waterhouse-Friderichsen syndrome (W.-F.S.). Acta Endocrinol (Copenh) 18:482–492, 1955.
11. Cooper MS, Stewart PM: Corticosteroid insufficiency in acutely ill patients. N Engl J Med 348:727–734, 2003.
12. Hamilton D, Harris MD, Foweraker J, et al: Waterhouse-Friderichsen syndrome as a result of non-meningococcal infection. J Clin Pathol 57:208–209, 2004.
*13. Pizarro CF, Troster EJ, Damiani D, et al: Absolute and relative adrenal insufficiency in children with septic shock. Crit Care Med 33:855–859, 2005.
14. Riordan FAI, Thomson APJ, Ratcliffe JM, et al: Admission cortisol and adrenocorticotrophic hormone levels in children with meningococcal disease: evidence of adrenal insufficiency? Crit Care Med 27:2257–2261, 1999.
*15. Adem PV, Montgomery CP, Husain AN, et al: Staphylococcus aureus sepsis and the Waterhouse-Friderichsen syndrome in children. N Engl J Med 353:1245–1251, 2005.
16. Guichelaar MMJ, Leenen LPH, Braams R: Transient adrenocortical insufficiency following traumatic bilateral adrenal hemorrhage. J Trauma 56:1135–1137, 2004.
17. Sivit CJ, Ingram JD, Taylor GA, et al: Posttraumatic adrenal hemorrhage in children: CT findings in 34 patients. AJR Am J Roentgenol 158:1299–1302, 1992.
18. Schwarz M, Horev G, Freud E, et al: Traumatic adrenal injury in children. Isr Med Assoc J 2:132–134, 2000.
19. Iuchtman M, Breitgand A: Traumatic adrenal hemorrhage in children: an indicator of visceral injury. Pediatr Surg Int 16:586–588, 2000.
20. Gabal-Shehab L, Alagiri M: Traumatic adrenal injuries. J Urol 173:1330-1331, 2005.
21. Perry R, Kecha O, Paquette J, et al: Primary adrenal insufficiency in children: twenty years experience at the Sainte-Justine Hospital, Montreal. J Clin Endocrinol Metab 90:3243–3250, 2005.
22. Ronghe MD, Barton J, Jardine PE, et al: The importance of testing for adrenoleucodystrophy in males with idiopathic Addison's disease. Arch Dis Child 86:185–189, 2002.
23. Henzen C, Suter A, Lerch E, et al: Suppression and recovery of adrenal response after short-term, high-dose glucocorticoid treatment. Lancet 355:542–545, 2000.
24. Omori K, Nomura K, Shimizu S, et al: Risk factors for adrenal crisis in patients with adrenal insufficiency. Endocr J 50:745–752, 2003.
25. Krasner AS: Glucocorticoid-induced adrenal insufficiency. JAMA 282:671–676, 1999.
26. Merke DP, Cutler DP: New approaches to the treatment of congenital adrenal hyperplasia. JAMA 277:1073–1076, 1997.
27. Werbel SS, Ober KP: Acute adrenal insufficiency. Endocrinol Metab Clin North Am 22:303–328, 1993.
28. Stanhope R: Management of adrenal crisis—how should glucocorticoids be administered? J Pediatr Endocrinol Metab 16:1099–1100, 2003.
29. Grinspoon KS, Biller BMK: Clinical review 62: laboratory assessment of adrenal insufficiency. J Clin Endocrinol Metab 79:923–931, 1994.
30. Sachdev S: Formulary adjunct. In Gunn VL, Nechyba C (eds): The Harriet Lane Handbook: A Manual for Pediatric House Officers, 16th ed. St. Louis: Mosby, 2002, p 907.
31. Sharkey I, Boddy AV, Wallace H, et al: Body surface area estimation in children using weight alone: application in paediatric oncology. Br J Cancer 85:23–28, 2001.

*Selected readings.

Chapter 109

Thyrotoxicosis

Ameer P. Mody, MD, MPH

Key Points

Thyrotoxicosis is an uncommon but important endocrine emergency.

The presentation of thyrotoxicosis ranges from mild hypermetabolism to thyroid storm.

Neonatal thyrotoxicosis may mimic sepsis.

β-Blockers and steroids are the mainstays of emergency management for children with thyroid storm.

Introduction and Background

Disorders of the thyroid gland are uncommon in children. However, the systemic effects of thyroid hormone and the occasional insidious onset of disease make these disorders an important part of pediatric emergency care. Thyroid hormone regulates overall metabolic activity. Thyrotoxicosis, the pathologic excess of thyroid hormone, can be due to a variety of etiologies that all result in similar symptoms of hypermetabolism. Thyrotoxicosis can develop in all pediatric age groups. Thyroid storm is a rare but life-threatening complication in patients with thyrotoxicosis and the most extreme form of hyperthyroidism.

Recognition and Approach

The three most common causes of pediatric thyrotoxicosis are Graves' disease and related autoimmune disorders, neonatal thyrotoxicosis, and inappropriate thyroid hormone ingestion.[1-13] Of these, the most common are Graves' disease and related autoimmune hyperthyroidism.[1-7] Graves' disease affects girls five times more often than boys.[2] Graves' disease is an autoimmune disorder in which antibodies are produced against the thyroid-stimulating hormone (TSH) receptor. The result is thyroid gland stimulation. Autoimmune disorders can commonly occur within multiple family members, and up to 50% of children with Graves' disease will have a family history of someone with an autoimmune disease.[1] Graves' disease also occurs more frequently in patients with other comorbid autoimmune disorders.[2] Neonatal thyrotoxi-cosis occurs in the setting of maternal Graves' disease.[10,11] Although TSH and thyroid hormone do not cross the placenta, maternal antibodies are occasionally transmitted, resulting in neonatal thyrotoxicosis. Symptoms are often present at birth, but may be delayed up to 6 weeks due to passage of maternal thyroid receptor–blocking antibodies or treatment of maternal disease. Approximately 20% of neonates with thyrotoxicosis develop high-output cardiac failure.[10] Thyroid replacement medication is used frequently in adult patients. When a child presents with symptoms of thyrotoxicosis, a history of thyroid replacement pills in the home may lead to the diagnosis of exogenous thyroid hormone ingestion.[12,13]

Other causes of thyrotoxicosis are rare. Patients with Hashimoto's thyroiditis can temporarily experience a hyperthyroid state from thyroid gland inflammation before developing the typical hypothyroidism. McCune-Albright syndrome is an uncommon condition characterized by a triad of polyostotic fibrous dysplasia, skin hyperpigmentation, and precocious puberty that often has accompanying hyperthyroidism.[14] TSH-secreting adenomas and thyroid masses are known causes of hyperthyroidism, but are rare in children.[2]

Thyroid storm is a rare, hyperacute presentation in patients with thyrotoxicosis. It is a complication that occurs in approximately 1% of patients with hyperthyroidism, often precipitated by infection, surgery, or trauma. Data on thyroid storm in children are limited to case reports,[15-17] but the adult literature suggests a mortality rate of 20%.[15,18]

Clinical Presentation

The clinical presentation of thyrotoxicosis is variable and somewhat age dependent. Of note, neonatal thyrotoxicosis may not be clinically apparent in the immediate postnatal period. These neonates may be discharged home from the nursery and present to the emergency department with symptoms developing as late as 6 weeks of age. Once apparent, goiter and exophthalmos are typically found in these neonates.[10,11] The most severely ill neonates may present with tachycardia, poor weight gain in the context of normal or supranormal feeding, congestive heart failure, and jaundice.[10,11] Neonatal thyrotoxicosis may present with vague symptoms initially indistinguishable from sepsis or other severe neonatal conditions. Children and adolescents with thyrotoxicosis have significant variability in presentation. The most common findings are goiter and exophthalmos.[1]

Other common symptoms include weight loss, tremors, polyphagia, and hyperhidrosis. Approximately one third of children and adolescents with thyrotoxicosis will have either psychological problems or a decline in school performance.[1]

Patients experiencing thyroid storm present with rapidly progressing, severe symptoms. Thyroid storm generally occurs in patients with previous underlying thyroid pathology exacerbated by surgery, trauma, or infection.[18] When thyroid storm is present, the manifestations of hyperthyroidism are present in an extreme form. Hyperthermia, as high as 41° C (105.8° F), diaphoresis, and tachycardia are characteristic. Mental status may be altered, and patients may experience seizures.[15] Hypertension with widened pulse pressure will also be present in the early phase of thyroid storm. If untreated, the significant hypermetabolic state can eventually lead to hypotension, cardiogenic shock, and death.[18]

The diagnostic evaluation of patients with acute thyrotoxicosis involves assessing thyroid function and monitoring for end-organ damage related to the hypermetabolic state. TSH level, thyroxine, free triiodothyronine (T_3), and T_3 resin uptake levels may be obtained to assist with the ongoing inpatient management.[2] A thyroid assay from the mother of a neonate with thyrotoxicosis may be helpful if the mother does not carry the diagnosis of a thyroid disorder.[11] Other studies may be indicated based on consultation with a pediatric endocrinologist. The diagnosis of thyroid storm is a clinical diagnosis, and thyroid levels will not alter the acute management of these patients. If thyroid storm is present, liver function enzymes, creatinine kinase, microscopic urinalysis, and an electrocardiogram are useful for emergency department management.[18] Urine toxicology screening may be helpful if ingestion of a sympathomimetic drug is high in the differential diagnosis.

Important Clinical Features and Considerations

The presentation of hyperthyroid states in children mimics many other conditions. Given the rarity of these conditions, it is often difficult to make these diagnoses in the emergency department. Situations in which thyrotoxicosis is relatively likely include cases in which a known thyroid disease is present in a child or mother of a young infant or exposure to exogenous thyroid hormone is suspected.

Management

The general goal of the emergency management of children presenting with thyrotoxicosis is to counteract the hyperadrenergic effects of thyroid hormone. Patients experiencing thyroid storm or neonatal thyrotoxicosis may present in extremis. For these patients, aggressive measures to restore homeostasis and evaluation for the inciting event are necessary. The initial approach to a child critically ill from thyrotoxicosis is similar to that to other critically ill children (see Chapter 1, Approach to Resuscitation and Advanced Life Support for Infants and Children; Chapter 8, Circulatory Emergencies: Shock; Chapter 11, Altered Mental Status/Coma; and Chapter 13, Sepsis). Patients with milder symptoms of thyrotoxicosis require symptomatic relief and initial diagnostic evaluation if necessary.

β-Blockers are the mainstay of treatment for symptomatic thyrotoxicosis, neonatal disease, and thyroid storm.[18] β-Blockers are effective in treating the majority of symptoms related to thyroid hormone excess. Propranolol given as a 10-mcg/kg infusion over 15 minutes is a reasonable first dose for most children. Additional doses of propranolol are typically indicated to achieve acceptable clinical improvement. A continuous infusion of esmolol is another option.[19]

Corticosteroids have also been utilized in the treatment of thyroid storm.[20] Studies of adult patients have shown increased survival with their use. Systemic steroids acutely inhibit thyroid hormone release and the conversion from thyroxine to free T_3 in the peripheral tissues.[20] Intravenous hydrocortisone given as a 5-mg/kg injection (up to 100 mg) is a reasonable option.

Propylthiouracil and methimazole are the main pharmacologic treatments for chronic hyperthyroidism. They act to prevent synthesis of thyroid hormone and prevent conversion of thyroxine to free T_3. These medications are particularly helpful in treating outpatients with hyperthyroidism.[2]

Summary

Thyrotoxicosis is an uncommon but important pediatric emergency. The widespread systemic effects of thyroid hormone create symptoms that may mimic other acute illnesses. Appropriate therapy of thyrotoxicosis should resolve symptoms, including behavioral changes, in a short period of time.

Patients with subacute thyrotoxicosis can likely be discharged with close primary and subspecialty care follow-up. Neonatal thyrotoxicosis and thyroid storm patients usually require pediatric intensive care unit admission for stabilization and monitoring.

REFERENCES

*1. Raza J, Hindmarsh PC, Brook CGD: Thyrotoxicosis in children: thirty years' experience. Acta Paediatr 88:937–941, 1999.
2. Zimmerman D, Lteif AN: Thyrotoxicosis in children. Endocrinol Metab Clin North Am 27:109–126, 1998.
3. Hung W, Sarlis NJ: Autoimmune and non-autoimmune hyperthyroidism in pediatric patients: a review and personal commentary on management. Pediatr Endocrinol Rev 2:21–38, 2004.
4. Kraiem Z, Newfield RS: Graves' disease in childhood. J Pediatr Endocrinol Metab 14:229–243, 2001.
5. Dotsch J, Rascher W, Dorr HG: Graves disease in childhood: a review of the options for diagnosis and treatment. Paediatr Drugs 5:95–102, 2003.
6. Forssberg M, Arvidsson CG, Engvall J 3rd, et al: Increasing incidence of childhood thyrotoxicosis in a population-based area of central Sweden. Acta Pediatr 93:25–29, 2004.
7. Hung W: Graves' disease in children. Curr Ther Endocrinol Metab 6:77–81, 1997.
8. Birrell G, Cheetham T: Juvenile thyrotoxicosis: can we do better? Arch Dis Child 89:745–750, 2004.
9. Perrild H, Jacobsen BB: Thyrotoxicosis in childhood. Eur J Endocrinol 134:678–679, 1996.
10. Ogilvy-Stuart AL: Neonatal thyroid disorders. Arch Dis Child Fetal Neonatal Ed 87:F165–F171, 2002.
11. Skuza KA, Sills IN, Stene M, et al: Prediction of neonatal hyperthyroidism in infants born to mothers with Graves' disease. J Pediatr 128:264–267, 1996.
12. Lewander WJ, Lacouture PG, Silva JE, et al: Acute thyroxine ingestion in pediatric patients. Pediatrics 84:262–265, 1989.

*Selected readings.

*13. Tsutaoka BT, Kim S, Santucci S: Seizure in a child after an acute ingestion of levothyroxine. Pediatr Emerg Care 21:857–859, 2005.

14. Volkl TM, Dorr HG: McCune-Albright syndrome: clinical picture and natural history in children and adolescents. J Pediatr Endocrinol Metab 19(Suppl 2):551–559, 2006.

15. Aiello DP, DuPlessis AJ, Pattishall EG, et al: Thyroid storm presenting with coma and seizures in a 3 year old girl. Clin Pediatr (Phila) 28:571–574, 1989.

16. Ho SC, Eng PH, Ding ZP, et al: Thyroid storm presenting as jaundice and complete heart block. Ann Acad Med Singapore 27:748–751, 1998.

17. Yoshida D: Thyroid storm precipitated by trauma. J Emerg Med 14:697–701, 1996.

*18. Pearce EN: Diagnosis and management of thyrotoxicosis. BMJ 332:1369–1373, 2006.

19. Brunette DD, Rothong C: Emergency department management of thyrotoxic crisis with esmolol. Am J Emerg Med 9:232–234, 1991.

20. Tsatsoulis A, Johnson EO, Kalogera CH, et al: The effect of thyrotoxicosis on adrenocortical reserve. Eur J Endocrinol 142:231–235, 2000.

Chapter 110

Dehydration and Disorders of Sodium Balance

Alan L. Nager, MD and Ian K. Maconochie, MBBS

Key Points

The most common cause of dehydration is diarrhea.

The initial estimation of dehydration is based on clinical critieria, not laboratory studies.

Treatments for dehydration include oral, nasogastric, and intravenous rehydration.

Clinically significant sodium disorders are uncommon in previously healthy children.

Introduction and Background

Dehydration is the result of a negative fluid balance. This results from decreased fluid intake, increased fluid output, or both. Dehydration occurs along a continuum from a clinically insignificant negative fluid balance to hypovolemic shock and death. The differential diagnosis of dehydration is extensive and heterogeneous (Table 110–1).

When laboratory testing is performed, dehydration is commonly classified according to the serum sodium concentration. A normal serum sodium ranges from 136 to 145 mmol/L (136 to 145 mEq/L).[1] The definition of *hyponatremia* is a "deficiency of sodium in the blood."[2] Similarly, the definition of *hypernatremia* is "excessive sodium in the blood."[3] These definitions lack clinical utility and contain no numeric values. It would be technically correct to define hyponatremia as a serum sodium less than 136 mmol/L (136 mEq/L) and hypernatremia as a serum sodium greater than 145 mmol/L (mEq/L). It is likely that clinically significant dysnatremia deviates further from normal than these numeric boundaries. One reasonable approach is to define hyponatremia, or "clinically significant hyponatremia," as a serum sodium less than 130 mmol/L (130 mEq/L).[4] Similarly, hypernatremia or "clinically significant hypernatremia" can be defined as a serum sodium greater than 150 mmol/L (150 mEq/L).[5] Dehydration occurring with a normal serum

sodium, or a serum sodium between 130 and 150 mmol/L (130 and 150 mEq/L), can be referred to as "isotonic" dehydration.

Recognition and Approach

In the United States, acute gastroenteritis remains the most significant cause of dehydration. More than 1.5 million outpatient visits occur annually, resulting in 200,000 hospitalizations and 300 deaths per year.[6] Worldwide, diarrheal disease remains the leading cause of morbidity and mortality, with 1.5 billion episodes and 1.5 to 2.5 million deaths occurring annually for patients younger than 5 years.[6]

The pathophysiology of dehydration and sodium homeostasis is based on the concept of intracellular and extracellular fluid "compartments." These compartments are idealized intellectual constructs that have some clinical utility. The intracellular compartment contains all of the fluids within cell membranes. These numerous tiny fluid collections are treated as if they are a unified fluid collection. Sodium levels are relatively low in this compartment. The extracellular compartment contains all of the fluids outside cell membranes. Plasma, interstitial fluid, and transcellular fluid are the major components of this compartment. Sodium levels are relatively high in this compartment.

These intracellular and extracellular compartments are useful for understanding the fluid shifts associated with dysnatremias and dehydration. Hyponatremic dehydration is present when the fluid lost contains relatively high levels of sodium. Water then shifts from the intracellular compartment into the extracellular compartment. This shift in water lowers the serum sodium. Hypernatremic dehydration is present with the fluid lost contains relatively low levels of sodium. Water then shifts from the extracellular space into the intracellular space. This shift in water raises the serum sodium. Isotonic dehydration occurs when the fluid lost is isotonic and substantial water shifting does not occur.

Clinical Presentation

For children at risk for dehydration, useful historical features include the environment in which symptoms developed, the presence of associated symptoms, and any prior treatment or home remedies. In addition, assessing the patient's input and output is useful. Attempting to quantify oral intake is helpful. Ascertaining the presence or absence of vomiting is important as vomiting can inhibit adequate oral intake. Output history includes the amount and frequency of urination, the presence of diarrhea and its quantity, and the presence of excessive sweating.[7] Other useful historical features include changes in the child's level of activity, the presence of fever, changes in mental status, difficulty swallowing, respiratory symptoms, skin changes (including periods of pallor or cyanosis), appetite or thirst changes, medication use (including antibiotics), the potential for a toxic ingestion, the travel history, and a change in weight.[8]

There are specific physical examination findings useful for assessing dehydration. Vital signs may reveal fever, tachycardia, tachypnea, and hypotension. Further evidence suggesting dehydration include listlessness or lethargy, a sunken fontanelle, sunken eyes or absent or diminished tears, dry or sticky mucous membranes, tachypnea, skin that is cool or mottled, delayed capillary refill time, and diminished pulses.

Ideally, the assessment of dehydration would be based on a comparison of the weight on presentation and the pre-illness weight.[9-14] Unfortunately, an accurate and recent pre-illness weight is seldom, if ever, available. Emergency physicians and others who care for children have come to use clinical criteria to assess dehydration in children[15] (Table 110–2). This type of estimation is useful, but imprecise.

When disorders of sodium are present, signs and symptoms directly related to the serum sodium level may be present. Signs and symptoms of hyponatremia depend on the serum sodium and the speed at which the sodium level falls. Symptoms primarily involve the central nervous or musculoskeletal systems. Neurologic symptoms include nausea, vomiting, headache, mental status changes, altered consciousness, diminished reflexes, hypothermia, pseudobulbar palsy, and seizures. Musculoskeletal symptoms include weakness, muscle cramps, and decreased movement. Signs and symptoms of hypernatremia include mental status changes, muscular weakness, ataxia, tremors, hyperreflexia, seizures, unresponsiveness, and intracerebral hemorrhage.

Routine laboratory testing for dehydration is controversial and has not been shown to be predictive of the degree to which a patient may be dehydrated. In addition, different mechanisms resulting in dehydration reveal varying laboratory abnormalities. Vomiting, for example, can cause a high bicarbonate level due to gastric acid losses or a low bicarbonate level due to volume contractions, lactic acidosis or starvation. Vomiting and diarrhea may lead to a variety of laboratory abnormalities, depending on the severity of vomiting or diarrhea, oral intake, and the duration of illness.[10] Several investigators have attempted to correlate severity of disease with various laboratory abnormalities by looking at bicarbonate, blood urea nitrogen, creatinine, sodium, uric acid, serum and urine anion gap, venous pH, urine specific gravity, and urine ketones.[7,15,16-19] No single laboratory test has been shown to be an accurate marker for dehydration. If a child is

Table 110–1	Differential Diagnosis of Dehydration

Decreased Intake

Eating disorders
Facial dysmorphism
Gastroesophageal reflux
Inappropriate feedings
Infantile nasal congestion
Lack of access to appropriate fluids
Malaise associated with an acute illness
Mechanical obstruction (e.g., pyloric stenosis)
Oral trauma
Pharyngitis
Stomatitis
Tachypnea interfering with feeding
Uncoordinated swallowing
Vomiting

Increased Output

Cerebral salt-wasting syndrome
Diabetes insipidis
Diabetic ketoacidosis
Diarrhea
Increased metabolism (e.g., fever)
Medication effects (e.g., diuretics)
Renal losses (e.g., nephrotic syndrome)
Tachypnea with respired losses

Table 110–2	Symptoms Associated with Dehydration		
Symptom	Minimal or No Dehydration (<3% Loss of Body Weight)	Mild to Moderate Dehydration (3–9% Loss of Body Weight)	Severe Dehydration (>9% Loss of Body Weight)
Mental status	Well, alert	Normal, fatigued or restless, irritable	Apathetic, lethargic, unconscious
Thirst	Normal, might refuse	Thirsty, eager to drink	Drinks poorly; unable to drink
Heart rate	Normal	Normal to increased	Tachycardia, ± bradycardia
Quality of pulses	Normal	Normal to decreased	Weak; thready, or impalpable
Breathing	Normal	Normal; fast	Deep
Eyes	Normal	Slightly sunken	Deeply sunken
Tears	Present	Decreased	Absent
Mouth and tongue	Moist	Dry	Parched
Skinfolds	Instant recoil	Recoil in <2 sec	Recoil in >2 sec
Capillary refill	Normal	Prolonged	Prolonged; minimal
Extremities	Warm	Cool	Cold; mottled; cyanotic
Urine output	Normal to decreased	Decreased	Minimal

Adapted from Duggan C, Santosham M, Glass RI: The management of acute diarrhea in children: oral rehydration, maintenance, and nutritional therapy. MMWR Recomm Rep 41(RR-16):1–20, 1992; and World Health Organization: The Treatment of Diarrhoea: A Manual for Physicians and Other Senior Health Workers. Geneva: World Health Organization, 1995.

Table 110–3	Conditions Altering Sodium and Total Body Water Balance		
	Serum Sodium		
Total Body H₂O (Vol)	**↑**	**Normal**	**↓**
↑	Excess saline infusion Bicarbonate intoxication Salt poisoning Hyperaldosteronism	Congestive heart failure Liver disease Nephrotic syndrome Renal failure SIADH Glucocorticoid deficiency	Congestive heart failure Liver disease Nephrotic syndrome Renal failure SIADH
Normal	Insensible losses (skin and respiratory) Diabetic insipidus (central or nephrogenic)	Mild–moderate GI losses	Water intoxication
↓	Insensible losses (skin and respiratory) Water deprivation Vomiting, diarrhea	Vomiting Diarrhea Diuretics	Vomiting/diarrhea Cystic fibrosis Diuretics Renal losses Burns/heat stroke Ascites

Abbreviations: GI, gastrointestinal; SIADH, syndrome of inappropriate secretion of antidiuretic hormone.

determined to be dehydrated based on clinical criteria, assessment of serum sodium can be helpful in generating an appropriate differential diagnosis (Table 110–3).

Important Clinical Features and Considerations

There is no universally accepted group of signs and symptoms that accurately estimates the degree of dehydration in children. Even though broad categories are often used (e.g., mild, moderate, severe), children may fail to fall into a single category.[15] Given the number of predictors examined, a child may fall into the mild category for some of them and the moderate category for others. This can be very confusing to families and clinicians. One strategy in dealing with this is to simply count the number of abnormal signs and symptoms. One suggested approach is to assess decreased skin elasticity, prolonged capillary refill time, general appearance, absence of tears, abnormal respirations, dry mucous membranes, sunken eyes, abnormal radial pulses, a heart rate greater than 150 beats/min, and decreased urine output. In one study, the presence of fewer than three of these signs and symptoms corresponded with mild dehydration, three to six signs or symptoms corresponded with moderate dehydration, and more than six signs or symptoms corresponded with severe dehydration.[9]

Another approach is to try to narrow the focus of the evaluation to those features most strongly associated with dehydration. One constellation of signs and symptoms suggested is general appearance, prolonged capillary refill time, dry mucous membranes, and reduced tears.[9] Another recommendation is that general appearance, sunken eyes, dry mucous membranes, and decreased tears be the focus of the evaluation.[20] Yet another recommendation includes deep breathing, decreased skin turgor, and decreased peripheral perfusion.[11,21] Still others have recommended focusing on prolonged capillary refill time as the sole factor used in estimated dehydration.[22-26] Because researchers and clinicians are using different groupings of signs and symptoms, it is problematic to compare research studies or standardize clinical care.

Management

The treatment of dehydration is based on the estimated degree of dehydration[12,14,27-34] (Table 110–4). In the last several years, a strong interest in utilizing oral rehydration in the emergency department has arisen.[28-31,35,36] It is conceivable that the increasingly widespread use of oral ondansetron in the pediatric emergency department has positively contributed to the acceptance and success of oral rehydration in this setting.[37] A few studies performed in the emergency department have shown success and effectiveness of nasogastric rehydration.[32,38-40] Although there is little controversy in initiating intravenous rehydration in severely dehydrated children, the exact point at which intravenous rehydration is preferred is unknown.

For children undergoing intravenous rehydration, determining the rate at which a child should be rehydrated is not always clear. Some children may receive one or two 20 mL/kg normal saline boluses, resume adequate oral intake, and be discharged home. For those requiring prolonged hydration due to poor oral intake or persistent vomiting, the "4-2-1" rule can be utilitized to calculate an appropriate rate at which to administer intravenous fluids: for the first 10 kg of weight, administer 4 ml/kg/hr; for the second 10 kg of weight, administer 2 ml/kg/hr; and for the remaining weight, administer 1 ml/kg/hr. Using this calculation results in the generally accepted rate for "maintenance fluids." To treat dehydrated children, it is customary to administer 1.5 times the maintenance rate. For a 26-kg child, the maintenance fluids would be administered at a rate of 66 ml/hr (40 + 20 + 6); thus 1.5 times the maintenance rate is 99 ml/hour (1.5 × 66). An order for 100 ml/hr would be appropriate for this 26-kg child.

The choice of fluid is controversial. Traditionally, hypotonic solutions have been selected, but some have advocated using isotonic solutions for ongoing intravenous infusions.[41] For previously healthy children who are not critically ill, hypotonic 0.45 normal saline with 5% dextrose and 20 mmol (20 mEq) potassium per liter run at 1.5 times the maintenance rate is a reasonable starting point. Neonates and young infants are customarily given 0.2 normal saline with added dextrose and potassium. These fluids are not intended for

Table 110–4   Treatment for Dehydration*

	Minimal	Mild to Moderate	Severe
Primary phase	PO	PO	IV
Secondary phase (if primary phase fails)	NG IV	NG IV	Central line Intraosseous (IO)
Tertiary phase (optional)	PO	PO	± PO after initial
Laboratory studies	None	None[†]	Electrolytes, blood urea nitrogen, creatinine, calcium, glucose, urine
Fluid amounts	<50 ml/kg	50–100 ml/kg	>100 ml/kg
Treatment length	<4 hr	1–4 hr	>4 hr
Discharge criteria	Baseline or near-baseline vital signs Urine output during hydrating period Moist oral mucosa Streaming tears No or minimal ongoing losses Able to tolerate PO fluids (optional)		Not applicable
Treatment failure	Admit or observation unit	Admit	

*PO: 5 ml (1 teaspoon) every 1–2 min; ↑ based on patient tolerance.
NG: 20 ml/kg/hr over 1–4 hr (ORS).
IV (moderate dehydration): 50–100 ml/kg over 1–4 hr (NS or LR).
IV (severe dehydration): 20 ml/kg over 5–30 min (NS or LR).
Aim for 60–100 ml/kg within the first hour. Contraindications include some forms of cardiac disease (e.g., cardiomyopathy) or neurologic disease.
[†]May need to obtain laboratory studies based on dietary history or disease state.
Abbreviations: IV, intravenous; LR, lactated Ringer's solution; NG, nasogastric; NS, normal saline; ORS, oral rehydration solution; PO, oral.

bolus therapy. Bolus therapy should be accomplished using normal saline without added glucose or potassium. Medically complicated children and those with conditions known to cause electrolyte abnormalities (e.g., children on dialysis) will require individualized approaches.

Treatment of mild derangements of sodium homeostasis can usually be accomplished by administering normal saline. Normal saline is hypertonic to hyponatremic serum and hypotonic to hypernatremic serum. Therefore, the administration of normal saline should be the appropriate treatment regardless of the serum sodium level. For more extreme sodium derangements, specific therapy may offer the opportunity for the best outcome. For symptomatic children with a serum sodium below 120 mmol/L (120 mEq/L), the administration of 5 ml/kg of 3% normal saline over several minutes can be used to treat seizures and other serious signs or symptoms. The goal for this type of treatment is to raise the serum sodium above the threshold for seizures or the concerning sign or symptom. Rapid correction of hyponatremia beyond this is to be avoided because permanent neurologic damage in the form of central pontine myelinolysis may occur. The treatment of hypernatremic dehydration should occur somewhat more slowly than that of hyponatremic or isotonic dehydration. Many times, providing an initial normal saline bolus followed by maintenance fluids (*not* 1.5 times maintenance) will be sufficient for the emergency department management of these children. Rapid rehydration may lead to cellular swelling and damage.

Summary

Dehydration is a common problem causing significant morbidity and mortality in children. With appropriate treatment, dehydration can be successfully treated in nearly all cases. Serious derangements of serum sodium are uncommon. With appropriate treatment, the prognosis of these electrolytes disturbances is excellent. An important task for the emergency physician is identifying the cause of the dehydration and initiating appropriate treatment for the underlying coexisting illness.

REFERENCES

1. Kratz A, Ferraro M, Sluss PM, et al: Laboratory reference values. N Engl J Med 351:1548–1563, 2004.
2. Anderson DM, Novak PD, Keith J, et al: Dorland's Illustrated Medical Dictionary, 30th ed. Philadelphia: WB Saunders, 2003, p 896.
3. Anderson DM, Novak PD, Keith J, et al: Dorland's Illustrated Medical Dictionary, 30th ed. Philadelphia: WB Saunders, 2003, p 884.
*4. Choong K, Kho ME, Menon K, et al: Hypotonic versus isotonic saline in hospitalised children: a systematic review. Arch Dis Child 91:828–835, 2006.
*5. King CK, Glass R, Bresee JS, et al: Managing acute gastroenteritis among children: oral rehydration, maintenance and nutritional therapy. MMWR Recomm Rep 52(RR-16):1, 2003.
6. Oddie S, Richmond S, Coulthard M: Hypernatraemic dehydration and breast feeding: a population study. Arch Dis Child 85:318–320, 2001.
7. Steiner MJ, DeWalt DA, Byerley JS: Is this child dehydrated? JAMA 291:2746–2754, 2004.
8. Porter SC, Fleisher GR, Kohane IS, et al: The value of parental report for diagnosis and management of dehydration in the emergency department. Ann Emerg Med 41:196–205, 2003.
*9. Gorelick MH, Shaw KN, Murphy KO: Validity and reliability of clinical signs in the diagnosis of dehydration in children. Pediatrics 99(5):e6, 1997.
10. Liebelt EL: Clinical and laboratory evaluation and management of children with vomiting, diarrhea and dehydration. Curr Opin Pediatr 10:461–469, 1998.
11. Mackenzie A, Shann F, Barnes G: Clinical signs of dehydration in children. Lancet 2:1529–1530, 1989.
12. Sharifi J, Ghavami F, Nowrouzi Z, et al: Oral versus intravenous rehydration therapy in severe gastroenteritis. Arch Dis Child 60:856–860, 1985.
13. Vega RM, Avner JR: A prospective study of the usefulness of clinical and laboratory parameters for predicting percentage of dehydration in children. Pediatr Emerg Care 13:179–182, 1997.

*Selected readings.

14. Vesikari T, Isolauri E, Baer M: A comparative trial of rapid oral and intravenous rehydration in acute diarrhea. Acta Pediatr Scand 76:300–305, 1987.

*15. Practice parameter: The management of acute gastroenteritis in young children. American Academy of Pediatrics, Provisional Committee on Quality Improvement Subcommittee on Acute Gastroenteritis. Pediatrics 97:424–436, 1996.

16. Bonadio WA, Hennes HH, Machi J, et al: Efficacy of measuring BUN in assessing children with dehydration due to gastroenteritis. Ann Emerg Med 18:755–757, 1989.

17. Narchi H: Serum bicarbonate and dehydration severity in gastroenteritis. Arch Dis Child 78:70–71, 1998.

18. Rothrock SG, Green SM, McArthur CL, et al: Detection of electrolyte abnormalities in children presenting to the emergency department: multicenter, prospective analysis. Acad Emerg Med 4:1025–1031, 1997.

19. Teach SJ, Yates EW, Feld LG: Laboratory predictors of fluid deficit in acutely dehydrated children. Clin Pediatr 36:395–400, 1997.

20. Friedman JN, Goldman RD, Srivastava R, et al: Development of a clinical dehydration scale for use in children between 1 and 36 months of age. J Pediatr 145:201–207, 2004.

21. Duggan C, Refit M, Hashem M, et al: How valid are clinical signs of dehydration in infants? J Pediatr Gastroenterol Nutr 22:56–61, 1996.

22. Gorelick MH, Shaw KN, Baker MD: Effect of ambient temperature on capillary refill in healthy children. Pediatrics 92:699–702, 1993.

23. Gorelick MH, Shaw KN, Murphy KD, et al: Effect of fever on capillary refill time. Pediatr Emerg Care 13:305–307, 1997.

24. Laron Z: Skin turgor as a quantitative index of dehydration in children. Pediatrics 19:816–822, 1957.

25. Saavedra JM, Harris GD, Li S, et al: Capillary refilling (skin turgor) in the assessment of dehydration. Am J Dis Child 145:296–298, 1991.

26. Shavit I, Brant R, Nijssen-Jordan C, et al: A novel imaging technique to measure capillary-refill time: improving diagnostic accuracy for dehydration in young children with gastroenteritis. Pediatrics 118:2402–2408, 2006.

27. Reid S, Bonadio WA: Outpatient rapid intravenous rehydration to correct dehydration and resolve vomiting in children with acute gastroenteritis. Ann Emerg Med 28:318–323, 1996.

28. Atherly-John YC, Cunningham SJ, Crain EF: A randomized trial of oral vs intravenous rehydration in a pediatric emergency department. Arch Pediatr Adolesc Med 156:1240–1243, 2002.

29. Bender BJ, Ozuah PO: Intravenous rehydration for gastroenteritis: how long does it really take? Pediatr Emerg Care 20:215–218, 2004.

30. Crocetti MT, Baron MA, Amin DD, et al: Pediatric observation status beds on an inpatient unit: an integrated care model. Pediatr Emerg Care 20:17–21, 2004.

31. Duggan C, Santosham M, Glass RI: The management of acute diarrhea in children: oral rehydration, maintenance and nutritional therapy. MMWR Recomm Rep 41(RR-16):1–20, 1992.

32. Mackenzie A, Barnes G: Randomized controlled trial comparing oral and intravenous rehydration therapy in children with diarrhoea. BMJ 303:393–396, 1991.

33. Phin SJ, McCaskill ME, Browne GJ, et al: Clinical pathway using rapid rehydration for children with gastroenteritis. J Paediatr Child Health 39:343–348, 2003.

34. Rahman O, Bennish ML, Alam AN, et al: Rapid intravenous rehydration by means of a single polyelectrolyte solution with or without dextrose. J Pediatr 113:654–660, 1988.

35. Fonseca BK, Holdgate A, Craig JC: Enteral vs intravenous rehydration therapy for children with gastroenteritis: a meta-analysis of randomized controlled trials. Arch Pediatr Adolesc Med 158:483–490, 2004.

36. Conners GP, Barker WH, Mushlin AL, et al: Oral versus intravenous rehydration preferences of pediatric emergency medicine fellowship directors. Pediatr Emerg Care 16:335–338, 2000.

37. Freedman SB, Adler M, Seshadri R, et al: Oral ondansetron for gastroenteritis in a pediatric emergency department. N Engl J Med 354:1698–1705, 2006.

38. Moineau G, Newman J: Rapid intravenous rehydration in the pediatric emergency department. Pediatr Emerg Care 6:186–188, 1990.

39. Gremse DA: Effectiveness of nasogastric rehydration in hospitalized children with acute diarrhea. J Pediatr Gastroenterol Nutr 21:145–148, 1995.

40. Nager AL, Wang VJ: Comparison of nasogastric and intravenous methods of rehydration in pediatric patients with acute dehydration. Pediatrics 109:566–572, 2002.

41. Hoorn EJ, Geary D, Robb M, et al: Acute hyponatremia related to intravenous fluid administration in hospitalized children: an observational study. Pediatrics 113:1279–1284, 2004.

Chapter 111

Metabolic Acidosis

John C. Brancato, MD

Key Points

Metabolic acidosis is commonly encountered in serious pediatric illnesses presenting to the emergency department.

The causes of metabolic acidosis can be categorized according to whether or not an elevation in the anion gap is present.

The treatment of metabolic acidosis is based on treatment of the underlying illness.

Administration of large volumes of normal saline can result in hyperchloremic acidosis.

Introduction and Background

Many of the more serious conditions for which children present to the emergency department manifest a metabolic acidosis. These include traumatic injuries,[1,2] ingestions,[3-6] inborn errors of metabolism,[7-9] diabetic ketoacidosis,[10-13] renal disorders,[13,14] dehydration due to diarrheal illness,[15] and septic shock.[16-18] Understanding metabolic acidosis is the foundation for understanding the clinical manifestations, diagnostic approach, and management of these myriad conditions.

Recognition and Approach

The human body is designed to keep a tightly controlled acid-base environment. However, the body also continually produces acids both when healthy and to an even greater extent in certain illnesses. Many of these acids are generated during the metabolism of the basic components of food. For example, lactic acid and ketoacids are generated during the metabolism of fat. Sulfuric acid and phosphoric acid are generated during the metabolism of proteins. Various homeostatic mechanisms promote the buffering and excretion of excess acids to allow tight control of the pH of the blood and interstitial fluids. When these homeostatic mechanisms become dysfunctional or are overwhelmed, acidosis develops.

Recognized for the last half century, one of the key homeostatic mechanisms involves carbonic acid (H_2CO_3).[19] H_2CO_3 is an intermediary in a bidirectional chemical reaction that converts water (H_2O) and carbon dioxide (CO_2) into a hydrogen ion (H^+) and bicarbonate (HCO_3^-) and vice versa. This homeostatic mechanism involving H_2CO_3 is the principal extracellular buffer allowing the body to accommodate fairly rapid, large increases in excess acid. When chemoreceptors in the brain encounter an increasingly acidic environment, increased respirations are generated to allow for greater expiration of CO_2. To some degree, this increase in ventilation compensates for metabolic acidosis (Fig. 111–1). At the same time, receptors in the kidney are triggered leading to increased excretion of H^+ and retention of HCO_3^- (Fig. 111–2).

Clinical Presentation

The clinical presentation of metabolic acidosis is dominated by the signs and symptoms of the underlying illness. However, there are some features common to many of these illnesses. In particular, deep, rapid respirations are often present. The paradigm for this is Kussmaul's respirations seen in children with diabetic ketoacidosis.[10] Dehydration, nausea, abdominal pain, vomiting, lethargy, and malaise are also common features in many cases of metabolic acidosis. In cases of inborn errors of metabolism, coma may dominate the presentation to the emergency department.[7] In some cases, such as seen with septic shock, the signs and symptoms of metabolic acidosis and those of septic shock are intimately intertwined.[18] As septic shock resolves, so does the metabolic acidosis. Determining if there are symptoms solely attributable to metabolic acidosis is of no clinical significance and not feasible.

The signs and symptoms of many of the conditions that cause metabolic acidosis are nonspecific and overlap. Given this, the emergency physician will encounter very ill patients for whom a metabolic acidosis has been identified, but for whom a specific diagnosis is not readily apparent.

One approach to refine the differential diagnosis for conditions presenting with a metabolic acidosis is to assess the serum for "unmeasured" anions. The term *unmeasured* is primarily of historical significance given that the measurement of important anions such as lactate is now routine. One approach to assessing serum for these excess anions is the anion gap.[13,20,21] The anion gap is calculated as follows:

$$\text{Anion gap} = [Na^+] + [K^+] - [Cl^-] - [HCO_3^-]$$

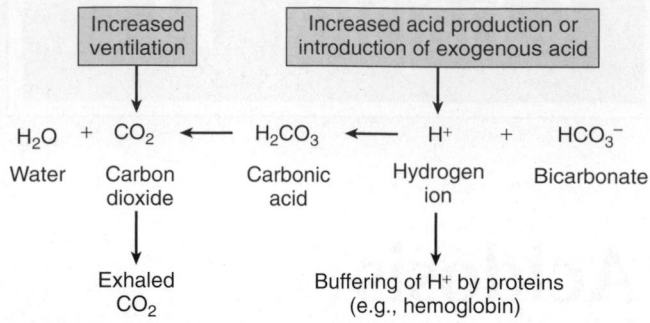

FIGURE 111–1. Simplified depiction of the basic chemical reactions involved in the immediate buffering of excess acids.

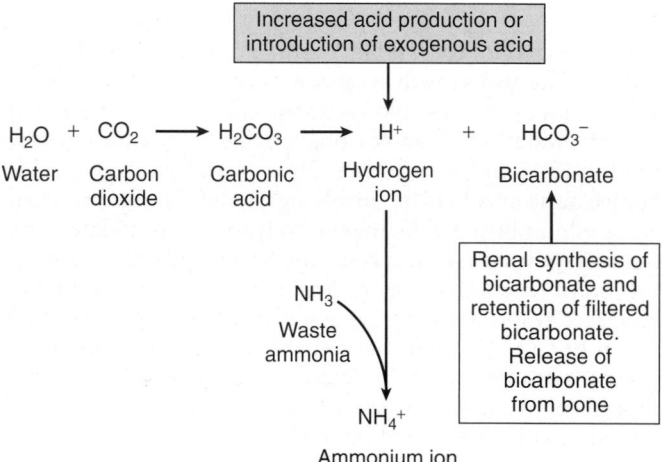

FIGURE 111–2. Simplified depiction of the basic chemical reactions involved in the renal excretion of excess acid.

where $[Na^+]$, $[K^+]$, and $[Cl^-]$ are the serum sodium, potassium, and chloride concentrations respectively.[13,20] The numerical values for these electrolytes are the same whether conventional units (mEq/L) or Système International d'Unites (SI) (mmol/L) are used. An alternative form of the anion gap does not include potassium in the sum.[22,23] There is not a universally agreed upon normal anion gap.[23] A reasonable approximation for a normal anion gap is in the range of 8 to 16.[24] Given differences in how individual hospital laboratories perform their electrolyte analyses, the exact values constituting a normal anion gap will vary.[24] Fortunately, many hospital laboratories report an anion gap along with their report on electrolyte measurements. The anion gap is useful in differentiating some relatively common and serious conditions that present to the emergency department with a metabolic acidosis (Table 111–1). One of the limitations of the anion gap is its inappropriate normalization in the setting of hypoalbuminemia.[13,20,25-28] Adjustments to the anion gap calculation to take abnormalities of serum albumin into account have been proposed.[26,27]

One alternative to the anion gap that adjusts for abnormalities in serum albumin is the strong ion gap.[20,29,30] The strong ion gap is calculated as follows:

$$\text{Strong ion gap} = [Na^+] + [K^+] - [Cl^-] - [HCO_3^-] - 2.8\,[\text{albumin (g/dL)}] - 0.6\,[\text{phosphate (mg/dL)}]$$

Table 111–1	Anion Gaps of Conditions Likely to Present to the Emergency Department with a Metabolic Acidosis
Increased Anion Gap	**Normal Anion Gap**
Diabetic ketoacidosis	Diarrhea with dehydration
Septic shock	Renal tubular acidosis
Ingestions*	Inborn errors of metabolism
Hemorrhagic shock	
Inborn errors of metabolism	

*Includes carbon monoxide, cyanide, toxic alcohols, iron, isoniazid, paraldehyde, metformin, salicylates, and theophylline.

A normal strong ion gap is zero. A falsely negative strong ion gap occurs in the setting of an elevated serum chloride. The role, if any, of the strong ion gap in evaluating children in the emergency department has not been determined. Another proposed alternative is the chloride:sodium ratio.[31]

Important Clinical Features and Considerations

Adequacy of the specimen used to determine the serum pH is an important concern. Although many blood gas analyses utilize arterial blood to assess oxygenation, arterial blood gases can be painful and technically difficult in children. If oxygenation can be assessed with pulse oximetry, a venous blood gas would be adequate to assess the serum pH. There is evidence to suggest that venous blood gases correlate very well with arterial specimens and accurately reflect the serum pH.[32,33] There is also evidence to support the use of capillary blood gases to assess the serum pH.[34,35] Initial specimens obtained from intraosseous access, before medications are instilled, may also yield an accurate assessment of the serum pH.[36]

Management

The key to treating a patient with a metabolic acidosis is to treat the underlying cause of the acidosis. Many children with metabolic acidosis will be dehydrated, intravascularly volume depleted, or both. Intravenous hydration with normal saline is generally indicated. It is useful to keep in mind that the administration of excessive volumes of parenteral normal saline may result in a hyperchloremic acidosis and an artificially normal anion gap.[37] For patients in shock, 20 ml/kg boluses of normal saline are indicated[16] (see Chapter 8, Circulatory Emergencies: Shock).

The administration of parenteral sodium bicarbonate is appropriate in some circumstances. For example, in the setting of tricyclic antidepressant overdose, sodium bicarbonate has been shown to be effective.[33] In conditions such as diabetic ketoacidosis, the use of sodium bicarbonate is controversial[11,12,38,39] (see Chapter 105, Diabetic Ketoacidosis). Similarly, in circumstances of severe hypoxic metabolic acidosis with excessive lactate formation, the use of sodium bicarbonate has not been shown to offer improved outcomes.[40,41]

Summary

Many serious conditions for which children present to the emergency department manifest a metabolic acidosis. Calculating the anion gap may be helpful in refining the differential diagnosis. Establishing adequate perfusion by administering intravenous fluids is frequently indicated. However, large volumes of normal saline can result in a hyperchloremic acidosis. Sodium bicarbonate should be administered when clearly indicated based on the underlying illness. Successful management of the child with metabolic acidosis is most dependent upon successfully treating the confirmed or presumptive underlying cause.

REFERENCES

*1. Kincaid EH, Chang MC, Letton RW, et al: Admission base deficit in pediatric trauma: a study using the National Trauma Data Bank. J Trauma 51:332–335, 2001.

2. Daniel SR, Morita SY, Yu M, et al: Uncompensated metabolic acidosis: an underrecognized risk factor for subsequent intubation requirements. J Trauma 57:993–997, 2004.

3. DeMars CS, Hollister K, Tomassoni A, et al: Citric acid ingestion: a life-threatening cause of metabolic acidosis. Ann Emerg Med 38:588–591, 2001.

4. Caravati EM, Heileson HL, Jones M: Treatment of severe pediatric ethylene glycol intoxication without hemodialysis. J Toxicol Clin Toxicol 42:255–259, 2004.

5. Rathi M, Sakhuja V, Jha V: Visual blurring and metabolic acidosis after ingestion of bootleg alcohol. Hemodial Int 10:8–14, 2006.

6. Ben-Abraham R, Szold O, Rudick V, et al: "Ecstacy" intoxication: life-threatening manifestations and resuscitative measures in the intensive care setting. Eur J Emerg Med 10:309–313, 2003.

*7. Calvo M, Artuch R, Macià E, et al: Diagnostic approach to inborn errors of metabolism in an emergency unit. Pediatr Emerg Care 16:405–408, 2000.

8. Mehta KC, Zxolway K, Osterhout KC, et al: Lessons from the late diagnosis of isovaleric acidemia in a five-year-old boy. J Pediatr 129:309–310, 1996.

9. Klose DA, Kölker S, Heinrich B, et al: Incidence and short-term outcome of children with symptomatic presentation of organic acid and fatty acid oxidation disorders in Germany. Pediatrics 110:1204–1211, 2002.

10. Garcia E, Abramo TJ, Okada P, et al: Capnometry for noninvasive continuous monitoring of metabolic status in pediatric diabetic keto-acidosis. Crit Care Med 31:2539–2543, 2003.

11. Green SM, Rothrock SG, Ho JD, et al: Failure of adjunctive bicarbonate to improve outcome in severe pediatric diabetic ketoacidosis. Ann Emerg Med 31:41–48, 1998.

*12. Glaser N, Barnett P, McCaslin I, et al: Risk factors for cerebral edema in children with diabetic ketoacidosis. The Pediatric Emergency Medicine Collaborative Research Committee of the American Academy of Pediatrics. N Engl J Med 344:264–269, 2001.

*13. Corey HE: The anion gap (AG): studies in the nephrotic syndrome and diabetic ketoacidosis (DKA). J Lab Clin Med 147:121–125, 2006.

14. Adedoyin O, Gottlieb B, Frank R, et al: Evaluation of failure to thrive: diagnostic yield of testing for renal tubular acidosis. Pediatrics 112:463–466, 2003.

15. Mallory MD, Kadish H, Zebrack M, et al: Use of a pediatric observation unit for treatment of children with dehydration caused by gastroenteritis. Pediatr Emerg Care 22:1–6, 2006.

*16. Carcillo JA, Davis AL, Zaritsky A: Role of early fluid resuscitation in pediatric septic shock. JAMA 266:1242–1245, 1991.

17. Han YY, Carcillo JA, Dragotta A, et al: Early reversal of pediatric-neo-natal septic shock by community physicians is associated with improved outcome. Pediatrics 112:793–799, 2003.

*18. Kellum JA: Metabolic acidosis in patients with sepsis: epiphenomenon or part of the pathophysiology? Crit Care Resusc 6:197–203, 2004.

19. Frazer SC, Stewart CP: Acidosis and alkalosis: a modern view. J Clin Pathol 12:195–206, 1959.

*20. Corey HE: Stewart and beyond: new models of acid-base balance. Kidney Int 64:777–787, 2003.

21. Story DA: Bench-to-bedside review: a brief history of clinical acid-base. Crit Care 8:253–258, 2004.

22. Gabow PA, Kaehny WD, Fennessey PV, et al: Diagnostic importance of an increased serum anion gap. N Engl J Med 303:854–858, 1980.

23. Witte DL, Rodgers JL, Barrett DA 2nd: The anion gap: its use in quality control. Clin Chem 22:643–646, 1976.

24. Moe OW, Fuster D: Clinical acid-base pathophysiology: disorders of plasma anion gap. Best Pract Res Clin Endocrinol Metab 17:559–574, 2003.

25. Hatherill M, Waggie Z, Purves L, et al: Correction of the anion gap for albumin in order to detect occult tissue anions in shock. Arch Dis Child 87:526–529, 2002.

26. Feldman M, Soni N, Dickson B: Influence of hypoalbuminemia or hyperalbuminemia on the serum anion gap. J Lab Clin Med 146:317–320, 2005.

27. Kellum JA: Determinants of plasma acid-base balance. Crit Care Clin 21:329–346, 2005.

28. Durward A, Mayer A, Skellet S, et al: Hypoalbuminaemia in critically ill children: incidence, prognosis, and influence on the anion gap. Arch Dis Child 88:419–422, 2003.

29. Gunnerson KJ, Kellum JA: Acid-base and electrolyte analysis in critically ill patients: are we ready for the new millennium? Curr Opin Crit Care 9:468–473, 2003.

30. Kellum JA, Kramer DJ, Pinsky MR: Strong ion gap: a methodology for exploring unexplained anions. J Crit Care 10:51–55, 1995.

31. Durward A, Skellett S, Mayer A, et al: The value of the chloride:sodium ratio in differentiating the aetiology of metabolic acidosis. Intensive Care Med 27:828–835, 2001.

32. Brandenburg MA, Dire DJ: Comparison of arterial and venous blood gas values in the initial emergency department evaluation of patients with diabetic ketoacidosis. Ann Emerg Med 31:459–465, 1998.

33. Eizadi-Mood N, Moein N, Saghaei M: Evaluation of relationship between arterial and venous blood gas values in the patients with tricyclic antidepressant poisoning. Clin Toxicol (Phila) 43:357–360, 2005.

34. Harrison AM, Lynch JM, Dean JM, et al: Comparison of simultaneously obtained arterial and capillary blood gases in pediatric intensive care unit patients. Crit Care Med 25:1904–1908, 1997.

35. McGillivray D, Ducharme FM, Charron Y, et al: Clinical decision making based on venous versus capillary blood gas values in the well-perfused child. Ann Emerg Med 34:58–63, 1999.

36. Abdelmoneim T, Kissoon N, Johnson L, et al: Acid-base status of blood from intraosseous and mixed venous sites during prolonged cardiopulmonary resuscitation and drug infusions. Crit Care Med 27:1923–1928, 1999.

37. Skellett S, Mayer A, Durward A, et al: Chasing the base deficit: hyperchloraemic acidosis following 0.9% saline fluid resuscitation. Arch Dis Child 83:514–516, 2000.

38. Viallon A, Zeni F, Lanford P, et al: Does bicarbonate therapy improve the management of severe diabetic ketoacidosis? Crit Care Med 27:2690–2693, 1999.

39. Okuda Y, Adrogue HJ, Field JB, et al: Counterproductive effects of sodium bicarbonate in diabetic ketoacidosis. J Clin Endocrinol Metab 81:314–320, 1996.

40. Lokesh L, Kumar P, Murki S, et al: A randomized controlled trial of sodium bicarbonate in neonatal resuscitation—effect on immediate outcome. Resuscitation 60:219–223, 2004.

41. Federiuk CS, Sanders AB, Kern KB, et al: The effect of bicarbonate on resuscitation from cardiac arrest. Ann Emerg Med 20:1173–1177, 1991.

*Selected readings.

Chapter 112

Metabolic Alkalosis

John C. Brancato, MD

Key Points

Metabolic alkalosis is a disturbance characterized by an increase in serum bicarbonate resulting from either a loss of hydrogen ions or a gain in bicarbonate.

Respiratory compensation for metabolic alkalosis is by hypoventilation.

Treatment depends on the underlying cause and the severity of the alkalosis.

Introduction and Background

Under normal circumstances, the body uses various homeostatic mechanisms to buffer and excrete the acid it produces daily. The carbonic acid system, for example, allows for large amounts of acid to be excreted through the ventilatory system as carbon dioxide (CO_2) and through the renal system as hydrogen ions (H^+) with conservation of bicarbonate (HCO_3^-).[1] However, either an excessive loss of H^+ or a gain of HCO_3^- results in alkalosis. As with acidosis, the alkalosis may be a primary metabolic process or it may be secondary to a respiratory derangement. In the latter instance, the retention of CO_2 is compensated for by an increased HCO_3^-. The excessive losses of H^+ that may lead to primary metabolic alkalosis can occur in several ways. Large amounts of gastric HCl may be lost through vomiting or nasogastric suctioning. Pyloric stenosis is often considered the prototype of processes characterized by gastric acid loss. Hyperaldosteronism or other mineralocorticoid excess causes an increase in renal sodium reabsorption with secretion of H^+ and potassium ions (K^+) into the tubular lumen.[2] Liddle's syndrome, through the action of a mutated sodium channel, and licorice ingestion, through the inhibition of cortisol metabolism, produce similar symptoms.[3-5]

An increase in HCO_3^- may occur through the administration of exogenous alkali as in antacid overdose, milk-alkali syndrome, large transfusions of blood with citrate anticoagulant, and parenteral therapy with acetate-, lactate-, or bicarbonate-containing fluids.[6-8] A loss of chloride-rich fluid as may occur from heavy vomiting, congenital chloride diarrhea, or thiazide and loop diuretics may lead to a decreased extracellular fluid volume.[9,10] The remaining HCO_3^- is effectively increased in concentration, producing a modest "contraction alkalosis."

Once it is established, multiple factors contribute to the maintenance of a metabolic alkalosis. An important one is increased activity by the renin-angiotensin-aldosterone system. Hypovolemia stimulates aldosterone production, in turn increasing the rate of sodium ion (Na^+) reabsorption and H^+ secretion. The addition of H^+ into the tubular lumen leads to the exchange of chloride ions (Cl^-) and HCO_3^-, enhancing the alkalosis. In the distal tubule, increased mineralocorticoid activity causes increased sodium/potassium (Na^+/K^+) exchange, leading to hypokalemia. When the extracellular potassium concentration drops, K^+ move out of the cells. The movement of H^+ intracellularly maintains charge balance but also stimulates renal HCO_3^- reabsorption.[11] The collecting duct responds to hypokalemia by holding onto K^+ but excretes H^+ in the process. Hypochloremia, from inadequate ingestion, cystic fibrosis or other losses, further stimulates the renin-angiotensin-aldosterone system and inhibits the kidney's ability to secrete HCO_3^- and retain H^+ via the chloride/bicarbonate (Cl^-/HCO_3^-) exchanger.[12,13] A reduced glomerular filtration rate due to hypovolemia, hypokalemia, or hypochloremia reduces the amount of HCO_3^- presented to the kidney and, therefore, available for excretion.[14]

Recognition and Approach

The causes of metabolic alkalosis are commonly classified by their responsiveness to saline therapy. Chloride-responsive alkaloses are those in which low extracellular fluid volume, hypochloremia, and hypokalemia predominate. Hyperaldosteronism occurs in these cases, but as a secondary process. Chloride-resistant alkaloses are those characterized by a primary increase in mineralocorticoid activity or by impaired chloride reabsorption. They are further divided into those causes with or without hypertension (Table 112–1).

Bartter's syndrome is a group of three inherited disorders caused by dysfunction of renal ion channels.[15] Classic Bartter's syndrome is caused by impaired sodium chloride reabsorption, resulting in hypokalemic metabolic alkalosis with hypercalciuria. Presentation is in infancy. Loop and thiazide diuretics have similar effects on the kidney and lead to similar electrolyte abnormalities. Gitelman's syndrome is also caused by a defect in a Na^+/Cl^- transporter but is clinically milder than Bartter's syndrome.[16] It is also

Table 112–1	Causes of Metabolic Alkalosis

Chloride Responsive

Congenital chloride diarrhea
Cystic fibrosis
Gastric fluid losses
Post-hypercapnic state
Thiazide and loop diuretic therapy

Chloride Resistant with Hypertension

Chewing tobacco ingestion
Cushing's syndrome
Hyperaldosteronism
Licorice ingestion
Liddle's syndrome
Renovascular hypertension

Chloride Resistant without Hypertension

Bartter's syndrome
Gitelman's syndrome
Severe hypokalemia

Other

Bicarbonate ingestion
Excess parenteral lactate or acetate
Milk-alkali syndrome
Organic acidosis recovery
Refeeding after prolonged fasting
Parenteral penicillin administration
Transfusion-related citrate administration

characterized by hypomagnesemia and hypocalciuria. Metabolic alkalosis, hypercalcemia, and renal insufficiency characterize the milk-alkali syndrome, more common prior to the development of proton pump inhibitors. Chronic ingestion of large amounts of calcium carbonate (e.g., antacid abuse, betel nut use) is the usual cause.[17]

Serious physiologic effects may ensue from metabolic alkalosis and the body's attempt to compensate through hypoventilation.[18] For example, an elevated pH shifts the oxyhemoglobin dissociation curve to the left, impeding oxygen delivery to the tissues.[19] Hypoventilation may worsen the hypoxemia. If alkalosis is secondary to protracted vomiting, significant dehydration and volume contraction are possible. Associated hypokalemia can cause muscle weakness and ventricular dysrhythmias. Secondary hypocalcemia may result from increased binding of calcium to serum proteins. Symptoms are most often related to the underlying process. Recognition rests with familiarity with likely clinical scenarios and subsequent laboratory testing.

Clinical Presentation

The history is important to the evaluation of a child with a suspected or confirmed metabolic alkalosis. Vomiting, regardless of etiology, is the most common cause in the emergency setting. A history of alkali ingestion may be present, and diuretic use, whether prescribed or surreptitious, should be determined. Weight gain and symptoms of hypertension may be present in conditions of elevated mineralocorticoid activity.

The physical examination may demonstrate weakness or neuromuscular excitability. An example of this is Chvostek's sign, spasm of the facial muscles brought on by tapping the patient's cheek in the area of the facial nerve near the parotid gland. Volume depletion is more common with chloride-

responsive alkaloses, while normovolemia or hypervolemia is seen with chloride-resistant alkaloses. Hypoventilation may be noted. The presence or absence of hypertension may narrow the differential diagnosis (see Table 112–1).

Laboratory tests are an important part of the evaluation of a child with a suspected metabolic alkalosis. Initial laboratory investigation with an extended serum chemistry panel is indicated. Key findings include hyponatremia, hypokalemia, hypochloremia, hypercalcemia, and hypomagnesemia. Results are not necessarily predictable. For example, pyloric stenosis may present with elevated, reduced, or normal potassium levels.[20,21] An arterial blood gas determination is helpful in identifying mixed acid-base disorders. For a primary metabolic process, a 0.7-mm Hg rise in arterial partial pressure of carbon dioxide ($PaCO_2$) is expected for each 1 mEq/L rise in HCO_3^-. An elevated $PaCO_2$ (>55 to 60 mm Hg) is likely to reflect a concomitant respiratory component to the acid-base derangement. Determination of the spot urine chloride (U_{Cl}) level allows classification of the process as chloride responsive or chloride resistant. A urine chloride level less than 10 mEq/L indicates a chloride-responsive process, while a level greater than 20 mEq/L indicates a chloride-resistant alkalosis.[9] Other values are indeterminate. However, diuretic use may give an unexpectedly elevated U_{Cl}.[22] In contrast to the U_{Cl}, the spot urine sodium (U_{Na}) level may not be useful in the setting of alkalosis as the kidney may excrete excess HCO_3^- as a sodium salt. Additional laboratory studies may further help identify the cause of the alkalosis, but the results seldom directly impact emergency department management. Examples of these include renin and aldosterone levels, fasting cortisol level, and a urine screen for diuretics.

Important Clinical Features and Considerations

For children with metabolic alkalosis, it is prudent to remember to treat the patient and not just the laboratory numbers. Many times, the cause of the metabolic alkalosis is evident from the initial emergency department history and physical examination. Although vomiting children undoubtedly have at least some degree of metabolic alkalosis, the metabolic derangement is seldom the focus of the management for these children. Aggressive pursuit and treatment of metabolic alkalosis is seldom indicated in previously healthy children.

Management

Patients with severe alkalosis may present with hypoventilation and hypoxemia. Those with hypokalemia and hypocalcemia are at risk for ventricular dysrhythmias. As patients with chloride-responsive alkaloses are likely to present with significant volume depletion and even shock, intravenous fluid resuscitation with normal saline is essential.[23] It is important to add potassium chloride and follow with K^+ levels for those children who are also hypokalemic (see Chapter 113, Hypokalemia). If the initial serum K^+ is critically low, no glucose should be added to initial fluids to avoid stimulation of an insulin response and subsequent driving of K^+ into the cells. When the degree of alkalosis is critical (i.e., if arterial pH > 7.55) or renal failure prevents adequate administration of crystalloid, the intravenous administration of HCl may be required. This situation is rare in children. When indicated, the administration of intravenous HCl may result in improved gas exchange and an increase in the arterial partial pressure of oxygen (PaO_2).[24]

Acetazolamide, a carbonic anhydrase inhibitor, is especially useful in chloride-resistant alkalosis. It blocks HCO_3^- reabsorption by the proximal renal tubules.[25] The increased flow of HCO_3^- to the collecting duct causes an increase in K^+ secretion. In absence of hyperkalemia, potassium chloride supplementation is indicated.

In cases of hyperaldosteronism or mineralocorticoid excess, spironolactone, a potassium-sparing diuretic, reverses the renal effects of the underlying process. Careful K^+ repletion is necessary to correct the alkalosis, though attention must be paid to avoid hyperkalemia. Other available potassium-sparing diuretics such as triamterene or amiloride may be used as well, and are the drugs of choice in Liddle's syndrome.[26] Bartter's and Gitelman's syndromes are both treated with these diuretics and potassium and magnesium supplements. Proton pump inhibitors are helpful to decrease acid production and subsequent ongoing losses in the setting of persistent vomiting or suctioning of gastric secretions.

Summary

Generating a differential diagnosis and assessing the severity of a metabolic alkalosis relies on the history, physical examination, extended serum electrolytes, arterial blood gas determinations, and a urine chloride level. Treatment should be directed at the likely causes, with particular emphasis on addressing hypoxia and dehydration. The disposition will depend on the likely cause of the acid-base disturbance, local medical resources, and the overall clinical condition of the child. Children with severe metabolic derangements often benefit from transfer to a pediatric intensive care unit.

REFERENCES

1. Narins RG, Kupin W, Faber MD, et al: Pathophysiology, classification and therapy of acid-base disturbances. *In* Arieff AI, DeFronzo RA (eds): Fluid, Electrolyte and Acid-Base Disorders. New York: Churchill-Livingstone, 1995, pp 105–198.
2. Sabatini S: The cellular basis of metabolic alkalosis. Kidney Int 49:906–917, 1996.
3. Hansson JH, Nelson-Williams C, Suzuki H, et al: Hypertension caused by a truncated epithelial sodium channel gamma subunit: genetic heterogeneity of Liddle syndrome. Nat Genet 11:76–82, 1995.
4. Jackson SN, Williams B, Houtman P, et al: The diagnosis of Liddle syndrome by identification of a mutation in the beta subunit of the epithelial sodium channel. J Med Genet 35:510–512, 1998.
*5. Heikens J, Fliers E, Endert E, et al: Liquorice-induced hypertension—a new understanding of an old disease: case report and brief review. Neth J Med 47:230–234, 1995.
*6. Fitzgibbons LJ, Snoey ER: Severe metabolic alkalosis due to baking soda ingestion: case reports of two patients with unsuspected antacid overdose. J Emerg Med 17:57–61, 1999.
7. Fiorino AS: Hypercalcemia and alkalosis due to the milk-alkali syndrome: a case report and review. Yale J Biol Med 69:517–523, 1996.
8. Kelleher SP, Schulman G: Severe metabolic alkalosis complicating regional citrate hemodialysis. Am J Kidney Dis 9:235–236, 1987.
9. Moseley RH, Hoglund P, Wu GD, et al: Downregulated in adenoma gene encodes a chloride transporter defective in congenital chloride diarrhea. Am J Physiol Gastrointest Liver Physiol 276:G185–G192, 1999.
10. Galla JH: Metabolic alkalois. J Am Soc Nephrol 11:369–375, 2000.
11. Capasso G, Unwin R, Rizzo M, et al: Bicarbonate transport along the loop of Henle: molecular mechanisms and regulation. J Nephrol 15(Suppl 5):S88–S96, 2002.
12. Roy S 3rd, Arant BS Jr: Hypokalemic metabolic alkalosis in normotensive infants with elevated plasma renin activity and hyperaldosteronism: role of dietary chloride deficiency. Pediatrics 67:423–429, 1981.
13. Mauri S, Pedroli G, Rudeberg A, et al: Acute metabolic alkalosis in cystic fibrosis: prospective study and review of the literature. Miner Electrolyte Metab 23:33–37, 1997.
14. Galla JH, Bonduris DN, Luke RG: Effects of chloride and extracellular fluid volume on bicarbonate reabsorption along the nephron in metabolic alkalosis in the rat: reassessment of the classical hypothesis of the pathogenesis of metabolic alkalosis. J Clin Invest 80:41–50, 1987.
15. Amirlak I, Dawson KP: Bartter syndrome: an overview. QJM 93:207–215, 2000.
16. Cruz DN, Shaer AJ, Bia MJ, et al: Gitelman's syndrome revisited: an evaluation of symptoms and health-related quality of life. Kidney Int 59:710–717, 2001.
*17. Nelson BS, Heischober B: Betel nut: a common drug used by naturalized citizens from India, Far East Asia, and the South Pacific Islands. Ann Emerg Med 34:238–243, 1999.
*18. Perrone J, Hoffman RS: Compensatory hypoventilation in severe metabolic alkalosis. Acad Emerg Med 3:981–982, 1996.
19. Brimioulle S. Kahn RJ: Effects of metabolic alkalosis on pulmonary gas exchange. Am Rev Respir Dis 141:1185–1189, 1990.
20. Oakley EA, Barnett PL: Is acid base determination an accurate predictor of pyloric stenosis? J Paediatr Child Health 36:587–589, 2000.
21. Schwartz D, Connelly NR, Manikantan P, et al: Hyperkalemia and pyloric stenosis. Anesth Analg 97:355–357, 2003.
22. Hropot M, Fowler N, Karlmark B, et al: Tubular action of diuretics: distal effects on electrolyte transport and acidification. Kidney Int 28:477–489, 1985.
23. Miozzari HH, Tonz M, von Vigier RO, et al: Fluid resuscitation in infantile hypertrophic pyloric stenosis. Acta Paediatr 90:511–514, 2001.
24. Brimioulle S, Berre J, Dufaye P, et al: Hydrochloric acid infusion for treatment of metabolic alkalosis associated with respiratory acidosis. Crit Care Med 17:232–236, 1989.
25. Marik PE, Kussman BD, Lipman J, et al: Acetazolamide in the treatment of metabolic alkalosis in critically ill patients. Heart Lung 20:455–459, 1991.
26. Assadi FK, Kimura RE, Subramanian U, et al: Liddle syndrome in a newborn infant. Pediatr Nephrol 17:609–611, 2002.

*Selected readings.

Chapter 113

Hypokalemia

Eric T. Carter, MD

Key Points

Excessive potassium losses, decreased potassium intake, and intracellular electrolyte shifts are the three main processes that lead to hypokalemia.

Hypokalemia is frequently associated with other electrolyte abnormalities.

The most common clinically evident signs and symptoms of hypokalemia are neuromuscular and cardiac.

In general, children tolerate mild to moderate degrees of hypokalemia well and do not require potassium replacement.

Successful treatment of hypokalemia needs to be undertaken in the context of the overall management of the child's medical condition and not just as an isolated process.

Introduction and Background

Potassium homeostasis is crucial to the normal cellular function of every cell in the human body.[1,2] The majority of potassium stores are located intracellularly.[1] Routine laboratory measurements of potassium only measure extracellular potassium. Therefore, routine laboratory testing may not correlate well with whole body stores. Hypokalemia refers to a lower than normal level of potassium in the blood and is defined as a serum or plasma level less than 3.5 mmol/L (3.5 mEq/L).[3] Although potassium homeostasis plays an important role in all cellular function, neuromuscular and cardiovascular manifestations appear to have the greatest clinical impact on patients.[1,2,4-8]

Recognition and Approach

The three general mechanisms through which hypokalemia may develop are excessive potassium losses, decreased potassium intake, and electrolyte shifts across cell membranes[9] (Table 113–1). Various medications are well known to cause hypokalemia. Some of these medications are very commonly used to treat children, including albuterol.[10-12] Common examples of how excessive losses may occur include vomiting, diarrhea, and excessive sweating.[1,6,13] Excessive renal losses of potassium may be due to primary renal disease (e.g., Bartter's syndrome, Gitelman's syndrome), medications, or excess mineralocorticoids (e.g., Cushing's syndrome, Conn's syndrome).[4,14,15] Hypokalemia may result from long-term inadequate oral intake of potassium. In one study of otherwise healthy young women with anorexia nervosa, nearly 20% were found to have hypokalemia.[16] Intracellular shifts of potassium from the extracellular spaces may result in decreased plasma levels in the face of either normal or abnormal whole body stores.[17-19] Examples of clinical conditions in which there is an intracellular shift of potassium include alkalemia, hypothermia, the administration of albuterol, and periodic hypokalemic paralysis[10-12,20,21] (see Chapter 47, Peripheral Neuromuscular Disorders). Traumatized children may have hypokalemia on laboratory testing.[22,23] The significance of this finding and its cause are unknown.

The recognition of clinically significant hypokalemia may result from the constellation of presenting signs or symptoms, a history of chronic disease such as diabetes mellitus, or chronic medication usage, or may occur as an incidental laboratory finding.[5,10-12,14,17-19,24] Useful diagnostic tests include a basic metabolic panel to evaluate for other clinically significant electrolyte abnormalities (e.g., hypomagnesemia, an elevated anion gap), an arterial or venous blood gas determination if an acid-base abnormality is suspected, and an electrocardiogram to detect cardiac conduction disturbances[7,8] (Table 113–2).

Clinical Presentation

In general, children with mild to moderate degrees of hypokalemia do not manifest clinically appreciable signs or symptoms. Clinical experience suggests that many children with vomiting and diarrhea have some degree of hypokalemia when laboratory testing is performed. For the majority of children with vomiting and diarrhea, the assessment of electrolytes is not indicated. It is likely that even those children who do not have laboratory testing performed also have some degree of hypokalemia that is clinically unimportant and requires no specific treatment. If evident, signs and symptoms of hypokalemia include muscle cramps, hyporeflexia,

Table 113–1	Important Causes of Hypokalemia

Decreased Intake

Eating disorders
Inappropriate preparation of total parenteral nutrition
Malnutrition

Excessive Losses

Congenital adrenal hyperplasia
Cushing's syndrome
Diabetic ketoacidosis
Dialysis
Diarrhea
Diuretic use
Hyperaldosteronism
Hyperhidrosis
Hypomagnesemia
Laxative use
Renal artery stenosis
Vomiting

Intracellular Shift

Alkalosis
Bartter's syndrome
Gitelman's syndrome
Hypomagnesemia
Hypothermia
Liddle's syndrome
Periodic hypokalemic paralysis
Renal tubular disorders

Medications

Amphotericin B
β-Agonists
Catecholamines
Diuretics
Gentamicin
Insulin
Laxatives
Mannitol
Penicillins
Steroids
Sympathomimetics
Theophylline
Verapamil

Table 113–2	Characteristic Electrocardiogram Findings Associated with Hypokalemia*

Low-voltage QRS complexes
Prolonged QT interval
Widening of QRS complexes
ST-segment depression
T-wave flattening or inversion
U waves
Ventricular dysrhythmias

*Absence of any or all of these findings does not exclude clinically significant hypokalemia.

and weakness.[1] More severe presentations may include bradycardia, arrhythmias, hypotension, respiratory muscle paralysis, and even cardiovascular collapse.[6-8,18-21]

Important Clinical Features and Considerations

Spuriously low potassium may occur if a blood specimen is drawn from a vein at a location proximal to an infusing intravenous line. Multiple low laboratory values from that same specimen may be a useful clue if this is suspected.[25,26]

Management

Hypokalemia can frequently be managed without primarily directing treatment at a specific potassium level. Clinical experience suggests that directing care at the underlying disease process usually leads to the proper identification of and treatment for hypokalemia. When indicated, potassium may be administered orally or intravenously. Some children, particularly those with renal disease, may require oral potassium supplementation when hypokalemia is identified. Coordinated care with a physician familiar with a particular child or with a pediatric nephrologist is prudent in many of these cases. There is no evidence-based potassium level at which oral potassium replacement should be initiated for children who were previously healthy and are not manifesting clinical findings attributable to hypokalemia. Clinical experience suggests that it is uncommon for children to present with a serum potassium level <2.5 to 3.0 mmol/L (2.5 to 3.0 mEq/L). This degree of hypokalemia may be a reasonable trigger point for pursuing a definitive diagnosis and initiating potassium replacement.

Intravenous potassium replacement needs to be provided in the context of overall fluid and electrolyte management. A good example of this is seen in the care of children with diabetic ketoacidosis (see Chapter 105, Diabetic Ketoacidosis). The American Diabetes Association has made specific recommendations regarding the management of potassium in children with diabetic ketoacidosis.[27] Although children with diabetic ketoacidosis typically have diminished whole body stores of potassium, the serum value may be high, low, or normal at the time the specimen is obtained. As fluid and insulin treatment is initiated, the serum potassium level will fall. In the context of hourly electrolyte assessments, the recommendation by the American Diabetes Association is for potassium replacement to be withheld if the serum potassium level is greater than 5 mmol/L (5 mEq/L), to replace potassium at 30 to 40 mmol/L (30 to 40 mEq/L) in the infusing intravenous fluids if the potassium level is between 3.5 and 5 mmol/L (3.5 and 5 mEq/L), and to replace potassium at 40 to 60 mmol/L (40 to 60 mEq/L) in the infusing intravenous fluids if the potassium level is between 2.5 and 3.5 mmol/L (2.5 and 3.5 mEq/L). In these instances, the potassium replacement should be performed using one third potassium phosphate (KPO_4) and two thirds potassium chloride (KCl). If the potassium level is less than 2.5 mmol/L (2.5 mEq/L), the potassium is to initially be replaced by 1 mmol/kg (1 mEq/kg) of KCl over 1 hour with insulin withheld until the potassium rises about 2.5 mmol/L (2.5 mEq/L).[27] This example illustrates how the treatment of hypokalemia needs to be undertaken in the context of the overall management of the child's condition. Infants and children receiving intravenous potassium replacement require continuous cardiac monitoring.

Summary

Hypokalemia is a relatively common electrolyte abnormality in children. The clinical importance of hypokalemia ranges from inconsequential to a life-threatening manifestation of many disease states. Understanding potassium homeostasis and its relation to disease processes allows for the appropriate evaluation and management of hypokalemia. Using readily obtained laboratory tests, the presenting signs and symptoms, and occasionally an electrocardiogram will allow the clinician to determine the significance of the hypokalemia and whether replacement is warranted. The disposition decision in cases of hypokalemia is seldom based solely on the potassium level. Instead, the disposition is usually based on the working diagnosis, the known underlying disease process, or the overall clinical status of the child.

REFERENCES

1. Reineck HJ: The control of potassium homeostasis. Kidney 12:13, 1979.
2. Choen JJ: Disorders of potassium balance. Hosp Pract 14:119, 1979.
3. Dorland's Illustrated Medical Dictionary, 30th ed. Philadelphia: WB Saunders, 2003, p 2184.
4. Weisber LS, Szerlip HM, Cox M: Disorders of potassium homeostasis in critically ill patients. Crit Care Clin 5:835–854, 1987.
5. Singhi S, Marudkar A: Hypokalemia in a pediatric intensive care unit. Indian Pediatr 33:9–14, 1996.
6. Uysal G, Sokmen A, Vidinlisan S: Clinical risk factors for fatal diarrhea in hospitalized children. Indian J Pediatr 67:329–333, 2000.
7. Cortesi C, Foglia PE, Bettinelli A, et al: Prevention of cardiac arrhythmias in pediatric patients with normotensive-hypokalemic tubulopathy: current attitude among European pediatricians. Pediatr Nephrol 18:729–730, 2003.
8. Calderari MZ, Vigier RO, Bettinelli A, et al: Electrocardiographic QT prolongation and sudden death in renal hypokalemic alkalosis. Nephron 91:762–763, 2002.
9. Jospe N, Forbes G: Fluids and electrolytes—clinical aspects. Pediatr Rev 17:395–404, 1996.
*10. Bodenhamer J, Bergstrom R, Brown D, et al: Frequently nebulized beta-agonists for asthma: effects on serum electrolytes. Ann Emerg Med 21:1337–1342, 1992.
*11. Rakhmanina NY, Kearns GL, Farrar HC: Hypokalemia in an asthmatic child from abuse of albuterol metered dose inhaler. Pediatric Emerg Care 14:145–147, 1998.

12. Leikin JB, Linowiecki KA, Soglin DF, Paloucek F: Hypokalemia after pediatric albuterol overdose: a case series. Am J Emerg Care 12:64–66, 1994.
13. Miozzari HH, Tonz M, von Vigier RO, Bianchetti MG: Fluid resuscitation in infantile hypertrophic pyloric stenosis. Acta Paediatr 90:511–514, 2001.
14. Khilnani P: Electrolyte abnormalities in critically ill children. Crit Care Med 20:241–250, 1992.
15. Vaisbich MH, Fujimura MD, Koch VH: Bartter syndrome: benefits and side effects of long-term treatment. Pediatr Nephrol 19:858–863, 2004.
16. Miller KK, Grinspoon SK, Ciampa J, et al: Medical findings in outpatients with anorexia nervosa. Arch Intern Med 165:561–566, 2005.
*17. Malone DR, McNamara RM, Malone RS, et al: Hypokalemia complicating fluid resuscitation in children. Pediatr Emerg Care 6:13–16, 1990.
18. Rosenbloom AL, Hanas R: Diabetic ketoacidosis (DKA): treatment guidelines. Clin Pediatr 35:261–266, 1996.
19. Jayashree M, Singhi S: Diabetic ketoacidosis: predictors of outcome in a pediatric intensive care unit of a developing country. Pediatr Crit Care Med 5:427–433, 2004.
20. Links TP, Smit AJ, Molenaar W, et al: Familial hypokalemic periodic paralysis: clinical, diagnostic, and therapeutic aspects. J Neurol Sci 122:33–43, 1994.
21. Deda G, Ekim M, Guven A, et al: Hypopotassemic paralysis: a rare presentation of proximal renal tubular acidosis. J Child Neurol 16:770–771, 2001.
*22. MacDonald JS, Atkinson CC, Mooney DP: Hypokalemia in acutely injured children: a benign laboratory abnormality. J Trauma 54:197–198, 2003.
23. Beal AL, Scheltema KE, Beilman GJ, Deuser WE: Hypokalemia following trauma. Shock 18:107–110, 2002.
24. Rothrock SG, Green SM, McArthur CL, et al: Detection of electrolyte abnormalities in children presenting to the emergency department: a multicenter, prospective analysis. Acad Emerg Med 4:1025–1031, 1997.
25. van Vonderen MG, Voerman BJ, Hensgens BE: Effect of intravenous infusions on laboratory results in blood specimens drawn proximal to the insertion site of an intravenous canula. Neth J Med 53:224–227, 1998.
26. Watson KR, O'Kell RT, Joyce JT: Data regarding blood drawing sites in patients receiving intravenous fluids. Am J Clin Pathol 79:119–121, 1983.
*27. Kitabchi AE, Umpierrez GE, Murphy MB, et al: Hyperglycemic crises in diabetes. Diabetes Care 27(Suppl 1):S94–S102, 2004.

---

*Selected readings.

Hyperkalemia

Eric T. Carter, MD

Introduction and Background

Hyperkalemia is an "abnormally high potassium concentration in the blood."[1] A normal serum potassium ranges from 3.5 to 5.0 mmol/L (3.5 to 5.0 mEq/L).[2] Therefore, by definition, a serum potassium greater than 5.0 mmol/L (5.0 mEq/L) is indicative of hyperkalemia. Hyperkalemia is seldom an isolated problem. The overall approach to hyperkalemia depends on the degree of hyperkalemia and the underlying cause.

Recognition and Approach

Potassium homeostasis is integral to normal cellular function. Most of the body's potassium is intracellular. Potassium is a major regulator of cellular resting membrane potentials. Clinical symptoms of hyperkalemia are most dramatic and serious when the cellular function of cardiac and neural tissues is disrupted.[3-8] The epidemiology of hyperkalemia is unknown, but clinical experience suggests it is rare in previously healthy children who have not sustained trauma such as large burns or a crush injury.[9,10]

Hyperkalemia may develop through three main processes (Table 114–1). The first process is decreased excretion of potassium. The kidneys are the dominant regulators of serum potassium levels. In particular, children who have poor renal function or end-stage renal disease are at risk for developing hyperkalemia through decreased excretion.[11] In neonates, hormonal alterations of the renal excretion of potassium occur in endocrinologic conditions such as congenital adrenal hyperplasia.[6,7] The second process is increased intake of potassium. Although excessive oral ingestion of potassium may lead to hyperkalemia,[3] the digestive process seems to offer substantial protection in this regard. Iatrogenic hyperkalemia due to inappropriate intravenous fluid, for example, is probably a more likely route for the increased intake of potassium. Transfusion of packed red blood cells through a small-gauge needle has been identified as a cause of increased potassium intake.[12] The third process is fluid and electrolyte shifts. If potassium shifts from the intracellular compartment to the extracellular compartment (e.g., the circulating blood), then hyperkalemia usually develops. Examples of when this type of potassium and fluid shifting occurs include diabetic ketoacidosis,[13] crush injuries,[9] and succinylcholine-induced hyperkalemia.[10] Because of this fluid and electrolyte shifting, hyperkalemia is not synonymous with increased total body stores of potassium.

Clinical Presentation

The clinical presentation of children with hyperkalemia is dominated by cardiac manifestations, neurologic manifestations, or the underlying illness. The most prominent cardiac manifestations are dysrhythmias.[5] The conduction disturbances roughly correspond to the degree of hyperkalemia. There is a classic progression through which the electrocardiogram changes as potassium values rise (Fig. 114–1). This progression is not universal and has substantial variability from one patient to the next.[14] Ventricular fibrillation and asystole occur with marked hyperkalemia.[4,6,15] Since an electrocardiogram usually can be obtained much more quickly than a set of electrolytes, an electrocardiogram is the most expeditious test in cases of suspected hyperkalemia. The neurologic manifestations include paresthesias and weakness. With regard to underlying illnesses and associated hyperkalemia, clinical experience suggests that hyperkalemia is more often identified during the workup for an underlying condition and less often the starting point of an evaluation. Since renal excretion plays such an important role in potassium homeostasis, obtaining tests of blood urea nitrogen and creatinine is reasonable in cases of suspected hyperkalemia.[11,16] The degree of hyperkalemia seen in children with renal insufficiency and end-stage renal disease roughly correlates with the degree of renal impairment.[11] Familiarity with the identification and management of specific conditions known

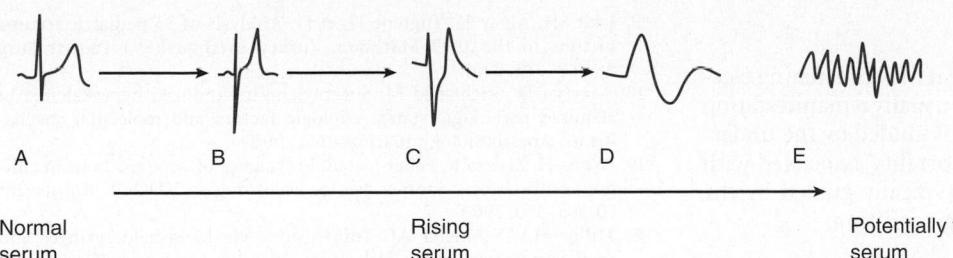

FIGURE 114–1. Hyperkalemia-associated electrocardiographic changes. **A,** Normal QRS complex. **B,** Peaked T waves. **C,** Widened QRS complex. **D,** Sine wave pattern. **E,** Ventricular fibrillation.

Table 114–1	Selected Causes of Hyperkalemia

Increased Intake

Inappropriate intravenous fluid preparation or administration
Medications containing potassium salts (e.g., penicillin)
Oral potassium ingestion
Transfusion of packed red blood cells through a small-gauge needle

Decreased Excretion

Congenital adrenal hyperplasia
Renal insufficiency or failure

Fluid and Electrolyte Shifts

Acidosis (e.g., diabetic ketoacidosis)
Burns involving a large body surface area
Crush injury
Heat stroke
Medications (e.g., succinylcholine)
Rhabdomyolysis
Tumor lysis syndrome

"Pseudohyperkalemia"

Hemolysis of the specimen
Laboratory error
Munchausen syndrome by proxy
Thrombocytosis

Table 114–2	Treatment Strategies for Hyperkalemia

Membrane Stabilization

- Calcium chloride (10%): 10–30 mg/kg per dose (0.1–0.3 ml/kg per dose) slowly IV (0.5–1 ml/min max), may repeat PRN. Not to exceed 5 ml (stop infusion if bradycardia develops).

Intracellular Shift

- Sodium bicarbonate: 1–2 mEq/kg per dose (1–2 ml/kg per dose of 1-mmol/ml solution) IV slowly. Incompatible with epinephrine, calcium, and atropine.
- Glucose and insulin: 0.5 g/kg (2 ml/kg) 25% dextrose solution + 0.1 unit/kg regular insulin IV
- Albuterol nebulized (unit dose); may repeat

Increased Elimination

- Furosemide: 0.5–2 mg/kg per dose IV; may increase by 1–2 mg/kg q6–8h. Limits: neonates, 2 mg/kg per dose; infants and children, 6 mg/kg per dose.
- Kayexalate: 0.5–1 g/kg PO or by retention enema
- Hemodialysis

Abbreviations: IV, intravenous; PO, per os (orally); PRN, as needed.

to be associated with hyperkalemia is prudent (see Chapter 88, Renal Disorders; Chapter 99, Rhabdomyolysis; and Chapter 105, Diabetic Ketoacidosis).

Important Clinical Features and Considerations

Serum potassium values obtained through laboratory testing may not reflect true hyperkalemia (see Table 114–1). One common cause of this "pseudohyperkalemia" is the hemolysis of laboratory specimens.[17] Since relatively small needles and catheters are used to draw pediatric blood specimens, the process may cause red blood cell rupture.[12] The release of intracellular potassium into the specimen tube will result in an elevated potassium value. Of course, this laboratory result does not reflect the potassium level in the patient's blood. Fortunately, laboratories report on whether or not specimens are hemolyzed.[17] In most instances, this allows the emergency physician to differentiate pseudohyperkalemia from true hyperkalemia. Hemolysis is particularly frustrating when there is a high likelihood of true hyperkalemia. In other circumstances, pseudohyperkalemia arises as a laboratory artifact because of other components of blood. For example, patients with thrombocytosis may have artificially elevated

potassium values on laboratory testing.[18,19] In a bizarre example of pseudohyperkalemia, a mother was suspected of adding urine to her child's blood tubes in a case of Munchausen syndrome by proxy.[20]

Management

The management of hyperkalemia depends on the underlying cause. An excellent example of this is the management of hyperkalemia identified during the evaluation of diabetic ketoacidosis. In this instance, the "treatment" of hyperkalemia is to simply avoid adding potassium to the intravenous fluids until the child demonstrates urinary output.[13] Since children experiencing diabetic ketoacidosis have a total body depletion of potassium, enhancing potassium excretion would lead to serious hypokalemia as treatment progressed (see Chapter 105, Diabetic Ketoacidosis). In another example, administering corticosteroids to neonates with congenital adrenal hyperplasia should lead to normalization of the potassium level.[6] For children with impeded excretion of potassium, particularly those with renal failure, temporizing measures will be followed by definitive care. The purpose of these temporizing measures is to stabilize cell wall electrical potentials, shift some of the serum potassium intracellularly, and enhance excretion (Table 114–2). Definitive care focuses on the prompt initiation of hemodialysis.

Summary

Hyperkalemia is a serious and potential life-threatening electrolyte abnormality. Hyperkalemia is usually a manifestation of another disease state. If treatment is guided by the underlying condition, the morbidity and mortality associated with hyperkalemia is low. Disposition is typically guided by the overall management of an underlying condition.

REFERNCES

1. Anderson DM, Novak PD, Keith J, et al: Dorland's Illustrated Medical Dictionary, 30th ed. Philadelphia: WB Saunders, 2003, p 882.
2. Kratz A, Ferraro M, Sluss PM, et al: Laboratory reference values. N Engl J Med 351:1548–1563, 2004.
*3. Parisi A, Alabiso A, Sacchetti M, et al: Complex ventricular arrhythmia induced by overuse of potassium supplementation in a young male football player. Case report. J Sports Med Phys Fitness 42:214–216, 2002.
4. Quick G, Bastani B: Prolonged asystolic hyperkalemic cardiac arrest with no neurologic sequelae. Ann Emerg Med 24:305–311, 1994.
*5. Webster A, Brady W, Morris F: Recognising signs of danger: ECG changes resulting from an abnormal serum potassium concentration. Emerg Med J 19:74–77, 2002.
6. Agarwal S, Deshpande G, Agarwal D, et al: Sudden cardiac arrest in a neonate with congenital adrenal hyperplasia. Pediatr Cardiol 26:686–689, 2005.
7. Giapros VI, Tsatsoulis AA, Drougia EA, et al: Rare causes of acute hyperkalemia in the first week of life: three case reports. Pediatr Nephrol 19:1046–1049, 2004.
8. Larach MG, Rosenberg H, Gronert GA, et al: Hyperkalemic cardiac arrest during anesthesia in infants and children with occult myopathies. Clin Pediatr 36:9–16, 1997.

---

*Selected readings.

9. Iskit SH, Alpay H, Tugtepe H, et al: Analysis of 33 pediatric trauma victims in the 1999 Marmara, Turkey earthquake. J Pediatr Surg 36:368–372, 2001.
*10. Martyn JA, Richtsfeld M: Succinylcholine-induced hyperkalemia in acquired pathologic states: etiologic factors and molecular mechanisms. Anesthesiology 104:158–169, 2006.
*11. Wong H, Mylrea K, Feber J, et al: Prevalence of complications in children with chronic kidney disease according to KDOQI. Kidney Int 70:585–590, 2006.
12. Miller MA, Schlueter AJ: Transfusions via hand-held syringes and small-gauge needles as risk factor for hyperkalemia. Transfusion 44:373, 2004.
13. Wolfsdorf J, Glaser N, Sperling MA, et al: Diabetic ketoacidosis in infants, children, and adolescents: a consensus statement from the American Diabetes Association. Diabetes Care 29:1150–1159, 2006.
14. Martinez-Vea A, Bardaji A, Garcia C: Severe hyperkalaemia with minimal electrocardiographic manifestations: a report of seven cases. J Electrocardiol 32:45–49, 1999.
15. Sever MS, Erek E, Vanholder R, et al: Serum potassium in the crush syndrome victims of the Marmara disaster. Clin Nephrol 59:326–333, 2003.
16. Kemper MJ, Harps E, Muller-Weifel DE: Hyperkalemia: therapeutic options in acute and chronic renal failure. Clin Nephrol 46:67–69, 1996.
17. Owens H, Siparsky G, Bajaj L, et al: Correction of factitious hyperkalemia in hemolyzed specimens. Am J Emerg Med 23:872–875, 2005.
18. Howard MR, Ashwell S, Bond LR, et al: Artefactual serum hyperkalaemia and hypercalcaemia in essential thrombocythaemia. J Clin Pathol 53:105–109, 2000.
19. Bakkaloglu SA, Soylemezoglu O, Karadeniz C, et al: Pseudohyperkalemia due to reactive thrombocytosis in an infant with yolk sac tumor. Pediatr Hematol Oncol 18:303–305, 2001.
20. Magen D, Skorecki K: Extreme hyperkalemia in Munchausen-by-proxy syndrome. N Engl J Med 340:1293–1294, 1999.

Hypocalcemia

Eric T. Carter, MD

Introduction and Background

Calcium is the most abundant mineral in the human body.[1] It is essential to cellular and enzymatic functions. Calcium is found primarily in bone, where 99% of the body's total calcium is stored. The remaining 1% either is bound to proteins or exists in the free ionized form. When a serum total calcium level is obtained, both the protein-bound and free ionized forms of calcium are measured. Ionized calcium is the physiologically active form of calcium. Calcium homeostasis is maintained by feedback loops that include parathyroid hormone, vitamin D, and calcitonin.[1] Parathyroid hormone acts to increase bone resorption and increase serum calcium. Vitamin D acts on the gastrointestinal tract to increase calcium absorption from the diet.[1] Calcitonin, in opposition to parathyroid hormone and vitamin D, acts to lower serum calcium levels. Magnesium and phosphate levels also directly affect calcium homeostasis. The normal range for total serum calcium is 2.2 to 2.6 mmol/L (9.0 to 10.5 mg/dl).[2] The normal range for ionized serum calcium is 1.1 to 1.4 mmol/L (4.5 to 5.6 mg/dl).[2] Since normal neonates may have a lower total serum calcium level than older children and adults, clinicians tend to use a somewhat lower age-specific threshold for defining hypocalcemia in neonates.[3]

Recognition and Approach

The multiple interconnected pathways associated with calcium regulation make recognition and diagnosis of the underlying process somewhat complex (Table 115–1). Once hypocalcemia has been identified, a more thorough investigation is warranted. The most important initial laboratory value in this setting is an ionized calcium level.[4,5] Low total serum calcium associated with a normal ionized calcium level suggests hypoproteinemia due to insufficient protein production (e.g., malabsorption, hepatic disease) or excessive protein loss (e.g., nephrotic syndrome).[6] Hypocalcemia in which both the total and ionized calcium levels are low suggests hypoparathyroidism, vitamin D deficiency, magnesium or phosphate abnormality, a medication effect, or an underlying disease process (e.g., malignancy, pancreatitis, sepsis).[6] Other laboratory studies helpful in identifying the cause of hypocalcemia include studies of renal and hepatic function, and magnesium, phosphate, and albumin levels.[5,7-10] Radiographs may be indicated, particularly in cases of suspected rickets, nonaccidental trauma, or pathologic fractures.[11]

Clinical Presentation

Because of calcium's ubiquitous involvement in many vital cellular functions, hypocalcemia results in a wide range of clinical presentations. Common neuromuscular manifestations seen with hypocalcemia include paresthesias, muscle cramping, carpopedal spasm, generalized weakness, tetany, Chvostek's sign (i.e., spasm of the facial muscles when the facial nerve is tapped near the parotid gland), Trousseau's phenomenon (i.e., spasms of muscles elicited by applying pressure to the nerves innervating them), and seizures.[11-13] Psychiatric manifestations include depression, anxiety, irritability, confusion, and progressive dementia. Cardiovascular manifestations include arrhythmias, hypotension, electrocardiographic changes including QT prolongation or ventricular dysrhythmias, and syncope.[14] Respiratory manifestations include laryngeal spasm, bronchospasm, stridor, respiratory distress, and apnea.[15,16] Gastrointestinal manifestations include abdominal distention, poor feeding, vomiting, excessive crying, and dysphagia. Chronic hypocalcemia leads to changes in the teeth, skin, and bones as well. Other diagnostic considerations include congenital syndromes, malnutrition, and neck surgery. A number of medications can affect calcium regulation, including phosphate-containing enemas[17,18] (see Table 115–1). Calcium chelation, as occurs with blood transfusions or renal failure, and altered protein-binding states (e.g., alkalosis, hypoalbuminemia) may also cause hypocalcemia.

Table 115–1	Common Causes of Hypocalcemia

Alkalosis
Blood transfusion (chelation)
Burns
DiGeorge syndrome
Hemosiderosis
Hepatic disease
Hyperphosphatemia
Hypoalbuminemia
Hypomagnesemia
Malabsorption
Medications*
Nephrotic syndrome
Pancreatitis
Parathyroid deficiency
Pseudohypoparathyroidism syndromes
Renal failure
Renal tubular disease
Rhabdomyolysis
Sepsis
Surgical/postoperative damage to parathyroid glands
Vitamin D deficiency
Wilson's disease

*Medications associated with hypocalcemia include aminoglycosides, amphotericin, calcitonin, calcium channel blockers, cimetidine, cisplatin, citrate, furosemide, glucagon, glucocorticoids, heparin, magnesium, phenobarbital, phenytoin, phosphates, protamine, and theophylline.

Important Clinical Features and Considerations

Clinical experience suggests that the child's history and physical examination are important keys to suspecting clinically significant hypocalcemia. The use of medications, recent blood transfusions, a history of neck surgery, a history of renal failure, and seizures in a neonate should all be considered "red flags" for hypocalcemia. Acknowledging the varied manifestations may allow the emergency physician to suspect hypocalcemia in clinical scenarios that are not intuitively obvious.[8,11] For example, physical examination findings such as wheezing and stridor, commonly associated with bronchiolitis and croup, have been described as being associated with hypocalcemia in children.[15,16]

Management

The management of a child with hypocalcemia is directed at identifying and treating the underlying cause. Given the varied causes of hypocalcemia, there is no standard approach to all children with hypocalcemia. Calcium replacement may be achieved via the oral route in mild or asymptomatic cases of hypocalcemia or in chronic disease states such as renal failure, vitamin D deficiency, and parathyroid hormone deficiency. Clinical experience suggests that appropriate follow-up with the patient's primary physician or endocrinologist should be arranged, and it is seldom, if ever, necessary to begin oral calcium therapy in the emergency department.

In contrast, life-threatening hypocalcemia should be treated in the emergency department. Cardiac monitoring is prudent given the known effects of hypocalcemia on ventricular function. Intravenous calcium chloride and calcium gluconate are both available for emergent calcium replacement. Calcium chloride, commonly stocked in "crash carts," contains three times the elemental calcium and is also more caustic to infuse in peripheral veins compared to calcium gluconate. Calcium chloride is typically available in a 10% solution and may be given intravenously at a dose of 0.2 to 0.3 ml/kg slowly over 5 to 20 minutes. Continuous cardiac monitoring during intravenous calcium replacement is indicated. Calcium gluconate, also typically available in a 10% solution, may be given intravenously at a dose of 0.5 to 1 ml/kg slowly over 5 to 20 minutes with continuous cardiac monitoring. Neonatal hypocalcemic seizures may be treated with 1 to 2 ml/kg of calcium gluconate over 5 to 10 minutes.[3]

Summary

Calcium is the most abundant element in the body, and its regulation is vital to cellular function. Calcium homeostasis is maintained via multiple interconnected metabolic pathways. Hypocalcemia affects multiple organ systems and therefore results in a wide range of clinical presentations. Intravenous replacement is indicated in life-threatening or severe hypocalcemia. Any child receiving intravenous calcium replacement warrants admission to the hospital and monitoring. Appropriate consultation and disposition are dependent on the suspected underlying cause of hypocalcemia and its clinical manifestations.

REFERENCES

1. Root AW, Harrison HE: Recent advances in calcium metabolism. I. Mechanisms of calcium homeostasis. J Pediatr 88:1–18, 1976.
2. Kratz A, Ferraro M, Sluss PM, et al: Laboratory reference values. N Engl J Med 351:1548–1563, 2004.
3. Kossoff EH, Silvia MT, Maret A, et al: Neonatal hypocalcemic seizures: a case report and literature review. J Child Neurol 17:236–239, 2002.
4. Kost GJ: The significance of ionized calcium in cardiac and critical care: availability and critical limits at US medical centers and children's hospitals. Arch Pathol Lab Med 117:890–896, 1993.
5. Guise TA, Mundy GR: Clinical Review 69: Evaluation of hypocalcemia in children and adults. J Clin Endocrinol Metab 80:1473–1478, 1995.
6. Root AW, Harrison HE: Recent advances in calcium metabolism. II. Disorders of calcium homeostasis. J Pediatr 88:177–199, 1976.
7. DeRubertis FR: Hypocalcemia: etiology and management. Hosp Med 3:88–118, 1985.
8. Cardenas-Rivero N, Chernow B, Stoiko MA, et al: Hypocalcemia in critically ill children. J Pediatr 114:946–951, 1989.
9. Khilnani P: Electrolyte abnormalities in critically ill children. Crit Care Med 20:241–250, 1992.
10. Zaloga GP, Chernow B: Hypocalcemia in critical illness. JAMA 256:1924–1929, 1986.
11. Bloom E, Klein EJ, Shushan D, Feldman KW: Variable presentations of rickets in children in the emergency department. Pediatr Emerg Care 20:126–130, 2000.
12. Duplechin RY, Nadkarni M, Schwartz RP: Hypocalcemic tetany in a toddler with undiagnosed rickets. Ann Emerg Med 34:399–402, 1999.
*13. Scarfone RJ, Pond K, Thompson K, Fall I: Utility of laboratory testing for infants with seizures. Pediatr Emerg Care 16:309–312, 2000.
14. Maffei FA, Kiaffas MG, Beerman LB: Three unusual causes of pediatric syncope: a reaffirmation for the screening electrocardiogram. Pediatr Emerg Care 14:342–344, 1998.
*15. Abrunzo TJ: An infant fatality associated with inspiratory and expiratory wheezing: another wheeze that wasn't asthma. Pediatr Emerg Care 11:48–51, 1995.
*16. Halterman JS, Smith SA: Hypocalcemia and stridor: an unusual presentation of vitamin D deficient rickets. J Emerg Med 16:41–43, 1998.
17. Marraffa JM, Hui A, Stork CM: Severe hyperphosphatemia and hypocalcemia following the rectal administration of a phosphate-containing Fleet pediatric enema. Pediatr Emerg Care 20:453–456, 2004.
*18. Walton DM, Thomas DC, Aly HZ, Short BL: Morbid hypocalcemia associated with phosphate enema in a six week-old infant. Pediatrics 106:e37, 2000.

*Selected readings.

Psychobehavioral Disorders

Thomas H. Chun, MD

Selected Diagnoses

Violent and/or agitated behavior
Psychosis
Other psychiatric conditions
   Behavioral disorders (attention-deficit/hyperactivity disorder, attention-deficit disorder)
   Pervasive developmental disorder
   Acute anxiety
   Obsessive-compulsive disorder
   Posttraumatic stress disorder
   Conduct disorders
Somatoform disorders
   Conversion disorder
   Munchausen syndrome
   Munchausen syndrome by proxy

Discussion of Individual Diagnoses

Violent and/or Agitated Behavior

Violent or agitated behavior is not a diagnosis unto itself but the final common pathway for a number of medical and psychiatric conditions.[1] Unfortunately, every year emergency department (ED) staff are injured or threatened by such patients. Violence has a much higher association with substance abuse than with mental illness in general. When it occurs with mental illness, it is greater in the presence of other acute psychiatric symptoms.[2,3]

Violent behavior includes verbal threats, destruction of property, and/or physical violence toward oneself or others. Agitation may present with these symptoms but may also present without any violence. Agitation can be so severe as to cause extreme distress or to impair the patient's ability cooperate.

Ensuring the safety of the patient, ED staff, and others is critical. All patients need to be carefully assessed for suicide (see Chapter 117, Major Depression and Suicidality), homicide, or plans for revenge, and any current violent thoughts or impulses. Equally important is identifying and treating potential organic etiologies of the behavior.

Management includes verbal, chemical, and physical restraint. Training in verbal restraint has been shown to decrease the need for chemical or physical restraint. Techniques common to all verbal restraint strategies include a calm, nonjudgmental manner; asking the patient to verbalize what is bothering him or her; active, empathetic listening; offering the patient as many treatment options as is reasonably possible while setting clear limits; and avoiding "bargaining" and punitive treatment(s).[4]

Many agents are available for chemical restraint (Table 116-1). None has been approved by the U.S. Food and Drug Administration for this purpose in pediatric patients. All, however, have been widely used and are considered safe and efficacious by experienced psychiatrists and emergency physicians. If a patient is already taking one of these medications, the current dose or a larger dose may be necessary. All medication doses should be rounded to the nearest half or whole milligram, or to the nearest whole-pill dose.[5-15]

A minimum of five personnel are needed to adequately physically restrain a patient, one to control each limb and one for the head. Padded leather restraints are recommended. The choice between positioning the patient supine or prone

Table 116–1	Chemical Restraint Medications		
Medication	**Starting Dose**	**Onset of Action (min)**	**Comments/Adverse Effect**
Diphenhydramine	1.25 mg/kg (IV/IM/PO) Adolescent: 25–50 mg	5–15 (IM/IV); 20–30 (PO)	
Hydroxyzine	0.5–1.0 mg/kg (IV/IM/PO) Adolescent: 25–50 mg	5–15 (IM/IV); 20–30 (PO)	
Lorazepam	0.05–0.1 mg/kg (IV/IM/PO) Adolescent: 0.07 mg/kg	5–15 (IM/IV); 20–30 (PO)	Slowly over 5 min (IV); may redose q60 min
Midazolam	0.05–0.15 mg/kg (IV/IM), 0.5–0.75 mg/kg (PO) Adolescent: 2–4 mg	5–15 (IM/IV); 20–30 (PO)	Over 2–3 min (IV); may redose q60 min
Haloperidol	0.1 mg/kg (PO) Adolescent: 1–5 mg (PO) or 2–5 mg per dose (IV/IM)	15–30 (IM); 30–60 (PO)	May redose q60 min; may prolong QTc
Risperidone	<12 yr: 0.5 mg (PO) Adolescent: 1 mg (PO)	45–60 (PO)	
Olanzapine	<12 yr: 2.5 mg (IM/PO) Adolescent: 5–10 mg (IM/PO)	30–60 (IM); 45–60 (PO)	
Quetiapine	25 mg/dose (PO)	45–60 (PO)	
Zisprasidone	<12 yr: 5 mg/dose (PO) Adolescent: 10–20 mg per dose (PO)	30–60 (IM); 60 (PO)	May prolong QTc

Abbreviations: IM, intramuscularly; IV, intravenously; PO, orally.
Adapted from Allen MH: Managing the agitated psychotic patient: a reappraisal of the evidence. J Clin Psychiatry 61(Suppl 14):11–20, 2000.

must be individualized to each patient. The prone position is safer but more restrictive than the supine position. Close observation and documentation of vital signs, assessment of behavioral status, and regularly offering food, water, and access to bathroom facilities are all mandated by law, as is regular reassessment of all parameters. Physical restraint is not without risk. A government analysis of a series of reported deaths following restraint identified three major risk factors for death: excessive weight being placed on the backs of prone patients, objects being used to cover patients' mouths to prevent spitting or biting, and airway obstructions due to placing patient's arms across their neck.[8,16]

The least restrictive means of treatment should always be tried first, a practice that represents an optimal clinical approach as well as compliance with the law. Once a patient has calmed, removal of physical restraints may be considered. There is no standard procedure for removing restraints. Some prefer removing one restraint at a time, to determine if the patient has regained control of him/herself. Others prefer to remove all restraints at once. The same type of personnel who were present when the restraints were placed should be present when they are removed, in case the restraints need to be reapplied.[8,16]

Psychosis

Psychosis specifically refers to a syndrome of significant alterations in cognition, perception, reality testing, mood, and/or impulse control, resulting in impaired social functioning. Psychosis can be seen in a large number of psychiatric and medical conditions (Table 116–2).

Classically the symptoms of psychosis include hallucinations and/or delusions, along with other changes in cognitive functioning, mood, and behavior. However, symptoms may vary considerably depending on the patient's developmental status and cultural background. In young children, it may be particularly challenging to differentiate between developmentally appropriate "magical thinking" and true psychosis.[17-19]

Table 116–2	Conditions That May Lead to Psychosis

Central Nervous System Lesions

Tumors
Brain abscess
Cerebral hemorrhage
Meningitis or encephalitis
Temporal lobe epilepsy

Cerebral Hypoxia

Pulmonary insufficiency
Severe anemia
Cardiac failure
Carbon monoxide poisoning

Drug Intoxications

Accidental ingestion
Drug abuse/experimentation
Alcohol abuse (alone or with other drugs)
Deliberate suicide attempt
Prescribed medications (toxicity/side effects/withdrawal)

Infections

Malaria
Typhoid fever
Subacute bacterial endocarditis

Metabolic and Endocrine Disorders

Electrolyte imbalance
Hypoglycemia
Hypocalcemia
Thyroid disease (hyper and hypo)
Adrenal disease (hyper and hypo)
Uremia
Hepatic failure
Diabetes mellitus
Porphyria

Rheumatic Diseases

Systemic lupus erythematosus
Polyarteritis nodosa

Miscellaneous Conditions

Wilson's disease
Reye's syndrome

Trauma

REFERENCES

1. Appelbaum PS, Robbins PC, Monahan J: Violence and delusions: data from the MacArthur Violence Risk Assessment Study. Am J Psychiatry 157:566–572, 2000.
2. Farrington DP, Loeber R: Epidemiology of juvenile violence. Child Adolesc Psychiatr Clin N Am 9:733–748, 2000.
3. Loeber R, Burke JD, Lahey BB, et al: Oppositional defiant and conduct disorder: a review of the past 10 years, part I. J Am Acad Child Adolesc Psychiatry 39:1468–1484, 2000.
4. Binder RL, McNiel DE: Contemporary practices in managing acutely violent patients in 20 psychiatric emergency rooms. Psychiatr Serv 50:1553–1554, 1999.
*5. Allen MH: Managing the agitated psychotic patient: a reappraisal of the evidence. J Clin Psychiatry 61(Suppl 14):11–20, 2000.
*6. Allen MH, Currier GW, Hughes DH, et al: The expert consensus guideline series: treatment of behavioral emergencies. Postgrad Med May(spec no.):1–88, 2001.
*7. American Academy of Child and Adolescent Psychiatry: Practice parameter for the prevention and management of aggressive behavior in child and adolescent psychiatric institutions, with special reference to seclusion and restraint. J Am Acad Child Adol Psychiatry 41(Suppl 2):4S–25S, 2002.
8. Currier GW, Allen MH: Physical and chemical restraint in the psychiatric emergency service. Psychiatr Serv 51:717–719, 2000.
9. Currier GW: Atypical antipsychotic medications in the psychiatric emergency service. J Clin Psychiatry 61(Suppl 14):21–26, 2000.
10. Dorfman DH: The use of physical and chemical restraints in the pediatric emergency department. Ped Emerg Care 16:355–360, 2000.
11. Green WH: Child and Adolescent Clinical Psychopharmacology, 3rd ed. Philadelphia: Lippincott Williams & Wilkins, 2001.
*12. McClellan JM, Werry JS: Evidence-based treatments in child and adolescent psychiatry: an inventory. J Am Acad Child Adolesc Psychiatry 42:1388–1400, 2003.
13. Riddle MA, Kastelic EA, Frosch E: Pediatric psychopharmacology. J Child Psychol Psychiatry 42:73–90, 2001.
14. Sorrentino A: Chemical restraints for the agitated, violent, or psychotic pediatric patient in the emergency department: controversies and recommendations. Curr Opin Pediatr 16.201–205, 2004.
15. Yildiz A, Sachs GS, Turgay A: Pharmacological management of agitation in emergency settings. Emerg Med J 20:339–346, 2003.
16. Busch AB, Shore MF: Seclusion and restraint: a review of the recent literature. Harvard Rev Psychiatry 8:261–270, 2000.
17. Reimherr JP, McClellan JM: Diagnostic challenges in children and adolescents with psychotic disorders. J Clin Psychiatry 65(Suppl 6):5–11, 2004.
18. Thomsen PS: Schizophrenia with childhood and adolescent onset: a nationwide register-based study. Acta Psychiatr Scand 94:187–193, 1996.
19. Volkmar FR: Childhood and adolescent psychosis: a review of the past 10 years. J Am Acad Child Adolesc Psychiatry 35:843–851, 1996.
20. American Academy of Child and Adolescent Psychiatry: Practice parameters for the assessment and treatment of children and adolescents with schizophrenia. J Am Acad Child Adolesc Psychiatry 40(Suppl):4S–23S, 2001.
21. Menezes NM, Milovan E: First-episode psychosis: a comparative review of diagnostic evolution and predictive variables in adolescents versus adults. Can J Psychiatry 45:710–716, 2000.
22. Werry JS, McClellan JM, Chard L: Childhood and adolescent schizophrenic, bipolar, and schizoaffective disorders: a clinical and outcome study. J Am Acad Child Adolesc Psychiatry 30:457–465, 1991.
23. Casidy LJ, Jellinek MS: Approaches to recognition and management of childhood psychiatric disorders in pediatric primary care. Pediatr Clin North Am 45:1037–1052, 1998.
24. Glascoe FP: Early detection of developmental and behavioral problems. Pediatr Rev 21:272–279, 2000.
25. Newcorn JH: New treatments and approaches for attention deficit hyperactivity disorder. Curr Psychiatry Rep 3:87–91, 2001.
26. Reiff MI, Stein MT: Attention-deficit/hyperactivity disorder: diagnosis and treatment. Adv Pediatr 51:289–327, 2004.
27. Goldson E: Autism spectrum disorders: an overview. Adv Pediatr 51:63–109, 2004.
28. Spence SJ, Sharifi P, Wiznitzer M: Autism spectrum disorder: screening, diagnosis, and medical evaluation. Semin Pediatr Neurol 11:186–195, 2004.
29. Volkmar FR, Lord C, Bailey A, et al: Autism and pervasive developmental disorders. J Child Psychol Psychiatry 45:135–170, 2004.
30. Arnold P, Banerjee SP, Bhandari R, et al: Childhood anxiety disorders and developmental issues in anxiety. Curr Psychiatry Rep 5:252–265, 2003.
31. Bernstein GA, Borchardt CM, Perwien AR: Anxiety disorders in children and adolescents: a review of the past 10 years. J Am Acad Child Adol Psychiatry 35:1110–1119, 1996.
32. American Psychiatric Association: Diagnostic and Statistical Manual of Mental Disorders, Fourth Edition, Text Revision. Washington, DC: American Psychiatric Press, 2000.
33. Varley CK, Smith CJ: Anxiety disorders in the child and teen. Pediatr Clin North Am 50:1107–1138, 2003.
34. Jenike MA: Clinical practice: obsessive-compulsive disorder. N Engl J Med 350:259–265, 2004.
35. March JS, Leonard HL: Obsessive-compulsive disorder in children and adolescents: a review of the past 10 years. J Am Acad Child Adolesc Psychiatry 35:1265–1273, 1996.
36. Piacentini J, Bergman RL: Obsessive-compulsive disorder in children. Psychiatr Clin North Am 23:519–533, 2000.
37. Davis L, Siegel LJ: Posttraumatic stress disorder in children and adolescents: a review and analysis. Clin Child Fam Psychol Rev 3:135–154, 2000.
38. Lonigan CJ, Phillips BM, Richey JA: Posttraumatic stress disorder in children: diagnosis, assessment, and associated features. Child Adolesc Psychiatry Clin N Am 12:171–194, 2003.
39. Pfefferbaum B: Posttraumatic stress disorder in children: a review of the past 10 years. J Am Acad Child Adolesc Psychiatry 36:1503–1511, 1997.
40. Boyle M, Offord D: Primary prevention of conduct disorders: issues and prospects. J Am Acad Child Adolesc Psychiatry 29:227–233, 1990.
41. Burke JD, Loeber R, Birmaher B: Oppositional defiant disorder and conduct disorder: a review of the past 10 years, part II. J Am Acad Child Adolesc Psychiatry 41:1275–1293, 2002.
42. Fritz GK, Fritsch S, Hagino O: Somatoform disorders in children and adolescents: a review of the past 10 years. J Am Acad Child Adolesc Psychiatry 36:1329–1338, 1997.
43. Silber TJ, Pao M: Somatization disorders in children and adolescents. Pediatr Rev 24:255–264, 2003.
44. Folks DG: Munchausen's syndrome and other factitious disorders. Neurol Clin 13:267–281, 1995.
45. Murray JB: Munchausen syndrome/Munchausen syndrome by proxy. J Psychol 131:343–352, 1997.

---

*Selected readings.

Chapter 117

Major Depression and Suicidality

Jacqueline Grupp-Phelan, MD, MPH and Sergio V. Delgado, MD

Key Points

The most common emergency department presentations of major depression in children are somatic complaints, and feeding disorders.

The most common emergency department presentations of major depression in adolescents are sleep disorders, aggressive/violent behavior, eating disorders, and superficial cutting on arms and/or legs.

Frequent reasons why children and adolescents present to the emergency department for treatment of major depression are fear of death, wish for problem relief, fear of reaction of parents, and suicidality.

The major focus of evaluation is assessment of suicidal risk, and the major focus of management is averting suicidal behavior and its acute consequences.

Introduction and Background

Major depression has become an important cause of emergency department (ED) utilization. The prevalence of depression increases throughout the lifespan, with approximately 1% of preschoolers, 2% of school-age children, and almost 8% of adolescents having major depression in the general population.[1-3] Depression in children is often unrecognized and inadequately treated.[4,5] The prevalence of mental illness in U.S. EDs has been increasing over the past decade, representing approximately 5% of all visits by children for mental health reasons.[6,7] The frequency of positive screens for depression across all age groups is about 4%.[8] The ED can play an important role in the detection and referral of children with depression.

Recognition and Approach

There is no single cause of depression; rather, a combination of predisposing factors, including genetics, neurobiologic factors, and environmental variables, is likely responsible.[9-11] Depressed children present differently according to age;

however, there is no gender differentiation until adolescence, where the incidence doubles for females.[5,12] Obsessive-compulsive disorder and learning disabilities are often precursors to major depression in children.[12-14] Suicide is the third leading cause of death in the 10- to 24-year-age group and has been increasing over the last decade. Suicide remains the most critical management issue for ED providers.[15]

Clinical Presentation

The clinical presentations for depressive disorders in children and adolescents are similar across health care venues and are similar to adult presentations with respect to irritable mood, failure to achieve, and significant weight gain or loss. However, the ED presentation of depressed school-age children does differ from that of adults in that children often present with somatic complaints or disorders of feeding. Adolescents are more likely to present with sleep disorders, aggressive behavior, and self-mutilation. Acute presentations in the adolescent age group include fear of death, wish for problem relief, fear of reaction of parents, and the most concerning presentation, suicidal ideation. Depressed preschoolers present with sadness or irritability, which is the most sensitive symptom, although lack of enjoyment or interest in play is the most specific symptom.[16-18]

The ED provider should be highly suspicious of depression when a younger child presents with extreme irritability, conflict with parents, fear of death, inappropriate guilt, or selective mutism. Older children display more traditional signs of depression, including dysthymia, hopelessness, self-mutilation, and suicidal ideation. Adolescents or their parents may report conflict in important social relationships. Finally, a significant change in weight or fears of returning home should cue ED providers to perform a mental health screen.[19] It is important to note that parents may underreport their childs' depression and not take the early signs seriously if it does not directly affect them.[20,21] For example, in these situations the child frequently reports that "my parents would be better off without me," and the parents feel "he/she has everything, I don't understand what he/she has to be depressed about."

Preschoolers and school-age children through the age of 14 are less able to accurately describe their internal state of sadness and often communicate in concrete terms: "I feel down, bad, sad." This explains the need for parental presence during the interview.

Table 117–1	Assessment of Suicidal Patients

Assessing Circumstances of an Attempt

Precipitating humiliating event
Preparatory actions: acquiring a method, putting affairs in order, suicide talk, giving away prized possessions, suicide note
Use of a more violent method
Precautions taken against discovery

Presenting Symptoms

Hopelessness
Depressed mood
Suicidal thoughts

Psychiatric Illness

Previous suicide attempt
Affective disorders
Alcoholism or substance abuse
Conduct disorder

Psychosocial History

Parents recently divorced
Multiple life stressors
Chronic medical history

Personality Factors

Impulsivity, hostility
Negativity
Borderline or antisocial personality disorder

Family History

Family history of suicidal behavior
Family history of affective disorder

Children with special health care needs are also at risk for depression and often are more difficult to assess. This group of children may present to the emergency department in a medical crisis, often after a period of noncompliance with medications. This may be a mechanism to ask for help and should prompt ED providers to perform a mental health screen.

The suicidal patient presents to the emergency department in crisis. A rigid algorithmic approach in the ED is unlikely to be beneficial due to the unique characteristics and risk factors of the individual patient. In the assessment of the suicidal patient, the emergency physician must utilize information about risk factors (Table 117–1) in consultation with a mental health professional to determine the appropriate disposition of the patient. Indications for psychiatric evaluation include acute suicidality, a combination of risk factors for suicide, recurrent ED visits over a short period of time, poor or nonexistent social and mental health supports, and a specific plan with lethal means.

As in any medical examination, the physician will start with the chief complaint and a review of present illness, including what brought the patient to the ED. Patients at high risk of suicide frequently present with nonspecific somatic complaints ranging from vague digestive problems and aches and pains to other symptoms more directly linked to depression—changes in appetite, fatigue, and insomnia. A staged suicide risk assessment with brief screening questions should be undertaken. Risk factors that increase the likelihood of suicide, such as recent drug use or trauma (domestic violence or rape), a previous suicide attempt, or gender identity issues, should prompt the ED provider to continue with a more in-depth assessment of suicidal risk (see Table 117–1). Unfortunately, structured instruments have shown high false-positive

and false-negative rates in general medical practice, requiring further research on the best way to classify patients with suicidal behavior.

A physical examination should be performed to rule out medical causes for psychiatric complaints. A mental status examination should be done evaluating mood, content of thought (hallucinations or delusions), and whether speech is pressured. Explicit questions about suicidal ideation, plans, attempts, and notes should be asked in a direct, compassionate, and confidential manner. Most importantly, the patients should be asked whether he or she can promise to contract for safety, control his or her behavior, and not act on impulses. Although confidentiality is imperative, patient safety may dictate the notification of family and psychiatric personnel even against the child's or adolescent's wishes.

Important Clinical Features and Considerations

Suspicion of suicidality or depression should be aroused when patients fear or are reluctant to allow a medical examination or discuss their problem with a nurse or physician. During the physical examination in children who present with risk factors for depression, it is important to ask and look for superficial cuts on arms and legs, particularly around the area of the thighs and hips. For children or adolescents being admitted for observation, it is important to completely check for abrasions or lacerations by performing a complete examination while the patient is in a hospital gown. Acute presentation to the ED is often in the evening, after parents return from work, after school hours, or anytime during the summer. In the review of systems, it is important to ask about preexisting or recent stressors that may have exacerbated an underlying depression, such as poor performance in school or a recent relationship difficulty (e.g., break up with a significant other). The educational level of parents has been found to be a risk factor associated with severe adolescent depression. Patients have a higher risk of depression if parents did not graduate from high school.[22] Pitfalls in the diagnosis may include dismissing somatic presentations of children who are high-achieving straight A students, described by their parents as "perfect" or "never angry." In a child with a bipolar disorder, a potential complication may be missing the depressive phase during which the risk for suicide is greatly increased.[23] It is important to ask about cycles of mania (not sleeping for days, hypersexuality, or spending sprees) and depression. Finally, there are a number of conditions that mimic acute depression in children and adolescents, including infections, neurologic disorders, and medication reactions[24] (Table 117–2).

Management

Although the child may be presenting for the first time with depressive complaints, it is mandatory to develop a biopsychosocial treatment plan beginning with the ED visit. Assessment of family willingness to participate in the treatment plan is essential for appropriate decisions with respect to the timeliness of the treatment plan and disposition. Individual psychotherapy, behavioral therapy, cognitive psychotherapy, and family therapy are the major nonpharmacologic treatments. Laying the groundwork for the initiation of

Table 117–2	Conditions Mimicking Depression in Children and Adolescents			
Infections	**Neurologic Disorders/Tumors**	**Endocrine**	**Medications**	**Others**
Infectious mononucleosis	Epilepsy	Diabetes	Antihypertensives	Alcohol abuse
Influenza	Postconcussion	Cushing's disease	Barbiturates	Drug abuse and withdrawal Cocaine Amphetamine Opiates
Encephalitis	Subarachnoid hemorrhage	Addison's disease	Benzodiazepines	Electrolyte abnormality Hypokalemia Hyponatremia
Subacute bacterial endocarditis	Cerebrovascular accident	Hypothyroidism	Corticosteroids	Failure to thrive
Pneumonia	Multiple sclerosis	Hyperthyroidism	Oral contraceptives	Anemia
Tuberculosis	Huntington's disease	Hyperparathyroidism	Cimetidine	Lupus
Hepatitis		Hypopituitarism	Aminophylline	Wilson's disease
Syphilis (CNS)			Anticonvulsants	Porphyria
AIDS			Clonidine	Uremia
			Digitalis	
			Thiazide diuretics	

Abbreviations: AIDS, acquired immunodeficiency syndrome; CNS, central nervous system.
Adapted from Wise MG, Rundell JR: Concise Guide to Consultation Psychiatry. Washington, DC: American Psychiatric Press, 1988.

therapy is an essential part of the ED management of acute depression.

Moderately to severely depressed children and adolescents should leave the emergency department with psychopharmacologic intervention. This is particularly important if there will not be urgent outpatient access to a child or adolescent psychiatrist. Mental health access has been a major problem in rural settings and increasingly has become a problem in urban centers. Thus, moderately depressed patients who are safe to go home are often unable to see a psychiatrist or psychologist for a full evaluation for weeks to months. For this reason, the emergency department visit may need to include the initiation of antidepressants in conjunction with mental health providers. Therefore, an understanding of the contraindications and potential complications regarding their use is imperative.

The most frequently prescribed pharmacologic agents for depression in children and adolescents continue to be the selective serotonin reuptake inhibitors (SSRIs), primarily because of their safety profile. Careful attention should be paid to U.S. Food and Drug Administration (FDA) "black box" warnings. Fluoxetine, at present, is the only medication approved for the use in major depressive disorders in children and adolescents.[25] Psychopharmacologic and psychotherapeutic approaches are often used together, with evidence supporting combination therapy.[26] Nevertheless, over 60% of depressed children have a positive response to the use of fluoxetine alone.

Of major concern in the initiation of SSRIs is the recent evidence surrounding increased adverse events in the initiation phase of therapy. Adverse events are defined as suicidal thinking or suicidal behavior. The average risk of adverse events in patients on SSRIs is 4%, twice the 2% risk in patients who received placebo in clinical trials. Although no deaths occurred, the FDA elected to present a black box warning, which mandates that clinicians have the duty to warn patients and their families about the risk associated with the medication, and to develop a clear way to follow up

and monitor the response to the medication. The monitoring should include "daily observations by families and frequent (weekly) contact with a physician during the first month of therapy."[25] Parents of children who receive antidepressant therapy with SSRIs must provide informed consent, recognizing that the FDA has not approved any of these medications for use in children for depression, aside from fluoxetine.[27] The primary goal is to maximize benefits and minimize potential side effects. Immediate consultation with a psychiatrist is highly recommended if using any other SSRI than fluoxetine.

An SSRI is contraindicated if the patient has known hypersensitivity or had received a monoamine oxidase inhibitor within the previous 2 weeks.[28] In general, tricyclic antidepressants may have serious cardiac effects and should be avoided.[29,30] Bupropion hydrochloride is contraindicated if the patient has a history of seizures.[28]

The emergency physician must gather information, weigh risk factors, and formulate a plan for managing suicidal behavior. The most important question is whether or not the patient can be managed as an inpatient or outpatient. Although hospitalization has no clear association with improved outcome in suicidal youth, it remains the most common risk management tool in the acute suicidal setting. For acutely suicidal patients who cannot contract for safely, inpatient care is mandatory. Suicidal patients are at risk for hurting themselves or eloping. As the number of suicidal and mentally ill youth increases, many EDs are investigating the use of locked rooms or psychiatric observation areas on site. Care must be taken to protect the patient from self-harm (see Chapter 154, The Child-Friendly Emergency Department: Practices, Policies, and Procedures). Some patients can be discharged from the ED based on absolute risk of suicide, the social and school supports available, and the availability of outpatient care. In all cases of patients who have a serious plan for suicide or who have made an attempt, psychiatric consultation is important in understanding an underlying psychiatric diagnosis, developing a confidential treatment plan, and managing the immediate psychiatric needs of the patient. Once patient safety is addressed and a decision regarding disposition is made, follow-up must be facilitated with the family.

Summary

For children and adolescents presenting with acute depression, referral to an outpatient therapist for patient and/or family counseling should ideally be arranged within 1 week. If a timely mental health evaluation is not possible, the ED physician should consider the initiation of psychopharmacologic treatment with return to the primary care physician for urgent follow-up of medication and therapeutic complications within several days.

For suicidal patients, emergency providers must be able to provide effective and appropriate identification and referral for mental, physical, and substance abuse disorders. In addition, the family must restrict access to highly lethal methods of suicide. Finally, a family-centered approach taking advantage of family and community support and support from ongoing medical and mental health care relationships is mandatory.

REFERENCES

1. Kashani JH, Sherma DD: Childhood depression: epidemiology, etiological models and treatment implications. Integr Psychiatry 6:1–8, 1988.
2. Birmaher B, Ryan ND, Williamson DE: Childhood and adolescent depression: a review of the past 10 years, part I. J Am Acad Child Adolesc Psychiatry 35:1427–1439, 1966
3. Birmaher B, Ryan ND, Williamson DE, et al: Childhood and adolescent depression: a review of the past 10 years, Part II. J Am Acad Child Adolesc Psychiatry 35:1575–1583, 1966
4. Costello EJ, Pine DS, Hammen C: Developmental and natural history of mood disorders. Biol Psychiatry 52:529–542, 2002.
5. Lewinsohn PM, Rohde P, Klein DN: Natural course of adolescent major depressive disorder: I. Continuing into young adulthood. J Am Acad Child Adolesc Psychiatry 38:56–63, 1999.
6. Grupp-Phelan J, Harman J, Kelleher K: Trends in mental health and chronic condition visits in children presenting for care at US emergency departments. Pub Health Rep 122:55–61, 2007.
*7. Sills M, Bland S: Summary statistics for pediatric psychiatric visits to US emergency departments, 1993–1999. Pediatrics 110:e40, 2002.
8. Grupp-Phelan J, Wade T, Ho M, Kelleher K: Mental health problems in children and caregivers in the emergency department setting. J Dev Behav Pediatr 28:16–21, 2007.
9. Beardslee WR, Bemporad J, Keller M: Children of parents with major affective disorder: a review. Am J Psychiatry 140:825–832, 1998.

*10. Lagges AM, Dunn DW: Depression in children and adolescents. Neurol Clin 21:953–960, 2003.
11. Rice F, Harold G, Thapar A: The genetic aetiology of childhood depression: a review. J Child Psychol Psychiatry 43:65–79, 2002.
12. Wade TJ, Cairney J: Age and depression in a nationally representative sample of Canadians: a preliminary look at the National Population Health Survey. Can J Public Health 88:297–302, 1997.
13. Kovacs M, Devlin B: Internalizing disorders in childhood. J Child Psychol Psychiatry 39:47–63, 1998.
14. Brent DA, Holder D: A clinical psychotherapy trial for adolescent depression comparing cognitive, family and supportive therapy. Arch Gen Psychiatry 54:877–885, 1997.
15. Fact Sheet on Adolescent Suicide. San Francisco: National Adolescent Health Information Center, University of California, 2000.
*16. Luby JL, Heffelfinger AK, Mrakotsky C, et al: The clinical picture of depression in preschool children. J Am Acad Child Adolesc Psychiatry 42:340–348, 2003.
17. Luby JL, Mrakotsky C, Heffelfinger AK, et al: Characteristics of depressed preschoolers with and without anhedonia: evidence for a melancholic depressive subtype in young children. Am J Psychiatry 161:1998–2004, 2004.
18. Weissman MM, Wolk S, Wickramaratne P, et al: Children with prepubertal-onset major depressive disorder and anxiety grown up. Arch Gen Psychiatry 56:794–801, 1999.
19. Sharp LK, Lipsky MS: Screening for depression across the lifespan: a review of measures for use in primary care settings. Am Fam Physician 66:1001–1008, 2002.
20. Logan DE, King CA: Parental identification of depression and mental health service use among depressed adolescents. J Am Acad Child Adolesc Psychiatry 41:296–304, 2002.
*21. Angold A, Messer SC, Stangl D, et al: Perceived parental burden and service use for child and adolescent psychiatric disorders. Am J Public Health 88:75–80, 1998.
22. Eley TC, Ling H, Plomin R, et al: Parental familial vulnerability, family enviroment and their interactions as predictors of depressive symptoms in adolescents. J Am Acad Child Adolesc Psychiatry 43:298–306, 2004.
23. Coyle JT, Pine DS, Charney DS, et al: Depression and Bipolar Support Alliance consensus statement on the unmet needs in diagnosis and treatment of mood disorders in children and adolescents. J Am Acad Child Adolesc Psychiatry 42:1494–1503, 2003.
24. Wise MG, Rundell JR: Concise Guide to Consultation Psychiatry. Washington, DC: American Psychiatric Press, 1988.
25. Center for Drug Evaluation and Research: FDA Public Health Advisory: Suicidality in Children and Adolescents Being Treated with Antidepressant Medications. Washington, DC: U.S. Food and Drug Administration, 2004.
*26. March J, Silva S, Petrycki S, et al: Fluoxetine, cognitive-behavior therapy, and their combination for adolescents with depression: Treatment for Adolescents with Depression Study (TADS) randomized controlled trial. JAMA 292:861–863, 2004.
27. Garland EJ: Facing the evidence: antidepressant treatment in children and adolescents. CMAJ 170:489–491, 2004.
28. Physicians' Desk Reference (PDR), 58th ed. Montvale, NJ: Thomson Healthcare, 2004.
29. Emslie GJ, Mayes TL: Mood disorders in children and adolescents: psychopharmacological treatment. Biol Psychiatry 49:1082–1090, 2001.
30. Ambrosini PJ, Bianchi MD, Rabinovich H, Elia J: Antidepressant treatments in children and adolescents I. Affective disorders. J Am Acad Child Adolesc Psychiatry 32:1–6, 1993.

*Selected readings.

Chapter 118

Sexual Abuse

Mathew A. Seibel, MD and Deborah Scott, RN, ARNP

Key Points

An understanding of normal prepubertal gynecologic anatomy can help distinguish abnormal anatomy associated with abuse from other genital complaints.

Due to the dynamics of prepubertal sexual abuse, children will often present with a variety of minor or superficial complaints masking the real problem

Many children who have been sexually abused will have normal examinations.

Knowledge of the differences between a purely medical examination and an examination in which forensic issues are to be considered is essential and can completely alter the provider's approach to diagnostics and documentation.

Introduction and Background

Physicians in the emergency department may be asked to evaluate and examine children and adolescents who may have been sexually abused. Such complaints evoke strong, emotional responses in professionals treating these patients and their families. Knowledge of sexual abuse in children has grown rapidly in the past 20 years. Numerous studies of normal genital findings, findings associated with genital trauma and abuse, where and when to perform sexual abuse exams, and what should be included in a complete sexual abuse examination have increased our understanding of the problem.[1-14] Many medical and community leaders are continually working to define protocols for medical and forensic evaluations.[15-20]

The dynamics of child sexual abuse are unique in the spectrum of human crisis response. Child sexual assault rarely involves "stranger danger." Currently available data from many sources indicate that over 80% of perpetrators are known to the child victim, and many sexually abused children are related to the perpetrator by blood or parental remarriage. Fathers are equally likely to be to perpetrators as stepfathers. Children also frequently report assault by other close relatives such as siblings, uncles, cousins, and grandfa-

thers. Perpetrators also include nonfamilial persons who are in a position of trust by the child and family, such as teachers, clergy, scoutmasters, coaches, and mentors. Less than 5% of reported child sexual assaults involve total strangers. The number is a bit higher for adolescents, though relatives and acquaintances remain the predominant source of origin. Interfamilial factors such as the divisiveness of allegations, denial, financial considerations, social isolation, loss of domicile, and threat of incarceration, make it difficult to assume that nonabusing parents and family members will step into the protective supportive roles that are readily seen in a family in crisis from a disease. Alternately, some children may present to the emergency department with a description of symptoms of sexual abuse that are aggressively pursued by a caregiver despite significant information to the contrary. The dynamics of this type of presentation may include factitious disorder, attempts to create custody barriers, and projection of the caregiver's own sexual abuse history onto the child. However, this scenario still leaves significant concerns for the emergency physician as to the physical and emotional safety of the child.

Recent articles have suggested that up to 1 of every 4 females and 1 of every 7 males will be a victim of some form of inappropriate sexual contact by the age of 18 years.[1] Some emergency physicians will experience contact with these types of cases monthly and others much less frequently. In either case, one must be aware of both the immediate medical treatment responsibilities and responsibilities to local law enforcement agencies, social services agencies, and the legal system. Many communities now have experts who specialize in evaluation of sexually abused children and adolescents. Under these conditions, recognition of the problem and appropriate referral is the standard of care. Other communities rely on emergency medical professionals to identify, evaluate, and treat these children at their most vulnerable time.

Recognition/Approach

Recognition of signs and symptoms of child sexual abuse involves an awareness of the types of behaviors that are typically reported by children to have occurred so as to better understand the types of findings that may or may not be present. Younger children will use terms and descriptions that make sense to them to explain incidents and events that have occurred. For example a child may describe an encounter as " 'X' put a stick in my butt." While the child may not have actually seen a stick, he or she may be trying to explain the insertion of a rigid, stick-sized object into the rectum and that this triggered a sharp sensation. A child may give details as simple as "white pee" or as involved as "choking his pee-pee by the neck until it throws up" to describe witnessing ejaculation. Many of the types of behavior described are physically noninjurious, and the examiner may be left with a feeling of helplessness in trying to evaluate something that does not create any physical findings.[14]

In male children, sexual abuse may involve fondling, pinching, squeezing, or oral manipulation of the penis, testicles, and anal area, or tying off of the penis with a ligature. It can also involve penetration of the anus or mouth. Children can be forced to assist in masturbating their assailants. In cases in which a boy is describing an event that happened in the past, a thorough external physical inspection of the child is typically all that is required. Cultures and DNA evidence are not typically necessary. The normalcy of the examination should be considered to be consistent with the child's statements, documented fully, and turned over to the legal and social services agencies for the remainder of the investigation.[10]

The approach to the evaluation of the sexually abused female child is more complicated and must be based on an understanding of normal pediatric and adolescent behavior as well as normal pediatric and adolescent genital anatomy and physiology (Fig. 118–1). In female sexual abuse, common complaints include touching, fondling, and putting things into various orifices such as the mouth, anus, and vagina. Again, the descriptions may involve the child's normal vocabulary to explain her perceptions and understandings of events beyond her full scope of comprehension. A detailed history of any symptoms that occurred at the time of this event will help to formulate an impression for different types of injuries and findings. Frequently the opportunity to clarify the initial description occurs during the actual examination.

Anatomic differences among newborn, prepubertal, and adolescent females are striking. Normal newborn female anatomy is strongly influenced by maternal hormones, and at birth the anatomic structures appear almost "adolescent like." The external labia and the prepuce are somewhat edematous, causing a more pronounced appearance. The clitoris is frequently prominent. The hymen is fuller and petaled or ruffled in appearance, and has a pale, whitewashed pink color. Physiologic leukorrhea is often present. As estrogen withdrawal progresses, discharge becomes serous in some infants. After several months, the anatomy changes and maternal hormone depletion allows the anatomy to become that of a prepubertal female. The labia, prepuce, and clitoris become smaller, and the minor labia and perivaginal structures become somewhat atrophic.[21]

Contrary to many layperson assumptions, an imperforate hymen is a medical anomaly, not the norm. The hymen is a ring of tissue that sits at the opening of the vagina and has a central opening creating an annular, crescentric, or fimbriated appearance. It often contains clefts and tags along the hymenal rim where longitudinal ridges form within the vagina to meet the hymen. The hymen itself can vary from thin and translucent to a thicker, more fascia-like appearance. Less frequently the hymenal opening may be divided by one or more bands of tissue, creating a septate appearance. Rarely the hymen may appear more like a solid sheet with multiple holes and areas of varied thickness, described as a cribiform hymen.[22,23]

During the peripubertal period, as external genitalia progress through the Tanner 2 and 3 stages, changes will also be noted in the appearance of the minor labia and the hymen. The labia begin to elongate until they meet posterior to the hymen (Tanner stages 4 and 5). The hymen becomes thicker and less translucent and develops a more rubbery appearance. The tissue continues to develop until it creates a mature, petaled or redundant mass that to varying extents occludes the opening of the vagina. It will again have a physiologic leukorrhea and a pale, whitewashed pink color. Children at the Tanner 2 and 3 stages may be aware of some vaginal discharge. Menarche ensues in late Tanner 3 to Tanner 4 stages of development.

Clinical Presentation

Sexually abused children and adolescents frequently present with a history of anogenital symptoms or trauma.[24] With toddlers, the disclosures frequently are triggered by

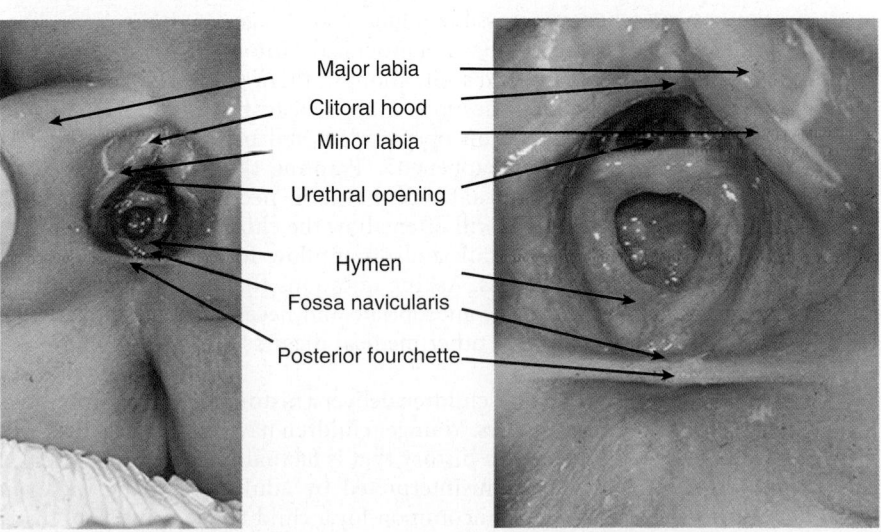

Major labia
Clitoral hood
Minor labia
Urethral opening

Hymen
Fossa navicularis
Posterior fourchette

FIGURE 118–1. Normal genital anatomy of the child (left) and adolescent (right).

Table 118–1	Typical Presenting Symptoms of Acute Sexual Abuse

Genital or rectal pain
Genital or rectal bleeding
Vaginal discharge
Genital or rectal inflammation or redness
History of abuse with or without symptoms
Constipation
Dysuria
Acute behavioral changes

discomfort in the genital area during bathing. After gathering more history, this is often determined to be the result of trauma that actually occurred at some time in the past. In these cases the emergency is more frequently a parental emergency, rather than an actual medical emergency. In other cases patients with genitourinary, rectal, or abdominal complaints have in fact been acutely sexually molested. Some may present with symptoms of anxiety (Table 118–1).

History should optimally be taken after one has established some type of rapport with the patient. The appearance of the interviewer (male vs. female, older vs. younger) can be an issue to the patient and may affect the quality of the history obtained. A quiet environment is preferable, and parties present must be supportive and nonjudgmental in their approach. Involved parties present during the interview or history may significantly affect the content of any history obtained. It is important to excuse all suspected or involved parties from the examination room throughout the evaluation. This may be a problem with special needs children or children who are minimally verbal. This can also trigger a very strong separation anxiety for the parent who is already feeling insecure in his or her ability to protect the child; however, there needs to be an opportunity for the child to provide his or her version of the history without cues, interruptions, or interjections by the adult. Along with providing an environment away from the parent or caregiver, the interviewer must be careful to limit his or her own emotional responses. Children frequently shut down communication when they notice that the information they are providing upsets the caregiver or interviewer.

Document accurately all historical statements made by the child. Include quotes and the exact wording of comments made by the patient whenever possible. Open-ended, age-appropriate questions are best, but may not provide the information needed to assess the child's situation if there is significant apprehension. Direct questions may need to be asked, and then followed up with an open-ended "tell me more about that" or "then what happened?" Framing the questions from the context of medical concern and the need to appropriately provide treatment will often allow the child to overcome initial reluctance to talk and often allow for inclusion in the future legal process. Asking questions that facilitate differential diagnostics are appropriate and necessary in these cases just as with any other medical diagnosis and should not be avoided.

It is important to understand how children deliver a history regarding emotionally difficult issues. Younger children have difficulty with time and often give a history that is factually correct but easily misleading or misinterpreted by adults when it seems to change. It is not uncommon for a child to mix several events that have occurred at different times and thus appear to give untruthful histories, when actually they are telling several "truths" simultaneously. Children can also give a history of events that did not occur due to suggestions by adults who may have secondary gain issues. These patients will have great difficulty with specifics and frequently be much less clear about the specific details of the allegations. Careful use of developmentally appropriate vocabulary and a simple question format can slow the history but is much more accurate.

When there are concerns for sexual abuse, the physical examination should be comprehensive.[25] By focusing on the patient's genitals alone, signs and symptoms pertinent to the final diagnosis may be overlooked, such as cutaneous injury, tonsilar contusions, grip marks, and abrasions. Sedation is only rarely necessary to complete the examination, but can be considered when fear or pain is severe enough to prevent a thorough medical examination. The need for collection of forensic evidence or to fully visualize or culture the vaginal orifice also increases the need for sedation. More often than not, time and a calming atmosphere is all that is necessary to perform an appropriate examination. When sedation is necessary, short-acting benzodiazepines or barbiturates are most frequently used.

Examine the perineum and the introitus in the supine lithotomy or frog leg position. Older texts defer the use of stirrups; however, many children are quite comfortable when the stirrups are shortened to accommodate the shorter leg length. Supine inspection should reveal most traumatic findings. The labia may appear either closed or gaping and need to be separated to reveal the vestibule and structures including the urethra and hymen. Use gentle outward and downward traction of the major labia to flatten the pelvic floor and allow optimal visualization of the vaginal area. Be careful not to pull laterally as this can sometimes tear posterior labial adhesions not initially recognized, causing pain or bleeding from the posterior fourchette. In prepubescent children, vaginal speculums are almost never required. Occasionally nasal speculums can be used to further spread the opening, but this should only occur under anesthesia and after carefully documenting the preprocedural state of the child's anatomy and the presence and location of any bleeding. This prevents the examination itself from clouding the diagnosis.

It is important to document the hymenal shape and configuration. The size of the hymenal opening is relatively unimportant. It is considered normal when there is a 1-mm rim of hymen present.[16,17] The anterior-posterior diameter can normally be elongated in overweight girls.

The vaginal examination can be enhanced by placing the child in the prone knee-chest position. Separating the buttocks upward and outward can provide the best view of the hymen. Loose or redundant hymens are also best visualized in this position. This position is not always required if the supine examination is adequate. The rectal examination can be performed supine but is best done in the prone knee-chest position. Separation of the buttocks will provide an excellent view of the rectum. Relaxation by the patient can allow dilation of the rectal opening. Visualization of the skin and mucosa inward to the dentate line is appropriate. Circumferential vascular congestion in the perianal area will increase during the examination and should not be confused with contusion. Instrumentation is rarely needed even for forensic sample collection. Sedation is necessary to evaluate and repair more extensive trauma, if suspected.

Examination of the adolescent female is essentially equivalent to the examination of an adult female. Tanner stage 3 through 5 females can be evaluated with a routine gynecologic examination, recognizing that this will be the first such exam in many traumatized girls. Detailed attention to the external and prevaginal anatomy should precede the speculum insertion. Translucent disposable speculums greatly facilitate the thorough inspection of the entire vaginal canal, as well as the cervix. Adolescents may be physiologically mature but emotionally immature or regressed during crisis, and these developmental and psychological issues need to be considered and accommodated prior to initiating the examination. Many locations have victim advocates who assist with this during the examination. In other locations, another staff person or a support person brought to the emergency department by the victim can assist in this role.

Penile examinations typically involve inspection only. Retraction of the foreskin in uncircumcised boys may reveal trauma to the glans. In circumstances in which repair is required, sedation will be necessary during repair and again at the time of suture removal to prevent further psychological trauma, especially if the initial injury involved any form of instrumentation. Certain physical findings are diagnostic of sexual abuse, while others only raise suspicion of sexual abuse (Table 118–2).

Photographic documentation of any abnormal finding is the standard of care for a forensic examination. This can be done using video or still photography. In specialized sexual trauma evaluation centers, colposcopes are frequently used, though a camera with a macro lens can also be used with excellent results. The purpose is to document a magnified image of any perineal, vaginal, penile, or rectal physical findings. Multiple images from different angles, with different amounts of traction, and while the child is in different positions are needed. This is due in part to medicolegal requirements and the desire to prevent a need for a second examination. Labeled drawings should also accompany the photographs as a part of the medical record.

Testing and treatment for sexually transmitted infection (STI) is not necessary or appropriate in *every* case. In the prepubescent child, data currently suggest a 1% to 5% STI transmission rate related to sexual abuse. STI testing should be reserved for children with acute vaginal injury, body fluid contamination, children who are symptomatic, and children who are found to be pregnant. Anytime a prepubescent child is determined to need testing, genital cultures should be obtained. Do not rely solely on polymerase chain reaction or DNA testing for a child, as many of the nonculture tests have been studied only in adults, causing a potential legal pitfall. With a cooperative child, a swab can be threaded into the vaginal orifice from an anterior angle, thus avoiding the highly sensitive posterior hymenal rim. Cultures can often be obtained with a cotton-tipped swab by obtaining cells from discharge external to the hymen. Infection with *Neisseria gonorrhoeae* will cause vaginitis, and cervical specimens are not needed in prepubescent children. The laboratory can be instructed to obtain a DNA analysis from a culture sample, but a culture cannot be obtained from a DNA specimen. This applies to both *N. gonorrhoeae* and Chlamydia testing. Genital herpes and Chlamydia can frequently be tested from the same specimen. Blood testing for syphilis (rapid plasma reagent) and human immunodeficiency virus (HIV) should also be obtained.[26]

In situations in which the history provided by the child indicates that the event was extremely recent, there may be DNA evidence from the assailant on the child's body. Suspected areas can be swabbed with a dry, cotton-tipped applicator to attempt evidence collection. Suspected areas can often be identified by the use of a black light. If the area being swabbed is already moist (i.e., a rectal vault, oral cavity, or a wet fold on the skin), using a dry cotton-tipped applicator is all that is necessary. It should be moved across the area in a gentle rolling motion to lift rather than smash the secretions onto the swab. If the area is already dried, moisten the swab with a small amount of sterile saline before collecting the evidence. Cultures and DNA collection are necessary only when the child describes a perpetrator's bodily fluid as having had contact with the skin, and there has been no time for the evidence to be removed through bathing, urinating, defecating, or eating or drinking, depending on the orifice involved.[27] DNA collection swabs should be fully dried prior to submitting the specimen to law enforcement. Specialized equipment for this process is commercially available. Detailed instructions for specimen collection are included in most evidentiary rape kits, but these are often based upon adult examinations. Only the portion of the kit that is medically indicated by history and physical examination findings should be utilized.

Important Clinical Features and Considerations

There are multiple emergency department presentations that may or may not represent child sexual abuse (Table 118–3).

Table 118–2	Physical Findings

Physical Findings DIAGNOSTIC of Sexual Abuse

Pregnancy in a child under the age of legal consent
Gonorrhea, syphilis, or HIV in a prepubescent child, other than a neonate
Semen in the vaginal vault of a child under the age of consent
Sperm, motile cells, or evidence of acid phosphatase
Acute laceration of the hymen with a history of sexual assault
A witnessed event of sexual assault
Photographic documentation of the sexual assault occurring

Physical Findings SUSPICIOUS FOR Sexual Abuse

Acute bruising of thigh, labia, and/or vestibule
Acute laceration of labia and/or external genitalia
Acute laceration of hymen
Nonacute hymenal changes
Presenting with genital inflammation and/or discharge
Acute and nonacute rectal findings
Penile injuries
Associated nongenital injuries
STIs
- *Chlamydia* and condylomata in children can be from abuse or present in children of up to 2–3 years of age from vertical transmission that has been dormant prior to presentation.
- Herpes can present from abuse or autoinfection.

Abbreviations: HIV, human immunodeficiency virus; STI, sexually transmitted infection.

Table 118–3	Signs and Symptoms Concerning for Possible Sexual Abuse

Bleeding (Rectal/Vaginal)

Nonsexual trauma—abrasions or lacerations of the vestibule or labia

Prolapsed urethra—seen as hemorrhagic tissue that often fills the area in front of the vestibule, obscuring the hymen

Straddle injury—seen as laceration or bleeding from the area of the posterior fourchette; often there is associated bruising

Precocious puberty—menstrual bleeding

Maternal estrogen withdrawal—neonates only

Gastrointestinal infections such as Shigella, Salmonella, or *Escherichia coli*

Rectal fissure—very common, especially in younger children

Hemorrhoid—not common in younger healthy children

Pain (Vaginal/Rectal/Penile)

Bacterial infections, such as with β-hemolytic streptococcus

UTI or urethritis

Perirectal abscess

Pinworms—can involve the rectum or vagina

Periurethral cyst

Nonsexual trauma with or without bruising

HSV infection—can be secondary to abuse or spread from oral lesions by patient

Discharge (Vaginal/Penile)

Nonspecific vaginitis—often seen with small amounts of green or yellow discharge

Balanitis

Hygiene—poor care can allow for nonspecific discharge

Physiologic leukorrhea

Foreign body—presents with recurrent discharge; sometimes examination under anesthesia is required for diagnosis

Redness or Swelling (Vaginal/Penile/Rectal)

Contact dermatitis

Thermal injury

Irritation from soaps, detergents

Infections such as yeast, staphylococcus, streptococcus

Laxative use causing perirectal burning

Lichen sclerosis—long-term irritation with itching

Abnormal Appearance (Vaginal/Rectal/Penile)

Septum—most often vertical but can also be horizontal

Gaping or "too big" vaginal opening

Dilated rectal opening when in knee-chest position

Imperforate anus with anterior fistula

Imperforate hymen

Labial adhesions—both posterior and anterior connections

Healed hymenal transection

Lesions—warts, molluscum contagiosum, Bartholin's gland cyst

Behavioral Changes "Suggestive of Sexual Activity"

Masturbation—many normal children masturbate

Inserting foreign objects into the vagina or rectum

Acting out of a sexual act with dolls, pets, or other children

Knowledge of Sexual Activity Abnormal for Age and Known Lifestyle Exposures

Abbreviations: HSV, herpes simplex virus; UTI, urinary tract infection.

Table 118–4	Circumstances in Sexual Abuse That Warrant Hospitalization

- Trauma so severe as to require surgical repair and postoperative observation
- Severe bleeding requiring observation for hemostasis
- Multidimensional trauma in which the need to care for other physical injuries, such as fractures, head injuries, dehydration, and chest and abdominal trauma, is a higher level of concern
- Social instability—the safety of the child in these situations is imperative and, if the social instability is potentially hazardous to this child, medical admission is appropriate; coding guidelines are inclusive of this.
- Treatment of unstable unassociated findings

physician may be better equipped to perform the differential evaluations for urinary tract infection, gastrointestinal bleed, constipation, hemorrhoids, diaper dermatitis, and other conditions.

Management

Management of a child who has been sexually assaulted or abused depends in large part on the community or geographic area where the patient is seen. While the specific wording may vary and different age cutoffs are used, all states mandate the reporting of cases in which there is a suspicion of child abuse and/or neglect. Failure to report is a crime that in some areas is punishable by fine and imprisonment. Awareness of the statutory requirements for the location is critical for both the physician's decision process and the legal process.

In areas in which specialized experts are not available, the emergency physician is the most accessible and appropriate person to evaluate and intervene on behalf of children who may be sexually abused. In areas in which specialized experts are available, the patient is stable, and forensic evidence will not be lost, referral to a trained specialist in a child advocacy center or other child abuse evaluation unit not only is appropriate for the child, but also frequently allows for more appropriate use of the emergency physician's time and resources. Admission to a medical facility is rarely medically necessary. Certain circumstances do warrant hospitalization. (Table 118–4).

Discharge from the emergency department is appropriate only after all evaluations are complete; the findings are documented; forensic evidence has been appropriately collected, labeled, and turned over to the appropriate law enforcement agency; and mandatory reports are made. Many areas have crisis intervention teams whose mission is to deal with sexual abuse victims. This evaluation should take place prior to discharge. Follow-up arrangements should be made for counseling, therapy, or immediate acute behavioral interventions. Arrangements should also be made for follow-up of culture results or other medical findings.

At this time the Centers for Disease Control and Prevention does not recommend HIV prophylaxis for all prepubescent sexual abuse victims. There is a move toward recommending a 1-month course of postexposure prophylaxis for the adolescent and adult sexual assault victim that is the same as the "needlestick" prophylaxis used in hospitals (see Chapter 156, Postexposure Prophylaxis). The local

As with any other medical evaluation, an appropriate differential diagnosis must be explored while fully assessing the child's symptoms, findings, and safety risk. In areas where an advocacy center or rape crisis center is available, the emergency department may defer forensic evaluation and focus strictly upon making sure that the patient is stable for transport to that center. In situations in which nonsexual sources of the complaint are the primary concern, the emergency pediatric infectious disease physician is an excellent resource for the most current recommendations for the prepubescent child and should be consulted in any case in which this is being considered. Decisions regarding the treatment of suspected STI need to be made on suspicion or likelihood of positive findings and likely ability for medical follow-up.

Law enforcement officers are often present in the emergency department. Communication with law enforcement is an integral part of the care of the sexual abuse/assault victim because of the criminal act involved and for maintaining a safe environment for the patient. The emergency physician should expect discussions with law enforcement and social services. The history and physical must be obtained and documented with the presumption that it will be reviewed by the law enforcement agent, the state prosecutor, a defense attorney, and a defense-sponsored medical expert. Deposition and criminal courtroom testimony by the examining physician will certainly occur when the child gives a positive history and/or when physical findings are present. Juvenile courts may also require testimony if an extended investigation shows a need to consider alternate living arrangements for the child.

Summary

Overall, medical prognosis from sexual abuse is excellent. Life-threatening injury is extremely rare. The psychological impact of these events is much more profound and, due to the fact that so many of these events are intrafamilial, the allegations alone will potentially permanently alter family dynamics and structure. Even under the best circumstances with widespread support of the victim, optimal medical care, available counseling, and swift and effective prosecution, many of these children will go on to have problems with interpersonal relationships and have a higher potential for self-destructive behaviors such as alcoholism, drug dependency, sexual promiscuity, and self-mutilation. These problems can present months or years later as posttraumatic stress disorder or other psychological abnormalities. The initial contact with the emergency department is often the place where the child's emotional healing can begin. As a medical authority figure, the emergency physician may be able to empower the victim to realize that he or she is not responsible for the actions of others, is healthy and "whole" as a person, and has a right to pursue a happy, fulfilling life. The emergency provider should take the time to communicate these basic tenants to the child whenever possible.

REFERENCES

1. Bays J, Jenny C: Genital and anal conditions confused with child sexual abuse trauma. Am J Dis Child 144:1319–1322, 1990.
2. Benton S: Child abuse or mimic—is there a medical explanation? Consultant for Pediatricians, Jan:2–5, 2003.
3. Berenson AB, Chacko MR, Wiemann CM, et al: Use of hymenal measurements in the diagnosis of previous penetration. Pediatrics 109:228–335, 2002.
4. Boos SC, Rosas AJ, Boyle C, McCann J: Anogenital injuries in child pedestrians run over by low-speed motor vehicles: four cases with findings that mimic child sexual abuse. Pediatrics 112(1 Pt 1):e77–e84, 2003.
5. Botash AS, Jean-Louis F: Imperforate hymen: congenital or acquired from sexual abuse? Pediatrics 108:e53, 2001.
*6. Christian CW, Lavelle JM, De Jong AR et al: Forensic evidence findings in prepubertal victims of sexual abuse. Pediatrics 106(1 Pt 1):100–104, 2000.
7. Heger AH, Ticson L, Guerra L, et al: Appearance of the genitalia in girls selected for nonabuse: review of hymenal morphology and nonspecific findings. J Pediatr Adolesc Gynecol 15:27–35, 2002.
8. Herrmann B, Crawford J: Genital injuries in prepubertal girls from inline skating accidents. Pediatrics 110(2 Pt 1):e16–e18, 2002.
9. Kadish HA, Schunk JE, Britton H: Pediatric male rectal and genital trauma: accidental and nonaccidental injuries. Pediatr Emerg Care 14:95–98, 1998.
10. McCann J: Use of the colposcope in child sexual abuse examinations. Pediatr Clin North Am 37:863–880, 1990.
11. McCann J, Voris J: Perianal injuries resulting from sexual abuse: a longitudinal study. Pediatrics 91:390–397, 1993.
12. Myhre AK, Berntzen K, Bratlid D: Genital anatomy in non-abused preschool girls. Acta Paediatr 92:1453–1462, 2003.
13. Emans SJ, Woods ER, Allred EN, Grace E: Hymenal findings in adolescent women: impact of tampon use and consensual sexual activity. J Pediatr 125:153–160, 1994.
14. Kellogg ND, Menard SW, Santos A: Genital anatomy in pregnant adolescents: "normal" does not mean "nothing happened." Pediatrics 113(1 Pt 1):e67–e69, 2004.
15. Terminology Subcommittee, APSAC Task Force on Medical Evaluation of Suspected Child Abuse, Adams J (chair): APSAC Practice Guidelines: Descriptive Terminology in Child Sexual Abuse Medical Evaluations. Charleston, SC: American Professional Society on the Abuse of Children. Available from *http://apsac.fmhi.usf.edu*
16. Adams J: Evolution of a classification scale: medical evaluation of suspected child sexual abuse. Child Maltreat 6:31–36, 2001.
17. Adams J: Medical evaluation of suspected child sexual abuse. J Pediatr Adolesc Gynecol 17:191–197, 2004.
*18. American Academy of Pediatrics, Committee on Child Abuse and Neglect: Guidelines for the evaluation of sexual abuse of children: subject review. Pediatrics 103:186–191, 1999.
19. American Academy of Pediatrics, Committee on Adolescence: Sexual assault and the adolescent. Pediatrics 94:761–765, 1994.
20. American Academy of Pediatrics, Committee on Adolescence: Sexually transmitted diseases. 94(4 Pt 1):568–572, 1994.
21. Botash AS: Evaluating Child Sexual Abuse: Education Manual for Medical Professionals. Baltimore: The John Hopkins University Press, 2000.
22. Girardin BW, Faugno DK, Seneski PC, et al: Color Atlas of Sexual Assault. St. Louis: Mosby, 1997.
23. Giardino AP, Datner E, Asher J, et al: Sexual Assault Victimization Across the Life Span: A Color Atlas. St. Louis: GW Medical Publishing, 2003.
24. Gordon S, Jaudes PK: Sexual abuse evaluations in the emergency department: is the history reliable? Child Abuse Negl 20:315–322, 1996.
25. Britton H: Emotional impact of the medical examination for child sexual abuse. Child Abuse Negl 22:573–579, 1998.
*26. Centers for Disease Control and Prevention: Sexually transmitted diseases treatment guidelines 2002. MMWR Recomm Rep 51(RR-6):1–78, 2002.
27. Ingram DL, Everett VD, Flick LA, et al: Vaginal gonococcal cultures in sexual abuse evaluation: evaluation of selected criteria for preteens. Pediatrics 99:e8, 1997.

*Selected readings.

Chapter 119

Physical Abuse and Child Neglect

Irene Tien, MD, MSc

Key Points

Physical abuse should always be considered in children presenting to the emergency department for a traumatic injury.

The American Academy of Pediatrics recommends that the evaluation of infants and young children for physical abuse should include a skeletal survey if the child is 2 years old or younger and retinal examination if 3 years old or younger. A head computed tomography scan should be considered if there is suspicion of abuse and the child has neurologic signs or symptoms, is under 6 months old, has fractures suggestive of abuse, or has bruises on the face.

A child may be neglected if his or her basic needs are not being met, including clothing, food, and shelter as well as adequate supervision, emotional needs, and education.

It is the ethical and legal obligation of health care providers to report cases of suspected child abuse or neglect to child protective services.

Introduction and Background

Of the 4.5 million children who were reported to child protective services (CPS) in 2002, 896,000 were abused.[1] Thirty-four percent of neglect and 10% of physical abuse cases were reported to CPS by medical professionals in 2002.[1] It is especially important that abused children are not misdiagnosed and are not returned to a dangerous environment, because abuse does not occur in isolation. Many abused children have a past history of hospitalization and many who are returned to the custody of their parents are subsequently abused.[2,3] Furthermore, studies have shown that some infants who are seen by a physician who did not recognize the diagnosis of abuse were subsequently re-injured, resulting in preventable deaths.[4] Abused children suffer higher in-hospital mortality and morbidity rates than children with accidental injuries.[5-7] Those who recover are more likely to have residual neurologic deficits, behavioral problems, mental health problems,

and substance abuse disorders, and to become adult abuse perpetrators or victims.[8-16]

The federal Child Abuse Prevention and Treatment Act (CAPTA) of 1976 established CPS agencies that were vested with the responsibility of investigating suspected child abuse and protecting children.[8,17] In the United States, all physicians are legally required to report cases of suspected abuse to their local CPS agency.[18] It is the ethical and legal obligation of all physicians to be aware of how to identify abused children and to know what to do when they think they are taking care of a child who has been injured from abuse.

During 2002, 61% of victims suffered physical abuse and 19% suffered neglect.[1] Federal legislation describes a minimum set of acts or behaviors that define child abuse and neglect: "any recent act or failure to act on the part of a parent or caretaker which results in death, serious physical or emotional harm, sexual abuse or exploitation or an act or failure to act which presents an imminent risk of serious harm."[19] Specific definitions of what constitutes abuse or neglect vary between states.

Recognition and Approach

History Gathering

The key to the diagnosis of physical abuse and child neglect is to always consider it in the differential diagnosis of childhood injury. The importance of a complete history cannot be overemphasized. The clinician must ask enough questions in order to clearly understand how an injury occurred and to resolve apparent discrepancies. In general, adults and children should be individually questioned in their primary language in a quiet, private space. Extended questioning of children is discouraged as they are especially vulnerable to distortions of memory. Children often perceive repeated questioning as a sign that their previous answers were wrong.[20] This may lead to a distortion of a child's account of his or her abuse during subsequent questioning by investigative officials. The approach should be supportive and neutral, using open-ended questions.[21] Appropriate preparation of the child for questioning is also necessary and important (Table 119–1).

General Approach to Physical Abuse

When evaluating any injured child, the clinician should consider the six core questions listed in Table 119–2. Answers to these questions will depend upon the understanding of the

Table 119–1	**Recommended Approach to History Gathering for Child Abuse Concerns**

Who Should Be Interviewed

- Parents and other witnesses to the injury or those present at the time when the injury was first noticed.
- Children, only if it is necessary to determine safety or immediate medical needs.

How To Conduct Interview

General considerations:

- Interview in the respondent's first language when possible. Use interpreter services.
- Use a quiet and private space.
- Interview the adults out of earshot of the child and vice versa.
- Give adolescents the option of being interviewed with or without the parents.
- Obtain the history of the events through open-ended statements, such as "Tell me why you are here."
- Avoid leading questions.
- Remain calm and sensitive.
- Minimize the number of interviews.

Special considerations for questioning children:

- Children are especially vulnerable to distortions in their recall of an event.
- Repeated questioning may be interpreted by the child that his or her previous answers were wrong.
- Do not question unless it is necessary for identification of immediate medical needs or assessment of safety in returning the child home from the emergency department.
- Interview in a supportive but neutral manner.
  - Do not suggest that you know what the child is thinking, how he or she should feel, or what has happened.
  - Show interest in the child's statements, and praise the effort in giving responses (not the content of the responses).
  - Use predominantly open-ended questions.
- Prepare the child for the interview.
  - Introduce yourself.
  - Give an age-appropriate explanation of what is going to happen.
  - Instruct the child that it is fine to say that he or she doesn't understand a question, doesn't know the answer, or doesn't wish to respond.

What Information Should Be Asked

- Obtain the details of who, what, when, where, and how.
- Ask enough questions that the story makes sense to you. For example, if the parent states that the child fell off of the bed, ask how they know that. Did they witness the fall? Did they find the child on the floor and presume the child fell?
- Obtain an extended social history.
  - Names, ages, addresses, and phone numbers of guardians, parents, other caregivers, and other children potentially at risk.
  - Details of the caregiving and custody arrangements for this child.
- Use screening questions for domestic violence (DV). There is concurrent DV in up to 50% of child physical abuse cases.[23]
  - Have you been hit, kicked, or punched by a partner in the past year?
  - Do you feel safe in your current relationship?
  - Is there a partner from a past relationship who is making you feel unsafe right now?
- Include other questions you feel necessary to ask to assess the child's immediate safety and the safety of other possibly involved children.

patterns of the presentation of abuse and the epidemiology, biomechanics, pathophysiology, and differential diagnosis of childhood injuries. A detailed history and physical examination are pivotal to arriving at an accurate conclusion about the likelihood of an injured child having been abused. This may differ from a more focused emergency department (ED) evaluation for other conditions.

General Approach to Neglect

Child neglect comes in many different forms, including emotional neglect, educational neglect, medical neglect, failure to provide health care, supervisory neglect, abandonment, inability to provide basic needs (food, shelter, clothing), inadequate protection from environmental hazards (e.g., failure to secure in a car seat, allowing access to a loaded gun), and drug exposure of neonates and children (Table 119–3).[22] An initial assessment of neglect should begin by answering the six core questions listed in Table 119–2.[22]

Filing with Child Protective Services

Definitive proof of abuse or neglect is not required to make a report to CPS. It is the job of CPS to follow up on all cases in which there is reasonable concern of abuse or neglect. Physicians are legally required to report suspicions of neglect.

This may include a report to law enforcement in addition to CPS. Specific procedures for reporting vary by state, and emergency physicians must be knowledgeable about these procedures. The Child Welfare Information Gateway provides information about reporting laws in each state on its web site (*www.childwelfare.gov/systemwide/laws_policies/search/index.cfm*).

Clinical Presentation

Physical Abuse

The identification of child abuse is very challenging. Health care providers traditionally begin their medical decision making based upon a gathered history. Children injured from abuse, however, often present for medical care without an accurate history.[23] Abused infants may present with vague signs and symptoms. Many of the injuries sustained from child abuse are also sustained through accidental mechanisms or may be confused with nontraumatic findings.[5,10,20,23-30] Clinicians must become familiar with the patterns of child abuse and neglect presentation and with recommendations for screening for occult injuries in order to identify abuse.[31,32] This requires that a detailed history and examination be performed in the evaluation of every injured child.

Table 119–2	Six Core Questions to Ask during an Assessment for Physical Abuse and Neglect

Physical Abuse

1. How did the injury happen?
   - A first-hand account by whoever witnessed the injury or the first signs of injury is preferable.
2. When did the injury happen?
3. Could it be abuse?
4. What medical and social considerations make you more or less concerned about abuse?
   - Consider the biomechanics and epidemiology of this injury for a child of this age given the mechanism described.
   - Consider the family's history of having been reported to child protective services (CPS) in the past; approximately 30% of families reported to CPS once will be reported again in 18 months.[48]
5. What is the medical prognosis for this child?
6. What is the safety prognosis for this child?

Neglect

1. Are the child's needs not being adequately met? Has this led to demonstrable harm? If not, what is the evidence of potential harm?
2. Has there been a pattern of neglect?
   - For how long?
   - What types?
   - Has CPS been involved?
3. What is contributing to the neglect? Consider child, parent, family, and community factors.
4. What strengths and resources are available?
5. What interventions have been tried? What were the results?
6. What is the likelihood that changes will occur?
   - Is the family motivated?
   - Do they understand the concern?
   - Are resources available?

Adapted from Dubowitz H, Giardino A, Gustavson E: Child neglect: guidance for pediatricians. Pediatr Rev 21:111–116, 2000.

There is no comprehensive list of historical indicators of physical abuse or child neglect. Patterns of presentation that should increase concern for child abuse include (1) a child who presents for medical care of a significant injury for which there is no history of trauma; (2) the history provided does not explain the injury based upon knowledge of the biomechanics and epidemiology of that injury; (3) the history of how the injury occurred changes significantly over time; (4) the history of self-inflicted injury does not correlate with the child's developmental abilities; (5) there is a delay in seeking medical care that is unexplained or unexpected; and (6) the child discloses abuse or neglect (Table 119–4).[23]

Worrisome historical indicators of abuse are not necessarily in themselves enough to result in a report to CPS. A detailed history and examination should be completed first. Considerations of cultural beliefs as well as specialized challenges associated with poverty or immigration should be taken into account. Reporting of suspected abuse or neglect should be based upon factual information and not "gut feelings," which are subject to personal biases. Biased reporting of child abuse has been shown to be affected by a reporter's perception of a family's ethnicity or socioeconomic status, type and severity of injury, age of the child and parents, and urban location.[23-25] The morbidity associated with reporting cases of nonabuse should be kept in mind. The need for social services support versus CPS investigation should be differentiated.

Child Neglect

Neglected children seek care in the ED for several reasons. Children left home alone may be reported by neighbors and brought into the ED by prehospital providers. Primary care pediatricians may be concerned about failure to thrive and refer children to the ED, or a child may become acutely ill because of dehydration associated with poor nutrition. A child may present with an acute injury related to poor supervision. Familiarity with the types of neglect will help identify cases of neglect (see Table 119–3).

Conditions That May Be Mistaken for Physical Abuse or Child Neglect

Many conditions have been mistaken for physical abuse or child neglect. These include ethnic therapies, mongolian spots, photodermatologic reactions, disorders leading to inadequate bone mineralization and increased susceptibility to fractures, organic causes of failure to thrive, organic causes of subdural hemorrhage, and organic causes of retinal hemorrhage (Table 119–5).

Important Clinical Features and Considerations

The frequent absence of an accurate history and the potential for confusion with nonabusive illness in cases of suspected child abuse require a more aggressive diagnostic evaluation that is not only based upon gathered history and examination findings, but also conducted with consideration of occult injuries (Table 119–6). The American Academy of Pediatrics (AAP) recently published guidelines recommending a skeletal survey in all cases of suspected abuse in children 2 years old or younger.[31] Approximately 15% of physically abused infants will have occult fractures diagnosed on skeletal survey. Thirty to 70% of infants with abusive head trauma will have a fracture on skeletal survey. Skeletal surveys may be considered in children up to 5 years of age, depending on the clinical scenario. For example, children with a predisposition to more easily broken bones (e.g., cerebral palsy) may be more likely to sustain abusive fractures than healthy children of the same age. Repeat skeletal surveys in 2 weeks may also be considered in cases of unclear findings or high risk. An additional 27% of children may have newly identified fractures on repeat skeletal survey.[33]

The AAP also recommends an ophthalmologic examination by an ophthalmologist familiar with retinal findings in child abuse in all children under 3 years of age who are suspected of having been physically abused.[32] As many as 65% to 90% of children with abusive head injury have retinal hemorrhages when examined by an ophthalmologist.[10,26,34-36] In one study, non-ophthalmologist retinal assessments were only accurate in identifying the presence or absence of retinal hemorrhages 87% of the time. An examination was attempted only in 63% of children, and 81% of these attempts resulted in a visualized retina.[37] Characterization of the type, number, and location of retinal hemorrhages is important when determining possible etiologies.[27,38-44]

Table 119-3   Types of Child Neglect*

Type	Definition	Example
Emotional neglect	Inadequate provision of affection, nurturance, or love.	Infant of a mentally ill mother who doesn't provide comfort when the infant cries.
Educational neglect	Failure to enroll a child in school, failure to assure adequate attendance at school without a satisfactory reason, or when special educational needs are not being met.	Teenager expelled from school, but parents do not enroll her in another school.
Medical neglect	Nonimplementation of health care recommendations leading to actual or potential significant harm.	Child with insulin-dependent diabetes not getting or taking prescribed treatments.
Failure or delay in getting health care	Delay or failure in getting health care that results in actual or probable significant harm.	Young child with second-degree burns to his hands who presents several days after the injury.
Supervisory neglect	Inadequate supervision in accordance with the child's developmental needs, resulting in clear risks to his or her health and well-being.	A toddler left unattended near a swimming pool; a preschooler left home alone.
Abandonment	Extreme form of supervisory neglect wherein children are not "claimed" within 2 days or teenagers are forced out of the home.	Parent gets angry at their 12-year-old child, locks him out of the house and does not allow him to return home.
Inability to provide basic needs†	Inadequate provision of food, clothing, shelter, or hygiene.	Child presents with failure to thrive (growth less than 5th percentile for age) for which no medical cause has been identified. Child inadequately dressed for the weather or dressed with poorly fitting clothes (e.g., no jacket in snowy weather; extremely tight-fitting, painful shoes). Child is homeless and sleeping on the street or in a car. Child repeatedly does not meet the basic standards of hygiene (e.g., obviously filthy, not just dirty).
Inadequate protection from environmental hazards	Failure to protect from avoidable environmental hazards.	Failure to use a car seat or seatbelt; riding a bike without a helmet; poisonous household substances left within reach of a child; access to a loaded gun.
Drug exposure of neonates and children	In utero exposure to illegal drugs and alcohol, indirect exposure in infants and older children.	Woman gives birth to a heroin-addicted baby; young child is exposed to second-hand marijuana smoke; child living in a home with a methamphetamine lab.

*A determination of the presence of neglectful behavior by a caregiver toward a child involves a degree of judgment on the part of the clinician. This table is not meant as an all-inclusive definition of child neglect, but rather should serve as a guide as to what could be considered neglectful behavior requiring consideration of a report to CPS.
†Please refer to your state statute for allowances made for poverty.

Table 119-4   Patterns of History or Injury That Should Increase Concern for Physical Abuse or Child Neglect*

Historical Patterns[20,23]

- Significant injuries for which no history is given.
- The history provided does not explain the injury identified. Take into consideration the biomechanics and epidemiology of the injury.
- The history of injury changes significantly over time.
- A history of self-inflicted trauma that doesn't correlate with the child's developmental abilities.
- Delay in seeking treatment for an injury or illness for which there is an inadequate or implausible explanation.
- Disclosure by the child that he or she has been physically, emotionally, or sexually abused by a caregiver.
- Frequently missed health care appointments that can reasonably be expected to result in additional injury to or illness in the child.

Injury Patterns

- Bruising in preambulatory children[49]
- Bruising in ambulatory children in areas not usually associated with normal activities (e.g., inner arms, inner thighs, buttocks, behind the ears, pinnae, trunk)[49]
- Laceration of the inferior or superior frenulum of the lips or the frenulum of the tongue
- Hematoma of the tragus of the ear[50]
- Scars or injuries in the shape of objects
- Traumatic intracranial injuries in children under 2 years for which there is no plausible mechanism, or in a child under 2 years in whom there is no external evidence of injury[51-56]
- Long bone or pelvic fractures in preambulatory children or for which there is no plausible explanation[57-67]
- Rib or metaphyseal fractures in young children[68-70]
- Multiple fractures or fractures of varying ages for which there is no plausible explanation
- Traumatic intra-abdominal injuries (e.g., pancreatic laceration, duodenal hematoma) without appropriate history
- Concerning patterns of burns[71-75]:
  - Bilateral burns of lower extremities
  - Burns localized to the perineal area or buttocks
  - Burns that are circumferential, have a clear tide mark, or do not present with splash marks if they were reported as liquid thermal burns
  - Burns in the shape of an object such as a cigarette or iron
  - "Doughnut sign"—an area of spared skin around which is scalded skin as a result of a child being held down in hot water where the part in contact with the bottom of the tub does not burn
  - Suspicious burns associated with restraint injuries on the upper limbs
- Infant or young child who is less than the 5th percentile on growth chart for weight, height, or head circumference for whom there is no medical history explaining failure to thrive or for whom there is an identified medical cause that the parent(s) are not appropriately managing

*These findings strongly suggest abuse or neglect. This is not intended to be an all-inclusive list of indicators of abuse or neglect.

Table 119–5	Nonabuse/Non-neglect Causes of Findings Mistaken for Abuse/Neglect	
Condition	**Examples**	**Differentiation from Abuse/Neglect**
Ethnic therapies	Coining	Characteristic diagonal bands of ecchymotic and/or petechial lesions in rows over the child's back measuring the approximate width of a coin.
	Cupping	Characteristic uniformly sized, round, ecchymotic and/or petechial lesions over the child's back.
Mongolian spots		Well-demarcated, blue-grey to deep brown or black, irregularly shaped skin lesions most commonly seen in babies of Asian, East Indian, Latino, or African descent. There may be multiple spots on the child that are most commonly seen on the buttocks and back but may be seen on the ankles and wrists. They have a normal overlying skin texture. They appear at birth or shortly after birth and often resolve by puberty. These do not resolve as a bruise would be expected to.
Phytophotodermatitis	Common offending substances: • Meadow grass • Parsley • Parsnips • Celery • Carrots • Limes	Refers to a cutaneous inflammatory rash caused by contact of the skin with a light-sensitizing botanical substance followed by exposure to ultraviolet light.[76] The rash begins as a delayed burning erythema 24–48 hr after exposure followed by frank blisters in 48–72 hr. Postinflammatory hyperpigmentation may last weeks to months. This reaction may be confused with a burn or injuries from being struck.
Increased susceptibility to fractures due to decreased bone mineralization	Rickets Premature or low birth weight infants (<1500 g) Osteogenesis imperfecta (OI) Hypophosphatemia Neuromuscular diseases Menkes' syndrome Osteoporosis	These children have a history consistent with a bone disease. Family history of bone disease should also be sought (OI). Menkes' syndrome is limited to boys and is associated with other problems, including poor tone, failure to thrive, and abnormal skin and hair. Bones of abnormal mineralization are identifiable on radiograph. Consultation with a pediatric radiologist is recommended when there is a concern for abuse and for abnormal bone mineralization.
Conditions with radiographic findings confused with abusive fractures[77]	Hypervitaminosis A	Diffuse periosteal reaction associated with pain and swelling. Child may have anorexia, irritability, and itching. Hard and tender swellings may be palpable over the extremities.
	Rickets	Cupping and fraying of the costochondral junctions and long bone metaphyses.
	Congenital syphilis	Destructive lesions of the metaphyses from osteomyelitis associated with symptoms from multiple organ systems.
	Skeletal dysplasias	May be associated with metaphyseal irregularities. Bones are otherwise not normal in appearance (shortened and dysplastic).
	Scurvy (vitamin C deficiency)	Usually seen in children older than 6 mo who receive milk formulas without vitamin supplements. Metaphyseal fractures and large calcific cloaks may be seen along long bone shafts.
	Copper deficiency	Rare. Associated with neurologic symptoms, pallor, neutropenia, anemia, and hepatosplenomegaly. Metaphyseal cupping and spurring and occasionally rib fractures may be seen.
Decreased intestinal absorption of nutrients, leading to failure to thrive (FTT)	Gluten-sensitive enteropathy Food allergies Gastroesophageal reflux Cystic fibrosis Lactose intolerance Enteric pathogens Renal tubular acidosis Urinary tract infections	Medical causes of FTT are often accompanied by signs and symptoms beyond simply poor growth. Poor growth will be identified at a young age in the vast majority of children presenting for regular medical care. An evaluation for FTT by the child's pediatrician should be initiated at the time of the identification of FTT. Discussion with the child's pediatrician will provide information important to the full evaluation of FTT concerns in the emergency department.
Nonabusive causes of subdural hemorrhages	Birth trauma	Subdural hemorrhages after birth trauma may be normal. These resolve by 3 wk of age and are not associated with neurologic signs/symptoms.[53]
	Ateriovenous malformations Glutaric aciduria type 1 Coagulation disorders	Other nonabusive causes of subdural hemorrhages may be differentiated based upon history, examination, and diagnostic studies.
Nonabusive causes of retinal hemorrhages	Birth trauma	Retinal hemorrhages commonly occur after birth. These should be resolved by 4 wk of age.
	Severe accidental head trauma Severe compressive chest trauma Coagulopathies Blood dyscrasias Meningitis Severe hypertension Vasculitis Thromboembolic phenomena Middle cerebral artery aneurysm	Other non–birth related causes of retinal hemorrhages have an associated history of severe trauma, illness, or laboratory findings suggestive of a blood dyscrasia.

Table 119–6	**Diagnostic Evaluation of Suspected Physical Abuse or Neglect**

Physical Abuse

- **Skeletal survey:** Recommended by the American Academy of Pediatrics (AAP) for all children under 2 yr of age when there is a suspicion of physical abuse. Skeletal survey may be performed selectively in children between 2 and 5 yr of age.[31] A 2-wk follow-up skeletal survey may be considered.[33]
- **Bone scan:** Bone scan may be a useful adjunct to skeletal survey when specifically attempting to delineate posterior rib fractures or other nonmetaphyseal fractures. It should not be used alone in evaluation of the skeleton in cases of suspected physical abuse.[78]
- **Retinal examination:** Recommended by the AAP in all children under 3 yr of age when there is a suspicion of physical abuse.[32] This should be performed by an ophthalmologist.
- **Computed tomography (CT):** In one series, 37% of infants meeting high risk criteria (rib fractures, multiple fractures, facial injury, or age < 6 mo) had an occult head injury.[46] Head CT should be strongly considered in infants meeting these high-risk criteria.
- **Magnetic resonance imaging (MRI):** Currently there are insufficient data to support routine use of MRI to identify abusive injuries. There is some evidence to support usefulness in differentiating abusive from accidental head injury.[79] There is no evidence to support routine MRI imaging of the cervical spine.[80]
- **Biochemical markers:** Currently there are insufficient data to reliably use biochemical markers in evaluation for abusive head trauma in children. Future studies will likely lead to usable markers.[81]
- **Hight's burn criteria:** (1) burn attributed to sibling; (2) unrelated adult seeking medical attention; (3) differing historical accounts; (4) treatment delay > 24 hr; (5) history of prior accidental injuries; (6) inappropriate affect of the parent; (7) inappropriate affect of the child; (8) history incompatible with physical examination; (9) burn incompatible with developmental age; (10) mirror-image burns; (11) localized burns of perineum, genitalia, and/or buttocks; (12) burn older than history given; and (13) other injuries. In one series, 37% of children with 1 criterion and 67% with 2 criteria had abusive burns.[47]

Neglect: Special Considerations for Evaluating Failure to Thrive (FTT)

- **Growth parameters:** Infants and young children in whom there is a concern for nutritional neglect should have their head circumference, length, and weight plotted on a growth chart. Data for other points on the growth chart, if available in the child's medical records or from the primary care physician, should also be included.
- **Documentation:** Documentation of previous FTT medical evaluations should be included. This information should be sought from the primary care physician and the child's medical records.
- **Preliminary ancillary testing for medical causes of FTT:** This may include complete blood count, electrolytes, lead, tuberculosis skin testing, and urinalysis and culture.[22] Additional testing is often beyond the scope of the emergency department visit. An admission to the hospital for a complete FTT evaluation and nutritional supplementation is warranted in severe cases.
- **Documentation of feeding issues:** Include information about what the child is fed, how much, how often, and by whom. Specifically ascertain the caregiver's perceptions of how feeding is going: Is the child a finicky eater? Does the caregiver often become frustrated with feeding time? Does the caregiver actively engage the child in feeding or is the child left with a plate of food and expect to feed him- or herself? Is there a feeding schedule?

Identification of abusive head injuries in infants can be very difficult. Significant numbers of infants are misdiagnosed because of a lack of history of trauma, vague or no neurologic symptoms, and no external evidence of trauma.[4,45,46] In one series, 37% of children under 2 years of age who met one of four "high risk" criteria, were admitted because of injuries suspicious for abuse, and underwent computed tomography (CT) of the head had an occult head injury.[46] "High risk" criteria included rib fractures, multiple fractures, facial injury, or age less than 6 months. Use of skeletal survey or retinal examination as a screening tool to identify the head-injured infants in this series was not effective. In another series of 38 children under 2 years old who were suspected of having been abused, 29% had traumatic intracranial injury without associated neurologic signs.[45] While there are no formal guidelines for when to perform a head CT in suspected abuse, the study should be performed any time there is suspicion of head injury, even if low, especially for children under 2 years of age.

Intentionally inflicted burns are more likely to be fatal than accidental burns.[28] Hight's burn criteria, a set of 13 factors based upon epidemiologic burn data, were determined to have a positive predictive value of 40% when any one criterion was present and 62% when any two criteria were present (see Table 119–6).[45,46] Consideration should be given to these criteria when evaluating children for burn injuries. One study demonstrated that inclusion of a checklist of Hight's criteria on an ED record increased reporting of suspicious burns to CPS from 3% to 12%.[30]

Management

Immediate Interventions

Evaluation and stabilization of the airway, breathing, and circulation occurs first. As soon as the patient is stable, a through examination should be completed because some cutaneous findings may progress or even disappear during the course of the child's stay in the ED. A focused, but detailed history as described in Table 119–1 must be done during the initial stages of evaluation. This will allow for follow-through by other members of the health care team as well as CPS and other investigative personnel, if they become involved.

Secondary Therapeutic Interventions

Once the child is medically stabilized, the situation should be evaluated on several levels. First, the clinician must make sure enough information has been gathered to form an opinion about the safety of the child as well as any other potentially vulnerable children. Second, appropriate medical, psychiatric, and social service referrals should be considered. Finally, a determination should be made as to whether a report should be filed with CPS. Types of responses by CPS will vary. Clinicians should be familiar with state statutes regarding the identification and reporting of child abuse.

Therapeutic Complications

One of the most dreaded consequences of considering child abuse in the differential diagnosis is addressing concerns with parents. The clinician should always consider that a family may become violent. The circumstances of this conversation with the family should be tailored to keep one's own personal safety and the safety of the staff in mind. It is preferable that discussions about concerns of abuse be conducted in a private, quiet environment. The clinician should be familiar with his or her rights as a physician over the legal guardian of a child in his or her care. A legal representative of the hospital may be consulted if necessary. Clinicians should become familiar with laws and hospital policies before there is an emergent issue.

There are some situations in which complete evaluation of a potentially abused child is not possible because of limitations in local resources. If specialized services, such as pediatric surgery, pediatric ophthalmology, or pediatric radiology, are required and not available, the child should be transferred to a hospital that does provide these pediatric-specific services. Transferring a child does not relieve the emergency physician of the resposibility of filing a report with CPS. Personnel at the accepting facility often are unable to obtain detailed information about what happened at the originating institution and information about the child's first presentation.

Documentation

Accurate, detailed documentation is paramount. Photographic documentation is especially helpful in circumstances in which cutaneous findings may be transiently visible, or may change over time. For example, if a child presents with an erythematous mark that resembles a handprint, it would be helpful to photograph the handprint because these types of injuries often fade over a few hours and may completely resolve before CPS or other investigators have an opportunity to examine and confirm the finding. The procedure for photographic documentation of this type varies between states and institutions. An overall algorithm for the approach to suspected child abuse and neglect is provided in Figure 119–1.

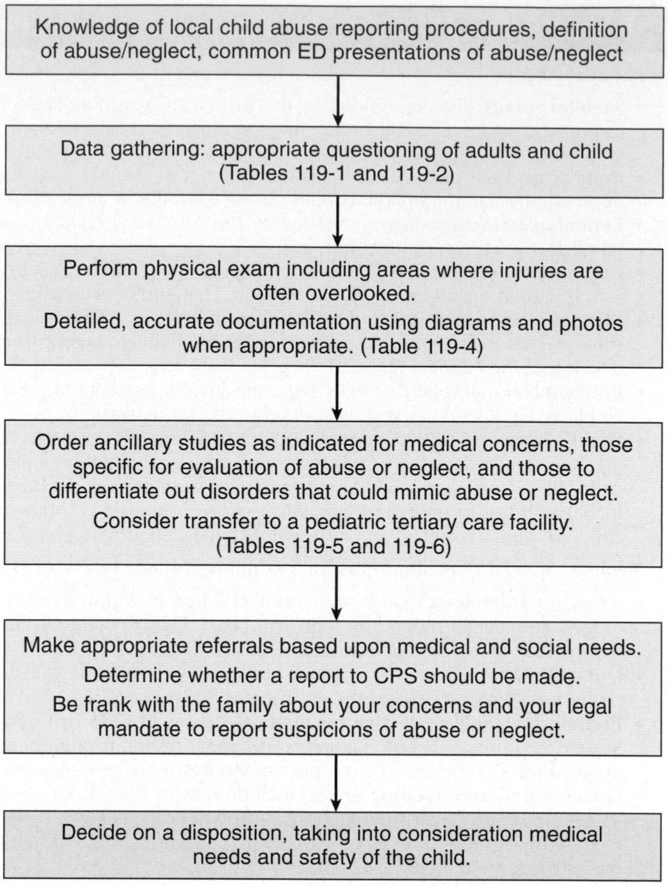

Summary

Prognosis

Abused children are more likely to suffer immediate and long-term medical and psychological consequences of greater severity than accidentally injured children. Abused children are also likely to be reabused if returned to the care of abusive caregivers. The key to protection of this vulnerable population is abuse prevention and prompt abuse and neglect recognition. Emergency physicians carry a large part of the burden of ensuring that abused children are placed in safe environments.

Disposition and Follow-up

Most children for whom the emergency physician has a concern of abuse or neglect may be safely sent home with a caregiver if the alleged perpetrator can be reliably kept away from the child, a safety plan can be established, and a report to CPS has been made. If there is concern that the child may return to an unsafe environment, an immediate response by CPS may be necessary to evaluate the home situation, or to establish temporary CPS custody in more severe cases. If there is concern about the immediate safety of the child and no mechanism by which CPS can respond to perform an

FIGURE 119–1. Algorithm for the emergency department (ED) evaluation and management of suspected child physical abuse or neglect. Abbreviation: CPS, child protective services.

immediate safety evaluation of the child's home situation, then the child should be admitted to the hospital. Admission is also indicated for medical or psychiatric care.

The emergency physician should communicate with the child's primary care physician to provide more reliable follow-up for the family. An initial determination of the family's psychosocial needs should be made in conjunction with a hospital social worker, if available. Appropriate medical follow-up should be discussed with the child's parents and CPS.

Future Directions

As CPS continues to strive to meet the prevention and investigation initiatives set forth to them by CAPTA, the medical community must continue to accumulate information that will allow for more timely and accurate identification of abused and neglected children. Studies of the epidemiology and biomechanisms of childhood injury, the use of radiographic studies, new biochemical markers for differentiating abusive and nonabusive head injuries, child abuse prevention measures, and improved physician education, among other topics, are being actively pursued.

REFERENCES

1. Administration on Children, Youth, and Families: Victims. *In* Child Maltreatment. Washington, DC: U.S. Department of Health and Human Services, 2002, pp 21–50.

2. Alexander R, Crabbe L, Sato Y: Serial abuse in children who are shaken. Am J Dis Child 144:58–60, 1990.

3. Ellaway BA, Payne EH, Rolfe K, et al: Are abused babies protected from further abuse? Arch Dis Child 89:845–846, 2004.

4. Jenny C, Hymel KP, Ritzen A, et al: Analysis of missed cases of abusive head trauma. JAMA 281:621–626, 1999.

*5. DiScala C, Sege R, Reece R: Child abuse and unintentional injuries: a ten year retrospective. Arch Pediatr Adolesc Med 154:16–22, 2000.

6. Irazuzta JE, McJunkin JE, Danadian K, et al: Outcome and cost of child abuse. Child Abuse Neglect 21:751–757, 1997.

7. Jayawant S, Rawlinson A, Gibbon F, et al: Subdural haemorrhages in infants: populations based study. BMJ 317:1558–1561, 1998.

8. English DJ: The extent and consequences of child maltreatment. Future Child 8(1):39–53, 1998.

9. Teicher MH: Scars that won't heal: the neurobiology of child abuse. Sci Am 286:68–75, 2002.

*10. Ewing-Cobbs L, Kramer L, Prasad M: Neuroimaging, physical, and developmental findings after inflicted and non-inflicted traumatic brain injury in young children. Pediatrics 102:300–307, 1998.

11. Erickson MR, Egeland B: A developmental view of the psychological consequences of maltreatment. School Psychol Rev 16:156–168, 1987.

12. Dodge KA, Bates JE, Pettit GS: Mechanisms in the cycle of violence. Science 250:1678–1683, 1990.

13. Salzinger S, Feldman RS, Hammer M, Rosario M: The effects of physical abuse on children's social relationships. Child Dev 64:169–187, 1993.

14. Pelcovitz D, Kaplan S, Goldernberg B, et al: Post-traumatic stress disorder in physically abused adolescents. J Am Acad Child Adolesc Psychiatry 33:305–312, 1994.

15. Kaufman J, Zigler E: Do abused children become abusive parents? Am J Orthopsychiatry 57:186–192, 1987.

16. DeBellis MD, Putnam FW: The psychobiology of child maltreatment. Child Adolesc Psychiatr Clin North Am 3:663–678, 1994.

17. Schene PA: Past, present, and future roles of child protective services. Future Child 8(1):23–38, 1998.

*18. National Clearinghouse on Child Abuse and Neglect: Definition of mandated reporter. Available at *http://nccanch.acf.hhs.gov/admin/glossarym.cfm*

*19. National Clearinghouse on Child Abuse and Neglect: What is child abuse and neglect? 2004. Available at *http://nccanch.acf.hhs.gov/pubs/factsheets/whatiscan.cfm*

20. Wissow LS: Current concepts: child abuse and neglect. JAMA 332:1425–1431, 1995.

21. Ceci SJ, Bruck M: Suggestibility of the child witness: a historical review and synthesis. Psychol Bull 113:403–439, 1993.

22. Dubowitz H, Giardino A, Gustavson E: Child neglect: guidance for pediatricians. Pediatr Rev 21:111–116, 2000.

*23. Christian CW: Assessment and evaluation of the physically abused child. Clin Fam Pract 5:21–46, 2003.

24. Kirschner RH, Stein RJ: The mistaken diagnosis of child abuse. Am J Dis Child 139:873–875, 1985.

25. Lane WG, Rubin DM, Monteith R, Christian CW: Racial differences in the evaluation of pediatric fractures for physical abuse. JAMA 288:1603–1609, 2002.

26. Bilmire ME, Myers PA: Serious head injury in infants: accident or abuse? Pediatrics 75:340–342, 1987.

27. Christian CW, Taylor AA, Hertle RW, Duhaime AC: Retinal hemorrhages caused by accidental trauma. J Pediatr 135:125–127, 1999.

28. Ayoub C, Pfeifer D: Burns as a manifestation of child abuse and neglect. Am J Dis Child 133:910–914, 1979.

29. Hight DW, Bakalar HR, Lloyd JR: Inflicted burns in children: recognition and treatment. JAMA 242:517–520, 1979.

30. Clark KD, Tepper D, Jenny C: Effect of a screening profile on the diagnosis of nonaccidental burns in children. Pediatric Emerg Care 13:259–261, 1997.

31. American Academy of Pediatrics, Section on Radiology: Diagnostic imaging of child abuse. Pediatrics 105:1345–1348, 2000.

32. American Academy of Pediatrics, Committee on Child Abuse and Neglect: Shaken baby syndrome. Pediatrics 108:508–512, 2001.

33. Kleinman PK, Nimkin K, Spevak MR: Follow-up skeletal surveys in suspected child abuse. AJR Am J Roentgenol 167:893–896, 1996.

34. Levin A: Ocular manifestations of child abuse. Ophthalmol Clin North Am 3:249–284, 1990.

35. Ludwig S, Warman M: Shaken baby syndrome: a review of 20 cases. Ann Emerg Med 13:104–107, 1984.

36. Hadley MN, Sonntag VK, Rekate HL, Murphy A: The infant whiplash-shake injury syndrome: a clinical and pathological study. Neurosurgery 24:536–540, 1989.

37. Morad Y, Kim Y, Mian M, et al: Nonophthalmologist accuracy in diagnosing retinal hemorrhages in the shaken baby syndrome. J Pediatr 142:431–434, 2003.

38. Pierre-Kahn V, Roche O, Dureau P, et al: Ophthalmologic findings in suspected child abuse victims with subdural hematomas. Ophthalmology 110:1718–1723, 2003.

39. Morad Y, Kim YM, Armstrong DC, et al: Correlation between retinal abnormalities and intracranial abnormalities in the shaken baby syndrome. Am J Ophthalmol 134:354–359, 2002.

40. Greenwald MJ, Weiss A, Oesterle CS, Friendly DS: Traumatic retinoschisis in battered babies. Ophthalmology 93:618–625, 1986.

41. Massicotte SJ, Folberg R, Torczynski E, et al: Vitreoretinal traction and perimacular retinal folds in the eyes of deliberately traumatized children. Ophthalmology 98:1124–1127, 1991.

42. Gaynon MW, Koh K, Marmor MF, Frankel LR: Retinal folds in the shaken baby syndrome. Am J Ophthalmol 106:423–425, 1988.

43. Schloff S, Mullaney PB, Armstrong DC, et al: Retinal findings in children with intracranial hemorrhage. Ophthalmology 109:1472–1476, 2002.

44. Odom A, Christ E, Kerr N, et al: Prevalence of retinal hemorrhages in pediatric patients after in-hospital cardiopulmonary resuscitation: a prospective study. Pediatrics 99(6):e3, 1997.

*45. Laskey AL, Holsti M, Runyan DK, Socolar RRS: Occult head trauma in young suspected victims of physical abuse. J Pediatr 144:719–722, 2004.

46. Rubin DM, Christian CW, Bilaniuk LT, et al: Occult head injury in high-risk abused children. Pediatrics 111:1382–1386, 2003.

47. Hammond J, Perez-Stable A, Ward CG: Predictive value of historical and physical characteristics for the diagnosis of child abuse. South Med J 84:166–168, 1991.

48. English DJ, Wingard T, Marshall D, et al: Alternative responses to child protective services: emerging issues and concerns. Child Abuse Neglect 24:375–388, 2000.

49. Sugar NF, Taylor JA, Feldman KW: Bruises in infants and toddlers: those who don't cruise rarely bruise. Arch Pediatr Adolesc Med 153:399–403, 1999.

50. Hanigan WC, Peterson RA, Njus G: Tin ear syndrome: rotational acceleration in pediatric head injuries. Pediatrics 87:618–627, 1987.

51. Duhaime AC, Alario AJ, Lewander WJ: Head injury in very young children: mechanisms, injury types, and ophthalmological findings in 100 hospitalized patients younger than 2 years of age. Pediatrics 90:179–185, 1992.

*52. Bechtel K, Stoessel K, Leventhal JM, et al: Characteristics that distinguish accidental from abusive injury in hospitalized young children with head trauma. Pediatrics 114:165–168, 2004.

53. Whitby EH, Griffiths PD, Rutter S, et al: Frequency and natural history of subdural haemorrhages in babies and relation to obstetric factors. Lancet 363:846–851, 2004.

54. Hymel KP, Abshire TC, Luckey DW, Jenny C: Coagulopathy in pediatric abusive head trauma. Pediatrics 99:371–375, 1997.

55. Keenan HT, Runyan DK, Marshall SW, et al: A population-based study of inflicted traumatic brain injury in young children. JAMA 290:621–626, 2003.

56. Morris MW, Smith S, Cressman J, Ancheta J: Evaluation of infants with subdural hematoma who lack external evidence of abuse. Pediatrics 105:549–553, 2000.

57. Brown D, Fisher E: Femur fractures in infants and young children. Am J Public Health 94:558–560, 2004.

58. Jones JCW, Feldman KW, Bruckner JD: Child abuse in infants with proximal physeal injuries of the femur. Pediatr Emerg Care 20:157–161, 2004.

59. Starling SP, Heller RM, Jenny C: Pelvic fractures in infants as a sign of physical abuse. Child Abuse Neglect 26:475–480, 2002.

60. Hymel KP, Jenny C: Abusive spiral fractures of the humerus: a videotaped exception. Arch Pediatr Adolesc Med 150:226–228, 1996.

61. Schwend RM, Werth C, Johnston A: Femur shaft fractures in toddlers and young children: rarely from child abuse. J Pediatr Orthop 20:475–481, 2000.

*Selected readings.

62. Rex C, Kay PR: Features of femoral fractures in nonaccidental injury. J Pediatr Orthop 20:411–413, 2000.

63. Grant P, Mata MB, Tidwell M: Femur fracture in infants: a possible accidental etiology. Pediatrics 108:1009–1012, 2001.

64. Mellick LB, Milker L, Egsieker E: Childhood accidental spiral tibial (CAST) fractures. Pediatr Emerg Care 15:307–309, 1999.

65. Mellick LB, Reesor K, Demers D, Reinker KA: Tibial fractures of young children. Pediatr Emerg Care 4:97–101, 1988.

66. Pierce MC, Bertocci GE, Vogeley E, Moreland MS: Evaluating long bone fractures in children: a biomechanical approach with illustrative cases. Child Abuse Neglect 28:505–524, 2004.

67. Leventhal JM, Thomas SA, Rosenfield NS, Markowitz RI: Fractures in young children: distinguishing child abuse from unintentional injuries. Am J Dis Child 147:87–92, 1993.

68. Bulloch B, Schubert CJ, Brophy PD, et al: Cause and clinical characteristics of rib fractures in infants. Pediatrics 105(4):e48, 2000.

69. Kleinman PK, Schlesinger AE: Mechanical factors associated with posterior rib fractures: laboratory and case studies. Pediatr Radiol 27:87–91, 1997.

70. Feldman KW, Brewer DK: Child abuse, cardiopulmonary resuscitation, and rib fractures. Pediatrics 73:339–342, 1984.

71. Andronicus M, Oates RK, Peat J, et al: Non-accidental burns in children. Burns 24:552–558, 1998.

72. Daria S, Sugar NF, Feldman KW, et al: Into hot water head first: distribution of intentional and unintentional immersion burns. Pediatr Emerg Care 20:302–310, 2004.

*73. Hettiaratchy S, Dziewulski P: ABC of burns: pathophysiology and types of burns. BMJ 328:1427–1429, 2004.

74. Titus MO, Baxter AL, Starling SP: Accidental scald burns in sinks. Pediatrics 111(2):e191, 2003.

75. Yeoh C, Nixon JW, Dickson W, et al: Patterns of scald injuries. Arch Dis Child 71:156–158, 1994.

76. Coffman K, Boyce WT, Hansen RC: Phytophotodermatitis simulating child abuse. Am J Dis Child 139:239–240, 1985.

77. Brill PW, Winchester P, Kleinman PK: Differential diagnosis I: diseases simulating abuse. In Kleinman PK (ed): Diagnostic Imaging of Child Abuse, 2nd ed. Philadelphia: Mosby, 1998, pp 178–196.

78. Mandelstam SA, Cook D, Fitzgerald M, Ditchfield MR: Complementary use of radiological skeletal survey and bone scintigraphy in detection of bony injuries in suspected child abuse. Arch Dis Child 88:387–390, 2003.

79. Stoodley N: Non-accidental head injury in children: gathering the evidence. Lancet 360:271–272, 2002.

80. Feldman KW, Weinberger E, Milstein JM, Fligner CL: Cervical MRI in abused infants. Child Abuse Neglect 21:199–205, 1997.

81. Berger RP, Kochanek PK, Pierce MC: Biochemical markers of brain injury: could they be used as diagnostic adjunct in cases of inflicted traumatic brain injury? Child Abuse Neglect 28:739–754, 2004.

Skin and Soft Tissue Infections

Michael J. Muszynski, MD

Key Points

Unusual pathogens may occur when skin infections are associated with human or animal bites, contaminated wounds, puncture wounds, or compromised hosts.

Resistant pathogens such as methicillin-resistant *Staphylococcus aureus* have become commonplace in skin and soft tissue infections in the community at large, leading to the need for more aggressive diagnostic approaches such as needle aspiration for culture.

In cases of moderate to severe disease or in cases demonstrating rapid clinical progression, accurate empirical therapy can be life saving.

The initial presentation of necrotizing fasciitis may be nondescript, suggesting more common and less serious conditions, such as cellulitis or benign muscular pain; unfortunately this may delay recognition and result in high mortality rates.

Selected Diagnoses

Cellulitis
Wound infections
Necrotizing fasciitis
Atopic dermatitis with bacterial superinfection
Eczema herpeticum
Folliculitis
Furuncles and carbuncles
Hidradenitis suppurativa
Lymphangitis

Discussion of Individual Diagnoses

Cellulitis

Cellulitis is a suppurative, inflammatory process of connective tissue within the subcutaneous space that has a varying degree of dermal involvement, and is most often infectious. The epidermis is generally spared. The process most commonly begins at the point of a wound or breach of the integu-ment, such as folliculitis or a furuncle. However, the portal of entry might not be obvious in some cases. Other mechanisms include extension from a deeper infectious focus, such as the teeth and paranasal sinuses, or from hematogenous seeding associated with systemic infection due to *Streptococcus pneumoniae*, *Streptococcus pyogenes* (group A streptococcus), *Staphylococcus aureus*, or *Haemophilus influenzae* type b. The latter is now rare due to the effectiveness of the *H. influenzae* type b conjugate vaccine.[1] The classic violaceous hue of *H. influenzae* type b cellulitis is rapidly approaching historical interest only. Hematogenously derived facial and periorbital cellulitis due to *S. pneumoniae* may clinically mimic that seen with *H. influenzae*. Other areas of the body may be involved as well, especially in patients with collagen vascular disorders or immune deficiency.[2]

Clinical Presentation

Cellulitis is clinically recognized as an area of erythema, edema, warmth, and tenderness with a gradual, tapered edge, distinguishing it from the abrupt, well-demarcated edge of erysipelas, which is an inflammatory condition of the epidermis. Cellulitis severity ranges from mild and limited to severe and extensive, and onset and progression can be slow or rapid. Presentation depends on multiple factors, which may be used as important predictors of severity (Table 120–1).

Wound cultures are strongly recommended, especially if methicillin-resistant *S. aureus* (MRSA) or unusual pathogens are suspected. Unusual pathogens may occur when skin infections are associated with human or animal bites, contaminated wounds, puncture wounds, or compromised hosts. Needle aspiration of the cellulitis site can be informative but is often not performed due to reported low yield of 5% to 36%.[3-5] Microbiologic yield does increase with disease severity. One study showed that aspiration identified bacterial etiologies in 4 of 7 patients with cellulitis and abscess (57%) compared to 9 of 56 patients with uncomplicated cellulitis (16%), and in 11 of 15 patients with necrotizing infections (73%).[6] Nonetheless, resistant pathogens such as MRSA have become commonplace in skin and soft tissue infections in the community at large,[7] leading to the need for more aggressive diagnostic approaches such as needle aspiration for culture. This is especially true in cases of moderate to severe disease or cases demonstrating rapid clinical progression, in which accurate empirical therapy can be life saving.

The needle aspiration procedure starts with cleansing the site with povidone-iodine solution and allowing the solution

Table 120–1	Factors Associated with Increased Severity of Soft Tissue Infections

Host

Young age (neonates, infants)
Immunocompromised states (congenital and acquired immune deficiency, asplenia, cancer, diabetes, renal disease, collagen vascular disease, burns)

Location

Head/neck (periorbital/orbital, facial/buccal, jugular)
Associated with deep structure infection (sinus, bone/joint, fascia, dental)

Disease Process

Bacteremia
Sepsis
Toxic shock syndrome
Human bite wound

Clinical Presentation

Fever
Toxic appearance
Extent of involvement (>5 cm in size)

Etiologic Agent

Group A streptococcus
Toxin-producing strains (group A streptococcus, *Staphylococcus aureus*)
Haemophilus influenzae type b
Vibrio species
Anaerobes

Table 120–2	Management Scheme for Skin and Soft Tissue Infections

Assess Need for Incision and Drainage

Obtain Culture Specimens

Wound
    Material from incision and drainage
    Consider needle aspiration of cellulitis
Blood
    If sepsis or bacteremia suspected

Assess Local MRSA Rate and Clindamycin Resistance Prevalence

Define Disease Severity

Mild (afebrile, healthy child with minor clinical findings)
Incision and drainage alone for abscesses if cellulitis < 5 cm
Incision and drainage plus antimicrobial therapy if cellulitis > 5 cm
    Cephalexin or amoxicillin/clavulanate
    If MRSA suspected, oral clindamycin (when community resistance rate < 10%) or trimethoprim-sulfamethoxazole, or doxycycline (if > 8 years of age)
Ensure follow-up
Moderate (febrile, healthy child or more extensive involvement)
Incision and drainage plus antimicrobial therapy as for mild disease; ensure follow-up
Incision and drainage, hospitalization, parenteral antimicrobial therapy if extensive cellulitis or poor adherence to therapy or follow-up suspected
Severe (toxicity, immune compromised, limb-threatening process, rapid progression, periorbital/facial, neonate)
Incision and drainage as needed, hospitalize for parenteral antimicrobial therapy
    Clindamycin if community clindamycin resistance rate < 10%, vancomycin if > 10%
    Add third-generation cephalosporin if periorbital/facial cellulitis or neonate
Critical (sepsis, shock, toxic shock syndrome)
Resuscitate, incision and drainage if focus of infection found, ICU admission, parenteral antimicrobial therapy
    Vancomycin plus nafcillin plus gentamicin regardless of local resistance rate data

Abbreviations: ICU, intensive care unit; MRSA, methicillin-resistant *Staphylococcus aureus*.

to dry. Locally injected anesthesia is generally avoided, since these agents have in vitro antibacterial activity; however, topical anesthesia is often employed. The area is aspirated using a 22-gauge needle for sites on the face and a 20-gauge needle elsewhere. The needle is attached to a 1- to 3-ml syringe with 0.5 ml of sterile, nonbacteriostatic saline. The saline is used to expel aspirated material from the needle and syringe hub onto plate media or a suitable transport vessel. Some authorities recommend aspirating the "leading edge" of the cellulitis, but a comparative study has shown that aspirating the point of maximal inflammation is superior in yield of the pathogen (45% versus 5% from the leading edge).[8] Blood cultures are recommended in seriously ill patients and anytime bacteremia is suspected.[9]

Management

The management of cellulitis is based on an assessment of risk factors, disease severity, and potential etiologies. As with other significant skin and soft tissue infections, patients should be risk-stratified for serious illness with consideration of hospitalization and intravenous therapy. Many cases of cellulitis are minor and will respond to local measures and oral antimicrobial therapy. Table 120–2 outlines a general management scheme for cellulitis, skin, and soft tissue infections. Empirical antibiotic choice depends on suspected pathogens, clinical presentation, patient age, and historical clues. Historically, antimicrobials active against *S. aureus*, group A streptococcus (e.g., first-generation cephalosporin [cephalexin], amoxicillin/clavulanate, or clindamycin) have been prescribed for uncomplicated and minor wound-associated infections. Dicloxacillin has also been used, but is difficult to prescribe as the suspension because of concentration and palatability issues. Mild infections due to MRSA may respond to antistaphylococcal agents demonstrating

poor in vitro MRSA activity. MRSA demonstrates a heterogeneity of susceptibility in infected sites. A subpopulation of bacteria at the site can be susceptible to an agent while the remainder of the bacterial inoculum is not. Thus, in mild infections, the antibiotic employed may simply decrease the total bacterial inoculum to the point at which immune responses can effect a cure.

Patients with simple abscesses and no surrounding cellulitis do not require antibiotics. Those who have cellulitis and an associated abscess require incision and drainage (see Chapter 166, Incision and Drainage and Supplemental Antibiotics).

Severely ill patients and moderately ill patients with extensive areas of involvement have always required intravenous antibiotic therapy. In these cases an antibiotic with activity against streptococci and *S. aureus*, including MRSA, is preferred. Seriously ill patients who may be infected with *S. aureus* should be empirically treated for MRSA with intravenous clindamycin,[10] provided that there are no risks for hospital-acquired MRSA (HA-MRSA) and local clindamycin resistance rates for community-associated MRSA (CA-MRSA) strains are less than 10%. Clinicians may obtain antibiotic susceptibility information for their community from local hospital infection control programs, local hospital laboratory antibiogram reports, local and state health departments, and the Centers for Disease Control and Prevention (*http://www.cdc.gov*). Local laboratories and clinicians must be aware that clindamycin resistance will be underestimated if the laboratory does not employ the "D test" for susceptibility testing. MRSA strains that are resistant to erythromycin and apparently sensitive to clindamycin by routine susceptibility assays may exhibit inducible resistance to clindamycin in vivo. Thus, when clindamycin is prescribed in these cases, resistance will emerge during therapy, which may lead to treatment failure. The D test utilizes an erythromycin disk placed 15 mm from a clindamycin disk on the susceptibility test agar plate. MRSA that exhibits inducible clindamycin resistance will show a zone of bacterial growth inhibition around the clindamycin disk affected by the presence of erythromycin that forms the shape of a "D" rather than the expected circle, hence the name "D test." Strains that form a circular shape of inhibition at a prescribed diameter are clindamycin sensitive without inducible resistance. Clindamycin therapy can be expected to be efficacious for infections due to these strains. Seriously ill patients infected with MRSA strains demonstrating any type of clindamycin resistance must be treated intravenously with an alternative agent such as vancomycin. This also includes all HA-MRSA cases and those with clindamycin resistant or inducible-resistant CA-MRSA. Antibiotic therapy choices for moderately ill patients and patients with potentially serious infections require coverage for CA-MRSA or HA-MRSA to avoid risk of mortality and serious morbidities. Serious infectious complications (shock, disseminated intravascular coagulation [DIC]), additional metastatic sites of infection, and death have been reported with delays in instituting an antibiotic effective against MRSA.[11]

CA-MRSA infection differs from HA-MRSA in that CA-MRSA is not associated with classic HA-MRSA risk factors (hospitalization, contact with a health care worker, dialysis, history of intensive care admission, recent surgery, long-term care facility residence).[12] CA-MRSA is also more likely than HA-MRSA to cause skin and soft tissue infections. CA-MRSA patients are more likely to have household members with similar infectious problems, such as recurrent boils and soft tissue infections. Infections due to CA-MRSA require surgical intervention more commonly than infections due to methicillin-sensitive *S. aureus* (MSSA). CA-MRSA is inherently resistant to antistaphylococcal β-lactams, cephalosporins, erythromycin, and quinolones. It is sensitive to vancomycin and linezolid and generally sensitive to clindamycin, trimethoprim-sulfamethoxazole, tetracyclines, and gentamicin. HA-MRSA is resistant to most antimicrobials except vancomycin and linezolid. Critically ill children with suspected *S. aureus* infection require the triple combination of vancomycin, nafcillin, and gentamicin.

Linezolid is an oxazolidinone with excellent activity against MRSA and MSSA, *S. pneumoniae* (penicillin/cephalosporin-sensitive and -resistant strains), group A streptococcus, and enterocci (including vancomycin-resistant strains). Linezolid has no gram-negative antibacterial activity. It has been shown to be safe and effective for uncomplicated skin and soft tissue infections in children.[13] It may become an attractive choice for the treatment of skin and soft tissue infections, since it is effective against both CA-MRSA and HA-MRSA by both intravenous and oral routes. Linezolid is costly, and experience with this drug as a first-line agent in children is somewhat limited, which leads some experts to discourage routine use, instead using an infectious disease expert for guidance for its application.[14]

Other Forms of Childhood Cellulitis

Several other forms of childhood cellulitis deserve specific mention. Periorbital cellulitis, buccal cellulitis, and cellulitis without an obvious wound precipitant generally require treatment with a parenteral third-generation cephalosporin plus clindamycin. Panniculitis of the cheek due to freeze injury, as can occur with popsicle eating in young children, mimics infectious buccal cellulitis.[15] Cellulitis of the face and neck of suspected odontogenic origin (e.g., tooth abscess) should be treated with antimicrobials effective against mouth anaerobes.[16] Oral amoxicillin/clavulanate or parenteral ampicillin/sulbactam are excellent choices. Pencillin-allergic patients may be treated with clindamycin either parenterally or orally as the situation requires.

ERYSIPELAS

Erysipelas is a superficial infection commonly involving the face or legs in children, although any area of the body can be affected. The involved skin has an orange peel appearance and is intensely red, warm, and very painful. The lesion displays significant edema with sharply defined and raised borders. Rapid spread is the rule, and blistering of the lesion can occur. Patients are commonly febrile and ill appearing. When positive, culture of aspiration of the lesion yields group A streptococcus. Patients tend to respond quickly to antibiotic therapy, but erysipelas must be respected as a potentially serious condition, especially in patients with immunodeficiency or malignancies such as lymphoma. The condition is especially worrisome in neonates and may be also due to group B streptococcus. Treatment with penicillin plus clindamycin is recommended for the most serious group A streptococcal infections and appears to be associated with a better clinical outcome than that seen with monotherapy.[17] Clindamycin inhibits bacterial protein synthesis and suppresses production of bacterial virulence factors, overcoming the deleterious effect of a large bacterial inoculum. It possesses a longer postantibiotic effect than penicillin (continued antibacterial effect after the antibiotic concentration falls below inhibitory levels in tissue). However, clindamycin cannot be used alone in serious group A streptococcal infections, since 1% to 2% of strains are resistant. Penicillin or cephalosporin resistance in group A streptococcus has not been described.

PERIANAL CELLULITIS

Perianal cellulitis or perianal dermatitis presents with rectal pain with sitting or defecation and is characterized by intense edema and erythema of perirectal tissues. The borders of inflammation are sharply demarcated, reminiscent of erysipelas, in an otherwise well-appearing child. Rectal swab cultures nearly always yield group A streptococcus.[18] There may be concomitant balanitis or vulvovaginitis.[19] Oral penicillin and cephalosporins are effective for perianal infection with or without genital involvement. Topical agents such as mupirucin and erythromycin ointment have also been used.[20] Relapses often require treatment with clindamycin or a combination of penicillin plus rifampin, or consideration of *S. aureus* as the cause (including MRSA).[21] Ongoing recurrences require inquiry for potential household or day care contacts with the same condition.[19, 22]

CELLULITIS OF THE EXTERNAL EAR

Cellulitis of the external ear may result from trauma, infected atopic dermatitis, or ear piercing. Infections of the earlobe tend to be relatively minor and are generally due to *S. aureus,* and respond to local measures of cleansing and warm compresses and oral antistaphylococcal antibiotics. More serious infections that involve the upper ear and its cartilage are associated with high risk for cosmetic deformation. Infections from ear cartilage piercing are most often due to *Pseudomonas aeruginosa.*[23] Wound culture is important to guide therapy. Empirical intravenous antibiotic coverage for *P. aeruginosa, S. aureus,* and group A streptococcus is often recommended to lessen the chance of a poor cosmetic result. Cefepime, piperacillin/tazobactam, or ceftazidime are good choices, but ceftazidime is a less potent gram-positive agent. Severe lesions or lesions failing to respond to initial therapy require consideration of MRSA as outlined for other forms of cellulitis.

BLISTERING DISTAL DACTYLITIS

Blistering distal dactylitis is a localized infection of the distal volar fat pad of the digits. Fingers are affected more commonly than toes. Most cases present in children 2 to 16 years of age. The condition has also been described in infants less than 9 months of age.[24] Patients develop superficial, tender bulla on the fat pad of the digit up to 2 cm in size. The process occasionally extends further up the fingers to involve the palms.[25] The primary etiology is group A streptococcus, which can be isolated from culture of the blisters. *S. aureus* has also been described, and may be more common with blisters on multiple digits or with more extensive disease.[25] Blistering distal dactylitis must be differentiated from herpetic whitlow, as the two conditions may have a similar appearance but differ greatly in management. Dactylitis is treated with antibiotics active against group A streptococcus and *S. aureus* (amoxicillin/clavulanate, a first-generation cephalosporin, or a macrolide), plus drainage of the blisters. Draining a herpetic whitlow is hazardous and will spread herpes simplex virus (HSV) found in the blisters more widely into surrounding tissue. The two conditions can be distinguished by the appearance of gram-positive cocci on Gram stain in blistering dactylitis and the presence of HSV by direct immunofluorescent antibody staining of cells from the base of a vesicle or blister in herpetic whitlow.[26] Although frequently recommended, the Tzanck smear is inferior when compared to direct fluorescent assays because of an unacceptable low sensitivity. A negative Tzanck preparation cannot definitively rule out herpes simplex infection.

Wound Infections

Wound care involving special circumstances, such as snake and spider envenomations, are described elsewhere in this text (see Chapter 141, Bites and Stings). Mammalian bite wounds sustained from unusual domesticated and wild animals are associated with particular organisms (see Table 120–5). Consider consulting an infectious disease specialist for management recommendations if such a situation is encountered. The same wound management principles discussed in this chapter and in Chapter 160 (Wound Management) apply to the management of wounds sustained from wild or domesticated animals and humans. Both common and unusual organisms may be present in infected bite wounds, and polymicrobial infections are the rule rather than the exception. Prophylactic treatment strategies depend on the type of bite sustained (see Table 120–6).

Classic water-contaminated wound pathogens include Aeromonas species, *P. aeruginosa,* a host of gram-negative enteric bacteria, and *Mycobacterium marinum.* The latter is also associated with skin injuries associated with maintaining home and commercial aquaria. *Chromobacterium violaceum* infections are related to stagnant, freshwater wounds mainly in the southeastern United States.[27] Marine water harbors the same list of potential pathogens as fresh water with the important addition of Vibrio species. Infected soil-contaminated wounds are characterized by a large number of etiologic possibilities and are often polymicrobial in nature. They present special challenges in the choice of empirical antimicrobial therapy. At the minimum, broad-spectrum coverage for organisms such as *S. aureus* and group A streptococcus, a variety of gram-negative enteric bacteria (especially Enterobacter species), enterococci, and anaerobes should be provided. If the contaminating soil was wet or mixed with vegetable matter, then *P. aeruginosa* and *Aeromonas hydrophila* must be kept in mind.[28] Soil also harbors Nocardia, Actinomyces, nontuberculous mycobacteria (especially *Mycobacterium fortuitum* complex), and a variety of fungi (Aspergillus, Zygomyces, Fusarium, Acremonium, Bipolaris). Wound cultures must be obtained before starting therapy and must employ specific media for the isolation of aerobic, anaerobic, mycobacterial, and fungal organisms. Empirical therapy for serious infections may include the broad-spectrum choices of imipenem (or meropenem), piperacillin/tazobactam, or clindamycin plus cefepime or ceftazidime. Each of these regimens covers the common anaerobic and aerobic bacteria, including Pseudomonas and Aeromonas. Therapy is based on the initial culture results as they become available. Simple wound infections with soil contamination can be managed with wound cleansing and oral antimicrobial therapy such as amoxicillin/clavulanate or a cephalosporin. Careful follow-up should be arranged for all cases. All patients should be evaluated for tetanus immunity and vaccinated if indicated.

Puncture wounds, particularly of the foot, are common emergency department presentations. These injuries are prone to infection due to the innate characteristics of the wound, specifically deep penetration, injury to underlying structures (fascia, vessels, muscle, tendons, cartilage, bones and joints), possible retained foreign body, and a small entrance with little chance of spontaneous drainage. The clinical presentation is the same as for any cellulitis with additional findings when other structures are affected (e.g., fasciitis, septic arthritis, osteomyelitis, deep abscesses, pyomyositis). The infecting agents are related to skin flora (staphylococci and streptococci) and contaminating material. Infected punctures of the foot through shoes, especially rubber-soled (e.g., tennis) shoes, are most likely due to *P. aeruginosa* and *S. aureus.* Rapid progression of infection is highly suggestive of a common bacterial etiology, whereas a subacute or delayed presentation raises suspicion for unusual pathogens such as nontuberculous mycobacteria, Nocardia, Actinomyces, and some fungi. Infectious disease consultation is helpful in these cases. As with all wound infections, cultures should be attempted before antibiotics are administered. Sonography is a sensitive and specific modality for evaluation for retained foreign bodies, especially wood.[29] Computed tomography (CT) and magnetic resonance imaging can provide additional information concerning extent of infection or purulent collections. Surgical or orthopedic consultation is commonly needed in these conditions to explore for foreign bodies, drain abscesses, and débride affected tissues. Pseudomonas infections due to puncture wounds of the foot require surgical intervention as the primary therapeutic approach, since cartilage and bone involvement is common. Aggressive surgical débridement of all infected material, including bone, combined with parenteral antipseudomonal therapy of just 7 days' duration, results in excellent clinical outcome.[30] The same is not true for other organisms, such as S. aureus. P. aeruginosa is a true opportunistic pathogen that can be effectively treated with short courses of antibiotics if the predisposing factor or infected nidus is removed.

Necrotizing Fasciitis

Necrotizing fasciitis is a rapidly spreading, fulminant infection in the subcutaneous space that involves the superficial fascia. The process initially spares adjacent muscle and overlying skin. Associated thrombosis of subcutaneous vasculature eventually leads to cutaneous gangrene and rapid destruction of deeper tissues. Missed diagnosis in the early phase can have disastrous consequences. This relatively rare but fearsome condition carries a mortality rate of about 25% even with application of modern therapeutic measures. Timely diagnosis followed by prompt surgical débridement and antibiotic therapy are required to save life and salvage limb.

Clinical Presentation

The initial presentation of necrotizing fasciitis may be nondescript, suggesting more common and less serious conditions such as cellulitis or benign muscular pain. Unfortunately this may delay recognition. One study of 39 pediatric cases found that 28% were missed at initial evaluation.[31] The most difficult challenge is to distinguish necrotizing fasciitis from benign inflammatory conditions during the early phase. Clues may come from the presence of underlying medical conditions or risk factors, suspected pathogenesis, and historical and clinical findings. Diabetes and peripheral vascular disease are common associations in adult patients, whereas typical predisposing conditions in children are malnutrition, neoplasia (especially leukemia), recent surgery (especially procedures in the inguinal region), omphalitis in infants, breast abscess in infants, and balanitis associated with circumcision. An association with Vibrio species has been reported in pediatric patients with iron overload.[32] Fasciitis has also been described after major trauma, soft tissue foreign bodies, minor injuries, and even insect bites. Fasciitis in the neck has been associated with lymphadenitis, dental infection, or tonsillopharyngitis. Some cases of necrotizing fasciitis have no predisposing factor. Of all associated conditions, chickenpox is the most important in childhood.[33] Varicella greatly increases the overall risk for invasive group A streptococcal disease, which is a major etiology of necrotizing fasciitis in children. In a large surveillance study, necrotizing fasciitis occurred in 4% of invasive group A streptococcus cases.[34] The varicella vaccine shows great promise in the prevention of the serious bacterial complications of chickenpox.

Use of nonsteroidal anti-inflammatory drugs (NSAIDs) has been suspected to increase the risk of developing necrotizing fasciitis with invasive group A streptococcal disease. Prospective studies have not borne this out; however, NSAIDs may increase risk of poor outcome in fasciitis by reducing pain and causing delay in seeking medical care. NSAID use is associated with the increased likelihood of renal failure as part of the systemic presentation of necrotizing fasciitis.[35]

Clinical manifestations of necrotizing fasciitis begin with pain followed by induration, edema, and erythema within 24 to 48 hours. In a report of 15 patients in whom group A streptoccal necrotizing fasciitis was missed at initial evaluation, unremitting pain out of proportion to physical findings was not appreciated.[36] Pain commonly extends beyond the area of suspected inflammation. Signs of necrosis such as purple skin coloration, ecchymosis, and blisters are seen much later. Presence of paresthesia or anesthesia is an ominous sign of severe underlying necrosis. Tissue crepitance is an infrequent but specific indicator of necrotizing fasciitis. Toxic appearance, generalized erythematous rash, and low platelet count or other findings suggestive of toxic shock are independent predictors of necrotizing fasciitis.[37] A scoring system termed the "Laboratory Risk Indicator for Necrotizing Fasciitis" was recently proposed as a tool to distinguish necrotizing fasciitis from other forms of cellulitis.[38] The scoring system uses total white cell count ($>15,000/mm^3$), hemoglobin (<11 to 13.5 g/dl), sodium (<135 mmol/L), glucose (<10 mmol/L), serum creatinine ($>141 \mu mol/L$), and C-reactive protein (>150 mg/L) as risk factors but awaits further validation, and it has not been applied to children. Ultrasound as a diagnostic tool for suspected necrotizing fasciitis has a sensitivity of 88%, a specificity of 93%, a positive predictive value of 83%, and a negative predictive value of 95%.[39] CT scan may also suggest the diagnosis, especially if air is seen in the tissues.[40] Contrast-enhanced magnetic resonance imaging has been shown to differentiate fasciitis from cellulitis and is helpful in evaluating deep structures and fascial layers,[41] but requires more to complete. Imaging should not be allowed to delay definitive surgical management of patients suspected to have necrotizing fasciitis. Tissue biopsy is the most accurate diagnostic method. Frozen surgical sections allow rapid decision making for proceeding with further exploration and aggressive débridement.[42]

Management

Prompt surgical intervention is paramount. In a report of 20 pediatric cases, all survivors had aggressive surgical débridement within 3 hours of admission. Delay in surgical management occurred in the five patients who died.[43] In another study of 29 patients, aggressive surgical approaches instituted within 24 hours of admission decreased the mortality rate from 25% to 6%.[44] Aerobic and anaerobic cultures of blood, wounds, and needle aspiration of compartments should be obtained when fasciitis is suspected and before starting antibiotic therapy. Gram stain should guide antibiotic choice when possible. Repeat cultures of the site are obtained at surgery. Fluid resuscitation with or without vasopressors, correction of electrolyte imbalances and hypoglycemia, and treatment of coagulopathy are often required for very ill patients. Polymicrobial infections are common, necessitating broad-spectrum antibiotic coverage including anaerobic bacteria. If S. aureus is suspected, vancomycin should be added. Antimicrobial choices are similar to those for serious

Table 120–3	Etiologic Considerations in Wound Infections

Associated Clinical Condition	Common Pathogens
Varicella	GABHS, MSSA, MRSA
Cervical adenitis	GABHS, MSSA, MRSA
Neck space infection	GABHS, MSSA, MRSA, anaerobes
Tonsillopharyngitis	GABHS, MSSA, MRSA
Jugular thrombosis	*Fusobacterium necrophorum*
Surgical wounds	
Uncomplicated	GABHS, MSSA, MRSA
Abdominal, inguinal, perineal, circumcision	GABHS, MSSA, MRSA, enteric gram-negative bacilli (esp. Proteus spp.), anaerobes
Omphalitis, breast abscess	MSSA, MRSA, group B streptococcus, GABHS, enteric gram-negative bacilli (esp. *Escherichia coli*), anaerobes
Traumatic wounds	GABHS, MSSA, MRSA
Aquatic	MSSA, MRSA, streptococci, *Pseudomonas aeruginosa,* Aeromonas spp., Vibrio spp. (salt water), *Chromobacterium violaceum* (stagnant freshwater)
Soil and wood	MSSA, MRSA, streptococci, gram-negative bacilli (esp. Enterobacter spp., *P. aeruginosa*), fungi (esp. Zygomycetes, Acremonium, Fusarium)
Neutropenia	Clostridia, gram-negative bacilli (esp. *P. aeruginosa*), GABHS, MSSA, MRSA
Neutrophil oxidative disorders	MSSA, MRSA, Serratia spp., *C. violaceum,* Pseudomonas spp.
Iron overload syndromes	Vibrio spp.
Vasculitis	*Streptococcus pneumoniae,* Serratia spp., GABHS, MSSA, MRSA
Injection drug use	Bacillus spp., *P. aeruginosa*

Abbreviations: GABHS, group A β-hemolytic streptococcus; MRSA, methicillin-resistant *Staphylococcus aureus;* MSSA, methicillin-sensitive *Staphylococcus aureus.*

or complicated cellulitis and are directed at potential causes related to the clinical situation (Table 120–3). When group A streptococcus is suspected, the combination of clindamycin and a β-lactam is optimal.[17] Early administration of intravenous immune globulin (0.5 to 1 g/kg) is recommended by some authorities, especially if there are signs of toxic shock due to group A streptococcus or *S. aureus.*[45]

Atopic Dermatitis with Bacterial Superinfection

Infectious complications of atopic dermatitis are common and present as bullous lesions, pustular lesions, increased erythema and discomfort, and increased oozing and crusting, as well as skin erosions and ulcerations. It is important to differentiate between possible bacterial and herpesvirus etiologies, since therapeutic misadventures can have significant consequences.

S. aureus and group A streptococcus are the most important bacterial causes of atopic dermatitis superinfection. Over 90% of individuals with atopic dermatitis are colonized with *S. aureus.* Increased colonization is known to correlate with increased disease severity, thus antistaphylococcal topical and oral antibiotic therapies are widely prescribed. As with other skin and soft tissue infections, CA-MRSA has become a major problem. Atopic dermatitis has clearly been identified as a risk factor for CA-MRSA infection.[46] Therefore, bacterial cultures are important to effective management. MSSA may be treated with topical mupirocin or oral antibiotics; cephalosporins and dicloxacillin are popular choices, but dicloxacillin suspension is especially unpalatable. Mupirocin cream and oral cephalexin have been shown to be equally effective; mupirocin is superior in reducing bacterial inoculum on the skin.[47] Cephalosporins may be used in patients with non–type I penicillin allergy, and clindamycin for patients with type I allergy. Trimethoprim-sulfamethoxazole should be used only in patients in whom *S. aureus* is the sole pathogen, due to lack of efficacy in group A streptococcus infections. Treatment and control of super-

infection also includes optimizing the treatment of atopic dermatitis using skin hydration and topical steroids. Nasal mupirocin therapy twice a day in each naris for 5 days is recommended by some authorities to reduce *S. aureus* carriage.

Disseminated viral infection is the other concern in atopic dermatitis superinfection. Molluscum contagiosum is a benign, self-limited skin condition in most children characterized by a few skin lesions. Patients with atopic dermatitis are more likely to exhibit widespread skin involvement with hundreds of lesions.[48] The latter has been termed *eczema molluscatum* and presents as a heavy concentration of 2- to 3-mm umbilicated, skin-colored papules in areas of affected skin with occasional scatter elsewhere. Patients are otherwise well appearing. The condition resolves on its own, except in individuals with T-cell immune deficiency, in particular that related to human immunodeficiency virus (HIV) infection. Curettage, cryotherapy, and laser vaporization have been used in minor cases. Patients with disseminated disease should be referred to a dermatologist, who may recommend topical imiquimod or related agents.[49]

Similarly, severe and disseminated varicella infection may occur in atopic dermatitis patients. Lesions similar to eczema herpeticum occur and are strikingly concentrated in areas with significant disease. Both of these viral infections have been termed *Kaposi's varicelliform eruptions.* Intravenous or oral acyclovir is indicated depending on disease severity. Infected atopic dermatitis that does not respond to standard therapy for a suspected etiology raises the possibility of a different or resistant pathogen, or a serious, previously unrecognized, underlying disorder (HIV infection, Wiskott-Aldrich syndrome, hyperimmunoglobulinemia E syndrome, histiocytosis, or zinc deficiency).

Eczema Herpeticum

HSV may infect eczema by auto-inoculation from oral lesions, by contact with HSV skin lesions (as seen in wrestlers), or from kissing. Crops of tiny vesicles develop in areas of eczema and become pustular, then ulcerated, and finally crusted. Normal skin tends to be spared. Constitutional symptoms are common. Eczema herpeticum is often misdiagnosed as bacterial superinfection. The vesicular and pustular appearance may be brief due to intense scratching by the patient. Concomitant bacterial infection may further confuse the clinician. Diagnosis is based on clinical appearance and the tendency for the lesions to recur on the same areas of the skin. Diagnosis is confirmed by viral culture of lesions or HSV direct fluorescent antibody immunostaining of cells scraped from the base of lesions.

Eczema herpeticum is a potentially severe condition. Systemic acyclovir therapy is required. For children under 12 years of age, the recommended dose is 750 mg/m^2 administered intravenously every 8 hours for 7 days. Oral acyclovir bioavailability is low, but this formulation can be prescribed as 20 mg/kg per dose four times daily for mild disease. Topical antivirals are ineffective.

Folliculitis

Folliculitis is a superficial infection of hair follicles that presents as small, discrete, pustules on an erythematous base. Skin irritation is a common cause. Usual etiologies are *S. aureus* and other staphylococcal species. Treatment with topical antiseptics (chlorhexidine, hexachlorophene, or clindamycin) suffices in most cases. More extensive presentations may require oral antibiotic therapy and consideration of MRSA. Chronic folliculitis responds to daily application of a benzoyl peroxide lotion or gel. Candida and *Malassezia furfur* may cause folliculitis in patients being treated with topical corticosteroids. Topical selenium sulfide, azoles, and tolnaftate have all been prescribed with success. Gram-negative organisms are found in patients with concomitant acne vulgaris. Standard therapies for acne are recommended in those cases. "Hot tub folliculitis" is due to *P. aeruginosa* found in hot tubs with suboptimal chemical maintenance. Lesions develop 8 to 48 hours after exposure and may be quite pruritic. Diagnosis is confirmed by culture of pustules. This is a benign, self-limited condition that resolves in 1 to 2 weeks, but treatment with an oral quinolone may be considered in teenagers and those with constitutional symptoms. Immunocompromised hosts may progress to more serious disease such as cellulitis, ecthyma, systemic infection, and even sepsis. Cancer patients and immune-deficient patients should avoid hot tubs. Immunocompromised children are frequently treated empirically with antipseudomonal agents (oral quinolones for well patients and parenteral agents in patients with illness or complications).

Furuncles and Carbuncles

Furuncles develop in a fashion similar to folliculitis but represent a more extensive infectious process in hair follicles. Furuncles may also develop as skin abscesses after minor skin injury. As the furuncle develops, infection progresses to deeper dermal levels with potential extension into subcutaneous tissues. Carbuncles are collections of two or more neighboring furuncles forming a confluence of purulent pockets, which eventually drain from several sites to the surface. As seen in folliculitis, furuncles and carbuncles have a predilection for hair-bearing skin and areas subject to rubbing and skin friction. Common sites in children are the buttocks, perineum, and axillae. The extremities are also commonly affected, resulting from minor, everyday skin trauma and insect bites. Furuncles present as painful areas of erythema with increasing edema. The discomfort can be distressing for the child. Lesions progress to abscess with eventual thinning of the overlying skin and rupture of the purulent contents. They often drain and heal spontaneously to leave a slightly depressed scar. In some cases lesions cause significant cellulitis and constitutional symptoms, including fever. Deeper underlying tissues may be threatened. Furuncles and carbuncles must be differentiated from a kerion of the scalp, inflamed epidermal and pilar cysts, acne vulgaris, and hidradenitis suppurativa.

S. aureus is the major cause of furunculosis. The incidence of furunculosis appears to be increasing due to the emergence of CA-MRSA.[7,50] These strains may also cause more severe skin disease and invasive infection due to ability to produce virulence factors, including Panton-Valentine leukocidin.[51] Outbreaks have occurred in day care and detention facilities and among competitive sports participants.[52] Wrestlers and rugby and football players have been increasingly affected, but the problem has occurred even in sports with little direct participant contact or physical trauma, such as fencing. An athletic outbreak can also be a marker of a community-wide outbreak.[53] Community and sports outbreaks have been shown to have been caused by specific CA-MRSA clones limited to a certain geographic area.[54] Because of epidemiologic and treatment implications, cultures of furunculosis and skin abscesses are mandatory in modern management.

Management

The treatment approach for furuncles and carbuncles is the same as that outlined for other potentially serious skin and soft tissue infections (see Table 120–2). As previously noted, furuncle management depends on clinical presentation, disease severity, and local antibiotic resistance rates. Simple incision and drainage alone suffices for the vast majority of cases. Patients often recover after incision and drainage even when no antibiotic is prescribed or an agent ineffective against CA-MRSA in vitro is used. A prospective study suggested that antimicrobial therapy is most likely to be helpful in cases in which cellulitis surrounding a furuncle is greater than 5 cm.[55] This group of patients were at risk for eventual hospitalization and parenteral therapy. This approach may not apply to infants and ill or immunocompromised patients, who are likely to require the most aggressive management, especially if they are febrile. Antibiotic choice depends on the severity of illness and local antibiotic resistance patterns (Table 120–4). The possibility of CA-MRSA infection should be considered when choosing. Seven to 10 days is the usual length of treatment.

Recurrent furunculosis is most often a benign condition and reflective of patient and familial colonization with a troublesome isolate of *S. aureus*. This, too, is becoming much more common with the rise of CA-MRSA. These patients tend to have heavy nasal colonization with *S. aureus* as well as colonization of other body sites. Nasal mupirocin (application into each naris twice daily or more for at least 5 days)[56] along with daily bathing with a chlorhexidine cleanser[57] has been recommended with some success. Oral rifampin has been used in combination with other antibiotics depending

Table 120–4	Antibiotics Useful in Skin and Soft Tissue Infections (see text)			
Drug	**Route**	**Dose**	**Max dose**	**Comments**
Dicloxacillin	PO	25–50 mg/kg/day in 4 doses	1–2 g/day	MSSA, GABHS; poorly palatable suspension
Penicillin VK	PO	25–50 mg/kg/day in 3–4 doses	2 g/day	GABHS, Eikenella, Pasteurella
Penicillin G	IV	250,000–400,000 U/kg/day in 4–6 doses	24 million U/day	
Amoxicillin/ clavulanate (14 : 1)	PO	90 mg/kg/day of amoxicillin in 2 doses	2 g/day	MSSA, GABHS, Haemophilus, Pneumococcus, Pastuerella, anaerobes
Ampicillin/ sulbactam	IV	3 mo–12 yr: 100–200 mg/kg/day of ampicillin in 4 doses Older: 200–400 mg/kg/day of ampicillin in 4 doses	6–12 g/day	MSSA, GABHS, Haemophilus, Pneumococcus, Pastuerella, anaerobes
Piperacillin/ tazobactam	IV	150–200 mg/kg/day of piperacillin in 3 doses	240 mg/dose	Not licensed for use in children; MSSA, GABHS, gram-negative enterics, Pseudomonas, anaerobes
Imipenem	IV	50–100 mg/kg/day in 4 doses	4 g/day	Many gram-negative and positive organisms, Aeromonas, Pseudomonas, anaerobes; no MRSA activity
Cefepime	IV	150 mg/kg/day in 3 doses	4 g/day	MSSA, GABHS, gram-negative enterics and Pseudomonas
Ceftazidime	IV	150–200 mg/kg/day in 3 doses	6 g/day	Gram-negative enterics and Pseudomonas, many Aeromonas; fair MSSA and GABHS coverage
Cephalexin	PO	25–50 mg/kg/day in 3–4 doses	1–4 g/day	MSSA, GABHS; no MRSA
Nafcillin	IV	150 mg/kg/day in 4 doses	12 g/day	MSSA, reasonable GABHS; no MRSA
Cefazolin	IV	50–100 mg/kg/day in 3 doses	6 g/day	MSSA, GABHS; no MRSA
Clindamycin	PO	25–40 mg/kg/day in 3–4 doses	2 g/day	MSSA, CA-MRSA, anaerobes, most GABHS, penicillin-resistant pneumococcus; no HA-MRSA
	IV	25–40 mg/kg/day in 3–4 doses	2.7 g/day	Do not use alone for serious GABHS infection (see text)
Linezolid	PO	20–30 mg/kg/day in 3 doses	1200 mg/day	MSSA, CA-MRSA, HA-MRSA, GABHS, Enterococcus (including vancomycin-resistant); no gram-negatives; very expensive
	IV	20 kg/day in 2 doses	1.2 g/day	
	IV	20–30 mg/kg/day in 3 doses	1200 mg/day	Expert infectious disease advice helpful
Trimethoprim-sulfamethoxazole		8–12 mg/kg/day of trimethoprim, 40–60 mg/kg/day of sulfa in 2 doses	300 mg/1.6 g per day	MSSA, CA-MRSA, Aeromonas; no GABHS
Doxycycline	PO	5 mg/kg/day in 1–2 doses	200 mg/day	CA-MRSA, Vibrio; limited to > 8 yr old
Ciprofloxacin	PO	30 mg/kg/day in 2 doses	1.0–1.5 g/day	Selective indications in children; expert infectious disease advice helpful
	IV	20–30 mg/kg/day in 2 doses	400–800 mg/day	Gram-negatives, Pseudomonas, Aeromonas; no anaerobes, poor MSSA
Azithromycin	PO	5–12 mg/kg once daily	600 mg/day	MSSA, GABHS; no MRSA; reserve for penicillin allergy
Vancomycin	IV	40 mg/kg/day in 3–4 doses; 40–60 mg/kg/day in 4 doses (severe cases)	2 g/day; 4 g/day	MSSA, CA-MRSA, HA-MRSA, GABHS, penicillin-resistant Pneumococcus
Rifampin	PO	10–20 mg/day in 1–2 doses	600 mg/day	Synergy against MSSA, CA-MRSA, HA-MRSA
Gentamicin	IV	3–7.5 mg/kg in 3 doses or 5–6 mg/kg every 24 hr	N/A	Used in combinations for synergy versus staphylococci, enterococci, Pseudomonas, gram-negative enterics

Abbreviations: GABHS, group A β-hemolytic streptococcus; CA-MRSA, community-acquired methicillin-resistant *Staphylococcus aureus;* HA-MRSA, hospital-acquired methicillin-resistant *Staphylococcus aureus;* MRSA, methicillin-resistant *Staphylococcus aureus;* MSSA, methicillin-sensitive *Staphylococcus aureus.*

on the antimicrobial susceptibility pattern of the patient's isolate in attempts to decolonize patients. Data are not currently sufficient to allow recommendation of such approaches as routine care. The emergency physician should seek infectious disease expertise in these situations.

Patients who do not respond to therapy or worsen despite use of effective antimicrobial agents, or continue to have significant recurrent disease, may have an underlying predisposing condition. *S. aureus* disease is most troublesome to patients with neutropenias (familial, cyclic, acquired), neutrophil disorders (oxidative burst deficiencies, myeloperoxidase deficiency, glucose-6-phosphate dehydrogenase deficiency, chemotactic disorders, leukocyte adhesion defects),

HIV-related immune deficiency, hyperimmunoglobulinemia E syndrome, and common variable immune deficiency.

Hidradenitis Suppurativa

Hidradenitis suppurativa is a chronic, often progressive, severe inflammatory disease of apocrine glands mainly in intertigenous areas such as the axillae, groin, perineum, and rectum. Disease severity is often cyclic and remitting; flare-ups can be debilitating. The spectrum of disease ranges from inflammatory nodules to nodules with draining wounds and sinus tracts. With each cycle of inflammation the extent of the lesions increases. The condition is commonly confused with furuncles and carbuncles, progressive folliculitis, and

Table 120–5	Organisms Associated with Unusual Domesticated and Wild Animal Bite Wounds	
Animal	**Organism**	**Treatment Should Include***
Horses	Similar to dog and cat	Amoxicillin/clavulanate
Pig/sheep	Dog/cat flora + *Francisella tularensis* and others	Amoxicillin/clavulanate, gentamycin
Rat	Dog/cat flora + *Streptobacillus moniliformis, Leptospira*	Amoxicillin/clavulanate
Ferret/gerbil	Rat flora + *Acinetobacter anitratus*	Antipseudomonal penicillin
Monkeys	Human flora + herpesvirus B	Antiviral therapy
Coyote	*Francisella tularensis*	Gentamycin
Wolf	*Pasteurella multocida*	Amoxicillin/clavulanate
Cougar	*Pasteurella multocida*	Amoxicillin/clavulanate
Panther	*Pasteurella multocida*	Amoxicillin/clavulanate
Lion	*Pasteurella multocida, Staphylococcus aureus, Escherichia coli*	Amoxicillin/clavulanate
Tiger	*Pasteurella multocida, Acinetobacter, Escherichia coli*, streptococci, staphylococci	Amoxicillin/clavulanate
Skunks	Rabies	RIG, HDCV
Raccons	Rabies	RIG, HDCV
Bats	Rabies	RIG, HDCV
Foxes	Rabies	RIG, HDCV
Opossum	*Pasteurella multocida*	Amoxicillin/clavulanate
Squirrel	*Francisella tularensis*	Gentamycin

*Consult with infectious disease specialist for total management strategy.
Abbreviations: HDCV, human diploid cell rabies vaccine; RIG, rabies immune globulin.

Table 120–6	Prophylactic Antimicrobial Strategy for Mammalian Bite Wounds (Domesticated Animals and Humans)			
	Commonly Associated Organisms	**First Choice**	**Other Choices**	**Penicillin-Allergic Patient***
Empirical therapy for most bites		Amoxicillin/clavulanate 25–40 mg/kg bid	Cefuroxime[†] 50 mg/kg divided bid *or* Ceftriaxone[†] 50–75 mg/kg IM qd × 2 3 days	Clindamycin 15 25 mg/kg divided tid *plus* Trimethoprim/sulfamethoxazole 6 12 mg/kg divided bid *or* Doxycycline[‡] 50–100 mg bid
Dog bites	*Pasteurella multocida* *Streptococcus* species *Staphylococcus aureus* *Neisseria* species Anaerobes: *Bacteroides, Fusobacterium* Other: *Eikenella, Capnocytophaga canimorsus*	Amoxicillin/clavulanate	Penicillin V 25–50 mg/kg divided tid–qid *or* Amoxicillin 40 mg/kg divided tid[§]	Clindamycin plus trimethoprim/ sulfamethoxazole *or* Doxycycline[‡]
Cat bites	*Pasteurella multocida* *Streptococcus* species *Staphylococcus aureus* *Neisseria* species Anaerobes: *Bacteroides, Fusobacterium* Other: *Eikenella, Capnocytophaga canimorsus*	Amoxicillin/clavulanate	Penicillin and/or dicloxicillin 25–50 mg/kg, divided qid for both	Clindamycin plus trimethoprim/ sulfamethoxazole *or* Doxycycline[‡]
Human bites	Many aerobic/anaerobic bacteria, esp. *Streptococcus, Staphylococcus, Eikenella corrodens, Corynebacterium, Bacteroides, Clostridium*	Amoxicillin/clavulanate	Penicillin and/or dicloxicillin	Clindamycin plus trimethoprim/ sulfamethoxazole *or* Doxycycline[‡] *or* Erythromycin[¶] *or* Macrolide

*Should consult with infectious disease expert.
[†]Effective against *S. aureus*, anaerobes, *E. corrodens*, and *P. multocida*.
[‡]Not for use in prepubertal children or pregnant women.
[§]Lower incidence of *P. multocida*.
[¶]*Pasturella multocida* only moderately sensitive, with known treatment failures; *Eikenella* with slightly increased sensitivity.

epidermoid or dermoid cysts. Hidradenitis suppurativa is differentiated from these other conditions by its chronicity, cyclic presentation, and progressive nature. Differentiation of perianal hidradenitis from perianal complications associated with inflammatory bowel disease may be difficult. Acne conglobata is similar in appearance to hidradenitis suppurativa but lacks cyclic features.

Over 98% of hidradenitis suppurativa cases present after the age of 11 years, and hormonal influences may play an important role. Oral contraceptives, pregnancy, and the latter portion of the menstrual cycle are known to worsen disease in females. Hidradenitis is more common in patients with a variety of endocrinopathies, including diabetes mellitus and adrenal gland diseases. The etiology of hidradenitis suppurativa remains largely undefined; however, apocrine gland duct obstruction and superinfection play roles in pathogenesis. A variety of organisms have been isolated from wound drainage, including Staphylococcus species, Streptococcus species, *Escherichia coli*, Klebsiella species, Proteus species, Corynebacteria, and anaerobes.[58,59]

Treatment of patients with flare-ups of hidradenitis involves warm baths, local antisepsis, and cleansing with mild antibacterial agents. Oral and topical antistaphyloccocal antimicrobial agents are commonly prescribed, with anaerobic coverage added in cases of perianal disease. Topical clindamycin or an oral tetracycline has some efficacy.[60] Oral clindamycin has also been used. Cultures should guide the ultimate antibiotic choice. There are no data to support a recommendation for chronic, suppressive antimicrobial therapy. Patients should be advised to wear loose-fitting clothes that will not rub and traumatize affected areas. Incision and drainage of lesions or unroofing of closed lesions to encourage marsupialization may speed healing, but has no effect on recurrence, prognosis, or disease severity. Referral to a dermatologist or surgeon is necessary since treatment with retinoids or immune-modulating medications such as cyclosporin, or local to wide surgical incision and even skin grafting, may be warranted.

Lymphangitis

Lymphangitis is an inflammatory process of the lymphatic system that drains an area of infection. Regional lymph nodes are often involved and may become suppurative at later stages. Physical examination reveals tender, erythematous streaks extending from the primary site of infection and along the tracts of the lymphatics. Group A streptococcus is the leading cause, with *S. aureus* implicated in most other cases; however, infection with a variety of other organisms may also present in a similar fashion. For example, lymphangitis may be seen with puncture and contaminated wound infections. Wound and blood cultures are recommended in children due to the risk of bacteremia and sepsis, especially when febrile. Therapy is directed against the primary infection and stratified by the general approach to soft tissue infections (see Table 120–2).

REFERENCES

1. Ambati B, Ambati J, Azar N, et al: Periorbital and orbital cellulitis before and after the advent of *Haemophilus influenzae* type b vaccination. Ophthalmology 107:1450–1453, 2000.
2. Patel M, Athrens JC, Moyer J, et al: Pneumococcal soft tissue infections: a problem deserving more recognition. Clin Infect Dis 19:149–151, 1994.
3. Newell PM, Norden CW: Value of needle aspiration in bacteriologic diagnosis of cellulitis in adults. J Clin Microbiol 26:401–404, 1988.
4. Sachs MK: Cutaneous cellulitis. Arch Dermatol 127:493–496, 1991.
5. Sigurdsson AF, Gudmundsson S: The etiology of bacterial cellulitis as determined by fine-needle aspiration. Scand J Infect Dis 21:537–542, 1989.
6. Lebre C, Girard-Pipau F, Roujeau JC, et al: Value of fine-needle aspiration in infectious cellulitis. Arch Dermatol 132:842–843, 1996.
7. Salgado CD, Farr BM, Calfee DP: Community acquired methicillin-resistant *Staphylococcus aureus*: a meta-analysis of prevalence and risk factors. Clin Infect Dis 36:131–139, 2003.
8. Howe PM, Eduardo-Fajardo J, Orcutt MA: Etiologic diagnosis of cellulitis: comparison of aspirates obtained from the leading edge and the point of maximal inflammation. Pediatr Infect Dis J 6:685–686, 1987.
9. Sadow KB, Chamberlain JM: Blood cultures in the evaluation of children with cellulitis. Pediatrics 101:e4, 1998.
10. Frank AL: Clindamycin treatment of methicillin-resistant *Staphylococcus aureus* infections in children. Pediatr Infect Dis J 21:530–534, 2002.
11. Centers for Disease Control and Prevention: Four pediatric deaths from community-acquired methicillin-resistant *Staphylococcus aureus*: Minnesota and North Dakota, 1997–1999. MMWR Morb Mortal Wkly Rep 37:2858–2862, 1999.
12. Herold BC, Immergluck LC, Maranan MC, et al: Community-acquired methicillin-resistant *Staphylococcus aureus* in children with no predisposing risk. JAMA 279:593–598, 1998.
13. Wible K, Tregnaghi M, Bruss J, et al: Linezolid versus cefadroxil in the treatment of skin and skin structure infections in children. Pediatr Infect Dis J 22:315–322, 2003.
14. Kaplan SL: Use of linezolid in children. Pediatr Infect Dis J 21:870–872, 2002.
15. Day S, Klein BL: Popsicle panniculitis. Pediatr Emerg Care 8:91–93, 1992.
16. Unkel JH, McKibben DH, Fenton SJ, et al: Comparison of odontogenic and nonodontogenic facial cellulitis in a pediatric hospital population. Pediatr Dent 19:476–479, 1997.
17. Zimbelman J, Palmer A, Todd J: Improved outcome of clindamycin compared with beta-lactam antibiotic treatment for invasive *Streptococcus pyogenes* infection. Pediatr Infect Dis J 18:1096–1100, 1999.
18. Mogielnicki NP, Schwartzman JD, Elliott JA: Perineal group A streptococcal disease in a pediatric practice. Pediatrics 106:276–281, 2000.
19. Nowicki MH, Bishop PR, Parker PH: Digital desquamation—a new finding in perianal streptococcal dermatitis. Clin Pediatr 39:237–239, 2000.
20. Paradisi M, Cianchini G, Angelo C: Efficacy of topical erythromycin in treatment of perianal streptococcal dermatitis. Pediatr Dermatol 10:297–298, 1993.
21. Montemarano AD, James WD: *Staphylococcus aureus* as a cause of perianal dermatitis. Pediatr Dermatol 10:259–262, 1993.
22. Hirschfeld AJ: Two family outbreaks of perianal cellulitis associated with group A beta-hemolytic streptococci. Pediatrics 46:799–802, 1970.
23. Keene WE, Markum AC, Samadpour M: Outbreak of *Pseudomonas aeruginosa* infections caused by commercial piercing of upper ear cartilage. JAMA 291:981–985, 2004.
24. Lyon M, Doehring MC: Blistering distal dactylitis: a case series in children under nine months of age. J Emerg Med 26:421–423, 2004.
25. Norcross MC Jr, Mitchell DF: Blistering distal dactylitis caused by *Staphylococcus aureus*. Cutis 51:353–354, 1993.
26. Zirn JR, Tompkins SD, Huie C, et al: Rapid detection and distinction of cutaneous herpesvirus infections by direct immunofluorescence. J Am Acad Dermatol 33:724–728, 1995.
27. Midani S, Rathore M: *Chromobacterium violaceum* infection. South Med J 91:464–466, 1998.
28. Vally H, Whittle A, Cameron S, et al: Outbreak of *Aeromonas hydrophila* wound infections associated with mud football. Clin Infect Dis 38:1084–1089, 2004.
29. Peterson JJ, Bancroft LW, Kransdorf MJ: Wooden foreign bodies: imaging appearance. AJR Am J Roentgenol 178:557–562, 2002.
30. Jacobs RF, McCarthy RE, Elser JM: *Pseudomonas* osteochondritis complicating puncture wounds of the foot in children: a 10-year evaluation. J Infect Dis 160:657–661, 1989.
31. Fustes-Morales A, Gutierrez-Castrellon P, Duran-McKinster C, et al: Necrotizing fasciitis: report of 39 pediatric cases. Arch Dermatol 138:893–899, 2002.

32. Miron D, Lev A, Colodner R, et al: *Vibrio vulnificus* necrotizing fasciitis of the calf presenting with compartment syndrome. Pediatr Infect Dis J 22:666–668, 2003.

33. Zerr DM, Alexander ER, Duchin JS, et al: A case-control study of necrotizing fasciitis during primary varicella. Pediatrics 103:783–790, 1999.

34. Laupland KB, Davies HD, Low DE, et al: Invasive group A streptococcal disease in children and association with varicella-zoster virus infection. Ontario Group A Streptococcal Study Group. Pediatrics 105: e60, 2000

35. Aronoff DM, Bloch KC: Assessing the relationship between the use of nonsteroidal antiinflammatory drugs and necrotizing fasciitis caused by group A streptococcus. Medicine 82:225–235, 2003.

36. Bisno AL, Cockerill FR 3rd, Bermudez CT: The initial outpatient-physician encounter in group A streptococcal necrotizing fasciitis. Clin Infect Dis 31:607–608, 2000

37. Hsieh T, Samson LM, Jabbour M, et al: Necrotizing fasciitis in children in eastern Ontario: a case-control study. CMAJ 163:393–396, 2000.

38. Wong C-H, Khin L-W, Heng K-S, et al: The LRINEC (Laboratory Risk Indicator for Necrotizing Fasciitis) score: a tool for distinguishing necrotizing fasciitis from other soft tissue infections. Crit Care Med 32:1535–1541, 2004.

39. Yen ZS, Wang HP, Ma HM, et al: Ultrasonographic screening of clinically-suspected necrotizing fasciitis. Acad Emerg Med 9:1448–1451, 2002.

40. Walshaw CF, Deans H: CT findings in necrotising fasciitis—a report of four cases. Clin Radiol 51:429–432, 1996.

41. Schmid MR, Kossman T, Duewell S: Differentiation of necrotizing fasciitis and cellulitis using MR imaging. AJR Am J Roentgenol 170:615–620, 1998.

42. Majeski J, Majeski E: Necrotizing fasciitis: improved survival with early recognition by tissue biopsy and aggressive surgical treatment. South Med J 90:1065–1068, 1997.

43. Moss RL, Musemeche CA, Kosloske AM: Necrotizing fasciitis in children: prompt recognition and aggressive therapy improve survival. J Pediatr Surg 31:1142–1146, 1996

44. Lille ST, Sato TT, Engrav LH, Jurkovich GJ: Necrotizing soft tissue infections: obstacles in diagnosis. J Am Coll Surg 182:7–11, 1996.

45. Cawley MJ, Briggs M, Haith LR Jr, et al: Intravenous immunoglobulin as adjunctive treatment for streptococcal toxic shock syndrome associated with necrotizing fasciitis: case report and review. Pharmacotherapy 19:1094–1098, 1999.

46. Sattler CA, Mason EO, Kaplan SL: Prospective comparison of risk factors and demographic and clinical characteristics of community-acquired, methicillin-resistant versus methicillin-susceptible *Staphylococcus aureus* infection in children . Pediatr Infect Dis J 21:910–917, 2002.

47. Rist T, Parish LC, Capin LR, et al: A comparison of the efficacy and safety of mupirocin cream and cephalexin in the treatment of secondarily infected eczema. Clin Exp Dermatol 27:14–20, 2002.

48. Wollenberg A, Wetzel S, Burgdorf WH, et al: Viral infections in atopic dermatitis: pathogenic aspects and clinical management. J Allergy Clin Immunol 112:683–685, 2003

49. Syed TA, Goswami J, Ahmadpour OA, et al: Treatment of molluscum contagiosum in males with an analog of imiquimod 1% in cream: a placebo-controlled, double-blind study. J Dermatol 25:309–313, 1998.

50. Iyer S, Jones DH: Community-acquired methicillin-resistant *Staphylococcus aureus* skin infection: a retrospective analysis of clinical presentation and treatment of a local outbreak. J Am Acad Dermatol 50:854–858, 2004.

51. Lina G, Piemont Y, Godail-Gamot F, et al: Involvement of Panton-Valentine leukocidin-producing *Staphylococcus aureus* in primary skin infections and pneumonia. Clin Infect Dis 29:1128–1132, 1999.

52. Centers for Disease Control and Prevention: Methicillin-resistant *Staphylococcus aureus* infections among competitive sports participants—Colorado, Indiana, Pennsylvania, and Los Angeles County, 2000–2003. MMWR Morb Mortal Wkly Rep 52:793–795, 2003.

53. Lindenmayer JM, Schoenfeld S, O'Grady R, et al: Methicillin-resistant *Staphylococcus aureus* in a high school wrestling team and the surrounding community. Arch Intern Med 158:895–899, 1998.

54. Kazakova SV, Hageman JC, Matava M: A clone of methicillin-resistant *Staphylococcus aureus* among professional football players. N Engl J Med 352:468–475, 2005.

55. Lee MC, Rios AM, Aten MF: Management and outcome of children with skin and soft tissue abscesses caused by community-acquired methicillin-resistant *Staphylococcus aureus*. Pediatr Infect Dis J 23:123–127, 2004.

56. Harbarth S, Dharan S, Liassine N, et al: Randomized, placebo-controlled, double-blind trial to evaluate the efficacy of mupirocin for eradicating carriage of methicillin resistant *Staphylococcus aureus*. Antimicrob Agent Chemother 43:1412–1416, 1999.

57. Watanakunakorn C, Axelson C, Bota B, et al: Mupirocin ointment with and without chlorhexidine baths in the eradication of *Staphylococcus aureus* nasal carriage in nursing home residents. Am J Infect Control 23:306–309, 1995.

58. Highet AS, Warren RE, Weekes AJ: Bacteriology and antibiotic treatment of perineal suppurative hidradenitis. Arch Dermatol 124:1047–1051, 1988.

59. Brook I, Frazier EH: Aerobic and anaerobic microbiology of axillary hidradenitis suppurativa. J Med Microbiol 48:103–105, 1999.

60. Jemec GB, Wendelboe P: Topical clindamycin versus systemic tetracycline in the treatment of hidradenitis suppurativa. J Am Acad Dermatol 39:971–974, 1998.

Chapter 121

Erythema Multiforme Major and Minor

Antonio E. Muñiz, MD

Introduction and Background

Erythema multiforme (EM) and Stevens-Johnson syndrome (SJS) are hypersensitivity syndromes that can be caused by infections, drugs, vaccinations, malignancy, and connective tissue disorders. EM is defined as an acute, self-limiting vesiculobullous disorder characterized by the formation of symmetrically distributed erythematous macules and papules, some of which evolve into the classic "target" lesions (Table 121–1).[1] On occasion it can involve one mucosal surface, particularly the oral mucosa.[2] It is seen most commonly in the second to fourth decade of life, but 20% of cases occur in children.

SJS is a potentially life-threatening condition with mortality up to 15%. By definition, it requires involvement of at least two mucous membranes, most often the conjunctivae and oropharynx, although the nasal, urethral, vaginal, and rectal mucosa can also be affected[3] (Table 121–2). The respiratory and gastrointestinal tracts are occasionally involved. As opposed to EM, mucosal and cutaneous involvement in SJS is severe with extensive necrosis. For many years EM was classified into minor and major forms, the major variant being SJS. However, recent consensus states that SJS is best

regarded as a different entity than EM, despite clinical and histologic similarities.[1,4] In addition, no one has been able to demonstrate that EM evolves into SJS.[4,5]

Recognition and Approach

The pathogenesis of EM is unknown, but it is considered to be a delayed hypersensitivity immune response to a number of different stimuli, particularly the herpes simplex virus (HSV) antigen in children.[6-8] Cytotoxic effector cells (CD8$^+$ T lymphocytes in the epidermis) induce apoptosis of scattered keratinocytes, which leads to cell necrosis. The diagnosis is often made by clinical assessment but can be confirmed by biopsy of a typical lesion, which shows T-lymphocyte infiltration.

Unlike EM, in SJS there is an excessive overexpression of tumor necrosis factor-α in the epidermis.[8,9] This may account for the greater degree of epidermal necrosis seen in SJS. Skin biopsy is characterized by a perivascular mononuclear infiltrate with some eosinophils in the dermis, variable hydrops degeneration of the basilar layer, and subepidermal blister formation in severe cases.

The list of putative trigger factors for EM and SJS in adults is an extensive one, but in children it seems that the majority of cases of EM are the result of a preceding recrudescence of HSV.[1,10] SJS in adults is usually drug induced, but in children it is associated with infections, especially *Mycoplasma pneumoniae*, as well as drugs, most notably antibiotics, anticonvulsants, and nonsteroidal anti-inflammatory drugs.[1,10-13]

Clinical Presentation

Erythema Multiforme

EM is often preceded by a herpes simplex infection, usually localized to the face but potentially occurring in any location. Prodromal symptoms are absent or mild and may consist of low-grade fever, cough, and anorexia. Myalgias or arthralgias are rare accompanying symptoms. Typically, crops of lesions develop over a few days in acral regions, especially the palms and dorsa of the hands, wrists, feet, and extensor surfaces of elbows and knees, and occasionally on the face. EM may manifest Koebner's phenomenon—target lesions appearing within areas of cutaneous trauma such as

Table 121–1	Clinical Features of Erythema Multiforme

- Benign, self-limited, and occasionally recurrent disorder
- Cutaneous lesions consisting of symmetric, fixed macules or papules evolving into "target" lesions
- Mucous membrane absent or limited only to the oral cavity
- Minimal or no prodromal symptoms
- Supportive treatment (antihistamines, acyclovir)

Table 121–2	Clinical Features of Stevens-Johnson Syndrome

- Prodromal symptoms
- Severe mucous membrane involvement (at least two)
- Much larger cutaneous involvement
- Treatment includes fluid and electrolyte replacement and meticulous skin care
- Other treatment may include corticosteroids and immune globulin
- Life threatening (mortality up to 15%)

Table 121–3	Differential Diagnosis of Erythema Multiforme

Giant urticaria
Drug reactions
Bullous pemphigoid
Chronic bullous dermatosis of childhood (CBDC)
Polymorphic light reaction
Systemic lupus erythematosus (SLE)
Urticarial vasculitis
Erythema annulare centrifugum

Table 121–4	Differential Diagnosis for Stevens-Johnson Syndrome

Burns or scalds
Staphylococcal scalded skin syndrome (SSSS)
Toxic epidermal necrolysis (TEN)
Kawasaki disease
Toxic shock syndrome
Acute graft-versus-host disease
Paraneoplastic pemphigus

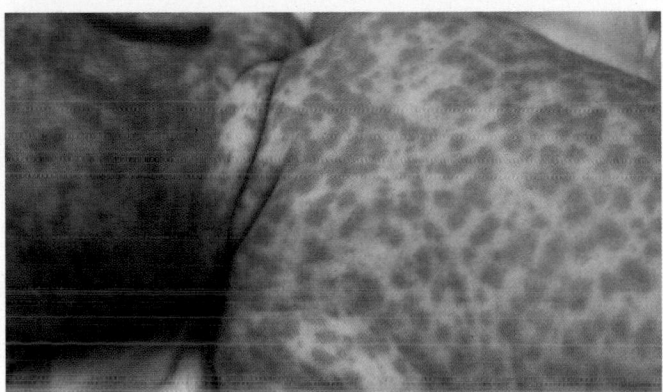

FIGURE 121–1. Typical target lesions in erythema multiforme.

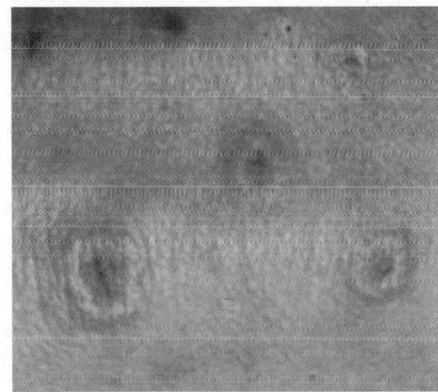

FIGURE 121–2. Concentric rings of target lesion in erythema multiforme.

scratches.[13,14] The cutaneous eruption of EM generally resolves in 1 to 2 weeks, but occasionally may be present for 4 weeks.

EM in childhood is frequently initially misdiagnosed as urticaria[14,15] (Table 121–3). The lesions in urticaria are transient and migratory and have a clear central zone, not a dusky one. In addition urticarial lesions will resolve with the administration of subcutaneous epinephrine, and EM will not.[14,15]

Stevens-Johnson Syndrome

SJS is usually preceded by a prodromal illness lasting up to 2 weeks and consisting of high fever, cough, coryza, sore throat, headache, chest pains, malaise, arthralgias, myalgias, vomiting, and diarrhea. Toxicity and generalized lymphadenopathy are common. Occasionally the child has hepatosplenomegaly or evidence of hepatitis. Myocarditis, pneumothorax, nephritis, and gastrointestinal bleeding are rare complications. After 1 to 14 days, the rash starts suddenly and occurs in the face, trunk, and limbs. Mucous membrane involvement, especially of the oral, conjunctival, and urethral mucosa, is typical and often severe. Oral mucous lesions may be confused with aphthous ulcers, herpes simplex infection, pemphigus, bullous pemphigoid, epidermolysis bullosa, and paraneoplastic pemphigus, and the differential diagnosis for SJS involves these and other serious disorders (Table 121–4).

Important Clinical Features and Considerations

Cutaneous lesions start as dull red macules or maculopapules, which may increase in size up to 3 cm in diameter within 24 to 48 hours. The lesions are usually asymptomatic, but some patients complain of itching. The lesions may evolve into target-shaped (or iris) plaques, which are the hallmark of EM[4] (Fig. 121–1). The target lesions consist of two or three concentric rings (Fig. 121–2). The central portion starts as a dusky red or purple macule before evolving into tense bullae with clear or hemorrhagic contents. There is usually a middle pale zone of edematous skin and an outer halo of well-demarcated erythema. As the name implies, there may be a variable pattern of lesions ranging from necrotic macules to an exclusively blistering disorder, but most have approximately 100 lesions[16] (Fig. 121–3). In SJS, depending on the severity, the

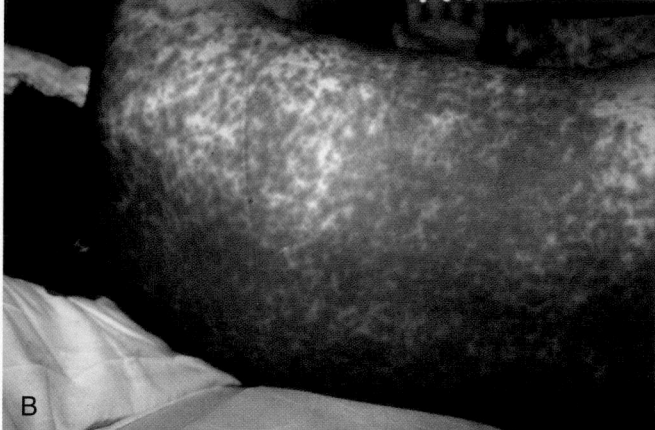

FIGURE 121–3. A, Close-up of extensive erythema multiforme. **B,** Stevens-Johnson syndrome demonstrating extensive skin lesions.

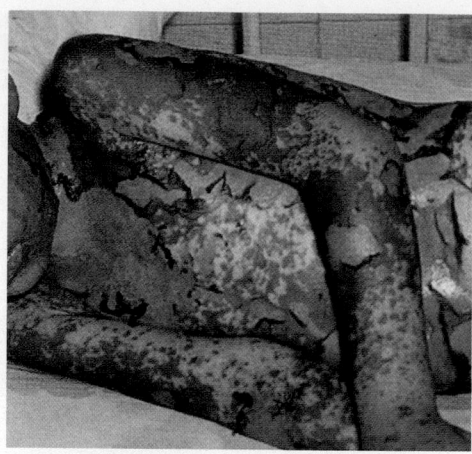

FIGURE 121–4. Large desquamation in Stevens-Johnson syndrome.

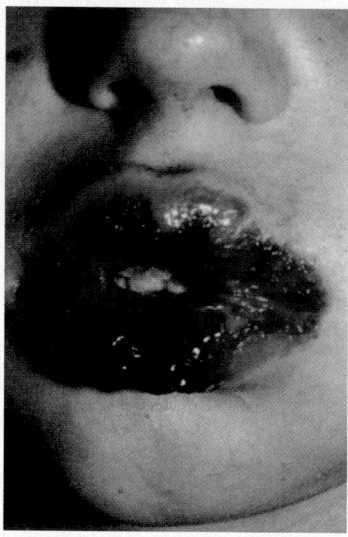

FIGURE 121–5. Hemorrhagic crusts of oral mucosa in Stevens-Johnson syndrome.

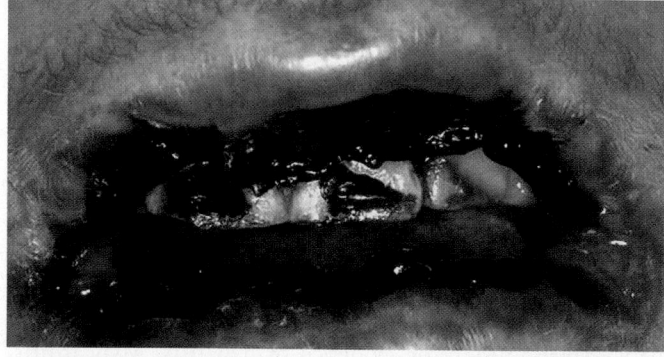

FIGURE 121–6. Extensive painful necrotic lesions of Stevens-Johnson syndrome.

epidermis begins to separate from the basal layer as a result of very minor frictional forces (Nikolsky's sign), and large flaccid blisters that resemble scalds rupture, leaving sheets of necrotic epidermis with a moist erythematous base (Fig. 121–4). Complications that occur with large areas of skin sloughing include fluid and electrolyte losses, secondary bacterial infections, scarring, and dyspigmentation.[1,17]

The primary oral lesion consists of an erythematous macule that evolves centrally into a thick-walled vesicle or bulla. The blisters last a brief period and, after rupture, leave the characteristic irregularly shaped ulcer with indistinct margins and a yellow necrotic base. Unlike EM, mucosal involvement in SJS is confluent and widespread. The lips are often covered with hemorrhagic crusts (Fig. 121–5). These lesions are extremely painful and may become covered with a pseudomembrane prior to healing. In severe cases, erosion of the pharynx and esophagus leads to necrotizing esophagitis (Fig. 121–6). Swallowing is so painful that dehydration is a common sequela.

Genital involvement induces urethritis, balanitis, and vulvovaginitis, which are associated with dysuria and purulent discharge (Fig. 121–7). The skin eruption consists of symmetric red macules that progress to central blister formation and extensive areas of epidermal necrosis. Erosions may also bleed. Genitourinary lesions may be so painful that urinary retention occurs. On occasion the rectal mucosa is also inflamed and ulcerated. Complications such as adhesions may develop.[18]

Ocular lesions constitute the most severe mucous membrane involvement. The early phase consists of a mucopurulent conjunctivitis with inflamed, edematous papillae and photophobia (Fig. 121–8). Focal ulcerations can occur and lead to formation of pseudomembranes and synechiae between the eyelids and conjunctiva. Other reported complications include entropion, keratitis, symblepharon,

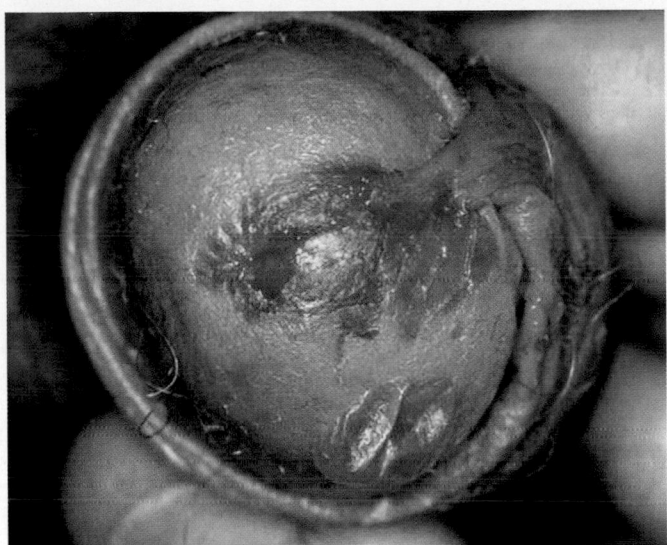

FIGURE 121–7. Penile mucosal involvement in Stevens-Johnson syndrome.

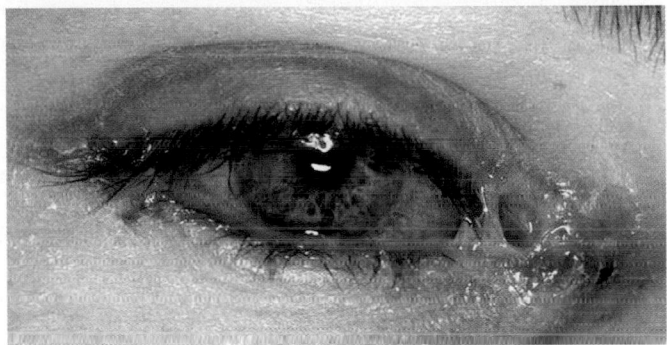

FIGURE 121–8. Involvement of the conjunctiva in Stevens-Johnson syndrome.

trichiasis, corneal pannus, uveitis, panophthalmos, and stricture of the lacrimal puncta.[19,20] Severe involvement may lead to loss of vision and even blindness.[21]

There are no specific laboratory abnormalities in EM, but SJS has been associated with elevated sedimentation rate, leukocytosis, eosinophilia, anemia, elevated hepatic transaminases, proteinuria, and hematuria.[1,22]

Management

Patients with EM require only symptomatic care, in addition to withdrawing any drugs suspected of initiating the eruption. If pruritus is prominent, oral antihistamines, calamine lotion, or oatmeal baths may be useful. Painful oral lesions may be treated with topical analgesic mouthwash (equal mixture of Maalox, 60 ml, and diphenhydramine, 15–30 ml), which is placed on the lesions with a Q-Tip. Viscous xylocaine should not be included since as little as 1–2 ml can be toxic to young children. HSV-associated EM does not usually respond to acyclovir, but prophylactic acyclovir, if given early enough, can prevent recurrences.[2,23,24]

Those patients with more extensive skin involvement, such as those with SJS, must be hospitalized for intravenous fluids,

correction of dehydration from transepidermal fluid losses, replacement of electrolytes, maintenance of nutrition, and pain control. These patients are best managed in a burn unit or pediatric intensive care unit with meticulous skin care for prevention of secondary bacterial infection, which can lead to sepsis, a leading cause of mortality. In addition, sulfonamide-containing ointments should be avoided since they have been implicated in causing these disorders.[18,25] Surgical débridement and whirlpool therapy to remove necrotic epidermis are recommended. Prompt withdrawal of the causative agent should be a priority since the course of the illness may be shortened.[26] Immediate ophthalmologic evaluation is mandatory if there are conjunctival lesions. Frequently applied lubrication with artificial tears and ophthalmic antibiotic drops or ointments (not containing sulfonamide) are necessary, with daily blunt disruption of synechiae.

The controversy over whether systemic corticosteroids should be used to attenuate progression of disease is still unresolved, since there are no large prospective, double-blind, multicenter controlled trials.[17,27] In small trials, corticosteroids have been shown to decrease the duration of fever and lesions.[27-29] Systemic corticosteroids do increase the risk of infection; however, their advocates suggest tapering the dose quickly once disease progression has ceased, and perhaps combining their use with a prophylactic antibiotic. High-dose intravenous immune globulins have been shown to improve some cases, with faster resolution of fever and skin lesions and shortened hospital stays.[30-33]

Summary

In EM, disease tends to be mild and attacks tend to subside within 1 to 3 weeks, usually without sequelae, except for an occasional pigmentary change. A follow-up visit in 24 to 48 hours is advisable to determine the progress of EM. In SJS, prognosis depends on prompt diagnosis and meticulous care for patients with extensive disease. Mortality is generally less for children than adults, but may be as high as 15%, and is worse with increasing body surface area involvement. In most cases recovery occurs within 3 to 6 weeks.

REFERENCES

*1. Lèautè-Labréze C, Lamireau T, Chawki D, et al: Diagnosis, classification and management of erythema multiforme and Stevens-Johnson syndrome. Arch Dis Child 83:347–352, 2000.
 2. Weston WL, Morelli JG, Rogers M: Target lesions on the lips: childhood herpes simplex associated with erythema multiforme mimics Stevens-Johnson syndrome. J Am Acad Dermatol 37:848–850, 1997.
 3. Wong KC, Kennedy PJ, Lee S: Clinical manifestations and outcomes of 17 cases of Stevens-Johnson syndrome and toxic epidermal necrolysis. Aust J Dermatol 40:131–134, 1999.
 4. Assier H, Bastuji-Garin S, Revuz J, Roujeau JC: Erythema multiforme with mucous membrane involvement and Stevens-Johnson syndrome are clinically different disorders with distinct causes. Arch Dermatol 131:539–543, 1995.
 5. Brice SL, Huff JC, Weston WL: Erythema multiforme minor in children. Curr Probl Dermatol 11:3–26, 1990.
 6. Weston WL, Stockert SS, Jester J, et al: Herpes simplex virus in childhood erythema multiforme. Pediatrics 89:32–34, 1992.
 7. Darragh TM, Egbert BM, Berger TG: Identification of herpes simplex virus DNA in lesions of erythema multiforme by the polymerase chain reaction. J Am Acad Dermatol 24:23–26, 1991.

*Selected readings.

8. Paquet P, Nikkels A, Arrese JE, et al: Macrophages and tumor necrosis factor alpha in toxic epidermal necrolysis. Arch Dermatol 130:605–608, 1994.

9. Ng PP, Sun YJ, Tan HH, Tan SH: Detection of herpes simplex virus genomic DNA in various subsets of erythema multiforme by polymerase chain reaction. Dermatology 207:349–353, 2003.

10. Aurelian L, Ono F, Burnett J: Herpes simplex virus (HSV)-associated erythema multiforme (HAEM): a viral disease with an autoimmune component. Dermatol Online J 9:1, 2003.

11. Tay YK, Huff JC, Weston WL: *Mycoplasma pneumoniae* infection is associated with Stevens-Johnson syndrome, not erythema multiforme (von Hebra). J Am Acad Dermatol 35:757–760, 1996.

12. Sullivan JR, Shear NH: The drug hypersensitivity syndrome: what is the pathogenesis? Arch Dermatol 137:357–364, 2001.

13. Huff JC, Weston WL: Isomorphic phenomenon in erythema multiforme. Clin Exp Dermatol 8:409–413, 1983.

14. Weston WL: What is erythema multiforme? Pediatr Ann 25:106–109, 1996.

15. Weston JA, Weston JL: The overdiagnosis of erythema multiforme. Pediatrics 89:802, 1992.

16. Huff JC, Weston WL: Recurrent erythema multiforme. Medicine 68:133–140, 1989.

17. Prendiville JS, Hebert AA, Greenwald MJ, et al: Management of Stevens-Johnson syndrome and toxic epidermal necrolysis. J Pediatr 115:881–887, 1989.

18. Hart R, Minto C, Creighton S: Vaginal adhesions caused by Stevens-Johnson syndrome. J Pediatr Adolesc Gynecol 15:151–152, 2002.

19. Ginsburg CM: Stevens-Johnson syndrome in children. Pediatric Infect Dis 1:155–158, 1982.

20. Lehman SS: Long-term ocular complications of Stevens-Johnson syndrome. Clin Pediatr 38:425–427, 1999.

21. Kompella VB, Sangwan VS, Bansal AK, et al: Ophthalmic complications and management of Stevens-Johnson syndrome at a tertiary eye care center in south India. Indian J Ophthalmol 50:283–286, 2002.

22. Wong KC, Kennedy PJ, Lee S: Clinical manifestations and outcomes of 17 cases of Stevens-Johnson syndrome and toxic epidermal necrolysis. Australas J Dermatol 40:131–134, 1999.

23. Schofield JK, Tatnall FM, Leigh IM: Recurrent erythema multiforme: clinical features and treatment in a large series of patients. Br J Dermatol 128:542–545, 1993.

24. Tatnall FM, Schofield JK, Leigh IM: A double-blind, placebo-controlled trial of continuous acyclovir therapy in recurrent erythema multiforme. Br J Dermatol 132:267–270, 1995.

25. Roujeau JC: Treatment of severe drug eruptions. J Dermatol 26:718–722, 1999.

26. Garcia-Doval I, LeCleach L, Bocquet H, et al: Toxic epidermal necrolysis and Stevens-Johnson syndrome: does early withdrawal of causative drugs decrease the risk of death? Arch Dermatol 136:323–327, 2000.

27. Kakourou T, Klontza D, Soteropoulou F, Kattamis C: Corticosteroid treatment of erythema multiforme major (Stevens-Johnson syndrome) in children. Eur J Pediatr 156:90–93, 1997.

28. Ayangco L, Rogers RS 3rd: Oral manifestations of erythema multiforme. Dermatol Clin 21:195–205, 2003.

*29. Prendiville JS: Erythema multiforme and steroids. Pediatr Dermatol 17:75–83, 2000.

30. Morici MV, Galen WK, Shetty AK, et al: Intravenous immunoglobulin therapy for children with Stevens-Johnson syndrome. J Rheumatol 27:2494–2497, 2000.

31. Metry DW, Jung P, Levy ML: Use of intravenous immunoglobulin in children with Stevens-Johnson syndrome and toxic epidermal necrolysis: seven cases and review of the literature. Pediatrics 112:1430–1436, 2003.

32. Prins C, Vittorio C, Padilla RS, et al: Effect of high-dose intravenous immunoglobulin in Stevens-Johnson syndrome: a retrospective, multicenter study. Dermatology 207:96–99, 2003.

33. Bachot N, Revuz J, Roujeau JC: Intravenous immunoglobulin treatment for Stevens-Johnson syndrome and toxic epidermal necrolysis: a prospective noncomparative study showing no benefit on mortality or progression. Arch Dermatol 139:33–36, 2003.

Henoch-Schönlein Purpura

Antonio E. Muñiz, MD

Introduction and Background

Henoch-Schönlein purpura (HSP), also known as anaphylactoid purpura or allergic vasculitis, is the most prevalent cause of leukocytoclastic vasculitis in children, particularly between 3 and 10 years of age. It can occur in adults but is associated with a worse prognosis, more renal involvement, and increased use of aggressive therapeutic regimens, including corticosteroids and cytotoxic drugs.[1,2] The disorder is characterized by a tetrad consisting of a distinctive purpuric rash, colicky abdominal pain, athralgias or arthritis, and in some cases renal disease.

Recognition and Approach

A history of an antecedent upper respiratory tract infection preceding the onset of illness, seen in up to 75% of cases, suggests a hypersensitivity reaction to a virus resulting in vascular damage. Other entities implicated in the pathogenesis have included drugs, foods, insect bites, immunizations, cold exposure, tumors, pregnancy, and chemical toxins.[3-5]

The disorder appears to be initiated by deposition of immune complexes on the basement membrane, mainly of the immunoglobulin A (IgA) class, which activates complement leading to systemic inflammation of small vessels in the upper dermis, gastrointestinal tract, synovial membranes, renal glomeruli, and occasionally the lungs and central nervous system.[6-8] The deposition of IgA occurs as a consequence of abnormal glycosylation of O-linked oligosaccharides of IgA1.[9]

Clinical Presentation

The eruption is frequently preceded by a prodrome consisting of fever, headache, malaise, nausea, and vomiting. Subsequently a characteristic rash, abdominal pain, and/or joint symptoms occur. In most children, HSP is a self-limited illness with no significant sequelae; however, in a small minority renal disease can occur.

The major diagnostic feature is that of palpable petechiae or purpura. Individual lesions vary in size from 2 to 10 mm in diameter. They are most commonly found in a symmetric distribution over the buttocks and extensor surfaces of the legs (Figs. 122–1, 122–2, and 122–3). Children younger than 2 years of age have lesions in atypical locations, such as the face, upper extremity, and trunk (Fig. 122–4). Individual lesions occur in successive crops, tend to fade after 5 days, and eventually are replaced by areas of brownish pigmentation, purpura, or ecchymosis. New crops of lesions frequently occur over the next 2 to 4 weeks over the fading lesions of a previous episode, thereby giving a polymorphous appearance to the disorder. Less than 5% of patients have associated edema of the hands, feet, or face, and few have lesions consisting of urticaria.[10]

The differential diagnosis of HSP is variable[3,4,11] (Table 122–1).

Important Clinical Features and Considerations

Fifty percent to 80% of affected children also have involvement of joints, gastrointestinal tract, and kidneys, with lesser involvement of the cardiopulmonary, genitourinary, and central nervous system (Table 122–2).

The diagnosis of HSP is made by clinical features. Confirmation of the diagnosis of HSP requires evidence of tissue deposition of IgA in the skin or kidney by IgA immunofluorescence microscopy. Biopsy of skin lesions demonstrates a leukocytoclastic vasculitis, or white blood cells surrounding dermal blood vessels. These are more prominent in the postcapillary venules.

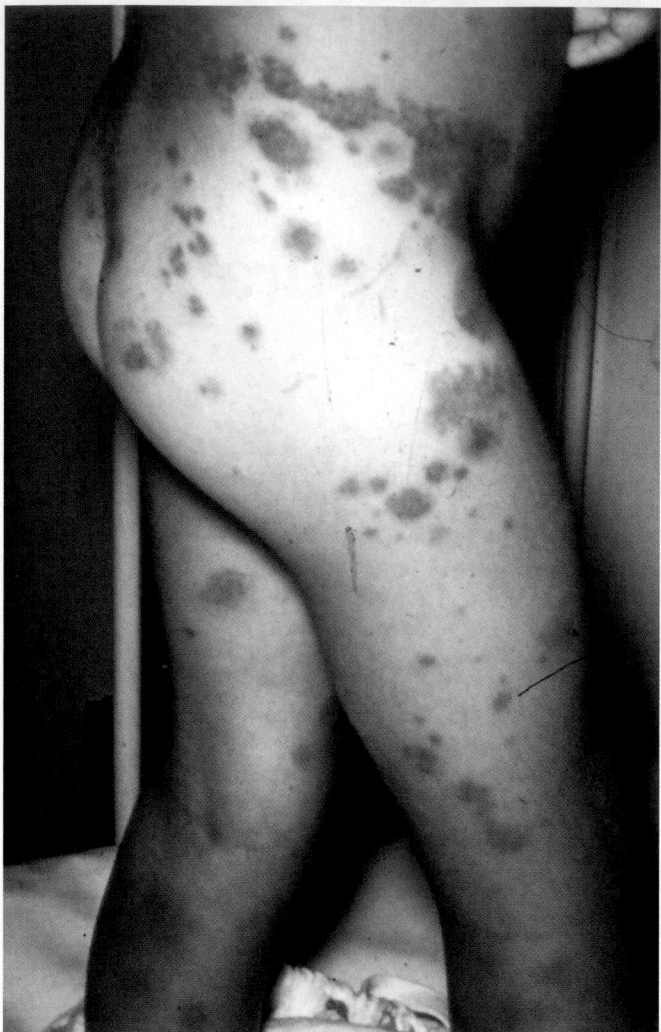

FIGURE 122–1. Typical purpuric lesions of the lower extremity.

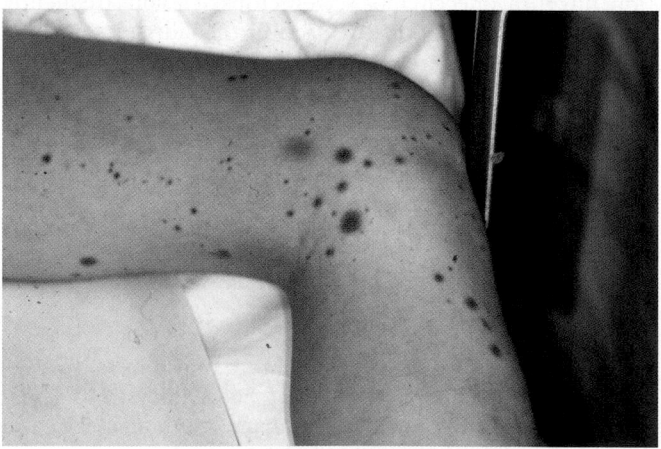

FIGURE 122–2. Typical purpuric lesions of the knee.

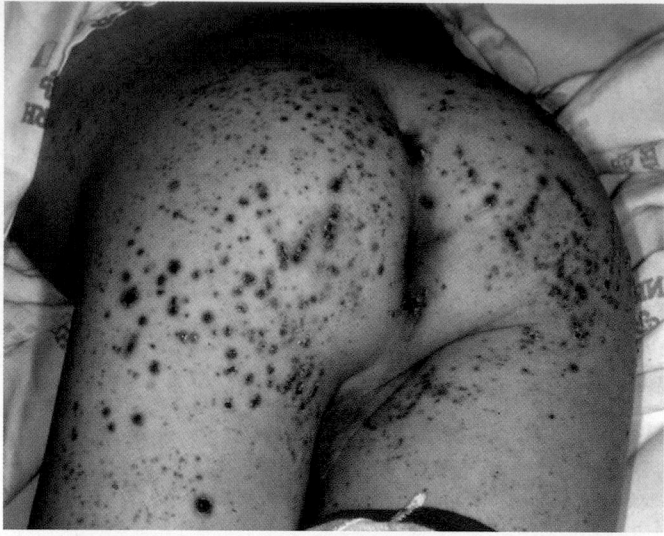

FIGURE 122–3. Typical purpuric lesions of the buttocks.

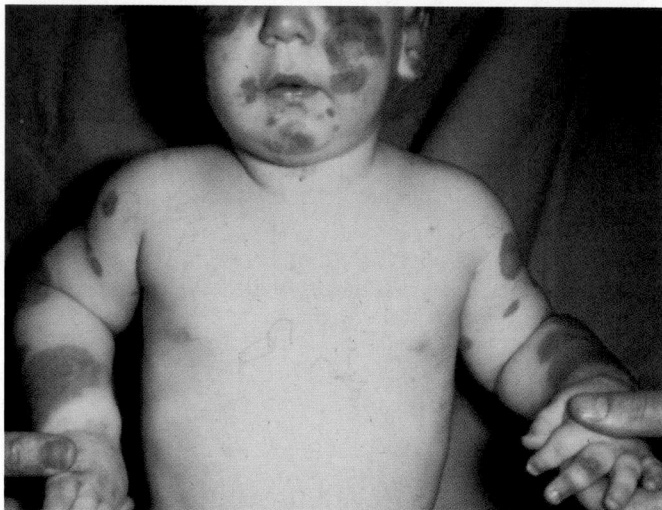

FIGURE 122–4. Atypical location of purpuric lesions in a young child.

Table 122–1	Differential Diagnosis of HSP

Juvenile rheumatoid arthritis (JRA)
Disseminated intravascular coagulation (DIC)
Acute glomerulonephritis
Idiopathic thrombocytopenic purpura (ITP)
Inflammatory bowel disease
Meningococcemia
Infectious mononucleosis
Systemic lupus erythematosus (SLE)
Thrombotic thrombocytopenic purpura (TTP)
Rocky Mountain spotted fever (RMSF)
Churg-Strauss syndrome
Chronic urticaria
Atypical measles
Staphylococcal sepsis
Pseudomonas sepsis
Subacute bacterial endocarditis
Gonococcemia
Mixed cryogobulinemia
Hypersensitivity vasculitis
Antiphospholipid syndrome
Wegener's granulomatosis
Trauma (including child abuse)

Table 122–2	Organ Systems Affected by HSP

Associated Features	Description
Joints (80%)	Warm, tender, and painful swelling of joints, with or without overlying purpura[11]
	Primarily in knees and ankles, but may be seen in elbows, hands, and feet
	Joint symptoms generally last a few days but have a high recurrence rate
Gastrointestinal symptoms (75%)	Symptoms from edema of the bowel wall, hemorrhage as a result of vasculitis, and thrombosis of the microvasculature
	Typically occur 1 wk after the rash but may precede in 14%–36%[31]
	Colicky abdominal pain, vomiting, visceral infarction or perforation, pancreatitis, cholecystitis, hydrops of the gallbladder, colitis, protein-losing enteropathy, appendicitis, pseudomembranous colitis, chronic intestinal obstruction with ileal stricture, intussusception, hemorrhage (melena or hematochezia), or shock[18,32-37]
	Location of intussusception is usually ileoileal and is diagnosed initially by ultrasound ("donut" or "pseudokidney" sign); may require surgical reduction but spontaneous reduction has occurred with conservative therapy, consisting of nasogastric drainage, corticosteroids, and intravenous fluids[38-40]
Kidney (25–50%)	Most serious cause of morbidity
	Occurs few days to 1 mo after onset
	May present with gross or, more commonly, microscopic hematuria, with or without casts and proteinuria
	Often self-limited; if proteinuria persists, may progress to advanced glomerular disease and acute or chronic renal failure
	Chronic renal disease in up to 15% with hematuria and proteinuria; if evidence of nephritis or nephrotic syndrome, end-stage renal disease in up to 50%[41]
	Overall, 1.7% of all patients develop chronic renal failure.[42] Children at higher risk for renal disease include those with hypertension, proteinuria > 1 g/L, elevations of serum blood urea nitrogen and creatinine, decreased fibrin-stabilizing factor (factor XIII) activity, glomerular crescents on biopsy, and rash greater than 1 month's duration.[41,43-48]
Central nervous system	Headache, diplopia, cerebral or cerebellar hemorrhage, subarachnoid hemorrhage, seizures, focal neurologic deficit, mononeuropathy, and coma[49-52]
Cardiopulmonary	Asymptomatic pulmonary infiltrate or recurrent episodes of pulmonary hemorrhage[53,54]
	Cardiac involvement is rare; may include myocarditis, coronary artery vasculitis resulting in acute myocardial ischemia or infarction, and cardiac tamponade[48,55,56]
Genitourinary (20%)	Scrotal hemorrhage may cause intense pain from severe scrotal swelling[57,58]
	Rare report of a simultaneous torsion of the testes; ultrasound or nuclear scan is recommended[59,60]

Management

Complete recovery occurs in 94% of children; therefore, most receive no specific therapy.[2] Bed rest and general supportive care are helpful. Analgesia with nonsteroidal anti-inflammatory drugs may reduce joint and soft tissue discomfort. For significant gastrointestinal hemorrhage, fluids and blood should be replaced as required. The degree to which diagnostic testing is performed in the emergency department depends on symptoms, but in all cases a urinalysis is warranted as a screening test for possible renal complications. Need for hospitalization is also dictated by severity of symptoms and the presence of complications. Most children can be managed as outpatients, but parents should be counseled that symptoms may wax and wane for several weeks before remitting entirely, and can be debilitating.

The efficacy of corticosteroids is controversial.[12-15] Although there is little evidence that corticosteroids alter the prognosis of HSP, they suppress and improve the acute manifestations, and hence may be justified for short periods in severe cases, especially those with significant gastrointestinal complications (except bleeding, perforation, intussusception) or chronic glomerulonephritis.[16,17] In this setting, a regimen of phased intravenous methylprednisolone followed by oral prednisone for 3 months may be beneficial.[18] This regimen is useful in reversing the anti-inflammatory process but not the IgA deposition. Dapsone, azathioprine, cyclophosphamide, cyclosporine, methotrexate, intravenous immune globulins, plasmapheresis, anticoagulation, and dipyridamole have been tried with varying success in severe and refractory cases.[8,19-28] Renal transplantation can be performed in those patients who progress to end-stage renal disease; however, recurrent disease can occur.[29,30] A pediatric nephrologist or rheumatologist should be consulted for guidance on the use of steroids and other medications.

Summary

HSP generally subsides within a few days to weeks, with some patients having recurrent attacks lasting weeks or months. The prognosis for most patients with HSP is excellent, with full recovery without sequelae in most cases. In children younger than 2 years of age, the disease is generally milder and of shorter duration, with fewer systemic complications.

Patients should be hospitalized if complications develop, such as significant bleeding, intussusception, renal disease (especially with hypertension), and pulmonary or central nervous system hemorrhages. All patients with an abnormal urinalysis should be referred for urgent follow-up so that the urine may continue to be frequently monitored.

REFERENCES

1. Garcia-Porra C, Calvino MC, Llorca J, et al: Henoch-Schönlein purpura in children and adults: clinical differences in a defined population. Semin Arthritis Rheum 32:149–156, 2002.
2. Blanco R, Martinez-Taboada VM, Rodriguez-Valverde V, et al: Henoch-Schönlein purpura in adulthood and childhood: two different expressions of the same syndrome. Arthritis Rheum 40:859–864, 1997.
3. Harper L, Ferreira MA, Howie AJ, et al: Treatment of vasculitic IgA nephropathy. J Nephrol 13:360–366, 2000.
4. Scott DG, Watts RA: Systemic vasculitis: epidemiology, classification and environmental factors. Ann Rheum Dis 59:161–163, 2000.

5. Campanile G, Hautmann G, Lotti TM: The etiology of cutaneous necrotizing vasculitis. Clin Dermatol 17:505–508, 1999.
6. Saulsbury FT: Henoch-Schönlein purpura. Pediatr Dermatol 1:195–201, 1984.
7. Saulsbury FT: IgA rheumatoid factor in Henoch-Schönlein purpura. J Pediatr 108:71–76, 1986.
8. Tarshish P, Bernstein J, Edelmann CM: Henoch-Schönlein purpura nephritis: course of disease and efficacy of cyclophosphamide. Pediatr Nephrol 19:51–56, 2003.
9. Saulsbury FT: Henoch-Schönlein purpura in children: report of 100 patients and review of the literature. Medicine 78:395–409, 1999.
10. Nussinovitch M, Prais D, Finkelstein Y, Varsano I: Cutaneous manifestations of Henoch-Schönlein purpura in young children. Pediatr Dermatol 15:426–428, 1998.
11. Sorenson SF, Slot O, Tvede N, Petersen J: A prospective study of vasculitis patients collected in a five year period: evaluation of the Chapel Hill nomenclature. Ann Rheum Dis 59:478–482, 2000.
12. Huber AM, King J, McLaine P, et al: A randomized, placebo controlled trial of prednisone in early Henoch-Schönlein purpura. BMC Med 2:7, 2004.
13. Mollica F, Li Volti S, Garozzo R, Russo G: Effectiveness of early prednisone therapy in preventing the development of nephropathy in anaphylactoid purpura. Eur J Pediatr 151:140–144, 1992.
14. Flynn JT, Smoyer WE, Bunchman TE, et al: Treatment of Henoch-Schönlein purpura glomerulonephritis in children with high-dose corticosteroids plus oral cyclophosphamide. Am J Nephrol 21:128–133, 2001.
15. Wyatt RJ, Hogg RJ: Evidence-based assessments of treatment options for children with IgA nephropathies. Pediatr Nephrol 16:156–167, 2001.
16. Rosenblum ND, Winter HS: Steroid effects in the course of abdominal pain in children with Henoch-Schönlein purpura. Pediatrics 79:1018–1021, 1987.
17. Niaudet P, Habib R: Methylprednisolone pulse therapy in the treatment of severe forms of Schönlein-Henoch purpura nephritis. Pediatr Nephrol 12:238–243, 1998.
19. Harries MJ, McWhinney P, Melsom R: Recurrent Henoch-Schönlein purpura controlled with cyclosporin. J R Soc Med 97:184–185, 2004.
20. Ronkainen J, Autio-Harmainen H, Nuutinen M: Cyclosporin A for the treatment of severe Henoch-Schönlein glomerulonephritis. Pediatr Nephrol 18:1138–1142, 2003.
21. Singh S, Devidayal, Kumar L, et al: Severe Henoch-Schönlein nephritis: resolution with azathioprine and steroids. Rheumatol Int 22:133–137, 2002.
22. Nakahata T, Tanaka H, Suzuki K, Ito E: Successful treatment with leukocytapheresis in refractory Henoch-Schönlein purpura: case report. Clin Rheumatol 22:248–250, 2003.
23. Tanaka H, Suzuki K, Nakahata T, et al: Early treatment with oral immunosuppresants in severe proteinuric purpura nephritis. Pediatr Nephrol 18:347–350, 2003.
24. Rettig P, Cron RQ: Methotrexate used as a steroid-sparing agent in non-renal chronic Henoch-Schönlein purpura. Clin Exp Rheumatol 21:767–769, 2003.
25. Bergstein J, Leiser J, Andreoli SP: Response of crescentic Henoch-Schönlein purpura to corticosteroid and azathioprine therapy. Clin Nephrol 49:9–14, 1998.
26. Oner A, Tinaztepe K, Erdogan O: The effect of triple therapy on rapidly progressive type of Henoch-Schönlein nephritis. Pediatr Nephrol 9:6–10, 1995.
27. Iijima K, Ito-Kariya S, Nakamura H, Yoshikawa N: Multiple combined therapy for severe Henoch-Schönlein nephritis in children. Pediatr Nephrol 12:244–248, 1998.
28. Hattori M, Ito K, Konomoto T, et al: Plasmapheresis as the sole therapy for rapidly progressive Henoch-Schönlein purpura nephritis in children. Am J Kidney Dis 33:427–433, 1999.
29. Nast CC, Ward HJ, Koyle MA, Cohen AH: Recurrent Henoch-Schönlein purpura following renal transplantation. Am J Kidney Dis 9:39–43, 1987.
30. Hasegawa A, Kawamura T, Ito H, et al: Fate of renal grafts with recurrent Henoch-Schönlein purpura nephritis in children. Transplant Proc 21:2130–2133, 1989.
31. Hattori M, Ito K, Konomoto T, et al: Plasmapheresis as the sole therapy for rapidly progressive Henoch-Schönlein purpura nephritis in children. Am J Kidney Dis 33:427–433, 1999.
32. Lombard KA, Shah PC, Thrasher TV, Grill BB: Ileal stricture as a late complication of Henoch-Schönlein purpura. Pediatrics 77:396–398, 1986.
33. Chen SY, Kong MS: Gastrointestinal manifestations and complications of Henoch-Schönlein purpura. Chang Gung Med J 27:175–181, 2004.
34. Lippl F, Huber W, Werner M, et al: Life-threatening gastrointestinal bleeding due to a jejunal lesion of Henoch-Schönlein purpura. Endoscopy 33:811–813, 2001.
35. Cho CS, Min JK, Park SH, et al: Protein losing enteropathy associated with Henoch-Schönlein in a patient with rheumatoid arthritis. Scand J Rheumatol 25:334–336, 1996.
36. Kumon Y, Hisatake K, Chikamori M, et al: A case of vasculitis cholecystitis associated with Schonlein-Henoch purpura in an adult. Gastroenterol Jpn 23:68–72, 1988.
37. Branski D, Gross V, Gross-Kieselstein E, et al: Pancreatitis as a complication of Henoch-Schönlein purpura. J Pediatr Gastroenterol Nutr 1:275–276, 1982.
38. Sonmez K, Turkyilmaz Z, Demirogullari B, et al: Conservative treatment for small intestinal intussusception associated with Henoch-Schönlein's purpura. Surg Today 32:1031–1034, 2002.
39. Connolly B, O'Halpin D: Sonographic evaluation of the abdomen in Henoch-Schonlein purpura. Clin Radiol 49:320–323, 1994.
40. Choong CK, Beasley SW: Intra-abdominal manifestations of Henoch-Schönlein purpura. J Paediatr Child Health 34:405–409, 1998.
41. Koskimies O, Mir S, Rapola J, Viska J: Henoch-Schönlein nephritis: long-term prognosis of unselected patients. Arch Dis Child 56:482–484, 1981.
42. Loirat C, Ehrich JH, Geerlings W, et al: Report on management of renal failure in children in Europe, XXIII, 1992. Nephrol Dial Transplant 1(Suppl):26–40, 1994.
43. Coppo R, Mazzucco G, Cagnoli L, et al: Long-term prognosis of Henoch-Schönlein nephritis in adults and children. Italian Group of Renal Immunopathology Collaborative Study on Henoch-Schönlein Purpura. Nephrol Dial Transplant 12:2277–2283, 1997.
44. Niaudet P, Murcia I, Beaufils H, et al: Primary IgA nephropathies in children: prognosis and treatment. Adv Nephrol Necker Hosp 22:121–140, 1993.
45. Riagnte D, Candelli M, Federico G, et al: Predictive factors of renal involvement or relapsing disease in children with Henoch-Schönlein purpura. Rheumatol Int 25:45–48, 2005.
46. Goldstein AR, White RH, Akuse R, Chantler C: Long-term follow-up of childhood Henoch-Schönlein nephritis. Lancet 339:280–282, 1992.
47. Rai A, Nast C, Adler S: Henoch-Schönlein purpura nephritis. J Am Soc Nephrol 10:2637–2644, 1999.
48. Kawasaki Y, Suzuki J, Sakai N, et al: Clinical and pathological features of children with Henoch-Schönlein purpura nephritis: risk factors associated with poor prognosis. Clin Nephrol 60:153–160, 2003.
49. Belman AL, Leicher CR, Moshe SL, Mezey AP: Neurologic manifestations of Schoenlein-Henoch purpura: report of three cases and a review of the literature. Pediatrics 75:687–692, 1985.
50. Chen CL, Chiou YH, Wu CY, et al: Cerebral vasculitis in Henoch-Schönlein purpura: case report with sequential magnetic resonance imaging changes and treated with plasmapheresis alone. Pediatr Nephrol 15:276–278, 2000.
51. Paolini S, Ciappetta P, Piattella MC, Domenicucci M: Henoch-Schönlein syndrome and cerebellar hemorrhage: report of an adolescent case and literature review. Surg Neurol 60:339–342, 2003.
52. Imai T, Okada H, Nanba M, et al: Henoch-Schönlein purpura with intracerebral hemorrhage. Brain Dev 24:115–117, 2002.
53. Chaussain M, de Boissieu D, Kalifa G, et al: Impairment of lung diffusing capacity in Schönlein-Henoch purpura. J Pediatr 121:12–16, 1992.
54. Besbas N, Duzova A, Topalogu R, et al: Pulmonary haemorrhage in a 6-year-old boy with Henoch-Schönlein purpura. Clin Rheumatol 20:293–296, 2001.
55. Gulati T, Kumar P, Dewan V, Anand VK: Henoch Schonlein purpura with rheumatic carditis. Indian J Pediatr 71:371–372, 2004.
56. Agraharkar M, Gokhale S, Le L, et al: Cardiopulmonary manifestations of Henoch-Schönlein purpura. Am J Kidney Dis 35:319–322, 2000.

57. Sakai N, Kawamoto K, Fukuoka H, et al: Acute scrotal swelling in Henoch-Schönlein purpura: a case report. Hinyokika Kiyo 46:739–741, 2000.
58. Ben-Sira L, Laor T: Severe scrotal pain in boys with Henoch-Schönlein purpura: incidence and sonography. Pediatr Radiol 30:125–128, 2000.
59. Turkish VJ, Traisman HS, Belman AB, et al: Scrotal swelling in the Schönlein-Henoch syndrome. J Urol 115:317–319, 1976.
60. Crosse JE, Soderdahl DW, Schamber DT: "Acute scrotum" in Henoch-Schönlein syndrome. Urology 7:66–67, 1976.

Classic Viral Exanthems

Antonio E. Muñiz, MD

Selected Diagnoses

Measles (rubeola, first disease)
Rubella (German measles, third disease)
Roseola infantum (exanthem subitum, sixth disease)
Erythema infectiosum (fifth disease, human parvovirus B19)
Herpes simplex (human herpesvirus 1 and human herpesvirus 2)
Varicella-zoster virus (human herpesvirus 3)
Coxsackievirus (hand-foot-and-mouth disease)

Introduction and Background

Any generalized cutaneous erythematous eruption associated with an acute viral syndrome is known as a viral exanthem. If the mucosa is involved, it is called an enanthem. The exact incidence of viral exanthems is unknown, and the most common are caused by enteroviruses.[1] A majority of childhood exanthems are nonspecific and cannot be accurately assigned to a discrete etiologic diagnosis. These exanthems are usually self-limited, resolving spontaneously in 1 week without long-term sequelae, and require only symptomatic therapy. Multiple viral agents are capable of causing a nonspecific exanthem, including nonpolio enteroviruses (i.e., cosackievirus, echovirus, and enterovirus) and respiratory viruses (i.e., rhinovirus, adenovirus, parainfluenza virus, respiratory syncytial virus, and influenza virus).[2,3] In general, most nonspecific exanthems occurring in the warmer months are caused the enteroviruses, and those occurring during the winter months by the respiratory viruses.

Discussion of Individual Diagnoses

Measles (Rubeola, First Disease)

Classic features of measles include a prodrome of fever, cough, coryza, conjunctivitis, and Koplik's spots, followed by an exanthematous phase. During the entire course of the illness, the child appears quite ill. Despite active immunization in the United States, outbreaks continue to occur.[4]

Measles is caused by an RNA virus, *Paramyxovirus*, that is highly contagious and is spread by direct contact with infectious droplets or, less commonly, by airborne spread. The incubation period, as defined by days prior to appearance of the rash, is 8 to 12 days. It is contagious 1 to 2 days before the prodrome and 4 days after the rash develops. It is most prevalent in late winter and spring. With the recommended two-dose vaccination schedule, first at 12 to 15 months and the second at 4 to 6 years of age, the incidence of measles in the United States has decreased to 100 cases per year.[5,6] Up to 67% are caused by importation of the virus from other countries.[7]

Typical measles infects the epithelial cells of the respiratory tract and binds to a cell surface glycoprotein, CD46.[8,9] This is followed by spread to lymphoid tissue, where it replicates, and eventually a primary viremia occurs. The virus disseminates to multiple sites, including skin, the liver, and the gastrointestinal tract tract.[10] Infection of the oral mucosa leads to the enanthem. The cutaneous eruption is related to the presence of the measles virus within keratinocytes and endothelial cells of the superficial dermal vessels.[11] The virus replicates within keratinocytes, leading to multinucleated giant cells, called Warthin-Finkeldey cells.[11] The clinical lesions are believed to be due to the host response to the virus within the skin.

Clinical Presentation

A prodrome occurs for 3 to 5 days of high fever, chills, systemic toxicity, headache, malaise, anorexia, and the "three Cs" (cough, coryza, and conjunctivitis). The cough is described as brassy or barking, and an initial diagnosis of croup or bronchitis may be made. The conjunctivitis is characterized by severe lacrimation with mild photophobia. The

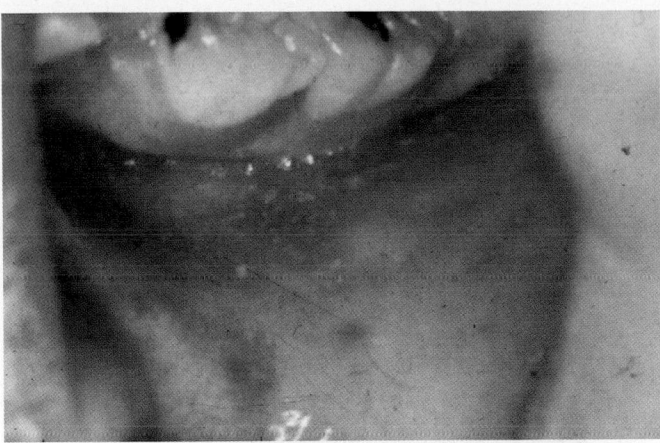

FIGURE 123–1. Koplik's spots on buccal mucosa seen in measles.

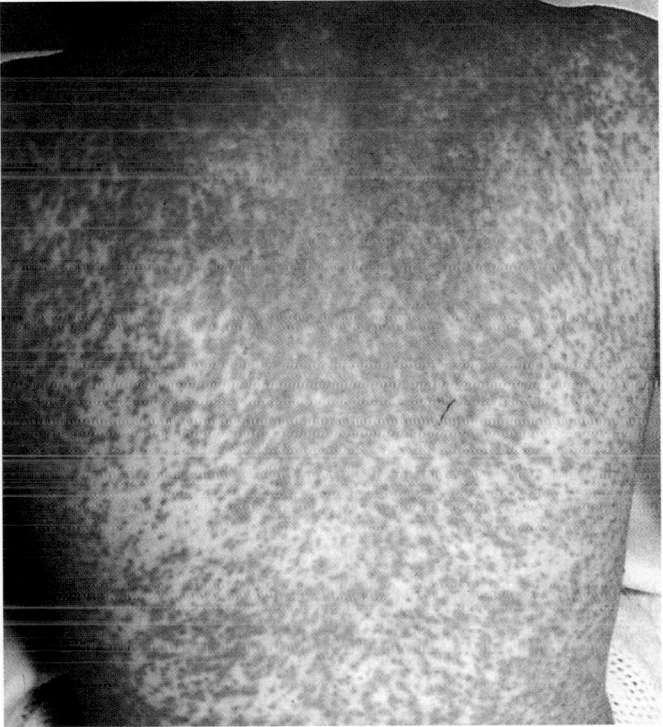

FIGURE 123–2. Erythematous macules and papules in measles.

Table 123–1	Differential Diagnosis of Morbilliform Rashes
Differential Diagnosis	**Causes**
Viruses	Measles
	Rubella
	Roseola infantum
	Erythema infectiosum
	Infectious mononucleosis
	Pityriasis rosea
	HIV (primary)
	Infectious hepatitis
Bacterial infections	Scarlet fever
	Rocky Mountain spotted fever
	Syphilis
Drug eruptions	Ampicillin, penicillin
	Nonsteroidal anti-inflammatory drugs
	Salicylic acid
	Phenytoin, barbiturates
	Phenothiazines
	Thiazide diuretics
	Isoniazid
Papulosquamous disorders	Guttate psoriasis
	Graft-versus-host disease
Reactive erythemas	Urticaria
	Papular urticaria
	Erythema multiforme
	Henoch-Schönlein purpura
	Kawasaki disease

Abbreviation: HIV, human immunodeficiency virus.

and desquamation, in the same order as it appeared. The rash fades by the 10th day ("10-day rash").

Complications of measles are infrequent but may be life threatening, especially in children less than 1 year of age, patients who are immunosuppressed, or the elderly.[12] Bacterial otitis media, bacterial pneumonia, bronchitis, laryngotracheobronchitis, diarrhea, myocarditis, and encephalitis may complicate measles.[1,13] Severe pneumonia and encephalitis are primary causes of death and are more likely to complicate measles in young infants and malnourished or immunocompromised children. Other rarely reported complications include thrombocytopenia, Stevens-Johnson syndrome, gangrenous stomatitis, appendicitis (lymphoid hyperplasia), hepatitis, laryngotracheal bronchitis, acute glomerulonephritis, pericarditis, lymphadenitis, and subacute sclerosing panencephalitis.[14] Mortality related to measles in the United States is estimated to be 1 per 1000.[4] Low vitamin A levels have been implicated in the severity of measles.[15]

The differential of morbilliform exanthems is vast and include viruses, bacterial infections, drug eruptions, papulosquamous disorders, and reactive erythema (Table 123–1). The typical features of measles are easily recognized. When the diagnosis is in doubt, viral isolation from mucosa or the nasopharynx, although difficult, will distinguish measles from other morbilliform exanthems. Acute and convalescent sera, obtained at 1 week and 3 weeks after the onset of the illness, showing a fourfold rise in immunoglobulin G antibodies assist with a retrospective diagnosis.[16] Laboratory diagnosis can be accomplished by serologic assays, including complement fixation, hemagglutination-inhibition (HAI) titer, direct immunofluorescence, and enzyme-linked immunosorbent assay (ELISA).[17] Leukocytosis is common.

coryza consists of copious mucopurulent discharge. Enlarged cervical and preauricular lymph nodes are present.

The exanthem follows the prodrome but is preceded by an enanthem. The enanthem is composed of intense erythema of the mucous membranes with focal 1- to 3-mm punctuate white-gray papules (Koplik's spots) usually adjacent to the lower premolars. These resemble a grain of salt on a red background (Fig. 123–1).

The exanthem begins at the hairline and behind the ears as blotchy erythema and spreads centrifugally and in a cephalocaudad direction to involve the face, trunk, and extremities, with multiple discrete macules and papules (Fig. 123–2). These gradually coalesce, and, by the third day, the entire body is involved and lesions are intensely erythematous, and at times purpuric (morbilliform). Usually by the fourth day, the rash begins to fade, with a coppery-brown discoloration

Management

No specific treatment is available, only supportive therapy in most cases. Using two doses of vitamin A (200,000 IU) on consecutive days is associated with a reduction in the risk of mortality in children under the age of 2 years as well as a reduction in the risk of pneumonia-specific mortality.[18] Those with suspected vitamin A deficiency should have a second dose on the following day and at 4 weeks. Others who should receive vitamin A include immunosuppressed or malnourished patients or those with impaired intestinal absorption, or patients recently emigrated from an area with high mortality due to measles. Vitamin A reduces mortality in hospitalized children up to 60%.[19] If bacterial pneumonia or otitis media occurs, appropriate antibiotics are indicated. Children with significant pulmonary symptoms or central nervous system (CNS) involvement should be hospitalized.

In areas where other patients are not immunized against measles, any patient with measles should be isolated during the contagious period, from onset of respiratory symptoms through the fourth day of the exanthem. Postexposure prophylaxis in susceptible individuals includes measles vaccine, if given within 72 hours of exposure, and immune globulin (0.25 ml/kg intramuscularly [IM]), which can be given up to 6 days following exposure to prevent disease or modify its course. Immune serum globulin should be administered to unimmunized infants less than 1 year of age or to those who are immunosuppressed at a dose of 0.5 ml/kg IM (maximum 15 ml) as soon as possible after exposure. Outbreaks should be reported to local public health authorities. Measles virus is susceptible in vitro to ribavirin, which has been given to patients with severe infection and immunocompromised children. Close follow-up should be arranged to observe for the development of severe pneumonia or encephalitis. Parents should be advised to return immediately if there is fever recurrence, headache, or a change in mental status, or if seizures or motor deficits develop.

Rubella (German Measles, Third Disease)

Rubella is a viral illness characterized by a maculopapular rash and enlargement of the posterior occipitocervical lymph nodes. Rubella is caused by an RNA virus, *Rubivirus*, that is transmitted by contact with aerosolized particles from an infected person. It can also be transmitted transplacentally. Rubella occurs most commonly in late winter and early spring, and the incubation period ranges from 14 to 21 days. The patient is contagious a few days before illness and up to 1 week after the onset of the rash. The primary site of infection is the nasopharynx, followed by spread to regional lymphatics and eventually viremia. Virus replicates in the reticuloendothelial system. The rash appears as the serum antibody titer is rising, suggesting a potential contribution of antigen-antibody interactions in the skin.

Clinical Presentation

Classic rubella is a mild illness in most children and usually not diagnosed unless an epidemic exists.[20] Rubella acquired postnatally in infants and children is accompanied by few or no prodromal symptoms, and up to 50% of rubella infections may be asymptomatic.[20,21] In children with clinical symptoms (10%), rubella presents insidiously with a mild prodrome of headache, low-grade fever, malaise, sore throat,

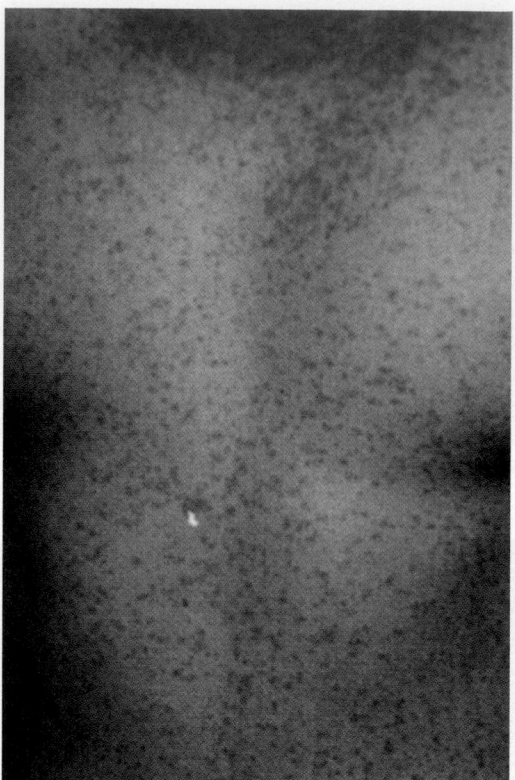

FIGURE 123–3. Rose-pink macular and papular eruption in rubella.

anorexia, conjunctivitis, cough, and coryza. These are more common in adolescents or adults.[20,21] Mild lymphadenopathy may precede the exanthem by several days and occurs in the occipital, posterior auricular, and posterior cervical lymph nodes. An enanthem characterized by erythematous and petechial macules on the soft palate (Forschheimer spots) may be present.

The rash occurs 1 to 5 days after onset of illness. A faint rose-pink, macular or papular eruption appears first on the face and spreads downward to the trunk and proximal extremities (Fig. 123–3). Within 48 hours, the face and trunk rash has faded and the eruption involves the distal extremities. Rarely, petechiae or purpura may be seen. In cases of extensive eruption, a fine, flaky desquamation may occur. The eruption is usually completely resolved by the third day ("3-day measles"), but occasionally may last 5 days. As opposed to measles, the child appears well.

A monoarticular arthritis or arthralgia may accompany rubella, especially in adolescent girls.[20,21] The fingers, wrists, and knees are most often affected, and symptoms resolve by 1 month. Occasionally the elbows, shoulders, and spine are involved. It may present as the so-called STAR (*s*ore *t*hroat, *a*rthritis, *r*ash) complex.[22] Other viruses associated with the STAR complex include human parvovirus B19, hepatitis B, adenovirus, echovirus, coxsackievirus, and Epstein-Barr virus. Other less common complications include encephalitis, myocarditis, pericarditis, hemolytic anemia, thrombocytopenic purpura, and hepatitis.

In distinguishing rubella from measles, the clinician should look for the absence of fever and toxicity. It may be difficult to distinguish rubella from enterovirus exanthems, infectious mononucleosis, cytomegalovirus, reovirus, adenovirus, measles, scarlet fever, roseola infantum, parvovirus B19, syphilis, toxoplasmosis, or mild drug reactions.[23] The diagnosis may be made from recovery of the organism from the nasal mucosa, blood, urine, or cerebrospinal fluid, but such tests are superfluous in most cases. Serologic diagnosis can be performed with the HAI titer, latex agglutination, direct immunofluorescence, ELISA, and passive HAI antibody test or by serologic acute and convalescent titers.[17] In infants with congenital rubella, the virus may be recovered from peripheral blood leukocytes, stool, or urine for months to years after birth. Leukopenia is common.

Rubella acquired during the first trimester of pregnancy may result in intrauterine transmission, and congenital rubella is seen 10% to 20% of cases.[23-25] The earlier in the pregnancy that the transmission occurs, the greater the risk to the fetus. The skin manifestations include purpura and petechiae from thrombocytopenia, and may recur any time during the first 5 years of life. Other features include sensorineural hearing loss, congenital heart defects (i.e., patent ductus arteriosus, pulmonary stenosis), cataract, retinopathy, glaucoma, pigmentary retinopathy, growth retardation, behavioral disorders, meningoencephalitis, pneumonia, intrauterine growth retardation (IUGR), psychomotor retardation, hepatosplenomegaly, hepatitis with jaundice, and "blueberry muffin" spots.[20,23-25]

Management

There is no specific treatment for rubella. If the patient is febrile, fever control measures will suffice. Oatmeal baths and antihistamines are helpful for pruritus. Nonsteroidal anti-inflammatory agents may be prescribed for arthritis. Administration of the rubella vaccine after exposure has not been demonstrated to ameliorate illness.

When a pregnant woman is exposed to rubella, a serum specimen should be obtained and tested for rubella antibody. If antibody is present, there is no risk of infection. If no rubella antibody is detectable, a second blood specimen should be obtained 2 or 3 weeks later. If antibody is present in the second specimen and not the first, infection is presumed to have occurred, and termination of pregnancy may be considered. If termination of pregnancy is not an option, serum immune globulin (0.55 ml/kg IM) should be given.

Roseola Infantum (Exanthem Subitum, Sixth Disease)

Roseola occurs predominantly in infants 6 months to 3 years of age, with a peak age of 6 to 7 months.[26-29] It is characterized by 2 to 3 days of sustained fever in an infant who otherwise appears well, after which the infant becomes afebrile and a pink, morbilliform exanthem appears transiently and fades within a few days. Roseola is caused by human herpesvirus 6 (HHV-6), a double-stranded DNA virus, and occasionally by human herpesvirus 7 (HHV-7).[30,31] It can occur at any time of the year, but is more common in the spring.[32] The incubation period is 5 to 15 days. Transmission is airborne and from contact with infected respiratory droplets and, rarely, transplacentally.[33]

Clinical Presentation

The illness begins with high fever that lasts 3 to 7 days, cough, and otitis media, but patients appear well.[26,27,34] Mild edema of the eyelids and posterior cervical lymphadenopathy

FIGURE 123–4. Rose-pink macules and papules in roseola infantum.

are occasionally seen. A seizure with the onset of fever is noted in 25% to 36% of cases.[27,29,35] A bulging fontanelle is also a common physical finding. An enanthem of erythematous papules on the mucosa of the soft palate and uvula (Nagayama's spots) may be seen in 65% of cases.[32]

The rash of roseola usually coincides with cessation of fever, or may follow it by 1 to 2 days. It is characterized by rose-pink macules and papules, and occurs predominantly on the neck and trunk, but occasionally involves the face and proximal extremities (Fig. 123–4). The eruption fades over a few days, rarely persisting for up to a week. Differential diagnosis may include other viruses (Table 123–2).

HHV-6 can be recovered from cultures of peripheral blood leukocytes, by serology with a fourfold increase in HHV-6 immunoglobulin G antibodies, by antigen detection by polymerase chain reaction (PCR) or immunofluorescence studies, or from skin lesions by molecular diagnosis.[34] Leukopenia with relative lymphocytosis develops on day 3 of illness.

Complications are uncommon and include seizures, hyperpyrexia, vomiting, diarrhea, cough, fulminant hepatitis, thrombocytopenia, disseminated infection, and hepatosplenomegaly. Rarely encephalitis or encephalopathy occurs.[36]

Management

There is no specific treatment for roseola. Antipyretics can be used for fever. Patients with severe disease or immunocompromised hosts may benefit from administration of ganciclovir, foscarnet, or cidofovir.[37,38] If an infant presents with a febrile seizure and the appropriate diagnostic studies reveal no source, it is prudent to inform parents that the child may have the roseola exanthem after the fever subsides.

Erythema Infectiosum (Fifth Disease)

Erythema infectiosum (fifth disease) is a viral infection caused by human parvovirus B19, which causes an intense,

Table 123–2	Differential Diagnosis of Roseola Infantum

Echovirus 16
Epstein-Barr virus
Adenovirus
Cytomegalovirus
Parvovirus B19
Rubella
Measles
Parainfluenza virus

confluent erythema on both cheeks, followed by a lacy rash on the rest of the body.[39] Human parvovirus B19, a single-stranded DNA virus, has been isolated within the skin lesions of patients with erythema infectiosum.[39] The organism replicates in erythroid bone marrow cells, accounting for its role in red-cell aplasia of immunodeficient patients or those with chronic hemolytic anemia.[40] It occurs more frequently in winter and spring. It can present at any age but is most common in children 4 to 10 years of age.[41] Transmission is via respiratory droplets or blood products, or vertically from mother to fetus. The incubation period is 6 to 14 days but can be as long as 21 days, and patients are contagious prior to the start of the eruption and up to 7 days posteruption.

Clinical Presentation

In most patients the first reported manifestation is the characteristic rash. Prodromal symptoms may occasionally occur, and include low-grade fever, coryza, headache, sore throat, chills, nausea, myalgias, and malaise. The exanthem of erythema infectiosum is divided into three stages. Initially a bright, fiery red macular erythema appears on the cheeks ("slapped-cheek" or "sunburned" appearance) (Fig. 123–5). It is often associated with a rim of sparing around the nose and mouth ("circumoral pallor"). The second stage occurs 1 to 4 days later when the rash may spread to involve the arms, legs, chest, and abdomen. It consists of a pink to dull red macular eruption. Fading of the central portion gives a lacy, reticulate pattern. Pruritus is unusual.[42] The third stage varies in duration from 1 week to several weeks and is characterized by waxing and waning intensity of the eruption. The exanthem generally lasts from 3 to 5 days, but may last up to 4 months.[39,40] The rash increases in intensity from vigorous exercise, overheating of the skin, sun exposure, or crying. Occasionally, morbilliform, vesicular, or purpuric skin eruptions are seen. A purpuric hand and foot eruption (purpuric gloves-and-socks syndrome) may develop.[39,43] The differential diagnosis may include drug reactions, other viral entities, and collagen vascular diseases (Table 123–3).

Diagnosis can be confirmed by analysis of serum obtained within 30 days of the onset of illness for the presence of immunoglobulin M B19 antibodies via ELISA or radioimmunoassay.[44] For immunocompromised hosts with chronic infection, nucleic acid hybridization or PCR assays are recommended.[45]

Symmetric arthritis of the hands, wrists, or knees has been described, especially in adolescent and adult females.[22,40,46] The STAR complex is caused by parvovirus B19 as often as by rubella.[22] Joint symptoms usually resolve by 1 to 2 months. Joint involvement worsens over the day.

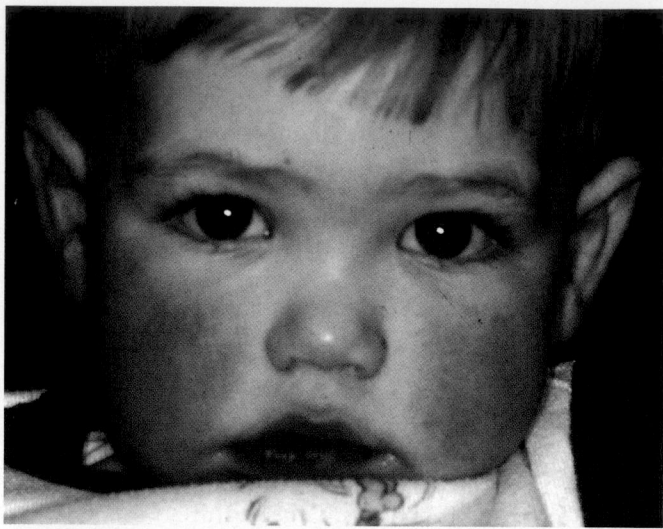

FIGURE 123–5. Slapped-cheek appearance of erythema infectiosum.

Table 123–3	Differential Diagnosis of Erythema Infectiosum	
Differential Diagnosis		**Causes**
Viruses		Echovirus
		Rubella
		Epstein-Barr virus
		Measles
		Coxsackievirus
		Dengue
		Hepatitis
Bacteria		Scarlet fever
Drug eruption		
Collagen vascular disease		
		Polyarteritis nodosa
		Lupus erythematosus
		Juvenile rheumatoid arthritis

Unusual complications may include encephalopathy, aseptic meningitis, neuropathy, cerebellar ataxia, seizures, myocarditis, and hepatitis.[47] In children with acquired or hereditary hemolytic anemias or any condition that results in red blood cell destruction (i.e., hereditary spherocytosis, sickle cell disease, glucose-6-phosphate dehydrogenase deficiency, pyruvate kinase deficiency) or decreased red blood cell production (i.e., iron deficiency anemia or thalassemia), parvovirus B19 is associated with a poorer prognosis and results in transient aplastic crisis.[40,48] It can occur under conditions of erythroid stress, such as during hemorrhage, during a state of iron deficiency anemia, and following kidney or bone marrow transplant. These episodes are accompanied by symptoms of anemia, such as dyspnea, lassitude, and confusion, and can last 10 to 15 days. Rarely congestive heart failure develops, which can be fatal.

In immunocompromised patients, such as those with human immunodeficiency virus infection, congenital immunodeficiencies, acute leukemia, organ transplants, or systemic lupus erythematosus, or in infants less that 1 year old, parvovirus B19 can cause a serious, prolonged chronic anemia due to persistent lysis of red blood cell precursors and bone marrow suppression. In pregnant women, parvovirus B19 infection may result in fetal anemia, high-output cardiac failure, pleural effusions, polyhydramnios, nonimmune hydrops fetalis, and fetal demise.[48-50] Fetal loss occurs in 8% to 10% of pregnancies complicated by parvovirus and is highest if infection is acquired prior to 20 weeks' gestation.[51,52]

Management

There is no specific treatment for erythema infectiosum. Isolation for 2 weeks of patients at risk for complications, such as pregnant women, immunosuppressed patients, or patients with chronic hemolytic anemia, is recommended. Administration of intravenous (IV) immune globulins may be used in these high-risk groups,[53] leading to a marked increase in reticulocyte counts and corresponding rise in hemoglobin. Blood transfusions may be required. Those with arthritis symptoms may gain relief with nonsteroidal anti-inflammatory drugs.

The risk of exposure should be explained to pregnant females, and serologic testing offered. If acute infection is confirmed, serial fetal ultrasonography should be performed, assessing for congestive heart failure, IUGR, or fetal hydrops. Management of severely affected fetuses has included in utero blood transfusion.

Herpes Simplex (Human Herpesvirus 1 and 2 Infections)

Grouped vesicles on an erythematous base are the characteristic lesions of herpes simplex virus (HSV) in the skin, regardless of location.[54] On mucous membranes, the blister roof is easily shed and an erosion is seen. The infection may be primary or recurrent.[54] Initial infection is termed *primary* if it occurs in a host with no prior HSV infection or *recurrent* in a host previously infected with HSV. Recurrent infections represent reactivation of latent herpesvirus.

Human herpesvirus 1 (HHV-1, or herpes simplex virus 1 [HSV-1]) and human herpesvirus 2 (HHV-2, or herpes simplex virus 2 [HSV-2]) are double-stranded DNA viruses. They are epidermotropic, and productive viral infection occurs within keratinocytes. Initial infection is characterized by viral replication at the initial site of contact, such as skin, mucous membranes, or eyes. The virus then travels along the regional nerves to the ganglia and establishes a latent infection, where it remains for life. The incubation period ranges from 2 days to 2 weeks. Transmission in neonates is during birth through contact with an infected maternal genital tract, or by direct contact with infected oral secretions or lesions.

Clinical Presentation

After initial exposure, HSV may persist in nerve ganglia and be reactivated by a number of factors, including fever, emotional disturbances, ultraviolet light, menses, and trauma.[54,55] Once recurrent skin involvement appears, the disease is contagious and can be transmitted to other areas of the skin or to other persons. Sites of involvement vary, but the most common are the lips, eyes, cheeks, and hands.[54,55] Regional lymphadenopathy may occur in all forms of herpes simplex. Distinct clinical features of the various types are listed in Table 123–4 and shown in Figures 123–6 through 123–9.

Herpes virus may be recovered from vesicles during the first 24 hours after their appearance. Other locations for recovery include conjunctivae, nasopharynx, rectum, urine, cerebrospinal fluid, and blood.[56] A Tzanck preparation (scraping from an intact blister treated with Geimsa or

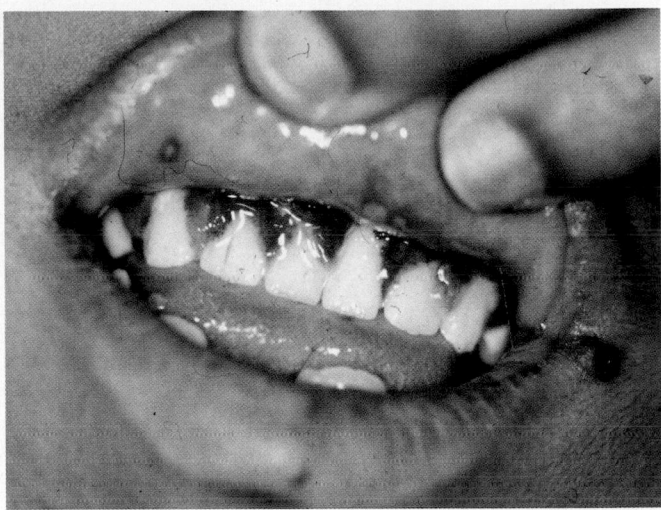

FIGURE 123–6. Herpetic gingivostomatitis: vesicular lesions on the lips and oral mucosa from herpes simplex virus.

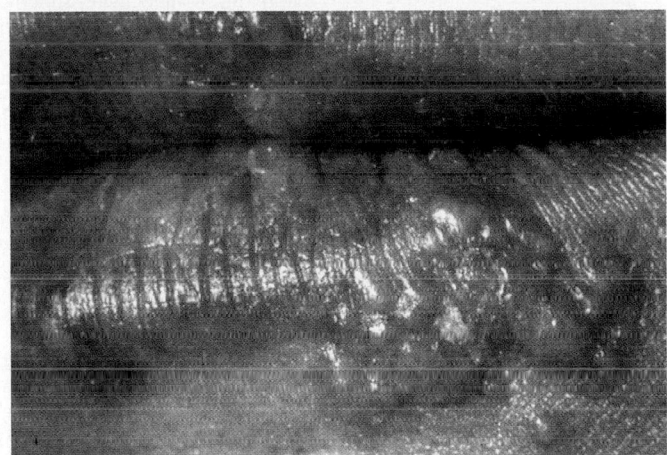

FIGURE 123–7. Herpes labialis: grouped vesicles on the lips.

Wright stain) will show the characteristic epidermal giant cells. Rapid diagnostic tests using direct fluorescent antibody or dye-labeled monoclonal antibodies are 90% accurate.[57] Some institutions may perform a PCR for detection of HSV DNA, especially in the setting of CNS infection.[58]

Many other viruses and diseases should be considered in the differential diagnosis of herpes simplex (Table 123–5).

The most common complication is secondary bacterial superinfection. Immunosuppressed patients or pregnant patients may have disseminated disease involving multiple organs, including the liver, lung, brain, heart, and adrenal glands. It presents as a sepsis-like syndrome with jaundice, progressive hepatosplenomegaly, hepatitis, poor feeding, dyspnea, pneumonia, adrenal necrosis, hypothermia, seizures, encephalitis, evidence of disseminated intravascular coagulopathy, and death, which may occur in 48 to 96 hours.

Management

Oral acyclovir, famciclovir, valcyclovir, or penciclovir, foscarnet, or cidofovir are specific therapies for localized cutaneous herpes simple infections[54] (Table 123–6). Antiviral

Table 123–4	Clinical Features of Herpes Simplex Virus (HSV) Disease in Children
Forms of HSV	**Clinical Features**
Herpes Gingivostomatitis (caused by HSV-1)	Most frequent clinical presentation of primary HSV infection in children (6 mo–5 yr)
	Transmitted by infectious saliva
	Incubation: 2–12 days
	Primary form: fever, irritability, malaise, refusal to eat or drink
	Vesicular lesions on tongue, buccal mucosa, gingiva, and palate (Fig. 123–6) become eroded and ulcerated, appearing as 1- to 3-mm shallow gray ulcers on a red base; gums become mildly swollen, red, ulcerated, exudative, and friable.
	Tender submandibular and cervical lymphadenopathy are common.
	Dehydration is the most common complication.[83]
	Acute disease lasts 3–7 days but may persist up to 3 wk.
Herpes Pharyngotonsillitis	Fever, malaise, odynophagia, and headache
Herpes Labialis (Fig. 123–7)	Vesiculoulcerative lesions develop on tonsils and pharynx.
	Recurrent infection of the lip
	Occurs in up to 20% of infants and children[54]
	Prodrome of pain, tingling, or itching
	Grouped vesicles on one portion of the lip, usually lower, typically follow an acute febrile illness or intense sun exposure.
	Lesions last up to 8 days.
Herpes Keratitis (Fig. 123–8)	Corneal involvement in <10% (must be ruled out in presence of any lesion around the eye)
	May lead to corneal scarring and permanent loss of vision
	Usually remains unilateral
	Blepharitis, conjunctivitis, superficial or deep keratitis, and anterior uveitis may occur.
	Pain, blurred vision, eyelid swelling, and itching
	May produce severe purulent conjunctivitis (edema, erythema, and vesicles with opacity and superficial erosion or ulceration of the cornea); dendritic ulcers may be seen.
	Ophthalmologic consultation is mandatory.
	Most lesions heal within 2 wk without residual damage.
Herpetic Whitlow (Fig. 123–9)	Occurs in 10% of patients with predilection for thumb sucking
	Inoculated into the skin
	Superficial vesiculopustules or extremely painful deep vesicular, bullous, or pustular eruption
	Often initially considered pyoderma or cellulitis
	Accompanied by regional lymphadenopathy
Herpes Facialis	Recurrent infection of grouped vesicles on the cheek or forehead
	May be confused with impetigo
	Acquired during wrestling (herpes gladiatorum)
	May result in endemic spread of HSV, with lesions more commonly on the head, neck, and shoulders[84]
Herpes Progenitalis (HSV-2)	Predominantly in adolescents and young adults[54]
	Appears 2–8 days following contact with infected individual
	Prodrome of fever, malaise, myalgias, and headaches
	Involves penile shaft and, less frequently, the glans, urethra, or scrotum. Single or multiple painful vesicles (2–4 mm) are transformed to painful shallow ulcers covered with exudates; these coalesce to form large ulcerations.
	Severe genital edema, ulceration, and pain
	Exclude gonococcal or chlamydial infection in presence of exudate.
	Recurrent case presents with a painful prodrome followed by eruption of grouped vesicles on an erythematous base in a localized area of genitalia.
	Contagious and sexually transmitted (in young children should raise question of abuse)
	Fever and symptoms last 5–7 days; lesions resolve in 10–14 days.
Herpes Vulvovaginitis	Severe pain associated with vulvovaginitis, urethritis, cervicitis, and cystitis
	Produces vesicles that coalesce to form large, painful ulcerations with edema of the genitalia
Herpes Encephalitis	From primary or recurrent infection
	Associated with fever, alteration in consciousness, personality changes, seizures, and focal neurologic findings
	Fulminant course leading to coma and death in untreated patients
Neonatal Herpes	Occurs in 10% of infants born to parents with active HSV-2 infection[85]
	Two thirds of cases caused by HSV-2, rest by HSV-1
	Grouped vesicles on an erythematous base may be present at birth or appear up to 7 days after birth.
	In severe cases, central nervous system involvement or dissemination may occur.[86,87]
	Can be localized to skin, eyes, and mouth (SEM disease)
	Oral mucous membrane involvement may manifest as vesicles, erosions, or ulcers and ocular involvement with conjunctivitis or keratitis.[88]
	If untreated, can lead to progression of more severe disease
	Neonates present with focal encephalitis or meningoencephalitis or nonspecific fever, decreased sensorium, irritability, poor feeding, seizures, bulging fontanelle, and lethargy or coma.[56] Skin manifestations are usually absent or develop late. Consider in differential of sepsis, especially with negative cultures and/or liver dysfunction.
	Cerebrospinal fluid shows lymphocytic pleocytosis.

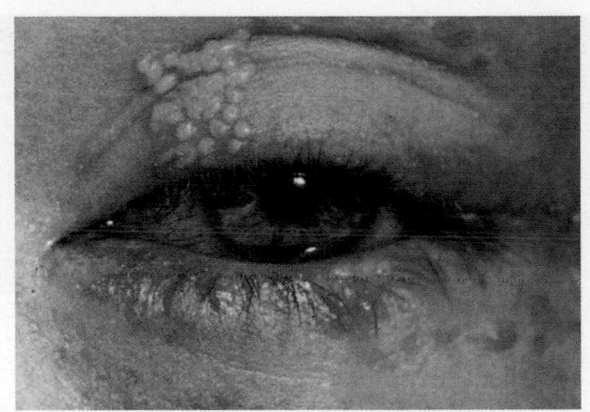

FIGURE 123–8. Herpes keratitis: grouped vesicles with crusting.

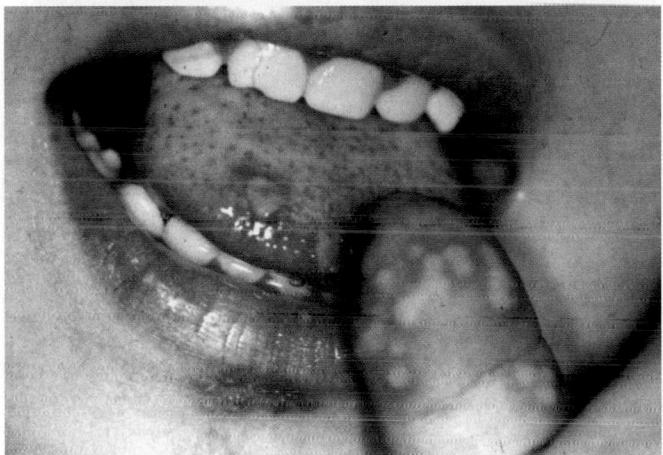

FIGURE 123–9. Herpetic whitlow: superficial vesiculopustules.

Table 123–5	Differential Diagnosis of Herpes Simplex Infection
Differential Diagnosis	**Causes**
Viruses	Varicella-zoster virus
	Coxsackievirus (herpangina)
	Orf
	Influenza
	Echovirus
	Variola
	Vaccinia
Disease	Erythema multiforme
	Aphthous ulcers
	Vincent's infection
	Behçet's syndrome
	Allergic contact dermatitis
	Impetigo
	Bacterial or other viral conjunctivitis
	Streptococcal blistering distal dactylitis
	Burns

agents given within 72 hours of the onset of the rash decrease severity or duration of the infection and are associated with less feeding difficulty and shorter duration of viral shedding. However, famciclovir, valcyclovir, foscarnet, and cidofovir are not approved for use in children.

In neonatal HSV, IV acyclovir is efficacious. The dose for preterm infants of 34 to 36 weeks' gestation is 10 mg/kg per dose IV every 8 hours, and that for premature infants less

Table 123–6	Antiviral Agents for Herpes Simplex Virus
Agents	**Doses**
Acyclovir	200 mg 5 times per day for 7 days
	30–80 mg/kg divided q8h IV
Valcyclovir (>12 yr)	1000 mg PO 1–2 times per day for 7–10 days
Abbreviations: IV, intravenously; PO, orally.	

than 34 weeks' gestation, 10 mg/kg per dose IV every 12 hours. The dose for term infants is 20 mg/kg per dose IV every 8 hours for 14 days. For infants with encephalitis or disseminated HSV, recommended treatment is up to 21 days. Although most neonates with encephalitis survive, most have substantial neurologic sequelae. Approximately 25% of neonates with disseminated disease die despite treatment. Supportive measures, such as fever control, maintenance of fluid and electrolyte balance, and thermal regulation, should be instituted immediately. Infected patients must be isolated as they shed virus. Pain relief should be provided for gingivostomatitis with acetaminophen and an analgesic mouth wash (equal parts of aluminum hydroxide and diphenhydramine plus viscous xylocaine added when age appropriate, but this should be done with extreme caution since as little as 1–2 ml may be toxic in young children), which is applied with a cotton swab onto lesions or, in older children, rinsed and expectorated. Patients should avoid citrus fruits and spicy or hot liquids.

Careful daily ophthalmologic follow up is required for ocular keratitis. Corticosteroid therapy, either topical or systemic, should be avoided. Topical corticosteroids may be required after several days of antiviral therapy in patients with marginal ulcers or associated stromal disease, but these agents should be given only in consultation with an ophthalmologist. Antiviral agents may include trifluridine (1%) drops, vidarabine (3%) ointment, 0.1% iododeoxyuridine, or acyclovir ophthalmic ointment. In severe cases, oral or IV acyclovir or vidarabine and a cycloplegic may be required.[59] Disseminated infections require hospitalization and intensive supportive therapy.

Treatment of genital herpes consists of warm sitz baths, topical anesthetics, oral analgesics, wet compresses with aluminum acetate (Burow's solution), and topical antibacterial ointment to prevent secondary infection. For severe cases, oral acyclovir can accelerate healing and shorten duration of symptoms and viral shedding.[60] The majority of children with HSV require supportive care, and follow-up is indicated in cases in which the lesions persist or in patients who are hospitalized with severe disease.

Varicella-Zoster Virus (Human Herpesvirus 3 Infections)

Varicella-zoster virus (VZV) or human herpesvirus 3 (HHV-3) is a double-stranded DNA virus producing an abrupt onset of crops of grouped vesicles.[61,62] It is highly contagious, with an incubation period of 14 to 16 days (range 10 to 21 days)[26] and occurs primarily in children from 2 to 8 years old, with 90% of cases occurring before the age of 14 years. It is most prevalent in late winter and early spring. The disease is spread through person-to-person contact and airborne spread, and occurs from 1 to 2 days before the onset of rash to 5 to 6 days after onset or when lesions have crusted.[62] Transplacental infection may also occur.

HHV-3 enters via the respiratory route and replicates in the lymph nodes. Viremia follows with entry into reticulo-endothelial cells. A second viremia results in spread into the skin and organs. In keratinocytes, HHV-3 produces ballooning degeneration of cells and an interepidermal blister. Primary infection is known as chickenpox. After an initial varicella infection, the VZV remains dormant in cells of the dorsal root ganglia or cranial nerve ganglia until reactivation. Subsequent propagation of the virus along the nerve to the skin gives rise to grouped vesicles. The reactivation stage is known as herpes zoster or shingles.[61,62] Reactivation may result from reexposure to varicella, physical trauma to the spinal column, radiation therapy, immunosuppressant drugs, cancer, leukemia, or Hodgkin's lymphoma.

Clinical Presentation

A prodrome consists of low-grade fever, malaise, headache, anorexia, cough, coryza, and sore throat. In normal children, systemic symptoms are mild and serious complications are rare. In immunocompromised patients, the disorder is more likely to be characterized by an extensive eruption that is often hemorrhagic, severe constitutional symptoms, and occasionally pneumonia and death.[63]

Individual lesions begin as faint erythematous macules that progress to edematous papules and then to delicate vesicles ("dewdrop on a rose petal") within 24 to 48 hours (Figs. 123–10 and 123–11). The exanthem usually begins on the scalp, face, and trunk and less commonly on the extremities. Intense pruritus commonly accompanies the vesicular stage of the rash. The vesicles develop moist crusts that dry and are shed, leaving a shallow erosion. Successive crops of lesions appear during the next 2 to 5 days, so that at any one time several stages of skin lesions can be seen concomitantly. The lesions spread centripetally. Lesions frequently involve mucous membranes, and isolated erosions may be seen in the conjunctiva, oral muscosa, or nasal cavity and occasionally in the vagina.[62] Lesions may vary from as few as 10 to greater than 100. The lesions disappear in 7 to 10 days and usually heal without scarring. In patients with thrombocytopenia, lesions may appear hemorrhagic.[64]

While smallpox has been eradicated, there is still concern regarding its use as a biological terrorism agent. In contrast to varicella, it causes a vesicular rash that evolves at the same rate for all lesions as opposed to the successive crops that occur with chickenpox.

Herpes zoster in prepubertal children is usually mild. Neuralgia, common in the elderly, is rarely seen in children and occasionally occurs in adolescents. Maternal varicella infection during pregnancy and varicella occurring in the newborn period represent risk factors for childhood herpes zoster. Malaise, headache, and fever may precede the rash, especially in young children. Herpes zoster is a unilateral eruption that involves one to three dermatomes, most commonly the thoracic and the ophthalmic branch of the trigeminal nerve (Fig. 123–12). Infection of the ophthalmic branch of the Vth cranial (trigeminal) nerve may involve the cornea with keratitis and uveitis and lead to permanent damage (zoster ophthalmicus). It is suspected when the nasociliary branch is involved and, accordingly, is present in those who have cutaneous involvement of the nose

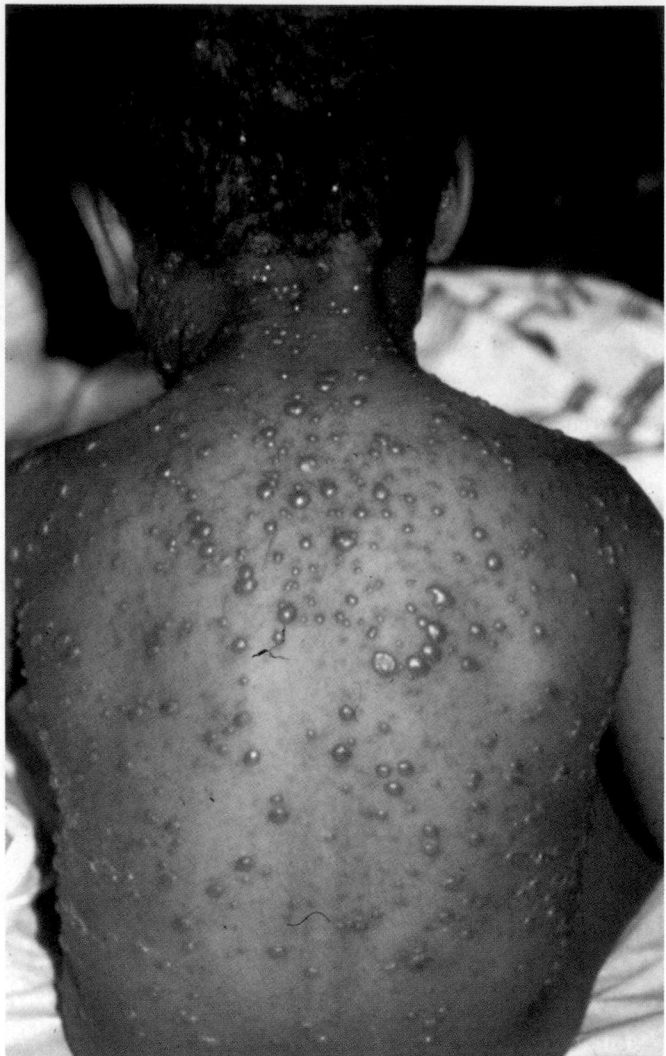

FIGURE 123–10. Papules, vesicles, and pustules seen in varicella-zoster virus infection.

(Hutchinson's sign). Involvement of the geniculate ganglion results in pain in the ear with vesicles on the pinnae, tongue, ear, and skin of the auditory canal. When accompanied by facial palsy and disturbances of hearing and equilibrium, it is part of the Ramsay Hunt syndrome (Fig. 123–13).

In herpes zoster, grouped lesions appear within several adjacent dermatomes. They begin as macules and edematous papules and progress to vesicles on an erythematous base. Intense pruritus occurs during the vesicular stage. As the eruption resolves, vesicles open up, become crusted, and slowly heal. The eruption tends to appear first at a point nearest the CNS and extends peripherally along the course of the nerve, thus producing the characteristic bandlike distribution of lesions. Generally the eruption is unilateral, but it may cross the midline and, at times, may involve the contralateral side. Successive crops continue to appear from 5 to 7 days. They resolve by crusting over in the course of another 7 to 10 days, and occasionally up to 3 weeks. In children, rarely dermatomal pain may precede the eruption.

Typical varicella is seldom confused with other illnesses, but some viruses may mimic the lesions (Table 123–7).

HHV-3 may be recovered from the vesicles during the first 72 hours after the onset of the eruption. A Tzanck

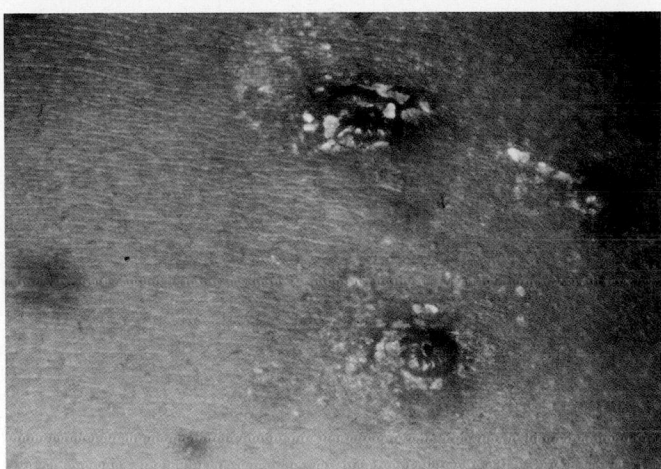

FIGURE 123–11. Different stages of lesions seen in varicella-zoster virus infection, consisting of macules, papules, vesicles ("dewdrop on a rose petal"), and crusting of vesicles.

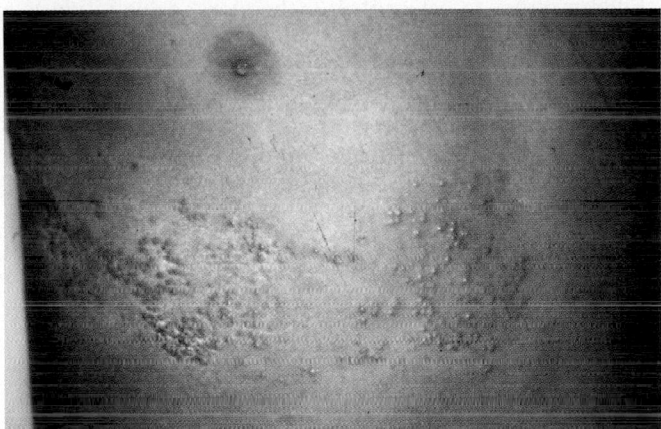

FIGURE 123–12. Herpes zoster in the thoracic dermatomal distribution.

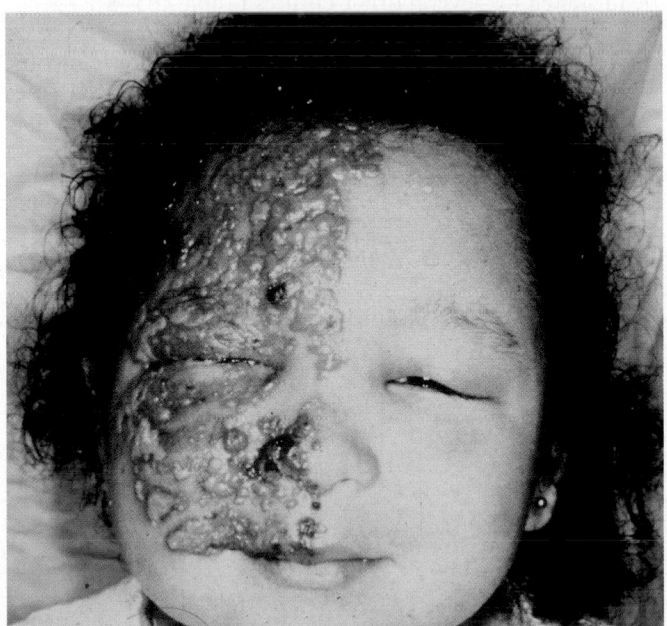

FIGURE 123–13. Ramsay Hunt syndrome with herpes zoster involving the ophthalmic branch of the trigeminal nerve.

Table 123–7	Differential Diagnosis of Varicella
Coxsackievirus (hand-foot-and-mouth disease)	
Herpes simplex virus	
Insect-bite reactions (popular urticaria)	
Erythema multiforme	
Parapsoriasis	
Rickettsialpox	
Dermatitis herpetiformis	
Smallpox (variola)	
Vaccinia	

preparation (scraping from an intact blister treated with Geimsa or Wright stain) will show the characteristic epidermal multinucleated giant cells containing intranuclear viral inclusions. Direct fluorescent antibody examination using a swab specimen taken from the base of a freshly opened lesion can distinguish HSV from HZV. Other laboratory tests include fluorescent antibody to membrane antigen, neutralization test, latex agglutination, ELISA, and demonstration of VZV DNA from vesicular fluid with PCR; identification of viral particles by direct electron microscopy; and serologic studies of acute and convalescent sera for VZV antibody.[65] Laboratory abnormalities usually show leukocytosis and elevated hepatic transaminases.

Secondary bacterial infection of varicella skin lesions is common.[66] It is generally caused by *Staphylococcus aureus* or group A β-hemolytic streptococci. The presence of fever after 4 or 5 days of illness or unusually indurated skin lesion should alert the clinician to the possibility of cellulitis. Life-threatening toxic shock syndrome, gangrenous cellulitis, and necrotizing fasciitis have all been described.[67] Data suggest that the use of ibuprofen may be associated with necrotizing fasciitis.[68] Pneumonia may complicate varicella, especially in adolescents. Other complications include otitis media, Reye's syndrome, acute postinfectious cerebellar ataxia, encephalitis, aseptic meningitis, transverse myelitis, Guillain-Barré syndrome, arthritis, nephritis, carditis, myositis, appendicitis, orchitis, nephritis, hepatitis, purpura fulminans, and thrombocytopenia.[69,70]

In immunocompromised patients or those with Hodgkin's lymphoma or leukemia, hematogenous spread of herpes zoster occurs 1 to 5 days after the dermatome infection begins.[71] This results in a generalized eruption. Most children recover without sequelae, but visceral involvement can occur. Some may have severe disease with high fever, encephalitis, pneumonia, hepatitis, or disseminated intravascular coagulation.[62] Congenital varicella syndrome occurs in 2% of infants in whom exposure to varicella occurred during the first or second trimester. It consists of IUGR, microcephaly, cortical atrophy, limb hypoplasia, microphthalmia, cataracts, micrognathia, chorioretinitis, and cutaneous scarring.[72]

Management

Healthy children with varicella do not require specific therapy. Treatment is supportive and aimed at decreasing pruritus and minimizing the risk of secondary infection. Wet dressing, soothing baths, and calamine lotion with oral antihistamines will provide symptomatic relief of pruritus.[73] Topical antihistamines containing diphenhydramine have the potential to cause sensitization and should probably be avoided. Acetaminophen can be used to control fever or pain; salicylates should be avoided due to the associated risk of

Reye's syndrome. Secondary bacterial infection is treated with antistaphylococcal drugs such as cephalexin, amoxicillin/clavulanate, or dicloxacillin. In penicillin-allergic patients, azithromycin, clarithromycin, or clindamycin can be used.

In immunocompetent hosts, most viral replication stops 72 hours after the onset of the eruption; however, it is extended in immunocompromised hosts. Oral acyclovir is not recommended for routine use in otherwise healthy children with varicella. Systemic antiviral agents, such as acyclovir and vidarabine, have been used with success in children.[74-76] If given within the first 24 hours of the exanthema, they can shorten the duration and magnitude of fever, accelerate healing time, and decrease the number of skin lesions. Since VZV is less sensitive to acyclovir than HSV, levels of acyclovir two to eight times greater are required. Oral acyclovir should be considered for patients at increased risk for moderate to severe varicella, such as those less than 6 months old or greater than 12 years old, those with chronic cutaneous or pulmonary disease, those on long-term salicylate therapy or corticosteroids, immunocompromised children, and children with ophthalmic involvement, Ramsay Hunt syndrome, disseminated zoster, and possible pregnancy. Children on corticosteroids or other immunosuppressive agents and exposed to varicella should have the dosages of these drugs reduced or discontinued whenever possible.

Passive immunization with varicella-zoster hyperimmune globulin has been shown to modify or prevent illness in high-risk individuals if given with 48 to 72 hours of exposure.[73,74] It is recommended for patients with immunodeficiencies, leukemia, or lymphoma, and in those receiving chemotherapy or other immunosuppressive agents, with seronegative pregnancy, or with disseminated disease. It is indicated for newborns whose mothers have developed primary varicella within 5 days before or 2 days after delivery and in neonates who develop varicella by the 10th day of life, as they are at increased risk of disseminated, fulminant infection.

In the rare case of postherpetic neuralgia, treatment consists solely of analgesics. Analgesics used primarily in adults have included tricyclic antidepressants, gabapentin, lidocaine patch, opioids, and capsacin, but none of these has been studied for use in children.[77]

All patients with complications such as fasciitis, Reyes's syndrome, pneumonia, or encephalitis should be hospitalized. The highly contagious nature of the infection should be emphasized, and child should be isolated until the lesions are crusted, which usually occurs 5 to 7 days after the eruption occurs. A follow-up visit within 48 hours should be scheduled for children who are discharged home from the emergency department to assess for any development of secondary bacterial infection. Children with disseminated zoster, ophthalmic zoster, or Ramsay Hunt syndrome should be seen daily until symptoms resolve.

Coxsackievirus (Hand-Foot-and-Mouth Disease)

Abrupt onset of scattered papules that progress to oval or linear vesicles in an acral distribution with oral involvement suggests hand-foot-and-mouth disease. The epidemic form is almost always caused by coxsackievirus A16 or enterovirus 71, but coxsackieviruses A2, A4 through A7, A9, A10, B1 through B3, and B5 have also been isolated.[78] The incubation period is 3 to 6 days, and patients are highly contagious from 2 days before to 2 days after onset of the eruption, with viral

excretion in feces persisting for 2 weeks. Coxsackievirus is transmitted transplacentally, by direct contact with nasal or oral secretions, through fecal material, or in aerosolized droplets. It is more prevalent during late summer or early fall. The virus enters the buccal or ileal mucosa and spreads to the lymph nodes. Viremia ensues with spread to the oral mucosa and skin. By day 7 after infection, serum antibody levels increase, and the virus disappears.

Clinical Presentation

A brief prodrome may occur, characterized by low-grade fever, anorexia, abdominal pain, cough, mouth soreness, and malaise, followed by the appearance of the enanthem and exanthem. The enanthem is the most characteristic finding and begins as small red macules that evolve into small vesicles, 1 to 3 mm to 2 cm in diameter, that rapidly rupture to leave behind erosions and ulcers superimposed on an erythematous base. They occur over the buccal mucosa and tongue as well as the palate, uvula, gingiva, and anterior tonsillar pillars (Fig. 123–14). These lesions are painful, and children refuse to eat or drink; therefore, dehydration is a common sequela.

The exanthem is maculopapular at first, then evolves into gray-white vesiculopustules ranging from 3 to 7 mm in diameter, with variable amounts of associated erythema. They are thin walled and contain a clear fluid, sometimes coalesce to form bullae, and are occasionally tender or pruritic. Lesions are usually elliptical or football shaped and surrounded by a red areola, and are found most commonly on the palms and soles, less often on the dorsal or lateral surfaces of the hands and feet, and occasionally on the buttocks and perineum (Fig. 123–15). Lesions clear within 2 to 7 days. Children with coxsackievirus infection are generally not ill appearing. Other findings include occasional lymphadenopathy in submandibular and cervical regions.

In the early nonvesicular stage, rubella and other morbilliform lesions must be considered, and in the vesicular stage the disease can be mistaken for varicella. The enanthem may be mistaken for several other entities (Table 123–8).

Occasionally coxsackievirus infections may cause myocarditis, pneumonia, meningoencephalitis, and aseptic meningitis.[79,80] In addition, there have been reports of fatal cases from enterovirus 71.[81] Infection in the first trimester may lead to spontaneous abortion or IUGR.

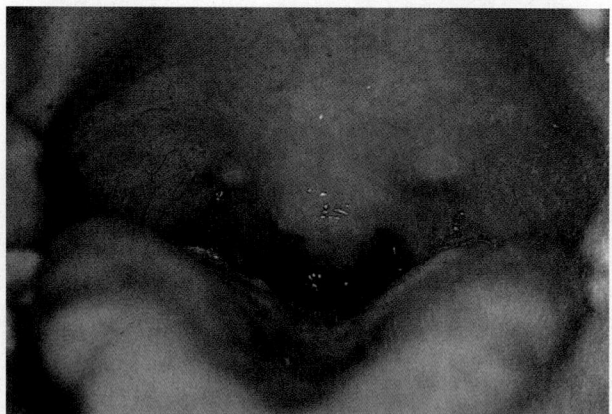

FIGURE 123–14. Vesicles and erosions seen on the palate in coxsackievirus infection (hand-foot-and-mouth syndrome).

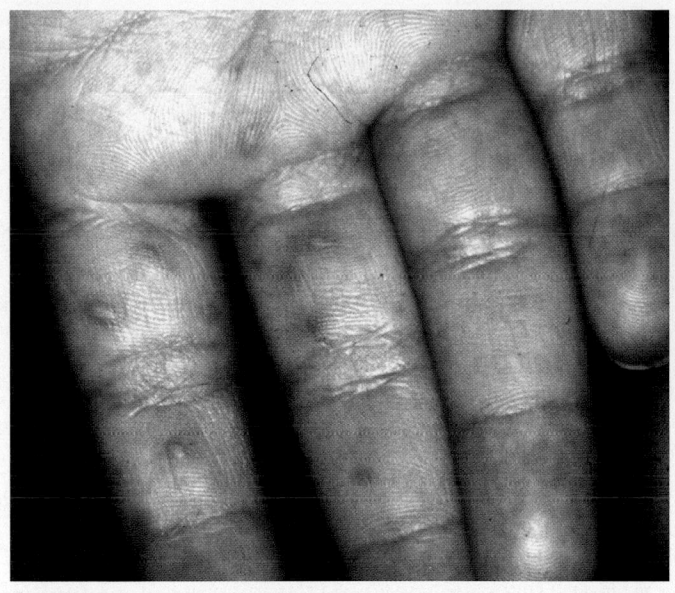
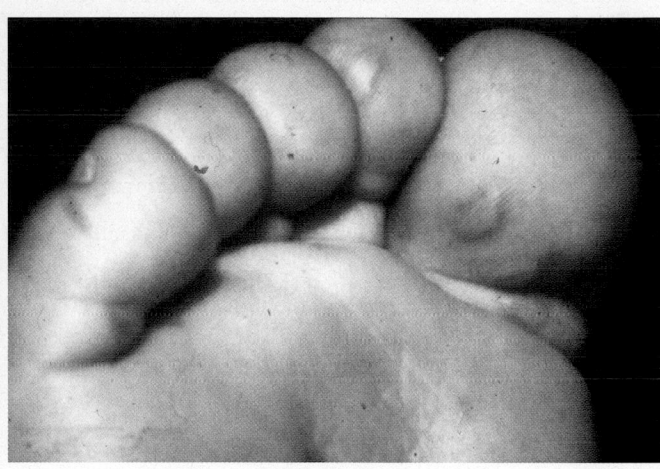

A   B

FIGURE 123–15. Elliptical vesicles seen on the hands **(A)** and feet **(B)** in coxsackievirus infection (hand-foot-and-mouth syndrome).

Table 123–8	Differential Diagnosis of the Enanthem of Coxsackievirus Infection

Varicella
Aphthous ulcers
Erythema multiforme
Herpes simplex virus
Herpangina

Management

No treatment is necessary in mild cases. Treatment is symptomatic and aimed at providing relief of painful oral lesions with topical agents, such as anesthetic mouth wash. In severe illness with enterovirus 71 infection, immune globulin or the antiviral agent pleconaril may be effective.[82]

REFERENCES

1. Mancini AJ: Exanthems in childhood: an update. Pediatr Ann 27:398, 1998.
2. Hogan PA: Viral exanthems in childhood. Aust J Dermatol 37:S14–S16, 1996.
3. Cherry JD, Feigin RD, Lobes LA Jr, et al: Atypical measles in children previously immunized with attenuated measles virus vaccines. Pediatrics 50:712–721, 1972.
4. Centers for Disease Control and Prevention: Measles—United States, 1999. MMWR Morb Mortal Wkly Rep 49:557, 2000.
5. Centers for Disease Control: Measles prevention: recommendations of the Immunization Practices Advisory Committee (AICP). MMWR Morb Mortal Wkly Rep 38:1–18, 1989.
6. Centers for Disease Control and Prevention: Final 1998 reports of notifiable disease. MMWR Morb Mortal Wkly Rep 48:749–753, 1999.
7. Papania MJ, Seward JF, Redd SB, et al: Epidemiology of measles in the United States, 1997–2001. J Infect Dis 189:SS61–S68, 2004.
8. Naniche D, Varior-Krishnan G, Cervoni F, et al: Human membrane cofactor protein (CD46) acts as a cellular receptor for measles virus. J Virol 67:6025–6232, 1993.
9. Schneider-Schaulies J, Meulen V, Schneider-Schaulies S: Measles infection of the central nervous system. J Neurovirol 9:247–252, 2003.
10. Schneider-Schaulies S, Meulen VT: Pathogenic aspects of measles virus infections. Arch Virol Suppl 15:139–158, 1999.
11. Dhiman N, Jacobson RM, Poland GA: Measles virus receptors: slam and CD46. Rev Med Virol 14:217–229, 2004.
12. Mason WH: Measles. Adolesc Med 6: 1–14, 1995.
*13. Perry RT, Halsey NA: The clinical significance of measles: a review. J Infect Dis 189:S4–S16, 2004.
14. Gold E: Almost extinct diseases: measles, mumps, rubella, and pertussis. Pediatr Rev 17:120–127, 1996.
15. West CE: Vitamin A and measles. Nutr Rev 58:S46, 2000.
16. Ratnam S, Tipples G, Head C, et al: Performance of indirect immunoglobulin M (IgM) serology tests and IgM capture assays for the laboratory diagnosis of measles. J Clin Microbiol 38:99–104, 2000.
17. Boyd AS. Laboratory testing in patients with morbilliform viral eruptions. Dermatol Clin 12:69–82, 1994.
18. Huiming Y, Chaomin W, Meng M: Vitamin A for treating measles in children. Cochrane Database Syst Rev (4):CD001479, 2005.
19. Villamor E, Fawzi WW: Vitamin A supplementation: implications for morbidity and mortality in children. J Infect Dis 182:S122–S133, 2000.
20. Rosa C: Rubella and rubeola. Semin Perinatol 22:318, 1998.
21. Sullivan EM, Burgess MA, Forrest JM: The epidemiology of rubella and congenital rubella in Australia, 1992 to 1997. Commun Dis Intell 23:209, 1999.
22. Jundt JW, Creager AH: STAR complexes: febrile illness associated with sore throat, arthritis and rash. South Med J 86:521, 1993.
23. Webster WS: Teratogen update: congenital rubella. Teratology 58:13, 1998.
24. Turner AJ: Surveillance of congenital rubella in Great Britain: rubella can be mistaken for parvovirus B19 infection. Br Med J 318:769, 1999.
25. Frey TK: Neurological aspects of rubella infection. Intervirology 40:167–175, 1997.
26. Myers MG, Hierholzer WJ: Incubation of varicella-zoster virus. Am J Dis Child 138:1155–1156, 1984.
27. Kosuge H: HHS-6 & 7 and their related diseases. J Dermatol Sci 22:205, 2000.
28. Leach CT: Human herpesvirus-6 and -7 infections in children: agents of roseola and other syndromes. Curr Opin Pediatr 12:269–274, 2000.
29. Hall CB, Long CE, Schnabel KC, et al: Human herpesvirus-6 infection in children: a prospective study of complications and reactivation. N Engl J Med 331:432–438, 1994.

*Selected readings.

30. Yamanishi K, Okuno T, Shiraki K, et al: Identification of human herpesvirus 6 as a casual agent for exanthema subitum. Lancet 1:1065–1067, 1988.
31. Tanaka K, Kondo T, Torigoe S, et al: Human herpesvirus 7: another casual agent for roseola (exanthema subitum). J Pediatr 125:1–5, 1994.
32. Asano Y, Yoshikawa T, Suga S, et al: Clinical features of infants with primary human herpesvirus 6 infection (exanthema subitum, roseola infantum). Pediatrics 93:104–108, 1994.
33. Adams O, Krempe C, Kogler G, et al: Congenital infections with human herpesvirus 6 infection in young children. N Engl J Med 326:1445–1450, 1992.
34. Teach SJ, Wallace HL, Evans MJ, et al: Human herpesvirus types 6 and 7 and febrile seizures. Pediatr Neurol 21:699–703, 1999.
35. Barone SR, Kaplan MH, Krilov LR: Human herpesvirus-6 infection in children with first febrile seizures. J Pediatr 127:95–97, 1995.
36. Yoshikawa T, Nakashima T, Suga S, et al: Human herpesvirus-6 DNA in cerebrospinal fluid in a child with exanthema subitum and meningoencephalitis. Pediatrics 89:888–890, 1992.
37. Burns WH, Sandford GR: Susceptibility of human herpesvirus 6 to antivirals in vitro. J Infect Dis 162:634–637, 1990.
38. Safrin S, Cherrington J, Jaffe HS: Clinical uses of cidofovir. Rev Med Virol 7:145–156, 1997.
39. Seishima M, Kanoh H, Izumi T: The spectrum of cutaneous eruptions in 22 patients with isolated serological evidence of infection by parvovirus B19. Arch Dermatol 135:1556–1557, 1999.
40. Barton RB: Parvovirus B19: twenty-five years in perspective. Pediatr Develop Pathol 2:296, 1999.
41. Anderson LJ: Role of parvovirus B19 in human disease. Pediatr Infect Dis 6:711–718, 1987.
42. Stiefel L: Erythema infectiosum (fifth disease). Pediatr Rev 16:474–475, 1995.
43. Ongradi J, Becker K, Horvath, A, et al: Simultaneous infection by human herpesvirus 7 and human parvovirus B19 in papular-purpuric gloves-and-socks syndrome. Arch Dermatol 136:672, 2000.
44. Chen MY, Lee KL, Hung CC: Imunoglobulin M and G immunoblots in the diagnosis of parvovirus B19 infection. J Formos Med Assoc 99:24, 2000.
45. Cherry JD: Parvovirus infections in children and adults. Adv Pediatr 46:245–269, 1999.
46. Moore TL: Parvovirus-associated arthritis. Curr Opin Rheumatol 12:289–294, 2000.
47. Heegaard ED, Hornsleth A: Parvovirus: the expanding spectrum of disease. Acta Paediatr 84:109–117, 1995.
*48. Heegaard ED, Brown KE: Human parvovirus B19. Clin Microbiol Rev 15:485–505, 2002.
49. Gilbert GL: Parvovirus B19 infection and its significance in pregnancy. Commun Dis Intell 24:69, 2000.
50. Anand A, Gray ES, Brown T, et al: Human parvovirus infection in pregnancy and hydrops fetalis. N Engl J Med 316:183–186, 1987.
51. Gratacos E, Torres PJ, Vidal J, et al: The incidence of human parvovirus B19 infection during pregnancy and its impact on perinatal outcome. J Infect Dis 171:1360–1363, 1995.
52. Miller E, Fairley CK, Cohen BJ, et al: Immediate and log term outcome of human parvovirus B19 infection in pregnancy. Br J Obstet Gynecol 105:174–178, 1998.
53. Koch WC, Massey G, Russell CE, et al: Manifestations and treatment of human parvovirus B19 infection in immunocompromised patients. J Pediatr 116:355–359, 1990.
54. Whitley RJ: Herpes simplex virus infection. Semin Pediatr Infect Dis 186(Suppl 1):S40–S46, 2002.
55. Jones VF, Badgett JT, Marshall GS: Repeated photoreactivation of herpes simplex virus type 1 in an extrafacial dermatomal distribution. Pediatr Infect Dis J 13:238, 1994.
56. Jacobs RF: Neonatal herpes simplex virus infections. Semin Perinatol 22:64–71, 1998.
57. Goodyear HM: Rapid diagnosis of cutaneous herpes simplex infections using specific monoclonal antibodies. Clin Exp Dermatol 19:294, 1994.
58. Troendle-Atkins J, Demmler GJ, Buffone GJ: Rapid diagnosis of herpes simplex virus encephalitis by using polymerase chain reaction. J Pediatr 123:376–380, 1993.
59. Flowers FB, Araujo OE, Turner LA: Recent advances in antiherpetic drugs. Int J Dermatol 27:612–616, 1988.
60. Mertz GJ, Critchlow CW, Benedetti J, et al: Double-blind placebo-controlled trial of oral acyclovir in first-episode genital herpes simplex virus infection. JAMA 252:1147–1151, 1984.
61. Takayama N, Takayama M, Takita J: Herpes zoster in healthy children immunized with varicella vaccine. Pediatr Infect Dis J 19:169, 2000.
62. Arvin AM: Chickenpox (varicella). Contrib Microbiol 3:96, 1999.
63. Feldman S, Hughes WT, Daniel CB: Varicella in children with cancer: seventy-seven cases. Pediatrics 56:388–397, 1975.
64. Charkes ND: Purpuric chickenpox: report of a case, review of the literature and classification by clinical features. Ann Intern Med 54:745, 1961.
65. Nahass GT, Goldstein BA, Zhu W-Y, et al: Comparison of Tzanck smear, viral culture, and DNA diagnostic methods in detection of herpes simplex and varicella-zoster infection. JAMA 268:2541, 1992.
66. Bullovwa JGM, Wishik SM: Complications of varicella. I. Their occurrence among 2,534 patients. Am J Dis Child 49:923, 1935.
67. Smith EWP, Garson A, Boyleston JA, et al: Varicella gangrenosa due to group A beta-hemolytic streptococcus. Pediatrics 57:306, 1976.
68. Zerr DM, Alexander ER, Duchin JS, et al: A case-control study of necrotizing fasciitis during primary varicella. Pediatrics 103:783–790, 1999.
69. Orlowski JP, Gilis J, Kilham HA: A catch in the Reye. Pediatrics 80:638–642, 1987.
70. Preblud SR, Orenstein WA, Bart KJ: Varicella: clinical manifestations, epidemiology and health impact in children. Pediatr Infect Dis 3:505, 1984.
71. Keiden SE, Mainwaring D: Association of herpes zoster with leukemia and lymphoma in children. Clin Pediatr 4:13–17, 1965.
72. Derrick CW Jr, Lord L: In utero varicella-zoster infections. South Med J 91:1064–1066, 1998.
73. Arvin AM: Management of varicella-zoster infections in children. Adv Exp Med Biol 458:167, 1999.
74. Lin F, Hadler JL: Epidemiology of primary varicella and herpes zoster hospitalization: the pre-varicella vaccine era. J Infect Dis 181:1897, 2000.
75. White R, Hilty M, Haynes R, et al: Vidarabine therapy of varicella in immunosuppressed patients. J Pediatr 101:125, 1982.
76. Prober CG, Kirk LE, Keeney RE: Acyclovir therapy of chickenpox in immunosuppressed children—a collaborative study. J Pediatr 101:622, 1982.
77. Dworkin RH, Schmader KE: Treatment and prevention of postherpetic neuralgia. Clin Infect Dis 36:877–882, 2003.
78. Lindenbaum JE, Van Dyck PC, Allen RG: Hand, foot and mouth disease associated with coxsackievirus group B. Scand J Infect Dis 7:161–163, 1975.
79. Tindall JP, Miller GD: Hand, foot, and mouth disease. Cutis 9:457–463, 1972.
80. Wright HT Jr, Landing BH, Lenette EH, et al: Fatal infection in an infant associated with Coxsackie virus group A type 16. N Engl J Med 268:1041–1044, 1963.
81. Shimizu H, Utama A, Yoshii K, et al: Enterovirus 71 from fatal and nonfatal cases of hand, foot, and mouth disease epidemics in Malaysia, Japan, and Taiwan in 1997–1998. Jpn J Infect Dis 52:12, 1999.
82. Robart HA, McCracken GH, Whitley RJ, et al: Clinical significance of enteroviruses in serious summer febrile illnesses of children. Pediatr Infect Dis J 18:869–874, 1999.
83. Amir J, Harel L, Smetana Z, et al: The natural history of primary herpes simplex type 1 gingivostomatitis in children. Pediatr Dermatol 16:259–263, 1999.
84. Dworkin MS, Shoemaker PC, Spitters C, et al: Endemic spread of herpes simplex virus type 1 among adolescent wrestlers and their coaches. Pediatr Infect Dis J 18:1108–1109, 1999.
85. ACOG practice bulletin: management of herpes in pregnancy. Clinical management guidelines for obstetrician-gynecologists. Int J Gynaecol Obstet 68:165–173, 2000.
86. Bale JF Jr: Human herpesvirus and neurological disorders of childhood. Semin Pediatr Neurol 6:278, 1999.
87. Kimberlin D: Herpes simplex virus, meningitis and encephalitis in neonates. Herpes 11(Suppl 2):65A–76A, 2004.
88. Kohl S: Neonatal herpes simplex virus infection. Clin Perinatol 24:129–150, 1997.

Dermatitis

Antonio E. Muñiz, MD

Selected Diagnoses

Atopic dermatitis
Diaper dermatitis
Seborrheic dermatitis
Contact dermatitis

Discussion of Individual Diagnoses

Atopic Dermatitis

Atopic dermatitis (AD) is a chronic, inherited, relapsing skin condition characterized by xerosis, pruritus, inflammation, and lichenification. Associated findings include a family history of AD, asthma, or allergic rhinitis. Eczema ("boiling over") in the acute setting refers to a morphology of erythema, scaling, vesicles, and crusts. In the chronic state, eczema refers to a morphology of scaling, lichenification, and pigmentary changes (either hypo- or hyperpigmentation). Eczematous lesions are found in conditions other than AD, including seborrheic dermatitis, contact dermatitis, scabies, autosensitization reactions, tinea pedis, immunodeficiencies, nummular eczema, dyshidrotic eczema, and lichen simplex chronicus. Eczema is essentially the morphologic skin finding to a number of different stimuli.

AD occurs during the first year of life in 60% of patients, generally appearing at 2 to 6 months of age. Approximately 70% to 95% develop AD by the age of 5 years. The lifetime prevalence of AD is 5% to 20% in children and 1% to 3% in adults.[1] There are three distinct phases of AD, in which both the location and morphology of the lesions change with age.[2-5] The infantile phase occurs in children up to 2 years of age; the childhood phase from 2 years of age to puberty; and the adult phase from puberty onward. The etiology of AD is still unknown; however, atopic dry skin is characterized by a decrease in skin lipids, an altered water-binding capacity of the stratum corneum, and increased transepidermal water loss with marked skin dehydration.[6] This impaired barrier function leads to increased skin irritability with subsequent scratching, which leads to the development of the typical lesions of AD. An immunologic etiology also has been suggested because many children with AD have chronic elevation of immunoglobulin E.[6a]

Clinical Presentation

INFANTILE PHASE

The quintessential feature and morbidity of AD is pruritus from dry skin, which may be unbearable and interferes with daily activity and normal sleep patterns. The eruption begins on the cheeks, forehead, scalp, and lateral aspects of the extensor surfaces of the legs[6] (Fig. 124–1). The trunk may also be involved (Fig. 124–2). The lesions are symmetric and ill defined, and consist of scaly, erythematous papules, patches, or vesicles that are sometimes covered with areas of crusting and excoriation. It spares the tip of the nose and the perioral and periorbital regions. Generalized xerosis is a prominent feature.

CHILDHOOD PHASE

The flexural areas are the sites of predilection. The antecubital and popliteal fossae are most affected, with the neck, flexural surfaces of the wrists and ankles, and buttock and thigh creases also commonly involved. The lesions are pruritic, ill-defined, scaly, erythematous patches, often covered with crusts and excoriations (Fig. 124–3). The childhood phase is when lichenification (thickening of the skin and accentuated skin markings) is first observed and is most prominent in the antecubital and popliteal fossae and around the wrists (Figs. 124–4 and 124–5). Nummular

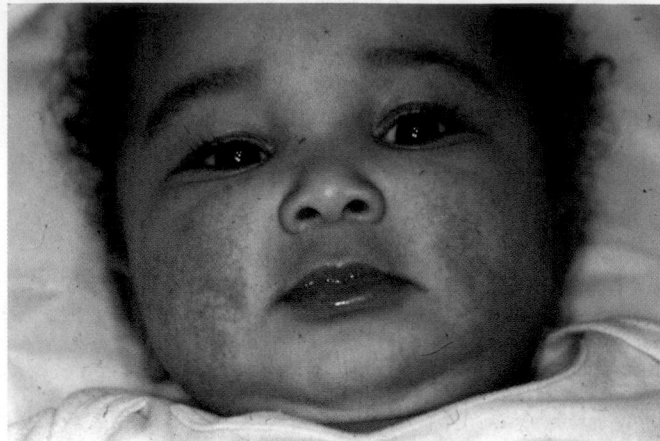

FIGURE 124–1. Symmetrical scaly, erythematous papules, patches, and vesicles on the cheeks seen in the infantile phase of atopic dermatitis.

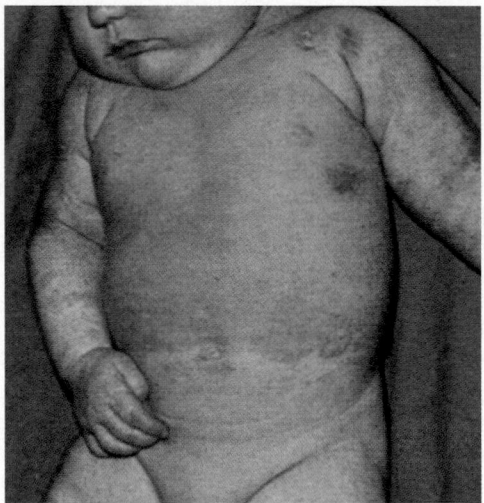

FIGURE 124–2. Symmetrical scaly, erythematous papules, patches, and vesicles on the cheeks and trunk seen in the infantile phase of atopic dermatitis.

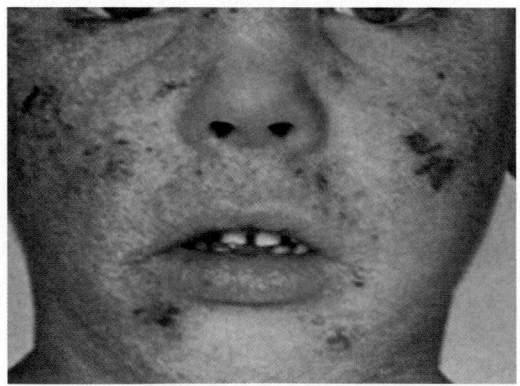

FIGURE 124–3. Scaly, erythematous patches covered with crusts and excoriations seen on childhood phase of atopic dermatitis.

(coin-shaped) exudative patches may be seen. The nails maybe shinny and buffed and the eyebrows sparse and broken off from constant rubbing. In dark skin, the lesions are more papular with follicular accentuation and hyperpigmentation.

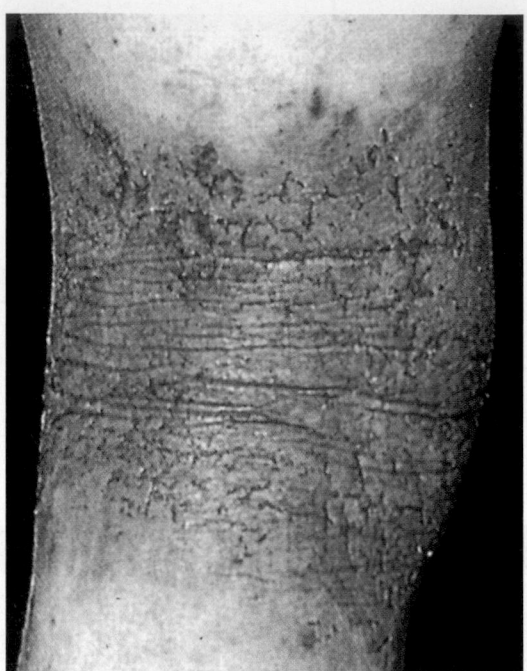

FIGURE 124–4. Lichenification seen in atopic dermatitis.

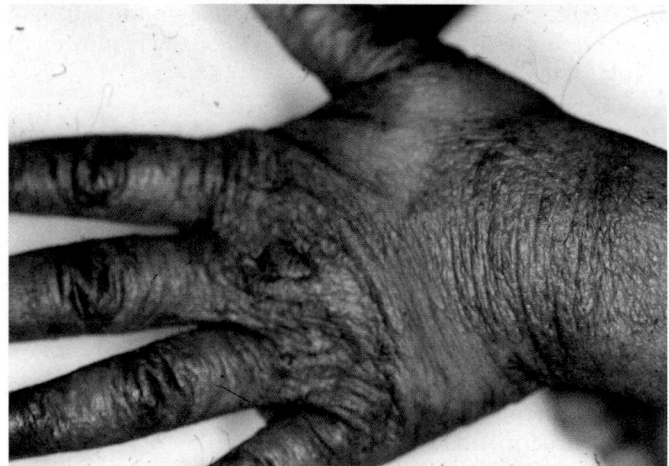

FIGURE 124–5. Lichenification seen in atopic dermatitis.

ADULT PHASE

After the child reaches puberty, the lesions are once again located on the face, neck, and body, with a more diffuse distribution with erythema and scaling, but with less exudation. Xerosis and lichenification are prominent features. The face continues to have a typical central pallor.

ASSOCIATED FINDINGS AND DIFFERENTIAL DIAGNOSIS

There are many associated findings with AD[7-12] (Table 124–1). Children with AD also have a tendency to develop secondary viral and bacterial skin infections. Herpes simplex virus infection is known as eczema herpeticum or Kaposi's varicelliform eruptions[13] (Fig. 124–6). The child is usually febrile and develops small, grouped vesicular lesions in the area of eczema, which subsequently spreads to normal skin. These vesicles form small erosions that crust over 24 to 48

Table 124–1	Associated Findings in Atopic Dermatitis (AD)
Findings	**Descriptions**
Ichthyosis vulgaris	Extensor surfaces of the extremities are dry, scaly, and hyperkeratotic.
Dennie-Morgan fold	Extra crease line found under the lower eyelid. Originally thought to be pathognomonic for AD, but may be seen with other inflammatory conditions around the eye or in Down syndrome.
Hertoghe's sign	Lateral thinning of eyebrows from rubbing
Allergic shiners	Hyperpigmentation under the eyes caused by chronic edema, lichenification, and postinflammatory hyperpigmentation
"Nasal salute"	Exaggerated linear nasal crease caused by frequent rubbing of the nose
Eye findings	Keratoconjunctivitis, which may occur in a painful form known as vernal conjunctivitis. Other eye findings include cataracts, keratoconus (elongation of corneal surface), and retinal detachment.
Keratosis pilaris	The lesions consist of asymptomatic hyperkeratotic follicular papules ("chicken-skin appearance"). It is found on extensor aspects of upper arms and anterior aspects of the thigh. It begins early in life and improves with age. In young children, the lateral aspects of the cheeks near the hairline are often involved, which may be mistaken for acne.
Pityriasis alba	Slightly scaly and dry hypopigmented patches on the cheeks and upper trunk. The lesions are ill defined and often misdiagnosed as tinea corporis. Mainly seen in children 6–12 years of age, especially in warm weather when the rest of the face is tanned
Dyshidrotic eczema	The lesions consist of small pruritic, multiloculated vesicles. These rupture, leaving crusts and scales with erythema. It affects the palms, soles, and sides of the fingers and toes and is associated with hyperhidrosis.
Juvenile plantar dermatitis	Scaling, cracking, and painful fissuring on both feet that markedly improves in puberty

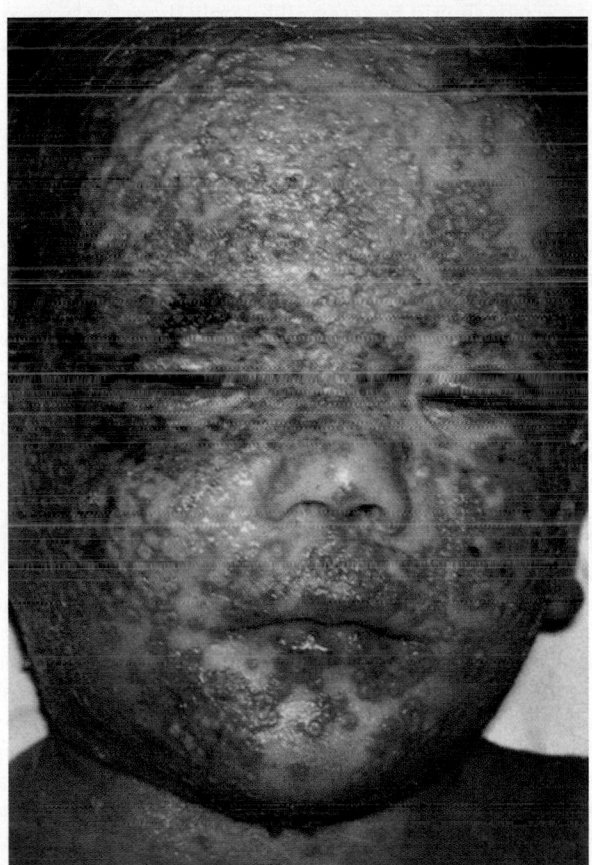

FIGURE 124–6. Infection with herpes simplex virus (eczema herpeticum) in a child with atopic dermatitis.

hours. Tzanck smears and viral cultures will confirm the diagnosis.

Ninety-three percent of patients with AD have significant *Staphylococcus aureus* colonization of the skin.[14] On occasion impetigo can occur in areas of eczema (Fig. 124–7). Widespread honey-colored crusting, erosions, oozing, follicular pustules, and furuncles suggest staphylococcal infection.

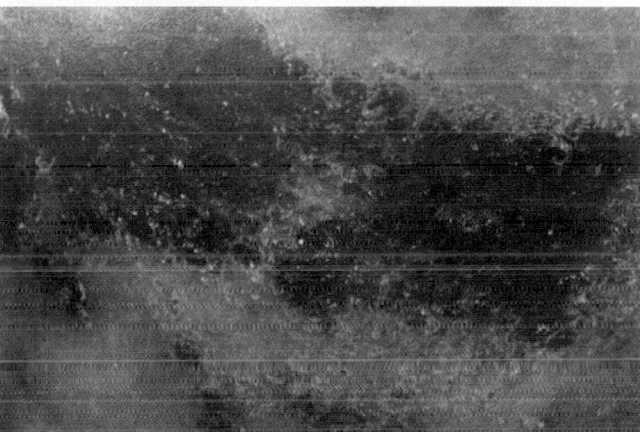

FIGURE 124–7. Secondary impetigo infection.

Chronic infection may lead to osteomyelitis. Infection with the nephritogenic M strain of streptococcus may lead to the development of glomerulonephritis.

The differential diagnosis of AD includes other eczematous disorders (Table 124–2).

Management

Effective management of AD hinges upon good rapport with the affected child and parents and education about the nature of the disease, potential aggravating factors to avoid, and treatment strategies.[15] Bubble baths and excessive exposure to soap, shampoo, and detergents aggravate dryness and should be discouraged. However, daily bathing is no longer considered to be harmful for atopic dry skin. Bathing in lukewarm water for 5 to 15 minutes rehydrates the stratum corneum, although benefits are only seen if an emollient is applied immediately after leaving the water to prevent evaporation.[16,17] Bathing once or twice daily is soothing during an acute flare, helps reduce bacterial counts, and aids in penetration of topical steroids applied after the bath. Soaps should be mild and unscented with a neutral pH (Dove, Oil of Olay, Caress, Camay, Aveeno, and Purpose). If soaps are too

Table 124–2	Differential Diagnosis of Atopic Dermatitis

Scabies
Seborrheic dermatitis
Contact dermatitis
Psoriasis
Acrodermatitis enteropathica
Agammaglobinemia
Ataxia-telangiectasia
Gluten-sensitive enteropathy
Langerhans cell histiocytosis
Hurler's syndrome
Hartnup syndrome
Leiner's disease
Omenn's syndrome
Phenylketonuria
Prolidase deficiency
Wiskott-Aldrich syndrome
Phenylketonuria
Job's syndrome
Letterer-Siwe disease
Mycosis fungoides
Secondary syphilis

irritating to the skin, hydrophobic lotions or creams (Cetaphil, Diprobase, and Unguentum Merck) may be used.

Many emollients are available that are suitable for use on atopic dry skin. These are best administered over slightly moistened skin, which seals in the moisture, rehydrates, lubricates, and moisturizes the skin and decreases inherent dryness and itchiness that appear to trigger the eczematous eruptions. They also aid in improving skin barrier function.[18] In general, ointments are better than creams and are more beneficial than lotions. Ointment-based emollients include Vaseline petroleum jelly, Aquaphor, and Elta. However, these can be too greasy for everyday use; cream-based alternatives include DML Forte, Moisturel, Aveeno, Curél, Purpose, Dermasil, Neutrogena, and Eucerin. Lotions are better tolerated but trap less water and are less effective than ointment. Lotions include many brands such as Nivea, Aveeno, Curél, Vaseline, Lubiderm, Neutrogena, Dermasil, Suave, Olay, Jergens, and Moisturel. The moisturizer should be applied two to three times daily and after steroid application, so as not to impede steroid absorption.

Topical corticoisteroids are the mainstay of treatment for AD.[19] In general, corticosteroids should be used intermittently to control exacerbations. Inflammation should be treated aggressively initially, with the aim of complete clearance. Topical steroids should be applied only in areas of acute exacerbation, while emollients should be used over the remainder of the skin. Topical steroid ointment preparations are preferable to creams as they penetrate more efficiently and produce less stinging. Ointments, however, tend to occlude eccrine pores and may induce sweat retention and pruritus, and are less tolerable during the summer months. Creams are more practical in warm, humid weather and for the scalp, although lotions and gels are more aesthetically acceptable; however, their alcohol content may produce burning and discomfort.

For mild cases of AD, a low-potency (class VI or VII) topical steroid should be used (Table 124–3). A 1% hydro-cortisone ointment is adequate for thin skin areas such as the face, neck, axilla, and groin, all areas prone to atrophy if more potent preparations are used. Potent steroids are not usually required, except for localized areas of long-standing dermatitis where significant lichenification has occurred. For moderate cases of AD, intermediate-potency (class III, IV, and V) topical steroids may be used for brief periods (<2 weeks) to control flares. The steroid preparation is applied one to three times daily until resolution. Once areas of inflammation have completely cleared, the steroid should be stopped and the skin moisturized regularly. For moderate to severe atopic dermatitis, maintenance therapy with application of topical steroid approximately twice weekly is effective.[17] Prolonged use of corticosteroids should be avoided since side effects are common, including skin atrophy, striae, telangiectasia, hypopigmentation, tachyphylaxis, hypothalamus-pituitary-adrenal axis suppression, Cushing's syndrome, intracranial hypertension, and growth delay.[20] Systemic steroids are rarely indicated in the management of chronic atopic dermatitis. Although a course of oral steroids will rapidly settle an acute flare, there is often a rebound flare after discontinuation. Oral steroids should be reserved for only those few extremely severe cases that cannot be controlled by other means, and the dose slowly tapered over time.

Wet dressings for 15 to 30 minutes three times a day (modified Burow's solution 1 : 40, 1 packet of Domeboro [aluminum acetate topical] powder per 12 ounces of water) are a useful adjunct to topical steroids during acute flares. The evaporation of water from the skin surface results in vasoconstriction and affords cooling to inflamed tissue, relief of pruritus, and débridement of crusts from the skin surface. Percutaneous penetration of topical steroids is increased, and the amount of steroids required to treat an acute flare is reduced, with wet dressings.

Localized infections should be treated during acute flares. Treatment with topical steroids has been shown to reduce the density of staphylococcal organisms on the skin, but the clinical course is improved only if combined with oral antibiotics effective against *S. aureus*,[21] such as cephalexin, dicloxacillin, and amoxicillin/clavulanate (Table 124–4). For penicillin-allergic patients, choices of antibiotics include azithromycin, clarithromycin, and clindamycin. Topical mupirocin can be used for impetigo involving a small surface area and is as effective as oral therapy.[22] Localized eczema herpeticum is treated with oral acyclovir, and more extensive skin involvement requires intravenous acyclovir.

Controlling the itch is also an important aspect in minimizing flares. A mild detergent should be used to wash clothes. Bleach, fabric softeners, and perfumed products should be avoided. Clothing is also an important factor in controlling pruritus. Cotton should be worn all year long. Synthetic fabrics and wool are irritating to the skin and should be avoided. Antihistamines have long been used in AD to prevent the scratch-itch cycle[23,24] (Table 124–5). Anecdotally, sedating antihistamines can be helpful in promoting sleep during a flare. Hydroxazine has excellent antihistaminic and antipruritic qualities with fewer tendencies to sedation. Overuse of these medications should be avoided since side effects may occur, such as paradoxical agitation, fatigue, and decreased attention, cognitive, motor, and intellectual performance.[25,26]

Table 124–3	Classification of Topical Steroids		
Steroid Potency	**Name**	**Preparation***	**Dosage**
Class I: highest potency	Betamethasone dipropionate (Diprolene) (0.05%)	oint, gel	qd–bid
	Clobetasol (Clobex, Embeline, Olux, Temovate) (0.05%)	crm, gel, oint	qd–bid
	Halobetasol (Ultravate) (0.05%)	crm, oint	qd–bid
Class II: high potency	Amcinonide topical (Cyclocort) (0.1%)	oint	bid–tid
	Betamethasone dipropionate (Diprosone) 0.05%	oint	qd–bid
	Desoximetasone topical (Topicort) 0.05%, 0.25%	crm, oint, gel	bid
	Diflorasone topical (ApexiCon, Maxiflor, Psorcon) 0.05%	oint	bid–tid
	Fluocinonide topical (Lidex) 0.05%	crm, gel, oint	qd–qid
	Halicinonide topical (Halog) 0.1%	crm	bid–tid
	Mometasone (Elocon) 0.1%	oint	qd
Class III: high/medium potency	Amcinonide topical (Cyclocort) 0.1%	crm, lot	bid–tid
	Betamethasone dipropionate (Diprosone) 0.05%	crm	qd–bid
	Betamethasone valerate 0.1%	oint	qd–bid
	Desoximethasone (Topicort) 0.05%	crm	bid
	Diflorasone topical (ApexiCon, Maxiflor, Psorcon) 0.05%	crm	bid–qid
	Fluticasone (Cutivate) 0.005%	oint	bid
	Fluocinonide topical (Lidex) 0.05%	lot	qd–qid
	Flurandrenolide (Cordran) 0.025%, 0.5%, 0.05%	lot, oint	qd–qid
	Halicinonide topical (Halog) 0.1%	oint, sol	bid–tid
	Triamcinolone (Aristocort A, Kenalog) 0.5%	crm, aerosol	qd–qid
Class IV: medium potency	Betamethasone valerate 0.1%	foam	bid
	Clocortolone (Cloderm) 0.1%	crm	tid
	Fluocinolone (Synalar) 0.025%	oint	bid–qid
	Hydrocortisone valerate (Westcort) 0.2%	oint	qd–qid
	Mometasone (Elocon) 0.1%	crm, lot	qd
	Prednicarbate (Dermatop) 0.1%	oint	bid
	Triamcinolone (Aristocort, Kenalog) 0.1%	crm	qd–qid
Class V: medium/low potency	Desonide (Tridesilon) 0.05%	oint	bid–tid
	Fluticasone (Cutivate) 0.05%	crm	bid
	Fluocinolone (Synalar) 0.025%	crm	bid–qid
	Hydrocortisone butyrate (Locoid) 0.1%	oint, sol	bid–tid
	Hydrocortisone valerate (Westcort) 0.2%	crm	qd–qid
	Triamcinolone (Aristocost, Kenalog) 0.1%	lot	bid–qid
Class VI: low potency	Alclometasone (Aclovate) 0.05%	crm, oint	bid–tid
	Desonide (Desowen, LoKara) 0.05%	crm, lot	bid–tid
	Fluocinolone (Synalar) 0.01%	crm, sol	bid–qid
	Triamcinolone (Aristocort, Kenalog) 0.025%	crm	qd–qid
Class VII: lowest potency	Hydrocortisone (Hytone) 1%, 2.5%	crm, oint	bid–qid
	Hydrocortisone/pramoxine (Pramosone) 1%/1%	crm	tid–qid
	Hydrocortisone/urea (Carmol HC) 1%/10%	crm	bid–qid

*Crm, cream; lot, lotion; oint, ointment; sol, solution.

The newest form of therapy includes the topical immuno-modulator agents. Tacrolimus ointment inhibits calcineurin, which results in decreased T-lymphocyte activation; especially CD4[+] cells, and suppression of cytokine release.[27-29] It has been safely used in children greater than 2 years of age, and results suggest it to be as effective as and possibly better than corticosteroids.[30-34] The main adverse effects are stinging, burning, and erythema on application.[35] It has been shown to result in over 90% improvement in skin lesions.[36] Because tacrolimus ointment does not cause skin atrophy, it may be safely used for prolonged periods on all skin areas, including the face and intertriginous areas. Pimecrolimus has the same mechanism as tacrolimus and has been shown to be effective in children older than 3 month of age but is approved for use in children over 2 years of age.[37-39] It is a cream that is less potent, but has less stinging upon application. The use of these agents early in flares has been shown to decrease the amount of corticosteroids required and has been more effective than corticosteroids and emollients.[40,41]

Table 124–4	Drugs for Secondary Bacterial Infections
Antimicrobials	**Dose**
Cephalexin	25–100 mg/kg/day PO divided q6h
Amoxicillin-clavulanate	25–45 mg/kg/day PO divided q12h
Dicloxacillin	12.5–25 mg/kg/day PO divided q6h
Azithromycin	5 mg/kg/day PO qd
Clarithromycin	15 mg/kg/day PO bid
Clindamycin	25–40 mg/kg/day divided q6-8h

Abbreviation: PO, orally.

Theoretically, the topical immunomodulators may increase the risk of cutaneous infections by altering local cutaneous response. However, controlled trials do not show an increase in bacterial, fungal, or viral infections.[42] Recently there has been a concern of an association between the development

Table 124–5	Common Antihistamines Used in Children
Antihistamine	**Dosage**
Diphenhydramine	5 mg/kg/day (maximum dose 300 mg/day and 50 mg per dose) divided q6h PO/IM/IV
Chlorpheniramine maleate	2–6 yr: 1 mg PO/IM/IV q4–6h (maximum dose 6 mg/day)
	6–12 yr: 2 mg PO q4–6h (maximum dose 12 mg/day)
	>12 yr: 4 mg PO q4–6h
Hydroxyzine	2–4 mg/kg/day PO divided q4–6h (maximum dose 400 mg/day)
	0.5–1 mg/kg IM q4–6h
Cetirizine	6 mo–2 yr: 2.5 mg PO qd
	2–5 yr: 2.5–5 mg PO qd
	≥6 yr: 5–10 mg PO qd
Loratadine	2–6 yr: 5 mg PO qd
	>6 yr: 10 mg PO qd
Fexofenadine	6–11 yr: 30 mg PO bid
	≥12 yr: 60 mg PO bid or 180 mg PO qd
Desloratidine	6–11 mo: 1 mg PO qd
	1–5 yr: 1.25 mg PO qd
	6–11 yr: 2.5 mg PO qd
	>12 yr: 5 mg PO qd

Abbreviations: IM, intramuscularly; IV, intravenously; PO, orally.

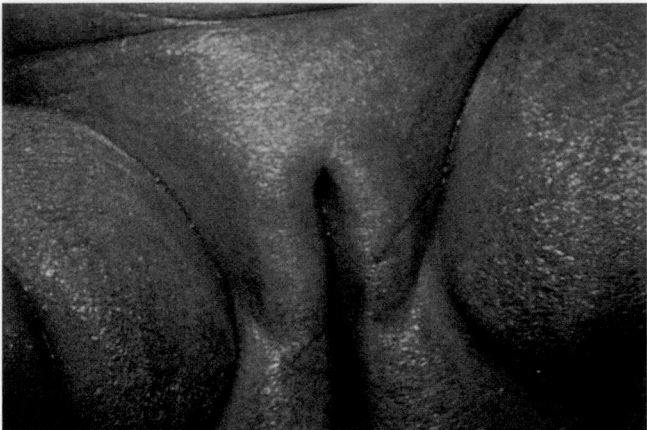

FIGURE 124–8. Friction diaper dermatitis.

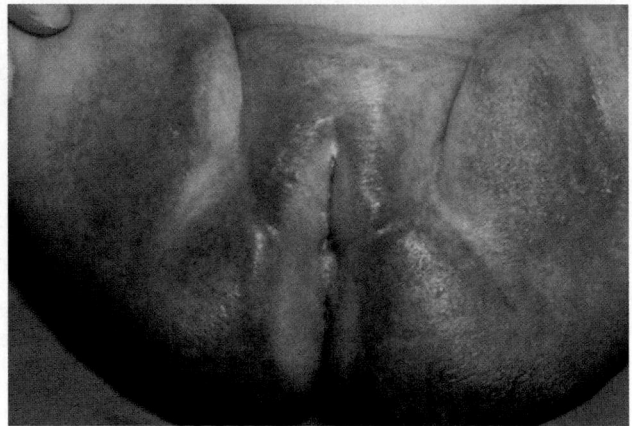

FIGURE 124–9. Irritant contact diaper dermatitis.

of skin cancer and lymphoma and use of these agents; therefore, they should be prescribed only if other therapies are ineffective or inappropriate and when patients have well-established follow-up care.[43]

Other agents tried for severe recalcitrant AD include cyclosporine, methotrexate, azathioprine, and phototherapy; however, their use is associated with significant adverse reactions such as renal damage, hypertension, infections, premature aging, and malignancy.[44-48] High-dose intravenous immune globulins have been used successfully in recalcitrant atopic dermatitis.[49]

Diaper Dermatitis

The term *diaper dermatitis* includes all inflammatory eruptions that occur in the area covered by the diaper. The etiology of irritant diaper dermatitis (IDD) is multifactorial and only partially understood, and includes recent antibiotic use, diarrhea, occlusion, overhydration of skin, maceration, prolonged contact with urine and feces, and the interaction of Candida and bacterial organisms.[50-53] The critical step in the development of diaper dermatitis is the occlusion of the skin under the diaper.[54] Infrequent diaper changes create overhydration and maceration of the stratum corneum, which makes the skin more sensitive to friction. Elevations in the pH of the diaper area from feces mixed with urine activate fecal lipases and proteases; this together with *Candida albicans* causes damage to the epidermis, resulting in loss of the barrier function and fostering increased susceptibility to irritation.[55] The incidence of IDD is equal between the sexes and begins around 3 to 18 months of age, peaking at 6 to 9 months of age. The prevalence in infants is 7% to 35%.[52,53,56]

Clinical Presentation

Friction dermatitis presents on areas where friction is most pronounced, such as the inner surfaces of thighs, genitalia, buttocks, and abdomen. It appears as a confluent shiny erythema with occasional papules that spares the intertriginous folds of the skin (Fig. 124–8).

Irritant contact dermatitis is generally asymptomatic and presents with erythema on the convex surface of the inner and upper thigh area, buttocks, and lower abdomen. The intertriginous creases are spared, as is the area over the mons pubis in boys. The eruption subsequently becomes deeply erythematous with a typical glistening or glazed appearance and with a wrinkled surface (Fig. 124–9). Papules, vesicles, and secondary erosions may occur in severe cases.

Candida diaper dermatitis presents with a diffuse erythematous patch extending over the genitalia with a peripheral scale. At the periphery of the patch it characteristically displays satellite red pustules or papules[54] (Fig. 124–10). The anterior perineal and perianal area are either both or separately involved, as are the intertriginous creases, which helps differentiate this from IDD. In cases in which diaper dermatitis has been present for 3 or more days, *C. albicans* has been isolated in up to 80% of infants.[54] Children with oropharyngeal candidiasis often have candidal diaper dermatitis due to excretion of *C. albicans* in the feces.[57] Candida growth is more common after taking antibiotics.

The differential diagnosis of diaper dermatitis is extensive (Table 124–6).

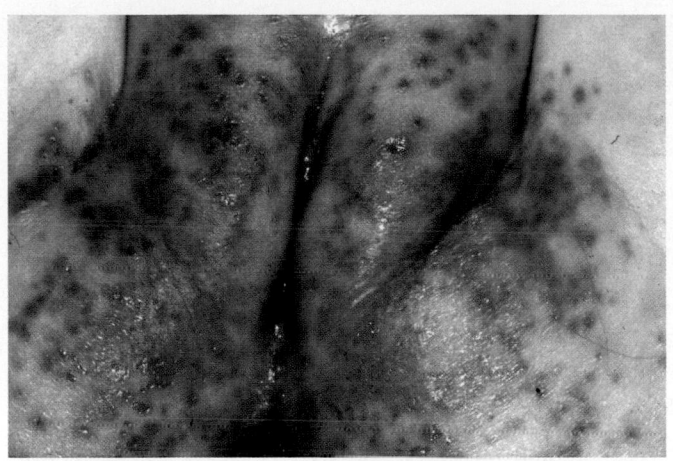

FIGURE 124–10. *Candida* diaper dermatitis.

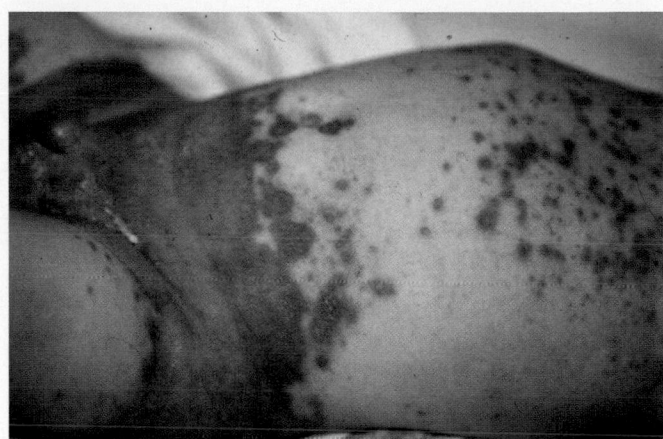

FIGURE 124–11. Id reaction from *Candida*.

Table 124–6	Differential Diagnosis of Diaper Dermatitis

Irritant contact dermatitis
Allergic contact dermatitis
Bullous impetigo
Seborrheic dermatitis
Psoriasis
Biotin deficiency
Jacquet's erosive diaper dermatitis
Langerhans cell histiocytosis (Letterer-Siwe disease)
Acrodermatitis enteropathica
Granuloma gluteale infantum
Congenital syphilis
Scabies
Urticaria
Miliaria
Herpes simplex virus
Varicella
Epidermolysis bullosa
Dermatitis herpetiformis
Chronic bullous dermatosis of childhood
Child abuse
Perianal cellulitis (streptococcal)

Table 124–7	Topical Antifungal Agents for *Candida* Diaper Dermatitis

Agents	Dosage
Nystatin (Mycostatin) cream, ointment, powder	bid or tid
Clotrimazole (Lotrimin) 1% cream, lotion, solution	bid
Econazole (Spectazole) 1% cream	bid
Sertaconazole (Ertaczo) 2% cream	bid
Sulconazole (Exelderm) 1% cream, solution	bid
Ciclopirox (Loprox) 0.77% cream, gel, suspension	bid
Miconazole (Micatin, Monistat-Derm) 2% cream, lotion, spray	bid

Table 124–8	Oral Antifungal Agents for *Candida* Diaper Dermatitis

Agents	Dosage
Nystatin	2 ml PO qid (1 ml in each side of mouth after feeding)
Fluconazole	6 mg/kg PO once, then 3 mg/kg/day PO (maximum 200 mg/day)

Abbreviation: PO, orally.

Candidal dermatitis with psoriaform id reaction represents a candidal infection in the diaper area followed by an explosive erythematous papulosquamous eruption resembling psoriasis on the cheeks and body[58] (Fig. 124–11). An id reaction occurs from generalized and symmetric response to severe local inflammation.

Management

Attempts should be made to prevent all inciting factors.[59] Frequent diaper changing is one of the most important factors in curing and preventing diaper dermatitis.[54,60] Using diapers made of sodium polyacrylate polymers that form a gel when hydrated to keep liquid away from the skin has been shown to decrease the incidence and severity of diaper dermatitis compared with the use of cloth diapers or other disposable diapers.[61] The diaper area should be gently cleaned at each diaper change. This is best done by immersing the area in lukewarm water in a basin. Harsh rubbing should be avoided. The area should be gently but completely dried. Use of cornstarch was believed to increase growth of *C. albicans*,

but recent studies refute this, and its use does decrease moisture.[62] Use of emollients, particularly zinc oxide preparations and petrolatum, will prevent overhydration of the skin and provides protection from urine and feces. Other topical barriers with proven efficacy include cod liver oil, dimethicone, and lanolin.[63] A nonfluorinated corticosteroid (hydrocortisone 1%), covered by the emollient, may be applied three times a day if emollients are ineffective. Their use, however, should be stopped after 14 days since overuse of corticosteroids can lead to skin atrophy or striae.[64]

Candidal superinfection is treated with topical anticandidal therapy, such as nystatin or an imidazole, two to three times daily in order to produce resolution in under 2 weeks (Table 124–7). If Candida is resistant to topical therapy or if there is evidence of Candida in the mouth as well as the perineal area, topical therapy may be supplemented with oral nystatin or fluconazole (Table 124–8). Adding hydrocortisone 1% to these agents may provide an anti-inflammatory effect and promote more rapid healing. The treatment of the id reaction involves a low-potency corticosteroid ointment on the face and a mid-potency corticosteroid ointment on the body (see Table 124–3).

Seborrheic Dermatitis

Seborrheic dermatitis refers to a chronic inflammatory disease with remissions and exacerbations, characterized by an erythematous, scaly, or crusting eruption that occurs primarily in the seborrheic areas, where the highest concentration of sebaceous glands exists. These areas include the scalp, face, and postauricular, presternal, axillary, and intertriginous folds. Seborrheic dermatitis is a disease of unknown etiology that affects infants from 3 weeks of age onward, is uncommon after 6 months of age, and usually clears by 12 months of age. It then can reoccur in adolescents.

The organism *Pityrosporum ovale* (*Malassezia furfur*) has been implicated in the etiology of adult seborrheic dermatitis, but its role in the infantile form of the disease is yet to be proven.[65-67] It has, however, been recovered more often in patients with seborrheic dermatitis than in controls.[68] In addition, some patients improve with topical or systemic ketoconazole.[69]

Clinical Presentation

The first area of involvement is generally the scalp. Here the lesions consists of diffuse greasy, yellow or white scales, frequently called "cradle cap" (retention hyperkeratosis) (Fig. 124–12).[69a] Lesions may spread to involve the face, especially the hairline and eyebrow area, where the scale is yellow and greasy and the underlying skin becomes erythematous (Fig. 124–13). The intertriginous, flexural, axillary, and postauricular areas and neck are involved in more severe cases, with scaling and linear erythema. In the diaper area, well-demarcated erythematous plaques are topped by a thin white scale or covered with thick, yellowish brown, greasy crusts. The lesions may become macerated, crusted, and superinfected with *C. albicans*. Pruritus is usually absent in comparison to AD. Infants are usually asymptomatic, and it is the parents who are dismayed by the cosmetic appearance. However, in one study up to 33% were seemingly itchy.[70]

In children between middle school age and puberty, seborrheic dermatitis may appear on the scalp as a dry, fine, flaky desquamation known as pityriasis sicca or dandruff. Erythema and scaling may also involve the supraorbital region, nasolabial crease, lips, pinna, retroauricular area, aural canal, and chest (Fig. 124–14). Pruritus is common.

The differential diagnosis of seborrheic dermatitis includes atopic dermatitis, contact dermatitis, tinea facialis, tinea capitis, psoriasis, Langerhans cell histiocytosis (Letterer-Siwe disease), and Leiner's disease.

Management

These lesions respond quickly to treatment with bathing in soothing oatmeal baths once or twice a day and shampooing with a tar shampoo daily. Shampoos containing salicylic acid should be avoided as they may be irritating and absorption may cause problems with salicylism. The use of ketoconazole

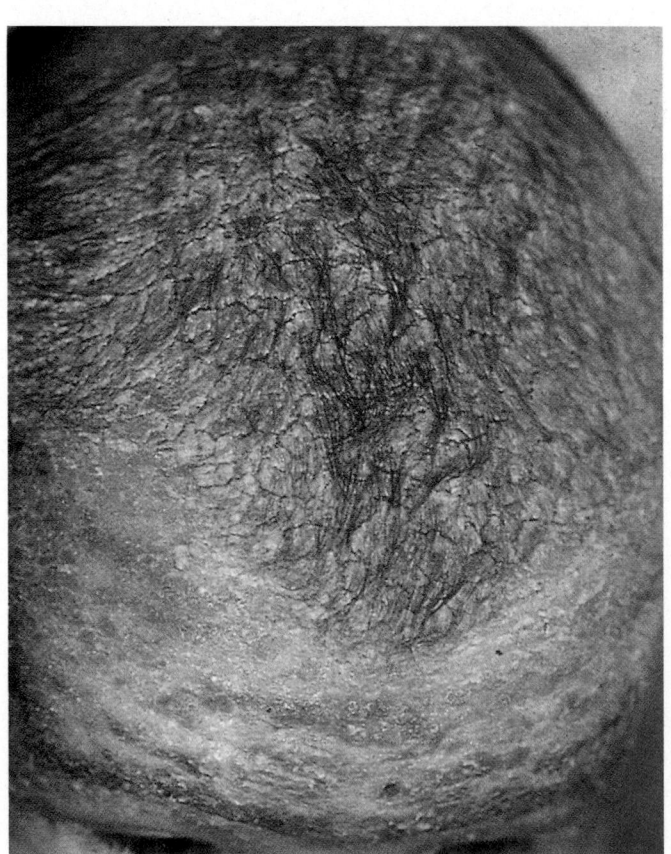

FIGURE 124–12. Seborrheic dermatitis ("cradle cap").

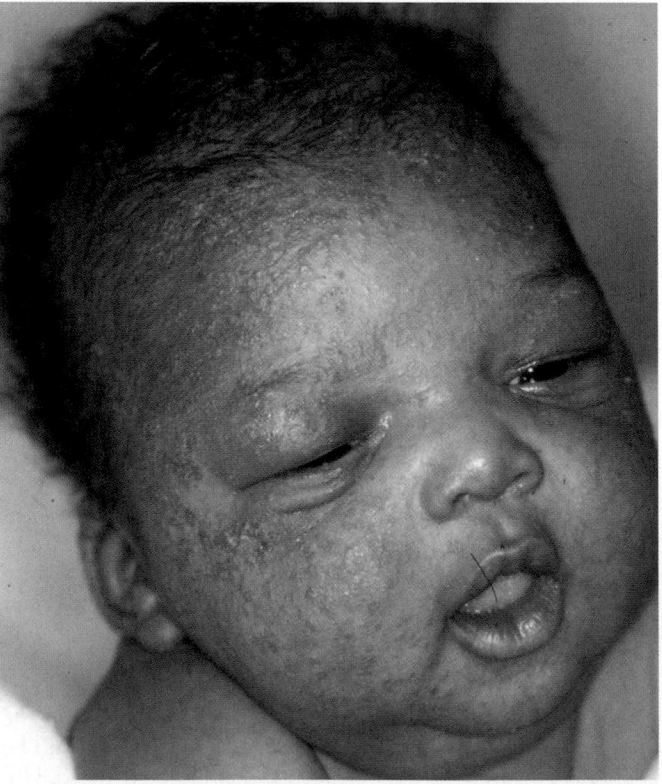

FIGURE 124–13. Yellow and greasy rash from seborrheic dermatitis.

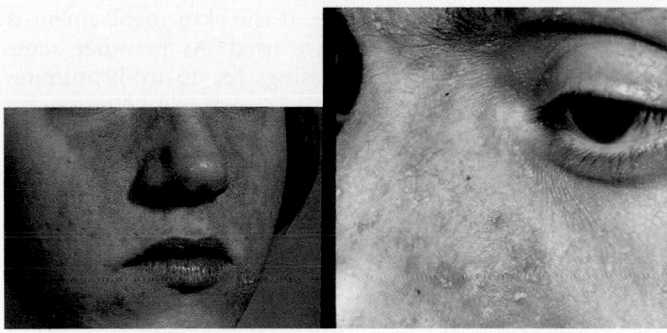

FIGURE 124–14. Erythematous scaly patches in an adolescent with seborrheic dermatitis.

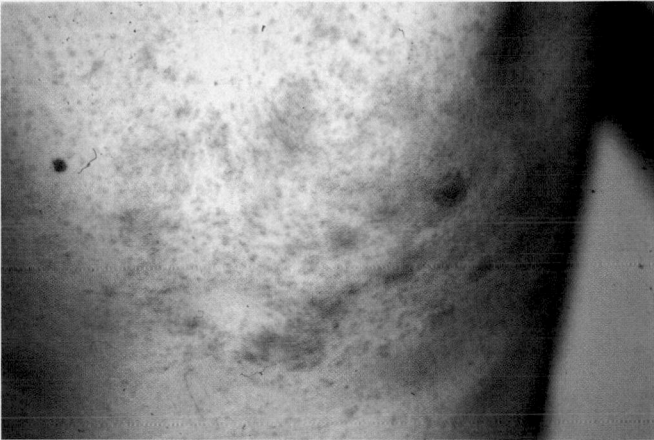

FIGURE 124–15. Allergic contact dermatitis from poison ivy.

2% results in clinical cure in patients with seborrheic dermatitis and has been found safe in infants.[71,72] Itraconazole has been shown to be effective in adults.[73] If the scale is extremely thick and adherent, it can be loosened by warmed mineral oil massaged into the scalp and then removed with a comb. In stubborn cases, a topical corticosteroid lotion may be used on the scalp one to three times daily.

Adolescents with seborrhea of the scalp may use antiseborrheic shampoos, which include zinc pyrithone (Head & Shoulders, DHS Zinc, Zincon, or XSeb), selenium sulfide (Exsel or Selsun), ketoconazole (Nizoral), corticosteroids (FS Shampoo), and tar (T/Gel). Recently, the immunomodulators pimecrolimus and tacrolimus have been shown to be effective in improving lesions of seborrheic dermatitis.[74,75] However, these agents have been associated with the development of dermal cancer and lymphoma and should be considered only for resistant cases.[43] Ciclopirox (Loprox) shampoo, which has anti-Malassezia activity, will improve lesions in seborrheic dermatitis. Topical lithium gluconate and topical metronidazole (MetroCream, MetroGel, MetroLotion, Noritate) have also been shown to be effective.[76,77]

Contact Dermatitis

Contact dermatitis may be defined as an eczematous eruption produced either by local exposure to a primary irritating substance (irritant contact dermatitis) or by an acquired allergic response to a sensitizing substance (allergic contact dermatitis).[78-80] Irritant contact dermatitis requires an irritant—any agent that is capable of producing cell damage in any individual if applied for sufficient time and in sufficient concentration. Common substances include harsh soaps, bleaches, detergents, acids, alkalis, solvents, fiberglass, bubble baths, certain foods, saliva, talcum, urine, feces, and intestinal secretions.

Allergic contact dermatitis (ACD) is unusual in children less than 10 years of age. It is a type IV hypersensitivity reaction only affecting previously sensitized individuals. There are two phases, the induction or sensitization phase and the elicitation phase.[78,80] During the induction phase, an allergen, or hapten, penetrates the epidermis, where a cascade of events causes T lymphocytes to become memory cells. The elicitation phase occurs when the sensitized individual is reexposed to the antigen. The antigen causes T lymphocytes to produce lymphokines that mediate the inflammatory response that is characteristic of an allergic contact dermatitis. The elicita-

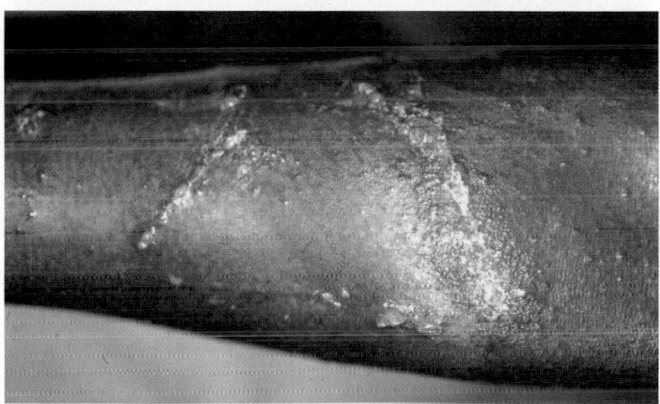

FIGURE 124–16. Köbner's phenomenon from contact dermatitis.

tion phase requires several hours to develop, and as a result symptoms are delayed. In infants, the only ACD seen with any frequency is nickel dermatitis, while in children ACD may include poison ivy, nickel, preservative or fragrances used in cosmetics, topical medications, and rubber (Figs. 124–15, 124–16, and 124–17). Teenagers may react to cosmetics and to formaldehyde used to size clothing. Flowers and pollens may all cause allergic reactions, but rarely in children. Adhesive tape reactions may occur in all ages.

Several dermatitis conditions in children have characteristic presentations (Table 124–9). The differential diagnosis of contact dermatitis is lengthy (Table 124–10).

Management

Once the diagnosis of contact dermatitis has been made and the causative agent elicited, elimination of the offending substance results in cure within 2 to 3 weeks, but during this time patients may be severely incapacitated. Symptomatic treatment should be initiated as soon as the diagnosis is made.

For relief of pruritus, antihistamines (see Table 124–5) can be given, and calamine lotion and oatmeal baths are soothing for the skin, but systemic corticosteroid therapy is the treatment of choice. If there is widespread skin involvement, corticosteroids should be given orally and tapered over 2 to 3

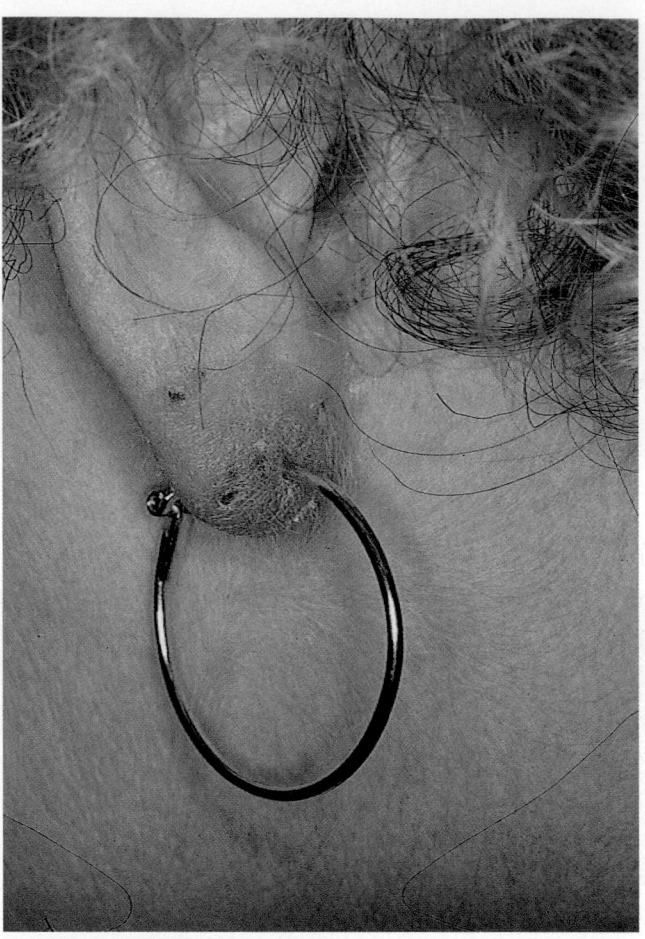

FIGURE 124–17. Contact dermatitis caused by nickel.

weeks to avoid a rebound flare. If the skin involvement is small, topical corticosteroids are used. As in other acute eczematous eruptions, wet dressings for 15 to 30 minutes three times a day (modified Burow's solution 1 : 40, 1 packet of Domeboro [aluminum acetate topical] powder per 12 ounces of water) are a useful adjunct to topical steroids. The crusts can be gently loosened from affected sites, followed by the application of a thin layer of emollient or antibacterial ointment.

Table 124–10	Differential Diagnosis of Contact Dermatitis
Angioedema	
Atopic dermatitis	
Burns	
Candidiasis	
Diaper dermatitis	
Dyshidrotic eczema	
Herpes simplex virus	
Impetigo	
Scabies	
Sunburns	
Tinea infections	
Pityriasis rosea	
Mycosis fungoides	
Psoriasis	
Systemic lupus erythematosus	
Varicella	
Zoster	

Table 124–9	Common Pediatric Dermatitis Conditions

Poison Ivy Dermatitis

- Most common ACD in children
- Caused by the plant of the *Rhus* or *Toxicodendron* genuses (poison ivy, oak, or sumac). Poison ivy occurs in all parts of the United States as a shrub or vine. Poison oak, an upright shrub, appears only on the West Coast. Poison sumac grows as a shrub or tree in Mississippi
- Sensitizing agent is an oleoresin (urushiol).
- Occurs in spring, summer, and autumn
- Sensitization may take 5–25 days and may be followed by the development of an acute pruritic dermatitis.
- Reexposure will always result in an eruption within 24–48 hours. Initial lesions consists of erythematous vesicular streaks mainly on the lower legs, but any area may be involved (see Fig. 124–15).
- A few hours to days later, other erythematous patches, papules, and bullae may develop.
- Linear distribution of papules or vesicles after minor epidermal trauma (Köbner's phenomenon) is highly characteristic of contact dermatitis (see Fig. 124–16).
- Allergen may be washed off within 20 minutes without causing an eruption.
- Oleoresin may remain in clothing for months to years, causing a typical dermatitis if contacted by a sensitized person.

Nickel Allergy

- Earrings with nickel result in bilateral dermatitis consisting of erythema, scaling, vesicles, and crusts on the back and less often on the front of the earlobe.
- Also widely used in bracelets, necklaces, watches, and rings as a hardening agent for gold (see Fig. 124–17).
- Area immediately below the umbilicus where the nickel snap on blue jeans comes in contact with the skin is commonly involved.[81]
- Areas of inflammation may become chronic with shiny lichenoid papules from constant rubbing.

Shoe Dermatitis

- Acute or subacute dermatitis along the dorsa of the toes and foot
- Erythema, lichenification, and, in severe cases, weeping and crusting
- Webs of the toes not involved
- Ball and heel also involved when rubber is the causative agent
- Most common cause is rubber, but other agents include chromates, adhesives, and dyes.
- Commonly misdiagnosed as tinea pedis (usually involves toe web spaces and is rarely seen prior to puberty).

REFERENCES

1. Laughter D, Istvan JA, Tofte SJ, Hanifin JM: The prevalence of atopic dermatitis in Oregon school children. J Am Acad Dermatol 43:649–655, 2000.
2. Mortz CG, Lauritsen JM, Bindslev-Jensen C, Andersen KE: Prevalence of atopic dermatitis, asthma, allergic rhinitis, hand and contact dermatitis in adolescents: The Odense Adolescent Cohort Study on Atopic Diseases and Dermatitis (TOACS). Br J Dermatol 144:523–532, 2001.
*3. Beltrani VS, Boguniewicz M: Atopic dermatitis. Dermatol Online J 9:1–24, 2003.
4. Foley P, Zuo Y, Plunkett A, Marks R: The frequency of common skin condition in preschool-age children in Australia: atopic dermatitis. Arch Dermatol 137:293–300, 2001.
5. William HC, Burney PG, Hay RJ, et al: The U.K. Working Party's diagnostic criteria for atopic dermatitis. I. Derivation of a minimum set of discriminators for atopic dermatitis. Br J Dermatol 131:383–396, 1994.
6. Aoki T, Fukuzumi T, Adachi J, et al: Re-evaluation of skin lesion distribution in atopic dermatitis: analysis of cases 0 to 9 years of age. Acta Derm Venereol Suppl 176:19–23, 1992.
6a. Stone KD: Atopic disease of childhood. Curr Opin Pediatr 15:495–511, 2003.
7. Uehara M, Hayashi S: Hyperlinear palm: association with ichthyosis and atopic dermatitis. Arch Dermatol 117:490–491, 1981.
8. Williams HC, Pembroke AC: Infraorbital crease, ethnic group, and atopic dermatitis. Arch Dermatol 132:51–54, 1996.
9. Gelmetti C: Extracutaneous manifestations of atopic dermatitis. Pediatr Dermatol 9:380–382, 1992.
10. Garrity JA, Liesegang TJ: Ocular complications of atopic dermatitis. Can J Ophthalmol 19:21–24, 1984.
11. Oshinskie L, Haine C: Atopic dermatitis and its ophthalmic complications. J Am Optom Assoc 53:889–894, 1982.
12. Takahashi M, Suzuma K, Inaba I, et al: Retinal detachment associated with atopic dermatitis. Br J Ophthalmol 80:54–57, 1996.
13. Goodyear HM, McLeish P, Randall S, et al: Immunological studies of herpes simplex virus infection in children with atopic eczema. Br J Dermatol 134:85–93, 1996.
14. Arslanagic N, Arslanagic R. Atopic dermatitis and Staphylococcus aureus. Med Arh 58:363–365, 2004.
15. Su JC, Kemp AS, Varigos GA, Nolan TM: Atopic eczema: its impact on the family and financial cost. Arch Dis Child 76:159–162, 1997.
16. Stender IM, Blichmann C, Serup J: Effects of oil and water baths on the hydration state of the epidermis. Clin Exp Dermatol 15:206–209, 1990.
17. Hanifin JM, Tofte SJ: Update on therapy for atopic dermatitis. J Allergy Clin Imunol 104:S123–S125, 1999.
18. Loden M, Andersson AC, Lindberg M: Improvement in skin barrier function in patients with atopic dermatitis after treatment with a moisturizing cream (Canoderm). Br J Dermatol 140:264–267, 1999.
19. Thomas KS, Armstrong S, Avery A, et al: Randomized controlled trial of short bursts of a potent topical corticosteroid versus prolonged use of a mild preparation for children with mild or moderate atopic dermatitis. BMJ 324:768, 2002.
20. Railian D, Wilson JK, Feldman SR, Fleischer AB: Pediatricians who prescribe clotrimazole-betamethasone dipropionate (Lotrisone) often utilize it in inappropriate settings regardless of their knowledge of the drug's potency. Dermatol Online J 8:3, 2002.
21. Nilsson EJ, Henning CG, Magnusson J: Topical corticosteroids and Staphylococcus aureus in atopic dermatitis. J Am Acad Dermatol 27:29–34, 1992.
22. Bass JW, Chan DS, Creamer KM, et al: Comparison of oral cephalexin, topical mupirocin and topical bacitracin for the treatment of impetigo. Pediatr Infect Dis J 16:708–710, 1997.
23. Klein PA, Clark RA: An evidence-based review of the efficacy of antihistamines in relieving pruritus in atopic dermatitis. Arch Dermatol 135:1522–1525, 1999.
24. Doherty V, Sylvester DG, Kennedy CT, et al: Treatment of itching in atopic eczema with antihistamines with a low sedative profile. BMJ 298:96, 1989.
25. Simons FE, Simons KJ: The pharmacology and use of H1-receptor-antagonist drugs. N Engl J Med 330:1663–1670, 1994.
26. Roth T, Roehrs T, Kosnorek G, et al: Sedative effects of antihistamines. J Allergy Clin Immunol 80:94–98, 1987.
27. Nakagawa H, Etoh T, Ishibashi Y, et al: Tacrolimus ointment for atopic dermatitis. Lancet 344:883, 1994.
28. Pascual JC, Fleisher AB: Tacrolimus ointment (Protopic) for atopic dermatitis. Skin Ther Lett 9:1–5, 2004.
29. Kapp A, Allen BR, Reitamo S: Atopic dermatitis management with tacrolimus ointment (Protopic). J Dermatol Treat 14(Suppl 1):5–16, 2003.
30. Paller A, Eichenfield LF, Leung DY, et al: A 12-week study of tacrolimus ointment for the treatment of dermatitis in pediatric patients. J Am Acad Dermatol 44(Suppl 1):S47–S57, 2001.
31. Bekersky I, Fitzsimmons W, Tanase A, et al: Nonclinical and early clinical development of tacrolimus ointment for the treatment of atopic dermatitis. J Am Acad Dermatol 44(1 Suppl):S17–S27, 2001.
32. Drake L, Prendergast M, Maher R, et al: The impact of tacrolimus ointment on health-related quality of life of adult and pediatric patients with atopic dermatitis. J Am Acad Dermatol 44(1 Suppl):S65–S72, 2001.
33. Kang S, Lucky AW, Pariser D, et al: Long-term safety and efficacy of tacrolimus ointment for the treatment of atopic dermatitis in children. J Am Acad Dermatol 44(1 Suppl):S58–S64, 2001.
34. Reitamo S, Harper J, Bos JD, et al; European Tacrolimus Ointment Group: 0.03% Tacrolimus ointment applied once or twice daily is more efficacious than 1% hydrocortisone acetate in children with moderate to severe atopic dermatitis: results of a randomized double-blind controlled trial. Br J Dermatol 150:554–562, 2004.
35. Ruzicka T, Bieber T, Schopf E, et al: A short-term trial of tacrolimus ointment for atopic dermatitis. N Engl J Med 337:816–821, 1997.
36. Thestrup-Pedersen K: Tacrolimus treatment of atopic eczema/dermatitis syndrome. Curr Opin Allergy Clin Immunol 3:359–362, 2003.
37. Eichenfield LF, Lucky AW, Boguniewicz M, et al: Safety and efficacy of pimecrolimus (ASM 981) cream 1% in the treatment of mild and moderate atopic dermatitis in children and adolescents. J Am Acad Dermatol 46:495–504, 2002.
38. Allen BR, Lakhanpaul M, Morris A, et al: Systemic exposure, tolerability, and efficacy of pimecrolimus cream 1% in atopic dermatitis patients. Arch Dis Child 88: 969–973, 2003.
39. Wolff K, Stuetz A: Pimecrolimus for the treatment of inflammatory skin disease. Expert Opin Pharmacother 5:643–655, 2004.
40. Torok HM, Mass-Irslinger R, Slayton RM: Clocortolone pivalate cream 0.1% used concomitantly with tacrolimus ointment 0.1% in atopic dermatitis. Cutis 72:161–166, 2003.
41. Nakahara T, Koga T, Fukagawa S, et al: Intermittent topical corticosteroid/tacrolimus sequential therapy improves lichenification and chronic papules more efficiently than intermittent topical corticosteroid/emollient sequential therapy in patients with atopic dermatitis. J Dermatol 31:524–528, 2003.
42. Fleischer AB Jr, Ling M, Eichenfield L, et al: Tacrolimus Ointment Study Group: Tacrolimus ointment for the treatment of atopic dermatitis is not associated with an increase in cutaneous infections. J Am Acad Dermatol 47:562–570, 2002.
43. Wooltorton E: Eczema drugs tacrolimus (Protopic) and pimecrolimus (Elidel): cancer concerns. CMAJ 172:1179–1180, 2005.
44. Jekler J, Larko O: Combined UVA-UVB versus UVB phototherapy for atopic dermatitis: a paired-comparison study. J Am Acad Dermatol 22:49–53, 1990.
45. Pasic A, Ceovic R, Lipozencic J, et al: Phototherapy in pediatric patients. Pediatr Dermatol 20:71–77, 2003.
46. de Prost Y, Bodemer C, Telliac D: Randomised double-blind placebo-controlled trial of local cyclosporin in atopic dermatitis. Acta Dermatol Venereol Suppl 144:136–138, 1989.
47. Buckley DA, Baldwin P, Rogers S: The use of azathioprine in severe adult atopic eczema. J Eur Acad Dermatol Venereol 11:137–140, 1998.
48. Lee SS, Tan AW, Giam YC: Cyclosporin in the treatment of severe atopic dermatitis: a retrospective study. Ann Acad Med Singapore 33:311–313, 2004.
49. Jolles S: A review of high-dose intravenous immunoglobulin treatment for atopic dermatitis. Clin Exp Dermatol 27:3–7, 2002.
50. Campbell RL, Bartlett AV, Sarbaugh FC, Pickering LK: Effects of diaper types on diaper dermatitis associated with diarrhea and antibiotic use in children in day-care centers. Pediatr Dermatol 5:83–87, 1988.

*Selected readings.

51. Seymour JL, Keswick BH, Milligan MC, et al: Clinical and microbial effects of cloth, cellulose core, and cellulose core/absorbent gel diapers in atopic dermatitis. Pediatrician 149(14 Suppl)1:39–43, 1987.

52. Ward DB, Fleischer AB Jr, Feldman SR, Krowchuk DP: Characterization of diaper dermatitis in the United States. Arch Pediatr Adolesc Med 154:943–946, 2000.

53. Visscher MO, Chatterjee R, Munson KA, et al: Development of diaper rash in the newborn. Pediatr Dermatol 17:52–57, 2000.

54. Hogan P: Irritant napkin dermatitis. Aust Fam Physician 28:385–386, 1999.

55. Berg RW: Etiology and pathophysiology of diaper dermatitis. Adv Dermatol 3:75–98, 1988.

*56. Kazaks EL, Lane AT: Diaper dermatitis. Pediatr Clin North am 47:909–919, 2000.

57. Hoppe J: Treatment of oropharyngeal candidiasis and candidal diaper dermatitis in neonates and infants: review and reappraisal. Pediatr Infect Dis J 16:885–894, 1997.

58. Fergusson AG, Fraser NG, Grant PW: Napkin dermatitis with psoriasiform "ide": a review of fifty-two cases. Br J Dermatol 78: 289–296, 1966.

59. Boiko S: Treatment of diaper dermatitis. Dermatol Clin 17:235–240, 1999.

60. Leyden JJ: Diaper dermatitis. Dermatol Clin 4:23–28, 1986.

61. Odio M, Friedlander SF: Diaper dermatitis and advances in diaper technology. Dermatology 12:342–346, 2000.

62. Leyden JJ: Corn starch, Candida albicans, and diaper rash. Pediatr Dermatol 1:322–325, 1984.

63. Wolf R, Wolf D, Tüzün B, Tüzün Y: Diaper dermatitis. Clin Dermatol 18:657–660, 2001.

64. De Zeeuwa R, van Praag MC, Oranje AP: Granuloma gluteale infantum: a case report. Pediatr Dermatol 17:141–143, 2000.

65. McGinley KJ, Leyden JJ, Marples RR, Kligman AM: Quantitative microbiology of the scalp in non-dandruff, dandruff, and seborrheic dermatitis. J Invest Dermatol 64:401–405, 1975.

66. Meshkinpour A, Sun J, Weinstein G: An open pilot study using tacrolimus ointment in the treatment of seborrheic dermatitis. J Am Acad Dermatol 49:145–147, 2003.

67. Tollesson A, Frithz A, Stenlund K: Malssezia furfur in infantile seborrheic dermatitis. Pediatr Dermatol 14:423–425, 1997.

68. Perez Chavarria EL, Castanon LR, Tamayo L, et al: Pityrosporum ovale in seborrheic dermatitis in children and in other dermatoses in children. Med Cutan Ibero Lat Am 17:98–102, 1989.

69. Pierard-Franchimont C, Pierard GE, Arrese JE, De Donker P: Effect of ketoconazole 1% and 2% shampoos on severe dandruff and seborrheic dermatitis: clinical, squamometric and mycological assessments. Dermatology 202:171–176, 2001.

69a. Gupta AK, Madzia SE, Batra R: Etiology and management of seborrheic dermatitis. Dermatology 208:89–93, 2004.

70. Yates VM, Kerr RE, Frier K, et al: Early diagnosis of infantile seborrheic dermatitis and atopic dermatitis—total and specific IgE levels. Br J Dermatol 108:639–645, 1983.

71. Mozzanica N: Pathogenic aspects of allergic and irritant contact dermatitis. Clin Dermatol 10:115–121, 1992.

72. Brodell R, Patel S, Venglarick J, et al: The safety of ketoconazole shampoo for infantile seborrheic dermatitis. Pediatr Dermatol 15:406–407, 1988.

73. Baysal V, Yildirim M, Ozcanli C, Ceyhan AM: Itraconazole in the treatment of seborrheic dermatitis: a new treatment modality. Int J Dermatol 43:63–66, 2004.

74. Rigopoulos D, Ioannides D, Kalogeromitros D, et al: Pimecrolimus cream 1% vs. betamethasone 17-valerate 0.1% cream in the treatment of seborrheic dermatitis: a randomized open-labeled clinical trial. Br J Dermatol 151:1071–1075, 2004.

75. Gupta AK, Bluhm R: Ciclopirox shampoo for treating seborrheic dermatitis. Skin Ther Lett 9:4–5, 2004.

76. Dreno B, Moyse D: Lithium gluconate in the treatment of seborrheic dermatitis: a multicenter, randomized, double-blind study versus placebo. Eur J Dermatol 12:549–552, 2002.

77. Parsad D, Pandhi R, Negi KS, Kumar B: Topical metronidazole in seborrheic dermatitis—double-blind study. Dermatology 202:35–37, 2001.

*78. Bruckner A, Weston WL: Allergic contact dermatitis in children: a practical approach to management. Skin Ther Lett 7:3–5, 2002.

79. Mortz CG, Andersen KE: Allergic contact dermatitis in children and adolescents. Contact Dermatitis 41:121–130, 1999.

80. Gawkroger DJ, Lewis FM, Shah M: Contact sensitivity to nickel and other metals in jewelry. J Am Acad Dermatol 43:31–36, 2000.

81. Weston WL, Bruckner A: Allergic contact dermatitis. Pediatr Clin North Am 47:897–907, 2000.

Infestations

Antonio E. Muñiz, MD

Selected Diagnoses

Scabies
Tick bites
Lyme disease
Rocky Mountain spotted fever
Pediculoses (louse infestations)

Discussion of Individual Diagnoses

Scabies

Scabies is a highly contagious, papular, pustulovesicular and occasionally crusting, pruritic eruption of the skin caused by the release of toxic or antigenic secretions of the eight-legged human female arachnid mite *Sarcoptes scabiei* var *hominis*.[1] The organism is an obligate parasite, requiring an appropriate host for survival. The life cycle begins with the mating of adult male and female mites, after which the adult male dies. The female mite tunnels into the stratum corneum and deposits up to 90 eggs during its life span of 30 to 40 days. The eggs reach maturity in 10 to 14 days, and a new cycle begins. The average patient is infected with about 10 to 15 live adult female mites.[2]

A delayed type IV hypersensitivity reaction to the mites, their eggs, or scybala (fecal pellets) that occurs approximately 30 days after infestation is responsible for the intense pruritus, the hallmark of the disease. Transmission of scabies requires prolonged human contact, although female mites can survive 2 to 3 days off the human body and theoretically lead to infestation by contact with objects or clothing containing the mites.[2]

Clinical Presentation

The earliest symptom is itching, especially at night. Primary lesions include burrows, papules, vesicles, and pustules (Fig. 125–1). Secondary lesions occur from scratching and include excoriated papules with honey-colored exudates and crusts (Figs. 125–2 and 125–3). Lesions are commonly located on the abdomen, dorsa of hands, flexural surfaces of the wrists and elbows, periaxillary skin, areolae, genitalia, ankles, feet, and interdigital web spaces of the hands.[2a] In infants, eczematous eruptions of the face and trunk are seen. In older children, adolescents, and adults, the head and neck regions are almost never involved. A few patients develop a nodular form of scabies, exhibiting firm, erythematous, pruritic, dome-shaped lesions 5 to 6 mm in diameter. The genitalia, groin, buttocks, and axillary folds are the usual sites of involvement. Some patients present with urticaria as the initial manifestations of scabies.[3]

S-shaped burrows are diagnostic, but not commonly seen in children[4] (Fig. 125–4). Occasionally the burrows are straight or curved, and they are usually 2 to 5 mm in length. A burrow is caused by the female mite when it tunnels into the skin, and appears as a white or gray threadlike, linear, wavy papule with a small vesicle at one end. It is most often found in the interdigital web spaces of the hand, flexural surfaces of the wrists and elbows, areolae in women, penis, scrotum, and belt line area.[5]

The term *scabies crustosa* (formerly known as Norwegian or crusted scabies) is used to describe heavy infections with severe cutaneous crusting and hundreds to thousands of adult mites on a patient's body.[6] Patients with this form of scabies are usually immunocompromised, debilitated, or developmentally disabled, but it has also been encountered among indigenous Australians with no known immune deficiency.[7] It begins with poorly defined erythematous patches that quickly develop a prominent scale. Any area may be affected, but the scalp, hands, and feet are particularly susceptible. Untreated, it spreads rapidly and may eventually involve the entire integument. Scales become warty and crusts appear.

Scabies may be confused with other pruritic conditions (Table 125–1).

The most common complication is secondary bacterial infection with *Staphylococcus aureus*, which is clinically suspected when there is pustule formation, bullous impetigo,

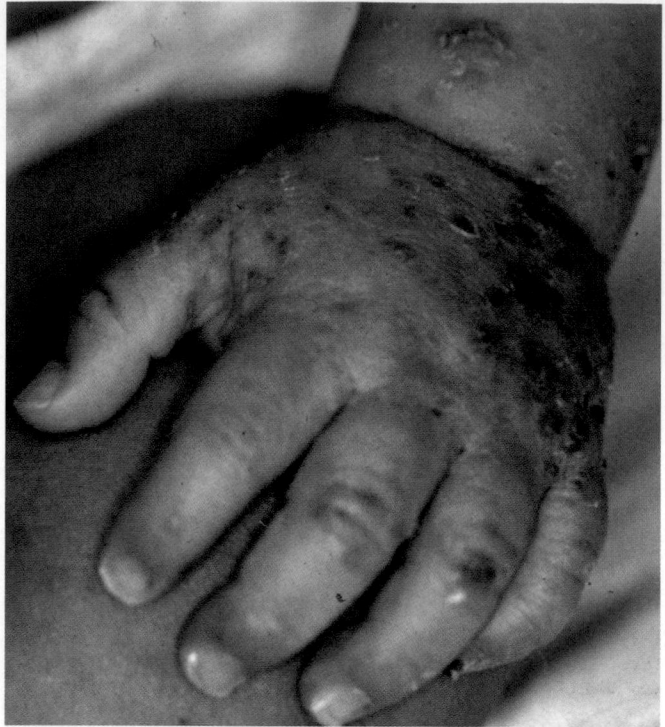

FIGURE 125–1. Excoriations, pustules, and vesicles on the hand from scabies.

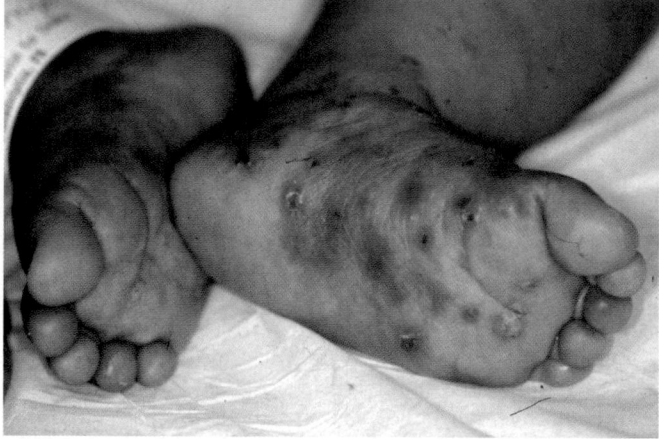

FIGURE 125–2. Excoriations, pustules, and vesicles on the feet from scabies.

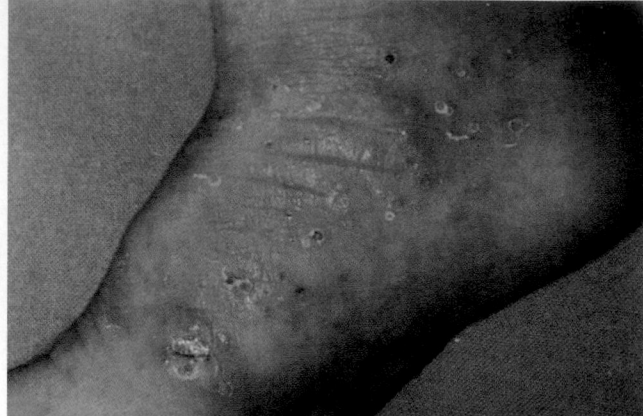

FIGURE 125–3. Scales and excoriations from scabies.

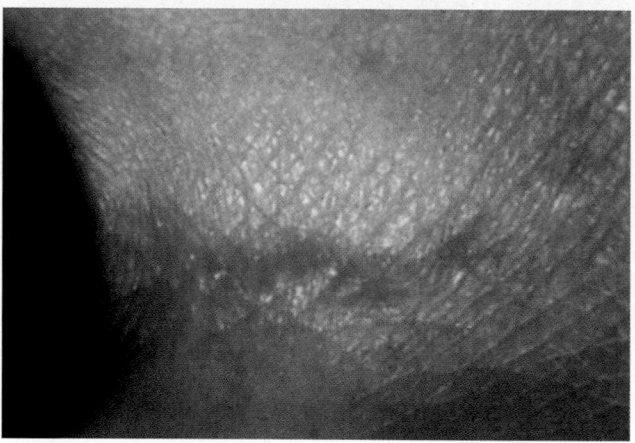

FIGURE 125–4. Burrows from scabies.

Table 125–1	Differential Diagnosis of Scabies
Atopic dermatitis	
Irritant or contact dermatitis	
Lichen planus	
Dermatitis herpetiformis	
Seborrheic dermatitis	
Urticaria	
Gianotti-Crosti syndrome	
Insect bites	
Papular urticaria	
Acropustulosis of infancy	
Dyshidrotic eczema	
Impetigo	
Letterer-Siwe disease (histiocytosis X)	

severe crusting, cellulitis, ecthyma, paronychia, or furunculosis.[8] Another organism causing secondary skin infection is *Streptococcus pyogenes.* Poststreptococcal glomerulonephritis may follow if nephritogenic strains of streptococci are involved.[9] Other complications may include lymphangitis, suppurative lymphadenitis, staphylococcal scalded skin syndrome, scarlet fever, rheumatic fever, osteomyelitis, septic arthritis, pneumonia, and sepsis.

The diagnosis of scabies is confirmed by scraping an unscratched burrow that is covered with a drop of microscopic immersion oil and placing the scrapings on a glass slide with a cover slip. Placing a drop of oil on the lesion prior to scraping with a number 15 scalpel blade improves the chance of obtaining a good specimen. Using the 10× magnification objective of the microscope, the female mite and/or its eggs or excreta (scybala) should be visible. Failure to find the mite does not rule out scabies, since it is difficult to obtain adequate scrapings from an uncooperative, crying and moving child or infant. Videodermatoscopy has been demonstrated to be an effective and sensitive diagnostic tool, allowing for noninvasive in vivo visualization of the skin at magnifications of up to 600 times to detect signs of infestations.[10]

Management

Treatment of scabies involves the control of symptoms, prevention of secondary infection, and eradication of the mites. Antihistamines, oatmeal baths, and calamine lotion may be used to help alleviate pruritus. Persistent itching after appropriate therapy may respond to topical corticosteroids. Secondary bacterial infections are treated with antistaphylococcal antibiotics.

Application of a scabicide (Table 125–2), such as 5% permethrin (Elimite) cream, is considered the treatment of choice.[1,4] It is recommended for infants older than 2 months of age but has been reported to be safe in neonates.[11] It can be used in pregnant patients and those who are breast-feeding. In children, the scabicide is applied to the entire body, including the scalp and face, and washed off in 8 to 14 hours. The treatment is repeated in 1 week to ensure complete eradication. In adults, the scabicide is applied to areas below the head, since scabies rarely involves the face; a 30-g tube is usually sufficient for an average adult. Permethrin produces a 98% cure rate.[1,11,12]

In the past, 1% gamma benzene hexachloride (lindane; Kwell) lotion has been used. Although equally effective in eradicating scabies, prolonged absorption or repetitive use of gamma benzene hexachloride, especially in infants less than 6 months of age, concentrates the compound in the central nervous system and may cause seizures and rarely death.[13,14] Other adverse effects include headache, nausea, vomiting, dizziness, restlessness, tremors, disorientation, weakness, twitching of eyelids, and respiratory failure.[15,16]

In addition to the patient, all family members and close contacts should be treated with a scabicide.[1,4] Normal laundering or dry cleaning of clothing is sufficient to prevent the potential reinfection with the mite. Potential fomites that cannot be laundered or dry cleaned should be sealed in plastic bags for 1 week, since the adult mite cannot survive more than 3 to 4 days when separated from humans.

For crusted scabies, crust and scale removal is necessary for scabicide penetration. Permethrin is the topical medication of choice, but when used by itself, topical treatment requires weeks of repeated application, and the failure rate is high. Oral ivermectin is rapidly becoming the treatment of choice for scabies crustosa[17] (see Table 125–2).

Follow-up within 2 weeks should be arranged to ascertain success of therapy. Many patients experience persistent symptoms for up to 2 weeks after curative treatment. This is likely due to the ongoing immune response to mite antigens. However, if symptoms persist beyond this period, one must consider other possibilities, such as an incorrect diagnosis, incorrect application of the topical scabicide, poor penetration of the agent into scaly skin, reinfection from untreated contacts or contaminated fomites, contact dermatitis from the topical agent, or drug-resistant infection.

Tick Bites

Tick bites are usually painless and inconspicuous in children and not noted until several hours to days later when pruritus becomes prominent. Tick bites are acquired when children play in woods or when ticks are transferred from animals to children. The tick attaches itself to the skin by its head in an effort to suck blood. The tick cuts the skin surface with chelicerae, introduces its proboscis, and secretes saliva into the wound. The saliva contains a cement substance, anesthetic, anti-inflammatory agent, and anticoagulant, and may also include a neurotoxin responsible for tick paralysis or other infections, such as agents for relapsing fever, rickettsial infections (Rocky Mountain spotted fever, typhus, trench fever, Q fever, ehrlichiosis, boutonneuse fever), Lyme disease, Colorado tick fever, babesiosis, and tularemia.

After a tick bite, a localized urticarial reaction occurs. The most common sites for tick attachment are the occiput, ear canal, axilla, groin, and vulva.[18,19] On rare occasions a systemic reaction consisting of fever, nausea, abdominal pain, and headache may occur. A persistent pruritic nodule with surrounding alopecia may be the result of an incompletely removed tick in which mouth parts remain in the skin.

Lyme Disease

Ticks may carry the spirochete *Borrelia burgdorferi,* which is responsible for Lyme disease (see Chapter 71, Selected Infectious Diseases). The predominant tick in the northeastern and midwestern United States is the deer tick, *Ixodes dammini* (or *Ixodes scapularis*). In the northwestern United States, *Ixodes pacificus* is the vector, and *Amblyomma americanum* (Lone Star tick) is the vector in the southern United States.[20]

Table 125–2	Medications for the Treatment of Scabies[64-66]	
Agent	**Application**	**Cautions**
Permethrin 5% (Elimite) cream	Apply and wash off in 8–14 hr; repeat in 1 wk	>2 mo old (reported safe in neonates), safe in pregnancy and breast-feeding
1% gamma benzene hexachloride (lindane; Kwell) lotion	Apply and wash off in 8–12 hr; repeat in 1 wk	Repeated use may cause seizures and death (<6 mo old); avoid if seizure disorder, pregnant, breast-feeding, or with extensive dermatitis
Precipitated sulfur (3–10%) in petrolatum ointment	Apply for 3 consecutive days; can be washed off after every 24 hr	Safe in pregnancy, breast-feeding and infants <2 mo of age; bad odor and messy; in hot or humid climate may lead to irritant dermatitis; less effective than permethrin
Crotamiton 10% (Eurax) cream or lotion	Apply and repeat in 24 hr, then washed off in 48 hr. Better results occur if applied for 5 days	Safe in pregnancy and infants; irritating in patients with eczema or with weeping wounds and associated with increased treatment failures
Benzyl benzoate (12.5–25%)	Apply three times in a 24-hr period, then wash off	Can cause irritant dermatitis
Ivermectin (Mectizan, Stromectol)	150–200 mcg/kg/day PO as a single dose; repeat 2 wk later	>5 yr old; not FDA approved; consider for treatment failures or immunosuppressed patients; deaths reported in elderly

Abbreviations: FDA, Food and Drug Administration; PO, orally.

Bacteria are introduced into the skin by a bite from an infected tick. It generally takes more that 24 hours of tick attachment for the transmission to occur.[21] Once in the skin, the spirochete can be overwhelmed and eliminated by host defense mechanisms, can remain viable but localized at the site of inoculation, or can disseminate via blood and lymphatics. Hematogenous spread can occur within days or weeks of the initial infection. The organism may travel to other parts of the skin, heart, joints, and central nervous system.

Three stages are usually described: stage I (early localized infection; onset days to weeks after infection), stage II (early disseminated infection; onset days to months), and stage III (late or persistent infection; onset months to many years). Early disseminated Lyme disease produces various neurologic syndromes, cardiac disease, multiple skin lesions, and sometimes early synovitis. Later manifestations are primarily neurologic and rheumatologic. Most tick bites occur from April through September. The highest attack rate occurs in children between 5 and 10 years of age.[22] The incubation period is 7 to 14 days. Only about one third of patients distinctly recall a tick bite.[18,23]

The pathognomonic skin manifestation of Lyme disease is erythema migrans (EM), formerly called erythema chronicum migrans. It begins as a red papule at the site of the bite, and then slowly enlarges over several weeks to form an annular ring with a flat red border, with less than 40% showing central clearing (Fig. 125–5).[23a] The most common lesion in the United States is round morphology with a homogeneous or central erythema.[24] Its size ranges from 5 cm up to 70 cm.[25,26] It is commonly found in the axilla, inguinal region, popliteal fossa or belt line. EM is usually asymptomatic, although it may itch or burn. Fifty percent will develop multiple secondary annular rings, which begin 1 to 6 days after the primary ring.[18] EM may spontaneously regress within weeks or months but may persist and spread. Patches remaining for 4 weeks or longer are referred to as erythema chronicum migrans. Two other less common skin findings, mostly seen in Europe, are borrelia lymphocytoma and acro-

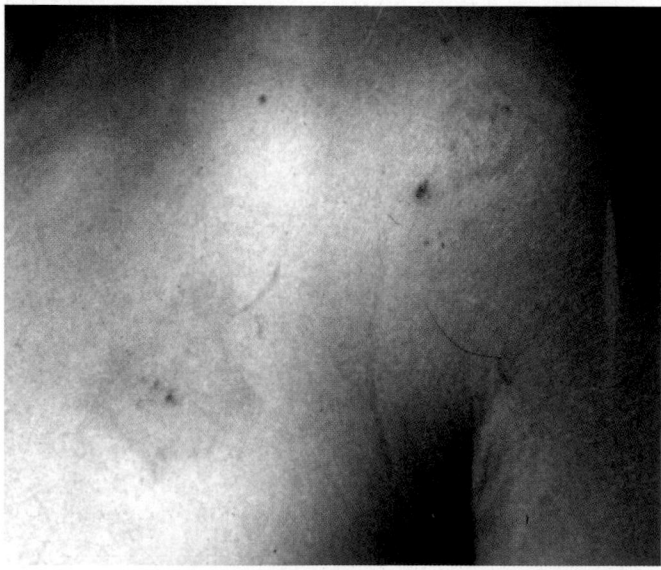

FIGURE 125–5. Acute erythema migrans.

dermatitis chronica atrophicans (ACA). Lymphocytoma consists of a bluish red papule, plaque, or nodule, most often located at the earlobe or nipples.[27] ACA is seen years after EM and is characterized by a bluish red discoloration, often with a doughy infiltration that progresses to atrophy of the skin, and is sometimes complicated by sclerodermic changes. It is usually found on the dorsal portion of the hand, elbow, foot, or knee.[28]

Other associated findings may include headaches, fatigue, malaise, myalgias, stiff neck, athralgias, low-grade fever, nausea, vomiting, sore throat, and lymphadenopathy.[18,29] Untreated, EM lasts about 3 to 4 weeks but may recur with arthritis, and in some cases neurologic or cardiologic complications occur.[27] Lyme arthritis is often monoarticular or oligoarticular, most commonly involving the knee joint. Neurologic manifestations occur in less than 10% of cases and consist of lymphocytic meningitis, encephalopathy, cerebritis, transverse myelitis, mononeuritis multiplex, and cranial nerve palsies, especially of cranial nerve VII.[22,30] Tertiary neuroborreliosis occurs in late disease and consist of encephalopathy, neurocognitive dysfunction, and peripheral neuropathy. Cardiac manifestations are less common, occurring in less than 10% of cases, and include electrocardiographic signs of myocarditis, such as atrioventricular block, left ventricular dysfunction, pericarditis, or fatal pancarditis.[31]

The expanding annular rings of EM may be confused with tinea corporis, urticaria, nummular eczema, erythema multiforme, erythema marginatum, erythema annulare centrifugum, granuloma annulare, fixed drug reaction, cellulitis, and insect or spider bites. The diagnosis of EM is purely clinical. Disseminated or late Lyme disease can be diagnosed by polymerase chain reaction detection of *B. burgdorferi* DNA, enzyme-linked immunosorbent assay, immunofluorescence antibody, and Western immunoblot assay.

Rocky Mountain Spotted Fever

Rocky Mountain spotted fever (RMSF) is caused by the obligate intracellular bacteria *Rickettsia rickettsii*. The clinical spectrum of human infection ranges from mild to fulminant disease. It is primarily a disease of the southeastern and south central United States, but has been reported in every state except Vermont. It also occurs in Canada, Mexico, Central America, and parts of South America. The ticks that serve as vectors and reservoirs include *Dermacentor variabilis* (American dog tick) in the eastern and south central United States, *Dermacentor andersoni* (wood tick) in the mountain states west of the Mississippi river, and *Amblyomma americanum* (Lone Star tick) in the southern United States.[32] It is transmitted by a bite from an infected tick or contamination of the skin when the arthropod is being crushed. It generally takes more than 6 hours of tick attachment for transmission. Occasionally the disease is transmitted by blood transfusions.

Following inoculation, *R. rickettsii* multiplies in the endothelial cells of small blood vessels and disseminates widely via the bloodstream. It attaches to and invades the vascular endothelial and smooth muscles cells of many organs, including the brain, liver, skin, lungs, kidneys, and gastrointestinal tract. The essential pathologic lesion is an anti-inflammatory reaction of the endothelium and smooth muscle of the arterioles and endothelia of capillaries. This leads to swelling, necrosis, thrombosis, and finally occlusion of the vascular lumen.

CLINICAL PRESENTATION

A history of a tick bite can be elicited in 50% to 80% of cases. The longer the infected tick feeds, the greater the chance of infection. The incubation period ranges from 2 to 12 days, with most cases occurring between 5 and 7 days after exposure. The symptoms of the prodrome phase include headache, malaise, anorexia, photophobia, conjunctival hyperemia, chills, low-grade fever, arthralgias, myalgias, nausea, vomiting, and abdominal pain. The presence of headache, fever, and myalgias should always alert one to the possibility of RMSF. Gastrointestinal involvement may be severe and lead to erroneous diagnoses such as cholecystitis, appendicitis, and even bowel obstruction.[33]

The classic triad includes fever, headache, and rash. The rash is seen in 90% of cases and occurs 1 to 4 days after onset of symptoms. It starts in the ankles and feet, and spreads within hours to the wrists and hands and then centripetally toward the head and trunk.[34] At first the rash is small, discrete, macular, and rose colored, with blanching on pressure. It soon becomes papular and assumes a darker hue. In 2 to 3 days, it develops a petechial or purpuric character[35] (Fig. 125–6). The rash may desquamate and leave hyperpigmented areas. Generalized nonpitting edema is present, especially in children.[36] Lymphadenopathy, hepatosplenomegaly, and nuchal rigidity may occur. The differential diagnosis is extensive (Table 125–3).

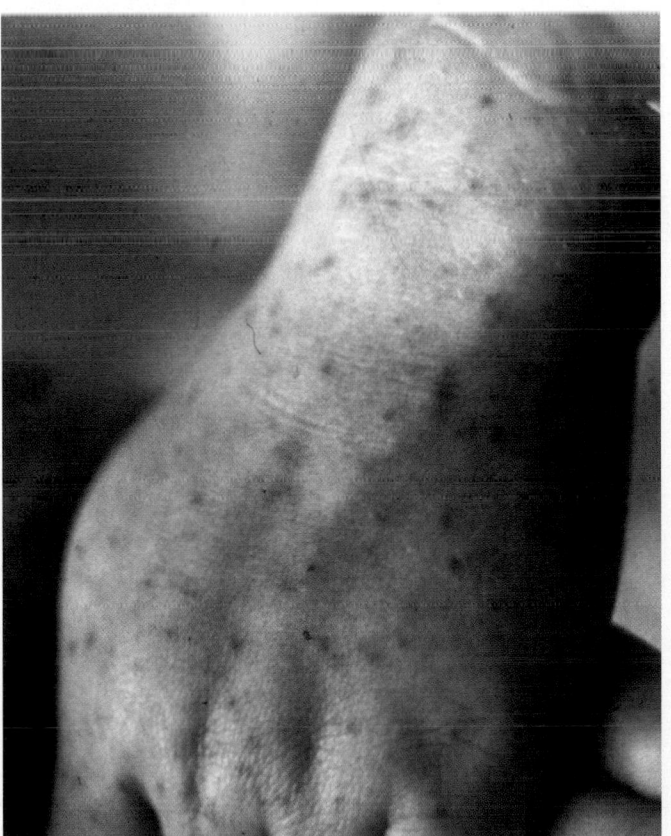

FIGURE 125–6. Petechial rash of Rocky Mountain spotted fever.

The diagnosis of RMSF is based largely on clinical presentation in a patient with history of tick exposure. There is no completely reliable diagnostic test in the early phases of illness when therapy should be initiated to prevent complications. Later, the diagnosis can be made by skin biopsy and confirmed serologically. Punch biopsy of the skin can be examined for Rickettsia using direct immunofluorescence or immunoenzyme methods. Serologic diagnosis includes a fourfold increase in acute and convalescent titers using indirect immunofluorescence antibody assay, enzyme immunoassay, complement fixation, latex agglutination, indirect hemagglutination, or microagglutination. Laboratory tests are nonspecific but might show anemia, an elevated or depressed white blood cell count, thrombocytopenia, coagulation abnormalities, elevated hepatic transaminases, an elevated blood urea nitrogen, and a lymphocytic cerebrospinal fluid pleocytosis.

Complications of RMSF include thrombocytopenia, disseminated intravascular coagulation, gangrene, acute disseminated encephalomyelitis, meningoencephalitis, seizures, coma, acute renal failure, aseptic monarticular arthritis, ataxia, hyperreflexia, paraparesis, hearing loss, peripheral neuropathy, pneumonia, respiratory failure, myocarditis, and bowel and bladder incontinence.[37,38]

MANAGEMENT

Removal of the tick is the treatment of choice. The preferred method of removal is with a blunt instrument, such as a forceps or tweezers, between the tick head and the child's skin. Gentle outward traction will cause the tick to be pulled out. This will prevent retention of tick parts within the skin. All methods that will injure the skin, such as burning the tick or using noxious substances on the skin, are not recommended. The body of the tick should not be squeezed; if there is a remnant of the tick in the skin, a simple surgical excision may be performed with local anesthetic.[39]

Routine administration of oral antibiotics after tick removal is not recommended for prophylaxis against Lyme disease since the infection rate is low.[40] However, one study showed that a single dose of doxycycline given within 72 hours after a tick bite can prevent the development of Lyme

Table 125–3	Differential Diagnosis of Rocky Mountain Spotted Fever

Meningococcemia
Coxsackievirus
Drug reactions
Echovirus
Cytomegalovirus
Epstein-Barr virus
Viral hemorrhagic fever
Disseminated gonococcal infections
Staphylococcus aureus septicemia
Idiopathic thrombocytopenic purpura
Thrombotic thrombocytopenic purpura
Viral hepatitis
Viral meningitis
Ehrlichiosis
Leptospirosis
Typhoid fever
Atypical measles
Secondary syphilis

disease.[41] If the child develops EM, then appropriate antibiotics, such as amoxicillin, azithromycin, doxycycline, or cefuroxime axetil for 10 days, should be given.[42,43] If the child develops fever, frontal headache, myalgias, and petechiae, then RMSF should be considered and doxycycline should be given. Early therapy of RMSF is important because delay beyond the fifth day of illness is associated with an increased risk of a fatal outcome.[44,45] The dose of doxycycline in children less than 45 kg is 0.9 mg/kg divided in two doses (maximum 200 mg/day), and in children greater than 45 kg, 2 mg/kg orally (PO) as a loading dose followed by 1 mg/kg PO every 12 hours. It should be given for 7 days or until 2 days after the patient becomes afebrile. Doxycycline does not stain the teeth when given for a short period of time. In pregnant patients with RMSF, chloramphenicol is the preferred drug, but it is associated with toxic effects on the baby (gray baby syndrome) when given close to delivery.[46]

Prevention is the best method for avoiding tick bites. Children should avoid tick habitats, such as dense brush or tall grass, and stay in the center of the path on wooded trails. They should wear protective clothing, such as long-sleeved tops, long pants, and caps, preferably of light color so ticks are easily seen, and should tuck pants into boots or socks. In endemic areas, regular and careful use of insect repellants during tick season is recommended. Caution should be exercised not to use DEET (*N,N*-diethyl-*m*-toluamide) on large areas of skin or in concentrations greater than 10% because of neurotoxicity.[47] Pretreatment of clothing with permethrin spray is also useful. Children and pets should be routinely inspected for ticks if they have been in wooded areas.

A follow-up visit in 2 weeks after a tick bite to observe for signs of EM should be considered in areas endemic for Lyme disease. Admission is indicated in all patients with RMSF with clinical evidence of toxicity, encephalitis, seizures, hypotension, thrombocytopenia, prolonged clotting factors, hyponatremia, or marked gastrointestinal symptoms. Patients who survive the initial episode generally go on to complete recovery and cure, although a small percentage of patients with severe RMSF develop long-term sequelae such as peripheral neuropathy, hemiparesis, or deafness.[48]

Pediculosis (Louse Infestations)

Pediculosis is an infestation of humans by lice. The human louse, an ectoparasite, is a six-legged insect. It attaches itself to the skin, ingests blood, and produces skin lesions by mechanical puncture and by injecting toxic substances.[49] The clinical signs and symptoms arise from host reaction to louse saliva injected at the time of feeding. The hallmark of all types of pediculosis is pruritus. There are two species of human lice, *Pediculus humanus* (body louse), which has subspecies *capitis* (head lice) and *corporis* (body lice), and *Pthirus pubis* (crab louse). The body louse is 2 to 4 mm in length, while the pubic louse is 1 to 2 mm in length. The female attaches to the hair and slides along it, laying eggs or nits that are white and less than 1 mm long. Nits are firmly attached to one side of the hair.[50] If hair is not available to the lice, clothing fibers are used.

The female produces new offspring every 2 weeks and up to 80 offspring during her life span. Newly hatched lice mate with older lice, and hundreds of nits result every 2 weeks. Transmission is by person-to-person contact or by fomites, such as hairbrushes, caps, clothing, or carpets.[51] Lice die

Table 125–4	Differential Diagnosis of Human Louse Infestations

Scabies
Atopic dermatitis
Allergic contact dermatitis
Irritant contact dermatitis
Drug reaction
Dermatitis herpetiformis
Neurotic excoriations
Folliculitis
Impetigo

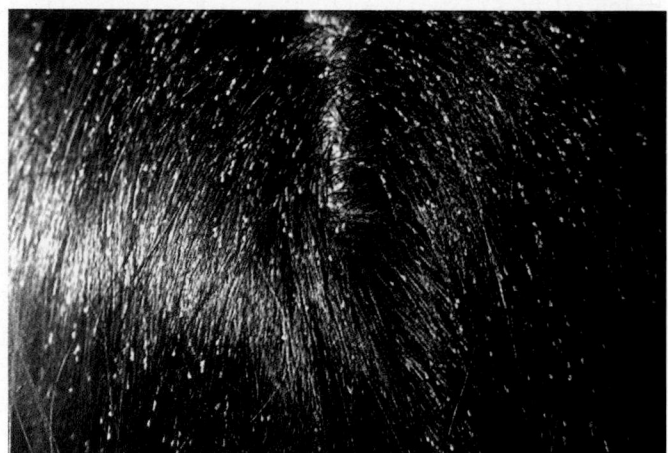

FIGURE 125–7. Head lice.

within 10 days of removal from their human host. Head lice are uncommon in African Americans because they have oval-shaped hair shafts that are harder for lice to grasp.[52]

The differential diagnosis of human louse infections is limited (Table 125–4).

Clinical Presentation

PEDICULOSIS CORPORIS

Pediculosis corporis is infestations of humans and their clothing by *P. humanus* (body louse). Body lice spend most of their lives in clothing and only go back to the body to feed. The lice lay their eggs on fibers in the fabric seams. The louse can carry *Bartonella,* can cause fever and endocarditis, and is a vector for relapsing fever, trench fever, and epidemic typhus.[53,54] The bites of body lice are relatively painless. Skin lesions include excoriated papules and pustules on the trunk and perineum. With chronic infestations, the skin may be thickened and hyperpigmented.[55] On occasion, the louse may be discovered by closely examining the seams of the patient's clothing.

PEDICULOSIS CAPITIS

Pediculosis capitis is an infestation of the scalp by *P. capitis.* The gelatinous nits of the head louse appear as white, ovoid bodies tightly adherent to the hair shafts (Fig. 125–7). The nits move away from the scalp as the hair grows. The nits fluoresce a pale blue color under a Wood's lamp and are usually located in the occipital and retroauricular areas. Patients present with nocturnal pruritus, excoriations, conjunctivitis, and posterior neck lymphadenopathy.[49,56] A hypersensitivity rash may mimic a viral exanthem.

PEDICULOSIS PUBIS

Pediculosis pubis is an infestation of the pubic hair with *P. pubis.* It is commonly spread as a sexually transmitted disease, and up to 30% of patients have another concomitant sexually transmitted infection.[57] The pubic (crab) louse may be seen crawling among pubic hair. It may also attach to eyelashes (pediculosis palpebrarum) and beard, mustache, and axillary hairs.[58] The lice lay their eggs at the base of hair fibers. Patients typically present with pruritus of the pubic region. On occasion there is a blue-black crusted macule (macula cerulea) in the pubic area, thighs, trunks, or upper arms.[50] Nits may be seen attached to pubic hair.

Management

Permethrin is the drug of choice for treatment of head lice,[59] although other agents are available (Table 125–5). After the hair has been washed with shampoo, rinsed with water, and towel dried, the scalp should be saturated with the pediculicide. Permethrin remains on the hair for 10 minutes before rinsing off with water. All agents can be repeated in 1 week to kill any newly hatched nymphs. Cutting of the child's hair should be avoided. Resistance of head lice to these agents has been reported, and ivermectin has been used with success in these cases.[60,61] Antihistamines are used to control itching.

Shampoo treatments will not remove the gelatinous nits. The use of warm, damp towels or towels saturated in white vinegar (dissolves chitin, which binds nits to hair shafts) for 30 minutes on the scalp will loosen nits and allow their mechanical removal with a fine toothed comb. Petroleum jelly massaged on the entire surface of the hair and scalp and left overnight with a shower cap has been shown to be effective by obstructing the respiratory spiracles of the louse, causing the lice to die of suffocation and desiccation.[62] Fine-toothed combs and brushes can be treated by soaking at least 5 minutes in hot water (>131° F or 55° C). Potential fomites such as towels, pillow cases, hats, and children's stuffed animals may benefit from washing in hot water. Because adult lice cannot survive more than 6 to 10 days when separated from humans, sealing potential fomites in plastic bags for 12 to 14 days is effective when they cannot be laundered or dry cleaned.

For treatment of body lice, the most important therapy is disinfection of all contaminated clothing and linens.[62a] The clothing may be dry cleaned, steam fumigated, or washed in hot water and dried on high heat. Furniture in the house should be sprayed with agents specifically approved for disinfecting lice, such as permethrin spray. The patient should be treated from head to toe with a pediculicide. Permethrin 5% topical cream is the safest agent and should be applied for 8 to 14 hours and repeated in 1 week to ensure appropriate cure.

Treatment of pubic lice with permethrin or pyrethrin applied for 10 minutes and repeated in 1 week is sufficient. Sexual contacts should be treated, and laboratory tests for other sexually transmitted infections should be performed.

The safest and most effective treatment for *P. pubis* of the eyelashes is petrolatum (Vaseline). The ointment is applied three to five times daily. Physostigmine 0.25% (Eserine) has been used successfully, but has the major drawback of miosis from an anticholinergic effect. For severe resistant cases, ivermectin has been successful.[62,63]

Human louse infection causes an annoying pruritic sensation. When treated with appropriate agents, the infection can easily be controlled.

Table 125 5 Treatment of Head Lice[67-72]

Agents	Instructions for Use	Precautions
Permethrin (Elimite 5%, Nix 1%) cream	Apply to hair for 10 min and wash; repeat in 1 wk	Approved for > 2 mo old
Piperonyl butoxide 4%/pyrethrins 0.33% (RID Mousse, RID shampoo, A-200 shampoo, R & C, Pronto, Clear lice system, End Lice)	Apply to hair for 10 min and wash; repeat in 1 wk	Approved for > 2 yr old; 80% cure rate
1% gamma benzene hexachloride shampoo and cream (lindane; Kwell, G-well)	Apply for no more than 4 min and wash; repeat in 1 wk	Not recommended due to neurotoxic adverse effects, such as seizures if used repeatedly; avoid if seizure disorder, pregnant, or breast-feeding
Malathion 0.5% (Ovide) lotion	Apply and leave for 8–12 hr, then wash; repeat in 1 wk	Approved for > 6 yr old; high alcohol content makes it flammable, may cause respiratory depression if ingested
Crotamiton 10% (Eurax) cream and lotion	Apply and leave for 24 hr, then wash	Not FDA approved and safety in children unknown
Ivermectin (Mectizan, Stromectal)	200 mcg/kg PO; repeat in 1 wk	Not FDA approved; use in resistant cases and if > 15 kg
Sulfamethoxazole/trimethoprim (co-trimoxazole)	8–10 mg/kg/day of trimethoprim q12h PO for 3 days; repeat in 1 wk	Not FDA approved; increased effectiveness if given with permethrin
Precipitated sulfur (3–10%) in petrolatum	Apply daily for several days	Safe in pregnancy, breast-feeding, and infants < 2 mo of age; bad odor and messy; in hot or humid climate may lead to irritant dermatitis; less effective than permethrin

Abbreviations: FDA, Food and Drug Administration; PO, orally.

REFERENCES

1. Meinking TL, Elgart GW: Scabies therapy for the millennium. Pediatr Dermatol 17:154–156, 2000.
2. Wendel K, Rompalo A: Scabies and pediculosis pubis: an update of treatment regimens and general review. Clin Infect Dis 35(Suppl 2): S146–S151, 2002.
2a. Huynh TH, Norman RA: Scabies and pediculosis. Dermatol Clin 22:7–11, 2004.
3. Witkowski JA, Parish LC: Scabies: a cause of generalized urticaria. Cutis 33:277–279, 1984.
4. Angel TA, Nigro J, Levy ML: Infestations in the pediatric patient. Pediatr Clin North Am 47:921–935, 2000.
5. Rasmmussen JE: Scabies. Pediatr Rev 15:100–114, 1994.
6. DelGiudice P, Carles M, Couppie P, et al: Successful treatment of crusted (Norwegian) scabies with ivermectin in two patients with human immunodeficiency virus infection. Br J Dermatol 135:494–495, 1996.
7. Gogna NK, Lee KC, Howe DW: Norwegian scabies in Australian Aborigines. Med J Aust 142:140–142, 1985.
8. Currie BJ, Carapetis JR: Skin infections and infestations in Aboriginal communities in northern Australia. Australas J Dermatol 41:139–143, 2000.
9. Svartman M, Finklea JF, Earle DP, Potter EV: Epidemic scabies and acute glomerulonephritis in Trinidad. Lancet 1:249–251, 1972.
10. Lacarruba F, Musumeci ML, Catabiano R, et al: High-magnification videodermatoscopy: a new noninvasive diagnostic tool for scabies in children. Pediatr Dermatol 18:439–441, 2001.
11. Quarterman MJ, Lasher JL Jr: Neonatal scabies treated with 5% permethrin cream. Pediatr Dermatol 11:264–266, 1994.
12. Usha V, Gopalakrishnan Nair TV: A comparative study of oral ivermectin and topical permethrin cream in the treatment of scabies. J Am Acad Dermatol 42:236–240, 2000.
13. Lee B, Groth P: Scabies transcutaneous poisoning during treatment. Pediatrics 59:643, 1977.
14. Diaz JE: Lindane toxicity is preventable. Acad Emerg Med 5:1126–1128, 1998.
15. Solomon LM, Fahrener L, West DP: Gamma benzene hexachloride toxicity: a review. Arch Dermatol 113:353–357, 1977.
16. Ramussen JE: The problem of lindane. J Am Acad Dermatol 5:507–516, 1981.
17. Taplin D, Meinking TL: Treatment of HIV-related scabies with emphasis on the efficacy of ivermectin. Semin Cutan Med Surg 16:235–240, 1997.
18. Gardner P: Long-term outcomes and management of patients with Lyme disease. JAMA 283:658–659, 2000.
19. Committee on Infectious Diseases, American Academy of Pediatrics: Prevention of Lyme disease. Pediatrics 105:142–147, 2000.
20. Spach DH, Liles WC, Campbell GL, et al: Tick-borne diseases in the United States. N Engl J Med 329:936–947, 1993.
21. Berger BW, Johnson RC, Kodner C, Coleman L: Cultivation of *Borrelia burgdorferi* from human tick bite site as guide to the risk of infection. J Am Acad Dermatol 32:184–187, 1995.
22. Edlow JA: Lyme disease and related tick-borne illnesses. Ann Emerg Med 33:680–693, 1999.
23. Orloski KA, Hayes EB, Campbell GL, Dennis DT: Surveillance for Lyme disease—United States, 1992–1998. Mor Mortal Wkly Rep CDC Surveill Summ 49:1–11, 2000.
23a. McGinley-Smith DE, Tsao SS: Dermatoses from ticks. J Am Acad Dermatol 49:363–392, 2003.
24. Smith RP, Schoen RT, Rahn DW, et al: Clinical characteristics and treatment of early Lyme disease in patients with microbiologically confirmed erythema migrans. Ann Intern Med 136:421–428, 2002.
*25. Edlow JA: Erythema migrans. Med Clin North Am 86:239–260, 2002.
26. Nadelman RB, Nowakowski J, Forseter G, et al: The clinical spectrum of early Lyme borreliosis in patients with culture-confirmed erythema migrans. Am J Med 100:502–508, 1996.
27. Pfister HW, Wilske B, Weber K: Lyme borreliosis: basic science and clinical aspects. Lancet 343:1013–1016, 1994.
28. Moreno C, Kutzner H, Palmedo G, et al: Intestinal granulomatous dermatitis with histiocytic pseudorosettes: a new histopathologic pattern in cutaneous borreliosis. Detection of *Borrelia burgdoferi* DNA sequences by a highly sensitive PCR-ELISA. J Am Acad Dermatol 48:376–384, 2003.
29. Steere AC, Dhar A, Hernandez J, et al: Systemic symptoms without erythema migans as the presenting picture of early Lyme disease. Am J Med 114:58–62, 2003.
30. Steere AC: Lyme disease. N Engl J Med 345:115–125, 2001.
31. Pinto DS: Cardiac manifestations of Lyme disease. Med Clin North Am 86:285–296, 2002.
32. Peters AH: Tick-borne typhus (Rocky Mountain spotted fever): epidemiology trends with particular reference to Virginia. JAMA 216:1003–1007, 1971.
33. Walker DH, Lesesne HR, Varma VA, Thacker WC: Rocky Mountain spotted fever mimicking acute cholecystitis. Arch Intern Med 145:2194–2196, 1985.
34. Myers SA, Sexton DJ: Dermatology manifestations of arthropod-borne diseases. Infect Dis Clin North Am 8:689–712, 1994.
35. Calhan EF, Adal KA, Tomecki KJ: Cutaneous (non-HIV) infections. Dermatol Clin 18:497–507, 2000.
36. Kelsey DS: Rocky Mountain spotted fever. Pediatr Clin North Am 26:367–376, 1979.
37. Kirkland KB, Marcom PK, Sexton DJ, et al: Rocky Mountain spotted fever complicated by gangrene: report of six cases and review. Clin Infect Dis 101:629–634, 1996.
38. Conlon PJ, Procop GW, Fowler V, et al: Predictors of prognosis and risk of acute renal failure in patients with Rocky Mountain spotted fever. Am J Med 101:621–626, 1996.
39. Needham GR: Evaluation of five popular methods for tick removal. Pediatrics 75:997–1002, 1985.
40. Warshafsky S, Nowakowski J, Naldelman RB, et al: Efficacy of antibiotic prophylaxis for prevention of Lyme disease. J Gen Intern Med 11:329–333, 1996.
41. Nadelman RB, Nowakowski J, Fish D, et al; Tick Bite Study Group: Prophylaxis with single-dose doxycycline for the prevention of Lyme disease after *Ixodes scapularis* tick bite. N Engl J Med 345:79–84, 2001.
42. Barsic B, Maretic T, Majerus L, Strugar J: Comparison of azithromycin and doxycycline in the treatment of erythema migrans. Infection 28:153–156, 2000.
43. Arnez M, Radsel-Medvescek A, Pleterski-Rigler D, et al: Comparison of cefuroxime axetil and phenoxymethyl penicillin in the treatment of children with solitary migrans. Wien Klin Wochenschr 111:916–922, 1999.
44. Kirkland KB, Wilkinson WE, Sexton DJ: Therapeutic delay and mortality in cases of Rocky Mountain spotted fever. Clin Infect Dis 20:1118–1121, 1995.
45. Centers for Disease Control and Prevention: Consequences of delayed diagnosis of Rocky Mountain spotted fever in children—West Virginia, Michigan, Tennessee, and Oklahoma, May–July 2000. MMWR Morb Mortal Wkly Rep 49:885–888, 2000.
46. Stallings SP: Rocky Mountain spotted fever and pregnancy: a case report and review of the literature. Obstet Gynecol Surv 56:37–42, 2001.
47. Fradin MG: Mosquitoes and mosquito repellants: a clinician's guide. Ann Intern Med 128:931–940, 1998.
48. Archibald LK, Sexton DJ: Long-term sequelae of Rocky Mountain spotted fever. Clin Infect Dis 20:1122–1125, 1995.
49. Chosidow O: Scabies and pediculosis. Lancet 355:819–826, 2000.
50. Burkhart CN, Burkhart CG, Pchalef I, Arbogast J: The adherent cylindrical nit structure and its chemical denaturation in vitro: an assessment with therapeutic implications for head lice. Arch Pediatr Adolesc Med 152:711–712, 1998.
51. Speare R, Buettner PG: Head lice in pupils of a primary school in Australia and implications for control. Int J Dermatol 38:285–290, 1999.
52. Frankowski BL, Weiner LB: Head lice. Pediatrics 110:638–643, 2002.
53. Spach DH, Kanter AS, Dougherty MJ, et al: *Bartonella (Rochalimaea) quintane* bacteremia in inner-city patients with chronic alcoholism. N Engl J Med 332:424–428, 1995.
54. Sunders KO, Haimanot AT: Epidemic of louse-borne relapsing fever in Ethiopia. Lancet 432:1213–1215, 1993.
55. Ko CJ, Elston DM: Pediculosis. J Am Acad Dermatol 50:1–12, 2004.
56. Elston DM: What's eating you? *Pediculus humanus* (head louse and body louse). Cutis 65:259–264, 1999.
57. Pierzchalski JL, Bretl DA, Matson SC: Phthirus pubis as a predictor from *Chlamydia* infections in adolscents. Sex Transm Dis 29:331–334, 2002.

*Selected readings.

58. Elgart ML: Pediculosis. Dermatol Clin 8:219–228, 1990.
59. Abramowicz M: Drugs for head lice. Med Lett Drugs Ther 39:3–7, 1997.
60. Burkhart CG, Burkhart CN, Burkhart KM: An assessment of topical and oral prescriptions and over-the-counter treatments for head lice. J Am Acad Dermatol 38:979–982, 1998.
61. Dawes M, Hicks NR, Fleminger M, et al: Evidence based case report: treatment for head lice. BMJ 318:385, 1999.
62. Schachner LA: Treatment resistant head lice: alternative therapeutic approaches. Pediatr Dermatol 14:409–410, 1997.
62a. Flinders DC, de Schweintz P: Pediculosis and scabies. Am Fam Physician 69:341–348, 2004.
63. Bukhart CN, Burkhart CG: Oral ivermectin therapy for phthiriasis palpebrum. Arch Ophthalmol 118:134–135, 2000.
64. Roos TC, Alam M, Roos S, et al: Pharmacotherapy of ectoparasitic infections. Drugs 61:1067–1088, 2001.
65. Meinking TL, Taplin D, Hermida JL, et al: The treatment of scabies with ivermectin. N Engl J Med 333:26–30, 1995.
66. Barkwell R, Shields S: Deaths associated with ivermectin treatment of scabies. Lancet 349:1144–1445, 1997.
67. Carson DS, Tribble PW, Weart CW: Pyrethrins combined with piperonyl butoxide (RID) vs. 1 per cent permethrin (Nix) in the treatment of head lice. Am J Dis Child 142:768–769, 1988.
68. Rassmussen JE: Pediculosis and the pediatrician. Pediatr Dermatol 2:74–79, 1984.
69. Tenenbein M: Seizures after lindane therapy. J Am Geriatr Soc 39:394–395, 1999.
70. Hipolito RB, Mallorca FG, Zuniga-Macaraig ZO, et al: Head lice infestation: single drug versus combination therapy with one percent permethrin and trimethoprim/sulfamethoxazole. Pediatrics 107:e30, 2001.
71. Glaziou P, Nguyen LN, Moulia-Pelat JP, et al: Efficacy of ivermectin for the treatment of head lice (pediculosis capitis). Trop Med Parasitol 45:253–254, 1994.
72. Burkhart CN, Burkhart CG: Another look at ivermectin in the treatment of cabbies and head lice [letter]. Int J Dermatol 38:235, 1999.

Chapter 126

Other Important Rashes

Antonio E. Muñiz, MD

Key Points

Scarlet fever is treated with penicillin to prevent local suppurative complications and the development of acute rheumatic fever.

Staphylococcal scalded skin syndrome and toxic shock syndrome require antistaphylococcal antibiotics, fluid and electrolyte replacement, and meticulous skin care.

Tinea capitis is the most common cause of hair loss in children and is usually treated with prolonged oral antifungal therapy.

Tinea corporis is the most common fungal skin infection in children and is usually treated with topical antifungal therapy.

Kawasaki disease is treated with aspirin and intravenous immune globulin to prevent formation of coronary artery aneurysms.

Selected Diagnoses

Scarlet fever (scarlatina, second disease)
Staphylococcal scalded skin syndrome
Staphylococcal toxic shock syndrome
Tinea capitis
Tinea corporis
Pityriasis versicolor
Molluscum contagiosum
Pityriasis rosea
Kawasaki disease (mucocutaneous lymph node syndrome)
Impetigo

Discussion of Individual Diagnoses

Scarlet Fever (Scarlatina, Second Disease)

Scarlet fever is a toxin-mediated disease characterized by fever, oral mucous membrane changes, and an exanthem. It occurs most often in children between 2 and 10 years of age.[1]

The disease is rare under 2 years of age presumably due to the presence of maternal antitoxin antibodies.

Most cases of scarlet fever are due to group A β-hemolytic streptococcal pyrogenic exotoxin–producing strains.[2] Occasionally cases are caused by strains of group C or G streptococci. Its highest incidence is in the late fall, winter, and early spring. Transmission occurs through person-to-person contact with infectious respiratory droplets. The incubation period prior to appearance of the rash is 2 to 5 days.

The most common infection that leads to scarlet fever is tonsillopharyngitis, but the rash develops in less than 10% of cases.[3] It can also occur after a streptococcal skin and soft tissue infection, or infection of surgical wounds (surgical scarlet fever) or the uterus (pubertal scarlet fever).

Clinical Presentation

The illness begins with nonspecific signs and symptoms: fever, headache, malaise, nausea, vomiting, abdominal pain, and myalgias. Exudative tonsillopharyngitis is characterized by an erythematous oral mucosa, petechiae, and punctate erythematous macules on the palate and uvula (Forschheimer spots). The tongue is covered initially by a yellowish white coat; protruding red papillae give it the appearance of a "white strawberry tongue." Within 2 to 4 days, disappearance of the white coating reveals a beefy red tongue with enlarged papillae known as a "red strawberry tongue" (Fig. 126–1).

The exanthem appears 24 to 48 hours afterward and consists of erythematous macules and papules, beginning on the neck, face, and upper trunk and spreading downward to the extremities over the next 1 to 2 days. Generalized erythroderma is punctuated by numerous pinpoint, erythematous, blanchable papules, imparting a sandpaper-like texture (Fig. 126–2). Occlusion of sweat glands produces the papular rash. In severe cases the exanthem may be petechial and worsened by the application of a tourniquet. Capillary fragility causes petechiae in a linear pattern along major skinfolds, such as the axilla, antecubital fossa, and inguinal fossa, known as Pastia's lines. The palms and soles are generally spared, and there is a facial flush with circumoral pallor. Generalized adenopathy is common, but particularly inguinal nodes and splenomegaly may occur.

The rash fades over 5 to 7 days, and is followed by fine superficial desquamation of the face, trunk, axilla, groin, and extremities. Desquamation may continue for weeks, especially in the hands and feet.

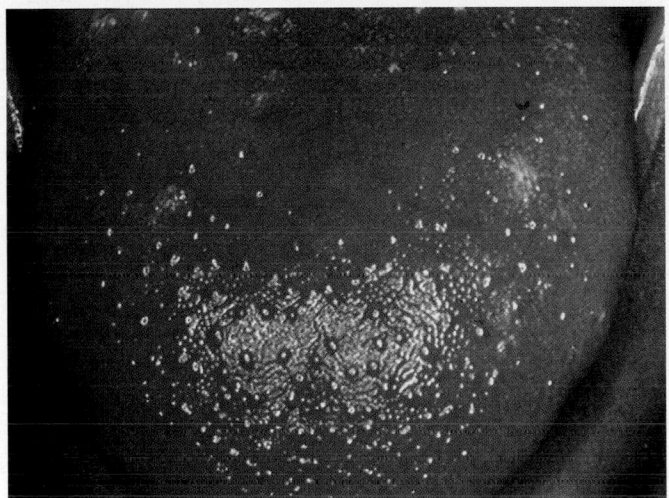

FIGURE 126–1. Red strawberry tongue in scarlet fever.

Table 126–1	Differential Diagnosis for Scarlet Fever

Staphylococcal scarlet fever
Viral hepatitis
Infectious mononucleosis
Kawasaki disease
Toxic shock syndrome
Measles
Rubella
Staphylococcal scalded skin syndrome
Roseola infantum
Erythema infectiosum
Echovirus 14
Drug-associated eruptions
Secondary syphilis
Juvenile rheumatoid arthritis
Streptobacillus moniliformis (rat bite fever)
Arcanobacterium haemolyticum

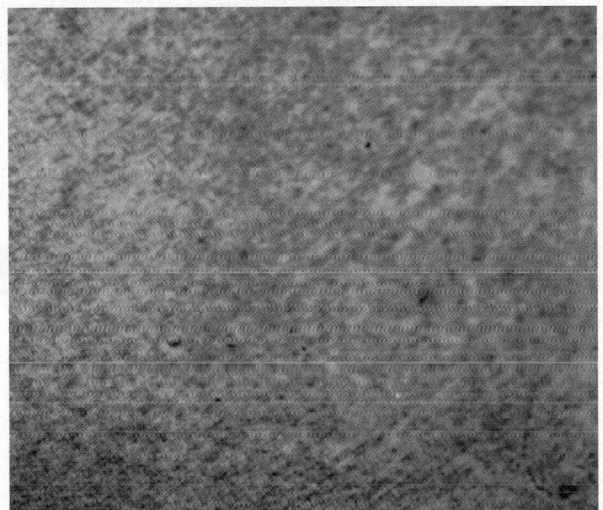

FIGURE 126–2. Papular rash in scarlet fever with sandpaper-like texture.

Table 126–2	Antimicrobial Agents Effective for Scarlet Fever

Antimicrobials	Doses
Penicillin V potassium	25–50 mg/kg/day qid PO for 10 days
Benzathine penicillin	Single daily dose:
	<1 mo old: 50,000 U/kg IM
	<27 kg: 600,000 units IM
	>27 kg: 1,200,000 units IM
Cephalexin	25–100 mg/kg/day qid PO for 10 days
Azithromycin	12 mg/kg/day qd PO for 5 days
Clarithromycin	15 mg/kg/day bid PO for 10 days

Abbreviations: IM, intramuscularly; PO, orally.

The differential diagnosis for scarlet fever includes other papular eruptions[4] (Table 126–1).

Complications of scarlet fever are unusual but include bacteremia, sepsis, pneumonia, myocarditis, hepatitis, otitis media, meningitis, and toxic shock syndrome (TSS). Late complications include acute rheumatic fever and acute poststreptococcal glomerulonephritis.[5]

Leukocytosis with a left shift is common, and eosinophilia may also occur. Diagnosis is generally made on clinical grounds and confirmed by culture of *Streptococcus pyogenes* from a focal infection such as the throat or skin. Highly specific rapid antigen detection technology is available for detection of *S. pyogenes*. False negatives can occur with a low level of infection and with infection caused by the non–group A streptococcus. Consequently, a negative antigen detection test should be followed up with a confirmatory throat culture. One can also confirm the diagnosis with an anti–streptolysin O titer that is noted to be rising.

Management

Early treatment of scarlet fever is associated with reduced infectivity, more rapid resolution of disease, and prevention of acute complications as well as acute rheumatic fever.[6] Penicillin is the treatment of choice; it can be given orally as penicillin VK for 10 days or intramuscularly as benzathine penicillin[7] (Table 126–2). Narrow-spectrum oral cephalosporins, such as cephalexin, are also effective therapies.[8] For penicillin-allergic patients, azithromycin, or clarithromycin is effective. Erythromycin should no longer be used for Group A Streptococcus infections due to resistance rates that approach 50%.

During the later stages of desquamation, antihistamines and bland ointments applied to wet skin will restore the skin integrity and ameliorate discomfort.

Staphylococcal Scalded Skin Syndrome

Staphylococcal scalded skin syndrome (SSSS) is a toxin-mediated disease characterized by cutaneous tenderness and widespread blistering and/or desquamation.[9] A spectrum of clinical presentations of SSSS is recognized, ranging from purely localized forms (bullous impetigo) to generalized involvement (Ritter's disease). It generally occurs in children less than 5 years of age, and is postulated to be due to reduced renal clearance and lack of immunity to the toxins. It has occurred in adults with immunosuppression, malignancy, chronic alcohol abuse, intravenous drug use, or renal impairment and is associated with greater than 50% mortality.[10-12] In children the mortality is approximately 4%.[13]

Staphylococcus aureus is an aerobic, gram-positive coccus that is ubiquitous and a virulent pathogen. It causes a wide range of infections from folliculitis and skin abscess to endocarditis and sepsis. SSSS is caused by phage II staphylococci, particularly strains 71 and 55, and occasionally strains 3A, 3B, and 3C.[14,15] *Staphylococcus aureus* elaborates two exotoxins, epidermolytic toxin A and epidermolytic toxin B, which are carried via the blood to the skin, where they act on the cell surface of the epidermal granular cells and activate serine proteinases.[16,17] Minor trauma to these keratinocytes results in intraepidermal separation of the cells within the granular layer and subsequent shedding of the skin.

Clinical Presentation

Foci of infection where the toxins are generated include the nasopharynx, umbilicus (neonates), urinary tract, cutaneous wounds, conjunctiva, and blood. Onset of the rash may be preceded by a prodrome of fever, malaise, and irritability. A faint erythematous eruption that resembles a sunburn begins, and is most intense on the central face, neck, axilla, and groin.[1,18] The skin rapidly becomes acutely tender, which is responsible for the marked irritability in many affected patients. The exfoliative phase is heralded by crusting around the mouth, eyes, and neck (Fig. 126–3). Often a purulent discharge emits from the eyes. Mild rubbing of the skin results in epidermal separation, leaving a shiny, moist, red surface (Nikolsky's sign).[18] Large fragments of crusts often become separated, leaving radial fissures surrounding the mouth that give the disorder its characteristic appearance. In infants and preschool children, lesions are usually limited to the upper body, while in newborns, the entire cutaneous surface may be involved (Ritter's disease) (Fig. 126–4). With severe involvement, large sheets of skin shear away, leaving a denuded oozing surface similar to the reaction that occurs after a burn or scald. Vesicles, pustules, and bullae can also occur during the exfoliative phase. Most children do well,

with resolution in 12 to 14 days with no residua. Intact bullae are consistently sterile. Occasionally the organism can be recovered from pyogenic foci on the skin, conjunctivae, or nasopharynx, from the stool, and rarely from the blood.

In the newborn, SSSS may be confused with diffuse cutaneous mastocytosis. In older children, the differential diagnosis is more broad (Table 126–3).

Complications may include sepsis and respiratory distress.[19]

Management

Therapy is directed against *S. aureus* to eliminate bacterial toxin production. For localized skin involvement, oral antibiotics such as cephalexin, amoxicillin-clavunalate, or dicloxacillin may be used. Those patients allergic to penicillin can be given azithromycin, clarithromycin, or clindamycin. Theoretically, clindamycin suppresses protein synthesis and further toxin production; therefore, its use may be more efficacious than bacterial cell wall inhibitor agents, such as β-lactamase antibiotics.[20] Neonates and infants less than 1 year old, and patients with extensive involvement, should be hospitalized and given parenteral antibiotics such as nafcillin or cefazolin. With the increasing prevalence of MRSA, consider administration of antibiotics effective against this organism (see Chapter 120, Skin and Soft Tissue Infections).

Replacement of fluid and electrolytes is required for patients with extensive skin involvement. The skin should be handled minimally, especially during the first 24 hours.

Table 126–3	Differential Diagnosis for SSSS
Drug-induced (toxic epidermal necrolysis, Stevens-Johnson syndrome)	
Diffuse cutaneous mastocytosis	
Exfoliative erythroderma	
Sunburn	
Thermal burn or scalds	
Toxic shock syndrome	
Streptococcal scarlet fever	
Scarlet fever	
Bullous impetigo	
Epidermolysis bullosa	
Epidermolytic hyperkeratosis	
Pemphigus foliaceus	

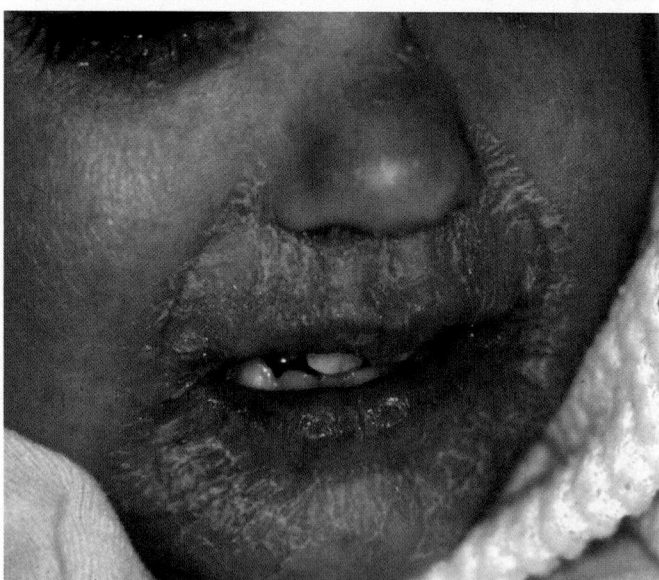

FIGURE 126–3. Exfoliative phase with crusting around mouth and eyes seen in staphylococcal scalded skin syndrome.

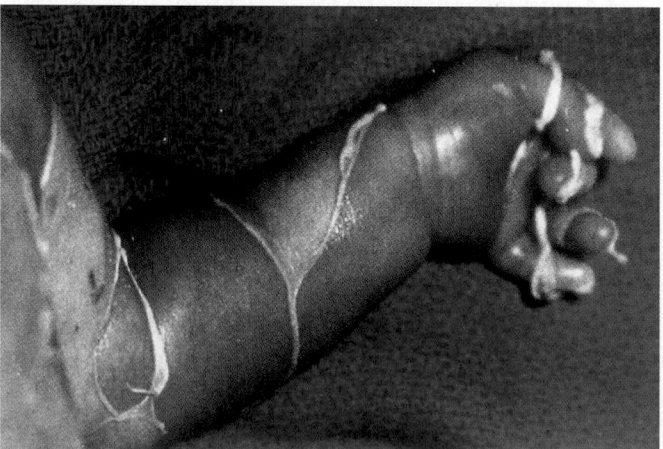

FIGURE 126–4. Scalded appearance from widespread desquamation seen in staphylococcal scalded skin syndrome.

Newborns may require burn therapy protocols, with careful attention to fluid and electrolyte losses and prevention of secondary infection.[17] During the desquamation stage, application of emollients twice a day may be helpful in restoring the skin surface and reducing dermal pain.

Staphyloccocal Toxic Shock Syndrome

Staphylococcal TSS is characterized by the acute onset of high fever, diffuse erythroderma followed by desquamation, hyperemic mucous membranes, hypotension, and multiorgan compromise. Prolonged tampon use with superinfection by *S. aureus* is the classic history, but many other sources have been implicated.

TSS is due to infection or colonization with a toxin-producing strain of *S. aureus,* especially phage types 29, 52, and 29/52 of phage group I, in a susceptible host with low to absent levels of specific antitoxin antibody.[21,22] The exotoxins include toxic shock syndrome toxin-1 (TSST-1), staphylococcal enterotoxin B (SEB), and staphylococcal enterotoxin C (SEC). TSST-1 occurs 75% of the time, SEB 25%, and SEC 2%. These toxins are associated with massive release of tumor necrosis factor-α (TNF-α) and interleukin-1. These substances have been shown to produce the features of TSS, including, fever, rash, hypotension, shock, and tissue injury.

Clinical Presentation

A typical presentation of TSS involves a menstruating adolescent female who presents with a high fever, generalized erythroderma, and hypotension.[1,23] Prominent desquamation of the palms and soles follows the acute eruption by 1 to 2 weeks. Additionally, in the nonmenstruating female or in males, sinusitis, otitis media, tracheitis, burns, minor skin infections, nasal packing, herpes zoster infection, cellulitis, osteomyelitis, bursitis, and uterine infection are sources for *S. aureus* to elaborate toxins.[24] Nonmenstrual TSS has less frequent central nervous system manifestations and anemia, but more frequent musculoskeletal involvement.[25]

High fever, malaise, chills, headache, myalgias, weakness, abdominal pain, vomiting, and diarrhea frequently precede the hypotensive state.[25] Hypotension ensues rapidly, leading to tissue ischemia and multiorgan injury.[26] The hypotension is caused by a decrease in systemic vascular resistance as well as nonhydrostatic leakage of fluid from the intravascular space to the interstitial space, both of which occur from massive cytokine release induced by the responsible exotoxins.[26] Patients typically present without focal neurologic or meningeal signs, but confusion and disorientation can occur, and may progress to seizures and coma. Persistent neuropsychological sequelae can develop, such as headaches, memory loss, and poor concentration.[27] Acute renal failure, adult respiratory distress syndrome (ARDS), myocardial dysfunction, hepatic dysfunction, and disseminated intravascular coagulation may be life threatening. Mortality occurs in up to 10% to 15% of cases without treatment and 3% to 5% with treatment.[23]

The rash develops in all patients within 1 to 3 days of the prodrome. A diffuse, macular, erythrodermic, scarlatiniform eruption develops on the trunk and spreads to the extremities[28] (Fig. 126–5). It resembles a sunburn that involves the palms and soles. Typically the rash fades over a few days, but on occasion it becomes petechial, purpuric, vesicular, or bullous.

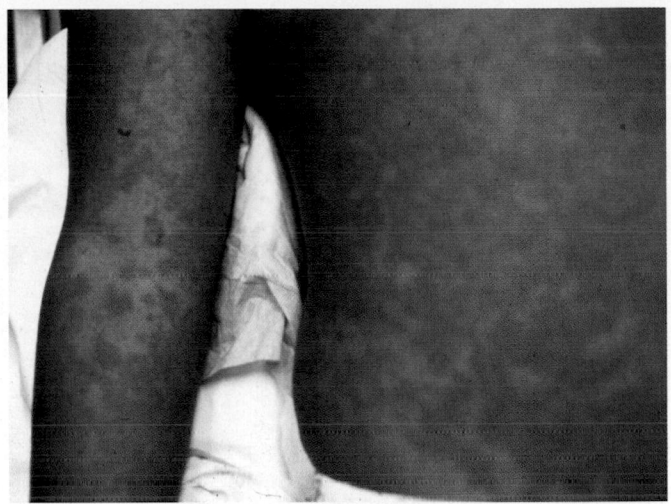

FIGURE 126–5. Diffuse erythrodermic rash seen in staphylococcal toxic shock syndrome.

Diffuse erythema of the pharyngeal, oral, conjunctival, and vaginal mucosa occurs and may progress to ulcerations.[23] A strawberry tongue and palatal petechiae may be seen.[29] One to 2 weeks after the onset of illness, approximately 50% of patients develop a diffuse, pruritic, maculopapular rash, which is sometimes urticarial, typically involving the palms and soles.[30] This secondary eruption lasts 2 to 7 days and is accompanied by edema of the face, hands, and feet as a consequence of increased interstitial fluid. Full-thickness desquamation of the skin, especially in the subungual, palm, and sole regions, occurs 10 to 21 days after onset of illness. The nails may be shed, and telogen effluvium or temporary cessation of hair growth may occur 2 months later.

Laboratory abnormalities reflect the multisystem involvement, shock, and endogenous cytokine release. They include low serum protein and albumin, leukocytosis with a left shift, anemia, thrombocytopenia, and evidence of disseminated intravascular coagulation. Renal abnormalities include reduced urine output, sterile pyuria, proteinuria, and elevated blood urea nitrogen and creatinine. Electrolyte abnormalities include hypocalcemia, hyponatremia, hypoalbuminemia, hypophosphatemia, and hypomagnesemia. Cerebrospinal fluid pleocytosis may occur. Hepatic enzymes, bilirubin, muscle creatinine, and serum lactate are elevated.

Diagnosis is usually based on the clinical features. *Staphylococcus aureus* is recovered from the cervix or vagina in more than 85% of patients with menstrual TSS and from the focus of infection in patients with nonmenstrual TSS. It is recovered from blood cultures in less than 5% of cases.[31]

The differential diagnosis for scarlet fever includes the entities listed in Table 126–4.

Complications include hypotension, myocardial dysfunction, acute renal failure, ARDS, disseminated intravascular coagulation, and fluid and electrolyte imbalances.

Management

Treatment of TSS centers on intensive supportive management of shock and multiorgan failure, identification and drainage of infection, and prompt institution of antibacterial therapy. Prompt replacement of fluids to correct hypotension

Table 126–4	Differential Diagnosis in Toxic Shock Syndrome

Rocky Mountain spotted fever
Meningococcemia
Leptospirosis
Ehrlichiosis
Staphylococcal scalded skin syndrome
Scarlet fever
Streptococcal toxic shock syndrome
Kawasaki disease
Infantile polyarteritis nodosa
Atypical measles
Stevens-Johnson syndrome
Typhoid fever
Dengue hemorrhagic fever
Toxic epidermal necrolysis
Septic shock
Drug reactions

Table 126–5	Antimicrobial Agents for Toxic Shock Syndrome	
Antimicrobials		**Doses**
Nafcillin		50–100 mg/kg divided q6h IV/IM
Cefazolin		25–100 mg/kg divided q8h IV/IM
Clindamycin		25–40 mg/kg divided q6–8h IV/IM
Azithromycin		5 mg/kg qd IV
Clarithromycin		15 mg/kg divided q12h PO

Abbreviations: IM, intramuscularly; IV, intravenously; PO, orally.

and shock is essential to achieve adequate tissue perfusion, as are other general supportive measures for shock. Treatment with an antistaphylococcal antibiotic is necessary to eliminate bacterial toxin production, but is unlikely to alter the acute course of the disease unless given early, before significant amounts of toxin can reach the circulation. The choice of antibiotics may include nafcillin or cefazolin (Table 126–5). Penicillin-allergic patients can be given azithromycin, clarithromycin, or clindamycin.[32] Theoretically, clindamycin suppresses protein synthesis and further toxin production; therefore, its use may be more efficacious than bacterial cell wall inhibitor agents, such as β-lactamase antibiotics.[20] Clindamycin is generally effective for patients with community-associated methicillin-resistant *S. aureus* (MRSA), and vancomycin is recommended for those with hospital-acquired MRSA.[33] Administration of intravenous immune globulin (IVIG) or TSST-1–specific monoclonal antibody may be considered for treatment of TSS with unrelenting shock and organ failure despite optimal management.[26,34-36] The use of high-dose corticosteroids, such as methylprednisolone 10 to 30 mg/kg/day for 2 to 3 days, is controversial. In a retrospective trial, corticosteroids reduced the severity of illness and duration of fever but had no effect on mortality.[37] If a tampon or nasal packing is present, it should be removed and the cavity irrigated in an effort to remove the organism, toxins, and possible retained pieces of tampon or packing. Drainage of a focus of infection is necessary to remove the offending *S. aureus*. Bland lubricants should be used on the desquamating skin.

Tinea Capitis

Tinea capitis is the most common dermatophytosis in children and is a fungal infection of the scalp characterized by scaling and alopecia. It is the most common cause of hair loss in children. Dermatophytes are fungi that invade and proliferate in the outer layer of the epidermis (stratum corneum). Some species can invade the hair and nails. Because of the annular appearance of the lesion, they are known as "ringworm." Dermatophytes can be of three types: geophilic organisms that live in the soil, zoophilic organisms that live on animals, and anthropophilic organisms that live on humans. These infections are common and increase with increasing age, in hot humid climates, and in crowded living conditions.[38,39] Hair involvement is usually seen in prepubertal children and is largely due to *Trichophyton tonsurans* and less often to *Microsporum audouinii* and *Microsporum canis*.[38,39] Each infection has a noninflammatory stage lasting 2 to 8 weeks, followed by an inflammatory stage.

Most cases occur in children ages 4 to 7 years with a prevalence of 2.5% in African Americans and less than 1% in whites.[34] The fungus is transmitted by person-to-person contact or animal-to-person contact.[40] The incubation period is 1 to 3 weeks, and the infection occurs more commonly in boys.[41]

Fungal infections of the scalp occur when hyphae invade the stratum corneum and then grow down a follicular wall between the skin and hair shaft until they reach the midfollicle. At this point they invade the hair itself and continue the downward invasion of the hair until they reach Adamson's fringe, where keratinization first occurs within the hair. If the infection is endothrix in nature, the hyphal element segments into arthroconidia inside the hair, which become replete with spores. These hairs are severely damaged, and tend to break off close to the scalp because of their fragility. In an ectothrix infection, the hyphae fragment into spores on the surface of the hair shaft, rather than within it.

Clinical Presentation

Hair loss is a regular feature of tinea capitis. *Microsporum canis* infections are noninflammatory and characterized by scaling and patchy hair loss. The infected areas are round, oval, or irregular and 1 to 6 cm in diameter, and multiple patches are common (Fig. 126–6). "Black dots," which are short (1- to 3-mm), broken-off hairs, may be noted in areas of alopecia. In some patients, no discrete hair loss is noted, and these cases may be misdiagnosed as seborrheic dermatitis or dandruff. Some hair follicles may be tinged gray as a result of the spores coating the outside of the hair shaft. Accompanying posterior cervical adenopathy is common.[42]

In contrast, *T. tonsurans* produces several distinct clinical presentations.[43] There is a "seborrheic" form in which scales occur without noticeable hair loss (Fig. 126–7). The inflammatory disease form is characterized by papules, pustules, erythema, and significant crusting (Fig. 126–8); it is very pruritic. An initial cluster of small follicular papules or pustules may gradually expand and coalesce, and at this stage the infection may be mistaken for folliculitis. Hair loss follows, which may be discrete and patchy or confluent. The most severe reaction consists of a tender, red, sometimes oozing, boggy mass known as a kerion (Fig. 126–9). The kerion may be misdiagnosed as a bacterial abscess. Severe

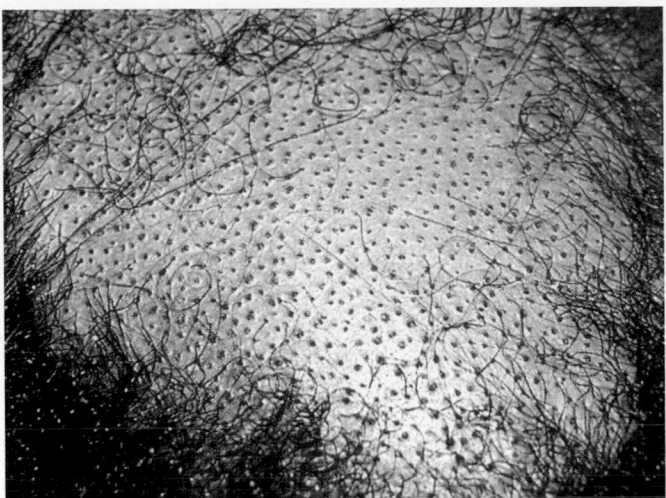

FIGURE 126–6. Annular patch of alopecia with scales and "black dots" seen in tinea capitis.

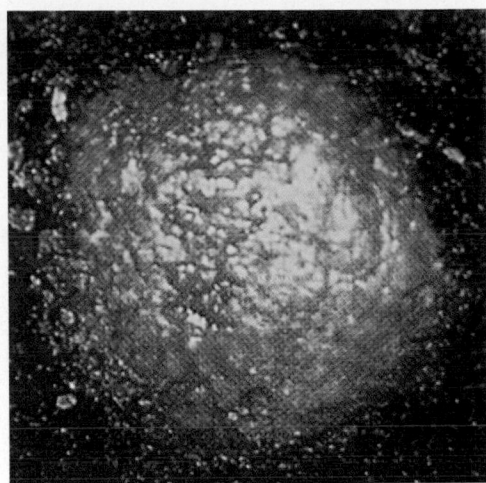

FIGURE 126–9. Kerion seen in tinea capitis.

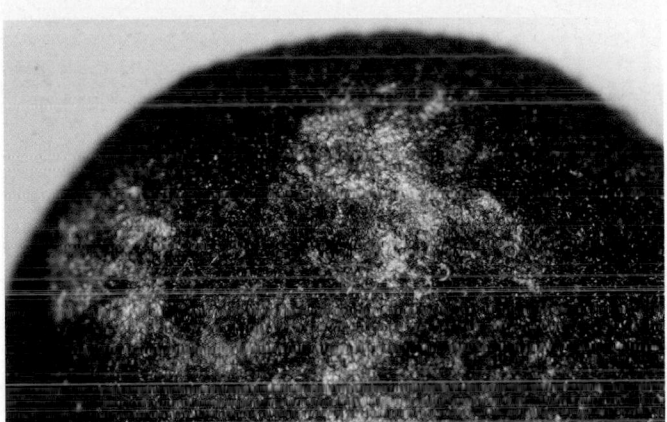

FIGURE 126–7. Patchy alopecia with scales in tinea capitis ("seborrheic" form).

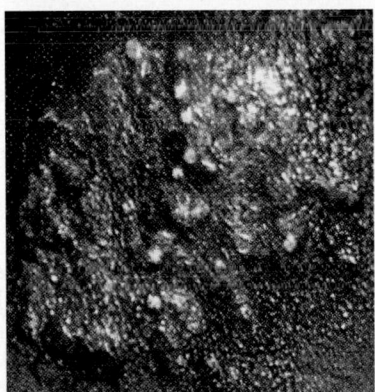

FIGURE 126–8. Inflammatory tinea capitis showing papules, pustules, erythema, and crusting.

scarring and permanent hair loss may occur even if proper therapy is given, but are more likely if therapy is delayed. A "black dot" variety of *T. tonsurans* infection is also seen. An extensive pruritic, eczema-like eruption on the trunk and extremities (dermatophytid or id reaction) may develop, especially after institution of antifungal therapy.[44] This occurs from an interaction between the host and fungal antigens.

Wood's lamp examination in Micosporum species is positive (fluoresces yellow-green) because it is an ectothrix infection of hairs, while *T. tonsurans,* an endothrix infection does not fluorescence. Culture in Sabouraud's agar is the "gold standard" for diagnosis. Potassium hydroxide (KOH) examination will reveal tiny arthrospores surrounding the hair shaft in Microsporum infection (ectothrix) and chains of arthrospores within the hair shaft (endothrix) in *T. tonsurans.* Dermatophyte test medium is a culture technique that changes color to deep red when the culture is positive.

The differential diagnosis includes alopecia areata, trichotillomania, traction alopecia, friction alopecia, seborrheic dermatitis, psoriasis, bacterial folliculitis, yeast folliculitis, impetigo, discoid lupus, and secondary syphilis.

Management

Topical therapy may be helpful, but is not sufficient to penetrate the hair shaft; therefore, systemic treatment is essential for eradication of the organism. Griseofulvin is still considered first-line therapy because of its efficacy, safety profile, and cost.[44a] However, a decreased sensitivity to this agent is emerging.[42] Increasing the dose to 20 to 25 mg/kg (maximum 1 g) of the microsize formulation has been shown to once again be efficacious.[45] Treatment consists of 6 to 12 weeks of therapy, and continuing for 2 weeks after clinical resolution. Accumulating experience with systemic terbinafine, itraconazole, and fluconazole indicates that they may be more effective and require shorter course of therapy[46,47,47a] (Table 126–6). Ketoconazole is the least effective agent and has a higher adverse effect profile, and is not recommended.

Rapid elimination of contagion risk is best achieved through systemic treatment in conjunction with twice-weekly use of a spore-inhibiting shampoo containing selenium sulfide, ketoconazole, or zinc pyrithione.[48] Contaminated hairbrushes, towels, pillowcases, or other fomites may spread infection and should be disinfected. Therefore, scalp grooming items and hats from infected patients should not be shared.

Table 126–6	Antifungal Therapy for Tinea Capitis	
Drug	**Dose**	**Duration**
Griseofulvin	20–25 mg/kg/day PO of microsize or 5–10 mg/kg/day PO of ultramicrosize qd or bid	6–12 wk; continue 2 wk after clinical resolution Take with fatty foods, eggs, or milk (improves absorption)
Terbinafine	3–6 mg/kg/day <20 kg: 62.5 mg/day 20–40 kg: 125 mg/day >40 kg: 250 mg/day	2–3 weeks *M. canis* may require 8 wk
Itraconazole	5 mg/kg/day PO qd or bid	2–4 wk
Fluconazole	8 mg/kg/day	2–4 wk

Abbreviation: PO, orally.

Treatment of the id reaction consists of topical or systemic corticosteroids. Kerions respond best by treating the underlying fungal disorder. Some advocate 3 to 4 weeks of oral corticosteroid therapy in patients with large and painful kerions; however, a randomized trial of corticosteroids plus oral antifungal agents versus antifungal agents alone showed no difference in cure rates.[49,50] If treated with oral antifungal agents, follow-up should occur in 2 to 3 months to ensure eradication of the infection.

Tinea Corporis

Tinea corporis, commonly known as "ringworm," is a dermatophyte infection of nonhairy (glabrous) surfaces, not otherwise designated as to specific area. It is more prevalent in warm or moist climates.[51] It may be caused by any of the dermatophytes making up the genera Trichophyton, Microsporum, and Epidermophyton.[52] In children the most common cause is *T. tonsurans*.[53] Sites of predilection include the nonhairy areas of the face, trunk, and limbs with exclusion of scalp (tinea capitis), bearded areas (t. barbae), hands (t. manuum), nails (onychomycosis), groin (t. cruris), and feet (t. pedis).

Clinical Presentation

Tinea corporis presents as one or more red, scaly papules. These papules spread and eventually coalesce into plaques that become scaly. The center of these plaques tends to clear, producing annular configurations and occasionally concentric rings (Fig. 126–10). Mild erythema, edema, vesicles, or even bulla formation may occur. If extensive crusting develops, the resulting plaques can resemble psoriasis. Itching may be prominent with inflammatory infections. Pustules and inflammation are more common with *M. canis*. A marked perifollicular or follicular granulomatous inflammatory response may occur, especially in patients inadvertently treated with topical corticosteroids. This disorder is termed *Majocchi's granuloma*; it is caused by *T. rubrum* and often requires oral antifungals.[54] The use of topical corticosteroids may mask the diagnosis by distorting the lesion (tinea incognito).

The diagnosis is made by demonstrating septate branching hyphae on KOH examination or cultured in Sabouraud's agar. The differential diagnosis includes nummular eczema, granuloma annulare, candidiasis, urticaria, erythema annulare centrifugum, psoriasis, pityriasis rosea, secondary syphilis, sarcoidosis, leprosy, and discoid lupus.

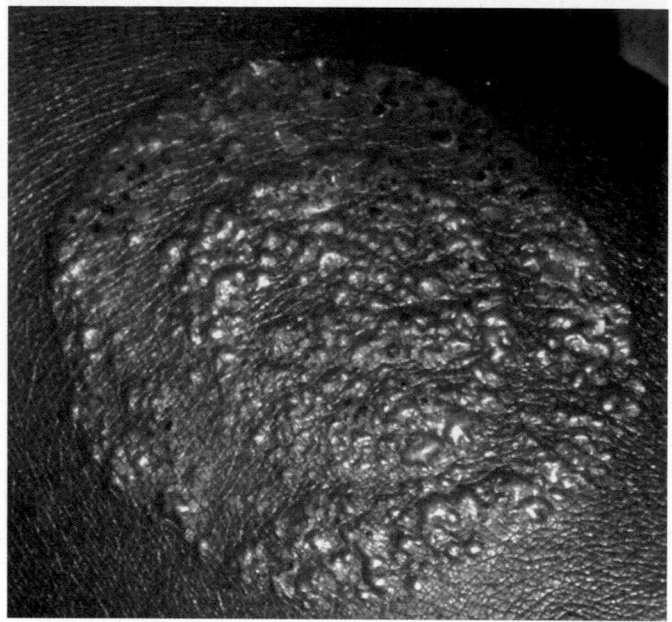

FIGURE 126–10. Annular plaque seen in tinea corporis.

Management

Many cases of tinea corporis resolve spontaneously; however, contagion is still an issue that compels treatment.[55] Topical treatment alone is usually effective in those patients with limited disease (Table 126–7). Treatment that involves the lesion and surrounding borders should be continued for about 1 week after apparent clinical eradication. In persistent cases or widespread disease, oral antifungals are used (Table 126–8). High-potency corticosteroids are likely to worsen the infection and are associated with substantial adverse effects.[56]

Imidazoles inhibit the enzyme lanosterol-14-α-demethylase, a cytochrome P-450–dependent enzyme that converts lanosterol to ergosterol. It results in unstable fungal cell wall and causes membrane leakage. Imidazoles include compounds such as econazole, miconazole, oxiconazole, and clotrimazole. All are broad-spectrum antifungal agents that have good activity against dermatophytes, Candida, and other yeasts. A second class of antifungals includes ciclopirox olamine, a pyridone ethanolamine salt that interferes with synthesis of cell membrane proteins. The allylamines are a

Table 126–7   Topical Drugs for Superficial Fungal Infections

Drugs	Strength	Formulations*	Application(s)/Day
Butenafine (Mentax, Lotrimin Ultra)	1%	C	1 or 2
Ciclopirox (Loprox)	0.77%	C	2
Clotrimazole (Lotrimin, Lotrimin AF, Mycelex)	1%	C, L, S	2
Econazole (Spectazole)	1%	C	1
Ketoconazole (Nizoral)	2%	C, Sh	2
Miconazole nitrate (Monistat-Derm, Micatin, Lotrimin AF spray)	2%	C, P, S, Sp	2
Naftifine (Naftin)	1%	C, G	2
Oxiconazole (Oxistat)	1%	C, L	1 or 2
Sulconazole (Exelderm)	1%	C, S	1 or 2
Terbinafine (Lamisil AT)	1%	C	1 or 2
Tolnaftate (Tinactin)	1%	C, P, S	2

*C, cream; G, gel; L, lotion; P, powder; S, solution; Sh, shampoo; Sp, spray; Su, suspension.

Table 126–8   Oral Drugs for Fungal Infections

Drugs	Doses
Griseofulvin microsize	20–25 mg/kg/day qd or bid
Griseofulvin ultramicrosize	5–10 mg/kg/day qd or bid
Terbinafine	3–6 mg/kg/day qd
	<20 kg: 62.5 mg/day qd
	20–40 mg/kg: 125 mg/day qd
	>40 kg: 250 mg/day qd
Itraconazole	5 mg/kg/day qd or bid
Fluconazole	8 mg/kg/day qd

third class of agents, which includes naftifine and terbinafine. They interfere with ergosterol synthesis through inhibition of squalene oxidase and are fungicidal in vitro. In addition, naftifine has anti-inflammatory properties that may be useful in severe inflammatory disease.[57] The older antifungal compounds, undecylenic acid and tolnaftate, are of limited value and have no activity against Candida. Haloprogin is somewhat useful against Candida and dermatophytes but has been supplanted by newer agents. Miconazole, clotrimazole, and terbinafine are available over the counter in topical formulations and are acceptable first-line agents for most uncomplicated fungal infections. Follow-up should occur in 2 to 4 weeks to ensure complete resolution of the infection.

Pityriasis Versicolor

Pityriasis versicolor is a condition caused by proliferation of pityrosporum filamentous yeast forms within the stratum corneum of human skin. It is characterized by hypopigmented and hyperpigmented macules and patches. The term *tinea* is inappropriate since this infection is caused by a yeast rather than a dermatophyte. It is most common in individuals 15 to 24 years of age.

Pityriasis versicolor is caused by *Malassezia furfur* (also known as *Pityrosporum orbiculare, Pityrosporum ovale,* and *Malasezzia ovalis*), a dimorphic lipophilic yeast that can reside on skin as a normal skin flora. However, it can also be an opportunistic pathogen, and under appropriate conditions, the benign yeast (spore) form can transform into an invasive filamentous (hyphal) phase. Factors that lead to the conversion of the saprophytic yeast to the parasitic mycelial morphologic form include a genetic predisposition, warm humid environments, immunosuppression, malnutrition, and Cushing's disease. Pityriasis is more common in areas of high heat and humidity because moisture promotes growth of the organism. The majority of cases occurs in adolescents and affect cutaneous areas where sebaceous glands are active. In children, up to one third have lesions on their faces.[58] It tends to be a chronic disease, and even with treatment, recurrences are common.[59]

Clinical Presentation

The organism produces dicarboxylic acids, such as azaleic acid, that inhibit melanogenesis and cause direct damage to melanocytes, which may account for the prolonged hypopigmentation that occurs following infection. Patients usually present for cosmetic reasons, but may also complain of pruritus. Children frequently have facial lesions that involve the forehead and temple. Adolescents and adults commonly have lesions on the upper back, chest, and arms. Other less common sites include the neck, axilla, legs, popliteal fossa, forearms, and genitalia.

Lesions of the face consist of ovoid macules that are hypopigmented with a faint scale. Lesions at other sites, as the name "versicolor" implies, can vary in color. Hypopigmented, faint pink, red, or tan to darker brown lesions may be present[59a] (Fig. 126–11). They consist of discrete and coalescent ovoid macules of varying size that have a fine, faint scale that is more noticeable upon scraping the area. They are often concentrated symmetrically over areas of high sebum content such as the upper chest and back. Papules and annular plaques are sometimes seen.

An inverse form of pityriasis versicolor exists in which the condition has an entirely different distribution, affecting the flexural regions, the face, or isolated areas of the extremities. It is usually seen in immunocompromised patients.

Microscopic examination of skin scrapings mounted in 10% KOH reveals both budding yeast and short, stubby hyphal forms ("spaghetti and meatballs") (Fig. 126–12). Culture can be performed in a media enriched with C12- or C14-sized fatty acids. Wood's lamp examination shows a yellowish brown or copper-orange fluorescence.

The differential diagnosis for pityriasis versicolor includes vitiligo, pityriasis alba, pityriasis rosea, pityriasis rotunda, tinea corporis, seborrheic dermatitis, atopic dermatitis, candidiasis, guttate psoriasis, erythrasma, secondary syphilis, pinta, and leprosy.

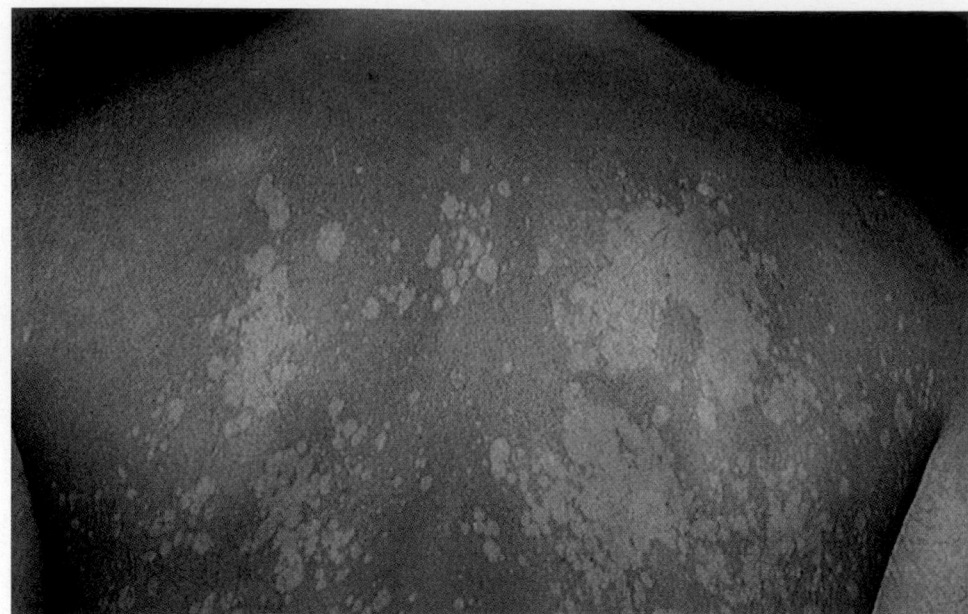

FIGURE 126–11. Hypopigmented macules seen in pityriasis versicolor.

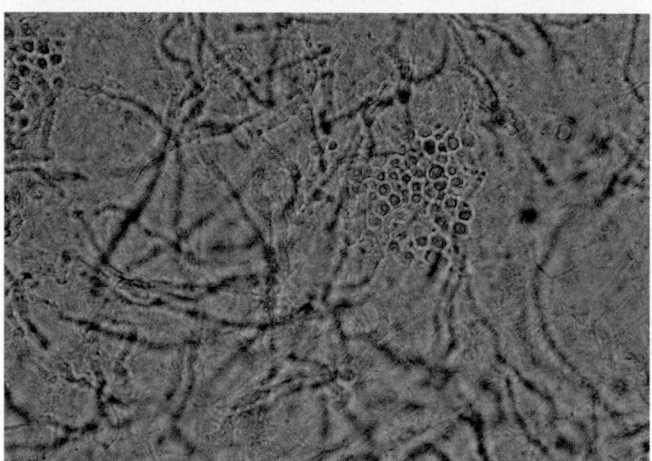

FIGURE 126–12. 10% KOH preparation showing the budding yeast and short, stubby hyphal form ("spaghetti and meatballs") of pityriasis versicolor.

Management

A number of topical agents are effective in the treatment of pityriasis versicolor (Table 126–9). Topical agents should be applied to the trunk, neck, arms, legs, and scalp to minimize spore count and possibility of relapse. Although selenium sulfide lotion applied for 5 to 10 minutes for 7 days is commonly utilized, the cosmetic problem and prolonged therapy required with this agent have led to the increasing use of therapeutic alternatives. Systemic therapy is generally indicated for extensive lesions resistant to topical treatment, or those with frequent relapse; however, oral therapy is not approved by the Food and Drug Administration in children (Table 126–10).

Molluscum Contagiosum

Molluscum contagiosum is a viral infection characterized by umbilicated papules. It is caused by poxvirus, a DNA virus.[60]

It can occur at any age, but infection is most common in young children, sexually active adults, and persons with impaired cellular immunity. Transmission is by person-to-person contact, contact with fomites, or autoinoculation. The incubation period ranges from 2 to 8 weeks, but has been noted to be as early as 1 week.[61]

Clinical Presentation

Children present because of the presence of visible bumps, pruritus, or soreness. The typical lesions are discrete, dome-shaped, umbilicated (central punctum) waxy papules[60] (Fig. 126–13). They may be skin colored, pink, or white. Lesions may appear to be vesicular because of a translucent quality. They also may appear as tiny, pinpoint papules simulating milia. Lesions vary in size from 1 to 5 mm, although they may be as large as 10 to 15 mm (giant molluscum). Secondary bacterial infection may occur producing crusting, redness, and pus formation.

Lesions may occur on any part of the body but, in young children, are most commonly on the axilla, side of the trunk, lower abdomen, thighs, and face. Lesions in the genital area that occur in adolescents or young adults are frequently sexually transmitted.[60] The presence of lesions in the genital area of young children is not usually a consequence of sexual abuse, but this possibility should be excluded. In this age group it is commonly a consequence of autoinoculation.

An eczematous eruption on the skin adjacent to molluscum ("molluscum dermatitis") occurs in 10% of cases.[62] Widespread cutaneous infection with hundreds of lesions has been reported in atopic dermatitis and in immunocompromised children.

Detection of the virus in skin lesions has been achieved using polymerase chain reaction.[63] Histologic examination by hematoxylin and eosin staining shows keratinocytes filled with intracytoplasmic inclusion bodies (Henderson-Paterson bodies), which are eosinophilic ovoid structures in the lower malpighian layer. These homogeneous molluscum inclusion bodies may also be demonstrated by smearing the cheesy

Table 126–9	Topical Agents Effective against Pityriasis Versicolor	
Agents		**Application**
Ketoconazole 2% (Nizoral) shampoo, cream		Once or twice daily for 3–14 days
Selenium sulfide shampoo (Selsun Blue, Excel, Head & Shoulders)		Once daily for 7–14 days
Terbinafine (Lamisil AT) cream, spray, solution		Twice daily for 5–7 days
Econazole 1% (Spectazole) cream		Once daily
Ciclopirox 0.77% (Loprox) cream, lotion, gel, suspension		Twice daily for 2–4 wk
Sulconazole 1% (Exelderm) cream, solution		Daily or twice daily for 3 wk
Clotrimazole 1% (Lotrimin) cream, solution		Twice daily for 2–4 wk
Butenafine 1% (Mentax) cream		Daily 14 days
Miconazole 2% (Monistat Derm, Micatin, Lotrimin AF Spray) cream, shampoo		Twice daily for 2–4 wk

Table 126–10	Oral Agents Effective against Pityriasis Versicolor
Agents	**Dose**
Ketoconazole	200–400 mg 3–7 days, then once a month
Itraconazole	200 mg 5–7 days
Fluconazole	400 mg once

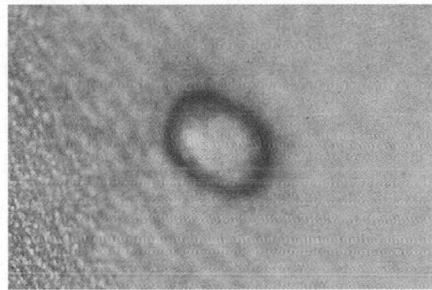

FIGURE 126–13. Dome-shaped, umbilicated waxy papule from molluscum contagiosum.

contents from a lesion onto a slide and staining with Gram, Giemsa, or Wright stain.[64] Electron microscopic examination shows the typical brick-shaped poxvirus particles.

The differential diagnosis includes verrucae, varicella, folliculitis, furunculosis, milia, juvenile xanthogranuloma, Spitz nevi, skin tags, and epidermal cysts.

Management

Molluscum infection, left untreated, nearly always resolves spontaneously, but resolution may take a few weeks to a few years. Therefore, treatment may not always be indicated.[65] In the case of bacterial superinfection, antistaphylococcal antibiotics should be administered. If treatment is considered, a large number of topical agents have been useful, such as tretinoin cream, benzoyl peroxide, podophyllum resin in tincture of benzoin, podofilox, salicylic acid, cantharidin, 10% KOH, and silver nitrate.[66-68a] Topical 3% cidofovir has been used successfully in children with immunodeficiency,[69,70] and oral cidofovir has been used in adults but is not approved in children.[71] Oral cimetidine has been reported to be effective.[72] In immunocompromised patients, ritonavir, cidofovir, saquinavir, lamivudine, and zidovudine have been used.[73-75] In resistant cases, imiquimod cream or intralesional interferon alfa has been used.[76,77] Cryotherapy (liquid nitrogen,

dry ice, or Frigiderm) applied to each lesion for a few seconds and repeated as needed in 2- to 3-week intervals has been effective.[78] For extensive lesions, ablative therapy may require general anesthesia with pulsed dye laser.[79]

An easy method to remove the lesion is eviscerating the core with an instrument such as a no. 11 scalpel blade, a needle, the edge of a glass slide, or superficial curettage.[80] Application of a eutectic mixture of prilocaine and lidocaine cream (EMLA) for at least 1 hour prior to treatment may help diminish the discomfort.[81] Scotch Tape applied one to three times daily on the lesion has also been successful.[80]

Pityriasis Rosea

Pityriasis rosea is an acute, self-limited papulosquamous disorder. Most cases occur between 10 and 35 years of age, with both sexes equally involved.[82] It is more prevalent in spring and autumn. The cause is unknown, but human herpesvirus 7 has been recovered from lesions of pityriasis rosea.[83]

Clinical Presentation

Pityriasis rosea begins with a scaly erythematous patch or plaque known as the herald patch in 50% to 80% of cases, which precedes and heralds the onset of widespread papulosquamous eruption by several days to up to 3 months. In a small number of cases, appearance of the herald patch coincides with the onset of the widespread eruption. The herald patch begins as a nondescript, smooth, erythematous macule or papule, which expands over 1 to 2 weeks to form an oval-shaped patch or plaque. Central clearing gives rise to an annular lesion. It can occur on any body part, and 5% of patients have more than one herald patch. Desquamation eventually occurs, creating a surface scale that is attached at the periphery with the free edge directed toward the center of the lesion ("collarette of scale"). The widespread eruption evolves bilaterally and symmetrically over 1 to 3 weeks on the trunk, neck, face, and proximal limbs (Fig. 126–14). The eruption consists of oval-shaped, erythematous papules or macules that enlarge to a maximum size of 5 to 30 mm. The lesions are initially smooth but quickly develop the typical collarette of scale on the surface. On the back, the long axis of these lesions runs parallel to the ribs, giving rise to the highly characteristic "Christmas tree" or "fir tree" pattern. The eruption is typically pruritic. Resolution occurs in 4 to 12 weeks and may be associated with postinflammatory hypopigmentation or hyperpigmentation.

A number of clinical variants have been seen. The eruption can have vesicular, pustular, purpuric, or erythema multiforme–like lesions.[84-87] The eruption can be localized to the

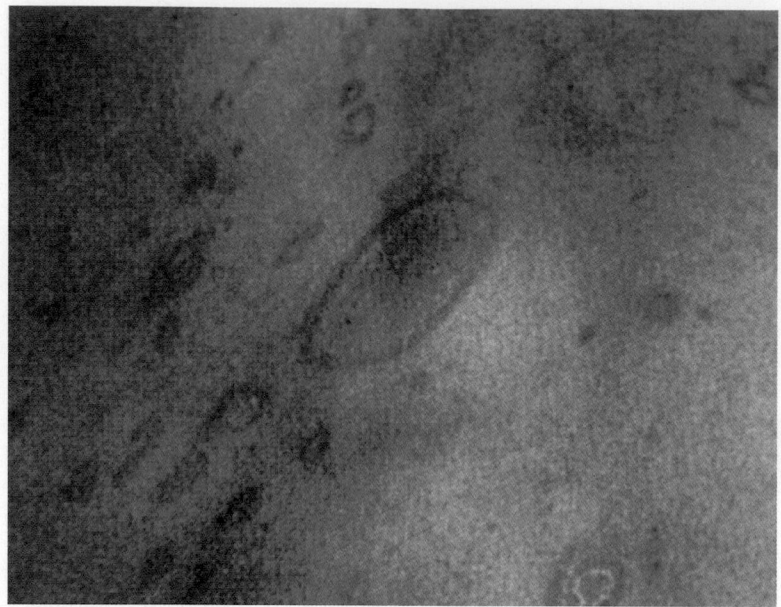

FIGURE 126–14. Oval-shaped, erythematous papules and macules with a collarette of scales seen in pityriasis rosea.

face and limbs with sparing of the trunk (inverse pityriasis rosea), localized to the axilla and groin as large plaques (pityriasis circinata et marginata of Vidal), or localized to one area of the body or one side of the body.[87,88] Oral lesions may occur during the course of disease and may consist of punctate petechiae, ulcerations, erythematous macules, plaques, vesicles, or bullae.[89]

On occasion a prodrome may occur consisting of headache, malaise, pharyngitis, and lymphadenopathy. The differential diagnosis for pityriasis rosea includes tinea corporis, guttate psoriasis, pityriasis lichenoides, lichen planus, drug eruptions, secondary syphilis, Lyme disease, human immunodeficiency virus seroconversion illness, and nummular eczema.

Management

In view of the self-limited nature of the eruption, treatment is only needed for patients with significant pruritus or cosmetic impairment. Treatment options for pruritus include antihistamines, topical emollients, calamine lotion, oatmeal bath, or colloidal starch. Others have used oral erythromycin, ultraviolet B (UVB) phototherapy, topical steroids, and oral steroids. Erythromycin has been shown to resolve lesions in 2 weeks in 73% of cases.[90] Daily erythemogenic doses of UVB phototherapy over 5 to 10 days can significantly improve the eruption, with variable degree in reduction of pruritus, but the course of the disease is not altered and this therapy may be associated with postinflammatory hyperpigmentation.[91] Corticosteroids may temporarily reduce pruritus without altering the course of the disease and, due to the widespread nature of the disease, can be associated with significant adverse effects.

Kawasaki Disease (Mucocutaneous Lymph Node Syndrome) (See Also Chapter 95)

Kawasaki disease (KD) is an acute febrile illness of unknown etiology with widespread vasculitis that affects children less than 5 years of age. It is a unique clinical symptom complex characterized by persistent high fever, bilateral nonexudative conjunctival injection, oropharyngeal mucosal changes, cervical lymphadenopathy, erythematous rash, and changes in peripheral extremities.[92] It is the most common cause of acquired heart disease in children in Japan and the United States.[93]

KD has been reported on all continents and in all ethnic groups; however, most cases are described in Japan.[94] It peaks at 9 to 11 months of age, with 55% of patients under 2 years of age and 80% to 85% under 5 years of age.[95] Adult cases are extremely rare.[96] There is a slightly higher prevalence in males. The mortality with treatment is 0.1% to 2%. Blood vessel damage appears to result from an aberrant immune response leading to endothelial cell injury and vessel wall damage.

Clinical Presentation

Infants in particular are usually very irritable, much more than seen with a simple viral cause of fever. If five or six of the principal symptoms are present (Table 126–11), the diagnosis of KD can be established after other diseases with similar findings are excluded.[96a] However, patients with only four or fewer of the six principal symptoms can be diagnosed as having KD when coronary artery aneurysm is recognized by two-dimensional echocardiography.

Other features of KD are less common, such as right upper quadrant pain, nausea, and vomiting caused by hydrops of the gallbladder, which can be confirmed by ultrasonography and resolves without surgical intervention. Other gastrointestinal manifestations include diarrhea, small bowel obstruction, ileus, hepatitis with hepatomegaly, and pancreatitis. Arthritis can occur in the first week in 30% of cases and is usually polyarticular, involving the knees, ankles, and hands and persisting for about 3 weeks. Sterile pyuria with monocytes is common. Dysuria may be associated with meatitis and cystitis. Evidence of aseptic meningitis may be seen in 50% of patients who undergo lumbar puncture. Rare finding include peripheral ischemia with resultant gangrene, pneumonitis, pleural effusion, testicular swelling, facial nerve palsy, and hemophagocytic syndrome.[97-99]

Table 126–11   Clinical Symptoms of Kawasaki Disease (KD)

Symptoms	Characteristics
Fever (95%)	• The illness starts and is suspected when fever of unknown etiology is present for more than 5 days. • Typically high spiking and remitting with peak temperature greater than 39° C. • Lasts 1–3 wk but subsides rapidly with intravenous immune globulin administration, and more so when aspirin is added. • The longer the fever, the higher incidence of coronary aneurysm formation.
Eye findings (87%–90%)	• Painless bulbar conjunctival injection with sparing of the limbus. • Occurs within 2–4 days from onset of disease (Fig. 126–15). • No purulent discharge (not "conjunctivitis"). • If a slit-lamp examination is performed, evidence of anterior uveitis or acute iridocyclitis is commonly seen.[133] • Usually subsides within 1 wk.
Oral changes (85%–95%)	• Dryness, redness, fissuring, peeling, cracking, and bleeding of the lips. • "Strawberry tongue" indistinguishable from streptococcal scarlet fever, with erythema and prominent papillae. • Diffuse erythema of the oropharyngeal mucosa seen 3–5 days after the onset of disease (Fig. 126–16). • Changes subside in 2 wk.
Lymph nodes (50%–70%)	• Swelling of cervical lymph nodes seen 1 day before the onset or concomitant with the fever (Fig. 126–17). • Child complains of pain and may have torticollis. • Swelling ranges from 1.5 to 5 cm in diameter without fluctuance or overlying skin erythema. • Seen in two thirds of children in Japan and only 50% in United States. • Swelling usually disappears with defervescence. • In children greater than 3 years old, cervical lymphadenopathy may be the most striking feature, and a misdiagnosis of adenitis may be made and antibiotic therapy given, which is ineffective. • KD should be suspected in patients with cervical adenitis, especially if unresponsive to antibiotic therapy.
Exanthem (85%–90%)	• From the first to fifth day after the onset of fever. • Polymorphous exanthem appears on the body and/or extremities (Fig. 126–18). • Morbilliform, maculopapular, scarlatiniform, urticarial with large erythematous plaques, or erythema multiforme–like with target or iris lesions. • Individual lesions are 5–13 mm in diameter and spread over the body and extremities within several days. • Each lesion becomes larger and may coalesce. • Rash may disappear over the next few days and may be recurrent. Erythema and desquamation in the perianal region often occurs.
Peripheral extremity changes (90%–95%)	• Reddening of palms and soles 2–5 days after onset of illness, at which time painful indurative edema occurs (Fig. 126–19). • Swelling resolves as the fever disappears. • At 10–15 days after onset, there is desquamation and fissuring between nails and tips of fingers, after which it spreads over palms and soles (Fig. 126–20). • Fingertip desquamation is one of the most important features of KD. From 1½ to 2 months later, transverse furrows appear in the nails (Beau's lines).

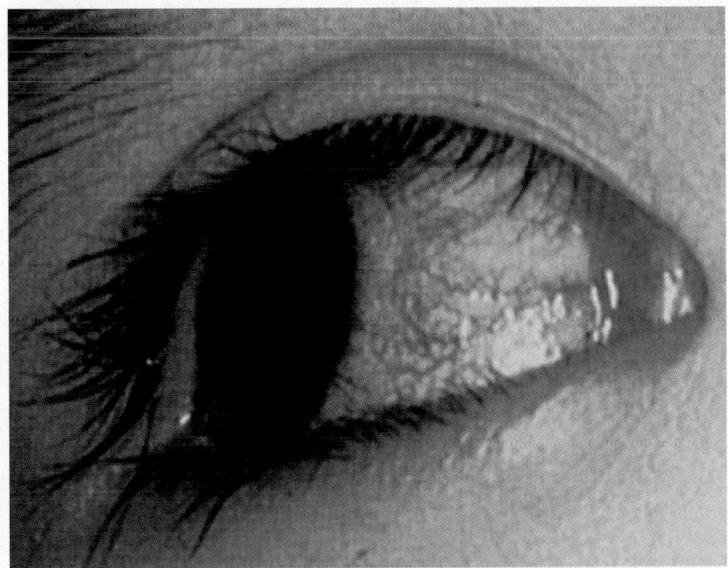

FIGURE 126–15. Bulbar conjunctival injection in Kawasaki disease.

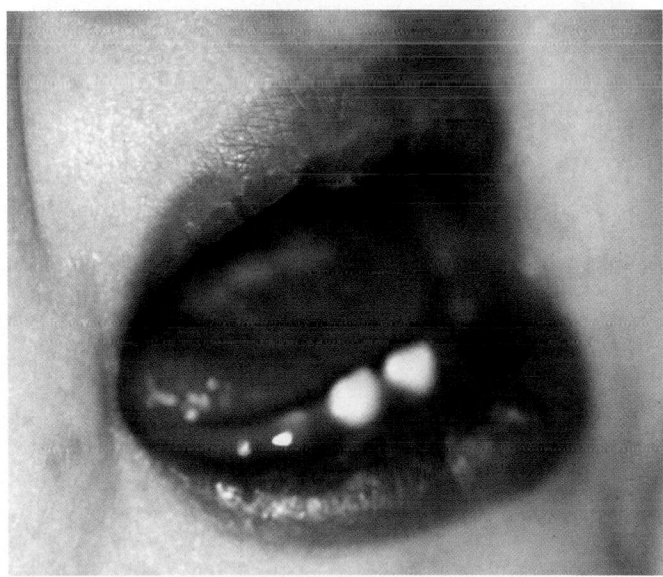

FIGURE 126–16. Diffuse erythema of oropharyngeal mucosa seen in Kawasaki disease.

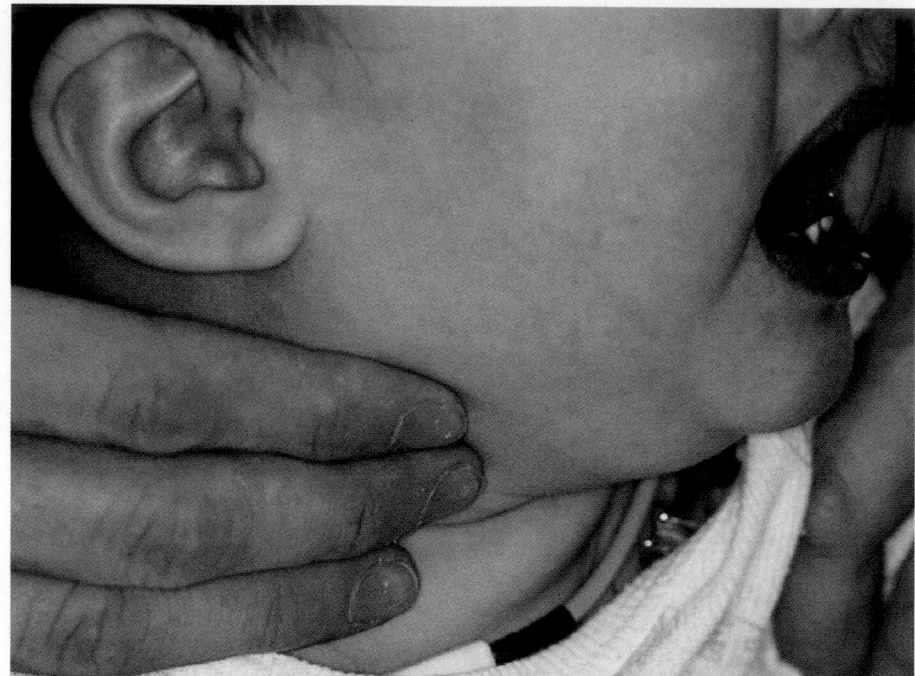

FIGURE 126–17. Enlarged lymph node seen in Kawasaki disease.

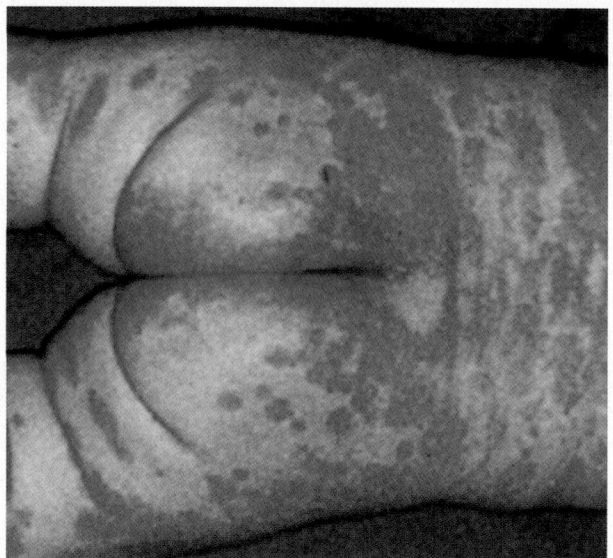

FIGURE 126–18. Erythematous maculopapular plaques seen in Kawasaki disease.

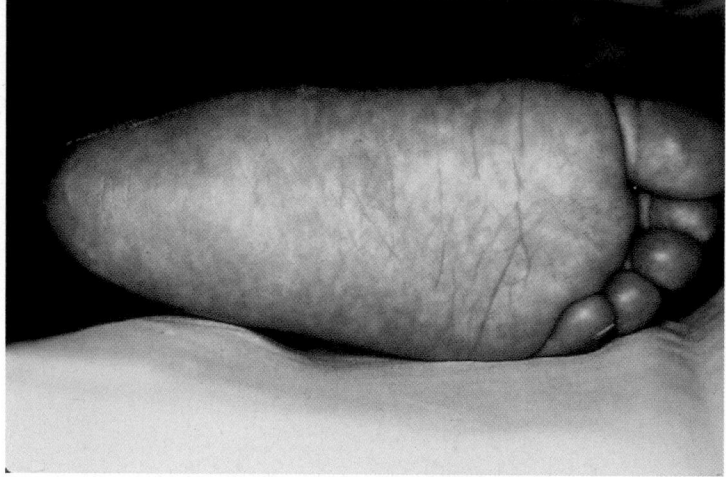

FIGURE 126–19. Indurative edema seen in Kawasaki disease.

The most important clinical complications affect the cardiovascular system, and may lead to myocardial ischemia and sudden death. Before the availability of IVIG, 15% to 25% of children developed coronary dilation or aneurysms; with therapy, this rate fell to 4%. Risk factors for developing coronary artery aneurysms include persistent fever, especially after IVIG therapy, low hemoglobin, low albumin, high white blood cell count, high band count, high C-reactive protein (CRP) or erythrocyte sedimentation rate (ESR), serum sodium less than 135 mEq/L, male sex, and age less than 1 year.[100,101] Children with giant coronary artery aneurysms (>8 mm in diameter) will have 50% stenosis and

obstruction, and two thirds will have evidence of myocardial ischemia.[102]

Other cardiac findings may include congestive heart failure, valvulitis (especially of the mitral valve), and pericardial effusion. The earliest cardiac changes occur within the first 10 days of onset and include endocarditis, myocarditis, and pericarditis. The formation of a coronary aneurysm may lead to turbulent flow and thrombus formation with coronary stenosis and subsequent myocardial ischemia, infarction, or sudden death.[103] Aneurysm may occur in other extraparenchymal muscular arteries such as the celiac, mesenteric, femoral, iliac, renal, axillary, and brachial arteries.[104]

Laboratory findings are nonspecific: leukocytosis with left shift, eosinophilia, and elevated ESR, CRP, and α_1-antitrypsin. Thrombocytosis, ranging from 500,000/mm^3 to greater

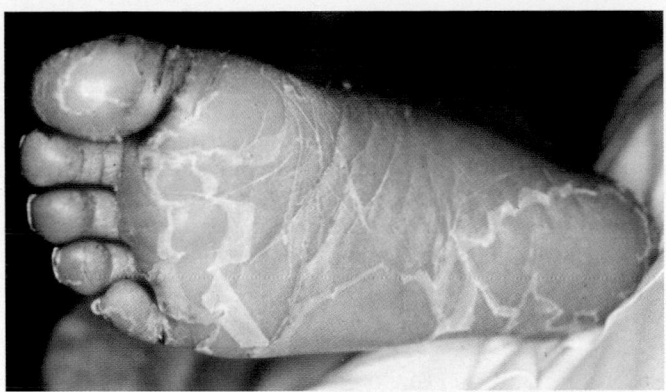

FIGURE 126–20. Desquamation seen in Kawasaki disease.

than 1,000,000/mm³, occurs on the second week of illness, and serum immunoglobulins may increase. A normochromic, normocytic anemia is frequent, and elevated hepatic transaminases and bilirubin may be seen. Urinalysis reveals sterile pyuria in a third of the patients. Arthrocentesis during the arthritis yields purulent-appearing fluid with a mean white blood cell count of 125,000/mm³ to 300,000/mm³, normal glucose level, and negative Gram stain and bacterial culture.[105] Cerebrospinal fluid may show a mononuclear pleocytosis without hypoglycorrhachia or elevated protein.

Abnormalities in serum lipids can occur, with increased triglycerides and low-density lipoproteins and decreased high-density lipoproteins.[106] Elevation of serum cardiac troponin I has been reported.[107] Electrocardiographic changes may include prolongation of the PR interval or QT interval and ST-segment and T-wave changes. The diagnosis of coronary artery aneurysm is accomplished by two-dimensional echocardiography. It is noninvasive and has a high sensitivity and specificity for detection of abnormalities in the coronary arteries. Other modalities used to diagnose coronary artery aneurysms have included magnetic resonance imaging, magnetic resonance angiography, and coronary angiography.[108]

The differential diagnosis for KD includes Stevens-Johnson syndrome, toxic shock syndrome, scarlet fever, measles, *Yersinia* pseudotuberculosis (Izumi fever), juvenile rheumatoid arthritis, drug eruption, serum sickness, Rocky Mountain spotted fever, infantile polyarteritis nodosa, acute adenovirus infection, measles, echovirus, leptospirosis, and mercury hypersensitivity reaction.[109]

Management

Treatment of KD in the acute phase is directed at decreasing inflammation in the coronary artery wall and preventing coronary thrombosis, whereas long-term therapy in patients who develop coronary aneurysms is aimed at preventing myocardial ischemia or infarction.

It is now clear that IVIG and aspirin combined therapy results in a more rapid anti-inflammatory effect and reduces coronary artery abnormalities more than aspirin alone. In the United States, it is recommended to give a single 2-g/kg infusion of IVIG over 8 to 12 hours and aspirin (80 to 100 mg/kg four times a day) within the first 10 days of onset, with the aspirin dose reduced (3 to 5 mg/kg) after defervescence.[112,111] In Japan, the initial aspirin dose is 30 to 50 mg/kg. Aspirin is discontinued if no coronary artery abnormalities

have been detected by 6 weeks after onset. Aspirin has been used to decrease inflammation and to inhibit platelet aggregation, although it has no effect on the development of coronary artery aneurysms.[112] Children who take salicylates while they are experiencing active infection with varicella or influenza are at risk of Reye's syndrome, and it has been reported in patients taking high-dose aspirin for a prolonged period after KD.[113] It is unclear whether the low-dose treatment increases the risk of Reye's syndrome. Nevertheless, children who are taking salicylates long term should receive an annual influenza vaccine. Those who cannot take aspirin should be given dipyridamole or clopidogrel. About 10% to 15% of patients treated with aspirin and IVIG will have persistent fever and are at higher risk of developing coronary artery aneurysms.[114,115] It is common practice to give a second dose of IVIG.[103,116] If fever persists, other options used successfully include pulsed intravenous methylprednisolone (30 mg/kg once daily for 2 to 3 days), cyclophosphamide and prednisone, cyclosporine, plasmapheresis, and etanercept or infliximab (monoclonal antibodies to TNF-α).[103,112,117,118] In Japan, other agents used include ulinstatin (human trypsin inhibitor) and abciximab (platelet glycoprotein IIb/IIIa receptor inhibitor).[119-121] Despite earlier reports that corticosteroids may worsen outcomes, a recent report shows that adding methylprednisolone to IVIG and aspirin had a faster resolution of fever, more rapid improvement in markers of inflammation, and shorter length of hospitalization.[118]

About 20% of patients who develop coronary artery aneurysms during the acute disease will develop coronary stenosis and might need treatment for myocardial ischemia, including percutaneous transluminal balloon angioplasty, coronary artery stenting, percutaneous transluminal coronary rotational ablation, coronary artery bypass grafting, and even cardiac transplantation.[122-124]

KD may be difficult to diagnosis when the classic features are not present. However, the diagnosis should be suspected in any child with fever greater than 5 days without a source. There should be follow-up with asymptomatic patients for repeat two-dimensional echocardiography in 2 weeks and at 6 to 8 weeks after onset of disease to detect dysrhythmias, heart failure, valvular insufficiency, or myocarditis.

Impetigo

Impetigo is a superficial vesiculopustular infection localized to the subcorneal epidermis and is the most common bacterial infection in children.[125] The peak incidence is between the ages of 2 and 6 years. The most common pathogen found on children's skin is *S. aureus* (70% to 80%), followed by *S. pyogenes*.[125-127] Microscopic breaks in the epidermal barrier, such as trauma from scratching dermatitic skin, predispose to impetigo, as these organisms penetrate the skin and proliferate. A warm, humid climate favors the development of impetigo. Impetigo has a high attack rate, and its spread is enhanced by crowding, poor socioeconomic conditions, and poor personal hygiene.

Impetigo can be subdivided into nonbullous (70%) and bullous forms. Bullous impetigo results from invasion by phage group II *S. aureus* onto the skin. The epidermolytic toxin disrupts epidermal cell attachment. An ulcerative form called ecthyma is due to group A β-hemolytic streptococcus. Group B streptococci can cause impetigo in neonates. Recent data from hospitalized patients demonstrate that *S. aureus*, Enterococcus species, coagulase-negative staphylococci, *Escherichia coli*, and *Pseudomonas aeruginosa* are the most prevalent pathogens in skin and soft tissue infections.[128]

Clinical Presentation

Erosions covered by moist, honey-colored crusts are suggestive of impetigo.[129] Impetigo begins as small (1- to 2-mm) erythematous macules, which soon develop into vesicles or bullae with friable roofs surrounded by red borders that are quickly lost. The vesicles rupture easily, with release of a thin, cloudy, yellow fluid. The serous discharge subsequently dries, with formation of thick, soft, honey-colored crusts, the hallmark of impetigo (Fig. 126–21). They occur mostly on the face, nares, and extremities. The exudates spread easily by autoinoculation and produce satellite lesions adjacent to areas of impetigo or other parts of the body. Fever and regional lymphadenopathy may be present.

The term *bullous impetigo* has been used to describe lesions with a central moist crust and an outer zone of blister formation. The blister is translucent, with a flaccid roof that is easily shed, such that bullous impetigo may be seen as shallow erosions, like a "scalded skin," with an outer rim of desquamation (Fig. 126–22).[126]

The differential diagnosis is shown in Table 126–12.

Poststreptococcal glomerulonephritis may follow impetigo if nephritogenic strains of streptococci are involved. This most commonly occurs in children 3 to 7 years of age, and is seen 18 to 21 days after the onset of impetigo. Other complications include cellulitis, lymphangitis, suppurative lymphadenitis, SSSS, scarlet fever, rheumatic fever, osteomyelitis, septic arthritis, pneumonia, and sepsis.

Management

Antibiotics effective against *S. aureus* are indicated in cases of impetigo. Choices include cephalexin, dicloxacillin, and amoxicillin-calvunalate (Table 126–13). Topical mupirocin can be used for impetigo involving a small surface area and is as effective as oral therapy.[130] For penicillin-allergic patients, choices of antibiotics include azithromycin, clarithromycin, and clindamycin. If *Haemophilus influenzae* is suspected, possible antibiotics include cefotaxime, ceftriaxone, and cefuroxime, and in those allergic to penicillin, clindamycin can be administered. Removal of the crust and scrubbing skin lesions with antibacterial soap has not been shown to be effective.[126] Use antibiotics effective against MRSA if there is a high prevalence of this organism in the community.

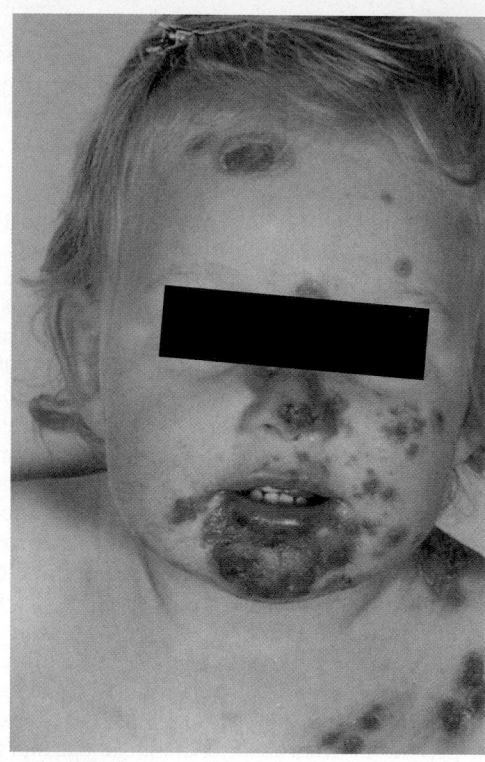

FIGURE 126–21. Erosions seen in impetigo.

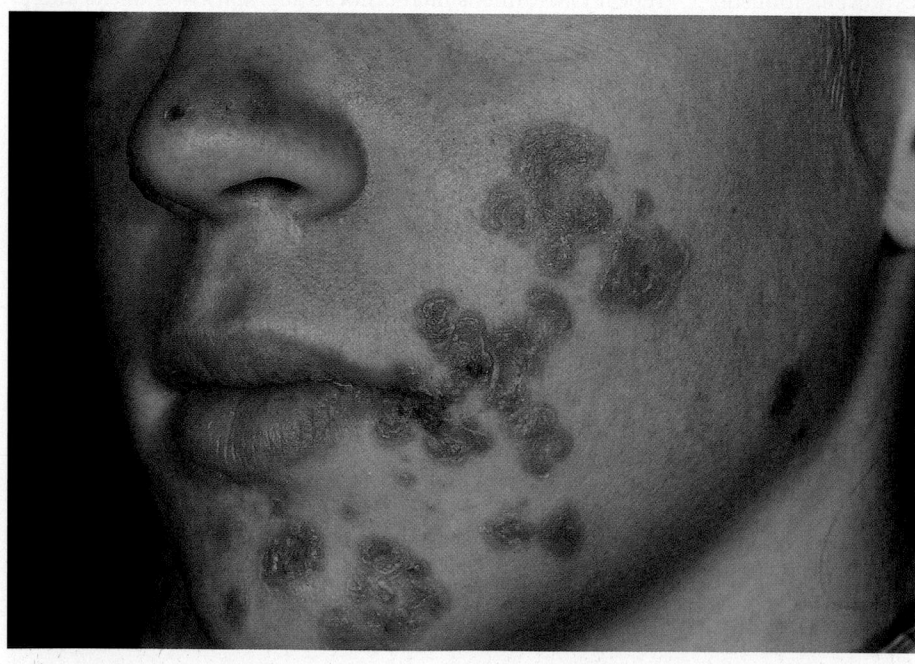

FIGURE 126–22. Bullous impetigo.

Table 126–12   Differential Diagnosis of Impetigo

Nummular dermatitis
Herpes simplex virus infection
Herpes zoster
Second-degree burns
Fixed drug eruptions
Linear Immunoglobulin A dermatosis
Bullous pemphigoid
Pemphigus vulgaris
Erythema multiforme
Staphylococcal scalded skin syndrome
Stevens-Johnson syndrome
Cellulitis
Lymphangitis
Thermal burns
Candidiasis
Scabies

Table 126–13   Antibiotics Effective against Impetigo

Antimicrobials	Dose
Cephalexin	25–100 mg/kg/day divided q6h PO
Amoxicillin–calvulanic acid	25–45 mg/kg/day divided q12h PO
Dicloxacillin	12.5–25 mg/kg/day divided q6h PO
Azithromycin	5 mg/kg/day qd PO
Clarithromycin	15 mg/kg/day bid PO
Clindamycin	25–40 mg/kg/day divided q6–8h PO/IV
Cefotaxime	100–200 mg/kg/day divided q6–8h IV/IM
Ceftriaxone	50–75 mg/kg/day divided q24h or q12h IV/IM
Cefuroxime	75–150 mg/kg/day divided q8h IV/IM
Mupirocin	Apply qd-tid
Trimethoprim [TMP]/ sulfamethoxazole	0–12 mg/kg/day of TMP divided bid

Abbreviations: IM, intramuscularly; IV, intravenously; PO, orally.

Hand washing with surgical soap and simple measures of good hygiene may reduce the likelihood of spread. A child with recurrent impetigo should be evaluated for carriage of *S. aureus*, especially in the nares, as this is the site of colonization three fourths of the time.[131] Nasal carriage of both methicillin-susceptible and methicillin-resistant strains of *S. aureus* has been eliminated in more than 90% of patients within 2 to 4 days through use of topical mupirocin three time daily.[132]

REFERENCES

1. Manders SM: Toxin-mediated streptococcal and staphylococcal disease. J Am Acad Dermatol 39:383–398, 1998.
2. Efstratiou A: Group A streptococci in the 1990s. J Antimicrob Chemother 45(Suppl):3S–12S, 2000.
3. Bialecji C, Feder HM Jr, Grant-Kels JM: The six classic childhood exanthems: a review and update. J Am Acad Dermatol 21:891–903, 1989.
4. Miller RA, Brancato F, Holmes KK: *Corynebacterium haemolyticum* as a cause of pharyngitis and scarlatiniform rash in young adults. Ann Intern Med 105:867–872, 1986.
5. Guven A: Hepatitis and hematuria in scarlet fever. Indian J Pediatr 69:985–986, 2002.
6. Randolph MF, Gerber MA, DeMeo KK, Wright L: Effect of antibiotic therapy on the clinical course of streptococcal pharyngitis. J Pediatr 106:870–875, 1985.
7. Bass JW, Person DA, Chan DS: Twice-daily oral penicillin for treatment of streptococcal pharyngitis: less is best. Pediatrics 105:423–424, 2000.
8. Pichichero ME: Cepahlosporins are superior to penicillin for treatment of streptococcal tonsillopharyngitis: is the difference worth it? Pediatr Infect Dis J 12:268–274, 1993.
9. Elias PM, Fritsch P, Epstein EH: Staphyloccocal scalded skin syndrome: clinical features, pathogenesis, and recent microbiological and biochemical developments. Arch Dermatol 113:207–219, 1977.
10. Sarai Y, Nakahara H, Ishikawa T, et al: A bacteriologic study on children with staphylococcal toxic epidermal necrolysis in Japan. Dermatologica 154:161–167, 1977.
11. Ridgway HB, Lowe NJ: Staphylococcal scalded skin syndrome in an adult with Hodgkin's disease. Arch Dermatol 115:589–590, 1979.
12. Cribier B, Piemont Y, Grosshans E: Staphylococcal scalded skin syndrome in adults: a clinical review illustrated with a new case. J Am Acad Dermatol 30:319–324, 1984.
*13. Patel GK, Finlay AY: Staphylococcal scalded skin syndrome: diagnosis and management. Am J Clin Dermatol 4:165–175, 2003.
14. Melish ME, Glasgow LA: Staphylococcal scalded skin syndrome: the expanded clinical syndrome. J Pediatr 78:958–967, 1971.
15. Ladhani S, Joannou CL, Lochrie DP, et al: Clinical, microbial, and biochemical aspects of exfoliative toxins causing staphylococcal scalded-skin syndrome. Clin Microbiol Rev 12:224–242, 1999.
16. Lina G, Gillet Y, Vandenesch F, et al: Toxin involvement in staphylococcal scalded skin syndrome. Clin Infect Dis 25:1369–1373, 1997.
17. Saiman L, Jakob K, Holmes KW, et al: Molecular epidemiology of staphylococcal scalded skin syndrome in premature infants. Pediatr Infect Dis J 17:329–334, 1998.
18. Ladhani S, Evans RW: Staphylococcal scalded skin syndrome. Arch Dis Child 78:85–88, 1998.
19. Loughead JL: Congenital staphylococcal scalded skin syndrome: report of a case. Pediatr Infect Dis J 11:413–414, 1992.
20. Schlievert PM, Kelly JA: Clindamycin-induced suppression of toxic-shock syndrome-associated exotoxins production. J Infect Dis 149:471, 1984.
21. Vergeront JM, Stolz SJ, Crass BA, et al: Prevalence of serum antibody to staphylococcal enterotoxin F among Wisconsin residents: implication for toxic shock syndrome. J Infect Dis 148:692–698, 1983.
22. Fjlertsen T, Jensen A, Lester A, Rosdahl VT: Epidemiology of toxic shock shock syndrome toxin-1 production in *Staphylococcus aureus* strains in Denmark 1959 and 1990. Scand J Infect Dis 26:599–604, 1994.
23. Kain KC, Schulzer M, Chow AW: Clinical spectrum of nonmenstrual toxic shock syndrome (TSS): comparison with menstrual TSS by multivariate discriminant analyses. Clin Infect Dis J 16:100–106, 1993.
24. Reingold AL: Nonmenstrual toxic shock syndrome: the growing picture. JAMA 249:932, 1983.
25. Chesney PJ, Davis JP, Purdy WK, et al: Clinical manifestations of toxic shock syndrome. JAMA 246:741–748, 1981.
26. Chesney PJ: Clinical aspects and spectrum of illness of toxic shock syndrome: overview. Rev Infect Dis 11(Suppl 1):S1–S7, 1989.
27. Rosene KA, Copass MK, Kasner LS, et al: Persistent neuropsychological sequelae of toxic shock syndrome. Ann Intern Med 96:865–870, 1982.
28. Hurwitz RM, Rivera HP, Gooch MH, et al: Toxic shock syndrome or toxic epidermal necrolysis? Case reports showing clinical similarity and histologic separation. J Am Acad Dermatol 7:246–254, 1982.
29. Bach MC: Dermatologic signs in toxic shock syndrome—clues to diagnosis. J Am Acad Dermatol 8:343–347, 1983.
30. Chesney PJ, Crass BA, Polyak MB, et al: Toxic shock syndrome: management and long-term sequelae. Ann Intern Med 96:847–851, 1982.
31. Reingold AL, Dan BB, Shands KN, Broome CV: Toxic-shock syndrome not associated with menstruation: a review of 54 cases. Lancet 1:1–4, 1982.
32. Annane D, Clair B, Salomon J: Managing toxic shock syndrome with antibiotics. Expert Opin Pharmacother 5:1701–1710, 2004.
33. Herold BC, Immergluck LC, Maranan MC, et al: Community-acquired methicillin-resistant *Staphylococcal aureus* in children. Pediatr Infect Dis J 279:593–598, 1998.

*Selected readings.

34. Tack DA, Fleishcer A Jr, McMichael A, Feldman S: The epidemic of tinea capitis disproportionately affects school-aged African Americans. Pediatr Dermatol 1:75, 1999.

35. Bonventre PF, Thompson MR, Adinolfi LE, et al: Neutralization of toxic shock syndrome toxin-1 by monoclonal antibodies in vitro and in vivo. Infect Immun 56:135–141, 1988.

36. Best GK, Scott DF, Kling JM, et al: Protection of rabbit in an infection model of toxic shock syndrome (TSS) by a TSS toxin-1-specific monoclonal antibody. Infect Immun 56:998–999, 1988.

37. Todd JK, Ressman M, Caston SA, et al: Corticosteroid therapy for patients with toxic shock syndrome. JAMA 252:399–402, 1984.

38. Aly R, Hay RJ, Del Palacio A, Galimberti R: Epidemiology of tinea capitis. Med Mycol 38(Suppl 1):S183–S188, 2000.

39. Frieden IJ: Tinea capitis: asymptomatic carriage of infection. Pediatr Infect Dis J 18:186–190, 1999.

40. Philpot C: Some aspects of the epidemiology of tinea. Mycopathologia 62:3–13, 1977.

41. Babel DE, Baugmans A: Evaluation of the adult carrier stage in juvenile tinea capitis caused by *Trichophyton tonsurans*. J Am Acad Dermatol 21:1209–1212, 1989.

42. Hubbard TW: The predictive value of symptoms in diagnosing childhood tinea capitis. Arch Pediatr Adolesc Med 153:1150–1153, 1999.

43. Pomeranz AJ, Sabnis SS: Tinea capitis: epidemiology, diagnosis, and management strategies. Paediatr Drugs 4:779–783, 2002.

44. Honig PJ, Caputo GL, Leyden JJ, et al: Treatment of kerions. Pediatr Dermatol 11:69–71, 1994.

44a. Fuller LC, Child FJ, Midgley G, Higgins EM: Diagnosis and management of scalp ringworm. BMJ 326:539–541, 2003.

45. Abdel-Rahman SM, Nahata MC, Powell DA: Response to initial griseofulvin therapy in pediatric patients with tinea capitis. Ann Pharmacother 31:406–410, 1997.

46. Gupta AK, Adam P, Dlova N, et al: Therapeutic options for the treatment of tinea capitis caused by *Trichophyton* species: griseofulvin versus the new oral antifungal agents, terbinafine, itraconazole, and fluconazole. Pediatr Dermatol 18:433–438, 2001.

47. Chan YC, Friedlander SF: New treatment for tinea capitis. Curr Opin Infect Dis 17:97–103, 2004.

47a. Gupta AK, Cooper EA, Ryder JE, Nicol KA: Optimal management of fungal infections of the skin, hair, and nails. Am J Clin Dermatol 5:225–237, 2004.

48. Allen H, Honig PJ, Leyden JJ, McGinley KJ: Selenium sulfide: adjunctive therapy for tinea capitis. Pediatrics 69:81–83, 1982.

49. Keipert JA: Beneficial effect of corticosteroid therapy in *Microsporum canis* kerion. Australas J Dermatol 25:127–130, 1984.

50. Hussain I, Muzaffar F, Rashid T, et al: A randomized, comparative trial of treatment of kerion celsi with griseofulvin plus oral prednisolone vs. griseofulvin alone. Med Mycol 37:97–99, 1999.

51. Laude TA, Shah BR, Lynfield Y: Tinea capitis in Brooklyn. Am J Dis Child 136:1047–1050, 1982.

52. Faergemann J, Mörk NJ, Hagland A, Ödegård A: A multicenter (double-blind) comparative study to assess the safety and efficacy of fluconazole and griseofulvin in the treatment of tinea corporis and tinea cruris. Br J Dermatol 136:575–577, 1997.

53. Bronson DM, Desai DR, Barsky S, Foley SM: An epidemic of infection with *Trichophyton tonsurans* revealed in a 20-year survey of fungal infections in Chicago. J Am Acad Dermatol 8:322–330, 1983.

54. Smith KJ, Neafie RC, Skelton HG 3rd, et al: Majocchi's granuloma. J Cutan Dermatol 18:28–35, 1991.

55. Jones HE, Reinhardt JH, Rinaldi MG: Acquired immunity to dermatophytes. Arch Dermatol 109:840–848, 1974.

56. Raynolds RD, Boiko S, Lucky AW: Exacerbation of tinea corporis during treatment with 1% clotrimazole/0.05% betamethasone diproprionate (Lotrisone). Am J Dis Child 145:1224–1225, 1991.

57. Solomon BA, Lee WL, Green SC, et al: Modification of neutrophils function by naftifine. Br J Dermatol 128:393–398, 1993.

58. Terragni L, Lasagni A, Oriani A: Pityriasis versicolor of the face. Mycoses 34:345–347, 1991.

59. Faergemann J: Pityrosporum species as a cause of allergy and infection. Allergy 54:413–419, 1999.

59a. Gupta AK, Batra R, Bluhm R, Faergemann J: Pityriasis versicolor. Dermatol Clin 21:413–429, 2003.

60. Diven DG: An overview of poxviruses. J Am Acad Dermatol 44:1–16, 2001.

61. Mandel MJ, Lewis RJ: Molluscum contagiosum of the newborn. Br J Dermatol 84:370–372, 1970.

62. Kipping HF: Molluscum dermatitis. Arch Dermatol 103:106–107, 1971.

63. Thompson CH: Identification and typing of molluscum contagiosum virus in clinical specimens by polymerase chain reaction. J Med Virol 53:205–211, 1997.

64. Brown ST, Nalley JF, Kraus SJ: Molluscum contagiosum. Sex Transm Dis 8:227–234, 1981.

65. Weston WL, Lane AT: Should molluscum be treated? Pediatrics 65:865, 1980.

66. Moed L, Shwayder TA, Chang MW: Cantharidin revisited: a blistering defense of an ancient medicine. Arch Dermatol 137:1357–1360, 2001.

67. Niizeki K, Hashimoto K: Treatment of molluscum contagiosum with silver nitrate paste. Pediatr Dermatol 16:395–397, 1999.

68. Silverberg NB, Sidbury R, Mancini AJ: Childhood molluscum contagiosum: experience with cantharidin therapy in 300 patients. J Am Acad Dermatol 43:503–507, 2000.

68a. Bikowski JB Jr: Molluscum contagiosum: the need for physician intervention and new treatment options. Cutis 73:202–206, 2004.

69. Davies EG, Thrasher A, Lacey K, Harper J: Topical cidofovir for severe molluscum contagiosum. Lancet 353:2042, 1999.

70. Zabawski EJ Jr: A review of topical and intralesional cidofovir. Dermatol Online J 6:3, 2000.

71. Meadows KP, Tyring A, Pavia AT, Rallis TM: Resolution of recalcitrant molluscum contagiosum virus lesions in human immunodeficiency virus infected patients treated with cidofovir. Arch Dermatol 133:987–990, 1997.

72. Yashar SS, Shamiri B: Oral cimetidine treatment of molluscum contagiosum. Pediatr Dermatol 16:493, 1999.

73. Hicks CB, Myers SA, Giner J: Resolution of intractable molluscum contagiosum in a human immunodeficiency virus-infected patient after institution of antiretroviral therapy with ritonavir. Clin Infect Dis 24:1023–1025, 1997.

74. Hurni MA, Bohlen L, Furrer H, Braathen LR: Complete regression of giant molluscum contagiosum lesions in an HIV-infected patient following combined antiretroviral therapy with saquinavir, zidovudine and lamivudine. AIDS 11:1784–1785, 1997.

75. Betlloch I, Pinazo I, Mestre F, et al: Molluscum contagiosum in human immunodeficiency virus infection: response to zidovudine. Int J Dermatol 28:351–352, 1989.

76. Theos AU, Cummins R, Silverberg NB, Paller AS: Effectiveness of imiguimid cream 5% for treating childhood molluscum contagiosum in a double-blind, randomized pilot trial. Cutis 74:134–138, 2004.

77. Nelson MR, Chard S, Barton SE: Intralesional interferon for the treatment of recalcitrant molluscum contagiosum in HIV antibody-positive individuals—a preliminary report. Int J STD AIDS 6:351–352, 1995.

78. Janniger CK, Schwartz RA: Molluscum contagiosum in children. Cutis 52:194–196, 1993.

79. Yoshinaga IG, Conrado LA, Schainberg SC, Grinblat M: Recalcitrant molluscum contagiosum in a patient with AIDS: combined treatment with CO_2 laser, trichloroacetic acid, and pulsed dye laser. Lasers Surg Med 27:291–294, 2000.

80. Scott PM: Curettage for molluscum contagiosum. JAAPA 15:53–54, 2002.

81. Ronnerfalt L, Fransson J, Wahlgren CF: EMLA cream provides rapid relief for the curettage of molluscum contagiosum in children with atopic dermatitis without causing serious application-site reactions. Pediatr Dermatol 15:309–312, 1998.

82. Parsons JM: Pityriasis rosea update: 1986. J Am Acad Dermatol 15:159–167, 1986.

83. Drago F, Ranieri E, Malaguti F, et al: Human herpesvirus 7 in patients with pityriasis rosea: electron microscopy investigations and polymerase chain reaction in mononuclear cells, plasma and skin. Dermatology 195:374–378, 1997.

84. Miranda SB, Lupi O, Lucas E: Vesicular pityriasis rosea: response to erythromycin treatment. J Eur Acad Dermatol Venerol 18:622–625, 2004.

85. Friedman SJ: Pityriasis rosea with erythema-multiforme-like lesions. J Am Acad Dermatol 17:135–136, 1987.

86. Pireson JC, Dijkstra JW, Elston DM: Purpuric pityriasis rosea. J Am Acad Dermatol 28:1021, 1993.

87. Imamura S, Ozaki M, Oguchi M, et al: Atypical pityriasis rosea. Dermatologica 171:474–477, 1985.

88. Ahmed I, Charles-Holmes R: Localized pityriasis rosea. Clin Exp Dermatol 25:624–626, 2000.

89. Vidimos AT, Camisa C: Tongue and cheek: oral lesions in pityriasis rosea. Cutis 50:276–280, 1992.

90. Sharma PK, Tadav TP, Gautam RK, et al: Erythromycin in pityriasis rosea: a double-blind placebo-controlled clinical trial. J Am Acad Dermatol 42:241–244, 2000.

91. Leenutaphong V, Jiamton S: UVB phototherapy for pityriasis rosea: a bilateral comparison study. J Am Acad Dermatol 33:996–999, 1995.

92. Kawasaki T: General review and problems in Kawasaki disease. Jpn Heart J 36:1–12, 1995.

93. Taubert KA, Rowley AH, Shulman ST: Nationwide survey of Kawasaki disease in children. Circulation 87:1776–1780, 1993.

94. Melish ME, Hicks RM, Larson EJ: Mucocutaneous lymph node syndrome in the United States. Am J Dis Child 130:599–607, 1976.

95. Chang LY, Chang IS, Lu CY, et al; Kawasaki Disease Research Group: Epidemiologic features of Kawasaki disease in Taiwan, 1996–2002. Pediatrics 114:e678–e682, 2004.

96. Rozo JC, Jefferies JL, Eidem BW, Cook PJ: Kawasaki disease in the adult: a case report and review of the literature. Tex Heart Inst J 31:160–164, 2004.

96a. Burns JC, Glodé MP: Kawasaki syndrome. Lancet 364:533–544, 2004.

97. Tomita S, Chung K, Mas M, et al: Peripheral gangrene associated with Kawasaki disease. Clinical Infect Dis 14:121–126, 1992.

98. Freeman AF, Crawford SE, Finn LS, et al: Inflammatory pulmonary nodules in Kawasaki disease. Pediatr Pulmonol 36:102–106, 2003.

99. Palazzi DL, McClain KL, Kaplan SL: Hemophagocytic syndrome after Kawasaki disease. Pediatr Infect Dis J 22:663–666, 2003.

100. Beiser AS, Takahashi M, Baker AL, et al: A predictive instrument for coronary artery aneurysms in Kawasaki disease. Am J Cardiol 81:1116–1120, 1998.

101. Nakamura Y, Yashiro M, Uehara R, et al: Use of laboratory data to identify risk factors of giant coronary aneurysms due to Kawasaki disease. Pediatr Int 46:33–38, 2004.

102. Hwong TM, Arifi AA, Wan IY, et al: Rupture of a giant coronary artery aneurysm due to Kawasaki disease. Ann Thorac Surg 78:693–695, 2004.

*103. Newburger JW, Takahashi M, Gerber MA, et al; Committee on Rheumatic Fever, Endocarditis, and Kawasaki Disease, Council on Cardiovascular Disease in the Young, American Heart Association: Diagnosis, treatment, and long-term management of Kawasaki disease: a statement for health professionals from the Committee on Rheumatic Fever, Endocarditis, and Kawasaki Disease, Council on Cardiovascular Disease in the Young, American Heart Association. Pediatrics 114:1708–1733, 2004. (Published erratum in: Pediatrics 115:1118, 2005)

104. Naoe S, Takahashi K, Masuda H, Tanaka N: Kawasaki disease: with particular emphasis on arterial lesions. Acta Pathol Jpn 41:785–797, 1991.

105. Hicks RV, Melish ME: Kawasaki syndrome: rheumatic complaints and analysis of salicylate therapy. Arthritis Rheum 22:621–622, 1979.

106. Newburger JW, Burns JC, Beiser AS, Loscalzo J: Altered lipid profile after Kawasaki syndrome. Circulation 84:625–631, 1991.

107. Kim M, Kim K: Elevation of cardiac troponin I in the acute stage of Kawasaki disease. Pediatr Cardiol 20:184–188, 1999.

108. Danias PG, Stuber M, Botnar RM, et al: Coronary MR angiography clinical applications and potential for imaging coronary artery disease. Magn Reson Imaging Clin N Am 11:81–99, 2003.

109. Sato K, Ouchi K, Taki M: Yersinia pseudotuberculosis infection in children resembling Izumi fever and Kawasaki syndrome. Pediatr Infect Dis 2:123–126, 1983.

110. Newburger JW, Takahashi M, Beiser AS, et al: A single intravenous infusion of gamma globulin as compared with four infusions in the treatment of acute Kawasaki syndrome. N Engl J Med 324:1633–1639, 1991.

111. Brogan PA, Bose A, Burgner D, et al: Kawasaki disease: an evidence based approach to diagnosis, treatment, and proposals for future research. Arch Dis Child 86:286–290, 2002.

112. Al-Mayouf SM: The use of corticosteroid therapy in refractory Kawasaki patients. Clin Rheumatol 23:11–13, 2004.

113. Lee JH, Hung HY, Huang FY: Kawasaki disease with Reye syndrome: report of one case. Zhonghua Min Guo Xiao Er Ke Yi Xue Hui Za Zhi 33:67–71, 1992.

114. Burns JC, Capparelli EV, Brown JA, et al: Intravenous gamma globulin treatment and retreatment in Kawasaki disease. US/Canadian Kawasaki Syndrome Study Group. Pediatr Infect Dis J 17:1144–1148, 1998.

115. Durongpisitkul K, Soongswang J, Laohaprasitiporn D, et al: Immunoglobulin failure and retreatment in Kawasaki disease. Pediatr Cardiol 24:145–148, 2003.

116. Miura M, Ohki H, Tsuchihashi T, et al: Coronary risk factors in Kawasaki disease treated with additional gammaglobulin. Arch Dis Child 89:776–780, 2004.

117. Wright DA, Newburger JW, Baker A, Sundel RP: Treatment of immune globulin-resistant Kawasaki disease with pulsed doses of corticosteroids. J Pediatr 123:146–149, 1996.

118. Weiss JE, Eberhard BA, Chowdhurry D, Gottlieb BS: Infliximab as a novel therapy for refractory Kawasaki disease. J Rheumatol 31:808–810, 2004.

119. Zaitsu M, Hamasaki Y, Tashiro K, et al: Ulinastatin, an elastase inhibitor, inhibits the increased mRNA expression of prostaglandin H_2 synthetase-type 2 in Kawasaki disease. J Infect Dis 181:1101–1109, 2000.

120. Williams RV, Wilke VM, Tani LY, Minich LL: Does abciximab enhance regression of coronary aneurysms resulting from Kawasaki disease? Pediatrics 109:e4, 2002.

121. Sundel RP, Baker AL, Fulton DR, Newburger JW: Corticosteroids in the initial treatment of Kawasaki disease: report of a randomized trial. J Pediatr 142:611–616, 2003.

122. Lee JY, Song JY, Kim SJ, et al: Coronary rotational ablation for calcific coronary artery stenosis in a young child. Int J Cardiol 99:349–350, 2005.

123. Tsuda E, Kitamura S; Cooperative Study of Japan: National survey of coronary artery bypass grafting for coronary stenosis caused by Kawasaki disease in Japan. Circulation 110:(11 Suppl 1):II61–II66, 2004.

124. Iliadis EA, Duvernoy CS: Stent placement for coronary stenosis in Kawasaki disease: case report and literature review. J Interv Cardiol 15:29–31, 2002.

125. Hayden GF: Skin diseases encountered in a pediatric clinic: a one-year prospective study. Am J Dis Child 139:36–38, 1985.

126. Brook I, Frazier EH, Yeager JK: Microbiology of nonbullous impetigo. Pediatr Dermatol 14:192–195, 1997.

127. Darmstadt GL: Oral antibiotic therapy for uncomplicated bacterial skin infections in children. Pediatr Infect Dis J 16:227–240, 1997.

128. Hogan P: Pediatric dermatology: impetigo. Aust Fam Physician 27:735–736, 1998.

129. Jones ME, Karlowsky JA, Draghi DC, et al: Epidemiology and antibiotic susceptibility of bacteria causing skin and soft tissue infections in USA and Europe: a guide to appropriate antimicrobial therapy. Int J Antimicrob Agents 22:406–419, 2003.

130. Bass JW, Chan DS, Creamer KM, et al: Comparison of oral cephalexin, topical mupirocin and topical bacitracin for the treatment of impetigo. Pediatr Infect Dis J 16:708–710, 1997.

131. Dancer SJ, Noble WC: Nasal, axillary, and perineal carriage of Staphylococcus aureus among women: identification of strains producing epidermolytic toxin. J Clin Pathol 44:681–684, 1991.

132. Doebbeling BN, Breneman DL, Neu HC, et al: Elimination of Staphylococcus aureus nasal carriage in health care workers: analysis of six clinical trials with calcium mupirocin ointment. Clin Infect Dis 17:466–474, 1993.

133. Burns JC, Joffe L, Sergeant RA, Glode MP: Anterior uveitis associated with Kawasaki syndrome. Pediatr Infect Dis 4:258–261, 1985.

Chapter 127

Sickle Cell Disease

Timothy G. Givens, MD

Introduction and Background

Sickle cell disease refers to a group of disorders resulting from mutations in the hemoglobin gene that can lead to deformation of the red blood cell (RBC) into a crescent, or sickle, shape. Hemoglobin S is formed when valine replaces glutamine at the sixth amino acid position of the beta chain of hemoglobin. Patients who inherit hemoglobin S in a homozygous autosomal recessive fashion (Hb SS) have sickle cell anemia, while those who are heterozygous have sickle trait (Hb AS).[1]

Sickle cell disease primarily affects persons of African, Mediterranean, Indian, and Middle Eastern descent. In the United States, African Americans are most affected, with approximately 0.15% having sickle cell anemia (Hb SS) and approximately 8% having sickle trait (Hb AS).[1,2] There is also a high incidence of sickle cell disease in Hispanic Americans from the Caribbean, Central America, and South America.[3,4] Children born in many hospitals in the United States are routinely screened in the neonatal period, and antenatal diagnosis is becoming more prevalent in at-risk populations. However, an index of suspicion is necessary when treating patients born outside U.S. hospitals or when results of the neonatal screen are unavailable.

Recognition and Approach

As the abnormal hemoglobin molecule is deoxygenated, it irreversibly forms a rigid polymer within the RBC, distorting its configuration. As a consequence, occlusion of small blood vessels, increased blood viscosity and concomitant stasis, and further tissue hypoxia follow. Sickle cell patients therefore develop symptoms related to impaired perfusion and ischemia, such as pain, impaired mental status, neurologic deficits, and tissue engorgement.

The rate and extent of sickling is related to three factors: the degree of cellular hypoxia, the hemoglobin concentration within the erythrocyte, and the presence (or absence) of fetal hemoglobin (Hb F).[5] Therapy for sickle cell disease is often directed at these three variables.

Clinical Presentations and Important Clinical Features

Complications of sickle cell disease present in one of four general ways: vaso-occlusive crisis, acute splenic sequestration crisis, acute aplastic crisis, and infection/sepsis.

Vaso-occlusive Crisis

Vaso-occlusive phenomena can occur in any tissue or organ system, as the microvasculature becomes clogged with sickled erythrocytes. Most commonly, this results in pain. As occlusion of small vessels occurs, tissue hypoxemia results, leading to further sickling in a cascade effect. Interruption of this vicious cycle with hydration, oxygen, and analgesia is the goal of therapy for vaso-occlusive pain crisis.

Virtually all patients with sickle cell disease experience acute pain to some degree. Coping abilities vary between patients, yet epidemiologic studies indicate that patients who seek medical care for pain have lower levels of fetal hemoglobin (Hb F) and higher steady state hemoglobin levels.[6] To expeditiously evaluate and manage a painful episode can be difficult. Painful crises may mimic a number of other disease states. A careful history and physical examination is key. The most frequently affected body regions are the lumbosacral spine, knee, shoulder, elbow, and femur. At times, pain episodes may be accompanied by localized tenderness, erythema, warmth, and swelling, raising a concern for osteomyelitis. Joint effusions are particularly common when the knees and elbows are involved. Often, however, there are no correlative physical findings, save for mild tachycardia and hypertension. The clinician must exercise caution not to dismiss all pain in patients with sickle cell disease as a vaso-occlusive crisis, as in doing so, one may overlook serious underlying pathology. In light of the range of clinical findings of vaso-occlusive pain crises, it is best to proceed conservatively in the emergency setting, taking the patient's pain at face value and yet maintaining an attitude of critical discernment for underlying disease.

Hand-Foot Syndrome

Often the first episode of vaso-occlusive pain occurs in infants and toddlers as acute swelling of the hands and feet (dactylitis).[1] It may provide the first indication that a child has sickle cell disease in the event that he or she has escaped detection by neonatal screening.[7] Hand-foot syndrome typically occurs symmetrically, involving the metacarpals and/or metatarsals. It may be unaccompanied by hematologic or radiographic abnormalities. When fever is present, osteomyelitis is difficult to exclude and may require a bone scan or MRI. Hand-foot syndrome should be treated as any other pain crisis, with regularly scheduled analgesia.

Acute Chest Syndrome

When the microcirculation of certain organ systems is compromised, life-threatening complications may result. One of these is acute chest syndrome, a leading cause of morbidity and mortality among patients with sickle cell disease. Pulmonary sequestration of erythrocytes and sickling leads to infarction of lung tissue and may progress to a full-blown acute respiratory distress syndrome picture. As with pain crises, the risk of developing acute chest syndrome is higher in sickle cell patients who are younger, have a lower concentration of Hb F, have a higher steady state hemoglobin concentration, or have a higher steady state leukocyte count.[8] Clinically, acute chest syndrome is a common manifestation of a variety of pathologic processes, which may be difficult to differentiate in a patient with Hb SS disease. Findings may include fever, cough, chest pain, dyspnea, productive cough or hemoptysis, hypoxia, leukocytosis, and new pulmonary infiltrates on chest radiograph. Hence, admission diagnoses in those patients found ultimately to have acute chest syndrome include fever, anemia, infection, nonpulmonary vaso-occlusive events, abdominal pain, asthma, heart failure, and orthopedic conditions.[9,10] In children, infection is somewhat more likely as a cause of acute chest syndrome than it is in adults, though often no etiologic agent is identified. When a pathogen is identified, the leading three organisms implicated are *Chlamydia, Mycoplasma,* and respiratory syncytial virus[10] (Table 127–1). While there are other minor differences in the presentation of acute chest syndrome between adults and children, these do not appreciably impact its management.

Cerebrovascular Accident

Cerebrovascular accidents (CVAs) are another serious complication of vaso-occlusive sickling. Strokes are more common in children with homozygous (Hb SS) disease, occurring in about 11% of patients by the age of 20 years.[11,12] Three quarters of CVAs are infarcts, and less than 10% are preceded by transient ischemic attacks. An association between recent and frequent episodes of acute chest syndrome and risk of CVA exists in children, perhaps because recurrent damage to the endothelium of the pulmonary vascular bed predicts

Table 127–1	Causes of Acute Chest Syndrome	
Cause	0–9 years N = 329 patients (%)	10–19 years N = 188 patients (%)
Infarction without known precipitant	50 (15.9%)	43 (22.9%)
Viral	36 (10.9%)	5 (2.7%)
Mycoplasma	29 (8.8%)	7 (3.7%)
Fat embolism ± infection	24 (7.3%)	16 (8.5%)
Chlamydia	19 (5.8%)	15 (8%)
Mixed infections	16 (4.9%)	3 (1.6%)
Bacteria	13 (4%)	12 (6.4%)
Mycobacterium (*tuberculosis* & *avium* complex)	3 (0.9%)	0
Unknown*	129 (41.3%)	79 (42%)

*The cause of episodes for which some or all of the diagnostic data were incomplete and no etiologic agent was identified was considered to be unknown.
From Vichinsky EP, Neumayr LD, Earles AN, et al; National Acute Chest Syndrome Study Group: Causes and outcomes of the acute chest syndrome in sickle cell disease. N Engl J Med 342:1855–1865, 2000.

damage to cerebral vasculature.[11,13] The diagnosis of stroke in patients with sickle cell disease can be challenging. Clinical signs are nonspecific and often subtle. Less than 10% of patients present with classic CVA symptoms, and headaches are common in sickle cell patients regardless of central nervous system involvement. Any sickle cell patient with focal neurologic signs, including seizure or hemiparesis, requires an intracranial imaging study and emergent intervention to limit ischemic injury (see Chapter 44, Central Nervous System Vascular Disorders).

Priapism

Males with sickle cell disease are susceptible to priapism, the presence of a persistent and often painful penile erection. Priapism may occur as a sustained episode lasting hours to weeks or as a series of repetitive, reversible erections with intervening detumescence ("stuttering"). Acute attacks of priapism sometimes follow sexual activity, but generally have no known precipitating event. In addition to the immediate effects of pain, cumulative ischemic damage with either a prolonged erection or recurrent priapism episodes over time puts the patient who suffers these episodes at risk of sexual dysfunction and impotence. Pediatric patients with priapism are more likely to respond to conservative measures such as analgesia and hydration, while management in adult patients usually requires a more aggressive approach, including surgery (see Chapter 89, Penile and Testicular Disorders).[3]

Acute Abdominal Pain

One of the most perplexing scenarios is the patient with sickle cell disease and acute abdominal pain. Intra-abdominal sickling and vaso-occlusion may occur and be difficult to distinguish from other myriad causes of intra-abdominal pathology. Analgesic therapy should not be withheld while pursuing a diagnosis in sickle cell patients with abdominal pain. Biliary colic and acute cholecystitis due to gallstones should always be considered. Sickled RBCs undergo chronic hemolysis, leading to hyperbilirubinemia and formation of bilirubin-containing gallstones. Patients are often asymptomatic, but the gallstones may cause abdominal pain due to obstruction or inflammation. The resultant right upper quadrant pain may be indistinguishable from intrahepatic sickling or pain due to lower lobe pneumonia. If gallstones are present, however, abdominal pain coupled with fever, nausea, and vomiting point to cholecystitis, and should be managed appropriately (see Chapter 85, Gallbladder Disorders).

Acute Sequestration Crisis

Young children with Hb SS disease whose spleens have not yet experienced recurrent infarctions and resultant fibrosis, as well as those with other hemoglobin S syndromes with spleens that remain enlarged into adult life, may undergo obstruction of splenic sinusoids with sickled cells. This may lead to sudden trapping of large amounts of blood and a massively enlarged spleen. The patient rapidly develops a precipitous drop in hemoglobin level and signs of circulatory collapse, requiring prompt intervention to reverse hypovolemic shock. While a specific causative agent is often hard to identify, infection is a frequent precipitant. Acute sequestration usually occurs in patients with Hb SS after 6 months of age (due to the protective effects of Hb F prior to this) and is rare after the age of 2 years.[3,7] It is a leading cause of morbidity and mortality among sickle cell patients in this age group.

Acute sequestration may also occur in the liver. Clinical signs include hepatomegaly and tenderness to palpation of the right upper quadrant, hyperbilirubinemia, anemia, and reticulocytosis. The liver is not as distensible as the spleen, however, so this presentation is seldom accompanied by cardiovascular collapse.

Acute Aplastic Crisis

The erythrocytes of patients with sickle cell disease have a shortened half-life (15 to 50 days) compared with normal erythrocytes (120 days). In the usual state, patients with Hb SS compensate for this by increasing marrow production of erythrocytes six- to eightfold.[1] However, any agent that can cause marrow suppression places the patient with sickle cell disease at risk of developing a profound anemia, as the hemoglobin concentration steadily falls by 10% to 15% per day without a compensatory reticulocytosis. Typically this phenomenon follows infection with parvovirus B19, although toxins, folate deficiency, and other viral and bacterial infections have been associated with erythropoietic suppression. While pallor and tachycardia are common features of an aplastic crisis, bone pain and hemodynamic instability are not. Patients may present with vague, nonspecific symptoms such as fever, headache, nausea and vomiting, fatigue, and dyspnea. The diagnosis is confirmed by noting the correlative laboratory values of anemia and absent reticulocyte production (i.e., reticulocyte count < 3%).

Infection/Sepsis

By far the most common cause of death in children with sickle hemoglobinopathies is infection. This is primarily related to splenic dysfunction. Both of the spleen's immunologic functions—removal of particulate matter from the intravascular space, and antibody synthesis—are impaired in sickle cell disease.[1] Additionally, the serum of patients with sickle cell disease is lacking in heat-labile opsonizing activity related to an abnormality of the properidin pathway, which is specific for phagocytosis of pneumococci.[14,15] Hence, Hb SS patients are at increased risk of sepsis from encapsulated organisms, particularly pneumococci. Outcomes for patients with sickle cell disease have been enhanced through the use of active immunization against *Streptococcus pneumoniae* and *Haemophilus influenzae* and through the use of prophylactic penicillin. Prophylactic penicillin is efficacious in reducing the incidence of pneumococcal sepsis and meningitis in children less than 5 years of age. After this age, this therapy shows no clinically beneficial effect and it is often discontinued.[16] Prophylactic penicillin should be continued indefinitely in children with prior pneumococcal sepsis, as they are at much higher risk of recurrent sepsis.[17] In spite of prophylactic penicillin use, the risk of sepsis is still great (see Chapter 13, Sepsis).

Management

Patients with sickle cell disease, like other emergency department patients, should first and foremost have their airway, breathing, and circulatory status addressed. Complications such as sequestration or sepsis can occur precipitously and become rapidly severe and even life-threatening. Frequent assessment of the patient is necessary to note subtle changes in physiologic status. Do not attribute tachycardia to baseline anemia in Hb SS patients and remember that, in the youngest patients, compensatory vasoconstriction can mask volume depletion and maintain blood pressure in the face of shock. In addition, ancillary tools for assessment of physiologic status may provide deceptive information. Pulse oximetry is not an accurate predictor of actual oxygen saturation in vaso-occlusive crisis, with true oxygen saturation averaging 5% higher than values measured by pulse oximetry.[18,19]

Vaso-occlusive Crisis

A complete history will catalog the frequency and nature of prior pain crises, medications required to control pain crises in the past and current medication use, and baseline laboratory values. Physical examination must be thorough and target the identification of acute infection or other precipitants of a vaso-occlusive crisis. The development of new neurologic signs or symptoms is of particular concern and mandates appropriate imaging studies. Laboratory tests beyond a baseline hemoglobin determination add little to management in patients who present with typical sickle crisis symptoms.[20,21] For patients with unusual presentations (e.g., worsening anemia, signs of joint or bone infection, fever, increased jaundice, or chest or abdominal pain) additional testing is generally required. Some clinicians routinely obtain a chest radiograph to screen for infection, though this practice in low-risk patients (i.e., those without fever, chills, or pulmonary signs or symptoms) is not supported by data.[22]

The cornerstones of therapy for vaso-occlusive episodes are hydration and provision of analgesia. Initial intravenous fluid is usually isotonic saline, particularly in patients with evidence of impaired circulation. There are theoretical benefits to use of hypotonic fluids, in that hyponatremia is known to interfere with the polymerization of hemoglobin S. One study demonstrated that hyponatremia induced by using desmopressin (DDAVP) in combination with a low-sodium diet and a diuretic correlated with a decline in the frequency and duration of painful crises.[23] However, there are no data to support the routine use of hypotonic fluids during acute vaso-occlusive crisis.

Analgesia is the other arm of mainstream therapy. Achieving adequate pain control while avoiding the complications of analgesic agents, such as opioids, is a clinical challenge. This is particularly true in pediatric patients who may not have developed tolerance to such agents. Oral analgesics are adequate for most patients with mild to moderate pain. Ibuprofen or acetaminophen with or without codeine is often adequate to control pain in children who are not yet of school age. Massage and local heat may also provide ancillary relief. Parenteral medications are generally reserved for those who cannot tolerate oral therapy or who are in severe pain. Ultimately, this is the majority of patients who seek emergency care. The experience of pain is multifactorial and difficult to objectively measure. By the teen years, many patients with Hb SS disease have experienced numerous pain crises, developed a level of opioid tolerance, and require high doses of opioid agents to relieve their acute pain. Medical personnel are often concerned about the chance of furthering drug dependence in these individuals with repeated provision of higher doses of medication. Unfortunately, there is little beyond subjective self-report by patients to inform the clinician about the level of their pain. In an effort to control the patient's pain adequately, analgesia must be titrated to patient need and not to artificially derived limits, while monitoring the patient appropriately for side effects. A fixed administration schedule, with an interval that maintains adequate analgesia, will foster a steady state drug level, improved pain control, and decreased patient anxiety.[3]

When using parenteral narcotics, morphine is preferred to meperidine (Demerol), which has a metabolite (normeperidine) that is epileptogenic and poorly metabolized in patients with sickle cell disease.[74] Also, morphine may be administered subcutaneously if venous access is problematic. A synergistic therapy is intravenous ketorolac (Toradol), which has a narcotic-sparing effect when administered for acute pain of various origins, including sickle cell disease.[25,26] Patient-controlled analgesia (PCA) is an effective method for administering narcotics to older children and adolescents. In addition to enabling titration of medication to pain severity, PCA provides patients with a sense of control and involvement in their own care (see Chapter 158, Approach to Pain Management).

Acute Chest Syndrome

Any patient with vaso-occlusive disease and demonstrated hypoxemia should receive supplemental oxygen therapy. While oxygen has been shown to reverse sickling in vitro, clinically it has not been shown to affect the incidence or course of vaso-occlusive episodes.[27,28] Paradoxically, oxygen can suppress erythropoietin levels and reticulocytosis, interfering with a compensatory response and increasing the mass of sickled cells. Also, empirical oxygen therapy in the child who is not hypoxic can mask the evolution of acute chest syndrome and delay its diagnosis.[1] At present, there are no conclusive data either supporting or contradicting the use of oxygen in this clinical setting, though it is traditionally provided to Hb SS patients in some centers.

Splinting due to pain and resultant atelectasis can exacerbate or even cause acute chest syndrome. Pain control is therefore an important facet of chest pain management in Hb SS patients. Nonetheless, judicious care must be exercised with opioids due to the attendant risks of pulmonary edema and respiratory depression. Incentive spirometry has been shown to be of use in limiting progression of acute chest syndrome.[29] These patients are also easily fluid overloaded and, once rehydrated, should receive fluid only at maintenance rates. Patients who have or are at risk of developing this complication often deteriorate quickly and require close monitoring, often in a pediatric intensive care unit. Hypoxemia is common and should be treated with supplemental oxygen. Because this disorder is difficult to distinguish from pneumonia, and because infection is a concomitant or antecedent factor in acute chest syndrome, empirical antibiotics are routinely given. Typically, a broad-spectrum cephalosporin such as cefuroxime and a macrolide to cover for atypical organisms are the recommended antimicrobial agents. Patients usually have hemoglobin levels 1 to 2 g/dl below their baseline and often respond well to simple transfusion of packed RBCs. In more severe cases, partial exchange transfusion should be considered. Guidelines for partial exchange transfusion include multilobar disease, rapidly progressive disease, marked respiratory distress, partial pressure of oxygen (Po_2) less than 70 mm Hg in a child, or a fall of 25% in baseline Po_2.[30] This is best accomplished in the intensive care setting.

Cerebrovascular Accident

Cerebrovascular events are managed with expeditious exchange transfusion. The goal in treatment of acute stroke is to limit further sickling by acutely decreasing the proportion of hemoglobin S to less than 30%. While doing so, it is advisable to avoid hyperviscosity by keeping the hematocrit in the 35% range. Seizures should be controlled with anticonvulsants. Intensive care monitoring is usually necessary, as some patients develop increased intracranial pressure requiring assisted ventilation and pharmacologic therapy. Because the recurrence rate for stroke is high (greater than two thirds of patients who are not chronically transfused), regular transfusions of packed erythrocytes at monthly intervals are employed to keep the hemoglobin S level below 30%. This approach has been shown to be effective in limiting further strokes.[11,12]

Priapism

Treatment of priapism is aimed at relieving pain, emptying the distended corpora cavernosa, and preventing impotence. The initial physical examination should include prostatic massage, which may cause detumescence. Minor repetitive episodes of priapism are often managed at home, with warm baths, exercise, and frequent bladder emptying. However, extremes of temperature should be avoided, as cold increases sickling and heat increases blood flow, compounding pain. If an individual episode persists for greater than 3 hours, patients should be encouraged to seek medical attention. Therapy of a more prolonged episode includes pain management with parenteral opioids, intravenous fluids, and, if needed, placement of a Foley catheter. As in stroke, reduction of the hemoglobin S level to less than 30% is the next immediate goal, via exchange transfusion. Complete detumescence may take weeks, but a response to exchange transfusion should see the onset of detumescence within a day or two.

If a response is not realized within that time frame, surgical intervention may be required, and a urologic consultation should be sought. Surgical techniques are seldom necessary in prepubertal boys, who usually respond to simpler maneuvers. The usual surgical procedure is the Winter procedure or one of its modifications, which may be performed under local anesthesia.[31] The Winter procedure is a corporospongiosum shunt performed by inserting a needle or scalpel through the glans into one of the corpora cavernosa and draining the viscous blood. The instrument is removed, the skin closed, and an ongoing drainage of cavernous blood into the systemic circulation occurs. Intermittently applied compression limits refilling of the corpora cavernosa. The shunt usually closes spontaneously after several weeks, permitting normal subsequent erectile function. Without intervention, severe priapism results in impotence in greater than 80% of cases, while with transfusions and surgery the incidence falls to between 25% and 50%.[3]

Acute Abdominal Pain

Management of patients with acute abdominal pain in sickle cell disease is like that of other patients with acute abdominal pain. Early involvement of a surgical consult is critical in the appropriate at-risk population, based upon history, physical examination, and laboratory and radiographic studies. If an Hb SS patient requires surgery, a simple or exchange transfusion should be performed prior to the operation if possible. Abdominal ultrasonography is an excellent imaging choice when considering gallstone disease in the differential diagnosis, as up to 50% of bilirubin stones are not radiopaque on plain radiographs. The clinician should be aware that the mere existence of gallstones in the presence of right upper quadrant pain and fever may not be indicative of acute cholecystitis. Often patients who have undergone cholecystectomy have been surprised to have their "cholecystitis" symptoms return.

Acute Sequestration Crisis

In the emergency setting, therapy for sequestration is directed at restoration of both intravascular volume and oxygen-carrying capacity via immediate transfusion of packed RBCs. Once normal hemodynamics are restored, patients improve quickly. If there is a delay in obtaining blood for transfusion, a bolus of isotonic saline may temporize and possibly mobilize some red cells from the spleen. However, in this situation, transfusion is life saving. Other general supportive measures are appropriate.

Splenic sequestration may recur, usually within a few months of the initial episode. On this basis, some hematologists have advocated elective splenectomy after the first instance of sequestration. Because asplenic patients have increased susceptibility to invasive disease from encapsulated organisms (e.g., *S. pneumoniae*), which primarily affect children under 2 years of age, splenectomy is ideally delayed until after the patient's second birthday.

Acute Aplastic Crisis

Most aplastic episodes are short lived and require no specific therapy beyond supportive measures. Transfusion of packed RBCs is primarily based on symptoms, though some recommend elective transfusion in patients whose hematocrit falls 20% to 25% below baseline values, or below an arbitrary

Table 127–2	**Criteria for Outpatient Treatment of Fever in Sickle Cell Disease (6 mo–12 yr of Age)**
Normal mental status	
Normal blood pressure/capillary refill	
Temperature ≤ 40° C (104° F)	
No prior pneumococcal sepsis	
Mild pain only	
No evidence of pneumonia	
WBC count 5000–30,000 cells/mm³	
Hemoglobin ≥ 5 gm/dl	
Platelets > 100,000/mm³	
Able to administer ceftriaxone 50 mg/kg IV/IM (no allergy)	
Reliable 24-hr follow-up	

Abbreviations: IM, intramuscularly; IV, intravenously; WBC, white blood cell.
From Wilimas JA, Flynn PM, Harris SC, et al: A randomized study of outpatient treatment with ceftriaxone for selected febrile children with sickle cell disease. N Engl J Med 329:472–476, 1993.

value such as 18%. During the aplastic episode, the patient with sickle cell disease is contagious and should be isolated from vulnerable groups such as pregnant women and the immunocompromised.

Infection/Sepsis

Because of the heightened risk of serious infection in sickle cell patients, the diagnostic approach to a young child who has fever without apparent source is fairly dogmatic. A thorough history and physical examination notwithstanding, a complete blood count, urinalysis, chest radiograph, and cultures of the blood, urine, and throat are generally obtained on febrile patients. Children who appear toxic or who have signs of meningitis should additionally have a lumbar puncture performed. All children who appear ill and all infants ≤ 6 months old require empirical parenteral antibiotics (e.g., ceftriaxone), even before the return of laboratory results, and admission to the hospital.[3] Well-appearing infants and children ≥ 6 months old who meet specific criteria (Table 127–2) may be treated as outpatients with closely coordinated follow-up.[32-35] It is prudent to confer with the patient's hematologist in making disposition decisions for sickle cell patients with fever.

All patients with a new infiltrate on chest radiograph, even if nontoxic appearing and with normal laboratory indices, require hospital admission due to the possibility of developing acute chest syndrome. Empirical antibiotics should be administered as previously described—a cephalosporin and a macrolide. Those with clinical findings suggestive of osteomyelitis require needle aspiration and culture of the offending lesion, and administration of empirical antibiotics directed against likely organisms (i.e., *Staphylococcus aureus*, *S. pneumoniae*, and *Salmonella*). Patients with urinary tract infections and pyelonephritis often develop papillary necrosis coincident with the infection, due to sickling in the renal papillae. The sloughing of the papillae may present clinically as hematuria. Urine cultures should guide antibiotic selection, and urologic consultation is recommended. Hydration should accompany intravenous antibiotic therapy in these instances, to ensure adequacy of renal perfusion.

Future Directions

Research continues into ways to cure sickle cell disease or prevent its complications. Some of these investigations are noted here. Hydroxyurea, an oral metabolite that promotes the synthesis of Hb F, has shown promise as a prophylactic agent to reduce the incidence of vaso-occlusive crises, acute chest syndrome, and stroke in pediatric patients with severe sickle cell disease.[36] Recent data have shown it to be safe, effective, and well tolerated by children over prolonged periods.[37] Bone marrow transplantation has been attempted and been curative in some cases of sickle cell disease. It is not without complications, however, and is expensive and not widely available. A substantial barrier to widespread use is the lack of human lymphocyte antigen–matched sibling donors.[38] Stem cell transplantation using cells harvested from cord blood may avoid the problems encountered by bone marrow transplantation, and this is being actively investigated.[39] Use of gene therapy is being explored as well. Angles of attack include attempts to inactivate the sickle gene, ways to increase expression of the Hb F gene, and introduction of genes whose protein products will block hemoglobin S polymerization.[40]

Summary

Infants and children with sickle cell disease are at risk for a variety of potentially life-threatening complications due to vaso-occlusive phenomena, profound anemia, or infection. Evaluation to exclude these and other complications is mandatory. Rapid identification of acute crises in sickle cell disease is essential to successful intervention and preservation of function. Prompt reversal of hypoxemia, restoration of perfusion and oxygen-carrying capacity, and administration of antibiotics targeted toward encapsulated organisms remain the cornerstones of emergency department management.

REFERENCES

1. Dover GJ, Platt OS: Sickle cell disease. *In* Nathan DG, Orkin SH (eds): Nathan and Oski's Hematology of Infancy and Childhood. Philadelphia: WB Saunders, 1998, pp 762–809.
*2. Minter KR, Gladwin MT: Pulmonary complications of sickle cell anemia: a need for increased recognition, treatment, and research. Am J Respir Crit Care Med 164:2016–2019, 2001.
3. National Heart, Lung and Blood Institute: The Management of Sickle Cell Disease (NIH Publication No. 02-2117). Bethsda, MD: National Institutes of Health, 2002.
*4. Steinberg MH: Management of sickle cell disease. N Engl J Med 340:1021–1030, 1999.
5. Bunn HF: Pathogenesis and treatment of sickle cell disease. N Engl J Med 337:762–769, 1997.
6. Platt OS, Brambilla DJ, Rosse WF, et al: Mortality in sickle cell disease: life expectancy and risk factors for early death. N Engl J Med 330:1639–1644, 1994.
7. Rodewald LE, Slovis CM, Palis J: Sickle cell syndromes: recognition and management of six crises. Emerg Med Rep 11:43–51, 1990.
8. Castro O, Brambilla DJ, Thorington B, et al: The acute chest syndrome in sickle cell disease: incidence and risk factors. Blood 84:643–649, 1994.
9. Quinn CT, Buchanan GR: The acute chest syndrome of sickle cell disease. J Pediatr 135:416–422, 1999.
10. Vichinsky EP, Neumayr LD, Earles AN, et al; National Acute Chest Syndrome Study Group: Causes and outcomes of the acute chest syndrome in sickle cell disease. N Engl J Med 342:1855–1865, 2000.
11. Adams RJ: Lessons from the Stroke Prevention Trial in Sickle Cell Anemia (STOP) study. J Child Neurol 15:344–349, 2000.
12. Adams RJ, McVie VC, Hsu L, et al: Prevention of a first stroke by transfusions in children with sickle cell anemia and abnormal results on transcranial Doppler ultrasonography. N Engl J Med 339:5–11, 1998.
13. Frempong KO, Weiner SJ, Sleeper LA, et al: Cerebrovascular accidents in sickle cell disease: rates and risk factors. Blood 91:288–294, 1998.
14. Winkelstein JA, Drachman RH: Deficiency of pneumococcal serum opsonizing activity in sickle-cell disease. N Engl J Med 279:459, 1968.
15. Johnston RB Jr, Newman SL, Struth AG: An abnormality of the alternate pathway of complement activation in sickle-cell disease. N Engl J Med 288:803–808, 1973.
16. Falletta JM, Woods GM, Verter JI, et al: Discontinuing penicillin prophylaxis in children with sickle cell anemia. Prophylactic Penicillin Study II. J Pediatr 27:685–690, 1995.
17. Hongeng S, Wilimas JA, Harris S, et al: Recurrent *Streptococcus pneumoniae* sepsis in children with sickle cell disease. J Pediatr 130:814–816, 1997.
18. Comber JT, Lopez BL: Evaluation of pulse oximetry in sickle cell anemia patients presenting to the emergency department in acute vaso-occlusive crisis. Am J Emerg Med 14:16–18, 1996.
*19. Blaisdell CJ, Goodman S, Clark K, et al: Pulse oximetry is a poor predictor of hypoxemia in stable children with sickle cell disease. Arch Pediatr Adolesc Med 154:900–903, 2000.
20. Lopez BL, Griswold SK, Navek A, Urbanski L: The complete blood count and reticulocyte count—are they necessary in the evaluation of acute vasoocclusive sickle-cell crisis? Acad Emerg Med 3:751–757, 1996.
21. Chapman JI, El-Shammaa EN, Bonsu BK: The utility of screening laboratory studies in pediatric patients with sickle cell pain episodes. Am J Emerg Med 22:258–263, 2004.
22. Ander DS, Vallee PA: Diagnostic evaluation for infectious etiology of sickle cell pain crisis. Am J Emerg Med 15:290–292, 1997.
23. Rosa RM, Bierer BE, Thomas R, et al: A study of induced hyponatremia in the prevention and treatment of sickle cell crises. N Engl J Med 303:1138–1143, 1980.
24. Barsan W, Hedges J: Meperidine usage in patients with sickle cell crisis. Ann Emerg Med 15:1506–1508, 1986.
25. Beiter JL Jr, Simon HK, Chambliss R, et al: Intravenous ketorolac in the emergency department management of sickle cell pain and predictors of its effectiveness. Arch Pediatr Adolesc Med 155:496–500, 2001.
26. Hardwick WE Jr, Givens TG, Monroe KW, et al: Effect of ketorolac in pediatric sickle cell vaso-occlusive pain crisis. Pediatr Emerg Care 15:179–182, 1999.
27. Robieux IC, Kellner JD, Coppes MJ: Analgesia in children with sickle cell crisis: comparison of intermittent opioids vs. continuous infusion of morphine and placebo controlled study of oxygen inhalation. Pediatr Hematol Oncol 9:317–326, 1992.
28. Zipursky A, Robieux IC, Brown EJ, et al: Oxygen therapy in sickle cell disease. Am J Pediatr Hematol Oncol 14:222–228, 1992.
29. Bellet PS, Kalinyak KA, Shukla R, et al: Incentive spirometry to prevent acute pulmonary complications in sickle cell diseases. N Engl J Med 333:699–703, 1995.
30. Vichinsky E, Lubin BH: Suggested guidelines for the treatment of children with sickle cell anemia. Hematol Oncol Clin North Am 1:483–501, 1987.
31. Winter CC, McDowell G: Experience with 105 patients with priapism: update review of all aspects. J Urol 140:980–983, 1988.
32. Rogers ZR, Morrison RA, Vedro DA, Buchanan GR: Outpatient management of febrile illness in infants and young children with sickle cell anemia. J Pediatr 117:736–739, 1990.
*33. Wilimas JA, Flynn PM, Harris SC, et al: A randomized study of outpatient treatment with ceftriaxone for selected febrile children with sickle cell disease. N Engl J Med 329:472–476, 1993.
34. West TB, West DW, Ohene-Frempong K: The presentation, frequency, and outcome of bacteremia among children with sickle cell disease and fever. Pediatr Emerg Care 10:141–143, 1994.
35. Williams LL, Wilimas JA, Harris SC, et al: Outpatient therapy with ceftriaxone and oral cefixime for selected febrile children with sickle cell disease. J Pediatr Hematol Oncol 18:257–261, 1996.
36. Scott JP, Hillery CA, Brown ER, et al: Hydroxyurea therapy in children severely affected with sickle cell disease. J Pediatr 128:820–828, 1996.

*Selected readings.

37. Zimmerman SA, Schultz WH, Davis JS, et al: Sustained long-term hematologic efficacy of hydroxyurea at maximum tolerated dose in children with sickle cell disease. Blood 103:2039–2045, 2004.

38. Walters MC, Patience M, Leisenring W, et al: Bone marrow transplantation for sickle cell disease. N Engl J Med 335:369–376, 1996.

39. Brichard B, Vermylen C, Ninane J, Cornu G: Persistence of fetal hemoglobin production after successful transplantation of cord blood stem cells in a patient with sickle cell anemia. J Pediatr 128:241–243, 1996.

40. Wethers DL: Sickle cell disease in childhood: Part II. Diagnosis and treatment of major complications and recent advances in treatment. Am Fam Physician 62:1309–1314, 2000.

Cancer and Cancer-Related Complications in Children

Peter D. Sadowitz, MD and Abdul-Kader Souid, MD, PhD

Key Points

Cancer remains a leading cause of death in children, accounting for approximately 10% of fatalities.

Febrile-neutropenic events are common in children receiving chemotherapy. Often the first sign of sepsis is fever (>38.0° C). The standard care for these patients includes *immediate* triage and clinical assessment, appropriate central venous line and peripheral blood cultures, administration of broad-spectrum antibiotics, and hospitalization.

Tumor lysis syndrome may produce hypercuricemia, hyperkalemia, hyperphosphatemia, hypocalcaemia, and renal failure. Patients with these complications require vigorous hydration, diuretics, and allopurinal or rasburicase. Potassium-containing solutions should be avoided.

Tumors compressing the airway, superior vena cava, or spinal cord require *immediate* assessment and urgent interventions.

Selected Diagnoses

Acute leukemias and lymphomas
Abdominal tumors
  Neuroblastoma
  Wilms' tumor
  Hepatoblastoma
Bone and tissue sarcomas
  Osteosarcoma
  Ewing's sarcoma (primitive neuroectodermal tumor)
  Rhabdomyosarcoma
Other tumors
  Hodgkin's lymphoma
  Retinoblastoma
  Germ cell tumors

Complications of chemotherapy
  Febrile neutropenia
  Acute tumor lysis syndrome
  Tumor-induced compression

Discussion of Individual Diagnoses

Acute Leukemias and Lymphomas

Acute leukemias and lymphomas account for approximately one third of childhood cancers. Children with immune deficiency (e.g., hypogammaglobulinemia, immunosuppressive therapy, human immunodeficiency virus infection) or constitutional chromosomal anomalies (e.g., trisomy 21) are particularly susceptible.

Acute lymphoblastic leukemia (ALL) accounts for approximately 85% of childhood leukemias. The disease peaks in early childhood. Malignant lymphoblasts originate from immature B cells in 80% of cases (B-cell precursor ALL), mature B cells in 5% of cases (B-cell or Burkitt's leukemia/lymphoma) and immature T cells in 15% of cases (T-cell leukemia/lymphoma). The term *lymphoma* is used when lymphoblasts arise primarily within lymph nodes, and the percentage of malignant cells in the bone marrow is less than 25%. Certain chromosomal abnormalities in lymphoblasts produce poor outcome, such as t(9;22)(q34;q11) or Philadelphia chromosome.[1]

Acute myelogenous leukemia (AML) accounts for approximately 15% of childhood leukemias. Its incidence is steady from birth to 18 years of age. Myeloblasts may originate from myeloid (M1 through M4), monocytic (M4 and M5), erythroid (M6), or megakaryocytic (M7) precursors.

Clinical Presentation

Patients may be asymptomatic, with leukemia detected on routine examination of blood smear or complete blood counts (CBCs). Symptoms and signs of leukemia (Table 128–1) occur when blasts proliferate in the bone marrow cavity (producing anemia, neutropenia, and/or thrombocytopenia) and other organs (producing lymphadenopathy, hepatomegaly, and splenomegaly). Clinical manifestations may also include fever (due to infection or leukemia itself), pallor, fatigue (due to anemia), bacterial infections (due to neutropenia), petechiae, and bruises (due to thrombocytopenia).

Table 128–1	Emergency Department Recognition, Workup and Management of Acute Lymphoblastic Leukemia (ALL) and Lymphoma

B-Cell Precursor (Common) ALL

Presentation
- Fever ($^1/_2$ of patients)
- Petechiae/bruises ($^1/_2$ of patients)
- Bone/joint pain ($^1/_3$ of patients), limp, refusal to walk
- Lymphadenopathy ($^2/_3$ of patients)
- Hepatomegaly ($^2/_3$ of patients)
- Splenomegaly ($^2/_3$ of patients)
- Pallor ($^1/_2$ of patients)

Workup
- CBC, type and screen, blood culture
- Serum electrolytes, BUN, creatinine, calcium, phosphate, uric acid, LDH, PT, PTT, TT, fibrinogen, AST, ALT, bilirubin
- Chest radiograph
- Urinalysis

Laboratory Findings
- Anemia, thrombocytopenia, neutropenia, and circulating blasts are common.
- White blood cell counts are $\leq 10 \times 10^3/mm^3$ in $^1/_2$ of the patients, $10–50 \times 10^3/mm^3$ in $^1/_4$ of the patients, and $> 50 \times 10^3/mm^3$ in $^1/_4$ of the patients.
- Hemoglobin concentrations are ≤ 7.5 g/dl in $^1/_2$ of the patients, 7.5–10 g/dl in $^1/_4$ of the patients, and > 10 g/dl in $^1/_4$ of the patients.
- Platelet counts are $< 20 \times 10^3/mm^3$ in $^1/_4$ of the patients, $20–100 \times 10^3/mm^3$ in $^1/_2$ of the patients, and $> 100 \times 10^3/mm^3$ in $^1/_4$ of the patients.
- LDH and uric acid are frequently elevated.

Management
- IVF (5% dextrose, 0.45% NaCl or 5% dextrose, 0.2% NaCl + 30 mEq/L NaHCO$_3$) at twice the maintenance rate
- IV antibiotics for febrile neutropenia (see Table 128–3)
- PRBC transfusion for hemoglobin concentration < 8.0 g/dl (see Chapter 132)
- Platelet transfusion for platelet count $< 20 \times 10^3/mm^3$ (see Chapter 132)
- Allopurinol (10 mg/kg/day in three divided doses) or rasburicase (single IV dose of 0.15–0.2 mg/kg/day, mixed in 50 ml of 0.9% NaCl, over 30 min)

T-Cell ALL/Lymphoma

Presentation
- Cough, wheezing, stridor
- Massive cervical or mediastinal lymphadenopathy

Workup
- Same as for B-cell precursor ALL
- CT scans of the neck and chest

Laboratory Findings
- Leukocytosis and circulating blasts are common. Hemoglobin concentration and platelet count are frequently normal.
- LDH and uric acid are markedly elevated.

Management
- Consultations with pediatric oncology, intensive care, and anesthesia services
- Careful airway management (e.g., may require steroid therapy and/or mediastinal radiation after pediatric oncology consultation to prevent life-threatening airway compromise)
- Frequent monitoring of vital signs and urine output, preferably in a pediatric intensive care unit (since intubation to secure the airway may be necessary)
- IVF and allopurinol or rasburicase as for B-cell precursor ALL

Burkitt's (B-Cell) Lymphoma

Presentation
- Abdominal involvement is common as the lymphoma cells infiltrate the various abdominal organs (e.g., abdominal mass, ascites, ileocecal intussusception, small bowel obstruction, mesenteric/retroperitoneal lymphadenopathy, renal infiltration and hepatosplenomegaly).
- Other sites of the disease include bone marrow and lymph nodes (including the tonsils).
- Spinal cord compression by a tumor occurs in ~10% of patients, producing paresis, neurogenic bladder, and lower extremity motor and sensory defects.

Workup
- Same as for B-precursor and T-cell leukemias
- Abdominal CT scan and spinal MRI (if neurologic findings are present)
- Peritoneal fluid (ascites) aspiration may be needed to obtain cells for diagnosis.

Laboratory Findings
- CBC could be normal if there is no bone marrow involvement.
- LDH and uric acid are markedly elevated.

Management
- Emergent consultations with pediatric oncology and surgery services are necessary.
- IVF and allopurinol or rasburicase as for B-cell precursor ALL

Abbreviations: ALT, alanine aminotransferase; AST, aspartate aminotransferase; BUN, blood urea nitrogen; CBC, complete blood count; CT, computed tomography; IV, intravenous(ly); IVF, intravenous fluids; LDH, lactate dehydrogenase; MRI, magnetic resonance imaging; PRBC, packed red blood cells; PT, prothrombin time; PTT, partial thromboplastin time; TT, thrombin time.

Bone pain (due to expanding leukemic clumps in the marrow cavity and infiltration into the subperiosteal space) is common, producing limp, refusal to walk, swollen joints, and arthralgias (mimicking juvenile rheumatoid arthritis).

Respiratory compromise with cough, wheezing, and stridor may result from airway compression by massive cervical, thoracic, and/or mediastinal lymphadenopathy (see Table 128–1). Superior vena cava compression produces venous congestion, swelling, and cyanosis in the upper chest, neck, and face. Eye examination is necessary to evaluate orbital masses (more common in AML) and retinal infiltration. Leukemic involvement of the testes should be carefully documented. Abdominal masses, ascites, and small bowel obstruction (e.g., ileocecal intussusception) can be seen in Burkitt's (B-cell) lymphoma (see Table 128–1).

The initial workup includes a CBC and examination of a blood smear (for blasts). Anemia, neutropenia, and thrombocytopenia are present in the majority of patients with B-cell precursor (common) ALL (see Table 128–1). The remaining workup includes a chest radiograph (a large thymus and mediastinal lymphadenopathy are common in T-cell leukemia/lymphoma); blood typing (for possible need of packed red blood cell and/or platelet transfusions); blood culture (in the presence of fever); prothrombin time, activated partial thromboplastin time, and thrombin time (all are prolonged in AML-induced disseminated intravascular coagulopathy [DIC]); fibrinogen (low in AML-induced DIC); serum electrolytes, creatinine, calcium, and phosphate (the initial value is often low due to phosphate uptake by the leukemia clone); lactate dehydrogenase and uric acid (both are usually elevated); and hepatic transaminases, bilirubin, and urinalysis.

All patients with suspected leukemia/lymphoma require admission for definitive evaluation, which includes a spinal tap to evaluate central nervous system (CNS) infiltration and a bone marrow examination to evaluate leukemic cell morphology, immunophenotyping, and cytogenetics. These procedures should be done after thrombocytopenia and coagulopathy are corrected. Cerebrospinal fluid (CSF) should be evaluated for cytology, cell count, protein, and glucose. CNS disease (present in approximately 5% of cases) is associated with an increased CSF white cell count (>5/mm^3) and leukemic blasts on a cytospin slide prepared shortly after CSF collection.

The differential diagnosis of acute leukemia includes juvenile rheumatoid arthritis, Epstein-Barr virus or cytomegalovirus infection, aplastic anemia, and bone marrow infiltration by metabolic cells (e.g., Gaucher's disease) or other neoplasms (blood smear frequently shows nucleated red blood cells and left shift).

Management

Intravenous antibiotics should be given for bacterial infections or febrile neutropenia. Packed red blood cell and platelet transfusions (using leukoreduced and irradiated products) may be necessary. The goals are to raise the hemoglobin concentration to greater than 8.0 g/dl and the platelet count to greater than 50×10^3/mm^3, especially prior to invasive procedures (e.g., spinal tap, central venous catheter placement). Patients with wheezing, cough, and/or respiratory distress due to a massive mediastinal or cervical lymphadenopathy may require emergent airway control. These patients should be admitted to the intensive care unit for observation. Immediate interventions (e.g., steroid therapy, mediastinal radiation) may be necessary. Other complications include tumor lysis syndrome (see "Complications of Chemotherapy" section),[2,3] renal failure (due to leukemic infiltrations and/or uric acid nephropathy), seizures (due to CNS leukemia, intracranial bleeding, or metabolic derangements), pleural effusion (due to leukemic infiltration), and DIC (seen in AML) (see Chapter 40, Seizures; Chapter 42, Conditions Causing Increased Intracranial Pressure; and Chapter 88, Renal Disorders).

Abdominal Tumors

Neuroblastoma

Neuroblastomas arise in the adrenal glands (~40% of cases) and abdominal (~25% of cases) or thoracic (~20% of cases) sympathetic ganglia. These tumors occur in children less than 5 years of age. Over 90% of tumors produce catecholamines (e.g., homovanillic acid [HVA], vanillylmandelic acid [VMA]).[8] These biochemical markers aid in establishing the diagnosis and in documenting a response to therapy. Patients may present with a large abdominal mass (potentially causing respiratory distress) or metastatic lesions to the orbits, bones, bone marrow, or lymph nodes. Tumors in the posterior mediastinum may be asymptomatic (discovered on a chest radiograph) or result in airway obstruction. Dumbbell-shaped tumors involving the intervertebral foramina may compress the spinal cord, causing paraplegia. Tumors involving the cervical sympathetic chain may produce Horner's syndrome (miosis, ptosis, enophthalmos, and anhydrosis). About 5% of the tumors produce cerebellar dysfunction, causing opsoclonus polymyoclonus syndrome (ataxia and dancing eyes). Periorbital metastases produce "raccoon eyes." Hypertension due to excess catecholamines may require antihypertensives. The workup includes a CBC; urine HVA/VMA; CT scans of the chest, abdomen, and pelvis; bone marrow examination; and technetium-99m (^{99m}Tc) bone scan. Spine MRI should be obtained if paraspinal tumors are suspected. Spinal cord compression requires immediate neurosurgical evaluation, radiation therapy, dexamethasone, or chemotherapy.

Wilms' Tumor

Wilms' tumors account for approximately 5% of the childhood cancer. Most children are less than 8 years old. Aniridia, hemihypertrophy, and Beckwith-Wiedemann syndrome (neonatal hypoglycemia, omphalocele, macroglossia, and visceromegaly) are highly associated with Wilms' tumors. Patients with any of these anomalies require regular abdominal ultrasounds for the first several years of life to detect tumor at an early stage. Urinary tract malformations (e.g., hypospadia, cryptorchidism, horseshoe kidney, ureteral duplication, polycystic kidney) are also associated with Wilms' tumors. Patients may present with a large abdominal mass, acute abdominal pain (due to tumor necrosis or hemorrhage), constipation, hypertension, microscopic hematuria, anemia, and rarely polycythemia. The workup includes abdominal and chest CT scans to evaluate the renal vein, inferior vena cava, right atrium (for tumor thrombus), regional lymph nodes (iliac, periaortic, and celiac), liver, opposite kidney, and lungs (lung metastasis occurs in approximately 15% of the cases). Nephrectomy is necessary for all tumors. More than 90% of children are cured with surgery plus chemotherapy (with or without radiation).[9]

Hepatoblastoma

Hepatoblastomas affect children in the first 2 years of life. They may occur in association with Beckwith-Wiedemann syndrome, hemihypertrophy, or extreme prematurity. Familial forms also occur in association with CNS anomalies, glycogen storage disease, and familial adenomatous polyposis.[10] Children usually present with a large abdominal mass. Lungs are a common metastatic site. Most tumors produce α-fetoprotein, which confirms the diagnosis and guides the treatment. The workup includes CBC, blood type (for possible need of packed red blood cell transfusion), serum α-fetoprotein and β-human choriogonadotrophin (βhCG), abdominal CT scan (shows large hepatic tumor), chest radiograph, and chest CT scan. The diagnosis is confirmed by tumor biopsy. The risk of tumor bleeding is high due to extensive tumor vascularity. As a consequence, tumor rupture can be produced by overzealous abdominal examination. The differential diagnosis includes hepatocellular carcinoma and hemangioma. The majority of patients are cured with chemotherapy followed by tumor resection.

Bone and Tissue Sarcomas

Osteosarcoma

Osteosarcoma (spindle cell tumor of the metaphysis) is the most common bone cancer.[11] The disease peaks between approximately 10 and 18 years of age (coinciding with the growth spurt). More than 80% of these tumors occur in the knee region (lower femur or upper tibia) and approximately 15% in the humerus. Lungs and bones are the most common metastatic sites. Typical presentations include localized pain with or without physical findings (e.g., firm, tender mass fixed to underlying bone) and pathologic fractures. A plain radiograph of involved bone shows poorly defined tumor margins, bone destruction, periosteal reaction, and calcification (reflecting new bone formation). In approximately 10% of cases, the lesion is purely osteolytic. In contrast, benign tumors are round, smooth, and well circumscribed, without cortical destruction or periosteal reaction. The workup includes MRI of the entire extremity (to detect skip lesions), ^{99m}Tc bone scan (to detect bone metastasis), chest radiography, and chest CT scan (to detect lung metastasis). The diagnosis is confirmed by open biopsy. The treatment involves preoperative chemotherapy followed by surgery (e.g., "en bloc" tumor resection with endprosthesis).[12]

Ewing's Sarcoma (Primitive Neuroectodermal Tumor)

Ewing's sarcomas are small round cell tumors of neuronal origin. The tumor arises in the diaphyses of long or flat bones and in soft tissues. Pelvic and femoral tumors account for approximately 50% of cases. Undifferentiated tumors are termed *Ewing's sarcoma*, and tumors exhibiting primitive neural characteristics are termed *peripheral primitive neuroectodermal tumors* (PNET). Ewing's sarcoma typically occurs after 10 years of age, with lungs, lymph nodes, bones, and bone marrow being the most common metastatic sites. The clinical presentation is similar to osteosarcoma. The tumors share common abnormalities involving chromosome 22 [t(11:22)(q24:q12) or t(21:22)(q 22:q 12)]. Successful treatment requires surgery and chemotherapy (with or without radiation).[13]

Rhabdomyosarcoma

Rhabdomyosarcomas arise from mesenchymal cells that normally differentiate to striated muscles. This tumor is the most common soft tissue sarcoma in children, accounting for approximately 50% of all sarcomas.[14] The disease may occur at any age. Tumors originate in the head and neck region (e.g., orbit, nasopharynx, sinuses, middle ear) in 40% of cases, genitourinary area (e.g., bladder, prostate, paratesticular, perineal, vaginal) in 20% of cases, extremities and trunk in 20% of cases, and retroperitoneum in 10% of cases. Parameningeal tumors may invade the CNS, causing cranial nerve palsies, increased intracranial pressure, and meningeal involvement. Lungs, lymph nodes, bones, bone marrow, and liver are common metastatic sites. The workup includes CBC, CT scan of involved sites, bone marrow examination, and ^{99m}Tc bone scan. Parameningeal tumors require brain or spine MRI and CSF cytology. The standard treatment involves chemotherapy, surgery, and radiation.

Other Tumors

Hodgkin's Lymphoma

Hodgkin's lymphoma is a neoplasm arising in the lymphatic system. Despite their undetermined origin, Reed-Sternberg cells are responsible for the disease.[15,16] Tumors spread from one nodal area to an adjacent nodal region. Extranodal spread (bone marrow, lungs, and bones) is rare. The disease is more common in adolescents. A typical presentation includes painless cervical, supraclavicular, or mediastinal lymphadenopathy, which progresses over several months. Symptoms such as fatigue, anorexia, weight loss, and night sweats may be present. The workup includes chest radiograph; CT scans of neck, chest, abdomen, and pelvis; and ^{99m}Tc and gallium bone scans. Lymph node biopsy is necessary to confirm the diagnosis. Treatment involves chemotherapy with or without radiation.[17] The cure rate is over 80%.

Retinoblastoma

Retinoblastomas are the most common primary eye tumor.[18] They arise from the outer layer of the retina. The mean age at diagnosis is approximately 17 months, with few cases occurring after 5 years of age. The most common presentations are leukocoria (white reflex within the eye), strabismus, and poor vision. The workup includes orbit MRI/CT scan, CSF cytology, bone marrow examination, and bone scan. Photocoagulation or cryotherapy is used for tumors less than 4 disk diameters in size, while larger tumors are treated with surgery or radiation. Chemotherapy is used for extensive local disease or distant metastasis. Enucleation is reserved for advanced unilateral disease. The current approach cures greater than 90% of patients. Children with a known family history of the disease need retinal examinations at regular intervals. Patients with the inherited form of retinoblastoma have increased risk of developing second malignancy (e.g., osteosarcoma).

Germ Cell Tumors

Germ cell tumors (germinoma, dysgerminoma, teratoma, endodermal sinus or yolk sac tumor, embryonal carcinoma, and choriocarcinoma) involve the gonads (testes and ovaries) and extragonadal regions (pineal gland, suprasellar area, anterior mediastinum, and sacrococcygeum).[19,20] Serum α-fetoprotein and βhCG are usually elevated, which confirms the diagnosis and guides the treatment. Clinical presentations vary depending on tumor location. Pineal/suprasellar tumors produce headache, upward paralysis, and poor coordination. Anterior mediastinal lesions produce cough and wheezing. Sacrococcygeal tumors occur in infants, who may present with constipation and a mass in the buttock or presacral region. Ovarian tumors occur in young girls and present with an abdominal or pelvic mass. Testicular tumors produce painless testicular swelling or torsion of the testis. Optimal therapy includes chemotherapy and, in some cases, radiation.

Complications of Chemotherapy

Febrile Neutropenia

Fever and neutropenia (febrile neutropenia) are common in children receiving chemotherapy (Table 128–2). In this setting, neutropenia is defined as an absolute neutrophil count (ANC) of less than 500/mm³, and determined as the total white blood cell count multiplied by the percentage of neutrophils plus bands. Fever is defined as temperature greater than 38.0° C (100.4° F). The risk of bacterial infection correlates with the severity of neutropenia and its duration. For example, life-threatening sepsis is more common when the ANC is less than 200/mm³ for more than 7 days. Other predictive parameters for invasive bacterial infections include high-dose chemotherapy (e.g., myeloablative therapy), young age, delayed capillary filling time (>3 seconds), tachycardia, hypotension, high temperature (>39° C), pneumonia (cough, short of breath, decreased hemoglobin-oxygen saturation, or abnormal chest radiograph), and compromised physical barriers due to oral mucositis or enterocolitis.[21-24]

Fever may the first and only sign of a life-threatening infection. Other clinical presentations may include headache, fatigue, chills, gastrointestinal symptoms (abdominal pain, nausea, vomiting, diarrhea, and perianal or perirectal cellulitis), mucositis or pain at central venous catheter or rectal region. All patients with fever and neutropenia require *immediate* clinical evaluation, appropriate cultures (blood cultures from central and peripheral venous catheter, and cultures of infected mucosal or skin lesions), prompt administration of broad-spectrum intravenous antibiotics, and hospitalization. The choice of empirical antibiotics (which should be administered as soon as intravenous access and cultures are obtained) is based on commonly isolated pathogens.[25] Gram-positive organisms include the low-virulence coagulase-negative *Staphylococcus* species and viridans streptococci (common contaminants of central venous catheters), and high-virulence α-hemolytic streptococci, enterococci, and *Streptococcus pneumoniae* (producing disseminated infections, such as meningitis). These organisms respond to vancomycin (15 mg/kg per dose intravenously every 8 hours). Common gram-negative organisms include *Escherichia coli, Pseudomonas* species, and *Klebsiella* species. These organisms respond to antipseudomonal cephalosporins (ceftazidime, cefoperazone, or cefepime) or aminoglycosides (e.g., amikacin, 5 mg/kg per dose every 8 hours) (see Table 128–2).

Table 128–2   Febrile Neutropenia

Definitions

- Neutropenia is defined as an absolute neutrophil count of < 500/mm³.
- Fever is defined as a temperature of ≥ 38.0° C (100.4° F).

Presentation

- Fever may be the only sign of a life-threatening infection.
- Other symptoms may include headache, lethargy, abdominal pain, nausea, vomiting, diarrhea, oral mucositis, perianal pain, and pain at central venous catheter site.

Workup

- CBC, type and screen, and blood cultures from the central venous catheter
- Peripheral blood cultures
- Cultures from infected mucosal or skin lesions

Monitoring

- All patients require *immediate* clinical evaluation, including frequent vital signs. Tachycardia and hypotension may reflect sepsis.
- Physical examination includes careful assessment of the cardiopulmonary-neurologic status, tissue perfusion, perianal region, oral mucosa, and central line site.
- Continuous patient monitoring is necessary for several hours following antibiotic administration, since endotoxin release may produce septic shock.

Management

- All patients with febrile neutropenia should be admitted and receive parenteral antibiotics.
- Hemodynamically unstable patients should be admitted to a pediatric intensive care unit.
- Vancomycin (15 mg/kg IV q8h) *plus* antipseudomonal cephalosporins (ceftazidime, cefoperazone or cefepime) or aminoglycosides (e.g., amikacin, 5 mg/kg q8h)
- Tachycardia, hypotension, and poor tissue perfusion require emergent fluid resuscitation (e.g., 0.9% NaCl or Ringer's lactate at 20–60 ml/kg). Dopamine may be required if fluid resuscitation does not improve perfusion and blood pressure.
- Packed red blood cell (if hemoglobin concentration < 8.0 g/dl) and platelet (if platelet count < 20 × 10³/mm³) transfusions are necessary. The products should be leukoreduced and irradiated (see Chapter 132).

Abbreviations: CBC, complete blood count; IV, intravenously.

Antifungal treatment is given for prolonged fever and neutropenia while on broad-spectrum antibiotics. *Aspergillus* species respond to voriconazole and *Candida* species respond to fluconazole.[26] All patients require admission. Hemodynamically unstable patients (tachycardia, hypotension, and poor tissue perfusion) require emergent intravenous fluid resuscitation (with 20 to 60 ml/kg of 0.9% NaCl or Ringer's lactate); vasoactive pressors (e.g., dopamine) may also be necessary. Stress-dose steroids may be required, especially in patients on steroid therapy. Careful physical evaluation, including overall appearance, vital signs (tachycardia and hypotension reflect sepsis), tissue perfusion, and perirectal, oral, and central catheter sites, is essential. Digital rectal examination and rectal temperatures should be avoided. Tachycardia and hypotension may reflect sepsis. Continuous monitoring is necessary, since septic shock may follow antibiotic administration. Packed red blood cell transfusion (~15 ml/kg over ~2 hours) improves tissue perfusion and may help correct tachycardia and hypotension in anemic patients. Platelet transfusion (1 apheresis unit, or ~15 ml/kg for infants, over 1 hour) may also be necessary in thrombocytopenic patients. Blood products should be leukoreduced and irradiated (see Chapter 132, Utilizing Blood Bank Resources/Transfusion Reactions and Complications). Patients with a history of a prior transfusion reaction (e.g., urticaria, chills, and fever) require premedication with acetaminophen (15 mg/kg orally), diphenhydramine (0.5 mg/kg orally or intravenously), methylprednisolone (1 mg/kg intravenously), and/or cimetidine (1 mg/kg; 25 mg maximum, intravenously) to decrease transfusion reactions. Granulocyte colony-stimulating factor decreases the incidence of febrile neutropenia and may be useful in severely neutropenic patients when documented bacterial infections cannot be controlled.[27]

Acute Tumor Lysis Syndrome

Acute tumor lysis syndrome may complicate the course of induction chemotherapy[2] (Table 128–3). The metabolic derangements include hyperuricemia (due to increased purine metabolism), hyperkalemia, and hyperphosphatemia. Hyperphosphatemia can produce hypocalcemia (cramps, tetany, and seizures). Phosphate and uric acid may precipitate in renal tubules, producing renal failure. Vigorous hydration to ensure production of dilute urine (specific gravity < 1.010) and adequate elimination of cellular debris (e.g., 5% dextrose + 0.45% NaCl [$D_{5^1/_2}$NS] or 5% dextrose + 0.2% NaCl [$D_{5^1/_4}$NS] *plus* 30 mEq/L NaHCO$_3$ at twice the maintenance rate) is necessary. If urine output is inadequate, diuretics (furosemide, 0.5 to 1.0 mg/kg) can be used. Potassium-containing solutions must absolutely be avoided. Urine alkalization (with intravenous NaHCO$_3$ or acetozolamide) is necessary in the presence of marked hyperuricemia. Allopurinol (300 mg/m^2/day or 10 mg/kg/day in three divided doses orally) or rasburicase[3] (a single dose of 0.15 to 0.2 mg/kg/day, mixed in 50 ml of 0.9% NaCl and infused intravenously over 30 minutes) should be administered to prevent uric acid formation. Rasburicase, a recombinant uricolytic agent (urate oxidase) derived from *Aspergillus,* converts uric acid to allatoin, which is easily excreted in the urine. By preventing uric acid nephropathy, phosphate and potassium excretion are also improved.[3] Hyperkalemia and symptomatic hypocalcemia require urgent corrections; patients with these complications require continuous cardiac monitoring. Dialysis is required for severe hyperkalemia and renal failure (see Chapter 114, Hyperkalemia; and Chapter 115, Hypocalcemia).

Tumor-Induced Compression

Tumor-induced *airway compression* produces cough, wheezing, stridor, dyspnea, and cyanosis. *Superior vena cava compression* produces face and neck swelling, dyspnea, cyanosis, and prominent chest wall veins. All patients will require admission, imaging (chest radiograph and CT), and a tissue diagnosis for confirmation. Management includes administration of oxygen, elevating the head of the bed, and observing the patient for airway compromise. Clinicians should be aware that sedation may further compromise the airway. Thus early involvement of pediatric intensive care, pediatric oncology, and anesthesia teams should be considered. Emer-

---

Table 128–3   Acute Tumor Lysis Syndrome

Definition

- The metabolic derangements (hyperuricemia, hyperkalemia, hyperphosphatemia, and hypocalcemia) that occur during induction chemotherapy from the destruction of tumor cells.

Complications

- Phosphate and uric acid may precipitate in renal tubules and can produce renal insufficiency or failure.
- Hyperphosphatemia may produce hypocalcemia, which may become symptomatic.

Management

- Hydration with 5% dextrose + 0.45% NaCl ($D_{5^1/_2}$NS) or 5% dextrose + 0.2% NaCl ($D_{5^1/_4}$NS) *plus* 30 mEq/L of NaHCO$_3$ at twice the maintenance rate. Intravenous boluses with 0.9% NaCl (20 ml/kg each) may be necessary in severely dehydrated patients. Potassium-containing solutions must be avoided.
- If urine output remains low (e.g., < 2 ml/kg/hr) after ~8 hr of adequate hydration, furosemide IV at 1 mg/kg IV should be administered.
- Allopurinol (300 mg/m^2/day or 10 mg/kg/day orally in three divided doses) or rasburicase (single IV dose of 0.15–0.2 mg/kg/day, mixed in 50 ml of 0.9% NaCl, given over 30 min)
- Dialysis is required for severe hyperkalemia and renal failure.

Monitoring

- Close monitoring of urine output and urine parameters is essential.
- Serum electrolytes, BUN, creatinine, phosphate, calcium, and uric acid should be repeated every 4–24 hr depending on the severity of tumor lysis.

Abbreviations: BUN, blood urea nitrogen; D, dextrose; IV, intravenously; NS, normal saline.

gent use of steroids or radiation may be necessary (although these modalities may obscure the diagnosis).

Spinal cord compression is most frequently caused by tumor extension through the neural foramina and may occur at any level of the cervical, thoracic, or lumbar spine. Most of these tumors distribute evenly throughout the cervical, thoracic, and lumbar spine. The mass can be intramedullary (e.g., astrocytoma, ependymoma, lipoma), intradural extramedullary (e.g., dermoid, neuroblastoma, neurofibroma, schwannoma, meningoma, PNET, hemangioepithelioma), or epidural (e.g., Ewing's sarcoma, neuroblastoma, ganglioneuroma, rhabdomyosarcoma, osteosarcoma, germ cell tumor, teratoma, lymphoma). Signs and symptoms of spinal cord compression include back pain, weakness, reflex changes, sensory deficit, atrophy, extremity pain, and incontinence. MRI (with and without gadolinium) of the involved region should be obtained. Consultations with neurosurgery, radiation therapy, and pediatric oncology are necessary. Dexamethasone (1 to 2 mg/kg intravenously) may decrease localized edema and swelling. In the absence of severe spinal cord compression, most tumors can be treated with chemotherapy or radiation. However, sarcomas usually require *immediate* surgical decompression.

REFERENCES

*1. Holleman A, Cheok MH, den Boer ML, et al: Gene expression in drug resistant acute lymphoblastic leukemia cells and response to treatment. N Engl J Med 351:533–542, 2004.

2. Davidson MB, Thakkar S, Hix JK, et al: Pathophysiology, clinical consequences and treatment of tumor lysis syndrome. Am J Med 116:546–554, 2004.

3. Lee AC, Li CH, So KT, et al: Treatment of impending tumor lysis with single-dose rasburicase. Ann Pharmacother 37:1614–1617, 2003.

4. Fang Z, Kulldorff M, Gregorio DI: Brain cancer mortality in the United States, 1986 to 1995: a geographic analysis. Neurooncology 6:179–187, 2004.

5. Baldwin RT, Preston-Martin S: Epidemiology of brain tumors in childhood—a review. Toxicol Appl Pharmacol 199:118–131, 2004.

6. Bucci MK, Maity A, Janss AJ, et al: Near complete surgical resection predicts a favorable outcome in pediatric patients with non-brainstem, malignant gliomas: results from a single center in the magnetic resonance imaging era. Cancer 101:817–824, 2004.

*7. The epidemiology of headache among children with brain tumor. Headache in children with brain tumors. The Childhood Brain Tumor Consortium. J Neurooncol 10:31–46, 1991.

*8. Riley RD, Heney D, Jones DR: A systematic review of molecular and biological tumor markers in neuroblastoma. Clin Cancer Res 10:4–12, 2004.

*9. Green DM: The treatment of stages I-IV favorable histology Wilms' tumor. J Clin Oncol 22:1366–1372, 2004.

10. Reynolds P, Urayama KY, Von Behren J, et al: Birth characteristics and hepatoblastoma risk in young children. Cancer 100:1070–1076, 2004.

11. Gorlick R, Anderson P, Andrulis I, et al: Biology of childhood osteogenic sarcoma and potential targets for therapeutic development: meeting summary. Clin Cancer Res 9:5442–5453, 2003.

12. Rao BN, Rodriguez-Galindo C: Local control in childhood extremity sarcomas: salvaging limbs and sparing function. Med Pediatr Oncol 41:584–587, 2003.

13. Krasin MJ, Rodriguez-Galindo C, Davidoff AM, et al: Efficacy of combined surgery and irradiation for localized Ewings sarcoma family of tumors. Pediatric Blood Cancer 43:229–236, 2004.

*14. Meyer WH, Spunt SL: Soft tissue sarcomas of childhood. Cancer Treat Rev 30:269–280, 2004.

15. Thorley-Lawson DA, Gross A: Persistence of the Epstein-Barr virus and the origins of associated lymphomas. N Engl J Med 350:1328–1337, 2004.

16. Thomas RK, Re D, Wolf J, et al: Part I: Hodgkin's lymphoma—molecular biology of Hodgkin and Reed-Sternberg cells. Lancet Oncol 5:11–18, 2004.

17. Diehl V, Thomas RK, Re D: Part II: Hodgkin's lymphoma—diagnosis and treatment. Lancet Oncol 5:19–26, 2004.

18. Castillo BV Jr, Kaufman L: Pediatric tumors of the eye and orbit. Pediatr Clin North Am 50:149–172, 2003.

19. Ueno T, Tanaka YO, Nagata M, et al: Spectrum of germ cell tumors: from head to toe. Radiographics 24:387–404, 2004.

20. Holzik MF, Rapley EA, Hoekstra HJ, et al: Genetic predisposition to testicular germ-cell tumors. Lancet Oncol 5:363–371, 2004.

21. Crawford J, Dale DC, Lyman GH: Chemotherapy-induced neutropenia: risks, consequences and new directions for its management. Cancer 100:228–237, 2004.

22. West DC, Marcin JP, Mawis R, et al: Children with cancer, fever and treatment-induced neutropenia: risk factors associated with illness requiring the administration of critical care therapies. Pediatr Emerg Care 20:79–84, 2004.

*23. Mullen CA: Ciprofloxacin in treatment of fever and neutropenia in pediatric cancer patients. Pediatr Infect Dis J 22:1138–1142, 2003.

24. Offidani M, Corvatta L, Malerba L, et al: Risk assessment of patients with hematologic malignancies who develop fever accompanied by pulmonary infiltrates: a historical cohort study. Cancer 101:567–577, 2004.

25. Vidal L, Paul M, Ben dor I, et al: Oral versus intravenous antibiotic treatment for febrile neutropenia in cancer patients: a systematic review and meta-analysis of randomized trials. J Antimicrob Chemother 54:29–37, 2004.

26. Neth O, Klein N: Febrile neutropenia: past, present and future. Adv Exp Med Biol 549:119–124, 2004.

27. Sung L, Nathan PC, Lange B, et al: Prophylactic granulocyte colony-stimulating factor and granulocyte-macrophage colony-stimulating factor decrease febrile neutropenia after chemotherapy in children with cancer: a meta-analysis of randomized controlled trials. J Clin Oncol 22:3350–3356, 2004.

*Selected readings.

Chapter 129

Acute Childhood Immune Thrombocytopenic Purpura and Related Platelet Disorders

Peter D. Sadowitz, MD and Abdul-Kader Souid, MD, PhD

Key Points

Acute childhood immune thrombocytopenic purpura is a common pediatric disease.

Children with profound thrombocytopenia (platelet counts $< 20 \times 10^3/mm^3$) and severe mucosal or cutaneous bleeding have significant risk of developing a life-threatening hemorrhage (intracranial, pulmonary, or upper airway). Patients with these findings should be admitted, and *promptly* treated with high-dose corticosteroids and anti-D antibody or immunoglobulin concentrates.

Aspirin and nonsteroidal anti-inflammatory drugs are *absolutely* contraindicated in children with thrombocytopenia.

Introduction and Background

Acute childhood immune thrombocytopenic purpura (ITP) is characterized by the sudden onset of profound thrombocytopenia in an otherwise healthy child.[1] The disease results from production of antiplatelet antibodies, which promote Fc/γ receptor–mediated platelet destruction in the spleen. Anti-D antibodies and immunoglobulins block these receptors.[2-4]

Recognition and Approach

Bruising and mild bleeding from minor trauma is common in active, healthy children and must be differentiated from serious or life-threatening disorders. To accurately diagnose ITP, clinicians must consider its diagnosis in all children with mucocutaneous bleeding that is either prolonged, profuse, in an unusual location, or inconsistent with the level of trauma.

In children with significant bleeding, the history, physical examination, and radiologic and laboratory screening are focused on discriminating between trauma (nonaccidental or accidental), blood vessel disorders, and hematologic disorders. Accidental trauma occurs in typical exposed areas with a history that is consistent with findings on physical examination. Children with nonaccidental trauma have bleeding or bruising that is inconsistent with the history given, while typical bony and soft tissues injuries are usually present (see Chapter 119, Physical Abuse and Child Neglect). Defects in coagulation are often associated with muscle, joint, or intracranial bleeding (see Chapter 130, Disorders of Coagulation). In contrast, platelet and vessel diseases (vasculitis) typically cause mucousal bleeding (e.g., epistaxis; gastrointestinal, gynecologic, or genitourinary) or purpura or petechiae. Importantly, other signs of systemic illness are often present in other serious causes of bleeding, while children with ITP are usually well appearing unless intracranial bleeding or significant blood loss is present.

In contrast to adults with ITP, males and females are affected with equal frequency. The median age of childhood ITP is 3 to 5 years, with most cases less than 10 years old. Childhood ITP is more likely to resolve spontaneously and to respond to treatment compared to adult cases.

Clinical Presentation

The typical clinical presentation of acute childhood ITP includes the sudden onset of bruises and petechiae in an otherwise healthy child. Often there is an antecedent viral illness. In a few patients, the thrombocytopenia follows infection with varicella virus, mumps, Epstein-Barr virus, cytomegalovirus, human immunodeficiency virus (HIV), viral hepatitis (A, B, or C), or vaccination (usually approximately 2 to 3 weeks following attenuated live virus immunization). The physical examination reveals a healthy-appearing child (unless there is significant blood loss or intracranial bleeding) with widespread bruises, petechiae, and purpuric lesions involving the skin (especially dependent areas). Mucous membrane bleeding (e.g., gingival or gastrointestinal bleed, epistaxis, menorrhagia) is also common with ITP. Intracranial bleeding, the most feared complication, occurs in less than 1% of cases. Lymphadenopathy, hepatomegaly, splenomegaly, bone or joint pain, fever, neutropenia, and anemia are characteristically absent; their presence suggests bone marrow infiltration by leukemia or solid tumor.

The complete blood count (including peripheral blood smear examination) demonstrates an isolated thrombocytopenia. The diagnosis of ITP should be considered if the platelet count is less than $150 \times 10^3/mm^3$; most patients have a platelet count of less than $20 \times 10^3/mm^3$. The platelets are typically large, reflecting production of fresh platelets. The hemoglobin concentration, white blood cell count, and differential are normal. Neutropenia, anemia, or circulating nucleated red blood cells, promyelocytes, metamyelocytes, or blasts are not found in ITP.

Bone marrow examination shows normal trilineage hematopoietic cells with increased megakaryocytes. This procedure (usually performed by a pediatric hematologist) is sometimes necessary to confirm the diagnosis of ITP (e.g., to exclude acute leukemia, which can be partially treated with corticosteroids).

The majority of children recover without recurrence. The platelet count usually becomes normal in 1 to 6 months. Recurrent thrombocytopenia occurs in approximately 10% of patients. Chronic ITP occurs in approximately 10% of children, and is defined as thrombocytopenia that persists more than 6 months. Patients with common variable immunodeficiency frequently develop ITP (alone or in combination with autoimmune hemolytic anemia, or Evans' syndrome). Thus it is recommended to measure immunoglobulin levels in patients with chronic ITP.[5] In some patients, eradicating *Helicobacter pylori* infection cures chronic ITP.[6,7] Thus it is also recommended to search for and treat *H. pylori* in patients with chronic ITP. Chronic ITP is more common in adolescents.[8] In these patients, other autoantibodies (e.g., antinuclear and anti-DNA antibodies) or autoimmune diseases (e.g., systemic lupus erythematosus) may be present or develop in the future.[8]

Important Clinical Features and Considerations

ITP should be distinguished from other causes of thrombocytopenia (Tables 129–1 and 129–2).[9] The most common entities are discussed in this section.

Acute leukemia often produces bone or joint pain, pallor, fever, and fatigue (in addition to bruising and petechiae). The physical examination usually reveals lymphadenopathy and hepatosplenomegaly. The blood smear may show circulating blasts. The complete blood count often shows abnormalities involving the leukocyte and erythroid lineages in addition to thrombocytopenia (e.g., anemia, reticulocytopenia, neutropenia, abnormal leukocyte differential) (see Chapter 128, Cancer and Cancer-Related Complications in Children).

Vasculitis (endothelial cell injury) produces microangiopathic intravascular hemolytic anemia (thrombocytopenia, circulating red blood cell fragments, hemoglobinemia, and hemoglobinuria). This process occurs in hemolytic-uremic syndrome (see Chapter 131, Hemolytic-Uremic Syndrome), thrombotic thrombocytopenic purpura, disseminated intravascular coagulation, and autoimmune vasculitis.

Table 129–1	Causes of Thrombocytopenia

Increased Platelet Destruction

Immune Mediated
- Immune thrombocytopenic purpura (ITP)
- Collagen vascular diseases (e.g., systemic lupus erythematosus)
- Post–viral infections (e.g., human immunodeficiency virus)
- Drug-induced thrombocytopenia
- Neonatal alloimmune thrombocytopenia (due to incompatibility between fetus and mother)[19]
- Neonatal thrombocytopenia due to maternal chronic ITP[19]

Non–Immune Mediated
- Hemolytic-uremic syndrome
- Thrombotic thrombocytopenic purpura
- Disseminated intravascular coagulation
- Prosthetic heart valve

Platelet Sequestration
- Hemangiomas (e.g., Kasabach-Merritt syndrome)
- Venous malformation
- Splenomegaly with hypersplenism

Decreased Platelet Production

Congenital
- Fanconi's aplastic anemia
- Thrombocytopenia and absent radii
- Amegakaryocytic thrombocytopenia
- Wiskott-Aldrich syndrome (X-linked, characterized by thrombocytopenia, severe eczema, and recurrent bacterial infections)
- Paroxysmal nocturnal hemoglobinuria

Acquired
- Bone marrow infiltration (e.g., leukemia, metastatic tumors, metabolic disorders)
- Drug induced
- Acquired aplastic anemia

Bruises with Normal Platelet Counts
- Child abuse
- Henoch-Schönlein purpura
- Increased vascular leak

Pseudothrombocytopenia

Bone marrow failure is associated with various severities of neutropenia, anemia, and thrombocytopenia (with small-size platelets) and a reduced number of megakaryocytes in the bone marrow.

Many *medications* (e.g., heparin, penicillin, cephalothin, sulfisoxazole, rifampin, phenytoin, valproic acid) produce destructive thrombocytopenia or decreased platelet production.

On rare occasions, platelets can be trapped and destroyed in capillary *hemangiomas,* producing thrombocytopenia (Kasabach-Merritt syndrome).

HIV infection is often associated with immune-mediated thrombocytopenia. The clinical presentation can be similar to that of acute ITP. Thus, HIV infection should be considered in high-risk patients (see Chapter 69, Human Immunodeficiency Virus Infection and Other Immunosuppressive Conditions).

Thrombocytopenia is common in infants with *congenital viral infections.* These infants usually have microcephaly, low birth weight, hepatosplenomegaly, and intracranial calcifications.

Henoch-Schönlein purpura is a systemic vasculitis associated with the development of painful symmetric, palpable purpura involving proximal regions of the extremities, particularly the legs and buttocks. There may be renal involvement with associated hematuria and proteinuria. Vasculitis

Table 129–2 Discriminating Features of Patients with Thrombocytopenia

Disorder	Clinical Findings	Laboratory Findings
ITP	Well-appearing child Generalized bruises and petechiae Absence of lymphadenopathy and hepatosplenomegaly	Isolated thrombocytopenia
Acute leukemia	Often appears ill Bone and/or joint pain, fever, etc. Lymphadenopathy and hepatosplenomegaly	Anemia Thrombocytopenia Neutropenia Circulating blasts
Bone marrow failure	Pallor, bruising, and fever Absence of hepatomegaly and lymphadenopathy	Pancytopenia of varying severity
Hemolytic-uremic syndrome	Pallor Petechiae and bruising Diarrhea Oliguria and hematuria	Thrombocytopenia Microangiopathic anemia Hemoglobinuria Elevated creatinine
DIC	Ill-appearing child Pallor with petechiae and purpura	Thrombocytopenia Microangiopathic anemia Prolonged PT, PTT, and TT Hypofibrinogenemia
Child abuse	Bruises of earlobes, back, buttocks, genitalia, etc.	Normal CBC, PT, PTT, and TT
Henoch-Schönlein purpura	Painful purpura involving the buttocks and lower extremities	Normal CBC Occasionally hematuria and proteinuria
Hypersplenism	Splenomegaly	Pancytopenia (cells are trapped in the spleen)

Abbreviations: CBC, complete blood count; DIC, disseminated intravascular coagulation; ITP, immune thrombocytopenic purpura; PT, prothrombin time; PTT, partial thromboplastin time; TT, thrombin time.

---

involving the intestinal tract can lead to intussusception. The platelet count is normal (see Chapter 122, Henoch-Schönlein Purpura).

Petechiae can result from increased *vascular leak/pressure* due to vomiting, coughing, or application of a tourniquet. The resulting petechiae mostly involve the upper chest and extremities. The platelet count is normal.

Child abuse should be considered in the presence of petechiae and bruises in certain locations (e.g., earlobes, back, buttocks) if the platelet count and coagulation studies are normal. The bruises are typically limited to contact sites (see Chapter 119, Physical Abuse and Child Neglect).

Rarely, platelets may agglutinate in blood tubes containing ethylenediaminetetraacetate (the anticoagulant used for blood counts), producing *pseudothrombocytopenia*. This possibility should be considered if the patient has no signs of thrombocytopenia. An estimation of the platelet count can be obtained by placing the patient's blood directly on a slide. Alternatively, the blood sample can be collected in a citrate-containing blood tube.

Management

Corticosteroids remain the best treatment option (Table 129–3).[10] Steroids increase vascular stability, decrease antiplatelet antibody production, and reduce clearance of the antibody-platelet complexes. Clinical improvement (e.g., decreased tendency to bruise) usually occurs before a rise in the platelet count. Conventional treatment is prednisone at 2 mg/kg/day (in three divided doses) for 14 days, followed by tapering and discontinuation by day 21. The efficacy of high-dose corticosteroids for 1 to 4 days (e.g., intravenous methylprednisolone at 6 mg/kg per dose over 30 minutes every 8 hours for approximately 2 days; pulsed dexamethasone

Table 129–3 Management of Childhood Acute ITP

Corticosteroids

Conventional Dose Options
- Prednisone, 2 mg/kg/day (in three divided doses) for 14 days, followed by tapering and discontinuation by day 21
- Prednisone, 4 mg/kg/day (in three divided doses) for 14 days, followed by tapering and discontinuation by day 21
- Prednisolone, 60 mg/m^2 (in three divided doses) for 14 days, followed by tapering and discontinuation by day 21

High-Dose Options
(Active bleeding—platelet count < 20 × 10^3/mm^3)
- Pulsed methylprednisolone, 30 mg/kg (maximum dose, 1 g) IV over 30 min q24h for two or three doses[20]
- Methylprednisolone, 6 mg/kg IV over 30 min q8h for 2–4 days
- Pulsed dexamethasone, 40 mg/day (maximum dose) orally for 4 days[11]

Immunoglobulins

Intravenous Anti-D Antibody (for patients who are Rh+):
- Rh$_0$(D) immune globulin, 50–75 mcg/kg IV over 5 min (one dose) (see text for appropriate precautions)

Intravenous IgG Concentrate Options (for patients who are Rh–):
- Conventional schedule: 0.4 g/kg/day IV over ~4 hr for 5 consecutive days
- Two-day schedule: 0.8–1 g/kg/day IV over ~4 hr for 2 consecutive days
- One-day schedule: 1 g/kg/day IV over ~4 hr for one dose (the most commonly used regimen)

Combined Corticosteroids and Immunoglobulins (for Severe ITP)

Conventional or high-dose steroid plus IV anti-D antibody or IgG concentrate

---

Abbreviations: IgG, immunoglobulin G; ITP, immune thrombocytopenic purpura; IV, intravenous(ly).

at 40 mg/day [maximum dose] orally for 4 days[11]; or dexamethasone 0.25 mg/kg every 6 hours orally for approximately 2 days) in severe acute ITP is well documented. This approach increases the platelet count to greater than $20 \times 10^3/mm^3$ by approximately 48 hours in the majority of patients.

Intravenous anti-D antibody, or human $Rh_0(D)$ immune globulin, is an effective treatment for patients who are Rh positive.[12] The dose is 50 to 75 mcg/kg intravenously over 5 minutes. In most patients, the platelet count rises to greater than $20 \times 10^3/mm^3$ within approximately 48 hours. Anti-D antibodies bind to red cells, promoting their destruction in the spleen. This process temporarily spares platelet destruction. Intravenous anti-D antibody is contraindicated in immunoglobulin A (IgA) deficiency and in patients with hemoglobin concentrations less than 8 g/dl. The immediate side effects include headache, chills (due to hemolysis of $Rh_0(D)$ antigen–positive red cells), nausea, vomiting, fever, hemolysis, and reduction in hemoglobin concentration. The hemoglobin concentration typically drops by 1 to 3 g/dl in approximately 24 hours. Marked drops in hemoglobin (requiring blood transfusion) and renal insufficiency (due to hemolysis) have been reported; however, their occurrence is very rare. Administration of methylprednisolone (1 mg/kg), acetaminophen, and ondansetron prior to anti-D antibody treatment may prevent fever, nausea, vomiting, and headache.

Intravenous polyvalent immunoglobulin G (IgG) concentrates (e.g., 1 g/kg intravenously over approximately 4 hours daily twice) represent an alternative treatment to anti-D antibody for patients who are Rh negative. IgG molecules block splenic Fc/γ receptors on macrophages (sites of platelet destruction). Disadvantages of IgG infusion include high cost and inconvenience (given over 4 hours). Adverse effects include headache (migraine like, lasting for 1 to 2 days), positive Coombs' tests, hemolytic anemia (due to high isoagglutinins), anaphylaxis (occurs in patients with IgA deficiency; IgA-depleted preparations are available), and viral transmission (e.g., hepatitis C).

Life-threatening hemorrhage (intracranial, pulmonary, and upper airway) may occur in children with platelet counts less than $20 \times 10^3/mm^3$.[3,13,14] The presence of severe mucosal, retinal, and cutaneous bleeding identifies patients at greatest risk for serious bleeding. These patients should be admitted and *promptly* treated with high-dose corticosteroids and anti-D antibody or immunoglobulin concentrates (see Table 129–3).

Danazol, mycophenolate mofetil, and rituximab (recombinant antibodies to the lymphocyte membrane antigen CD20) are used in refractory ITP.[15-17] Emergency splenectomy is considered for life-threatening, refractory bleeding. Platelets should be administered in active, life-threatening bleeding. Platelet survival is improved if they are transfused soon after immunoglobulin infusion.

Aspirin, aspirin-containing compounds, nonsteroidal anti-inflammatory drugs, and anticoagulants are *absolutely* contraindicated. Intramuscular injections should be avoided. For venous access, the dorsa of the hands and feet are the most suitable sites. Antecubital fossa, jugular, and femoral veins should be avoided to prevent neurovascular compromise if excessive bleeding occurs. After a venipuncture, pressure should be applied to the site for 5 to 10 minutes. Arterial punctures are *absolutely* contraindicated.

The risk for significant bleeding should be carefully assessed. Patients with potential complications related to thrombocytopenia require prompt treatment (see Table 129–3) and admission for observation. For example, patients with significant head injury require combined therapy (see Table 129–3) and hospitalization (even if a head computed tomography scan is normal). Similarly, patients with significant trauma (e.g., blunt trauma from a car accident) should also receive combined therapy and be admitted for observation. In patients with suspected meningitis, antibiotics should be administered and the spinal tap deferred until the platelet count is approximately $50 \times 10^3/mm^3$. Major trauma with the need for emergent surgery (e.g., chest, abdominal, central nervous system, orthopedic) requires aggressive combined therapy (see Table 129–3) and immediate consultations with a hematologist and surgeon. A hematology consultation should be considered for assistance in confirming the diagnosis or, in the patient with known stable ITP, arranging disposition and follow-up care, if appropriate.

Children should be kept away from sports and playground activities until the platelet count is approximately $50 \times 10^3/mm^3$. Protective equipment should be used during activities to prevent trauma, especially head injury (e.g., wearing a helmet).

Summary

Acute childhood ITP is a self-limited disease in the majority of children. The diagnosis requires a careful medical history, a thorough physical examination, and complete blood counts (including a careful review of the blood smear) to exclude other etiologies of thrombocytopenia. Physicians outside tertiary care centers can diagnose and treat children with acute ITP based on clinical and laboratory evaluations. Consultation and referral to a tertiary care center are necessary for children who deviate from the "typical" features of this entity.[18]

REFERENCES

1. Blanchette VS, Carcao M: Childhood acute immune thrombocytopenic purpura: 20 years later. Semin Thromb Hemost 29:605–617, 2003.
2. Beardsley DJ, Tang C, Chen BG, et al: The disulfide-rich region of platelet glycoprotein (GP) IIIa contains hydrophilic peptide sequences that bind anti-GPIIIa autoantibodies from patients with immune thrombocytopenic purpura (ITP). Biophys Chem 105:503–515, 2003.
3. Cooper N, Heddle NM, Haas M, et al: Intravenous (IV) anti-D and IV immunoglobulin achieve acute platelet increases by different mechanisms: modulation of cytokine and platelet responses to IV anti-D by FcγRIIa and FcγRIIIa polymorphisms. Br J Haematol 124:511–518, 2004.
4. Hansen RJ, Balthasar JP: Mechanisms of IVIG action in immune thrombocytopenic purpura. Clin Lab 50:133–140, 2004.
5. Michel M, Chanet V, Galicier L, et al: Autoimmune thrombocytopenic purpura and common variable immunodeficiency: analysis of 21 cases and review of the literature. Medicine (Baltimore) 83:254–263, 2004.
6. Kurtoglu E, Kayacetin E, Ugur A: *Helicobacter pylori* infection in patients with autoimmune thrombocytopenic purpura. World J Gastroenterol 10:2113–2115, 2004.
7. Michel M, Cooper N, Jean C, et al: Does *Helicobater pylori* initiate or perpetuate immune thrombocytopenic purpura? Blood 103:890–896, 2004.
8. Buchanan GR, Journeycake JM, Adix L: Severe chronic idiopathic thrombocytopenic purpura during childhood: definition, management and prognosis. Semin Thromb Hemost 29:595–603, 2003.

*9. Kaplan RN, Bussel JB: Differential diagnosis and management of thrombocytopenia in childhood. Pediatr Clin North Am 51:1109–1140, 2004.

10. Bolton-Maggs P, Tarantino MD, Buchanan GR, et al: The child with immune thrombocytopenic purpura: is pharmacotherapy or watchful waiting the best initial management? A panel discussion from the 2002 meeting of the American Society of Pediatric Hematology/Oncology. J Pediatr Hematol Oncol 26:146–151, 2004.

11. Cheng Y, Wong RS, Soo YO, et al: Initial treatment of immune thrombocytopenic purpura with high-dose dexamethasone. N Engl J Med 349:831–836, 2003.

12. Moser AM, Shalev H, Kapelushnik J: Anti-D exerts a very early response in childhood acute idiopathic thrombocytopenic purpura. Pediatr Hematol Oncol 19:407–411, 2002.

13. Butros L, Bussel JB: Intracranial hemorrhage in immune thrombocytopenic purpura: a retrospective analysis. J Pediatr Hematol Oncol 25:660–664, 2003.

*14. Thomas K, Buchanan GR, Zimmerman S: A prospective comparative study of 2540 infants and children with newly diagnosed idiopathic thrombocytopenic purpura (ITP) from the Intercontinental Childhood ITP Study Group. J Pediatr 143:605–608, 2003.

15. Maloisel F, Andres E, Zimmer J, et al: Danazol therapy in patients with chronic idiopathic thrombocytopenic purpura: long-term results. Am J Med 116:590–594, 2004.

16. Narang M, Penner JA, Williams D: Refractory autoimmune thrombocytopenic purpura: responses to treatment with a recombinant antibody to lymphocyte membrane antigen CD20 (rituximab). Am J Hematol 74:263–267, 2003.

17. Imbach P, Kuhne T, Zimmerman S: New developments in idiopathic thrombocytopenic purpura (ITP): cooperative, prospective studies by the Intercontinental Childhood ITP Study Group. J Pediatr Hematol Oncol 25:S74–S76, 2003.

*18. Modak SI, Bussel JB: Treatment of children with immune thrombocytopenic purpura: are we closer to resolving the dilemma? J Pediatr 133:313–314, 1998.

19. Bussel JB: Fetal and neonatal cytopenias: what have we learned? Am J Perinatol 20:425–431, 2003.

20. Kelton JG: Management of the pregnant patient with idiopathic thrombocytopenic purpura. Ann Intern Med 99:796–800, 1983.

*Selected readings.

Chapter 130

Disorders of Coagulation

Abdul-Kader Souid, MD, PhD

Key Points

Regarding the need for a product replacement, the clinician should remember: when in doubt, infuse.

The product of choice for patients with factor VIII deficiency is recombinant factor VIII, and for patients with factor IX deficiency, recombinant factor IX.

For factor VIII deficiency, 20 to 30 units/kg are infused for mild to moderate bleeding, and 50 to 75 units/kg for moderate to severe bleeding. Follow-up infusions may be necessary.

For factor IX deficiency, 40 to 60 units/kg are infused for mild to moderate bleeding, and 80 to 100 units/kg for moderate to severe bleeding.

Inherited thrombophilia underlies a large percentage of venous thromboembolic events in children. Other risk factors include estrogen therapy, central venous catheters, congenital heart disease, and nephrotic syndrome.

Selected Diagnoses

Factor VIII deficiency (hemophilia A or classic hemophilia)
Factor IX deficiency (hemophilia B or Christmas disease)
Factors VIII and IX inhibitors
von Willebrand's disease
Venous thromboembolism

Discussion of Individual Diagnoses

Factor VIII Deficiency (Hemophilia A or Classic Hemophilia)

Factor VIII deficiency is the most common inherited (X-linked recessive) disorder involving secondary hemostasis (affecting approximately 1 in 5000 to 10,000 males). Normal plasma levels of factor VIII are 50 to 150 units/dl. Male patients and female carries who have factor VIII levels greater than 30 units/dl generally have normal hemostasis. Patients with levels less than 1 unit/dl have severe disease (60% of total patients), those with levels of 1 to 5 units/dl have moderate disease, and those with levels greater than 5 units/dl have mild disease (mild and moderate disease comprise 40% of all patients). Patients with severe disease have frequent bleeding episodes (spontaneously or following trauma), particularly into the joints and muscles. Patients with moderate disease experience bleeding after minor trauma. Patients with mild disease experience bleeding after significant trauma or surgery. Some female carriers have factor levels less than 30 units/dl, and may exhibit symptoms of mild hemophilia (symptomatic carriers).

The half-life of endogenous factor VIII is approximately 8 to 12 hours. The half-life of infused factor VIII should be measured in each patient at the time of starting a new product. For repetitive infusions, factor VIII is usually given every 8 to 12 hours. Some patients receive prophylactic infusions (e.g., two to three times per week). Most patients, however, receive on-demand treatment (e.g., following trauma or symptoms related to bleeding). The average cost of factor VIII concentrates is about $1.00 per unit. Most patients with moderate and severe disease have a supply of factor at home. Young children with severe hemophilia usually have an intravenous access device to facilitate infusions (see Chapter 170, Access of Ports and Catheters and Management of Obstruction). Self-infusion education usually begins after about 10 years of age.

Clinical Presentation

Patients with hemophilia A are typically males. Their symptoms may begin at the time of crawling and walking. Almost all severely affected patients are diagnosed by about 1 year of age. It should be noted that normal screening coagulation tests—prothrombin time (PT), activated partial thromboplastin time (aPTT), and thrombin time (TT)—exclude a clinically significant coagulation factor deficiency (including hemophilias).

The diagnosis of hemophilia A should be suspected in children with a family history of the disease or a bleeding event (e.g., prolonged bleeding from circumcision, medical procedure, surgery, dental extraction, hemarthrosis, or hematoma) associated with a prolonged PTT. A positive family history for the disease is present in only two thirds of patients; the remaining cases have de novo mutations. Infants with hemophilia may tolerate circumcision without excessive bleeding. Thus a history of uneventful circumcision does not exclude the presence of a severe bleeding disorder.

The hallmarks of factor VIII deficiency are joint and muscle hemorrhages.[1] The initial symptoms of hemarthrosis are warmth and a tingling sensation (these complaints require immediate factor infusion). As blood fills the joint space, swelling, pain, and limitation of movement occur. Bleeding into a target joint (a joint that the patient bleeds into repetitively due to synovitis; defined as 4 bleeding episodes in 6 months, 8 bleeding episodes in 12 months or 20 total bleeding episodes) produces progressive synovitis, hemophilic arthropathy, and chronic arthritis. The latter complication is progressive and irreversible. Thus joint bleeding should be treated at the onset of the earliest symptoms and prior to the development of physical findings. The joint should be immobilized with no weight bearing by using crutches for weight-bearing joints or splinting for joint support. Management includes elevating the limb, applying ice packs, and wrapping the joint.[1] Joint bleeding is common in severe and less common in mild hemophilia. Thus some patients with severe hemophilia receive prophylactic factor infusion to prevent chronic arthritis.

Patients with hematomas present with pain and limited mobility. Iliopsoas bleeding causes pain in the right lower quadrant, resembling appendicitis or hip disease. Muscle bleeding at this site (after heavy weight lifting or strenuous exercise) causes leg flexion, pain in the anterior surface of the thigh due to femoral nerve compression, and inability to extend the leg. Abdominal cavity bleeding (into the liver, spleen, pancreas, or retroperitoneum) produces falling hemoglobin and abdominal or back pain. Buttock, thigh, deltoid, and forearm bleeding may produce neurovascular compression and compartment syndrome. Neck or oral hematoma may cause dyspnea and dysphagia and compromise the airway. Gastrointestinal (GI) bleeding causes melena and bloody vomiting. Each of these scenarios requires immediate (major-dose) factor infusion, rest, close observation, and consultation with a hematologist.

Bleeding in the gum, tooth, frenulum, tongue, throat, or pharynx may last a few days. It responds to factor infusions, antifibrinolytic therapy (aminocaproic acid), and diet instructions (using soft/cool diet, such as jello, soft drinks, baby foods, and spaghetti; avoiding hard foods, such as chips, popcorn, and tacos).

Painless hematuria is treated by increased fluid intake and bed rest for several days. Factor infusions (for 2 to 4 days) are necessary for persistent painless hematuria. Painless hematuria should be distinguished from hematuria with flank pain. Painful hematuria (e.g., abdominal or flank pain) requires renal ultrasound to assess renal parenchymal bleed and to rule out clots obstructing the ureter, bed rest, and factor infusions for a few days, depending on severity of the bleeding. Antifibrinolytic agents should be avoided due to their ability to cause clots that may obstruct the ureter.

Intracranial bleeding is the leading cause of death. Central nervous system (CNS) bleeding may be spontaneous. Head trauma or any signs or symptoms of intracranial hemorrhage (e.g., headache, irritability, vomiting, seizure, ocular or visual problems, focal deficits, stiff neck, change of consciousness) require *immediate* treatment with a major-dose factor infusion prior to any diagnostic imaging or lengthy clinical evaluation. The onset of neurologic signs or symptoms following head trauma may be delayed due to the slowly oozing nature of hemophiliac bleeding.

Hemophilia A is diagnosed by prolonged aPTT and low factor VIII activity (<50 units/dl). PT and TT are normal. There is no need to repeat these tests in the emergency department (ED) in patients with known hemophilia. A postinfusion factor VIII level is necessary in severe bleeding or if inhibitors to factor VIII are suspected. This test assures adequate factor dosing and confirms that factor VIII is at the desired level. A postinfusion aPTT level is not sensitive for assessing adequate replacement, since the aPTT is normal with factor VIII levels greater than 30 units/dl.

Management

Hemophilia A treatment involves infusing recombinant factor VIII (produced by cell lines transfected with human factor VIII gene).[2-4] The dose, frequency, and duration of infusions vary depending on the site and severity of bleeding. The required in vivo level of factor VIII for mild to moderate bleeding (e.g., early joint, muscle, lip, or dental bleed; laceration; persistent hematuria) is 40 to 60 units/dl, and that for moderate to severe bleeding (e.g., surgery; major trauma; intracranial, retroperitoneal, advanced joint, pharyngeal, neck, or GI bleed) is 100 to 150 units/dl. In theory, each unit per kilogram of factor VIII results in an approximately 2-units/dl rise in plasma level (e.g., a 20-kg patient with bleeding requiring a factor VIII level of approximately 60 units/dl needs: 20 kg × 60 units/dl ÷ 2 units/dl = 600 units). Thus 20 to 30 units/kg should be infused for mild to moderate bleeding and 50 to 75 units/kg for moderate to severe bleeding (Table 130–1). The infusion is repeated as necessary. Instructions on factor reconstitution are found on the drug insert. The lot number(s), expiration date, trade name, and total number of units infused should be documented (empty boxes should be given to the patient). Most patients bring unmixed factor to the ED to minimize treatment delay and cost. Mixed products are stable for approximately 3 hours. The contents of all reconstituted vials for an infusion should be used (reconstituted factor should not be wasted). Further evaluation is necessary if the patient experiences increasing joint pain and swelling within 24 hours after multiple (e.g., greater than two) adequate factor infusions. It this occurs, the clinician should assess the patient for inhibitors, obtain radiographs looking for a fracture, and consider tapping the joint if infection is highly suspected.

Aminocaproic acid (Amicar), an antifibrinolytic agent, is administered for oral, gingival, or dental bleeding (see Table 130–1). The dose is 25 to 100 mg/kg every 6 to 8 hours for approximately 7 days.[5] The intravenous and oral preparations contain 250 mg/ml. The tablets are 500 mg or 1000 mg each. Aminocaproic acid should be avoided in patients with hematuria.

In patients with mild factor VIII deficiency and minor bleeding, desmopressin acetate (1-deamino-8-D-arginine vasopressin, or DDAVP) is the treatment of choice.[6-8] Desmopressin increases factor VIII (and von Willebrand factor) levels by three- to fivefold within 30 to 60 minutes.[5] A test dose is recommended. DDAVP is not likely to achieve adequate hemostasis if baseline factor VIII levels are less than 10%. Desmopressin (DDAVP Injection) is given intravenously at 0.3 mcg/kg in 50 ml normal saline over 30 minutes. Intravenous administration is preferred in acute bleeding and prior to surgery. Desmopressin (DDAVP Injection) can also be given subcutaneously at 0.3 mcg/kg. Intranasal des-

Table 130–1	Treatment of Hemophilias and von Willebrand Disease		
Deficiency	**Treatment**	**Preparation**	**Dosing**
Factor VIII	Factor VIII concentrates	Recombinant factor VIII	Mild to moderate bleeding: 20–30 units/kg*
			Moderate to severe bleeding: 50–75 units/kg*
	Desmopressin	DDAVP Injection	0.3 mcg/kg IV or subQ (single daily dose)[†]
		Stimate Nasal Spray	One or two sprays (single daily dose)[†]
	Aminocaproic acid	Amicar	25–100 mg/kg q6–8h for ~7 days
Factor IX	Factor IX concentrates	Recombinant factor IX	Mild to moderate bleeding: 50–70 units/kg[‡]
			Moderate to severe bleeding: 100–120 units/kg[‡]
	Aminocaproic acid	Amicar	25–100 mg/kg q6–8h for ~7 days
von Willebrand factor	Desmopressin	DDAVP Injection	0.3 mcg/kg IV or subQ (single daily dose)[2]
		Stimate Nasal Spray	One or two sprays (single daily dose)[2]
	Aminocaproic acid	Amicar	25–100 mg/kg q6–8h for ~7 days
	Intermediate-purity factor VIII concentrates	Humate-P	~50 vWF:RCof units/kg IV q8–12h

*For repetitive infusions, factor VIII is commonly given every 8 to 12 hours.
[†]The same dose can be repeated once a day for 3 to 5 days if necessary.
[‡]For repetitive infusions, factor IX is commonly given every 12 to 24 hours.
Abbreviations: IV, intravenously; subQ, subcutaneously; vWF:RCof, von Willebrand factor: Ristocetin Cofactor.

mopressin (Stimate Nasal Spray), one spray (150 mcg) if the patient's weight is less than 110 lb or two sprays (300 mcg) if weight is greater than 110 lb, is also effective.[8]

If factor VIII concentrates are unavailable and bleeding is unresponsive to desmopressin, or for those patients with severe disease who are not candidates for desmopressin, fresh frozen plasma (20 ml/kg) or cryoprecipitate (1 to 4 units/ 10 kg, 8 to 12 bags for adults) can be administered. If appropriate replacement is unavailable, transfer the patient to a center that has factor VIII concentrates. It should be noted that fresh frozen plasma and cryoprecipitate do not undergo virus inactivation (see Chapter 132, Utilizing Blood Bank Resources/Transfusion Reactions and Complications).

Intramuscular injections, aspirin, and aspirin-containing compounds (e.g., Pepto-Bismol, Exedrin, Percodan) are contraindicated. Aspiration of the joint should be avoided. Acetaminophen can be used for mild pain, while narcotics may be required for severe acute pain.

A hematologist should be consulted prior to surgery or invasive procedures (e.g., spinal tap). The surgeon should be familiar with hemophilia. The pharmacy should have adequate recombinant factor VIII. Prior to a major surgery, 50 units/kg should be infused at least every 8 hours; plasma levels greater than 50 units/dl should be maintained for 7 to 10 days after surgery. Prior to spinal tap, 50 units/kg should be infused every 8 to 12 hours for at least 24 hours.

For venous access, the limb with the joint or muscle bleeding should be avoided. As a rule, proximal, deep, and noncompressible venous access sites (e.g., jugular, femoral, and subclavian veins) should also be avoided, as bleeding at these sites can lead to a neurovascular compromise. The dorsa of the hands and feet are the most suitable sites. After needle stick, pressure and a bandage are applied for a few minutes. Arterial punctures are contraindicated.

Patients with severe bleeding require hospital admission and close observation for progression of symptoms. Those with significant head trauma or neurologic findings require admission for continuation of factor infusion and observation. Depending on the clinical situation, patients with moderate bleeding may require admission or close follow-up with a hematologist. Most patients with mild bleeding are

discharged with instructions and a follow-up appointment. For patients who are discharged, caregivers should be instructed to observe for clinical deterioration, continued bleeding, or progressive symptoms. For patients with mild head injury who are discharged, caregivers should be instructed to observe for signs of CNS bleeding for at least 2 weeks since late signs and symptoms may develop. For patients with joint bleeding, the discharge instructions should include rest, compression (Ace wraps), elevation of an affected limb, and use of splinting for joint support for at least 24 hours. In all patients who are discharged, consultation with a hematologist is necessary for possible need for follow-up factor infusions. When a patient or the family is traveling, regional hemophilia treatment centers can be located on the National Center on Birth Defects and Developmental Disabilities website at *www.cdc.gov/ncbddd/hbd/ care_model.htm.*

Risks of acquisition of hepatitis B or C virus, human immunodeficiency virus, parvovirus B19, and human T-lymphotropic virus type I are eliminated with the use of recombinant factors. Recombinant factor products that are completely free of all human and animal proteins (e.g., Advate) are available.[4] The risk of viral transmission via cryoprecipitate is the same as that for other blood components (see Chapter 132, Utilizing Blood Bank Resources/ Transfusion Reactions and Complications).

Early application of factor infusions (prophylaxis or intense-on-demand) prevents joint destruction and the need for repetitive infusions.[1] The majority of hospitalizations are for joint and soft tissue bleeding, especially in patients with inhibitors.[9] Psychological and economic problems remain major issues.

Factor IX Deficiency (Hemophilia B or Christmas Disease)

Factor IX deficiency is a heterogeneous X-linked recessive disorder involving secondary hemostasis (affecting approximately 1 in 60,000 males). Normal plasma levels of factor IX are 50 to 150 units/dl. Patients with levels less than 1 unit/dl have severe disease, those with levels of 1 to 5 units/dl moderate disease, and those with levels greater than 5 units/dl mild disease. The half-life of factor IX is approximately 18 to 24 hours. For repetitive infusions, factor IX is commonly given every 12 to 24 hours. About one third of patients have de novo mutations.

The clinical presentation is indistinguishable from that of hemophilia A. Patients with hemophilia B are also males. Their initial symptoms frequently begin at the time of crawling and walking. The diagnosis of hemophilia B should be suspected in children with positive family history for the disease (in two thirds of patients) or a bleeding event associated with prolonged aPTT.

The diagnostic tests show prolonged aPTT and low factor IX activity (<50 units/dl). PT and TT are normal. There is no need to routinely repeat these tests in the ED. In severe or refractory bleeding or in patients with known or suspected factor IX inhibitors, the factor IX level should be measured immediately following the infusion (see discussion for hemophilia A). A postinfusion aPTT level is not sensitive for assessing adequate replacement, since the aPTT is normal with factor IX levels greater than 35 units/dl.

Treatment involves infusing recombinant factor IX. The dose, frequency, and duration of infusion vary depending on the site and severity of bleeding. The required plasma level of factor IX for mild to moderate bleeding (e.g., early joint or muscle bleed, persistent hematuria) is 40 to 60 units/dl, and that for moderate to severe bleeding (e.g., surgery; major trauma; intracranial, retroperitoneal, advanced joint, pharyngeal, neck, or GI bleeding) is 80 to 100 units/dl. In theory, each unit per kilogram of factor IX (e.g., recombinant factor IX, or Benefix) results in an approximately 0.8-units/dl rise in plasma level (e.g., a 20-kg patient with bleeding requiring a factor IX level of approximately 60 units/dl needs: 20 kg × 60 units/dl ÷ 0.8 = 1500 units). Thus 50 to 70 units/kg of recombinant factor IX should be infused for mild to moderate bleeding and 100 to 120 units/kg for moderate to severe bleeding (see Table 130–1). The infusion should be repeated as necessary. When repeated factor IX infusions are administered for serious bleeding, plasma levels should be measured immediately after the infusion (peak) and just before the next infusion (trough). Peak levels should be kept at approximately 100 units/dl and trough levels at greater than 50 units/dl.

Prior to surgery, the patient's factor IX level should be increased to 100 units/dl and maintained by infusions every 12 to 24 hours for 7 to 10 days, depending on the type of surgery. In addition to factor IX infusions, aminocaproic acid can be administered for oral, gingival, or dental bleed (see Table 130–1 and section on factor VIII deficiency). Desmopressin is ineffective in hemophilia B.

If factor IX concentrates are unavailable, fresh frozen plasma (20 ml/kg) can be considered (see Chapter 132, Utilizing Blood Bank Resources/Transfusion Reactions and Complications). The patient should then be transferred to a center that has factor IX concentrates. It should be noted that fresh frozen plasma does not undergo virus inactivation.

Factors VIII and IX Inhibitors

Inhibitors to factors VIII and IX are more common in severely affected patients.[10] These antibodies neutralize the activity of infused factors. The presence of inhibitors should be suspected if the bleeding does not stop after two adequate infusions. The patient, family, and treating hematologist should inform the ED staff if inhibitors have been present in the past.

Inhibitors are quantified by measurements of factor VIII or IX activity in mixes of serial dilutions of patients' plasma with normal plasma. Levels of the inhibitor are expressed in Bethesda inhibitor units (BIU). One BIU causes 50% reduction in the factor activity. Patients with low-titer (low-responding) inhibitors (<10 BIU) can be treated with increased factor VIII or IX dosing (e.g., using two to three times the recommended dose). In patients with high-titer (high-responding) inhibitors (>10 BIU), a factor infusion stimulates further rise in BIU. For these patients, management requires infusion of products that bypass the missing factor in the clotting cascade. These preparations include recombinant factor VIIa (90 mcg/kg of NonoSeven) or activated prothrombin complex concentrate (APCC) (75 to 100 units/kg of FEIBA).[11,12] The patient's hematologist should be consulted prior to using these preparations. FEIBA should not be used in patients with factor IX deficiency who have inhibitors associated with known history of anaphylaxis. Moreover, APCC can produce thrombosis and disseminated intravascular coagulation. The response to NonoSeven and FEIBA is evaluated clinically (no laboratory tests are necessary).

von Willebrand's Disease

Von Willebrand's disease (vWD) is the most common inherited hemorrhagic disorder (prevalence is ~1%). Its inheritance is mostly autosomal dominant. The disease is heterogeneous, produced by a deficiency (types 1 and 3) or dysfunction (type 2) of Willebrand factor (vWF). vWF is an adhesive, multimeric glycoprotein produced by platelets and endothelial cells. It is present in plasma and subendothelial surfaces. It mediates platelet adhesion to exposed subendothelial collagen and platelet-platelet spreading and aggregation. vWF carries factor VIII, preventing its premature activation by factor IX and proteolysis by protein C. Acquired vWD due to accelerated vWF consumption (e.g., autoimmune diseases, cancer, aortic stenosis) occurs rarely; the treatment is the same as discussed here in addition to correcting the underlying cause.

The diagnosis and treatment of vWD can improve the lifestyle of patients and allow their surgeries to be safer. The clinical history is the most sensitive screen for vWD. Diversity exists in the clinical and laboratory findings within each family whose affected members have the same genetic defect. Repeated laboratory testing may be necessary to confirm the diagnosis.

Clinical Presentation

The clinical presentation is usually mild. Patients characteristically bleed from the mucous membranes (most notably, epistaxis and menorrhagia). Recurrent epistaxis occurs in more than two thirds of the patients. However, most children presenting to the ED with epistaxis have normal hemostasis. Among patients referred for hematology evaluation for recurrent epistaxis, 20% have vWD, 10% have another coagulopathy, and 70% have normal hemostasis.[13] Impaired primary or secondary hemostasis is present in 10% to 30% of adolescents with menorrhagia.[5,14-17] Thus hemostatic evaluation (Table 130–2) is indicated in patients with recurrent epistaxis or menorrhagia. Other presentations include bleeding following

Table 130–2	Treatment of von Willebrand Disease Based on Bleeding Site
Bleeding Site	**Treatment**
Easy bruising	Requires no treatment.
Prolonged nose bleeding	1. Stimate Nasal Spray on the side that is not bleeding.
	2. If no response within 1 hour, administer IV DDAVP Injection.
	3. If no response, request ENT consult and consider Humate-P.
Oral bleeding	Stimate Nasal Spray and aminocaproic acid are the treatment of choice.
Dental extraction	Aminocaproic acid (starting the evening before the procedure) plus desmopressin (Stimate Nasal Spray or DDAVP Injection) just before the procedure.
Menorrhagia	DDAVP Injection. Discharge the patient on aminocaproic acid and Stimate Nasal Spray (one spray in each nostril every day for ~5 days). If refractory, request gynecologic consultation and consider contraceptives pills.
Bleeding after surgery	Mild bleeding: DDAVP Injection and aminocaproic acid.
	Severe bleeding: Humate-P (~50 vWF:RCof units/kg IV q8–12h).
Minor surgery or procedure	DDAVP Injection and aminocaproic acid.
Major surgery or procedure	Humate-P (~50 vWf:RCof units/kg IV every 8–12 hr) for 7–10 days.

Abbreviations: ENT, otorhinolaryngology; IV, intravenously; vWF:RCof, von Willebrand factor: Ristocetin Cofactor.

surgery (most notably, tonsillectomy), dental extraction (greater than half of the patients diagnosed with vWD), mild trauma, spontaneous ecchymoses (more common in females), and GI bleeding (more common in adults). Hemarthroses and muscular bleeding do not occur with vWD.

For patients with known vWD disease, no specific tests are necessary in the ED. Bleeding time has limited clinical use and should be avoided. For patients with bleeding disorders who are undiagnosed, complete blood counts, PT, aPTT, and TT are usually performed in the ED. The aPTT is abnormal in severe vWD (type 3). The platelet function analyzer (PFA) is available acutely at many hospitals and has replaced the bleeding time. This test generally takes less than 15 minutes to perform. Pediatric studies have found the PFA to be sensitive and specific for detecting impaired primary hemostasis due to vWD or qualitative platelet abnormalities.[18] Inpatient studies that confirm the diagnosis of vWD include a vWF multimer assay, low-dose ristocetin-induced platelet aggregation, and cryoprecipitate-induced platelet aggregation.

Management

Treatment of vWD depends on severity and site of bleeding (see Table 130–2). Desmopressin acetate stimulates the release of stored vWF, increasing its plasma level approximately threefold within about 30 minutes. Desmopressin increases vWF secretion from Weibel-Palade bodies in endothelial cells through the cyclic AMP signaling pathway. It is the drug of choice for most patients with vWD (see Tables 130–1 and 130–2).[5-8] Patients with type 2 vWD may have a suboptimal response to desmopressin.[5]

The DDAVP Injection preparation (4 mg/ml) is given intravenously (0.3 mcg/kg in 50 ml normal saline over 30 minutes) or subcutaneously (0.3 mcg/kg). The intravenous route is more effective.[5] The intranasal preparation (Stimate Nasal Spray, 1.5 mg/ml) is given as one spray (150 mcg) if the patient weights less than 110 lb or one spray per nostril (300 mcg) if the patient weights greater than 110 lb. Testing the response to DDAVP is important. DDAVP Nasal Spray (0.1 mg/ml) is a different preparation given for nocturnal enuresis, and is ineffective in vWD. Adverse effects of desmopressin are water retention, facial flushing, nausea, headache, tachycardia, hypertension, angioedema, and tachyphylaxis (due to depletion of vWF stores). Desmopressin is contraindicated in heart failure, unstable coronary artery disease, polydipsia, and pregnancy (the drug crosses the placenta). Rarely, hyponatremic seizures occur due to water intoxication (e.g., in patients receiving large volumes of hypotonic fluids during anesthesia), especially in infants with repetitive intravenous fluid administration.[5] Fluid restriction is recommended during and immediately following DDAVP treatment.

Aminocaproic acid (Amicar) inhibits plasminogen activators and plasmin activity. This agent is used for dental and nasal bleeding. The dose is 25 to 100 mg/kg every 6 to 8 hours for 7 to 10 days (see Tables 130–1 and 130–2). The intravenous and oral preparations contain 250 mg/ml. The tablets are 500 mg or 1000 mg each.

Humate-P, an intermediate-purity factor VIII concentrate (pasteurized, i.e., heated at 60° C for 10 hours to inactivate blood-borne viruses), is rich in vWf (containing two- to threefold more vWf than factor VIII).[5] This product contains approximately 2 to 3 units of von Willebrand factor: Ristocetin Cofactor (vWF:RCof) per unit of factor VIII, and retains high-molecular-weight vWF multimers. It is widely used for serious or refractory bleeding. It is indicated for all types of vWD if desmopressin and aminocaproic acid are inadequate or inappropriate. The dose is approximately 50 vWF:RCof units/kg intravenously every 8 to 12 hours, as necessary (see Tables 130–1 and 130–2). Each unit of vWF:RCof per kilogram raises plasma level by 1.5 units/dl (or 1.5%). For minor bleeding, one to two doses are sufficient. Significant bleeding (e.g., CNS trauma, refractory bleeding) requires infusions for 3 to 10 days. In these situations, trough vWF:RCof levels greater than 50% should be maintained.

Humate-P is labeled as a "triple safety net" product (donor self-referral, rigorous testing, and virucidal treatment). If Humate-P is unavailable and the patient has active bleeding despite intravenous desmopressin and aminocaproic acid, fresh frozen plasma (20 to 25 ml/kg) or cryoprecipitate (1 to 4 units/10 kg, 8 to 12 bags for adults) can be considered.[5] The patient should then be transferred to a center that has Humate-P. It should be noted that fresh frozen plasma and cryoprecipitate do not undergo virus inactivation (see Chapter 130, Utilizing Blood Bank Resources/Transfusion Reactions and Complications).

Severe patients (type 3 vWD) may experience muscle or joint bleeding and should be treated like those with hemophilia A.[5] Nonsteroidal anti-inflammatory drugs are contraindicated. Criteria for admission include postoperative (e.g., tonsillectomy, adenoidectomy) bleeding (these patients must receive aminocaproic acid and desmopressin), uncontrolled bleeding, head trauma, and neurovascular compromise.

Most patients with vWD present to the ED with epistaxis, menorrhagia, or excessive postoperative bleeding (e.g., following tonsillectomy or dental extraction). The treatment of choice includes desmopressin and aminocaproic acid. Humate-P is mostly used for patients with vWF:RCof levels less than 10 units/dl or with refractory or serious bleeding. If a diagnostic procedure is necessary, it should be performed after treatment. Routine laboratory tests are not indicated. Successful treatment depends on consultative dialogues among the ED physician, hematologist, and patient/family. Follow-up with the treating hematologist within 24 hours is necessary.

Venous Thromboembolism

Inherited thrombophilia underlies a large percentage of the venous thromboembolic events in children. Common entities include factor V Leiden, prothrombin mutation, antithrombin deficiency, proteins C and S deficiencies, hyperhomocystinemia, and elevated lipoprotein (a). Other less common inherited disorders of thrombosis include elevated factor VIII, dysfibrinogenemias, plasminogen deficiency, and paroxysmal nocturnal hemoglobinuria. The genes for factors V and antithrombin are located on the long arm of chromosome 1, which allows for co-inheritance of both mutations. The risk of thrombosis markedly increases in compound heterozygous states, emphasizing that venous thrombosis is a multigene disorder.[19-28]

Acquired causes of thrombosis include estrogen therapy, pregnancy, diabetes mellitus, hyperlipidemia, congestive heart failure, nephrotic syndrome (due to urinary losses of antithrombin and free protein S), immobilization (e.g., postoperative period), vertebral artery dissection (due to neck trauma), central venous catheter, and antiphospholipid syndrome (causes prolonged aPTT). These acquired conditions (Table 130–3) markedly increase the risk of thrombosis in the presence of an inherited disorder (e.g., factor V Leiden and birth control pills).[21] Thus estrogen therapy is contraindicated in the presence of inherited thrombophilia.[19-28]

Clinical Presentation

The medical history should include precipitating factors, recurrent episodes, involved sites, patient ethnicity, sickle cell disease, metabolic disorders, and familial thromboembolic diseases (including early stroke or heart attack). Upper venous system thrombosis is relatively common in children with central venous catheters.[25] One study found that the majority of infected central venous devices contained clots.[29] Presenting features of deep venous thrombosis (DVT) in the lower extremity include progressive pain, swelling, erythema, and limping. Importantly, DVT may not be noticed until pulmonary embolism (PE) occurs.[22,23] Shortness of breath, chest pain, tachycardia, tachypnea, and unexplained syncope are prominent features of PE in adults, and can be expected to be present in children.[30] In one pediatric study, up to 50% of patients who died from PE had no symptoms attributable

Table 130–3   Risk Factors in Children with Deep Venous Thrombosus or Pulmonary Embolism

Risk Factor	Percent*
Central venous catheter	33
Cancer	23
Congenital heart disease	15
Trauma	15
Total parenteral nutrition administration	8
Infection	7
Nephrotic syndrome	6
Surgery	6
Birth control pills	5
Obesity	3
Systemic lupus erythematosus	2
Sickle cell anemia	2
Liver failure	2
Other	4
No risk factors	4

*Numbers add up to > 100% as many patients have more than one risk factor.
Data from Andrew M, David M, Adams M, et al: Venous thromboembolic (VTE) complications in children: first analysis of the Canadian Registry of VTE. Blood 83:1251–1257, 1994.

to PE, and the diagnosis was suspected in only 15%.[31] In another study, hypoxia (Po_2 35 to 80 mm Hg) was present in all 17 children with PE.[32] In adults with PE, nonspecific complaints such as fever (present in 14%), cough (37%), and wheezing (13%) may lead to an erroneous diagnosis.[33]

Children with renal vein thrombosis may present with flank (or abdominal) pain, flank mass, hematuria, proteinuria, and hypertension. With inferior vena cava thrombosis, the legs are often cold, cyanotic, and edematous; a chronic obstruction also causes development of collateral veins in the abdomen and thighs.[34] Predisposing conditions include severe dehydration, polycythemia, cyanotic congenital heart disease, septicemia, nephrotic syndrome, and systemic lupus erythematosus.[30]

A detailed neurologic examination is necessary to detect thrombi involving the CNS.[35] Important historical features include head and neck trauma, hypertension, migraine, dehydration, polycythemia, drug abuse, oral contraceptive use, and prior radiation therapy or chemotherapy. Other risk factors include sickle cell anemia and metabolic (e.g., hyperhomocystinemia, hyperlipidemia, mitochondrial diseases, Fabry's disease, urea cycle defects), infectious (e.g., varicella, meningitis, cat-scratch fever), and autoimmune (e.g., vasculitis, antiphospholipid antibody syndrome, systemic lupus erythematosus) diseases. Sinus vein thrombosis produces headache, blurred or double vision (with or without cranial nerve palsy), and increased intracranial pressure. Cerebral venous or arterial thrombosis can produce an acute headache, slurred speech, facial drooping, blurred or double vision, cranial nerve palsies, ataxia, head tilt, hemiparesis, altered mental status, and increased intracranial pressure (see Chapter 44, Central Nervous System Vascular Disorders).

Purpura fulminans (disseminated thrombi) occurs in neonates with homozygous protein C or S deficiency. In these patients, ecchymoses occur on the head, trunk, and extremities, often accompanied by cerebral thrombosis.[35] In older children, purpura fulminans occurs with sepsis or high-dose warfarin (due to rapid depletion of protein C and S).

EVALUATION

A complete blood count, PT, aPTT, TT, and type and screen are required for patients receiving heparin or warfarin. Antifactor Xa is required for those patients on low-molecular-weight heparin, and fibrinogen and fibrin split products for those on thrombolytics. Further inpatient testing will be directed by the admitting physician or consultant and may include factor II (prothrombin), factor VIII, fibrinogen, immunogenic and functional assays for protein C, immunologic and functional assays for protein S (total and free), antithrombin immunologic and functional assays, plasminogen, lipoprotein (a), cholesterol, triglyceride, serum creatinine, albumin, urinalysis, fasting plasma homocysteine, antiphospholipid antibodies (lupus-like anticoagulants), anticardiolipin antibodies, and genetic testing for factor V Leiden (Q506R) and antithrombin (G to A at 20210 locus) mutations. Patients with factor V Leiden show resistance to activated protein C (APC) in an aPTT-based assay (APC resistance). D-dimer assay is elevated in more than 60% of children with arterial or venous thrombosis; however, this test has limited specificity.[30,36] Some of the tests mentioned here need to be requested in the ED prior to starting anticoagulant therapy. Otherwise, genetic testing is most appropriately ordered by the admitting physician.

RADIOLOGIC IMAGING

Diagnostic imaging is required to confirm the presence and extent of thrombi.[33] Doppler ultrasound detects almost all DVTs of the lower extremities and axillary and internal jugular veins.[37] However, proximal upper extremity clots (e.g., subclavian vein, innominate vein, superior vena cava) can be missed by ultrasound and require contrast venography or computed tomography (CT).[22] Multidetector helical CT (CT angiography) identifies most subclavian, superior vena cava and internal jugular venous clots.[38] Renal vein thrombi are detected by doppler ultrasound, CT angiography, and magnetic resonance (MR) venography.[28,39,39a] Echocardiography identifies clots in the right atrium.

In cerebral vein and venous sinus thrombi, CT during the acute phase may show hyperdense blood at the site of thrombosis.[40] A linear hyperdense area may be seen with a cerebral vein thrombosis or an abnormally shaped hyperdense area with a venous sinus thrombosis (e.g., dense triangle sign consistent with thrombosis of the posterior aspect of the superior sagittal sinus). Beyond 2 weeks, this area may appear isodense and is easily missed. Acutely, magnetic resonance imaging (MRI) may show hypointense areas on T2-weighted images with venous sinus thrombi. Subacutely (after 3 to 5 days), MRI may show hyperintense areas on T1- and T2-weighted images.[40] MR venography will show abnormal flow signal of the sinus and changes within the brain's parenchyma.[25-28]

In one study, plain chest radiographs were normal in 88% of children with PE, while 12% had small infiltrates.[32] The frequency of other radiologic findings of PE in pediatric patients (e.g., atelectasis, pleural effusion, wedge-shaped defect, consolidation) is still unknown. Pulmonary angiography, once considered the procedure of choice, has a high interobserver disagreement for diagnosing subsegmental PE.[41] CT angiography, in contrast, is equally accurate. With increased acquisition speed, the entire chest can be imaged with thinner (0.6-mm or 1.25-mm) collimation, which improves the resolution and quality of images. The use of thin section widths (1 to 1.25 mm) results in a greater interobserver agreement and improvement in identifying peripheral pulmonary arterial clots.[41,42] While CT angiography has become the standard diagnostic test for PE in adults, no pediatric series have compared its accuracy to that of pulmonary angiography or ventilation/perfusion (V/Q) scanning. If V/Q scanning is employed, clinicians should realize that this test is often nonspecific and its accuracy in children is extrapolated from that in adults. In adults, a normal V/Q scan signifies that the patient has a less than 5% chance of PE, an abnormal but nondiagnostic scan signifies the patient has at least a 15% chance of PE, and a diagnostic scan signifies the patient has at least an 85% chance of PE.[43]

Management

The guidelines published by the American College of Chest Physicians give specific recommendations for neonates and children with thrombosis.[44] National referral services (1-800-NO CLOTS) are available for phone consultation. Whenever possible, a pediatric hematologist should be consulted. Patients with newly diagnosed DVT require continuous cardiac and oxygen saturation monitoring. Supplemental oxygen is required for patients with hypoxia or respiratory difficulties. The underlying thrombotic defect predicts the risk of recurrent events and determines the length of anticoagulant therapy.[27] Patients with two or more thrombotic episodes or one life-threatening thromboembolic event should receive anticoagulant therapy for life (warfarin or low-molecular-weight heparin).

HEPARIN INFUSION

Infants require higher heparin dosing than older children and adults. Heparin therapy typically involves an intravenous bolus dose followed by continuous infusion (Table 130-4). An aPTT should be checked 4 hours after the loading dose, and the infusion rate should be adjusted to keep the aPTT between 60 and 85 seconds (the rate is increased or decreased by 10% to 15% to achieve this goal) (see Table 130-4). A heparin level (measured by an anti-factor Xa assay) of 0.35 to 0.7 units/ml assures that the aPTT reflects heparin concentration. The heparin infusion is continued for at least 5 days. Intramuscular injections, arterial punctures, acetylsalicylic acid, and nonsteroidal anti-inflammatory drugs should be avoided. Maintenance warfarin or low-molecular-weight heparin can begin on day 2 or 3 of heparin therapy.

The half-life of heparin is approximately 60 minutes. Thus, if the drug needs to be stopped for bleeding or other clinical needs, discontinuation of the infusion is usually sufficient. If an immediate antidote is necessary, intravenous protamine sulfate will neutralize heparin within 5 minutes (see Table 130-4). The side effects of protamine include hypersensitivity reaction and hypotension (associated with rapid infusions). Contraindications to heparin include active bleeding, severe hypertension, recent CNS neoplasm, recent trauma or surgery, prior heparin-induced thrombocytopenia, recent GI bleeding, and hemorrhagic stroke.

LOW-MOLECULAR-WEIGHT HEPARIN THERAPY

Enoxaparin (Lovenox) contains 110 anti-factor X units/mg and is the most commonly used product.[34] The drug is

Table 130–4   Dosing for Local and Systemic Anticoagulation in Children*

Heparin

Loading dose: 75 units/kg IV over 10 min
Maintenance dose:
- Infant < 1 yr old: 28 units/kg/hr
- Child ≥ 1 yr old: 20 units/kg/hr
Adjustment: adjust heparin to maintain aPTT at 60–85 sec, assuming that this is equivalent to anti-factor Xa level of 0.35–0.7
Check initial aPTT 4 hr after loading dose:
- aPTT < 50 sec, rebolus with 50 units/kg IV over 10 min and ↑ rate 10%
- aPTT 50–59 sec, ↑ rate 10%
- aPTT 60–85 sec, do not alter rate
- aPTT 86–95 sec, ↓ rate 10%
- aPTT 96–120 sec, hold maintenance for 30 min, then ↓ rate 10%
- aPTT > 120 sec, hold maintenance for 30 min, then ↓ rate 15%

Protamine (reversal for heparin, partial reversal for LMWH†)

If time since last heparin dose is
- <30 min: administer 1 mg protamine IV for every 100 units heparin received
- 30–60 min: administer 0.5–0.75 mg protamine IV for every 100 units heparin received
- 60–120 min: administer 0.375–0.5 mg protamine IV for every 100 units heparin received
Maximum dose: 50 mg
Infusion rate 10 mg/ml; solution should not exceed 5 mg/min
For LMWH: a dose of 1 mg protamine per 100 units LMWH can be used if protamine is given within 3–4 hours of LMWH.

Reviparin (LMWH)

Weight < 5 kg
- Treatment dose: 150 units/kg q12h
- Prophylactic dose: 50 units/kg q12h
Weight ≥ 5 kg
- Treatment dose: 100 units/kg q12h
- Prophylactic dose: 30 units/kg q12h

Enoxaparin (LMWH)

Age < 2 mo
- Treatment dose: 1.5 mg/kg q12h
- Prophylactic dose: 0.75 mg/kg q12h
Age ≥ 2 mo
- Treatment dose: 1 mg/kg q12h
- Prophylactic dose: 0.5 mg/kg q12h

Alteplase‡ (t-PA)

Local instillation for CVL:
- If < 10 kg: Dilute 0.5 mg in 0.9% NaCl to the volume required to fill the line.
- If ≥ 10 kg: Mix 1 mg in 1 ml 0.9% NaCl. Instill the amount required to fill the volume of the line to a maximum of 2 ml (= 2 mg).
- Use the same amount above for each lumen if a double-lumen CVL is present.
Local instillation for subcutaneous port:
- If < 10 kg: Dilute 0.5 mg with 0.9% NaCl to 3 ml
- If ≥ 10 kg: Dilute 2 mg with 0.9% NaCl to 3 ml
Systemic dosing: 0.1–0.6 mg/kg/hr for 6 hr. Monitor fibrinogen, thrombin clotting time, prothrombin time, and activated partial thromboplastin time.

Urokinase

Load 4400 units/kg, then infuse 4400 units/kg/hr for 6–12 hr. Monitor fibrinogen, thrombin clotting time, prothrombin time, and activated partial thromboplastin time.

Streptokinase

Load 2000 units/kg, then infuse 2000 units/kg/hr for 6–12 hr. Monitor fibrinogen, thrombin clotting time, prothrombin time, and activated partial thromboplastin time.

*Based on the 7th ACCP Conference on Antithrombotic and Thrombolytic Therapy.[34,45]
†Administered subcutaneously.
‡Consider concurrent administration of heparin (10 units/kg/hr) and administration of fresh frozen plasma (10 units/kg) prior to systemic t-PA administration.
Abbreviations: aPTT, activated partial thromboplastin time; CVL, central venous line; IV, intravenously; LMWH, low-molecular-weight heparin; t-PA, tissue-type plasminogen activator.
From Rothrock SG (ed): Tarascon Pediatric Emergency Pocketbook, 5th ed. Lompoc, CA: Tarascon Publishing, 2006.

administered subcutaneously every 12 hours (see Table 130–4). For therapeutic treatment, the goal is to maintain an anti-factor Xa level between 0.5 and 1.0 units/ml in a sample taken 4 to 6 hours following subcutaneous injection. For prophylactic treatment, the goal is to maintain an anti-factor Xa level between 0.2 and 0.4 units/ml in a sample taken 4 to 6 hours following subcutaneous injection. Osteoporosis is a potential long-term side effect. Protamine sulfate does not completely reverse enoxaparin. Nevertheless, if it is necessary to reverse an enoxaparin dose that is given within the prior 3 to 4 hours, 1 mg protamine sulfate per milligram enoxaparin can be given intravenously over 10 minutes.

WARFARIN THERAPY

The administration of the oral anticoagulant warfarin (Coumadin) typically begins 2 to 3 days after starting heparin infusion, and continues for at least 3 months. Patients with liver dysfunction or direct hyperbilirubinemia require less dosing. Thus baseline liver functions and direct bilirubin should be checked prior to initiating warfarin treatment. To decrease toxicity, the diet should contain ≤ 1 μg/kg/day of vitamin K. Warfarin should be avoided in neonates. Infants on exclusively breast milk need at least 4 oz of formula (usually contains 30 μg/L vitamin K) as a steady supplement of low-dose vitamin K. The PT and international normalized ratio (INR) are elevated by warfarin. The starting dose of warfarin is usually 0.1 to 0.2 mg/kg (maximum initial dose should not exceed 10 mg), and subsequent doses should be based on the INR. The INR should be maintained between 2 and 3. Warfarin antidotes include vitamin K (subcutaneous injection of 0.5 to 5 mg, depending on patient's size and clinical history), fresh frozen plasma (20 ml/kg), or factor IX concentrate (50 units/kg). Rapid intravenous infusion of vitamin K can produce anaphylactic shock. Warfarin should be withheld for at least 72 hours prior to invasive procedures.

SYSTEMIC THROMBOLYTIC THERAPY

Thrombolytic agents (tissue-type plasminogen activator [t-PA], urokinase, and streptokinase) convert plasminogen to plasmin, the major protease that degrades fibrin. The use of t-PA (Alteplase) is preferred. The decision to use t-PA is made after careful consultation with an experienced pediatric hematologist. Indications for systemic t-PA include massive PE, arterial occlusion, and extensive DVT (e.g., acute superior vena cava syndrome, extensive DVT with a possibility of limb gangrene, bilateral renal vein thrombi with renal insufficiency). Contraindications to t-PA include active bleeding, surgery within the prior 10 days, neurosurgery within the prior 3 weeks, thrombocytopenia, and prematurity. Complications include bleeding (e.g., intracranial hemorrhage), especially in preterm infants. One protocol administers t-PA at 0.5 mg/kg/hr for 6 hours plus heparin infusion at 10 units/kg/hr during t-PA infusion plus fresh frozen plasma (ensures adequate plasminogen and fibrinogen levels) at 10 ml/kg over 30 minutes given 30 minutes prior to t-PA (see Table 130–4). In cases of severe bleeding, t-PA infusion should be stopped, and cryoprecipitate (1 unit/5 kg for fibrinogen levels < 100 mg/dl), protamine sulfate, or aminocaproic acid (100 mg/kg intravenous bolus dose) may be necessary.

SURGICAL INTERVENTIONS

Surgical thrombectomy and the use of temporary venous interruption devices (e.g., inferior vena cava filters) have not been fully investigated in children.

BLOCKED VENOUS ACCESS DEVICES

Depending on the clinical situation, blocked central venous catheters, manifested by a failure to infuse or draw back, require investigation by linogram or venogram. A linogram or contrast study through the catheter may identify a clot at the tip of the line, a leakage due to tear, or retrograde flow due to large vessel occlusion. However, venograms remain the procedure of choice to identify large vessel occlusion. An abnormal venogram requires removal of the line and initiation of anticoagulant therapy. For local thrombi confined to the line, t-PA (Alteplase, 1 mg/ml) can be administered (see Table 130–4). To avoid systemic leakage, the dose of Alteplase (in milliliters) should be equivalent to estimated intraluminal volume (usually approximately 1 to 2 ml) (see Table 130–4). The dose is instilled for 30 to 120 minutes, followed by aspiration (see Chapter 170, Access of Ports and Catheters and Management of Obstruction).

REFERENCES

1. Soucie JM, Cianfrini C, Janco RL, et al: Joint range-of-motion limitations among young males with hemophilia: prevalence and risk factors. Blood 103:2467–2473, 2004.
2. Ananyeva N, Khrenov A, Darr F, et al: Treating hemophilia A with recombinant blood factors: a comparison. Expert Opin Pharmacother 5:1061–1070, 2004.
3. Farrugia A: Safety and supply of haemophilia products: worldwide perspectives. Haemophilia 10:327–333, 2004.
4. The World Federation of Hemophilia's third global forum on the safety and supply of hemophilia treatment products, 22–23 September 2003, Budapest, Hungary. Haemophilia 10:290–294, 2004.
*5. Mannucci PM: Drug therapy: treatment of von Willebrand's disease. N Engl J Med 351:683–694, 2004.
*6. Gill JC, Ottum M, Schwartz B: Evaluation of high concentration intranasal and intravenous desmopressin in pediatric patients with mild hemophilia A or mild-to-moderate type 1 von Willebrand disease. J Pediatr 140:595–599, 2002.
7. De La Fuente B, Kasper CC, Rickles F, et al: Response of patients with mild and moderate hemophilia A and von Willebrand disease to treatment with desmopressin. Ann Intern Med 103:6–13, 1985.
8. Warrier AL, Lusher JM: DDAVP: a useful alternative to blood components in moderate hemophilia A and von Willebrand's disease. J Pediatr 102:228–233, 1983.
9. Wong WY, Donfield SM, Rains E, et al: Frequency and causes of hospitalization in HIV-negative children and adolescents with haemophilia A or B and its effect on academic achievement. Haemophilia 10:27–33, 2004.
10. Hay CR, Baglin TP, Collins PW, et al: The diagnosis and management of factor VIII and IX inhibitors: a guideline from the UK Haemophilia Centre Doctors' Organization (UKHCDO). Br J Haematol 111:78–90, 2000.
11. O'Connell N, McMahon C, Smith J, et al: Recombinant factor VIIa in the management of surgery and acute bleeding episodes in children with haemophilia and high responding inhibitors. Br J Haematol 116:632–635, 2002.
12. Goodnough LT, Lublin DM, Zhang L, et al: Transfusion medicine service policies for recombinant factor VIIa administration. Transfusion 44:1325–1331, 2004.
*13. Sandoval C, Dong S, Visintainer P, et al: Clinical and laboratory features of 178 children with recurrent epistaxis. J Pediatr Hematol Oncol 24:47–49, 2002.
*14. Bevan JA, Maloney KW, Hillery CA, et al: Bleeding disorders: a common cause of menorrhagia in adolescents. J Pediatr 138:856–861, 2001.
15. Kadir RA, Economides DL, Sabin CA, et al: Frequency of inherited bleeding disorders in women with menorrhagia. Lancet 351:485–489, 1998.
16. Diley A, Drews C, Miller C, et al: Von Willebrand disease and other inherited bleeding disorders in women with diagnosed menorrhagia. Obstet Gynecol 97:630–636, 2001.
17. Kadir RA, Economides DL, Sabin CA, et al: Assessment of menstrual blood loss and gynecological problems in patients with inherited bleeding disorders. Haemophilia 5:40–48, 1999.
18. Cariappa R, Wilhite TR, Parvin CA, Luchtman-Jones L: Comparison of PFA-100 and bleeding time testing in pediatric patients with suspected hemorrhagic problems. J Pediatr Hematol Oncol 25:474–479, 2003.
19. Andrew M, David M, Adams M, et al: Venous thromboembolic (VTE) complications in children: first analysis of the Canadian Registry of VTE. Blood 83:1251–1257, 1994.

*Selected readings.

20. Stein PD, Kayali F, Olson RE: Incidence of venous thromboembolism in infants and children: data from the National Hospital Discharge Survey. J Pediatr 145:563–565, 2004.

21. van Ommen CH, Peters M: Venous thromboembolic disease in childhood. Semin Thromb Hemost 29:391–403, 2003.

22. Anton N, Massicotte MP: Venous thromboembolism in pediatrics. Semin Vasc Med 1:111–122, 2001.

23. Journeycake JM, Manco-Johnson MJ: Thrombosis during infancy and childhood: what we know and what we do not know. Hematol Oncol Clin North Am 18:1315–1338, 2004.

24. Kuhle S, Massicotte P, Chan A, et al: Systemic thromboembolism in children. Thromb Haemost 92:722–728, 2004.

25. Nowack-Gottl U, Kosch A, Schlegel N: Thromboembolism in newborns, infants and children. Thromb Haemost 86:464–474, 2001.

26. Nowack-Gottl U, Kosch A, Schlegel N, et al: Thromboembolism in children. Curr Opin Hematol 9:448–453, 2002.

27. Revel-Vilk S, Chan A, Bauman M, Massicotte P: Prothrombotic conditions in an unselected cohort of children with venous thromboembolic disease. J Thromb Haemost 1:915–921, 2003.

28. Richardson MW, Allen GA, Monahan PE: Thrombosis in children: current perspective and distinct challenges. Thromb Haemost 88:900–911, 2002.

29. Lordick F, Hentrick M, Decker T, et al: Ultrasound screening for internal jugular vein thrombosis aids the detection of central venous catheter-related infections in patients with haemato-oncological diseases: a prospective observational study. Br J Haematol 120:1073–1078, 2003.

30. Nowack-Gottl U, Kosch A: Factor VIII, D-dimer, and thromboembolism in children. N Engl J Med 351:1051–1053, 2004.

31. Derish MT, Smith DW, Frankel LR: Venous catheter thrombus formation and pulmonary embolism in children. Pediatr Pulmonol 20:349–354, 1995.

32. Udeerzo C, Rovelli FA, Marchi PF, et al: Pulmonary thromboembolism in childhood leukemia: 8 years experience in a pediatric hematology center. J Clin Oncol 13:2805–2812, 1995.

33. Merli G: Diagnostic assessment of deep vein thrombosis and pulmonary embolism. Am J Med 118(Suppl 8A):3S–12S, 2005.

*34. Monagle P, Chan A, Chalmers E, Michelson AD: Antithrombotic therapy in children: the Seventh ACCP Conference on Antithrombotic and Thrombolytic Therapy. Chest 126:645S–675S, 2004.

35. Sutor AH, Chan KC, Massicotte P: Low molecular weight heparin in pediatric patients. Semin Thromb Hemost 30:31–39, 2004.

*36. Goldenberg NA, Knapp-Clevenger R, Manco-Johnson MJ: Elevated plasma factor VIII and D-dimer levels as predictors of poor outcomes of thrombosis in children. N Engl J Med 351:1081–1088, 2004.

37. Babyn PS, Gahunia HK, Massicotte P: Pulmonary thromboembolism in children. Pediatr Radiol 35:258–274, 2005.

38. Qanadli SD, El Hajjam M, Bruckert F, et al: Helical CT phlebography of the superior vena cava: diagnosis and evaluation of venous obstruction. AJR Am J Roentgenol 172:1327–1333, 1999.

39. O'Neill WC, Baumgarten DA: Imaging. Am J Kid Dis 42:601–604, 2003.

39a. Pedrosa I, Rofsky NM: MR imaging in abdominal emergencies. Radiol Clin North Am 41:1243–1247, 2003.

40. Visrutaratna P, Oranratanachai K, Likasitwattanakul S: Clinics in Diagnostic Imaging (103): dural sinus thrombosis with cerebral venous infarction. Singapore Med J 46:238–245, 2005.

41. Gulsun M, Goodman LR, Washington L: Venous thromboembolic disease: where does multidetector computed tomography fit? Cardiol Clin 21:631–638, 2003.

42. Quiroz R, Kucher N, Zou KH, et al: Clinical validity of a negative computed tomography scan in patients with suspected pulmonary embolism: a systematic review. JAMA 293:2012–2017, 2005.

43. PIOPED Investigators: Value of the ventilation/perfusion scan in acute pulmonary embolism: results of the Prospective Investigation of Pulmonary Embolism Diagnosis (PIOPED). JAMA 263:2753–2759, 1990.

44. Male C, Chait P, Ginsberg JS, et al: Comparison of venography and ultrasound for the diagnosis of asymptomatic deep vein thrombosis in the upper body in children: results of the PARKAA study. Prophylactic Antithrombin Replacement in Kids with ALL treated with Asparaginase. Thromb Haemost 87:593–598, 2002.

45. Ronghe MD, Halsey C, Gouldon JL: Anticoagulation therapy in children. Paediatr Drugs 5:803–820, 2003.

Chapter 131

Hemolytic-Uremic Syndrome

Boura'a Bou Aram, MD and Abdul-Kader Souid, MD, PhD

Key Points

Hemolytic-uremic syndrome is characterized by the acute onset of nonimmune microangiopathic hemolytic anemia (circulating red cell fragments, hemoglobinemia, and hemoglobinuria), consumptive thrombocytopenia, and renal insufficiency or failure.

Although the disease usually follows infectious enteritis (e.g., *Escherichia coli* serotype O157:H7), up to 10% of cases occur without a diarrheal prodrome.

Severity of acute symptoms (anuria, hypertension, and seizure) is the main predictor of a complicated course.

Management includes observation and supportive care (e.g., plasmapheresis, dialysis, packed red blood cell transfusion).

Introduction and Background

Hemolytic-uremic syndrome (HUS) is a leading cause of acute renal failure in children under 5 years of age. Its hallmarks are the acute onset of nonimmune microangiopathic (thrombotic microangiopathy) hemolytic anemia (circulating red cell fragments, hemoglobinemia, and hemoglobinuria), consumptive thrombocytopenia, and renal insufficiency or failure. The disease is sporadic, peaking in the summer and early fall. It usually follows acute infectious hemorrhagic colitis (vomiting, bloody diarrhea, and abdominal pain). This stage lasts 2 to 14 days before the onset of HUS. Bacterial contamination may occur from water supplies, undercooked meat, yogurt, unpasteurized milk, apple cider made from unwashed apples, and vegetables grown in a garden fertilized with cow manure. Bacteria can also be transmitted by person-to-person contact.[1,2] Outbreaks and multiple relapses are well known.

Recognition and Approach

Diarrhea-associated (typical or epidemic) HUS accounts for approximately 90% of cases. The disease mainly affects children between 7 months and 5 years of age. It is best described as a thrombotic microangiopathy that is produced by a 71-kDa protein termed *verotoxin* or *Shiga toxin* (produced by *Shigella dysenteriae*). Verotoxin binds to high-affinity glycosphyngolipid surface (GB₃) receptors on endothelial cells, causing vasculitis. The toxin is frequently produced by the enterohemorrhagic strains of *Escherichia coli* (especially serotype O157:H7). Other responsible organisms include *S. dysenteriae*, *Campylobacter jejunae*, *Salmonella*, *Streptococcus pneumoniae*, and viruses. The incidence of HUS in children with enteritis caused by *E. coli* O157:H7 ranges from 6% to 15%. Complete recovery occurs in 1 to 2 weeks in greater than 95% of cases.

Non–diarrhea-associated (atypical, hereditary, or familial) HUS accounts for approximately 10% of cases. This form of the disease occurs in all ages, any time of the year, and without a diarrheal prodrome. It has a higher incidence of relapses. It is also more likely to produce end-stage renal disease, proteinuria, and hypertension.

Rare forms occur in association with systemic disease (e.g., systemic lupus erythematosus, transplant rejection, pregnancy) or medications (e.g., cyclosporin A, tacrolimus).

Pathogenesis

The development of thrombotic microangiopathy is preceded by verotoxin-induced endothelial cell injury (vasculitis), platelet aggregation, augmented thrombin generation, and impaired fibrinolysis.[3-7] Acquired or congenital deficiency of a specific von Willebrand factor–cleaving metalloproteinase (factor H, or ADAMTS13) produces persistent, extremely large von Willebrand factor multimers, which induce platelet aggregation at sites with high levels of intravascular shear stress.[7,8] Verotoxin also directly activates platelets.[9,10] These prothrombotic disturbances (intravascular platelet aggregation and fibrin clot formation) involve multiple organs, but are more prominent in the kidneys and central nervous system. Intravascular red blood cell destruction occurs as blood passes through involved organs (mechanical stress).

Clinical Presentation

The diagnosis of HUS is based on clinical features (simultaneous acute anemia with circulating red cell fragments, hemoglobinemia, hemoglobinuria, thrombocytopenia, and increased serum creatinine). The clinical presentation usually begins ~2-14 days after the onset of diarrhea. Other prodromes include upper respiratory tract infection, abdominal pain, bloody diarrhea or heme-positive stools.

Acute symptoms of HUS are related to renal failure, hypertension, volume overload (due to anuria/oliguria), dehydration (due to diarrhea, decreased intake, and renal disease), profound anemia (due to intravascular hemolysis), congestive heart failure (due to anemia, hypertension, and volume overload), bleeding (due to thrombocytopenia), central nervous system thrombosis (seizures, strokes, alterations of consciousness, abnormal muscle tone, and cerebral edema, all due to thrombosis), hyperkalemia (due to acute renal failure), and acidosis (due to HCO_3^- loss in the diarrhea and decreased H^+ excretion due to renal failure). Rare complications include bowel perforation and/or necrosis, rectal prolapse (due to colitis), hepatitis, pancreatitis, and diabetes mellitus.[1] Chronic complications include end-stage renal disease, hypertension, and long-term central nervous system insults (due to thrombosis or bleeding).

The natural history of HUS varies markedly. More than 95% of affected children recover from the acute illness in 1 to 2 weeks. In mild forms, urine output may remain normal, and renal insufficiency resolves spontaneously without intervention. In more severe cases, plasmapheresis, dialysis, packed red blood cell transfusion, and long-term supportive care are necessary.

Recovery is reflected by improvements in urine output, renal function, platelet count, and hemoglobin concentration. Patients with severe disease develop chronic hypertension, renal failure, and persistent proteinuria. Poor outcome is associated with older age at onset of the disease, marked leukocytosis ($>20 \times 10^3/mm^3$), central nervous system involvement (e.g., stroke, seizure), and prolonged anuria (>7 days) or oliguria (>14 days). Relapses lead to hypertension and end-stage renal disease.

Laboratory Evaluation

A complete blood count often shows normocytic anemia and thrombocytopenia (Table 131–1). The plasma is pink-red, reflecting hemoglobinemia. The blood smear shows red cell fragments and thrombocytopenia. Blood typing is necessary because of a potential need for packed red blood cell transfusion. Serum electrolytes, blood urea nitrogen (BUN), creatinine, phosphate, and uric acid levels may show disturbances produced by diarrhea (hyperchloremic metabolic acidosis with normal anion gap) or acute renal failure (increase serum

creatinine, hyperkalemia, hyperphosphatemia, elevated uric acid, and metabolic acidosis). Lactate dehydrogenase is markedly elevated due to red cell hemolysis and microangiopathy. Indirect bilirubin is mildly elevated due to the hemolysis. Urinalysis shows hemoglobinuria (without red blood cells) and, sometimes, granular casts. A centrifuged urine sample remains pink-red, containing free hemoglobin molecules. In contrast, hematuria due to the presence of red blood cells produces clear urine supernatant.

Normal tests in HUS include direct and indirect antiglobulin (Coombs') tests, partial thromboplastin time, prothrombin time, thrombin time, and fibrinogen. Antinuclear antibodies, anti-DNA antibodies, and C3 and C4 are negative (as evidence against the presence of systemic lupus erythematosus and membranoproliferative glomerulonephritis). Other frequently abnormal but nonspecific laboratory tests include serum albumin, amylase, lipase, glucose, triglyceride, and liver transaminases.

Stool culture may identify the infectious agent (important for reporting outbreaks). However, routine stool cultures may not identify *E. coli*. A rapid screening test for *E. coli* (based on failure to ferment on sorbitol) has been developed; a positive reaction should be confirmed by commercially available agglutination tests. Positive results are more common within 7 days of the onset of diarrhea. Verotoxin can be identified in stool samples by polymerase chain reaction or other readily available laboratory techniques.

Differential Diagnosis

Thrombotic thrombocytopenic purpura (TTP) has a presentation similar to HUS (Table 131–2). TTP usually develops in adolescents and adults. It produces more prominent neurologic deterioration than renal involvement. Prompt recognition is essential, since this entity requires immediate plasmapheresis.

Autoimmune hemolytic anemia may produce intravascular hemolysis (more commonly seen in cold agglutinin disease and paroxysmal cold hemoglobinuria). In these entities, platelet count and renal function are normal. In cold agglutinin disease, immunoglobulin M–coated red blood cells activate the hemolytic complement cascade, causing intravascular hemolysis (red blood cell fragments, hemoglobinemia, and hemoglobinuria). Acrocyanosis and hemolysis follow exposure to cold. A direct antiglobulin test is positive with the reagent containing anticomplement antibodies. Par-

Table 131–1	**Interpretation of Laboratory Results in Hemolytic-Uremic Syndrome**
Laboratory Tests	**Interpretation/Purpose**
CBC	Anemia and thrombocytopenia.
Peripheral blood smear	Red blood cell fragments.
Urinalysis	Hemoglobinuria.
Serum electrolytes, BUN, creatinine, phosphate, and uric acid	Metabolic derangements (e.g., hyperkalemia, metabolic acidosis) are common.
Lactate dehydrogenase and bilirubin	Elevated levels reflect hemolysis.
Stool culture and other stool studies	Used to detect *E. coli*, verotoxin, or other causative pathogens.
Antiglobulin (Coombs') tests	Normal, positive results suggest autoimmune hemolytic anemia and not HUS as cause of symptoms.
aPTT, PT, TT, and fibrinogen	Normal, prolonged results suggest DIC and not HUS as cause of symptoms.
Antinuclear antibodies, anti-DNA antibodies, C3 and C4	Normal, positive results suggest systemic lupus erythematosus or membranoproliferative glomerulonephritis and not HUS as cause of symptoms.

Abbreviations: aPTT, activated partial thromboplastin time; BUN, blood urea nitrogen; CBC, complete blood count; DIC, disseminated intravascular coagulation; HUS, hemolytic-uremic syndrome; PT, prothrombin time; TT, thrombin time.

Table 131-2	Differential Diagnosis of Hemolytic-Uremic Syndrome
Disorder	**Clinical Features**
HUS	Prodrome manifestations include diarrhea, abdominal pain, and bloody or heme-positive stools. Simultaneous occurrence of acute anemia with circulating red cell fragments, hemoglobinemia, hemoglobinuria, thrombocytopenia, and increased serum creatinine.
TTP	Clinical presentation similar to HUS. More prominent neurologic deterioration than renal involvement. Immediate plasmapheresis is necessary.
ITP	Normal renal function; absence of hematuria; normal hemoglobin (see Chapter 129).
Autoimmune hemolytic anemia	Acute hemolytic anemia with positive Coombs' tests. Platelet count and renal function are normal.
Renal disease	Normal platelet count and absence of microangiopathic hemolytic anemia.
DIC	Prolonged PT, aPTT, and TT; hypofibrinogenemia.
Henoch-Schönlein purpura	Painful symmetric, palpable purpura involving proximal regions of the extremities, particularly legs and buttocks. Petechiae/purpura with normal platelet count.

Abbreviations: aPTT, activated partial thromboplastin time; DIC, disseminated intravascular coagulation; HUS, hemolytic-uremic syndrome; ITP, immune thrombocytopenic purpura; PT, prothrombin time; TT, thrombin time; TTP, thrombotic thrombocytopenic purpura.

oxysmal cold hemoglobinuria is produced by immunoglobulin G antibodies (Donath-Landsteiner cold autoantibodies), having biphasic thermal activities. These antibodies fix to red blood cell membranes in the cold (4° C) and activate the hemolytic complement cascade at 37° C.

Thrombocytopenia (see Chapter 129, Acute Childhood Immune Thrombocytopenic Purpura and Related Platelet Disorders) may occur as a result of immune-mediated destruction (acute childhood immune thrombocytopenic purpura), after a viral infection (human immunodeficiency virus, chicken pox, and postimmunization), drugs, vasculitis (systemic lupus erythematosus), intravascular destruction (disseminated intravascular coagulation and prosthetic heart valve), platelet trapping (venous malformation, hemangiomas, and hypersplenism), and decreased platelet production (aplastic anemia, thrombocytopenia–absent radius syndrome, amegakaryocytic thrombocytopenia, and Wiscott-Aldrich syndrome).

In *disseminated intravascular coagulation*, fibrinogen is low. Renal parenchymal disease is usually associated with a normal platelet count and absence of microangiopathic hemolytic anemia.

Important Clinical Features and Considerations

Clinicians should be aware that HUS might reoccur. While debate exists as to causation or worsening of disease with antibiotic administration,[11,12] clinicians should avoid their use unless absolutely necessary (e.g., proven bacterial infection, bowel perforation). Renal manifestations including hematuria, oliguria, and hypertension many herald the onset of renal failure. Neurologic findings include altered mental status, seizures, and coma. The skin features include pallor (due to anemia), petechiae, and purpura.

Management

All patients require hospitalization for observation and appropriate interventions. Treatment is mainly supportive[2] (Table 131-3). Dehydration due to diarrhea and decreased intake must be corrected while avoiding volume overload. Acute hypertension is treated with short-acting oral agents if asymptomatic or intravenous agents for encephalopathy or other hypertensive emergencies (see Chapter 65, Hyper-

Table 131-3	Management of Hemolytic-Uremic Syndrome

1. Correct dehydration due to diarrhea while avoiding fluid overload
2. Adequately treat hypertension using intravenous agents (e.g., nicardipine, sodium nitroprusside) for hypertensive emergencies.
3. Avoid platelet transfusions.
4. Use antibiotics only for proven infections or suspected bowel perforation.
5. Dialysis is indicated if patient develops anuria, severe oliguria, hyperkalemia unresponsive to conventional therapy, severe azotemia (e.g., encephalopathy), fluid overload, or pulmonary edema.
6. Administer packed red blood cells to keep hemoglobin ~8.0 g/dl.
7. Plasma infusion (10 ml/kg over 2–4 hr) or plasmapheresis is indicated in patients with central nervous system involvement or severe renal disease.
8. Patients with seizures require emergent imaging to exclude intracranial pressure or bleeding. Promptly treat seizures with standard agents (e.g., lorazepam followed by fosphenytoin).
9. Early consultations with nephrology, hematology, and plasmapheresis teams to assist with clinical care and to expedite interventions (e.g., dialysis, plasmapheresis).
10. Admit patients to a floor that can adequately monitor vital signs and fluid intake/output, and observe for acute deterioration (e.g., seizures).

tensive Emergencies). Packed red blood cells should be administered to maintain hemoglobin concentrations above approximately 8.0 g/dl. Seizures should be investigated with computed tomography or magnetic resonance imaging of the brain and treated appropriately (see Chapter 40, Seizures).

Platelet transfusion should be avoided and antibiotics reserved for suspected bowel perforation or documented bacterial infection. Dialysis is indicated in the presence of anuria (>24 hours), severe oliguria, uncontrollable hyperkalemia, severe azotemia (e.g., encephalopathy, BUN >100 mg/dl), or fluid overload with pulmonary edema. Once fluid deficit is corrected, total fluid intake should be limited to replacing insensible water loss (pure water at ~50% of estimated maintenance fluid therapy), measured urine output, and measured ongoing fluid loss from the diarrhea.

Plasma infusion or plasmapheresis is indicated in patients with central nervous system involvement or severe renal disease (e.g., oliguria, hypertension, hyperkalemia, hypervolemia, pulmonary edema). Treatment frequency varies from daily to twice weekly.[2] Consultations include those to nephrology, hematology, and plasmapheresis teams. Controversial therapies include tissue-type plasminogen activator (Alteplase) and aspirin (platelet inhibitor).

Summary

Children with mild to moderate HUS can be treated with supportive care only. Children with moderate to severe HUS are more likely to need plasmapheresis and dialysis (especially if neurologic and severe renal involvements are present). TTP has a presentation similar to HUS; it occurs in adolescents and requires aggressive treatment, particularly with plasmapheresis. Antibiotics may increase the release of verotoxin and should be avoided unless they are absolutely indicated. Platelet transfusion may lead to thrombosis, and should be avoided in the absence of a life-threatening hemorrhage.

REFERENCES

1. Siegler RL: Management of hemolytic uremic syndrome. J Pediatr 112:1014–1020, 1988.
*2. Chandler WL, Lelacic S, Boster DR, et al: Prothrombotic coagulation abnormalities preceding the hemolytic-uremic syndrome. N Engl J Med 345:23–32, 2002.

---

*Selected readings.

*3. Bergstein JM, Riley M, Bang NU: Role of plasminogen-activator inhibitor type 1 in the pathogenesis and outcome of the hemolytic uremic syndrome. N Engl J Med 327:755–759, 1992.
4. Nevard CH, Blann AD, Jurd KM, et al: Markers of endothelial cell activation and injury in childhood hemolytic uremic syndrome. Pediatr Nephrol 13:487–492, 1999.
5. Moake JL, Rudy CK, Troll JH, et al: Unusually large plasma factor VIII:von Willebrand factor multimers in chronic relapsing thrombotic thrombocytopenic purpura. N Engl J Med 307:1432–1435, 1982.
6. Moake JL, Byrnes JJ, Troll JH, et al: Abnormal VIII:von Willebrand factor patterns in the plasma of patients with the hemolytic uremic syndrome. Blood 64:592–598, 1984.
7. Furlan M, Robles R, Galbusera M, et al: Von Willebrand factor-cleaving protease in thrombotic thrombocytopenic purpura. N Engl J Med 339:1578–1584, 1998.
8. Veyradier A, Obert B, Houllier A, et al: Specific von Willebrand factor-cleaving protease in thrombotic microangiopathies: a study of 111 cases. Blood 98:765–772, 2001.
9. Karpman D, Papadopoulou D, Nilsson K, et al: Platelet activation by Shiga toxin and circulatory factors as a pathogenic mechanism in the hemolytic uremic syndrome. Blood 97:3100–3108, 2001.
10. Tsai H, Chandler WL, Sarode R, et al: Von Willebrand factor and von Willebrand factor-cleaving metalloprotease activity in *Escherichia coli* O157:H7-associated hemolytic uremic syndrome. Pediatr Res 49:653–659, 2001.
11. Wong CS, Jelacic S, Habeeb RL, et al: The risk of the hemolytic-uremic syndrome after antibiotic treatment of *Escherichia coli* O157:H7 infections. N Engl J Med 342:1930–1936, 2000.
12. Safdar N, Said A, Gangnon RE, et al: Risk of hemolytic uremic syndrome after antibiotic treatment of *Escherichia coli* O157:H7 enteritis: a meta-analysis. JAMA 288:996–1001, 2002.

Utilizing Blood Bank Resources/ Transfusion Reactions and Complications

Abdul-Kader Souid, MD, PhD, Lazaro G. Rosales, MD, and Boura'a Bou Aram, MD

Key Points

A transfusion should be recommended only after the risks and benefits are carefully considered.

Most transfusion fatalities occur as a result of ABO incompatibility due to an error in identifying the patient or a unit of blood.

Leukocyte-depleted blood components are recommended for patients requiring chronic transfusion.

Irradiated blood components are recommended for immune-compromised patients.

Permission with informed consent to transfuse should be obtained for each patient.

Blood Bank Resources

Collecting Donated Blood and Testing Blood Components Prior to Use

Blood products obtained for medical use are donated by healthy volunteers under federal and state regulations.[1,2] Donated blood is tested for infectious disease markers, such as syphilis, hepatitis B surface and human immunodeficiency virus type 1 (HIV-1) p24 antigens, and hepatitis B core, human T-cell lymphotropic virus types I and II (HTLV-I and HTLV-II), hepatitis C, HIV-1, and HIV type 2 (HIV-2) antibodies. Polymerase chain reaction is performed for HIV and hepatitis C virus. Risk of missing the detection of infectious agents occurs in the "window period" between exposure and positive testing. A high risk especially involves hepatitis B

virus due to its long window period; vaccination for hepatitis B virus reduces this risk. Other rare viruses and diseases include West Nile virus, herpesviruses, parvovirus B19, variant Creutzfeldt-Jakob disease, and severe acute respiratory syndrome. Current standard testing does not detect these infections; nevertheless, viral transmission via blood components is very rare.[3,4]

The blood groups routinely tested for donors and recipients are the ABO and Rh systems. The ABO blood group is determined because anti-A and/or anti-B immunoglobulin M (IgM) alloantibodies in the recipient's serum produce rapid hemolysis of donor red cells. Commercially available anti-A and anti-B antibodies are used to determine ABO blood type. These IgM molecules bind to A group and B group red cell antigens, respectively, producing direct (macroscopic) agglutination. Moreover, incubating the recipient's serum with commercially available group A and group B red cells demonstrates the presence of specific alloantibodies, confirming the ABO blood type. For example, blood type A shows the recipient's red cell agglutination with commercial anti-A antibodies and commercial group A red cell agglutination with the recipient's serum. Commercially available (modified) anti-Rh immunoglobulin G (IgG) can directly agglutinate (macroscopically visible) D-positive (or Rh_0) red blood cells.

The Rh blood group is determined because D antigen, the major determinant of the Rh system, is a strong immunogen, producing anti-D antibodies in Rh-negative recipients. An Rh-negative woman who is immunized to D antigen by transfusion or pregnancy is at risk of delivering a newborn with severe hemolysis. Thus individuals who are Rh-negative, especially females of childbearing age, require Rh-negative blood and platelets to prevent Rh sensitization.

For Rh-negative recipients, the decision to stay with Rh-negative blood versus switching to Rh-positive components is based on the anticipated need for future red blood cell (RBC) transfusion, availability of Rh-negative components, and urgency of transfusing other Rh-negative patients. As soon as it becomes apparent that the Rh-negative patient will receive massive transfusion (more than the patient's blood volume in 24 hours; blood volume is estimated as 100 ml/kg for preterm neonates, 85 ml/kg for term neonates, and 75 ml/kg for children >1 month of age) that will exceed the Rh-negative blood inventory, the patient should be switched to Rh-positive components. The problem with giving O-positive red cells immediately without antibody screening in an emergency is the potential for developing hemolytic transfusion in patients who have anti-D antibodies.

Detecting blood group antibodies (isoagglutinins) directed against non-ABO blood group antigens is also performed prior to blood transfusion. This antibody screening test is performed using recipient serum against a panel of "group O" RBCs of known antigenic composition. The term *antibody screening test* is sometimes used synonymously with the term *indirect antiglobulin (Coombs) test* (IAT). If the test is positive (hemolysis or agglutination), further tests to determine specific antibodies will be performed.

The IAT is performed by incubating the recipient's serum (at 37° C) with commercially available red blood cells of known antigen type. Unbound antibodies are removed by washing RBCs with 0.9% NaCl. An antiglobulin reagent (rabbit anti-human IgG or IgG plus complement) is then added. A positive test shows red cell agglutination, reflecting the presence of allo- or autoantibodies. Allo- versus autoantibodies are determined by a commercially available panel of red cells, varying with antigen phenotype. Agglutination of all red cell panels indicates autoantibodies (e.g., patients with autoimmune hemolytic anemia). By contrast, specific reactivity indicates alloantibodies (e.g., patients with alloimmunization). The direct antiglobulin (Coombs') test detects antibodies or complement on the surface of red cells. Washed recipient's red cells are incubated with antiglobulin reagent (rabbit anti-human IgG or IgG plus complement) as in the IAT. Agglutination is observed if antibodies or complement are present on the surface of red cells. A crossmatch with an ABO- and Rh-compatible unit of blood determines whether the recipient's serum contains unexpected antibodies to the donor's red cell antigens.

Whenever red cell products are requested, ABO and Rh typing, antibody screening, and a full crossmatch are routinely performed. If the antibody screen is negative, the patient may be transfused the appropriate ABO/Rh type. An immediate spin crossmatch (mixing the patient's serum with RBCs from a unit selected for transfusion and observing for hemolysis or agglutination) provides added safety. If the antibody screen is positive, the specificity of the antibody is identified; if clinically significant, only red cells negative for the relevant antigen will be transfused. A full crossmatch is also performed. Additional time is required to identify the antibodies, find antigen-negative red cells, and perform full crossmatch tests. This may take hours or days if multiple antibodies are present (Table 132–1).

In an emergency situation, blood may need to be transfused before standard testing is completed. In these circumstances, physicians are asked to sign an "emergency release form" to document the reason for the urgent need and to acknowledge that the blood is not fully crossmatched at the time of transfusion. O-negative red cells are available for immediate transfusion to any patient, but should be used only when the patient's blood type is not known and there is no time to determine it. This situation sometimes occurs in

Table 132–1	Estimated Times for Blood Bank to Release Units of Red Blood Cells
Test/Product	**Time to Completion**
O⁻	Immediate
ABO and Rh typing	10 min
Type and screen	15 min
Type and crossmatch	45 min
Leukocyte-reduced PRBCs	Typically performed at the time of blood collection or at the bedside using a filter
Irradiated PRBCs	10 min

Abbreviation: PRBCs, packed red blood cells.

the setting of trauma and should apply to the first few units transfused.

Packed Red Blood Cell (Red Cell Concentrate) Transfusion

Packed red blood cell (PRBCs) transfusions are used to improve blood oxygen-carrying capacity and restore blood volume. Units are prepared from whole blood by removing most of the plasma (producing an average hematocrit value of 70%). This procedure reduces the transfusion volume and the isoagglutinin load. Each unit usually contains approximately 200 ml of RBCs, 70 ml of plasma, and 100 ml of additive nutrient solution (e.g., citrate [as an anticoagulant], phosphate, dextrose, and ATP). Clinical citrate toxicity (hypocalcemia due to calcium chelation) is rare, occurring only with massive transfusions (e.g., exchange transfusion), and responds to calcium supplements. Prolonged storage produces a leakage of potassium into the plasma, which is usually clinically insignificant. Blood should be infused through a filter (170 to 260 μm) to remove debris caused by storage.[1,2]

Transfusion is usually given if the symptoms of anemia or blood loss are severe and further delay might result in significant disability or death. Selected indications for transfusion include acute bleeding, high-dose chemotherapy, severe prematurity, sickle cell disease (e.g., splenic sequestration, severe acute chest syndrome), thalassemia major, aplastic anemia, pure red cell aplasia, and severe autoimmune hemolytic anemia (using the most compatible unit).[2] Transfusing 10 to 15 ml/kg of PRBCs in a child raises the hemoglobin concentration by 2 to 3 g/dl and the hematocrit by 6% to 9% (Table 132–2).[1,5] Transfusion is usually given at 15 ml/kg over 2 to 4 hours. Faster transfusion may be necessary to replace acute blood loss. If the intention is to transfuse small amounts (e.g., in infants), a unit can be divided into several aliquots.

Leukocyte-reduced PRBCs are prepared by passing the unit through a filter that removes 85% to 90% of the white blood cells; the procedure is frequently performed at the time of blood collection. This type of product produces fewer nonhemolytic febrile reactions, which are mediated by antibodies against the donor's white cell antigens as well as by cytokines produced during component storage. This product also produces less alloimmunization and viral (e.g., cytomegalovirus) transmission. It is indicated for patients who need chronic transfusion (e.g., children on chemotherapy or with hemoglobinopathy) or who have prior exposure to blood antigens (e.g., multiparous females).[1]

Table 132–2	Blood Component Transfusion*			
Product	**Indication**	**Crossmatch**	**Dose**	**Expected Rise**

PRBCs
    Leukocyte-reduced PRBCs
    Irradiated PRBCs
    Washed PRBCs
	Improving blood oxygen-carrying
	    capacity and restoring blood volume
	Chronic PRBC transfusions
	Immune-compromised patients
	Persistent allergic reactions
		Complete	10–15 ml/kg	Hemoglobin concentration
				    increases by 2–3 g/dl[†]

Platelets (whole blood
    derived)
	Thrombocytopenia	ABO	1 unit/10 kg; 4–6
			    units for adults[‡]
				Platelet count increases by
				    25–50 × 10³/mm³

Platelets (apheresis)	Chronic platelet transfusions	ABO	10 ml/kg; 1 unit for adults[§]	

FFP	Acquired coagulopathy, reversal of
	    warfarin, clotting factor (II, X, XI
	    and XIII) deficiency, TTP and HUS
		ABO	10–25 ml/kg	Each coagulation factor
				    increases by 10%–20%[¶]

Cryoprecipitate	Rich in fibrinogen, von Willebrand's
	    factor, and factor VIII
		ABO	1–4 units/10 kg;
			    8–12 units for
			    adults**
				Plasma fibrinogen increases
				    by 60–100 mg/dl

*Modified from Pisciotto P (ed): Pediatric Hemotherapy Data Card. Bethesda, MD: American Association of Blood Banks, 2002.
[†]Increments depend on anticoagulant-preservative solution.
[‡]Each unit contains 5.5 × 10¹⁰ platelets in 50 ml of plasma.
[§]Each unit contains 3.0 × 10¹¹ platelets in 250 ml of plasma.
[¶]Different recovery for each factor (depending on circulatory half-lives).
**Each unit contains approximately 250 mg of fibrinogen.
Abbreviations: FFP, fresh frozen plasma; HUS, hemolytic-uremic syndrome; PRBC(s), packed red blood cell(s); TTP, thrombotic thrombocytopenic purpura.

Irradiated PRBCs are prepared by exposing the unit to 2500 cGy of radiation. This treatment inactivates the donor's T cells, which reduces the risk of a graft-versus-host reaction in the recipient. This type of product is recommended for immune-compromised patients (e.g., children on chemotherapy).[1]

Washed PRBCs are prepared by washing red cells with 0.9% NaCl, which removes most of the plasma. This type of product is used for patients who have severe allergic reactions (e.g., cough, wheezing, swollen lips, and urticaria) to transfusion despite antihistamine administration. Immunoglobulin E antibodies against the donor's plasma proteins mediate this adverse reaction. This product is also used for patients with immunoglobulin A (IgA) deficiency who have developed IgA antibodies.[2]

Platelet Transfusion

Platelets are the principal mediator of hemostasis and are constantly required to support endothelial functions. Bleeding (e.g., petechiae, epistaxis, melena, hematemesis, menorrhagia, hematuria) is common when the platelet count is 10,000/mm³ or less. Moreover, life-threatening hemorrhage (e.g., into the airway, lungs, central nervous system, and gastrointestinal tract) becomes more likely when the platelet count is 5000/mm³ or less. Thus profound thrombocytopenia (defined as a platelet count < 20,000/mm³) due to decreased production (e.g., patients on chemotherapy or with aplastic anemia) should be promptly treated with platelet transfusion. A prophylactic transfusion is recommended when the platelet count is less than 20,000/mm³. A therapeutic transfusion, in contrast, is given to treat any significant bleeding even if the platelet count is greater than 20,000/mm³.[2]

Platelet concentrates are prepared from routinely donated whole blood by centrifugation, producing platelet-rich plasma that, on further centrifugation and separation of the supernatant plasma, yields a platelet concentrate (unit) of 50 ml. A single unit (prepared from 1 unit of whole blood) should contain greater than 5.5 × 10¹⁰ platelets, which raises the platelet count by 6 to 10 × 10³/mm³ in adults. Transfusing 4 to 6 pooled random-donor units of platelets for adults and children greater than 20 kg (1 unit/10 kg for children < 20 kg) raises the platelet count by 25 to 50 × 10³/mm³ (see Table 132–2),[5] which is usually adequate for supporting hemostasis (see Table 132–2).[5] Platelets are also prepared from blood from a single donor with the use of blood cell separator machines, yielding a platelet product (apheresis) equivalent to that of 5 random units. For adults and children greater than 20 kg, a platelet transfusion requires 1 single-donor apheresis unit (10 ml/kg for children < 20 kg) (see Table 132–2).[1,5] This type of product (apheresis unit of platelets) aims to minimize donor exposure and is recommended for patients requiring chronic transfusion.[5] If the intention is to transfuse a small volume (e.g., in infants), an apheresis unit of platelets can be divided into two aliquots.

Platelet survival (normal, 9.6 ± 0.6 days) is shorter in patients with profound thrombocytopenia (platelets are normally consumed in the spleen and blood vessels), alloimmunization, fever, infection, and splenomegaly. ABO-compatible, single-donor apheresis, leukocyte-depleted and irradiated platelets are less likely to produce alloimmunization, and are therefore recommended for patients requiring chronic transfusion. Other indications for leukocyte-depleted and irradiated products are as discussed for PRBC transfusion. Platelet transfusion is not recommended in patients with hemolytic-uremic syndrome, thrombotic thrombocytopenic purpura, heparin-induced thrombocytopenia, and idiopathic thrombocytopenic purpura. Any medication that could inhibit platelet function (e.g., salicylates and nonsteroidal anti-inflammatory drugs) should be avoided in thrombocytopenic patients.

Fresh Frozen Plasma and Cryoprecipitate Transfusion

Fresh frozen plasma (FFP) is prepared from whole blood; it should be frozen at less than 18° C within 6 hours of collection. This procedure preserves the activities of labile proteins, such as factors V and VII. It is a nonconcentrated source of clotting factors and is used for acquired coagulopathy (e.g., liver disease and disseminated intravascular coagulation), rapid reversal of warfarin, congenital coagulation factor deficiency (e.g., factors II, X, XI, XIII), thrombotic thrombocytopenic purpura, and hemolytic-uremic syndrome (see Chapter 129, Acute Childhood Immune Thrombocytopenic Purpura and Related Platelet Disorders; and Chapter 131, Hemolytic-Uremic Syndrome). The dose ranges from 10 to 25 ml/kg, repeated as necessary (see Table 132–2).[5] The product should be ABO compatible. Potential complications include viral transmission (e.g., HIV, hepatitis), anaphylactic reaction, urticaria, and alloimmunization. Because of the risk of viral transmission, FFP should be used only if absolutely necessary.

Cryoprecipitate is prepared from FFP by thawing at 4° C. The precipitate is then suspended in 15 ml plasma and refrozen at less than 18° C. It is rich in fibrinogen (each unit contains approximately 250 mg), factor VIII, and von Willebrand's factor. It is used to treat bleeding due to fibrinogen deficiency, such as severe liver disease, disseminated intravascular coagulation, and afibrinogenemia (rare). The recommended dose is 1 to 4 units (bags) per 10 kg (8 to 12 units for adults), which raises plasma fibrinogen to by 60 to 100 mg/dl (see Table 132–2).[5] Due to the risk of viral transmission and availability of safer products, cryoprecipitate should not be used to treat patients with hemophilia A or von Willebrand's disease.

Transfusion Reactions

Hemolytic Transfusion Reactions

ABO incompatibility produces severe immune-mediated hemolytic reactions. The anti-A and/or anti-B IgM alloantibodies in the recipient's plasma produce intravascular hemolysis (circulating RBC fragments, hemoglobinemia, and hemoglobinuria) of the donor's RBCs. The symptoms include rigors, headache, fever, chest tightness, flank pain, red/black urine, hypotension, nausea, and vomiting. Serious progression may be fatal due to shock and organ failure. Management includes immediately stopping the transfusion and administering isotonic fluid (0.9% NaCl) and mannitol (0.25 g/kg intravenously) to induce diuresis. Careful monitoring (respiratory and circulatory status, urine output, and urine color), supportive care (intravenous fluid, diuretics, and oxygen) and appropriate consultations (blood bank, nephrology, and hematology) are necessary. The blood bag and blood sample from the recipient should be returned to the blood bank for retyping.

Nonimmune hemolytic reaction occurs when RBCs are damaged prior to transfusion (e.g., exposed to improper temperature during shipping or storage, mishandling during transfusion). Hemoglobinemia and hemoglobinuria are present in the recipient without symptoms. This complication requires no treatment.

Nonhemolytic Transfusion Reactions

Febrile reactions are caused by cytokines (produced by the donor's leukocytes) accumulated in stored blood. These molecules produce fever, rigors, tachycardia, and dyspnea. Management consists of stopping the transfusion and excluding a hemolytic transfusion reaction (repeat crossmatching of the unit of blood and performing Coombs' tests). The symptoms usually subside within 30 minutes of stopping the transfusion. Premedication with acetaminophen is usually helpful.

Allergic symptoms (rash and urticaria, pruritus, flushing, and, rarely, angioedema) follow the recipient's exposure to the donor's plasma proteins or other substances (e.g., medications taken by the donor). This reaction can be ameliorated by premedicating with diphenhydramine (0.5 to 1 mg/kg) and methylprednisolone (0.5 to 1 mg/kg). A severe form of allergic reaction (anaphylactic) can occur in recipients who are IgA deficient. Management of urticaria consists of discontinuing the transfusion and administering diphenhydramine and methylprednisolone. Anaphylaxis requires intravenous fluids, steroids, and subcutaneous or intravenous epinephrine administration depending upon the severity.

Transfusion-related acute lung injury is a noncardiogenic pulmonary edema associated with passive transfusion of donor granulocyte antibodies. The reaction occurs when the donor's antileukocyte antibodies (e.g., in multiparous or previously transfused donors) react with the recipient's leukocytes, which are then aggregated and activated in the lung microvasculature, producing altered vascular permeability and pulmonary capillary leak syndrome, resembling acute respiratory distress syndrome (ARDS). It should be managed similarly to ARDS.

Circulatory overload (cough, precordial pain, tachycardia, tachypnea, dyspnea, and hypoxia) may follow rapid transfusion. This complication is more common in patients with cardiac or renal disease, hypertension, or profound anemia (hemoglobin concentration < 5.0 g/dl). Treatment includes stopping the transfusion, oxygen supplementation, and administration of furosemide (0.5 to 1 mg/kg intravenously). Volume overload can be avoided by transfusing half of the desired transfusion over 4 hours, followed by administration of intravenous furosemide (0.5 to 1 mg/kg), followed by the second half of the transfusion over 4 hours.

Rare acute complications include bacterial contamination (most notably from platelet transfusion), citrate-induced hypocalcemia, and hyperkalemia (due to ruptured red cells).

Delayed Transfusion Reactions

Viral contamination with cytomegalovirus, HIV, and hepatitis A, B, and C virus remains a serious complication. Posttransfusion hepatitis is of particular concern because donors are usually asymptomatic. The risk of HIV transmission is almost negligible (probably 1 in 8 million transfusions).

Alloimmunization (developing alloantibodies against red cell, platelet, and leukocyte antigens) results from multiple exposures to donor antigens. Every transfusion has the potential to induce alloimmunization.

Posttransfusion graft-versus-host reaction occurs in patients on chemotherapy or with immunodeficiency. It also occurs in newborns and young infants who receive transfusion from blood relatives. Donor T cells attack recipient tissues, producing skin rash, increased transaminases, and diarrhea. Gamma irradiation of blood components eliminates this risk.

Iron overload results from repeated PRBC transfusions. Long-term complications of hemochromatosis include cirrhosis, fibrosis of the pancreas, and cardiomyopathy. Chelation therapy with deferoxamine mesylate (Desferol) is necessary for patients receiving long-term transfusions.

Summary

Viral transmission through transfusion occurs very rarely, and the risk of developing acquired immunodeficiency syndrome from a blood transfusion is almost negligible. Nevertheless, the risk of not receiving a transfusion should always outweigh the potential adverse effects. Serious transfusion reactions can be avoided by verifying each patient's identification and the blood groups of recipients and donors. Blood

components should be transfused slowly in the first 15 minutes, with the patient being closely monitored. Diphenhydramine (0.5 to 1 mg/kg), methylprednisolone (1 mg/kg), and acetaminophen can be given for minor allergic and/or febrile reactions. These medications also can be used as prophylaxis for patients with prior adverse reactions to transfusion. Leukocyte-reduced and irradiated blood components produce less adverse reactions.

REFERENCES

1. Gorlin JB (ed): Standards for Blood Banks and Transfusion Services, 21st ed. Bethesda, MD: American Association of Blood Banks, 2002.
2. Roseff AD, Luban NLC, Manno CS: Guidelines for assessing appropriateness of pediatric transfusion. Transfusion 42:1398–1413, 2002.
3. Ceccherini-Nelli L, Filipponi F, Mosca F, Campa M: The risk of contracting an infectious disease from blood transfusion. Transplant Proc 36:680–682, 2004.
4. Pealer LN, Marfin AA, Petersen LR, et al: Transmission of West Nile virus through blood transfusion in the United States in 2002. N Engl J Med 349:1236–1245, 2003.
5. Pisciotto P (ed): Pediatric Hemotherapy Data Card. Bethesda, MD: American Association of Blood Banks, 2002.

Chapter 133

Common Pediatric Overdoses

Deborah J. Mann, MD and Richard M. Cantor, MD

Key Points

Specific medications are harmful to children, even in small amounts.

Cyanosis unresponsive to supplemental oxygen may be a sign of methemoglobinemia.

Exposure to long-acting oral hypoglycemics often necessitates overnight admission for glucose monitoring.

Serum acetaminophen and aspirin levels are mandatory in all intentional overdose cases.

Acetaminophen levels drawn before 4 hours postingestion do not reflect or predict potential toxicity or the need for *N*-acetylcysteine therapy.

Introduction and Background

Epidemiology of Pediatric Poisonings

Exposure to toxins represents a large subset of pediatric emergencies, both within the home and in emergency departments. Poisoning is ranked as the third leading cause of mortality following motor vehicle accidents and farm injuries. Poisoning was the underlying cause of death for 18,549 people in the United States in 1998.[1,2]

Analysis of Poison Control Center national data reveals that 75% of exposures occur within the home. In the pediatric subgroup, 85% to 90% of exposures are unintentional. There is a peak age under 5 years with parallel rises at ages 12, 13 to 19, the 20s, and the 30s. As children enter adolescence, accidental exposures become rare and intentional exposures more common. Seventy-five percent of exposures are ingestions, followed by dermal, inhalation, and ocular exposures. Commonly involved agents and reported fatalities are listed in Tables 133–1 and 133–2.[3,4]

Parents often underestimate the motor skills of children. Children are curious about their environment. They explore using hand-to-mouth behavior. Children's higher respiratory rates impart greater susceptibility to toxic gases and aspira-

tion. Enhanced skin permeability of children is a factor in absorption as well.

The average 2-year-old places nonfood items in his or her mouth at a rate that approximates three events per hour; however, most pediatric ingestions are benign in nature. A small percentage of pediatric patients (12%) will develop signs and symptoms following ingestion.[3,4] Current annual estimates suggest that 2000 patients less than 6 years of age will develop life-threatening events as a result of intoxication. Approximately 20 fatal cases are reported from toxic exposure each year.[1-4]

Ingestion involves a complex interplay of variables that include the child, the substance, and the environment. The typical child is unable to discriminate safe from unsafe, and is observant of the ritual of self-medication in other family members. The child often mistakes the substance for an edible ingredient, when in fact it is a medication (as in "look-a-like medications") (Table 133–3). The environment may be unsafe for children, with poor storage techniques of toxicants within the household (Table 133–4). A common pitfall is storage of a harmful substance within a recognizable container (i.e., kerosene or gasoline in a soda bottle). Many poisonings are a result of poor parental supervision.

The Individual Encounter

An ingestion should be suspected when a preverbal child is found with an open container, when a classic toxidrome is present, or in cases of unexplained multiorgan system abnormality.

Liquids or pelleted materials are more likely to be ingested in larger amounts than aerosols or powders. Flavoring or irritant additives have little to do with determining whether the product was actually ingested. The volume of the swallow is a function of body mass. The volume of a swallow is 0.27 ml/kg, or roughly 1 teaspoon, for a 2-year-old, 1 tablespoon for an adult female, and 1 to 2 tablespoons for an adult male.

The situation of an unwitnessed disappearance of the contents of a container of a toxic substance often presents poison centers with difficult management decisions. When the amount of toxicant ingested is difficult to estimate, the physician must default to the assumption that the child may have consumed the full container of the toxicant involved. When two children are involved in an ingestion, it must be assumed that each took the entire amount. The classic concept of sharing may not apply.

Table 133–1   Nationally Reported Ingestions

All Calls to the Poison Center		Children ≤ 6 Yr Old	
Substance	Percent	Substance	Percent
Analgesics	10.5	Cosmetics	13.3
Cleaning products	9.5	Cleaning products	10.5
Cosmetics	9.4	Analgesics	7.2
Foreign bodies	5.0	Foreign bodies	6.8
Plants	4.9	Plants	6.6
Cold and cough medicines	4.5	Topical agents	6.3
Bites and envenomations	4.2	Cold and cough medicines	5.3
Sedatives and hypnotics	4.1	Pesticides	4.1
Topical agents	4.1	Vitamins	3.6
Pesticides	4.0	GI preparations	3.2

Table 133–2   Nationally Reported Fatalities

All Calls Groups		Children ≤ 6 Yr Old	
Substance	Percent	Substance	Percent
Analgesics	44	Carbon monoxide	15
Antidepressants	26	Iron	7
Sedatives and hypnotics	24	Analgesics	7
Stimulants and street drugs	20	Cleaning substances	6
Cardiovascular drugs	12	Cardiovascular agents	6
Toxic alcohols	11	Antidepressants	6
		Insecticides/pesticides	5

While most pediatric exposures are benign in nature, there are some toxins that are dangerous even when presented in the form of a small taste, lick, or swallow (Table 133–5).

Selected Pediatric Overdoses

Nonsteroidal anti-inflammatory drugs
Oral hypoglycemics
Agents causing methemoglobinemia
Iron poisoning
Acetaminophen
Aspirin (salicylate)
Selected comments on other pharmaceuticals

Discussion of Individual Pediatric Overdoses

Nonsteroidal Anti-Inflammatory Drugs

The nonsteroidal anti-inflammatory drugs (NSAIDs) are a group of medications that have antipyretic, anti-inflammatory, and analgesic properties. With their widespread availability and increasing use in the United States, NSAIDs represent some of the most common medications involved in the overdose setting. Fortunately, most NSAID exposures cause minimal morbidity and mortality. The most prevalent complications are therapeutic side effects, specifically gastrointestinal (GI) bleeding.

NSAIDs exert their pharmacologic effect by inhibiting cyclooxygenases, which are involved in prostaglandin synthesis.[5,6] NSAIDs are rapidly and almost completely absorbed. They are weak acids, highly protein bound, and metabolized by the cytochrome P-450 system. More than half of the drug is excreted unchanged in the urine.

NSAIDs seldom cause serious toxicity, even in large doses. At this time, there are inadequate data defining the minimum toxic or lethal dose.[7] Following acute overdose, most children are asymptomatic or develop only mild GI symptoms. Specific signs and symptoms are summarized in Table 133–6. Generally, full recovery can be expected within 6 to 24 hours. In contrast, phenylbutazone and its active metabolite oxyphenbutazone can cause coma, seizures, shock, respiratory alkalosis, and metabolic acidosis. Within 24 hours, hepatic necrosis may develop. Urine discoloration due to a metabolite may result in a red hue.

The emergency department evaluation consists of standard supportive care and GI decontamination. Gastrointestinal bleeding should be treated by standard measures for hemodynamic support. Activated charcoal remains the preferred method of GI decontamination.[7]

Oral Hypoglycemics

Diabetes mellitus is the most common endocrine disorder in our country today and is frequently managed with oral agents. Oral medications including sulfonylureas, meglitinides, biguanides, and thiazolidinediones. Of all these drug classes, only the sulfonylureas and meglitinides are truly hypoglycemic agents (Table 133–7).

Most poisonings from oral hypoglycemic agents involve sulfonylureas, with most of the fatalities involving biguanides.[8-10] Their primary mechanism of action is the release of endogenous insulin. Glyburide has the highest incidence of hypoglycemia and is the most widely utilized of these agents. Most hospitalizations are due to overdose of long-acting agents. In the overdose setting, hypoglycemia typically occurs within the first several hours after ingestion. Delayed hypoglycemia has also been reported in some cases. In a retrospective pediatric study, 96% of children exposed to oral

Table 133–3	Pharmaceuticals Toxic to Children

Analgesics

Acetaminophen
Nonsteroidal anti-inflammatory drugs
Salicylates

Anesthetics

Benzocaine
Lidocaine

Anticholinergics

Cyproheptadine
Diphenhydramine
Dimenhydrinate
Hydroxyzine
Hyoscyamine
Orphenadrine
Scopolamine

Anticonvulsants

Barbiturates
Carbamazepine
Phenytoin

Antidepressants/Antipsychotics

Chlorpromazine
Clozapine
Cyclic antidepressants
Lithium
Monoamine oxidase inhibitors
Sertraline
Thioridazine

Antihypertensives/Antidysrhythmics

Captopril
Clonidine
Digoxin
Nifedipine
Verapamil

Antimalarials

Chloroquine
Quinines

Antituberculosis Drugs

Isoniazid

Bronchodilators

Albuterol
Caffeine
Ephedrine
Theophylline

Fluoride

Ammonium fluoride, befluoride

Hypoglycemics

Sulfonylureas

Iron

Prenatal hematinics

Methylxanthines

Caffeine
Theophylline

Opioids

Codeine
Diphenoxylate
Hydrocodone
Methadone
Pentazocine
Propoxyphene

Sedatives

Triazolam

Sympathomimetics

Amphetamine
Cocaine
Nasal/ocular imidazoline
Phencyclidine
Phenylpropanolamine
Pseudoephedrine

Table 133–4	Household Products and Plants Toxic to Children

Acid/Alkali Products

Boric acid
Bowl cleansers
Clinitest tablet
Disc battery

Alcohols

Ethanol
Ethylene glycol
Isopropyl alcohol
Methanol

Antiseptics

Camphor
Cantharidin
Hydrogen peroxide
Phenol
Pine oil

Cyanide

Hydrocarbons

Industrial Chemicals

Butyrolactone (solvent for acrylate polymers)
Methylene chloride (paint thinner)
Selenious acid (gun blueing)
Zinc chloride (soldering flux)

Mothballs

Naphthalene

Nail Products

Acetone (polish remover)
Acetonitrile (sculptured nail remover)
Methacrylic acid (artificial nail primer)
Nitromethane (artificial nail remover)

Organophosphates

Carbamate

Plants

Aconite
Castor bean
Clove oil
Comfrey
Foxglove
Ma huang
Mushrooms (specific)
Nutmeg
Oleander
Pennyroyal oil

Rodenticides

Arsenic
Hydroxycoumarin
Indanediones
Strychnine

Weed/Bug Killers

Lindane
Nicotine
Paraquat

hypoglycemics had a drop in their blood sugar within 8 hours.[11]

The biguanide class includes metformin and phenformin. Phenformin was removed from U.S. distribution as a result of fatal lactic acidosis. Metformin is the only biguanide in common use today. It increases insulin sensitivity, decreases hepatic gluconeogenesis, and diminishes intestinal glucose absorption. Insulin secretion remains unaffected. Therefore, metformin will correct hypoglycemia in diabetics but will

Table 133–5	Medicinal Preparations Fatal to a 10-kg Toddler		
Drug	**Minimal Potential Fatal Dose (per kg weight)**	**Maximal Unit Dose Available**	**Amount Causing Fatality**
Camphor	100 mg	1 g/5 ml	1 tsp
Chloroquine	20 mg	500 mg	<1 tbsp
Hydroxychloroquine	20 mg	200 mg	1 tbsp
Imipramine	15 mg	150 mg	1 tbsp
Desipramine	15 mg	75–150 mg	1 tbsp
Quinine	80 mg	650 mg	1–2 tbsp
Methyl salicylate	200 mg	1.4 g/ml	<1 tsp
Theophylline	8.4 mg	500 mg	<1 tbsp
Thioridazine	15 mg	200 mg	<1 tbsp
Chlorpromazine	25 mg	200 mg	1–2 tbsp

Ingestion of small quantities of antidysrhythmics, calcium channel blockers, clonidine (especially patches), lidocaine (e.g., viscous preparations), sulfonylureas, lindane, nicotine patches, and long-acting narcotics (e.g., fentanyl patches, methadone, oxycontin, MS Contin) also may be life-threatening.
Abbreviations: tbsp, tablespoon; tsp, teaspoon.

Table 133–6	Clinical Effects of NSAID Toxicity
Organ System	**Sign/Symptom**
GI	Nausea, vomiting, anorexia, abdominal pain, gastritis, GI bleeding, cholestasis
Neurologic	Dizziness, nystagmus, diploplia, blurred vision, headache, tinnitus, lethargy, ataxia, confusion, seizures
Respiratory	Hyperventilation, respiratory depression, apnea
Cardiovascular	Hypotension, bradycardia
Renal	Sodium retention and edema, proteinuria, hematuria, renal failure
Hematologic	Decreased platelet aggregation, elevated PTT and PT
Other	Metabolic acidosis

Abbreviations: GI, gastrointestinal; NSAID, nonsteroidal anti-inflammatory drug; PT, prothrombin time; PTT, partial thromboplastin time.

Table 133–7	Pharmacokinetics of Hypoglycemic Agents		
Generic Name	**Trade Name**	**Peak (hr)**	**Duration (hr)**
First-Generation Sulfonylureas			
Chlorpropamide	Diabinese	3–6	24–72
Acetohexamide	Dymelor	3	12–24
Tolbutamide	Orinase	5–8	6–12
Second-Generation Sulfonylureas			
Glipizide	Glucotrol	1–3	12–24
Glipizide ER	Glucotrol XL	6–12	24
Glyburide	Micronase	2–6	24
Meglitinides			
Repaglinide	Prandin	0.5–1	1
Nateglinide	Starlix	1	1.5
Biguanides			
Metformin	Glucophage	2–3	5–6
alpha-Glucosidase Inhibitors			
Acarbose	Precose	NA	NA
Thiazolidinediones			
Rosiglitazone	Avandia	1–3	3–4

not induce hypoglycemia in nondiabetics. Lactic acidosis is the most serious side effect associated with metformin.[12]

Hypoglycemia affects many organ systems. Autonomic symptoms are prominent and result from excessive adrenergic tone. Symptoms and signs include anxiety, diaphoresis, palpitations, irritability, and tremor. Neurologic symptoms include dizziness, tingling, and faintness. Simultaneous therapy with β-blockers may mask the autonomic symptoms. Hypoglycemia may also cause focal neurologic deficits.

Emergency department management involves standard gastrointestinal decontamination techniques. Intravenous (IV) dextrose remains the first line of therapy for hypoglycemia. Children should receive 2 to 4 ml/kg of 25% dextrose. Euglycemia maintenance may require an infusion of 5% to 10% dextrose. Infusions of higher concentrations of dextrose may require the use of a large-bore or central venous catheter. All children who are symptomatic or potentially ingested long-acting agents require admission and prolonged observation for hypoglycemia.

Refractory hypoglycemia may be treated with either diazoxide or octreotide. Diazoxide inhibits pancreatic insulin release. The dose is 1 to 3 mg/kg IV in children (to a maximum of 150 mg). Octreotide inhibits pancreatic insulin secretion and has a well established place in the management of sulfonylurea-induced refractory hypoglycemia. Clinical trials

have clearly demonstrated its effectiveness.[13] The suggested dose is 4 to 5 mcg/kg/day divided every 6 hours in children (maximum dose should not exceed 1500 mcg/24 hr).

Agents Causing Methemoglobinemia

Methemoglobinemia is caused by the conversion of iron molecules in hemoglobin from the ferrous to ferric state. Under normal conditions, methemoglobin levels are less than 1% to 2% of a child's total hemoglobin. Oxyhemoglobin is red and methemoglobin is dark brown, creating its characteristic chocolate brown color. At least 5 g of hemoglobin per deciliter of blood must be oxidized to methemoglobin to cause clinical cyanosis. Methemoglobin is incapable of transporting oxygen. This induces a leftward shift in the oxyhemoglobin dissociation curve. The final result is a global decrease in tissue oxygenation accompanied by metabolic acidosis.

Mammalian red blood cells contain enzymes that are capable of reducing methemoglobin back to oxyhemoglobin. The vast majority of this reduction is carried out by the transfer of electrons from NADH (NADH-dependent methemoglobin reductase). In the normal resting state, the

Table 133–8	Agents Known to be Associated with Methemoglobinemia

Acetanalid
Amyl nitrate
Aniline dyes
Benzocaine
Chlorates
Dapsone
Dinitrophenol
EMLA
Flutamide
Hydrazines
Lidocaine
Local anesthetics
Methylene blue
Metoclopramide
Napthalene
Nitrates
Nitrites
Nitroglycerin
Phenacetin
Phenols
Prilocaine
Primaquine
Pyridine
Quinones
Sulfonamides
Sulfones
Trinitrotoluene

enzymatic reduction of methemoglobin keeps up with its spontaneous formation. In the neonate, any oxygen stress may cause methemoglobinemia due to decreased reducing ability.[14,15]

Many agents have been known to result in acquired methemoglobinemia (Table 133–8). The mechanisms for their causation are varied, either involving direct oxidant stress or a secondary effect of their metabolites. The most commonly reported substances associated with methemoglobinemia are local anesthetics such as benzocaine. These may be delivered parenterally or topically (as in teething gels). Other prescribed medications implicated in methemoglobinemia include metoclopramide, phenazopyridine, and diaminodiphenylsulfone. Environmental factors include analine dyes and exposure to either nitrates or nitrites. Well water is a common source of nitrites. Recreational use of inhaled nitrites has also been associated with cases of methemoglobinemia. Finally, acute diarrheal conditions in infants have also been associated with methemoglobinemia.[16]

As methemoglobin levels exceed 10%, patients present with unexplained cyanosis and often no other symptoms. At levels from 15% to 35%, headache, shortness of breath, tachypnea, and tachycardia may occur. As levels rise further, central nervous system (CNS) signs and symptoms include confusion, coma, seizures, and apnea. Death occurs with levels over 70%.[14,15]

Patients with methemoglobinemia remain cyanotic even with administration of supplemental oxygen. Arterial oxygen levels are normal or elevated. Bedside pulse oximetry[15] is unreliable in most cases. Venous blood will turn brown when exposed to room air.

All patients with suspected methemoglobinemia should be placed on supplemental oxygen. This will ensure oxygen delivery to the fraction of hemoglobin that is functional. Most patients with levels less than 30% will not require any additional treatment. Methylene blue should be administered to symptomatic patients, those with levels above 30%, those with electrocardiogram changes, or those with metabolic acidosis. The recommended dose is 2 mg/kg given IV over 3 to 5 minutes. Most patients resolve their cyanosis within 15 minutes. In refractory cases, repeat doses may be given. The total dose of methylene blue during the first 2 to 3 hours should not exceed 5 to 7 mg/kg. Methylene blue is contraindicated in patients with known glucose-6-phosphate dehydrogenase (G6PD) deficiency since hemolysis may occur. There is an increased incidence of G6PD deficiency in individuals of African and Mediterranean descent.

Treatment with hyperbaric oxygen or exchange transfusion may be effective for patients with G6PD deficiency or those who are resistant to methylene blue. All patients with methemoglobinemia should be admitted to a monitored setting for observation. A toxicologist or poison control center should be consulted in difficult-to-manage cases.

Iron Poisoning

Iron poisoning is the leading cause of accidental death from pharmaceutical agents in young children. There are over 30,000 iron ingestions annually.[1,2] Iron is readily available in the home, with many preparations resembling chewable candy. Toxicity is dependent on the amount of elemental iron ingested. Ingestion of greater than 20 mg/kg will often produce GI upset. Exposures above 50 mg/kg are potentially fatal. Exposure to children's chewable vitamins rarely causes severe iron poisoning.

Free unbound iron is toxic to tissues. The body protects itself by binding iron to ferritin. Iron is transported globally bound to transferrin. The total iron-binding capacity (TIBC) represents the amount of iron that transferrin can bind. Normally, the TIBC far exceeds the serum iron concentration, resulting in no circulating unbound iron.

Iron is a corrosive with the potential to cause hemorrhage, hypovolemia, and GI perforation. Systemic effects occur if enough iron is absorbed. Iron disrupts oxidative phosphorylation and promotes the formation of free radicals, contributing to cell death. Iron is also a vasodilator. The net effect is shock and metabolic acidosis.

Traditionally, clinicians have attempted to characterize iron poisoning by clinical stages according to symptoms. However, the emergency physician must be aware of overlapping presentations.[17] The first stage of iron poisoning occurs within the first few hours and is characterized by abdominal pain, vomiting, and diarrhea. Significant GI bleeding may occur. The second stage involves resolution of GI symptoms, with silent absorption of toxic amounts of iron. This may last up to 36 hours after exposure, giving a false sense of clinical improvement. Clinically evident systemic iron poisoning heralds the third stage. Shock and metabolic acidosis will occur because of shifts of fluid out of the vasculature. Liver failure may result. Scarring of the gastric outlet or small bowel represents the fourth stage. This may occur several weeks after the acute event.

Serum iron concentrations usually peak 2 to 6 hours after exposure. A normal serum iron level drawn very early or late after ingestion does not exclude toxicity. Previous management favored the use of white blood cell or serum glucose levels to predict severity. This has been proven to be unreliable.[17] Plain radiographs of the abdomen may demonstrate opacities in severe poisoning and confirm the suspicion of iron poisoning.

Most symptomatic patients, or those with a history of ingesting more than 20 mg/kg, are referred to emergency departments by poison control centers. Activated charcoal does not bind iron and is of no use in a pure ingestion. Gastric lavage is ineffective as well. There are no data supporting the use of bicarbonate or phosphate solutions to prevent absorption. Whole bowel irrigation (WBI) has been shown to be effective in reducing toxicity and is especially effective if tablets are seen on plain radiography. Patients undergoing WBI must be awake and alert without evidence of GI dysfunction (e.g., intractable vomiting, ileus, significant bleeding, obstruction, or perforation). Elevate the head of the bed to 45 degrees. Administer 25–40 ml/kg per hour of polyethylene glycol by nasogastric tube until effluent clear and radiography no longer shows any iron tablets.

Patients who are asymptomatic after 6 hours with normal serum iron levels (50–150 mcg/dl) may be discharged. Patients who develop emesis or diarrhea, or have evidence of hypovolemia, tablets seen on plain radiography, serum iron levels > 350 mcg/dl, or serum iron levels > TIBC should receive fluids and chelation with deferoxamine mesylate. Chelation should not be delayed while waiting for serum iron levels in ill patients. Administration of 20 to 40 ml/kg of crystalloid or more may be necessary. The dose of deferoxamine is 15 mg/kg/hr, administered IV until all symptoms and signs of toxicity have resolved, serum iron is <100 mcg/dl plus 24 hours after vin rose urine disappears. Rapid administration can be associated with histamine release and hypotension. If this occurs, administer IV fluids, lower the rate of administration and administer antihistamines for histamine symptoms.

Acetaminophen

Acetaminophen is one of the most popular medications used to treat pain and fever in children and comes in many forms, including tablets, elixirs, and rectal suppositories. With its popularity and ready availability in homes, acetaminophen overdoses, both intentional and unintentional, are common. Over 60,000 acetaminophen-only exposures and approximately 150 acetaminophen-induced deaths were reported by the American Association of Poison Control Centers in 2003. More than 40,000 of these exposures occurred in patients less than 19 years old. Fortunately, most acute one-time accidental ingestions in small children are associated with lower risks of toxicity than in adults due to difference in metabolism.[18] However, significant morbidity and mortality may occur after repeated supratherapeutic dosing.[19]

Acetaminophen is metabolized by the liver primarily through glucuronidation and sulfation. A small percentage of acetaminophen is metabolized by the cytochrome P-450 mixed function oxidase pathway into a toxic intermediate compound, N-acetyl-p-benzoquinoneimine (NAPQI). At recommended doses of acetaminophen, NAPQI is conjugated with glutathione, making it nontoxic and allowing its excretion in the urine and bile. With overdoses and repeated supratherapeutic doses of acetaminophen, glutathione stores are depleted. The toxic metabolite, NAPQI, then accumulates and binds to hepatocytes, causing centrilobular necrosis.

Patients taking medications that induce cytochrome P-450 activity (e.g., anticonvulsants) may be at increased risk of hepatoxicity following an acetaminophen overdose, as are those with depleted glutathione stores (e.g., alcoholics and acquired immunodeficiency syndrome patients).[20-22] The clinical presentation of acetaminophen toxicity can be divided into four stages. Symptoms of stage I are vague and may include anorexia, nausea, vomiting, and pallor. These symptoms, if present, typically resolve in the first 12 to 24 hours. Stage II occurs at 24 to 48 hours postingestion, and clinical signs of hepatotoxicity may be present, such as right upper quadrant abdominal pain and elevation of liver transaminases and bilirubin. Even without treatment, most of these patients will recover without sequelae. By days 3 to 4 postingestion, some patients will progress to stage III with signs of fulminant hepatic failure, including metabolic acidosis, coagulopathy, jaundice, renal failure, encephalopathy, and recurrent GI symptoms. Stage IV occurs 4 to 14 days postingestion, and patients either make a full recovery or die from complete liver failure or its complications.[6]

Clinical Presentation

Early recognition of patients with acetaminophen poisoning and treatment with N-acetylcysteine (NAC) limit morbidity and mortality. This is challenging since patients are often asymptomatic at the time of presentation. All patients with suspected overdose should be screened for acetaminophen.[23] Important historical factors to determine are the time of acute ingestion, repeated supratherapeutic dosing, formulation (immediate release versus extended release), amount of acetaminophen ingested, and co-ingestants. Dose history is not always reliable, especially in situations in which the ingestion is not witnessed, there is suspected drug abuse, or the patient's intent is self-harm.

During initial evaluation, the patient should be placed in one of the following categories for acetaminophen exposure: acute acetaminophen ingestion within 24 hours; acute ingestion for which the time is unknown or greater than 24 hours; ingestion of extended-release acetaminophen; ingestion of repeated supratherapeutic doses; and signs or symptoms of hepatic injury (Fig. 133–1).

When used properly, the acetaminophen nomogram is an excellent screening tool for assessing potential acetaminophen toxicity (Fig. 133–2). The acetaminophen nomogram applies only to acetaminophen levels obtained between 4 and 24 hours postingestion. It is important to precisely define the time at which the ingestion occurred; if this is not possible, the earliest possible time of ingestion should be used. If the level falls below the treatment line on the nomogram, then no NAC therapy is needed.

ACUTE ACETAMINOPHEN INGESTION WITHIN 24 HOURS

An acute acetaminophen overdose is defined as a single ingestion of at least 7.5 g in an adult or 150 mg/kg in a child and should be considered possible in any patient who presents with a history of another overdose or altered mental status.[23-25] In these patients, a serum acetaminophen level should be acquired 4 hours postingestion or as soon thereafter and plotted on the acetaminophen nomogram (see Fig. 133–2). If the serum acetaminophen level falls above the treatment line on the nomogram, therapy with NAC is started. If the acetaminophen level will not be available within 8 hours of ingestion, NAC should be started and then discontinued if the acetaminophen level falls below the treatment line when plotted on the nomogram.

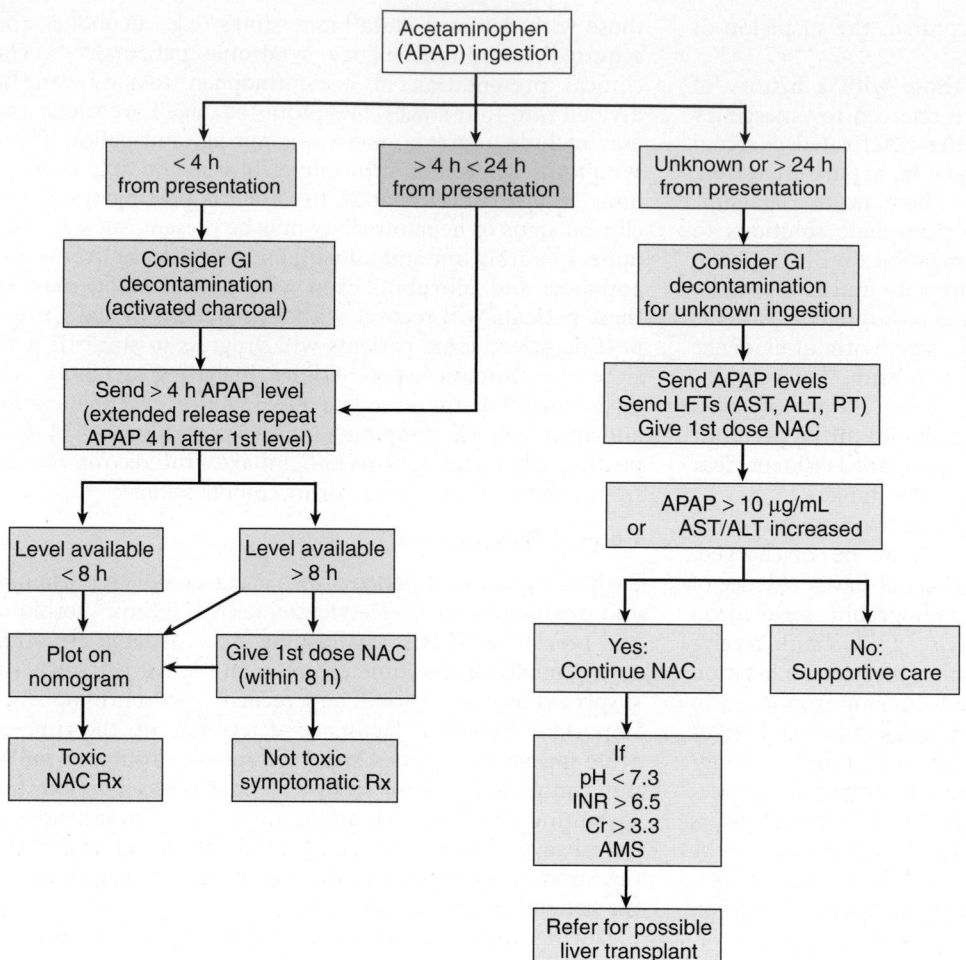

FIGURE 133–1. Treatment guidelines for acetaminophen ingestion. All times noted are postingestion. Abbreviations: ALT, alanine aminotransferase; AMS, altered mental status; APAP, acetaminophen; AST, aspartate aminotransferase; Cr, creatinine; GI, gastrointestinal; INR, international normalized ratio; LFTs, liver function tests; NAC, *N*-acetylcysteine; PT, prothrombin time; Rx, treatment.

If the patient presents within 4 hours of the acetaminophen ingestion or there is a history of a co-ingestant, oral activated charcoal can be given. There is no evidence that administering activated charcoal will interfere with oral NAC therapy.[26] In patients who present greater than 8 hours postingestion with serum acetaminophen levels that plot above the treatment line, liver function tests (aspartate aminotransferase [AST] and alanine aminotransferase [ALT]) should be ordered before and after NAC therapy[27] (see Fig. 133–1).

ACUTE ACETAMINOPHEN INGESTION WITH UNKNOWN TIME OR GREATER THAN 24 HOURS POSTINGESTION

It may be challenging to obtain the exact time of acetaminophen ingestion, but with a careful history obtained from the patient, family, and others, a time window can often be established. If the time of ingestion cannot be determined or it has been greater than 24 hours, a serum acetaminophen level and liver function tests (AST and ALT) should be drawn immediately. The acetaminophen nomogram cannot be used. Potential toxicity must be assumed and NAC therapy started (see Fig. 133–1).

EXTENDED RELEASE ACETAMINOPHEN INGESTION

For patients presenting after an overdose of an extended-release acetaminophen, a serum acetaminophen level is drawn 4 hours postingestion and repeated again in 4 hours.

The acetaminophen levels are plotted on the acetaminophen nomogram.[24,28] If either of the acetaminophen levels drawn falls above the treatment line, NAC therapy is started (see Fig. 133–1).

REPEATED SUPRATHERAPEUTIC ACETAMINOPHEN DOSING

Although death has rarely been reported in children less than 6 years old with a single overdose of acetaminophen, there have been multiple reports of hepatotoxicity and death associated with repeated supratherapeutic doses of acetaminophen in children.[29] Many studies have investigated what factors may put children at increased risk of hepatoxicity with repeated supratherapeutic dosing, such as febrile illness, starvation states, total dose given, duration of acetaminophen therapy, and use of P-450–inducing medications. Although there have been more cases of hepatoxicity and death in children with febrile illness who received supratherapeutic doses of acetaminophen than in nonfebrile children, it is not clear what role fever plays. Prevention of future overdoses may be accomplished with adequate therapy instructions or education during well-child visits. All recommendations for acetaminophen therapy should include the dose, frequency, duration of therapy, and specific strength and formulation for the individual child.

Chronic acetaminophen toxicity should be considered in any child with a history of acetaminophen doses of

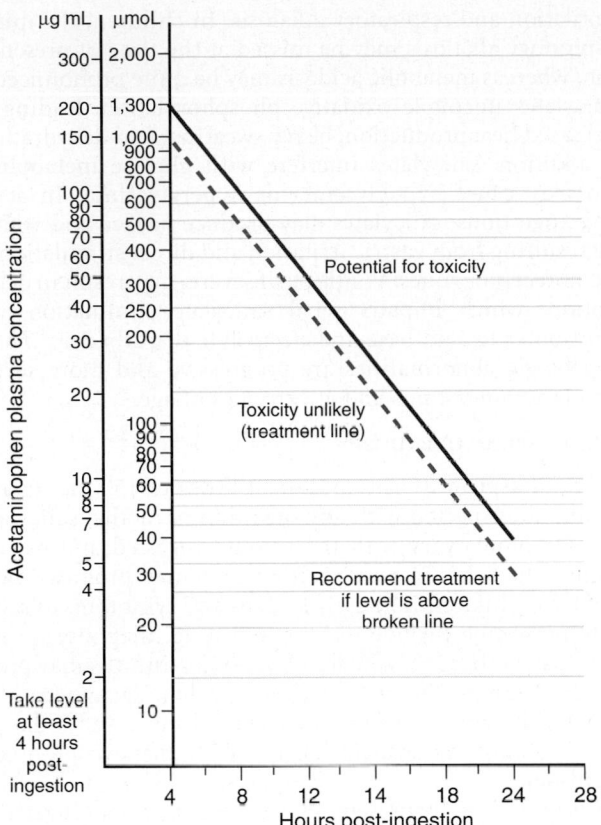

FIGURE 133–2. Acetaminophen nomogram: serum acetaminophen concentration versus time after ingestion. (From Management of Acetaminophen Overdose. Raritan, NJ: McNeil Consumer Products, 1986.)

150 mg/kg/day for more than 2 days or in an adult with a history of acetaminophen doses of 4 g/day for more than 2 days, as well as in a patient who presents with signs of hepatic dysfunction.

In patients with signs or symptoms of hepatic injury, acetaminophen levels should be drawn immediately. Additional laboratory workup should include liver function tests (AST and ALT), international normalized ratio (INR) for prothrombin time, bilirubin, glucose, blood urea nitrogen, creatinine, lactate, phosphate, electrolytes, and arterial blood gases. With repeated doses, the physician should assume the ingestion to begin from the time of the first dose, and use this to plot the level on the acetaminophen nomogram. Laboratory tests should be repeated every 12 to 24 hours.[30] NAC therapy should be started if the acetaminophen level is greater than 10 µg/ml or if the acetaminophen level is not detectable but the liver function test results are elevated (see Fig. 133–1).

Treatment of Acetaminophen Toxicity

The treatment of acetaminophen toxicity consists of GI decontamination with activated charcoal, supportive care, and the timely administration of the antidote, NAC.[31] Activated charcoal may be given orally or by nasogastric tube (1 g/kg) if the patient presents within 4 hours or if co-ingestants are suspected. More aggressive GI decontamination, with orogastric lavage and whole bowel irrigation, is not recommended for isolated acetaminophen toxicity because of acetaminophen's rapid absorption and the effectiveness of NAC as an antidote. Aggressive forms of GI decontamination

should be reserved for potentially life-threatening polydrug overdoses.

NAC is the mainstay of therapy for acetaminophen toxicity, although its mechanisms of action are not fully understood. One of several ways that NAC prevents hepatoxicity is through its conversion to cysteine, which repletes glutathione stores. Secondly, NAC binds directly to NAPQI, creating a nontoxic metabolite. Thirdly, it provides a substrate for sulfonation and thus promotes nontoxic metabolism of acetaminophen. These mechanisms of action promote the early administration of NAC (within 24 hours of acetaminophen overdose) to prevent hepatoxicity, but there is evidence that IV NAC is also effective in late acetaminophen overdose (>24 hours postingestion) and in fulminant hepatic failure.[32] Proposed mechanisms for this benefit in late toxicity include an antioxidant effect, decreased neutrophil accumulation, improved oxygen delivery to tissues, and improved microcirculatory changes in the liver.

Both the oral and IV treatment protocols are nearly 100% effective in preventing hepatoxicity when given within 8 hours of ingestion, and lessen the risk of hepatoxicity when given within the first 24 hours. The 72-hour oral NAC regimen had been the standard of care for acetaminophen toxicity in the United States, but the Food and Drug Administration approved IV NAC in January of 2004.

The standard 72-hour oral NAC regimen is a loading dose of 140 mg/kg followed by maintenance doses of 70 mg/kg every 4 hours for 17 additional doses. Few side effects are associated with oral NAC except for nausea and vomiting, which are aggravated by oral NAC's foul rotten egg odor. In order to mask its unpleasant odor, the standard 10% to 20% NAC solution may diluted to a 5% concentration in a chilled beverage, and served from a covered cup with a straw. Beverages that may mask the odor are soft drinks and fruit juice. If this is not enough to prevent nausea and vomiting, then an antiemetic such as metaclopromide or ondansetron can be given. In cases in which the nausea and vomiting cannot be controlled or oral NAC is contraindicated because of a caustic ingestion, IV NAC should be considered. The IV solution is well tolerated by most patients and considered safe when administered properly. The most common complication of IV NAC is an anaphylactoid reaction producing flushing, urticaria, angioedema, and bronchospasm. Most of these reactions are mild and related to the infusion rate. Symptoms can be controlled by slowing down the rate of infusion, or by treatment with an antihistamine or epinephrine if needed.[33] There is the potential for severe hyponatremia in small children when following the manufacturer's guidelines, since the amount of NAC received is weight based but the amount of fluid is constant for all patients: 1700 ml of free water over 20 hours. When using the 20-hour IV NAC protocol, a concentration of 40 mg/ml should be used in children less than 40 kg in order to avoid hyponatremia[34] (Table 133–9).

Fulminant Hepatic Failure

Unfortunately, a small percentage of acetaminophen overdose patients do develop fulminant hepatic failure. The mortality rate without NAC therapy is greater than 50%. NAC increases a patient's chances for survival even in the setting of fulminant hepatic failure. Predictors of poor outcome, including death and the need for a liver transplant, are as follows: serum pH less than 7.3 after fluid resuscitation, INR

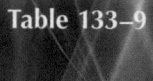

Table 133–9	Intravenous NAC (Acetadote) Pediatric Dosing (weight < 40 kg)/ Fluid Restrictions

Prepare 4% Concentration in D5W

- Mix 50 ml of NAC (20% solution) with 200 ml of D5W (remove 50 ml from a 250-ml bag of D5W) to obtain 40 mg/ml (4% concentration)

Loading Dose

- 150 mg/kg infused over NOT LESS THAN 15 min
- Infuse 3.75 ml/kg over NOT LESS THAN 15 min

First Maintenance Infusion

- 50 mg/kg infused over 4 hr
- Infuse 1.25 ml/kg over 4 hr (0.31 ml/kg/hr)

Second Maintenance Infusion

- 100 mg/kg infused over 16 hr
- Infuse 2.5 ml/kg over 16 hr (0.16 ml/kg/hr)

Abbreviations: D5W, dextrose 5% in water; NAC, N-acetylcysteine.
Adapted from package insert for Acetadote (2004) and Sung et al.[34]

greater than 6.5, grade III or IV encephalopathy; creatinine greater than 3.3 mg/dL (275 micromol/L), lactate greater than 25 mg/dl (3.0 mmol/L) after fluid resuscitation, and phosphorus greater than 3.8 mg/dl (1.2 mmol/L) after fluid resuscitation.[30]

Patients with acetaminophen-induced fulminant hepatic failure should receive early referral to a liver transplant center. The treatment of patients with fulminant hepatic failure includes correction of metabolic acidosis, correction of coagulopathy, and close monitoring and aggressive treatment of cerebral edema. In addition, IV NAC therapy is preferable to oral NAC therapy and should be continued until the patient improves, receives a liver transplant, or dies.

Aspirin (Salicylate)

The use of childproof containers, aspirin alternatives such as acetaminophen, and education to avoid the use of aspirin in children because of Reye's syndrome have reduced the incidence of unintentional salicylate poisoning in the United States. The American Association of Poison Control Centers' Toxic Exposure Surveillance System reported approximately 20,000 salicylate exposures and 60 salicylate-related deaths in the United States in 2003. Approximately half of these exposures occurred in people less than 19 years old.

Serious intoxications continue to occur because people are often unaware that over-the-counter medications such as Pepto-Bismol contain salicylate (1 ml contains 8.77 mg of aspirin), or that topical ointments or liniments used in hot vaporizers contain methyl salicylate (oil of wintergreen). Topical ointments may cause toxicity with extensive application. Even more dangerous is the consumption of oil of wintergreen. It contains 1440 mg/ml of salicylate, and even a small ingestion of 1 to 2 ml may be fatal for a young child.[35] Aspirin continues to be readily available, and serious salicylate toxicity may result from suicide attempts in adolescents and adults.

Clinical Presentation

The toxic effect of salicylates is complex. Salicylates stimulate the respiratory center of the brainstem, causing early hyper-

ventilation and respiratory alkalosis. In children, the initial respiratory alkalosis may be missed at the time of presentation, whereas metabolic acidosis may be quite pronounced.[36] Salicylates uncouple oxidative phosphorylation, leading to increased heat production, heavy sweating, and dehydration. In addition, salicylates interfere with glucose metabolism and may cause hypoglycemia or hyperglycemia. In acute large ingestions, salicylates may produce nausea and vomiting resulting from gastric irritation and direct stimulation of chemoreceptor zones. Vomiting, if severe, may result in dehydration, which impairs renal salicylate elimination and contributes to acid-base and electrolyte disturbances. These physiologic abnormalities are progressive and more severe with larger ingestions and at extremes of age.

ACUTE ASPIRIN OVERDOSE

Potential aspirin toxicity occurs at doses of 150 mg/kg and should be suspected with any ingestion of methyl salicylate. The symptoms vary with the amount ingested, but usually begin 3 to 8 hours postingestion and may progress more rapidly in children. The earliest signs and symptoms of salicylate poisoning include nausea, vomiting, diaphoresis, and tinnitus. As the CNS salicylate levels rise, tinnitus may progress to deafness. Other CNS effects include tachypnea, disorientation, agitation, delirium, convulsions, and lethargy. Coma is rare and usually occurs with massive or mixed overdoses.

Children usually present with an unintentional ingestion, and symptoms occur within a few hours of ingestion. Children less than 4 years of age typically present with metabolic acidosis, whereas older children and adults typically present with a mixed disturbance of respiratory alkalosis and increased anion gap metabolic acidosis. Sweating, dehydration, tachypnea, and fever are often attributed to the underlying illness for which the patient is taking aspirin or aspirin-containing products, and not correctly attributed to salicylate toxicity. The clinical presentation of salicylate toxicity may be indistinguishable from septic shock with multiple organ failure, encephalopathy, and acute respiratory distress syndrome.

Adult and adolescent salicylate toxicity typically occurs after an intentional overdose and often mixed with substances such as CNS depressants, which impair hyperpneic response. This produces a respiratory acidosis rather than the expected respiratory alkalosis. Salicylate and acetaminophen levels must be obtained for all intentional overdoses.

CHRONIC ASPIRIN TOXICITY

Chronic toxicity occurs most commonly in the elderly, with symptoms that overlap with those of acute ingestion. However, symptoms of chronic toxicity are typically milder at the time of presentation and have a more gradual onset. These patients are more difficult to diagnose and often have a worse prognosis.[37]

Diagnosis and Treatment of Salicylate Toxicity

The differential diagnosis of salicylate toxicity in all age groups includes infection, sepsis, diabetic ketoacidosis, and other causes of increased anion gap metabolic acidosis.

If potential salicylate toxicity is suspected in an asymptomatic patient, a urine ferric chloride test should be obtained. Do not rely on a serum salicylate level unless it is obtained at least 6 hours post-ingestion. Chronic toxicity and sustained release tablets may cause problems in interpreting serum levels. The salicylate level is repeated in 1 hour to obtain a trend, and at intervals of every 2 to 4 hours based on the patient's clinical condition until the serum salicylate level is ≤ 15 mg/dL.

If the patient is symptomatic, vital signs and mental status should be monitored and the following laboratory studies obtained: serum salicylate level, electrolytes, and arterial blood gases. The serum salicylate level should be repeated in 1 hour and every 2 to 4 hours thereafter as clinically indicated. If the patient requires intubation, the same degree of hyperventilation needed prior to intubation should be maintained, since failure to do so may cause rapid deterioration of the patient.[38] Failure to hyperventilate the patient causes respiratory acidosis and the rapid shift of salicylate into the CNS.

Supportive care includes hydration at 1.5 to 2 times maintenance to compensate for dehydration and fluid losses brought on by salicylates. Glucose must be monitored closely and should be administered in all cases of altered mental status, even if there is peripheral euglycemia. CNS hypoglycemia can occur despite peripheral euglycemia.[39] Gastric decontamination with multiple doses of activated charcoal should be used to prevent further salicylate absorption in doses of 1 to 2 g/kg without sorbitol. Although there is no true antidote for salicylate toxicity, alkalinization therapy is crucial. Alkalinizing the blood and urine traps salicylate (a weak acid) in the blood, preventing CNS toxicity. Alkalinization also increases urinary excretion of the salicylate ion. The recommended dosage of $NaHCO_3$ is 1 to 2 mEq/kg as an IV bolus followed by an infusion of 3 ampules of $NaCHO_3$ (containing 44 mEq $NaHCO_3$ each) in 1 L of dextrose 5% in water at 1.5 to 2 times maintenance. (The bolus of $NaHCO_3$ can be omitted if blood pH is > 7.45.) This fluid may replace the hydration fluid discussed previously. Alkalinization is successful when the blood pH is 7.45 to 7.55 and the urine pH is greater than 7. Potassium should be monitored and supplemented prophylactically since the increasing pH causes intracellular shifting of potassium and may cause hypokalemia, which will limit urinary alkalinization.[36,40] Acetazolamide and other carbonic anhydrase inhibitors are dangerous and should not be used since they achieve urinary alkalinization at the expense of blood acidification, which promotes salicylate movement into the CNS.[41,42] Hemodialysis is indicated in acute overdoses when the salicylate level is 100 mg/dl or rapidly approaching such levels. It is also indicated if acidosis is refractory to alkalinization, CNS symptoms are already present, there is progressive deterioration despite appropriate treatment, there are signs of pulmonary edema, or the patient has severe cardiac disease or renal failure. In chronic overdoses, hemodialysis should be considered if the salicylate level is greater than 30 mg/dl and the patient is symptomatic.

Selected Comments on Other Pharmaceuticals

Chloroquine and *quinine* are antimalarial medications. Toxic symptoms include immediate epigastric discomfort, nausea, vomiting, and diarrhea followed by CNS stimulation or seizures.

Imidazoline products are sympathetic amines present in ocular drops and nasal sprays. Toxicity occurs rapidly with CNS stimulation and/or depression and either hypertension and tachycardia or hypotension and bradycardia. Naloxone is indicated for altered sensorium, atropine or isoproterenol for bradycardia, and dopamine for hypotension refractory to fluid administration.

Theophylline, once a mainstay of asthma therapy, is a xanthine producing GI manifestations, generalized major motor seizures, tachydysrhythmias, hypotension, hypokalemia, hyperglycemia, and acidosis. Whole bowel irrigation alone or whole bowel irrigation combined with activated charcoal will greatly enhance elimination. Seizures may occur and should be managed with standard protocols.

Acetonitrile is an artificial nail removing compound that causes cyanide toxicity. Gastrointestinal manifestations herald the onset of CNS alterations and the cardiac manifestations of cyanide. Utilization of the cyanide antidote kit is indicated.

Camphor is contained in over-the-counter liniments. Patients present with GI disturbances followed by CNS excitation and seizures.

Hydrocarbons are common ingredients in household cleaning products, solvents, and gasoline. Emesis and lavage are contraindicated. Patients may present with transient CNS or GI disturbances followed by bronchospasm, seizures, or dysrhythmias.

Summary

The details of individual toxic ingestions can vary considerably, and the guidelines and therapies may change over time. Therefore, calling a regional Poison Control Center (1-800-222-1222) for consultation should always be considered.

REFERENCES

*1. Watson WA, Lovitz TL, Rodgers GC Jr, et al: 2002 Annual Report of the American Association of Poison Control Centers Toxic Exposure Surveillance System. Am J Emerg Med 21:353–421, 2003.
*2. Litovitz TL, Klein-Schwartz W, Rodgers GC Jr, et al: 2001 Annual Report of the American Association of Poison Control Centers Toxic Exposure Surveillance System. Am J Emerg Med 20:391–452, 2002.
*3. Koren G: Medications which can kill a toddler with a tablet or teaspoonful. J Toxicol Clin Toxicol 31:407–412, 1993.
4. Emery D: Highly toxic ingestions for toddlers: when a pill can kill. Pediatr Emerg Med Rep 3:111–122, 1998.
5. Brater DC: Clinical pharmacology of NSAIDs. J Clin Pharmacol 28:518–523, 1988.
6. Hawkey CJ: COX-2 inhibitors. Lancet 353:307–314, 1999.
7. Vale JA, Meredith TJ: Acute poisoning due to non-steroidal anti-inflammatory drugs: clinical features and management. Med Toxicol 1:12–31, 1986.
8. Harrigan RA, Nathan MS, Beattie P: Oral agents for the treatment of type 2 diabetes mellitus: pharmacology, toxicity, and treatment. Ann Emerg Med 38:68–78, 2001.
*9. Quadrani DA, Spiller HA, Widder P: Five year retrospective evaluations of sulfonylurea ingestion in children. J Toxicol Clin Toxicol 34:267–270, 1996.
10. Spiller HA, Villalobos D, Krenzelok EP, et al: Prospective multicenter study of sulfonylurea ingestion in children. J Pediatr 131:141–146, 1997.
11. Burkhart KK: When does hypoglycemia develop after sulfonyurea ingestion? Ann Emerg Med 31:771–772, 1998.
12. Bailey CJ, Turner RC: Metformin. N Engl J Med 334:574–579, 1996.
13. McLaughlin SA, Crandall CS, McKinney PE: Octreotide: an antidote for sulfonylurea-induced hypoglycemia. Ann Emerg Med 36:133–138, 2000.

———————
*Suggested readings.

14. Curry S: Methemoglobinemia. Ann Emerg Med 11:214–221, 1982.

15. Kulick RM: Pulse oximetry. Pediatr Emerg Care 3:127–130, 1987.

16. Yano SS, Danish EH, Hsia YE: Transient methemoglobinemia with acidosis in infants. J Pediatrics 100:415–418, 1982.

17. Mills KC, Curry SC: Acute iron poisoning. Emerg Med Clin North Am 12:397–413, 1994.

18. Penna A, Buchanan N: Paracetamol poisoning in children and hepatotoxicity. Br J Clin Pharmacol 32:143–149, 1991.

*19. Sztajnkrycer M, Bond G: Chronic acetaminophen overdosing in children: risk assessment and management. Curr Opin Pediatr 13:177–182, 2001.

20. Brackett C, Bloch J: Phenytoin as a possible cause of acetaminophen hepatotoxicity: case report and review of the literature. Pharmacotherapy 20:229, 2000.

21. Bray G, Harrison P, O'Grady J, et al: Long-term anticonvulsant therapy worsens outcome in paracetamol-induced fulminant hepatic failure. Hum Exp Toxicol 11:265, 1992.

*22. American Academy of Pediatrics, Committee on Drugs: Acetaminophen toxicity in children. Pediatrics 108:1020–1024, 2001.

23. Ashbourne J, Olson K, Khayam-Bashi H: Value of rapid screening for acetaminophen in all patients with intentional overdose. Ann Emerg Med 18:1035, 1989.

24. Bizovi K, Smilkstein M: Acetaminophen. In Goldfrank L, Flomenbaum N, Lewin N, et al (eds): Goldfrank's Toxicologic Emergencies, 7th ed. New York: McGraw-Hill, 2002, pp 480–501.

25. Roth B, Woo O, Blanc P: Early metabolic acidosis and coma after acetaminophen ingestion. Ann Emerg Med 33:452–456, 1999.

26. Spiller H, Krenzelok E, Grande G, et al: A prospective evaluation of the effect of activated charcoal before the oral N-acetylcysteine in acetaminophen overdose. Ann Emerg Med 23:519, 1994.

27. Smilkstein M, Knapp G, Kulig K, Rumack B: Efficacy of oral N-acetylcysteine in the treatment of acetaminophen overdose. N Engl J Med 319:1557–1562, 1988.

28. Bizovi K, Aks S, Paloucek F, et al: Late increase in acetaminophen concentration after overdose of Tylenol Extended Relief. Ann Emerg Med 28:549–551, 1996.

29. Sztajnkrycer M, Bond G: Chronic acetaminophen overdosing in children: risk assessment and management. Curr Opin Pediatr 13:177–182, 2001.

30. O'Grady J, Alexander G, Hayllar K, Williams R: Early indicators of prognosis in fulminant hepatic failure. Gastroenterology 97:439–445, 1989.

31. Linden C, Rumack B: Acetaminophen overdose. Emerg Clin North Am 2:103–119, 1984.

32. Tucker JR: Late-presenting acute acetaminophen toxicity and the role of N-acetylcysteine. Pediatr Emerg Care 14:424–426, 1998.

33. Bailey B, McGuigan M: Management of anaphylactoid reactions to intravenous N-acetylcysteine. Ann Emerg Med 31:710–715, 1998.

34. Sung L, Simons J, Dayneka N: Dilution of intravenous N-acetylcysteine as a cause of hyponatremia. Pediatrics 100:389–391, 1997.

35. Chan TY: Medicated oils and severe salicylate poisoning: quantifying the risk based on methyl salicylate content and bottle size. Vet Hum Toxicol 38:133–134, 1996.

36. Flomenbaum N: Salicylates. In Goldfrank L, Flomenbaum N, Lewin N, et al (eds): Goldfrank's Toxicologic Emergencies, 7th ed. New York: McGraw-Hill, 2002, pp 507–518.

37. Anderson R, Potts D, Gabow P, et al: Unrecognized adult salicylate intoxication. Ann Intern Med 85:745–748, 1976.

38. Gabow P, Anderson R, Potts D, Schrier R: Acid-base disturbances in the salicylate-intoxicated adult. Arch Intern Med 138:1481–1484, 1978.

39. Thurston J, Pollock P, Warren S, Jones E: Reduced brain glucose with normal plasma glucose in salicylate poisoning. J Clin Invest 49:2139–2145, 1970.

40. Goldberg M, Barlow C, Roth L: The effects of carbon dioxide on the entry and accumulation of drugs in the central nervous system. J Pharmacol Exp Ther 131:308–318, 1961.

41. Hill JB: Experimental salicylate poisoning: observations on the effects of altering blood pH on tissue and plasma salicylate concentrations. Pediatrics 47:658–665, 1971.

42. Kaplan S, del Carmen F: Experimental salicylate poisoning: observations on the effects of carbonic anhydrase inhibitor and bicarbonate. Pediatrics 21:762–770, 1958.

Chapter 134

Toxic Alcohols

Kevin C. Osterhoudt, MD, MSCE

Key Points

Ethanol intoxication may cause hypoglycemia in young children.

Isopropyl alcohol poisoning does not typically cause acidosis, but may cause profound central nervous system depression.

Methanol poisoning causes metabolic acidosis and may lead to blindness, encephalopathy, and/or multisystem organ failure.

Ethylene glycol poisoning causes metabolic acidosis and may lead to renal failure and/or multisystem organ failure.

Ethanol or fomepizole, both of which inhibit alcohol dehydrogenase, are important emergency antidotes for methanol or ethylene glycol poisoning.

Selected Diagnoses

Ethanol intoxication
Isopropanol poisoning
Methanol poisoning
Ethylene glycol poisoning

Discussion of Individual Diagnoses

Ethanol Intoxication

Ethanol is nearly ubiquitous in American homes as a constituent of beverages, mouthwashes, and cleaning products. In 2003, over 19,000 pediatric ethanol exposure cases were reported to the American Association of Poison Control Centers (AAPCC).[1] Of note, these statistics do not represent the formidable health hazards associated with driving while intoxicated, or other risk behaviors associated with inebriation and impaired decision making.

An ethanol dose of 0.7 g/kg produces a blood alcohol concentration of approximately 0.1 g/dl (100 mg/dl). This equates to ingestion of 17.5 ml (slightly more than one tablespoon) of 80-proof vodka by a 10-kg toddler. Ethanol is a central nervous system (CNS) depressant. Intoxication initially manifests through loss of inhibition, incoordination, slurred speech, and stupor. The examiner may note flushing of the face, dysarthria, and/or nystagmus. As blood ethanol levels approach 0.3 g/dl, coma, inhibition of airway-protective reflexes, and respiratory depression ensue. Aspiration pneumonia is a frequent complication, as is gastritis.

Hepatic alcohol dehydrogenase is the primary metabolic pathway for ethanol; dependent upon differences in individual enzyme phenotypes and ethanol tolerance, ethanol may be metabolized at a rate of 10 to 30 mg/dl/hr.[2] The enzymatic activity of alcohol dehydrogenase requires the cofactor nicotinamide adenine dinucleotide, oxidized (NAD+), and the consumption of this cofactor inhibits gluconeogenesis. As a result, young children, with reduced glycogen stores, are at risk for profound hypoglycemia.[3] This most often presents with CNS depression in the morning hours after the overnight fast.

Ethanol intoxication may be suspected based upon clinical history, physical examination findings, hypoglycemia, or an elevated osmolal gap (Table 134-1). It can be confirmed by measurement of the blood alcohol concentration.

Careful attention to the patient's airway, breathing, and circulation will be sufficient treatment for most cases of ethanol intoxication. There is no evidence to support a correlation between the Glasgow Coma Scale score and a need for endotracheal intubation after alcohol poisoning, so individual risks and benefits should be considered. Rapid bedside blood glucose concentration should be performed on any obtunded patient, and hypoglycemia should be treated as indicated (see Chapter 106, Hypoglycemia). Due to the diuretic nature of ethanol, hypovolemia may warrant intravenous fluid administration. Hemodialysis effectively eliminates ethanol from the bloodstream, and may be considered in severe cases of ethanol-induced coma and respiratory depression, but is rarely indicated. The possibility of concomitant traumatic injury, or co-ingestion, should be considered in any intoxicated adolescent. Alcohol withdrawal seizures and delirium tremens are rare among pediatric patients, but may complicate hospitalization of chronic high-level alcohol-abusing teens. A pattern of chronic alcohol abuse would warrant activation of social services.

Isopropanol Poisoning

Isopropyl alcohol, also known as "rubbing alcohol," is a widely used solvent and is commonly found within the home

Table 134–1	Estimation of Alcohol and Glycol Levels from the Osmolal Gap*	
Toxic Alcohol		**Conversion Factor**
Methanol		3.2
Ethanol		4.6
Isopropanol		6.0
Ethylene glycol		6.2

*[Osmolal gap (mOsm/L) × conversion factor] estimates alcohol concentration (mg/dl).
Osmolal gap = measured − calculated osmolality.
Calculated osmolality = 2[Na (mEq/L)] + [glucose (mg/dl)]/18 + [BUN (mg/dl)]/2.8.

Table 134–2	Antidotal Therapy for Methanol Poisoning

Alcohol Dehydrogenase Inhibition
Ethanol (10% ethanol in D5W IV or 40% ethanol by NG)
• 600 mg/kg load, then
• 100 mg/kg/hr infusion*
Or
Fomepizole
• 15 mg/kg IV load, then
• 10 mg/kg IV q12h × 4 doses, then 15 mg/kg q12h†
Folate
• 1 mg/kg (max: 50mg) IV q4h

*Titrate ethanol infusion to achieve blood ethanol concentration of 100 mg/dl. During hemodialysis, the infusion rate may need to be doubled (or ethanol may be added to dialysate).
†During hemodialysis, fomepizole should be dosed every 4 hours.
Abbreviations: D5W, dextrose 5% in water; IV, intravenously; NG, nasogastric tube.

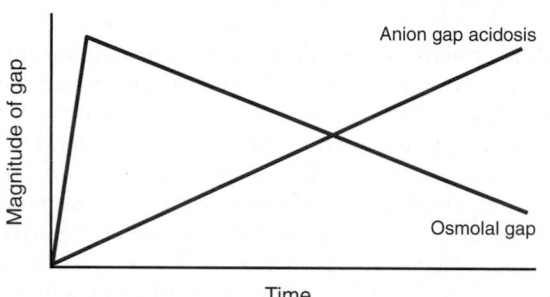

FIGURE 134–1. Relationship of osmolal gap to anion gap acidosis.

as the cooling ingredient among topical liniments. Over 12,000 isopropanol exposures among children up to 19 years of age were reported to the AAPCC in 2003.[1] Isopropyl alcohol toxicity may occur via the dermal and inhalation routes, such as may result during misguided sponge baths for fever.

Isopropanol is twice as potent as ethanol in terms of CNS depression. Altered mental status, when it occurs, typically manifests within 2 hours of ingestion.[4] Hypotension may occur due to diuresis, peripheral vasodilation, and myocardial depression. In addition to an osmolal gap (see Table 134–1), ketonemia or ketonuria may occur. Isopropyl alcohol is metabolized to acetone by alcohol dehydrogenase without the production of significant metabolic acidosis but may lead to hypoglycemia in young children, as was described for ethanol. Gastritis is common after ingestion. Patient care is supportive. The risks and benefits of hemodialysis may be considered for comatose patients with blood isopropanol levels exceeding 500 mg/dl.

Methanol Poisoning

Methanol poisoning may result from the ingestion of windshield washer fluid, gasoline additives, duplicating fluids, canned cooking fuels, and a variety of other products found in the home and workplace. Over 1000 pediatric exposures were reported to the AAPCC in 2003.[1]

Ingestion of greater than 100 mg/kg of methanol should be deemed potentially toxic. Therefore, even a single swallow of windshield washer fluid, with 40% methanol, is to be considered dangerous. Methanol is less inebriating than ethanol or ethylene glycol, so patients may appear well shortly after ingestion. As methanol is osmotically active, an increased osmolal gap is sometimes evident on initial laboratory testing (see Table 134–1), but disappears as methanol is metabolized (Fig. 134–1). The presence of an increased osmolal gap has good positive predictive value, but the absence of an osmolal gap is not sensitive enough to screen for methanol poisoning.[5] Blood methanol levels greater than 50 mg/dl, obtained soon after ingestion, should be regarded with concern.[6] Unfortunately, blood methanol levels are not available on an immediate basis in many emergency departments, mandating that clinical decisions be based on a combination of history, examination, and laboratory factors.

Gastritis and/or pancreatitis sometimes occur after acute ingestion of methanol. Methanol is slowly metabolized by alcohol dehydrogenase into formaldehyde, which is further metabolized to formic acid. Hypoglycemia may occur as was described for ethanol. After several hours, profound metabolic acidosis, with a wide anion gap (see Chapter 111, Metabolic Acidosis), is common. Clinical evidence of toxicity may be further delayed if ethanol has also been ingested. Formic acid is directly toxic to the retina, and may lead to blindness.[7] Patients may describe the initial visual disturbance as being akin to "standing in a snowfield." Funduscopic examination may reveal a hyperemic optic disc and venous engorgement. Severe poisoning may progress to seizures, coma, and possibly persistent encephalopathy.

Emergency management of methanol poisoning should first focus upon support of airway patency, breathing, circulation, and glycemic control. Endotracheal intubation, if performed, should be accompanied by mechanical ventilation to match the patient's physiologic hyperventilation to prevent worsening acidemia. Intravenous fluids should be administered to reverse hypovolemia, and sodium bicarbonate is a useful adjunct in the face of metabolic acidosis[6] (and may reduce the penetration of formic acid through the blood-brain barrier). Specific antidotal therapies for methanol poisoning are summarized in Table 134–2. Fomepizole, as an alcohol dehydrogenase inhibitor, may be easier to use than ethanol therapy as it is not inebriating, does not cause hypoglycemia, and does not require a continuous infusion.[8] However, fomepizole is more expensive than ethanol, and its use in pediatrics is off-label. Alcohol dehydrogenase inhibition should be continued until all metabolic acidosis is corrected and the blood methanol level falls below 20 mg/dl. The

Table 134–3	Relative Indications for Hemodialysis after Methanol or Ethylene Glycol Poisoning

Methanol or ethylene glycol level >50 mg/dl PLUS one or more of the following:
- Visual disturbance or renal failure
- Acidemia not corrected with bicarbonate therapy
- Coma
- Difficulty maintaining adequate alcohol dehydrogenase inhibition
- Long elimination half-life, which portends prolonged, intensive hospitalization

Table 134–4	Antidotal Therapy for Ethylene Glycol Poisoning

Alcohol Dehydrogenase Inhibition
- As described in Table 134–2 for methanol

Thiamine
- 50 mg IV/IM q6h

Pyridoxine
- 50 mg IV/IM q6h

Abbreviations: IM, intramuscularly; IV, intravenously.

relative indications for hemodialysis are listed in Table 134–3.

Ethylene Glycol Poisoning

Ethylene glycol is a sweet-tasting common constituent of automobile antifreeze, and the similarly toxic diethylene glycol is commonly used as a glycerin substitute in commercial products. Sporadic epidemics of diethylene glycol–tainted medications and beverages still occur. Over 1400 pediatric ethylene glycol exposures were reported to poison control centers in 2003.[1]

Ethylene glycol is inebriating, and ingestion may first manifest with vomiting, somnolence, nystagmus, and/or incoordination. As described for methanol, ethylene glycol in the bloodstream may produce an osmolal gap (see Table 134–1), but metabolism to glycolic and oxalic acids by alcohol dehydrogenase leads to metabolic acidosis as the osmolal gap recedes (see Fig. 134–1). Calcium oxalate crystals in the urine and urine fluorescence under Wood's lamp illumination (due to fluorscein added to some commercial antifreezes) have been advocated as screens for ethylene glycol poisoning; but neither is sensitive or specific enough to be recommended clinically.[9,10] Hypocalcemia may be noted after severe poisoning due to calcium and oxalic acid complex formation. Hypoglycemia, dehydration, and pancreatitis are common complications. However, metabolic acidosis, encephalopathy, and especially renal failure are complications of ethylene glycol poisoning. Blood ethylene glycol levels greater than 50 mg/dl should warrant concern.

The principles of management of ethylene glycol poisoning are similar to those presented for methanol. Appropriate ventilation must be maintained to compensate for metabolic acidosis, intravenous fluid hydration is commonly warranted, and blood glucose, renal function, and clinical manifestations of hypocalcemia must be closely monitored. Sodium bicarbonate can be useful to alleviate metabolic acidosis. Specific antidotal therapy for ethylene glycol poisoning is presented in Table 134–4, and alcohol dehydrogenase inhibition should be continued until the blood ethylene glycol concentration is below 20 mg/dl and acidosis is resolved. The indications for hemodialysis are presented in Table 134–3.

REFERENCES

*1. Watson WA, Litovitz TL, Klein-Schwartz W, et al: 2003 Annual report of the American Association of Poison Control Centers Toxic Exposure Surveillance System. Am J Emerg Med 22:335–404, 2004.
*2. Brennan DF, Betzelos S, Reed R, Falk JL: Ethanol elimination rates in an ED population. Am J Emerg Med 13:276–280, 1995.
3. Marks V, Teale JD: Drug-induced hypoglycemia. Endocrinol Metab Clin North Am 28:555–577, 1999.
4. Stremski E, Hennes H: Accidental isopropanol ingestion in children. Pediatr Emerg Care 16:238–240, 2000.
5. Hoffman RS, Smilkstein MJ, Howland MA, Golfrank LR: Osmol gaps revisited: normal values and limitations. J Toxicol Clin Toxicol 31:81–93, 1993.
*6. Barceloux DG, Bond GR, Krenzelok EP, et al: American Academy of Clinical Toxicology practice guidelines on the treatment of methanol poisoning. J Toxicol Clin Toxicol 40:415–446, 2002.
7. Treichel JL, Murray TG, Lewandowski MF, et al: Retinal toxicity in methanol poisoning. Retina 24:309–312, 2004.
8. Brent J, McMartin K, Phillips S, et al: Fomepizole for the treatment of methanol poisoning. N Engl J Med 344:424–429, 2001.
9. Jacobsen D, Akesson I, Shefter E: Urinary calcium oxalate monohydrate crystals in ethylene glycol poisoning. Scand J Clin Lab Invest 42:231–234, 1982.
10. Casavant MJ, Shah MN, Battels R: Does fluorescent urine indicate antifreeze ingestion by children? Pediatrics 107:113–114, 2001.

*Suggested readings.

Chapter 135

Drugs of Abuse

John A. Tilelli, MD

Key Points

One should always treat the patient, not the poison. Supportive care is the first priority in the setting of drug abuse.

Drug abuse histories are unreliable and laboratory testing is only minimally helpful.

Polydrug ingestion is common in the setting of drug abuse.

Drug diluents and vehicles may be more toxic than the ingested drug.

Introduction and General Principles

Patterns of Abuse

Drug abuse is largely a phenomenon of the young. Drug experimentation and use achieves significant proportions by adolescence and peaks in the early 20s.[1] By age 30, the rate of use of and addiction to all substances of abuse declines, and continues to do so throughout adulthood.

It is clear that specific socioeconomic status correlates exist among all drugs of abuse, and that certain drugs are more prevalent in one age population as opposed to another.[2] Inhalant abuse, for example, begins to appear at age 10, peaks by age 14, and declines thereafter. Tobacco use appears at age 10 and increases throughout adolescence. Alcohol, marijuana, amphetamine, cocaine, and hallucinogen use follow a similar pattern. Age-related incidences of each class of drug may reflect drug availability, perception of safety, financial independence, peer interactions, or parental control of children and permissiveness.

General Approach to the Intoxicated Patient

The intoxicated patient generally presents with acute symptoms that may at first suggest an illness unrelated to intoxication. The agitated, hyperthermic patient might be considered to have encephalitis or meningitis. Focal neurologic symptoms secondary to stroke might be suggestive of a clotting disorder or embolic event. Similarly, seizures, loss of consciousness, ataxia, peripheral neuropathy, tremor, weakness,

acute psychosis, chest pain, palpitations, and respiratory distress have extensive differential diagnoses of diseases unrelated to poisoning. Similarly, many common complaints have toxic diagnoses. A brief, and by no means comprehensive, list of drugs of abuse associated with common complaints is provided in Table 135–1.

Finally, the patient experiencing withdrawal from a substance of abuse may present with a confusing array of symptoms that may mimic another intoxication. Withdrawal toxidromes are discussed later.

Detection of Drugs of Abuse

All laboratory tests have intrinsic sensitivity and specificity, as well as timeliness and cost-effectiveness constraints. Testing for drugs of abuse is no exception. Compared to the number of potential intoxicants comprising the drugs of abuse, few analytic techniques of value are available. Definitive assays are often time consuming and unavailable on an emergency basis. Screening techniques are often insensitive to intoxicants at clinically significant concentrations, and may be masked by or detected as a cross-reacting substance present in the sample.

Commonly tested substrates for substances of abuse include blood, urine, and gastric aspirate. The latter should be inspected, as gastric contents may contain pill fragments suggestive of a particular intoxicant. Although medical management issues should take priority, it should be recalled that a crime might have been committed. Specimen collection should be done, if appropriate, in a manner that will make the laboratory assays useful in subsequent legal proceedings, by preservation of the chain of custody, retention of the specimen, and processing. Frequently, forensic specimens, when obtained, are separated from those destined for clinical use, and are handled by law enforcement officers present. The emergency department should have policies in place for the collection of specimens compliant with the National Institute on Drug Abuse Guidelines.[3,4]

The commonly available drug assays rely upon either immunologic or chromatographic techniques to determine the presence of a drug or its metabolite. Other techniques rely upon specific physical-chemical properties of the compound, such as atomic absorption spectra. The sensitivity and specificity of both techniques are method specific.[5]

Serum testing is available for barbiturates and ethanol, but most of the commonly tested substances are assayed in urine. Table 135–2 summarizes the tests commonly provided by hospital laboratory services on site. Notably absent from this list, or missed by assay techniques, are lysergic acid diethylamide (LSD) and the other hallucinogens, methylenedioxymethamphetamine (MDMA) and other substituted amphetamines, toxic inhalants, nitrates and nitrites, γ-hydroxybutyrate (GHB), anabolic steroids, and the botanical agents (except Ma Huang).

Laboratory techniques, then, can be incorrect, misleading, or irrelevant. Not uncommonly, the intoxicated patient may have another substance present more toxic than the compound detected in testing. The caveat is, therefore, that one should *always treat the patient, not the poison.* A positive laboratory test should not deter the clinician from considering an alternative etiology to the substance detected in screening, nor persuade the clinician that another cannot be present. In the emergency setting, managing the patient in accordance with the symptoms is less fraught with risk than an approach reliant upon analytic techniques.

Withdrawal

Many of the drugs of abuse are associated with some form of tolerance and dependence. Irrespective of the agent, *tolerance* is caused by pharmacologic or pharmacodynamic alterations

Table 135–1	Drugs of Abuse Associated with Common Complaints
If the Patient Demonstrates	**Consider**
Depressed LOC, somnolence	Narcotics, sedative-hypnotics, toxic inhalants, GHB, ketamine, nitrous oxide, amphetamine withdrawal
Delirium, agitation	Phencyclidine, amphetamines, MDMA, cocaine
Hypertension, stroke, chest pain	Cocaine, phencyclidine, amphetamine, MDMA
Hyperpyrexia	Cocaine, phencyclidine, amphetamine, LSD, anticholinergics, narcotic and sedative withdrawal
Hallucinations	LSD, MDMA, other organic hallucinogens
Cyanosis/priapism	Nitrates

Abbreviations: GHB, γ-hydroxybutyrate; LOC, level of consciousness; LSD, lysergic acid diethylamide; MDMA, methylenedioxymethamphetamine.

necessitating increasing the dose of a drug to achieve an equivalent desired effect. *Withdrawal* is a constellation of symptoms that appear after a period of drug abstinence and represent a displacement of homeostasis that occurs when a drug is administered. The two processes are linked, and, generally speaking, one occurs in the context of the other.

Both stimulant and depressant drugs are associated with symptomatic withdrawal. Like drugs tend to produce similar symptoms in abstinence. Withdrawal from both narcotics and sedative-hypnotic drugs is associated with restlessness, hypertension, and tachycardia (see Table 135–3 for their similarities and differences).

Considerable overlap exists between the two presentations, but the presence of seizures, hyperpyrexia, and agitated delirium strongly suggest sedative withdrawal. Sedative-hypnotic withdrawal and alcohol withdrawal seem to be similarly mediated, by down-regulation of the central nervous system inhibitory transmitter γ-aminobutyric acid (GABA). Alcohol withdrawal presents also with tremor, diaphoresis, irritability, restlessness, nausea, vomiting, hallucinations, insomnia, and agitation, but hyperpyrexia and hypertension are uncommon.[6] Hallucinations associated with alcohol withdrawal may be the consequence of depleted thiamine stores.[7] Symptoms of alcohol withdrawal seem to be related to the intensity of drinking and duration, and the age of onset of problem drinking behavior. Alcoholics who began drinking before age 20 were more likely to experience symptomatic withdrawal upon cessation than older drinkers, notwithstanding a substantial difference in duration of the behavior.[8] Delirium tremens has been reported in a child who was 10 years old and had a history of alcohol consumption for 3 years.[9] There is a strong similarity between the alcohol abstinence syndrome and that of benzodiazepines, barbiturates, hydrocarbon inhalants, and GABA. It is strongly suggested that therapeutic effects as well as symptoms of withdrawal are mediated by GABA.[10] A strategy for therapy, then, would include, in addition to basic stabilization measures, augmentation of GABA with either a benzodiazepine or barbiturate. There are no studies comparing one approach to the other; both have been reported effective.[11] A recent double-blind, controlled study comparing the use of the benzodiazepine antagonist flumazenil to oxazepam in the treatment of symptomatic withdrawal found that flumazenil does not precipitate withdrawal in tolerant subjects, and is effective at modulating symptoms.[12]

Table 135–2	Commonly Used Screening Tests for Drugs of Abuse		
Drug or Class	**Sensitivity**	**Cross-Reacting Substance**	**Misses**
Cannabinoids	Good	None	
Opioids	Fair	Dextromethorphan*	Dextromethorphan,* all synthetic narcotics, notably fentanyl
Phencyclidine	Fair	Dextromethorphan	PCP congeners
Cocaine	Good	None	
Benzodiazepines	Fair	None	Many congeners unrelated to oxazepam† (especially flunitrazepam)
Barbiturates	Good	None	None
Amphetamine	Poor	Pseudoephedrine, ephedrine‡	MDMA and congeners

*Dextromethorphan may (when detected) be from a cough suppressant and confused for an abused drug. On the other hand, many assays are of insufficient sensitivity to detect dextromethorphan, which also may confound PCP assays.
†Benzodiazepines detected by urinary screens include chlordiazepoxide, oxazepam, diazepam, temazepam.
‡Over-the-counter decongestants are most commonly confused with abused amphetamines.
Abbreviations: MDMA, methylenedioxymethamphetamine; PCP, phencyclidine.

Table 135–3	Manifestations of Narcotic versus Sedative-Hypnotic Withdrawal	
	Narcotics	**Sedative-Hypnotics**
Blood pressure	Hypertension	Hypertension
Pulse	Tachycardia	Tachycardia
Respiratory rate	Elevated	Elevated
Temperature	NORMAL	ELEVATED
Mental status	Normal (or restless)	Restless, irritable, DISORIENTED
Miscellaneous	Piloerection	Tremor
	Nausea	SEIZURES
	Diarrhea	
	Myalgias	

Adapted from Hamilton RJ: Substance withdrawal. In Goldfrank LR, Flomenbum NE, Lewin NA, et al (ed): Goldfrank's Toxicologic Emergencies, 7th ed. New York: McGraw-Hill, 2002, pp 1059–1074.

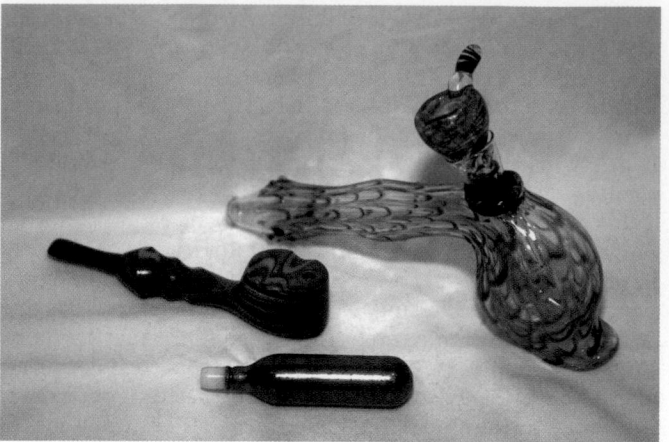

FIGURE 135–1. Drug paraphernalia. Pipes commonly used in the smoking of crack cocaine and hashish. Nitrous oxide whippet.

Opiate withdrawal differs from sedative-hypnotic withdrawal, as it is not commonly associated with seizures or hyperpyrexia, and psychosis is rarely seen. Opiate effects and withdrawal symptoms are mediated by specific receptor proteins in the brain and spinal cord that are down-regulated with the administration of an agonist drug. These receptors are closely linked central α_2 receptors that may be stimulated by the centrally acting agent clonidine. Symptoms of withdrawal, while uncomfortable, are rarely life threatening. A strategy of symptomatic relief from opiate withdrawal would consist of basic stabilization and the administration of a pure narcotic agonist or clonidine to modulate symptoms.[13-15] Rapid opiate withdrawal techniques use general anesthesia to subdue symptoms and accelerate the course of withdrawal.[16] It has been used successfully in a child.[17] Experience is too limited to make a general recommendation on the utility of this technique.

A syndrome of excessive somnolence, craving, depression, and lethargy has been identified with the discontinuation of amphetamines and hallucinogens. It has been identified in children after discontinuation of stimulant medications and in neonates exposed to amphetamines in utero.[18,19] While symptoms are not life threatening, drug craving may precipitate a relapse or exploration of the use of another drug. Recently bupropion has been used successfully to modulate the symptoms of amphetamine withdrawal.[20]

Selected Drugs of Abuse

Marijuana
Opioids
Sedative-hypnotics
    Barbiturates
    Benzodiazepines
Cocaine
Amphetamines
Lysergic acid diethylamide
"Club drugs"
    Ketamine and phencyclidine
    Flunitrazepam
    γ-Hydroxybutyrate
Inhalants
    Volatile nitrogen oxides

Miscellaneous agents
    Over-the-counter drugs
    Botanicals and natural products
    Anabolic steroids

Discussion of Individual Agents

Marijuana

Marijuana is the most commonly encountered drug of abuse among children and adolescents after tobacco and alcohol. As many as 20 million Americans may use this drug on a regular basis.

Marijuana is the popular term for the substances obtained from the plant *Cannabis sativa* that grows wild and is cultivated, both domestically and abroad, for recreational purposes. The principles of *Cannabis* horticulture are easily available on the Internet. As a consequence, availability is widespread and difficult to eradicate. All parts of the plant, including leaves and flowers, contain the active alkaloids known as cannabinoids. The most important of these is Δ9-tetrahydrocannabinol (THC), which is present in its highest concentration in the buds. The leaves are dried and ground into a mass resembling oregano or tobacco. The buds may be compressed into a fine powder or resin ("hashish" or "hash"), prized for its potency. Marijuana is conventionally smoked, but is effective orally. Hashish is smoked in small pipes resembling those used for crack cocaine abuse, while marijuana is rolled into cigarettes (Fig. 135–1). Occasionally, its use may be ritualized, inhaling the drug through an elaborate water pipe or "bong."

The subjective sense attendant to marijuana use is dose dependent, but also varies among individuals. The widespread belief is that naive users do not appreciate its effect as much as those who have prior extensive drug experience. The user generally describes a state of dreamy intoxication, in which sensory perception, especially to color and sound, seems enhanced. Increased appetite is commonly expressed. Conjunctival injection is commonly present. Judgment, especially that which is required for complex or subtle activities such as driving, is significantly impaired, a finding that may persist as long as 24 hours after use.[21] The concurrent use of ethanol with marijuana appears to impair judgment more than either drug alone. Acute psychosis and panic attacks are infrequent, but have been described. Pneumomediastinum and pneumothorax may occur as a consequence of the widespread practice of taking the drug by deep inhalation and retaining the breath to encourage absorption of the drug.

Chronic effects of marijuana include chronic lung disease and gynecomastia, caused by diminished testosterone levels associated with its use.[22] It may appear after relatively brief use.[23] There is debate over a relationship to psychiatric disease, cognitive impairment, or a chronic amotivational state attributed to its use, but unequivocal data are lacking.[24] Neuropsychiatric effects attributed to the chronic use of marijuana may be attendant to preexistent psychopathology. Marijuana is advocated for a variety of medical indications, including cachexia, glaucoma, and chemotherapy-induced nausea, none of which has been rigorously investigated.[25-29] Its legalization in various states has been the subject of great public debate.[30] The precise clinical role, if any, for marijuana in the medical center has not yet been well defined. Some analgesic potential for marijuana may exist, but its role in pain management is uncertain.

Severe intoxication due to marijuana use is rare. The patient who presents to the emergency department with complaints directly related to its use can be often managed by removal to a nonthreatening environment and emotional support. Occasionally an especially anxious or agitated patient may benefit from the administration of a benzodiazepine. Marijuana is frequently adulterated with other compounds of greater potency. The user may be unaware of the presence of excipients, added to alter or increase the effect of the drug. Among these are phencyclidine, LSD, amphetamines, anticholinergics, narcotics, and benzodiazepines. The presence of severe hypertension and tachycardia, mydriasis, miosis, frank hallucinations, hyperthermia, depressed level of consciousness, or respiratory depression should alert the caregiver to the possibility of an occult co-intoxicant.

Opioids

In the simplest terms, opioids (narcotics) are a class of drugs characterized by the production of analgesia, miosis, sedation, and respiratory depression; in overdose they are treated with supportive care. The term *narcotic*, however, is misleading, as these drugs produce analgesia better than sleep. The generic term *narcotic* is used to connote a group of drugs that alter the perception of pain, notwithstanding that many of these drugs bear no structural similarity. The drugs most commonly identified with the narcotics are the natural and semisynthetic alkaloids of the poppy that have been used throughout the ages for recreational and religious purposes. The natural poppy alkaloids are morphine, thebane, and papaverine. Alteration of the chemical structure was undertaken in an attempt to modulate the undesirable properties of the drug without altering analgesic strength. Heroin (diacetyl morphine) was the first such semisynthetic derivative. Codeine, dihydromorphone (Dilaudid), and oxycodone (OxyContin) are the three other semisynthetic derivatives of poppy alkaloids, the latter being a thujone derivative. Other commonly used narcotic analgesics, such as dextromethorphan, pentazocine, meperidine, fentanyl, methadone, and propoxyphene, are synthetic.

Opioids are absorbed by the oral, parenteral, and inhalational routes. Intravenous abuse of narcotics in the 1950s has given way to abuse by smoking or intranasal insufflation. Effects are noted shortly after administration, and peak 10 minutes after an intravenous dose and 30 minutes after administration by another route. Some addicts may introduce the drug by the subclavian vessels (a so-called "pocket shot") to increase the effect, a technique associated with air embolism, subclavian vessel thrombosis, and pulmonary thromboembolism.[31] Generally, however, an intravenous abuser will self-administer the drug until a subjective effect is perceived (the "flash"), and then stop. This practice may lead to fatal overdose if the drug is of unanticipated potency.[32,33]

Abused opioids are inevitably adulterated with extraneous substances, some of which have pharmacologic activity. Heroin is often diluted with quinine, manitol, lactose, talc, bicarbonate, acetaminophen, lidocaine, phenobarbital, methaqualone, caffeine, antihistamines, or phencyclidine.[34] The specific pattern of adulterants may be of forensic value in determining the source of the drug.[35] As a consequence, the original bag of drug, and any paraphernalia with the patient, should be saved with the protection of the chain of custody for later use by law enforcement. As these are nonsterile, they are often contaminated by biologic agents, including *Clostridium* species, *Bacillus,* and others.[36] Intravenous users typically prepare heroin for consumption by dissolving the drug in a spoon and heating it with a flame. It is then aspirated through a cotton ball into a syringe. The cotton is subsequently reused, causing "cotton fever,"[37] the etiology of which is obscure. Inhalation of heroin fumes is called "chasing the dragon."

Tolerance develops to all effects of narcotics except miosis. The central nervous system effects include tolerance to pain, suppression of anxiety, sedation, suppression of the cough reflex, and euphoria. The therapeutic index of narcotic agonists varies considerably depending on the relative potency of the drug and the experience of the user. Cross-tolerance is the rule, and resistance to one narcotic generally implies resistance to all others. In overdose, therapeutic symptoms are exaggerated. Pupils may become dilated in the presence of hypoxia or with overdose of meperidine, pentazocine, diphenoxylate/atropine (Lomotil), propoxyphene or nonnarcotic coingestants. Respiratory depression and hypoxia are generally the mechanism for death. Orthostatic hypotension and syncope may occur as a consequence of histamine release observed uniquely with morphine. Noncardiogenic pulmonary edema may occur, although rarely at therapeutic doses. Seizures rarely occur except uniquely after the abuse of pentazocine or propoxyphene. Similarly, meperidine has an active metabolite that is capable of causing seizures. The naturally occurring and semisynthetic opioids may be detected in the urine by a commonly available and rapid urinary immunofluorescent assay. Morphine, heroin, oxycodone, and codeine are all detected, but many assays are not of sufficient sensitivity to detect agents such as dextromethorphan, and drugs with unrelated structures, such as meperidine and fentanyl, are not detected at all.[38] Definitive drug testing and confirmation of positive drug screens may be accomplished by chromatographic techniques such as gas chromatography–mass spectrometry.

Basic stabilization is the mainstay of therapy. The presence of an adequate airway should be assured in all patients with a depressed level of consciousness and/or lack of airway-protective reflexes. Noncardiogenic pulmonary edema should be managed by the administration of oxygen and positive airway pressure. The use of narcotic antagonists is controversial, as they may precipitate withdrawal symptoms. They may have a role in the diagnostic assessment of the patient. Partial response may indicate the presence of another drug, such as a sedative-hypnotic, or hypoxia.

Naloxone, a pure opioid antagonist, reverses all effects of opiates, including analgesia, miosis, respiratory depression, and sedation. It is unknown if it protects against seizures encountered with some opiates such as propoxyphene, but appears to do so in animal models. It does not appear to reverse pulmonary edema. It has a half-life of 20 to 30 minutes. The initial dose is 0.01 mg/kg IV or SQ. Give a subsequent dose of 0.1 mg/kg if there is an inadequate response. Higher doses may be required for the reversal of some drugs such as propoxyphene and dextromethorphan. If the use of naloxone is undertaken, it should be remembered that the half-life of the abused substance may exceed that of the antagonist, and that continued observation of the patient, and possibly repeated or continuous administration, is indicated. Recently, a shortage of naloxone has been reported, mitigating against its prolonged use except in unusual circumstances. Nalmefene, a newer agent, has a half-life of 10.3 to 12.9 hours, and appears to be safe and potent.

Bowel decontamination of ingested drugs may be occasionally indicated. Polyethylene glycol catharsis may be useful for the removal of packets of drugs from body packers or body stuffers when bowel obstruction is not present. Gastrointestinal hypomotility may prolong the gastric retention of the ingested substance.

Some of the acute and chronic complications of narcotic abuse are listed in Table 135–4. Infectious complications are especially common among intravenous drug abusers. Infective endocarditis, hepatitis, human immunodeficiency virus (HIV) infection, and abscess formation are commonplace among them.[36-38] Patients may present with a complication attendant to their habit and symptoms only peripherally suggestive of an acute complication of narcotic abuse, with chronic illness acquired as the result of a high-risk behavior, or both. Malnutrition and accessory diseases unrelated to the intoxication, but related to the lifestyle of a drug-addicted individual (e.g., tuberculosis, sexually transmitted disease) are also common.

The general belief is that some tolerance occurs after both the therapeutic and nontherapeutic use of all narcotic agonists, usually after the administration of successively higher doses over several weeks. However, some tolerance begins after the first dose, especially with the more potent drugs, such as fentanyl. The course is similar for all opiates, with the time course compressed for the more potent and shorter acting drugs. The initial stage of withdrawal begins with drug craving and anxiety. Later, yawning, mydriasis, lacrimation, rhinorrhea, piloerection (from which is derived the term "*cold turkey*"), twitching, nausea, vomiting, diarrhea, and abdominal pain are observed. Dehydration, fever, hyperglycemia, and spontaneous erections may occur. Symptom intensity seems to correlate with the duration and dose of the abused drug. The administration of opioid agonists is effective in modulating the symptoms of withdrawal, and may be required in significant doses. Fear of enhancing the patient's

Table 135–4	**Complications of Narcotic Abuse**
Infection	
HIV	
Hepatitis B, C, and D	
Soft tissue infection	
Bacterial sepsis	
Cardiovascular	
Bacterial endocarditis	
Thrombophlebitis	
Pulmonary	
Pneumonia	
Aspiration	
Nontuberculous granulomas	
Dermatologic	
Abscess formation	
Cellulitis	
Neurologic	
Cerebral edema	
Transverse myelitis	
Seizures	
Polyneuritis	
Brain abscess	
Hepatic	
Cirrhosis	
Liver abscess	
Renal	
Nephritis	
Hematologic	
Thrombocytopenia	
Leukopenia	
Musculoskeletal	
Myositis ossificans	
Osteomyelitis	
Miscellaneous	
False-positive VDRL	

Abbreviations: HIV, human immunodeficiency virus; VDRL, Venereal Disease Research Laboratory (test).

addiction to a narcotic should not prevent the clinician from administering them to the individual with symptomatic withdrawal. Recently, centrally acting α_2 agonist drugs such as clonidine have been reported effective as well. The effects of clonidine and opiates, including respiratory depression and sedation, are additive. Sedative agents, such as the benzodiazepines, may assist in relieving the agitation and anxiety that accompany narcotic withdrawal, but do not reverse the autonomic effects.[14]

Sedative-Hypnotics

The first of the sedative-hypnotic drugs, the barbiturates, appeared in the early 20th century. The barbiturates, and associated drugs such as the benzodiazepines, whose principal manifestations are anxiolysis and sedation, have been widely used in medicine and as targets for illicit abuse. Between 1950 and 1970, they were the most common cause of drug-induced death. The replacement of barbiturates with drugs of wider therapeutic index, and a general trend of decline in illicit drug use of sedative-hypnotics, have significantly reduced mortality associated with these agents. Numerous agents unrelated to the barbiturates and benzodiazepines are used for their sedative properties. The clinical effects and unique toxicities of some of these agents are summarized here.

The barbiturates and benzodiazepines are used, often in combination with other drugs, to treat anxiety, pain, and sleep disorders. They also have important use in the acute and chronic treatment of seizure disorders, and are used as anesthetic agents.[39] Barbiturates all share a common nucleus, the modification of which alters its pharmacologic properties but not its effects, which are common to all drugs of this class. All barbiturates are absorbed well by the intestine. The rate of elimination among them varies considerably. The half-life of these agents depends on their lipophilicity, and thus volume of distribution. More lipophilic agents, such as thiopental, are classified as ultra-short acting, while longer acting drugs such as phenobarbital are more water soluble. Shorter acting agents are eliminated by hepatic metabolism. Only the longer acting barbiturates have substantial renal clearance. Toxic doses are generally seen at five times the therapeutic dose, and toxicity is an extension of the therapeutic effects.

Benzodiazepines are among the most commonly prescribed drugs. Over 3000 have been synthesized and over 50 are marketed worldwide. As a group, they account for the majority of toxic exposures to sedative-hypnotic agents. Like barbiturates, all drugs of this class share a common chemical nucleus, but unlike the barbiturates, each varies slightly in effects. Some, such as flunitrazepam and midazolam, are more commonly associated with amnesia and hallucinations than other benzodiazepines. They are metabolized in the liver. Many have active metabolites, the notable exception being lorazepam, which is metabolized to solely inactive compounds.

Both the barbiturates and benzodiazepines have sedative, hypnotic, amnestic, anxiolytic, and anticonvulsant properties.[40] Additionally, the benzodiazepines are muscle relaxants, and are often prescribed for that purpose. Although specific benzodiazepine and barbiturate receptors probably exist, both appear to exert their sedative and anticonvulsant effects by exerting an effect on the inhibitory neurotransmitter GABA.

The effects of sedative-hypnotic drugs are related to dose and prior drug experience. The onset and duration of symptoms depend on the type and amount of drug ingested.[39] While short-acting agents have an onset of symptoms 15 to 20 minutes after ingestion, the effects of longer acting agents may be delayed as much as 18 hours. The early stage of intoxication may resemble the effects of alcohol, a substance commonly co-ingested with sedative agents. Patients with mild intoxication may appear stuporous but responsive. More impaired patients become unresponsive, and eventually anemic, arreflexic, and hypotensive. Pupils generally demonstrate miosis in early coma, but are dilated later. Respiratory depression is common in symptomatic ingestion. Hypoglycemia and hypothermia are occasionally observed. Cardiovascular instability with hypotension and shock is more characteristic of barbiturate than benzodiazepine overdose, but the effects of both drugs are similar in type if not degree.[41]

Tolerance and dependence on sedative-hypnotics are well recognized.[42] An abstinence syndrome of restlessness, insomnia, irritability, agitation, seizures, tremors, tachycardia, and hypertension may be seen, its intensity and duration being dependent on the type and amount of the substance abused. Hyperpyrexia, uncommon in narcotic withdrawal, is observed in the sedative-hypnotic abstinence syndrome.[43]

The treatment of sedative-hypnotic overdose relies heavily on supportive measures. Protection of the airway and the support of respiration with adequate oxygenation is the cornerstone of management of the seriously intoxicated patient. Hypotension is mediated by vasodilation, and may be managed with the administration of volume expansion and vasopressor drugs such as dopamine and norepinephrine. Pure inotropic agents such as dobutamine and milrinone are rarely necessary except in the most severe circumstances, as many sedatives do not lend themselves to enhanced elimination. Phenobarbital, which has a smaller volume of distribution than many of the other agents, is the exception, and has been reported as being successfully treated with dialysis.[44] The effects of the benzodiazepines may be reversed by the specific antagonist flumazenil. It may provoke seizures and withdrawal symptoms in the patient who chronically uses a benzodiazepine either therapeutically or as a recreational drug,[45] or in the patient who has an underlying seizure diathesis.[46] A recent study concluded that flumazenil was not cost effective compared to supportive therapy, nor did it improve outcome.[47] It does not reverse the sedative effects of other drugs with similar manifestations such as the barbiturates. Its use in the acutely intoxicated patient may be of diagnostic benefit. Failure to respond may imply the presence of another substance, hypoxic encephalopathy, or the postictal state. Its half-life is shorter than that of many benzodiazepines, and repeated administration may be necessary. Flumazenil should not be considered a replacement for supportive therapy.

Barbiturates

Massive oral overdose of barbiturates is associated with bezoar formation, which may be observable on plain film or demonstrable by endoscopy. Drug removal may be hastened by lavage or endoscopic removal. The detection of barbiturates may be accomplished by either serum or urine screens. The presence of a therapeutically administered drug such as phenobarbital may obfuscate the presence of another barbiturate. The management of barbiturate overdose may necessitate prolonged mechanical ventilation for a long-acting drug. Drug elimination may be hastened by the administration of multiple doses of activated charcoal.[48] Barbiturate intoxication may precipitate noncardiogenic pulmonary edema, necessitating the administration of positive pressure ventilation.[49] The unique manifestation of cutaneous bulla formation is occasionally seen with massive barbiturate poisoning.[50]

Benzodiazepines

Generally speaking, the manifestations of benzodiazepine intoxication are less severe than barbiturate overdose. Death after the sole oral ingestion of a benzodiazepine is rare. Benzodiazepines are, however, additive to the effects of other depressant medications, such as narcotics and alcohol.[51] Death is more commonly the result of a multiple drug ingestion. The exception may be flunitrazepam. A series of deaths were reported over a 2-year period in which flunitrazepam appeared to be the sole or principal precipitating agent.[52] The most commonly abused agents at the time of this writing are diazepam and lorazepam. Both of these drugs are easily obtainable from offshore sources, and are frequently sought from legitimate sources in drug-seeking behavior. Most benzodiazepines are detectable by urinary screening assay, but some, such as flunitrazepam, may be present in a sufficiently small quantity to render screening techniques ineffective. This latter drug deserves special mention as it has achieved a reputation for producing amnesia, sexual arousal, and euphoria, making it a target drug for date rape (see the "Club Drugs" section later). The treatment of patients intoxicated with a benzodiazepine is supportive, as outlined previously. The usefulness of the benzodiazepine antagonist flumazenil in the management of benzodiazepine intoxication is at best limited. Recovery without sequelae is the rule in the absence of hypoxic encephalopathy acquired antecedent to the initiation of supportive management.

Cocaine

Cocaine is the alkaloid of the *Erythroxylon coca,* which grows wild in many South American countries. It has been advocated as an aid to psychotherapy, an analeptic, and an anesthetic agent. It has been considered a controlled substance in the United States since the passage of the Harrison Narcotic Act of 1914.

Legal cocaine manufacture is strictly controlled. Illicit use in the United States, after a long period of relative quiescence, has increased dramatically over the past 20 years. As many as 11% of Americans over 11 years of age report having used cocaine at least once in their lifetime; 0.7% of children 12 to 17 years of age admitted using it at least twice per week.[53] Cocaine intended for abuse is smuggled into the country by a variety of routes, the most important of which medically is the practice of "body packing," in which condoms filled with drug are ingested orally with the intention of later passage through the gastrointestinal tract[54] (Fig. 135–2).

Children have been used as "mules" to assist in the illicit transport of cocaine. One such child was reported to have ingested 53 packets of cocaine, recovering after rupture of a packet.[55] Bowel obstruction of ingested packets may occur, and accidental rupture of a packet may prove fatal. Oral polyethylene glycol administration has been advocated as a relatively safe method to expedite the passage of ingested packets. Bowel obstruction may necessitate surgical removal.[56]

Cocaine is absorbed by all routes—by ingestion, inhalation, intranasal absorption, or the intravenous route. Orally, its potency is about one tenth that of the intranasal route. A high vaporization temperature renders the hydrochloride salt unacceptable for smoking.[57] The typical intranasal dose is between 30 and 45 mg. Cocaine is frequently adulterated with lidocaine, ephedrine, and caffeine,[58] which are included to mimic the anticipated effects and suggest a higher potency drug to the user. The diagnosis of cocaine intoxication may be suggested in the appropriate clinical context by the finding of drug paraphernalia at the scene or a white residue on the nose.

"Freebase" and "crack," extractions of free cocaine from the hydrochloride salt, have a lower temperature of vaporization and are therefore better suited for smoking. The latter acquires its name from the popping sound when smoked. It is supplied as brown crystalline pebble wrapped in tin foil, which is ignited over a screen placed in the bottom of a pipe.

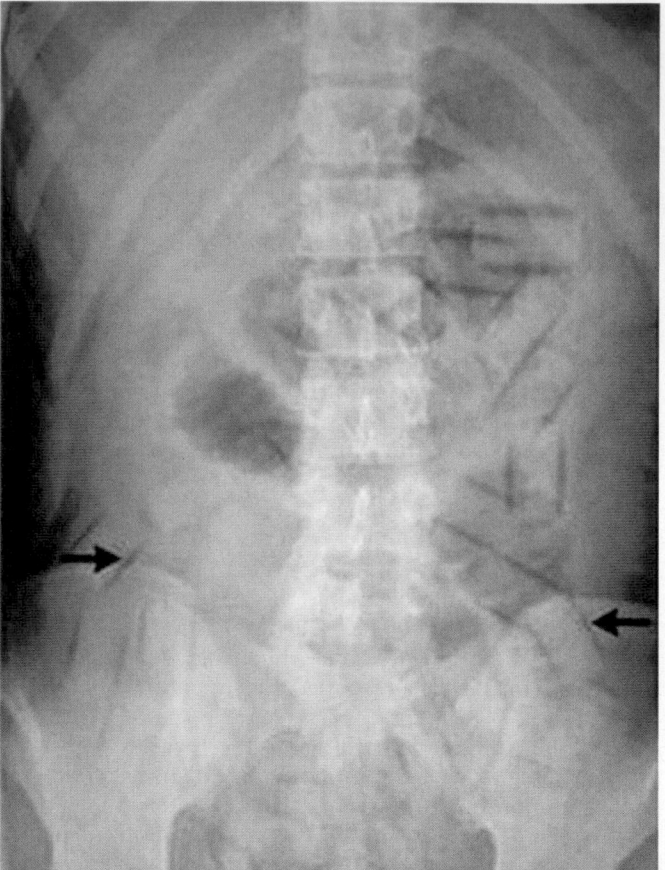

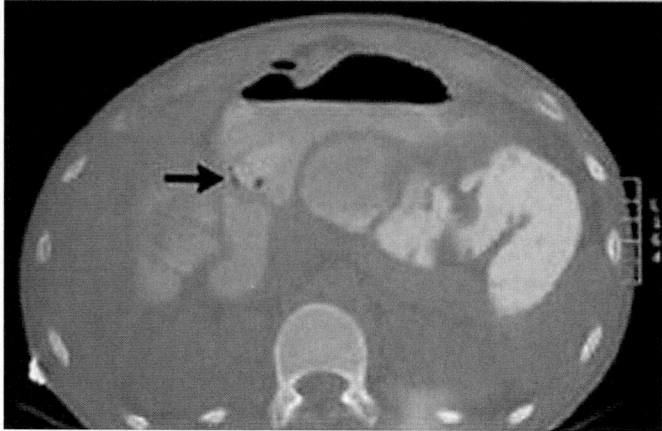

FIGURE 135–2. Computed tomographic scan of a body packer. Arrows indicate air trapped within, and outlining packets. (From Traub SJ, Hoffman RS, Nelson LS: Body packing—the internal concealment of illicit drugs. N Engl J Med 349:2519, 2003.)

The usual dose is 5 to 10 mg. Inhalation of the smoked vapors provides a more direct route for the drug to the circulation compared to the intranasal route, thereby amplifying its effect; both provide levels approximately two-thirds that of intravenously administered drug.[59] Accidental fatal ingestion of crack cocaine by a child has been reported.[60]

Cocaine is the benzoic acid ester of ecgonine, with anesthetic and central stimulatory properties. Conventional detection techniques utilize enzyme-amplified immunofluo-

Table 135–5	Symptoms of Cocaine Intoxication

Phase 1: Early

- Euphoria, elation, garrulousness, emotional lability, pseudohallucinations, sense of impending doom
- Tics
- Hypertension
- Cold sweats
- Mydriasis
- Hyperpyrexia
- Premature ventricular contractions
- Increased respiratory rate

Phase II: Advanced

- Unresponsiveness to voice
- Hyperreflexia, convulsions, status epilepticus
- Incontinence
- Severe hypertension giving way to hypotension
- Cyanosis
- Central nervous system hemorrhage
- Congestive heart failure
- Irregular respirations

Phase III: Depressive

- Flaccid paralysis
- Coma
- Fixed pupils
- Arreflexia
- Ventricular tachycardia and fibrillation, cardiac arrest
- Apnea
- Pulmonary edema

Adapted from Comerci GD, Schwebel R: Substance abuse: an overview. Adolesc Med 11:79–101, 2000.

rescent techniques to detect one or another metabolite in urine.

Cocaine is a potent central nervous system stimulant and anesthetic. It exerts its principal effects by blocking the reuptake of norepinephrine, serotonin, and other neurotransmitters at nerve endings. Administration is accompanied shortly by a sense of euphoria, elation, garrulousness, and restlessness. Intranasal use is attended by local anesthesia, termed "*the freeze*", The pulse is usually elevated, but may be transiently depressed by reflex vagal effects. The blood pressure is usually elevated. Mydriasis and myoclonic twitching can be noted. The patient can experience auditory or visual hallucinations, or tactile hallucinations known as "*cocaine bugs*." Toxic psychosis may occur. In more advanced intoxication, the patient becomes unresponsive and hyperreflexic. Seizures may occur. Hypertension or hypotension may be present, and arrhythmias, especially atrial and ventricular tachycardia, could occur. Irregular respirations may give way to apnea. Greater toxicity is accompanied by flaccid paralysis, coma, fixed pupils, ventricular fibrillation, and death. Symptoms are summarized in Table 135–5.[57]

Cardiac complications of cocaine use include myocardial ischemia, infarction, accelerated atherosclerosis, and cardiomyopathy.[61,62] Rhabdomyolysis and renal failure may occur as a consequence of hyperpyrexia.[63] Cocaine-associated chest pain may mimic a myocardial infarction and merits monitored observation.[64] Neurologic complications include central nervous system hemorrhage, ischemic infarction, and seizures. Headache in the patient who presents after cocaine exposure may be the result of sympathetic stimulation, migraine, impending stroke, or hemorrhage, and may occur during cocaine withdrawal. Concern for cerebrovascular injury should strongly suggest appropriate neuroimaging studies for all patients with altered mental status, focal neurologic signs, or severe headache. Smoking crack cocaine has been associated with pneumothorax.[65] Chronic use has been associated with renal insufficiency and hypertension,[66] chronic cognitive defects,[67] nasal septal perforation, sinusitis, and a necrotizing vasculitis.[68,69] Cocaine is likely a teratogen, with cardiac, urogenital, central nervous system, and gastrointestinal anomalies in 7% to 26% of exposed infants.[70] Cocaine metabolites may be detected in meconium and infants' hair.

Treatment of cocaine intoxication is largely supportive. Elimination techniques are generally of no benefit, although activated charcoal absorbs cocaine and may have some role in the management of the body packer. There is no antidote of proven value. Airway control should be undertaken in patients with compromised mental status. Hyperthermia should be aggressively treated (see Chapter 139, Hyperthermia). The risk of rhabdomyolysis probably contraindicates the use of depolarizing muscle relaxants in rapid sequence intubation.[71] Sedation with benzodiazepines has been demonstrated beneficial for the management of fever, seizures, hypertension, and agitation.[72] Butyrophenones and other major tranquilizers may be associated with worse outcome.[73] Rhabdomyolysis should be managed by the administration of intravenous fluids, and maintaining urine flow at 3 ml/kg/hr. Hypertension is usually responsive to the administration of sedatives. Occasionally, antihypertensive agents are indicated. Nitroprusside, nitroglycerine, or other vasodilators are effective.[74] Beta-blocking agents such as labetalol may worsen hypertension by failing to reverse α-mediated vasoconstriction, and do not reverse coronary vasoconstriction.[75,76] They should be avoided in the management of cocaine intoxication. Anticoagulation for cocaine-induced thrombosis is not well studied. Most cocaine-associated arrhythmias respond to sedation. Ventricular tachycardia occurring shortly after exposure may result from the local anesthetic property of cocaine and should be managed similarly to intoxication with class IA or IC agents, with the administration of bicarbonate.[77] Lidocaine in this circumstance may exacerbate seizures and arrhythmias and therefore is contraindicated.[72,77] Conversely, ventricular arrhythmias occurring several hours after exposure are likely the result of ischemia, and may be managed safely with lidocaine.[78] Pulmonary edema may be of cardiac or noncardiogenic origin and is managed with positive pressure ventilation. There is no consensus for the management of cocaine-associated congestive heart failure. Postmortem examination suggests a direct toxic effect of cocaine on the heart,[79] correlating clinically with the development of a dilated cardiomyopathy.[80] Management of the low cardiac output state would be directed at inotropic support and afterload reduction.

Amphetamines

The amphetamines are a group of substituted noncatecholamine phenylamines with diverse central nervous system stimulant and hallucinatory properties (Fig. 135–3). They were first synthesized in the late 19th century and were quickly recognized for their biologic effects. Amphetamines are still used in the management of attention deficit/hyperactivity disorder and narcolepsy and in weight control, and for these indications they are widely prescribed. Use migrated to the recreational market in the 1960s, when "speed freaks"

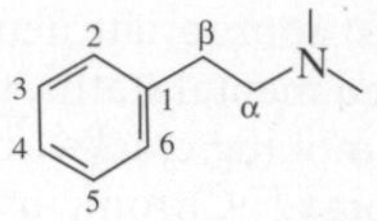

FIGURE 135–3. Amphetamine ring.

would engage in serial use, often consuming thousands of milligrams over days ("the rush"), to be terminated by a period of lethargy and somnolence during withdrawal ("the crash"). The introduction of substituted amphetamines as drugs of abuse began in 1968 with MDMA, known first as "Adam" and later as "Ecstasy," which was, for a brief time, legally sold without prescription. What followed was a series of drugs, each replacing the one before, as the sale of prior agents was restricted or discredited by the community of users. The substituted amphetamines, then, became the first "designer" drugs. This process was interrupted in 1986 with the passage of the Controlled Substances Act.[81] Notwithstanding their proscription, their popularity has not waned and they remain popular in the club culture as one of the so-called rave drugs (see later). It has been estimated that as many as 6.8 million individuals have used Ecstasy.[82]

Amphetamine is often abused orally, but may be used intravenously. In this form it may be used with heroin, known as a "speedball." Tolerance develops to the drug, and users may take hundreds of milligrams at a time. The hydrochloride salt of amphetamine is smokable, and is known as "ice." It is occasionally mixed with lidocaine to mimic the "freeze" of cocaine, and sold as that drug. Amphetamine is well absorbed orally and by inhalation, and has a large volume of distribution. It undergoes some hepatic metabolism, but substantial amounts are excreted in the urine. The half-life of amphetamine is dependent on urine pH, and is between 12 and 34 hours, an alkaline urine prolonging its retention.[83]

The clinical effects of amphetamine are caused by the release of norepinephrine, dopamine, and serotonin at nerve endings. A wide variety of signs and symptoms may be present.[84] The intoxicated patient appears restless, hypervigilant, and agitated. Anxiety, paranoia, and delusions are common. Hallucinations, frequently visual, are also common. The seriously intoxicated patient may exhibit toxic psychosis, suicidal ideation, or aggressive behavior. Mydriasis may be present. Seizures, cerebral edema, intraventricular hemorrhage, and cerebral infarction occur. The patient may experience tightness in the chest, or chest pain, and a sense of impending doom. Hypertension is common and may be severe. A dilated cardiomyopathy may be present, to which sudden death in amphetamine abuse has been attributed.[85] Renal failure, hyperpyrexia, rhabdomyolysis, and vasculitis are also reported. The intravenous user is subject to all the complications of the abuse of drugs by that route, including HIV and hepatitis. Additionally, pulmonary granulomas may occur as a consequence of the intravenous administration of dissolved pills containing talc.[86,87]

MDMA (Ecstasy) use has increased more rapidly than any other drug.[88] It has acquired a place among the "club drugs," used to enhance social experiences, along with flunitrazepam, ketamine, and GHB. Increasing use has been reported among 8th, 10th, and 12th graders.[89] It has a reputation as a harmless drug and is easily synthesized in clandestine laboratories. Tablets typically contain 50 to 150 mg of the drug,

and are often imprinted in different colors with a popular icon. Common adulterants include aspirin, other amphetamines, ketamine, LSD, and dextromethorphan.[90] Drug paraphernalia includes a pacifier, used to control bruxism common with MDMA use, and Vicks Vapo-Rub, inhaled through a surgical mask, which has a reputation for enhancing the effect of the drug. MDMA has both stimulant and hallucinogenic properties. Effects begin 30 minutes after ingestion, and include euphoria, increased libido, altered visual perception, and a distorted sense of time. Tachycardia is observed, and peaks 1 to 2 hours after administration.[91] Ecstasy did not reliably increase the body temperature of volunteers,[92] but life-threatening hyperpyrexia has been reported.[93] Elevations in body temperature may be attendant to activities undertaken during its use that produce dehydration, but a relationship to the serotonin syndrome has also been proposed.[94] Persistent cognitive defects have been reported after prolonged use.[95]

Side effects of Ecstasy are similar to those of other amphetamines. MDMA decreases thirst, and concurrent activity may cause dehydration. Hyponatremic dehydration has been reported.[96] Cerebral infarction[97] and myocardial infarction[98] have been reported as a cause of death. In a recently reported series of Ecstasy-related deaths with a review of the literature, two thirds were attributable to aortic dissection, disseminated intravascular coagulation, rhabdomyolysis, myocardial infarction, hyperpyrexia, or sudden collapse, presumably due to arrhythmia.[99] One third of deaths were due to blunt trauma or gunshot wounds. A relationship between inhibition of hepatic cytochromes by antiretroviral drugs and sudden death attendant to simultaneous use of Ecstasy has been proposed.[100]

Detection of the amphetamine-intoxicated patient is based on history and symptoms. Immunofluorescent screening of the urine may be of assistance. False-positive screens may be caused by ephedrine-containing over-the-counter medications. MDMA is detected by high-sensitivity urinary assays.[101,102] Evaluation of the patient should include a search for commonly present co-intoxicants, such as fentanyl, GHB, and flunitrazepam. A diagnostic survey for occult injury should be performed. Diagnostic tests may include serum electrolytes, an electrocardiogram, and cardiac enzymes. Management of the patient who is intoxicated with an amphetamine congener is largely supportive. As symptoms usually are noted more than 1 hour after ingestion, there is little role for the use of activated charcoal or gastric lavage. The comatose patient should be intubated. Neuroimaging should be performed on patients with altered mental status or severe headache. There is no antidote, but most symptoms can be controlled with the aggressive administration of benzodiazepines. Dehydration and electrolyte abnormalities, especially hyponatremia, should be corrected. Hyperthermia should be aggressively controlled, and neuromuscular blockade may be required to control shivering that may contribute to heat production. Dantrolene may be helpful.[103] A relationship between MDMA and the serotonin syndrome has been proposed, prompting the suggestion that cyproheptidine may also be of use.[94,104] No clinical trials of either therapy have been conducted. Rhabdomyolysis with myoglobinuria mandates alkaline diuresis, to maintain a urine flow greater than 3 ml/kg/hr.[88] Concern over prolongation of the excretion time of MDMA should not deter one from urinary alkalinization. Hypertension may be severe, but is frequently controlled with satisfactory sedation. A vasodilator, such as nitroprusside, should be considered in those patients with refractory hypertensive urgency. Seizures are also usually responsive to benzodiazepines, but may be caused by hyponatremia, which, once again, should be corrected.[105]

Lysergic Acid Diethylamide

LSD is one of a class of drugs abused for their perception-altering qualities. It is an indole derivative and was first synthesized by Hoffman in 1946 from a rye fungus (ergot). Several other compounds share the neuropsychiatric characteristics of LSD and are similarly abused, or misrepresented as LSD. Among them are psilocybin, dimethyltryptamine, and dimethyoxy methylamphetamine (known as DOM or STP). The latter is a hallucinogenic amphetamine congener (see previous section). The piperidine derivatives ketamine and phencyclidine are also hallucinogens. Use of LSD peaked in the 1960s and then waned, with reemergence in the 1990s among high school students.[106] It is sold in thin gelatin squares, on colored paper, or as tablets that may be crushed.

LSD is commonly taken orally. Symptoms begin 30 to 90 minutes after ingestion, and persist for 2 to 4 hours. There is no clinically useful laboratory test for detection. There is a wide variation in clinical effect, but the most common experience is altered visual perception, including the unusual description of crossed sensory experience, or synesthesia, in which the subject believes he or she can smell a color or see a sound.[107] Sympathomimetic effects such as mydriasis, flushing, tremor, hyperthermia, tachycardia, hypertension, and piloerection are seen, and a syndrome resembling neuroleptic malignant syndrome has been described.[108] Depression, mood swings, and altered body perception may occur. Persistent or recurrent perceptual alterations, or "flashbacks," are reported, and LSD may exacerbate preexisting psychosis.[109] Panic attacks or "bad trips" are the most common reason for presentation to the emergency department.

Most patients who present after LSD ingestion may be managed conservatively. There is no antidote, and elimination techniques are not of assistance. Vital signs should be monitored and the presence of other intoxicants ruled out. Patients with psychotic reactions frequently may be managed by removal to quiet surroundings and verbal reassurance. Benzodiazepines may occasionally be of use, but phenothiazines may potentiate seizures and has been associated with cardiovascular collapse.[110,111] Clonazepam may be of assistance in the management of persistent hallucinations.[112]

"Club Drugs"

A group of drugs has become popular at all-night dance parties called "raves." The so-called club drugs are used recreationally in social settings, frequently among young people.[113] Among them are MDMA (see earlier), phencyclidine, ketamine, GHB, and flunitrazepam. They are considered safe by the population of individuals who use them, and consumption, especially of Ecstasy, is increasing among adolescents, as reported by the Drug Awareness Warning Network and the Monitoring the Future studies.[114]

Ketamine and Phencyclidine

Phencyclidine and ketamine are related piperidine derivatives with analgesic, amnestic, and dissociative properties.

Both have been used as anesthetic agents, and ketamine is still widely used for procedural sedation. They are termed *dissociative,* in that the patient may remain semiconscious but indifferent to surroundings.[115] Phencyclidine was first synthesized in the 1950s and appeared as a substance of abuse in the 1970s. It is commonly sold as a powder or pill that is ingested, or laced in marijuana and smoked. Impurities such as benzocaine, ephedrine, caffeine, and other piperidine derivatives are common.[116] Ketamine may be smoked or taken orally or intravenously. It is formulated for legal use as an intravenous drug, and entry to the illicit market is by diversion from legitimate sources. Pediatric intoxication after accidental ingestion has been reported.[117] Phencyclidine and ketamine may be detected by a urinary immunofluorescent assay that is both sensitive and relatively specific.

Phencyclidine and ketamine are agonists of N-methyl-D-aspartate, an excitatory neurotransmitter. A typical dose of phencyclidine is 0.01 mg/kg, which causes distorted body image and a sense of depersonalization; 10 mg causes total disorientation and catatonic stupor. Ketamine is given in doses typically of 1 mg/kg, which causes stupor and depersonalization. Higher doses are associated with progressive unconsciousness and respiratory arrest. Patients present with a combination of central nervous system stimulation and depression, as well as cholinergic and anticholinergic effects. Nystagmus, often rotatory, and hypertension are the most commonly noted findings.[118] Miosis, an unusual finding in association with an excitatory drug, may be observed. Patients present with confusion, disorientation, agitation, or violence and behavior indistinguishable from acute schizophrenia.[119,120] The level of consciousness may vary from alert to comatose. Hypertension, hyperthermia, and rigidity with opisthotonus may occur but are rarely severe. Rhabdomyolysis may attend violent behavior in both ketamine and phencyclidine abuse.[121,122] Death in phencyclidine intoxication is commonly due to behavioral mishap, such as violent trauma, suicide, or bizarre behavior.[123] Asphyxial death attendant to the restraint of a violent or uncooperative patient has been reported.[124] A prior history of psychiatric disease is common among fatal cases.[113]

The management of phencyclidine and ketamine intoxication is supportive. There is no antidote, and elimination techniques are of little value. Accidental therapeutic administration of ketamine in as much as 100 times the intended dose has been associated with a favorable outcome.[125] Comatose patients, or those with depressed respirations, should undergo intubation. The avoidance of depolarizing muscle relaxants that may transiently raise vagal tone or exacerbate hyperthermia seems prudent. Physical restraint of the severely agitated or combative patient should be avoided; a nonthreatening environment and chemical restraint would be better utilized, a benzodiazepine being the drug of choice. Rhabdomyolysis should be managed with intravenous fluids and attention to electrolyte balance. Patients should be observed for several hours until the return of normal mental status. Rhabdomyolysis, seizures, persistent psychosis, or injuries are indications for hospitalization. In a series of 20 patients presenting to the emergency department after ketamine abuse, 18 were discharged from the emergency department without admission.[122]

Flunitrazepam

Flunitrazepam, marketed as Rohypnol, is a potent benzodiazepine that is marketed legally in South America, although its sale in the United States and Canada has been restricted. It is 10 times as potent as diazepam, and shares amnestic properties with other benzodiazepines.[126] Its potency and ability to produce amnesia has led to its misuse in facilitating sexual assault, giving it the reputation of being a "date rape drug."[127,128] It is available under a variety of street names including "rookie," "circle," "rope," and "forget-me," as a 1- or 2-mg scored pill that may be colored to obscure its identity. The pills are inexpensive, and thus thought of as a "cheap high." They are imported illegally through the mail, and are acquired over the Internet from offshore sources. Although benzodiazepines may be detected by urine screen, flunitrazepam is generally taken at a dose below the detection limits of most assays.[129]

At low doses, flunitrazepam is an anxiolytic, muscle relaxant, and sedative-hypnotic. At higher doses, behavioral inhibition, amnesia, and unconsciousness occur, as may respiratory depression. Its effects are potentiated by the concurrent use of alcohol. Disinhibition may lead to motor vehicle accidents, other trauma, violent behavior, or sexual assault,[130] and flunitrazepam has been implicated in the occurrence of violent crime.[131] Fatal intoxication has been reported with the concurrent use of alcohol; rarely, death associated solely with the ingestion of flunitrazepam may occur.[52]

Management of flunitrazepam intoxication is largely supportive. Neurologic impairment, amnesia, and respiratory depression, which may begin as early as 30 minutes after ingestion, generally last for 8 to 12 hours and are dose related.[132] Support of the patient with a jeopardized airway is indicated. Gastric lavage and activated charcoal are likely to be of little benefit, unless the patient presents shortly after the ingestion. The benzodiazepine antagonist flumazenil may reverse respiratory depression, but should be used with caution as it may precipitate benzodiazepine withdrawal, manifested as tremor, irritability, and seizures.[133] Supportive care with airway protection and mechanical ventilation until the patient is fully awake is the safest approach.

γ-Hydroxybutyrate

GHB was introduced to the mass market as a dietary supplement that could enhance muscle growth. Reports of intoxication and death appeared soon thereafter.[134,135] Sale as a dietary supplement was restricted, but reports began appearing in 1997 of its use as a rave drug. Of 72 patients in a reported cohort, 20 were admitted to intensive care with coma or apnea; there was one death.[136] Its reputation for increasing libido and producing amnesia increased its popularity. The prior restriction of its sale resulted in the appearance of two congeners, γ-butyrolactone (GBL) and 1,4-butanediol (1,4-BD) with similar properties. It is easily manufactured, and instructions for production can be obtained on the Internet.[137] In addition to increasing reports of acute toxicity, it has been recognized, along with flunitrazepam, as a date or acquaintance rape drug.[128]

GHB is a naturally occurring analogue of GABA, an inhibitory neurotransmitter. It is supplied as a white powder that has a soapy taste when dissolved. It is rapidly absorbed after oral administration, and effects are observed within 15 to 30 minutes. There is no clinically useful laboratory assay detection or confirmation of the poisoning. Central nervous system effects include euphoria, headache, dizziness, ataxia, miosis, and hallucinations. The effect is dose dependent, and at higher doses euphoria gives way to somnolence and coma. Apnea is rare, but vomiting and salivation are common.[138] Seizures have occasionally been noted. A withdrawal syndrome consisting of toxic psychosis, severe agitation, and seizures has been reported[139] after compulsive repeated use.[140]

There is no antidote for GHB intoxication. Most patients may be treated supportively. Induced emesis is contraindicated because of the possibility of rapidly occurring loss of consciousness or seizures. There are no data on the use of activated charcoal or gastric lavage, but neither is likely to be effective in a symptomatic intoxication. Comatose patients should have their airway protected. Evacuation of the stomach by nasogastric suction may offer some protection against aspiration. Seizures may be treated with benzodiazepines. Most patients recover within 8 hours. There is no consensus on the treatment of GHB withdrawal syndrome, but high-dose benzodiazepines and barbiturates have been advocated.

Inhalants

The abuse of volatile substances is appealing to the drug-seeking adolescent. Inhalation is associated with rapid onset and predictable euphoria, quickly dissipating, which allows the child to engage in the practice while unobserved. They are often legally obtained, readily available, and inexpensive. A national annual survey of drug abuse trends among schoolchildren has reported that the lifetime prevalence of inhalant abuse among 8th graders is 20%. The only more commonly abused substances are nicotine and alcohol.[141] A wide variety of inhalant substances and sources are reported (Table 135–6).

Table 135–6	Commonly Abused Volatile Substances	
Family	**Substance**	**Source**
Aliphatic hydrocarbons	Propane	Bottled fuel
	Butane	Cigarette lighter fluid
	Gasoline	Automotive fuel
	n-Hexane	Model glue, rubber cement
Alkyl halides	1,1,1-Trochloroethane	Correction fluid, degreaser
	Trichloroethylene	Dry cleaning fluid
	Trichorofl[u]romethane	Freon refrigerant
	Dichlormethane	Paint stripper
Aromatic hydrocarbons	Benzene	Resins, varnishes
	Toluene	Spray paint, glues
	Xylene	Paint thinner, glue
	Naphthalene	Mothballs
Ethers	Diethyl ether	Solvent
Ketones	Actone	Nail polish remover
	Butanone	Adhesives
	Methyl n-butyl ketone	Paint
	Methyl isobutyl ketone	Spray paint
Nitrogen oxides	Butyl/isobutyl nitrite	Room air freshener
	Amyl nitrate	Coronary vasodilator
	Nitrous oxide	Whipped cream

Inhalants are often abused by a group, but may be engaged in as a solitary activity. Typically, the agent is sprayed into a bag, which is placed over the face and inhaled (so-called "bagging"), or sprayed into a rag, which is then placed over the face ("huffing"). Some agents are supplied in characteristic dispensers such as whippets or glass beads (see below). Intoxicated individuals frequently present with altered mental status, rendering history difficult, but the identification of an offending substance may be facilitated by inquiring among others present, or an inspection of the surroundings. Emergency medical services personnel should be instructed to retrieve items such as paint cans, rags, or other paraphernalia. These items, along with the patient's clothing, should be brought in an airtight container along with the patient. Examination of the patient may be of assistance: the child may have a suggestive odor, or the presence of residue such as paint or correction fluid on the face. Mucous membrane irritation, especially perioral (termed a "*huffer's rash*"), and swelling may be present. Cyanosis unresponsive to oxygen therapy suggests methemoglobinemia secondary to nitrite abuse.

Inhalant abuse is a hazardous activity. Death, although uncommon, may result from cardiac arrhythmia or asphyxia.[142] Severe burns have been reported after ignition of a volatile substance concurrent with cigarette smoking.[143] Sudden death is associated with the abuse of butane, propane, and halogenated hydrocarbons. It has been attributed to the sensitization of myocardium to circulating catecholamines,[144] and is suggested by the history of cardiac arrest following vigorous physical activity after inhalant abuse. Most recently, it has been described with the abuse of typewriter correction fluid, which contains 1,1,1-trichloroethylene, and spray containers using Freon propellants.[145,146]

Solvent inhalation generally produces central nervous system depression, which may impair ventilation and airway reflexes. Subjective effects and symptoms are dose dependent and are subject to considerable individual variation. Patients may be lethargic, disinhibited, ataxic, dysarthric, or comatose.[147] Hallucinations may occur. Seizures have been reported.[148] The duration of symptoms is dependent on the individual agent. Most solvents produce euphoria after 15 to 20 inhalations. Rebreathing the substance by bagging may produce hypoxia that enhances its effects.[149] Duration of symptoms depends on the lipid solubility of the substance. Gasoline sniffing will produce sedation for as long as 8 hours. Patients may wake with headache, dizziness, palpitations, vomiting, and weakness. These symptoms, although unpleasant, are rarely life threatening. Tolerance to the acute effects of hydrocarbon inhalants, especially with toluene and 1,1,1-trichloroethylene abuse, has been described after as little as 3 months' regular use.[150-152] An acute withdrawal syndrome characterized by tremor, agitation, insomnia, and delirium tremens has also been described.[153] Acute methylene chloride exposure may produce the unique problem of carboxyhemoglobinemia, developing hours after exposure, as a consequence of carbon monoxide generated in its metabolism.[154]

Chronic solvent inhalant abuse produces a wide range of organ system injuries, summarized in Table 135–7. The most common neurologic sequelae are polyneuropathy and dementia.[155-158] Gasoline sniffing presents unique problems. The chronic multifocal polyneuropathy associated with its chronic abuse may worsen after cessation of the practice.[159]

Table 135–7	Chronic Effects of Inhalant Abuse	
Organ System	**Manifestation**	**Associated with:**
Neurologic	Cerebellar ataxia	Toluene
	Electroencephalographic slowing	n-Hexane
	Peripheral neuropathy	n-Hexane
	Trigeminal neuralgia	1,1,1-Trichloroethylene
	Parkinsonism	Gasoline additive
Psychiatric	Dementia, memory loss	Multiple
Renal	Renal tubular acidosis	Toluene
Cardiovascular	Myocarditis	Gasoline
Pulmonary	Chemical pneumonitis	Multiple
	Emphysema	Gasoline
Hepatotoxicity	Chemical hepatitis	Chlorinated hydrocarbons
Hematologic	Carboxyhemoglobinemia	Methylene chloride
	Leukemia, aplastic anemia	Benzene

Adapted from Brouette T, Anton R: Clinical review of inhalants. Am J Addict 10:79–94, 2001.

Additionally, acute and chronic lead encephalopathy has been reported.[160]

Volatile Nitrogen Oxides

Nitrous oxide, still used as an anesthetic gas, has been increasingly reported as a drug of abuse. As many as 10% of adolescent youths in some populations may use nitrous oxide regularly; one third of adolescents surveyed at a correctional institution reported use, beginning at a median age of 13 years.[161] It is readily available in health care facilities and restaurants, but in the pediatric population it has been obtained in the form of "whippets," which are sold for the production of whipped cream. They can be obtained at grocery stores and at specialty shops specializing in drug paraphernalia, often sold with a device to puncture and evacuate the canister. The gas is expended into a balloon, which may be passed around in a group setting. Many first-time users experience nausea, chest tightness, or no effect; however, some report a sense of dreamlike anesthesia shortly after inhalation.

Nitrous oxide, like other inhaled drugs of abuse, readily crosses the alveolus to the bloodstream and thereafter penetrates the blood-brain barrier. After termination of exposure, nitrous oxide in the bloodstream is rapidly excreted by the lungs. Its lifetime in the central nervous system is longer than its circulatory half-life. It has the reputation of being a clean and safe drug, but deaths, principally in the workplace, have been reported,[162] attendant to asphyxia during the inhalation of high concentrations. Death has not been reported with the use of nitrous oxide whippets; however, impaired driving skills were observed after brief recreational exposure.[163] Chronic intermittent inhalation has been associated with a diffuse polyneuropathy, commonly more sensory than motor, which is caused by inactivation of vitamin B_{12}. Ataxia and lower extremity weakness are often noted.[164,165] Megaloblastic anemia, leukopenia, and thrombocytopenia are also occasionally observed.[166]

Organic nitrites have been abused by inhalation since the 1970s, when they acquired the reputation of being a sexual stimulant, particularly among homosexuals. Popularity waned with their unproven association with the acquisition of acquired immunodeficiency syndrome. Similarly, an alleged association of nitrite abuse with Kaposi's sarcoma is unproven, and is more likely the result of promiscuous unprotected sex.[167] Abuse of amyl nitrate and butyl nitrite, although less common than in the past, continues to be occasionally seen.

Amyl, butyl, and isobutyl nitrite are potent vasodilators and have narcotic effects similar to nitrous oxide. Alkyl nitrites are also found as the propellant in a variety of cleaning products and sold as a "locker room deodorant," to be bagged or huffed. Amyl nitrite is distributed in glass beads called "poppers," which are broken and the contents inhaled. Inhalation is accompanied by sexual arousal and a dreamy, euphoric state. Onset is within seconds, but the effect last only minutes. The pattern of abuse is repeated inhalation, often dozens of times.

Patients may present with flushing reactions that can be attributed to nitrite-induced vasodilation or allergy. The principal severe toxicities associated with volatile nitrite abuse, however, are consequent to oxidative stress, as nitrite-induced methemoglobin formation may overwhelm NADH- and NADPH-dependent reduction pathways. Hemolytic anemia, often associated with congenital glucose-6-phosphate dehydrogenase (G6PD) deficiency, has been reported.[168] Methemoglobinemia is rare but may be life threatening. The diagnosis is suggested by the presentation of cyanosis unresponsive to 100% oxygen, and is confirmed by co-oximetry. Pulse oximeters do not detect methemoglobin and may falsely report satisfactory oxygen saturation in the presence of severe disease. Manifestations are those of acute anemia. Symptomatic tachycardia develops with a methemoglobin level over 30%. Neurologic symptoms, including headache, lethargy, and coma, are noted at a level over 55%. Arrhythmias and cardiovascular collapse occur at this level, and a concentration over 70% is frequently fatal. Symptomatic patients should be treated with methylene blue, 1 to 2 g of 1% solution.[169] Unresponsiveness to therapy may indicate G6PD deficiency. Occasionally, exchange transfusion may be required.

Miscellaneous Agents

Over-the-Counter Drugs

Over-the-counter medications are frequently abused by children and adolescents. A recent report from the Utah poison control system identified 2214 contacts over a 10-year period, asserting the inappropriate use of medications by children 6 to 19 years old.[170] Most common among them were the anticholinergic decongestants, caffeine, dextromethorphan, and stimulants.[38] Two thirds of the children were brought to a health care facility. There were no deaths.

Caffeine is a methylxanthine, chemically related to theophylline and a ubiquitous substance in the Western diet. Caffeine is a stimulant that elevates blood pressure, pulse, and respiratory rate. It is used clinically in the management of neonatal apnea. At doses near therapeutic, it may produce palpitations, sweating, and a sense of anxiety. In overdose, tremors, fasciculations, and seizures are observed. Fatal caffeine poisoning has been reported.[171] Caffeine dependence in childhood has been described, and a withdrawal syndrome consisting of somnolence and a decline in motor perfor-

mance 24 hours after the discontinuation of caffeinated beverages has been recognized.[172] The acutely poisoned patient should be observed for the abrupt onset of seizures. Peritoneal dialysis was reported to be effective in accelerating the removal of caffeine from one seriously poisoned child.[173]

Ephedrine and pseudoephedrine are noncatecholamine stimulants chemically related to amphetamines, with biologic effects similar to that group of compounds. Ephedrine is a naturally occurring alkaloid and has been sold in herbal form (see later). It was sold as an over-the-counter stimulant, anorectic, and bronchodilator. Its sale was prohibited in 2004 after a series of deaths were reported,[174] but it is still available by mail order from offshore sources. Pseudoephedrine is present in many decongestants, frequently with diphenhydramine or dextromethorphan, and is still widely sold. Both are abused by adolescents for their stimulant properties and as anorectic agents. Like caffeine, they are sold under the misrepresentation of being other illicit substances. At therapeutic doses, both ephedrine and pseudoephedrine produce tachycardia, hypertension, increased respirations, sweating, salivation, mydriasis, nausea, and palpitations. Tolerance develops rapidly, and increasing doses are required for the user to achieve the desired effect. The urine drug screen for amphetamines may be positive, rendering the distinction from methamphetamine or MDMA intoxication difficult. In acute overdose, arrhythmias, myocardial infarction, hypertension, hyperpyrexia, seizures, and death have been reported.[175] A chronic dilated cardiomyopathy has been reported in adolescents using ephedrine as an anorectic.[176-178] An acute toxic psychosis has been reported in children ingesting the combination of pseudoephedrine and dextromethorphan.[179,180] An abstinence syndrome consisting of excessive somnolence and lethargy has been recognized.[181]

Dextromethorphan is a semisynthetic opioid with poor analgesic properties used commonly as a cough suppressant (e.g., Coricidin Cough and Cold whose street name is triple C's). It is commonly sold in combination with acetaminophen, diphenhydramine, or pseudoephedrine. Sedation and relaxation are noted at recommended doses, but increasing amounts are associated with hallucinations and psychosis.[182] The serotonin syndrome, consisting of confusion, ataxia, hyperthermia, and rigidity, has been associated with the use of dextromethorphan.[183] The abuse potential of dextromethorphan has been long recognized.[184] Dependence and death have been also associated with abuse.[185] Recently, reports have appeared suggesting the increased abuse of Coricidin HBP, apparently because of its high dextromethorphan content.[186] In 92 reported patients, the most common symptoms were tachycardia, hypertension, lethargy, mydriasis, agitation, ataxia, and dizziness. Most patients were treated in the emergency department and released. All patients recovered.

Diphenhydramine, an antihistamine, is a common constituent of cough and cold remedies and is also sold as a sleep aid. Literally hundreds of over-the-counter formulations exist. Much of its therapeutic potential is obtained from its anticholinergic potential. Dry mouth, tachycardia, sedation, and mydriasis are observed. Its abuse potential has been long recognized,[185,187] and unintentional intoxication in the therapeutic setting has been reported.[188] Diphenhydramine has been used in intentional poisoning of children.[189] A syndrome of diphenhydramine dependence has been recently recognized,[190] and chronic abuse may manifest as adolescent depression.[68] Diphenhydramine is commonly taken orally, but it may occasionally be used intravenously or smoked with marijuana.[191] In overdose, diphenhydramine produces symptoms of acute anticholinergic poisoning: fever, seizures, coma, agitation, toxic psychosis, and tachyarrythmias. A wide-complex tachycardia resembling torsades de pointes may be observed.[192] There is no clinically useful laboratory assay, and the diagnosis must be made by history and physical examination with a high index of suspicion. Most patients recover with conservative management. Benzodiazepines may be used for agitation and seizures. Bicarbonate has been reported to be therapeutic in the treatment of wide-complex tachycardia. The use of physostigmine as an antidote for anticholinergic poisoning is controversial but has been reported effective.[193,194] Its use is contraindicated if tricyclic antidepressant poisoning is considered in the differential diagnosis of the intoxicated child.

Botanicals and Natural Products

A wide variety of naturally occurring products are used as alternative medical therapies and substances of abuse. Many herbal remedies are available as dietary aids at health food stores and sold as stimulants, appetite suppressants, antidepressants, and dietary aids. They are subject to limited regulation, and neither purity nor safety nor consistent formulation can be assured. Common contaminants of herbal products include pesticides, metals, orthodox drugs such as phenylbutazone or salicylate, and microbial substances and toxins.[195] Some substances of abuse are harvested as wild or locally grown plants. It is beyond the scope of this chapter to comprehensively review the botanical substances of abuse, but those of importance to the pediatric emergency physician are presented herein.

Ephedrine, a precursor of methamphetamine, is the active alkaloid of the plant *Ephedra vulgaris,* which has been used in China for centuries as the herb Ma Huang. Ma Huang was extensively marketed as a stimulant and weight loss product, and is popular among adolescents. In this formulation, it was subject to the variations in purity and potency of other herbal products. Its sale, and that of other ephedrine-containing products, has recently been restricted by the Food and Drug Administration after the appearance of reports of adverse cardiovascular events, including stroke, myocardial infarction, and sudden death.[175,196] The acute toxicity of ephedra-containing compounds is similar to that of other stimulants. Patients are restless, agitated, diaphoretic, tachycardic, and often hypertensive. Mydriasis is common. Seizures and unresponsiveness have been reported.[197] A toxic psychosis has been reported.[198] Chronic effects including vasculitis, myocarditis, hepatotoxicity, and a fixed drug eruption have been reported with the use of Ma Huang, possibly the result of unidentified additives to the preparation.[199-201]

Ginseng is prepared from the root of *Panax quinquefolium,* and is advocated as a stimulant and general aid to well-being (Fig. 135–4). The active ingredients are poorly characterized saponins. It is widely popular and supplied as herbal tea, chewing gum, and dietary supplements. Few medical problems have been described specifically; however, a syndrome of hypertension, restlessness, and diarrhea has been attributed to heavy use.[202]

Many decorative and wild plants are sought as drugs of abuse. Two such common agents are angel's trumpet and

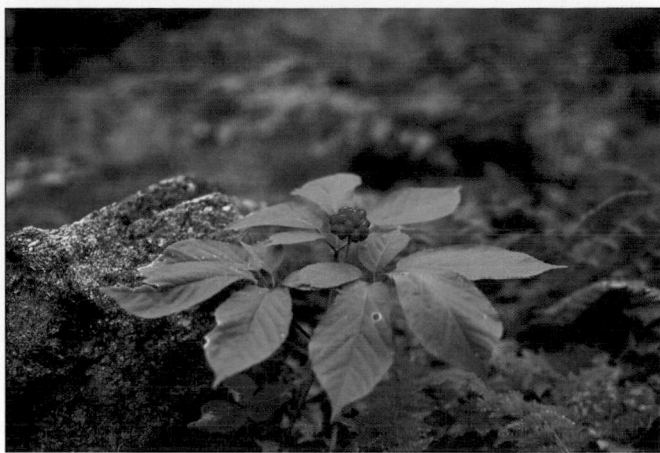

FIGURE 135–4. Wild ginseng.

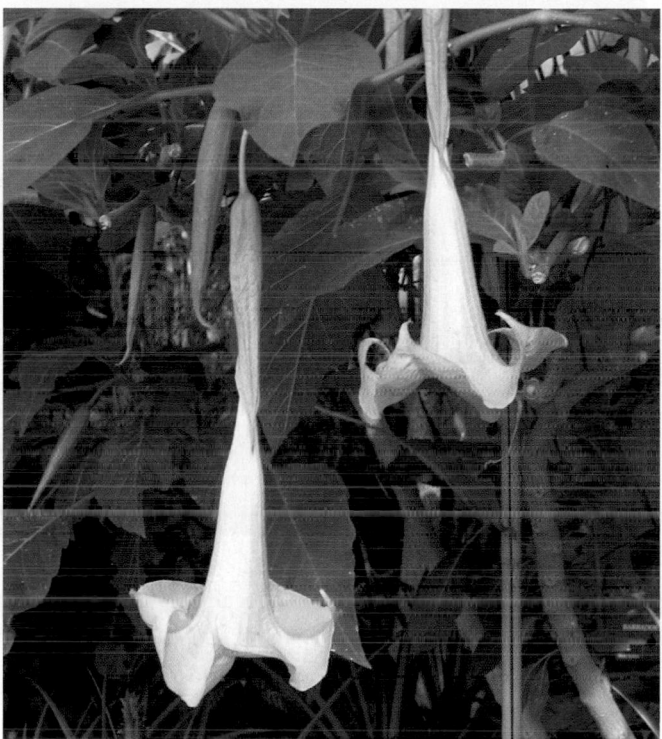

FIGURE 135–5. Angel's trumpet.

jimsonweed. They are related *Datura* species, and both are cultivated as a decorative plant and grow as weeds. Synonyms are "devil's weed," and "thorn apple," and they contain solanine alkaloids that are potent anticholinergic substances. They appear as graceful, trumpet-shaped yellow or white flowers becoming thorny seedpods in the autumn (Figs. 135–5 and 135–6). All parts of the plant are toxic. It is commonly harvested, dried, and either smoked or ingested as a soup or tea. Intoxicated patients present with agitation, delirium, hyperthermia, dry mouth, tachycardia, and mydriasis.[203] In a reported series of 35 patients, all had mydriasis, 88% had delirium, and 33% had tachycardia. Symptoms were prolonged (18 to 29 hours). No patient had seizures or arrhythmias, and none died.[204] Conservative management, with sedation and occasionally airway protection, is indicated. In

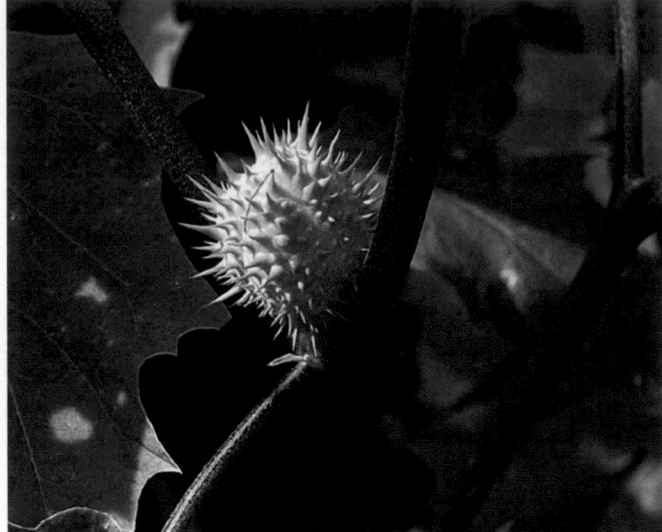

FIGURE 135–6. Jimsonweed.

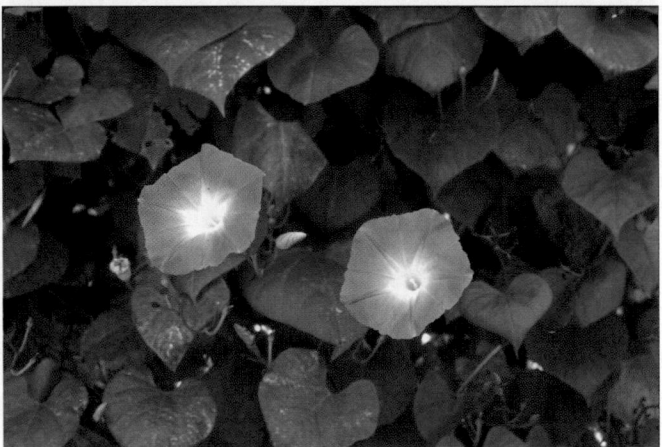

FIGURE 135–7. Morning glory.

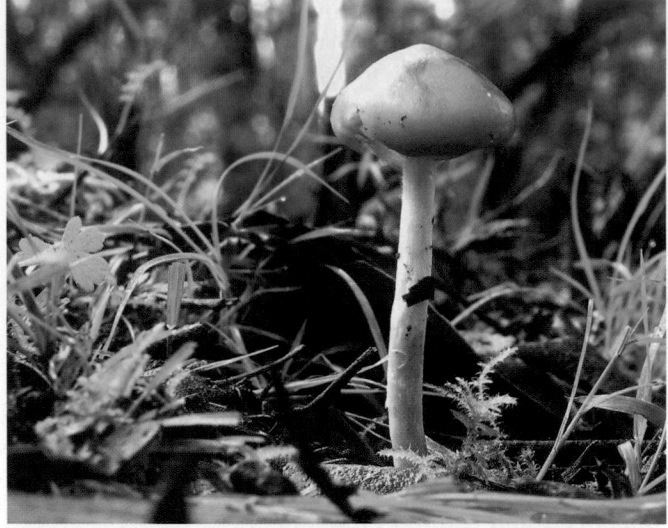

A

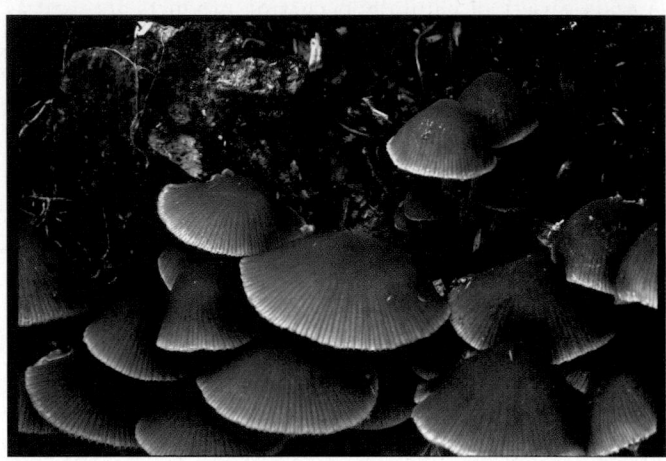

B

FIGURE 135–8. A and B, *Psilocybe* mushrooms.

one reported case of severe anticholinergic syndrome secondary to angel's trumpet abuse, physostigmine was of benefit.[205]

Several botanical agents are used for their hallucinogenic properties. Among these are the morning glory, mimosa, and peyote cactus. The seeds of the morning glory, of the *Convolvulaceae* family, produce an alkaloid similar to LSD that causes altered perception and hallucinations when ingested (Fig. 135–7). The seeds are first obtained from the mature plant or in garden supply stores. They are ground, soaked, and filtered before consumption. Synesthesia, visual hallucinations, and mydriasis are common signs and symptoms. The effect lasts about 60 minutes.[206] Medical complications are rare, and death has not been reported.[207] Dimethyltryptamine is a serotonin agonist contained in snuff manufactured from the seeds and bark of *Justia pectoralis, Mimosa hostilis,* and other plants. They are collected wild and are available by mail order. Abuse is by inhalation of the ground powder or by smoking. Intoxication closely resembles LSD. The treatment is supportive. Pharmacologic management of agitation may be undertaken with benzodiazepines. A powder ground from the seeds of the spice nutmeg is used as a hal-

lucinogen similar to LSD. Myristicin, the active alkaloid, is present in a concentration of 0.2 mg/g of spice. Ingestion of 5 g of ground nutmeg induces hallucinations and arousal.[208] Symptoms are said to resemble acute anticholinergic poisoning, with mydriasis, tachycardia, palpitations, and a feeling of impending doom.[209] Uncomplicated recovery with supportive care is the rule, but death, presumably secondary to tachyarrythmia, has been reported.[210]

The use of mushrooms and cactus as hallucinogenic agents dates back to antiquity. *Psilocybe cubensis* is found in moist southeastern climates and produces the alkaloids psilocybin and psilocin, which closely resemble dimethyl tryptamine, a serotonin analogue (Fig. 135–8). The active agent is stable and retains potency when boiled. It is foraged by amateur mushroom hunters and is sold as a street drug frequently misrepresented as LSD. It is commonly ingested as a soup or tea, but occasionally has been abused intravenously.[211] Ingestion is accompanied by symptoms closely resembling those of other hallucinogens, with hallucinations, altered color perception, tachycardia, hypertension, and mydriasis. Patients may present with an agitated delirium or paranoid delusions. Symptoms begins shortly after ingestion and last

3 to 4 hours. Medical complications are rare, but convulsions and myocardial infarction have been reported.[212,213] A principal danger is the misidentification of a more toxic species, such as *Amanita* species.[214] Treatment is supportive. An attempt should be made to formally identify the mushroom if it is available. Peyote is the common name of the cactus *Lophophora williamsii,* from which the active alkaloid, mescaline, is extracted. It grows wild in the Southwest and is still used legally in religious ceremonies. As a drug of abuse, it is produced from buttons of the dried cactus, which are consumed as a tea. It is often misrepresented as LSD or phencyclidine. Effects begin 30 minutes after ingestion. A gastrointestinal phase is accompanied by nausea, vomiting, diaphoresis, and mydriasis, to be followed by a psychoactive phase closely resembling that of LSD. Prolonged psychosis and fatal intoxication have been reported.[215,216] Treatment is once again supportive. Pharmacologic management of agitation is better accomplished with benzodiazepines rather than phenothiazines, which may contribute to hyperpyrexia.[217]

Anabolic Steroids

Not all drugs are abused for their mind-altering properties. Androgenic steroids are frequently used by athletes to increase muscle mass and improve performance. They are structurally related to testosterone, and, in addition to masculinization, increase muscle mass (anabolism). Their use has increased among adolescents seeking to improve athletic performance. Two recent surveys of high-school children reported prevalence of anabolic steroid use in all students as 2.8% and 5.8%. One third of those who admitted use indicated that they abused these drugs parenterally.[218] The use of anabolic agents, along with stimulants, hormones such as erythropoietin and growth hormone, and blood doping, is officially proscribed. In 1990, Congress enacted the Anabolic Steroid Control Act, which placed them on Schedule III of controlled substances, but acquisition is easily accomplished through illicit sources. Surreptitious use is accomplished by taking them in cycles to avoid detection. Athletes tend to use more than one agent and cycle their use to modulate drug tolerance. Numerous complications of anabolic steroid use have been reported and include toxic hepatitis, overuse injuries, gynecomastia, cerebral hemorrhage, and pulmonary embolism.[219-223] Anabolic steroids lower high-density lipoprotein and increase platelet adhesiveness. Cardiac effects include myocardial infarction and sudden death.[224] Athletes who parenterally abuse anabolic steroids are subject to the infectious and noninfectious complications of nonsterile administration, including hepatitis, HIV, and abscesses, but at a rate that may be lower than that of intravenous drug users.[225]

REFERENCES

*1. Comerci GD, Schwebel R: Substance abuse: an overview. Adolesc Med 11:79–101, 2000.
2. Newcomb MD: Identifying high-risk youth: prevalence and patterns of adolescent drug abuse. NIDA Res Monogr 156:7–38, 1995.
3. Du Mont J, Parnis D: The doctor's dilemma: caregiving and medicolegal evidence collection. Med Law 23:515–529, 2004.
4. Hoyt CA: Evidence recognition and collection in the clinical setting. Crit Care Nurs Q 22:19–26, 1999.

*5. Ferrara SD, Tedeschi L, Frison G, et al: Drugs-of-abuse testing in urine: statistical approach and experimental comparison of immuno-chemical and chromatographic techniques. J Anal Toxicol 18:278–291, 1994.
6. Mann K: Pharmacotherapy of alcohol dependence: a review of the clinical data. CNS Drugs 18:485–504, 2004.
7. Holzbach E: Thiamine absorption in alcoholic delirium patients. J Stud Alcohol 57:581–584, 1996.
8. Lee GP, DiClimente CC: Age of onset versus duration of problem drinking on the Alcohol Use Inventory. J Stud Alcohol 46:398–402, 1985.
9. Sherwin D, Mead B: Delirium tremens in a nine-year-old child. Am J Psychiatry 132:1210–1212, 1975.
10. Beckstead MJ, Weiner JL, Eger EI 2nd, et al: Glycine and gamma-aminobutyric acid^A receptor function is enhanced by inhaled drugs of abuse. Mol Pharmacol 57:1199–1205, 2000.
11. Martin PR, Bhushan CM, Kapur BM, et al: Intravenous phenobarbital therapy in barbiturate and other hypnosedative withdrawal reactions: a kinetic approach. Clin Pharmacol Ther 26:256–264, 1979.
12. Gerra G, Zaimovic A, Giusti F, et al: Intravenous flumazenil versus oxazepam tapering in the treatment of benzodiazepine withdrawal: a randomized, placebo-controlled study. Addict Biol 7:385–395, 2002.
13. Gonzalez G, Oliveto A, Kosten TR: Combating opiate dependence: a comparison among the available pharmacological options. Expert Opin Pharmacother 5:713–725, 2004.
14. Raith K, Hochhaus G: Drugs used in the treatment of opioid tolerance and physical dependence: a review. Int J Clin Pharmacol Ther 42:191–203, 2004.
15. Gowing L, Farrell M, Ali R, White J: Alpha2 adrenergic agonists for the management of opioid withdrawal. Cochrane Database Syst Rev (2), CD002024, 2001.
16. Kienbaum P, Scherbaum N, Thurauf N, et al: Acute detoxification of opioid-addicted patients with naloxone during propofol or methohexital anesthesia: a comparison of withdrawal symptoms, neuroendocrine, metabolic, and cardiovascular patterns. Crit Care Med 28:969–976, 2000.
17. Greenberg M: Ultrarapid opioid detoxification of two children with congenital heart disease. J Addict Dis 19:53–58, 2000.
18. Chomchai C, Na Manorom N, Watanarungsan P, et al: Methamphetamine abuse during pregnancy and its health impact on neonates born at Siriraj Hospital, Bangkok, Thailand. Southeast Asian J Trop Med Public Health 35:228–231, 2004.
19. Nolan EE, Gadow KD, Sprafkin J: Stimulant medication withdrawal during long-term therapy in children with comorbid attention-deficit hyperactivity disorder and chronic multiple tic disorder. Pediatrics 103:730–737, 1999.
20. Tardieu S, Poirier Y, Micallef J, Blin O: Amphetamine-like stimulant cessation in an abusing patient treated with bupropion. Acta Psychiatr Scand 109:75–77; discussion 77–78, 2004.
21. Selden BS, Clark RF, Curry SC: Marijuana. Emerg Med Clin North Am 8:527–539, 1990.
22. Evans DL, Pantanowitz L, Dezube BJ, Aboulafia DM: Breast enlargement in 13 men who were seropositive for human immunodeficiency virus. Clin Infect Dis 35:1113–1119, 2002.
23. Dardick KR: Holiday gynecomastia related to marijuana? Ann Intern Med 119:253, 1993.
24. Iversen L: Cannabis and the brain. Brain 126:1252–1270, 2003.
25. Carter GT, Ugalde V: Medical marijuana: emerging applications for the management of neurologic disorders. Phys Med Rehabil Clin N Am 15:943–954, 2004.
26. Carter GT, Weydt P, Kyashna-Tocha M, Abrams DI: Medicinal cannabis: rational guidelines for dosing. IDrugs 7:464–470, 2004.
27. Hall PW, Christie PM, Currow D: Cannabinoids and cancer: causation, remediation, and palliation. Lancet Oncol 6:35–42, 2005.
28. Rhee DJ, Katz LJ, Spaeth GL, Myers JS: Complementary and alternative medicine for glaucoma. Surv Ophthalmol 46:43–55, 2001.
29. Smith PF: Medicinal cannabis extracts for the treatment of multiple sclerosis. Curr Opin Investig Drugs 5:727–730, 2004.
*30. Hall W, Degenhardt L: Medical marijuana initiatives: are they justified? How successful are they likely to be? CNS Drugs 17:689–697, 2003.
31. McCarroll KA, Roszler MH: Lung disorders due to drug abuse. J Thorac Imaging 6:30–35, 1991.
32. Chaturvedi AK, Rao NG, Baird JR: A death due to self-administered fentanyl. J Anal Toxicol 14:385–387, 1990.

*Selected readings.

33. Smialek JE, Levine B, Chin L, et al: A fentanyl epidemic in Maryland 1992. J Forensic Sci 39:159–164, 1994.

34. Kaa E: Impurities, adulterants and diluents of illicit heroin: changes during a 12-year period. Forensic Sci Int 64:171–179, 1994.

35. Kaa E: Changes in place of origin of heroin seized in Denmark from 1981 to 1986: "chemical fingerprint" of 138 samples. Z Rechtsmed 99:87–94, 1987.

36. Cushman P Jr.: Methadone maintenance: long-term follow-up of detoxified patients. Ann N Y Acad Sci 311:165–172, 1978.

37. Harrison DW, Walls RM: "Cotton fever": a benign febrile syndrome in intravenous drug abusers. J Emerg Med 8:135–139, 1990.

38. Baker SD, Borys DJ: A possible trend suggesting increased abuse from Coricidin exposures reported to the Texas Poison Network: comparing 1998 to 1999. Vet Hum Toxicol 44:169–171, 2002.

39. Matthew H: Barbiturates. Clin Toxicol 8:495–513, 1975.

40. Roehrs T, Roth T: Hypnotics: an update. Curr Neurol Neurosci Rep 3:181–184, 2003.

41. Bertino JS Jr, Reed MD: Barbiturate and nonbarbiturate sedative hypnotic intoxication in children. Pediatr Clin North Am 33:703–722, 1986.

42. Chouinard G: Issues in the clinical use of benzodiazepines: potency, withdrawal, and rebound. J Clin Psychiatry 65(Suppl 5):7–12, 2004.

*43. Jenkins DH: Substance abuse and withdrawal in the intensive care unit: contemporary issues. Surg Clin North Am 80:1033–1053, 2000.

44. Jacobs F, Brivet FG: Conventional haemodialysis significantly lowers toxic levels of phenobarbital. Nephrol Dial Transplant 19:1663–1664, 2004.

45. Haverkos GP, DiSalvo RP, Imhoff TE: Fatal seizures after flumazenil administration in a patient with mixed overdose. Ann Pharmacother 28:1347–1349, 1994.

46. Schulze-Bonhage A, Elger CE: Induction of partial epileptic seizures by flumazenil. Epilepsia 41:186–192, 2000.

*47. Barnett R, Grace M, Boothe P, et al: Flumazenil in drug overdose: randomized, placebo-controlled study to assess cost effectiveness. Crit Care Med 27:78–81, 1999.

48. Mohammed Ebid AH, Abdel-Rahman HM: Pharmacokinetics of phenobarbital during certain enhanced elimination modalities to evaluate their clinical efficacy in management of drug overdose. Ther Drug Monit 23:209–216, 2001.

49. Roquefeuil B, Lefebvre F, Kienlein J, Du Cailar J: [Acute pulmonary edema in barbiturate poisoning (a propos of 3 cases)]. Poumon Coeur 26:975–980, 1970.

50. Hoffbrand BI, Ridley CM: Bullous lesions in poisoning. Br Med J 2:295, 1972.

51. Koski A, Ojanpera I, Vuori E: Alcohol and benzodiazepines in fatal poisonings. Alcohol Clin Exp Res 26:956–959, 2002.

52. Drummer OH, Syrjanen ML, Cordner SM: Deaths involving the benzodiazepine flunitrazepam. Am J Forensic Med Pathol 14:238–243, 1993.

53. Warner EA: Cocaine abuse. Ann Intern Med 119:226–235, 1993.

54. Dunne JW: Drug smuggling by internal bodily concealment. Med J Aust 2:436–439, 1983.

*55. Traub SJ, Hoffman RS, Nelson LS: Body packing—the internal concealment of illicit drugs. N Engl J Med 349:2519–2526, 2003.

56. Traub SJ, Kohn GL, Hoffman RS, Nelson LS: Pediatric "body packing." Arch Pediatr Adolesc Med 157:174–177, 2003.

57. Hall WC, Talbert RL, Ereshefsky L: Cocaine abuse and its treatment. Pharmacotherapy 10:47–65, 1990.

58. Fucci N, De Giovanni N: Adulterants encountered in the illicit cocaine market. Forensic Sci Int 95:247–252, 1998.

59. Foltin RW, Fischman MW: Smoked and intravenous cocaine in humans: acute tolerance, cardiovascular and subjective effects. J Pharmacol Exp Ther 257:247–261, 1991.

60. Havlik DM, Nolte KB: Fatal "crack" cocaine ingestion in an infant. Am J Forensic Med Pathol 21:245–248, 2000.

61. Loper KA: Clinical toxicology of cocaine. Med Toxicol Adverse Drug Exp 4:174–185, 1989.

62. Mouhaffel AH, Madu EC, Satmary WA, Fraker TD Jr: Cardiovascular complications of cocaine. Chest 107:1426–1434, 1995.

63. Horowitz BZ, Panacek EA, Jouriles NJ: Severe rhabdomyolysis with renal failure after intranasal cocaine use. J Emerg Med 15:833–837, 1997.

64. Weber JE, Shofer FS, Larkin GL, et al: Validation of a brief observation period for patients with cocaine-associated chest pain. N Engl J Med 348:510–517, 2003.

65. Lieberman ME, Shepard H, Reynolds F, Christopher, T: Bilateral spontaneous pneumothorax after cocaine inhalation. Am J Emerg Med 8:466–467, 1990.

66. Norris KC, Thornhill-Joynes M, Robinson C, et al: Cocaine use, hypertension, and end-stage renal disease. Am J Kidney Dis 38:523–528, 2001.

67. Rogers RD, Robbins TW: Investigating the neurocognitive deficits associated with chronic drug misuse. Curr Opin Neurobiol 11:250–257, 2001.

68. Gardner DM, Kutcher S: Dimenhydrinate abuse among adolescents. Can J Psychiatry 38:113–116, 1993.

69. Neugebauer P: Sinuorbital complications after intranasal cocaine abuse. Strabismus 12:205–209, 2004.

70. Boghdadi MS, Henning RJ: Cocaine: pathophysiology and clinical toxicology. Heart Lung 26:466–483, 1997.

71. Halliday NJ: Malignant hyperthermia. J Craniofac Surg 14:800–802, 2003.

72. Derlet RW, Albertson TE, Rice P: The effect of haloperidol in cocaine and amphetamine intoxication. J Emerg Med 7:633–637, 1989.

73. Derlet RW, Albertson TE: Diazepam in the prevention of seizures and death in cocaine-intoxicated rats. Ann Emerg Med 18:542–546, 1989.

74. Brogan WC 3rd, Lange RA, Kim AS, et al: Alleviation of cocaine-induced coronary vasoconstriction by nitroglycerin. J Am Coll Cardiol 18:581–586, 1991.

75. Boehrer JD, Moliterno DJ, Willard JE, et al: Influence of labetalol on cocaine-induced coronary vasoconstriction in humans. Am J Med 94:608–610, 1993.

76. Sybertz EJ, Zimmerman BG: The role of alpha receptors in the facilitation of the chemoreflex and inhibition of the carotid occlusion reflex by clonidine. Clin Exp Hypertens 2:955–972, 1980.

77. Beckman KJ, Parker RB, Hariman RJ, et al: Hemodynamic and electrophysiological actions of cocaine: effects of sodium bicarbonate as an antidote in dogs. Circulation 83:1799–1807, 1991.

78. Shih RD, Hollander JE, Burstein JL, et al: Clinical safety of lidocaine in patients with cocaine-associated myocardial infarction. Ann Emerg Med 26:702–706, 1995.

79. Karch SB, Billingham ME: The pathology and etiology of cocaine-induced heart disease. Arch Pathol Lab Med 112:225–230, 1988.

80. Peng SK, French WJ, Pelikan PC: Direct cocaine cardiotoxicity demonstrated by endomyocardial biopsy. Arch Pathol Lab Med 113:842–845, 1989.

81. Buchanan JF, Brown CR: "Designer drugs": a problem in clinical toxicology. Med Toxicol Adverse Drug Exp 3:1–17, 1988.

82. Landry MJ: MDMA: a review of epidemiologic data. J Psychoactive Drugs 34:163–169, 2002.

83. Cook CE, Jeffcoat AR, Hill JM, et al: Pharmacokinetics of methamphetamine self-administered to human subjects by smoking S-(+)-methamphetamine hydrochloride. Drug Metab Dispos 21:717–723, 1993.

84. Albertson TE, Derlet RW, Van Hoozen BE: Methamphetamine and the expanding complications of amphetamines. West J Med 170:214–219, 1999.

85. Nishida N, Ikeda N, Kudo K, Esaki R: Sudden unexpected death of a methamphetamine abuser with cardiopulmonary abnormalities: a case report. Med Sci Law 43:267–271, 2003.

86. Ward S, Heyneman LE, Reittner P, et al: Talcosis associated with IV abuse of oral medications: CT findings. AJR Am J Roentgenol 174:789–793, 2000.

87. Williams J, Wilhoite S, Manos P, et al: Pulmonary talc granulomatosis due to intravenous ritalin. J Tenn Med Assoc 81:560–561, 1988.

88. Smith KM, Larive LL, Romanelli F: Club drugs: methylenedioxymethamphetamine, flunitrazepam, ketamine hydrochloride, and gamma-hydroxybutyrate. Am J Health Syst Pharm 59:1067–1076, 2002.

89. Wallace JM Jr, Bachman JG, O'Malley PM, et al: Tobacco, alcohol, and illicit drug use: racial and ethnic differences among U.S. high school seniors, 1976–2000. Public Health Rep 117(Suppl 1):S67–S75, 2002.

90. Baggott M, Heifets B, Jones RT, et al: Chemical analysis of ecstasy pills. JAMA 284:2190, 2000.

91. Cole JC, Sumnall HR: Altered states: the clinical effects of Ecstasy. Pharmacol Ther 98:35–58, 2003.

92. Mas M, Farre M, de la Torre R, et al: Cardiovascular and neuroendocrine effects and pharmacokinetics of 3,4-methylenedioxymethamphetamine in humans. J Pharmacol Exp Ther 290:136–145, 1999.

93. Logan AS, Stickle B, O'Keefe N, Hewitson H: Survival following "Ecstasy" ingestion with a peak temperature of 42 degrees C. Anaesthesia 48:1017–1018, 1993.

94. Parrott AC: Recreational Ecstasy/MDMA, the serotonin syndrome, and serotonergic neurotoxicity. Pharmacol Biochem Behav 71:837–844, 2002.

95. Fox HC, Parrott AC, Turner JJ: Ecstasy use: cognitive deficits related to dosage rather than self-reported problematic use of the drug. J Psychopharmacol 15:273–281, 2001.

96. Ben-Abraham R, Szold O, Rudick V, Weinbroum AA: 'Ecstasy' intoxication: life-threatening manifestations and resuscitative measures in the intensive care setting. Eur J Emerg Med 10:309–313, 2003.

97. Manchanda S, Connolly MJ: Cerebral infarction in association with Ecstasy abuse. Postgrad Med J 69:874–875, 1993.

98. Rella JG, Murano T: Ecstasy and acute myocardial infarction. Ann Emerg Med 44:550–551; author reply 551, 2004.

99. Gill JR, Hayes JA, deSouza IS, et al: Ecstasy (MDMA) deaths in New York City: a case series and review of the literature. J Forensic Sci 47:121–126, 2002.

100. de la Torre R, Ortuno J, Mas M, et al: Fatal MDMA intoxication. Lancet 353:593, 1999.

101. Kunsman GW, Levine B, Kuhlman JJ, et al: MDA-MDMA concentrations in urine specimens. J Anal Toxicol 20:517–521, 1996.

102. Ramseier A, Siethoff C, Caslavska J, Thormann W: Confirmation testing of amphetamines and designer drugs in human urine by capillary electrophoresis-ion trap mass spectrometry. Electrophoresis 21:380–387, 2000.

103. Fiege M, Wappler F, Weisshorn R, et al: Induction of malignant hyperthermia in susceptible swine by 3,4-methylenedioxymethamphetamine ("ecstasy"). Anesthesiology 99:1132–1136, 2003.

104. Demirkiran M, Jankovic J, Dean JM: Ecstasy intoxication: an overlap between serotonin syndrome and neuroleptic malignant syndrome. Clin Neuropharmacol 19:157–164, 1996.

105. Holmes SB, Banerjee AK, Alexander WD: Hyponatraemia and seizures after ecstasy use. Postgrad Med J 75:32–33, 1999.

106. Schwartz RH: LSD: its rise, fall, and renewed popularity among high school students. Pediatr Clin North Am 42:403–413, 1995.

107. Kulig K: LSD. Emerg Med Clin North Am 8:551–558, 1990.

108. Bakheit AM, Behan PO, Prach AT, et al: A syndrome identical to the neuroleptic malignant syndrome induced by LSD and alcohol. Br J Addict 85:150–151, 1990.

109. Abraham HD, Aldridge AM: Adverse consequences of lysergic acid diethylamide. Addiction 88:1327–1334, 1993.

110. Solursh LP, Clement WR: Use of diazepam in hallucinogenic drug crises. JAMA 205:644–645, 1968.

111. Solursh LP, Clement WR: Hallucinogenic drug abuse: manifestations and management. Can Med Assoc J 98:407–410, 1968.

112. Lerner AG, Gelkopf M, Skladman I, et al: Clonazepam treatment of lysergic acid diethylamide-induced hallucinogen persisting perception disorder with anxiety features. Int Clin Psychopharmacol 18:101–105, 2003.

113. Heilig SM, Diller J, Nelson FL: A study of 44 PCP-related deaths. Int J Addict 17:1175–1184, 1982.

114. Yacoubian GS Jr: Tracking ecstasy trends in the United States with data from three national drug surveillance systems. J Drug Educ 33:245–258, 2003.

115. Giannini AJ, Loiselle RH, Giannini MC, Price WA: Phencyclidine and the dissociatives. Psychiatr Med 3:197–217, 1985.

116. Shesser R, Jotte R, Olshaker J: The contribution of impurities to the acute morbidity of illegal drug use. Am J Emerg Med 9:336–342, 1991.

117. Schwartz RH, Einhorn A: PCP intoxication in seven young children. Pediatr Emerg Care 2:238–241, 1986.

118. McCarron MM: Phencyclidine intoxication. NIDA Res Monogr 64:209–217, 1986.

119. Baldridge EB, Bessen HA: Phencyclidine. Emerg Med Clin North Am 8:541–550, 1990.

120. Barton CH, Sterling ML, Vaziri ND: Phencyclidine intoxication: clinical experience in 27 cases confirmed by urine assay. Ann Emerg Med 10:243–246, 1981.

121. Reddy SK, Kornblum RN: Rhabdomyolysis following violent behavior and coma. J Forensic Sci 32:550–553, 1987.

122. Weiner AL, Vieira L, McKay CA, Bayer MJ: Ketamine abusers presenting to the emergency department: a case series. J Emerg Med 18:447–451, 2000.

123. Garey RE: PCP (phencyclidine): an update. J Psychedelic Drugs 11:265–275, 1979.

124. Mercy JA, Heath CW Jr, Rosenberg ML: Mortality associated with the use of upper-body control holds by police. Violence Vict 5:215–222, 1990.

125. Green SM, Clark R, Hostetler MA, et al: Inadvertent ketamine overdose in children: clinical manifestations and outcome. Ann Emerg Med 34:492–497, 1999.

126. McKay AC, Dundee JW: Effect of oral benzodiazepines on memory. Br J Anaesth 52:1247–1257, 1980.

127. Anglin D, Spears KL, Hutson HR: Flunitrazepam and its involvement in date or acquaintance rape. Acad Emerg Med 4:323–326, 1997.

128. Schwartz RH, Weaver AB: Rohypnol, the date rape drug. Clin Pediatr (Phila) 37:321, 1998.

129. ElSohly MA, Salamone SJ: Prevalence of drugs used in cases of alleged sexual assault. J Anal Toxicol 23:141–146, 1999.

130. Calhoun SR, Wesson DR, Galloway GP, Smith DE: Abuse of flunitrazepam (Rohypnol) and other benzodiazepines in Austin and south Texas. J Psychoactive Drugs 28:183–189, 1996.

131. Druid H, Holmgren P, Ahlner J: Flunitrazepam: an evaluation of use, abuse and toxicity. Forensic Sci Int 122:136–141, 2001.

132. Smith KM: Drugs used in acquaintance rape. J Am Pharm Assoc (Wash) 39:519–525, 1999.

133. Martin WR, Sloan JW, Wala E: Precipitated abstinence in orally dosed benzodiazepine-dependent dogs. J Pharmacol Exp Ther 255:744–755, 1990.

134. Centers for Disease Control: Multistate outbreak of poisonings associated with illicit use of gamma hydroxy butyrate. MMWR Morb Mortal Wkly Rep 39:861–863, 1990.

135. Lane RB: Gamma hydroxy butyrate (GHB). JAMA 265:2959, 1991.

136. Centers for Disease Control and Prevention: Gamma hydroxy butyrate use—New York and Texas, 1995–1996. MMWR Morb Mortal Wkly Rep 46:281–283, 1997.

137. Shannon M, Quang LS: Gamma-hydroxybutyrate, gamma-butyrolactone, and 1,4-butanediol: a case report and review of the literature. Pediatr Emerg Care 16:435–440, 2000.

138. Dyer JE: γ-Hydroxybutyrate: a health-food product producing coma and seizurelike activity. Am J Emerg Med 9:321–324, 1991.

139. McDonough M, Kennedy N, Glasper A, Bearn J: Clinical features and management of gamma-hydroxybutyrate (GHB) withdrawal: a review. Drug Alcohol Depend 75:3–9, 2004.

140. Dyer JE, Roth B, Hyma BA: Gamma-hydroxybutyrate withdrawal syndrome. Ann Emerg Med 37:147–153, 2001.

141. Kurtzman TL, Otsuka KN, Wahl RA: Inhalant abuse by adolescents. J Adolesc Health 28:170–180, 2001.

142. Steffee CH, Davis GJ, Nicol KK: A whiff of death: fatal volatile solvent inhalation abuse. South Med J 89:879–884, 1996.

143. Cox MJ, Hwang JC, Himel HN, Edlich RF: Severe burn injury from recreational gasoline use. Am J Emerg Med 14:39–42, 1996.

144. Bass M: Sudden sniffing death. JAMA 212:2075–2079, 1970.

145. King GS, Smialek JE, Troutman WG: Sudden death in adolescents resulting from the inhalation of typewriter correction fluid. JAMA 253:1604–1606, 1985.

146. Wason S, Gibler WB, Hassan M: Ventricular tachycardia associated with non-freon aerosol propellants. JAMA 256:78–80, 1986.

147. Brouette T, Anton R: Clinical review of inhalants. Am J Addict 10:79–94, 2001.

148. Allister C, Lush M, Oliver JS, Watson JM: Status epilepticus caused by solvent abuse. Br Med J (Clin Res Ed) 283:1156, 1981.

149. Watson JM: Solvent abuse: presentation and clinical diagnosis. Hum Toxicol 1:249–256, 1982.

150. Bushnell PJ, Oshiro WM: Behavioral components of tolerance to repeated inhalation of trichloroethylene (TCE) in rats. Neurotoxicol Teratol 22:221–229, 2000.

151. Funada M, Sato M, Makino Y, Wada K: Evaluation of rewarding effect of toluene by the conditioned place preference procedure in mice. Brain Res Brain Res Protoc 10:47–54, 2002.

152. Oshiro WM, Krantz QT, Bushnell PJ: Characterizing tolerance to trichloroethylene (TCE): effects of repeated inhalation of TCE on performance of a signal detection task in rats. Neurotoxicol Teratol 23:617–628, 2001.

153. Henretig F: Inhalant abuse in children and adolescents. Pediatr Ann 25:47–52, 1996.
154. Horowitz BZ: Carboxyhemoglobinemia caused by inhalation of methylene chloride. Am J Emerg Med 4:48–51, 1986.
155. Ashton CH: Solvent abuse. BMJ 300:135–136, 1990.
156. Filley CM, Halliday W, Kleinschmidt-DeMasters BK: The effects of toluene on the central nervous system. J Neuropathol Exp Neurol 63:1–12, 2004.
157. Fornazzari L, Pollanen MS, Myers V, Wolf A: Solvent abuse-related toluene leukoencephalopathy. J Clin Forensic Med 10:93–95, 2003.
158. Hormes JT, Filley CM, Rosenberg NL: Neurologic sequelae of chronic solvent vapor abuse. Neurology 36:698–702, 1986.
159. Burns TM, Shneker BF, Juel VC: Gasoline sniffing multifocal neuropathy. Pediatr Neurol 25:419–421, 2001.
160. Fortenberry JD: Gasoline sniffing. Am J Med 79:740–744, 1985.
161. McGarvey EL, Clavet GJ, Mason W, Waite D: Adolescent inhalant abuse: environments of use. Am J Drug Alcohol Abuse 25:731–741, 1999.
162. Suruda AJ, McGlothlin JD: Fatal abuse of nitrous oxide in the workplace. J Occup Med 32:682–684, 1990.
163. Moyes D, Cleaton-Jones P, Lelliot J: Evaluation of driving skills after brief exposure to nitrous oxide. S Afr Med J 56:1000–1002, 1979.
164. Diamond AL, Diamond R, Freedman SM, Thomas FP: "Whippets"-induced cobalamin deficiency manifesting as cervical myelopathy. J Neuroimaging 14:277–280, 2004.
165. Miller MA, Martinez V, McCarthy R, Patel MM: Nitrous oxide "whippit" abuse presenting as clinical B12 deficiency and ataxia. Am J Emerg Med 22:124, 2004.
166. Temple WA, Beasley DM, Baker DJ: Nitrous oxide abuse from whipped cream dispenser chargers. N Z Med J 110:322–323, 1997.
167. Romanelli F, Smith KM, Thornton AC, Pomeroy C: Poppers: epidemiology and clinical management of inhaled nitrite abuse. Pharmacotherapy 24:69–78, 2004.
168. Neuberger A, Fishman S, Golik A: Hemolytic anemia in a G6PD-deficient man after inhalation of amyl nitrite ("poppers"). Isr Med Assoc J 4:1085–1086, 2002.
169. Coleman MD, Coleman NA: Drug-induced methaemoglobinaemia: treatment issues. Drug Saf 14:394–405, 1996.
170. Crouch BI, Caravati EM, Booth J: Trends in child and teen nonprescription drug abuse reported to a regional poison control center. Am J Health Syst Pharm 61:1252–1257, 2004.
171. Shum S, Seale C, Hathaway D, et al: Acute caffeine ingestion fatalities: management issues. Vet Hum Toxicol 39:228–230, 1997.
172. Bernstein GA, Carroll ME, Dean NW, et al: Caffeine withdrawal in normal school-age children. J Am Acad Child Adolesc Psychiatry 37:858–865, 1998.
173. Walsh I, Wasserman GS, Mestad P, Lanman RC: Near-fatal caffeine intoxication treated with peritoneal dialysis. Pediatr Emerg Care 3:244–249, 1987.
174. Centers for Disease Control and Prevention: Adverse events associated with ephedrine-containing products—Texas, December 1993–September 1995. MMWR Morb Mortal Wkly Rep 45:689–693, 1996.
175. Haller CA, Benowitz NL: Adverse cardiovascular and central nervous system events associated with dietary supplements containing ephedra alkaloids. N Engl J Med 343:1833–1838, 2000.
176. Naik SD, Freudenberger RS: Ephedra-associated cardiomyopathy. Ann Pharmacother 38:400–403, 2004.
177. To LB, Sangster JF, Rampling D, Cammens I: Ephedrine-induced cardiomyopathy. Med J Aust 2:35–36, 1980.
178. Roberge RJ, Hirani KH, Rowland PL 3rd, et al: Dextromethorphan- and pseudoephedrine-induced agitated psychosis and ataxia: case report. J Emerg Med 17:285–288, 1999.
179. Hall RC, Beresford TP, Stickney SK, et al: Psychiatric reactions produced by respiratory drugs. Psychosomatics 26:605–608, 615–616, 1985.
180. Sauder KL, Brady WJ Jr, Hennes H: Visual hallucinations in a toddler: accidental ingestion of a sympathomimetic over-the-counter nasal decongestant. Am J Emerg Med 15:521–526, 1997.
181. Loosmore S, Armstrong D: Do-Do abuse. Br J Psychiatry 157:278–281, 1990.
182. Price LH, Lebel J: Dextromethorphan-induced psychosis. Am J Psychiatry 157:304, 2000.
183. Bodner RA, Lynch T, Lewis L, Kahn D: Serotonin syndrome. Neurology 45:219–223, 1995.
184. Craig DF: Psychosis with Vicks Formula 44-D abuse. CMAJ 146:1199–1200, 1992.
185. Murray S, Brewerton T: Abuse of over-the-counter dextromethorphan by teenagers. South Med J 86:1151–1153, 1993.
186. Banerji S, Anderson IB: Abuse of Coricidin HBP cough & cold tablets: episodes recorded by a poison center. Am J Health Syst Pharm 58:1811–1814, 2001.
187. Brown JH, Sigmundson HK: Delirium from misuse of dimenhydrinate. Can Med Assoc J 101:49–50, 1969.
188. McGann KP, Pribanich S, Graham JA, Browning DG: Diphenhydramine toxicity in a child with varicella: a case report. J Fam Pract 35:210, 213–214, 1992.
189. Arnold SM, Arnholz D, Garyfallou GT, Heard K: Two siblings poisoned with diphenhydramine: a case of factitious disorder by proxy. Ann Emerg Med 32:256–259, 1998.
190. Cox D, Ahmed Z, McBride AJ: Diphenhydramine dependence. Addiction 96:516–517, 2001.
191. Brower KJ: Smoking of prescription anticholinergic drugs. Am J Psychiatry 144:383, 1987.
192. Farrell M, Heinrichs M, Tilelli JA: Response of life threatening dimenhydrinate intoxication to sodium bicarbonate administration. J Toxicol Clin Toxicol 29:527–535, 1991.
193. Padilla RB, Pollack ML: The use of physostigmine in diphenhydramine overdose. Am J Emerg Med 20:569–570, 2002.
194. Rinder CS, D'Amato SL, Rinder HM, Cox PM: Survival in complicated diphenhydramine overdose. Crit Care Med 16:1161–1162, 1988.
195. Chan K: Some aspects of toxic contaminants in herbal medicines. Chemosphere 52:1361–1371, 2003.
196. Samenuk D, Link MS, Homoud MK, et al: Adverse cardiovascular events temporally associated with ma huang, an herbal source of ephedrine. Mayo Clin Proc 77:12–16, 2002.
197. Kockler DR, McCarthy MW, Lawson CL: Seizure activity and unresponsiveness after hydroxycut ingestion. Pharmacotherapy 21:647–651, 2001.
198. Walton R, Manos GH: Psychosis related to ephedra-containing herbal supplement use. South Med J 96:718–720, 2003.
199. Zaacks SM, Klein L, Tan CD, et al: Hypersensitivity myocarditis associated with ephedra use. J Toxicol Clin Toxicol 37:485–489, 1999.
200. Matsumoto K, Mikoshiba H, Saida T: Nonpigmenting solitary fixed drug eruption caused by a Chinese traditional herbal medicine, ma huang (Ephedra hebra), mainly containing pseudoephedrine and ephedrine. J Am Acad Dermatol 48:628–630, 2003.
201. Nadir A, Agrawal S, King PD, Marshall JB: Acute hepatitis associated with the use of a Chinese herbal product, ma-huang. Am J Gastroenterol 91:1436–1438, 1996.
202. Siegel RK: Ginseng abuse syndrome: problems with the panacea. JAMA 241:1614–1615, 1979.
203. Greene GS, Patterson SG, Warner E: Ingestion of angel's trumpet: an increasingly common source of toxicity. South Med J 89:365–369, 1996.
204. Isbister GK, Oakley P, Dawson AH, Whyte IM: Presumed Angel's trumpet (Brugmansia) poisoning: clinical effects and epidemiology. Emerg Med (Fremantle) 15:376–382, 2003.
205. Hall RC, Popkin MK, McHenry LE: Angel's trumpet psychosis: a central nervous system anticholinergic syndrome. Am J Psychiatry 134:312–314, 1977.
206. Brady ET Jr: A note on morning glory seed intoxication. Am J Hosp Pharm 25:88–89, 1968.
207. Whelan FJ, Bennett FW, Moeller WS: Morning glory seed intoxication: a case report. J Iowa Med Soc 58:946–948, 1968.
208. Hallstrom H, Thuvander A: Toxicological evaluation of myristicin. Nat Toxins 5:186–192, 1997.
209. Abernethy MK, Becker LB: Acute nutmeg intoxication. Am J Emerg Med 10:429–430, 1992.
210. Stein U, Greyer H, Hentschel H: Nutmeg (myristicin) poisoning—report on a fatal case and a series of cases recorded by a poison information centre. Forensic Sci Int 118:87–90, 2001.
211. Curry SC, Rose MC: Intravenous mushroom poisoning. Ann Emerg Med 14:900–902, 1985.
212. Borowiak KS, Ciechanowski K, Waloszczyk P: Psilocybin mushroom (Psilocybe semilanceata) intoxication with myocardial infarction. J Toxicol Clin Toxicol 36:47–49, 1998.
213. McCawley EL, Brummett RE, Dana GW: Convulsions from psilocybe mushroom poisoning. Proc West Pharmacol Soc 5:27–33, 1962.

214. O'Brien BL, Khuu: A fatal Sunday brunch: amanita mushroom poisoning in a Gulf Coast family. Am J Gastroenterol 91:581–583, 1996.
215. Brown RT, Braden NJ: Hallucinogens. Pediatr Clin North Am 34:341–347, 1987.
216. Reynolds PC, Jindrich EJ: A mescaline associated fatality. J Anal Toxicol 9:183–184, 1985.
217. Haddad LM: Management of hallucinogen abuse. Am Fam Physician 14:82–87, 1976.
218. Melia P, Pipe A, Greenberg L: The use of anabolic-androgenic steroids by Canadian students. Clin J Sport Med 6:9–14, 1996.
219. Liow RY, Tavares S: Bilateral rupture of the quadriceps tendon associated with anabolic steroids. Br J Sports Med 29:77–79, 1995.
220. de Luis DA, Aller R, Cuellar LA, et al: [Anabolic steroids and gynecomastia: review of the literature]. An Med Interna 18:489–491, 2001.
221. Stimac D, Milic S, Dintinjana RD, et al: Androgenic/anabolic steroid-induced toxic hepatitis. J Clin Gastroenterol 35:350–352, 2002.
222. Kennedy C: Myocardial infarction in association with misuse of anabolic steroids. Ulster Med J 62:174–176, 1993.
223. Robinson RJ, White S: Misuse of anabolic drugs. BMJ 306:61, 1993.
224. Dickerman RD, McConathy WJ, Schaller F, Zachariah NY: Cardiovascular complications and anabolic steroids. Eur Heart J 17:1912, 1996.
225. Rich JD, Dickinson BP, Feller A, et al: The infectious complications of anabolic-androgenic steroid injection. Int J Sports Med 20:563–566, 1999.

Chapter 136

Adverse Effects of Anticonvulsants and Psychotropic Agents

Paul Kolecki, MD and Richard D. Shih, MD

Introduction and Background

Seizures and status epilepticus (SE) are common pediatric emergencies. Approximately 60,000 patients suffer from SE annually.[1] Prompt pharmacologic treatment of pediatric seizures and SE is necessary to terminate the seizures and avoid permanent and potentially fatal neurologic damage.

Antipsychotics are medications used to reduce and potentially terminate hallucinations, delusions, and other mental and behavioral disturbances. Many child and adolescent psychiatrists prescribe antipsychotics on both an inpatient and outpatient basis.[2] In addition, many antipsychotics may cause significant adverse effects, including death.

Typical pediatric anticonvulsant agents (Table 136–1) and typical pediatric antipsychotic agents (Table 136–2) are discussed.

Selected Pediatric Overdoses

Anticonvulsant agents
Antipsychotic agents
    Phenothiazines
    Butyrophenones
    Atypical antipsychotics

Discussion of Individual Overdoses

Anticonvulsant Agents

Phenytoin (Dilantin)

Phenytoin is a first-line anticonvulsant used for most seizure disorders, except for absence seizures. Phenytoin's anticonvulsant activity stems from its ability to block neural sodium channels. Unlike the benzodiazepines and other anticonvulsants, phenytoin does not cause sedation in therapeutic doses. Phenytoin can be given orally and intravenously. Therapeutic levels are 10 to 20 mg/L.

Adverse effects associated with phenytoin use can be subdivided based on acute use versus chronic use. Idiosyncratic adverse effects can also occur.

Adverse effects associated with acute use include nystagmus, ataxia, dizziness, diplopia, and dyskinesia-like movements. Rapid intravenous (IV) phenytoin administration can cause significant hypotension, bradycardia, atrioventricular conduction delays, ventricular tachycardia, ventricular fibrillation, and asystole. Extravasation of IV phenytoin can produce local skin irritation, skin and soft tissue necrosis, compartment syndrome, gangrene, and amputation. A delayed bluish discoloration of the effected extremity (purple glove syndrome) followed by erythema, edema, vesicles, bullae, and local tissue ischemia, can also occur. These cardiovascular and soft tissue side effects from IV administration occur secondary to phenytoin's diluent (propylene glycol).

Adverse effects associated with long-term phenytoin use include gingival hyperplasia, facial coarsening, peripheral neuropathy, collagen disturbances, bone diseases, hypovitaminosis D, and megaloblastic anemia (secondary to folic acid deficiency). Idiosyncratic reactions include leukopenia, thrombocytopenia, aplastic anemia, agranulocytosis, and a hypersensitivity syndrome.[3]

The treatment of the adverse effects with both acute and chronic phenytoin use is mainly supportive. No specific antidote exists for phenytoin poisoning. Serial phenytoin levels are necessary when treating overdose patients. Activated charcoal binds phenytoin well, and multiple doses of activated charcoal should be considered for patients with rising phenytoin levels. Oral overdoses of phenytoin rarely produce

Table 136–1	Pediatric Anticonvulsant Agents

Benzodiazepines (Ativan, Valium)
Carbamazepine (Tegretol)
Clonazepam (Klonopin)
Ethosuximide (Zarontin)
Felbamate (Felbatol)
Fosphenytoin (Cerebyx)
Gabapentin (Neurontin)
Lamotrigine (Lamictal)
Levetiracetam (Keppra)
Oxcarbazepine (Trileptal)
Phenobarbital (Luminal)
Phenytoin (Dilantin)
Primidone (Mysoline)
Tiagabine (Gabitril)
Topiramate (Topamax)
Valproate (Depakote)
Vigabatrin (Sabril)
Zonisamide (Zonegran)

Table 136–2	Pediatric Anticonvulsant Agents

Phenothiazines

Aripiprazole (Abilify)
Chlorpromazine (Thorazine)
Fluphenazine (Prolixin)
Loxapine (Loxitane)
Mesoridazine (Serentil)
Molindone (Moban)
Perphenazine (Trilafon)
Pimozide (Orap)
Thioridazine (Mellaril)
Thiothixene (Navane)
Trifluoperazine (Stelazine)

Butyrophenones

Droperidol (Inapsine)
Haloperidol (Haldol)

Atypicals

Clozapine (Clozaril)
Olanzapine (Zyprexa)
Quetiapine (Seroquel)
Risperidone (Risperdal)
Ziprasidone (Geodon)

cardiovascular complications, thus cardiac monitoring is not routinely recommended. Admission should be considered for patients suffering severe ataxia or dizziness. Patients with mild and moderate symptoms can be discharged and observed closely by responsible individuals. Discharged patients need timely follow-up with their primary care physician and/or neurologist. Intravenous phenytoin–induced hypotension is best avoided with slow infusions (<15 to 20 mg/kg over 20 minutes) and continuous cardiac and blood pressure monitoring. Treatment includes the discontinuation of the infusion and the administration of IV boluses of normal saline solution. Skin and soft tissue toxicity secondary to phenytoin extravasation is best avoided with close observation of the extremity during IV infusion.

Fosphenytoin (Cerebyx)

Fosphenytoin is a water-soluble derivative of phenytoin that can be given intramuscularly (IM) and IV. Fosphenytoin's anticonvulsant activity stems from its ability to block neural sodium channels.

The adverse effects and their respective treatments associated with fosphenytoin are very similar to those of phenytoin.[4] However, skin and soft tissue toxicity is rarely seen with fosphenytoin use.

Carbamazepine (Tegretol)

Carbamazepine, an oral agent, is a potent anticonvulsant used to treat many seizure disorders, except absence seizures. Carbamazepine blocks neural sodium channels. In addition, carbamazepine has strong anticholinergic activity.[5] Therapeutic levels are 4 to 12 mg/L.

Acute carbamazepine toxicity can produce neurologic and cardiovascular adverse effects. The neurologic effects include nystagmus, ataxia, dysarthria, lethargy, seizures (including SE), and fluctuating coma.[5] The cardiovascular effects include tachycardia, hypotension, QRS widening, prolonged QTc interval, and conduction abnormalities. Interestingly, pediatric toxicity compared to adult toxicity is more commonly associated with dystonic reactions, choreoathetosis, seizures, and a lower serum concentration.[3,5] Acute carbamazepine overdoses can form gastric concretions with a resultant delay in levels or signs and symptoms. In addition, the formation of an active metabolite also contributes to delayed toxicity.[5]

Chronic carbamazepine toxicity can produce headaches, diplopia, ataxia, and hyponatremia (secondary to increased vasopressin stimulation).[5-7]

Neuropsychiatric adverse effects include irritability, impaired concentration, and memory impairment. Idiosyncratic reactions include rashes, hepatitis, drug-induced systemic lupus erythematosus, leukopenia, and aplastic anemia.[3]

The treatment of adverse effects with both acute and chronic carbamazepine use is mainly supportive. No specific antidote exists for carbamazepine poisoning. Serial carbamazepine levels are necessary when treating overdose patients. Activated charcoal binds carbamazepine well, and multiple doses of activated charcoal should be considered for patients with rising carbamazepine levels or concretions. Cardiac monitoring is recommended, and IV sodium bicarbonate should be considered for QRS widening of greater than 100 msec. Carbamazepine-induced seizures respond well to benzodiazepines.[8] Serum electrolytes should be followed, especially in severe overdoses. Admission to an intensive care unit is recommended for poisoned patients with severe neurologic and/or cardiovascular toxicity. Admission should also be considered for patients suffering severe ataxia or dizziness. Patients with mild and moderate symptoms can be discharged and observed closely by responsible individuals. Discharged patients need timely follow-up with their primary care physician and/or neurologist.

Valproate (Depakote)

Valproate is an oral and IV anticonvulsant agent used to treat a wide range of seizure disorders. Valproate also blocks neural sodium channels. In addition, it prevents the metabolism of the inhibitory neurotransmitter γ-aminobutyric acid (GABA). Therapeutic levels typically are in the 50- to 100-mg/L range.

There are many adverse hepatic effects associated with valproate use. Hepatoxicity can present as transient reversible aminotransferase elevation, reversible hyperammonemia, toxic hepatitis, Reye's-like syndrome, and fulminant hepatitis. Gastrointestinal symptoms, anorexia, and seizures may precede liver failure. Age less than 2 years is a risk factor for valproate-induced liver failure. Other adverse effects include pancreatitis, hypoglycemia, metabolic acidosis, alopecia, respiratory depression, and coma.[3] Leukopenia, thrombocytopenia, and anemia may occur, all of which typically are reversible.

The treatment of valproate toxicity is mainly supportive. Serial valproate levels are necessary when treating overdose patients. Activated charcoal binds valproate well, and multiple doses of activated charcoal should be considered for patients with rising valproate levels. Naloxone (Narcan) has been reported to reverse valproate-induced central nervous system (CNS) depression. Admission to an intensive care unit is recommended for poisoned patients with severe neurologic, hepatic, and/or metabolic toxicity. Carnitine has been recommended as an antidote for patients with valproate-induced hepatic dysfunction or hyperammonemia. Supplemental carnitine has also been recommended for pediatric patients less than 2 who are receiving valproate. Hemodialysis and hemoperfusion have been successfully used for patients with severe valproate toxicity (levels > 1000 mg/L). Patients with mild and moderate symptoms can be discharged and observed closely by responsible individuals. Discharged patients need timely follow-up with their primary care physician and/or neurologist.

Gabapentin (Neurontin)

Gabapentin is a derivative of the inhibitory neurotransmitter GABA and is used mainly for the treatment of partial seizures. Gabapentin levels are not readily available in most hospital laboratories. The recommended therapeutic level for seizure control is 2 to 15 mg/L.

Sedation, ataxia, and slurred speech can occur after an overdose of gabapentin. Adverse effects associated with gabapentin use include somnolence, dizziness, ataxia, fatigue, nystagmus, weight gain, headache, and rhinitis.[9] Compare to many other anticonvulsants, the adverse effects associated with gabapentin use are relatively benign. The treatment of gabapentin overdose is mainly supportive. No specific antidote exists.

Felbamate (Felbatol)

Felbamate is a sodium channel–blocking anticonvulsant. Felbamate levels are not readily available in most hospital laboratories. Overdoses may cause mild CNS depression and mild gastrointestinal irritation, and treatment is supportive. Chronic felbamate use is associated with significant hepatic toxicity and aplastic anemia.[4]

Lamotrigine (Lamictal)

Lamotrigine is an anticonvulsant used for the treatment of partial seizures. Lamotrigine is also a sodium channel–blocking anticonvulsant. Lamotrigine levels are not readily available in most hospital laboratories. Acute poisoning with lamotrigine may cause lethargy, ataxia, nystagmus, slurred speech, and QRS prolongation. Acute pediatric lamotrigine poisoning may cause seizures.[10] Chronic lamotrigine use can cause rashes, Stevens-Johnson syndrome, elevations in the hepatic aminotransferases, and elevations in creatine phosphokinase.[4]

The treatment of lamotrigine poisoning is supportive. Cardiac monitoring is recommended, and sodium bicarbonate may resolve QRS durations greater than 100 msec. Sei-

zures secondary to lamotrigine poisoning can be treated with benzodiazepines. Admission to a monitored unit is recommended for poisoned patients with moderate or severe neurologic and/or cardiovascular toxicity. Patients with mild symptoms can be discharged and observed closely by responsible individuals. Discharged patients need timely follow-up with their primary care physician and/or neurologist.

Topiramate (Topamax)

Topiramate is an anticonvulsant used mainly for adults with partial seizures. Topiramate's precise mechanism of action is unclear. Topiramate levels are not readily available in most hospital laboratories. Large overdoses are presumed to cause neurologic impairment, cardiac conduction abnormalities, metabolic acidosis, electrolyte disturbances, ataxia, slurred speech, hallucinations, and possibly seizures.[11,12] Adverse effects associated with the chronic use of topiramate include lethargy, confusion, somnolence, dizziness, ataxia, diplopia, paresthesias, weight loss, and the formation of kidney stones.[4,9]

The treatment of a topiramate overdose is mainly supportive. Cardiac and electrolyte monitoring are recommended. Admission to a monitored unit is recommended for poisoned patients with moderate or severe neurologic, metabolic, and/or cardiovascular toxicity. Patients with mild symptoms can be discharged and observed closely by responsible individuals. Discharged patients need timely follow-up with their primary care physician and/or neurologist.

Tiagabine (Gabitril)

Tiagabine, a new anticonvulsant, blocks the uptake of GABA. Tiagabine levels are not readily available in most hospital laboratories. Large tiagabine ingestions may cause seizures.[13] Other adverse effects include dizziness, tremor, and difficulty concentrating.[4] Admission is recommended for poisoned patients with moderate or severe neurologic toxicity. Discharged patients need timely follow-up with their primary care physician and/or neurologist.

Levetiracetam (Keppra)

Levetiracetam, a new anticonvulsant, is generally well tolerated. The mechanism of action is unknown. Levetiracetam levels are not readily available in most hospital laboratories. Reported adverse effects include dizziness, asthenia, flulike syndrome, headache, rhinitis, and somnolence.[4,14,15] Treatment of overdose is supportive care.

Oxcarbazepine (Trileptal)

Oxcarbazepine, a sodium channel–blocking anticonvulsant, is structurally related to carbamazepine.[15] Oxcarbazepine levels are not readily available in most hospital laboratories. Reported adverse effects include vomiting, somnolence, fatigue, dizziness, nausea, rash (Stevens-Johnson syndrome), and hyponatremia.[4,9,16] Treatment of overdose is supportive care.

Zonisamide (Zonegran)

Zonisamide, a sodium channel– and calcium channel–blocking anticonvulsant, is a sulfonamide derivative. Zonisamide levels are not readily available in most hospital laboratories Reported adverse effects include ataxia, somnolence, agitation, anorexia, psychosis, nephrolithiasis, oligohydrosis, rash (Stevens-Johnson syndrome), and hyperthermia.[4,17-19]

Treatment of overdose is supportive care. Zonisamide is contraindicated in patients allergic to sulfonamides.[9]

Vigabatrin (Sabril)

Vigabatrin is a new anticonvulsant that decreases the metabolism of the neurotransmitter GABA. Vigabatrin levels are not readily available in most hospital laboratories. The major adverse effects are depression, psychosis, and visual field deficits.[4]

Antipsychotic Agents

Phenothiazines

Phenothiazines are used to treat a variety of psychiatric conditions. The mechanism of action is central and peripheral dopaminergic blockade. Many of the phenothiazines have anticholinergic, α receptor–blocking, sodium channel–blocking, and potassium channel–blocking properties. These properties cause the clinical manifestations listed in the following paragraph. Phenothiazine levels are not readily available in most hospital laboratories. These medications are given orally, IM, or IV.

Numerous adverse effects are associated with phenothiazine use. The first is orthostatic hypotension. QRS and QT interval prolongation can occur along with tachycardia, conduction abnormalities, and anticholinergic toxicity.[20,21] Movement disorders (acute dystonia, parkinsonism, akathisia, and tardive dyskinesia) frequently are seen with phenothiazine use. Acute dystonic reactions (oculogyric crisis, torticollis, retrocollis, and opisthotonos) typically occur within 24 to 72 hours of phenothiazine use. Akathisia, the sensation of restlessness and the inability to sit still, also occurs rapidly. Phenothiazine-induced parkinsonism and tardive dyskinesia are delayed, typically 1 month to years after initiating therapy.

The treatment for phenothiazine toxicity is predominantly supportive. Activated charcoal and/or gastric lavage should be considered for an acute symptomatic overdose, as long as the airway is protected. No specific antidote exists for phenothiazine poisoning. Hypotensive patients should receive IV fluids and vasopressors if necessary. Cardiac monitoring is recommended, and IV sodium bicarbonate should be considered for QRS widening of greater than 100 msec. Admission to an intensive care unit is recommended for poisoned patients with severe neurologic and/or cardiovascular toxicity. Discharged patients need timely follow-up with their primary care physician and/or psychiatrist.

Acute dystonic reactions rapidly resolve with anticholinergic agents (diphenhydramine 1 mg/kg IM or IV; benztropine 1 to 2 mg IV or IM) and typically do not require hospital admission. To prevent a recurrence of the dystonic reactions, all treated patients should receive several days of anticholinergic therapy. Akathisia also resolves with anticholinergic therapy. Phenothiazine-induced parkinsonism and tardive dyskinesia are more difficult to treat, often necessitating a reduction in phenothiazine dosage.

Butyrophenones

Butyrophenones, like the phenothiazines, block central and peripheral dopaminergic receptors. These medications typically are given orally, IM, or IV. Butyrophenone levels are not readily available in most hospital laboratories.

Severe cardiac toxicity may occur with high-dose butyrophenone use, mainly cardiac dysrhythmias including prolonged QT-associated torsades de pointes.[20,21] Dystonic reactions can also occur following butyrophenone use.

The treatment for butyrophenone overdose is mainly supportive. Activated charcoal and/or gastric lavage should be considered for an acute symptomatic overdose, as long as the airway is protected. No specific antidote exists for butyrophenone poisoning. Cardiac monitoring is recommended. Treatment options for torsades de pointes include magnesium (25 to 50 mg/kg IV or IM), isoproterenol (0.05 to 2 mcg/kg/min IV), and overdrive pacing. Admission to an intensive care unit is recommended for poisoned patients with cardiovascular toxicity. Discharged patients need timely follow-up with their primary care physician and/or psychiatrist.

Dystonic reactions rapidly resolve with anticholinergic agents (diphenhydramine or benztropine) and typically do not require hospital admission. To prevent a recurrence of the dystonic reactions, all treated patients should receive several days of anticholinergic therapy.

Atypical Antipsychotics

The atypical antipsychotics have effects mainly at the dopaminergic and serotonergic receptors. Clozapine and olanzapine have strong anticholinergic properties. All of these agents can be given orally, IM, or IV.

Several adverse acute effects are associated with the atypical antipsychotics. Clozapine and olanzapine, when taken as an overdose, can cause CNS depression and seizures mainly from their anticholinergic properties. Interestingly, olanzapine poisoning has been reported to cause miosis and not mydriasis.[22] Acute risperidone, quetiapine, and ziprasidone poisoning may cause obtundation, respiratory depression, and cardiac conduction abnormalities. Acute dystonic reactions may also occur.[23,24] Chronic clozapine use has been reported to cause agranulocytosis.

The treatment for an atypical antipsychotic adverse effect is mainly supportive. Airway and cardiac monitoring are recommended.

REFERENCES

1. Bebin M: The acute management of seizures. Pediatr Ann 28:225–229, 1999.
2. Findling RL, Schultz SC, Reed MD, Blumer JL: The antipsychotics: a pediatric perspective. Pediatr Clin North Am 45:1205–1232, 1998.
3. Doyon S: Anticonvulsants. In Goldfrank LR, Flomenbum NE, Lewin NA, et al (eds): Goldfrank's Toxicologic Emergencies, 7th ed. New York: McGraw-Hill, 2002, pp 614–630.
4. Begin AM, Connolly M: New antiepileptic drug therapies. Neurol Clin 20:1163–1182, 2002.
5. Spiller HA: Management of carbamazepine overdose. Pediatr Emerg Care 17:452–456, 2001.
6. Schmidt S, Schmitz-Buhl M: Signs and symptoms of carbamazepine overdose. J Neurol 242:169–173, 1995.
7. Seymour JF: Carbamazepine overdose: features in 33 cases. Drug Saf 8:81–88, 1993.
8. Stremski ES, Brady WB, Prasad K, et al: Pediatric carbamazepine intoxication. Ann Emerg Med 25:624–630, 1995.
9. Kopec K: New anticonvulsants for use in pediatric patients. J Pediatr Health Care 15:81–86, 2001.
10. Thundiyil J, Stuart P, Anderson IB, Olson KR: Lamotrigine-induced seizures in a pediatric patient [Abstract]. J Toxicol Clin Toxicol 42:716–717, 2004.
11. Marquardt KA, Alsop JA, Albertson TE: Unreported symptoms seen in a series of topiramate overdose [Abstract]. J Toxicol Clin Toxicol 42:726–727, 2004.

12. Lin G, Lawrence R: Topamax toxicity in the pediatric population [Abstract]. J Toxicol Clin Toxicol 42:718–719, 2004.

13. Kazzi Z, Jones C, Hamilton E, Morgan B: Tiagabine overdose in a toddler resulting in seizure activity [Abstract]. J Toxicol Clin Toxicol 42:721, 2004.

14. Cereghino JJ, Biton V, Abou-Khalil B, et al: Levetiracetam for partial seizures: results of a double-blind, randomized clinical trial. Neurology 55:236–242, 2000.

15. McAuley JW, Biederman TS, Smith JC, Moore JL: Newer therapies in the drug treatment of epilepsy. Ann Pharmacother 36:119–129, 2002.

16. Barcs G, Walker EB, Elger CE, et al: Oxcarbazepine placebo-controlled, dose ranging trial in refractory period epilepsy. Epilepsia 41:1597–1607, 2000.

17. Chadwick DW, Marson AG: Zonisamide for drug-resistant partial epilepsy. Cochrane Database Syst Rev (2):CD001416, 2000.

18. Kubota M, Nishi-Nagase M, Sakakihara Y, et al: Zonisamide-induced urinary lithiasis in patients with intractable epilepsy. Brain Dev 22:230–233, 2000.

19. Prescribing information: Zonegran (zonisamide). San Francisco, CA: Elan Pharmaceuticals, 2000.

20. Wolbrette DL: Drugs that cause torsades de pointes and increase the risk of sudden cardiac death. Curr Cardiol Reps 6:379–384, 2004.

21. LoVecchio F, Lewin NA: Antipsychotics. In Goldfrank LR, Flomenbum NE, Lewin NA, et al (eds): Goldfrank's Toxicologic Emergencies, 7th ed. New York: McGraw-Hill, 2002, pp 875–884.

22. Stewart SK, Doyon S: One-dose dangers in pediatric patients. Crit Decisions Emerg Med 18(11):15–21, 2004.

23. Adamou M, Hale AS: Extrapyramidal syndrome and long-acting injectable risperadone. Am J Psychiatry 161:756–757, 2004.

24. Remington G, Kapur S: Atypical antipsychotics: are some more atypical than others? Psychopharmacology 148:3–15, 2000.

Chapter 137

Cardiovascular Agents

John A. Tilelli, MD

Key Points

Most antihypertensive and antiarrhythmic poisoning is treated with supportive measures (i.e., fluid replacement, correction of electrolyte abnormalities, and inotropic support).

Intoxicated patients may present with an array of symptoms not related to the heart, such as vomiting, lethargy, ataxia, weakness, tinnitus, and visual disturbance.

Digoxin Fab antidote is indicated for unstable arrhythmias and hyperkalemia. It may be given for acute and chronic intoxications.

Specific therapies, when available, should not substitute for stabilization with supportive care.

Children may present with either intoxication with their own medication, or, more commonly from ingestion of a caregiver's pills. Ingestion of medications, such as quinidine and digoxin, can have a high morbidity and mortality even with a single pill.

Introduction and Background

The emergency physician frequently encounters children with toxicity from cardiovascular medications. Antiarrhythmic, inotropic, and antihypertensive medications are commonly prescribed for children with congenital and acquired cardiac and renal diseases, and are often used in a context of multiple therapies. Altered drug clearance, a change in the underlying disease, or the addition or alteration of another therapy may provoke drug toxicity. The symptoms of intoxication may be difficult to distinguish from an acceleration of the underlying condition or intercurrent illness, leading to uncertainty as to whether or not a symptom is the consequence of the disease or of the therapy. The pitfall for the emergency physician is the failure to consider that new symptoms, such as vomiting or mental status change, might represent drug toxicity. Children may also present with the ingestion of a medication intended for an adult. Accidental antihypertensive ingestion is among the most common of pediatric intoxications. More than 20,000 exposures to cardiovascular medications were reported to poison control centers in 2003.[1] The therapeutic index of these drugs may be sufficiently narrow such that the ingestion of 1 pill may provoke toxicity in a child. The emergency physician also commonly uses these drugs in clinical practice. A general understanding of the acute toxicity of these agents is essential to their safe use in the emergency department (ED).

A broad overview of cardiac drugs leads one to approach them in two distinct classes: antihypertensives and antiarrhythmics. While this approach may provide some cognitive separation, it is of less practical use, as many drugs serve in both roles. The calcium channel blockers and β-blockers, for example, serve both roles. Some drugs, such as the nitrate vasodilators, bipyridine inotropes, amrinone, and milrinone, are rarely encountered in the outpatient setting but deserve individual mention. Digoxin, the most commonly prescribed cardiac glycoside, is important because of its widespread use as an inotrope and antiarrhythmic. In this overview of the cardiac medications, emphasis is placed on toxicity rather than therapeutic utility.

Selected Pediatric Overdoses

Antiarrhythmics
Antihypertensives
  Clonidine
  Angiotensin-converting enzyme inhibitors
  Vasodilators
  Diuretics
Digoxin
Miscellaneous agents
  Amrinone and milrinone
  Adenosine

Discussion of Individual Overdoses

Antiarrhythmics

Antiarrhythmic drugs affect cardiac automaticity by altering the flux of sodium, potassium, and calcium as they cross the myocardial cell membrane during an action potential. These agents are classified by the component of the action potential altered. Class IA agents, for example, decrease sodium conductance during depolarization, thereby decreasing automaticity, additionally slowing calcium flux, and thereby impairing contractility. Class IB agents decrease sodium and potassium flux. A basic understanding of the mechanism of each class of agent is helpful in predicting an agent's toxicity and planning for the therapeutic interventions.

Class IA Drugs: Quinidine, Procainamide, and Disopyramide

Quinidine, procainamide, and disopyramide comprise the drugs in class IA. Their low therapeutic index and idiosyncratic pharmacokinetics limit their usefulness. They are still widely prescribed, however, and are used in both adult and pediatric patients for the control of atrial arrhythmias. All class 1A agents inhibit fast sodium channels and decrease the rate of rise of the action potential, inhibiting automaticity of the heart. QRS and QT prolongation may be observed at therapeutic doses.[2] All drugs of this class, but most importantly disopyramide, have negative inotropic effects and may exacerbate heart failure. Side effects of these drugs, especially quinidine, are significant and may limit their utility. "Quinidine syncope" and hypersensitivity are potentially life threatening. Procainamide is associated with drug-induced lupus.[3]

Quinidine is well absorbed orally and widely distributed. Its metabolism is by hepatic hydroxylation. Both its therapeutic effect and toxicity are related to the concentration, but therapeutic drug monitoring is not usually performed. Quinidine's potential for toxicity increases when additional medications that inhibit hepatic oxidation are used. Such drugs include ketoconazole, cimetidine, and drugs that affect sodium influx, such as macrolide antibiotics, neuroleptics, and tricyclic antidepressants.[4]

Similarly, procainamide is well absorbed orally and distributed widely. Its plasma half-life is approximately 3 hours. It is both excreted unchanged in the urine and metabolized by hepatic acylation; the metabolite is excreted at a lower rate than the parent compound. The rate of acylation is genetically determined. Both the plasma concentration of procainamide and that of of its acylated metabolite are commonly available for therapeutic drug monitoring.

Disopyramide is well absorbed orally and has a small volume of distribution. It is also metabolized by renal excretion and hepatic metabolism.

Manifestations of toxicity due to class IA antiarrhythmic drugs are numerous and frequently life threatening. Most characteristic is a polymorphic ventricular tachyarrhythmia termed *torsades de pointes,* in which the QRS complexes appear to twist about an isoelectric line (Fig. 137–1). Polymorphic ventricular tachycardia appears to be the cause of quinidine syncope. It may occur at therapeutic levels.[5] Its etiology is not completely understood, but it is likely due to transient arrhythmias that spontaneously resolve. Patients who experience syncope should be considered toxic. Prolongation of the QRS complex is common with quinidine therapy, but an increase of 25% over baseline may be considered evidence of toxicity.[6] Depression of myocardial function is dose related. Severe overdose is accompanied by hypotension and shock. The acylated metabolite of procainamide is capable of causing torsades in the absence of accumulation of the parent compound. Disopyramide has more negative inotropic potential than either quinidine or procainamide.

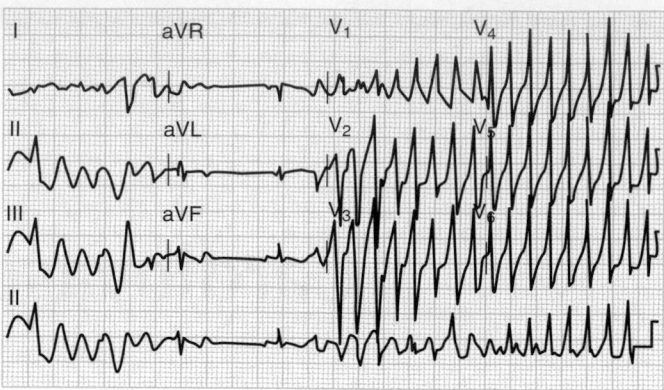

FIGURE 137–1. Torsades de pointes.

Overdoses of all three agents are accompanied by cardiovascular collapse and ventricular arrhythmias.

Extracardiac manifestations of quinidine toxicity include cinchonism, a syndrome consisting of tinnitus, vertigo, blurry vision with altered color perception, and confusion.[7] Procainamide at therapeutic doses may cause hallucinations and anticholinergic side effects. Gastrointestinal side effects are common. Hypersensitivity reactions and blood dyscrasias, most commonly agranulocytosis, are commonly associated with quinidine. Fever may appear shortly after the initiation of a class IA medication, and may be accompanied by rash and eosinophilia. Both quinidine and procainamide are associated with the development of antinuclear antibodies and drug-induced systemic lupus erythematosus. Rarely, antiphospholipid antibodies may be associated with thrombosis.[8]

Because of the narrow therapeutic index of these agents, intoxication in a child may accompany the accidental ingestion of 1 pill. Therefore, decontamination with activated charcoal is indicated in all patients suspected of exposure, irrespective of symptoms. All patients should be admitted for observation.[9] Hypokalemia and hypomagnesemia may provoke the development of torsades, and should be corrected. Intoxication with any of the class IA agents may present with dramatic, life-threatening torsades de pointes. Magnesium sulfate and sodium bicarbonate are the first-line treatment of drug-induced torsades.[10] Their efficacy is multifactorial, altering intracellular potassium concentration and increasing protein binding of the drug. Treatment should be undertaken in patients with ventricular tachyarrhythmias. Magnesium may assist in preventing the early afterdepolarizations that are thought to initiate torsades.[11] Lidocaine has been recommended for the treatment of torsades, but should be undertaken, if at all, with caution, as it may be proarrhythmic (see the next section). Overdrive pacing has also been used successfully.[12]

Class 1B Drugs: Lidocaine, Tocainide, and Mexiletine

Lidocaine is the most commonly used drug among the class IB antiarrhythmic drugs, both as an antiarrhythmic and an analgesic. Intoxication, however, is relatively uncommon. Life-threatening events (LTEs) have been observed after the accidental administration of an intravenous overdose. More commonly, they are observed during the administration of therapeutic doses in the context of impaired clearance, as in the case of congestive heart failure, or intravenous injection of a local anesthetic. LTEs are occasionally observed after the topical administration of analgesic jelly to a mucous membrane.

Although oral lidocaine is poorly bioavailable, oral intoxication has been reported.[13] Mexiletine and tocainide are both well absorbed. All undergo extensive hepatic metabolism. The half-life of lidocaine is between 1.5 and 2 hours, but may be altered in the face of hepatic disease, circulatory disturbances, or heart failure.[14] Therapeutic drug monitoring of lidocaine is widely available.

Central nervous system manifestations of lidocaine toxicity include dysarthria, tremors, seizures, respiratory depression, and coma.[15] Similar toxicity has been reported with mexiletine and tocainide. Cardiovascular toxicity of class IB agents includes sinus bradycardia, conduction disturbances, heart block, and asystole.[16] Arrhythmias may occur at therapeutic doses in patients with underlying rhythm disturbances. Ventricular tachycardia, ventricular fibrillation, and torsades de pointes have been observed. None of the class IB agents alters the QT interval or affects the QRS duration.

Management of class IB intoxication consists of discontinuation of the drug, and, in the case of ingestion of tocainide or mexiletine, decontamination of the bowel with activated charcoal. Stabilization of the comatose patient should be undertaken with endotracheal intubation and mechanical ventilation. Seizures may be treated with benzodiazepines or barbiturates. Symptomatic bradyarrhythmias necessitate cardiac pacing. Hypotension may be due both to cardiac depression and vasodilation, and should be treated with fluid administration and vasopressor agents, such as dopamine and epinephrine. Extracorporeal support may be considered in severe cases.[17]

Class IC Drugs: Flecainide, Encainide, and Propafenone

Poisoning with the class IC antiarrhythmic drugs, flecainide and encainide, has rarely been reported in childhood. An infant who ingested 1 pill of encainide was reported to have ventricular tachycardia.[18] Seizures have been reported with flecainide toxicity.[19] Decontamination of the potentially exposed child with activated charcoal is standard. Supportive management and therapy for arrhythmias and hypotension is the same as with class IA and IB agents. Extracorporeal membrane removal of the class 1C drugs has been suggested for the seriously intoxicated patient.[20]

Class II Drugs: β-Blockers

β-Blocking agents are widely used in children and adults to control hypertension and arrhythmias. Additionally, they are used in the management of congestive heart failure, cardiomyopathies, and (in adults) angina. Their common mechanism is the blockade of membrane β receptors, modulating calcium-mediated excitation-contraction. Clinical effects are expressed by the location of the receptor, and the affinity of the drug for it. Classically, two receptors exist; β_1-receptors are located in the myocardium, kidney, and eye, while β_2-receptors are found in smooth and skeletal muscle, pancreas, liver, and adipose tissue. Stimulation of the former receptors increases cardiac chronotropy and inotropy, while stimulation of the latter receptors relaxes smooth muscle in the

bronchial tree, uterus, and blood vessels. β-blockers may also have centrally mediated effects as well as membrane-stabilizing ability, which is apparent in overdose. Some have intrinsic sympathomimetic activity.[21]

β-Blocker toxicity manifests as decreased cardiac contractility and conduction delay. Sinus bradycardia is common in most ingestions, but may be absent in overdose of agents with partial agonist activity. QRS prolongation and conduction abnormalities may be present, especially in poisoning with propranolol. Hypotension, often profound, is secondary to negative inotropy. Paradoxical hypertension secondary to partial agonist activity may occur.

Depressed level of consciousness and seizures may occur, especially with propranolol overdose.[22] Respiratory depression may be centrally mediated. Bronchospasm is common, especially in agents that are not β_1 selective. Patients with underlying reversible obstructive airway disease may experience worsening symptoms at therapeutic doses.[23] Hypoglycemia may occur in toxicity with nonselective agents such as atenolol and propranolol.[24]

Overdose in children is relatively common. Despite its frequency, serious intoxication is rare. No case of fatal β-blocker intoxication in a child has been documented in the literature.[25] In a review of self-poisonings, all patients who developed toxicity did so within 6 hours of ingestion.[26] The seriously intoxicated patient may present a significant therapeutic challenge. Basic measures for the treatment of overdose should be undertaken, including decontamination with activated charcoal. Enhanced elimination techniques such as dialysis may be feasible for selected agents with a small volume of distribution and little protein binding. Seizures may be treated with conventional agents such as benzodiazepines and barbiturates. Hypoglycemia, if present, should be corrected. Respiratory failure may be treated with conventional supportive therapy, including mechanical ventilation and inhaled bronchodilators. Catecholamines have been a mainstay of therapy for β-blocker overdose, with variable results.[27] Isoproterenol, a pure β-agonist, is rational therapy but is not uniformly successful at restoring blood pressure. Epinephrine has been used in high doses, beginning at 1 mg/kg/min.[28] Optimal dosing should be determined by blood pressure and tissue perfusion. Dobutamine has not been well studied. Glucagon has been reported useful as a noncatecholamine inotrope with a mechanism unrelated to catecholamines, but has not been subjected to clinical trials. A review of the case literature reports a total of seven adult patients given between 1 and 80 mg of glucagon, all of whom survived.[29] If used, experts recommend a starting dose of 50 mcg/kg diluted and infused over 1–2 minutes × 1–2 doses, then begin an infusion of 50 mcg/kg/min. The impact of glucagon on survival, however, has been questioned.[30] Atropine is safe, but rarely effective at improving the heart rate. The experience with amrinone in augmenting cardiac output is limited. Transvenous pacing may be attempted, but capture may not be possible.[31]

Class III Drugs: Sotalol and Amiodarone

Amiodarone and sotalol, class III antiarrhythmic drugs, are being used with increasing frequency in the pediatric setting. Amiodarone, in particular, has become more prominent in the management of arrhythmias refractory to other agents. All class III agents prolong the action potential without affecting depolarization. These drugs may be proarrhythmic and should be used in the context of defined indications.[32,33] Amiodarone acts by inhibiting the slow outward current of potassium, delaying intraventricular conduction and reducing cardiac automaticity. Significant childhood poisoning has been rarely reported. Overdose of both class III drugs has generally been accompanied by an exaggeration of the primary effects. Massive overdose has been accompanied by bradycardia, hypotension, and cardiovascular collapse.[34] The level of consciousness may be unimpaired in the absence of symptomatic bradycardia. The electrocardiogram generally shows bradycardia and, rarely, heart block or QT interval prolongation. Prolongation of the PR interval is considered a therapeutic and not a toxic effect. Symptoms are related to the plasma level and generally disappear within 12 hours. Torsades de pointes has been described as occurring with both drugs,[35,36] and has been successfully treated with lidocaine. Hypotension is associated with amiodarone administration and is generally the result of rapid intravenous administration. The hypotension is attributed to the benzyl alcohol additive. Oral amiodarone has no hypotensive effect.

Chronic amiodarone administration is associated with multiple problems. In children followed during amiodarone therapy for an average of 1.5 years, toxicity was reported in 29%. Complaints included cataracts, thyroid abnormalities, pulmonary fibrosis, hypertension, rash, peripheral neuropathy, and vomiting. Skeletal dysplasia has been reported, but its significance may have been overestimated.[37] These problems resolved with reduction of the dose or cessation of the drug. Emergency physicians should be aware of the possible relationship of these complaints to the administration of amiodarone.

Acute intoxication with a class III antiarrhythmic agent rarely presents with life-threatening problems. Activated charcoal significantly reduces the bioavailability of both amiodarone and sotalol. Cholestyramine may shorten the half-life of amiodarone by interrupting its enterohepatic circulation.[34] An unstable rhythm such as profound bradycardia, attributed to amiodarone, may be treated with the cautious administration of magnesium or potassium. Lidocaine may be helpful in the therapy of torsades de pointes. The treatment of hypotension during intravenous administration of amiodarone is supportive. Class IA agents are contraindicated.

Class IV Drugs: Calcium Channel Blockers

Calcium channel–blocking agents are a chemically diverse group of drugs used in the treatment of hypertension and arrhythmias. Verapamil, diltiazem, and nifedipine are three of the most commonly prescribed and have different structures. They act by inhibiting calcium flux through low-voltage channels in cardiac and smooth muscle, as well as pacemaker cells in the sinoatrial and atrioventricular nodes. Therefore, all share the properties of vasodilation, myocardial depression, and slowed atrioventricular nodal conduction. Each, however, has characteristics that render one effect more prominent than others. None of the currently available agents has a demonstrated effect on skeletal muscle. They are poorly bioavailable and undergo principally hepatic metabolism, and drugs that inhibit hepatic cytochromes may increase calcium channel blocker bioavailability and potentiate toxicity.[38] Many are marketed in sustained-release preparations.

In childhood, they are used in the management of hypertension and the control of supraventriular tachycardia. In adults, they are used additionally in the management of angina.

Poisoning in childhood is relatively common. In 2003, the American Association of Poison Control Centers reported 9650 exposures, 57 of which resulted in death.[1] Little agreement exists on the toxic dose or time to onset of symptoms. As these drugs are intended to lower blood pressure, it would be expected that symptoms might occur at or near the therapeutic dose. In a recent review of calcium channel blocker poisoning in children, the majority of symptomatic children ingested doses at or near what might be considered the therapeutic range.[39] Symptoms generally develop within 5 hours of ingestion, but may be delayed as long as 15 hours in the event of the ingestion of a sustained-release product. Their effects are additive with other antihypertensive agents, and may be aggravated by hypovolemia, as may occur with concurrent diuretic administration, or a concurrent disease such as gastroenteritis.

Symptoms of intoxication consist of an exaggeration of the effects of the drug. Cardiovascular collapse with hypotension, which may be profound, and bradycardia resistant to conventional therapy may occur. Noncardiogenic pulmonary edema has been reported.[40] Lethargy, nausea, and vomiting have been observed, but severe central nervous system depression is usually present only in the context of cardiovascular collapse. Electrolyte abnormalities are not generally present. Metabolic acidosis is observed as a consequence of low cardiac output, and, if severe or unremitting, carries a poor prognosis.

Therapy for the child who has ingested a calcium channel blocker is largely supportive. One study suggests that children who ingest less than 12 mg/kg of verapamil or 2.7 mg/kg of nifedipine may be monitored at home.[39] The same study indicates that children who are asymptomatic 3 hours after ingestion of a regular-release product or 14 hours after ingestion of a sustained-release product may be discharged. Activated charcoal has been advocated for all patients, but gastric lavage and emesis should be undertaken with caution, if at all, as the resulting vagal maneuver may worsen preexisting bradycardia. Multiple doses of activated charcoal should be considered in the patient who has ingested a sustained-release preparation. Correction of hypovolemia should be a priority. Calcium salts have been advocated as specific therapy, although reports of benefit are conflicting.[41] Administration of calcium salts to maintain at least normal calcium is reasonable. Alternately, administer calcium gluconate at 20–40 mg/kg (0.2–0.4 ml/kg of 10% solution) IV over 5 minutes, with an infusion of 20–40 mg/kg/hr if there is a favorable response. Care should be undertaken to avoid extravasations of peripherally administered calcium, and monitor carefully its serum concentration, especially in the context of concurrent digoxin administration. Insulin and glucagon have both been recommended for calcium channel blocker overdose. The latter is thought to directly affect myocardial contractility. If used, administer a regular insulin bolus of 1.0 U/kg, followed by an infusion of 1.0 U/kg/hr for the first hour, then 0.5 U/kg/hr until toxicity resolves. At the same time a 0.5 g/kg bolus of glucose is administered with an additional 0.5 g/kg/hr until insulin is discontinued. Frequent monitoring of glucose (hourly during treatment and hourly until 6 hours after treatment) and potassium is required with this regimen.

Supportive care of the child with a calcium channel blocker intoxication is challenging. Many strategies have been advocated with varying success. Fluid replacement should be undertaken with caution to avoid pulmonary edema. Inotropic support with dopamine, epinephrine, or norepinephrine may be required; however, myocardium and vascular smooth muscle may be resistant to conventional doses. No consensus exists regarding the superiority of one drug over another. Amrinone in conjunction with glucagon was reported successful in treating one patient with refractory hypertension secondary to verapamil overdose.[42] No controlled studies have been published to date suggesting their routine use. Atropine may be administered for appropriate arrhythmias, although its benefit is unproven. Cardiac pacing may be undertaken for bradyarrhythmias resistant to therapy.[43] Both intra-aortic balloon counterpulsation and cardiopulmonary bypass have been reported as successful in restoring hemodynamic stability.[44] A retrospective study of patients with symptomatic calcium channel blocker overdose reported that both calcium and dopamine were effective in restoring blood pressure and cardiac rhythm to all patients who received them.[45]

Antihypertensives

Clonidine

Clonidine is a centrally acting antihypertensive agent. Its mechanism of action is the stimulation of central α receptors. It has no peripheral α receptor activity. It is widely used in the treatment of hypertension, and is useful in the management of narcotic withdrawal. Its widespread use makes it a frequent source of pediatric poisonings. α-Methyldopa, another clinically useful centrally acting antihypertensive, is far more infrequently prescribed and is therefore uncommonly accidentally ingested.

Clonidine therapy in adults is commonly initiated at a dose of 0.1 mg, and 1 tablet may be sufficient to cause symptoms in a small child. Overdose may occur when a small child has access to the pills of a parent or caregiver, or as the result of an intentional overdose in an older child. Symptomatic clonidine overdose presents as bradycardia, hypotension, lethargy, coma, and miosis. Respiratory depression sufficient to require mechanical ventilation is common in severely intoxicated patients. Hypotension may be modest or absent, but may occasionally require therapy. A large review of 10,060 clonidine exposures reported to the American Association of Poison Control Centers revealed that 60% of the patients were symptomatic, lethargy being the most common symptom (80%).[46] Bradycardia, hypotension, and respiratory depression were each observed, in decreasing frequency.

Basic management of clonidine poisoning includes decontamination with activated charcoal. Airway protection and mechanical ventilation are needed in the unconscious or severely lethargic patient. Hypothermia may be corrected with surface warming. Hypotension is usually responsive to fluid administration. Occasionally, vasopressor agents may be indicated. As the mechanism of clonidine resembles that of opioid (narcotic) agonists, naloxone has occasionally been recommended.[47] It may be diagnostically useful, but supportive measures will frequently be satisfactory until the drug is eliminated. Tolazoline, an α-adrenergic antagonist,

has been considered as theoretically useful[48] but has also failed to be of benefit in individual case reports.[49] The outcome of conservatively managed clonidine overdose is generally good, and death is rare.

Angiotensin-Converting Enzyme Inhibitors

Angiotensin-converting enzyme (ACE) inhibitors are among the most commonly prescribed drugs in the management of hypertension and congestive heart failure in adults, and are frequently used in combination with other agents such as β-blockers and centrally acting agents. Captopril and enalapril are commonly used in children for these indications. Symptomatic hypotension is rare, but acute overdose may be accompanied by profound and prolonged hypotension.[50] ACE inhibitors reduce systemic vascular resistance, but may induce renal insufficiency.[51] Hyperkalemia has been observed at therapeutic doses, and renal insufficiency may occur as a consequence of ACE inhibition.[52] The emergency physician should be mindful of the possibility that preexisting disease and concurrent therapy in the patient prescribed an ACE inhibitor may compound the risk for renal insufficiency and hyperkalemia.[53]

Hypotension in the patient who has acutely ingested an ACE inhibitor is frequently responsive to fluid administration. Vasopressors are occasionally required.[54] Hypotension encountered in the patient who is using an ACE inhibitor for therapeutic purposes is similarly managed, keeping in mind that symptoms of congestive heart failure may be worsened in doing so. Hyperkalemia and renal insufficiency should be addressed with the appropriate laboratory studies and acute interventions. There is no accepted antidotal therapy.

Vasodilators

Oral vasodilators are less commonly prescribed in the management of hypertension in children and adults, and, therefore, infrequently seen as causes of pediatric poisonings. Hydralazine overdose has only been reported in the adult literature. Hypotension is the predominant symptom, but electrocardiographic changes suggestive of ischemia are also described.[55] There is no consensus on therapy, but the aforementioned patient, who was additionally ethanol intoxicated, responded to conservative management. Hydralazine has been implicated in drug-induced lupus, which is characterized by arthralgia, myalgia, pleurisy, rashes, fever, and a positive antinuclear antibody screen. Procainamide, and to a lesser extent β-blockers, methyldopa, quinidine, and numerous other drugs, have also been implicated.[56] Recognition by the emergency physician is important, as resolution of the syndrome occurs within a few weeks of discontinuation of the drug.

Nitrates are used in the management of angina, congestive heart failure, and hypertension in adults. Children who have ingested an oral nitrate preparation may present with flushing, headache, tachycardia, and hypotension resulting in syncope. As the effect is short lived, the symptomatic patient may improve prior to arrival in the ED. Management is similar to that of other vasodilators. In addition to inadvertent overdose, the nitrates are also drugs of abuse (see Chapter 135, Drugs of Abuse). Methemoglobinemia and hemolytic anemia have been reported.[57,58] The intoxicated patient presents with cyanosis and acidosis, but normal external oxygen tension. Diagnosis is confirmed by the demonstration of an elevated methemoglobin concentration by co-oximetry. Hereditary deficiency in the enzyme glucose-6-phosphate dehydrogenase may predispose the individual to this occurrence. Limited experience with nitrite-induced methemoglobinemia suggests that it responds to the administration of methylene blue in a manner similar to other etiologies[59] (see Chapter 133, Common Pediatric Overdoses).

Nitroprusside is widely used in the management of a hypertensive emergency. Chronic complications include methemoglobinemia and hemolytic anemia, which are not encountered in the acute overdose, and are unlikely to be seen in the emergency management of children. The degradation of nitroprusside releases cyanide, which is once again rarely problematic in the ED. Thiocyanate is formed with the degradation of nitroprusside after administration. Levels are of no use in predicting nitroprusside toxicity. Hypotension is treated by decreasing or discontinuing the medication, which has a half-life of minutes.[60]

Minoxidil is a potent vasodilator prescribed for the treatment of severe hypertension. It is rarely used in childhood. Hirsuitism is a side effect that accompanies its chronic use and, it has been marketed as an over-the-counter drug intended for topical use. Overdose in childhood has rarely been observed, but intentional ingestion of the hair treatment by an adult produced severe hypotension and tachycardia that required massive fluid administration, vasopressor support, and mechanical ventilation.[61]

Diuretics

Diuretics are widely used in both children and adults in the management of hypertension and congestive heart failure. Their availability makes them frequently seen in accidental overdose. Additionally, the emergency physician may be called upon to evaluate a child with a preexisting illness for which diuretic therapy has been undertaken.

Diuretics are commonly classified as either potassium wasting or potassium sparing. The former consist of the potent loop diuretics, including furosemide and ethacrynic acid, and the thiazide diuretics. Potassium wasting is commonplace, and secondary metabolic alkalosis is frequently seen as a consequence of attendant urinary hydrogen ion excretion. Calciuria also occurs with the loop agents, but hypocalcemia is rarely a problem in the acute setting. Potassium-sparing agents include the aldosterone antagonist spironolactone, and acetazolamide, a carbonic anhydrase inhibitor. As their classification implies, therapeutic use of these drugs is not accompanied by hypokalemia.

The child with acute overdose is rarely a therapeutic challenge. Ingestion of loop diuretics and thiazides present more acute problems than do the potassium-sparing agents. Dehydration may occasionally be seen, as well as electrolyte disturbances. Hyponatremia is generally mild. Hypokalemia may be present after an acute ingestion, but is more common with chronic therapeutic use. Appropriate fluid and electrolyte replacement should be undertaken.[62]

Chronic complications of diuretic use include hypokalemia, severe metabolic alkalosis, and, with loop diuretic use, hypocalcemia. Occasionally tetany may be seen, requiring the cautious administration of intravenous calcium (see Chapter 115, Hypocalcemia). Seizures and hypocalcemic prolongation of the QT interval are rarely seen.[63] Chronic use of loop diuretics is associated with pancreatitis.[64] Renal insufficiency may be worsened by diuretic therapy when administered concurrently with an ACE inhibitor.[65] Caution should be undertaken in the fluid replacement of a child who presents with diuretic-induced dehydration, renal insufficiency, and the concurrent use of a loop diuretic and potassium-sparing agent.

Acetazolamide is infrequently used as a diuretic, but more commonly prescribed in the control of intraocular pressure and pseudotumor cerebri. Acetazolamide toxicity may present with significant metabolic acidosis, manifesting as lethargy and Kussmaul's respirations. A toddler reported to have ingested 10 g of acetazolamide recovered completely with the administration of sodium bicarbonate.[66]

Digoxin

Digoxin is a member of a group of glycosides derived from the foxglove plant and increases cardiac contractility and automaticity. Digoxin and digitoxin are the sole agents currently in use. Therefore, they are still widely used in the management of congestive heart failure and arrhythmias in both children and adults. They have a narrow therapeutic index, and poisoning is common both in the setting of clinical use and in accidental ingestion. Cardiac glycosides are found in many common decorative plants such as yellow oleander, and accidental ingestion presents with symptoms similar to digitalis poisoning. Because of its prolonged kinetics, digoxin therapy is frequently initiated by a loading dose, commonly 35 to 50 mcg/kg, given in divided doses over several days, followed by maintenance therapy of 7 to 10 mcg/kg/dose every 12 hours. The dose is adjusted in the face of renal insufficiency.

Digoxin has a large volume of distribution, being concentrated in the muscle mass. Bioavailability after oral ingestion is variable, depending substantially on the manufacturer. For that reason Lanoxin is the most widely prescribed agent, in which nearly 90% of an oral dose is absorbed. Onset of effect is between 1.5 and 6 hours. It is slowly excreted intact by the kidneys. A decrease in renal function or significant dehydration may provoke digoxin intoxication in the patient who has previously been safely taking a given dose. In this setting, peritoneal dialysis may be useful in addition to the other measures undertaken to treat digitalis intoxication.[67] Digoxin impairs the Na^+/K^+ membrane pump, increasing intracellular sodium and impairing Na^+-Ca^{2+}-dependent egress of calcium from the cell, thereby enhancing contractility. The transmembrane potential is raised, increasing automaticity. Digoxin also increases cardiac vagal tone, slowing the heart rate and delaying atrioventricular nodal conduction. As digoxin's effect is dependent on its membrane-bound fraction, serum digoxin levels, although widely available, are poor prognostic indicators for the development of digitoxicity.[68] Intracellular electrolytes, although not widely available, may be a sensitive indicator of the risk for digitoxicity.[69] Therapeutic drug monitoring may be more useful in specific settings, such as the management of congestive heart failure in a patient with renal impairment. Elevated digoxin levels in the correct clinical setting may be of assistance in establishing the diagnosis of digitoxicity, but too great an overlap exists between therapeutic and toxic levels to use the digoxin level as a sole index of toxicity.[70]

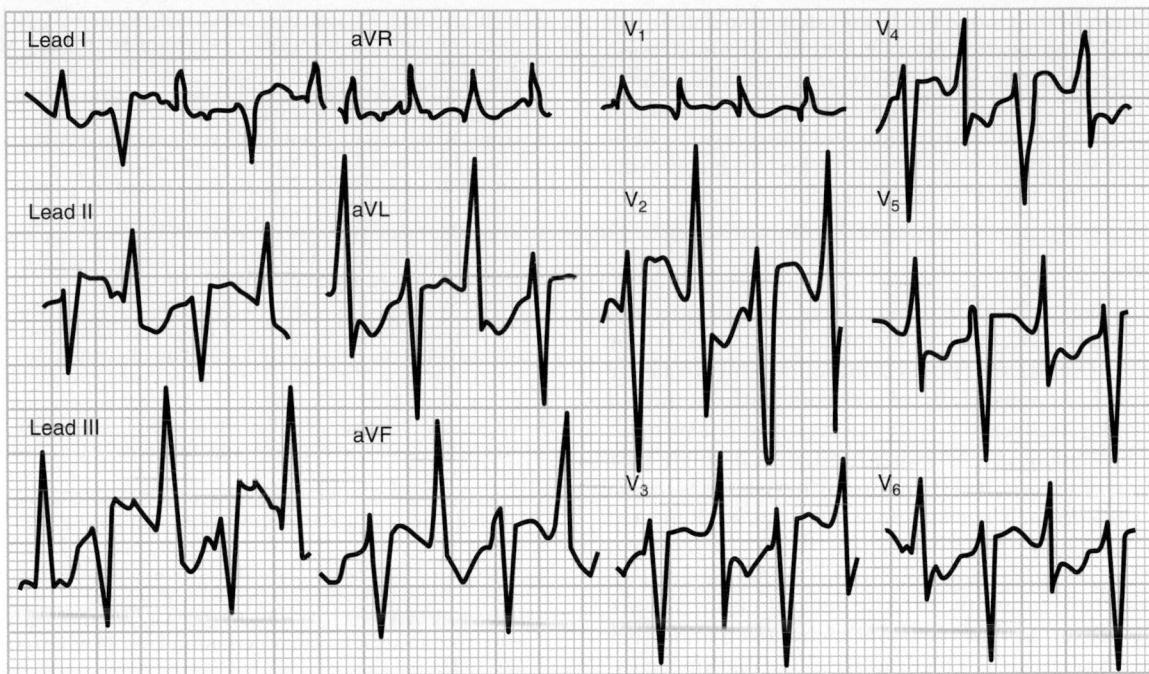

FIGURE 137–2. Bidirectional ventricular tachycardia.

Acute digoxin poisoning presents with vomiting, bradycardia, and arrhythmias, frequently heart block and bradycardia, although virtually any cardiac rhythm disturbance may be attributed to digitalis poisoning. Hyperkalemia is frequently observed and may be life threatening. Chronic digoxin poisoning may present with an array of bizarre complaints, including vomiting, anorexia, weakness, altered mental status, and visual disturbances such as altered color perception. Cardiac manifestations of poisoning include ventricular arrhythmias, heart block, and nodal escape rhythms. Rhythm disturbances commonly manifest some form of myocardial irritability with delayed conduction. Bidirectional ventricular tachycardia is thought to be particularly characteristic of digitalis poisoning[71] (Fig. 137–2).

Emesis is not recommended in digoxin poisoning, as it may increase vagal tone, exacerbating bradycardia. Activated charcoal binds digoxin well, and should be given. Multiple-dose activated charcoal is not clearly beneficial.[72] There are no data on the efficacy of catharsis. Dialysis is of no benefit.

The development of digoxin-specific antibody fragments (Fab) has significantly altered the management of digoxin poisoning. Administration rapidly reverses bradycardia, arrhythmias, and hyperkalemia associated with digoxin poisoning and related, naturally occurring, cardiac glycosides.[73,74] It is effective in the treatment of poisoning due to digoxin, digitoxin, and congeners, as well as the naturally occurring glycosides.[75] Fab should be given to patients with any dysrrhythmia causing hemodynamic compromise or with a serum potassium level greater than 10 mEq/L.[76] It should be given after ingestion of more than 4 mg in a child without underlying disease, and may be given intravenously or by the intraosseous route. The amount administered may be determined by the following formula if the dose taken is known[77]:

Number of Fab vials (38 mg/vial) = amount ingested (mg)
× 0.48 (mg neutralized/vial)

If the dose is unknown, the amount given may be determined by the steady state serum digoxin concentration 6 hours after the ingestion:

Number of Fab vials = serum digoxin level (ng/ml)
× body weight (kg)/100

Fab is also useful in the treatment of chronic digoxin intoxication. The previous equation may be used, obtaining the steady state concentration. If the dose ingested is unknown, 5 vials may be given to a child, 10 to 20 vials to an acutely intoxicated adult, or 10 vials to an adult with chronic toxicity.

Atropine is useful as an antidote and is indicated for severe bradycardia. Phenytoin and lidocaine were both previously considered primary therapy for the treatment of ventricular dysrhythmias, and may still be useful in the absence of Fab, or as adjunctive therapy.[78] Amiodarone has been reported to be of assistance in the conversion of ventricular fibrillation.[79] Magnesium has occasionally been reported to be of assistance in the conversion of ventricular arrhythmias attendant to chronic digitalis poisoning.

Miscellaneous Agents

Amrinone and Milrinone

Amrinone and milrinone are bipyridine derivatives useful in the management of congestive heart failure, and have both inotropic and vasodilator properties. Although commonly used in inpatient settings for the management of shock and low cardiac output postoperative states, they are also used in the outpatient setting and may rarely present as an overdose. Oral overdose is usually well tolerated. Amrinone is associated with thrombocytopenia. Milrinone, which is not associated with this adverse effect, is more commonly prescribed.

Administration of milrinone has been rarely associated with hypotension. Vasopressor support and fluid administration may rarely be required. One fatality was reported after a massive intravenous overdose,[80] manifesting as hypotension unresponsive to fluid administration and vasopressors. Peritoneal dialysis was ineffective. An adult who had tachycardia attributed to milrinone was successfully treated with β-blockers.[81]

Adenosine

Adenosine is useful in the conversion of supraventricular tachyarrhythmias sustained by atrioventricular reentry by prolonging atrioventricular nodal conduction time. In a large series of cardioversions, 72% of patients with presumed supraventricular tachycardia were successfully converted.[82] The half-life of adenosine is short, limited to a single pass through the circulation. It is therefore administered by rapid intravenous injection. The usual dose is 0.1 mg/kg. Repeated administration may be undertaken, with incremental increases of 0.05 mg/kg, to a dose of 0.2 mg/kg or until an effect is observed. In another study, 96% of children were successfully converted, but recurrent tachycardia and other significant complications, including atrial fibrillation, accelerated ventricular tachycardia, apnea, and asystole, occurred.[83] Continuous monitoring and equipment should be available in this event. Prolonged heart block and ventricular fibrillation may be encountered in the setting of administration of adenosine with digoxin, calcium channel blockers, or class IA antiarrhythmics.[84,85] Adenosine can cause cardiac arrest in de-inervated hearts (post-transplant), high degree heart block in patients who already have second degree heart block or who are on carbemazepine, and bronchospasm in asthmatics (especially if they are taking theophylline preparations).

Summary

Complications of cardiac drugs are fortunately infrequent. When they do occur, they are frequently managed in the ED. The principles of management revolve around attention to basic hemodynamic stabilization, followed by specific therapy based on knowledge of the drug. Correction of hypotension, restoration of a stable rhythm, attention to fluid and electrolyte balance, and support of ventilation will optimize therapy directed toward an individual agent.

REFERENCES

*1. Watson WA, Litovitz TL, Klein-Schwartz W, et al: 2003 Annual report of the American Association of Poison Control Centers Toxic Exposure Surveillance System. Am J Emerg Med 22:335–404, 2004.
*2. Roden DM: Drug Therapy: Drug-induced prolongation of the QT interval. N Engl J Med 350:1013–1022, 2004.
3. Lin JC, Quasny HA: QT prolongation and development of torsades de pointes with the concomitant administration of oral erythromycin base and quinidine. Pharmacotherapy 17:626–630, 1997.
*4. Trujillo TC, Nolan PE: Antiarrhythmic agents: drug interactions of clinical significance. Drug Saf 23:509–532, 2000.
5. Jenzer HR, Hagemeijer F: Quinidine syncope: torsades de pointes with low quinidine plasma concentrations. Eur J Cardiol 4:447–451, 1976.
6. Kim SY, Benowitz NL: Poisoning due to class IA antiarrhythmic drugs—quinidine, procainamide and disopyramide. Drug Saf 5:393–420, 1990.
7. Wolf LR, Otten EJ, Spadafora MP: Cinchonism: two case reports and review of acute quinine toxicity and treatment. J Emerg Med 10:295–301, 1992.
8. Bateman DN, Dyson EH: Quinine toxicity. Adverse Drug React Acute Poisoning Rev 5:215–233, 1986.
9. Hruby K, Missliwetz J: Poisoning with oral antiarrhythmic drugs. Int J Clin Pharmacol Ther Toxicol 23:253–257, 1985.
10. Gowda RM, Khan IA, Wilbur SL, et al: Torsade de pointes: the clinical considerations. Int J Cardiol 96:1–6, 2004.
11. Bailie DS, Inoue H, Kaseda S, et al: Magnesium suppression of early afterdepolarizations and ventricular tachyarrhythmias induced by cesium in dogs. Circulation 77:1395–1402, 1988.
12. Pinski SL, Eguia LE, Trohman RG: What is the minimal pacing rate that prevents torsades de pointes? Insights from patients with permanent pacemakers. Pacing Clin Electrophysiol 25:1612–1615, 2002.
13. Hess GP, Walson PD: Seizures secondary to oral viscous lidocaine. Ann Emerg Med 17:725–727, 1988.
14. Denaro CP, Benowitz NL: Poisoning due to class 1B antiarrhythmic drugs: lignocaine, mexiletine and tocainide. Med Toxicol Adverse Drug Exp 4:412–428, 1989.
15. Ryan CA, Robertson M, Coe JY: Seizures due to lidocaine toxicity in a child during cardiac catheterization. Pediatr Cardiol 14:116–118, 1993.
16. Edgren B, Tilelli J, Gehrz R: Intravenous lidocaine overdosage in a child. J Toxicol Clin Toxicol 24:51–58, 1986.
17. Freedman MD, Gal J, Freed CR: Extracorporeal pump assistance—novel treatment for licocaine poisoning. Eur J Clin Pharmacol 22:129–135, 1982.
18. Mortensen ME, Bolon CE, Kelley MT, et al: Encainide overdose in an infant. Ann Emerg Med 21:998–1001, 1992.
19. Kennerdy A, Thomas P, Sheridan DJ: Generalized seizures as the presentation of flecainide toxicity. Eur Heart J 10:950–954, 1989.
20. Pond SM: Extracorporeal techniques in the treatment of poisoned patients. Med J Aust 154:617–622, 1991.
21. Frishman W, Jacob H, Eisemberg E, et al: Clinical pharmacology of the new beta-adrenergic blocking drugs. Am Heart J 98:798–811, 1979.
22. Lifshitz M, Zucker N, Zalzstein E: Acute dilated cardiomyopathy and central nervous sytem toxicity following propranolol intoxication. Pediatr Emerg Care 15:262–263, 1999.
23. Boskabady MH, Snashall PD: Bronchial responsiveness to beta-adrenergic stimulation and enhanced beta-blockade in asthma. Respirology 5:111–118, 2000.
24. Hesse B, Pederson JT: Hypoglycaemia after propranolol in children. Acta Med Scand 193:551–552, 1973.
25. Love JN, Silka N: Are 1-2 tablets dangerous? Beta-blocker exposure in toddlers. J Emerg Med 26:309–314, 2004.
26. Reith DM, Dawson AH, Epid D, et al: Relative toxicity of beta blockers in overdose. J Toxicol Clin Toxicol 34:273–278, 1996.
27. Langemeijer JJ, de Wildt DJ, de Groot G, Sangster B: Intoxication with beta-sympathicolytics. Neth J Med 40:308–315, 1992.
28. Kerns W, Kline J, Ford MD: Beta-blocker and calcium channel blocker toxicity. Emerg Med Clin North Am 12:365–390, 1994.
29. Boyd R, Gosh A: Glucagon for the treatment of symptomatic β blocker overdose. Emerg Med J 20:266–267, 2003.
30. Bailey B: Glucagon in beta-blocker and calcium channel blocker overdoses: a systematic review. J Toxicol Clin Toxicol 41:595–602, 2003.
31. Lane AS, Woodward AC, Goldman MR: Massive propranolol overdose poorly responsive to pharmacologic therapy: use of the intra-aortic balloon pump. Ann Emerg Med 16:1381–1383, 1987.
32. Hohnloser SH: Proarrhythmia with class III antiarrhythmic drugs: types, risks, and management. Am J Cardiol 80:82G–89G, 1997.
33. Hohnloser SH, Woosley RL: Sotalol. N Engl J Med 331:31–38, 1994.
*34. Leatham EW, Holt DW, McKenna WJ: Class III antiarrhythmics in overdose: presenting features and management principles. Drug Saf 9:450–462, 1993.
35. Assimes TL, Malcolm I: Torsade de pointes with sotalol overdose treated successfully with lidocaine. Can J Cardiol 14:753–756, 1998.
36. Hohnloser SH, Klingenheben T, Singh BN: Amiodarone-associated proarrhythmic effects: a review with special reference to torsade de pointes tachycardia. Ann Intern Med 121:529–535, 1994.
37. Guccione P, Paul T, Garson A Jr: Long-term follow-up of amiodarone therapy in the young: continued efficacy, unimpaired growth, moderate side effects. J Am Coll Cardiol 15:1118–1124, 1990.
38. Abernathy DR, Schwartz JB: Calcium-antagonist drugs. N Engl J Med 341:1447–1457, 1999.

---

*Suggested readings.

39. Belson MG, Gorman SE, Sullivan K, Geller RJ: Calcium channel blocker ingestions in children. Am J Emerg Med 18:581–586, 2000.

40. Brass BJ, Winchester-Penny S, Lipper BL: Massive verapamil overdose complicated by noncardiogenic pulmonary edema. Am J Emerg Med 14:459–461, 1996.

41. Salhanick SD, Shannon MW: Management of calcium channel antagonist overdosage. Drug Saf 26:65–79, 2003.

42. Wolf LR, Spadafora MP, Otten EJ: Use of amrinone and glucagons in a case of calcium channel blocker overdose. Ann Emerg Med 22:1225–1228, 1993.

43. Proano L, Chiang WK, Wang RY: Calcium channel blocker overdose. Am J Emerg Med 13:444–450, 1995.

44. Durward A, Guerguerian AM, Lefebvre M, Shemie SD: Massive diltiazem overdose treated with extracorporeal membrane oxygenation. Pediatr Crit Care Med 4:372–376, 2003.

45. Ramoska EA, Spiller HA, Winter M, Borys D: A one-year evaluation of calcium channel blocker overdoses: toxicity and treatment. Ann Emerg Med 22:196–200, 1993.

46. Klein Schwartz W: Trends and toxic effects from pediatric clonidine exposures. Arch Pediatr Adolesc Med 156:392–396, 2002.

47. Kappagoda C, Schell DN, Hanson RM, Hutchins P: Clonidine overdose in childhood: implications of increased prescribing. J Paediatr Child Health 34:508–512, 1998.

48. Anderson RJ, Hart GR, Crumpler CP, Lerman MJ: Clonidine overdose: report of six cases and review of the literature. Ann Emerg Med 10:107–112, 1981.

49. Olsson JM, Priutt AW: Management of clonidine ingestion in children. J Pediatr 103:646–650, 1983.

50. Barr CS, Payne R, Newton RW: Profound prolonged hypotension following captopril overdose. Postgrad Med J 67:953–954, 1991.

51. Navis G, Faber HJ, de Zeeuw D, de Jong PE: ACE inhibitors and the kidney: a risk-benefit assessment. Drug Saf 15:200–211, 1996.

52. Warner NJ, Rush JE: Safety profiles of the angiotensin-converting enzyme inhibitors. Drugs 35(Suppl 5):89–97, 1988.

53. Rimmer JM, Horn JF, Gennari FJ: Hyperkalemia as a complication of drug therapy. Arch Intern Med 147:867–869, 1987.

54. Lip GY, Ferner RE: Poisoning with antihypertensive drugs: angiotensin converting enzyme inhibitors. J Hum Hypertens 9:711–715, 1995.

55. Smith BA, Ferguson DB: Acute hydralazine overdose: marked ECG abnormalities in a young adult. Ann Emerg Med 21:326–330, 1992.

56. Price EJ, Venables PJ: Drug-induced lupus. Drug Saf 12:283–290, 1995.

57. Stainikowicz R, Amitai Y, Bentur Y. Aphrodisiac drug-induced hemolysis. J Toxicol Clin Toxicol 42:313–316, 2004.

58. Romanelli F, Smith KM, Thornton AC, Pomeroy C: Poppers: epidemiology and clinical management of inhaled nitrite. Pharmacotherapy 24:69–78, 2004.

59. Modarai B, Kapadia YK, Kerins M, Terris J: Methylene blue: a treatment for severe methaemoglobinaemia secondary to misuse of amyl nitrite. Emerg Med J 19:271–272, 2002.

60. Curry SC, Arnold-Capell P: Toxic effects of drugs used in the ICU: nitroprusside, nitroglycerin, and angiotensin-converting enzyme inhibitors. Crit Care Clin 7:555–581, 1991.

61. Farrell, SE, Epstein SK: Overdose of Rogaine Extra Strength for Men topical minoxidil. J Toxicol Clin Toxicol 37:781–783, 1999.

62. Lip GYH, Ferner RE: Poisoning with antihypertensive drugs: diuretics and potassium supplements. J Hum Hypertens 9:295–301, 1995.

63. Chvilicek JP, Hurlbert BJ, Hill GE: Diuretic-induced hypokalaemia inducing torsades de pointes. Can J Anaesth 42:1137–1139, 1995.

64. Lankisch PG, Droge M, Gottesleben F: Drug induced acute pancreatitis: incidence and severity. Gut 37:565–567, 1995.

*65. Loboz KK, Shenfield GM: Drug combinations and impaired renal function—the 'triple whammy.' Br J Clin Pharmacol 59:239–243, 2005.

66. Baer E, Reith DM: Acetazolamide poisoning in a toddler. J Paediatr Child Health 37:411–412, 2001.

67. Berkovitch M, Akilesh MR, Gerace R, et al: Acute digoxin overdose in a newborn with renal failure: use of digoxin immune Fab and peritoneal dialysis. Ther Drug Monit 16:531–533, 1994.

68. McCormick W, Ingelfinger JA, Isakson G, Goldman P: Errors in measuring drug concentrations. N Engl J Med 299:1118–1121, 1978.

69. Loes MW, Singh S, Lock JE, Mirkin BL: Relation between plasma and red-cell electrolyte concentrations and digoxin levels in children. N Engl J Med 299:501–504, 1978.

70. Biddle TL, Weintraub M, Lasagna L: Relationship of serium and myocardial digoxin concentration to electrocardiographic estimation of digoxin intoxication. J Clin Pharmacol 18:10–15, 1978.

71. Ma G, Brady WJ, Pollack M, Chan TC: Electrocardiographic manifestations: digitalis toxicity. J Emerg Med 20:145–152, 2001.

72. Position statement and practice guidelines on the use of multi-dose activated charcoal in the treatment of acute poisoning. American Academy of Clinical Toxicology; European Association of Poison Control Centres and Clinical Toxicologists. J Toxicol Clin Toxicol 37:731–751, 1999.

73. Antman EM, Wenger TL, Butler VP, et al: Treatment of 150 cases of life-threatening digitalis intoxication with digoxin-specific Fab antibody fragments: final report of a multicenter study. Circulation 81:1774–1752, 1990.

74. Cheung K, Urech R, Taylor L, et al: Plant cardiac glycosides and digoxin Fab antibody. J Paediatr Child Health 27:312–313, 1991.

75. Flanagan RJ, Jones AL: Fab antibody fragments: some applications in clinical toxicology. Drug Saf 27:1115–1133, 2004.

76. Marchlinski FE, Hook BG, Callans DJ: Which cardiac disturbances should be treated with digoxin immune Fab (ovine) antibody? Am J Emerg Med 9(2 Suppl 1):24–28, 1991.

77. Heard K: Digoxin and therapeutic cardiac glycosides. In Dart R, Caravati EM, et al (eds): Medical Toxicology, 3rd ed. Philadelphia: JB Lippincott, 2004, pp 700–706.

78. Rumack BH, Wolfe RR, Gilfrich H: Phenytoin treatment of massive digoxin overdose. Br Heart J 36:405–408, 1974.

79. Nicholls DP, Murtagh JG, Holt DW: Use of amiodarone and digoxin specific Fab antibodies in digoxin overdosage. Br Heart J 53:462–464, 1985.

80. Lebovitz DJ, Lawless ST, Weise KL: Fatal amrinone overdose in a pediatric patient. Crit Care Med 23:977–980, 1995.

81. Alhashemi JA, Hooper J: Treatment of milrinone-associated tachycardia with beta-blockers. Can J Anaesth 45:67–70, 1998.

82. Losek JD, Endom E, Dietrich A, et al: Adenosine and pediatric supraventricular tachycardia in the emergency department: multicenter study. Ann Emerg Med 33:185–191, 1999.

83. Crosson JE: Therapeutic and diagnostic utility of adenosine during tachycardia evaluation in children. Am J Cardiol 74:155–160, 1994.

84. Mulla N, Karpawich PP: Ventricular fibrillation following adenosine therapy for supraventricular tachycardia in a neonate with concealed Wolff-Parkinson-White syndrome treated with digoxin. Pediatr Emerg Care 11:238–239, 1995.

85. Lowenstein SR, Laperin BD, Reiter MJ: Paroxysmal supraventricular tachycardias. J Emerg Med 14:39–51, 1996.

SECTION V

Approach to Environmental Illness and Injury

Chapter 138

Near Drowning and Submersion Injuries

T. Kent Denmark, MD and Steven C. Rogers, MD

Key Points

The literature predicting outcome of submersion injury is contradictory.

Rare, evidence-based, guideline-defying recoveries occur.

Technological advances have not affected outcomes.

Patients who remain asymptomatic for 4 to 6 hours may be discharged home.

Introduction and Background

While more common in temperate climates, submersion injuries and drowning will be encountered and managed by every emergency physician at some point during his or her career. Drowning deaths occur throughout the United States, in decreasing order, from the South, West, Midwest, and Mid-Atlantic to New England.[1] Drowning is the second leading cause of injurious deaths in children 1 to 14 years of age. The Centers for Disease Control estimates that over 2000 children less than 4 years of age seek medical attention for near drowning per year. In addition, 1000 children ages 5 to 14 years, and approximately 900 adolescents, will also be treated for near drowning.[2] The most dangerous water exposures occur with children less than 4 years of age in either pools or bathtubs.[3-5] In contrast to the exploratory behavior of children, adolescents who have submersion injuries or drown are usually intoxicated and swimming at lakes or rivers.[6] Adolescent incidents tend to occur while swimming or boating and are usually witnessed.[3] There is an additional sense of tragedy when these cases are encountered in the emergency department (ED) because drowning is one of the most preventable causes of morbidity and mortality.

Drowning and submersion injuries continue to occur in large part due to lack of recognition of the danger on the part of parents and caregivers. A study of parental beliefs and practices regarding home safety showed that the potential injury severity and extent of effort required to implement the safety practices determined which precautions were undertaken.[7] Parents simply do not believe their particular child is at risk, and their assumptions about the inherent safety of an above-ground pool are inaccurate.[7] Partial preventative efforts may not be enough to prevent submersion or drowning from occurring. For example, two thirds of 4-year-olds can scale a smooth 48-inch barrier in less than 2 minutes.[8] Appreciation of this information may enable emergency physicians to serve as an important resource for home safety education.[9]

One of the most distressing decisions in managing a patient who has drowned is the decision to discontinue the resuscitation. While clinical guidelines exist, several cases have been reported in the medical literature and in the popular media that defy these guidelines. First documented by Kvittingen in 1963, there are several reports of "near drownings" in patients who fully recovered from significant submersion events of up to 66 minutes.[10,11] Therefore, family members' expectations of resuscitation outcome may be inaccurate and overly optimistic. The media have contributed to these beliefs by focusing on the dichotomous outcomes from arrest while completely ignoring the severe neurologic impairment that may result from a significant cardiopulmonary arrest.[12] The reality is that hospitalized near-drowning victims in the United States have a high case fatality rate (~25%) and high rate of subsequent sequelae (10%).[4] This is consistent with a comprehensive study in the British Isles that found that greater than one third of admitted patients either expired or had residual neurologic deficits following a near-drowning incident.[13] Therefore, the treating physician should be mindful of these faulty beliefs when informing the family about management decisions. In spite of an increase in understanding of the pathophysiology of submersion injuries and advances in therapy, the mortality has not significantly decreased, but the number of neurologically impaired children who survive may be increasing.[4,14,15]

Recognition and Approach

The physiologic response to submersion has been studied extensively. The initial response to a cold water submersion is tachypnea, tachycardia, and hypertension for 1 to 2 minutes followed by apnea 3 minutes after submersion and finally hypotension and asystole between 6 and 8 minutes postsubmersion.[16-18] Either electroencephalographic silence or seizure activity occurs with hypotension prior to asystole.[18] The rapidity of significant physiologic changes in submersion victims underscores the necessity of supervisory vigilance and prevention.

Some children survive prolonged submersions, and a number of explanations for this phenomenon have been offered. The diving reflex, defined as apnea, generalized marked peripheral vasoconstriction, and bradycardia, is well described in marine mammals and has been generally accepted as the mechanism for survival.[19] However, given that breath-holding duration is decreased by 25% upon rapid exposure to water colder than 15° C, the theory of the diving reflex as an explanation for remarkable recoveries is questionable.[17,20] In addition, it has been proven that, even with the greater body surface area of infants, surface cooling does not occur quickly enough to be cerebroprotective.[21-23] Hypothermia is only protective if the central nervous system (CNS) temperature drops by greater than 7° C in 10 minutes.[24] Aspiration of cold water causes rapid cooling when compared to submersion.[16]

Dog studies have shown that rapid, involuntary respirations occur following submersion for a little more than a minute.[25] Extremely rapid core cooling can occur within 2 minutes of submersion when cold water is aspirated, leading to rapid core cooling to protective levels, which occurs about 1 minute before cardiac arrest.[16,18] Microaspiration with initial tachypnea will cause rapid cooling of circulation, which is preferentially shunted to the CNS.[19] Animals resuscitated with cold solutions following 20 minutes of arrest have good functional recovery compared those resuscitated with room-temperature fluids.[26] Pulmonary vasoconstriction and pulmonary hypertension following aspiration are attenuated when cold fluid is aspirated.[27] This may help explain the miraculous cases of full recovery from extended submersions.

Studies of military and competitive swimmers show that even body-only immersion increases cardiac preload and pulmonary arterial pressure from peripheral vasoconstriction.[28] Subsequently, ventilation-perfusion (V/Q) mismatch, hypoxemia, and pulmonary vasoconstriction will lead to a decrease in functional residual capacity.[28] This clinically manifests itself as tachypnea to compensate for inefficient gas exchange. Swimming-induced pulmonary edema occurs in about 2% of healthy competitive swimmers and presents with dyspnea, cough, and hemoptysis.[29] The effects may still be detected on pulmonary function tests for up to a week.[29] Patients who are actually submerged have more extensive sequelae. Surfactant loss or inactivation decreases pulmonary compliance, and there may be significant V/Q mismatch, with 75% of blood flow to nonventilated areas.[30,31]

Clinical Presentation

In most cases, the history of submersion is known or apparent as relayed by rescue personnel, parents, or bystanders. History can be especially helpful in a witnessed event when trying to differentiate between primary submersion injury and an event secondary to another process such as seizure or arrhythmia. While seizures can occur from anoxia, seizure activity prior to submersion or in a patient with a history of epilepsy should raise concern for a primary neurologic process.[18] Patients with a history of seizures or epilepsy have a 10-fold increased risk for drowning.[32] Typical epileptic submersion victims are older than 5 years of age and in the bathtub, although children and adolescents with epilepsy are also at increased risk of drowning in pools.[32] Patients with a known seizure disorder should never be left unattended near water. In particular, patients with a history of febrile seizures should not be left unattended while receiving "cooling measures" in the bathtub.

Complaints of palpitations prior to submersion or a history of arrhythmia should prompt a more thorough cardiac investigation. In teenagers, a significant percentage of submersion injuries involve alcohol or other drugs.[6,15] This potentially complicates mental status assessment and evaluation for associated trauma. A serum alcohol level and urine drug screen should be obtained in all adolescents with submersion injury to aid in management decisions. Cervical spine injuries in adolescents do not occur without a significant mechanism; the routine activation of the trauma team without a suspicious mechanism (such as diving or submersion in ocean surf) is not useful, nor are routine cervical spine radiographs in nontraumatic submersions.[33]

A subpopulation at high risk for associated traumatic injuries are those patients who are submersed in bathtubs. In a landmark study, two thirds of bathtub drownings seen at one facility over a 10-year period had historical findings consistent with neglect and one third had physical findings of child abuse.[34] In this population, 49% either expired or had significant neurologic sequelae.[34] It is therefore prudent to have concern for abuse and/or neglect in these patients.

Chest radiographs do not predict disposition or clinical course.[35,36] Specifically, the presence or absence of radiographic findings does not correlate with clinical findings, pulse oximetry, or length of oxygen requirement and is not useful. Although electrolyte disturbances do occur, the presence of an abnormality does not automatically necessitate hospitalization, and should not alter initial fluid resuscitation. Similarly, the initial pH is not prognostic in predicting morbidity or mortality, so that routinely obtaining blood gases in submersion patients is not beneficial.[35,36] However, patients who have been intubated should be monitored appropriately, including regular evaluation of arterial blood gases and electrolytes.

Management

Immediate airway management and initiation of CPR are unequivocally the most effective interventions for the submersion victim (Table 138–1). Bystander cardiopulmonary resuscitation (CPR) has been shown to significantly affect patient survival, and even rescue breathing or cardiac compressions alone are superior to no intervention.[37-39]

All patients should be transported to the hospital for evaluation. Basic life support protocols and standard trauma protocols must be followed, including cervical spine immobilization when there is a history suggestive of an injury or suspicion of a traumatic mechanism.[33] Wet clothing should be removed to minimize heat loss. Airway protection must be a high priority due to the high frequency of vomiting (up to 86%) with chest compressions.[40] Early placement of a

Table 138–1	Clinical Pearls and Pitfalls

Pearls

- "Just do something": chest compressions and assisted ventilation improve outcome in asphyxial arrest.[37]
- Cardiopulmonary resuscitation prior to Emergency Medical Services arrival is associated with significantly better neurologic outcome.[38,39,69]

Pitfalls

- Ending a resuscitation too soon risks an inadequate chance for return of spontaneous circulation in very cold water submersions.[55-57]
- Continuing resuscitation too long creates neurologically devastated survivors.[4]
- Decrease in core temperature during rewarming is not necessarily a sign of inadequate therapy.[45]
- Pulse oximetry does not always correlate with hypoxemia in severe hypothermia.[44]

Table 138–2	Complications of Submersion Injury

Acute respiratory distress syndrome
Arrhythmias
Aspiration
Cerebral edema
Chronic pulmonary dysfunction
Disseminated intravascular coagulopathy
Hyperthermia
Hypotension
Neurologic impairment
Renal impairment
Sepsis

nasogastric tube to decompress the stomach will decrease the risk of vomiting in patients who have received rescue breaths. Early tracheal intubation is recommended for airway protection, to ensure removal of any foreign material from the airway, and to institute continuous positive airway pressure or positive end-expiratory pressure as needed for respiratory failure.[40] Once the airway is controlled, hypoxia and acidosis are better tolerated than hypoxia and hypotension. Permissive hypercapnia is preferable to avoid hypotension secondary to high mean airway pressures, which impede preload.[41]

No literature specifically addresses the use of bronchodilators for wheezing in a submersion victim. A reasonable approach is a one-time trial of bronchodilator therapy, with repeated treatments for the patients who improve clinically. In patients with a history of reactive airways disease or asthma, bronchodilators should be considered beneficial despite a dearth of evidence to support this recommendation.

Pediatric submersion victims are frequently hypothermic upon arrival to the ED. Due to significant peripheral vasoconstriction, rectal temperature lags behind true core temperature.[16,18] Jugular bulb temperature reflects body temperature, not true CNS temperature, but determining true CNS temperature is impossible without invasive monitoring.[42] An exaggerated response to warming occurs, making hyperthermia after resuscitation common.[43] When monitoring the hypothermic patient, the clinician should remember that pulse oximetry is not reliable under 27° C.[44]

"Afterdrop" is a phenomenon that occurs during rewarming when a patient experiences a drop in core temperature secondary to mobilization of cold blood from the peripheral circulation. Afterdrop has been associated with sudden death in otherwise intact hypothermia survivors.[45] Care must be taken not to be overly aggressive during the rewarming process. Rewarming with forced air (Bair Hugger) can increase temperature at a safe rate of 1.7° C/hr.[46] This method requires circulation to be effective. In cases of severe hypothermia or cardiac arrest, extracorporeal rewarming may be beneficial.[11] This technique has been available outside the surgical suite since 1993.[47] Extracorporeal rewarming has a 50% intact survival rate for adults with severe accidental nonsubmersion hypothermia but presents obvious logistic difficulties for ED care.[48]

Alternatively, therapeutic hypothermia is potentially beneficial and neuroprotective for submersion victims.[49,50] The stipulation is that the hypothermia must occur within 7 minutes of hypoxemia to be beneficial.[24] However, hypothermia can also decrease peripheral circulation and may inhibit adequate distribution of rescue medications. Caution must be exercised to not overmedicate based on lack of effect at time of administration in patients with compromised circulation or peripheral vasoconstriction.

Multiple secondary therapeutic interventions have been investigated. High-dose barbiturate therapy has been shown to help control intracranial pressure (ICP), but neither barbiturate therapy nor ICP monitoring appears to improve neurologic outcome.[40,51] Prophylactic steroids and antibiotics have been studied extensively and do not increase the odds of survival[52] (see Chapter 9, Cerebral Resuscitation).

Patients who are initially hypothermic must be continually monitored to gauge the success of intervention and to guard against hyperthermia. An initial decrease in temperature as a result of afterdrop is not uncommon and should not be equated with inadequate rewarming.[45] During rewarming from profound hypothermia, care must be taken so that rewarming does not occur too quickly and precipitate arrhythmias. Overly rapid rewarming also leads to hypotension from peripheral vasodilation, hypoxemia, and sinus bradycardia.[53]

Aspiration, whether of gastric contents or from the body of water, is a risk in any patient with an altered level of consciousness (Table 138–2). Tachypnea secondary to the pulmonary effects of submersion and the possibility that some rescuers will perform the Heimlich maneuver increases the odds of an aspiration.

Awake, alert patients who are asymptomatic after 4 to 6 hours of observation may be safely discharged home.[35,36] Historically, there have been reports of "secondary drowning" in otherwise normal-appearing patients, but similar cases have not been seen in subsequent research. Upon review, such cases were not clinically subtle or suitable for discharge.[54]

Patients who are clinically symptomatic after 6 hours require inpatient care in a monitored bed. The emergency physician should communicate early with pediatric intensivists and/or referral centers for children with persistent symptoms or severe initial condition to arrange for admission or transport to a capable facility. Bathtub drownings or other cases suspicious for nonaccidental injury or neglect should be evaluated in conjunction with social work and law enforcement in accordance with local protocols. As noted earlier, maintaining high concern for abuse and/or neglect is the key to identifying these cases.

When a patient has a clear traumatic mechanism of injury associated with submersion, surgical consultants should be involved in evaluation and management. Other subspecialty services should be consulted as needed for patients with identifiable predisposing factors such as seizures or arrhythmias. If possible, the emergency physician should contact the patients' primary care physician to identify any unknown history and to arrange for adequate follow-up or ongoing care of more severe patients. The primary care physician may also be helpful in assisting the family in making important decisions about termination of life support when neurologic devastation is apparent.

Consensus exists for poor prognostic signs and symptoms, yet it is important to acknowledge that there will be outlying cases that defy all predictions of survival despite meeting all poor prognostic criteria.[55-57] These cases occur very rarely and must be weighed against the more frequent occurrence of survival with neurologic devastation.

There are no absolutely reliable indicators of intact survival with cold water submersions.[58] Positive prognostic indicators include submersion time less than 10 minutes, no evidence of aspiration, and body core temperature less than 35° C.[58] Younger age of the victim as a positive prognosticator is supported in some studies but not others.[58-60] Hypothermia that is delayed 15 minutes does not have the same protective effect (only moderate disability) as immediate hypothermia.[61] Severe acidosis, with a pH as low as 6.33, has been reported with full recovery, reinforcing the poor prognostic value of this particular test.[62] Mean time to return of spontaneous circulation for hypothermic submersion patients requiring CPR upon arrival at the ED is 58 minutes.[63] It seems prudent to continue resuscitation of the hypothermic patient from a cold water submersion for a total of at least 1 hour.

In the ED, outcome of patients who have spontaneous circulation without spontaneous respirations cannot be reliably predicted. Children may experience an unexpected full recovery following a prolonged vegetative state.[64] Dilated pupils 6 hours after injury and seizures 24 hours after admission have been associated with poor outcome, but again, case reports with exceptions have been published.[13,55,57,65] The Pediatric Risk of Mortality (PRISM) score is somewhat helpful, but often does not differentiate neurologically intact survival among patients with median scores.[14,66,67] There is universally poor neurologic outcome for patients who were normothermic, pulseless, and apneic upon arrival in the ED, although some still recommend continued support for 24 hours.[63] The prognosis for children requiring CPR regardless of etiology is poor, and patients requiring more than two doses of epinephrine or resuscitation longer than 20 minutes also have a very poor prognosis.[39,68] All patients with spontaneous respirations on presentation to the ED recover, and reactive pupils support a good prognosis.[13]

Summary

Submersion injuries in children are common and are likely to be seen in geographically diverse practice settings. Patients who are asymptomatic 4 to 6 hours after submersion may be discharged home, while all others require admission to a monitored bed. Since near-drowning patients may be difficult to ventilate, it is prudent to expeditiously transfer symptomatic patients to a tertiary care facility.

In spite of advances in knowledge and technology, the prognosis of near-drowning patients has not changed. While there is a possible role for therapeutic hypothermia, the most effective strategy in minimizing morbidity and mortality from drowning is obviously prevention. Once a near drowning has occurred, immediate bystander CPR is the most effective intervention.

REFERENCES

1. Brenner RA, Trumble AC, Smith GS, et al: Where children drown, United States, 1995. Pediatrics 108:85–89, 2001.
2. Gilchrist J, Gotsch K, Ryan G: Nonfatal and fatal drownings in recreational water settings—United States, 2001–2002. MMWR Morb Mortal Wkly Rep 53:447–452, 2004.
3. Quan L, Cummings P: Characteristics of drowning by different age groups. Inj Prev 9:163–168, 2003.
4. Joseph MM, King WD: Epidemiology of hospitalization for near-drowning. South Med J 91:253–255, 1998.
5. O'Carroll PW, Akron E, Weiss B: Drowning mortality in Los Angeles County, 1976–1984. JAMA 260:380–383, 1988.
6. Quan L, Gore EJ, Wentz K, et al: Ten-year study of pediatric drownings and near-drownings in King County, Washington: lessons in injury prevention. Pediatrics 83:1035–1040, 1989.
7. Morrongiello BA, Kiriakou S: Mothers' home-safety practices for preventing six types of childhood injuries: what do they do, and why? J Pediatr Psychol 29:285–297, 2004.
8. Ridenour MV: Climbing performance of children: is the above-ground pool wall a climbing barrier? Percept Mot Skills 92:1255–1262, 2001.
9. Posner JC, Hawkins LA, Garcia-Espana F, et al: A randomized, clinical trial of a home safety intervention based in an emergency department setting. Pediatrics 113:1603–1608, 2004.
10. Kvittingen TD, Naess A: Recovery from drowning in fresh water. Br Med J 1:1315–1317, 1963.
11. Bolte RG, Black PG, Bowers RS, et al: The use of extracorporeal rewarming in a child submerged for 66 minutes. JAMA 260:377–379, 1988.
12. Diem SJ, Lantos JD, Tulsky JA: Cardiopulmonary resuscitation on television—miracles and misinformation. N Engl J Med 334:1578–1582, 1996.
13. Kemp AM, Sibert JR: Outcome in children who nearly drown: a British Isles study. BMJ 302:931–933, 1991.
14. Spack L, Gedeit R, Splaingard M, et al: Failure of aggressive therapy to alter outcome in pediatric near-drowning. Pediatr Emerg Care 13:98–102, 1997.
15. Cummings P, Quan L: Trends in unintentional drowning: The role of alcohol and medical care. JAMA 281:2198–2202, 1999.
16. Conn AW, Miyasaka K, Katayama M, et al: A canine study of cold water drowning in fresh versus salt water. Crit Care Med 23:2029–2037, 1995.
17. Hayward JS, Eckerson JD: Physiological responses and survival time prediction for humans in ice water. Aviat Space Environ Med 55:206–211, 1984.
18. Gilbertson L, Safar P, Stezowski X, et al: Pattern of dying during cold water drowning in dogs. Crit Care Med 4:216, 1982.
19. Golden F: Mechanisms of body cooling in submersed victims. Resuscitation 35:107–109, 1997.
20. Gooden BA: Why some people do not drown: hypothermia versus the diving response. Med J Aust 157:629–632, 1992.
21. Xu X, Tikuisis P, Giesbrecht G: A mathematical model for human brain cooling during cold-water near-drowning. J Appl Physiol 86:265–272, 1999.
22. Mohri H, Dillard DH, Crawford EW, et al: Method of surface induced deep hypothermia for open-heart surgery in infants. J Thorac Cardiovasc Surg 58:262–270, 1969.
23. Zeiner A, Holzer M, Sterz F, et al: Mild resuscitative hypothermia to improve neurological outcome after cardiac arrest. Stroke 31:86–94, 2000.
24. Stern WE, Good RG: Studies of the effects of hypothermia upon cerebrospinal fluid oxygen tension and carotid blood flow. Surgery 48:13–30, 1960.
25. Fainer DC, Martin CG, Ivy AC: Resuscitation of dogs from fresh water drowning. J Appl Physiol 3:417–426, 1951.

26. Behringer W, Prueckner S, Safar P, et al: Rapid induction of mild cerebral hypothermia by cold aortic flush achieves normal recovery in a dog outcome model with 20-minute exsanguinations cardiac arrest. Acad Emerg Med 7:1341–1348, 2000.

27. Colebatch HJH, Halmagyi DJF: Effect of vagotomy and vagal stimulation on lung mechanics and circulation. J Appl Physiol 18:881–887, 1963.

28. Lund KL, Mahon RT, Tanen DA, Bakhda S: Swimming-induced pulmonary edema. Ann Emerg Med 41:251–256, 2003.

29. Adir R, Shupak A, Gil A, et al: Swimming-induced pulmonary edema: clinical presentation and serial lung function. Chest 126:394–399, 2004.

30. Halmagyi DFJ, Colebatch HJH: Ventilation and circulation after fluid aspiration. J Appl Physiol 16:35–40, 1961.

31. Bergquist RE, Vogelhut MM, Modell JH, et al: Comparison of ventilatory patterns in the treatment of freshwater near-drowning in dogs. Anaesthesiology 52:142–148, 1980.

32. Diekema DS, Quan L, Holt VL: Epilepsy as a risk factor for submersion injury in children. Pediatrics 91:612–616, 1993.

33. Hwang V, Shofer FS, Durbin DR, et al: Prevalence of traumatic injuries in drowning and near drowning in children and adolescents. Arch Pediatr Adolesc Med 157:50–53, 2003.

*34. Lavelle JM, Shaw KN, Seidl T: Ten-year review of pediatric bathtub near-drownings: evaluation for child abuse and neglect. Ann Emerg Med 25:344–348, 1995.

*35. Causey AL, Tilelli JA, Swanson ME: Predicting discharge in uncomplicated near-drowning. Am J Emerg Med 18:9–11, 2000.

36. Noonan L, Howrey R, Ginsburg CM: Freshwater submersion injuries in children: a retrospective review of seventy-five hospitalized patients. Pediatrics 98:368–371, 1996.

37. Berg RA, Hilwig RW, Kern KB, et al: "Bystander" chest compressions and assisted ventilation independently improve outcome from piglet asphyxial pulseless "cardiac arrest." Circulation 101:1743–1748, 2000.

38. Kyriacou DN, Arcinue EL, Peek C, et al: Effect of immediate resuscitation on children with submersion injury. Pediatrics 94(2 Pt 1):137–142, 1994.

39. Sirbaugh PE, Pepe PE, Shook JE, et al: A prospective, population-based study of the demographics, epidemiology, management, and outcome of out-of-hospital pediatric cardiopulmonary arrest. Ann Emerg Med 33:174–184, 1999.

40. Kloeck W, Cummins R, Chamberlain D, et al: Special resuscitation situations: an advisory statement from the International Liaison Committee on Resuscitation. Circulation 95:2196–2210, 1997.

41. Bender TM, Johnston JA, Manepalli AN, et al: Correlation of brain tissue pH with histopathology in a piglet model of perinatal asphyxia. Pediatrics 100:494, 1997.

42. Rumana CS, Gopinath SP, Rzura M, et al: Brain temperature exceeds systemic temperature in head-injured patients. Crit Care Med 26:562–567, 1998.

43. Hickey RW, Kochanek PM, Ferimer H, et al: Hypothermia and hyperthermia in children after resuscitation from cardiac arrest. Pediatrics 106:118–122, 2000.

44. Iyer P, McDougall P, Loughnan P, et al: Accuracy of pulse oximetry in hypothermic neonates and infants undergoing cardiac surgery. Crit Care Med 24:507–511, 1996.

45. Nuckton TJ, Claman DM, Goldreich D, et al: Hypothermia and afterdrop following open water swimming: the Alcatraz/San Francisco swim study. Am J Emerg Med 18:703–707, 2000.

46. Kornberger E, Schwarz B, Lindner KH, et al: Forced air surface rewarming in patients with severe accidental hypothermia. Resuscitation 41:105–111, 1999.

47. Waters DJ, Belz M, Lawse D, et al: Portable cardiopulmonary bypass: resuscitation from prolonged ice-water submersion and asystole. Ann Thorac Surg 57:1018–1019, 1994.

48. Walpoth BH, Walpoth-Aslan BN, Mattle HP, et al: Outcome of survivors of accidental deep hypothermia and circulatory arrest treated with extracorporeal blood warming. N Engl J Med 337:1500–1505, 1997.

49. Holzer M, Behringer W, Schörkhuber W, et al: Mild hypothermia and outcome after CPR. Acta Anaesthesiol Scand 111(Suppl):55–58, 1997.

50. Thoresen M, Bagenholm R, Loberg EM, et al: Posthypoxic cooling of neonatal rats provides protection against brain injury. Arch Dis Child 74:F3–F9, 1996.

51. Bohn DJ, Biggar WD, Smith CR, et al: Influence of hypothermia, barbiturate therapy, and intracranial pressure monitoring on morbidity and mortality after near-drowning. Crit Care Med 14:529–534, 1986.

52. Modell JH, Graves SA, Ketover A: Clinical course of 91 consecutive near-drowning victims. Chest 70:231–238, 1976.

53. Thoresen M, Whitelaw A: Cardiovascular changes during mild therapeutic hypothermia and rewarming in infants with hypoxic-ischemic encephalopathy. Pediatrics 106:92–99, 2000.

54. Pearn JH: Secondary drowning in children. BMJ 281:1103–1105, 1980.

55. Modell JH, Idris AH, Pineda JA, et al: Survival after prolonged submersion in freshwater in Florida. Chest 125:1948–1951, 2004.

56. Associated Press: "Dead" boy survived drowning. Boise, ID: May 28, 2004.

57. Yi D, Mena J: Near drowning: toddler resuscitated 40 minutes after being declared dead. LA Times, Nov 8, 2003.

58. Bierens JJ, van der Velde EA, van Berkel M, et al: Submersion in the Netherlands: prognostic indicators and results of resuscitation. Ann Emerg Med 19:1390–1395, 1990.

59. Suominen PK, Korpela RE, Silfvast TGO, et al: Does water temperature affect outcome of nearly drowned children? Resuscitation 35:111–115, 1997.

60. Suominen P, Baillie C, Korpela R, et al: Impact of age, submersion time and water temperature on outcome in near-drowning. Resuscitation 52:247–254, 2002.

61. Kuboyama K, Safar P, Radovsky A, et al: Delay in cooling negates the beneficial effect of mild resuscitative cerebral hypothermia after cardiac arrest in dogs: a prospective, randomized study. Crit Care Med 21:1348–1358, 1993.

62. Opdahl H: Survival put to the acid test: Extreme arterial blood acidosis (pH 6.33) after near drowning. Crit Care Med 25:1431–1436, 1997.

63. Biggart MJ, Bohn DJ: Effect of hypothermia and cardiac arrest on outcome of near-drowning accidents in children. J Pediatr 117(2 Pt 1):179–183, 1990.

64. Quan L, Wentz KR, Gore EJ, et al: Outcome and predictors of outcome in pediatric submersion victims receiving prehospital care in King County, Washington. Pediatrics 86:586–593, 1990.

65. Christensen DW, Janesen P, Perkin RM: Outcome and acute care hospital costs after warm water near drowning in children. Pediatrics 99:715–721, 1997.

66. Gonzales-Luis G, Pons M, Cambra FJ: Use of the Pediatric Risk of Mortality score as predictor of death and serious neurologic damage in children after submersion. Pediatr Emerg Care 17:405–409, 2001.

67. Zuckerman GB, Gregory PM, Santos-Diamiani SM: Predictors of death and neurologic impairment in pediatric submersion injuries. Arch Pediatr Adolesc Med 152:134–140, 1998.

68. Young KD, Seidel JS: Pediatric cardiopulmonary resuscitation: A collective review. Ann Emerg Med 33:195–205, 1999.

69. Schindler MB, Bohn D, Cox PN, et al: Outcome out-of-hospital cardiac or respiratory arrest in children. N Engl J Med 335:1473–1479, 1996.

*Selected readings.

Chapter 139

Hyperthermia

Paul Ishimine, MD

Key Points

The hallmark of heatstroke is central nervous system dysfunction, but children with heatstroke may only have subtle neurologic findings and may be sweating profusely.

Cooling measures should be initiated immediately in patients with heatstroke even in the prehospital environment.

Heatstroke should be considered in children who collapse while exercising, even if their temperature is minimally elevated upon emergency department presentation.

Introduction and Background

Heat-related illness results from excessive heat stress. This may occur from an increased environmental burden or from an inability of the body to dissipate endogenous heat. The spectrum of heat illness ranges from minor to life threatening. Heat-related morbidity and mortality increase significantly during periods of high environmental temperature[1-3] Heat-related morbidity and mortality also increases in the presence of comorbid disease and increasing age; the highest rate of death is in the elderly population.[4,5] However, children are also susceptible to heat-related morbidity and mortality because of unique anatomic and physiologic characteristics.

Recognition and Approach

The human body is remarkably homeostatic and constantly regulates body temperature through a balance of heat production, absorption, and dissipation. Heat transfer occurs by four mechanisms: evaporation, convection, radiation, and conduction. Evaporation is the conversion of a liquid into a gas. The *evaporation* of sweat is the primary means of heat loss as ambient temperature rises, but this mechanism of heat transfer becomes less effective as ambient humidity increases. Additionally, dehydration results in decreased skin blood flow and increased rate of sweating, which in turn results in a decrease in evaporative cooling. *Convection* is the transfer of heat from skin to circulating air and water vapor molecules. Convective heat loss directly varies with wind velocity, and once the air temperature exceeds the skin temperature, convection results in heat gain. *Radiation* refers to the transfer of heat between the body and its surroundings by electromagnetic waves, and this represents a substantial source of heat gain in hot environments. *Conduction* is the transfer of heat from warmer to cooler objects via direct physical contact. This generally represents a minimal source of heat transfer, unless the skin is in contact with water.

Heat regulation is mediated by thermosensors, a central integrative area, and thermoregulatory effectors. Thermosensors are located peripherally in the skin and centrally in the preoptic area of the anterior hypothalamus, brainstem and spinal cord, and abdominal viscera. The central integrative area interprets information from the thermosensors and regulates thermoregulatory effectors. The thermoregulatory effectors stimulate sweating, vasodilation, and cold-seeking behavior, which are the main means by which heat loss is accelerated.

Several key anatomic and physiologic differences exist between children and adults. Children have a higher surface area–to-mass ratio, resulting in a greater rate of heat loss by convection than adults. In extreme conditions this results in a higher rate of heat absorption in hot environments. Children have both a smaller absolute blood volume and a smaller blood volume relative to body mass and surface area, which limits potential heat transfer from the body core to the body surface, where it can be dissipated.[6] Children have a lower rate of sweating than adults as a result of a lower sweat rate per gland,[7] and they take longer than adults to acclimatize to hot environments.[8] Children have higher energy expenditure and heat production compared with adults. Exercising children, who are dehydrated, have a greater rise in rectal temperature than adults who are exercising in the heat even when corrected for body weight.[9] They inadequately replenish fluid losses during exercise.[10] Children are also susceptible to heat-related illness because of an inability to escape from hot environments. Young children are at high risk for morbidity and mortality when left unattended in vehicles, as intravehicular temperatures rapidly rise to dangerous levels.[11,12] Heavily bundled young children have also died from hyperthermia while in bed.[13] Teenage athletes are another group that is at high risk for exertional heat-related illness.

Clinical Presentation

The degree to which children develop signs and symptoms from heat stress depends on a number of factors. Much of the risk for heat illness is attributable to the environment, such as the ambient temperature and humidity level. However, individual variables also place the child at risk for heat-related disease. Children with special health care needs are especially vulnerable to heat-related illness (Table 139–1).

Miliaria ("prickly heat" or "heat rash") is an inflammatory rash resulting from blockage and subsequent rupture of sweat glands. Miliaria crystallina occurs typically in neonates and in sunburned areas. This rash is characterized by clear, small, sweat-filled vesicles. Miliaria rubra is an erythematous papular rash typically seen in intertriginous areas or in truncal areas covered by clothing. The sweat glands enlarge and rupture within the lower epidermis, resulting in an erythematous rash.

Heat cramps are muscle cramps that usually occur several hours after exertion and commonly involve the large muscle groups of the legs. These are thought to occur because of dilutional hyponatremia from rehydration with free water but not salt, but the exact etiology is unclear.[14] While these can be quite uncomfortable, heat cramps do not lead to significant morbidity. Heat cramps are often confused with *heat tetany*, which is caused by hyperventilation associated with heat stress, resulting in respiratory alkalosis, circumoral and extremity paresthesias, and carpopedal spasm.

Heat edema and *heat syncope* are heat-related conditions found more commonly in the elderly than in children. Heat edema, which causes swelling of the hands and feet, results from vasodilation and pooling of increased interstitial fluid in dependent extremities, as well as an increase in aldosterone and antidiuretic hormone secretion. Heat syncope results from volume depletion, peripheral vasodilation, and decreased vasomotor tone.

Heat exhaustion is characterized by volume depletion, and is usually (but not always) associated with a slightly elevated body temperature. Heat exhaustion can be further subclassified as water-depletion heat exhaustion (characterized by inadequate water replacement) or salt-depletion heat exhaustion (characterized by salt loss and replacement by hypotonic solution), but most patients have combined water-salt depletion. Symptoms are nonspecific and include thirst, weakness, fatigue, dizziness, irritability, headache, nausea, and vomiting. Patients with water-depletion heat exhaustion typically have elevated sodium and chloride levels, while those patients with salt-depletion heat exhaustion have hyponatremia and hypochloremia.

Heatstroke is typically defined as a core temperature $\geq 40° C$ and central nervous system (CNS) dysfunction. This must be continuously monitored with a rectal probe thermometer that is accurate to high temperatures. While anhidrosis is commonly present, this is not an absolute criterion for making this diagnosis.[15] Signs of heatstroke may occur abruptly. Classic heatstroke arises from environmental exposure to heat and is more common in younger children who are unable to escape from hot environments. Exertional heatstroke results from strenuous exercise and is more common in older children and adolescents. The differential diagnosis for heatstroke is presented in Table 139–2.

Heatstroke is associated with a systemic inflammatory response, with a predominance of CNS symptoms. While CNS symptoms may be subtle and manifest as impaired judgment or inappropriate behavior, children commonly present with more significant neurologic symptoms such as seizures, delirium, hallucinations, ataxia, or coma. Anhidrosis results from severe dehydration and sweat gland dysfunction, but profuse sweating may precede anhidrosis. Patients are tachycardic and tachypneic. Vomiting, diarrhea, and gastrointestinal bleeding are thought to be consequences of impaired perfusion to the mesentery. Patients may be incontinent and have hematuria, oliguria, or anuria. Coagulopathies may result in purpura, subconjunctival hemorrhage, and other signs of bleeding.

Table 139–1	Risk Factors for Heat Illness[31]

Excessive Fluid Loss

Febrile illness
Gastrointestinal illness
Dehydration
Diabetes
Burns

Sweating Dysfunction

Cystic fibrosis[32-34]
Spina bifida
Sweating insufficiency syndrome
Ectodermal dysplasia

Diminished Fluid Intake

Developmental delay
Young children

Thermoregulatory Dysfunction

Anorexia nervosa
Previous heat-related illness

Multifactorial

Obesity
Medications (e.g., anticholinergic agents, pseudoephedrine, amphetamines, cocaine,[35] alcohol)
Prepubescent age
Lack of fitness or acclimatization
Sickle cell disease[36-38]

Table 139–2	Differential Diagnosis of Heat Stroke

Infectious

Central nervous system infections
Sepsis

Neurologic

Status epilepticus
Intracranial hemorrhage
Hypothalamic dysfunction

Drug Related

Anticholinergic medications
Stimulants (e.g., amphetamines, cocaine)
Salicylates
Drug withdrawal (e.g., ethanol)
Serotonin syndrome
Neuroleptic malignant syndrome
Malignant hyperthermia

Endocrine

Thyroid storm

Miscellaneous

Hemorrhagic shock and encephalopathy syndrome[39-42]

Patients with heatstroke have abnormal laboratory tests, reflecting the systemic inflammatory response and end-organ damage as a result of heat stress. Hematologic findings include hemoconcentration and elevated white blood cell count. Thrombocytopenia and disseminated intravascular coagulation are seen frequently in heatstroke, although these findings are seen 18 to 36 hours after the initial heat stress.[16,17] Electrolytes disturbances are frequent. Patients are usually hypokalemic but may be hyperkalemic. While hypernatremia may be present, normal sodium levels are common as well. Serum calcium levels can be either high or low. Elevated blood urea nitrogen and creatinine levels indicate acute renal failure, which occurs from a combination of factors, including dehydration and direct renal injury. Rhabdomyolysis, with an accompanying rise in creatine kinase, contributes to renal failure. Patients can be hyper-, normo-, or hypoglycemic. Metabolic acidosis is the most commonly observed acid-base disturbance and is associated with the degree of hyperthermia; respiratory alkalosis is seen frequently as well.[18] Elevation of liver enzymes is common in heatstroke,[19] but liver failure is much less common. The presence of hepatic injury has been suggested as a criterion to distinguish between heat exhaustion and heatstroke. A computed tomography scan of the head should be obtained if a child has persistently altered mental status despite cooling, or if a neurologic cause of hyperthermia (e.g., intracranial hemorrhage) is suspected.

Important Clincial Features and Considerations

The diagnosis of heat illness is usually straightforward with the acute onset of symptoms in the setting of heat stress, but may be more difficult in other circumstances. In the presence of elevated body temperature and nonspecific symptoms, these patients are sometimes misdiagnosed as having infectious illnesses. The diagnosis may be difficult or missed when children undergo cooling interventions in the prehospital setting, as they may arrive in the emergency department with near-normal body temperature. There is some overlap of symptoms between heat exhaustion and heatstroke. While the distinction between heat exhaustion and heatstroke is sometimes unclear, the hallmark of heatstroke is CNS dysfunction. Children with elevated body temperature and CNS abnormalities should always be treated as having heatstroke, given the significant morbidity and mortality associated with this condition. Heat stroke must be distinguished from malignant hyperthermia and neuroleptic malignant syndrome which are induced by medications (phenothiazines, anesthetics, succinylcholine) and cause fever and muscle rigidity.

While complications with minor heat illness are uncommon, patients with heatstroke are prone to many significant complications. Heatstroke patients have hyperdynamic cardiovascular systems with low peripheral vascular resistance. This low peripheral resistance persists even after cooling, leading to speculation that this is similar to a postshock or sepsis state, and this can lead to high-output cardiac failure. Heatstroke patients frequently have pulmonary edema, which is likely due to a combination of capillary leak and overaggressive fluid resuscitation, and this may progress to acute respiratory distress syndrome. Rhabdomyolysis and oliguric renal failure are common findings in heatstroke as well. The gastrointestinal system plays a key role in the pathogenesis of heat injury. Intestinal mucosal injury from heat stress, with subsequent release of toxic substances into the circulation, is thought to contribute to the systemic response to heat injury.[20] For patients with heatstroke-associated liver failure, hepatic transplantation has been performed, but experience in children and young adults is limited. Two case reports described unsuccessful liver transplantation in teenagers.[21-23] Both liver dysfunction and coagulation abnormalities are seen in a delayed fashion after the initial heat injury.

Management

Most patients with minor heat illness can be treated and discharged home. Treatment for miliaria entails allowing the skin to dry, use of lightweight clothing, and avoidance of further sweating. Superinfection of miliaria occasionally occurs and should be treated with antistaphylococcal antibiotics. Heat cramps are usually treated sufficiently with oral salt solutions, although some patients may need intravenous normal saline. The treatment for heat tetany is removal from the heat, which allows the patient to cease hyperventilation. Treatment for heat edema entails elevation and compressive stockings as well as removal from the heat source. Heat syncope is usually treated with either oral or intravenous fluids depending on the degree of symptoms. Heat exhaustion should be treated with cooling measures and hydration. Correction of fluid and electrolyte abnormalities with replacement of free water deficit and electrolyte losses is the therapeutic goal.

Children with heatstroke need to be treated aggressively since the extent of CNS damage is related to the duration of hyperthermia. After the usual resuscitative maneuvers addressing airway, breathing, and circulation, heatstroke patients need aggressive cooling measures. The most commonly utilized modalities for rapid cooling are evaporative cooling and cold water immersion. The goal of therapeutic cooling is to bring the core temperature down to 40° C as quickly as possible. Treatment should always be initiated in the prehospital setting if possible.

Immediate therapeutic interventions include removal of the patient from the heat source and removal of all clothing. Evaporative cooling is quickly accomplished by spraying tepid water (to minimize shivering) over patients and then using high-flow fans to circulate air to facilitate evaporation. Both spray bottles and fans are usually available from hospital housekeeping services. Cold water immersion of the trunk and extremities is an effective cooling mechanism as well.[24] Children can be immersed in wading pools that are commonly found in supplies used for chemical decontamination. Logistically, however, monitoring and performing interventions on submerged patients is challenging. Additional methods of cooling include covering patients in ice, and selective application of ice packs to the neck, axillae, and groin. The latter technique can be used in conjunction with evaporative cooling techniques.[25]

Theoretically, the most effective method of lowering the core body temperature quickly is the use of cardiopulmonary bypass. Cold water gastric[26,27] and peritoneal[28] lavage have been proposed as additional means of invasive cooling, but these techniques have not been well studied in humans. Consider dantrolene administration (2–3 mg/kg IV to maximum of 10 mg) if malignant hyperthermia or neuroleptic malignant syndrome are a consideration.[29] There is no role for isopropyl alcohol sponge baths or antipyretic medications in the heatstroke patient. Anticipate and treat rhabdomyolysis as needed (see Chapter 99, Rhabdomyolysis).

Care must be taken to prevent shivering, since this physiologic response will increase endogenous heat production. Shivering is best treated with benzodiazepines. Another complication associated with cooling measures is overshoot hypothermia. A decrease in measured body temperatures generally lags behind the actual drop in core temperature, and for this reason, cooling measures are generally stopped once the core temperature reaches 40° C. While heatstroke patients are generally dehydrated, they also have low peripheral resistance because of cutaneous vasodilation and may be hypotensive. Consequently, these patients often receive large amounts of fluids, which may lead to pulmonary edema if these fluids are not administered judiciously.

Simple preventive measures may forestall significant complications associated with excessive heat. Children become dehydrated when exercising in hot environments, even when allowed to drink water freely.[9,10] Flavoring water and adding both carbohydrates and sodium chloride may eliminate hypohydration.[30] Restricting physical activity during hot times of the day and wearing loose-fitting, light-colored clothing reduces the risk of heat-related illness. Children should be encouraged to drink approximately 10 ml/kg prior to engaging in a period of intense exercise in hot ambient temperatures and to maintain hydration at 5 ml/kg/hr throughout the duration of the exercise.

Summary

Most patients with heat-related illness have minor symptoms that are correctable in the emergency department and can thus be discharged home. Some patients with heat exhaustion may need to be admitted to the hospital if they have significant electrolyte abnormalities or if there is a concern about recurrence.

All children with heatstroke must be admitted to the hospital. Patients with heatstroke generally have dysfunction of multiple organ systems and therefore need to be monitored closely. Specifically, these patients need close hemodynamic and neurologic monitoring. Because of these monitoring requirements and the potential for delayed complications (e.g., coagulopathies, hepatic dysfunction), these patients may require transfer to a pediatric critical care facility.

The prognosis in patients with heatstroke is directly related to the duration of hyperthermia, and for this reason, heatstroke must be treated aggressively. Poor prognostic indicators include persistent CNS dysfunction despite cooling and persistent hypotension despite adequate fluid resuscitation.

REFERENCES

1. Dematte JE, O'Mara K, Buescher J, et al: Near-fatal heat stroke during the 1995 heat wave in Chicago. Ann Intern Med 129:173–181, 1998.
2. Kaiser R, Rubin CH, Henderson AK, et al: Heat-related death and mental illness during the 1999 Cincinnati heat wave. Am J Forensic Med Pathol 22:303–307, 2001.
3. Naughton MP, Henderson A, Mirabelli MC, et al: Heat-related mortality during a 1999 heat wave in Chicago. Am J Prev Med 22:221–227, 2002.
4. Centers for Disease Control and Prevention: Heat-related deaths—four states, July–August 2001, and United States, 1979–1999. MMWR Morb Mortal Wkly Rep 51:567–570, 2002.
5. Centers for Disease Control and Prevention: Heat-related deaths—Chicago, Illinois, 1996–2001, and United States, 1979–1999. MMWR Morb Mortal Wkly Rep 52:610–613, 2003.
*6. Falk B, Bar-Or O, Calvert R, et al: Effects of thermal stress during rest and exercise in the paediatric population. Sports Med 25:221–240, 1998.
7. Falk B, Bar-Or O, Calvert R, et al: Sweat gland response to exercise in the heat among pre-, mid-, and late-pubertal boys. Med Sci Sports Exerc 24:313–319, 1992.
*8. Wagner JA, Robinson S, Tzankoff SP, et al: Heat tolerance and acclimatization to work in the heat in relation to age. J Appl Physiol 33:616–622, 1972.
9. Bar-Or O, Dotan R, Inbar O, et al: Voluntary hypohydration in 10- to 12-year-old boys. J Appl Physiol 48:104–108, 1980.
*10. Bar-Or O, Wilk B: Water and electrolyte replenishment in the exercising child. Int J Sport Nutr 6:93–99, 1996.
11. King K, Negus K, Vance JC: Heat stress in motor vehicles: a problem in infancy. Pediatrics 68:579–582, 1981.
12. Roberts KB, Roberts EC: The automobile and heat stress. Pediatrics 58:101–104, 1976.
13. Krous HF, Nadeau JM, Fukumoto RI, et al: Environmental hyperthermic infant and early childhood death: circumstances, pathologic changes, and manner of death. Am J Forensic Med Pathol 22:374–382, 2001.
*14. Noakes TD: Fluid and electrolyte disturbances in heat illness. Int J Sports Med 19:S146–S149, 1998.
*15. Bouchama A, Knochel JP: Heat stroke. N Engl J Med 346:1978–1988, 2002.
16. Bouchama A, Hammami MM, Haq A, et al: Evidence for endothelial cell activation/injury in heatstroke. Crit Care Med 24:1173–1178, 1996.
17. Bouchama A, Bridey F, Hammami MM, et al: Activation of coagulation and fibrinolysis in heatstroke. Thromb Haemost 76:909–915, 1996.
18. Bouchama A, De Vol EB: Acid-base alterations in heatstroke. Intensive Care Med 27:680–685, 2001.
19. Hassanein T, Razack A, Gavaler JS, et al: Heatstroke: its clinical and pathological presentation, with particular attention to the liver. Am J Gastroenterol 87:1382–1389, 1992.
20. Eshel GM, Safar P, Stezoski W: The role of the gut in the pathogenesis of death due to hyperthermia. Am J Forensic Med Pathol 22.100–104, 2001.
21. Hadad E, Ben-Ari Z, Heled Y, et al: Liver transplantation in exertional heat stroke: a medical dilemma. Intensive Care Med 30:1474–1478, 2004.
22. Berger J, Hart J, Millis M, et al: Fulminant hepatic failure from heat stroke requiring liver transplantation. J Clin Gastroenterol 30:429 431, 2000.
23. Pastor MA, Perez-Aguilar F, Ortiz V, et al: [Acute hepatitis due to heatstroke]. Gastroenterol Hepatol 22:398–399, 1999.
24. Gaffin SL, Gardner JW, Flinn SD: Cooling methods for heatstroke victims. Ann Intern Med 132:678–679, 2000.
25. Eshel GM, Safar P, Stezoski W: Evaporative cooling as an adjunct to ice bag use after resuscitation from heat-induced arrest in a primate model. Pediatr Res 27:264–267, 1990.
26. White JD, Riccobene E, Nucci R, et al: Evaporation versus iced gastric lavage treatment of heatstroke: comparative efficacy in a canine model. Crit Care Med 15:748–750, 1987.
27. Syverud SA, Barker WJ, Amsterdam JT, et al: Iced gastric lavage for treatment of heatstroke: efficacy in a canine model. Ann Emerg Med 14:424–432, 1985.
28. White JD, Kamath R, Nucci R, et al: Evaporation versus iced peritoneal lavage treatment of heatstroke: comparative efficacy in a canine model. Am J Emerg Med 11:1–3, 1993.
29. Bouchama A, Cafege A, Devol EB, et al: Ineffectiveness of dantrolene sodium in the treatment of heatstroke. Crit Care Med 19:176–180, 1991.
30. Wilk B, Bar-Or O: Effect of drink flavor and NaCl on voluntary drinking and hydration in boys exercising in the heat. J Appl Physiol 80:1112–1117, 1996.
*31. Climatic heat stress and the exercising child and adolescent. American Academy of Pediatrics, Committee on Sports Medicine and Fitness. Pediatrics 106:158–159, 2000.

*Selected readings.

32. Orenstein DM, Henke KG, Costill DL, et al: Exercise and heat stress in cystic fibrosis patients. Pediatr Res 17:267–269, 1983.

33. Bar-Or O, Blimkie CJ, Hay JA, et al: Voluntary dehydration and heat intolerance in cystic fibrosis. Lancet 339:696–699, 1992.

34. Kriemler S, Wilk B, Schurer W, et al: Preventing dehydration in children with cystic fibrosis who exercise in the heat. Med Sci Sports Exerc 31:774–779, 1999.

35. Martinez M, Devenport L, Saussy J, et al: Drug-associated heat stroke. South Med J 95:799–802, 2002.

36. Kerle KK, Nishimura KD: Exertional collapse and sudden death associated with sickle cell trait. Mil Med 161:766–767, 1996.

37. Kark JA, Posey DM, Schumacher HR, et al: Sickle-cell trait as a risk factor for sudden death in physical training. N Engl J Med 317:781–787, 1987.

38. Wirthwein DP, Spotswood SD, Barnard JJ, et al: Death due to microvascular occlusion in sickle-cell trait following physical exertion. J Forensic Sci 46:399–401, 2001.

39. Levin M, Hjelm M, Kay JD, et al: Haemorrhagic shock and encephalopathy: a new syndrome with a high mortality in young children. Lancet 2:64–67, 1983.

40. Chaves-Carballo E, Montes JE, Nelson WB, et al: Hemorrhagic shock and encephalopathy: clinical definition of a catastrophic syndrome in infants. Am J Dis Child 144:1079–1082, 1990.

41. Ince E, Kuloglu Z, Akinci Z: Hemorrhagic shock and encephalopathy syndrome: neurologic features. Pediatr Emerg Care 16:260–264, 2000.

42. Bacon CJ, Bell SA, Gaventa JM, et al: Case control study of thermal environment preceding haemorrhagic shock encephalopathy syndrome. Arch Dis Child 81:155–158, 1999.

Hypothermia

Paul Ishimine, MD

Introduction and Background

Hypothermia is defined as a core temperature of less than 35° C (95° F).[1] Primary ("accidental") hypothermia is a result of environmental exposure, while secondary hypothermia is a result of underlying disease. Hypothermia is more frequently seen in cold environments and in winter months,[2,3] but children may become hypothermic in any location or climate. While the role of therapeutically induced hypothermia is an area of ongoing investigation for a number of different medical conditions,[4-12] this discussion focuses on accidental hypothermia.

Recognition and Approach

Hypothermia is further categorized as mild (32.2° C to 35° C), moderate (28° C to 32.1° C), and severe (<28° C) hypothermia.[1] This represents a continuum of illness; the patient is able to compensate to some degree in mild and moderate hypothermia, but with severe hypothermia, the patient's compensatory mechanisms have failed. Cold stimuli sensed by thermoreceptors, located both in the skin and centrally, lead to compensatory responses mediated by the hypothalamus and include shivering, autonomic nervous system responses (primarily vasoconstriction), and endocrinologic and adaptive behavioral changes.[13,14]

The rate of hypothermia-associated death increases with age, and the majority of patients who die from hypothermia are elderly.[2,15] While children are less likely to have some of the risk factors associated with hypothermia in adults (e.g., alcohol use, homelessness, mental illness), children have certain anatomic, physiologic, and behavioral differences from adults that place them at higher risk for hypothermia. Because heat transfer between the body and environment is related to the exposed body surface area (BSA), the increased BSA-to-mass ratio in children leads to relatively greater heat loss than in adults. Young children have less subcutaneous tissue than adults, leading to less insulation of the body core. Shivering increases the metabolic rate to five to six times than that observed at rest, and this involuntary muscle contraction leads to heat production.[16] Young children are unable to shiver, precluding this highly effective mechanism of endogenous heat production. Young infants increase thermogenesis by lipolysis of brown adipose tissue. Depending on a child's age and developmental level, he or she may not be able to adapt behaviorally to cold stimuli, such as seeking a warmer environment or putting on additional clothing.

Clinical Presentation

Frequently, the diagnosis of hypothermia is suspected when there is a history of environmental exposure, but the diagnosis can be subtle, especially in preverbal children. Paradoxically, the signs and symptoms may be even more difficult to appreciate with decreasing body temperature. In addition to feeling cold, patients may complain of lethargy or confusion. Other vague symptoms include dizziness, nausea, or hunger.

Hypothermia affects all of the organ systems and leads to numerous physical examination abnormalities. The severity of symptoms generally correlates with the degree of hypothermia, and the most prominently affected systems are the cardiovascular and neurologic systems. Patients who are hypothermic initially present with tachycardia and peripheral vasoconstriction. As they become more hypothermic, bradycardia develops with an accompanying decrease in mean arterial pressure and cardiac output. The drop in body temperature typically leads to atrial fibrillation or atrial flutter with slow ventricular response rates, which is then followed by ventricular fibrillation and asystole. This risk is most pronounced when the core temperature drops below 30° C.

Hypothermia depresses the central nervous system, resulting in decreased cerebral metabolism. This results in impaired judgment and memory as well as depressed mental status. Paradoxical undressing has been noted in hypothermic patients.[17] Hyperreflexia is followed by hyporeflexia, ultimately resulting in the loss of reflexes in severely hypothermic patients. Fine motor control is lost early in hypothermia. Shivering is initially stimulated with mild hypothermia, but as hypothermia progresses, shivering thermogenesis ceases and patients become poikilothermic. Because hypothermia depresses cerebral metabolism, this offers some degree of cerebral protection, but the amount of this protection is difficult to predict clinically.

Other organ systems are also involved. The respiratory rate in patients with mild hypothermia initially increases, but is followed by a progressive decline in minute ventilation as hypothermia worsens. Hypothermia also induces bronchorrhea, decreased ciliary motility, and noncardiogenic pulmonary edema. With the accompanying decrease in mental status, patients are at risk for aspiration pneumonia. Peripheral vasoconstriction initially leads to relative central hypervolemia. This phenomenon, along with a decrease in renal concentrating ability and a decrease in antidiuretic hormone, is thought to contribute to cold-induced diuresis. There is an accompanying shift of intravascular fluid to the extravascular space, and this contributes to the development of hypovolemia. Gastrointestinal effects of hypothermia result in poor intestinal motility, leading to ileus and abdominal distention. Hepatic dysfunction and pancreatitis are also seen with hypothermia.

Multiple hematologic derangements are associated with hypothermia. Activated clotting factors are depressed by cold, and, along with thrombocytopenia that accompanies hypothermia, this can lead to significant coagulopathy Conversely, blood viscosity increases after diuresis, leading to increased rates of thromboembolic phenomena. Disseminated intravascular coagulation may occur as well. Musculoskeletal findings include increased tone, shivering, and muscular rigidity. Dermatologic findings include erythema, pallor, cold urticaria, and frostbite.

In neonates, common presenting complaints include refusal to eat and drowsiness. Physical examination findings include coldness to touch, extremity edema, and a ruddy appearance. Bradycardia, hypotension, and periodic breathing with apneic episodes are commonly noted upon initial presentation.[18] The newly born are at particularly high risk for hypothermia, especially those born in the prehospital or emergency department setting. Half of these patients are hypothermic when their rectal temperatures are initially taken.[19,20]

The definitive diagnostic test for hypothermia is accurate measurement of the core temperature. The core temperature must be measured with a low-temperature–reading thermometer and is most commonly obtained by rectal measurements, although these measurements are not as accurate as esophageal measurements. Other diagnostic tests may yield additional information, but the core temperature is the cornerstone in making this diagnosis.

The white blood count and platelet counts are commonly low or normal in hypothermia, and the hematocrit is elevated because of hemoconcentration. Coagulation studies may be normal because blood is warmed in the laboratory when prothrombin and partial thromboplastin times are measured. This will not reflect the coagulopathy caused by cold-induced inhibition of the enzymes of the clotting cascade.

Serum electrolytes can be abnormal. Both hypokalemia and hyperkalemia are seen in hypothermic patients. The blood urea nitrogen and creatinine levels are often elevated. Initially, patients may develop hyperglycemia, as cold cells are initially insulin resistant, but this is followed by hypoglycemia. A urine toxicology screen may be helpful when drug exposure is a consideration. Patients who are hypothermic can be acidotic or alkalotic, and arterial blood gases should be interpreted without correction for temperature.[21]

The electrocardiogram (ECG) reveals prolongation of the PR, QRS, and QT intervals. The J wave ("Osborn wave") is an extra deflection noted at the junction of the QRS complex and the beginning of the ST segment. This finding is seen frequently in hypothermic patients, and the amplitude of this wave is inversely correlated with the core temperature[22] (Fig. 140–1). However, the J wave is not pathognomic of hypothermia,[23] and may persist in hypothermic patients who have been rewarmed to normothermia.[24] Muscle tremor artifact is seen commonly, resulting in fine oscillation of the ECG baseline, even in the absence of clinically evident shivering.

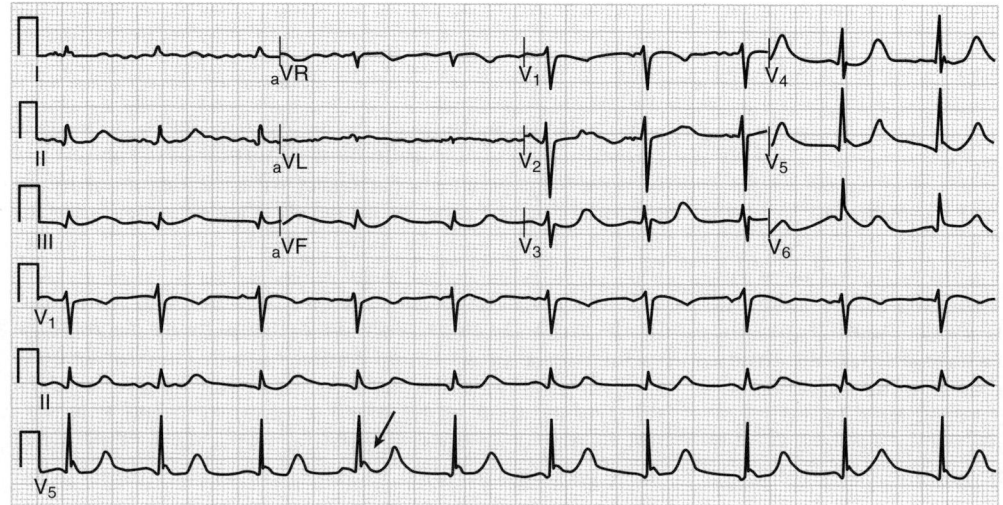

FIGURE 140–1. Hypothermia. Electrocardiogram in a patient with a core temperature of 30° C featuring bradycardia, Osborne waves *(arrow)*, and prolongation of the QRS complex and QT interval.

Table 140–1	Causes of Hypothermia

Cold Exposure

Environmental exposure
Near drowning
Iatrogenic (e.g., fluid resuscitation, exposure of undressed patient)

Infectious

Sepsis
Central nervous system infections

Endocrinologic/Metabolic

Hypoglycemia
Hyponatremia
Malnutrition
Anorexia nervosa
Hypothyroidism
Addison's disease
Hypopituitarism

Central Nervous System Dysfunction

Intracranial hemorrhage
Birth asphyxia
Tumors
Prader-Willi syndrome[53]

Drug Induced

Ethanol
Benzodiazepines
Barbiturates
Narcotics
Oral hypoglycemics

Integumentary Dysfunction

Burns
Exfoliative dermatitis

Miscellaneous

Child maltreatment[54,55]
Episodic spontaneous hypothermia with hyperhidrosis[56]

Important Clinical Features and Considerations

Hypothermia in children can develop rapidly in the setting of environmental stressors. Appropriately, these patients need interventions to increase core temperature. Conversely, a common pitfall is focusing solely on warming interventions without addressing the underlying etiology of the hypothermia. While most children who are hypothermic are hypothermic from environmental causes, there are many other etiologies (Table 140–1). Warming interventions will not be successful without treatment of underlying precipitants, such as sepsis or hypoglycemia. Additionally, hypothermia is frequently iatrogenic; during the course of treating a sick child, an unclothed patient in an emergency department treatment area may quickly become hypothermic.

Management

Many recommendations generated for the treatment of hypothermia have been derived from case series, animal models, or small laboratory investigations with healthy human (almost always adult) volunteers, and the recommendations for management of hypothermic children should be interpreted with these limitations in mind.

Initial management of the hypothermic patient entails assessment of airway patency and adequacy of ventilation. The pulse and respiratory rates in patients with significant hypothermia will generally be slow and difficult to detect. The airway needs to be secured in hypothermic patients as with any other patients. There is little evidence to support the contention that endotracheal intubation precipitates ventricular fibrillation,[3] but patients should be handled carefully, as the hypothermic myocardium is irritable and prone to dysrhythmias. Because these patients may be profoundly bradycardic, the clinician must search for a pulse for at least 1 minute before initiating cardiopulmonary resuscitation. Alternatively, if a cardiac monitor reveals a nonperfusing rhythm, defibrillation and cardiopulmonary resuscitation should be initiated as indicated. Patients in ventricular fibrillation should initially receive one shock. If the patient is severely hypothermic (<30° C), current guidelines suggest deferring further shocks until the core temperature rises, as hypothermia may contribute to refractory ventricular fibrillation.[25]

Hypothermic patients need to be rewarmed, and the general presumption is that rapid rewarming (as opposed to gradual rewarming) is desired. Three categories of warming interventions exist: passive rewarming, active external rewarming, and active core rewarming. In general, active core rewarming techniques raise core temperature faster than active external techniques, which, in turn, are more effective than passive measures. For these reasons, colder children require more aggressive warming techniques.

Children with mild hypothermia can be treated with passive rewarming techniques. These interventions include maintaining a warm environment, drying patients who are wet, removing wet clothing, and covering patients with insulating material in order to minimize heat loss. Especially in neonates, large amounts of heat are lost from the head, and during passive rewarming of the young child, a head covering is helpful in preventing heat loss.[26] A significant limitation of passive rewarming techniques is that they are dependent on endogenous heat production in order to be successful. Hypothermic patients stop shivering and become functionally poikilothermic as their core temperature drops, and therefore passive rewarming is ineffective in more severely hypothermic patients.

Active external rewarming entails utilization of an external heat source on the body surface and is used primarily for mild hypothermia. A commonly used technique is forced air rewarming through specialized blankets. Heated air is forced through semi-closed blanket covers and exits onto the patient, allowing for convective heat transfer and limitation of radiant heat loss. This technique has been used successfully in the emergency department without core temperature afterdrop.[27-29] Immersion in warm water is an effective, albeit impractical, method of active external rewarming.

Active core rewarming entails application of heat to internal surfaces and is used for moderate and severe hypothermia. Inhalation of heated air is typically accomplished by the use of nebulizers and ventilators with the capacity to heat and humidify air. This technique minimizes respiratory heat loss. Controversy persists as to the efficacy of airway rewarming, and the role of this technique is most appropriate as an adjunct to other warming techniques.[30,31] Hypothermic patients are frequently hypovolemic and require fluid resuscitation. Intravenous infusion devices with countercurrent heat exchangers may be used to warm intravenous fluids.[32]

Alternatively, intravenous fluids that are warmed in microwave ovens[33,34] may be used if prewarmed fluids are not available. Irrigation of the stomach through nasogastric or orogastric tubes, or gastrointestinal decontamination tubing, can be used to rewarm the core by gastric lavage with warmed fluids. Similarly, bladder irrigation with warm fluids may be used. However, the relatively small surface area available for heat exchange limits these warming techniques. Peritoneal lavage with warmed fluids has been used in the treatment of severe hypothermia.[35] Using standard open or closed techniques for diagnostic peritoneal lavage, a large catheter is placed into the peritoneal cavity, and warmed fluid is infused into the abdominal cavity and then withdrawn. Pleural irrigation has also been used in the treatment of hypothermia in children.[36] This treatment requires placement of two chest tubes; one is placed anteriorly in the second intercostal space in the midclavicular line, and the second is placed in the posterior axillary line at the level of the fifth intercostal space. Warm fluid is infused in the anterior tube and suctioned or drained out of the posterior tube. Thoracotomy with mediastinal lavage has been described as a warming technique in adults.

The treatment of choice in patients with hypothermic cardiopulmonary arrest is extracorporeal warming via cardiopulmonary bypass.[37] Typically this is achieved with femoral-femoral bypass, although in younger children, circulatory access may be more easily achieved via median sternotomy.[38-40] In patients with adequate perfusion pressures, continuous arteriovenous warming with countercurrent heat exchangers interposed between femoral artery and femoral vein catheters is another option, as is standard hemodialysis.

There is a strong association between hypothermia and sepsis in young infants, and empirical therapy with broad-spectrum antibiotics in this age group is warranted.[18,41] While hypothyroidism and adrenal insufficiency are associated with hypothermia, empirical treatment with levothyroxine or steroids is not indicated, as these are rare causes of hypothermia in children.

Therapeutic Complications

When the core temperature continues to decline after initiation of warming maneuvers, this phenomenon is known as core temperature afterdrop. The temperature gradient between the warmer core and cooler periphery contributes to this drop as the cooler blood returns to the core. This is coupled with a drop in the mean arterial pressure and peripheral vascular resistance.[42]

Atrial and ventricular arrhythmias are common in patients with hypothermia, but these generally convert spontaneously during rewarming. Ventricular dysrhythmias occur frequently as well. The drug of choice for treatment of ventricular fibrillation remains unclear. The most recent American Heart Association guidelines recommend withholding antiarrhythmic medications if the core temperature is less than 30° C, and to give medications at longer intervals for temperatures above 30° C. Bretylium is no longer recommended.[25] Alternative medications such as vasopressin[43,44] and amiodarone,[45,46] which are now recommended for treatment of normothermic ventricular fibrillation, have been proposed as treatment modalities for hypothermia, but results from experimental studies have been inconclusive.

Summary

Predicting which patients will survive severe hypothermia is difficult. Patients with significant underlying medical illness, longer duration of cold exposure, lower core temperature, and depressed mental status, as well as those failing to rewarm rapidly and those requiring cardiopulmonary resuscitation, are thought to have a lower likelihood of survival,[3,47] but dramatic cases of hypothermic patients surviving prolonged cardiac arrest have been described.[38,48,49]

Nonetheless, most patients who present in cardiopulmonary arrest from hypothermia are not successfully resuscitated.[47,50] Patients who sustained a lethal insult prior to the onset of accidental hypothermia will not be resuscitated with warming therapy. Evidence of intravascular thrombosis, elevated ammonia, and severe hypokalemia have been suggested as markers for death in patients with hypothermia.[47,50,51] However, while some people are indeed "dead when they're cold and dead,"[52] there are no consistently accurate variables that predict an irreversible state in hypothermic patients in cardiopulmonary arrest. In a resuscitation, clinicians must also recognize that hypothermia occurs secondary to prolonged cardiac arrest from other etiologies and should consider that prolonged resuscitation under these circumstances may not be warranted.

Children with mild environmental hypothermia can be discharged home from the emergency department after correction of the core temperature. Neonates and hypothermic children who require more aggressive warming techniques, those who have significant laboratory abnormalities, and those in whom the etiology of the hypothermia cannot be identified should be admitted to the hospital for further evaluation, monitoring, and treatment.

REFERENCES

1. Danzl DF, Pozos RS: Accidental hypothermia. N Engl J Med 331:1756–1760, 1994.
2. Centers for Disease Control and Prevention: Hypothermia-related deaths—United States, 2003. MMWR Morb Mortal Wkly Rep 53:172–173, 2004.
*3. Danzl DF, Pozos RS, Auerbach PS, et al: Multicenter hypothermia survey. Ann Emerg Med 16:1042–1055, 1987.
4. Bernard SA, Gray TW, Buist MD, et al: Treatment of comatose survivors of out-of-hospital cardiac arrest with induced hypothermia. N Engl J Med 346:557–563, 2002.
5. Broderick JP, Hacke W: Treatment of acute ischemic stroke: Part II: Neuroprotection and medical management. Circulation 106:1736–1740, 2002.
6. Clifton GL, Miller ER, Choi SC, et al: Lack of effect of induction of hypothermia after acute brain injury. N Engl J Med 344:556–563, 2001.
7. Gadkary CS, Alderson P, Signorini DF: Therapeutic hypothermia for head injury. Cochrane Database Syst Rev (4):CD001048, 2004.
8. Jacobs S, Hunt R, Tarnow-Mordi W, et al: Cooling for newborns with hypoxic ischaemic encephalopathy. Cochrane Database Syst Rev (4): CD003311, 2003.
9. McIntyre LA, Fergusson DA, Hebert PC, et al: Prolonged therapeutic hypothermia after traumatic brain injury in adults: a systematic review. JAMA 289:2992–2999, 2003.
10. Niermeyer S, Kattwinkel J, Van Reempts P, et al: International guidelines for neonatal resuscitation: an excerpt from the Guidelines 2000 for Cardiopulmonary Resuscitation and Emergency Cardiovascular Care: International Consensus on Science. Contributors and Reviewers for the Neonatal Resuscitation Guidelines. Pediatrics 106:e29, 2000.

*Selected readings.

11. Polderman KH: Application of therapeutic hypothermia in the ICU: opportunities and pitfalls of a promising treatment modality. Part 1: Indications and evidence. Intensive Care Med 30:556–575, 2004.
12. The Hypothermia after Cardiac Arrest Study Group: Mild therapeutic hypothermia to improve the neurologic outcome after cardiac arrest. N Engl J Med 346:549–556, 2002.
13. Danzl DF: Accidental hypothermia. In Auerbach PS (ed): Wilderness Medicine, 4th ed. St. Louis: Mosby, 2001, pp 135–177.
14. Mallet ML: Pathophysiology of accidental hypothermia. QJM 95:775–785, 2002.
15. Centers for Disease Control and Prevention: Hypothermia-related deaths—Utah, 2000, and United States, 1979–1998. MMWR Morb Mortal Wkly Rep 51:76–78, 2002.
16. Stocks JM, Taylor NA, Tipton MJ, Greenleaf JE: Human physiological responses to cold exposure. Aviat Space Environ Med 75:444–457, 2004.
17. Sivaloganathan S: Paradoxical undressing due to hypothermia in a child. Med Sci Law 25:176–178, 1985.
18. Dagan R, Gorodischer R: Infections in hypothermic infants younger than 3 months old. Am J Dis Child 138:483–485, 1984.
19. Moscovitz HC, Magriples U, Keissling M, Schriver JA: Care and outcome of out-of-hospital deliveries. Acad Emerg Med 7:757–761, 2000.
20. Wyckoff MH, Perlman JM: Effective ventilation and temperature control are vital to outborn resuscitation. Prehosp Emerg Care 8:191–195, 2004.
21. Delaney KA, Howland MA, Vassallo S, Goldfrank LR: Assessment of acid-base disturbances in hypothermia and their physiologic consequences. Ann Emerg Med 18:72–82, 1989.
22. Vassallo SU, Delaney KA, Hoffman RS, et al: A prospective evaluation of the electrocardiographic manifestations of hypothermia. Acad Emerg Med 6:1121–1126, 1999.
23. Patel A, Getsos JP, Moussa G, Damato AN: The Osborn wave of hypothermia in normothermic patients. Clin Cardiol 17:273–276, 1994.
24. Okada M, Nishimura F, Yoshino H, et al: The J wave in accidental hypothermia. J Electrocardiol 16:23–28, 1983.
*25. Part 10.4: Hypothermia. Circulation 112(24 suppl):IV-136–138, 2005.
26. Elabbassi EB, Chardon K, Bach V, et al: Head insulation and heat loss in naked and clothed newborns using a thermal mannequin. Med Phys 29:1090–1096, 2002.
27. de Caen A: Management of profound hypothermia in children without the use of extracorporeal life support therapy. Lancet 360:1394–1395, 2002.
28. Kornberger E, Schwarz B, Lindner KH, Mair P: Forced air surface rewarming in patients with severe accidental hypothermia. Resuscitation 41:105–111, 1999.
*29. Steele MT, Nelson MJ, Sessler DI, et al: Forced air speeds rewarming in accidental hypothermia. Ann Emerg Med 27:479–484, 1996.
30. Goheen MSL, Ducharme MB, Kenny GP, et al: Efficacy of forced-air and inhalation rewarming by using a human model for severe hypothermia. J Appl Physiol 83:1635–1640, 1997.
31. Weinberg AD: The role of inhalation rewarming in the early management of hypothermia. Resuscitation 36:101–104, 1998.
32. Barcelona SL, Vilich F, Cote CJ: A comparison of flow rates and warming capabilities of the level 1 and rapid infusion system with various-size intravenous catheters. Anesth Analg 97:358–363, 2003.
33. Anshus JS, Endahl GL, Mottley JL: Microwave heating of intravenous fluids. Am J Emerg Med 3:316–319, 1985.
34. Leaman PL, Martyak GG: Microwave warming of resuscitation fluids. Ann Emerg Med 14:876–879, 1985.
35. Papenhausen M, Burke L, Antony A, Phillips JD: Severe hypothermia with cardiac arrest: complete neurologic recovery in a 4-year-old child. J Pediatr Surg 36:1590–1592, 2001.
36. Kangas E, Niemela H, Kojo N: Treatment of hypothermic circulatory arrest with thoracotomy and pleural lavage. Ann Chir Gynaecol 83:258–260, 1994.
*37. Walpoth BH, Walpoth-Aslan BN, Mattle HP, et al: Outcome of survivors of accidental deep hypothermia and circulatory arrest treated with extracorporeal blood warming. N Engl J Med 337:1500–1505, 1997.
38. Bolte RG, Black PG, Bowers RS, et al: The use of extracorporeal rewarming in a child submerged for 66 minutes. JAMA 260:377–379, 1988.
39. Vretenar DF, Urschel JD, Parrott JC, Unruh HW: Cardiopulmonary bypass resuscitation for accidental hypothermia. Ann Thorac Surg 58:895–898, 1994.
40. Wollenek G, Honarwar N, Golej J, Marx M: Cold water submersion and cardiac arrest in treatment of severe hypothermia with cardiopulmonary bypass. Resuscitation 52:255–263, 2002.
41. Sofer S, Benkovich E: Severe infantile hypothermia: short- and long-term outcome. Intensive Care Med 26:88–92, 2000.
42. Giesbrecht GG, Goheen MS, Johnston CE, et al: Inhibition of shivering increases core temperature afterdrop and attenuates rewarming in hypothermic humans. J Appl Physiol 83:1630–1634, 1997.
43. Schwarz B, Mair P, Raedler C, et al: Vasopressin improves survival in a pig model of hypothermic cardiopulmonary resuscitation. Crit Care Med 30:1311–1314, 2002.
44. Sumann G, Krismer AC, Wenzel V, et al: Cardiopulmonary resuscitation after near drowning and hypothermia: restoration of spontaneous circulation after vasopressin. Acta Anaesthesiol Scand 47:363–365, 2003.
45. Schwarz B, Mair P, Wagner-Berger H, et al: Neither vasopressin nor amiodarone improve CPR outcome in an animal model of hypothermic cardiac arrest. Acta Anaesthesiol Scand 47:1114–1118, 2003.
46. Stoner J, Martin G, O'Mara K, et al: Amiodarone and bretylium in the treatment of hypothermic ventricular fibrillation in a canine model. Acad Emerg Med 10:187 191, 2003.
47. Hauty MG, Esrig BC, Hill JG, Long WB: Prognostic factors in severe accidental hypothermia: experience from the Mt. Hood tragedy. J Trauma 27:1107–1112, 1987.
48. Southwick FS, Dalglish PH Jr: Recovery after prolonged asystolic cardiac arrest in profound hypothermia: a case report and literature review. JAMA 243:1250–1253, 1980.
49. Thompson DA, Anderson N: Successful resuscitation of a severely hypothermic neonate. Ann Emerg Med 23:1390–1393, 1994.
50. Mair P, Kornberger E, Furtwaengler W, et al: Prognostic markers in patients with severe accidental hypothermia and cardiocirculatory arrest. Resuscitation 27:47–54, 1994.
51. Schaller MD, Fischer AP, Perret CH: Hyperkalemia: a prognostic factor during acute severe hypothermia. JAMA 264:1842–1845, 1990.
52. Auerbach PS: Some people are dead when they're cold and dead. JAMA 264:1856–1857, 1990.
53. Watanabe T, Iwabuchi H, Oishi M: Accidental hypothermia in an infant with Prader-Willi syndrome. Eur J Pediatr 162:550–551, 2003.
54. Ludwig S, Warman M: Shaken baby syndrome: a review of 20 cases. Ann Emerg Med 13:104–107, 1984.
55. Wahl NG, Woodall BN: Hypothermia in shaken infant syndrome. Pediatr Emerg Care 11:233–234, 1995.
56. Greenberg RA, Rittichier KK: Pediatric nonenvironmental hypothermia presenting to the emergency department: episodic spontaneous hypothermia with hyperhidrosis. Pediatr Emerg Care 19:32–34, 2003.

Chapter 141

Snake and Spider Envenomations

Sean P. Bush, MD and James A. Moynihan, MS, DO

Key Points

First, do no harm: Many historically recommended interventions add insult to injury when applied to snakebite. Make sure that the potential benefits exceed risk.

Antivenom is the definitive treatment for serious snake envenomation. The sooner antivenom is given, the more likely that irreversible damage can be prevented.

Envenomation is an uncommon occurrence, so available resources (such as regional poison centers) should be consulted as necessary.

The diagnosis of spider bite is overused for wounds of uncertain etiology. There is no accepted specific treatment for brown recluse spider bite in the United States.

Envenomations and the treatment of such can cause severe allergic reactions, so be prepared to treat these potentially life-threatening complications.

Selected Diagnoses

Snakebites
Spider bites
    Widow spider bites
    Recluse and other spider bites

Discussion of Individual Diagnoses

The general principles of envenomation medicine are similar around the world, although the availability of resources varies widely. A comprehensive discussion of all available antivenoms is beyond the scope of this chapter, so the discussion will focus on U.S. antivenoms.[1] However, readers are encouraged to become familiar with the prescribing information for the antivenom(s) available in their area(s) of practice for the envenomations they may encounter.

Snakebites

Introduction and Background

Snakebite is a particularly challenging clinical problem because of the wide variety of toxic effects. Children with snakebites may suffer little more than a fang puncture mark or they may develop multisystem failure and die.[2,3] In part this is due to the extreme variability of snake venom, even within the same species.[4] Unfortunately, it is difficult to predict at the time of the bite which patients will have relatively mild symptoms and which will develop a rapidly progressive and potentially fatal envenomation syndrome.

Snakebite envenomation syndromes can be loosely associated with snake families. Viperidae includes old world vipers and pit vipers (collectively referred to as "viperids"). The vast majority of snakebites in the United States are inflicted by pit vipers, which include rattlesnakes, cottonmouths (also known as water moccasins), and copperheads.[5] All pit vipers have a heat-sensing pit between the eye and nostril.[6] Elapidae ("elapids") includes the cobras, coral snakes, kraits, and mambas.[7] Their venom effects can be as diverse as the species that comprise this family of snakes. Cobras are hooded, high-profile snakes inhabiting Africa and southern Asia. The coral snakes of the Americas and kraits of Asia and India are often small, shy, colorfully banded snakes. Mambas in Africa are long, lean, and fast-moving. Australian elapids can be large and nondescript. Sea snakes are found in waters around Southeast Asia and Australia. Sea snakes possess some of the world's most toxic snake venom, although few bites occur, mostly because of this family of snakes' marine distribution and nonaggressive temperament. Most snakes from the Colubridae family ("colubrids") are considered harmless, although many species possess venom and some have primitively specialized teeth to facilitate venom delivery. Some, such as the boomslang in Africa, are considered dangerous to humans, and antivenom is produced.

It is often stated that children are more severely affected by snakebite than adults.[8] Indeed, some preliminary data suggests that smaller patients present with increased severity. However, there is not much in terms of evidence to support the assertion that outcomes for children are worse than those for adults. For example, of the 104,750 exposures and 23 deaths described by the American Association of Poison Control Centers (AAPCC) since its first report in 1983, there have only been 2 deaths described in pediatric patients.[9] In some respects, children are no different than adults when it comes to snakebite. For instance, antivenom dosing is not based on the patient's weight.[10,11] Yet there are a few concerns specific to pediatric patients. For example, young children may not be able to give a good description of the snake or circumstances so that it is unclear whether a venomous snake has bitten them.

Although viper and pit viper venom composition varies from snake to snake, components can lead to capillary leak, abnormal clotting, inefficient muscle movement, or neurotoxicity. Capillary leak and abnormal clotting can lead to tachycardia, hypotension, or even hemorrhagic shock. Neurotoxicity or inefficient muscle movement can lead to respiratory difficulty or distress.[12] Meanwhile, proteolytic enzymes, predominant in viper and pit viper venoms, digest tissue. The longer that enzymatic components of venom have time to work, the more tissue damage is sustained. Therefore, "time is tissue."[13] The sooner that antivenom can be started, the sooner irreversible injury can be prevented.[14] However, once tissue is injured by way of digestion, antivenom will not reverse the damage—it will require time to heal.[15] Myotoxicity and rhabdomyolysis can also ensue.

Envenomation by most elapids is notable for severe neurologic dysfunction, such as cranial nerve abnormalities, paralysis, and respiratory arrest. However, the venom of some elapids (such as spitting and monocellate cobras) can cause local necrosis as well. Most elapid envenomations do not induce coagulopathy. Other symptoms and signs may include swelling, lethargy, vomiting, chest pain, and shock. Some cobras and cobra-like species can "spit" venom toward the face of an antagonist, which can result in eye pain and visual impairment. Sea snake envenomation can cause profound neurotoxicity and myotoxicity but generally does not induce coagulopathy or result in serious local injury. Additionally, some individuals may experience anaphylactic or anaphylactoid reactions to venom.[16,17] Finally, some responses can be attributed to anxiety, although this should be a diagnosis of exclusion.[6]

Clinical Presentation

Immediately after a snakebite, the only apparent manifestation may be fang puncture wounds. If a patient presents very early, an envenomation syndrome might not have developed yet. Symptoms and signs can begin very rapidly or they may be insidious. Generally, the more severe an envenomation, the more rapidly it progresses. However, even a slowly progressing envenomation can lead to severe sequelae. If a patient presents very late, the envenomation could have already run its course and antivenom will not be as effective.[14]

Typically snakebites by pit vipers and vipers cause pain around the bite site as tissues distort with swelling (Fig. 141–1). There may or may not be associated taste changes. Difficulty breathing can follow many types of venomous snakebites and can progress to respiratory distress or failure in some cases. Patients may experience nausea, vomiting, or diarrhea, and venom-induced coagulopathies (often associated with viper and pit viper envenomation) can lead to hematemesis and/or hematochezia. Certain snakebites (such as those inflicted by most elapids and some populations of rattlesnakes) can also be associated with neurologic symptoms, such as ptosis, motor weakness, or paresthesias. Syncope or lethargy can result from severe or prolonged hypotension.[6]

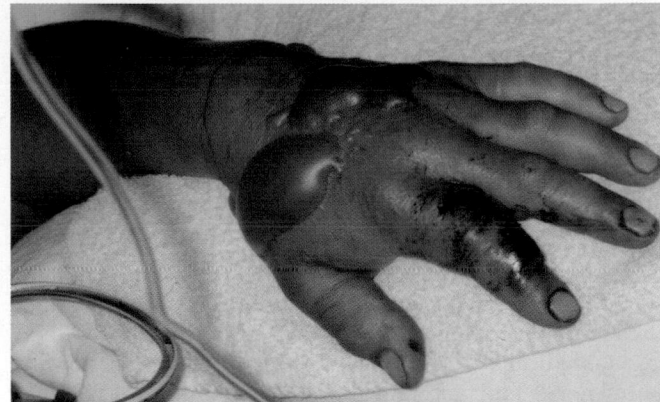

FIGURE 141–1. Tissue distortion and swelling on site of pit-viper bite.

Vital signs may reflect tachycardia, hypo- or hypertension, tachypnea, or hypoventilation. On physical examination, there may be one, two, or more fang puncture wounds or there may be none discernable. There is usually tenderness and swelling surrounding the bite site, which expands as the venom spreads locally. Other local signs can include erythema, ecchymosis, and bullae after viperid envenomation. Systemic viperid envenomation may manifest in many ways. There may be abnormal bleeding, such as prolonged bleeding from fang puncture wounds or intravenous line sites. Patients may have epistaxis or gingival bleeding. Serious and potentially life-threatening bleeding may manifest as gastrointestinal tract or intracranial hemorrhage. In extremely rare instances, snakebite can also cause hypercoagulability, which can lead to infarcts. Additionally, there may be neurologic signs, such as ptosis and muscle fasciculations.[6]

Initial laboratory studies after pit viper or viper envenomation should include a complete blood count, prothrombin time, international normalized ratio (INR), fibrinogen, and a type and screen. Venom-induced coagulopathies are common after many types of viperid envenomations (although not after elapid or sea snake envenomations) and are most typically characterized by thrombocytopenia and hypofibrinogenemia. Venom-induced coagulopathies can develop late, recur, or persist. Repeat laboratory testing is often used to gauge response to treatment. The same laboratory tests as initially drawn should be ordered, plus creatine kinase (CK), electrolytes, blood urea nitrogen, and creatinine. Patients with just about any kind of snakebite can develop rhabdomyolysis, which usually responds to aggressive fluid hydration but can require dialysis if myoglobinuria leads to renal failure. In certain regions, such as Australia, venom detection kits (such as enzyme-linked immunosorbent assays) may be available to help identify species and guide specific antivenom selection. Other diagnostic studies may be indicated on the basis of a patient's past medical history or special circumstances.[6]

It is possible that a snakebite might be mistaken for a puncture wound from another etiology (e.g., plant thorn) if the patient presents very early or if the envenomation is very mild, or if there are difficulties obtaining a reliable history. If there is any question about whether a patient has been bitten by a venomous snake, an observation period and diagnostic studies may help clarify the diagnosis. Patients with snakebites usually progress if significant envenomation has occurred. Certain signs (e.g., ecchymosis), symptoms (e.g., local paresthesias), and laboratory data (e.g., thrombocytopenia or hypofibrinogenemia) are fairly consistent with viperid envenomation. If a bite by an elapid is suspected, envenomation should be assumed.

Management

The factors that most reduce snakebite-related injury and mortality in the United States are rapid transport, intensive care, and antivenom.[18] All patients with snakebites should be transported to the hospital as expeditiously as safely possible, preferably by calling 911 where available to activate Emergency Medical Services. The following measures are not recommended for first aid: incision, suction, tourniquets, electric shock, ice directly on the wound, alcohol, or folk therapies.[19-21] Insufficient evidence exists for splinting and/or positioning (e.g., above or below the level of the heart). Therefore, the extremity should initially be maintained in a neutral position of comfort.

The Australian technique of pressure immobilization resulted in significantly longer survival, but higher intracompartmental pressures, after artificial intramuscular western diamondback rattlesnake envenomation in a pig model.[22] This technique involves immediately wrapping the entire snakebitten extremity, starting at the bite site and proceeding proximally, with an elastic Ace wrap or crepe bandage as tightly as one would for a sprain, then splinting and immobilizing the extremity. While pressure immobilization is not recommended widely, certain scenarios may warrant its use. It is generally not recommended for most viper bites or for bites by spitting cobras, but is recommended for most types of Australian fauna, cape cobras, kraits, coral snakes, mambas, and sea snakes. Once pressure immobilization is instituted, it should not be removed until antivenom is ready to infuse (if asymptomatic) or infusing (if symptomatic) because of a potential bolus effect after its removal.

Although it is difficult to predict snakebite severity at the time of the bite, certain factors may reflect increased likelihood of a more severe envenomation: large snake size, dangerous snake species, small patient size, prolonged fang contact, previous snakebites (treated or not) or exposures to snakes, or delays in medical care. All emergency personnel should be able to distinguish a venomous from a nonvenomous snake. If there is uncertainty about whether a particular snake is venomous or not, consider taking photographs of the snake from a safe distance of at least 6 feet away using a digital or instantly developing camera. These images can be seen immediately and may aid in clinical decision making. Although it may be helpful to identify the species of snake,[15,23] transporting it (alive or dead) is discouraged because of inherent dangers. On scene, snakes should only be moved or contained if absolutely necessary. A snake hook or long shovel may be helpful to move the snake into a large, empty trash canister where it can be recovered by a professional, such as an animal control agent.

Appropriate airway support should be provided as needed. Severe respiratory difficulty may require intubation and mechanical ventilation. Vital signs should be checked frequently, oxygen provided, and monitors placed. Two intravenous lines should be started, and central venous or intraosseous access should be considered if peripheral access proves difficult to achieve and maintain. However, the clinician should avoid placing a central line in a noncompressible site (e.g., subclavian) after viperid envenomation because of the risk of bleeding from venom-induced coagulopathy. A 20-ml/kg normal saline fluid bolus should be given. If there is evidence of shock, a second 20-ml/kg fluid bolus of normal saline should be given. Because viperid envenomation can induce coagulopathy and bleeding, transfusion may be required after treatment with two fluid boluses; 10 ml/kg packed red blood cells should be given for acute, life-threatening blood loss. Persistent hypotension may require vasopressors. Urine output of 1 to 2 ml/kg/hr for infants and young children and 0.5 to 1 ml/kg/hr for older children and adolescents may be used as a measure of adequate hydration. The patient should take nothing by mouth until it has been determined that he/she will not need to be mechanically ventilated.

After pit viper or viper envenomation, any rings or other constricting jewelry and clothing should be removed in anticipation of severe swelling. The expanding area of swelling and tenderness can be used to follow the progression of viperid envenomations. Tenderness is more sensitive than swelling for detecting progression. By palpating until the advancing edge of tenderness is found, marking this leading edge with a permanent marker and the time, and repeating this every 15 to 20 minutes initially, progression can be gauged. Once antivenom is started, the advancing edge of tenderness should still be followed every 1 to 2 hours. Serial measurements of circumference may be helpful as well.

ANTIVENOM

All hospitals should stock at least enough antivenom to treat a patient. This should be arranged ahead of time if possible, although sometimes there are antivenom shortages and other resource challenges. Two agents are available in the United States for treatment of pit viper envenomation: Crotalidae Polyvalent Immune Fab (Ovine), which goes by the trade name CroFab, and Antivenin Crotalidae Polyvalent (Equine).[24] CroFab is manufactured by Protherics Inc. (Nashville, TN) and distributed by Fougera (Melville, NY; 1-800-231-0206). A similar formulation is produced for European vipers. Antivenin Crotalidae Polyvalent, manufactured by Wyeth-Ayerst, is still available on the shelves of many hospital pharmacies, but is no longer being produced. Coral snake antivenom manufacture was reportedly discontinued by Wyeth-Ayerst in 2004; however, a new antivenom is being developed. Several manufacturers produce antivenom for elapid bites in Africa, Asia, Europe, and Australia (e.g., Commonwealth Serum Laboratories in Melbourne, *http://www.allergytest.com/index.cfm*) and in the Americas (e.g., Instituto Bioclon in Mexico, *http://www.bioclon.com.mx*; Instituto Clodomiro Picado in Costa Rica, *http://www.icp.ucr.ac.cr/indice.shtml*; and the Butantan Institute, *http://bernard.pitzer.edu/~lyamane/butantan.htm*). A polyvalent sea snake antivenom (Commonwealth Serum Laboratories) is the drug of choice for sea snake envenomation. Haffkine Institute in Bombay, India, produces an alternate sea snake antivenom.

A new resource recently became available for assistance in managing exotic envenomations: the Online Antivenom Index (OAI), developed by the AAPCC and the American Zoo and Aquarium Association. By calling any regional poison control center (1-800-222-1222), the OAI can be accessed, and antivenom stocked by zoos for exotic snakes can be emergently located. This will facilitate determining, locating, and obtaining exotic antivenoms in a timely manner, potentially improving the care of patients with uncommonly encountered and very challenging envenomations. Additionally, zoos can continuously update the OAI with their antivenom stock and have access to contact information, replacing a 7-year old hardcopy reference.

Fifty or more non-native, venomous snake exposures are reported to U.S. poison centers each year, a third of which result in serious clinical effects, including deaths. Exotic snakes are easily obtained, both legally and illegally, at trade shows or via the Internet. The AAPCC Toxic Exposure Surveillance System reported more bites from exotic venomous snakes than from native U.S. coral snakes last year. Antivenom may not always be available for all species. Supplies have limited shelf life and may be expensive, and several are no longer in production. The Food and Drug Administration considers foreign antivenoms investigational and/or unapproved. Information on antivenom should be researched ahead of time, and practitioners should be familiar with sources and administration techniques for the antivenoms available. Each antivenom has varying specificity, efficacy, and safety. Some antivenoms developed for one species may have some efficacy against other closely related species.

If antivenom is unavailable, a patient with an elapid or sea snake envenomation may need ventilatory support for days or even weeks. Hypotension should be treated with intravenous fluids, then vasopressors. Edrophonium may temporarily improve weakened muscles of respiration after elapid envenomation while awaiting antivenom (after pretreatment with atropine). The need for antivenom must be determined in each patient. Many grading scales are available, but it is better to treat a patient based on envenomation progression or potential. Grading scales should not be used for elapid or sea snake envenomations. Antivenom should be given promptly for best results, although it may have benefit for days to weeks after an envenomation. Any time antivenom is given, allergic reactions should be anticipated. It may be helpful to know whether the patient has allergies or previous exposures to serums or other agents used to make antivenom. Informed consent must be obtained, and the potential for an allergic reaction discussed with the patient and caregivers.

Because many of the principles are similar for other antivenoms (although dosing may vary), the technique for administering CroFab is given as an example. A starting dose of CroFab is 4 to 6 vials.[25] There is no change in the dose for children, although fluid volume may need to be adjusted for very small infants and children. Each vial is reconstituted with 10 ml of sterile water for injection. It can take anywhere from 10 to 30 minutes to go into solution. It is best to swirl or roll the vials between the hands rather than shake them. Once each vial goes into solution, it should be further diluted into a total volume of 250 ml of normal saline. No skin test is recommended for CroFab, although manufacturers of many other types of antivenom recommend skin testing. With CroFab, the infusion is started slowly, at a rate of 25 to 50 ml/hr for the first 10 minutes. While the infusion is started, a physician skilled in resuscitation should be immediately available. Equipment for a difficult airway, epinephrine and diphenhydramine, and a histamine$_2$ (H$_2$)-blocker

(such as cimetidine) should also be readily available. As the infusion is initiated, the physician should watch for signs of any adverse reaction (see later). If the infusion is tolerated for the first 10 minutes without evidence of an adverse reaction, the rate should be increased to a maximum of 250 ml/hr.

If there is a problem at any time, the infusion should be stopped and the adverse reaction treated accordingly, with reassessment of the need to continue antivenom treatment. A physician should be nearby at all times during the remainder of the infusion. The infusion is repeated with 4- to 6-vial increments until initial control is achieved. "Initial control" is defined as the arrest of progression of any and all components of the envenomation syndrome (i.e., no further advancement of swelling, improvement of systemic effects, and improving coagulopathy). The patient should be assessed at up to 1 hour after each dose. After initial control is achieved, a maintenance dose of 2 vials of CroFab every 6 hours for three doses is recommended.[26] The package insert may be consulted for additional details.[25]

Important Clinical Features and Considerations

For pharmacokinetic reasons that are not entirely understood, recurrence phenomena are often associated with antivenoms.[27-29] "Local recurrence" is the return of new progressive swelling after initial control; that is, the leading edge of tenderness or swelling begins to advance again. An additional 2 vials of CroFab should be given as soon as progressive swelling recurs, and more antivenom may be needed to regain control. Patients with rattlesnake bites commonly develop thrombocytopenia and hypofibrinogenemia, which can resolve with CroFab and then recur ("coagulopathy recurrence"). Indications for an additional 2 vials of CroFab are serious abnormal bleeding, fibrinogen less than 50 µg/ml, platelet count less than 25,000/mm^3, INR greater than 3.0, multicomponent coagulopathy, worsening trend in a patient with prior severe coagulopathy, high-risk behavior for trauma, or comorbid conditions that increase bleeding risk. Coagulopathy can recur as late as 2 weeks or more after treatment.

The patient should be transfused if antivenom does not correct coagulopathy or if there is an imminent risk of serious bleeding. Transfusion of the appropriate blood product is generally recommended for life-threatening bleeding, platelets less than 10,000 to 30,000/mm^3, or hemoglobin less than 7 g/dl. Additionally, fresh frozen plasma and/or platelets may be required to treat venom-induced coagulopathy if antivenom does not promptly resolve. Computed tomography of the brain should be considered if the patient has a severe headache or an altered level of consciousness with a severe coagulopathy.

Ocular exposure to venom necessitates prompt and copious irrigation and an ophthalmologist's evaluation.

Pain relief is provided with an opioid while maintaining a respiratory rate and blood pressure that is appropriate for age. Nonsteroidal anti-inflammatory drugs are contraindicated for approximately 2 weeks after viper and pit viper envenomation because they can contribute to venom-induced coagulopathy and bleeding. Tetanus prophylaxis should be updated as appropriate.

Prophylactic antibiotics are unnecessary. However, if an infection develops, aerobic and anaerobic wound cultures should be obtained. Empirical therapy should then be started pending culture and sensitivity results. If an abscess occurs, it should be drained in standard fashion. A suggested outpatient regimen would include amoxicillin-clavulanate plus a dose of ceftriaxone. For penicillin-allergic patients, an extended-spectrum cephalosporin or trimethoprim-sulfamethoxazole plus clindamycin should be selected. An infected snakebite should prompt a further examination of the wounds for potential retained teeth or fangs.[5]

Envenomations by vipers and pit vipers are remarkable for the amount of swelling they can produce. With prompt and adequate antivenom treatment, surgical intervention is rarely indicated, even after severe viperid envenomation.[30-33] Compartment syndrome is diagnosed using clinical examination and compartment pressure, and treated with additional antivenom and pressure monitoring. Antivenom has been shown to limit the decrease in perfusion pressure associated with compartment syndrome.[34] Surgical consultation may be needed. Fasciotomy and/or digit dermotomy should be considered a last resort. It may be difficult to distinguish compartment syndrome from the effects of envenomation. Similar to compartment syndrome, viperid envenomation may cause a bluish discoloration of the skin or pallor (because of subcutaneous bruising), severe swelling, paresthesias, and pain. If effects are only caused by envenomation and the patient does not have compartment syndrome, capillary refill should be normal and compartmental pressures should not be elevated.

Antivenoms can induce immediate anaphylactic (type I hypersensitivity) or anaphylactoid reactions, which can be rapidly life threatening. Airway swelling, wheezing, shock, and/or urticaria characterize these reactions. Anaphylactic and anaphylactoid reactions are treated with antihistamines, H₂-blockers, epinephrine, steroids, and ventilatory/circulatory support as needed. Antivenoms can also cause serum sickness, a delayed (type III hypersensitivity) reaction characterized by fever, urticaria, lymphadenopathy, and polyarthralgias days to weeks after treatment. Although serum sickness can be a very uncomfortable experience, it is usually benign and self-limited and is treated on an outpatient basis with antihistamines and steroids. Adverse reactions are much less common after treatment with Fab-based antivenoms than they are with whole immunoglobulin formulations.[14] All commercially available antivenoms in the United States use mercury (in the form of thimerosal) as a preservative, which in high doses can cause nerve and kidney toxicities in small children.[25] The manufacturer of CroFab is investigating alternative preservatives and plans to remove thimerosal from its product sometime in the near future. The AAPCC may assist in management of envenomations. A regional poison control center may be contacted at 1-800-222-1222.

All children with snake envenomations should be admitted to the hospital. Serious effects can be delayed and can recur even after treatment with antivenom. Therefore, a regimen of very close observation with monitoring, frequent measurements of swelling/tenderness, and neurologic checks for at least 24 hours is recommended. This degree of monitoring may require transfer to a pediatric intensive care unit. Some hospitals may have intermediate intensive care units or observation units that may be appropriate for patients with less severe envenomations. Patients with bites by less toxic vipers, such as copperheads, are probably best managed as inpatients as well, although this may change as more experience is gained with safer, more effective antivenoms.[35] Patients believed to have "dry bites" in which no venom effects develop should be observed for at least 8 hours.[6] Several reports in the literature have documented instances in which patients who initially were discharged with apparent nonenvenomations or mild envenomations returned in several hours with significant injury and required antivenom and admission.

Upon discharge, the patient should be instructed to return immediately for further swelling, severe pain, abnormal bleeding or bruising, dark tarry stools, petechiae, or severe headache. Also, patients should be given wound care instructions and told to return for signs of wound infection. Signs of serum sickness should be outlined, and the patient should return or follow up if these signs deveop any time in the few weeks after treatment with antivenom. The patient should be told not to take nonsteroidal anti-inflammatory drugs for 2 weeks after a pit viper or viper bite. Instead, acetaminophen with or without a combined opioid analgesic should be prescribed. The patient should not engage in contact sports or schedule any elective surgery or dental work for 2 weeks after viperid bites. The patient should be instructed to drink plenty of liquids and warned to return for decreased urination or cola-colored urine.

Some patients may need referral to a physical therapist. Blisters, blebs, and bullae should be left in place, but may need débridement along with necrotic tissue after several days, so surgical referral as appropriate is suggested.[30] Skin grafting is sometimes necessary. If the patient was bitten on the foot or leg, crutches and crutch training should be provided. However, the patient should be encouraged to bear weight and mobilize the extremity as tolerated. In some cases, a next-day wound check may be appropriate. Otherwise, the patient should return or follow up in a few days.[28] At that time, laboratory tests may need to be repeated, depending on the clinical scenario. The patient should be re-treat with antivenom as needed. Most patients recover fully after snakebite. However, viperid envenomation results in tissue loss, deformity, or loss of function in a clinically significant percentage of patients.[8]

Preventative measures should be explained to parents and children. Children should be taught to leave snakes alone. They should never touch, handle, or try to kill venomous snakes. Many people are bitten when they are intentionally interacting with the snake. Even after a snake is believed to be dead, fangs still can inject venom. Snakes that were presumed dead have bitten many people and delivered serious, even fatal, envenomations. Additionally, a snake can strike faster and farther than one might think—about half its body length—so children should be warned to stay at least "two giant steps" away from snakes. If a child finds a snake, he/she should tell an adult. Additionally, children should be told not to reach or step into places that they cannot see into. Wearing boots and jeans may prevent some (but not all) snakebites. Emergency physicians practicing in a snake territory should inform the patient population that, although there is no way to completely eliminate exposure to snakes, there are a few things that may make a property less appealing for snakes. For example, one can eliminate places where snakes can hide (e.g., log piles or heavy vegetation). Children should be educated about what to do if a snake bites them (i.e., it is very important that they tell an adult right away).

Spider Bites

Widow Spider Bites

Widow spiders belong to the genus *Latrodectus* and are represented in the United States by the black widows, the brown widow, and the red-legged widow.[36] The redback spider is endemic to Australia. Other species, such as the kara kurt and black button spider, are found in other parts of the world, including Europe, South America, and South Africa. The adult female black widow spider is approximately 2 cm in length and shiny black with a red-orange hourglass or spot on the ventral abdomen. The male is much smaller, brown, and much less commonly implicated in human envenomation. Juvenile females are also brown, with yellow and white markings, but have the general body morphology of the adult. Males and juveniles have a pale hourglass shape, similar to adult females. Webs are irregular, low-lying, and commonly seen in garages, barns, outhouses, and foliage. Other widow spiders around the world are generally black but may have red spots, such as the kara kurt, or a dorsal red stripe, such as the redback spider. The brown widow is brown with red and yellow markings. Similar species include the false black widow or cupboard spider (*Steatoda* species), which can produce symptoms that are similar in character to but milder in intensity than widow spiders. No deaths caused by widow spider envenomation have been reported to the AAPCC since its first annual report in 1983. However, recent deaths have been reported elsewhere.[37,38]

CLINICAL PRESENTATION

The envenomation syndrome caused by the various species of widow spiders around the world is similar.[39,40] The predominant clinical effects are neurologic and autonomic. Typically, the bite site has a "target" appearance. There may be a central reddened, indurated area around fang puncture site(s) surrounded by an area of blanching and an outer halo of redness (Fig. 141–2). The findings around the bite wound may be quite subtle, and the wound does not become necrotic. The predominant symptoms frequently involve painful muscle cramping. If the patient is bitten on the lower extremity, pain usually progresses from the foot, up the leg, and into the back and abdomen. If bitten on the upper extremity, pain usually progresses from the hand, up the arm, and into the chest and abdomen. Abdominal pain may be so severe as to mimic an acute abdomen, with tenderness and rigidity.[41]

Diaphoresis locally around the bite site is distinctive for widow spider envenomation, although diaphoresis may be diffuse and profuse, or it may manifest in unusual patterns remote from the bite site. Local piloerection is sometimes seen. Patients may exhibit "*Latrodectus* facies" (Fig. 141–3), characterized by spasm of facial muscles, edematous eyelids, and lacrimation, which may be mistaken for an allergic reaction. Other common symptoms and signs include high blood pressure, rapid heart rate, nausea, vomiting, headache, and anxiety. In a typical progression, symptoms begin within an hour, reach maximum intensity by about 12 hours, and can last for days to weeks. Unusual presentations have been described following widow spider envenomation, including pulmonary edema, myocarditis, and priapism.[37,42]

It has been suggested that there may be increased danger to pediatric patients with widow spider bites and that this population may require more aggressive treatment and hospitalization, although this assertion has been challenged.[43] Very little evidence supports either argument. The only recent documented fatalities from widow spider envenomation involved a healthy 19-year-old woman and an elderly male.

Rhabdomyolysis has been reported after widow spider envenomation,[42] so CK should be determined if severe envenomation develops. If the patient has respiratory difficulty, a chest radiograph should be obtained. Electrocardiography or echocardiography may detect the rare case of venom-induced myocarditis in a critically ill patient. Otherwise, diagnostics are not particularly helpful. If the diagnosis is uncertain, evaluation should be aimed uncovering other etiologies (such as an acute abdomen). Misdiagnosing an acute abdomen in a patient with a widow spider envenomation could lead to unnecessary surgery.

MANAGEMENT

In the prehospital setting, the airway, breathing, and circulation should be supported with oxygen, monitors, and intravenous access as necessary. First aid is not particularly helpful for widow spider envenomation. Electric shock and various folk and herbal remedies lack therapeutic value and are potentially harmful. There are two basic definitive treatment options: antivenom, or a combination of pain medications and sedatives. There are risks and benefits associated with

FIGURE 141–2. "Target appearance" of widow spider bite.

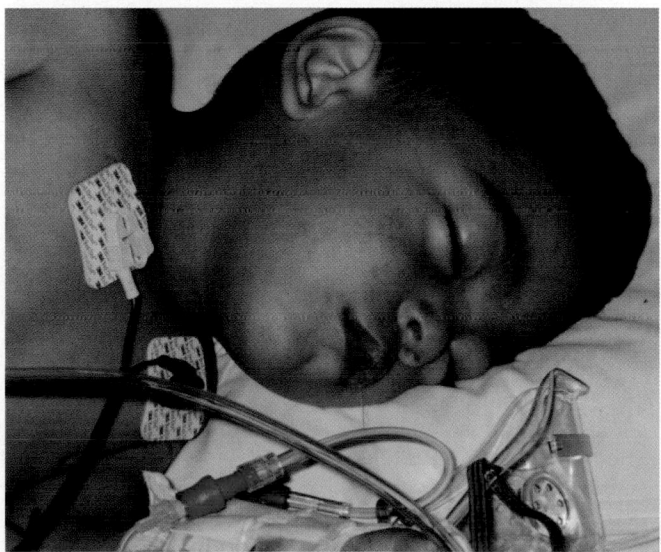

FIGURE 141–3. "*Latrodectus* facies" resulting from widow spider bite.

each alternative. Management with an opioid analgesic and a benzodiazepine is generally considered safe. However, this treatment option is purely palliative, and symptoms may persist for days or even weeks. The pain and discomfort associated with widow spider envenomation can be quite severe.

In contrast, antivenom is remarkably effective. Unfortunately it can be associated with very severe side effects, including death.[44] Because death is so rare after widow spider envenomation, it may be argued that the treatment is more dangerous than the bite itself. Historically, intravenous calcium was recommended, although it is believed to be ineffective.[44] Several antivenoms have been manufactured, including Black Widow Spider Antivenin (Equine) in the United States; Australia Red-back spider Antivenom, USSR Monovalent (*L. tredecimguttatus*); and South Africa spider antivenom (button spider).[1] Indications for antivenom use and routes of administration vary around the world. To give Black Widow Spider Antivenin according to the package insert, one vial should be reconstituted in 2.5 ml of the sterile diluent supplied. It is further diluted into a volume of 10 to 50 ml saline and administered intravenously over 15 minutes. Patients usually experience dramatic relief within an hour of treatment with one vial, although sometimes two and rarely three vials are needed. It may be effective days, weeks, or possibly even months after the envenomation.[45] The risk of allergy to antivenom must be weighed against the benefit of relieving prolonged discomfort, avoiding hospitalization, and preventing complications.

Although most widow spider envenomations can be managed with opioid analgesics and benzodiazepines, antivenom may be indicated for patients who have severe envenomations with pain refractory to these measures. Antivenom should be given if there is an imminent risk of a severe complication of envenomation. Factors that could increase the risk of antivenom include allergy or previous exposure to horse serum, or a past medical history of reactive airways.[46]

Serious, even fatal, adverse reactions have been documented after treatment with black widow spider antivenom. Anaphylactic and anaphylactoid reactions to antivenom can occur and may even be more life threatening than the envenomation itself. Skin testing, by injecting 0.02 ml of the test material supplied intradermally and observing for an urticarial wheal in 10 minutes, variably predicts immediate hypersensitivity to antivenom and may influence the decision regarding its administration. Increasing the volume of dilution and slowing the rate of infusion may reduce the chance that an allergic (anaphylactoid) reaction will occur. Additionally, premedication with antihistamines (H_1- and H_2-blockers) may reduce the likelihood that an acute allergic reaction will occur. Serum sickness, characterized by fever, urticaria, lymphadenopathy, and polyarthralgias, can occur days to weeks after treatment and is treated with antihistamines and steroids.

Antibiotics are not indicated for widow spider envenomation. Tetanus prophylaxis should be updated as appropriate. The regional poison control center may be helpful with management of widow spider envenomations and can be contacted at 1-800-222-1222.

Because it so effectively resolves symptoms, antivenom has been shown to decrease the need for hospitalization after widow spider envenomation. Admission to the hospital and possibly the pediatric intensive care unit is prudent for severely symptomatic children, those with intractable pain and contraindications to antivenom, those with unusual complications of envenomation, and those who develop anaphylaxis to antivenom. Patients who experience relief with opioid analgesics, benzodiazepines, and/or antivenom may be discharged. Upon discharge, signs of serum sickness should be outlined and the patient should return or follow up if these signs show up any time in the few weeks after treatment with antivenom. The envenomation syndrome usually resolves completely, with or without treatment, and does not leave the patient with long-term sequelae. Death is very rare.

Spider bites may be prevented by eliminating the spider's food and habitat; by shaking sheets, shoes, and clothing before donning; by keeping a child's bed away from the wall; and by brushing spiders off rather than crushing them. Safer, effective antivenoms are being developed and investigated.

Recluse and Other Spider Bites

The diagnosis of brown recluse spider bite is overused for dermonecrotic wounds of uncertain etiology.[47] In addition, reports of presumptive brown recluse spider bites reinforce improbable diagnosis in regions of North America where the spider is not endemic.[48] There are so many published accounts of "suspected," "presumed," or "possible" spider bites that it has led to a poor understanding of the true pathophysiology of spider envenomation. The literature on the topic is contradictory, and little is evidence based. Fewer than 100 recluse spider bites have been confirmed and documented in the literature. The true incidence, morbidity, and mortality are unknown. Reported deaths are questionable.[49] This overdiagnosis of spider bites occurs in pandemic proportions in many parts of the world, including the Americas, Australia, Africa, and Europe. The primary toxin in recluse spider venom is sphingomyelinase D.

CLINICAL PRESENTATION

Brown recluse spider (*Loxosceles reclusa*) bites are thought to produce a dry, irregular, sinking blue-gray/white patch with ragged edges, surrounded by erythema—the "red, white, and blue" sign. After a bite, the typical progression is thought to start with mild stinging for 6 to 8 hours followed by aching. The lesion develops a violacious center, with a ring of pallor and a halo of erythema and edema. There may be a gravity-influenced eccentric ring of redness. After about 24 to 72 hours, an eschar forms. After approximately 2 to 5 weeks, it sloughs, leaving an ulcer. Systemic loxoscelism has been described, but it is rare and very poorly understood.

No routine laboratory tests are indicated in the evaluation of a spider bite. Experimental venom detection assays are in development. Because so many things can be mistaken for spider bites, diagnostics should be used as necessary to evaluate for other conditions. Appearances can be deceiving. It is difficult (if not impossible) to diagnose a recluse spider bite just by looking at the wound. Dozens of conditions resemble a spider bite, and many conditions, including treatable ones, have been misdiagnosed as a brown recluse bite (cellulitis, necrotizing faciitis, Lyme disease, cancer, cutaneous anthrax, sporotrichosis, chemical burns, vasculitis, stasis ulcerations, poison ivy dermatitis, and many more).[50]

Certain features make it less likely that a recluse spider caused a lesion. The spider's range should be taken into account. If an unexplained wound developed in a geographic area where there are no native recluse spiders or populations, then it is much less likely to be a recluse spider bite. It is possible that spiders may occasionally be transported out of their range, but this happens much less often than could account for the number of lesions attributed to these spiders.[48,51] In the absence of recluse spiders in the Pacific Northwest of the United States, the hobo spider (*Tegenaria agrestis*) became the scapegoat for idiopathic lesions and grew to urban legend proportions. However, there is no evidence that hobo spiders cause necrotic wounds at all.[52] Similar extrapolation to other spiders has occurred in Australia with the black house spider (*Badumna insignis*) and the white-tailed spider (*Lampona cylindrata*). Other spiders possibly implicated in necrotic wounds in other parts of the world include the sac and running spiders (*Cheiracanthium* species) as well as the six-eyed spiders (*Sicarius* species) in South Africa. Bites from the vast majority of spiders do not cause necrotic wounds.[53]

Spider behavior should be taken into account as well when considering the likelihood that a spider caused a wound. For example, because spiders are not parasitic and generally only bite humans out of defense, multiple lesions are suggestive of an etiology other than spider bites. Recluse spiders are non-aggressive, and there are reports of people living in homes infested with hundreds, even thousands, of brown recluse spiders with no bites. Certain wound features should move a spider bite lower in the differential diagnosis. Large (>10 cm in diameter) ulcers are less likely to be spider bites. Early ulceration, within a week, is suggestive of an etiology other than spider bite.[54] If a spider is caught in the act of biting, it may be helpful to identify it or have it identified by an entomologist or arachnologist (if available). Recluse spiders have 6 eyes grouped in pairs, whereas most other spiders have 8 eyes.

MANAGEMENT

Electric shock was once proposed as a treatment for brown recluse spider bite, but no benefit has been shown from it and it can injure the patient. Treatment recommendations in the literature vary widely. Most agree that routine wound care is standard. If there is any question regarding the diagnosis, the actual etiology should be sought and treated. Sphingomyelinase D activity may be attenuated with cooling measures and augmented with heat. Therefore, a cooling pack may reduce the effects of recluse spider envenomation, although cold-induced injury should be avoided. Conversely, factors that increase warmth to the area, such as infection, should be treated. Although a spider bite itself is not infectious, antibiotics are indicated if a wound appears infected. Dapsone has been recommended for treatment of confirmed brown recluse spider bites, but it is not approved for this use, has serious side effects (such as methemoglobinemia and hemolysis), and is contraindicated in children. Furthermore, its efficacy is unclear. Similarly, hyperbaric oxygen has been suggested on a theoretical basis, but there is no evidence that it is effective for treatment of spider bites.[55,56] Surgical excision may be necessary once a necrotic lesion declares itself. However, early surgical excision (i.e., to prevent venom effects) is strongly discouraged. Skin grafting may be needed for wound defects. Steroids are not helpful for cutaneous loxoscelism. Antivenom is available for *Loxosceles laeta* (Peru Antiloxoscelico).[1] An investigational Fab antivenom has been developed in the United States, but it has to be given within 4 hours to be effective. This is generally not clinically practical. Venom detection tests are being researched. One such assay is sensitive enough to tell if a patient has a venomous arthropod bite, but it is nonspecific such that false positives occur with venoms of many other spider species and even scorpion species.[54]

Most patients with suspected or actual recluse spider bites can be managed on an outpatient basis. However, because of the difficulties associated with diagnosis, it is important for patients with suspected spider bites to follow up closely for further evaluation. The vast majority of spider bites heal completely, although a small percentage can develop into a chronic, ulcerative or necrotic wound. However, many chronic idiopathic wounds of other etiologies are attributed to spider bites, and so the actual prognosis is hard to estimate.

A tarantula may have a formidable, intimidating appearance, and its bite may be painful, but it is not particularly dangerous to humans. Basic wound care and tetanus prophylaxis are generally all that is needed. However, urticating hairs flicked from the abdomen can irritate the eyes, skin, and mucous membranes. Ocular exposure can necessitate removal of the hairs by an ophthalmologist.

REFERENCES

1. Boyer DM: Antivenom Index. Bethesda, MD: American Zoo and Aquarium Association, 1999.
2. Bush SP, Jansen PW: Severe rattlesnake envenomation with anaphylaxis and rhabdomyolysis. Ann Emerg Med 25:845 848, 1995.
3. Bush SP, Thomas TL, Chin ES: Envenomations in children. Pediatr Emerg Med Rep 2:1–12, 1997.
4. French WJ, Hayes WK, Bush SP, et al: Mojave toxin in venom of *Crotalus helleri* (southern Pacific rattlesnake): molecular and geographic characterization. Toxicon 44:781–791, 2004.
5. Norris RL Jr, Bush SP: North American venomous reptile bites. *In* Auerbach PS (ed): Wilderness Medicine, 4th ed. St. Louis: Mosby, 2001, pp 896–926.
*6. Gold BS, Dart RC, Barish RA: Bites of venomous snakes. N Engl J Med 347:347–356, 2002.
7. Norris RL Jr, Minton SA: Non-North American venomous reptile bites. *In* Auerbach PS (ed): Wilderness Medicine, 4th ed. St. Louis: Mosby, 2001, pp 927–951.
8. Dart RC, McNally JT, Spaite DW, et al: The sequelae of pit viper poisoning in the United States. *In* Campbell JA, Brodie ED (eds): Biology of the Pitvipers. Selva: Tyler, 1992, pp 395–404.
9. Watson WA, Litovitz TL, Klein-Schwartz W, et al: 2003 annual report of the American Association of Poison Control Centers toxic exposure surveillance system. Am J Emerg Med 22:335–404, 2004.
10. Behm MO, Kearns GL, Offerman S, et al: Crotaline Fab antivenom for treatment of children with rattlesnake envenomation [Letter]. Pediatrics 112:1458–1459, 2003.
*11. Offerman SR, Bush SP, Moynihan JA, et al: Crotaline Fab antivenom for the treatment of children with rattlesnake envenomation. Pediatrics 110:968–971, 2002.
12. Bush SP, Siedenburg E: Neurotoxicity associated with suspected southern Pacific rattlesnake (*Crotalus viridis helleri*) envenomation. Wilderness Environ Med J 10:247–249, 1999.
13. Dart RC, Waeckerle JF: Introduction: "Advances in the management of snakebite" symposium. Ann Emerg Med 37:166–167, 2001.
*14. Dart RC, McNally J: Efficacy, safety, and use of snake antivenoms in the United States. Ann Emerg Med 37:181–188, 2001.
15. Bush SP, Green SM, Moynihan JA, et al: Crotalidae Polyvalent Immune Fab (Ovine) antivenom is efficacious for envenomations by southern Pacific rattlesnakes (*Crotalus helleri*). Ann Emerg Med 40:619–624, 2002.

*Selected readings.

16. Hinze JD, Barker JA, Jones TR, et al: Life-threatening upper airway edema caused by a distal rattlesnake bite. Ann Emerg Med 38:79–82, 2001.

17. Camilleri C, Offerman S: Anaphylaxis after rattlesnake bite [Letter]. Ann Emerg Med 43:784–785, 2004.

18. Hardy DL: Fatal rattlesnake envenomation in Arizona: 1969–1984. Clin Toxicol 24:1–10, 1986.

19. Bush SP, Hegewald K, Green SM, et al: Effects of a negative pressure venom extraction device (Extractor™) on local tissue injury after artificial rattlesnake envenomation in a porcine model. Wilderness Environ Med J 11:180–188, 2000.

*20. Bush SP: Snakebite suction devices don't remove venom—they just suck [Editorial]. Ann Emerg Med 43:187–188, 2004.

21. Bush SP, Hardy DL Sr: Immediate removal of Extractor is recommended [Letter]. Ann Emerg Med 38:607–608, 2001.

22. *Bush SP, Green SM, Laack TA, et al: Pressure-immobilization delays mortality and increases intra-compartmental pressure after artificial intramuscular rattlesnake envenomation in a porcine model. Ann Emerg Med 44:599–604, 2004.

23. Bush SP, Cardwell MD: Mojave rattlesnake (*Crotalus scutulatus scutulatus*) identification. Wilderness Environ Med J 10:6–9, 1999.

24. Dart RC, Seifert SA, Carroll L, et al: Affinity-purified, mixed monospecific crotalid antivenom ovine Fab for treatment of crotalid venom poisoning. Ann Emerg Med 30:33–39, 1997.

*25. Prescribing Information: CroFab™. Nashville, TN: Protherics, Inc., 2000.

*26. Dart RC, Seifert SA, Boyer LV, et al: A randomized multicenter trial of crotaline polyvalent immune Fab (ovine) antivenom for the treatment for crotaline snakebite in the United States. Arch Intern Med 161:2030–2036, 2001.

27. Seifert SA, Boyer LV: Recurrence phenomena after immunoglobulin therapy for snake envenomations: Part 1. Pharmacokinetics and pharmacodynamics of immunoglobulin antivenoms and related antibodies. Ann Emerg Med 37:189–195, 2001.

28. Boyer LV, Seifert SA, Cain JS: Recurrence phenomena after immunoglobulin therapy for snake envenomations: Part 2. Guidelines for clinical management with crotaline Fab antivenom. Ann Emerg Med 37:196–201, 2001.

29. Bush SP, Wu VH, Corbett SW: Rattlesnake venom-induced thrombocytopenia response to Antivenin (Crotalidae) Polyvalent. Acad Emerg Med 7:181–185, 2000.

*30. Hall EL: Role of surgical intervention in the management of crotaline snake envenomation. Ann Emerg Med 37:175–180, 2001.

31. Gold BS, Barish RA, Dart RC, et al: Resolution of compartment syndrome after rattlesnake envenomation utilizing non-invasive measures. J Emerg Med 24:285–288, 2003.

32. Rosen PB, Leiva J, Ross C: Delayed antivenom treatment for a patient after envenomation by *Crotalus atrox*. Ann Emerg Med 35:86–88, 2000.

33. Tanen DA, Ruha AM, Graeme KA, Curry SC: Epidemiology and hospital course of rattlesnake envenomations cared for at a tertiary referral center in central Arizona. Acad Emerg Med 8:177–182, 2001.

34. Tanen DA, Danish DC, Clark RF: Crotalidae Polyvalent Immune Fab antivenom limits the decrease in perfusion pressure of the anterior leg compartment in a porcine crotaline envenomation model. Ann Emerg Med 41:384–390, 2003.

*35. Lavonas EJ, Gerardo CJ, O'Malley G, et al: Initial experience with crotaline Fab antivenom in the treatment of copperhead snakebite. Ann Emerg Med 43:200–206, 2004.

36. Boyer LV, McNally JT, Binford GJ: Spider bites. *In* Auerbach PS (ed): Wilderness Medicine, 4th ed. St. Louis: Mosby, 2001, pp 807–838.

37. Pneumatikos IA, Galiatsou E, Goe D, et al: Acute fatal toxic myocarditis after a black widow spider envenomation. Ann Emerg Med 41:158, 2003.

38. Bush SP: Why no antivenom? [Letter]. Ann Emerg Med 42:431–432, 2003.

39. Graudins A, Padula M, Broady K, Nicholson GM: Red-back spider (*Latrodectus hasselti*) antivenom prevents the toxicity of widow spider venoms. Ann Emerg Med 37:154–160, 2001.

40. Daly FFS, Hill RE, Bogdan GM, Dart RC: Neutralization of *Latrodectus hesperus* venom by antivenom raised against *L. hasselti* in a murine model [Abstract]. Ann Emerg Med 35:S57–S58, 2000.

41. Bush SP: Black widow spider envenomation mimicking cholecystitis [Letter]. Am J Emerg Med 17:315, 1999.

42. Cohen J, Bush SP: Compartment syndrome after a suspected black widow spider bite. Ann Emerg Med 45:414–416, 2005.

43. Woestman R, Perkin R, Van Stralen D: The black widow: is she deadly to children? Pediatr Emerg Care 12:360–364, 1996.

*44. Clark RF, Wethern-Kestner S, Vance MV, Gerkin R: Clinical presentation and treatment of black widow spider envenomation: a review of 163 cases. Ann Emerg Med 21:782–787, 1992.

45. Allen RC, Norris RL: Delayed use of widow spider antivenin. Ann Emerg Med 26:393–394, 1995.

46. Bush SP, Naftel J, Farstad D: Injection of a whole black widow spider [Letter]. Ann Emerg Med 27:532–533, 1996.

*47. Vetter RS, Bush SP: The diagnosis of brown recluse spider bite is overused for dermonecrotic wounds of uncertain etiology [Editorial]. Ann Emerg Med 39:544–546, 2002.

48. Vetter RS, Bush SP: Reports of presumptive brown recluse spider bites reinforce logistically improbable diagnoses in non-endemic North America [Editorial]. Clin Infect Dis 35:442–445, 2002.

49. Langley RL, Morrow WE: Deaths resulting from animal attacks in the United States. Wild Environ Med 8:8–16, 1997.

50. Vetter RS, Bush SP: Chemical burn misdiagnosed as brown recluse spider bite [Letter]. Am J Emerg Med 20:68–69, 2002.

51. Maugh TH II: L.A. spider survey finds a tropical brown widow. Los Angeles Times, February 8:A14, 2003.

*52. Vetter RS, Isbister GK: Do hobo spider bites cause dermonecrotic injuries? Ann Emerg Med 44:605–607, 2004.

53. Bush SP, Giem P, Vetter R: Green lynx spider (*Peucetia viridans*) envenomation. Am J Emerg Med 18:64–66, 2000.

54. Gomez HF, Krywko DM, Stoecker WV: A new assay for the detection of *Loxosceles* species (brown recluse) spider venom. Ann Emerg Med 39:469–474, 2002.

55. Bush SP: Hyperbaric oxygen treatments' utility should be confirmed [Letter]. Wilderness Med Lett 14:12, 1997.

56. Hobbs GD, Anderson AR, Greene TJ, Yealy DM: Comparison of hyperbaric oxygen and dapsone therapy for *Loxosceles* envenomation. Acad Emerg Med 3:758–761, 1996.

Chapter 142

Electrical Injury

Kenneth T. Kwon, MD and Carl H. Schultz, MD

Key Points

Blunt traumatic and multisystem injuries can be associated with electrical injury in children.

Alternating current electrical injuries have a much higher fluid requirement than dictated by standard burn formulas.

Oral cavity burns in infants and small children may require reconstructive surgery.

Proper triaging of a multivictim lightening injury scene involves caring for victims in cardiopulmonary arrest first.

Introduction and Background

Electrical injuries from natural causes have existed since ancient times, but it was not until the worldwide distribution of man-made electricity beginning in the late 1800s that electrical injuries became commonplace. Electricity can be divided into alternating current (AC) and direct current (DC). Household electrical current is AC with a standard frequency of 60 Hertz (Hz) in the United States. Examples of DC include lightning, medical defibrillation, and batteries. Although some believe that lightning is unique and not specifically DC, it will be categorized as DC for purposes of this chapter. Lightning strikes the United States approximately 25 million times per year.[1]

Children are especially prone to electrical injuries. The skin is thinner with higher water content, which predisposes them to greater internal tissue damage than adults. The oral and exploratory nature of toddlers makes them prone to electrical cord and outlet injuries. Adolescents and young adults have a high rate of electrical injuries due to their increased risk-taking behavior in electrical environments and at work relative to other age groups. Throughout their young lives, frequent outdoor group recreational activities expose children to lightning injuries in inclement weather.

Recognition and Approach

In the United States, electrical injuries comprise over 20,000 emergency department (ED) visits per year and account for up to 4% of all admissions to major burn centers.[2] In 2001, there were 409 deaths attributable to electric current, with 10% of victims less than 20 years of age, and 44 lightning deaths, with 8 (18%) under 20 years of age.[3] Lightning injury statistics are poorly tracked, but it is believed that 70% to 80% of lightning strike victims survive, two thirds of whom are left with permanent sequelae.[4] Most injuries in younger children are due to mouthing a live electrical cord or placing a metallic object into an outlet.[5-7] High-voltage injuries tend to occur in older children while exploring building or utility structures, or with specific recreational activities such as kite-flying.[8]

The pathophysiology of these injuries is best appreciated by reviewing electricity physics. Electrical energy is defined using Ohm's law, $V = I \times R$, or voltage (energy possessed by each electron, in volts) = current (number of electrons moving per time, in amperes) × resistance (ability of a material to slow electron flow, in ohms). Each component contributes to the severity of injury, as does the type of current, duration of contact, and surface area exposed to the current.

Voltage is usually the only variable that is readily known at the time of injury. Typically, high voltage is defined as greater than 1000 volts (V), although some use a lower cutoff of 500 V. Most U.S. household circuits use 110 V, with some larger appliances using 220 V. In comparison, residential power lines carry greater than 7000 V. A lightning strike is estimated to carry up to 100 million V. In general, high voltage is more dangerous than low voltage. Current flow determines heat production and is considered the greatest danger to life of all components, but cannot be quantified during an acute injury. Current follows the path of least resistance, and tissues more susceptible to injury are somewhat predictable. Different body tissues offer different degrees of resistance to current flow. In decreasing order of resistance, they are bone > fat > tendon > skin > muscle > blood vessels > nerves. Skin resistance, however, is extremely variable depending on moisture, thickness, and age. Wet skin can decrease resistance by over 100-fold,[5] and a neonate's skin provides relatively lower resistance due to its thinness and high water content. Resistance will also determine the pathway of current, with the most dangerous circuit being from hand to hand with heart involvement, or head to toe with brain and respiratory drive involvement.

The type of current, AC or DC, also plays a major factor in determining injury severity. AC current is generally more dangerous due to the "locked-on" phenomenon. This results from simultaneous tetanic contractions of both hand flexors and extensors. Since the flexors are stronger, the hand cannot be opened and gets "locked on" the electricity source. This phenomenon is associated with standard 60-Hz household current and increases duration of contact. Lightning has an extremely short duration of contact (<0.001 second) and generally imparts less energy to its victims than AC shock. Blunt traumatic injuries are more common with lightning and high-voltage AC due to victims being thrown from the source of contact by muscular contractions. Lastly, surface area of contact will also determine burn type and severity. A small area of contact, such as current passing through a hand, will create more localized heat production and more severe local injury. A large area of contact, such as bathtub electrocution, can result in no localized injury but significant systemic effects.

Lightning can strike a victim by different mechanisms. Aside from a *direct strike*, in which the victim is the primary point of contact of the electrical discharge, lightning can create a *side flash* when it hits a nearby object and then discharges from object to person. Lightning can also cause *step voltage*, or *stride potential*, when it spreads along the ground and flows into one foot, through the body, and out the other foot. Side flash and step voltage can explain why lightning injuries occur in groups. Lastly, lightning can cause *flashover*, which is rapid heating of skin moisture and vaporization. Wet clothes can be blown off, shoes can explode, and blunt trauma may result from the blast effect.

Clinical Presentation

Electrical burns can be categorized into several different types. A true electrical burn, or *conductive burn*, is caused by electron flow through tissue with resultant heat generation. Temperatures have been measured up to thousands of degrees Celsius. Conductive burns can cause cellular damage or coagulation necrosis of surrounding tissues. Entrance wounds, exit wounds, or both are frequently seen, but may be absent or inconspicuous. Entrance wounds tend to take on a smaller charred appearance, with exit wounds more extensive and sometimes explosive in nature. The amount of damage to underlying tissues and organs is not always evident by looking at the skin, as the path of current flow cannot be determined. Conductive burns should be considered as a crush-type injury, because they cause more swelling than a true thermal burn. An *arc burn* is caused by electrons moving through the air instead of through the body, and injury occurs when the body contacts the arc. Arc burns can generate temperatures up to 4000° C. A *flame burn* occurs with ignition of clothing by arcs or sparks, causing direct thermal injury. Both arc and flame burns are usually seen with high-voltage injuries.

Lightning strikes can present with unique characteristic burns. Linear burns are due to the vaporization of sweat; this phenomenon can also blow articles of clothing off victims. Punctate burns can be seen, which appear like cigarette burns 3 to 10 mm in diameter. Feather burns, also called Lichtenberg figures, are not actual burns but staining of the skin caused by a shower of electrons creating a branch or fernlike pattern. These feather burns fade within 24 hours of injury and are considered pathognomonic for lightning injury.

Electrical injuries tend to affect multiple organ systems (Table 142–1). With significant AC injury, the typical presentation includes transient loss of consciousness with possible apnea or ventricular fibrillation, neurologic symptoms or deficits, and external evidence of trauma. Fractures or dislocations, particularly of the shoulder, are commonly seen due to the tetanic forces caused by AC electricity. The conductive burns can be deep and extensive, causing coagulation necrosis and predisposing to compartment syndrome and infection. Rhabdomyolysis and cardiac dysrhythmias may ensue and need to be considered early in management.

Table 142–1	Patterns of Electrical Injuries	
	AC Current	**Lightning (DC Current)**
Cardiac	Dysrhythmias including ventricular fibrillation, asystole, MI (rare)	Dysrhythmias including asystole, hypertension (transient)
Neurologic	Apnea, LOC or mental status changes, motor paralysis/paresis/paresthesia, seizure, intracranial hemorrhage, cerebral edema Delayed symptoms: ascending paralysis, transverse myelitis, ALS-like syndrome	Apnea, LOC or mental status changes, keraunoparalysis*, autonomic instability, seizure, intracranial hemorrhage, antegrade amnesia, peripheral neuropathy
Musculoskeletal	Compartment syndrome, tendon rupture, fracture/dislocation	Compartment syndrome (rare)
Cutaneous	Entrance/exit wounds, flexor crease burn, oral commissure burn	Linear, punctate, and feather burns, serious burns (rare)
Pulmonary	Diaphragm/thoracic muscle tetany, ARDS, pneumothorax, aspiration	Diaphragm/thoracic muscle tetany, ARDS, pneumothorax, aspiration
Gastrointestinal	Ileus, bowel perforation, GI bleeding, solid organ injury, stress ulcers	Blunt abdominal trauma
Renal	Rhabdomyolysis, acute renal failure	Rhabdomyolysis (rare)
Vascular	Vasospasm (transient), thrombosis, progressive amputations	Vasospasm (transient)
HEENT	Fixed/dilated pupils (transient), visual changes, optic neuritis, intraocular hemorrhage, cataract	Fixed/dilated pupils (transient), tympanic membrane rupture, tinnitus, cataract, corneal lesion

*Keraunoparalysis is a syndrome consisting of limb paralysis, mottled skin, and pulselessness.
Abbreviations: AC, alternating current; ALS, amyotrophic lateral sclerosis; ARDS, acute respiratory distress syndrome; DC, direct current; GI, gastrointestinal; HEENT, head, ears, eyes, nose, and throat; LOC, loss of consciousness; MI, myocardial infarction.

Lightning injuries have several differences from AC injury patterns. Asystole is the usual life-threatening rhythm. If treated quickly, patients have an excellent prognosis, unlike other causes of asystole. When asystole resolves spontaneously, it usually does so prior to the return of spontaneous respirations. Autonomic dysfunction can be quite marked in lightning strikes, causing transient absence of extremity pulses or even hypertension. Keraunoparalysis is an early manifestation of autonomic instability characterized by bilateral lower extremity paralysis associated with mottled or pulseless extremities, which usually resolves within a few hours. Although paraplegia is characteristic, unilateral hemiplegia is unusual and should be aggressively investigated for another acute cerebrovascular cause. The single muscular contraction effect of DC energy can powerfully throw a victim; thus blunt trauma is more likely associated with lightning injuries. Severe burns rarely occur, and extensive local tissue damage and rhabdomyolosis are not commonly seen. Tympanic membrane rupture is a characteristic examination finding following lightning injury. Although previously thought to be the result of the lightning's blast effect, rupture is now considered to be the result of direct conductive damage.[9]

Because electrical injuries are usually evident based on historical factors, an exhaustive differential diagnosis or etiologic search is usually not necessary. Exceptions can occur with bathtub electrical injury, in which circumstances may be unclear and external evidence of injuries are usually minimal, and with high voltage injury, in which a victim may be thrown far enough away from the source as to create confusion as to the cause of injury.

Important Clinical Features and Considerations

Contact burns to the mouth and lips, especially the oral commissure, are commonly seen in infants and toddlers. The mouth was the second most frequent site of injury, after the extremities, in pediatric burn admissions in one retrospective review,[2] while another study found 38% of hospitalized pediatric burn patients were admitted due to oral burns.[5] Extension cords are the most common source, with injury occurring either by biting into the cord itself or by mouthing the female live end of a connected cord. Saliva significantly lowers the resistance of the oral mucosa and lips, and tissue damage occurs from a combination of direct conductive and arc mechanisms. Commissure burns are usually full thickness, initially appearing as a painless, pale, yellow-gray coagulated patch with a depressed center and surrounding edema and erythema (Fig. 142–1). Bleeding almost never occurs at the time of presentation. Delayed bleeding of the labial artery can occur as the eschar sloughs off 1 to 4 weeks postinjury. The rate of this complication in oral burns is up to 23%.[10] Granulation tissue fills the wound, but disfiguring scarring and loss of function can be seen, often necessitating reconstructive plastic surgery. Other late complications of oral burns include dental devitalization, microstomia, oral adhesions, and speech problems.

Pregnant patients, both teenagers and adults, deserve special consideration. Fetal skin has much less resistance than postnatal skin, and, combined with a gravid uterus filled with amniotic fluid, makes the fetus particularly sus-

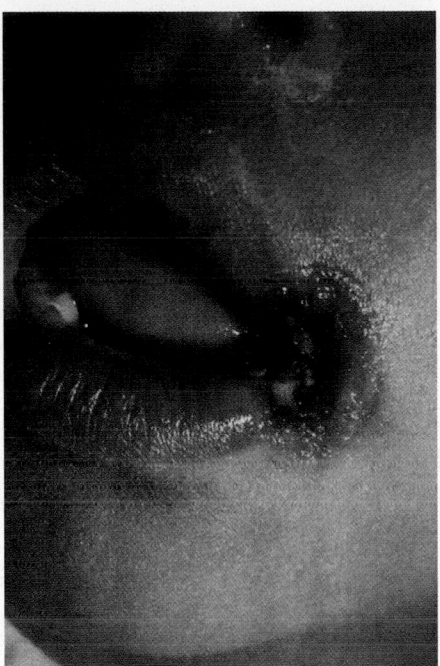

FIGURE 142–1. Oral commissure burn.

ceptible to serious injury. Because of limited studies with small numbers and unknown exposure data, the significance of electrical injury in pregnancy remains unclear. A review of 15 pregnant victims of AC injury showed minimal harm to mothers but fetal death in the majority of cases.[11] Fetal demise has been reported after lightning injuries as well.[4,12] Of note is that emergent iatrogenic DC cardioversion in pregnant patients is generally considered safe because the current path does not include the pelvic area.

Management

In the prehospital setting, rescuers need to ensure their own safety while providing care. Any source of electricity needs to be shut off, and the voltage and type of current should be determined. The child victim should be evacuated from a higher to lower risk area when possible, particularly during a lightning storm. In the case of multiple victims and suspected lightning injury, normal mass casualty triage guidelines should be reversed, with initial focus on those in cardiopulmonary and respiratory arrest. Whether cardiac activity returns spontaneously or due to intervention, it is likely to restart prior to respirations, so early and proper respiratory management is of paramount importance. Because lightning and high-voltage injuries can result in transient autonomic dysfunction, fixed and dilated pupils, apnea, and absent pulses on scene are not reliable indicators for death. Any child with suspected major electrical injury should be treated similar to a multisystem trauma victim in the field and ED setting.

In the ED, diagnostic evaluation of the moderately to severely injured child should include a complete blood count, electrolytes, blood gases, urinalysis, and urine myoglobin. Urine testing may reveal the classic finding of heme in the absence of red blood cells suggestive of myoglobinuria and rhabdomyolysis. Blood creatine phosphokinase (CPK) is frequently obtained to help determine the degree of muscle breakdown, but CPK levels have no relationship to burn severity or overall prognosis.[2] Radiographic studies should be obtained as indicated. Cardiac monitoring, electrocardiogram (ECG), and cardiac enzyme tests should be initiated if a transthoracic electrical current is suspected.

In children with minor household electrical injuries or isolated burns, the need for diagnostic studies and cardiac monitoring is controversial. Some authors suggest that routine cardiac monitoring is not required in most children sustaining household electrical injuries.[13-16] However, an ECG and cardiac monitoring should be considered in cases in which there was loss of consciousness, tetany, wet skin, or current flow crossing the chest.[13] A retrospective review suggested that pediatric victims of minor low-voltage household current who are asymptomatic or have only minor burns do not require cardiac monitoring or laboratory evaluation of any kind and can be safely discharged home.[15]

Initial ED treatment should focus on burn care and fluid management. Patients with high-voltage AC injuries should be aggressively fluid resuscitated, as they tend to have substantial third spacing and tissue swelling. Traditional burn formulas will grossly underestimate the fluid requirement in these patients. Therefore, maintaining urine output at a rate of at least 1 ml/kg/hr should dictate the amount of intravenous crystalloid fluid administered. Placement of a central venous pressure catheter should be considered. If rhabdomyolysis is suspected, urine alkalinization should be undertaken. Sodium bicarbonate can be used, first as a bolus of 1 mEq/kg, followed by one to two ampules (50 to 100 mEq) in 1 L of 5% dextrose in water at a rate to maintain adequate urine output and a urine pH ≥ 7.45. Diuretics such as mannitol (0.25 to 1 g/kg) or furosemide (1 mg/kg) can be used intermittently to ensure adequate urine output, assuming hypotension is not a concern (see Chapter 99, Rhabdomyolysis). Electrical burn wounds should be loosely dressed in sterile gauze per standard burn care management (see Chapter 26, Burns), and tetanus prophylaxis administered as needed. Extremity injuries should be carefully monitored, as compartment syndrome and the need for emergent fasciotomy occasionally occur (see Chapter 22, Compartment Syndrome). With high-voltage AC injuries, vascular thrombosis may necessitate progres-sive amputations of an extremity over the course of 7 to 10 days, so parents should be informed early of this possible complication.

Lightning injuries usually do not involve as much tissue swelling or fluid shifts as AC-type injuries, thus aggressive fluid resuscitation is usually not necessary. Similarly, fasciotomies are rarely needed in lightning injuries, and compartment pressures should be checked prior to performing a fasciotomy, as the absence of extremity pulses may be due to lightning-induced autonomic instability (i.e., keraunoparalysis).

Summary

All high-voltage and lightning injuries in children require hospitalization, as do low-voltage exposures with significant burns or associated injuries. Admission with cardiac monitoring or in an intensive care setting is indicated with any suspected transthoracic current injury, history of cardiopulmonary arrest or dysrhythmias in the field or ED, large or deep burns, altered mental status, hypotension, severe acidosis, or rhabdomyolysis. When possible, transfer to a specialized inpatient burn center is recommended, especially in young children. All patients with viable pregnancies need fetal monitoring and obstetric consultation, as these mothers will be considered high risk for the remainder of their pregnancies.

Low-voltage household injuries in children who are asymptomatic or have just minor burns can usually be managed as outpatients. The utility of cardiac monitoring in the ED is limited. Clinical experience suggests it is reasonable to observe these patients for dysrhythmias or symptoms in the ED for 2 to 4 hours prior to discharge. Exceptions would include patients with an abnormal initial ECG, loss of consciousness during the event, voltage exposure greater than 240 V, or a known cardiac condition. Admission and monitoring for at least 24 hours is recommended in these cases.[14] Oral commissure burns not involving deeper oral structures can generally be discharged home with strict parental instructions concerning delayed bleeding complications and with close plastic surgery follow-up.

Prevention of electrical injuries centers on parental supervision, childproofing measures at home, and education about lightning safety guidelines. The increased use of ground fault circuit interrupters and outlet protectors has helped reduce household injuries, although not all outlet protectors are failsafe, and they may give parents a false sense of security.[6,17] During a lightning storm, expert consensus recommends the following: seek cover in large enclosed structures, such as a house or office building, or in a car with the windows rolled up; avoid being near or in water, areas near tall structures, open fields, open structures, or open vehicles; seek the lowest spot and get in a curled position if outdoors, and disperse when in a group.[1,18]

REFERENCES

1. Zimmermann C, Cooper MA, Holle RL: Lightning safety guidelines. Ann Emerg Med 39:660–664, 2002.
*2. Wallace BH, Cone JB, Vanderpool RD, et al: Retrospective evaluation of admission criteria for paediatric electrical injuries. Burns 21:590–593, 1995.
3. National Center for Health Statistics: Total deaths for each cause by 5-year age groups, United States, 2001. Available at *http://www.cdc.gov/nchs/datawh/statab/unpubd/mortabs/gmwki10.htm* (accessed December 6, 2004).
4. Cooper MA: Lightning injuries: prognostic signs for death. Ann Emerg Med 9:134–138, 1980.
5. Zubair M, Besner GE: Pediatric electrical burns: management strategies. Burns 23:413–420, 1997.
*6. Rai J, Jeschke M, Barrow RE, Herndon DN: Electrical injuries: a 30-year review. J Trauma 46:933–936, 1999.
7. Lee JW, Jang UC, Oh SJ: Paediatric electrical burn: outlet injury caused by steel chopstick misuse. Burns 30:244–247, 2004.
*8. Tiwari VK, Sharma D: Kite-flying: a unique but dangerous mode of electrical injury in children. Burns 25:537–539, 1999.
9. Redleaf MI, McCabe BF: Lightning injury of the tympanic membrane. Ann Otol Rhinol Laryngol 102:867–869, 1993.
*10. Canady JW, Thompson SA, Bardach J: Oral commissure burns in children. Plast Reconstr Surg 97:738–743, 1996.
*11. Fatovich DM: Electric shock in pregnancy. J Emerg Med 11:175–177, 1993.
12. Pierce MR, Henderson RA, Mitchell JM: Cardiopulmonary arrest secondary to lightning injury in a pregnant woman. Ann Emerg Med 15:597–599, 1986.

----

*Selected readings.

*13. Bailey B, Gaudreault P, Thivierge RL, Turgeon JP: Cardiac monitoring in children with household electrical injuries. Ann Emerg Med 25:612–617, 1995.

14. Bailey B, Gaudreault P, Thivierge RL: Experience with guidelines for cardiac monitoring after electrical injury in children. Am J Emerg Med 18:671–675, 2000.

15. Garcia CT, Smith GA, Cohen DM, Fernandez K: Electrical injuries in a pediatric emergency department. Ann Emerg Med 26:604–608, 1995.

*16. Wilson CM, Fatovich DM: Do children need to be monitored after electric shocks? J Paediatr Child Health 34:474–476, 1998.

17. Ridenour MV: Age appropriateness and safety of electric outlet protectors for children. Percept Mot Skills 84:387–392, 1997.

*18. Cherington M, Martorano FJ, Siebuhr L, et al: Childhood lightning injuries on the playing field. J Emerg Med 12:39–41, 1994.

Chapter 143

Inhalation Exposures

Mark A. Hostetler, MD, MPH

Key Points

The main mechanisms by which inhalation exposures cause injury are asphyxia, direct injury to the pulmonary tree, and systemic toxicity.

Inhalation injury patterns are closely related to volatility, water solubility, and viscosity.

Volatile agents more easily vaporized, making them subject to inhalation.

Highly water-soluble agents are more rapidly absorbed in the upper airway and produce immediate local irritation; water-insoluble agents are not readily absorbed, and produce lower respiratory tract symptoms that are usually delayed.

Aspiration risk is inversely proportional to viscosity: low-viscosity agents have the highest aspiration risk.

Selected Inhalation Exposures

Smoke
Carbon monoxide
Cyanide
Chlorine gas

Discussion of Individual Inhalation Exposures

Smoke

Inhalation injury occurs when the respiratory tract is exposed to one or more toxic substances (toxicants) with resultant anatomic or physiologic damage. Although these toxicants are primarily gases, volatilized products of combustion and inhaled particulate matter also cause injury. Oxygen depletion and direct thermal injury also play a role in inhalation injuries. House fires are a major cause of serious smoke inhalation injuries[1,2] (see Chapter 26, Burns). Mortality rates,

particularly in children, have declined over the last 2 decades.[3] Still, approximately 4000 Americans die each year in residential fires.[4] Most of these fatalities occur in adults.[1] Approximately 25% of these fatalities occur in children younger than 18 years, with 17% occurring in children younger than 5 years.[1] Inhalation injury is a primary contributor to pediatric burn mortality.[5,6] Many cases of smoke inhalation involve exposure to a mixture of gases as well as particulate matter and heat.[7] The most common fatal gas involved in smoke inhalation is carbon monoxide (CO). Other toxic gases are hydrogen cyanide (HCN), and hydrochloric acid (HCl). HCl is commonly released when polyvinyl chloride is burned. Polyvinyl chloride is found in many household products and construction materials, including flooring and siding. When polyvinyl chloride is burned, HCl is released as a dense white smoke. As polyvinyl chloride continues to burn, white smoke is followed by a dense black smoke with a very high CO content.

Clinical Presentation

Physical examination may reveal facial burns, singed nasal hairs, pharyngeal soot, and carbonaceous sputum. The clinician should evaluate the airway for thermal injury and monitor the patient for impending airway obstruction (Table 143–1). Before respiratory failure occurs, intubation for airway protection is prudent in many cases. Signs of respiratory distress may be delayed for 12 to 24 hours, but may include tachypnea, cough, and stridor. Auscultatory abnormalities may include wheezing, rales, and rhonchi. Acute respiratory failure may occur at any point. Pneumonia may develop days after the initial insult and carries a high mortality rate.[8-10] Pulse oximetry can be falsely reassuring in patients poisoned by CO. This has been called the "pulse oximetry gap."[11] When CO is suspected, arterial blood gas analysis should be performed with co-oximetry to measure carboxyhemoglobin (COHb). The presence of hypoxemia, hypercarbia, and an elevated COHb level are hallmarks of smoke inhalation. Metabolic acidosis may be due to respiratory insufficiency, or cellular asphyxia due to CO or HCN may lead to a metabolic acidosis.[8,12]

A chest radiograph obtained shortly after exposure is an insensitive indicator of smoke inhalation injury.[8,13] Auscultatory abnormalities may precede abnormalities on chest radiography by 12 to 24 hours. When present, radiographic abnormalities include diffuse interstitial infiltration or local areas of atelectasis and edema.

Table 143–1	Management of Inhalation Injuries

Initial Management

Remove patient from contaminated environment
Rapid cardiopulmonary assessment
Cardiopulmonary resuscitation as needed
Provide humidified 100% supplemental oxygen
Primary survey—ABCDEs (airway, breathing, circulation, disability, exposure)
Assess for other injuries

Diagnostic Evaluation

Arterial/venous blood gas analysis (co-oximetry)
Carboxyhemoglobin level
Complete blood count, electrolytes
Urinalysis for myoglobin
Chest radiograph

Continuous Cardiopulmonary Monitoring

Heart rate
Electrocardiogram
Respiratory rate
Blood pressure
Pulse oximetry

Treatment

Humidified 100% oxygen
Continuously re-evaluate for airway edema, obstruction, failure
Meticulous pulmonary toilette
β_2-Agonist bronchodilator therapy
Fluid therapy to maintain urine output > 1 ml/kg/hr
Consider antidotal therapy as indicated

Management

When burned children with inhalation injuries receive mechanical ventilation, permissive hypercapnia may minimize barotrauma.[14] Continuous positive airway pressure or positive end-expiratory pressure (5 to 15 cm H_2O) is recommended for refractory hypoxemia.[8,9] Inhaled β_2-agonist bronchodilators are useful for acute bronchospasm. There is no documented benefit from steroids or prophylactic antibiotics.[8,12]

All symptomatic children should be admitted to the hospital. Clinical experience suggests observing asymptomatic children for a minimum of 4 to 6 hours and admitting them to the hospital if signs or symptoms of inhalation injury develop during this observation period. Family members who survive house fires should be encouraged to develop an emergency plan and use smoke and CO detectors in their homes.

Carbon Monoxide

CO is a colorless, odorless, tasteless, and nonirritating gas formed as a by-product of incomplete combustion of fossil fuels or materials such as wood or charcoal. CO poisoning is most commonly due to smoke inhalation, but also occurs from exposure to malfunctioning or improperly vented heating and cooking appliances, automobile exhaust fumes, and methylene chloride (found in paint strippers). CO exerts its potentially lethal effects via several different mechanisms. CO binds to hemoglobin 250 times as tenaciously as oxygen; therefore, it greatly reduces the ability of hemoglobin to carry oxygen. CO also shifts the oxyhemoglobin dissociation curve to the left, making it more difficult for oxygen to be released from hemoglobin to the cells. As a result of binding to myoglobin, there is impaired diffusion of oxygen to cardiac and

skeletal muscles, resulting in the victim's reduced ability to move and escape.[7]

Analysis of data from the National Center for Health Statistics for the years 1994 to 1998 identified an average of 516 annual deaths from unintentional non–fire-related CO poisoning in the United States.[15] These fatality figures do not include intentional poisoning and deaths from fire and smoke inhalation, some of which were undoubtedly the result of CO toxicity. Unintentional CO toxicity and deaths are more common in northern climates and during the winter months. The mortality rate among patients with severe CO poisoning is about 30%. Most patients who die do so at the scene of exposure. Up to 11% of survivors develop persistent gross neurologic or psychiatric deficits. A larger number may develop more subtle pathology such as personality changes or memory impairment. Up to 25% of treated patients will experience delayed neurologic deterioration following a period of apparent recovery. Although most delayed sequelae will resolve, the course may span years.[16]

Clinical Presentation

Clinical signs and symptoms of CO poisoning are relatively nonspecific and correlate only roughly with the COHb level. The longer the interval between exposure and evaluation in the emergency department, the more likely that the symptoms and COHb level will be discordant. Many patients with relatively mild CO intoxication complain of flulike symptoms with headache, nausea, and fatigue. More severe symptoms include unexplained alterations of mental status, neurologic abnormalities, syncope, and metabolic acidosis. In infants, the only suggestion of toxicity may be irritability or feeding difficulties. COHb levels do not correlate with clinical signs and symptoms in children.[17]

COHb levels are measured using co-oximetry. COHb levels are adequately reflected in both arterial and venous samples. Chest radiography is not indicated unless there is clinical evidence of pulmonary edema or a concern about related smoke inhalation injury. A urinalysis and serum creatine kinase are indicated for patients with prolonged unconsciousness or those otherwise at risk for rhabdomyolysis (see Chapter 99, Rhabdomyolysis). Computed tomography may be performed for other indications (see Chapter 9, Cerebral Resuscitation), but is not specifically indicated in the acute management of suspected CO poisoning.[16,18]

Management

The cornerstone of treatment is high-flow supplemental oxygen. The short-term administration of high concentrations of oxygen is indicated as soon as the diagnosis of CO poisoning is suspected as this treatment offers little, if any, risk to most patients. In the awake patient, a fraction of inspired oxygen (FiO_2) of nearly 100% can be achieved using a tight-fitting non-rebreathing mask with a reservoir. The half-life of COHb is approximately 3 to 4 hours while breathing room air, 60 minutes while breathing 100% oxygen, and 20 minutes breathing hyperbaric oxygen (HBO) at 2.5 atmospheres of pressure.

HBO treatment of CO poisoning is controversial. Traditional recommendations for HBO treatment were based on COHb levels. This approach is no longer advocated.[19-21] It is not currently clear that HBO treatment is beneficial for patients for CO poisoning.[19-21] Until these treatment issues are resolved, a hyperbaric specialist or poison control center it is reasonable to consult for cases of severe CO toxicity. U.S. emergency physicians can find the location of the nearest hyperbaric chamber by calling the Divers Alert Network (DAN), Duke University, Durham, NC, at 1-919-684-8111 (see Chapter 144, Dysbarism). An absolute contraindication to HBO treatment is an untreated pneumothorax. Complications of HBO treatment include rare seizures, vascular gas emboli, and barotrauma to the ears, sinuses, and lungs. The use of HBO typically involves transport to another facility with the inherent risks incurred during transport.

Clinical experience suggests that CO-exposed patients who are asymptomatic or manifest mild, flulike symptoms may be discharged if a repeat CO level is less than 5 mg/dl after 4 hours receiving 100% FiO$_2$. All other patients with CO exposures should be admitted. Severely ill children should be transferred to a pediatric tertiary care center.

Summary

CO poisoning is common, but the diagnosis is not always obvious. It should be suspected when multiple victims or family members present with headache and vague flulike symptoms. Accurate testing requires co-oximetry, which can accurately be performed on arterial or venous blood. A hyperbaric specialist or poison control center should be consulted for severe cases.

Cyanide

Cyanide is a cellular asphyxiant. Cyanide binds with the ferric ion of mitochondrial cytochrome oxidase enzymes and halts aerobic cellular respiration. This shift to anaerobic metabolism results in a severe lactic acidosis. Cyanide also shifts the oxygen-hemoglobin dissociation curve to the left, further impairing oxygen delivery to the tissues. HCN gas is formed when wool, silk, synthetic fabrics, and some building materials catch fire. It is estimated that up to 35% of all house fire victims may have been exposed to cyanide.[22] Cyanide also is used in the mining and photographic chemical recycling industries. Industrial firms in the United States manufacture over 300,000 tons of cyanide each year. As a terrorist weapon, cyanide gas could be generated in an enclosed space via the addition of an acid to a solid cyanide salt, but is highly volatile and rapidly disperses in air. In the 10-year period between 1993 and 2002, the Toxic Exposure Surveillance System compiled by the American Association of Poison Control Centers recorded 3165 human exposures to cyanide.[23] Eighty (2.5%) of these exposures resulted in death and 413 (13%) resulted in serious morbidity. In the Union Carbide pesticide plant disaster in Bhopal, India, there were an estimated 1800 to 5000 deaths and almost 200,000 injuries.[24]

Clinical Presentation

The onset of symptoms following inhalation exposure to HCN gas is immediate. Low concentrations (e.g., < 50 parts per million) cause restlessness, anxiety, palpitations, dyspnea, and headache. Very high concentrations result in marked tachypnea, immediately followed by severe respiratory depression, convulsions, respiratory arrest, and death.[7] Patients who are alert may hyperventilate and complain of breathlessness. Since cyanide prevents tissue extraction of oxygen from the blood, the oxygen content of venous blood approaches that of arterial blood, resulting in the brightening of venous blood. The typical seriously poisoned patient is hyperventilating, hypotensive, and bradycardic without cyanosis.

There is no rapid or readily available diagnostic test for cyanide exposure. In the absence of a known cyanide exposure, the diagnosis must be made empirically (e.g., smoke inhalation with high lactate, enclosed space, or mass casualty). A high anion gap metabolic acidosis and plasma lactate levels greater than 10 mmol/L (90 mg/dl) are consistent with cyanide toxicity.[25] Comparing arterial and venous blood gases may demonstrate a diminished arterial-venous O$_2$ difference.

Management

The mainstay of therapy for cyanide poisoning is aggressive supportive care (see Table 143–1) and prompt administration of the cyanide antidote kit (Table 143–2). The antidotal action of the cyanide antidote kit is at least in part due to nitrites causing methemoglobinemia. Caution must be used in the administration of the cyanide antidote kit to fire victims with possible simultaneous CO and cyanide poisoning. Since COHb does not carry oxygen, the creation of methemoglobin can further decrease oxygen delivery. In this situation, sodium thiosulfate should be used alone.[26] The reported death of a child from methemoglobinemia following aggressive treatment of a nonlethal ingestion has led to the recommendation of adjusting the pediatric dose of sodium nitrite according to the patient's hemoglobin level (Table 143–3).

Side effects of nitrite administration include headache, blurred vision, nausea, vomiting, and hypotension. Methemoglobin levels of 20% to 30% are associated with symptoms of headache and nausea. Weakness, dyspnea, and tachycardia occur at levels of 30% to 50%. Dysrhythmias, central nervous system depression, and seizures occur at levels of 50% to 70%. Death typically occurs at methemoglobin levels above 70%. In contrast to the nitrites, thiosulfate has few if any side effects other than burning at the injection site, localized muscle cramping, and occasional nausea and vomiting.[27] There are limited data on hydroxocobalamin use in children.

Table 143–2	Cyanide Antidote Kit: Contents and General Instructions for Usage	
Antidote	**Quantity/Form Supplied**	**Pediatric Dose**
Amyl nitrite	12 perles (0.3 ml/perle)	Crush 1–2 perles in gauze and hold under patient's nose or over ET tube for 15–30 sec every minute until sodium nitrite is infusing
Sodium nitrite	2 ampules of 3% solution (300 mg/10 ml)	0.3 ml/kg (9 mg/kg), not to exceed 10 ml (300 mg), IV at 2.5 ml/min, or over 30 min, in smoke inhalation victims with CO poisoning
Sodium thiosulfate	2 ampules of 25% solution (12.5 g/50 ml)	1.6 ml/kg (400 mg/kg), up to 50 ml (12.5 g), at rate of 3–5 ml/min

Abbreviations: CO, carbon monoxide; ET, endotracheal; IV, intravenously.

Table 142–3	Dose Adjustment Recommendations for Sodium Nitrite Based on Hemoglobin Level	
Hemoglobin Level (g/dl)	3% Sodium Nitrate (NaNO$_2$) (ml/kg)	25% Sodium Thiosulfate (Na$_2$S$_2$O$_3$) (ml/kg)*
7	0.19	1.65
8	0.22	1.65
9	0.25	1.65
10	0.27	1.65
11	0.30	1.65
12	0.33	1.65
13	0.36	1.65
14	0.39	1.65

*There is a uniform dose for sodium thiosulfate for all hemoglobin levels.

Chlorine Gas

Chlorine gas is a pulmonary irritant. Pulmonary irritants are among the most common toxic inhalants. Chlorine is a yellow-green gas that is slightly water soluble and has a pungent, irritating odor. With a density almost twice that of air, it descends and remains near ground level. Chlorine gas is 20 times more potent and irritating than HCl. When chlorine gas and mucosal water react, HCl and hypochlorous acid (HOCl) are produced and are responsible for the caustic effects. As particle size and water solubility decrease, progressively lower regions of the airways are affected, and resultant symptoms are more insidious and severe. The potential sources of exposure to chlorine are multiple and include industrial operations, inappropriate mixing of household cleaning agents, emissions during transport, school chemistry experiments, and mishaps in the chlorinating of swimming pools. Chlorine is shipped widely by truck, train, and barge, making transportation and storage accidents ever-present dangers.

Chlorine exposures are most frequently due to industrial (pulp mills), household cleaner, and swimming pool exposures.[28] Children and adolescents younger than 18 years constitute the majority and most severely affected of patients.[29,30] The medical literature is replete with household exposures involving cleaning agents. Household ammonia and bleach are two of the most common cleaning agents. Combining them releases chloramine gas. When inhaled, chloramine gas reacts with the moisture of the respiratory tract to release ammonia, HCl, and oxygen free radicals. Typically, exposures to low concentrations of chloramines produce only mild respiratory tract irritation. In higher concentrations, the combination of HCl, ammonia, and oxygen free radicals may cause corrosive effects and cellular injury, resulting in pneumonitis and edema.[31,32] Aside from the initial cough and irritation, serious morbidity is rare and no deaths have been reported from household cleaning agents.[31,32]

Toxic manifestations of chlorine gas may be significant, and occur within seconds or minutes of exposure, depending on the concentration. Upper airway symptoms include irritation of the eyes, nose, and throat. Stridor and upper airway swelling leading to obstruction may occur. Lower airway manifestations include cough, shortness of breath, chest pain, and wheezing. Pulmonary edema and death may occur with significant exposure. Burns and corneal abrasions have resulted from skin and eye exposures. Various nonspecific symptoms, such as headache and nausea, may be present.[30,31] Clinical manifestations are predictable and typically resolve within 6 hours after mild exposures. Blood gases are generally normal. Mild hypoxemia and hypercarbia or respiratory alkalosis may be seen.[30,32,33] Chest radiographs are generally normal.[33]

Standard treatment of acute chlorine gas exposure includes removal of the patient from the source and respiratory support measures as needed. Eye and skin exposure requires copious irrigation with water or saline. Bronchospasm usually responds to standard β$_2$-agonists (e.g., albuterol). Corticosteroids and nebulized sodium bicarbonate have no clear efficacy and are not recommended.[30,33] Long-term effects after acute and chronic exposures to chlorine do not appear to be clinically significant, and the risk of reactive airways disease is undefined.[28,33]

Exposures to chlorine gas and other pulmonary irritants are relatively common. Symptoms are usually acute and short lived. Humidified oxygen and β-agonist applications are the best supportive therapy for chlorine gas exposure. Acute household cleaning agent exposures are generally benign. More severe injuries are possible with industrial exposures to more highly concentrated chemicals.

REFERENCES

*1. Marshall SW, Runyan CW, Bangdiwala SI, et al: Fatal residential fires: who dies and who survives? JAMA 279:1633–1637, 1998.
2. Feck GA, Baptise MS, Tate CLJ: Burn injuries: epidemiology and prevention. Accid Anal Prev 11:129–136, 1983.
*3. Sheridan RL, Remensnyder JP, Schnitzer JJ, et al: Current expectations for survival in pediatric burns. Arch Pediatr Adolesc Med 154:245–249, 2000.
4. Karter MJ: 1996 U.S. fire loss. NFPA J Sep/Oct:77–83, 1997.
*5. Barrow RE, Spies M, Barrow LN, et al: Influence of demographics and inhalation injury on burn mortality in children. Burns 30:72–77, 2004.
6. Wolf SE, Rose JK, Desai MH, et al: Mortality determinants in massive pediatric burns: an analysis of 103 children with ≥ 80% TBSA burns (≥ 70% full-thickness). Ann Surg 225:554–569, 1997.
7. Alarie Y: Toxicity of fire smoke. Crit Rev Toxicol 32:259–289, 2002.
8. Herndon DN, Langner F, Thompson P, et al: Pulmonary injury in burned patients. Surg Clin North Am 67:31–46, 1987.
9. Heimbach DM, Waeckerle JF: Inhalation injuries. Ann Emerg Med 17:1316–1320, 1988.
10. Shirani KZ, Pruitt BA, Mason AD. The influence of inhalation injury and pneumonia on burn mortality. Ann Surg 205:82–87, 1987.
*11. Bozeman WP, Myers RA, Barish RA: Confirmation of the pulse oximetry gap in carbon monoxide poisoning. Ann Emerg Med 30:608–611, 1997.
12. Parish RA: Smoke inhalation and carbon monoxide poisoning in children. Pediatr Emerg Care 2:36–39, 1986.
13. Wittram C, Kenny JB: The admission chest radiograph after acute inhalation injury and burns. Br J Radiol 67:751–754, 1994.
14. Sheridan RL, Kacmarek RM, McEttrick MM, et al: Permissive hypercapnia as a ventilatory strategy in burned children: effect of barotrauma, pneumonia, and mortality. J Trauma 39:854–859, 1995.
15. Mah JC: Non-Fire Carbon Monoxide Deaths Associated with the Use of Consumer Products: 1998 Estimates. Bethesda, MD: Consumer Products Safety Commission, 1998.
16. Parkinson RB, Hopkins RO, Cleavinger HB, et al: White matter hyperintensities and neuropsychological outcome following carbon monoxide poisoning. Neurology 58:1525–1532, 2002.
17. Crocker PJ, Walker JS: Pediatric carbon monoxide toxicity. J Emerg Med 3:443–448, 1985.
18. Gale SD, Hopkins RO: Effects of hypoxia on the brain: neuroimaging and neuropsychological findings following carbon monoxide poi-

*Selected readings.

soning and obstructive sleep apnea. J Int Neuropsychol Soc 10:60–71, 2004.

*19. Gilmer B, Kilkenny J, Tomaszewski C, et al: Hyperbaric oxygen does not prevent neurologic sequelae after carbon monoxide poisoning. Acad Emerg Med 9:1–8, 2002.

20. Juurlink D, Buckley N, Stanbrook M, et al: Hyperbaric oxygen for carbon monoxide poisoning. Cochrane Database Syst Rev (4): CD002041, 2005.

21. Weaver LK, Hopkins RO, Chan KJ, et al: Hyperbaric oxygen for acute carbon monoxide poisoning. N Engl J Med 347:1057–1067, 2002.

22. Sauer SW, Keim ME: Hydroxocobalamin: improved public health readiness for cyanide disasters. Ann Emerg Med 37:635–641, 2001.

23. American Association of Poison Control Centers: Toxic Exposure Surveillance System. Annual Reports 1993–2002. Available at *http://www.aapcc.org/poison.htm*.

24. Mehta PS, Mehta AS, Mehta SJ, et al: Bhopal tragedy's health effects: a review of methyl isocyanate toxicity. JAMA 264:2781–2187, 1990.

25. Baud FJ, Barriot P, Toffis V, et al: Elevated blood cyanide concentrations in victims of smoke inhalation. N Engl J Med 325:1761–1766, 1991.

26. Kulig K: Cyanide antidotes and fire toxicology. N Engl J Med 325: 1801–1802, 1991.

27. Forsyth JC, Mueller PD, Becker CE, et al: Hydroxocobalamin as a cyanide antidote: safety, efficacy and pharmacokinetics in heavily smoking normal volunteers. J Toxicol Clin Toxicol 31:277–294, 1993.

28. Vohra R, Clark RF: Chlorine-related inhalation injury from a swimming pool disinfectant in a 9-year-old girl. Pediatr Emerg Care 22: 254–257, 2006.

29. Agabiti N, Ancona C, Forastiere F, et al: Short term respiratory effects of acute exposure to chlorine due to a swimming pool accident. Occup Environ Med 58:399–404, 2001.

30. Fleta J, Calvo C, Zuniga J, et al: Intoxication of 76 children by chlorine gas. Hum Toxicol 5:99–100, 1986.

31. Tanen DA, Graeme KA, Raschke R: Severe lung injury after exposure to chloramines gas from household cleaners. N Engl J Med 341: 848–849, 1999.

32. Mrvos R, Dean BS, Krenzelok EP: Home exposures to chlorine/chloramines gas: review of 216 cases. South Med J 86:654–657, 1993.

33. Sexton JD, Pronchik DJ: Chlorine inhalation: the big picture. J Toxicol Clin Toxicol 36:87–93, 1998.

Dysbarism

John P. Santamaria, MD

Introduction and Background

Dysbarism is a term for any clinical syndrome caused by a difference between the atmospheric pressure and the total gas pressure in a body tissue, fluid, or cavity.[1] Although the term could be applied to changes in atmospheric pressure such as occurs during a space walk,[2] the most common situations in which emergency physicians will encounter children and adolescents with dysbarism is either at high altitudes in mountainous regions (see Chapter 145, High Altitude–Associated Illnesses) or after scuba diving.

Given that the symptoms of diving-related illnesses can arise several hours after a dive and that patients may present days after diving, emergency physicians working several hours' travel from the coast may occasionally see patients with diving-related illnesses. Although many interesting and serious conditions can arise from spending time in the ocean[3] (see Chapter 140, Hypothermia), this discussion focuses on those conditions related to changes in atmospheric pressure associated with scuba diving.

Recognition and Approach

The vast majority of scuba divers are middle-aged adults.[4-8] Not surprisingly, most dive-related injuries and fatalities occur in middle-aged adults.[4-8] However, increasingly younger children have been accepted into scuba certification courses and encouraged to dive. In 2000, diving certification organizations lowered the minimum training age from 12 to 8

years.[9,10] Although still relatively rare, serious pediatric diving injuries and fatalities occur. Of 423 diving-related fatalities reported to the Divers Alert Network from 1999 through 2003, 7 (2%) occurred in children ≤ 19 years[4-8] (Table 144–1). From data on citizens of the United States and Canada, the age of the youngest child to sustain a diving injury is 11 years and the age of the youngest child to suffer a diving fatality is 14 years.[3]

Emotional maturity, appropriate training, and tight supervision appear to be key components to successful pediatric diving. Many children and adolescents are intellectually capable of completing and excelling in the cognitive portions of scuba diving classes. The concern is that a child or adolescent will react badly to unexpected, uniquely stressful experiences under water or take unnecessary, dangerous risks. Poor decision making, lack of proper training, ignoring proper procedures for safe diving, and panicking at a critical moment are recurrent themes in fatal adolescent dives (see Table 144–1).

The pathophysiology of dysbarism falls into two general categories. The first category involves pressure changes in relatively fixed body spaces. These disorders are generally referred to as "barotrauma." These types of injuries are reasonably straightforward and based on a well-described physical principle, Boyle's law.[11,12] Boyle's law states that, at a constant temperature, volume and pressure are inversely proportional. Every 10 meters of sea water in depth adds 1 additional atmosphere of pressure. So, if an air-filled ball is taken down 10 m in the ocean, the volume of the ball would be half of its volume at the surface because the air in the ball would be exposed to twice the atmospheric pressure. The same principles apply to body cavities such as sinuses. Unfortunately, the bony walls of a sinus cannot easily accommodate large changes in volume. The signs and symptoms will reflect the body cavity involved.

The second category in the pathophysiology of dysbarism involves gases dissolved in liquids. Affecting one or more body regions, the constellation of problems arising from nitrogen dissolving in body tissues is typically referred to as "decompression illness."[4,11] The relevant physical law in this instance is Henry's law.[13] Henry's law states that the amount of gas dissolved in a liquid is proportional to the partial pressure of that gas in contact with the liquid.[13] The higher the pressure, the more gas dissolved in that liquid. When diving, the higher atmospheric pressure drives nitrogen into the body tissues. Since nitrogen is not metabolized by the body,

Table 144–1			Deaths Associated with Scuba Diving by Children and Adolescents ≤ 19 Years, 1999–2003	
Year	Age (yr)	Gender	Prior Diving Experience	Circumstances
2003	18	Male	Certified for 18 mo; 130 dives completed	Shore-entry night dive using nitrox. Third dive of the day. Depth to 93 feet of sea water (28 m) for 25 min. Rapid ascent after running out of breathing gas. Unconscious upon surfacing.
2001	19	Male	Completed open water certification the morning of the day he died	Without prior planning, separated from an instructor and entered an underwater cave with 35-yr-old diving buddy. Ran out of air after becoming lost in the cave.
2001	17	Male	No formal dive training or experience	Did not dive with a buddy. Did not use a buoy or any other mark for his location. When his body was found 2 days later, his tank was empty.
2001	17	Female	No formal dive training or experience	Collecting sand dollars at a depth of 10 feet. Did not wear fins. Began with a partially empty tank. Was holding hands with another equally inexperienced diver during the dive, but let go at the surface. Her body was found 8 hr later.
2001	19	Female	Completed certification course; participating in her first dive after certification and first dive in cold water	Strong current and poor visibility. Planned a dive to 50 feet of sea water (15 m), but descended to 200 feet of sea water (60 m). She lost consciousness after appearing to panic and have difficulty with her buoyancy compensator. She was too heavy for the dive buddy to lift. Her body was never recovered.
2000	16	Male	Certified by an organization with no national affiliation 1 year prior	Second dive of the day that went past 200 feet of sea water (60 m). Shot an extremely large fish and attached it to his buoyancy compensation device. Struggle with the fish resulted in him being hit in the face and neck. Unconscious when his dive buddy reached him. Went beyond maximum for depth and time based on buddy's dive computer.
1999	19	Male	Open-water certified for 2 wk	Made a dive to 227 feet of sea water (69 m) with two other divers. Ascended to 190 feet of sea water (57.8 m). He ran out of air and began to buddy breath with one of the other divers. Then made a rapid ascent to the surface from 170 feet of sea water. Pronounced dead at a local hospital.

Data source: Divers Alert Network: Report on Decompression Illness, Diving Fatalities and Project Dive Exploration (2001 through 2005 editions). Available at http://www.DiversAlertNetwork.org.

if ascent is too rapid, the nitrogen may be released rapidly from tissues and bubbles may form. These bubbles can obstruct arteries, veins, and lymphatics or distort local tissue architecture. The signs, symptoms, and clinical syndrome relate to the body parts involved.

Clinical Presentation

The feature most strongly affecting the clinical presentation and severity of dysbarism is the body part affected. The degree to which the dysbarism is life threatening can be deduced directly from the body part involved. Overall, the most common symptoms reported by divers are pain and paresthesias.[4] The most immediately life-threatening conditions involve loss of consciousness or loss of motor function while underwater.

Brain

The most serious manifestations of dysbarism in the brain are acute stroke, altered mental status, and loss of consciousness.[14] An acute stroke arises when a bubble of gas (i.e., a gas embolism) occludes a critical artery supplying the brain. The symptoms will reflect the area of brain injured (see Chapter 44, Central Nervous System Vascular Disorders). Unconsciousness may be the dominant sign and is often fatal if this occurs while the diver is underwater (see Table 144–1). Patients with a patent foramen ovale are at increased risk for strokes from arterial gas emboli.[15-17] Arterial gas emboli occur during ascent. Another condition affecting the brain is nitrogen narcosis. At depths of 30 m or greater, dissolved nitrogen

alters the ionic conductance through neuronal membranes.[11] This leads to a clinical condition similar to alcohol intoxication. Impaired judgment, clumsiness, light-headedness, euphoria, and disorientation are common symptoms. Divers may misuse their equipment, fail to acknowledge low air in their tanks, become trapped, or go deeper and lose consciousness. Nitrogen narcosis occurs during the deepest portions of a dive.

Spinal Cord

The spinal cord is particularly vulnerable to decompression sickness.[18] Symptoms can range from limb paresthesias to paraplegia. Spinal cord injuries occur during ascent.

Inner Ear

Vertigo, nausea, vomiting, unsteadiness, tinnitus, and hearing loss are common symptoms of inner ear decompression sickness.[19] In adults, the onset of symptoms is usually within the first hour or two after a dive, but symptoms may arise after more than 5 hours.[19] Inner ear decompression sickness occurs during ascent.

Middle Ear and Ear Canal

If a diver's eustachian tubes are partially or completely occluded, spontaneous equalization of the pressure in the middle ear with the environmental pressure encountered during a dive will be impaired. This condition is the most common form of dysbarism, affecting 30% of new divers on their first dive and 10% of experienced divers.[20] This condition is commonly referred to as "barotitis media" or "middle ear squeeze." Signs and symptoms of barotitis media include ear pain, tympanic membrane injury or rupture, and blood in the ear canal. If the tympanic membrane ruptures, cold water may enter the middle ear and lead to life-threatening severe vertigo and disorientation during a dive. A similar phenomenon may occur if ear plugs or a wax plug completely occlude the external ear canal, creating a pocket of air.[21] Middle ear and canal injuries more frequently occur during descent, but may occur during ascent.

Sinuses

If the sinus ostia are occluded, spontaneous equalization of the pressure in a sinus with the environmental pressure encountered during a dive will be impaired. The maxillary sinus is the most frequently affected. The most common symptoms are facial pain and epistaxis. Decreased facial sensation in the area innervated by the infraorbital nerve may also occur.[22] Sinus barotrauma is also known as "sinus squeeze."[13] Sinus barotrauma occurs twice as frequently during descent as ascent.

Teeth

Air pockets may be present in teeth due to recent dental work or from pathology such as cavities. Pressure changes during a dive may cause pain with or without tooth fracture.[23] This condition is referred to as "barodontalgia" or "tooth squeeze." Barodontalgia typically occurs during descent.

Tongue

An arterial gas embolism may leave a well-circumscribed area of pallor on the tongue. This physical finding is also called Liebermeister's sign.[24]

Lungs

Pulmonary barotrauma is the most life-threatening form of barotrauma. The classic example of pulmonary barotrauma occurs when a diver takes a breath at depth and then rapidly ascends while holding his or her breath. As the diver ascends, the pressure and volume of gas in the lungs will progressively increase due to the continually decreasing environmental pressure as the diver approaches the surface. Resulting injuries include simple pneumothorax, tension pneumothorax, pneumomediastinum, alveolar rupture, and the release of gas emboli into the central circulation. Signs and symptoms include chest pain, dyspnea, cardiovascular collapse, stroke, hemoptysis, and unconsciousness.[11] Divers with uncontrolled asthma or wheeze precipitated by exercise, cold, or emotion are at increased risk for pulmonary barotrauma.[25] Pulmonary barotrauma occurs during ascent.

Gastrointestinal Tract

The gastrointestinal tract is a distensible tube containing air and liquid. As the environmental pressure changes during a dive, the air in the gastrointestinal tract will contract or expand. Although serious conditions such as rupture of the stomach have been reported,[26] most cases of gastrointestinal dysbarism result in crampy abdominal pains or dyspepsia. Gastrointestinal dysbarism occurs during ascent.

Skin

Cutaneous manifestations of decompression illness most commonly occur on the torso. Itching is the most common symptom.[12] Examination of the skin may reveal an erythematous, macular rash or patchy mottling.[12]

Localized lymphedema may be present.[11] The onset of cutaneous manifestations of decompression illness is variable, but may occur after a dive has concluded.

Extremities

Deep, aching pains in the extremities due to decompression illness may occur up to an hour after surfacing from a dive.[11] The severity is variable, but the pain may be severe. A common name for this syndrome is "the bends." The bends occurs after resurfacing.

Face

When a mask is tightly adhered to a diver's face at the surface, this air-filled space is vulnerable to dysbarism. If a diver does not properly ventilate his or her mask by exhaling through the nose during descent, a "mask squeeze" may occur.[27,28] Signs and symptoms of a mask squeeze include periorbital pain, conjunctival and periorbital edema, subconjunctival hemorrhages, periorbital ecchymoses, and petechial hemorrhages in the distribution of the mask on the face.[28] Mask squeeze occurs during descent.

Important Clinical Features and Considerations

When a diver presents to the emergency department after a dive, reviewing his or her dive table may have some utility. The risk for dysbarism is directly related to the duration and depth of a dive. Dive tables offer a rough estimate of safe dive plans based on duration and depth.[29] Identifying a diver who has substantially deviated from a published dive table helps risk-stratify that patient. However, divers are notorious for underestimating and underreporting depth and "bottom times." There are significant differences among various decompression tables that are used by different dive agencies and in different parts of the world. Dive computers used during a dive to estimate the duration and depth of a dive extrapolate values from various dive tables. This, in turn, results in more bottom time and a greater risk of dysbarism.

Management

The management of dysbarism is based on the clinical syndrome. In general, serious signs and symptoms warrant the immediate application of high-flow oxygen and transfer to the care of a dive specialist at a facility capable of recompression therapy in a hyperbaric chamber.[30] In anticipation of transfer, the only test indicated is a chest radiograph to identify a pneumothorax. If a patient with a small, unrecognized pneumothorax undergoes recompression therapy, the patient may develop a tension pneumothorax in the hyperbaric chamber. Identifying a pneumothorax and placing a thoracostomy tube (see Chapter 168, Thoracostomy) allows the patient to undergo recompression therapy more safely. The performance of other tests that do not clearly meet other indications (e.g., a glucose check in a known diabetic diver) only delays recompression therapy without offering the patient additional benefit. Unconsciousness after a rapid ascent or acute stroke symptoms are obvious indication for recompression therapy. Other indications for consultation with a dive specialist regarding recompression therapy that are less obvious to emergency physicians who do not dive are numbness and tingling in the extremities, dizziness and vertigo, crampy extremity pains, joint pains, Liebermeister's sign, and skin mottling. Inexperienced divers may not associate their symptoms with dysbarism. Experienced divers may minimize their symptoms. A dive specialist should be consulted if these or other vague symptoms arise within days of a dive. Untreated dysbarism can lead to permanent injuries, particularly to the central nervous system. Recommendations regarding returning to diving should be deferred to a dive specialist.

Relatively minor diving injuries, including the "squeezes," rarely require emergent treatment. Barotitis media should be treated symptomatically, and follow-up arranged with a primary care doctor. Tympanic membrane rupture may be an indication for follow-up with an otolaryngologist. Barodontalgia, including most dental fractures, should also be treated symptomatically. The patient can follow up with a dentist at his or her convenience. Mask squeeze and sinus squeeze should be treated symptomatically.

Summary

An increase in the number of children and adolescents experiencing dysbarism is expected given the recent lowering of the minimum scuba training age. Emotional maturity, appropriate training, and tight supervision appear to be key components to successful pediatric diving. Poor decision making, lack of proper training, ignoring proper procedures for safe diving, and panicking at a critical moment are recurrent themes in fatal adolescent dives. Signs and symptoms of dysbarism, although often dramatic and unmistakable, may also be subtle. Children and adolescents with dysbarism may present to emergency departments far from the coast days after diving.

REFERENCES

1. Anderson DM, Novak PD, Keith J, et al: Dorland's Illustrated Medical Dictionary, 30th ed. Philadelphia: WB Saunders, 2003, p 573.
2. Conkin J, Powell MR, Gernhardt ML: Age affects severity of venous gas emboli on decompression from 14.7 to 4.3 psia. Aviat Space Environ Med 74:1142–1150, 2003.
3. Armoni M, Ohali M, Hay E, et al: Severe dyspnea due to jellyfish envenomation. Pediatr Emerg Care 19:84–86, 2003.
4. Divers Alert Network: Report on Decompression Illness, Diving Fatalities and Project Dive Exploration. 2005. Available at *http://www.DiversAlertNetwork.org* (accessed May 8, 2006).
5. Divers Alert Network: Report on Decompression Illness, Diving Fatalities and Project Dive Exploration. 2004. Available at *http://www.DiversAlertNetwork.org* (accessed May 8, 2006).
6. Divers Alert Network: Report on Decompression Illness, Diving Fatalities and Project Dive Exploration. 2003. Available at *http://www.DiversAlertNetwork.org* (accessed May 8, 2006).
7. Divers Alert Network: Report on Decompression Illness, Diving Fatalities and Project Dive Exploration. 2002. Available at *http://www.DiversAlertNetwork.org* (accessed May 8, 2006).
8. Divers Alert Network: Report on Decompression Illness, Diving Fatalities and Project Dive Exploration. 2001. Available at *http://www.DiversAlertNetwork.org* (accessed May 8, 2006).
9. Tsung JW, Chou KJ, Martinez C, et al: An adolescent scuba diver with 2 episodes of diving-related injuries requiring hyperbaric oxygen recompression therapy: a case report with medical considerations for child and adolescent scuba divers. Pediatr Emerg Care 21:681–686, 2005.
10. Table of programs offering scuba diving training courses for children aged 8 to 15 years. Available at *http://dive.scubadiving.com/html/200110Childcert_chart.html* (accessed May 8, 2006).
11. DeGorordo A, Vallejo-Manzur F, Chanin K, et al: Diving emergencies. Resuscitation 59:171–180, 2003.
12. Smith DJ: Diagnosis and management of diving accidents. Med Sci Sports Exerc 28:587–590, 1996.
13. Clenney TL, Lassen LF: Recreational scuba diving injuries. Am Fam Physician 53:1761–1774, 1996.
14. Carstairs S: Arterial gas embolism in a diver using a closed-circuit oxygen rebreathing diving apparatus. Undersea Hyperb Med 28:229–231, 2001.
15. Torti SR, Billinger M, Schwerzmann M, et al: Risk of decompression illness among 230 divers in relation to the presence and size of patent foramen ovale. Eur Heart J 25:1014–1020, 2004.
16. Schwerzmann M, Seiler C, Lipp E, et al: Relation between directly detected patent foramen ovale and ischemic brain lesions in sport divers. Ann Intern Med 134:21–24, 2001.
17. Bove AA: Risk of decompression sickness with patent foramen ovale. Undersea Hyperb Med 25:175–178, 1998.
18. Chesire WP Jr, Ott MC: Headache in divers. Headache 41:235–247, 2001.
19. Hills BA: Spinal decompression sickness: hydrophobic protein and lamellar bodies in spinal tissue. Undersea Hyperb Med 20:3–16, 1993.
20. Nachum Z, Shupak A, Spitzer O, et al: Inner ear decompression sickness in sport compressed-air diving. Laryngoscope 111:851–856, 2001.
21. Brown M, Jones J, Krohmer J: Pseudoephedrine for the prevention of barotitis media: a controlled clinical trial in underwater divers. Ann Emerg Med 21:849–852, 1992.
22. Butler FK, Bove AA: Infraorbital hypesthesia after maxillary sinus barotrauma. Undersea Hyperb Med 26:257–259, 1999.
23. Robichaud , McNally ME: Barodontalgia as a differential diagnosis: symptoms and findings. J Can Dent Assoc 71:39–42, 2005.
24. Decompression Sickness. Available at *http://www.ukdivers.net/physiology/dcs.htm* (accessed May 10, 2006).
25. British Thoracic Society Fitness to Dive Group, Subgroup of the British Thoracic Society Standards of Care Committee: British Thoracic Society guidelines on respiratory aspects of fitness for diving. Thorax 58:3–13, 2003.
26. Yeung P, Crowe P, Bennett M: Barogenic rupture of the stomach: a case for non-operative management. Aust N Z J Surg 68:76–77, 1998.
27. Butler FK, Gurney N: Orbital hemorrhage following face-mask barotrauma. Undersea Hyperb Med 28:31–34, 2001.
28. Rudge FW: Ocular barotrauma caused by mask squeeze during a scuba dive. South Med J 87:749–750, 1994.
29. Van Liew HD, Flynn ET: Decompression tables and dive-outcome data: graphical analysis. Undersea Hyperb Med 32:187–198, 2005.
30. Brubakk A: Hyperbaric oxygen therapy: oxygen and bubbles. Undersea Hyperb Med 31:73–79, 2004.

Chapter 145

High Altitude–Associated Illnesses

William M. McDonnell, MD, JD and Mark G. Roback, MD

Key Points

A history of rapid onset of nonspecific symptoms shortly after ascent to high altitude suggests acute mountain sickness.

It is important to rapidly recognize acute mountain sickness, because it may progress to the life-threatening conditions of high-altitude pulmonary edema and high-altitude cerebral edema.

Preventative strategies are available for acute mountain sickness.

Severe complications of acute mountain sickness can be treated effectively with transport to lower elevation, and less effectively with supportive care and pharmacotherapy.

Selected Diagnoses

Acute mountain sickness
High-altitude pulmonary edema
High-altitude cerebral edema

Discussion of Individual Diagnoses

Acute Mountain Sickness

Altitude illness historically affected explorers and a few extreme sport adventurers, with little impact on the broader population. However, with increasing access to high-altitude recreation and tourism destinations, there is increasing potential for altitude-related illness in the general population, including children. Substantial research has been done regarding the incidence, etiology, treatment, and prevention of altitude-related illness in adults. However, little has been reported in these areas with respect to children. Therefore, pediatric health care providers, in many cases, must care for their pediatric patients based on elements of adult practice.

Although quite variable,[1] the incidence of altitude illness is approximately 25% in travelers to altitudes above 6500 feet (2000 m),[2] and up to 60% above 14,000 feet (4200 m).[3] Both hypoxia and the lower atmospheric pressure contribute to acute mountain sickness (AMS).[4] A history of travel to altitude is the most important factor in recognizing altitude illness. The most common of the acute altitude illnesses, AMS includes the nonspecific symptoms of headache, anorexia, nausea, dyspnea, sleep disturbance, low-grade fever, and malaise. In young children, AMS may manifest as tachypnea,[5] increased fussiness, sleep disturbance, decreased playfulness, and decreased appetite.[6] Symptoms in both adults and children typically develop within 1 to 2 days of exposure to altitude, with the majority of those affected first experiencing symptoms within 12 hours of arrival at altitude.[2,6]

The primary risk factors for developing AMS are rapid rate of ascent to high altitude, lack of acclimatization at moderate altitude, and previous altitude illness.[7] Strenuous exercise at altitude may result in increased incidence and severity of AMS.[8] Dehydration also increases the risk of AMS and worsens its symptoms. Dehydration stimulates increased renal sodium and bicarbonate reabsorption, and the resulting relative metabolic alkalosis reduces the patient's ability to compensate for the hypoxia of altitude with an appropriately increased ventilatory response.[9] Although obesity has been associated with a greater risk for the development of AMS,[10] physical fitness does not appear to be protective.[7]

It is uncertain whether children are at greater risk of developing AMS than adults. One study observed a higher rate of AMS symptoms among children ages 6 to 48 months than among adolescents and adults.[11] This study also noted more pronounced hypoxemia among the children with AMS than among the adults and adolescents with the same condition. However, other studies have found no significant difference in the incidence of AMS between preverbal children and adults.[6,12] Nevertheless, it is clear that children can and do develop AMS.

Clinical Presentation

A history of rapid onset of headache and other symptoms such as anorexia, nausea, dyspnea, sleep disturbance, low-grade fever, and malaise shortly after travel to high altitude strongly suggests AMS, which may progress to the more severe acute altitude illnesses, high-altitude pulmonary edema (HAPE) and high-altitude cerebral edema (HACE). Evaluation of the patient should include a careful assessment of vital signs, and a physical examination with particular scrutiny of respiratory, cardiovascular, and neurologic status.

Physical examination findings common in AMS include mild temperature elevation, tachypnea, tachycardia, and mild hypoxia. Chest auscultation may reveal diminished aeration, diffuse crackles, or both.

AMS may mimic conditions commonly encountered in lower altitude settings, including pneumonitis of viral, bacterial, fungal, or chemical etiologies; dehydration; intracranial hemorrhage or infarction; cerebral edema; and migraine headache. Many of these diagnoses remain in the differential diagnosis, and may be systematically distinguished from altitude illness.

An extensive laboratory and radiologic evaluation is rarely warranted. A chest radiograph may help identify the progression of AMS to HAPE, but the findings of AMS or HAPE may be difficult to distinguish from pneumonia. Pulse oximetry helps in assessing the degree of respiratory compromise.

Management

For all patients with AMS, further ascent is contraindicated, and patients should promptly descend to lower altitude if symptoms worsen. Indications for immediate descent to lower altitude include hypoxia unresponsive to supplemental oxygen, worsening dyspnea, ataxia, and mental status changes. Children's AMS symptoms resolve quickly after return to lower elevation.[6] Moreover, brief AMS from high-altitude exposure produces no lasting neuropsychological impairment or anatomic changes of the brain.[13]

Patients with mild AMS symptoms may be treated at altitude. Therapy consists of supportive care. Rest and oral hydration are frequently sufficient treatment for mild AMS. As dehydration has been noted to worsen AMS, rehydration with intravenous normal saline may be indicated. However, progression to pulmonary edema is a risk of AMS, and it is prudent to avoid excessive fluid administration. Analgesics such as acetaminophen and ibuprofen typically provide effective relief from the headaches and nausea generally associated with AMS.[14,15] However, common migraine headache therapies such as sumatriptan are not effective in treating high-altitude headaches.[15]

Prevention of AMS is more effective than treatment. The best preventative strategy for AMS is gradual ascent, allowing time for acclimatization. A few days' acclimatization at altitude generally allows resolution of mild AMS symptoms and may prevent progression of symptoms. An overnight stay at an intermediate altitude has been shown to reduce the incidence of subsequent AMS symptoms.[2] The acclimatization effect is generally attributed to increased ventilation and diuresis.[16] Similar acclimatization effects have been observed in subjects exposed to brief simulated intermittent altitude exposures in a hypobaric chamber over a period of 3 weeks.[17]

Acetazolamide has been demonstrated to be useful in preventing AMS, with treated adult subjects showing a decrease in symptoms and greater oxygen saturation levels at altitude.[18-20] However, no specific data regarding efficacy or dosing recommendations exist for children. Low-dose glucocorticoids hold promise for prophylaxis against AMS,[21] and one adult study has shown that prophylactic acetazolamide in combination with low-dose dexamethasone is more effective in preventing AMS than is acetazolamide alone.[22] Another adult study investigating the use of prophylactic nifedipine to prevent HAPE also found a significant reduction in AMS symptoms.[23]

Although there is some evidence that the use of the herbal supplement ginkgo biloba before and during ascent may reduce the severity of AMS symptoms in healthy adults,[24] this finding is not conclusive. A recent large, prospective, randomized controlled study concluded that ginkgo is not effective in reducing either the incidence or severity of AMS, and there are some indications that ginkgo may worsen AMS symptoms.[20]

Summary

Generalized, nonspecific symptoms following ascent to high altitude suggest AMS. The primary risk factors for AMS are rapid ascent to high altitude and a prior history of AMS. Although AMS is generally self-limited, and responds well to acclimatization, as many as 5% to 10% of patients with AMS may develop the more serious altitude illnesses of HAPE or HACE if they do not promptly return to lower altitude.[1]

High-Altitude Pulmonary Edema

With extended exposure to high altitude, a patient with AMS may develop HAPE, with progression to severe hypoxemia. HAPE is a form of rapidly progressive hydrostatic pulmonary edema.[25,26] HAPE is characterized by the marked elevation of pulmonary artery and capillary pressures, and changes in left ventricular diastolic function.[26-28] Insufficient hypoxic ventilatory response at high altitude, combined with impaired gas exchange resulting from pulmonary edema, produces the severe hypoxemia seen with HAPE.[16] Untreated, HAPE may rapidly progress to respiratory failure and death. Although the reported incidence of HAPE is somewhat variable, most individuals will probably experience HAPE if the rate of ascent, maximum elevation attained, and physical exertion are great enough.[29] People who exhibit an increased pulmonary artery pressure response to exercise are more likely also to have an increased pulmonary artery pressure response to altitude-related hypoxia, and thus are more prone to develop HAPE.[30] It may be possible to identify these individuals at increased risk of developing HAPE by Doppler echocardiography during strenuous exercise.[30] For children, the risk of developing HAPE is exacerbated by a concomitant upper respiratory viral infection, while adults seem to face no such increased risk.[31]

Clinical Presentation

The usual progression to HAPE includes the typical nonspecific signs and symptoms of AMS, and the development of a cough that may be productive of blood-tinged mucus, increasing tachypnea, dyspnea at rest, and marked hypoxia.[28] Crackles and wheezes are often detected on chest auscultation. Some patients with HAPE have described a "gurgling" sensation in their chests.[32]

When HAPE is suspected, the patient's respiratory, hemodynamic, and neurologic status are the focus of the evaluation. Preparations for transport to lower elevation are indicated. As with AMS, only limited laboratory and imaging studies are needed. Chest radiographs show dilation of the central pulmonary arteries, and patchy, peripheral, bilateral or unilateral infiltrates that are often asymmetric.[33] Electrocardiography may show evidence of right ventricular strain, with extensive T-wave negativity in precordial leads,[34] which is consistent with autopsy studies that have demonstrated right ventricular dilation.[35]

Management

With the progression of AMS to HAPE, further ascent is absolutely contraindicated. Appropriate treatment includes supplemental oxygen at the maximum available concentration, stabilization of hemodynamic status, and prompt descent to lower elevation. Although some patients with mild HAPE may be treated at moderate altitudes (below 10,000 feet/3000 m) with bed rest and supplemental oxygen, any significant deterioration requires immediate transport to lower elevation.[36] Portable fabric hyperbaric chambers can be used to provide increased atmospheric pressure while awaiting transport or en route to a lower altitude. With the progression of substantial pulmonary edema, some patients may develop inadequate ventilation and severe hypoxia despite supplemental oxygen, requiring endotracheal intubation and positive pressure ventilation.

High pulmonary artery pressure is key to the development of HAPE.[26,28] In adults with HAPE, nifedipine reduces pulmonary vascular resistance and pulmonary artery pressures, and thereby reduces symptoms such as dyspnea and chest pain, as well as improving oxygen saturation.[37] Although transport to lower elevation remains the definitive treatment for HAPE, nifedipine is generally accepted as an appropriate temporizing therapy in adults when transport is unavoidably delayed. The benefits of nifedipine therapy in children with HAPE have not been established.

The signs and symptoms of HAPE typically reverse completely after patients are transferred to low altitude.[26] However, patients who have experienced HAPE are at an increased risk of recurrence on return to high altitude.[23] Prophylactic inhalation of a β-adrenergic agonist (e.g., albuterol) may reduce the risk of recurrence of HAPE.[38] The prophylactic use of nifedipine has also been shown to be effective in preventing HAPE in adults.[73] Some victims of HAPE may slowly reascend after a few days at lower altitude and after complete resolution of their symptoms, without recurrence.[39] However, such patients should immediately descend at the first sign of recurrence.

In summary, patients with AMS who remain at high altitude may develop the worsening pulmonary symptoms of HAPE. Although unrecognized HAPE may be fatal, prompt recognition and transport to lower elevation typically results in complete resolution of symptoms.

High-Altitude Cerebral Edema

Patients with AMS who remain at high altitude or who continue to climb may progress to HACE. HACE is generally considered to be the end-stage progression of AMS, and is characterized by reversible brain white matter edema, particularly in the corpus callosum.[32,40] The mechanism appears to be vasogenic, with movement of fluid and proteins out of the vascular compartment.[40] There is some evidence that patients with early AMS are already experiencing minor cerebral edema, which can be demonstrated by subtle cognitive changes on psychomotor testing.[41]

HACE is usually preceded by the generalized, nonspecific symptoms of AMS. Signs and symptoms of HACE include severe headache, cognitive-behavioral changes, and ataxia, which may quickly progress to obtundation and coma.[32] Patients may experience vivid hallucinations.[32] The time period for progression from mild neurologic symptoms to deep coma is variable, from hours to days.[33] HACE is often comorbid with HAPE.[32,35]

Management

As with AMS and HAPE, the initial approach to a patient with HACE includes careful evaluation and stabilization of respiratory and circulatory functions, including securing the patient's airway in the case of significant depression of mental status. Supplemental oxygen is indicated, and preparations for immediate medical evacuation to lower altitude should be started. Pulse oximetry and arterial blood gases may be useful in evaluating respiratory function. As in any setting of altered mental status, evaluating serum glucose levels is appropriate. Brain imaging studies of HACE patients reveal a picture of cerebral edema. Computed tomography shows diffuse edema, with a paucity or absence of sulci, small ventricles, and diffuse low density of white matter.[32,42] Brain magnetic resonance imaging shows increased T2 signal in the white matter, with a characteristic marked increased signal in the corpus callosum.[32,40] HACE can usually be diagnosed based on a history of ascent to high elevation and the progression of signs and symptoms, making brain imaging studies unnecessary.

HACE is a potentially fatal, but easily reversible, illness. The optimal and definitive management includes immediate transport to lower elevation. After prompt return to low altitude, HACE patients typically have no appreciable residual central nervous system impairment on brain magnetic resonance imaging and neuropsychological testing.[13] However, when transport to lower elevation is delayed, HACE may progress to brain herniation and death. Accordingly, transport should not be delayed by any therapy other than assuring adequate respiratory and circulatory function. In the event that transport is unavoidably delayed, oral or parenteral dexamethasone may be of benefit.[32,40,41] As with HAPE, portable hyperbaric chambers may be used to simulate lower elevation while awaiting transport.

In summary, the development of neurologic signs in a patient with AMS signals the onset of HACE. Although unrecognized and untreated HACE can be fatal, patients who are promptly transported to lower elevation typically have complete resolution of their HACE without sequelae. Immediate transport to lower elevation is universally indicated in cases of HACE.

REFERENCES

1. Hackett PH, Rennie D, Levine HD: The incidence, importance, and prophylaxis of acute mountain sickness. Lancet 308:1149–1155, 1976.
2. Honigman B, Theis MK, Koziol-McLain J, et al: Acute mountain sickness in a general tourist population at moderate altitudes. Ann Intern Med 118:587–592, 1993.
3. Ziaee V, Yunesian M, Ahmadinejad Z, et al: Acute mountain sickness in Iranian trekkers around Mount Damavand in Iran. Wilderness Environ Med 14:214–219, 2003.
4. Roach RC, Loeppky JA, Icenogle MV, et al: Acute mountain sickness: increased severity during simulated altitude compared with normobaric hypoxia. J Appl Physiol 81:1908–1910, 1996.
*5. Yaron M, Niermeyer S, Lindgren KN, et al: Physiologic response to moderate altitude exposure among infants and young children. High Alt Med Biol 4:53–59, 2003.

*Selected readings.

*6. Yaron M, Waldman N, Niermeyer S, et al: The diagnosis of acute mountain sickness in preverbal children. Arch Pediatr Adolesc Med 152:683–687, 1998.

7. Schneider M, Bernasch D, Weymann J, et al: Acute mountain sickness: influence of susceptibility, preexposure, and ascent rate. Med Sci Sports Exerc 34:1886–1891, 2002.

8. Roach RC, Maes D, Sandoval D, et al: Exercise exacerbates acute mountain sickness at simulated high altitude. J Appl Physiol 88:581–585, 2000.

9. Cumbo TA, Basnyat B, Graham J, et al: Acute mountain sickness, dehydration, and bicarbonate clearance: preliminary field data from the Nepal Himalaya. Aviat Space Environ Med 73:898–901, 2002.

10. Ri-Li G, Chase PJ, Witkowski S, et al: Obesity: associations with acute mountain sickness. Ann Intern Med 139:253–258, 2003.

*11. Moraga FA, Osorio JD, Vargas ME: Acute mountain sickness in tourists with children at Lake Chungara (4400 m) in northern Chile. Wilderness Environ Med 13:31–35, 2002.

*12. Yaron M, Niermeyer S, Lindgren KN, et al: Evaluation of diagnostic criteria and incidence of acute mountain sickness in preverbal children. Wilderness Environ Med 13:21–26, 2002.

13. Anooshiravani M, Dumont L, Mardirosoff C, et al: Brain magnetic resonance imaging (MRI) and neurological changes after a single high altitude climb. Med Sci Sports Exerc 31:969–972, 1999.

14. Harris NS, Wenzel RP, Thomas SH: High altitude headache: efficacy of acetaminophen vs. ibuprofen in a randomized, controlled trial. J Emerg Med 24:383–387, 2003.

15. Burtscher M, Likar R, Nachbauer W, et al: Ibuprofen versus sumatriptan for high-altitude headache. Lancet 346:254–255, 1995.

16. Bartsch P, Swenson ER, Paul A, et al: Hypoxic ventilatory response, ventilation, gas exchange, and fluid balance in acute mountain sickness. High Alt Med Biol 3:361–376, 2002.

17. Beidleman BA, Muza SR, Fulco CS, et al: Intermittent altitude exposures reduce acute mountain sickness at 4300 m. Clin Sci 106:321–328, 2004.

*18. Basnyat B, Gertsch JH, Johnson EW, et al: Efficacy of low-dose acetazolamide (125 mg BID) for the prophylaxis of acute mountain sickness: a prospective, double-blind, randomized, placebo-controlled trial. High Alt Med Biol 4:45–52, 2003.

19. Carlsten C, Swenson ER, Ruoss S: A dose-response study of acetazolamide for acute mountain sickness prophylaxis in vacationing tourists at 12,000 feet (3630 m). High Alt Med Biol 5:33–39, 2004.

20. Gertsch JH, Basnyat B, Johnson EW, et al: Randomised, double blind, placebo controlled comparison of ginkgo biloba and acetazolamide for prevention of acute mountain sickness among Himalayan trekkers: the Prevention of High Altitude Illness Trial (PHAIT). BMJ 328:797, 2004.

21. Basu M, Sawhney RC, Kumar S, et al: Glucocorticoids as prophylaxis against acute mountain sickness. Clin Endocrinol 57:761–767, 2002.

22. Bernhard WN, Schalick LM, Delaney PA, et al: Acetazolamide plus low-dose dexamethasone is better than acetazolamide alone to ameliorate symptoms of acute mountain sickness. Aviat Space Environ Med 69:883–886, 1998.

23. Bartsch P, Maggiorini M, Ritter M, et al: Prevention of high-altitude pulmonary edema by nifedipine. N Engl J Med 325:1284–1289, 1991.

24. Gertsch JH, Seto TB, Mor J, et al: Ginkgo biloba for the prevention of severe acute mountain sickness (AMS) starting one day before rapid ascent. High Alt Med Biol 3:29–37, 2002.

*25. Swenson ER, Maggiorini M, Mongovin S, et al: Pathogenesis of high-altitude pulmonary edema: inflammation is not an etiologic factor. JAMA 287:2228–2235, 2002.

26. Maggiorini M: Cardio-pulmonary interactions at high altitude: pulmonary hypertension as a common denominator. Adv Exp Med Biol 543:177–189, 2003.

27. Allemann Y, Rotter M, Hutter D, et al: Impact of acute hypoxic pulmonary hypertension on LV diastolic function in healthy mountaineers at high altitude. Am J Physiol Heart Circ Physiol 286:H856–H862, 2004.

28. Maggiorini M, Melot C, Pierre S, et al: High-altitude pulmonary edema is initially caused by an increase in capillary pressure. Circulation 103:2078–2083, 2001.

29. Cremona G, Asnaghi R, Baderna P: Pulmonary extravascular fluid accumulation in recreational climbers: a prospective study. Lancet 359:303–309, 2002.

30. Grunig E, Mereles D, Hildebrandt W, et al: Stress Doppler echocardiography for identification of susceptibility to high altitude pulmonary edema. J Am Coll Cardiol 35:980–987, 2000.

31. Durmowicz AG, Noordeweir E, Nicholas R, et al: Inflammatory processes may predispose children to high-altitude pulmonary edema. J Pediatr 130:838–840, 1997.

32. Yarnell PR, Heit J, Hackett PH: High-altitude cerebral edema (HACE): The Denver/Front Range experience. Semin Neurol 20:209–217, 2000.

33. Vock P, Fretz C, Franciolli M, et al: High-altitude pulmonary edema: findings at high-altitude chest radiography and physical examination. Radiology 170:661–666, 1989.

34. Fiorenzano G, Papalia MA, Parravicini M, et al: Prolonged ECG abnormalities in a subject with high altitude pulmonary edema (HAPE). J Sports Med Phys Fitness 37:292–296, 1997.

35. Hultgren HN, Wilson R, Kosek JC: Lung pathology in high-altitude pulmonary edema. Wilderness Environ Med 8:218–220, 1997.

36. Zafren K, Reeves JT, Schoene R: Treatment of high-altitude pulmonary edema by bed rest and supplemental oxygen. Wilderness Environ Med 7:127–132, 1996.

37. Oelz O, Ritter M, Jenni R, et al: Nifedipine for high altitude pulmonary oedema. Lancet 334:1241–1244, 1989.

38. Sartori C, Allemann Y, Duplain H, et al: Salmeterol for the prevention of high-altitude pulmonary edema. N Engl J Med 346:1631–1636, 2002.

39. Litch JA, Bishop RA: Reascent following resolution of high altitude pulmonary edema (HAPE). High Alt Med Biol 2:53–55, 2001.

*40. Hackett PH, Yarnell PR, Hill R: High-altitude cerebral edema evaluated with magnetic resonance imaging: clinical correlation and pathophysiology. JAMA 280:1920–1925, 1998.

41. Lafleur J, Giron M, Demarco M: Cognitive effects of dexamethasone at high altitude. Wilderness Environ Med 14:20–23, 2003.

42. Kobayashi T, Koyoma S, Kubo K, et al: Clinical features of patients with high-altitude pulmonary edema in Japan. Chest 92:814–821, 1987.

The Practice Environment

Chapter 146

The Sick or Injured Child in a Community Hospital Emergency Department

Alfred Sacchetti, MD, John A. Brennan, MD, and Neil Schamban, MD

Key Points

Tertiary children's hospitals and community hospitals have different available resources.

Different diagnostic and therapeutic strategies exist in a children's hospital emergency department versus a community hospital's emergency department.

The lack of tertiary pediatric services in a community hospital is countered by increased capabilities within the community emergency department.

Appropriate interactions with consultants from a children's hospital will favorably impact the care of a critically injured or ill child.

Pediatric emergency medicine leadership is very important in a community-based emergency department.

Introduction and Background

There are over 31 million pediatric emergency department (ED) visits per year, most of which are treated in facilities that may be described as community hospitals.[1] Many of these visits will be for relatively minor ambulatory complaints, although an important minority will be critically ill or injured children. The principles of resuscitation and stabilization do not vary between a tertiary children's hospital and a community ED, although the manner in which these fundamentals are accomplished can differ dramatically.

Issues and Solutions

Institutional Differences

Tertiary children's hospitals and community hospitals are intrinsically different.[2] One of the hallmarks of a children's hospital is immediate access to subspecialists from almost every discipline. More importantly, pediatric anesthesiologists, intensivists, and surgeons maintain a continuous presence in the hospital for assistance with resuscitation attempts. By contrast, the community ED frequently has limited subspecialty resources available, and resuscitation attempts are the exclusive domain of ED personnel.[3,4] Ironically, this clinical situation mandates a greater degree of individual competence in the community ED than is required at the tertiary care center. Stated more simply, the ED capabilities of any hospital are an inverse function of the hospital's inpatient capabilities. This rule of ED functional capacity is applicable to any area of medicine and is summarized in Figure 146–1. The ability of the community ED to deliver care equivalent to that of a tertiary care hospital requires motivated clinicians with access to appropriate equipment, medications, diagnostic studies, and timely transfers.

The qualifications and roles of ED personnel needed to optimize pediatric care are contained in the joint American Academy of Pediatrics–American College of Emergency Physicians publication "Care of Children in the Emergency Department: Guidelines for Preparedness."[5] To provide appropriate care with good outcomes, though, any group of clinicians will require appropriate institutional support. It is important to recognize the need for specialized pediatric equipment in the emergency department, even in facilities with no inpatient pediatric capabilities (see Chapter 154, The Child Friendly Emergency Department: Practices, Policies, and Procedures).

These same considerations need to be given to medications not typically contained in the formulary of a nonpediatric hospital. Because of its responsibility in the extended stabilizations of critical children, the ED requires access to a wider assortment of procedural sedation and resuscitation medications. The best example of such a need might be the use of prostaglandin E to reopen the ductus arteriosus in a cyanotic neonate. Unless specifically requested by the ED, no hospital without obstetric services is likely to stock this medication.

Procedural sedation medications must be given special consideration in EDs with expanded pediatric responsibilities.

$$\text{ED capabilities} = f(1/\text{Hospital capabilities})$$

FIGURE 146–1. Law of emergency department (ED) functional capacity. To optimize patient outcomes, the capabilities of the ED vary inversely with the capabilities of the hospital.

Table 146–1	Essential Procedural Sedation Medications
Propofol or methohexital	
Etomidate	
Ketamine	
Fentanyl	
Rocuronium	
Vecuronium	

Simple sedation for diagnostic imaging, analgesia for painful conditions, procedural sedation for invasive procedures, or extended sedation for ventilator cooperation all require unrestricted access to an extended formulary to optimize patient outcomes. At the very least, emergency physicians should be granted privileges for and unrestricted access to the medications listed in Table 146–1.[6,7]

Diagnostic studies unique to the ED must also be available to accommodate unusual pediatric presentations. In particular, the ability to handle microsized specimens for blood counts, electrolytes, and basic metabolic analysis must be assured. The introduction of single-drop blood analyzers can resolve this issue for institutions hesitant to purchase expensive pediatric-specific laboratory equipment.[8] Radiology departments may also be required to provide pediatric-specific imaging studies applicable only to ED pediatric patients. Although it is unreasonable to expect a hospital to purchase expensive equipment simply for a potential ED need, it is appropriate to request basic pediatric imaging capabilities. In some institutions the problem may not be with the technical component of an imaging study, but with the staff radiologist, who may be uncomfortable interpreting certain pediatric studies. This problem may be solved through the use of teleradiology to a remote pediatric center.[9-11] For some EDs, access to appropriate diagnostic studies may just not be possible. In these instances, the emergency physician may be required to transfer a child to a pediatric center for a simple diagnostic study to exclude a potential disease condition.

The expanded responsibilities of the ED or emergency personnel may require modifications of hospital policies. If patient outcomes are to be optimized, then the ED must be equipped and the emergency physicians must be credentialed to perform all of the initial stabilization activities not provided by the remainder of the hospital. This credentialing of emergency physicians for procedures reserved only for hospital subspecialists may be the only way to assure that a critical child receives all of the necessary support in a timely manner. Credentialing for deep sedation, ultrasonography, fluoroscopy, and fiberoptic evaluations must be provided for the emergency physicians or be immediately available from other members of the medical staff.

Finally, emergency physicians may find themselves in the role of children's advocate at hospitals that lack any in-patient pediatric services. As the sole providers for this "orphaned" subset of patients, they will need to compete for hospital resources that may not be shared by other departments or medical staff. In these institutions a representative emergency physician will need to assume a leadership position in the acute management of the sick or injured child. Fortunately, this is a role that emergency physicians are uniquely qualified to assume.

Clinical Skills

Maintenance of clinical capabilities is a problem in all aspects of medicine. In certain surgical specialties, evidence exists that a minimum number of procedures must be performed annually to assure successful outcomes.[12-17] The ED is unique in that emergency physicians do not have the ability to arrange elective patient encounters to maintain certain skills. However, unlike studies involving surgeons or other interventionalists, there are no data to indicate any outcome differences in children managed in EDs with limited pediatric encounters.

The clinical skills of any practitioner are a function of his or her past experiences and ongoing patient encounters. General emergency physicians may draw on their ability to perform resuscitative procedures on adults to assist them in performing the same procedures in children. Arguments about children not being small adults aside, procedural differences between adults and children are relatively minor and easily incorporated into clinical practice. Recognition of the subtle signs of diseases can be difficult for clinicians with limited pediatric exposures. Ongoing contact with ambulatory children remains the best means to improve recognition of a sick child. However, in critically ill children, the degree of distress will generally be obvious and unlikely to be missed.

Unique Clinical Aspects of Community ED Stabilization

The principles of pediatric stabilization do not change, although the manner in which the care is delivered can vary greatly between institutions. For a number of reasons, treatment in a community ED trends towards more aggressive management of critical children.

For facilities without an onsite pediatric intensive care unit (PICU), extended observation is not an option. Immediate access to tertiary care support provides an opportunity to initially provide more conservative care in a critical care setting and withhold interventions until they are unavoidable. In contrast, the need for an actual physical transfer requires immediate reversal of any downward physiologic trends in order to minimize the risk of decompensation once the child leaves the sending hospital. The concept of waiting to see if a child turns around on his or her own is unrealistic for anyone anticipating an extended ground or air transport. The actual performance of a resuscitative procedure is also more easily accomplished in a hospital setting than in a moving transport vehicle.

An in-house PICU also provides another set of hands to assure expedient management of the child regardless of the point at which the child decompensates. In contrast, in an ED with only one physician, and no in-house critical care backup, watchful waiting can jeopardize the care of the child if a sudden change occurs and multiple procedures are immediately required, or if a second emergent patient presents to the ED.

An underappreciated aspect of the single-coverage community ED, which directly affects the timing of procedures,

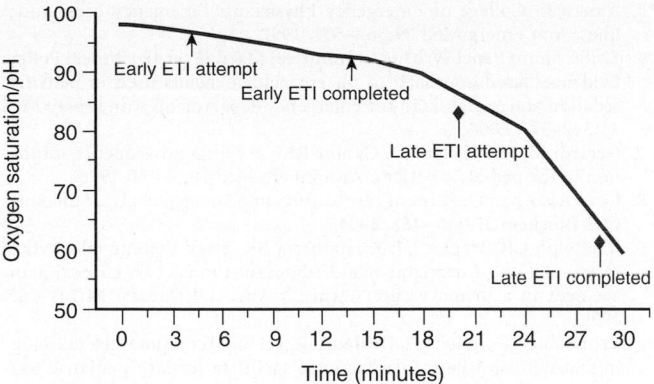

FIGURE 146–2. Loss of reserves in a child with progressive respiratory failure. Initiation of endotracheal intubation (ETI) attempt early will permit completion of even a very difficult procedure while the child still has acceptable physiologic parameters. A late intubation attempt may lead to exhaustion of any reserves and cardiac arrest prior to completion.

is the continuing responsibility for all patients within the department. Early completion of potential procedures permits a lone emergency physician to manage a critically ill child from a distance. For example, a ventilated child with secure vascular access and proper electronic monitoring may be managed by a bedside nurse who can relay information back and forth to a physician elsewhere in the department. The same child, with less aggressive care, will require a near-continuous bedside presence from that single attending physician regardless of what other patient responsibilities may arise.

Earlier procedure attempts also increase the odds of successful outcomes, particularly in children with rapidly evolving findings. As a child's condition deteriorates so, too, do his or her reserves. Figure 146–2 presents the physiologic decline of a child progressing from respiratory failure toward respiratory arrest. If endotracheal intubation is begun before the child's pH and oxygen saturation have begun to drop, even a time-consuming, difficult intubation will be completed before premorbid physiologic conditions develop. However, if airway attempts are delayed until the child is severely hypoxic and acidotic, then that same time-consuming intubation may not be completed until the child has progressed on to a cardiac arrest.

Aggressive medical management will also help define further treatment options when care is relinquished to the tertiary care facility. Defining what has been attempted and what has not worked places an accepting physician much further along a treatment algorithm than if only first-line therapies were applied. Determining that benzodiazepines and barbiturates failed to control a child's seizures moves the consultant immediately to more advanced interventions without having to recommend each of the earlier treatments and waiting to see an effect.

Managing Patient Transfers and Consultation

Like every other aspect of patient care in a community ED, the transfer of a patient must be coordinated with other ongoing activities in the department. The extent to which the transfer process can be streamlined will impact greatly the amount of time nurses and physicians will be diverted from direct patient care. Ideally, clinicians should be involved only in conversations related to patient management while support

personnel address administrative and logistic issues. Development of transfer agreements with specific institutions and internal policies governing individual ED staff responsibilities during patient transfers decreases medical errors and improves patient outcomes.

The degree of interaction between the sending and receiving medical staffs will be determined by the nature of the transfer. In some instances the management of a child is straightforward and the transfer is strictly for services unavailable at the community hospital. A stable child with an isolated femur fracture being moved to a hospital with inpatient pediatric facilities exemplifies such a transfer. The communication between the emergency physician and receiving physician will likely be minimal and focus primarily on the logistics of the transfer. In other instances the emergency physician may require management consultations as well as transfer arrangements. In these instances the emergency physician and consultant interactions may become as important as the management of the patient.

All tertiary care institutions have protocols in place to assist facilities transferring patients. Depending on the receiving facility, a call to initiate a transfer is coordinated by a nurse, a transfer center, a resident or fellow in training, or a subspecialty attending physician. If immediate management advice is required, it is important for the emergency physician to gain access to the necessary consultant as efficiently as possible. Valuable time can be wasted with extended delays on telephone hold or working up through a resident hierarchy to reach the consultant needed. Transfer agreements or policies to assist unit secretaries in locating the appropriate personnel at the receiving hospital can help to resolve these types of problems.

When discussing the specifics of the clinical scenario with a consultant, it is imperative for the sending emergency physician to direct the conversation. In presenting the case, the sending emergency physician should begin with the suspected diagnosis and a very succinct summary of care to that point. This can be followed by any questions or solicitations for recommendations. The more focused the sending emergency physician can keep the conversation, the quicker patient care issues can be addressed. An example of a concise presentation might be: "We have a 9-month-old male with septic shock, diffuse purpura, intubated, fluid resuscitated with 60 ml/kg of NSS, on a 10-mcg/kg dopamine infusion, with a blood pressure of 60/20, who has received 100 mg/kg of ceftriaxone. We are preparing to begin a neosynephrine infusion; do you wish to change this?" This presentation sets the tone for a very efficient conversation. In addition, the description of the interventions and management of the case cues the consultant as to the capabilities of the clinicians in the sending ED. This is useful in helping the consultant determine the sophistication of the advice to be given. In contrast, a less effective conversation may begin "We have a 9-month-old who's been less active for 2 days and then developed a slight fever yesterday." Such an introduction takes far too long to move the consultant to the current point in the child's treatment and will provide extraneous information not needed for the immediate care. A consultant can always ask for additional information or clarification as the conversation progresses.

Once a consultant has been contacted, determination of a child's ongoing treatment is by mutual agreement. It is perfectly reasonable for a sending physician to ask for justification for unusual recommendations, just as it is appropriate for a consultant to request specific procedures be accomplished prior to transfer.

The logistics of the actual transfer will vary with the complexity of the case, the arrangements between the sending and receiving facilities, and the degree of stabilization accomplished at the community hospital.

Summary

Community hospital EDs manage the majority of critically sick or injured children presenting for acute care. The community hospital ED must be appropriately equipped with physicians and nurses capable of caring for these children. Community EDs provide the key management link between their community and a tertiary children's hospital care.

REFERENCES

*1. Gausche-Hill M, Fuchs S, Yamamoto L (eds): APLS: The Pediatric Emergency Medicine Resource, 4th ed. Sudbury, MA: Jones & Bartlett, 2004.
2. Goldfrank L, Henneman PL, Ling LJ, et al: Emergency center categorization standards. Acad Emerg Med 6:638–655, 1999.
3. Sacchetti AD, Brennan J, Kelly-Goodstein N, et al: Should pediatric emergency care be decentralized? An out of hospital destination model for critically ill children. Acad Emerg Med 7:787–791, 2000.
4. Sacchetti AD, Warden T, Moakes ME, et al: Can sick children tell time? Emergency department presentation patterns of critically ill children. Acad Emerg Med 6:906–910, 1999.

---

*Selected readings.

*5. American College of Emergency Physicians: Emergency care guidelines. Ann Emerg Med 29:564–571, 1997.
*6. EMSC Grant Panel Writing Committee; Mace SE, et al: Clinical Policy: Evidence-based approach to pharmacologic agents used in pediatric sedation and analgesia in the emergency department. Ann Emerg Med 44:342–377, 2004.
7. Gerardi MJ, Sacchetti AD, Cantor RM, et al: Rapid-sequence intubation in the pediatric patient. Ann Emerg Med 28:55–74, 1996.
8. Rossi AF, Khan D: Point of care testing: improving pediatric outcomes. Clin Biochem 37:456–461, 2004.
9. Randolph GR, Hagler DJ, Khandheria BK, et al: Remote telemedical interpretation of neonatal echocardiograms: impact on clinical management in a primary care setting. J Am Coll Cardiol 34:241–245, 1999.
10. Yamamoto LG, Inaba AS, DiMauro R: Personal computer teleradiology interhospital image transmission to facilitate tertiary pediatric telephone consultation and patient transfer: soft-tissue lateral neck and elbow radiographs. Pediatr Emerg Care 10:273–277, 1994.
11. Krupinski E, Nypaver M, Poropatich R, et al: Telemedicine/telehealth: an international perspective. Clinical applications in telemedicine/telehealth. Telemed J E Health 8:13–34, 2002.
12. Birkmeyer JD, Stukel TA, Siewers AE, et al: Surgeon volume and operative mortality in the United States. N Engl J Med 349:2117–2127, 2003.
13. Jollis JG, Peterson ED, DeLong ER, et al: The relation between the volume of coronary angioplasty procedures at hospitals treating Medicare beneficiaries and short-term mortality. N Engl J Med 331:1625–1629, 1994.
14. Birkmeyer JD, Dimick JB: Potential benefits of the new Leapfrog standards: effect of process and outcomes measures. Surgery 135:569–575, 2004.
15. National Center of Healthcare Leadership (NCHL) web site. Available at http://www.nchl.org/ns/about/aboutnchl.asp
*16. Gausche-Hill M, Johnson RW, Warden CR, et al: The role of the emergency physician in emergency medical services for children. Ann Emerg Med 42:206–215, 2003.
17. The Institute of Family Centered Care web site. Available at http://www.familycenteredcare.org/about-us-frame.html

Chapter 147

Emergency Medical Services and Transport

Michael G. Tunik, MD and George L. Foltin, MD

Key Points

Physicians, nurses, and other practitioners should understand the components and capabilities of their Emergency Medical Services (EMS) system, which plays a critical role in caring for acutely ill or injured children.

Improving the EMS system will improve the care of ill or injured children.

Appropriate EMS equipment and protocols and a quality program are essential components of a successful EMS program.

Effective communications with and transfer of care from the out-of-hospital setting to the emergency department are essential components of a successful EMS program.

Introduction and Background

Definitions

Emergency Medical Services (EMS) System

Emergency Medical Services (EMS) systems are groups of organizations responsible for delivering emergency care in the out-of-hospital setting. The collaboration of these organizations delivers appropriate out-of-hospital care, triage, and transport of children who are acutely ill or injured.

Medical Control

Off-line, or indirect, medical control includes the development and modification of equipment lists, treatment protocols, criteria for dispatch, the system's quality and safety programs, and triage.

On-line, or direct, medical control is the real-time communication between EMS care providers and authorized medical personnel who assist out-of-hospital providers with interventions, triage, and transport decisions. Communica-

tion is usually by radio or telephone. Medical personnel are typically based in the receiving hospital, or a centralized EMS system communications facility.

Protocols for Out-of-Hospital Care

Out-of-hospital protocols are written guidelines that are the standing medical orders directing the interventions, triage, and transport of acutely ill or injured children. These protocols are written by physicians participating in off-line or indirect medical control.

Emergency Medical Services for Children (EMSC)

Emergency Medical Services for Children (EMSC) is not a separate EMS system, but is the integration of the special needs of children into existing EMS system. The components of an EMS system that may need specific modifications for children[1] are listed in Table 147–1.

Trauma System

A trauma system is a system of care involving out-of-hospital stabilization, care, triage (based on trauma severity scores), and transport to trauma centers capable of addressing the unique needs of traumatized patients, including emergency care, surgical care, anesthesia care, critical care, and rehabilitation.

Transport

Primary transport is the movement of a patient from the out-of-hospital location of an injury or illness to a hospital emergency department (ED). Secondary transport occurs when the patient is moved from the ED or hospital ward to a specialty center (e.g., trauma center, burn center) or definitive care center.

Issues

History of EMS

The need for systemized EMS was first identified in the 1960s.[2,3] Surgeons returning from Korea and Vietnam observed the inadequate care that victims of vehicular trauma were receiving in comparison to the care of injured military personnel. This resulted in the publication of a milestone

Table 147–1	Components of an EMS System

Personnel
Training
Communications
Medical control
Transportation
Transfer of patients
Facilities
Critical care units
Public safety agencies
Disaster linkage
Mutual aid agreements
Consumer participation
Consumer education
Access to care
Medical record keeping
Independent review (continuous quality improvement)

Table 147–2	Personnel Providing EMS for Children

Parents (medical home)
Public
Primary care physician
"911" operators/medical dispatch
Out-of-hospital personnel (first responder, EMT, paramedic)
Medical control physicians (direct and indirect)
Emergency department physicians, nurses
Hospital inpatient physicians, nurses, respiratory therapists, and
    other health care providers
Secondary transportation team
Pediatric critical care/trauma center
Rehabilitation team

paper, "Accidental Death and Disability: The Neglected Disease of Modern Society" which explicitly delineated the inadequate level of EMS.[4] This publication stimulated the development of a systems approach to EMS.

Pioneering work in EMS systems development was taking place in the late 1960s and early 1970s funded by the Department of Transportation and the Robert Wood Johnson Foundation, among others. The federal government provided funding for the development of EMS systems with the Emergency Medical Services Act of 1973 (PL 93-154). The program specified patient populations that would benefit from specialized care at regional hospitals within an integrated EMS system. This included seven populations: patients with trauma, cardiac disease, burns, spinal cord injuries, poisonings, and behavioral emergencies, and those requiring neonatal care.[5] Neonatal care patients were the first nonmilitary population in which the process of regionalization, specialty transport, and secondary transport was successfully utilized.

The EMS system components developed included manpower, training, communications, transportation, facilities, critical care units, public safety agencies, consumer participation, access to care, patient transfer, coordinated patient record keeping, public information and education, review and evaluation, and disaster planning. These components were to be found in a spectrum of independent organizations, and the success of a given EMS system was a result of these organizations' ability to work interdependently.[6]

Ill and injured children were *not* initially included as a target population for regionalized care, nor did developing EMS systems recognize their special needs. No pediatric specialists other than neonatologists became involved at that time.[7] Studies of children's needs and outcome after EMS care were not available; children were simply overlooked.

To effectively provide care for children, their needs must be identified and methods to provide for those special needs integrated into already existing EMS systems. Adult needs that have been demonstrated to improve outcome include rapid defibrillation of ventricular dysrhythmias, and immobilization and rapid transport of multisystem trauma patients to definitive care. Recent studies have also demonstrated that adults benefit from advanced life support (ALS) for complaints of chest pain and respiratory difficulty.[8,9]

A goal for EMS for children is to identify the etiologies of morbidity and mortality and to incorporate interventions into the already existing EMS system that will improve outcome.

Models of Care

The trauma model of out-of-hospital care is to provide a patent airway and adequate ventilation, to control hemorrhage, and to transport the patient to an appropriate trauma center, which provides definitive care. Out-of-hospital interventions should not prolong transport time, as this may be deleterious to patient outcome.[7]

In the medical (cardiac) model of care, the priority in adults includes rapid delivery of defibrillation to treat ventricular dysrhythmias and reverse sudden cardiac death.

Emergency Medical Services for Children

Historical Perspective

The needs of children in EMS systems were not initially addressed. In 1985 the federal government recognized the need for improved EMSC and passed legislation that funded the EMSC program. Senator Daniel Inoue (D–Hawaii), his aide Patrick DeLeon, and Calvin Sia, MD, provided the impetus for EMS. Senators Orrin Hatch (R–Utah) and Lowell Weicker (R–Connecticut) joined Senator Inouye in writing the EMSC legislation (PL 98-555), which established a national EMSC program.

Other organizations have also targeted resources and personnel toward improved EMSC; these include but are not limited to the American Academy of Pediatrics (Committee on Pediatric Emergency Medicine), the American College of Emergency Physicians (Section on Pediatric Emergency Medicine), the Ambulatory Pediatric Association (Special Interest Group on Pediatric Emergency Medicine), the National Association of EMS Physicians (Pediatric Committee), and the National Association of Emergency Medical Technicians.

To be effective in integrating EMSC into EMS, individuals and members of organizations must be involved in improving EMSC care based on their area of expertise (Table 147–2). The process of education about the special needs of children and the provision of formal education are critical steps to ensure that all these individuals deliver the best care possible.

Pediatric Model of Care

Respiratory distress, failure, and arrests are relatively infrequent events in the out-of-hospital care of children. However, recent studies demonstrate a high rate of respiratory arrest in children, compared to cardiac arrest, with the rate and absolute numbers of survivors from respiratory arrest far surpassing the rate and absolute numbers of survivors from pediatric cardiac arrests.[10-12] Airway management skills are critical for out-of-hospital providers caring for children. The pediatric out-of-hospital care model should be conservative (providing basic life support [BLS] care, focusing on airway and ventilation, and on transport to pediatric-capable hospital EDs) yet permissive (providing ALS) when the life-saving benefits are clearly present (e.g., treating ventricular dysrhythmias with defibrillation, reactive airways disease with bronchodilators, and anaphylaxis with epinephrine).[7]

Solutions: EMSC System Development

Epidemiology

The epidemiology of pediatric illness and injury encountered by the EMS system dictates the training, equipment, and protocols for treatment, triage, and transfer, as well as the capabilities of the transport system. Studies of the epidemiology of illness and injury in the out-of-hospital setting have demonstrated similar patterns.

Children are frequently transported by their caregivers for emergency evaluation, which accounts for approximately one third of all ED visits nationally. In the out-of-hospital setting, children account for approximately 6% to 10% of all ambulance runs.[13-15] The acuity level for pediatrics in the out of hospital setting is lower than for adults. Approximately 0.3% to 0.5% of transported children require tertiary care, and 5% of these cases involve life- or limb-threatening problems. Most children are transported between 12 noon and 12 midnight.[13] Children present in a bimodal age distribution, with the most frequent transports for ages less than 2 years and greater than 10 years. Younger children frequently present with medical problems; above age 2 years, trauma predominates. Most pediatric patients are managed by first responders and emergency medical technicians (EMTs) providing BLS, and about one third are managed by paramedics and receive ALS. Children transported to emergency departments by EMS personnel are three to four times more likely to require admission than are those who arrive by other methods.[16]

Injury mechanisms include motor vehicle accidents (including vehicle occupant, pedestrian struck, or bicyclist struck), burns, and falls. Medical complaints include seizures, respiratory difficulty (choking, stridor, lower airway disease, apnea), submersion injuries, and poisonings. Other problems include pregnancy-related problems, out-of-hospital births, and abdominal pain. These patterns of illness and injury are different than adult patterns, requiring education and treatment protocols that meet the needs of children.[13,17]

Early EMSC System Development

In 1978, Los Angeles County EMS developed guidelines for out-of-hospital care of pediatric emergencies, a pediatric equipment list for out-of-hospital care providers, a curriculum for the education of paramedics in pediatric emergencies, and a plan for integration of EMSC into the existing EMS system. Through their work, guidelines for a two-tiered system developed with facilities designated as Emergency Departments Approved for Pediatrics (EDAPs) or Pediatric Critical Care Centers (PCCCs). EDAPs are emergency facilities that provide basic emergency services and also voluntarily meet minimum standards for staffing, education, equipment, supplies, and protocols appropriate for the initial care and stabilization of critically ill and injured children. PCCCs must meet EDAP criteria and, in addition, have specialized pediatric services, including a pediatric intensive care unit and dedicated pediatric medical and surgical specialists.[18]

Others cities were also involved in improving EMSC (Mobile, Alabama; New York City; and Milwaukee, Wisconsin) through cooperative efforts initiated by and involving pediatricians, emergency physicians, and EMS physicians in the area.[7,10,19] The Maryland Institute for Emergency Medical Service Systems (MIEMSS) also became a model for a successful and fully integrated EMS/trauma system and was one of the first to incorporate pediatric trauma receiving hospitals.

EMS System Stages of Care

There are seven stages of care for children in EMS systems: entry (recognition and activation), response, treatment and triage, transport, hospital, rehabilitation, and prevention.

Entry (Recognition and Activation) Phase

A parent, teacher, sibling, or bystander must recognize the urgency of signs and symptoms in ill or injured children that begin the entry stage of care. Advice on when to activate the EMS system is readily available.[20] In many regions, a "911" or a "911"-enhanced telephone system exists and provides direct access to the EMS system. Parents, caregivers, and schools should be familiar with this number and its correct use.[21] Physicians should provide information for parents regarding when to contact the physicians' office versus "911"[20] (Table 147–3), as well as which EDs are most appropriate for children. A call to "911" for a minor ailment can cause potentially life-threatening delays in the EMS response to a serious injury requiring emergent care.

Table 147–3	Example Situations Requiring Activation of the EMSC System

Acting strangely, less alert
Less and less of a response when you talk to your child
Unconsciousness or lack of response
Rhythmic jerking and loss of consciousness (a seizure)
Increasing trouble with breathing
Skin or lips that look blue, purple, or gray
Neck stiffness or rash with fever
Increasing or severe persistent pain
A cut or burn that is large or deep, or involves the head, chest, or abdomen
Bleeding that does not stop after applying pressure for 5 minutes
A burn that is large or involves the hands, groin, or face
Any loss of consciousness, confusion, headache, or vomiting after a head injury

Response Phase

The response phase includes activation of the "911" system to elicit an ambulance dispatch, which should be medically directed and coordinated. EMS systems may be one, two, or three tiered, composed of first responders, BLS, and/or ALS units. The type of unit dispatched, and the priority of the dispatch (high, medium, or low priority, response with lights and sirens, etc.) should be based on predetermined guidelines developed by a regional medical control physician.[22,23] Standardized dispatch protocols include standard prearrival instructions, allowing the dispatcher to assist the on-scene parent, caregiver, or bystander to deliver optimal care. Adult-oriented ambulance dispatching may not adequately triage pediatric calls in determining which patient requires an ALS unit versus a BLS unit.[16] More research is needed to determine the optimal dispatch protocols for children as these should be part of every EMS-EMSC integrated system.

There are five levels of EMS providers with regard to training and care. First responders can clear and maintain the airway, perform assisted ventilations and cardiopulmonary resuscitation (CPR), and establish hemorrhage control. Emergency Medical Technicians–Basic (EMT-Bs) provide these skills and, in addition, perform patient assessment, administer oxygen, assist ventilation using a bag-mask device, immobilize the spine, and transport patients. In some EMS systems, EMTs are trained to assist in administering autoinjected epinephrine to treat anaphylaxis, and to administer inhaled bronchodilators. EMT-Ds (providers of BLS) possesses all the skills of EMT-Bs, and are also trained to use an automated external defibrillator and defibrillate. EMT-Intermediates (EMT-Is) are trained to an intermediate level between EMT-Ds and paramedics. The level of training varies with the state and EMS system. EMT-Is may perform endotracheal intubation and obtain vascular access. Paramedics (EMT-Ps) are trained to obtain vascular access and deliver medications via inhaled, intraosseous, intravenous, intramuscular, and endotracheal routes. Paramedics perform endotracheal intubation, and in some EMS systems are trained to perform intubation using sedative and paralytic medications. Care by EMS providers (first responder, EMT, paramedic) includes a scene assessment and assessment of the child (standard assessment approach now includes the Pediatric Assessment Triangle; see Chapter 2, Respiratory Distress and Respiratory Failure). Initial interventions include maintenance of the airway, adequate ventilation, and circulation. Other interventions depend on the particular medical illness or traumatic injury. Treatments are determined by the training of EMS providers (assessment skills, technical skills), as well as protocols for allowable interventions, appropriate equipment on the ambulance, and on-line medical control communication to guide therapy and transportation decisions.

Treatment and Triage Phase

The National Association of EMS Physicians (NAEMSP) has developed model protocols for out-of-hospital care of children. The conditions covered are listed in Table 147–4. Protocols and policies are available from NAEMSP at *http://www. naemsp.org* and from the American College of Emergency Physicians (ACEP) at *http://www.acep.org.* Recommended pediatric equipment lists have also been published[24,25] (Table

Table 147–4	Model Pediatric Protocols
General patient care	
Trauma	
Burns	
Foreign body obstruction	
Respiratory distress, failure, or arrest	
Bronchospasm	
Neonatal resuscitation	
Bradycardia	
Tachycardia	
Nontraumatic cardiac arrest	
Ventricular fibrillation or pulseless ventricular tachycardia	
Asystole	
Pulseless electrical activity	
Altered mental status	
Seizures	
Nontraumatic hypoperfusion (shock)	
Anaphylactic shock/allergic reaction	
Toxic exposure	
Near drowning	
Pain management	
Sudden infant death syndrome	

147–5). Other priorities include maintenance of temperature, triage decisions (based on severity of illness or injury), and primary transport to a hospital ED or pediatric critical care or trauma center. The scope of training necessary for EMS personnel to appropriately care for children has been developed through a national consensus process. Recommended curriculum content for paramedics[26] can be found in Table 147–6. Paramedic skills necessary for caring for children[26] are listed in Table 147–7. Treatment priorities include airway maintenance, providing oxygen, assisting ventilation, spinal immobilization, prevention of hypothermia, and transport to definitive care.

Triage includes the identification of an appropriate hospital destination and method of transport and is based on the patient's age and medical problem or type of trauma, an objective measure of the acuity of the condition, and the distance from an ED. Triage decisions can be made by protocol or with direct (on-line) medical control. An important aspect of an EMSC system is having trained physicians, nurses, and EMTs to provide direct medical control for the unique issues that arise in the care of children in the field. These include pediatric treatment protocols, medication dosing, and triage protocols. Validated pediatric trauma scores exist (e.g., Pediatric Trauma Score), though currently no triage score for medical illness has been developed or validated for children in the out-of-hospital setting. Very few systems currently triage children for medical problems based on severity. Preliminary studies suggest that, whether their problems are medical or traumatic, children have improved outcomes when triaged and transported to tertiary care facilities.[14]

Transport Phase

Transport to a hospital involves triage decisions to determine the type of facility the child should be transported to, and the type of transportation used (ground ambulance vs. helicopter vs. fixed-wing aircraft). Most pediatric EMS transports are by ground ambulance. When severity of the child's condition dictates transport in a short period of time, the use of a helicopter may be required. For greater distances, fixed-

Table 147–5 — Basic Life Support (BLS) and Advanced Life Support (ALS) Ambulance Equipment for Children

BLS Equipment and Supplies

Essential
Oropharyngeal airways: infant, child, adult (sizes 00–5)
Self-inflating resuscitation bag-valve devices: child and adult sizes
Masks for bag-valve resuscitation devices: infant, child, and adult sizes
Oxygen masks: infant, child, and adult sizes
Non-rebreathing masks: pediatric and adult sizes
Stethoscope
Backboard
Cervical immobilization devices: infant, child, and adult sizes
Blood pressure cuffs: infant, child, and adult sizes
Portable suction unit with regulator
Suction catheters: tonsil-tip and 6F–14F
Extremity splints: pediatric sizes
Bulb syringe
Obstetric pack
Thermal blanket
Water-soluble lubricant

Desirable
Infant car seat
Nasopharyngeal airways: sizes 18F–34F, or 4.5 mm–8.5 mm
Glasgow Coma Scale reference
Pediatric Trauma Score reference
Small stuffed toy
Computer w/CD ROM capability and EMSC training CDs at base station for pediatric continuing medical education

ALS Equipment and Supplies

ALS ambulance equipment includes everything on the BLS list, plus the following items:

Essential
Transport monitor
Defibrillator with adult and pediatric paddles
Monitoring electrodes: pediatric sizes
Laryngoscope with straight blades (0–2) and curved blades (2–4)
Endotracheal tube stylets: pediatric and adult sizes
Endotracheal tubes: uncuffed sizes 2.5–6.0, cuffed sizes 6.0–8.0
Magill forceps: pediatric and adult sizes
Nasogastric tubes: 8F–16F
Nebulizer
Intravenous catheters: 16–24 gauge
Intraosseous needles
Length/weight-based drug dose chart or tape (e.g., Broselow tape)
Needles: 20–25 gauge
Resuscitation drugs and intravenous fluids that meet local standards of practice

Desirable
Blood glucose analysis system
Disposable CO_2 detection device

Table 147–6 — Out-of-Hospital Pediatric Curriculum Content

Patient Assessment
Growth and Development
Emergency Medical Services for Children
Illness and Injury Prevention
Respiratory Emergencies (Airway and Breathing Problems)
　Respiratory distress, respiratory failure, respiratory arrest
　Possible causes of respiratory emergencies:
　　Airway obstruction (upper airway and lower airway obstruction)
　　Fluid in the lungs
Cardiovascular/Circulatory Emergencies
　Shock (compensated and decompensated shock)
　Rate and rhythm disturbances, cardiopulmonary arrest
Altered Mental Status
　Possible causes: airway/breathing problems, shock, seizures, poisoning, metabolic, occult trauma, serious infection
Trauma
Burns
Child Abuse and Neglect
Behavioral Emergencies
　Suicide, aggressive behavior
Child-Family Communications
Critical Incident Stress Management
Fever
Medicolegal Issues
　Do Not Resuscitate (DNR) order, consent, guardianship, refusal of care
Newborn Emergencies
Near Drowning
Pain Management
Poisoning
SIDS and Death in the Field
Transport Considerations
　Destination issues, methods for transport (safety seats and parental transport)
Infants and Children with Special Needs
　Technically Assisted Children (TAC): tracheostomy care, apnea monitors, central lines, chronic illness, gastrostomy tubes, home artificial ventilators and shunts

cerns. To make ambulance transport safer, guidelines are currently being developed. A list of recomendations is available from the EMSC program[27] and includes the following:

1. Drive cautiously at safe speeds, observing traffic laws.
2. Tightly secure all monitoring devices and other equipment.
3. Ensure that available restraint systems are used by EMTs and other occupants, including the patient.
4. Transport children who are not patients, properly restrained, in an alternate passenger vehicle whenever possible.
5. Encourage utilization of the Department of Transportation National Highway Traffic Safety Administration Emergency Vehicle Operating Course (EVOC), National Standard Curriculum.

Ongoing therapy and reassessment are performed during transport. Radio or telephone communication with a medical control physician or the receiving facility is not standardized, but communication with direct medical control may be optimal in certain circumstances. Contact with poison control centers for instructions on correct management of a pediatric poisoning during transport is a good example. Once at the receiving hospital, EMS providers report the child's current status, detailed information from the scene, treatments performed en route, and changes in the child's

wing aircraft are needed. Paramedics providing ALS should be available in such circumstances. Additional treatments, including vascular access and fluid resuscitation for shock, are frequently provided en route or if there is unavoidable transport delay due to an extrication problem. Occasionally, when prolonged transport times are anticipated, endotracheal intubation or vascular access may be performed prior to transport as these procedures are more difficult to perform in a moving vehicle.

Ambulance transportation of children has risks. Principles of transport should include a balance between the risk of transportation and the benefit of rapid arrival. High speeds and the use of lights and sirens, which potentially results in ambulance crashes that may injure or cause the death of patients, providers, pedestrians, or other motor vehicle occupants, are con-

Table 147–7	Out-of-Hospital Pediatric Skills for Paramedics

Assessment of infants and children
Use of a length-based resuscitation tape
Airway management
   Mouth-to-mouth barrier devices
   Oropharyngeal airway
   Nasopharyngeal airway
   Oxygen delivery system
   Bag-mask ventilation
   Endotracheal intubation
     Endotracheal placement confirmation devices (CO_2 detection)
     Optional: rapid sequence induction
   Foreign body removal with Magill forceps
   Needle thoracostomy
   Nasogastric or orogastric tubes
   Suctioning
   Tracheostomy management
Monitoring
   Cardiorespiratory monitoring
   Pulse oximetry
   End-tidal CO_2 monitoring and/or CO_2 detection
Vascular access
   Intravenous line placement
   Intraosseous line placement
Fluid/medication administration
   Endotracheal
   Intramuscular
   Intravenous
   Nasogastric
   Nebulized
   Oral
   Rectal
   Subcutaneous
Cardioversion
Defibrillation
Drug dosing in infants and children
Immobilization/extrication
   Car seat extrication
   Spinal immobilization

Table 147–8	Prevention of Critical Injury in EMSC

Child restraints in motor vehicles
   Infant seats, booster seats, seat belts
Safe driving for teens
   Driver's education
   Education regarding dangers of alcohol and driving
Burn prevention
   Smoke detectors
   Limitation of hot water temperature
Bicycle safety
   Bicycle helmets
   Educational programs
Drowning
   Mandatory pool fencing
   Boating safety
Poisoning
   Education
   Safety caps on containers
Falls
   Mandatory window guards

status during transport. Patient care is then transferred to hospital personnel, which begins the next stage of care.

Hospital Phase

The hospital phase includes stabilization in a hospital ED and, if needed, transfer (secondary transport) to a pediatric-capable trauma center or critical care center. Hospital care also includes definitive therapy, which may be in an operating room, an intensive care unit, or an inpatient hospital ward. Hospitals capable of caring for critically ill or severely injured children are pre-identified. Preferential transport to these hospitals should be part of written triage protocols and/or included in on-line medical control communications and triage. EMS systems contain hospitals with varying levels of pediatric capability and resources. Improvements in the care of children within EMS systems have been achieved through regionalization of pediatric care. Other approaches include improving the pediatric capability of all EDs in the EMS system. ED guidelines to improve pediatric preparedness exist.[28-31] Unfortunately, there is evidence that not all hospitals follow available guidelines.[32-34]

Rehabilitation Phase

Appropriate physical or mental rehabilitation is needed to allow patient to continue receiving care for illness or injury in a family-centered care environment whenever possible.

Prevention Phase

Emergency and intensive care to treat critically ill and injured children is expensive in terms of both personal anguish and societal cost.[35] Prevention is the least expensive intervention possible and has the best outcome. A functioning EMS system should be involved in identifying, developing, improving, and supporting successful prevention aactivities. The key to prevention is education. Parents, children, the lay public, pediatricians, family physicians, and emergency physicians, nurses, and EMS providers can all be involved in this phase by delivering anticipatory information concerning prevention in many areas (Table 147–8). Parents can be taught CPR, how to recognize significant illness and injury, what to do for particular medical emergencies, when to call for help ("911"), and what to do until help arrives.

The EMSC Program and Improvements in EMSC

The EMSC program has facilitated significant changes in EMS systems and EMS organizations in the United States. Some of these include educational programs for out-of-hospital providers in pediatrics. The EMSC Program's National Education of Out-of-Hospital Providers Task Force makes recommendations for EMS educational curricula.[26] Pediatric out-of-hospital education programs developed based on this model include the following:

1. Teaching Resource for Instructors in Prehospital Pediatrics (TRIPP) and Paramedic TRIPP from the Center for Pediatric Emergency Medicine (*http://www.cpem.org*)[36,37]
2. Pediatric Education for Prehospital Professionals (PEPP) course (*http://www.PEPPsite.com*) from the American Academy of Pediatrics (*http://www.aap.org*)[38]
3. Pediatric Prehospital Care (PPC) course from the National Association of EMTs (*http://www.naemt.org*)[39]

The Institute of Medicine's report on EMSC published in 1993 recognized these improvements and recommended further changes in access to care, equipment, educational programs, and research.[34] The National Association of EMS Physicians, supported by the EMSC program, developed model protocols for out-of-hospital care of children (see

Table 147–4). Ambulance equipment was recommended by a multidisciplinary committee for out-of-hospital care of children[24] (see Table 147–5). Guidelines for EDs to prepare for pediatric patients have been developed by several national organizations.[28-31] The EMSC program has also supported a landmark study, one of the few randomized controlled trials in out-of-hospital care for children. This study examined the outcomes of children who had out-of-hospital endotracheal intubation versus bag-mask ventilation performed by paramedics in California and showed that there were no outcome differences in patients who were intubated versus those who had appropriate bag-valve-mask ventilation performed.[9]

Despite these accomplishments, not all EMS systems or EDs are prepared to care for children.[32,33] Emergency physicians and pediatricians must continue to provide leadership for local EMS systems and receiving hospitals so that the resources, guidelines, and products designed for children are used and incorporated into all EMS systems and EDs in the United States.

Summary

The development of resources, products, system changes, and research networks has improved the care children receive in our nation's EMS systems. More research is needed to demonstrate the positive impact that many EMSC programs and initiatives have already produced. Maintaining the collaboration of national, public, and government organizations and programs that have concentrated on improving children's out-of-hospital and emergency care will ensure continued improvements in the outcome of children cared for in our EMS system.

REFERENCES

1. History of emergency medical services for children. *In* Seidel JS, Henderson DP (eds): Emergency Medical Services for Children: A Report to the Nation. Washington, DC: National Center for Education in Maternal and Child Health, 1991.
2. Pantridge JF, Geddes JS: Cardiac arrest after myocardial infarction. Lancet 1:807–808, 1966.
3. Mustalish A: Emergency medical services: twenty years of growth and development. N Y State J Med 86:414–420, 1986.
*4. National Research Council: Accidental Death and Disability: The Neglected Disease of Modern Society. Washington, DC: National Academy of Sciences, 1966.
*5. Seidel JS: EMS-C in urban and rural areas: The California experience. *In* Haller JA Jr (ed): Emergency Medical Services for Children: Report of the Ninety-Seventh Ross Conference on Pediatric Research. Columbus, OH: Ross Laboratories, 1989, pp 22–30.
6. Luten RC: Educational overview. *In* Luten RC, Foltin G (eds): Pediatric Resources for Prehospital Care, 2nd ed. Elk Grove Village, IL: American Academy of Pediatrics, 1990, pp 16–24.
*7. Foltin G, Salomon M, Tunik M, et al: Developing prehospital advanced life support for children: the New York City experience. Pediatr Emerg Car 6:141–144, 1990.
*8. Stiell I, Wells G, Spaite D, et al for the OPALS Study Group: Multicenter controlled clinical trial to evaluate the impact of advanced life support on out-of-hospital respiratory distress patients. Acad Emerg Med 9:357, 2002.
9. Stiell IG, Nesbitt L, Wells GA, et al for the OPALS Study Group: Multicenter controlled clinical trial to evaluate the impact of advanced life support on out-of-hospital chest pain patients. Acad Emerg Med 10:501–502, 2003.

*10. Gausche M, Lewis RJ, Stratton SJ, et al: Effect of out-of-hospital pediatric endotracheal intubation on survival and neurological outcome: a controlled clinical trial. JAMA 283:783–790, 2000.
11. Foltin G, Galea S, Treiber M, et al: Pediatric Pre Hospital Evaluation of New York Cardiorespiratory Survival (PHENYCS): a large, prospective population based study of cardiac and respiratory arrest. Analysis of cardiac arrests. Acad Emerg Med 12(5 Suppl 1):107–108, 2005
12. Tunik M, Richmond N, Treiber M, et al: Pediatric Pre Hospital Evaluation of New York Cardiorespiratory Survival (PHENYCS): a large, prospective population based study of cardiac and respiratory arrest. Analysis of respiratory arrests. Acad Emerg Med 12(5 Suppl 1):107–108, 2005.
13. Tsai A, Kallsen G: Epidemiology of pediatric prehospital care. Ann Emerg Med 16:284–292, 1987.
14. Seidel JS, Hornbein M, Yoshiyama K, et al: Emergency medical services and the pediatric patient: Are the needs being met? Pediatrics 73:769–772, 1984.
15. Babl FE, Vinci RJ, Bauchner H, Mottley L: Pediatric pre-hospital advanced life support care in an urban setting. Pediatr Emerg Care 17:5–9, 2001.
*16. Foltin G, Pon S, Tunik M, et al: Pediatric ambulance utilization in a large American city: a systems analysis approach. Pediatr Emerg Care 14:254–258, 1998.
*17. Systems approach to care of ill and injured children. *In* Seidel JS, Henderson DP (eds): Emergency Medical Services for Children: A Report to the Nation. Washington, DC: National Center for Education in Maternal and Child Health, 1991.
18. Seidel JS, Henderson DP (eds): Prehospital Care of Pediatric Emergencies. Los Angeles: Los Angeles Pediatric Society, 1987, pp 102–106.
19. Ramenofsky ML, Luterman A, Curreri PW, et al: EMS for pediatrics: optimum treatment or unnecessary delay? J Pediatr Surg 18:498–504, 1983.
20. American Academy of Pediatrics: Injury prevention program TIPP. http://www.aap.org/family/tipp-ems.htm
21. Luten RC, Foltin G, Pons P: Access to optimal care. *In* Luten RC, Foltin G (eds): Pediatric Resources for Prehospital Care, 2nd ed. Elk Grove Village, IL: American Academy of Pediatrics, 1990, pp 1–15.
22. Clawson JJ: Emergency medical dispatching. *In* Roush WR (ed): Principles of EMS Systems. Dallas: American College of Emergency Physicians Press, 1989, pp 127–128.
23. Foltin GL, Schneiderman WJ, Dieckmann RA: 911 and ambulance dispatch. *In* Dieckmann RA (ed): Pediatric Emergency Care and Systems: Planning and Management. Baltimore: Williams & Wilkins, 1992, pp 109–116.
24. Seidel JS, Glaeser P, Zimmerman L, et al: Guidelines for pediatric equipment and supplies for basic and advanced life support ambulances. Ann Emerg Med 28:699–701, 1996.
25. Seidel JS, Tittle S, Henderson DP, et al: Guidelines for pediatric equipment and supplies for emergency departments. Ann Emerg Med 31:54–57, 1998.
26. Gausche M, Henderson DP, Brownstein D, Foltin G: The education of out-of-hospital medical personnel in pediatrics: report of a national task force. Ann Emerg Med 31:58–63, 1998; and Prehosp Emerg Care 2:56–61, 1998.
*27. EMS for Children National Resource Center: The Do's and Don'ts of Transporting Children in an Ambulance. Available at *http://www.ems-c.org/products/frameproducts.htm*
28. American Medical Association, Commission on Emergency Medical Services: Pediatric emergencies: an excerpt from "Guidelines for Categorization of Hospital Emergency Capabilities." Pediatrics 85:879–887, 1990.
29. American College of Emergency Physicians: Emergency care guidelines. Ann Emerg Med 29:564–571, 1997.
*30. American Academy of Pediatrics, Committee on Pediatric Emergency Medicine: Guidelines for pediatric emergency care facilities. Pediatrics 96:526–537, 1995.
*31. American Academy of Pediatrics, Committee on Pediatric Emergency Medicine; American College of Emergency Physicians, Pediatric Committee: Care of children in the emergency department: guidelines for preparedness. Pediatrics 107:777–781, 2001; and Ann Emerg Med 37:423–427, 2001.
32. Athey J, Dean JM, Ball J, et al: Ability of hospitals to care for pediatric emergency patients. Pediatr Emerg Care 17:170–174, 2001.

*Selected readings.

33. McGillivray D, Nijssen-Jordan C, Kramer MS, et al: Critical pediatric equipment availability in Canadian hospital emergency departments. Ann Emerg Med 37:371–376, 2001.

34. Durch JS, Lohr KN (eds): Emergency Medical Services for Children. Washington, DC: National Academy Press, 1993.

35. Division of Injury Control, Centers for Disease Control: Childhood injuries in the United States. Am J Dis Child 144:627–644, 1990.

36. Foltin GL, Tunik MG, Cooper A, et al (eds): Teaching Resource for Instructors in Prehospital Pediatrics (EMT-Basic). New York: Maternal and Child Health Bureau, 1998.

37. Foltin GL, Tunik MG, Cooper A, et al (eds): Paramedic Teaching Resource for Instructors in Prehospital Pediatrics. New York: Center for Pediatric Emergency Medicine, 2002.

*38. Dieckmann RA, Brownstein D, Gausche-Hill M (eds): Pediatric Education for Prehospital Professionals. Sudbury, MA: Jones and Bartlett, 2000.

39. Markenson D (ed): Pediatric Prehospital Care. Upper Saddle River, NJ: Prentice-Hall, 2002.

Chapter 148

End-of-Life Issues

Jill M. Baren, MD, MBE

Key Points

It is the responsibility of the emergency physician to develop prognostic information and to convey it, accurately and comprehensively, to children and families so that the most well-informed decisions can be made at the end of life.

Physicians should never delegate the task of death notification to another emergency department (ED) staff member.

Implementing palliative care in the ED can alleviate the feeling that "there is nothing we can do" for dying children.

Introduction and Background

Each year in the United States, approximately 53,000 children die.[1] Pediatric deaths can be delineated into three categories: the deaths of infants (babies born prematurely through 1 year of age), deaths from illness, and traumatic deaths. Of these, the most likely to occur in emergency departments (EDs) are traumatic deaths. Almost 17,000 children die each year from traumatic injuries.[1] Sudden infant death syndrome continues to be the leading cause of postneonatal infant death, accounting for about 25% of all deaths between 1 month and 1 year of age, and many of these infants are pronounced dead in the ED.[2] The epidemiology of pediatric death from medical illness in the ED is not well studied.

Decision making about the goals of care immediately following traumatic injury is rarely complicated. For a previously healthy child who sustains injuries in a motor vehicle crash or from a gunshot wound, a fall, blunt force trauma, or any other cause, all efforts to cure are made under most circumstances. Decisions about whether cure is possible may arise, but generally occur after the patient is admitted to the hospital. The same principles apply in the case of cardiopulmonary arrest or critical illness such as meningitis or sepsis. When a child is dying from a chronic illness in the ED, such as cancer, muscular dystrophy, cystic fibrosis, or another previously diagnosed condition, as opposed to an acute infectious process, the clinical picture—especially whether cure is possible—is often not clear upon presentation. The difficult question confronting the ED staff is, "What is the appropriate goal for this child at this time?"

For children with life-threatening conditions in the ED, several factors must be considered in decision making:
- What were the goals of treatment or care, if any, before the child came to the ED?
- Who is aware of these goals?
- Are these goals appropriate given the child's pathophysiology at this time?
- How do these goals fit with this child's current visit to the ED?
- Who is appropriate and available for decision making?
- What can and should the ED staff do to facilitate these goals?

A framework for answering these questions is provided in this chapter.

Issues

Death occurs more frequently in the ED compared with many other health care environments, even in the pediatric population. Many barriers make the provision of empathic and timely end-of-life care more difficult to provide in the ED. Care in the ED is characterized by rapid turnover of patients and complex interactions both within and outside of the ED. ED patients frequently experience acute changes in their condition, and there may be little available information and little time for gathering additional information before decision making. The impact of this incomplete physiologic database may be further complicated by medical conditions that render ED patients incapable of participating in the process of decision making. Furthermore, appropriate surrogate decision makers may be unknown, unprepared, or unavailable, which, in the case of children, is the major issue.

The lack of a prior physician-patient-family relationship contributes to the complexity of the emotionally and medically difficult situations of dying children. The unpredictability of conditions in the ED at any given time leads to great difficulty in establishing relationships between clinicians and patients and among clinicians with different areas of expertise and different clinical end points. This may be the greatest barrier in establishing effective care for dying patients as it these relationships that provide the necessary foundation of trust.

Despite these limitations, it remains the responsibility of emergency physicians to provide high-quality and compassionate care and support to terminally ill and acutely dying patients and their families. Professional organizations have strongly endorsed this concept by creating codes of ethics and professional statements. The Code of Ethics for Emergency Physicians, established by the American College of Emergency Physicians in 1997, acknowledges that the fundamental moral responsibility of emergency physicians includes embracing patient welfare as the primary professional responsibility; respecting the rights and best interests of patients, particularly those most vulnerable and those unable to make treatment choices due to diminished decision-making capacity; and communicating truthfully with patients.[3] This code establishes the obligation that emergency physicians have to be "patient and family focused" in situations in which there is the greatest need for this level of commitment.[4]

Solutions

To arrive at the best possible solutions for the difficult issues raised in the care of dying patients in the pediatric ED, an informed, structured, and empathetic approach is needed in the clinical practice of pediatric emergency medicine. Three particularly important aspects of this approach are communication, palliation, and education. Excellence in these three areas is likely to lead to a high degree of professional and family satisfaction regardless of clinical outcome.

Communication

Most adults have never confronted the death or dying of a child. This applies not only to families, but also to health care providers. Physicians, nurses, social workers, chaplains, and others may lack the skills to engage in conversations about such deaths. A belief that children do not/should not die often results in an extremely aggressive pursuit of an extremely improbable or even impossible cure. As with adults, the burdens to the child must be weighed against the likelihood of benefit. Clinicians should engage in this calculation before bringing the discussion to the family and the child if appropriate. While this suggestion is often met with protestations—"That's the family's decision, not ours!"—part of the decision does lie with clinicians. Any clinical decision exists only in the context of physiologic parameters. It is the responsibility of providers, even in the ED, to develop this information and to convey it accurately and comprehensively to children and families, so that the most well-informed decisions can be made.

Adults faced with critical illness or injury may have established advance directives as a mechanism to formulate and communicate health care preferences. Advance directives have two components: (1) naming a surrogate decision maker, and (2) conveying information to guide health care decision making if the patient is unable to, or chooses not to, participate. Living wills, durable powers of attorney for health care, Do Not Resuscitate (DNR) or Do Not Attempt Resuscitation (DNAR) orders, and informal documents are all widely accepted types of advance directives.

Certain advance directives apply to more than end-of-life situations. Most, however, are prepared with considerations of what one wants or does not want when dying. In clinical practice, advance directives are often not helpful for a number of reasons. Many advance directives (especially living wills) are written with categorical statements (I ____ do/do not want ____ . . .) that are difficult to apply to a specific clinical situation. Similarly, advance directives are also likely to contain well-meaning but murky phrases such as "no heroic measures" or "no extraordinary means." While the author may have had some notion of what was intended, in reality these statements cannot be construed as a comprehensible conveyal of the patient's preferences for health care.

More importantly for this discussion, advance directives are not intended to be written by, or used for children, at least from a legal perspective. A return to the intent of advance directives, however, reveals a way that advance directives can be wisely and appropriately used with and for children.

For most children who come to the ED, the goal is to save lives. However, there will be children for whom all the best curative efforts are not enough to restore or prolong life.[1] These children either will die, or will live with sequelae (physical, psychological, and/or cognitive) of the illness or injury. Second, for certain children, the goals of care, and of medical interventions, must shift from cure to comfort.

From a clinical perspective, children may have the wherewithal to make informed decisions about their care at the end of life. It has been demonstrated that dying children, even of preschool age, know they are dying.[5] Often, the adults involved in dying children's lives are slower to recognize the inevitability of the death. The responsibility of health care providers is to be honest about prognosis, with ourselves, and with our patients and their families. Often this is not the case. Not only are prognoses calculated inaccurately, but there is a tendency to convey more optimistic data about prognosis than is truly believed.[6] If objective criteria lead to the conclusion that a patient has a poor prognosis, clinicians should not attempt to find a reason why that poor prognosis does not apply, nor should they allow that to dominate the conversation.

Before a parent, guardian, and even a child is engaged in a discussion about end of life, the providers must be clear about the prognosis. In the ED, a team approach often makes this difficult activity more feasible. When an infant or child presents to the ED in cardiopulmonary arrest, parents should receive information in a stepwise fashion, hearing first that the situation is grave but that everything possible is being done. This information can be delivered by a social worker, nurse, or caring and trained administrative person prior to the clinician meeting with the family. When it becomes inevitable that death is the outcome, the physician involved in the child's care should deliver that message. Physicians should never delegate this task to another ED staff member.

In the unusual case of a dying child or adolescent who is capable of speaking with the clinician, it is often helpful to pose the following question, "What do you think is going on with your disease?" When given the opportunity, children will often speak at length about their feelings and what they know. If a child does wish to discontinue life-prolonging therapies, the child's experienced-based knowledge allows one to consider him/her an informed and appropriate decision maker. What must be assessed is whether the child understands the decision about which he/she is being asked; if the child understands the burdens/costs and benefits of the treatment being offered, or of refusing the treatment; and whether the child responds consistently in conveying the decision. Many children who have lived with life-threatening illnesses or the sequelae of injuries do have this expertise, perhaps with a stronger base in reality than the adults around them.

Palliation

Understanding of palliative care has evolved markedly over the past decade. Palliative care is now understood as distinct from hospice, though many of the same concepts apply. Palliative care, like hospice, focuses on the patient's life being lived as well as is possible. What distinguishes them is that hospice care is provided with and for patients whose expected life span is limited. Prognosis is often difficult to develop and even more difficult to convey. Calculating life expectancy is more difficult still in the case of children.[1] Palliative care refers to aggressive symptom management across the trajectory of disease. Palliative care can and should be pursued concurrently with curative therapies.

Palliative care for children in the ED includes aggressive symptom management while pursuing whatever goals of treatment are physiologically indicated. Dying children often have a high symptom burden.[7] When children come to the ED, palliative care must be considered. Fear and lack of knowledge often result in children's pain being grossly undertreated.[8,9] The claim that one cannot manage pain and other symptoms because of a need to assess and diagnose is frequently misapplied and results in undue burden of suffering. In most cases, optimal pain management will not interfere with an assessment of level of consciousness. The American Academy of Pediatrics, in conjuction with the Canadian Pediatric Society and the American Pain Society, have developed guidelines for the management of pain and stress in neonates, children, and adolescents.[8,9]

In the most difficult cases when a child is dying, parents are often told, "We've done everything we can. There is nothing else we can do." To the contrary, there is always something else that can be done. Understanding palliative care as a mandate for broad-based, aggressive symptom management shapes interventions with dying children. Whether the death of a child is from a progressive neurodegenerative disease, advanced cancer, or trauma, a focus on relieving pain, dyspnea, anxiety, and other symptoms benefits both the child and the family. Most providers are not trained in these skills in the context of dying. Developing a paradigm shift toward implementing palliative care in the ED can alleviate the feeling that "there is nothing we can do."

Emergency physicians have a duty to preserve life, but must recognize that there are key differences between withholding and withdrawing treatment in the pediatric emergency setting that may differ from the moral equivalence that has been afforded to these actions in other medical settings.[10] From a societal viewpoint, there is an expectation that emergency physicians will act to preserve life in the absence of a few well-established conditions (rigor mortis, decapitation, failed cardiopulmonary resuscitation [CPR]). The withholding of treatment often feels like a public event and has been described as the most traumatic of all decisions in the practice of emergency medicine.[10]

From a practical standpoint, the lack of information about a child presenting to an ED is a frequent characteristic in life-threatening situations. Clinicians have little insight regarding patient identity, wishes, and prognosis, and there-fore aggressive therapy aimed at preserving life should be immediately instituted with one exception—the intervention is unequivocally judged to be nonbeneficial or futile. If and when surrogate decision makers or additional information become available, treatment options can be discussed and modified. Terminally ill children who are actively dying, who do not possess advance directives or other clearly articulated wishes for their care, who are not accompanied to the ED by surrogate decisions makers, or who have multiple surrogate decision makers in conflict about withholding specific interventions should have life-saving care initiated until additional information is available and conflict can be mediated. This does not imply that such care will always be successful in reversing the life-threatening condition. Withdrawal of life support in the ED *is* a viable option depending on the subsequent information and circumstances. Treatments should be chosen and implemented within the context of what is physiologically indicated.

A vast array of ethical issues surrounds the process of CPR in children. Fortunately, pediatric cardiopulmonary arrest is rare. Outcomes from pediatric cardiac arrest are well documented in the literature and are dismal.[11,12] The underlying medical condition of the patient, the presenting cardiac rhythm, and response to prehospital advanced life support measures are important factors affecting both the outcome of CPR and medical decisions surrounding CPR.[13] Approximately one to two traumatic or medical pediatric cardiopulmonary arrests occur in busy EDs per month, thus the skills involved are not easily practiced let alone perfected.

In the early stages of resuscitation, when few to no data are available, the emergency physician must be primarily concerned with the restoration of circulation and life of the patient. As additional data are gathered, medical decision making can be broadened to include new information such as the underlying condition of the patient and the likelihood of survival. An important but often overlooked part of the resuscitation process is the need for lessening the guilt of survivors and providing a sense of closure. This involves developing important skills for incorporation into resuscitation protocols: recognition of futility, procedures for stopping the resuscitation, and ability to communicate with families.

Numerous studies in the emergency medicine literature indicate that patients, families, and health care providers believe that a supported, structured environment for the presence of family members during resuscitation and other medical encounter is both feasible and desirable.[14,15] Although this concept has been fraught with controversy and resisted in many health care environments, there appears to be a general trend in many institutions toward the development of protocols to allow families to be present, albeit with assistance (see Chapter 153, Family Presence).

Mishandling the events surrounding a pediatric death can set the stage for an abnormal bereavement for survivors. To facilitate a family's recovery, various postmortem activities have been suggested for ED staff. Surveys of families whose children were either pronounced dead on arrival or underwent unsuccessful resuscitation showed the following activities to be highly desired and helpful[16]: strong preference that the news of a patient's death be delivered by a physician, viewing the body, having the child's clothing be returned to them even after it was used as part of the investigation of the cause of death, having a physical memento such as a lock of hair or a mold or print of the baby's hand, and a follow-up phone call from the ED after the death.[16] These are not things that parents are capable of thinking about during the acute event, so there should be processes in place to make sure they are offered.

These activities can be time consuming but could be accomplished by a few dedicated individuals. Although the impact of such practices on bereavement and long-term coping by survivors has not been studied, they may at the very least contribute significantly to the perception that the ED, the hospital, and its health care providers are caring entities.

Request for Autopsy and Organ/Tissue Donation

Request for autopsy and organ/tissue donation is often viewed by physicians as one of the more difficult tasks in the death of a patient in the ED. Some of the barriers inherent in asking for an autopsy, when it is not required by law, are fear of offending the family, fear of legal retribution for care that resulted in death, and avoidance of contact with the family after the death notification has occurred. Autopsies are mandated by law whenever an unexpected death has occurred or when there are suspicious circumstances surrounding the death (suicide, homicide, child abuse). Emergency physicians must be aware of the specific cases that need to be referred to their local medical examiner's office.

Learning the results of an autopsy can be extremely helpful for grieving families, providing them with closure or some explanation for a terribly tragic and seemingly inexplicable event. In addition, there are some myths regarding autopsy that should be dispelled. The autopsy is not disfiguring and will not interfere with funeral arrangements as it is typically performed within 24 to 48 hours. Autopsy is not disallowed by most major religions; families should be encouraged to consult with hospital chaplains or their own religious advisors to confirm this. Finally, the performance of an autopsy does not result in additional cost to the family. The cost is absorbed by either the hospital or the medical examiner. The emergency physician can offer to meet with the family to go over the results; alternatively, the results can be forwarded to the pediatrician or family physician for discussion. Physicians should not discount how valuable autopsy results are for their own closure and continued medical knowledge.

Request for organ/tissue donation has a different set of associated issues. Many states have laws mandating the request for organ/tissue donation. In the case of a beating heart potential donor, and in some cases a non–beating heart donor, trained specialists from organ procurement agencies can be dispatched to the ED to make the request in person. These individuals have expertise in the language necessary to obtain permission for donation and the knowledge to answer difficult questions when they arise. In addition, having the request come from someone distinct from the patient care team can provide valuable separation of the death and the events that must occur for organ harvest. The initial idea, however, must be introduced by the emergency physician. Many families view organ donation as a way to bring about some good from a bad situation, and may be waiting for the opportunity to be asked; therefore, both organ/tissue donation and autopsy requests should be a standard part of the death encounter.

Education

There is much evidence to support the fact that physicians in training and in practice still feel relatively uneducated and largely unsupported on issues of death and dying. In 1993, the American Medical Association reported that only 26% of primary care residencies offered training in the care of dying patients.[17] Yet studies have indicated that exposure to dying patients is high, with pediatric residents caring for an average of 35 dying children during the first 2.5 years of residency training. The specific exposure of emergency physicians to dying patients is not known. However, neither high nor low exposure rates will necessarily be associated with a greater level of comfort in dealing with death and dying for any given physician. Training must not only address knowledge and skills to improve interactions with families, but examine personal reactions as well.

Programs such as Education for Physicians on End-of-Life Care (EPEC), End of Life Nursing Education Consortium (ELNEC), and Toolkit for Nursing Excellence at End of Life Transition (TNEEL) are formal, albeit relatively brief mechanisms for education. If knowledge and skills are lacking, both children and families will suffer, physically and otherwise. Education, however, is not enough in that it does not always translate into practice. Optimal end-of-life care must be integrative. There must be an expectation of excellence within institutions, at the levels of attending physicians, clinical directors, and chief medical and nursing officers. There must be integration into practice at the levels of staff nurses, house officers, and beginning providers. Real excellence will require a change in culture within disciplines and health care systems. Death should not be viewed as a failure, and excellence in the provision of end-of-life care is the responsibility of all providers in an ED.

Summary

The death of a child is not a common event, but there remain variations across populations, geography, and socioeconomic status. For most people, however, the death of a child is almost unheard of and leaves the family at risk for complicated bereavement.[18] While the provision of excellent end-of-life care for children is not likely to alter families' grief significantly, the absence of excellence will leave families with memories and impressions of their child's suffering. The knowledge and skills exist to provide excellent end-of-life care to children even, and perhaps especially, in the ED.

REFERENCES

1. Children's International Project on Palliative/Hospice Services (ChIPPS) Administrative/Policy Workgroup of the National Hospice and Palliative Care Organization: A Call for Change: Recommendations to Improve the Care of Children Living with Life-Threatening Conditions. National Hospice and Palliative Care Organization. Available at *www.nhpco.org* (accessed May 3, 2002).
2. Mathews TJ, Menacker F, MacDorman MF; U.S. Centers for Disease Control and Prevention, National Center for Health Statistics: Infant mortality statistics from the 2002 period: linked birth/infant death data set. Natl Vital Stat Rep 53:1–29, 2004.
*3. Code of ethics for emergency physicians. American College of Emergency Physicians. Ann Emerg Med 30:365–372, 1997.

---

*Selected readings.

4. Iserson KV: Principles of biomedical ethics. Emerg Med Clin North Am 17:283–306, 1999.

5. Bluebond-Langner M: The Private Worlds of Dying Children. Princeton, NJ: Princeton University Press, 1978.

6. Christakis NA: Death Foretold: Prophecy and Prognosis in Medical Care. Chicago: University of Chicago Press, 1999.

7. Wolfe J, Grier HE, Klar N, et al: Symptoms and suffering at the end of life in children with cancer. N Engl J Med 342:326–333, 2000.

8. American Academy of Pediatrics & Canadian Paediatric Society: Prevention and management of pain and stress in the neonate. Pediatrics 105:454–461, 2000.

*9. American Academy of Pediatrics & American Pain Society: The assessment and management of acute pain in infants, children, and adolescents. Pediatrics 108:793–797, 2001.

10. Iserson KV: Withholding and withdrawing medical treatment: an emergency medicine perspective. Ann Emerg Med 28:51–54, 1996.

11. Young KD, Seidel JS: Pediatric cardiopulmonary resuscitation: a collective review. Ann Emerg Med 33:195–205, 1999.

12. Young KD, Gausche-Hill M, McClung CD, Lewis RJ: A prospective, population-based study of the epidemiology and outcome of out-of-hospital pediatric cardiopulmonary arrest. Pediatrics 114:157–164, 2004.

*13. Marco CA: Ethical issues of resuscitation. Emerg Med Clin North Am 17:527–538, 1999.

14. Meyers T, Eichhorn DJ, Guzzetta CE: Do families want to be present during CPR? A retrospective survey. J Emerg Nurs 24:400–405, 1998.

15. Boudreaux ED, Francis JL, Loyacano T: Family presence during invasive procedures and resuscitations in the emergency department: a critical review and suggestions for future research. Ann Emerg Med 40:193–205, 2002.

16. Aherns WR, Hart RG: Emergency physicians' experience with pediatric death. Am J Emerg Med 15:642–643, 1997.

17. Hill TP: Treating the dying patient: the challenge for medical education. Arch Intern Med 155:1265–1269, 1995.

18. Rando T: Treatment of complicated mourning. Champaign, IL: Research Press, 1993.

Chapter 149

Patient Safety, Medical Errors, and Quality of Care

David P. John, MD, John A. Brennan, MD, Nancy E. Holecek, RN,
and Patricia Sweeney-McMahon, RN, MS

Key Points

The "culture of blame" has done little to improve quality and patient safety. Malpractice litigation, morbidity and mortality rounds, and physician profiling drive errors underground. A "just culture" error reporting system with data tracking must be in place in order to understand, categorize, and decrease system failures.

Individual institutions should use data to understand the problems within their health care system.

Hospitals' administration, physician, and nursing leadership should be directly involved and drive these changes. However, true culture change occurs with staff involvement.

Quality and safety initiatives should focus on system re-evaluation that ensures safe, effective, patient-centered, efficient, timely, and equitable health care for all patients.

Pediatric patients are particularly prone to medication errors secondary to miscalculations.

- Between 44,000 and 98,000 Americans die from medical errors annually.[3-5]
- Medication-related errors for hospitalized patients cost roughly $2 billion annually.[3,6]
- The lag between the discovery of more effective forms of treatment and their incorporation into routine patient care averages 17 years.[7,8]

Now, however, the public, health care regulatory agencies, and the federal government are aware of the shortcomings in quality and safety in medicine. Additionally, the Agency for Healthcare Research and Quality, the Institute of Healthcare Improvement, and Six Sigma have also been instrumental in addressing the patient safety and quality process change and developing best practices (Table 149–1).

Joseph M. Juran and W. Edwards Deming pioneered quality improvement in industry. In post–World War II Japan, "Made in Japan" was synonymous with inexpensive, mass-produced, poor-quality goods. Under the guidance of Deming and Juran, Japan redesigned systems and developed a culture of quality in their businesses. Companies such as Sony and Toyota equaled, and perhaps surpassed, some of their American counterparts.

In the 1960s, 1 in 1000 airline takeoffs had some form of system flaw. Many of these resulted in crashes, causing loss of human life, loss of million-dollar aircraft, and countless dollar losses in profit to the industry.[9,10] "Aviation safety was not built on evidence that certain practices reduced the frequency of crashes. Instead it relied on the widespread implementation of hundreds of small changes in procedures, equipment, training, and organization that aggregated to establish an incredibly strong safety culture and amazingly effective practices."[3]

Over the last 20 years, the specialty of anesthesia has reduced its death rate from 1 in 20,000 to 1 in 200,000. Anesthesiologists developed processes that helped them better understand and measure the effectiveness of their systems.[11-13] With this basic knowledge, they standardized procedures, orders, monitoring capabilities, competencies, and recovery room criteria. Their systems became simpler, with multiple checks and balances to help avoid adverse events. Standardizing anesthesiology carts and making it mechanically impossible to hook up the wrong gas to the

Introduction and Background

Quality and safety in medicine have not evolved to anywhere near the standards of other industries. Medicine has always been viewed as a "calling" or "art" rather than a business. As such, it has not been subject to the scrutiny of the business model (productivity, efficiency, and quality) . . . until now.[1] An Institute of Medicine (IOM) report[2] and pay-for-performance initiatives have suddenly made quality and patient safety top priorities in medicine. The IOM report *To Err is Human: Building a Safer Health System*[3] brought to light what most health care workers already know: errors occur and patients are harmed, and occasionally die.

Table 149–1	Emergency Medicine Best Practice Resources
Organization Name	**Web Site**
Agency for Healthcare Research and Quality (AHRQ)	www.ahrq.gov
American Academy of Pediatrics (AAP)	www.aap.org
American College of Emergency Physicians (ACEP)–Clinical Policies	www.acep.org
American College of Quality	www.asq.org
American College of Surgeons	www.acs.org
American Society for Healthcare Risk Management	www.ashrm.org
Hospital Quality Incentive Demonstration Project (Premier and CMS)	www.cms.gov
Institute for Safe Medication Practices (ISMP) Voluntary Reporting of Medication Errors	www.ismp.org
Institute of Healthcare Improvement (IHI)	www.ihi.org
Joint Commission on Accreditation of Healthcare Organizations (JCAHO)	www.jcaho.org
Leapfrog Group	www.leapfroggroup.org
National Committee on Quality Assurance (NCQA)	www.ncqa.org
National Guideline Clearinghouse (NGC)	www.ngc.org
National Hospital Voluntary Reporting Initiative Consensus Standards for Hospital Care	www.cms.gov
National Patient Safety Foundation	www.npsf.org
National Quality Forum (NQF)	www.qualityforum.org
Physician Consortium for Performance Improvement (AMA)	www.ama-assn.org

Table 149–2	Impact of Overcrowding on Quality and Safety Outcomes

Medication errors
Inability to provide standard level of care for high-acuity patients
Continuity of care threatened
Inability to meet quality core measure best practices
Miscommunication
Delay in diagnostics
Patient and staff dissatisfaction

wrong tube are just two examples of how system changes can prevent adverse events.

In emergency medicine, the development of the color-coded tape is one of the first pediatric safety initiatives. Medication dosing and equipment size are based on the weight and length of the child. Calculations are difficult, cumbersome, and not readily available during an emergency, and errors can result in patient harm. To help prevent this, a color scheme based on the length of the child was developed to aid in accessing the proper-sized equipment and medication doses for the child. These length-based, color-coded systems have been placed in many emergency departments (EDs) in the country because[14]

- The system is easy to use.
- It is not prohibitively expensive.
- It improves patient outcomes.

Issues

Since the IOM report *To Err is Human*, quality and patient safety issues have come to light in the media, in hospital boardrooms, and among consumers. This report, as well the IOM's report *Crossing the Quality Chasm: A New Health System for the 21st Century*,[2] has refocused the government, regulatory agencies, and private payers on health care reform.

The Joint Commission on Accreditation of Healthcare Organizations, along with state and federal governments, has recently implemented a mandatory reporting system for medical errors. This initiative, like the current medical liability system, seems intuitively to drive disclosure underground. Why would a health care provider openly report a medical error in this system? The individual reporting the error could be sued, lose his or her ability to practice medicine, and be publicly reported. The airline industry has a "just culture" with mandatory error reporting and they study "near misses" and malfunctions in an effort to improve quality and safety.

No medical practitioner intends to harm patients. Providers of emergency care work in a chaotic environment. They are overworked, understaffed, and overcrowded. They handle numerous sound bytes of information from every direction and, not unusually, the unexpected occurs.[15] These events occur in every ED across the country every day. To prevent adverse events, one needs to understand what went wrong, categorize it, collect data on it, and then, most importantly, put systems in place to prevent or minimize harm to patients.[16] Some of the chief impediments to reporting errors include the fear of punishment by state licensing boards and regulatory agencies, embarrassment, and being branded as a troublemaker. In order to analyze and decrease errors, a just culture environment must be created.

Evidence-based clinical guidelines and pathways have been shown to improve quality and patient safety.[17,18] Like the Emergency Medical Treatment Act and Labor Act, quality and patient safety are largely unfunded mandates. In a time of decreasing reimbursement, who is going to pay for the infrastructure changes needed to implement sweeping reforms and new technology? Despite the financial implications, emergency medicine needs to embrace this concept in all aspects of patient care. As Karl Albrecht noted, "You seldom improve quality by cutting costs, but you can often cut costs by improving quality."

EDs are frequently in an overcapacity state. This was referred to initially as ED overcrowding when it was actually a systems issue within the individual hospital. The unintended consequence of overcapacity is ambulance diversion. Ambulances are asked to take sick patients to other hospitals, often a distance away. The quality and safety issues inherent in this situation are numerous (Table 149–2). Diversion is a symptom of, not a solution to, overcrowding. Numerous problems have an impact on crowding, but one of the most critical is access of care (Table 149–3). Emergency departments are the last safe harbor for economically challenged parents with children, the frail elderly, and patients with urgent needs whose doctors cannot see them.

When the ED/hospital is over capacity, waiting times increase, the number of patients who have "Left Without Being Seen" increases, and the fixed staff cannot provide the type of care that they have been trained to give. In an overcapacity situation, the criteria for a disaster or mass casualty incident are often met but not matched with a prescribed action plan. Additionally, hours and even days go by without

Table 149–3	Reasons for Lack of Access to Health Care

Doctor's offices are full.
Doctor's offices are closed.
Offices are not accepting new Medicare patients.
Patient cannot afford outpatient care or prescription drugs.
The "clinic system" has failed.

Table 149–4	Selected Hospital-Related Opportunities to Decrease Overcrowding

- Measure each step of the admission process to identify the opportunities for improvement.
- Include key members of the multidisciplinary team in all process improvement discussions.
- Create units that can expand to accept greater number of patients and avoid adding nonclinical ancillary personnel.
- Improve the accuracy of forecasting beds for elective surgery and the resources to support it.
- Expand the elective surgery schedule for nonpeak hours; negotiate with the surgical staff to comply.
- Assign accountability for timely discharges, efficient room turnover, and adequate resources for timely transportation.
- Assign executive leadership to adopt or "own" a project or process.
- Analyze operational data as they relate to quality and safety outcomes and report regularly.

Table 149–5	Emergency Department (ED) "Real-Time" Dashboard: Reflects the Current Condition in the ED

Patients Currently in the ED

Capture Time at Door	Seen by a provider
	Triaged and waiting for screening examination
	Waiting to be triaged
Current Resources Assigned to Patient Care	Physicians
	Mid-level practitioners
	Registered nurses
	Ancillary staff: clerks, technicians, registrars etc.
	Total
Turnaround Time (TAT)	Average chemistry TAT: order to result
	Average microbiology TAT: order to result
	Average radiology plain film TAT: order to film
	Average radiology CT TAT: order to result

Patients Holding in the ED

Patient	Admitting Physician	Acuity (CC, Tele, Regular, OB)	Bed Assigned	Comments
Patient 1				
Patient 2				
Patient 3				
Etc.				

Abbreviations: CC, critical care; CT, computed tomography; OB, obstetric; Tele, telephone.

any relief, giving the impression that overcrowding is "status quo" for the ED. As a result, quality and safety are compromised, and hospital-related opportunities to decrease overcrowding should be strategically discussed and accountability assigned (Table 149–4).

EDs/hospitals must have an overcapacity or surge plan that includes the ability to increase resources and obtain additional staff. The senior management of the ED/hospital must streamline and reallocate resources throughout the hospital, including the canceling of elective surgeries, to focus on the overcapacity. They must establish the importance and priority of the ED, prior to overcapacity, as part of a strategic plan. Additional areas of the hospital must be opened up for patient care, including the creation of transition areas for admitted and discharged patients. Preparation for overcapacity and the prevention of the errors resulting from overcapacity includes education planning and the hospital's commitment to patient safety and quality. This preparation is mandatory, and the operational effort required to implement an overcapacity plan must be simple and administratively supported. At the very least, there should be an "ED dashboard" or mechanism in place to communicate the real-time current condition of the ED to all members of the management team responsible for patient throughput (Table 149–5).

Solutions

Benchmarking quality indicators, measuring them, and making system changes to improve compliance are fundamental components of an ED quality improvement program. It is necessary to understand best practices and share successes to improve the way care is delivered. The department must do away with the "culture of blame," and develop an environment in which "near misses" are reviewed in a just culture reporting system and systems are put into place to prevent harm.

In order to implement national best practices, there must be a complete facility buy-in to achieve the desired quality and/or safety outcomes. The Institute for Healthcare Improvement describes one such example as the "Plan-Do-Study-Act" cycle. This process tests a quality/safety change in the real work setting—by planning it, trying it, observing the results, and acting on what is learned. This is the scientific method used for action-oriented learning.

The department focuses on a desired outcome that is presently challenging and maps the process to help define critical steps that are captured and measured for analysis. A multidisciplinary team is selected that best represents key stakeholders, and changes for improvement are defined. A trial is implemented and the results are used to support a permanent change in process or policy.

All successful quality programs must have the support of their hospital's leadership. As stated by L. L. Leape, "Management must 'manage' for patient safety and quality just as they manage for efficiency and profit maximization. Safety must become part of what a hospital or healthcare organization prides itself on."[19] Successful organizations have implemented the following practices and created a culture of quality and safety:

Collaborative Environment: Create an environment in which every member of the patient care team is empowered to provide information, ask questions, and question orders or a patient disposition.

Just Culture Error Reporting Systems: Incident reports must be simple to complete. Root-cause analysis must be completed to understand system errors. An anonymous reporting system provides practitioners with a "safe harbor" reporting environment. Staff education will raise the level of awareness about medication errors and near misses.

Dashboard: An ED dashboard should reflect the current/real-time condition of the ED and be accessible to all appropriate leadership via a shared computer hard drive or Intranet. This report should help facilitate the appropriate actions to decompress the ED and allocate the appropriate resources to meet patient care demands (see Table 149–4).

Report card: The ED report card must include financial, operational, quality, and satisfaction data, with the appropriate benchmarks to provide leadership with the insight to identify opportunities for improvement and processes that are successful. The data points selected to create the measurement should adequately reflect the processes of the department and the results should be validated (Table 149–6).

Clinical Information System: Electronic information systems should facilitate easy documentation of assessments, care, and treatment of ED patients and access to that information in an organized and retrievable format. Additionally, they should provide tools to prevent error, improve the staff's ability to communicate, and provide up-to-date clinical best practices to drive quality outcomes.

Quality Program: The most successful quality programs include executive leadership with multidisciplinary representation, evidence-based care paths, the appropriate tools to assure successful implementation, and a process to measure outcomes and communicate them to all departments involved in the care path.

Safety Program: A successful safety program is one that promotes a collaborative and patient-centric culture throughout the entire organization.

Patient Callbacks: Radiology discrepancies, positive cultures, and patients who left without being seen all provide useful quality and follow-up data.

Clinical Guidelines and Pathways: Best practices should be developed for frequent and high-risk/complex patient presentations. Asthma, fever, and dehydration are examples for which specific evidence-based medicine protocols should be tracked and linked to outcomes.

Sign Out/Change of Shift: Every patient must have a physician and nurse who understand his or her problem and treatment plan. A policy on how a patient's care is transitioned from one health care provider to another is critical to prevent errors.

Improvement of All Communications: Improving written and verbal exchange of imformation applies to how one communicates to other medical personnel as well as to the patients and their families.
- Written:
  Utilize electronic ordering systems where possible.
  Safety protocols implemented at the institution should include:
    Discontinuing the use of all error prone abbreviations.
    Never using a trailing "0" (1.00 mg/kg).
    Always using a leading "0" (0.1 mg/kg).
  Do not write or accept poorly written orders or charts.
  Always customize discharge instructions to include a simple but explicit follow-up plan regarding outpatient care and medication. To enhance understanding, choose the appropriate language and grade level for all people involved in the care.

Table 149–6	**Selected Emergency Department (ED) Report Card Measurements: Monitoring of the ED Over Time**		
Financial	**Quality & Safety**	**Operational**	**Satisfaction**

Volume
• Month to date (MTD)
• Year to date (YTD)
• Include % increase and decrease
• Expected vs. actual
• Track specialty service utilization
  • Fast track
  • Orthopedics
	Core Measure Outcomes Driven by Care in the ED
	• AMI
	• Pneumonia
	• Infectious disease
	Monitor changes to the course of treatment implemented in the ED vs. inpatient and link to outcomes
		Turnaround Times
		• Admitted
		• Discharged
		• ED area
		  • Fast track
		  • Pediatrics
		• Laboratory
		• Radiology
			Patient Satisfaction
			• By question
			• By time of day
			• By staff member

Resource Utilization • Patients per physician hour • Patients per provider hour	**Safety Culture Measurement (CUSP)**	**Quality-Linked Operations** • Door to ECG • Door to PCI • Door to thrombolytics	**Employee Satisfaction** • By discipline within the department • By shift
Charge Capture: Assure adequate resources are available to maintain quality: • Adequate central line kits to support recommendations to decrease central line–associated primary bloodstream infections • Foley kits with urimeter attached to catheter to prevent UTIs associated with breaking the sterile field	**Physician- and Nurse-to-Patient Ratios** • Measure by acuity • In real time, by time of day Map to outcomes	**Admission Process** • Process map each step • Analyze by service • Analyze by destination	**Medical Staff Satisfaction** • Monitor formally with a survey that reflects the distinction between ED and hospital process • Allow for ongoing monitoring

Abbreviations: AMI, acute myocardial infarction; ECG, electrocardiogram; PCI, patient controlled infusion; UTIs, urinary tract infections.

- Verbal:
  Use appropriate time-out policy during procedures.
  Minimize use of verbal orders. Always do a read back of a verbal order.
  Introduce yourself and know your coworkers.
  Create a collaborative, not hierarchical, working environment.
  Identify high-risk or very unstable patients.
  When speaking to a patient, always follow verbal instructions with a written version.

Emergency Medicine–Specific Quality Guidelines: Develop indicators based on chief complaint or clinical presentations versus the diagnosis.

Patient-Centered Care: Historically, the environment of care was based on staff convenience (nursing stations, lack of test availability at night, etc.). The focus needs to change to "what is best for the patient."

Telephone and Verbal Orders: Limit these wherever possible and have them repeated and confirmed.

ED Medications: Institute measures to prevent medication errors:

- Reduce the number of medications with similar indications.
- Consider having a pharmacist in the ED to mix all medications, similar to the intensive care unit.
- Place concentrated electrolyte solutions from the ED in secured areas.
- Clearly label medications and do not store look-alike/sound-alike medications near each other.
- Limit interruptions, if possible, during medication preparation and administration.

On-Call Specialist and Follow-up Care: The hospital administration and physician leadership must ensure that there is adequate subspecialty care and follow-up.

Table 149–1 is a resource for finding EM best practices. Systems must be in place to minimize human factors. As stated by W. A. Foster, "Quality is never an accident. It is always the result of high intention, sincere effort, intelligent direction, and skilled execution."

Summary

Individual EDs need to use the evidence, information, and technology that have already been demonstrated to improve patient outcomes. If the hospital administration is not visibly advocating for quality and patient safety, they must be motivated to become involved. Joseph Juran stated that "every successful quality revolution has included the participation of upper management. We know of no exception." This is a cultural change and requires hospital-wide participation.

Health care providers need to be patient advocates and provide patient-centered care. As with patient satisfaction, it is not enough to be good clinicians; they must make the system work for their patients. As Aristotle noted several centuries ago, "We are what we repeatedly do. Excellence, then, is not an act but a habit." Continuous improvement in patient care must be embraced by the entire health care industry.[20]

REFERENCES

1. Laffe G, Blumenthal D: The case for using industrial quality management science in health care organizations. JAMA 262:2869–2873, 1989.
*2. Institute of Medicine: Crossing the Quality Chasm: A New Health System for the 21st Century. Washington, DC: National Academy Press, 2001.
*3. Institute of Medicine; Kohn LT, Corrigan JM, Donaldson MS (eds): To Eerr is Human: Building a Safer Health System. Washington, DC: National Academy Press, 2000.
4. Thomas EJ, Studdert DM, Burstin HR, et al: Incidence and types of adverse events and negligent care in Utah and Colorado [Comment]. Med Care 38:261–271, 2000.
5. Thomas EJ, Studdert DM, Newhouse JP, et al: Costs of medical injuries in Utah and Colorado. Inquiry 36:255–264, 1999.
6. Bates DW, Spell N, Cullen DJ, et al: The costs of adverse drug events in hospitalized patients. Adverse Drug Events Prevention Study Group. JAMA 277:307–311, 1997.
7. Balas EA: Information systems can prevent errors and improve quality [Comment]. J Am Med Inform Assoc 8:398–399, 2001.
*8. Greiner AC, Knebel E (eds): Health Professions Education: A Bridge to Quality. Washington, DC: National Academy Press, 2003.
9. Layton C, Smith PJ, McCoy CE: Design of a cooperative problem-solving system for en-route flight planning: an empirical evaluation. Hum Factors 36:94–119, 1994.
10. Weick KE, Roberts KH: Collective mind and organizational reliability: the case of flight operations on an aircraft carrier deck. Adm Sci Q 38:357–381, 1993.
11. Gaba DM, Maxwell MS, DeAnda A: Anesthetic mishaps: breaking the chain of accident evolution. Anesthesiology 66:670–676, 1987.
12. Gaba DM, Howard SK, Jump B: Production pressure in the work environment: California anesthesiologists' attitudes and experiences. Anesthesiology 81:488–500, 1994.
13. Howard SK, Gaba DM, Fish KJ, et al: Anesthesia crisis resource management training: teaching anesthesiologists to handle critical incidents. Aviat Space Environ Med 63:763–770, 1992.
*14. Broselow JB: Color coding kids . . . a patient safety initiative. Quality Improvement and Patient Safety Section News, Vol 4, July 2003.
*15. Chisolm CD, Collison EK, Nelson DR, Cordell WH: Emergency department workplace interruptions: are emergency physicians "interrupt driven" and "multitasking"? Acad Emerg Med 7:1239–1243, 2000.
16. Grabowski M, Roberts KH: Risk mitigation in large-scale systems: lessons from high reliability organizations. Calif Manage Rev 39(4), Summer 1997.
17. Hauck LD, Adler LM, Mulla ZD: Clinical pathway care improves outcomes among patients hospitalized for community-acquired pneumonia. Ann Epidemiol 14:669–675, 2004.
18. Benenson R, Magalski A, Cavanaugh S, Williams E: Effects of a pneumonia clinical pathway on time to antibiotic treatment, length of stay, and mortality. Acad Emerg Med 6:1243–1248, 1999.
*19. Leape LL, Berwick DM: Safe health care: are we up to it? BMJ 320:725–726, 2000.
*20. Berwick DM: Continuous improvement as an ideal in health care. N Engl J Med 320:53–56, 1989.

*Suggested readings.

Chapter 150

Emergency Medical Treatment and Labor Act (EMTALA)

Todd B. Taylor, MD

Key Points[1]

The original intent of the Emergency Medical Treatment and Labor Act (EMTALA) is consistent with standards of medical care.

The EMTALA obligation is voluntarily accepted by hospitals as part of the Medicare Conditions of Participation Agreement. Physicians are duty bound by EMTALA, by virtue of their voluntary agreement with the hospital, to serve on call and/or by agreement or contract with the hospital to provide emergency services

EMTALA requires Medicare-participating hospitals with emergency departments to provide screening for and treatment of emergency medical conditions in a nondiscriminatory manner to any individual regardless of ability to pay, insurance status, national origin, race, creed, color, and the like.

EMTALA requires individuals with similar medical complaints or conditions to be treated similarly. It applies to all individuals at Medicare-participating hospitals, not just those covered by Medicare.

As a federal statute, EMTALA supersedes state and local laws, including peer-review protections, certain tort reform limitations, and statutes of limitations. It grants every individual a federal right to emergency care and creates additional rights when hospitals or physicians fail to comply.

EMTALA violations can result in significant penalties for hospitals and physicians, including civil monetary penalties of up to $50,000 per violation and/or Medicare participation termination.

EMTALA is an unfunded mandate and does not require health insurance companies, governments, or individuals to pay for mandated emergency services.

Emergency physicians on average provide $138,300 of uncompensated EMTALA-related medical care each year, and one third of emergency physicians provide more than 30 hours of EMTALA-related care each week.[2]

Introduction and Background

EMTALA's Original Intent

A hospital is charged only with the responsibility of providing an adequate first response to a medical crisis [which] means the patient must be evaluated and, at a minimum, provided with whatever medical support services and/or transfer arrangements that are consistent with the capability of the institution and the well-being of the patient.[3]

The Emergency Medical Treatment and Labor Act (EMTALA) was enacted by Congress in 1986 as part of the Consolidated Omnibus Budget Reconciliation Act of 1985 (42USC§1395dd). Often referred to as the patient "anti-dumping" law, it was originally designed to prevent hospitals from transferring uninsured or Medicaid patients to public hospitals without, at a minimum, providing a medical screening examination (MSE) and treatment to assure that such transfers could be done safely.

The concern for patient safety at that time was not unwarranted. Studies showed that, in the early 1980s, of transfers to public or Veterans Administration hospitals, 87% were for economic reasons. Only 6% of patients gave informed consent, 24% of patients were unstable at the time of transfer, mortality was three times that of other patients, and 250,000 such transfers were occurring annually.[4-7]

Congress has amended and expanded the scope of EMTALA five times. For example, until 1989, EMTALA did not require hospitals or physicians to provide on-call services, nor did it require hospitals with specialized services to accept patients in transfer. Over the years, additional amendments enhanced the ability to impose fines, increased penalties, provided whistle-blower protections, and expanded the reach of the law and the mandated duties of providers.

Despite passage in 1986, there was little enforcement of EMTALA for the first 10 years.[8,9] Enforcement increased significantly after the Centers for Medicare & Medicaid Services (CMS; formerly the Health Care Financing Administration) published rules for the enforcement of EMTALA in the Code of Federal Regulations (CFR) in 1994 [42CFR§489.xx]. (The full statute and definitions of terms are available at *http://www.gpoaccess.gov/cfr/index.html.*) By 1999, there had been more than 2000 EMTALA investigations and more than 1000 confirmed violations.[10]

In June 1996, a diverse national EMTALA Task Force was formed to clarify the regulations with new Interpretive Guidelines published in July 1998. The Interpretive Guidelines did not carry the force of law and, while well intentioned, left many issues vague. As a result, federal and state civil courts continued to have a significant influence on EMTALA interpretation. Consequently, EMTALA now has little resemblance to its original intent of regulating economically motivated transfers.[11]

On November 10, 2003, CMS published a final rule revising the 1994 EMTALA CFR. In large part, these revised rules simply codified interim CMS guidance, but in addition they revised the definition of an "emergency department," clarified what is considered "hospital property," recognized certain limitations of on-call specialists and on-call panels, added a "prudent layperson" standard with regard to the request for services, and clarified applicability to hospital-owned ambulances. In addition, although EMTALA has never applied to inpatients, the new rules drew a "bright line" at admission for when the EMTALA obligation ends [42CFR§489.24(d)(2)]. Once a patient is admitted, other Medicare Conditions of Participation requirements apply, making EMTALA superfluous for hospital inpatients [42CFR§482.55].

While EMTALA is a complex law with many ambiguities, one would need to read no further if only one principle were adopted for EMTALA compliance: "Take care of the patient." EMTALA is a "medical anti-discrimination" law. Anytime one considers treating any patient differently for other than a good medical reason, EMTALA is in jeopardy of being violated. The difficulty comes in properly documenting such reasoning and in achieving technical compliance. EMTALA is of special concern to hospitals with limited, focused, and special capabilities, such as pediatric-only hospitals and general hospitals that provide "specialized" pediatric services (e.g., a pediatric emergency department [ED]).

This chapter presents the basics of EMTALA, drawing heavily upon the actual statutory language. It has been written primarily for physicians, and additional references and CRF and United States Code (USC) citations are provided for more detailed reading and study.

Issues: Implications of EMTALA for American Health Care

According to Rep. Pete Stark (D-CA), co-sponsor of EMTALA:

> Patient dumping is but a symptom of a much larger problem. Thirty-seven million Americans [47 million in 2005] are without health insurance. Low income sick people are finding it increasingly difficult to get needed health care, and the burden of caring for them is falling on fewer and fewer hospitals.[12]

> Access should be the government's responsibility at the federal, state, and local levels. We cannot and should not expect hospitals to be this nation's National Health Service.[13]

From a legal perspective, EMTALA's original purpose was simply to create a duty to provide an MSE to assure that either no emergency medical condition (EMC) exists or, if an EMC is present, it is "stabilized" prior to the patient's transfer to a public hospital. With significant changes in payment mechanisms in the early 1980s (e.g., "diagnosis-related groups"), the onslaught of managed care, and increasing numbers of uninsured patients, private hospitals felt compelled to limit their exposure to revenue losses from uninsured and Medicaid patients. This led to a "wallet biopsy" being performed prior to offering even emergency care. Ultimately, this mistreatment of patients prompted the creation of a clever "voluntary" governmental solution we now know as EMTALA.

EMTALA was the first time Congress had used the Medicare statute to create public policy extending beyond Medicare recipients. As a result, it became a national standard of care for emergency services and a federal right to emergency care.[11] While noble in its intent, and representing what most would find to be ethical and a standard of medical care obligation, in the ensuing years the EMTALA statute and regulations resulted in many unintended and even untoward consequences.

EMTALA now regulates virtually every aspect of care provided on hospital property, but by design has no bearing on payment. It allowed local and state governments to abdicate responsibility for charity care, thereby shifting this public responsibility to the private sector. Subsequently, many public "free" clinics were closed due to budgetary concerns, and public hospitals use EMTALA as a shield against accepting indigent patients. In essence, EMTALA made every Medicare-participating hospital a "public" hospital. EMTALA has become the de facto national health care policy for emergency care and for the uninsured. It also forced America's EDs to become the safety net of the health care system.[14-17]

Until recently, the federal government had never accepted any direct financial responsibility for EMTALA. The Medicare Modernization Act of 2003[18] for the first time provides financial relief to hospitals burdened with undocumented aliens due to EMTALA. Nevertheless, the financial strain of EMTALA continues to plague hospitals and their associated physicians with over $25 billion in uncompensated care annually,[19] and "55 percent of emergency services go[ing] uncompensated."[20] Furthermore, the traditional cost-shifting mechanism to compensate for this burden has largely been eliminated by managed care, and many managed care practices are irreconcilable with the requirements of EMTALA.

The direct and indirect impact of EMTALA continues to mount. Specialists are fleeing hospital medical staffs to avoid ED on-call duties, hospitals are limiting the scope of services or creating "specialty" hospitals to carve out a niche with less EMTALA exposure, efforts are made to "manage" the financial risk with ED "triage-out" procedures for "nonurgent" conditions, and medical repatriation programs have been devised for foreign nationals; these are but a few examples.

After more than two decades of EMTALA, two fundamental principles are clear:

1. How health care is funded (and litigated) drives health care availability and delivery.
2. America cannot solve the EMTALA conundrum until it addresses the reason EMTALA exits—a failure to appropriately fund and provide for indigent and uncompensated emergency medical care.

General EMTALA Duty

EMTALA creates a duty that otherwise would not exist for hospitals. Ethical duty aside, prior to enactment of EMTALA, there was no legal duty for a hospital to provide medical care (even emergency care) to anyone not already accepted as a patient. EMTALA was specifically design to create such a duty for any "individual" that arrived on hospital property and requested treatment for a "medical condition." It should be noted that the statute does not say "emergency medical condition." Whether the medical condition is an "emergency" must be determined by an MSE, and, if an EMC is present, additional EMTALA obligations are imposed.

Under EMTALA, hospitals voluntarily accept this duty by virtue of their "contract" with Medicare, called the Medicare Conditions of Participation. In doing so, they agree to be investigated, sanctioned, and fined for noncompliance without due process. Physicians do not have a similar Medicare requirement; therefore, EMTALA is the sole burden of Medicare-participating hospitals. Nonparticipating hospitals, such as the Veterans Administration, certain military hospitals, non-hospital owned urgent care centers, and the like, are not obligated under EMTALA.

Since EMTALA applies only to hospitals, administration must make arrangements to provide physician services as part of this duty. Ironically, EMTALA provides no formal mechanism or requirement for this to be accomplished. So, while the law mandates that hospitals provide on-call physicians, it does not require physicians to provide on-call services. As a result, most hospitals do so via contract (e.g., with emergency physicians or employed physicians) or by imposing duties by voluntary participation in the medical staff and the ED on-call roster. Because EMTALA is "voluntary" (i.e., hospitals can choose not to participate in Medicare and physicians can choose not to be on the medical staff or choose not to take ED call), it avoids the U.S. Constitution's XIIIth Amendment prohibition against involuntary servitude and slavery.

Voluntary or not, EMTALA often creates opportunities for discord between hospitals, between a hospital and its medical staff, and among the medical staff itself, particularly between the ED and on-call physicians. This discord is often exacerbated by the threat of fines and sanctions, which are equally onerous for physicians as for hospitals.

Statutory Definitions

Increasingly, EMTALA is now controlled by statutory definitions that often have little basis in medical science [42CFR§489.24(b)]. Table 150–1 lists the potential sanctions and fines. Table 150–2 lists the regulatory agencies overseeing EMTALA.

EMTALA-Mandated Responsibilities for Hospitals and Physicians

As a federal statute, EMTALA supersedes conflicting and contradictory state and local laws [42USC§1395dd(f)], including peer-review protections, certain tort reform limitations, and statutes of limitations. It grants every individual a federal right to emergency care and creates additional rights when hospitals or physicians fail to comply.

Table 150–1   Potential EMTALA Sanctions and Fines (42CFR§1003.102)

Action	Amount/Duration	Comment	Regulation
Medicare & Medicaid program termination	Up to 2 yr	This can be a financial "death sentence" for any hospital or physician.	42CFR§489.24(g) & 42CFR§1003.105
Civil monetary penalties	Up to $50,000 for each violation (not each patient)	A malpractice insurance carrier may cover defense of the action, but fines are almost never covered without an EMTALA rider.	42CFR§1003.103(e) & 42CFR§1003.106
Hospital vs. hospital	A hospital "dumped on" can recover all costs for the patient's care.		42USC§1395dd(d)(2)(B)
Private cause of action	Depends on proven damages	Allows a civil case to be brought in federal court under "strict compliance with the law." Strict liability is less open to "expert" defense and easier to prove.	42USC§1395dd(d)(2)(A)
Injunctions		The court may impose an injunction requiring certain remedies to correct future violations or public notice of nondiscrimination policies.	
Hill-Burton Act funds	Varies	EMTALA violations may result in government action to recover loans and grants made to the facility.	
Civil rights	Fines and/or incarceration	EMTALA violation based on discrimination may result in referral to the Civil Rights Division of DHHS, resulting in criminal prosecution under the Civil Rights Act.	State Operations Manual: Appendix V—Interpretive Guidelines[25]

Abbreviation: DHHS, Department of Health and Human Services.

Table 150–2	EMTALA Regulating Entities

Centers for Medicare & Medicaid Services (CMS)
Office of the Inspector General (OIG)
The courts
   Federal Administrative Courts
   Civil state or federal courts

Duty to Provide an "Appropriate" Medical Screening Examination [42CFR§489.24(a)(1) & (a)(1)(i)]

The sole purpose of the MSE is to determine if an EMC exists. If the ED has the ability to rule out an EMC and documents this in the medical record, then EMTALA no longer applies. At that point the patient may be dispositioned in accordance with community standards of medical care, hospital policy, and local regulations. It is important to recognize that, even if EMTALA no longer applies, other regulations may, and many states have passed similar and even more stringent regulations regarding emergency care.

The MSE is all encompassing and includes all the available hospital resources necessary to make a determination of an EMC, including on-call specialists. However, hospitals are not required to provide all services 24 hours a day, if these services are not routinely provided after hours.

Application of the EMTALA MSE requirement now depends upon "where" the individual presents on hospital property. If they present to the "dedicated emergency department" and request examination or treatment for a "medical condition," this duty applies. If they present anywhere else, the duty only applies if the request is for what may be an EMC. In actual practice, this differentiation is only important for legal defense purposes, but documentation to that effect may assist in such defense. Although not necessarily required by EMTALA, the safest course of action may be to take any individual who presents with anything remotely resembling a request for medical care to the appropriate area in the hospital (i.e., ED, pediatric ED, obstetrics triage, psychiatry, etc.) for a formal MSE.

Perhaps the easiest way to train staff in this regard is to instruct them to ask such individuals, "Do you want to see a doctor?" If the answer is "yes," then the individual should be taken to the ED or other appropriate department. If the answer is "no," then staff should inquire further as to what the individual wants or needs. If there is any uncertainty, the safest course of action is to let the ED sort it out.

Pediatric EDs, particularly those that are part of a pediatric hospital, must understand their obligation to medically screen and stabilize any "individual" (regardless of age) that "comes to the emergency department" and requests evaluation for a medical condition. While such a facility is only required to provide such screening and stabilization that is within their capacity and capability, it is assumed that any hospital ED can and will do as much as they can while making arrangements for transfer to a more appropriate facility. If an EMC cannot be ruled out, then the patient should be considered "unstable" for the purposes of transfer and an "appropriate" formal EMTALA transfer accomplished.

Special Circumstances Related to the MSE

NO DELAY IN PROVIDING A MEDICAL SCREENING EXAMINATION OR TREATMENT [42CFR§489.24(d)(4)]

The "no delay" provision is often a misconstrued requirement. Some hospitals have taken the approach that, to be completely "safe," no insurance information may be obtained until the MSE has been initiated. Clearly this is not a requirement and may itself delay treatment since managed care often utilizes certain specialty consultants that may be unknown until insurance information is available. Nevertheless, whatever information is obtained cannot alter the usual course of examination and treatment.

This provision clearly prohibits prior authorization for at least the initial MSE and treatment. Also, the determination as to whether a patient has an EMC or is stable remains the purview of the on-site examining physician. Therefore, it is not appropriate for an off-site managed care gatekeeper to make such a determination.

Once the MSE has determined that there is no EMC or the EMC has been stabilized, then authorization (e.g., for admission or nonemergent testing) may be obtained if necessary. However, this may become a very delicate situation when authorization for admission is denied and an "economic transfer" is requested by the health plan. For truly "stable" patients this should not be an EMTALA issue, but "stability" is often reviewed retrospectively if anything adverse occurs during or even after the transfer. Under strict EMTALA statute interpretation, an "economic transfer" is allowable, but the physician must always be correct about "stability." In the current EMTALA and medical-legal climate, such transfers should be severely limited (i.e., to the absolutely most stable patients) or initiated after admission once stability is assured and EMTALA clearly no longer applies.

If such "economic transfers" are to be contemplated, it is prudent to identify additional legitimate reasons for the transfer, such as "continuity of care," and to assess the patient's desire to be transferred to an in-network facility by his or her formal request to be transferred. Emergency physicians compelled by the hospital to initiate economic transfers for the hospital's benefit may wish to seek indemnification by the hospital for any untoward EMTALA or other legal action.

Regardless, it is always prudent to clearly document that the patient is "stable" and that he or she is aware of the reasons for transfer along with the risks and benefits. The following acknowledgment statement has been recommended: *The physician has determined that my condition is stable and that there is no significant risk to my being transferred. I want the cost of further treatment to be covered by my health plan. My health plan has agreed to cover the cost of treatment at the receiving facility, but denied payment for services at this facility.*

AVAILABILITY OF ON-CALL PHYSICIANS [42CFR§489.24(j)]

On-call specialty coverage for EDs and hospital inpatients has emerged as a major health care issue[21,22] but is beyond the scope of this chapter. While EMTALA is neither the cause nor the solution, along with other stresses in the health care system it continues to have a significant impact on ED specialty coverage.[23] Increasingly, hospitals are finding it necessary to compensate or employ physician specialists in order to comply with the EMTALA mandate. Under EMTALA, the hospital and not its medical staff or individual physicians is responsible for maintaining an on-call roster for the ED [42 USC§1395cc(a)(1)(I)(i) & (iii)]. EMTALA case law requires hospitals to cajole, force, or otherwise negotiate and procure physician services to operate their EDs and provide on-call specialty care.[24]

USE OF DEDICATED EMERGENCY DEPARTMENT FOR NONEMERGENCY SERVICES [42CFR§489.24(c)]

If an individual comes to a hospital's dedicated ED and a request is made on his or her behalf for examination or treatment for a medical condition, but the nature of the request makes it clear that the medical condition is not of an emergency nature, the hospital is required only to perform such screening as would be appropriate for any individual presenting in that manner, to determine that the individual does not have an EMC. This clarifies that hospitals are not required to provide EMTALA-related services for "nonemergencies." However, this is a "chicken and egg" conundrum and in no way alleviates hospitals from performing an appropriate MSE for what may seem at triage to be the most trivial complaint yet later turns out to be an EMC.

QUALIFIED MEDICAL PERSON PERFORMING THE MSE [42CFR§489.24(a)(1)(i)]

A hospital must formally determine who is qualified to perform the initial MSE, that is, a "qualified medical person" (see also "Duty to Transfer" section). While it is permissible for a hospital to designate a nonphysician practitioner as the qualified medical person, the designated nonphysician practitioners must be set forth in a document that is approved by the governing body of the hospital. Following governing body approval, those health practitioners designated to perform MSEs are to be identified in the hospital bylaws or in the rules and regulations governing the medical staff. It is not acceptable for the hospital to allow the medical director of the ED to make what may be informal personnel appointments that could frequently change.

Duty to Stabilize [42CFR§489.24(a)(1)(ii) & 489.24(d)]

If the MSE determines that an EMC exists, then additional EMTALA duties apply. However, it should be noted that the statutory definition of "emergency" medical condition is quite restrictive, in that it requires that the "absence of immediate medical attention" will result in bad things happening. This fact is useful from a legal defense perspective, but from a practical standpoint almost any acute medical condition should be treated to an appropriate conclusion in the ED prior to discharge. While not required by EMTALA, this approach is prudent in light of aggressive CMS EMTALA enforcement, the impact of an EMTALA investigation, the potential severity of penalties, and the current medial-legal climate. It should also be noted that other Medicare Conditions of Participation, state regulations, and general medical liability may apply even if EMTALA does not.

Furthermore, a failure to follow hospital policy is often considered a per se EMTALA violation, even if the policy in question is not otherwise required by the EMTALA statute. Therefore, hospitals should construct their policies and procedures with extraordinary care to assure universal compli-

ance. For example, an ED triage policy that requires every patient to be triaged within 5 minutes of arrival may be unrealistic in the current overcrowded ED environment. A requirement for on-call physicians to arrive within 30 minutes is unrealistic for most communities. Nevertheless, under EMTALA, 6 minutes to triage or 31 minutes for the specialist to arrive could both be potential violations for failing to comply with hospital policy.

As with the MSE requirement, the duty to stabilize is all encompassing, including necessary on-call specialists. If the EMC can be resolved in the ED and is documented as such, then EMTALA no longer applies. If the EMC cannot be resolved in the ED and the hospital has inpatient services appropriate to resolve it, then the patient must be admitted. At the point of admission, the EMTALA obligation ends and is superseded by other Medicare Conditions of Participation requirements [42CFR§489.24(a)(1)(ii) & (d)(2)].

If the hospital does not have inpatient or emergency services (i.e., capacity and/or capability) necessary to stabilize the EMC, then an appropriate formal EMTALA transfer must be accomplished unless refused by the patient.

Duty to Transfer [42CFR§489.24(e)]

There are only three circumstances under which a patient may be transferred.
1. The patient is "stable" under the statutory EMTALA definition, in which case theoretically EMTALA does not apply.

This is theoretical because transferring a "stable" patient for admission or for further ED workup begs the question as to why the patient is being transferred instead of simply being discharged home. Again, this makes for an excellent legal argument when a transfer "goes bad," but in practice can be risky. While not required by EMTALA, it is prudent to document a legal "appropriate" transfer on all patients not otherwise being routinely discharged from the ED. While in many instances transferred patients will be declared "stable," if in retrospect the patient deteriorates, the transfer documentation will help protect the transferring hospital. In addition, some states require similar documentation on all transfers regardless of stability.

In an ill-conceived ploy, some have tried to circumvent EMTALA by "discharging" a patient with instructions to "go to the 'county' hospital." For EMTALA purposes, a "discharge" is a transfer, and such behavior invariably raises suspicion and results in an investigation.
2. The individual (or legal representative) requests to be transferred and accepts, in writing, the documented risks.

EMTALA does not empower hospitals to force involuntary treatment, admission, or transfer. However, it does require specific documentation and informed risk should a patient request to be transferred or refuse transfer, examination, or treatment. While this may seem relatively straightforward, an EMTALA conundrum can be created when a patient requests to be transferred to a hospital that then refuses to accept him or her based on the premise that the sending facility has the ability to treat. If the patient cannot be dissuaded, the best course of action is to have him or her sign out "against medical advice"; complete as much of the transfer documentation as is possible, including sending medical records; and notify the receiving facility of the situation.

3. The transfer is medically indicated (i.e., the risk of transfer is outweighed by the benefits) as certified by a physician (or qualified medical person in consultation with an off-site physician).

If the ED does not have the ability (capacity or capability) to determine if an EMC exists or to stabilize an identified EMC, then the patient should be considered unstable and an "appropriate" formal EMTALA transfer to a hospital with ability should occur unless refused by the patient.

"Appropriate" Formal EMTALA Transfer [42CFR§489.24(e)(2)]

This section of the EMTALA statute lists the four required elements of an "appropriate transfer":

1. Ongoing medical treatment until transfer
2. Confirmation of capability, capacity, and acceptance at the receiving facility
3. Sending of all available pertinent medical records
4. Assurance that the transfer is effected through qualified personnel and equipment

Once the decision to transfer has been made, ongoing treatment and monitoring are required within the ability of the transferring facility until the transfer can be effected. This includes all available services, including on-call specialists even if they will not ultimately admit the patient. If the on-site physician requests the presence of an on-call specialist to help care for a patient while waiting for transfer, the specialist is required by EMTALA to come in within a "reasonable" time. There is a requirement to provide the name of any on-call physician that failed to appear whether or not that is the inciting reason for the transfer.

Documentation that the receiving facility has the ability and has acknowledged acceptance of the transfer is required. While it is perhaps good medical practice under many circumstances, there is no specific requirement that a physician be contacted or accept the patient in transfer at the receiving facility. Anyone authorized at the receiving facility to accept the patient may do so, even a clerk in the admitting office.

As with all medical encounters, documentation is important. For example, failure to document that medical records were sent is a per se EMTALA violation whether they were actually sent or not.

The method of transport will depend upon the situation, but in most cases an ambulance is required. If for some reason an "unstabilized" patient is not being sent by ambulance (such as an eye injury sent with family to an ophthalmologist's office with better equipment), careful documentation as to the reason for and safety of such method of transfer should be done.

Documenting the required elements of an "appropriate transfer" in the medical record is sufficient, but difficult to consistently accomplish. While an EMTALA "Transfer Form" is not required, it is perhaps the best method to ensure technical compliance in documenting the three elements of a transfer: (1) request for transfer, (2) consent to transfer, and (3) certification of stability and/or risk/benefits of transfer.

Special Circumstances Related to Transfers

REFUSAL TO CONSENT TO TRANSFER [42CFR§489.24(d)(5)]

A hospital meets the EMTALA requirements if the hospital offers to transfer the individual to another medical facility and informs the individual (or a person acting on his or her behalf) of the risks and benefits of the transfer, but the individual does not consent to the transfer. The hospital must take all reasonable steps to secure the individual's written informed refusal.

Duty to Accept Transfers

Recipient Hospital Responsibilities [42CFR§489.24(f)]

A participating hospital that has specialized capabilities or facilities—including, but not limited to, facilities such as burn units, shock-trauma units, neonatal intensive care units, or (with respect to rural areas) regional referral centers—may not refuse to accept from a referring hospital within the boundaries of the United States an appropriate transfer of an individual who requires such specialized capabilities or facilities if the receiving hospital has the capacity to treat the individual.

The "duty to accept" is an often misunderstood and perhaps poorly defined requirement. The operative words are "including, but not limited to" and "if the receiving hospital has the capacity." Pediatric hospitals, hospitals with pediatric EDs, and community hospitals that provide inpatient pediatric services should all be considered "hospitals with specialized services."

With increasing hospital ED and inpatient capacity issues, it is not uncommon for hospitals with "specialized services" to lack "capacity." The issue becomes how to document such transfer refusals for individuals who never become patients. Another issue is who does this documentation if private on-call specialists screen these calls. There is no accepted standard and, in fact, most hospitals rely upon the good will of the calling facility to do this documentation for them. Nevertheless, some facilities have established "transfer coordinators" who document these calls and file a nonaccepted patient form by date of call for retrieval if necessary.

Transfers Between the Same Hospital's Departments or Facilities[25]

The movement of the individual between hospital departments is not considered an EMTALA transfer since the individual is simply being moved from one department of a hospital to another department or facility of the same hospital.

Transfer Agreements

Although transfer agreements are not required by EMTALA, they are mentioned in the State Operations Manual Interpretive Guidelines. They have been suggested as a way for specialized hospitals, such as pediatric hospitals, to expedite appropriate transfers of adults when necessary. They are useful because they allow for an established, well thought-out process before it is needed in the "heat of the moment." However, transfer agreements are not the panacea that some may hope. First, there may be little incentive, and perhaps a disincentive, for a receiving hospital to cooperate without payment issues being addressed. Second, having a transfer agreement does not guarantee acceptance of a patient, because EMTALA requires services (i.e., inpatient beds) to be granted on a "first come, first served basis." It is fundamentally discriminatory to give preference to one hospital over another in accepting transfers, and "holding beds" for this purpose will likely be construed as a violation of the section on "recipient hospital responsibilities" [42CFR§489.24(f)]. For these and other reasons, transfer agreements are rarely executed.

Other EMTALA Duties for Medicare-Participating Hospitals

Duty to Report [42CFR§489.20(m)]

A hospital must report to CMS or the state survey agency any time it has reason to believe it may have received an individual who has been transferred in an unstable EMC from another hospital in violation of EMTALA.

Whistle-Blower Protection [42CFR§489.24(e)(3)]

A participating hospital may not penalize or take adverse action against a physician or a qualified medical person because he or she refuses to authorize the transfer of an individual with an EMC who has not been stabilized, or against any hospital employee because the employee reports an EMTALA violation.

Only *hospitals* have the duty to report suspect violations, and then only for patients transferred *to them* (i.e., not for a refusal to accept an outgoing transfer). Although permitted to do so, physicians and hospital employees do not have a duty to report under EMTALA. However, they may have an obligation to report to hospital administration under hospital policy. Regardless, a hospital cannot take an adverse action against a physician or employee for complying with EMTALA or voluntarily reporting.

Signage Requirement [42CFR§489.20(q)(1)]

Hospitals must post conspicuously in any ED or in a place or places likely to be noticed by all individuals entering the ED, as well as those individuals waiting for examination and treatment in areas other than traditional EDs (i.e., entrance, admitting area, waiting room, treatment area), a sign specifying rights of individuals under EMTALA with respect to examination and treatment for EMCs and women in labor. Also, they must post conspicuously information indicating whether or not the hospital or rural primary care hospital participates in the Medicaid program under a state plan approved under Title XIX.

Maintenance of Information [42CFR§489.20(r)(1)]

Medical records related to individuals transferred to or from the hospital must be maintained for a period of 5 years from the date of the transfer. Also, a list of physicians who are on call for duty after the initial examination to provide treatment necessary to stabilize an individual with an EMC must be maintained, as well as a central log on each individual who comes to the ED seeking assistance and whether he or she refused treatment, was refused treatment, or was transferred, admitted and treated, stabilized and transferred, or discharged. Although perhaps not intuitively obvious, the "list of physicians on-call" must identify specific physicians' names (i.e., not the group name and not a mid-level provider taking "first call").

Although most hospitals keep medical records indefinitely, the statute of limitations for an EMTALA violation is 2 years [42USC§1395dd(d)(2)(C)], although penalties may be assessed up to 6 years [42USC§1320a-7(a)(c)(l)] after the incident.

State Operations Manual Interpretive Guidelines

The interpretive guidelines serve to interpret and clarify the responsibilities of Medicare participating hospitals in emergency cases. They contain authoritative interpretations and clarifications of statutory and regulatory requirements and are to be used to assist in making consistent determinations about a provider's compliance with the requirements. These interpretive guidelines merely define or explain the relevant statutes and regulations and do not impose any requirements that are not otherwise set forth in the statutes or regulations. The revised guidelines clarify and provide detailed interpretation of the EMTALA provisions located at 42CFR§489.24 and parts 489.20 (l), (m), (q), and (r).[26]

The Interpretative Guidelines assist state surveyors (those who investigate potential EMTALA violations) and providers to better understand how CMS will enforce EMTALA and conduct investigations. The Guidelines do not carry the force of law and are ignored by the courts. Nevertheless, they are an important resource in avoiding an EMTALA citation. There are a few areas in which the Guidelines appear to overreach the EMTALA statutes.

EMTALA Enforcement

An EMTALA investigation, and the resulting citation process, can be quite complicated and is beyond the scope of this chapter. However, it should be noted that defending oneself in an EMTALA action can be expensive, often exceeding the amount of the potential civil monetary penalty. Furthermore, Medicare participation termination is a reality for both hospitals and physicians and a potential financial "death sentence."

EMTALA enforcement is fundamentally a complaint-driven process, so the principle objective in managing EMTALA risk should be to avoid being investigated. This requires that hospitals take an aggressive, yet very conservative approach to EMTALA compliance and at times implement policies more restrictive than technically required by the statute. Also, because of its complexity, the challenge for EMTALA is to achieve fail-safe compliance, but not interrupt the usual and reasonable ED process (Tables 150–3 and 150–4).

Summary: Ten Strategies for Successful EMTALA Compliance

EMTALA continues to represent an ever-changing paradigm shift in how hospitals and physicians deliver emergency care and requires new ways of thinking, planning, and documentation.[11] Regardless of its complexities, solutions are relatively straightforward:

1. Hospitals and physicians must acknowledge EMTALA's existence and pervasiveness.
2. Area hospitals and medical staffs must act cooperatively because EMTALA compliance is impossible without cooperation from the medical staff leadership and hospital administration.

Table 150-3 EMTALA Principles for Hospital Staff and Emergency Physicians

Inquiries about Any Medical Condition on Hospital Property
- Ask, "Do you want to see a doctor?"
- If "Yes," take individual to the ED.

In the ED
- Log ALL patients.
- Provide MSE for ALL patients by a physician or a "qualified medical person."
- If not, document why (i.e., left without treatment, refused MSE and/or treatment).
- Treat ALL patients to a reasonable disposition in the ED.

Transfers
- Obtain acceptance from the receiving facility and complete a transfer form on ALL patients not otherwise being routinely discharged.
- Accept ALL transfers if the hospital has the capacity (bed available and ever done it before) to treat the presenting problem. If not, document why.

Reporting
- Set up a system for reporting suspicious transfers.
- Report ALL suspicious transfers to you.
- Document ALL incoming and outgoing transfers.

Table 150-4 EMTALA Principles for Medical Staff Physicians*

If you are called, you are chosen.
- Respond appropriately.
- The emergency physician dictates appropriateness unless or until you assume care of the patient.

Transfers
- Accept ALL incoming transfers if the hospital has the capacity (bed available and ever done it before) to treat the presenting problem. If not, document why.

ED Patient Outpatient Follow-Up
- Do what you agreed to do in your office or risk being required to always come to the ED.
- Do not demand payment up front or refer back to the ED if the patient is unable to pay or is a member of a noncontracted health plan. Do what the patient needs that day and make definitive arrangements for further care if necessary.
- **The best response to any inquiry from a hospital emergency department is, "How can I help you with this patient?"**

*These principles only apply when the physician is on call for the hospital emergency department.

3. Hospital EMTALA compliance policies and procedures, including forms, medical staff on-call responsibilities, and acceptance of patients in transfer, must be developed with extreme care.
4. Hospitals should require EMTALA education for anyone who may come into contact with individuals seeking medical care, including all hospital employees (nursing, ancillary, security, cafeteria, and administrative) and all medical staff.
5. Hospitals and physicians must document using the EMTALA paradigm, including appropriate legal terminology, new definitions of medical terms, and required norms and practices.
6. Hospital capabilities, including on-call services, must be defined and reviewed on a regular basis.
7. An in-house EMTALA compliance program should be created as part of the regular quality improvement process, and an EMTALA "hot line" should be established.
8. EMTALA issues must be addressed aggressively as they occur. It is not if, but when, so staff should prepare for an EMTALA investigation BEFORE it occurs by identifying resources. Preparing a model "corrective plan of action" may be worthwhile.
9. The emergency physicians are the hospital's first, best, and final defense against an EMTALA violation. They must be empowered to do whatever is necessary to mitigate a developing EMTALA situation at the time it occurs.
10. Hospitals and physicians should always "take care of the patient" first.

REFERENCES

1. American College of Emergency Physicians: EMTALA Fact Sheet. Dallas: American College of Emergency Physicians, 2005.
2. Kane CK: The impact of EMTALA on physician practices. AMA PCPS Report from 2001. Chicago: American Medical Association, 2003.
3. Testimony of Sen. Bob Dole (R–KS), co-sponsor of EMTALA. Congressional Record 28569, October 23, 1985.
4. Schiff RL, Ansell DA, Schlosser JE, et al: Transfers to a public hospital: a prospective study of 467 patients. N Engl J Med 314:552–557, 1986.
5. Himmelstein DU, Woolhandler S, Harnly M, et al: Patient transfers: medical practice as social triage. Am J Public Health 74:494–497, 1984.
6. Kerr HD, Byrd JC: Community hospital transfers to a VA Medical Center. JAMA 262:70–73, 1989.
7. Ansell DA, Schiff RL: Patient dumping: status, implications, and policy recommendations. JAMA 257:1500–1502, 1987.
8. Levine RJ, Guisto JA, Meislin HW, Spaite DW: Analysis of federally imposed penalties for violations of the Consolidated Omnibus Reconciliation Act. Ann Emerg Med 28:45–50, 1996.
9. Schiff RL, Ansell D: Federal anti-patient-dumping provisions: the first decade [Editorial]. Ann Emerg Med 28:77–78, 1996.
10. Centers for Medicare & Medicaid Services: Central Office Investigation Logs, June 2001. Washington, DC: Centers for Medicare & Medicaid Services, 2001.
*11. Bitterman RA: Providing Emergency Care Under Federal Law: EMTALA. Dallas: American College of Emergency Physicians, 2000.
12. Testimony of Rep. Pete Stark (D–CA), co-sponsor of EMTALA. Congressional Record 13903, October 23, 1985.
13. Testimony of Sen. David Durenberger (R–MN). Congressional Record 13903, October 23, 1985.
14. Nolan L, Vaquerano L, Regenstein M, Jones K: An assessment of the safety net in Phoenix, Arizona. In Walking a Tightrope: The State of the Safety Net in 10 U.S. Communities. Washington, DC: George Washington University School of Public Health and Health Services, Urgent Matters Program, 2004.
15. Richardson LD, Hwang U: America's health care safety net: intact or unraveling? Acad Emerg Med 8:1056–1063, 2001.
16. Fields W (ed): Defending America's Safety Net: 1998–99 Safety Net Task Force Report. Dallas: American College of Emergency Physicians, 1999.
17. Shactman D, Altman SH: Utilization & overcrowding of hospital emergency departments. Paper presented at the Council on the Economic Impact of Heath System Change, January 2002, Waltham, MA.
18. Medicare Modernization Act of 2003, PL 108-173, Sec. 1011: Payment for EMTALA services for undocumented aliens.
19. American Hospital Association: Annual Survey of Hospitals, 2003. Chicago: American Hospital Association, 2003.

*Selected readings.

20. American College of Emergency Physicians: Fact Sheet: Costs of Emergency Care. Dallas: American College of Emergency Physicians, 2003.
21. Vanlandingham B: On-Call Specialist Coverage in U.S. Emergency Departments—ED Director Survey. Dallas: American College of Emergency Physicians, 2004.
22. Johnson LA, Taylor TB, Lev R: The emergency department on-call backup crisis: finding remedies for serious public health problems. Ann Emerg Med 37:495–499, 1999.
23. Bitterman RA: Explaining the EMTALA paradox. Ann Emerg Med 40:470–475, 2002.
24. Burditt v U.S. Department of Health and Human Services, 934 F2d 1362 (5th Cir 1991).
25. Centers for Medicare & Medicaid Services: Appendix V. Interpretive Guidelines. *In* State Operations Manual. Washington, DC: Centers for Medicare & Medicaid Services, 2004.
26. Centers for Medicare & Medicaid Services: Revised Appendix V. Interpretive Guidelines: Responsibilities of Medicare Participating Hospitals in Emergency Cases—Introductory Letter, May 13, 2004. *In* State Operations Manual. Washington, DC: Centers for Medicare & Medicaid Services, 2004.

Chapter 151

Issues of Consent, Confidentiality and Minor Status

Cynthia R. Jacobstein, MD, MSCE

Key Points

Consent for medical care of minors may be waived in four general situations: emergency need for care, emancipated minor status, conditions covered by minor treatment statutes, and cases involving mature minor doctrines.

Minor treatment statutes and definitions of emancipation vary from state to state. The emergency physician should be familiar with the specific regulations of his or her state(s) of practice.

Minors are more likely to seek health care when they are assured of confidentiality. The provision of confidential care, when appropriate, should be practiced in the emergency department treatment of minors.

Psychosocial assessment is a key portion of the emergency department evaluation of most minors.

Introduction and Background

Minors commonly present to the emergency department (ED) for medical care. While adult guardians frequently accompany them, minors may also seek care in the ED on their own or without legal guardians. A 1991 study looking at ED visits by minors to pediatric and general EDs found that approximately 3% of the visits by minors were unaccompanied.[1] More recently, it has been estimated that this number may be even higher.[2] In addition, the reasons for which minors seek care in the ED often involve complex psychosocial issues, such as sexually transmitted infection (STI) or undiagnosed pregnancy. Thus, it is imperative that the emergency physician is knowledgeable about the issues related to consent in the treatment of minors.

A minor is defined as an individual who is younger than the age of consent. This age is 18 years in all but four states.[3] It is generally expected that informed consent by a parent or legal guardian will be obtained prior to medical treatment of minors. This requirement is not always easily or readily accomplished in the ED setting as minor patients may present alone or with adults other than their parents, such as teachers or day care providers.

Consent for medical care of minors may be waived for multiple reasons. Minors may be treated without the consent of a parent or guardian if they present with an emergency medical condition.[2-8] Emergency medical conditions include those with potential threat to life or limb, as well as conditions in which extreme pain is present or in which the potential for a harmful outcome exists if the condition is not immediately treated. Furthermore, there are a number of presenting complaints or conditions for which minors may seek and be granted health care without parental consent. These categories include mental health care; testing and treatment for STIs, including human immunodeficiency virus; contraceptive services; and drug and alcohol dependency treatment.[2-5,9] It is important to note that there are state-by-state variations with respect to the provision of confidential care for these treatment categories. The ED physician should be familiar with the laws of his or her state of practice regarding the treatment of such conditions. The GovSpot web site (Table 151–1) or individual state government web sites may serve as resources for this information. The Guttmacher Institute web site includes a table that lists the specific consent regulations for all 50 states.[3]

A subset of minors who may give their own consent for medical care are emancipated minors. Emancipated minors have living situations that suggest some degree of independence.[2-6,8-10] Examples of reasons for emancipation include marriage, military service, legal ruling, financial independence and residence apart from parents, and parenthood. As with the specific medical conditions for which minors may seek care without parental consent, the definition of emancipation varies from state to state. The GovSpot web site (see Table 151–1) or individual state government web sites may serve as resources for this information.

A further category of minors who may be allowed to consent to medical care is that of the mature minor.[2-7,9,10] A mature minor is generally 14 years of age or older and deemed mature enough to understand the risks, benefits, and treatment options of a given medical condition. Other factors

1062

Table 151–1	Web Sites/Links to Guidelines, Policies, and Laws on Minor Consent Issues
Web Site	**Organization**
www.ama-assn.org	American Medical Association (click on Policy Finder)
www.aap.org	American Academy of Pediatrics
www.saem.org	Society of Academic Emergency Medicine
www.guttmacher.org	The Guttmacher Institute: "The Alan Guttmacher Institute (AGI) is a nonprofit organization focused on sexual and reproductive health research, policy analysis and public education."
www.govspot.com	"GovSpot.com is a non-partisan government information portal designed to simplify the search for the best and most relevant government information online."

Note: The Guttmacher Institute site is included as a source of factual reference material only and does not represent the opinions of the authors and editors of this text.

that should be considered when deciding if a patient qualifies as a mature minor include the seriousness of the illness and the risks and benefits of potential therapies.

The provision of confidentiality in the treatment of minors in the ED is of utmost importance. The American Medical Association published a guideline for confidential health services for adolescents that outlines many of the important issues and recommendations regarding this topic.[11] In addition, a number of medical societies, including the American College of Obstetricians and Gynecologists, the American Academy of Pediatrics, and the American Academy of Family Physicians, support the provision of confidentiality to adolescents seeking health care.[17] The American College of Emergency Physicians also recognizes the importance of confidentiality in patient care but refers to confidentiality and the care of minors as a "problem area."[13,14]

Adolescents are more likely to seek medical care and provide a complete and true history if their confidentiality is respected.[11,15] Parents or guardians should be asked to leave the adolescent patient's room when sensitive areas of the history are being obtained. A discussion of the availability and limits of confidentiality should be held with all minors and their guardians prior to asking potentially personal information as part of the medical history. Reasons that confidentiality may be breeched include cases of potential injury to self (suicidality) or others (homicidality) or abuse. These exceptions should be included in discussions of confidentiality.

Issues

While the provision of confidentiality is of utmost importance to minors seeking care in the emergency department, situations often arise in which inclusion of a parent or guardian is essential to ensuring the best care for the minor. One example of such a scenario is the new diagnosis of pregnancy in a young adolescent. The treating physician may believe that it is in the minor's best interest to involve a mature adult

in the ongoing evaluation and care of such an issue. In cases such as this, the emergency physician should try to work with the teen to find a way to discuss the diagnosis with a parent or guardian. Possible solutions include having the physician tell the parent about the diagnosis with the adolescent's permission, involving another mature relative (e.g., older sister or aunt) who may help the minor with the issues at hand, or involving a social worker to help with the discussion and follow-up.

Other situations in which confidentiality may be inadvertently breached involve events that occur after the minor has been discharged from the ED. When there are pending test results at the time of discharge (e.g., STI results), it is important to discuss a follow-up plan with the adolescent. This may involve obtaining a mobile phone or pager number or some other way to reach the teen directly to discuss test results. Adolescent patients who are using the family insurance card should also be informed that their parents or guardians might receive an itemized bill that may contain specific information about the care provided, such as pregnancy or STI testing.

One difficult situation that may arise in the care of minors in the ED is the request by a parent or guardian to have their child tested for drug use. There are some situations in which ED testing for drug use is appropriate. It is reasonable to test for substance use when the goal to be achieved is the diagnosis of and subsequent referral for treatment for substance abuse. In such cases, it is expected that the adolescent would give informed consent regarding the testing to be performed. In general, involuntary testing in an adolescent who is thought to be capable of making informed judgments is not approved or recommended by the American Academy of Pediatrics.[16] Involuntary testing may be considered in cases in which the minor "lacks decision-making capacity" or in which "there are strong medical indications or legal requirements to do so."[16] Medical need for involuntary drug testing implies that identification of a particular substance would potentially avoid harm to the affected individual.

Solutions

The psychosocial assessment of minors in the ED is an extremely important part of their medical care. A thorough psychosocial interview often uncovers significant stressors or problems that might not otherwise be brought up by the adolescent patient, including but not limited to depression and suicidality. The mnemonics HEADSS (home, education, activities, drug use and abuse, sexual behavior, and suicidality and depression) and SHADSSS (school, home, activities, depression/self-esteem, substance abuse, sexuality, and safety) are helpful reminders of the important issues to be considered and discussed when providing medical care to minors in the emergency department.[17,18] The emergency physician must decide how much of the psychosocial assessment is necessary for any given patient care episode. At a minimum, it is important to consider the topics of safety, depression, and suicidality.

Summary

Treatment of minors in the ED often requires the emergency physician to consider and apply a number of legal and ethical principles that are unique to this patient population. The emergency physician needs to be familiar with consent and confidentiality issues with respect to the treatment of minors. These issues take on even greater importance with a number of more sensitive patient complaints, such as STIs, pregnancy, and mental health issues. It is vital that the physician be aware of the specific exceptions to standard consent issues when a minor presents for emergency care so that these may be incorporated into practice. Likewise, the importance of confidential care for adolescent minors, when appropriate, cannot be overemphasized. However, this should not preclude involving a parent or responsible adult in the care of minors when it is important to ensure the best possible outcome for the given problem. The emergency physician may need to work with the teen and other support personnel to find the best way to involve an adult in the care when it is deemed necessary.

REFERENCES

1. Treloar DJ, Peterson E, Randall J, et al: Use of emergency services by unaccompanied minors. Ann Emerg Med 20:297–301, 1991.
*2. American Academy of Pediatrics, Committee on Pediatric Emergency Medicine: Consent for emergency medical services for children and adolescents. Pediatrics 111:703–706, 2003.
3. Boonstra H, Nash E: Minors and the right to consent to health care. Guttmacher Rep Public Policy 3:4–8, 2000.

*4. Kassutto Z, Vaught W: Informed decision making and refusal of treatment. Clin Ped Emerg Med 4:285–291, 2003.
5. Jacobstein CR, Baren JM: Emergency department treatment of minors. Emerg Med Clin North Am 17:341–352, 1999.
6. Guertler AT: The clinical practice of emergency medicine. Emerg Med Clin North Am 15:303–313, 1997.
7. Sullivan DJ: Minors and emergency medicine. Emerg Med Clin North Am 11:841–851, 1993.
8. Tsai AK, Schafermeyer RW, Kalifon D, et al: Evaluation and treatment of minors: reference on consent. Ann Emerg Med 22:1211–1217, 1993.
9. Kuther TL: Medical decision-making and minors: issues of consent and assent. Adolescence 38:343–358, 2003.
10. English A: Treating adolescents: legal and ethical considerations. Med Clin North Am 74:1097–1112, 1990.
*11. American Medical Association, Council on Scientific Affairs: Confidential health services for adolescents. JAMA 269:1420–1424, 1993.
12. American College of Obstetricians and Gynecologists: ACOG Statement of Policy: Confidentiality in Adolescent Health Care. Washington, DC: American College of Obstetricians and Gynecologists, 1988.
13. American College of Emergency Physicians: Patient confidentiality. Ann Emerg Med 24:1209, 1994.
14. Larkin GL, Moskop J, Sanders A, et al: The emergency physician and patient confidentiality: a review. Ann Emerg Med 24:1161–1167, 1994.
15. Proimos J: Confidentiality issues in the adolescent population. Curr Opin Pediatr 9:325–328, 1997.
16. American Academy of Pediatrics, Committee on Substance Abuse: Testing for drugs of abuse in children and adolescents. Pediatrics 98:305–307, 1996.
17. Cohen E, Mackenzie RG, Yates GL: HEADSS, a psychosocial risk assessment instrument: implications for designing effective intervention programs for runaway youth. J Adolesc Health 12:539–544, 1991.
18. Clark LR, Ginsburg KR: How to talk to your teenage patients. Contemp Adolesc Gynecol Winter:23–27, 1995.

*Selected readings.

Chapter 152

Disaster Preparedness for Children

Stuart B. Weiss, MD and Ryan S. McCormick, BS, EMT-P

Key Points

Physicians caring for children during a mass casualty event will face challenges due to the unique anatomic, physiologic, cognitive, and behavioral characteristics of children.

The needs for pediatric mass casualty care are often inadequately addressed in hospital and community disaster plans.

All hospitals must adopt an incident management system that seamlessly integrates with community response agencies.

All facilities are equally at risk to receive large influxes of children during a disaster, so all emergency department staff must receive adequate education and training in mass casualty pediatric care.

Introduction and Background

Children are commonly involved as victims of both natural and man-made disasters. However, in many instances, hospital and community planners have not considered disasters that generate large numbers of sick or injured children.[1] Hospitals run exercises utilizing adult patient scenarios and rarely exercise with scenarios that include a pediatric patient surge. Government plans often lack specific sections that deal with the unique characteristics of mass casualty care for children.[2] As children constitute approximately 29% of the population in the United States, we can expect significant pediatric casualties in natural disasters.[3-11]

The growing problem with school violence has led to an increase in pediatric mass casualty events as well. In Columbine High School in Littleton, Colorado, on April 20, 1999, two students utilizing a combination of guns and homemade improvised explosive devices killed 14 students, seriously injured 23 others, and terrorized an entire community.[12] Since then, concern about school violence and incidents involving weapons being brought into schools has been increasing. It is reported that 17% of high school students carry a weapon (knife, gun, or club) to school and 5% carried a gun to school in the past month.[13]

With large numbers of children involved in natural disasters and increasing risk to children from terrorist events or school violence, it is imperative that emergency physicians play an active role in developing hospital and community plans that include policies and procedures for delivering care to large numbers of affected children

Emergency Medical Services (EMS) field triage may not distribute children to the correct receiving facility. Inadequate or incorrect triage of children may result in a mismatch of injuries to health care assets. In the Avianca Airline crash of 1990, for example, pediatric survivors were neither adequately triaged nor transported to appropriate facilities that could have optimized their care.[14]

Issues

Unique Characteristics of Children in Disasters

Children are uniquely susceptible to terrorist events and disasters due to a combination of anatomic, physiologic, developmental, and psychological characteristics.[2,15,16] Additional factors that complicate pediatric care include caregiver issues and facility issues.

Anatomic and Physiologic Differences

Children are shorter and therefore are closer to the ground, resulting in high doses of some chemicals and radiation. Many chemical agents (including some that are commonly listed as potential terrorist agents, such as Sarin, mustard, chlorine, and phosgene) are heavier than air[16] and would have a higher concentration closer to ground level. In addition, radiologic fallout material settles on the ground, emitting more radiation to children whose vital organs are closer to the particles. With certain types of cancer (e.g., thyroid cancer), children are especially more susceptible than adults.[17] In both of these cases, children would receive a higher dose of the agent than adults.

Children also have a proportionately larger body surface area–to-mass ratio than adults. For those agents that are absorbed through the skin, this results in a higher concentration per kilogram in an exposed child. Additionally, due to the larger surface area, children have a much higher risk for rapid body cooling and hypothermia if cold water is used during decontamination or if rapid drying and sheltering do not occur when decontamination is performed in cold environments.

Children's skin is less keratinized than adults' skin, resulting in potentially greater injury from vesicants and corrosives. In addition, children have an increased respiratory rate as compared with adults. This increased minute ventilation results in more rapid uptake and higher accumulated doses of a chemical, biologic, or radiologic agent by the lungs as well as a more rapid onset of effects.

Developmental and Psychological Differences

Due to physical developmental limitations, infants, toddlers, and young children may lack the motor skills to escape from the site of the disaster. For example, in the 2004 disaster in India and East Africa caused by tsunamis, young children were unable to grab onto stationary objects to prevent themselves from being swept underwater. Older children who may possess the motor skills to walk or evade the disaster may lack the cognitive ability to understand the events around them or appreciate the need to flee. Older children may also be frightened by the circumstances around them and refuse to cooperate with rescuers or will not take necessary protective actions, such as wearing a mask. Finally, curious children may actually migrate toward an event to better see a pretty colored gas, or to investigate noise or other chaos.

Caregiver Issues

Efforts are often made to keep children with their caregivers. This may result in pediatric emergency departments caring for adult patients or adult emergency departments caring for pediatric patients. In addition, most children older than 4 to 5 years spend most of their days away from their parents or caregivers in school or day care. In the devastating daytime earthquake in Armenia in December 1988, approximately 32,000 children were temporarily evacuated and had to be reunited with their parents at a later time.[18] Tremendous logistical challenges are involved with reuniting displaced children with their parents. Young children may not know their last name or address and may not have any identifying items on them. Finally, issues related to treating minors without parental consent must be addressed in advance.

Operational Issues

In a large-scale disaster, especially one with a multiagency response, an incident management system or incident command system (ICS) must be utilized to manage the many problems that arise and the varied resources that come into play. Several incident management systems have been developed and utilized. The system that has been most widely adopted for health care facilities has been the Hospital Incident Command System (HICS). It is vital that hospital systems adopt some type of formal incident management system so that they seamlessly integrate into the community ICS structure.

NIMS and ICS

The National Incident Management System (NIMS) is a federally mandated structure designed to assist responders with coordination and resource management during a disaster. One component of NIMS is the ICS, a standardized framework for organizing resources during an event. ICS was developed for the fire service in the 1970s based on sound, tested business practices adapted for the changing needs of emergency services. This version of ICS (fire ICS) has been widely adopted by fire departments and other public agencies across the country. To meet the needs of hospitals, in 1993 the HICS was developed.[19] Fire ICS and HICS are based on many of the same principles; however, HICS applies only to hospitals and was not widely adopted by other response agencies. Under a federal mandate issued in 2003, all response agencies must adopt the NIMS.[20] The HICS system is currently being adapted to meet NIMS requirements.[21]

ICS in Hospitals

During a public health emergency or disaster, hospitals may find themselves inundated with patients, medical professionals, and resources. If each is not managed effectively, chaos, misuse of resources, or poor patient care may result. Management practices and systems in place during daily operations may not be adequate to manage a disaster, which often requires higher levels of coordination, control, and communication. It also may be necessary for hospital leadership to work with and direct the actions of personnel and agencies they do not typically oversee. In order to effectively manage incidents, hospital leadership must utilize a standardized management and organizational system such as NIMS or HICS. The use of such a system will allow for easier integration of outside resources and leadership into the hospital organizational structure.

Several regulatory bodies require the adoption of an ICS. The Joint Commission on Accreditation of Healthcare Organizations requires that facilities adopt a command structure that links with that of the community.[22] Also, while the 2003 federal NIMS mandate does not specifically require hospitals to adopt NIMS, it does link future federal funding to NIMS compliance. Use of an ICS by hospital personnel assures that the hospital will better interface with local, state, and federal agencies during a crisis. Training in NIMS and the ICS is available in many formats, including self-study and on-line courses from the Federal Emergency Management Agency at *http://www.fema.gov/nims.*

Benefits of Adopting Standardized ICS

There are several advantages to adopting a standard ICS. First, an ICS utilizes a common vocabulary and terminology across all responding agencies. This eliminates any confusion about job titles and responsibilities. Similar positions in fire, police, EMS, or the hospital have the same job title and similar responsibilities.

Secondly, the ICS creates a uniform reporting hierarchy and employs a standardized set of job action sheets. HICS, for example, manages hospital responsibilities through predefined jobs with clearly written job action sheets. Job action sheets clearly outline the roles and responsibilities of each position in the HICS structure. When disasters occur, designated responders can quickly read an assigned job action sheet and immediately understand what is required of them.

Finally, the ICS provides a method for expanding and contracting the command staff based on the requirements of the crisis.

Facility Issues

While children make up 29% of the U.S. population,[7] they are essentially healthy and do not utilize a similar proportion of health care resources. In addition, while pediatric cases make up approximately 20% of emergency department volume,[23] few facilities have excess pediatric capacity to cover a pediatric patient surge. This results in fewer pediatric beds, fewer pediatric specialists, and less overall experience in pediatric critical care. Thus, in many regions of this country, a true pediatric disaster would result in a critical shortage of pediatric resources.[1]

Patient Care Issues

Change in Level of Patient Care

During a true disaster, a fundamental change in the level of patient care delivered within an affected region must take place. This unavoidable change must occur when the medical needs of the affected population overwhelm the available medical resources. In this scenario, caregivers must shift from their normal practice mode, in which maximal care is given to few people, to a disaster mode, in which minimal care is given to many people. This transition is difficult to achieve when dealing with adult victims and even more challenging with pediatric casualties. Clinicians must plan to implement true pediatric triage and a decreased level of care during a disaster. Some children who require significant health care resources, and might otherwise be saved, may not be resuscitated during a true disaster. This transition in level of care is extremely difficult for emergency department staff to make and must be discussed and practiced well in advance of a disaster.

Triage

In disasters that produce many casualties, it is necessary to quickly determine which patients have the most severe injuries and require immediate treatment versus those who have minor injuries and can wait for medical attention. This process of categorizing patients is called *triage*, a French word meaning "to sort." During a disaster, a more rapid type of triage is instituted to allow for the accelerated classification, treatment, and transport of patients.

The main goal of triage is to determine where the limited medical resources available during a disaster would best be applied. If triage is not performed properly, critical patients may be overlooked while less acute patients receive minor treatment. A clinical staff member should be assigned the role of triage as soon as multiple patients are discovered. This staff member does not necessarily have to be the most highly trained medical professional available. Triage can be effectively performed by a physician, a nurse, an emergency medical technician, or other allied health professionals trained in triage methods. There are two widely recognized triage systems in use today, Simple Triage and Rapid Treatment (START) for adult patients and JumpSTART for pediatric patients. Both triage systems use a combination of respiratory function, pulse, and neurologic function to determine triage classification. The original START system (Fig. 152–1) was developed for adults at Hogue Memorial Hospital in California.[24] It is universally used by EMS and other first responders to classify patients. Due to physiologic and cognitive differences between adults and children, the START system was modified to be appropriate for pediatric patients. This modified system is called JumpSTART[25] (Fig. 152–2). Both systems require training and practice prior to an actual disaster to be efficient (see Chapter 155, Triage).

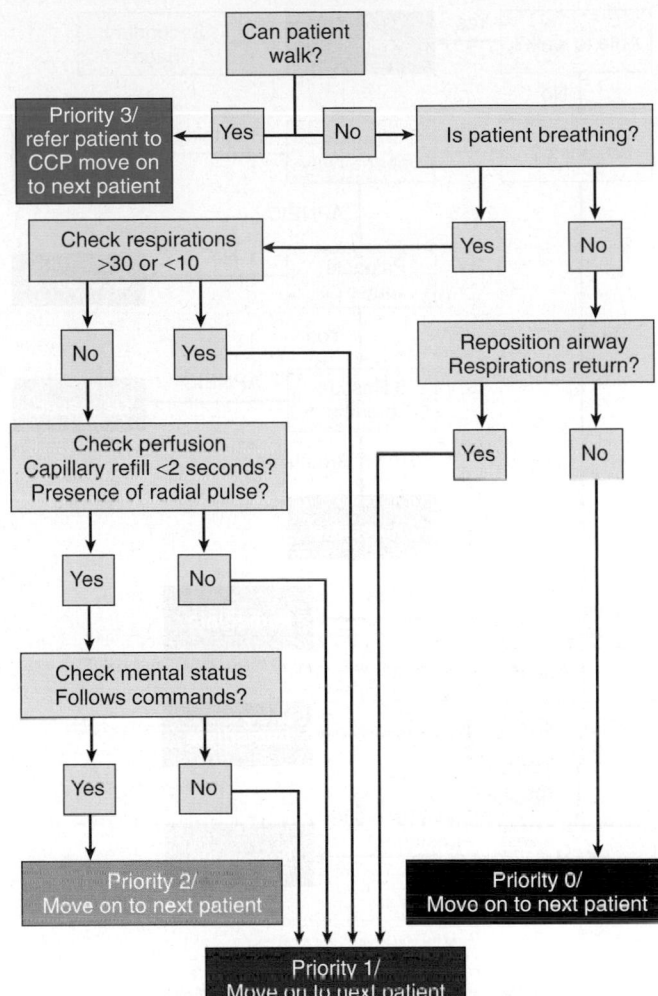

FIGURE 152–1. The Simple Triage and Rapid Treatment system (START) was developed by the Newport Beach Fire Department and Hoag Memorial Hospital. The system uses clinically significant objective findings to sort patients into four categories based on severity. Abbreviation: CCP, casualty collection point.

Chemical, Biologic, and Radiologic Agents

For quite some time, bacteria, viruses, biologic toxins, and toxic chemicals have been used by military forces to gain an advantage over an enemy.[26] Currently, considerable concern surrounds their possible use on civilian populations.[27-29] A chemical attack tends to be an acute, obvious event. Typically, the onset of signs and symptoms is rapid, the event is quickly recognized, and there is a "lights and sirens" response from traditional first responders (police, fire, and EMS). In contrast, a covert biologic attack would occur as a slow, insidious event that would present as a public health crisis. Depending on the incubation period of the agent utilized, there may be some delay in onset of illness. As a result, people may travel far from the initial release site and, if the disease is contagious, may transmit it to others. First responders in this case will be emergency departments, clinics, pediatricians, and other physicians. Radiologic events may have characteristics of either a chemical or a biologic event depending on the method of dispersement of the radioactive material. Events involving an explosive dispersal of radioactive material will have an obvious, sudden onset. Events in which

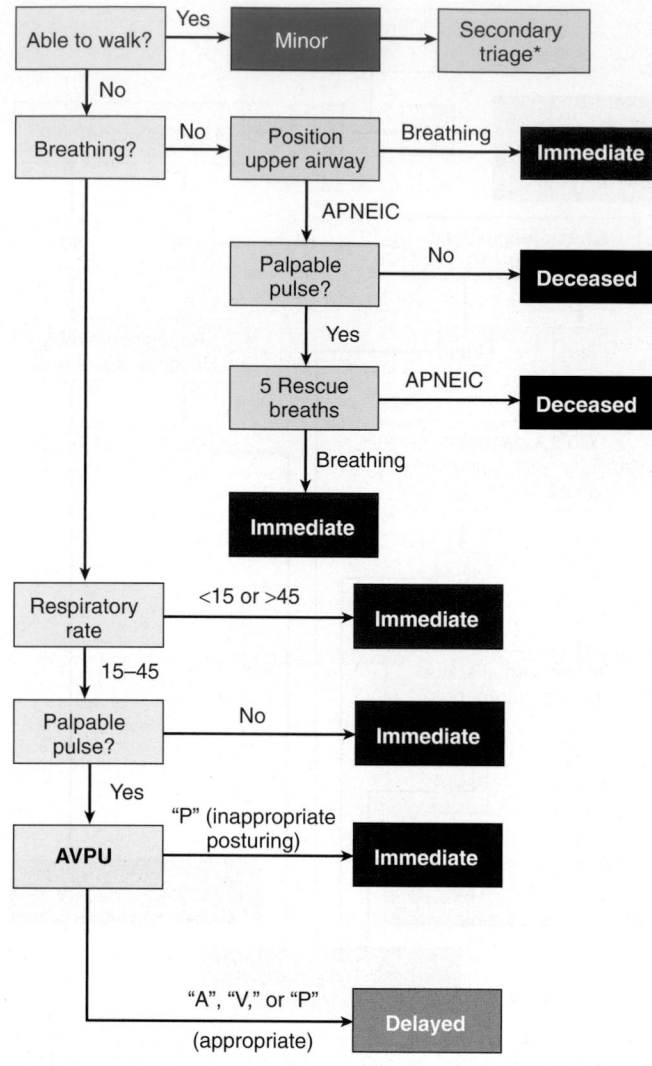

*Evaluate infants first in secondary triage using the entire JS algorithm

FIGURE 152–2. The JumpSTART Triage algorithm was designed as a method to triage pediatric patients. The system can be used for any patient 1 to 8 years of age. Abbreviation: AVPU, alert, responsive to verbal stimuli, inappropriate posturing, unresponsive.

radioactive material is surreptitiously spread in the environment may appear insidiously, similar to a biologic event.

Emergency physicians caring for childhood victims of biologic, chemical, or radiologic attacks will encounter some pediatric-specific problems. For example, many of the drugs helpful in treating casualties are not commonly used in children, while others are not available in pediatric formulations or have relative contraindications. There is also a lack of widely accepted pediatric-specific guidelines for the treatment of these victims.

Biologic Agents

Biologic agents have the potential to create large numbers of casualties that could quickly overwhelm the medical delivery system. In the past, large numbers of people have died as a result of naturally occurring disease outbreaks. Intentional outbreaks could have similar results. While virtually any microorganism could be used as a biologic weapon, most

would be difficult to weaponize and disseminate effectively. A Centers for Disease Control and Prevention (CDC) working group has considered which biologic agents would constitute the gravest threats to public health and classified the agents into three groups.[30] This categorization is based on a combination of factors including availability, potential for morbidity and mortality, and ease of dissemination.[31] Category A agents have the highest potential for use as a biologic weapon, and category C agents have the lowest. These agents are listed in Table 152–1.

Most of the category A agents have been the subject of comprehensive reviews. Treatment recommendations for all agents are evolving. The CDC maintains a web site (*http://www.bt.cdc.gov*) and a 24-hour hot line (1-770-488-7100) that provide the latest disease reviews and treatment recommendations.

Fluoroquinolones and/or tetracyclines are considered drugs of choice for the treatment of anthrax, plague, and tularemia. Although there may be some hesitation in using these antibiotics in pediatric patients, considerable recent experience has demonstrated their appropriateness in selected serious pediatric infections.[32-34] Ciprofloxacin use in children had been questioned due to a theoretical risk of cartilage damage based on animal studies; however, this medication appears to be relatively free from this adverse effect. Doxycycline was also questioned due to its potential to stain teeth. However, this risk also appears to be low. Overall, the potential morbidity and mortality from these category A agents far outweighs the minor risks associated with the short-term use of these medications.[35]

Chemical Agents

Chemical warfare dates back to antiquity. Chemical agents are classified into several broad classes as listed in Table 152–2. Many of these chemicals are used in industry and are transported on our roadways on a daily basis. For others, there are recipes readily available on the Internet and in published books. The toxic effect of these chemicals may occur through topical injury to skin, eyes, or mucous membranes, or through systemic absorption via dermal or respiratory means.[2]

When treating chemically contaminated patients, the initial crucial step is to determine what level of personal protective equipment (PPE) is required by health care workers. In previous chemical events, health care workers have been injured by chemical vapors from victim's clothing.[36] Before initiating treatment in these circumstances, proper PPE must be utilized. EMS crews must not be allowed to bring contaminated victims into the emergency department. Once the proper PPE is worn, resuscitation and decontamination efforts can begin. Removing clothing eliminates between 75% and 90% of contaminate.[37] This can then be followed by showering with warm water and soap. There is no proven benefit to the use of diluted bleach solution over soap and water, as bleach may act as a skin irritant.[26] It should not be used in civilian decontamination efforts.

To reduce the risk of hypothermia in children, warm water must be used in the decontamination process. In addition, there must be the ability to rapidly dry and warm pediatric victims if decontamination is occurring in a cold environment.

Contaminated clothing must be double-bagged and either placed outside or far away from the decontamination process.

Table 152–1   Potential Bioterrorism Agents

Category A

The U.S. public health system and primary health care providers must be prepared to address varied biologic agents, including pathogens that are rarely seen in the United States. High-priority agents include organisms that pose a risk to national security because they:
- can be easily disseminated or transmitted person-to-person
- cause high mortality, with potential for major public health impact
- might cause public panic and social disruption
- require special action for public health preparedness

Category A agents include:
- Anthrax (*Bacillus anthracis*)
- Botulism *(Clostridium botulinum* toxin)
- Plague (*Yersinia pestis*)
- Smallpox (variola major)
- Tularemia (*Francisella tularensis*)
- Viral hemorrhagic fevers
- Filoviruses
  - Ebola hemorrhagic fever
  - Marburg hemorrhagic fever
- Arenaviruses
  - Lassa (Lassa fever)
  - Junin (Argentine hemorrhagic fever)
  - Machupo (Bolivian hemorrhagic fever)
  - Guanarito (Venezuelan hemorrhagic fever)
  - Sabia (Brazilian hemorrhagic fever)

Category B

Second highest priority agents include those that:
- are moderately easy to disseminate
- cause moderate morbidity and low mortality
- require specific enhancements of CDC's diagnostic capacity
- require enhanced disease surveillance

Category B agents include:
- *Brucellosis (Brucella* species)
- Epsilon toxin of *Clostridium perfringens*
- Glanders (*Burkholderia malle*)
- Melioidosis (*Burkholderia pseudomallei*)
- Psittacosis (*Chlamydia psittaci*)
- Q fever (*Coxiella burnetti*)
- Ricin toxin from *Ricinus communis* (castor beans)
- Staphylococcal enterotoxin B
- Typhus fever (*Rickettsia prowazekii*)
- Viral encephalitis (alphaviruses)
  - Venezuelan encephalomyelitis
  - Eastern and Western equine encephalomyelitis

A subset of List B agents includes pathogens that are food- or waterborne. These pathogens include but are not limited to:
- *Salmonella* species
- *Shigella dysenteriae*
- *Escherichia coli* O157:H7
- *Vibrio cholerae*
- *Cryptosporidium parvum*

Category C

Third highest priority agents include emerging pathogens that could be engineered for mass dissemination in the future because of:
- availability
- ease of production and dissemination
- potential for high morbidity and mortality and major health impact

Category C agents include:
- Nipah virus
- Hantaviruses
- Multidrug-resistant tuberculosis
- Tickborne hemorrhagic fever viruses
- Tickborne encephalitis viruses
- Yellow fever

Preparedness for List C agents requires ongoing research to improve disease detection, diagnosis, treatment, and prevention. Knowing in advance which newly emergent pathogens might be employed by terrorists is not possible; therefore, linking bioterrorism preparedness efforts with ongoing disease surveillance and outbreak response activities as defined in CDC's emerging infectious disease strategy is imperative.

Abbreviation: CDC, Centers for Disease Control and Prevention.
Modified from Centers for Disease Control and Prevention: Bioterrorism Agents/Diseases. Available at *http://www.bt.cdc.gov/agent/agentlist-category.asp* (accessed September 2005).

These clothes may have trapped chemicals on them that could pose a continuing threat to health care workers.

The major classes of chemical agents that have been used or are likely to be used are listed in Table 152–2, which includes examples of each chemical and common antidotes. Although these chemicals are often listed as potential terrorist agents, there are many tons of equally harmful industrial chemicals in our communities that could be intentionally or accidentally released. Some of the largest chemical events in the past have resulted from the accidental release of industrial chemicals used in manufacturing (methylisocyanate in Bhopal, India; hydrofluoric acid release in Texas, etc.). In order to adequately assess risks in the community and plan for chemical disasters, it is important to perform an analysis of industry in the area. Companies are required to disclose the types and quantities of dangerous chemicals that are used. This information is available through the local Office of Emergency Management. By utilizing this information, the proper level of PPE can be selected, antidotes can be identified, and required resources can be determined.

One of the major categories of agents that has received much attention recently is nerve agents. These agents are organophosphate compounds that act as potent inhibitors of acetylcholinesterase, similar in action to organophosphate insecticides.[16] Common cholinergic signs and symptoms are listed in Table 152–3. Overall treatment focuses on airway and ventilatory support, aggressive use of antidotes, prompt control of seizures, and decontamination. Treatment for nerve agents includes atropine, pralidoxime, and a benzodiazepine (for control of seizures in significant exposures). While there is a commonly discussed and widely stocked nerve agent antidote kit for adult exposure (MARK I kit), a similar kit for children is not available in the United States.

In 2003, the Food and Drug Administration (FDA) approved a pediatric atropine autoinjector.[38] The AtroPen now comes in three strengths: AtroPen 2 mg (green) for adults and children weighing over 90 pounds, AtroPen 1 mg (dark red) for children weighing 40 to 90 pounds (generally 4 to 10 years of age), and AtroPen 0.5 mg (blue) for children weighing 15 to 40 pounds (generally 6 months to 4 years).[39] Currently, there is no approved pediatric 2-PAM autoinjector. While it would be optimal to use the appropriate AtroPen for the size of the child, most EMS agencies in the United States only stock the adult MARK I kits, which contain the 2-mg AtroPen autoinjector. In dire circumstances, the use of adult MARK I kits (with 0.8-inch needles and 2 mg of atropine and 600 mg of pralidoxime) might be useful in children older than 2 to 3 years of age or weighing more than 13 kg.[26] During the Gulf War in 1991, 240 Israeli children, none of whom was exposed to nerve agents, were evaluated due to accidental atropine injection by an autoinjector. While some had systemic anticholinergic effects, there were no deaths, severe dysrhythmias, or seizures.[40] The use of adult MARK I kits in children during extreme emergencies is summarized in Table 152–4.

Although nerve agents are most often discussed and MARK I kits are stocked by first response agencies across the United States, there may be multiple other chemicals present in the community that pose a risk to the population. As treatment guidelines for chemical exposures continue to evolve, there are several sources of valuable information. The CDC

Table 152–2 Potential Chemical Agents for Use in Chemical Terrorism*

Class	Examples	Interventions[†]	Antidotes
Nerve agents	Tabun Sarin Soman VX	Respiratory support, skin decontamination	Atropine, pralidoxime, diazepam
Vesicants	Mustard gas	Respiratory support, skin and eye decontamination	
	Nitrogen mustard	Respiratory support, skin and eye decontamination	Nebulized albuterol
Irritants/corrosives	Chlorine Bromine Ammonia		
Choking agents	Phosgene	Respiratory support	
Cyanogens	Hydrogen cyanide	Cardiorespiratory support	Amyl nitrate, sodium nitrite, sodium thiosulfate
Incapacitating agents			
CNS depressants	Cannabinoids Barbiturates	Respiratory support	
Anticholinergics	3-Quinuclidinyl benzilate (BZ)		Physostigmine
Lacrimators	Capsaicin		

*Chemical agents that might be used by terrorists range from warfare agents to toxic chemicals commonly used in industry. Criteria for determining the high-priority chemical agents include chemical agents already known to be used as weaponry, agents that are available to potential terrorists, agents likely to cause major morbidity or mortality, agents with a high potential for causing public panic and social disruption, and agents that require special action for public health preparedness.
[†]Note: Decontamination includes rapid removal of clothing and washing with soap and warm water. Health care workers must protect themselves adequately from the chemical agent before initiating patient care.

Table 152–3 Cholinergic Signs and Symptoms

Muscarinic Effects

Glands (increased secretions)
 Saliva (drooling)
 Tears
 Airway secretions
 Runny nose
 Sweating
 Gastrointestinal secretions (diarrhea)
Smooth muscles
 Eyes: miosis (pinpoint pupils)
 Airways: bronchoconstriction
 Gastrointestinal: hyperactivity (nausea, vomiting, diarrhea)

Nicotinic Effects

Skeletal muscles
 Fasciculations
 Twitching
 Weakness
 Paralysis
Ganglia
 Tachycardia
 Hypertension

Other

Cardiovascular
 Tachycardia or bradycardia
 Arrhythmias
Central Nervous System
 Loss of consciousness
 Seizures
 Apnea
 Prolonged psychological effects

maintains a 24-hour hot line for health care providers at 1-770-488-7100 and a website at *http://www.bt.cdc.gov.* In addition, one may consult the local poison control center at 1-800-222-1222 (same number everywhere in the United States).

Radiologic Agents

Radiologic exposure can be either accidental or intentional. Accidental exposures include nuclear power plant releases and unintentional exposure to radiologic sources. Intentional acts may result from terrorism or military conflict.

Radiologic disasters can be grouped into four categories:

Detonation of a nuclear weapon. While this is possible, it is considered unlikely due to the sophistication of such devices and the intrinsic difficulties in producing a successful nuclear fission explosion.

Damage to a facility that contains radioactive material (such as nuclear power plants, facilities that make radioactive materials for medical use, and nuclear waste reprocessing plants). This may result in the release of radioactive substances into the environment.

Explosion of a radiologic dispersal device ("dirty bomb"). These devices use conventional explosives to spread radioactive material over a large area. This is considered to be the most likely terrorist scenario involving radiologic materials.

Radiologic source left unshielded in a public place. Many highly radioactive materials are used in industry. For example, potent radiologic agents are used to examine pipe welds. There have been examples of the accidental loss of these agents with the subsequent radiologic exposure of unsuspecting people.

Proper management of a child with a radiologic injury depends on the type of exposure (whole body or partial), the amount of radiation exposure, and the presence of other associated injuries. An important early step in managing a radiologic exposure victim is determining whether the victim is simply exposed, or contaminated and exposed. An exposed victim is one who receives a dose of radiation without coming into physical contact with the source material. Once

Table 152–4   MARK I Autoinjector Usage

Note: Each MARK I kit contains 2 autoinjectors (0.8-inch needle insertion depth), one each of atropine 2 mg (0.7 ml) and pralidoxime 600 mg (2 ml). While not approved for pediatric use, they should be used as initial treatment in circumstances for children with severe, life-threatening nerve agent toxicity for whom intravenous treatment is not possible or available or for whom more precise intramuscular (mg/kg) dosing would be logistically impossible. Suggested dosing guidelines are offered below; note potential excess of initial atropine and pralidoxime dosage for age/weight, although within general guidelines for recommended total over first 60 to 90 minutes of therapy for severe exposures. Although this table describes usage of the MARK I kit for children 3 years and older based on adherence to recommended dosages for atropine and pralidoxime, following an actual nerve agent exposure if a MARK I kit is the only available source of atropine and pralidoxime, it should not be withheld from even the youngest child based on weight-based dosing guidelines.

Approximate Age (yr)	Approximate Weight (kg)	No. of Autoinjectors (Each Type)	Atropine Dosage Range (mg/kg)	Pralidoxime Dosage Range (mg/kg)
3–7	13–25	1	0.08–0.13	24–46
8–14	26–50	2	0.08–0.13	24–46
>14	>51	3	0.11 or less	35 or less

- Atropine: 0.05 mg/kg IV, IM (min. 0.1 mg, max. 5 mg), repeat q2–5min prn for marked secretions, bronchospasm
- Pralidoxime: 25 mg/kg IV, IM* (max. 1 g IV; 2 g IM), may repeat within 30–60 min prn, then again q1h for 1 or 2 doses; 0.2 mg/kg prn for persistent weakness, high atropine requirement
- Diazepam: 0.3 mg/kg (max. 10 mg) IV
- Lorazepam: 0.1 mg/kg IV, IM (max. 4 mg)
- Midazolam: 0.2 mg/kg (max. 10 mg) IM prn for seizures or severe exposure

*Pralidoxime is reconstituted to 50 mg/ml (1 g in 20 ml water) for IV administration, and the total dose is infused over 30 minutes, or may be given by continuous infusion (loading dose 25 mg/kg over 30 minutes, then 10 mg/kg/hr). For IM use, it might be diluted to a concentration of 300 mg/ml (1 g added to 3 ml water—by analogy to the U.S. Army's MARK I autoinjector concentration), to effect a reasonable volume for injection.
Adapted from Henretig FM, Cieslak TJ, Eitzen EM: Biological and chemical terrorism. J Pediatr 141:311–326, 2002.

this person is removed from the source of radiation, they are no longer subject to irradiation. A good example of this would be patients who have had a chest radiograph taken. While they are exposed to x-ray radiation, they are not contaminated, are not radioactive, and do not pose a threat to health care workers. These patients do not require decontamination as they do not have any radioactive material on them.

Contaminated victims, in contrast, actually have radioactive material on them and continue to be exposed to radiation even when removed from the event site. They may contaminate other surfaces or health care workers and must be decontaminated to reduce the risk to themselves and others. As with adults, the first step in decontamination of children is removing clothing. In many cases, this will eliminate up to 90% of contaminated particles. Contaminated clothing must be moved as far away from health care workers and victims as possible so as not to further expose individuals to radiation. It is important to remember that putting this clothing in a plastic bag is not an adequate shield from the radiation. In addition, it is important not to create a large pile of contaminated clothing as this will create a large irradiating source.

The initial care of the radiologically injured patient involves treating any associated trauma or medical problems. Caring for his or her radiation injuries is secondary to the other medical needs. One caveat to remember is that all necessary surgery must be completed within 48 hours of a large exposure before immunosuppression and wound healing impairment prevents surgical intervention for up to 3 months.[41]

Table 152–5 lists commonly used treatments for radiation injuries. Consultation in the care of radiologically injured patients can be obtained at any time from the Radiation Emergency Assistance Center/Training Site at the Oak Ridge Institute for Science and Education at 1-865-576-1005.

Table 152–5   Radionuclide Treatment Options

Radionuclide	Radioprotectant
Americium (^{241}Am)	Diethylenetriamine pentaacetic acid (DTPA)
Californium (^{252}Cf)	DTPA
Cesium (^{137}Cs)	Prussian blue, sodium polystyrene sulfonate
Cobalt (^{60}Co)	Laxatives*
Curium (^{244}Cm)	DTPA
Iodine (^{131}I)	Potassium iodide (KI)
Iridium (^{192}Ir)	Unknown
Plutonium (^{238}Pu; ^{239}Pu)	DTPA
Radium (^{226}Ra)	Common antacids, barium sulfate
Strontium (^{90}Sr)	Common antacids, barium sulfate
Technetium (^{99m}Tc)	DTPA
Thallium (^{201}Tl)	Prussian blue
Uranium (^{235}U; ^{238}U)	Common antacids
High radiation dose	Filgrastim, amifostine, antiemetics, Neumune, 5-AED
Gastrointestinal uptake of radionuclides	Laxatives, sodium polystyrene sulfonate

*Little information is available on treatment options. One should also consider EDTA, N-acetyl-L-cysteine, or penicillamine.
From New Jersey Center for Public Health Preparedness: Radiological Countermeasures: Candidates for Inclusion in a State Stockpile. White paper, 2005.

There are some additional issues concerning potassium iodide (KI). Many people are under the misconception that KI is indicated as a general radiation antidote. There has been much press about this medication in the past few years. The only indication for this medication is in the prevention of thyroid cancer in releases of radioactive iodine (^{131}I). Radioactive iodine is most likely to be released from a nuclear reactor accident. For this reason, the Nuclear Regulatory Commission has directed that KI be included in the emergency planning for the residents in areas 10 miles around a nuclear plant.[42] This is in order to facilitate the rapid administration of KI to affected residents. It is unlikely that radiologic dispersal devices or "dirty bombs" will contain ^{131}I due to the difficulty in obtaining large quantities of radioactive iodine and the short half-life of the material. Therefore, in these exposures, KI is not indicated.

KI blocks the uptake of radioactive iodine by saturating the thyroid with nonradioactive iodine. In order for KI to be effective, the correct dose must be taken quickly, preferably within 2 hours of exposure. The protective effect of KI lasts approximately 24 hours, so additional doses may be required if continuing exposure to radioactive iodine is expected.

Current recommendations for the safe and effective use of KI to prevent the uptake of radioiodine by the thyroid are based on a review of data from the Chernobyl nuclear accident in 1986 where large amounts of ^{131}I were released into the atmosphere. Following the event, thyroid cancers in Belarus, Ukraine, and the Russian Federation skyrocketed. In neighboring Poland, where KI was used in 10.5 million children less than 16 years old and in 7 million adults, there was a significant decrease in cancer rates. As the risk of thyroid cancer is inversely proportional to age, it is essential to make KI available to children.[43]

Table 152–6 lists the current FDA recommendations for the use of KI during an emergency. The following caveats should be kept in mind:

1. Neonates who receive KI must be monitored for hypothyroidism by measuring thyroid-stimulating hormone and free thyroxine. Thyroid hormone replacement must be initiated in cases in which hypothyroidism develops to protect critical neurologic development.

2. Pregnant females should be given KI for their own protection and for that of the fetus, as iodine readily crosses the placenta. However, because of the risk of blocking fetal thyroid function with excess stable iodine, repeat dosing with KI should be avoided. Lactating females should be given KI for their own protection and potentially to reduce the concentration of radioiodine in their breast milk, but not as a means to deliver KI to infants, who should get their KI directly. Iodine as a component of breast milk may also pose a risk of hypothyroidism in nursing neonates. Therefore, repeat dosing of KI should be avoided in lactating mothers, except during continuing severe contamination. If repeat dosing of the mother is necessary, the nursing neonate should be monitored for hypothyroidism as noted above.

Tables 152–7 and 152–8 outline methods for preparing KI solutions for children using the 130-mg tablets and the 65-mg tablets, respectively.[44] During an emergency, high accuracy in dosing is less important than rapidly administering KI to affected populations.

Solutions

Caring for children during a mass casualty event or disaster poses many challenges. Whether childhood casualities are the result of an accident, a natural phenomenon, or an inten-

Table 152–6	Threshold Thyroid Radioactive Exposures and Recommended Doses of KI for Different Risk Groups—U.S. Food and Drug Administration (FDA)				
	Predicted Thyroid Exposure(cGy)	KI Dose (mg)	# of 130-mg Tablets	# of 65-mg Tablets
Adults >40 yr	≥500	130	1	2
Adults >18–40 yr	≥10	130	1	2
Pregnant or lactating women	≥5	130	1	2
Adolescents >12–18 yr*	≥5	65	$1/2$	1
Children >3–12 yr	≥5	65	$1/2$	$1/4$
Over 1 mo–3 yr	≥5	32	$1/4$	$1/2$
Birth–1 mo	≥5	16	$1/8$	$1/4$

*Adolescents approaching adult size (≥ 70 kg) should receive the full adult dose (130 mg).

The protective effect of KI lasts approximately 24 hours. For optimal prophylaxis, KI should therefore be dosed daily, until a risk of significant exposure to radioiodines by either inhalation or ingestion no longer exists. Individuals intolerant of KI at protective doses, and neonates and pregnant and lactating women (in whom repeat administration of KI raises particular safety issues; see below) should be given priority with regard to other protective measures (i.e., sheltering, evacuation, and control of the food supply).

Note that adults over 40 need to take KI only in the case of a projected large internal radiation dose to the thyroid (>500 cGy) to prevent hypothyroidism.

These recommendations are meant to provide states and local authorities as well as other agencies with the best current guidance on safe and effective use of KI to reduce thyroidal radioiodine exposure and thus the risk of thyroid cancer. FDA recognizes that, in the event of an emergency, some or all of the specific dosing recommendations may be very difficult to carry out given their complexity and the logistics of implementation of a program of KI distribution. The recommendations should therefore be interpreted with flexibility as necessary to allow optimally effective and safe dosing given the exigencies of any particular emergency situation. In this context, we offer the following critical general guidance: ***across populations at risk for radioiodine exposure, the overall benefits of KI far exceed the risks of overdosing, especially in children, though we continue to emphasize particular attention to dose in infants.***

These FDA recommendations differ from those put forward in the World Health Organization (WHO) 1999 guidelines[†] for iodine prophylaxis in two ways. WHO recommends a 130-mg dose of KI for adults and adolescents (over 12 years). For the sake of logistical simplicity in the dispensing and administration of KI to children, FDA recommends a 65-mg dose as standard for all school-age children while allowing for the adult dose (130 mg, 2 × 65-mg tablets) in adolescents approaching adult size. The other difference lies in the threshold for predicted exposure of those up to 18 years of age and of pregnant or lactating women that should trigger KI prophylaxis. WHO recommends a threshold of 1 cGy for these two groups. As stated earlier, FDA has concluded from the Chernobyl data that the most reliable evidence supports a significant increase in the risk of childhood thyroid cancer at exposures of 5 cGy or greater.

[†]World Health Organization: Guidelines for Prophylaxis Following Nuclear Accidents: Update. Geneva: World Health Organization, 1999.
Modified from Food and Drug Administration, Center for Drug Evaluation and Research: Guidance: Potassium Iodide as a Thyroid Blocking Agent in Radiation Emergencies. Washington, DC: Food and Drug Administration, 2001.

Table 152–7	Preparation of Potassium Iodide Solution for Children

Preparation Using 130-mg Potassium Iodide Tablet

1. Put **one** 130-mg potassium iodide tablet into a small bowl and grind it into a fine powder using the back of the metal teaspoon against the inside of the bowl. The powder should not have any large pieces.
2. Add four teaspoonfuls (20 ml) of water to the potassium iodide powder in the small bowl. Use a spoon to mix them together until the potassium iodide powder is dissolved in the water.
3. Add four teaspoonfuls of raspberry syrup, low-fat chocolate milk, juice, or flat soda* to the potassium iodide powder and water mixture described in Step 2.

The amount of potassium iodide in the drink is 16.25 mg per teaspoon (5 ml).

Dosing Guidelines

(This is the amount for **one** dose. Repeat daily doses may be indicated.)

Newborn–1 mo of age: Give 1 teaspoon (5 ml)
2 mo–3 yr of age: Give 2 teaspoons (10 ml)
4–17 yr of age: Give 4 teaspoons (20 ml)
Children over 70 kg (154 pounds) should receive one 130-mg tablet or 8 teaspoons.

Notes

*To see what worked best to disguise the taste of potassium iodide, FDA asked adults to taste the following six mixtures of potassium iodide and drinks: water, low-fat white milk, low-fat chocolate milk, orange juice, flat soda (e.g., cola), and raspberry syrup. The mixture of potassium iodide with raspberry syrup disguised the taste of potassium iodide best. The mixtures of potassium iodide with low-fat chocolate milk, orange juice, and flat soda generally had an acceptable taste. Low-fat white milk and water did not hide the salty taste of potassium iodide.

   Potassium iodide in any of the six drinks listed above and in infant formulas will keep for up to 7 days in the refrigerator. FDA recommends that the potassium iodide drink mixtures be prepared weekly; unused portions should be discarded.

Table 152–8	Preparation of Potassium Iodide Solution for Children

Preparation Using 65-mg Potassium Iodide Tablet

1. Put **one** 65-mg potassium iodide tablet into a small bowl and grind it into a fine powder using the back of the metal teaspoon against the inside of the bowl. The powder should not have any large pieces.
2. Add four teaspoonfuls (20 ml) of water to the potassium iodide powder in the small bowl. Use a spoon to mix them together until the potassium iodide powder is dissolved in the water.
3. Add four teaspoonfuls of raspberry syrup, low-fat chocolate milk, juice, or flat soda* to the potassium iodide powder and water mixture described in Step 2.

The amount of potassium iodide in the drink is 8.125 mg per teaspoon (5 ml).

Dosing Guidelines

(This is the amount for **one** dose. Repeat daily doses may be indicated.)

Newborn–1 mo of age: Give 2 teaspoons (10 ml)
2 mo–3 yr of age: Give 4 teaspoons (20 ml)
4–17 yr of age: Give 8 teaspoons (40 ml) or one 65-mg tablet
Children over 70 kg (154 pounds) should receive two 65-mg tablet or 16 teaspoons.

Notes

*To see what worked best to disguise the taste of potassium iodide, FDA asked adults to taste the following six mixtures of potassium iodide and drinks: water, low-fat white milk, low-fat chocolate milk, orange juice, flat soda (e.g., cola), and raspberry syrup. The mixture of potassium iodide with raspberry syrup disguised the taste of potassium iodide best. The mixtures of potassium iodide with low-fat chocolate milk, orange juice, and flat soda generally had an acceptable taste. Low-fat white milk and water did not hide the salty taste of potassium iodide.

   Potassium iodide in any of the six drinks listed above and in infant formulas will keep for up to 7 days in the refrigerator. FDA recommends that the potassium iodide drink mixtures be prepared weekly; unused portions should be discarded.

tional attack, there are several general planning principles that must be addressed when preparing for pediatric mass casualties:

1. Understand how the facility fits into the overall emergency management plan for the community. Most communities in this country have a Local Emergency Planning Committee. This committee is responsible for developing the emergency management plans for the community. Assess whether there is adequate representation of medical professionals on this committee and, more specifically, medical professionals with pediatric expertise. In addition, have planning discussions with local industry. It is important to determine what community medical risks are posed by industry and what emergency plans exist. There have been occasions when local hospitals have been included in industry emergency response plans without their knowing it. Finally, review the hospital disaster command structure to guarantee that it utilizes an ICS that is NIMS compliant, to seamlessly interface with local response agencies.

2. Review community plans to ensure that the needs of pediatric patients will be met. Unfortunately, for a variety of reasons, pediatric needs are often overlooked in government and community planning. It is vital that emergency physicians bring their expertise in caring for children to the planning table. In addition, children spend the majority of their days in school. It is vital that adequate plans are in place to address the care of children when they are not with their parents.

3. Review hospital plans to ensure that they address the needs of pediatric patients. Apply the plan to a fictitious influx of children during an exercise to assess how it functions. Train the staff so they are comfortable in mass casualty care of children. If the emergency department is segregated into adult and pediatrics sections, ensure that all staff are cross-trained to care for all patients. Finally, educate and drill the adult and pediatric emergency department staff in pediatric disaster triage.

4. Review antidotes for the most likely agents and plan how to administer them to pediatric patients. If premade kits are not available for children, develop plans to obtain necessary medications and devise ways to formulate them for administration to children. This may involve having the pharmacy mix antidotes into cherry syrup, and crush pills. Determine the hazards in the community and plan for any needed medications to treat victims of these hazards.

5. Develop community-wide transfer agreements and procedures to distribute injured or sick children across a region. Consider matching needed pediatric resources with the nature and severity of a child's injuries.

6. Work with day care centers and schools to ensure that they have adequate disaster management plans in place. Check that those plans integrate into the community's plans and the hospital's plan.

7. Encourage family disaster planning. Many resources are available to help families plan for disaster. These resources can be downloaded from ready.gov or obtained from the American Red Cross.

Summary

Children make up approximately 29% of our population and will invariably be involved in disasters. Many community disaster plans presently do not adequately address the needs of large numbers of critically injured or sick children. As discussed, there are distinctive characteristics and challenges involved in providing mass casualty care for children. It is imperative that emergency physicians share this information with local emergency planners to guarantee that community plans include policies and procedures to provide optimal care for childhood victims of disasters.

REFERENCES

*1. Freishtat RJ: Issues in children's hospital disaster preparedness. Clin Pediatr Emerg Med 3:224–230, 2002.

2. Redlener I, Markenson D: Disaster and terrorism preparedness: what pediatricians need to know. Dis Mon 50:6–40, 2004.

*3. American Academy of Pediatrics, Committee on Environmental Health and Committee on Infectious Disease: Chemical-biological terrorism and its impact on children: a subject review. Pediatrics 105:662–670, 2000.

4. UNICEF Executive Director statement. New York Times, December 28, 2004.

5. United States Geological Survey: Most Recent Natural Disasters Were Not the Century's Worst. Available at *http://geography.about.com/library/misc/blcenturyworst.htm* (accessed December 31, 2004).

6. Azarian A: Baseline assessment of children traumatized by the Armenia earthquake. Child Psychol Hum Dev 29:29–41, 1996.

7. U.S. Census Bureau: 2000 Census Data. Washington, DC: U.S. Census Bureau, 2000.

8. Hogan DE, Waeckerle JF: Emergency department impact of the Oklahoma City terrorist bombings. Ann Emerg Med 34:160–167, 1999.

9. Beslan School Crisis Assistance. Available at *www.moscowhelp.org/en/index.html* (accessed December 30, 2004).

10. Satter D: A small town in Russia. Wall Street Journal, September 7, 2004.

11. Waisman Y, Aharonson-Daniel L, Mor M, et al: The impact of terrorism on children: a two-year experience. Prehosp Disaster Med 18:242–248, 2003.

12. Timeline of Recent Worldwide School Shootings. Available at *www.infoplease.com/ipa/a0777958.html*

13. Centers for Disease Control and Prevention: Youth risk behavior surveillance. MMWR Mrob Mortal Wkly Rep 49:1–94, 2000.

14. Van Amerogen RH, Fine JS: The Avianca plane crash: an emergency medical system's response to pediatric survivors of a disaster. Pediatrics 92:105–110, 1993.

15. White SR, Henretig FM: Medical management of vulnerable populations and co-morbid conditions of victims of bioterrorism. Emerg Med Clin North Am 20:365–392, 2002.

*16. Franz DR, Sidell FR, Takafuji ET: Meciala Aspects of Chemical and Biological Warfare. *In* Textbook of Military Medicine, Part 1: Warfare, Weaponry, and the Casualty. Washington, DC: Borden Institute, Walter Reed Army Medical Center, 1997.

17. Food and Drug Administration: Center for Drug Evaluation and Research: Guidance: Potassium Iodide as a Thyroid Blocking Agent in Radiation Emergencies. Washington, DC: Department of Health and Human Services, 2001.

18. Azarian A, Skriptchenko-Gregorian V: Children in Natural Disasters: An Experience of the 1988 Earthquake in Armenia. American Academy of Experts in Traumatic Stress web site. Available at *www.aaets.org/arts/art38.htm*

*19. California Emergency Medical Services Authority: The Hospital Emergency Incident Command System. Available at *http://www.emsa.cahwnet.gov/dms2/heics_main.asp* (accessed January 14, 2004).

20. Bush GW: Management of domestic incidents. Homeland Security Presidential Directive, Feb. 28, 2003. Washington, DC: Department of Homeland Security.

21. California Emergency Medical Services Authority: The HEICS 4 Project. Available at *http://www.emsa.cahwnet.gov/dms2/heics4project.asp*

22. Joint Commission on the Accreditation of Healthcare Organizations: Emergency Management Standards, E.C.1.4 and E.C. 2.9.1. January 1, 2003. Available at *http://www.jcrinc.com/subscribers/perspectives.asp?durki=2914&site=10&return=2897* (accessed January 2, 2005).

23. McCaig LF, Burt CW: National Hospital Ambulatory Medical Care Survey: 2002 emergency department summary. Adv Data (340):1–34, 2004.

24. Super G, Groth S, Hook R: START: A Triage Training Module. Newport Beach, CA: Hoag Memorial Hospital Presbyterian, 1984.

25. Romig LE: Pediatric triage: a system to JumpSTART your triage of young patients at MCIs. JEMS 27(7):52–63, 2002.

26. Henretig FM, Cieslak TJ, Eitzen EM: Biological and chemical terrorism. J Pediatr 141:311–326, 2002.

27. Centers for Disease Control and Prevention: Update: investigation of bioterrorism related anthrax and interim guidelines for clinical evaluation of persons with possible anthrax. MMWR Morb Mortal Wkly Rep 50:941–948, 2001.

28. Centers for Disease Control and Prevention: Investigation of anthrax associated with intentional exposure and interim public health guidelines. MMWR Morb Mortal Wkly Rep 50:889–893, 2001.

29. Torok TJ, Tauxe RV: A large community outbreak of salmonellosis caused by intentional contamination of restaurant salad bars. JAMA 278:389–395, 1997.

*30. Centers for Disease Control and Prevention, Strategic Planning Group: Biological and chemical terrorism: strategic plan for preparedness and response. MMWR Morb Mortal Wkly Rep 49(RR-4):1–14, 2000.

31. Cieslak TJ: Bioterrorism: agents of concern. J Public Health Manag Pract 6(4):19–29, 2000.

32. Bowlware KL, Stull T: Antibacterial agents in pediatrics. Infect Dis Clin North Am 18:513–531, 2004.

33. American Academy of Pediatrics: Fluoroquinolones, tetracyclines. *In* Pickering LK (ed): 2000 Red Book: Report of the Committee on

---

*Suggested readings.

Infectious Diseases, 25th ed. Elk Grove Village, IL: American Academy of Pediatrics, 2000, pp 645–646.

34. Freifeld A, Pizzo P: Use of fluoroquinolones for empirical management of febrile neutropenia in pediatric cancer patients. Pediatr Infect Dis 16:140–145, 1997.

35. Centers for Disease Control and Prevention: Update: interim recommendations for antimicrobial prophylaxis for children and breastfeeding mothers and treatment of children with anthrax. MMWR Morb Mortal Wkly Rep 50:1014–1016, 2001.

36. Okumura T, Takasu N: Report on 640 victims of the Tokyo subway sarin attack. Ann Emerg Med 28:129–135, Aug 1996.

37. Macintyre AG, Christopher GW, Eitzen E: Weapons of mass destruction events with contaminated casualties: effective planning for health care facilities. JAMA 283:242–249, 2000.

38. Food and Drug Administration: FDA approves pediatric doses of AtroPen. Talk Paper 03-45, June 20, 2003. Washington, DC: Department of Health and Human Resources, 2003.

39. AtroPen Package Insert NDA 17-106/S-028. Columbia, MD: Meridian Medical Technologies, 2004.

40. Amitai Y, Almog S, Singer R, et al: Atropine Poisoning in Children During the Persian Gulf Crisis: A National Survey in Israel. JAMA 268:630–632, 1992.

41. U.S. Army Soldier and Biological Chemical Command (SBCCOM): Domestic Preparedness Training Program (DPT-8), p M5-33. Natick, MA: SBCCOM.

42. U.S. Nuclear Regulatory Commission: Policy Issue Paper: Status of Potassium Iodide Activities (SECY-01-0208). Rockville, MD: U.S. Nuclear Regulatory Commission.

43. Food and Drug Administration: Potassium Iodide as a Thyroid Blocking Agent in Radiation Emergencies. December 2001. Available at *http://www.fda.gov/cder/guidance/4825fnl.htm*

44. Food and Drug Administration: Home Preparation Procedure for Emergency Administration of Potassium Iodide Tablets to Infants and Small Children. Available at *http://www.fda.gov/cder/drugprepare/kiprep.htm*

Family Presence

Mirna M. Farah, MD

Introduction and Background

The concept of family presence during resuscitation emerged in the mid-1980s when the emergency department staff at a Michigan hospital questioned a policy that excluded families from the resuscitation room.[1] Initially opinions about family presence were mixed; however, the trend of subsequent literature has moved toward acceptance of the process.[2] Currently, several organizations promote family presence, including the American Academy of Pediatrics, the American Heart Association, the Emergency Nurses Association, and the federally funded Emergency Medical Services for Children program.[3-6]

Parents play an integral role in the health and well-being of their child. Supporting and integrating the family into the emergency care process is vital to meeting the full spectrum of the patient's needs. The fear that family presence would hinder medical care can be eliminated by properly assessing and preparing families prior to entering the resuscitation room. The more experience health care providers (HCPs) have with family presence and dealing with distressed families, and the more comfort they have in their clinical skills, the higher the acceptance and success of family presence.

Issues

There are several compelling reasons to consider offering the option for family presence (Table 153–1). Including the family in the care plan, promotes collaboration among medical providers, patients, and family members. Both pediatric patients and their parents are significantly less distressed when the parents are present during a procedure.[7-9] Regardless of the patient's condition, parents seem to focus on their child comforting role rather than the logistics of medical care.[10] The patient becomes less anxious, and therefore more compliant, so the procedure has the potential to go more smoothly.[11] Even if the parents decide not to be at their child's bedside, knowing that they have that option fosters trust and positive communication.

Even when the patient is likely to die, family presence remains extremely beneficial.[11] Family presence allows parents to be by their loved one until the last minute. Parents can touch their child, express their love, and say good-bye while there is still a chance that the patient can hear. Family presence brings a sense of reality to the treatment efforts and clinical status of the patient, avoiding a prolonged period of denial.[12] Parents can see for themselves the tremendous effort put into the resuscitation attempt, and this has far more meaning then being told: "Everything possible was done."[1] Family presence facilitates the grieving process, and may be one of the most powerful interventions that can be offered to a grieving family.[1,13-16] The manner in which HCPs care for and respect the wishes of both the dying patient and their parents is crucial in helping the family accept the death and deal with the crisis.

There are many perceived barriers to family presence.[17] It often represents breaking a tradition. Family presence challenges basic assumptions and long-standing practices. In the past, parents were routinely excluded from visitation and were never permitted to view resuscitations. The more informed HCPs are about the process of family presence, the higher the acceptance for family presence.[12,18-20] There are concerns that family presence may increase staff anxiety or hinder performance. Patient care is always a top priority, and it may be harder for a resuscitation team to work with an audience.[1] Confidence in procedural and cardiopulmonary resuscitation (CPR) skills, and experience with family presence, quickly decrease the anxiety level.[12] The majority of HCPs who offer family presence do not report a change in their performance or a change in the outcome of the procedure or CPR.[7-9,11,12]

Worries that family presence may distract staff or obstruct medical care are unfounded. Disruptions and occurrences of family members becoming physically involved in the resuscitation attempt have not been consistently reported.[13,21] Most family members are awed by the activity in the resuscitation room and frequently have to be led to the bedside

Table 153–1	Rationale for Offering the Option for Family Presence

- Promotes collaboration and fosters trust between medical providers, patients, and family members
- Reduces anxiety and sense of helplessness
- Allows parents to comfort and support their child
- Meets the family's need of being informed and feeling accepted
- Facilitates the grieving process
- Allows families to be by their loved one until the last minute and be able to say good-bye
- Brings a sense of reality to the treatment efforts and clinical status of the patient

and encouraged to touch and speak with their loved ones.[21] Regardless of their background, family members understand the need for appropriate behavior so that their presence does not impede the care of the person they are trying to help.

It may be harder to end an unsuccessful resuscitation when family members are expressing grief.[21] Stressing that every possible intervention has been done, and allowing time for family members to say what they need to say before ending the resuscitation, may help them accept the death. Witnessing CPR helps family members understand how grave the patient's condition is, and allows them to feel confident that everything was done to save the patient.[1,12,21]

Staff may be traumatized by witnessing the family grieving, bringing emotions to the surface and making it harder to forget and move on. However, this is unavoidable, and taking the time after a resuscitation to talk and vent these feelings can make the circumstances easier to deal with.[21] Family presence may also be very traumatic for the family. No matter how often people see HCPs providing CPR on television, witnessing these procedures on a loved one is not the same. Family presence should be offered as a choice so parents can participate in the decision about their presence. Being present during invasive procedures or resuscitation is not something all families want. Patients who choose not to have family members present, or family members who desire not to participate, must be supported in their decision without judgment. Even though a parents' desire to stay decreases as procedures becomes more invasive, the majority still wish to be present.[22] Even family members who have witnessed CPR say that they would participate again.[12,13,15,23]

It may be difficult to teach trainees in the presence of family members. We must remain professional and careful with our choice of words in the presence of family. Family presence should be viewed as an opportunity to learn about how to address and support distressed parents. Family presence during resuscitation and procedures does not increase litigation.[24,25] In fact, family presence may decrease disputes by improving communication, increasing openness, and decreasing doubt about the adequacy of care.[26,27] Family presence should be presented as an option by letting parents know that they can leave the room any time if they wish to avoid further stress.

Solutions

Institutional/Systems Requirements

Family presence requires the availability of critical staff members and institutional resources to succeed. A family

presence program needs a family presence champion who will write guidelines that are institution specific, delineate roles and responsibilities, survey and educate staff members, and monitor progress and provide feedback. A family support person (FSP) is an individual who will provide most or all of the clinical support when family presence occurs. This individual must understand grief reactions, be competent at supporting distressed families, and have training in the explanation of medical care and in assessment and preparation of family members. The designated FSP can be a social worker, nurse, or chaplain who has no direct patient care responsibility, and is assigned exclusively to assist the family. Duties will include screening and preparing families prior to entering the treatment area, and remaining present with the family at all times in the resuscitation room.

Follow-up services, especially when death occurs, should be established. Staff can be defused or debriefed, informally or through a critical incident stress management program. Security personnel should be available at all times to prevent serious disruption by family members. A family room adjacent to the resuscitation room works well as a staging area, and there must be adequate space in the treatment room. Any family presence program should have dedicated resources and funding for staff education and a mechanism for feedback.

Setting Up a Family Presence Program

One or more family presence champions must first be identified. These are individuals who believe in the benefits of family presence and have good knowledge of the literature. They are committed to initiate and motivate change and act as the driving force behind the establishment of the family presence program. They help to increase awareness and role model family support interventions. A project team assists the family presence champion and should be assembled from a number of disciplines to assure consideration of all perspectives. Input is sought from a broad constituency, including nursing, medicine (emergency department, trauma, critical care, anesthesia, residents, fellows), transport personnel, social work, pastoral care, child life, administration, risk management, respiratory therapy, and technicians. Family member representation on the team should be encouraged. Team members meet regularly and help develop and implement the family presence program.

Next, barriers to family presence within the institution should be identified. The project team should assess institutional resources and identify root causes that prevent the practice of family presence. They should survey a broad group of colleagues for suggestions, concerns, and educational needs. Based on this information, guidelines that are institution specific can be written. These should help delineate staff roles and responsibilities during a family presence event. Support procedures must be addressed for all hours of the day. HCP involvement in both resuscitation situations and invasive procedures that vary in complexity and need for personnel should be specified. The guidelines should balance the staff's concerns about providing care and the families' need to be present in the treatment room. They also need to stress that family presence should remain an option both for the family and for the staff and that the decision to participate must be supported without judgment. A sample guideline is provided in Table 153–2.

Table 153–2	Guidelines for Family Presence during Invasive Procedures and Resuscitations

Family Support Person (FSP)

Prior to Patient's Arrival:
- Inquire about patient's status and anticipated interventions
- Prepare the space where family members will stay

Patient and Family Assessment:
- Promptly communicate known information about the patient's status to the family.
- Assess the family's reaction:
  - Acceptable behaviors for family presence:
    - Quiet
    - Distressed, crying but consolable
    - Distracted but able to focus and answer questions
    - Anxious or angry but cooperative and follows instructions
  - Worrisome behaviors:
    - Uncooperative
    - Physically aggressive, combative
    - Threatening and argumentative
    - Extremely unstable emotionally, hysterical, loud, cannot be redirected or calmed
    - Altered mental status, intoxicated

A family member's ability to participate can progress or regress throughout their presence in the emergency department. Continuous assessment and intervention are critical for the success of family presence.

- Assess the patient's desire for family members to be present when applicable.
- Assess the family's desire/willingness to participate, and comfort with being present from previous experiences with similar situations (blood draws, procedures performed on a loved one, etc.).
- Inform the HCP of the family's arrival and request to be present in the treatment area.

Preparation of the Patient and Family:

Prior to entering the treatment room:
- Families should be told:
  - How many family members may enter the room at one time
  - Where they will stand/sit initially and when they will be able to move to the bedside
  - That they may leave the room if they feel the need to step out, and that they are welcome to reenter
  - Why they may be **asked to step out of the room:**
    - At the request of the HCP
    - Obstruction of care: violent behavior, uncontrolled outbursts, etc. Security will join the FSP in moving the family out of the treatment area.
    - Need for medical assistance: fainting, chest pain, etc. In this case an HCP not involved in the care of their child will assist them.

In the treatment room:
- During resuscitations, an FSP must always remain with the family in the treatment area. During invasive procedures, the HCP will assign an FSP as needed.
- The family must be clearly informed of the status of their loved one and be prepared for the interventions that are in progress.
  - Explain the procedures being performed.
  - Potential responses the patient may exhibit.
  - Explain the patient's role during the procedure (i.e,, holding still etc.).
  - Family members' role in providing comfort and reassurance.
  - Interpret medical jargon.
  - Provide opportunity to ask questions and clarify details: The FSP should mainly describe the procedures performed. The physicians will explain indications and outcomes.

Health Care Professional (HCP)

Attending Physician:
- Communicates with the FSP known information about the patient's status and anticipated plan of care.
- Approves/disapproves family presence, indicates to the FSP when to bring the family in.
  - The attending physician and the trauma chief will retain the option to allow the family to enter the treatment room or be escorted away from the bedside and/or out of the room if deemed necessary.
- Notifies family of outcome of procedures and/or resuscitation as soon as practical.

Emergency Department Charge Nurse:
- Assures FSP is contacted for resuscitation situations.
- Designates a staff member to act in the FSP role until support staff arrives.
- Provides the FSP with clinical information and helps answering questions.

All Care Providers:
- Interact with the family as soon as practical.
- Address the patient by name.
- Offer and provide comfort measures: Assist the family in making phone calls, provide a place to sit down, water, tissues, etc.
- Use terminology appropriate to the person's level of understanding.
- Provide opportunities for the family to see and speak with the patient.
- Provide for patient and family privacy.
- Maintain professional behavior and language at all times.

Situational Constraints

- When space is critically limited, it may be necessary to limit the number of family members to one at a time, or ask the family to step out temporarily.
- When multiple patients need the resuscitation room simultaneously, family members may not be allowed in the room. Accommodations to bring the family to the bedside should be made as soon as practical, even if only briefly.

Educating staff is a large part of the creation of a family presence program. The purpose of this education is to provide the skills necessary to support distressed families, become familiar with grief reactions, and introduce the guidelines and respective roles of the staff. Support personnel need to have a strong psychosocial background and some understanding of common invasive procedures and CPR. Other personnel need to be comfortable assessing families' needs and initiating appropriate interventions and consultation. A variety of formats may be used, including lectures and workshops, role play exercises, videotaped presentations, self-study modules, and case reviews.

A date should be designated for the program to begin. Implementation of a family presence program will take time and will require a shift in the culture of the department. Assessing staff readiness and ensuring adequate resources are essential steps in changing practice and integrating a family-centered care approach. Once the program is in place, the project team should monitor progress, provide feedback, and customize the guidelines. Evaluation is an essential step to validate the efficacy of the strategies implemented. Input should be sought from HCPs, support staff, and families. This helps to identify further educational needs, problems, and potential revisions of the guidelines. The mechanisms for evaluation may include surveys, postevent questionnaires, interviews, and open forum discussions. The timing of the evaluation should take into consideration the clinical situation and outcome. Opinions from staff may be solicited within days of an event and after several weeks to months from families who lost a loved one. Knowledge of the program should be spread within and outside the institution among all parties, including prehospital care providers.

Summary

Due to perceptions, attitudes, previous exposures, and biases, many HCPs overlook the benefits of family presence. When planned properly, family presence helps meet the family's needs without disrupting medical care. However, this type of change requires great commitment, adequate resources, continuing education, careful planning, and time. The greater the depth of experience with family presence, the greater the likelihood of supporting the process. As patient advocates, HCPs should strive for widespread establishment of family presence.

REFERENCES

*1. Doyle CJ, Post H, Burney RE, et al: Family participation during resuscitation: an option. Ann Emerg Med 16:673–675, 1987.

*2. Boudreaux ED, Francis JL, Loyacano T: Family presence during invasive procedures and resuscitations in the emergency department: a critical review and suggestions for future research. Ann Emerg Med 40:193–205, 2002.

3. American Academy of Pediatrics Committee on Pediatric Emergency Medicine, American College of Emergency Physicians Pediatric Emergency Medicine Committee, O'Malley P, Broun K, Mace SE: Patient and family centered care and the role of the emergency physician providing care to a child in the emergency department. Pediatrics 118:2242–2244, 2006.

4. Emergency Nurses Association: Family Presence at the Bedside During Invasive Procedures and/or Resuscitations, 2nd ed, 2001. Available at http://www.ena.org

5. Henderson DP, Knapp JF: Report of the national consensus conference on Family Presence during Pediatric Cardio pulmonary Resuscitation and Procedures. J Emerg Nurs 32(1):23–29, 2006.

6. Guidelines 2000 for cardiopulmonary resuscitation and emergency cardiovascular care. Circulation 102(8):I-19, 2000.

*7. Wolfram RW, Turner ED, Philput C: Effects of parental presence during young children's venipuncture. Pediatr Emerg Care 13:325–328, 1997.

8. Bauchner H, Vinci R, Bak S, et al: Parents and procedures: a randomized controlled trial. Pediatrics 98:861–867, 1996.

9. Powers KS, Rubenstein JS: Family presence during invasive procedures in the pediatric intensive care unit. Arch Pediatr Adolesc Med 153:955–958, 1999.

10. Barratt F, Wallis DN: Relatives in the resuscitation room: their point of view. J Accid Emerg Med 15:109–111, 1998.

*11. Sacchetti A, Lichenstein R, Carraccio CA, et al: Family member presence during pediatric emergency department procedures. Pediatr Emerg Care 12:268–271, 1996.

*12. Meyers TA, Eichhorn DJ, Guzzetta CE, et al: Family presence during invasive procedures and resuscitation. Am J Nurs 100(2):32–43, 2000.

*13. Belanger MA, Reed S: A rural community hospital's experience with family-witnessed resuscitation. J Emerg Nurs 23:238–239, 1997.

14. Williams AG, O'Brien DL, Laughton KJ, et al: Improving services to bereaved relatives in the emergency department: making health care more human. Med J Aust 173:480–483, 2000.

15. Robinson SM, Mackenzie-Ross S, Campbell Hewson GL, et al: Psychological effect of witnessed resuscitation on bereaved relatives. Lancet 352:614–617, 1998.

16. Eichhorn DJ, Meyers TA, Mitchell TG, Guzzetta CE: Opening the doors: family presence during resuscitation. J Cardiovasc Nurs 10:59–70, 1996.

17. Helmer SD, Smith SR, Dort JM, et al: Family presence during trauma resuscitation: a survey of AAST and ENA members. J Trauma 48:1015–1024, 2000.

*18. Bassler PC: The impact of education on nurses' beliefs regarding family presence in a resuscitation room. J Nurses Staff Dev 15(3):126–131, 1999.

*19. Mitchell MH, Lynch MB: Should relatives be allowed in the resuscitation room? J Accid Emerg Med 14:366–369, 1997.

20. Sacchetti A, Carraccio C, Leva E, et al: Acceptance of family member presence during pediatric resuscitations in the emergency department: effects of personal experience. Pediatr Emerg Care 16:85–87, 2000.

*21. Hanson C, Strawser D: Family presence during cardiopulmonary resuscitation: Foote Hospital emergency department's nine-year perspective. J Emerg Nurs 18:104–106, 1992.

*22. Boie ET, Moore GP, Brummett C, et al: Do parents want to be present during invasive procedures performed on their children in the emergency department? A survey of 400 parents. Ann Emerg Med 34:70–74, 1999.

23. Meyers TA, Eichhorn DJ, Guzzetta CE: Do families want to be present during CPR? A retrospective survey. J Emerg Nurs 24:400–405, 1998.

24. Forster H, Schwartz J, Derenzo E: Reducing legal risk by practicing patient-centered medicine. Arch Intern Med 162:1217–1219, 2002.

25. Brown JR: Letting the family in during a code: legally it makes good sense. Nursing 19(3):46, 1989.

26. Tsai E: Should family members be present during cardiopulmonary resuscitation? N Engl J Med 346:1019–1021, 2002.

27. Trout A, Magnusson R, Hedges JR: Patient satisfaction investigations and the emergency department: what does the literature say? Acad Emerg Med 7:695–709, 2000.

---

*Selected readings.

Chapter 154

The Child-Friendly Emergency Department: Practices, Policies, and Procedures

Susan Fuchs, MD

Key Points

There are suggested minimum pediatric emergency department (ED) equipment, supplies, and medication.

There are many different staff training options.

Continuous quality improvement and creating a safe environment are essential for any pediatric ED.

Key pediatric policies, procedures and external agreements must be available 24 hours a day, 7 days a week in all pediatric EDs.

Introduction and Background

What is Emergency Department Preparedness?

Emergency department (ED) preparedness means that the "Emergency Department must have the staff and resources to evaluate all persons presenting to the ED."[1] However, when it comes to pediatric patients, this is not always the case. A national survey concluded that only 10% of U.S. hospitals have a pediatric intensive care unit, 25% of hospitals without a pediatric trauma service admit critically injured children, and 7% of hospitals without a pediatric ward admit children.[2] A Canadian study of ED preparedness demonstrated deficiencies in equipment needed to resuscitate a critically ill pediatric patient.[3]

Not all children are, or need to be, seen in a pediatric ED. In fact, of the approximately 35 million pediatric ED visits per year, only 10% seek care initially in a children's hospital/pediatric ED. What this means is that the other 31.5 million children seek care in general and community EDs, which have varying abilities to care for them. In most community EDs, pediatric patients account for 20% to 35% of the patient visits. This chapter reviews the issues involved in prepared-ness, possible solutions, suggested policies and procedures, and additional information that may prove beneficial to create an ED appropriately prepared for infants, children, and adolescents.

Facility Categorization

While most physicians and nurses are familiar with terms such as a Level I trauma center or a burn center, the terminology for pediatric centers is new, and often varies from state to state, if it exists at all. "Categorization is the assessment of a facility based on its ability to manage certain categories of patients."[4] The levels of categorization are usually based upon state (e.g., Level I vs. II adult/pediatric trauma center) or national (e.g., burn center) standards. This can lead to a "designation," or the assignment of responsibility for care of certain categories of patients to specific institutions based upon compliance with standards as well as on their catchment area.[4] The designation is conferred by an outside agency once the facility has gone through a site survey or other process to verify that it meets the existing standards. A hospital can also voluntarily agree to adopt a set of standards as its own, without an outside agency involved, and can be "confirmed."[4]

Another important distinction is the method by which states categorize hospitals and EDs. In many states there are comprehensive EDs. This is an ED with at least one physician available 24 hours a day, 7 days a week (24/7), with specialty services, and with ancillary services such as radiology, laboratory, and pharmacy staffed at all times.[5] A basic ED has at least one physician 24/7, limited specialty services, and ancillary services staffed or "on call." A standby ED has a registered nurse, nurse practitioner, or physician's assistant available for emergency services 24/7, and a physician who is "on call."[5]

Issues

In 1995, the American Academy of Pediatrics (AAP) issued guidelines for pediatric emergency care facilities. This document established four levels of care: standby, basic, general emergency facilities, and comprehensive regional pediatric center.[6] It included recommendations on personnel, medical specialist consultants, surgical specialists, equipment and supplies, and facilities for each level. It also covered topics such as access, triage, transfer and transport, education, training, research, quality assessment and improvement, administrative support and hospital commitment.[6] This guideline added the requirement that the physician be competent in the care of pediatric emergencies. This could be demonstrated by the successful completion of Pediatric Advanced Life Support (PALS) or Advanced Pediatric Life Support (APLS) courses.[6] This set the foundation for the development of a national policy statement in 2001 (see later).[7]

In February 1995, the American College of Emergency Physicians (ACEP) issued a policy statement on pediatric equipment guidelines. These were recommended for equipment of pediatric patients in a general ED. This list included monitoring devices, vascular access supplies and equipment, respiratory equipment and supplies, medications, related supplies/equipment, miscellaneous equipment, specialized pediatric trays, and fracture management devices.[8] The equipment and medications listed in this document and the AAP 1995 document are similar.

In 1998, the Committee on Pediatric Equipment and Supplies for Emergency Departments of the National Emergency Medical Services for Children Resource Alliance developed a consensus statement regarding pediatric resuscitation medication and minimum equipment and supplies.[9] They based their recommendations on previously published lists, including the two documents by the AAP and ACEP.[6,8] The article mentioned that the ED may choose to modify this list, and that ED health care providers should be trained in the use of all equipment and supplies. The committee also took into account financial factors when recommending items, and occasionally provided some equipment options.

In 2001, the AAP and ACEP, along with the federal Emergency Medical Services for Children (EMSC) program, developed a joint policy statement: "Care of Children in the Emergency Department: Guidelines for Preparedness."[7] In addition to these organizations, this statement was supported by numerous national organizations and agencies. While this document does list medications, equipment, and supplies (adapted from the 1998 list[9]), its strength lies in the agreement on personnel staffing and training, administration and coordination for pediatric emergency care, quality improvement (QI), and ED policies, procedures, protocols, and support services. The information in this policy provides a framework for many of the areas to be discussed in the "Solutions" section later in this chapter.

State Guidelines

In 1994, the California Emergency Medical Services Authority compiled a list of recommended equipment, supplies, and medications for the care of pediatric patients in the ED.[10] In 1999, the Los Angeles County Department of Health Services' Emergency Medical Services (EMS) division published Emergency Department Approved for Pediatrics (EDAP) standards.[4,11] These standards include administration, coordination, personnel, policies, procedures and protocols, QI, support services, equipment, supplies, and medications. Pediatric Critical Care Center (PCCC) was another category

designation that was added. This designation is achieved if a hospital meets requirements for an EDAP, has a trauma center, and has a California Children's Services–approved pediatric intensive care unit.[11] In 2004, there were 57 EDAPs and 9 PCCCs in Los Angeles County.[11]

In 2002, the State of Illinois added a section to the Emergency Medical Services and Trauma Center Code to include facility recognition criteria for EDAPs and the Standby Emergency Department Approved for Pediatrics (SEDP).[12,13] Although this is a voluntary process, since these rules have been in effect the EMSC facility recognition process has recognized 114 (out of a possible 200) hospitals. These criteria cover topics similar to the Los Angeles County criteria, but include recommended equipment lists as well as professional staff (nurse, physician, nurse practitioner, physician assistant) qualifications, continuing medical education (CME) requirements, a multidisciplinary QI committee, and a pediatric continuous QI liaison.[12-14] Another important part of this document was the development of interfacility pediatric trauma and critical care consultation and/or transfer guidelines.[15]

Solutions

Triage

When a child enters an ED with his or her parent(s), the first encounter they have with a health professional is at triage. It is important for that person to be comfortable assessing a child, to have the necessary equipment (e.g., scales, thermometer, appropriate-sized blood pressure cuffs, and pulse oximeter probes), as well as to have some criteria on which to base the child's triage category assessment. Published criteria for children are based upon age-related norms, signs, and symptoms, and are divided into three or five categories.[16-18] Triage criteria provide a guide as to the level of acuity of the patient, which in turn provide a time frame in which the patient should be seen (see Chapter 155, Triage).

Physical Space (Child Friendly)

While a designated pediatric care area is not feasible in many facilities, it may be possible to make the ED child friendly in several simple ways. Just separating pediatric patients from adult patients in the waiting room may protect them from some of the sights, language, and other inappropriate behavior of adults. It can also provide some separation between children who may have a contagious disease and elderly adults, who are very susceptible to these illnesses. It is important to childproof the waiting room by avoiding sharp corners on chairs and tables, locking cabinets, covering electrical outlets, and covering trash cans.[19] If pediatric-size furniture is available, it is important to keep it clean after use. This is also true of any toys used in a play area. Some simple solutions are to provide coloring books and crayons, or books to read, all of which can be taken home.

If a separate pediatric room or care area is available, simple decorations can brighten the room and provide distractions for children. This can be a cheerful wall border, hanging pictures, or ceiling drawings. While one could argue that a teenager will not enjoy being in a room decorated with Mickey Mouse or Sesame Street characters, they can still provide distractions during an examination. This room should also be childproofed by placing all medical equipment out of reach of a child, providing bed rails with child guards, and assuring that there are no sharp objects or corners at an infant or roaming child level. Another option is to provide a TV/VCR/DVD player in the room. The TV can have limited channels, and the VCR or DVD can be utilized to view cartoons, movies, or even educational tapes.[19] As a convenience to parents, having diapers, skin wipes, and blankets in the room can help them provide care or comfort for their child while waiting to be seen.

Staffing

Creating a child-friendly environment should involve the staff. While many pediatric hospitals allow brightly colored shirts/blouses/scrub tops, these may not look professional to an adult entering the ED. Each hospital has dress code regulations that determine the use of scrubs outside of the operating room. The ability of clerical, ED, and ancillary staff to deal with patients of various ages cannot be overstressed. Education and training sessions on how to communicate and interact with pediatric patients should be available to all the staff involved in their care.

Many emergency nurses work in different hospital locations before they seek employment in the ED, but their exposure to pediatrics may have been limited to nursing school rotations. If there is a pediatrics ward in the hospital, having them spend some time with pediatric nurses (and vice versa) can be an invaluable experience. There are specific CME courses, including the Emergency Nurse Pediatric Course (ENPC) offered through the Emergency Nurses Association, APLS, and PALS, that can help them improve their assessment, technical, and treatment skills.[20] The specific number of staff is based upon the hospital designation (comprehensive vs. standby) as well as the usual census, but will include at least one nurse present 24/7.

Physician attitude and training are also crucial. Once again, depending upon the physician's specialty, his or her last exposure to pediatrics may have been in medical school. Residency-trained emergency physicians are trained in the acute and emergent care of pediatric patients. Additionally, each state may have additional CME requirements for physicians, some being specific for topics such as pain management, end-of-life issues (California), and child maltreatment (New York). Specific physician staffing is based upon hospital designation (e.g., for a standby hospital, the physician may be on call but promptly available, whereas a basic facility has an emergency physician present 24/7). The ACEP emergency care guidelines contains specific staffing and credentialing requirements for physicians and nurses.[9]

The availability of specialists (surgical and medical) varies based upon the hospital designation. The AAP guidelines for pediatric emergency care facilities include a table that lists these physicians, and whether they are essential in the hospital or promptly available, based on hospital designation.[6]

Competency

The issue of developing staff competency is difficult to define. Courses that do exist do not guarantee competency, but provide certification that one has completed the course. Becoming competent requires experience, ongoing training, practice, and education. There are no set number of times a

physician must suture a laceration, or a nurse must start an intravenous line, to prove he or she is competent. The requirements for board certification in all medical specialties are undergoing change to include the following: physicians must maintain active licensure, pass a written examination, read current literature, obtain CME credits, and receive an evaluation of their practice performance. While this does not prove competency either, it is a multilayered process that is more rigorous than previous requirements.

For those staff who do not have pediatric experience, available courses can help educate them about common pediatric illnesses and injuries, resuscitation skills, and procedural techniques. These classes include ENPC and APLS or PALS for nurses, and PALS or APLS for physicians.[18,20,21]

Equipment/Supplies

Even with all of the expertise and training of the staff, an ill infant cannot be cared for appropriately if the right-size equipment is not present. This can include basic equipment such as a sphygmomanometer with an infant-sized blood pressure cuff, or a 22- or 24-gauge intravenous catheter, or a 10F chest tube. While there are several published equipment lists, the equipment/supply list published by the AAP and ACEP is based upon the consensus of many organizations[7] (Table 154–1).

Medications

The majority of the medications required in the ED can be used in children.[1,9] However, there are some unique concentrations for children, such as sodium bicarbonate (4.2%), and dextrose (10%, 25%).[9] It is important to have frequently used medications readily available in the ED, and a process for obtaining those used less frequently in a short time frame (Table 154–2).

Quality Improvement

The Joint Commission on Accreditation of Healthcare Organizations (JCAHO) requires that hospitals improve patient safety and perform QI activities. Each year JCAHO establishes national patient safety goals and quality indicators.[22] Common ED QI monitors include deaths, transfers, and ED returns visits within 48 or 72 hours. Additional pediatric QI indicators can include pediatric resuscitations, intubations, and patients admitted to the general pediatric ward who require transfer to a pediatric intensive care unit. More specific QI ideas can include timing to administration of antipyretics, or pain assessment and management.[23] It is important to include some out-of-hospital QI indicators such as appropriate airway management (airway adjunct or assisted ventilation), delivery of 100% oxygen to a child in respiratory distress, establishment of vascular access, appropriate immobilization for trauma, and appropriate sized equipment used. The Institute of Health Care Improvement has defined the four essential components of a high-performing quality program as follows: (1) focus on identifying appropriate indicators, developing a plan for improvement (plan); (2) implement this plan (do); (3) collect and analyze the data (study); and (4) reach conclusions and make recommendations (act). It is also important to have a multidisciplinary QI team, as different perspectives will be obtained and many lessons learned (see Chapter 149, Patient Safety, Medical Errors, and Quality of Care).

Table 154–1	Recommended Equipment and Supplies

Monitoring

- Cardiorespiratory monitor with strip recorder
- Defibrillator (0–400 J) with pediatric (4.5-cm) and adult (8-cm) paddles or corresponding adhesive pads
- Pediatric and adult monitor electrodes
- Pulse oximeter with sensors for children
- Sphygmomanometer
- Doppler blood pressure device
- Blood pressure cuffs (neonatal, infant, child, adult arm and thigh cuffs)
- Stethoscope
- Thermometer (must be able to measure from 25° C to 44° C)
- Endotracheal tube placement monitor (disposable CO_2 detector, electronic waveform or measurement, or for children ≥ 20 kg or ≥5 yr, esophageal detector device)

Airway Management

- Portable oxygen regulators/canisters
- Oxygen masks
  - clear simple face masks—neonatal, infant, child, adult
  - Venturi masks—neonatal, infant, child, adult
  - partial non-rebreathing masks—neonatal, infant, child
  - rebreathing masks—child, adult
- Oropharyngeal airways (sizes 0–5)
- Nasopharyngeal airways (sizes 12F–30F)
- Bag-valve-mask resuscitator—self-inflating (450- and 1000-ml sizes)
- Nasal cannulae (infant, child, adult)
- Endotracheal tubes
  - uncuffed (sizes 2.5, 3.0, 3.5, 4.0, 4.5, 5.0, 5.5, and 6.0 mm)
  - cuffed (sizes 6.5, 7.0, 7.5, 8.0, and 9.0 mm)
- Stylets (pediatric and adult)
- Laryngoscope handle (pediatric and adult)
- Laryngoscope blades: straight/Miller (sizes 0, 1, 2, and 3) and curved/Macintosh (sizes 2 and 3)
- Magill forceps (pediatric and adult)
- Nasogastric/feeding tubes (sizes 5F–18F)
- Suction catheters—flexible (sizes 6F–16F)
- Yankauer suction tip
- Bulb syringe

Vascular Access

- Butterfly needles (sizes 19G–25G)
- Catheter-over-needle devices (sizes 14G–24G)
- Intraosseous needles (two sizes, between 13G and 18G)

- Intravenous fluids
- Rate-limiting infusing device and tubing
- Fluid/blood warmer

Fracture Management

- Cervical immobilization equipment (backboard with straps, and head immobilizer)
- Semi-rigid cervical collars (sizes to fit infant, child, and adolescent)

Miscellaneous Equipment

- Length-based resuscitation tape (precalculated drug or equipment list based on weight)
- Pediatric urinary catheters (sizes 5F–16F)
- Infant and standard scales
- Towel rolls, blanket rolls
- Resuscitation board
- Medical photography capability

Specialized Pediatric Trays

- Lumbar puncture
- Tube thoracotomy with water seal drainage capability
- Venous cutdown kit
- Needle cricothyrotomy tray

Essential Equipment That Can Be Shared (Nursery, Floor, Operating Room), but Is Readily Available to the Emergency Department

- Umbilical vein catheters (3.5F, 5F [but size 5F feeding tube can also be used])
- Chest tubes (sizes 8F–40F)
- Seldinger vascular access technique kit (3F, 5F, 8F)
- Extremity splints
- Femur splints (child and adult)
- Tracheostomy tubes (sizes 00–6)
- Obstetrics pack
- Newborn delivery kit
- Umbilical vessel cannulation supplies
- Surgical airway kit (tracheostomy or surgical cricothyrotomy kit)
- Infant formula and oral rehydrating solutions
- Heating source (infrared lamps or overhead warmer)
- Sterile linen

Equipment That Is Desirable

- Laryngeal mask airways (sizes 1, 1.5, 2, 2.5, 3, 4, and 5)

Adapted from American Academy of Pediatrics, Committee on Pediatric Emergency Medicine; and American College of Emergency Physicians, Pediatric Committee: Care of children in the emergency department: guidelines for preparedness. Pediatrics 107:777–781, 2001.

Table 154–2	Recommended Medications

Activated charcoal
Adenosine
Antibiotics (parenteral)
Anticonvulsants
Antidotes
Antipyretics
Atropine
Bronchodilators
Calcium chloride
Corticosteroids
Dextrose (25%, 50%)
Epinephrine (1:1000, 1:10,000)
Inotropic agents
Lidocaine
Naloxone hydrochloride
Neuromuscular blocking agents
Oxygen
Sedatives
Sodium bicarbonate (4.2%, 8.4%)

Transfer Criteria

While many ill and injured children can be cared for in local EDs and hospitals, some require transfer to a specialized care center. There are hospitals that offer specialized care for newborns, critical care services, pediatric trauma, and burns. They offer 24-hour consultation with the appropriate specialist, and may have their own interfacility transport service. The decision to transfer pediatric patients depends upon the ED and hospital capabilities, but guidelines have been developed to help physicians identify which patients would benefit from specialized care. It is important for the referring physician to consult with the receiving physician, so the appropriate method of transport and the required personnel can be determined. Transfer guidelines can be based upon physiologic criteria, anatomic criteria, burn criteria, or diagnostic criteria. An example of these guidelines has been developed for the Illinois EMSC program.[24]

Policies and Procedures

Policies, procedures, and protocols that specifically deal with the emergency care of children should be developed for use in the ED and hospital. These include policies on child maltreatment and consent issues. Other protocols may be integrated into ED/hospital policies, procedures, and protocols, but pediatric-specific components should be included. This includes policies on death in the ED, do-not-resuscitate orders, injury and illness triage, sedation and analgesia, immunization status, mental health emergencies, physical or chemical restraint of patients, family issues (e.g., family presence during care), communication with the patient's primary care provider, and transfer policies.[7]

Restraints (Chemical and Physical)

JCAHO has behavioral health care restraint and seclusion standards that apply to patients in the ED who are being restrained or secluded for behavioral health reasons.[25] Restraint, whether chemical or physical, should be a method of last resort. It should never be used as a means of discipline, coercion, or retaliation or for convenience. Restraint is often considered when the patient's or another's safety is a concern. Included in this policy should be the use of seclusion. When restraint or seclusion is considered, the patient's caregivers should be involved in the treatment decision. If this is not possible, they should be notified.

Each use of restraint or seclusion must be based on the patient's needs, age, and past medical history. The restraint policy should cover definitions and exceptions to restraints (e.g., intravenous infusion armboards, temporary immobilization for procedures). When restraint or seclusion is utilized, there need to be written orders by a physician, time limits for the written orders, patient assessment parameters (constant visualization, vital signs, nutrition, hydration, and safety every 15 minutes), and a re-evaluation time for renewal of the restraint order.[25] During restraint or seclusion, documentation should include a physician order, completion of a nursing or trained staff form/flowsheet, notification of the patient's legal guardian, and documentation of monitoring/vital signs. All staff are required to have ongoing education in the proper use of restraint devices and seclusion techniques, as well as alternative methods for handling behaviors that may lead to the use of restraint or seclusion. The ED medical records of those patients who require restraint or seclusion should be reviewed as part of the department's QI plan.

Procedural Sedation and Analgesia

The use of sedation and analgesia for pediatric procedures should be standard in the ED. According to JCAHO and the American Society of Anesthesiologists (ASA), there are only two levels that are appropriate for the ED: minimal sedation (anxiolysis), and moderate sedation/analgesia ("procedural sedation").[26] The fact that two children may respond differently to the same dose of medication necessitates advanced planning on the part of the ED staff. The procedural sedation and analgesia policy should include the following: preparation (patient history and physical examination, information about allergies, prior sedation and analgesia procedures, last meal and liquids), monitoring parameters, "nothing by mouth" guidelines, appropriate candidates for sedation (ASA

Physical Status Classification classes I and II), parental consent, and discharge criteria.[26] Depending upon the level of sedation planned, the monitoring parameters may change, as will the equipment available in the room and the personnel present[26-29] (see Chapter 159, Procedural Sedation and Analgesia).

Drug Testing

The use of drug testing for alcohol, drugs of abuse, controlled substance, or other toxins should be written in an ED policy. In some states, the state police can request that a physician perform this test, even without the patient's consent. In some states, the emergency physician is required to obtain drug testing if the physician believes the patient was given a controlled substance without his or her consent. If it is unclear that the patient was given a drug, then asking the patient for consent is appropriate. The consent form for a toxicology screen should be completed by the patient/legal guardian, and witnessed, timed, and dated. It may also be possible for the patient/legal guardian to sign the consent later, and to revoke the consent (both within 48 hours).

Health Care–Acquired Infection

One of the 2004 JCAHO safety parameters is to reduce the risk of health care–acquired infection.[22] This can be accomplished by complying with the Centers for Disease Control and Prevention (CDC) hand hygiene guidelines.[30] Items in these guidelines include limiting the use of artificial nails, keeping natural nails short, and using alcohol-based hand cleaners.[22,30] In addition, nosocomial infections that result in unanticipated death or major permanent loss of function should be managed as sentinel events.[22]

Infectious Diseases

In the United States, state laws and regulations mandate which diseases are reportable, and this varies from state to state. Local and/or state departments of health collect this information. The CDC maintains a list of notifiable infectious diseases that is released every year that allows the CDC to follow trends in reportable disease across the United States during a given year, and from year to year. This list currently contains 60 diseases such as acquired immunodeficiency syndrome, anthrax, gonorrhea, hepatitis (types A, B, and C), Lyme disease, meningococcal disease, pertussis, salmonellosis, shigellosis, smallpox, syphilis, and tuberculosis.[31,32] Recently, diseases such as erhlichosis, giardiasis, severe acute respiratory syndrome (SARS), smallpox, and vancomycin-intermediate and -resistant *Staphylococcus aureus* have been added.[31]

The use of standard precautions took on a heightened awareness during the early days of acquired immunodeficiency syndrome/human immunodeficiency virus infection, and this has continued. In order to reduce the number of needle sticks, there has been an increased use of needleless systems and retractable needles. With new and emerging infections such as SARS, this has progressed to include special respiratory masks (N-95), rather than simple paper/procedure masks.

The ED should have policies regarding the use of isolation rooms, negative pressure rooms (if available), and patient decontamination. There should also be a policy regarding exposure to potential blood-borne pathogens, which includes reporting, testing, and prophylaxis.

EMTALA

The Emergency Medical Treatment and Labor Act (EMTALA) is a federal law that forbids a hospital, physician, dentist, or other health care provider to refuse to provide emergency care based upon a patient's inability to pay[33] (see Chapter 150, Emergency Medical Treatment and Labor Act [EMTALA]). This legislation, often referred to as the Comprehensive Omnibus Budget Reconciliation Act or "anti-dumping" legislation, is included in Title XVII of the Social Security Act. Any hospital that received Medicare funding must comply with these regulations, even for non-Medicare patients. A hospital can be fined up to $50,000 per violation, and the hospital's or physicians' Medicare and Medicaid agreements may be terminated by the Centers for Medicare & Medicaid Services.[33,34]

EMTALA applies when a person comes to a hospital with an ED and requests care for an emergency medical condition. It also applies if a parent is requesting care for his or her child. An emergency medical condition is an illness or injury that manifests itself by acute symptoms requiring immediate attention to avoid placing the health of the person in serious jeopardy.[33] In terms of a woman in labor, this constitutes inadequate time to transfer her prior to delivery. However, the existence of an "emergency medical condition" is based upon the definition of a prudent layperson, not a health care professional.[33]

In order to fulfill the EMTALA obligation, a patient must be screened and, if necessary, stabilized. If a patient cannot be stabilized, he or she must be transferred to an appropriate facility, with the receiving facility aware of and accepting the transfer.[33]

The ED and hospital should have an EMTALA policy that addresses items such as what constitutes a screening examination, who can perform the screening examination, which parts of the hospital/main campus qualify under EMTALA, and who responds to medical emergencies outside of the ED.[33,34]

A revised aspect of EMTALA is the "on-call" requirement. Each hospital must have an on-call schedule and written policies related to the schedule, including response times. This policy applies to emergency physicians as well as medical and surgical specialists[34] (see Chapter 150, Emergency Medical Treatment and Labor Act [EMTALA]).

Transfer Policies and Procedures

A transfer policy should be in place for hospitals that do not have pediatric intensive care units, inpatient beds, or pediatric trauma capabilities/specialists, or when specialized pediatric care is not available. It is helpful to have a list of referral hospitals and contact numbers placed prominently in the ED. It is preferable to have transfer agreements with several hospitals in the region for similar or different categories of patients (e.g., trauma vs. medical). These agreements should be signed by the hospital chief executive officer and updated as needed. In some cases, these agreements are extremely important for reimbursement if the transfer involves crossing state lines. In rare cases, the receiving facility may have no available beds, but can assist the transferring hospital in finding another appropriate

facility. Before the patient is transferred, there should be physician-to-physician and nurse-to-nurse communication. Written documentation, including consent to transfer, method of transfer, and reason for transfer, should be included.[35]

Hospital Overcrowding

In 2003, there were nearly 114 million ED visits, a 26% increase over the last 10 years.[36] Yet at the same time, the number of EDs decreased by 10%.[36] This is just one of the many causes of hospital overcrowding, a situation in which the identified need for emergency services exceeds the available resources in the ED.[37] This problem can affect child-friendly EDs and can result in ambulance diversion, where an ED does not have the capability to accept an EMS/ambulance patient, and prolonged ED stays after admission or transfer decisions are made due to a lack of inpatient beds ("ED boarders").[37,38] This may mean that an ill child will be transported by EMS to another ED that may be further away, and perhaps not child friendly. It can also mean that, even after an ill or injured child has been stabilized, there may be no available beds at the pediatric centers. While there are no easy solutions to this problem, utilizing QI indicators to track time on EMS diversion, ED boarding time, ED waiting room time, the number of patients who left without being seen, and the number of times when patients could not be transferred in a timely manner will help those outside the ED realize there is a problem, and help advocate for change.

Summary

The process of developing ED preparedness for children is not a new issue. Over the last 20 years, the goal of the EMSC program was to assure that children were included in the entire scope of care, including out-of-hospital care, the ED, and hospital care. Many of the policies and programs developed over the past 10 years were the result of this initiative.[7,9,12-15] By being inclusive rather than exclusive, many national organizations have supported the idea of pediatric ED guidelines for preparedness. It is unrealistic to expect that a rural community hospital that lacks pediatric inpatient beds would have the same ED equipment and supplies as a large suburban community hospital with pediatric inpatient beds, or even an urban, freestanding children's hospital. The goal is to provide some ideas, solutions, and examples that will improve the care of children everywhere.

The Future: An ACEP/AAP Implementation Kit

The AECP, through a grant from the federal EMSC program, is developing an implementation kit for ED preparedness.[39] This kit contains information such as a copy of the AAP/ACEP paper "Care of Children in Emergency Departments: Guidelines for Preparedness"[7]; 12 model emergency department policies for care of children, including child maltreatment, consent, and death in the ED; relevant ACEP and AAP pediatric clinical care guidelines and policies; a pediatric medication calculator; and a pediatric preparedness checklist. Prior to wide dissemination, the implementation kit is currently being evaluated, and will be refined based on evidence generated (Table 154–3).

Table 154–3 **ACEP/AAP Implementation Kit for ED Preparedness**

- A copy of "Care of Children in the Emergency Department: Guidelines for Preparedness."[7]
- 12 model ED policies for the care of children
- Pediatric Medication Calculator
- Pediatric Preparedness Checklist

Abbreviations: AAP, American Academy of Pediatrics; ACEP, American College of Emergency Physicians; ED, emergency department.

REFERENCES

*1. American College of Emergency Physicians: Emergency care guidelines. Ann Emerg Med 29:564–571, 1997.

2. Athey J, Dean JM, Ball J, et al: Ability of hospitals to care for pediatric emergency patients. Pediatr Emerg Care 17:170–174, 2001

3. McGillivray D, Nijssen-Jordan C, Kramer MS, et al: Critical pediatric equipment availability in Canadian hospital emergency departments. Ann Emerg Med 37:371–376, 2001.

4. The community hospital emergency department. *In* Seidel JS, Knapp JF (eds): Childhood Emergencies in the Office, Hospital, and Community: Organizing Systems of Care. Elk Grove Village, IL: American Academy of Pediatrics, 2000, pp 133–150.

5. State of Illinois, Administrative Code: Illinois Department of Public Health, Emergency Services and Highway Safety, Section 515.100: Definitions. Available at *http://www.ilga.gov/commission/jcar/admincode/077/077005150A01000R.html*

*6. Committee on Pediatric Emergency Medicine, American Academy of Pediatrics: Guidelines for pediatric emergency care facilities. Pediatrics 96:526–537, 1995.

*7. American Academy of Pediatrics, Committee on Pediatric Emergency Medicine; and American College of Emergency Physicians, Pediatric Committee: Care of children in the emergency department: guidelines for preparedness. Pediatrics 107:777–781, 2001. [also published in Ann Emerg Med 37:423–427, 2001]

*8. American College of Emergency Physicians. Pediatric equipment guidelines. Ann Emerg Med 25:307–309, 1995.

*9. Committee on Pediatric Equipment and Supplies for Emergency Departments, National Emergency Medical Services for Children Resource Alliance: Guidelines for pediatric equipment and supplies for emergency departments. Ann Emerg Med 31:54–57, 1998.

10. State of California, Health and Welfare Agency, Emergency Medical Services Authority: Administration, Personnel and Policy Guidelines for the Care of Pediatric Patients in the Emergency Department (EMSA#182). Sacramento: Emergency Medical Services Authority, 1994.

11. Los Angeles County Department of Health Services, Emergency Medical Services Agency. Available at *http://www.dhs.co.la.ca.us/ems*

12. State of Illinois, Administrative Code: Illinois Department of Public Health, Emergency Services and Highway Safety, Section 515.4000: Facility Recognition Criteria for the Emergency Department Approved for Pediatrics (EDAP). Available at *http://www.luhs.org/depts/emsc/EDAPres/02crf515.400.doc*

13. State of Illinois, Administrative Code: Illinois Department of Public Health, Emergency Services and Highway Safety, Section 515.4010: Facility Recognition Criteria for the Standby Emergency Department Approved for Pediatrics (SEDP). Available at *http://www.luhs.org/depts/emsc/EDAPres/03sec515.4010.doc*

14. State of Illinois, Administrative Code: Illinois Department of Public Health, Emergency Services and Highway Safety, Section 515: Appendix L, Pediatric Equipment Recommendations for Emergency Departments. Available at *http://www.luhs.org/depts/emsc/stndrd-ed-guideline.htm*

15. State of Illinois, Administrative Code: Illinois Department of Public Health, Emergency Services and Highway Safety, Section 515: Appendix M, Interfacility Pediatric Trauma and Critical Care Consultations and/or Transfer Guideline. Available at *http://www.luhs.org/depts/emsc/stndrd-transfer.htm*

*16. Triage Curriculum. Emergency Nurses Association web site. Aailable at *http://www.ena.org*

17. Emergency Severity Index (ESI). Emergency Nurses Association web site. Available at *http://www.ena.org*

*18. Seidel J, Knapp JF: Preparedness for pediatric emergencies. *In* Gausche-Hill M, Fuchs SD, Yamamoto L (eds): APLS: The Pediatric Emergency Medicine Resource, 4th ed. Boston: Jones and Bartlett, 2004, pp 1–17.

19. Making the environment child friendly. *In* Seidel JS, Knapp JF (eds): Childhood Emergencies in the Office, Hospital, and Community: Organizing Systems of Care. Elk Grove Village, IL: American Academy of Pediatrics, 2000, pp 151–158.

20. Emergency Nurses Pediatric Care Course. Emergency Nurses Association web site. Available at *http://www.ena.org*

21. Illinois Emergency Medical Services for Children: Pediatric Educational Recommendations for Professional Healthcare Providers. Available at *http://www.luhs.org/depts/emsc/stndrd-edu.htm*

*22. 2004 National Patient Safety Goals. Joint Commission on Accreditation of Healthcare Organizations web site. Available at *http://www.jointcommission.org/PatientSafety/NationalPatientSafetyGoals/2004_npsgs.htm*

23. Illinois Emergency Medical Services for Children. Continuous Quality Improvement. *http://www.luhs.org/depts/emsc/quality.htm*.

24. Illinois Emergency Medical Services for Children. Interfacility Pediatric Trauma and Critical Care Consultation and/or Transfer Guideline. *http://www.luhs.org/depts/emsc/stndrd-transfer.htm*.

25. Behavioral Health Care Standards on Restraint and Seclusion. Joint Commission on Accreditation of Healthcare Organizations web site: *http://www.jointcommission.org/accreditationprograms/behavioralhealthcare/standards*

26. Sacchetti A: Procedural sedation and analgesia. *In* Gausche-Hill M, Fuchs SD, Yamamoto L (eds): APLS: The Pediatric Emergency Medicine Resource, 4th ed. Boston: Jones and Bartlett, 2004, pp 498–523.

27. American Academy of Pediatrics, Committee on Drugs: Guidelines for monitoring and management of pediatric patients during and after diagnostic and therapeutic procedures. Pediatrics 89:1110–1115, 1992.

*28. Mace SE, Barata IA, Cravero JP, et al: Clinical policy: Evidence-based approach to pharmacologic agents used in pediatric sedation and analgesia in the emergency department. Ann Emerg Med 44:342–377, 2004.

29. American Society of Anesthesiologists Task Force on Sedation and Anesthesia by Non-Anesthesiologists: Practice guidelines for sedation and analgesia by non-anesthesiologists. Anesthesiology 94:1004–1017, 2002.

30. Centers for Disease Control and Prevention: Guidelines for hand hygiene in health care settings: recommendations of the Healthcare Infection Control Practices Advisory Committee and the HICPAC/SHEA/APIC/IDSA Hand Hygiene Task Force. MMWR Morb Mortal Wkly Rep 51(RR-16): 26–34, 2002.

31. Centers for Disease Control and Prevention. Nationally Notifiable Infectious Diseases, United States, 2005. Available at *http://www.cdc.gov/epo/dphsi/PHS/infdis2005.htm*

32. Centers for Disease Control and Prevention: Case definition for infectious conditions under public health surveillance. MMWR Recomm Rep 46(RR-10):1–55, 1997. (Also available at *http://www.cdc.gov/epo/dphsi/casedef/index.htm*)

33. Emergency Medical Treatment and Labor Act (EMTALA). Fed Reg 68(174):53222, 2003.

34. CMS Interpretive Guidelines on EMTALA. Centers for Medicare & Medicaid Services web site. Available at *http://www/cms/hhs.gov/providers/emtala*

35. The pediatric critical care center. *In* Seidel JS, Knapp JF (eds): Childhood Emergencies in the Office, Hospital, and Community: Organizing Systems of Care. Elk Grove Village, IL: American Academy of Pediatrics, 2000, pp 159–172.

36. McCraig LF, Burt CW: National Hospital Ambulatory Medical Care Survey: 2003 emergency department summary. Adv Data 358:1–38, 2005.

37. American Academy of Pediatrics, Committee on Pediatric Emergency Medicine: Overcrowding crisis in our nation's emergency departments: Is our safety net unraveling? Pediatrics 114:878–888, 2004.

*38. American College of Emergency Physicians, Crowding Resources Task Force: Responding to Emergency Department Crowding: A Guidebook for Chapters. Dallas: American College of Emergency Physicians, 2002.

39. American College of Emergency Physicians. Care of Children in the Emergency Department: Guidelines for Preparedness-Implementation Kit. Available at *http://host.acep.org.tmp3.secure-xp.net/aapacep*

---

*Suggested readings.

Chapter 155

Triage

Sharon E. Mace, MD and Thom A. Mayer, MD

Key Points

Triage is the prioritization of care based on illness/injury, severity, prognosis, and resource availability.

Triage identifies patients who cannot wait to be seen, prioritizes all patients, and initiates diagnostic and therapeutic measures.

Disaster triage differs from emergency department triage. During a disaster with limited resources, patients with little or no chance of survival are not resuscitated.

The disaster triage categories are red (most urgent, first priority), yellow (urgent, second priority), green (nonurgent, walking wounded, third priority), and black (dead or catastrophic).

Introduction and Background

Triage is the prioritization of patient care (or victims during a disaster) based on illness/injury, severity, prognosis, and resource availability. The purpose of triage is to identify patients needing immediate resuscitation; to assign patients to a predesignated patient care area, thereby prioritizing their care; and to initiate diagnostic/therapeutic measures as appropriate.

The term *triage* originated from the French verb *trier* which means to sort. During the time of Napoleon, the French military used triage to serve as a battlefield clearing hospital for wounded soldiers. The U.S. military's first use of triage was during the Civil War. Triage on the battlefield was a distribution center from which injured soldiers were sorted or distributed to various hospitals. For the military during World Wars I and II, triage was the procedure that determined which injured soldiers were able to be returned to the battlefield. Military triage continued to evolve during the Korean and Vietnam wars with the tenet of doing the "greatest good for the greatest number of wounded and injured."[1] Refinements in battlefield medicine and military triage have continued during more recent conflicts, including Iraq.

Other situations in which the triage process has been employed, in addition to the battlefield, are during disasters, following mass casualty incidents (MCI), and in emergency departments (EDs). Triage during a disaster involves field triage, which sorts disaster victims into categories ranging from the walking wounded to those with injuries who are salvageable to the unsalvageable and the dead.

Issues and Solutions

The Triage Process

The nurse assesses and determines priority of care (triages) based not only on the patient's physical, developmental, and psychosocial needs but also on parameters of patient flow in the emergency care system and of health care access. According to the Emergency Nurses Association (ENA), triage should be done by an experienced nurse with competency in triage.[2,3] The nurse should accomplish the following during triage: take history appropriate to the severity of the complaint, obtain vital signs, ask predetermined ED/hospital-required screening questions, and assign patient priority. Triage may be either focused or comprehensive. Comprehensive triage refers to taking a complete history, checking vital signs, determining allergies, and, where appropriate, performing a physical examination. Focused triage is generally used for more minor illnesses or injuries and includes a more limited history and screening prior to assessing patient priority. Triage bypass, which is addressed more fully later in this chapter, refers to an approach that places patients directly into ED rooms at times when space and staffing allow, and triage is performed at the bedside.

The advantages of comprehensive triage include immediate identification of patients with life-threatening or emergent conditions and administration of basic first aid measures. In addition, the patient (and family) are met by an experienced nurse who can address the patient/family's physical, psychosocial, and emotional issues.

One criticism of a comprehensive triage system is that it takes too much time, thereby creating a "logjam" of patients backed up waiting to be seen by the triage nurse.[4] This has led to a two-tier triage system with the triage nurse determining, from the chief complaint and an observation or "across the room" assessment, who is taken immediately to the patient care area versus waiting for additional assessment and registration. The two-tiered triage system includes a primary nurse and a sorter nurse, and may be used to achieve comprehensive triage during high-volume periods.

Pediatric and geriatric patients take more time to triage than other patients. Comprehensive triage is said to take only 2 to 5 minutes, although one study found that this occurred only 22% of the time.[5] A concern has been expressed that this 2- to 5-minute time frame for triage may be unrealistic.[4] There have also been studies indicating inconsistency in triage assessment among experienced triage personnel and between nurses and physicians.[6-10] Whether focused triage, comprehensive triage, or triage bypass is used, performance improvement data should be monitored to assess efficacy.

Triage Categories

Emergency department triage has several functions, including (1) identification of patients who should not wait to be seen, and (2) prioritization of incoming patients. This is accomplished by determining the patient's illness/injury severity or acuity. Acuity is the degree to which the patient's condition is life- or limb-threatening and whether immediate treatment is needed to alleviate symptoms.

There are various triage acuity systems ranging from two to five levels (Table 155–1). In the United States, a three-level triage system is most commonly used (69%), with 12% of EDs using a four-level system, 3% using a five-level model, and 16% using no acuity system or nonresponding according to an ENA survey done in 2001.[11] There is some evidence that a five-level triage system is more effective than a three-level triage system.[12]

Specific Triage Systems

Various triage systems have been used throughout the world: the Australian Triage Scale, the Manchester Triage Scale, the Canadian Triage and Acuity Scale, and the Emergency Severity Index (ESI)[13-21] (Table 155–2). All four of these scales have been validated for reliability and validity in adults.[14-17]

Emergency Severity Index

The ESI is a five-level triage system developed in the United States that uses a flowchart-based triage algorithm.[18-21] The ESI uses patient acuity (stability of vital signs, degree of distress), as well as expected resource intensity and timeliness (expected staff response, time to disposition), to define the five categories (Table 155–3).

Pediatric Triage

Of the approximately 110.2 million patients seen in EDs in the United States in 2002, about 30% were pediatric patients, with 85% of those seen in general EDs.[22] Furthermore, there is some evidence that, in a general ED, adults may be "seen sooner than equally ill pediatric patients, resulting in unacceptable waiting times for seriously ill pediatric patients" unless triage criteria are modified for pediatric patients.[23] Improvement in pediatric patient flow with an increase in pediatric triage acuity levels (e.g., a significant increase in the emergent and urgent pediatric patients) resulted from incorporating specific pediatric acuity markers and from posting age-specific abnormal signs and symptoms.[23]

Issues relevant to pediatric triage include inapplicability of adult triage criteria to pediatric patients; the often subtle and difficult-to-recognize signs and symptoms of illness/injury in young children and infants, especially those less than 1 to 2 years of age; the frequent unreliability of the clinical impression (even with experienced triage personnel); physiology and behavior in children and infants, particularly in infants, different from that in adults; greater morbidity and mortality in pediatric patients than in adults for similar diseases; and symptom variability during a given illness. Because

---

Table 155–1 Triage Acuity Systems by Level

2 Levels	3 Levels	4 Levels	5 Levels	5 Levels
Emergent	Emergent	Life threatening	Resuscitation	Critical
Nonemergent	Urgent	Emergent	Emergent	Emergent
	Nonurgent	Urgent	Urgent	Urgent
		Nonurgent	Nonurgent	Nonurgent
			Referred	Fast track

Table 155–2 International Triage Systems

Australasian		Manchester (United Kingdom)		Canadian		Emergency Severity Index	
Level	Physician/ Staff Response Time (min)	Level	Physician/ Staff Response Time (min)	Level	Physician/ Staff Response Time (min)	Level	Physician/ Staff Response Time (min)
1 = Resuscitation	0 (Immediate)	1 = Immediate (Red)	0 (Immediate)	1 = Resuscitation	0 (Immediate)	1 = Unstable	0 (Immediate)
2 = Emergency	≤10	2 = Very Urgent (Orange)	≤10	2 = Emergent	≤15	2 = Threatened	Minutes
3 = Urgent	≤30	3 = Urgent (Yellow)	≤60	3 = Urgent	≤30	3 = Stable	≤60
4 = Semi-Urgent	≤60	4 = Standard (Green)	≤120	4 = Less Urgent	≤60	4 = Stable	Could be delayed
5 = Nonurgent	≤120	5 = Nonurgent (Blue)	≤240	5 = Nonurgent	≤120	5 = Stable	Could be delayed

Table 155–3	Emergency Severity Index (ESI)				
	ESI-1	**ESI-2**	**ESI-3**	**ESI-4**	**ESI-5**
Stability of vital functions (ABCs)	Unstable	Threatened	Stable	Stable	Stable
Life threat or organ threat	Obvious	Reasonably likely	Unlikely (possible)	No	No
Requires resuscitation	Immediately	Sometimes	Seldom	No	No
Severe pain or severe distress	Yes	Yes (sufficient, but not necessary for this category)	No	No	No
Expected resource intensity	Maximum: staff at bedside continuously; mobilization of outside resources	High: multiple, often complex diagnostic studies; frequent consultation; continuous (remote) monitoring	Medium: multiple diagnostic studies; or brief period of observation; or complex procedure	Low: one simple diagnostic study; or one simple procedure	Low: examination only
Physician/staff response	Immediate team effort	Minutes	Up to 1 hr	Could be delayed	Could be delayed
Expected time to disposition	1.5 hr	4 hr	6 hr	2 hr	1 hr
Examples	Cardiac arrest, intubated trauma patient, severe drug overdose	Most chest pain, stable trauma (mechanism concerning), elderly pneumonia patient, altered mental status, behavioral disturbance (potential violence)	Most abdominal pain, dehydration, esophageal food impaction, hip fracture	Closed extremity trauma, simple laceration, cystitis, typical migraine	Sore throat, minor burn, recheck

of the difficulties in determining acuity for infants less than 6 months old, some have recommended that EDs that see relatively few pediatric patients assign all children less than 6 months old to the emergent category.[24]

Triage Categories and Triage Systems for Pediatric Patients

Various acuity systems for specific diseases, illnesses, and injuries in pediatric patients have been developed. Multiple pediatric trauma scoring systems exist.[25] Scoring systems for specific respiratory diseases, such as "Croup Scores," have also been developed.[26] Various scales for assessment of the young infant with fever, such as the Yale observational scale, have been used to specifically evaluate the febrile infant.[27] Unfortunately, a comprehensive pediatric triage assessment tool that applies to all types of pediatric illnesses and injuries throughout the entire range of pediatric age groups (newborns, infants, toddlers, preschool age, early school years, and adolescence) has yet to be developed and validated in extensive numbers of pediatric patients.[24] However, several pediatric triage and/or assessment tools are available.

A commonly used triage acuity classification for pediatric patients uses four levels[28]:

Class 1—critical: life- or limb-threatening illness/injury that needs immediate care

Class 2—acute: significant alteration in physical or mental health that could potentially become life or limb threatening and needs intervention as soon as possible

Class 3—urgent: significant physical or mental health problems that are not life threatening and need intervention in a timely fashion

Class 4—nonurgent: may receive care when convenient

These are similar to the adult four-level acuity classifications. More recently, a five-level system has been suggested, again similar to the adult five-level acuity classifications: level 1 = critical, level 2 = emergent, level 3 = urgent, level 4 = nonurgent, and level 5 = fast track[29] (see Table 155–1).

Several important caveats have also been suggested. All immunocompromised pediatric patients should be considered as being seriously ill even if their presenting symptoms are not critical.[30] Immunocompromised patients include those on corticosteroids or immunosuppressives; patients with chronic illnesses, malignancy, and sickle cell disease; and the very young (particularly young infants), who may not have the typical signs and symptoms of a serious or life-threatening illness early during the course of their illness. Such high-risk patients, including patients with a history of premature birth, chronic illness, and being immunocompromised, may initially "look well" and then rapidly deteriorate.

Child maltreatment should be considered in the differential diagnosis of all pediatric complaints. Key elements of the suspected child abuse or neglect (SCAN) triage interview include detailed documentation of a thorough history with quotes, and an exact description of findings and observations.[28,31]

Many of the specific pediatric triage systems are based on the primary survey (airway, breathing, and circulation [ABCs]) and a secondary survey from the American College of Surgeons Committee on Trauma[28,32,33] (Tables 155–4 and 155–5). A primary and secondary pediatric triage survey using an A-to-J alphabetized mnemonic is included in the Emergency Nursing Pediatric Course[28] (see Table 155–4).

All of these various triage systems, whether adult or pediatric, need to be validated for reliability and validity in large numbers of pediatric patients. There is evidence that application of the adult triage systems (see Table 155–2) may not be valid for pediatric patients without the addition of pediatric clinical observations and pediatric vital signs, which may lead to a more reliable triage of younger children.[23,34-36]

Table 155–4   Primary and Secondary Pediatric Triage Survey

	Primary		Secondary
A = Airway	✔ Patency, positioning for air entry, audible sounds, airway obstruction (blood, mucus, edema, foreign body)	F = Find	Find out underlying history of current illness or injury
B = Breathing	✔ Increased or decreased work of respiration, quality of breath sounds; nasal flaring; use of accessory muscles; pattern; quality; rate	G = Get vital signs	Obtain vital signs, obtain orthostatic vital signs if condition warrants
C = Circulation	✔ Color and temperature of skin; capillary refill; strength and rate of peripheral pulses	H = Head-to-toe assessment	Perform a head-to-toe assessment for a complete and thorough examination
C = Cervical collar	Placement of a cervical collar when indicated	I = Initiate	Initiate the Triage Documentation Record
C = Consciousness	✔ Level of consciousness (Glasgow Coma Scale); response to environment; muscle tone; pupil response	I = Isolate	Assess patient for rashes, communicable diseases, or immunosuppression, and place in appropriate isolation
D = Dextrose	✔ Serum glucose level in patients with altered mental status	I = Intervention	Perform triage interventions (first aid, medication administration, diagnostic studies)
E = Expose	Expose patient by undressing to identify underlying injuries	J = Judgment	Make appropriate triage classification of patient acuity

Table 155–5   Triage Observation Tool

Triage Observation Tool (No/Yes)	
Airway	Obstructed airway (blood, vomit, foreign bodies, facial burn)
	Allergic reaction
Breathing	Increased respiratory effort
	Fatigue, nasal flaring
	Tachypnea
	Tracheal tug, chest recession
	Wheeze, stridor, grunting
	Bradypnea, hypoventilation
	O₂ saturation higher than expected for degree of respiratory effort
Circulation	Tachycardia, bradycardia
	Capillary return >2 sec
	Pale, mottled, or cyanosed
	Peripheral pulses or perfusion
	Obvious bleeding out
	Sunken eyes, dry oral mucosa
	Decreased feeding, decreased urine output
Disability	Irritable or drowsy and hard to wake
	Responds only to pain
	High-pitched cry
	Obvious pain
Expose	Purpura
	Chickenpox or measles
Risk Factors	Oncology patient or immunosuppressed
	Cardiac history
	Infant <3 mo old
	Diabetic or metabolic illness
	Central line or Port-A-Cath

Training and pediatric experience may also play a role in nursing triage assessment of pediatric patients.[37,38]

PEDIATRIC ASSESSMENT TRIANGLE

The pediatric assessment triangle refers to an "across-the-room" assessment or a quick "eyeball" assessment of the pediatric patient.[33] This is done while the triage nurse obtains the history and chief complaint. The assessment triangle includes evaluation of the infant or child's overall appearance (look, cry or speech, hygiene/dress), breathing (respiratory effort and rate), and skin circulation (color, appearance)[33] (see Chapter 10, General Approach to Poisoning).

SAVE-A-CHILD GUIDE

A pediatric triage mnemonic—"SAVE-a-CHILD"—was designed to aid in recognizing a seriously ill pediatric patient.[24] SAVE stands for the skin, activity, ventilation, and eye contact. SAVE is based on observations made before touching the child. The "CHILD" component stands for cry, heat, immune system, level of consciousness, and dehydration; this information is obtained from the parent (or caregiver) and a brief examination[24] (Fig. 155–1).

Pediatric Triage Assessment and Interventions

Pediatric assessment may use any one or a combination of techniques (e.g., pediatric assessment triangle, SAVE-a-CHILD, primary/secondary survey using ABCs). Important elements in the triage history include the chief complaint, history of present illness or injury, allergies, medications, immunizations, and past medical history.

Several mnemonics for the history have been suggested. CIAMPEDS stands for chief complaint, immunizations or isolation (communicable disease exposure), allergies, medications, past medical history, events surrounding the illness or injury, diet or diapers (bowel/bladder history), and symptoms associated with the illness/injury. Alternatively, the OLDCART mnemonic has also been used (onset of symptoms, location of problem, duration of symptoms, characteristics of symptoms, aggravating factors, relieving factors, and treatment before arrival). For patients in pain, PQRST has been used: precipitating factors, quality of pain, region/radiation of pain, severity, and time of pain onset.

A problem-oriented method, the SOAPIE format, has been recommended by the ENA for comprehensive triage documentation. SOAPIE follows the steps in the comprehensive triage process from obtaining the history and vital signs, to assigning a triage category, to determining and

Save-A-Child	
Recognition of the seriously ill pediatric patient	
Skin	Mottled? Cyanotic? Petechiae? Pallor?
Activity	Needs assistance/ Not ambulating? Responsive?
Ventilation	Retractions? Head bobbing? Drooling? Nasal flaring? Slow rate? Fast rate? Stridor? Wheezing?
Eye Contact	Glassy stare? Fails to engage/focus?
Abuse	Unexplained bruising/injuries? Inappropriate parent?
Cry	High pitched, cephalic? Irritable?
Heat	High fever (>41°)? Hypothermia (36°)?
Immune System	Sickle cell? AIDS? Corticosteroids?
Level of Consciousness	Irritable? Lethargic? Pain only? Convulsing? Unresponsive?
Dehydration	Hollow eyes? Capillary refill? Cold hands, feet? Voiding? Severe diarrhea? Vomiting: projectile, bilious, persistent? Dry mucous membranes?
SAVE: Observations made prior to touching the child **CHILD**: History from caretaker and brief exam	

FIGURE 155–1. SAVE-a-CHILD triage system for recognition of the seriously ill pediatric patient.

implementing diagnostic/therapeutic measures and reassessing the patient. SOAPIE stands for *s*ubjective data (chief complaint); *o*bjective data such as vital signs; *a*nalysis of data, leading to assigning acuity; *p*lan, or what is to be done; *i*nitiating diagnostic/therapeutic interventions per protocols and nursing practice; and *e*valuation, which indicates that triage is a dynamic process with constant evaluation and re-evaluation.

Triage interventions range from beginning diagnostic studies, such as radiologic studies and an electrocardiogram, to initiating therapeutic measures, including giving oral pain medications and antipyretics and applying dressings. Other triage measures include applying topical anesthetics to wounds (to be sutured later) and to potential intravenous sites for children and infants who will likely needs intravenous fluids and/or medications. Such treatment interventions in triage have been shown to decrease ED turnaround time, thereby improving ED flow. Triage-initiated protocols can expedite care and improve patient/family satisfaction.

Customer Service at Triage

Customer service has become an increasingly emphasized aspect of the provision of emergency medical care, and is especially pertinent to the care of children. Virtually every hospital in the country has some patient satisfaction tool, which is used to assess the patient's and family's perception of the care that they received in the ED. While the axiom "You never get a second chance to make a first impression" was not meant to specifically describe ED triage, it might well have been. Nearly 75% of patients presenting to the ED undergo triage, which is their first contact with the medical care system. For that reason, triage nurses and other personnel assisting in the process should be trained in the importance of delivering customer service excellence at the earliest appropriate time. Mayer and Cates have suggested that this comprises three elements[39]:

- Making the customer service diagnosis as well as the clinical diagnosis
- Negotiating agreement and resolution of expectations
- Building moments of truth into the clinical encounter

By way of simple example, one of the most common clinical presentations in the pediatric and general ED is the child with fever. While the clinical diagnosis is often apparent, even at triage, the customer service diagnosis comprises the fear of more serious illness on the part of the parents and perhaps even the child. Addressing those concerns at triage by providing reassurance at the earliest time is an extremely important part of maximizing patient satisfaction. Similarly, the parent's expectations are often dramatically different from those of experienced health care providers, since the parents often are concerned that the child may have seizures, meningitis, or another life-threatening illness, whereas an experienced clinician may understand from simple observation of the child that these diagnoses are not likely. In order to assure that the best customer service is provided, negotiating these expectations is important, and can also begin at triage.

Finally, the concept of "moments of truth" was originally described by Jan Carlzon in a book of that same name. Carlzon pointed out that customer perceptions are usually not based on technical aspects, but rather comprise what he described as "50,000 Moments of Truth per day, created by the service provider himself."[40] Thus the institution is not assessed so much on the detailed provision of clinical care, but on the moments of truth provided by the nurses, physicians, technicians, and other ED personnel. For example, simple statements ("scripts") can be made, such as, "I have three children of my own, and I remember how concerned I was the first time one of them developed a fever in the middle of the night." Delivering excellent customer service and assuring patient satisfaction require the same proactive approach that one would apply to clinical guidelines or protocols. The customer service aspects of triage should be discussed among the providers of clinical care, so that such scripts and procedures can be proactively developed.

Newer Concepts of Triage

Virtually all EDs encounter times when they are severely capacity constrained. A number of creative process improvements have been made to help assure that triage functions expeditiously, even at times when there are a large number of patients to be seen. These include advanced triage/advanced initiatives (AT/AI), Team Triage and Treatment, triage bypass, Triage Away, and secondary triage. Each of these is designed to be used in various ways and addresses the substantial capacity constraint issues faced by many EDs, including both general and pediatric EDs.

AT/AI consists of a set of medically approved standing orders and initiatives that may be implemented at the triage area at times when rooms are not available in the treatment area. These include protocols for minor extremity trauma, urinary tract infections, abdominal pain, neutropenic patients with fever, and pretreatment of lacerations with topical anesthetic agents. Each of these protocols is discussed in advance between the medical and nursing staff of the ED, approved jointly, and implemented after training of the triage nurses.

Triage bypass is utilized at times when several patients have presented to triage, but there are adequate numbers of physicians, nurses, and support personnel in the treatment area to care for such patients in a timely fashion. Since these patients will be seen by the same ED staff in the same treatment areas, they bypass triage, are registered in the room, and are triaged and treated by the same nurses and physicians who will be caring for them. Because of the nature of patient flow and the fact that most EDs become capacity constrained by the mid-morning or afternoon hours, triage bypass is predominantly utilized during the early to mid-morning hours.

Team Triage and Treatment is a unique and innovative approach to dealing with capacity constraints by assigning an emergency physician (or physician assistant/nurse practitioner), nurse, technician, and, in some cases, registrar to the triage area at times when there are predictable delays in patient care due to the number of treatment rooms available. Following initial triage by the triage nurse, acutely ill or injured patients are sent directly back to the treatment area. Similarly, patients with minor (fast track) problems are sent to such an area. The remainder of the patients are then evaluated at the triage area by the team triage members. In a busy level I trauma center that sees over 80,000 patients per year, team triage is utilized approximately 8 hours per day and substantially decompresses patient waiting times, improves patient satisfaction, improves patient safety, and offers better access to care for patients (T. Mayer, personal communication, May 2005). These data indicate that one third of such patients are evaluated, treated, and have their treatment completed at the triage area, including patients with sufficient severity of abdominal pain to warrant an abdominal computed tomography scan. While this program requires an investment in resources, the reduction in patients left without treatment and the capacity for increasing volume more than offset the cost of the investment in the program.

Triage Away is a program used in some EDs that have chosen to evaluate patients at triage and, when it is determined that they have a minor illness or injury, simply triage them away to other facilities. In some communities such programs can be effective; however, it does require a clearly specified primary health clinic or public health facility to which the patients can be safely and efficiently triaged. Such Triage Away programs are unusual, precisely because the safety net capacity of the ED is not backed up by such primary care or public health facilities in most communities.

Secondary triage refers to the combined effort of the emergency physicians and nurses to re-triage patients who are already in treatment rooms either to alternate rooms or to hallway spaces at times when their workup and treatment have not been completed, but additional patients are in need of treatment areas in which they can be evaluated. Emergency physicians and nurses should prospectively design protocols and procedures to assure that such secondary triage is safe, efficient, and in the patient's best interest.

Legal Considerations

According to the Consolidated Omnibus Budget Reconciliation Act passed in 1985, hospitals receiving Medicare funds are mandated to evaluate all patients who arrive in the ED and treat anyone with an emergent medical problem or any woman in active labor. In addition, any transferred patients must be stabilized and the receiving institution must have agreed to accept the patient. Under the Emergency Medical Treatment and Labor Act (EMTALA), patients can be transferred only when they need a higher level of care (or a service not provided at the institution at which they present) and only after an appropriate "screening" evaluation and stabilization (see Chapter 150, Emergency Medical Treatment and Labor Act [EMTALA]). It is inappropriate for a nurse or any other medical personnel to arbitrarily triage a patient to another facility. After an appropriate medical screening examination, usually by the responsible physician, it is possible that triage nurses, while following written protocols, could redirect patients to predesignated areas such as an outpatient clinic. However, precise documentation and preestablished written protocols are mandatory. Indeed, many experts recommend that a chart be generated for any patient presenting to the ED regardless of whether or not they are evaluated and treated.

Prehospital Triage

Field triage by Emergency Medical Services (EMS) personnel is the assessment of individual patients with the purpose of determining the most appropriate receiving facility. The development of trauma systems led to trauma triage in prehospital care. This is based on the principle that patients with life-threatening or serious multisystem injuries from trauma have a better outcome when transported directly to a facility staffed and equipped to provide resuscitation and definitive treatment. The aim is to send all seriously injured patients to a trauma center without overwhelming the resources of the trauma center by over-triaging. Occasionally a trauma patient may bypass the closest hospital to be transported directly to the trauma center. System-wide prehospital EMS trauma protocols provide guidelines to prehospital care providers for differentiating which trauma patient is transported to the trauma center or to the closest hospital for treatment.

With the advent of more sophisticated therapies and specialized hospitals, such as chest pain centers with around-the-clock cardiac catheterization capabilities or stroke centers capable of delivering organ/region-specific thrombolytics, the expansion and increased importance of "prehospital" or "field" triage are likely.

Disaster Triage

A disaster is an event that exceeds the capabilities of the response (e.g., the need is greater than the resources), resulting in disruption of normal function.[41,42] In order to more concisely describe and reflect the degree (or stage) of disaster, the Potential Injury Causing Event (PICE) nomenclature has been developed.[43]

Triage during a disaster is different from ED triage. The purpose of ED triage is to identify critically ill patients and assure that they receive immediate resuscitation, while the principle of disaster management is to "do the most good for the most people."[1] It is possible during a disaster with limited response resources that, in order to maximize care for the majority of victims, some patients who have little or no chance of survival will not be not resuscitated.[44] It is often a difficult concept for health care providers to ration resources and not expend efforts to resuscitate patients who are considered near death in order to save others. Comfort care should be provided to the dying patients when resources become available.

As with ED triage, there is no universally accepted standardized system for disaster or MCI triage, although several triage systems have been suggested. One MCI/disaster triage tool is the Simple Triage and Rapid Treatment (START) technique.[45] This is based on a rapid assessment of respiration, perfusion, and mental status (RPM). Casualties who are ambulatory are asked to move away from the immediate area of the incident. These "walking wounded" are categorized as "green" or minor. The remaining patients are sorted into unsalvageable, immediate, and delayed (Fig. 155–2). If the patient has a patent airway and is breathing, by assessing the respiratory rate (>30 per minute or < 30 per minute), the radial pulse (present or absent), and the mental status (follows commands: yes or no), the patient can be categorized. Unsalvageable patients are patients who are not breathing even after positioning their airway and are classified "black" or deceased. "Red" (immediate) patients have an immediate threat to life or limb but, if given immediate care, will probably survive. Examples include a patient with altered mental status, labored respirations, or shock. "Yellow" (delayed) patients have significant injuries but can probably tolerate a 45- to 60-minute wait without undue risk.

This color-coded four-category system is probably the most common disaster/MCI triage system in the United States. "Red" casualties are the first priority and are "most urgent." Patients classified "Yellow" are the second priority and are "urgent." "Green" patients comprise the "walking

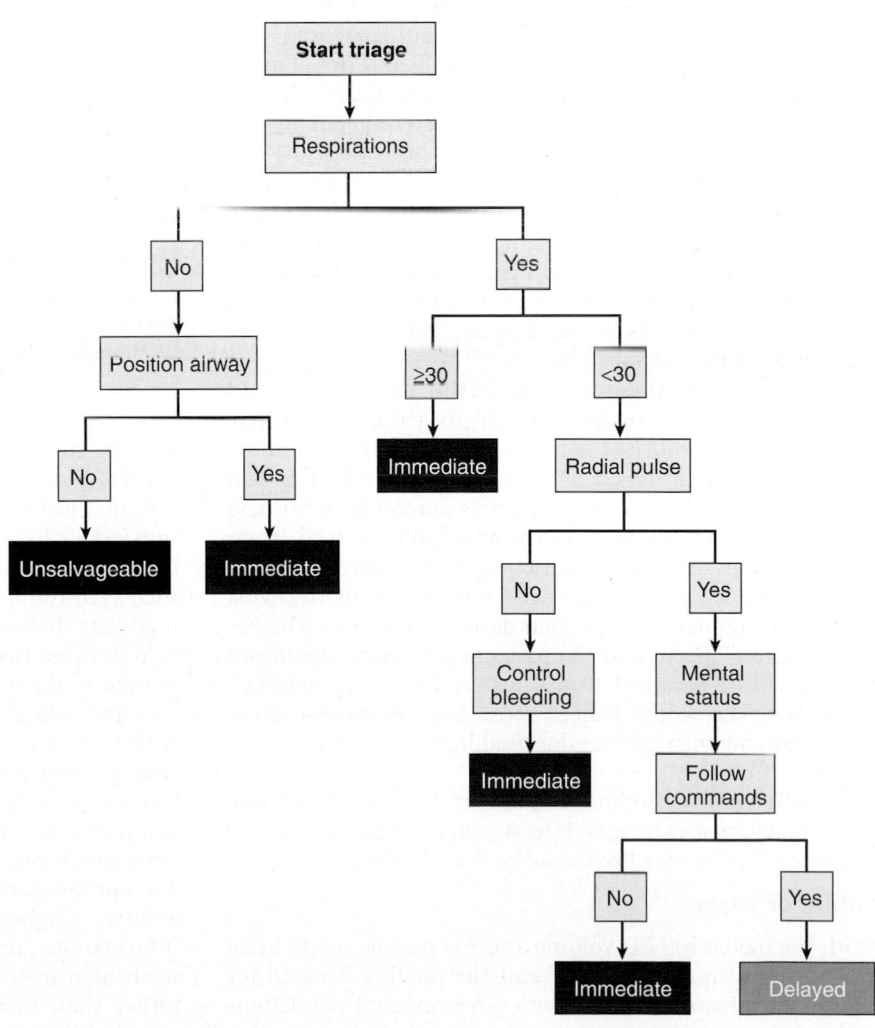

FIGURE 155–2. Simple Triage and Rapid Treatment (START) tool.

wounded" or "nonurgent" and are the third priority. Dead patients and catastrophically injured patients with a negligible chance of survival belong to the "Black" triage category.

The MASS triage model has been used by the U.S. military in order to quickly assign large numbers of casualties into treatment categories.[42] MASS triage incorporates the processes of "move, access, sort, and send." Patients are grouped into four categories based on the "ID-ME" mnemonic: "immediate, delayed, minimal, and expectant."[42] Minimal patients are stable patients with minor injuries, such as contusions and minor lacerations, whose medical care could be delayed for days without any untoward effect from the delay. At the disaster or MCI scene, the triage officer should request that "Everyone who can hear me [the triage officer] and needs medical attention should move to the area with the green flag." This will separate out the ambulatory "minimal" group or walking wounded.

The "delayed" patients need definitive medical care but will quickly decompensate if their care is delayed initially. Patients with open fractures, deep lacerations with pulses/distal circulation, hemodynamically stable abdominal injuries, or stable head injuries belong to the "delayed" category. To sort this delayed group of patients after separating out the ambulatory walking wounded, the "MOVE" command is to ask the remaining casualties to raise a hand (or leg) so that they can be helped.

After separating out the "minimal" and "delayed" groups, the rescuers proceed immediately to those who are left. These patients are in the immediate or expectant categories. The immediate patients are patients with an obvious threat to life or limb. These casualties generally have a problem with the ABCs, such as shock, respiratory distress, altered mental status, or a severe abdominal, chest, or head injury. These patients often need immediate life-saving care. The expectant patients are patients near death who probably will not survive no matter what treatment is rendered. A patient in traumatic arrest, a patient with a penetrating chest wound in shock, or a trauma patient who is not breathing would be classified as "expectant" since they are near death and have a minimal chance of surviving.

The Secondary Assessment of Victim Endpoint (SAVE) triage system was developed to identify patients who have the greatest possibility of benefit from care delivered under austere field conditions.[46] SAVE is employed when patient transport to a definitive care facility is not available for days and treatment within the "golden hour" at a medical center is nonexistent.[45] The three patient groups according to the SAVE triage are: (1) patients who will die no matter what treatment is rendered, (2) patients destined to survive whether or not care is given, and (3) patients for whom significant benefit will be obtained from "austere field interventions." Casualties who would benefit most from early evacuation (e.g., a patient with intra-abdominal hemorrhage) are designated as "first out."

JumpSTART is a modification of the START disaster triage for pediatric patients ages 1 to 8 years[47] (Fig. 155–3) (see Chapter 152, Disaster Preparedness for Children).

Future of Triage

With the increasing ED volume and ED patient acuity in an era of diminishing resources, and the public's demand for more rapid treatment along with governmental regulations

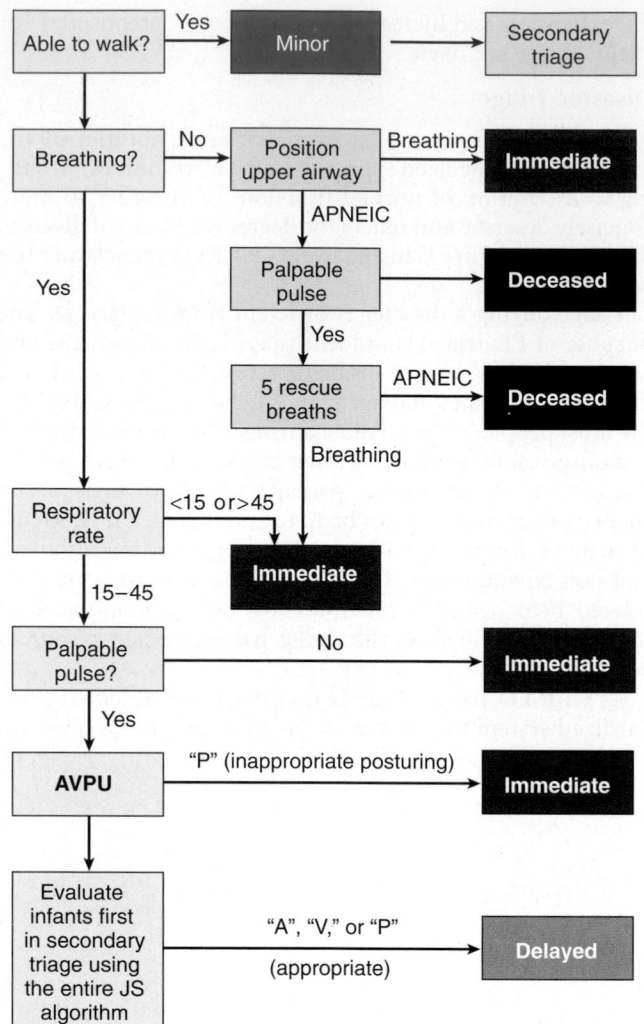

FIGURE 155–3. JumpSTART pediatric mass casualty incident triage. Abbreviations: AVPU, alert, responsive to *voice*, responsive to *posturing*, or *unresponsive*. (From Romig LE: Pediatric triage: a system to Jump START your triage of young patients at MCIs. J Emerg Med Serv 27(7):52–58, 60–63, 2002.)

and the focus on patient safety and quality, triage will be expected to perform an even more complex and important role in the future.[48,49] Triage in the redesigned ED of the future will have new systems and processes and expanded technology to streamline patient flow. Current technology such as in-room registration and discharge by mobile patient registrars using laptop computers may be replaced by hand-held devices. Registrars may not even need to be physically present in the room to interview patients but could use videoconferencing techniques. More elaborate instantaneous patient tracking systems are possible. Real-time communication via cell phones/walkie-talkies or microchip tracking technology will allow the triage nurse to instantly see and communicate with patients and families in the waiting room and other areas. Patient pagers can be distributed to patients and families (and to ED staff) to notify them of room availability, radiology, and other testing availability. Medical information, including medications, allergies, and past medical history, will be automatically available via computer, rather than manually entered, in a fashion that protects patient confidentiality according to the Health Information Portability and Accountability Act. Individual patient data will be connected to patient data banks within and between hospitals so clinical information for purposes of research and new therapies as well as syndromic surveillance (for new diseases or bioterrorist threats) is available while maintaining individual patient confidentiality and patient rights.[50] The ED of the future will also incorporate the principles of family-centered care so that the ED provision of care occurs in a caring, comfortable environment attentive to the emotional, social, and cultural needs of patients and families. Such advances, however, are dependent on the necessary financial resources and continuing technological advances.

Summary

Triage is a critical and necessary component of ED care. Triage is essential for the early recognition of the seriously ill patient and rapid initiation of therapy, which reduces morbidity and mortality. Early initiation of therapy not only saves lives, but also decreases hospital and intensive care unit length of stay, and lowers morbidity, ultimately decreasing health care costs. An efficient triage can expedite patient care, improve ED flow, and increase patient and family satisfaction, thereby decreasing litigation, and, most importantly, improve patient care and outcome by rapidly initiating care to the seriously ill or injured.

REFERENCES

1. Auf der Heide E: Triage. *In* Disaster Response: Principles of Preparation and Coordination. St. Louis: CV Mosby, 1989.
2. Thompson JD, Dains JE: Comprehensive Triage: A Manual for Developing and Implementing a Nursing Care System. Reston, VA: Reston Publishing Co, 1982.
*3. Emergency Nurses Association: Standards of Emergency Nursing Practice, 4th ed. Des Plains, IL: Emergency Nurses Association, 1999, p 23.
4. Gilboy N: The evolution of triage. *In* Gilboy N, Tanabe P, Travers DA, et al: The Emergency Severity Index Implementation Handbook: A Five-Level Triage System. Des Plaines, IL: Emergency Nurses Association, 2003, pp 2–5.
5. Travers D: Triage: how long does it take? How long should it take? J Emerg Nurs 25:238–240, 1999.
6. Wuerz R, Fernandez CMB, Alarcon J: Inconsistency of emergency department triage. Ann Emerg Med 32:431–435, 1998.
7. Gill JM, Reese CL 4th, Diamond JJ: Disagreement among health care professionals about the urgent care needs of emergency department patients. Ann Emerg Med 28:474–479, 1996.
8. Brillman JC, Doezema D, Tandberg D, et al: Triage: limitations in predicting need for emergent care and hospital admission. Ann Emerg Med 27:493–500, 1996.
9. Bergeron S, Gouin S, Bailey B, et al: Comparison of triage assessments among pediatric registered nurses and pediatric emergency physicians. Acad Emerg Med 9:1397–1401, 2002.
10. Nakagawa J, Ouk S, Schwartz B, et al: Interobserver agreement in emergency department triage. Ann Emerg Med 41:191–195, 2003.
11. MacLean S: 2001 ENA National Benchmark Guide: Emergency Departments. Des Plaines, IL: Emergency Nurses Association, 2001.
*12. Travers DA, Waller AE, Bowling JM, et al: Five-level triage system: more effective than three-level in tertiary emergency department. J Emerg Nurs 28:395–400, 2002.
13. Australasian College for Emergency Medicine: National triage scale. Emerg Med Australas 6:145–146, 1994.
14. Cameron PA, Bradt DA, Ashby R: Emergency medicine in Australia. Ann Emerg Med 28:342–346, 1996.
15. Cronin JG: The introduction of the Manchester Triage Scale to an emergency department in the Republic of Ireland. Accid Emerg Nurs 11:121–125, 2003.
16. Beveridge R, Ducharme J, Janes L, et al: Reliability of the Canadian emergency department Triage and Acuity Scale: interrater agreement. Ann Emerg Med 34:155–159, 1999.
17. Beveridge RC, Ducharme J: Emergency department triage and acuity: development of a national model [Abstract]. Acad Emerg Med 4:475, 1997.
18. Zimmerman PG: The case for a universal reliable 5-tier triage acuity scale for U.S. emergency departments. J Emerg Nurs 27:246–254, 2001.
19. Wuerz RC, Milne LW, Eitel DR, et al: Reliability and validity of a new five-level triage instrument. Acad Emerg Med 7:236–242, 2000.
20. Wuerz RC, Travers D, Gilboy N, et al: Implementation and refinement of the Emergency Severity Index. Acad Emerg Med 8:170–176, 2001.
*21. Tanabe P, Gimbel R, Yarnold PR, et al: Reliability and validity of scores on the Emergency Severity Index version 3. Acad Emerg Med 11:59–65, 2004.
22. National Center for Health Statistics: Injury Data and Resources—National Hospital Ambulatory Medical Care Survey, 2002 Emergency Department Summary. Centers for Disease Control and Prevention web site, 2000. Available at *http://www.cdc.gov*
23. Cain P, Waldrop RD, Jones J: Improved pediatric patient flow in a general emergency department by altering triage criteria. Acad Emerg Med 3:65–71, 1996.
24. Wiebe RA, Rosen LM: Triage in the emergency department. Emerg Med Clin North Am 9:491–505, 1991.
25. Marcin JP, Pollack MM: Triage scoring systems, severity of illness measures, and mortality prediction models in pediatric trauma. Crit Care Med 30:S456–S467, 2002.
26. Macfarlane PI, Suri S: Steroids in the management of croup. BMJ 312:510, 1996.
27. McCarthy PL, Sharpe MR, Spiesel SZ, et al: Observation scales to identify serious illness in febrile children. Pediatrics 70:802–809, 1982.
*28. Murphy KA: Introduction to pediatric triage. *In* Pediatric Triage Guidelines. St. Louis: CV Mosby, 1997, pp 1–7.
29. O'Neill KA, Molczan K: Pediatric triage: a 2-tier, 5-level system in the United States. Pediatr Emerg Care 19:285–290, 2003.
30. Rambler CL, Mohammed N: Triage. *In* Kitt S, Selfridge-Thomas J, Proehl JA, et al (eds): Emergency Nursing: A Physiologic and Clinical Perspective. Philadelphia: WB Saunders, 1994, pp 19–27.
31. Mace SE: Child physical abuse: a state-of-the-art approach. Pediatr Emerg Med Pract 2:1–20, 2004.
32. Selfridge-Thomas J: Patient assessment and priority setting. *In* Manual of Emergency Nursing. Philadelphia: WB Saunders, 1995, pp 3–18.
33. Thomas DO: Special considerations for the emergency department. Nurs Clin North Am 37:145–159, 2002.
*34. Browne GJ: Paediatric emergency departments: old needs, new challenges and future opportunities. Emerg Med 13:409–417, 2001.
35. Phillips S, Rond PC, Kelly SM, et al: The need for pediatric-specific triage criteria: results from the Florida trauma triage study. Pediatr Emerg Care 12:394–399, 1996.
36. Gorelick MH, Lee C, Cronan K: Pediatric Emergency Assessment Tool (PEAT): a risk-adjustment measure for pediatric emergency patients. Acad Emerg Med 8:156–162, 2001.
37. Durojaiye L, O'Meara M: A study of triage of paediatric patients in Australia. Emerg Med 14:67–76, 2003.
38. Crellin DJ, Johnston L: Who is responsible for pediatric triage decisions in Australian emergency departments? A description of the educational and experimental preparation of general and pediatric emergency nurses. Pediatr Emerg Care 18:382–388, 2002.
39. Mayer TA, Cates RJ: Leadership for Great Customer Service. Chicago: Health Administration Press, 2004.
40. Carlzon J: Moments of Truth: New Strategies for Today's Customer-Driven Economy. New York: Harper Collins, 1987.
41. Aghababian RV: Pediatric Disaster Life Support–PDLS: Caring for Children during Disaster. Boston: University of Massachusetts Medical School, 1995.
42. All-hazards course overview and disaster paradigm. *In* Pepe PE, Schwartz RB (eds): Basic Disaster Life Support BDLS Provider Manual. 2004, pp 1–28.
43. Koenig KL, Dinerman N, Kuehl AE: PICE nomenclature: a new system to describe disaster. Prehospital Disaster Med 9:S65, 1994.

44. Waeckerle JF: Disaster planning and response. N Engl J Med 324:815–821, 1991.

45. Schultz CH, Koenig KL, Noji EK: A medical disaster response to reduce immediate mortality after an earthquake. N Engl J Med 334:438–444, 1996.

46. Benson M, Koenig KL, Schultz CH: Disaster triage: START, then SAVE—a new method of dynamic triage for victims of a catastrophic earthquake. Prehospital Disaster Med 11:117–124, 1996.

47. Romig LE: Pediatric triage: a system to Jump START your triage of young patients at MCIs. J Emerg Med Serv 27(7):52–58, 60–63, 2002.

*48. Fields W (Chair, Safety Net Task Force): Defending America's safety net. American College of Emergency Physicians web site, April 2000. Available at *http://www.acep.org*

*49. Richardson LD, Asplin BR, Lowe RA: Emergency department crowding as a health policy issue: past development, future directions. Ann Emerg Med 40:388–393, 2002.

50. Barthell EN, Aaronsky D, Cochrane DG, et al; Frontlines Work Group: The Frontlines of Medicine Project progress report: standardized communication of emergency department triage data for syndromic surveillance. Ann Emerg Med 44:247–252, 2004.

Chapter 156

Postexposure Prophylaxis

Esther H. Chen, MD

Key Points

Children and adolescents are most likely to acquire human immunodeficiency virus (HIV) through perinatal transmission, high-risk sexual contact, and needle sharing. Contact sports activities, human bites, or casual mucosal contacts generally have almost no risk of transmission.

Postexposure prophylaxis with a three-drug regimen (zidovudine, lamivudine, and nelfinavir) should be initiated for high-risk situations within 72 hours of the exposure and continued for 28 days, but only if counseling and follow-up with an infectious disease specialist can be ensured.

All health care providers are required to report new HIV seroconversions and acquired immunodeficiency syndrome cases.

Introduction and Background

Exposure to blood or body fluids prompts most people to seek immediate medical attention in an emergency department (ED). These exposures have an associated risk of hepatitis B virus (HBV), hepatitis C virus (HCV), and human immunodeficiency virus (HIV) transmission. However, because all children currently receive the HBV vaccine series (neonates born to hepatitis B surface antigen–positive mothers receive concurrent HBV immunoglobulin)[1] and prophylactic antiviral therapy has not been shown to be effective following HCV exposure,[2] postexposure prophylaxis (PEP) is reserved for secondary prevention against HIV. This chapter focuses primarily on the transmission risks of HIV in the pediatric population and discusses current available recommendations for pediatric PEP.

PEP is classified into occupational and nonoccupational exposures. Occupational exposures, defined as any percutaneous injury or contact of mucous membrane or nonintact skin with any blood, tissue, or body fluid that is potentially infectious, occur in health care workers (HCWs) and are managed using established public health guidelines.[2] In contrast, no established guidelines exist for nonoccupational exposures (percutaneous penetration and mucous membrane and nonintact skin contact with potentially infectious body fluids, and sexual exposures [discrete penetrative acts involving vaginal, anal, penile, and/or oral contact]),[3] although several states now have their own recommendations.[4,5]

There are even fewer recommendations for adolescents and children except for the use of chemoprophylaxis to prevent perinatal and postnatal transmission.[6] Antepartum use of zidovudine (ZDV) can decrease the HIV transmission rate from 25.5% (for infants receiving placebo) to 8.3%[7]; use of elective cesarean delivery further reduces the rate to 1.8%.[8] Results from these clinical trials led to current recommendations that all pregnant HIV-infected women receive full clinical, immunologic, and virologic evaluation, with initiation of chemoprophylaxis after the first trimester.

Children and adolescents commonly present after nonoccupational exposures, consisting of bite injuries, sexual assault, consensual unprotected sex, needle sharing, or unintentional needle sticks. In a recent study of PEP use in an urban ED, pediatric patients were more likely to present with a sexual exposure compared to adult non-HCWs (37% vs. 6%), with the majority caused by sexual abuse (71%).[9] Rates of nonsexual exposures were similar in both pediatric and adult patients, with human bites occurring most frequently, followed by needle stick injuries and blood splashes. However, compared to adult non-HCWs, PEP was less likely to be initiated in adolescents and children for needle stick injuries (29% vs. 18%), blood and body fluid splashes (9% vs. 0%), and human bites (<1% vs. 0%).[9]

Issues

Determining the Risk of Transmission

A patient's risk of viral transmission depends on the probability that the source patient has HIV infection and that transmission of a sufficient amount of virus has occurred. The probability that the source patient has HIV may be determined directly from prior HIV testing or indirectly from assessing the patient's risk (i.e., medical history, intravenous drug use, sexual history). In contrast, the probability of viral transmission depends on the type and volume of source material, concentration and viability of virus in the source material, and mode of contact.

All body fluids are not equally infectious. Any blood or blood-contaminated body fluid from an HIV-infected person

Table 156–1	Transmission Risk by Exposure Type		
Type of Exposure	**Transmission Risk per Exposure**	**Exposure Risk Category**	**Suggested Approach**
Perinatal exposure[7]	25.5%	High	Recommend PEP
Cutaneous exposure: body fluid splash on intact skin[11]	Almost 0%	No risk	No PEP
Sexual contact			
Receptive anal intercourse[13]	0.82%	High	Recommend PEP
Receptive vaginal intercourse[14]	0.15%	Intermediate	Consider PEP
Insertive anal intercourse[13]	0.06%	Intermediate	Consider PEP
Insertive vaginal intercourse[14]	0.09%	Intermediate	Consider PEP
Mucous membrane exposure			
Kissing/oral-genital contact[11]	Almost 0%	No risk	No PEP
Breast-feeding[11]	0.004%	Low	Consider PEP
Percutaneous injury			
Scratch from discarded needle[11]	Almost 0%	No risk	No PEP
Needle sharing (injection drug use)[21]	0.67%	High risk	Recommend PEP
Occupational needle stick injury[10]	0.3%	Intermediate risk	Recommend PEP

has the highest risk of transmission. Less infectious materials include semen or vaginal secretions, body fluids (cerebrospinal, synovial, peritoneal, pericardial, amniotic), human milk, and unfixed body tissue. Least likely to be infectious are urine, feces, saliva, and vomitus.[2] Furthermore, exposure to a large volume of infectious material carries a greater risk of transmission than a small exposure. For example, the transmission risk of a percutaneous injury from a large hollow-bore needle is four times higher than from a solid suture needle.[10]

Another important determinant of transmission risk is the characteristic of the virus in the infected material, such as its concentration and viability. Percutaneous exposure to blood from a patient with a high viral load increases transmission risk by more than fivefold.[10] Antiretroviral therapy use in these patients decreases their viral load, thereby decreasing their risk of transmission. This risk is further influenced by the viability of the virus in the infected fluid, which depends largely on its environment. HIV is susceptible to drying, so a needle immediately withdrawn from an infected patient would have a higher concentration of live virus than a contaminated syringe that had been discarded several hours ealier.[10]

A final consideration in determining transmission risk is the mode of contact. Blood transfusion carries the highest transmission risk, followed by perinatal transmission, breast-feeding, sexual exposure, percutaneous injury, and human bites[11] (Table 156–1).

Transmission Rates and Management by Type of Exposure

Cutaneous Exposure to Body Fluids

Cutaneous or mucous membrane exposure to body fluids usually carries a low risk of transmission. Kissing, body fluid splashes on intact skin, bites that causes no skin breaks, and close athletic contact in school are considered to have almost no risk of transmission.[11,12] Oral-genital sex and body fluid splashes to the eye or mouth are also considered low-risk incidents. PEP is not recommended for these exposures.[11] Routine wound care should be administered, including flushing the exposed site with water or saline solution and administration of antibiotics and a tetanus booster.

Sexual Contact

Adolescents have the highest rate of HIV from sexual transmission of any group, particularly from sexual assault and rape (5 per 1000 adolescents annually).[4] Even though there are established management guidelines for classic sexually transmitted illnesses (STIs) in sexual assault victims, they do not include use of PEP for HIV prevention.[4] The risk of HIV transmission from sexual exposure varies significantly, according to the type and frequency of contact. In addition, the presence of a concurrent STI increases the risk of HIV acquisition. Receptive anal intercourse with a known HIV-infected partner has the highest per-contact risk of transmission (0.82%),[13] followed by receptive vaginal intercourse (0.15%).[13,14] Insertive vaginal and anal intercourse are lower risk activities, with transmission rates of 0.09%[14] and 0.06%, respectively.[13] Factors that increase transmission risk are local infection at the exposure site, presence of foreskin, use of an intrauterine device contraception, presence of cervical ectopy, genital tract trauma, active menstruation, and source patient's stage of HIV infection.[15] Use of condoms and antiretroviral therapy significantly decreases infectivity.[15]

PEP use after sexual abuse is extrapolated from adult data, even though a pediatric exposure might result in a higher transmission rate because children often are repeatedly abused by the same person over a period of time. PEP should be considered for patients presenting within 72 hours of the exposure (although optimally within 4 hours), if the assailant has known HIV disease, and if the type of exposure is considered high risk (i.e., concurrent genital tissue injury, presence of STI, receptive anal intercourse).[16] PEP is not recommended for patients participating in ongoing consensual sexual exposure to HIV.

Breast-feeding

Breast-feeding is a leading source of mother-to-child HIV transmission, with an overall risk of 16.2%, the majority of which (75%) occurs within 6 months of feeding.[17] In addition, there is an associated increased risk of mortality in the mother.[18] Assuming that an infant breast-feeds 6 to 10 times daily, his or her transmission risk is estimated to be 0.001% to 0.004% per episode.[11] Risk factors for transmission include longer duration of breast-feeding, maternal characteristics (e.g., higher parity, lower CD4+ count, higher blood viral load, breast/nipple infections or lesions), infant characteristics (i.e., oral candidiasis), and milk characteristics (e.g., higher viral load).[19] According to the American Academy of Pediatrics, HIV-infected mothers should avoid breast-feeding if replacement feeding is readily available.[19] If replacement feedings are not available, interventions that decrease transmission include early weaning, decreasing viral load in the milk through antiretroviral therapy or breast milk pasteurization, treating breast infections, and treating infant oral candidiasis.[19]

The transmission risk after a single exposure to infected breast milk is magnitudes lower than that for other mucous membrane exposures, so PEP is not recommended (although it may be considered in high-risk situations).[11] Management after a single exposure includes flushing the infant's mucous membranes with water or saline solution.

Percutaneous Injury

Percutaneous exposures include not only accidental needle injuries, but also needle sharing and human bite wounds. HIV seroconversion from exposure to discarded needles has been reported in the pediatric population.[12] Adolescents, however, represent a unique group because new HIV cases are usually associated with injection drug use (including anabolic steroids) and associated risky sexual behavior. An estimated 14% of new HIV infections in teenage girls are caused by injection drug use.[20]

The transmission risk is related to the severity of the injury, the initial concentration of HIV on the needle, and the time interval since the needle was in contact with the source patient. Factors associated with a higher risk of infectivity are deep wounds, presence of blood on the needle, hollow-bore needles, and needles recently in the source patient's vein or artery.[11] The risk of a puncture wound sustained from a discarded needle appears to be lower than that for an occupational needle stick injury, perinatal exposure, or blood transfusion.[11] However, needle sharing during injection drug use has a higher infection risk per injection compared to occupational percutaneous injury in HCWs (0.67%[21] vs. 0.3%[10]).

The decision to initiate PEP depends on the risk of transmission through the wound. A superficial scratch with a discarded needle or body piercing is considered to have almost no risk, so PEP is not recommended. Injuries caused by discarded needles are also considered low risk, so PEP should not be initiated unless the needle or syringe has visible blood and the source is known to be HIV infected. Testing the syringe is low yield and not recommended. Cases of needle sharing during injection drug use should be treated with PEP, except for cases of repeated consensual contact.[11]

Another percutaneous injury incurred by children is bite wounds. Although the HIV transmission risk of human bites is relatively low, cases of seroconversion have been reported in the literature, specifically in police officers and HCWs. A needle transmits 20 times more HIV-infected cells than a human bite.[22] PEP is not recommended if blood is absent in the saliva and the bite wound. Even if there is potential blood exchange, transmission is still extremely rare. Large, deep, bloody wounds caused by an HIV-infected patient poses a greater risk, so PEP may be more strongly indicated.[11]

All percutaneous exposure sites should also be thoroughly assessed for the presence of a potential foreign body or associated crush injury. Initial management includes washing thoroughly with soap and water, followed by irrigation with saline in the ED.[23]

Mandatory Reporting for Seroconversion

Treatment of adolescents in the ED setting should follow state and local confidentiality laws.[11] Significant exposures (where PEP is initiated) used to be reported to the nonoccupational HIV PEP registry, which was completed and closed on October 31, 2004. All states require health care providers to report new cases of HIV infection and AIDS to the state health department. Although protocols vary by state, the majority place the responsibility on both the health care provider and the laboratory to report new cases.[24]

Use of Antiretrovirals in Children

Because there are no studies to date that evaluate the effectiveness of PEP in reducing the transmission rate in nonoccupational exposures, the benefit of PEP is extrapolated from animal studies, PEP use in occupational settings, and perinatal studies.[11] A recent survey of ED health care providers showed that 68% have ever prescribed PEP, mostly for HCW needle stick injuries (92%), and only 19% have ever prescribed PEP for pediatric patients, mainly for sexual assault (69%) and needle stick injuries (31%).[25]

PEP for perinatal exposure and occupational injury is now standard practice. There is growing evidence supporting PEP for sexual assault (with subsequent mucosal or cutaneous injury), significant needle stick injury with obvious mixing of blood, and needle sharing (during injection drug use). There are few contraindications. Absolute contraindications are known allergy to the medications and known HIV infection. Relative contraindications have been proposed in the literature, such as exposures with no likelihood of transmission and recurrent risky behavior.[12,26]

Before treatment, draw baseline HIV, CBC, liver and renal function, βhCG and hepatitis B antibody titers. CBC, liver and renal tests will be repeated in 2 weeks and HIV in 6 and 12 weeks. If source patient is available, draw rapid HIV if such testing is available. Discontinue treatment of exposed individual if rapid HIV test is negative.

One approach to determine whether to initiate PEP in adolescents and children is shown in Figure 156–1. Once the decision to start PEP has been made, choosing the best regimen for nonoccupational exposures in children and adolescents may be difficult. Medications that might be considered are shown in Table 156–2. Even though monotherapy with ZDV has been extensively studied, triple therapy with ZDV, lamivudine, and nelfinavir is now thought to be more effective (although this is based primarily on the chemoprophylaxis guidelines for occupational exposures). Theoretically, using two nucleoside analogue reverse transcriptase inhibitors and a protease inhibitor should more effectively suppress viral replication than monotherapy or dual therapy.[11]

PEP use in the pediatric group may be problematic for several reasons. Compliance with a three-drug combination therapy is very difficult. Recent data suggest that only 25% of patients were able to finish a 28-day regimen.[27] Reasons cited for this noncompliance were financial hardship, side

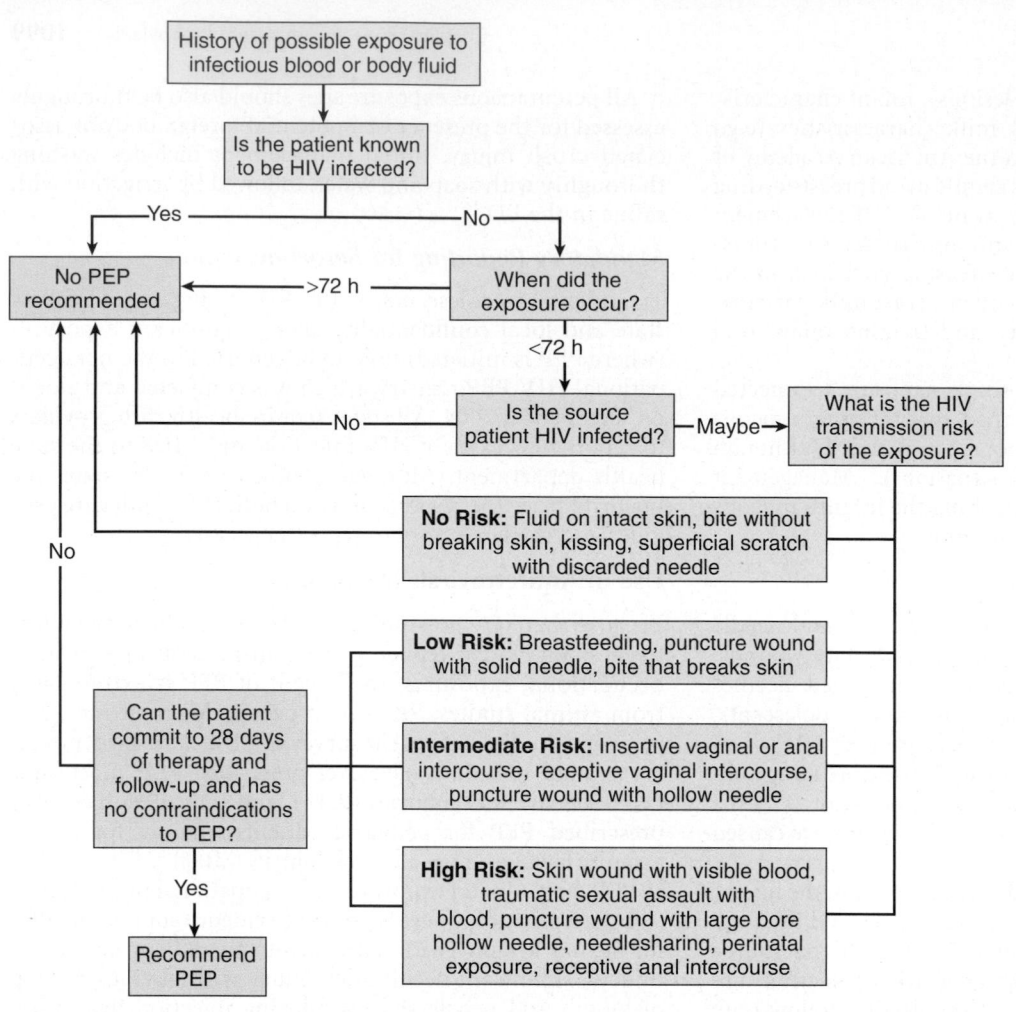

FIGURE 156–1. Decision algorithm: determining initiation of postexposure prophylaxis (PEP) for potential human immunodeficiency virus (HIV) exposures.[11,12]

Table 156–2	Antiretroviral Medications Used for PEP[11,12,28]	
Medication	**Pediatric Dosage**	**Major Side Effects**
Nucleoside Reverse Transcriptase Inhibitors		
First-Line Therapy		
Zidovudine (ZDV, AZT, Retrovir)	Birth–4 wk: 1–2 mg/kg/dose IV q12h 4 wk–12 yr: 160 mg/m²/dose PO q8h >13 yr–adult: 200 mg q8h or 300 mg PO q12h	Granulocytopenia, lactic acidosis, steatosis
Lamivudine (Epivir, 3TC)	Birth–4 wk: 2 mg/kg/dose q12h <50 kg: 4 mg/kg/dose q12h ≥50 kg: 150 mg/dose q12h or 300 mg q24h	Pancreatitis, peripheral neuropathy, steatosis
Alternatives		
Abacavir (Ziagen, ABC)	Birth–3 mo: not recommended 3 mo–16 yr: 8 mg/kg/dose q12h >16 yr: 300 mg/dose q12h	Fatal hypersensitivity reaction
Didanosine (Videx, DDI, dideoxyinosine)	1–3 mo: 50 mg/m²/dose q12h 3 mo–12 yr: 90–150 mg/m²/dose q12h >13 yr: <60 kg, 125 mg q12h ≥60 kg, 200 mg q12h	Severe hepatomegaly
Stavudine (Zerit, d4T)	<30 kg: 1 mg/kg/dose q12h 30–60 kg: 30 mg q12h >60 kg: 40 mg q12h	Severe hepatomegaly
Protease Inhibitor		
Indinavir (Crixivan, IDV)	Neonates: not recommended Pediatric: 500 mg/m²/dose q8h Adult: 800 mg/m²/dose q8h	Hyperbilirubinemia, nephrolithiasis
Nelfinavir (Viracept, NPV)	1 mo–12 yr: 20–30 mg q8h ≥13 yr: 750–1250 mg q12h	Spontaneous bleeding, hypoglycemia, ketoacidosis
Ritonavir (Norvir, RTV)	3 mo–12 yr: 400 mg/m²/dose q12h ≥13 yr: 600 mg q12h	Spontaneous bleeding, hypoglycemia, ketoacidosis

Combivir = ZDV 300 mg + Epivir 150 mg.
Most cases will require a 2 drug regimen, seven cases may require 3 drugs; consult with pediatric infectious disease expert for specific recommendations.
Abbreviations: IV, intravenously; PO, orally.

effects, and admission or transfer to another health care facility.[27] Therefore, in patients for whom compliance might be an issue, a two-drug regimen might be a more reasonable option.[13] Moreover, fewer medications may mean fewer associated side effects, which are commonly reported to be nausea, vomiting, and abdominal pain.[27] More serious side effects are listed in Table 156–2. Symptoms usually resolve after medications are discontinued.

The safety profile of these drugs has not been extensively studied in children. Abacavir sulfate potentially causes severe hypersensitivity reactions. Indinavir may be associated with nephrolithiasis, and therefore requires extra hydration and should be avoided in children. Liquid amprenavir contains propylene glycol in concentrations that might be toxic for infants and are not recommended for children under 4 years old. Nevirapine has been associated with life-threatening hepatotoxicity and should also be avoided.

Solutions

Health care professionals should not manage potentially exposed patients without consulting an infectious disease specialist familiar with using these medications in the pediatric population. EDs should have clear, easy-to-use protocols for PEP use in both adult and pediatric patients and provide "starter kits" of 3 days of medications for immediate initiation of therapy. Follow-up in these patients is especially important to ensure compliance, schedule repeated HIV testing, monitor toxicity, and provide psychological counseling. Referral to specialists in HIV care is paramount to ensuring adequate follow-up clinical care.

The dearth of standardized guidelines for PEP use in children has spawned a flurry of initiatives by the American Academy of Pediatrics and several states to make practical recommendations for clinicians. The University of California–San Francisco has a hotline (1-888-HIV-4911) supported by the Centers for Disease Control and Prevention that is staffed 24 hours a day to answer questions and provide guidance.[12] Data collected from the nonoccupational HIV PEP registry should lead to national guidelines in the near future.

Summary

Children and adolescents may be exposed to HIV-infected blood or body fluids through perinatal transmission, breast-feeding, sexual contact, injection drug use, and human bites. High-risk sexual behaviors are the leading cause of seroconversion in adolescents. PEP with dual or triple combination therapy may be initiated for high-risk exposures, such as perinatal exposure, sexual contact with mucosal injury or concurrent STI, and injection drug use, and continued for 28 days. Follow-up counseling and monitoring of side effects should be provided by infectious disease specialists. More studies on the efficacy and safety profiles of these medications in children will enable standardized guidelines to be developed and implemented.

REFERENCES

1. Mast EE, Margolis HS, Fiore AE, et al: A comprehensive immunization strategy to eliminate transmission of hepatitis B virus infection in the United States: recommendations of the Advisory Committee on Immunization Practices (ACIP), Part 1. Immunization of infants, children, and adolescents. MMWR Recomm Rep 54(RR-16):1–31, 2005.

*2. Centers for Disease Control and Prevention: Updated U.S. Public Health Service guidelines for the management of occupational exposures to HBV, HCV, and HIV and recommendations for postexposure prophylaxis. MMWR Recomm Rep 50(RR-11):1–67, 2001.

*3. Centers for Disease Control and Prevention: Management of possible sexual, injection-drug-use, or other nonoccupational exposures to HIV, including considerations related to antiretroviral therapy. MMWR Recomm Rep 47(RR-17):1–19, 1998.

4. Kaplan DW, Feinstein RA, Fisher MM, et al: Care of the adolescent sexual assault victim. Pediatrics 107:1476–1479, 2001.

5. Merchant RC, Mayer KH, Browning CA: Nonoccupational Human Immunodeficiency Virus Postexposure Prophylaxis: Guidelines for Rhode Island Healthcare Practitioners. Providence, RI: Brown University AIDS Program and Rhode Island Department of Health, 2002.

6. Mofenson LM: U.S. Public Health Service Task Force recommendations for use of antiretroviral drugs in pregnant HIV-1-infected women for maternal health and interventions to reduce perinatal HIV-1 transmission in the United States. MMWR Recomm Rep 51(RR-18):1–38, 2002.

7. Connor EM, Sperling RS, Gelber R, et al: Reduction of maternal-infant transmission of human immunodeficiency virus type 1 with zidovudine treatment. Pediatric AIDS Clinical Trials Group Protocol 076 Study Group. N Engl J Med 331:1173–1180, 1994.

8. Elective caesarean-section versus vaginal delivery in prevention of vertical HIV-1 transmission: a randomised clinical trial. The European Mode of Delivery Collaboration. Lancet 353:1035–1039, 1999.

9. Merchant RC, Becker BM, Mayer KH, et al: Emergency department blood or body fluid exposure evaluations and HIV postexposure prophylaxis usage. Acad Emerg Med 10:1345–1353, 2003.

10. Cardo DM, Culver DH, Ciesielski CA, et al: A case-control study of HIV seroconversion in health care workers after percutaneous exposure. Centers for Disease Control and Prevention Needlestick Surveillance Group. N Engl J Med 337:1485–1490, 1997.

*11. Havens PL: Postexposure prophylaxis in children and adolescents for nonoccupational exposure to human immunodeficiency virus. Pediatrics 111(6 Pt 1):1475–1489, 2003.

12. Merchant RC, Keshavarz R: Human immunodeficiency virus postexposure prophylaxis for adolescents and children. Pediatrics 108:e38, 2001.

13. Vittinghoff E, Douglas J, Judson F, et al: Per-contact risk of human immunodeficiency virus transmission between male sexual partners. Am J Epidemiol 150:306–311, 1999.

14. Mastro TD, de Vincenzi I: Probabilities of sexual HIV-1 transmission. AIDS 10(Suppl A):S75–S82, 1996.

15. Royce RA, Sena A, Cates W Jr, Cohen MS: Sexual transmission of HIV. N Engl J Med 336:1072–1078, 1997.

16. Gostin LO, Lazzarini Z, Alexander D, et al: HIV testing, counseling, and prophylaxis after sexual assault. JAMA 271:1436–1444, 1994.

17. Nduati R, John G, Mbori-Ngacha D, et al: Effect of breastfeeding and formula feeding on transmission of HIV-1: a randomized clinical trial. JAMA 283:1167–1174, 2000.

18. Nduati R, Richardson BA, John G, et al: Effect of breastfeeding on mortality among HIV-1 infected women: a randomised trial. Lancet 357:1651–1655, 2001.

*19. Read JS: Human milk, breastfeeding, and transmission of human immunodeficiency virus type 1 in the United States. American Academy of Pediatrics Committee on Pediatric AIDS. Pediatrics 112:1196–1205, 2003.

20. Centers for Disease Control and Prevention: HIV/AIDS Surveill Rep 12:1–43, 2000.

21. Kaplan EH, Heimer R: A model-based estimate of HIV infectivity via needle sharing. J Acquir Immune Defic Syndr Hum Retrovirol 5:1116–1118, 1992.

22. Richman KM, Rickman LS: The potential for transmission of human immunodeficiency virus through human bites. J Acquir Immune Defic Syndr Hum Retrovirol 6:402–406, 1993.

23. McCarthy GM, Ssali CS, Bednarsh H, et al: Transmission of HIV in the dental clinic and elsewhere. Oral Dis 8(Suppl 2):126–135, 2002.

—————

*Selected readings.

24. Centers for Disease Control: HIV reporting—United States. MMWR Morb Mortal Wkly Rep 38:496–499, 1989.

25. Merchant R, Keshavarz R: Emergency prophylaxis following needlestick injuries and sexual exposures: Results from a survey comparing New York emergency department practitioners with their national colleagues. Mt Sinai J Med 70(5):338–343, 2003.

26. Olshen E, Samples CL: Postexposure prophylaxis: an intervention to prevent human immunodeficiency virus infection in adolescents. Curr Opin Pediatr 15:379–384, 2003.

27. Babl FE, Cooper ER, Damon B, et al: HIV postexposure prophylaxis for children and adolescents. Am J Emerg Med 18:282–287, 2000.

*28. The Working Group on Antiretroviral Therapy and Medical Management of HIV-infected Children: Guidelines for the use of antiretroviral agents in pediatric HIV infection. Available at *http://aidsinfo.nih. gov/guidelines/pediatric/PED_113004.html* (accessed December 28, 2004).

Chapter 157

Interpersonal and Intimate Partner Violence

Joel A. Fein, MD, MPH and Megan H. Bair-Merritt, MD, MSCE

Key Points

Children can be exposed to and be victims of violence in homes, in schools, and on the streets; many who experience violence in one setting also experience it in another.

The emergency department clinician should perform a safety and risk assessment of violently injured patients.

The American Academy of Pediatrics recommends that pediatric practitioners routinely screen for intimate partner violence (IPV).

Child abuse and IPV co-occur in 30% to 70% of families.

Introduction and Background

Youth violence is defined as any intentional assault on another person by one or more young people ages 12 to 19 years. Although the emergency practitioner is most often confronted with patients who have physical injuries after an assault, the broad definition of youth violence also includes emotional and psychological violence. Youth violence is unfortunately part of many American children's routine daily activities. Despite an overall decrease in firearm mortality in the past decade, the prevalence and severity of this problem in American adolescents remains high, especially in impoverished areas. Age-adjusted rates of assault-related trauma for 10- to 19-year-olds were 5 per 100,000 deaths and 1035 per 100,000 nonfatal injuries in 2002.[1] Although advances in trauma care may reduce mortality, the level of self-reported violent behaviors by adolescents and young adults has not declined.[2]

When faced with a patient who is injured through community violence, emergency physicians can either "treat or street," or can "screen and intervene." In order to accomplish the latter, the clinician must recognize the injury mechanism, assess the youth's risk factors for violent injury, and implement interventions or referrals on his or her behalf.

Exposure to intimate partner violence (IPV) is an equally common and damaging life experience for children. Every year in the United States, between 2 and 4 million women are abused by an intimate partner.[3] Children are overrepresented in homes in which this occurs. In particular, families with current IPV are significantly more likely than families without IPV to have children less than 5 years of age living in the home.[4] Current literature cites that between 3.3 and 10 million children witness IPV each year.[5-9] These numbers are extrapolated from population-based surveys,[10] and are potentially an underestimate of the overall prevalence. One cross-sectional survey conducted with a convenience sample of mothers in an urban pediatric emergency department (ED) determined that 32% of women had been physically abused by a spouse or boyfriend over their lifetime, and 9% had been physically abused by a spouse or boyfriend within the past year.[11] The authors of this study theorized that abused women preferentially select ED care for their children secondary to the availability of 24-hour service and to the perceived anonymity of this environment.

Children who are exposed to IPV are at increased risk for poor mental, behavioral, and physical health outcomes. For example, children in homes with IPV are more likely than their peers to be depressed, to have anxiety disorders, to suffer from posttraumatic stress disorder, and to become involved in risky behaviors, such as alcohol and drug abuse, during adolescence.[12-14] The physical health consequences have been somewhat less clearly delineated. However, a large, retrospective cohort study has suggested an independent association between childhood IPV exposure and a variety of poor physical health outcomes in adulthood.[15-19] Additionally, multiple studies have cited a large overlap between child abuse and IPV, with the co-occurrence of both forms of violence 30% to 70% of the time.[20-22] Recognizing the scale and the impact of childhood exposure to IPV, the American Academy of Pediatrics (AAP) established guidelines in 1998 entitled "The Role of the Pediatrician in Recognizing and Intervening on Behalf of Abused Women." In these guidelines, the AAP stated, "identifying and intervening on behalf of battered women may be one of the most effective means of preventing child abuse."[6] They recommend routine screening for IPV in the pediatric setting.

Issues

Most ED clinicians believe that they can recognize violent injury, and feel comfortable referring to a social worker, chaplain, or other external resource.[23,24] However, many clinicians report that they do not fully assess safety and risk factors in violently injured patients.[24]

Although male gender is a consistently reported single risk factor for violent injury, both genders are at risk for youth violence.[25] Males and females may, however, present to the ED with different stories and physical complaints. Girls who come to the ED with nonfatal injures are more likely than males to suffer a contusion or human bite injury rather than a gunshot wound or laceration.[26] Younger girls (under 14) are more likely than boys to be injured in or around the home, and to have had a previous fight with the other person(s) involved.[27] Although most patients are forthcoming with the details of their violence-related injuries, some will not admit to the nature of their injuries. For example, one can assume that, if the patient is involved in illegal activities, or is in an intimate relationship with the offender, he or she could be less likely to disclose the full story. As discussed later, an appropriate safety assessment relies on the details of the actual injury-related events.

The violently injured patient may exhibit a range of emotional responses, such as anger, sadness, or apparent indifference. Younger children are often just as frightened about the impact of their injuries as they are about the manner in which they were incurred. It is known that violently injured youth are at risk for developing posttraumatic stress symptoms after the event, although there is significant variability in the expression of these symptoms.[28,29] Traumatic stress symptoms include reexperiencing the event, avoidance, hyperarousal, and dissociation. Most patients experience relief of these symptoms over weeks to months.

Screening for IPV

Just as assessing safety and risk factors in violently injured patients can assist in recognizing traumatic stress symptoms and in providing comprehensive care, screening for IPV in the patient's caregiver may improve the ED provider's understanding of the child's current illness, home environment, and ability to follow physician recommendations. In addition to the AAP recommendations for routine IPV screening, the American College of Emergency Physicians, the Joint Commission on Accreditation of Healthcare Organizations, and the American Medical Association all have policies or statements advocating routine screening of women. However, in 2004, the United States Preventive Services Taskforce (USPSTF) published guidelines stating that insufficient evidence exists to recommend either for or against routine IPV screening.[30] Critiques of these guidelines include the following: 1) the concept of a "screening" test for IPV had been misapplied, and asking about IPV should instead be viewed as a routine behavioral health inquiry; 2) benefits of screening may extend beyond simply decreasing violent episodes, and these should be considered in evaluating the merits of screening; and 3) IPV is a complex issue, and qualitative research or studies outside of the traditional medical literature should be considered.[31-33] Benefits and risks for children related to screening mothers for IPV therefore remain uninvestigated.

With the neutral position on screening from the USPSTF, the evidence-based clinician is left in somewhat of a quandary. Alternatives to routine screening include not screening at all or performing targeted screening. In the pediatric setting, targeted screening would naturally include children in whom concern exists for child abuse and neglect. However, with a targeted approach, many female victims of IPV will not be identified. As a general rule, inquiring about IPV provides important data about behavioral risk factors. Importantly, women generally support routine IPV screening in the pediatric setting.[5]

In considering screening, decisions must be made by the institution and by the provider about what method will be used (face-to-face, pen and paper survey, computer/technology-assisted questionnaire), and what questions will be asked. Numerous methods have been tested and compared and each has advantages and disadvantages, with no clear consensus regarding which is preferred.[34-36] With face-to-face screening, women appear to be equally comfortable with physician and nurse screening, but are less at ease when screening is performed in triage.[37]

Numerous sets of screening questions have been studied for appropriateness and effectiveness in the adult ED setting.[38,39] One of the more commonly used screens is the three-question Partner Violence Screen described by Feldhaus et al.[40] (Table 157–1). The efficacy of specific screening questions for female caregivers in a pediatric ED has not been studied.

In the pediatric setting, concern has been raised about performing direct screening in the presence of children over the age of 3.[34] In a qualitative study of former abuse victims, Zink and Jacobson detailed women's concern that screening in front of older children may lead the children to inadvertently relay the conversation to the abuser, thereby potentially increasing abuse.[34] When an older child is present, Zink and Jacobson suggested that providers attempt to separate the caregiver and child. If this cannot occur, they suggested that the provider ask general questions such as "Do you feel safe in your current relationship?" and "In general, how would you describe your relationship: a lot of tension, some tension, or no tension?" If there is continued concern based upon the response or the reaction to these questions, the provider should attempt to interview the woman alone to pursue more specific questions.

A second controversy relevant to screening for IPV in the pediatric ED setting is documentation. Unlike in the adult

---

Table 157–1	Partner Violence Screen

1. Have you been hit, kicked, punched, or otherwise hurt by someone within the past year? If so, by whom?
2. Do you feel safe in your current relationship?
3. Is there a partner from a previous relationship who is making you feel unsafe now?

Adapted from Feldhaus K, Koziol-McLain J, Amsbury H, et al: Accuracy of 3 brief screening questions for detecting partner violence in the emergency department. JAMA 277:1357–1361, 1997.

ED, where providers are directly screening their patients and the chart reflects care for the female adult patient, in the pediatric setting, the child is the patient and both legal guardians can access the medical record. If the perpetrator is the child's father, he has access to the chart and could become aware of the IPV conversation, thereby potentially increasing the risk of violence. In contrast, it may be legally beneficial to document the abuse in case the victim requires this information in court. While the risks of documentation are more theoretical than evidence based, it is important to discuss the risks and benefits of documentation with the victim, and abide by her wishes.

When a patient's caregiver discloses IPV in the ED setting, the response should entail the following: (1) a statement supporting the woman for her disclosure, and emphasizing that the abuse is not her fault and that she does not deserve to be treated that way; (2) an assessment of the woman's and child's current safety (including questions about escalation of violence and weapons) and comfort going home; (3) careful questioning and examination for child abuse and injury to the child or children; (4) the offer of social work and/or national and local IPV resources; and (5) safety planning, as needed.[39]

Mandated Reporting

As evidenced by the aforementioned dilemmas about screening and documentation, screening for IPV in a pediatric setting poses unique challenges. One of the important issues to consider and to discuss is mandated reporting. Pediatric providers are obligated to report to child protective services any concern for child abuse or neglect, or concern that the child is in a situation of imminent danger (see Chapter 119, Physical Abuse and Child Neglect). With any disclosure of IPV, a careful assessment of the child's well being and safety is essential. While adult health care providers may be mandated reporters of IPV, pediatric providers generally are not responsible for reporting injury to the child's mother when the practitioner is not actually providing medical care to the woman.[39]

Currently, some states have mandated reporting laws for childhood exposure to IPV. Staying current with requirements for reporting is essential. If practicing in a state *with* mandated reporting laws for childhood exposure to IPV, your response should include the following: (1) inform the mother of your responsibility to report, (2) encourage the mother to also file a report herself (which often lessens later accusations of "failure to protect"), (3) provide child protective services with all relevant information, and (4) ensure that the safety needs of the mother are met.[39] If practicing in a state with less specific reporting laws, consider each situation individually to determine what is best for that child and mother.

While proponents of mandated reporting state that it is justified secondary to the negative sequelae of childhood exposure to IPV, many in the field of IPV are concerned about such requirements. Apprehension about mandated reporting for exposure stems from fear that reporting is punitive to the victim, implying that she failed to protect the child. Universal reporting also incorrectly assumes that all children are affected in the same way by IPV exposure, and may increase demands on an already overburdened child protective services system. There are also concerns that man-

dated reporting decreases women's likelihood of disclosing and seeking help.[39]

Solutions

There are no easy solutions for preventing violence in the lives of children and adolescents. For the individual patient who presents to the ED, the standard of care is to address patient safety and emotional needs. It is crucial to recognize the mindset of some urban youth regarding the role of violence in settling conflicts and to understand what sociologic phenomena govern many inner-city interactions and behaviors.[41]

For the adolescent patient, the clinician should clarify any issues of confidentiality before interviewing the patient about sensitive topics, such as emotions, safety, and sexuality. Specifically, the practitioner could state: "Our conversation will remain private unless you tell me something that makes me believe that you or someone else will suffer serious harm." This short statement helps to establish trust on which the clinician can perform a brief risk assessment and develop a safety plan with the youth. At all costs, the clinician should avoid the perception that he or she is blaming the youth for his or her situation. This will invariably destroy the trust that is required to gather important information, and will sabotage potential interventions on the part of the health care system.

The ED clinician should assess the immediate safety issues related to the violent event, asking questions regarding the patient's safety concerns, his or her relationship with the other involved persons, and if the incident was reported to the police or other authorities. Intuitively, if the other involved person is a complete stranger, as in a robbery incident, the potential for retaliation seems less. Likewise, it seems unlikely that a juvenile who reports an incident to the police would incite a retaliation event. Mandatory reporting of gunshot wounds is a controversial topic and varies by jurisdiction; it is prudent to know the laws and regulations in your practice setting.[42-44]

If the patient knows the other involved person(s), the ED clinician should ask directly if he or she thinks that the argument or fight is over and will remain so. It is important to assess any ongoing rivalries that could lead to further injury. This line of questioning should include asking about friends or family members who may plan to retaliate. To assess overall safety concerns, the clinician can ask the simple question, "Will you feel safe when you leave today?" If needed, strategies for safety planning can then be made in conjunction with social workers, police, or other community resources. This may also be an opportune time to assess and counsel about weapon carrying and use.

Many violently injured patients will experience emotional and psychological ramifications, irrespective of injury severity. Family and patient education about the signs and symptoms of posttraumatic stress provide support to the patient. Information about posttraumatic stress disorder is available through various national organizations such as the National Child Traumatic Stress Network (*http://www.nctsnet.org*), the International Society for Traumatic Stress Studies (*http://www.istss.org*), and the National Center for Post-Traumatic Stress Disorder (*http://www.ncptsd.org*).

Although a safety and risk analysis is within the domain of ED care, interventions for violence are often more aptly situated in the patient's community. It may be helpful to share any concerns with the patient's primary care provider, and encourage the family to involve the patient's school counselors, if applicable. Hospital social workers may be helpful in linking the patient with school-based or community-based organizations that range from after-school programs, external support programs (such as Big Brother/Big Sister), or Rites of Passage programs. In some areas, community organizations such as the Police Athletic League and Boys' and Girls' Clubs have specific programs for troubled youth.[45] Older adolescents may benefit from job training and placement programs, General Education Development services, and alcohol or drug rehabilitation services. It is not possible, or even necessary, to link all violently injured patients with a community-based intervention. However, safety assessment, risk factor analysis, and intuition will identify the most concerning patients. A well-suited referral can alter the trajectory of a few youth who otherwise may present to the ED time and time again with violence-related injury.

Children who are not obviously injured may still have significant violence exposure risks, including exposure to IPV. Ideally, every ED should develop a protocol surrounding IPV identification, documentation, and management. Development of this protocol should include input from physicians, nurses, social workers, and IPV advocates. Potential solutions for issues about screening in front of children include providing a pen-and-paper or computer-based questionnaire, or starting with more general safety questions and pursuing more specific IPV questions with the woman alone if concerned. A code known by members of the department, but not otherwise obvious, can be created for IPV documentation. For management, each department should consider state laws as well as available resources. In the absence of a departmental protocol, providers must make a personal decision about when and how to screen for IPV in the pediatric ED. At a minimum, one should be aware of the high co-occurrence of IPV with child abuse. Additionally, ready access to IPV resources such as posters and numbers with IPV hotlines can provide an essential service for women in abusive relationships.

Additional information can be obtained through reading the AAP clinical guidelines, or through contact with the Family Violence Prevention Fund, whose publications include "Identifying and Responding to Domestic Violence: Consensus Recommendations for Child and Adolescent Health" (*http://www.endabuse.org*).[6,39]

Summary

Consideration of both youth and family violence is essential when treating children. Youth violence is a public health problem that permeates most EDs. The multifactorial nature of violence should not dissuade ED practitioners from performing a safety and risk assessment for violently injured patients, or from attempting to link patients and families with social and emotional support resources. IPV is prevalent and is frequently comorbid with child abuse, and exposure to IPV may lead to poor mental, behavioral, and physical health outcomes in children. After IPV is disclosed, an empathetic response may be an intervention in and of itself. A careful assessment of the child's and the caregiver's safety and an offer of resources are of utmost importance. Practi-

tioners should be aware of state laws with regard to mandated reporting of IPV exposure.

REFERENCES

1. National Center for Injury Prevention and Control (NCIPC): WISQARS™ (Web-based Injury Statistics Query and Reporting System). Available at *http://www.cdc.gov/ncipc/wisqars/default.htm* (accessed March 12, 2005).
2. U.S. Department of Health and Human Services: Youth Violence: A Report of the Surgeon General, 2001. Available at *http://www.surgeongeneral.gov/library/youthviolence* (accessed March 12, 2005).
3. Novello A, Rosenberg M, Saltzman L, et al: From the Surgeon General, U.S. Public Health Service. JAMA 267:3132, 1992.
4. Fantuzzo J, Boruch R, Beriama A, et al: Domestic violence and children: prevalence and risk in five major U.S. cities. J Am Acad Child Adolesc Psychiatry 36:116–122, 1997.
5. Dowd D, Kennedy C, Knapp J, et al: Mothers' and health care providers' perspectives on screening for intimate partner violence in a pediatric emergency department. Arch Pediatr Adolesc Med 156:794–799, 2002.
6. American Academy of Pediatrics: The role of the pediatrician in recognizing and intervening on behalf of abused women. Pediatrics 101:1091–1092, 1998.
7. Berger R, Bogan D, Dulani T, et al: Implementation of a program to teach pediatric residents and faculty about domestic violence. Arch Pediatr Adolesc Med 156:804–810, 2002.
8. Kerker B, Horwitz S, Leventhal J, et al: Identification of violence in the home: pediatric and parental reports. Arch Pediatr Adolesc Med 154:457–462, 2000.
9. Knapp J, Dowd M: Family violence: implications for the pediatrician. Pediatr Rev 19:316–321, 1998.
10. Fantuzzo J, Mohr W: Prevalence and effects of child exposure to domestic violence. Future Child 9:21–32, 1999.
11. Duffy S, McGrath M, Becker B, et al: Mothers with histories of domestic violence in a pediatric emergency department. Pediatrics 103:1007–1013, 1999.
12. Wolfe D, Crooks C, Lee V, et al: The effects of children's exposure to domestic violence: a meta-analysis and critique. Clin Child Family Psychol Rev 16:171–187, 2003.
13. Kitzmann K, Gaylord N, Holt A, et al: Child witnesses to domestic violence: a meta-analytic review. J Consult Clin Psychol 71:339–352, 2003.
14. Kolbo J: Risk and resilience among children exposed to family violence. Violence Vict 11:113–128, 1996.
15. Hillis S, Anda R, Dube S, et al: The association between adverse childhood experiences and adolescent pregnancy, long-term psychosocial consequences, and fetal death. Pediatrics 113:320–327, 2004.
16. Dube S, Anda R, Felitti V, et al: Exposure to abuse, neglect, and household dysfunction among adults who witnessed intimate partner violence as children: implications for health and social services. Violence Vict 17:3–17, 2002.
17. Hillis S, Anda R, Felitti V, et al: Adverse childhood experiences and sexually transmitted diseases in men and women: a retrospective study. Pediatrics 106:e11, 2000.
18. Hillis S, Anda R, Felitti V, et al: Adverse childhood experiences and sexual risk behaviors in women: a retrospective cohort study. Family Plann Perspect 33:206–211, 2001.
19. Anda R, Croft J, Felitti V, et al: Adverse childhood experiences and smoking during adolescence and adulthood. JAMA 282:1652–1658, 1999.
20. Edleson J: The overlap between child maltreatment and woman battering. Violence Against Women 5:134–154, 1999.
21. Hazen A, Connelly C, Kelleher K, et al: Intimate partner violence among female caregivers of children reported for child maltreatment. Child Abuse Neglect 28:301–319, 2004.
22. Appel A, Holden G: The Co-occurence of spouse and physical child abuse: a review and appraisal. J Family Psychol 12:578–599, 1998.
23. Fein JA, Ginsburg KR, McGrath ME, et al: Violence prevention in the emergency department: clinician attitudes and limitations. Arch Pediatr Adolesc Med 154:495–498, 2000.
24. Wilkinson D, Kurtz E, Lane P, et al: The emergency department approach to violently injured youth: a regional survey. Injury Prevent 11:206–208, 2005.

25. Chan L, Kipke M, Schneir A, et al: Preventing Violence and Related Health-Risking Social Behaviors in Adolescents (AHRQ Publication No. 04-E032-1). Rockville, MD: Agency for Healthcare Research and Quality, 2004.

26. Mollen C, Fein J, Vu T, et al: Gender differences in injuries and event characteristics resulting from youth violence. Pediatr Emerg Care 19:379–384, 2003.

27. Mollen C, Fein J, Localio A, et al: Characterization of interpersonal violence events involving young adolescent girls vs. events involving young adolescent boys. Arch Pediatr Adolesc Med 158:545–550, 2004.

28. Fein JA, Kassam-Adams N, Vu TN, et al: Acute stress disorder symptoms in violently injured youth in the emergency department. Ann Emerg Med 38:391–396, 2001.

29. Fein J, Kassam-Adams N, Gavin M, et al: Persistence of posttraumatic stress in violently injured youth seen in the emergency department. Arch Pediatr Adolesc Med 156:836–840, 2002.

30. Nelson H, Nygren P, McInerney Y, et al: Screening women and elderly adults for family and intimate partner violence: a review of the evidence for the U.S. Preventive Services Task Force. Ann Intern Med 140:387–396, 2004.

31. Lachs M: Screening for family violence: what's an evidence-based doctor to do? Ann Intern Med 140:399–400, 2004.

32. Soler E, Campbell J: Screening for family and intimate partner violence. Ann Intern Med 141:82, 2004.

33. Warshaw C, Alpert E: Integrating routine inquiry about domestic violence into daily practice. Ann Intern Med 131:619–620, 1999.

34. Zink T, Jacobson J: Screening for intimate partner violence when children are present. J Interpersonal Violence 18:872–890, 2003.

35. Furbee P, Sikora R, Williams J, et al: Comparison of domestic violence screening methods: a pilot study. Ann Emerg Med 31:495–501, 1998.

36. McFarlane J, Christoffel K, Bateman L, et al: Assessing for abuse: self-report versus nurse interview. Public Health Nurs 8:245–250, 1991.

37. Hayden S, Barton E, Hayden M: Domestic violence in the emergency department: how do women prefer to disclose and discuss the issues? J Emerg Med 15:447–451, 1997.

38. Heron S, Thompson M, Jackson E, et al: Do responses to an intimate partner violence screen predict scores on a comprehensive measure of intimate partner violence in low-income black women? Ann Emerg Med 42:483–491, 2003.

39. McAlister Groves B, Augustyn M, Lee D, et al: Identifying and responding to domestic violence: consensus recommendations for child and adolescent health. In Family Violence Prevention Fund. Available at *http://endabuse.org/programs/display.php3?DocID=231* (accessed March 12, 2005).

40. Feldhaus K, Koziol-McLain J, Amsbury H, et al: Accuracy of 3 brief screening questions for detecting partner violence in the emergency department. JAMA 277:1357–1361, 1997.

41. Anderson E: Code of the Street: Decency, Violence, and the Moral Life of the Inner City. New York: WW Norton, 1999.

42. Ovens H: Why mandatory reporting of gunshot wounds is necessary: a response from the OMA's Executive of the Section on Emergency Medicine. CMAJ 170:1256–1257, 2004.

43. Carlisle J: Mandatory reporting of gunshot wounds to police not as simple as it seems. Health Law Can 25:1–10, 2004.

44. Pauls M, Downie J: Shooting ourselves in the foot: why mandatory reporting of gunshot wounds is a bad idea. CMAJ 170:1255–1256, 2004.

45. Zun LS, Downey L, Rosen J: An emergency department-based program to change attitudes of youth toward violence. J Emerg Med 26:247–251, 2004.

Chapter 158

Approach to Pain Management

Kelly D. Young, MD, MS

Key Points

Pain management in the emergency department (ED) is increasingly recognized as an important topic: in clinical practice, in the research literature, and among accrediting organizations.

Pain needs to be assessed, managed, and reassessed routinely in the ED. Achieving this goal requires a multidisciplinary approach.

Successful pain management includes both pharmacologic and nonpharmacologic techniques, as well as modifications to the ED environment and "culture."

Introduction and Background

Pain is often inadequately assessed and addressed in emergency departments (EDs), and this is especially true for pediatric patients.[1] As recently as a few decades ago, the myth that young children did not feel pain was widely believed. Since then, there has been a burst of literature on the pediatric pain experience, but a gap remains between knowledge and clinical practice.[2,3] Nevertheless, improved pain management is increasingly recognized as an important goal. Congress has declared the current decade as the "Decade of Pain Control and Research" as of 2001.[4] The Joint Commission, formally known as the Joint Commission on Accreditation of Healthcare Organizations (JCAHO) has also set standards for pain assessment and management.[5] Research has shown that, in addition to acute pain itself, other consequences of undertreated pain include decreased parent and patient satisfaction, adverse effects such as hypoxemia and poor healing, and possible long-term effects such as increased risk for chronic pain syndromes, decreased pain tolerance, and avoidance of medical care.[1,6] Consequences to staff include stress and career dissatisfaction from having to inflict pain on children during procedures.

Issues and Barriers

Perpetuation of several myths regarding the pediatric pain experience and available treatments has been a barrier to improved pain management.[7] Young children cannot self-report their pain, and ED practitioners are often less comfortable with pediatric medication dosages, and may be more wary of potential adverse effects. Whereas adult patients who are dissatisfied with pain management can complain, and such complaints are likely to result in changes in practice, children require adult advocates. Parents focused on diagnosis and management of the primary condition (e.g., otitis media) may be satisfied with an antibiotic prescription, while the child's related pain goes untreated. Parents recalling procedures performed on themselves when they were children may not realize that advances in procedural pain and anxiety management exist.

The ED environment is busy and chaotic and has a constantly changing staff. ED flow is an important factor in clinicians' decision making and practice. Overcoming these barriers requires a multidisciplinary team, composed of physicians, nurses, child life specialists if available, pharmacists, and any other interested parties, to work together to educate health care workers, create pain management policies that do not significantly interfere with ED flow, perform quality improvement projects, and work toward a change in the "culture" of the ED to emphasize good pain management.[1,8] Table 158–1 outlines some of the major barriers to adequate pain management in the pediatric ED.

Parental presence during pediatric procedures is an increasingly discussed topic (see Chapter 153: Family Presence). While evidence on whether parental presence actually results in lower child self-reported pain scores, pain behaviors, and anxiety is mixed, it is clear that children prefer to have their parents present.[9] Health care workers are often uncomfortable with parental presence, citing concerns about interference and decreased procedural success. These concerns are not evidence based. Each unique situation should be assessed depending on the individual parent and child's preference, but an overall policy of allowing parental presence is recommended.[1,6]

Solutions

The greatest barriers to adequate pain management in health care systems are lack of support from administration, lack of coordination of improvement efforts, and lack of accountability.[5] The Joint Commission has set standards related to pain management as of 2001 (Table 158–2).[5] Increased regulatory scrutiny should provide the impetus for strong

Table 158–1	Ten Barriers to Adequate Pediatric Pain Management in the Emergency Department (ED)

1. Belief that children do not feel pain, or that pain is a beneficial "life lesson" of childhood
2. Difficulty in assessing pain in children
3. Myth that pain medication use (especially opiates) will result in addiction, or carries an exceptionally high risk of adverse effects in children
4. Concern that ED flow will be slowed considerably by using pain management methods
5. Lack of health care worker knowledge of effective pain management techniques, especially nonpharmacologic techniques
6. Belief that children prefer "one needle" to the two needles required for local anesthetic injection, and belief that rapid completion of the procedure, using forceful restraint if necessary, is less stressful than prolonging the procedure for use of pain management techniques
7. Staff and parents more focused on diagnosis and management of primary condition and/or believe that pain treatment will interfere with diagnosis
8. Staff uncomfortable with parental presence during pediatric procedures
9. Lack of coordination between various health care workers in efforts to reduce pain
10. Lack of health care provider accountability and feedback regarding pain management practices

Table 158–2	Joint Commission Standards

1. Recognize the right of patients to appropriate assessment and treatment of pain.
2. Assess the presence, intensity, and nature of pain in all patients.
3. Record the results of the assessment such that regular reassessment is promoted.
4. Evaluate and establish staff competency in pain assessment and management.
5. Establish polices that support appropriate prescription and recommendation of pain medications.
6. Ensure that pain does not interfere with patients' ability to participate in rehabilitation.
7. Educate patients and their families about effective pain management and its significance.
8. Address patient needs for pain management in the discharge planning process.
9. Incorporate pain management into quality performance activities and assessments.

Adapted from National Pharmaceutical Council, Inc: Pain: Current Understanding of Assessment, Management, and Treatments [monograph]. Available at *http://www.jcaho.org/news+room/ health+care+issues/pm+monographs.htm* (accessed January 19, 2005).

institutional commitment to focus on pain management. Thus the first step is to establish institutional pain management standards and to empower a pain management "czar" and/or multidisciplinary pain management team to work toward meeting these standards.

Education of health care workers to improve pain assessment is one important goal for the pain management team. Many methods for pediatric pain assessment exist, broadly categorized as self-report, behavioral measures, and physiologic measures[6,10] (Table 158–3). Self-report is considered the "gold standard," but children younger than 3 years are generally not able to differentiate levels of pain. Behavioral

measures, looking at such factors as facial expression, torso movements, resistance, and crying, may be used in young children and noncommunicating developmentally delayed children. Physiologic measures should be used as corroborative evidence only. The pain management team should review available measures, choose one appropriate measure for each age group or patient type, educate all health care workers on using the selected methods, and make the assessment tools widely available in the triage and patient care areas. Redesign of patient care triage forms and computer entry interfaces to include routine pain assessment may improve the frequency of pain assessment.[8]

Both pharmacologic and nonpharmacologic pain management methods exist. Health care providers may be unfamiliar with pediatric dosing for pain medications, or may be overly concerned about potential adverse effects. The pain management team can provide pocket card references of commonly used pain medications[5,11,12] (Table 158–4); education regarding the incidence, prevention, and treatment of potential adverse effects; and follow-up data on the actual occurrence of any significant adverse effects seen in the ED. Nurse-driven standing-order protocols allowing pain medication administration in triage will improve the rapidity with which pain relief is provided.[13]

The World Health Organization developed a three-step Pain Relief Ladder for management of cancer pain; the concepts behind this ladder are also applicable in the ED setting.[14] Using the ladder, a nonopiate is first given for mild to moderate pain. If pain persists, a weak opiate is added. If pain continues to persist, a stronger opiate is given. Adjunctives such as muscle relaxants, antianxiety agents, anticonvulsants or antidepressants for chronic neuropathic pain, and nonpharmacologic methods can be added. For severe pain, the clinician may choose to start higher on the ladder and give an opiate immediately. Treatment should be multimodal, given preemptively when pain is expected (e.g., for a procedure), and given around the clock rather than on an as-needed basis (to avoid a cycle of breakthrough pain due to undermedication, then overmedication, then breakthrough pain again).

Health care providers may be unfamiliar with the adjunctives, topical agents, and nonpharmacologic methods available (Table 158–5).[1,6] The literature strongly supports decreased pain for minor needle procedures with use of topical anesthetics.[15,16] Studies have demonstrated the efficacy of pretreatment of lacerations with topical anesthetics at triage,[17-19] and the ability of triage nurses to predict the need for intravenous cannulation and thus place topical anesthetic at triage.[20] In this study, the majority of intravenous cannulations were performed more than 60 minutes after triage, allowing for full efficacy of topical anesthetics. Orally administered sucrose, 2 ml of a 24% to 30% solution given 2 minutes prior to the procedure and/or during the procedure, is an effective pain reducer in neonates.[21] Commercial solutions are available, or the pharmacy may prepare them. One group reports mixing a standard packet of table sugar with 10 ml of water.[22] Pain management teams should work with pharmacists to ensure availability of topical anesthetics and sucrose, and institute protocols for their routine use.

Distraction has been definitively shown to be effective in reducing procedural pain and distress.[23] Child life

Table 158–3 Pediatric Pain Assessment

Method	Examples	Validated Age Range	Comments
Self-report			Gold standard
Faces scales	Bieri faces[32] Wong-Baker faces[33]	3 yr–adult	Preferred by children, young children may tend to choose extremes, minimum clinically significant difference = 1 face
Visual analog scale	10-cm line labeled "no pain" at one end, "worst pain possible" at other end	7 yr–adult	Best validated for research purposes, minimally clinically significant difference 10–13 mm[34,35]
Oucher	Combination of 0–10 numeric scale for older children and faces scale for younger children	3–12 yr	African American, Hispanic, and white versions validated[36–38]
Others	Colored analog scale, pain ladder, poker chip tool, pain thermometer	Variable	
Behavioral			For preverbal and noncommunicating children
Preverbal children	Children's Hospital of Eastern Ontario Pain Scale (CHEOPS),[39] Faces, Legs, Activity, Cry, Consolability (FLACC)[40,41]	1–7 yr 0–7 yr	Based on pain behaviors such as facial expression, torso movements, kicking, verbal protest, need for restraint
Developmentally delayed children	Noncommunicating Children's Pain Checklist,[42,43] University of Wisconsin Children's Hospital Pain Scale for Preverbal and Nonverbal Children[44]	3–18 yr All ages	
Neonates	Neonatal Facial Coding System (NCFS)[45]	Neonates	Facial expressions most valid indicator of neonatal pain
	CRIES[46] Modified Behavioral Pain Scale[47]	Neonates Birth–6 mo	
Physiologic			Least reliable, should be used as corroborative data only
Heart rate		All ages	
Blood pressure		All ages	
Salivary cortisol		All ages	Increases 20 min after painful procedures[48]

Table 158–4 Pharmacologic Pediatric Pain Management Methods[5,11,12]

Medication	Indication	Dosage Guidelines and Comments
Nonopiate Analgesics	Mild to moderate pain	Potential adverse effects include gastric upset, renal insufficiency, hypersensitivity reaction, platelet dysfunction.
Acetaminophen	Mild to moderate pain	15 mg/kg (max 650 mg per dose or 4 g/day, whichever is less) PO or PR q4–6h; antipyretic also.
Ibuprofen	Mild to moderate pain	10 mg/kg (max 800 mg per dose or 2400 mg/day) PO q6–8h; anti-inflammatory and antipyretic also.
Naproxen	Mild to moderate pain	5–7 mg/kg PO q8–12h for children 2 yr or older, max 1250 mg/day; anti-inflammatory also.
Ketorolac	Moderate pain, short-term use (<5 days)	0.5 mg/kg IV or IM (max 30 mg per dose or 90 mg/day) q6h; anti-inflammatory, particularly effective for renal colic.
Opiates	Moderate to severe pain	Potential adverse effects include nausea, constipation, pruritis, respiratory depression, sedation, and hypotension. Tolerance and dependence are very unlikely with acute use and appropriate doses in children. Naloxone 0.1 mg/kg (max 2 mg) IV, IM, subQ, or ET may reverse adverse effects. If one opiate is ineffective, switching to another may be effective.
Morphine	Severe pain	0.1 mg/kg IV or IM (max 15 mg) q1–2h; 0.5 mg/kg PO (max 30 mg for adult size) q4–6h
Fentanyl	Severe pain	1 mcg/kg IV or IM (max 100 mcg) q30–60 min; shorter duration of action.
Hydromorphone	Severe pain	0.015 mg/kg IV (max 1 mg) q4–6h; 0.05 mg/kg PO (max 5 mg) q4–6h; less pruritis than morphine.
Meperidine	Severe pain	1 mg/kg IV or IM (max 100 mg) q3–4h; high incidence of dysphoria, agitation; not preferred.
Codeine	Moderate pain	1 mg/kg PO (max 60 mg) q4–6h. Often given with acetaminophen in premixed preparations: elixir, 12 mg codeine and 120 mg acetaminophen in 5 ml; Tylenol #2, 325 mg acetaminophen/15 mg codeine; Tylenol #3, 325/30; Tylenol #4, 325/60. Must be metabolized to be effective; 10% or more of patients may not be able to metabolize to effective metabolite.
Oxycodone	Moderate pain	0.1 mg/kg PO (max 5 mg) q4–6h. Often given with acetaminophen in premixed preparations: 325 mg acetaminophen + 5 mg oxycodone (Percocet) most common form.
Hydrocodone	Moderate pain	0.15 mg/kg PO (max 10 mg) q4–6h. Often given with acetaminophen in premixed preparation of 500 mg acetaminophen + 5 mg hydrocodone (Vicodin) or 7.5 mg hydrocodone (Vicodin ES), or premixed with ibuprofen 200 mg + 7.5 mg hydrocodone (Vicoprofen).

Abbreviations: ET, endotracheally; IM, intramuscularly; IV, intravenously; PO, orally; PR, rectally; subQ, subcutaneously.

Table 158–5   Adjunctive and Nonpharmacologic Pediatric Pain Management Methods[6,12]

Antianxiety Agent

Midazolam	Adjunctive	0.05–0.1 mg/kg IV (max 2 mg) q3–5 min for up to three doses, titrated to effect; 0.5–0.75 mg/kg PO (max 10 mg). Antianxiety and amnestic only; no analgesia. Flumazenil may reverse respiratory depression: 0.01 mg/kg IV (max 0.2 mg) q1min to max of 1 mg, then q20min to max of 3 mg.

Topical Agents

Eutectic mixture of local anesthetics (EMLA)	Procedural pain	1–2 g topical cream per 10-cm^2 area of intact skin; cover with occlusive dressing; gives 4- to 5-mm depth of anesthesia after 45–60 min on skin. Maximum doses: Birth–3 mo: 1 g 3–12 mo: 2 g 1–6 yr: 10 g 7–12 yr: 20 g
4% Liposomal lidocaine (LMX4)	Procedural pain	Apply as for EMLA; no occlusive dressing needed; anesthesia within 20–30 min; available without a prescription.
Vapocoolants (ethyl chloride, flouromethane)	Procedural (injection) pain	Spray onto area of injection immediately prior to injection; cold sensation may be unpleasant to some children.
Lidocaine iontophoresis (Numby Stuff, LidoSite)	Procedural (injection) pain	Uses iontophoresis of lidocaine to provide 5- to 7-mm depth of anesthesia within 10 min. Requires initial investment in equipment.
Lidocaine 4%, epinephrine 1 : 2000, and tetracaine 0.5% gel (LET)	Laceration repair	Apply 3 ml directly into wound using a cotton ball (not gauze) for 15–30 min prior to laceration repair with sutures, staples, tissue adhesive, or prior to additional local anesthetic infiltration if needed. Not for areas where epinephrine is contraindicated.
Lidocaine jelly 2%	Urethral catheterization,[49] nasogastric tube insertion[50]	Instill 0.5–2 ml into urethra 2 mins before procedure (may instill up to three times). Use 5 ml in an adult for lubricant when inserting nasogastric tube.

Nonpharmacologic Methods

Distraction	Procedural pain	Age appropriate selection: pacifier/non-nutritive sucking, bubbles, toys, songs, pop-up books, party blower, kaleidoscope, videos, video games, puzzles, stories, jokes, counting, music, nonprocedural conversation
Sucrose	Procedural pain	Effective for young infants <6 mo; 2 ml of 30% sucrose or glucose solution, half 2 min prior to procedure and half during the procedure.
Counter-irritation	Injection pain	Rub on the surrounding skin during local anesthetic infiltration or injections; Shot Blocker device (http://www.bionix.com) stimulates surrounding skin, leaving a center hole for inserting the needle.
Tissue adhesives	Laceration repair	Dermabond or Indermil can be used to painlessly repair simple lacerations
Blowing, deep breathing	Procedural pain	Have child blow out imaginary candles, "blow away the pain," or use a party blower. Have child take slow deep breaths.
Suggestion	Procedural pain, visceral or headache pain	Suggest the child place a "magic glove" or "magic invisible cream" that removes the pain of a procedure, or turn a "pain switch" to off position. Works best with suggestible preschool-age children.
Heat or cold	Muscular pain, visceral or ear or headache pain	Apply cold in the first 24 hr after a muscular injury; apply warm compresses to other sources of pain.

specialists can work with health care providers to ensure that distraction items are available and used. Health care providers can always use nonprocedural conversation, such as asking the child questions about school, sports, or favorite television shows, or even allowing demonstration of math skills, to distract the child without the need for special equipment.[6]

Table 158–5 lists other effective yet uncommonly used nonpharmacologic methods to reduce pain in the ED. Pain management teams can provide education, demonstration, and encouragement to use these methods. They can ensure, for example, that sucrose for use with young infants undergoing painful procedures,[21,24] and tissue adhesives for laceration repairs,[25] are available in the ED, and that health care providers are comfortable with their use. A "train-the-trainer" approach, utilizing shift leaders who undergo educational sessions and then teach the rest of the health care workers on their shift, may be used. Similarly, one physician or nurse in

a group may attend a continuing education presentation or undergo training, and then teach the technique to others in the group.

Table 158–6 lists pain management approaches to several common pediatric procedural and medical situations seen in the ED[1,26] (see Chapter 159, Procedural Sedation and Analgesia). Because clinicians tend to concentrate on diagnosis and management of the primary condition, rather than the associated pain, the pain management team must emphasize pain control. Education of health care providers, inclusion of pain management in patient aftercare handouts, and inclusion of pain assessment and management in clinical practice guidelines for specific complaints will improve attention to pain management.[8] Patients and parents may inadequately treat children's pain due to false beliefs about the importance of being stoic, fears of addiction or side effects from pain medications, and lack of education on medication dosing and alternative therapies.[5] Discharge instructions should empha-

Table 158–6	Management of Specific Emergency Department Pediatric Pain Situations

Situation	Management Options
Mildly painful procedure (e.g., venipuncture)	Distraction + topical or local anesthesia
Moderately painful procedure (e.g., laceration repair, lumbar puncture, nail avulsion)	Distraction + topical or local anesthesia Distraction + topical or local anesthesia + midazolam Nitrous oxide Procedural sedation and analgesia
Moderately to severely painful procedure (e.g., abscess incision and drainage, fracture reduction, chest thoracostomy)	Procedural sedation and analgesia (most commonly fentanyl + midazolam or ketamine)[51,52]
Injections	Topical anesthetic cream, counter-irritation
Intravenous catheter placement	Topical anesthetic cream
Urethral catheterization	Viscous lidocaine placed in urethral opening 2 min prior to catheterization, with additional viscous lidocaine used as lubricant for the catheter[49]
Nasogastric tube placement	Lidocaine jelly placed in nasopharynx and used as lubricant; vasoconstrictor (phenylephrine) adjuvant; lidocaine solution in nasopharynx and oropharynx and/or cetacaine spray in oropharynx, or nebulized lidocaine[50]
Laceration repair	Topical anesthetic, evaluation for tissue adhesive. Inject local anesthetic that is warmed and buffered; inject slowly with smallest gauge needle available
Infant lumbar puncture	Topical anesthetic cream, infiltrated local anesthetic
Burns	Depending on severity of pain, nonopiate analgesics or opiates. For dressing changes, procedural sedation and analgesia may be necessary
Otitis media pain	Nonopiate analgesics, weak opiate oral analgesics, topical anesthetic otic solution, warm compresses
Pharyngitis pain	Nonopiate analgesics, weak opiate oral analgesics, anesthetic sprays and lozenges, salt water gargles, dexamethasone
Viral stomatitis pain	Nonopiate analgesics, "magic mouthwash" with topical anesthetic, sucralfate, bland diet
Musculoskeletal pain	Rest, ice, compression, elevation, nonopiate analgesics (especially nonsteroidal anti-inflammatory drugs)
Chest pain	If musculoskeletal (e.g., costochondritis): nonopiate analgesic (especially nonsteroidal anti-inflammatory drugs). If due to gastroesophageal reflux: antacid therapy
Mild abdominal pain	Nonopiate analgesics; relieve any constipation present
Acute abdominal pain	Short-acting opiate (fentanyl); no reason to delay pain treatment for consulting specialist examination[53]
Renal colic	Ketorolac, opiate for severe pain
Fracture pain	Acutely: strong opiate parenterally may be required, then nonopiate analgesic or weak opiate oral analgesic, immobilization
Headache	Nonopiate analgesics, opiates, migraine therapies if indicated

size the importance of pain management to the healing process, appropriate medication dosing and around-the-clock administration, and the need for the patient to return if pain is inadequately controlled.

Overcoming myths regarding pediatric pain is an important educational goal. For example, generations of clinicians have been previously taught that use of local anesthetics for infant lumbar puncture actually increases pain due to the use of a "second needle," and that it may interfere with the success of the procedure. A recent study confirms that 68% of pediatric ED physicians still do not use routine analgesia for neonatal lumbar punctures.[27] The literature does not support these myths; use of local anesthesia results in decreased pain behaviors and has no effect on the success of the procedure.[28,29] There are no physiologic data to support a different standard of care for infants versus older children and adults—that is to say, if the myth were true, why wouldn't adults also prefer just one needle? For clinicians still concerned about procedural success, use of topical anesthetic cream offers an alternative, although the depth of anesthesia is less.[30] These and other myths will expire only when the next generation of emergency physicians, pediatricians, and family practitioners are no longer exposed to them by the current generation.

An important barrier to overcome is the overall "culture" of the ED.[6] Because the ED is a busy and often hectic environment, health care providers may feel that changes are impossible, and that patients must accept the ED as it is. However, the pain management team can use education, newsletters, positive feedback, examples, policies, and even rewards to promote change.[8] Change will not be instantaneous, and the team must be patient and persistent. Table 158–7 lists changes to the ED environment to improve children's experiences with procedures.[6] Table 158–8 summarizes policies and projects that can be used to provide solutions to barriers in improving pediatric pain management in the ED.[1,8,31]

Summary

Adequate pain management is increasingly recognized as a significant factor in patient well-being and satisfaction. Inadequate pain management has both short-term (suffering, decreased healing, dissatisfaction with care, possible decreased compliance with other treatments) and long-term (chronic pain syndromes, increased pain sensitivity, avoidance of medical care) consequences. Regulatory agencies are emphasizing pain management, and research advances are rapidly occurring. EDs need multidisciplinary pain management teams to collect, assimilate, and then disseminate information on pain assessment and management to health care providers. The "culture" of the ED must promote

Table 158-7   Emergency Department Cultural Characteristics that Promote Reduction of Pediatric Procedural Pain[6]

Providing Information and Preparing the Parent and Child

- Give step-by-step information as to what will occur during the procedure.
- Give sensory information about what the child will see, hear, and feel.
- Use age-appropriate language and terminology and avoid medical jargon.
- Avoid high-anxiety words such as pain, hurt, cut, and shot. Use words such as poking, freezing, squeezing, bothering, or bugging you instead.
- Do not insinuate that the procedure will definitely hurt.
- Be aware of possible misinterpretations of words and phrases such as "dye" or "put to sleep."
- Address children's concerns (e.g., "taking all my blood").
- Consider using books describing the procedure that the child can read with the parents.
- Give information both before and during the procedure.
- Be honest.

Parental Involvement

- Ask the parents how much distress they expect from the child.
- Allow parents to remain present.
- Do not ask the parent to help restrain the child.
- Instruct the parent not to threaten the child (e.g., with additional shots).
- Instruct the parent on coping-promoting behaviors (e.g., distraction) and to avoid distress-promoting behaviors (e.g., reassurance).

Health Care Worker Behavior

- Be calm, confident, and in control.
- Avoid reassurance, apology, and criticism.

- Avoid conversation with other health care workers and parents that may be distressing (e.g., describing possible adverse events) in front of the child.
- Teach students how to perform the procedure outside the room to minimize discussion in front of the child.

Health Care Setting

- Maintain a quiet, calm environment.
- Avoid stressors such as beeping monitors.
- Avoid long delays between informing the child of the procedure and performing it.
- Avoid situations in which children can see or hear procedures performed on other children.

Procedural Details

- Allow comfort items such as favorite stuffed animals or blankets.
- For venipunctures and intravenous cannulation in thumb-sucking children, avoid the arm of the preferred thumb.
- Don't force the child to lay down if he or she doesn't want to and isn't required to.
- Consider giving the child a "job" (e.g., holding a gauze).
- Give the child choices to increase the perception of control (e.g., right arm or left).
- For long procedures (e.g., burn dressing changes), allow the child "time-outs" of a predetermined number and duration (e.g., three 20-second time-outs).
- Allow the child to "count down" from 10 to 1 before a brief procedure.
- Use automatic lancets for fingersticks.
- Venipuncture, when feasible, may be less painful than heel lance.
- Do not allow the child to see the larger needle used to draw up local anesthetic.

Table 158-8   Solutions to Barriers in Reducing Pediatric Pain in the Emergency Department (ED)

Barrier	Solution
Lack of organization in approach to pain, lack of coordination and education of health care workers, failure of health care system to make pain relief a priority	Appointment of a "pain czar" and/or a multidisciplinary "pain management team" to establish standards and target goals for improvement, provide health care worker education, devise policies and procedures to improve pain management, perform ongoing quality assessments, and test interventions
Need for health care worker education, need to stop perpetuation of myths regarding pediatric pain	Variety of educational methods, including lectures, workshops, in-services, continuing medical education meetings, journal clubs to review particular pain management solutions, distribution of review articles, periodic newsletters from the pain management team, and appointment of shift leaders who disseminate and teach new policies and procedures
Lack of assessment of pain	Multidisciplinary team reviews existing pain assessment methods, chooses a few methods that cover all ages and situations to use, educates all health care providers in using these methods, posts the methods in the triage and patient care areas
Delay in pain medication due to time spent in triage, registration, and waiting to be seen	Nurse-driven protocols allowing standing orders for nonopiate analgesic administration for moderate pain, and automatic contact of physicians to prescribe analgesics in triage for severe pain
Analgesics not used effectively	Educate health care workers and encourage use of preemptive analgesia, multimodal analgesia (World Health Organization Pain Relief Ladder), around-the-clock dosing rather than PRN dosing.
Disruption to ED flow when topical anesthetics requiring 20–60 min for effect are applied	Nurse-driven protocols allowing placement of topical anesthetics in triage for lacerations judged by nurses to require repair, or patients judged by nurses likely to require phlebotomy, intravenous catheterization, lumbar puncture, or other needle procedure. Placement of topical anesthetic cream by physician or registered nurse at time of placing order for phlebotomy, intravenous access, or lumbar puncture setup.
Lack of availability of items for distraction; health care provider discomfort with parental presence	Put together "distraction baskets" for each room, with items appropriate for all ages. Put together a preprinted brief instruction booklet for parents on how to help their child through a procedure, and how to use the distraction items.
Busy health care providers concentrating on diagnosis and management of primary condition	Redesign patient care forms and charts to include preprinted spaces for pain assessment, reassessment, and pain management recommendations at discharge. Redesign computer interfaces to include automatic prompts for pain assessment and treatment.
Health care providers' lack of knowledge regarding pain medication doses and nonpharmacologic methods available	Multidisciplinary team to formulate a pocket reference card for all health care providers with medication doses, equianalgesic doses for opiates, protocols for nonpharmacologic methods
Patients and health care providers concentrating on primary condition and not knowledgeable about importance of managing pain	Revise patient aftercare handouts to emphasize the importance of pain management to adequate healing and of appropriate and around-the-clock medication dosing, or formulate separate handouts.
Lack of accountability for pain management practices	Conduct quality assessment projects, and give both positive feedback and suggestions for improvement to health care providers. Consider periodic rewards to individual health care workers demonstrating superior pain management practices.
Lack of availability of literature-supported pain management methods	Pain management team to include pharmacist representative, with goals of making available topical anesthetics, oral sucrose solutions for use with infants, etc. Pain management team to conduct in-services and educational workshops to educate health care providers on the use of these methods.

an environment conducive to good pain management practices.

REFERENCES

1. Zempsky WT, Cravero JP: Relief of pain and anxiety in pediatric patients in emergency medical systems. Pediatrics 114:1348–1356, 2004.
2. Howard RF: Current status of pain management in children. JAMA 290:2464–2469, 2003.
3. Cousins MJ, Brennan F, Carr DB: Pain relief: a universal human right. Pain 112:1–4, 2004.
4. Ashburn MA: The role of APS in the decade of pain control and research [President's Message]. May/June 2001. Available at *http://www.ampainsoc.org/pub/bulletin/may01/pres1.htm* (accessed January 19, 2005).
5. National Pharmaceutical Council, Inc: Pain: Current Understanding of Assessment, Management, and Treatments [monograph]. Available at *http://www.jcaho.org/news+room/health+care+issues/pm+monographs.htm* (accessed January 19, 2005).
6. Young KD: Pediatric procedural pain. Ann Emerg Med 45:160–171, 2005.
7. Walco GA, Cassidy RC, Schechter NL: Pain, hurt, and harm: the ethics of pain control in infants and children. N Engl J Med 331:541–544, 1994.
8. Joint Commision on Accreditation of Healthcare Organizations: Improving the Quality of Pain Management through Measurement and Action [monograph]. Available at *http://www.jcaho.org/news+room/health+care+issues/pm+monographs.htm* (accessed January 19, 2005).
9. Boudreaux ED, Francis JL, Loyacano T: Family presence during invasive procedures and resuscitations in the emergency department: a critical review and suggestions for future research. Ann Emerg Med 40:193–205, 2002.
10. Franck LS, Greenberg CS, Stevens B: Pain assessment in infants and children. Pediatr Clin North Am 47:487–512, 2000.
11. Blackburn P, Vissers R: Pharmacology of emergency department pain management and conscious sedation. Emerg Med Clin North Am 18:803–827, 2000.
12. Tobias JD, Deshpande JK (eds): Pediatric Pain Management, 2nd ed. Elk Grove Village, IL: American Academy of Pediatrics, 2005.
13. Meunier-Sham J, Ryan K: Reducing pediatric pain during ED procedures with a nurse-driven protocol: an urban pediatric emergency department's experience. J Emerg Nurs 29:127–132, 2003.
14. World Health Organization: WHO's Pain Relief Ladder. Available at *http://www.who.int/cancer/palliative/painladder/en/* (accessed January 19, 2005).
15. Fetzer SJ: Reducing venipuncture and intravenous insertion pain with eutectic mixture of local anesthetic: a meta-analysis. Nurs Res 51:119–124, 2002.
16. Taddio A, Ohlsson A, Einarson TR, et al: A systematic review of lidocaine-prilocaine cream (EMLA) in the treatment of acute pain in neonates. Pediatrics 101:e1, 1998.
17. Singer AJ, Stark MJ: LET versus EMLA for pretreating lacerations: a randomized trial. Acad Emerg Med 8:223–230, 2001.
18. Singer AJ, Stark MJ: Pretreatment of lacerations with lidocaine, epinephrine, and tetracaine at triage: a randomized double-blind trial. Acad Emerg Med 7:751–756, 2000.
19. Priestley S, Kelly AM, Chow L, et al: Application of topical local anesthetic at triage reduces treatment time for children with lacerations: a randomized controlled trial. Ann Emerg Med 42:34–40, 2003.
20. Fein JA, Callahan JM, Boardman CR, Gorelick MH: Predicting the need for topical anesthetic in the pediatric emergency department. Pediatrics 104:e19, 1999.
21. Stevens B, Yamada J, Ohlsson A: Sucrose for analgesia in newborn infants undergoing painful procedures. Cochrane Database Syst Rev (3):CD001069, 2001.
22. Reis EC, Roth EK, Syphan JL, et al: Effective pain reduction for multiple immunization injections in young infants. Arch Pediatr Adolesc Med 157:1115–1120, 2003.
23. Kleiber C, Harper DC: Effects of distraction on children's pain and distress during medical procedures: a meta-analysis. Nurs Res 48:44–49, 1999.
24. Grazel R: Neonatal pain management with oral sucrose: 2003 update. Online J Knowl Synth Nurs 10:7C, 2003.
25. Farion KJ, Osmond MH, Hartling L, et al: Tissue adhesives for traumatic lacerations: a systematic review of randomized controlled trials. Acad Emerg Med 10:110–118, 2003.
26. Zempsky WT, Schechter NL: Office-based pain management: the 15-minute consultation. Pediatr Clin North Am 47:601–615, 2000.
27. Baxter AL, Welch JC, Burke BL, Isaacman DJ: Pain, position, and stylet styles: infant lumbar puncture practices of pediatric emergency attending physicians. Pediatr Emerg Care 20:816–820, 2004.
28. Carraccio C, Feinberg P, Hart LS, et al: Lidocaine for lumbar punctures: a help not a hindrance. Arch Pediatr Adolesc Med 150:1044–1046, 1996.
29. Pinheiro JM, Furdon S, Ochoa LF: Role of local anesthesia during lumbar puncture in neonates. Pediatrics 91:379–382, 1993.
30. Kaur G, Gupta P, Kumar A: A randomized trial of eutectic mixture of local anesthetics during lumbar puncture in newborns. Arch Pediatr Adolesc Med 157:1065–1070, 2003.
31. American Academy of Pediatrics Task Force on Pain in Infants, Children, and Adolescents: The assessment and management of acute pain in infants, children, and adolescents. Pediatrics 108:793–797, 2001.
32. Bieri D, Reeve RA, Champion GD, et al: The Faces Pain Scale for the self-assessment of the severity of pain experienced by children: development, initial validation, and preliminary investigation for ratio scale properties. Pain 41:139–150, 1990.
33. Wong DL, Baker CM: Pain in children: comparison of assessment scales. Pediatr Nurs 14:9–17, 1988.
34. Gallagher EJ, Liebman M, Bijur PE: Prospective validation of clinically important changes in pain severity measured on a visual analog scale. Ann Emerg Med 38:633–638, 2001.
35. Powell CV, Kelly AM, Williams A: Determining the minimum clinically significant difference in visual analog pain score for children. Ann Emerg Med 37:28–31, 2001.
36. Beyer JE, Denyes MJ, Villarruel AM: The creation, validation, and continuing development of the Oucher: a measure of pain intensity in children. J Pediatr Nurs 7:335–346, 1992.
37. Beyer JE, Knott CB: Construct validity estimation for the African-American and Hispanic versions of the Oucher Scale. J Pediatr Nurs 13:20–31, 1998.
38. Jordan-Marsh M, Yoder L, Hall D, Watson R: Alternate Oucher form testing: gender, ethnicity, and age variations. Res Nurs Health 17:111–118, 1994.
39. McGrath PJ, Johnson G, Goodman JT, et al: CHEOPS: a behavioral scale for rating postoperative pain in children. Adv Pain Res Ther 9:395–402, 1983.
40. Merkel SI, Voepel-Lewis T, Shayevitz JR, Malviya S: The FLACC: a behavioral scale for scoring postoperative pain in young children. Pediatr Nurs 23:293–297, 1997.
41. Voepel-Lewis T, Merkel S, Tait AR, et al: The reliability and validity of the Face, Legs, Activity, Cry, Consolability observational tool as a measure of pain in children with cognitive impairment. Anesth Analg 95:1224–1229, 2002.
42. Breau LM, McGrath PJ, Camfield CS, Finley GA: Psychometric properties of the Non-communicating Children's Pain Checklist–Revised. Pain 99:349–357, 2002.
43. Breau LM, Finley GA, McGrath PJ, Camfield CS: Validation of the Non-communicating Children's Pain Checklist–Postoperative Version. Anesthesiology 96:528–535, 2002.
44. Soetenga D, Frank J, Pellino TA: Assessment of the validity and reliability of the University of Wisconsin Children's Hospital Pain Scale for Preverbal and Nonverbal Children. Pediatr Nurs 25:670–676, 1999.
45. Craig KD, Hadjistavropoulos HD, Grunau RV, Whitfield MF: A comparison of two measures of facial activity during pain in the newborn child. J Pediatr Psychol 19:305–318, 1994.
46. Krechel SW, Bildner J: CRIES: a new neonatal postoperative pain measurement score. Initial testing of validity and reliability. Paediatr Anaesth 5:53–61, 1995.
47. Taddio A, Nulman I, Koren BS, et al: A revised measure of acute pain in infants. J Pain Symptom Manage 10:456–463, 1995.
48. Lewis M, Thomas D: Cortisol release in infants in response to inoculation. Child Dev 61:50–59, 1990.

49. Gerard LL, Cooper CS, Duethman KS, et al: Effectiveness of lidocaine lubricant for discomfort during pediatric urethral catheterization. J Urol 170:564–567, 2003.
50. Gallagher EJ: Nasogastric tubes: hard to swallow. Ann Emerg Med 44:138–141, 2004.
51. Krauss B, Green SM: Sedation and analgesia for procedures in children. N Engl J Med 342:938–945, 2000.
52. Flood RG, Krauss B: Procedural sedation and analgesia for children in the emergency department. Emerg Med Clin North Am 21:121–139, 2003.
53. Kim MK, Strait RT, Sato TT, Hennes HM: A randomized clinical trial of analgesia in children with acute abdominal pain. Acad Emerg Med 9:281–287, 2002.

Procedures, Sedation, Pain Management and Devices

SECTION VII

Chapter 159

Procedural Sedation and Analgesia

PART 1 ■ PRINCIPLES AND PRACTICE

Steven M. Green, MD and Baruch Krauss, MD, EdM

Key Points

Successful and safe application of procedural sedation and analgesia requires careful patient selection, customization of therapy to the type of procedure and the specific needs of the patient, and careful patient monitoring for prevention of adverse events.

The most important element of procedural sedation and analgesia monitoring is close and continuous patient observation by an individual capable of recognizing adverse events prior to the development of complications.

Current sedation state terminology includes moderate sedation, deep sedation, and dissociative sedation. Although historically popular, the widely misinterpreted and misused term *conscious sedation* has fallen into disfavor and has been replaced with the term *moderate sedation*.

For nondissociative agents, intravenous titration to patient response is the most effective method of obtaining rapid and safe analgesia and/or sedation.

Recent food intake is not a contraindication for administering procedural sedation and analgesia, but should be considered in choosing the depth and sedation end point.

requires careful patient selection, customization of therapy to the specific needs of the patient, and continuous patient monitoring for adverse events. Emergency physicians must ensure that all patients receive pain relief and sedation commensurate with their individual needs during any procedure.

The most common pediatric PSA indications include diagnostic imaging, fracture reduction, and laceration repair, as well as a variety of other painful and/or anxiety producing procedures. There are two absolute PSA contraindications: severe clinical instability requiring immediate attention, and refusal by a competent patient or his or her parents or guardians. Relative contraindications include hemodynamic or respiratory compromise, abnormal airway, altered sensorium, or inability to monitor side effects. However, even in many of these circumstances, appropriate agents can be given to provide analgesia and sedation while minimizing the chances for further deterioration. Although safely sedating infants and young children is challenging and requires additional care, age is not a contraindication to PSA.

In all but the most emergent situations, a directed history and physical examination should precede PSA. If this evaluation suggests additional risk, the advisability of PSA should be reconsidered. High-risk cases may be better managed in the more controlled environment of an operating room. The decision to proceed with PSA should be a thoughtful process in which the urgency of the procedure is considered together with the associated risks identified by the presedation evaluation. PSA is contraindicated when the risks outweigh the expected benefits.

Indications and Contraindications

Procedural sedation and analgesia (PSA), is the use of analgesic, dissociative, and sedative agents to relieve the pain and anxiety associated with diagnostic and therapeutic procedures. Successful and safe application of PSA

Preparation and Consent

The practice of PSA has four sequential phases: the presedation evaluation; medication administration, and where appropriate, titration to a specific sedation end point; maintenance of appropriate level of sedation during the procedure; and postprocedure recovery and patient discharge from the emergency department (ED). Presedation assessments are a requirement of the Joint Commission on Accreditation of Healthcare Organizations (JCAHO),[1] and most hospitals have developed specific forms to facilitate consistent

Portions of this chapter were adapted from Green SM, Krauss B: Procedural sedation and analgesia. In Roberts JR, Hedges JR (eds): Clinical Procedures in Emergency Medicine, 4th ed. Philadelphia: W.B. Saunders, 2004, pp 596–620.

documentation of the involved items. Except in emergency situations, the risks, benefits, and limitations of any PSA should be discussed with the parents or guardians in advance and verbal agreement obtained. Written consent is not required (unless it is a local institutional requirement), though documentation, as discussed, is essential.

General

Physicians should assess the type and severity of any underlying medical problems. A common tool used for this purpose is the American Society of Anesthesiologists' physical status classification, which is used for preoperative risk stratification (Table 159–1).[2] Current medications and allergies should be verified. It is advisable to inquire regarding prior adverse experiences with PSA or anesthesia.

Airway

The airway should be inspected to determine if there are abnormalities that might impair airway management (e.g., severe obesity, short neck, small mandible, large tongue, trismus).

Cardiovascular

Cardiac auscultation should be performed to assess for rhythm disturbance or other abnormality. In patients with known cardiovascular disease, their degree of reserve should be evaluated, as most PSA agents can cause vasodilation and hypotension.

Respiratory

Lung auscultation should be performed to assess for active pulmonary disease, especially obstructive lung disease and active upper respiratory infections that may predispose to airway reactivity.

Gastrointestinal

Although pulmonary aspiration of gastric contents is a serious complication of vomiting when protective airway reflexes are impaired, there is no evidence that a specific fasting duration is necessary prior to PSA.[3,4] Two large, prospective ED series have failed to show any association between fasting and adverse effects.[5,6] However, aspiration is not an acceptable PSA outcome, and clinicians must remain consistently and aggressively vigilant in its prevention. A case-by-case risk:benefit assessment is more consistent with the current literature than setting an arbitrary fasting period,

and clinicians should avoid sedation depth where protective airway reflexes might be impaired unless the expected benefits outweigh the additional risk. Great care should be taken to avoid inducing respiratory depression necessitating assisted ventilation, because such ventilation insufflates the stomach and may induce emesis.[3,4]

Hepatic/Renal

The implications of delayed metabolism or excretion of PSA agents in infants less than 6 months of age, in the elderly, and in the presence of hepatic or renal abnormality should be carefully evaluated.

Equipment and Monitoring

Personnel and Interactive Monitoring

The most important element of PSA monitoring is close and continuous patient observation by an individual capable of recognizing adverse events during PSA. This person must be able to continuously observe the patient's face, mouth, and chest wall motion, and equipment or sterile drapes must not interfere with such visualization. This careful observation will allow prompt detection of adverse events such as respiratory depression, apnea, upper airway obstruction, laryngospasm, emesis, and hypersalivation.

PSA personnel should understand the pharmacology of analgesic and sedative agents and their respective reversal agents, and be proficient at maintaining airway patency and assisting ventilation if needed. PSA requires a minimum of two experienced individuals, most frequently one physician and one nurse or respiratory therapist. The physician typically oversees drug administration and performs the procedure, while the nurse or respiratory therapist continuously monitors the patient for potential adverse events and documents administration of medication, response to sedation, and periodic vital signs. The nurse or respiratory therapist may assist with minor, interruptible tasks; however, their ability to remain focused on the patient's cardiopulmonary status must not be impaired. An individual with advanced life-support skills should be immediately available, a requisite easy to fulfill in the ED setting.

During deep sedation (Table 159–2), the individual dedicated to patient monitoring should be experienced with this depth of sedation and have no other responsibilities that would interfere with the advanced level of monitoring and documentation appropriate for this sedation level.[7] Individual

Table 159–1	American Society of Anesthesiologist's (ASA) Physical Status Classification		
ASA Class	Description	Examples	Suitability for Sedation
1	A normally healthy patient	Unremarkable past medical history	Excellent
2	A patient with mild systemic disease—no functional limitation	Mild asthma, controlled seizure disorder, anemia, controlled diabetes mellitus	Generally good
3	A patient with severe systemic disease—definite functional limitation	Moderate to severe asthma, poorly controlled seizure disorder, pneumonia, poorly controlled diabetes mellitus, moderate obesity	Intermediate to poor; consider benefits relative to risks
4	A patient with severe systemic disease that is a constant threat to life	Severe bronchopulmonary dysplasia, sepsis; advanced degrees of pulmonary, cardiac, hepatic, renal, or endocrine insufficiency	Poor, benefits rarely outweigh risks
5	A moribund patient who is not expected to survive without the operation	Septic shock, severe trauma	Extremely poor

From Krauss B, Green SM: Sedation and analgesia for procedures in children. N Engl J Med 342:938–945, 2000.

Table 159–2	PSA Terminology and Definitions

General

- **Analgesia:** Relief of pain without intentional production of an altered mental state such as sedation. An altered mental state may be a secondary effect of medications administered for this purpose.[14]
- **Anxiolysis:** A state of decreased apprehension concerning a particular situation in which there is no change in a patient's level of awareness.[14]
- **Procedural Sedation and Analgesia (PSA):** A technique of administering sedatives, analgesics, and/or dissociative agents to induce a state that allows the patient to tolerate unpleasant procedures while maintaining cardiorespiratory function. PSA is intended to result in a depressed level of consciousness but one that allows the patient to maintain airway control independently and continuously. Specifically, the drugs, doses, and techniques used are not likely to produce a loss of protective airway reflexes.[15]

Specific Sedation States

- **Minimal sedation (anxiolysis):** A drug-induced state during which patients respond normally to verbal commands. Although cognitive function and coordination may be impaired, ventilatory and cardiovascular functions are unaffected.[1]
- **Moderate sedation** (formerly "conscious sedation"): A drug-induced depression of consciousness during which patients respond purposefully to verbal commands, either alone or accompanied by light tactile stimulation. Reflex withdrawal from a painful stimulus is not considered a purposeful response. No interventions are required to maintain a patent airway, and spontaneous ventilation is adequate. Cardiovascular function is usually maintained.[1]
- **Dissociative Sedation:** A trancelike cataleptic state induced by the dissociative agent ketamine, characterized by profound analgesia and amnesia, with retention of protective airway reflexes, spontaneous respirations, and cardiopulmonary stability.[16]
- **Deep sedation:** A drug-induced depression of consciousness during which patients cannot be easily aroused but respond purposefully following repeated or painful stimulation. The ability to independently maintain ventilatory function may be impaired. Patients may require assistance in maintaining a patent airway, and spontaneous ventilation may be inadequate. Cardiovascular function is usually maintained.[1]
- **General anesthesia:** A drug-induced loss of consciousness during which patients are not arousable, even by painful stimulation. The ability to independently maintain ventilatory function is often impaired. Patients often require assistance in maintaining a patent airway, and positive pressure ventilation may be required because of depressed spontaneous ventilation or drug-induced depression of neuromuscular function. Cardiovascular function may be impaired.[1]

hospital-wide sedation policies may have additional requirements for how and when deep sedation is administered, based upon their specific needs and available expertise.

For situations in which sedation is initiated by the intramuscular (IM), oral, nasal, inhalational, or rectal routes, it is not mandatory to have intravenous (IV) access, although this may be preferred based upon anticipated depth of sedation and on comorbidity, or for the convenience of additional drug titration. When sedation is performed without IV access, an individual skilled in initiating such access should be immediately available.

Mechanical Monitoring

The routine use of mechanical monitoring has greatly enhanced the safety of PSA. With current technology, oxygenation (pulse oximetry), ventilation (capnography), and hemodynamics (blood pressure and electrocardiography [ECG]) can all be monitored noninvasively in spontaneously breathing patients. Although continuous ECG monitoring cannot be considered mandatory in the absence of cardiovascular disease, such monitoring is simple, inexpensive, and readily available. PSA mechanical monitoring should include continuous pulse oximetry with an audible signal (if available). Pulse oximetry measures the percentage of hemoglobin that is bound to oxygen and is not a substitute for monitoring ventilation, as there is a variable lag time between the onset of hypoventilation or apnea and a change in oxygen saturation of hemoglobin molecules.

Capnography provides a continuous, breath-by-breath measure of respiratory rate and CO_2 exchange and provides the earliest detection of respiratory failure.[8] Hypoventilation and respiratory depression result in a progressive decrease in respiratory rate, an increase in the end-tidal CO_2, and a change in the shape of the CO_2 waveform. Apnea, upper airway obstruction, and laryngospasm result in an almost instantaneous loss of the CO_2 waveform. Early detection of respiratory compromise is especially important in infants

and toddlers, who have smaller functional residual capacity and greater oxygen consumption relative to older children and adults.[9,10] In the ED setting, capnography has been shown to identify respiratory depression undetectable by pulse oximetry.[8] Capnography should be added where available, as it can alert practitioners to respiratory depression and apnea before hypoxemia develops, especially if the patient is on supplemental oxygen.

The sedation area should include all necessary age-appropriate equipment for airway management and resuscitation, including oxygen, a bag-valve mask, suction, and drug reversal agents. A defibrillator should be available for subjects with significant cardiovascular disease.

The need for supplemental oxygen during PSA, and its benefits, have not been studied. Although this intervention will decrease the incidence and severity of hypoxemia due to airway complications, it will also delay the detection of apnea with pulse oximetry.[11,12] If oxygen is administered and capnography is not available, continual visual inspection of chest-wall motion and air movement is especially important. Supplemental oxygen cannot be considered mandatory at this time and remains an option best left to the physician's preference.

Vital signs should be periodically measured at individualized intervals, in most cases including measurements at baseline, after drug administration, on completion of the procedure, during early recovery, and at completion of recovery. During deep sedation, it is advisable to assess vital signs every 5 minutes. Patients are at highest risk of complications 5 to 10 minutes following IV medications and during the immediate postprocedure period when external stimuli are discontinued.

Standards and Guidelines

Terminology

The progression from minimal sedation to general anesthesia represents a continuum. Low doses of opioids or benzodiazepines induce mild analgesia or sedation, respectively, with little danger of adverse events. If clinicians continue administering additional medication beyond this initial level, progressively altered consciousness ensues with a proportionately increased risk of respiratory and airway complications. At a certain point on the continuum, protective airway reflexes are lost and general anesthesia is ultimately reached. This sedation continuum is not drug specific, as varying states from mild sedation to general anesthesia can be achieved with virtually all nondissociative PSA agents (e.g., opioids, sedative-hypnotics).

A key recent development in the field of PSA has been the revision of the original 1985 sedation-state terminology and the adoption of clearer descriptions of varying types and degrees of sedation (see Table 159–2).[1,13-16] Although historically popular, the widely misinterpreted and misused term *conscious sedation* is an inaccurate descriptor[13] and has been replaced with the term *moderate sedation*.[1] Despite improvements in PSA terminology, there is still not an objective method for assessing sedation depth. Levels of responsiveness are crude surrogate markers of respiratory drive and retention of protective airway reflexes. This is especially true for all levels of sedation in young children who do not understand or who cannot reliably follow verbal commands. Although respiratory depression and respiratory arrest can be quickly detected using standard interactive and mechanical monitoring, there is no safe and practical method to assess the status of protective airway reflexes.

PSA Standards and Guidelines

There are numerous sets of PSA guidelines created by various specialty societies, with the intent of better standardizing the manner in which PSA is performed in order to enhance patient safety. Those most pertinent to emergency physicians are those from the American College of Emergency Physicians,[15,17] the American Academy of Pediatrics,[7,18] and the American Society of Anesthesiologists.[11,12] In the early 1990s, the JCAHO took a special interest in PSA, with the central theme that the standard of sedation care provided should be comparable throughout a given hospital.[1] Thus patients sedated in the ED should not receive a significantly different level of attention or monitoring than those sedated for a similar-level procedure in the operating room. To ensure this, the JCAHO requires specific PSA protocols that apply consistently throughout each institution. These hospital-wide sedation policies will vary from site to site based upon the specific needs and expertise available within each institution.[1]

At each hospital accreditation survey, the JCAHO will look to see if practitioners practice PSA consistent with their hospital-wide sedation policy, and whether they provide sufficient documentation of such compliance. Physicians must be familiar with their hospital's sedation policies, and should work with their medical staff to ensure that such policies are suitably detailed, yet reasonable and realistic. Unduly restrictive policies do a disservice to patients by discouraging appropriate use of analgesia and anxiolysis. Most hospitals pattern their sedation policies after JCAHO standards and definitions. It is important to note that the unique ketamine dissociative state is incompatible with existing JCAHO definitions of sedation and anesthesia.[16] A ready solution adopted by some hospitals is the assignment of a distinct definition for "dissociative sedation" (see Table 159–2).

The JCAHO requires that PSA practitioners who are permitted to administer deep sedation must be qualified to rescue patients from general anesthesia,[1] a standard readily met by emergency physicians. Emergency physicians will typically perform all levels of sedation except general anesthesia. Moderate sedation suffices for the majority of procedures in cooperative children, although it will not be adequate for painful procedures (e.g., fracture reduction, cardioversion). Deep sedation can facilitate these, but at greater risk of cardiorespiratory depression than moderate sedation. Moderate sedation is frequently insufficient for effective anxiolysis and immobilization in younger, frightened children. In this instance, deep and dissociative sedation are possible alternatives.

Techniques

Therapeutic mistakes resulting in inadequate analgesia and sedation include using the wrong agent, the wrong dose, and the wrong route and frequency of administration, and poor use of adjunctive agents. With proper training and technique, adequate PSA can be provided under almost any circumstance. Understanding titration principles is critical to providing safe and effective PSA. Physicians must have a thorough knowledge of the pharmacokinetics, dosing, administration, and potential complications of the PSA agents that they use. Onset time from injection to initial observed effect must be appreciated, especially when using drugs in combination, to avoid stacking of drug doses resulting in oversedation.

The correct agent (or combination of agents) and the route and timing of administration depend on the following factors: How long will the procedure last? Will it be seconds (e.g., simple relocation of a dislocated joint, incision and drainage of a small abscess, cardioversion), minutes (e.g., complex fracture manipulation for reduction, breaking up loculations in a large abscess and then packing it), or prolonged (e.g., complex facial laceration repair)? How likely is it that the procedure will need to be repeated (e.g., fracture reduction)? Can topical, local, or regional anesthesia be used as an adjunct? Does the patient only require sedation for a noninvasive diagnostic imaging study?

Prior to drug administration, every effort should be made, pharmacologically and nonpharmacologically, to minimize a child's anxiety and distress. The emotional state of a patient on induction strongly correlates with the degree of distress on emergence and in the immediate days following the procedure.[19-22]

Emergency physicians must avoid being pressured by consultants to cut corners or rush PSA. During the presedation preparation, discuss the sedation plan and length of time required to safely prepare and sedate the patient with the consultant to avoid risks associated with a hurried sedation.

Routes of Administration

For nondissociative agents, IV titration to patient response is the best method to obtain rapid and safe analgesia and/or sedation. When using opioids, doses administered in 2- to 3-minute increments, while observing for side effects such as miosis, somnolence, decreased responsiveness to verbal stimuli, minimally impaired speech, and diminished pain on questioning, are appropriate initial end points. For sedative-hypnotics, similar end points such as ptosis (rather than miosis), somnolence, slurred speech, and gaze alteration should be sought. Repeated doses may be given in a titrated fashion based on the patient's response during the procedure.

Oral, transmucosal (i.e., nasal, rectal), and IM routes are convenient means of administration when IV access is not necessary. However, they cannot be titrated to a desired response. The efficacy of intranasal drug administration in particular is operator dependent. The main advantage of these other routes is their usefulness for children in whom IV access may be problematic, for procedures that may require only minimal sedation in conjunction with the use of local anesthetics, and for diagnostic imaging.

With the exception of ketamine, agents administered IM have erratic absorption and a variable onset of action. As such, prolonged preprocedural and postprocedural observation may be necessary. When required because of limitations in obtaining IV access, the IM route offers little advantage over oral or transmucosal administration.

Another PSA route is via inhalation using nitrous oxide. This gas can either be delivered by a demand-flow system using a handheld mask, or delivered to young children by a continuous-flow system under close physician supervision using a nose mask.

Because individual needs may vary widely, application of arbitrary ceiling doses of analgesic and sedative regimens is unwarranted. The true ceiling dose of an agent is that dose that provides adequate pain relief or sedation without major cardiopulmonary side effects such as respiratory depression, apnea, bradycardia, or hypotension.

Alternatives

Many ED nonpainful, or minimally painful, procedures in older children and cooperative young children can be performed without PSA. Skilled practitioners can frequently combine a calm, reassuring bedside manner with distraction techniques and careful local or regional anesthesia.[23,24] Should such techniques fail, then PSA can be used. The traditional alternative of performing painful and/or anxiety-provoking ED procedures in children using forcible restraint alone is strongly discouraged.

Complications

The principal adverse effect of most PSA agents is cardiopulmonary depression, and this can be identified through interactive and mechanical monitoring practices as described earlier. Other drug-specific adverse effects are discussed in the second part of this chapter.

Postprocedure Care and Disposition

All children receiving PSA should be monitored until they are no longer at risk for cardiorespiratory depression. To be discharged, they should be alert and oriented (or returned to age-appropriate baseline), and vital signs should be stable. Many hospitals have chosen to use standardized recovery-scoring systems similar to those used in their surgical post-

anesthesia recovery areas (Table 159–3). A reliable adult must be available to observe these children for postprocedure complications after discharge. Instructions should be given regarding appropriate diet, medications, and level of activity (Table 159–4). To be eligible for safe discharge, children are not required to demonstrate that they can tolerate an oral

Table 159–3 Modified Aldrete Recovery Scoring System

Vital Signs	
Stable	1
Unstable	0
Respirations	
Normal	2
Shallow respirations/tachypnea	1
Apnea	0
Level of Consciousness	
Alert, oriented/returned to preprocedural level	2
Arousable, giddy, agitated	1
Unresponsive	0
Oxygen Saturation	
95–100% of preprocedural level	2
90–94%	1
<90%	0
Color	
Pink/preprocedural color	2
Pale/dusky	1
Cyanotic	0
Activity	
Moves on command/preprocedural level	2
Moves extremities/uncoordinated walking	1
No spontaneous movement	0

Sedation Score	Action
>8	Consider discharge if all scores > 0 and total score > 8
7–8	Vital signs q20min
4–6	Vital signs q10min
0–3	Vital signs q5min—consider further evaluation if prolonged

From Krauss B, Brustowicz R (Eds): Pediatric Procedural Sedation and Analgesia. Philadelphia: Lippincott Williams & Wilkins, 1999, pp 148, 157.

Table 159–4 Sample Pediatric Disposition Instructions after PSA

Your child has been given medicine for sedation and/or pain control. These medicines may cause your child to be sleepy and less aware of his or her surroundings, making it easier for accidents to happen as he or she walks or crawls. Because of these side effects, your child should be watched closely for the next few hours. We suggest the following:
1. No eating or drinking for the next 2 hours. If your child is an infant, you may resume half normal feedings when they are hungry.
2. No playing for the next day that requires normal coordination, such as bike riding or jungle gym activities.
3. No playing without an adult to watch and supervise.
4. No baths, showers, cooking, or use of potentially dangerous electrical appliances unless supervised by an adult.

If you notice anything unusual about your child, please consider returning to the emergency department for re-evaluation.

challenge (most PSA agents are emetogenic, and forcing fluids postsedation can lead to emesis pre- and/or postdischarge), nor are they required to walk unaided. The American Academy of Pediatrics guidelines only stipulate that "the patient can talk (if age-appropriate)" and "the patient can sit up unaided (if age-appropriate)."[7] A recent study has demonstrated that primary adverse events did not occur 30 minutes beyond final drug administration in children sedated with either ketamine or midazolam.[25]

REFERENCES

1. Joint Commission on Accreditation of Healthcare Organizations: Accreditation Manual for Hospitals. Oakbrook Terrace, IL: Joint Commission on Accreditation of Healthcare Organizations, 2001.
*2. Krauss B, Green SM: Sedation and analgesia for procedures in children. N Engl J Med 342:938–945, 2000.
*3. Green SM: Fasting is a consideration—not a necessity—for emergency department procedural sedation and analgesia [Editorial]. Ann Emerg Med 42:647–650, 2003.
4. Green SM, Krauss B: Pulmonary aspiration risk during ED procedural sedation—an examination of the role of fasting and sedation depth. Acad Emerg Med 9:35–42, 2002.
5. Agrawal D, Manzi SF, Gupta R, Krauss B: Preprocedural fasting state and adverse events in children undergoing procedural sedation and analgesia in a pediatric emergency department. Ann Emerg Med 42:636–646, 2003.
6. Roback MG, Bajaj L, Wathen JE, Bothner J: Preprocedural fasting and adverse events in procedural sedation and analgesia in a pediatric emergency department: are they related? Ann Emerg Med 44:454–459, 2004.
*7. American Academy of Pediatrics, Committee on Drugs: Guidelines for monitoring and management of pediatric patients during and after sedation for diagnostic and therapeutic procedures. Pediatrics 89:1110–1115, 1992.
8. Miner JR, Heegaard W, Plummer D: End-tidal carbon dioxide monitoring during procedural sedation. Acad Emerg Med 9:275–280, 2002.
9. Patel R, Lenczyk M, Hannallah RS, McGill WA: Age and the onset of desaturation in apnoeic children. Can J Anaesth 41:771–774, 1994.
10. Farmery AD, Roe PG: A model to describe the rate of oxyhaemoglobin desaturation during apnoea. Br J Anaesth 76:284–291, 1996.

*Selected readings.

11. American Society of Anesthesiologists: Practice guidelines for sedation and analgesia by non-anesthesiologists. Anesthesiology 96:1004–1017, 2002.
12. American Society of Anesthesiologists: Practice guidelines for sedation and analgesia by non-anesthesiologists. Anesthesiology 84:459–471, 1996.
13. Green SM, Krauss B: Procedural sedation terminology: moving past "conscious sedation" [Editorial]. Ann Emerg Med 39:433–435, 2002.
14. Sacchetti A, Schafermeyer R, Gerardi M, et al: Pediatric analgesia and sedation. Ann Emerg Med 23:237–250, 1994.
*15. American College of Emergency Physicians: Clinical policy for procedural sedation and analgesia in the emergency department. Ann Emerg Med 31:663–677, 1998.
16. Green SM, Krauss B: The semantics of ketamine [Editorial]. Ann Emerg Med 36:480–482, 2000.
17. American College of Emergency Physicians: Clinical policy: evidence-based approach to pharmacologic agents used in pediatric sedation and analgesia in the emergency department. Ann Emerg Med 44:342–377, 2004.
18. American Academy of Pediatrics, Committee on Drugs: Guidelines for monitoring and management of pediatric patients during and after sedation for diagnostic and therapeutic procedures: addendum. Pediatrics 110:836–838, 2002.
19. Kain ZN, Mayes LC, O'Connor TZ, Cicchetti DV: Preoperative anxiety in children: predictors and outcomes. Arch Pediatr Adolesc Med 150:1238–1245, 1996.
20. Kain Z, Mayes L, Caramico L, Hofstadter M: Distress during induction of anesthesia and postoperative behavioral outcomes. Anesth Analg 88:1042–1047, 1999.
21. Kain Z, Mayes L, Caramico L, et al: Postoperative behavioral outcomes in children: effects of sedative premedication. Anesthesiology 90:758–765, 1999.
22. McCann ME, Kain ZN: The management of preoperative anxiety in children: an update. Anesth Analg 93:98–105, 2001.
23. Chen E, Joseph MH, Zeltzer LK: Behavioral and cognitive interventions in the treatment of pain in children. Pediatr Clin North Am 47:513–525, 2000.
24. Kennedy RM, Luhmann JD: The "ouchless emergency department." Getting closer: advances in decreasing distress during painful procedures in the emergency department. Pediatr Clin North Am 46:1215–1247, 1999.
25. Newman DH, Azer MM, Pitetti RD, Singh S: When is a patient safe for discharge after procedural sedation? The timing of adverse effect events in 1,367 pediatric procedural sedations. Ann Emerg Med 42:627–635, 2003.

PART 2 ■ DRUG SELECTION

Steven M. Green, MD and Baruch Krauss, MD, EdM

Key Points

Emergency physicians should tailor their drug selection strategies to the specific needs of the procedure at hand (i.e., analgesia, anxiolysis, and/or immobilization).

Intravenous pentobarbital appears to be the most effective agent to facilitate nonpainful diagnostic imaging studies such as computed tomography or magnetic resonance imaging scanning, although many centers use oral chloral hydrate, particularly in children less than 18 months of age.

Midazolam can be effectively used for moderate and deep sedation through careful intravenous (IV) titration to effect, typically together with fentanyl.

When administered IV, the ultra-short-acting sedatives propofol, etomidate, thiopental, and methohexital can rapidly induce potent sedation followed by relatively rapid awakening, but with a greater risk of respiratory depression.

Ketamine produces a unique state of cortical dissociation that permits painful procedures to be performed more consistently and effectively than with other agents.

Nitrous oxide can be administered via a self-administered demand mask in cooperative children, or by a continuous-flow face mask in the uncooperative child.

Drug Selection Strategies

The majority of emergency department (ED) procedures in older children can be performed without procedural sedation and analgesia (PSA). Skilled practitioners can frequently combine a calm, reassuring bedside manner with distraction techniques and/or careful local or regional anesthesia.[1,2] Many procedures, however, cannot be technically or humanely performed without PSA, especially in younger children. These situations can be divided into three categories:

Insufficient Analgesia—Regardless of the level of cooperation, for some procedures it is impossible to achieve effective pain control with local or regional anesthesia. Examples of procedures requiring systemic PSA include fracture reductions, dislocation reductions, large loculated abscess incision and drainage, wounds that require scrubbing (e.g., "road rash"), bone marrow aspiration/biopsy, and extensive burn débridement.

Insufficient Anxiolysis—Some patients will be so frightened despite effective local or regional anesthesia that procedures cannot be technically or humanely performed without PSA. Young children requiring laceration repair are frequently terrified, and older children may be highly anxious in anticipation of laceration repairs in sensitive and/or personal regions (e.g., face, genitalia, perineum).

Insufficient Immobilization—Despite effective local or regional anesthesia and anxiolysis, PSA may be indicated to prevent excessive motion during procedures that require substantial immobilization (e.g., repair of complex facial lacerations). Immobilization is most commonly an issue with young or mentally disabled children.

Clinicians must therefore customize their drug selection based upon the unique needs of the patient (i.e., anxiolysis, analgesia, immobilization) and their individual level of experience with specific agents. A risk:benefit analysis should be performed prior to every administration of sedation and analgesia. The benefits of reducing anxiety and controlling pain should be carefully weighed against the risks of respiratory depression and airway compromise.

Cooperative Older Children

Minor procedures can usually be managed with topical, local, or regional anesthesia. Systemic PSA is typically unnecessary, although mild anxiolysis (nitrous oxide, oral midazolam) can make some of these patients more comfortable.

For longer procedures, supplementation of topical, local, or regional anesthesia with either nitrous oxide, or intravenous (IV) midazolam and fentanyl permits customization of sedation depth and pain relief to the specific needs of each patient.

Uncooperative Children

Minor procedures (e.g., small lacerations, IV cannulation, venipuncture, superficial foreign body removal) in uncooperative children can frequently be managed by skilled practitioners using a combination of nonpharmacologic techniques (e.g., distraction, guided imagery, hypnosis, comforting, breathing techniques; see Chapter 158, Approach to Pain Management) in conjunction with topical anesthesia, careful local anesthesia, and—when necessary—brief physical restraint (by personnel or by a restraining device). In other cases, supplementing nonpharmacologic techniques with topical or local anesthesia and anxiolysis with oral midazolam may be sufficient. Although oral midazolam administration is most popular and least invasive, the nasal or rectal routes can also be used depending upon operator experience and preference.

Major painful procedures (fracture reduction, large loculated abscess incision and drainage, arthrocentesis of a major joint) require systemic PSA, as do essentially all procedures in uncooperative children in whom satisfactory immobilization cannot be achieved. Options include IV fentanyl/midazolam, intramuscular (IM) or IV ketamine, or an ultra-short-acting sedative such as IV propofol.

Selection Strategies and Dosing Recommendations

Drug selection strategies are summarized in Table 159–5, and dosing recommendations for PSA drugs are shown in Table 159–6. Specialized protocols for midazolam/fentanyl and ketamine are shown later in Tables 159–7 and 159–8, respectively. Individual agents are discussed in the following sections.

Sedative-Hypnotic Agents

Chloral Hydrate

Pharmacology

Chloral hydrate is a pure sedative-hypnotic agent without analgesic properties. When administered orally, the average time to peak sedation is approximately 30 minutes, with a recovery time of an additional 1 to 2 hours.[3,4] Residual motor imbalance and agitation may persist for several hours beyond this.[5] Rectal administration is erratically absorbed and therefore not recommended.

Pediatric Use

Chloral hydrate is widely used as a sedative to facilitate non-painful diagnostic procedures such as electroencephalography[3] and computed tomography (CT) or magnetic resonance imaging (MRI).[6-10] Pentobarbital IV appears to be more effective for the latter indication than chloral hydrate,[11] although many centers prefer chloral hydrate in younger children (e.g., <18 months) simply to avoid the need for IV access.[7,8,11]

Adverse Effects

Despite a wide margin of safety, chloral hydrate can cause airway obstruction and respiratory depression, especially at higher doses (75 to 100 mg/kg).[3,5,7,9,10,12] The incidence was 0.6% in one large series.[3] There is not a known dosage threshold of chloral hydrate below which this potential

---

Table 159–5 PSA Indications and Sedation Strategies*

Clinical Situation	Indication	Procedural Requirements	Suggested Sedation Strategies
Noninvasive procedures	Computed tomography Echocardiography Electroencephalography Magnetic resonance imaging Ultrasonography	Motion control	Comforting alone Chloral hydrate PO (in patients <3 yr of age) Pentobarbital IV or IM Methohexital PR Midazolam IV
Procedure associated with low pain and high anxiety	Dental procedures Flexible fiberoptic laryngoscopy Foreign body removal, simple Intravenous cannulation Laceration repair, simple Lumbar puncture Ocular irrigation Phlebotomy Slit-lamp examination Nasogastric tube Urethral catheterization	Sedation Anxiolysis Motion control	Comforting and topical/local anesthesia Midazolam PO/IN/PR/IV Nitrous oxide Propofol IV
Procedures associated with high level of pain, high anxiety, or both	Abscess incision and drainage Arthrocentesis Bone marrow aspiration/biopsy Burn débridement Cardioversion Central line placement Endoscopy Foreign body removal, complicated Fracture/dislocation reduction Hernia reduction Interventional radiology procedures Laceration repair, complex Lumbar puncture Paracentesis Paraphimosis reduction Sexual assault examination Thoracentesis Thoracostomy tube placement	Sedation Anxiolysis Analgesia Amnesia Motion control	Midazolam and fentanyl IV Ketamine IM/IV ± midazolam Propofol IV

*This table is intended as a general overview. Sedation strategies should be individualized. Although the pharmacopeia is large, clinicians should familiarize themselves with a few agents that are flexible enough to be used for the majority of procedures. In all cases it is assumed that practitioners are fully trained in the technique, appropriate personnel and monitoring are used as detailed in this chapter, and specific drug contraindications are absent.
Abbreviations: IM, intramuscular; IN, intranasal; IV, intravenous; PO, oral; PR, rectal.
Modified from Krauss B, Green SM: Sedation and analgesia for procedures in children. N Engl J Med 342:938–945, 2000.

Table 159–6   PSA Drug Dosing Recommendations*

Drug	Clinical Effects	Indications	Pediatric Dose	Onset (min)	Duration (min)	Comments
Sedative-Hypnotics						
Chloral hydrate	Sedation, motion control, anxiolysis. No analgesia. Not reversible.	Diagnostic imaging (age <3 yr)	PO: 25–100 mg/kg, after 30 min may repeat 25–50 mg/kg. Max total dose: 2 g or 100 mg/kg whichever is less. Single use only in neonates.	PO: 15–30	PO: 60–120	Effects unreliable if age > 3 yr. Avoid in patients with significant cardiac, hepatic, or renal disease. Rectal absorption erratic. May produce paradoxical excitement. Since drugs cannot be titrated with the oral route, monitor closely for oversedation.
Etomidate (Amidate)	Sedation, motion control, anxiolysis. No analgesia. Not reversible.	Procedures requiring sedation and/or anxiolysis	IV (caution, limited research): 0.15–0.2 mg/kg	IV: <1	IV: 5–15	**See warnings in text.** Adverse effects include respiratory depression, myoclonus, nausea, and vomiting. Adrenocortical suppression occurs, but is rarely of clinical significance. Not FDA approved in children.
Midazolam† (Versed)	Sedation, motion control, anxiolysis. No analgesia. Reversible with flumazenil.	Procedures requiring sedation and/or anxiolysis	IV (0.5–5 yr): Initial 0.05–0.1 mg/kg, then titrated to max 0.5 mg/kg. IV (6–12 yr): Initial 0.025–0.05 mg/kg, then titrated to max 0.4 mg/kg. IM: 0.1–0.15 mg/kg. PO: 0.5–0.75 mg/kg. IN: 0.2–0.5 mg/kg. PR: 0.25–0.5 mg/kg	IV: 2–3, IM: 10–20, PO: 15–30, IN: 10–15, PR: 10–30	IV: 45–60, IM: 60–120, PO: 60–90, IN: 60, PR: 60–90	Reduce dose when used in combination with opioids. May produce paradoxical excitement. Since drugs cannot be titrated with the oral/rectal/intranasal routes, monitor closely for oversedation.
Methohexital (Brevital)	Sedation, motion control, anxiolysis. No analgesia. Not reversible.	Diagnostic imaging	PR: 25 mg/kg. IV (caution, limited research): 0.5–1 mg/kg	PR: 10–15	PR: 60	**See warnings for IV use in text.** Avoid in patients with temporal lobe epilepsy or porphyria. Since drugs cannot be titrated with the rectal route, monitor closely for oversedation.
Pentobarbital (Nembutal)	Sedation, motion control, anxiolysis. No analgesia. Not reversible.	Diagnostic imaging	IV: 1–6 mg/kg, titrated in increments of 1–2 mg/kg to desired effect. IM: 2–6 mg/kg, max 100 mg. PO/PR (<4 yr): 3–6 mg/kg, max 100 mg. PO/PR (>4 yr): 1.5–3 mg/kg, max 100 mg	IV: 3–5, IM: 10–15, PO/PR: 15–60	IV: 1–45, IM: 60–120, PO/PR: 60–240	May produce paradoxical excitement. Avoid in patients with porphyria. Since drugs cannot be titrated with the oral/rectal routes, monitor closely for oversedation.
Propofol (Diprivan)	Sedation, motion control, anxiolysis. No analgesia. Not reversible.	Procedures requiring sedation and/or anxiolysis	IV: 1 mg/kg over 20–30 sec, followed with similar repeat 0.5 mg/kg doses PRN to maintain sedation.	IV: <1	IV: 5–15	**See warnings in text.** Frequent respiratory depression and hypotension. Avoid with egg or soy allergies.
Thiopental (Pentothal)	Sedation, motion control, anxiolysis. No analgesia. Not reversible.	Diagnostic imaging	PR: 25 mg/kg	PR: 10–15	PR: 60–120	Avoid in patients with porphyria. Since drugs cannot be titrated with the rectal route, monitor closely for oversedation.

Table continued on following page

Table 159–6   PSA Drug Dosing Recommendations* (Continued)

Drug	Clinical Effects	Indications	Pediatric Dose	Onset (min)	Duration (min)	Comments
Analgesic‡						
Fentanyl (Sublimaze)	Analgesia. Reversible with naloxone.	Procedures of moderate to severe pain	IV: 1.0 mcg/kg/dose, may repeat q3–10min, titrate to effect	IV: 3–5	IV: 30–60	Reduce dosing when combined with midazolam.
Dissociative Agent						
Ketamine (Ketalar)	Analgesia, dissociation, amnesia, motion control. Not reversible.	Procedures of moderate to severe pain or requiring immobilization	IV: 1–1.5 mg/kg slowly over 1–2 min, may repeat ½ dose q10min PRN; IM: 4–5 mg/kg, may repeat after 10 min (full or ½ dose without additional atropine)	IV: 1; IM: 3–5	IV: dissociation 15; recovery 60; IM: dissociation 15–30; recovery 90–150	Multiple contraindications (see Table 159–8). Risk of unpleasant hallucinations and dreams if age > 15 yr (rare if younger) that may be blunted with midazolam. No apparent advantage to routine coadministration of midazolam in children. Hypersalivation can be minimized with concurrent atropine 0.01 mg/kg IM/IV (min 0.1 mg, max 0.5 mg), although such coadministration does not appear mandatory.
Inhalational Agent						
Nitrous oxide (Nitronox)	Anxiolysis, analgesia, sedation, amnesia (all mild).	Procedures requiring mild analgesia or sedation (age > 4 yr)	Preset mixture with minimum 40% O$_2$ self-administered by demand-valve mask for cooperative child; continuous-flow nasal mask in uncooperative child with close monitoring.	<5	<5 min following discontinuation	Requires specialized apparatus and gas scavenger capability. Several contraindications.§ Synergistic effect with recent opioids or sedative-hypnotics—use with caution in this setting.
Reversal Agents (Antagonists)						
Naloxone (Narcan)	Opioid reversal	Opioid toxicity	IV: 0.01 mg/kg, may repeat 0.1 mg/kg if inadequate response, may use IM/SC/ET route if IV unavailable	IV: 2	IV: 20–40; IM: 60–90	If shorter acting than the reversed drug, serial doses may be required.
Flumazenil (Romazicon)	Benzodiazepine reversal	Benzodiazepine toxicity	IV: 0.02 mg/kg/dose, may repeat q1min up to 1 mg	IV: 1–2	IV: 30–60	If shorter acting than the reversed drug, serial doses may be required. Do not use in patients receiving chronic benzodiazepines, cyclosporine, isoniazid, lithium, propoxyphene, theophylline, tricyclic antidepressants.

*Alterations in dosing may be indicated based upon the clinical situation and the practitioner's experience with these agents. Individual dosages may vary when used in combination with other agents, especially when benzodiazepines are combined with opioids.

†Midazolam is preferred to other benzodiazepines (e.g., diazepam, lorazepam) for PSA due to its shorter duration of action and multiple routes of administration.

‡Fentanyl is preferred to other opioids (e.g., morphine, meperidine) for PSA due to its faster onset, shorter recovery, and lack of histamine release.

§Generally accepted contraindications to nitrous oxide: pregnancy (patient or personnel); preexisting nausea/vomiting; trapped gas pockets (e.g., middle ear infection, pneumothorax, bowel obstruction).

Abbreviations: FDA, Food and Drug Administration; IM, intramuscular; IN, intranasal; IV, intravenous; PRN, as needed; PO, oral; PR, rectal.

Adapted from Krauss B, Green SM: Sedation and analgesia for procedures in children. N Engl J Med 342:938–945, 2000.

Table 159–7	Procedure for Moderate to Deep Sedation with Intravenous Midazolam and Fentanyl

Caveats

- Do not consider this procedure if you do not have experience with the drugs or the time to perform it properly. Do not attempt the procedure if the pulse oximeter, suction, oxygen, or bag-valve-mask is not working, the intravenous (IV) access is not secured, or the room is too small or not set up for procedural sedation and analgesia.
- This is a two-person procedure, one to monitor the patient and one to perform the procedure.
- Individual response to the drugs is variable and dependent upon the patient's underlying physiologic state and the presence of concomitant drugs/medication.
- Maximum drug effect occurs 2–3 minutes following administration. Proceed slowly and patiently, allowing the medication to take full effect before giving the next dose.
- Have naloxone and flumazenil immediately available for oversedation and/or respiratory depression.
- If the patient seems overly sedated, begin the procedure. The pain of the procedure often stimulates respiration and lessens sedation.

Contraindications—Absolute (Risks Essentially Always Outweigh Benefits)

- Active hemodynamic instability
- Active respiratory distress or hypoxemia

Contraindications—Relative (Risks May Outweigh Benefits)

- Respiratory depression or altered level of consciousness
- Anticipated difficulty if ventilatory assistance should become necessary (e.g., facial deformity or trauma, small mandible, large tongue, trismus)

Protocol

- Establish IV access.
- Connect appropriate monitoring equipment to the patient.
- Pulse, respiratory rate, blood pressure, and level of consciousness should all be recorded initially, and periodically throughout the procedure depending on the depth of sedation.
- Suction equipment, oxygen, a bag-valve-mask, and reversal agents should be immediately available. An age-appropriate resuscitation cart with oral and nasal airways, endotracheal tubes, and a functioning laryngoscope must be nearby.
- The order of the drugs is one of personal preference. The ratio of analgesia to sedation is determined by the nature of the procedure. Some procedures require primary analgesia and secondary anxiolysis/sedation (e.g., abscess incision and drainage, bone marrow aspiration, arthrocentesis, burn débridement, central catheter placement), while others require primary anxiolysis/sedation with secondary analgesia (e.g., lumbar puncture, simple foreign body removal).
- Administer local anesthesia if indicated (this often serves to help gauge effectiveness of systemic analgesia).
- Perform the procedure. Additional doses of fentanyl or midazolam may be required if further pain or anxiety is noted based on the response and length of the procedure.
- If hypoxemia, oversedation, or slowed respirations are seen during or after procedure, the patient should be first stimulated while oxygen is applied and the airway repositioned. If the patient's response is insufficient, assist ventilations with a bag-valve-mask. Reversal agents should be considered if there is not a prompt response to assisted ventilation.
- Continue close observation until the patient is awake and alert, and release the patient with a friend, parent, or relative only after a sufficient discharge score has been attained.

complication can be consistently avoided,[9,12] and accordingly standard interactive and mechanical monitoring precautions apply to chloral hydrate as they do to other PSA agents.

Despite reports of potential carcinogenicity, the American Academy of Pediatrics has judged that the evidence is currently insufficient to avoid single doses of chloral hydrate for this reason alone.[13]

Midazolam

Pharmacology

Benzodiazepines are a group of highly lipophilic agents that possess anxiolytic, amnestic, sedative, hypnotic, muscle relaxant, and anticonvulsant properties. They lack direct analgesic properties, and thus are commonly coadministered with opioids. Caution must be exercised when using benzodiazepines and opioids together, since the risks of hypoxia and apnea are significantly greater than when either is used alone.[14]

Midazolam is by far the most common benzodiazepine used for PSA, and is preferred over the longer acting lorazepam and diazepam unless unavailable. The time to peak effect for midazolam is approximately 2 to 3 minutes when given IV. Unlike diazepam, midazolam and lorazepam are water soluble, making parenteral administration less painful and mucosal absorption more rapid.

Pediatric Use

Midazolam can be effectively used for moderate and deep sedation through careful IV titration to effect, typically together with fentanyl (Table 159–7). The advantage of midazolam over other benzodiazepines is its availability in multiple routes of administration. Some children require larger doses than would be typical for adults on a milligram-per-kilogram basis,[15] and paradoxical responses (e.g., hyperexcitability) are not infrequent.[5,16,17]

To avoid the need for IV access in frightened or uncooperative children, midazolam has been alternatively administered via the IM,[18] oral,[17,19-23] intranasal,[23-27] and rectal[28,29] routes. However, the inability to effectively titrate using these routes dictates that a reliable depth of sedation cannot be predictably or regularly achieved. Thus these routes are primarily reserved for pure anxiolysis and/or minimally painful procedures. Respiratory depression can also occur via these routes.[21]

Adverse Effects

When administered by skilled practitioners using standard precautions (see Table 159–7), the safety profile for midazolam is excellent.[30-33] However, when administering benzodiazepines, one must maintain continuous vigilance for respiratory depression.[5,12,14,32] Such respiratory depression is dose dependent and greatly enhanced in the presence of ethanol or other depressive drugs, especially opioids. Deaths from undetected apnea have occurred in non-ED settings,[14] underscoring the critical role for continuous interactive and mechanical monitoring.

Benzodiazepines induce mild cardiovascular depression. Although hypotension can occur, it is rare when the agents are carefully titrated.

Pentobarbital

Pharmacology

Pentobarbital is a barbiturate capable of profound sedation, hypnosis, amnesia, and anticonvulsant activity in a dose-dependent fashion. It has no inherent analgesic properties. When carefully titrated IV, sedation is evident within 5 minutes with a duration of approximately 30 to 40 minutes.[34]

Pediatric Use

Pentobarbital is the IV sedative of choice in many centers for diagnostic imaging in children.[8,11,34-37] It is regarded as superior to midazolam[11,34,35] or chloral hydrate[11] for this indication. Pentobarbital, like midazolam, is available in multiple routes of administration.

Adverse Effects

Like other barbiturates, pentobarbital can lead to respiratory depression and hypotension, as it is a negative inotrope.[8,11,34,35]

Ultra-Short-Acting Sedatives

The current ultra-short-acting sedatives used in ED PSA are propofol, etomidate, thiopental, and methohexital. When administered IV, all can rapidly produce potent sedation and result in rapid awakening (<5 minutes) following drug discontinuation. As described later, rectal thiopental and methohexital also have established safety and efficacy for pediatric neuroimaging.

Substantial controversy surrounds the IV administration of these agents for ED PSA.[38] Proponents cite their extremely rapid onset and recovery as advantages over other sedatives. Critics cite the need for continuous vigilance required to achieve a desired effect while simultaneously avoiding significant respiratory depression as a distinct disadvantage. Patients receiving these agents can exhibit rapid swings in level of consciousness. An additional dedicated physician (separate from the individual performing the procedure) is widely believed to be required to oversee medication administration and patient monitoring; however, oversedation may not be reliably avoided despite this precaution. Currently, data from case series do not sufficiently quantify depth of sedation, and it is unclear whether some subjects experienced periods of general anesthesia. Although profound obtundation creates superlative procedural conditions, it also presents a greater aspiration risk than traditional sedatives.[38,39]

Propofol

Pharmacology

Propofol exhibits numerous exceptionally desirable characteristics of a PSA agent. First, its clinical effect is essentially immediate following IV administration ("one arm-brain circulatory time"). Second, its marked potency reliably produces effective PSA conditions, even for very painful procedures. Third, recovery following sedation is extremely short, typically 5 to 15 minutes. Finally, patient satisfaction is high, as propofol has antiemetic and euphoric properties.[38]

Pediatric Use

Two large ED series[40,41] and several smaller ones[36,42-46] demonstrated that propofol can be administered to children in the ED with a high level of efficacy, with apparent safety, and with rapid recovery. The depth of sedation achieved in these reports is not well described, but frequently appears to be at or past levels consistent with deep sedation.

If it is ultimately shown that emergency physicians can consistently administer this drug in a manner that avoids oversedation and respiratory depression, propofol could potentially become the IV PSA sedative agent of choice.

Adverse Effects

The most serious adverse effect of propofol is potent respiratory depression, and apnea can occur suddenly and without warning. Rates of respiratory depression range widely by study (8% to 30%)[38] and thus the technique appears more operator dependent than does sedation with longer acting agents.

Propofol can also produce hypotension (by direct negative inotropy as well as arterial and venodilation), although this adverse effect is typically so transient as to be of little clinical importance in healthy patients.[38]

Etomidate

Pharmacology

Etomidate produces sedation, anxiolysis, and amnesia equal to that of barbiturates, but with significantly fewer adverse hemodynamic effects. Its onset of action and recovery are similar to those of thiopental and methohexital.

Pediatric Use

Etomidate is widely administered as the induction agent of choice for rapid sequence intubation in both children and adults, especially for patients with head trauma or marginal blood pressure. As with the other ultra-short-acting agents, preliminary reports describe rapid recovery and a high level of efficacy using IV etomidate for pediatric PSA.[47-49] Similarly, the depth of sedation achieved in these reports is not well described, but appears to frequently be at or past levels consistent with deep sedation.

Adverse Effects

The primary adverse effects of etomidate are respiratory depression, myoclonus, nausea, and vomiting.[47-50] Etomidate appears to be a less desirable PSA choice than propofol, given that it induces myoclonus and emesis. Transient adrenal suppression occurs with etomidate, but appears to lack clinical significance when used in single doses.[51]

Thiopental and Methohexital

Pharmacology

When given IV, both thiopental and methohexital produce sedation within 1 minute. Clinical recovery is rapid (approximately 15 minutes) and reflects the rapid redistribution of these agents from the central nervous system to the periphery. Because of their lipid solubility, barbiturates are rapidly absorbed rectally.

Pediatric Use

When administered rectally, thiopental and methohexital can reliably produce anxiolysis and sedation suitable for CT or MRI scanning.[52-57] IV methohexital has been administered for brief PSA in children with excellent procedural success.[58,59] The depth of sedation achieved in these small series is not well described, but appears to be at or past levels consistent with deep sedation.

Adverse Effects

Although respiratory depression is unusual when using rectal thiopental or methohexital in typical doses (see Table 159–6), it can rarely occur.[52-56] Standard interactive and mechanical monitoring are warranted as with any PSA.

When these agents are administered IV, they exhibit potent respiratory depression in the same manner as propofol and etomidate.[58-60] Barbiturates frequently can cause hypotension at typical IV doses, so their use should be avoided whenever possible in patients with volume depletion or cardiovascular compromise.

Analgesic Agents

Fentanyl

Fentanyl is the most common opioid used for PSA due to its rapid onset, brief duration of action, and lack of histamine release.[61] Morphine and meperidine are instead preferred for pure pain control due to their longer duration of action. Children in the ED frequently receive morphine or meperidine initially for acute analgesia, and then later are administered shorter acting agents to facilitate a needed procedure. Although longer acting opioids can be readily used for analgesia during PSA, they will be associated with longer recovery times. Fentanyl is preferred unless unavailable.

Pharmacology

Fentanyl is 75 to 125 times more potent than morphine and has no intrinsic anxiolytic or amnestic properties. A single dose given IV has rapid onset (<30 seconds), with a peak at 2 to 3 minutes and brief clinical duration (20 to 40 minutes). This increase in potency and onset of action is in part related to its greater lipid solubility, which facilitates its passage across the blood-brain barrier. The effects of fentanyl can be reversed with opioid antagonists (i.e., naloxone, nalmefene).

Pediatric Use

Because of its pharmacokinetics, IV fentanyl is an ideal agent when analgesia is required for painful procedures, because it can be easily and rapidly titrated.[61] As anxiolysis and sedation do not occur at low doses of fentanyl (1 to 2 mcg/kg), the concurrent administration of a pure sedative, most commonly midazolam, is advisable (see Table 159–7). The combination of fentanyl and midazolam remains a popular PSA sedation regimen in children, with a strong safety and efficacy profile when both drugs are carefully titrated to effect.[31-33,62,63] Any level of mild, moderate, or deep sedation can be achieved using these agents.

Fentanyl is also available in an oral transmucosal preparation. Although this novel and noninvasive delivery route obviates the need for IV access, titration is difficult and efficacy is variable.[64] Furthermore, the incidence of emesis is high (31% to 45%),[64,65] and this formulation has never become popular for PSA.

Adverse Effects

Like all opioids, fentanyl can cause respiratory depression.[31-33,61-63] When used for PSA, standard interactive and mechanical monitoring are required. As the opioid effect is most pronounced on the central nervous system respiratory centers, apnea can precede loss of consciousness. If apnea should occur, verbal or tactile stimulation should be attempted prior to administration of opioid antagonists. As discussed earlier, caution must be exercised when using benzodiazepines and opioids together, since the risks of hypoxia and apnea are significantly greater than when either is used alone.[14,30]

In the absence of significant ethanol intoxication, hypovolemia, or concomitant drug ingestion, hypotension is rare. Because of its safe hemodynamic profile, fentanyl is an ideal analgesic agent for use in critically ill or injured patients. Additionally, nausea and vomiting are rare compared to morphine and meperidine. A commonly observed reaction to fentanyl is facial pruritus, with patients frequently scratching their nose.[61]

A rare side effect of fentanyl that has the potential to cause respiratory compromise is chest wall rigidity. This complication is related to higher doses (>5 mcg/kg as a bolus dose) than those used for PSA, and has not been reported in ED series.[31,61-63] If chest wall rigidity occurs, it usually can be reversed with opioid antagonists and/or positive pressure ventilation. Equipment for urgent pharmacologic paralysis should be available in case antagonist reversal and positive pressure ventilation are unsuccessful.

Other Short-Acting Opioids

Sufentanil, alfentanil, and remifentanil are other short-acting opioids that have a potential role in PSA in the future. However, currently there is insufficient published experience to warrant their routine use. Although intranasal sufentanil 0.75 mcg/kg appeared promising when combined with midazolam in one small pediatric trial,[66] in another study doses of 1.5 mcg/kg resulted in oxygen desaturation in 8 of 10 children studied.[26] This low toxic:therapeutic ratio and inability to titrate limit the utility of intranasal sufentanil. In the one published report of IV remifentanil with midazolam for PSA, there was an unacceptably high incidence of hypoxemia.[67] Currently there does not appear to be a clinically important advantage to these drugs compared to fentanyl.

Ketamine

Pharmacology

Ketamine produces a unique state of cortical dissociation that permits painful procedures to be performed more consistently and effectively than with other PSA agents. This state of "dissociative sedation" is characterized by profound analgesia, sedation, amnesia, and immobilization, and can be rapidly and reliably produced with IV or IM administration. Ketamine has been widely used worldwide since its introduction in 1970 and has demonstrated a remarkable safety profile in a variety of settings.[31,68-72] In 1999, the Joint Commission on Accreditation of Healthcare Organizations confirmed that ED ketamine administration is fully compliant with their standards when administered according to protocol.[73] Clinicians administering ketamine must be especially knowledgeable about the unique actions of this drug and the numerous contraindications to its use (Table 159–8).

Ketamine differs from all other PSA agents in several important ways. First, it uniquely preserves cardiopulmonary stability. Upper airway muscular tone and protective airway reflexes are maintained. Spontaneous respiration is preserved, although, when administered IV, ketamine must be given slowly (over 1 to 2 minutes) to prevent respiratory depression. Second, it differs from other agents in that it lacks the characteristic dose-response continuum to progressive titration. At doses below a certain threshold, ketamine produces analgesia and sedation. However, once a critical dosage threshold (approximately 1 to 1.5 mg/kg IV or 3 to 4 mg/kg IM) is achieved, the characteristic dissociative state abruptly appears. This dissociation has no observable levels of depth, and thus the only value of ketamine "titration" is to maintain the presence of the state over time. Finally, the dissociative state is not consistent with formal definitions of moderate sedation, deep sedation, or general anesthesia, and therefore must be considered from a different perspective than agents that exhibit the classical sedation continuum.[68,74]

Ketamine is most effective and reliable when given IV or IM. Ketamine has a one arm-brain circulation time when given IV, with onset of dissociation noted within 1 minute and effective procedural conditions lasting for about 10 to 15 minutes. When given IM, the same effect is achieved within 5 minutes, with effective procedural conditions lasting 15 to 30 minutes. The typical duration from dosing until dischargeable recovery is 50 to 110 minutes when given IV, and 60 to 140 minutes when given IM.[69,71,75]

Like benzodiazepines, ketamine undergoes substantial first-pass hepatic metabolism. Therefore, oral and rectal administration results in less predictable effectiveness and requires substantially higher doses. Clinical onset and recovery are substantially longer than when given parenterally, and thus these routes are rarely used in the ED.[28,29,76]

Ketamine can induce salivation, and anticholinergics have traditionally been routinely coadministered to prevent this effect. Atropine is most commonly chosen in emergency medicine due to its ready familiarity to physicians and nurses, although glycopyrrolate is an equally acceptable but not superior alternative. However, a recent trial noted similar hypersalivation scores between children who did and did not receive concurrent atropine,[77] indicating that anticholinergics may not be considered mandatory with ketamine. Another author anecdotally described no difficulty with administration of ketamine without an anticholinergic to approximately 1100 children.[78]

Pediatric Use

Ketamine is an ideal agent to facilitate short, painful procedures in children. The safety and efficacy of ketamine for this indication have been widely documented.[30,31,68,69,71,75] The IM route is simple and effective. Venous access is unnecessary, and atropine can be concurrently administered in the same syringe.[69] Intravenous administration is attractive because a lower cumulative dose can be used, and recovery is more rapid than with the IM route. The primary caution is that, with this route, ketamine must be administered slowly (each dose over 1 to 2 minutes) or respiratory depression and transient apnea can occur.[75]

Unpleasant recovery reactions are uncommon in children and teenagers, and are typically mild.[68,79,80] There is no evidence of any benefit from the prophylactic administration of concurrent benzodiazepines in children,[79,80] and their role should be confined to treating unpleasant reactions if they occur.

Adverse Effects

In the largest published ED series (1022 patients), the following adverse airway events were noted: airway malalignment (0.7%), transient laryngospasm (0.4%), and transient apnea or respiratory depression (0.3%). All were quickly identified and treated, and there were no sequelae.[69]

Vomiting was noted in 6.7% of patients from the same series, and in most cases it occurred well into recovery.[69] The incidence was age related, occurring in 12.1% of children age 5 years or older, and 3.5% in those younger than 5 years.[70] There was no evidence of aspiration[69]; indeed, in 30 years of regular use there have been no documented reports of clinically significant ketamine-associated aspiration in patients without established contraindications. Because of its unique preservation of protective airway reflexes, ketamine may be preferred over other agents for urgent or emergent procedures when fasting is not assured.[30,69,71]

Mild agitation during recovery (whimpering or crying) was noted in 17.6% of children from the same series, with more pronounced agitation in 1.6%. The incidence was age related, with agitation occurring in 12.1% of children age 5 years or older, and 22.5% in those younger than 5 years.[70] Only 2 of 1022 children had reactions that treating physicians judged severe enough to require treatment, and both children responded promptly to small doses of midazolam.[69] Another study quantified the degree of recovery agitation using a 0 to 100-millimeter visual analog scale; the median rating of recovery agitation was a 5, likely below the threshold of clinical importance.[79]

Nitrous Oxide

Pharmacology

Inhaled nitrous oxide provides anxiolysis and mild analgesia. It is commonly dispensed at concentrations between 30% and 50%, with oxygen composing the remainder of the mixture. Nitrous oxide quickly diffuses across biologic membranes and accordingly has a rapid onset of action (30 to 60 seconds). Maximum effect occurs after about 5 minutes, and the clinical effect wears off quickly upon discontinuation. At typical PSA concentrations there is preservation of hemodynamic status, spontaneous respirations, and protective airway reflexes.[81-84] Nitrous oxide is widely used in dentistry at higher concentrations.[85]

Nitrous oxide has an excellent safety profile; however, as a sole agent it cannot reliably produce adequate procedural conditions.[81-84] Given its relatively weak analgesic properties, in many cases nitrous oxide will need to be supplemented with an IV opioid and/or local anesthesia.

Table 159–8	Procedure for Dissociative Sedation with Ketamine

Purpose

- To define the guidelines for patient selection, administration, monitoring, and recovery for emergency department dissociative sedation.

Definition of Dissociative Sedation

- A trancelike cataleptic state induced by the dissociative agent ketamine, characterized by profound analgesia and amnesia, with retention of protective airway reflexes, spontaneous respirations, and cardiopulmonary stability.

Characteristics of the Ketamine "Dissociative State"

- *Dissociation*—Following administration of ketamine, the patient passes into a fugue state or trance. The eyes may remain open but the patient does not respond ("the lights are on, but no one's home").
- *Catalepsy*—Normal or slightly enhanced muscle tone is maintained. On occasion the patient may move or be moved into a position that is self-maintaining. Occasional muscular clonus may be noted.
- *Analgesia*—Analgesia is typically substantial or complete.
- *Amnesia*—Total amnesia is typical.
- *Maintenance of Airway Reflexes*—Upper airway reflexes remain intact and may be slightly exaggerated. Intubation is unnecessary, but occasional repositioning of the head may be necessary for optimal airway patency. Suctioning of hypersalivation may occasionally be necessary.
- *Cardiovascular Stability*—Blood pressure and heart rate are not decreased, and typically are mildly increased.
- *Nystagmus*—Nystagmus is typical.

Indications

- Short, painful procedures, especially those requiring immobilization (e.g., facial laceration, burn débridement, fracture reduction, abscess incision and drainage, central line placement, tube thoracostomy).
- Examinations judged likely to produce excessive emotional disturbance (e.g., pediatric sexual assault examination).

Contraindications—Absolute (Risks Essentially Always Outweigh Benefits)

- Age less than 3 months (higher risk of airway complications)
- Known or suspected psychosis, even if currently stable or controlled with medications (can exacerbate condition)

Contraindications—Relative (Risks May Outweigh Benefits)

- Age 3 to 12 months (higher risk of airway complications)
- Procedures involving stimulation of the posterior pharynx (higher risk of laryngospasm)
- History of airway instability, tracheal surgery, or tracheal stenosis (presumed higher risk of airway complications)
- Active pulmonary infection or disease, including upper respiratory infection or asthma (higher risk of laryngospasm)
- Known or suspected cardiovascular disease, including angina, heart failure, or hypertension (exacerbation due to sympathomimetic properties of ketamine). Avoid ketamine in patients who are already hypertensive, and in older adults with risk factors for coronary artery disease.
- Head injury associated with loss of consciousness, altered mental status, or emesis (elevated intracranial pressure with ketamine)
- Central nervous system masses, abnormalities, or hydrocephalus (elevated intracranial pressure with ketamine)
- Glaucoma or acute globe injury (elevated intraocular pressure with ketamine)
- Porphyria, thyroid disorder, or thyroid medication (enhanced sympathomimetic effect)

Personnel

- Dissociative sedation is a two-person procedure, one (e.g., nurse) to monitor the patient and one (e.g., physician) to perform the procedure. Both must be knowledgeable regarding the unique characteristics of ketamine.
- Avoid dissociative sedation when personnel are not experienced with ketamine or may not have time to perform such sedation properly.

Presedation (See Part 1 of Chapter)

- Perform a standard presedation assessment.
- Educate accompanying family regarding the unique characteristics of the dissociative state, especially if they will be present during the procedure and/or recovery.
- Frame the dissociative encounter as a positive experience. Consider encouraging older children to "plan" specific, pleasant dream topics in advance of sedation (believed to decrease unpleasant recovery reactions). Emphasize, especially to school-age children and teenagers, that ketamine delivers sufficient analgesia so there will be no pain.

Ketamine Administration—General

- If a consultant physician is performing the procedure, discuss with him or her in advance the goal and anticipated depth of sedation and ensure that he or she is aware of the unique features of dissociative sedation.
- Ketamine is not administered until the physician is ready to begin the procedure, as onset of dissociation typically occurs within 5 min.
- Ketamine is initially administered as a single intramuscular (IM) injection or IV loading dose. There is no benefit from attempts to titrate to effect.
- The IM route is especially useful in those settings in which IV access cannot be consistently obtained with minimal upset to the child and for patients who are uncooperative and/or combative (e.g., the mentally disabled).
- IV access is unnecessary in children receiving IM ketamine. Since unpleasant recovery reactions are more common in adults, IV access is desirable in older teenagers to permit rapid treatment of these reactions should they occur.

Ketamine Administration—IM Route

- Administer ketamine 4–5 mg/kg IM.
- Repeat ketamine dose (full or half dose IM) if sedation is inadequate after 5–10 minutes (unusual) or if additional doses are required.

Ketamine Administration—IV Route

- Administer a loading dose of 1.5 mg/kg IV over 60 sec; 100 mg is a typical adult dose. More rapid administration produces high central nervous system levels and has been associated with respiratory depression.
- Additional incremental doses of ketamine may be given (0.5–1.0 mg/kg) if initial sedation is inadequate, or if repeated doses are necessary to accomplish a longer procedure.

Table continued on following page

Table 159–8	Procedure for Dissociative Sedation with Ketamine (Continued)	
Route of Administration	**IM**	**IV**
Advantages	No IV access necessary	Ease of repeat dosing Slightly faster recovery
Peak concentrations and clinical onset	5 min	1 min
Typical duration of effective dissociation	20–30 min	5–10 min
Typical time from dose to discharge	60–140 min	50–110 min

Coadministered Medications

- Concurrent anticholinergics have been traditionally administered with the intent of minimizing ketamine-associated hypersalivation, although recent evidence suggests that this recommendation has been overstated.
- If atropine is used, the typically recommended dose is 0.01 mg/kg (minimum 0.1 mg, maximum 0.5 mg). Atropine can either be given IV just prior to ketamine, or mixed with ketamine in the same syringe for IM injection.
- Glycopyrrolate is an acceptable alternative to atropine at equipotent doses; however, there is no evidence that it is more effective or in any way advantageous.
- In children, benzodiazepine coadministration does not appear to decrease unpleasant recovery reactions. However, a benzodiazapine should be readily available to treat such rare reactions should they occur.

Procedure

- Adjunctive physical immobilization may be needed occasionally to control random motion.
- Adjunctive local anesthetic is usually unnecessary when using dissociative dose.

Interactive Monitoring

- Mandatory close observation of airway and respirations by an experienced health care professional is maintained until recovery is well established. THE PATIENT IS NEVER LEFT ALONE.
- Drapes should be positioned such that airway and chest motion can be visualized at all times.
- Occasional repositioning of the head may be indicated for optimal airway patency.
- Occasional suctioning of the anterior pharynx may be necessary.

Mechanical Monitoring

- Suction equipment, oxygen, a bag-valve-mask, and age-appropriate equipment for advanced airway management should be immediately available.
- Maintain continuous pulse oximetry until recovery is well established.
- Maintain continuous cardiac monitoring until recovery is well established.
- Maintain continuous capnography, if available, until recovery is well established.
- Pulse and respiratory rate should all be recorded periodically throughout the procedure. Blood pressure measurements following the initial value are generally unnecessary, as ketamine stimulates catecholamine release and does not depress the cardiovascular system in healthy patients.

Potential Side Effects

- Airway misalignment requiring repositioning of head (0.7%)
- Transient laryngospasm (0.4%)
- Transient apnea or respiratory depression (0.3%)
- Hypersalivation (1.7%)
- Emesis while sedated (0.8%)
- Emesis well into recovery (5.9%)
- Recovery agitation (mild in 17.6%, moderate or severe in 1.6%)
- Muscular hypertonicity and random, purposeless movements are common.
- Clonus, hiccupping, and/or rash may occur.

Recovery

- Maintain minimal physical contact or other sensory disturbance.
- Maintain a quiet area with dim lighting if possible.
- Advise parents or caregivers not to stimulate patient prematurely.

Discharge Criteria

- Return to pretreatment level of verbalization and awareness
- Return to pretreatment level of purposeful neuromuscular activity
- A predischarge requirement of tolerating oral fluids is not necessary or recommended after dissociative sedation.

Discharge Instructions

- Nothing by mouth for approximately 2 hr
- Careful family observation and no independent ambulation for approximately 2 hr

From Green SM, Krauss B: Clinical practice guideline for emergency department ketamine dissociative sedation in children. Ann Emerg Med 44:460–471, 2004.

Cooperative Child Use

The safest method of nitrous oxide administration is via a self-administered demand-valve mask.[82-84] The patient must generate a negative pressure of 3 to 5 cm H_2O within the handheld mask or mouthpiece to activate the flow of gas. Patients can thus self-titrate by inhaling at will through the mask. This will only be effective when the patient is cooperative. This technique provides a built-in fail-safe mechanism. If the patient becomes somnolent, the mask will fall from the face and gas delivery will cease.

Nitrous oxide can be used as an adjunctive anxiolytic during mildly painful procedures, or during local or regional anesthesia administration for other procedures. Administration may also be useful during difficult pelvic examinations, attempts at difficult IV access, and the like.

A double-tank system is commonly used to deliver the nitrous oxide–O_2 mixture. The system relies on a mixing valve preset to deliver a fixed ratio that will only deliver gas when O_2 is flowing. The double-tank system contains a fail-safe device that automatically stops the flow of nitrous oxide when the O_2 supply is depleted.

Uncooperative Child Use

The primary limitation of self-administration is that it is ineffective in uncooperative patients, including most frightened young children. Continuous-flow nitrous oxide has been used in this population using a mask strapped over the nose, or over the nose and mouth.[86-89] Nitrous oxide can effectively produce moderate or deep sedation when administered in this manner; however, this technique necessitates an additional physician dedicated to continuous gas titration to avoid oversedation. Additionally, the continuous-flow technique is associated with more frequent emesis (10%)[86,88,89] than self-administration (0% to 4%),[81-84] posing a potential hazard when a mask is strapped over the child's mouth. Finally, the requirement of a mask hinders procedures involving parts of the face that are covered.[89]

Adverse Effects and Precautions

A number of generally minor adverse effects may be seen, including nausea, dizziness, voice change, euphoria, and laughter.[81-84] Nitrous oxide should be avoided in patients with potential closed-space diseases such as bowel obstruction, middle ear disease, pneumothorax, or pneumocephaly. Because it is highly diffusible, nitrous oxide has the potential to increase the size of the closed space. This should be clinically unimportant for most short-term uses in typical PSA concentrations.

A scavenging system must be in place to collect exhaled nitrous oxide, and care must be taken to ensure compliance with occupational safety regulations. Care should also be taken to avoid nitrous oxide exposure in pregnant ED staff members as nitrous oxide is a known teratogen and mutagen.

Although the potential for abuse by ED staff exists, such abuse should be rare if simple steps are taken. As with other agents, a strict protocol of accountability should be in place. A simple locking device can be added to the cylinders of gas. In addition, the delivery valve or mouthpiece may be locked in the same location as controlled substances.

Other PSA Agents

Historically a popular PSA cocktail was the IM combination of meperidine, promethazine, and chlorpromazine ("DPT," "Dem compound"). However, this regimen cannot be titrated, is frequently ineffective, and is associated with prolonged recovery times.[90,91] Its use can no longer be recommended.

Antagonists

Reversal agents should not be routinely administered following administration of opioids or benzodiazepines for PSA, but rather should be reserved for rare situations of oversedation or respiratory depression. When administered, caution should be taken to avoid resedation after discharge by continuing to monitor patients until the effects of the PSA agents (which may last longer than the antagonist) wear off.

Naloxone

Naloxone is an antagonist that competitively displaces opioids from opiate receptors. It rapidly reverses the analgesic and respiratory depressant effects of opioids. It may be administered IV, IM, subcutaneously, or even sublingually if needed,[92] and dosing has been standardized for infants and children.[93] Naloxone will not induce systemic opioid withdrawal symptoms in a patient without preexisting physiologic dependence. However, some patients will experience nausea with opioid reversal, and those patients with persistent pain following their procedure will be quite uncomfortable. Rapid reversal also may lead to return of anxiety and sympathetic stimulation. If the situation permits, careful titration of small amounts of naloxone may permit partial rather than complete reversal. The only absolute contraindication to the use of naloxone is administration to a neonate born to an opioid-dependent mother due to the risk of precipitating life-threatening opioid withdrawal.

Flumazenil

Flumazenil is a benzodiazepine antagonist that can promptly reverse benzodiazepine-induced sedation and respiratory depression.[12,61,94] Flumazenil lowers the seizure threshold and may lead to life-threatening seizures. It should be avoided or used with extreme caution in settings of benzodiazepine dependence, seizure disorder, cyclic antidepressant overdose, and elevated intracranial pressure.[95] It should also be given cautiously to patients who are on medications known to lower the seizure threshold (cyclosporine, tricyclic antidepressants, propoxyphene, theophylline, isoniazid, lithium).[95] Rapid reversal also may lead to return of anxiety and sympathetic stimulation. If the situation permits, careful titration of small amounts of flumazenil may permit partial rather than complete reversal.

REFERENCES

1. Chen E, Joseph MH, Zeltzer LK: Behavioral and cognitive interventions in the treatment of pain in children. Pediatr Clin North Am 47:513–525, 2000.
2. Kennedy RM, Luhmann JD: The "ouchless emergency department." Getting closer: advances in decreasing distress during painful procedures in the emergency department. Pediatr Clin North Am 46:1215–1247, 1999.

3. Olson DM, Sheehan MG, Thompson W, et al: Sedation of children for electroencephalograms. Pediatrics 108:163–165, 2001.

4. Binder LS, Leake LA: Chloral hydrate for emergent pediatric procedural sedation: a new look at an old drug. Am J Emerg Med 9:530–534, 1991.

5. Malviya S, Voepel-Lewis T, Prochaska G, Tait AR: Prolonged recovery and delayed side effects of sedation for diagnostic imaging studies in children. Pediatrics 105:e42, 2000.

6. D'Agostino J, Terndrup TE: Chloral hydrate versus midazolam for sedation of children for neuroimaging: a randomized clinical trial. Pediatr Emerg Care 16:1–4, 2000.

7. Greenberg SB, Faerber EN, Aspinall CL, Adams RC: High-dose chloral hydrate sedation for children undergoing MR imaging: safety and efficacy in relation to age. AJR Am J Roentgenol 161:639–641, 1993.

8. Hubbard AM, Markowitz RI, Kimmel B, et al: Sedation for pediatric patients undergoing CT and MRI. J Comput Assist Tomogr 16:3–6, 1992.

9. Malviya S, Voepel-Lewis T, Tait AR: Adverse events and risk factors associated with the sedation of children by nonanesthesiologists. Anesth Analg 85:1207–1213, 1997.

10. Vade A, Sukhani R, Dolenga M, Habisohn-Schuck C: Chloral hydrate sedation in children undergoing CT and MR imaging: safety as judged by American Academy of Pediatrics (AAP) guidelines. AJR Am J Roentgenol 165:905–909, 1995.

11. Pereira JK, Burrows PE, Richards HM, et al: Comparison of sedation regimens for pediatric outpatient CT. Pediatr Radiol 23:341–344, 1993.

12. Cote CJ, Karl HW, Notterman DA, et al: Adverse sedation events in pediatrics: a critical incident analysis of contributing factors. Pediatrics 105:805–814, 2000.

13. American Academy of Pediatrics, Committee on Drugs: Use of chloral hydrate for sedation in children. Pediatrics 92:471–473, 1993.

14. Bailey PL: Frequent hypoxemia and apnea after sedation with midazolam and fentanyl. Anesthesiology 73:826, 1990.

15. Karl HW, Coté CJ, McCubbin MM, et al: Intravenous midazolam for sedation of children undergoing procedures: an analysis of age- and procedure-related factors. Pediatr Emerg Care 15:167–172, 1999.

16. Massanari M, Novitsky J, Reinstein LJ: Paradoxical reactions in children associated with midazolam use during endoscopy. Clin Pediatr 36:681–684, 1997.

17. Davies FC, Waters M: Oral midazolam for conscious sedation of children during minor procedures. J Accid Emerg Med 15:244–248, 1998.

18. McGlone RG, Fleet T, Durham S, Hollis S: A comparison of intramuscular ketamine with high dose intramuscular midazolam with and without intranasal flumazenil in children before suturing. Emerg Med J 18:34–38, 2001.

19. Fatovich DM, Jacobs IG: A randomized, controlled trial of oral midazolam and buffered lidocaine for suturing lacerations in children (the SLIC trial). Ann Emerg Med 25:209–214, 1995.

20. Feld LH, Negus JB, White PF: Oral midazolam preanesthetic medication in pediatric outpatients. Anesthesiology 73:831–834, 1990.

21. Younge PA, Kendall JM: Sedation for children requiring wound repair: a randomized controlled double blind comparison of oral midazolam and oral ketamine. Emerg Med J 18:30–33, 2001.

22. Haas DA, Nenniger SA, Yacobi R, et al: A pilot study of the efficacy of oral midazolam for sedation in pediatric dental patients. Anesth Prog 43:1–8, 1996.

23. Connors K, Terndrup TE: Nasal versus oral midazolam for sedation of anxious children undergoing laceration repair. Ann Emerg Med 24:1074–1079, 1994.

24. Theroux MC, West DW, Corddry DH, et al: Efficacy of intranasal midazolam in facilitating suturing of lacerations in preschool children in the emergency department. Pediatrics 91:624–627, 1993.

25. McGlone RG, Ranasinghe S, Durham S: An alternative to "brutacaine": a comparison of low dose intramuscular ketamine with intranasal midazolam in children before suturing. J Accid Emerg Med 15:231–236, 1998.

26. Abrams R, Morrison JE, Villasenor A, et al: Safety and effectiveness of intranasal administration of sedative medications (ketamine, midazolam, or sufentanil) for urgent brief pediatric dental procedures. Anesth Prog 40:63–66, 1993.

27. Ackworth JP, Purdie D, Clark RC: Intravenous ketamine plus midazolam is superior to intranasal midazolam for emergency paediatric procedural sedation. Emerg Med J 18:39–45, 2001.

28. Roelofse JA, Joubert JJ, Roelofse PGR: A double-blind randomized comparison of midazolam alone and midazolam combined with ketamine for sedation of pediatric dental patients. J Oral Maxillofac Surg 54:838–844, 1996.

29. Tanaka M, Sato M, Saito A, Nishikawa T: Reevaluation of rectal ketamine premedication in children: comparison with rectal midazolam. Anesthesiology 93:1217–1224, 2000.

*30. Krauss B, Green SM: Sedation and analgesia for procedures in children. N Engl J Med 342:938–945, 2000.

*31. Pena BMG, Krauss B: Adverse events of procedural sedation and analgesia in a pediatric emergency department. Ann Emerg Med 34:483–490, 1999.

32. Kennedy RM, Porter FL, Miller JP, Jaffe DM: Comparison of fentanyl/midazolam with ketamine/midazolam for pediatric orthopedic emergencies. Pediatrics 102:956–963, 1998.

33. Pitetti RD, Singh S, Pierce MC: Safe and efficacious use of procedural sedation and analgesia by nonanesthesiologists in a pediatric emergency department. Arch Pediatr Adolesc Med 157:1090–1096, 2003.

34. Moro-Sutherland DM, Algren JT, Louis PT, et al: Comparison of intravenous midazolam with pentobarbital for sedation for head computed tomography imaging. Acad Emerg Med 7:1370–1375, 2000.

35. Strain JD, Campbell JB, Harvey LA, Foley LC: IV Nembutal: safe sedation for children undergoing CT. AJR Am J Roentgenol 151:975–979, 1988.

36. Bloomfield EL, Masaryk TJ, Caplin A, et al: Intravenous sedation for MR imaging of the brain and spine in children: pentobarbital versus propofol. Radiology 186:93–97, 1993.

37. Egelhoff JC, Ball WS Jr, Koch BL, et al: Safety and efficacy of sedation in children using a structured sedation program. AJR Am J Roentgenol 168:1259–1262, 1997.

38. Green SM, Krauss B: Propofol in emergency medicine: pushing the sedation frontier [Editorial]. Ann Emerg Med 42:792–797, 2003.

*39. Green SM: Fasting is a consideration—not a necessity—for emergency department procedural sedation and analgesia [Editorial]. Ann Emerg Med 42:647–650, 2003.

40. Bassett KE, Anderson JL, Pribble CG, Guenther E: Propofol for procedural sedation in children in the emergency department. Ann Emerg Med 42:773–782, 2003.

41. Guenther E, Pribble CG, Junkins EP, et al: Propofol sedation by emergency physicians for elective pediatric outpatient procedures. Ann Emerg Med 42:783–791, 2003.

42. Havel CJ, Strait RT, Hennes H: A clinical trial of propofol vs midazolam for procedural sedation in a pediatric emergency department. Acad Emerg Med 6:989–997, 1999.

43. Swanson ER, Seaberg DC, Mathias S: The use of propofol for sedation in the emergency department. Acad Emerg Med 3:234–238, 1996.

44. Lowrie L, Weiss AH, Lacombe C: The pediatric sedation unit: a mechanism for pediatric sedation. Pediatrics 102:e30, 1998.

45. Hertzog JH, Campbell JK, Dalton HJ, Hauser GJ: Propofol anesthesia for invasive procedures in ambulatory and hospitalized children: experience in the pediatric intensive care unit. Pediatrics 103:657, 1999.

46. Hertzog JH, Dalton HJ, Anderson BD, et al: Prospective evaluation of propofol anesthesia in the pediatric intensive care unit for elective oncology procedures in ambulatory and hospitalized children. Pediatrics 106:742–747, 2000.

47. Dickinson R, Singer AJ, Carrion W: Etomidate for pediatric sedation prior to fracture reduction. Acad Emerg Med 8:74–77, 2001.

48. Ruth WJ, Burton JH, Bock AJ: Intravenous etomidate for procedural sedation in emergency department patients. Acad Emerg Med 8:13–18, 2001.

49. Yealy DM: Safe and effective . . . maybe: etomidate in procedural sedation/analgesia [Editorial]. Acad Emerg Med 8:68–69, 2001.

50. Burton JH, Bock AJ, Strout TD, Marcolini EG: Etomidate and midazolam for reduction of anterior shoulder dislocation: a randomized, controlled trial. Ann Emerg Med 40:496–504, 2002.

51. Schenarts CL, Burton JH, Riker RR: Adrenocortical dysfunction following etomidate induction in emergency department patients. Acad Emerg Med 8:1–7, 2001.

52. Pomeranz ES, Chudnofsky CR, Deegan TJ, et al: Rectal methohexital sedation for computed tomography imaging of stable pediatric emergency department patients. Pediatrics 105:1110–1114, 2000.

*Selected readings.

53. Manuli MA, Davies L: Rectal methohexital for sedation of children during imaging procedures. AJR Am J Roentgenol 160:577–580, 1993.

54. O'Brien JF, Falk JL, Carey BE, Malone LC: Rectal thiopental compared with intramuscular meperidine, promethazine, and chlorpromazine for pediatric sedation. Ann Emerg Med 20:644–647, 1991.

55. Daniels AL, Cote CJ, Polaner DM: Continuous oxygen saturation monitoring following rectal methohexitone induction in paediatric patients. Can J Anaesth 39:27–30, 1992.

56. Beekman RP, Hoorntje TM, Beek FJ, Kuijten RH: Sedation for children undergoing magnetic resonance imaging: efficacy and safety of rectal thiopental. Eur J Pediatr 155:820–822, 1996.

57. Glasier CM, Stark JE, Brown R, et al: Rectal thiopental sodium for sedation of pediatric patients undergoing MR and other imaging studies. AJNR Am J Neuroradiol 16:111–114, 1995.

58. Sedik H: Use of intravenous methohexital as a sedative in pediatric emergency departments. Arch Pediatr Adolesc Med 155:665–668, 2001.

59. Schwanda AE: Brief unconscious sedation for painful pediatric oncology procedures: intravenous methohexital with approrpirate monitoring is safe and effective. Am J Pediatr Hematol Oncol 15:370, 1993.

60. Lerman B, Yoshida D, Levitt MA: A prospective evaluation of the safety and efficacy of methohexital in the emergency department. Am J Emerg Med 14:351–354, 1996.

61. Chudnofsky CR, Wright SW, Dronen SC, et al: The safety of fentanyl use in the emergency department. Ann Emerg Med 18:635–639, 1989.

62. Billmire DA, Neale HW, Gregory RO: Use of IV fentanyl in the outpatient treatment of pediatric facial trauma. J Trauma 25:1079–1080, 1985.

63. Pohlgeers AP, Friedland LF, Keegan-Jones L: Combination fentanyl and diazepam for pediatric conscious sedation. Acad Emerg Med 2:879–883, 1995.

64. Schechter NL, Weisman SJ, Rosenblum M, et al: The use of oral transmucosal fentanyl citrate for painful procedures in children. Pediatrics 95:335–339, 1995.

65. Schutzman SA, Liebelt E, Wisk M, Burg J: Comparison of oral transmucosal fentanyl citrate and intramuscular meperidine, promethazine, and chlorpromazine for conscious sedation of children undergoing laceration repair. Ann Emerg Med 28:385–390, 1996.

66. Bates BA, Schutzman SA, Fleisher GR: A comparison of intranasal sufentanil and midazolam to intramuscular meperidine, promethazine, and chlorpromazine for conscious sedation in children. Ann Emerg Med 24:646–651, 1994.

67. Litman RS: Conscious sedation with remifentanil and midazolam during brief painful procedures in children. Arch Pediatr Adolesc Med 153:1085–1088, 1999.

68. Green SM, Krauss B: Clinical practice guideline for emergency department ketamine dissociative sedation in children. Ann Emerg Med 44:460–471, 2004.

69. Green SM, Rothrock SG, Lynch EL, et al: Intramuscular ketamine for pediatric sedation in the emergency department: safety profile with 1,022 cases. Ann Emerg Med 31:688–697, 1998.

70. Green SM, Kupperman N, Rothrock SG, et al: Predictors of adverse events with ketamine sedation in children. Ann Emerg Med 35:35–42, 2000.

71. Green SM, Johnson NE: Ketamine sedation for pediatric procedures, Part 2: review and implications. Ann Emerg Med 19:1033–1046, 1990.

72. Green SM, Clem KJ, Rothrock SG: Ketamine safety profile in the developing world—survey of practitioners. Acad Emerg Med 3:598–604, 1996.

73. Joint Commission on Accreditation of Healthcare Organizations: Care of Patients: Examples of Compliance. Oakbrook Terrace, IL: Joint Commission on Accreditation of Healthcare Organizations, 1999, pp 87–91.

74. Green SM, Krauss B: The semantics of ketamine [Editorial]. Ann Emerg Med 36:480–482, 2000.

75. Green SM, Rothrock SG, Harris T, et al: Intravenous ketamine for pediatric sedation in the emergency department: safety and efficacy with 156 cases. Acad Emerg Med 5:971–976, 1998.

76. Qureshi F, Mellis PT, McFadden MA: Efficacy of oral ketamine for providing sedation and analgesia to children requiring laceration repair. Pediatr Emerg Care 11:93–97, 1995.

77. Brown L, Green SM, Sherwin TS, et al: Ketamine with and without atropine: what's the risk of excessive salivation? [abstract]. Acad Emerg Med 10:482–483, 2003.

78. Epstein FB: Ketamine dissociative sedation in pediatric emergency medical practice. Am J Emerg Med 11:180–182, 1993.

79. Sherwin TS, Green SM, Khan A, et al: Does adjunctive midazolam reduce recovery agitation after ketamine sedation for pediatric procedures? A randomized, double-blind, placebo-controlled trial. Ann Emerg Med 35:239–244, 2000.

80. Wathen JE, Roback MG, Mackenzie T, Bothner JP: Does midazolam alter the clinical effects of intravenous ketamine sedation in children? A double-blind, randomized, controlled emergency department trial. Ann Emerg Med 36:579–588, 2000.

81. Annequin D, Carbajal R, Chauvin P, et al: Fixed 50% nitrous oxide oxygen mixture for painful procedures: a French survey. Pediatrics 105:e47, 2000.

82. Wattenmaker I, Kasser JR, McGravey A: Self-administered nitrous oxide for fracture reduction in children in an emergency room setting. J Orthop Trauma 4:35–38, 1990.

83. Hennrikus WL, Shin AY, Klingelberger CE: Self-administered nitrous oxide and a hematoma block for analgesia in the outpatient reduction of fractures in children. J Bone Joint Surg Am 77:335–339, 1995.

84. Burton JH, Auble TE, Fuchs SM: Effectiveness of 50% nitrous oxide/50% oxygen during laceration repair in children. Acad Emerg Med 5:112–117, 1998.

85. Wilson S. A survey of the American Academy of Pediatric Dentistry membership: nitrous oxide and sedation. Pediatr Dent 18:287–293, 1996.

86. Gamis AS, Knapp JF, Glenski JA: Nitrous oxide analgesia in a pediatric emergency department. Ann Emerg Med 18:177–181, 1989.

87. Luhmann JD, Kennedy RM, Jaffe DM, McAllister JD: Continuous-flow delivery of nitrous oxide and oxygen: a safe and cost-effective technique for inhalation analgesia and sedation of pediatric patients. Pediatr Emerg Care 15:388–392, 1999.

88. Luhmann JD, Kennedy RM, Porter FL, et al: A randomized clinical trial of continuous-flow nitrous oxide and midazolam for sedation of young children during laceration repair. Ann Emerg Med 37:20–27, 2001.

89. Krauss B: Continuous-flow nitrous oxide: Searching for the ideal procedural anxiolytic for toddlers. Ann Emerg Med 37:61–62, 2001.

90. Nahata MC, Clotz MA, Krogg EA: Adverse effects of meperidine, promethazine, and chlorpromazine for sedation in pediatric patients. Clin Pediatr 24:558–560, 1985.

91. American Academy of Pediatrics, Committee on Drugs: Reappraisal of lytic cocktail/demerol, phenergan, and thorazine (DPT) for the sedation of children. Pediatrics 95:598–602, 1995.

92. Barsan WG, Seger D, Danzl DF, et al: Duration of antagonistic effects of nalmefene and naloxone in opiate-induced sedation for emergency department procedures. Am J Emerg Med 7:155–161, 1989.

93. American Academy of Pediatrics, Committee on Drugs: Naloxone dosage and route of administration for infants and children: addendum to emergency drug doses for infants and children. Pediatrics 86:484–485, 1990.

94. Shannon M, Albers G, Burkhart K, et al: Safety and efficacy of flumazenil in the reversal of benzodiazepine-induced conscious sedation. J Pediatr 131:582–586, 1997.

95. Sugarman JM, Paul RI: Flumazenil: a review. Pediatr Emerg Care 10:37–43, 1994.

Chapter 160

Wound Management

Jason E. Bernad, MD and James M. Callahan, MD

Key Points

Providing proper anesthesia will allow for a complete evaluation, thorough irrigation, and meticulous repair of wounds.

Thorough cleaning and careful examination will identify and prevent most complications associated with wounds.

Proper lighting, adequate hemostasis, and examining the injured area through a complete range of motion will aid in identifying deep tissue trauma (e.g., tendon, joint injury).

Removal of nonviable tissue and foreign bodies is vital to ensure infection does not develop.

Indications

In 2002, there were 110 million emergency department (ED) visits in the United States. Of these, 39.2 million were injury related, with patients under 18 years of age accounting for approximately 3.5 million.[1] Over the last 10 years, there has been a significant decline in open wound–related visits in the pediatric population.[1] Still, the number of pediatric patients with open wound injuries is quite large, and clinicians must have a solid foundation regarding wound types and their proper management.

Wounds are sustained after a mechanical force has been applied to the skin; the types of forces that can produce injury are compression, shear, and tension type forces. These forces, whether alone or in combination, act to produce one of six types of wounds:

- *Abrasions:* loss of epidermis due to forces acting in different directions (e.g., "road rash")
- *Lacerations:* tearing of the tissue secondary to shear forces (e.g., a knife cut)
- *Crush wounds:* result of an object impacting tissue, notably over a bone surface, which compresses the overlying tissue

- *Avulsions:* tissue is completely separated, and will be either in a flap configuration with a small base or completely lost
- *Puncture:* small area whose depth is unknown
- Any combination of abrasion, laceration, crush, avulsion, and puncture

Proper wound management revolves around five fundamental principles:

- Providing proper anesthesia
- Cleaning and careful examination for associated tendon, bone, or neurovascular injury
- Removal of nonviable tissue and foreign bodies
- Closure
- Protection

Equipment

The equipment that should be available for wound management is shown in Figure 160–1.

Wound Preparation

Preparation for wound exploration and closure begins with a history that includes the mechanism of injury and the patient's tetanus immunization status and allergies. Important points to address include any factors that may put the patient at risk for infection or impaired wound healing. This includes, but is not limited to, end-stage renal disease, diabetes mellitus, malnutrition, and compromised immune status. Subsequently, a thorough examination is performed to evaluate tendons, neurovascular status, and bone or joint involvement. Then, a sterile field is established and local anesthesia provided. At that time, a more meticulous examination of the wound is undertaken.

Adequate anesthesia is paramount to obtaining a good examination, and allowing proper irrigation and exploration. Local anesthetics comprise two major classes: the esters and the amides. Lidocaine is one of the most popular of the amides. Prior to infiltration, it is necessary to ascertain whether your patient is allergic to the anesthetic you plan to use. There is little to no cross-reactivity between the two classes. However, patients may also be allergic to the preservative methylparaben, which is used in multidose vials. This preservative is similar in structure to one of the degradation products of the ester anesthetics and may cause problems.[2] In patients with allergies to both classes of local anesthetics,

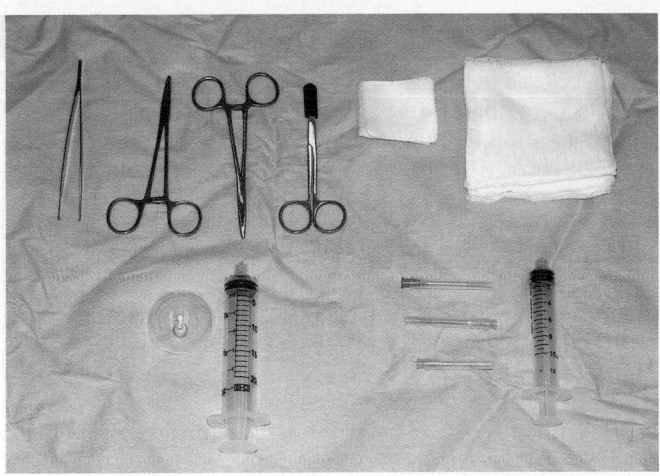

FIGURE 160–1. Equipment used during wound management.

Table 160–1	Maximum Dose of Local Anesthetics (with) and Without Epinephrine
Lidocaine (Xylocaine)*	4 mg/kg (7 mg/kg)
Bupivicaine (Marcaine, Sensorcaine)†	2.5 mg/kg (3 mg/kg)
Mepivicaine (Carbocaine)	4 mg/kg (7 mg/kg)
Prilocaine (never use in patient < 3–6 mo old)	5.5 mg/kg (8.5 mg/kg)

*The maximum dose is 3 mg/kg for intravenous (IV) regional anesthesia (Bier blocks), and even less for a mini-Bier block. Preservative-free lidocaine without epinephrine should be used for Bier or hematoma blocks.
†Due to cardiac toxicity, never use for IV regional anesthesia or hematoma block, do not use <12 years old.

alternatives include the use of cardiac lidocaine (which does not contain a preservative) or the injection of diphenhydramine (which must be injected in a 1% solution to avoid tissue necrosis and has been shown to be more painful than injection of lidocaine).[2-5] Once an agent is chosen, the maximum safe dose is calculated (Table 160–1).

The pain associated with local infiltration of anesthetic is often thought of as a "necessary evil" in wound management, but many options exist for easing this discomfort. These include the use of topical anesthetic prior to infiltration, buffering the lidocaine with sodium bicarbonate in a 1 : 10 solution, warming the lidocaine, infiltration of anesthetic into wound edges instead of outside the wound, use of small needles, and slow infiltration.[2-6]

LET gel (a combination of lidocaine, epinephrine, and tetracaine) has been shown to be effective and equivalent to the infiltration of lidocaine when applied to the face and scalp. If it is applied upon presentation to triage, use of this agent can reduce ED wait times and improve patient (and parent) satisfaction.[7,8] When administering LET, the gel is applied directly into the wound and the wound is covered with cotton for 20 to 30 minutes. Gauze should not be used to cover the wound, since this material will absorb the gel and diminish the amount of LET present within the wound. After 20 to 30 minutes, wound edges that are blanched are likely to have good local anesthesia. At this time, the wound edges are re-evaluated for any missed areas that do not blanch. Some authors have recommended additional infiltration of local

anesthetic, citing the fact that any interruption during the repair process would lead to lost time and decreased patient satisfaction.[7] As with any epinephrine-containing compound, LET gel should not be applied to any area containing an end artery (fingers, nose, toes, ears, and the tip of the penis) or devitalized tissue.

Following achievement of good local anesthesia, the wound is copiously irrigated. The goal of irrigation is to decrease the potential bacterial concentration so that it can be handled by host defenses.[9-13] Normal saline is the irrigating fluid of choice in this situation, although studies have shown no difference in infection rates between saline and tap water irrigation.[12,13] A syringe (preferably 30 to 60 ml) with an attached 18- to 19-gauge angiocatheter or splash guard (to avoid splatter and exposure to bodily fluids) is used for irrigation. Use of constant steady pressure will ensure proper irrigation; very high pressures have been shown to cause trauma to the tissue. The amount of fluid necessary for proper irrigation is tailored to the patient, location of the wound, amount of contamination, and underlying cause of the wound. Wounds should be irrigated with at least 50 to 100 ml of fluid per centimeter of wound.[4] Wounds of the face and scalp (highly vascularized areas with low incidence rates of infection) deserve special mention in this regard. Infection rates and cosmetic appearance do not differ whether these wounds are irrigated or washed with normal saline and gauze if they are noncontaminated and nondevitalized, and patients present within 6 hours of injury.[10]

The use of antiseptic solutions, such as povidone-iodine and hydrogen peroxide, on wounds continues to be an area of controversy. Multiple studies have shown them to be effective at controlling the growth of microorganisms in wounds when used at low concentrations. However, at high concentrations they are cytotoxic and may actually hinder the healing process.[14] Cell death and necrotic tissue left from this process may actually lead to infection. They are primarily useful for cleansing the skin surrounding the wound in preparation for further wound management, but should not routinely be used to irrigate wounds. If used to clean the inside of a wound, the solution needs to be diluted with saline and thoroughly rinsed out of the wound before further wound management and closure.

Techniques

Once a sterile field is established, the clinician should provide local anesthesia and irrigate and thoroughly examine the wound. Proper lighting should always be used to perform the examination. Achieving hemostasis will help maintain a dry field. Techniques that can be employed to ensure hemostasis include direct pressure or a blood pressure cuff placed proximal to the wound and inflated to 20 to 30 mm Hg above the patient's systolic blood pressure. If the wound is on a digit, the clinician can place a sterile glove over the hand, cut off the tip of the glove on the corresponding digit, and roll the glove to the base of the digit.[3,5]

Careful examination of the wound includes putting the area in question through a full range of motion, paying careful attention to those wounds overlying joints and tendons. Any suspected tendon injury or joint involvement will require orthopedic consultation and possibly operative intervention. Clinicians must always exclude a retained foreign body by directly examining wounds and obtaining radiographic studies if there is any suspicion of a retained foreign body (see Chapter 162, Foreign Body Removal).

Hair in the area of the wound should be removed as this has been shown to be a source of contamination.[3,5] Hair should be clipped or cut, since shaving injures the hair follicles and allows greater access to bacteria, increasing infection rates. The eyebrows should never be clipped or shaved as they may not grow back.

During the examination, the clinician should determine if there is any nonviable tissue. This tissue should be excised since nonviable tissue impairs resistance to bacterial infection.[2,4,15] No more tissue should be removed than is necessary. This is especially important in areas with high tension (joints, digits) and areas where cosmetic outcome is significant (e.g., the face). If an extensive area is contaminated, crushed, or devitalized, high-pressure irrigation should be used initially and the tissue then re-evaluated. The option always exists for operative débridement, depending again on the wound's size, location, and degree of contamination. For wounds with jagged edges, conversion to a straight line may improve cosmetic outcome.[15]

Primary closure of wounds can be performed on most patients who present to the ED. While there is a direct relation between the time from injury to wound closure and infection rate, that precise time beyond which wounds should not be closed is controversial.[2,3,5,15-17] Each wound should be considered on an individual basis depending on time of injury, location, contamination, infection risk, and importance of cosmetic appearance.[2,5] For wounds that are highly contaminated, in areas of poor vascular supply, or if the patient is immunocompromised, primary closure should be performed within 6 hours.[3] Clean facial and scalp wounds can be closed up to 24 hours after injury.

Sutures are the most universally used wound closure material. They provide the greatest tensile strength and lowest risk of dehiscence.[5] The proper choice of suture material is dependent on the type of wound, location, depth, and cosmetic goals. While evaluating the wound, the clinician should make note of the depth as well as the tension at the wound edges. Deep sutures should be considered to close deep wounds, diminish dead space and hematoma formation, and decrease tension at the surface of wounds. Deep sutures should be avoided in highly contaminated wounds and in fat due to increased risk of infection.[2,3,5,15] Suture size and timing of suture removal varies with location of wounds (Table 160–2).

Choice of suture material is highly wound dependent (Table 160–3). In general, monofilament and synthetic

Table 160–2 Suture Size and Location

	Face	Scalp	Torso	Extremities	Joints	Oral
Suture size	6-0 to 7-0	3-0 to 5-0	3-0 to 4-0	4-0 to 5-0	3-0 to 4-0	3-0 to 5-0
Suture removal*	3–5 days	7 days	10 days	7–10 days	10–14 days	Absorbable

*Sutures under high tension may need to stay in place longer than the specified time.

Table 160–3 Properties of Various Suture Materials

Suture Material (s)	Absorbable	Synthetic	Properties
Surgical gut (chromic or not)	Yes	No	Plain gut is used for rapidly healing tissues and suturing subcutaneous fatty tissue, fast-absorbing gut is for epidermal use only, and chromic has tensile strength for 10–14 days with a slower absorption rate (due to chromium) and may be used in the presence of infection.
Polyglactin 910 (Vicryl)	Yes	Yes	Multifilament and coated with lactide to slow loss of tensile strength and calcium stearate to permit easy tissue passage and precise knots and tying. Tensile strength is $^2/_3$ by 14 days after use. Causes only minimal tissue reaction; may be used if infection is present, and for soft tissue approximation and vessel ligation. Dexon II has similar properties.
Poliglecaprone 25 (Monocryl)	Yes	Yes	Monofilament with good pliability and handling. Used for subcuticular closure, soft tissue approximation and ligations.
Polydioxanone (PDS II)	Yes	Yes	Monofilament polyester suture with only slight tissue reaction with wound support up to 6 wk. It is used for soft tissue approximations.
Surgical silk, cotton, and steel	No	No	These are rarely used in ED wounds.
Nylon Monofilament (Ethilon/Dermalon)			
Braided (Nurolon/Surgilon)	No	Yes	Pliable, elastic, and good for skin closures. Stronger than silk and minimal tissue inflammatory reaction.
Polybutester (Novofil)	No	Yes	Very elastic and low coefficient of friction, allowing for surface closure while permitting tissue edema and detumesence.
Polyester fiber Uncoated (Mersilene/Dacron)			
Coated (Ethibond/Ti-cron)	No	Yes	Polybutylate coating or silicone coating reduces friction for easy tissue passage and tying. Only minimal tissue reaction. Mostly used for vessel closure and tying prosthesis.
Polypropylene (Prolene)	No	Yes	Monofilament suture that does not adhere to tissues and is easy to pull out/remove. It also holds knots better than other monofilament materials. Can be used in contaminated and infected wounds.

materials are preferable to braided and natural materials because they result in lower infection rates. The optimal suture material is easy to work with and has good tensile strength, minimal tissue reactivity, and excellent knot security. Based on the wound, the clinician must decide whether deep sutures will be placed. If so, an absorbable material should be used. In general, synthetic absorbable materials carry lower infection rates, less tissue reactivity, and more tensile strength than natural material. Polyglactin (Vicryl) is an example of a synthetic absorbable suture, and surgical or chromic gut are examples of natural material. The use of absorbable material need not be limited to the deep structures, as using them for superficial wound closure in children will avoid the traumatic experience of having those sutures removed. Fast-absorbing plain gut sutures are rapidly broken down and are even acceptable for use on the face in children. Cosmetic outcome is excellent as long as families are instructed in the care of the wound and they comply with these instructions. The wound should be gently cleansed with hydrogen peroxide two to three times per day using a cotton-tipped applicator and then bacitracin ointment applied to the wound. This leads to rapid breakdown of the absorbable sutures and decreased scar formation.

Nonabsorbable material (e.g., nylon and polypropylene) is often used for skin closure. This material maintains its tensile strength for more than 60 days and is relatively nonreactive. These sutures require removal.

Suture Technique

Wound closure requires attention to good cosmetic outcome. Simple interrupted sutures can be used for wounds with minimal tension. A suturing technique that allows for a slight eversion of wound edges should be used. This can be accomplished by taking a slightly wider bite at the depth of the wound compared to the surface (Fig. 160–2). During healing and skin remodeling, the wound will flatten out as the tissue below it contracts. Without eversion, the patient will be left with a depressed scar. Also, the suture should be tied in such as way as to approximate the edges, but not so tightly as to cause necrosis due to swelling. When tying deep sutures, the knots should be buried to avoid any further tissue reactivity (Fig. 160–3).

Running sutures can be used to quickly close long wounds that are already well approximated (Fig. 160–4). Running locked sutures can be used for wounds with tension and minimal to moderate bleeding (Fig. 160–5). Since they can impair circulation, they are best suited for areas where cosmesis is less important (e.g., scalp, torso, extremities).

Corner sutures are used to approximate a laceration with a flap. The initial bite begins on the side of the wound on

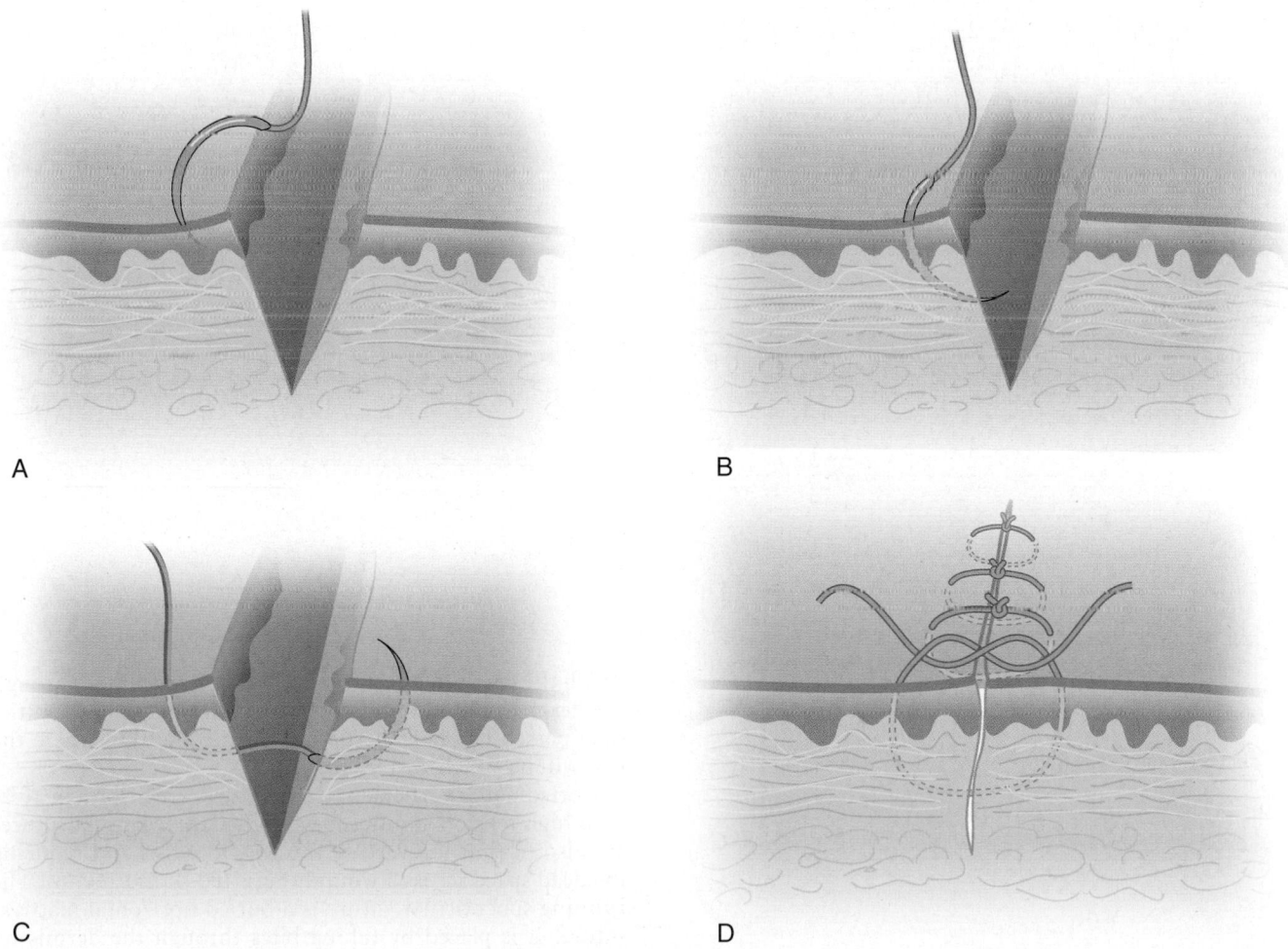

A

B

C

D

FIGURE 160–2. Simple interrupted sutures.

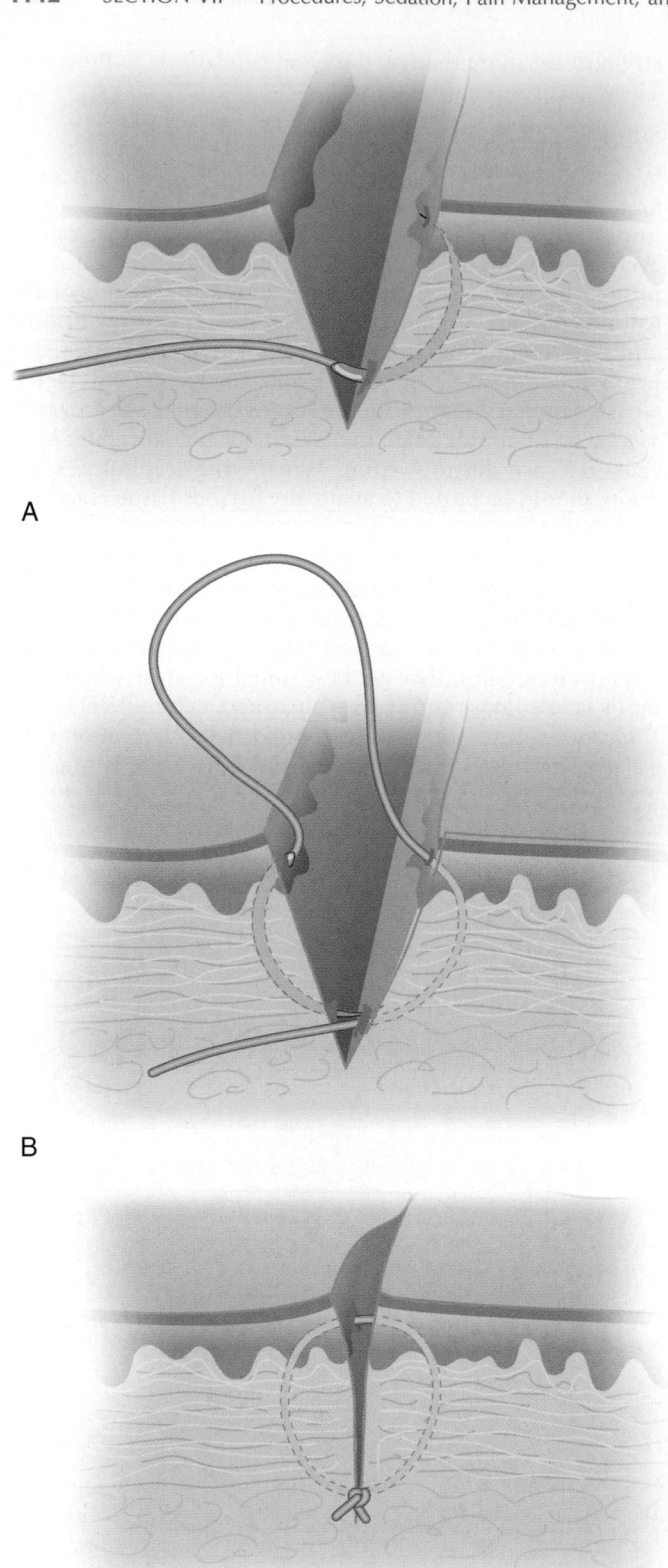

A

B

C

FIGURE 160–3. Deep absorbable sutures with buried knot.

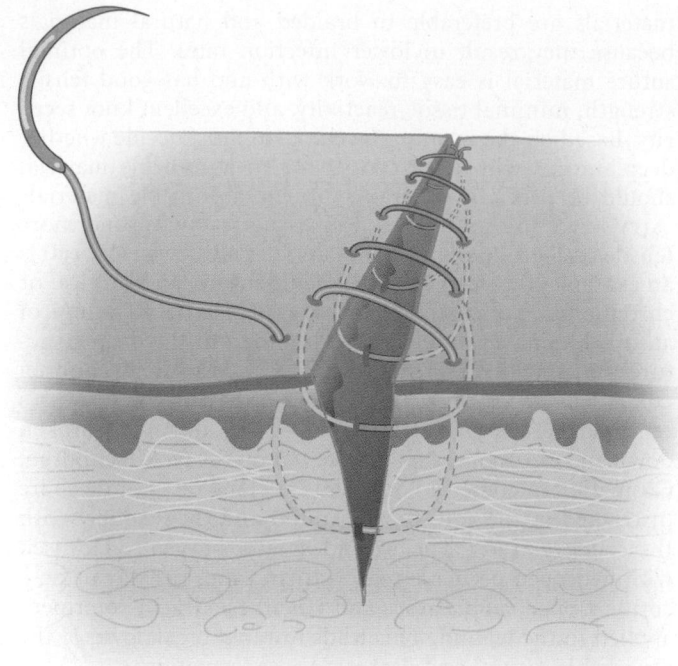

FIGURE 160–4. Running sutures.

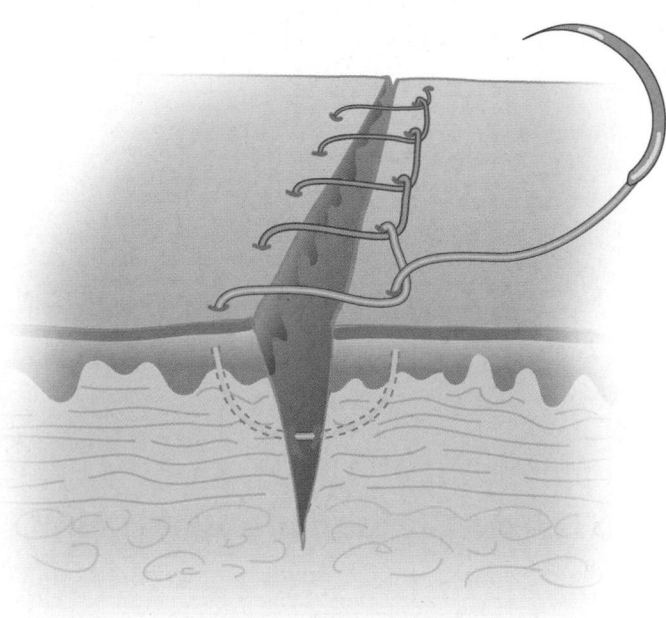

FIGURE 160–5. Running locked sutures.

which the flap is to be attached. The suture is placed through the dermis of the wound edge to the dermis of the flap tip, then passed through the flap to reenter the skin where the flap will be attached (Fig. 160–6).

Horizontal or vertical mattress sutures are helpful in areas with high tension across the wound edges. Mattress sutures are also helpful in everting the wound edges and reducing the dead space across a wound (Figs. 160–7 and 160–8). The running subcuticular suture is a buried horizontal mattress suture. It is placed by taking bites through the dermis on alternating sides of the wound (Fig. 160–9). This technique

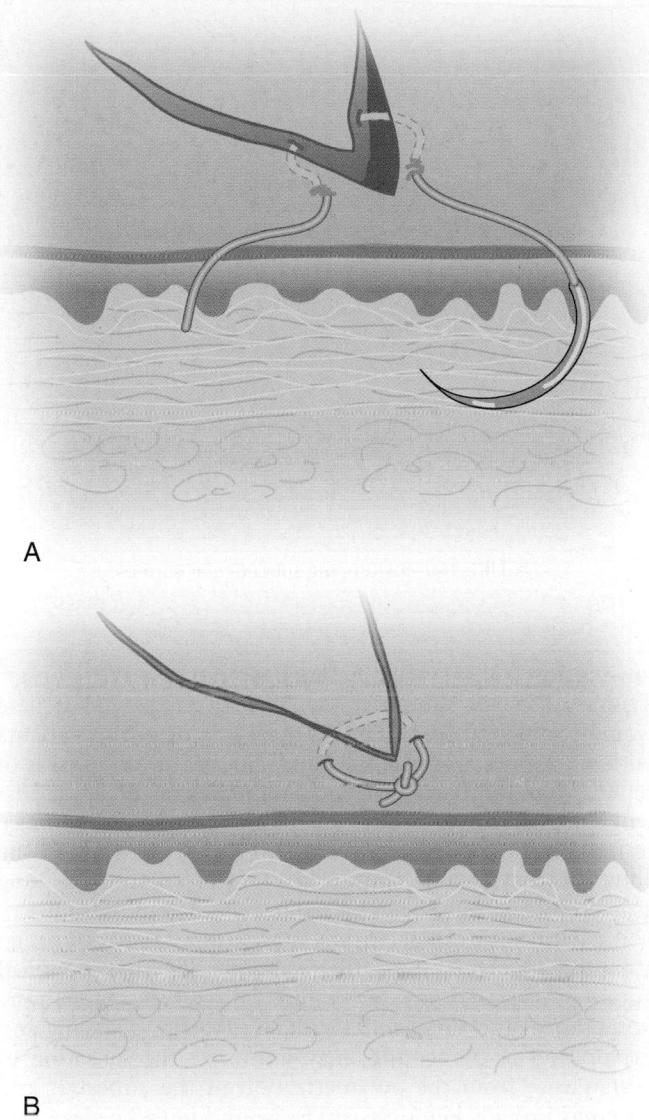

FIGURE 160–6. Corner sutures.

leaves no suture marks, and the suture may be left in place for several weeks.

Alternatives

Staples are an alternative to closure with sutures that offer a more rapid application time and are associated with decreased foreign body reactions and infection rates. This method is useful for wounds of the scalp, trunk, and extremities; they are also useful for very long wounds and situations in which a mass casualty incident may require triage-type wound management until definitive treatment can take place. Their placement is not as esthetically pleasing, and they are not suited for the hands, feet, or face.

Tissue adhesives are cost effective, and allow decreased ED wait times and improved patient and parent satisfaction. They are low risk as no sharp instruments are used, and they require no dressing, have antimicrobial properties against gram-positive organisms, and offer a cosmetic outcome as good as or better than suturing. In addition, there is no need

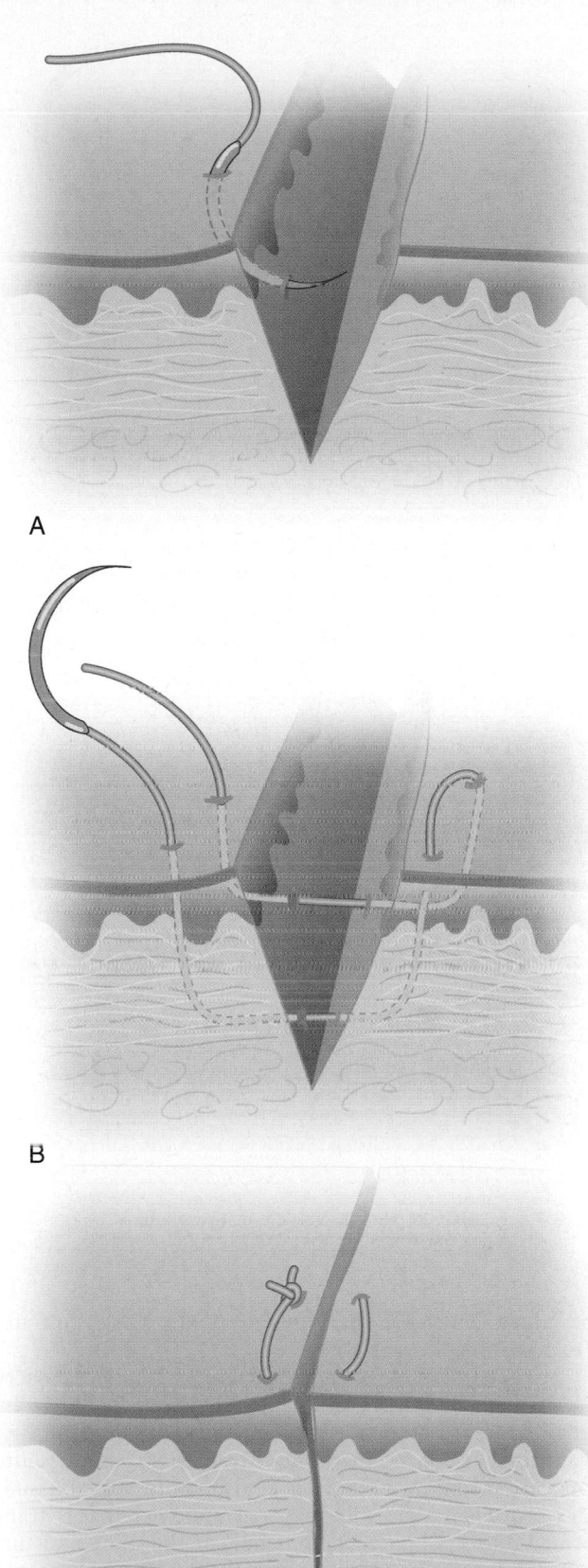

FIGURE 160–7. Horizontal mattress sutures.

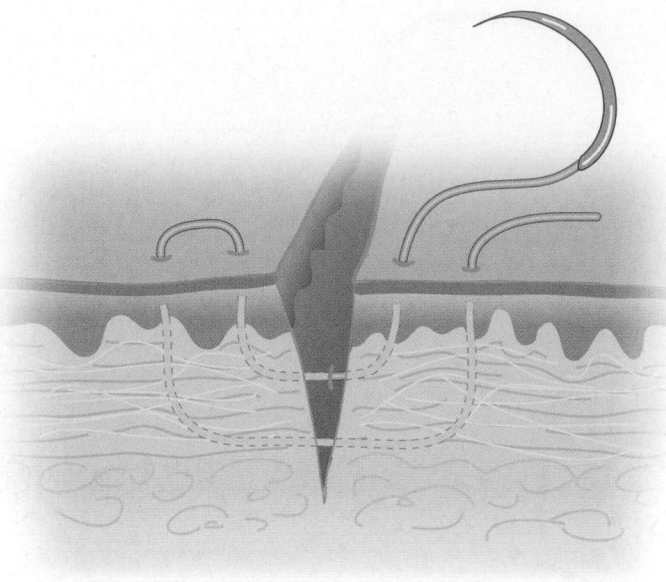

A

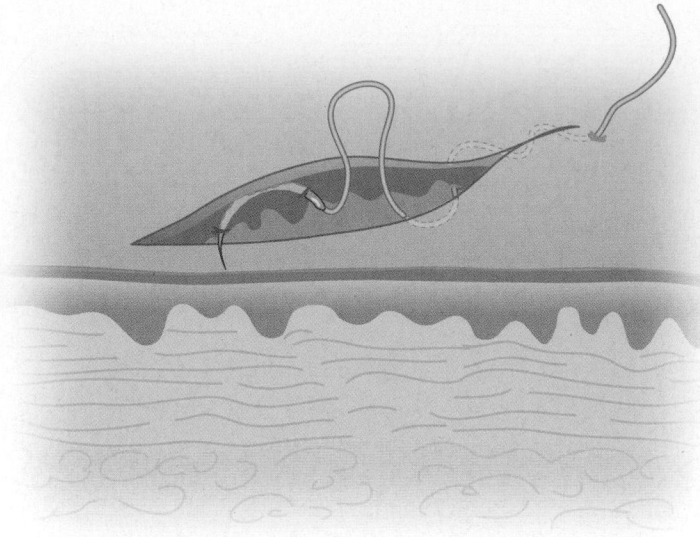

FIGURE 160–9. Running subcuticular sutures.

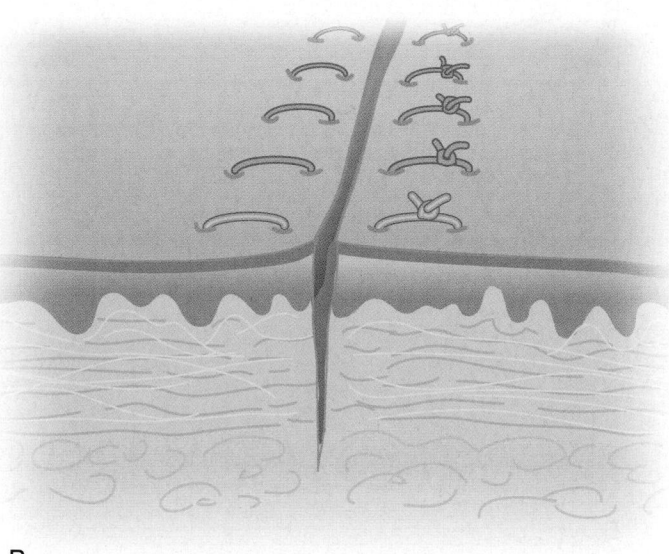

B

FIGURE 160–8. Verticle mattress sutures.

for suture removal as the adhesive usually sloughs off after 7 to 10 days.[3,18-22]

The tissue adhesive most widely used is 2-octylcyanoacrylate (Dermabond; Ethicon). This adhesive is less toxic and provides greater strength than previous adhesives. 2-Octylcyanoacrylate reaches maximum strength $2^1/_2$ minutes after application, and its strength is equivalent to healed tissue 7 days postrepair. The adhesive is a monomer that is transformed into a polymer when it contacts the skin's moisture. This polymer forms a link between the two wound edges and allows healing to occur below. The change from monomer to polymer is exothermic and may be felt by patients. It is best to warn patients that the adhesive will feel warm and may be uncomfortable for young children.

Tissue adhesives are best used for wounds on the face, extremities, or trunk. Wounds that are short (<6 cm) and low tension (<0.5-cm gap between wound edges) are best.[23] Tissue adhesives should be avoided in jagged or stellate wounds, mucosal surfaces, and the axilla or groin. Patients with wounds that overlie the hands, joints, or other areas of repetitive motion are not good candidates as the epidermis will slough prior to proper healing. If used in these areas, immobilization is indicated to ensure proper healing. Tissue adhesives may also be appropriate for deep wounds as long as deep sutures have been placed to reduce skin tension.

As with suture placement, application requires special attention to detail. It is still recommended that a topical anesthetic be used for any wound. This serves several purposes. Local anesthesia will facilitate adequate cleansing and exploration of the wound, may minimize the sensation of heat release from the polymerization of the adhesive, and also may provide hemostasis. The wound must be clean and dry for the adhesive to work properly. After anesthesia and hemostasis, the wound is cleaned and evaluated. The area around the wound is dried, and the tissue edges are carefully aligned. Tissue adhesives are not bioabsorbable—the body will not break them down. Therefore, any adhesive that makes its way into the wound not only will prevent epithelialization, but can provoke foreign body reactions (inflammation, necrosis, and infection).[18,24,25] After good tissue approximation, the plastic vial is cracked and the applicator tip is saturated. New devices have recently become available that are basically a pen with a needle-tipped applicator, which allows for a more precise application. The adhesive is applied in even strokes along the length of the wound in a layered manner, allowing 15 seconds between layers. Four layers are suitable for proper healing. When complete, the wound edges are held together for 30 to 60 seconds for drying.[4] The skill of applying adhesive in a smooth, even manner without extensive runoff or dripping is attained with practice. All drips and runoff should be wiped up immediately. The clinician should pay careful attention when applying tissue adhesive to the forehead, protecting the eyes with gauze pads or applying a Tegaderm dressing over the eye for protection during application.

A wound dressing is unnecessary at this time. Patients and caregivers should be instructed to keep the area clean and dry. Petroleum jelly or antibiotic ointment should not be applied to the wound as either will advance breakdown of the adhesive. Importantly, these agents can be used to remove errantly placed adhesive. After application, the adhesive will slough off in 7 to 10 days with the top layer of skin. An adhesive bandage over the wound may prevent younger children from picking at the tissue adhesive and increase the time until it sloughs off. When placing a bandage over the wound, ensure that the tissue adhesive has completely dried and that only the gauze portion of the bandage comes in contact with the tissue adhesive.

An alternative to complete wound closure is open management. Wounds left to heal on their own will develop more inflammation and edge contraction than wound with edges that are approximated with sutures or tissue adhesives. This may lead to worse cosmetic outcome and possibly loss of function. This is especially true in areas with less vascular supply than the face or scalp. Also, the healing process may be unable to adequately heal an area that has little mobile tissue (i.e., the scalp). One small study found that hand lacerations (<2 cm in length) treated openly had cosmetic outcome at 3 months equivalent to suturing, had less pain during the procedure, and experienced no loss of function.[23] Open management may be considered in situations in which, after adequate irrigation and exploration, the wound is still considered to be highly contaminated and at risk for infection if closed. Puncture wounds, wounds more than 24 hours old, and wounds exposed to organic matter, soil, or feces are often appropriately left open. Wound that are left open can remain open until healing takes place, or they may be closed in a delayed fashion (delayed primary closure). In this instance, the clinician should administer oral antibiotics, cleanse the wound daily, and close the wound 2 to 5 days after the injury.

Finally, wounds that require extensive débridment, prolonged suturing times (e.g., >30 minutes), or meticulous alignment of involved structures (e.g., eyelids, philtrum) or that cover extensive areas may require plastic surgery consultation and possible management under general anesthesia.

Complications

Despite the large number of wounds treated in EDs every year, the rate of infection is extremely low (<1%). Most wound infections are due to poor cleansing and exploration, improper sterile technique, noncompliance with discharge instructions, or selection of dirty wounds that required delayed primary closure or healing by secondary intention. Potentially infected wounds in patients who return to the ED require gentle compression and the removal of enough sutures to allow for drainage. If purulent material is expressed from the wound, more extensive exploration, irrigation, and hospital admission may be required. The sutures may remain in place with one end of the wound remaining open to allow for further drainage. For deep or obviously tense wounds, the clinician should remove sutures and incise the wound (after proper local anesthesia), irrigate it, and pack it with gauze. The gauze is removed in 2 to 3 days and the wound left to heal by secondary intention.[26]

Based on the anatomic location and extent of infection, an intravenous (IV) dose of antibiotics effective against suspected organisms should be administered. The decision to admit or discharge the patient will be based on many factors. These include anatomic location and the extent of infection: whether the infection is localized to the wound area, whether there is significant erythema or purulent drainage, and whether the patient is immunocompromised or is febrile, which may indicate systemic seeding. For localized infections, a single dose of IV antibiotics is administered followed by a course of oral antibiotics. Then, the wound is properly dressed and treated by delayed primary closure. In this case, the patient should return for a wound check and dressing change in 24 hours. If systemic signs of infection develop, the clinician should administer IV antibiotics and admit the patient to the hospital.

Wound dehiscence is usually caused by wounds closed under tension, formation of a hematoma or abscess, or placement of an inadequate number or size of sutures. If dehiscence is noted, the original sutures should be left in place. At the time of standard removal, alternating sutures are removed, leaving the others in place for an additional few days.[26] If dehiscence is noted when the remaining sutures are finally removed, skin tape can be placed until the wound heals. Resuturing is not recommended.

When patients return to the ED for reevaluation, the clinician should always consider the possibility of a missed foreign body, tendon injury, or bone injury. Radiographic examination may be required as well as reexploration of the wound if there is a high suspicion that a foreign body is present.

If there is any question of tendon injury after examination and exploration, the clinician should consider closing the wound, splinting the site and adjacent joints, and arranging orthopedic follow-up. Acute repair of tendon injuries in the ED setting may be associated with an increased complication rate. Repair of tendon or vascular injuries is often safely delayed for 1 to 3 days after closure. The use of microscopic instruments by an experienced operator in the operative setting is often associated with better outcomes and decreased rates of unintentional injuries to nearby nerves or other structures.

Postprocedure Care and Disposition

For all wounds, the clinician must consider whether the patient will need tetanus immunization (see Chapter 103, Tetanus Prophylaxis) or prophylactic antibiotics. Fortunately, less than 1% of all wounds become infected. For this reason, antibiotic use is not routinely recommended.[27] The decision to administer antibiotics is based on the mechanism and extent of injury, as well as the extent of contamination and the patient's immune status. Antibiotics are indicated for human, dog, and cat bites, open fractures, intraoral lacerations, and devitalized or severely contaminated wounds (see Chapter 120, Skin and Soft Tissue Infection).

Following wound repair, placement of a dressing is indicated in all but facial wounds. Optimal dressings will protect the wound from bacteria and foreign material, absorb exudate from the wound, prevent heat and fluid loss from the wound; in addition, they are are nonadherent and provide a warm, moist, occluded environment to maximize epithelialization and minimize pain.[28] The patient should be instructed to keep the initial bandage in place for the first 24 to 48 hours to allow for epithelialization of the initial skin layer.[5] After 72 hours, wounds are resistant to infection from external contamination and dressings are not necessary.[4] The patient may gently wash the wound after the first 72 hours, but should be instructed not to scrub it, as this may disrupt the healing process. Application of antibiotic ointment will help to keep the wound moist and may decrease the likelihood of infection.[3,4] Topical antibiotics should be avoided if tissue adhesives are applied. Sutures on the face may be removed in 3 to 5 days, and those on extremities and most other areas of the body in 7 to 10 days (see Table 160–2).

Areas with high tension and mobility (i.e., joints and digits) should be immobilized. This will allow for proper healing without tension on the wound edges. Extremities should be splinted in their position of function. Sutures in these high stress areas may be removed in 10 to 14 days.

Patients are instructed to return for pain, erythema, drainage, or any evidence that the wound may have become infected. Following suture removal, patients should be instructed to apply sunblock to the healed area whenever they are outside for the next 6 to 12 months, as this will prevent the healed area from becoming hyperpigmented.

Summary

All wounds require anesthesia to allow for careful and thorough cleaning and examination. Foreign bodies, tendon, bone, and neurovascular injury should always be excluded before closing any wound. Choosing the most appropriate technique for closure and then appropriately protecting the wound during the healing process will lead to decreased rates of infection, decreased scarring, and increased patient comfort and satisfaction.

REFERENCES

1. McCaig LF, Burt CW: National Hospital Ambulatory Medicine Care Survey: 2002 emergency department summary. Adv Data 340:1–34, 2004.
*2. Hollander JE, Singer AJ: State of the art laceration management. Ann Emerg Med 34:356–367, 1999.
*3. Singer AJ, Hollander JE, Quinn JV: Evaluation and management of traumatic lacerations. N Engl J Med 337:1142–1148, 1997.
4. Knapp JF: Updates in wound management for the pediatrician. Pediatr Clin North Am 46:201–213, 1999.
5. Capellan O, Hollander JE: Management of lacerations in the emergency department. Emerg Med Clin North Am 21:205–231, 2003.

6. Brogan GX, Giarrusso E, Hollander JE, et al: Comparison of plain, warmed, and buffered lidocaine for anesthesia of traumatic wounds. Ann Emerg Med 26:121–125, 1995.
7. Priestley S: Application of topical local anesthetic at triage reduces treatment time for children with lacerations: a randomized controlled trial. Ann Emerg Med 42:34–40, 2003.
8. Singer AJ, Stark MJ: Pretreatment of lacerations with LET at triage: a randomised double-blind trial. Acad Emerg Med 7:751–756, 2000.
9. Edlich RF: Wound irrigation. Ann Emerg Med 24:88–90, 1994.
10. Hollander JE, Richman PB, Werblud M, et al: Irrigation in facial and scalp lacerations: does it alter outcome? Ann Emerg Med 31:73–77, 1998.
11. Singer AJ, Hollander JE, Subramanian S, et al: Pressure dynamics of various irrigation techniques commonly used in the emergency department. Ann Emerg Med 24:36–40, 1994.
12. Moscati R, Mayrose J, Fincher L, et al: Comparison of normal saline with tap water for wound irrigation. Am J Emerg Med 16:379–381, 1998.
13. Valente JH: Wound irrigation in children: saline solution or tap water? Ann Emerg Med 41:609–616, 2003.
*14. Drosou A, Falabella A, Kirsner RS: Antiseptics on wounds: an area of controversy. Wounds 15:149–166, 2003.
15. Key SJ, Thomas DW, Shepherd JP: The management of soft tissue facial wounds. Br J Oral Maxillofac Surg 33:76–85, 1995.
16. Hollander JE, Singer AJ, Valentine S: Comparison of wound care practices in pediatric and adult lacerations repaired in the emergency department. Pediatr Emerg Care 14:15–18, 1998.
17. Baker MD, Lanuti M: The management and outcome of lacerations in urban children. Ann Emerg Med 19:1001–1005, 1990.
18. Bruns TB, Worthington JM: Using tissue adhesive for wound repair: a practical guide to Dermabond. Am Fam Physician 61:1383–1388, 2000.
19. Singer AJ, Hollander JE, Valentine SM, et al: Prospective randomized controlled trial of tissue adhesive (2-octylcyanoacrylate) vs standard wound closure techniques for laceration repair. Acad Emerg Med 5:94–99, 1998.
20. Quinn JV, Drzewiecki A, Li MM, et al: A randomized, controlled trial comparing a tissue adhesive with suturing in the repair of pediatric facial lacerations. Ann Emerg Med 22:23–28, 1993.
21. Quinn J, Wells G, Sutcliffe T, et al: Tissue adhesive versus suture wound repair at 1 year randomized clinical trial correlating early, 3-month, and 1-year cosmetic outcome. Ann Emerg Med 32:645–649, 1998.
22. Holger J: Cosmetic outcomes of facial lacerations repaired with tissue-adhesive, absorbable, and nonabsorbable sutures. Am J Emerg Med 22:254–257, 2004.
23. Quinn J, Cummings S, Callaham M, Sellers K: Suturing versus conservative management of lacerations of the hand: randomised controlled trial. BMJ 325:299, 2002.
24. Quinn J, Wells G, Sutcliffe T, et al: A randomized trial comparing octylcyanoacrylate tissue adhesive and sutures in the management of lacerations. JAMA 277:1527–1530, 1997.
*25. Reece TB, Maxey TS, Kron IL: A prospectus on tissue adhesives. Am J Surg 182:s40–s44, 2001.
26. Arpey CJ: Postsurgical wound management. Dermatol Clin 19:787–797, 2001.
27. Cummings P, Del Beccaro MA: Antibiotics to prevent infection of simple wounds: a meta-analysis of randomized studies. Am J Emerg Med 13:396–400, 1995.
28. Lionelli GT, Lawrence WT: Wound dressings. Surg Clin North Am 83:617–638, 2003.

*Selected readings.

Vascular Access

Frances M. Nadel, MD, MSCE

Selected Procedures

Peripheral intravenous line placement
Intraosseous needle placement
Central venous access
Umbilical vessel cannulation

Discussion of Individual Procedures

Peripheral Intravenous Line Placement

Peripheral intravenous (PIV) access is a rapid, safe method of delivering medications, fluids, and blood products to the circulating blood system. In children, resuscitation medications given through PIVs have an onset of action and concentration similar to those delivered centrally. The volume of flush following a medication appears to be more important than the type of access.[1]

Venous access should be avoided in areas distal to an injury, such as a fractured limb, because of the possibility of disrupted vasculature and difficulty monitoring for complications associated with extravasated infusions. When possible, areas with edema, overlying burns, or cellulitis should also be avoided. A vein that is scarred from frequent use may be difficult to access.

Families and children are often very anxious about PIV insertion. If time is available, the clinician should explain the procedure prior to insertion as well as during each step. Children should be informed honestly about the painfulness of the insertion to prevent future mistrust. Separating a child from the guardian during a painful procedure may increase the child's anxiety. Instructing parents who are willing to stay for the procedure on how to convey support may be particularly helpful. Families of chronically ill children may have helpful hints regarding access.

Anatomy and Physiology

The smaller vessel diameter and pudginess of infants and young children can make vascular access challenging. In young infants, vessels are more superficial than in adults. PIVs can be inserted in the forearm, hands, feet, scalp, and external jugular veins. On the forearm, the medially located cephalic vein and proximal basilic veins and their branches on the dorsum of the hand are the vessels most commonly used. The cephalic vein that courses over the proximal radius is often overlooked. Since it is firmly fixed to the underlying fascia, it is a reliable site. The radial and ulnar arteries should not be punctured if the veins on the ventral aspect of the wrist are used. The antecubital veins are useful sites when emergency access is required or there is a suspicion of intra-abdominal injury. On the foot, the saphenous vein is another site that is firmly affixed to the underlying tissue. This vessel predictably is located along the anterior aspect of the medial malleous and can be accessed blindly. On the dorsum of the foot, the lateral and medial median and dorsal arch vessels can be accessed as well.

In infants less than 9 months old, the scalp veins can be used. The superficial temporal vein and frontal veins are easily located and relatively large. The superficial temporal vein courses down from the midparietal region to anterior to the ear. The frontal vein is found in the midline of the forehead. Scalp arteries can be differentiated from veins by their tortuosity, presence of a pulse, and flow away from the heart. Fluids or medications injected into an artery will also cause blanching and require removal.

The physician may choose to peripherally access the external jugular vein when other sites have been unsuccessful. It is a large vessel that is easily visible as it passes posteriorly over the sternomastoid muscle from the angle of the jaw. This vessel is harder to cannulate because of its loose affixation to the underlying fascia and the presence of valves. The patient should be placed in Trendelenburg position with lateral neck rotation. Such positioning is contraindicated in a patient with a known or suspected cervical spine injury or in a patient in whom it would interfere with airway management.

Finally, the femoral vein can be accessed via peripheral and central techniques.

There are many commercially available topical anesthetics, such as ELA-max (liposomal lidocaine) and EMLA (lidocaine/prilocaine), that can be used to decrease the pain associated with PIV insertion in the nonemergent setting.[2] The major drawback is that these agents can take up to 30 to 60 minutes to work, though newer products are being developed that may have a quicker onset of action.[3] Additionally, a triage nurse or family member of chronically ill children can be trained to apply the cream when it is suspected that a PIV will be inserted. The cream should be placed on the dorsa of both hands in case the first attempt fails. Injecting buffered lidocaine with sodium bicarbonate in a 9 : 1 ratio at the proposed puncture site can provide immediate anesthesia. However, this requires two punctures, which may be less preferable to families and may serve to obscure the vessel. The use of topical anesthetic or lidocaine is contraindicated in children allergic to any of the components of the medications. Other methods such as iontophoresis, nitrous oxide, and distraction are currently under investigation.[4,5]

Equipment for PIV Insertion

- Retractable needle catheters (14 to 26 gauge)
- Topical antiseptic
- Alcohol swabs
- Tourniquet, rubber band
- Normal saline flush
- Gloves (nonsterile)
- T connectors
- Transparent tape
- Transparent occlusive dressing
- Arm board
- Warm packs, handheld illuminators
- Sharps disposal unit

The operator should have all the equipment easily available prior to starting the procedure. The tape should be cut to the appropriate size and the occlusive dressing removed from the package before beginning insertion. Two health care providers are usually necessary, especially for the young child who will likely need restraint.

Site Identification and Procedure

If the patient is in extremis, the physician should use the largest vessel than can be most easily accessed without interfering with other life-saving procedures.[6] Patients undergoing less emergent access should be placed in a comfortable position and possible sites identified. Normal venous flow distal to the site should be assessed, and, if time permits, topical anesthetic should be applied to likely sites. Warm packs on the distal extremities, tapping the vein, placing the vein in a dependent position, rubbing the site with alcohol, light illumination under the vein, and having older children open and close the hand can help increase peripheral vasodilation and identification of sites.

A tourniquet is applied proximal to the intended site, making sure that the tourniquet does not impede arterial flow. For scalp veins, a rubber band placed around the baby's head can serve as a tourniquet. This scalp tourniquet is easier to remove if two pieces of tape are wrapped around the rubber band to form two pull tabs.

Universal precautions and antiseptic technique must be followed to prevent blood-borne pathogen exposure and catheter-related infections.[7] Gloves do not need to be sterile.[7] Antiseptic is applied in a circular fashion over the proposed site and surrounding area. Chlorhexidine, povidone-iodine, or 70% alcohol can be used for site preparation,[7] waiting 20 to 30 seconds for the area to dry. Wiping away the povidine with an alcohol swab may help visualization.

With an assistant restraining the extremity proximally, and using the nondominant hand, the extremity is held distal to the site. It is best to select the most distal site so that, if necessary, more proximal sites can still be used. With the bevel side of the needle facing upwards, the skin is punctured just below the vessel at a 30- to 45-degree angle. The needle is advanced with catheter until a flashback of blood is seen. Once there is flashback, the needle and catheter are advanced only slightly to make sure the catheter is in the vein. The catheter is angled parallel to the skin and slowly advanced into the vessel, while withdrawing the metal stylet. The plastic portion should slide easily into the vein. Placing a finger just proximal to the catheter tip will help staunch blood return. In infants, young children, and severely hypovolemic patients, there may not be blood return after the initial flashback. In this case, the tourniquet is loosened and the catheter slowly flushed with a small amount of saline. If the PIV flushes easily and no extravasation of fluid is evident, the line is useable. A T connector is attached to the hub of the catheter. A Vacutainer or syringe attached to the T connector can be used to collect blood. For smaller catheters, it may be easiest to allow the blood to drip directly into the specimen tube from the catheter hub. The use of a needleless cap placed on the T connector can reduce further needle exposure. If the first attempt is unsuccessful, the needle portion should not be placed back in the catheter for repositioning as this may cause shearing of the catheter. A new PIV catheter should be used with every attempt.

A semipermeable polyurethane dressing or gauze is used to secure the line.[7] Though the risk of infection is equivalent, the transparent dressing offers better visualization of the site. Before applying the dressing, blood should be cleaned from the area and the skin around the catheter dried to reduce the risk of infection. A tincture of iodine or chlorohexidine may be helpful as well. One method of stabilizing the PIV is taping the hub of the catheter using a chevron configuration (Fig. 161–1).

If the PIV stops flushing after it is taped, gentle traction should be applied to the PIV to locate a functional position, and the PIV retaped. The T connector tubing should be taped separately from the catheter to prevent accidental dislodgement. The PIV can be further protected by placing a soft splint on the extremity on the side opposite the PIV, taped above and below the insertion site, with the limb in a comfortable, functional position. A small limb restraint that encircles the site can further serve to protect the PIV.

Complications

Serious complications are rare.[8] Dislodgement, hematomas, and intravenous infiltrates are common complications. Compression of a hematoma may help decrease swelling, and if associated with a lot of swelling, distal extremity perfusion should be monitored. The volume and type of infiltrate will determine necessary interventions. Small infiltrates of non-

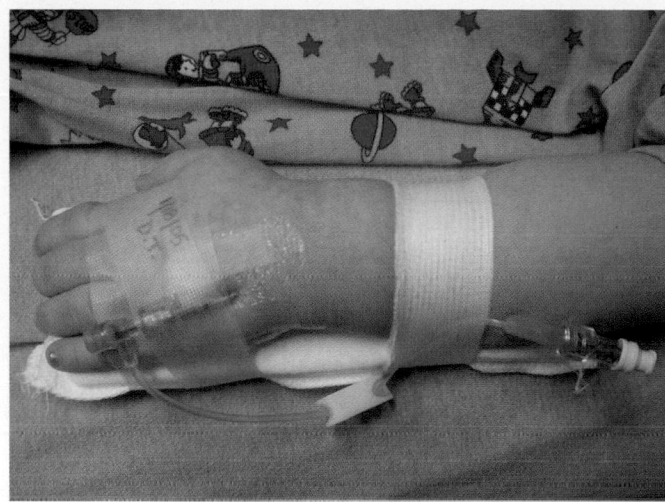

FIGURE 161–1. Peripheral intravenous catheter with a chevron anchor, tape, and board.

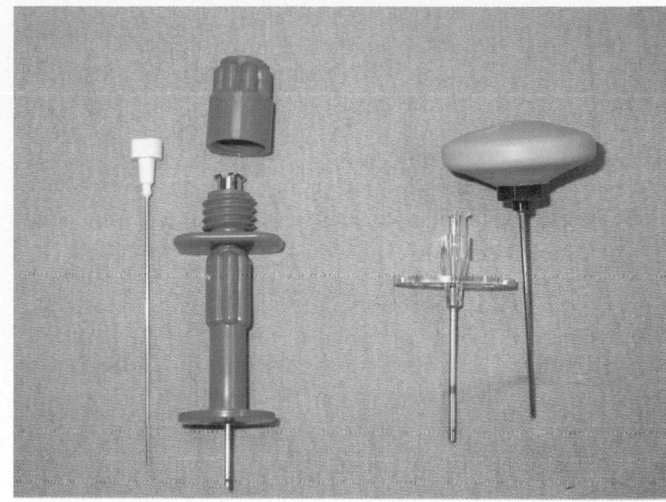

FIGURE 161–2. Jamshidi and Cook catheters. The trocars have been removed.

sclerotic medications usually require compression and elevation alone. Some specific infiltrates may be toxic to the underlying tissue (e.g., vasopressors, promethazine, phenytoin), and specific antidotes may diminish damage. A pharmacist should be consulted for specific medications that may require such therapy (e.g., phentolamine for vasopressors). Arterial puncture, phlebitis, cellulitis, thrombus formation, tendon injury, and nerve injury are less common problems. If infection is suspected, the physician should remove the PIV and administer antibiotics directed at the suspected organism.

Intraosseous Needle Placement

Intraosseous (IO) needle placement is an excellent method for rapidly obtaining vascular access in children with cardiac collapse or arrest.[6] Intraosseous access should be considered in other critically ill or injured children if access is needed emergently and other routes were unsuccessful or would delay therapy. An IO line can be used in any age group, though it may be more difficult to penetrate the thicker cortex of older children and adults. During resuscitation, the onset of action and peak concentrations of medications through the IO route are comparable to the vascular route.[6] Though IO access has been shown to be useful in the neonate and older infant, it is not commonly used in newly born infants because the umbilical vein is more accessible, the small bones are fragile, and the intraosseous space is small in a premature infant.[9,10] Intraosseous access can be used as an alternative route for medications and volume expansion if umbilical or other direct venous access is not readily attainable.[7] For those physicians who infrequently perform neonatal resuscitation, the IO route may be a more rapid method of access than the umbilical route.[11]

Intraosseous lines should not be placed in children with osteogenesis imperfecta or osteopetrosis, and bones that are fractured or infected should not be used. An overlying cellulitis or burn is a relative contraindication. If cannulation was unsuccessful in a bone because the needle went through both cortices, subsequent attempts should not be made in that same location.

Anatomy and Physiology

Blood in the marrow cavity reaches the central circulation through a rich venous network that drains from the central venous sinus into the emissary and nutrient vessels. The rigid marrow cavity is noncollapsible so that it can be accessed even with circulatory failure or hypovolemia. Though the marrow vasculature in the young child is much richer than in older children and adults, IO lines have been used successfully in all age groups. Blood obtained from IO aspiration can be used to assess serum pH, hemoglobin, and blood glucose, and sent for type and crossmatch. As with a central line, an IO line can be used for any medication or blood product.

Equipment for IO Needle Placement

- Antiseptic swabs
- Gloves (sterile if time permits)
- Needle with a trocar: IO/bone aspiration needles (16 to 18 gauge), 20-gauge spinal needle
- Syringe (5 to 10 ml)
- Saline flush
- Tubing
- Hemostat
- Tape
- 1% Lidocaine
- 25- to 27-gauge needle and syringe

The Jamshidi and Cook catheters are two of the most commonly used IO needles (Fig. 161–2). Both have distinct advantages, and individual preference is the primary reason for selection of one system over another. Threaded IO needles offer little advantage over straight needles and may make it difficult to feel the bone give when the marrow space is entered.[13] There are newer IO needles that use a spring-loaded device that injects the needle into bone.[14] This may be particularly helpful in thicker bones, although spring-loaded needles have not been extensively studied in children.

Site Selection and Procedure

Site selection is based primarily on the age of the patient as an estimate of cortical thickness of the bone. In infants less than 2 months of age, the distal femur is preferred as the proximal tibia is often too thin. The proximal tibia is an excellent site until about 3 to 4 years of age, when the cortex becomes more difficult to penetrate. For older child and adults, the area just proximal to the medial malleolus or the anterior iliac spine is thin enough to use for an IO access site. Though the sternum in adults has been successfully used, this location is dangerous in children and not recommended. For the distal femur site, the IO catheter is inserted midline, 2 to 3 cm above the femoral epicondyles. The proximal tibial site is medial and 1 to 2 cm distal to the tibial tuberosity, on the flat part of the tibia.[15] The distal tibial site is entered approximately 1 cm superior to the medial malleolus, on the flat part of the tibia (Fig. 161–3).

If time permits, the physician should glove and sterilely prepare the site. In the conscious or semiconscious child, the skin and periosteum are locally anesthetized with 1% lidocaine using a 25- to 27-gauge needle and syringe. Before inserting the IO needle, the physician should make sure that the trocar is easily removed from the needle and then replaced. Placing the knob of the needle into the palm of the hand, using the dominant hand, the needle is held approximately 1 to 2 cm above the tip using the thumb and index finger. The extremity is grasped with the other hand, making sure the hand is not behind the insertion site. The needle is placed over the desired spot, either at an angle pointed away from the joint/growth plate or perpendicular to the bone. With a gentle clockwise-and-counterclockwise twisting motion, the needle is drilled into the bone until a sudden release of resistance is felt, indicating access into the marrow. Insertion is stopped immediately, the Luer-Lok connector of the needle is held in the nondominant hand, and the trocar is removed by unscrewing it. Confirmation of proper placement includes (1) a needle that stands firmly without moving, (2) aspiration of bone marrow, and (3) easy flushing with saline. Bone marrow can only be aspirated from a properly inserted IO about half of the time. Aspirated marrow can be sent for all the usual laboratory tests except a complete blood count.[16] Though a properly placed IO will stand on its own, it should be secured to avoid accidental dislodgement. One method is to place a hemostat around the needle where it enters the skin and taped as depicted in Figure 161–4.

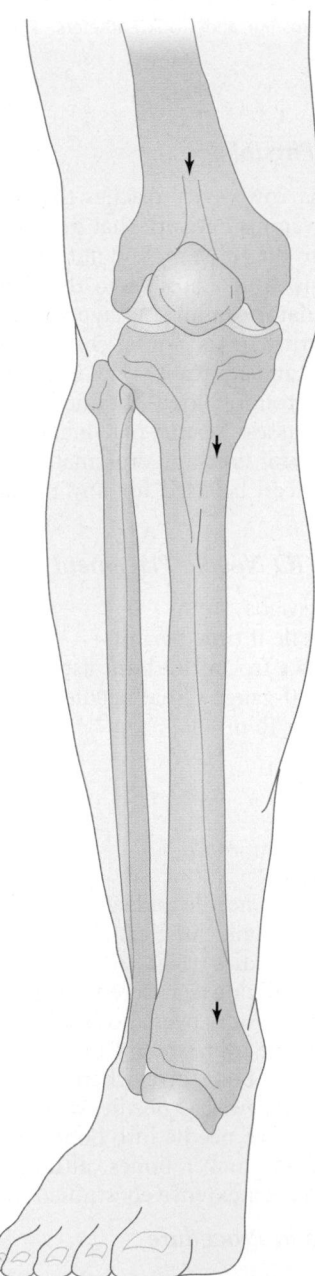

FIGURE 161–3. Common intraosseous needle sites.

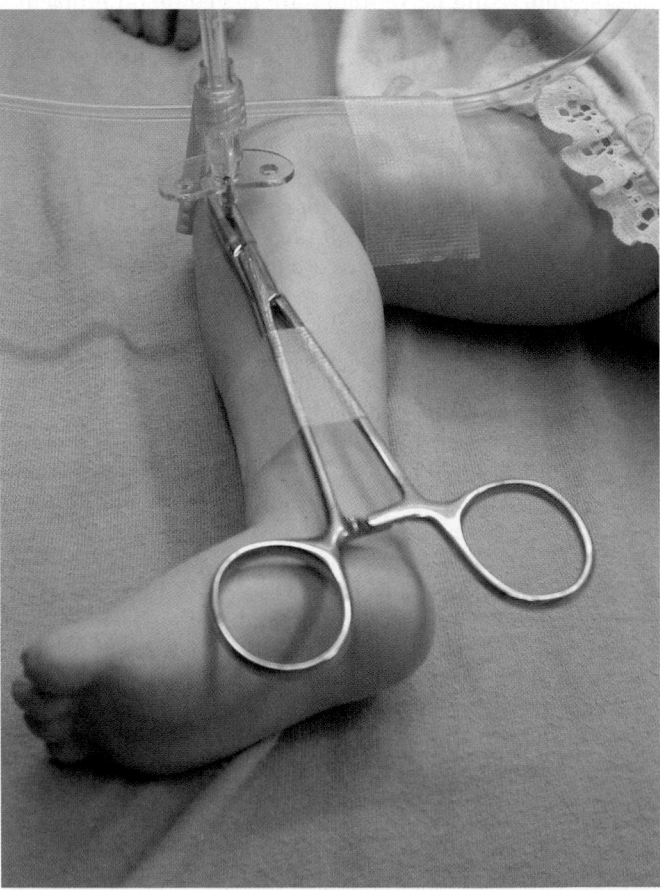

FIGURE 161–4. Securing an intraosseous line with a hemostat on a mannequin model. Note the tubing is taped separately.

Complications

The most immediate complication is the inability to place an IO line because the needle cannot penetrate the bone or the needle went into and through the bone. Subcutaneous infiltration of a large volume of fluid or medications in an improperly placed IO catheter may cause compartment syndrome. The area around and posterior to the IO site should be carefully monitored for swelling that may indicate fluid extravasation. Later complications may include osteomyelitis and cellulitis. The risk of infection is directly related to the duration of IO use. For this reason, the needle should be removed promptly when more definitive access is obtained. Fat embolism and growth plate injury are theoretical risks of the procedure of unknown clinical significance.

Central Venous Access

Central venous access should be considered in critically ill or injured children who require large-volume resuscitation or multiple infusions, medications, or hypertonic solutions that can only be delivered centrally, or who require central venous monitoring. Central venous access is also used in children who require immediate intervention due to critical illness and in whom peripheral access cannot be obtained.

Central venous lines should not be placed in abnormal vasculature such as a scarred or thrombosed vessel, or if perfusion distal to the proposed site is compromised. Relative contraindications to femoral access include an ipsilateral femoral hernia, abdominal trauma, or an abdominal tumor. In general, known or suspected injury to a limb or vasculature proximal to the proposed site, as well as overlying burns, cellulitis, or edema, are relative contraindications. Acquired and congenital bleeding disorders are relative contraindications, especially in the internal jugular and subclavian veins where hemostasis may be difficult to obtain or may result in airway obstruction.

Anatomy

In children, the femoral site offers many advantages over subclavian or jugular veins, including the high rate of success for relatively inexperienced physicians, visible/palpable landmarks, the low risk of serious complications, and the lack of interference with airway management and chest compressions.[17,18] The femoral vein is located in the femoral sheath medial to the femoral artery and nerve. It becomes the external iliac vein as it passes under the inguinal ligament.

The smaller neck area and difficulty in identifying landmarks make the jugular veins difficult to use in children. The internal jugular vein lies in the carotid sheath, alongside the carotid artery and vagus nerve. It courses vertically down the neck and empties into the subclavian vein behind the sternoclavicular joint. The right internal jugular is easier to cannulate because it follows a straight course to the subclavian vein, whereas the left joins at a more acute angle. The subclavian vein lies behind the middle third of the clavicle in the lower part of the supraclavicular triangle. It lies medial to the posterior sterncleidomastoid (SCM) muscle and lateral to the anterior border of the trapezius muscle. It begins at the outer border of the first rib, extending to the sternal border of the clavicle, where it joins the internal jugular vein.

The subclavian approach is made more difficult because the chest shape in small children may make them more susceptible to a pneumothorax and the subclavian vein is smaller in diameter compared to the internal jugular vein.[19] If subclavian lines are attempted, the right side of the neck is preferred because of the lower right pleural dome and the smaller right thoracic duct. However, under the age of 1 year, the right subclavian vein angles more acutely than in older children, first arching superiorly (cephalad) before coursing centrally and caudally into the superior vena cava.[19] This acute angle may make placement of a right subclavian central catheter into the superior vena cava difficult in infants less than 1 year old, and the left side may easier to cannulate at this age.

Procedural sedation should be considered in awake or semiconscious patients. Specific medications will depend on the physician's preference and the patient's condition.

Equipment for Central Venous Access

It is important that all the equipment is ready before the procedure starts. Prepackaged, commercially available central line kits simplify the gathering of equipment. Many emergency departments have designed additional trays with the necessary equipment not included in the commercially available kits:

- Antiseptic solution
- Sterile gloves, gowns, and masks
- Sterile drapes, gauze
- Lidocaine 1%, syringe, and 23- to 27-gauge needle
- Central line catheter
- Guidewire
- Introducer needle and syringe
- Heparinized saline
- Suture material (3-0 or 4-0 silk)
- Needle driver
- Scalpel
- Dressing material
- Blood sample collection tubes

A child's age, weight, or height can be used to guide selection of appropriate catheter sizes and depth (Tables 161–1 and 161–2).

Pulse oximetry and cardiorespiratory and blood pressure monitoring are required for all patients undergoing central venous line placement. Additional monitoring may be necessary based on the patient's condition and whether or not procedural sedation is being used. If attempting subclavian or internal jugular vein access, equipment necessary to decompress a pneumothorax should be readily accessible.

Procedure

The methods below describe central line insertion using the Seldinger technique, in which the catheter is passed over a guidewire. This technique is a safe, rapid means of central venous access in the emergency department.

In appropriate patients, the physician should obtain consent and consider procedural sedation. All necessary equipment is placed nearby to minimize contamination by the operator, assistants, or patient. An appropriate catheter size is chosen based on the patient's age and weight. The kit is opened, all lines are flushed with saline, and the dressing material is placed nearby. Universal precautions are used throughout the procedure. A sterile gown, gloves, and mask should be used when possible, though there is no evidence that this decreases the risk of infection.[7]

Table 161–1	Right Internal Jugular and Right Subclavian Vein Central Venous Catheter Depth (in cm)*		
	Height < 100 cm		**Height 100 ≥ cm**
Initial catheter insertion based on patient height/length†	Initial catheter depth = Height (cm)/10 − 1 cm		Initial catheter depth = Height (cm)/10 − 2 cm
	Approx. Age	**Weight (kg)**	**Length/Depth (cm)**
Initial catheter insertion based on patient weight‡	0–2 mo	3.0–4.9	5
	>2–5 mo	5.0–6.9	6
	6–11 mo	7.0–9.9	7
	1–2 yr	10.0–12.9	8
	>2–6 yr	13.0–19.9	9
	>6–9 yr	20–29.9	10
	>9–12 yr	30–39.9	11
	>12–14 yr	40–50	12

*Adapted from Andropoulos DB, Bent ST, Skjonsby B, Stayer SA: The optimal length of insertion of central venous catheters for pediatric patients. Anesth Analg 93:883–886, 2001. Formulas will place 97% to 98% of catheters above right atrium.
†If height is less than 100 cm, skin for SC vein is punctured 1 cm lateral to the midclavicle, if height is greater than 100 cm, it is punctured 2 cm lateral.
‡Note: chart and formula are based on patient's weight when known, and age is only approximated based on patient weight.

Table 161–2	Central Venous Catheter Size Based on Patient Age, Length/Height and Weight		
Age	**Weight (kg)**	**Length/Height (cm)**	**French Size**
Premature	≤2.5	<50	2.0–2.5
Birth–30 days	3–4	50–55	3.0
>1 mo–1 yr	4.5–10	55–75	3.0–4.0
>1–7 yr	11–25	76–120	4.0–5.0
>7–15 yr	26–60	125–175	5.0–8.0

POSITIONING

For femoral access, the child's hip is abducted and externally rotated. To improve exposure and create a firmer surface, a rolled towel can be placed under the ipsilateral hip. For the jugular and subclavian veins, the patient should be positioned supine, arms at the side, with the head down at about a 15-degree angle and rotated away from the proposed site. The head-down, or Trendelenburg, position is used to decrease the risk of air embolus as well as distend the vessels. Over-rotation of the head past 30 degrees may cause the internal jugular vein to be compressed. For subclavian access, there is some controversy on optimal positioning in children. Though the cross-sectional area of the vein appears to be largest with the child's head in a neutral position with the chin midline, tilting the head toward the puncture site may improve the success rate of right subclavian access.[20,21]

SITE IDENTIFICATION

The femoral vein is the preferred central venous access site in children, while either the internal jugular, subclavian, or femoral veins are appropriate for adolescents. Unlike in adults, use of the femoral vein is not associated with an increased rate of catheter-related infections compared to other central venous sites.[21]

The femoral vein is located 1 to 2 cm medial to the femoral arterial pulse. When there is a weak or absent pulse, the femoral vein can be assumed to be located halfway between the pubic tubercle and the anterior iliac spine. The entry needle is inserted at a 10- to 20-degree angle for infants and a 30- to 45-degree angle for children. Needle entry should be 1 to 2 cm below the inguinal ligament to prevent inadvertent peritoneal perforation.

The median portion of the internal jugular vein is located lateral to the carotid artery, at the apex of the triangle formed by the sternal and clavicular heads of the SCM muscle (Fig. 161–5). More precise localization can be accomplished by using a vascular probe (within a sterile glove) during bedside ultrasonography. Moreover, needle insertion and advancement relative to the internal jugular vein can be monitored if bedside ultrasonography is available. Using the middle internal jugular approach, the child's head is rotated to the contralateral side. The needle is inserted just below this apex, at a 30-degree angle, directed toward the ipsilateral nipple. Using the posterior internal jugular approach, the needle is inserted just superior to the external jugular vein as it crosses the posterior border of the sternomastoid (see Fig. 161–5). The needle is directed caudally and medially toward the sternal notch under the lateral border of the sternomastoid. Using this approach, the internal jugular vein will be punctured before the carotid artery and the pleural dome will be avoided.

The external jugular vein (EJV) is used only when it can be visualized directly or by ultrasound. The EJV is accessed as it crosses over the SCM muscle. Because it is not firmly fixed to the underlying fascia, it is helpful to apply tension above the puncture site to stabilize the vessel. Using an angiocatheter instead of an entry needle may prevent through-and-through EJV perforation. The angiocatheter is inserted at a 10- to 20-degree angle, and when flashback is obtained, the needle is withdrawn and the guidewire inserted through the plastic catheter. Prior to insertion, the operator should check that the guidewire will pass through the plastic catheter.

An infraclavivular or supraclavicular approach can be used to access the subclavian vein. Use of the patient's right side is preferred due to the lower pleural dome, because there is a more direct route to the superior vena cava, and because the thoracic duct will not be injured since it is on the left side. In the infraclavicular approach, the needle is inserted infe-

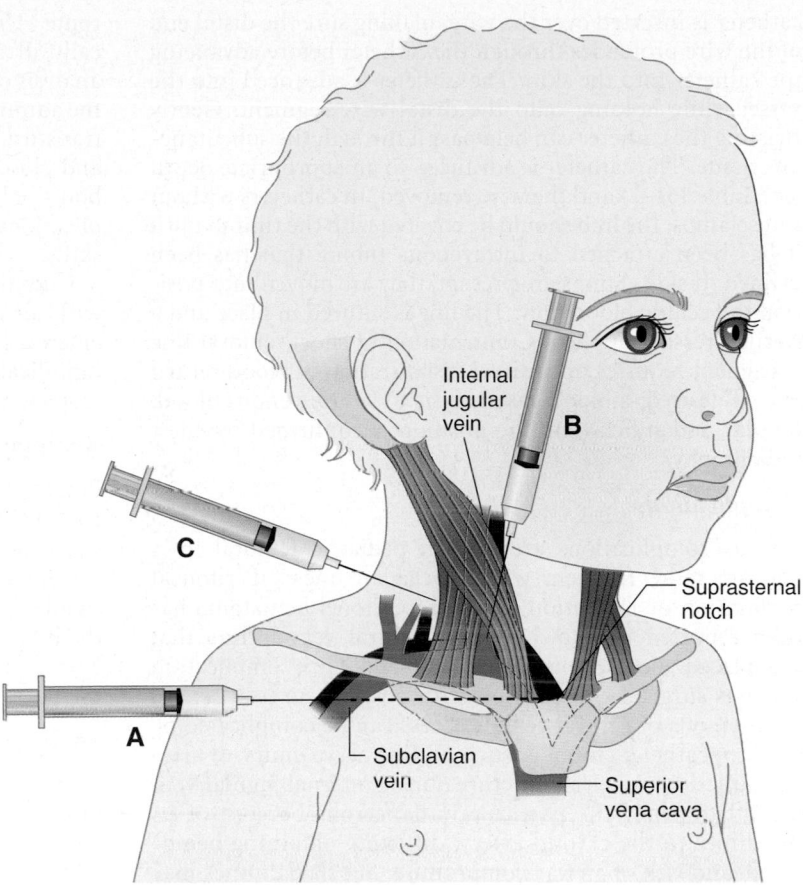

FIGURE 161–5. Insertion sites for **(A)** subclavian vein infraclavicular approach, **(B)** middle internal jugular vein approach, and **(C)** posterior internal jugular vein approach.

rior to the midclavicle (see Fig. 161–5). The needle should be maintained in the horizontal plane, and directed toward the sternal notch. In the supraclavicular approach, the needle is inserted superior to the clavicle at the point where the lateral border of the clavicular head of the SCM muscle joins the clavicle. The bevel of the needle should be directed medially and the needle advanced toward the contralateral nipple, parallel to the clavicle.

Technique

For internal jugular and subclavian approaches, the patient is placed in Trendelenburg position and the head is turned to the contralateral side. In awake or semiconscious patients, the skin and subcutaneous area are locally anesthetized with lidocaine. If desired, a small-gauge (23- or 25-gauge) finder needle and syringe can be used to locate the vessel. This needle can be left in place to guide the path of the entry needle or removed and the same path cannulated with the entry needle. Prior to use, the entry needle should be flushed with heparinized saline. The needle and syringe are slowly advanced while gently aspirating until there is blood return, continuing to advance the needle just slightly while maintaining negative pressure. If blood return stops, this may mean the posterior wall of the vessel was perforated. The needle is gently withdrawn while aspirating until there is free-flowing blood again. If no blood return is obtained, the physician should withdraw the needle to just below the skin entry site, reconfirm landmarks, and reattempt cannulation.

Once there is good blood return, the syringe is removed from the entry needle, placing a thumb over the hub to prevent excessive blood loss or air embolus. If the blood is bright red or pulsating, it is likely that the artery has been cannulated, and the needle should be removed and pressure applied over the site. If it is difficult to determine if the vein or artery has been accessed, an arterial blood gas analysis may be helpful.

Next, the guidewire is inserted. The wire may be straight or have a flexible curved proximal end that is encased in a plastic sheath. Curved wires, or J wires, are particularly helpful in negotiating more tortuous vessels such as the EJV. The sheath is inserted into the hub, slowly advancing the wire. If resistance is met, it suggests that the vessel has not been properly cannulated or the wire is frayed. If this occurs, the wire should be removed and inspected. If there is no fraying, the physician should make sure blood flow is easily aspirated.

The distal end of the wire should always be visible to prevent its full insertion into the vessel. The wire is advanced to an appropriate depth, a little more than one half to three fourths of its total length. Then the index finger of the nondominant hand is placed at the entry site while the dominant hand removes the entry needle and sheath together. The physician should press down on the wire at the entry site during this process to ensure that it is not removed as well.

To allow easy passage of the more fragile plastic catheter, the entry site is enlarged with a scalpel. The blade is inserted over the wire and, with the sharp side pointed away from the patient, a 0.5-cm line is incised up through the subcutaneous tissue and skin. Next, a single-lumen dilator is inserted over the wire to enlarge the tract for the catheter. Then the plastic catheter is inserted over the wire, making sure the distal end of the wire protrudes through the catheter before advancing the catheter into the skin. The catheter is advanced into the vessel while holding onto the distal wire segment. Gently twisting the catheter can help pass it through the subcutaneous tissue. The catheter is advanced to an appropriate depth (see Table 161–1) and the wire removed. In catheters without slide clamps, the hub should be covered with the thumb until it has been attached to intravenous tubing that has been primed. If side clamps are present, they are moved into position to occlude blood flow. The line is sutured in place and a sterile dressing applied. Confirmation of short femoral line placement requires only direct visualization of blood return and, if desired, a blood gas analysis to assure venous blood. Jugular and subclavian line position is confirmed by chest radiography.

Complications

Serious complications are rare in pediatric femoral lines and are more frequent with subclavian lines.[17] Peritoneal perforation or formation of a retroperitonel hematoma has been reported due to a femoral central venous line that was placed above the inguinal ligament. This complication requires surgical consultation with possible surgical repair. All methods of central venous access can be complicated by an air or catheter embolus, surrounding nerve injury, or arterial puncture. Arterial puncture during internal jugular vein cannulation may be particularly dangerous because of its proximity to the carotid artery, difficulty obtaining hemostasis, and risk of airway compromise. Subclavian lines may be also be complicated by pneumothoraces, thoracic duct injury, dysrhythmias, and cardiac tamponade. Vessel wall perforation and erosion are rare complications; proper catheter positioning and appropriate sizing decreases these risks.

Thrombosis and catheter-related infections are delayed complications. Thrombosis may be prevented by use of heparinized solutions or flushes and rapid removal of the catheter. Recent studies have not shown an increase risk of clinically significant thrombosis with femoral lines.[17,18] Aseptic technique in placement and caring for the catheter may decrease the risk of infection. Unlike in adults, pediatric femoral lines are not more likely to become infected than lines at other sites.[7,22] There is growing evidence that an antiseptic sponge dressing and catheters impregnated or coated with antimicrobial or antiseptic agents may decrease the risk of catheter-related infection.[7] It is unclear if an antimicrobial ointment applied at the insertion site prevents infection, and it may cause emergence of bacterial resistance. Some ointments may cause breakdown of the catheter, and compatibility should be assessed before using them.

Umbilical Vessel Cannulation

Umbilical vessel cannulation can be a rapid means of obtaining vascular access in the critical ill newly born infant in the emergency department. Umbilical venous catherization (UVC) should be considered in newborns up to 2 weeks of age who are critically ill and require intravenous fluids, medications, or blood products when alternative means of access are not readily obtainable. In the neonate who has not responded to tracheally administered epinephrine, or who requires volume expansion, UVC is the next recommended

route.[9] Umbilical arterial catherization is indicated for critically ill neonates who require frequent arterial blood gas analysis or blood pressure monitoring. It can also be used for the administration of fluids and medications, or for exchange transfusions. Oxygen causes the umbilical artery to spasm and close, so insertion is best accomplished in the first 24 hours of life. Umbilical access is associated with serious complications and requires considerable experience and advanced skills.

Umbilical cannulation must not be attempted in neonates with an omphalocele, omphalitis, suspicion of necrotizing enterocolitis, inadequate bowel perfusion, or peritonitis. An umbilical arterial catheter must not be placed if there is a suspicion of vascular compromise of the lower extremities.

Anatomy and Physiology

Prenatally, the umbilical vessels serve as a blood exchange conduit between the fetus and placenta. Most infants have two umbilical arteries and one umbilical vein. The arteries are usually located above the vein and have a thicker wall and smaller lumen. The artery enters the abdominal aorta through the internal iliac artery. The umbilical vein is approximately 2 to 3 cm in length and joins the central circulation through the portal vein.

Equipment for Umbilical Vessel Catheterization

A great deal of specialized equipment is required for umbilical cannulation. Emergency departments planning to perform such a procedure should have prepackaged kits with all the required materials available. In addition, this procedure should be done under a radiant heater with temperature monitoring since the critically ill neonate is especially vulnerable to hypothermia.

- Radiant warmer
- Sterile gown, gloves, mask, cap
- Antiseptic solution
- Sterile drapes and gauze
- Umbilical tape
- Scalpel
- Curved, smooth iris forceps
- Two curved mosquito hemostats
- Straight Crile forceps
- Iris scissors
- Needle holder
- Umbilical catheters (3.5, 4, and 8 French)
- 3-0 and 4-0 silk suture on a needle, or with a needle driver
- 10-ml syringe
- Saline flush
- Intravenous tubing, pump
- Three-way stopcock
- Needle (20 to 22 gauge)
- Cardiac monitor, pulse oximeter
- Tape measure

Patients undergoing umbilical catherization require constant cardiorespiratory monitoring. Often it is helpful to have a second person responsible for monitoring since the physician may be primarily focused on the procedure. Besides visually assessment, continuous electrocardiography, pulse oximetry, and patient temperature should be monitored. Other monitoring will depend on the patient's specific condition.

Procedure

The procedure varies slightly depending on the urgency of access needs. For emergent access, the umbilical vein is catherized first. A stopcock is attached to the catheter and flushed with (heparinized) saline, making sure there is no air in the system and the stopcock is in the off position to the patient. The procedure should be performed as sterilely as possible and, at a minimum, the stump and abdomen cleaned with povidone-iodine solution. If time permits or there is a lot of bleeding from the stump, the stump base should be encircled with the umbilical tape and the tape tied with a single knot. The tape should be placed around the skin and not the actual cord, and the knot should not be tied so tight as to impede passage of a catheter or so loose as to allow constant blood oozing. The stump is grasped and the distal part cut off horizontally about 1 to 2 cm above the base. The umbilical catheter is inserted until there is free flow of blood, usually about 1 to 2 cm below the skin. If no blood returns at this depth, the catheter is flushed and aspirated back. This lower position assures that the catheter is not in the liver, and it can be used immediately without need for radiologic confirmation of position.

In the stabilized, critically ill patient, the umbilical artery often is accessed first. The patient is placed supine under a radiant warmer in a frog leg position. The necessary equipment should be in an easily accessible place that minimizes cross contamination. The physician should don a mask and gown and sterilely prepare the stump and abdomen. An eyelet drape may be particularly helpful. Umbilical tape is used and the cord incised as described for umbilical vein catheterization.

For arterial catherization, the edges of the stump are grasped near the artery with the two curved hemostats, or a single hemostat is used to grasp a single edge to further expose the artery, being sure not to crush the artery. Using the curved iris forceps, the artery is dilated by gently opening and closing the forceps until the tip easily passes to about a depth of 1 cm. Keeping the forceps open and in the artery, the catheter is inserted. Resistance encountered before passing beyond the abdominal wall may indicate that the umbilical tape is too tight and should be loosened. Resistance may also occur at the abdominal wall where the vessel turns caudally. Gently pulling the stump up and toward the infant's head may help. Resistance may also be felt at about 5 to 6 cm of insertion depth. Gently twisting the catheter may help bypass this junction of the umbilical artery to the internal iliac artery. The catheter is inserted to the predetermined length (see later) and aspirated for blood. Lack of blood flow may indicate a false track, and the line should be removed.

To secure this line, the stump is encircled with a purse-string suture and tied tightly around the catheter at the entry site. A bridge can then be constructed from tape to further stabilize the line (Fig. 161–6).

For UVC the procedure is similar, though the vessel often does not need to be dilated. The umbilical vein is larger than the arteries and is often collapsed on itself. Visible clots should be removed. A 5.0 catheter is usually sufficient for most infants, but for large infants an 8.0 French catheter may be needed.

UMBILICAL LINE POSITION

Umbilical arterial lines can be placed above or below the diaphragm (high or low positions). High umbilical arterial lines have less clinically obvious ischemic complications, a reduced incidence of aortic thrombosis, and a longer duration of catheter usability without an increase in serious complications.[23] To estimate insertion depth, the distance from the patient's umbilicus to the shoulder is measured. A quick approximation of a high umbilical arterial position is adding 1 cm to the umbilical stump–to-shoulder distance. The low

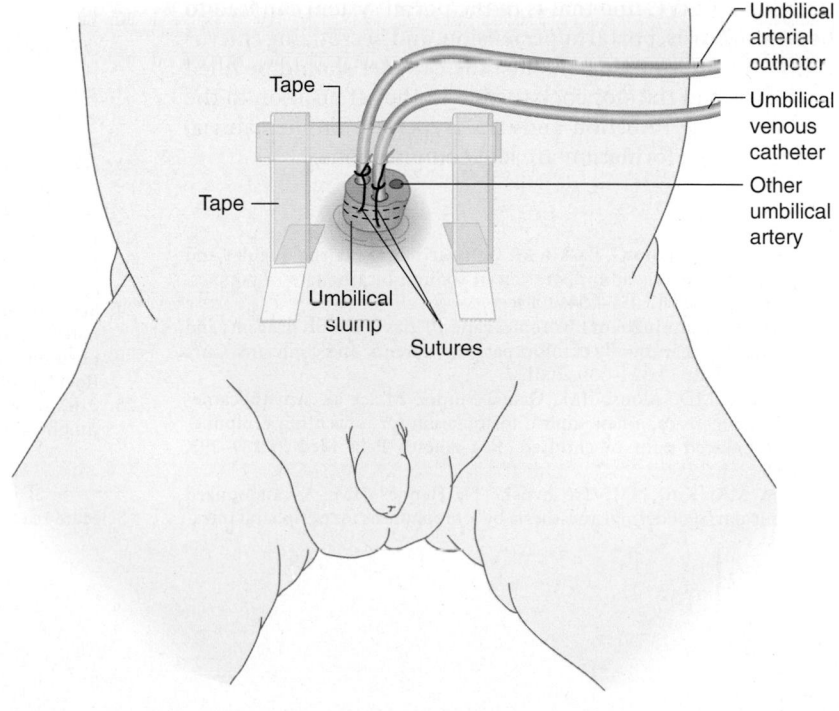

FIGURE 161–6. Umbilical vessel cannulation.

position can be approximated by advancing the catheter 1 cm beyond the point where blood is first obtained. UVC insertion depth is approximately two thirds of the shoulder-to-umbilicus distance, not including the stump length.

Though subject to error, line position should initially be assessed with radiographs.[24,25] Often an anteroposterior radiograph is sufficient, but a lateral radiograph may be helpful when it is difficult to establish position. The umbilical artery enters at the umbilicus and courses caudally in the internal iliac artery before ascending in the aorta, posterior to the vein. The umbilical vein line enters at the umbilicus and travels cephalad. The catheter tip of a "high" arterial is above the diaphragm, between the sixth and ninth thoracic vertebral bodies on a radiograph. A low arterial line lies between the third and fifth vertebral bodies on a radiograph. The umbilical vein line should be at the right atrium–inferior vena cava junction, which corresponds to the eighth and ninth thoracic vertebral bodies on a radiograph. A catheter that is in the portal system should be removed. If a catheter is too low, it should be removed rather than pushing the nonsterile distal portion into the patient. Echocardiography may provide a more accurate assessment of line position.[25]

Complications

Insertion may result in false tract formation, or perforation of a vessel or the pericardium or peritoneum. Gentle pressure with insertion and use of the correct catheter size and location can help prevent these complications. Sterile procedure in placement and use of the lines may help prevent infectious complications such as bacteremia, line sepsis, and omphalitis. Catheter hemorrhage can occur if the connections are not secure or the stopcock is left open when not in use. Dysrhythmias may occur if the catheter tip is inserted too high. Blanching and cyanosis of an extremity can occur soon after line placement and is usually due to either vasospasm or vessel obstruction from an oversized catheter. If the perfusion does not improve after 15 minutes of warming the contralateral extremity, the line should be removed to prevent limb loss. A UVC line that is in the portal system can lead to hepatic necrosis, portal hypertension, and necrotizing enterocolitis. To prevent air embolus, the catheter should be filled with fluid and the stopcock turned in the off position to the patient during insertion and use. Hypertension, hematuria, and thrombus formation are late complications.

REFERENCES

1. Fleisher G, Caputo G, Baskin M: Comparison of external jugular and peripheral venous administration of sodium bicarbonate in puppies. Crit Care Med 17:251–254, 1989.
2. Chen BK, Cunningham BB: Topical anesthetics in children: agents and techniques that equally comfort patients, parents, and clinicians. Curr Opin Pediatr 13:324–330, 2001.
3. Carceles MD, Alonso JM, Garcia-Munoz M, et al: Amethocaine-lidocaine cream, a new topical formulation for preventing venipuncture-induced pain in children. Reg Anesth Pain Med 27:289–295, 2002.
4. Kim MK, Kini NM, Troshynski TJ, Hennes HM: A randomized clinical trial of dermal anesthesia by iontophoresis for peripheral intra-
venous catheter placement in children. Ann Emerg Med 33:395–399, 1999.
5. Wolf AR, Stoddart PA, Murphy PJ, Sasada M: Rapid skin anaesthesia using high velocity lignocaine particles: a prospective placebo controlled trial. Arch Dis Child 86:309–312, 2002.
6. Guidelines 2000 for Cardiopulmonary Resuscitation and Emergency Cardiovascular Care, Part 10: pediatric advanced life support. The American Heart Association in collaboration with the International Liaison Committee on Resuscitation. Circulation 102(Suppl I):I305–I306, 2000.
7. Centers for Disease Control and Prevention: Guidelines for the prevention of intravascular catheter-related infections. MMWR Morb Mortal Wkly Rep 51:1–26, 2002.
8. Garland JS, Dunne WM Jr, Havens P, et al: Peripheral intravenous catheter complications in critically ill children: a prospective study. Pediatrics 89(6 Pt 2):1145–1150, 1992.
9. Niermeyer S, Kattwinkel J, Van Reempts P, et al: International guidelines for neonatal resuscitation: an excerpt from the Guidelines 2000 for Cardiopulmonary Resuscitation and Emergency Cardiovascular Care: International Consensus on Science. Guidelines. Pediatrics 106: e29, 2000.
10. Ellemunter H, Simma B, Trawoger R, Maurer H: Intraosseous lines in preterm and full term neonates. Arch Dis Child Fetal Neonatal Ed 80: F74–F75, 1999.
11. Abe KK, Blum GT, Yamamoto LG: Intraosseous is faster and easier than umbilical venous catheterization in newborn emergency vascular access models. Am J Emerg Med 18:126–129, 2000.
12. Fiser DH: Intraosseous infusion. N Engl J Med 322:1579–1581, 1990.
13. Jun H, Haruyama AZ, Chang KS, Yamamoto LG: Comparison of a new screw-tipped intraosseous needle versus a standard bone marrow aspiration needle for infusion. Am J Emerg Med 18:135–139, 2000.
14. Lindsey J: Ready, aim, fire! New IO device simplifies vascular access in severe cases. J Emerg Med Serv 28:97–98, 2003.
15. Boon JM, Gorry DL, Meiring JH: Finding an ideal site for intraosseous infusion of the tibia: an anatomical study. Clin Anat 16:15–18, 2003.
16. Johnson L, Kissoon N, Fiallos M, et al: Use of intraosseous blood to assess blood chemistries and hemoglobin during cardiopulmonary resuscitation with drug infusions. Crit Care Med 27:1147–1152, 1999.
17. Chiang VW, Baskin MN: Uses and complications of central venous catheters inserted in a pediatric emergency department. Pediatr Emerg Care 16:230–232, 2000.
18. Venkataraman ST, Thompson AE, Orr RA: Femoral vascular catheterization in critically ill infants and children. Clin Pediatr 36:311–319, 1997.
19. Cobb LM, Vinocur WC, Wagner CW, Weintraub WH: The central venous anatomy in infants. Surg Gynecol Obstet 165:230–234, 1987.
20. Lukish J, Valladares E, Rodriguez C, et al: Classical positioning decreases subclavian vein cross-sectional area in children. J Trauma Injury Infect Crit Care 53:272–275, 2002.
21. Jung CW, Bahk JH, Kim MW, et al: Head position for facilitating the superior vena caval placement of catheters during right subclavian approach in children. Crit Care Med 30:297–299, 2002.
*22. O'Grady NP, Alexander M, Dellinger P, et al: Guidelines for prevention of intravascular infections. Guidelines for prevention of catheter related infections. Pediatrics 110:e51, 2002.
23. Barrington KJ: Umbilical artery catheters in the newborn: effects of position of the catheter tip (Cochrane Review). Cochrane Database Syst Rev (1):CD000505, 2005.
24. Schlesinger AE, Braverman RM, DiPietro MA: Pictorial essay. Neonates and umbilical venous catheters: normal appearance, anomalous positions, complications, and potential aid to diagnosis. AJR Am J Roentgenol 180:1147–1153, 2003.
25. Ades A, Sable C, Cummings S, et al: Echocardiographic evaluation of umbilical venous catheter placement. J Perinatol 23:24–28, 2003.

*Selected reading.

Chapter 162

Foreign Body Removal

Ruth Ann Pannell, MD and Joe Pagane, MD

Selected Procedures

Ear foreign body removal
Nose foreign body removal
Fishhook removal
Piercing removal
Ring removal
Subcutaneous foreign body removal

Discussion of Individual Procedures

Ear Foreign Body Removal

Parents and children with otic foreign bodies are often unaware that the foreign body is the cause of the symptoms. Sometimes, only a thorough physical examination will elicit the cause of the problem because many patients will not freely offer the examiner an adequate history. Presenting symptoms may include ear pain, increased cerumin, purulent drainage, hearing loss, and external inflammation.[1]

Anatomy

The external auditory canal has an oval cylindrical shape, is approximately 2.5 cm long in adults, is short and straight in infancy, and forms an "S" shape as one matures to adulthood. Sensitive epithelium lines the canal. Two narrowings in the canal, one in the osseous portion close to the tympanic membrane and another at the medial end of the cartilaginous area of the canal, are areas where objects frequently lodge.[2]

Common foreign bodies removed from the ear include beads, paper, popcorn kernels, insects, and small toys. The object's size, shape, material, and location present different challenges regarding removal.[1,3,4] Tissue damage may occur from the foreign body itself, prior removal attempts, or the removal process. The presence of any tissue damage before manipulation should be documented. If there is concern regarding hearing damage, a pre-removal assessment should be performed prior to manipulation.[1]

Few foreign bodies require immediate removal except those associated with significant infection and alkaline (button/disk) batteries. Alkaline batteries should be removed immediately because of the risk of tissue destruction due to pressure necrosis, liquefaction necrosis, and tissue electrolysis.[5,6] Patients with previous unsuccessful removal attempts who meet certain criteria (Table 162–1) are less likely to have successful removal under direct visualization in the ED. Further manipulation in the ED is often unsuccessful and unnecessary. These patients usually require referral to otolaryngologists.[4,7]

Evaluation

Imaging is rarely necessary in the evaluation of patients with an otic foreign body. Computed tomography (CT) or magnetic resonance imaging (MRI) may be indicated in order to characterize significant associated infection (e.g., mastoiditis) or erosive damage, or if other serious complications are suspected. MRI should be avoided if metallic foreign bodies are suspected.

Some children with foreign bodies require sedation or general anesthesia for removal because of location. The medial portion of the canal is narrow, and even minor manipulation can cause intense pain.[7] Topical anesthetics inadequately anesthetize the canal due to their poor absorption at this site. Local injection of anesthetics is painful and difficult to perform in uncooperative patients. Frequently, successful removal requires immobilization with restraint by assistants or wrapping a sheet around the child.[1] Procedural sedation allows for a high (84%) success rate for foreign body removal by emergency physicians.[8]

Equipment

Useful tools for removing foreign bodies include[1,7,9-11]

- Otoscope
- Forceps
- Curettes
- Hooks
- Hemostats
- Dental pick
- Baron suction
- Fogarty or Foley catheters
- Cyanoacrylate glue (Superglue)
- Saline
- 10- to 20-ml syringe
- Plastic catheter
- Mineral oil
- Lidocaine 2%, 4%
- Acetone

Table 162–1	Indications for Direct Referral for Otomicroscopic Removal
Object type	Spherical, sharp-edged, disk battery, vegetable matter
History	In canal greater than 24 hr
	Prior removal attempt(s)
Location	Adjacent to tympanic membrane
Patient	Age < 4 yr, agitated, and/or difficulty with visualization

Depending on what technique is used to immobilize or sedate the patient, cardiac telemetry and oxygen saturation monitoring may be required.

Techniques

Emergency physicians should be acquainted with several techniques and use the most appropriate approach based on equipment available, personal skill, cooperation of the patient, and the location, size, shape, and material of the foreign object.[1] For direct visualization, an otoscope is the instrument of choice for optimal magnification and lighting. In order to straighten the canal and inspect the foreign body, the pinna is grasped and retracted in a superior and posterior direction to provide good visualization.[12] The tympanic membrane should be inspected for any signs of rupture. The hand holding the otoscope should be stabilized against the patient's head to prevent injury if the patient moves unexpectedly.

Alligator forceps, hooks, a hemostat, or a dental pick may be used to manually remove foreign bodies. Objects with a leading edge or small rounded objects can be removed with alligator forceps or a hemostat if forceps are unavailable (Fig. 162–1A). Hooks, loops, or suction can be used to remove larger spherical objects or objects without a leading edge. A hook or loop can be placed behind the object, rotated 90 degrees, and used to pull the object outward (Fig. 162–1B). For soft foreign bodies, a stout hook can be used to spear the foreign body and withdraw it (Fig. 162–1C). For spherical, round, or light mobile objects, suction may be successful

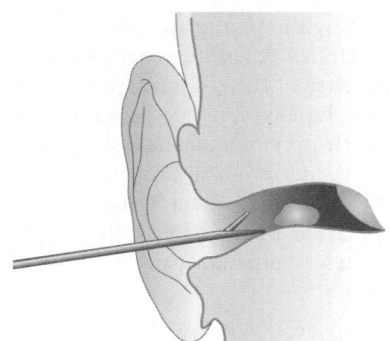
A. Removal with alligator forceps: open forceps and grasp object

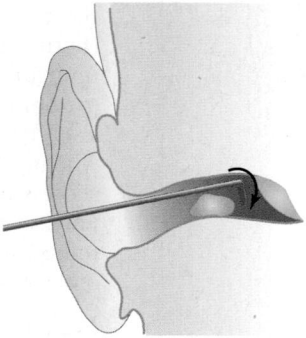
B. Removal with hook or loop: place behind object and rotate

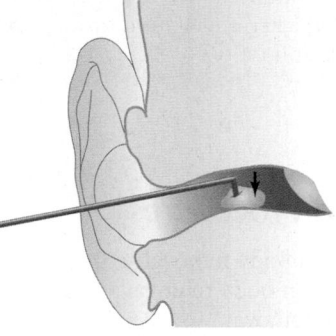
C. Removal with hook: spear object and remove

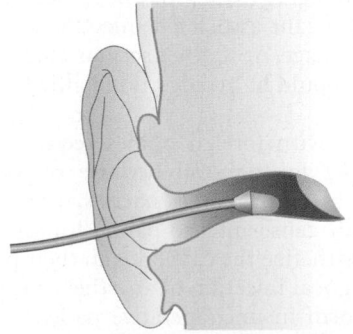
D. Removal with suction tip catheter: place tip on object with suction and withdraw

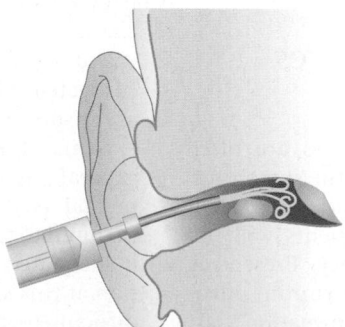
E. Irrigation technique: inject water at periphery of object to flush object outward

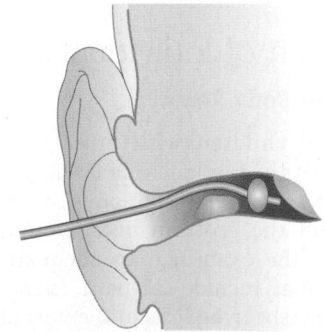
F. Catheter removal: placed behind object, inflated then withdrawn

FIGURE 162–1. Techniques for removing foreign bodies from the ear.

alone. A suction-tip catheter is placed against the object, suction is turned on, then the catheter and object are slowly removed (Fig. 162–1D).

Irrigation can be a safe technique for removing certain otic foreign bodies. However, irrigation should never be used with vegetable matter that can expand, with button batteries, or if there is a possibility of tympanic membrane perforation.[4] Warm water is instilled using a 10- to 20-ml syringe attached to the plastic tubing of a catheter. The water is gently injected toward the periphery of the object so that the water will go past the object, hit the tympanic membrane, and flush the object outward via posterior pressure[13] (Fig. 162–1E).

The tip of a small Fogarty or Foley catheter can be placed carefully behind the object. Then, the balloon is inflated distal to the object in the canal. The foreign body is removed as the catheter balloon is pulled from the external auditory canal (Fig. 162–1F).

Another approach includes the application of cyanoacrylate glue (Superglue) to the end of a paperclip or swab. A small amount of rapidly drying glue is placed against the foreign body, the glue is given a few seconds to dry, and the bonded object is withdrawn from the canal. This method is effective but imposes the risk of contaminating the canal with glue that is difficult to remove.[13,14]

A Styrofoam impaction was successfully removed in one case by direct application of 0.1 ml of pure acetone via a 22-gauge catheter and 1-ml syringe. This caused the Styrofoam to shrink in, allowing for easy extraction. To minimize the possibility of ototoxicity, a minimal amount of acetone should be instilled, and the ear canal should be irrigated after the procedure.[11]

Insects in the external auditory canal can cause great discomfort and distress. It is important to kill the insect to provide relief from its movement and to aid with extraction. Mineral oil and 2% or 4% lidocaine kill insects within 1 minute.[9,10] Lidocaine should not be used if the tympanic membrane is perforated since it can cause vertigo.[15] When the insect stops moving, it may be mechanically extracted with forceps or suction.[13]

Before beginning manipulation of an external auditory canal foreign body, the physician must decide how many attempts are reasonable before stopping and referring to an otolaryngologist. In general, not more than two to three attempts should be made, and efforts should be discontinued if external auditory canal damage occurs or sedation and immobilization are inadequate. This will prevent frustration from causing unnecessary attempts and avoid iatrogenic damage. It is important to appropriately refer patients at risk for local complications (e.g., perforation, alkaline injury) if the object is not easily removable (see Table 162–1). In most cases, allowing foreign bodies to stay in the external auditory canal while the patient waits for referral is safe. Exceptions to this are foreign bodies associated with infection and presence of a button/disk battery.[1]

Complications

Complications of foreign body extraction can occur from the removal procedure or from the foreign body. These include tympanic membrane perforation, canal wall laceration, bleeding or canal abrasions, hematomas, otitis externa, and otitis media.[1,4,7]

Postprocedure Care and Disposition

In patients in whom cutaneous damage is present, a topical antibiotic is prescribed and the parents and patient are instructed to keep the canal clean and dry. Treatment of any associated infection or complication (e.g., otitis media) is initiated, and follow-up for unremovable foreign bodies is arranged. No follow-up is warranted following removal of uncomplicated foreign bodies. A complete examination of the nose and the opposite ear is essential prior to discharge.

Nose Foreign Body Removal

Nasal foreign bodies can be difficult to identify since children rarely relay a history of placing the foreign body in their nose.[4] Children often present with a unilateral malodorous nasal discharge. Children with nasal objects also can present with symptoms consistent with sinusitis, the common cold, allergic rhinitis, tumor, or halitosis, as well as recurrent epistaxis.[16]

Anatomy

The nose consists of the nares, nasal septum, vestibule, and lateral walls.[2] On the lateral walls lie the superior, middle, and inferior nasal conchae with corresponding meatuses. Nasal foreign bodies are frequently found on the floor of the nose just below the inferior turbinate or immediately anterior to the middle turbinate.[17] The types of foreign bodies that have been found in children's noses include rubber erasers, paper, pebbles, beads, beans, peanuts, marbles, sponges, small toys, and chalk.[18-21]

Damage to the nose may occur from the foreign body, inflammation, or the removal process. Complications include pressure necrosis, mucosal erosion, epistaxis, formation of rhinoliths, and the promotion of infections in the surrounding structures, including sinusitis and otitis media.[5,17,19]

Few foreign bodies of the nasal canal require emergent removal, and some have remained for years without significant complications.[17] Exceptions to this include foreign bodies with any associated infection and alkaline batteries (button/disk) within the nose.[20] Foreign bodies adjacent to the cribiform plate (superior and medial to the middle turbinate) require otolaryngology removal.

Structures contiguous to an intranasal foreign body are not as easily damaged and are not as sensitive as the ear canal. Therefore, the need for consultation for removal is less likely. If necessary, procedural sedation is used to assist with nasal foreign body removal (see Chapter 159, Procedural Sedation and Analgesia).[8] If there is concern for posterior displacement into the airway, removal under general anesthesia may be necessary.[17,19]

Evaluation

Imaging is rarely necessary in the evaluation of children with a nasal foreign body. CT or MRI may be indicated to characterize associated infections, erosive damage, or other associated serious complications.

Proper examination of the nares involves placing the patient in the "sniffing" position while he or she is sitting upright. It may be helpful to tilt the head back slightly. A nasal head speculum is used to spread the naris in an inferior-to-superior direction.[17] Any nasal damage should be documented prior to manipulation.

In many cases, mucosal edema may obstruct viewing and hinder removal of nasal foreign bodies. Prior to removal, the nasal mucosa may be sprayed with an available vasoconstrictor such as phenylephrine or oxymetazoline to shrink the mucosa, and a local anesthetic agent such as benzocaine spray.[17,21]

Equipment

Removal tools and agents include[21-23]
- Nasal speculum
- Topical vasoconstrictor
- Topical anesthetic
- Right-angle forceps
- Right-angle probe
- Suction catheter
- Alligator forceps
- Fogarty/Foley catheter
- Ambu bag

Depending on what technique is used to immobilize the patient, oxygen saturation and cardiac monitoring and airway rescue devices may be required.

Technique

Many nasal foreign bodies can be removed with manual instrumentation (Table 162–2). Alligator forceps or bayonet forceps can retrieve anteriorly lodged foreign bodies if they have edges that can be grasped. Wire loops and right-angle hooks can be carefully passed by the object and rotated 90 degrees, then used to easily spoon out the object.[22] Number 4 or 5 Fogarty catheters or 5F to 6F Foley catheters can be used by inserting them carefully beyond the object, slowly inflating the balloon, and gently pulling the object outward.[21]

For suctioning spherical or smooth objects, a suction-tip catheter is placed in the nose until the tip is in contact with the object. Suction is turned on and the object retrieved while the catheter removed.[21]

A positive air pressure technique, similar to mouth-to-mouth resuscitation, is a safe and effective method for nasal foreign body removal. While digitally obstructing the nasal canal opposite the foreign body, air is exhaled through a child's mouth until resistance is felt (closing of the epiglottis). Air is then exhaled briskly into the child's mouth, producing an outward pressure that repositions the foreign object so it can be grasped or is dislodged. A modified version involves placing an Ambu bag over the child's mouth that is then squeezed forcefully[18,23] (Fig. 162–2). Alternately, cooperative patients can be instructed to take a deep breath and exhale through the nose while the unobstructed nostril is occluded.[17]

Otolaryngology consultation is required if the foreign body cannot be removed in the ED. Button batteries or foreign bodies with significant mucosal damage, prolonged impaction, or infection warrant quick removal and consultation in the ED.[20]

Table 162–2	Best Techniques for Removing Nasal Foreign Bodies With Respect to Object Position and Properties	
Technique	**Position**	**Object Properties**
Forceps	Anteriorly lodged	Objects with leading edges
Wire loops and right-angle hoops	Anteriorly lodged	Any type, texture
Fogarty/Foley catheter	Posteriorly lodged	Any type, texture
Suction	Anteriorly lodged	Spherical, smooth, round
Positive air pressure	Posteriorly lodged	Any type, texture

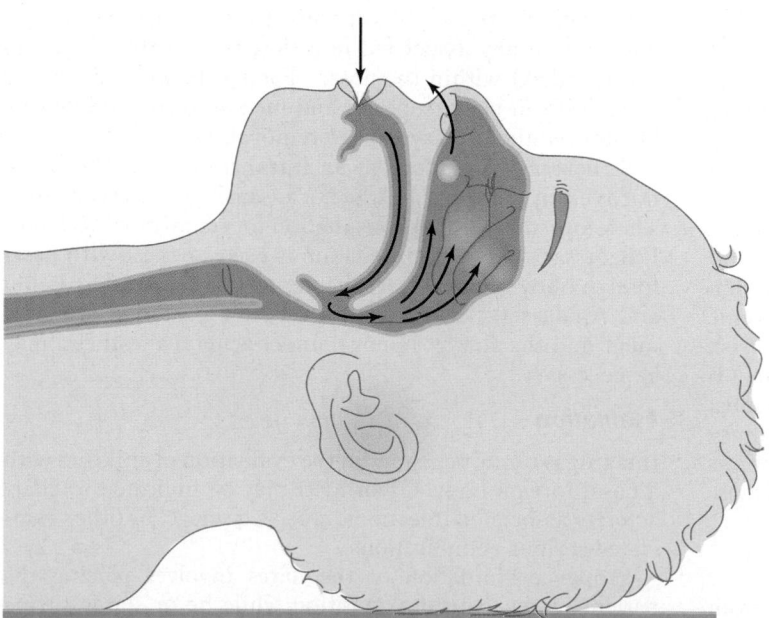

Air is exhaled through mouth until resistance is felt. Then air is exhaled briskly into child's mouth which forces air into patient's posterior nares. Outward pressure then drives the foreign object into a new anterior position or out of the nares.

FIGURE 162–2. Use of positive pressure ventilation to dislodge nasal foreign bodies.

Complications

Complications from nasal foreign body removal include epistaxis from direct mucosal trauma and infection.[17] With the air pressure technique, overzealous blowing theoretically can result in barotrauma to the tympanic membrane.[18] Importantly, superiorly located foreign bodies can be lodged next to the cribiform plate, placing the patient at risk for intracranial trauma from removal attempts or intracranial extension of infection. Otolaryngology consultation is required for removal of these foreign bodies.

The most significant complication with nasal foreign bodies is the potential for posterior displacement leading to aspiration or airway obstruction. This complication can be avoided by using familiar removal techniques, appropriate equipment, lighting, and adequate visualization. Removal should be attempted only in children who are cooperative, adequately immobilized, or sedated. A small percentage of nasal foreign bodies may require removal under general anesthesia with the patient intubated to protect the airway.[20]

Postprocedure Care and Disposition

Most patients will not require follow-up after removal of a nasal foreign body. Associated infection or complications (e.g., otitis media) require treatment and follow-up. If significant epistaxis or mucosal trauma is present, the patient should avoid nose blowing. The physician should always perform an examination of other orifices prior to discharging the patient.

Fishhook Removal

The choice of method to remove a fishhook will depend on the type of fishhook, location of the injury, and depth of penetration. Three main types of fishhooks exist: simple single-barbed, multiple barbed, and treble barbed fishhooks. Fishhooks should be left in place if they penetrate the orbital area, involve the eye, or place the eye at risk for injury during removal. In these cases, ophthalmology consultation is indicated.[24,25]

Evaluation

Before attempting to remove a fishhook, any neurologic deficits or tissue damage should be recorded. Involvement of the bone, tendon, and vessels should be evaluated, and radiographs should be considered to evaluate the depth of penetration and the location of the barb, and to determine the type of fishhook involved.[24] CT scan should be considered for precise identification, localization, and determination of associated tissue injury in cases of orbital fishhooks. A local anesthetic or a nerve block can be used for pain control if needed.[26]

Equipment

Equipment for removal may include
- Antiseptic solution
- Tape
- String or suture
- Scissors
- 18-gauge or larger needle
- Scalpel
- Needle driver
- Pliers

Removal is initiated by cleaning the site with povidone-iodine or hexachlorophene and removing debris by irrigating with saline. Fishhooks with more than one uninvolved point (hook) should be covered with tape prior to removal.[24,26]

Technique

Occasionally, more than one removal technique may be required for fishhook removal. There are four standard techniques for removal of fishhooks: the retrograde, string-yank, needle cover, and advance-and-cut procedures (Table 162–3). The retrograde technique is simple, causes minimal tissue damage, and works best for barbless and superficial hooks.[24,27] Gentle downward pressure is applied to the shank of the hook in order to disengage the barb while backing the hook out along the entry path (Fig. 162–3A). If resistance is met, an alternate technique should be considered.

The string-yank technique works well with small to medium fishhooks and with fishhooks that are deeply embedded. Material such as fishing line or silk suture is tied around the midpoint of the fishhook bend. The area is stabilized with the hook against a flat surface. The shank of the fishhook is depressed while holding the string tightly several inches away. As the shank is depressed, a firm quick jerk is then applied to the string while holding the string parallel to the shank (Fig. 162–3B). If the fishhook disengages, it may come out rapidly, placing the physician and bystanders at risk for trauma from the fishhook.[28]

The needle cover technique works well with single barbs and large hooks, especially when the barb is superficially embedded and can be easily reached by a needle. An 18-gauge or larger needle is inserted along the entry pathway and used to cover and disengage the barb. The fishhook and needle covering the barb are removed as a unit simultaneously (Fig. 162–3C). A modification of this technique involves incising with a no. 11 blade along the wound to the point of the fishhook. This incision allows the fishhook to be backed out by creating room for the point and barb.[24,27]

The advance-and-cut technique is usually successful, although it may produce tissue trauma. Using pliers or a needle driver, the tip of the hook is advanced through the skin. The sharp point is anchored with a clamp to avoid injury and then cut with pliers or another cutting tool. Then, the rest of the fishhook is backed out (Fig. 162–3D) If the fishhook has multiple barbs, the eye of the fishhook should be removed, then the shank and barbs advanced[26,29] (Fig. 162–3E).

Table 162–3	Standard Techniques for Fishhook Removal		
Technique	**Location**	**Hook Size**	**Barb Number**
Retrograde	Superficial	Any	Single
String-yank	Embedded	Small to medium	Single
Needle cover	Superficial	Large	Single
Advance-and-cut barb	Embedded	Any	Single
Advance-and-cut eye	Embedded	Any	Multiple

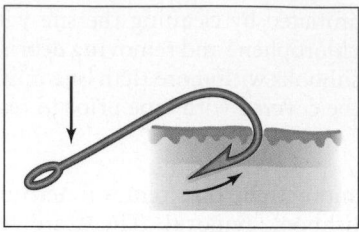
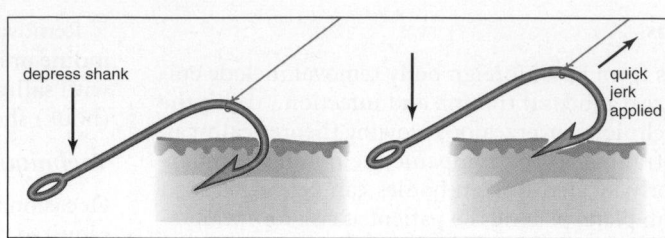

A. Retrograde technique.
Apply downward pressure to shank in order to disengage barb while backing out hook along entry path.

B. String yank.
Tie string around midpoint of bend. Depress shank while holding string firmly. Apply quick jerk while string taught and parallel to shank.

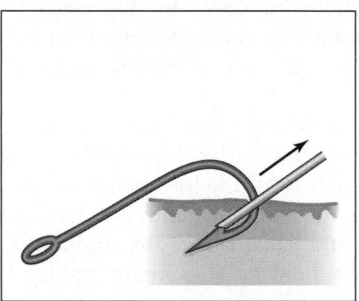
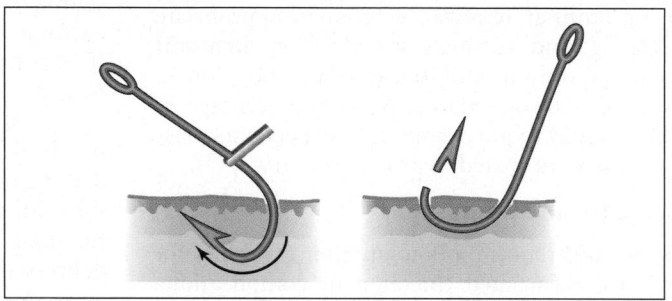

C. Needle cover technique.
Insert needle along entry pathway to cover and disengage barb. Position bevel of needle toward inside of curve of barb. Back out needle and hook as a unit.

D. Advance and cut.
Advance fishhook through skin. Cut off barb and back out remaining portion of fishhook.

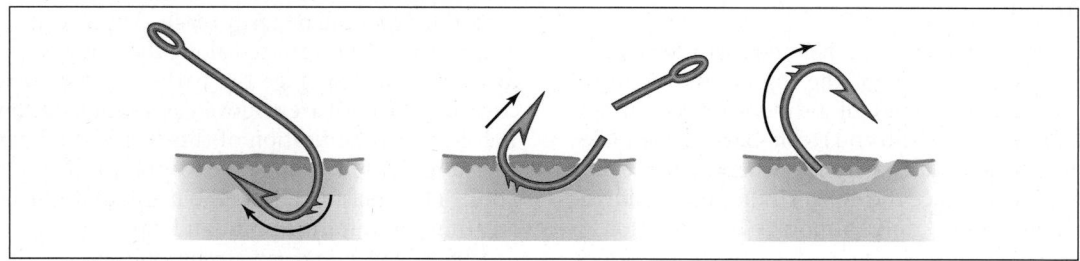

E. For multi-barbed fishhooks, advance hook until barb is visible. Cut off eye and complete extraction.

FIGURE 162–3. Techniques for removing embedded fishhooks.

Consultation is necessary for fishhooks that involve the orbit or orbital area, where removal may damage the eye. Consultation for removal may also be warranted for fishhooks associated with infection or if they involve bone, tendons, blood vessels, and nerves. Complications of fishhook removal include infection, abscess formation, scarring, and injury to surrounding structures.[24]

Postprocedure Care and Disposition

Tetanus prophylaxis should be administered if needed. The wound should be explored for any foreign bodies. The wound can be left open and treated with antibiotic ointment and a simple dressing. Systemic antibiotics are generally not indicated, but prophylactic antibiotic therapy should be considered for patients with immunosuppression, poor wound healing (i.e., diabetes, peripheral vascular disease), or involvement of deep structures.[26] Follow-up care is generally not required except in complicated cases to ensure proper healing and absence of infection.

Piercing Removal

Jewelry may need to be removed in order to perform a procedure (e.g., Foley catheter insertion, intubation, electrocautery), to prevent damage to nearby structures, and to avoid interference with reading plain radiographs, CT scans, and MRI images.[23,30] A complete examination of the site should be performed and preexisting infection, trauma, and neurological deficits documented prior to manipulation. Radiography is indicated if swelling or infection obstructs viewing of the ornament.[31] To remove some piercings, a local anesthetic block of the pierced area may be necessary for pain control.[32]

There are numerous types of body jewelry, including barbells, capture bar rings, labrets, rubes, flared eyelet flesh funnels, safety pins, and studs. The barbell is either straight or curved, and the ball on the barbell can be internally or externally threaded. The capture ball rings are circular rings that contain spheres that are held in place by tension. Labret-type jewelry has a threaded ball or cone on one side and a flat surface on the other. Tubes and flared eyelet flesh tunnels are used to enlarge a pierced hold. Studs have a removable back that slides off.[19]

Ear piercing frequently uses capture ball jewelry or studs and can be placed in any portion of the ear or ear lobe. The nose may be pierced at the septum, nostril, or bridge using curved barbells, studs, or capture ball jewelry. Labret-type jewelry is used in lip piercing, with the flat surface of the jewelry resting inside the mouth. The tongue, navel, nipple, and genitalia can be pierced horizontally or vertically using barbell or capture ball ring jewelry.[30]

Equipment

Specific tools available for removing jewelry include ring-closing and ring-opening pliers, which are available from commercial suppliers. If unavailable, hemostats, needle drivers, or surgical clamps may be used.[30] Use of a wire cutter for removal should be avoided since this instrument can create sharp edges and cause soft tissue trauma.

Technique

Barbell jewelry can be removed by unscrewing the removable ball attached to one end using pliers, clamps, or a hemostat. The removable ball is grasped while holding the opposite side still and turned counter clockwise to loosen it. When the ball is detached, the straight end of the bar can be pulled toward the stationary ball and removed.[30] Capture ball rings can be removed by inserting ring-opening pliers or clamps into the middle of the ring and prying the ring open. This will allow the ball to drop out, and the ring can be removed.[33]

One newly described method for removing navel piercing involves opening the jewelry and placing the tip of a close-fitting intravenous catheter (14 or 16 gauge), without the needle, over the threaded tip of the bar. Advancing the catheter will push the jewelry out of the skin tract. The jewelry is then removed while leaving the catheter in place.[33]

Studs are removed by grasping the stationary stud with clamps and pulling the removable back in an opposite direction, which may also warrant the use of clamps for a tight grasp. Flared eyelet flesh tunnels may be removed by holding the tissue stationary while either pushing or pulling the jewelry through the piercing to remove it.

Depending on piercing location, consultation with surgical subspecialists may be warranted if piercing is associated with infection or swelling that obstructs visualization and removal. Patients with serious associated infections may require hospital admission, surgical débridement, and treatment with intravenous antibiotics.[31]

Complications

Short-term complications of removal include closure of the subcutaneous tissue tract, which could cause emotional stress to the patient.[30] If jewelry is associated with local infection, it is important to consider gauze or wick placement within the tract after jewelry removal to avoid abscess formation. Any complication associated with the piercing or removal requires prompt follow-up (e.g., in 1 to 2 days) to ensure adequate healing and response to treatment.[35,36]

Ring Removal

Injuries to the fingers, such as sprains, fracture, or bee sting, can cause significant edema, and rings can impair circulation and cause ischemia if swelling is significant.[37,38] Prior to ring removal, a neurologic, vascular, and tendon examination of the digit should be documented. Radiographs may be warranted if bony injury is suspected.[37] Occasionally a digital block may be necessary before ring removal.

Equipment

Necessary equipment for ring removal may include[38-40]
- Ice
- Water-soluble lubricant
- 0 or 1-0 silk
- Manual ring cutter
- Battery-operated ring cutter
- Surgical gloves
- Ear curette
- Scissors
- Hemostats or a ring spreader

Technique

Before resorting to more involved techniques for ring removal, simple methods such as elevating the patient's arm above the heart and application of ice to the finger should be considered. Next, the physician can lubricate the finger and attempt manual ring removal. If the ring does not slip off, it will be necessary to employ another technique.[38]

The string wrap method is initiated by wrapping a wide tourniquet around the finger, distal to the ring. The tourniquet is left in place for approximately 5 minutes and then removed. Then, 20 to 25 inches of umbilical tape, 0 or 1-0 silk, or another type of atraumatic thread is fed under the ring using a forceps, hemostat, or metal ear curette. The string's proximal end is tightly grasped and the distal end wrapped clockwise around the finger, avoiding gaps. The string is unwrapped by pulling on the proximal end slowly, and the ring will be removed as the string is unwrapped[40,41] (Fig. 162–4A).

Another method involving the finger of a surgical glove can be used with burned, traumatized, or fractured fingers, for which the string wrap method may be too painful or traumatic. The glove finger can be cut off cylindrically and the cut end passed between the patient's finger and the ring using small forceps. The segment of the rubber behind the ring is then pulled toward the fingertip with a twisting motion on the ring[39] (Fig. 162–4B).

If the ring cannot be removed with these methods, it must be cut off. Manual cutters work best with thin to moderately thick rings. The least ornate part of the ring should be selected and the manual ring cutter guard placed under the ring. The thumbscrew is then turned clockwise. This technique may take several attempts in order to saw through the ring. If the ring is thick or cannot be cut manually, a battery-powered cutting device can be used, following the manufacturer's instructions. Once the ring is cut, hemostat or a ring spreader is used to open and remove the ring.[38]

Complications

If rings are not removed from entrapped digits expeditiously, permanent, irreversible tendon, nerve, or vascular compromise can occur. Complications from ring removal include soft tissue (vascular, nerve, or tendon) and bony injury with resulting infection and loss of function.[37] Patients with entrapped rings require close monitoring to ensure that

A. String wrap method for ring removal.

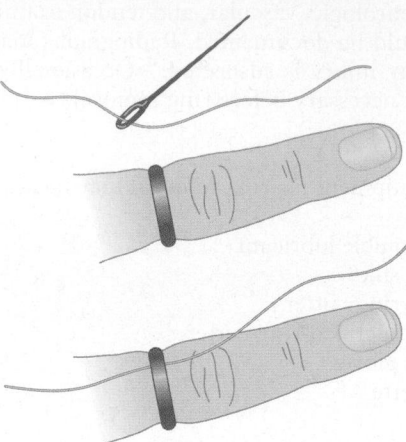

Wrap a wide tourniquet around the distal end of the finger and leave in place for five minutes before beginning technique. Umbilical tape or atraumatic thread should be fed under the ring using forceps, hemostat, or metal ear curotic.

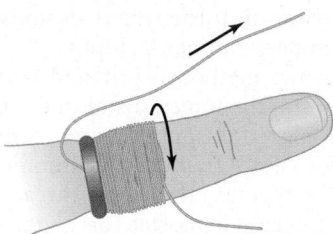

Tightly grasp the string's proximal end and wrap the distal end clockwise around the finger.

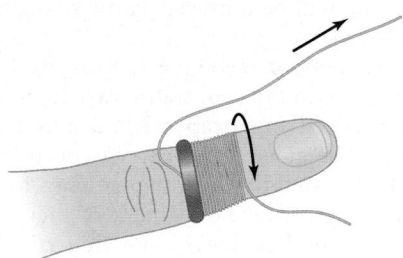

Unwrap by pulling on the proximal end slowly and the ring will be removed as the string is unwrapped.

B. Glove method for ring removal.

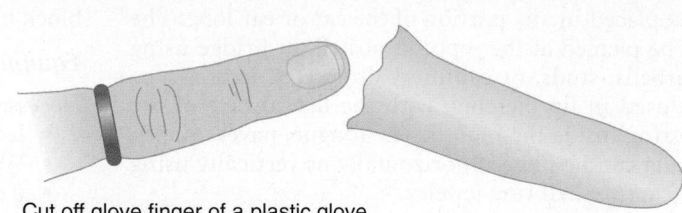

Cut off glove finger of a plastic glove.

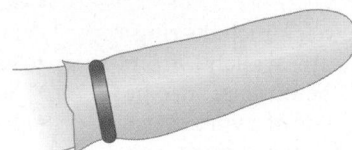

Pass the cut ends between the patient's finger and ring using small forceps.

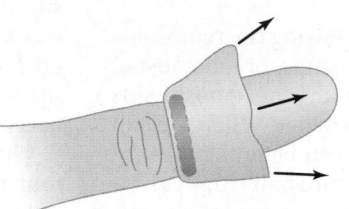

Pull segment of rubber behind the ring forward toward the fingertip with a twisting motion on the ring for removal.

FIGURE 162–4. Techniques for removing rings from fingers.

vascular flow returns and infection does not develop. In general, antibiotics are not indicated unless significant tissue damage has occurred.

Subcutaneous Foreign Body Removal

A significant percentage of wounds treated in pediatric emergency departments involve retained foreign bodies.[42-44] The presence of these foreign bodies places patients at risk for many complications, including infection, neurologic compromise, and increased scarring. In addition, retained foreign bodies continue to be a major source of malpractice claims against emergency physicians.

Anatomy and Physiology

The variability of a foreign body's reactivity with the host immune system can result in destruction and extrusion of the foreign body or chronic inflammation with granuloma formation. The presence of a foreign body can be relatively asymptomatic or can cause chronic inflammation depending on the retained foreign body material or its reactivity.[43-47] Eighty percent of all foreign bodies are glass, wood, or metal.[43-47] Wood and vegetable material produce more of an immune response than do metallic or glass foreign bodies. Vegetable matter foreign bodies can also introduce fungal organisms.[45,47] The rubber in the sole of a sneaker or tennis shoe is a good medium for *Pseudomonas* growth leading to perichondritis and osteomyelitis. Some anatomic areas, including the hand and foot, are associated with a higher complication rate and more technically difficult foreign body removal. Their complex anatomy, with proximity of tendon, bone, muscle, and neurovascular structures, places these areas at increased risk of tissue injury, infection, and missed foreign body. Small radiopaque foreign bodies in these areas may not be visualized because of proximity to bone.[45,46,48] One of the most difficult steps in managing wounds is to determine if a foreign body is present. Historical clues to the presence of a foreign body include a puncture mechanism; scalp, face, or foot wounds; and involvement in a motor vehicle collision.[49]

Particulate matter (e.g., dirt, rust, skin, sock, vegetable matter) can be tracked into a wound if a shoe is penetrated by a sharp object such as a nail. This is especially true if the penetrating object is 4.5 mm or greater.[50] A history of prior attempts at removal of wood foreign body or a nonhealing foot infection is highly suggestive of a retained foreign body.

Evaluation

Lacerations less than 0.5 mm in depth have been shown to very rarely contain glass foreign body.[51] Physical examination findings suggestive of retained foreign body include excessive wound pain, tenderness to palpation over the wound, pain with passive movement, or a painful mass. A preverbal or apprehensive child can make these examination findings very difficult to uncover. Therefore, a slowly resolving or recurrent cellulitis, chronic drainage, culture-negative abscess, or any radiographic evidence of infection (lytic lesion, periosteal reaction, joint destruction) may require further evaluation, CT or MRI, or consultation with a surgical subspecialist for evaluation of a retained foreign body.

Plain radiographs can identify most metal and glass foreign bodies.[48] Embedded aluminum is also usually seen; however, ingested aluminum is usually not seen on plain radiographs.[52] Plain radiographs may not identify glass or metal foreign body less than 2 mm in diameter in certain projections.[48] Wood, plastic, and vegetable foreign bodies are typically not visualized with plain films. Air within wood may be visible on plain films up to 48 hours, at which time body fluids absorbed into the wood make it the same density as soft tissue on radiographs.[46,50] Ultrasound can be helpful in identifying foreign bodies and is especially helpful for identifying nonradiographic foreign bodies. CT and MRI can be extremely helpful to identify foreign bodies when a more exact anatomic location is needed.[53]

Technique

First, the foreign body must be identified and localized. If foreign bodies cannot be directly visualized, radiologic studies must be used to localize the foreign body's anatomic location. Before any manipulation or exploration is performed, nerve and tendon function as well as vascular status are examined and documented. This examination should be performed throughout a complete range of motion of to identify all possible entry points and wound tracts, and to identify associated neurovascular or tendon injuries. To gain optimal visualization, complete immobilization, adequate anesthesia or sedation, and proper lighting are needed. If a tourniquet is needed, a blood pressure cuff inflated to 20 mm Hg above systolic blood pressure will provide needed hemostasis.

Once a foreign body is identified and the area is properly prepped and draped, the removal procedure can begin. If the foreign body is not visualized, extension of the wound with a small scalpel (no. 15 blade) should be considered. The risk of damaging underlying structures will be minimized if only the superficial skin layers (epidermis and dermis) are incised. When possible, the wound should be extended parallel to Langer's lines, the natural skin creases. In small children, vital structures are close to one another and to the skin surface, placing them at an increased risk of injury during extension and manipulation. Therefore, all explorations should be performed by gentle spreading of the tissues with a hemostat, avoiding blind probing. When the foreign body is located, its proximity to other structures and its anatomic position are noted. The foreign body can then be grasped with a hemostat and removed.

After removal of the foreign body, the wound is reexplored to check for retained foreign bodies or damage to nearby structures. If no remaining foreign body is identified, and the wound appears clean and is less than 24 hours old, primary closure after irrigation can be performed. If the wound contains particulate matter, identifiable injured structures, or devitalized tissue, further management such as delayed primary closure, placement of a drain, and antibiotic therapy should be planned in consultation with a surgical subspecialist.

Long, thin foreign bodies, such as needles or glass, embedded parallel to the skin surface and superficial to deep structures can be removed by a slightly different technique. An incision is made in the skin perpendicular to the midpoint of the foreign body's long axis. Then, the tissue is gently spread with a hemostat until the foreign body is identified. The foreign body is grasped with the hemostat and pushed out through the original entrance wound or a wound created along the foreign body's initial tract. The wound should be examined for retained foreign body, and primary closure considered. Antibiotics should be administered for contaminated or infected wounds, wounds with retained foreign body, and wounds over 24 hours old.[43,47,50,54]

Deciding whether or not to remove a retained foreign body can be difficult. Generally, foreign bodies with the following features should be removed: those that contain reactive materials, are likely to cause inflammation or infection, have heavy bacterial contamination, are toxic (spines with venom), impinge on or can damage tendons/vessels/nerves, impair mechanical function, are intra-articular, are proximate to fractured bone, can potentially migrate toward important anatomic structures, are intravascular, cause persistent pain, have established inflammation or infection, cause an allergic reaction, alter cosmesis, or cause psychological distress.[50] If the decision is made to leave a foreign body in place, the treating physician should explain the reasoning to the patient and the family. Then, the patient should be referred to a surgical subspecialist for further management. Discharge instructions should include this referral as well as aftercare instructions for wound care.

Contraindications to removal of a foreign body in the ED include an abnormal location. Foreign bodies in the chest, abdomen, and neck require surgical consultation as removal of foreign bodies in these locations could result in excessive bleeding from a previously tamponaded blood vessel, or damage to the plural space or abdominal cavity. Time constraints for exploration and removal should also prompt the emergency physician to consult a surgical subspecialist. In general, an attempt in the ED should not exceed 30 minutes; further exploration and tourniquet time place nerves and vessels at greater risk.

Complications

Complications of a retained foreign body as well as of foreign body removal after exploration include wound infection, cellulitis, abscess formation, septic arthritis, osteomyelitis, and chronically draining wounds.[43,48,50,54] Wound exploration and foreign body removal can injure adjacent structures or cause scarring. Complications associated with hemostasis, whether by tourniquets or by the use of vasoactive agents, include vascular damage, neurapraxia, and thrombosis. These complications can be greatly reduced by keeping tourniquet time to 20 to 30 minutes and by not using vasoactive agents on devitalized tissue or at end-organ sites.[50,54,55]

Summary

The ability to assess, manage, identify, and remove foreign bodies is an important skill. Proper preparation, patient selection, technique selection, antibiotic use, and hemostasis and appropriate consultation with surgical subspecialists will improve outcome, while reducing complication rates.

REFERENCES

1. Bressler K, Shelton C: Ear foreign-body removal. Laryngoscope 103:367–370, 1993.
2. Gray H: Anatomy. Stamford, CT: Longmeadow Press, 1991, pp. 550–553, 567–572.
3. Ansley J, Cunningham M: Treatment of aural foreign bodies in children. Pediatrics 101:638–641, 1998.
*4. Schulze S, Kerschner J, Beste D: Pediatric external auditory canal foreign bodies: a review of 698 cases. Otolaryngology 127:73–78, 2002.
5. Capo J, Lucente F: Alkaline battery foreign bodies of the ear and nose. Arch Otolaryngol Head Neck Surg 112:562–563, 1986.
6. Lin Y, Daniel S, Papsin B: Button batteries in the ear, nose, and upper aerodigestive tract. Int J Pediatr Otorhinolaryngol 68:473–479, 2004.
7. Thompson S, Wein R, Dutcher P: External auditory canal foreign body removal: management practices and outcomes. Laryngoscope 113:1912–1915, 2003.
8. Brown L, Denmark T, Wittlake W, et al: Procedural sedation use in the ED: management of pediatric ear and nose foreign bodies. Am J Emerg Med 22:310–314, 2004.
9. Antonelli P, Ahmadi A, Prevatt A: Insecticidal activity of common reagents for insect foreign bodies of the ear. Laryngoscope 111:15–20, 2001.
10. Leffler S, Cheney P, Tandberg D: Chemical immobilization and killing of intra-aural roaches: an in vitro comparative study. Ann Emerg Med 22:1795–1798, 1993.
11. White S, Broner S: The use of acetone to dissolve a styrofoam impaction of the ear. Ann Emerg Med 23:580–582, 1994.
12. Burke M: Small things from small places. Aust Fam Physician 28:132–133, 1999.
13. Thompson M: Removing objects from the external auditory canal. N Engl J Med 311:1635, 1984.
14. McLaughlin R, Ullah R, Heylings D: Comparative prospective study of foreign body removal from external auditory canals of cadavers with right angle hook or cyanoacrylate glue. Emerg Med J 19:43–45, 2002.
15. Cantrell H: More on removing cockroaches from the auditory canal. N Engl J Med 314:720, 1986.
16. Myer C, Cotton R: Nasal obstruction in the pediatric patient. Pediatrics 72:766–777, 1983.
*17. Kalan A, Tariq M: Foreign bodies in the nasal cavities: a comprehensive review of the aetiology, diagnostic pointers, and therapeutic measures. Postgrad Med J 76:484–487, 2000.
18. Fallis G, Ferguson K, Waldman M: Simple technique for removing foreign objects from the nose. Am Fam Physician 46:1046, 1992.
19. Balbani A, Sanchez T, Butugan O, et al: Ear and nose foreign body removal in children. Int J Pediatr Otorhinolaryngol 46:37–42, 1998.
20. Leach A: Evidenced based problem solving in general practice: the foreign body in the nose. J R Army Med Corps 146:31–32, 2000.
21. Kadish H, Corneli H: Removal of nasal foreign bodies in the pediatric population. Am J Emerg Med 15:54–56, 1997.
22. McMaster W: Removal of foreign body from the nose. JAMA 213:1905, 1970.
23. Cohen H, Goldberg E, Horev Z: Removal of nasal foreign bodies in chidren. Clin Pediatr 32:192, 1993.
*24. Gammons M, Jackson E: Fishhook removal. Am Fam Physician 63:2231–2236, 2001.
25. Swanson J, Augustine J: Penetrating intracranial trauma from a fishhook. Ann Emerg Med 21:568–571, 1992.
26. Lantsberg L, Blintsovovsky E, Hoda J: How to extract an indwelling fishhook. Am Fam Physician 45:2589–2590, 1992.
27. Doser C, Cooper W, Ediger W, et al: Fishhook injuries: a prospective evaluation. Am J Emerg Med 9:413–415, 1991.
28. Terrill P: Fishhook removal. Am Fam Physician 47:1372, 1993.
29. Eldad S, Amiram S: Embedded fishhook removal. Am J Emerg Med 18:736–737, 2000.
30. Larkin B: The ins and outs of body piercing. AORN J 79:333–342, 2004.
31. Shacham R, Zaguri A, Librus H, et al: Tongue piercing and its adverse effects. Oral Surg Oral Med Oral Pathol Oral Radiol Endod 95:274–276, 2003.
32. Gleeson A, Gray A: Management of retained ear-rings using an ear block. J Accid Emer Med 12:199–201, 1995.
33. Muensterer O: Temporary removal of navel piercing jewelry for surgery and imaging studies. Pediatrics 114:384–386, 2004.
34. Stirn A: Body piercing: medical consequences and psychological motivations. Lancet 361:1205–1215, 2003.
35. Keogh I, O'Leary G: Serious complications of tongue piercing. J Laryngol Otol 15:233–234, 2001.
36. Biber J: Oral piercing: the hole story. Northwest Dent 82:13–17, 2003.
37. Rubman M: A rapid method for emergency ring removal. Am J Orthop 25:42–44, 1996.
38. Ramponi D: Don't get uptight about ring removal. Nursing 32:56–57, 2002.
39. Inoue S, Akazawa S, Fukuda H, et al: Another simple method for ring removal. Anesthesiology 83:1133–1134, 1995.
*40. Mizrahi S, Lunski I: A simplified method for ring removal from an edematous finger. Am J Surg 151:412–413, 1986.
41. Rubio P: A simplified method for ring removal from an edematous finger. Am J Surg 153:A42, 1987.
42. Baker MD, Lanuti M: The management and outcome of lacerations in urban children. Ann Emerg Med 19:1001–1006, 1990.
43. Chisolm CD, Schlesser JF: Plantar puncture wounds: controversies and treatment recommendations. Ann Emerg Med 18:1352–1357, 1989.
44. Fitzgerald RH, Cowan JD: Puncture wounds of the foot. Orthop Clin North Am 6:965–972, 1975.
45. Brewer Jr TE, Leonard RB: Detection of retained wood following trauma. North Carolina Med J 47:575–577, 1986.
46. Flom LL, Ellis GL: Radiologic evaluation of foreign bodies. Emerg Med Clin North Am 10:163–177, 1992.
47. Hedrick J: Acute bacterial skin infections in pediatric medicine: current issues in presentation and treatment. Paediatr Drugs 5(Suppl 1):35–46, 2003.

---

*Selected readings.

48. Courter BJ: Radiographic screening for glass foreign bodies—what does a "negative" foreign bodies series really mean? Ann Emerg Med 19:997–1000, 1990.

49. Montano JB, Steele MR, Watson WA: Foreign body retention in glass-caused wounds. Ann Emerg Med 21:1360–1363, 1992.

*50. Lammers RL, Magill T: Detection and management of foreign bodies in soft tissue. Emerg Med Clin North Am 10:767–781, 1992.

51. Avner JR, Baker D: Lacerations involving glass. Am J Dis Child 146:600–602, 1992.

52. Bodne D, Quinn SF, Cochran CF: Imaging foreign glass and wooden bodies of the extremities with CT and MR. J Comput Assist Tomogr 12:608–611, 1988.

53. Bikowski J: Secondarily infected wounds and dermatoses: a diagnosis and treatment guide. J Emerg Med 17:197–206, 1999.

54. Dove A, Clifford R: Ischemia after use of a finger tourniquet. Br Med J 284:256, 1982.

55. Pedowitz RA: Limb tourniquets during surgery. Acta Orthop Scand Suppl 245:17–33, 1991.

Chapter 163

Enterostomy Tubes

Andrew D. Mason, MD and Kelly A. Keogh, MD

Key Points

Most problems with enterostomy tubes can be managed by emergency physicians.

Prior to removing and replacing a clogged enterostomy tube, the clinician should attempt to unclog the tube by flushing it with warm water or a carbonated beverage.

One should never attempt to place an enterostomy tube into an immature tract.

Maintaining patency of the fistula is a priority if the tube is dislodged. If replacement tubes are unavailable and the tract is mature, placement of a Foley catheter should be considered to maintain tract patency.

Indications and Contraindications

The use of enteral feeding tubes has become common in the management of children with medical and surgical problems who require long-term enteral feeding.[1] Children who require short-term enteral feeding (<2 to 3 months) are frequently managed with a feeding tube passed through the nose, with the tip of the tube being placed in the stomach (nasogastric tube) or the jejunum (nasojejunal tube). Complications of prolonged nasal tube use include sinusitis, reflux, aspiration, and esophageal strictures.[2]

Enterostomy tubes are placed if prolonged enteral feeding is required. A feeding catheter is placed through the abdominal wall into the stomach (gastrostomy tube, or G tube), or further down the gastrointestinal (GI) tract (gastrojejunostomy tube, or GJ tube, and jejunostomy tube, or J tube). GJ tubes and J tubes have the advantage of a lower incidence of reflux, aspiration, and GI bleeding compared to G tubes. However, GJ tubes and J tubes have a higher rate of obstruction, migration, and intussusception than G tubes.

Several different types of feeding catheters are in use today (Fig. 163–1). Most are made of silicone. A pigtail/loop, balloon, button, or collapsible wing is used to keep the distal end of the tube in place. A bumper or disk may be attached to the tube at the skin surface in order to prevent the tube from migrating inward. After 8 weeks, when the fistula tract matures, the tube may be replaced by a low-profile "button," which is cosmetically superior and eliminates the potential complication of inward migration of the catheter. Options for placement of enterostomy tubes include surgically placed G tubes; tubes placed using percutaneous endoscopy, or percutaneous endoscopic gastrostomy (PEG) tubes; and tubes placed by percutaneous insertion under fluoroscopy without endoscopy, or percutaneous radiologic gastrostomy (PRG) tubes. In patients who are candidates for PEG tube placement, this method of insertion is safer and more cost effective than surgical placement.[3]

Children with existing enterostomy tubes commonly develop problems requiring replacement of the tube. Indications for replacement include tubes that are dislodged, malpositioned, damaged, or occluded (if the occlusion cannot be corrected). Contraindications to replacing enterostomy tubes include recently placed tubes with an immature fistula tract (within 8 weeks of initial operative procedure), a fistula tract that is no longer freely patent, and the presence of peritoneal signs. In these cases, the surgeon, gastroenterologist, or interventional radiologist who originally placed the tube is consulted. Surgery consultation is always required if peritoneal signs are present. If the appropriate consultant is not immediately available, intravenous access is obtained to administer fluids and medication. Enterostomy tubes distal to the stomach (GJ and J tubes) must be replaced endoscopically.

Preparation and Consent

If the tube is dislodged, it must be expeditiously replaced to prevent the fistula tract from closing. Dislodged tubes should be replaced with the same type of tube, and often parents will carry an "extra" with them. If there is no replacement tube immediately available, a Foley catheter can be inserted to preserve fistula patency.

A thorough history should be obtained, including the original date of enterostomy tube placement and prior enterostomy tube complications. Physical examination is performed to ensure that there are no peritoneal signs and that there is no localized infection. The procedure is explained to the patient and family, and informed consent is obtained.

Several types of catheters are currently in use, and each comes with instructions for replacement. Equipment must be

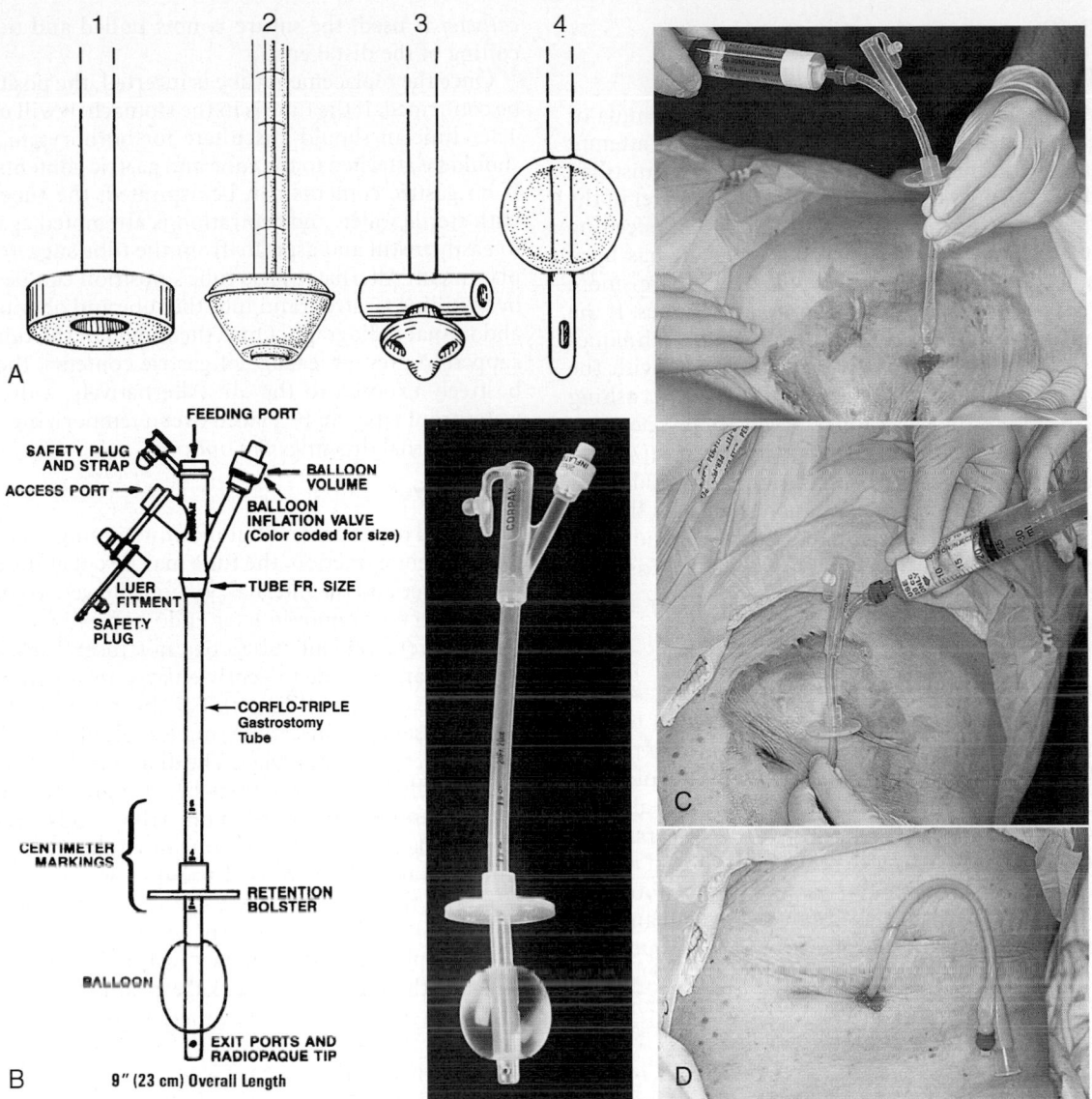

FIGURE 163–1. Various types of gastrostomy tubes. From left to right: coil loop gastrostomy tube (Cook Mac-Loc); balloon gastrostomy tube with a sliding retention disk (MIC, Kimberly Clark), and MIC-Key low-profile gastrostomy feeding tube with antireflux valve.

checked prior to the procedure. For balloon catheters that will be removed, an adaptable syringe (i.e., Luer-Lok) is checked to ensure that it fits the balloon port of the old gastrostomy tube. The integrity of the new balloon is checked. For collapsible wing or mushroom catheters, the clinician should ensure that the stylet or obturator fully distends the distal tip and allows narrowing for passage through the stoma. The child will need to be placed supine and restrained or sedated if unable to cooperate (see Chapter 159, Procedural Sedation and Analgesia).

Equipment

- Replacement tube of the same size as the old tube, *or*
- Temporizing balloon-tipped Foley catheter (one size smaller than the existing enterostomy tube)
- 5-ml syringe for balloon
- Lubricant (i.e., viscous lidocaine or K-Y Jelly)
- 20 ml normal saline
- Stethoscope
- Waterproof tape
- Adaptable syringe or Luer-Lok syringe (for balloon port of old enterostomy tube)
- Benzoin
- Gauze
- Absorbent dressing
- Obturator for stylet of dysfunctional tube (depending on type of tube used)
- Dilators (e.g., Hegar uterine dilators)

Monitoring

Monitoring devices are not necessary for a child simply requiring tube removal or replacement, unless the child is sedated (see Chapter 159, Procedural Sedation and Analgesia).

Techniques

Unblocking an Obstructed Enterostomy Tube

Tubes may become blocked when occluded with formula or undissolved medication. If the tube is blocked, an attempt should be made to unblock it. Warm water is gently instilled into the tube while pushing and pulling on the plunger of the syringe, allowing the water to flow in and out of the feeding tube repeatedly until patency is reestablished. It has been reported anecdotally that carbonated drinks are more effective than noncarbonated fluids for clearing tubes. If the tube remains blocked, then it must be replaced. Techniques to prevent future obstruction should be reviewed with the family, such as avoiding thick suspensions and fully crushing and dissolving tablets in warm water. Medications known to have a high incidence of tube obstruction include corn starch, lactulose, cholestyramine, kayexalate, magnesium oxide, ciprofloxacin, and clarithromycin. The tube should be flushed with at least 10 ml of sterile water after each use, and every 4 hours when the patient is receiving continuous feeds.

Removal of Dysfunctional G Tubes With a Mature Fistula Tract

First, the stoma site is liberally lubricated with water-soluble lubricant or lidocaine gel. If the old tube is balloon tipped, an adaptable syringe is attached to the balloon port of the old tube and the balloon contents are withdrawn. If the old tube has a loop, there is a suture at the skin surface that allowed the distal aspect of the tube to coil, preventing expulsion. This suture should be cut prior to removal. If the old tube is a collapsible wing or mushroom type, a stylet or obturator (which came with the catheter) is inserted to extend and collapse the distal tip within the stomach wall. A cooperative child can be asked to take a deep breath and hold it. As the child takes a breath, the tube is removed by gentle, constant traction.

Replacement of G Tubes With a Mature Fistula Tract

Several types of catheters are currently in use, and each comes with specific instructions for replacement. The stoma site is liberally lubricated prior to introducing the new catheter. The catheter is inserted into the stoma perpendicular to the abdominal wall. Holding the tip of the catheter between the thumb and index finger and placing the heel of the hand on the abdominal wall will stabilize it. The tip of the catheter is passed into the stoma with steady, firm pressure directed posteriorly, perpendicular to the abdominal wall. It may take 30 to 45 seconds of this steady pressure to stretch the site enough to permit entry. Intermittent or jerky movements should be avoided. Constant gentle, firm pressure directed posteriorly will maximize success. When the stomach is entered, the resistance suddenly decreases. The catheter should be advanced further to ensure placement in the stomach.

If a *balloon-tipped catheter* is used, the balloon is inflated with saline or water, and then pulled gently outward until the balloon contacts the stomach wall. If a *mushroom or collapsible wing type of catheter* is used, the obturator or stylet is now fully removed. The collapsible wing tube is gently pulled outward until the wings contact the stomach wall. If a *loop*

catheter is used, the suture is now pulled and tied to allow coiling of the distal end.

Once the replacement tube is inserted, the position should be confirmed. If the tube is in the stomach, it will move freely. The clinician should auscultate for borborygmi. A syringe should be attached to the tube and gastric contents aspirated. If no gastric contents can be aspirated, the tube is flushed with sterile water, and aspiration is attempted again. Failure to easily instill and aspirate from the tube suggests incorrect placement. Alternately, the tube's position can be confirmed by instilling Gastrografin into the tube and obtaining a plain abdominal radiograph. Once the lumen of the tube has been capped to prevent leakage of gastric contents, the tube may be freely exposed to the air. Alternatively, a dressing with waterproof tape can be placed over a temporizing Foley catheter. External dressings are optional.

Alternatives

If removal of the current but malfunctioning tube is not possible by gentle traction, the tube may be cut at the abdominal wall surface and the internal portion allowed to pass through the GI tract, or removed later endoscopically.

If the replacement tube does not insert successfully, an attempt can be made to gently enlarge the mature tract with dilators (e.g., Hegar dilators). For this purpose, the clinician should first gently insert the smallest blunt dilator that easily fits completely into the tract. The dilator is then gently rotated to gradually increase the tract size. Progressively larger dilators are inserted into the tract until the tract is an appropriate size for the replacement enterostomy tube. During dilation, clinicians must be sure that the dilators are in the correct tract and that trauma to the site is minimal. Alternately, a temporizing Foley catheter can be inserted into the tract. If the fit is not snug, the patency of the fistula will be maintained, although excessive leakage around the tube may limit the catheter's use for feeds or medications.

Complications

Complications are divided into those that occur soon after an enterostomy tube is manipulated or replaced, and delayed complications of enterostomy tube placement and utilization (Table 163–1).

Immediate Complications

Unsuccessful Replacement

In the event that the catheter will not advance into the stoma, or if the child is in extreme distress, the clinician should assume that the fistula is no longer patent. In this case, endoscopic or surgical placement of a new tube may be necessary. Intravenous access is obtained to administer fluids and medications pending definitive management.

Peritonitis

Peritonitis is an uncommon but serious complication after initial radiologic placement of a G tube, with an estimated incidence of up to 3%.[4] When replacing a G tube, the fistula can become disrupted, creating a false lumen into the peritoneum. This complication is more common with immature fistulas. If excessive force is used, perforation of the stomach or bowel may occur. Instillation of formula into an improperly positioned tube or perforated viscus can cause chemical

Table 163–1	Enterostomy Tube Complications and Management	
Complication	**Possibility**	**Management**
Tube dislodged < 8 wk after placement	If tube < 8 wk old, an immature fistula is present.	Do not replace tube percutaneously. Endoscopic or surgical replacement may be needed.
Tube dislodged > 8 wk after placement	Mature fistula is likely.	Replace tube or insert Foley catheter (one size smaller if needed). Dilators (e.g., Hegar cervical dilators) may be needed to gently enlarge tract. Confirm position by aspirating gastric contents. If unable, consider contrast confirmation.
Tube cannot be used for medicine or feeds	Tube is blocked from medications or inadequate postuse flushing.	Flush tube with warm water or carbonated beverage using small syringe under high pressure. Push and pull on the plunger of the syringe, allowing the water to flow in and out of the feeding tube repeatedly until patency is reestablished.
Tube leakage	Tube may be broken, or tube may be intact and leakage may be from around tube.	If tube is leaking, replace with similar-size tube. If unable to replace, seal tube with tape. If tube is intact and leakage is around site, see below.
Tube site redness, discharge, or irritation	Tube may be too mobile or loose, gastric contents may be leaking, infection may be present, granulation tissue may be forming, or tape allergy may be present.	Tube mobility—secure tube with tape Leaking gastric contents—apply antacids or barrier cream to site Infection—cleanse, administer antimicrobials Granulation tissue—soak with saline or apply silver nitrate sticks as needed Tape allergy—use hypoallergenic tape.
Tube migration	Tube is too mobile.	Secure tube to skin and consider disk to stabilize if needed.
Vomiting with gastrostomy tube	Balloon migration to duodenum with obstruction.	Measure tube length and reposition or pull back.
Vomiting with gastrojejunostomy tube	Gastric coil leak Migration into stomach Intussusception	Diagnose with contrast study (via tube). Ultrasound may diagnose intussusception. Removal is required if coil leak or migration is present, with air contrast enema for intussusception.
Formula-like diarrhea	Enterocolonic fistula	Diagnose with contrast study. Surgery may be required.

or bacterial peritonitis. Patients with peritonitis may present with vomiting, fever, and abdominal pain and distention. Management includes discontinuation of tube use, empirical antibiotic administration, and surgical consultation.

Malpositioned Enterostomy Tube

If the new tube is not advanced far enough, the distal tip will be in the fistula tract rather than the stomach. Pain and leakage will occur during instillation of materials through the tube. If this occurs, the tube should be advanced further.

Gastric Outlet Obstruction

If the catheter is not properly secured, it can migrate proximally or distally in the GI tract, resulting in esophageal migration, gastric outlet obstruction, or intestinal obstruction. Management consists of withdrawing the G tube to the appropriate position.

Delayed Complications

Major Complications

Major complications include aspiration of feeds with resulting pneumonia, peritonitis, or GI hemorrhage, and fistula formation, requiring discontinuation of enterostomy tube use and administration of intravenous hydration and medications as required.

Aspiration of feeds is a common problem in children whose oromotor pathology predisposes them to aspiration and pneumonia. Patients present with respiratory distress. Acute treatment may include antibiotics, bronchodilators, and steroids. Preventative measures include medications to reduce gastroesophageal reflux, and positioning of the tube distal to the pylorus (J tube).

Gastrointestinal hemorrhage is relatively uncommon but may be secondary to ulceration at the enterostomy site and gastritis. Following acute resuscitation, treatment may include discontinuation of tube use, administration of medications to reduce gastric acid production, and removal of the tube.

Fistulas may develop in patients with enteral feeding tubes. Fistulas may connect to the skin (enterocutaneous) or to the bowel (enterocolonic). Children with enterocolonic fistulas may present with liquid stools. Contrast studies may be helpful to delineate the fistula tract.

Vomiting (bilious or nonbilious) in patients with enterostomy tubes may indicate partial or complete bowel obstruction. Often a radiographic contrast study is helpful. Common causes include

- Inward migration of the balloon into the pylorus. This may be relieved by applying traction to pull the balloon back against the gastric wall, and securing it in place.
- Development of intussusception around GJ tubes. This requires radiologic evaluation. Shortening the length of the tube or replacing it entirely will usually relieve the intussusception. This procedure is usually performed by interventional radiology.

Other common causes of vomiting include gastritis, ulcers, and systemic infection.

Buried bumper syndrome occurs in patients whose internal bumper erodes through the gastric mucosa. As the erosion re-epithialines over the bumper, it becomes "buried." Patient's symptoms frequently begin several months after placement of the tube, and include pain with feeding, resistance to flow, and irritability with movement or rotation of the tube. Replacement of the tube is curative.

Minor Complications

Minor complications of enterostomy tube use are common, and are often considered "routine maintenance problems." These include blocked tubes (see Techniques section), dislodged tubes, and stoma site problems.

DISLODGED TUBE

Dislodged enteral tubes require expeditious attention since the fistula tract between the skin and stomach may close within hours. If it has been less than 8 weeks since insertion of the enterostomy tube, the fistula tract is immature, and the tube is NOT replaced in the emergency department. The clinician who inserted the tube is consulted. With a mature fistula tract, however, the enterostomy tube may be replaced, or a Foley catheter may be used to maintain fistula patency. For J tubes, a Foley catheter is inserted to maintain fistula patency until the tube can be replaced by an interventional radiologist.

STOMA SITE PROBLEMS

Stoma erythema must be differentiated into infectious and noninfectious causes. *Stoma site infection* may cause erythema, induration, tenderness, and local discharge. Infections are usually polymicrobial, predominately staphylococcal and streptococcal organisms. Minor infections often respond to topical antimicrobial ointment. Cellulitis is treated with systemic antibiotics. Yeast superinfection may present with typical "satellite" lesions. Wound cultures may be helpful for definitive diagnosis, especially in patients who are unresponsive to initial therapy or who are at risk for infection with resistant microorganisms (e.g., methicillin-resistant *Staphylococcus aureus*).

Noninfectious causes of stoma site erythema include irritation from leakage of gastric contents around the tube, mechanical irritation due to friction from movement of the tube, allergy to tape, and formation of granulation tissue. Many skin problems respond to saline-soaked dressings changed three times a day, barrier creams, hypoallergenic tape, and tighter affixing of the tube to the skin to prevent excessive movement. If these techniques are ineffective, definitive treatment may require shortening of the tube or conversion to another type of enterostomy tube.

Dermatitis from leakage of gastric contents may occur if there is excessive space between the fistula tract and the catheter. Barrier cream is applied to protect the abdominal wall. Medications to decrease gastric acid production and local application of antacids may be beneficial. Persistent leakage of gastric contents may respond to discontinuation of tube use and connection to low suction for a time. If unsuccessful, the tube may require endoscopic replacement with a larger tube.

Granuloma formation at the enterostomy tube site appears as a pink or red cauliflower-like protuberance. This may regress with measures to decrease local irritation, such as saline-soaked dressings, and minimizing excessive movement of the tube. Bleeding is treated with the application of direct pressure, or cauterization with silver nitrate.

Postprocedure Care and Disposition

Patients are advised to return to the emergency department for potential complications of enterostomy tube placement, including abdominal pain, vomiting, fever, GI bleeding, and respiratory distress. Parents are advised that the best way to avoid tube obstruction is with proper flushing of the tube before and after each use. Parents should also be reassured that blockage, malpositioned tubes, cellulitis, and granuloma formation are not necessarily the result of incorrect technique, but rather are common and often unavoidable complications of enteral feeding tubes.

REFERENCES

1. Campos ACL, Marchesini JB: Recent advances in the placement of tubes for enteral nutrition. Curr Opin Clin Metab Care 2:265–269, 1999.
2. Hamaoui E, Kodsi R: Complications of enteral feedings and their prevention. In Rombeau JL, Rolandelli R (eds): Clinical Nutrition: Enteral and Tube Feeding. Philadelphia: WB Saunders 1997, pp 554–574.
3. Wollman BS, D'Agostino HB, Walus-Wigle JR, et al: Radiologic, endoscopic, and surgical gastrostomy: an institutional evaluation and meta-analysis of the literature. Radiology 197:699–704, 1995.
4. Friedman JN, Ahmed S, Connolly B, et al: Complications associated with image-guided gastrostomy and gastrojejunostomy tubes in children. Pediatrics 114:458–461, 2004.

Chapter 164

Replacing a Tracheostomy Tube

Jill C. Posner, MD, MSCE

Key Points

Respiratory distress in a patient with a tracheostomy indicates tube obstruction until proven otherwise.

It is important to ascertain and understand the indication for patient's tracheostomy.

All equipment (including rescue devices) should be prepared prior to initiating the procedure.

Parents and/or home care nurses are excellent sources for information and assistance.

The clinician should recognize when help is needed and call for assistance and/or backup (otorhinolaryngology, anesthesia).

Indications and Contraindications

In children, tracheostomies are indicated for respiratory insufficiency due to a variety of disorders, most commonly bronchopulmonary dysplasia and airway anomalies, including congenital anomalies and subglottic stenosis. Relatively common indications are neuromuscular or central diseases such as a brain tumor or Chiari malformation.[1-3] A child with a tracheostomy may or may not require additional ventilatory assistance.

Routine care for the child with an artificial airway includes periodic replacement of the tracheostomy tube. Commonly, trained family members or skilled home care nurses carry out this procedure in the child's home. However, in crisis situations or when acute medical issues arise, families will seek assistance from an emergency department or other health care personnel. The indications for tracheostomy tube replacement are *cannula obstruction* and *cannula dislodgement*. A child with a tracheostomy and respiratory distress is assumed to have airway compromise until proven otherwise.[4]

Patients may present with bleeding from the tracheostomy tube. Intratracheal bleeding most commonly results from drying and friability of the tracheal mucosa due to inadequate humidification. However, even a small amount of bleeding from the tracheostomy tube may indicate a rare but life-threatening condition: erosion of the distal aspect of the tube into an innominate vessel. Large amounts of bleeding may ensue, making it difficult to secure the airway if the tracheostomy tube is removed. For this reason, tracheostomy tube change is relatively contraindicated in patients with bleeding depending upon the suspicion of arterial erosion and the severity of the patient's symptoms.

Preparation and Consent

Ideally, there should be at least two people available for the procedure, one to secure the patient and remove the old cannula and a second person who is responsible for placing the new tube. All the equipment necessary to complete a cannula replacement should be on hand, as should airway adjuncts, suction devices, and other rescue devices. Formal informed consent procedures are not necessary when managing an airway emergency; however, it is important to keep patients, caregivers, and nurses informed about management plans.

Equipment

Many caregivers of children with tracheostomy tubes are taught to carry "go-bags" or "emergency boards" containing all of the equipment required to perform an emergent tracheostomy tube change with them at all times. This includes a bag-mask ventilation device, oxygen source, replacement cannula, endotracheal tubes of the same diameter and smaller, lubricant, scissors, securing ties, and padding.[5] If such a bag/board is not available, all the necessary equipment should be gathered prior to initiating the procedure.

Tracheostomy Tube Features

Some characteristics of a patient's tracheostomy tube of importance in the emergent setting are its size, whether it is cuffed or uncuffed, if it has an inner cannula, and if it is fenestrated. Tracheostomy tubes are *sized* according to three dimensions: the inner diameter, the outer diameter, and the length. The inner diameter is standardized among the many manufacturers of tracheostomy tubes, whereas the other dimensions may vary considerably among manufacturers. All or some of the dimensions of an individual tube are generally imprinted on that tube's flanges. In addition,

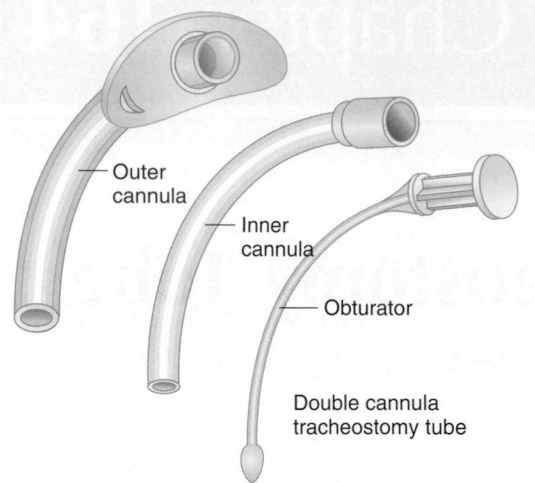

Outer
cannula

Inner
cannula

Obturator

Double cannula
tracheostomy tube

FIGURE 164–1. Use of double-cannula tracheostomy tube. Insertion of a double-cannula tracheostomy tube requires an outer cannula, an inner cannula, and an obturator.

tracheostomy tubes may be *cuffed* or *uncuffed*. The general guideline that the use of a cuffed tube is reserved for children over 8 years old does *not* hold true for children with tracheostomy tubes. Younger children, and even infants, may have a cuffed tracheostomy tube in place (e.g., if there is an airway anomaly); therefore, it is always important to look for the presence of a cuff for any age child and be sure to deflate it prior to removal of the trachestomy tube.

Some tubes have a single cannula with a removable obturator, while others have a double cannula with an outer and and an *inner cannula* (Fig. 164–1). This type of tube commonly is used for children with especially precarious airways, for whom routine tracheostomy tube changes could prove particularly threatening. With this type of tube, the inner cannula can be removed and cleaned while the outer cannula remains in place, providing a secure airway at all times. Importantly, the manual resuscitator bag cannot be attached directly to the outer cannula, and the inner cannula must be in place for hand ventilation. Finally, a *fenestrated* tube has a hole in the posterior aspect of the tube that allows the child to vocalize by forcing air retrograde through the vocal cords.[4,6,7]

Monitoring

The monitoring of patients undergoing tracheostomy tube replacement parallels that which is routinely performed for other airway emergencies. Careful observation of cardiorespiratory function and gas exchange is performed noninvasively via cardiorespiratory and pulse oximetry monitoring. The detection of end-tidal carbon dioxide ($ETCO_2$) by colorimetric (yellow = yes, blue = bad) or capnography devices assists in the assessment of proper tube position.

Techniques

Assessment of Tube Position and Patency

The immediate management of patients presenting in respiratory distress with a tracheotomy tube seemingly in place is to assess tube position and patency. The clinician should keep in mind that a tracheostomy tube positioned in the stoma does not necessarily indicate that it is positioned in the trachea, as false passage into the paratracheal soft tissues may have resulted in prior replacement attempts either at home or en route to the hospital. High-flow humidified oxygen should be supplied while rapidly evaluating tube positioning by physical examination and noninvasive monitoring techniques.

Clearing an Obstructed Tracheostomy Tube

Removal of obstructing secretions by careful suctioning may negate the need for emergent tracheostomy tube replacement. One to 2 ml of normal saline is placed into the tube to loosen secretions. The largest size suction catheter that will fit is inserted into the tube 2 to 3 inches into the cannula. If the child starts to cough, the catheter is in deep enough. Suction is applied for 3 to 5 seconds—and never for more than 10 seconds—with a portable machine set to 100 mm Hg or less. Heart rate and pulse oximetry should always be monitored,[6,8] and suctioning should be stopped if the patient develops bradycardia or cyanosis. If suctioning equipment is not available, the clinician may try clearing the tube of secretions by inserting the obturator or a smaller sized endotracheal tube. If the tube cannot be cleared and respiratory distress continues, the tracheostomy tube should be changed.

Replacing a Tracheostomy Tube

Positioning the Patient

The patient should be lying supine with the neck in slight extension, fully exposing the tracheostomy tube and stoma. A rolled towel can be placed under the patient's shoulders to further optimize the view of the tracheal stoma. At least two people should be available to execute the tracheostomy tube change. One has the responsibility of securing the patient's head and removing the old tube, while the other's focus is on placing the new tube.

Removing the Old Tube

Before removing the existing tube, it is necessary to check for a balloon, indicating the tube has a cuff, and deflate it by aspirating until the balloon is flat (cutting the balloon will *not* deflate the cuff). Securing tape or ties are unfastened or cut. The tube is removed by withdrawing it out and down in an arclike motion.

Inserting the New Tube

After lubricating the tube and with the obturator in place, the tip of the cannula is gently placed into the stoma, pushing it posteriorly and down (again, in an arclike motion) using gentle pressure. The clinician should avoid scraping the posterior aspect of the trachea. The tube is pushed in until the flanges are flush against the patient's neck. The obturator is removed, and the inner cannala inserted and connected to the bag-valve circuit (Fig. 164–2). The cuff is then inflated if used.

Confirmation of Tube Positioning

Physical examination clues (e.g., improvement in respiratory distress, equal breath sounds over the anterior and lateral

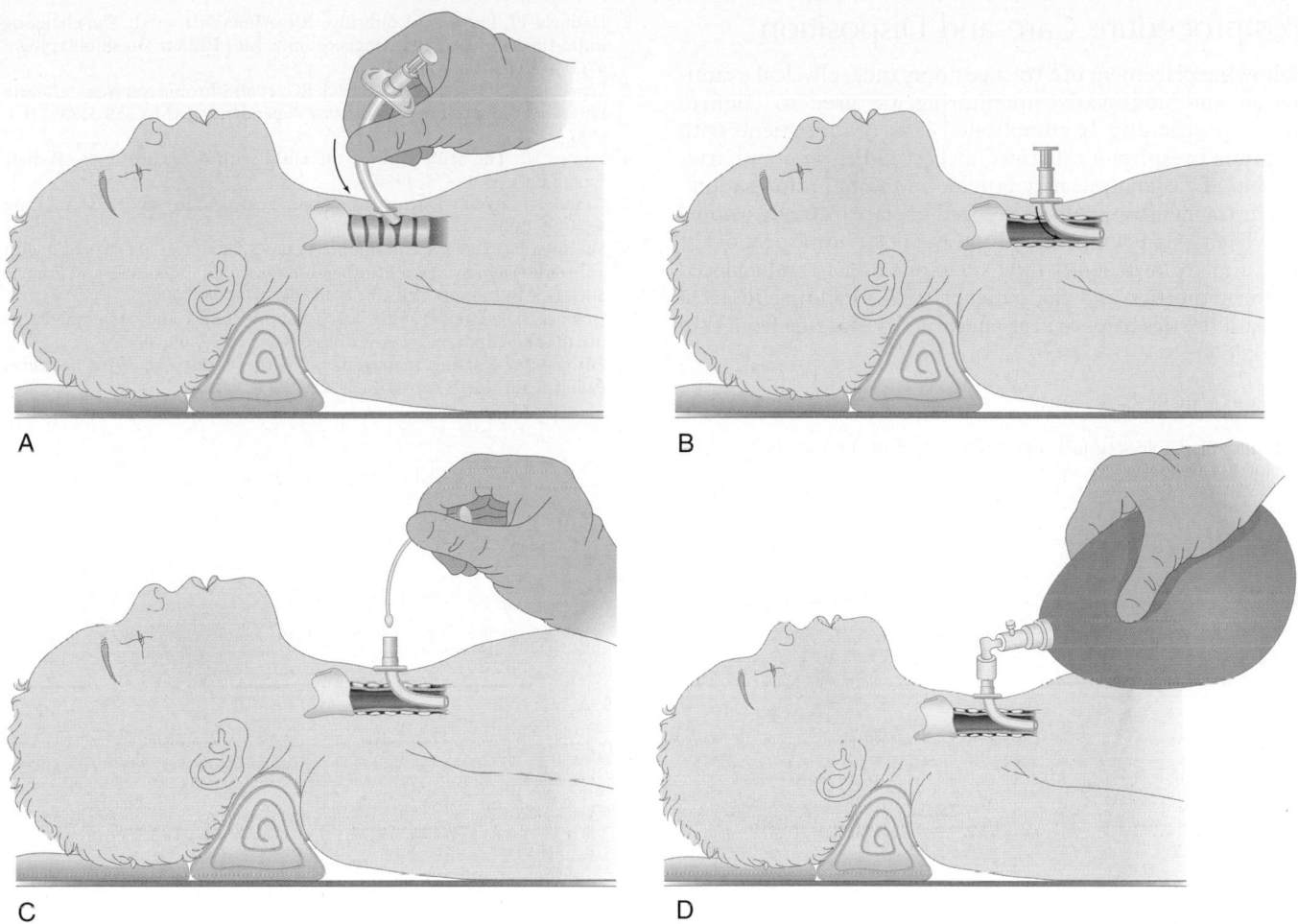

FIGURE 164–2. Placement of a trachestomy tube. Using an arclike motion and with the obturator inserted, the tracheostomy tube is gently guided into the tracheal stoma **(A)** until the flanges are flush against the skin of the neck **(B).** The obturator is removed **(C)** and the resuscitor bag attached to the trachestomy tube **(D),** thereby facilitating manual ventilation.

chest walls, symmetric chest rise) and $ETCO_2$ monitoring are used to confirm placement into the trachea. The tube is then secured using tracheostomy tube ties and padded sufficiently to avoid neck irritation.

Alternatives

Constriction tends to occur when the tracheal stoma is left unstented, a condition that may make it difficult to pass a replacement tube of the patient's usual size. In these instances, the airway should be secured with the largest size tube that the stoma will accommodate. Generally, a tracheostomy tube one-half size smaller is sufficient. Alternatively, a smaller sized endotracheal tube is placed and then the stoma is dilated to its original size through serial insertions of progressively larger endotracheal tubes.

If false passage into the paratracheal soft tissues occurs, it may be helpful to use an oxygen catheter, or an endotracheal intubating stylet with an internal oxygen source (e.g., Frova), or gum elastic bougie as a guide for the tracheostomy tube insertion using the Seldinger technique. The catheter is placed into the tracheal stoma and the patient is oxygenated. The oxygen source is separated from the catheter or stylet. The connector tip is cut off if an oxygen catheter is

used, or the intubating stylet is disconnected from its oxygen source. Next, the tracheostomy tube is slid over the catheter/stylet into the trachea. Then, the catheter or stylet is removed.

Finally, if attempts to secure the airway via the stoma fail, traditional bag-valve-mask techniques (the stoma should be covered with a gloved finger) may be applied, or the airway may be secured using oral-tracheal methods. The indication for the patient's tracheostomy should be considered before electing to administer neuromuscular blocking agents. In cases of airway anomalies (e.g., a tracheal shelf), the anatomic landmarks commonly used in direct laryngoscopy may be obscured or absent, thereby impeding a successful intubation. In such cases, it may be prudent for the clinician to provide support of the patient's own respiratory effort and call for anesthesia or otorhinolaryngology assistance.

Complications

The most common complications encountered during the replacement of a tracheostomy tube are the inability to replace the tube and the false passage of the tube into a paratracheal soft tissue tract. In addition, pneumothorax can occur with manual or mechanical ventilation.

Postprocedure Care and Disposition

Following placement of a tracheostomy tube, physical examination and noninvasive monitoring are used to confirm proper positioning. In complicated cases or for patients with continued respiratory distress, a chest radiograph and arterial blood gas analysis may provide additional information.

The tracheostomy tube is secured in place by tracheostomy ties. The ties are wrapped around the posterior aspect of the neck and are sufficiently tight when one finger can be placed between the ties and the patient's neck.[6] Padding inserted beneath the ties helps to keep the neck dry and free from skin breakdown.

REFERENCES

1. Pilmer SL: Prolonged mechanical ventilation in children. Pediatr Clin North Am 41:473–512, 1994.
2. Hadfield PJ, Lloyd-Faulconbridge RV, Almeyda J, et al: The changing indications for paediatric tracheostomy. Int J Pediatr Otorhinolaryngol 67:7–10, 2003.
3. Schreiner MS, Downes JJ, Kettrick RG, et al: Chronic respiratory failure in infants with prolonged ventilator dependency. JAMA 258:3398–3404, 1987.
4. Posner JC: The acute care of the child with a tracheostomy. Pediatr Emerg Care 15:49–54, 1999.
5. Gracey K, Fiske E: Tracheostomy home care guide. Adv Neonatal Care 4:54–55, 2004.
6. Sherman JM, Davis S, Albamonte-Petris S, et al: Care of the child with a chronic tracheostomy: the official statement of the American Thoracic Society. Am J Respir Crit Car Med 161:297–308, 2000.
7. Downes JJ, Schreiner MS: Tracheostomy tubes and attachments in infants and children. Int Anesthesiol Clin 23:37–60, 1985.
8. Fitton CM: Nursing management of the child with a tracheotomy. Pediatr Clin North Am 41:513–523, 1994.

Ventilator Considerations

John A. Tilelli, MD

Indications

Mechanical ventilation of children with respiratory insufficiency, once a procedure solely found in the intensive care unit, is now increasingly performed in the outpatient setting. As such, patients now come to the emergency department for the management of complications of home ventilation. Furthermore, the application of mechanical ventilation in the emergency department in support of the child in need of airway control or ventilatory assistance is increasing. Emergency physicians must be familiar with the techniques of home mechanical ventilation and of the practical considerations of initiating mechanical ventilation in the patient who presents with an acute illness.

Mechanical ventilation is used most frequently to augment minute ventilation of the patient in whom airflow is impaired by weakness, fatigue, altered lung mechanics, or loss of respiratory drive, and for the application of positive pressure to the airway to improve lung volume and thereby favorably affect oxygenation. Related indications are found in the management of extrapulmonary diseases in which control of ventilation or decreasing the work of breathing might be important, such as the control of carbon dioxide tension in head injury, or the management of congestive heart failure (Table 165–1).

Occasionally, mechanical ventilation may be instituted for the delivery of medications to the airway, such as nitric oxide, helium-oxygen mixtures, bronchodilators, or antibiotics. Mechanical ventilation may be instituted as an aid to pulmonary toilet in the patient with impaired secretion clearance.

Strictly speaking, there are no contraindications to mechanical ventilation for the patient in whom the airway is controlled. Many of the issues that physicians confront in the decision to secure the airway embrace the question of whether or not mechanical ventilation should be undertaken. For infants and children with terminal disease, family members and primary care physicians can assist with decisions regarding the appropriateness of instituting mechanical ventilation (see Chapter 148, End-of-Life Issues).

Preparation and Consent

If time permits, consent for mechanical ventilation is obtained in conjunction with that for airway control. However, in the emergency department, most children requiring intubation and mechanical ventilation are critically ill, and consent is implied based on the existence of an emergency. Mechanical ventilation involves many of the same risks as that of intubation, and is often seen as an extension of the latter procedure. Special risks attributable to mechanical ventilation include the need for deeper and more prolonged sedation, the acquisition of ventilator-associated pneumonia, muscular weakness resulting from disuse, and barotrauma-induced lung disease, possibly necessitating prolonged mechanical assistance.

Preparation for mechanical ventilation involves the choice of a mechanical ventilator, and assembly of the circuit.[1] The ventilator used depends to some extent on the mode of ventilation provided. While most modern ventilators offer a choice of volume- or pressure-regulated, assisted and controlled modes, some neonatal ventilators may not be able to deliver a volume-controlled breath. Ventilators designed for adults may not be sufficiently sensitive to detect inspiration in an infant, or able to deliver a reliably small-volume breath, and thus function poorly as a child ventilator. Monitoring devices should be at the bedside and calibrated.

Table 165–1	Indications for Mechanical Ventilation

Impaired Minute Ventilation

- *Increased work of breathing:* pneumonia, pulmonary fibrosis, small airways disease, impaired chest wall compliance such as in burns
- *Decreased ability to sustain the work of breathing:* neuromuscular disease, electrolyte disturbances characterized by weakness (e.g., hypokalemia, hypocalcemia)
- *Altered control of breathing:* trauma, sedative drugs, postictal state, congenital or acquired diseases of respiratory control such as apnea of prematurity

Alteration of Lung Mechanics

- *Positive pressure ventilation:* atelectasis, acute respiratory distress syndrome, tracheomalacia with airway closure, ascites or chest wall injury, extraventilatory air or pleural effusions

Adjunctive Management of Extrapulmonary Disease

- *Hyperventilation:* head trauma, ↑ intracranial pressure (primarily a temporizing measure)
- *Decrease work of breathing:* congestive heart failure
- *Improvement of cardiopulmonary interactions:* shock, sepsis, hypovolemia, pulmonary hypertension

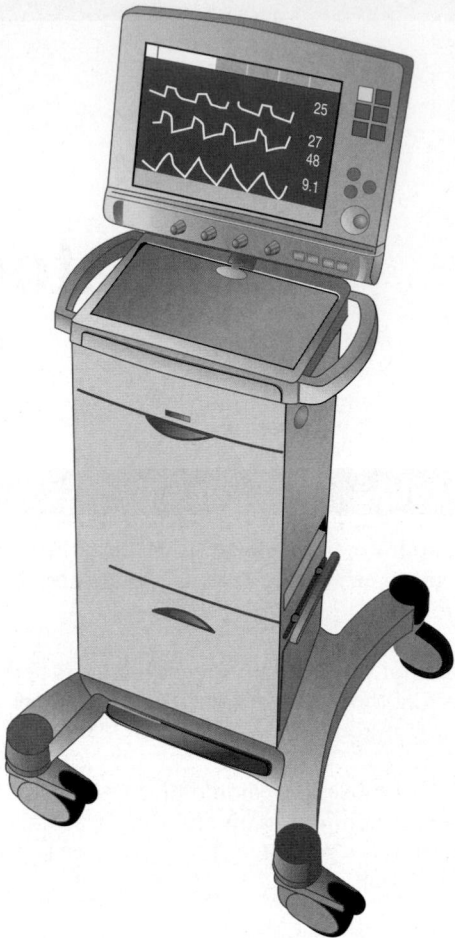

FIGURE 165–1. Servo-i ventilator. All controls are accessible from the simple panel surrounding the display screen. (Photo courtesy of Maquet.)

Patients who come with their own mechanical ventilator offer an opportunity for the physician to assess the mode of ventilation that best suits the patient. Assessment of these patients requires the determination of the goal of home ventilation, the equipment that was being used, and the settings that were applied prior to arrival at the emergency room. The physician should understand whether the patent was being ventilated for the delivery of oxygen, augmentation of minute ventilation, or improvement of lung mechanics. An understanding of the underlying disease of the child is mandatory.[2] The review of the medical record of a child who has previously been ventilated may provide valuable insight into optimum ventilator settings. If the patient is to be ventilated using a device brought from home, it should be inspected by an individual familiar with its assembly and operation to assure that it is functioning properly.

The airway will have been secured prior to the institution of ventilation (see Chapter 3, Rapid Sequence Intubation; and Chapter 4, Intubation, Rescue Devices, and Airway Adjuncts). Endotracheal intubation is the most common method, but occasionally mechanical ventilation may be applied to the patient via a laryngeal mask airway or an occlusive mask device.[3] After intubation, placement of a nasogastric tube may be required to relieve abdominal distention, a maneuver that may improve respiratory mechanics. Bagging the patient will give information on the compliance of the lungs and chest wall. A patient with decreased compliance may be difficult to bag, predicting the need for high mean airway pressures and difficulty with pressure-regulated ventilation. Auscultation of the patient during bagging is of further assistance in determining the initial ventilator settings. Expiratory wheezes as the result of small airways disease might suggest that a ventilatory technique of prolonging expiration would be helpful in reducing gas trapping. Symmetric breath sounds provide some assurance that the airway is secured in a manner in which both lungs can be ventilated equally, but may be deceptive. Review of a chest radiograph with the patient on the mechanical ventilator will confirm satisfactory

tube placement, equal lung ventilation, the absence of gas trapping, and satisfactory tidal volume.

Sedation is almost always required for mechanical ventilation, except in the patient who arrives in stable condition having been chronically mechanically ventilated. Frequently, the same agents that were administered during intubation may be continued during mechanical ventilation. The need for neuromuscular relaxation should be judged by the possible benefits to respiratory mechanics of paralysis, versus the loss of a neurologic examination.[4] Whether or not paralysis is initiated, analgesics, anxiolytics, and sedatives should be administered based on the clinical condition of the patient. Benzodizaepines and narcotics are appropriate. With or without neuromuscular relaxation, satisfactory sedation can be maintained in the great majority of patients with these agents alone.[5] Etomidate and propofol, while unsatisfactory for prolonged sedation, may be useful in the emergency setting.[6,7]

Equipment

A wide array of mechanical ventilators is available for clinical use. Some generalities can be made. The Servo-i is prototypic of a modern mechanical ventilator (Fig. 165–1). Air movement is provided by compressed gas, and a microprocessor controls delivery. Medical oxygen and air connections are required. The ventilator is connected to the patient via a low-compliance circuit (i.e., one that does not distend appreciably during a respiratory cycle). Delivered air is humidified with a heated reservoir in line with the circuit. At the patient end of the circuit, a port may be present to facilitate suctioning. Uninterrupted power is recommended, unless the ventilator is equipped with a battery backup. Scavenger gas collection is necessary if the administration of anesthetic gases is anticipated.

Monitoring

All patients who are mechanically ventilated require continuous monitoring. Measurement of heart rate, respirations, and blood pressure should be routinely performed. Oxygen saturation via pulse oximetry is also routine. End-tidal carbon dioxide determination provides important insurance that the ventilator is attached to the patient and is functioning properly, and may decrease the need for repeated blood gas determinations[8] (see Chapter 5, Monitoring in Critically Ill Children). Ventilators are manufactured with alarms to detect changes in airway pressure and changes in delivered volume; these should always be turned on and have appropriate tolerances for the ventilator settings. Additionally, many modern mechanical ventilators continuously display information relevant to the delivery of gas. Airway pressure, gas flow, delivered volume, and inspired oxygen concentration are typical of the parameters that are displayed. Likewise, the temperature of humidified air is monitored. The size of a modern emergency room may not be conducive to prompt detection of an alarm. As a result, central monitoring is desirable.

Notwithstanding the degree of assurance provided by automated alarm systems, all patients should be located in an area where they may be continuously observed and intervention promptly undertaken if the need arises. Supervising personnel should have a working knowledge of the ventilator alarms, and the appropriate interventions if the patient deteriorates or if there is a malfunction.

Technique

Modern mechanical ventilation offers a variety of modes, each useful under a given set of circumstances.[9] The emergency physician should have a working knowledge of the basic modes, realizing that the desired result is delivery of satisfactory minute ventilation and the improvement of lung mechanics.

Conceptual Framework

The conceptual framework of mechanical ventilation is as follows.

Tidal Volume

The volume of a single breath, either spontaneously or provided by the ventilator, is termed the *tidal volume*. It represents the total of the effective ventilation (i.e., alveolar, and wasted ventilation or dead space). Volume lost in the ventilator circuit due to its compliance characteristics is generally not included in the determination of tidal volume.

Minute Volume

The volume of gas moved in 1 minute, totaling that spontaneously inspired by the patient plus the sum of the assisted breaths, is the *minute volume*. Its relative magnitude is an estimate of the degree to which ventilation is supported by the mechanical ventilator itself.

Mandatory Ventilation

The ventilator may initiate a breath at a predetermined volume or pressure, at an appointed rate. It may be coordinated with a patient breath, initiated to correspond to an inspiratory effort (synchronized) either intermittently or continuously. The ventilator senses patient effort as a negative pressure on the airway, typically −1 to −3 cm H_2O. The sensitivity of the ventilator is determined by adjusting the negative pressure required to initiate a ventilator breath. If the sensitivity is set too low, the patient may not exert enough force to trigger a breath. If the ventilator is too sensitive, ventilator breaths may be initiated one on top of another, leaving insufficient time for exhalation. Synchronized intermittent mandatory ventilation is the most common mode employed in the acute setting.

Assisted Ventilation

The ventilator may assist a patient breath by providing airflow and pressure during an inspiratory effort. This assisted breath is initiated by patient effort, as a negative inspiratory pressure, similar to that provided by a synchronized mandatory breath. In contrast, assisted breaths are limited to the augmentation of respiration by adding supplemental pressure to the airway as the patient needs it. Patients are more comfortable and have improved distribution of ventilation in assisted as opposed to mandatory modes.[10] Pressure support gives assistance to the patient to overcome the airway resistance of an endotracheal tube, and is customarily administered at 10 cm water pressure.[11]

Mode of Ventilation

The ventilator may provide air during an inspiratory cycle by delivering gas either at a fixed volume of air irrespective of the pressure required to give that breath, or at a fixed pressure over time, without control of the total volume delivered. Each mode carries risks and benefits. Volume-controlled modes provide a predictable volume, while pressure-regulated ventilation may reduce the risk of pneumothorax and barotrauma.[12]

PRESSURE-CONTROLLED/TIME-CYCLED VENTILATION

In pressure-controlled ventilation, gas is delivered at a fixed pressure applied to the airway for a determined period of time, thereby allowing the lung to fill. The tidal volume is measured by calculating the volume of expired gas. A change in the compliance of the lung will result in a change in the delivered tidal volume. Extraventilatory air, patient agitation, or occlusive secretions may dramatically decrease the delivered gas volume.

VOLUME-CONTROLLED VENTILATION

Gas may be provided to the airway regardless of the pressure and the lung allowed to fill to a calculated volume. In this mode of ventilation, tidal volume is preserved regardless of changes in patient lung compliance. Delivered volume is more predictable, but the risk of pneumothorax and barotrauma may be higher.[13] The first manifestation of a pneumothorax in this mode may be a rise in the pressure observed during the inspiration of a tidal volume.

PRESSURE-REGULATED/VOLUME-CONTROLLED VENTILATION

It is possible to combine pressure- and volume-regulated modes. Gas is delivered to the airway until a maximum pressure is achieved, and inspiration is prolonged until a predetermined tidal volume is delivered. If the tidal volume cannot be delivered by the end of an inspiratory period, it is wasted. Barotrauma is limited in this mode, and the risk of the development of extraventilatory air is modulated.[14]

End-Expiratory Pressure

At the end of inspiration, positive distending pressure may be applied continuously during exhalation. Positive end-expiratory pressure (PEEP) is useful in maintaining alveolar volume and airway patency throughout the respiratory cycle. PEEP is also useful in overcoming airway resistance in patients who are on pressure-controlled ventilation without pressure support.

Compliance

The volume of air moved with the application of a given pressure to the airway is termed *compliance*. It may be determined during active inspiration (termed *dynamic compliance*) or with no air movement (*static compliance*). Poorly compliant lungs are "stiff" and require high pressures to ventilate. This may be the case in acute respiratory distress syndrome or pulmonary fibrosis, or may be due to alterations in chest wall rigidity, as occur with ascites or scoliosis.

Airway Resistance

Resistance is defined by the airflow produced by the application of pressure to the airway. High pressure generating low airflow is characteristic of increased resistance. The product of resistance and compliance is termed the *time constant*, which determines the ideal rate of filling of the lung. Airway resistance is not constant throughout the respiratory cycle. During inspiration, positive pressure dilates the airway. Airway diameter decreases during exhalation, increasing the resistance to airflow. As a result, the presence of small airway narrowing (e.g., status asthmaticus) may necessitate the prolongation of the expiratory phase to allow for complete exhalation of a ventilator breath.

Ventilation/Perfusion Mismatch

Inspired gas must be delivered to an alveolus with an adjacent perfused capillary for gas exchange to occur. The delivery of gas to unperfused alveoli results in increased dead space and ineffective ventilation. On the other hand, failure to ventilate a perfused alveolus results in unoxygenated blood returned to the heart with accompanying obligatory cyanosis. Ventilation/perfusion (V/Q) mismatching results from the maldistribution of ventilation, perfusion, or both, with resulting hypoxemia and hypercarbia. It may be a consequence of hypovolemia, overdistention, atelectasis, or airway occlusion.[15] Its solution is in the restoration of circulation and optimization of lung volume and airflow.

Inspiratory Time and Gas Flow

Inspiration must be long enough for air to enter the lung and distribute to the alveoli evenly. In volume-controlled modes, gas is given at a specific flow rate over a given time. Pressure-controlled modes deliver gas at a fixed pressure over a preset time. Short inspiratory times (usually < 0.7 seconds) may cause turbulent airflow, which interferes with gas delivery and distribution. Prolongation of inspiration increases mean airway pressure, and may improve gas exchange in the low-compliance lung. The inspiration:expiration (I : E) ratio expresses the duration of inspiration with respect to exhalation. In the ventilation of a lung with near-normal compliance and diffusion characteristics, the I : E ratio is typically near 0.5. In the poorly compliant lung with impaired diffusion, inspiration may be prolonged to an I : E ratio of 2 to 3. In this circumstance, the I : E ratio is termed *inverted*. Prolongation of inspiration is not without consequences. At a given rate, as inspiration is prolonged, exhalation is shortened. The resulting increase in mean airway pressure may decrease cardiac output. Shortened exhalation, especially in small airways disease, may lead to overdistention and gas trapping.[16]

Goal of Mechanical Ventilation

The goal of mechanical ventilation is to provide satisfactory alveolar ventilation to the patient at a predictable pressure, limiting the mismatch of ventilation and perfusion. Commonly, ventilation is initiated by estimating the respiratory rate, end-expiratory pressure, amount of pressure support given to spontaneous breaths, and inspired oxygen concentration. The mode of ventilation is determined by the therapeutic goal. In the presence of low-compliance lung disease, such as acute respiratory distress syndrome, mean airway pressure is more easily manipulated with pressure-controlled ventilation. As small tidal volumes may be difficult to reliably deliver, neonates and infants may be more satisfactorily ventilated with this technique. Volume-controlled modes more predictably manipulate minute volume and thereby may be appropriate in the patient with hypercarbic respiratory failure. If pressure-controlled ventilation is performed, the peak pressure and flow are ordered. If volume-controlled ventilation is used, a tidal volume is ordered. Typical settings differ based on patient age, underlying disease, and the specific ventilator used (Table 165–2).

Table 165–2	Initial Ventilator Settings			
	Infant	**Toddler**	**Child**	**Adolescent**
Tidal volume	8–10 ml/kg	10 ml/kg	8 ml/kg	6–8 ml/kg
Rate	20 bpm	16 bpm	12 bpm	10 bpm
Peak pressure	25–30 cm H_2O	25–30 cm H_2O	25–30 cm H_2O	25–30 cm H_2O
Peak end-expiratory pressure	5 cm H_2O	5 cm H_2O	5 cm H_2O	5 cm H_2O
Pressure support	10 cm H_2O	10 cm H_2O	10 cm H_2O	10 cm H_2O
Inspiratory time	0.8 sec	0.9 sec	1.0 sec	1.0 sec

Optimum flow characteristics are dependent on the circuit and the size of the patient's airway. Significant volume may be lost in the tubing and humidifier.[17] Adequacy of ventilation is determined by observing chest rise, and verifying air entry by auscultating breath sounds. A chest radiograph is useful in demonstrating that overdistention or collapse is not present. It must be emphasized that the final determination of adequacy of ventilation is made by blood gas analysis (see Chapter 5, Monitoring in Critically Ill Children). Hypercarbia generally requires an increase in alveolar ventilation, by increasing tidal volume or rate, or controlling overdistention. Hypoxemia is responsive to increased inspired oxygen concentration or techniques aimed at reducing V/Q mismatching, such as increased PEEP.

In the face of severe lung disease, it may not be possible to achieve normal arterial blood gas tension in the ventilated patient. This is especially true in the patient with respiratory failure due to small airways disease such as status asthmaticus. Overaggressive ventilation with an excessively large tidal volume or short expiratory time in the face of severe pulmonary parenchymal disease may worsen gas trapping and increase the risk of pneumothorax. In this circumstance, limiting ventilatory support and tolerating increased carbon dioxide tension with the intention to maintain an arterial pH over 7.2 and partial pressure of carbon dioxide of 60 to 70 mm Hg may modulate these risks without jeopardy to the patient. This technique, termed *permissive hypercapnea,* has been demonstrated effective in the management of congenital diaphragmatic hernia.[18] It is likewise useful in other forms of restrictive and obstructive airways disease and in modulating barotrauma.[19]

Alternatives

In the absence of a mechanical ventilator, bag-valve-mask ventilation may be undertaken for as long as the patient is in the emergency room. Mechanical ventilation is primarily performed in conjunction with airway management in the form of endotracheal intubation or tracheostomy. The patient with respiratory insufficiency due to neuromuscular weakness or obstructive apnea who has not been intubated, however, may benefit from nasally applied bilevel positive airway pressure (BiPAP), a noninvasive form of intermittent, pressure-controlled ventilation.[20] This technique has also been reported useful in the management of chronic lung disease, tracheomalacia, sleep apnea, pulmonary edema, and acute respiratory distress syndrome.[21] It may provide transitional support in the process of weaning a child from mechanical ventilation.[22] BiPAP is being used with increasing frequency in the outpatient setting.[23] Initiation of BiPAP is similar to that of pressure-controlled ventilation. The peak pressure is typically between 8 and 15 cm H_2O, and the end-expiratory pressure is near 3 to 5 cm H_2O. Tidal volume is not measured. Continuous gas flow between 1 and 5 L of oxygen per minute is applied as a bias at the end of the airway. Breaths may be triggered by patient effort, or provided at a constant backup rate. BiPAP carries risks to the intubated patient beyond those of mechanical ventilation. Abdominal distention may complicate BiPAP, as some air may be forced down the esophagus. The airway is not protected, and emesis caries an increased risk of aspiration. Children may not tolerate the tightly fitting nasal mask. Patient agitation may interfere with minute ventilation.

Several techniques not customarily included in the discussion of conventional mechanical ventilation deserve mention. High-frequency ventilation administers breaths at a very high rate, 400 breaths per minute or more. A pulse of pressure is applied to the airway with active or passive expiration. The usual pressure change during a cycle is approximately 30 to 40 cm H_2O. The mean airway pressure is held constant, usually greater than 20 cm H_2O. The physiology of high-frequency ventilation is not well understood, but the technique has been demonstrated to be useful in oxygenating and ventilating children with pulmonary parenchymal disease too noncompliant for conventional ventilation, and in the setting of extraventilatory air.[24,25]

Helium-oxygen mixtures may improve ventilation in patients with critically large or small airway resistance (e.g., croup or asthma).[26] It may be delivered via ambient air, or via the mechanical ventilator. As the density of the helium-oxygen mixture is lower than that of air, the ventilator must be calibrated for its use.

Nitric oxide, a pulmonary vasodilator, may assist in the management of pulmonary hypertension and acute respiratory distress syndrome with V/Q mismatch.[27] It is applied through the ventilator circuit at a concentration of 1 to 20 ppm, and requires exhaled air to be processed through a scavenger gas system. Its use requires the pretreatment determination of pulmonary artery pressure by echocardiography. Methemoglobinemia may accompany prolonged use at high concentrations.

Negative pressure ventilation is another noninvasive technique used in patients with high-compliance lungs, in which the driving force is generated by a cuirasse or jacket that generates negative pressure on the chest wall. It is useful in children with chronic neuromuscular diseases or cardiac conditions in which positive pressure ventilation might be poorly tolerated.[28]

Complications

The complications of mechanical ventilation are manifold (Table 165–3). The true incidence of acute complications arising from the institution of mechanical ventilation is unknown. Overdistention contributes to hypoxemic dead space, and the incidence of pneumothorax.[29] Excessive intrathoracic preassure, caused by high mean airway pressures or PEEP, interferes with cardiac output.[30] Careful attention to sterile technique during intubation and suctioning clearly reduces the incidence of ventilator-associated pneumonia.[31]

Table 165–3	Complications of Mechanical Ventilation
Acute	
Extraventilatory air (pneumothorax, pneumomediastinum)	
Overdistention	
Interference with cardiac output	
Infection (ventilator-induced pneumonia)	
Chronic	
Tracheomalacia and other forms of airway injury	
Fibrosis (barotrauma)	
Infection	

Of these complications, pneumothorax is the most life threatening. A high index of suspicion must be maintained, and pneumothorax must be entertained in all patients with a sudden decline in tidal volume with increased airway pressure, especially in the context of recent bagging, suctioning, or small airways disease. It is signaled by a deterioration of pulmonary compliance, hypoxemia, and tachycardia leading to eventual bradycardia. Unattended, or aggravated by continued ventilation or bagging, air will accumulate by ball-valve effect. Ultimately, cardiac arrest will occur. Resuscitative efforts will be unsuccessful without the evacuation of accumulated air.

Given the complexity of mechanical ventilation, it is surprising that the overall complication rate is low. In a study of 23 chronically ventilator-dependent children, only 1 child died in a 2-year study period.[32] Other studies have reported a 5-year survival rate of 65%.[33] Patients will frequently present with complications of ventilation, the most important of which is ventilator-associated pneumonia. Commonly occurring organisms are gram-negative organisms such as *Pseudomonas* and *Klebsiella pneumoniae,* and gram-positive organism such as *Staphylococcus aureus* and *Enterococcus faecalis.*

Postprocedure Care and Disposition

Early identification of complications of mechanical ventilation and maintenance of a secure airway require continuous patient monitoring until patients are transferred to inpatient units. Repeated examination, assessment of vital signs, chest radiography, and arterial blood gas analysis will guide ongoing care.

Occasionally, a patient who is intubated and mechanically ventilated acutely in the emergency department may improve sufficiently before admission to consider the discontinuation of ventilatory support. This may be the case, for example, in the patient intubated for respiratory failure in the postictal state who quickly recovers respiratory drive. Parameters for weaning from mechanical ventilation include the demonstration of stable blood gases, normal respiratory rate for age, satisfactory air entry on auscultatory examination, and the absence of manifestations of respiratory distress such as tachycardia or retractions. Support is generally withdrawn by decreasing one of the ventilator parameters at a time, and then observing the patient to be stable for a period of hours before making further changes. The discontinuation of mechanical ventilation may be contemplated when the mandatory ventilation rate is near 5 breaths/min, the end-expiratory pressure is 5 cm H_2O, the mean airway pressure is under 18 cm H_2O, and the fraction of inspired oxygen is less than 35%. The ability to wean the patient to continuous positive airway pressure with pressure support only—that is, with no mandatory rate—has been advocated as predictive of successful extubation in adults,[34] but has been found unnecessary in children.[35]

REFERENCES

1. Ivanyi ZA, Rademacher PB, Kuhlen RC, Calzia EB: How to choose a mechanical ventilator. Curr Opin Crit Care 11:50–55, 2005.
2. Edwards EA, O'Toole M, Wallis C: Sending children home on tracheostomy-dependent ventilation: pitfalls and outcomes. Arch Dis Child 89:251–255, 2004.
3. Chmielewski C, Snyder-Clickett S: The use of the laryngeal mask airway with mechanical positive pressure ventilation. AANA J 72:347–351, 2004.
4. Papastamelos C, Panitch HB Allen JL: Chest wall compliance in infants and children with neuromuscular disease. Am Rev Respir Crit Care Med 154:1045–1048, 1996.
5. Playfor SD, Thomas DA, Choonra I, Jarvis A: Quality of sedation during mechanical ventilation. Paediatr Anaesth 10:195–199, 2000.
6. Tobias JD: Sedation and analgesia in paediatric intensive care units: a guide to drug selection and use. Paediatr Drugs 1:109–126, 1999.
7. Tobias JD, Berkenbosch JW: Sedation during mechanical ventilation in infants and children: dexmetomidate versus midazolam. South Med J 97:451–455, 2004.
8. Berkenbosch JW, Lam J, Burd RS, Tobias JD: Noninvasive monitoring of carbon dioxide during mechanical ventilation in older children: end-tidal versus transcutaneous techniques. Anesth Analg 92:1427–1431, 2001.
*9. Tobin MJ: Advances in mechanical ventilation. N Engl J Med 344:1986–1996, 2001.
10. Putensen C, Hering R, Muders T, Wrigge H: Assisted breathing is better in acute respiratory failure. Curr Opin Crit Care 11:63–68, 2005.
11. Putensen C, Hering R, Wrigge H: Controlled versus assisted mechanical ventilation. Curr Opin Crit Care 8:51–57, 2002.
12. MacDonald KD, Johnson SR: Volume and pressure modes of mechanical ventilation in pediatric patients. Respir Care Clin N Am 2:607–618, 1996.
13. Amato MBP, Barbas CSV, Medeiros DM, et al: Effect of a protective-ventilation strategy on mortality in the acute respiratory distress syndrome. N Engl J Med 338:347–354, 1998.
14. The Acute Respiratory Distress Syndrome Network: Ventilation with lower tidal volumes as compared with traditional tidal volumes for acute lung injury and the acute respiratory distress syndrome. N Engl J Med 342:1301–1308, 2000.
*15. Calzia E, Rademacher P: Alveolar ventilation and pulmonary blood flow: the VA/Q concept Intensive Care Med 29:1229–1232, 2003.
16. Sabato K, Hanson JH: Mechanical ventilation for children with status asthmaticus. Respir Care Clin N Am 6:171–188, 2000.
17. Cheifetz IM: Invasive and nonivasive pediatric mechanical ventilation. Respir Care 48:442–453, 2003.
18. Boloker J, Bateman DA, Wung JT, Stolar CJ: Congenital diaphragmatic hernia in 120 infants treated consectively with permissive hypercapnea/spontaneous respiration/elective repair. J Pediatr Surg 37:357–366, 2002.
19. Laffey JG, O'Croinin D, McLoughlin P, et al: Permissive hypercapnea—role in protective lung ventilatory strategies. Intensive Care Med 30:347–356, 2003.
20. Mossa F, Gonsalez S, Laverty A, et al: The use of nasal continuous positive airway pressure to treat obstructive sleep apnoea. Arch Dis Child 87:438–443, 2002.
21. Fortenberry JD, Del Toro J, Jefferson LS, et al: Management of pediatric acute hypoxemic respiratory insufficiency with bilevel positive pressure (BiPAP) nasal mask ventilation. Chest 108:1059–1064, 1995.
22. Keogh S, Courtney M, Coyer F: Weaning from ventilation in paediatric intensive care: an intervention study. Intensive Crit Care Nurs 19:186–197, 2003.
23. Tibballis J, Henning RD: Noninvasive ventilatory strategies in the management of a newborn infant and three children with congenital central hypoventilation syndrome. Pediatr Pulmonol 36:544–548, 2003.
24. Ventre KM, Arnold JH: High frequency oscillatory ventilation in acute respiratory failure. Paediatr Respir Rev 5:323–332, 2004.
25. Clark RH: High-frequency ventilation. J Pediatr 124:661–670, 1994.
26. Schaeffer EM, Pohlman A, Morgan S, Hall JB: Oxygenation in status asthmaticus improves during ventilation with helium-oxygen. Crit Care Med 27:2666–2670, 1999.
27. Abman SH, Kinsella JP: Inhaled nitric oxide therapy for pulmonary disease in pediatrics. Curr Opin Pediatr 10:236–242, 1998.
28. Thompson A: The role of negative pressure ventilation. Arch Dis Child 77:454–458, 1997.
29. Nève V, Leclerc F, Dumas de la Roque E, et al: Overdistention in ventilated children. Crit Care 5:196–203, 2001.
30. Shekerdemian L, Bohn D: Cardiovascular effects of mechanical ventilation. Arch Dis Child 80:475–480, 1999.

*Selected readings.

31. Rello J, Diaz E, Roque M, Vallés J: Risk factors for developing pneumonia within 48 hours of intubation. Am J Respir Crit Care Med 159:1742–1748, 1998.

32. Fields AI, Coble DH, Pollack MM, Kaufman J: Outcome of home care for technology-dependent children: success of an independent, community-based case management model. Pediatr Pulmonol 11:310–317, 1991.

33. Frates RC, Splaingard ML, Smith EO, Harrison GM: Outcome of home mechanical ventilation in children. J Pediatr 106:850–856, 1985.

34. Leitch EA, Moran JL, Grealy B: Weaning and extubation in the intensive care unit: clinical or index-driven approach? Intensive Care Med 22:752–759, 1996.

35. Tapia JL, Bancalari A, Gonzalez A, Mercado ME: Does continuous positive airway pressure (CPAP) during weaning from intermittent mandatory ventilation in very low birth weight infants have risks or benefits? A controlled trial. Pediatr Pulmonol 19:269–274, 1995.

Chapter 166

Incision and Drainage

Sean F. Isaak, MD and John F. O'Brien, MD

Indications and Contraindications

Localized skin infections may develop in any area of the body, and are a frequent result of local breakdown of epidermal defense mechanisms, with invasion by normal resident bacterial flora. Such infections often follow abrasions, lacerations, various dermatitides, insect bites, or skin maceration (e.g., from diapers).[1] Infections of the soft tissue often begin as cellulitis, with some bacteria causing tissue necrosis, liquefaction, and accumulation of leukocytes as well as debris within a walled-off area of purulent fluid. The natural course of an untreated abscess is gradual cavity enlargement with spreading through tissue planes until final release of contents into an external or internal surface.[2]

The distinction between a cutaneous abscess and cellulitis is often difficult to make clinically. A cutaneous abscess must be drained because it may extend to compress or injure nearby structures, may contributes to bacteremia with possible sepsis, and will not resolve with antibiotic therapy alone. Decompression of an abscess may alleviate pain. Conversely, incision and drainage (I&D) of cellulitis will not improve and may even worsen outcome. Both cellulitis and abscesses may cause localized erythema, pain, and induration, although a superficial abscess is distinguished by local fluctuance. If the distinction is not clear (e.g., deeper abscesses), sterile aspiration with an 18-gauge needle may return purulent fluid, indicating a need for I&D.

Recently, ultrasound has been used to confirm the presence of a cutaneous abscess in difficult cases,[3] and to exclude mimics such as mycotic aneurysms. Typical sonographic findings of an abscess include a mass that is totally or partially anechoic and a deformable fluid collection upon compression, which may have sharp margins and distorted subcutaneous tissue[4] (see Fig. 166–1). Sonographically directed aspiration and drainage may also simplify the procedure. Plain radiography can be used to exclude radiopaque foreign bodies.

There are circumstances in which drainage of an abscess in the emergency care setting is not appropriate. An abscess may require drainage in the operating room under general anesthesia if sufficient sedation and analgesia cannot be achieved, if patient cooperation cannot be accomplished, if the abscess appears complex due to size or relation to vital structures, or if there is the possibility that an alternate, more serious diagnosis is present. In particular, the possibility of a mycotic aneurysm or pseudoaneurysm may mandate careful operating room management. Consultation with a surgeon is warranted in any circumstance in which more than a simple I&D procedure is anticipated.

Preparation and Consent

I&D has been described as one of the most painful procedures performed in the emergency department,[5] in part due to the difficulty in obtaining adequate local anesthesia. A large tender area and unfavorable local conditions for anesthesia make this process challenging. Several options exist to achieve optimal anesthesia (see Chapter 172, Local and Regional Anesthesia).

1. Topical anesthesia with various agents may suffice for small abscesses. Topical lidocaine, epinephrine, and tetracaine (LET) gel, lidocaine/prilocaine (EMLA) cream, and lidocaine by iontophoresis[6] have been used to locally anesthetize small abscesses. Use of topical ethyl chloride or fluoromethane spray in this setting should be discouraged, as the resulting short duration of anesthesia is usually insufficient.

2. Local anesthetics may be injected intradermally along the path of the proposed incision site. However, this technique will only help alleviate the pain of incision, not the discomfort associated with disruption of loculations, manipulation of inflamed tissue, or wound packing. Infiltration of high-concentration, buffered

and warmed lidocaine or similar local anesthetic using a small-gauge (27- to 30-gauge) needle with slow injection rate minimizes pain related to anesthesia.[7]

3. Ring or field block anesthesia, in which infiltration of anesthetic is advanced 1 cm beyond the periphery of the erythematous tissue, may be effective in conjunction with injection of the incision site. This method may require a large amount of anesthesia, and close adherence to maximal dosing must be observed.

4. Regional block is the anesthetic of choice if the abscess is in an anatomically suitable location.

5. Procedural sedation and analgesia is an effective alternative method of anesthesia for I&D (see Chapter 159, Procedural Sedation and Analgesia).

Special situations, including multiple abscesses as well as large abscess size, should prompt calculation of maximal anesthetic dose and increased consideration for general anesthesia (see Chapter 160, Wound Management). Preprocedural antibiotics should be used in patients at risk for bacterial endocarditis or distant infection of prosthetic material by possible transient bacteremia from abscess I&D, and should follow American Heart Association (AHA) recommendations[8] (see Chapter 64, Pericarditis, Myocarditis, and Endocarditis). Antibiotic choice should be dictated by the likely organism in the anatomic region of the abscess.

Equipment

Various scalpel blades may be utilized depending on characteristics of the abscess, with the no. 11 blade usually most suitable. Large abscesses (>5 cm diameter) may be managed with a no. 10 blade. Other equipment required for abscess drainage includes hemostats, forceps, scissors, and packing materials. Several different packing materials are available, with the $1/4$- to 1-inch iodoform gauze most commonly used. Various balloon catheters (e.g., Word catheter) and other pliable drainage catheters (e.g., Pezzer catheters) may obviate the need for packing material changes during abscess follow-up.

Techniques

The involved area is cleaned with an antiseptic solution (e.g., povidone-iodine) and draped with sterile towels. For healthy patients, I&D is the definitive treatment and cultures are not warranted. There are certain conditions in which wound culturing is important. Examples include gas-containing abscesses, infections that involve fascia or muscle, abscesses that penetrate the abdominal cavity, or anatomic locations that may involve deep structures (e.g., central triangle of the face, which drains into the cavernous sinus).[9] Some patients with cutaneous abscess may benefit from Gram stain and culture to direct antibiotic therapy. These include the immunocompromised, parenteral drug users, and those with systemic involvement or extensive areas of cellulitis. Some experts also recommend routine cultures to determine the prevalence of organisms (e.g., methicillin-resistant *Staphylococcus aureus* [MRSA]) and the development of antibiotic resistance patterns in communities.[10] If indicated, obtain cultures by needle aspiration through sterile prepared skin or aspirate without delay after the incision is made to improve anaerobic yield.[11]

To optimize cosmetic results, the incision should be made parallel to Langer's lines. A no. 11 blade is usually suitable to make a stab incision at the edge of greatest fluctuance (Fig. 166–1a), which is extended the entire length of the area of purulence to maximize drainage. Inadequate incisions lead to insufficient drainage and limited access to the wound cavity. Use of elliptical incisions may aid drainage, but should not be used in cosmetically important areas due to their tendency to leave unattractive scars. An elliptical incision should be considered when the skin overlying the abscess is necrotic or includes draining sinuses.[11] Cruciate incisions rarely improve drainage success, and may cause more wound edge necrosis and lead to poor cosmetic results.

Loculations may exist within the abscess cavity with isolated areas of purulent material. To disrupt loculations, the area is probed gently with either a hemostat or gloved finger (Fig. 166–1b and 166–1c). Caution should be used when probing with a gloved finger as fractured bone or sharp foreign bodies may be present in the abscess. The deep wall of the abscess should not be aggressively manipulated since this may lead to bleeding or damage to nearby structures.[12] Saline irrigation of the abscess cavity facilitates removal of remaining purulent material and necrotic debris (Fig. 166–1d). Curettage is reserved for clearing the abscess of debris not removed by irrigation. However, no study has demonstrated that irrigation or curettage is necessary or improves outcome in the management of abscesses. The wound is loosely filled with a single continuous piece of iodoform gauze, petrolatum gauze, or other packing material, leaving one end exiting the wound to assist later removal (Fig. 166–1e). Other drainage devices may be substituted for gauze at the discretion of the operator. Finally, the wound is covered with dry, sterile dressings sufficiently absorbent to contain significant drainage.

Alternatives

Alternative treatments for cutaneous abscess include needle aspiration, marsupialization, and abscess resection, as well as incision with curettage and primary suturing under antibiotic coverage. Needle aspiration alone is seldom appropriate for abscess management as it rarely provides adequate drainage. However, breast abscesses have been managed by sonographically guided aspiration (often repeated one or more times) with irrigation and local instillation of antibiotics without placing indwelling drains.[13] Marsupialization refers to suturing the abscess walls open, with granulation and secondary closure of the abscess cavity, and is occasionally used for Bartholin's gland abscesses. Complete abscess resection may be curative for epidermoid cysts when the entire wall of the abscess cavity may be visualized and safely removed. Incision with curettage of abscesses followed by primary suturing and appropriate antibiotic coverage has been utilized with limited success.[14] Use of antibiotics without drainage of cutaneous abscess will fail unless adequate spontaneous drainage occurs. However, spontaneous drainage of abscesses is often inadequate, and frequently requires further I&D to facilitate cure.

Complications

The main complications of abscess management arise from inadequate incision size and incomplete drainage. Incisions

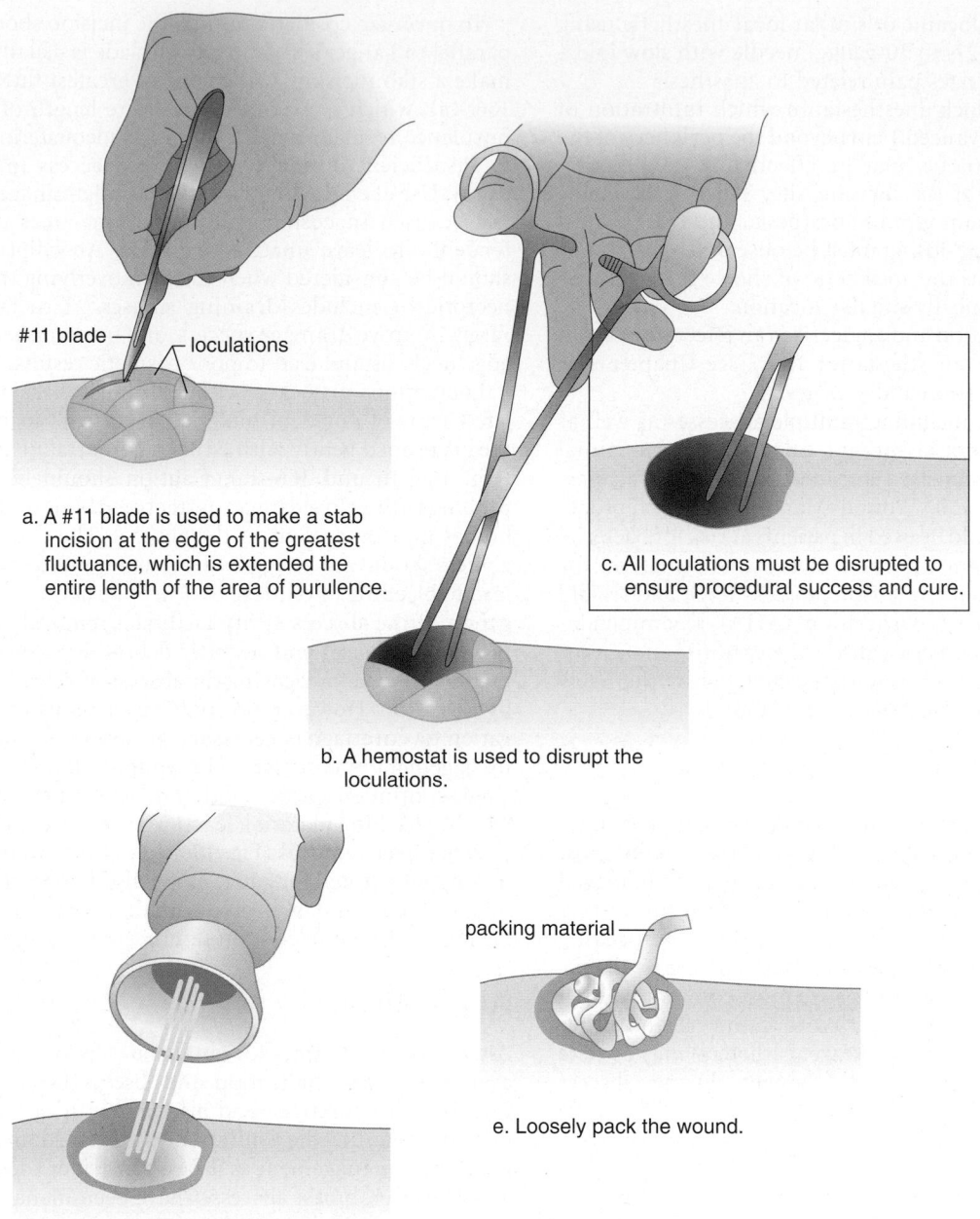

#11 blade — loculations

a. A #11 blade is used to make a stab incision at the edge of the greatest fluctuance, which is extended the entire length of the area of purulence.

b. A hemostat is used to disrupt the loculations.

c. All loculations must be disrupted to ensure procedural success and cure.

d. Irrigate the wound.

packing material —

e. Loosely pack the wound.

FIGURE 166–1. Technique for incision and drainage.

that are too small limit the amount of drainage and access to the interior of the abscess. Failure to attain sufficient incision length may be secondary to an underestimate of the size of the abscess or inability to provide adequate analgesia to accomplish the procedural goal. Incomplete abscess drainage may lead to osteomyelitis, tenosynovitis, septic thrombophlebitis, necrotizing fasciitis, and fistula formation.[2] In addition, infection may become systemic with resultant bacteremia or endocarditis. Incisions that are too deep or excessively large may result in injury to adjacent structures or poor cosmetic results.

Bleeding is a frequent complication from the incision of inflamed tissue at an abscess site, and is in general easily resolved with a few minutes of local tissue compression. This should be distinguished from rare but more serious complications related to laceration of a major vessel or neurovascular bundle, which should prompt immediate surgical consultation.

Postprocedure Care and Disposition

Most patients with normal host defenses do not need antibiotics unless there is an associated cellulitis. Postprocedure antibiotics have not been shown to affect the outcome of cutaneous abscesses. MRSA has been identified as a major pathogen in skin and soft tissue infections in the emergency department.[15] Even the rising prevalence of community-acquired MRSA among healthy children does not change the fact that I&D without any antibiotics cure most abscesses.[16,17]

A single dose of appropriate antibiotic is indicated as preprocedure prophylaxis in patients who are at high or moderate risk of infective endocarditis as defined by AHA guidelines.[8] Patients who may require more extensive antibiotic therapy include children with cellulitis, signs of systemic involvement (fever, toxicity, or significant tachycardia), and immunocompromised states (see Chapter 120, Skin and Soft Tissue Infections).

Organisms causing abscesses can be predicted based on anatomic location.[9,18-20] This knowledge may guide initial antibiotic therapy when indicated. Selective use of Gram stains may also assist in appropriate antibiotic choices. Overall, *S. aureus* is the most common organism isolated from cutaneous abscesses. Children tend to have a large number of anaerobes in cutaneous abscesses that are perirectal, adjacent to mucous membranes, and on the head or fingers, particularly at nail bed areas.[19] The antibiotic chosen should be based on the most likely causative organism.[21] For cutaneous abscesses, consider an antistaphylococcal penicillin or first-generation cephalosporin. In the penicillin-allergic patient, clindamycin may be useful and extends anaerobic coverage. Trimethoprim-sulfamethoxazole, rifampin, clindamycin, doxycycline (if the patient is >8 years old), or linezolid may be required in areas with a known high prevalence of MRSA.[10] Vancomycin or clindamycin should be used in patients suspected to have community-associated MRSA bacteremia, and gram-negative or extended anaerobic coverage may be necessary based on anatomic considerations.[10]

The American Academy of Pediatrics has published an algorithm for managing abscesses and furuncles in areas of high MRSA prevalence[10] (Fig. 166–2). Hospital admission is required for cutaneous abscess in children who need general anesthesia for drainage, or those with systemic toxicity, immunocompromised states (e.g., diabetes), and abscesses in vulnerable locations (hand, face, perineal region) or involving deep structures (tendon sheaths, fascia, or muscles).

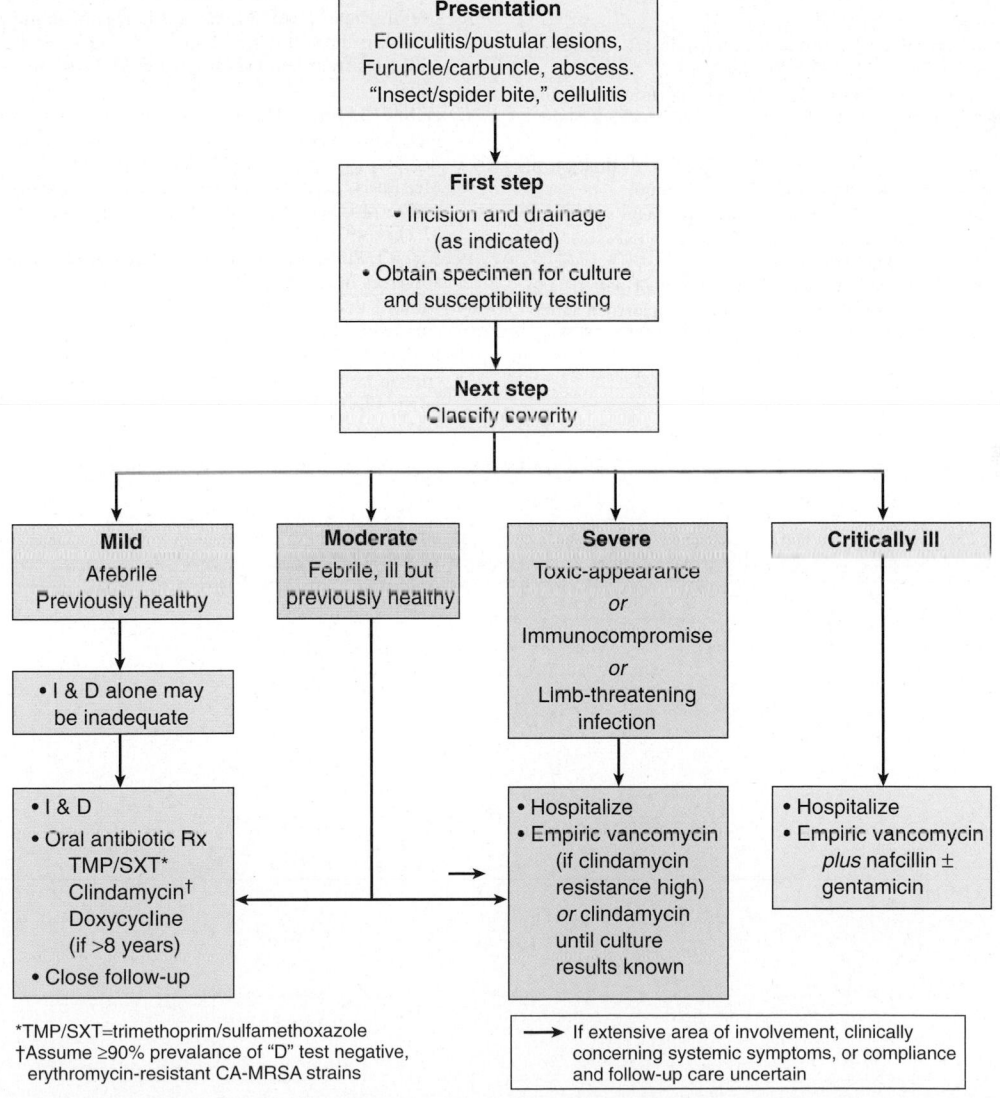

FIGURE 166–2. Algorithm for managing children with suspected community-associated methicillin-resistant *Staphylococcus aureus* (CA-MRSA) skin and soft tissue infections suggested by the American Academy of Pediatrics. Initial outpatient management of suspected infections is schematically illustrated and assumes CA-MRSA strains are prevalent in the community. Data from Baker CJ, Frenck RW Jr: Change in management of skin/soft tissue infections needed. AAP News 25:10, 2004. (From Kaplan SL. Implications of *Staphylococcus aureus* as a community acquired pathogen in pediatric patients. Infect Dis North Am 19: 747–757, 2005.)

Following I&D, the child should return for a recheck visit in 24 hours for facial abscesses or up to 48 hours for other cutaneous abscesses. At this time, packing material is removed and the wound reassessed for signs of healing and evidence of ongoing drainage. Packing should not be left in place longer than 48 hours. If the wound continues to drain, it should be repacked and reexamined in 24 to 48 hours. If the wound has minimal or no drainage, and has decreased surrounding cellulitis, then the patient should begin warm soaks approximately four times a day until the wound closes. Repeated examination is not necessary once the wound exhibits signs of healing. Most cutaneous abscess incisions will heal within 7 to 10 days.

Antibiotic therapy, if indicated, is usually necessary for only 5 to 7 days. Postoperative pain management should always be provided when necessary, with recognition that I&D alone generally reduces pain significantly. On rare occasion, immobilization of the incised area may reduce pain and protect the wound.

REFERENCES

*1. Bikowski J: Secondarily infected wounds and dermatoses: a diagnosis and treatment guide. J Emerg Med 17:197–206, 1999.

2. Halvorson GD, Halvorson JE, Iserson KV: Abscess incision and drainage in the emergency department—Part I. J Emerg Med 3:227–232, 1985.

*3. Chao H, Syh-Jae L, Yhu-Chering H, et al: Sonographic evaluation of cellulitis in children. J Ultrasound Med 19:743–749, 2000.

4. Loyer E, DuBrow R, David C, et al: Imaging of superficial soft-tissue infections: sonographic findings in cases of cellulitis and abscess. AJR Am J Roentgenol 166:149–152, 1996.

5. Singer A, Richman P, Kowalska A, et al: Comparison of patient and practitioner assessments of pain from commonly performed emergency department procedures. Ann Emerg Med 33:652–658, 1999.

6. DeCou J, Abrams R, Hammond J, et al: Iontophoresis: a needle-free, electrical system of local anesthesia delivery for pediatric surgical office procedures. J Pediatr Surg 34:946–949, 1999.

7. Gunter JB: Benefit and risks of local anesthetics in infants and children. Paediatr Drugs 4:649–672, 2002.

8. Dajani A, Taubert K, Wilson W, et al: Prevention of bacterial endocarditis: recommendations by the American Heart Association. JAMA 277:1794–1801, 1997.

9. Meislin H: Pathogen identification of abscesses and cellulites. Ann Emerg Med 15:329–332, 1986.

10. Kaplan SL: Implications of *Staphylococcus aureus* as a community acquired pathogen in pediatric patients. Infect Dis North Am 19:747–757, 2005.

11. Meislin H, McGehee M, Rosen P: Management and microbiobiology of cutaneous abscesses. JACEP 7:186–191, 1978.

12. Burney R: Incision and drainage procedures: soft tissue abscesses in the emergency service. Emerg Med Clin North Am 4:527–542, 1986.

13. Leborgne F, Leborgne F: Treatment of breast abscesses with sonographically guided aspiration, irrigation, and instillation of antibiotics. AJR Am J Roentgenol 181:1089–1091, 2003.

14. Blick P, Flowers M, Marsden A, et al: Antibiotics in surgical treatment of acute abscesses. Br Med J 281:111–112, 1980.

*15. Frazee B, Lynn J, Charlebois E, et al: High prevalence of methicillin-resistant *Staphylococcus aureus* in emergency department skin and soft tissue infections. Ann Emerg Med 45:311–320, 2005.

16. Lee M, Rios A, Aten M, et al: Management and outcome of children with skin and soft tissue abscess caused by community-acquired methicillin-resistant *Staphylococcus aureus*. Pediatr Infect Dis J 23:123–127, 2004.

17. Herold B, Immergluck L, Maranan M, et al: Community-acquired methicillin-resistant *Staphylococcus aureus* in children with no identified predisposing risk. JAMA 279:593–598, 1998.

18. Meislin H, Lerner S, Graves M, et al: Cutaneous abscesses: anaerobic and aerobic bacteriology and outpatient management. Ann Intern Med 87:145–149, 1977.

19. Brook I, Finegold S: Aerobic and anaerobic bacteriology of cutaneous abscesses in children. Pediatrics 67:891–895, 1981.

20. Brook I, Frazier E: Aerobic and anaerobic bacteriology of wounds and cutaneous abscesses. Arch Surg 125:1445–1451, 1990.

21. Hedrick J: Acute bacterial skin infections in pediatric medicine: current issues in presentation and treatment. Paediatr Drugs 5(Suppl 1):35–46, 2003.

*Selected readings.

Chapter 167

Ventriculoperitoneal and Other Intracranial Shunts

Russell Migita, MD and Tony Woodward, MD, MBA

Key Points

Infants and children with shunt malfunction can present with nonspecific symptoms.

Parents should be asked if current symptoms are similar to those that occurred with previous shunt malfunctions.

Shunt infection is uncommon. If it occurs, it is most likely to happen during the first weeks to months after shunt placement or revision.

Shunt malfunction can rarely be definitively ruled out with a single test or finding.

Shunt tap or burr hole puncture can be life saving in a patient with impending herniation.

Indications and Contraindications

Cerebrospinal fluid (CSF) shunts are placed in patients to drain fluid from ventricles, cysts, and subdural collections to areas that are able to absorb that fluid, such as the peritoneum or atrium. CSF shunt placement is the most common neurosurgical procedure performed in the United States.[1] Shunts are most commonly placed in pediatric patients for actual or potential hydrocephalus/fluid space collections due to spina bifida or intraventricular hemorrhage and have improved mortality from these conditions. Unfortunately, CSF shunts may fail, with potentially life-threatening consequences.[2,3] Up to 39% of patients have shunt failure during the first year after placement, and 80% of patients require revision within 12 years of shunt placement or revision.[4-8] All infants and children with the possibility of shunt failure or infection require evaluation of the shunt.

A child with a shunt malfunction may initially present with nonspecific symptoms such as irritability, vomiting, personality change, or headache.[9] Other features include swelling around the external shunt hardware (valves, reservoir, and tubing), bulging fontanelle, gait disturbance, and vision changes.[10] Late signs include altered mental status, seizures, posturing, coma, and hemiparesis. During the first 5 months after placement, the strongest indicators of shunt failure include nausea and vomiting (positive predictive value [PPV], 79%; likelihood ratio [LR], 10.4), irritability (PPV 78%, LR 9.8), decreased level of consciousness (PPV 100%), erythema (PPV 100%), and bulging fontanelle (PPV 92%, LR 33.1).[11] In addition, parents should be asked if the current symptoms resemble those of prior obstructive episodes.[12] Shunts may fail due to hardware failure, kinks in the tubing, disconnection,[13] blockage of the shunt by blood or proteinaceous or infectious material, or migration of the shunt at either the proximal or distal end. They may also fail due to CSF overdrainage, which can cause ventricular collapse and parenchymal blockage.[14]

Shunt infection is usually secondary to contamination encountered at the time of surgery, and 90% of infections will present within the first 6 months after placement, most commonly during the first 2 to 3 months.[15] A recent population-based study found an overall infection rate of 2.7% per procedure.[16] Infants have the highest risk, with infection rates of 15.7%.[17] Patients with infected shunts usually present with low-grade fever and may also show signs of shunt obstruction.[18,19]

Shunts consist of four main components: (1) a proximal catheter that is placed in the obstructed or fluid-filled (cyst) central nervous system site; (2) a reservoir, which may consist of one (single) or two (double) chambers; (3) a valve that controls the rate of CSF drainage (differential pressure, flow control, gravitational, programmable, or siphon type); and (4) a distal catheter that drains into a site that allows absorption of the fluid. Newer shunts may have an electronically (externally) programmable component that prevents overdrainage of CSF.[20]

An evaluation of shunt function should be performed for any suspected obstruction or infection. The shunt reservoir or tubing may be entered with a needle to attempt to relieve pressure and withdraw CSF. This shunt puncture procedure may be indicated when infection is suspected or when it is necessary to measure an opening pressure.[21] Burr hole puncture involves inserting a needle directly through the skull burr hole into the CSF space to relieve pressure. Some reservoirs are located within the burr hole, and puncture of these shunts will generally damage the shunt mechanism. This procedure carries a risk of morbidity but may be life saving in instances of cerebral herniation after medical interventions have been maximized.

Preparation and Consent

In addition to the physical examination of the patient and underlying shunt apparatus, evaluation of shunt function is generally augmented by radiographic examination with both plain radiographs and computed tomography (CT). Plain radiographs assess shunt continuity and roughly establish the locations of the proximal and distal ends of the shunt. CT scans assess ventricular size and brain parenchyma. Prior CT scans are valuable to compare ventricular/fluid cyst size, though up to one third of CT scans are not able to rule out shunt malfunction.[22] Unless circumstances warrant immediate life-saving intervention, informed consent should be obtained prior to invasive shunt evaluation or management.

Equipment

No special equipment is required for the external evaluation of the shunt. Shunt puncture and burr hole puncture require universal precautions and preparation (sterile gloves, goggles, mask, gown), topical antiseptic (isopropyl alcohol, Betadine, povidone) to clean the skin, a medical razor to shave hair immediately around the puncture site, and sterile towels to ensure a sterile surgical site. Ventricular shunt puncture is performed under sterile conditions with a 23- or 25-gauge butterfly needle, while burr hole puncture uses a 3.5-inch, 22-gauge spinal needle with stylet.

Monitoring

All patients at risk for increased intracranial pressure (ICP) require continuous visual and electronic monitoring. Vital sign changes that may indicate increased ICP include apnea and Cushing's triad (bradycardia, hypertension, and decreased/variable respiratory effort and rate). Patients require cardiorespiratory monitoring with apnea alarms and pulse oximetry. Vital signs should be measured regularly.

Techniques

Clinical Examination

Many different types of shunt systems exist. The most common types include the single-reservoir and double-reservoir ("double-bubble") shunts. The clinician should be familiar with the different types of shunts that are in use at his or her hospital, and should be aware of other types of shunts that may be encountered in transferred or out-of-area patients. First, the skin is inspected over the shunt for erythema or swelling, and palpated for discontinuity. Swelling suggests a shunt disconnection, while overlying erythema and warmth along the shunt track suggest infection.

Pumping the Shunt

The utility and consideration of "pumping the shunt" is controversial. Shunts are constructed with reservoirs that serve as a site of entry for fluid retrieval and evaluation. These reservoirs have also historically been used as a means to manipulate flow as well as quickly and noninvasively evaluate the shunt at the bedside. Longitudinal studies show that pumping the shunt has a sensitivity of 11% to 20% and a specificity of 63% to 99% for detecting obstruction.[11,23,24] One author found a PPV of only 17% to 21%; however, others have described a PPV of 80% to 86% for pumping the shunt. The negative predictive value in these studies ranged from 65% to 81%. Pumping the shunt should be considered as a potential adjunct to the comprehensive history, physical evaluation, and radiographic evaluation of the suspected malfunctioning shunt. Some shunt valves cannot be evaluated by pumping. The technique cannot be used to definitively rule in or rule out malfunction (Fig. 167–1).

Shunt Puncture

To perform a shunt puncture, the child is positioned in a reclining position. The reservoir is identified, and the surrounding area is cleaned with isopropyl alcohol, and shaved if necessary. The area is prepped with povidone or Betadine. Sterile gloves must be used and a sterile field established. Most reservoirs are dome shaped and should be entered tangentially to a depth of a few millimeters. The reservoir is entered with a 23-gauge butterfly needle until a pop is felt (Fig. 167–2). Care is needed to avoid advancing the needle too far so that it does not become embedded in the back wall of the reservoir. The needle may need to be adjusted until flow is achieved. Button-type Rickham-style reservoirs are situated in the burr hole and are punctured perpendicular to the scalp. The opening pressure is measured by holding the butterfly tubing upright and measuring the distance from the external auditory meatus to the top of the fluid column.[25] Opening pressure has a poor specificity for shunt obstruction.[26] Ideally, fluid is collected by gravitational or pressure-backed free flow, or if necessary, by gently aspirating with a syringe. CSF is sent for routine CSF studies. For diagnostic taps, a volume of 5 to 10 ml is generally sufficient. If the shunt is being tapped due to cerebral herniation, fluid is removed until the patient's condition improves. This quantity is generally 50 to 100 ml for children with signs of cerebral herniation.

Burr Hole

Emergency department burr hole puncture is reserved for children with signs of herniation in situations in which medical management and interventions have been maximized and operative options are not readily available. The hair and scalp are prepped, the burr hole is palpated, and a 3.5-inch, 22-gauge needle is introduced through the burr hole perpendicular to the scalp. The needle is advanced slowly, removing the stylet periodically until CSF flow is achieved. The ventricle is generally reached by a depth of 5 cm. The stylet is removed and fluid is allowed to drain until the pressure has been released. Burr hole puncture will often damage the shunt, and patients will require definitive operative revision (Fig. 167–3).

Complications

The risk of iatrogenic infection is approximately 1% after a shunt tap.[21] The most common pathogen encountered is

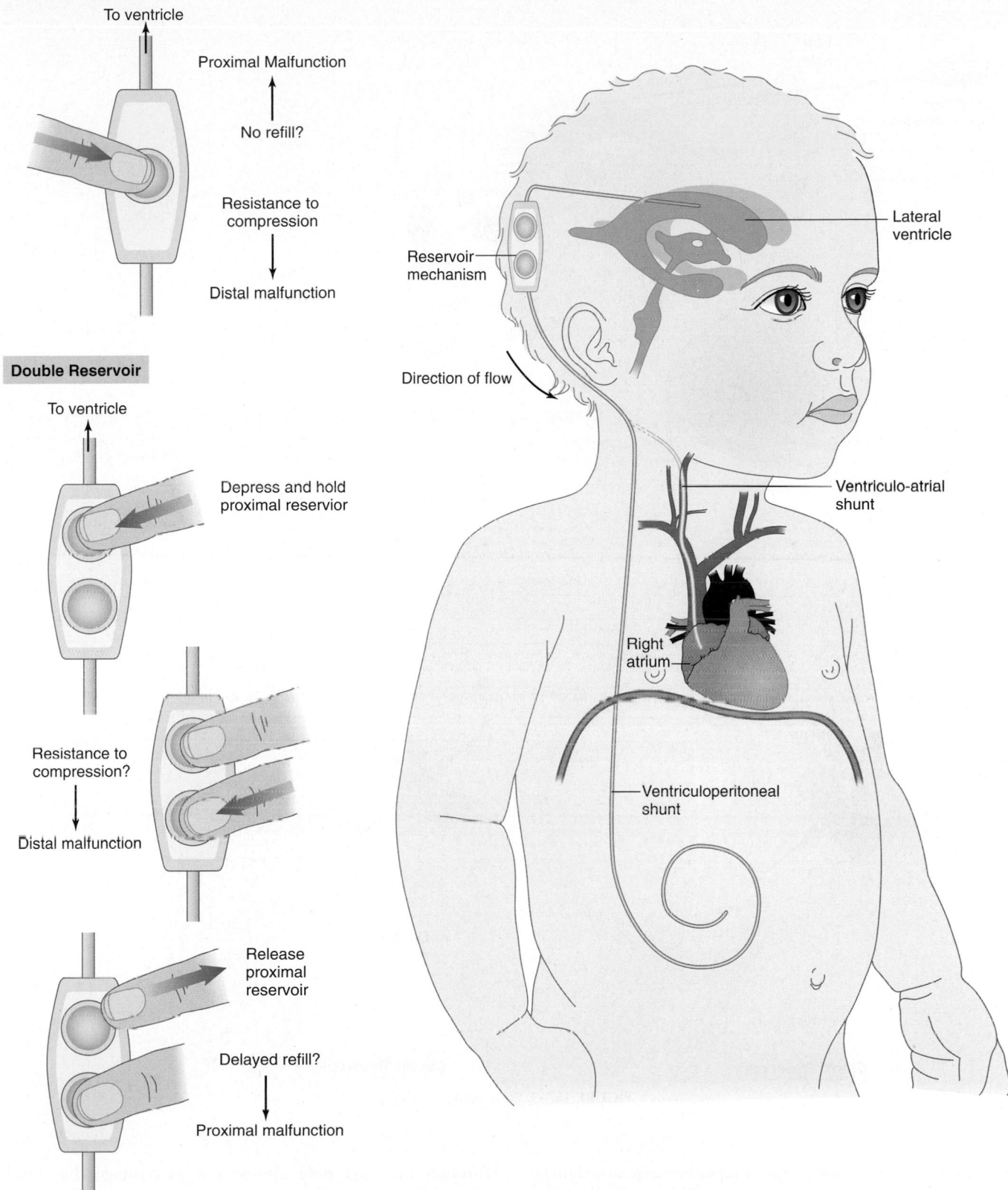

Single Reservoir

To ventricle

Proximal Malfunction

No refill?

Resistance to compression

Distal malfunction

Double Reservoir

To ventricle

Depress and hold proximal reservoir

Resistance to compression?

Distal malfunction

Release proximal reservoir

Delayed refill?

Proximal malfunction

Lateral ventricle

Reservoir mechanism

Direction of flow

Ventriculo-atrial shunt

Right atrium

Ventriculoperitoneal shunt

FIGURE 167–1. Pumping double- and single-bubble shunts.

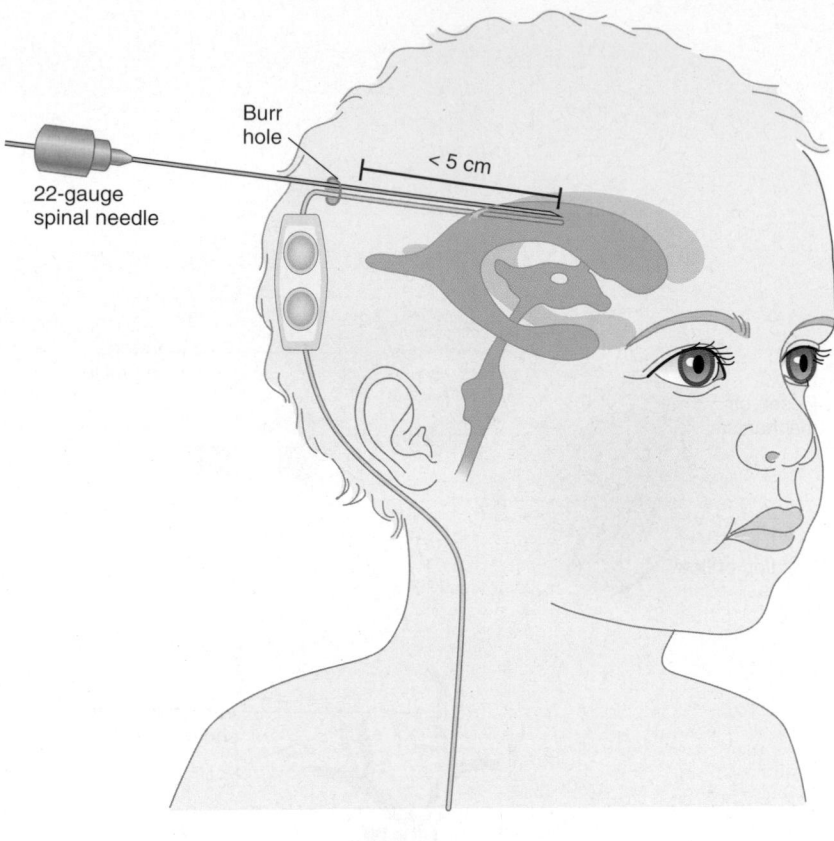

FIGURE 167–2. Shunt puncture.

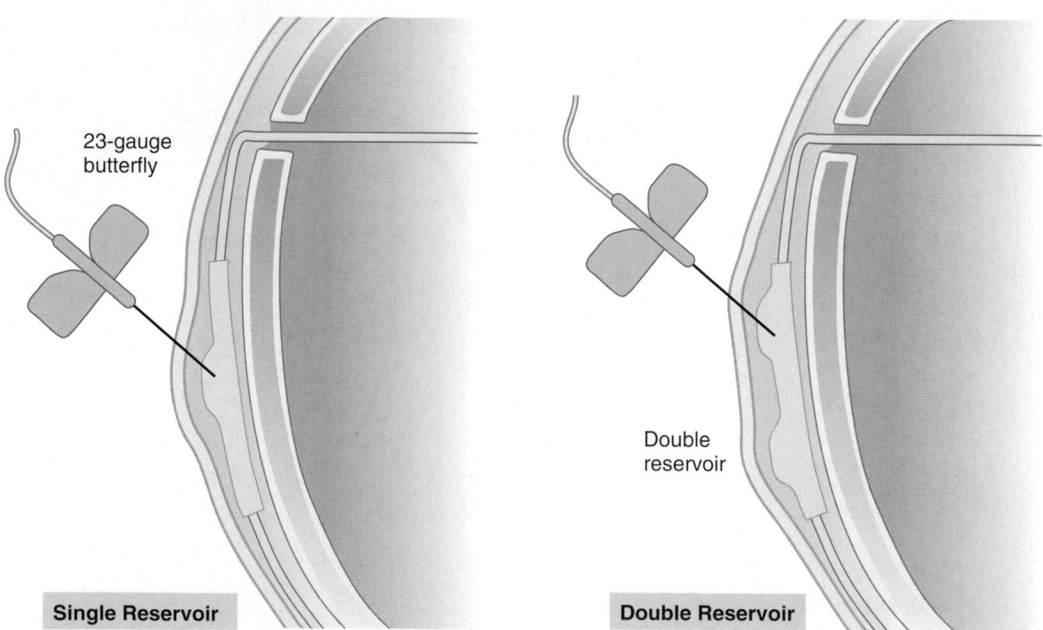

FIGURE 167–3. Burr hole puncture.

Staphylococcus epidermidis. Shunt taps also can cause damage to the shunt mechanism if not performed properly. Burr hole puncture carries the added risk of infection or direct parenchymal or vascular injury, such as intracranial abscess formation. A burr hole puncture also can cause sudden changes of ICP that can lead to fluid shifts, subdural hematoma, intracerebral hemorrhage, and edema. Ventricular punctures through the burr hole almost always damage the shunt mechanism.

Postprocedure Care and Disposition

Neurosurgical evaluation, and continous cardiopulmonary observation with frequent assessment of neurologic status will be required in symptomatic patients after shunt evaluation. A negative (easy compression and reinflation of reservoir; no erythema, edema, or palpable separation along the shunt tract) noninvasive evaluation of the shunt does not completely rule out the possibility of malfunction. Further evaluation may include shunt tap, plain radiographs, CT scan, magnetic resonance imaging, and shunt flow studies. After a shunt tap, the results of laboratory evaluation of the CSF must be followed, including results of the CSF culture. Patients who require burr hole puncture almost always require operative shunt revision. Prophylactic antibiotics are generally not required.

REFERENCES

1. Bondurant C, Jimenez D: Epidemiology of cerebrospinal fluid shunting. Pediatr Neurosurg 23:254–258, 1995.
2. Bryant M, McEniery J, Walker D, et al: Preliminary study of shunt related death in paediatric patients. J Clin Neurosci 11:614–615, 2004.
3. Kang J, Lee I: Long-term follow-up of shunting therapy. Childs Nerv Sys 15:711–717, 1999.
4. Borgbjerg B, Gjerris F, Albeck M, et al: Frequency and causes of shunt revisions in different cerebrospinal fluid shunt types. Acta Neurochir 136:189–194, 1995.
5. Kestle J, Drake J, Milner R, et al: Long-term follow-up data from the shunt design trial. Pediatr Neurosurg 33:230–236, 2000.
*6. Key C, Rothrock S, Falk J: Cerebrospinal fluid shunt complications: an emergency medicine perspective. Pediatr Emerg Care 11:265–273, 1995.
7. Raimondi AJ, Robinson JS, Kuwamura K: Complications of ventriculoperitoneal shunting and a critical comparison of the three-piece and one-piece systems. Childs Brain 3:321–342, 1977.
8. Sainte-Rose C, Piatt J, Renier D, et al: Mechanical complications in shunts. Pediatr Neurosurg 17:2–9, 1991–1992.
9. Barnes N, Jones S, Hayward R, et al: Ventriculoperitoneal shunt block: what are the best predictive clinical indicators? Arch Dis Child 87:198–201, 2002.
10. Kraus R, Hanigan WC, Kattah J, et al: Changes in visual acuity associated with shunt failure. Childs Nerv Syst 19:226–231, 2003.
*11. Garton H, Kestle J, Drake J: Predicting shunt failure on the basis of clinical symptoms and signs in children. J Neurosurg 94:202–210, 2001.
*12. Isaacman D, Poirier M, Hegenbarth M, et al: Ventriculoperitoneal shunt management. Pediatr Emerg Care 19:119–125, 2003.
13. Aldrich E, Harmann P: Disconnection as a cause of ventriculoperitoneal shunt malfunction in multicomponent shunt systems. Pediatr Neurosurg 16:309–312, 1990–1991.
14. Faulhauer K, Schmitz P: Overdrainage phenomena in shunt treated hydrocephalus. Acta Neurochir (Wien) 45:89–101, 1978.
15. Renier D, Lacombe J, Pierre-Kahn A, et al: Factors causing acute shunt infection: computer analysis of 1174 operations. J Neurosurg 61:1072–1078, 1984.
16. Enger P, Svendsen F, Wester K: CSF shunt infections in children: experiences from a population-based study. Acta Neurochir (Wien) 145:243–248, 2003.
17. Pople I, Bayston R, Hayward R: Infection of cerebrospinal fluid shunts in infants: a study of etiological factors. J Neurosurg 77:29–36, 1992.
18. Lan C, Wong T, Chen S, et al: Early diagnosis of ventriculoperitoneal shunt infections and malfunctions in children with hydrocephalus. J Microbiol Immunol Infect 36:47–50, 2003.
*19. Lozier A, Sciacca R, Romagnoli M, et al: Ventriculostomy-related infections: a critical review of the literature. Neurosurgery 51:170–182, 2002.
20. Yamashita N, Kamiya K, Yamada K: Experience with a programmable valve shunt system. J Neurosurg 91:26–31, 1999.
21. Noetzel M, Baker R: Shunt fluid examination: risks and benefits in the evaluation of shunt malfunction and infection. J Neurosurg 61:328–332, 1984.
22. Iskandar B, McLaughlin C, Mapstone T, et al: Pitfalls in the diagnosis of ventricular shunt dysfunction: radiology reports and ventricular size. Pediatrics 101:1031–1036, 1998.
23. Piatt J: Physical examination of patients with cerebrospinal fluid shunts: is there useful information in pumping the shunt? Pediatrics 89:470–473, 1992.
24. Piatt J: Pumping the shunt revisited: a longitudinal study. Pediatr Neurosurg 25:73–77, 1996.
25. Naradzay J, Browne B, Rolnick M, et al: Cerebral ventricular shunts. J Emerg Med 17:311–322, 1999.
26. Sood S, Kim S, Ham S, et al: Useful components of the shunt tap test for evaluation of shunt malfunction. Childs Nerv Syst 9:157–162, 1993.

*Selected readings.

Chapter 168

Thoracostomy

Nicole P. Carbonell, MD and Thomas E. Terndrup, MD

Key Points

Needle decompression must be performed immediately for suspected tension pneumothorax.

Local and systemic anesthesia should be used during insertion of tube thoracostomies.

Complications from tube thoracostomy can be minimized by following appropriate technique, including sterility, attention to anatomic landmarks, and confirmation by radiography following placement.

Indications and Contraindications

Abnormal Pleural Collections

Tube thoracostomy is a bedside procedure that allows drainage of a variety of abnormal collections from the thoracic cavity. A pneumothorax is a collection of air in the pleural space. In a simple pneumothorax, air in the pleural space separates the lung and pleura, while a tension pneumothorax results in intrapleural air trapping, potentially causing decreased venous return and shock if sufficiently severe. An open pneumothorax occurs when injury produces a full-thickness chest wall defect that connects the pleural cavity to the body surface. If the chest wall defect has less resistance to airflow than the airways, air preferentially passes in and out of the chest wall defect when the patient takes a breath, interfering with inspiratory airflow. An open pneumothorax with ingress of air is called a "sucking" chest wound.

A tension pneumothorax develops when the volume of air trapped in the pleural spaces increases positive intrapleural pressure. Increased intrapleural pressure may shift the mediastinum, compress the vena cava, and lead to decreased cardiac preload, hypotension, shock, and death.[1,2] While the most common etiology of tension pneumothorax is secondary to complications from positive pressure ventilation, other causes include bronchial or major parenchymal injury, the inadvertent sealing of a sucking chest wound, or as a complication of a spontaneous pneumothorax.

A hemothorax, or blood in the pleural cavity, results from intrathoracic hemorrhage from lacerated lung parenchyma, the heart, great vessels or their branches, the diaphragm, or intercostal or chest wall vessels. Up to 40% of a patient's total blood volume may be lost into the pleural cavity.[1] A combination of air and blood in the pleural space is a hemopneumothorax.

Other abnormal pleural collections requiring tube thoracostomy include chylothorax, pulmonary effusion, and empyema. A chylothorax results from a disruption of the thoracic duct. An effusion is fluid in the pleural cavity, and an empyema is a purulent collection. Pulmonary effusions can often be treated with thoracentesis alone, but the presence of an empyema necessitates tube thoracostomy.

Indications

The significance of these abnormal pleural collections is their interference with respiratory and cardiovascular mechanics. Management depends on several factors, including the etiology and size of the lesion, condition of the patient, need for patient transport, and need for positive pressure ventilation. All tension pneumothoraces are life threatening and should be treated with immediate needle decompression followed by tube thoracostomy.

Tube thoracostomy is indicated for any collection that requires continuous drainage over time. Large or symptomatic simple pneumothoraces, open pneumothoraces, recurrent pleural effusions, empyema, and chylothorax should all be managed with tube thoracostomy. Tube thoracostomy may also be indicated in patients with pulmonary contusion or subcutaneous emphysema who undergo prolonged transports, general anesthesia, or positive pressure ventilation, because such patients are at high risk for developing a tension pneumothorax. Less commonly, tube thoracostomy may be used therapeutically for rapid rewarming of pleural structures during intensive management of severe hypothermia, for thoracoscopy to evaluate pleural lesions, or for instillation of agents used to promote scarring or healing of recurrent pneumothoraces.

For the hemothorax, tube thoracostomy drains blood that may interfere with respiratory mechanics and may serve as a nidus of infection. It also allows precision measurement of blood loss, monitors the rate of hemorrhage, and helps to prevent organization of the hematoma into a fibrothorax.[2] Aggressive fluid resuscitation and administration of blood products are important for patients with massive hemothorax before significant evacuation is begun. An existing hemothorax may tamponade a briskly bleeding vessel, and clinically significant hypotension may result if the tube thoracostomy is performed before volume resuscitation.[3,4] An initial amount of blood drainage of 15 ml/kg or subsequent drainage of 3 to 4 ml/kg/hr for 4 hours is an indication for open thoracotomy.[5] Commercial devices exist to collect, filter, anticoagulate, and autotransfuse blood drained by tube thoracostomy.

An open pneumothorax is managed first with occlusion of the chest wall defect with a three-sided dressing, followed rapidly by tube thoracostomy at an alternate site. The dressing creates a flutter-type valve that prevents air entry during inspiration, but allows trapped air to escape during expiration. Tube thoracostomy followed by repair of the chest wall defect is the treatment of an open pneumothorax.

Contraindications

There are no absolute contraindications to tube thoracostomy. Relative contraindications include a local dermatologic disorder or a coagulopathy. The site of chest tube insertion can be modified to avoid a problematic skin lesion. Coagulopathies should be corrected, but life-saving procedures should not be withheld. Other relative contraindications include multiple adhesions or blebs, recurrent pneumothoraces mandating surgical treatment, massive hemothorax without adequate volume replacement, or the need for an immediate open thoracotomy. It is widely recommended that a chest tube not be inserted at the site of a penetrating chest wound.

Preparation and Consent

Anatomy and Physiology

The anatomy and physiology of an infant's or child's thorax affects the pathophysiology and management of abnormal pleural collections. A child's chest wall is less ossified and much more elastic than that of an adult, thus rib fractures are uncommon and severe chest injury may be masked by the absence of external clinical findings. Other intrathoracic injuries, such as pulmonary contusions, occur frequently. A child's mediastinum is also more mobile, thus mediastinal shift with resultant tracheal and caval angulation is more common in a child.[1,2,6,7] The shorter, smaller diameter, and more compressible trachea worsens the potential pathophysiologic consequences of small airway and chest wall injuries.[2] Finally, the distal airways are relatively narrow, which creates increased peripheral airway resistance. Greater positive airway pressures required for mechanical ventilation in children also increase the risk of iatrogenic barotrauma.

Neonates seem to have the greatest incidence of spontaneous pneumothorax, probably due to the dramatic changes in pulmonary physiology that occur during and immediately after birth.[8] Mechanical obstruction of alveoli can occur in the setting of meconium aspiration. Compression of the chest wall in the birth canal puts the respiratory muscles at a mechanical disadvantage. With the first extrauterine breath, the transpulmonary pressure rises from 40 cm H_2O to as much as 100 cm H_2O. Transmission of this increased pressure to alveoli can lead to overdistention, rupture of alveoli, and development of a pneumothorax.[8-10]

History and Physical

The history of a child with an abnormal pleural collection should include the details of the incident, the child's past medical and surgical history, medications, and allergies. Detailed information regarding the mechanism of the trauma and the use of personal protective gear or restraints helps the physician predict the pattern of injury. Nonaccidental trauma, falls, motor vehicle collisions, and other transport-related mechanisms such as roller blades and skateboards account for most of the blunt trauma resulting in thoracic injury.

Physical examination findings in patients with pleural collections include increased work of breathing and abnormal or diminished breath sounds. The physical examination in a child is not as predictive of thoracic injury as that of an adult. External signs of chest wall trauma may be absent due to the increased compliance of the thoracic cage. In the setting of a tension pneumothorax, one would expect cyanosis, diminished breath sounds, and hyperresonance on the affected side. Contralateral deviation of the trachea and jugular venous distention are late and uncommon findings in children. The shorter neck and wide transmission of breath sounds across the thorax of the child render abnormal auscultatory findings less obvious. Therefore, the sole presentation of a tension pneumothorax in a child may be respiratory distress followed by overt signs of shock.

Diagnostic Evaluation

The chest radiograph is the primary screening study in the evaluation of all abnormal pleural collections. In the setting of suspected tension pneumothorax in a severely compromised infant or child, it is inappropriate to delay decompression for chest radiography. It is helpful to divide the collections into traumatic and nontraumatic to direct the diagnostic evaluation. For the noninjured patient without a tension pneumothorax, posteroanterior and lateral radiographs of the chest should be obtained to determine whether the collection contains air or fluid. For infants, anteroposterior (AP) and decubitus radiographs are normally required, and when uncertainty exists about an occult pneumothorax, expiratory chest films or chest computed tomography (CT) may be required. Radiographic signs of a pneumothorax include an asymmetric lucency extending beyond lung markings, sharply outlined mediastinal structures, and a shifted mediastinum.[2] If the AP radiograph shows fluid, lateral decubitus radiographs should be obtained. All effusions may require thoracentesis to further delineate whether they are transudative, exudative, or purulent, as well as to provide symptomatic relief when substantial. A chest CT is often helpful when the chest radiograph is completely "whited out" to distinguish whole lung consolidation from a free-flowing or a loculated effusion.[11] Disadvantages of a CT scan include increased radiation exposure, cost, the associated risks of sedation, and the possibility that the CT scan may miss a multiloculated collection. Thoracic ultrasound is useful to identify air or fluid in the pleural cavity and to delineate the extent of loculation and organization of the effusion or empyema.[11] Such information is very useful in determining whether the collection can be treated at the bedside with tube thoracostomy or whether surgical intervention is necessary.

In the setting of trauma, the supine AP chest radiograph is taken early during the secondary survey. In this position, air layers anteriorly, and radiographic signs of a pneumothorax may be subtle or absent. Researchers have shown that CT better describes the characteristics and extent of injury than chest radiographs, but is not clear that this extra information changes patient management.[12-17] Occult pneumothoraces are often an unexpected finding on an abdominal CT scan of pediatric trauma patients. A prospective study of 538 pediatric trauma patients undergoing both chest radiography and abdominal CT found that 55% of pneumothoraces found on the CT (11 of 20) were not identified on the initial chest radiograph. However, only 1 of the 11 occult pneumothoraces required tube thoracostomy.[18] This study validates the notion that the increased information obtained with the CT may not alter patient management, and that not all occult traumatic pneumothoraces require tube thoracostomy.

Consent

Informed consent for tube thoracostomy in minors should be obtained from parents or the most appropriate legal guardian if available. Emergency consent is implied for lifesaving procedures. Assent by the child is normally required in children age 7 years or older.

Pain Management and Sedation

Proactive and effective pain management in children should be a priority for all practitioners who care for infants and children. Tube thoracostomy is painful regardless of who is performing the procedure. If the patient is awake, infiltrative local anesthetic is clinically prudent. Intravenous opioids, dissociative agents, and anxiolytics should be used early in management, with small, titrated doses depending upon the individual needs of the patient.[19] Using a small-gauge needle, preferentially 27 or 30 gauge, as well as buffering the lidocaine with bicarbonate, substantially decreases the pain associated with the infiltration of subcutaneous and local lidocaine anesthetic.

Equipment

The contents of a typical prepackaged tube thoracostomy tray are listed in Table 168–1. Other adjunctive supplies include adhesive tape, tincture of benzoin, antiseptic solution, proper-sized chest tubes, and a drainage apparatus with sterile water for water seal, plastic tubing, and connectors. All equipment should be assembled and inspected before beginning the procedure. The size of the chest tubes will vary with the patient's size and type of collection to be drained. Larger tubes are used to drain blood or pus; smaller tubes drain air (Table 168–2). The appropriate-sized chest tube can

Table 168–1	Contents of a Typical Tube Thoracostomy Tray

Sterile gauze
Kelly clamps
Large suture and Mayo scissors
Local anesthetic
Multiple syringes and needles
Needle driver
No. 0 silk sutures
Scalpel
Sterile towels

be estimated from the patient's weight. The clinician should ensure adequate lighting, monitoring equipment, and assistant personnel.

Drainage Systems

All chest tubes need a fluid drainage system, except for those with flutter valves used periodically for simple pneumothoraces. With the extrathoracic end of the tube placed underwater at a level below the chest, air under positive intrapleural pressure escapes into the bottle and cannot reenter the pleural space. A single bottle system works only for the drainage of air. If fluid is draining in a single-bottle system, it will build up in the bottle, increase pressure of the water seal system, and render it ineffective. A two-bottle system allows fluid to collect in the second bottle while still providing an escape for pressurized intrapleural air. Suction improves the rate of drainage of fluid or air, but can damage the lung parenchyma or pleura if applied directly to the system. Adding a third bottle to the two-bottle system connected to the water seal bottle and filled to a level corresponding to the desired level of suction (usually 15 to 20 cm H_2O) avoids this problem. The vent allows the entrance of air from the environment when the wall suction applied is greater than the set level. Commercially available plastic chest tube drainage units usually employ the three-bottle system (Fig. 168–1).

Table 168–2	Determination of Appropriate Chest Tube Size by Patient Age and Weight	
Patient Age	Weight (kg)	Tube Size (French)
Premature	3	10–14
0–6 mo	3.5	12–18
6–12 mo	7	14–20
1–3 yr	10–12	14–24
4–7 yr	16–18	20–32
8–10 yr	24–30	28–38

From Extremes of trauma: Pediatric trauma. In American College of Surgeons Advanced Trauma Life Support For Doctors: Student Course Manual, 7th ed. Chicago: American College of Surgeons, 2004, pp 243–262.

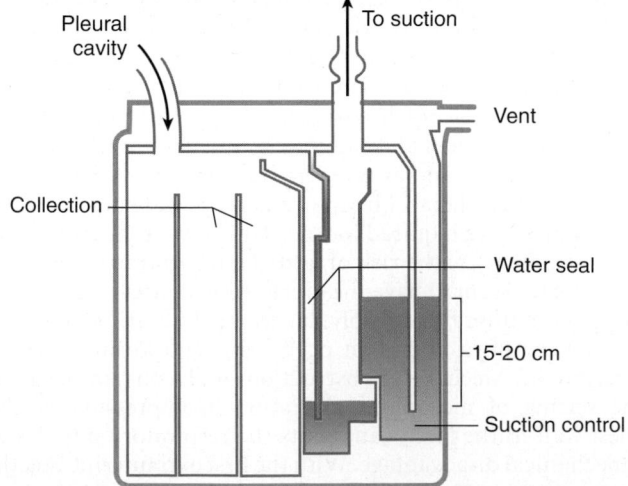

FIGURE 168–1. Commercial three-bottle system. (From Connors KM, Terndrup TE: Tube thoracostomy and needle decompression of the chest. In Henretig FM, King C [eds]: Textbook of Pediatric Emergency Procedures. Baltimore: Williams & Wilkins, 1997, p 404.)

Monitoring

Patients with chest tubes need continuous cardiac and pulse oximetry monitoring. Once analgesia or sedation is administered, continuous monitoring for efficacy and complications is necessary. Routine assessment of respiratory rate and effort, arterial blood pressure, and level of consciousness is performed, and oxygen is monitored continuously. Guidelines promulgated by the American College of Emergency Physicians and American Academy of Pediatrics should be incorporated into institutional guidelines for monitoring during tube thoracostomy (see Chapter 159, Procedural Sedation and Analgesia).

Technique

Needle Decompression

Needle decompression is the first step for the direct treatment of a tension pneumothorax. Endotracheal intubation and positive pressure ventilation in severely ill patients with an undiagnosed pneumothorax may worsen the patient's condition, and immediate decompression is required. The patient is positioned in supine with the head of the bed elevated 30 degrees. The insertion site is swabbed with antiseptic, and a local infiltrative anesthetic is used if time permits. A large-gauge needle or angiocatheter is inserted perpendicularly over the superior aspect of the third rib, and walked over the rib into the lower portion of the second intercostal space at the midclavicular line (Fig. 168–2). A rush of air is usually heard or felt as the pleural space is entered and pressurized air is evacuated. When using an angiocatheter, it should be

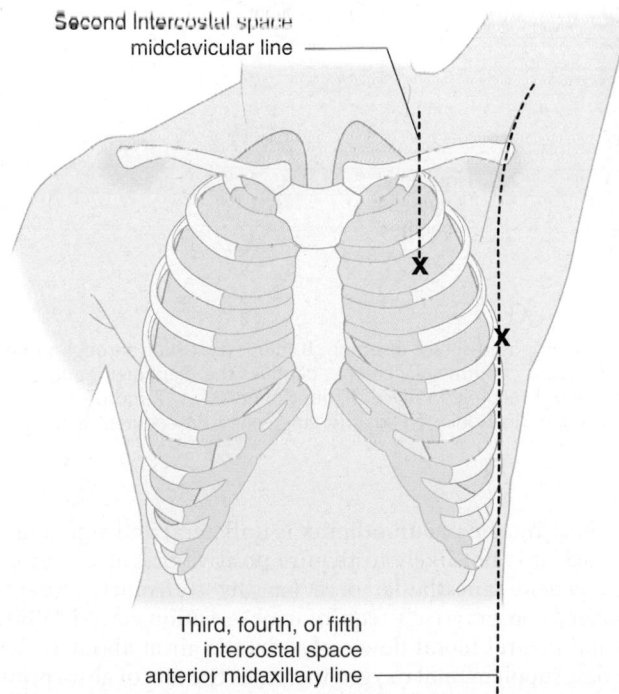

FIGURE 168–2. Sites of needle decompression and tube thoracostomy. (From Connors KM, Terndrup TE: Tube thoracostomy and needle decompression of the chest. In Henretig FM, King C [eds]: Textbook of Pediatric Emergency Procedures. Baltimore: Williams & Wilkins, 1997, p 399.)

advanced into the pleural space, then the needle is removed and the catheter left in place.

Tube Thoracostomy

The patient is positioned in supine with the head of the bed elevated 30 degrees. The preferred insertion site is the fourth or fifth intercostal space at the anterior or midaxillary line[20-22] (see Fig. 168–2). Using universal precautions, the insertion site is prepared and sterilely draped. A generous wheal of local anesthetic is made over the rib below the insertion site, anesthetizing the subcutaneous tissue overlying the upper rib, the periosteum, and the pleura. To anesthetize the pleura, the needle is advanced into the pleural space where air or fluid can easily be aspirated. Then, it is withdrawn slowly while aspirating until no air or fluid returns. At this point, injected lidocaine should anesthetize the pleura. Caution should be used not to exceed 5 mg/kg of total lidocaine to avoid systemic toxicity.

An incision is made with a scalpel through the skin and subcutaneous tissue at the site of the skin wheal. In an infant or a small child, a 0.5- to 1-cm incision will be adequate, while in a larger child or adolescent, a 2- to 4-cm incision may be necessary. Next, blunt dissection is performed through the subcutaneous tissue by opening and closing a Kelly clamp. Tunneling over the next rib provides a better seal against air leaks while the tube is in place, and may help to prevent pleural fistulas when it is removed. Dissection is continued to the upper surface of the upper rib, avoiding the neurovascular structures located on the inferior margin of the rib. Next, the tip of the clamp is slid over the superior rib margin through the intercostal muscles and parietal pleura with firm but controlled pressure. A "pop" or sudden loss of resistance and a rush of air or fluid should be felt when the pleura is punctured. The tip of the clamp is placed 1 cm into the thoracic cavity and spread widely to open the pleura. The clamp is then withdrawn and the pleural space checked with a finger to confirm placement and strip any adhesions between the lung and parietal pleura. The chest tube is guided into the pleural space with the finger or with a Kelly clamp inserted through the tip of the chest tube. If the patient is large, the probing finger is left in the pleural space and the tube is guided along the track of the finger while attached to a curved clamp (Fig. 168–3).

For a fluid collection, the chest tube is directed posteriorly and superiorly. For pneumothorax alone, it is directed anteriorly and superiorly. It is critical to insert the chest tube far enough that all the side holes lie within the pleural space. The tube is connected to a drainage system, and secured with a suture. A purse-string type suture placed around the chest tube where it enters the chest wall secures the tube and closes the incision when the tube is removed. After suturing, an occlusive dressing with petrolatum gauze is placed around the base of the tube as it enters the skin. This is covered with two pieces of gauze that are each cut from the middle of one side to the center and oriented 90 degrees to each other. Then the area and the tube are securely taped down.

Chest tube placement should be verified by a chest radiograph as soon as possible. Serial radiographs confirm the resolution of the collection. Any sudden change in the patient's cardiorespiratory status should be considered to be a recurrence of the collection until proven otherwise. Patients receiving mechanical ventilation are especially at risk for

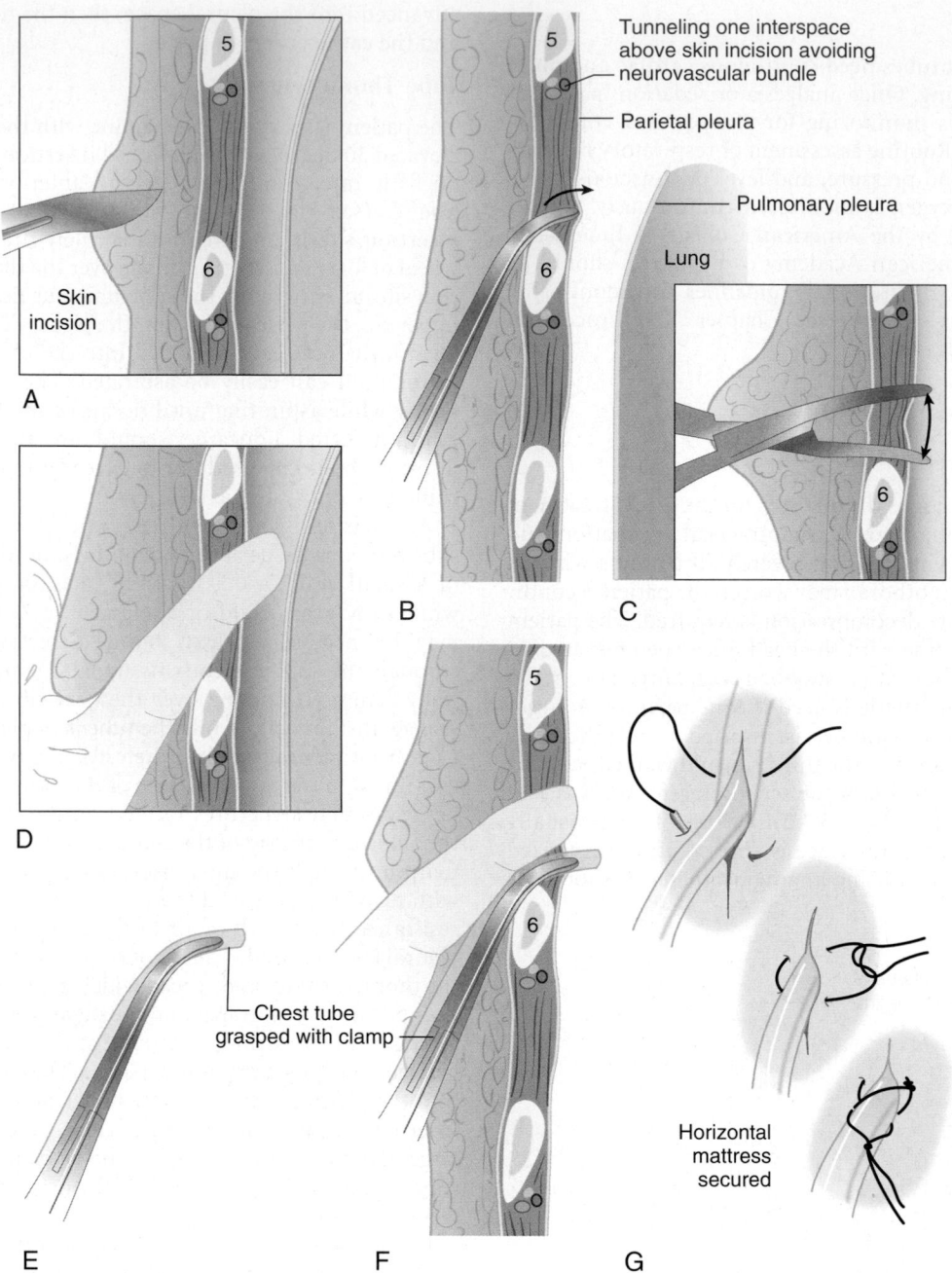

FIGURE 168-3. Blunt dissection technique. **A,** Incision made one interspace below proposed site of insertion. **B,** Blunt dissection throughout the subcutaneous tissue. **C,** Clamp spread after entering the pleural space. **D,** Probing finger confirms placement, identifies the diaphragm, and strips adhesions. **E** and **F,** Chest tube grasped with clamp and inserted. **G,** Chest tube sutured securely in place. (From Connors TM, Terndrup TE: Tube thoracostomy and needle decompression of the chest. In Henretig FM, King C [eds]: Textbook of Pediatric Emergency Procedures. Baltimore: Williams & Wilkins, 1997, p 401.)

recurrence of the original collection or the development of a new pneumothorax.

Alternatives

Conservative Management

Children with a simple, iatrogenic, or occult traumatic pneumothorax are often asymptomatic.[23,24] A few studies suggest that conservative management may be safe in children.[18] Observation alone is appropriate when the patient is other-wise healthy, the pneumothorax is unilateral and small, and the patient is not likely to require positive pressure ventilation, general anesthesia, or a lengthy transport. Patients managed conservatively require an observation period. While normal pleural blood flow reabsorbs the air at about 1.25% per day, supplemental oxygen increases the rate of absorption by as much as sixfold.[25] Therefore, the patient should be placed on a pure oxygen mask or nasal oxygen immediately and continuously until the appropriate end point is reached. Serial radiography monitors the progression of the collection. Estimating the size of a pneumothorax is often inaccurate, but most authorities agree that a small pneumothorax occupies less than 10% to 20% of the thoracic cavity.[20,26]

Catheter Aspiration

Larger, simple spontaneous or iatrogenic pneumothoraces may be managed by catheter aspiration. Catheter aspiration has several advantages over tube thoracostomy. It is simpler to perform, less traumatic, leaves a smaller scar, and generally results in less patient discomfort.[25,27,28] Trauma patients with a tension pneumothorax, hemothorax, persistent air leak, hemodynamic instability, or other serious injuries are not candidates for this procedure. Underlying lung pathology (e.g., restrictive or reactive lung diseases) is also a relative contraindication for catheter aspiration.

Complications

Patients undergoing tube thoracostomy infrequently have serious complications.[29] Complications from incorrect insertion include damage to local anatomic structures, ineffective drainage, and infection. Damage to the thoracic nerve and intercostal arteries may lead to bleeding and a winged scapula. Injury to the intercostal nerve results in continued pain or numbness at the thoracostomy site. Blunt dissection and avoiding the neurovascular bundle on the inferior margin of the rib minimizes the risk of neurovascular injury. Foley catheter tamponade of hemorrhage from a lacerated intercostal artery has been reported in a neonate.[30] Other complications include damage to thoracic or abdominal organs. The blunt dissection technique minimizes this risk by providing an easy passage for the tube. Using a finger to explore the tract and pleural space also minimizes the risk of diaphragm penetration or subcutaneous placement. A high-lying diaphragm occurs in the setting of forced expiration, hemidiaphragm paralysis, previous thoracotomy, intra-abdominal injuries, and the supine position. Abdominal placement of a chest tube can occur in this setting.[31] If a high-lying diaphragm is suspected, sit the patient upright to reduce the possibility of injury.

A chest tube inserted too far presses against the pleura or thoracic structures and causes rare but serious complications. Cardiogenic shock secondary to right atrial compression can occur.[32] Horner's syndrome due to pressure on the inferior cervical ganglion has been reported.[33,34] Diaphragm paralysis due to phrenic nerve injury has also been reported.[35] A chest tube not inserted far enough for all drainage holes to lie within the pleural cavity increases the risk of an air leak and subcutaneous emphysema. Correcting the position of the chest tube and applying suction under a water seal is the treatment for both air leaks and subcutaneous emphysema.[36]

Complications can result even with a properly placed tube. The tube itself may move or become disconnected. Re-expansion pulmonary edema and hypotension have been described following drainage of large, long-standing effusions in young patients.[25,37] Treatment for re-expansion pulmonary edema is supportive. Finally, significant scarring can occur at the insertion site. Placing a chest tube in the midclavicular line or even too high in the anterior axillary line of premature neonates has resulted in severe breast deformities.[38] Lateral placement of the chest tube minimizes the cosmetic impact of scarring.

Finally, infectious complications may occur. Splinting due to pain at the insertion site may lead to pneumonia or atelectasis. Intercostal nerve blocks, intravenous opioids, and use of incentive spirometry help prevent these complications. Infection at the insertion site is minimized by good sterile technique. The role of prophylactic antibiotics for tube thoracostomy is unclear. The adult literature is inconclusive, but one study demonstrated a benefit of fewer infectious complications and a shorter hospital stay resulting from the administration of a first generation cephalosporin during tube thoracostomy.[39] Despite this research, most authorities do not recommend prophylactic antibiotics for tube thoracostomy in children.[40]

Postprocedure Care and Disposition

All patients with a chest tube need admission for observation, serial radiography, and eventual removal of the chest tube following resolution of their injury or illness. The exception to this is the rare case of simple pneumothorax drained with a catheter aspiration and a flutter valve that might be safely managed on an outpatient basis with close follow-up. In the emergency department, patients must be continually monitored for further deterioration from their illness or injury. Ongoing management of hemodynamic, neurologic, respiratory, analgesia-sedation, and other patient care needs must be maintained throughout the course of the patient's acute clinical problems.

REFERENCES

1. Grisoni ER, Volsko TA: Thoracic injuries in children. Respir Care Clin N Am 7:25–38, 2001.
2. Bliss D, Silen M: Pediatric thoracic trauma. Crit Care Med 30(11 Suppl):s409–3415, 2002.
3. Rhea JT, Deluca SA, Greene RE: Determining the size of pneumothorax in the upright patient. Radiology 144:733, 1982.
4. Bayne CG: Pulmonary complications of the McSwain dart. Ann Emerg Med 11:136, 1982.
5. Cullen ML: Pulmonary and respiratory complications of pediatric trauma. Respir Care Clin N Am 7:59–77, 2001.
6. Stafford PW, Blinman TA, Nance ML: Practical points in evaluation and resuscitation of the injured child. Surg Clin North Am 82:273–301, 2002.
7. Beaver BL, Laschinger JC: Pediatric thoracic trauma. Semin Thorac Cardiovasc Surg 4:255–262, 1992.
8. Yu VY, Lieu SW, Robertson NR: Pneumothorax in the newborn: changing patterns. Arch Dis Child 50:449, 1975.
9. Monin P, Vert P: Pneumothorax. Clin Perinatol 5:535, 1978.
10. Wigglesworth JS: Pathology of the lung in the fetus and neonate, with particular reference to problems of growth and maturation. Histopathology 11:671–689, 1987.
11. Lewis RA, Feigin RD: Current issues in the diagnosis and management of pediatric empyema. Semin Pediatr Infect Dis 13:280–288, 2002.
12. Brasel KJ, Stafford RE, Weigelt JA, et al: Treatment of occult pneumothoraces from blunt trauma. J Trauma 46:987–990, 1999.
13. Rhea JT, Noveline RA, Lawrason J, et al: The frequency and significance of thoracic injuries detected on abdominal CT scans of multiple trauma patients. J Trauma 29:502–505, 1989.
14. Hill SL, Edmisten T, Holtzman G, et al: The occult pneumothorax: an increasing entity in trauma. Am Surg 65:254–258, 1999.
15. Sivit CJ, Taylor GA, Eichelberger MR: Chest injury in children with blunt abdominal trauma: evaluation with CT. Radiology 171:815–818, 1989.
16. Bridges KG, Welch G, Silver M, et al: CT detection of occult pneumothorax in multiple trauma patients. J Emerg Med 11:179–186, 1993.
17. Furnival RA: Controversies in pediatric thoracic and abdominal trauma. Clin Pediatr Emerg Med 2:48–62, 2001.

*18. Holmes JF: A clinical decision rule for identifying children with thoracic injuries after blunt torso trauma. Ann Emerg Med 39:492–499, 2002.

19. Murat I, Gall O, Tourniaire B: Procedural pain in children: evidence-based best practice and guidelines. Reg Anesth Pain Med 28:561–572, 2003.

*20. Iberti TJ, Stern PM: Chest tube thoracostomy. Crit Care Clin 8:879–894, 1992.

21. Symbas PN: Chest drainage tubes. Surg Clin North Am 69:41–46, 1989.

22. Miller KS, Sahn SA: Chest tubes: indications, technique, management and complications. Chest 91:258–264, 1987.

23. Collins JC, Levine G, Waxman K: Occult traumatic pneumothorax: immediate tube thoracostomy versus expectant management. Am Surg 58:743–746, 1992.

24. Wolfman NT, Gilpin JW, Bechtold RE, et al: Occult pneumothorax in patients with abdominal trauma: CT studies. J Comput Assist Tomogr 17:56–59, 1993.

25. Baumann MH, Strange C: Treatment of spontaneous pneumothorax: a more aggressive approach? Chest 112:789–804, 1997.

26. Vukick DJ: Diseases of the pleural space. Emerg Med Clin North Am 7:309–324, 1989.

27. Minami H, Saka H, Senda K, et al: Small catheter drainage for spontaneous pneumothorax. Am J Med Sci 304:345–347, 1992.

28. Conces DJ, Tarver RD, Gray WC, et al: Treatment of pneumothoraces utilizing small caliber chest tubes. Chest 94:55–57, 1988.

29. Ernst A: Interventional pulmonary procedures: Guidelines from the American College of Chest Physicians. Chest 123:1693–1717, 2003.

30. McElroy SJ: Foley catheter tamponade of intercostals hemorrhage in preterm infants. J Pediatr 145:241, 2004.

31. Foresti V, Villa A, Casati O, et al: Abdominal placement of tube thoracostomy due to lack of recognition of paralysis of hemidiaphragm. Chest 102:29, 1992.

32. Kolleff MH, Dothager DW: Reversible cardiogenic shock due to chest tube compression of the right ventricle. Chest 99:976–980, 1991.

33. Mahfood S, Hix WR, Aaron BL, et al: Reexpansion pulmonary edema. Ann Thorac Surg 45:340, 1988.

34. Cook T, Kietzman L, Leibold R: "Pneumo-ptosis" in the emergency department. Am J Emerg Med 10:431–434, 1992.

35. Nahum E: Acute diaphragmatic paralysis caused by chest-tube trauma to phrenic nerve. Pediatr Radiol 31:444–446, 2001.

36. Cerfolio RJ: Advances in thoracostomy tube management. Surg Clin North Am 82:833–848, vii, 2002.

37. Bertino RE, Wesbey GE, Johnson R: Horner syndrome occurring as a complication of chest tube placement. Radiology 164:745, 1987.

38. Rainer C, Gardetto A, Fruhwirth M, et al: Breast deformity in adolescence as a result of pneumothorax drainage during neonatal intensive care. Pediatrics 111:80–86, 2003.

39. Gonzales RP, Holevar MR: Role of prophylactic antibiotics for tube thoracostomy in chest trauma. Am Surg 65:617–621, 1998.

40. Mollitt DL: Infection control: avoiding the inevitable. Surg Clin North Am 82:365–378, 2002.

*Suggested readings.

Chapter 169

Hernia Reduction

Mark C. Clark, MD and John A. Brennan, MD

Key Points

Indirect inguinal hernias present with a mass at the internal ring of the inguinal canal (vs. other inguinal and scrotal masses).

Hydroceles are usually smooth, nontender, and mobile; have brilliant transillumination (bowel can transilluminate); and do not extend into the internal ring of the inguinal canal.

Even with irreducible incarcerated inguinal hernias, strangulation is rare.

Most attempts at reduction of an incarcerated inguinal hernia should be successful.

Irreducible inguinal hernias in girls may be an incarcerated ovary.

Evidence of bowel obstruction is not a contraindication to manual reduction of an inguinal hernia.

Indications and Contraindications

When to Reduce an Inguinal Hernia

Unless the child is extremely ill appearing with signs of toxicity from gangrenous bowel, manual reduction should be attempted.[1] In a survey of 40 senior pediatric surgeons, 100% would attempt manual reduction in clinically stable patients without signs of peritoneal irritation.[2] The advantages of early reduction of an incarcerated inguinal hernia are that it prevents strangulation from occurring, decreases the risk of testicular atrophy, and stabilizes the child before surgery. Pediatric surgeons have an increased complication rate when operating on an incarcerated inguinal hernia compared to nonincarcerated hernias[3] (see Chapter 84, Abdominal Hernias).

In the past, evidence of bowel obstruction has been considered a contraindication for a manual reduction of a hernia. In one study in which 12 of 14 infants less than 2 years old showed radiographic evidence of bowel obstruction, the success of manual reduction was not affected by this finding. In a survey, 75% of pediatric surgeons replied they would still attempt manual reduction for incarcerated inguinal hernias even if the child had abdominal distention and radiographic evidence of intestinal obstruction.[2]

When Not to Reduce an Inguinal Hernia

Manual reduction should not be attempted by the emergency physician in a child who appears toxic or febrile or has bloody diarrhea, entrapped viscera that are black or blue, peritoneal signs, or leukocytosis greater than $15,000/mm^3$.[1,2] Even though it is considered nearly impossible to reduce a necrotic bowel, cases have been reported.[4]

Preparation and Consent

Preparation

Hernia reduction requires minimal preparation unless the practitioner decides to use procedural sedation. Some physicians may elect to use parental analgesia, such as intravenous or intramuscular morphine, but often manual reduction can be accomplished relatively easily and quickly so that the need for parental sedation and analgesia would be unnecessary. If the manual reduction cannot be achieved easily, then procedural sedation and analgesia should be strongly considered.

Consent

Parents should be given a description of the procedure about to be performed and the potential for complications. Since this not a surgical procedure, signed consent for treatment given during patient registration is adequate.

Equipment

The use of ice packs to decrease swelling and possibly decrease pain may make it easier to reduce an incarcerated hernia, but this has never been studied. A bed that can place a child in Trendelenberg positioning may be helpful, but again it is only a theoretical technique. Monitoring and resuscitation equipment will be needed if procedural sedation is performed (see Chapter 159, Procedural Sedation and Analgesia).

Monitoring

Most children with an incarcerated hernia are not ill unless their examination suggests dehydration from vomiting or

Table 169–1	Procedural Summary

1. Be certain it is a hernia.
2. Be sure the hernia is not strangulated.
3. Consider sedation; many would use this on the first attempt at hernia reduction.
4. Warm your hands.
5. Apply gentle, firm bimanual pressure along the entire inguinal canal, using the hand most distal to "milk out" the contents or gas within the incarcerated bowel.
6. After reducing the contents of the incarcerated bowel, pressure should be increased distally as compared to the proximal inguinal canal.
7. If the bowel fails to reduce after 5 minutes of continuous pressure, use sedation with the patient in the Trendelenburg position, and place an ice pack on the groin.
8. Repeat the above bimanual technique, hopefully after the child has fallen asleep.
9. If successful or unsuccessful reduction occurs, call the pediatric surgeon.
10. Admit nearly all patients who presented with an incarcerated inguinal hernia.

toxicity from strangulation. In the typical patient with an incarcerated hernia, monitoring vital signs beyond what is customary for a pediatric emergency patient is not necessary. If procedural sedation or analgesia is given, then appropriate monitoring will need to be instituted (see Chapter 159, Procedural Sedation and Analgesia).

Techniques

No prospective study has examined the success rate of different techniques for manual reduction. Instead, most authors report using some combination of sedation, ice packs, elevation, and gentle manual reduction (Table 169–1). The patient's leg should be externally rotated and abducted. When pediatric surgeons were surveyed, they used gentle manipulation 95% of the time, sedation 75%, elevation 55%, and ice packs in only 18% of cases.[2] The technique for manual reduction is to apply bimanual pressure along the inguinal canal and use the hand most distal to "milk out" the gas or contents of the incarcerated bowel (Fig. 169–1). After reducing the contents

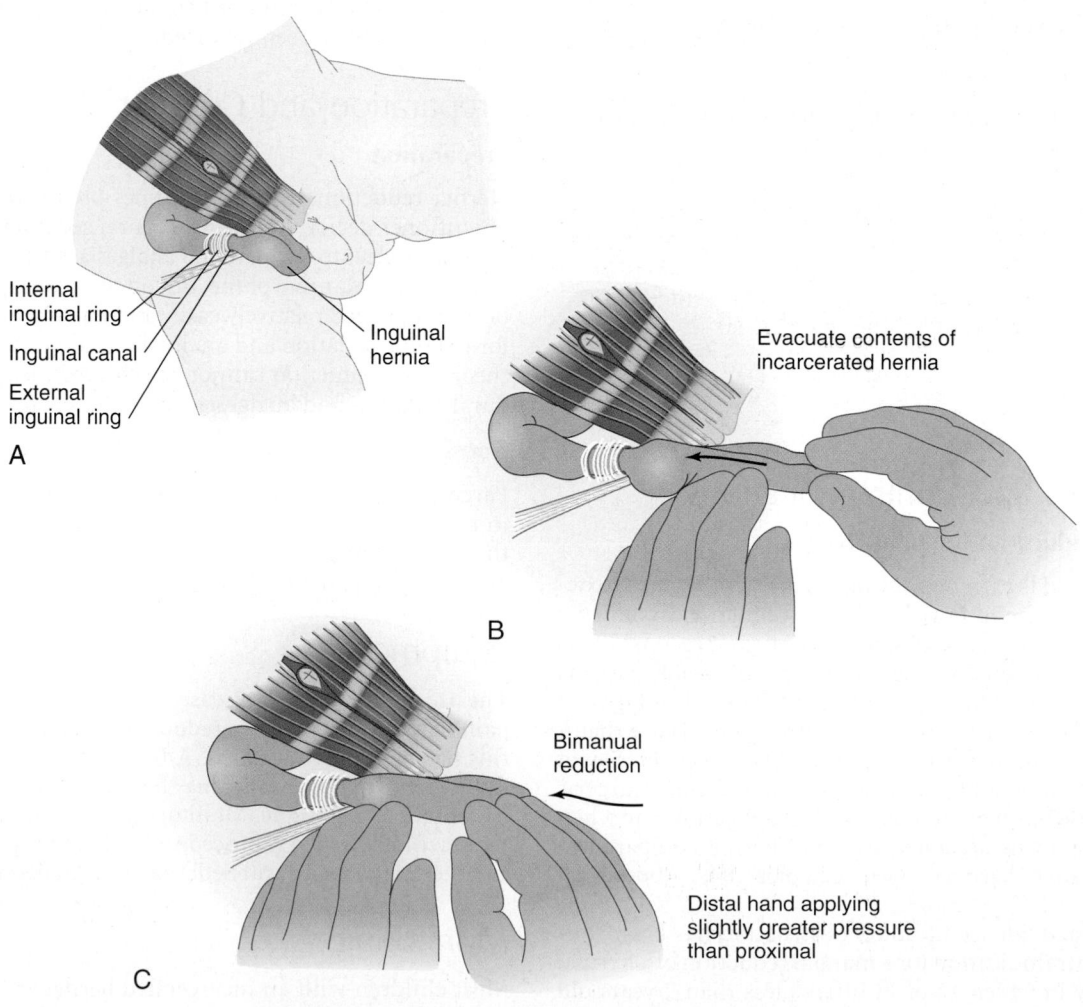

FIGURE 169–1. Bimanual reduction of an inguinal hernia.

of the incarcerated bowel, pressure should be slightly increased over the distal hernia as compared to the proximal aspect to reduce the bowel. The pressure should be held constant up to 5 minutes. If this fails, most would recommend—and many would use even on the first attempt—sedation, Trendelenburg positioning, and a covered ice pack or cold pack to the groin. When the child relaxes, or ideally falls asleep, gentle pressure as described should be attempted again[1,2,4-7] (see Chapter 159, Procedural Sedation and Analgesia).

In recent years there has been gradual improvement in the manual reduction rate of incarcerated inguinal hernias. Most recently, two studies have had 95.5% (151 of 158) and 100% (30 of 30) success rates in reduction of incarcerated inguinal hernia in children less than 2 years old (the age group in which incarceration occurs most commonly).[5,6] Earlier studies had reported successful reductions in the 70% to 80% range.[3,7]

Alternatives

Placing the child in Trendelenberg position with parenteral sedation has been described. The sedated child is placed in Trendelenberg position and then observed for up to 1 hour. The success rate has been reported to be as high as 75%.

Complications

Reducing a Strangulated Hernia

The most serious complication of manual reduction of an incarcerated inguinal hernia is reduction of necrotic or strangulated bowel. It is uncommon to find gangrenous bowel even in an irreducible incarcerated inguinal hernia. The incidence of intestinal infarction is extremely low. Between 1960 and 1965, the intestinal resection rate among 351 patients with incarcerated inguinal hernias was 1.4%. A review of three series published since 1978 indicated no resection of bowel in 221 patients with incarcerated inguinal hernias. Still, there have been reported cases of a necrotic bowel being reduced.[4,8]

Incomplete Hernia Reduction

After reducing an inguinal hernia, the physician should be sure the inguinal canal is empty, especially the internal ring. There have been reports of an incompletely reduced bowel, such as Richter's hernia (one wall of the bowel still incarcerated), resulting in a necrotic bowel.[9] Most experts recommend that children with a reduced incarcerated inguinal hernia be admitted to the hospital to observe for such complications and to schedule for semi-elective repair of the hernia. It is known that a previously incarcerated bowel has a propensity to recur relatively soon after the last incarceration.[2,3,5,7,9-13]

Incarcerated Ovary

In a female, if an incarcerated inguinal hernia will not reduce, an incarcerated ovary is likely.[7] It was previously thought that an asymptomatic irreducible ovary could be managed by elective surgical reduction. It is now known that there is a relatively high incidence of future torsion with strangulation in this situation. For this reason, females with incarcerated ovaries require urgent surgical correction.[7,14]

Testicular Infarction

The vascular supply to the testis can be compromised by the incarcerated inguinal hernia, resulting in ischemic necrosis and atrophy of the testis. Ischemic changes in the testes are relatively common with incarcerated inguinal hernias, but the rate of infarction is actually low. Children most at risk for this complication are premature infants, infants less than 6 months of age, and those who have unsuccessful manual reduction who require emergency herniotomy.[5,7,15,16]

Irreducible Inguinal Hernia

Two factors influence the success of an attempted hernia reduction. The longer the duration of symptoms at the time of presentation and the younger the child, the higher the incidence of nonreduction.[7] The complication rate for irreducible inguinal hernias is 22% to 33% with emergency surgery as opposed to 1.7% to 4.5% for manually reduced hernias followed by elective repair.[3,12] Children with irreducible incarcerated inguinal hernias need emergent surgery consultation, usually intravenous broad-spectrum antibiotics, correction of fluid and electrolyte abnormalities, and nasogastric suctioning if severe vomiting, abdominal distention, or bowel obstruction is present. Emergency herniotomy will have to be performed.[12,17] The primary reason pediatric surgeons now admit children with reduced incarcerated inguinal hernia for early semi-elective repair is to prevent the future possibility of recurrent incarceration and irreducibility with their associated complications.[2,3,5,7,9-13]

Postprocedure Care and Disposition

Parents should be taught how to reduce an inguinal hernia and to return to the physician if the hernia becomes incarcerated. All children should have a referral to a pediatric surgeon. Some pediatric surgeons believe that, if an inguinal hernia becomes incarcerated and reduced, admission for urgent herniorrhaphy is necessary since recurrent incarceration is a substantial risk.

REFERENCES

*1. Grosfeld JL: Current concepts in inguinal hernia in infants and children. World J Surg 13:506–515, 1989.
2. Rowe MI, Marchildon MB: Inguinal hernia and hydrocele in infants and children. Surg Clin North Am 61:1137–1145, 1981.
3. Rowe MI, Clatworthy HW: Incarcerated and strangulated hernias in children. Arch Surg 101:136–137, 1970.
*4. Klein BL, Ochsenschlager DW: A scrotal masses in children and adolescents: A review for the emergency physician. Pediatr Emerg Care 9:351–361, 1993.
5. Puri P, Guiney EJ, O'Donnell L:. Inguinal hernia in infants: The fate of the testis following incarceration. J Pediatr Surg 19:44–46, 1984.
6. Stringer MD, Higgins M, Capps ANJ, Holmes SJK: Irreducible inguinal hernia. Br J Surg 78:504–505, 1991.
7. Davies N, Najmaldin A, Burge DM: Irreducible inguinal hernia in children below two years of age. Br J Surg 77:1291–1292, 1990.
8. Lynn HB, Johnson WW: Inguinal herniorrhaphy in children. Arch Surg 83:573, 1961.
9. Sparnon AL, Kiely EM, Spitz L: Incarcerated inguinal hernia in infants. BMJ 293:376–377, 1986.
10. Skinner MA, Grosfeld JL: Inguinal and umbilical hernia repair in infants and children. Surg Clin North Am 73:439–449, 1993.
11. Moss RL, Hatch EI: Inguinal hernia repair in early infancy. Am J Surg 161:596–599, 1991.

*Selected readings.

12. Rescorla FJ, Grosfeld JL: Inguinal hernia repair in the perinatal period and early infancy: Clinical considerations. J Pediatr Surg 19:832–837, 1984.

*13. Stylianos S, Jacir NN, Harris BH: Incarceration of inguinal hernia in infants prior to elective repair. J Pediatr 28:582–583, 1993.

14. Boley SJ, Cahn D, Lauer T, et al: The irreducible ovary: A true emergency. J Pediatr Surg 26:1035–1038, 1991.

15. Friedman D, Schwartzbard A, Velcek FT, et al: The government and the inguinal hernia. J Pediatr Surg 14:356–359, 1979.

16. Sloman JG, Mylius RE: Testicular infarction in infancy: Its association with irreducible inguinal hernia. Med J Aust 1:242–244, 1958.

17. Nakayama DK, Rowe MI: Inguinal hernia and the acute scrotum in infants and children. Pediatr Rev 11:87–93, 1989.

Chapter 170

Access of Ports and Catheters and Management of Obstruction

Stacey Murray-Taylor, MD and Neil Schamban, MD

Preparation and Consent

Although the majority of children who require intravenous access in the emergency department receive it via peripheral vein cannulation, an increasing number of children arrive with long-term vascular access in place. The most common access agents are catheters and ports.

Chronic Venous Access Catheters

Silastic central venous catheters are also known as Hickman and Broviac catheters (Fig. 170–1). The Hickman is a modification of the Broviac catheter.[1] The difference between the two is minor, and they function in very similar manners; they remain the most popular long-term, indwelling catheters in children. They range in size from 2.7 to 12 French.[2] They are implanted surgically and are tunneled underneath the skin to an exit point on the wall of the anterior chest or abdomen. The subcutaneous portion possesses a Dacron cuff that forms an anchor and creates a barrier to help prevent the spread of bacteria from the skin.[1] As the tissue heals, it also allows for the fixation of the catheter without the need for external immobilizing sutures. This may account for the lower rates of thrombus and infection in these catheters. The catheter may possess one or two lumens. Each lumen is composed of its own inner core with a cuff and its own heparin lock–style cap.

Implantable Venous Access Devices

Currently the most commonly used ports are Port-A-Cath, Infuse-A-Port, and MediPort ports. These implantable access ports were developed for long-term access. They are surgically placed in the subcutaneous tissue and tunneled a short distance to a central vein (Fig. 170–2). The reservoir is a small region, either stainless steel or firm plastic, usually implanted just over the pectoralis major muscle. The side facing the skin consists of a thick rubber membrane. The diaphragm of the port may be punctured up to 2000 times prior to replacement.[2] The ports also contain a self-sealing silicone septum, thereby decreasing the risk of infection.

Consent

The general consent signed by the patient or guardian is generally all that is needed to access these catheters and ports.

Equipment and Technique

Chronic Venous Access Catheters

Hickman and Broviac catheters are easily accessible via sterile technique. The dressing is removed from the catheter. Next, the exit site should be cleaned with standard aseptic technique, followed by clamping the catheter and removing the cap. A 10-ml syringe is attached to the port and the catheter may then be unclamped. Approximately 5 ml of blood is removed and discarded. Then, using a new syringe, blood samples are obtained and/or medications are infused. The catheter is reclamped when this process is complete. A heparin solution is flushed and a new injection cap is placed. It cannot be overstated that these catheters require meticulous aseptic techniques when accessing and handling the device.

Implantable Venous Access Devices

To access implantable ports, a special needle containing a side hole (Huber needle) is required. To access the port, the subcutaneous reservoir is palpated. The overlying skin is cleansed with standard aseptic technique. Then, a 10-ml syringe is attached to extension tubing, which is in turn attached to a 20- to 22-gauge Huber needle. The needle is

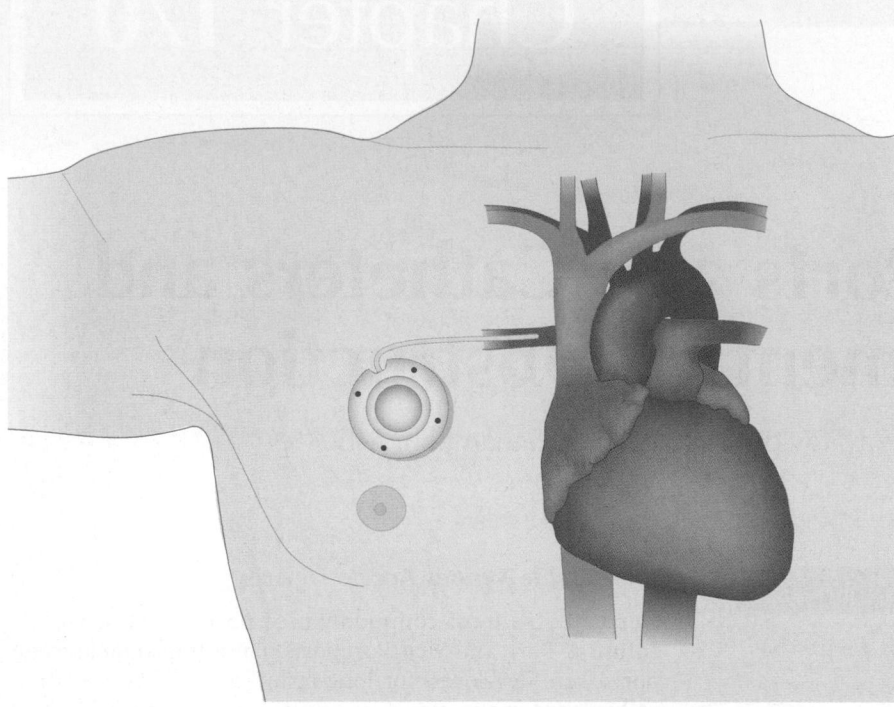

FIGURE 170–1. Implantable venous access device (ports).

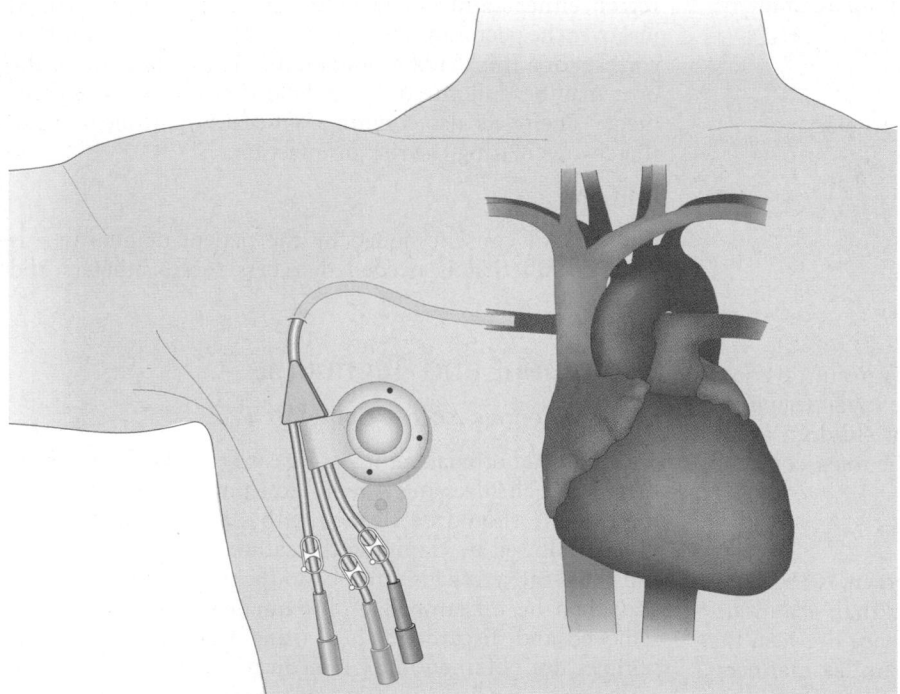

FIGURE 170–2. Chronic venous access catheters (Hickman and Broviac).

inserted through skin and aspirated until blood is returned. Fluids can then be infused. The Huber needle is stabilized with sterile gauze and transparent dressing.

Complications

Maintenance

The requirement of daily catheter maintenance for the Hickman or Broviac catheters is one of the main disadvantages. These catheters are external to the skin and require daily cleaning and dressing changes with washing. This can be time consuming and may require additional education for health care providers and the family. Ports are subcutaneous. As a result, they require no daily maintenance. They can be washed like any other part of the body, with frequent visual inspections to observe for signs of infection.

Emotional Impact

A subtle but equally important aspect to consider is the disfigurement and psychological effects on a young child or adolescent. As mentioned above, ports are subcutaneous. Visually, there is simply a bump under the skin while Hickman and Broviac catheters are external and more apparent.[3]

Common Complications

Common complications that may occur include infection, malpositioning, excessive negative pressure, and clot formation. Many children with VADs are immunocompromised increasing their risk for infections with atypical pathogens (e.g., Pseudomonas in patients with neutropenia). Importantly, the close approximation of these devices to the skin increases the risk for infections with skin flora (e.g., *S. aureus* and *S. epidermidis*). Thus, antibiotic coverage for children with infections and VADs must take into consideration organisms associated with their underlying disease and skin flora. Clot formation[4] and resulting catheter obstruction are two of the most serious complications. Infection is a very serious complication as well. Stringent aseptic technique must be used when accessing catheters, and proper cleaning and maintenance are vital. Visual inspection of the catheter site is also important to ascertain early signs of a skin infection around the catheter site. Fever, chills, and malaise should always be taken seriously, and a workup to exclude catheter infection is appropriate.

For all indwelling vascular access devices, clotting can be a major complication.[5] Clotting should be suspected if an attempt to draw blood produces a dry tap or if infusing and flushing the catheter or port is difficult. Helpful maneuvers to obtain blood include raising the patient's arm above the head, Valsalva maneuvers, reverse Trendelenburg positioning, and gentle traction on the catheter. If occlusion is suspected, increasing the pressure to the syringe should not be attempted as catheter rupture may occur. Prior to using heparin or fibrinolytic agents to declot a catheter that is not working, a chest radiograph should be obtained to verify that the catheter tip is in the correct location and has not been dislodged or migrated. If the location of the catheter tip is still in question, a dye study can be helpful to localize it.

Once the catheter is known to be obstructed, declotting measures will need to be undertaken.[6] It is advisable to obtain an early consultation with the specialist who placed and cares for the catheter. Clotted catheters may need to be replaced, which is a major procedure for the patient. If no blood can be aspirated, 2 ml of 1:1000 heparin solution should be instilled into each lumen and allowed to dwell for 1 hour. If the line still remains obstructed, a fibrinolytic agent will need to be used. Tissue plasminogen activator is currently the agent of choice. For children less than 2 years of age, 2 mg/ml is infused into the line. For younger children, 0.03 to 0.1 mg/kg is infused.[7] The fibrinolytic agent should be allowed to dwell for 20 minutes to 1 hour before aspiration is attempted.[2,8] Usually the occlusion is dissolved at least partially. If this is not successful, an additional attempt may be made in 1 hour (see Chapter 130, Disorders of Coagulation).

REFERENCES

*1. King D, Conway E: Vascular access. Pediatr Ann 25:693–698, 1996.
*2. Gauderer M: Vascular access techniques and devices in the pediatric patient. Surg Clin North Am 72:1267–1283, 1992.
*3. Wesenberg F, Flaatten H, Janssen CW: Central venous catheter with subcutaneous injection port (Port-A-Cath): 8 years of clinical follow up with children. Pediatr Hematol Oncol 10:233–239, 1993.
4. Glaser MD, Medeiros D, Rollins N, et al: Catheter related thrombosis in children with cancer. J Pediatr 138:255–259, 2001.
5. Stokes DC, Rao BN, Mirro J, et al: Early detection and simplified management of obstructed Hickman and Broviac catheters. J Pediatric Surg 24:257–262, 1989.
6. Choi M, Massicotte MP, Marzinotto V, et al: The use of alteplase to restore patency of central venous lines in pediatric patients: a cohort study. J Pediatr 139:152–156, 2001.
7. Manco-Johnson M, Grabowski EF, Hellgreen M, et al: Recommendations for tPA thrombolysis in children. Thromb Haemost 88:157–158, 2002.
8. Miller R, Leno T: Advances in pediatric emergency department procedures. Emerg Med Clin North Am 3:639–653, 1991.

*Suggested readings.

Chapter 171

Lumbar Puncture

Kathleen Brown, MD and Deena Berkowitz MD, MPH

Indications and Contraindications

Lumbar puncture (LP) is most often performed in the emergency department as a diagnostic test. Cerebrospinal fluid (CSF) obtained from an LP can be used to diagnose central nervous system infections, including bacterial, viral, fungal, protozoan, and mycobacterial infections. CSF analysis also allows for immunologic confirmation of certain diseases (e.g., Guillain-Barré syndrome, multiple sclerosis, Lyme disease) as well as verification of subarachnoid hemorrhage and CSF malignancies. For children with pseudotumor cerebri, the opening pressure during LP is a valuable diagnostic tool and the withdrawal of spinal fluid is therapeutic. An LP is indicated when any of these diagnoses is in question.

Patients with hemodynamic or pulmonary instability should not undergo LP until they are stabilized. Other contraindications to performing LP include suspicion of increased intracranial pressure (ICP), local celluitis, and bleeding disorder.[1] Physical examination findings such as markedly decreased level of consciousness, focal neurologic findings, and papilledema have been noted in reported cases of cerebral herniation after LP.[2] Computed tomography (CT) scan is sometimes used to assess for the possibility of increased ICP in patients with suspected meningitis. While some patients with CT evidence of increased ICP have undergone LP without herniation, CT findings of increased ICP place patients at a dramatically increased risk for herniation if an LP is performed. Therefore, LP should be avoided when any signs of increased ICP are seen on CT. In contrast, a normal CT does not guarantee that herniation will not occur. While cerebral edema may cause slitlike lateral and third ventricles, generalized low attenuation of the white matter, and obliteration of the basilar and suprachiasmatic cisterns, there is considerable variation in ventricular and cisternal size, diminishing the accuracy of a single CT scan in the setting of increased ICP.[2-4] Most experts agree that infants and children with a normal mental status, no papilledema, a normal neurologic examination, normal pupils, and no history of intracranial mass or shunt can safely undergo LP without a CT scan.[5,6]

None of these relative contraindications should prevent the practitioner from administering antibiotic therapy if there is a strong suspicion of bacterial meningitis. The time period in which the CSF becomes sterilized varies by etiologic agent.[7] In cases in which LP must be deferred for a significant amount of time, antigen studies may be helpful in detecting the etiologic agent.

Preparation and Consent

Once the patient is deemed stable for LP, the procedure should be carefully explained to the patient or legal guardian. This includes the risks of infection and traumatic injuries and benefits of the procedure itself, and if necessary, the risks and benefits of sedative medication to facilitate the LP. The patient/guardian should be aware that a nurse or other hospital personnel will be assisting with the procedure. The family should be given the option of being present for the procedure.[8-10] Written informed consent should be documented in the chart prior to the start of the procedure.

An LP is a painful procedure, and thus all patients regardless of age should receive some form of analgesia. Lidocaine infiltration is commonly used in older patients and can be used in all age groups. The belief that local infiltration will "obscure landmarks" and make the procedure more difficult is not supported in studies.[11,12] Alternative or complementary methods of providing local anesthesia include topical mixtures such as a eutectic mixture of local anesthetics (EMLA).[13,14] Sucrose is effective in reducing pain in neonates and young infants undergoing painful procedures.[15]

LP may provoke anxiety in children. Both pharmacologic and nonpharmacologic methods of reducing anxiety should be considered. Allowing family members to be present may reduce anxiety in both the child and the family members.[8-10] Pharmacologic sedation may be necessary, especially in preschool and younger school-age children who are not able to understand the procedure and may struggle and make positioning more difficult. There are many reports in the literature of LPs in children facilitated by various pharmacologic agents.[16] Practitioners should use those agents that they are most familiar with and that are most appropriate for the individual patient (see Chapter 159, Procedural Sedation and Analgesia; and Chapter 172, Local and Regional Anesthesia).

Equipment

Gloves, mask, and gown should be used for the procedure. Prepackaged LP kits are available in infant, pediatric, or adult sizes. The kits include

  CSF manometers
  Spinal needles—22-gauge, 1.5-inch for infants; 22-gauge, 2.5-inch for toddlers through early school-age children; and 22-gauge, 3.5-inch for older children and adolescents
  Three-way stopcock
  Sterile drapes
  Chlorhexidine solution
  Sterile gauze pads
  3 to 4 specimen tubes
  1% lidocaine
  Syringe and injection needles

The needle used for puncturing the dura should contain a stylet. The use of a "butterfly" needle or any needle without a stylet is associated with an increased risk of the development of epidermoid tumors after lumbar puncture.[17,18]

Monitoring

Patients with increased work of breathing, concerns for apnea, the newly born, infants, and those on mechanical ventilation should be on a cardiorespiratory monitor during the procedure. An LP should not be performed on patients with hypotension or respiratory distress. For infants and toddlers who are often held firmly in the fetal position, the assistant restraining the patient should periodically check that the patient's airway is not being compromised. Consideration should be given to cardiorespiratory and oximeter monitoring for all patients being held in the fetal position.

Techniques

Lateral Decubitus Position

The gurney should be flat and the patient should be lying on his or her side (Fig. 171–1). The patient's body should be perfectly perpendicular to the bed. The patient should assume the fetal position. In young patients, the assistant should maximally flex the spine without compromising the airway. This is usually accomplished by using one hand to flex the neck and the other to hold the knees flexed into the abdomen. The desired sites for lumbar puncture are the interspaces between L3-4 or L4-5. To locate these spaces, the apex of the pelvic bone (the iliac crests) is identified. On an imaginary

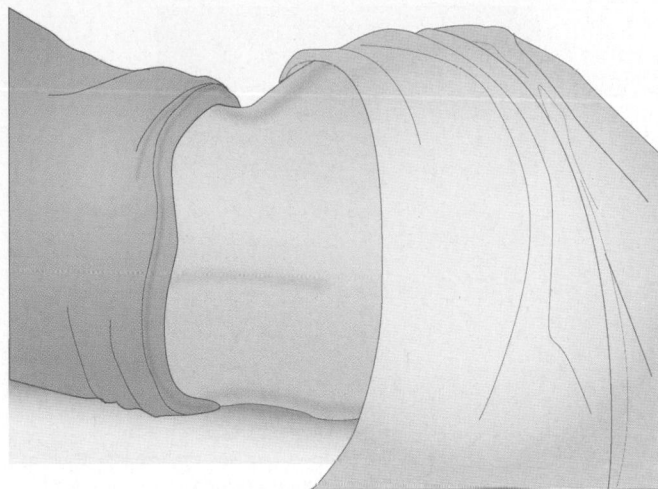

FIGURE 171–1. Lateral decubitus technique with patient lying on his or her side on the flat gurney.

line running from one iliac crest to the other, the interspace will be palpable in the center of this line.

Using sterile technique, the skin is cleaned with chlorhexidine and then the child is draped beneath the flank and around the entry site. The site is infiltrated with 1% lidocaine, being careful not to enter the spinal canal or blood vessel with the anesthetic. Once the entry area between the two spinous processes is located, the spinal needle's stylet is checked to see that it is secure. The spinal needle is introduced with the bevel facing up toward the ceiling. The needle is inserted slowly, aiming cephalad toward the umbilicus and making sure that the needle's trajectory is parallel to the spinous process. Needle entry into the subarachnoid space is often preceded by a pop. If this occurs and no fluid returns, the bevel should be rotated 90 degrees; if fluid still does not return, the needle should be withdrawn 2 to 3 mm. If still unsuccessful, landmarks should be examined with the needle in place to determine the optimal location for needle placement with subsequent attempts.[19-23]

To obtain opening pressures, the manometer is attached to the needle's hub once the CSF is flowing. The column of fluid is allowed to rise until it is stable and varies with respiration, at which point the pressure should be read. Some authors suggest that the reading should be taken in the lateral decubitus position with the legs extended and that flexion may falsely elevate the reading. However, there is little evidence to support this assertion.[24]

At least three sample tubes are filled with CSF, collecting 1 ml of fluid in each tube. The stylet is reinserted and the needle removed, applying pressure if needed. The iodine solution is cleaned off the puncture site and a Band-Aid applied. CSF samples should be isolated, labeled, and removed from the field before discarding the LP kit.

Sitting Position

The patient should be positioned in a seated position on the edge of the gurney with maximum spinal flexion. The patient's feet are placed on a chair so that the legs are bent, the hips are flexed, and the knees are together. This will serve to open the interspinous spaces. The assistant should flex the patient's neck with one hand while holding the arms between

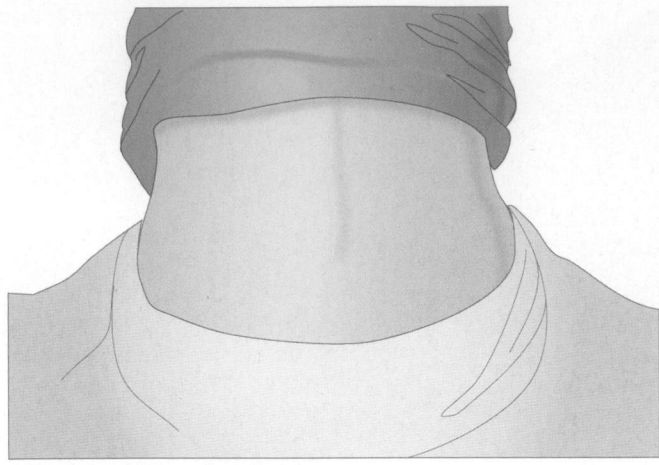

FIGURE 171–2. Sitting position.

the trunk to stabilize the patient. Older patients and those with respiratory disorders often find this position more comfortable (Fig. 171–2). The correct insertion site should be identified and the needle inserted just above either the L4 or L5 interspace. Opening pressures should not be measured from this position. Sedation may be required for a safe LP to be performed (see Chapter 159, Procedural Sedation and Analgesia).

Complications

Common complications of the procedure include a positional or "spinal headache," nonpositional headaches, local pain, and backache. Positional headaches occur in about one third of adults who undergo an LP. A recent prospective study of children ages 2 to 16 years who underwent diagnostic LP found a 40% incidence of backache, 27% incidence of any type of headache, and 9% incidence of positional headache. Frequency of complaints was higher in older children. Among children greater than 10 years old, complaints were more frequent in girls.[25] Using the smallest needle gauge possible and ensuring the appropriate bevel orientation should help reduce the rate of postprocedure "spinal headaches."

Less common complications include spinal cord bleeding, infection, apnea, and ecchymosis where the child was restrained too forcefully. Rare complications include cerebral herniation, transient ocular muscle palsy, subarachnoid or subdural hemorrhage, and acute neurologic deterioration.

Postprocedure Care and Disposition

First, the clinician should document the procedure and how it was tolerated by patient. The patient and caregiver should be reminded of the possibility of headache and backache. Post-LP headaches usually last 2 to 7 days. Pain is relieved by lying flat, drinking plenty of fluids, and taking acetaminophen or ibuprofen. If the symptoms are severe and are not relieved within a few days, an epidural blood patch may be necessary.[26]

Prophylactic bed rest is often prescribed in an attempt to prevent positional headaches after an LP. However, a recent study in children and adolescents who had undergone diagnostic LPs found that patients who were randomized to 24 hours of bed rest had a significantly higher incidence of headaches and backaches than those allowed free mobility.[27] Studies in adults also have not shown a benefit from prophylactic bed rest.[28]

REFERENCES

1. Faillace WJ, Warrier I, Canedy AL: Paraplegia after lumbar puncture in an infant with previously undiagnosed hemophilia. Clin Pediatr 28:136–138, 1989.
2. Rennick G, Shann F, de Campo J: Cerebral herniation during bacterial meningitis in children. BMJ 306:953–955, 1993.
*3. Hasbun R, Abrahams J, Jekel J, Quagliarello VJ: Computed tomography of the head before lumbar puncture in adults with suspected meningitis. N Engl J Med 345:1727–1733, 2001.
4. Shetty, AK, Deselle B C, Craver RD, Steele RW: Fatal cerebral herniation after lumbar puncture in a patient with a normal computed tomography scan. Pediatrics 103:1284–1287, 1999.
5. Oliver WJ, Shope TC, Kuhns LR: Fatal lumbar puncture: fact versus fiction—an approach to a clinical dilemma. Pediatrics 112:e174–e176, 2003.
*6. Riordan FAI, Cant AJ: When to do a lumbar puncture. Arch Dis Child 87:235–237, 2002.
*7. Kanegaye JT, Soliemanzadeh P, Bradley JS: Lumbar puncture in pediatric bacterial meningitis: defining the time interval for recovery of cerebrospinal fluid pathogens after parenteral antibiotic pretreatment. Pediatrics 108:1169–1174, 2001.
8. Tan M, Tan H, Buyukavci M, Karakelleoglu C: Parents' attitudes toward performance of lumbar puncture on their children. J Pediatr 144:400–402, 2004.
9. Eppich WJ, Arnold LD: Family member presence in the pediatric emergency department. Curr Opin Pediatr 15:294–298, 2003.
10. Haimi-Cohen Y, Amir J, Harel L, et al: Parental presence during lumbar puncture: anxiety and attitude toward the procedure. Clin Pediatr 35:2–4, 1996.
11. Pinheiro JMB, Furdon S, Ochoa LF: Role of local anesthesia during lumbar puncture in neonates. Pediatrics 91:379–382, 1993.
12. Carraccio C, Feinberg P, Hart LS, et al: Lidocaine for lumbar punctures: a help not a hinderance. Arch Pediatr Adolesc Med 150:1044–1046, 1996.
13. Kaur G, Gupta P, Kumar A: A randomized trial of eutectic mixture of local anesthetics during lumbar puncture in newborns. Arch Pediatr Adolesc Med 157:1065–1070, 2003.
14. Enad D, Salvador A, Brodsky NL, Hurt H: Safety and efficacy of eutectic mixture of local anesthetics (EMLA) for lumbar puncture in newborns. Pediatr Res 37:204A, 1995.
15. Stevens B, Yamada J, Ohlsson A: Sucrose for analgesia in newborn infants undergoing painful procedures. Cochrane Database Syst Rev (4):CD001069, 2004.
*16. Quinn M, Carraccio C, Sacchetti A: Pain, punctures and pediatricians. Pediatr Emerg Care 9:12–14, 1993.
17. McDonald JV, Klump TE: Epidermoid spinal cord tumors caused by lumbar puncture. Arch Neurol 43:936–939, 1986.
18. Batnitzky S, Keucher TR, Mealey J, et al: Iatrogenic intraspinal epidermoid tumors. JAMA 237:148–150, 1977.
*19. Baxter AL, Welch JC, Burke BL, Isaacman DJ: Pain position and stylet styles: infant lumbar puncture practices of pediatric emergency attending physicians. Pediatr Emerg Care 20:816–820, 2004.
20. Craig F, Stroobant J, Winrow A, Davies H: Depth of insertion of a lumbar puncture needle. Arch Dis Child 77:450–452, 1997.
21. Baonadio W, Smith D, Metrou M, Debwitz B: Estimating lumbar-puncture depth in children. N Engl J Med 319:952–953, 1988.
22. Hasan M, Howard R, Lloyd-Thomas A: Depth of epidural space in children. Anesthesia 49:1085–1087, 1994.
23. Shenkman Z, Rathaus V, Jedeikin R, et al: The distance from the skin to the subarachnoid space can be predicted in premature and former-premature infants. Can J Anaesth 51:160–162, 2004.
24. Abbrescia KL, Brabson TA, Dalsey WC, et al: The effect of lower-extremity position on cerebrospinal fluid pressures. Acad Emerg Med 8:8–12, 2001.

*Suggested readings.

25. Ebinger F, Kosel C, Pietz J, Rating D: Headache and backache after lumbar puncture in children and adolescents: A prospective study. Pediatrics 113:1588–1592, 2004.

26. Ylonen P, Kokki H: Management of postdural puncture headache with epidural blood patch in children. Paediatr Anaesth 12:526–529, 2002.

*27. Ebinger F, Kosel C, et al: Strict bed rest following lumbar puncture in children and adolescents is of no benefit. Neurology 62:6–8, 2004.

28. Thoennissen J, Herkner H, Lang W, et al: Does bed rest after cervical or lumbar puncture prevent headache? A systematic review and meta-analysis. CMAJ 165:1311–1316, 2001.

Chapter 172

Local and Regional Anesthesia

Kimberly R. Roth, MD and Christopher King, MD

TOPICAL ANESTHESIA
Indications and Contraindications

Topical anesthesia offers a noninvasive way of providing local anesthesia. This essentially painless method is particularly beneficial for pediatric patients, as the fear of "getting a needle" is eliminated.

Topical anesthetics can be used for relatively small wounds—and in certain circumstances, for intact skin—to provide anesthesia for simple procedures. In randomized clinical trials, topical anesthetics have been shown to be as efficacious as lidocaine infiltration for the repair of certain minor lacerations in children.[1-3] These agents also offer a few key advantages over infiltration anesthesia. First, eliminating pain with administration often improves cooperation and decreases the need for restraint and sedation in young children.[4] Furthermore, a more positive experience by the child with laceration repair can make subsequent suture removal easier to perform.[1] Another advantage is that topical agents do not distort wound edges and thereby may enhance tissue approximation and cosmetic outcome. Finally, the simplicity

of using topical agents makes it possible for nurses to administer the anesthesia for certain wounds, potentially reducing the length of stay for a patient in the emergency department.[5]

The main disadvantage to topical anesthetics is that they are slow in onset compared with infiltration anesthesia. For this reason, topical agents are contraindicated in situations in which anesthesia is needed quickly. Additionally, topical anesthetics are less effective when used for lacerations in areas of the body that have less subcutaneous vasculature, such as the extremities. However, even in these areas, prior application of topical anesthesia to a laceration has been shown to reduce the pain associated with subsequent infiltration anesthesia.[5]

Preparation and Consent

Before using topical anesthesia, it is important to know the patient's past medical history, current medications, allergies, and previous experience with anesthetic agents. In selecting a topical agent, the clinician must take these patient factors, as well as the nature of the procedure to be performed, into consideration so that complications are avoided.

Tetracaine, Adrenaline, and Cocaine

A solution of tetracaine 0.5%, adrenaline 1:2000, and cocaine 11.8% (TAC) can be used as a topical anesthetic agent for the repair of minor lacerations in children. Its utility was first demonstrated in 1980.[1] TAC was at one time the preferred topical anesthetic agent for most lacerations. However, misuse of TAC (e.g., on mucous membranes or extensively abraded skin) has caused serious complications, including prolonged seizures and death, primarily due to cocaine toxicity.[6,7] As a result, the popularity of TAC has waned significantly in recent years and it is no longer recommended.

Lidocaine, Epinephrine, and Tetracaine

A solution of lidocaine 4%, epinephrine 1:2000, and tetracaine 0.5% (LET) is as effective as TAC.[7,8] LET is also less expensive and safer, and avoids the controlled substance issues associated with TAC. LET is indicated for open wounds that do not involve mucous membranes, as excessive absorption of lidocaine, while not as dangerous as excessive cocaine absorption, may result in toxicity. Because it contains epinephrine, LET is contraindicated in areas with end arterial supply (penis, digits, pinna of ear). It is available both as a solution and in gel form. The two preparations are equally efficacious, but the gel is easier to apply and has less of a tendency to run off into mucosal surfaces or the eyes.[9]

EMLA Cream

A eutectic mixture of local anesthetics (EMLA 5% cream) was approved by the Food and Drug Administration in 1992. The active ingredients are lidocaine and prilocaine. EMLA is indicated for use on intact skin for simple procedures such as venipuncture, accessing MediPort catheters, and lumbar puncture. It provides a maximal depth of analgesia to needle insertion of 5 mm.[10] The main limitation to the use of EMLA in the emergency department is its slow onset. It is effective in 65% of individuals after application for 60 minutes, but it is more effective if left in place for 90 to 120 minutes.[10] While some studies suggest that EMLA may be safe and effective for open wounds, it is not currently approved for this indication.[11,12]

L.M.X.4

L.M.X.4, or 4% liposomal lidocaine (formerly called ELA-Max) is indicated for intact skin and requires a 30-minute application. No occlusive dressing is necessary to achieve full effect; however, an occlusive dressing may help the cream stay localized and prevent accidental ingestion or mucous membrane deposition in toddlers. Randomized trials comparing a 30-minute application of L.M.X.4 to a 60-minute application of EMLA found no difference between the two agents.[13,14] L.M.X.4 also has the advantage of producing a longer duration of analgesia, as the lipid carrier helps maintain a prolonged localization of the lidocaine.[15]

Equipment

Depending on the topical anesthetic to be used, the following equipment is needed:
- LET solution: cotton-tipped applicator, cotton ball, gauze, and adhesive tape
- LET gel: cotton-tipped applicator, gauze, and adhesive tape
- EMLA (5-g tube): occlusive dressing (Tegaderm or plastic wrap)
- L.M.X.4 (5-g tube): occlusive dressing if desired (Tegaderm or plastic wrap)

Techniques

Prior to the administration of the topical anesthetic, the neurovascular status of the involved area must be assessed. All necessary supplies should be readily available. Although the procedure is painless, the clinician should consider whether a child may require restraint by an assistant, papoose board, or both.

LET Solution

Whenever possible, any debris or clotted blood should be removed from the wound. The solution is first "painted" into the laceration using a cotton-tipped applicator. A ball of cotton that has been soaked with the solution is then placed over the wound and secured with gauze and adhesive tape for 20 to 30 minutes.

Table 172–1	Maximum Doses for EMLA	
Age	**Weight**	**Dose**
0–2 mo *or*	<5 kg	1 g over maximum of 10 cm²
3–11 mo *and*	>5 kg	2 g over maximum of 20 cm²
1–5 yr *and*	>10 kg	10 g over maximum of 100 cm²
6–11 yr *and*	>20 kg	20 g over maximum of 200 cm²

LET Gel

As with the solution, any debris or clotted blood should be removed from the wound when possible. The gel is applied using a cotton-tipped applicator or gloved finger. Gel should cover the wound and extend for a 1-cm perimeter around the wound. The area is then covered with gauze and adhesive tape for 20 to 30 minutes.

EMLA Cream

A layer is applied to the intact skin (¼-inch thick, or approximately 2.5 g—half of the standard 5-g tube—for children >12 months). The EMLA is then covered with an occlusive dressing and left in place for 60 to 90 minutes. Application time should not exceed 4 hours. Recommendations for maximum dose by age are as follows: 1 g for children birth to 2 months of age, 2 g for those 3 to 11 months, 10 g for those 1 to 5 years, and 20 g for those 6 years and older[16] (Table 172–1).

L.M.X.4

A ¼-inch thick layer, or approximately 2.5 g (half of the standard 5-g tube), is applied to the intact skin. An occlusive dressing is not necessary, but the area may be covered to prevent spread of the cream if desired. L.M.X.4 should be left in place for 30 minutes to achieve full effect.

Alternatives

The primary alternative to topical anesthesia is infiltration anesthesia. Infiltration anesthesia generally has an onset of less than 5 minutes, which represents a significant advantage in the emergency department. Investigators are currently searching for new ways to provide rapid topical anesthesia. Recent research in adult volunteers suggests that cutaneous analgesia with EMLA cream can be achieved in as little as 5 minutes after a brief pretreatment of the area with a low-energy ultrasound device.[17] Further study of this method is needed in pediatric patients.

Complications

Local anesthetics can produce toxicity when large amounts are systemically absorbed. Reports of systemic toxicity from topical anesthetic agents have involved mucous membrane application of large concentrations or accidental ingestion by toddlers. Thus the likelihood of causing systemic toxicity can be minimized by taking care not to apply any topical agents to mucous membranes and by not exceeding maximum recommended drug dosages.[7]

The most common complications of topical anesthetic agents are local skin reactions. The vast majority of reactions are mild and self-limited. Skin reactions to EMLA are common and virtually always benign. Reactions include transient blanching of the skin, pallor, and edema, which occur in approximately 50% of patients. Although not a frequent reaction, clinicians should be aware that a petechial or purpuric local eruption can occur following EMLA administration and should resolve without sequelae.[18]

Although rare, administration of EMLA may cause methemoglobinemia due to the prilocaine component. In prospective studies using a one-time age-appropriate dose of EMLA, increases in serum methemoglobin levels were small and of no clinical significance.[16,19,20] However, infants less than 3 months of age may be at greater risk due to decreased activity of methemoglobin reductase. For these patients, EMLA should be used with appropriate caution.[18] In addition, patients younger than 12 months of age who are taking other potential methemoglobin-inducing agents (e.g., sulfonamides, phenytoin) should not receive EMLA due to possible additive effects.[16] Glucose-6-phosphate dehydrogenase deficiency is a contraindication to EMLA use.

INFILTRATION ANESTHESIA
Indications and Contraindications

Infiltration anesthesia is a local injection of anesthetic directly into tissues. Indications for this procedure include incision and drainage of abscesses, repair of certain lacerations, and removal of soft tissue foreign bodies. For large wounds, especially when located in areas such as the plantar aspect of the foot, infiltration anesthesia may not be appropriate because the patient will experience excessive pain and/or the maximum dose of the anesthetic will be exceeded. Local infiltration may also distort wound edges and obscure important anatomic landmarks; therefore, it is relatively contraindicated for wounds in which tissue distortion would hinder optimal wound closure and cosmetic outcome (e.g., lacerations through the vermilion border).

Local anesthetic agents share a common basic structure consisting of an aromatic ring attached to an amine group by an intermediate chain. The intermediate chain is either an ester linkage (–COO–) or an amide linkage (–CONH–). Local anesthetics are classified into two groups based on this intermediate chain: "esters" (procaine, tetracaine) and "amides" (lidocaine, prilocaine, bupivacaine). Esters are very rapidly metabolized by pseudocholinesterase and therefore have less inherent toxicity. Amides undergo slower enzymatic degradation in the liver.

Large wounds requiring more than the recommended dose of anesthetic should be closed under general anesthesia or using a regional block with analgesia and sedation (Table 172–2). Moreover, allergy to one class of anesthetic (amide or ester) precludes use of other drugs in the same class. Lidocaine is the most commonly used local anesthetic. Reactions to this agent are usually due to the methyparaben (MPB) preservative, which is not present in dental injectors and cardiac forms of this drug. Patients with prior allergy to *para*-aminobenzoic acid (PABA) are at risk for allergy to anesthetics with MPB preservatives since they have similar chemical structures.

Preparation and Consent

Before administering infiltration anesthesia, it is important to know the patient's past medical history, current medications, allergies, and previous experience with anesthetic agents. The choice of an appropriate anesthetic should be based on these patient factors as well as the anticipated duration of the procedure. Table 172–3 is a summary of infiltration anesthetic agents commonly used in children.

Lidocaine is the most commonly used agent for infiltration anesthesia. It has a rapid onset and a duration of action that is suitable for most minor procedures performed in the emergency department. Lidocaine has also been shown to produce less pain on injection when compared to other local anesthetics.[21] When epinephrine is added to lidocaine, it facilitates hemostasis and limits vascular "washout" of the anesthetic from the injection site, thereby providing a longer duration of effect. Epinephrine also permits larger doses of anesthetic to be given safely, because the "release" of lidocaine into the blood occurs gradually as the vasoconstrictive effect of the epinephrine slowly wanes. It is acceptable to use lidocaine with epinephrine at all sites except those near end-arterial

Table 172–2	Maximum Dose of Local Anesthetics Without (and With) Epinephrine
Anesthetic	**Maximum Dose**
Bupivicaine (Marcaine, Sensorcaine)*†	2.5 mg/kg (3 mg/kg)
Lidocaine (Xylocaine)‡	5 mg/kg (7 mg/kg)
Mepivicaine (Carbocaine)	4 mg/kg (7 mg/kg)
Prilocaine	5.5 mg/kg (8.5 mg/kg)

*Due to cardiac toxicity, never use for intravenous regional anesthesia or hematoma block.
†Not recommended for use in children under 12 years old.
‡For intravenous regional anesthesia (Bier blocks), the maximum lidocaine dose is 3 mg/kg, with even less for mini-Bier block. Use preservative-free lidocaine without epinephrine for Bier or hematoma blocks.

Table 172–3	Local Anesthetic Agents Used for Infiltration Anesthesia			
Anesthetic Agent	**Class**	**Onset (min)**	**Relative Potency**	**Duration (min)**
Procaine	Ester	5–10	1	15–30
Chloroprocaine	Ester	2–5	1	15–30
Lidocaine	Amide	2–5	2	30–90
Prilocaine	Amide	2–5	2	30–90
Mepivacaine	Amide	2–5	2	45–90
Etidocaine	Amide	2–5	6	120–180
Bupivacaine	Amide	5–10	8	120–360

Table 172–4	Example of How to Calculate Appropriate Anesthetic Dose

Anesthetic solutions are typically labeled with drug concentration as a percentage. This example uses 1% lidocaine for laceration repair in a 10-kg child.

1% solution = 1 g drug/100 ml of solution
1 g drug/100 ml = 1000 mg/100 ml = 10 mg/ml

Remember: the maximum dose of lidocaine is 5 mg/kg. If the child weighs 10 kg, the maximum dose allowed would be 50 mg.
Remember: 1% lidocaine is 10 mg/ml. Therefore, 50 mg lidocaine = 5 ml lidocaine.
Maximum dose for this patient is 5 ml of 1% lidocaine.

distributions (i.e., digits, penis, ear pinna, tip of nose) and areas of decreased perfusion (i.e., narrow wound flaps, infected wounds). The maximum recommended dose of lidocaine without epinephrine is 5 mg/kg; the addition of epinephrine allows for a maximum dose of 7 mg/kg. Anesthetic solutions are manufactured with drug concentration expressed as percentages. Physicians and other health care providers should become familiar with how to use these percentages to calculate the appropriate weight-based anesthetic dose for a child (Table 172–4).

Bupivacaine is another commonly used agent in the emergency department. It has a longer duration of action and is useful when prolonged anesthesia is desired. This agent can significantly reduce the amount of pain experienced after wound repair for at least 6 hours.[22] The maximum recommended dose is 2.5 mg/kg. Bupivacaine is an inherent vasoconstrictor, and the addition of epinephrine confers no advantage.[23] The toxicity profile is among the worst of the amide anesthetics, and bupivacaine-induced toxicity can be highly resistant to standard resuscitative measures.

If a patient reports an allergy to local anesthetics, the circumstances of this should be carefully assessed. True allergic reactions to local anesthetics are rare. Most reported reactions reflect unintentional intravenous injection or the absorption of epinephrine, which may produce dizziness, headache, or agitation.[24] In fact, less than 1% of adverse reactions caused by local anesthetics are attributed to true allergies.[25] True hypersensitivity may manifest as urticaria, bronchospasm, anaphylaxis, and in extreme cases, cardiovascular collapse. Individuals are more likely to develop an allergy to agents in the ester group that form *para*-aminobenzoic acid (PABA) derivatives. Amide anesthetics, such as lidocaine, have a much lower risk of allergic reaction, although this complication has been reported.[25]

While testing for an anesthetic allergy is useful, it is not feasible to perform in the emergency department. Therefore, when the history of allergy is convincing, local anesthetics should be avoided. An alternative to lidocaine for local infiltration is diphenhydramine. Antihistamines are structurally similar to lidocaine; however, allergic cross-reactivity has not been reported.[26] A randomized trial comparing 1% lidocaine with 1% diphenhydramine for local injection prior to laceration repair showed no difference in anesthetic efficacy.[27] Diphenhydramine may also be used for large lacerations after the maximal lidocaine dose has been reached. However, diphenhydramine causes pain on injection, requires dilution, and can cause traumatic discoloration of the skin.

Equipment

Alcohol swab or antimicrobial solution
1% lidocaine (with or without epinephrine depending on the location)
5- or 10-ml syringe
27- or 30-gauge, 1.5-inch needle
Gauze
Sodium bicarbonate

Technique

There are two methods of infiltration anesthesia: direct infiltration and field block. Preparation is the same for both methods. A careful neurovascular examination of the area should be performed prior to administration of the anesthetic. An effort should be made to keep the needle and syringe from the child's view if possible. Young children may require manual restraint by an assistant, restraint using a papoose board, or both. Once the child is properly positioned, the skin around the wound should be cleansed with an antimicrobial solution or an alcohol swab.

Direct infiltration involves inserting the needle through the open wound to administer anesthetic along the length of the wound edges. This method is indicated for most minimally contaminated wounds. Injection into the wound is less painful than injecting through intact skin. The needle is inserted just beneath the dermis at the junction of the superficial fascia (subcutaneous tissue). In this tissue plane, there is less resistance and the anesthetic is quickly distributed to the sensory nerves. As the needle is advanced, a small amount of anesthetic should be injected, forming a wheal in the skin. Alternatively, the needle can be fully advanced on insertion and anesthetic slowly injected as the needle is withdrawn. The needle is then removed and the procedure is repeated at an adjacent site, entering the skin just at the margin of anesthesia provided by the previous injection. This is continued until all edges and corners of the wound are anesthetized. Aspiration is generally unnecessary with this technique since only a small amount of local anesthetic is injected at any given point while the needle is either advancing or withdrawing. Aspiration is recommended when injecting in areas of major blood vessels or when injecting deeper than the subcutaneous space. With this technique, full anesthetic effect of lidocaine is usually achieved within 2 to 5 minutes. The needle tip can be used to lightly touch the wound edges as a test for adequate anesthesia.

Field block (or parallel margin infiltration) requires creating an area of anesthesia that encircles the entire wound. This method is preferred in areas of gross contamination (e.g., incision and drainage of an infected wound or abscess) to prevent tracking of debris into the surrounding tissues. Preparation is the same as for direct infiltration up to the point of needle insertion. For this method, the needle is inserted through intact skin approximately 1 to 2 cm from the wound or abscess. For lacerations, the needle is directed parallel to the wound edge and fully advanced into the subcutaneous tissue plane. For all lesions, anesthetic is slowly injected as the needle is withdrawn, forming a small wheal in the skin. The needle is then reinserted at the end of the first wheal where the skin is anesthetized. This is repeated until the circumference around the lesion has been completely infiltrated.

Full anesthetic effect of lidocaine is usually achieved in 2 to 5 minutes.

Although intended to reduce the pain of simple procedures, the injection of a local anesthetic can be painful itself. Several techniques can help minimize the pain of injection. First, a slow rate of injection produces less tissue distention, which is the main reason for pain and burning on injection. The rate of injection can be effectively controlled by using a long, small-gauge needle (27- or 30-gauge, 1.5-inch needle). Buffering lidocaine with sodium bicarbonate also reduces the pain of injection with no increase in wound infection rates.[28,29] Anesthetics are not manufactured with buffering agents because it reduces their shelf life. Sodium bicarbonate can be added to lidocaine prior to infiltration using 1 ml of 1 mEq/ml sodium bicarbonate to 9 ml of lidocaine. Of note, sodium bicarbonate may precipitate bupivacaine and, therefore, is not generally used with this agent. Warming lidocaine has also been shown to significantly reduce pain with infiltration.[28] In the emergency department, this can be accomplished by placing the lidocaine in a fluid warmer. Finally, distraction techniques can be very effective in children undergoing minor procedures.[30] Distraction can be provided by the person performing the procedure, an assistant, or the parent. Many pediatric emergency departments have child life specialists on staff. These specialists are a very valuable resource in helping children overcome the anxiety of an emergency department procedure.

Alternatives

In general, infiltration anesthesia is safe, effective, and easy to perform. However, there are several adjuncts and alternatives to this method that may prove useful. Application of topical anesthetics should be considered for non–mucous membrane sites, if time permits. As mentioned previously, this has been shown to make a subsequent lidocaine injection less painful. Procedural sedation may also be a helpful adjunct in infants and young children undergoing lengthy procedures or repair of wounds that necessitate significant patient cooperation. Finally, nerve block anesthesia is an alternative when adequate local infiltration would require an excessive dose of lidocaine, inflict excessive pain, compromise blood flow (e.g., fingertip), or distort important anatomic landmarks.

Iontophoresis is a needle-free system in which a small electrical current draws ionized lidocaine through the skin and into the underlying soft tissues. Although further research is needed, small trials in children have shown that lidocaine iontophoresis can achieve dermal anesthesia in less than 15 minutes and reduce the discomfort associated with venipuncture and minor procedures.[31-33]

Complications

Minor complications of infiltration anesthesia include bleeding and infection. Bleeding is usually minor and easily controlled by direct pressure. The addition of epinephrine to lidocaine enhances local hemostasis. Lidocaine does have some antibacterial activity in vitro; the injection of anesthetic prior to obtaining wound cultures should be avoided if possible, as it may lead to false-negative culture results. Although local anesthetics may hinder growth of cultures, there is no evidence that they prevent wound infections. Conversely, clinical trials have shown that local anesthetics, epinephrine, and buffering agents do not increase the risk of wound infection.[29]

Systemic toxicity is the most serious potential complication of local anesthetics, occurring in approximately 0.1% to 0.4% of administrations. Systemic toxicity is determined by total dose and the rate of absorption into the blood. It is imperative that physicians and other health care providers be familiar with the weight-based dosage limits for infants and children. Furthermore, recommended dosages are based on appropriate deposition of the anesthetic within the subcutaneous tissue. Unintentional intravascular injection may produce toxic effects even at a dose below the maximum "safe dose."

Infants are at increased risk of systemic toxicity from local anesthetics compared with adults. Infants less than 6 months of age have decreased activity of the enzymes responsible for metabolism and degradation of local anesthetics.[24,34] Infants also have decreased concentrations of the serum proteins that bind local anesthetics, primarily α1-acid glycoprotein and albumin. With decreased protein binding, the free fraction may be elevated and contribute to systemic toxicity even when the total plasma concentration is within an acceptable range.[35] However, for local administration of infiltration anesthesia that does not result in inadvertent intravascular injection, this likely bears no clinical significance.

Although there is variation among individuals, signs of toxicity generally develop in an orderly progression from central nervous system (CNS) effects to cardiovascular involvement.[36] Early signs are numbness of the tongue and mouth, metallic taste, light-headedness, tinnitus, visual disturbance (e.g., nystagmus), and slurring of speech. This may progress to muscle twitching, confusion, unconsciousness, and seizures. Seizures are a warning sign of impending cardiac toxicity. Cardiac effects include ectopy, atrioventricular conduction disturbances, hypotension, dysrhythmias, and cardiac arrest.[24]

If a patient does not inform the physician of the early symptoms, seizure may be the first sign of toxicity. This is especially relevant to pediatric patients, as infants and young children are often developmentally unable to communicate symptoms of early toxicity. A child's agitation from early toxicity may be mistakenly interpreted as pain or anxiety during the procedure. Furthermore, if children are receiving adjunctive procedural sedation, the early signs of toxicity may be suppressed and therefore difficult or impossible to identify.

If early symptoms of toxicity develop, use of the local anesthetic agent should be discontinued and the patient should be monitored closely. Treatment of CNS toxicity is necessary only if the patient develops seizure activity. In the case of toxicity due to inadvertent intravenous administration, seizures are usually brief as the drug is redistributed from the CNS. In the case of toxicity due to an excessive dose, seizures may be prolonged or recurrent until the anesthetic is metabolized. Intravenous lorazepam is usually highly effective for terminating seizures caused by lidocaine toxicity. Prolonged seizures may actually exacerbate toxicity because of the resulting metabolic acidosis that often occurs. Acidosis causes local anesthetics to dissociate from serum binding proteins, resulting in additional unbound or free anesthetic being delivered to the brain and heart.[23,34,37]

Bupivacaine-induced cardiac toxicity can be highly resistant to standard resuscitative measures and carries a mortality rate as high as 50%.[37] Recent animal studies show that diazepam may prolong the half-life of bupivacaine and preferentially raise cardiac levels of the anesthetic. Consequently, some authors now recommend phenytoin for treatment of bupivacaine-induced seizures.[34,37] Phenytoin and fosphenytoin may also have a role in treating bupivacaine-induced dysrhythmias. The use of phenytoin (a class I$_B$ anti-dysrhythmic agent) to successfully terminate ventricular dysrhythmias in bupivacaine-toxic infants has been reported.[38,39]

In summary, significant morbidity and mortality from local anesthetics is quite rare. The vast majority of reports result from excessive dose of the anesthetic agent. Physicians and other health care providers should obtain an accurate weight on the patient, be familiar with dosage guidelines, and monitor patients closely for toxicity when nearing the maximum recommended dose of a local anesthetic.

NERVE BLOCK (REGIONAL) ANESTHESIA

Indications and Contraindications

Nerve blocks produce regional anesthesia by injection of a local anesthetic near a nerve or nerve group supplying a specific area. Among the indications for nerve block anesthesia are: (1) extensive wounds for which local infiltration would require multiple injections or would exceed the maximum recommended dose of anesthetic; (2) wounds for which local infiltration would distort wound edges; (3) areas in which local infiltration would be excessively painful (e.g., plantar surface of the foot[40]); and (4) areas in which local infiltration may compromise blood flow (e.g., fingertip). Nerve blocks are relatively contraindicated in patients with a known coagulation disorder due to the possible risk of arterial puncture and significant bleeding during the procedure. They also are relatively contraindicated in areas of the body with preexisting neurologic deficits because of the potential for causing further nerve damage during the procedure.[41]

Preparation and Consent

The clinician should review the area of distribution of a nerve to ensure that the block will provide adequate anesthesia at the site where the procedure will be performed (Table 172–5). Of note, successful anesthesia may require blocking two or more nerves depending on the area involved. Accurate needle placement obviously depends on a clear understanding of the location of surface landmarks in relation to the underlying neural anatomy.

Adequate sensory anesthesia will generally be provided by administration of 1% lidocaine for most procedures performed in the emergency department. Lidocaine with epinephrine is typically not used for nerve blocks due to the close proximity to arteries. In addition to systemic effects, intra-arterial injection of epinephrine may cause severe local vasospasm that could further compromise injured tissue. Epinephrine is contraindicated in areas with end-arteriolar supply, such as the digits. If significant postprocedure pain is anticipated, 0.25% bupivacaine may be used to provide a longer duration of anesthesia. The recommended maximum weight-based dose of anesthetic should not be exceeded.

Table 172–5	Nerve Blocks Commonly Performed in the Emergency Department
Type of Nerve Block	**Indicated for Procedures in the Following Locations**
Supraorbital and supratrochlear nerves	Forehead, anterior scalp
Infraorbital nerve	Upper lip, lateral-inferior portion of nose
Mental nerve	Lower lip
Digital nerves	Fingers or toes
Median nerve	Palmar aspect of lateral three and one-half fingers, radial half of palm
Ulnar nerve	Ulnar aspect of medial one and one-half fingers, ulnar half of palm and dorsum of hand
Radial nerve	Radial aspect of dorsum of hand, variable area of dorsum of lateral three fingers
Sural nerve	Posterolateral ankle and heel, plantar surface lateral foot and fifth toe
Posterior tibial nerve	Plantar surface medial foot, sole, and toes one through four

Modified from Roberts J, Hedges J: Clinical Procedures in Emergency Medicine, 4th ed. Philadelphia: Elsevier Saunders, 2004.

Equipment

Alcohol swab or antimicrobial solution
1% lidocaine (typically without epinephrine) or 0.25% bupivacaine
10-ml syringe
27- or 30-gauge needle for initial skin wheal
22- or 25-gauge needle for injecting deeper structures
Standard resuscitation equipment (in the emergency department)

Techniques

The details of each nerve block depend on the specific block to be performed (see Table 172–5). In general, pertinent bony landmarks and neural anatomy should be reviewed. Once the patient is properly positioned, the skin at the injection site should be cleansed with alcohol or an antimicrobial solution. Aseptic technique should be used throughout the procedure. While palpating the surface landmarks, the clinician should determine the likely course of the underlying nerve. A 27- or 30-gauge needle is inserted into the subcutaneous tissue and anesthetic is injected to form a superficial skin wheal. The needle is withdrawn and changed to a 22- or 25-gauge needle. This needle is then reinserted through the skin wheal in close proximity to the nerve. The plane of the needle bevel should be parallel to the long axis of the nerve when possible to minimize potential trauma to the nerve.[42] After the needle has been inserted to the appropriate depth, aspiration is performed by applying suction with the syringe. If no blood is aspirated, the anesthetic can be slowly injected. Any blanching of an extremity at this point suggests intra-arterial injection. If this occurs, no further anesthetic should be injected, the needle should be withdrawn slightly, and then anesthetic should be slowly injected again.

Paresthesias elicited with either insertion of the needle or injection of the anesthetic may indicate penetration of the needle tip into the nerve bundle. If this occurs, the needle should be repositioned (usually by withdrawing slightly) until paresthesias are no longer experienced by the patient. Whenever a nerve block is performed, the anesthetic should be administered slowly both to minimize the pain of injection and to allow the clinician to detect signs of systemic toxicity (i.e., due to inadvertent intravascular injection) before a large dose of anesthetic has been injected.

Unlike infiltration anesthesia, which is effective almost immediately, the onset of nerve block anesthesia is influenced by the proximity of the deposited anesthetic solution to the nerve for which the block is intended. In other words, diffusion of the anesthetic through the tissues plays an important role. Onset may be within a few minutes if the anesthetic is injected adjacent to the nerve. However, the full effect of a nerve block may take 15 to 30 minutes if the anesthetic is deposited more than a few millimeters from the nerve. Thus a nerve block that seems to have "failed" after several minutes may in fact prove to be highly effective once more time passes.

Alternatives

Alternatives include local infiltration anesthesia, intravenous regional anesthesia (Bier block), deep sedation (usually with ketamine) in the emergency department, and operative intervention under general anesthesia.

Complications

Specific complications will vary with the particular nerve block being performed. In general, complications are rare and usually result from poor technique. While there are no data regarding the complication rate for nerve blocks performed in the emergency department, studies from the anesthesiology literature report a complication rate less than 1% for distal nerve blocks.

Nerve blocks can fail when needle placement is inaccurate. This complication probably occurs most frequently with nerve blocks of the ankle because the landmarks used are relatively imprecise. Needle breakage may occur if a patient moves suddenly during injection. For this reason, a 22- or 25-gauge needle is recommended when injecting anesthetic. A hematoma may form if a vessel is unintentionally punctured. Local infection is another possible complication; therefore, the needle should be inserted through noninfected skin and aseptic technique should always be used.

Intraneuronal injection can damage the nerve, resulting in pain and/or various degrees of nerve dysfunction. The exact origin of the injury is not well understood. Three factors may contribute: direct trauma from the needle, microvascular injury resulting in nerve ischemia, or direct toxicity of the anesthetic agent.[43] The risk of nerve injury can be minimized by properly positioning the needle, avoiding excessive needle movement, and repositioning the needle if paresthesias occur. Concentrated anesthetics can produce a chemical irritation of the nerve. For this reason, 1% lidocaine or 0.25% bupivacaine are recommended for nerve blocks.

Systemic toxicity from the anesthetic agent can occur as a result of an excessive dosage or inadvertent intravascular injection. Nerve structures are often in close proximity to blood vessels, and thus particular care must be taken to avoid intravascular injection when performing nerve blocks. Aspiration of the syringe should be performed prior to injecting anesthetic every time the needle is repositioned.

Postprocedure Care

The anesthetized area is at risk of injury until sensation has returned to normal. Caution must be taken when applying heat, ice, or circumferential dressings because patients may not be able to sense impending problems while still anesthetized. For distal extremity blocks, patients should be informed that they may not have full control of the extremity until the anesthetic wears off. For this reason, patients who have had an ankle block performed should be advised not to drive until sensation is fully recovered.[42]

INTRAVENOUS REGIONAL ANESTHESIA

Intravenous regional anesthesia (Bier block) can be used in the emergency department to provide anesthesia of the distal arm for repair of wounds, reduction of fractures and dislocations, and débridement of burns. While a detailed description of this method is beyond the scope of this text, the basic concept involves exsanguination of the distal extremity using elevation and the application of a tourniquet, followed by administration of intravenous lidocaine distal to the tourniquet (Table 172–6). With proper technique, Bier block provides rapid, safe, and satisfactory anesthesia.

Table 172–6	Technique for Mini-Bier Block—Regional Anesthesia

Indication: fracture reduction below the elbow
Medication: 0.5% lidocaine without epinephrine, without preservatives
Technique:
- Apply cardiac monitor.
- Insert intravenous (IV) line in dorsum of ipsilateral hand ± contralateral arm for resuscitation.
- Place a double pneumatic or two single pneumatic tourniquets above elbow.
- Exsanguinate limb by elevation for few minutes or by elevation + wrapping arm with Esmarch rubber or Ace elastic bandage in distal-to-proximal fashion.
- With extremity elevated, inflate proximal cuff 50 mm Hg above systolic blood pressure (BP).
- Remove bandage and lower extremity back to horizontal.
- Tourniquet pressure must be maintained 50 mm Hg > systolic BP throughout.
- Infuse 1.5 mg/kg of lidocaine diluted to total of 10 ml into hand IV over 60–90 sec.
- Successful block may manifest as blanching skin with erythematous patches.
- As paresthesia/warmth spreads proximally, the lower/distal cuff is inflated to 50 mm Hg above systolic BP, followed by deflation of the proximal cuff. The tourniquet pressure is now exerted over an already anesthetized area. Anesthesia is usually complete by 10 min, with muscle relaxation. Tactile and proprioceptive sensation, with some motor function, may be retained.
- Infuse additional 0.5 mg/kg of 0.5% lidocaine if anesthesia is poor at 15 min.
- Do not exceed maximum dose of 100 mg IV.
- Once adequate anesthesia reached, remove IV and bandage site.
- Leave tourniquet in place at least 15–20 min and no more than 60–90 min after infusion. When procedure is finished, completely deflate the cuff in cycles for 5 sec, then reinflate for 2 min. Repeat inflation/deflation (5 sec/2 min) several times until capillary refill is normal. Observe patient for at least 1 hr before discharge.

REFERENCES

1. Pryor GJ, Kilpatrick WR, Opp DR, et al: Local anesthesia in minor lacerations: topical TAC vs. lidocaine infiltration. Ann Emerg Med 9:568–571, 1980.
2. Anderson AB, Colecchi C, Baronoski R, DeWitt TG: Local anesthesia in pediatric patients: topical TAC versus lidocaine. Ann Emerg Med 19:519–522, 1990.
3. Ernst AA, Marvez-Valls E, Nick TG, et al: Topical lidocaine adrenaline tetracaine (LAT gel) versus injectable buffered lidocaine for local anesthesia in laceration repair. West J Med 167:79–81, 1997.
4. Pierluisi GJ, Terndrup TE: Influence of topical anesthesia on the sedation of pediatric emergency department patients with lacerations. Pediatr Emerg Care 5:211–215, 1989.
5. Singer AJ, Stark MJ: Pretreatment of lacerations with lidocaine, epinephrine, and tetracaine at triage: a randomized double-blind trial. Acad Emerg Med 7:751–756, 2000.
6. Barnett P: Cocaine toxicity following dermal application of adrenaline-cocaine preparation. Pediatr Emerg Care 14:280–281, 1998.
7. Ernst AA, Marvez E, Nick TG, et al: Lidocaine adrenaline tetracaine gel versus tetracaine adrenaline cocaine gel for topical anesthesia in linear scalp and facial lacerations in children aged 5 to 17 years. Pediatrics 95:255–258, 1995.
8. Schilling CG, Bank DE, Borchert BA, et al: Tetracaine, epinephrine, and cocaine versus lidocaine, epinephrine, and tetracaine for anesthesia of lacerations in children. Ann Emerg Med 25:203–208, 1995.
9. Resch K, Schilling C, Borchert BD, et al: Topical anesthesia for pediatric lacerations: a randomized trial of lidocaine-epinephrine-tetracaine solution versus gel. Ann Emerg Med 32:693–697, 1998.
*10. Russell SC, Doyle E: A risk-benefit assessment of topical percutaneous local anaesthetics in children. Drug Safety 16:279–287, 1997.
11. Zempsky WT, Karasic RB: EMLA versus TAC for topical anesthesia of extremity wounds in children. Ann Emerg Med 30:163–166, 1997.
*12. Singer AJ, Stark MJ: LET versus EMLA for pretreating lacerations: a randomized trial. Acad Emerg Med 8:223–230, 2001.
*13. Kleiber C, Sorenson M, Whiteside K, et al: Topical anesthetics for intravenous insertion in children: a randomized equivalency study. Pediatrics 110:758–761, 2002.
14. Eichenfield LF, Funk A, Fallon-Friedlander S, et al: A clinical study to evaluate the efficacy of ELA-Max (4% liposomal lidocaine) as compared with eutectic mixture of local anesthetics cream for pain reduction of venipuncture in children. Pediatrics 109:1093–1099, 2002.
15. Chen BK, Cunningham BB: Topical anesthetics in children: agents and techniques that equally comfort patients, parents, and clinicians. Curr Opin Pediatr 13:324–330, 2001.
16. Lillieborg S, Otterborn I, Ahlen K: Topical anaesthesia in neonates, infants and children [Comment]. Br J Anaesth 92:450–451, 2004.
*17. Katz NP, Shapiro DE, Herrmann TE, et al: Rapid onset of cutaneous anesthesia with EMLA cream after pretreatment with a new ultrasound-emitting device. Anesth Analg 98:371–376, 2004.
18. Calobrisi, SD, Drolet BA, Esterly NB: Petechial eruption after the application of EMLA cream. Pediatrics 101:471–473, 1998.
19. Brisman M, Ljung BML, Otterbom I, et al: Methaemoglobin formation after the use of EMLA cream in term neonates. Acta Paediatr 87:1191–1194, 1998.
20. Frayling IM, Addison GM, Chattergee K, et al: Methaemoglobinaemia in children treated with prilocaine-lignocaine cream. BMJ 301:153–154, 1990.
21. Morris R, McKay W, Mushlin P: Comparison of pain associated with intradermal and subcutaneous infiltration with various local anaesthetic solutions. Anesth Analg 66:1180–1182, 1987.
22. Spivey WH, McNamara RM, MacKenzie RS, et al: A clinical comparison of lidocaine and bupivacaine. Ann Emerg Med 16:752–757, 1987.
23. Wilder RT: Local anesthetics for the pediatric patient. Pediatr Clin North Am 47:545–558, 2000.
24. Berde CB: Toxicity of local anesthetics in infants and children. J Pediatr 122(5 Pt 2):S14–S20, 1993.
25. Chiu C, Lin T, Hsia S, et al: Systemic anaphylaxis following local lidocaine administration during a dental procedure. Pediatr Emerg Care 20:178–180, 2004.
*26. Pollack CV Jr, Swindle GM: Use of diphenhydramine for local anesthesia in "caine"-sensitive patients. J Emerg Med 7:611–614, 1989.
27. Ernst AA, Anand P, Nick T, Wassmuth S: Lidocaine versus diphenhydramine for anesthesia in the repair of minor lacerations. J Trauma 34:354–357, 1993.
*28. Brogan GX, Giarrusso E, Hollander JE, et al: Comparison of plain, warmed, and buffered lidocaine for anesthesia of traumatic wounds. Ann Emerg Med 26:121–125, 1995.
*29. Brogan GX, Singer AJ, Valentine SM, et al: Comparison of wound infection rates using plain versus buffered lidocaine for anesthesia of traumatic wounds. Am J Emerg Med 15:25–28, 1997.
30. Lal MK, McClelland J, Phillips J, et al: Comparison of EMLA cream versus placebo in children receiving distraction therapy for venepuncture. Acta Paediatr 90:154–159, 2001.
31. Galinkin JL, Rose JB, Harris K, Watcha MF: Lidocaine iontophoresis versus eutectic mixture of local anesthetics (EMLA) for IV placement in children. Anesth Analg 94:1484–1488, 2002.
32. Rose JB, Galinkin JL, Jantzen EC, et al: A study of lidocaine iontophoresis for pediatric venipuncture. Anesth Analg 94:867–871, 2002.
*33. DeCou JM, Abrams RS, Hammond JH, et al: Iontophoresis: a needle-free, electrical system of local anesthesia delivery for pediatric surgical office procedures. J Pediatr Surg 34:946–949, 1999.
*34. Yaster M, Tobin JR, Fisher QA, Maxwell LG: Local anesthetics in the management of acute pain in children. J Pediatr 124:165–176, 1994.
*35. Gunter JB: Benefit and risks of local anesthetics in infants and children. Paediatr Drugs 4:649–672, 2002.
36. Scott DB: Toxic effects of local anaesthetic agents on the central nervous system. Br J Anaesth 58:732–735, 1986.
37. Yan AC, Newman RD: Bupivacaine-induced seizures and ventricular fibrillation in a 13-year-old girl undergoing wound debridement. Pediatr Emerg Care 14:354–355, 1998.
38. Maxwell LG, Martin LD, Yaster M: Bupivacaine-induced cardiac toxicity in neonates: successful treatment with intravenous phenytoin. Anesthesiology 80:682–686, 1994.
39. Reiz S, Nath S: Cardiotoxicity of local anaesthetic agents. Br J Anaesth 58:736–746, 1986.
40. Ferrera PC, Chandler R: Anesthesia in the emergency setting: Part I. Hand and foot injuries. Am Fam Physician 50:569–573, 1994.
*41. Murphy MF: Regional anesthesia in the emergency department. Emerg Med Clin North Am 6:783–810, 1988.
42. Locke RK, Locke SE: Nerve blocks of the foot. JACEP 5:698–701, 1976.
43. Selander D, Dhuner K, Lundborg G: Peripheral nerve injury due to injection needles used for regional anesthesia. Acta Anaesth Scand 21:182–188, 1977.

*Suggested readings.

Chapter 173

Digital Injuries and Infections

PART 1 ■ INJURIES

Gloria Cecelia C. Jacome, MD, Jennifer L. Waxler, DO, and
Patricia Sweeney-McMahon, RN, MS

Key Points

Subungual hematomas result from crush injuries or
blunt trauma to the distal phalanx and are manifested
by throbbing pain and dark red to black discoloration.
Greater than 30% blood collection between the nail
and the vascular nail bed warrants evacuation as
persistent pain is usually only relieved by this
maneuver.

Subungual hematomas greater than one-half the size of
the nail are associated with fractures of the distal
phalanx and have nail bed lacerations that may or may
not require repair.

Nail avulsion not appropriately treated can lead to
morbidity.

Onychocryptosis is commonly referred to as an
ingrown nail. An ingrown toenail occurs when the nail
plate impinges upon, and then pierces, the lateral nail
fold epithelium. It can be caused by improperly
performed nail trimming, repetitive trauma, and tight-
fitting shoes.

The fingernail rests on the nail bed, also termed the *matrix*.
The distal nail covers the sterile matrix; the proximal nail
arises from and covers the germinal matrix. The tissue adherent to the proximal dorsal nail is the eponychium (also
termed the *cuticle*), and the potential space between the nail
and the eponychium is the nail fold (Figs. 173–1 and 173–2).

SUBUNGUAL HEMATOMA

Indications and Contraindications

Nail regeneration following injury varies with age, climate,
and the involved digit. Relatively rapid growth occurs in the
adolescent and young adult, in warm weather, and in the
middle and index fingers.[1] To gain optimal nail regeneration,
early and precise repair of the disrupted bed and fold is
required.[1] Crush injuries to the fingertip result in compression of the nail bed between the nail and underlying bone,
often creating a straight, stellate, or tearing laceration.[2] The
blood usually remains fluid for 24 to 36 hours and is easily
expressed with slight pressure (Fig. 173–3).

Nearly 10–25% of these injuries are associated with a tuft
fracture. Simple lacerations in the middle or distal third of
the nail bed are the highest in frequency; distal tuft fractures
that accompany subungual hematomas are usually comminuted, but reduction is seldom necessary.[2,3]

Equipment

The most commonly used equipment includes
    Chlorhexadine
    Normal saline
    Anesthesia for digital block
    Oversized heated paper clip
    No. 11 scalpel blade
    Handheld electrocautery device
    Splint
    Sterile dressing

Techniques

Decompression of the hematoma is the goal of therapy; it can
be achieved with the following techniques. Care should be
taken, no matter which methodology, is used to make multiple holes or a single hole that is large enough to allow continued drainage.

Handheld Electrocautery Device

The cautery is a sterile, disposable, lightweight device generating temperatures up to 2200° F.[4,5] This permits rapid and
painless penetration of the nail plate without significant pressure.[4] Variations of the cautery involve different tips (fine,
loop, elongated) and different temperature ranges (700° F to
2250° F) for specialized needs. The unit comes prepackaged
in a sterile envelope for single use, and the power source is
contained in the unit (Fig. 173–4).

One can modify the electrocautery device to burn a larger
hole by "fattening" the end of the wire loop and rotating the
device slowly as the nail is penetrated, or by using it to remove

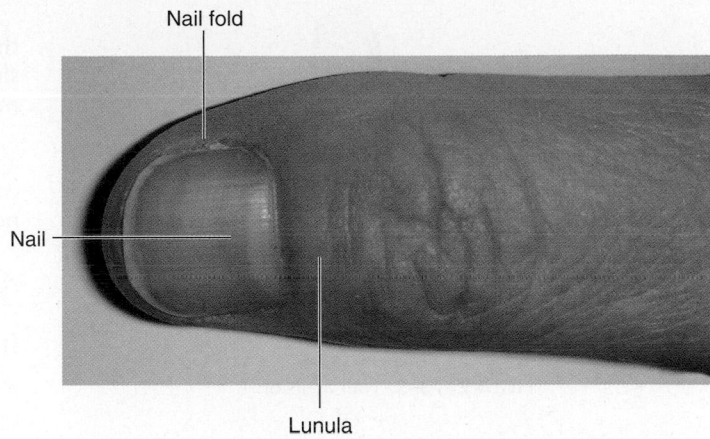

FIGURE 173–1. Anatomy of the fingernail.

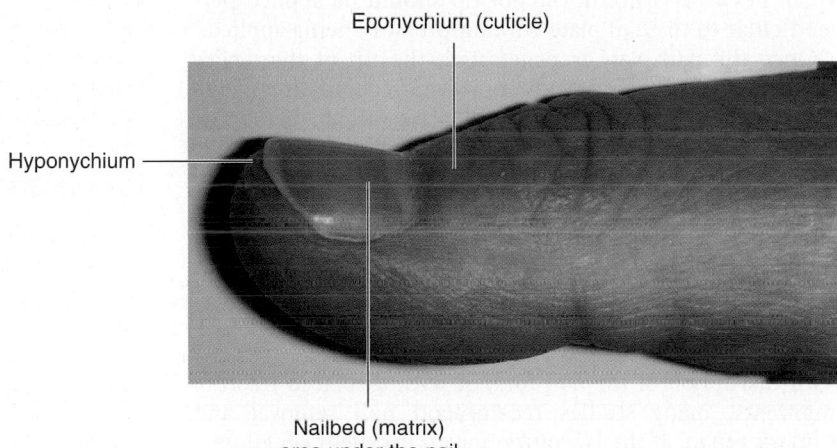

FIGURE 173–2. Anatomy of the nail bed.

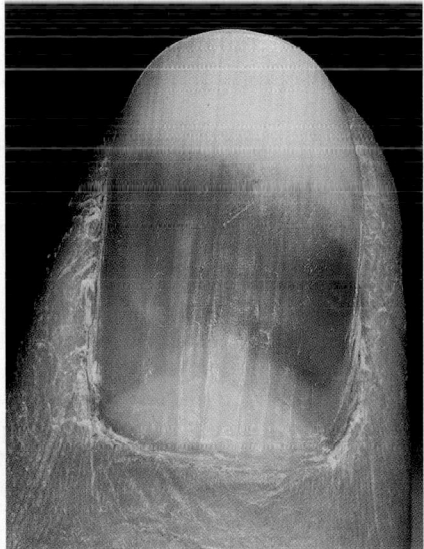

FIGURE 173–3. Subungual hematoma.

a small rectangle of nail. In addition to convenience, this device is desirable because the wire stays hotter longer, thus enhancing nail penetration.

Trephination of the Nail

Trephining the nail by drainage requires making an incision beneath the distal end of the nail. This can be accomplished

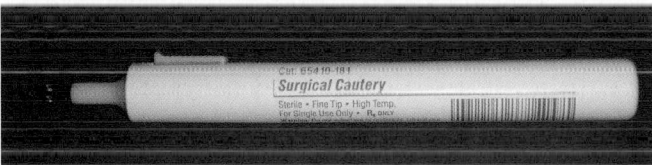

FIGURE 173–4. Surgical cautery.

with a no. 11 scalpel blade, a 19-gauge needle, or a fine-point hand drill. Because of the pain involved and the pressure required to produce the hole in the nail, a digital anesthetic block is often needed with this methodology.[4,6-8]

Heated Paper Clip Method

Heat penetration of the nail can occur with a heated, unfolded paper clip. Care must be taken not to sear the underlying tissue, which would plug the hole, thereby defeating the purpose of the treatment.[4,7]

Procedure

The same general procedure is used with each of the previously described techniques. Patients must wash their hands thoroughly with an antimicrobial agent from the affected area to the elbow prior to the procedure. The nail is prepped with chlorhexadine and allowed to dry completely. A site is selected for maximum evacuation of blood and wiped with an alcohol swab just prior to incision. No matter

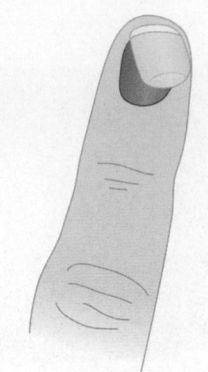

FIGURE 173–5. Nail avulsion.

which device is utilized, the hot tip should be applied perpendicular to the nail plate without pressure being applied.[5]

Once the nail plate is penetrated, the tip of the device should be withdrawn quickly to prevent coagulation of the hematoma or burning of the nail plate or nail bed.[5] The trapped blood will evacuate rapidly through the small hole, and light pressure to the nail should permit total evacuation of the hematoma. The wound should be dressed with absorbent gauze, and a splint should be applied only if there is an underlying fracture.

Alternatives

With disruption of the nail fold, or with displaced fracture fragments, many studies recommend nail removal and primary repair of the laceration for an excellent prognosis.[1] However, nail removal and nail bed exploration are not warranted or justified with subungual hematoma and an intact nail and nail margin.[2,4,9]

Complications

Subungual hematoma is associated with fractures of the distal phalanx in 10% to 25% of patients. Nail loss is possible but less likely when the evacuation of hematoma is undertaken within 24 hours of injury. If the nail is lost, there will be nail regeneration, possibly with an abnormal shape. While infection is uncommon, osteomyelitis of the tuft fracture is a theoretical complication. The value of routine antibiotic prophylaxis in such cases is unproven.[4]

If immediate drainage does not occur, pain may last for days and discoloration will last until the involved nail grows out in 3 to 6 months or is shed. There may be some residual horizontal white markings, called *leukonychia*, that have no structural or functional consequences.

Postprocedure Care and Disposition

Because of the potential for a secondary infection, the finger should be soaked three times a day using an antimicrobial soap, until the underlying space has closed. An Alumafoam splint or a bulky dressing can be applied to protect the fingertip for up to 3 days until the tenderness subsides. For those injuries associated with a fracture, 2 to 3 weeks of immobilization is recommended to allow the distal tuft to heal.

In cases of delayed presentation of a subungual hematoma, there may be damage to the nail bed and matrix. Parents should be warned of the possibility of onycholysis, nail deformity, and infection.

A distal phalangeal tuft fracture in combination with a subungual hematoma requires a nonurgent orthopedic consultation, but should not preclude evacuation, if necessary.

NAIL AVULSION

Indications and Contraindications

A traumatic injury to the distal portion of the nail may necessitate partial or complete removal of the nail. Avulsion of the nail at its base is usually caused by a forceful blow to the distal end of the nail. Because the proximal border lies free and is covered by an eponychial rim, the nail is torn away from the germinal matrix (Fig. 173–5). There may also be a tearing away from the underlying nongerminal matrix and/or a fracture of the distal phalanx.

Preparation and Consent

Before performing any procedure or treatment, a radiograph should be obtained to look for a fracture. A digital anesthetic block may be necessary for pain control and to facilitate the procedure.

Equipment

Anesthetic for digital block
Chlorhexadine
Clamp
Normal saline for irrigation
Absorbable suture material
Xeroform gauze dressing

Techniques

A digital block is performed (see Chapter 122, Local and Regional Anesthesia), and the injured and adjacent digits are cleaned with chlorhexidine solution and draped appropriately. A straight, closed clamp is inserted under the distal nail margin. When it reaches the area where the nail is free because of the avulsion, the jaws are spread. The nail can then be eased away without distraction of the wound or any fracture, and the hematoma irrigated. The nail bed can then be sutured (Fig. 173–6). Usually the sutures adequately stabilize any fracture. If the nail is removed after the injury, consideration should be given to placing a "splint" such as sterile petroleum gauze under the eponychium to prevent premature closing of this space, which would interfere with new nail growth.

Alternatives

As an alternative, the nail may be fixed with a fine Kirschner wire or 5-0 colored, monofilament nylon on a fine P-3 or PRE-2 needle.[1,7] The suture should be snug but not tight, and may be tied over Xeroform gauze to prevent adherence to the nail bed.[7] A small piece of Xeroform gauze may also be placed

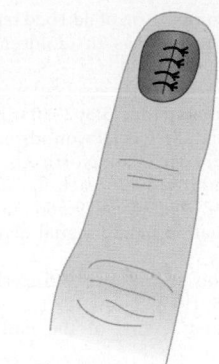

FIGURE 173–6. Nail bed repair.

between the nail bed and the eponychial fold to prevent adherence.

Complications

There is some evidence that leaving the nail in place may act as a splint, but this technique may delay healing and lead to a severe deformity and is therefore not recommended. The hematoma should be removed by gentle irrigation so that it does not act as a nidus for infection. A free-floating proximal nail may be a chronic irritant and may cause mechanical disruption of new nail growth.

Postprocedure Care and Disposition

Sutures are removed at about 1 week. Ten days after injury, the nail bed becomes hard and nontender, and no dressing is required. The new nail grows in over a 3- to 4-month period.

ONYCHOCRYPTOSIS

Indications and Contraindications

Treatment of onychocryptosis is primarily based upon the subjective discomfort of the patient and the history of acute versus chronic infection. The clinical presentation of onychocryptosis can be divided into three stages[10] (Fig. 173–7):

  Stage I: tenderness and swelling of the lateral nail fold that occurs when the nail impinges upon the structure
  Stage II: accumulation of granulation tissue, accompanied by sharp pain, erythema, and more swelling, as the nail pierces the lateral nail fold
  Stage III: ingrown toenail, in which epithelial tissue develops over the granulation tissue, making it difficult to lift the nail out above the lateral nail groove

The type of treatment chosen is based on clinical stage at presentation.

Equipment

  Chlorhexadine
  Peroxide
  Normal saline and sterile water
  Anesthetic for digital block
  Cotton-tipped applicators

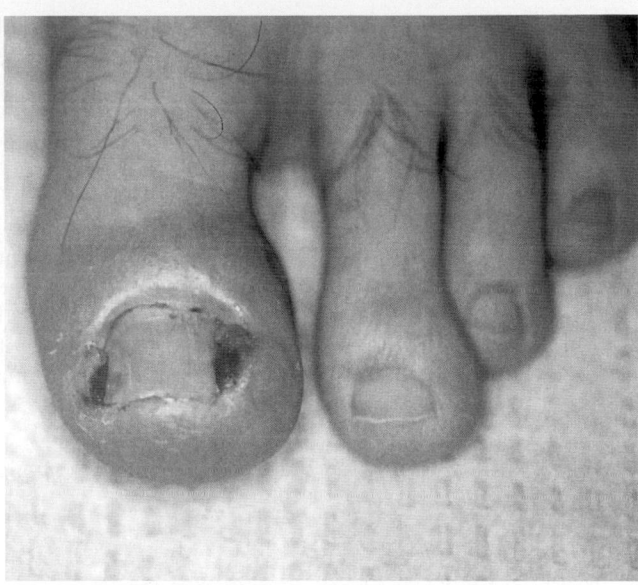

FIGURE 173–7. Onychocryptosis.

  Nail splitter
  Scalpel blade (no. 11 or 15)
  Small hemostat or clamp
  Phenol solution 88% or silver nitrate Q-tip cautery
  Antibiotic ointment
  Nonadherent dressing material, or dry dressing
  Postoperative shoe

Techniques

Conservative Treatment

A cotton wedge is used to lift the nail plate up out of the nail groove. This should be repeated daily by the patient. Frequent warm soaks in antibiotic solutions are helpful, with expected resolution within 1 to 2 weeks.

When the accumulation of granulation tissue prevents the nail plate from being lifted, cauterization with silver nitrate should be considered. Steroid treatment, either intralesionally or with topical rich-potency steroids over a period of 1 to 2 days, is an effective adjunct treatment.

Surgical Treatment

Surgical treatment involves removal of the nail spicule and débridement of hyperkeratosis. This procedure is primarily reserved for ingrown toenails with minimal inflammation and a small amount of incurvation.

Partial nail removal (88% phenol solution application) is indicated for ingrown toenails associated with chronic inflammation, severe pain, and infection (with the exception of paronychiae). The patient should be referred to a foot care specialist (e.g., podiatrist or orthopedic surgeon) for this procedure.

Complications

Complications include regrowth of the ingrown toenail, infection, and a postsurgical reaction to the remaining cuticle or nail. An inclusion cyst may also form around the nail remnants; curettage of the nail groove and posterior nail fold may be necessary. Total nail removal is indicated when there is extensive infection.

If infection has been present for more than 1 month, osteomyelitis should be considered and radiographs obtained.

Postprocedure Care and Disposition

A nonadherent dressing should be applied and the patient instructed to avoid tight, poorly fitting shoes. In addition, the patient should be instructed to trim the nails in a horizontal fashion. Systemic antibiotics are indicated only if significant cellulitis is present or if the patient is at high risk for infection.

REFERENCES

1. Melone CP Jr: Primary care of fingernail injuries. Emerg Med Clin North Am 3:255–261, 1985.
2. Roser SE, Gellman H: Comparison of nail bed repair versus nail trephination for subungual hematomas in children. J Hand Surg [Am] 24:1166–1170, 1999.
3. Simon RR: Subungual hematoma: association with occult laceration requiring repair. Am J Emerg Med 5:302–304, 1987.
4. Chudnofsky CR, Sebastian S: Special wounds: nail bed, plantar puncture, and cartilage. Emerg Med Clin North Am 10:801–822, 1992.
5. Palamarchuk HJ: An improved approach to evacuation of subungual hematoma. J Am Podiatr Med Assoc 79:566–568, 1989.
6. Wee GC: Painless evacuation of subungual hematoma. Surg Gynecol Obstet 131:531, 1970.
7. Newmeyer WL: Common injuries of the fingernail and nail bed. Am Fam Physician 16:93–95, 1977.
8. Goettmann S: Pigmented lesions of the nail apparatus. Rev Prat 50:2246–2250, 2000.
9. Kaya TI: Extra-fine insulin syringe needle: an excellent instrument for the evacuation of subungual hematoma. Dermatol Surg 29:1141–1143, 2003.
10. Aksakal AB: Minimizing postoperative drainage with 20% ferric chloride after chemical matricectomy with phenol. Dermatol Surg 27:158–160, 2001

PART 2 ■ INFECTIONS

Gloria Cecelia C. Jacome, MD, Jennifer L. Waxler, DO, and Patricia Sweeney-McMahon, RN, MS

Key Points

Paronychia, one of the most common infections of the hand, is a collection of pus in the potential space between the cuticle and proximal fingernail. Although usually limited to this area, it may occasionally spread to include tissue under the nail as well, forming a subungual abscess.

Paronychial infection develops when a disruption occurs between the seal of the proximal nail fold and the nail plate that allows a portal of entry for invading organisms.

A felon is an abscess of the distal pulp or pad of the fingertip, most often following a penetrating injury, that rapidly progresses from mild cellulitis to extensive necrosis and nerve degeneration. The most common pathogen is *Staphylococcus aureus,* although gram-negative organisms have also been described.

Pain caused by a felon is usually more intense than that caused by paronychia.

A felon will not extend proximal to the distal interphalangeal joint.

Herpetic whitlow is an infection of the distal phalanx caused by an invasion of the herpes simplex virus through broken skin, causing severe pain. When vesicular fluid is cloudy, herpetic whitlow may mimic a pyogenic bacterial infection. Surgical intervention is contraindicated as this may potentiate a secondary bacterial infection and delay healing.

Herpetic whitlow is commonly reported in adult women with genital herpes and children with coexistent herpetic gingivostomatitis. Health care workers exposed to oral secretions (e.g., dental hygienists, respiratory therapists) are at increased risk for developing herpetic whitlow.

Predisposing factors for onychomycosis include increasing age, immunosuppression, poor peripheral circulation, smoking, and tinea pedis. Spontaneous resolution is rare and is less likely as the nail plate become more extensively involved and thickened.

PARONYCHIA

Indications and Contraindications

Clinically, paronychia presents as either an acute or a chronic condition. Acute paronychia (AP) most commonly results from minor trauma with or without a foreign body present. Nail biting, thumb sucking, aggressive manicuring, and hangnails may allow entry of bacteria into the soft tissue of the nail fold.[1] Patients typically present with a red, swollen, painful area around the nail.

Chronic paronychia (CP) resembles AP clinically, but the cause is multifactorial with a different pathogenesis.[2] CP often is caused by *Candida albicans,* and may respond to treatment with a topical antifungal/steroid agent.[1-4] Chronic insults such as frequent exposure to wet conditions, or situations in which the person is not properly protected against predisposing factors such as chemicals or cleaners, destroy the normal epidermal barrier.

Antibiotics are not indicated if drainage is complete or if the surrounding area of cellulitis is minimal. If the infection has produced purulence beneath the dorsal roof of the nail, a portion of the nail must be removed to ensure complete drainage.

Equipment

The most commonly used equipment includes
Chlorhexadine
Normal saline
Anesthesia for digital block
No. 11 scalpel
Splint and sterile dressing

Techniques

The patient should wash the hand thoroughly with an antimicrobial agent from the affected area to the elbow prior to the procedure. The affected area is prepped with chlorhexadine and allowed to dry completely.

Drainage may be accomplished without anesthesia in selected patients but frequently requires a digital nerve block. Softening the eponychium by soaking is sometimes advised to facilitate separation from the nail. The nail is separated by placing the flat portion of a no. 11 scalpel on top of the nail with the point of the blade directed toward the center of the abscess. The blade is gently guided between the nail and the eponychial (cuticle) fold so that the tip of the blade reaches the center of the most raised portion of the abscess. Without further advancement, the scalpel should be rotated 90 degrees, with the sharp side toward the nail, gently lifting the eponychium from its attachment to the nail (Figs. 173–8 and 173–9). Pus should extrude from the abscess cavity. Because the skin is not cut, no bleeding should occur.[5,6]

After the pus is expressed, the abscess is irrigated and packed with a small piece of plain gauze. The finger is placed in a splint for protection. A wick of gauze can be placed beneath the eponychium for 48 hours to ensure continued drainage.

Optimal management of CP includes protective measures to avoid exposure to environmental causes and topical steroids to reduce the inflammatory reaction. Topical steroids are the best treatment of CP, producing improvement or cure in up to 88% of patients.[2]

Alternatives

Milder cases of AP may be treated with warm soaks for 15 minutes two to four times daily, with or without systemic antibiotics.[7] If infection persists, warm soaks in addition to an oral antistaphylococcal antibiotic and splint protection of the affected part are indicated.[5]

Complications

Direct incision and drainage of the cuticle is not recommended.[3] Complications include osteomyelitis of the distal phalanx and a chronic, indolent infection of the paronychium. Occasionally surgery may be indicated. Difficulty in avoiding or limiting exposure to predisposing environmental factors explains why clinical improvement is more frequent than clinical cure.[2] A primary squamous cell carcinoma of the nail fold may masquerade as a paronychia and should be considered in unusual, refractory cases. These cases need to be referred to a specialist.[1]

Postprocedure Care and Disposition

Most paronychiae will resolve in 5 to 10 days. One or two postprocedure visits should be scheduled to evaluate healing and reinforce home care. In 24 hours, the patient may be started on frequent soaks in warm tap water. The patient may easily remove the packing after the first soak, and cover the

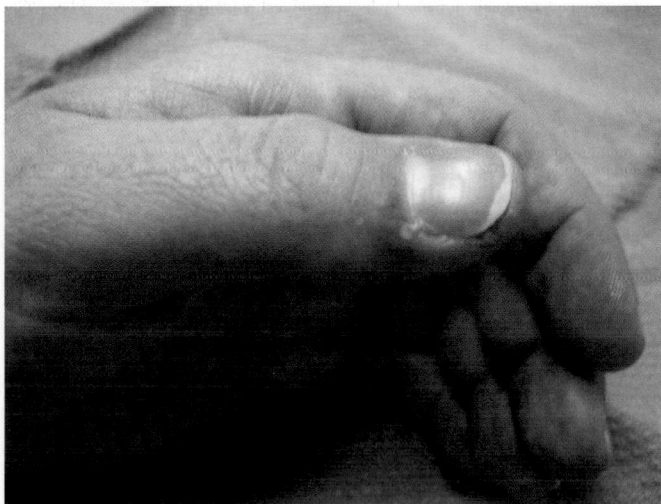

FIGURE 173–8. Paronychia.

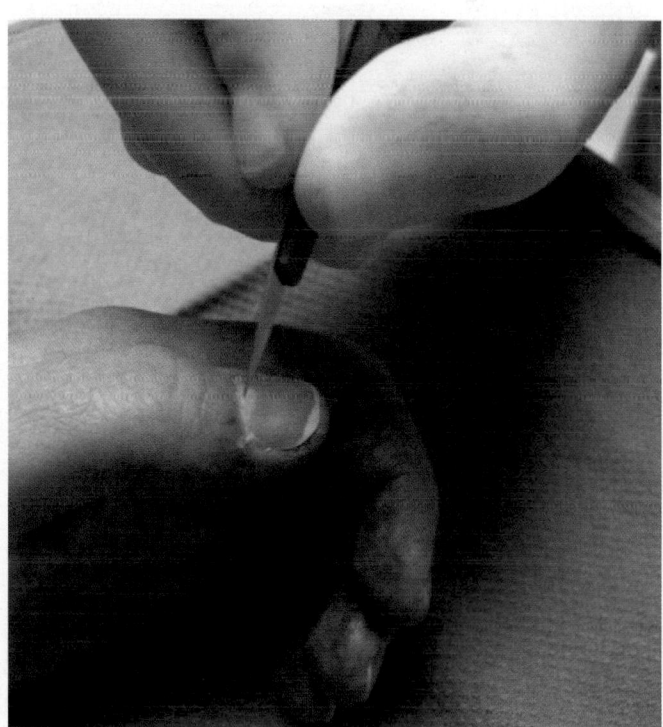

FIGURE 173–9. Paronychia drainage.

area with a dry, absorbent dressing. An antibiotic ointment or antifungal agent may be used on the site for a few days.

Counseling the patient to avoid predisposing factors is paramount in the aftercare instructions for chronic paronychiae. For chronic infections, after aerobic and anaerobic cultures are obtained, an antistaphylococcal penicillin or a first-generation cephalosporin should be given. Clindamycin or amoxicillin–clavulanate potassium may be considered if anaerobes and/or *Escherichia coli* are suspected organisms.

A tetanus booster should be administered when appropriate.

FELON

Indications and Contraindications

A felon occurs in stages. The initial stage consists of mild pain; fibrous septa limit swelling in the closed pulp space. The intermediate stage includes swelling and redness, which become clinically obvious. The entire pulp is very tender (Figs. 173–10 and 173–11). The late stage occurs with cessation of pain due to extensive necrosis and nerve degeneration.

The most commonly affected digits are the thumb and index finger. Common predisposing causes include wooden splinters, glass, abrasions, and other minor puncture wounds. A felon also may arise when an untreated paronychia spreads into the pad of the fingertip. Felons have been reported following multiple finger stick blood tests.

Fibrous septa extend from the volar skin of the fat pad to the periosteum of the phalanx. These subdivide and com-

partmentalize the pulp area, making a felon a closed-space infection. Occasionally, the high pressure in the fingertip pad will cause a felon to spontaneously drain, resulting in a visible sinus.

Preparation and Consent

Mechanism of injury should be determined. The patient should understand the complications of the specific surgical modality used for treatment. Appropriate anesthesia must be provided (see Chapter 172, Local and Regional Anesthesia).

Equipment

Equipment commonly used includes
   Bupivacaine
   1.25-cm Penrose drain
   No. 11 scalpel
   Finger tourniquet
   Hemostat
   Gauze pack
   Finger splint
   Tape
   Chlorhexadine
   Normal saline

Techniques

If diagnosed in the early stages of cellulitis, a felon may be amenable to treatment with elevation, oral antibiotics, and warm water or saline soaks.[3,8,9] Radiographs should be obtained to evaluate for osteomyelitis or a foreign body. Tetanus prophylaxis should be administered when necessary.

If fluctuance is present, incision and drainage are appropriate. The incision is performed under digital anesthesia with a long-acting agent (i.e., bupivacaine). Simple longitudinal incision in the midline accomplishes this most effectively and has the fewest complications.[3,8,9] A tourniquet may be applied to enhance visualization of the surgical field.

Of two commonly used techniques, the volar longitudinal incision and the high lateral incision, the former is preferred. An incision is made 3 to 5 mm from the distal interphalan-

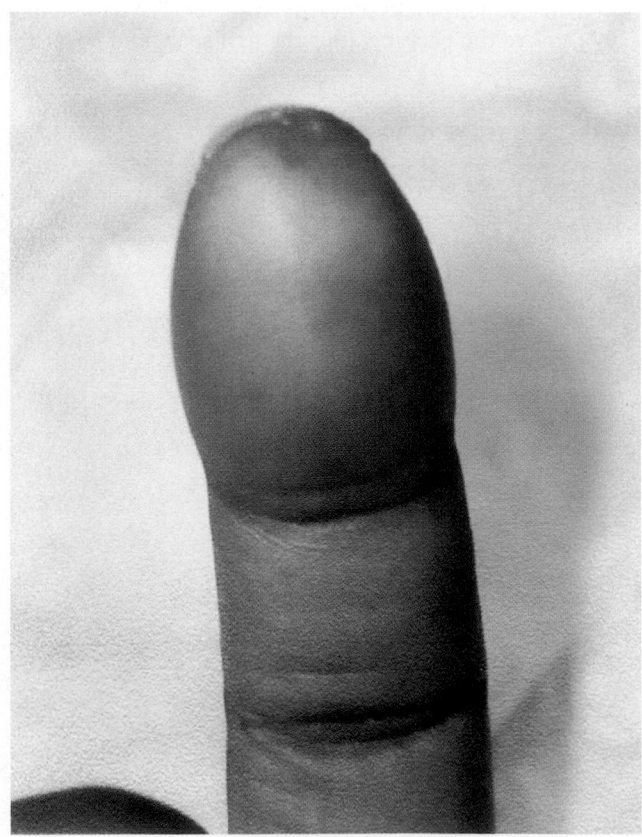

FIGURE 173–10. Felon (palmar view).

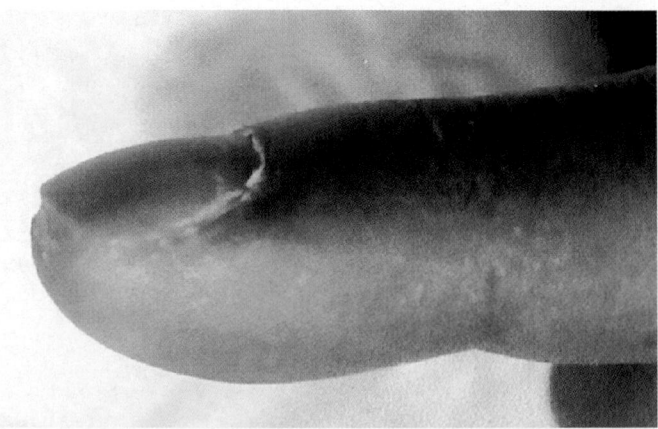

FIGURE 173–11. Felon (lateral view).

geal (DIP) joint flexor crease and extend to the end of the distal phalanx. The depth of the incision is to the dermis. The subcutaneous tissues are gently dissected and explored with a small hemostat. Necrotic skin edges are excised, and the abscess is decompressed and irrigated.

A high lateral incision is made on the nonoppositional side of the appropriate digit (ulnar side of the index, middle, and ring fingers, and radial aspect of the thumb and fifth digit) starting 5 mm distal to the flexor DIP crease and continuing parallel to the lateral border of the nail plate, maintaining approximately 5 mm between the incision and the nail plate border. This distance should allow for avoiding the more volar neurovascular structures. The incision is extended to just distal to the unattached portion of the nail plate. The subcutaneous tissue is sharply dissected just volar to the cortex of the distal phalanx. The wound is explored by disecting bluntly and decompressing and irrigating any absess. This procedure allows complete visualization and débridement of necrotic tissue. However, it will require a long time to heal and can produce a sizable scar and an unstable finger pulp.

With both techniques, the wound is packed with sterile gauze. The gauze should be removed in approximately 24 to 48 hours, and the wound allowed to close by secondary intention. Gram staining should guide initial antibiotic therapy. The most commonly isolated organism is *Staphylococcus aureus*. An empirical antibiotic (first-generation cephalosporin or antistaphylococcal penicillin) should be prescribed for an uncomplicated felon for 5 to 14 days, depending on the clinical response and severity of infection.[8] Methicillin-resistant *S. aureus* has been reported in felons, and therefore the clinical response, as well as bacterial cultures, should be followed closely.[9] A snug dressing and splint should be applied. Discharge instructions and medications should include elevation, opioid analgesics, and a follow-up appointment in 2 to 3 days.

Alternatives

Incision techniques not recommended include the "fish-mouth" incision, the "hockey stick" (or "J") incision, and the transverse palmar incision.[3,8] Fish-mouth incisions may destroy the blood supply to the fingertip.[9] Longitudinal midline incisions on the volar surface may leave scars over an important area for sensation but do not have the other disadvantages of lateral incisions. Any incision that is made too deeply and proximally can injure the flexor tendon sheath and initiate a tenosynovitis.

Complications

Potential complications of a felon and felon drainage include an anesthetic fingertip, a neuroma, and an unstable finger pad. Because the septa attach to the periosteum of the distal phalanx, spread of infection to the underlying bone can result in osteomyelitis.[8]

If untreated, the expanding abscess can extend toward the phalanx, producing an osteitis or osteomyelitis, or toward the skin, causing necrosis and a sinus tract on the palmar surface of the digital pulp. Other complications include soft tissue and bony-tuft necrosis, septic arthritis of the DIP joint, and flexor tenosynovitis.

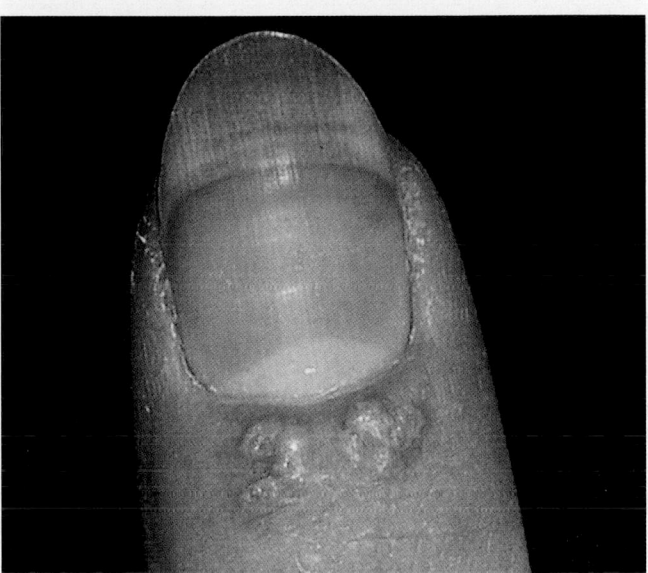

FIGURE 173–12. Herpetic whitlow.

Postprocedure Care and Disposition

Postprocedure care includes antibiotics, loose packing, splinting, and elevation of the hand for approximately 24 hours. Dry dressing changes with twice-daily saline soaks, range-of-motion activities, and, eventually, scar massage may accelerate return to normal activity.[8]

HERPETIC WHITLOW

Indications and Contraindications

This condition is characterized by the presence of erythema, swelling, pain, and the presence of vesicular or pustular lesions (Fig. 173–12). Patients may also experience fever, lymphadenitis, and epitrochlear or axillary lymphadenopathy. Usually there is a slow response to treatment and a tendency for recurrence. Herpetic whitlow is a self-limited condition that resolves in 2 to 3 weeks.[10]

Preparation

A thorough history, including a history of localized trauma to the nail cuticle as well as occupational history, may be helpful in distinguishing herpetic whitlow from paronychia.

Equipment

Equipment commonly used to treating herpetic whitlow includes culture swab and dry dressing material.

Techniques

A Tzanck smear that demonstrates multinucleated giant cells in a scraping taken from the base of an unroofed vesicle, or a positive herpes culture, will confirm the diagnosis. Because viral shedding continues until the epidermal lesion is healed, contact with the lesion should be avoided by keeping the affected digit covered with a dry dressing.[3]

Treatment within the first 48 hours of symptom onset with acyclovir, famciclovir, or valacyclovir may lessen the severity of infection, but randomized controlled trials have not been performed.[3] Treatment with antivirals may be beneficial for recurrent herpetic whitlow if initiated during the prodromal stage.[3]

Alternatives

Oral acyclovir has a role in the treatment of immunocompromised patients and patients with recurrent infections, but its role in healthy patients is less clear. Topical acyclovir has not been shown to be effective in either the treatment or prophylaxis of this disorder. Serologic tests are not helpful.

Complications

Surgical intervention such as incision and drainage of the herpetic lesion is contraindicated as this may potentiate a secondary bacterial infection and delay healing.

Postprocedure Care and Disposition

Strict infection-control precautions should be followed. Health care workers should refrain from patient contact until all lesions have crusted over and viral shedding has stopped. Patients should be advised that the infection recurs in 30% to 50% of cases, but the initial infection is typically the most severe.

ONYCHOMYCOSIS

Indications and Contraindications

Onychomycosis is most frequently caused by members of the *Trichophyton* species: *Trichophyton rubrum* and *Trichophytum mentagrophytes*.[11] Four types of onychomycosis, characterized according to clinical presentation and the route of invasion, are recognized (Fig. 173–13).[12,13]

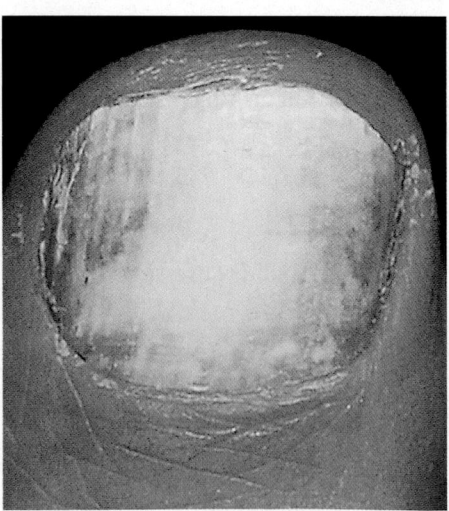

FIGURE 173–13. Onychomycosis.

- Distal subungual onychomycosis (DSO): the most common form; characterized by the invasion of the nail bed and underside of the nail plate beginning at the eponychium
- Proximal subungual onychomycosis (PSO): uncommon subtype; organisms invade the nail unit via the proximal nail fold through the cuticle area, penetrate the newly formed nail plate, and migrate distally
- White subungual onychomycosis (WSO): less common than DSO; occurs when certain fungi invade the superficial layers of the nail plate directly
- *Candida* onychomycosis: occurs in patients with chronic mucocutaneous candidiasis; caused invasion of the entire nail plate by *C. albicans*

Onychomycosis can also be caused by trauma, which is more frequently seen in the hallux and fifth toenails, where the greatest shoe friction occurs. However, in younger children (less than 7 years of age), there maybe a higher prevalence in the fingernails.[14]

Preparation and Consent

The clinical appearance of the nail (subungual hyperkeratosis, yellowish brown discoloration, onycholysis) and the patient's history (older age, hyperhidrosis, onychogryposis, poor peripheral circulation, immunosuppression, nail trauma) will help differentiate fungal from nonfungal etiologies of nail dystrophies.

Mycologic confirmation of the diagnosis should be performed before starting treatment to avoid unnecessary exposure to systemic antifungals.

Equipment

Common equipment used to treat onychomycosis includes KOH preparation, culture swab, nail clipper, and dry dressing material.

Techniques

Direct microscopy of the sampled material serves as a screening test for the presence or absence of fungi and can provide clues about the identity of the microorganism. However, careful matching of the microscopic and culture results is necessary for accurate diagnosis and appropriate therapy. Histologic examination of nail clippings stained with periodic acid–Schiff provides a permanent record of the specimen.

For fungal infections limited to the distal nail, simple surface nail plate filling with topical anti-tinea therapy is often effective (e.g., ciclopirox, terbinafine, bifonazole, and amorolfine creams). With more extensive involvement, oral antifungal medications are indicated (e.g., fluconazole, itraconazole, and terbinafine). When the nail matrix is involved, the hypertrophy becomes fixed and the condition is usually irreversible.

Alternatives

Although nail surgery is useful in some cases, it is painful and disfiguring, and should be limited to one or only a few nails if used at all.[13] Surgical approaches to treatment of chronic onychomycosis include nail plate avulsion with nail bed débridement and periodic limited débridement of the involved nail using a Dremel tool.

Complications

Recurrent inflammation and secondary bacterial infection are the most common complications. There is a 20% treatment failure rate caused by inaccurate diagnosis, misidentification of the pathogens, or the presence of a second disorder such as psoriasis, as well as characteristics of the nail (slow growth and excessive thickness), presence of a high fungal inoculum, drug-resistant microorganisms, and the presence of diabetes, poor circulation, or immunodeficiency disorder.[15]

Postprocedure Care and Disposition

In addition to specific drug therapies, patients may benefit from several hygiene measures that may prevent relapses. Patient should wear thong sandals in public showers and slippers in hotel rooms and should rest their shoes periodically to limit exposure to infectious fungi. Antifungal powders should be used once a week to help keep shoes free from pathogens. Certain individuals seem to have a genetic predisposition to fungal infections, and may experience relapses despite careful care and effective therapy.

REFERENCES

1. Hochman L: Paronychia: more than just an abscess. Int J Dermatol 34:385–386, 1995.
2. Tosti A, Piraccini BM, Ghetti E, Colombo MD: Topical steroids versus systemic antifungals in the treatment of chronic paronychia: an open, randomized double blind and double dummy study. J Am Acad Dermatol 47:73, 2002.
3. Clark DC: Common acute hand infections. Am Fam Physician 68:2167–2176, 2003.
4. Loo DS: Cutaneous fungal infections in the elderly. Dermatol Clin North Am 22:33–50, 2004.
5. Rockwell PG: Acute and chronic paronychiae. Am Fam Physician 63:1113, 2001.
6. Roberts J, Hedges J: Clinical Procedures in Emergency Medicine, 4th ed. Philadelphia: Elsevier Saunders, 2004, pp 739–744.
7. Mayeaux EJ Jr: Nail disorders. Primary Care 27:333–351, 2000.
8. Bhumbra NA, McCullough SG: Skin and subcutaneous infections. Prim Care 30:1–24, 2003.
9. Kilgore ES, Brown LG, Newmeyer WL, et al: Treatment of felons. Am J Surg 130:194–198, 1975.
10. Walker LG, Simmons BP, Lovallo JL: Pediatric herpetic hand infections. J Hand Surg (Am) 15:176, 1990.
11. Ghannoum MA, Hajjeh RA, Scher R, et al: A large-scale North American study of fungal isolates from nails: the frequency of onychomycosis, fungal distribution, and antifungal susceptibility patterns. J Am Acad Dermatol 43:641–648, 2000.
12. Faergemann J, Baran R: Epidemiology, clinical presentation and diagnosis of onychomycosis. Br J Dermatol 149:1–4, 2003.
13. Elewski BE: Onychomycosis: pathogenesis, diagnosis, and management. Clin Microbiol Rev 11:415–429, 1998.
14. Gupta AK, Skinner AR: Onychomycosis in children: a brief overview with treatment strategies. Pediatr Dermatol 21:74–79, 2004.
15. Minisini AM: Taxane-induced nail changes: incidence, clinical preservation and outcome. Ann Oncol 14:333–337, 2003.

Chapter 174

Epistaxis Control

Kenneth B. Briskin, MD

Key Points

The overall assessment of the patient is the first priority in patients with epistaxis.

Adequate lighting and universal precautions are essential for effective treatment.

Posterior packing is associated with significant morbidity and discomfort. These patients should be admitted.

Beware of blood streaming down the posterior pharynx following anterior packing, indicating inadequate packing or a posterior source of epistaxis.

Indications and Contraindications

Epistaxis occurs at all ages, but in children it is most common between the ages of 2 and 10 years. It can cause significant anxiety in both patients and parents. Typically most parents have tried first aid measures prior to presenting to the emergency department. The specific procedure to control epistaxis will depend on the history. The approach to nosebleeds should be in an orderly, stepwise fashion. There are no specific contraindications to the procedures for epistaxis control, but most cases can be treated with simple measures, avoiding unnecessary discomfort for the patient[1] (see Chapter 49, Epistaxis).

Preparation and Consent

The patient who presents with epistaxis needs to be approached in a logical and consistent fashion (Fig. 174–1). The initial evaluation should include the history of bleeding, especially the duration and laterality. Factors in identifying the etiology of epistaxis include frequency of epistaxis, other abnormal bleeding, bruising, recent infection, history of trauma, surgery, and exposure to chemicals.[2,3] Patients may have a history of hypertension or antiplatelet medications (e.g., aspirin or nonsteroidal anti-inflammatory drugs). The patient's overall condition and vital signs should be evaluated and treated initially.

The pertinent anatomy needs to be understood in order to appropriately treat epistaxis. The most common site of epistaxis is from Kiesselbach's plexus on the anterior nasal septum. The septum is fed from both the internal and external carotid systems. The sphenopalatine artery, facial artery, and anterior and posterior ethmoid arteries all contribute to the nasal blood supply and can be the source of epistaxis.[4]

The frequency of bleeding, which nostril is involved, history of trauma, past medical history, current medications, and family history are important initial points to plan treatment.[5,6] An examination of the nose with good lighting should be performed, if possible. Blood should be drawn and sent for hemoglobin, platelets, coagulations studies, and possible type and cross, if severe bleeding is present or if a bleeding disorder is suspected[2] (see Chapter 49, Epistaxis; Chapter 129, Acute Childhood Immune Thrombocytopenic Purpura and Related Platelet Disorders; and Chapter 130, Disorders of Coagulation). Premedication with a topical vasoconstrictor, such as oxymetazoline (Afrin) or neosynephrine mixed with 4% topical lidocaine, will help with anesthesia and initial bleeding control.

Consent should be obtained, outlining the plan for treatment. The patient and parents need to understand the rationale involved with each stage of treatment. It should be made clear that further surgical procedures may be necessary if initial maneuvers to control the bleeding fail. The risks of the procedure, as outlined later, need to be clearly conveyed.

Equipment

The equipment for control of nosebleeds should be kept together in an epistaxis tray at all times (Table 174–1). Keeping this tray complete obviates the need to spend time looking for separate pieces of equipment in the emergency department and other parts of the hospital. This can expedite the control of the bleed and ease the anxiety of the patient, family, nurse, and physician. A good, working headlight is invaluable to help in identification of the bleeding site. A strong suction with a Frazier tip is necessary to keep the field clear. Universal precautions must be observed by all personnel using protective face shields, gowns, and gloves. Rarely, if bleeding is uncontrollable, intubation may be necessary. All of this equipment should be in place prior to attempting to treat the nose. Dislodging the nasal clot without the proper equipment available can accelerate bleeding and turn a difficult situation into a crisis.[7]

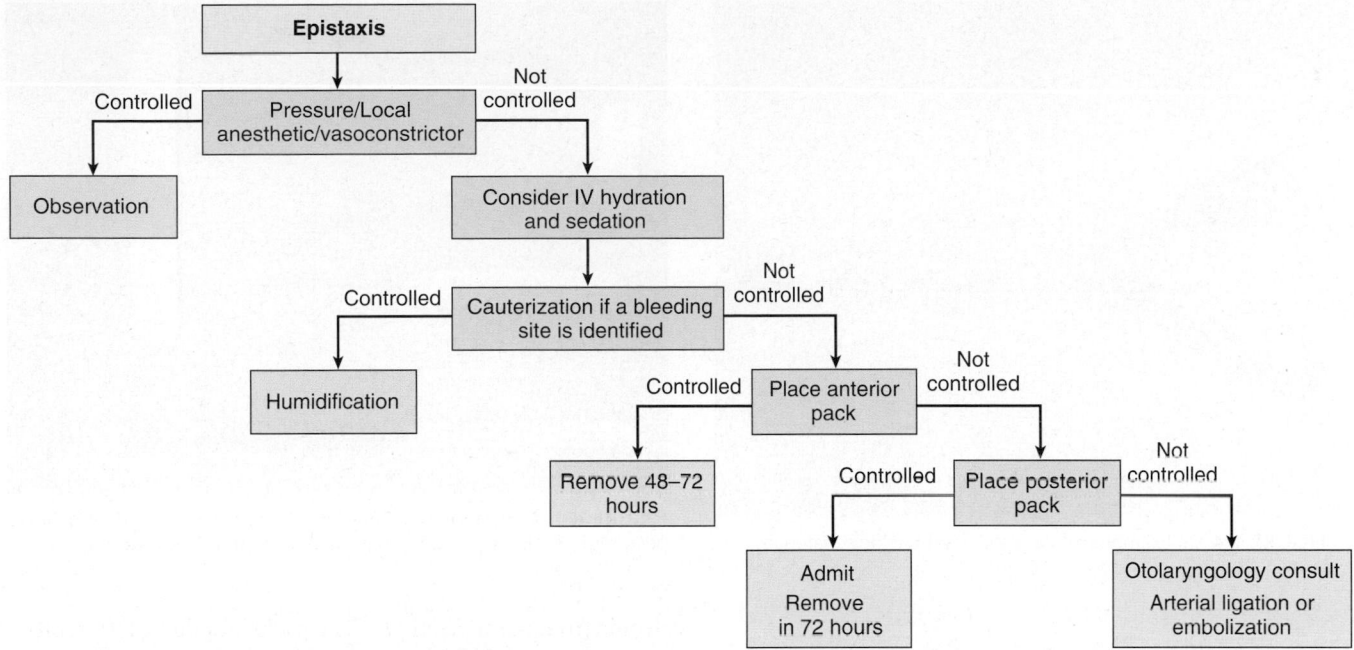

FIGURE 174–1. Emergency department management of epistaxis.

Table 174–1	Epistaxis Tray

4% topical lidocaine
Oxymetazoline nasal spray (Afrin)
Cotton balls
Medicine cup
Nasal speculum
Bayonet forceps
Frazier suction tips (8F and 10F)
Yankauer suction tip
Scissors
Tongue blades (wood and metal)
4 × 4 gauze sponges
10-ml syringes
1-inch tape
Bactroban
Gelfoam
Surgicel
Silver nitrate sticks
Petrolatum gauze, {1/2} inch × 72 inches
Self-expanding packs (small, medium, large)
Epistat double balloon catheter
Additional equipment if posterior pack (Epistat) not available:
  Foley catheter (30 ml)
  C-clamp
  Endotracheal tube size 6, cut into 2.5-cm sections

Monitoring

The degree and method of monitoring patients with epistaxis depends on the history of bleeding, patient cooperation, and past medical history. An initial assessment is made, and those patients who have a history of excessive bleeding require cardiac monitoring. Uncooperative patients and those who require posterior packing will need sedation. These patients need cardiac and blood pressure monitoring, and pulse oximetry.[8,9] Patients who are stable and cooperative do not require monitoring during epistaxis control.

Techniques

The procedures for controlling epistaxis should be approached in a stepwise fashion (see Fig. 174–1). First aid measures are initially employed. Patients should use digital compression, applying pressure with the thumb and index finger to the nares directly inferior to the nasal bones. Ice can be applied to the nasal dorsum, but there is little evidence to support this practice. The patient should be encouraged to bend forward to avoid swallowing large amounts of blood.[10]

If first aid measures are not successful, cautery is the next step in treatment. Sedation may be necessary for the anxious child. A headlight and suction are necessary to identify the bleeding point. Cotton pledgets soaked in oxymetazoline and 2% lidocaine, placed in each nostril, provide for topical anesthetic and vasoconstriction. The nasal speculum is placed into the nose and the blades opened. The clot should be suctioned, and the interior of the nose examined. Most bleeding comes from Kiesselbach's plexus on the anterior septum, and this area should be examined first. When the bleeding site is identified, a silver nitrate stick is placed over the site and held for about 10 seconds.[1,11] Once the bleeding is controlled, a small piece of absorbable gelatin sponge (Gelfoam) can be placed over the site. Cauterizing both sides of the septum at the same time can deprive the septal cartilage of blood supply. This can lead to a perforation and should be avoided. Patients should use nasal saline spray twice a day for the week following this procedure.

If the patient continues to bleed after cauterization, or the bleeding is too profuse to identify the site, nasal packing is necessary. Cotton pledgets with vasoconstrictor and anesthetic are placed. Many self-expanding packs are now available that put pressure on the bleeding site (Fig. 174–2). These nasal packs are quickly and easily inserted even by those with little experience. These packs should be coated with an antibiotic ointment prior to insertion. This lubricates the packs

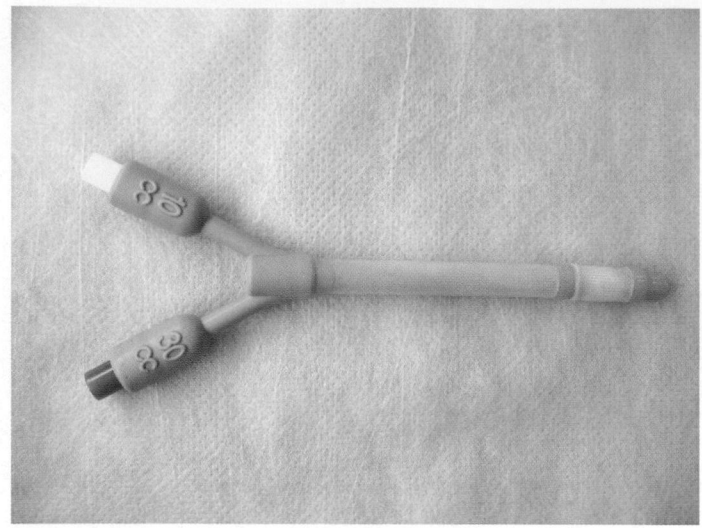

FIGURE 174–2. Examples of anterior nasal packing materials.

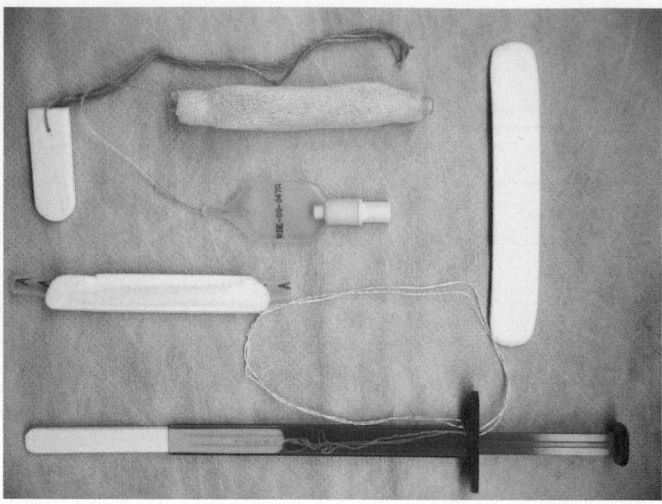

FIGURE 174–4. Posterior packing can be achieved with a dual-balloon pack more easily than traditional methods with a Foley catheter.

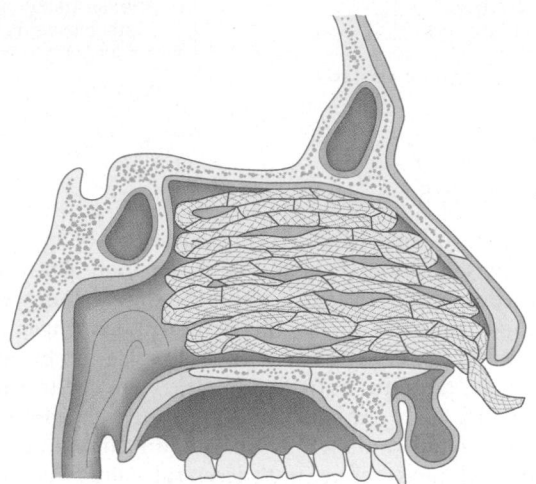

FIGURE 174–3. Anterior nasal packing. Note the layering of packing in the nasal cavity from the floor to the roof.

and may help to avoid complications of rhinosinusitis and toxic shock syndrome.[12,13]

Petrolatum-impregnated strip gauze is the more traditional pack used for persistent epistaxis. This provides for more pressure at the bleeding site, but requires more experience to place properly. This packing can be very uncomfortable for the patient during placement and may require more sedation. To place the gauze, it is grasped approximately 7 cm from the end with a bayonet forceps. The gauze is inserted all the way back in the nasal cavity along the floor of the nose. The end of the gauze should slightly drape out of the nostril. The gauze is then regrasped about 7 cm from where it exits the nose and is placed on top of the first layer to the back of the nasal cavity. This process is repeated until the entire nasal cavity is filled on that side (Fig. 174–3). Both free ends of the gauze should protrude from the nose. This helps to prevent the pack from falling into the nasopharynx.[2]

Oral antibiotics such as amoxicillin-clavulanate or clindamycin are generally recommended while the packing is in place. The packs block the exit of sinus secretions and sinusitis can develop. There have been reports of toxic shock syndrome from nasal packing.[13] The packs should be left in place for approximately 72 hours.[14]

If properly placed anterior packs are not successful in stopping the epistaxis, posterior packs may need to be placed. Fortunately, the need for this type of packing is rare in the pediatric population. The patient will likely need sedation and analgesia because placement of posterior packs is uncomfortable. In the past, either gauze or a Foley catheter was placed in the posterior nasopharynx as a buttress to pack against. These can be very difficult to place.[2] More recently, balloon catheter packs have become available that are much easier to insert (Fig. 174–4). These packs have two balloons, one anterior and one posterior. The nose is anesthetized as previously described. The catheter is lubricated with antibiotic ointment and inserted into the nostril back to the nasopharynx. The balloons, one in the nasopharynx and one in the nasal cavity, are filled with saline. This puts pressure on the bleeding site. Posterior nasal packs can be associated with hypoxia and hypercapnia. These patients should therefore be admitted and closely observed. Packing is generally removed in 48 to 72 hours.[1,7]

Alternative Techniques

If the patient continues to bleed despite these maneuvers or rebleeds after packing removal, other interventions are necessary. An otolaryngologist should be consulted for consideration of arterial ligation. In the past, transantral internal maxillary artery ligation had been advocated. More recently, the endoscopic ligation of the sphenopalatine artery has been effective.[15,16] Angiography with arterial embolization is another technique used to control these difficult cases. This has been used with great success and minimal morbidity.[17]

REFERENCES

1. Wuman LH, Sack JG, Flannery JV, Lipsman RA: The management of epistaxis. Am J Otolaryngol 13:193–209, 1992.
*2. Tan LK, Calhoun KH: Epistaxis. Med Clin North Am 83:43–56, 1999.

*Selected readings.

3. Jackson KR, Jackson RT: Factors associated with active, refractory epistaxis. Arch Otolaryngol Head Neck Surg 114:862–865, 1988.

*4. Alvi A, Joyner-Triplett N: Acute epistaxis: how to spot the source and stop the flow. Postgrad Med 99:83–96, 1996.

5. Katsanis E, Luke KH, Hsu E, et al: Prevalence and significance of mild bleeding disorders in children with recurrent epistaxis. J Pediatr 113:73–76, 1998.

6. Herkner H, Laggner AN, Mullner M, et al: Hypertension in patients presenting with epistaxis. Ann Emerg Med 35:126–130, 2000.

*7. Shaw CB, Wax MK, Wetmore SJ: Epistaxis: a comparison of treatment. Otolaryngol Head Neck Surg 109:60–65, 1993.

8. Viducich RA, Blanda MP, Gerson LW: Posterior epistaxis: clinical features and acute complications. Ann Emerg Med 25:592–596, 1995.

9. Murray AB, Milner RA: Allergic rhinitis and recurrent epistaxis in children. Ann Allergy Asthma Immunol 74:30–33, 1995.

10. Mcgarry GW, Moulton C: Epistaxis first aid. Arch Emerg Med 10:298–300, 1993.

11. Pollice PA, Yoder MG: Epistaxis: A retrospective review of hospitalized patients. Otolaryngol Head Neck Surg 117:49–53, 1997.

12. Pringle MB, Beasley P, Brightwell AP: The use of Merocel nasal packs in the treatment of epistaxis. J Laryngol 110:543–546, 1996.

13. Breda SD, Jacobs JB, Lebowitz AS, et al: Toxic shock syndrome in nasal surgery: a physiochemical and microbiologic evaluation of Merocel and NuGauze nasal packing. Laryngoscope 97:1388–1391, 1986.

*14. Fairbanks DNF: Complications of nasal packing. Otolaryngol Head Neck Surg 94:412–415, 1986.

15. El-Guindy A: Endoscopic transeptal sphenopalatine artery ligation for intractable posterior epistaxis. Ann Otol Rhinol Laryngol 107:1033–1037, 1998.

16. Scaramuzzi N, Walsh RM, Brennan P, Walsh M: Treatment of intractable epistaxis using arterial embolization. Clin Otolaryngol 26:307–309, 2001.

17. Siniluoto TM, Leinonen AS, Karttunen AI, et al: Embolization for the treatment of posterior epistaxis: an analysis of 31 cases. Arch Otolaryngol Head Neck Surg 119:837–841, 1993.

Chapter 175

Removal of Ocular Foreign Bodies

Gregory Garra, DO

Examination

Extraocular foreign bodies often present with symptoms of irritation or pain. The standard evaluation of a patient presenting with a complaint of a foreign body in the eye consists of a thorough external examination, while maintaining a high index of suspicion for globe or corneal perforation. Signs and symptoms of globe or corneal perforation may be subtle. Up to 20% of patients with globe perforation will report no discomfort, and vision may not be impaired. External inspection with a slit lamp may reveal focal conjictival swelling or hemorrhage, scleral hemorrhage, hyphema, pupil irregularity, iris prolapse, a positive Seidel's test (streaming of fluoroscein stain from the site of penetration), loss of contour of the cornea, or a shallow anterior chamber. It is not only important to appreciate the presence of such an injury but also to prevent further damage by avoiding unnecessary examination techniques. In cases in which the patient's behavioral disposition prohibits such careful examination, it may be necessary to administer procedural sedation or involve an ophthalmologist for examination under general anesthesia.

Examination of the eye should begin with measurement of monocular and binocular visual acuity. In children younger than 3 years or in nonverbal children, vision assessment is accomplished by evaluating the child's ability to fix and follow interesting objects. Picture tests, such as Allen figures or LEA symbols, may be used to determine visual acuity in children 2 to 4 years old. Snellen letters or numbers may be utilized for children older than 4 years.[1] Testing at 10 feet is recommended for all visual acuity tests. In children of appropriate age in whom visual acuity cannot be obtained, finger counting, presence of shadows, or light perception should be ascertained.

The external ocular examination should consist of a general inspection of the lids and periorbital soft tissue. It is important to note the position of the globe relative to its surrounding bony structure. Injuries to the lids should be inspected for full-thickness injury, margin involvement, or injury to the lacrimal drainage system.

The pupil must be examined for size, shape, and response to light. An irregularly shaped pupil in the setting of trauma may represent corneal or scleral rupture. Likewise, the presence of an afferent pupillary defect in the injured eye is a poor prognostic sign in the setting of ocular trauma.[2]

Foreign bodies are frequently trapped between the inner surface of the lids and the globe. Therefore, it is important that all patients presenting with foreign body sensation have their lids everted and inspected. Lower lid eversion is easily accomplished by instructing the patient to gaze upward while the examiner applies gentle downward and inward traction of the lower lid. Examination of the upper lid and superior fornix is facilitated by instructing the patient to gaze downward. The examiner, grasping the lid margin and eyelashes, exerts a downward and outward traction on the upper lid while using a cotton-tipped applicator as a fulcrum for everting the tarsal plate.

Examination of the sclera, conjictiva, cornea, and anterior chamber is best accomplished with the illuminated magnification of a slit lamp. It is important to proceed in a stepwise manner, progressing through the anterior segment structures: lid margins, palpebral conjunctiva, bulbar conjunctiva, scleral surface, cornea, anterior chamber, and iris. The examiner should resist the temptation to examine the site of pathology first as concomitant injuries may be overlooked. Evaluation of the lid margins and conjunctiva is accomplished by moving the slit lamp in a sweeping motion across the surface. The sclera and overlying conjunctiva should be examined for the presence of swelling, focal hemorrhages, or discoloration. The cornea is examined in a similar fashion, scanning across the surface assessing for the presence of inflammation, infiltrates, or defects. If a foreign body is identified, the examiner should make attempts at assessing the depth of penetration. Depth perception is facilitated by adjusting the light source so that it strikes the area of interest at a 45-degree angle. Objects violating the full thickness of the cornea should be referred to ophthalmology for treatment. Fluoroscein staining of the cornea will facilitate diagnosis of corneal epithelial defects. Focusing the slit lamp further into the anterior chamber, the aqueous humor is inspected for layering of red blood cells (hyphema), white blood cells (hypopyon), or the presence of cell flare. The iris is assessed for regularity or defects.

In situations in which a perforated cornea or ruptured globe is suspected, further diagnostic maneuvers that may inflict additional damage on the eye should not be attempted. The affected eye should be covered with a protective shield and secured in a fashion that prevents pressure to the globe. The patient should be maintained with the head elevated at a 45-degree angle. Analgesics, antiemetics, and antibiotics should be administered while awaiting emergent ophthalmology evaluation.

Indications and Contraindications

Suspected globe rupture or corneal perforation is an absolute contraindication for emergency department foreign body removal. The examiner should be vigilant in protecting the eye from further injury. Deeply embedded or multiple foreign bodies should be referred to ophthalmology to minimize corneal damage. Removal of a foreign body should not be attempted if the patient is unable to cooperate with positioning.

Preparation and Consent

Topical anesthesia should be administered to facilitate examination, diagnosis, and treatment. Tetracaine 0.5% or proparacaine 0.5% may be instilled into the lower lid fornix. Anesthesia generally lasts up to 30 minutes. Proparacaine reportedly causes less discomfort on instillation[3] and may be the superior alternative in the pediatric population. In patients who are allergic to ester anesthetics such as tetracaine or proparacaine, a suitable alternative for ocular anesthesia would be lidocaine 2% to 4% topical solution or gel.

Equipment

    Slit lamp
    Sterile cotton-tipped applicators
    Antibiotic ointment
    Foreign body spuds or 25- to 27-gauge needle attached to
      a syringe

Monitoring

No specific monitoring is required for routine slit-lamp examination.

Techniques

The technique used for removal largely depends upon whether the foreign body is embedded into the cornea. Loosely adherent foreign bodies may be removed by using gentle irrigation. The patient should be placed in Fowler's position with the

head turned to the side of the affected eye. Using a sterile, isotonic, buffered solution, the eye should be gently irrigated in an attempt to displace the foreign body.

Conjuctival or scleral foreign bodies may be amenable to removal by swabbing the surface with a cotton-tip applicator moistened with saline or a thin layer of ophthalmic ointment.

Patients with adherent superficial or more deeply embedded corneal foreign bodies benefit from localization with slit-lamp magnification and removal using a foreign body spud (Fig. 175–1) or needle. Patient cooperation is essential for successful foreign body removal using a slit lamp and foreign body spud. An explanation of the purpose of the slit lamp may serve to alleviate fear. The patient should be comfortable seated in front of the slit-lamp apparatus. Smaller children are best placed in a caregiver's lap to provide reassurance and aid with positioning in the slit lamp.

After the cornea is anesthetized, the patient is seated with his or her chin nestled firmly in the chin rest and propped forward such that the forehead is stabilized against the forehead band (Fig. 175–2). The eyes should be at the same level as the black stripe (eye-level guide) on the chin rest support pole. The head and body can be further stabilized by having

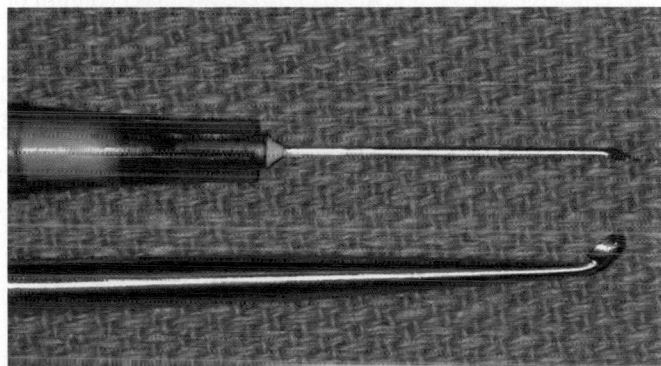

FIGURE 175–1. Foreign body spud (commercial [bottom] and self-fabricated [top]).

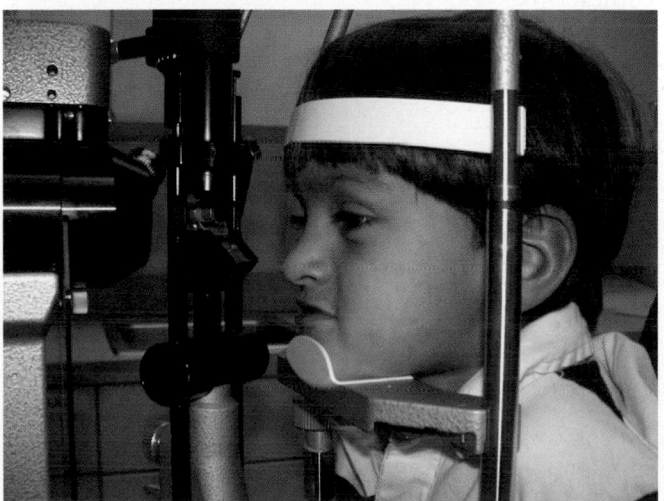

FIGURE 175–2. Patient positioning in slit lamp apparatus.

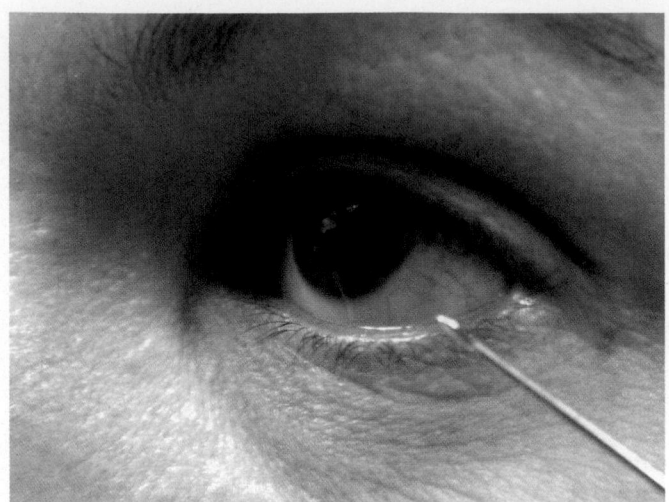

FIGURE 175–3. Approach to foreign body removal utilizing a sterile needle.

the child grasp the handholds on the slit lamp and having the caregiver apply a gentle, reassuring pressure to the back of the head. Ocular play can be eliminated by having the patient fixate on a stabilized object such as the examiner's ear. Once the foreign body is visualized, the main column of the slit lamp can be stabilized by tightening the screw on the base. This will allow the examiner to work with both hands, one to keep the patient's eye open and the other to remove the foreign body. Stabilization of the operating hand (and foreign body spud or needle) is accomplished by resting the dorsal surface of the forth and fifth digits against the patient's cheekbone. This technique will reduce the chance of inadvertent globe perforation should the patient move unexpectedly. Using a foreign body spud or a medium-bore needle (22- to 25-gauge) attached to a tuberculin syringe, the foreign body is approached tangentially from the lateral aspect of the orbit under direct visualization (Fig. 175–3). As the needle edge approaches the foreign body, further manipulation of the needle should be attempted under visualization through the binoculars of the slit lamp. The beveled edge of the needle is used to gently tease away or lift the foreign body off the cornea.

Reexamination with a slit lamp should follow foreign body removal to ascertain the presence of another foreign body, residual damage, or rust ring deposition.

Alternatives

Examination under general anesthesia is a reasonable alternative for examination and treatment of an uncooperative patient. Emergent ophthalmology consultation is warranted in all cases of globe rupture for definitive diagnosis and treatment.

Complications

Patients with corneal foreign bodies generally have a concomitant abrasion resulting from the foreign body itself. Attempts at removal can cause further abrasions or injury. Most corneal abrasions will heal within 24 to 72 hours.[4]

Interruption of the corneal epithelium may predispose the patient to infection, ulceration, scarring, or posttraumatic corneal erosions. The most serious complication of foreign body removal is a corneal perforation. This is minimized by using the described technique in which the examiner's hand is stabilized on the patient's cheek. Immediate ophthalmology consultation should be obtained for suspected corneal perforation or laceration.

Metallic objects that become embedded into the cornea will often leave a rust deposit. Rust rings can result in further corneal inflammation, staining, or scarring. Removal of the rust ring is accomplished by scraping away the stained epithelium with the edge of a small-gauge needle or using a handheld ophthalmic drill.[5] In general, residual rust rings can be assessed and treated during follow-up with an ophthalmologist.

Postprocedure Care and Disposition

A slit-lamp examination must be repeated after foreign body removal to evaluate for residual foreign bodies or rust ring and to ensure no additional trauma occurred during the procedure. Corneal abrasions resulting from ocular foreign bodies should be treated with antibiotic ointment and pain medication. Eye patching does not appear to speed the healing of corneal abrasions or provide greater benefit in pain reduction.[6] Mydriatics are no longer recommended for the treatment of pain in patients with corneal abrasions.[7] Topical antibiotic ointments serve two purposes, antimicrobial activity and lubricant. Bacitracin, erythromycin, or gentamycin is a reasonable first-line treatment option. Ointment is more lubricating than drops. Contact lens wearers should be prescribed an antipseudomonal antibiotic and instructed to avoid contact lens use until resolution of the corneal abrasion.[8] Pain management should be considered paramount and treated with either nonsteroidal anti-inflammatory drugs or narcotic analgesics.

Following removal of the foreign body, peripheral or small abrasions should be referred to ophthalmology for re-evaluation in 3 to 5 days, unless symptoms worsen. Large or central abrasions should be re-evaluated in 24 hours to assess corneal re-epithelialization. Residual rust rings should be referred to ophthalmology for re-evaluation in 24 hours. Incomplete removal of the foreign body will result in continued corneal inflammation and delay healing of the epithelium. The epithelium may slough off and heal or grow over the foreign body, leaving a scar or corneal opacity.

REFERENCES

*1. American Academy of Pediatrics, Committee on Practice and Ambulatory Medicine and Section on Ophthalmology: Eye examination in infants, children, and young adults by pediatricians. Pediatrics 111:902–907, 2003.

*2. Pieramici DJ, Eong KG, Sternberg P Jr, Marsh MJ: The prognostic significance of a system for classifying mechanical injuries of the eye (globe) in open-globe injuries. J Trauma 54:750–754, 2003.

3. Bartfield JM, Holmes TJ, Raccio-Robak N: A comparison of proparacaine and tetracaine eye anesthetics. Acad Emerg Med 4:364–367, 1994.

4. Dua HS, Forrester JV: Clinical patterns of corneal epithelial wound healing. Am J Ophthalmol 104:481–489, 1987.

─────────

*Selected readings.

5. Liston RL, Olson RJ, Mamalis N: A comparison of rust-ring removal methods in a rabbit model: small gauge hypodermic needle versus electric drill. Ann Ophthalmol 23:24–27, 1991.

*6. Michael JG, Hug D, Dowd MD: Management of corneal abrasions in children: a randomized clinical trial. Ann Emerg Med 40:6772, 2002.

7. Carley F, Carley S: Towards evidence based emergency medicine: best BETs from the Manchester Royal Infirmary. Mydriatics in corneal abrasion. Emerg Med J 18:273, 2001.

8. Wilson SA, Last A: Management of corneal abrasions. Am Fam Physician 70:123–128, 2004.

Chapter 176

Pacemakers and Internal Defibrillators

Alfred Sacchetti, MD and Steve Levi, MD

Key Points

Placing an external magnet over the pulse generator of a pacemaker turns off all programmed functions and forces the pacemaker to pace at a fixed rate (asynchronous mode).

If placing an external magnet does not lead to a paced rhythm, undersensing, a dead battery, fractured pacer leads, or pacing device component malfunction may be the cause.

Symptomatic patients with pacer dysfunction can be managed by placing a transcutaneous pacer.

Oversensing can lead to significant bradycardia or asystole when the pacemaker inappropriately senses electrical activity that is not an atrial or ventricular depolarization and does not pace. Treatment consists of placing a magnet over the pacer and converting the pacer to asynchronous mode.

Selected Technical Issues

Pacemakers
  Evaluation of pacemaker function
  Battery failure
  Failure to capture
  Failure to pace (output failure)
  Oversensing
  Undersensing
  Pacemaker syndrome
  Pacemaker-mediated tachycardia
  Runaway pacemaker
  Infection
  Defibrillation and cardioversion in patient with pacemaker
Internal defibrillators
  Evaluation of internal defibrillators
  Failure to convert arrhythmia
  Discharge of defibrillator (appropriate and inappropriate)

Discussion of Individual Technical Issues

Pacemakers

Cardiac pacemakers are becoming an increasingly common component in the care of children with cardiac diseases. As with adult patients, the most common indication for pacemaker insertion in children is symptomatic bradycardia. In patients with complete or partial heart block, the site of the block, type of escape rhythm, and permanence of the block are also factors. Patients with a block below the atrioventricular (AV) node or who are symptomatic regardless of the site of block should receive a permanent pacemaker. Heart block may originate from congenital problems in any portion of the conduction system, from channelopathies, or from surgical damage stemming from repair of structural anomalies. Children with dilated cardiomyopathies or bundle branch blocks may utilize multiple-chamber pacing patterns to synchronize atrial and/or ventricular activities. In children with anatomic repairs and univentricular heart syndromes, multilead ventricular pacing has been used to coordinate mechanical heart activity and thus maximize cardiac output. Rate control devices are also placed for overdrive pacing of intra-atrial reentrant tachycardias, a common arrhythmia in children following atrial surgeries.[1-5]

In general, pacemakers are described by four or five letters (Table 176–1). The first letter describes the chamber or chambers being paced. The second letter describes the chambers being sensed. The third letter describes the action taken on a sensed event. For example, the most common mode is DDD. In this mode, both chambers are paced and sensed and, for each sensed atrial or ventricular event, the pacemaker both inhibits the chamber sensed and paces the other chamber. The fourth letter describes rate modulation. A rate-responsive pacemaker has a motion or temperature sensor that raises or lowers the rate of the pacemaker to match heart rate and metabolic demands by increasing cardiac output.[6] The fifth letter describes the anti-tachydysrhythmia functions.

Pacer leads may be placed transvenously into the endocardial surface of the heart chamber or coronary sinus. They may also be screwed into the epicardium of the heart. Epicardial leads are more common in children because of the

Table 176–1	North American Society of Pacing and Electrophysiology Generic Pacemaker Code			
I **Chamber Paced**	**II** **Chamber Sensed**	**III** **Response to Sensing**	**IV** **Programmability,** **Rate Modulation**	**V** **Anti-tachydysrhythmia** **Functions**
O—none A—atrium (A) V—ventricle (V) D—dual (A and V)	O—none A—atrium V—ventricle D—dual (A and V)	O—none T—triggered I—inhibited D—dual (A triggered and A + V inhibited)	O—none P—simple programmable M—multiprogrammable C—communicating	O—none P—pacing S—antidysrhythmia shock D—dual pacing and shock

difficulties in maneuvering transvenous leads within the heart of patients with complex anatomic repairs. Whenever possible, the pulse generator for the pacemaker is placed in an infraclavicular pocket on the child's anterior chest wall. An abdominal wall insertion may be used in very small children or those requiring epicardial leads. Recently, femoral vein approaches to transvenous pacemakers have been developed that also utilize an abdominal wall site for the pulse generator. Pacemakers placed in a small child generally contain redundant lead length to accommodate the growth of the child.[7-14]

All characteristics of a permanent pacemaker may be set via a dedicated programmer device. Unfortunately, each company has a unique programmer that only functions with their devices. However, all pacemakers respond to placement of an external magnet. Placement of a magnet over the pulse generator of a pacemaker turns off all programmed functions and forces the pacemaker to pace at a fixed rate regardless of the heart's activity.

Evaluation of Pacemaker Function

Evaluation of pacemaker activity and function is through surface monitoring of cardiac electrical activity. Because a pacemaker's impulse is transmitted through the myocardium and not along any specialized conduction pathways, the wave front spreads slowly, leading to wide, bizarre-appearing QRS complexes on electrocardiograms (ECGs) and cardiac monitors. The pacemaker impulse appears as a very thin spike on the monitoring device, generally followed by depolarization of one or more chambers. Newer cardiac monitors have the ability to isolate the pacemaker spikes and highlight them specifically on the monitor screen.

Pacemakers have two general functions: sensing and pacing. The sensing function of a pacemaker describes its ability to detect electrical activity within a given chamber of the heart. The interval between intrinsic electrical events is used to calculate the child's heart rate and determine the need for pacing activity. Pacemakers placed to treat bradyarrhythmias will initiate pacing when the native heart rate falls below the desired rate, while those implanted to treat tachyarrhythmias begin activity when too rapid a heart rate is detected. The sensing function of a pacemaker can be estimated through observation of a continuous cardiac monitor. Initiation of pacemaker activity when the native rate falls below or exceeds threshold settings indicates proper pacer sensing. Initiation of pacing activity while the heart rate is still within an acceptable range indicates failure of the pacemaker to properly sense or analyze electrical activity in the heart.

Assessment of capture requires pacer activity to determine if the impulses generated by the pacemaker produce mechan-ical activity in the heart. Proper capture is confirmed by demonstration of appropriate heart activity following each pacer spike. In a child whose native heart rate is within his or her defined range, no pacer activity should be evident and no evaluation of the pacemaker's capture will be possible. In these patients, the pacemakers may be placed into the asynchronous mode by placement of the magnet over the pulse generator to suppress the sensing function and begin pacing at a fixed interval. Pacer spikes should be evident on the cardiac monitor with associated QRS complexes. No QRS complexes in the presence of pacemaker activity indicate failure to capture. The complete absence of pacer spikes indicates a malfunction in either the lead or the pulse generator.

An accurate history and physical examination associated with a 12-lead ECG are the first steps in the evaluation of a child with a pacemaker. Chest radiography is obtained to ensure that all components and leads are connected. Relevant questions include the indications for the pacemaker, the number of leads, the age of the pacemaker, and the name of the company that produces the device. The name of the company is necessary should a pacer representative need to be called to interrogate the pacemaker. All of this information is contained on wallet cards provided when the pacemaker is inserted. Family members may need to be asked specifically about this card.

Battery Failure

A pacemaker's battery life varies from 3 years in a dual-chamber pacemaker for a small child to 15 years for a large single-chamber pacemaker that works infrequently. When the battery starts to fail, there is a gradual slowing of the paced rate if the pacemaker is pacing continuously. When the battery nears complete failure, there may be failure to capture or failure to pace.

Failure to Capture

Failure to capture indicates that a pacing spike is present on the ECG without associated cardiac depolarization. Causes of failure to capture include high thresholds with an inadequately programmed output, pacemaker component failure, disconnection or dislodgment, impending battery depletion, air in the pulse generator pocket with a unipolar pacemaker, and elevated thresholds due to drugs or metabolic abnormality. A patient's cardiac rhythms will revert to the specific arrhythmia for which the pacemaker was inserted. For children with underlying bradyarrhythmias, this may lead to complaints of syncope, light-headedness, and fatigue. In children with pacemakers inserted for overdrive pacing, complaints of palpitations, syncope, or nervousness may be noted. The diagnosis of capture failure is confirmed by placing the pacer into its fixed mode and demonstrating a pulse generation without associated myocardial activity. Emergency department (ED) treatment of capture failure depends on the clinical scenario.

If use of a magnet does not generate a pacing rhythm with myocardial activity and palpable pulses, a number of possibilities must be considered. If pacer spikes appear on the monitor without capture, then scar tissue may have formed at the lead insertion site, requiring a stronger impulse to initiate capture. Treatment is through the reprogramming of the pulse generator to increase lead output. If no pacer spike is noted on the monitor, the device may not have any battery function remaining. Treatment of these patients requires replacement of the pulse generator. An absent pacer spike may also indicate a fracture of the pacer lead or insulation. Chest radiographs should be obtained on these patients to search for lead fractures. Regardless of the cause, any symptomatic patient with a pacemaker dysfunction requires transcutaneous pacing or placement of a temporary transvenous pacemaker. Consultation with an electrophysiologist for pacemaker evaluation and definitive treatment is prudent.

Failure to Pace (Output Failure)

Failure to pace, or failure to output, is often due to oversensing and inhibition of output. It could also be due to true failure to output from the pacemaker or circuit interruption that prevents the electrical signal from reaching the heart. The reasons for failure to output are circuit failure, pacemaker component failure, fracture or dislodgement, total battery depletion, oversensing of noncardiac activity, cross talk (atrial pacing output is sensed by the ventricular sensing circuit, with subsequent inhibition), air in the pocket of a unipolar device, and unipolar pacemaker not in the pocket.

Oversensing

Oversensing occurs when the pacemaker inappropriately senses electrical activity that is not an atrial or ventricular depolarization. This oversensing may result from lead fracture, insulation breakdown, or lead placement in proximity to skeletal muscle. Because oversensing creates the impression of cardiac activity when none is present, it can lead to suppression of pacer activity and clinical asystole. Oversensing is easily treated with conversion of the pacer to an asynchronous mode through placement of a magnet.

Undersensing

Undersensing occurs when the pacemaker fails to detect or sense normal cardiac activity. Children may be asymptomatic or may complain of palpitations. The ECG may be normal or may not show a normal response to electrical signals (e.g., a DDD system showing P waves without corresponding QRS signals). Functional undersensing occurs when a normal cardiac depolarization is not sensed because it falls within a programmed refractory period. Sensing abnormalities can be seen secondary to insulation defects, component failure, or normally functioning pacing systems that fail to detect atrial or ventricular extrasystoles. Other causes include a new bundle branch block, ventricular and atrial arrhythmias, lead problems, battery failures, and programming errors (too high of a sensing threshold).

Fusion beats and pseudofusion occur as a result of superimposition of an ineffective pacemaker stimulus on a spontaneously occurring P wave or QRS complex. Fusion beats occur when a paced beat is superimposed upon a normal cardiac depolarization. Pseudofusion occurs when the normal cardiac beat morphology is altered by the superimposed pacing artifact. This usually occurs when the pacing rate and the intrinsic rate are similar. Pseudofusion also can be due to delayed activation due to intraventricular conduction abnormalities.

Reprogramming the pacemaker's sensing threshold to allow the extrasystoles to be sensed can resolve undersensing. Alternately, leads may need to be repositioned. In the ED, placing a magnet over the pacemaker may convert resulting abnormal rhythms to a relatively stable fixed rate.

Pacemaker Syndrome

Pacemaker syndrome occurs with suboptimal pacing modes or programming that leads to abnormal AV synchrony (especially with VVI or VVO pacers) or AV dyssynchrony (with increased atrial pressure, cannon a waves, etc.). When this occurs, there is no atrial contribution to cardiac output. Patients may have diminished cardiac output, hypotension, syncope, and shortness of breath. Management consists of reprogramming, repair, or replacement of the pacemaker.

Pacemaker-Mediated Tachycardia

Reentry tachycardia can occur with dual-chamber pacers with atrial sensing and the pacemaker acting as part of the reentry circuit. The rate is variable but cannot rise above the programmed upper limit of the pacer. Application of a magnet usually stops this reentry circuit. Adenosine, carotid massage, and external pacing (pulse width of 40 msec) are alternative ways to end this tachycardia if the rhythm is refractory to magnet application.

Runaway Pacemaker

A runaway pacemaker occurs when inappropriate rapid discharges occur, potentially leading to ventricular tachycardia or fibrillation. It is most commonly due to pacemaker component failure. Applying a magnet may slow the rate, and emergency pacemaker interrogation and reprogramming will be required. If magnet application is unsuccessful, surgery may be needed to disconnect the leads.

Infection

As with all implanted foreign objects, any portion of a pacemaker may become infected. Intravascular components, such as pacer leads, behave essentially the same as bacterial endocarditis when infected. Infections of the pulse generator appear as inflammation over the insertion site with erythema, swelling, and tenderness. Regardless of how benign such infections appear, any inflammation in this area should be treated aggressively with blood cultures, intravenous antibiotics, and immediate consultation with an electrophysiologist and surgeon.[15]

Defibrillation and Cardioversion in Patients with Pacemakers

If electrical cardioversion or defibrillation is required in a patient with a pacemaker or defibrillator, the paddles should be placed as far from the pulse generator as possible. Also, paddles should be placed perpendicular to the axis of the pacemaker generator and electrodes (usually anteroposterior placement). An external pacemaker must be ready after any cardioversion/defibrillation since the electrical shock may disrupt the internal pacemaker and external pacing may be required.

Internal Defibrillators

Tachyarrhythmias are a common problem in pediatric patients either as congenital reentry tracts, ion channel abnormalities, or disruptions of normal conduction pathways secondary to corrective anatomic surgery. Some atrial arrhythmias may be treatable with overdrive pacing but, for many tachyarrhythmias, cardioversion remains the only effective means of termination.[1,2]

Automated implantable defibrillator (AID) is a generic term used to describe all devices that convert cardiac rhythms through myocardial depolarization. Unlike surface paddles, which depolarize the entire heart, AIDs utilize specifically placed electrodes to depolarize only a strategic portion of the heart to effect rhythm conversion. Modern defibrillation leads employ large-surface-area coils located in the chambers they are trying to defibrillate, which is almost always the ventricles. This configuration, in combination with a biphasic waveform, has drastically reduced the defibrillation thresholds of energy needed to terminate arrhythmias.[16]

Evaluation of Internal Defibrillators

As with pacemakers, it is best to have an electrophysiologist and a technician perform a formal interrogation of the AID when evaluating its performance. Unless an arrhythmia occurs during the ED visit while the patient is monitored, it will be difficult for ED personnel to assess the AID's sensing or rhythm conversion functions. Similarly, inappropriate discharge can be recognized only if the device discharges while the child is monitored and in a stable rhythm. Unlike with a pacemaker, placement of a magnet on an AID simply inactivates all functions in the device rather than placing it in a fixed mode.

The clinical presentation of a child with a malfunctioning AID depends on the indication for the device and the nature of the problem. Internal defibrillator dysfunction generally presents as either a failure to convert a dysrhythmia or inappropriate discharge when a tachyarrhythmia is not present.

Failure to Convert Arrhythmia

Failure to convert an arrhythmia will generally result in an ED complaint of palpitations, syncope, or, if a lethal arrhythmia occurs, cardiac arrest. Conversion failure may stem from an inability of the AID to recognize the presence of the tachyarrhythmia. If the rate of the rhythm is below the threshold for which the AID is programmed, the arrhythmia will not be recognized and cardioversion will not be attempted. Alternately, not every discharge of the AID will result in a rhythm conversion, and even a properly functioning defibrillator may not successfully convert an arrhythmia. Finally, as with pacemakers, lead fracture can also be a source of conversion failure.

Discharge of Defibrillator (Appropriate and Inappropriate)

Inappropriate discharge of an AID is impossible to determine without a formal interrogation of the device. The child may complain of feeling the device discharge without any of the sensations typically associated with his or her arrhythmia. However, it is still possible that the AID converted the arrhythmia before the patient became symptomatic. If the device is observed to discharge inappropriately in the ED, a magnet should be secured in place over the device to prevent any further discharges until formal interrogation and reprogramming can be performed.

A child who has had an appropriate discharge of the AID requires evaluation for underlying malignant arrhythmias. This may involve an evaluation for electrolyte abnormalities, anemia, and hypoxia, and a new and old medications review. Most children will require admission for continued cardiac monitoring and correction of the underlying disease.

Summary

As with every child, the ED disposition of children with pacemakers or internal defibrillators will be a function of the underlying condition, the presenting complaint, and the degree to which the problem was resolved during the ED visit. If the treating clinicians can assure that the child's device is functioning correctly at the end of the ED visit, then a discharge to home is appropriate. In some patients, evaluation of the device may prove entirely normal in the ED and the cause of the child's complaints will not be evident. In these children, discharge to home may still be considered if the underlying problem is relatively minor, such as a supraventricular tachycardia with no associated symptoms. Arrangements for an outpatient Holter monitor and close outpatient follow-up are prudent. In children with more severe underlying rhythm disturbances, such as syncope associated with heart block or ventricular fibrillation, hospital admission or formal consultation with an electrophysiologist will be required.

REFERENCES

*1. Walsh EP, Cecchin F: Recent advances in pacemaker and implantable defibrillator therapy for young patients. Curr Opin Cardiol 19:91–96, 2004.

2. Bevilacqua LM, Berul CI: Advances in pediatric electrophysiology. Curr Opin Pediatr 16:494–499, 2004.

*3. Berul CI, Cecchin F; American Heart Association; American College of Cardiology: Indications and techniques of pediatric cardiac pacing. Expert Rev Cardiovasc Ther 1:165–176, 2003.

4. Bostan OM, Celiker A, Karagoz T, et al: Dual chamber cardiac pacing in children: single chamber pacing dual chamber sensing cardiac pacemaker or dual chamber pacing and sensing cardiac pacemaker? Pediatr Int 44:635–640, 2002.

5. Karpawich PP: Chronic right ventricular pacing and cardiac performance: the pediatric perspective. Pacing Clin Electrophysiol 27(6 Pt 2):844–849, 2004.

6. Zeigler VL, Gillette PC, Kratz J: Is activity sensored pacing in children and young adults a feasible option? Pacing Clin Electrophysiol 13(12 Pt 2):2104–2107, 1990.

*7. Swygman C, Wang PJ, Link MS, et al: Advances in implantable cardioverter defibrillators. Curr Opin Cardiol 17:24–28, 2002.

8. Costa R, Filho MM, Tamaki WT, et al: Transfemoral pediatric permanent pacing: long-term results. Pacing Clin Electrophysiol 26(1 Pt 2):487–491, 2003.

*9. Cohen MI, Rhodes LA, Spray TL, et al: Efficacy of prophylactic epicardial pacing leads in children and young adults. Ann Thorac Surg 78:197–202, 2004.

10. Sliz NB Jr, Johns JA: Cardiac pacing in infants and children. Cardiol Rev 8:223–239, 2000.

*Suggested readings.

11. Bauersfeld U, Nowak B, Molinari L, et al: Low-energy epicardial pacing in children: the benefit of autocapture. Ann Thorac Surg 68:1380–1383, 1999.

12. Gillette PC, Edgerton J, Kratz J, et al: The subpectoral pocket: the preferred implant site for pediatric pacemakers. Pacing Clin Electrophysiol 14:1089–1092, 1991.

13. Cabrera ME, Portzline G, Aach S, et al: Can current minute ventilation rate adaptive pacemakers provide appropriate chronotropic response in pediatric patients? Pacing Clin Electrophysiol 25:907–914, 2002.

14. Ragonese P, Guccione P, Drago F, et al: Efficacy and safety of ventricular rate responsive pacing in children with complete atrioventricular block. Pacing Clin Electrophysiol 17(4 Pt 1):603–610, 1994.

15. Cohen MI, Bush DM, Gaynor JW, et al: Pediatric pacemaker infections: twenty years of experience. J Thorac Cardiovasc Surg 124:821–827, 2002.

16. Epstein AE: An update on implantable cardioverter-defibrillator guidelines. Curr Opin Cardiol 19:23–25, 2004.

Paraphimosis Reduction

Fred Schwartz, MD

Indications and Contraindications

In children, paraphimosis most commonly occurs after a parent has fully retracted the foreskin of the son (Fig. 177–1). The condition may also follow urethral catheterization if the practitioner fails to return the retracted foreskin back to its normal position.

Preparation and Consent

Examination will typically reveal swelling of the retracted foreskin that constricts the neck of the penis. This interferes with venous drainage from the glans, resulting in glans enlargement to the point that the prepuce cannot be retracted over it. Pain may or may not be present. If left untreated, necrosis may develop, the signs of which include blackened areas on the glans or prepuce.

No diagnostic testing is required prior to paraphimosis reduction.

Analgesic medications are required prior to reduction. Local analgesia consists of lidocaine 2.5%, and prilocaine 2.5% cream applied to the glans and distal penis. Often, procedural sedation is also required. Although dorsal penile blocks are sometimes used in adults, it is more appropriate to utilize sedation in the pediatric population.

Equipment

Glove
Bucket of ice
Lidocaine 2% gel, or lidocaine/prilocaine (2.5/2.5%) cream, or lidocaine 1% without epinephrine
27-gauge needle with syringe for local anesthetic
18- or 20-gauge needle with syringe
Babcock tissue clamps
Tuberculin syringe
Hyaluronidase, 150 units/ml (1 ml)
4 × 4 gauze
No. 11 blade scalpel (if dorsal slit is considered)

Monitoring

Monitoring of the patient is necessary only if the patient undergoes sedation (see Chapter 159, Procedural Sedation and Analgesia).

Technique

Decreasing Edema

Local anesthesia is administered alone or in combination with parenteral sedation with analgesia. Prior to manual or surgical attempts at reducing a paraphimosis, an attempt at decreasing penile edema is indicated. A latex or rubber glove is partially filled with ice and water. The partially filled glove is then placed around the glans and distal swollen penis so that it conforms to the shape of these structures. At least 15 to 20 minutes are allowed to pass before manual reduction attempts. Another method for reducing edema is the injection of hyaluronidase (~1 ml) directly into the connective tissue. This agent causes fluid to cross tissue planes and quickly decreases edema.[1]

Manual Procedures

Manual reduction is attempted after anesthesia, analgesia with sedation, and local measures to reduce edema. Prior to attempting foreskin manual reduction, the foreskin should be compressed manually with 4 × 4 gauze or the distal penis wrapped with an elastic or Kerlix bandage for 10 to 15 minutes. To reposition the foreskin, direct pressure is applied on the glans with the thumbs of both hands while pulling the prepuce forward with the index and middle fingers. Gentle, steady pressure is maintained until the foreskin

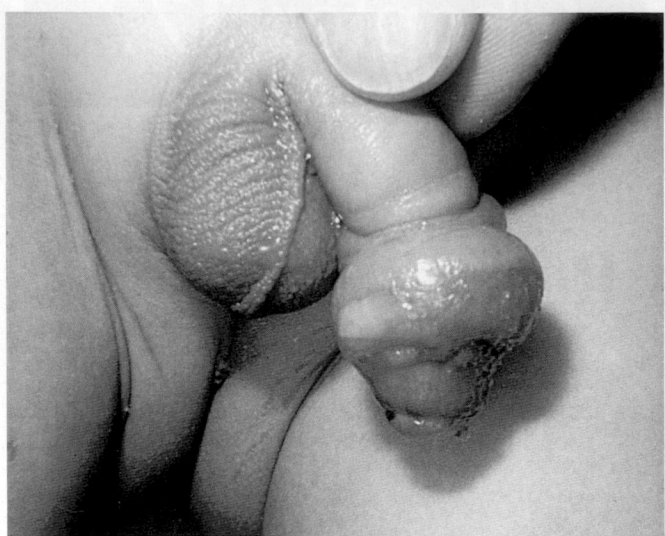

FIGURE 177–1. Paraphismosis. The foreskin has been retracted proximal to the glans penis and has become markedly swollen secondary to venous congestion. (From Urologic disorders in infants and children. *In* Nelson's Textbook of Pediatrics, 17th ed. p 18114.)

returns to its normal position, completely covering the glans (Fig. 177–2).

If this maneuver is unsuccessful, the retracted foreskin is grasped with the Babcock clamps. Traction is gently applied to reduce the foreskin over the glans (Fig. 177–3).

Alternatives

Puncture Technique

To perform this technique, an 18- or 21-gauge hypodermic needle is inserted into the edematous foreskin at several sites to release the trapped fluid. External drainage can improve edema, with subsequent manual reduction of the foreskin.[2,3]

Dorsal Slit

If a severely constricting band of tissue cannot be reduced by conservative or minimally invasive therapy, an emergency bedside dorsal slit procedure can be performed, followed by a delayed circumcision. Ideally, this procedure is performed in the operating room. However, if timely consultation is unavailable and there is concern about impending necrosis, emergency department (ED) performance of this procedure is appropriate. To perform this procedure, a dorsal nerve block or local anesthesia is administered at the site of intended incision and sedation with analgesia is administered. An incision is made vertically through the foreskin while avoiding the glans and dartos fascia, which lies just under the skin. Finally, the distal and proximal end of the incision are approximated with absorbable sutures (Fig. 177–4).

Complications

If the paraphimosis is not successfully reduced, gangrene or permanent damage to the penis may develop. A urologist should be emergently consulted.[4]

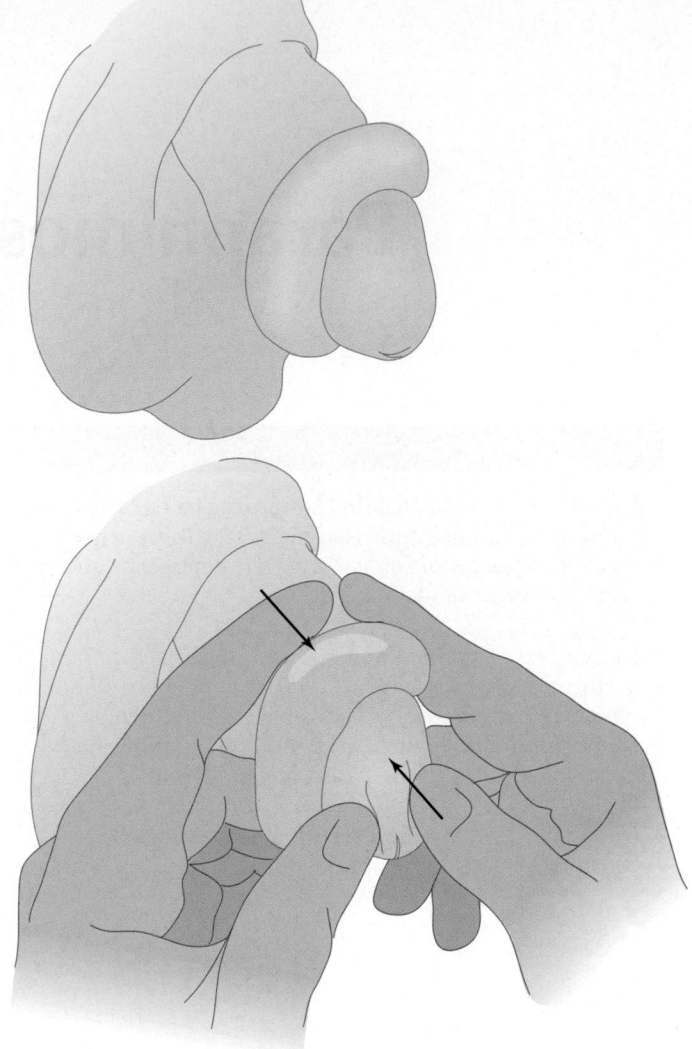

FIGURE 177–2. Manual reduction technique.

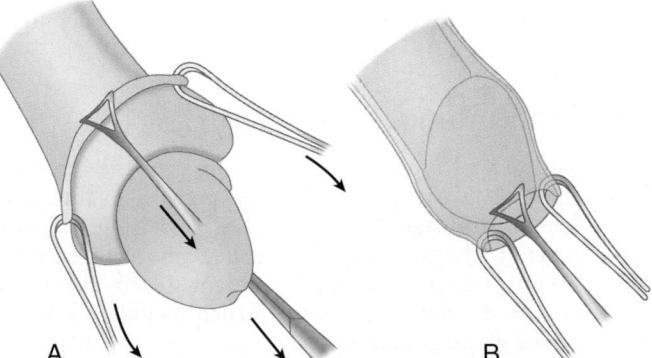

FIGURE 177–3. A, Application of Babcock clamps to reduce paraphimosis. **B,** Foreskin reduced. (From Skoglund RW, Chapman WH: Reduction of paraphimosis. J Urol 104:137, 1970. Reproduced by permission. © Williams & Wilkins, 1970.)

FIGURE 177-4. Anesthetizing the penis for surgical treatment of paraphimosis. **A,** Line of infiltration of local anesthesia used before performing dorsal slit. **B,** Incision for paraphimosis. A diamond-shaped defect results from incision of the foreskin. **C,** The two apices of the dorsal slit (*a* and *b*) are approximated after the foreskin is reduced. (From Roberts J, Hedges J: Clinical Procedures in Emergency Medicine, 4th ed. Philadelphia: Elsevier Saunders, 2004, pp 739–744.)

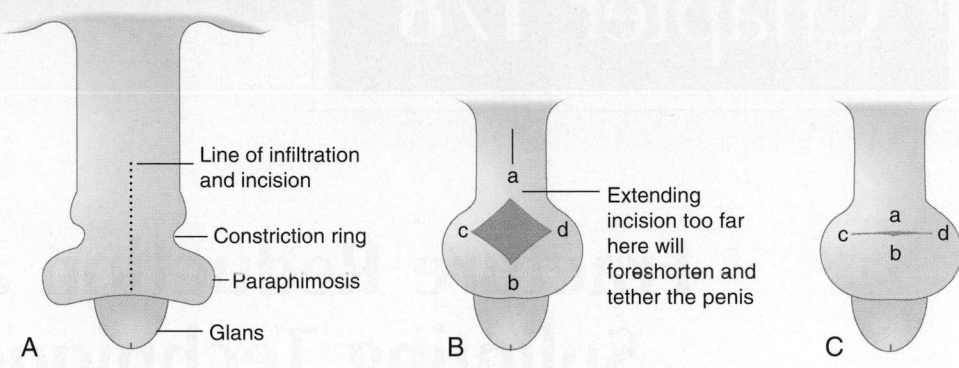

Postprocedure Care and Disposition

Once the paraphimosis is reduced, the patient may be safely discharged home. The outcome is usually excellent, with rapid return to normal function. The length of the ED stay is generally determined by the duration of the sedation only. A urology follow-up should be arranged for possible elective circumcision to prevent recurrences.

REFERENCES

1. Devries CR, Miller AK, Packer MG: Reduction of paraphimosis with hyaluronidase. Urology 48:464–465, 1996.
2. Barone JG, Fleisher MH: Treatment of paraphimosis using the "puncture" technique. Pediatr Emerg Care 9:298–299, 1993.
3. Kumar V, Javle P: Modified puncture technique for reduction of paraphimosis. Ann R Coll Surg Engl 83:126–127, 2001.
4. Turner CD, Kim HL, Cromie WJ: Dorsal band traction for reduction of paraphimosis. Urology 54:917–918, 1999.

Chapter 178

Fracture Reduction and Splinting Techniques

Gregory Garra, DO

Indications and Contraindications

Indications for orthopedic consultations vary between institutions. An accurate clinical and radiographic interpretation is essential for formulating an appropriate treatment plan. Description of the injury should include the status of the overlying skin (open vs. closed, with or without tenting of the skin), orientation of the fracture line, anatomic location of the fracture, amount of displacement, degree of angulation, presence of shortening or malrotation, involvement of joint or growth plate, and neurovascular status. Generally accepted indications for emergent orthopedic consultation include open fractures, grossly unstable or unacceptably displaced fractures, irreducible dislocations, and injuries with associated vascular compromise or compartment syndromes. In emergency departments (EDs) with teleradiology, information provided by electronically transmitted radiographs to orthopedic specialists may help to further improve treatment plans.[1] Splinting is used to temporarily stabilize an unstable fracture in the ED or to immobilize an injury that requires orthopedic follow-up.

Immediate reduction is indicated for all dislocations that are associated with absent or diminished pulses. Open dislocations often need reduction in the operating room with thorough irrigation of the involved joint and débridement of devitalized tissue. In addition, hip dislocations must be performed within 1 hour—for every minute they are out, the avascular necrosis rate rises 1% in adults; more time is allowed for children. Most other simple, closed dislocated joints can be reduced in the ED.

Preparation and Consent

As with any procedure, proper preparation is paramount. The extremity should be completely exposed. The extremity should be free of potential tourniquets such as jewelry, pant legs, or shirt sleeves. All materials must be measured and cut to size prior to formation of the splint. The length can be estimated by laying the dry splint next to the area to be splinted. The width of the splint should be slightly greater than the diameter of the limb to be immobilized. Elastic bandages should be open and readily available to secure the splint in place. Tape should be available to secure the elastic bandages. Splints involving the fingers or toes should have padding placed between digits to prevent maceration of interdigitary surfaces.

Safe and effective management of fracture-related pain in the ED reduces patient distress during initial evaluation and often facilitates definitive management of the fracture.[2] Analgesics should be given in almost all cases of musculoskeletal injury. Administration of medicine should occur as early as possible to prevent unnecessary suffering. Procedural sedation should be considered for fractures and dislocations that require manipulation. In anticipation of procedural sedation, patients should be instructed by nursing personnel to refrain from oral intake until further notification.

Equipment

Plaster Slabs

Nearly any splint can be fabricated from cotton bandages (Webril), plaster, and elastic bandages. Most splints can be formed by "sandwiching" plaster between two layers of padding. The first layer of padding will rest atop the patient's skin and should be six to eight sheets thick. This is especially important over bony prominences where pressure sores can result. The padding should be slightly longer and wider than the plaster to avoid contact with the skin and prevent irritation. The middle layer is composed of plaster, which will maintain position and immobility. Thickness of the plaster layer depends upon the extremity being immobilized. As a general rule, splints applied to the lower extremity should be constructed of 12 to 15 layers of plaster sheeting to be of adequate strength. Splints to the upper extremity can be constructed of 8 to 10 layers of plaster sheeting. The third or top layer consists of a thin layer of padding (two to three sheets) to prevent the elastic bandage from adhering to the plaster and losing compressibility.

Prefabricated Molds

Although limited in scope and application, prefabricated molds may have some application in the management of pediatric fractures.[3] The most commonly available prefabricated molds are finger splints, volar wrist splints, knee immobilizers, inflatable ankle molds, and posterior ankle molds.

Prefabricated Splinting Material

Products that combine fiberglass and polypropylene padding into a single preparation are commercially available. They generally cost more than plaster rolls and cotton bandages but reduce the amount of preparation time and are quite versatile.

Fluoroscopy

Although not routinely available to most emergency physicians, portable fluoroscopy equipment may facilitate reduction of fractures and dislocation by providing real-time visualization of the bony structures.

Radiology: Pre- and Postreduction Needs

Evidence on simple anterior shoulder dislocation suggests that one set of radiographs may be sufficient.[4-6] Few data exist on the need for pre- and postreduction radiographs of simple dislocations involving the patella or interphalangeal joints. Dislocations of other joints and fracture/dislocations should have both pre- and postmanipulation radiographs.

Monitoring

Vascular function should be assessed both before and after reduction maneuvers. Signs of vascular compromise such as delayed capillary refill or weak/absent pulses require emergent intervention. Significant swelling within a closed space can result in increased pressure and further compromise of blood flow. Systolic pressure measurement using Doppler ultrasound is a sensitive predictor for arterial injury. When compared to the unaffected extremity, the arterial pressure should be more than 0.9 times the contralateral value. A value less than 0.9 has a sensitivity of 95% and a specificity of 97% for major arterial injury.[7] Angiography is useful in confirming a suspected arterial injury.

Nerve injuries may result from fractures, dislocations, or manipulation of an orthopedic injury. Proper neurologic evaluation should focus on motor and sensory function of the individual peripheral nerves supplying the injured extremity. Although nerve injuries are not immediately reversible, documentation and follow-up are important.

Techniques

Reductions

Shoulder

Numerous methods for shoulder reduction are described. Each method has its advantages.

EXTERNAL ROTATION

The external rotation technique is a gentle technique that may obviate the need for procedural sedation.[8] With the elbow flexed at 90 degrees, gentle, slow external rotation is applied to the humeral head. Most reductions will occur between 70 and 110 degrees of external rotation. If unsuccessful, applying longitudinal traction on the humerus while abducting the humeral head may facilitate reduction.

SCAPULAR MANIPULATION

This technique involves rotating the inferior border of the scapula medially while applying longitudinal traction to a 90-degree flexed shoulder. The patient may be positioned prone on the gurney or sitting upright.[9]

STIMSON TECHNIQUE

This technique is performed with the patient positioned prone with the affected arm hanging off the stretcher. A 10- to 15-pound weight is strapped to the distal forearm or wrist and allowed to hang for 20 to 30 minutes. Gentle external rotation of the humeral head may facilitate reduction. This technique may be combined with scapular manipulation in failed cases.[10]

Nursemaid's Elbow (Radial Head Subluxation)

Nursemaid's elbow is a common injury of young children and usually results from sudden traction of the distal forearm/wrist applied to an extended elbow. Two methods of reduction are available. In both methods, the child should be placed in the parent's lap so that both the parent and child are facing the physician. The parent is instructed to hold the uninjured arm. The physician embraces the child's hand as in a handshake, placing the other hand on the radial head. Reduction is accomplished by recreating the forces that resulted in the injury. Gentle longitudinal traction is applied at the elbow, the wrist is supinated, and pressure is applied to the volar aspect of the radial head. Flexion at the elbow is the final maneuver that serves to reduce the radial head. If this maneuver is unsuccessful, the physician may attempt an alternative technique that involves wrist hyperpronation with elbow flexion. Both methods are reported to have equal success. However, the hyperpronation method may be less painful.[11]

Fingers and Toes

Dorsal dislocations of the interphalangeal joints of the hand are commonly encountered in the ED. Reduction of the second to fifth digits is easily accomplished by applying longitudinal traction and slight hyperextension of the affected digit, followed by flexion of the affected joint. In simple dislocations that do not involve an avulsion fracture or entrapment of the volar plate of the interphalangeal joint, the physician will feel the dislocation slide smoothly over the rounded surface of the head of the phalanx.

Reduction should always be followed by an appropriate examination of ligamentous integrity as well as neurovascular function. Injury to the central slip of the extensor tendon may result in the formation of a boutonnière deformity. Signs suggestive of central slip injury are swelling and ecchymosis at the base of the middle phalanx. Tendon injury should be suspected if the patient loses more than 15 to 20 degrees of active extension of the affected finger with the wrist and metacarpophalyngeal joints in full flexion.[12] All patients with suspected central slip injury should be treated with a dorsal finger splint across the proximal interphalangeal (PIP) joint in extension, leaving the distal interphalangeal (DIP) joint free. Follow-up evaluation with a hand surgeon is warranted.

Hip

Hip reductions should be done in consultation with an orthopedic surgeon as they are frequently associated with other injuries to the lower extremity or pelvis. Hip dislocations should be corrected within 6 hours of the injury to minimize the incidence of avascular necrosis of the femoral head[13] and sciatic neuropathy.[14] Two types of dislocations can result: anterior and posterior. Both injuries require procedural sedation. Anterior hip dislocations are treated by applying in-line traction with flexion and internal rotation of the hip. Multiple methods for reducing posterior hip dislocations are described.[15] One of the more commonly employed methods (the Allis maneuver) places the patient in a supine position. An assistant stabilizes the pelvis by applying a downward force over the bilateral iliac crests. Longitudinal traction is applied to the femur in the direct line of the deformity, followed by gentle flexion of the hip to 90 degrees, followed by gentle internal and external rotation of the hip until reduced.

Knee

Many knee dislocations may reduce spontaneously. Therefore, physicians must maintain a high index of suspicion in patients who report such an event or present with injury to three or more of the major knee ligaments.[16] These injuries are often associated with injuries to the popliteal artery and peroneal nerve. Most authorities recommend angiography to assess vascular integrity in all suspected knee dislocations. However, a thorough physical examination, checking foot pulses and the ankle-brachial index, may obviate the need for such studies.[17] Prompt reduction is important to prevent further neurovascular injury. Knee reductions should be performed in consultation with an orthopedic surgeon. Both anterior and posterior knee dislocations uniformly involve disruption of ligamentous structures, resulting in a highly unstable joint. Reduction is accomplished by applying in-line traction to the lower extremity, with manipulation of the proximal tibia according to the direction of the dislocation.[16] For anterior dislocations, the femur is lifted, while for posterior dislocations, the proximal tibia is lifted while an assistant applies countertraction. The injured extremity should be immobilized and elevated. The patient should be admitted for serial neurovascular examinations.

Patella

Dislocations of the patella usually result in its lateral displacement. Most dislocations reduce spontaneously with terminal knee extension. For those patients presenting with patellar dislocation, reduction is accomplished in the supine position by flexing the hip to 90 degrees, extending the knee to 180 degrees, and applying gentle pressure on the patella directed toward the midline. Following reduction, evaluation of the major knee ligaments is necessary to rule out a concurrent injury. The joint should be immobilized in full extension. Orthopedic follow-up is important to assess for osteochondral fractures and factors that predispose to recurrent dislocations.[18]

Ankle and Elbow

Dislocations of the ankle generally result from high-energy trauma and therefore are frequently associated with fractures and significant soft tissue injury. As with other dislocations, injuries associated with neurovascular compromise must be treated immediately. Radiographs are necessary to determine the direction of the dislocation and associated injuries and will facilitate reduction techniques. Although no specific method is described, reduction is typically accomplished by applying longitudinal traction to the foot with gentle manipulation. For dorsal dislocations, the foot is plantar flexed. For anterior dislocations, the foot is dorsiflexed. Immobilization with a posterior mold is necessary until definitive fixation can be arranged.

The elbow is the most commonly dislocated joint in the pediatric population, and dislocations frequently result from a fall on an outstretched hand. As a result of the mechanism, most elbow dislocations are posterior. Soft tissue injuries and associated fractures are common. Prereduction radiographs are necessary to determine the direction of the dislocation, identify associated injuries, and direct management. Elbow dislocations with associated bony fractures generally require treatment with open reduction and internal fixation. Several methods for reduction are described. One such method is reported to be simple and safe, requiring no anesthesia or assistant. The patient is placed supine and the affected limb is draped across the chest. The physician palpates the olecranon and gently pushes it into position while applying traction on the forearm and flexion to the elbow.[19] As with other injuries, neurovascular assessment is important. The most commonly injured neurovascular structure is the ulnar nerve. Vascular injuries are rare.[20]

Splinting

The choice of splinting techniques used to protect and immobilize fractures and reduced dislocations is extensive. Often, more than one technique can be used for the same injury. Clinicians must keep in mind that the purpose of the splint is to immobilize injuries so that deforming rotational and flexion/extension forces have minimal effect on the fracture site. For this reason, specific angles of flexion/extension and degrees of supination/pronation are often recommended for particular fractures (Table 178–1).

Upper Extremity

SLING AND SWATHE

This device is available as a commercially prepared product or can be fashioned by placing the patient's arm in a shoulder

Table 178–1	Splinting Positions for Various Fracture Types
Fracture Type	**Preferred Splinting Position***
Clavicle fracture	Sling; a figure-of-eight bandage is rarely used
Proximal and middle humerus fracture	Long arm handing cast, coaptation splint, or sling and swathe
Elbow trauma	For undiagnosed injury at elbow, splint elbow at 20–30 degrees of flexion until radiography
Elbow dislocation—postreduction	Long arm posterior splint with elbow flexed 90 degrees
Supracondylar fracture	Type I (nondisplaced or humeral line intersects capitellum)—elbow at 90 degrees of flexion and forearm/wrist neutral or pronated
Lateral condyle fracture	If less than 2–4 mm displacement, long arm splint with elbow flexed 90 degrees, and neutral or supinated forearm
Medial epicondyle fracture	If less than 5 mm displacement, posterior splint or long arm cast with elbow flexed 90 degrees
Olecranon fracture	If ≤ 2 mm displaced, posterior splint with elbow flexed to less than 75 to 80 degrees
Radius fracture	• Proximal radius—long arm cast or sugar-tong splint with forearm supinated • Middle radius—long arm cast or sugar-tong splint with forearm neutral • Distal radius—sugar-tong splint with forearm pronated For each of these fractures, make sure that the distal fragment is immobilized in a degree of rotation such that it is aligned with the bicipital tuberosity.
Radioulnar fracture (fracture of both bones of forearm)	• Fractures with the apex of the fracture in volar position and distal fragment angulated dorsally—reduce by pronating and splint in pronation • Fractures with the apex of the fracture in dorsal position and distal fragment angulated volarly—reduce by supinating and splint in supination Splint both fractures with flexed elbow and wrist in supination or pronation as described. For unstable fractures, splint elbow in extension.
Metacarpal neck fracture	Splint with metacarpophalangeal joint in maximum flexion, and interphalangeal joints extended
Metacarpal shaft fracture	"Beer (or soda) can" position with metacarpophalangeal joint flexed 70 degrees
First metacarpal, scaphoid, and first proximal phalanx fractures	Thumb spica splint
Knee dislocation—postreduction	Long leg splint with knee flexed 15 degrees
Patella dislocation	Long leg splint with knee in full extension
Tibia spine fracture	Long leg splint with knee flexed 10–20 degrees
Proximal tibia fracture	Long leg splint with knee in full extension
Distal tibia spiral fracture (toddler's fracture)	Long leg splint with knee flexed 30–40 degrees
Distal tibia fracture	
Ankle tibiotalar dislocation—postreduction	Long leg splint with ankle flexed 90 degrees

*Splint positions assume fractures are nondisplaced or minimally displaced. The exact amount of displacement, degree of angulation, and rotation differ for each fracture type and differ among different experts. Fractures that are more displaced often require pinning or surgery.

sling and securing it against the chest by wrapping the torso with an elastic bandage. The sling serves to support the upper extremity while the swathe limits range of motion at the shoulder and elbow.

SHOULDER IMMOBILIZER

These commercially available devices maintain immobilization of the shoulder, humerus, and elbow by fastening the distal humerus and forearm to a strap that encircles the chest.

SUGAR-TONG SPLINT

This splint is used to immobilize fractures of the wrist and distal forearm, minimizing flexion/extension of the elbow and supination/pronation of the wrist. The splint is applied to the volar and dorsal surfaces of the forearm and hand, extending from the palmar aspect of the midhand around the elbow to the dorsal aspect of the midhand. Proper positioning should maintain 90 degrees of flexion at the elbow and slight extension at the wrist (Fig. 178–1). The splint should not impede flexion of the fingers at the metacarpophalangeal joint and should allow full range of motion of the thumb.

VOLAR SPLINT

This splint has limited applicability and has been largely replaced with prefabricated molds. The splint serves only to limit flexion and extension at the wrist. As a result of the

limited immobilization, volar splints should only be used for stable fractures, such as torus fractures or sprains.

THUMB SPICA SPLINT

This splint is used to immobilize injuries to the first proximal phalynx, first metacarpal, or scaphoid bone. There are multiple variations of a thumb spica splint; however, any variation should accomplish immobilization of the first metacarpophalangeal joint, metacarpal-carpal joint, and wrist. The splint is applied to the dorsum of the forearm and hand and encapsulates the thumb. Proper positioning should maintain slight dorsiflexion at the wrist, thumb abduction, and slight flexion at the interphalangeal joint, extending from the interphalangeal joint of the thumb to the proximal third of the forearm (Fig. 178–2).

LONG ARM SPLINT

The posterior long arm splint is used for the management of injuries to the elbow or proximal forearm. The splint is applied to the ulnar aspect of the forearm, extending from the distal third of the humerus to the midhand. Appropriate positioning maintains the elbow at 90° of flexion with slight extension or neutral positioning of the wrist (Fig. 178–3). The forearm may be maintained in either supination or pronation.

ULNAR GUTTER SPLINT

This splint is used to immobilize fractures of the fourth and fifth metacarpals. A variation of the splint, the radial gutter

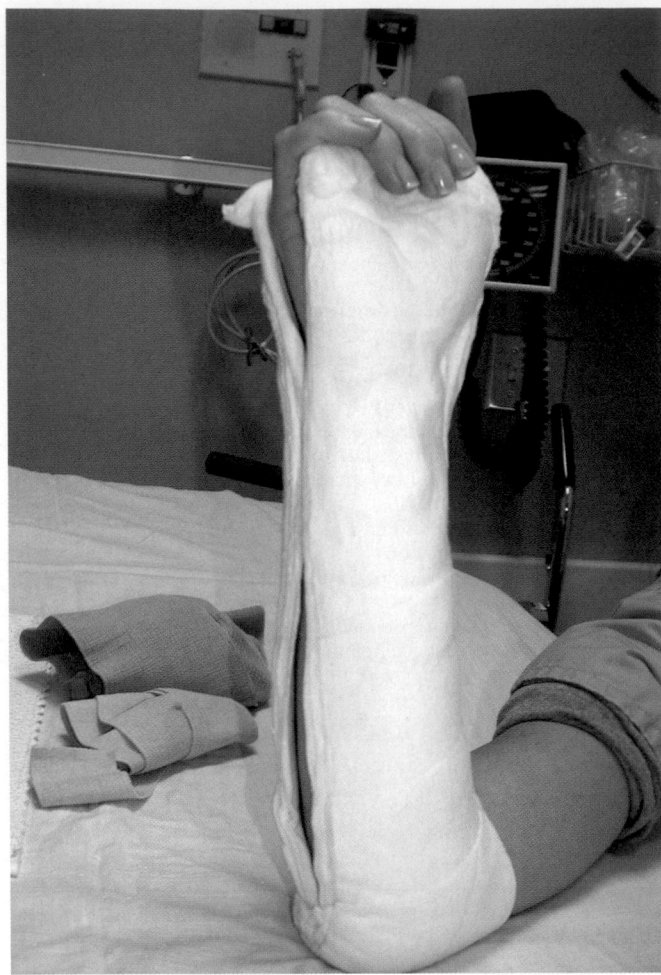

FIGURE 178–1. Sugar-tong splint.

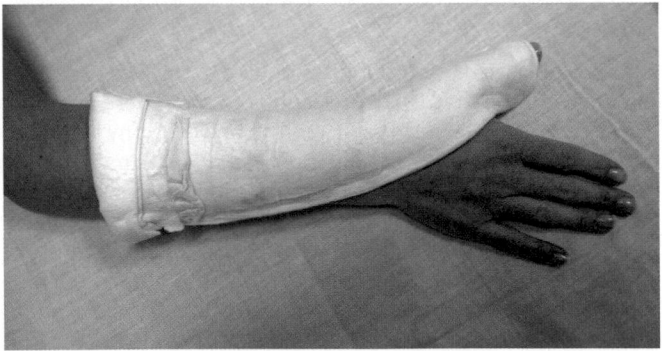

FIGURE 178–2. Thumb spica splint.

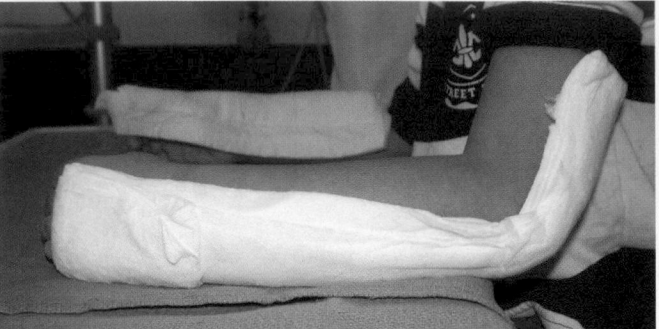

FIGURE 178–3. Long arm splint.

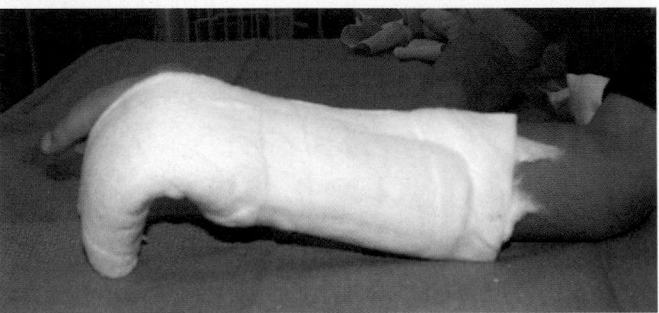

FIGURE 178–4. Ulnar gutter splint.

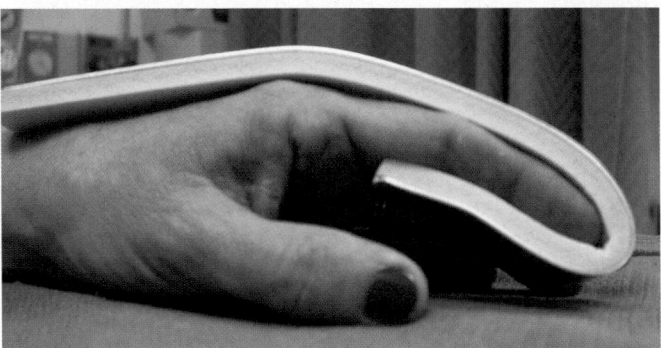

FIGURE 178–5. Finger splint.

splint, can be used for management of second and third metacarpal fractures. The splint is applied to the ulnar aspect of the forearm, extending from the tip of the fingers to the proximal forearm (Fig. 178–4). Proper positioning maintains slight flexion at the interphalangeal joints, 90-degree flexion at the metacarpophalangeal joint, and slight extension at the wrist.

FINGER SPLINT

Finger splints are available as commercially prepared products that are generally fashioned from aluminum and foam.

The splint is applied to the dorsal aspect of the finger, extending from the fingertip to the dorsum of the wrist. The proper positioning should maintain slight flexion at the interphalangeal joints (Fig. 178–5). Flexion contracture of the PIP joint is a frequent complication following ligamentous injury, especially after immobilization in more than 20 degrees of finger flexion.[21] Treatment of a mallet finger injury (avulsion fracture of the dorsal surface of the base of the distal phalanx) is slightly different, requiring hyperextension of the DIP joint only. Commercially prepared products are available or can be fashioned from aluminum and foam.

Lower Extremity

JONES DRESSING

Although not technically a splint, this bulky dressing does create substantial immobilization of the ankle joint. The dressing is fabricated from cotton and elastic bandages. The lower extremity is wrapped with cotton bandage in a bulky

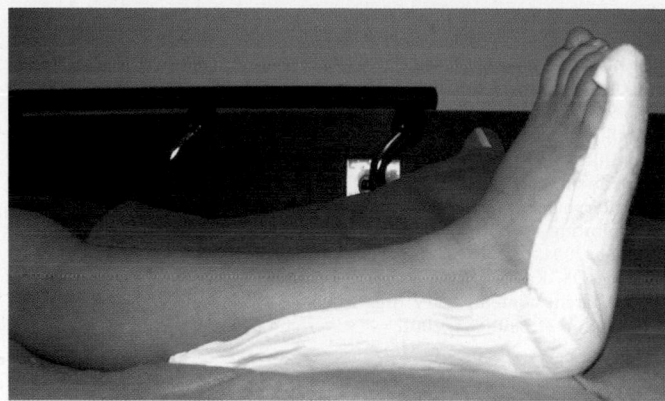

FIGURE 178–6. Posterior ankle mold.

fashion from the proximal aspect of the lower extremity to the forefoot. The cotton bandage is covered with a compressive, elastic bandage. Proper positioning will maintain 90 degrees of angulation at the ankle joint.

POSTERIOR ANKLE MOLD

This splint is used to immobilize injuries of the ankle, hindfoot, or midfoot. The splint is applied to the dorsal surface of the leg extending from the proximal third of the leg around the heel to the plantar surface of the forefoot. Proper positioning maintains the foot at a 90-degree angle to the tibia (Fig. 178–6).

Alternatives

The major alternative to splinting with either plaster slabs, prefabricated molds, or commercially prepared prefabricating splinting material is to place the injured extremity in a cast. Pinning and open reduction with internal fixation may be required if splinting/immobilization does not keep a fracture aligned appropriately.

Complications

Complications arising from application of a splint are uncommon. However, clinicians must be aware of the potential for problems such as pressure sores, allergic reactions, joint stiffness, infections, thermal burns, thrombophlebitis, compartment syndrome, and neurovascular compromise from a tightly fitted splint.

Compartment syndrome is a clinical condition characterized by elevated pressure within a confined fascial space causing circulatory compromise, swelling, and tissue necrosis.[22] Increased pressure within closed tissue spaces results from intrinsic or extrinsic factors. Intrinsic factors such as bleeding, soft tissue injury or swelling, tissue toxins, or venous stasis result in increased compartment size and pressure. Extrinsic factors such as constrictive dressings or casts, excessive traction on a fracture limb, or thermal injuries and frostbite exert compressive forces on the closed tissues and reduce compartment size (see Chapter 22, Compartment Syndrome).

Maceration of the skin caused by sweating may result in a breakdown of skin integrity, predisposing to bacterial or fungal skin infections. Pressure sores and skin necrosis typi-

cally result from extrinsic circumferential compression over inadequately or improperly padded bony prominences. Patients with complaints of persistent pain or burning under a splint should be promptly inspected for complications.

Postprocedure Care and Disposition

Discharge instructions should include recommendations for rest, icing, and elevation. In the first 24 to 48 hours, elevation and icing of the injured extremity will limit swelling and prevent untoward events. Patients with upper extremity splints should be instructed to use a sling for comfort and to maintain elevation of the fingers relative to the elbow. Patients with lower extremity splints should limit activity for the first 48 hours and utilize crutches for ambulation. Patients should be educated on the signs and symptoms of neurovascular compromise, and instructed to loosen the splint and return immediately to the emergency department for increased pain or tingling of the extremity. Patients should be encouraged to leave the splint in place until follow-up evaluation with a specialist.

As with any ED visit, appropriate follow-up should be arranged. Although no clear guidelines exist, patients with injuries that are likely to require operative intervention or further manipulation should be seen by an orthopedist within 48 hours. Stable, nondisplaced, nonangulated fractures and simple dislocations of the shoulder, patella, and interphalangeal joints may be re-evaluated within 1 week.

REFERENCES

*1. Ricci WM, Borrelli J: Teleradiology in orthopaedic surgery: impact on clinical decision making for acute fracture management. J Orthop Trauma 16:1–6, 2002.
*2. Kennedy RM, Luhmann JD, Luhmann SJ: Emergency department management of pain and anxiety related to orthopedic fracture care: a guide to analgesic techniques and procedural sedation in children. Paediatr Drugs 6:11–31, 2004.
3. Davidson JS, Brown DJ, Barnes SN, Bruce CE: Simple treatment for torus fractures of the distal radius. J Bone Joint Surg Br 83:1173–1175, 2001.
4. Shuster M, Abu-Laban RB, Boyd J: Prereduction radiographs in clinically evident anterior shoulder dislocation. Am J Emerg Med 17:653–658, 1999.
5. Hendey GW, Kinlaw K: Clinically significant abnormalities in postreduction radiographs after anterior shoulder dislocation. Ann Emerg Med 28:399–402, 1996.
6. Hendey GW: Necessity of radiographs in the emergency department management of shoulder dislocations. Ann Emerg Med 36:108–113, 2000.
7. Johansen K, Lynch K, Paun M, et al: Non-invasive vascular tests reliably exclude occult arterial trauma in injured extremities. J Trauma 31:515–522, 1991.
8. Plummer D, Clinton J: The external rotation method for reduction of acute anterior shoulder dislocation. Emerg Med Clin North Am 7:165–175, 1989.
9. Doyle WL, Ragar T: Use of the scapular manipulation method to reduce an anterior shoulder dislocation in the supine position. Ann Emerg Med 27:92–94, 1996.
10. Kothari RU, Dronen SC: Prospective evaluation of the scapular manipulation technique in reducing anterior shoulder dislocations. Ann Emerg Med 21:1349–1352, 1992.
11. McDonald J, Whitelaw C, Goldsmith LJ: Radial head subluxation: comparing two methods of reduction. Acad Emerg Med 7:715–718, 1999.

12. Coons MS, Green SM: Boutonniere deformity. Hand Clinics 11:387–402, 1995.

13. Rodriguez-Merchan EC: Osteonecrosis of the femoral head after traumatic hip dislocation in the adult. Clin Orthop Relat Res 377:68–77, 2000.

14. Cornwall R, Radomisli TE: Nerve injury in traumatic dislocation of the hip. Clin Orthop Relat Res 377:84–91, 2000.

*15. Yang EC, Cornwall R: Initial treatment of traumatic hip dislocations. Clin Orthop Relat Res 377:24–31, 2000.

16. Knee dislocations: management of the multiligament-injured knee. Am J Orthop 33:553–559, 2004.

17. Klineberg EO, Crites BM, Flinn WR, et al: The role of arteriography in assessing popliteal artery injury in knee dislocations. J Trauma 56:786–790, 2004.

18. Hinton RY: Acute and recurrent patellar instability in the young athlete. Orthop Clinic North Am 34:385–396, 2003.

19. Kumar A, Ahmed M: Closed reduction of posterior dislocation of the elbow: a simple technique. J Orthop Trauma 13:58–59, 1999.

*20. Burra G, Andrew JR: Acute shoulder and elbow dislocation in the athlete. Orthop Clin North Am 33:479–495, 2002.

21. Arora R, Lutz M, Fritz D, et al: Dorsolateral dislocation of the proximal interphalangeal joint: closed reduction and early active motion or static splinting—a retrospective study. Arch Orthop Trauma Surg 124:486–488, 2004.

22. Bae DS, Kadiyala RK, Water PM: Acute compartment syndrome in children: contemporary diagnosis, treatment and outcome. J Pedia Orthop 21:680–688, 2001.

Chapter 179

Ultrasonography

Barry G. Gilmore, MD and Jay Pershad, MD

Key Points

Bedside ultrasonography (US) in the emergency department is considered an extension of the physical examination.

The utility of ultrasonography in assessing blunt abdominal trauma in pediatric patients is currently limited by trends in nonoperative management for injuries that result in hemoperitoneum.

Ultrasonography can be used in the setting of cardiac arrest to detect the presence or absence of cardiac motion or cardiac tamponade.

Vascular access can be facilitated by US.

Ultrasonography can facilitate suprapubic aspiration when catheterization is unsuccessful.

Indications and Contraindications

Over the past decade, focused bedside ultrasonography (US) has gained wide acceptance as a tool for advanced trauma care by emergency physicians, and its use is now part of the guidelines for Advanced Trauma Life Support.[1] Currently, there are six main uses of US by pediatric emergency physicians: assessment of patients who have experienced blunt abdominal trauma, assessment of patients who are experiencing cardiopulmonary arrest, visualization of a target vein during vessel cannulation, identifying intrauterine pregnancy/exclusion of ectopic pregnancy (see Chapter 90, Ectopic Pregnancy), visualization of the bladder during suprapubic bladder aspiration or prior to urethral catheterization, and localization and removal of foreign bodies in subcutaneous tissue.

Bedside US is noninvasive and inherently safe for patients of any age. There are no contraindications to the performance of US except those related to interference with a lifesaving procedure (intubation, needle thoracostomy, etc.).

Preparation and Consent

Bedside US is a painless procedure that requires little patient preparation other than age-appropriate explanations, the heating of transducer gel, and, occasionally, patient positioning. Because bedside US is an extension of the physical examination and because virtually no risks are associated with this imaging method, no specific consent separate from the general consent for emergency care is required.

Equipment

Sonographic machines come in all sizes and shapes, from the large complex instruments commonly seen in radiology departments to small, shoebox-sized, handheld machines. Most machines have numerous options and abilities unnecessary for the evaluation of most cases in the emergency department. The primary requirements for a bedside instrument are portability to the bedside, a screen of sufficient size (5 to 7 inches) and resolution (64 to 256 shades of gray), transducers (also known as probes) of different frequencies (3.5 to 7.5 MHz), sufficient image storage, and a printer.

If the personnel operating the device have adequate training and experience, the main consideration in using the device is the selection of the appropriate transducer for the task at hand. The main shapes of transducers and their operating frequencies are listed in Table 179–1.

As the transducer frequency increases (3.5 to 7.5 MHz), the resolution or clarity of the screen image will improve. However, the depth of the sound waves' penetration into the tissue will decrease, and the deeper structures will not be visualized. The choice of the best transducer is based on the balance between clarity and depth.

Once US has been completed, the key images must be documented on continuous videotape or as static pictures or digital images. The ability to review images is essential in establishing and maintaining a program of continuous quality improvement and in providing feedback to trainees.

Monitoring

There is no specific additional monitoring required during US.

Techniques

Focused Assessment Sonography for Trauma

The purpose of focused assessment sonography for trauma (FAST) is to rapidly detect intraperitoneal fluid in patients who have experienced blunt trauma to the torso (see Chapter

Table 179–1	Types of Transducers and Their Features	
Transducer Frequency	**Shape of Transducer**	**Situations of Recommended Use**
3.5 MHz	Curvilinear (convex)	Adolescent/young adult blunt abdominal trauma
		Adolescent/young adult cardiac arrest
5 MHz	Curvilinear (convex or microconvex)	Infant/child blunt abdominal trauma
		Infant/child cardiac arrest
7.5 MHz	Linear	Vascular access
		Suprapubic aspiration
		Foreign body localization and management
5–7.5 MHz	Endovaginal (microconvex)	Intrauterine pregnancies
		Vaginal bleeding or cramping during the first trimester of pregnancy
		Pelvic pain

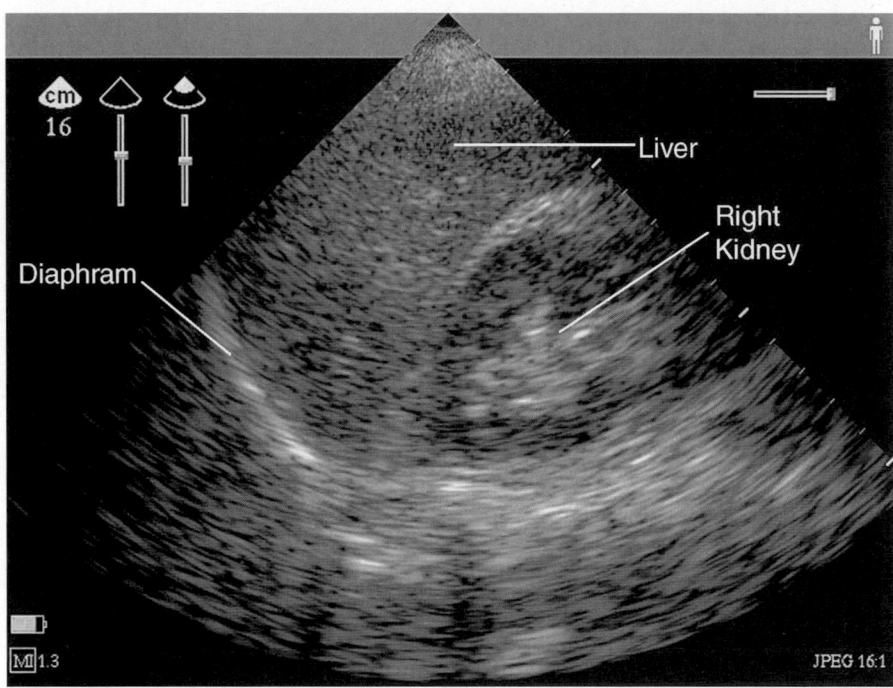

FIGURE 179–1. A positive FAST showing free fluid that appears as a black (anechoic) stripe between the liver and kidney (Morison's pouch). (From Rose JS: Ultrasound in abdominal trauma. Emerg Med Clin North Am 22:581–599, 2004.)

25, Abdominal Trauma). When conducted by trained emergency physicians, FAST has a sensitivity between 80% and 90% and a specificity between 95% and 100%.[2-5] Ultrasonography can consistently detect 200 to 650 ml of free fluid, whereas computed tomography (CT) can detect 100 to 250 ml.[5,6] FAST has greater sensitivity in the evaluation of hemodynamically unstable patients than in the evaluation of stable ones. In one study, US had 100% sensitivity and specificity in detecting hemoperitoneum related to intra-abdominal injury.[7]

FAST is usually performed immediately after the primary trauma survey and should not take longer than 3 to 5 minutes to complete. FAST is particularly useful for patients who are hemodynamically unstable, have an associated head injury or distracting injury that makes the physical examination unreliable, have progressive hypotension of unknown causes, or are unable to undergo CT.[8] Because of the current trend toward nonoperative management of parenchymal injury (with or without hemoperitoneum) in pediatric trauma patients, the exact role of FAST has been the subject of controversy.[9] However, US is easier to conduct in children than in adults, because children have smaller body habitus and less

mesenteric fat. Because of the dynamic behavior of abdominal injuries, serial US examinations can also be performed easily. For these reasons, FAST may assist in triage and prioritization of imaging studies for stable patients. At some institutions, protocols for blunt abdominal trauma recommend a careful physical examination, observation, and serial FAST for stable patients.[7,10] In standard FAST, four views are used: a subxiphoid view can reveal pericardial fluid, a right intercostal view can show fluid in Morison's pouch and the right paracolic gutter, a left intercostal view permits examination of the perisplenic space and the left paracolic gutter, and a suprapubic view permits examination of the bladder, pouch of Douglas, and uterus (Fig. 179–1).

Limitations and Technical Challenges

Several limitations and technical challenges are associated with FAST. First, the results of FAST are operator dependent. Second, FAST does not generally indicate the source of the intraperitoneal fluid or permit adequate evaluation of injuries in the retroperitoneum, bowel wall or viscus, pancreas, or renal pedicle. Third, FAST is often ineffective in visualizing the splenic recess, which is between the spleen and kidney, but visualization can be improved by placing the transducer at the level of the eight or ninth intercostal space along the posterior axillary line. Fourth, US may fail to detect free intraperitoneal fluid in some patients, because its collection depends on patient positioning. Placement of the patient in a slight Trendelenburg position may enhance the chance of detecting abnormal fluid collections, as will serial FAST.

Focused Cardiac Ultrasonography in the Setting of Cardiac Arrest

Focused cardiac US (C-US) is an important noninvasive bedside adjunct to the physical examination in assessing cardiac contractility and determining whether pericardial effusion is present. Emergency physician–directed echocardiography during cardiac arrest is used to diagnose pericardial tamponade and confirm (or refute) a diagnosis of pulseless electrical activity (PEA)[11-14] (see Chapter 1, Approach to Resuscitation and Advanced Life Support for Infants and Children).

A single subcostal cardiac view is included in the FAST protocol of the ATLS course.[1] Doppler echocardiography, which is a recommended component of the Pediatric Advanced Life Support (PALS) guidelines created by the American Heart Association, has been shown to distinguish true PEA from "pseudo" PEA.[15] The detection of cardiac activity by US may promote a concerted search for reversible causes. As a corollary, the absence of organized wall motion portends a futile resuscitation. Data from adult subjects in pulseless arrest suggest that bedside C-US discriminates apparent electrical asystole from underlying ventricular fibrillation, which is amenable to electrical countershock.[16]

The optimal technique for C-US involves the use of a cardiac transducer with an appropriate frequency (see Table 179–1). The subcostal or parasternal long axis view permits adequate assessment of pericardial effusion and wall motion (Fig. 179–2). The standard subcostal view requires placement of the transducer in the subxiphoid region, aimed extremely superiorly, with the beam directed toward the left side (i.e., with the imaging marker [notch] toward the left side). If the beam is directed to the right, the inferior vena cava entering the right atrium is visualized. The subcostal view is relatively easy to obtain in young children with a thin abdominal wall.

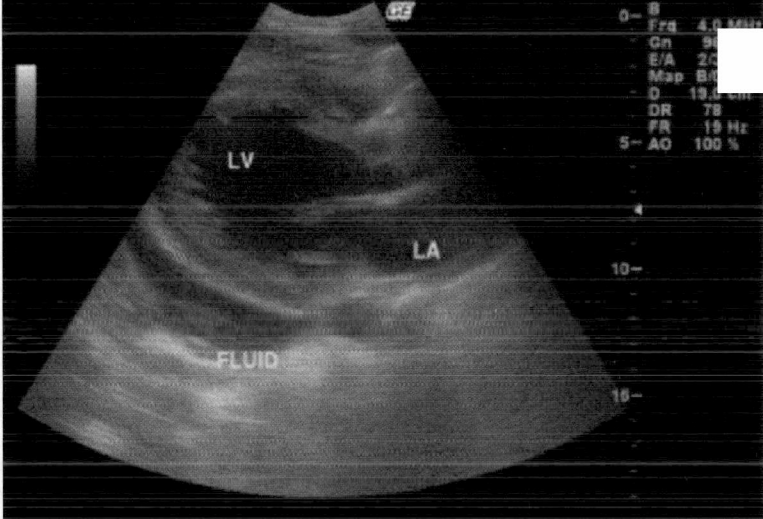

A

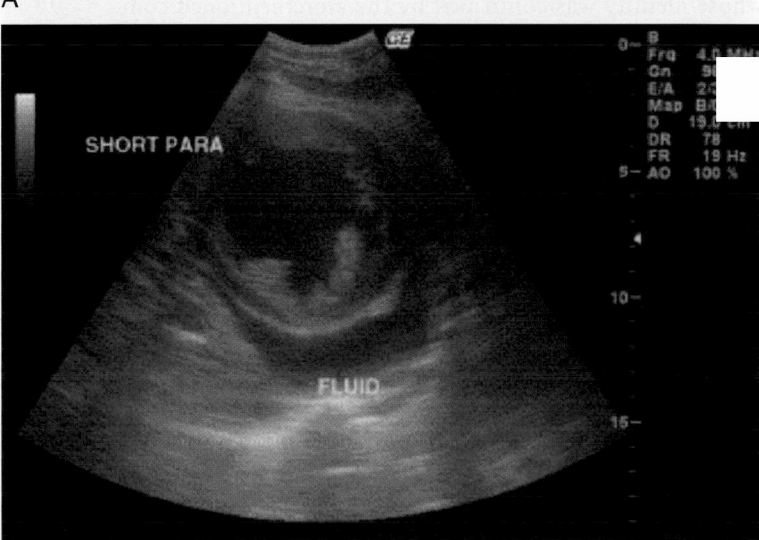

B

FIGURE 179–2. Focused C-US using the **(A)** parasternal long axis and **(B)** short axis views detected a large pericardial effusion (PE). Abbreviations: LA, left atrium; LV, left ventricle. (From Tang A: Emergency department ultrasound and echocardiography. Emerg Med Clin North Am 23:1179–1194, 2005.)

Ultrasonography in Attaining Vascular Access

Establishing central or peripheral vascular access in infants and children is a challenge, even in the best of circumstances. Compared with the traditional landmark-based practice, bedside US has the potential to significantly improve the speed and accuracy of vessel cannulation.[17] In 2001, the Agency for Healthcare Research and Quality cited ultrasonogram-guided central line placement as one of its 11 evidence-based practices that should be widely implemented.[18] To date there have been only a few studies of ultrasonogram-assisted venous access in children. Although limited by small sample size, these studies, which did not include emergency department patients, showed 85% and 73% reductions in the relative risk of failure and complications, respectively.[19-21]

Ultrasonography is most commonly used in the cannulation of the internal and external jugular veins, the subclavian vein, the femoral vein, and the brachial and cephalic veins, although theoretically any visualized vein could be cannulated[22,23] (see Chapter 161, Vascular Access). The two main methods of ultrasonogram-guided venous access (the indirect and direct methods) are described here.

Indirect Method

The indirect method is more commonly used than the direct method and provides less true "guidance." Once US has located the vessel of interest, a mark that corresponds to the vessel's location beneath the surface is made on the skin. The optimal situation is usually one in which the mark is between the center of the transducer and the center of the vessel of interest. Before cannulation begins, a "compression" test (one in which the operator applies light pressure to the transducer) should always be conducted to confirm that the vessel is a vein (which easily compresses) rather than an artery (which resists compression). The indirect method requires only one person to perform it and does not involve any special preparations or equipment such as a sterile transducer sleeve or sterile gel.

A variation of the indirect method is one in which two marks (one proximal and one distal, about 1 cm apart) are made on the skin above a vein that was located by US and whose identity was confirmed by the aforementioned compression test. This approach allows the person attempting cannulation to "connect the dots." When this variation of the indirect method is performed, the patient should be placed in the appropriate position for cannulation before the vessel is marked. Any movement after marking will change the location of the vessel.

Direct Method

In the direct method, US is used to directly visualize the placement of the needle in "real time." This method can be done with one or two operators, and requires different preparation and equipment than does the indirect method. A sterile sheath or cover whose tip is filled with transducer gel is rolled up over the probe and secured. Great care needs to be taken to ensure that the gel contains no air bubbles, which can distort the image. The transducer is placed over the selected area and the vessel located. If the image of the vessel is centered on the monitor's screen, the transducer can function as the directional guide. Once the skin is punctured, the needle can be visualized by its "ring-down" effect. Just before the needle enters the vessel, it will appear to "tent" or become temporarily deformed.[24]

The US transducer used to guide cannulation of a central or peripheral vessel should be a high-frequency (7.5-MHz) linear one. If unavailable, then the available probe with the highest frequency and smallest footprint should be selected. If a convex or curvilinear transducer is used, the image will be pie-shaped and its edges distorted. The orientation of the transducer (longitudinal or transverse) is a matter of preference and procedure. The longitudinal orientation gives information about depth and slope and helps with needle orientation, whereas the transverse orientation provides information about structures surrounding the vessel of interest.

Ultrasonography in Suprapubic Bladder Aspiration or Prior to Catheterization

Compared to urethral catheterization, suprapubic bladder aspiration (SPA) has an important advantage. The risk of contamination during SPA is minimal; therefore, urine obtained in this way yields fewer false-positive cultures. Moreover, when urethral catheterization is technically difficult, as in uncircumcised male neonates or female neonates with labial adhesions, SPA is useful. However, one limitation of SPA performed in the absence of real-time imaging has been the low success rate of the procedure.

Bedside US can serve as a useful adjunct to SPA. Bladder distention as well as position can be easily confirmed by this imaging method. In several studies, US increased the success rates of SPA: the lowest reported success rate in the absence of US was 36%, whereas the highest success rate of US-guided SPA was 100%.[25-28] Ultrasonography reduces the number of unsuccessful attempts of SPA; hence, the discomfort of patients is reduced.

In US-guided SPA, the transducer is placed in the transverse plane of the suprapubic area: the operator approaches from the midline of the pelvis and angles the transducer toward the patient's feet. The bladder will appear as an anechoic (black) structure. If the bladder appears distended, SPA can be performed relatively easily with very little risk to the patient (Fig. 179–3). A transverse diameter of the bladder greater than 3 cm has been associated with high success rates.[29]

Ultrasonography can be used to determine whether or not a bladder is full and if urethral catheterization will be successful in infants. A bladder index (anterior-posterior diameter × transverse diameter) greater than 2.4 cm^2 identifies infants with at least 2 ml of urine that can be obtained by urethral catheterization with near 100% accuracy.[30] When the bladder index is less than 2.4 cm^2, obtaining at least 2 ml of urine during catheterization is unlikely.

Ultrasonography in Foreign Body Localization and Management

The most common approach to locating foreign bodies in extremity wounds has been plain radiography (see Chapter 162, Foreign Body Removal). The limitation of plain radiography is that only radiopaque foreign objects (e.g., metal, stone, and glass fragments larger than 2 or 3 mm) are detectable.[31] However, US can overcome this limitation.

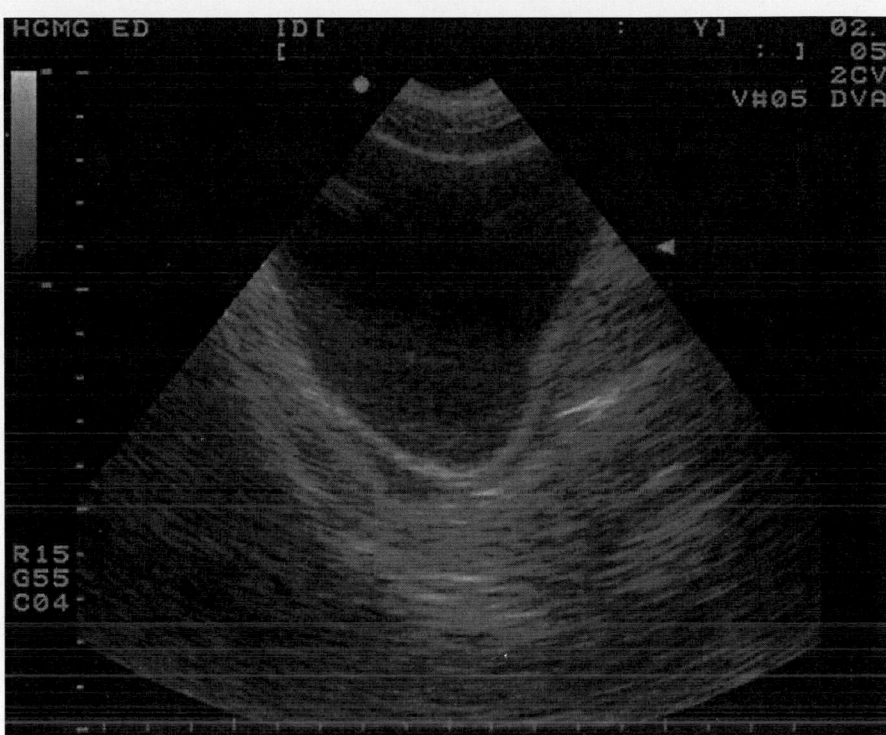

FIGURE 179–3. Suprapubic view of a distended bladder. (From Tibbles CD: Procedural applications of ultrasound. Emerg Med Clin North Am 22:797–815, 2004.)

Several clinical studies have demonstrated the utility of US in locating foreign bodies in extremity wounds.[32,33] What has also been shown is that the skill and experience of the clinician and the size of the object play significant roles in successful detection.[34] In general, a high-frequency (7.5-MHz or higher) linear transducer is preferred because most foreign bodies are usually less than 2 cm from the surface. If a lower frequency transducer, which focuses on deeper structures, is used, a stand-off pad can improve the device's ability to detect an embedded foreign object. Stand-off pads are "invisible" to the transducer and serve to raise it to a level where it can focus more closely on the tissue surface. These pads are available commercially or can be created by filling the finger of a glove with transducer gel.

Most foreign bodies are hyperechoic: metal appears to have a "comet tail," glass appears as a scattered "muddy" image, and rocks appear as "gallstone-like" images. Wood and plastic give fainter and less distinct images that are more challenging to detect.

Alternatives

Despite the convenience and immediate feedback that bedside US gives, it is unable to provide the necessary level of information regarding solid organ, hollow viscus, and retroperitoneal injuries. Hence, abdominal CT remains the imaging study of choice for stable patients with abdominal trauma.

Complications

Although patients may sustain complications from procedures conducted during US or from their overall clinical circumstances, complications directly attributable to US are essentially nonexistent.

Postprocedure Care and Disposition

Patients may require postprocedure care because of the nature of the procedure performed in conjunction with US, but there is no special care is required after US alone.

REFERENCES

1. American College of Surgeons: ATLS® (Advanced Trauma Life Support® for Doctors), 6th ed. Chicago: American College of Surgeons, 1997, pp 301–302.
2. Rowland JL, Kuhn M, Bonnin RL, et al: Accuracy of emergency department bedside ultrasonography. Emerg Med 13(3):305–313, 2001.
3. Akgur FM, Aktug T, Olguner M, et al: Prospective study investigating routine usage of ultrasonography as the initial diagnostic modality for the evaluation of children sustaining blunt abdominal trauma. J Trauma 42:626–628, 1997.
4. Liu M, Lee CH, P'eng FK: Prospective comparison of diagnostic peritoneal lavage, computed tomographic scanning, and ultrasonography for the diagnosis of blunt abdominal trauma. J Trauma 35:267–270, 1993.
5. Branney SW, Wolfe RE, Moore EE, et al: Quantitative sensitivity of ultrasound in detecting free intraperitoneal fluid. J Trauma 39:375–380, 1995.
6. Gracias VH, Frankel HL, Gupta R, et al: Defining the learning curve for the Focused Abdominal Sonogram for Trauma (FAST) examination: implications for credentialing. Am Surg 67:364–368, 2001.
7. Soudack M, Epelman M, Maor R, et al: Experience with focused abdominal sonography for trauma (FAST) in 313 pediatric patients. J Clin Ultrasound 32:53–61, 2004.
8. Scalea TM, Rodriguez A, Chiu WC, et al: Focused Assessment with Sonography for Trauma (FAST): results from an international consensus conference. J Trauma 46:466–472, 1999.
9. Coley BD, Mutabagani KH, Martin LC, et al: Focused abdominal sonography for trauma (FAST) in children with blunt abdominal trauma. J Trauma 48:902–906, 2000.
10. Holmes JF, Brant WE, Bond WF, et al: Emergency department ultrasonography in the evaluation of hypotensive and normotensive children with blunt abdominal trauma. J Pediatr Surg 36:968–973, 2001.

11. American College of Emergency Physicians: ACEP emergency ultrasound guidelines—2001. Ann Emerg Med 38:470–481, 2001.

12. Mandavia DP, Hoffner RJ, Mahaney K, et al: Bedside echocardiography by emergency physicians. Ann Emerg Med 38:377–382, 2001.

13. Milner D, Losek JD, Schiff J, et al: Pediatric pericardial tamponade presenting as altered mental status. Pediatr Emerg Care 19:35–37, 2003.

14. Plummer D, Dick C, Ruiz E, et al: Emergency department two-dimensional echocardiography in the diagnosis of nontraumatic cardiac rupture. Ann Emerg Med 23:1333–1342, 1994.

15. Zaritski AL, Nadkarni V, Hickey RW, et al: PALS Provider Manual. Dallas: American Heart Association, 2002, pp 127–147.

16. Amaya SC, Langsam A: Ultrasound detection of ventricular fibrillation disguised as asystole. Ann Emerg Med 33:344–346, 1999.

17. Hind D, Calvert N, McWilliams R, et al: Ultrasonic locating devices for central venous cannulation: meta-analysis. BMJ 327:361–367, 2003.

18. Agency for Healthcare Research and Quality: Making Health Care Safer: A Critical Analysis of Patient Safety Practices [Summary] (AHRQ Publication No. 01-E058). Evid Rep Technol Assess No. 43, pp i–x, 1–668, 2001.

19. Alderson PJ, Burrows FA, Stemp LI, et al: Use of ultrasound to evaluate internal jugular vein anatomy and to facilitate central venous cannulation in paediatric patients. Br J Anaesth 70:145–148, 1993.

20. Verghese ST, McGill WA, Patel RI, et al: Ultrasound-guided internal jugular venous cannulation in infants: a prospective comparison with the traditional palpation method. Anesthesiology 91:71–77, 1999.

21. Verghese ST, McGill WA, Patel RI, et al: Comparison of three techniques for internal jugular vein cannulation in infants. Paediatr Anaesth 10:505–511, 2000.

22. Nee PA, Picton AJ, Ralston DR, Perks AG: Facilitation of peripheral intravenous access: an evaluation of two methods to augment venous filling. Ann Emerg Med 24:944–946, 1997.

23. Keyes LE, Frazee BW, Snoey ER, et al: Ultrasound-guided brachial and basilic vein cannulation in emergency department patients with difficult intravenous access. Ann Emerg Med 34:711–714, 1999.

24. Donaldson JS, Morello FP, Junewick JJ, et al: Peripherally inserted central venous catheters: US-guided vascular access in pediatric patients. Radiology 197:542–544, 1995.

25. Gochman RF, Karasic RB, Heller MB: Use of portable ultrasound to assist urine collection by suprapubic aspiration. Ann Emerg Med 20:631–635, 1991.

26. Kiernan SC, Pinckert TL, Keszler M: Ultrasound guidance of suprapubic bladder aspiration in neonates. J Pediatr 123:789–791, 1993.

27. Munir V, Barnett P, South M: Does the use of volumetric bladder ultrasound improve the success rate of suprapubic aspiration of urine? Pediatr Emerg Care 18:346–349, 2002.

28. Ramage IJ, Chapman JP, Hollman AS, et al: Accuracy of clean-catch urine collection in infancy. J Pediatr 135:765–767, 1999.

29. Garcia-Nieto V, Navarro JF, Sanchez-Almeida E, et al: Standards for ultrasound guidance of suprapubic bladder aspiration. Pediatr Nephrol 11:607–609, 1997.

30. Milling TJ, Van Amerongen R, Melville L, et al: Use of ultrasonography to identify infants for whom urinary catheterization will be unsuccessful because of insufficient urine volume: validation of the urinary bladder index. Ann Emerg Med 45:510–513, 2005.

31. Ginsburg MJ, Ellis GL, Flom LL: Detection of soft-tissue foreign bodies by plain radiography, xerography, computed tomography, and ultrasonography. Ann Emerg Med 19:701–703, 1990.

32. Turner J, Wilde CH, Hughes KC, et al: Ultrasound-guided retrieval of small foreign objects in subcutaneous tissue. Ann Emerg Med 29:731–734, 1997.

33. Bray PW, Mahoney JL, Campbell JP: Sensitivity and specificity of ultrasound in the diagnosis of foreign bodies in the hand. J Hand Surg [Am] 20:661–666, 1995.

34. Orlinsky M, Knittel P, Feit T, et al: The comparative accuracy of radiolucent foreign body detection using ultrasonography. Am J Emerg Med 18:401–403, 2000.

Chapter 180

Pericardiocentesis

Robert Steele, MD and Andrea Thorp, MD

Indications and Contraindications

In an unstable patient, needle percutaneous pericardiocentesis is the treatment of choice for emergent drainage of a pericardial effusion causing hemodynamic decompensation.[1-3] In a stable patient, bedside ultrasound-guided pericardiocentesis is the preferred technique because of decreased rates of morbidity and mortality relative to blind needle pericardiocentesis.[2,4-7] Surgical techniques such as pericardiotomy, pericardial window, or thoracotomy for drainage of pericardial effusions are indicated when percutaneous pericardiocentesis has failed or the patient is hemodynamically stable enough to wait for surgical preparation and management.[1,2,8] The placement of a percutaneous drainage catheter (pigtail catheter) after pericardiocentesis is associated with higher morbidity and mortality but is indicated if the effusion is at high risk for reaccumulation.[2,9]

There are no absolute contraindications for blind needle pericardiocentesis in a patient with hemodynamic decompensation secondary to pericardial effusion.[10,11] Relative contraindications to pericardiocentesis include myocardial rupture, aortic dissection, and blood dyscrasias.[10,11] Blind needle percutaneous pericardiocentesis is relatively contraindicated when the patient is stable enough to tolerate the time needed to set up an ultrasound-guided pericardiocentesis.[2,9] Immediate thoracotomy is an important alternative in patients with penetrating injuries to the chest. An asymptomatic pericardial effusion can be medically managed with observation and fluids. Fluids should be the initial intervention as they help to increase preload and increase right atrial pressures, and may buy time while setting up for the pericardiocentesis. Dialysis may also be an appropriate alternate therapy in patients with renal failure.[12]

Patients with cardiac tamponade may present with shock, chest pain, abdominal pain, or dyspnea. Signs of cardiac tamponade include tachycardia, hypotension, tachypnea, narrow pulse pressure, and pulsus paradoxus.[13] The combination of Beck's triad (muffled heart tones, jugular venous distention, and hypotension) is uncommon in clinical practice (see Chapter 64, Pericarditis, Myocarditis, and Endocarditis).

Preparation and Consent

Prior to performing a pericardiocentesis, clinicians should assess anatomic landmarks and underlying factors that might affect the procedure. Prior chest or abdominal surgery or underlying lung disease might displace or alter landmarks. Patients with bleeding diatheses (e.g., coagulopathy, thrombocytopenia) may require fresh frozen plasma, platelets, or other factors prior to or concurrent with performance of the procedure. Placement of a nasogastric tube should be considered if there is abdominal distention, to reduce the possibility of abdominal trauma during the procedure.

All patients undergoing emergent pericardiocentesis require continuous cardiac monitoring, airway support, and supplemental oxygen. Rescue airway equipment and a defibrillator should be at the immediate bedside in case the patient deteriorates. While preparing the patient for pericardiocentesis, one or more fluid boluses with saline should be administered at 20 ml/kg. If the patient can tolerate the position, he or she should sit upright at 45 degrees to bring the heart closer to the inner aspect of the anterior chest wall and to make the fluid gravitate to a more dependent position. If patients are unable to tolerate sitting upright, they should be placed supine with the bed in a slight reverse Trendelenburg (head up) position. Emergency physicians with available bedside ultrasonography should prepare the machine with a sterile cover over the ultrasound probe. The anterior chest and xiphoid areas should be cleansed with an antiseptic solution (e.g., povidone-iodine or alcohol). The site of insertion should be as sterile as possible, with sterile towels draped around the insertion site. In the hemodynamically unstable pericardial effusion, blind needle pericardiocentesis should be performed immediately. Consent may be obtained if time permits, but medical intervention should take priority.

If time permits, bedside ultrasonography should be performed to confirm the presence and the size of the effusion. In this situation, verbal consent should be obtained from the parents and the pericardiocentesis should be performed under sterile technique with ultrasound guidance.

Equipment

Commercially available kits include sterile drapes, an 18-gauge angiocatheter needle, syringes in 10- and 20-ml sizes, a three-way stopcock, and an electrocardiogram (ECG) alligator clip. The essential equipment, if a kit is unavailable, includes an 18-gauge central line needle or Angiocath with a 20-ml syringe. Use of a 22-gauge spinal needle has been suggested for infants.[14] Protective gear such as sterile gloves, gown, and a face mask will be needed. A local anesthetic agent such as 1% lidocaine should be used, but additional systemic sedation for a young child may be needed. If a drain will be left in the pericardial space after the pericardiocentesis is performed, the additional equipment includes a floppy-tipped guidewire with a pigtail catheter. A bedside ultrasound machine should be used if rapidly available. If ultrasound or fluoroscopic techniques will be used to confirm placement of needle and catheter, agitated saline or contrast medium may be helpful.

Monitoring

The patient should be attached to continuous cardiorespiratory monitoring, with a member of the medical staff dedicated to monitor vital signs closely during the procedure. An ECG monitor should be readily available.

Techniques

Subxiphoid Approach

For the blind needle pericardiocentesis technique using the subxiphoid approach, the xiphoid process is located and local lidocaine is injected to the inferior and left of the xiphoid. The pericardiocentesis needle is inserted at a 30- to 45-degree angle to the chest wall and aimed toward either the substernal notch or the left shoulder (Fig. 180–1). The syringe is aspirated until fluid is obtained in the needle. Once fluid is obtained, the syringe is removed, the sheath advanced, and the needle removed.[10]

Parasternal Approach

With this technique, the pericardiocentesis needle is introduced in the fifth intercostal space, just lateral to the left border of the sternum, and directed 90 degrees from the skin. Autopsy studies of transthoracic pacemakers in adults show that this approach is less likely to injure important vascular structures (e.g., internal mammary artery) than an approach puncturing the fifth intercostal space 4 to 6 cm from the sternal margin.[15] However, this approach has not been studied

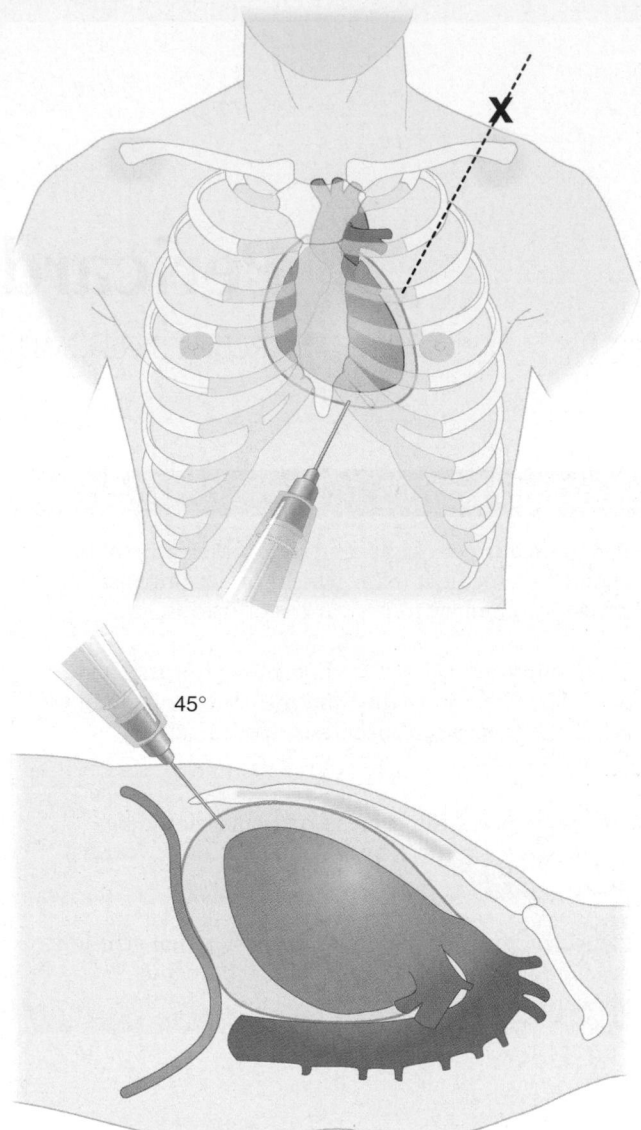

FIGURE 180–1. Subxiphoid approach of pericardiocentesis needle into the pericardial space.

in children and cannot be recommended unless anatomic or patient factors (e.g., scar tissue, trauma in the subxiphoid region) preclude use of the subxiphoid approach.

Alternatives

Many alternatives exist for this procedure. The clinical status of the patient, personal experience, and availability of equipment often dictate which technique is used.

Using the Commercially Available Kit

The three-way stopcock is attached to the needle, the 20-ml syringe to the side of the stopcock, and the transducer to the end of the stopcock. The V_1 ECG lead is attached with an alligator clip to the metal aspect of the needle. The needle is advanced as previously described until fluid is aspirated out the syringe. Ventricular wall contact causes ST-segment elevation, PR-segment depression, or premature ventricular beats. Atrial wall puncture causes PR-segment depression, atrial arrhythmias, and atrioventricular dissociation.[10] If any of these abnormalities is noted on the ECG monitor, the needle should be withdrawn and repositioned, and needle advancement repeated.

Ultrasound-Guided Procedure

Bedside ultrasonography can be used to confirm the location of the effusion and provide real-time visualization of needle advancement. The ultrasound probe is placed in the subxiphoid window or the anterior transthoracic window to view needle insertion. When the equipment is available to the emergency physician, this is the preferred method.[2,4-7] In a small child in whom the transthoracic echocardiographic probe would obstruct most of the field, transesophageal echocardiography has been described in the literature.[16] Echocardiographic evidence of cardiac tamponade includes right atrial compression, right ventricular collapse, or a swinging heart.[6]

Echocardiographic, Fluoroscopic, or Computed Tomographic Confirmation

If blood is aspirated during advancement of the needle or the placement of the needle is in question, 2 ml of agitated saline or contrast material (Echovist) can be injected under radiographic/ultrasonographic visualization.[17,18] If the contrast or agitated saline quickly dissipates, the needle is in the ventricle. If the contrast enhances the cardiac silhouette, the needle is in the pericardial sac. Once placement is confirmed, continued radiographic visualization is no longer necessary. Agitated saline can be obtained by attaching two 10-ml syringes filled with 9 ml of sterile saline and 1 ml of air to a three-way stopcock. Saline and air are rapidly injected from one syringe into the other via the three-way stopcock. This creates bubbles, or agitated saline, that can be injected into the pericardial space to confirm placement of the needle.[17,18]

Placement of Drainage Catheter after Pericardiocentesis

A soft-tipped guidewire can be advanced through the needle or Angiocath sheath and advanced until wrapping around the heart. A 5- to 7-French dilator is advanced over the wire. A 5- to 7-French pigtail catheter is then advanced and the guidewire is removed.

Surgical Techniques

The techniques available if pericardiocentesis fails or the patient is hemodynamically decompensating include thoracotomy, pericardial window, and single- or double-balloon pericardiotomy.

Complications

The complications depend on the technique being used. Blind needle pericardiocentesis has a high morbidity rate of 15% to 20%.[19,20] Ultrasound guidance in elective pericardiocentesis decreases the incidence of complication to 0.5% to 3.7%.[21,22] One of the most common complications in blind needle pericardiocentesis is puncture of a cardiac chamber. Inadvertent puncture of the left ventricle seldom, if ever, causes clinically significant bleeding. A puncture of the right ventricle carries an increased risk of bleeding due to the

thinner wall but rarely is clinically significant.[9,23] If there is a laceration of either ventricle or the patient becomes hemodynamically unstable, thoracotomy is indicated for surgical repair.[13] Inadvertent puncture of the coronary artery or vein is a rare complication of pericardiocentesis, and treatment of coronary perforation involves urgent surgical intervention.[13] Pneumothorax is also a rare complication that can be treated with placement of a chest tube. Acute left ventricular failure with pulmonary edema is seen when large effusions have been drained. This is due to the rapid increase in venous return to the left heart after the cardiac compression is released. Treatment involves draining the fluid slowly and monitoring the patient's fluid balance after the procedure. Ventricular or atrial ectopic beats are common, but serious arrhythmias such as PEA can occur and should be treated according to Advanced Cardiac Life Support protocols. Other complications include air embolism, pneumoperitoneum, supppurative pericarditis, and cardiac tamponade due to trauma. Using the presence or absence of "nonclotting blood" to determine if aspirated blood is from the pericardium or ventricle is inaccurate and has been disproved as a useful discriminatory technique.

Postprocedure Care and Disposition

After completion of the pericardiocentesis, the patient should continue on cardiorespiratory monitoring for arrhythmias and evidence of heart failure. Monitoring for symptoms of recurrent effusion accumulation is needed. If reaccumulation occurs, the emergency physician should either repeat pericardiocentesis or attempt a surgical technique.[1,2]

REFERENCES

1. Bastian A, Meissner A, Lins M, et al: Pericardiocentesis: differential aspects of a common procedure. Intensive Care Med 26:572–576, 2000.
2. Kirkland LL, Taylor RW: Pericardiocentesis. Crit Care Clin 8:699–712, 1992.
3. Markiewicz W, Borovik R, Ecker S: Cardiac tamponade in medical patients: treatment and prognosis in the echocardiographic era. Am Heart J 111:1138–1142, 1986.
4. Callahan JA, Seward JB: Pericardiocentesis guided by two-dimensional echocardiography. Echocardiography 14:497–504, 1997.
5. Callahan JA, Seward JB, Rajik AJ: Cardiac tamponade: pericardiocentesis directed by two-dimensional echocardiography. Mayo Clin Proc 60:344–347, 1985.
6. Cho BC, Kang SM, Kim DH, et al: Clinical and echocardiographic characteristics of pericardial effusion in patients who underwent echocardiographically guided pericardiocentesis. Yonsei Med J 45:462–468, 2004.
7. Salem K, Mulhi A, Lonn E: Echocardiographically guided pericardiocentesis—the gold standard for the management of pericardial effusion and cardiac tamponade. Can J Cardiol 15:1251–1255, 1999.
8. Allen KB, Faber LP, Warren WH, Shaar CJ: Pericardial effusion: subxiphoid pericardiostomy versus percutaneous catheter drainage. Ann Thorac Surg 67:437–440, 1999.
9. Tsang T, El-Najdawi E, Seward J, et al: Percutaneous echocardiographically guided pericardiocentesis in pediatric patients: evaluation of safety and efficacy. J Am Soc Echocardiogr 11:1072–1077, 1998.
10. Spodick DH: The technique of pericardiocentesis: when to perform it and how to minimize complications. J Crit Illness 10:807–812, 1995.
11. Kirkland LL, Taylor RW: Pericardiocentesis. Crit Care Clin 8:699–712, 1992.
12. Callam M: Pericardiocentesis in traumatic and nontraumatic cardiac tamponade. Ann Emerg Med 13:924–945, 1984.
13. Spodick DH: Acute pericarditis: current concepts and practice. JAMA 289:1150, 2003.

14. Anthony CL, Crawford EW, Morgan BC: Management of cardiac and respiratory arrest in children. Clin Pediatr 8:647, 1969.

15. Brown CG, Gurley HT, Hutchins GM, et al: Injuries associated with percutaneous placement of transthoracic pacemakers. Ann Emerg Med 14:223–228, 1985.

16. Chen TH, Chan KC, Cheng YJ, et al: Bedside pericardiocentesis under the guidance of transesophageal echocardiography in a 13 month old boy. J Formos Med Assoc 100:620–621, 2001.

17. Muhler EG, Engelhardt W, VonBermuth G: Pericardial effusions in infants and children: injection of echo contrast medium enhances the safety of echocardiographically-guided pericardiocentesis. Cardiol Young 8:506–508, 1998.

18. Watzinger N, Brussee J, Fruhwalk FM, et al: Pericardiocentesis guided by contrast echocardiography. Echocardiography 15:635–640, 1998.

19. Wong B, Murphy J, Chiang CJ, et al: The risk of pericardiocentesis. Am J Cardiol 44:1110, 1979.

20. Bishop LH, Estes EH, McIntosh HD: Electrocardiogram as a safeguard in pericardiocentesis. JAMA 162:264, 1956.

21. Duvernoy O, Borowiec J, Helmius G, et al: Complications of percutaneous pericardiocentesis under fluoroscopic guidance. Acta Radiol 33:309, 1992.

22. Tsang T, Barnes M, Hayes S, et al: Clinical and echocardiographic characteristics of significant pericardial effusions following cardiothoracic surgery and outcomes of echo-guided pericardiocentesis for management. Chest 116:322, 1999.

23. Chiang HT, Lin M: Pericardiocentesis guided by two dimensional contrast echocardiography. Echocardiography 10:465–469, 1993.

Quick Looks

Chapter 181

Headaches

A Quick Look at Headache

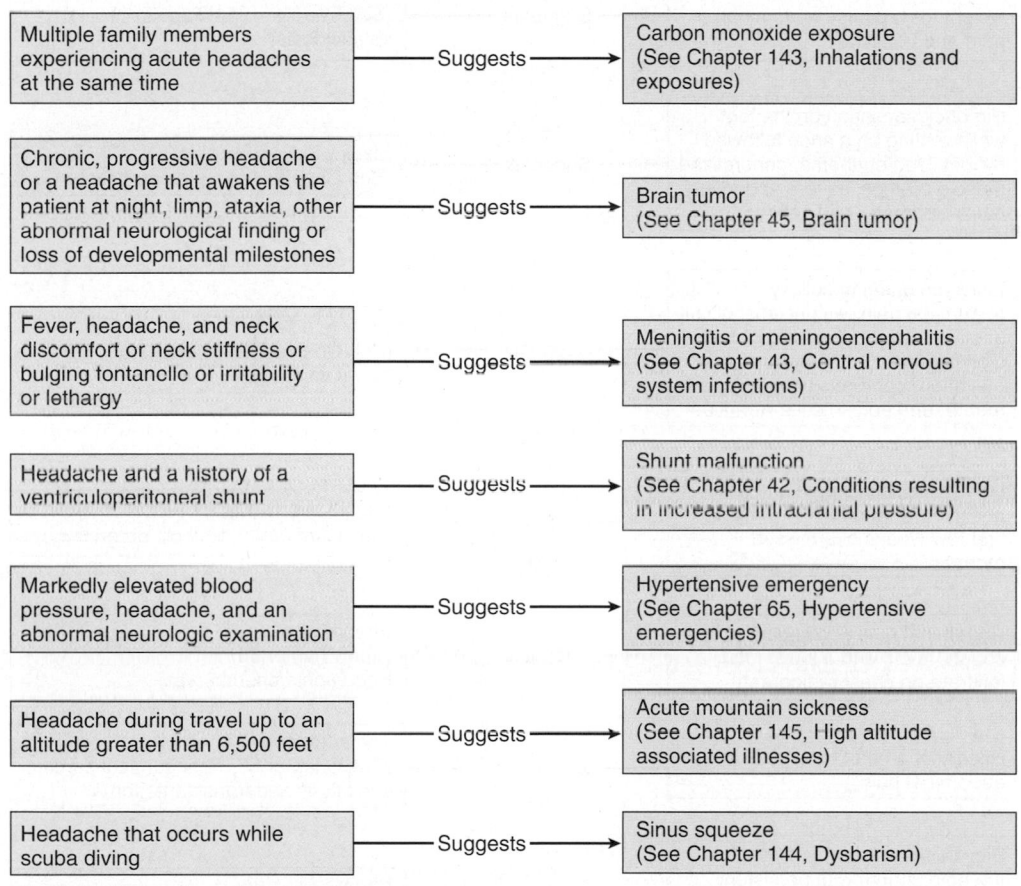

Multiple family members experiencing acute headaches at the same time	Suggests	Carbon monoxide exposure (See Chapter 143, Inhalations and exposures)
Chronic, progressive headache or a headache that awakens the patient at night, limp, ataxia, other abnormal neurological finding or loss of developmental milestones	Suggests	Brain tumor (See Chapter 45, Brain tumor)
Fever, headache, and neck discomfort or neck stiffness or bulging fontanelle or irritability or lethargy	Suggests	Meningitis or meningoencephalitis (See Chapter 43, Central nervous system infections)
Headache and a history of a ventriculoperitoneal shunt	Suggests	Shunt malfunction (See Chapter 42, Conditions resulting in increased intracranial pressure)
Markedly elevated blood pressure, headache, and an abnormal neurologic examination	Suggests	Hypertensive emergency (See Chapter 65, Hypertensive emergencies)
Headache during travel up to an altitude greater than 6,500 feet	Suggests	Acute mountain sickness (See Chapter 145, High altitude associated illnesses)
Headache that occurs while scuba diving	Suggests	Sinus squeeze (See Chapter 144, Dysbarism)

For information on common and serious causes of headache, please also see:
Chapter 17 Head trauma
Chapter 41 Headaches
Chapter 44 Central nervous system vascular disorders

Chapter 182

Abdominal Pain

A Quick Look at Abdominal Pain

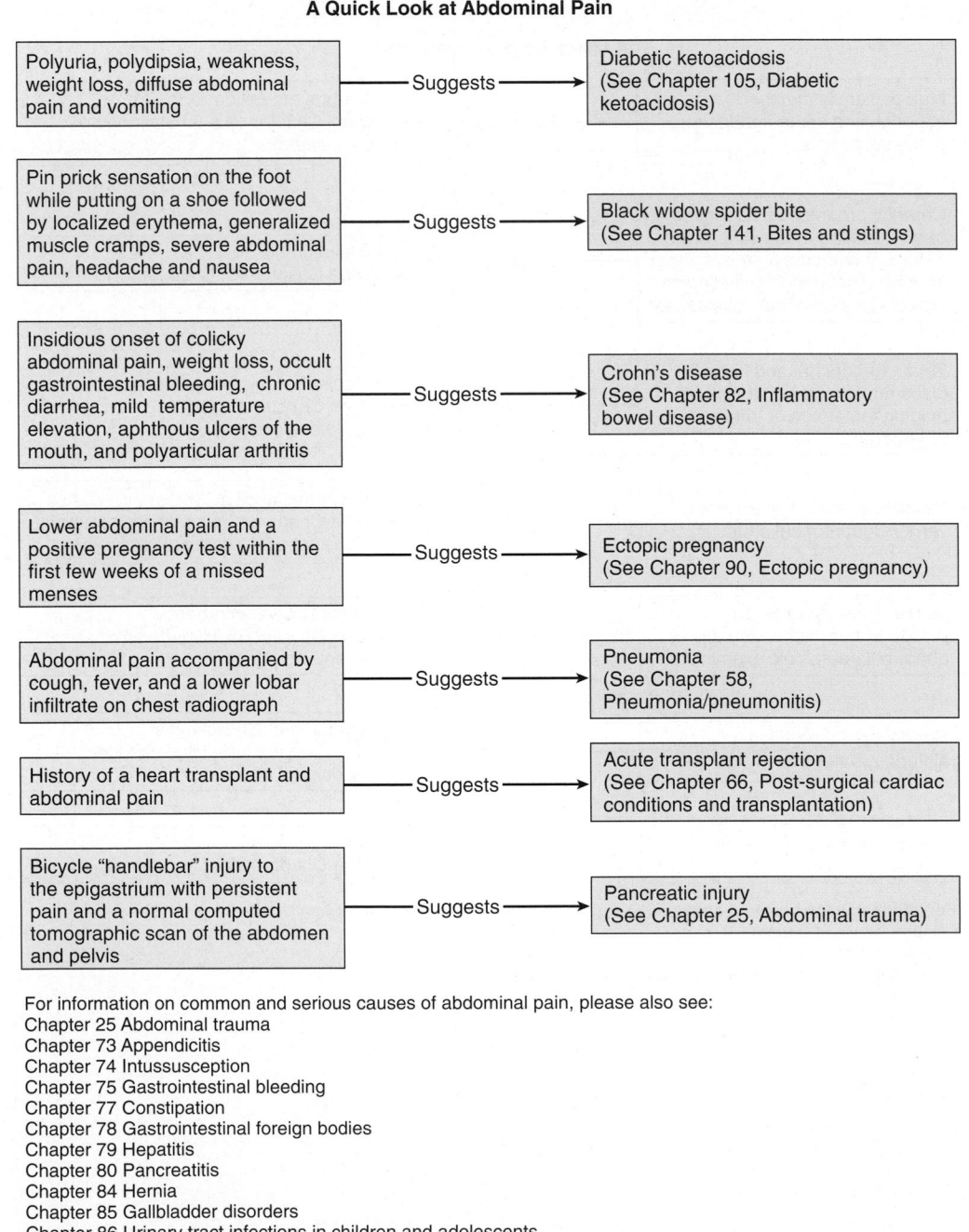

Polyuria, polydipsia, weakness, weight loss, diffuse abdominal pain and vomiting	— Suggests →	Diabetic ketoacidosis (See Chapter 105, Diabetic ketoacidosis)
Pin prick sensation on the foot while putting on a shoe followed by localized erythema, generalized muscle cramps, severe abdominal pain, headache and nausea	— Suggests →	Black widow spider bite (See Chapter 141, Bites and stings)
Insidious onset of colicky abdominal pain, weight loss, occult gastrointestinal bleeding, chronic diarrhea, mild temperature elevation, aphthous ulcers of the mouth, and polyarticular arthritis	— Suggests →	Crohn's disease (See Chapter 82, Inflammatory bowel disease)
Lower abdominal pain and a positive pregnancy test within the first few weeks of a missed menses	— Suggests →	Ectopic pregnancy (See Chapter 90, Ectopic pregnancy)
Abdominal pain accompanied by cough, fever, and a lower lobar infiltrate on chest radiograph	— Suggests →	Pneumonia (See Chapter 58, Pneumonia/pneumonitis)
History of a heart transplant and abdominal pain	— Suggests →	Acute transplant rejection (See Chapter 66, Post-surgical cardiac conditions and transplantation)
Bicycle "handlebar" injury to the epigastrium with persistent pain and a normal computed tomographic scan of the abdomen and pelvis	— Suggests →	Pancreatic injury (See Chapter 25, Abdominal trauma)

For information on common and serious causes of abdominal pain, please also see:
Chapter 25 Abdominal trauma
Chapter 73 Appendicitis
Chapter 74 Intussusception
Chapter 75 Gastrointestinal bleeding
Chapter 77 Constipation
Chapter 78 Gastrointestinal foreign bodies
Chapter 79 Hepatitis
Chapter 80 Pancreatitis
Chapter 84 Hernia
Chapter 85 Gallbladder disorders
Chapter 86 Urinary tract infections in children and adolescents
Chapter 91 Pregnancy-related complications
Chapter 92 Menstrual disorders
Chapter 93 Ovarian disorders

Chapter 183

Cyanosis

A Quick Look at Cyanosis

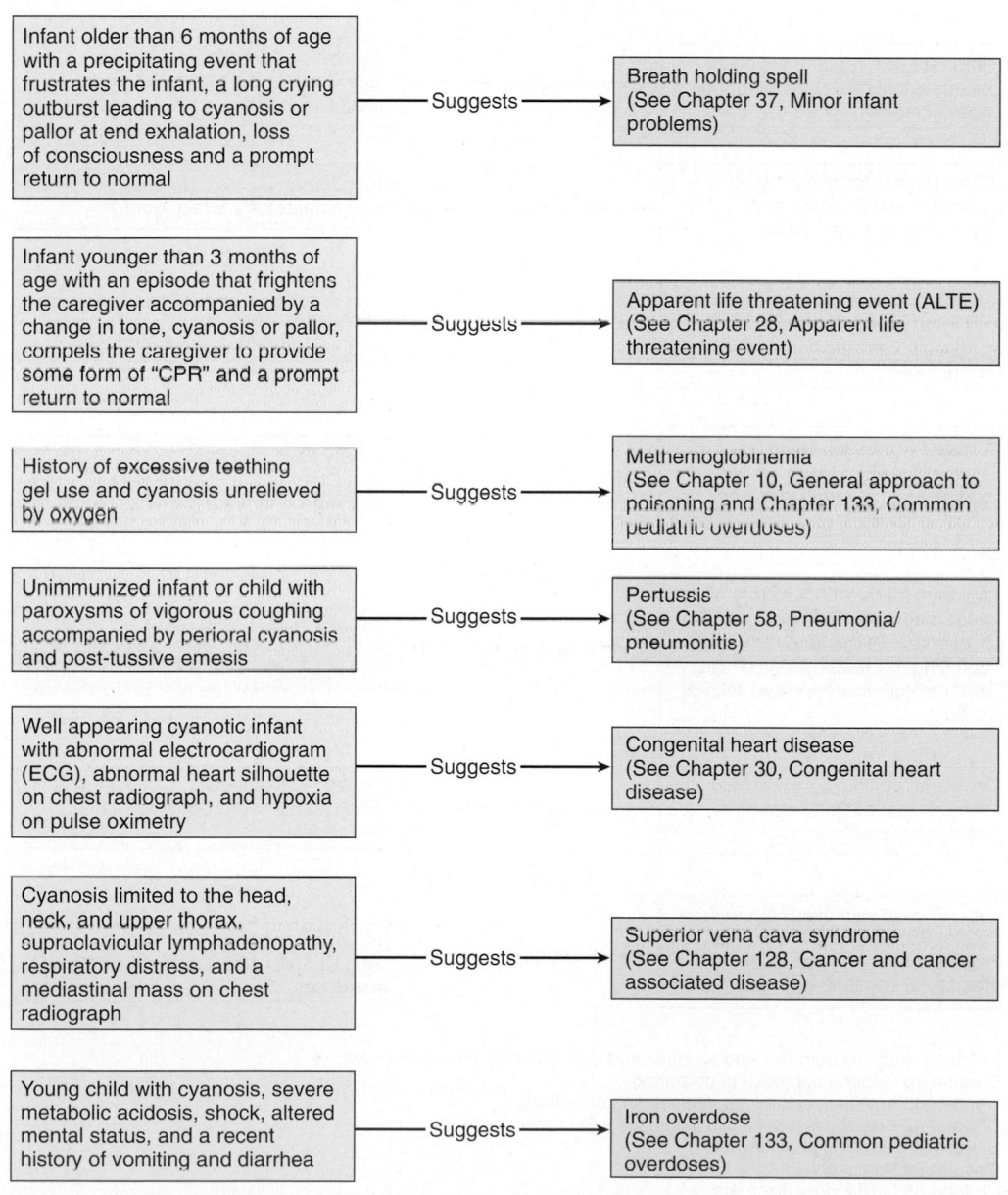

Infant older than 6 months of age with a precipitating event that frustrates the infant, a long crying outburst leading to cyanosis or pallor at end exhalation, loss of consciousness and a prompt return to normal	Suggests	Breath holding spell (See Chapter 37, Minor infant problems)
Infant younger than 3 months of age with an episode that frightens the caregiver accompanied by a change in tone, cyanosis or pallor, compels the caregiver to provide some form of "CPR" and a prompt return to normal	Suggests	Apparent life threatening event (ALTE) (See Chapter 28, Apparent life threatening event)
History of excessive teething gel use and cyanosis unrelieved by oxygen	Suggests	Methemoglobinemia (See Chapter 10, General approach to poisoning and Chapter 133, Common pediatric overdoses)
Unimmunized infant or child with paroxysms of vigorous coughing accompanied by perioral cyanosis and post-tussive emesis	Suggests	Pertussis (See Chapter 58, Pneumonia/pneumonitis)
Well appearing cyanotic infant with abnormal electrocardiogram (ECG), abnormal heart silhouette on chest radiograph, and hypoxia on pulse oximetry	Suggests	Congenital heart disease (See Chapter 30, Congenital heart disease)
Cyanosis limited to the head, neck, and upper thorax, supraclavicular lymphadenopathy, respiratory distress, and a mediastinal mass on chest radiograph	Suggests	Superior vena cava syndrome (See Chapter 128, Cancer and cancer associated disease)
Young child with cyanosis, severe metabolic acidosis, shock, altered mental status, and a recent history of vomiting and diarrhea	Suggests	Iron overdose (See Chapter 133, Common pediatric overdoses)

For information on common and serious causes of cyanosis, please also see:
Chapter 11 Altered mental status
Chapter 30 Congenital heart disease
Chapter 143 Inhalation exposures

Chapter 184

Vomiting

A Quick Look at Vomiting

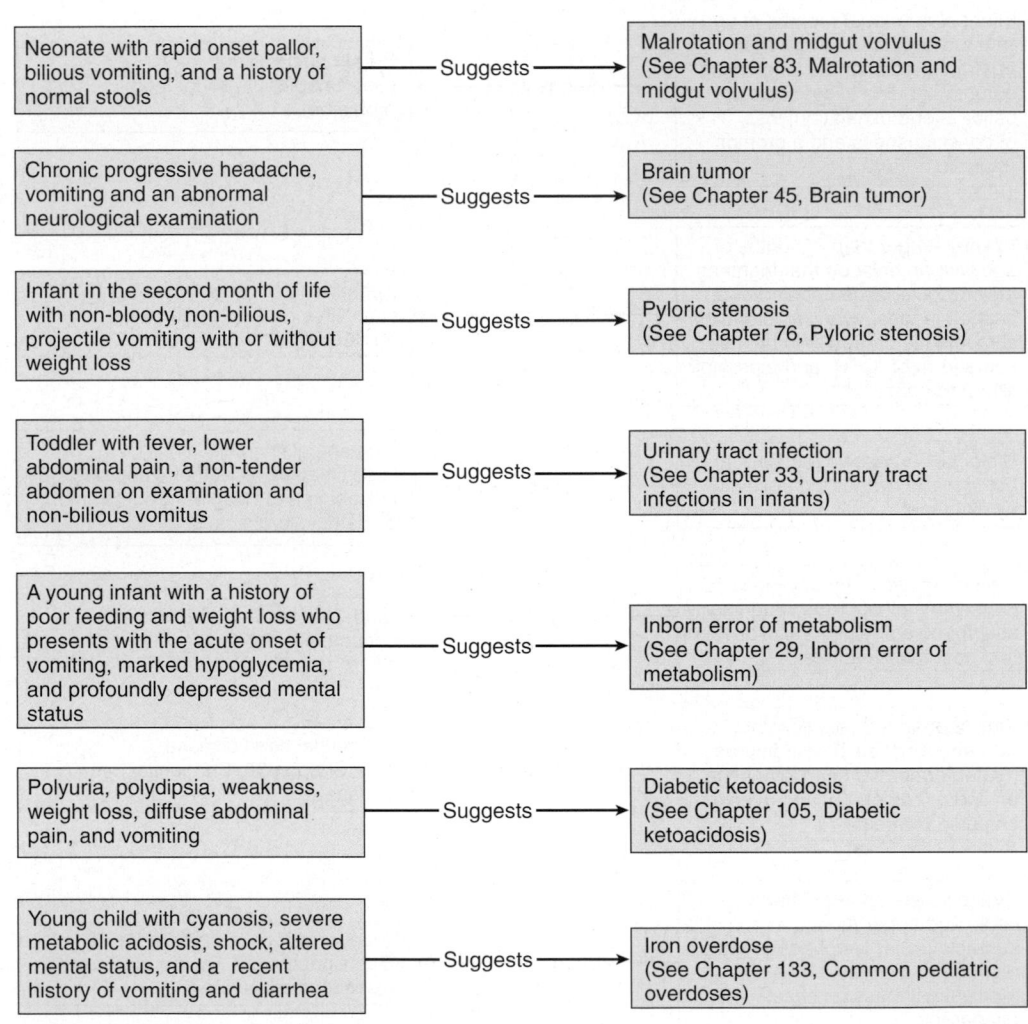

Neonate with rapid onset pallor, bilious vomiting, and a history of normal stools	— Suggests →	Malrotation and midgut volvulus (See Chapter 83, Malrotation and midgut volvulus)
Chronic progressive headache, vomiting and an abnormal neurological examination	— Suggests →	Brain tumor (See Chapter 45, Brain tumor)
Infant in the second month of life with non-bloody, non-bilious, projectile vomiting with or without weight loss	— Suggests →	Pyloric stenosis (See Chapter 76, Pyloric stenosis)
Toddler with fever, lower abdominal pain, a non-tender abdomen on examination and non-bilious vomitus	— Suggests →	Urinary tract infection (See Chapter 33, Urinary tract infections in infants)
A young infant with a history of poor feeding and weight loss who presents with the acute onset of vomiting, marked hypoglycemia, and profoundly depressed mental status	— Suggests →	Inborn error of metabolism (See Chapter 29, Inborn error of metabolism)
Polyuria, polydipsia, weakness, weight loss, diffuse abdominal pain, and vomiting	— Suggests →	Diabetic ketoacidosis (See Chapter 105, Diabetic ketoacidosis)
Young child with cyanosis, severe metabolic acidosis, shock, altered mental status, and a recent history of vomiting and diarrhea	— Suggests →	Iron overdose (See Chapter 133, Common pediatric overdoses)

For information on common and serious causes of vomiting, please also see:
Chapter 10 General approach to poisoning
Chapter 35 Vomiting, spitting up, and feeding difficulties
Chapter 42 Conditions resulting in increased intracranial pressure
Chapter 72 Vomiting and diarrhea
Chapter 80 Pancreatitis
Chapter 85 Gallbladder disorders
Chapter 91 Pregnancy-related complications

Chapter 185

Chest Pain

A Quick Look at Chest Pain

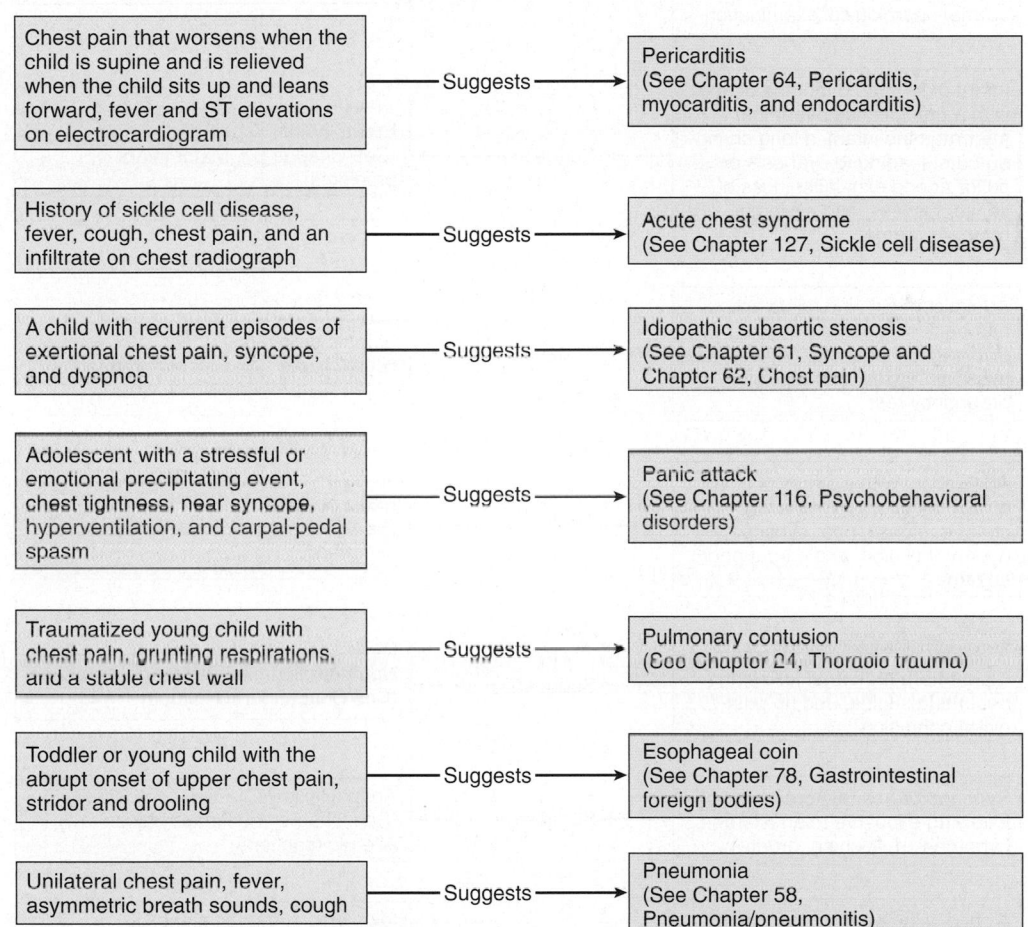

Chest pain that worsens when the child is supine and is relieved when the child sits up and leans forward, fever and ST elevations on electrocardiogram	— Suggests →	Pericarditis (See Chapter 64, Pericarditis, myocarditis, and endocarditis)
History of sickle cell disease, fever, cough, chest pain, and an infiltrate on chest radiograph	— Suggests →	Acute chest syndrome (See Chapter 127, Sickle cell disease)
A child with recurrent episodes of exertional chest pain, syncope, and dyspnea	— Suggests →	Idiopathic subaortic stenosis (See Chapter 61, Syncope and Chapter 62, Chest pain)
Adolescent with a stressful or emotional precipitating event, chest tightness, near syncope, hyperventilation, and carpal-pedal spasm	— Suggests →	Panic attack (See Chapter 116, Psychobehavioral disorders)
Traumatized young child with chest pain, grunting respirations, and a stable chest wall	— Suggests →	Pulmonary contusion (See Chapter 24, Thoracic trauma)
Toddler or young child with the abrupt onset of upper chest pain, stridor and drooling	— Suggests →	Esophageal coin (See Chapter 78, Gastrointestinal foreign bodies)
Unilateral chest pain, fever, asymmetric breath sounds, cough	— Suggests →	Pneumonia (See Chapter 58, Pneumonia/pneumonitis)

For information on common and serious causes of chest pain, please also see:
Chapter 24 Thoracic trauma
Chapter 56 Acute asthma
Chapter 62 Chest pain

Chapter **186**

Near Syncope/Syncope

A Quick Look at Near Syncope and Syncope

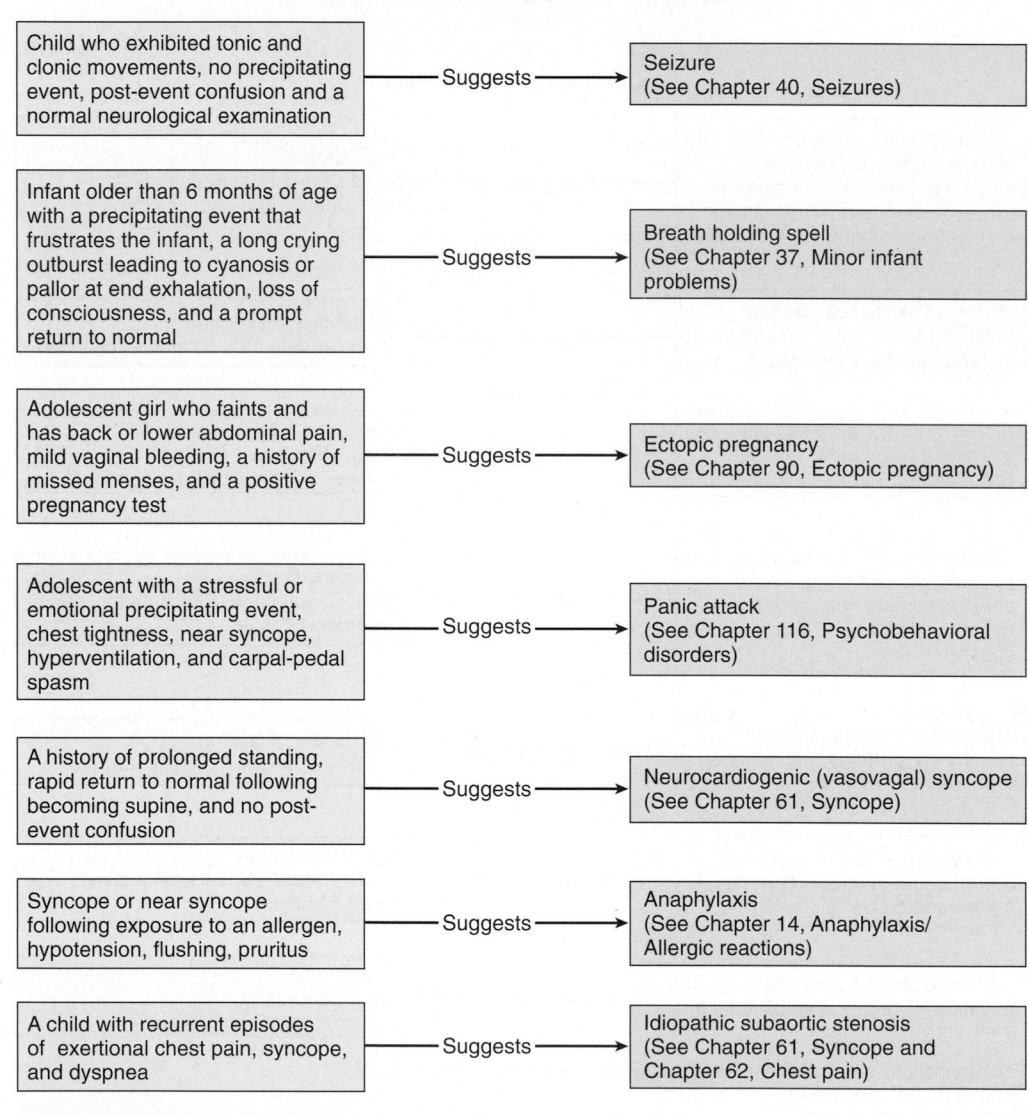

Child who exhibited tonic and clonic movements, no precipitating event, post-event confusion and a normal neurological examination	— Suggests →	Seizure (See Chapter 40, Seizures)
Infant older than 6 months of age with a precipitating event that frustrates the infant, a long crying outburst leading to cyanosis or pallor at end exhalation, loss of consciousness, and a prompt return to normal	— Suggests →	Breath holding spell (See Chapter 37, Minor infant problems)
Adolescent girl who faints and has back or lower abdominal pain, mild vaginal bleeding, a history of missed menses, and a positive pregnancy test	— Suggests →	Ectopic pregnancy (See Chapter 90, Ectopic pregnancy)
Adolescent with a stressful or emotional precipitating event, chest tightness, near syncope, hyperventilation, and carpal-pedal spasm	— Suggests →	Panic attack (See Chapter 116, Psychobehavioral disorders)
A history of prolonged standing, rapid return to normal following becoming supine, and no post-event confusion	— Suggests →	Neurocardiogenic (vasovagal) syncope (See Chapter 61, Syncope)
Syncope or near syncope following exposure to an allergen, hypotension, flushing, pruritus	— Suggests →	Anaphylaxis (See Chapter 14, Anaphylaxis/ Allergic reactions)
A child with recurrent episodes of exertional chest pain, syncope, and dyspnea	— Suggests →	Idiopathic subaortic stenosis (See Chapter 61, Syncope and Chapter 62, Chest pain)

For information on common and serious causes of syncope, please also see:
Chapter 10 General approach to poisoning
Chapter 11 Altered mental status
Chapter 17 Head trauma
Chapter 28 Apparent life-threatening events
Chapter 44 Central nervous system vascular disorders
Chapter 61 Syncope
Chapter 63 Dysrhythmias
Chapter 67 Valvular heart disease
Chapter 106 Hypoglycemia
Chapter 110 Dehydration and disorders of sodium balance
Chapter 134 Toxic alcohols
Chapter 137 Cardiovascular agents
Chapter 139 Hyperthermia

Chapter 187

Muscular Weakness/Paralysis

A Quick Look at Muscular Weakness and Paralysis

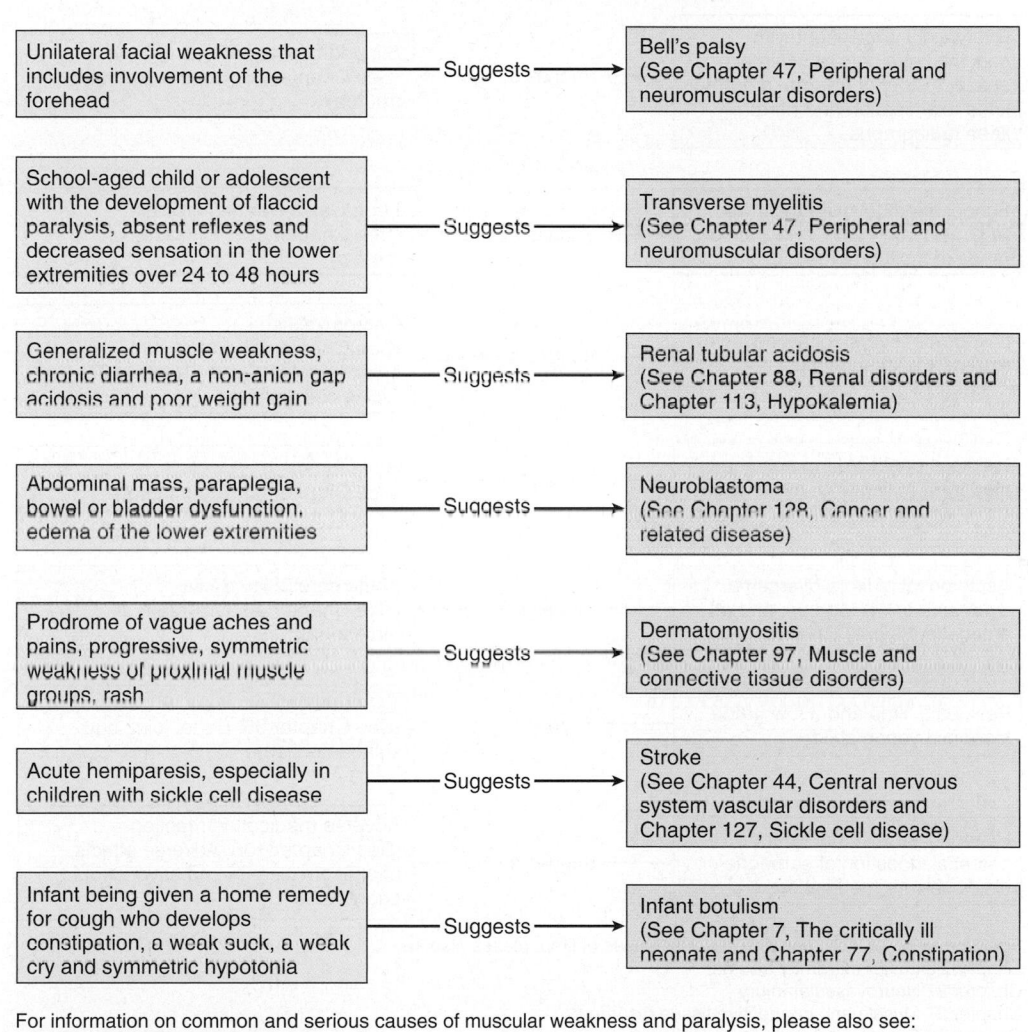

Unilateral facial weakness that includes involvement of the forehead	— Suggests →	Bell's palsy (See Chapter 47, Peripheral and neuromuscular disorders)
School-aged child or adolescent with the development of flaccid paralysis, absent reflexes and decreased sensation in the lower extremities over 24 to 48 hours	— Suggests →	Transverse myelitis (See Chapter 47, Peripheral and neuromuscular disorders)
Generalized muscle weakness, chronic diarrhea, a non-anion gap acidosis and poor weight gain	— Suggests →	Renal tubular acidosis (See Chapter 88, Renal disorders and Chapter 113, Hypokalemia)
Abdominal mass, paraplegia, bowel or bladder dysfunction, edema of the lower extremities	— Suggests →	Neuroblastoma (See Chapter 128, Cancer and related disease)
Prodrome of vague aches and pains, progressive, symmetric weakness of proximal muscle groups, rash	— Suggests →	Dermatomyositis (See Chapter 97, Muscle and connective tissue disorders)
Acute hemiparesis, especially in children with sickle cell disease	— Suggests →	Stroke (See Chapter 44, Central nervous system vascular disorders and Chapter 127, Sickle cell disease)
Infant being given a home remedy for cough who develops constipation, a weak suck, a weak cry and symmetric hypotonia	— Suggests →	Infant botulism (See Chapter 7, The critically ill neonate and Chapter 77, Constipation)

For information on common and serious causes of muscular weakness and paralysis, please also see:
Chapter 19 Upper extremity trauma
Chapter 20 Lower extremity trauma
Chapter 22 Compartment syndrome
Chapter 23 Spinal trauma
Chapter 27 Neurovascular injuries
Chapter 40 Seizures
Chapter 44 Central nervous system vascular disorders
Chapter 46 Disorders of movement
Chapter 47 Peripheral and neuromuscular disorders
Chapter 99 Rhabdomyolysis
Chapter 107 The steroid dependent child
Chapter 116 Psychobehavioral disorders

Chapter 188

Limp

A Quick Look at Limp

Overweight adolescent with nagging knee pain, a minimal or absent history of trauma, a normal knee examination and normal knee radiographs	— Suggests — →	Slipped-capital femoral epiphysis (See Chapter 20, Lower extremity trauma)
School-aged boy with a chronic limp, mild thigh pain, and limited range of motion at the hip	— Suggests — →	Legg-Calvé-Perthes disease (See Chapter 100, Diseases of the hip)
Low-grade fevers, localized lower extremity pain and limp	— Suggests — →	Osteomyelitis (See Chapter 96, Bone, joint, and spine infections and Chapter 127, Sickle cell disease)
Insidious onset of limp accompanied by vomiting and headaches	— Suggests — →	Brain tumor (See Chapter 45, Brain tumor)
Acute onset of limp, dysmetria, dysarthria or nystagmus, and an antecedent febrile illness	— Suggests — →	Acute cerebellar ataxia (See Chapter 46, Disorders of movement)
Back pain, limp and a low grade fever in a young child	— Suggests — →	Vertebral osteomyelitis or discitis (See Chapter 96, Bone, joint, and spine infections)
History of seizure disorder or potential ingestion of someone else's seizure medication	— Suggests — →	Adverse medication reaction (See Chapter 136, Adverse effects of anticonvulsants and psychotropic agents)

For information on common and serious causes of limp, please also see:
Chapter 20 Lower extremity trauma
Chapter 27 Neurovascular injury
Chapter 97 Muscle and connective tissue disorders
Chapter 98 Overuse syndromes and inflammatory conditions

Chapter 189

Lymphadenopathy

A Quick Look at Lymphadenopathy

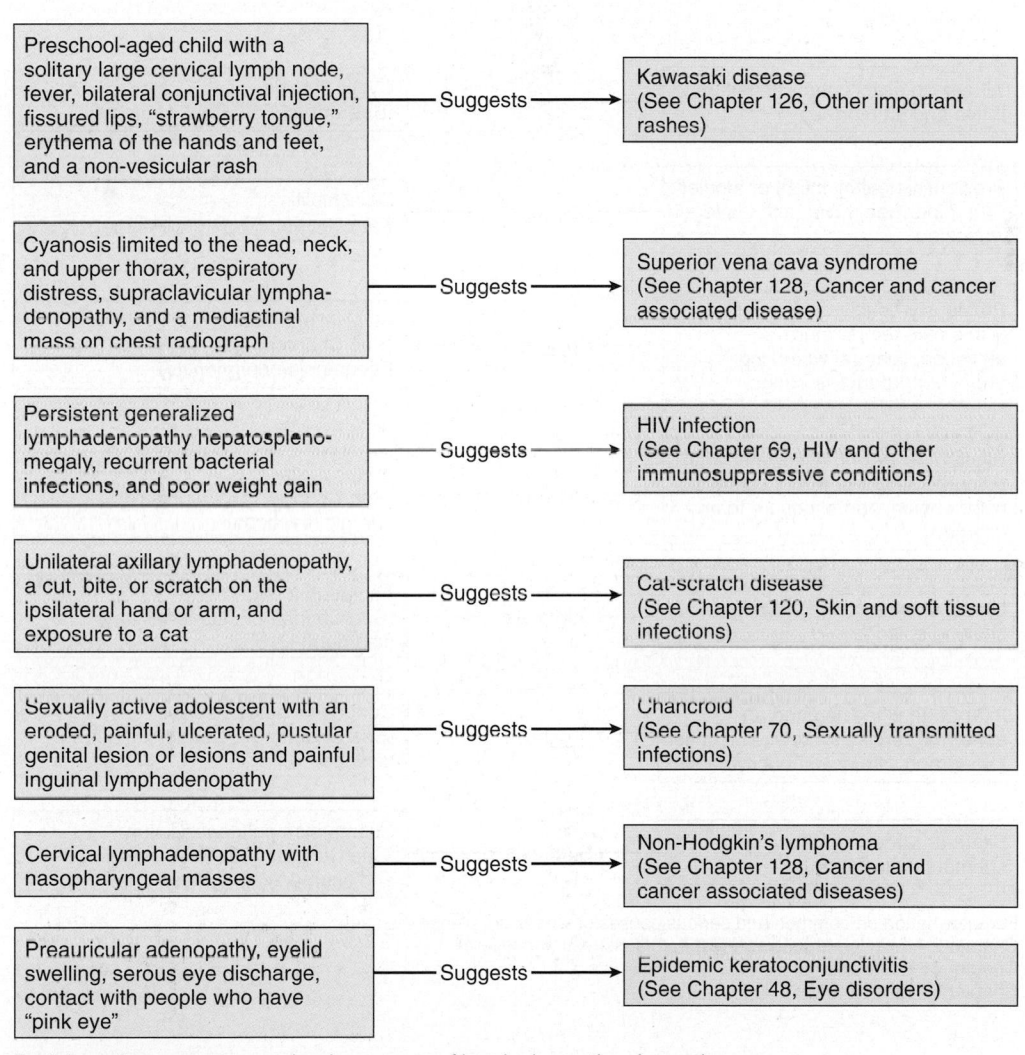

Preschool-aged child with a solitary large cervical lymph node, fever, bilateral conjunctival injection, fissured lips, "strawberry tongue," erythema of the hands and feet, and a non-vesicular rash	Suggests	Kawasaki disease (See Chapter 126, Other important rashes)
Cyanosis limited to the head, neck, and upper thorax, respiratory distress, supraclavicular lymphadenopathy, and a mediastinal mass on chest radiograph	Suggests	Superior vena cava syndrome (See Chapter 128, Cancer and cancer associated disease)
Persistent generalized lymphadenopathy hepatosplenomegaly, recurrent bacterial infections, and poor weight gain	Suggests	HIV infection (See Chapter 69, HIV and other immunosuppressive conditions)
Unilateral axillary lymphadenopathy, a cut, bite, or scratch on the ipsilateral hand or arm, and exposure to a cat	Suggests	Cat-scratch disease (See Chapter 120, Skin and soft tissue infections)
Sexually active adolescent with an eroded, painful, ulcerated, pustular genital lesion or lesions and painful inguinal lymphadenopathy	Suggests	Chancroid (See Chapter 70, Sexually transmitted infections)
Cervical lymphadenopathy with nasopharyngeal masses	Suggests	Non-Hodgkin's lymphoma (See Chapter 128, Cancer and cancer associated diseases)
Preauricular adenopathy, eyelid swelling, serous eye discharge, contact with people who have "pink eye"	Suggests	Epidemic keratoconjunctivitis (See Chapter 48, Eye disorders)

For information on common and serious causes of lymphadenopathy, please also see:
Chapter 54 Neck infections
Chapter 55 Neck masses
Chapter 71 Selected infectious diseases
Chapter 128 Cancer and cancer associated disease

Chapter 190

Wheezing

A Quick Look at Wheezing

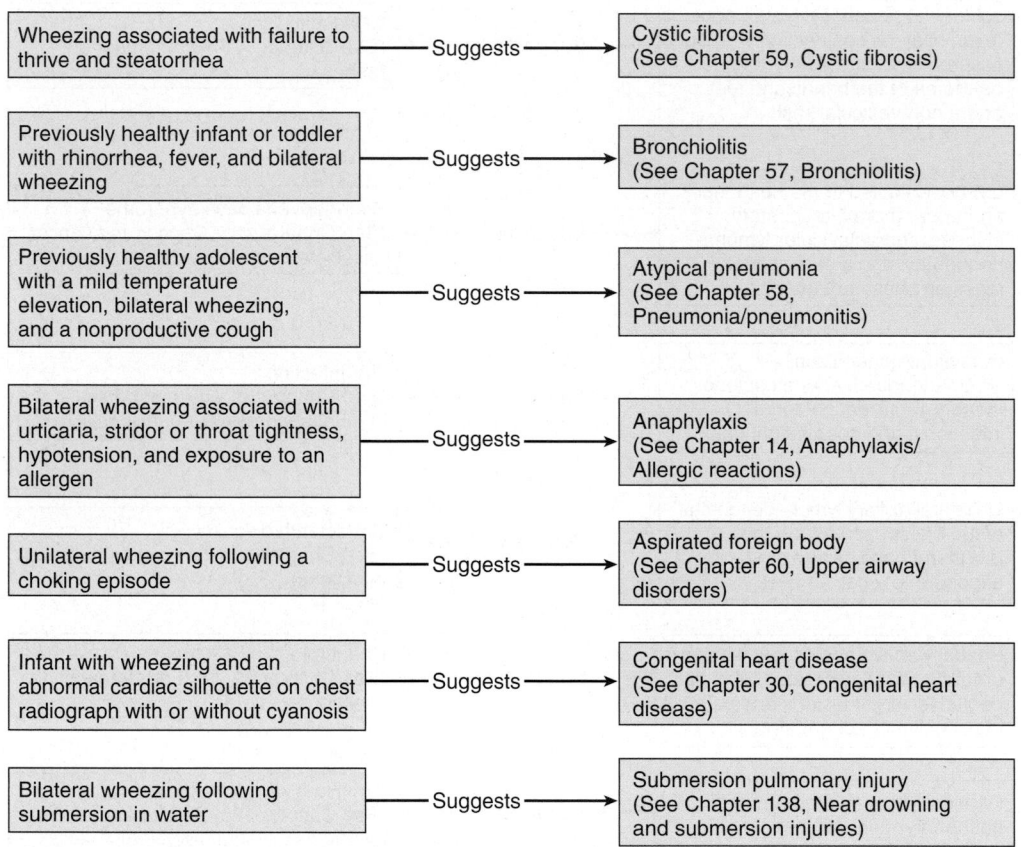

Wheezing associated with failure to thrive and steatorrhea	Suggests	Cystic fibrosis (See Chapter 59, Cystic fibrosis)
Previously healthy infant or toddler with rhinorrhea, fever, and bilateral wheezing	Suggests	Bronchiolitis (See Chapter 57, Bronchiolitis)
Previously healthy adolescent with a mild temperature elevation, bilateral wheezing, and a nonproductive cough	Suggests	Atypical pneumonia (See Chapter 58, Pneumonia/pneumonitis)
Bilateral wheezing associated with urticaria, stridor or throat tightness, hypotension, and exposure to an allergen	Suggests	Anaphylaxis (See Chapter 14, Anaphylaxis/ Allergic reactions)
Unilateral wheezing following a choking episode	Suggests	Aspirated foreign body (See Chapter 60, Upper airway disorders)
Infant with wheezing and an abnormal cardiac silhouette on chest radiograph with or without cyanosis	Suggests	Congenital heart disease (See Chapter 30, Congenital heart disease)
Bilateral wheezing following submersion in water	Suggests	Submersion pulmonary injury (See Chapter 138, Near drowning and submersion injuries)

For information on common and serious causes of wheezing, please also see:
Chapter 2 Airway emergencies: Respiratory distress and failure
Chapter 56 Acute asthma
Chapter 57 Bronchiolitis

Chapter 191

Hematuria

A Quick Look at Hematuria

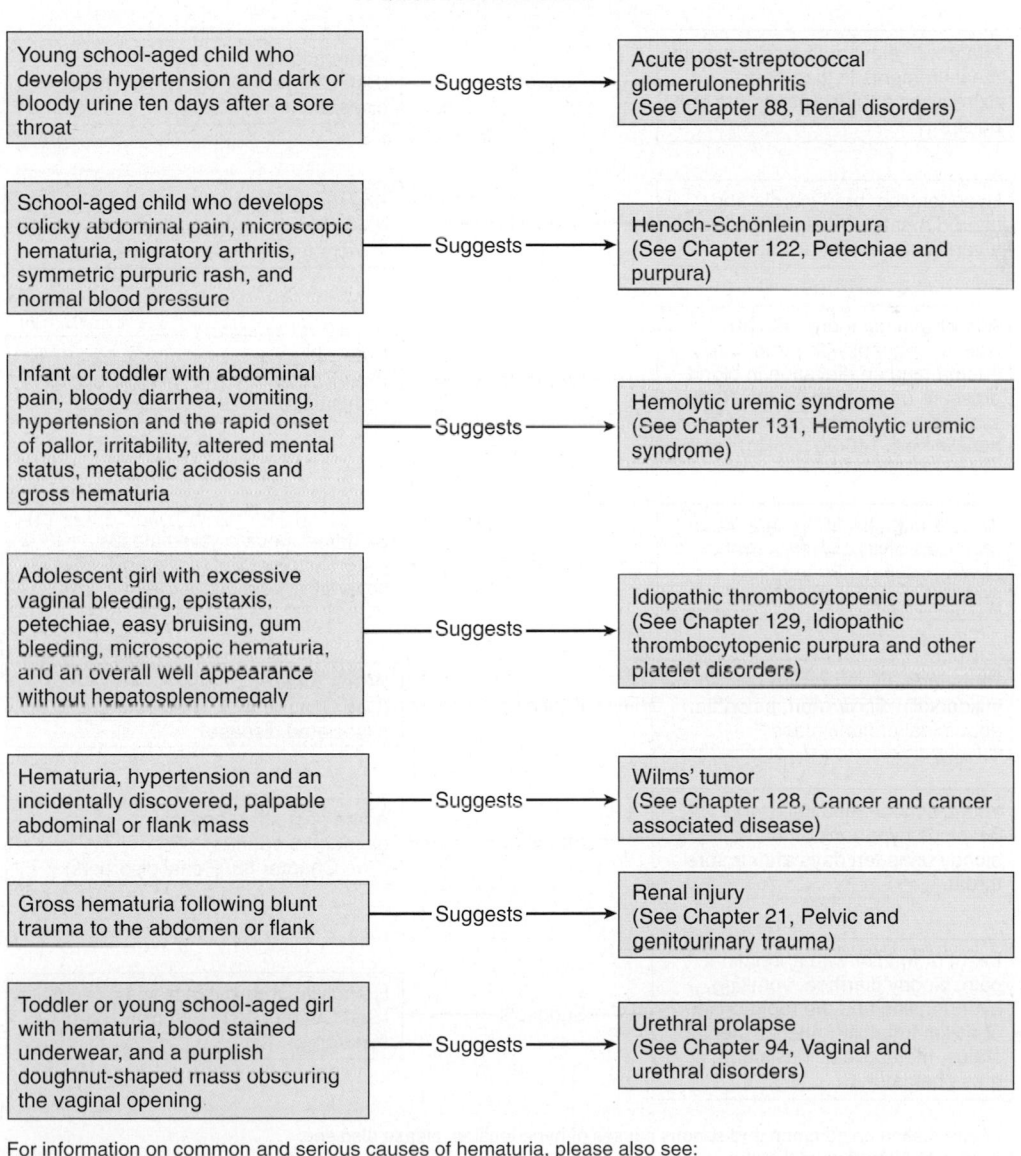

Young school-aged child who develops hypertension and dark or bloody urine ten days after a sore throat	Suggests	Acute post-streptococcal glomerulonephritis (See Chapter 88, Renal disorders)
School-aged child who develops colicky abdominal pain, microscopic hematuria, migratory arthritis, symmetric purpuric rash, and normal blood pressure	Suggests	Henoch-Schönlein purpura (See Chapter 122, Petechiae and purpura)
Infant or toddler with abdominal pain, bloody diarrhea, vomiting, hypertension and the rapid onset of pallor, irritability, altered mental status, metabolic acidosis and gross hematuria	Suggests	Hemolytic uremic syndrome (See Chapter 131, Hemolytic uremic syndrome)
Adolescent girl with excessive vaginal bleeding, epistaxis, petechiae, easy bruising, gum bleeding, microscopic hematuria, and an overall well appearance without hepatosplenomegaly	Suggests	Idiopathic thrombocytopenic purpura (See Chapter 129, Idiopathic thrombocytopenic purpura and other platelet disorders)
Hematuria, hypertension and an incidentally discovered, palpable abdominal or flank mass	Suggests	Wilms' tumor (See Chapter 128, Cancer and cancer associated disease)
Gross hematuria following blunt trauma to the abdomen or flank	Suggests	Renal injury (See Chapter 21, Pelvic and genitourinary trauma)
Toddler or young school-aged girl with hematuria, blood stained underwear, and a purplish doughnut-shaped mass obscuring the vaginal opening	Suggests	Urethral prolapse (See Chapter 94, Vaginal and urethral disorders)

For information on common and serious causes of hematuria, please also see:
Chapter 21 Pelvic and genitourinary trauma
Chapter 25 Abdominal trauma
Chapter 26 Burns
Chapter 33 Urinary tract infection in infants
Chapter 86 Urinary tract infections in children and adolescents
Chapter 99 Rhabdomyolysis
Chapter 130 Coagulation disorders

Chapter 192

Hypertension

A Quick Look at Hypertension

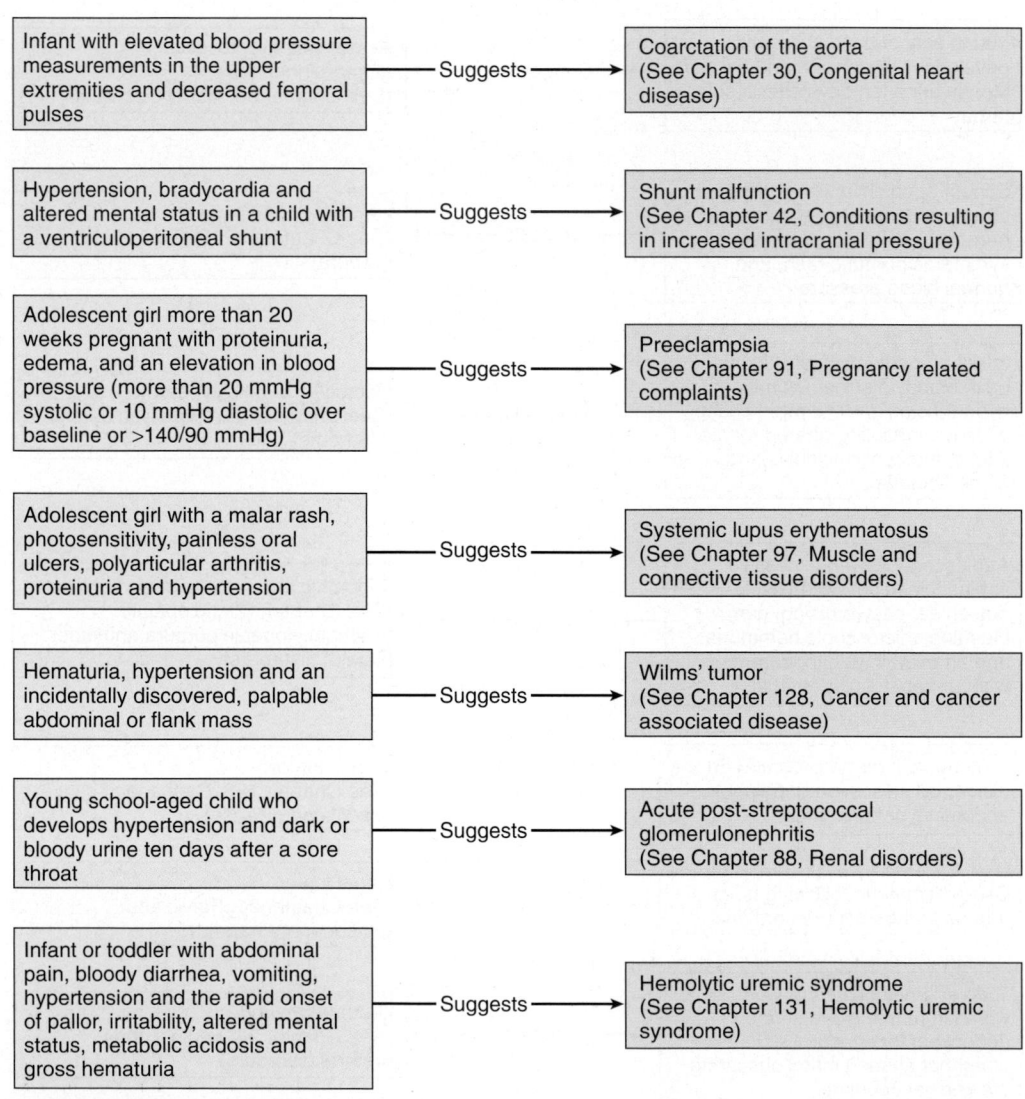

Infant with elevated blood pressure measurements in the upper extremities and decreased femoral pulses	—— Suggests —→	Coarctation of the aorta (See Chapter 30, Congenital heart disease)
Hypertension, bradycardia and altered mental status in a child with a ventriculoperitoneal shunt	—— Suggests —→	Shunt malfunction (See Chapter 42, Conditions resulting in increased intracranial pressure)
Adolescent girl more than 20 weeks pregnant with proteinuria, edema, and an elevation in blood pressure (more than 20 mmHg systolic or 10 mmHg diastolic over baseline or >140/90 mmHg)	—— Suggests —→	Preeclampsia (See Chapter 91, Pregnancy related complaints)
Adolescent girl with a malar rash, photosensitivity, painless oral ulcers, polyarticular arthritis, proteinuria and hypertension	—— Suggests —→	Systemic lupus erythematosus (See Chapter 97, Muscle and connective tissue disorders)
Hematuria, hypertension and an incidentally discovered, palpable abdominal or flank mass	—— Suggests —→	Wilms' tumor (See Chapter 128, Cancer and cancer associated disease)
Young school-aged child who develops hypertension and dark or bloody urine ten days after a sore throat	—— Suggests —→	Acute post-streptococcal glomerulonephritis (See Chapter 88, Renal disorders)
Infant or toddler with abdominal pain, bloody diarrhea, vomiting, hypertension and the rapid onset of pallor, irritability, altered mental status, metabolic acidosis and gross hematuria	—— Suggests —→	Hemolytic uremic syndrome (See Chapter 131, Hemolytic uremic syndrome)

For information on common and serious causes of hypertension, please also see:
Chapter 11 Altered mental status
Chapter 17 Head trauma
Chapter 41 Headache
Chapter 44 Central nervous system vascular disorders
Chapter 65 Hypertensive emergencies

Chapter 193

Jaundice

A Quick Look at Jaundice

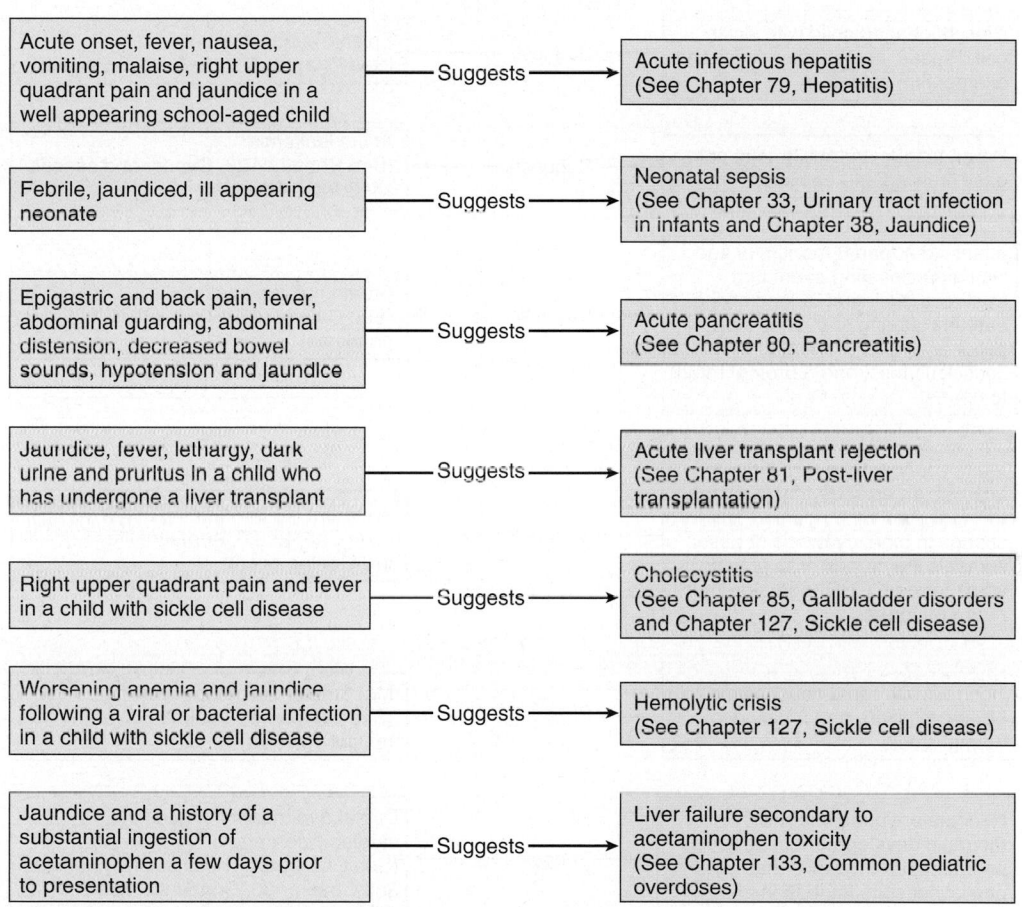

Acute onset, fever, nausea, vomiting, malaise, right upper quadrant pain and jaundice in a well appearing school-aged child — Suggests → Acute infectious hepatitis (See Chapter 79, Hepatitis)

Febrile, jaundiced, ill appearing neonate — Suggests → Neonatal sepsis (See Chapter 33, Urinary tract infection in infants and Chapter 38, Jaundice)

Epigastric and back pain, fever, abdominal guarding, abdominal distension, decreased bowel sounds, hypotension and jaundice — Suggests → Acute pancreatitis (See Chapter 80, Pancreatitis)

Jaundice, fever, lethargy, dark urine and pruritus in a child who has undergone a liver transplant — Suggests → Acute liver transplant rejection (See Chapter 81, Post-liver transplantation)

Right upper quadrant pain and fever in a child with sickle cell disease — Suggests → Cholecystitis (See Chapter 85, Gallbladder disorders and Chapter 127, Sickle cell disease)

Worsening anemia and jaundice following a viral or bacterial infection in a child with sickle cell disease — Suggests → Hemolytic crisis (See Chapter 127, Sickle cell disease)

Jaundice and a history of a substantial ingestion of acetaminophen a few days prior to presentation — Suggests → Liver failure secondary to acetaminophen toxicity (See Chapter 133, Common pediatric overdoses)

For information on common and serious causes of jaundice, please also see:
Chapter 7 The critically ill neonate
Chapter 38 Jaundice
Chapter 71 Selected infectious diseases
Chapter 85 Gallbladder disorders
Chapter 132 Utilizing blood bank resources/transfusion reactions and complications

Chapter 194

Pallor

A Quick Look at Pallor

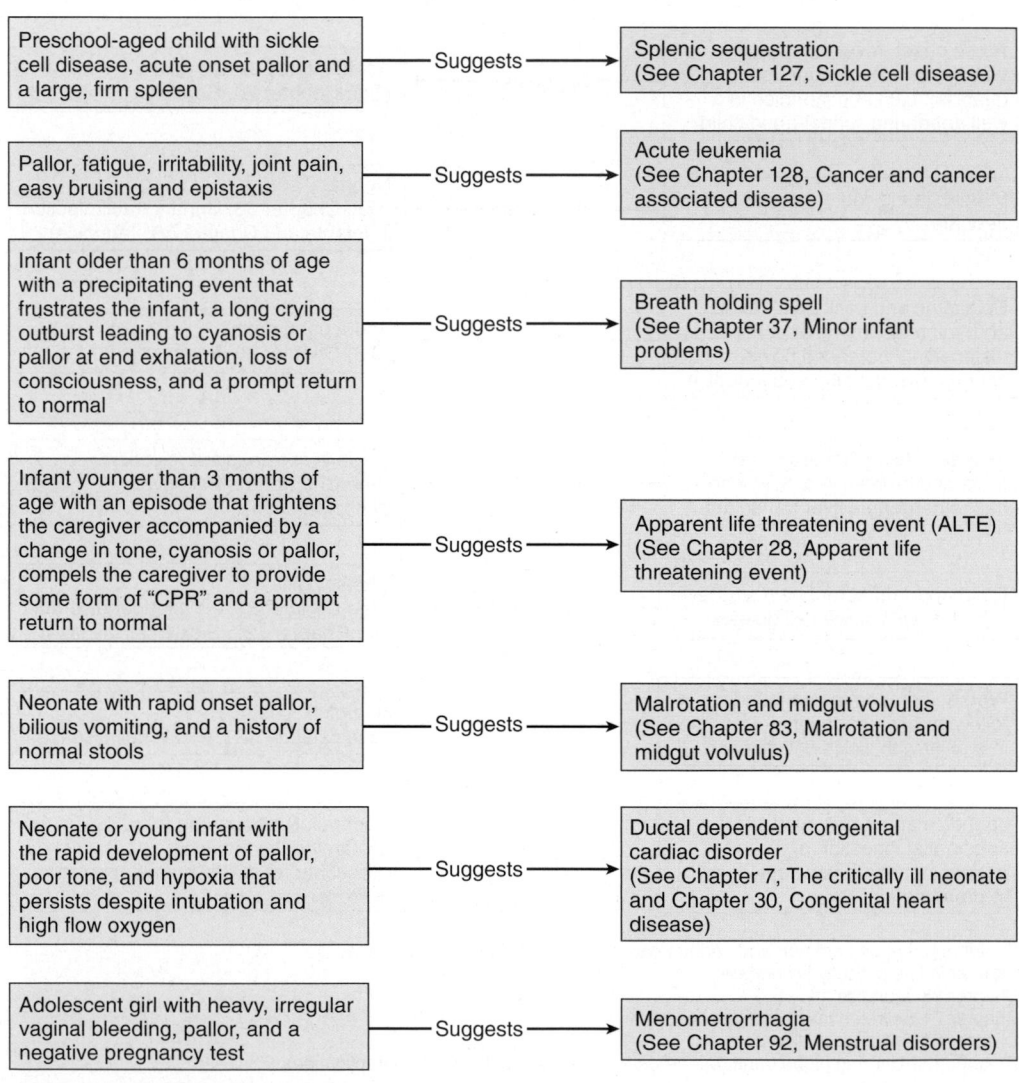

Preschool-aged child with sickle cell disease, acute onset pallor and a large, firm spleen — Suggests → Splenic sequestration (See Chapter 127, Sickle cell disease)

Pallor, fatigue, irritability, joint pain, easy bruising and epistaxis — Suggests → Acute leukemia (See Chapter 128, Cancer and cancer associated disease)

Infant older than 6 months of age with a precipitating event that frustrates the infant, a long crying outburst leading to cyanosis or pallor at end exhalation, loss of consciousness, and a prompt return to normal — Suggests → Breath holding spell (See Chapter 37, Minor infant problems)

Infant younger than 3 months of age with an episode that frightens the caregiver accompanied by a change in tone, cyanosis or pallor, compels the caregiver to provide some form of "CPR" and a prompt return to normal — Suggests → Apparent life threatening event (ALTE) (See Chapter 28, Apparent life threatening event)

Neonate with rapid onset pallor, bilious vomiting, and a history of normal stools — Suggests → Malrotation and midgut volvulus (See Chapter 83, Malrotation and midgut volvulus)

Neonate or young infant with the rapid development of pallor, poor tone, and hypoxia that persists despite intubation and high flow oxygen — Suggests → Ductal dependent congenital cardiac disorder (See Chapter 7, The critically ill neonate and Chapter 30, Congenital heart disease)

Adolescent girl with heavy, irregular vaginal bleeding, pallor, and a negative pregnancy test — Suggests → Menometrorrhagia (See Chapter 92, Menstrual disorders)

For information on common and serious causes of pallor, please also see:
Chapter 8 Circulatory emergencies: Shock
Chapter 75 Gastrointestinal bleeding
Chapter 90 Ectopic pregnancy
Chapter 91 Pregnancy-related complications
Chapter 130 Coagulation disorders
Chapter 139 Hyperthermia
Chapter 140 Hypothermia

Chapter 195

Arthralgias/Arthritis

A Quick Look at Arthralgias and Arthritis

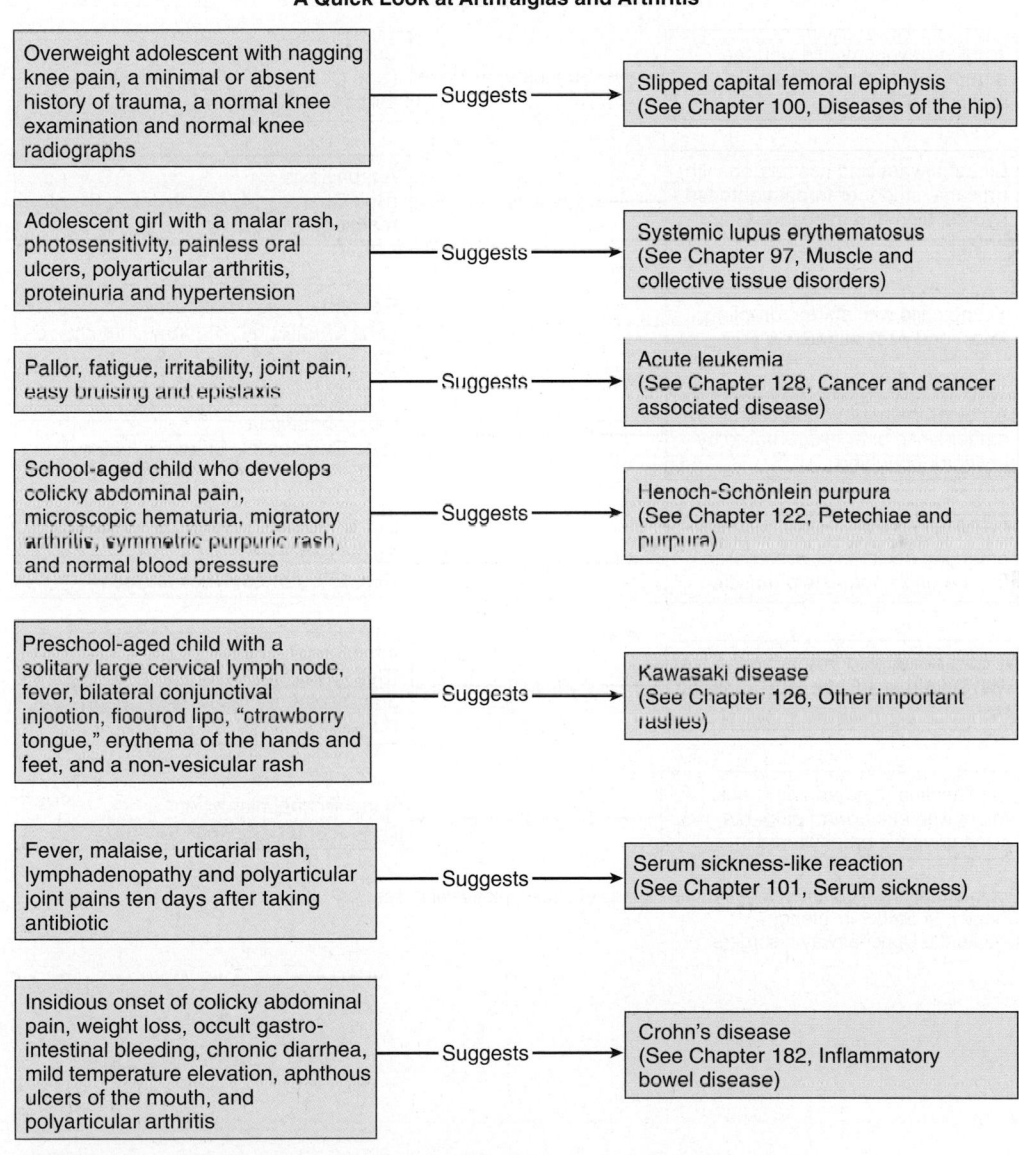

Overweight adolescent with nagging knee pain, a minimal or absent history of trauma, a normal knee examination and normal knee radiographs — Suggests → Slipped capital femoral epiphysis (See Chapter 100, Diseases of the hip)

Adolescent girl with a malar rash, photosensitivity, painless oral ulcers, polyarticular arthritis, proteinuria and hypertension — Suggests → Systemic lupus erythematosus (See Chapter 97, Muscle and collective tissue disorders)

Pallor, fatigue, irritability, joint pain, easy bruising and epistaxis — Suggests → Acute leukemia (See Chapter 128, Cancer and cancer associated disease)

School-aged child who develops colicky abdominal pain, microscopic hematuria, migratory arthritis, symmetric purpuric rash, and normal blood pressure — Suggests → Henoch-Schönlein purpura (See Chapter 122, Petechiae and purpura)

Preschool-aged child with a solitary large cervical lymph node, fever, bilateral conjunctival injection, fissured lips, "strawberry tongue," erythema of the hands and feet, and a non-vesicular rash — Suggests → Kawasaki disease (See Chapter 126, Other important rashes)

Fever, malaise, urticarial rash, lymphadenopathy and polyarticular joint pains ten days after taking antibiotic — Suggests → Serum sickness-like reaction (See Chapter 101, Serum sickness)

Insidious onset of colicky abdominal pain, weight loss, occult gastro-intestinal bleeding, chronic diarrhea, mild temperature elevation, aphthous ulcers of the mouth, and polyarticular arthritis — Suggests → Crohn's disease (See Chapter 182, Inflammatory bowel disease)

For information on common and serious causes of arthralgias and arthritis, please also see:
Chapter 95 Musculoskeletal disorders in systemic diseases
Chapter 96 Bone, joint, and spine infections
Chapter 97 Muscle and connective tissue disorders
Chapter 98 Overuse syndromes and inflammatory conditions
Chapter 99 Rhabdomyolysis
Chapter 102 Vaccination-related complaints and side effects
Chapter 107 The steroid dependent child

Chapter 196

Stridor

A Quick Look at Stridor

Toddler or young child with the abrupt onset upper chest pain, stridor and drooling	Suggests →	Esophageal coin (See Chapter 78, Gastrointestinal foreign bodies)
Bilateral wheezing associated with urticaria, stridor or throat tightness, hypotension and exposure to an antigen	Suggests →	Anaphylaxis (See Chapter 14, Anaphylaxis/Allergic reaction)
Young child with stridor, drooling, fever, and neck stiffness	Suggests →	Retropharyngeal abscess (See Chapter 34, Stridor in infancy and Chapter 54, Neck infections)
An older infant or young child with stridor since birth exacerbated by crying or coughing	Suggests →	Laryngomalacia (See Chapter 34, Stridor in infancy)
Infant with stridor and a unilateral, enlarging neck mass posterior to the sternocleidomastoid muscle	Suggests →	Cystic hygroma (See Chapter 55, Neck masses)
A child evacuated from a house fire with singed facial hair, oral soot and stridor	Suggests →	Inhalational airway injury (See Chapter 2, Respiratory distress and respiratory failure and Chapter 26, Burns)
"Clothesline" type anterior neck injury with stridor and palpable subcutaneous emphysema	Suggests →	Blunt tracheal disruption (See Chapter 18, Neck trauma)

For information on common and serious causes of stridor, please also see:
Chapter 34 Stridor in infancy
Chapter 60 Upper airway disorders

Chapter 197

Vaginal Bleeding

A Quick Look at Vaginal Bleeding

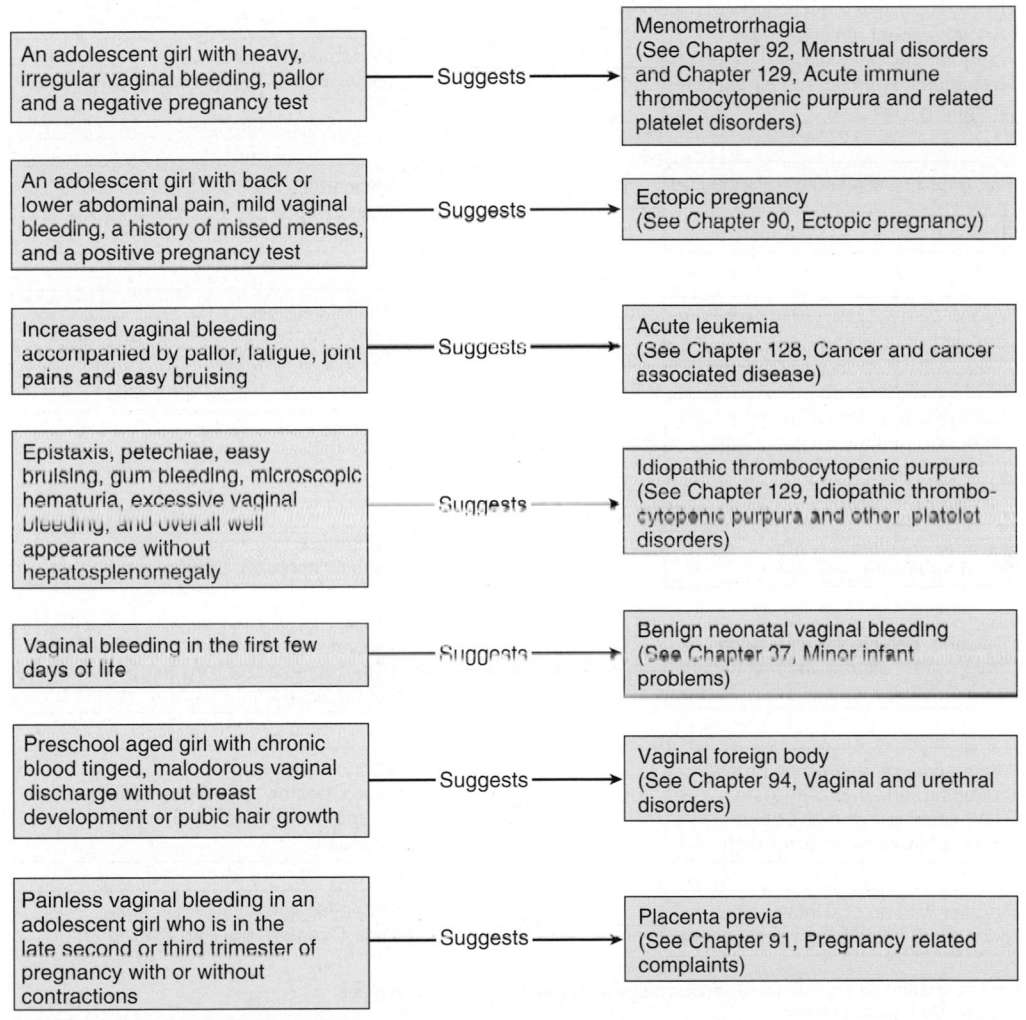

An adolescent girl with heavy, irregular vaginal bleeding, pallor and a negative pregnancy test	— Suggests —	Menometrorrhagia (See Chapter 92, Menstrual disorders and Chapter 129, Acute immune thrombocytopenic purpura and related platelet disorders)
An adolescent girl with back or lower abdominal pain, mild vaginal bleeding, a history of missed menses, and a positive pregnancy test	— Suggests —	Ectopic pregnancy (See Chapter 90, Ectopic pregnancy)
Increased vaginal bleeding accompanied by pallor, fatigue, joint pains and easy bruising	— Suggests —	Acute leukemia (See Chapter 128, Cancer and cancer associated disease)
Epistaxis, petechiae, easy bruising, gum bleeding, microscopic hematuria, excessive vaginal bleeding, and overall well appearance without hepatosplenomegaly	— Suggests —	Idiopathic thrombocytopenic purpura (See Chapter 129, Idiopathic thrombocytopenic purpura and other platelet disorders)
Vaginal bleeding in the first few days of life	— Suggests —	Benign neonatal vaginal bleeding (See Chapter 37, Minor infant problems)
Preschool aged girl with chronic blood tinged, malodorous vaginal discharge without breast development or pubic hair growth	— Suggests —	Vaginal foreign body (See Chapter 94, Vaginal and urethral disorders)
Painless vaginal bleeding in an adolescent girl who is in the late second or third trimester of pregnancy with or without contractions	— Suggests —	Placenta previa (See Chapter 91, Pregnancy related complaints)

For information on common and serious causes of vaginal bleeding, please also see:
Chapter 21 Pelvic and genitourinary trauma
Chapter 37 Minor infant problems
Chapter 70 Sexually transmitted infections
Chapter 92 Menstrual disorders
Chapter 118 Sexual abuse

Chapter 198

Weakness

A Quick Look at Weakness

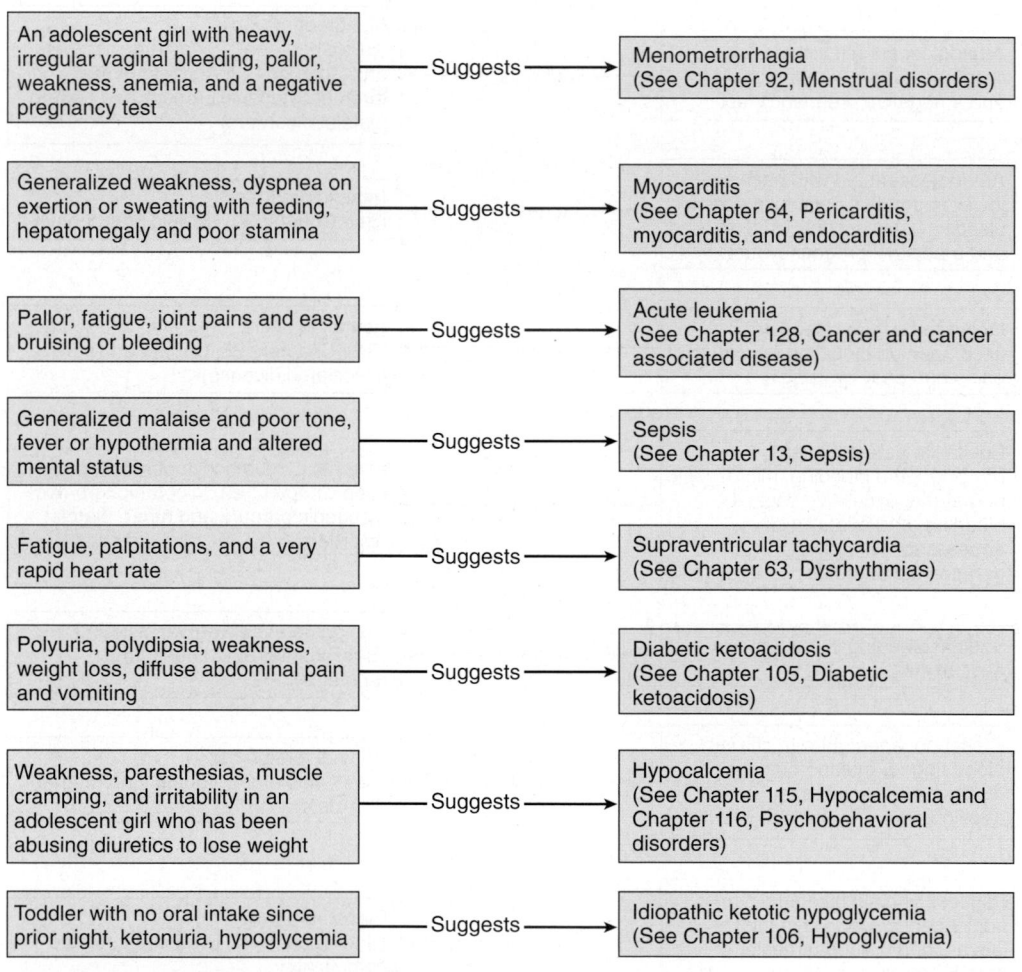

An adolescent girl with heavy, irregular vaginal bleeding, pallor, weakness, anemia, and a negative pregnancy test	Suggests	Menometrorrhagia (See Chapter 92, Menstrual disorders)
Generalized weakness, dyspnea on exertion or sweating with feeding, hepatomegaly and poor stamina	Suggests	Myocarditis (See Chapter 64, Pericarditis, myocarditis, and endocarditis)
Pallor, fatigue, joint pains and easy bruising or bleeding	Suggests	Acute leukemia (See Chapter 128, Cancer and cancer associated disease)
Generalized malaise and poor tone, fever or hypothermia and altered mental status	Suggests	Sepsis (See Chapter 13, Sepsis)
Fatigue, palpitations, and a very rapid heart rate	Suggests	Supraventricular tachycardia (See Chapter 63, Dysrhythmias)
Polyuria, polydipsia, weakness, weight loss, diffuse abdominal pain and vomiting	Suggests	Diabetic ketoacidosis (See Chapter 105, Diabetic ketoacidosis)
Weakness, paresthesias, muscle cramping, and irritability in an adolescent girl who has been abusing diuretics to lose weight	Suggests	Hypocalcemia (See Chapter 115, Hypocalcemia and Chapter 116, Psychobehavioral disorders)
Toddler with no oral intake since prior night, ketonuria, hypoglycemia	Suggests	Idiopathic ketotic hypoglycemia (See Chapter 106, Hypoglycemia)

For information on common and serious causes of weakness, please also see:
Chapter 36 Failure to thrive
Chapter 44 Central nervous system vascular disorders
Chapter 97 Muscle and connective tissue disorders

Chapter 199

Weight Loss

A Quick Look at Weight Loss

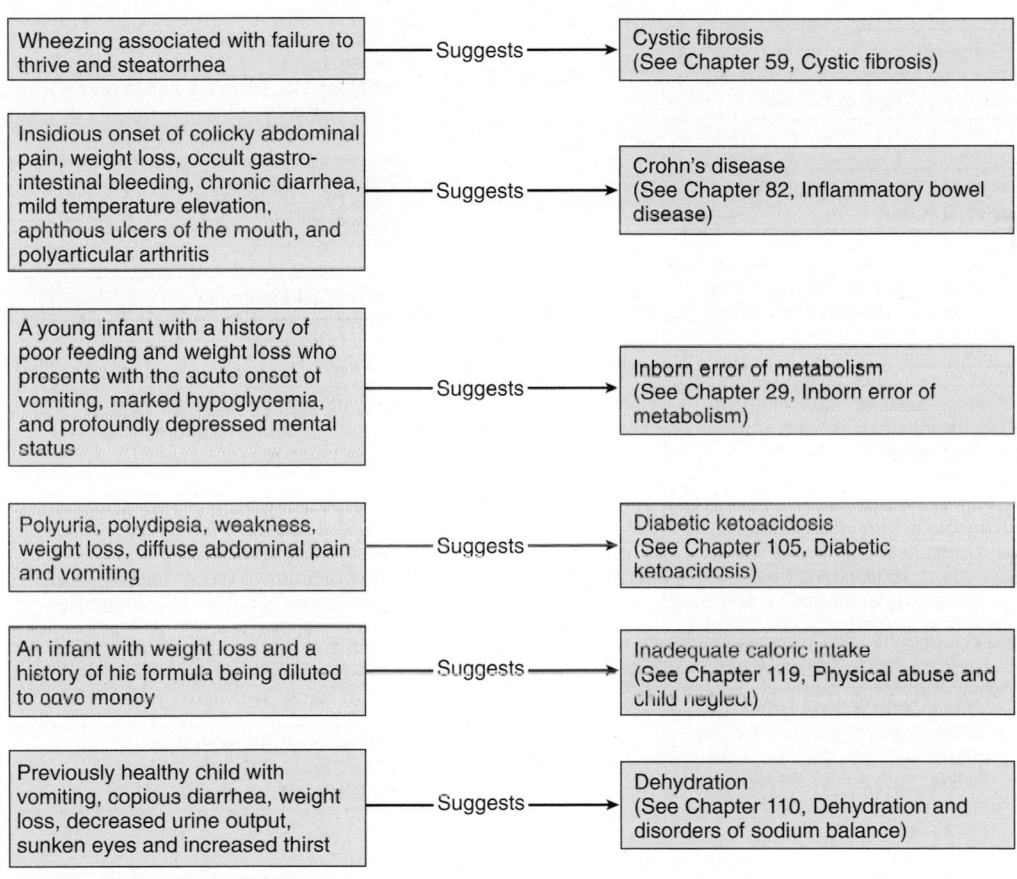

Wheezing associated with failure to thrive and steatorrhea	Suggests	Cystic fibrosis (See Chapter 59, Cystic fibrosis)
Insidious onset of colicky abdominal pain, weight loss, occult gastro-intestinal bleeding, chronic diarrhea, mild temperature elevation, aphthous ulcers of the mouth, and polyarticular arthritis	Suggests	Crohn's disease (See Chapter 82, Inflammatory bowel disease)
A young infant with a history of poor feeding and weight loss who presents with the acute onset of vomiting, marked hypoglycemia, and profoundly depressed mental status	Suggests	Inborn error of metabolism (See Chapter 29, Inborn error of metabolism)
Polyuria, polydipsia, weakness, weight loss, diffuse abdominal pain and vomiting	Suggests	Diabetic ketoacidosis (See Chapter 105, Diabetic ketoacidosis)
An infant with weight loss and a history of his formula being diluted to save money	Suggests	Inadequate caloric intake (See Chapter 119, Physical abuse and child neglect)
Previously healthy child with vomiting, copious diarrhea, weight loss, decreased urine output, sunken eyes and increased thirst	Suggests	Dehydration (See Chapter 110, Dehydration and disorders of sodium balance)

For information on common and serious causes of weight loss, please also see:
Chapter 35 Vomiting, spitting up and feeding difficulties
Chapter 36 Failure to thrive
Chapter 69 Human immunodeficiency virus infection and other immunosuppressive conditions
Chapter 72 Vomiting and diarrhea
Chapter 109 Thyrotoxicosis
Chapter 116 Psychobehavioral disorders
Chapter 117 Major depression and suicidality
Chapter 128 Cancer and cancer associated disease
Chapter 135 Drugs of abuse

Chapter 200

The Septic-Appearing Child

A Quick Look at the Septic Appearing Child

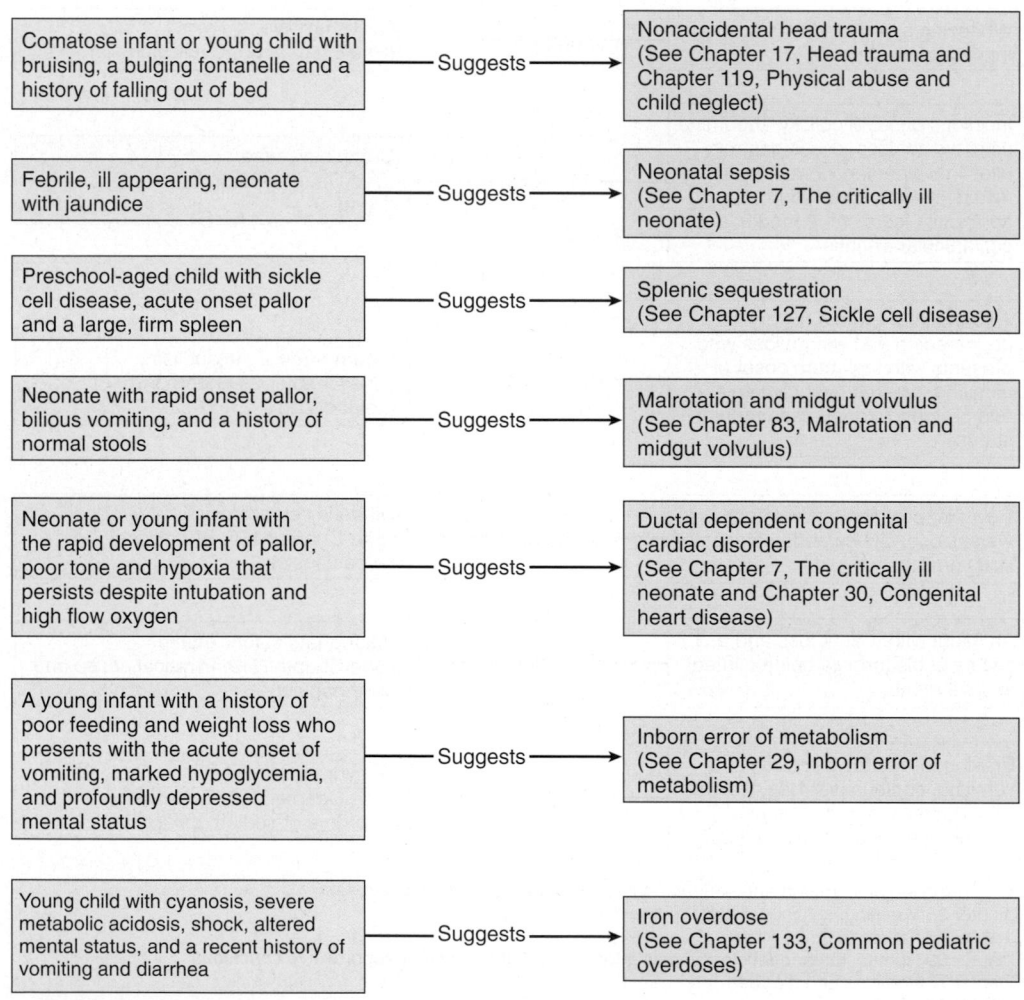

Comatose infant or young child with bruising, a bulging fontanelle and a history of falling out of bed	— Suggests →	Nonaccidental head trauma (See Chapter 17, Head trauma and Chapter 119, Physical abuse and child neglect)
Febrile, ill appearing, neonate with jaundice	— Suggests →	Neonatal sepsis (See Chapter 7, The critically ill neonate)
Preschool-aged child with sickle cell disease, acute onset pallor and a large, firm spleen	— Suggests →	Splenic sequestration (See Chapter 127, Sickle cell disease)
Neonate with rapid onset pallor, bilious vomiting, and a history of normal stools	— Suggests →	Malrotation and midgut volvulus (See Chapter 83, Malrotation and midgut volvulus)
Neonate or young infant with the rapid development of pallor, poor tone and hypoxia that persists despite intubation and high flow oxygen	— Suggests →	Ductal dependent congenital cardiac disorder (See Chapter 7, The critically ill neonate and Chapter 30, Congenital heart disease)
A young infant with a history of poor feeding and weight loss who presents with the acute onset of vomiting, marked hypoglycemia, and profoundly depressed mental status	— Suggests →	Inborn error of metabolism (See Chapter 29, Inborn error of metabolism)
Young child with cyanosis, severe metabolic acidosis, shock, altered mental status, and a recent history of vomiting and diarrhea	— Suggests →	Iron overdose (See Chapter 133, Common pediatric overdoses)

For information on common and serious causes of the septic appearing child, please also see:
Chapter 7 The critically ill neonate
Chapter 8 Circulatory emergencies: Shock
Chapter 13 Sepsis
Chapter 74 Intussusception

Index

Note: Page numbers followed by "f" indicate figures; those followed by "t" indicate tables.